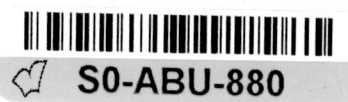
S0-ABU-880

SAUNDERS

2007

ICD-9-CM

Volumes 1, 2, & 3

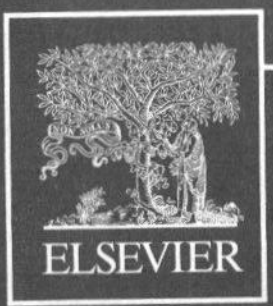
ELSEVIER

evolve

To access your Student Resources, visit:

http://evolve.elsevier.com/Buck/icd

Evolve® Student Resources for ***Buck: Saunders 2007 ICD-9-CM, Volumes 1, 2, & 3,*** offer the following features:

Student Resources

- **Content Updates**
  Download any updates for the ICD-9-CM as changes are released.
- **Updates to ICD-9-CM Official Guidelines for Coding and Reporting**
  Download the latest government guidelines for the ICD-9-CM, available in PDF.
- **Industry Updates**
  Get the latest news on ICD-10, links to the websites with the latest coding information, quarterly updates for ICD-9-CM, and more!
- **Links by Body System**
  Get connected to numerous websites with information on the very latest disease entities, diagnostic procedures, therapeutic techniques, and other advancements in medicine. Organized to follow the ICD-9-CM Table of Contents.

SAUNDERS

2007

ICD-9-CM

Volumes 1, 2, & 3

CAROL J. BUCK
MS, CPC, CPC-H, CCS-P
Program Director, Retired
Medical Secretary Programs
Northwest Technical College
East Grand Forks, Minnesota

Technical Assistant
KAREN D. LOCKYER
BA, RHIT, CPC
Consultant
Southlake, Texas

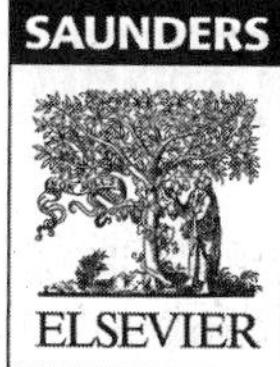

SAUNDERS
ELSEVIER

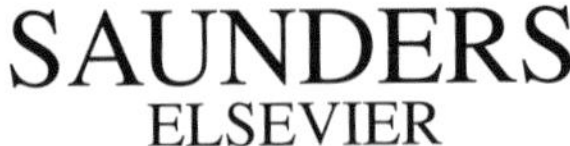

11830 Westline Industrial Drive
St. Louis, Missouri 63146

SAUNDERS 2007 ICD-9-CM, VOLUMES 1, 2, & 3

ISBN-13: 978-1-4160-4040-8
ISBN-10: 1-4160-4040-4

Copyright © 2007, 2006, 2005, 2004, 2003, 2002, 2001, 2000 by Saunders, an imprint of Elsevier Inc.

All rights reserved. No part of this publication may be reproduced or transmitted in any form or by any means, electronic or mechanical, including photocopying, recording, or any information storage and retrieval system, without permission in writing from the publisher.

Permissions may be sought directly from Elsevier's Health Sciences Rights Department in Philadelphia, USA: phone: (+1) 215 239 3804, fax: (+1) 215 239 3805, email: healthpermissions@elsevier.com. You may also complete your request on-line via the Elsevier homepage (http://www.elsevier.com), by selecting "Customer Support" and then "Obtaining Permissions."

Notice

Knowledge and best practice in this field are constantly changing. As new research and experience broaden our knowledge, changes in practice, treatment, and drug therapy may become necessary or appropriate. Readers are advised to check the most current information provided (i) on procedures featured or (ii) by the manufacturer of each product to be administered, to verify the recommended dose or formula, the method and duration of administration, and contraindications. It is the responsibility of the practitioner, relying on his or her own experience and knowledge of the patient, to make diagnoses, to determine dosages and the best treatment for each individual patient, and to take all appropriate safety precautions. To the fullest extent of the law, neither the Publisher nor the Author assumes any liability for any injury and/or damage to persons or property arising out of or related to any use of the material contained in this book.

The Publisher

Current Procedural Terminology (CPT) is copyright 2005 American Medical Association. All Rights Reserved. No fee schedules, basic units, relative values, or related listings are included in CPT. The AMA assumes no liability for the data contained herein. Applicable FARS/DFARS restrictions apply to government use.

ISBN-13: 978-1-4160-4040-8
ISBN-10: 1-4160-4040-4

Publisher: Michael S. Ledbetter
Senior Developmental Editor: Melissa K. Boyle
Associate Developmental Editor: Josh Rapplean
Publishing Services Manager: Melissa Lastarria
Designer: Andrea Lutes

Printed in the United States of America

Last digit is the print number: 9 8 7 6 5 4 3 2

Working together to grow libraries in developing countries

www.elsevier.com | www.bookaid.org | www.sabre.org

ELSEVIER BOOK AID International Sabre Foundation

CONTENTS

GUIDE TO USING THE SAUNDERS 2007 ICD-9-CM, VOLUMES 1, 2, & 3 vii

SYMBOLS AND CONVENTIONS ix

GUIDE TO 2007 ICD-9-CM UPDATES xv

UNIT ONE ICD-9-CM 1

Part I Introduction 3

ICD-9-CM BACKGROUND 3
COORDINATION AND MAINTENANCE COMMITTEE 3
CHARACTERISTICS OF THE ICD-9-CM 3
The Disease Classification 4
ICD-9-CM OFFICIAL GUIDELINES FOR CODING AND REPORTING 4

Part II Alphabetic Index Volume 2 43

Section I Index to Diseases 44
Section II Table of Drugs and Chemicals 488
Section III Index to External Causes of Injury (E Code) 566

Part III Diseases: Tabular List Volume 1 591

1. Infectious and Parasitic Diseases (001–139) 591
2. Neoplasms (140–239) 616
3. Endocrine, Nutritional and Metabolic Diseases, and Immunity Disorders (240–279) 638
4. Diseases of the Blood and Blood-forming Organs (280–289) 650
5. Mental Disorders (290–319) 656
6. Diseases of the Nervous System and Sense Organs (320–389) 669
7. Diseases of the Circulatory System (390–459) 704
8. Diseases of the Respiratory System (460–519) 721
9. Diseases of the Digestive System (520–579) 731
10. Diseases of the Genitourinary System (580–629) 752
11. Complications of Pregnancy, Childbirth, and the Puerperium (630–677) 769
12. Diseases of the Skin and Subcutaneous Tissue (680–709) 785
13. Diseases of the Musculoskeletal System and Connective Tissue (710–739) 794
14. Congenital Anomalies (740–759) 808
15. Certain Conditions Originating in the Perinatal Period (760–779) 824
16. Symptoms, Signs, and Ill-defined Conditions (780–799) 831
17. Injury and Poisoning (800–999) 844

V-Codes—Supplementary Classification of Factors Influencing Health Status and Contact with Health Services 882
E-Codes—Supplementary Classification of External Causes of Injury and Poisoning 901
Appendix A—Morphology of Neoplasms 937
Appendix B—Glossary of Mental Disorders (Deleted as of October 1, 2004) 944

Appendix C—Classification of Drugs by American Hospital Formulary Services List Number and Their ICD-9-CM Equivalents 945
Appendix D—Classification of Industrial Accidents According to Agency 948
Appendix E—List of Three-Digit Categories 950

Part IV Procedures Volume 3 963

Index to Procedures 964
Tabular List of Procedures 1070

0. Procedures and Interventions, Not Elsewhere Classified (00) 1070
1. Operations on the Nervous System (01–05) 1075
2. Operations on the Endocrine System (06–07) 1079
3. Operations on the Eye (08–16) 1081
4. Operations on the Ear (18–20) 1087
5. Operations on the Nose, Mouth, and Pharynx (21–29) 1089
6. Operations on the Respiratory System (30–34) 1093
7. Operations on the Cardiovascular System (35–39) 1097
8. Operations on the Hemic and Lymphatic System (40–41) 1109
9. Operations on the Digestive System (42–54) 1111
10. Operations on the Urinary System (55–59) 1125
11. Operations on the Male Genital Organs (60–64) 1130
12. Operations on the Female Genital Organs (65–71) 1133
13. Obstetrical Procedures (72–75) 1138
14. Operations on the Musculoskeletal System (76–84) 1140
15. Operations on the Integumentary System (85–86) 1151
16. Miscellaneous Diagnostic and Therapeutic Procedures (87–99) 1155

UNIT TWO 2006 INPATIENT PROCEDURES 1171

2006 Inpatient Procedures 1173

GUIDE TO USING THE SAUNDERS 2007 ICD-9-CM, Volumes 1, 2, & 3

Medical coding has long been a part of the health care profession. Through the years medical coding systems have become more complex and extensive. Today, medical coding is an intricate and immense process that is present in every health care setting. The increased use of electronic submissions for health care services only increases the need for coders who understand the coding process.

Saunders 2007 ICD-9-CM, Volumes 1, 2, & 3 was developed to help meet the needs of students preparing for a career in medical coding by offering a comprehensive coding text at a reasonable price. This text combines the official coding guidelines and all three volumes of the ICD-9-CM in one book.

All material strictly adheres to the latest government versions available at the time of printing.

ILLUSTRATIONS AND ITEMS

The ICD-9-CM, Volume 1, Tabular List contains illustrations, pictures, and items to assist you in understanding difficult terminology, diseases/conditions, or coding in a specific category. Items are always printed in ▬ ink so the added material is not mistaken for official notations or instructions. Your ideas on what other descriptions or illustrations should be in future editions of this text are always appreciated.

Annotated

Throughout this text revisions and additions are indicated by the following symbols:

- **Revised:** Revisions within the line or code from the previous edition are indicated by the black arrow.

- ◀ **New:** Additions to the previous edition are indicated by the color triangle.

The revision and addition symbols are the only symbols that appear in the ICD-9-CM indexes.

ICD-9-CM, Volume 1, Tabular List Symbols

- ● **Not a Principal Diagnosis:** These codes have a black dot before them. These codes give additional information or describe the circumstances affecting the health care encounter but are unacceptable as principal diagnosis for inpatient admission.

- ❶ **First Listed:** The number 1 inside a circle appears before V codes that may be listed as the first code.

- 1/2 **First Listed or Additional:** The 1/2 inside a circle appears before V codes that may be listed as the first code and may also be listed as an additional V code.

- ❷ **Additional Only:** The number 2 inside a circle appears before V codes that may only be listed as an additional code. These codes may not be listed as a first code.

- ● **Use Additional Digit(s):** The color dot cautions you that the code requires additional digit(s) to ensure the greatest specificity.

- ❑ **Nonspecific Code:** These have a square before the code. Although these codes are valid as a principal diagnosis, they are usually too general to be used as a principal diagnosis for Medicare, and you should continue to seek a code that is more specific.

ICD-9-CM, Volume 3, Tabular List Symbols

● **Use Additional Digit(s):** The color dot cautions you that the code requires additional digit(s) to ensure the greatest specificity.

✖ **Valid O.R. Procedure:** The color "x" is placed before a code that is a valid operating room (O.R.) procedure according to the DRG grouper.

In addition to the symbols, the official ICD-9-CM conventions appear throughout the text. Refer to the illustrations of conventions on the following pages and to the Introduction for further information on conventions.

SYMBOLS AND CONVENTIONS

ICD-9-CM, Volumes 1, 2, & 3
Symbols Used in All Volumes of ICD-9-CM to Identify New or Revised Material

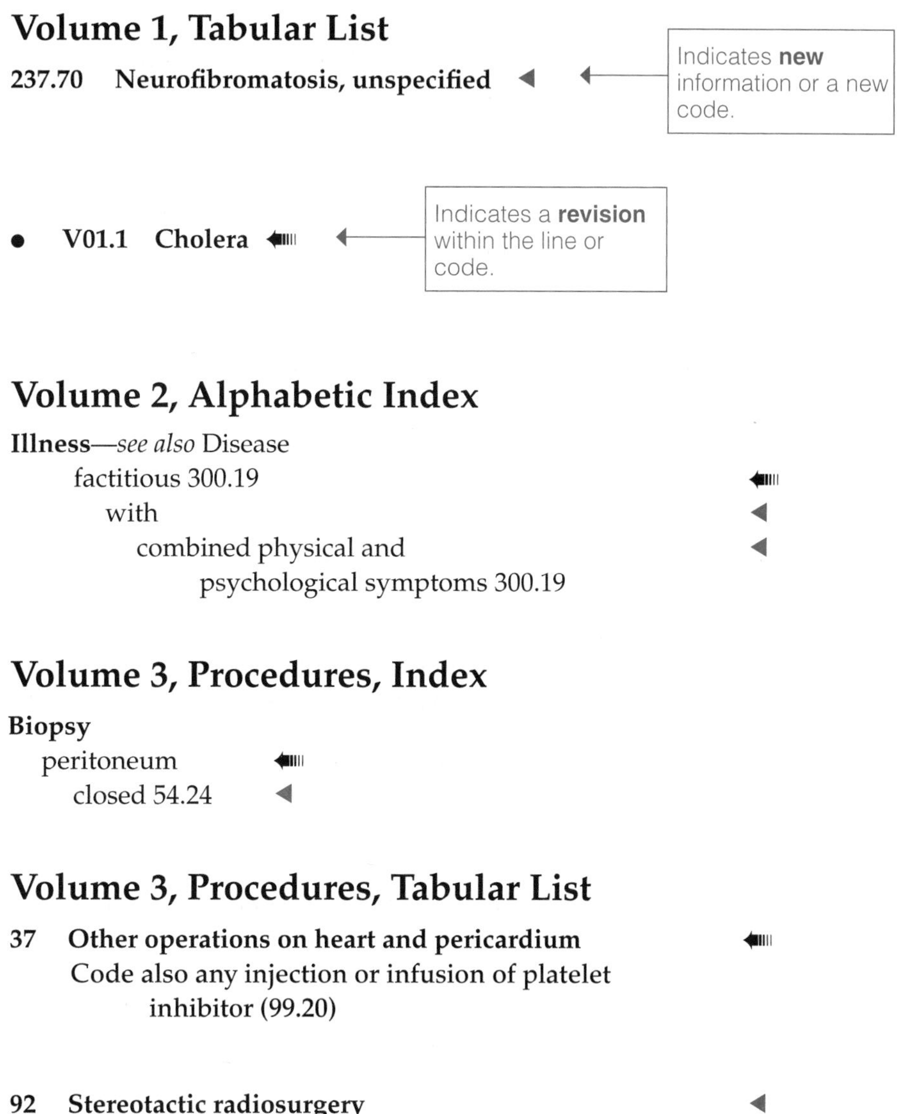

Volume 1, Tabular List
237.70 Neurofibromatosis, unspecified
Indicates **new** information or a new code.
● V01.1 Cholera
Indicates a **revision** within the line or code.
Volume 2, Alphabetic Index
Illness—*see also* Disease
factitious 300.19
with
combined physical and
psychological symptoms 300.19
Volume 3, Procedures, Index
Biopsy
peritoneum
closed 54.24
Volume 3, Procedures, Tabular List
37 Other operations on heart and pericardium
Code also any injection or infusion of platelet
inhibitor (99.20)
92 Stereotactic radiosurgery

Symbols for Volume 1, Tabular List

Use Additional Digit(s): The color dot cautions you that the code requires additional digit(s) to ensure the greatest specificity.

● **237.7 Neurofibromatosis**
von Recklinghausen's disease
❑ **237.70 Neurofibromatosis, unspecified**

Not a Principal Diagnosis: These codes have a black dot before them. These codes give additional information or describe the circumstances affecting the health care encounter but are unacceptable as principal diagnosis for inpatient admission.

Nonspecific Code: These codes have a square before them. Although these codes are valid as a principal diagnosis, they are usually too general to be used as a principal diagnosis for Medicare, and you should continue to seek a code that is more specific

● *284.2 Myelophthisis*

❶ **V46.13 Encounter for weaning from respirator [ventilator]**

First Listed: This symbol appears before V codes/categories/subcategories that are only acceptable as first listed.

1/2 **V46.14 Mechanical complication of respirator [ventilator]**

First Listed or Additional: This symbol appears before V codes/categories/subcategories that may be either first listed or additional codes.

Additional Only: This symbol appears before V codes/categories/subcategories that may only be used as additional codes, not first listed.

❷ **V46.11 Dependence on respirator, status**

Conventions for Volume 1, Tabular List

2. NEOPLASMS (140–239)

Notes define terms or give coding instructions.

Notes
1. Content
This chapter contains the following broad groups:
140–195 Malignant neoplasms, stated or presumed to be primary, of specified sites, except of lymphatic and hematopoietic tissue.

510 Empyema
Use additional code to identify infectious organism (041.0–041.9)

"Use additional digit(s)" directs you to use an additional code to give a more complete picture of the diagnosis.

"*Code first*" is used in those categories not intended as the principal diagnosis. In such cases, the code, title, and instructions appear in italics. The note requires that the underlying disease (etiology) be sequenced first.

366.4 Cataract associated with other disorders
366.41 Diabetic cataract
Code first diabetes (250.5)

A code with this note may be principal if no causal condition is applicable or known

428 Heart failure
Code, if applicable, heart failure due to hypertension first (402.0–402.9, with fifth-digit 1 or 404.0–404.9 with fifth-digit 1 or 3)

474 **Chronic disease of tonsils and adenoids**

"and" indicates a code that can be assigned if either of the conditions is present or if both of the conditions are present.

366.4 **Cataract associated with other disorders**

"with" indicates a code that can only be used if both conditions are present.

The "Includes" note appears immediately under a code to further define, or give example of, the contents of the code.

087 **Relapsing fever**
Includes: recurrent fever

420.0 ***Acute pericarditis in disease classified elsewhere***

Italicized type is used for all exclusion notes and to identify those codes that are not usually sequenced as the principal diagnosis.

Terms following the word "Excludes" are to be coded elsewhere. The term "Excludes" means "Do Not Code Here."

150.2 **Abdominal esophagus**
Excludes: *recurrent fever*

244.8 **Other specified acquired hypothyroidism**
Secondary hypothyroidism NEC

NEC means Not Elsewhere Classifiable and is to be used only when the information at hand specifies a condition but there is no more specific code for that condition.

Bold type is used for all codes and titles.

159.0 **Intestinal tract, part unspecified**
Intestine NOS

NOS means Not Otherwise Specified and is the equivalent of "unspecified."

426.89 **Other**
Dissociation:
atrioventricular [AV]

Brackets are used to enclose synonyms, alternative wording, or explanatory phrases.

158.8 **Specified parts of peritoneum**
Cul-de-sac (of Douglas)
Mesentery

Parentheses are used to enclose supplementary words that may be present or absent in the statement of a disease without affecting the code.

628.4 **Of cervical or vaginal origin**
Infertility associated with:
anomaly of cervical mucus
congenital structural anomaly

A colon is used after an incomplete term that needs one or more of the modifiers that follow in order to make it assignable to a given category.

Conventions for Volume 2, Alphabetic Index

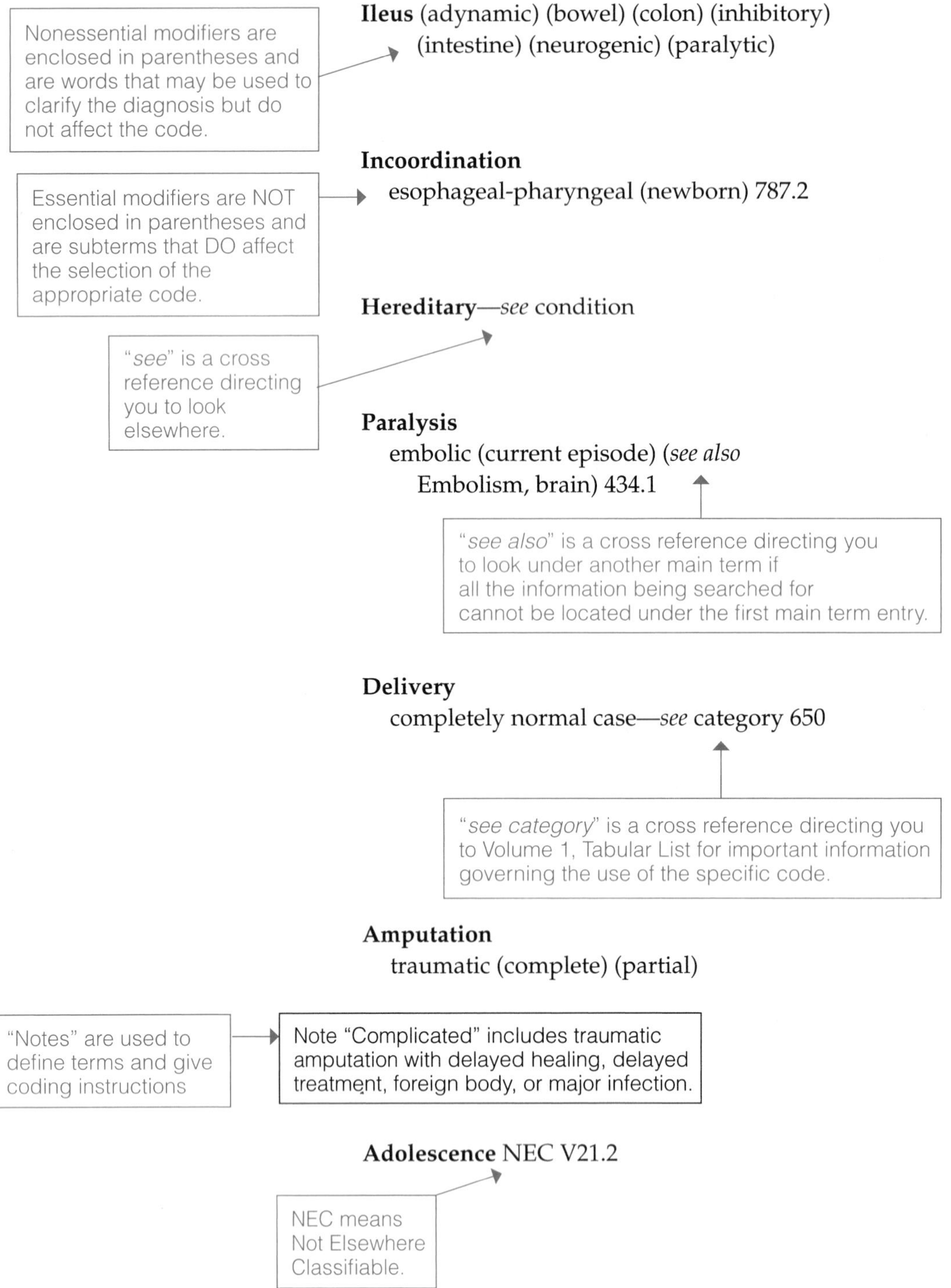
Ileus (adynamic) (bowel) (colon) (inhibitory)
(intestine) (neurogenic) (paralytic)
Nonessential modifiers are enclosed in parentheses and are words that may be used to clarify the diagnosis but do not affect the code.
Incoordination
esophageal-pharyngeal (newborn) 787.2
Essential modifiers are NOT enclosed in parentheses and are subterms that DO affect the selection of the appropriate code.
Hereditary—*see* condition
"*see*" is a cross reference directing you to look elsewhere.
Paralysis
embolic (current episode) (*see also*
Embolism, brain) 434.1
"*see also*" is a cross reference directing you to look under another main term if all the information being searched for cannot be located under the first main term entry.
Delivery
completely normal case—*see* category 650
"*see category*" is a cross reference directing you to Volume 1, Tabular List for important information governing the use of the specific code.
Amputation
traumatic (complete) (partial)
"Notes" are used to define terms and give coding instructions
Note "Complicated" includes traumatic amputation with delayed healing, delayed treatment, foreign body, or major infection.
Adolescence NEC V21.2
NEC means Not Elsewhere Classifiable.

Conventions for Volume 3, Procedures Index

Arthrotomy 80.10
as operative approach—*omit code*

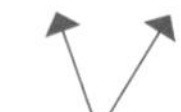

"*omit code*" identifies procedures or services that are included in another larger procedure or service. For example, an incision that is part of the main surgical procedure is not coded separately.

Ileal
bladder
closed 57.87 [*45.51*]

For some operative procedures it is necessary to record the individual components of the procedure. These procedures are termed **"synchronous procedures"** and are listed together in the Index. The codes are sequenced in the same order as displayed in the Index.

Operation
Thompson
cleft lip repair 27.54
correction of lymphedema 40.9
quadricepsplasty 83.86

Eponyms are operations named for people and are listed in the Index both under the eponym and under the term "Operation."

Thompson operation
cleft lip repair 27.54
correction of lymphedema 40.9
quadricepsplasty 83.86

Volume 3, Index to Procedures, also contains "*see*," "*see also*," "*see* category," "essential modifiers," "nonessential modifiers," "notes," NEC, and NOS as in Volume 2, Alphabetic Index.

Symbols for Volume 3, Procedures, Tabular List

Use Additional Digit(s): The color dot cautions you that the code requires additional digit(s) to ensure the greatest specificity.

Valid O.R. Procedure: The red X is placed before a code that is a valid operating room (O.R.) procedure according to the DRG grouper.

● **31.9 Other operations on larynx and trachea**

✖ **31.91 Division of laryngeal nerve**

Conventions for Volume 3, Procedures, Tabular List

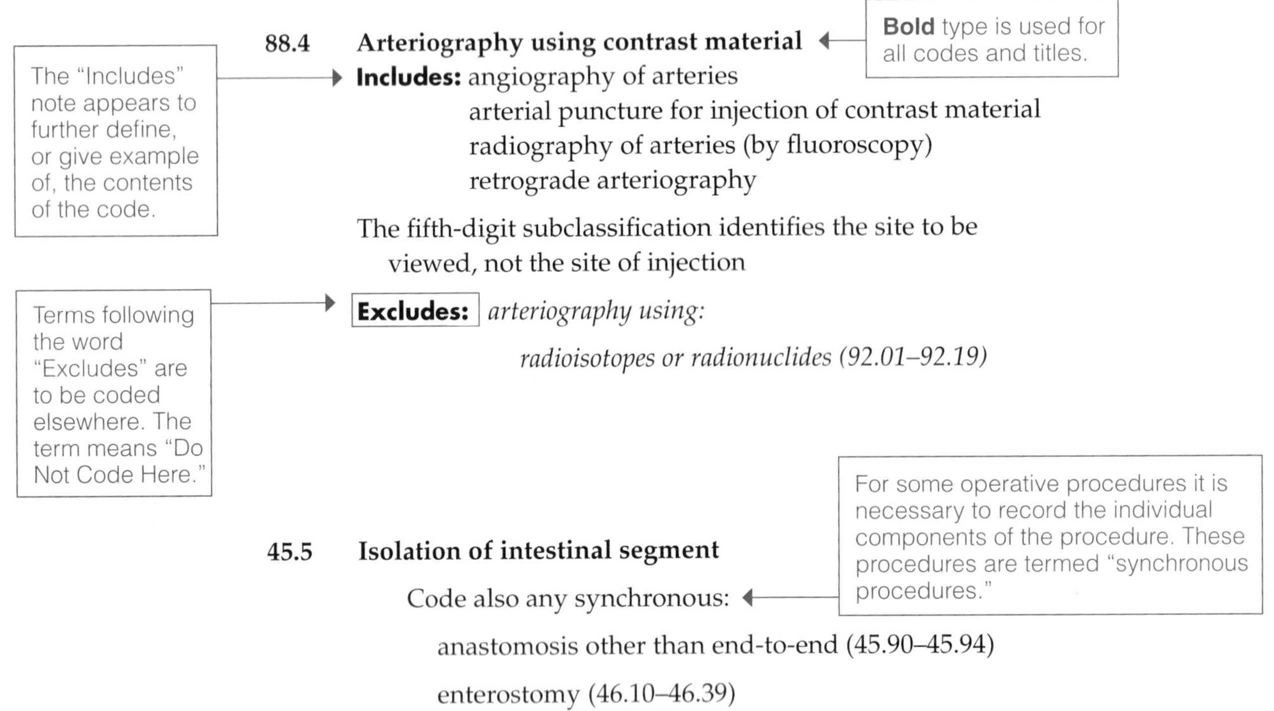
Bold type is used for all codes and titles.
88.4 Arteriography using contrast material
The "Includes" note appears to further define, or give example of, the contents of the code.
Includes: angiography of arteries
arterial puncture for injection of contrast material
radiography of arteries (by fluoroscopy)
retrograde arteriography
The fifth-digit subclassification identifies the site to be viewed, not the site of injection
Terms following the word "Excludes" are to be coded elsewhere. The term means "Do Not Code Here."
Excludes: arteriography using:
radioisotopes or radionuclides (92.01–92.19)
For some operative procedures it is necessary to record the individual components of the procedure. These procedures are termed "synchronous procedures."
45.5 Isolation of intestinal segment
Code also any synchronous:
anastomosis other than end-to-end (45.90–45.94)
enterostomy (46.10–46.39)

GUIDE TO THE 2007 ICD-9-CM UPDATES

VOLUME 1 CHANGES EFFECTIVE OCTOBER 1, 2006, AND CLASSIFICATION OF DISEASES AND E CODES

1. INFECTIOUS AND PARASITIC DISEASES (001–139)

052 Chickenpox

New Code **052.2 Postvaricella myelitis**

Postchickenpox myelitis

053 Herpes zoster

053.1 With other nervous system complications

New Code **053.14 Herpes zoster myelitis**

054 Herpes simplex

054.7 With other specified complications

New Code **054.74 Herpes simplex myelitis**

136 Other and unspecified infectious and parasitic diseases

136.3 Pneumocystosis

Add Pneumonia due to Pneumocystis jiroveci

2. NEOPLASMS (140–239)

151 Malignant neoplasm of stomach

Add **Excludes** *malignant stromal tumor of stomach (171.5)*

152 Malignant neoplasm of small intestine, including duodenum

Add **Excludes** *malignant stromal tumor of small intestine (171.5)*

171 Malignant neoplasm of connective and other soft tissue

Add **Includes:** malignant stromal tumors

Excludes *connective tissue:*

Revise *internal organs (except stromal tumors) – code to malignant neoplasm of the site [e.g., leiomyosarcoma of stomach, 151.9]*

174 Malignant neoplasm of female breast

Add Use additional code to identify estrogen receptor status (V86.0, V86.1)

175 Malignant neoplasm of male breast

Add Use additional code to identify estrogen receptor status (V86.0, V86.1)

202 Other malignant neoplasms of lymphoid and histiocytic tissue

202.0 Nodular lymphoma

Delete ~~Reticulosarcoma, follicular or nodular~~

211 Benign neoplasm of other parts of digestive system

Add **Excludes** *benign stromal tumors of digestive system (215.5)*

215 Other benign neoplasm of connective and other soft tissue

215.5 Abdomen

Add Benign stromal tumors of abdomen

233 Carcinoma in situ of breast and genitourinary system

233.1 Cervix uteri

Add Cervical intraepithelial glandular neoplasia

Revise **Excludes** *cytologic evidence of malignancy without histologic confirmation (795.06)*

235 Neoplasm of uncertain behavior of digestive and respiratory systems

Add **Excludes** *stromal tumors of uncertain behavior of digestive system (238.1)*

238 Neoplasm of uncertain behavior of other and unspecified sites and tissues

238.1 Connective and other soft tissue

Add Stromal tumors of digestive system

238.7 Other lymphatic and hematopoietic tissues

Delete ~~Disease:~~

~~lymphoproliferative (chronic) NOS~~

~~myeloproliferative (chronic) NOS~~

~~Idiopathic thrombocythemia~~

~~Megakaryocytic myelosclerosis~~

~~Myelodysplastic syndrome~~

~~Myelosclerosis with myeloid metaplasia~~

~~Panmyelosis (acute)~~

~~Refractory anemia~~

Add **Excludes** *acute myelogenous leukemia (205.0)*

Add *chronic myelomonocytic leukemia (205.1)*

Revise *myelofibrosis (289.83)*

New code **238.71 Essential thrombocythemia**

Essential hemorrhagic thrombocythemia

Essential thrombocytosis

Idiopathic (hemorrhagic) thrombocythemia

Primary thrombocytosis

New code **238.72 Low grade myelodysplastic syndrome lesions**

Refractory anemia (RA)

Refractory anemia with ringed sideroblasts (RARS)

Refractory cytopenia with multilineage dysplasia (RCMD)

Refractory cytopenia with multilineage dysplasia and ringed sideroblasts (RCMD-RS)

New code **238.73 High grade myelodysplastic syndrome lesions**

Refractory anemia with excess blasts-1 (RAEB-1)

Refractory anemia with excess blasts-2 (RAEB-2)

New code **238.74 Myelodysplastic syndrome with 5q deletion**

5q minus syndrome NOS

Excludes *constitutional 5q deletion (758.39)*
high grade myelodysplastic syndrome with 5q deletion (238.73)

New code **238.75 Myelodysplastic syndrome, unspecified**

New code **238.76 Myelofibrosis with myeloid metaplasia**

Agnogenic myeloid metaplasia

Idiopathic myelofibrosis (chronic)

Myelosclerosis with myeloid metaplasia

Primary myelofibrosis

Excludes *myelofibrosis NOS (289.83)*
myelophthisic anemia (284.2)
myelophthisis (284.2)
secondary myelofibrosis (289.83)

New code **238.79 Other lymphatic and hematopoietic tissues**

Lymphoproliferative disease (chronic) NOS

Megakaryocytic myelosclerosis

Myeloproliferative disease (chronic) NOS

Panmyelosis (acute)

3. ENDOCRINE, NUTRITIONAL AND METABOLIC DISEASES, AND IMMUNITY DISORDERS (240–279)

255 Disorders of adrenal glands

255.1 Hyperaldosteronism

Revise **255.10 ~~Primary aldosteronism~~ Hyperaldosteronism, unspecified**

Delete ~~Hyperaldosteronism, unspecified~~

Add Primary aldosteronism, unspecified

277 Other and unspecified disorders of metabolism

277.3 Amyloidosis

Delete ~~Amyloidosis:~~

Delete ~~NOS~~

Delete ~~inherited systemic~~

Delete ~~nephropathic~~

Delete ~~neuropathic (Portuguese) (Swiss)~~

Delete ~~secondary~~

Delete ~~Benign paroxysmal peritonitis~~

Delete ~~Familial Mediterranean fever~~

Delete ~~Hereditary cardiac amyloidosis~~

New Code **277.30 Amyloidosis, unspecified**

Amyloidosis NOS

New Code **277.31 Familial Mediterranean fever**

Benign paroxysmal peritonitis
Hereditary amyloid nephropathy
Periodic familial polyserositis
Recurrent polyserositis

New Code **277.39 Other amyloidosis**

Hereditary cardiac amyloidosis
Inherited systemic amyloidosis
Neuropathic (Portuguese) (Swiss) amyloidosis
Secondary amyloidosis

278 Overweight, obesity, and other hyperalimentation

278.0 Overweight and obesity

Revise Use additional code to identify Body Mass Index (BMI), if known (~~V85.21-V85.4~~ V85.0–V85.54)

4. DISEASES OF THE BLOOD AND BLOOD-FORMING ORGANS (280–289)

281 Other deficiency anemias

281.3 Other specified megaloblastic anemias not elsewhere classified

Delete ~~**Excludes** *refractory megaloblastic anemia (238.7)*~~

Revise **284 Aplastic anemia and other bone marrow failure syndromes**

284.0 Constitutional aplastic anemia

Delete ~~Aplasia, (pure) red cell:~~
~~congenital~~
~~of infants~~
~~primary~~
~~Blackfan-Diamond syndrome~~
~~Familial hypoplastic anemia~~
~~Fanconi's anemia~~
~~Pancytopenia with malformations~~

New code **284.01 Constitutional red blood cell aplasia**

Aplasia, (pure) red cell:
congenital
of infants
primary
Blackfan-Diamond syndrome
Familial hypoplastic anemia

New code **284.09 Other constitutional aplastic anemia**

Fanconi's anemia
Pancytopenia with malformations

New code **284.1 Pancytopenia**

Excludes *pancytopenia (due to) (with):*
aplastic anemia NOS (284.9)
bone marrow infiltration (284.2)
constitutional red blood cell aplasia (284.01)
drug induced (284.8)
hairy cell leukemia (202.4)
human immunodeficiency virus disease (042)
leukoerythroblastic anemia (284.2)
malformations (284.09)
myelodysplastic syndromes (238.72–238.75)
myeloproliferative disease (238.79)
other constitutional aplastic anemia (284.09)

New code **284.2 Myelophthisis**

Leukoerythroblastic anemia
Myelophthisic anemia
Code first the underlying disorder, such as:
malignant neoplasm of breast (174.0–174.9, 175.0–175.9)
tuberculosis (015.0–015.9)

Excludes *idiopathic myelofibrosis (238.76)*
myelofibrosis NOS (289.83)
myelofibrosis with myeloid metaplasia (238.76)
primary myelofibrosis (238.76)
secondary myelofibrosis (289.83)

284.8 Other specified aplastic anemias

Delete ~~Pancytopenia (acquired)~~

284.9 Aplastic anemia, unspecified

Revise **Excludes** *refractory anemia (238.72)*

285 Other and unspecified anemias

285.0 Sideroblastic anemia

Revise **Excludes** *refractory sideroblastic anemia (238.72)*

Revise **285.2 Anemia ~~in~~ of chronic ~~illness~~ disease**

Add Anemia in other chronic illness

Revise **285.29 Anemia of chronic ~~illness~~ disease**

Add Anemia in other chronic illness

285.8 Other specified anemias

Anemia:

Delete ~~Leukoerythroblastic~~

287 Purpura and other hemorrhagic conditions

Revise **Excludes** *hemorrhagic thrombocythemia (238.79)*

288 Diseases of white blood cells

Revise **288.0 ~~Agranulocytosis~~ Neutropenia**

Add Decreased Absolute Neutrophil Count (ANC)

Delete ~~Infantile genetic agranulocytosis~~
~~Kostmann's syndrome~~
~~Neutropenia:~~
~~NOS~~
~~cyclic~~
~~drug-induced~~
~~immune~~
~~periodic~~
~~toxic~~
~~Neutropenic splenomegaly~~

Delete ~~Use additional E code to identify drug or other cause~~

Add Use additional code for any associated fever (780.6)

Add **Excludes** *neutropenic splenomegaly (289.53)*

New code **288.00 Neutropenia, unspecified**

New code **288.01 Congenital neutropenia**

Congenital agranulocytosis
Infantile genetic agranulocytosis
Kostmann's syndrome

New code **288.02 Cyclic neutropenia**

Cyclic hematopoiesis
Periodic neutropenia

New code **288.03 Drug induced neutropenia**

Use additional E code to identify drug

New code 288.04 **Neutropenia due to infection**

New code 288.09 **Other neutropenia**
Agranulocytosis
Neutropenia:
immune
toxic

New code 288.4 **Hemophagocytic syndromes**
Familial hemophagocytic lymphohistiocytosis
Familial hemophagocytic reticulosis
Hemophagocytic syndrome, infection-associated
Histiocytic syndromes
Macrophage activation syndrome

New sub-category 288.5 **Decreased white blood cell count**
Excludes *neutropenia (288.01–288.09)*

New code 288.50 **Leukocytopenia, unspecified**
Decreased leukocytes, unspecified
Decreased white blood cell count, unspecified
Leukopenia NOS

New code 288.51 **Lymphocytopenia**
Decreased lymphocytes

New code 288.59 **Other decreased white blood cell count**
Basophilic leukopenia
Eosinophilic leukopenia
Monocytopenia
Plasmacytopenia

New sub-category 288.6 **Elevated white blood cell count**
Excludes *eosinophilia (288.3)*

New code 288.60 **Leukocytosis, unspecified**
Elevated leukocytes, unspecified
Elevated white blood cell count, unspecified

New code 288.61 **Lymphocytosis (symptomatic)**
Elevated lymphocytes

New code 288.62 **Leukemoid reaction**
Basophilic leukemoid reaction
Lymphocytic leukemoid reaction
Monocytic leukemoid reaction
Myelocytic leukemoid reaction
Neutrophilic leukemoid reaction

New code 288.63 **Monocytosis (symptomatic)**
Excludes *infectious mononucleosis (075)*

New code 288.64 **Plasmacytosis**

New code 288.65 **Basophilia**

New code 288.69 **Other elevated white blood cell count**

288.8 **Other specified disease of white blood cells**

Delete ~~Leukemoid reaction:~~
~~lymphocytic~~
~~monocytic~~
~~myelocytic~~
~~Leukocytosis~~
~~Lymphocytopenia~~
~~Lymphocytosis (symptomatic)~~
~~Lymphopenia~~
~~Monocytosis (symptomatic)~~
~~Plasmacytosis~~

Add **Excludes** *decreased white blood cell counts (288.50–288.59)*
elevated white blood cell counts (288.60–288.69)

289 **Other diseases of blood and blood-forming organs**

289.4 **Hypersplenism**

Revise **Excludes** *primary splenic neutropenia (289.53)*

289.5 **Other diseases of spleen**

New code 289.53 **Neutropenic splenomegaly**

289.8 **Other specified diseases of the blood and blood-forming organs**

New code 289.83 **Myelofibrosis**
Myelofibrosis NOS
Secondary myelofibrosis
Code first the underlying disorder, such as:
malignant neoplasm of breast (174.0–174.9, 175.0–175.9)

Excludes *idiopathic myelofibrosis (238.76)*
leukoerythroblastic anemia (284.2)
myelofibrosis with myeloid metaplasia (238.76)
myelophthisic anemia (284.2)
myelophthisis (284.2)
primary myelofibrosis (238.76)

289.89 **Other specified diseases of blood and blood-forming organs**

Delete ~~Myelofibrosis~~

5. MENTAL DISORDERS (290–319)

305 **Nondependent abuse of drugs**

305.1 **Tobacco use disorder**

Add **Excludes** *smoking complicating pregnancy (649.0)*
tobacco use disorder complicating pregnancy (649.0)

307 **Special symptoms or syndromes, not elsewhere classified**

307.8 **Pain disorders related to psychological factors**

307.89 **Other**

Revise Code first to type or site of pain

309 **Adjustment reaction**

309.8 **Other specified adjustment reactions**

309.81 **Posttraumatic stress disorder**

Add Post-Traumatic Stress Disorder (PTSD)

6. DISEASES OF THE NERVOUS SYSTEM AND SENSE ORGANS (320–389)

323 **Encephalitis, myelitis, and encephalomyelitis**

Revise **Includes:** myelitis (~~acute~~):

Add **Excludes** *acute transverse myelitis NOS (341.20)*
acute transverse myelitis in conditions classified elsewhere (341.21)
idiopathic transverse myelitis (341.22)

Revise 323.0 **Encephalitis, myelitis, and encephalomyelitis in viral diseases classified elsewhere**

Delete ~~**Excludes** *encephalitis (in):*~~
~~*arthropod-borne viral (062.0–064)*~~
~~*herpes simplex (054.3)*~~
~~*mumps (072.2)*~~
~~*other viral diseases of central nervous system (049.8–049.9)*~~
~~*poliomyelitis (045.0–045.9)*~~
~~*rubella (056.01)*~~
~~*slow virus infections of central nervous system (046.0–046.9)*~~
~~*viral NOS (049.9)*~~

New code 323.01 **Encephalitis and encephalomyelitis in viral diseases classified elsewhere**

Excludes *encephalitis (in):*
arthropod-borne viral (062.0–064)
herpes simplex (054.3)
mumps (072.2)
other viral diseases of central nervous system (049.8–049.9)
poliomyelitis (045.0–045.9)
rubella (056.01)
slow virus infections of central nervous system (046.0–046.9)
viral NOS (049.9)
West Nile (066.41)

New code — **323.02 Myelitis in viral diseases classified elsewhere**

Excludes *myelitis (in):*
herpes simplex (054.74)
herpes zoster (053.14)
poliomyelitis (045.0–045.9)
rubella (056.01)
other viral diseases of central nervous system (049.8–049.9)

Revise — **323.1 Encephalitis, myelitis, and encephalomyelitis in rickettsial diseases classified elsewhere**

Revise — **323.2 Encephalitis, myelitis, and encephalomyelitis in protozoal diseases classified elsewhere**

Revise — **323.4 Other encephalitis, myelitis, and encephalomyelitis due to infection classified elsewhere**

Delete — ~~**Excludes** *encephalitis (in):*~~
~~*meningococcal (036.1)*~~
~~*syphilis:*~~
~~*NOS (094.81)*~~
~~*congenital (090.41)*~~
~~*toxoplasmosis (130.0)*~~
~~*tuberculosis (013.6)*~~
~~*meningoencephalitis due to free-living ameba [Naegleria] (136.2)*~~

New code — **323.41 Other encephalitis and encephalomyelitis due to infection classified elsewhere**

Excludes *encephalitis (in):*
meningococcal (036.1)
syphilis:
NOS (094.81)
congenital (090.41)
toxoplasmosis (130.0)
tuberculosis (013.6)
meningoencephalitis due to free-living ameba [Naegleria] (136.2)

New code — **323.42 Other myelitis due to infection classified elsewhere**

Excludes *myelitis (in):*
syphilis (094.89)
tuberculosis (013.6)

Revise — **323.5 Encephalitis, myelitis, and encephalomyelitis following immunization procedures**

Delete — ~~Encephalitis postimmunization or postvaccinal~~
~~Encephalomyelitis postimmunization or postvaccinal~~

New Code — **323.51 Encephalitis and encephalomyelitis following immunization procedures**
Encephalitis postimmunization or postvaccinal
Encephalomyelitis postimmunization or postvaccinal

New Code — **323.52 Myelitis following immunization procedures**
Myelitis postimmunization or postvaccinal

Revise — **323.6 Postinfectious encephalitis, myelitis, and encephalomyelitis**

Delete — ~~Infectious acute disseminated encephalomyelitis (ADEM)~~

Delete — ~~**Excludes** *encephalitis:*~~
~~*postchickenpox (052.0)*~~
~~*postmeasles (055.0)*~~

New code — **323.61 Infectious acute disseminated encephalomyelitis (ADEM)**
Acute necrotizing hemorrhagic encephalopathy

Excludes *noninfectious acute disseminated encephalomyelitis (ADEM) (323.81)*

New code — **323.62 Other postinfectious encephalitis and encephalomyelitis**

Excludes *encephalitis:*
postchickenpox (052.0)
postmeasles (055.0)

New code — **323.63 Postinfectious myelitis**

Excludes *postchickenpox myelitis (052.2)*
herpes simplex myelitis (054.74)
herpes zoster myelitis (053.14)

Revise — **323.7 Toxic encephalitis, myelitis, and encephalomyelitis**

New code — **323.71 Toxic encephalitis and encephalomyelitis**

New code — **323.72 Toxic myelitis**

Revise — **323.8 Other causes of encephalitis, myelitis, and encephalomyelitis**

Delete — ~~Noninfectious acute disseminated encephalomyelitis (ADEM)~~

New code — **323.81 Other causes of encephalitis and encephalomyelitis**
Noninfectious acute disseminated encephalomyelitis (ADEM)

New code — **323.82 Other causes of myelitis**
Transverse myelitis NOS

Revise — **323.9 Unspecified cause of encephalitis, myelitis, and encephalomyelitis**

326 Late effects of intracranial abscess or pyogenic infection

Revise — Note: This category is to be used to indicate conditions whose primary classification is to 320-325 [excluding 320.7, 321.0-321.8, 323.01–323.42, 323.61–323.72] as the cause of late effects, themselves classifiable elsewhere…

Add — **ORGANIC SLEEP DISORDERS (327)**

327 Organic sleep disorders

327.5 Organic sleep related movement disorders

Revise — **Excludes** *restless legs syndrome (333.94)*

331 Other cerebral degenerations

331.8 Other cerebral degeneration

New code — **331.83 Mild cognitive impairment, so stated**

Excludes *altered mental status (780.97)*
cerebral degeneration (331.0–331.9)
change in mental status (780.97)
cognitive deficits following (late effects of) cerebral hemorrhage or infarction (438.0)
cognitive impairment due to intracranial or head injury (850–854, 959.01)
cognitive impairment due to late effect of intracranial injury (907.0)
dementia (290.0–290.43, 294.8)
mild memory disturbance (310.8)
neurologic neglect syndrome (781.8)
personality change, nonpsychotic (310.1)

333 Other extrapyramidal disease and abnormal movement disorders

Revise — **333.6 ~~Idiopathic~~ Genetic torsion dystonia**

Revise — **333.7 ~~Symptomatic~~ Acquired torsion dystonia**

Delete — ~~Athetoid cerebral palsy [Vogt's disease]~~

Delete — ~~Double athetosis (syndrome)~~

Delete — ~~Neuroleptic induced acute dystonia~~

Delete — ~~Use additional E code to identify drug, if drug-induced~~

New Code — **333.71 Athetoid cerebral palsy**
Double athetosis (syndrome)
Vogt's disease

Excludes *infantile cerebral palsy (343.0–343.9)*

New Code **333.72 Acute dystonia due to drugs**
Acute dystonic reaction due to drugs
Neuroleptic induced acute dystonia
Use additional E code to identify drug

Excludes *blepharospasm due to drugs (333.85)*
orofacial dyskinesia due to drugs (333.85)
secondary Parkinsonism (332.1)
subacute dyskinesia due to drugs (333.85)
tardive dyskinesia (333.85)

New Code **333.79 Other acquired torsion dystonia**
333.8 Fragments of torsion dystonia
333.81 Blepharospasm
Add **Excludes** *blepharospasm due to drugs (333.85)*
333.82 Orofacial dyskinesia
Delete ~~Neuroleptic-induced tardive dyskinesia~~
Add **Excludes** *orofacial dyskinesia due to drugs (333.85)*

New Code **333.85 Subacute dyskinesia due to drugs**
Blepharospasm due to drugs
Orofacial dyskinesia due to drugs
Tardive dyskinesia
Use additional E code to identify drug

Excludes *acute dystonia due to drugs (333.72)*
acute dystonic reaction due to drugs (333.72)
secondary Parkinsonism (332.1)

333.9 Other and unspecified extrapyramidal diseases and abnormal movement disorders
333.92 Neuroleptic malignant syndrome
Add **Excludes** *neuroleptic induced Parkinsonism (332.1)*

New code **333.94 Restless legs syndrome (RLS)**
333.99 Other
Delete ~~Restless legs~~
336 Other disease of spinal cord
336.9 Unspecified disease of spinal cord
Revise **Excludes** *myelitis (323.02, 323.1, 323.2, 323.42, 323.52, 323.63, 323.72, 323.82, 323.9)*

337 Disorders of the autonomic nervous system
337.1 Peripheral autonomic neuropathy in disorders classified elsewhere
Code first underlying disease, as:
Revise amyloidosis (277.30–277.39)

Add **PAIN (338)**
New Category **338 Pain, not elsewhere classified**

Use additional code to identify:
pain associated with psychological factors (307.89)

Excludes *generalized pain (780.96)*
localized pain, unspecified type – code to pain by site
pain disorder exclusively attributed to psychological factors (307.80)

New code **338.0 Central pain syndrome**
Déjérine-Roussy syndrome
Myelopathic pain syndrome
Thalamic pain syndrome (hyperesthetic)
New sub-category **338.1 Acute pain**
New code **338.11 Acute pain due to trauma**
New code **338.12 Acute post-thoracotomy pain**
Post-thoracotomy pain NOS
New code **338.18 Other acute postoperative pain**
Postoperative pain NOS
New code **338.19 Other acute pain**

Excludes *neoplasm related acute pain (338.3)*

New sub-category **338.2 Chronic pain**

Excludes *causalgia (355.9)*
lower limb (355.71)
upper limb (354.4)
chronic pain syndrome (338.4)
myofascial pain syndrome (729.1)
neoplasm related chronic pain (338.3)
reflex sympathetic dystrophy (337.20–337.29)

New code **338.21 Chronic pain due to trauma**
New code **338.22 Chronic post-thoracotomy pain**
New code **338.28 Other chronic postoperative pain**
New code **338.29 Other chronic pain**
New code **338.3 Neoplasm related pain (acute) (chronic)**
Cancer associated pain
Pain due to malignancy (primary) (secondary)
Tumor associated pain
New code **338.4 Chronic pain syndrome**
Chronic pain associated with significant psychosocial dysfunction
341 Other demyelinating diseases of central nervous system
New sub-category **341.2 Acute (transverse) myelitis**

Excludes *acute (transverse) myelitis (in) (due to):*
following immunization procedures (323.52)
infection classified elsewhere (323.42)
postinfectious (323.63)
protozoal diseases classified elsewhere (323.2)
rickettsial diseases classified elsewhere (323.1)
toxic (323.72)
viral diseases classified elsewhere (323.02)
transverse myelitis NOS (323.82)

New code **341.20 Acute (transverse) myelitis NOS**
New code **341.21 Acute (transverse) myelitis in conditions classified elsewhere**
Code first underlying condition
New code **341.22 Idiopathic transverse myelitis**
343 Infantile cerebral palsy
Add **Excludes** *athetoid cerebral palsy (333.71)*
hereditary cerebral paralysis, such as:
Revise *Vogt's disease (333.71)*
Revise **345 Epilepsy and recurrent seizures**
345.1 Generalized convulsive epilepsy

Excludes *convulsions:*
Revise *NOS (780.39)*
Revise *infantile (780.39)*

Revise **345.4** ~~**Partial epilepsy, with impairment of consciousness**~~ **Localization-related (focal) (partial) epilepsy and epileptic syndromes with complex partial seizures**
Epilepsy:
partial:
Add with impairment of consciousness
Revise **345.5** ~~**Partial epilepsy, without mention of impairment of consciousness**~~ **Localization-related (focal) (partial) epilepsy and epileptic syndromes with simple partial seizures**
Epilepsy:
partial NOS:
Add without impairment of consciousness
Revise **345.8 Other forms of epilepsy and recurrent seizures**
345.9 Epilepsy, unspecified
Add Recurrent seizures NOS
Add Seizure disorder NOS

Add **Excludes** *convulsion (convulsive) disorder (780.39)*
Revise *convulsive seizures or fit NOS (780.39)*
Add *recurrent convulsions (780.39)*

348 Other conditions of brain
348.3 Encephalopathy, not elsewhere classified
348.31 Metabolic encephalopathy
Add — **Excludes** *toxic metabolic encephalopathy (349.82)*

349 Other and unspecified disorders of the nervous system
349.8 Other specified disorders of nervous system
349.82 Toxic encephalopathy
Add — Toxic metabolic encephalopathy

357 Inflammatory and toxic neuropathy
357.4 Polyneuropathy in other diseases classified elsewhere
Code first underlying disease, as:
Revise — amyloidosis (277.30–277.39)
Add — chronic uremia (585.9)
Revise — uremia NOS (586)

359 Muscular dystrophies and other myopathies
359.6 Symptomatic inflammatory myopathy in diseases classified elsewhere
Code first underlying disease, as:
Revise — amyloidosis (277.30–277.39)

360 Disorders of the globe
360.0 Purulent endophthalmitis
Add — **Excludes** *bleb associated endophthalmitis (379.63)*
360.1 Other endophthalmitis
Add — **Excludes** *bleb associated endophthalmitis (379.63)*

377 Disorders of optic nerve and visual pathways
377.4 Other disorders of optic nerve
New code — **377.43 Optic nerve hypoplasia**

379 Other disorders of eye
New subcategory — **379.6 Inflammation (infection) of postprocedural bleb, unspecified**
Postprocedural blebitis
New code — **379.60 Inflammation (infection) of postprocedural bleb, unspecified**
New code — **379.61 Inflammation (infection) of postprocedural bleb, stage 1**
New code — **379.62 Inflammation (infection) of postprocedural bleb, stage 2**
New code — **379.63 Inflammation (infection) of postprocedural bleb, stage 3**
Bleb associated endophthalmitis

389 Hearing loss
389.1 Sensorineural hearing loss
Revise — **389.11 Sensory hearing loss, bilateral**
Revise — **389.12 Neural hearing loss, bilateral**
Revise — **389.14 Central hearing loss, bilateral**
New code — **389.15 Sensorineural hearing loss, unilateral**
New code — **389.16 Sensorineural hearing loss, asymmetrical**
Revise — **389.18 Sensorineural hearing loss of combined types, bilateral**

7. DISEASES OF THE CIRCULATORY SYSTEM (390–459)

Revise — **403 Hypertensive chronic kidney disease**
Delete — ~~Use additional code to identify the stage of chronic kidney disease (585.1–585.6), if known~~
The following fifth-digit subclassification is for use with category 403:
Revise — 0 ~~without chronic kidney disease~~ with chronic kidney disease stage I through stage IV, or unspecified
Add — Use additional code to identify the stage of chronic kidney disease (585.1–585.4, 585.9)
Revise — 1 with chronic kidney disease stage V or end stage renal disease
Add — Use additional code to identify the stage of chronic kidney disease (585.5, 585.6)

Revise — **404 Hypertensive heart and chronic kidney disease**
Delete — ~~Use additional code to identify the stage of chronic kidney disease (585.1–585.6), if known~~
The following fifth-digit subclassification is for use with category 404:
Revise — 0 without heart failure ~~or chronic kidney disease~~ and with chronic kidney disease stage I through stage IV, or unspecified
Add — Use additional code to identify the stage of chronic kidney disease (585.1–585.4, 585.9)
Revise — 1 with heart failure and with chronic kidney disease stage I through stage IV, or unspecified
Add — Use additional code to identify the stage of chronic kidney disease (585.1–585.4, 585.9)
Revise — 2 without heart failure and with chronic kidney disease stage V or end stage renal disease
Add — Use additional code to identify the stage of chronic kidney disease (585.5, 585.6)
Revise — 3 with heart failure and chronic kidney disease stage V or end stage renal disease
Add — Use additional code to identify the stage of chronic kidney disease (585.5–585.6)

420 Acute pericarditis
420.0 Acute pericarditis in diseases classified elsewhere
Code first underlying disease, as:
Add — chronic uremia (585.9)
Revise — uremia NOS (586)

425 Cardiomyopathy
425.7 Nutritional and metabolic cardiomyopathy
Code first underlying disease, as:
Revise — amyloidosis (277.30–277.39)

429 Ill-defined descriptions and complications of heart disease
429.8 Other ill-defined heart diseases
New Code — **429.83 Takotsubo syndrome**
Broken heart syndrome
Reversible left ventricular dysfunction following sudden emotional stress
Stress induced cardiomyopathy
Transient left ventricular apical ballooning syndrome

440 Atherosclerosis
440.2 Of native arteries of the extremities
440.24 Atherosclerosis of the extremities with gangrene
Add — Use additional code for any associated ulceration (707.10–707.9)

445 Atheroembolism
445.8 Of other sites
445.81 Kidney
Revise — Use additional code for any associated ~~kidney~~ acute renal failure or chronic kidney disease (584, 585)

8. DISEASES OF THE RESPIRATORY SYSTEM (460–519)

478 Other diseases of upper respiratory tract
478.1 Other diseases of nasal cavity and sinuses
Delete — ~~Abscess of nose (septum)~~
Delete — ~~Necrosis of nose (septum)~~
Delete — ~~Ulcer of nose (septum)~~
Delete — ~~Cyst or mucocele of sinus (nasal)~~
Delete — ~~Rhinolith~~
New Code — **478.11 Nasal mucositis (ulcerative)**
Use additional E code to identify adverse effects of therapy, such as:
antineoplastic and immunosuppressive drugs (E930.7, E933.1)
radiation therapy (E879.2)

New Code **478.19 Other diseases of nasal cavity and sinuses**
Abscess of nose (septum)
Necrosis of nose (septum)
Ulcer of nose (septum)
Cyst or mucocele of sinus (nasal)
Rhinolith

496 Chronic airway obstruction, not elsewhere classified
Excludes *chronic obstructive lung disease [COPD] specified (as) (with):*
Add *decompensated (491.21)*

514 Pulmonary congestion and hypostasis
Add **Excludes** *hypostatic pneumonia due to or specified as a specific type of pneumonia – code to the type of pneumonia (480.0–480.9, 481, 482.0–482.49, 483.0–483.8, 485, 486, 487.0)*

517 Lung involvement in conditions classified elsewhere
517.8 Lung involvement in other diseases classified elsewhere
Code first underlying disease, as:
Revise amyloidosis (277.30–277.39)

518 Other diseases of lung
New code **518.7 Transfusion related acute lung injury (TRALI)**

519 Other diseases of respiratory system
519.1 Other diseases of trachea and bronchus, not elsewhere classified
Delete ~~Calcification of bronchus or trachea~~
~~Stenosis of bronchus or trachea~~
~~Ulcer of bronchus or trachea~~
New code **519.11 Acute bronchospasm**
Bronchospasm NOS
Excludes *acute bronchitis with bronchospasm (466.0)*
asthma (493.00–493.92)
exercise induced bronchospasm (493.81)
New code **519.19 Other diseases of trachea and bronchus**
Calcification of bronchus or trachea
Stenosis of bronchus or trachea
Ulcer of bronchus or trachea

9. DISEASES OF THE DIGESTIVE SYSTEM (520–579)

520 Disorders of tooth development and eruption
520.6 Disturbances in tooth eruption
Teeth:
Add prenatal

521 Diseases of hard tissues of teeth
521.0 Dental caries
521.06 Dental caries pit and fissure
Add Primary dental caries, pit and fissure origin
521.07 Dental caries of smooth surface
Add Primary dental caries, smooth surface origin
521.08 Dental caries of root surface
Add Primary dental caries, root surface
521.8 Other specified diseases of hard tissues of teeth
Delete ~~Irradiated enamel~~
Delete ~~Sensitive dentin~~
New code **521.81 Cracked tooth**
Excludes *asymptomatic craze lines in enamel – omit code*
broken tooth due to trauma (873.63, 873.73)
fractured tooth due to trauma (873.63, 873.73)
New code **521.89 Other specified diseases of hard tissues of teeth**
Irradiated enamel
Sensitive dentin

523 Gingival and periodontal diseases
523.0 Acute gingivitis
New code **523.00 Acute gingivitis, plaque induced**
Acute gingivitis NOS
New code **523.01 Acute gingivitis, non-plaque induced**
523.1 Chronic gingivitis
Gingivitis (chronic):
Delete ~~NOS~~
Delete ~~Gingivostomatitis~~
New code **523.10 Chronic gingivitis, plaque induced**
Chronic gingivitis NOS
Gingivitis NOS
New code **523.11 Chronic gingivitis, non-plaque induced**
Revise **523.3 Aggressive and ~~A~~acute periodontitis**
Delete ~~Paradontal abscess~~
Delete ~~Periodontal abscess~~
New code **523.30 Aggressive periodontitis, unspecified**
New code **523.31 Aggressive periodontitis, localized**
Periodontal abscess
New code **523.32 Aggressive periodontitis, generalized**
New code **523.33 Acute periodontitis**
523.4 Chronic periodontitis
Delete ~~Alveolar pyorrhea~~
New code **523.40 Chronic periodontitis, unspecified**
New code **523.41 Chronic periodontitis, localized**
New code **523.42 Chronic periodontitis, generalized**

524 Dentofacial anomalies, including malocclusion
524.0 Major anomalies of jaw size
524.07 Excessive tuberosity of jaw
Add Entire maxillary tuberosity
524.2 Anomalies of dental arch relationship
Add Anomaly of dental arch
Revise **524.21 Malocclusion, Angle's class I**
Revise **524.22 Malocclusion, Angle's class II**
Revise **524.23 Malocclusion, Angle's class III**
524.24 Open anterior occlusal relationship
Add Anterior open bite
524.25 Open posterior occlusal relationship
Add Posterior open bite
524.26 Excessive horizontal overlap
Add Excessive horizontal overjet
524.27 Reverse articulation
Add Crossbite
524.29 Other anomalies of dental arch relationship
Add Other anomalies of dental arch
524.3 Anomalies of tooth position of fully erupted teeth
524.33 Horizontal displacement of teeth
Add Tipped teeth
524.34 Vertical displacement of teeth
Add Extruded tooth
Add Intruded tooth
Revise **524.35 Rotation of tooth/teeth**
524.36 Insufficient interocclusal distance of teeth (ridge)
Add Lack of adequate intermaxillary vertical dimension
524.37 Excessive interocclusal distance of teeth
Add Excessive intermaxillary vertical dimension
524.5 Dentofacial functional abnormalities
Add **524.54 Insufficient anterior guidance**
Insufficient anterior occlusal guidance
Add **524.55 Centric occlusion maximum intercuspation discrepancy**
Centric occlusion of teeth discrepancy

Add **524.56 Non-working side interference**
Balancing side interference

525 Other diseases and conditions of the teeth and supporting structures

New sub-category **525.6 Unsatisfactory restoration of tooth**
Defective bridge, crown, fillings
Defective dental restoration

Excludes *dental restoration status (V45.84)*
unsatisfactory endodontic treatment (526.61–526.69)

New code **525.60 Unspecified unsatisfactory restoration of tooth**
Unspecified defective dental restoration

New code **525.61 Open restoration margins**
Dental restoration failure of marginal integrity
Open margin on tooth restoration

New code **525.62 Unrepairable overhanging of dental restorative materials**
Overhanging of tooth restoration

New code **525.63 Fractured dental restorative material without loss of material**

Excludes *cracked tooth (521.81)*
fractured tooth (873.63, 873.73)

New code **525.64 Fractured dental restorative material with loss of material**

Excludes *cracked tooth (521.81)*
fractured tooth (873.63, 873.73)

New code **525.65 Contour of existing restoration of tooth biologically incompatible with oral health**
Dental restoration failure of periodontal anatomical integrity
Unacceptable contours of existing restoration
Unacceptable morphology of existing restoration

New code **525.66 Allergy to existing dental restorative material**
Use additional code to identify the specific type of allergy

New code **525.67 Poor aesthetics of existing restoration**
Dental restoration aesthetically inadequate or displeasing

New code **525.69 Other unsatisfactory restoration of existing tooth**

526 Diseases of the jaws

New sub-category **526.6 Periradicular pathology associated with previous endodontic treatment**

New code **526.61 Perforation of root canal space**

New code **526.62 Endodontic overfill**

New code **526.63 Endodontic underfill**

New code **526.69 Other periradicular pathology associated with previous endodontic treatment**

528 Diseases of the oral soft tissues, excluding lesions specific for gingiva and tongue

Revise **528.0 Stomatitis and mucositis (ulcerative)**

Delete ~~Stomatitis:~~
~~NOS~~
~~ulcerative~~
~~Vesicular stomatitis~~

Add **Excludes** *cellulitis and abscess of mouth (528.3)*
diphtheritic stomatitis (032.0)
epizootic stomatitis (078.4)
gingivitis (523.0–523.1)
oral thrush (112.0)
Stevens-Johnson syndrome (695.1)

New code **528.00 Stomatitis and mucositis, unspecified**
Mucositis NOS
Ulcerative mucositis NOS
Ulcerative stomatitis NOS
Vesicular stomatitis NOS

New code **528.01 Mucositis (ulcerative) due to antineoplastic therapy**
Use additional E code to identify adverse effects of therapy, such as:
antineoplastic and immunosuppressive drugs (E930.7, E933.1)
radiation therapy (E879.2)

New code **528.02 Mucositis (ulcerative) due to other drugs**
Use additional E code to identify drug

New code **528.09 Other stomatitis and mucositis (ulcerative)**

528.3 Cellulitis and abscess

Revise **Excludes** *gingivitis (523.00–523.11)*

528.7 Other disturbances of oral epithelium, including tongue

528.71 Minimal keratinized residual ridge mucosa
Add Minimal keratinization of alveolar ridge mucosa

528.72 Excessive keratinized residual ridge mucosa
Add Excessive keratinization of alveolar ridge mucosa

528.79 Other disturbances of oral epithelium, including tongue
Add Other oral epithelium disturbances

Revise DISEASES OF ESOPHAGUS, STOMACH, AND DUODENUM (530–538)

536 Disorders of function of stomach

536.8 Dyspepsia and other specified disorders of function of stomach
Add Tachygastria

New code **538 Gastrointestinal mucositis (ulcerative)**
Use additional E code to identify adverse effects of therapy, such as:
antineoplastic and immunosuppressive drugs (E930.7, E933.1)
radiation therapy (E879.2)

Excludes *mucositis (ulcerative) of mouth and oral soft tissue (528.00–528.09)*

567 Peritonitis and retroperitoneal infections

Excludes *peritonitis:*
Revise *benign paroxysmal (277.31)*
Revise *periodic familial (277.31)*

567.2 Other suppurative peritonitis

567.23 Spontaneous bacterial peritonitis

Add **Excludes** *bacterial peritonitis NOS (567.29)*

NEPHRITIS, NEPHROTIC SYNDROME, AND NEPHROSIS (580–589)

Revise **Excludes** *hypertensive ~~renal~~ chronic kidney disease (403.00–403.91, 404.00–404.93)*

573 Other disorders of liver

Revise **Excludes** *amyloid or lardaceous degeneration of liver (277.39)*

10. DISEASES OF THE GENITOURINARY SYSTEM (580–629)

581 Nephrotic syndrome

581.8 With other specified pathological lesion in kidney

581.81 Nephrotic syndrome in diseases classified elsewhere
Code first underlying disease, as:
Revise amyloidosis (277.30–277.39)

582 Chronic glomerulonephritis
582.8 With other specified pathological lesion in kidney
582.81 Chronic glomerulonephritis in diseases classified elsewhere
Code first underlying disease, as:
Revise amyloidosis (277.30–277.39)
583 Nephritis and nephropathy, not specified as acute or chronic
583.8 With other specified pathological lesion in kidney
583.81 Nephritis and nephropathy, not specified as acute or chronic, in diseases classified elsewhere
Code first underlying disease, as:
Revise amyloidosis (277.30–277.39)
585 Chronic kidney disease (CKD)
Delete **Excludes** ~~*that with any condition classified to 401 (403.0–403.9 with fifth-digit 1)*~~
Add Code first hypertensive chronic kidney disease, if applicable, (403.00–403.91, 404.00–404.94)
585.5 Chronic kidney disease, stage V
Add **Excludes** *chronic kidney disease, stage V requiring chronic dialysis (585.6)*
585.6 End stage renal disease
Add Chronic kidney disease requiring chronic dialysis
599 Other disorders of urethra and urinary tract
599.6 Urinary obstruction
Delete **Excludes** ~~*urinary obstruction due to hyperplasia of prostate (600.0–600.9 with fifth-digit 1)*~~
599.69 Urinary obstruction, not elsewhere classified
Add Code, if applicable, any causal condition first, such as: hyperplasia of prostate (600.0–600.9 with fifth-digit 1)
600 Hyperplasia of prostate
Add **Includes:** enlarged prostate
Delete ~~Use additional code to identify urinary incontinence (788.30–788.39)~~
600.0 Hypertrophy (benign) of prostate
Revise **600.00 Hypertrophy (benign) of prostate without urinary obstruction and other lower urinary tract symptoms (LUTS)**
Revise **600.01 Hypertrophy (benign) of prostate with urinary obstruction and other lower urinary tract symptoms (LUTS)**
Add Use additional code to identify symptoms:
incomplete bladder emptying (788.21)
nocturia (788.43)
straining on urination (788.65)
urinary frequency (788.41)
urinary hesitancy (788.64)
urinary incontinence (788.30–788.39)
urinary obstruction (599.69)
urinary retention (788.20)
urinary urgency (788.63)
weak urinary stream (788.62)
600.2 Benign localized hyperplasia of prostate
Revise **600.20 Benign localized hyperplasia of prostate without urinary obstruction and other lower urinary tract symptoms (LUTS)**
Revise **600.21 Benign localized hyperplasia of prostate with urinary obstruction and other lower urinary tract symptoms (LUTS)**
Add Use additional code to identify symptoms:
incomplete bladder emptying (788.21)
nocturia (788.43)
straining on urination (788.65)
urinary frequency (788.41)
urinary hesitancy (788.64)
urinary incontinence (788.30–788.39)
urinary obstruction (599.69)
urinary retention (788.20)
urinary urgency (788.63)
weak urinary stream (788.62)
600.9 Hyperplasia of prostate, unspecified
Revise **600.90 Hyperplasia of prostate, unspecified, without urinary obstruction and other lower urinary symptoms (LUTS)**
Revise **600.91 Hyperplasia of prostate, unspecified, with urinary obstruction and other lower urinary symptoms (LUTS)**
Add Use additional code to identify symptoms:
incomplete bladder emptying (788.21)
nocturia (788.43)
straining on urination (788.65)
urinary frequency (788.41)
urinary hesitancy (788.64)
urinary incontinence (788.30–788.39)
urinary obstruction (599.69)
urinary retention (788.20)
urinary urgency (788.63)
weak urinary stream (788.62)
608 Other disorders of male genital organs
608.2 Torsion of testis
Delete ~~Torsion of:~~
~~epididymis~~
~~spermatic cord~~
~~testicle~~
New code **608.20 Torsion of testis, unspecified**
New code **608.21 Extravaginal torsion of spermatic cord**
New code **608.22 Intravaginal torsion of spermatic cord**
New code **608.23 Torsion of appendix testis**
New code **608.24 Torsion of appendix epididymis**
616 Inflammatory disease of cervix, vagina, and vulva
616.8 Other specified inflammatory diseases of cervix, vagina, and vulva
Delete ~~Caruncle, vagina or labium~~
~~Ulcer, vagina~~
New Code **616.81 Mucositis (ulcerative) of cervix, vagina, and vulva**
Use additional E code to identify adverse effects of therapy, such as:
antineoplastic and immunosuppressive drugs (E930.7, E933.1)
radiation therapy (E879.2)
New Code **616.89 Other inflammatory disease of cervix, vagina and vulva**
Caruncle, vagina or labium
Ulcer, vagina
618 Genital prolapse
618.8 Other specified genital prolapse
New code **618.84 Cervical stump prolapse**
629 Other disorders of female genital organs
629.2 Female genital mutilation status
Add Female genital cutting
629.20 Female genital mutilation status, unspecified
Add Female genital cutting status, unspecified
629.21 Female genital mutilation Type I status
Add Female genital cutting Type I status
629.22 Female genital mutilation Type II status
Add Female genital cutting Type II status
629.23 Female genital mutilation Type III status
Add Female genital cutting Type III status

New code 629.29 **Other female genital mutilation status**
Female genital cutting Type IV status
Female genital mutilation Type IV status
Other female genital cutting status

629.8 **Other specified disorders of female genital organs**

New code 629.81 **Habitual aborter without current pregnancy**
Excludes *habitual aborter with current pregnancy (646.3)*

New code 629.89 **Other specified disorders of female genital organs**

629.9 **Unspecified disorder of female genital organs**
Delete ~~Habitual aborter without current pregnancy~~

11. COMPLICATIONS OF PREGNANCY, CHILDBIRTH, AND THE PUERPERIUM (630–677)

Revise COMPLICATIONS MAINLY RELATED TO PREGNANCY (640–649)

Revise The following fifth-digit subclassification is for use with categories 640–649 to denote the current episode of care.

641 **Antepartum hemorrhage, abruptio placentae, and placenta previa**
641.3 **Antepartum hemorrhage associated with coagulation defects**
Add **Excludes** *coagulation defects not associated with antepartum hemorrhage (649.3)*

642 **Hypertension complicating pregnancy, childbirth, and the puerperium**
642.2 **Other pre-existing hypertension complicating pregnancy, childbirth, and the puerperium**
Hypertensive:
Revise heart and ~~renal~~ chronic kidney disease specified as complicating, or as a reason for obstetric care during pregnancy, childbirth, or the puerperium
Revise ~~renal~~ chronic kidney disease specified as complicating, or as a reason for obstetric care during pregnancy, childbirth, or the puerperium

646 **Other complications of pregnancy, not elsewhere classified**
646.8 **Other specified complications of pregnancy**
Delete ~~Uterine size-date discrepancy~~

648 **Other current conditions in the mother classifiable elsewhere, but complicating pregnancy, childbirth, or the puerperium**
648.4 **Mental disorders**
Revise Conditions classifiable to 290–303, 305.0, 305.2–305.9, 306–316, 317–319

New Category 649 **Other conditions or status of the mother complicating pregnancy, childbirth, or the puerperium**

New subcategory 649.0 [0-4] **Tobacco use disorder complicating pregnancy, childbirth, or the puerperium**
Smoking complicating pregnancy, childbirth, or the puerperium

New subcategory 649.1 [0-4] **Obesity complicating pregnancy, childbirth, or the puerperium**
Use additional code to identify the obesity (278.00, 278.01)

New subcategory 649.2 [0-4] **Bariatric surgery status complicating pregnancy, childbirth, or the puerperium**
Gastric banding status complicating pregnancy, childbirth, or the puerperium
Gastric bypass status for obesity complicating pregnancy, childbirth, or the puerperium
Obesity surgery status complicating pregnancy, childbirth, or the puerperium

New subcategory 649.3 [0-4] **Coagulation defects complicating pregnancy, childbirth, or the puerperium**
Conditions classifiable to 286
Use additional code to identify the specific coagulation defect (286.0–286.9)
Excludes *coagulation defects causing antepartum hemorrhage (641.3)*
postpartum coagulation defects (666.3)

New subcategory 649.4 [0-4] **Epilepsy complicating pregnancy, childbirth, or the puerperium**
Conditions classifiable to 345
Use additional code to identify the specific type of epilepsy (345.00–345.91)
Excludes *eclampsia (642.6)*

New subcategory 649.5 [0,1,3] **Spotting complicating pregnancy**
Excludes *antepartum hemorrhage (641.0–641.9)*
hemorrhage in early pregnancy (640.0–640.9)

New subcategory 649.6 [0-4] **Uterine size date discrepancy**

666 **Postpartum hemorrhage**
666.1 **Other immediate postpartum hemorrhage**
Revise Atony of uterus with hemorrhage
Add **Excludes** *atony of uterus without hemorrhage (669.8)*

12. DISEASES OF THE SKIN AND SUBCUTANEOUS TISSUE (680–709)

692 **Contact dermatitis and other eczema**
692.3 **Due to drugs and medicines in contact with skin**
Revise **Excludes** *allergy NOS due to drugs (995.27)*

693 **Dermatitis due to substances taken internally**
Revise **Excludes** *adverse effect NOS of drugs and medicines (995.20)*

13. DISEASES OF THE MUSCULOSKELETAL SYSTEM AND CONNECTIVE TISSUE (710–739)

713 **Arthropathy associated with other disorders classified elsewhere**
713.7 **Other general diseases with articular involvement**
Code first underlying disease, as:
Revise amyloidosis (277.30–277.39)
Revise familial Mediterranean fever (277.31)

729 **Other disorders of soft tissues**

New subcategory 729.7 **Nontraumatic compartment syndrome**
Excludes *compartment syndrome NOS (958.90)*
traumatic compartment syndrome (958.90–958.99)

New code 729.71 **Nontraumatic compartment syndrome of upper extremity**
Nontraumatic compartment syndrome of shoulder, arm, forearm, wrist, hand and fingers

New code 729.72 **Nontraumatic compartment syndrome of lower extremity**
Nontraumatic compartment syndrome of hip, buttock, thigh, leg, foot and toes

New code 729.73 **Nontraumatic compartment syndrome of abdomen**

New code 729.79 **Nontraumatic compartment syndrome of other sites**

730 Osteomyelitis, periostitis, and other infections involving bone

730.0 Acute osteomyelitis

Add Use additional code to identify major osseous defect, if applicable (731.3)

730.1 Chronic osteomyelitis

Add Use additional code to identify major osseous defect, if applicable (731.3)

730.2 Unspecified osteomyelitis

Add Use additional code to identify major osseous defect, if applicable (731.3)

731 Osteitis deformans and osteopathies associated with other disorders classified elsewhere

New code **731.3 Major osseous defects**

Code first underlying disease, if known, such as:
- aseptic necrosis (733.40–733.49)
- malignant neoplasm of bone (170.0–170.9)
- osteomyelitis (730.00–730.29)
- osteoporosis (733.00–733.09)
- peri-prosthetic osteolysis (996.45)

733 Other disorders of bone and cartilage

733.0 Osteoporosis

Add Use additional code to identify major osseous defect, if applicable (731.3)

733.4 Aseptic necrosis of bone

Add Use additional code to identify major osseous defect, if applicable (731.3)

14. CONGENITAL ANOMALIES (740–759)

743 Congenital anomalies of eye

743.8 Other specified anomalies of eye

Add **Excludes** *optic nerve hypoplasia (377.43)*

15. CERTAIN CONDITIONS ORIGINATING IN THE PERINATAL PERIOD (760–779)

768 Intrauterine hypoxia and birth asphyxia

Add **Excludes** *acidemia NOS of newborn (775.81)*
acidosis NOS of newborn (775.81)
cerebral ischemia NOS (779.2)
hypoxia NOS of newborn (770.88)
mixed metabolic and respiratory acidosis of newborn (775.81)
respiratory arrest of newborn (770.87)

Revise **768.3 Fetal distress first noted during labor and delivery, in liveborn infant**

Revise Fetal metabolic acidemia first noted during labor and delivery, in liveborn infant

768.5 Severe birth asphyxia

Add **Excludes** *hypoxic-ischemic encephalopathy (HIE) (768.7)*

768.6 Mild or moderate birth asphyxia

Add **Excludes** *hypoxic-ischemic encephalopathy (HIE) (768.7)*

New code **768.7 Hypoxic-ischemic encephalopathy (HIE)**

768.9 Unspecified birth asphyxia in liveborn infant

Delete ~~Hypoxia NOS, in liveborn infant~~

770 Other respiratory conditions of fetus and newborn

770.8 Other respiratory problems after birth

Add **Excludes** *mixed metabolic and respiratory acidosis of newborn (775.81)*

New code **770.87 Respiratory arrest of newborn**

New code **770.88 Hypoxemia of newborn**

Hypoxia NOS of newborn

775 Endocrine and metabolic disturbances specific to the fetus and newborn

Revise **775.8 Other ~~transitory~~ neonatal endocrine and metabolic disturbances**

Delete ~~Amino-acid metabolic disorders described as transitory~~

New code **775.81 Other acidosis of newborn**

Acidemia NOS of newborn
Acidosis of newborn NOS
Mixed metabolic and respiratory acidosis of newborn

New code **775.89 Other neonatal endocrine and metabolic disturbances**

Amino-acid metabolic disorders described as transitory

776 Hematologic disorders of fetus and newborn

776.7 Transient neonatal neutropenia

Revise **Excludes** *congenital neutropenia (nontransient) (288.01)*

779 Other and ill-defined conditions originating in the perinatal period

779.2 Cerebral depression, coma, and other abnormal cerebral signs

Add Cerebral ischemia NOS of newborn

Add **Excludes** *cerebral ischemia due to birth trauma (767.0)*
intrauterine cerebral ischemia (768.2–768.9)
intraventricular hemorrhage (772.10–772.14)

779.8 Other specified conditions originating in the perinatal period

New code **779.85 Cardiac arrest of newborn**

16. SYMPTOMS, SIGNS, AND ILL-DEFINED CONDITIONS (780–799)

780 General symptoms

780.3 Convulsions

Revise **780.31 Febrile convulsions (simple), unspecified**

Revise Febrile seizure NOS

New code **780.32 Complex febrile convulsions**

Febrile seizure:
- atypical
- complex
- complicated

Excludes *status epilepticus (345.3)*

780.39 Other convulsions

Add Recurrent convulsions NOS

780.5 Sleep disturbances

780.58 Sleep related movement disorder, unspecified

Revise **Excludes** *restless legs syndrome (333.94)*

780.6 Fever

Add Code first underlying condition when associated fever is present, such as with:
- leukemia (codes from categories 204–208)
- neutropenia (288.00–288.09)
- sickle-cell disease (282.60–282.69)

780.9 Other general symptoms

Revise **780.95 ~~Other e~~Excessive crying of child, adolescent, or adult**

New code **780.96 Generalized pain**

Pain NOS

New code **780.97 Altered mental status**

Change in mental status

Excludes *altered level of consciousness (780.01–780.09)*
altered mental status due to known condition- code to condition
delirium NOS (780.09)

780.99 Other general symptoms

Delete ~~Generalized pain~~

781 Symptoms involving nervous and musculoskeletal systems

781.2 Abnormality of gait

Excludes *ataxia:*

Delete ~~*difficulty in walking (719.7)*~~

Add *difficulty in walking (719.7)*

783 Symptoms concerning nutrition, metabolism, and development

783.2 Abnormal loss of weight and underweight

Revise — Use additional code to identify Body Mass Index (BMI), if known (V85.0–V85.54)

784 Symptoms involving head and neck

784.3 Aphasia

Add — **Excludes** *aphasia due to late effects of cerebrovascular disease (438.11)*

784.9 Other symptoms involving head and neck

Delete — ~~Choking sensation~~
~~Halitosis~~
~~Mouth breathing~~
~~Sneezing~~

New code — **784.91 Postnasal drip**

New code — **784.99 Other symptoms involving head and neck**

Choking sensation
Halitosis
Mouth breathing
Sneezing

785 Symptoms involving cardiovascular system

785.52 Septic shock

Code first:

Delete — ~~systemic inflammatory response syndrome due to noninfectious process with organ dysfunction (995.94)~~

788 Symptoms involving urinary system

Add — **Excludes** *urinary obstruction (599.60, 599.69)*

788.2 Retention of urine

Delete — ~~**Excludes** *urinary retention due to hyperplasia of prostate (600.0–600.9 with fifth-digit 1)*~~

Add — Code, if applicable, any causal condition first, such as: hyperplasia of prostate (600.0–600.9 with fifth-digit 1)

788.3 Urinary incontinence

Code, if applicable, any causal condition first, such as:

Add — hyperplasia of prostate (600.0–600.9 with fifth-digit 1)

788.4 Frequency of urination and polyuria

Add — Code, if applicable, any causal condition first, such as:
hyperplasia of prostate (600.0–600.9 with fifth-digit 1)

788.6 Other abnormality of urination

Add — Code, if applicable, any causal condition first, such as:
hyperplasia of prostate (600.0–600.9 with fifth-digit 1)

New code — **788.64 Urinary hesitancy**

New code — **788.65 Straining on urination**

790 Nonspecific findings on examination of blood

Excludes *abnormalities of:*

Revise — *white blood cells (288.00–288.9)*

790.2 Abnormal glucose

790.29 Other abnormal glucose

Add — Hyperglycemia NOS

790.6 Other abnormal blood chemistry

Abnormal blood level of:

Add — lead

Add — **Excludes** *lead poisoning (984.0–984.9)*

793 Nonspecific abnormal findings on radiological and other examination of body structure

793.8 Breast

793.81 Mammographic microcalcification

Add — **Excludes** *mammographic calcification (793.89)*
mammographic calculus (793.89)

793.89 Other abnormal findings on radiological examination of breast

Add — Mammographic calcification

Add — Mammographic calculus

793.9 Other

Delete — ~~Abnormal:~~
~~placental finding by x-ray or ultrasound method~~
~~radiological findings in skin and subcutaneous tissue~~

New code — **793.91 Image test inconclusive due to excess body fat**

Use additional code to identify Body Mass Index (BMI), if known (V85.0–V85.54)

New code — **793.99 Other nonspecific abnormal findings on radiological and other examinations of body structure**

Abnormal:
placental finding by x-ray or ultrasound method
radiological findings in skin and subcutaneous tissue

795 Other and nonspecific abnormal cytological, histological, immunological, and DNA test findings

795.0 Abnormal Papanicolaou smear of cervix and cervical HPV

795.04 Papanicolaou smear of cervix with high grade squamous intraepithelial lesion (HGSIL)

Delete — ~~Cytologic evidence of carcinoma~~

New code — **795.06 Papanicolaou smear of cervix with cytologic evidence of malignancy**

795.7 Other nonspecific immunological findings

Add — **Excludes** *abnormal tumor markers (795.81–795.89)*
elevated prostate specific antigen [PSA] (790.93)
elevated tumor associated antigens (795.81–795.89)

New subcategory — **795.8 Abnormal tumor markers**

Elevated tumor associated antigens [TAA]
Elevated tumor specific antigens [TSA]

Excludes *elevated prostate specific antigen [PSA] (790.93)*

New code — **795.81 Elevated carcinoembryonic antigen [CEA]**

New code — **795.82 Elevated cancer antigen 125 [CA 125]**

New code — **795.89 Other abnormal tumor markers**

799 Other ill-defined and unknown causes of morbidity and mortality

799.4 Cachexia

Add — Code first underlying condition, if known

Delete — ~~**Excludes** *nutritional marasmus (261)*~~

17. INJURY AND POISONING (800–999)

873 Other open wound of head

873.6 Internal structures of mouth, without mention of complication

Revise — **873.63 Tooth (broken) (fractured) (due to trauma)**

Add — **Excludes** *cracked tooth (521.81)*

873.7 Internal structures of mouth, complicated

Revise — **873.73 Tooth (broken) (fractured) (due to trauma)**

Add — **Excludes** *cracked tooth (521.81)*

958 Certain early complications of trauma

New subcategory — **958.9 Traumatic compartment syndrome**

Excludes *nontraumatic compartment syndrome (729.71–729.79)*

New code — **958.90 Compartment syndrome, unspecified**

New code 958.91 **Traumatic compartment syndrome of upper extremity**
Traumatic compartment syndrome of shoulder, arm, forearm, wrist, hand, and fingers
New code 958.92 **Traumatic compartment syndrome of lower extremity**
Traumatic compartment syndrome of hip, buttock, thigh, leg, foot, and toes
New code 958.93 **Traumatic compartment syndrome of abdomen**
New code 958.99 **Traumatic compartment syndrome of other sites**

POISONING BY DRUGS, MEDICINAL AND BIOLOGICAL SUBSTANCES (960–979)

Excludes *adverse effects…*
Revise *adverse effect NOS (995.20)*

995 Certain adverse effects not elsewhere classified
Revise **995.2 Other and u~~U~~nspecified adverse effect of drug, medicinal and biological substance**
New code **995.20 Unspecified adverse effect of unspecified drug, medicinal and biological substance**
New code **995.21 Arthus phenomenon**
Arthus reaction
New code **995.22 Unspecified adverse effect of anesthesia**
New code **995.23 Unspecified adverse effect of insulin**
New code **995.27 Other drug allergy**
Drug allergy NOS
Drug hypersensitivity NOS
New code **995.29 Unspecified adverse effect of other drug, medicinal and biological substance**
995.3 Allergy, unspecified
Revise **Excludes** *allergic reaction NOS to correct medicinal substance properly administered (995.27)*
Add *allergy to existing dental restorative materials (525.66)*

995.4 Shock due to anesthesia
Revise **Excludes** *unspecified adverse effect of anesthesia (995.22)*

995.9 Systemic inflammatory response syndrome (SIRS)
Delete ~~Code first underlying systemic infection~~
Revise **995.91 Sepsis ~~Systemic inflammatory response syndrome due to infectious process without organ dysfunction~~**
~~Sepsis~~
Add Systemic inflammatory response syndrome due to infectious process without acute organ dysfunction
Add Code first underlying infection
Add **Excludes** *sepsis with acute organ dysfunction (995.92)*
sepsis with multiple organ dysfunction (995.92)
severe sepsis (995.92)

Revise **995.92 Severe sepsis ~~Systemic inflammatory response syndrome due to infectious process with organ dysfunction~~**
Delete ~~Severe sepsis~~
Add Sepsis with acute organ dysfunction
Add Sepsis with multiple organ dysfunction (MOD)
Add Systemic inflammatory response syndrome due to infectious process with acute organ dysfunction
Add Code first underlying infection
Revise Use additional code to specify acute organ dysfunction, such as:
Add disseminated intravascular coagulopathy (DIC) syndrome (286.6)
Revise **995.93 Systemic inflammatory response syndrome due to noninfectious process without acute organ dysfunction**
Add Code first underlying conditions, such as:
acute pancreatitis (577.0)
trauma
Add **Excludes** *systemic inflammatory response syndrome due to noninfectious process with acute organ dysfunction (995.94)*
Revise **995.94 Systemic inflammatory response syndrome due to noninfectious process with acute organ dysfunction**
Add Code first underlying condition, such as:
acute pancreatitis (577.0)
trauma
Revise Use additional code to specify acute organ dysfunction, such as:
Add disseminated intravascular coagulopathy (DIC) syndrome (286.6)
Delete ~~septic shock (785.52)~~
Add **Excludes** *severe sepsis (995.92)*

COMPLICATIONS OF SURGICAL AND MEDICAL CARE, NOT ELSEWHERE CLASSIFIED (996–999)

996 Complications peculiar to certain specified procedures
996.4 Mechanical complication of internal orthopedic device, implant, and graft
996.45 Peri-prosthetic osteolysis
Add Use additional code to identify major osseous defect, if applicable (731.3)
996.7 Other complications of internal (biological) (synthetic) prosthetic device, implant and graft
Add Use additional code to identify complication, such as:
pain due to presence of device, implant or graft (338.18–338.19, 338.28–338.29)
997 Complications affecting specified body systems, not elsewhere classified
997.3 Respiratory complications
Add **Excludes** *transfusion related acute lung injury (TRALI) (518.7)*

998 Other complications of procedures, not elsewhere classified
998.5 Postoperative infection
Add **Excludes** *bleb associated endophthalmitis (379.63)*
999 Complications of medical care, not elsewhere classified
Revise **Excludes** *postvaccinal encephalitis (323.51)*
999.8 Other transfusion reaction
Add **Excludes** *transfusion related acute lung injury (TRALI) (518.7)*

V CODES

Revise SUPPLEMENTARY CLASSIFICIATION OF FACTORS INFLUENCING HEALTH STATUS AND CONTACT WITH HEALTH SERVICES (V01–V86)

V07 Need for isolation and other prophylactic measures
V07.39 Other prophylactic chemotherapy
Revise **Excludes** *maintenance chemotherapy following disease (V58.11)*

V18 Family history of certain other specific conditions
V18.5 Digestive disorders
New code **V18.51 Colonic polyps**
Excludes *family history of malignant neoplasm of gastrointestinal tract (V16.0)*
New code **V18.59 Other digestive disorders**
V20 Health supervision of infant or child
V20.2 Routine infant or child health check
Add Initial and subsequent routine newborn check
V26 Procreative management
V26.2 Investigation and testing
V26.21 Fertility testing
Revise **Excludes** *genetic counseling and testing (V26.31–V26.39)*
V26.3 Genetic counseling and testing
Add **Excludes** *nonprocreative genetic screening (V82.71, V82.79)*
Revise **V26.31 Testing of female for genetic disease carrier status**
Revise **V26.32 Other genetic testing of female**
Add Use additional code to identify habitual aborter (629.81, 646.3)
New code **V26.34 Testing of male for genetic disease carrier status**
New code **V26.35 Encounter for testing of male partner of habitual aborter**
New code **V26.39 Other genetic testing of male**
Revise **V28 Encounter for ~~A~~antenatal screening of mother**
V45 Other postprocedural states
V45.3 Intestinal bypass or anastomosis status
Add **Excludes** *bariatric surgery status (V45.86)*
gastric bypass status (V45.86)
obesity surgery status (V45.86)
V45.7 Acquired absence of organ
V45.77 Genital organs
Revise **Excludes** *female genital mutilation status (629.20–629.29)*
V45.8 Other postprocedural status
New code **V45.86 Bariatric surgery status**
Gastric banding status
Gastric bypass status for obesity
Obesity surgery status
Excludes *bariatric surgery status complicating pregnancy, childbirth or the puerperium (649.2)*
intestinal bypass or anastomosis status (V45.3)
V54 Other orthopedic aftercare
V54.1 Aftercare for healing traumatic fracture
Add **Excludes** *aftercare for amputation stump (V54.89)*
V58 Encounter for other and unspecified procedures and aftercare
Revise **V58.3 Attention to ~~surgical~~ dressings and sutures**
Delete ~~Change of dressings~~
Delete ~~Removal of sutures~~
Add Change or removal of wound packing
Add **Excludes** *attention to drains (V58.49)*
planned postoperative wound closure (V58.41)
New code **V58.30 Encounter for change or removal of nonsurgical wound dressing**
Encounter for change or removal of wound dressing NOS
New code **V58.31 Encounter for change or removal of surgical wound dressing**
New code **V58.32 Encounter for removal of sutures**
Encounter for removal of staples

V58.4 Other aftercare following surgery
V58.41 Encounter for planned postoperative wound closure
Add **Excludes** *encounter for dressings and suture aftercare (V58.30–V58.32)*
V58.49 Other specified aftercare following surgery
Add Change or removal of drains
V65 Other persons seeking consultation
V65.3 Dietary surveillance and counseling
Add Use additional code to identify Body Mass Index (BMI), if known (V85.0–V85.54)
V65.4 Other counseling, not elsewhere classified
Revise **Excludes** *counseling (for):*
genetic (V26.31–V26.39)

Revise PERSONS WITHOUT REPORTED DIAGNOSIS ENCOUNTERED DURING EXAMINATION AND INVESTIGATION OF INDIVIDUALS AND POPULATIONS (V70–V82)
V72 Special investigations and examinations
V72.1 Examination of ears and hearing
New code **V72.11 Encounter for hearing examination following failed hearing screening**
New code **V72.19 Other examination of ears and hearing**
V82 Special screening for other conditions
New sub-category **V82.7 Genetic screening**
Add **Excludes** *genetic testing for procreative management (V26.31–V26.32)*
New code **V82.71 Screening for genetic disease carrier status**
New code **V82.79 Other genetic screening**
Add GENETICS (V83–V84)
Add BODY MASS INDEX (V85)
Revise **V85 Body Mass Index [BMI]**
New subcategory **V85.5 Body Mass Index, pediatric**
Add Note: BMI pediatric codes are for use for persons age 2–20 years old. These percentiles are based on the growth charts published by the Centers for Disease Control and Prevention (CDC)
New code **V85.51 Body Mass Index, pediatric, less than 5th percentile for age**
New code **V85.52 Body Mass Index, pediatric, 5th percentile to less than 85th percentile for age**
New code **V85.53 Body Mass Index, pediatric, 85th percentile to less than 95th percentile for age**
New code **V85.54 Body Mass Index, pediatric, greater than or equal to 95th percentile for age**
Add ESTROGEN RECEPTOR STATUS (V86)
New Category **V86 Estrogen receptor status**
Code first malignant neoplasm of breast (174.0–174.9, 175.0–175.9)
New code **V86.0 Estrogen receptor positive status [ER+]**
New code **V86.1 Estrogen receptor negative status [ER-]**

VOLUME 3 CHANGES EFFECTIVE OCTOBER 1, 2006

Tabular List

New code **00.44 Procedure on vessel bifurcation**
Note: this code is to be used to identify the presence of a vessel bifurcation; it does not describe a specific bifurcation stent. Use this code only once per operative episode, irrespective of the number of bifurcations in vessels.

00.50 Implantation of cardiac resynchronization pacemaker without mention of defibrillation, total system [CRT-P]

Add note — NOTE: Device testing during procedure – *omit code*

Add inclusion term — Biventricular pacemaker

Add inclusion term — BiV pacemaker

00.51 Implantation of cardiac resynchronization defibrillator, total system [CRT-D]

Add note — NOTE: Device testing during procedure – *omit code*

Add inclusion term — BiV defibrillator

Add inclusion term — Biventricular defibrillator

Add inclusion term — BiV ICD

Add inclusion term — BiV pacemaker with defibrillator

Add inclusion term — BiV pacing with defibrillator

00.53 Implantation or replacement of cardiac resynchronization pacemaker pulse generator only [CRT-P]

Add note — NOTE: Device testing during procedure – *omit code*

00.54 Implantation or replacement of cardiac resynchronization defibrillator pulse generator device only [CRT-D]

Add note — NOTE: Device testing during procedure – *omit code*

00.55 Insertion of drug-eluting peripheral vessel stent(s)

Code also any:

Add code also note — procedure on vessel bifurcation (00.44)

New code — **00.56 Insertion or replacement of implantable pressure sensor (lead) for intracardiac hemodynamic monitoring**

Code also any associated implantation or replacement of monitor (00.57)

Excludes *circulatory monitoring (blood gas, arterial or venous pressure, cardiac output and coronary blood flow) (89.60–89.69)*

New code — **00.57 Implantation or replacement of subcutaneous device for intracardiac hemodynamic monitoring**

Implantation of monitoring device with formation of subcutaneous pocket and connection to intracardiac pressure sensor (lead)

Code also any associated insertion or replacement of implanted pressure sensor (lead) (00.56)

00.61 Percutaneous angioplasty or atherectomy of precerebral (extracranial) vessel(s)

Code also any:

Add code also note — procedure on vessel bifurcation (00.44)

00.62 Percutaneous angioplasty or atherectomy of intracranial vessel(s)

Code also any:

Add code also note — procedure on vessel bifurcation (00.44)

00.63 Percutaneous insertion of carotid artery stent(s)

Code also any:

Add code also note — procedure on vessel bifurcation (00.44)

00.64 Percutaneous insertion of other precerebral (extracranial) artery stent(s)

Code also any:

Add code also note — procedure on vessel bifurcation (00.44)

00.65 Percutaneous insertion of intracranial vascular stent(s)

Code also any:

Add code also note — procedure on vessel bifurcation (00.44)

00.66 Percutaneous transluminal coronary angioplasty [PTCA] or coronary atherectomy

Code also any:

Add code also note — procedure on vessel bifurcation (00.44)

00.70 Revision of hip replacement, both acetabular and femoral components

Code also any:

Revise code — type of bearing surface, if known (00.74–00.77)

00.71 Revision of hip replacement, acetabular component

Code also any:

Revise code — type of bearing surface, if known (00.74–00.77)

00.72 Revision of hip replacement, femoral component

Code also any:

Revise code — type of bearing surface, if known (00.74–00.77)

00.73 Revision of hip replacement, acetabular liner and/or femoral head only

Code also any:

Revise code — type of bearing surface, if known (00.74–00.77)

New code — **00.77 Hip replacement bearing surface, ceramic-on-polyethylene**

Revise code title — **00.8 Other knee and hip procedures**

New code — **00.85 Resurfacing hip, total, acetabulum and femoral head**

Hip resurfacing arthroplasty, total

New code — **00.86 Resurfacing hip, partial, femoral head**

Hip resurfacing arthroplasty, NOS

Hip resurfacing arthroplasty, partial, femoral head

Excludes *that with resurfacing of acetabulum (00.85)*

New code — **00.87 Resurfacing hip, partial, acetabulum**

Hip resurfacing arthroplasty, partial, acetabulum

Excludes *that with resurfacing of femoral head (00.85)*

Revise code title — **01.26 Insertion of catheter(s) into cranial cavity or tissue**

Add exclusion term — **Excludes** *placement of intracerebral catheter(s) via burr hole(s) (01.28)*

Revise code title — **01.27 Removal of catheter(s) from cranial cavity or tissue**

New code — **01.28 Placement of intracerebral catheter(s) via burr hole(s)**

Convection enhanced delivery

Stereotactic placement of intracerebral catheter(s)

Code also infusion of medication

Excludes *insertion of catheter(s) into cranial cavity or tissue(s) (01.26)*

02.93 Implantation or replacement of intracranial neurostimulator lead(s)

Revise code — Code also any insertion of neurostimulator pulse generator 86.94–~~86.96~~ 86.98

03.93 Implantation or replacement of spinal neurostimulator lead(s)

Revise code — Code also any insertion of neurostimulator pulse generator 86.94– ~~86.96~~ 86.98

04.92 Implantation or replacement of peripheral neurostimulator lead(s)

Revise code — Code also any insertion of neurostimulator pulse generator 86.94- ~~86.96~~ 86.98

13.7 Insertion of prosthetic lens [pseudophakos]

Add exclusion term — **Excludes** *implantation of intraocular telescope prosthesis (13.91)*

New subcategory — **13.9 Other operations on lens**

New code — **13.90 Operation on lens, Not Elsewhere Classified**

New code — **13.91 Implantation of intraocular telescope prosthesis**
Includes: removal of lens, any method
Implantable miniature telescope
Excludes *secondary insertion of ocular implant (16.61)*

14.74 Other mechanical vitrectomy
Add inclusion term — Posterior approach

New code — **32.23 Open ablation of lung lesion or tissue**

New code — **32.24 Percutaneous ablation of lung lesion or tissue**

New code — **32.25 Thoracoscopic ablation of lung lesion or tissue**

New code — **32.26 Other and unspecified ablation of lung lesion or tissue**

32.28 Endoscopic excision or destruction of lesion or tissue of lung
Add exclusion term — **Excludes** *ablation of lung lesion or tissue:*
open (32.23)
other (32.26)
percutaneous (32.24)
thoracoscopic (32.25)

32.29 Other local excision or destruction of lesion or tissue of lung
Add exclusion term — **Excludes** *ablation of lung lesion or tissue:*
open (32.23)
other (32.26)
percutaneous (32.24)
thoracoscopic (32.25)

New subcategory — **33.7 Endoscopic insertion, replacement and removal of therapeutic device or substances in bronchus or lung**
Biologic Lung Volume Reduction (BLVR)
Excludes *insertion of tracheobronchial stent (96.05)*

New code — **33.71 Endoscopic insertion or replacement of bronchial valve(s)**
Endobronchial airflow redirection valve
Intrabronchial airflow redirection valve

New code — **33.78 Endoscopic removal of bronchial device(s) or substances**

New code — **33.79 Endoscopic insertion of other bronchial device or substances**
Biologic Lung Volume Reduction NOS (BLVR)

34.92 Injection into thoracic cavity
Add inclusion term — Instillation into thoracic cavity

Revise code title — **35.53 Repair of ventricular septal defect with prosthesis, open technique**

New code — **35.55 Repair of ventricular septal defect with prosthesis, closed technique**

36.03 Open chest coronary artery angioplasty
Code also any:
Add code also note — procedure on vessel bifurcation (00.44)

36.04 Intracoronary artery thrombolytic infusion
Revise exclusion term — **Excludes** *that associated with any procedure in ~~00.66~~, 36.03*

36.06 Insertion of non-drug-eluting coronary artery stent(s)
Code also any:
Add code also note — procedure on vessel bifurcation (00.44)

36.07 Insertion of drug-eluting coronary artery stent(s)
Code also any:
Add code also note — procedure on vessel bifurcation (00.44)

36.09 Other removal of coronary artery obstruction
Code also any:
Add code also note — procedure on vessel bifurcation (00.44)

36.32 Other transmyocardial revascularization
Delete inclusion term — ~~Percutaneous transmyocardial revascularization~~
Delete inclusion term — ~~Thoracoscopic transmyocardial revascularization~~

New code — **36.33 Endoscopic transmyocardial revascularization**
Robot-assisted transmyocardial revascularization
Thoracoscopic transmyocardial revascularization

New code — **36.34 Percutaneous transmyocardial revascularization**
Endovascular transmyocardial revascularization

New code — **37.20 Noninvasive programmed electrical stimulation [NIPS]**
Excludes *that as part of intraoperative testing – omit code*
catheter based invasive electrophysiologic testing (37.26)
device interrogation only without arrhythmia induction (bedside check) (89.45–89.49)

Revise code title — **37.26 ~~Cardiac electrophysiologic stimulation and recording studies~~ Catheter based invasive electrophysiologic testing**
Delete inclusion term — ~~Non-invasive programmed electrical stimulation (NIPS)~~
Delete inclusion term — ~~Programmed electrical stimulation~~
Add exclusion term — **Excludes** *that as part of intraoperative testing – omit code*
Add exclusion term — *noninvasive programmed electrical stimulation (NIPS) (37.20)*

37.66 Insertion of implantable heart assist system
Add 2nd note — Note: This device can be used for either destination therapy (DT) or bridge-to-transplant (BTT)

Revise title — **37.7 Insertion, revision, replacement and removal of ~~pacemaker~~ leads; insertion of temporary pacemaker system; or revision of cardiac device pocket**

37.75 Revision of lead [electrode]
Revise inclusion term — Repositioning of lead(s) (AICD) (cardiac device) (CRT-D) (CRT-P) (defibrillator) (pacemaker) (pacing) (sensing) [electrode]

37.79 Revision or relocation of cardiac device pocket
Add inclusion term — Insertion of loop recorder
Add inclusion term — Removal of cardiac device/pulse generator without replacement
Add inclusion term — Removal of the implantable hemodynamic pressure sensor (lead) and monitor device
Add inclusion term — Removal without replacement of cardiac resynchronization defibrillator device
Add inclusion term — Repositioning of implantable hemodynamic pressure sensor (lead) and monitor device
Add inclusion term — Repositioning of pulse generator
Add inclusion term — Revision of cardioverter/defibrillator (automatic) pocket
Add inclusion term — Revision of pocket for intracardiac hemodynamic monitoring
Add inclusion term — Revision or relocation of CRT-D pocket
Add exclusion term — **Excludes** *removal of loop recorder (86.05)*

37.8 Insertion, replacement, removal, and revision of pacemaker device

Add note — NOTE: Device testing during procedure – *omit code*

37.94 Implantation or replacement of automatic cardioverter/defibrillator, total system [AICD]

Implantation of defibrillator with leads (epicardial patches), formation of pocket (abdominal fascia) (subcutaneous), any transvenous leads, intraoperative procedures for evaluation of lead signals, and obtaining defibrillator threshold measurements

Delete inclusion term — ~~(electrophysiologic studies [EPS])~~

Add note — NOTE: Device testing during procedure – *omit code*

37.96 Implantation of automatic cardioverter/defibrillator pulse generator only

Add note — NOTE: Device testing during procedure – *omit code*

37.97 Replacement of automatic cardioverter/defibrillator lead(s) only

Add exclusion term — **Excludes** *replacement of epicardial lead [electrode] into epicardium (37.74)*

Add exclusion term — *replacement of transvenous lead [electrode] into left ventricular coronary venous system (00.52)*

37.98 Replacement of automatic cardioverter/defibrillator pulse generator only

Add note — NOTE: Device testing during procedure – *omit code*

37.99 Other

Delete inclusion term — ~~Removal of cardioverter/defibrillator pulse generator only without replacement~~

Delete inclusion term — ~~Removal without replacement of cardiac resynchronization defibrillator device [CRT-D]~~

Delete inclusion term — ~~Repositioning of lead(s) (sensing) (pacing) [electrode]~~

Delete inclusion term — ~~Repositioning of pulse generator~~

Delete inclusion term — ~~Revision of cardioverter/defibrillator (automatic) pocket~~

Delete inclusion term — ~~Revision or relocation of CRT-D pocket~~

Add exclusion term — **Excludes** *repositioning of pulse generator (37.79)*

Add exclusion term — *revision of lead(s) (37.75)*

Add exclusion term — *revision or relocation of pacemaker, defibrillator or other implanted cardiac device pocket (37.79)*

38 Incision, excision, and occlusion of vessels

Revise exclusion term — **Excludes** *that of coronary vessels (00.66 ~~(36.01–36.99)~~ 36.03, 36.04, 36.09, 36.10–36.99)*

38.0 Incision of vessel

Add exclusion term — **Excludes** *endovascular removal of obstruction from head and neck vessel(s) (39.74)*

38.1 Endarterectomy

Add code also note — Code also any:
procedure on vessel bifurcation 00.44

38.4 Resection of vessel with replacement

Add inclusion term — Partial resection with replacement

39.50 Angioplasty or atherectomy of other non-coronary vessel(s)

Code also any:

Add note — procedure on vessel bifurcation (00.44)

39.72 Endovascular repair or occlusion of head and neck vessels

Add exclusion term — **Excludes** *mechanical thrombectomy of pre-cerebral and cerebral vessels (39.74)*

New code — **39.74 Endovascular removal of obstruction from head and neck vessel(s)**

Endovascular embolectomy
Endovascular thrombectomy of pre-cerebral and cerebral vessels
Mechanical embolectomy or thrombectomy

Code also:
any injection or infusion of thrombolytic agent (99.10)
number of vessels treated (00.40–00.43)
procedure on vessel bifurcation (00.44)

Excludes *endarterectomy of intracranial vessels and other vessels of head and neck (38.11–38.12)*
occlusive endovascular repair of head or neck vessels (39.72)
open embolectomy or thrombectomy (38.01–38.02)

39.90 Insertion of non-drug-eluting peripheral vessel stent(s)

Code also any:

Add code also note — procedure on vessel bifurcation (00.44)

New code — **50.23 Open ablation of liver lesion or tissue**

New code — **50.24 Percutaneous ablation of liver lesion or tissue**

New code — **50.25 Laparoscopic ablation of liver lesion or tissue**

New code — **50.26 Other and unspecified ablation of liver lesion or tissue**

50.29 Other destruction of lesion of liver

Add exclusion term — **Excludes** *ablation of liver lesion or tissue:*
laparoscopic (50.25)
open (50.23)
other (50.26)
percutaneous (50.24)

New code — **55.32 Open ablation of renal lesion or tissue**

New code — **55.33 Percutaneous ablation of renal lesion or tissue**

New code — **55.34 Laparoscopic ablation of renal lesion or tissue**

New code — **55.35 Other and unspecified ablation of renal lesion or tissue**

55.39 Other local excision or destruction of renal lesion or tissue

Add exclusion term — **Excludes** *ablation of renal lesion or tissue:*
laparoscopic (55.34)
open (55.32)
other (55.35)
percutaneous (55.33)

Revise code title — **68.39 Other and unspecified subtotal abdominal hysterectomy**

New subcategory — **68.4 Total abdominal hysterectomy**

Code also any synchronous removal of tubes and ovaries (65.31–65.64)

Excludes *laparoscopic total abdominal hysterectomy (68.41)*
radical abdominal hysterectomy, any approach (68.61–68.69)

New code — **68.41 Laparoscopic total abdominal hysterectomy**

Total laparoscopic hysterectomy [TLH]

New code — **68.49 Other and unspecified total abdominal hysterectomy**

Hysterectomy:
Extended

Revise code title — **68.59 Other and unspecified vaginal hysterectomy**

New subcategory — **68.6 Radical abdominal hysterectomy**
Code also any synchronous:
lymph gland dissection (40.3, 40.5)
removal of tubes and ovaries (65.31–65.64)

New code — **68.61 Laparoscopic radical abdominal hysterectomy**
Laparoscopic modified radical hysterectomy
Total laparoscopic radical hysterectomy [TLRH]

New code — **68.69 Other and unspecified radical abdominal hysterectomy**
Modified radical hysterectomy
Wertheim's operation

Excludes *laparoscopic total abdominal hysterectomy (68.41)*
laparoscopic radical abdominal hysterectomy (68.61)

New subcategory — **68.7 Radical vaginal hysterectomy**
Code also any synchronous:
lymph gland dissection (40.3, 40.5)
removal of tubes and ovaries (65.31–65.64)

Excludes *abdominal hysterectomy, any approach (68.31–68.39, 68.41–68.49, 68.61–68.69, 68.9)*

New code — **68.71 Laparoscopic radical vaginal hysterectomy [LRVH]**

New code — **68.79 Other and unspecified radical vaginal hysterectomy**
Hysterocolpectomy
Schauta operation

68.9 Other and unspecified hysterectomy
Hysterectomy, NOS

Revise exclusion term — **Excludes** *abdominal hysterectomy, any approach (68.31–68.39, 68.41–68.49, 68.61–68.69)*

Revise exclusion term — *vaginal hysterectomy, any approach (68.51–68.59, 68.71–68.79)*

80.51 Excision of intervertebral disc

Add exclusion term — **Excludes** *that with corpectomy, (verterbral) (80.99)*

84.59 Insertion of other spinal devices

Add inclusion term — Insertion of non-fusion spinal stabilization device

84.73 Application of hybrid external fixator device

Add inclusion term — Computer (assisted) (dependent) external fixator device

86.28 Nonexcisional debridement of wound, infection, or burn

Add inclusion term — Water scalpel (jet)

89.45 Artificial pacemaker rate check

Revise exclusion term — **Excludes** ~~*electrophysiologic studies [EPS]*~~
catheter based invasive electrophysiologic testing (37.26)
noninvasive programmed electrical stimulation [NIPS]

Revise exclusion term — *(arrhythmia induction) (~~37.26~~ 37.20)*

89.49 Automatic implantable cardioverter/defibrillator (AICD) check

Revise exclusion term — **Excludes** ~~*electrophysiologic studies [EPS]*~~
catheter based invasive electrophysiologic testing (37.26)
noninvasive programmed electrical stimulation [NIPS]

Revise exclusion term — *(arrhythmia induction) (~~37.26~~ 37.20)*

89.6 Circulatory monitoring

Add exclusion term — **Excludes** *implantation or replacement of subcutaneous device for intracardiac hemodynamic monitoring (00.57)*

Add exclusion term — *insertion or replacement of implantable pressure sensor (lead) for intracardiac hemodynamic monitoring (00.56)*

93.11 Assisting exercise

Revise exclusion term — **Excludes** *assisted exercise in pool (93.31)*

93.59 Other immobilization, pressure and attention to wound

Add inclusion term — Strapping (non-traction)

96.05 Other intubation of respiratory tract

Add exclusion term — **Excludes** *endoscopic insertion or replacement of bronchial device or substance (33.71, 33.79)*

99.10 Injection or infusion of thrombolytic agent

Add inclusion term — Alteplase
Add inclusion term — Anistreplase
Add inclusion term — Reteplase
Add inclusion term — Tenecteplase

99.28 Injection or infusion of biological response modifier [BRM] as an antineoplastic agent

Add inclusion term — **Includes:** infusion of cintredekin besudotox

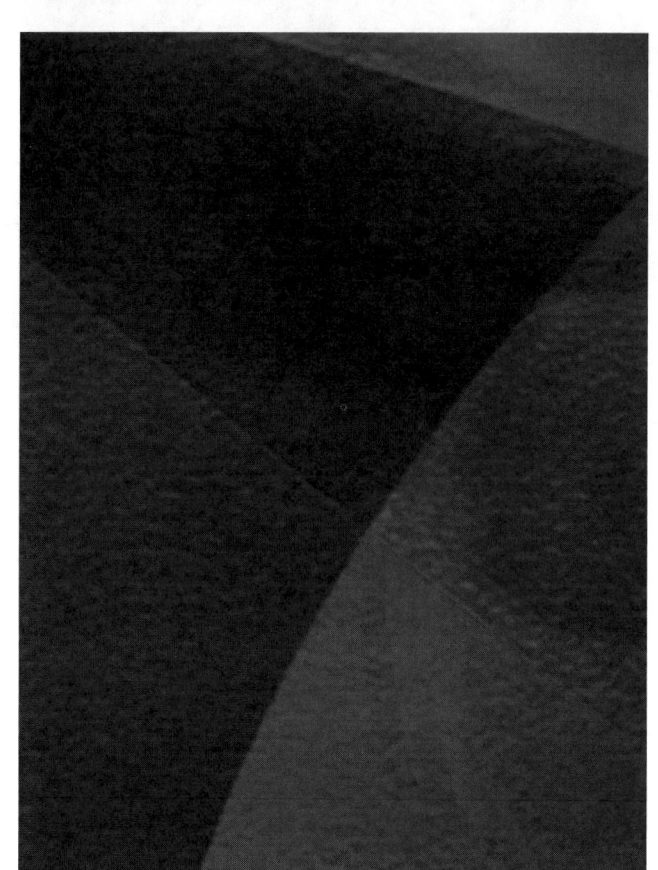

UNIT ONE

ICD-9-CM

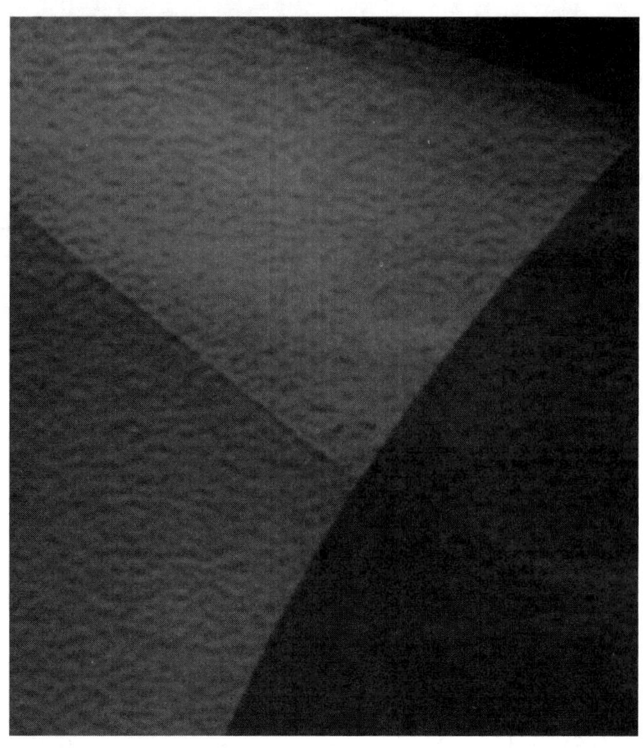

PART I

Introduction

ICD-9-CM BACKGROUND

The International Classification of Diseases, 9th Revision, Clinical Modification (ICD-9-CM) is based on the official version of the World Health Organization's 9th Revision, International Classification of Diseases (ICD-9). ICD-9 is designed for the classification of morbidity and mortality information for statistical purposes, and for the indexing of hospital records by disease and operations, for data storage and retrieval. The historical background of the International Classification of Diseases may be found in the Introduction to ICD-9 (Manual of the International Classification of Diseases, Injuries, and Causes of Death, World Health Organization, Geneva, Switzerland, 1977).

ICD-9-CM is a clinical modification of the World Health Organization's International Classification of Diseases, 9th Revision (ICD-9). The term "clinical" is used to emphasize the modification's intent: to serve as a useful tool in the area of classification of morbidity data for indexing of medical records, medical care review, and ambulatory and other medical care programs, as well as for basic health statistics. To describe the clinical picture of the patient, the codes must be more precise than those needed only for statistical groupings and trend analysis.

COORDINATION AND MAINTENANCE COMMITTEE

Annual modifications are made to the ICD-9-CM through the ICD-9-CM Coordination and Maintenance Committee (C&M). The Committee is made up of representatives from two Federal Government agencies, the National Center for Health Statistics and the Health Care Financing Administration. The Committee holds meetings twice a year which are open to the public. Modification proposals submitted to the Committee for consideration are presented at the meetings for public discussion. Those modification proposals which are approved are incorporated into the official government version of the ICD-9-CM and become effective for use October 1 of the year following their presentation. The C&M also prepares updates for use April 1 of each year. To date, no April 1 updates have been released.

CHARACTERISTICS OF ICD-9-CM

ICD-9-CM far exceeds its predecessors in the number of codes provided. The disease classification has been expanded to include health-related conditions and to provide greater specificity at the fifth-digit level of detail. These fifth digits are not optional; they are intended for use in recording the information substantiated in the clinical record.

Volume I of ICD-9-CM contains five appendices:

Appendix A	Morphology of Neoplasms
Appendix B	Glossary of Mental Disorders (Deleted in 2004)
Appendix C	Classification of Drugs by American Hospital Formulary Service List Number and Their ICD-9-CM Equivalents
Appendix D	Classification of Industrial Accidents According to Agency
Appendix E	List of Three-Digit Categories

These appendices are included as a reference to the user in order to provide further information about the patient's clinical picture, to further define a diagnostic statement, to aid in classifying new drugs, or to reference three-digit categories.

Volume 2 of ICD-9-CM contains many diagnostic terms which do not appear in Volume 1 since the index includes most diagnostic terms currently in use.

The Disease Classification

ICD-9-CM is totally compatible with its parent system, ICD-9, thus meeting the need for comparability of morbidity and mortality statistics at the international level. A few fourth-digit codes were created in existing three-digit rubrics only when the necessary detail could not be accommodated by the use of a fifth-digit subclassification. To ensure that each rubric of ICD-9-CM collapses back to its ICD-9 counterpart the following specifications governed the ICD-9-CM disease classification:

Specifications for the Tabular List

1. Three-digit rubrics and their contents are unchanged from ICD-9.
2. The sequence of three-digit rubrics is unchanged from ICD-9.
3. Unsubdivided three-digit rubrics are subdivided where necessary to:
   a) Add clinical detail
   b) Isolate terms for clinical accuracy
4. The modification in ICD-9-CM is accomplished by the addition of a fifth digit to existing ICD-9 rubrics.
5. The optional dual classification in ICD-9 is modified.
   a) Duplicate rubrics are deleted:
      1) Four-digit manifestation categories duplicating etiology entries.
      2) Manifestation inclusion terms duplicating etiology entries.
   b) Manifestations of diseases are identified, to the extent possible, by creating five-digit codes in the etiology rubrics.
   c) When the manifestation of a disease cannot be included in the etiology rubrics, provision for its identification is made by retaining the ICD-9 rubrics used for classifying manifestations of disease.
6. The format of ICD-9-CM is revised from that used in ICD-9.
   a) American spelling of medical terms is used.
   b) Inclusion terms are indented beneath the titles of codes.
   c) Codes not to be used for principal tabulation of disease are printed with the notation, "Code first underlying disease."

Specifications for the Alphabetic Index

1. Format of the Alphabetic Index follows the format of ICD-9.
2. When two codes are required to indicate etiology and manifestation, the manifestation code appears in brackets, e.g., diabetic cataract 250.5X [366.41]. The etiology code is always sequenced first followed by the manifestation code.

ICD-9-CM Official Guidelines for Coding and Reporting

Effective December 1, 2005
Narrative changes appear in bold text
Items underlined have been moved within the guidelines since April 2005
The guidelines include the updated V Code Table

The Centers for Medicare and Medicaid Services (CMS) and the National Center for Health Statistics (NCHS), two departments within the U. S. Federal Government's Department of Health and Human Services (DHHS) provide the following guidelines for coding and reporting using the International Classification of Diseases, 9th Revision, Clinical Modification (ICD-9-CM). These guidelines should be used as a companion document to the official version of the ICD-9-CM as published on CD-ROM by the U.S. Government Printing Office (GPO).

These guidelines have been approved by the four organizations that make up the Cooperating Parties for the ICD-9-CM: the American Hospital Association (AHA), the American Health Information Management Association (AHIMA), CMS, and NCHS. These guidelines are included on the official government version of the ICD-9-CM, and also appear in "*Coding Clinic for ICD-9-CM*" published by the AHA.

These guidelines are a set of rules that have been developed to accompany and complement the official conventions and instructions provided within the ICD-9-CM itself. These guidelines are based on the coding and sequencing instructions in Volumes I, II and III of ICD-9-CM, but provide additional instruction. Adherence to these guidelines when assigning ICD-9-CM diagnosis and procedure codes is required under the Health Insurance Portability and Accountability Act (HIPAA). The diagnosis codes (Volumes 1-2) have been adopted under HIPAA for all healthcare settings. Volume 3 procedure codes have been adopted for inpatient procedures reported by hospitals. A joint effort between the healthcare provider and the coder is essential to achieve complete and accurate documentation, code assignment, and reporting of diagnoses and procedures. These guidelines have been developed to assist both the healthcare provider and the coder in identifying those diagnoses and procedures that are to be reported. The importance of consistent, complete documentation in the medical record cannot be overemphasized. Without such documentation accurate coding cannot be achieved. The entire record should be reviewed to determine the specific reason for the encounter and the conditions treated.

The term encounter is used for all settings, including hospital admissions. In the context of these guidelines, the term provider is used throughout the guidelines to mean physician or any qualified health care practitioner who is legally accountable for establishing the patient's diagnosis. Only this set of guidelines, approved by the Cooperating Parties, is official.

The guidelines are organized into sections. Section I includes the structure and conventions of the classification and general guidelines that apply to the entire classification, and chapter-specific guidelines that correspond to the chapters as they are arranged in the classification. Section II includes guidelines for selection of principal diagnosis for non-outpatient settings. Section III includes guidelines for reporting additional diagnoses in non-outpatient settings. Section IV is for outpatient coding and reporting.

ICD-9-CM Official Guidelines for Coding and Reporting.................................. 4

Section I. Conventions, General Coding Guidelines, and Chapter-Specific Guidelines 7

A. Conventions for the ICD-9-CM 7
   1. Format:.. 7
   2. Abbreviations 7
      a. Index abbreviations.......................... **7**
      b. Tabular abbreviations **7**
   3. Punctuation 7
   4. Includes and Excludes Notes and Inclusion terms 8
   5. Other and Unspecified codes 8
      a. "Other" codes **8**
      b. "Unspecified" codes **8**
   6. Etiology/manifestation convention ("code first", "use additional code", and "in diseases classified elsewhere" notes) 8
   7. "And" 8
   8. "With" 8
   9. "See" and "See Also"............................. 9
B. General Coding Guidelines.......................... 9
   1. Use of Both Alphabetic Index and Tabular List....................................... 9
   2. Locate each term in the Alphabetic Index 9
   3. Level of Detail in Coding........................ 9
   4. Code or codes from 001.0 through V84.8 9
   5. Selection of codes 001.0 through 999.9.......... 9
   6. Signs and symptoms 9
   7. Conditions that are an integral part of a disease process 9
   8. Conditions that are not an integral part of a disease process 9
   9. Multiple coding for a single condition 9
   10. Acute and Chronic Conditions 10
   11. Combination Code............................. 10
   12. Late Effects.................................... 10
   13. Impending or Threatened Condition......... 10
C. Chapter-Specific Coding Guidelines 10
   1. Chapter 1: Infectious and Parasitic Diseases (001-139)............................... 10
      a. Human Immunodeficiency Virus (HIV) Infections.............................. **10**
      b. Septicemia, Systemic Inflammatory Response Syndrome (SIRS), Sepsis, Severe Sepsis, and Septic Shock............ **11**
   2. Chapter 2: Neoplasms (140-239)............... 13
      a. Treatment directed at the malignancy..... **13**
      b. Treatment of secondary site **13**
      c. Coding and sequencing of complications **13**
      d. Primary malignancy previously excised... **14**
      e. Admissions/Encounters involving chemotherapy, immunotherapy, and radiation therapy **14**
      f. Admission/encounter to determine extent of malignancy **14**
      g. Symptoms, signs, and ill-defined conditions listed in Chapter 16............ **14**
   3. Chapter 3: Endocrine, Nutritional, and Metabolic Diseases and Immunity Disorders (240-279) 14
      a. Diabetes mellitus **14**
   4. Chapter 4: Diseases of Blood and Blood Forming Organs (280-289).............. 15
      a. Anemia of chronic disease................. 15
   5. Chapter 5: Mental Disorders (290-319) 16
      Reserved for future guideline expansion
   6. Chapter 6: Diseases of Nervous System and Sense Organs (320-389)................... 16
      Reserved for future guideline expansion
   7. Chapter 7: Diseases of Circulatory System (390-459) 16
      a. Hypertension................................ **16**
      b. Cerebral infarction/stroke/ cerebrovascular accident (CVA) **17**
      c. Postoperative cerebrovascular accident **17**
      d. Late Effects of Cerebrovascular Disease **17**
      e. Acute myocardial infarction (AMI) 17

8. Chapter 8: Diseases of Respiratory System (460-519) 17
   a. Chronic Obstructive Pulmonary Disease [COPD] and Asthma **17**
   b. Chronic Obstructive Pulmonary Disease [COPD] and Bronchitis..... **18**
9. Chapter 9: Diseases of Digestive System (520-579)..... 18
   Reserved for future guideline expansion
10. Chapter 10: Diseases of Genitourinary System (580-629) 18
   a. Chronic kidney disease 18
11. Chapter 11: Complications of Pregnancy, Childbirth, and the Puerperium (630-677) 19
   a. General Rules for Obstetric Cases **19**
   b. Selection of OB Principal or First-listed Diagnosis..... **19**
   c. Fetal Conditions Affecting the Management of the Mother **20**
   d. HIV Infection in Pregnancy, Childbirth, and the Puerperium **20**
   e. Current Conditions Complicating Pregnancy **20**
   f. Diabetes mellitus in pregnancy **20**
   g. Gestational diabetes..... **20**
   h. Normal Delivery, Code 650..... **20**
   i. The Postpartum and Peripartum Periods..... **21**
   j. Code 677, Late effect of complication of pregnancy **21**
   k. Abortions..... **21**
12. Chapter 12: Diseases Skin and Subcutaneous Tissue (680-709) 21
   Reserved for future guideline expansion
13. Chapter 13: Diseases of Musculoskeletal and Connective Tissue (710-739) 22
   Reserved for future guideline expansion
14. Chapter 14: Congenital Anomalies (740-759)..... 22
   a. Codes in categories 740-759, Congenital Anomalies **22**
15. Chapter 15: Newborn (Perinatal) Guidelines (760-779) 22
   a. General Perinatal Rules..... **22**
   b. Use of codes V30-V39 ..... **22**
   c. Newborn transfers..... **23**
   d. Use of category V29 ..... **23**
   e. Use of other V codes on perinatal records **23**
   f. Maternal Causes of Perinatal Morbidity..... **23**
   g. Congenital Anomalies in Newborns **23**
   h. Coding Additional Perinatal Diagnoses..... **23**
   i. Prematurity and Fetal Growth Retardation..... **23**
   j. Newborn sepsis..... **23**
16. Chapter 16: Signs, Symptoms, and Ill-Defined Conditions (780-799) 24
   Reserved for future guideline expansion
17. Chapter 17: Injury and Poisoning (800-999)..... 24
   a. Coding of Injuries **24**
   b. Coding of Fractures **24**
   c. Coding of Burns **24**
   d. Coding of Debridement of Wound, Infection, or Burn..... **25**
   e. Adverse Effects, Poisoning, and Toxic Effects **25**
   f. Complications of care 26
18. Classification of Factors Influencing Health Status and Contact with Health Service (Supplemental V01-V84)..... 27
   a. Introduction..... **27**
   b. V codes use in any healthcare setting..... **27**
   c. V Codes indicate a reason for an encounter **27**
   d. Categories of V Codes..... **27**
   e. V Code Table 33
19. Supplemental Classification of External Causes of Injury and Poisoning (E-codes, E800-E999) 35
   a. General E Code Coding Guidelines..... **36**
   b. Place of Occurrence Guideline..... **36**
   c. Adverse Effects of Drugs, Medicinal and Biological Substances Guidelines..... **36**
   d. Multiple Cause E Code Coding Guidelines..... **37**
   e. Child and Adult Abuse Guideline..... **37**
   f. Unknown or Suspected Intent Guideline **37**
   g. Undetermined Cause..... **37**
   h. Late Effects of External Cause Guidelines..... **37**
   i. Misadventures and Complications of Care Guidelines..... **38**
   j. Terrorism Guidelines..... **38**

Section II. Selection of Principal Diagnosis..... 38

A. Codes for symptoms, signs, and ill-defined conditions..... 38
B. Two or more interrelated conditions, each potentially meeting the definition for principal diagnosis 38

C. Two or more diagnoses that equally meet the definition for principal diagnosis 38
D. Two or more comparative or contrasting conditions 38
E. A symptom(s) followed by contrasting/ comparative diagnoses 39
F. Original treatment plan not carried out 39
G. Complications of surgery and other medical care 39
H. Uncertain Diagnosis 39
I. Admission from Observation Unit 39
1. Admission Following Medical Observation 39
2. Admission Following Post-Operative Observation 39
J. Admission from Outpatient Surgery 39

Section III. Reporting Additional Diagnoses........................... 39

A. Previous conditions 40
B. Abnormal findings 40
C. Uncertain Diagnosis 40

Section IV. Diagnostic Coding and Reporting Guidelines for Outpatient Services... 40

A. Selection of first-listed condition 40
1. Outpatient Surgery 40
2. Observation Stay 40
B. Codes from 001.0 through V84.8 40
C. Accurate reporting of ICD-9-CM diagnosis codes 40
D. Selection of codes 001.0 through 999.9 41
E. Codes that describe symptoms and signs 41
F. Encounters for circumstances other than a disease or injury 41
G. Level of Detail in Coding 41
1. ICD-9-CM codes with 3, 4, or 5 digits 41
2. Use of full number of digits required for a code 41
H. ICD-9-CM code for the diagnosis, condition, problem, or other reason for encounter/visit 41
I. "Probable", "suspected", "questionable", "rule out", or "working diagnosis" 41
J. Chronic diseases 41
K. Code all documented conditions that coexist 41
L. Patients receiving diagnostic services only 41
M. Patients receiving therapeutic services only 41
N. Patients receiving preoperative evaluations only 41
O. Ambulatory surgery 42
P. Routine outpatient prenatal visits 42

Section I. Conventions, General Coding Guidelines, and Chapter-Specific Guidelines

The conventions, general guidelines, and chapter-specific guidelines are applicable to all health care settings unless otherwise indicated.

A. Conventions for the ICD-9-CM

The conventions for the ICD-9-CM are the general rules for use of the classification independent of the guidelines. These conventions are incorporated within the index and tabular of the ICD-9-CM as instructional notes. The conventions are as follows:

1. Format:

The ICD-9-CM uses an indented format for ease in reference

2. Abbreviations

a. Index abbreviations

NEC "Not elsewhere classifiable"
This abbreviation in the index represents "other specified" when a specific code is not available for a condition the index directs the coder to the "other specified" code in the tabular.

b. Tabular abbreviations

NEC "Not elsewhere classifiable"
This abbreviation in the tabular represents "other specified". When a specific code is not available for a condition the tabular includes an NEC entry under a code to identify the code as the "other specified" code (See Section I.A.5.a. "Other" codes).

NOS "Not otherwise specified"
This abbreviation is the equivalent of unspecified. (See Section I.A.5.b., "Unspecified" codes)

3. Punctuation

[ ] Brackets are used in the tabular list to enclose synonyms, alternative wording or explanatory phrases. Brackets are used in the index to identify manifestation codes. (See Section I.A.6. "Etiology/manifestations")

( ) Parentheses are used in both the index and tabular to enclose supplementary words that may be present or absent in the statement of a disease or procedure without affecting the code number to which it is assigned. The terms within the parentheses are referred to as nonessential modifiers.

: Colons are used in the Tabular list after an incomplete term which needs one or more of the modifiers following the colon to make it assignable to a given category.

4. **Includes and Excludes Notes and Inclusion terms**

   Includes: This note appears immediately under a three-digit code title to further define, or give examples of, the content of the category.

   Excludes: An excludes note under a code indicates that the terms excluded from the code are to be coded elsewhere. In some cases the codes for the excluded terms should not be used in conjunction with the code from which it is excluded. An example of this is a congenital condition excluded from an acquired form of the same condition. The congenital and acquired codes should not be used together. In other cases, the excluded terms may be used together with an excluded code. An example of this is when fractures of different bones are coded to different codes. Both codes may be used together if both types of fractures are present.

   Inclusion terms: List of terms is included under certain four and five digit codes. These terms are the conditions for which that code number is to be used. The terms may be synonyms of the code title, or, in the case of "other specified" codes, the terms are a list of the various conditions assigned to that code. The inclusion terms are not necessarily exhaustive. Additional terms found only in the index may also be assigned to a code.

5. **Other and Unspecified codes**

   a. **"Other" codes**

      Codes titled "other" or "other specified" (usually a code with a 4th digit 8 or 5th digit 9 for diagnosis codes) are for use when the information in the medical record provides detail for which a specific code does not exist. Index entries with NEC in the line designate "other" codes in the tabular. These index entries represent specific disease entities for which no specific code exists so the term is included within an "other" code.

   b. **"Unspecified" codes**

      Codes (usually a code with a 4th digit 9 or 5th digit 0 for diagnosis codes) titled "unspecified" are for use when the information in the medical record is insufficient to assign a more specific code.

6. **Etiology/manifestation convention ("code first", "use additional code", and "in diseases classified elsewhere" notes)**

   Certain conditions have both an underlying etiology and multiple body system manifestations due to the underlying etiology. For such conditions, the ICD-9-CM has a coding convention that requires the underlying condition be sequenced first followed by the manifestation. Wherever such a combination exists, there is a "use additional code" note at the etiology code, and a "code first" note at the manifestation code. These instructional notes indicate the proper sequencing order of the codes, etiology followed by manifestation.

   In most cases the manifestation codes will have in the code title, "in diseases classified elsewhere." Codes with this title are a component of the etiology/manifestation convention. The code title indicates that it is a manifestation code. "In diseases classified elsewhere" codes are never permitted to be used as first listed or principal diagnosis codes. They must be used in conjunction with an underlying condition code and they must be listed following the underlying condition.

   There are manifestation codes that do not have "in diseases classified elsewhere" in the title. For such codes a "use additional code" note will still be present and the rules for sequencing apply.

   In addition to the notes in the tabular, these conditions also have a specific index entry structure. In the index both conditions are listed together with the etiology code first followed by the manifestation codes in brackets. The code in brackets is always to be sequenced second.

   The most commonly used etiology/manifestation combinations are the codes for Diabetes mellitus, category 250. For each code under category 250 there is a use additional code note for the manifestation that is specific for that particular diabetic manifestation. Should a patient have more than one manifestation of diabetes, more than one code from category 250 may be used with as many manifestation codes as are needed to fully describe the patient's complete diabetic condition. The **category** 250 diabetes codes should be sequenced first, followed by the manifestation codes.

   "Code first" and "Use additional code" notes are also used as sequencing rules in the classification for certain codes that are not part of an etiology/manifestation combination. See - Section I.B.9. "Multiple coding for a single condition".

7. **"And"**

   The word "and" should be interpreted to mean either "and" or "or" when it appears in a title.

8. **"With"**

   The word "with" in the alphabetic index is sequenced immediately following the main term, not in alphabetical order.

9. **"See" and "See Also"**

The "see" instruction following a main term in the index indicates that another term should be referenced. It is necessary to go to the main term referenced with the "see" note to locate the correct code.

A "see also" instruction following a main term in the index instructs that there is another main term that may also be referenced that may provide additional index entries that may be useful. It is not necessary to follow the "see also" note when the original main term provides the necessary code.

B. **General Coding Guidelines**

1. **Use of Both Alphabetic Index and Tabular List**

Use both the Alphabetic Index and the Tabular List when locating and assigning a code. Reliance on only the Alphabetic Index or the Tabular List leads to errors in code assignments and less specificity in code selection.

2. **Locate each term in the Alphabetic Index**

Locate each term in the Alphabetic Index and verify the code selected in the Tabular List. Read and be guided by instructional notations that appear in both the Alphabetic Index and the Tabular List.

3. **Level of Detail in Coding**

Diagnosis and procedure codes are to be used at their highest number of digits available.

ICD-9-CM diagnosis codes are composed of codes with either 3, 4, or 5 digits. Codes with three digits are included in ICD-9-CM as the heading of a category of codes that may be further subdivided by the use of fourth and/or fifth digits, which provide greater detail.

A three-digit code is to be used only if it is not further subdivided. Where fourth-digit subcategories and/or fifth-digit subclassifications are provided, they must be assigned. A code is invalid if it has not been coded to the full number of digits required for that code. For example, Acute myocardial infarction, code 410, has fourth digits that describe the location of the infarction (e.g., 410.2, Of inferolateral wall), and fifth digits that identify the episode of care. It would be incorrect to report a code in category 410 without a fourth and fifth digit.

ICD-9-CM Volume 3 procedure codes are composed of codes with either 3 or 4 digits. Codes with two digits are included in ICD-9-CM as the heading of a category of codes that may be further subdivided by the use of third and/or fourth digits, which provide greater detail.

4. **Code or codes from 001.0 through V84.8**

The appropriate code or codes from 001.0 through V84.8 must be used to identify diagnoses, symptoms, conditions, problems, complaints, or other reason(s) for the encounter/visit.

5. **Selection of codes 001.0 through 999.9**

The selection of codes 001.0 through 999.9 will frequently be used to describe the reason for the admission/encounter. These codes are from the section of ICD-9-CM for the classification of diseases and injuries (e.g., infectious and parasitic diseases; neoplasms; symptoms, signs, and ill-defined conditions, etc.).

6. **Signs and symptoms**

Codes that describe symptoms and signs, as opposed to diagnoses, are acceptable for reporting purposes when a related definitive diagnosis has not been established (confirmed) by the provider. Chapter 16 of ICD-9-CM, Symptoms, Signs, and Ill-defined conditions (codes 780.0-799.9) contain many, but not all codes for symptoms.

7. **Conditions that are an integral part of a disease process**

Signs and symptoms that are integral to the disease process should not be assigned as additional codes.

8. **Conditions that are not an integral part of a disease process**

Additional signs and symptoms that may not be associated routinely with a disease process should be coded when present.

9. **Multiple coding for a single condition**

In addition to the etiology/manifestation convention that requires two codes to fully describe a single condition that affects multiple body systems, there are other single conditions that also require more than one code. "Use additional code" notes are found in the tabular at codes that are not part of an etiology/manifestation pair where a secondary code is useful to fully describe a condition. The sequencing rule is the same as the etiology/manifestation pair—"use additional code" indicates that a secondary code should be added.

For example, for infections that are not included in chapter 1, a secondary code from category 041, Bacterial infection in conditions classified elsewhere and of unspecified site, may be required to identify the bacterial organism causing the infection. A "use additional code" note will normally be found at the infectious disease code, indicating a need for the organism code to be added as a secondary code.

"Code first" notes are also under certain codes that are not specifically manifestation codes but may be due to an underlying cause. When a "code first" note is present and an underlying condition is present the underlying condition should be sequenced first.

"Code, if applicable, any causal condition first", notes indicate that this code may be assigned as a principal diagnosis when the causal condition is unknown or not applicable. If a causal condition is known, then the code for that condition should be sequenced as the principal or first-listed diagnosis.

Multiple codes may be needed for late effects, complication codes, and obstetric codes to more fully describe a condition. See the specific guidelines for these conditions for further instruction.

10. Acute and Chronic Conditions

If the same condition is described as both acute (subacute) and chronic, and separate subentries exist in the Alphabetic Index at the same indentation level, code both and sequence the acute (subacute) code first.

11. Combination Code

A combination code is a single code used to classify:
Two diagnoses, or
A diagnosis with an associated secondary process (manifestation)
A diagnosis with an associated complication

Combination codes are identified by referring to subterm entries in the Alphabetic Index and by reading the inclusion and exclusion notes in the Tabular List.

Assign only the combination code when that code fully identifies the diagnostic conditions involved or when the Alphabetic Index so directs. Multiple coding should not be used when the classification provides a combination code that clearly identifies all of the elements documented in the diagnosis. When the combination code lacks necessary specificity in describing the manifestation or complication, an additional code should be used as a secondary code.

12. Late Effects

A late effect is the residual effect (condition produced) after the acute phase of an illness or injury has terminated. There is no time limit on when a late effect code can be used. The residual may be apparent early, such as in cerebrovascular accident cases, or it may occur months or years later, such as that due to a previous injury. Coding of late effects generally requires two codes sequenced in the following order: The condition or nature of the late effect is sequenced first. The late effect code is sequenced second.

An exception to the above guidelines are those instances where the code for late effect is followed by a manifestation code identified in the Tabular List and title, or the late effect code has been expanded (at the fourth and fifth-digit levels) to include the manifestation(s). The code for the acute phase of an illness or injury that led to the late effect is never used with a code for the late effect.

13. Impending or Threatened Condition

Code any condition described at the time of discharge as "impending" or "threatened" as follows:

If it did occur, code as confirmed diagnosis.
If it did not occur, reference the Alphabetic Index to determine if the condition has a subentry term for "impending" or "threatened" and also reference main term entries for "Impending" and for "Threatened."
If the subterms are listed, assign the given code.
If the subterms are not listed, code the existing underlying condition(s) and not the condition described as impending or threatened.

C. Chapter-Specific Coding Guidelines

In addition to general coding guidelines, there are guidelines for specific diagnoses and/or conditions in the classification. Unless otherwise indicated, these guidelines apply to all health care settings. Please refer to Section II for guidelines on the selection of principal diagnosis.

1. Chapter 1: Infectious and Parasitic Diseases (001-139)

a. Human Immunodeficiency Virus (HIV) Infections

1) Code only confirmed cases

Code only confirmed cases of HIV infection/illness. This is an exception to the hospital inpatient guideline Section II, H.

In this context, "confirmation" does not require documentation of positive serology or culture for HIV; the provider's diagnostic statement that the patient is HIV positive, or has an HIV-related illness is sufficient.

2) Selection and sequencing of HIV codes

(a) Patient admitted for HIV-related condition

If a patient is admitted for an HIV-related condition, the principal diagnosis should be 042, followed by additional diagnosis codes for all reported HIV-related conditions.

(b) Patient with HIV disease admitted for unrelated condition

If a patient with HIV disease is admitted for an unrelated condition (such as a traumatic injury), the code for the unrelated condition (e.g., the nature of injury code) should be the principal diagnosis. Other diagnoses would be 042 followed by additional diagnosis codes for all reported HIV-related conditions.

(c) Whether the patient is newly diagnosed

Whether the patient is newly diagnosed or has had previous admissions/encounters for HIV conditions is irrelevant to the sequencing decision.

(d) Asymptomatic human immunodeficiency virus

V08 Asymptomatic human immunodeficiency virus [HIV] infection, is to be applied when the patient without any documentation of symptoms is listed as being "HIV positive," "known HIV," "HIV test positive," or similar terminology. Do not use this code if the term "AIDS" is used or if the patient is treated for any HIV-related illness or is described as having any condition(s) resulting from his/her HIV positive status; use 042 in these cases.

(e) Patients with inconclusive HIV serology

Patients with inconclusive HIV serology, but no definitive diagnosis or manifestations of the illness, may be assigned code 795.71, Inconclusive serologic test for Human Immunodeficiency Virus [HIV].

(f) Previously diagnosed HIV-related illness

Patients with any known prior diagnosis of an HIV-related illness should be coded to 042. Once a patient has developed an HIV-related illness, the patient should always be assigned code 042 on every subsequent admission/encounter. Patients previously diagnosed with any HIV illness (042) should never be assigned to 795.71 or V08.

(g) HIV Infection in Pregnancy, Childbirth, and the Puerperium

During pregnancy, childbirth or the puerperium, a patient admitted (or presenting for a health care encounter) because of an HIV-related illness should receive a principal diagnosis code of 647.6X, Other specified infectious and parasitic diseases in the mother classifiable elsewhere, but complicating the pregnancy, childbirth, or the puerperium, followed by 042 and the code(s) for the HIV-related illness(es). Codes from Chapter 15 always take sequencing priority.

Patients with asymptomatic HIV infection status admitted (or presenting for a health care encounter) during pregnancy, childbirth, or the puerperium should receive codes of 647.6X and V08.

(h) Encounters for testing for HIV

If a patient is being seen to determine his/her HIV status, use code V73.89, Screening for other specified viral disease. Use code V69.8, Other problems related to lifestyle, as a secondary code if an asymptomatic patient is in a known high risk group for HIV. Should a patient with signs or symptoms or illness, or a confirmed HIV related diagnosis be tested for HIV, code the signs and symptoms or the diagnosis. An additional counseling code V65.44 may be used if counseling is provided during the encounter for the test.

When a patient returns to be informed of his/her HIV test results use code V65.44, HIV counseling, if the results of the test are negative.

If the results are positive but the patient is asymptomatic use code V08, Asymptomatic HIV infection. If the results are positive and the patient is symptomatic use code 042, HIV infection, with codes for the HIV related symptoms or diagnosis. The HIV counseling code may also be used if counseling is provided for patients with positive test results.

b. Septicemia, Systemic Inflammatory Response Syndrome (SIRS), Sepsis, Severe Sepsis, and Septic Shock

1) Sepsis as principal diagnosis or secondary diagnosis

(a) Sepsis as principal diagnosis

If sepsis is present on admission, and meets the definition of principal diagnosis, the underlying systemic infection code (e.g., 038.xx, 112.5, etc) should be assigned as the principal diagnosis, followed by code 995.91, Systemic inflammatory response syndrome due to infectious process without organ dysfunction, as required by the sequencing rules in the Tabular List. Codes from subcategory 995.9 can never be assigned as a principal diagnosis.

(b) Sepsis as secondary diagnoses

When sepsis develops during the encounter (it was not present on admission), the sepsis codes may be assigned as secondary diagnoses, following the sequencing rules provided in the Tabular List.

(c) Documentation unclear as to whether sepsis present on admission

If the documentation is not clear whether the sepsis was present on admission, the provider should be queried. After provider query, if sepsis is determined at that point to have met the definition of principal diagnosis, the underlying systemic infection (038.xx, 112.5, etc) may be used as principal diagnosis along with code 995.91, Systemic inflammatory response syndrome due to infectious process without organ dysfunction.

2) Septicemia/Sepsis

In most cases, it will be a code from category 038, Septicemia, that will be used in conjunction with a code from subcategory 995.9 such as the following:

(a) Streptococcal sepsis

If the documentation in the record states streptococcal sepsis, codes 038.0 and code 995.91 should be used, in that sequence.

(b) Streptococcal septicemia

If the documentation states streptococcal septicemia, only code 038.0 should be assigned, however, the provider should be queried whether the patient has sepsis, an infection with SIRS.

(c) Sepsis or SIRS must be documented

Either the term sepsis or SIRS must be documented, to assign a code from subcategory 995.9.

3) Terms sepsis, severe sepsis, or SIRS

If the terms sepsis, severe sepsis, or SIRS are used with an underlying infection other than septicemia, such as pneumonia, cellulitis, or a nonspecified urinary tract infection, a code from category 038 should be assigned first, then code 995.91, followed by the code for the initial infection. The use of the terms sepsis or SIRS indicates that the patient's infection has advanced to the point of a systemic infection so the systemic infection should be sequenced before the localized infection. The instructional note under subcategory 995.9 instructs to assign the underlying systemic infection first.

Note: The term urosepsis is a nonspecific term. If that is the only term documented then only code 599.0 should be assigned based on the default for the term in the ICD-9-CM index, in addition to the code for the causal organism if known.

4) Severe sepsis

For patients with severe sepsis, the code for the systemic infection (e.g., 038.xx, 112.5, etc) or trauma should be sequenced first, followed by either code 995.92, Systemic inflammatory response syndrome due to infectious process with organ dysfunction, or code 995.94, Systemic inflammatory response syndrome due to noninfectious process with organ dysfunction. Codes for the specific organ dysfunctions should also be assigned.

5) Septic shock

(a) Sequencing of septic shock

Septic shock is a form of organ dysfunction associated with severe sepsis. A code for the initiating underlying systemic infection followed by a code for SIRS (code 995.92) must be assigned before the code for septic shock. As noted in the sequencing instructions in the Tabular List, the code for septic shock cannot be assigned as a principal diagnosis.

(b) Septic Shock without documentation of severe sepsis

Septic shock cannot occur in the absence of severe sepsis. A code from subcategory 995.9 must be sequenced before the code for septic shock. The use additional code notes and the code first note provide sequencing instructions.

6) Sepsis and septic shock associated with abortion

Sepsis and septic shock associated with abortion, ectopic pregnancy, and molar pregnancy are classified to category codes in Chapter 11 (630-639).

7) **Negative or inconclusive blood cultures**

Negative or inconclusive blood cultures do not preclude a diagnosis of septicemia or sepsis in patients with clinical evidence of the condition, however, the provider should be queried.

8) **Newborn sepsis**

See Section I.C.15.j for information on the coding of newborn sepsis.

9) **Sepsis due to a Postprocedural Infection**

Sepsis resulting from a postprocedural infection is a complication of care. For such cases code 998.59, Other postoperative infections, should be coded first followed by the appropriate codes for the sepsis. The other guidelines for coding sepsis should then be followed for the assignment of additional codes.

10) **External cause of injury codes with SIRS**

An external cause code is not needed with codes 995.91, Systemic inflammatory response syndrome due to infectious process without organ dysfunction, or code 995.92, Systemic inflammatory response syndrome due to infectious process with organ dysfunction.

Refer to Section I.C.19.a.7 for instruction on the use of external cause of injury codes with codes for SIRS resulting from trauma.

2. **Chapter 2: Neoplasms (140-239)**

<u>General guidelines</u>

Chapter 2 of the ICD-9-CM contains the codes for most benign and all malignant neoplasms. Certain benign neoplasms, such as prostatic adenomas, may be found in the specific body system chapters. To properly code a neoplasm it is necessary to determine from the record if the neoplasm is benign, in-situ, malignant, or of uncertain histologic behavior. If malignant, any secondary (metastatic) sites should also be determined.

The neoplasm table in the Alphabetic Index should be referenced first. However, if the histological term is documented, that term should be referenced first, rather than going immediately to the Neoplasm Table, in order to determine which column in the Neoplasm Table is appropriate. For example, if the documentation indicates "adenoma," refer to the term in the Alphabetic Index to review the entries under this term and the instructional note to "see also neoplasm, by site, benign." The table provides the proper code based on the type of neoplasm and the site. It is important to select the proper column in the table that corresponds to the type of neoplasm. The tabular should then be referenced to verify that the correct code has been selected from the table and that a more specific site code does not exist.

See Section I. C. 18.d.4. for information regarding V codes for genetic susceptibility to cancer.

a. **Treatment directed at the malignancy**

If the treatment is directed at the malignancy, designate the malignancy as the principal diagnosis.

b. **Treatment of secondary site**

When a patient is admitted because of a primary neoplasm with metastasis and treatment is directed toward the secondary site only, the secondary neoplasm is designated as the principal diagnosis even though the primary malignancy is still present.

c. **Coding and sequencing of complications**

Coding and sequencing of complications associated with the malignancies or with the therapy thereof are subject to the following guidelines:

1) **Anemia associated with malignancy**

When admission/encounter is for management of an anemia associated with the malignancy, and the treatment is only for anemia, the **appropriate** anemia **code (such as code 285.22, Anemia in neoplastic disease)** is designated at the principal diagnosis and is followed by the appropriate code(s) for the malignancy.

Code 285.22 may also be used as a secondary code if the patient suffers from anemia and is being treated for the malignancy.

2) **Anemia associated with chemotherapy, <u>immunotherapy, and radiation therapy</u>**

When the admission/encounter is for management of an anemia associated with chemotherapy, **immunotherapy**, or radiotherapy and the only treatment is for the anemia, the anemia is sequenced first followed by **code E933.1. The appropriate neoplasm code should be assigned as an additional code.**

3) **Management of dehydration due to the malignancy**

When the admission/encounter is for management of dehydration due to the malignancy or the therapy, or a combination of both, and only the dehydration is being treated (intravenous rehydration), the dehydration is sequenced first, followed by the code(s) for the malignancy.

4) **Treatment of a complication resulting from a surgical procedure**

When the admission/encounter is for treatment of a complication resulting from a surgical procedure, designate the complication as the principal or first-listed diagnosis if treatment is directed at resolving the complication.

d. **Primary malignancy previously excised**

When a primary malignancy has been previously excised or eradicated from its site and there is no further treatment directed to that site and there is no evidence of any existing primary malignancy, a code from category V10, Personal history of malignant neoplasm, should be used to indicate the former site of the malignancy. Any mention of extension, invasion, or metastasis to another site is coded as a secondary malignant neoplasm to that site. The secondary site may be the principal or first-listed with the V10 code used as a secondary code.

e. **Admissions/Encounters involving chemotherapy, immunotherapy, and radiation therapy**

1) **Episode of care involves surgical removal of neoplasm**

When an episode of care involves the surgical removal of a neoplasm, primary or secondary site, followed by adjunct chemotherapy or radiation treatment **during the same episode of care**, the neoplasm code should be assigned as principal or first-listed diagnosis, using codes in the 140-198 series or where appropriate in the 200-203 series.

2) **Patient admission/encounter solely for administration of chemotherapy, immunotherapy, and radiation therapy**

If a patient admission/encounter is solely for the administration of chemotherapy, **immunotherapy** or radiation therapy **assign** code V58.0, Encounter for radiation therapy, or **V58.11**, Encounter for **antineoplastic** chemotherapy, **or V58.12, Encounter for antineoplastic immunotherapy as** the first-listed or principal diagnosis. If a patient receives **more than one of these therapies during the same admission more than one of these codes may be assigned, in any sequence.**

3) **Patient admitted for radiotherapy/chemotherapy and develops complications**

When a patient is admitted for the purpose of radiotherapy, **immunotherapy**, or chemotherapy and develops complications such as uncontrolled nausea and vomiting or dehydration, the principal or first-listed diagnosis is V58.0, Encounter for radiotherapy, or V58.11, **Encounter for antineoplastic chemotherapy, or V58.12, Encounter for antineoplastic immunotherapy** followed by any codes for the complications.

See Section I.C.18.d.7. for additional information regarding aftercare V codes.

f. **Admission/encounter to determine extent of malignancy**

When the reason for admission/encounter is to determine the extent of the malignancy, or for a procedure such as paracentesis or thoracentesis, the primary malignancy or appropriate metastatic site is designated as the principal or first-listed diagnosis, even though chemotherapy or radiotherapy is administered.

g. **Symptoms, signs, and ill-defined conditions listed in Chapter 16**

Symptoms, signs, and ill-defined conditions listed in Chapter 16 characteristic of, or associated with, an existing primary or secondary site malignancy cannot be used to replace the malignancy as principal or first-listed diagnosis, regardless of the number of admissions or encounters for treatment and care of the neoplasm.

See section I.C.18.d.14, Encounter for prophylactic organ removal

3. **Chapter 3: Endocrine, Nutritional, and Metabolic Diseases and Immunity Disorders (240-279)**

a. **Diabetes mellitus**

Codes under category 250, Diabetes mellitus, identify complications/manifestations associated with diabetes mellitus. A fifth-digit is required for all category 250 codes to identify the type of diabetes mellitus and whether the diabetes is controlled or uncontrolled.

1) **Fifth-digits for category 250:**

The following are the fifth-digits for the codes under category 250:

0 type II or unspecified type, not stated as uncontrolled

1 type I, [juvenile type], not stated as uncontrolled

Assign code 642.3x for transient hypertension of pregnancy.

9) **Hypertension, Controlled**

Assign appropriate code from categories 401-405. This diagnostic statement usually refers to an existing state of hypertension under control by therapy.

10) **Hypertension, Uncontrolled**

Uncontrolled hypertension may refer to untreated hypertension or hypertension not responding to current therapeutic regimen. In either case, assign the appropriate code from categories 401-405 to designate the stage and type of hypertension. Code to the type of hypertension.

11) **Elevated Blood Pressure**

For a statement of elevated blood pressure without further specificity, assign code 796.2, Elevated blood pressure reading without diagnosis of hypertension, rather than a code from category 401.

b. **Cerebral infarction/stroke/cerebrovascular accident (CVA)**

The terms stroke and CVA are often used interchangeably to refer to a cerebral infarction. The terms stroke, CVA, and cerebral infarction NOS are all indexed to the default code 434.91, Cerebral artery occlusion, unspecified, with infarction. Code 436, Acute, but ill-defined, cerebrovascular disease, should not be used when the documentation states stroke or CVA.

c. **Postoperative cerebrovascular accident**

A cerebrovascular hemorrhage or infarction that occurs as a result of medical intervention is coded to 997.02, Iatrogenic cerebrovascular infarction or hemorrhage. Medical record documentation should clearly specify the cause-and-effect relationship between the medical intervention and the cerebrovascular accident in order to assign this code. A secondary code from the code range 430-432 or from a code from subcategories 433 or 434 with a fifth digit of "1" should also be used to identify the type of hemorrhage or infarct.

This guideline conforms to the use additional code note instruction at category 997. Code 436, Acute, but ill-defined, cerebrovascular disease, should not be used as a secondary code with code 997.02.

d. **Late Effects of Cerebrovascular Disease**

1) **Category 438, Late Effects of Cerebrovascular disease**

Category 438 is used to indicate conditions classifiable to categories 430-437 as the causes of late effects (neurologic deficits), themselves classified elsewhere. These "late effects" include neurologic deficits that persist after initial onset of conditions classifiable to 430-437. The neurologic deficits caused by cerebrovascular disease may be present from the onset or may arise at any time after the onset of the condition classifiable to 430-437.

2) **Codes from category 438 with codes from 430-437**

Codes from category 438 may be assigned on a health care record with codes from 430-437, if the patient has a current cerebrovascular accident (CVA) and deficits from an old CVA.

3) **Code V12.59**

Assign code V12.59 (and not a code from category 438) as an additional code for history of cerebrovascular disease when no neurologic deficits are present.

e. **Acute myocardial infarction (AMI)**

1) **ST elevation myocardial infarction (STEMI) and non ST elevation myocardial infarction (NSTEMI)**

The ICD-9-CM codes for acute myocardial infarction (AMI) identify the site, such as anterolateral wall or true posterior wall. Subcategories 410.0-410.6 and 410.8 are used for ST elevation myocardial infarction (STEMI). Subcategory 410.7, Subendocardial infarction, is used for non ST elevation myocardial infarction (NSTEMI) and nontransmural MIs.

2) **Acute myocardial infarction, unspecified**

Subcategory 410.9 is the default for the unspecified term acute myocardial infarction. If only STEMI or transmural MI without the site is documented, query the provider as to the site, or assign a code from subcategory 410.9.

3) **AMI documented as nontransmural or subendocardial but site provided**

If an AMI is documented as nontransmural or subendocardial, but the site is provided, it is still coded as a subendocardial AMI. If NSTEMI evolves to STEMI, assign the STEMI code. If STEMI converts to NSTEMI due to thrombolytic therapy, it is still coded as STEMI.

8. Chapter 8: Diseases of Respiratory System (460-519)

a. **Chronic Obstructive Pulmonary Disease [COPD] and Asthma**

1) **Conditions that comprise COPD and Asthma**

The conditions that comprise COPD are obstructive chronic bronchitis, subcategory 491.2, and emphysema, category 492. All asthma codes are under category 493, Asthma. Code 496, Chronic airway obstruction, not elsewhere classified, is a nonspecific code that should only be used when the documentation in a medical record does not specify the type of COPD being treated.

2) **Acute exacerbation of chronic obstructive bronchitis and asthma**

The codes for chronic obstructive bronchitis and asthma distinguish between uncomplicated cases and those in acute exacerbation. An acute exacerbation is a worsening or a decompensation of a chronic condition. An acute exacerbation is not equivalent to an infection superimposed on a chronic condition, though an exacerbation may be triggered by an infection.

3) **Overlapping nature of the conditions that comprise COPD and asthma**

Due to the overlapping nature of the conditions that make up COPD and asthma, there are many variations in the way these conditions are documented. Code selection must be based on the terms as documented. When selecting the correct code for the documented type of COPD and asthma, it is essential to first review the index, and then verify the code in the tabular list. There are many instructional notes under the different COPD subcategories and codes. It is important that all such notes be reviewed to assure correct code assignment.

4) **Acute exacerbation of asthma and status asthmaticus**

An acute exacerbation of asthma is an increased severity of the asthma symptoms, such as wheezing and shortness of breath. Status asthmaticus refers to a patient's failure to respond to therapy administered during an asthmatic episode and is a life threatening complication that requires emergency care. If status asthmaticus is documented by the provider with any type of COPD or with acute bronchitis, the status asthmaticus should be sequenced first. It supersedes any type of COPD including that with acute exacerbation or acute bronchitis. It is inappropriate to assign an asthma code with 5th digit 2, with acute exacerbation, together with an asthma code with 5th digit 1, with status asthmatics. Only the 5th digit 1 should be assigned.

b. **Chronic Obstructive Pulmonary Disease [COPD] and Bronchitis**

1) **Acute bronchitis with COPD**

Acute bronchitis, code 466.0, is due to an infectious organism. When acute bronchitis is documented with COPD, code 491.22, Obstructive chronic bronchitis with acute bronchitis, should be assigned. It is not necessary to also assign code 466.0. If a medical record documents acute bronchitis with COPD with acute exacerbation, only code 491.22 should be assigned. The acute bronchitis included in code 491.22 supersedes the acute exacerbation. If a medical record documents COPD with acute exacerbation without mention of acute bronchitis, only code 491.21 should be assigned.

9. **Chapter 9: Diseases of Digestive System (520-579)**

Reserved for future guideline expansion

10. **Chapter 10: Diseases of Genitourinary System (580-629)**

a. **Chronic kidney disease**

1) **Stages of chronic kidney disease (CKD)**

The ICD-9-CM classifies CKD based on severity. The severity of CKD is designated by stages I-V. Stage II, code 585.2, equates to mild CKD; stage III, code 585.3, equates to moderate CKD; and stage IV, code 585.4, equates to severe CKD. Code 585.6, End stage renal disease (ESRD), is assigned when the provider has documented end-stage-renal disease (ESRD).

If both a stage of CKD and ESRD are documented, assign code 585.6 only.

2) **Chronic kidney disease and kidney transplant status**

Patients who have undergone kidney transplant may still have some form of CKD because the kidney transplant may not fully restore kidney function. Code V42.0 may be assigned with the appropriate CKD code for patients who are status post kidney transplant, based on the patient's post-transplant stage. The use additional code note under category 585 provides this instruction.

Use of a 585 code with V42.0 does not necessarily indicate transplant rejec-

tion or failure. Patients with mild or moderate CKD following a transplant should not be coded as having transplant failure, unless it is documented in the medical record. For patients with severe CKD or ESRD it is appropriate to assign code 996.81, Complications of transplanted organ, kidney transplant, when kidney transplant failure is documented. If a post kidney transplant patient has CKD and it is unclear from the documentation whether there is transplant failure or rejection it is necessary to query the provider.

3) Chronic kidney disease with other conditions

Patients with CKD may also suffer from other serious conditions, most commonly diabetes mellitus and hypertension. The sequencing of the CKD code in relationship to codes for other contributing conditions is based on the conventions in the tabular list.

See I.C.3.a.4 for sequencing instructions for diabetes.

See I.C.4.a.1. for anemia in CKD.

See I.C.7.a.3 for hypertensive kidney disease.

See I.C.17.f.1.b. Transplant complications, for instructions on coding of documented rejection or failure.

11. Chapter 11: Complications of Pregnancy, Childbirth, and the Puerperium (630-677)

a. General Rules for Obstetric Cases

1) Codes from chapter 11 and sequencing priority

Obstetric cases require codes from chapter 11, codes in the range 630-677, Complications of Pregnancy, Childbirth, and the Puerperium. Chapter 11 codes have sequencing priority over codes from other chapters. Additional codes from other chapters may be used in conjunction with chapter 11 codes to further specify conditions. Should the provider document that the pregnancy is incidental to the encounter, then code V22.2 should be used in place of any chapter 11 codes. It is the provider's responsibility to state that the condition being treated is not affecting the pregnancy.

2) Chapter 11 codes used only on the maternal record

Chapter 11 codes are to be used only on the maternal record, never on the record of the newborn.

3) Chapter 11 fifth-digits

Categories 640-648, 651-676 have required fifth-digits, which indicate whether the encounter is antepartum, postpartum and whether a delivery has also occurred.

4) Fifth-digits, appropriate for each code

The fifth-digits, which are appropriate for each code number, are listed in brackets under each code. The fifth-digits on each code should all be consistent with each other. That is, should a delivery occur all of the fifth-digits should indicate the delivery.

b. Selection of OB Principal or First-listed Diagnosis

1) Routine outpatient prenatal visits

For routine outpatient prenatal visits when no complications are present codes V22.0, Supervision of normal first pregnancy, and V22.1, Supervision of other normal pregnancy, should be used as the first-listed diagnoses. These codes should not be used in conjunction with chapter 11 codes.

2) Prenatal outpatient visits for high-risk patients

For prenatal outpatient visits for patients with high-risk pregnancies, a code from category V23, Supervision of high-risk pregnancy, should be used as the principal or first-listed diagnosis. Secondary chapter 11 codes may be used in conjunction with these codes if appropriate.

3) Episodes when no delivery occurs

In episodes when no delivery occurs, the principal diagnosis should correspond to the principal complication of the pregnancy, which necessitated the encounter. Should more than one complication exist, all of which are treated or monitored, any of the complications codes may be sequenced first.

4) When a delivery occurs

When a delivery occurs, the principal diagnosis should correspond to the main circumstances or complication of the delivery. In cases of cesarean delivery, the selection of the principal diagnosis should correspond to the reason the cesarean delivery was performed unless the reason for admission/encounter was unrelated to the condition resulting in the cesarean delivery.

5) Outcome of delivery

An outcome of delivery code, V27.0-V27.9, should be included on every maternal record when a delivery has occurred. These codes are not to be used on subsequent records or on the newborn record.

c. Fetal Conditions Affecting the Management of the Mother

1) Codes from category 655

Known or suspected fetal abnormality affecting management of the mother, and category 656, Other fetal and placental problems affecting the management of the mother, are assigned only when the fetal condition is actually responsible for modifying the management of the mother, i.e., by requiring diagnostic studies, additional observation, special care, or termination of pregnancy. The fact that the fetal condition exists does not justify assigning a code from this series to the mother's record.

2) In utero surgery

In cases when surgery is performed on the fetus, a diagnosis code from category 655, Known or suspected fetal abnormalities affecting management of the mother, should be assigned identifying the fetal condition. Procedure code 75.36, Correction of fetal defect, should be assigned on the hospital inpatient record.

No code from Chapter 15, the perinatal codes, should be used on the mother's record to identify fetal conditions. Surgery performed in utero on a fetus is still to be coded as an obstetric encounter.

d. HIV Infection in Pregnancy, Childbirth, and the Puerperium

During pregnancy, childbirth or the puerperium, a patient admitted because of an HIV-related illness should receive a principal diagnosis of 647.6X, Other specified infectious and parasitic diseases in the mother classifiable elsewhere, but complicating the pregnancy, childbirth or the puerperium, followed by 042 and the code(s) for the HIV-related illness(es).

Patients with asymptomatic HIV infection status admitted during pregnancy, childbirth, or the puerperium should receive codes of 647.6X and V08.

e. Current Conditions Complicating Pregnancy

Assign a code from subcategory 648.x for patients that have current conditions when the condition affects the management of the pregnancy, childbirth, or the puerperium. Use additional secondary codes from other chapters to identify the conditions, as appropriate.

f. Diabetes mellitus in pregnancy

Diabetes mellitus is a significant complicating factor in pregnancy. Pregnant women who are diabetic should be assigned code 648.0x, Diabetes mellitus complicating pregnancy, and a secondary code from category 250, Diabetes mellitus, to identify the type of diabetes.

Code V58.67, Long-term (current) use of insulin, should also be assigned if the diabetes mellitus is being treated with insulin.

g. Gestational diabetes

Gestational diabetes can occur during the second and third trimester of pregnancy in women who were not diabetic prior to pregnancy. Gestational diabetes can cause complications in the pregnancy similar to those of pre-existing diabetes mellitus. It also puts the woman at greater risk of developing diabetes after the pregnancy. Gestational diabetes is coded to 648.8x, Abnormal glucose tolerance. Codes 648.0x and 648.8x should never be used together on the same record.

Code V58.67, Long-term (current) use of insulin, should also be assigned if the gestational diabetes is being treated with insulin.

h. Normal Delivery, Code 650

1) Normal delivery

Code 650 is for use in cases when a woman is admitted for a full-term normal delivery and delivers a single, healthy infant without any complications antepartum, during the delivery, or postpartum during the delivery episode. Code 650 is always a principal diagnosis. It is not to be used if any other code from chapter 11 is needed to describe a current complication of the antenatal, delivery, or perinatal period. Additional codes from other chapters may be used with code 650 if they are not related to or are in any way complicating the pregnancy.

2) Normal delivery with resolved antepartum complication

Code 650 may be used if the patient had a complication at some point during her pregnancy, but the complication is not present at the time of the admission for delivery.

3) V27.0, Single liveborn, outcome of delivery

V27.0, Single liveborn, is the only outcome of delivery code appropriate for use with 650.

i. The Postpartum and Peripartum Periods

1) Postpartum and peripartum periods

The postpartum period begins immediately after delivery and continues for six weeks following delivery. The peripartum period is defined as the last month of pregnancy to five months postpartum.

2) Postpartum complication

A postpartum complication is any complication occurring within the six-week period.

3) Pregnancy-related complications after 6 week period

Chapter 11 codes may also be used to describe pregnancy-related complications after the six-week period should the provider document that a condition is pregnancy related.

4) Postpartum complications occurring during the same admission as delivery

Postpartum complications that occur during the same admission as the delivery are identified with a fifth digit of "2." Subsequent admissions/encounters for postpartum complications should be identified with a fifth digit of "4."

5) Admission for routine postpartum care following delivery outside hospital

When the mother delivers outside the hospital prior to admission and is admitted for routine postpartum care and no complications are noted, code V24.0, Postpartum care and examination immediately after delivery, should be assigned as the principal diagnosis.

6) Admission following delivery outside hospital with postpartum conditions

A delivery diagnosis code should not be used for a woman who has delivered prior to admission to the hospital. Any postpartum conditions and/or postpartum procedures should be coded.

j. Code 677, Late effect of complication of pregnancy

1) Code 677

Code 677, Late effect of complication of pregnancy, childbirth, and the puerperium is for use in those cases when an initial complication of a pregnancy develops a sequelae requiring care or treatment at a future date.

2) After the initial postpartum period

This code may be used at any time after the initial postpartum period.

3) Sequencing of Code 677

This code, like all late effect codes, is to be sequenced following the code describing the sequelae of the complication.

k. Abortions

1) Fifth-digits required for abortion categories

Fifth-digits are required for abortion categories 634-637. Fifth-digit 1, incomplete, indicates that all of the products of conception have not been expelled from the uterus. Fifth-digit 2, complete, indicates that all products of conception have been expelled from the uterus prior to the episode of care.

2) Code from categories 640-648 and 651-659

A code from categories 640-648 and 651-659 may be used as additional codes with an abortion code to indicate the complication leading to the abortion.

Fifth digit 3 is assigned with codes from these categories when used with an abortion code because the other fifth digits will not apply. Codes from the 660-669 series are not to be used for complications of abortion.

3) Code 639 for complications

Code 639 is to be used for all complications following abortion. Code 639 cannot be assigned with codes from categories 634-638.

4) Abortion with Liveborn Fetus

When an attempted termination of pregnancy results in a liveborn fetus assign code 644.21, Early onset of delivery, with an appropriate code from category V27, Outcome of Delivery. The procedure code for the attempted termination of pregnancy should also be assigned.

5) Retained Products of Conception following an abortion

Subsequent admissions for retained products of conception following a spontaneous or legally induced abortion are assigned the appropriate code from category 634, Spontaneous abortion, or 635 Legally induced abortion, with a fifth digit of "1" (incomplete). This advice is appropriate even when the patient was discharged previously with a discharge diagnosis of complete abortion.

12. Chapter 12: Diseases Skin and Subcutaneous Tissue (680-709)

Reserved for future guideline expansion

13. **Chapter 13: Diseases of Musculoskeletal and Connective Tissue (710-739)**

    Reserved for future guideline expansion

14. **Chapter 14: Congenital Anomalies (740-759)**

    a. **Codes in categories 740-759, Congenital Anomalies**

    Assign an appropriate code(s) from categories 740-759, Congenital Anomalies, when an anomaly is documented. A congenital anomaly may be the principal/first listed diagnosis on a record or a secondary diagnosis.

    When a congenital anomaly does not have a unique code assignment, assign additional code(s) for any manifestations that may be present.

    When the code assignment specifically identifies the congenital anomaly, manifestations that are an inherent component of the anomaly should not be coded separately. Additional codes should be assigned for manifestations that are not an inherent component.

    Codes from Chapter 14 may be used throughout the life of the patient. If a congenital anomaly has been corrected, a personal history code should be used to identify the history of the anomaly. **Although present at birth, a congenital anomaly may not be identified until later in life. Whenever the condition is diagnosed by the physician, it is appropriate to assign a code from codes 740-759.**

    For the birth admission, the appropriate code from category V30, Liveborn infants, according to type of birth should be sequenced as the principal diagnosis, followed by any congenital anomaly codes, 740-759.

15. **Chapter 15: Newborn (Perinatal) Guidelines (760-779)**

    For coding and reporting purposes the perinatal period is defined as **before** birth through the 28th day following birth. The following guidelines are provided for reporting purposes. Hospitals may record other diagnoses as needed for internal data use.

    a. **General Perinatal Rules**

    1) **Chapter 15 Codes**

    They are <u>never</u> for use on the maternal record. Codes from Chapter 11, the obstetric chapter, are never permitted on the newborn record. Chapter 15 code may be used throughout the life of the patient if the condition is still present.

    2) **Sequencing of perinatal codes**

    Generally, codes from Chapter 15 should be sequenced as the principal/first-listed diagnosis on the newborn record, with the exception of the appropriate V30 code for the birth episode, followed by codes from any other chapter that provide additional detail. The "use additional code" note at the beginning of the chapter supports this guideline. If the index does not provide a specific code for a perinatal condition, assign code 779.89, Other specified conditions originating in the perinatal period, followed by the code from another chapter that specifies the condition. Codes for signs and symptoms may be assigned when a definitive diagnosis has not been established.

    3) **Birth process or community acquired conditions**

    If a newborn has a condition that may be either due to the birth process or community acquired and the documentation does not indicate which it is, the default is due to the birth process and the code from Chapter 15 should be used. If the condition is community-acquired, a code from Chapter 15 should not be assigned.

    4) **Code all clinically significant conditions**

    All clinically significant conditions noted on routine newborn examination should be coded. A condition is clinically significant if it requires:

    - clinical evaluation; or
    - therapeutic treatment; or
    - diagnostic procedures; or
    - extended length of hospital stay; or
    - increased nursing care and/or monitoring; or
    - has implications for future health care needs

    Note: The perinatal guidelines listed above are the same as the general coding guidelines for "additional diagnoses", except for the final point regarding implications for future health care needs. Codes should be assigned for conditions that have been specified by the provider as having implications for future health care needs. Codes from the perinatal chapter should not be assigned unless the provider has established a definitive diagnosis.

    b. **Use of codes V30-V39**

    When coding the birth of an infant, assign a code from categories V30-V39, according to the type of birth. A code from this series is assigned as a principal diagnosis, and assigned only once to a newborn at the time of birth.

c. Newborn transfers

If the newborn is transferred to another institution, the V30 series is not used at the receiving hospital.

d. Use of category V29

1) Assigning a code from category V29

Assign a code from category V29, Observation and evaluation of newborns and infants for suspected conditions not found, to identify those instances when a healthy newborn is evaluated for a suspected condition that is determined after study not to be present. Do not use a code from category V29 when the patient has identified signs or symptoms of a suspected problem; in such cases, code the sign or symptom.

A code from category V29 may also be assigned as a principal code for readmissions or encounters when the V30 code no longer applies. Codes from category V29 are for use only for healthy newborns and infants for which no condition after study is found to be present.

2) V29 code on a birth record

A V29 code is to be used as a secondary code after the V30, Outcome of delivery, code.

e. Use of other V codes on perinatal records

V codes other than V30 and V29 may be assigned on a perinatal or newborn record code. The codes may be used as a principal or first-listed diagnosis for specific types of encounters or for read missions or encounters when the V30 code no longer applies.

See Section I.C.18 for information regarding the assignment of V codes.

f. Maternal Causes of Perinatal Morbidity

Codes from categories 760-763, Maternal causes of perinatal morbidity and mortality, are assigned only when the maternal condition has actually affected the fetus or newborn. The fact that the mother has an associated medical condition or experiences some complication of pregnancy, labor, or delivery does not justify the routine assignment of codes from these categories to the newborn record.

g. Congenital Anomalies in Newborns

For the birth admission, the appropriate code from category V30, Liveborn infants according to type of birth, should be used, followed by any congenital anomaly codes, categories 740-759. Use additional secondary codes from other chapters to specify conditions associated with the anomaly, if applicable.

Also, see Section I.C.14 for information on the coding of congenital anomalies.

h. Coding Additional Perinatal Diagnoses

1) Assigning codes for conditions that require treatment

Assign codes for conditions that require treatment or further investigation, prolong the length of stay, or require resource utilization.

2) Codes for conditions specified as having implications for future health care needs

Assign codes for conditions that have been specified by the provider as having implications for future health care needs.

Note: This guideline should not be used for adult patients.

3) Codes for newborn conditions originating in the perinatal period

Assign a code for newborn conditions originating in the perinatal period (categories 760-779), as well as complications arising during the current episode of care classified in other chapters, only if the diagnoses have been documented by the responsible provider at the time of transfer or discharge as having affected the fetus or newborn.

i. Prematurity and Fetal Growth Retardation

Providers utilize different criteria in determining prematurity. A code for prematurity should not be assigned unless it is documented. The 5th digit assignment for codes from category 764 and subcategories 765.0 and 765.1 should be based on the recorded birth weight and estimated gestational age.

A code from subcategory 765.2, Weeks of gestation, should be assigned as an additional code with category 764 and codes from 765.0 and 765.1 to specify weeks of gestation as documented by the provider in the record.

j. Newborn sepsis

Code 771.81, Septicemia [sepsis] of newborn, should be assigned with a secondary code from category 041, Bacterial infections in conditions classified elsewhere and of unspecified site, to identify the organism. It is not necessary to use a code from subcategory 995.9, Systemic inflammatory response syndrome (SIRS), on a newborn record. A code from category 038, Septicemia, should not be used on a newborn record. Code 771.81 describes the sepsis.

16. **Chapter 16: Signs, Symptoms, and Ill-Defined Conditions (780-799)**

    Reserved for future guideline expansion

17. **Chapter 17: Injury and Poisoning (800-999)**

    a. **Coding of Injuries**

    When coding injuries, assign separate codes for each injury unless a combination code is provided, in which case the combination code is assigned. Multiple injury codes are provided in ICD-9-CM, but should not be assigned unless information for a more specific code is not available. These codes are not to be used for normal, healing surgical wounds or to identify complications of surgical wounds.

    The code for the most serious injury, as determined by the provider and the focus of treatment, is sequenced first.

    1) **Superficial injuries**

    Superficial injuries such as abrasions or contusions are not coded when associated with more severe injuries of the same site.

    2) **Primary injury with damage to nerves/blood vessels**

    When a primary injury results in minor damage to peripheral nerves or blood vessels, the primary injury is sequenced first with additional code(s) from categories 950-957, Injury to nerves and spinal cord, and/or 900-904, Injury to blood vessels. When the primary injury is to the blood vessels or nerves, that injury should be sequenced first.

    b. **Coding of Fractures**

    The principles of multiple coding of injuries should be followed in coding fractures. Fractures of specified sites are coded individually by site in accordance with both the provisions within categories 800-829 and the level of detail furnished by medical record content. Combination categories for multiple fractures are provided for use when there is insufficient detail in the medical record (such as trauma cases transferred to another hospital), when the reporting form limits the number of codes that can be used in reporting pertinent clinical data, or when there is insufficient specificity at the fourth-digit or fifth-digit level. More specific guidelines are as follows:

    1) **Multiple fractures of same limb**

    Multiple fractures of same limb classifiable to the same three-digit or four-digit category are coded to that category.

    2) **Multiple unilateral or bilateral fractures of same bone**

    Multiple unilateral or bilateral fractures of same bone(s) but classified to different fourth-digit subdivisions (bone part) within the same three-digit category are coded individually by site.

    3) **Multiple fracture categories 819 and 828**

    Multiple fracture categories 819 and 828 classify bilateral fractures of both upper limbs (819) and both lower limbs (828), but without any detail at the fourth-digit level other than open and closed type of fractures.

    4) **Multiple fractures sequencing**

    Multiple fractures are sequenced in accordance with the severity of the fracture. The provider should be asked to list the fracture diagnoses in the order of severity.

    c. **Coding of Burns**

    Current burns (940-948) are classified by depth, extent, and by agent (E code). Burns are classified by depth as first degree (erythema), second degree (blistering), and third degree (full-thickness involvement).

    1) **Sequencing of burn and related condition codes**

    Sequence first the code that reflects the highest degree of burn when more than one burn is present.

    a. **When the reason for the admission or encounter is for treatment of external multiple burns, sequence first the code that reflects the burn of the highest degree.**

    b. **When a patient has both internal and external burns, the circumstances of admission govern the selection of the principal diagnosis or first-listed diagnosis.**

    c. **When a patient is admitted for burn injuries and other related conditions such as smoke inhalation and/or respiratory failure, the circumstances of admission govern the selection of the principal or first-listed diagnosis.**

    2) **Burns of the same local site**

    Classify burns of the same local site (three-digit category level, 940-947) but of different degrees to the subcategory identifying the highest degree recorded in the diagnosis.

3) **Non-healing burns**

Non-healing burns are coded as acute burns. Necrosis of burned skin should be coded as a non-healed burn.

4) **Code 958.3, Posttraumatic wound infection**

Assign code 958.3, Posttraumatic wound infection, not elsewhere classified, as an additional code for any documented infected burn site.

5) **Assign separate codes for each burn site**

When coding burns, assign separate codes for each burn site. Category 946 Burns of Multiple specified sites, should only be used if the location of the burns are not documented. Category 949, Burn, unspecified, is extremely vague and should rarely be used.

6) **Assign codes from category 948, Burns**

Burns classified according to extent of body surface involved, when the site of the burn is not specified or when there is a need for additional data. It is advisable to use category 948 as additional coding when needed to provide data for evaluating burn mortality, such as that needed by burn units. It is also advisable to use category 948 as an additional code for reporting purposes when there is mention of a third-degree burn involving 20 percent or more of the body surface.

In assigning a code from category 948:

Fourth-digit codes are used to identify the percentage of total body surface involved in a burn (all degree).

Fifth-digits are assigned to identify the percentage of body surface involved in third-degree burn.

Fifth-digit zero (0) is assigned when less than 10 percent or when no body surface is involved in a third-degree burn.

Category 948 is based on the classic "rule of nines" in estimating body surface involved: head and neck are assigned nine percent, each arm nine percent, each leg 18 percent, the anterior trunk 18 percent, posterior trunk 18 percent, and genitalia one percent. Providers may change these percentage assignments where necessary to accommodate infants and children who have proportionately larger heads than adults and patients who have large buttocks, thighs, or abdomen that involve burns.

7) **Encounters for treatment of late effects of burns**

Encounters for the treatment of the late effects of burns (i.e., scars or joint contractures) should be coded to the residual condition (sequelae) followed by the appropriate late effect code (906.5-906.9). A late effect E code may also be used, if desired.

8) **Sequelae with a late effect code and current burn**

When appropriate, both a sequelae with a late effect code, and a current burn code may be assigned on the same record (when both a current burn and sequelae of an old burn exist).

d. **Coding of Debridement of Wound, Infection, or Burn**

Excisional debridement involves an excisional debridement (surgical removal or cutting away), as opposed to a mechanical (brushing, scrubbing, washing) debridement.

For coding purposes, excisional debridement is assigned to code 86.22.

Nonexcisional debridement is assigned to code 86.28.

e. **Adverse Effects, Poisoning, and Toxic Effects**

The properties of certain drugs, medicinal and biological substances, or combinations of such substances, may cause toxic reactions. The occurrence of drug toxicity is classified in ICD-9-CM as follows:

1) **Adverse Effect**

When the drug was correctly prescribed and properly administered, code the reaction plus the appropriate code from the E930-E949 series. Codes from the E930-E949 series must be used to identify the causative substance for an adverse effect of drug, medicinal and biological substances, correctly prescribed and properly administered. The effect, such as tachycardia, delirium, gastrointestinal hemorrhaging, vomiting, hypokalemia, hepatitis, renal failure, or respiratory failure, is coded and followed by the appropriate code from the E930-E949 series.

Adverse effects of therapeutic substances correctly prescribed and properly administered (toxicity, synergistic reaction, side effect, and idiosyncratic reaction) may be due to (1) differences among patients, such as age, sex, disease, and genetic factors, and (2) drug-related factors, such as type of drug, route of administration, duration of therapy, dosage, and bioavailability.

2) **Poisoning**

(a) **Error was made in drug prescription**

Errors made in drug prescription or in the administration of the drug by provider, nurse, patient, or other person, use the appropriate poisoning code from the 960-979 series.

(b) **Overdose of a drug intentionally taken**

If an overdose of a drug was intentionally taken or administered and resulted in drug toxicity, it would be coded as a poisoning (960-979 series).

(c) **Nonprescribed drug taken with correctly prescribed and properly administered drug**

If a nonprescribed drug or medicinal agent was taken in combination with a correctly prescribed and properly administered drug, any drug toxicity or other reaction resulting from the interaction of the two drugs would be classified as a poisoning.

(d) **Sequencing of poisoning**

When coding a poisoning or reaction to the improper use of a medication (e.g., wrong dose, wrong substance, wrong route of administration) the poisoning code is sequenced first, followed by a code for the manifestation. If there is also a diagnosis of drug abuse or dependence to the substance, the abuse or dependence is coded as an additional code.

See Section I.C.3.a.6.b. if poisoning is the result of insulin pump malfunctions and Section I.C.19 for general use of E-codes.

3) **Toxic Effects**

(a) **Toxic effect codes**

When a harmful substance is ingested or comes in contact with a person, this is classified as a toxic effect. The toxic effect codes are in categories 980-989.

(b) **Sequencing toxic effect codes**

A toxic effect code should be sequenced first, followed by the code(s) that identify the result of the toxic effect.

(c) **External cause codes for toxic effects**

An external cause code from categories E860-E869 for accidental exposure, codes E950.6 or E950.7 for intentional self-harm, category E962 for assault, or categories E980-E982, for undetermined, should also be assigned to indicate intent.

f. **Complications of care**

1) **Transplant complications**

(a) **Transplant complications other than kidney**

Codes under subcategory 996.8, Complications of transplanted organ, are for use for both complications and rejection of transplanted organs. A transplant complication code is only assigned if the complication affects the function of the transplanted organ. Two codes are required to fully describe a transplant complication, the appropriate code from subcategory 996.8 and a secondary code that identifies the complication.

Pre-existing conditions or conditions that develop after the transplant are not coded as complications unless they affect the function of the transplanted organs.

Post-transplants surgical complications that do not relate to the function of the transplanted organ are classified to the specific complication. For example, a surgical wound dehiscence would be coded to the wound dehiscence, not as a transplant complication.

Post-transplant patients who are seen for treatment unrelated to the transplanted organ should be assigned a code from category V42, Organ or tissue replaced by transplant, to identify the transplant status of the patient. A code from category V42 should never be used with a code from subcategory 996.8.

(b) Kidney transplant and chronic kidney disease

Patients with chronic kidney disease (CKD) following a transplant should not be assumed to have transplant failure or rejection unless it is documented by the provider. If documentation supports

the presence of failure or rejection, then it is appropriate to assign code 996.81, Complications of transplanted organs, kidney followed by the appropriate CKD code.

18. **Classification of Factors Influencing Health Status and Contact with Health Service (Supplemental V01-V84)**

Note: The chapter specific guidelines provide additional information about the use of V codes for specified encounters.

a. **Introduction**

ICD-9-CM provides codes to deal with encounters for circumstances other than a disease or injury. The Supplementary Classification of Factors Influencing Health Status and Contact with Health Services (V01.0-V84.8) is provided to deal with occasions when circumstances other than a disease or injury (codes 001-999) are recorded as a diagnosis or problem.

There are four primary circumstances for the use of V codes:

1) A person who is not currently sick encounters the health services for some specific reason, such as to act as an organ donor, to receive prophylactic care, such as inoculations or health screenings, or to receive counseling on health related issues.
2) A person with a resolving disease or injury, or a chronic, long-term condition requiring continuous care, encounters the health care system for specific aftercare of that disease or injury (e.g., dialysis for renal disease; chemotherapy for malignancy; cast change). A diagnosis/symptom code should be used whenever a current, acute, diagnosis is being treated or a sign or symptom is being studied.
3) Circumstances or problems influence a person's health status but are not in themselves a current illness or injury.
4) Newborns, to indicate birth status

b. **V codes use in any healthcare setting**

V codes are for use in any healthcare setting. V codes may be used as either a first listed (principal diagnosis code in the inpatient setting) or secondary code, depending on the circumstances of the encounter. Certain V codes may only be used as first listed, others only as secondary codes. See Section I.C.18.e, **V Code Table.**

c. **V Codes indicate a reason for an encounter**

They are not procedure codes. A corresponding procedure code must accompany a V code to describe the procedure performed.

d. **Categories of V Codes**

1) **Contact/Exposure**

Category V01 indicates contact with or exposure to communicable diseases. These codes are for patients who do not show any sign or symptom of a disease but have been exposed to it by close personal contact with an infected individual or are in an area where a disease is epidemic. These codes may be used as a first listed code to explain an encounter for testing, or, more commonly, as a secondary code to identify a potential risk.

2) **Inoculations and vaccinations**

Categories V03-V06 are for encounters for inoculations and vaccinations. They indicate that a patient is being seen to receive a prophylactic inoculation against a disease. The injection itself must be represented by the appropriate procedure code. A code from V03-V06 may be used as a secondary code if the inoculation is given as a routine part of preventive health care, such as a well-baby visit.

3) **Status**

Status codes indicate that a patient is either a carrier of a disease or has the sequelae or residual of a past disease or condition. This includes such things as the presence of prosthetic or mechanical devices resulting from past treatment.

A status code is informative, because the status may affect the course of treatment and its outcome. A status code is distinct from a history code. The history code indicates that the patient no longer has the condition.

A status code should not be used with a diagnosis code from one of the body system chapters, if the diagnosis code includes the information provided by the status code. For example, code V42.1, Heart transplant status, should not be used with code 996.83, Complications of transplanted heart. The status code does not provide additional information. The complication code indicates that the patient is a heart transplant patient.

The status V codes/categories are:

V02 Carrier or suspected carrier of infectious diseases

Carrier status indicates that a person harbors the specific

organisms of a disease without manifest symptoms and is capable of transmitting the infection.

V08 Asymptomatic HIV infection status

This code indicates that a patient has tested positive for HIV but has manifested no signs or symptoms of the disease.

V09 Infection with drug-resistant microorganisms

This category indicates that a patient has an infection that is resistant to drug treatment. Sequence the infection code first.

V21 Constitutional states in development

V22.2 Pregnant state, incidental

This code is a secondary code only for use when the pregnancy is in no way complicating the reason for visit. Otherwise, a code from the obstetric chapter is required.

V26.5x Sterilization status

V42 Organ or tissue replaced by transplant

V43 Organ or tissue replaced by other means

V44 Artificial opening status

V45 Other postsurgical states

V46 Other dependence on machines

V49.6 Upper limb amputation status

V49.7 Lower limb amputation status

V49.81 Postmenopausal status

V49.82 Dental sealant status

V49.83 Awaiting organ transplant status

V58.6 Long-term (current) drug use

This subcategory indicates a patient's continuous use of a prescribed drug (including such things as aspirin therapy) for the long-term treatment of a condition or for prophylactic use. It is not for use for patients who have addictions to drugs.

Assign a code from subcategory V58.6, Long-term (current) drug use, if the patient is receiving a medication for an extended period as a prophylactic measure (such as for the prevention of deep vein thrombosis) or as treatment of a chronic condition (such as arthritis) or a disease requiring a lengthy course of treatment (such as cancer). Do not assign a code from subcategory V58.6 for medication being administered for a brief period of time to treat an acute illness or injury (such as a course of antibiotics to treat acute bronchitis).

V83 Genetic carrier status

Genetic carrier status indicates that a person carries a gene, associated with a particular disease, which may be passed to offspring who may develop that disease. The person does not have the disease and is not at risk of developing the disease.

V84 Genetic susceptibility status

Genetic susceptibility indicates that a person has a gene that increases the risk of that person developing the disease.

Codes from category V84, Genetic susceptibility to disease, should not be used as principal or first-listed codes. If the patient has the condition to which he/she is susceptible, and that condition is the reason for the encounter, the code for the current condition should be sequenced first. If the patient is being seen for follow-up after completed treatment for this condition, and the condition no longer exists, a follow-up code should be sequenced first, followed by the appropriate personal history and genetic susceptibility codes. If the purpose of the encounter is genetic counseling associated with procreative management, a code from subcategory V26.3, Genetic counseling and testing, should be assigned as the first-listed code, followed by a code from category V84.

Additional codes should be assigned for any applicable family or personal history. <u>See Section I.C. 18.d.14 for information on prophylactic organ removal due to a genetic susceptibility.</u>

Note: Categories V42-V46, and subcategories V49.6, V49.7 are for use only if there are no complications or malfunctions of the organ or tissue replaced, the amputation site or the equipment on which the patient is dependent. These are always secondary codes.

4) History (of)

There are two types of history V codes, personal and family. Personal history codes explain a patient's past medical condition that no longer exists and is not receiving any treatment, but that has the potential for recurrence, and therefore may require continued monitoring. The exceptions to this general rule are category V14, Personal history of allergy to medicinal agents, and subcategory V15.0, Allergy, other than to medicinal agents. A person who has had an allergic episode to a substance or food in the past should always be considered allergic to the substance.

Family history codes are for use when a patient has a family member(s) who has had a particular disease that causes the patient to be at higher risk of also contracting the disease.

Personal history codes may be used in conjunction with follow-up codes and family history codes may be used in conjunction with screening codes to explain the need for a test or procedure. History codes are also acceptable on any medical record regardless of the reason for visit. A history of an illness, even if no longer present, is important information that may alter the type of treatment ordered.

The history V code categories are:

V10 Personal history of malignant neoplasm

V12 Personal history of certain other diseases

V13 Personal history of other diseases

Except: V13.4, Personal history of arthritis, and V13.6, Personal history of congenital malformations. These conditions are life-long so are not true history codes.

V14 Personal history of allergy to medicinal agents

V15 Other personal history presenting hazards to health

Except: V15.7, Personal history of contraception.

V16 Family history of malignant neoplasm

V17 Family history of certain chronic disabling diseases

V18 Family history of certain other specific diseases

V19 Family history of other conditions

5) Screening

Screening is the testing for disease or disease precursors in seemingly well individuals so that early detection and treatment can be provided for those who test positive for the disease. Screenings that are recommended for many subgroups in a population include: routine mammograms for women over 40, a fecal occult blood test for everyone over 50, an amniocentesis to rule out a fetal anomaly for pregnant women over 35, because the incidence of breast cancer and colon cancer in these subgroups is higher than in the general population, as is the incidence of Down's syndrome in older mothers.

The testing of a person to rule out or confirm a suspected diagnosis because the patient has some sign or symptom is a diagnostic examination, not a screening. In these cases, the sign or symptom is used to explain the reason for the test.

A screening code may be a first listed code if the reason for the visit is specifically the screening exam. It may also be used as an additional code if the screening is done during an office visit for other health problems. A screening code is not necessary if the screening is inherent to a routine examination, such as a pap smear done during a routine pelvic examination.

Should a condition be discovered during the screening then the code for the condition may be assigned as an additional diagnosis.

The V code indicates that a screening exam is planned. A procedure code is required to confirm that the screening was performed.

The screening V code categories:

V28	Antenatal screening
V73-V82	Special screening examinations

6) Observation

There are two observation V code categories. They are for use in very limited circumstances when a person is being observed for a suspected condition that is ruled out. The observation codes are not for use if an injury or illness or any signs or symptoms related to the suspected condition are present. In such cases the diagnosis/symptom code is used with the corresponding E code to identify any external cause.

The observation codes are to be used as principal diagnosis only. The only exception to this is when the principal diagnosis is required to be a code from the V30, Live born infant, category. Then the V29 observation code is sequenced after the V30 code. Additional codes may be used in addition to the observation code but only if they are unrelated to the suspected condition being observed.

The observation V code categories:

V29	Observation and evaluation of newborns for suspected condition not found For the birth encounter, a code from category V30 should be sequenced before the V29 code.
V71	Observation and evaluation for suspected condition not found

7) Aftercare

Aftercare visit codes cover situations when the initial treatment of a disease or injury has been performed and the patient requires continued care during the healing or recovery phase, or for the long-term consequences of the disease. The aftercare V code should not be used if treatment is directed at a current, acute disease or injury, the diagnosis code is to be used in these cases. Exceptions to this rule are codes V58.0, Radiotherapy, and **codes from subcategory** V58.1, **Encounter for** chemotherapy **and immunotherapy for neoplastic conditions**. These codes are to be first listed, followed by the diagnosis code when a patient's encounter is solely to receive radiation therapy or chemotherapy for the treatment of a neoplasm. Should a patient receive both chemotherapy and radiation therapy during the same encounter code V58.0 and V58.1 may be used together on a record with either one being sequenced first.

The aftercare codes are generally first listed to explain the specific reason for the encounter. An aftercare code may be used as an additional code when some type of aftercare is provided in addition to the reason for admission and no diagnosis code is applicable. An example of this would be the closure of a colostomy during an encounter for treatment of another condition.

Certain aftercare V code categories need a secondary diagnosis code to describe the resolving condition or sequelae, for others, the condition is inherent in the code title.

Additional V code aftercare category terms include, fitting and adjustment, and attention to artificial openings.

Status V codes may be used with aftercare V codes to indicate the nature of the aftercare. For example code V45.81, Aortocoronary bypass status, may be used with code V58.73, Aftercare following surgery of the circulatory system, NEC, to indicate the surgery for which the aftercare is being performed. Also, a transplant status code may be used following code V58.44, Aftercare following organ transplant, to identify the organ transplanted. A status code should not be used when the aftercare code indicates the type of status, such as using V55.0, Attention to tracheostomy with V44.0, Tracheostomy status.

The aftercare V category/codes:

V52	Fitting and adjustment of prosthetic device and implant
V53	Fitting and adjustment of other device
V54	Other orthopedic aftercare
V55	Attention to artificial openings
V56	Encounter for dialysis and dialysis catheter care
V57	Care involving the use of rehabilitation procedures
V58.0	Radiotherapy
V58.11	**Encounter for antineoplastic chemotherapy**
V58.12	**Encounter for antineoplastic immunotherapy**

2 type II or unspecified type, uncontrolled
3 type I, [juvenile type], uncontrolled

The age of a patient is not the sole determining factor, though most type I diabetics develop the condition before reaching puberty. For this reason type I diabetes mellitus is also referred to as juvenile diabetes.

2) Type of diabetes mellitus not documented

If the type of diabetes mellitus is not documented in the medical record the default is type II.

3) Diabetes mellitus and the use of insulin

All type I diabetics must use insulin to replace what their bodies do not produce. However, the use of insulin does not mean that a patient is a type I diabetic. Some patients with type II diabetes mellitus are unable to control their blood sugar through diet and oral medication alone and do require insulin. If the documentation in a medical record does not indicate the type of diabetes but does indicate that the patient uses insulin, the appropriate fifth-digit for type II must be used. For type II patients who routinely use insulin, code V58.67, Long-term (current) use of insulin, should also be assigned to indicate that the patient uses insulin. Code V58.67 should not be assigned if insulin is given temporarily to bring a type II patient's blood sugar under control during an encounter.

4) Assigning and sequencing diabetes codes and associated conditions

When assigning codes for diabetes and its associated conditions, the code(s) from category 250 must be sequenced before the codes for the associated conditions. The diabetes codes and the secondary codes that correspond to them are paired codes that follow the etiology/manifestation convention of the classification (See Section I.A.6., Etiology/manifestation convention). Assign as many codes from category 250 as needed to identify all of the associated conditions that the patient has. The corresponding secondary codes are listed under each of the diabetes codes.

(a) Diabetic retinopathy/diabetic macular edema

Diabetic macular edema, code 362.07, is only present with diabetic retinopathy. Another code from subcategory 362.0, Diabetic retinopathy, must be used with code 362.07. Codes under subcategory 362.0 are diabetes manifestation codes, so they must be used following the appropriate diabetes code.

5) Diabetes mellitus in pregnancy and gestational diabetes

(a) For diabetes mellitus complicating pregnancy, see Section I.C.11.f., Diabetes mellitus in pregnancy.

(b) For gestational diabetes, see Section I.C.11, g., Gestational diabetes.

6) Insulin pump malfunction

(a) Underdose of insulin due insulin pump failure

An underdose of insulin due to an insulin pump failure should be assigned 996.57, Mechanical complication due to insulin pump, as the principal or first listed code, followed by the appropriate diabetes mellitus code based on documentation.

(b) Overdose of insulin due to insulin pump failure

The principal or first listed code for an encounter due to an insulin pump malfunction resulting in an overdose of insulin, should also be 996.57, Mechanical complication due to insulin pump, followed by code 962.3, Poisoning by insulins and antidiabetic agents, and the appropriate diabetes mellitus code based on documentation.

4. Chapter 4: Diseases of Blood and Blood Forming Organs (280-289)

a. Anemia of chronic disease

Subcategory 285.2, Anemia in chronic illness, has codes for anemia in chronic kidney disease, code 285.21; anemia in neoplastic disease, code 285.22; and anemia in other chronic illness, code 285.29. These codes can be used as the principal/first listed code if the reason for the encounter is to treat the anemia. They may also be used as secondary codes if treatment of the anemia is a component of an encounter, but not the primary reason for the encounter. When using a code from subcategory 285 it is also necessary to use the code for the chronic condition causing the anemia.

1) **Anemia in chronic kidney disease**

When assigning code 285.21, Anemia in chronic kidney disease. It is also necessary to assign a code from category 585, Chronic kidney disease, to indicate the stage of chronic kidney disease. See I.C.10.a. Chronic kidney disease (CKD)

2) **Anemia in neoplastic disease**

When assigning code 285.22, Anemia in neoplastic disease, it is also necessary to assign the neoplasm code that is responsible for the anemia. Code 285.22 is for use for anemia that is due to the malignancy, not for anemia due to antineoplastic chemotherapy drugs, which is an adverse effect.
See I.C.2.c.1 Anemia associated with malignancy
See I.C.2.c.2 Anemia associated with chemotherapy, immunotherapy, and radiation therapy
See I.C.17.e.1. Adverse effects

5. **Chapter 5: Mental Disorders (290-319)**

Reserved for future guideline expansion

6. **Chapter 6: Diseases of Nervous System and Sense Organs (320-389)**

Reserved for future guideline expansion

7. **Chapter 7: Diseases of Circulatory System (390-459)**

a. **Hypertension**

<u>**Hypertension Table**</u>
The Hypertension Table, found under the main term, "Hypertension", in the Alphabetic Index, contains a complete listing of all conditions due to or associated with hypertension and classifies them according to malignant, benign, and unspecified.

1) **Hypertension, Essential, or NOS**

Assign hypertension (arterial) (essential) (primary) (systemic) (NOS) to category code 401 with the appropriate fourth digit to indicate malignant (.0), benign (.1), or unspecified (.9). Do not use either .0 malignant or .1 benign unless medical record documentation supports such a designation.

2) **Hypertension with Heart Disease**

Heart conditions (425.8, 429.0-429.3, 429.8, 429.9) are assigned to a code from category 402 when a causal relationship is stated (due to hypertension) or implied (hypertensive). Use an additional code from category 428 to identify the type of heart failure in those patients with heart failure. More than one code from category 428 may be assigned if the patient has systolic or diastolic failure and congestive heart failure.

The same heart conditions (425.8, 429.0-429.3, 429.8, 429.9) with hypertension, but without a stated causal relationship, are coded separately. Sequence according to the circumstances of the admission/encounter.

3) **Hypertensive <u>Kidney</u> Disease**

Assign codes from category 403, Hypertensive **kidney** disease, when conditions classified to categories 585-587 are present. Unlike hypertension with heart disease, ICD-9-CM presumes a cause-and-effect relationship and classifies renal failure with hypertension as hypertensive **kidney** disease.

4) **Hypertensive Heart and <u>Kidney</u> Disease**

Assign codes from combination category 404, Hypertensive heart and **kidney** disease, when both hypertensive **kidney** disease and hypertensive heart disease are stated in the diagnosis. Assume a relationship between the hypertension and the **kidney** disease, whether or not the condition is so designated. Assign an additional code from category 428, to identify the type of heart failure. More than one code from category 428 may be assigned if the patient has systolic or diastolic failure and congestive heart failure.

5) **Hypertensive Cerebrovascular Disease**

First assign codes from 430-438, Cerebrovascular disease, then the appropriate hypertension code from categories 401-405.

6) **Hypertensive Retinopathy**

Two codes are necessary to identify the condition. First assign the code from subcategory 362.11, Hypertensive retinopathy, then the appropriate code from categories 401-405 to indicate the type of hypertension.

7) **Hypertension, Secondary**

Two codes are required: one to identify the underlying etiology and one from category 405 to identify the hypertension. Sequencing of codes is determined by the reason for admission/encounter.

8) **Hypertension, Transient**

Assign code 796.2, Elevated blood pressure reading without diagnosis of hypertension, unless patient has an established diagnosis of hypertension.

V58.3	Attention to surgical dressings and sutures
V58.41	Encounter for planned postoperative wound closure
V58.42	Aftercare, surgery, neoplasm
V58.43	Aftercare, surgery, trauma
V58.44	Aftercare involving organ transplant
V58.49	Other specified aftercare following surgery
V58.7x	Aftercare following surgery
V58.81	Fitting and adjustment of vascular catheter
V58.82	Fitting and adjustment of nonvascular catheter
V58.83	Monitoring therapeutic drug
V58.89	Other specified aftercare

8) Follow-up

The follow-up codes are used to explain continuing surveillance following completed treatment of a disease, condition, or injury. They imply that the condition has been fully treated and no longer exists. They should not be confused with aftercare codes that explain current treatment for a healing condition or its sequelae. Follow-up codes may be used in conjunction with history codes to provide the full picture of the healed condition and its treatment. The follow-up code is sequenced first, followed by the history code.

A follow-up code may be used to explain repeated visits. Should a condition be found to have recurred on the follow-up visit, then the diagnosis code should be used in place of the follow-up code.

The follow-up V code categories:

V24	Postpartum care and evaluation
V67	Follow-up examination

9) Donor

Category V59 is the donor codes. They are used for living individuals who are donating blood or other body tissue. These codes are only for individuals donating for others, not for self donations. They are not for use to identify cadaveric donations.

10) Counseling

Counseling V codes are used when a patient or family member receives assistance in the aftermath of an illness or injury, or when support is required in coping with family or social problems. They are not necessary for use in conjunction with a diagnosis code when the counseling component of care is considered integral to standard treatment.

The counseling V categories/codes:

V25.0	General counseling and advice for contraceptive management
V26.3	Genetic counseling
V26.4	General counseling and advice for procreative management
V61	Other family circumstances
V65.1	Person consulted on behalf of another person
V65.3	Dietary surveillance and counseling
V65.4	Other counseling, not elsewhere classified

11) Obstetrics and related conditions

See Section I.C.11., the Obstetrics guidelines for further instruction on the use of these codes.

V codes for pregnancy are for use in those circumstances when none of the problems or complications included in the codes from the Obstetrics chapter exist (a routine prenatal visit or postpartum care). Codes V22.0, Supervision of normal first pregnancy, and V22.1, Supervision of other normal pregnancy, are always first listed and are not to be used with any other code from the OB chapter.

The outcome of delivery, category V27, should be included on all maternal delivery records. It is always a secondary code.

V codes for family planning (contraceptive) or procreative management and counseling should be included on an obstetric record either during the pregnancy or the postpartum stage, if applicable.

Obstetrics and related conditions V code categories:

V22	Normal pregnancy
V23	Supervision of high-risk pregnancy Except: V23.2, Pregnancy with history of abortion. Code 646.3, Habitual aborter, from the OB chapter is required to indicate a history of abortion during a pregnancy.

V24 Postpartum care and evaluation

V25 Encounter for contraceptive management

Except V25.0x (See Section I.C.18.d.11, Counseling)

V26 Procreative management

Except V26.5x, Sterilization status, V26.3 and V26.4 (See Section I.C.18.d.11., Counseling)

V27 Outcome of delivery

V28 Antenatal screening

(See Section I.C.18.d.6., Screening)

12) Newborn, infant and child

See Section I.C.15, the Newborn guidelines for further instruction on the use of these codes.

Newborn V code categories:

V20 Health supervision of infant or child

V29 Observation and evaluation of newborns for suspected condition not found (See Section I.C.18.d.7, Observation).

V30-V39 Liveborn infant according to type of birth

13) Routine and administrative examinations

The V codes allow for the description of encounters for routine examinations, such as, a general check-up, or, examinations for administrative purposes, such as, a pre-employment physical. The codes are for use as first listed codes only, and are not to be used if the examination is for diagnosis of a suspected condition or for treatment purposes. In such cases the diagnosis code is used. During a routine exam, should a diagnosis or condition be discovered, it should be coded as an additional code. Pre-existing and chronic conditions and history codes may also be included as additional codes as long as the examination is for administrative purposes and not focused on any particular condition.

Pre-operative examination V codes are for use only in those situations when a patient is being cleared for surgery and no treatment is given.

The V codes categories/code for routine and administrative examinations:

V20.2 Routine infant or child health check

Any injections given should have a corresponding procedure code.

V70 General medical examination

V72 Special investigations and examinations

Except V72.5 and V72.6

14) Miscellaneous V codes

The miscellaneous V codes capture a number of other health care encounters that do not fall into one of the other categories. Certain of these codes identify the reason for the encounter, others are for use as additional codes that provide useful information on circumstances that may affect a patient's care and treatment.

Prophylactic Organ Removal

For encounters specifically for prophylactic removal of breasts, ovaries, or another organ due to a genetic susceptibility to cancer or a family history of cancer, the principal or first listed code should be a code from subcategory V50.4, Prophylactic organ removal, followed by the appropriate genetic susceptibility code and the appropriate family history code.

If the patient has a malignancy of one site and is having prophylactic removal at another site to prevent either a new primary malignancy or metastatic disease, a code for the malignancy should also be assigned in addition to a code from subcategory V50.4. A V50.4 code should not be assigned if the patient is having organ removal for treatment of a malignancy, such as the removal of the testes for the treatment of prostate cancer.

Miscellaneous V code categories/codes:

V07 Need for isolation and other prophylactic measures

V50 Elective surgery for purposes other than remedying health states

V58.5 Orthodontics

V60 Housing, household, and economic circumstances

V62 Other psychosocial circumstances

V63 Unavailability of other medical facilities for care

V64 Persons encountering health services for specific procedures, not carried out

V66 Convalescence and Palliative Care

V68 Encounters for administrative purposes

V69 Problems related to lifestyle

15) **Nonspecific V codes**

Certain V codes are so non-specific, or potentially redundant with other codes in the classification, that there can be little justification for their use in the inpatient setting. Their use in the outpatient setting should be limited to those instances when there is no further documentation to permit more precise coding. Otherwise, any sign or symptom or any other reason for visit that is captured in another code should be used.

Nonspecific V code categories/codes:

V11 Personal history of mental disorder

A code from the mental disorders chapter, with an in remission fifth-digit, should be used.

V13.4 Personal history of arthritis

V13.6 Personal history of congenital malformations

V15.7 Personal history of contraception

V23.2 Pregnancy with history of abortion

V40 Mental and behavioral problems

V41 Problems with special senses and other special functions

V47 Other problems with internal organs

V48 Problems with head, neck, and trunk

V49 Problems with limbs and other problems

Exceptions:

V49.6 Upper limb amputation status

V49.7 Lower limb amputation status

V49.81 Postmenopausal status

V49.82 Dental sealant status

V49.83 Awaiting organ transplant status

V51 Aftercare involving the use of plastic surgery

V58.2 Blood transfusion, without reported diagnosis

V58.9 Unspecified aftercare

V72.5 Radiological examination, NEC

V72.6 Laboratory examination

Codes V72.5 and V72.6 are not to be used if any sign or symptoms, or reason for a test is documented. See Section IV.K. and Section IV.L. of the Outpatient guidelines.

e. V Code Table

<u>Items in bold indicate a change from the April 2005 table</u>

<u>Items underlined have been moved within the table since April 2005</u>

FIRST LISTED: V codes/categories/subcategories which are only acceptable as principal/first listed.

Codes:

V22.0 Supervision of normal first pregnancy

V22.1 Supervision of other normal pregnancy

V46.12 Encounter for respirator dependence during power failure

V46.13 Encounter for weaning from respirator [ventilator]

V56.0 Extracorporeal dialysis

V58.0 Radiotherapy

V58.0 and V58.11 may be used together on a record with either one being sequenced first, when a patient receives both chemotherapy and radiation therapy during the same encounter code.

V58.11 Encounter for antineoplastic chemotherapy

V58.0 and **V58.11** may be used together on a record with either one being sequenced first, when a patient receives both chemotherapy and radiation therapy during the same encounter code.

V58.12 Encounter for antineoplastic immunotherapy

Categories/Subcategories:

V20 Health supervision of infant or child

V24 Postpartum care and examination

V29 Observation and evaluation of newborns for suspected condition not found

Exception: A code from the V30-V39 may be sequenced before the V29 if it is the newborn record.

V30-V39 Liveborn infants according to type of birth

V57	Care involving use of rehabilitation procedures
V59	Donors
V66	Convalescence and palliative care Exception: V66.7 Palliative care
V68	Encounters for administrative purposes
V70	General medical examination Exception: V70.7 Examination of participant in clinical trial
V71	Observation and evaluation for suspected conditions not found
V72	Special investigations and examinations Exceptions: **V72.4 Pregnancy examination or test** V72.5 Radiological examination, NEC V72.6 Laboratory examination **V72.86 Encounter for blood typing**

FIRST OR ADDITIONAL: V code categories/subcategories which may be either principal/first listed or additional codes

Codes:

V15.88	**History of fall**
V43.22	Fully implantable artificial heart status
V46.14	**Mechanical complication of respirator [ventilator]**
V49.81	Asymptomatic postmenopausal status (age-related) (natural)
V49.84	**Bed confinement status**
V49.89	Other specified conditions influencing health status
V70.7	Examination of participant in clinical trial
V72.5	Radiological examination, NEC
V72.6	Laboratory examination
V72.86	**Encounter for blood typing**

Categories/Subcategories:

V01	Contact with or exposure to communicable diseases
V02	Carrier or suspected carrier of infectious diseases
V03-06	Need for prophylactic vaccination and inoculations
V07	Need for isolation and other prophylactic measures
V08	Asymptomatic HIV infection status
V10	Personal history of malignant neoplasm
V12	Personal history of certain other diseases
V13	Personal history of other diseases Exception: V13.4 Personal history of arthritis V13.69 Personal history of other congenital malformations
V16-V19	Family history of disease
V23	Supervision of high-risk pregnancy
V25	Encounter for contraceptive management
V26	Procreative management Exception: V26.5 Sterilization status
V28	Antenatal screening
V45.7	Acquired absence of organ
V49.6x	Upper limb amputation status
V49.7x	Lower limb amputation status
V50	Elective surgery for purposes other than remedying health states
V52	Fitting and adjustment of prosthetic device and implant
V53	Fitting and adjustment of other device
V54	Other orthopedic aftercare
V55	Attention to artificial openings
V56	Encounter for dialysis and dialysis catheter care Exception: V56.0 Extracorporeal dialysis
~~V57~~	~~Care involving use of rehabilitation procedures~~
V58.3	Attention to surgical dressings and sutures
V58.4	Other aftercare following surgery
~~V58.6~~	~~Long-term (current) drug use~~
V58.7	Aftercare following surgery to specified body systems, not elsewhere classified
V58.8	Other specified procedures and aftercare
V61	Other family circumstances
V63	Unavailability of other medical facilities for care
V65	Other persons seeking consultation without complaint or sickness
V67	Follow-up examination
V69	Problems related to lifestyle
V72.4	**Pregnancy examination or test**
V73-V82	Special screening examinations
V83	Genetic carrier status

ADDITIONAL ONLY: V code categories/subcategories which may only be used as additional codes, not principal/first listed

Codes:

V13.61	Personal history of hypospadias
V22.2	Pregnancy state, incidental
V46.11	**Dependence on respirator, status**
V49.82	Dental sealant status
V49.83	Awaiting organ transplant status
V66.7	Palliative care

Categories/Subcategories:

V09	Infection with drug-resistant microorganisms

V14 Personal history of allergy to medicinal agents

V15 Other personal history presenting hazards to health

Exception:

V15.7 Personal history of contraception

V15.88 History of fall

V21 Constitutional states in development

V26.5 Sterilization status

V27 Outcome of delivery

V42 Organ or tissue replaced by transplant

V43 Organ or tissue replaced by other means

Exception: V43.22 Fully implantable artificial heart status

V44 Artificial opening status

V45 Other postsurgical states

Exception: Subcategory V45.7 Acquired absence of organ

V46 Other dependence on machines

Exception:

V46.12 Encounter for respirator dependence during power failure

V46.13 Encounter for weaning from respirator [ventilator]

V49.6x Upper limb amputation status

V49.7x Lower limb amputation status

V58.6 Long-term current drug use

V60 Housing, household, and economic circumstances

V62 Other psychosocial circumstances

V64 Persons encountering health services for specified procedure, not carried out

V84 Genetic susceptibility to disease

V85 Body Mass Index

NONSPECIFIC CODES AND CATEGORIES:

V11 Personal history of mental disorder

V13.4 Personal history of arthritis

V13.69 Personal history of congenital malformations

V15.7 Personal history of contraception

V40 Mental and behavioral problems

V41 Problems with special senses and other special functions

V47 Other problems with internal organs

V48 Problems with head, neck, and trunk

V49.0 Deficiencies of limbs

V49.1 Mechanical problems with limbs

V49.2 Motor problems with limbs

V49.3 Sensory problems with limbs

V49.4 Disfigurements in limbs

V49.5 Other problems with limbs

V49.9 Unspecified condition influencing health status

~~V49 Problems with limbs and other problems~~

Exceptions:

~~V49.6 Upper limb amputation status~~

~~V49.7 Lower limb amputation status~~

~~V49.81 Postmenopausal status (age-related) (natural)~~

~~V49.82 Dental sealant status~~

~~V49.83 Awaiting organ transplant status~~

V51 Aftercare involving the use of plastic surgery

V58.2 Blood transfusion, without reported diagnosis

V58.5 Orthodontics

V58.9 Unspecified aftercare

V72.5 Radiological examination, NEC

V72.6 Laboratory examination

19. Supplemental Classification of External Causes of Injury and Poisoning (E-codes, E800-E999)

Introduction: These guidelines are provided for those who are currently collecting E codes in order that there will be standardization in the process. If your institution plans to begin collecting E codes, these guidelines are to be applied. The use of E codes is supplemental to the application of ICD-9-CM diagnosis codes. E codes are never to be recorded as principal diagnoses (first-listed in non-inpatient setting) and are not required for reporting to CMS.

External causes of injury and poisoning codes (E codes) are intended to provide data for injury research and evaluation of injury prevention strategies. E codes capture how the injury or poisoning happened (cause), the intent (unintentional or accidental; or intentional, such as suicide or assault), and the place where the event occurred.

Some major categories of E codes include:

transport accidents
poisoning and adverse effects of drugs, medicinal substances, and biologicals
accidental falls
accidents caused by fire and flames
accidents due to natural and environmental factors
late effects of accidents, assaults, or self injury
assaults or purposely inflicted injury
suicide or self inflicted injury

These guidelines apply for the coding and collection of E codes from records in hospitals, outpatient clinics, emergency departments, other ambulatory care settings and provider offices, and nonacute care settings, except when other specific guidelines apply.

a. General E Code Coding Guidelines

1) Used with any code in the range of 001-V84.8

An E code may be used with any code in the range of 001-V84.8, which indicates an injury, poisoning, or adverse effect due to an external cause.

2) Assign the appropriate E code for all initial treatments

Assign the appropriate E code for the initial encounter of an injury, poisoning, or adverse effect of drugs, **not for subsequent treatment.**

3) Use the full range of E codes

Use the full range of E codes to completely describe the cause, the intent and the place of occurrence, if applicable, for all injuries, poisonings, and adverse effects of drugs.

4) Assign as many E codes as necessary

Assign as many E codes as necessary to fully explain each cause. If only one E code can be recorded, assign the E code most related to the principal diagnosis.

5) The selection of the appropriate E code

The selection of the appropriate E code is guided by the Index to External Causes, which is located after the alphabetical index to diseases and by Inclusion and Exclusion notes in the Tabular List.

6) E code can never be a principal diagnosis

An E code can never be a principal (first listed) diagnosis.

7) External cause code(s) with systemic inflammatory response syndrome (SIRS)

An external cause code(s) may be used with codes 995.93, Systemic inflammatory response syndrome due to noninfectious process without organ dysfunction, and 995.94, Systemic inflammatory response syndrome due to noninfectious process with organ dysfunction, if trauma was the initiating insult that precipitated the SIRS. The external cause(s) code should correspond to the most serious injury resulting from the trauma. The external cause code(s) should only be assigned if the trauma necessitated the admission in which the patient also developed SIRS. If a patient is admitted with SIRS but the trauma has been treated previously, the external cause codes should not be used.

b. Place of Occurrence Guideline

Use an additional code from category E849 to indicate the Place of Occurrence for injuries and poisonings. The Place of Occurrence describes the place where the event occurred and not the patient's activity at the time of the event.

Do not use E849.9 if the place of occurrence is not stated.

c. Adverse Effects of Drugs, Medicinal and Biological Substances Guidelines

1) Do not code directly from the Table of Drugs

Do not code directly from the Table of Drugs and Chemicals. Always refer back to the Tabular List.

2) Use as many codes as necessary to describe

Use as many codes as necessary to describe completely all drugs, medicinal or biological substances.

3) If the same E code would describe the causative agent

If the same E code would describe the causative agent for more than one adverse reaction, assign the code only once.

4) If two or more drugs, medicinal or biological substances

If two or more drugs, medicinal or biological substances are reported, code each individually unless the combination code is listed in the Table of Drugs and Chemicals. In that case, assign the E code for the combination.

5) When a reaction results from the interaction of a drug(s)

When a reaction results from the interaction of a drug(s) and alcohol, use poisoning codes and E codes for both.

6) If the reporting format limits the number of E codes

If the reporting format limits the number of E codes that can be used in reporting clinical data, code the one most related to the principal diagnosis. Include at least one from each category (cause, intent, place) if possible.

There are different fourth digit codes in the same three digit category, use the code for "Other specified" of that category. If there is no "Other specified" code in that category, use the appropriate "Unspecified" code in that category.

If the codes are in different three digit categories, assign the appropriate E code for other multiple drugs and medicinal substances.

7) **Codes from the E930-E949 series**

Codes from the E930-E949 series must be used to identify the causative substance for an adverse effect of drug, medicinal and biological substances, correctly prescribed and properly administered. The effect, such as tachycardia, delirium, gastrointestinal hemorrhaging, vomiting, hypokalemia, hepatitis, renal failure, or respiratory failure, is coded and followed by the appropriate code from the E930-E949 series.

d. Multiple Cause E Code Coding Guidelines

If two or more events cause separate injuries, an E code should be assigned for each cause. The first listed E code will be selected in the following order:

E codes for child and adult abuse take priority over all other E codes. See Section I.C.19.e., Child and Adult abuse guidelines

E codes for terrorism events take priority over all other E codes except child and adult abuse

E codes for cataclysmic events take priority over all other E codes except child and adult abuse and terrorism.

E codes for transport accidents take priority over all other E codes except cataclysmic events and child and adult abuse and terrorism.

The first-listed E code should correspond to the cause of the most serious diagnosis due to an assault, accident, or self-harm, following the order of hierarchy listed above.

e. Child and Adult Abuse Guideline

1) **Intentional injury**

When the cause of an injury or neglect is intentional child or adult abuse, the first listed E code should be assigned from categories E960-E968, Homicide and injury purposely inflicted by other persons, (except category E967). An E code from category E967, Child and adult battering and other maltreatment, should be added as an additional code to identify the perpetrator, if known.

2) **Accidental intent**

In cases of neglect when the intent is determined to be accidental E code E904.0, Abandonment or neglect of infant and helpless person, should be the first listed E code.

f. Unknown or Suspected Intent Guideline

1) **If the intent (accident, self-harm, assault) of the cause of an injury or poisoning is unknown**

If the intent (accident, self-harm, assault) of the cause of an injury or poisoning is unknown or unspecified, code the intent as undetermined E980-E989.

2) **If the intent (accident, self-harm, assault) of the cause of an injury or poisoning is questionable**

If the intent (accident, self-harm, assault) of the cause of an injury or poisoning is questionable, probable or suspected, code the intent as undetermined E980-E989.

g. Undetermined Cause

When the intent of an injury or poisoning is known, but the cause is unknown, use codes: E928.9, Unspecified accident, E958.9, Suicide and self-inflicted injury by unspecified means, and E968.9, Assault by unspecified means.

These E codes should rarely be used, as the documentation in the medical record, in both the inpatient, outpatient, and other settings, should normally provide sufficient detail to determine the cause of the injury.

h. Late Effects of External Cause Guidelines

1) **Late effect E codes**

Late effect E codes exist for injuries and poisonings but not for adverse effects of drugs, misadventures and surgical complications.

2) **Late effect E codes (E929, E959, E969, E977, E989, or E999.1)**

A late effect E code (E929, E959, E969, E977, E989, or E999.1) should be used with any report of a late effect or sequela resulting from a previous injury or poisoning (905-909).

3) **Late effect E code with a related current injury**

A late effect E code should never be used with a related current nature of injury code.

4) **Use of late effect E codes for subsequent visits**

Use a late effect E code for subsequent visits when a late effect of the initial injury or poisoning is being treated. There is no late effect E code for adverse effects of drugs. Do not use a late effect E code for subsequent visits for follow-up care (e.g., to assess healing, to receive rehabilitative therapy) of the injury or poisoning when no late effect of the injury has been documented.

i. Misadventures and Complications of Care Guidelines

1) Code range E870-E876

Assign a code in the range of E870-E876 if misadventures are stated by the provider.

2) Code range E878-E879

Assign a code in the range of E878-E879 if the provider attributes an abnormal reaction or later complication to a surgical or medical procedure, but does not mention misadventure at the time of the procedure as the cause of the reaction.

j. Terrorism Guidelines

1) Cause of injury identified by the Federal Government (FBI) as terrorism

When the cause of an injury is identified by the Federal Government (FBI) as terrorism, the first-listed E-code should be a code from category E979, Terrorism. The definition of terrorism employed by the FBI is found at the inclusion note at E979. The terrorism E-code is the only E-code that should be assigned. Additional E codes from the assault categories should not be assigned.

2) Cause of an injury is suspected to be the result of terrorism

When the cause of an injury is suspected to be the result of terrorism a code from category E979 should not be assigned. Assign a code in the range of E codes based circumstances on the documentation of intent and mechanism.

3) Code E979.9, Terrorism, secondary effects

Assign code E979.9, Terrorism, secondary effects, for conditions occurring subsequent to the terrorist event. This code should not be assigned for conditions that are due to the initial terrorist act.

4) Statistical tabulation of terrorism codes

For statistical purposes these codes will be tabulated within the category for assault, expanding the current category from E960-E969 to include E979 and E999.1.

Section II. Selection of Principal Diagnosis

The circumstances of inpatient admission always govern the selection of principal diagnosis. The principal diagnosis is defined in the Uniform Hospital Discharge Data Set (UHDDS) as "that condition established after study to be chiefly responsible for occasioning the admission of the patient to the hospital for care."

The UHDDS definitions are used by hospitals to report inpatient data elements in a standardized manner. These data elements and their definitions can be found in the July 31, 1985, Federal Register (Vol. 50, No, 147), pp. 31038-40.

Since that time the application of the UHDDS definitions has been expanded to include all non-outpatient settings (acute care, short term, long term care, and psychiatric hospitals; home health agencies; rehab facilities; nursing homes, etc).

In determining principal diagnosis the coding conventions in the ICD-9-CM, Volumes I and II take precedence over these official coding guidelines. (See Section I.A., Conventions for the ICD-9-CM).

The importance of consistent, complete documentation in the medical record cannot be overemphasized. Without such documentation the application of all coding guidelines is a difficult, if not impossible, task.

A. Codes for symptoms, signs, and ill-defined conditions

Codes for symptoms, signs, and ill-defined conditions from Chapter 16 are not to be used as principal diagnosis when a related definitive diagnosis has been established.

B. Two or more interrelated conditions, each potentially meeting the definition for principal diagnosis.

When there are two or more interrelated conditions (such as diseases in the same ICD-9-CM chapter or manifestations characteristically associated with a certain disease) potentially meeting the definition of principal diagnosis, either condition may be sequenced first, unless the circumstances of the admission, the therapy provided, the Tabular List, or the Alphabetic Index indicate otherwise.

C. Two or more diagnoses that equally meet the definition for principal diagnosis

In the unusual instance when two or more diagnoses equally meet the criteria for principal diagnosis as determined by the circumstances of admission, diagnostic workup, and/or therapy provided, and the Alphabetic Index, Tabular List, or another coding guidelines does not provide sequencing direction, any one of the diagnoses may be sequenced first.

D. Two or more comparative or contrasting conditions.

In those rare instances when two or more contrasting or comparative diagnoses are documented as "either/or" (or similar terminology), they are coded as if the diagnoses were confirmed and the diagnoses are sequenced according to the circumstances of the admission. If no further determination can be made as to which diagnosis should be principal, either diagnosis may be sequenced first.

E. **A symptom(s) followed by contrasting/comparative diagnoses**

When a symptom(s) is followed by contrasting/comparative diagnoses, the symptom code is sequenced first. All the contrasting/comparative diagnoses should be coded as additional diagnoses.

F. **Original treatment plan not carried out**

Sequence as the principal diagnosis the condition, which after study occasioned the admission to the hospital, even though treatment may not have been carried out due to unforeseen circumstances.

G. **Complications of surgery and other medical care**

When the admission is for treatment of a complication resulting from surgery or other medical care, the complication code is sequenced as the principal diagnosis. If the complication is classified to the 996-999 series and the code lacks the necessary specificity in describing the complication, an additional code for the specific complication should be assigned.

H. **Uncertain Diagnosis**

If the diagnosis documented at the time of discharge is qualified as "probable", "suspected", "likely", "questionable", "possible", or "still to be ruled out", code the condition as if it existed or was established. The bases for these guidelines are the diagnostic workup, arrangements for further workup or observation, and initial therapeutic approach that correspond most closely with the established diagnosis.

Note: This guideline is applicable only to short-term, acute, long-term care and psychiatric hospitals.

I. **Admission from Observation Unit**

1. **Admission Following Medical Observation**

   When a patient is admitted to an observation unit for a medical condition, which either worsens or does not improve, and is subsequently admitted as an inpatient of the same hospital for this same medical condition, the principal diagnosis would be the medical condition which led to the hospital admission.

2. **Admission Following Post-Operative Observation**

   When a patient is admitted to an observation unit to monitor a condition (or complication) that develops following outpatient surgery, and then is subsequently admitted as an inpatient of the same hospital, hospitals should apply the Uniform Hospital Discharge Data Set (UHDDS) definition of principal diagnosis as "that condition established after study to be chiefly responsible for occasioning the admission of the patient to the hospital for care."

J. **Admission from Outpatient Surgery**

When a patient receives surgery in the hospital's outpatient surgery department and is subsequently admitted for continuing inpatient care at the same hospital, the following guidelines should be followed in selecting the principal diagnosis for the inpatient admission:

- **If the reason for the inpatient admission is a complication, assign the complication as the principal diagnosis.**
- **If no complication, or other condition, is documented as the reason for the inpatient admission, assign the reason for the outpatient surgery as the principal diagnosis.**
- **If the reason for the inpatient admission is another condition unrelated to the surgery, assign the unrelated condition as the principal diagnosis.**

Section III. Reporting Additional Diagnoses

GENERAL RULES FOR OTHER (ADDITIONAL) DIAGNOSES

For reporting purposes the definition for "other diagnoses" is interpreted as additional conditions that affect patient care in terms of requiring:

clinical evaluation; or
therapeutic treatment; or
diagnostic procedures; or
extended length of hospital stay; or
increased nursing care and/or monitoring.

The UHDDS item #11-b defines Other Diagnoses as "all conditions that coexist at the time of admission, that develop subsequently, or that affect the treatment received and/or the length of stay. Diagnoses that relate to an earlier episode which have no bearing on the current hospital stay are to be excluded." UHDDS definitions apply to inpatients in acute care, short-term, long term care and psychiatric hospital setting. The UHDDS definitions are used by acute care short-term hospitals to report inpatient data elements in a standardized manner. These data elements and their definitions can be found in the July 31, 1985, Federal Register (Vol. 50, No, 147), pp. 31038-40.

Since that time the application of the UHDDS definitions has been expanded to include all non-outpatient settings (acute care, short term, long term care and psychiatric hospitals; home health agencies; rehab facilities; nursing homes, etc).

The following guidelines are to be applied in designating "other diagnoses" when neither the Alphabetic Index nor the Tabular List in ICD-9-CM provide direction. The listing of the diagnoses in the patient record is the responsibility of the attending provider.

A. **Previous conditions**

If the provider has included a diagnosis in the final diagnostic statement, such as the discharge summary or the face sheet, it should ordinarily be coded. Some providers include in the diagnostic statement resolved conditions or diagnoses and status-post procedures from previous admission that have no bearing on the current stay. Such conditions are not to be reported and are coded only if required by hospital policy.

However, history codes (V10-V19) may be used as secondary codes if the historical condition or family history has an impact on current care or influences treatment.

B. **Abnormal findings**

Abnormal findings (laboratory, x-ray, pathologic, and other diagnostic results) are not coded and reported unless the provider indicates their clinical significance. If the findings are outside the normal range and the attending provider has ordered other tests to evaluate the condition or prescribed treatment, it is appropriate to ask the provider whether the abnormal finding should be added.

Please note: This differs from the coding practices in the outpatient setting for coding encounters for diagnostic tests that have been interpreted by a provider.

C. **Uncertain Diagnosis**

If the diagnosis documented at the time of discharge is qualified as "probable", "suspected", "likely", "questionable", "possible", or "still to be ruled out", code the condition as if it existed or was established. The bases for these guidelines are the diagnostic workup, arrangements for further workup or observation, and initial therapeutic approach that correspond most closely with the established diagnosis.

Note: This guideline is applicable only to short-term, acute, long-term care and psychiatric hospitals.

Section IV. Diagnostic Coding and Reporting Guidelines for Outpatient Services

These coding guidelines for outpatient diagnoses have been approved for use by hospitals/providers in coding and reporting hospital-based outpatient services and provider-based office visits.

Information about the use of certain abbreviations, punctuation, symbols, and other conventions used in the ICD-9-CM Tabular List (code numbers and titles), can be found in Section IA of these guidelines, under "Conventions Used in the Tabular List." Information about the correct sequence to use in finding a code is also described in Section I.

The terms encounter and visit are often used interchangeably in describing outpatient service contacts and, therefore, appear together in these guidelines without distinguishing one from the other.

Though the conventions and general guidelines apply to all settings, coding guidelines for outpatient and provider reporting of diagnoses will vary in a number of instances from those for inpatient diagnoses, recognizing that:

The Uniform Hospital Discharge Data Set (UHDDS) definition of principal diagnosis applies only to inpatients in acute, short-term, long-term care and psychiatric hospitals.

Coding guidelines for inconclusive diagnoses (probable, suspected, rule out, etc.) were developed for inpatient reporting and do not apply to outpatients.

A. **Selection of first-listed condition**

In the outpatient setting, the term first-listed diagnosis is used in lieu of principal diagnosis.

In determining the first-listed diagnosis the coding conventions of ICD-9-CM, as well as the general and disease specific guidelines take precedence over the outpatient guidelines.

Diagnoses often are not established at the time of the initial encounter/visit. It may take two or more visits before the diagnosis is confirmed.

The most critical rule involves beginning the search for the correct code assignment through the Alphabetic Index. Never begin searching initially in the Tabular List as this will lead to coding errors.

1. **Outpatient Surgery**

When a patient presents for outpatient surgery, code the reason for the surgery as the first-listed diagnosis (reason for the encounter), even if the surgery is not performed due to a contraindication.

2. **Observation Stay**

When a patient is admitted for observation for a medical condition, assign a code for the medical condition as the first-listed diagnosis.

When a patient presents for outpatient surgery and develops complications requiring admission to observation, code the reason for the surgery as the first reported diagnosis (reason for the encounter), followed by codes for the complications as secondary diagnoses.

B. **Codes from 001.0 through V84.8**

The appropriate code or codes from 001.0 through V84.8 must be used to identify diagnoses, symptoms, conditions, problems, complaints, or other reason(s) for the encounter/visit.

C. **Accurate reporting of ICD-9-CM diagnosis codes**

For accurate reporting of ICD-9-CM diagnosis codes, the documentation should describe the patient's condition, using terminology which includes specific diagnoses as well as symptoms, problems, or reasons for the encounter. There are ICD-9-CM codes to describe all of these.

D. Selection of codes 001.0 through 999.9

The selection of codes 001.0 through 999.9 will frequently be used to describe the reason for the encounter. These codes are from the section of ICD-9-CM for the classification of diseases and injuries (e.g. infectious and parasitic diseases; neoplasms; symptoms, signs, and ill-defined conditions, etc.).

E. Codes that describe symptoms and signs

Codes that describe symptoms and signs, as opposed to diagnoses, are acceptable for reporting purposes when a diagnosis has not been established (confirmed) by the provider. Chapter 16 of ICD-9-CM, Symptoms, Signs, and Ill-defined conditions (codes 780.0–799.9) contain many, but not all codes for symptoms.

F. Encounters for circumstances other than a disease or injury

ICD-9-CM provides codes to deal with encounters for circumstances other than a disease or injury. The Supplementary Classification of factors Influencing Health Status and Contact with Health Services (V01.0-V84.8) is provided to deal with occasions when circumstances other than a disease or injury are recorded as diagnosis or problems.

G. Level of Detail in Coding

1. ICD-9-CM codes with 3, 4, or 5 digits

ICD-9-CM is composed of codes with either 3, 4, or 5 digits. Codes with three digits are included in ICD-9-CM as the heading of a category of codes that may be further subdivided by the use of fourth and/or fifth digits, which provide greater specificity.

2. Use of full number of digits required for a code

A three-digit code is to be used only if it is not further subdivided. Where fourth-digit subcategories and/or fifth-digit subclassifications are provided, they must be assigned. A code is invalid if it has not been coded to the full number of digits required for that code. See also discussion under Section I.b.3., General Coding Guidelines, Level of Detail in Coding.

H. ICD-9-CM code for the diagnosis, condition, problem, or other reason for encounter/visit

List first the ICD-9-CM code for the diagnosis, condition, problem, or other reason for encounter/visit shown in the medical record to be chiefly responsible for the services provided. List additional codes that describe any coexisting conditions. In some cases the first-listed diagnosis may be a symptom when a diagnosis has not been established (confirmed) by the physician.

I. "Probable", "suspected", "questionable", "rule out", or "working diagnosis"

Do not code diagnoses documented as "probable", "suspected," "questionable," "rule out," or "working diagnosis". Rather, code the condition(s) to the highest degree of certainty for that encounter/visit, such as symptoms, signs, abnormal test results, or other reason for the visit. **Please note:** This differs from the coding practices used by short-term, acute care, long-term care and psychiatric hospitals.

J. Chronic diseases

Chronic diseases treated on an ongoing basis may be coded and reported as many times as the patient receives treatment and care for the condition(s)

K. Code all documented conditions that coexist

Code all documented conditions that coexist at the time of the encounter/visit, and require or affect patient care treatment or management. Do not code conditions that were previously treated and no longer exist. However, history codes (V10-V19) may be used as secondary codes if the historical condition or family history has an impact on current care or influences treatment.

L. Patients receiving diagnostic services only

For patients receiving diagnostic services only during an encounter/visit, sequence first the diagnosis, condition, problem, or other reason for encounter/visit shown in the medical record to be chiefly responsible for the outpatient services provided during the encounter/visit. Codes for other diagnoses (e.g., chronic conditions) may be sequenced as additional diagnoses.

For outpatient encounters for diagnostic tests that have been interpreted by a physician, and the final report is available at the time of coding, code any confirmed or definitive diagnosis(es) documented in the interpretation. Do not code related signs and symptoms as additional diagnoses.

Please note: This differs from the coding practice in the hospital inpatient setting regarding abnormal findings on test results.

M. Patients receiving therapeutic services only

For patients receiving therapeutic services only during an encounter/visit, sequence first the diagnosis, condition, problem, or other reason for encounter/visit shown in the medical record to be chiefly responsible for the outpatient services provided during the encounter/visit. Codes for other diagnoses (e.g., chronic conditions) may be sequenced as additional diagnoses.

The only exception to this rule is that when the primary reason for the admission/encounter is chemotherapy, radiation therapy, or rehabilitation, the appropriate V code for the service is listed first, and the diagnosis or problem for which the service is being performed listed second.

N. Patients receiving preoperative evaluations only

For patients receiving preoperative evaluations only, sequence **first** a code from category V72.8, Other specified examinations, to describe the pre-op consultations. Assign a code for the condition to describe the reason for the surgery as an additional diagnosis. Code also any findings related to the pre-op evaluation.

O. Ambulatory surgery

For ambulatory surgery, code the diagnosis for which the surgery was performed. If the postoperative diagnosis is known to be different from the preoperative diagnosis at the time the diagnosis is confirmed, select the postoperative diagnosis for coding, since it is the most definitive.

P. Routine outpatient prenatal visits

For routine outpatient prenatal visits when no complications are present, codes V22.0, Supervision of normal first pregnancy, or V22.1, Supervision of other normal pregnancy, should be used as the principal diagnosis. These codes should not be used in conjunction with chapter 11 codes.

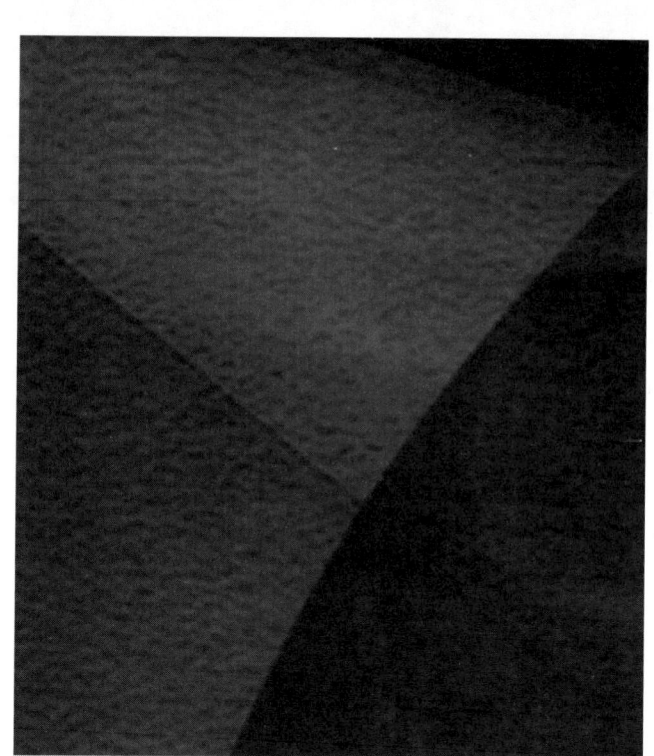

PART II

Alphabetic Index Volume 2

SECTION I INDEX TO DISEASES

A

AAT (alpha-1 antitrypsin) deficiency 273.4
AAV (disease) (illness) (infection) - *see* Human immunodeficiency virus (disease) (illness) (infection)
Abactio - *see* Abortion, induced
Abactus venter - *see* Abortion, induced
Abarognosis 781.99
Abasia (-astasia) 307.9
  atactica 781.3
  choreic 781.3
  hysterical 300.11
  paroxysmal trepidant 781.3
  spastic 781.3
  trembling 781.3
  trepidans 781.3
Abderhalden-Kaufmann-Lignac syndrome (cystinosis) 270.0
Abdomen, abdominal - *see also* condition
  accordion 306.4
  acute 789.0
  angina 557.1
  burst 868.00
  convulsive equivalent (*see also* Epilepsy) 345.5
  heart 746.87
  muscle deficiency syndrome 756.79
  obstipum 756.79
Abdominalgia 789.0
  periodic 277.31 (Revised)
Abduction contracture, hip or other joint - *see* Contraction, joint
Abercrombie's syndrome (amyloid degeneration) 277.39 (Revised)
Aberrant (congenital) - *see also* Malposition, congenital
  adrenal gland 759.1
  blood vessel NEC 747.60
    arteriovenous NEC 747.60
    cerebrovascular 747.81
    gastrointestinal 747.61
    lower limb 747.64
    renal 747.62
    spinal 747.82
    upper limb 747.63
  breast 757.6
  endocrine gland NEC 759.2
  gastrointestinal vessel (peripheral) 747.61
  hepatic duct 751.69
  lower limb vessel (peripheral) 747.64
  pancreas 751.7
  parathyroid gland 759.2
  peripheral vascular vessel NEC 747.60
  pituitary gland (pharyngeal) 759.2
  renal blood vessel 747.62
  sebaceous glands, mucous membrane, mouth 750.26
  spinal vessel 747.82
  spleen 759.0
  testis (descent) 752.51
  thymus gland 759.2
  thyroid gland 759.2
  upper limb vessel (peripheral) 747.63
Aberratio
  lactis 757.6
  testis 752.51
Aberration - *see also* Anomaly
  chromosome - *see* Anomaly, chromosome(s)
  distantial 368.9

Aberration *(Continued)*
  mental (*see also* Disorder, mental, nonpsychotic) 300.9
Abetalipoproteinemia 272.5
Abionarce 780.79
Abiotrophy 799.89
Ablatio
  placentae - *see* Placenta, ablatio
  retinae (*see also* Detachment, retina) 361.9
Ablation
  pituitary (gland) (with hypofunction) 253.7
  placenta - *see* Placenta, ablatio
  uterus 621.8
Ablepharia, ablepharon, ablephary 743.62
Ablepsia - *see* Blindness
Ablepsy - *see* Blindness
Ablutomania 300.3
Abnormal, abnormality, abnormalities - *see also* Anomaly
  acid-base balance 276.4
    fetus or newborn - *see* Distress, fetal
  adaptation curve, dark 368.63
  alveolar ridge 525.9
  amnion 658.9
    affecting fetus or newborn 762.9
  anatomical relationship NEC 759.9
  apertures, congenital, diaphragm 756.6
  auditory perception NEC 388.40
  autosomes NEC 758.5
    13 758.1
    18 758.2
    21 or 22 758.0
    D_1 758.1
    E_3 758.2
    G 758.0
  ballistocardiogram 794.39
  basal metabolic rate (BMR) 794.7
  biosynthesis, testicular androgen 257.2
  blood level (of)
    cobalt 790.6
    copper 790.6
    iron 790.6
    lead 790.6 (New)
    lithium 790.6
    magnesium 790.6
    mineral 790.6
    zinc 790.6
  blood pressure
    elevated (without diagnosis of hypertension) 796.2
    low (*see also* Hypotension) 458.9
      reading (incidental) (isolated) (nonspecific) 796.3
  bowel sounds 787.5
  breathing behavior - *see* Respiration
  caloric test 794.19
  cervix (acquired) NEC 622.9
    congenital 752.40
    in pregnancy or childbirth 654.6
      causing obstructed labor 660.2
        affecting fetus or newborn 763.1
  chemistry, blood NEC 790.6
  chest sounds 786.7
  chorion 658.9
    affecting fetus or newborn 762.9
  chromosomal NEC 758.89
    analysis, nonspecific result 795.2
    autosomes (*see also* Abnormal, autosomes NEC) 758.5
    fetal (suspected), affecting management of pregnancy 655.1
    sex 758.81

Abnormal, abnormality, abnormalities *(Continued)*
  clinical findings NEC 796.4
  communication - *see* Fistula
  configuration of pupils 379.49
  coronary
    artery 746.85
    vein 746.9
  cortisol-binding globulin 255.8
  course, Eustachian tube 744.24
  dentofacial NEC 524.9
    functional 524.50
    specified type NEC 524.89
  development, developmental NEC 759.9
    bone 756.9
    central nervous system 742.9
  direction, teeth 524.30
  dynia (*see also* Defect, coagulation) 286.9
  Ebstein 746.2
  echocardiogram 793.2
  echoencephalogram 794.01
  echogram NEC - *see* Findings, abnormal, structure
  electrocardiogram (ECG) (EKG) 794.31
  electroencephalogram (EEG) 794.02
  electromyogram (EMG) 794.17
    ocular 794.14
  electro-oculogram (EOG) 794.12
  electroretinogram (ERG) 794.11
  erythrocytes 289.9
    congenital, with perinatal jaundice 282.9 *[774.0]*
  eustachian valve 746.9
  excitability under minor stress 301.9
  fat distribution 782.9
  feces 787.7
  fetal heart rate - *see* Distress, fetal
  fetus NEC
    affecting management of pregnancy - *see* Pregnancy, management affected by, fetal
    causing disproportion 653.7
      affecting fetus or newborn 763.1
      causing obstructed labor 660.1
        affecting fetus or newborn 763.1
  findings without manifest disease - *see* Findings, abnormal
  fluid
    amniotic 792.3
    cerebrospinal 792.0
    peritoneal 792.9
    pleural 792.9
    synovial 792.9
    vaginal 792.9
  forces of labor NEC 661.9
    affecting fetus or newborn 763.7
  form, teeth 520.2
  function studies
    auditory 794.15
    bladder 794.9
    brain 794.00
    cardiovascular 794.30
    endocrine NEC 794.6
    kidney 794.4
    liver 794.8
    nervous system
      central 794.00
      peripheral 794.19
    oculomotor 794.14
    pancreas 794.9

◀ New ⟸ Revised

Abnormal, abnormality, abnormalities *(Continued)*
function studies *(Continued)*
placenta 794.9
pulmonary 794.2
retina 794.11
special senses 794.19
spleen 794.9
thyroid 794.5
vestibular 794.16
gait 781.2
hysterical 300.11
gastrin secretion 251.5
globulin
cortisol-binding 255.8
thyroid-binding 246.8
glucagon secretion 251.4
glucose 790.29
in pregnancy, childbirth, or puerperium 648.8
fetus or newborn 775.0
non-fasting 790.29
gravitational (G) forces or states 994.9
hair NEC 704.2
hard tissue formation in pulp 522.3
head movement 781.0
heart
rate
fetus affecting liveborn infant
before the onset of labor 763.81
during labor 763.82
unspecified as to time of onset 763.83
intrauterine
before the onset of labor 763.81
during labor 763.82
unspecified as to time of onset 763.83
newborn
before the onset of labor 763.81
during labor 763.82
unspecified as to time of onset 763.83
shadow 793.2
sounds NEC 785.3
hemoglobin (*see also* Disease, hemoglobin) 282.7
trait - *see* Trait, hemoglobin, abnormal
hemorrhage, uterus - *see* Hemorrhage, uterus
histology NEC 795.4
increase
in
appetite 783.6
development 783.9
involuntary movement 781.0
jaw closure 524.51
karyotype 795.2
knee jerk 796.1
labor NEC 661.9
affecting fetus or newborn 763.7
laboratory findings - *see* Findings, abnormal
length, organ or site, congenital - *see* Distortion
loss of height 781.91
loss of weight 783.21
lung shadow 793.1
mammogram 793.80
calcification 793.89 ◀
calculus 793.89 ◀
microcalcification 793.81
Mantoux test 795.5

Abnormal, abnormality, abnormalities *(Continued)*
membranes (fetal)
affecting fetus or newborn 762.9
complicating pregnancy 658.8
menstruation - *see* Menstruation
metabolism (*see also* condition) 783.9
movement 781.0
disorder NEC 333.90
sleep related, unspecified 780.58
specified NEC 333.99
head 781.0
involuntary 781.0
specified type NEC 333.99
muscle contraction, localized 728.85
myoglobin (Aberdeen) (Annapolis) 289.9
narrowness, eyelid 743.62
optokinetic response 379.57
organs or tissues of pelvis NEC
in pregnancy or childbirth 654.9
affecting fetus or newborn 763.89
causing obstructed labor 660.2
affecting fetus or newborn 763.1
origin - *see* Malposition, congenital
palmar creases 757.2
Papanicolaou (smear)
cervix 795.00
with
atypical squamous cells
cannot exclude high grade squamous intraepithelial lesion (ASC-H) 795.02
of undetermined significance (ASC-US) 795.01
cytologic evidence of malignancy 795.06 ◀
high grade squamous intraepithelial lesion (HGSIL) 795.04
low grade squamous intraepithelial lesion (LGSIL) 795.03
nonspecific finding NEC 795.09
other site 795.1
parturition
affecting fetus or newborn 763.9
mother - *see* Delivery, complicated
pelvis (bony) - *see* Deformity, pelvis
percussion, chest 786.7
periods (grossly) (*see also* Menstruation) 626.9
phonocardiogram 794.39
placenta - *see* Placenta, abnormal
plantar reflex 796.1
plasma protein - *see* Deficiency, plasma, protein
pleural folds 748.8
position - *see also* Malposition
gravid uterus 654.4
causing obstructed labor 660.2
affecting fetus or newborn 763.1
posture NEC 781.92
presentation (fetus) - *see* Presentation, fetus, abnormal
product of conception NEC 631
puberty - *see* Puberty
pulmonary
artery 747.3
function, newborn 770.89
test results 794.2
ventilation, newborn 770.89
hyperventilation 786.01
pulsations in neck 785.1
pupil reflexes 379.40
quality of milk 676.8

Abnormal, abnormality, abnormalities *(Continued)*
radiological examination 793.99 ⬅
abdomen NEC 793.6
biliary tract 793.3
breast 793.89
mammogram NOS 793.80
mammographic ⬅
calcification 793.89
calculus 793.89
microcalcification 793.81 ◀
gastrointestinal tract 793.4
genitourinary organs 793.5
head 793.0
image test inconclusive due to excess body fat 793.91 ◀
intrathoracic organ NEC 793.2
lung (field) 793.1
musculoskeletal system 793.7
retroperitoneum 793.6
skin and subcutaneous tissue 793.99 ⬅
skull 793.0
red blood cells 790.09
morphology 790.09
volume 790.09
reflex NEC 796.1
renal function test 794.4
respiration signs - *see* Respiration
response to nerve stimulation 794.10
retinal correspondence 368.34
rhythm, heart - *see also* Arrhythmia
fetus - *see* Distress, fetal
saliva 792.4
scan
brain 794.09
kidney 794.4
liver 794.8
lung 794.2
thyroid 794.5
secretion
gastrin 251.5
glucagon 251.4
semen 792.2
serum level (of)
acid phosphatase 790.5
alkaline phosphatase 790.5
amylase 790.5
enzymes NEC 790.5
lipase 790.5
shape
cornea 743.41
gallbladder 751.69
gravid uterus 654.4
affecting fetus or newborn 763.89
causing obstructed labor 660.2
affecting fetus or newborn 763.1
head (*see also* Anomaly, skull) 756.0
organ or site, congenital NEC - *see* Distortion
sinus venosus 747.40
size
fetus, complicating delivery 653.5
causing obstructed labor 660.1
gallbladder 751.69
head (*see also* Anomaly, skull) 756.0
organ or site, congenital NEC - *see* Distortion
teeth 520.2
skin and appendages, congenital NEC 757.9
soft parts of pelvis - *see* Abnormal, organs or tissues of pelvis
spermatozoa 792.2

- **Abnormal, abnormality, abnormalities** *(Continued)*
  - sputum (amount) (color) (excessive) (odor) (purulent) 786.4
  - stool NEC 787.7
    - bloody 578.1
      - occult 792.1
    - bulky 787.7
    - color (dark) (light) 792.1
    - content (fat) (mucus) (pus) 792.1
    - occult blood 792.1
  - synchondrosis 756.9
  - test results without manifest disease - *see* Findings, abnormal
  - thebesian valve 746.9
  - thermography - *see* Findings, abnormal, structure
  - threshold, cones or rods (eye) 368.63
  - thyroid-binding globulin 246.8
  - thyroid product 246.8
  - toxicology (findings) NEC 796.0
  - tracheal cartilage (congenital) 748.3
  - transport protein 273.8
  - ultrasound results - *see* Findings, abnormal, structure
  - umbilical cord
    - affecting fetus or newborn 762.6
    - complicating delivery 663.9
    - specified NEC 663.8
  - union
    - cricoid cartilage and thyroid cartilage 748.3
    - larynx and trachea 748.3
    - thyroid cartilage and hyoid bone 748.3
  - urination NEC 788.69
    - psychogenic 306.53
    - stream
      - intermittent 788.61
      - slowing 788.62
      - splitting 788.61
      - weak 788.62
    - urgency 788.63
  - urine (constituents) NEC 791.9
  - uterine hemorrhage (*see also* Hemorrhage, uterus) 626.9
    - climacteric 627.0
    - postmenopausal 627.1
  - vagina (acquired) (congenital)
    - in pregnancy or childbirth 654.7
      - affecting fetus or newborn 763.89
      - causing obstructed labor 660.2
        - affecting fetus or newborn 763.1
  - vascular sounds 785.9
  - vectorcardiogram 794.39
  - visually evoked potential (VEP) 794.13
  - vulva (acquired) (congenital)
    - in pregnancy or childbirth 654.8
      - affecting fetus or newborn 763.89
      - causing obstructed labor 660.2
        - affecting fetus or newborn 763.1
  - weight
    - gain 783.1
      - of pregnancy 646.1
        - with hypertension - *see* Toxemia, of pregnancy
    - loss 783.21
  - x-ray examination - *see* Abnormal, radiological examination
- **Abnormally formed uterus** - *see* Anomaly, uterus
- **Abnormity** (any organ or part) - *see* Anomaly
- **ABO**
  - hemolytic disease 773.1
  - incompatibility reaction 999.6
- **Abocclusion** 524.20
- **Abolition, language** 784.69
- **Aborter, habitual or recurrent NEC**
  - without current pregnancy 629.81
  - current abortion (*see also* Abortion, spontaneous) 634.9
    - affecting fetus or newborn 761.8
  - observation in current pregnancy 646.3
- **Abortion** (complete) (incomplete) (inevitable) (with retained products of conception) 637.9

> Note Use the following fifth-digit subclassification with categories 634-637:
>
> 0 unspecified
> 1 incomplete
> 2 complete

  - with
    - complication(s) (any) following previous abortion - *see* category 639
    - damage to pelvic organ (laceration) (rupture) (tear) 637.2
    - embolism (air) (amniotic fluid) (blood clot) (pulmonary) (pyemic) (septic) (soap) 637.6
    - genital tract and pelvic infection 637.0
    - hemorrhage, delayed or excessive 637.1
    - metabolic disorder 637.4
    - renal failure (acute) 637.3
    - sepsis (genital tract) (pelvic organ) 637.0
      - urinary tract 637.7
    - shock (postoperative) (septic) 637.5
    - specified complication NEC 637.7
    - toxemia 637.3
    - unspecified complication(s) 637.8
    - urinary tract infection 637.7
  - accidental - *see* Abortion, spontaneous
  - artificial - *see* Abortion, induced
  - attempted (failed) - *see* Abortion, failed
  - criminal - *see* Abortion, illegal
  - early - *see* Abortion, spontaneous
  - elective - *see* Abortion, legal
  - failed (legal) 638.9
    - with
      - damage to pelvic organ (laceration) (rupture) (tear) 638.2
      - embolism (air) (amniotic fluid) (blood clot) (pulmonary) (pyemic) (septic) (soap) 638.6
      - genital tract and pelvic infection 638.0
      - hemorrhage, delayed or excessive 638.1
      - metabolic disorder 638.4
      - renal failure (acute) 638.3
      - sepsis (genital tract) (pelvic organ) 638.0
        - urinary tract 638.7
      - shock (postoperative) (septic) 638.5
      - specified complication NEC 638.7
      - toxemia 638.3
      - unspecified complication(s) 638.8
      - urinary tract infection 638.7
  - fetal indication - *see* Abortion, legal
  - fetus 779.6
  - following threatened abortion - *see* Abortion, by type

- **Abortion** *(Continued)*
  - habitual or recurrent (care during pregnancy) 646.3
    - with current abortion (*see also* Abortion, spontaneous) 634.9
      - affecting fetus or newborn 761.8
    - without current pregnancy 629.81
  - homicidal - *see* Abortion, illegal
  - illegal 636.9
    - with
      - damage to pelvic organ (laceration) (rupture) (tear) 636.2
      - embolism (air) (amniotic fluid) (blood clot) (pulmonary) (pyemic) (septic) (soap) 636.6
      - genital tract and pelvic infection 636.0
      - hemorrhage, delayed or excessive 636.1
      - metabolic disorder 636.4
      - renal failure 636.3
      - sepsis (genital tract) (pelvic organ) 636.0
        - urinary tract 636.7
      - shock (postoperative) (septic) 636.5
      - specified complication NEC 636.7
      - toxemia 636.3
      - unspecified complication(s) 636.8
      - urinary tract infection 636.7
    - fetus 779.6
  - induced 637.9
    - illegal - *see* Abortion, illegal
    - legal indications - *see* Abortion, legal
    - medical indications - *see* Abortion, legal
    - therapeutic - *see* Abortion, legal
  - late - *see* Abortion, spontaneous
  - legal (legal indication) (medical indication) (under medical supervision) 635.9
    - with
      - damage to pelvic organ (laceration) (rupture) (tear) 635.2
      - embolism (air) (amniotic fluid) (blood clot) (pulmonary) (pyemic) (septic) (soap) 635.6
      - genital tract and pelvic infection 635.0
      - hemorrhage, delayed or excessive 635.1
      - metabolic disorder 635.4
      - renal failure (acute) 635.3
      - sepsis (genital tract) (pelvic organ) 635.0
        - urinary tract 635.7
      - shock (postoperative) (septic) 635.5
      - specified complication NEC 635.7
      - toxemia 635.3
      - unspecified complication(s) 635.8
      - urinary tract infection 635.7
    - fetus 779.6
  - medical indication - *see* Abortion, legal
  - mental hygiene problem - *see* Abortion, legal
  - missed 632
  - operative - *see* Abortion, legal
  - psychiatric indication - *see* Abortion, legal
  - recurrent - *see* Abortion, spontaneous
  - self-induced - *see* Abortion, illegal
  - septic - *see* Abortion, by type, with sepsis

Abortion *(Continued)*
- spontaneous 634.9
  - with
    - damage to pelvic organ (laceration) (rupture) (tear) 634.2
    - embolism (air) (amniotic fluid) (blood clot) (pulmonary) (pyemic) (septic) (soap) 634.6
    - genital tract and pelvic infection 634.0
    - hemorrhage, delayed or excessive 634.1
    - metabolic disorder 634.4
    - renal failure 634.3
    - sepsis (genital tract) (pelvic organ) 634.0
      - urinary tract 634.7
    - shock (postoperative) (septic) 634.5
    - specified complication NEC 634.7
    - toxemia 634.3
    - unspecified complication(s) 634.8
    - urinary tract infection 634.7
  - fetus 761.8
  - threatened 640.0
    - affecting fetus or newborn 762.1
- surgical - *see* Abortion, legal
- therapeutic - *see* Abortion, legal
- threatened 640.0
  - affecting fetus or newborn 762.1
- tubal - *see* Pregnancy, tubal
- voluntary - *see* Abortion, legal

Abortus fever 023.9
Aboulomania 301.6
Abrachia 755.20
Abrachiatism 755.20
Abrachiocephalia 759.89
Abrachiocephalus 759.89
Abrami's disease (acquired hemolytic jaundice) 283.9
Abramov-Fiedler myocarditis (acute isolated myocarditis) 422.91
Abrasion - *see also* Injury, superficial, by site
- cornea 918.1
- dental 521.20
  - extending into
    - dentine 521.22
    - pulp 521.23
  - generalized 521.25
  - limited to enamel 521.21
  - localized 521.24
- teeth, tooth (dentifrice) (habitual) (hard tissues) (occupational) (ritual) (traditional) (wedge defect) (*see also* Abrasion, dental) 521.20

Abrikossov's tumor (M9580/0) - *see also* Neoplasm, connective tissue, benign
- malignant (M9580/3) - *see* Neoplasm, connective tissue, malignant

Abrism 988.8
Abruption, placenta - *see* Placenta, abruptio
Abruptio placentae - *see* Placenta, abruptio
Abscess (acute) (chronic) (infectional) (lymphangitic) (metastatic) (multiple) (pyogenic) (septic) (with lymphangitis) (*see also* Cellulitis) 682.9
- abdomen, abdominal
  - cavity 567.22
  - wall 682.2
- abdominopelvic 567.22
- accessory sinus (chronic) (*see also* Sinusitis) 473.9

Abscess *(Continued)*
- adrenal (capsule) (gland) 255.8
- alveolar 522.5
  - with sinus 522.7
- amebic 006.3
  - bladder 006.8
  - brain (with liver or lung abscess) 006.5
  - liver (without mention of brain or lung abscess) 006.3
    - with
      - brain abscess (and lung abscess) 006.5
      - lung abscess 006.4
  - lung (with liver abscess) 006.4
    - with brain abscess 006.5
  - seminal vesicle 006.8
  - specified site NEC 006.8
  - spleen 006.8
- anaerobic 040.0
- ankle 682.6
- anorectal 566
- antecubital space 682.3
- antrum (chronic) (Highmore) (*see also* Sinusitis, maxillary) 473.0
- anus 566
- apical (tooth) 522.5
  - with sinus (alveolar) 522.7
- appendix 540.1
- areola (acute) (chronic) (nonpuerperal) 611.0
  - puerperal, postpartum 675.1
- arm (any part, above wrist) 682.3
- artery (wall) 447.2
- atheromatous 447.2
- auditory canal (external) 380.10
- auricle (ear) (staphylococcal) (streptococcal) 380.10
- axilla, axillary (region) 682.3
  - lymph gland or node 683
- back (any part) 682.2
- Bartholin's gland 616.3
  - with
    - abortion - *see* Abortion, by type, with sepsis
    - ectopic pregnancy (*see also* categories 633.0-633.9) 639.0
    - molar pregnancy (*see also* categories 630-632) 639.0
  - complicating pregnancy or puerperium 646.6
  - following
    - abortion 639.0
    - ectopic or molar pregnancy 639.0
- bartholinian 616.3
- Bezold's 383.01
- bile, biliary, duct or tract (*see also* Cholecystitis) 576.8
- bilharziasis 120.1
- bladder (wall) 595.89
  - amebic 006.8
- bone (subperiosteal) (*see also* Osteomyelitis) 730.0
  - accessory sinus (chronic) (*see also* Sinusitis) 473.9
  - acute 730.0
  - chronic or old 730.1
  - jaw (lower) (upper) 526.4
  - mastoid - *see* Mastoiditis, acute
  - petrous (*see also* Petrositis) 383.20
  - spinal (tuberculous) (*see also* Tuberculosis) 015.0 *[730.88]*
    - nontuberculous 730.08

Abscess *(Continued)*
- bowel 569.5
- brain (any part) 324.0
  - amebic (with liver or lung abscess) 006.5
  - cystic 324.0
  - late effect - *see* category 326
  - otogenic 324.0
  - tuberculous (*see also* Tuberculosis) 013.3
- breast (acute) (chronic) (nonpuerperal) 611.0
  - newborn 771.5
  - puerperal, postpartum 675.1
  - tuberculous (*see also* Tuberculosis) 017.9
- broad ligament (chronic) (*see also* Disease, pelvis, inflammatory) 614.4
  - acute 614.3
- Brodie's (chronic) (localized) (*see also* Osteomyelitis) 730.1
- bronchus 519.19
- buccal cavity 528.3
- bulbourethral gland 597.0
- bursa 727.89
  - pharyngeal 478.29
- buttock 682.5
- canaliculus, breast 611.0
- canthus 372.20
- cartilage 733.99
- cecum 569.5
  - with appendicitis 540.1
- cerebellum, cerebellar 324.0
  - late effect - *see* category 326
- cerebral (embolic) 324.0
  - late effect - *see* category 326
- cervical (neck region) 682.1
  - lymph gland or node 683
  - stump (*see also* Cervicitis) 616.0
- cervix (stump) (uteri) (*see also* Cervicitis) 616.0
- cheek, external 682.0
  - inner 528.3
- chest 510.9
  - with fistula 510.0
  - wall 682.2
- chin 682.0
- choroid 363.00
- ciliary body 364.3
- circumtonsillar 475
- cold (tuberculous) - *see also* Tuberculosis, abscess
  - articular - *see* Tuberculosis, joint
- colon (wall) 569.5
- colostomy or enterostomy 569.61
- conjunctiva 372.00
- connective tissue NEC 682.9
- cornea 370.55
  - with ulcer 370.00
- corpus
  - cavernosum 607.2
  - luteum (*see also* Salpingo-oophoritis) 614.2
- Cowper's gland 597.0
- cranium 324.0
- cul-de-sac (Douglas') (posterior) (*see also* Disease, pelvis, inflammatory) 614.4
  - acute 614.3
- dental 522.5
  - with sinus (alveolar) 522.7

Abscess *(Continued)*
dentoalveolar 522.5
with sinus (alveolar) 522.7
diaphragm, diaphragmatic 567.22
digit NEC 681.9
Douglas' cul-de-sac or pouch (*see also* Disease, pelvis, inflammatory) 614.4
acute 614.3
Dubois' 090.5
ductless gland 259.8
ear
acute 382.00
external 380.10
inner 386.30
middle - *see* Otitis media
elbow 682.3
endamebic - *see* Abscess, amebic
entamebic - *see* Abscess, amebic
enterostomy 569.61
epididymis 604.0
epidural 324.9
brain 324.0
late effect - *see* category 326
spinal cord 324.1
epiglottis 478.79
epiploon, epiploic 567.22
erysipelatous (*see also* Erysipelas) 035
esophagostomy 530.86
esophagus 530.19
ethmoid (bone) (chronic) (sinus) (*see also* Sinusitis, ethmoidal) 473.2
external auditory canal 380.10
extradural 324.9
brain 324.0
late effect - *see* category 326
spinal cord 324.1
extraperitoneal - *see* Abscess, peritoneum
eye 360.00
eyelid 373.13
face (any part, except eye) 682.0
fallopian tube (*see also* Salpingo-oophoritis) 614.2
fascia 728.89
fauces 478.29
fecal 569.5
femoral (region) 682.6
filaria, filarial (*see also* Infestation, filarial) 125.9
finger (any) (intrathecal) (periosteal) (subcutaneous) (subcuticular) 681.00
fistulous NEC 682.9
flank 682.2
foot (except toe) 682.7
forearm 682.3
forehead 682.0
frontal (sinus) (chronic) (*see also* Sinusitis, frontal) 473.1
gallbladder (*see also* Cholecystitis, acute) 575.0
gastric 535.0
genital organ or tract NEC
female 616.9
with
abortion - *see* Abortion, by type, with sepsis
ectopic pregnancy (*see also* categories 633.0-633.9) 639.0
molar pregnancy (*see also* categories 630-632) 639.0
following
abortion 639.0
ectopic or molar pregnancy 639.0

Abscess *(Continued)*
genital organ or tract *(Continued)*
female *(Continued)*
following *(Continued)*
puerperal, postpartum, childbirth 670
male 608.4
genitourinary system, tuberculous (*see also* Tuberculosis) 016.9
gingival 523.30
gland, glandular (lymph) (acute) NEC 683
glottis 478.79
gluteal (region) 682.5
gonorrheal NEC (*see also* Gonococcus) 098.0
groin 682.2
gum 523.30
hand (except finger or thumb) 682.4
head (except face) 682.8
heart 429.89
heel 682.7
helminthic (*see also* Infestation, by specific parasite) 128.9
hepatic 572.0
amebic (*see also* Abscess, liver, amebic) 006.3
duct 576.8
hip 682.6
tuberculous (active) (*see also* Tuberculosis) 015.1
ileocecal 540.1
ileostomy (bud) 569.61
iliac (region) 682.2
fossa 540.1
iliopsoas 567.31
tuberculous (*see also* Tuberculosis) 015.0 *[730.88]*
infraclavicular (fossa) 682.3
inguinal (region) 682.2
lymph gland or node 683
intersphincteric (anus) 566
intestine, intestinal 569.5
rectal 566
intra-abdominal (*see also* Abscess, peritoneum) 567.22
postoperative 998.59
intracranial 324.0
late effect - *see* category 326
intramammary - *see* Abscess, breast
intramastoid (*see also* Mastoiditis, acute) 383.00
intraorbital 376.01
intraperitoneal 567.22
intraspinal 324.1
late effect - *see* category 326
intratonsillar 475
iris 364.3
ischiorectal 566
jaw (bone) (lower) (upper) 526.4
skin 682.0
joint (*see also* Arthritis, pyogenic) 711.0
vertebral (tuberculous) (*see also* Tuberculosis) 015.0 *[730.88]*
nontuberculous 724.8
kidney 590.2
with
abortion - *see* Abortion, by type, with urinary tract infection
calculus 592.0
ectopic pregnancy (*see also* categories 633.0-633.9) 639.8
molar pregnancy (*see also* categories 630-632) 639.8

Abscess *(Continued)*
kidney *(Continued)*
with *(Continued)*
complicating pregnancy or puerperium 646.6
affecting fetus or newborn 760.1
following
abortion 639.8
ectopic or molar pregnancy 639.8
knee 682.6
joint 711.06
tuberculous (active) (*see also* Tuberculosis) 015.2
labium (majus) (minus) 616.4
complicating pregnancy, childbirth, or puerperium 646.6
lacrimal (passages) (sac) (*see also* Dacryocystitis) 375.30
caruncle 375.30
gland (*see also* Dacryoadenitis) 375.00
lacunar 597.0
larynx 478.79
lateral (alveolar) 522.5
with sinus 522.7
leg, except foot 682.6
lens 360.00
lid 373.13
lingual 529.0
tonsil 475
lip 528.5
Littre's gland 597.0
liver 572.0
amebic 006.3
with
brain abscess (and lung abscess) 006.5
lung abscess 006.4
due to Entamoeba histolytica 006.3
dysenteric (*see also* Abscess, liver, amebic) 006.3
pyogenic 572.0
tropical (*see also* Abscess, liver, amebic) 006.3
loin (region) 682.2
lumbar (tuberculous) (*see also* Tuberculosis) 015.0 *[730.88]*
nontuberculous 682.2
lung (miliary) (putrid) 513.0
amebic (with liver abscess) 006.4
with brain abscess 006.5
lymph, lymphatic, gland or node (acute) 683
any site, except mesenteric 683
mesentery 289.2
lymphangitic, acute - *see* Cellulitis
malar 526.4
mammary gland - *see* Abscess, breast
marginal (anus) 566
mastoid (process) (*see also* Mastoiditis, acute) 383.00
subperiosteal 383.01
maxilla, maxillary 526.4
molar (tooth) 522.5
with sinus 522.7
premolar 522.5
sinus (chronic) (*see also* Sinusitis, maxillary) 473.0
mediastinum 513.1
meibomian gland 373.12
meninges (*see also* Meningitis) 320.9
mesentery, mesenteric 567.22
mesosalpinx (*see also* Salpingo-oophoritis) 614.2
milk 675.1

Abscess *(Continued)*
- Monro's (psoriasis) 696.1
- mons pubis 682.2
- mouth (floor) 528.3
- multiple sites NEC 682.9
- mural 682.2
- muscle 728.89
  - psoas 567.31
- myocardium 422.92
- nabothian (follicle) (*see also* Cervicitis) 616.0
- nail (chronic) (with lymphangitis) 681.9
  - finger 681.02
  - toe 681.11
- nasal (fossa) (septum) 478.19
  - sinus (chronic) (*see also* Sinusitis) 473.9
- nasopharyngeal 478.29
- nates 682.5
- navel 682.2
  - newborn NEC 771.4
- neck (region) 682.1
  - lymph gland or node 683
- nephritic (*see also* Abscess, kidney) 590.2
- nipple 611.0
  - puerperal, postpartum 675.0
- nose (septum) 478.19
  - external 682.0
- omentum 567.22
- operative wound 998.59
- orbit, orbital 376.01
- ossifluent - *see* Abscess, bone
- ovary, ovarian (corpus luteum) (*see also* Salpingo-oophoritis) 614.2
- oviduct (*see also* Salpingo-oophoritis) 614.2
- palate (soft) 528.3
  - hard 526.4
- palmar (space) 682.4
- pancreas (duct) 577.0
- paradontal 523.30
- parafrenal 607.2
- parametric, parametrium (chronic) (*see also* Disease, pelvis, inflammatory) 614.4
  - acute 614.3
- paranephric 590.2
- parapancreatic 577.0
- parapharyngeal 478.22
- pararectal 566
- parasinus (*see also* Sinusitis) 473.9
- parauterine (*see also* Disease, pelvis, inflammatory) 614.4
  - acute 614.3
- paravaginal (*see also* Vaginitis) 616.10
- parietal region 682.8
- parodontal 523.30
- parotid (duct) (gland) 527.3
  - region 528.3
- parumbilical 682.2
  - newborn 771.4
- pectoral (region) 682.2
- pelvirectal 567.22
- pelvis, pelvic
  - female (chronic) (*see also* Disease, pelvis, inflammatory) 614.4
    - acute 614.3
  - male, peritoneal (cellular tissue) - *see* Abscess, peritoneum
  - tuberculous (*see also* Tuberculosis) 016.9
- penis 607.2
  - gonococcal (acute) 098.0
    - chronic or duration of 2 months or over 098.2

Abscess *(Continued)*
- perianal 566
- periapical 522.5
  - with sinus (alveolar) 522.7
- periappendiceal 540.1
- pericardial 420.99
- pericecal 540.1
- pericemental 523.30
- pericholecystic (*see also* Cholecystitis, acute) 575.0
- pericoronal 523.30
- peridental 523.30
- perigastric 535.0
- perimetric (*see also* Disease, pelvis, inflammatory) 614.4
  - acute 614.3
- perinephric, perinephritic (*see also* Abscess, kidney) 590.2
- perineum, perineal (superficial) 682.2
  - deep (with urethral involvement) 597.0
  - urethra 597.0
- periodontal (parietal) 523.31
  - apical 522.5
- periosteum, periosteal (*see also* Periostitis) 730.3
  - with osteomyelitis (*see also* Osteomyelitis) 730.2
    - acute or subacute 730.0
    - chronic or old 730.1
- peripleuritic 510.9
  - with fistula 510.0
- periproctic 566
- periprostatic 601.2
- perirectal (staphylococcal) 566
- perirenal (tissue) (*see also* Abscess, kidney) 590.2
- perisinuous (nose) (*see also* Sinusitis) 473.9
- peritoneum, peritoneal (perforated) (ruptured) 567.22
  - with
    - abortion - *see* Abortion, by type, with sepsis
    - appendicitis 540.1
    - ectopic pregnancy (*see also* categories 633.0-633.9) 639.0
    - molar pregnancy (*see also* categories 630-632) 639.0
  - following
    - abortion 639.0
    - ectopic or molar pregnancy 639.0
  - pelvic, female (*see also* Disease, pelvis, inflammatory) 614.4
    - acute 614.3
  - postoperative 998.59
  - puerperal, postpartum, childbirth 670
  - tuberculous (*see also* Tuberculosis) 014.0
- peritonsillar 475
- perityphlic 540.1
- periureteral 593.89
- periurethral 597.0
  - gonococcal (acute) 098.0
    - chronic or duration of 2 months or over 098.2
- periuterine (*see also* Disease, pelvis, inflammatory) 614.4
  - acute 614.3
- perivesical 595.89
- pernicious NEC 682.9
- petrous bone - *see* Petrositis
- phagedenic NEC 682.9
  - chancroid 099.0

Abscess *(Continued)*
- pharynx, pharyngeal (lateral) 478.29
- phlegmonous NEC 682.9
- pilonidal 685.0
- pituitary (gland) 253.8
- pleura 510.9
  - with fistula 510.0
- popliteal 682.6
- postanal 566
- postcecal 540.1
- postlaryngeal 478.79
- postnasal 478.19
- postpharyngeal 478.24
- posttonsillar 475
- posttyphoid 002.0
- Pott's (*see also* Tuberculosis) 015.0 *[730.88]*
- pouch of Douglas (chronic) (*see also* Disease, pelvis, inflammatory) 614.4
- premammary - *see* Abscess, breast
- prepatellar 682.6
- prostate (*see also* Prostatitis) 601.2
  - gonococcal (acute) 098.12
    - chronic or duration of 2 months or over 098.32
- psoas 567.31
  - tuberculous (*see also* Tuberculosis) 015.0 *[730.88]*
- pterygopalatine fossa 682.8
- pubis 682.2
- puerperal - *see* Puerperal, abscess, by site
- pulmonary - *see* Abscess, lung
- pulp, pulpal (dental) 522.0
  - finger 681.01
  - toe 681.10
- pyemic - *see* Septicemia
- pyloric valve 535.0
- rectovaginal septum 569.5
- rectovesical 595.89
- rectum 566
- regional NEC 682.9
- renal (*see also* Abscess, kidney) 590.2
- retina 363.00
- retrobulbar 376.01
- retrocecal 567.22
- retrolaryngeal 478.79
- retromammary - *see* Abscess, breast
- retroperineal 682.2
- retroperitoneal 567.38
  - postprocedural 998.59
- retropharyngeal 478.24
  - tuberculous (*see also* Tuberculosis) 012.8
- retrorectal 566
- retrouterine (*see also* Disease, pelvis, inflammatory) 614.4
  - acute 614.3
- retrovesical 595.89
- root, tooth 522.5
  - with sinus (alveolar) 522.7
- round ligament (*see also* Disease, pelvis, inflammatory) 614.4
  - acute 614.3
- rupture (spontaneous) NEC 682.9
- sacrum (tuberculous) (*see also* Tuberculosis) 015.0 *[730.88]*
  - nontuberculous 730.08
- salivary duct or gland 527.3
- scalp (any part) 682.8
- scapular 730.01
- sclera 379.09
- scrofulous (*see also* Tuberculosis) 017.2
- scrotum 608.4

Abscess *(Continued)*
seminal vesicle 608.0
amebic 006.8
septal, dental 522.5
with sinus (alveolar) 522.7
septum (nasal) 478.19
serous (*see also* Periostitis) 730.3
shoulder 682.3
side 682.2
sigmoid 569.5
sinus (accessory) (chronic) (nasal) (*see also* Sinusitis) 473.9
intracranial venous (any) 324.0
late effect - *see* category 326
Skene's duct or gland 597.0
skin NEC 682.9
tuberculous (primary) (*see also* Tuberculosis) 017.0
sloughing NEC 682.9
specified site NEC 682.8
amebic 006.8
spermatic cord 608.4
sphenoidal (sinus) (*see also* Sinusitis, sphenoidal) 473.3
spinal
cord (any part) (staphylococcal) 324.1
tuberculous (*see also* Tuberculosis) 013.5
epidural 324.1
spine (column) (tuberculous) (*see also* Tuberculosis) 015.0 *[730.88]*
nontuberculous 730.08
spleen 289.59
amebic 006.8
staphylococcal NEC 682.9
stitch 998.59
stomach (wall) 535.0
strumous (tuberculous) (*see also* Tuberculosis) 017.2
subarachnoid 324.9
brain 324.0
cerebral 324.0
late effect - *see* category 326
spinal cord 324.1
subareolar - *see also* Abscess, breast
puerperal, postpartum 675.1
subcecal 540.1
subcutaneous NEC 682.9
subdiaphragmatic 567.22
subdorsal 682.2
subdural 324.9
brain 324.0
late effect - *see* category 326
spinal cord 324.1
subgaleal 682.8
subhepatic 567.22
sublingual 528.3
gland 527.3
submammary - *see* Abscess, breast
submandibular (region) (space) (triangle) 682.0
gland 527.3
submaxillary (region) 682.0
gland 527.3
submental (pyogenic) 682.0
gland 527.3
subpectoral 682.2
subperiosteal - *see* Abscess, bone
subperitoneal 567.22
subphrenic - *see also* Abscess, peritoneum 567.22
postoperative 998.59
subscapular 682.2
subungual 681.9

Abscess *(Continued)*
suburethral 597.0
sudoriparous 705.89
suppurative NEC 682.9
supraclavicular (fossa) 682.3
suprahepatic 567.22
suprapelvic (*see also* Disease, pelvis, inflammatory) 614.4
acute 614.3
suprapubic 682.2
suprarenal (capsule) (gland) 255.8
sweat gland 705.89
syphilitic 095.8
teeth, tooth (root) 522.5
with sinus (alveolar) 522.7
supporting structures NEC 523.30
temple 682.0
temporal region 682.0
temporosphenoidal 324.0
late effect - *see* category 326
tendon (sheath) 727.89
testicle - *see* Orchitis
thecal 728.89
thigh (acquired) 682.6
thorax 510.9
with fistula 510.0
throat 478.29
thumb (intrathecal) (periosteal) (subcutaneous) (subcuticular) 681.00
thymus (gland) 254.1
thyroid (gland) 245.0
toe (any) (intrathecal) (periosteal) (subcutaneous) (subcuticular) 681.10
tongue (staphylococcal) 529.0
tonsil(s) (lingual) 475
tonsillopharyngeal 475
tooth, teeth (root) 522.5
with sinus (alveolar) 522.7
supporting structure NEC 523.30
trachea 478.9
trunk 682.2
tubal (*see also* Salpingo-oophoritis) 614.2
tuberculous - *see* Tuberculosis, abscess
tubo-ovarian (*see also* Salpingo-oophoritis) 614.2
tunica vaginalis 608.4
umbilicus NEC 682.2
newborn 771.4
upper arm 682.3
upper respiratory 478.9
urachus 682.2
urethra (gland) 597.0
urinary 597.0
uterus, uterine (wall) (*see also* Endometritis) 615.9
ligament (*see also* Disease, pelvis, inflammatory) 614.4
acute 614.3
neck (*see also* Cervicitis) 616.0
uvula 528.3
vagina (wall) (*see also* Vaginitis) 616.10
vaginorectal (*see also* Vaginitis) 616.10
vas deferens 608.4
vermiform appendix 540.1
vertebra (column) (tuberculous) (*see also* Tuberculosis) 015.0 *[730.88]*
nontuberculous 730.0
vesical 595.89
vesicouterine pouch (*see also* Disease, pelvis, inflammatory) 614.4
vitreous (humor) (pneumococcal) 360.04

Abscess *(Continued)*
vocal cord 478.5
von Bezold's 383.01
vulva 616.4
complicating pregnancy, childbirth, or puerperium 646.6
vulvovaginal gland (*see also* Vaginitis) 616.3
web-space 682.4
wrist 682.4
Absence (organ or part) (complete or partial)
acoustic nerve 742.8
adrenal (gland) (congenital) 759.1
acquired V45.79
albumin (blood) 273.8
alimentary tract (complete) (congenital) (partial) 751.8
lower 751.5
upper 750.8
alpha-fucosidase 271.8
alveolar process (acquired) 525.8
congenital 750.26
anus, anal (canal) (congenital) 751.2
aorta (congenital) 747.22
aortic valve (congenital) 746.89
appendix, congenital 751.2
arm (acquired) V49.60
above elbow V49.66
below elbow V49.65
congenital (*see also* Deformity, reduction, upper limb) 755.20
lower - *see* Absence, forearm, congenital
upper (complete) (partial) (with absence of distal elements, incomplete) 755.24
with
complete absence of distal elements 755.21
forearm (incomplete) 755.23
artery (congenital) (peripheral) NEC (*see also* Anomaly, peripheral vascular system) 747.60
brain 747.81
cerebral 747.81
coronary 746.85
pulmonary 747.3
umbilical 747.5
atrial septum 745.69
auditory canal (congenital) (external) 744.01
auricle (ear) (with stenosis or atresia of auditory canal), congenital 744.01
bile, biliary duct (common) or passage (congenital) 751.61
bladder (acquired) V45.74
congenital 753.8
bone (congenital) NEC 756.9
marrow 284.9
acquired (secondary) 284.8
congenital 284.09
hereditary 284.09
idiopathic 284.9
skull 756.0
bowel sounds 787.5
brain 740.0
specified part 742.2
breast(s) (acquired) V45.71
congenital 757.6
broad ligament (congenital) 752.19
bronchus (congenital) 748.3
calvarium, calvaria (skull) 756.0

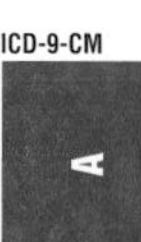
ICD-9-CM
A
Vol. 2

Absence *(Continued)*
canaliculus lacrimalis, congenital 743.65
carpal(s) (congenital) (complete) (partial) (with absence of distal elements, incomplete) (*see also* Deformity, reduction, upper limb) 755.28
with complete absence of distal elements 755.21
cartilage 756.9
caudal spine 756.13
cecum (acquired) (postoperative) (posttraumatic) V45.72
congenital 751.2
cementum 520.4
cerebellum (congenital) (vermis) 742.2
cervix (acquired) (uteri) V45.77
congenital 752.49
chin, congenital 744.89
cilia (congenital) 743.63
acquired 374.89
circulatory system, part NEC 747.89
clavicle 755.51
clitoris (congenital) 752.49
coccyx, congenital 756.13
cold sense (*see also* Disturbance, sensation) 782.0
colon (acquired) (postoperative) V45.72
congenital 751.2
congenital
lumen - *see* Atresia
organ or site NEC - *see* Agenesis
septum - *see* Imperfect, closure
corpus callosum (congenital) 742.2
cricoid cartilage 748.3
diaphragm (congenital) (with hernia) 756.6
with obstruction 756.6
digestive organ(s) or tract, congenital (complete) (partial) 751.8
acquired V45.79
lower 751.5
upper 750.8
ductus arteriosus 747.89
duodenum (acquired) (postoperative) V45.72
congenital 751.1
ear, congenital 744.09
acquired V45.79
auricle 744.01
external 744.01
inner 744.05
lobe, lobule 744.21
middle, except ossicles 744.03
ossicles 744.04
ossicles 744.04
ejaculatory duct (congenital) 752.89
endocrine gland NEC (congenital) 759.2
epididymis (congenital) 752.89
acquired V45.77
epiglottis, congenital 748.3
epileptic (atonic) (typical) (*see also* Epilepsy) 345.0
erythrocyte 284.9
erythropoiesis 284.9
congenital 284.01 ⇐
esophagus (congenital) 750.3
eustachian tube (congenital) 744.24
extremity (acquired)
congenital (*see also* Deformity, reduction) 755.4

Absence *(Continued)*
extremity (acquired) *(Continued)*
lower V49.70
upper V49.60
extrinsic muscle, eye 743.69
eye (acquired) V45.78
adnexa (congenital) 743.69
congenital 743.00
muscle (congenital) 743.69
eyelid (fold), congenital 743.62
acquired 374.89
face
bones NEC 756.0
specified part NEC 744.89
fallopian tube(s) (acquired) V45.77
congenital 752.19
femur, congenital (complete) (partial) (with absence of distal elements, incomplete) (*see also* Deformity, reduction, lower limb) 755.34
with
complete absence of distal elements 755.31
tibia and fibula (incomplete) 755.33
fibrin 790.92
fibrinogen (congenital) 286.3
acquired 286.6
fibula, congenital (complete) (partial) (with absence of distal elements, incomplete) (*see also* Deformity, reduction, lower limb) 755.37
with
complete absence of distal elements 755.31
tibia 755.35
with
complete absence of distal elements 755.31
femur (incomplete) 755.33
with complete absence of distal elements 755.31
finger (acquired) V49.62
congenital (complete) (partial) (*see also* Deformity, reduction, upper limb) 755.29
meaning all fingers (complete) (partial) 755.21
transverse 755.21
fissures of lungs (congenital) 748.5
foot (acquired) V49.73
congenital (complete) 755.31
forearm (acquired) V49.65
congenital (complete) (partial) (with absence of distal elements, incomplete) (*see also* Deformity, reduction, upper limb) 755.25
with
complete absence of distal elements (hand and fingers) 755.21
humerus (incomplete) 755.23
fovea centralis 743.55
fucosidase 271.8
gallbladder (acquired) V45.79
congenital 751.69
gamma globulin (blood) 279.00
genital organs
acquired V45.77
congenital
female 752.89
external 752.49
internal NEC 752.89
male 752.89
penis 752.69

Absence *(Continued)*
genitourinary organs, congenital NEC 752.89
glottis 748.3
gonadal, congenital NEC 758.6
hair (congenital) 757.4
acquired - *see* Alopecia
hand (acquired) V49.63
congenital (complete) (*see also* Deformity, reduction, upper limb) 755.21
heart (congenital) 759.89
acquired - *see* Status, organ replacement
heat sense (*see also* Disturbance, sensation) 782.0
humerus, congenital (complete) (partial) (with absence of distal elements, incomplete) (*see also* Deformity, reduction, upper limb) 755.24
with
complete absence of distal elements 755.21
radius and ulna (incomplete) 755.23
hymen (congenital) 752.49
ileum (acquired) (postoperative) (posttraumatic) V45.72
congenital 751.1
immunoglobulin, isolated NEC 279.03
IgA 279.01
IgG 279.03
IgM 279.02
incus (acquired) 385.24
congenital 744.04
internal ear (congenital) 744.05
intestine (acquired) (small) V45.72
congenital 751.1
large 751.2
large V45.72
congenital 751.2
iris (congenital) 743.45
jaw - *see* Absence, mandible
jejunum (acquired) V45.72
congenital 751.1
joint, congenital NEC 755.8
kidney(s) (acquired) V45.73
congenital 753.0
labium (congenital) (majus) (minus) 752.49
labyrinth, membranous 744.05
lacrimal apparatus (congenital) 743.65
larynx (congenital) 748.3
leg (acquired) V49.70
above knee V49.76
below knee V49.75
congenital (partial) (unilateral) (*see also* Deformity, reduction, lower limb) 755.31
lower (complete) (partial) (with absence of distal elements, incomplete) 755.35
with
complete absence of distal elements (foot and toes) 755.31
thigh (incomplete) 755.33
with complete absence of distal elements 755.31
upper - *see* Absence, femur
lens (congenital) 743.35
acquired 379.31
ligament, broad (congenital) 752.19

Absence *(Continued)*
limb (acquired)
congenital (complete) (partial) (*see also* Deformity, reduction) 755.4
lower 755.30
complete 755.31
incomplete 755.32
longitudinal - *see* Deficiency, lower limb, longitudinal
transverse 755.31
upper 755.20
complete 755.21
incomplete 755.22
longitudinal - *see* Deficiency, upper limb, longitudinal
transverse 755.21
lower NEC V49.70
upper NEC V49.60
lip 750.26
liver (congenital) (lobe) 751.69
lumbar (congenital) (vertebra) 756.13
isthmus 756.11
pars articularis 756.11
lumen - *see* Atresia
lung (bilateral) (congenital) (fissure) (lobe) (unilateral) 748.5
acquired (any part) V45.76
mandible (congenital) 524.09
maxilla (congenital) 524.09
menstruation 626.0
metacarpal(s), congenital (complete) (partial) (with absence of distal elements, incomplete) (*see also* Deformity, reduction, upper limb) 755.28
with all fingers, complete 755.21
metatarsal(s), congenital (complete) (partial) (with absence of distal elements, incomplete) (*see also* Deformity, reduction, lower limb) 755.38
with complete absence of distal elements 755.31
muscle (congenital) (pectoral) 756.81
ocular 743.69
musculoskeletal system (congenital) NEC 756.9
nail(s) (congenital) 757.5
neck, part 744.89
nerve 742.8
nervous system, part NEC 742.8
neutrophil 288.00 ◄Revised
nipple (congenital) 757.6
nose (congenital) 748.1
acquired 738.0
nuclear 742.8
ocular muscle (congenital) 743.69
organ
of Corti (congenital) 744.05
or site
acquired V45.79
congenital NEC 759.89
osseous meatus (ear) 744.03
ovary (acquired) V45.77
congenital 752.0
oviduct (acquired) V45.77
congenital 752.19
pancreas (congenital) 751.7
acquired (postoperative) (posttraumatic) V45.79
parathyroid gland (congenital) 759.2
parotid gland(s) (congenital) 750.21
patella, congenital 755.64
pelvic girdle (congenital) 755.69

Absence *(Continued)*
penis (congenital) 752.69
acquired V45.77
pericardium (congenital) 746.89
perineal body (congenital) 756.81
phalange(s), congenital 755.4
lower limb (complete) (intercalary) (partial) (terminal) (*see also* Deformity, reduction, lower limb) 755.39
meaning all toes (complete) (partial) 755.31
transverse 755.31
upper limb (complete) (intercalary) (partial) (terminal) (*see also* Deformity, reduction, upper limb) 755.29
meaning all digits (complete) (partial) 755.21
transverse 755.21
pituitary gland (congenital) 759.2
postoperative - *see* Absence, by site, acquired
prostate (congenital) 752.89
acquired V45.77
pulmonary
artery 747.3
trunk 747.3
valve (congenital) 746.01
vein 747.49
punctum lacrimale (congenital) 743.65
radius, congenital (complete) (partial) (with absence of distal elements, incomplete) 755.26
with
complete absence of distal elements 755.21
ulna 755.25
with
complete absence of distal elements 755.21
humerus (incomplete) 755.23
ray, congenital 755.4
lower limb (complete) (partial) (*see also* Deformity, reduction, lower limb) 755.38
meaning all rays 755.31
transverse 755.31
upper limb (complete) (partial) (*see also* Deformity, reduction, upper limb) 755.28
meaning all rays 755.21
transverse 755.21
rectum (congenital) 751.2
acquired V45.79
red cell 284.9
acquired (secondary) 284.8
congenital 284.01 ◄Revised
hereditary 284.01 ◄Revised
idiopathic 284.9
respiratory organ (congenital) NEC 748.9
rib (acquired) 738.3
congenital 756.3
roof of orbit (congenital) 742.0
round ligament (congenital) 752.89
sacrum, congenital 756.13
salivary gland(s) (congenital) 750.21
scapula 755.59
scrotum, congenital 752.89
seminal tract or duct (congenital) 752.89
acquired V45.77

Absence *(Continued)*
septum (congenital) - *see also* Imperfect, closure, septum
atrial 745.69
and ventricular 745.7
between aorta and pulmonary artery 745.0
ventricular 745.3
and atrial 745.7
sex chromosomes 758.81
shoulder girdle, congenital (complete) (partial) 755.59
skin (congenital) 757.39
skull bone 756.0
with
anencephalus 740.0
encephalocele 742.0
hydrocephalus 742.3
with spina bifida (*see also* Spina bifida) 741.0
microcephalus 742.1
spermatic cord (congenital) 752.89
spinal cord 742.59
spine, congenital 756.13
spleen (congenital) 759.0
acquired V45.79
sternum, congenital 756.3
stomach (acquired) (partial) (postoperative) V45.75
with postgastric surgery syndrome 564.2
congenital 750.7
submaxillary gland(s) (congenital) 750.21
superior vena cava (congenital) 747.49
tarsal(s), congenital (complete) (partial) (with absence of distal elements, incomplete) (*see also* Deformity, reduction, lower limb) 755.38
teeth, tooth (congenital) 520.0
with abnormal spacing 524.30
acquired 525.10
with malocclusion 524.30
due to
caries 525.13
extraction 525.10
periodontal disease 525.12
trauma 525.11
tendon (congenital) 756.81
testis (congenital) 752.89
acquired V45.77
thigh (acquired) 736.89
thumb (acquired) V49.61
congenital 755.29
thymus gland (congenital) 759.2
thyroid (gland) (surgical) 246.8
with hypothyroidism 244.0
cartilage, congenital 748.3
congenital 243
tibia, congenital (complete) (partial) (with absence of distal elements, incomplete) (*see also* Deformity, reduction, lower limb) 755.36
with
complete absence of distal elements 755.31
fibula 755.35
with
complete absence of distal elements 755.31
femur (incomplete) 755.33
with complete absence of distal elements 755.31

Absence *(Continued)*
toe (acquired) V49.72
congenital (complete) (partial) 755.39
meaning all toes 755.31
transverse 755.31
great V49.71
tongue (congenital) 750.11
tooth, teeth (congenital) 520.0
with abnormal spacing 524.30
acquired 525.10
with malocclusion 524.30
due to
caries 525.13
extraction 525.10
periodontal disease 525.12
trauma 525.11
trachea (cartilage) (congenital) (rings) 748.3
transverse aortic arch (congenital) 747.21
tricuspid valve 746.1
ulna, congenital (complete) (partial) (with absence of distal elements, incomplete) (*see also* Deformity, reduction, upper limb) 755.27
with
complete absence of distal elements 755.21
radius 755.25
with
complete absence of distal elements 755.21
humerus (incomplete) 755.23
umbilical artery (congenital) 747.5
ureter (congenital) 753.4
acquired V45.74
urethra, congenital 753.8
acquired V45.74
urinary system, part NEC, congenital 753.8
acquired V45.74
uterus (acquired) V45.77
congenital 752.3
uvula (congenital) 750.26
vagina, congenital 752.49
acquired V45.77
vas deferens (congenital) 752.89
acquired V45.77
vein (congenital) (peripheral) NEC (*see also* Anomaly, peripheral vascular system) 747.60
brain 747.81
great 747.49
portal 747.49
pulmonary 747.49
vena cava (congenital) (inferior) (superior) 747.49
ventral horn cell 742.59
ventricular septum 745.3
vermis of cerebellum 742.2
vertebra, congenital 756.13
vulva, congenital 752.49
Absentia epileptica (*see also* Epilepsy) 345.0
Absinthemia (*see also* Dependence) 304.6
Absinthism (*see also* Dependence) 304.6
Absorbent system disease 459.89
Absorption
alcohol, through placenta or breast milk 760.71
antibiotics, through placenta or breast milk 760.74
anticonvulsants, through placenta or breast milk 760.77
antifungals, through placenta or breast milk 760.74

Absorption *(Continued)*
anti-infective, through placenta or breast milk 760.74
antimetabolics, through placenta or breast milk 760.78
chemical NEC 989.9
specified chemical or substance - *see* Table of Drugs and Chemicals
through placenta or breast milk (fetus or newborn) 760.70
alcohol 760.71
anticonvulsants 760.77
antifungals 760.74
anti-infective agents 760.74
antimetabolics 760.78
cocaine 760.75
"crack" 760.75
diethylstilbestrol [DES] 760.76
hallucinogenic agents 760.73
medicinal agents NEC 760.79
narcotics 760.72
obstetric anesthetic or analgesic drug 763.5
specified agent NEC 760.79
suspected, affecting management of pregnancy 655.5
cocaine, through placenta or breast milk 760.75
drug NEC (*see also* Reaction, drug)
through placenta or breast milk (fetus or newborn) 760.70
alcohol 760.71
anticonvulsants 760.77
antifungals 760.74
anti-infective agents 760.74
antimetabolics 760.78
cocaine 760.75
"crack" 760.75
diethylstilbestrol (DES) 760.76
hallucinogenic agents 760.73
medicinal agents NEC 760.79
narcotics 760.72
obstetric anesthetic or analgesic drug 763.5
specified agent NEC 760.79
suspected, affecting management of pregnancy 655.5
fat, disturbance 579.8
hallucinogenic agents, through placenta or breast milk 760.73
immune sera, through placenta or breast milk 760.79
lactose defect 271.3
medicinal agents NEC, through placenta or breast milk 760.79
narcotics, through placenta or breast milk 760.72
noxious substance - *see* Absorption, chemical
protein, disturbance 579.8
pus or septic, general - *see* Septicemia
quinine, through placenta or breast milk 760.74
toxic substance - *see* Absorption, chemical
uremic - *see* Uremia
Abstinence symptoms or syndrome
alcohol 291.81
drug 292.0
Abt-Letterer-Siwe syndrome (acute histiocytosis X) (M9722/3) 202.5
Abulia 799.89
Abulomania 301.6
Abuse
adult 995.80
emotional 995.82

Abuse *(Continued)*
adult *(Continued)*
multiple forms 995.85
neglect (nutritional) 995.84
physical 995.81
psychological 995.82
sexual 995.83
alcohol (*see also* Alcoholism) 305.0
dependent 303.9
nondependent 305.0
child 995.50
counseling
perpetrator
non-parent V62.83
parent V61.22
victim V61.21
emotional 995.51
multiple forms 995.59
neglect (nutritional) 995.52
physical 995.54
shaken infant syndrome 995.55
psychological 995.51
sexual 995.53
drugs, nondependent 305.9

Note Use the following fifth-digit subclassification with the following codes: 305.0, 305.2-305.9:

0 unspecified
1 continuous
2 episodic
3 in remission

amphetamine type 305.7
antidepressants 305.8
anxiolytic 305.4
barbiturates 305.4
caffeine 305.9
cannabis 305.2
cocaine type 305.6
hallucinogens 305.3
hashish 305.2
hypnotic 305.4
inhalant 305.9
LSD 305.3
marijuana 305.2
mixed 305.9
morphine type 305.5
opioid type 305.5
phencyclidine (PCP) 305.9
sedative 305.4
specified NEC 305.9
tranquilizers 305.4
spouse 995.80
tobacco 305.1
Acalcerosis 275.40
Acalcicosis 275.40
Acalculia 784.69
developmental 315.1
Acanthocheilonemiasis 125.4
Acanthocytosis 272.5
Acanthokeratodermia 701.1
Acantholysis 701.8
bullosa 757.39
Acanthoma (benign) (M8070/0) - *see also* Neoplasm, by site, benign
malignant (M8070/3) - *see* Neoplasm, by site, malignant
Acanthosis (acquired) (nigricans) 701.2
adult 701.2
benign (congenital) 757.39
congenital 757.39
glycogenic
esophagus 530.89

Acanthosis *(Continued)*
juvenile 701.2
tongue 529.8
Acanthrocytosis 272.5
Acapnia 276.3
Acarbia 276.2
Acardia 759.89
Acardiacus amorphus 759.89
Acardiotrophia 429.1
Acardius 759.89
Acariasis 133.9
sarcoptic 133.0
Acaridiasis 133.9
Acarinosis 133.9
Acariosis 133.9
Acarodermatitis 133.9
urticarioides 133.9
Acarophobia 300.29
Acatalasemia 277.89
Acatalasia 277.89
Acatamathesia 784.69
Acataphasia 784.5
Acathisia 781.0
due to drugs 333.99
Acceleration, accelerated
atrioventricular conduction 426.7
idioventricular rhythm 427.89
Accessory (congenital)
adrenal gland 759.1
anus 751.5
appendix 751.5
atrioventricular conduction 426.7
auditory ossicles 744.04
auricle (ear) 744.1
autosome(s) NEC 758.5
21 or 22 758.0
biliary duct or passage 751.69
bladder 753.8
blood vessels (peripheral) (congenital) NEC (*see also* Anomaly, peripheral vascular system) 747.60
cerebral 747.81
coronary 746.85
bone NEC 756.9
foot 755.67
breast tissue, axilla 757.6
carpal bones 755.56
cecum 751.5
cervix 752.49
chromosome(s) NEC 758.5
13-15 758.1
16-18 758.2
21 or 22 758.0
autosome(s) NEC 758.5
D_1 758.1
E_3 758.2
G 758.0
sex 758.81
coronary artery 746.85
cusp(s), heart valve NEC 746.89
pulmonary 746.09
cystic duct 751.69
digits 755.00
ear (auricle) (lobe) 744.1
endocrine gland NEC 759.2
external os 752.49
eyelid 743.62
eye muscle 743.69
face bone(s) 756.0
fallopian tube (fimbria) (ostium) 752.19
fingers 755.01
foreskin 605
frontonasal process 756.0
gallbladder 751.69

Accessory *(Continued)*
genital organ(s)
female 752.89
external 752.49
internal NEC 752.89
male NEC 752.89
penis 752.69
genitourinary organs NEC 752.89
heart 746.89
valve NEC 746.89
pulmonary 746.09
hepatic ducts 751.69
hymen 752.49
intestine (large) (small) 751.5
kidney 753.3
lacrimal canal 743.65
leaflet, heart valve NEC 746.89
pulmonary 746.09
ligament, broad 752.19
liver (duct) 751.69
lobule (ear) 744.1
lung (lobe) 748.69
muscle 756.82
navicular of carpus 755.56
nervous system, part NEC 742.8
nipple 757.6
nose 748.1
organ or site NEC - *see* Anomaly, specified type NEC
ovary 752.0
oviduct 752.19
pancreas 751.7
parathyroid gland 759.2
parotid gland (and duct) 750.22
pituitary gland 759.2
placental lobe - *see* Placenta, abnormal
preauricular appendage 744.1
prepuce 605
renal arteries (multiple) 747.62
rib 756.3
cervical 756.2
roots (teeth) 520.2
salivary gland 750.22
sesamoids 755.8
sinus - *see* Condition
skin tags 757.39
spleen 759.0
sternum 756.3
submaxillary gland 750.22
tarsal bones 755.67
teeth, tooth 520.1
causing crowding 524.31
tendon 756.89
thumb 755.01
thymus gland 759.2
thyroid gland 759.2
toes 755.02
tongue 750.13
tragus 744.1
ureter 753.4
urethra 753.8
urinary organ or tract NEC 753.8
uterus 752.2
vagina 752.49
valve, heart NEC 746.89
pulmonary 746.09
vertebra 756.19
vocal cords 748.3
vulva 752.49
Accident, accidental - *see also* condition
birth NEC 767.9
cardiovascular (*see also* Disease, cardiovascular) 429.2
cerebral (*see also* Disease, cerebrovascular, acute) 434.91

Accident, accidental *(Continued)*
cerebrovascular (current) (CVA) (*see also* Disease, cerebrovascular, acute) 434.91
embolic 434.11
healed or old V12.59
hemorrhagic - *see* Hemorrhage, brain
impending 435.9
ischemic 434.91
late effect - *see* Late effect(s) (of) cerebrovascular disease
postoperative 997.02
thrombotic 434.01
coronary (*see also* Infarct, myocardium) 410.9
craniovascular (*see also* Disease, cerebrovascular, acute) 436
during pregnancy, to mother, affecting fetus or newborn 760.5
heart, cardiac (*see also* Infarct, myocardium) 410.9
intrauterine 779.89
vascular - *see* Disease, cerebrovascular, acute
Accommodation
disorder of 367.51
drug-induced 367.89
toxic 367.89
insufficiency of 367.4
paralysis of 367.51
hysterical 300.11
spasm of 367.53
Accouchement - *see* Delivery
Accreta placenta (without hemorrhage) 667.0
with hemorrhage 666.0
Accretio cordis (nonrheumatic) 423.1
Accretions on teeth 523.6
Accumulation secretion, prostate 602.8
Acephalia, acephalism, acephaly 740.0
Acephalic 740.0
Acephalobrachia 759.89
Acephalocardia 759.89
Acephalocardius 759.89
Acephalochiria 759.89
Acephalochirus 759.89
Acephalogaster 759.89
Acephalostomus 759.89
Acephalothorax 759.89
Acephalus 740.0
Acetonemia 790.6
diabetic 250.1
Acetonglycosuria 982.8
Acetonuria 791.6
Achalasia 530.0
cardia 530.0
digestive organs, congenital NEC 751.8
esophagus 530.0
pelvirectal 751.3
psychogenic 306.4
pylorus 750.5
sphincteral NEC 564.89
Achard-Thiers syndrome (adrenogenital) 255.2
Ache(s) - *see* Pain
Acheilia 750.26
Acheiria 755.21
Achillobursitis 726.71
Achillodynia 726.71
Achlorhydria, achlorhydric 536.0
anemia 280.9
diarrhea 536.0
neurogenic 536.0
postvagotomy 564.2

Achlorhydria, achlorhydric *(Continued)*
psychogenic 306.4
secondary to vagotomy 564.2
Achloroblepsia 368.52
Achloropsia 368.52
Acholia 575.8
Acholuric jaundice (familial) (splenomegalic) (*see also* Spherocytosis) 282.0
acquired 283.9
Achondroplasia 756.4
Achrestic anemia 281.8
Achroacytosis, lacrimal gland 375.00
tuberculous (*see also* Tuberculosis) 017.3
Achroma, cutis 709.00
Achromate (congenital) 368.54
Achromatopia 368.54
Achromatopsia (congenital) 368.54
Achromia
congenital 270.2
parasitica 111.0
unguium 703.8
Achylia
gastrica 536.8
neurogenic 536.3
psychogenic 306.4
pancreatica 577.1
Achylosis 536.8
Acid
burn - *see also* Burn, by site
from swallowing acid - *see* Burn, internal organs
deficiency
amide nicotinic 265.2
amino 270.9
ascorbic 267
folic 266.2
nicotinic (amide) 265.2
pantothenic 266.2
intoxication 276.2
peptic disease 536.8
stomach 536.8
psychogenic 306.4
Acidemia 276.2
arginosuccinic 270.6
fetal
affecting management of pregnancy 656.3
before onset of labor, in liveborn infant 768.2
during labor and delivery, in liveborn infant 768.3 (Revised)
intrauterine 656.3
newborn 775.81 (New)
unspecified as to time of onset, in liveborn infant 768.4
pipecolic 270.7
Acidity, gastric (high) (low) 536.8
psychogenic 306.4
Acidocytopenia 288.59 (Revised)
Acidocytosis 288.3
Acidopenia 288.59 (Revised)
Acidosis 276.2
diabetic 250.1
fetal
affecting management of pregnancy 656.8
affecting newborn 775.81 (Revised)
kidney tubular 588.89
lactic 276.2
metabolic NEC 276.2
with respiratory acidosis 276.4
of newborn 775.81 (New)
late, of newborn 775.7
newborn 775.81 (New)

Acidosis *(Continued)*
renal
hyperchloremic 588.89
tubular (distal) (proximal) 588.89
respiratory 276.2
complicated by
metabolic acidosis 276.4
of newborn 775.81 (New)
metabolic alkalosis 276.4
Aciduria 791.9
arginosuccinic 270.6
beta-aminoisobutyric (BAIB) 277.2
glutaric
type I 270.7
type II (type IIA, IIB, IIC) 277.85
type III 277.86
glycolic 271.8
methylmalonic 270.3
with glycinemia 270.7
organic 270.9
orotic (congenital) (hereditary) (pyrimidine deficiency) 281.4
Acladiosis 111.8
skin 111.8
Aclasis
diaphyseal 756.4
tarsoepiphyseal 756.59
Acleistocardia 745.5
Aclusion 524.4
Acmesthesia 782.0
Acne (pustular) (vulgaris) 706.1
agminata (*see also* Tuberculosis) 017.0
artificialis 706.1
atrophica 706.0
cachecticorum (Hebra) 706.1
conglobata 706.1
conjunctiva 706.1
cystic 706.1
decalvans 704.09
erythematosa 695.3
eyelid 706.1
frontalis 706.0
indurata 706.1
keloid 706.1
lupoid 706.0
necrotic, necrotica 706.0
miliaris 704.8
neonatal 706.1
nodular 706.1
occupational 706.1
papulosa 706.1
rodens 706.0
rosacea 695.3
scorbutica 267
scrofulosorum (Bazin) (*see also* Tuberculosis) 017.0
summer 692.72
tropical 706.1
varioliformis 706.0
Acneiform drug eruptions 692.3
Acnitis (primary) (*see also* Tuberculosis) 017.0
Acomia 704.00
Acontractile bladder 344.61
Aconuresis (*see also* Incontinence) 788.30
Acosta's disease 993.2
Acousma 780.1
Acoustic - *see* condition
Acousticophobia 300.29
Acquired - *see* condition
Acquired immune deficiency syndrome - *see* Human immunodeficiency virus (disease) (illness) (infection)

Acquired immunodeficiency syndrome - *see* Human immunodeficiency virus (disease) (illness) (infection)
Acragnosis 781.99
Acrania 740.0
Acroagnosis 781.99
Acroasphyxia, chronic 443.89
Acrobrachycephaly 756.0
Acrobystiolith 608.89
Acrobystitis 607.2
Acrocephalopolysyndactyly 755.55
Acrocephalosyndactyly 755.55
Acrocephaly 756.0
Acrochondrohyperplasia 759.82
Acrocyanosis 443.89
newborn 770.83
meaning transient blue hands and feet - *omit code*
Acrodermatitis 686.8
atrophicans (chronica) 701.8
continua (Hallopeau) 696.1
enteropathica 686.8
Hallopeau's 696.1
perstans 696.1
pustulosa continua 696.1
recalcitrant pustular 696.1
Acrodynia 985.0
Acrodysplasia 755.55
Acrohyperhidrosis (*see also* Hyperhidrosis) 780.8
Acrokeratosis verruciformis 757.39
Acromastitis 611.0
Acromegaly, acromegalia (skin) 253.0
Acromelalgia 443.82
Acromicria, acromikria 756.59
Acronyx 703.0
Acropachy, thyroid (*see also* Thyrotoxicosis) 242.9
Acropachyderma 757.39
Acroparesthesia 443.89
simple (Schultz's type) 443.89
vasomotor (Nothnagel's type) 443.89
Acropathy thyroid (*see also* Thyrotoxicosis) 242.9
Acrophobia 300.29
Acroposthitis 607.2
Acroscleriasis (*see also* Scleroderma) 710.1
Acroscleroderma (*see also* Scleroderma) 710.1
Acrosclerosis (*see also* Scleroderma) 710.1
Acrosphacelus 785.4
Acrosphenosyndactylia 755.55
Acrospiroma, eccrine (M8402/0) - *see* Neoplasm, skin, benign
Acrostealgia 732.9
Acrosyndactyly (*see also* Syndactylism) 755.10
Acrotrophodynia 991.4
Actinic - *see also* condition
cheilitis (due to sun) 692.72
chronic NEC 692.74
due to radiation, except from sun 692.82
conjunctivitis 370.24
dermatitis (due to sun) (*see also* Dermatitis, actinic) 692.70
due to
roentgen rays or radioactive substance 692.82
ultraviolet radiation, except from sun 692.82
sun NEC 692.70
elastosis solare 692.74
granuloma 692.73

Actinic *(Continued)*
  keratitis 370.24
  ophthalmia 370.24
  reticuloid 692.73
Actinobacillosis, general 027.8
Actinobacillus
  lignieresii 027.8
  mallei 024
  muris 026.1
Actinocutitis NEC (*see also* Dermatitis, actinic) 692.70
Actinodermatitis NEC (*see also* Dermatitis, actinic) 692.70
Actinomyces
  israelii (infection) - *see* Actinomycosis
  muris-ratti (infection) 026.1
Actinomycosis, actinomycotic 039.9
  with
    pneumonia 039.1
  abdominal 039.2
  cervicofacial 039.3
  cutaneous 039.0
  pulmonary 039.1
  specified site NEC 039.8
  thoracic 039.1
Actinoneuritis 357.89
Action, heart
  disorder 427.9
    postoperative 997.1
  irregular 427.9
    postoperative 997.1
    psychogenic 306.2
Active - *see* condition
Activity decrease, functional 780.99
Acute - *see also* condition
  abdomen NEC 789.0
  gallbladder (*see also* Cholecystitis, acute) 575.0
Acyanoblepsia 368.53
Acyanopsia 368.53
Acystia 753.8
Acystinervia - *see* Neurogenic, bladder
Acystineuria - *see* Neurogenic, bladder
Adactylia, adactyly (congenital) 755.4
  lower limb (complete) (intercalary) (partial) (terminal) (*see also* Deformity, reduction, lower limb) 755.39
    meaning all digits (complete) (partial) 755.31
    transverse (complete) (partial) 755.31
  upper limb (complete) (intercalary) (partial) (terminal) (*see also* Deformity, reduction, upper limb) 755.29
    meaning all digits (complete) (partial) 755.21
    transverse (complete) (partial) 755.21
Adair-Dighton syndrome (brittle bones and blue sclera, deafness) 756.51
Adamantinoblastoma (M9310/0) - *see* Ameloblastoma
Adamantinoma (M9310/0) - *see* Ameloblastoma
Adamantoblastoma (M9310/0) - *see* Ameloblastoma
Adams-Stokes (-Morgagni) disease or syndrome (syncope with heart block) 426.9
Adaptation reaction (*see also* Reaction, adjustment) 309.9
ADEM (acute disseminated encephalomyelitis)(postinfectious) 136.9 *[323.61]* (Revised)
  infectious 136.9 *[323.61]* (Revised)
  noninfectious 323.81 (Revised)
Addiction - *see also* Dependence
  absinthe 304.6
  alcoholic (ethyl) (methyl) (wood) 303.9
    complicating pregnancy, childbirth, or puerperium 648.4
      affecting fetus or newborn 760.71
    suspected damage to fetus affecting management of pregnancy 655.4
  drug (*see also* Dependence) 304.9
  ethyl alcohol 303.9
  heroin 304.0
  hospital 301.51
  methyl alcohol 303.9
  methylated spirit 303.9
  morphine (-like substances) 304.0
  nicotine 305.1
  opium 304.0
  tobacco 305.1
  wine 303.9
Addison's
  anemia (pernicious) 281.0
  disease (bronze) (primary adrenal insufficiency) 255.4
    tuberculous (*see also* Tuberculosis) 017.6
  keloid (morphea) 701.0
  melanoderma (adrenal cortical hypofunction) 255.4
Addison-Biermer anemia (pernicious) 281.0
Addison-Gull disease - *see* Xanthoma
Addisonian crisis or melanosis (acute adrenocortical insufficiency) 255.4
Additional - *see also* Accessory
  chromosome(s) 758.5
    13-15 758.1
    16-18 758.2
    21 758.0
    autosome(s) NEC 758.5
    sex 758.81
Adduction contracture, hip or other joint - *see* Contraction, joint
Adenasthenia gastrica 536.0
Aden fever 061
Adenitis (*see also* Lymphadenitis) 289.3
  acute, unspecified site 683
    epidemic infectious 075
  axillary 289.3
    acute 683
    chronic or subacute 289.1
  Bartholin's gland 616.89 (Revised)
  bulbourethral gland (*see also* Urethritis) 597.89
  cervical 289.3
    acute 683
    chronic or subacute 289.1
  chancroid (Ducrey's bacillus) 099.0
  chronic (any lymph node, except mesenteric) 289.1
    mesenteric 289.2
  Cowper's gland (*see also* Urethritis) 597.89
  epidemic, acute 075
  gangrenous 683
  gonorrheal NEC 098.89
  groin 289.3
    acute 683
    chronic or subacute 289.1
  infectious 075
  inguinal (region) 289.3
    acute 683
    chronic or subacute 289.1
  lymph gland or node, except mesenteric 289.3
Adenitis *(Continued)*
  lymph gland or node, except mesenteric *(Continued)*
    acute 683
    chronic or subacute 289.1
    mesenteric (acute) (chronic) (nonspecific) (subacute) 289.2
  mesenteric (acute) (chronic) (nonspecific) (subacute) 289.2
    due to Pasteurella multocida (P. septica) 027.2
  parotid gland (suppurative) 527.2
  phlegmonous 683
  salivary duct or gland (any) (recurring) (suppurative) 527.2
  scrofulous (*see also* Tuberculosis) 017.2
  septic 289.3
  Skene's duct or gland (*see also* Urethritis) 597.89
  strumous, tuberculous (*see also* Tuberculosis) 017.2
  subacute, unspecified site 289.1
  sublingual gland (suppurative) 527.2
  submandibular gland (suppurative) 527.2
  submaxillary gland (suppurative) 527.2
  suppurative 683
  tuberculous - *see* Tuberculosis, lymph gland
  urethral gland (*see also* Urethritis) 597.89
  venereal NEC 099.8
  Wharton's duct (suppurative) 527.2
Adenoacanthoma (M8570/3) - *see* Neoplasm, by site, malignant
Adenoameloblastoma (M9300/0) 213.1
  upper jaw (bone) 213.0
Adenocarcinoma (M8140/3) - *see also* Neoplasm, by site, malignant

> Note The list of adjectival modifiers below is not exhaustive. A description of adenocarcinoma that does not appear in this list should be coded in the same manner as carcinoma with that description. Thus, "mixed acidophil-basophil adenocarcinoma" should be coded in the same manner as "mixed acidophil-basophil carcinoma," which appears in the list under "Carcinoma."
>
> Except where otherwise indicated, the morphological varieties of adenocarcinoma in the list below should be coded by site as for "Neoplasm, malignant."

  with
    apocrine metaplasia (M8573/3)
    cartilaginous (and osseous) metaplasia (M8571/3)
    osseous (and cartilaginous) metaplasia (M8571/3)
    spindle cell metaplasia (M8572/3)
    squamous metaplasia (M8570/3)
  acidophil (M8280/3)
    specified site - *see* Neoplasm, by site, malignant
    unspecified site 194.3
  acinar (M8550/3)
  acinic cell (M8550/3)

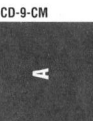

Adenocarcinoma *(Continued)*
adrenal cortical (M8370/3) 194.0
alveolar (M8251/3)
and
epidermoid carcinoma, mixed (M8560/3)
squamous cell carcinoma, mixed (M8560/3)
apocrine (M8401/3)
breast - *see* Neoplasm, breast, malignant
specified site NEC - *see* Neoplasm, skin, malignant
unspecified site 173.9
basophil (M8300/3)
specified site - *see* Neoplasm, by site, malignant
unspecified site 194.3
bile duct type (M8160/3)
liver 155.1
specified site NEC - *see* Neoplasm, by site, malignant
unspecified site 155.1
bronchiolar (M8250/3) - *see* Neoplasm, lung, malignant
ceruminous (M8420/3) 173.2
chromophobe (M8270/3)
specified site - *see* Neoplasm, by site, malignant
unspecified site 194.3
clear cell (mesonephroid type) (M8310/3)
colloid (M8480/3)
cylindroid type (M8200/3)
diffuse type (M8145/3)
specified site - *see* Neoplasm, by site, malignant
unspecified site 151.9
duct (infiltrating) (M8500/3)
with Paget's disease (M8541/3) - *see* Neoplasm, breast, malignant
specified site - *see* Neoplasm, by site, malignant
unspecified site 174.9
embryonal (M9070/3)
endometrioid (M8380/3) - *see* Neoplasm, by site, malignant
eosinophil (M8280/3)
specified site - *see* Neoplasm, by site, malignant
unspecified site 194.3
follicular (M8330/3)
and papillary (M8340/3) 193
moderately differentiated type (M8332/3) 193
pure follicle type (M8331/3) 193
specified site - *see* Neoplasm, by site, malignant
trabecular type (M8332/3) 193
unspecified type 193
well differentiated type (M8331/3) 193
gelatinous (M8480/3)
granular cell (M8320/3)
Hürthle cell (M8290/3) 193
in
adenomatous
polyp (M8210/3)
polyposis coli (M8220/3) 153.9
polypoid adenoma (M8210/3)
tubular adenoma (M8210/3)
villous adenoma (M8261/3)
infiltrating duct (M8500/3)
with Paget's disease (M8541/3) - *see* Neoplasm, breast, malignant

Adenocarcinoma *(Continued)*
infiltrating duct *(Continued)*
specified site - *see* Neoplasm, by site, malignant
unspecified site 174.9
inflammatory (M8530/3)
specified site - *see* Neoplasm, by site, malignant
unspecified site 174.9
in situ (M8140/2) - *see* Neoplasm, by site, in situ
intestinal type (M8144/3)
specified site - *see* Neoplasm, by site, malignant
unspecified site 151.9
intraductal (noninfiltrating) (M8500/2)
papillary (M8503/2)
specified site - *see* Neoplasm, by site, in situ
unspecified site 233.0
specified site - *see* Neoplasm, by site, in situ
unspecified site 233.0
islet cell (M8150/3)
and exocrine, mixed (M8154/3)
specified site - *see* Neoplasm, by site, malignant
unspecified site 157.9
pancreas 157.4
specified site NEC - *see* Neoplasm, by site, malignant
unspecified site 157.4
lobular (M8520/3)
specified site - *see* Neoplasm, by site, malignant
unspecified site 174.9
medullary (M8510/3)
mesonephric (M9110/3)
mixed cell (M8323/3)
mucinous (M8480/3)
mucin-producing (M8481/3)
mucoid (M8480/3) - *see also* Neoplasm, by site, malignant
cell (M8300/3)
specified site - *see* Neoplasm, by site, malignant
unspecified site 194.3
nonencapsulated sclerosing (M8350/3) 193
oncocytic (M8290/3)
oxyphilic (M8290/3)
papillary (M8260/3)
and follicular (M8340/3) 193
intraductal (noninfiltrating) (M8503/2)
specified site - *see* Neoplasm, by site, in situ
unspecified site 233.0
serous (M8460/3)
specified site - *see* Neoplasm, by site, malignant
unspecified site 183.0
papillocystic (M8450/3)
specified site - *see* Neoplasm, by site, malignant
unspecified site 183.0
pseudomucinous (M8470/3)
specified site - *see* Neoplasm, by site, malignant
unspecified site 183.0
renal cell (M8312/3) 189.0
sebaceous (M8410/3)
serous (M8441/3) - *see also* Neoplasm, by site, malignant

Adenocarcinoma *(Continued)*
serous *(Continued)*
papillary
specified site - *see* Neoplasm, by site, malignant
unspecified site 183.0
signet ring cell (M8490/3)
superficial spreading (M8143/3)
sweat gland (M8400/3) - *see* Neoplasm, skin, malignant
trabecular (M8190/3)
tubular (M8211/3)
villous (M8262/3)
water-clear cell (M8322/3) 194.1
Adenofibroma (M9013/0)
clear cell (M8313/0) - *see* Neoplasm, by site, benign
endometrioid (M8381/0) 220
borderline malignancy (M8381/1) 236.2
malignant (M8381/3) 183.0
mucinous (M9015/0)
specified site - *see* Neoplasm, by site, benign
unspecified site 220
prostate 600.20
with ⬅
other lower urinary tract symptoms (LUTS) 600.21 ◀
urinary ◀
obstruction 600.21 ◀
retention 600.21 ◀
serous (M9014/0)
specified site - *see* Neoplasm, by site, benign
unspecified site 220
specified site - *see* Neoplasm, by site, benign
unspecified site 220
Adenofibrosis
breast 610.2
endometrioid 617.0
Adenoiditis 474.01
acute 463
chronic 474.01
with chronic tonsillitis 474.02
Adenoids (congenital) (of nasal fossa) 474.9
hypertrophy 474.12
vegetations 474.2
Adenolipomatosis (symmetrical) 272.8
Adenolymphoma (M8561/0)
specified site - *see* Neoplasm, by site, benign
unspecified 210.2
Adenoma (sessile) (M8140/0) - *see also* Neoplasm, by site, benign

Note Except where otherwise indicated, the morphological varieties of adenoma in the list below should be coded by site as for "Neoplasm, benign."

acidophil (M8280/0)
specified site - *see* Neoplasm, by site, benign
unspecified site 227.3
acinar (cell) (M8550/0)
acinic cell (M8550/0)
adrenal (cortex) (cortical) (functioning) (M8370/0) 227.0
clear cell type (M8373/0) 227.0

- **Adenoma** *(Continued)*
  - adrenal *(Continued)*
    - compact cell type (M8371/0) 227.0
    - glomerulosa cell type (M8374/0) 227.0
    - heavily pigmented variant (M8372/0) 227.0
    - mixed cell type (M8375/0) 227.0
  - alpha cell (M8152/0)
    - pancreas 211.7
    - specified site NEC - *see* Neoplasm, by site, benign
    - unspecified site 211.7
  - alveolar (M8251/0)
  - apocrine (M8401/0)
    - breast 217
    - specified site NEC - *see* Neoplasm, skin, benign
    - unspecified site 216.9
  - basal cell (M8147/0)
  - basophil (M8300/0)
    - specified site - *see* Neoplasm, by site, benign
    - unspecified site 227.3
  - beta cell (M8151/0)
    - pancreas 211.7
    - specified site NEC - *see* Neoplasm, by site, benign
    - unspecified site 211.7
  - bile duct (M8160/0) 211.5
  - black (M8372/0) 227.0
  - bronchial (M8140/1) 235.7
    - carcinoid type (M8240/3) - *see* Neoplasm, lung, malignant
    - cylindroid type (M8200/3) - *see* Neoplasm, lung, malignant
  - ceruminous (M8420/0) 216.2
  - chief cell (M8321/0) 227.1
  - chromophobe (M8270/0)
    - specified site - *see* Neoplasm, by site, benign
    - unspecified site 227.3
  - clear cell (M8310/0)
  - colloid (M8334/0)
    - specified site - *see* Neoplasm, by site, benign
    - unspecified site 226
  - cylindroid type, bronchus (M8200/3) - *see* Neoplasm, lung, malignant
  - duct (M8503/0)
  - embryonal (M8191/0)
  - endocrine, multiple (M8360/1)
    - single specified site - *see* Neoplasm, by site, uncertain behavior
    - two or more specified sites 237.4
    - unspecified site 237.4
  - endometrioid (M8380/0) - *see also* Neoplasm, by site, benign
    - borderline malignancy (M8380/1) - *see* Neoplasm, by site, uncertain behavior
  - eosinophil (M8280/0)
    - specified site - *see* Neoplasm, by site, benign
    - unspecified site 227.3
  - fetal (M8333/0)
    - specified site - *see* Neoplasm, by site, benign
    - unspecified site 226
  - follicular (M8330/0)
    - specified site - *see* Neoplasm, by site, benign
    - unspecified site 226
  - hepatocellular (M8170/0) 211.5
- **Adenoma** *(Continued)*
  - Hürthle cell (M8290/0) 226
  - intracystic papillary (M8504/0)
  - islet cell (functioning) (M8150/0)
    - pancreas 211.7
    - specified site NEC - *see* Neoplasm, by site, benign
    - unspecified site 211.7
  - liver cell (M8170/0) 211.5
  - macrofollicular (M8334/0)
    - specified site NEC - *see* Neoplasm, by site, benign
    - unspecified site 226
  - malignant, malignum (M8140/3) - *see* Neoplasm, by site, malignant
  - mesonephric (M9110/0)
  - microfollicular (M8333/0)
    - specified site - *see* Neoplasm, by site, benign
    - unspecified site 226
  - mixed cell (M8323/0)
  - monomorphic (M8146/0)
  - mucinous (M8480/0)
  - mucoid cell (M8300/0)
    - specified site - *see* Neoplasm, by site, benign
    - unspecified site 227.3
  - multiple endocrine (M8360/1)
    - single specified site - *see* Neoplasm, by site, uncertain behavior
    - two or more specified sites 237.4
    - unspecified site 237.4
  - nipple (M8506/0) 217
  - oncocytic (M8290/0)
  - oxyphilic (M8290/0)
  - papillary (M8260/0) - *see also* Neoplasm, by site, benign
    - intracystic (M8504/0)
  - papillotubular (M8263/0)
  - Pick's tubular (M8640/0)
    - specified site - *see* Neoplasm, by site, benign
    - unspecified site
      - female 220
      - male 222.0
  - pleomorphic (M8940/0)
  - polypoid (M8210/0)
  - prostate (benign) 600.20
    - with (Revised)
      - other lower urinary tract symptoms (LUTS) 600.21 ◀
      - urinary ◀
        - obstruction 600.21 ◀
        - retention 600.21 ◀
  - rete cell 222.0
  - sebaceous, sebaceum (gland) (senile) (M8410/0) - *see also* Neoplasm, skin, benign
    - disseminata 759.5
  - Sertoli cell (M8640/0)
    - specified site - *see* Neoplasm, by site, benign
    - unspecified site
      - female 220
      - male 222.0
  - skin appendage (M8390/0) - *see* Neoplasm, skin, benign
  - sudoriferous gland (M8400/0) - *see* Neoplasm, skin, benign
  - sweat gland or duct (M8400/0) - *see* Neoplasm, skin, benign
  - testicular (M8640/0)
    - specified site - *see* Neoplasm, by site, benign
- **Adenoma** *(Continued)*
  - testicular *(Continued)*
    - unspecified site
      - female 220
      - male 222.0
  - thyroid 226
  - trabecular (M8190/0)
  - tubular (M8211/0) - *see also* Neoplasm, by site, benign
    - papillary (M8460/3)
    - Pick's (M8640/0)
      - specified site - *see* Neoplasm, by site, benign
      - unspecified site
        - female 220
        - male 222.0
  - tubulovillous (M8263/0)
  - villoglandular (M8263/0)
  - villous (M8261/1) - *see* Neoplasm, by site, uncertain behavior
  - water-clear cell (M8322/0) 227.1
  - wolffian duct (M9110/0)
- **Adenomatosis** (M8220/0)
  - endocrine (multiple) (M8360/1)
    - single specified site - *see* Neoplasm, by site, uncertain behavior
    - two or more specified sites 237.4
    - unspecified site 237.4
  - erosive of nipple (M8506/0) 217
  - pluriendocrine - *see* Adenomatosis, endocrine
  - pulmonary (M8250/1) 235.7
    - malignant (M8250/3) - *see* Neoplasm, lung, malignant
  - specified site - *see* Neoplasm, by site, benign
  - unspecified site 211.3
- **Adenomatous**
  - cyst, thyroid (gland) - *see* Goiter, nodular
  - goiter (nontoxic) (*see also* Goiter, nodular) 241.9
    - toxic or with hyperthyroidism 242.3
- **Adenomyoma** (M8932/0) - *see also* Neoplasm, by site, benign
  - prostate 600.20
    - with (Revised)
      - other lower urinary tract symptoms (LUTS) 600.21 ◀
      - urinary ◀
        - obstruction 600.21 ◀
        - retention 600.21 ◀
- **Adenomyometritis** 617.0
- **Adenomyosis** (uterus) (internal) 617.0
- **Adenopathy** (lymph gland) 785.6
  - inguinal 785.6
  - mediastinal 785.6
  - mesentery 785.6
  - syphilitic (secondary) 091.4
  - tracheobronchial 785.6
    - tuberculous (*see also* Tuberculosis) 012.1
      - primary, progressive 010.8
  - tuberculous (*see also* Tuberculosis, lymph gland) 017.2
    - tracheobronchial 012.1
      - primary, progressive 010.8
- **Adenopharyngitis** 462
- **Adenophlegmon** 683
- **Adenosalpingitis** 614.1
- **Adenosarcoma** (M8960/3) 189.0
- **Adenosclerosis** 289.3

Adenosis
breast (sclerosing) 610.2
vagina, congenital 752.49
Adentia (complete) (partial) (*see also* Absence, teeth) 520.0
Adherent
labium (minus) 624.4
pericardium (nonrheumatic) 423.1
rheumatic 393
placenta 667.0
with hemorrhage 666.0
prepuce 605
scar (skin) NEC 709.2
tendon in scar 709.2
Adhesion(s), adhesive (postinfectional) (postoperative)
abdominal (wall) (*see also* Adhesions, peritoneum) 568.0
amnion to fetus 658.8
affecting fetus or newborn 762.8
appendix 543.9
arachnoiditis - *see* Meningitis
auditory tube (Eustachian) 381.89
bands - *see also* Adhesions, peritoneum
cervix 622.3
uterus 621.5
bile duct (any) 576.8
bladder (sphincter) 596.8
bowel (*see also* Adhesions, peritoneum) 568.0
cardiac 423.1
rheumatic 398.99
cecum (*see also* Adhesions, peritoneum) 568.0
cervicovaginal 622.3
congenital 752.49
postpartal 674.8
old 622.3
cervix 622.3
clitoris 624.4
colon (*see also* Adhesions, peritoneum) 568.0
common duct 576.8
congenital - *see also* Anomaly, specified type NEC
fingers (*see also* Syndactylism, fingers) 755.11
labium (majus) (minus) 752.49
omental, anomalous 751.4
ovary 752.0
peritoneal 751.4
toes (*see also* Syndactylism, toes) 755.13
tongue (to gum or roof of mouth) 750.12
conjunctiva (acquired) (localized) 372.62
congenital 743.63
extensive 372.63
cornea - *see* Opacity, cornea
cystic duct 575.8
diaphragm (*see also* Adhesions, peritoneum) 568.0
due to foreign body - *see* Foreign body
duodenum (*see also* Adhesions, peritoneum) 568.0
with obstruction 537.3
ear, middle - *see* Adhesions, middle ear
epididymis 608.89
epidural - *see* Adhesions, meninges
epiglottis 478.79
Eustachian tube 381.89

Adhesion(s) *(Continued)*
eyelid 374.46
postoperative 997.99
surgically created V45.69
gallbladder (*see also* Disease, gallbladder) 575.8
globe 360.89
heart 423.1
rheumatic 398.99
ileocecal (coil) (*see also* Adhesions, peritoneum) 568.0
ileum (*see also* Adhesions, peritoneum) 568.0
intestine (postoperative) (*see also* Adhesions, peritoneum) 568.0
with obstruction 560.81
with hernia - *see also* Hernia, by site, with obstruction
gangrenous - *see* Hernia, by site, with gangrene
intra-abdominal (*see also* Adhesions, peritoneum) 568.0
iris 364.70
to corneal graft 996.79
joint (*see also* Ankylosis) 718.5
kidney 593.89
labium (majus) (minus), congenital 752.49
liver 572.8
lung 511.0
mediastinum 519.3
meninges 349.2
cerebral (any) 349.2
congenital 742.4
congenital 742.8
spinal (any) 349.2
congenital 742.59
tuberculous (cerebral) (spinal) (*see also* Tuberculosis, meninges) 013.0
mesenteric (*see also* Adhesions, peritoneum) 568.0
middle ear (fibrous) 385.10
drum head 385.19
to
incus 385.11
promontorium 385.13
stapes 385.12
specified NEC 385.19
nasal (septum) (to turbinates) 478.19 ⇐
nerve NEC 355.9
spinal 355.9
root 724.9
cervical NEC 723.4
lumbar NEC 724.4
lumbosacral 724.4
thoracic 724.4
ocular muscle 378.60
omentum (*see also* Adhesions, peritoneum) 568.0
organ or site, congenital NEC - *see* Anomaly, specified type NEC
ovary 614.6
congenital (to cecum, kidney, or omentum) 752.0
parauterine 614.6
parovarian 614.6
pelvic (peritoneal)
female (postoperative) (postinfection) 614.6
male (postoperative) (postinfection) (*see also* Adhesions, peritoneum) 568.0

Adhesion(s) *(Continued)*
pelvic *(Continued)*
postpartal (old) 614.6
tuberculous (*see also* Tuberculosis) 016.9
penis to scrotum (congenital) 752.69
periappendiceal (*see also* Adhesions, peritoneum) 568.0
pericardium (nonrheumatic) 423.1
rheumatic 393
tuberculous (*see also* Tuberculosis) 017.9 *[420.0]*
pericholecystic 575.8
perigastric (*see also* Adhesions, peritoneum) 568.0
periovarian 614.6
periprostatic 602.8
perirectal (*see also* Adhesions, peritoneum) 568.0
perirenal 593.89
peritoneum, peritoneal (fibrous) (postoperative) 568.0
with obstruction (intestinal) 560.81
with hernia - *see also* Hernia, by site, with obstruction
gangrenous - *see* Hernia, by site, with gangrene
duodenum 537.3
congenital 751.4
female (postoperative) (postinfective) 614.6
pelvic, female 614.6
pelvic, male 568.0
postpartal, pelvic 614.6
to uterus 614.6
peritubal 614.6
periureteral 593.89
periuterine 621.5
perivesical 596.8
perivesicular (seminal vesicle) 608.89
pleura, pleuritic 511.0
tuberculous (*see also* Tuberculosis, pleura) 012.0
pleuropericardial 511.0
postoperative (gastrointestinal tract) (*see also* Adhesions, peritoneum)
eyelid 997.99
surgically created V45.69
pelvic, female 614.9
pelvic, male 568.0
urethra 598.2
postpartal, old 624.4
preputial, prepuce 605
pulmonary 511.0
pylorus (*see also* Adhesions, peritoneum) 568.0
Rosenmüller's fossa 478.29
sciatic nerve 355.0
seminal vesicle 608.89
shoulder (joint) 726.0
sigmoid flexure (*see also* Adhesions, peritoneum) 568.0
spermatic cord (acquired) 608.89
congenital 752.89
spinal canal 349.2
nerve 355.9
root 724.9
cervical NEC 723.4
lumbar NEC 724.4
lumbosacral 724.4
thoracic 724.4
stomach (*see also* Adhesions, peritoneum) 568.0

- **Adhesion(s)** *(Continued)*
  - subscapular 726.2
  - tendonitis 726.90
    - shoulder 726.0
  - testicle 608.89
  - tongue (congenital) (to gum or roof of mouth) 750.12
    - acquired 529.8
  - trachea 519.19 ⬅
  - tubo-ovarian 614.6
  - tunica vaginalis 608.89
  - ureter 593.89
  - uterus 621.5
    - to abdominal wall 614.6
      - in pregnancy or childbirth 654.4
        - affecting fetus or newborn 763.89
  - vagina (chronic) (postoperative) (postradiation) 623.2
  - vaginitis (congenital) 752.49
  - vesical 596.8
  - vitreous 379.29
- **Adie** (-Holmes) syndrome (tonic pupillary reaction) 379.46
- **Adiponecrosis neonatorum** 778.1
- **Adiposa dolorosa** 272.8
- **Adiposalgia** 272.8
- **Adiposis**
  - cerebralis 253.8
  - dolorosa 272.8
  - tuberosa simplex 272.8
- **Adiposity** 278.02
  - heart (*see also* Degeneration, myocardial) 429.1
  - localized 278.1
- **Adiposogenital dystrophy** 253.8
- **Adjustment**
  - prosthesis or other device - *see* Fitting of
  - reaction - *see* Reaction, adjustment
- **Administration, prophylactic**
  - antibiotics V07.39
  - antitoxin, any V07.2
  - antivenin V07.2
  - chemotherapeutic agent NEC V07.39
  - chemotherapy NEC V07.39
  - diphtheria antitoxin V07.2
  - fluoride V07.31
  - gamma globulin V07.2
  - immune sera (gamma globulin) V07.2
  - passive immunization agent V07.2
  - RhoGAM V07.2
- **Admission** (encounter)
  - as organ donor - *see* Donor
  - by mistake V68.9
  - for
    - adequacy testing (for)
      - hemodialysis V56.31
      - peritoneal dialysis V56.32
    - adjustment (of)
      - artificial
        - arm (complete) (partial) V52.0
        - eye V52.2
        - leg (complete) (partial) V52.1
      - brain neuropacemaker V53.02
      - breast
        - implant V52.4
        - prosthesis V52.4
      - cardiac device V53.39
        - defibrillator, automatic implantable V53.32
        - pacemaker V53.31
          - carotid sinus V53.39
- **Admission** *(Continued)*
  - for *(Continued)*
    - adjustment (of) *(Continued)*
      - catheter
        - non-vascular V58.82
        - vascular V58.81
      - cerebral ventricle (communicating) shunt V53.01
      - colostomy belt V55.3
      - contact lenses V53.1
      - cystostomy device V53.6
      - dental prosthesis V52.3
      - device, unspecified type V53.90
        - abdominal V53.5
        - cardiac V53.39
          - defibrillator, automatic implantable V53.32
          - pacemaker V53.31
        - carotid sinus V53.39
        - cerebral ventricle (communicating) shunt V53.01
        - insulin pump V53.91
        - intrauterine contraceptive V25.1
        - nervous system V53.09
        - orthodontic V53.4
        - other device V53.99
        - prosthetic V52.9
          - breast V52.4
          - dental V52.3
          - eye V52.2
          - specified type NEC V52.8
        - special senses V53.09
        - substitution
          - auditory V53.09
          - nervous system V53.09
          - visual V53.09
        - urinary V53.6
      - dialysis catheter
        - extracorporeal V56.1
        - peritoneal V56.2
      - diaphragm (contraceptive) V25.02
      - growth rod V54.02
      - hearing aid V53.2
      - ileostomy device V55.2
      - intestinal appliance or device NEC V53.5
      - intrauterine contraceptive device V25.1
      - neuropacemaker (brain) (peripheral nerve) (spinal cord) V53.02
      - orthodontic device V53.4
      - orthopedic (device) V53.7
        - brace V53.7
        - cast V53.7
        - shoes V53.7
      - pacemaker
        - brain V53.02
        - cardiac V53.31
        - carotid sinus V53.39
        - peripheral nerve V53.02
        - spinal cord V53.02
      - prosthesis V52.9
        - arm (complete) (partial) V52.0
        - breast V52.4
        - dental V52.3
        - eye V52.2
        - leg (complete) (partial) V52.1
        - specified type NEC V52.8
      - spectacles V53.1
      - wheelchair V53.8
    - adoption referral or proceedings V68.89
    - aftercare (*see also* Aftercare) V58.9
      - cardiac pacemaker V53.31
- **Admission** *(Continued)*
  - for *(Continued)*
    - aftercare *(Continued)*
      - chemotherapy V58.11
      - antineoplastic
        - chemotherapy V58.11
        - immunotherapy V58.12
      - dialysis
        - extracorporeal (renal) V56.0
        - peritoneal V56.8
        - renal V56.0
      - fracture (*see also* Aftercare, fracture) V54.9
      - medical NEC V58.89
      - organ transplant V58.44
      - orthopedic V54.9
        - specified care NEC V54.89
      - pacemaker device
        - brain V53.02
        - cardiac V53.31
        - carotid sinus V53.39
        - nervous system V53.02
        - spinal cord V53.02
      - postoperative NEC V58.49
        - wound closure, planned V58.41
      - postpartum
        - immediately after delivery V24.0
        - routine follow-up V24.2
      - postradiation V58.0
      - radiation therapy V58.0
      - removal of
        - non-vascular catheter V58.82
        - vascular catheter V58.81
      - specified NEC V58.89
      - surgical NEC V58.49
        - wound closure, planned V58.41
    - antineoplastic
      - chemotherapy V58.11
      - immunotherapy V58.12
    - artificial insemination V26.1
    - attention to artificial opening (of) V55.9
      - artificial vagina V55.7
      - colostomy V55.3
      - cystostomy V55.5
      - enterostomy V55.4
      - gastrostomy V55.1
      - ileostomy V55.2
      - jejunostomy V55.4
      - nephrostomy V55.6
      - specified site NEC V55.8
        - intestinal tract V55.4
        - urinary tract V55.6
      - tracheostomy V55.0
      - ureterostomy V55.6
      - urethrostomy V55.6
    - battery replacement
      - cardiac pacemaker V53.31
    - blood typing V72.86
      - Rh typing V72.86 ◀
    - boarding V65.0
    - breast
      - augmentation or reduction V50.1
      - removal, prophylactic V50.41
    - change of
      - cardiac pacemaker (battery) V53.31
      - carotid sinus pacemaker V53.39
      - catheter in artificial opening - *see* Attention to, artificial, opening
      - drains V58.49 ◀
      - dressing ⬅
        - wound V58.30 ◀
          - nonsurgical V58.30 ◀
          - surgical V58.31 ◀

◀ **New** ⬅ **Revised**

Admission *(Continued)*
for *(Continued)*
change of *(Continued)*
fixation device
external V54.89
internal V54.01
Kirschner wire V54.89
neuropacemaker device (brain) (peripheral nerve) (spinal cord) V53.02
nonsurgical wound dressing V58.30 ◀
pacemaker device
brain V53.02
cardiac V53.31
carotid sinus V53.39
nervous system V53.02
plaster cast V54.89
splint, external V54.89
Steinmann pin V54.89
surgical wound dressing V58.31 ⬅
wound packing V58.30 ◀
nonsurgical V58.30 ◀
surgical V58.31 ◀
traction device V54.89
checkup only V70.0
chemotherapy, antineoplastic V58.11
circumcision, ritual or routine (in absence of medical indication) V50.2
clinical research investigation (control) (normal comparison) (participant) V70.7
closure of artificial opening - *see* Attention to, artificial, opening
contraceptive
counseling V25.09
emergency V25.03
postcoital V25.03
management V25.9
specified type NEC V25.8
convalescence following V66.9
chemotherapy V66.2
psychotherapy V66.3
radiotherapy V66.1
surgery V66.0
treatment (for) V66.5
combined V66.6
fracture V66.4
mental disorder NEC V66.3
specified condition NEC V66.5
cosmetic surgery NEC V50.1
following healed injury or operation V51
counseling (*see also* Counseling) V65.40
without complaint or sickness V65.49
contraceptive management V25.09
emergency V25.03
postcoital V25.03
dietary V65.3
exercise V65.41
for
nonattending third party V65.19
pediatric pre-birth visit for expectant mother V65.11
victim of abuse
child V61.21
partner or spouse V61.11
genetic V26.33
gonorrhea V65.45
HIV V65.44

Admission *(Continued)*
for *(Continued)*
counseling *(Continued)*
human immunodeficiency virus V65.44
injury prevention V65.43
insulin pump training V65.46
procreative management V26.4
sexually transmitted disease NEC V65.45
HIV V65.44
specified reason NEC V65.49
substance use and abuse V65.42
syphilis V65.45
desensitization to allergens V07.1
dialysis V56.0
catheter
fitting and adjustment
extracorporeal V56.1
peritoneal V56.2
removal or replacement
extracorporeal V56.1
peritoneal V56.2
extracorporeal (renal) V56.0
peritoneal V56.8
renal V56.0
dietary surveillance and counseling V65.3
drug monitoring, therapeutic V58.83
ear piercing V50.3
elective surgery
breast
augmentation or reduction V50.1
removal, prophylactic V50.41
circumcision, ritual or routine (in absence of medical indication) V50.2
cosmetic NEC V50.1
following healed injury or operation V51
ear piercing V50.3
face-lift V50.1
hair transplant V50.0
plastic
cosmetic NEC V50.1
following healed injury or operation V51
prophylactic organ removal V50.49
breast V50.41
ovary V50.42
repair of scarred tissue (following healed injury or operation) V51
specified type NEC V50.8
end-of-life care V66.7
examination (*see also* Examination) V70.9
administrative purpose NEC V70.3
adoption V70.3
allergy V72.7
at health care facility V70.0
athletic team V70.3
camp V70.3
cardiovascular, preoperative V72.81
clinical research investigation (control) (participant) V70.7
dental V72.2
developmental testing (child) (infant) V20.2
donor (potential) V70.8
driver's license V70.3
ear V72.19 ⬅
employment V70.5
eye V72.0

Admission *(Continued)*
for *(Continued)*
examination *(Continued)*
follow-up (routine) - *see* Examination, follow-up
for admission to
old age home V70.3
school V70.3
general V70.9
specified reason NEC V70.8
gynecological V72.31
health supervision (child) (infant) V20.2
hearing V72.19 ⬅
following failed hearing screening V72.11 ◀
immigration V70.3
infant, routine V20.2 ◀
insurance certification V70.3
laboratory V72.6
marriage license V70.3
medical (general) (*see also* Examination, medical) V70.9
medicolegal reasons V70.4
naturalization V70.3
pelvic (annual) (periodic) V72.31
postpartum checkup V24.2
pregnancy (possible) (unconfirmed) V72.40
negative result V72.41
positive result V72.42
preoperative V72.84
cardiovascular V72.81
respiratory V72.82
specified NEC V72.83
preprocedural V72.84
cardiovascular V72.81
general physical V72.83
respiratory V72.82
specified NEC V72.83
prison V70.3
psychiatric (general) V70.2
requested by authority V70.1
radiological NEC V72.5
respiratory, preoperative V72.82
school V70.3
screening - *see* Screening
skin hypersensitivity V72.7
specified type NEC V72.85
sport competition V70.3
vision V72.0
well baby and child care V20.2
exercise therapy V57.1
face-lift, cosmetic reason V50.1
fitting (of)
artificial
arm (complete) (partial) V52.0
eye V52.2
leg (complete) (partial) V52.1
biliary drainage tube V58.82
brain neuropacemaker V53.02
breast V52.4
implant V50.1
prosthesis V52.4
cardiac pacemaker V53.31
catheter
non-vascular V58.82
vascular V58.81
cerebral ventricle (communicating) shunt V53.01
chest tube V58.82
colostomy belt V55.2
contact lenses V53.1
cystostomy device V53.6

Admission *(Continued)*
for *(Continued)*
fitting *(Continued)*
dental prosthesis V52.3
device, unspecified type V53.90
abdominal V53.5
cerebral ventricle (communicating) shunt V53.01
insulin pump V53.91
intrauterine contraceptive V25.1
nervous system V53.09
orthodontic V53.4
other device V53.99
prosthetic V52.9
breast V52.4
dental V52.3
eye V52.2
special senses V53.09
substitution
auditory V53.09
nervous system V53.09
visual V53.09
diaphragm (contraceptive) V25.02
fistula (sinus tract) drainage tube V58.82
growth rod V54.02
hearing aid V53.2
ileostomy device V55.2
intestinal appliance or device NEC V53.5
intrauterine contraceptive device V25.1
neuropacemaker (brain) (peripheral nerve) (spinal cord) V53.02
orthodontic device V53.4
orthopedic (device) V53.7
brace V53.7
cast V53.7
shoes V53.7
pacemaker
brain V53.02
cardiac V53.31
carotid sinus V53.39
spinal cord V53.02
pleural drainage tube V58.82
prosthesis V52.9
arm (complete) (partial) V52.0
breast V52.4
dental V52.3
eye V52.2
leg (complete) (partial) V52.1
specified type NEC V52.8
spectacles V53.1
wheelchair V53.8
follow-up examination (routine) (following) V67.9
cancer chemotherapy V67.2
chemotherapy V67.2
high-risk medication NEC V67.51
injury NEC V67.59
psychiatric V67.3
psychotherapy V67.3
radiotherapy V67.1
specified surgery NEC V67.09
surgery V67.00
vaginal pap smear V67.01
treatment (for) V67.9
combined V67.6
fracture V67.4
involving high-risk medication NEC V67.51
mental disorder V67.3
specified NEC V67.59

Admission *(Continued)*
for *(Continued)*
hair transplant, for cosmetic reason V50.0
health advice, education, or instruction V65.4
hormone replacement therapy (postmenopausal) V07.4
hospice care V66.7
immunotherapy, antineoplastic V58.12
insertion (of)
subdermal implantable contraceptive V25.5
insulin pump titration V53.91
insulin pump training V65.46
intrauterine device
insertion V25.1
management V25.42
investigation to determine further disposition V63.8
isolation V07.0
issue of
medical certificate NEC V68.0
repeat prescription NEC V68.1
contraceptive device NEC V25.49
kidney dialysis V56.0
lengthening of growth rod V54.02
mental health evaluation V70.2
requested by authority V70.1
nonmedical reason NEC V68.89
nursing care evaluation V63.8
observation (without need for further medical care) (*see also* Observation) V71.9
accident V71.4
alleged rape or seduction V71.5
criminal assault V71.6
following accident V71.4
at work V71.3
foreign body ingestion V71.89
growth and development variations, childhood V21.0
inflicted injury NEC V71.6
ingestion of deleterious agent or foreign body V71.89
injury V71.6
malignant neoplasm V71.1
mental disorder V71.09
newborn - *see* Observation, suspected, condition, newborn
rape V71.5
specified NEC V71.89
suspected disorder V71.9
abuse V71.81
accident V71.4
at work V71.3
benign neoplasm V71.89
cardiovascular V71.7
exposure
anthrax V71.82
biological agent NEC V71.83
SARS V71.83
heart V71.7
inflicted injury NEC V71.6
malignant neoplasm V71.1
mental NEC V71.09
neglect V71.81
specified condition NEC V71.89
tuberculosis V71.2
tuberculosis V71.2
occupational therapy V57.21
organ transplant, donor - *see* Donor

Admission *(Continued)*
for *(Continued)*
ovary, ovarian removal, prophylactic V50.42
palliative care V66.7
Papanicolaou smear
cervix V76.2
for suspected malignant neoplasm V76.2
no disease found V71.1
routine, as part of gynecological examination V72.31
to confirm findings of recent normal smear following initial abnormal smear V72.32
vaginal V76.47
following hysterectomy for malignant condition V67.01
passage of sounds or bougie in artificial opening - *see* Attention to, artificial, opening
paternity testing V70.4
peritoneal dialysis V56.32
physical therapy NEC V57.1
plastic surgery
cosmetic NEC V50.1
following healed injury or operation V51
postmenopausal hormone replacement therapy V07.4
postpartum observation
immediately after delivery V24.0
routine follow-up V24.2
poststerilization (for restoration) V26.0
procreative management V26.9
specified type NEC V26.8
prophylactic
administration of
antibiotics V07.39
antitoxin, any V07.2
antivenin V07.2
chemotherapeutic agent NEC V07.39
chemotherapy NEC V07.39
diphtheria antitoxin V07.2
fluoride V07.31
gamma globulin V07.2
immune sera (gamma globulin) V07.2
RhoGAM V07.2
tetanus antitoxin V07.2
breathing exercises V57.0
chemotherapy NEC V07.39
fluoride V07.31
measure V07.9
specified type NEC V07.8
organ removal V50.49
breast V50.41
ovary V50.42
psychiatric examination (general) V70.2
requested by authority V70.1
radiation management V58.0
radiotherapy V58.0
reforming of artificial opening - *see* Attention to, artificial, opening
rehabilitation V57.9
multiple types V57.89
occupational V57.21
orthoptic V57.4
orthotic V57.81
physical NEC V57.1

Admission *(Continued)*
for *(Continued)*
rehabilitation *(Continued)*
specified type NEC V57.89
speech V57.3
vocational V57.22
removal of
cardiac pacemaker V53.31
cast (plaster) V54.89
catheter from artificial opening - *see* Attention to, artificial, opening
cerebral ventricle (communicating) shunt V53.01
cystostomy catheter V55.5
device
cerebral ventricle (communicating) shunt V53.01
fixation
external V54.89
internal V54.01
intrauterine contraceptive V25.42
traction, external V54.89
drains V58.49 ◀
dressing ⬅
wound V58.30 ◀
nonsurgical V58.30 ◀
surgical V58.31 ◀
fixation device
external V54.89
internal V54.01
intrauterine contraceptive device V25.42
Kirschner wire V54.89
neuropacemaker (brain) (peripheral nerve) (spinal cord) V53.02
nonsurgical wound dressing V58.30 ◀
orthopedic fixation device
external V54.89
internal V54.01
pacemaker device
brain V53.02
cardiac V53.31
carotid sinus V53.39
nervous system V53.02
plaster cast V54.89
plate (fracture) V54.01
rod V54.01
screw (fracture) V54.01
splint, traction V54.89
staples V58.32 ◀
Steinmann pin V54.89
subdermal implantable contraceptive V25.43
surgical wound dressing V58.31 ⬅
sutures V58.32 ⬅
traction device, external V54.89
ureteral stent V53.6
wound packing V58.30 ◀
nonsurgical V58.30 ◀
surgical V58.31 ◀
repair of scarred tissue (following healed injury or operation) V51
reprogramming of cardiac pacemaker V53.31
respirator [ventilator] dependence
during
mechanical failure V46.14
power failure V46.12
for weaning V46.13
restoration of organ continuity (poststerilization) (tuboplasty) (vasoplasty) V26.0

Admission *(Continued)*
for *(Continued)*
Rh typing V72.86 ◀
sensitivity test - *see also* Test, skin
allergy NEC V72.7
bacterial disease NEC V74.9
Dick V74.8
Kveim V82.89
Mantoux V74.1
mycotic infection NEC V75.4
parasitic disease NEC V75.8
Schick V74.3
Schultz-Charlton V74.8
social service (agency) referral or evaluation V63.8
speech therapy V57.3
sterilization V25.2
suspected disorder (ruled out) (without need for further care) - *see* Observation
terminal care V66.7
tests only - *see* Test
therapeutic drug monitoring V58.83
therapy
blood transfusion, without reported diagnosis V58.2
breathing exercises V57.0
chemotherapy, antineoplastic V58.11
prophylactic NEC V07.39
fluoride V07.31
dialysis (intermittent) (treatment)
extracorporeal V56.0
peritoneal V56.8
renal V56.0
specified type NEC V56.8
exercise (remedial) NEC V57.1
breathing V57.0
immunotherapy, antineoplastic V58.12
long-term (current) drug use NEC V58.69
antibiotics V58.62
anticoagulants V58.61
anti-inflammatories, non-steroidal (NSAID) V58.64
antiplatelets V58.63
antithrombotics V58.63
aspirin V58.66
insulin V58.67
steroids V58.65
occupational V57.21
orthoptic V57.4
physical NEC V57.1
radiation V58.0
speech V57.3
vocational V57.22
toilet or cleaning
of artificial opening - *see* Attention to, artificial, opening
of non-vascular catheter V58.82
of vascular catheter V58.81
tubal ligation V25.2
tuboplasty for previous sterilization V26.0
vaccination, prophylactic (against)
arthropod-borne virus, viral NEC V05.1
disease NEC V05.1
encephalitis V05.0
Bacille Calmette-Guérin (BCG) V03.2
BCG V03.2

Admission *(Continued)*
for *(Continued)*
vaccination, prophylactic *(Continued)*
chickenpox V05.4
cholera alone V03.0
with typhoid-paratyphoid (cholera + TAB) V06.0
common cold V04.7
dengue V05.1
diphtheria alone V03.5
diphtheria-tetanus-pertussis (DTP) (DTaP) V06.1
with
poliomyelitis (DTP + polio) V06.3
typhoid-paratyphoid (DTP + TAB) V06.2
diphtheria-tetanus [Td] [DT] without pertussis V06.5
disease (single) NEC V05.9
bacterial NEC V03.9
specified type NEC V03.89
combinations NEC V06.9
specified type NEC V06.8
specified type NEC V05.8
viral NEC V04.89
encephalitis, viral, arthropod-borne V05.0
Hemophilus influenzae, type B [Hib] V03.81
hepatitis, viral V05.3
immune sera (gamma globulin) V07.2
influenza V04.81
with
Streptococcus pneumoniae [pneumococcus] V06.6
Leishmaniasis V05.2
measles alone V04.2
measles-mumps-rubella (MMR) V06.4
mumps alone V04.6
with measles and rubella (MMR) V06.4
not done because of contraindication V64.09
pertussis alone V03.6
plague V03.3
pneumonia V03.82
poliomyelitis V04.0
with diphtheria-tetanus-pertussis (DTP + polio) V06.3
rabies V04.5
respiratory syncytial virus (RSV) V04.82
rubella alone V04.3
with measles and mumps (MMR) V06.4
smallpox V04.1
specified type NEC V05.8
Streptococcus pneumoniae [pneumococcus] V03.82
with
influenza V06.6
tetanus toxoid alone V03.7
with diphtheria [Td] [DT] V06.5
and pertussis (DTP) (DTaP) V06.1
tuberculosis (BCG) V03.2
tularemia V03.4
typhoid alone V03.1
with diphtheria-tetanus-pertussis (TAB + DTP) V06.2

- **Admission** *(Continued)*
  - for *(Continued)*
    - vaccination, prophylactic *(Continued)*
      - typhoid-paratyphoid alone (TAB) V03.1
      - typhus V05.8
      - varicella (chicken pox) V05.4
      - viral encephalitis, arthropod-borne V05.0
      - viral hepatitis V05.3
      - yellow fever V04.4
    - vasectomy V25.2
    - vasoplasty for previous sterilization V26.0
    - vision examination V72.0
    - vocational therapy V57.22
    - waiting period for admission to other facility V63.2
      - undergoing social agency investigation V63.8
    - well baby and child care V20.2
    - x-ray of chest
      - for suspected tuberculosis V71.2
      - routine V72.5
- **Adnexitis** (suppurative) (*see also* Salpingo-oophoritis) 614.2
- **Adolescence** NEC V21.2
- **Adoption**
  - agency referral V68.89
  - examination V70.3
  - held for V68.89
- **Adrenal gland** - *see* condition
- **Adrenalism** 255.9
  - tuberculous (*see also* Tuberculosis) 017.6
- **Adrenalitis, adrenitis** 255.8
  - meningococcal hemorrhagic 036.3
- **Adrenarche, precocious** 259.1
- **Adrenocortical syndrome** 255.2
- **Adrenogenital syndrome** (acquired) (congenital) 255.2
  - iatrogenic, fetus or newborn 760.79
- **Adrenoleukodystrophy** 277.86
  - neonatal 277.86
  - x-linked 277.86
- **Adrenomyeloneuropathy** 277.86
- **Adventitious bursa** - *see* Bursitis
- **Adynamia** (episodica) (hereditary) (periodic) 359.3
- **Adynamic**
  - ileus or intestine (*see also* Ileus) 560.1
  - ureter 753.22
- **Aeration lung, imperfect, newborn** 770.5
- **Aerobullosis** 993.3
- **Aerocele** - *see* Embolism, air
- **Aerodermectasia**
  - subcutaneous (traumatic) 958.7
    - surgical 998.81
  - surgical 998.81
- **Aerodontalgia** 993.2
- **Aeroembolism** 993.3
- **Aerogenes capsulatus infection** (*see also* Gangrene, gas) 040.0
- **Aero-otitis media** 993.0
- **Aerophagy, aerophagia** 306.4
  - psychogenic 306.4
- **Aerosinusitis** 993.1
- **Aerotitis** 993.0
- **Affection, affections** - *see also* Disease
  - sacroiliac (joint), old 724.6
  - shoulder region NEC 726.2
- **Afibrinogenemia** 286.3
  - acquired 286.6
- **Afibrinogenemia** *(Continued)*
  - congenital 286.3
  - postpartum 666.3
- **African**
  - sleeping sickness 086.5
  - tick fever 087.1
  - trypanosomiasis 086.5
    - Gambian 086.3
    - Rhodesian 086.4
- **Aftercare** V58.9
  - amputation stump V54.89 ◀
  - artificial openings - *see* Attention to, artificial, opening
  - blood transfusion without reported diagnosis V58.2
  - breathing exercise V57.0
  - cardiac device V53.39
    - defibrillator, automatic implantable V53.32
    - pacemaker V53.31
      - carotid sinus V53.39
  - carotid sinus pacemaker V53.39
  - cerebral ventricle (communicating) shunt V53.01
  - chemotherapy session (adjunctive) (maintenance) V58.11
  - defibrillator, automatic implantable cardiac V53.32
  - exercise (remedial) (therapeutic) V57.1
    - breathing V57.0
  - extracorporeal dialysis (intermittent) (treatment) V56.0
  - following surgery NEC V58.49
    - for
      - injury V58.43
      - neoplasm V58.42
      - organ transplant V58.44
      - trauma V58.43
    - joint replacement V54.81
    - of
      - circulatory system V58.73
      - digestive system V58.75
      - genital system V58.76
      - genitourinary system V58.76
      - musculoskeletal system V58.78
      - nervous system V58.72
      - oral cavity V58.75
      - respiratory system V58.74
      - sense organs V58.71
      - skin V58.77
      - subcutaneous tissue V58.77
      - teeth V58.75
      - urinary system V58.76
    - wound closure, planned V58.41
  - fracture V54.9
    - healing V54.89
      - pathologic
        - ankle V54.29
        - arm V54.20
          - lower V54.22
          - upper V54.21
        - finger V54.29
        - foot V54.29
        - hand V54.29
        - hip V54.23
        - leg V54.24
          - lower V54.26
          - upper V54.25
        - pelvis V54.29
        - specified site NEC V54.29
        - toe(s) V54.29
        - vertebrae V54.27
        - wrist V54.29
      - traumatic
        - ankle V54.19
        - arm V54.10
- **Aftercare** *(Continued)*
  - fracture *(Continued)*
    - healing *(Continued)*
      - traumatic *(Continued)*
        - arm *(Continued)*
          - lower V54.12
          - upper V54.11
        - finger V54.19
        - foot V54.19
        - hand V54.19
        - hip V54.13
        - leg V54.14
          - lower V54.16
          - upper V54.15
        - pelvis V54.19
        - specified site NEC V54.19
        - toe(s) V54.19
        - vertebrae V54.17
        - wrist V54.19
    - removal of
      - external fixation device V54.89
      - internal fixation device V54.01
    - specified care NEC V54.89
  - gait training V57.1
    - for use of artificial limb(s) V57.81
  - internal fixation device V54.09
  - involving
    - dialysis (intermittent) (treatment)
      - extracorporeal V56.0
      - peritoneal V56.8
      - renal V56.0
    - gait training V57.1
      - for use of artificial limb(s) V57.81
    - growth rod
      - adjustment V54.02
      - lengthening V54.02
    - internal fixation device V54.09
    - orthoptic training V57.4
    - orthotic training V57.81
    - radiotherapy session V58.0
    - removal of
      - drains V58.49 ◀
      - dressings ⬅
        - wound packing V58.30 ◀
          - nonsurgical V58.30 ◀
          - surgical V58.31 ◀
      - fixation device
        - external V54.89
        - internal V54.01
      - fracture plate V54.01
      - nonsurgical wound dressing V58.30 ◀
      - pins V54.01
      - plaster cast V54.89
      - rods V54.01
      - screws V54.01
      - staples V58.32 ◀
      - surgical wound dressings V58.31 ⬅
      - sutures V58.32 ⬅
      - traction device, external V54.89
      - wound packing V58.30 ◀
        - nonsurgical V58.30 ◀
        - surgical V58.31 ◀
  - neuropacemaker (brain) (peripheral nerve) (spinal cord) V53.02
  - occupational therapy V57.21
  - orthodontic V58.5
  - orthopedic V54.9
    - change of external fixation or traction device V54.89
    - following joint replacement V54.81
    - internal fixation device V54.09
    - removal of fixation device
      - external V54.89
      - internal V54.01

◀ New ⬅ Revised

Aftercare *(Continued)*
orthopedic *(Continued)*
specified care NEC V54.89
orthoptic training V57.4
orthotic training V57.81
pacemaker
brain V53.02
cardiac V53.31
carotid sinus V53.39
peripheral nerve V53.02
spinal cord V53.02
peritoneal dialysis (intermittent) (treatment) V56.8
physical therapy NEC V57.1
breathing exercises V57.0
radiotherapy session V58.0
rehabilitation procedure V57.9
breathing exercises V57.0
multiple types V57.89
occupational V57.21
orthoptic V57.4
orthotic V57.81
physical therapy NEC V57.1
remedial exercises V57.1
specified type NEC V57.89
speech V57.3
therapeutic exercises V57.1
vocational V57.22
renal dialysis (intermittent) (treatment) V56.0
specified type NEC V58.89
removal of non-vascular cathether V58.82
removal of vascular catheter V58.81
speech therapy V57.3
stump, amputation V54.89 ◀
vocational rehabilitation V57.22
After-cataract 366.50
obscuring vision 366.53
specified type, not obscuring vision 366.52
Agalactia 676.4
Agammaglobulinemia (*see also* Agranulocytosis) 288.09 ⬅
with lymphopenia 279.2
acquired (primary) (secondary) 279.06
Bruton's X-linked 279.04
infantile sex-linked (Bruton's) (congenital) 279.04
Swiss-type 279.2
Aganglionosis (bowel) (colon) 751.3
Age (old) (*see also* Senile) 797
Agenesis - *see also* Absence, by site, congenital
acoustic nerve 742.8
adrenal (gland) 759.1
alimentary tract (complete) (partial) NEC 751.8
lower 751.2
upper 750.8
anus, anal (canal) 751.2
aorta 747.22
appendix 751.2
arm (complete) (partial) (*see also* Deformity, reduction, upper limb) 755.20
artery (peripheral) NEC (*see also* Anomaly, peripheral vascular system) 747.60
brain 747.81
coronary 746.85
pulmonary 747.3
umbilical 747.5
auditory (canal) (external) 744.01

Agenesis *(Continued)*
auricle (ear) 744.01
bile, biliary duct or passage 751.61
bone NEC 756.9
brain 740.0
specified part 742.2
breast 757.6
bronchus 748.3
canaliculus lacrimalis 743.65
carpus NEC (*see also* Deformity, reduction, upper limb) 755.28
cartilage 756.9
cecum 751.2
cerebellum 742.2
cervix 752.49
chin 744.89
cilia 743.63
circulatory system, part NEC 747.89
clavicle 755.51
clitoris 752.49
coccyx 756.13
colon 751.2
corpus callosum 742.2
cricoid cartilage 748.3
diaphragm (with hernia) 756.6
digestive organ(s) or tract (complete) (partial) NEC 751.8
lower 751.2
upper 750.8
ductus arteriosus 747.89
duodenum 751.1
ear NEC 744.09
auricle 744.01
lobe 744.21
ejaculatory duct 752.89
endocrine (gland) NEC 759.2
epiglottis 748.3
esophagus 750.3
Eustachian tube 744.24
extrinsic muscle, eye 743.69
eye 743.00
adnexa 743.69
eyelid (fold) 743.62
face
bones NEC 756.0
specified part NEC 744.89
fallopian tube 752.19
femur NEC (*see also* Absence, femur, congenital) 755.34
fibula NEC (*see also* Absence, fibula, congenital) 755.37
finger NEC (*see also* Absence, finger, congenital) 755.29
foot (complete) (*see also* Deformity, reduction, lower limb) 755.31
gallbladder 751.69
gastric 750.8
genitalia, genital (organ)
female 752.89
external 752.49
internal NEC 752.89
male 752.89
penis 752.69
glottis 748.3
gonadal 758.6
hair 757.4
hand (complete) (*see also* Deformity, reduction, upper limb) 755.21
heart 746.89
valve NEC 746.89
aortic 746.89
mitral 746.89
pulmonary 746.01
hepatic 751.69

Agenesis *(Continued)*
humerus NEC (*see also* Absence, humerus, congenital) 755.24
hymen 752.49
ileum 751.1
incus 744.04
intestine (small) 751.1
large 751.2
iris (dilator fibers) 743.45
jaw 524.09
jejunum 751.1
kidney(s) (partial) (unilateral) 753.0
labium (majus) (minus) 752.49
labyrinth, membranous 744.05
lacrimal apparatus (congenital) 743.65
larynx 748.3
leg NEC (*see also* Deformity, reduction, lower limb) 755.30
lens 743.35
limb (complete) (partial) (*see also* Deformity, reduction) 755.4
lower NEC 755.30
upper 755.20
lip 750.26
liver 751.69
lung (bilateral) (fissures) (lobe) (unilateral) 748.5
mandible 524.09
maxilla 524.09
metacarpus NEC 755.28
metatarsus NEC 755.38
muscle (any) 756.81
musculoskeletal system NEC 756.9
nail(s) 757.5
neck, part 744.89
nerve 742.8
nervous system, part NEC 742.8
nipple 757.6
nose 748.1
nuclear 742.8
organ
of Corti 744.05
or site not listed - *see* Anomaly, specified type NEC
osseous meatus (ear) 744.03
ovary 752.0
oviduct 752.19
pancreas 751.7
parathyroid (gland) 759.2
patella 755.64
pelvic girdle (complete) (partial) 755.69
penis 752.69
pericardium 746.89
perineal body 756.81
pituitary (gland) 759.2
prostate 752.89
pulmonary
artery 747.3
trunk 747.3
vein 747.49
punctum lacrimale 743.65
radioulnar NEC (*see also* Absence, forearm, congenital) 755.25
radius NEC (*see also* Absence, radius, congenital) 755.26
rectum 751.2
renal 753.0
respiratory organ NEC 748.9
rib 756.3
roof of orbit 742.0
round ligament 752.89
sacrum 756.13
salivary gland 750.21

Agenesis *(Continued)*
scapula 755.59
scrotum 752.89
seminal duct or tract 752.89
septum
atrial 745.69
between aorta and pulmonary artery 745.0
ventricular 745.3
shoulder girdle (complete) (partial) 755.59
skull (bone) 756.0
with
anencephalus 740.0
encephalocele 742.0
hydrocephalus 742.3
with spina bifida (*see also* Spina bifida) 741.0
microcephalus 742.1
spermatic cord 752.89
spinal cord 742.59
spine 756.13
lumbar 756.13
isthmus 756.11
pars articularis 756.11
spleen 759.0
sternum 756.3
stomach 750.7
tarsus NEC 755.38
tendon 756.81
testicular 752.89
testis 752.89
thymus (gland) 759.2
thyroid (gland) 243
cartilage 748.3
tibia NEC (*see also* Absence, tibia, congenital) 755.36
tibiofibular NEC 755.35
toe (complete) (partial) (*see also* Absence, toe, congenital) 755.39
tongue 750.11
trachea (cartilage) 748.3
ulna NEC (*see also* Absence, ulna, congenital) 755.27
ureter 753.4
urethra 753.8
urinary tract NEC 753.8
uterus 752.3
uvula 750.26
vagina 752.49
vas deferens 752.89
vein(s) (peripheral) NEC (*see also* Anomaly, peripheral vascular system) 747.60
brain 747.81
great 747.49
portal 747.49
pulmonary 747.49
vena cava (inferior) (superior) 747.49
vermis of cerebellum 742.2
vertebra 756.13
lumbar 756.13
isthmus 756.11
pars articularis 756.11
vulva 752.49
Ageusia (*see also* Disturbance, sensation) 781.1
Aggressiveness 301.3
Aggressive outburst (*see also* Disturbance, conduct) 312.0
in children or adolescents 313.9
Aging skin 701.8
Agitated - *see* condition
Agitation 307.9
catatonic (*see also* Schizophrenia) 295.2
Aglossia (congenital) 750.11
Aglycogenosis 271.0
Agnail (finger) (with lymphangitis) 681.02
Agnosia (body image) (tactile) 784.69
verbal 784.69
auditory 784.69
secondary to organic lesion 784.69
developmental 315.8
secondary to organic lesion 784.69
visual 784.69
developmental 315.8
secondary to organic lesion 784.69
visual 368.16
developmental 315.31
Agoraphobia 300.22
with panic disorder 300.21
Agrammatism 784.69
Agranulocytopenia 288.0
Agranulocytosis (angina) 288.09 ⇐ Revised
chronic 288.09 ◄
cyclical 288.02 ◄
genetic 288.01 ◄
infantile 288.01 ◄
periodic 288.02 ◄
pernicious 288.09 ◄
Agraphia (absolute) 784.69
with alexia 784.61
developmental 315.39
Agrypnia (*see also* Insomnia) 780.52
Ague (*see also* Malaria) 084.6
brass-founders' 985.8
dumb 084.6
tertian 084.1
Agyria 742.2
Ahumada-del Castillo syndrome (nonpuerperal galactorrhea and amenorrhea) 253.1
AIDS 042
AIDS-associated retrovirus (disease) (illness) 042
infection - *see* Human immunodeficiency virus, infection
AIDS-associated virus (disease) (illness) 042
infection - *see* Human immunodeficiency virus, infection
AIDS-like disease (illness) (syndrome) 042
AIDS-related complex 042
AIDS-related conditions 042
AIDS-related virus (disease) (illness) 042
infection - *see* Human immunodeficiency virus, infection
AIDS virus (disease) (illness) 042
infection - *see* Human immunodeficiency virus, infection
Ailment, heart - *see* Disease, heart
Ailurophobia 300.29
Ainhum (disease) 136.0
Air
anterior mediastinum 518.1
compressed, disease 993.3
embolism (any site) (artery) (cerebral) 958.0
with
abortion - *see* Abortion, by type, with embolism
ectopic pregnancy (*see also* categories 633.0-633.9) 639.6
molar pregnancy (*see also* categories 630-632) 639.6
Air *(Continued)*
embolism *(Continued)*
due to implanted device - *see* Complications, due to (presence of) any device, implant, or graft classified to 996.0-996.5 NEC
following
abortion 639.6
ectopic or molar pregnancy 639.6
infusion, perfusion, or transfusion 999.1
in pregnancy, childbirth, or puerperium 673.0
traumatic 958.0
hunger 786.09
psychogenic 306.1
leak (lung) (pulmonary) (thorax) 512.8
iatrogenic 512.1
postoperative 512.1
rarefied, effects of - *see* Effect, adverse, high altitude
sickness 994.6
Airplane sickness 994.6
Akathisia, acathisia 781.0
due to drugs 333.99
neuroleptic-induced acute 333.99
Akinesia algeria 352.6
Akiyami 100.89
Akureyri disease (epidemic neuromyasthenia) 049.8
Alacrima (congenital) 743.65
Alactasia (hereditary) 271.3
Alagille syndrome 759.89
Alalia 784.3
developmental 315.31
receptive-expressive 315.32
secondary to organic lesion 784.3
Alaninemia 270.8
Alastrim 050.1
Albarrán's disease (colibacilluria) 791.9
Albers-Schönberg's disease (marble bones) 756.52
Albert's disease 726.71
Albinism, albino (choroid) (cutaneous) (eye) (generalized) (isolated) (ocular) (oculocutaneous) (partial) 270.2
Albinismus 270.2
Albright (-Martin) (-Bantam) disease (pseudohypoparathyroidism) 275.49
Albright (-McCune) (-Sternberg) syndrome (osteitis fibrosa disseminata) 756.59
Albuminous - *see* condition
Albuminuria, albuminuric (acute) (chronic) (subacute) 791.0
Bence-Jones 791.0
cardiac 785.9
complicating pregnancy, childbirth, or puerperium 646.2
with hypertension - *see* Toxemia, of pregnancy
affecting fetus or newborn 760.1
cyclic 593.6
gestational 646.2
gravidarum 646.2
with hypertension - *see* Toxemia, of pregnancy
affecting fetus or newborn 760.1
heart 785.9
idiopathic 593.6
orthostatic 593.6
postural 593.6
pre-eclamptic (mild) 642.4

◄ New ⇐ Revised

Albuminuria, albuminuric *(Continued)*
pre-eclamptic *(Continued)*
affecting fetus or newborn 760.0
severe 642.5
affecting fetus or newborn 760.0
recurrent physiologic 593.6
scarlatinal 034.1
Albumosuria 791.0
Bence-Jones 791.0
myelopathic (M9730/3) 203.0
Alcaptonuria 270.2
Alcohol, alcoholic
abstinence 291.81
acute intoxication 305.0
with dependence 303.0
addiction (*see also* Alcoholism) 303.9
maternal
with suspected fetal damage affecting management of pregnancy 655.4
affecting fetus or newborn 760.71
amnestic disorder, persisting 291.1
anxiety 291.89
brain syndrome, chronic 291.2
cardiopathy 425.5
chronic (*see also* Alcoholism) 303.9
cirrhosis (liver) 571.2
delirium 291.0
acute 291.0
chronic 291.1
tremens 291.0
withdrawal 291.0
dementia NEC 291.2
deterioration 291.2
drunkenness (simple) 305.0
hallucinosis (acute) 291.3
induced
circadian rhythm sleep disorder 291.82
hypersomnia 291.82
insomnia 291.82
mental disorder 291.9
anxiety 291.89
mood 291.89
sexual 291.89
sleep 291.82
specified type 291.89
parasomnia 291.82
persisting
amnestic disorder 291.1
dementia 291.2
psychotic disorder
with
delusions 291.5
hallucinations 291.3
sleep disorder 291.82
insanity 291.9
intoxication (acute) 305.0
with dependence 303.0
pathological 291.4
jealousy 291.5
Korsakoff's, Korsakov's, Korsakow's 291.1
liver NEC 571.3
acute 571.1
chronic 571.2
mania (acute) (chronic) 291.9
mood 291.89
paranoia 291.5
paranoid (type) psychosis 291.5
pellagra 265.2
poisoning, accidental (acute) NEC 980.9
specified type of alcohol - *see* Table of Drugs and Chemicals

Alcohol, alcoholic *(Continued)*
psychosis (*see also* Psychosis, alcoholic) 291.9
Korsakoff's, Korsakov's, Korsakow's 291.1
polyneuritic 291.1
with
delusions 291.5
hallucinations 291.3
related disorder 291.9
withdrawal symptoms, syndrome NEC 291.81
delirium 291.0
hallucinosis 291.3
Alcoholism 303.9

Note Use the following fifth-digit subclassification with category 303:

0 unspecified
1 continuous
2 episodic
3 in remission

with psychosis (*see also* Psychosis, alcoholic) 291.9
acute 303.0
chronic 303.9
with psychosis 291.9
complicating pregnancy, childbirth, or puerperium 648.4
affecting fetus or newborn 760.71
history V11.3
Korsakoff's, Korsakov's, Korsakow's 291.1
suspected damage to fetus affecting management of pregnancy 655.4
Alder's anomaly or syndrome (leukocyte granulation anomaly) 288.2
Alder-Reilly anomaly (leukocyte granulation) 288.2
Aldosteronism (primary) 255.10
congenital 255.10
familial type I 255.11
glucocorticoid-remediable 255.11
secondary 255.14
Aldosteronoma (M8370/1) 237.2
Aldrich (-Wiskott) syndrome (eczema-thrombocytopenia) 279.12
Aleppo boil 085.1
Aleukemic - *see* condition
Aleukia
congenital 288.09 ⬅ Revised
hemorrhagica 284.9
acquired (secondary) 284.8
congenital 284.09 ⬅ Revised
idiopathic 284.9
splenica 289.4
Alexia (congenital) (developmental) 315.01
secondary to organic lesion 784.61
Algoneurodystrophy 733.7
Algophobia 300.29
Alibert's disease (mycosis fungoides) (M9700/3) 202.1
Alibert-Bazin disease (M9700/3) 202.1
Alice in Wonderland syndrome 293.89
Alienation, mental (*see also* Psychosis) 298.9
Alkalemia 276.3
Alkalosis 276.3
metabolic 276.3
with respiratory acidosis 276.4
respiratory 276.3
Alkaptonuria 270.2

Allen-Masters syndrome 620.6
Allergic bronchopulmonary aspergillosis 518.6
Allergy, allergic (reaction) 995.3
air-borne substance (*see also* Fever, hay) 477.9
specified allergen NEC 477.8
alveolitis (extrinsic) 495.9
due to
Aspergillus clavatus 495.4
cryptostroma corticale 495.6
organisms (fungal, thermophilic actinomycete, other) growing in ventilation (air conditioning systems) 495.7
specified type NEC 495.8
anaphylactic shock 999.4
due to food - *see* Anaphylactic shock, due to, food
angioneurotic edema 995.1
animal (cat) (dog) (epidermal) 477.8
dander 477.2
hair 477.2
arthritis (*see also* Arthritis, allergic) 716.2
asthma - *see* Asthma
bee sting (anaphylactic shock) 989.5
biological - *see* Allergy, drug
bronchial asthma - *see* Asthma
conjunctivitis (eczematous) 372.14
dander, animal (cat) (dog) 477.2
dandruff 477.8
dermatitis (venenata) - *see* Dermatitis
diathesis V15.09
drug, medicinal substance, and biological (any) (correct medicinal substance properly administered) (external) (internal) 995.27 ⬅ Revised
wrong substance given or taken NEC 977.9
specified drug or substance - *see* Table of Drugs and Chemicals
dust (house) (stock) 477.8
eczema - *see* Eczema
endophthalmitis 360.19
epidermal (animal) 477.8
existing dental restorative material 525.66 ◀ New
feathers 477.8
food (any) (ingested) 693.1
atopic 691.8
in contact with skin 692.5
gastritis 535.4
gastroenteritis 558.3
gastrointestinal 558.3
grain 477.0
grass (pollen) 477.0
asthma (*see also* Asthma) 493.0
hay fever 477.0
hair, animal (cat) (dog) 477.2
hay fever (grass) (pollen) (ragweed) (tree) (*see also* Fever, hay) 477.9
history (of) V15.09
to
eggs V15.03
food additives V15.05
insect bite V15.06
latex V15.07
milk products V15.02
nuts V15.05
peanuts V15.01
radiographic dye V15.08
seafood V15.04
specified food NEC V15.05
spider bite V15.06

Allergy, allergic *(Continued)*
horse serum - *see* Allergy, serum
inhalant 477.9
dust 477.8
pollen 477.0
specified allergen other than pollen 477.8
kapok 477.8
medicine - *see* Allergy, drug
migraine 346.2
milk protein 558.3
pannus 370.62
pneumonia 518.3
pollen (any) (hay fever) 477.0
asthma (*see also* Asthma) 493.0
primrose 477.0
primula 477.0
purpura 287.0
ragweed (pollen) (Senecio jacobae) 477.0
asthma (*see also* Asthma) 493.0
hay fever 477.0
respiratory (*see also* Allergy, inhalant) 477.9
due to
drug - *see* Allergy, drug
food - *see* Allergy, food
rhinitis (*see also* Fever, hay) 477.9
due to food 477.1
rose 477.0
Senecio jacobae 477.0
serum (prophylactic) (therapeutic) 999.5
anaphylactic shock 999.4
shock (anaphylactic) (due to adverse effect of correct medicinal substance properly administered) 995.0
food - *see* Anaphylactic shock, due to, food
from serum or immunization 999.5
anaphylactic 999.4
sinusitis (*see also* Fever, hay) 477.9
skin reaction 692.9
specified substance - *see* Dermatitis, due to
tree (any) (hay fever) (pollen) 477.0
asthma (*see also* Asthma) 493.0
upper respiratory (*see also* Fever, hay) 477.9
urethritis 597.89
urticaria 708.0
vaccine - *see* Allergy, serum
Allescheriosis 117.6
Alligator skin disease (ichthyosis congenita) 757.1
acquired 701.1
Allocheiria, allochiria (*see also* Disturbance, sensation) 782.0
Almeida's disease (Brazilian blastomycosis) 116.1
Alopecia (atrophicans) (pregnancy) (premature) (senile) 704.00
adnata 757.4
areata 704.01
celsi 704.01
cicatrisata 704.09
circumscripta 704.01
congenital, congenitalis 757.4
disseminata 704.01
effluvium (telogen) 704.02
febrile 704.09
generalisata 704.09
hereditaria 704.09
marginalis 704.01
Alopecia *(Continued)*
mucinosa 704.09
postinfectional 704.09
seborrheica 704.09
specific 091.82
syphilitic (secondary) 091.82
telogen effluvium 704.02
totalis 704.09
toxica 704.09
universalis 704.09
x-ray 704.09
Alpers' disease 330.8
Alpha-lipoproteinemia 272.4
Alpha thalassemia 282.49
Alphos 696.1
Alpine sickness 993.2
Alport's syndrome (hereditary hematuria-nephropathy-deafness) 759.89
Alteration (of), altered
awareness 780.09
transient 780.02
consciousness 780.09
persistent vegetative state 780.03
transient 780.02
mental status 780.97 (Revised)
amnesia (retrograde) 780.93
memory loss 780.93
Alternaria (infection) 118
Alternating - *see* condition
Altitude, high (effects) - *see* Effect, adverse, high altitude
Aluminosis (of lung) 503
Alvarez syndrome (transient cerebral ischemia) 435.9
Alveolar capillary block syndrome 516.3
Alveolitis
allergic (extrinsic) 495.9
due to organisms (fungal, thermophilic actinomycete, other) growing in ventilation (air conditioning systems) 495.7
specified type NEC 495.8
due to
Aspergillus clavatus 495.4
Cryptostroma corticale 495.6
fibrosing (chronic) (cryptogenic) (lung) 516.3
idiopathic 516.3
rheumatoid 714.81
jaw 526.5
sicca dolorosa 526.5
Alveolus, alveolar - *see* condition
Alymphocytosis (pure) 279.2
Alymphoplasia, thymic 279.2
Alzheimer's
dementia (senile)
with behavioral disturbance 331.0 *[294.11]*
without behavioral disturbance 331.0 *[294.10]*
disease or sclerosis 331.0
with dementia - *see* Alzheimer's, dementia
Amastia (*see also* Absence, breast) 611.8
Amaurosis (acquired) (congenital) (*see also* Blindness) 369.00
fugax 362.34
hysterical 300.11
Leber's (congenital) 362.76
tobacco 377.34
uremic - *see* Uremia
Amaurotic familial idiocy (infantile) (juvenile) (late) 330.1
Ambisexual 752.7
Amblyopia (acquired) (congenital) (partial) 368.00
color 368.59
acquired 368.55
deprivation 368.02
ex anopsia 368.00
hysterical 300.11
nocturnal 368.60
vitamin A deficiency 264.5
refractive 368.03
strabismic 368.01
suppression 368.01
tobacco 377.34
toxic NEC 377.34
uremic - *see* Uremia
Ameba, amebic (histolytica) - *see also* Amebiasis
abscess 006.3
bladder 006.8
brain (with liver and lung abscess) 006.5
liver 006.3
with
brain abscess (and lung abscess) 006.5
lung abscess 006.4
lung (with liver abscess) 006.4
with brain abscess 006.5
seminal vesicle 006.8
spleen 006.8
carrier (suspected of) V02.2
meningoencephalitis
due to Naegleria (gruberi) 136.2
primary 136.2
Amebiasis NEC 006.9
with
brain abscess (with liver or lung abscess) 006.5
liver abscess (without mention of brain or lung abscess) 006.3
lung abscess (with liver abscess) 006.4
with brain abscess 006.5
acute 006.0
bladder 006.8
chronic 006.1
cutaneous 006.6
cutis 006.6
due to organism other than Entamoeba histolytica 007.8
hepatic (*see also* Abscess, liver, amebic) 006.3
nondysenteric 006.2
seminal vesicle 006.8
specified
organism NEC 007.8
site NEC 006.8
Ameboma 006.8
Amelia 755.4
lower limb 755.31
upper limb 755.21
Ameloblastoma (M9310/0) 213.1
jaw (bone) (lower) 213.1
upper 213.0
long bones (M9261/3) - *see* Neoplasm, bone, malignant
malignant (M9310/3) 170.1
jaw (bone) (lower) 170.1
upper 170.0
mandible 213.1
tibial (M9261/3) 170.7
Amelogenesis imperfecta 520.5
nonhereditaria (segmentalis) 520.4

Amenorrhea (primary) (secondary) 626.0
due to ovarian dysfunction 256.8
hyperhormonal 256.8
Amentia (*see also* Retardation, mental) 319
Meynert's (nonalcoholic) 294.0
alcoholic 291.1
nevoid 759.6
American
leishmaniasis 085.5
mountain tick fever 066.1
trypanosomiasis - *see* Trypanosomiasis, American
Ametropia (*see also* Disorder, accommodation) 367.9
Amianthosis 501
Amimia 784.69
Amino acid
deficiency 270.9
anemia 281.4
metabolic disorder (*see also* Disorder, amino acid) 270.9
Aminoaciduria 270.9
imidazole 270.5
Amnesia (retrograde) 780.93
auditory 784.69
developmental 315.31
secondary to organic lesion 784.69
dissociative 300.12
hysterical or dissociative type 300.12
psychogenic 300.12
transient global 437.7
Amnestic (confabulatory) syndrome 294.0
alcohol-induced persisting 291.1
drug-induced persisting 292.83
posttraumatic 294.0
Amniocentesis screening (for) V28.2
alphafetoprotein level, raised V28.1
chromosomal anomalies V28.0
Amnion, amniotic - *see also* condition
nodosum 658.8
Amnionitis (complicating pregnancy) 658.4
affecting fetus or newborn 762.7
Amoral trends 301.7
Amotio retinae (*see also* Detachment, retina) 361.9
Ampulla
lower esophagus 530.89
phrenic 530.89
Amputation
any part of fetus, to facilitate delivery 763.89
cervix (supravaginal) (uteri) 622.8
in pregnancy or childbirth 654.6
affecting fetus or newborn 763.89
clitoris - *see* Wound, open, clitoris
congenital
lower limb 755.31
upper limb 755.21
neuroma (traumatic) - *see also* Injury, nerve, by site
surgical complication (late) 997.61
penis - *see* Amputation, traumatic, penis
status (without complication) - *see* Absence, by site, acquired
stump (surgical) (posttraumatic)
abnormal, painful, or with complication (late) 997.60
healed or old NEC - *see also* Absence, by site, acquired
lower V49.70
upper V49.60
Amputation *(Continued)*
traumatic (complete) (partial)

Note "Complicated" includes traumatic amputation with delayed healing, delayed treatment, foreign body, or infection.

arm 887.4
at or above elbow 887.2
complicated 887.3
below elbow 887.0
complicated 887.1
both (bilateral) (any level(s)) 887.6
complicated 887.7
complicated 887.5
finger(s) (one or both hands) 886.0
with thumb(s) 885.0
complicated 885.1
complicated 886.1
foot (except toe(s) only) 896.0
and other leg 897.6
complicated 897.7
both (bilateral) 896.2
complicated 896.3
complicated 896.1
toe(s) only (one or both feet) 895.0
complicated 895.1
genital organ(s) (external) NEC 878.8
complicated 878.9
hand (except finger(s) only) 887.0
and other arm 887.6
complicated 887.7
both (bilateral) 887.6
complicated 887.7
complicated 887.1
finger(s) (one or both hands) 886.0
with thumb(s) 885.0
complicated 885.1
complicated 886.1
thumb(s) (with fingers of either hand) 885.0
complicated 885.1
head 874.9
late effect - *see* Late, effects (of), amputation
leg 897.4
and other foot 897.6
complicated 897.7
at or above knee 897.2
complicated 897.3
below knee 897.0
complicated 897.1
both (bilateral) 897.6
complicated 897.7
complicated 897.5
lower limb(s) except toe(s) - *see* Amputation, traumatic, leg
nose - *see* Wound, open, nose
penis 878.0
complicated 878.1
sites other than limbs - *see* Wound, open, by site
thumb(s) (with finger(s) of either hand) 885.0
complicated 885.1
toe(s) (one or both feet) 895.0
complicated 895.1
upper limb(s) - *see* Amputation, traumatic, arm
Amputee (bilateral) (old) - *see* Absence, by site, acquired V49.70
Amusia 784.69
developmental 315.39
secondary to organic lesion 784.69
Amyelencephalus 740.0
Amyelia 742.59
Amygdalitis - *see* Tonsillitis
Amygdalolith 474.8
Amyloid disease or degeneration 277.30
heart 277.39 *[425.7]*
Amyloidosis (familial) (general) (generalized) (genetic) (primary) 277.39
with lung involvement 277.39 *[517.8]*
cardiac, hereditary 277.39
heart 277.39 *[425.7]*
nephropathic 277.39 *[583.81]*
neuropathic (Portuguese) (Swiss) 277.39 *[357.4]*
pulmonary 277.39 *[517.8]*
secondary 277.39
systemic, inherited 277.39
Amylopectinosis (brancher enzyme deficiency) 271.0
Amylophagia 307.52
Amyoplasia congenita 756.89
Amyotonia 728.2
congenita 358.8
Amyotrophia, amyotrophy, amyotrophic 728.2
congenita 756.89
diabetic 250.6 *[358.1]*
lateral sclerosis (syndrome) 335.20
neuralgic 353.5
sclerosis (lateral) 335.20
spinal progressive 335.21
Anacidity, gastric 536.0
psychogenic 306.4
Anaerosis of newborn 770.88
Analbuminemia 273.8
Analgesia (*see also* Anesthesia) 782.0
Analphalipoproteinemia 272.5
Anaphylactic shock or reaction (correct substance properly administered) 995.0
due to
food 995.60
additives 995.66
crustaceans 995.62
eggs 995.68
fish 995.65
fruits 995.63
milk products 995.67
nuts (tree) 995.64
peanuts 995.61
seeds 995.64,
specified NEC 995.69
tree nuts 995.64
vegetables 995.63
immunization 999.4
overdose or wrong substance given or taken 977.9
specified drug - *see* Table of Drugs and Chemicals
serum 999.4
following sting(s) 989.5
purpura 287.0
serum 999.4
Anaphylactoid shock or reaction - *see* Anaphylactic shock
Anaphylaxis - *see* Anaphylactic shock
Anaplasia, cervix 622.10
Anarthria 784.5
Anarthritic rheumatoid disease 446.5
Anasarca 782.3
cardiac (*see also* Failure, heart 428.0
fetus or newborn 778.0

ICD-9-CM A Vol. 2

Anasarca *(Continued)*
lung 514
nutritional 262
pulmonary 514
renal (*see also* Nephrosis) 581.9
Anaspadias 752.62
Anastomosis
aneurysmal - *see* Aneurysm
arteriovenous, congenital NEC (*see also* Anomaly, arteriovenous) 747.60
ruptured, of brain (*see also* Hemorrhage, subarachnoid) 430
intestinal 569.89
complicated NEC 997.4
involving urinary tract 997.5
retinal and choroidal vessels 743.58
acquired 362.17
Anatomical narrow angle (glaucoma) 365.02
Ancylostoma (infection) (infestation) 126.9
americanus 126.1
braziliense 126.2
caninum 126.8
ceylanicum 126.3
duodenale 126.0
Necator americanus 126.1
Ancylostomiasis (intestinal) 126.9
Ancylostoma
americanus 126.1
caninum 126.8
ceylanicum 126.3
duodenale 126.0
braziliense 126.2
Necator americanus 126.1
Anders' disease or syndrome (adiposis tuberosa simplex) 272.8
Andersen's glycogen storage disease 271.0
Anderson's disease 272.7
Andes disease 993.2
Andrews' disease (bacterid) 686.8
Androblastoma (M8630/1)
benign (M8630/0)
specified site - *see* Neoplasm, by site, benign
unspecified site
female 220
male 222.0
malignant (M8630/3)
specified site - *see* Neoplasm, by site, malignant
unspecified site
female 183.0
male 186.9
specified site - *see* Neoplasm, by site, uncertain behavior
tubular (M8640/0)
with lipid storage (M8641/0)
specified site - *see* Neoplasm, by site, benign
unspecified site
female 220
male 222.0
specified site - *see* Neoplasm, by site, benign
unspecified site
female 220
male 222.0
unspecified site
female 236.2
male 236.4
Android pelvis 755.69
with disproportion (fetopelvic) 653.3
Android pelvis *(Continued)*
with disproportion *(Continued)*
affecting fetus or newborn 763.1
causing obstructed labor 660.1
affecting fetus or newborn 763.1
Anectasis, pulmonary (newborn or fetus) 770.5
Anemia 285.9
with
disorder of
anaerobic glycolysis 282.3
pentose phosphate pathway 282.2
koilonychia 280.9
6-phosphogluconic dehydrogenase deficiency 282.2
achlorhydric 280.9
achrestic 281.8
Addison's (pernicious) 281.0
Addison-Biermer (pernicious) 281.0
agranulocytic 288.09
amino acid deficiency 281.4
aplastic 284.9
acquired (secondary) 284.8
congenital 284.01
constitutional 284.01
due to
chronic systemic disease 284.8
drugs 284.8
infection 284.8
radiation 284.8
idiopathic 284.9
myxedema 244.9
of or complicating pregnancy 648.2
red cell (acquired) (with thymoma) 284.8
congenital 284.01
pure 284.01
specified type NEC 284.8
toxic (paralytic) 284.8
aregenerative 284.9
congenital 284.01
asiderotic 280.9
atypical (primary) 285.9
autohemolysis of Selwyn and Dacie (type I) 282.2
autoimmune hemolytic 283.0
Baghdad Spring 282.2
Balantidium coli 007.0
Biermer's (pernicious) 281.0
blood loss (chronic) 280.0
acute 285.1
bothriocephalus 123.4
brickmakers' (*see also* Ancylostomiasis) 126.9
cerebral 437.8
childhood 282.9
chlorotic 280.9
chronica congenita aregenerativa 284.01
chronic simple 281.9
combined system disease NEC 281.0 *[336.2]*
due to dietary deficiency 281.1 *[336.2]*
complicating pregnancy or childbirth 648.2
congenital (following fetal blood loss) 776.5
aplastic 284.01
due to isoimmunization NEC 773.2
Heinz-body 282.7
hereditary hemolytic NEC 282.9
nonspherocytic
type I 282.2
type II 282.3
Anemia *(Continued)*
congenital *(Continued)*
pernicious 281.0
spherocytic (*see also* Spherocytosis) 282.0
Cooley's (erythroblastic) 282.49
crescent - *see* Disease, sickle-cell
cytogenic 281.0
Dacie's (nonspherocytic)
type I 282.2
type II 282.3
Davidson's (refractory) 284.9
deficiency 281.9
2,3 diphosphoglycurate mutase 282.3
2,3 PG 282.3
6-PGD 282.2
6-phosphogluronic dehydrogenase 282.2
amino acid 281.4
combined B_{12} and folate 281.3
enzyme, drug-induced (hemolytic) 282.2
erythrocytic glutathione 282.2
folate 281.2
dietary 281.2
drug-induced 281.2
folic acid 281.2
dietary 281.2
drug-induced 281.2
G-6-PD 282.2
GGS-R 282.2
glucose-6-phosphate dehydrogenase (G-6-PD) 282.2
glucose-phosphate isomerase 282.3
glutathione peroxidase 282.2
glutathione reductase 282.2
glyceraldehyde phosphate dehydrogenase 282.3
GPI 282.3
G SH 282.2
hexokinase 282.3
iron (Fe) 280.9
specified NEC 280.8
nutritional 281.9
with
poor iron absorption 280.9
specified deficiency NEC 281.8
due to inadequate dietary iron intake 280.1
specified type NEC 281.8
of or complicating pregnancy 648.2
pentose phosphate pathway 282.2
PFK 282.3
phosphofructo-aldolase 282.3
phosphofructokinase 282.3
phosphoglycerate kinase 282.3
PK 282.3
protein 281.4
pyruvate kinase (PK) 282.3
TPI 282.3
triosephosphate isomerase 282.3
vitamin B_{12} NEC 281.1
dietary 281.1
pernicious 281.0
Diamond-Blackfan (congenital hypoplastic) 284.01
dibothriocephalus 123.4
dimorphic 281.9
diphasic 281.8
diphtheritic 032.89
Diphyllobothrium 123.4
drepanocytic (*see also* Disease, sickle-cell) 282.60

- **Anemia** *(Continued)*
  - due to
    - blood loss (chronic) 280.0
      - acute 285.1
    - defect of Embden-Meyerhof pathway glycolysis 282.3
    - disorder of glutathione metabolism 282.2
    - fetal blood loss 776.5
    - fish tapeworm (D. latum) infestation 123.4
    - glutathione metabolism disorder 282.2
    - hemorrhage (chronic) 280.0
      - acute 285.1
    - hexose monophosphate (HMP) shunt deficiency 282.2
    - impaired absorption 280.9
    - loss of blood (chronic) 280.0
      - acute 285.1
    - myxedema 244.9
    - Necator americanus 126.1
    - prematurity 776.6
    - selective vitamin B_{12} malabsorption with proteinuria 281.1
  - Dyke-Young type (secondary) (symptomatic) 283.9
  - dyserythropoietic (congenital) (types I, II, III) 285.8
  - dyshemopoietic (congenital) 285.8
  - Egypt (*see also* Ancylostomiasis) 126.9
  - elliptocytosis (*see also* Elliptocytosis) 282.1
  - enzyme deficiency, drug-induced 282.2
  - epidemic (*see also* Ancylostomiasis) 126.9
  - EPO resistant 285.21
  - erythroblastic
    - familial 282.49
    - fetus or newborn (*see also* Disease, hemolytic) 773.2
      - late 773.5
  - erythrocytic glutathione deficiency 282.2
  - erythropoietin-resistant (EPO resistant anemia) 285.21
  - essential 285.9
  - Faber's (achlorhydric anemia) 280.9
  - factitious (self-induced bloodletting) 280.0
  - familial erythroblastic (microcytic) 282.49
  - Fanconi's (congenital pancytopenia) 284.09
  - favism 282.2
  - fetal, following blood loss 776.5
  - fetus or newborn
    - due to
      - ABO
        - antibodies 773.1
        - incompatibility, maternal/fetal 773.1
        - isoimmunization 773.1
      - Rh
        - antibodies 773.0
        - incompatibility, maternal/fetal 773.0
        - isoimmunization 773.0
    - following fetal blood loss 776.5
  - fish tapeworm (D. latum) infestation 123.4
  - folate (folic acid) deficiency 281.2
    - dietary 281.2
    - drug-induced 281.2

- **Anemia** *(Continued)*
  - folate malabsorption, congenital 281.2
  - folic acid deficiency 281.2
    - dietary 281.2
    - drug-induced 281.2
  - G-6-PD 282.2
  - general 285.9
  - glucose-6-phosphate dehydrogenase deficiency 282.2
  - glutathione-reductase deficiency 282.2
  - goat's milk 281.2
  - granulocytic 288.09
  - Heinz-body, congenital 282.7
  - hemoglobin deficiency 285.9
  - hemolytic 283.9
    - acquired 283.9
      - with hemoglobinuria NEC 283.2
      - autoimmune (cold type) (idiopathic) (primary) (secondary) (symptomatic) (warm type) 283.0
      - due to
        - cold reactive antibodies 283.0
        - drug exposure 283.0
        - warm reactive antibodies 283.0
      - fragmentation 283.19
      - idiopathic (chronic) 283.9
      - infectious 283.19
        - autoimmune 283.0
        - non-autoimmune 283.10
      - toxic 283.19
      - traumatic cardiac 283.19
    - acute 283.9
      - due to enzyme deficiency NEC 282.3
      - fetus or newborn (*see also* Disease, hemolytic) 773.2
        - late 773.5
      - Lederer's (acquired infectious hemolytic anemia) 283.19
    - autoimmune (acquired) 283.0
    - chronic 282.9
      - idiopathic 283.9
    - cold type (secondary) (symptomatic) 283.0
    - congenital (spherocytic) (*see also* Spherocytosis) 282.0
      - nonspherocytic - *see* Anemia, hemolytic, nonspherocytic, congenital
    - drug-induced 283.0
      - enzyme deficiency 282.2
    - due to
      - cardiac conditions 283.19
      - drugs 283.0
      - enzyme deficiency NEC 282.3
        - drug-induced 282.2
      - presence of shunt or other internal prosthetic device 283.19
      - thrombotic thrombocytopenic purpura 446.6
    - elliptocytotic (*see also* Elliptocytosis) 282.1
    - familial 282.9
    - hereditary 282.9
      - due to enzyme deficiency NEC 282.3
      - specified NEC 282.8
    - idiopathic (chronic) 283.9
    - infectious (acquired) 283.19
    - mechanical 283.19
    - microangiopathic 283.19
    - nonautoimmune 283.10

- **Anemia** *(Continued)*
  - hemolytic *(Continued)*
    - nonspherocytic
      - congenital or hereditary NEC 282.3
        - glucose-6-phosphate dehydrogenase deficiency 282.2
        - pyruvate kinase (PK) deficiency 282.3
        - type I 282.2
        - type II 282.3
      - type I 282.2
      - type II 282.3
    - of or complicating pregnancy 648.2
    - resulting from presence of shunt or other internal prosthetic device 283.19
    - secondary 283.19
      - autoimmune 283.0
    - sickle-cell - *see* Disease, sickle-cell
    - Stransky-Regala type (Hb-E) (*see also* Disease, hemoglobin) 282.7
    - symptomatic 283.19
      - autoimmune 283.0
    - toxic (acquired) 283.19
    - uremic (adult) (child) 283.11
    - warm type (secondary) (symptomatic) 283.0
  - hemorrhagic (chronic) 280.0
    - acute 285.1
  - HEMPAS 285.8
  - hereditary erythroblast multinuclearity-positive acidified serum test 285.8
  - Herrick's (hemoglobin S disease) 282.61
  - hexokinase deficiency 282.3
  - high A_2 282.49
  - hookworm (*see also* Ancylostomiasis) 126.9
  - hypochromic (idiopathic) (microcytic) (normoblastic) 280.9
    - with iron loading 285.0
    - due to blood loss (chronic) 280.0
      - acute 285.1
    - familial sex linked 285.0
    - pyridoxine-responsive 285.0
  - hypoplasia, red blood cells 284.8
    - congenital or familial 284.01
  - hypoplastic (idiopathic) 284.9
    - congenital 284.01
    - familial 284.01
    - of childhood 284.09
  - idiopathic 285.9
    - hemolytic, chronic 283.9
  - in
    - chronic illness NEC 285.29
    - chronic kidney disease 285.21
    - end-stage renal disease 285.21
    - neoplastic disease 285.22
  - infantile 285.9
  - infective, infectional 285.9
  - intertropical (*see also* Ancylostomiasis) 126.9
  - iron (Fe) deficiency 280.9
    - due to blood loss (chronic) 280.0
      - acute 285.1
    - of or complicating pregnancy 648.2
    - specified NEC 280.8
  - Jaksch's (pseudoleukemia infantum) 285.8
  - Joseph-Diamond-Blackfan (congenital hypoplastic) 284.01
  - labyrinth 386.50
  - Lederer's (acquired infectious hemolytic anemia) 283.19

Anemia *(Continued)*
leptocytosis (hereditary) 282.49
leukoerythroblastic 284.2
macrocytic 281.9
nutritional 281.2
of or complicating pregnancy 648.2
tropical 281.2
malabsorption (familial), selective B_{12} with proteinuria 281.1
malarial (*see also* Malaria) 084.6
malignant (progressive) 281.0
malnutrition 281.9
marsh (*see also* Malaria) 084.6
Mediterranean (with hemoglobinopathy) 282.49
megaloblastic 281.9
combined B_{12} and folate deficiency 281.3
nutritional (of infancy) 281.2
of infancy 281.2
of or complicating pregnancy 648.2
refractory 281.3
specified NEC 281.3
megalocytic 281.9
microangiopathic hemolytic 283.19
microcytic (hypochromic) 280.9
due to blood loss (chronic) 280.0
acute 285.1
familial 282.49
hypochromic 280.9
microdrepanocytosis 282.49
miners' (*see also* Ancylostomiasis) 126.9
myelopathic 285.8
myelophthisic (normocytic) 284.2
newborn (*see also* Disease, hemolytic) 773.2
due to isoimmunization (*see also* Disease, hemolytic) 773.2
late, due to isoimmunization 773.5
posthemorrhagic 776.5
nonregenerative 284.9
nonspherocytic hemolytic - *see* Anemia, hemolytic, nonspherocytic
normocytic (infectional) (not due to blood loss) 285.9
due to blood loss (chronic) 280.0
acute 285.1
myelophthisic 284.2
nutritional (deficiency) 281.9
with
poor iron absorption 280.9
specified deficiency NEC 281.8
due to inadequate dietary iron intake 280.1
megaloblastic (of infancy) 281.2
of childhood 282.9
of chronic
disease NEC 285.29
illness NEC 285.29
of or complicating pregnancy 648.2
affecting fetus or newborn 760.8
of prematurity 776.6
orotic aciduric (congenital) (hereditary) 281.4
osteosclerotic 289.89
ovalocytosis (hereditary) (*see also* Elliptocytosis) 282.1
paludal (*see also* Malaria) 084.6
pentose phosphate pathway deficiency 282.2

Anemia *(Continued)*
pernicious (combined system disease) (congenital) (dorsolateral spinal degeneration) (juvenile) (myelopathy) (neuropathy) (posterior sclerosis) (primary) (progressive) (spleen) 281.0
of or complicating pregnancy 648.2
pleochromic 285.9
of sprue 281.8
portal 285.8
posthemorrhagic (chronic) 280.0
acute 285.1
newborn 776.5
postoperative
due to blood loss 285.1
other 285.9
postpartum 648.2
pressure 285.9
primary 285.9
profound 285.9
progressive 285.9
malignant 281.0
pernicious 281.0
protein-deficiency 281.4
pseudoleukemia infantum 285.8
puerperal 648.2
pure red cell 284.8
congenital 284.01
pyridoxine-responsive (hypochromic) 285.0
pyruvate kinase (PK) deficiency 282.3
refractoria sideroblastica 238.72
refractory (primary) 238.72
with
excess
blasts-1 (RAEB-1) 238.73
blasts-2 (RAEB-2) 238.73
hemochromatosis 238.72
ringed sideroblasts (RARS) 238.72
megaloblastic 281.3
sideroblastic 238.72
sideropenic 280.9
Rietti-Greppi-Micheli (thalassemia minor) 282.49
scorbutic 281.8
secondary (to) 285.9
blood loss (chronic) 280.0
acute 285.1
hemorrhage 280.0
acute 285.1
inadequate dietary iron intake 280.1
semiplastic 284.9
septic 285.9
sickle-cell (*see also* Disease, sickle-cell) 282.60
sideroachrestic 285.0
sideroblastic (acquired) (any type) (congenital) (drug-induced) (due to disease) (hereditary) (primary) (secondary) (sex-linked hypochromic) (vitamin B_6 responsive) 285.0
refractory 238.72
sideropenic (refractory) 280.9
due to blood loss (chronic) 280.0
acute 285.1
simple chronic 281.9
specified type NEC 285.8
spherocytic (hereditary) (*see also* Spherocytosis) 282.0
splenic 285.8
familial (Gaucher's) 272.7

Anemia *(Continued)*
splenomegalic 285.8
stomatocytosis 282.8
syphilitic 095.8
target cell (oval) 282.49
thalassemia 282.49
thrombocytopenic (*see also* Thrombocytopenia) 287.5
toxic 284.8
triosephosphate isomerase deficiency 282.3
tropical, macrocytic 281.2
tuberculous (*see also* Tuberculosis) 017.9
vegan's 281.1
vitamin
B_6-responsive 285.0
B_{12} deficiency (dietary) 281.1
pernicious 281.0
von Jaksch's (pseudoleukemia infantum) 285.8
Witts' (achlorhydric anemia) 280.9
Zuelzer (-Ogden) (nutritional megaloblastic anemia) 281.2
Anencephalus, anencephaly 740.0
fetal, affecting management of pregnancy 655.0
Anergasia (*see also* Psychosis, organic) 294.9
senile 290.0
Anesthesia, anesthetic 782.0
complication or reaction NEC 995.22
due to
correct substance properly administered 995.22
overdose or wrong substance given 968.4
specified anesthetic - *see* Table of Drugs and Chemicals
cornea 371.81
death from
correct substance properly administered 995.4
during delivery 668.9
overdose or wrong substance given 968.4
specified anesthetic - *see* Table of Drugs and Chemicals
eye 371.81
functional 300.11
hyperesthetic, thalamic 338.0
hysterical 300.11
local skin lesion 782.0
olfactory 781.1
sexual (psychogenic) 302.72
shock
due to
correct substance properly administered 995.4
overdose or wrong substance given 968.4
specified anesthetic - *see* Table of Drugs and Chemicals
skin 782.0
tactile 782.0
testicular 608.9
thermal 782.0
Anetoderma (maculosum) 701.3
Aneuploidy NEC 758.5
Aneurin deficiency 265.1
Aneurysm (anastomotic) (artery) (cirsoid) (diffuse) (false) (fusiform) (multiple) (ruptured) (saccular) (varicose) 442.9

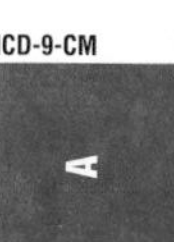
ICD-9-CM
A
Vol. 2

Aneurysm *(Continued)*
abdominal (aorta) 441.4
ruptured 441.3
syphilitic 093.0
aorta, aortic (nonsyphilitic) 441.9
abdominal 441.4
dissecting 441.02
ruptured 441.3
syphilitic 093.0
arch 441.2
ruptured 441.1
arteriosclerotic NEC 441.9
ruptured 441.5
ascending 441.2
ruptured 441.1
congenital 747.29
descending 441.9
abdominal 441.4
ruptured 441.3
ruptured 441.5
thoracic 441.2
ruptured 441.1
dissecting 441.00
abdominal 441.02
thoracic 441.01
thoracoabdominal 441.03
due to coarctation (aorta) 747.10
ruptured 441.5
sinus, right 747.29
syphilitic 093.0
thoracoabdominal 441.7
ruptured 441.6
thorax, thoracic (arch) (nonsyphilitic) 441.2
dissecting 441.01
ruptured 441.1
syphilitic 093.0
transverse 441.2
ruptured 441.1
valve (heart) (*see also* Endocarditis, aortic) 424.1
arteriosclerotic NEC 442.9
cerebral 437.3
ruptured (*see also* Hemorrhage, subarachnoid) 430
arteriovenous (congenital) (peripheral) NEC (*see also* Anomaly, arteriovenous) 747.60
acquired NEC 447.0
brain 437.3
ruptured (*see also* Hemorrhage, subarachnoid) 430
coronary 414.11
pulmonary 417.0
brain (cerebral) 747.81
ruptured (*see also* Hemorrhage, subarachnoid) 430
coronary 746.85
pulmonary 747.3
retina 743.58
specified site NEC 747.89
acquired 447.0
traumatic (*see also* Injury, blood vessel, by site) 904.9
basal - *see* Aneurysm, brain
berry (congenital) (ruptured) (*see also* Hemorrhage, subarachnoid) 430
brain 437.3
arteriosclerotic 437.3
ruptured (*see also* Hemorrhage, subarachnoid) 430
arteriovenous 747.81
acquired 437.3

Aneurysm *(Continued)*
brain *(Continued)*
arteriovenous *(Continued)*
acquired *(Continued)*
ruptured (*see also* Hemorrhage, subarachnoid) 430
ruptured (*see also* Hemorrhage, subarachnoid) 430
berry (congenital) (ruptured) (*see also* Hemorrhage, subarachnoid) 430
congenital 747.81
ruptured (*see also* Hemorrhage, subarachnoid) 430
meninges 437.3
ruptured (*see also* Hemorrhage, subarachnoid) 430
miliary (congenital) (ruptured) (*see also* Hemorrhage, subarachnoid) 430
mycotic 421.0
ruptured (*see also* Hemorrhage, subarachnoid) 430
nonruptured 437.3
ruptured (*see also* Hemorrhage, subarachnoid) 430
syphilitic 094.87
syphilitic (hemorrhage) 094.87
traumatic - *see* Injury, intracranial
cardiac (false) (*see also* Aneurysm, heart) 414.10
carotid artery (common) (external) 442.81
internal (intracranial portion) 437.3
extracranial portion 442.81
ruptured into brain (*see also* Hemorrhage, subarachnoid) 430
syphilitic 093.89
intracranial 094.87
cavernous sinus (*see also* Aneurysm, brain) 437.3
arteriovenous 747.81
ruptured (*see also* Hemorrhage, subarachnoid) 430
congenital 747.81
ruptured (*see also* Hemorrhage, subarachnoid) 430
celiac 442.84
central nervous system, syphilitic 094.89
cerebral - *see* Aneurysm, brain
chest - *see* Aneurysm, thorax
circle of Willis (*see also* Aneurysm, brain) 437.3
congenital 747.81
ruptured (*see also* Hemorrhage, subarachnoid) 430
ruptured (*see also* Hemorrhage, subarachnoid) 430
common iliac artery 442.2
congenital (peripheral) NEC 747.60
brain 747.81
ruptured (*see also* Hemorrhage, subarachnoid) 430
cerebral - *see* Aneurysm, brain, congenital
coronary 746.85
gastrointestinal 747.61
lower limb 747.64
pulmonary 747.3
renal 747.62
retina 743.58
specified site NEC 747.89
spinal 747.82
upper limb 747.63
conjunctiva 372.74

Aneurysm *(Continued)*
conus arteriosus (*see also* Aneurysm, heart) 414.10
coronary (arteriosclerotic) (artery) (vein) (*see also* Aneurysm, heart) 414.11
arteriovenous 746.85
congenital 746.85
syphilitic 093.89
cylindrical 441.9
ruptured 441.5
syphilitic 093.9
dissecting 442.9
aorta 441.00
abdominal 441.02
thoracic 441.01
thoracoabdominal 441.03
syphilitic 093.9
ductus arteriosus 747.0
embolic - *see* Embolism, artery
endocardial, infective (any valve) 421.0
femoral 442.3
gastroduodenal 442.84
gastroepiploic 442.84
heart (chronic or with a stated duration of over 8 weeks) (infectional) (wall) 414.10
acute or with a stated duration of 8 weeks or less (*see also* Infarct, myocardium) 410.9
congenital 746.89
valve - *see* Endocarditis
hepatic 442.84
iliac (common) 442.2
infective (any valve) 421.0
innominate (nonsyphilitic) 442.89
syphilitic 093.89
interauricular septum (*see also* Aneurysm, heart) 414.10
interventricular septum (*see also* Aneurysm, heart) 414.10
intracranial - *see* Aneurysm, brain
intrathoracic (nonsyphilitic) 441.2
ruptured 441.1
syphilitic 093.0
jugular vein 453.8
lower extremity 442.3
lung (pulmonary artery) 417.1
malignant 093.9
mediastinal (nonsyphilitic) 442.89
syphilitic 093.89
miliary (congenital) (ruptured) (*see also* Hemorrhage, subarachnoid) 430
mitral (heart) (valve) 424.0
mural (arteriovenous) (heart) (*see also* Aneurysm, heart) 414.10
mycotic, any site 421.0
without endocarditis - *see* Aneurysm, by site ◄
ruptured, brain (*see also* Hemorrhage, subarachnoid) 430
myocardium (*see also* Aneurysm, heart) 414.10
neck 442.81
pancreaticoduodenal 442.84
patent ductus arteriosus 747.0
peripheral NEC 442.89
congenital NEC (*see also* Aneurysm, congenital) 747.60
popliteal 442.3
pulmonary 417.1
arteriovenous 747.3
acquired 417.0
syphilitic 093.89

Aneurysm *(Continued)*
pulmonary *(Continued)*
valve (heart) (*see also* Endocarditis, pulmonary) 424.3
racemose 442.9
congenital (peripheral) NEC 747.60
radial 442.0
Rasmussen's (*see also* Tuberculosis) 011.2
renal 442.1
retinal (acquired) 362.17
congenital 743.58
diabetic 250.5 *[362.01]*
sinus, aortic (of Valsalva) 747.29
specified site NEC 442.89
spinal (cord) 442.89
congenital 747.82
syphilitic (hemorrhage) 094.89
spleen, splenic 442.83
subclavian 442.82
syphilitic 093.89
superior mesenteric 442.84
syphilitic 093.9
aorta 093.0
central nervous system 094.89
congenital 090.5
spine, spinal 094.89
thoracoabdominal 441.7
ruptured 441.6
thorax, thoracic (arch) (nonsyphilitic) 441.2
dissecting 441.01
ruptured 441.1
syphilitic 093.0
traumatic (complication) (early) - *see* Injury, blood vessel, by site
tricuspid (heart) (valve) - *see* Endocarditis, tricuspid
ulnar 442.0
upper extremity 442.0
valve, valvular - *see* Endocarditis
venous 456.8
congenital NEC (*see also* Aneurysm, congenital) 747.60
ventricle (arteriovenous) (*see also* Aneurysm, heart) 414.10
visceral artery NEC 442.84
Angiectasis 459.89
Angiectopia 459.9
Angiitis 447.6
allergic granulomatous 446.4
hypersensitivity 446.20
Goodpasture's syndrome 446.21
specified NEC 446.29
necrotizing 446.0
Wegener's (necrotizing respiratory granulomatosis) 446.4
Angina (attack) (cardiac) (chest) (effort) (heart) (pectoris) (syndrome) (vasomotor) 413.9
abdominal 557.1
accelerated 411.1
agranulocytic 288.03 ⬅
aphthous 074.0
catarrhal 462
crescendo 411.1
croupous 464.4
cruris 443.9
due to atherosclerosis NEC (*see also* Arteriosclerosis, extremities) 440.20
decubitus 413.0
diphtheritic (membranous) 032.0
erysipelatous 034.0

Angina *(Continued)*
erythematous 462
exudative, chronic 476.0
faucium 478.29
gangrenous 462
diphtheritic 032.0
infectious 462
initial 411.1
intestinal 557.1
ludovici 528.3
Ludwig's 528.3
malignant 462
diphtheritic 032.0
membranous 464.4
diphtheritic 032.0
mesenteric 557.1
monocytic 075
nocturnal 413.0
phlegmonous 475
diphtheritic 032.0
preinfarctional 411.1
Prinzmetal's 413.1
progressive 411.1
pseudomembranous 101
psychogenic 306.2
pultaceous, diphtheritic 032.0
scarlatinal 034.1
septic 034.0
simple 462
stable NEC 413.9
staphylococcal 462
streptococcal 034.0
stridulous, diphtheritic 032.3
syphilitic 093.9
congenital 090.5
tonsil 475
trachealis 464.4
unstable 411.1
variant 413.1
Vincent's 101
Angioblastoma (M9161/1) - *see* Neoplasm, connective tissue, uncertain behavior
Angiocholecystitis (*see also* Cholecystitis, acute) 575.0
Angiocholitis (*see also* Cholecystitis, acute) 576.1
Angiodysgensis spinalis 336.1
Angiodysplasia (intestinalis) (intestine) 569.84
with hemorrhage 569.85
duodenum 537.82
with hemorrhage 537.83
stomach 537.82
with hemorrhage 537.83
Angioedema (allergic) (any site) (with urticaria) 995.1
hereditary 277.6
Angioendothelioma (M9130/1) - *see also* Neoplasm, by site, uncertain behavior
benign (M9130/0) (*see also* Hemangioma, by site) 228.00
bone (M9260/3) - *see* Neoplasm, bone, malignant
Ewing's (M9260/3) - *see* Neoplasm, bone, malignant
nervous system (M9130/0) 228.09
Angiofibroma (M9160/0) - *see also* Neoplasm, by site, benign
juvenile (M9160/0) 210.7
specified site - *see* Neoplasm, by site, benign
unspecified site 210.7

Angiohemophilia (A) (B) 286.4
Angioid streaks (choroid) (retina) 363.43
Angiokeratoma (M9141/0) - *see also* Neoplasm, skin, benign
corporis diffusum 272.7
Angiokeratosis
diffuse 272.7
Angioleiomyoma (M8894/0) - *see* Neoplasm, connective tissue, benign
Angioleucitis 683
Angiolipoma (M8861/0) (*see also* Lipoma, by site) 214.9
infiltrating (M8861/1) - *see* Neoplasm, connective tissue, uncertain behavior
Angioma (M9120/0) (*see also* Hemangioma, by site) 228.00
capillary 448.1
hemorrhagicum hereditaria 448.0
malignant (M9120/3) - *see* Neoplasm, connective tissue, malignant
pigmentosum et atrophicum 757.33
placenta - *see* Placenta, abnormal
plexiform (M9131/0) - *see* Hemangioma, by site
senile 448.1
serpiginosum 709.1
spider 448.1
stellate 448.1
Angiomatosis 757.32
bacillary 083.8
corporis diffusum universale 272.7
cutaneocerebral 759.6
encephalocutaneous 759.6
encephalofacial 759.6
encephalotrigeminal 759.6
hemorrhagic familial 448.0
hereditary familial 448.0
heredofamilial 448.0
meningo-oculofacial 759.6
multiple sites 228.09
neuro-oculocutaneous 759.6
retina (Hippel's disease) 759.6
retinocerebellosa 759.6
retinocerebral 759.6
systemic 228.09
Angiomyolipoma (M8860/0)
specified site - *see* Neoplasm, connective tissue, benign
unspecified site 223.0
Angiomyoliposarcoma (M8860/3) - *see* Neoplasm, connective tissue, malignant
Angiomyoma (M8894/0) - *see* Neoplasm, connective tissue, benign
Angiomyosarcoma (M8894/3) - *see* Neoplasm, connective tissue, malignant
Angioneurosis 306.2
Angioneurotic edema (allergic) (any site) (with urticaria) 995.1
hereditary 277.6
Angiopathia, angiopathy 459.9
diabetic (peripheral) 250.7 *[443.81]*
peripheral 443.9
diabetic 250.7 *[443.81]*
specified type NEC 443.89
retinae syphilitica 093.89
retinalis (juvenilis) 362.18
background 362.10
diabetic 250.5 *[362.01]*
proliferative 362.29
tuberculous (*see also* Tuberculosis) 017.3 *[362.18]*

◀ **New** ⬅ **Revised**

Angiosarcoma (M9120/3) - *see* Neoplasm, connective tissue, malignant
Angiosclerosis - *see* Arteriosclerosis
Angioscotoma, enlarged 368.42
Angiospasm 443.9
  brachial plexus 353.0
  cerebral 435.9
  cervical plexus 353.2
  nerve
    arm 354.9
      axillary 353.0
      median 354.1
      ulnar 354.2
    autonomic (*see also* Neuropathy, peripheral, autonomic) 337.9
    axillary 353.0
    leg 355.8
      plantar 355.6
    lower extremity - *see* Angiospasm, nerve, leg
    median 354.1
    peripheral NEC 355.9
    spinal NEC 355.9
    sympathetic (*see also* Neuropathy, peripheral, autonomic) 337.9
    ulnar 354.2
    upper extremity - *see* Angiospasm, nerve, arm
  peripheral NEC 443.9
  traumatic 443.9
    foot 443.9
    leg 443.9
  vessel 443.9
Angiospastic disease or edema 443.9
Angle's
    class I 524.21
    class II 524.22
    class III 524.23
Anguillulosis 127.2
Angulation
  cecum (*see also* Obstruction, intestine) 560.9
  coccyx (acquired) 738.6
    congenital 756.19
  femur (acquired) 736.39
    congenital 755.69
  intestine (large) (small) (*see also* Obstruction, intestine) 560.9
  sacrum (acquired) 738.5
    congenital 756.19
  sigmoid (flexure) (*see also* Obstruction, intestine) 560.9
  spine (*see also* Curvature, spine) 737.9
  tibia (acquired) 736.89
    congenital 755.69
  ureter 593.3
  wrist (acquired) 736.09
    congenital 755.59
Angulus infectiosus 686.8
Anhedonia 302.72
Anhidrosis (lid) (neurogenic) (thermogenic) 705.0
Anhydration 276.51
  with
    hypernatremia 276.0
    hyponatremia 276.1
Anhydremia 276.52
  with
    hypernatremia 276.0
    hyponatremia 276.1
Anidrosis 705.0
Aniridia (congenital) 743.45
Anisakiasis (infection) (infestation) 127.1
Anisakis larva infestation 127.1
Aniseikonia 367.32
Anisocoria (pupil) 379.41
  congenital 743.46
Anisocytosis 790.09
Anisometropia (congenital) 367.31
Ankle - *see* condition
Ankyloblepharon (acquired) (eyelid) 374.46
  filiforme (adnatum) (congenital) 743.62
  total 743.62
Ankylodactly (*see also* Syndactylism) 755.10
Ankyloglossia 750.0
Ankylosis (fibrous) (osseous) 718.50
  ankle 718.57
  any joint, produced by surgical fusion V45.4
  cricoarytenoid (cartilage) (joint) (larynx) 478.79
  dental 521.6
  ear ossicle NEC 385.22
    malleus 385.21
  elbow 718.52
  finger 718.54
  hip 718.55
  incostapedial joint (infectional) 385.22
  joint, produced by surgical fusion NEC V45.4
  knee 718.56
  lumbosacral (joint) 724.6
  malleus 385.21
  multiple sites 718.59
  postoperative (status) V45.4
  sacroiliac (joint) 724.6
  shoulder 718.51
  specified site NEC 718.58
  spine NEC 724.9
  surgical V45.4
  teeth, tooth (hard tissues) 521.6
  temporomandibular joint 524.61
  wrist 718.53
Ankylostoma - *see* Ancylostoma
Ankylostomiasis (intestinal) - *see* Ancylostomiasis
Ankylurethria (*see also* Stricture, urethra) 598.9
Annular - *see also* condition
  detachment, cervix 622.8
  organ or site, congenital NEC - *see* Distortion
  pancreas (congenital) 751.7
Anodontia (complete) (partial) (vera) 520.0
  with abnormal spacing 524.30
  acquired 525.10
    causing malocclusion 524.30
    due to
      caries 525.13
      extraction 525.10
      periodontal disease 525.12
      trauma 525.11
Anomaly, anomalous (congenital) (unspecified type) 759.9
  abdomen 759.9
  abdominal wall 756.70
  acoustic nerve 742.9
  adrenal (gland) 759.1
  Alder (-Reilly) (leukocyte granulation) 288.2
  alimentary tract 751.9
    lower 751.5
    specified type NEC 751.8
    upper (any part, except tongue) 750.9
      tongue 750.10
        specified type NEC 750.19
Anomaly, anomalous *(Continued)*
  alveolar 524.70
    ridge (process) 525.8
    specified NEC 524.79
  ankle (joint) 755.69
  anus, anal (canal) 751.5
  aorta, aortic 747.20
    arch 747.21
    coarctation (postductal) (preductal) 747.10
    cusp or valve NEC 746.9
    septum 745.0
    specified type NEC 747.29
  aorticopulmonary septum 745.0
  apertures, diaphragm 756.6
  appendix 751.5
  aqueduct of Sylvius 742.3
    with spina bifida (*see also* Spina bifida) 741.0
  arm 755.50
    reduction (*see also* Deformity, reduction, upper limb) 755.20
  arteriovenous (congenital) (peripheral) NEC 747.60
    brain 747.81
    cerebral 747.81
    coronary 746.85
    gastrointestinal 747.61
      acquired - *see* Angiodysplasia
    lower limb 747.64
    renal 747.62
    specified site NEC 747.69
    spinal 747.82
    upper limb 747.63
  artery (*see also* Anomaly, peripheral vascular system) NEC 747.60
    brain 747.81
    cerebral 747.81
    coronary 746.85
    eye 743.9
    pulmonary 747.3
    renal 747.62
    retina 743.9
    umbilical 747.5
  arytenoepiglottic folds 748.3
  atrial
    bands 746.9
    folds 746.9
    septa 745.5
  atrioventricular
    canal 745.69
    common 745.69
    conduction 426.7
    excitation 426.7
    septum 745.4
  atrium - *see* Anomaly, atrial
  auditory canal 744.3
    specified type NEC 744.29
      with hearing impairment 744.02
  auricle
    ear 744.3
      causing impairment of hearing 744.02
    heart 746.9
      septum 745.5
  autosomes, autosomal NEC 758.5
  Axenfeld's 743.44
  back 759.9
  band
    atrial 746.9
    heart 746.9
    ventricular 746.9
  Bartholin's duct 750.9
  biliary duct or passage 751.60
    atresia 751.61

Anomaly, anomalous *(Continued)*
bladder (neck) (sphincter) (trigone) 753.9
specified type NEC 753.8
blood vessel 747.9
artery - *see* Anomaly, artery
peripheral vascular - *see* Anomaly, peripheral vascular system
vein - *see* Anomaly, vein
bone NEC 756.9
ankle 755.69
arm 755.50
chest 756.3
cranium 756.0
face 756.0
finger 755.50
foot 755.67
forearm 755.50
frontal 756.0
head 756.0
hip 755.63
leg 755.60
lumbosacral 756.10
nose 748.1
pelvic girdle 755.60
rachitic 756.4
rib 756.3
shoulder girdle 755.50
skull 756.0
with
anencephalus 740.0
encephalocele 742.0
hydrocephalus 742.3
with spina bifida (*see also* Spina bifida) 741.0
microcephalus 742.1
toe 755.66
brain 742.9
multiple 742.4
reduction 742.2
specified type NEC 742.4
vessel 747.81
branchial cleft NEC 744.49
cyst 744.42
fistula 744.41
persistent 744.41
sinus (external) (internal) 744.41
breast 757.9
broad ligament 752.10
specified type NEC 752.19
bronchus 748.3
bulbar septum 745.0
bulbus cordis 745.9
persistent (in left ventricle) 745.8
bursa 756.9
canal of Nuck 752.9
canthus 743.9
capillary NEC (*see also* Anomaly, peripheral vascular system) 747.60
cardiac 746.9
septal closure 745.9
acquired 429.71
valve NEC 746.9
pulmonary 746.00
specified type NEC 746.89
cardiovascular system 746.9
complicating pregnancy, childbirth, or puerperium 648.5
carpus 755.50
cartilage, trachea 748.3
cartilaginous 756.9
caruncle, lacrimal, lachrymal 743.9
cascade stomach 750.7

Anomaly, anomalous *(Continued)*
cauda equina 742.59
cecum 751.5
cerebral - *see also* Anomaly, brain vessels 747.81
cerebrovascular system 747.81
cervix (uterus) 752.40
with doubling of vagina and uterus 752.2
in pregnancy or childbirth 654.6
affecting fetus or newborn 763.89
causing obstructed labor 660.2
affecting fetus or newborn 763.1
Chédiak-Higashi (-Steinbrinck) (congenital gigantism of peroxidase granules) 288.2
cheek 744.9
chest (wall) 756.3
chin 744.9
specified type NEC 744.89
chordae tendineae 746.9
choroid 743.9
plexus 742.9
chromosomes, chromosomal 758.9
13 (13-15) 758.1
18 (16-18) 758.2
21 or 22 758.0
autosomes NEC (*see also* Abnormal, autosomes) 758.5
deletion 758.39
Christchurch 758.39
D_1 758.1
E_3 758.2
G 758.0
mitochondrial 758.9
mosaics 758.89
sex 758.81
complement, XO 758.6
complement, XXX 758.81
complement, XXY 758.7
complement, XYY 758.81
gonadal dysgenesis 758.6
Klinefelter's 758.7
Turner's 758.6
trisomy 21 758.0
cilia 743.9
circulatory system 747.9
specified type NEC 747.89
clavicle 755.51
clitoris 752.40
coccyx 756.10
colon 751.5
common duct 751.60
communication
coronary artery 746.85
left ventricle with right atrium 745.4
concha (ear) 744.3
connection
renal vessels with kidney 747.62
total pulmonary venous 747.41
connective tissue 756.9
specified type NEC 756.89
cornea 743.9
shape 743.41
size 743.41
specified type NEC 743.49
coronary
artery 746.85
vein 746.89
cranium - *see* Anomaly, skull
cricoid cartilage 748.3
cushion, endocardial 745.60
specified type NEC 745.69

Anomaly, anomalous *(Continued)*
cystic duct 751.60
dental arch 524.20 ◀
specified NEC 524.29 ◀
dental arch relationship 524.20
angle's class I 524.21
angle's class II 524.22
angle's class III 524.23
articulation
anterior 524.27
posterior 524.27
reverse 524.27
disto-occlusion 524.22
division I 524.22
division II 524.22
excessive horizontal overlap 524.26
interarch distance (excessive) (inadequate) 524.28
mesio-occlusion 524.23
neutro-occlusion 524.21
open
anterior occlusal relationship 524.24
posterior occlusal relationship 524.25
specified NEC 524.29
dentition 520.6
dentofacial NEC 524.9
functional 524.50
specified type NEC 524.89
dermatoglyphic 757.2
Descemet's membrane 743.9
specified type NEC 743.49
development
cervix 752.40
vagina 752.40
vulva 752.40
diaphragm, diaphragmatic (apertures) NEC 756.6
digestive organ(s) or system 751.9
lower 751.5
specified type NEC 751.8
upper 750.9
distribution, coronary artery 746.85
ductus
arteriosus 747.0
Botalli 747.0
duodenum 751.5
dura 742.9
brain 742.4
spinal cord 742.59
ear 744.3
causing impairment of hearing 744.00
specified type NEC 744.09
external 744.3
causing impairment of hearing 744.02
specified type NEC 744.29
inner (causing impairment of hearing) 744.05
middle, except ossicles (causing impairment of hearing) 744.03
ossicles 744.04
ossicles 744.04
prominent auricle 744.29
specified type NEC 744.29
with hearing impairment 744.09
Ebstein's (heart) 746.2
tricuspid valve 746.2
ectodermal 757.9
Eisenmenger's (ventricular septal defect) 745.4
ejaculatory duct 752.9
specified type NEC 752.89

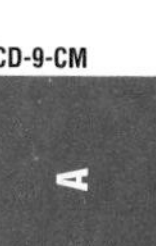
ICD-9-CM
A
Vol. 2

Anomaly, anomalous *(Continued)*
elbow (joint) 755.50
endocardial cushion 745.60
specified type NEC 745.69
endocrine gland NEC 759.2
epididymis 752.9
epiglottis 748.3
esophagus 750.9
specified type NEC 750.4
Eustachian tube 744.3
specified type NEC 744.24
eye (any part) 743.9
adnexa 743.9
specified type NEC 743.69
anophthalmos 743.00
anterior
chamber and related structures 743.9
angle 743.9
specified type NEC 743.44
specified type NEC 743.44
segment 743.9
combined 743.48
multiple 743.48
specified type NEC 743.49
cataract (*see also* Cataract) 743.30
glaucoma (*see also* Buphthalmia) 743.20
lid 743.9
specified type NEC 743.63
microphthalmos (*see also* Microphthalmos) 743.10
posterior segment 743.9
specified type NEC 743.59
vascular 743.58
vitreous 743.9
specified type NEC 743.51
ptosis (eyelid) 743.61
retina 743.9
specified type NEC 743.59
sclera 743.9
specified type NEC 743.47
specified type NEC 743.8
eyebrow 744.89
eyelid 743.9
specified type NEC 743.63
face (any part) 744.9
bone(s) 756.0
specified type NEC 744.89
fallopian tube 752.10
specified type NEC 752.19
fascia 756.9
specified type NEC 756.89
femur 755.60
fibula 755.60
finger 755.50
supernumerary 755.01
webbed (*see also* Syndactylism, fingers) 755.11
fixation, intestine 751.4
flexion (joint) 755.9
hip or thigh (*see also* Dislocation, hip, congenital) 754.30
folds, heart 746.9
foot 755.67
foramen
Botalli 745.5
ovale 745.5
forearm 755.50
forehead (*see also* Anomaly, skull) 756.0
form, teeth 520.2
fovea centralis 743.9
frontal bone (*see also* Anomaly, skull) 756.0

Anomaly, anomalous *(Continued)*
gallbladder 751.60
Gartner's duct 752.41
gastrointestinal tract 751.9
specified type NEC 751.8
vessel 747.61
genitalia, genital organ(s) or system
female 752.9
external 752.40
specified type NEC 752.49
internal NEC 752.9
male (external and internal) 752.9
epispadias 752.62
hidden penis 752.65
hydrocele, congenital 778.6
hypospadias 752.61
micropenis 752.64
testis, undescended 752.51
retractile 752.52
specified type NEC 752.89
genitourinary NEC 752.9
Gerbode 745.4
globe (eye) 743.9
glottis 748.3
granulation or granulocyte, genetic 288.2
constitutional 288.2
leukocyte 288.2
gum 750.9
gyri 742.9
hair 757.9
specified type NEC 757.4
hand 755.50
hard tissue formation in pulp 522.3
head (*see also* Anomaly, skull) 756.0
heart 746.9
auricle 746.9
bands 746.9
fibroelastosis cordis 425.3
folds 746.9
malposition 746.87
maternal, affecting fetus or newborn 760.3
obstructive NEC 746.84
patent ductus arteriosus (Botalli) 747.0
septum 745.9
acquired 429.71
aortic 745.0
aorticopulmonary 745.0
atrial 745.5
auricular 745.5
between aorta and pulmonary artery 745.0
endocardial cushion type 745.60
specified type NEC 745.69
interatrial 745.5
interventricular 745.4
with pulmonary stenosis or atresia, dextraposition of aorta, and hypertrophy of right ventricle 745.2
acquired 429.71
specified type NEC 745.8
ventricular 745.4
with pulmonary stenosis or atresia, dextraposition of aorta, and hypertrophy of right ventricle 745.2
acquired 429.71
specified type NEC 746.89
tetralogy of Fallot 745.2
valve NEC 746.9
aortic 746.9

Anomaly, anomalous *(Continued)*
heart *(Continued)*
valve *(Continued)*
aortic *(Continued)*
atresia 746.89
bicuspid valve 746.4
insufficiency 746.4
specified type NEC 746.89
stenosis 746.3
subaortic 746.81
supravalvular 747.22
mitral 746.9
atresia 746.89
insufficiency 746.6
specified type NEC 746.89
stenosis 746.5
pulmonary 746.00
atresia 746.01
insufficiency 746.09
stenosis 746.02
infundibular 746.83
subvalvular 746.83
tricuspid 746.9
atresia 746.1
stenosis 746.1
ventricle 746.9
heel 755.67
Hegglin's 288.2
hemianencephaly 740.0
hemicephaly 740.0
hemicrania 740.0
hepatic duct 751.60
hip (joint) 755.63
hourglass
bladder 753.8
gallbladder 751.69
stomach 750.7
humerus 755.50
hymen 752.40
hypersegmentation of neutrophils, hereditary 288.2
hypophyseal 759.2
ileocecal (coil) (valve) 751.5
ileum (intestine) 751.5
ilium 755.60
integument 757.9
specified type NEC 757.8
interarch distance (excessive) (inadequate) 524.28
intervertebral cartilage or disc 756.10
intestine (large) (small) 751.5
fixational type 751.4
iris 743.9
specified type NEC 743.46
ischium 755.60
jaw NEC 524.9
closure 524.51
size (major) NEC 524.00
specified type NEC 524.89
jaw-cranial base relationship 524.10
specified NEC 524.19
jejunum 751.5
joint 755.9
hip
dislocation (*see also* Dislocation, hip, congenital) 754.30
predislocation (*see also* Subluxation, congenital, hip) 754.32
preluxation (*see also* Subluxation, congenital, hip) 754.32
subluxation (*see also* Subluxation, congenital, hip) 754.32
lumbosacral 756.10

Anomaly, anomalous *(Continued)*
joint *(Continued)*
lumbosacral *(Continued)*
spondylolisthesis 756.12
spondylosis 756.11
multiple arthrogryposis 754.89
sacroiliac 755.69
Jordan's 288.2
kidney(s) (calyx) (pelvis) 753.9
vessel 747.62
Klippel-Feil (brevicollis) 756.16
knee (joint) 755.64
labium (majus) (minus) 752.40
labyrinth, membranous (causing impairment of hearing) 744.05
lacrimal
apparatus, duct or passage 743.9
specified type NEC 743.65
gland 743.9
specified type NEC 743.64
Langdon Down (mongolism) 758.0
larynx, laryngeal (muscle) 748.3
web, webbed 748.2
leg (lower) (upper) 755.60
reduction NEC (*see also* Deformity, reduction, lower limb) 755.30
lens 743.9
shape 743.36
specified type NEC 743.39
leukocytes, genetic 288.2
granulation (constitutional) 288.2
lid (fold) 743.9
ligament 756.9
broad 752.10
round 752.9
limb, except reduction deformity 755.8
lower 755.60
reduction deformity (*see also* Deformity, reduction, lower limb) 755.30
specified type NEC 755.69
upper 755.50
reduction deformity (*see also* Deformity, reduction, upper limb) 755.20
specified type NEC 755.59
lip 750.9
harelip (*see also* Cleft, lip) 749.10
specified type NEC 750.26
liver (duct) 751.60
atresia 751.69
lower extremity 755.60
vessel 747.64
lumbosacral (joint) (region) 756.10
lung (fissure) (lobe) NEC 748.60
agenesis 748.5
specified type NEC 748.69
lymphatic system 759.9
Madelung's (radius) 755.54
mandible 524.9
size NEC 524.00
maxilla 524.90
size NEC 524.00
May (-Hegglin) 288.2
meatus urinarius 753.9
specified type NEC 753.8
meningeal bands or folds, constriction of 742.8
meninges 742.9
brain 742.4
spinal 742.59
meningocele (*see also* Spina bifida) 741.9
acquired 349.2
mesentery 751.9

Anomaly, anomalous *(Continued)*
metacarpus 755.50
metatarsus 755.67
middle ear, except ossicles (causing impairment of hearing) 744.03
ossicles 744.04
mitral (leaflets) (valve) 746.9
atresia 746.89
insufficiency 746.6
specified type NEC 746.89
stenosis 746.5
mouth 750.9
specified type NEC 750.26
multiple NEC 759.7
specified type NEC 759.89
muscle 756.9
eye 743.9
specified type NEC 743.69
specified type NEC 756.89
musculoskeletal system, except limbs 756.9
specified type NEC 756.9
nail 757.9
specified type NEC 757.5
narrowness, eyelid 743.62
nasal sinus or septum 748.1
neck (any part) 744.9
specified type NEC 744.89
nerve 742.9
acoustic 742.9
specified type NEC 742.8
optic 742.9
specified type NEC 742.8
specified type NEC 742.8
nervous system NEC 742.9
brain 742.9
specified type NEC 742.4
specified type NEC 742.8
neurological 742.9
nipple 757.6
nonteratogenic NEC 754.89
nose, nasal (bone) (cartilage) (septum) (sinus) 748.1
ocular muscle 743.9
omphalomesenteric duct 751.0
opening, pulmonary veins 747.49
optic
disc 743.9
specified type NEC 743.57
nerve 742.9
opticociliary vessels 743.9
orbit (eye) 743.9
specified type NEC 743.66
organ
of Corti (causing impairment of hearing) 744.05
or site 759.9
specified type NEC 759.89
origin
both great arteries from same ventricle 745.11
coronary artery 746.85
innominate artery 747.69
left coronary artery from pulmonary artery 746.85
pulmonary artery 747.3
renal vessels 747.62
subclavian artery (left) (right) 747.21
osseous meatus (ear) 744.03
ovary 752.0
oviduct 752.10
palate (hard) (soft) 750.9
cleft (*see also* Cleft, palate) 749.00
pancreas (duct) 751.7

Anomaly, anomalous *(Continued)*
papillary muscles 746.9
parathyroid gland 759.2
paraurethral ducts 753.9
parotid (gland) 750.9
patella 755.64
Pelger-Huët (hereditary hyposegmentation) 288.2
pelvic girdle 755.60
specified type NEC 755.69
pelvis (bony) 755.60
complicating delivery 653.0
rachitic 268.1
fetal 756.4
penis (glans) 752.69
pericardium 746.89
peripheral vascular system NEC 747.60
gastrointestinal 747.61
lower limb 747.64
renal 747.62
specified site NEC 747.69
spinal 747.82
upper limb 747.63
Peter's 743.44
pharynx 750.9
branchial cleft 744.41
specified type NEC 750.29
Pierre Robin 756.0
pigmentation 709.00
congenital 757.33
specified NEC 709.09
pituitary (gland) 759.2
pleural folds 748.8
portal vein 747.40
position tooth, teeth 524.30
crowding 524.31
displacement 524.30
horizontal 524.33
vertical 524.34
distance
interocclusal
excessive 524.37
insufficient 524.36
excessive spacing 524.32
rotation 524.35
specified NEC 524.39
preauricular sinus 744.46
prepuce 752.9
prostate 752.9
pulmonary 748.60
artery 747.3
circulation 747.3
specified type NEC 748.69
valve 746.00
atresia 746.01
insufficiency 746.09
specified type NEC 746.09
stenosis 746.02
infundibular 746.83
subvalvular 746.83
vein 747.40
venous
connection 747.49
partial 747.42
total 747.41
return 747.49
partial 747.42
total (TAPVR) (complete) (subdiaphragmatic) (supradiaphragmatic) 747.41
pupil 743.9
pylorus 750.9
hypertrophy 750.5
stenosis 750.5

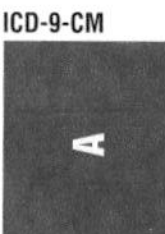
ICD-9-CM
A
Vol. 2

Anomaly, anomalous *(Continued)*
rachitic, fetal 756.4
radius 755.50
rectovaginal (septum) 752.40
rectum 751.5
refraction 367.9
renal 753.9
vessel 747.62
respiratory system 748.9
specified type NEC 748.8
rib 756.3
cervical 756.2
Rieger's 743.44
rings, trachea 748.3
rotation - *see also* Malrotation
hip or thigh (*see also* Subluxation, congenital, hip) 754.32
round ligament 752.9
sacroiliac (joint) 755.69
sacrum 756.10
saddle
back 754.2
nose 754.0
syphilitic 090.5
salivary gland or duct 750.9
specified type NEC 750.26
scapula 755.50
sclera 743.9
specified type NEC 743.47
scrotum 752.9
sebaceous gland 757.9
seminal duct or tract 752.9
sense organs 742.9
specified type NEC 742.8
septum
heart - *see* Anomaly, heart, septum
nasal 748.1
sex chromosomes NEC (*see also* Anomaly, chromosomes) 758.81
shoulder (girdle) (joint) 755.50
specified type NEC 755.59
sigmoid (flexure) 751.5
sinus of Valsalva 747.29
site NEC 759.9
skeleton generalized NEC 756.50
skin (appendage) 757.9
specified type NEC 757.39
skull (bone) 756.0
with
anencephalus 740.0
encephalocele 742.0
hydrocephalus 742.3
with spina bifida (*see also* Spina bifida) 741.0
microcephalus 742.1
specified type NEC
adrenal (gland) 759.1
alimentary tract (complete) (partial) 751.8
lower 751.5
upper 750.8
ankle 755.69
anus, anal (canal) 751.5
aorta, aortic 747.29
arch 747.21
appendix 751.5
arm 755.59
artery (peripheral) NEC (*see also* Anomaly, peripheral vascular system) 747.60
brain 747.81
coronary 746.85
eye 743.58
pulmonary 747.3

Anomaly, anomalous *(Continued)*
specified type NEC *(Continued)*
artery *(Continued)*
retinal 743.58
umbilical 747.5
auditory canal 744.29
causing impairment of hearing 744.02
bile duct or passage 751.69
bladder 753.8
neck 753.8
bone(s) 756.9
arm 755.59
face 756.0
leg 755.69
pelvic girdle 755.69
shoulder girdle 755.59
skull 756.0
with
anencephalus 740.0
encephalocele 742.0
hydrocephalus 742.3
with spina bifida (*see also* Spina bifida) 741.0
microcephalus 742.1
brain 742.4
breast 757.6
broad ligament 752.19
bronchus 748.3
canal of Nuck 752.89
cardiac septal closure 745.8
carpus 755.59
cartilaginous 756.9
cecum 751.5
cervix 752.49
chest (wall) 756.3
chin 744.89
ciliary body 743.46
circulatory system 747.89
clavicle 755.51
clitoris 752.49
coccyx 756.19
colon 751.5
common duct 751.69
connective tissue 756.89
cricoid cartilage 748.3
cystic duct 751.69
diaphragm 756.6
digestive organ(s) or tract 751.8
lower 751.5
upper 750.8
duodenum 751.5
ear 744.29
auricle 744.29
causing impairment of hearing 744.02
causing impairment of hearing 744.09
inner (causing impairment of hearing) 744.05
middle, except ossicles 744.03
ossicles 744.04
ejaculatory duct 752.89
endocrine 759.2
epiglottis 748.3
esophagus 750.4
eustachian tube 744.24
eye 743.8
lid 743.63
muscle 743.69
face 744.89
bone(s) 756.0
fallopian tube 752.19
fascia 756.89

Anomaly, anomalous *(Continued)*
specified type NEC *(Continued)*
femur 755.69
fibula 755.69
finger 755.59
foot 755.67
fovea centralis 743.55
gallbladder 751.69
Gartner's duct 752.89
gastrointestinal tract 751.8
genitalia, genital organ(s)
female 752.89
external 752.49
internal NEC 752.89
male 752.89
penis 752.69
scrotal transposition 752.81
genitourinary tract NEC 752.89
glottis 748.3
hair 757.4
hand 755.59
heart 746.89
valve NEC 746.89
pulmonary 746.09
hepatic duct 751.69
hydatid of Morgagni 752.89
hymen 752.49
integument 757.8
intestine (large) (small) 751.5
fixational type 751.4
iris 743.46
jejunum 751.5
joint 755.8
kidney 753.3
knee 755.64
labium (majus) (minus) 752.49
labyrinth, membranous 744.05
larynx 748.3
leg 755.69
lens 743.39
limb, except reduction deformity 755.8
lower 755.69
reduction deformity (*see also* Deformity, reduction, lower limb) 755.30
upper 755.59
reduction deformity (*see also* Deformity, reduction, upper limb) 755.20
lip 750.26
liver 751.69
lung (fissure) (lobe) 748.69
meatus urinarius 753.8
metacarpus 755.59
mouth 750.26
muscle 756.89
eye 743.69
musculoskeletal system, except limbs 756.9
nail 757.5
neck 744.89
nerve 742.8
acoustic 742.8
optic 742.8
nervous system 742.8
nipple 757.6
nose 748.1
organ NEC 759.89
of Corti 744.05
osseous meatus (ear) 744.03
ovary 752.0
oviduct 752.19
pancreas 751.7

Anomaly, anomalous *(Continued)*
specified type NEC *(Continued)*
parathyroid 759.2
patella 755.64
pelvic girdle 755.69
penis 752.69
pericardium 746.89
peripheral vascular system NEC (*see also* Anomaly, peripheral vascular system) 747.60
pharynx 750.29
pituitary 759.2
prostate 752.89
radius 755.59
rectum 751.5
respiratory system 748.8
rib 756.3
round ligament 752.89
sacrum 756.19
salivary duct or gland 750.26
scapula 755.59
sclera 743.47
scrotum 752.89
transposition 752.81
seminal duct or tract 752.89
shoulder girdle 755.59
site NEC 759.89
skin 757.39
skull (bone(s)) 756.0
with
anencephalus 740.0
encephalocele 742.0
hydrocephalus 742.3
with spina bifida (*see also* Spina bifida) 741.0
microcephalus 742.1
specified organ or site NEC 759.89
spermatic cord 752.89
spinal cord 742.59
spine 756.19
spleen 759.0
sternum 756.3
stomach 750.7
tarsus 755.67
tendon 756.89
testis 752.89
thorax (wall) 756.3
thymus 759.2
thyroid (gland) 759.2
cartilage 748.3
tibia 755.69
toe 755.66
tongue 750.19
trachea (cartilage) 748.3
ulna 755.59
urachus 753.7
ureter 753.4
obstructive 753.29
urethra 753.8
obstructive 753.6
urinary tract 753.8
uterus 752.3
uvula 750.26
vagina 752.49
vascular NEC (*see also* Anomaly, peripheral vascular system) 747.60
brain 747.81
vas deferens 752.89
vein(s) (peripheral) NEC (*see also* Anomaly, peripheral vascular system) 747.60
brain 747.81
great 747.49

Anomaly, anomalous *(Continued)*
specified type NEC *(Continued)*
vein(s) *(Continued)*
portal 747.49
pulmonary 747.49
vena cava (inferior) (superior) 747.49
vertebra 756.19
vulva 752.49
spermatic cord 752.9
spine, spinal 756.10
column 756.10
cord 742.9
meningocele (*see also* Spina bifida) 741.9
specified type NEC 742.59
spina bifida (*see also* Spina bifida) 741.9
vessel 747.82
meninges 742.59
nerve root 742.9
spleen 759.0
Sprengel's 755.52
sternum 756.3
stomach 750.9
specified type NEC 750.7
submaxillary gland 750.9
superior vena cava 747.40
talipes - *see* Talipes
tarsus 755.67
with complete absence of distal elements 755.31
teeth, tooth NEC 520.9
position 524.30
crowding 524.31
displacement 524.30
horizontal 524.33
vertical 524.34
distance
interocclusal
excessive 524.37
insufficient 524.36
excessive spacing 524.32
rotation 524.35
specified NEC 524.39
spacing 524.30
tendon 756.9
specified type NEC 756.89
termination
coronary artery 746.85
testis 752.9
thebesian valve 746.9
thigh 755.60
flexion (*see also* Subluxation, congenital, hip) 754.32
thorax (wall) 756.3
throat 750.9
thumb 755.50
supernumerary 755.01
thymus gland 759.2
thyroid (gland) 759.2
cartilage 748.3
tibia 755.60
saber 090.5
toe 755.66
supernumerary 755.02
webbed (*see also* Syndactylism, toes) 755.13
tongue 750.10
specified type NEC 750.19
trachea, tracheal 748.3
cartilage 748.3
rings 748.3
tragus 744.3
transverse aortic arch 747.21

Anomaly, anomalous *(Continued)*
trichromata 368.59
trichromatopsia 368.59
tricuspid (leaflet) (valve) 746.9
atresia 746.1
Ebstein's 746.2
specified type NEC 746.89
stenosis 746.1
trunk 759.9
Uhl's (hypoplasia of myocardium, right ventricle) 746.84
ulna 755.50
umbilicus 759.9
artery 747.5
union, trachea with larynx 748.3
unspecified site 759.9
upper extremity 755.50
vessel 747.63
urachus 753.7
specified type NEC 753.7
ureter 753.9
obstructive 753.20
specified type NEC 753.4
obstructive 753.29
urethra (valve) 753.9
obstructive 753.6
specified type NEC 753.8
urinary tract or system (any part, except urachus) 753.9
specified type NEC 753.8
urachus 753.7
uterus 752.3
with only one functioning horn 752.3
in pregnancy or childbirth 654.0
affecting fetus or newborn 763.89
causing obstructed labor 660.2
affecting fetus or newborn 763.1
uvula 750.9
vagina 752.40
valleculae 748.3
valve (heart) NEC 746.9
formation, ureter 753.29
pulmonary 746.00
specified type NEC 746.89
vascular NEC (*see also* Anomaly, peripheral vascular system) 747.60
ring 747.21
vas deferens 752.9
vein(s) (peripheral) NEC (*see also* Anomaly, peripheral vascular system) 747.60
brain 747.81
cerebral 747.81
coronary 746.89
great 747.40
specified type NEC 747.49
portal 747.40
pulmonary 747.40
retina 743.9
vena cava (inferior) (superior) 747.40
venous return (pulmonary) 747.49
partial 747.42
total 747.41
ventricle, ventricular (heart) 746.9
bands 746.9
folds 746.9
septa 745.4
vertebra 756.10
vesicourethral orifice 753.9
vessels NEC (*see also* Anomaly, peripheral vascular system) 747.60
optic papilla 743.9
vitelline duct 751.0

Anomaly, anomalous *(Continued)*
- vitreous humor 743.9
  - specified type NEC 743.51
- vulva 752.40
- wrist (joint) 755.50

Anomia 784.69
Anonychia 757.5
- acquired 703.8

Anophthalmos, anophthalmus (clinical) (congenital) (globe) 743.00
- acquired V45.78

Anopsia (altitudinal) (quadrant) 368.46
Anorchia 752.89
Anorchism, anorchidism 752.89
Anorexia 783.0
- hysterical 300.11
- nervosa 307.1

Anosmia (*see also* Disturbance, sensation) 781.1
- hysterical 300.11
- postinfectional 478.9
- psychogenic 306.7
- traumatic 951.8

Anosognosia 780.99
Anosphrasia 781.1
Anosteoplasia 756.50
Anotia 744.09
Anovulatory cycle 628.0
Anoxemia 799.02
- newborn 770.88

Anoxia 799.02
- altitude 993.2
- cerebral 348.1
  - with
    - abortion - *see* Abortion, by type, with specified complication NEC
    - ectopic pregnancy (*see also* categories 633.0-633.9) 639.8
    - molar pregnancy (*see also* categories 630-632) 639.8
  - complicating
    - delivery (cesarean) (instrumental) 669.4
    - ectopic or molar pregnancy 639.8
    - obstetric anesthesia or sedation 668.2
  - during or resulting from a procedure 997.01
  - following
    - abortion 639.8
    - ectopic or molar pregnancy 639.8
  - newborn (*see also* Distress, fetal, liveborn infant) 770.88
- due to drowning 994.1
- fetal, affecting newborn 770.88
- heart - *see* Insufficiency, coronary
- high altitude 993.2
- intrauterine
  - fetal death (before onset of labor) 768.0
    - during labor 768.1
  - liveborn infant - *see* Distress, fetal, liveborn infant
- myocardial - *see* Insufficiency, coronary
- newborn 768.9
  - mild or moderate 768.6
  - severe 768.5
- pathological 799.02

Anteflexion - *see* Anteversion
Antenatal
- care, normal pregnancy V22.1
  - first V22.0
- screening of mother (for) V28.9
  - based on amniocentesis NEC V28.2
    - chromosomal anomalies V28.0
    - raised alphafetoprotein levels V28.1
  - chromosomal anomalies V28.0
  - fetal growth retardation using ultrasonics V28.4
  - isoimmunization V28.5
  - malformations using ultrasonics V28.3
  - raised alphafetoprotein levels in amniotic fluid V28.1
  - specified condition NEC V28.8
  - Streptococcus B V28.6

Antepartum - *see* condition
Anterior - *see also* condition
- spinal artery compression syndrome 721.1

Antero-occlusion 524.24
Anteversion
- cervix - *see* Anteversion, uterus
- femur (neck), congenital 755.63
- uterus, uterine (cervix) (postinfectional) (postpartal, old) 621.6
  - congenital 752.3
  - in pregnancy or childbirth 654.4
    - affecting fetus or newborn 763.89
    - causing obstructed labor 660.2
      - affecting fetus or newborn 763.1

Anthracosilicosis (occupational) 500
Anthracosis (lung) (occupational) 500
- lingua 529.3

Anthrax 022.9
- with pneumonia 022.1 *[484.5]*
- colitis 022.2
- cutaneous 022.0
- gastrointestinal 022.2
- intestinal 022.2
- pulmonary 022.1
- respiratory 022.1
- septicemia 022.3
- specified manifestation NEC 022.8

Anthropoid pelvis 755.69
- with disproportion (fetopelvic) 653.2
  - affecting fetus or newborn 763.1
  - causing obstructed labor 660.1
    - affecting fetus or newborn 763.1

Anthropophobia 300.29
Antibioma, breast 611.0
Antibodies
- maternal (blood group) (*see also* Incompatibility) 656.2
  - anti-D, cord blood 656.1
    - fetus or newborn 773.0

Antibody deficiency syndrome
- agammaglobulinemic 279.00
- congenital 279.04
- hypogammaglobulinemic 279.00

Anticoagulant, circulating (*see also* Circulating anticoagulants) 286.5
Antimongolism syndrome 758.39
Antimonial cholera 985.4
Antisocial personality 301.7
Antithrombinemia (*see also* Circulating anticoagulants) 286.5
Antithromboplastinemia (*see also* Circulating anticoagulants) 286.5
Antithromboplastinogenemia (*see also* Circulating anticoagulants) 286.5
Antitoxin complication or reaction - *see* Complications, vaccination
Anton (-Babinski) syndrome (hemiasomatognosia) 307.9
Antritis (chronic) 473.0
- maxilla 473.0
  - acute 461.0
- stomach 535.4

Antrum, antral - *see* condition
Anuria 788.5
- with
  - abortion - *see* Abortion, by type, with renal failure
  - ectopic pregnancy (*see also* categories 633.0-633.9) 639.3
  - molar pregnancy (*see also* categories 630-632) 639.3
- calculus (impacted) (recurrent) 592.9
  - kidney 592.0
  - ureter 592.1
- congenital 753.3
- due to a procedure 997.5
- following
  - abortion 639.3
  - ectopic or molar pregnancy 639.3
- newborn 753.3
- postrenal 593.4
- puerperal, postpartum, childbirth 669.3
- specified as due to a procedure 997.5
- sulfonamide
  - correct substance properly administered 788.5
  - overdose or wrong substance given or taken 961.0
- traumatic (following crushing) 958.5

Anus, anal - *see* condition
Anusitis 569.49
Anxiety (neurosis) (reaction) (state) 300.00
- alcohol-induced 291.89
- depression 300.4
- drug-induced 292.89
- due to or associated with physical condition 293.84
- generalized 300.02
- hysteria 300.20
- in
  - acute stress reaction 308.0
  - transient adjustment reaction 309.24
- panic type 300.01
- separation, abnormal 309.21
- syndrome (organic) (transient) 293.84

Aorta, aortic - *see* condition
Aortectasia 441.9
Aortitis (nonsyphilitic) 447.6
- arteriosclerotic 440.0
- calcific 447.6
- Döhle-Heller 093.1
- luetic 093.1
- rheumatic (*see also* Endocarditis, acute, rheumatic) 391.1
- rheumatoid - *see* Arthritis, rheumatoid
- specific 093.1
- syphilitic 093.1
  - congenital 090.5

Apathetic thyroid storm (*see also* Thyrotoxicosis) 242.9
Apepsia 536.8
- achlorhydric 536.0
- psychogenic 306.4

Aperistalsis, esophagus 530.0
Apert's syndrome (acrocephalosyndactyly) 755.55
Apert-Gallais syndrome (adrenogenital) 255.2

Apertognathia 524.20
Aphagia 787.2
psychogenic 307.1
Aphakia (acquired) (bilateral) (postoperative) (unilateral) 379.31
congenital 743.35
Aphalangia (congenital) 755.4
lower limb (complete) (intercalary) (partial) (terminal) 755.39
meaning all digits (complete) (partial) 755.31
transverse 755.31
upper limb (complete) (intercalary) (partial) (terminal) 755.29
meaning all digits (complete) (partial) 755.21
transverse 755.21
Aphasia (amnestic) (ataxic) (auditory) (Broca's) (choreatic) (classic) (expressive) (global) (ideational) (ideokinetic) (ideomotor) (jargon) (motor) (nominal) (receptive) (semantic) (sensory) (syntactic) (verbal) (visual) (Wernicke's) 784.3
developmental 315.31
syphilis, tertiary 094.89
uremic - *see* Uremia
Aphemia 784.3
uremic - *see* Uremia
Aphonia 784.41
clericorum 784.49
hysterical 300.11
organic 784.41
psychogenic 306.1
Aphthae, aphthous - *see also* condition
Bednar's 528.2
cachectic 529.0
epizootic 078.4
fever 078.4
oral 528.2
stomatitis 528.2
thrush 112.0
ulcer (oral) (recurrent) 528.2
genital organ(s) NEC
female 629.89
male 608.89
larynx 478.79
Apical - *see* condition
Apical ballooning syndrome 429.83
Aplasia - *see also* Agenesis
alveolar process (acquired) 525.8
congenital 750.26
aorta (congenital) 747.22
aortic valve (congenital) 746.89
axialis extracorticalis (congenital) 330.0
bone marrow (myeloid) 284.9
acquired (secondary) 284.8
congenital 284.01
idiopathic 284.9
brain 740.0
specified part 742.2
breast 757.6
bronchus 748.3
cementum 520.4
cerebellar 742.2
congenital (pure) red cell 284.01
corpus callosum 742.2
erythrocyte 284.8
congenital 284.01
extracortical axial 330.0
eye (congenital) 743.00
fovea centralis (congenital) 743.55
germinal (cell) 606.0
iris 743.45

Aplasia *(Continued)*
labyrinth, membranous 744.05
limb (congenital) 755.4
lower NEC 755.30
upper NEC 755.20
lung (bilateral) (congenital) (unilateral) 748.5
nervous system NEC 742.8
nuclear 742.8
ovary 752.0
Pelizaeus-Merzbacher 330.0
prostate (congenital) 752.89
red cell (with thymoma) 284.8
acquired (secondary) 284.8
congenital 284.01
hereditary 284.01
of infants 284.01
primary 284.01
pure 284.01
round ligament (congenital) 752.89
salivary gland 750.21
skin (congenital) 757.39
spinal cord 742.59
spleen 759.0
testis (congenital) 752.89
thymic, with immunodeficiency 279.2
thyroid 243
uterus 752.3
ventral horn cell 742.59
Apleuria 756.3
Apnea, apneic (spells) 786.03
newborn, neonatorum 770.81
essential 770.81
obstructive 770.82
primary 770.81
sleep 770.81
specified NEC 770.82
psychogenic 306.1
sleep 780.57
with
hypersomnia, unspecified 780.53
hyposomnia, unspecified 780.51
insomnia, unspecified 780.51
sleep disturbance 780.57
central, in conditions classified elsewhere 327.27
obstructive (adult) (pediatric) 327.23
organic 327.20
other 327.29
primary central 327.21
Apneumatosis newborn 770.4
Apodia 755.31
Apophysitis (bone) (*see also* Osteochondrosis) 732.9
calcaneus 732.5
juvenile 732.6
Apoplectiform convulsions (*see also* Disease, cerebrovascular, acute) 436
Apoplexia, apoplexy, apoplectic (*see also* Disease, cerebrovascular, acute) 436
abdominal 569.89
adrenal 036.3
attack 436
basilar (*see also* Disease, cerebrovascular, acute) 436
brain (*see also* Disease, cerebrovascular, acute) 436
bulbar (*see also* Disease, cerebrovascular, acute) 436
capillary (*see also* Disease, cerebrovascular, acute) 436
cardiac (*see also* Infarct, myocardium) 410.9

Apoplexia, apoplexy, apoplectic *(Continued)*
cerebral (*see also* Disease, cerebrovascular, acute) 436
chorea (*see also* Disease, cerebrovascular, acute) 436
congestive (*see also* Disease, cerebrovascular, acute) 436
newborn 767.4
embolic (*see also* Embolism, brain) 434.1
fetus 767.0
fit (*see also* Disease, cerebrovascular, acute) 436
healed or old V12.59
heart (auricle) (ventricle) (*see also* Infarct, myocardium) 410.9
heat 992.0
hemiplegia (*see also* Disease, cerebrovascular, acute) 436
hemorrhagic (stroke) (*see also* Hemorrhage, brain) 432.9
ingravescent (*see also* Disease, cerebrovascular, acute) 436
late effect - *see* Late effect(s) (of) cerebrovascular disease
lung - *see* Embolism, pulmonary
meninges, hemorrhagic (*see also* Hemorrhage, subarachnoid) 430
neonatorum 767.0
newborn 767.0
pancreatitis 577.0
placenta 641.2
progressive (*see also* Disease, cerebrovascular, acute) 436
pulmonary (artery) (vein) - *see* Embolism, pulmonary
sanguineous (*see also* Disease, cerebrovascular, acute) 436
seizure (*see also* Disease, cerebrovascular, acute) 436
serous (*see also* Disease, cerebrovascular, acute) 436
spleen 289.59
stroke (*see also* Disease, cerebrovascular, acute) 436
thrombotic (*see also* Thrombosis, brain) 434.0
uremic - *see* Uremia
uteroplacental 641.2
Appendage
fallopian tube (cyst of Morgagni) 752.11
intestine (epiploic) 751.5
preauricular 744.1
testicular (organ of Morgagni) 752.89
Appendicitis 541
with
perforation, peritonitis (generalized), or rupture 540.0
with peritoneal abscess 540.1
peritoneal abscess 540.1
acute (catarrhal) (fulminating) (gangrenous) (inflammatory) (obstructive) (retrocecal) (suppurative) 540.9
with
perforation, peritonitis, or rupture 540.0
with peritoneal abscess 540.1
peritoneal abscess 540.1
amebic 006.8
chronic (recurrent) 542
exacerbation - *see* Appendicitis, acute
fulminating - *see* Appendicitis, acute
gangrenous - *see* Appendicitis, acute
healed (obliterative) 542

Appendicitis *(Continued)*
interval 542
neurogenic 542
obstructive 542
pneumococcal 541
recurrent 542
relapsing 542
retrocecal 541
subacute (adhesive) 542
subsiding 542
suppurative - *see* Appendicitis, acute
tuberculous (*see also* Tuberculosis) 014.8
Appendiclausis 543.9
Appendicolithiasis 543.9
Appendicopathia oxyurica 127.4
Appendix, appendicular - *see also* condition
Morgagni (male) 752.89
fallopian tube 752.11
Appetite
depraved 307.52
excessive 783.6
psychogenic 307.51
lack or loss (*see also* Anorexia) 783.0
nonorganic origin 307.59
perverted 307.52
hysterical 300.11
Apprehension, apprehensiveness (abnormal) (state) 300.00
specified type NEC 300.09
Approximal wear 521.10
Apraxia (classic) (ideational) (ideokinetic) (ideomotor) (motor) 784.69
oculomotor, congenital 379.51
verbal 784.69
Aptyalism 527.7
Aqueous misdirection 365.83
Arabicum elephantiasis (*see also* Infestation, filarial) 125.9
Arachnidism 989.5
Arachnitis - *see* Meningitis
Arachnodactyly 759.82
Arachnoidism 989.5
Arachnoiditis (acute) (adhesive) (basic) (brain) (cerebrospinal) (chiasmal) (chronic) (spinal) (*see also* Meningitis) 322.9
meningococcal (chronic) 036.0
syphilitic 094.2
tuberculous (*see also* Tuberculosis, meninges) 013.0
Araneism 989.5
Arboencephalitis, Australian 062.4
Arborization block (heart) 426.6
Arbor virus, arbovirus (infection) NEC 066.9
ARC 042
Arches - *see* condition
Arcuatus uterus 752.3
Arcus (cornea)
juvenilis 743.43
interfering with vision 743.42
senilis 371.41
Arc-welders' lung 503
Arc-welders' syndrome (photokeratitis) 370.24
Areflexia 796.1
Areola - *see* condition
Argentaffinoma (M8241/1) - *see also* Neoplasm, by site, uncertain behavior
benign (M8241/0) - *see* Neoplasm, by site, benign
malignant (M8241/3) - *see* Neoplasm, by site, malignant
syndrome 259.2
Argentinian hemorrhagic fever 078.7
Arginosuccinicaciduria 270.6
Argonz-del Castillo syndrome (nonpuerperal galactorrhea and amenorrhea) 253.1
Argyll-Robertson phenomenon, pupil, or syndrome (syphilitic) 094.89
atypical 379.45
nonluetic 379.45
nonsyphilitic 379.45
reversed 379.45
Argyria, argyriasis NEC 985.8
conjunctiva 372.55
cornea 371.16
from drug or medicinal agent
correct substance properly administered 709.09
overdose or wrong substance given or taken 961.2
Arhinencephaly 742.2
Arias-Stella phenomenon 621.30
Ariboflavinosis 266.0
Arizona enteritis 008.1
Arm - *see* condition
Armenian disease 277.31 ⇐
Arnold-Chiari obstruction or syndrome (*see also* Spina bifida) 741.0
type I 348.4
type II (*see also* Spina bifida) 741.0
type III 742.0
type IV 742.2
Arousals
confusional 327.41
Arrest, arrested
active phase of labor 661.1
affecting fetus or newborn 779.85 ⇐
any plane in pelvis
complicating delivery 660.1
affecting fetus or newborn 763.1
bone marrow (*see also* Anemia, aplastic) 284.9
cardiac 427.5
with
abortion - *see* Abortion, by type, with specified complication NEC
ectopic pregnancy (*see also* categories 633.0-633.9) 639.8
molar pregnancy (*see also* categories 630-632) 639.8
complicating
anesthesia
correct substance properly administered 427.5
obstetric 668.1
overdose or wrong substance given 968.4
specified anesthetic - *see* Table of Drugs and Chemicals
delivery (cesarean) (instrumental) 669.4
ectopic or molar pregnancy 639.8
surgery (nontherapeutic) (therapeutic) 997.1
fetus or newborn 779.85 ⇐
following
abortion 639.8
ectopic or molar pregnancy 639.8
postoperative (immediate) 997.1
long-term effect of cardiac surgery 429.4
cardiorespiratory (*see also* Arrest, cardiac) 427.5
Arrest, arrested *(Continued)*
deep transverse 660.3
affecting fetus or newborn 763.1
development or growth
bone 733.91
child 783.40
fetus 764.9
affecting management of pregnancy 656.5
tracheal rings 748.3
epiphyseal 733.91
granulopoiesis 288.09 ⇐
heart - *see* Arrest, cardiac
respiratory 799.1
newborn 770.87 ⇐
sinus 426.6
transverse (deep) 660.3
affecting fetus or newborn 763.1
Arrhenoblastoma (M8630/1)
benign (M8630/0)
specified site - *see* Neoplasm, by site, benign
unspecified site
female 220
male 222.0
malignant (M8630/3)
specified site - *see* Neoplasm, by site, malignant
unspecified site
female 183.0
male 186.9
specified site - *see* Neoplasm, by site, uncertain behavior
unspecified site
female 236.2
male 236.4
Arrhinencephaly 742.2
due to
trisomy 13 (13-15) 758.1
trisomy 18 (16-18) 758.2
Arrhythmia (auricle) (cardiac) (cordis) (gallop rhythm) (juvenile) (nodal) (reflex) (sinus) (supraventricular) (transitory) (ventricle) 427.9
bigeminal rhythm 427.89
block 426.9
bradycardia 427.89
contractions, premature 427.60
coronary sinus 427.89
ectopic 427.89
extrasystolic 427.60
postoperative 997.1
psychogenic 306.2
vagal 780.2
Arrillaga-Ayerza syndrome (pulmonary artery sclerosis with pulmonary hypertension) 416.0
Arsenical
dermatitis 692.4
keratosis 692.4
pigmentation 985.1
from drug or medicinal agent
correct substance properly administered 709.09
overdose or wrong substance given or taken 961.1
Arsenism 985.1
from drug or medicinal agent
correct substance properly administered 692.4
overdose or wrong substance given or taken 961.1
Arterial - *see* condition
Arteriectasis 447.8

Arteriofibrosis - *see* Arteriosclerosis
Arteriolar sclerosis - *see* Arteriosclerosis
Arteriolith - *see* Arteriosclerosis
Arteriolitis 447.6
necrotizing, kidney 447.5
renal - *see* Hypertension, kidney
Arteriolosclerosis - *see* Arteriosclerosis
Arterionephrosclerosis (*see also* Hypertension, kidney) 403.90
Arteriopathy 447.9
Arteriosclerosis, arteriosclerotic (artery) (deformans) (diffuse) (disease) (endarteritis) (general) (obliterans) (obliterative) (occlusive) (senile) (with calcification) 440.9
with
gangrene 440.24
psychosis (*see also* Psychosis, arteriosclerotic) 290.40
ulceration 440.23
aorta 440.0
arteries of extremities - *see* Arteriosclerosis, extremities
basilar (artery) (*see also* Occlusion, artery, basilar) 433.0
brain 437.0
bypass graft
coronary artery 414.05
autologous artery (gastroepiploic) (internal mammary) 414.04
autologous vein 414.02
nonautologous biological 414.03
of transplanted heart 414.07
extremity 440.30
autologous vein 440.31
nonautologous biological 440.32
cardiac - *see* Arteriosclerosis, coronary
cardiopathy - *see* Arteriosclerosis, coronary
cardiorenal (*see also* Hypertension, cardiorenal) 404.90
cardiovascular (*see also* Disease, cardiovascular) 429.2
carotid (artery) (common) (internal) (*see also* Occlusion, artery, carotid) 433.1
central nervous system 437.0
cerebral 437.0
late effect - *see* Late effect(s) (of) cerebrovascular disease
cerebrospinal 437.0
cerebrovascular 437.0
coronary (artery) 414.00
graft - *see* Arteriosclerosis, bypass graft
native artery 414.01
of transplanted heart 414.06
extremities (native artery) NEC 440.20
bypass graft 440.30
autologous vein 440.31
nonautologous biological 440.32
claudication (intermittent) 440.21
and
gangrene 440.24
rest pain 440.22
and
gangrene 440.24
ulceration 440.23
and gangrene 440.24
ulceration 440.23
and gangrene 440.24
gangrene 440.24
rest pain 440.22
and
gangrene 440.24
ulceration 440.23
and gangrene 440.24

Arteriosclerosis, arteriosclerotic *(Continued)*
extremities (native artery) NEC *(Continued)*
specified site NEC 440.29
ulceration 440.23
and gangrene 440.24
heart (disease) - *see also* Arteriosclerosis, coronary
valve 424.99
aortic 424.1
mitral 424.0
pulmonary 424.3
tricuspid 424.2
kidney (*see also* Hypertension, kidney) 403.90
labyrinth, labyrinthine 388.00
medial NEC (*see also* Arteriosclerosis, extremities) 440.20
mesentery (artery) 557.1
Mönckeberg's (*see also* Arteriosclerosis, extremities) 440.20
myocarditis 429.0
nephrosclerosis (*see also* Hypertension, kidney) 403.90
peripheral (of extremities) - *see* Arteriosclerosis, extremities
precerebral 433.9
specified artery NEC 433.8
pulmonary (idiopathic) 416.0
renal (*see also* Hypertension, kidney) 403.90
arterioles (*see also* Hypertension, kidney) 403.90
artery 440.1
retinal (vascular) 440.8 *[362.13]*
specified artery NEC 440.8
with gangrene 440.8 *[785.4]*
spinal (cord) 437.0
vertebral (artery) (*see also* Occlusion, artery, vertebral) 433.2
Arteriospasm 443.9
Arteriovenous - *see* condition
Arteritis 447.6
allergic (*see also* Angiitis, hypersensitivity) 446.20
aorta (nonsyphilitic) 447.6
syphilitic 093.1
aortic arch 446.7
brachiocephalica 446.7
brain 437.4
syphilitic 094.89
branchial 446.7
cerebral 437.4
late effect - *see* Late effect(s) (of) cerebrovascular disease
syphilitic 094.89
coronary (artery) - *see also* Arteriosclerosis, coronary
rheumatic 391.9
chronic 398.99
syphilitic 093.89
cranial (left) (right) 446.5
deformans - *see* Arteriosclerosis
giant cell 446.5
necrosing or necrotizing 446.0
nodosa 446.0
obliterans - *see also* Arteriosclerosis
subclavicocarotica 446.7
pulmonary 417.8
retina 362.18
rheumatic - *see* Fever, rheumatic
senile - *see* Arteriosclerosis
suppurative 447.2

Arteritis *(Continued)*
syphilitic (general) 093.89
brain 094.89
coronary 093.89
spinal 094.89
temporal 446.5
young female, syndrome 446.7
Artery, arterial - *see* condition
Arthralgia (*see also* Pain, joint) 719.4
allergic (*see also* Pain, joint) 719.4
in caisson disease 993.3
psychogenic 307.89
rubella 056.71
Salmonella 003.23
temporomandibular joint 524.62
Arthritis, arthritic (acute) (chronic) (subacute) 716.9
meaning Osteoarthritis - *see* Osteoarthrosis

Note Use the following fifth-digit subclassification with categories 711-712, 715-716:

0 site unspecified
1 shoulder region
2 upper arm
3 forearm
4 hand
5 pelvic region and thigh
6 lower leg
7 ankle and foot
8 other specified sites
9 multiple sites

allergic 716.2
ankylosing (crippling) (spine) 720.0 *[713.2]*
sites other than spine 716.9
atrophic 714.0
spine 720.9
back (*see also* Arthritis, spine) 721.90
Bechterew's (ankylosing spondylitis) 720.0
blennorrhagic 098.50 *[711.6]*
cervical, cervicodorsal (*see also* Spondylosis, cervical) 721.0
Charcôt's 094.0 *[713.5]*
diabetic 250.6 *[713.5]*
syringomyelic 336.0 *[713.5]*
tabetic 094.0 *[713.5]*
chylous (*see also* Filariasis) 125.9 *[711.7]*
climacteric NEC 716.3
coccyx 721.8
cricoarytenoid 478.79
crystal (-induced) - *see* Arthritis, due to crystals
deformans (*see also* Osteoarthrosis) 715.9
spine 721.90
with myelopathy 721.91
degenerative (*see also* Osteoarthrosis) 715.9
idiopathic 715.09
polyarticular 715.09
spine 721.90
with myelopathy 721.91
dermatoarthritis, lipoid 272.8 *[713.0]*
due to or associated with
acromegaly 253.0 *[713.0]*
actinomycosis 039.8 *[711.4]*
amyloidosis 277.39 *[713.7]* ⇐ Revised
bacterial disease NEC 040.89 *[711.4]*
Behçet's syndrome 136.1 *[711.2]*
blastomycosis 116.0 *[711.6]*

Arthritis, arthritic *(Continued)*
due to or associated with *(Continued)*
brucellosis (*see also* Brucellosis) 023.9 *[711.4]*
caisson disease 993.3
coccidioidomycosis 114.3 *[711.6]*
coliform (Escherichia coli) 711.0
colitis, ulcerative - (*see also* Colitis, ulcerative) 556.9 *[713.1]*
cowpox 051.0 *[711.5]*
crystals -(*see also* Gout)
dicalcium phosphate 275.49 *[712.1]*
pyrophosphate 275.49 *[712.2]*
specified NEC 275.49 *[712.8]*
dermatoarthritis, lipoid 272.8 *[713.0]*
dermatological disorder NEC 709.9 *[713.3]*
diabetes 250.6 *[713.5]*
diphtheria 032.89 *[711.4]*
dracontiasis 125.7 *[711.7]*
dysentery 009.0 *[711.3]*
endocrine disorder NEC 259.9 *[713.0]*
enteritis NEC 009.1 *[711.3]*
infectious (*see also* Enteritis, infectious) 009.0 *[711.3]*
specified organism NEC 008.8 *[711.3]*
regional (*see also* Enteritis, regional) 555.9 *[713.1]*
specified organism NEC 008.8 *[711.3]*
epiphyseal slip, nontraumatic (old) 716.8
erysipelas 035 *[711.4]*
erythema
epidemic 026.1
multiforme 695.1 *[713.3]*
nodosum 695.2 *[713.3]*
Escherichia coli 711.0
filariasis NEC 125.9 *[711.7]*
gastrointestinal condition NEC 569.9 *[713.1]*
glanders 024 *[711.4]*
Gonococcus 098.50
gout 274.0
H. influenzae 711.0
helminthiasis NEC 128.9 *[711.7]*
hematological disorder NEC 289.9 *[713.2]*
hemochromatosis 275.0 *[713.0]*
hemoglobinopathy NEC (*see also* Disease, hemoglobin) 282.7 *[713.2]*
hemophilia (*see also* Hemophilia) 286.0 *[713.2]*
Hemophilus influenzae (H. influenzae) 711.0
Henoch (-Schönlein) purpura 287.0 *[713.6]*
histoplasmosis NEC (*see also* Histoplasmosis) 115.99 *[711.6]*
hyperparathyroidism 252.00 *[713.0]*
hypersensitivity reaction NEC 995.3 *[713.6]*
hypogammaglobulinemia (*see also* Hypogammaglobulinemia) 279.00 *[713.0]*
hypothyroidism NEC 244.9 *[713.0]*
infection (*see also* Arthritis, infectious) 711.9
infectious disease NEC 136.9 *[711.8]*
leprosy (*see also* Leprosy) 030.9 *[711.4]*
leukemia NEC (M9800/3) 208.9 *[713.2]*
lipoid dermatoarthritis 272.8 *[713.0]*

Arthritis, arthritic *(Continued)*
due to or associated with *(Continued)*
Lyme disease 088.81 *[711.8]*
Mediterranean fever, familial 277.31 *[713.7]* (Revised)
meningococcal infection 036.82
metabolic disorder NEC 277.9 *[713.0]*
multiple myelomatosis (M9730/3) 203.0 *[713.2]*
mumps 072.79 *[711.5]*
mycobacteria 031.8 *[711.4]*
mycosis NEC 117.9 *[711.6]*
neurological disorder NEC 349.9 *[713.5]*
ochronosis 270.2 *[713.0]*
O'Nyong Nyong 066.3 *[711.5]*
parasitic disease NEC 136.9 *[711.8]*
paratyphoid fever (*see also* Fever, paratyphoid) 002.9 *[711.3]*
Pneumococcus 711.0
poliomyelitis (*see also* Poliomyelitis) 045.9 *[711.5]*
Pseudomonas 711.0
psoriasis 696.0
pyogenic organism (E. coli) (H. influenzae) (Pseudomonas) (Streptococcus) 711.0
rat-bite fever 026.1 *[711.4]*
regional enteritis (*see also* Enteritis, regional) 555.9 *[713.1]*
Reiter's disease 099.3 *[711.1]*
respiratory disorder NEC 519.9 *[713.4]*
reticulosis, malignant (M9720/3) 202.3 *[713.2]*
rubella 056.71
salmonellosis 003.23
sarcoidosis 135 *[713.7]*
serum sickness 999.5 *[713.6]*
Staphylococcus 711.0
Streptococcus 711.0
syphilis (*see also* Syphilis) 094.0 *[711.4]*
syringomyelia 336.0 *[713.5]*
thalassemia 282.49 *[713.2]*
tuberculosis (*see also* Tuberculosis, arthritis) 015.9 *[711.4]*
typhoid fever 002.0 *[711.3]*
ulcerative colitis - (*see also* Colitis, ulcerative) 556.9 *[713.1]*
urethritis
nongonococcal (*see also* Urethritis, nongonococcal) 099.40 *[711.1]*
nonspecific (*see also* Urethritis, nongonococcal) 099.40 *[711.1]*
Reiter's 099.3 *[711.1]*
viral disease NEC 079.99 *[711.5]*
erythema epidemic 026.1
gonococcal 098.50
gouty (acute) 274.0
hypertrophic (*see also* Osteoarthrosis) 715.9
spine 721.90
with myelopathy 721.91
idiopathic, blennorrheal 099.3
in caisson disease 993.3 *[713.8]*
infectious or infective (acute) (chronic) (subacute) NEC 711.9
nonpyogenic 711.9
spine 720.9
inflammatory NEC 714.9
juvenile rheumatoid (chronic) (polyarticular) 714.30
acute 714.31

Arthritis, arthritic *(Continued)*
juvenile rheumatoid *(Continued)*
monoarticular 714.33
pauciarticular 714.32
lumbar (*see also* Spondylosis, lumbar) 721.3
meningococcal 036.82
menopausal NEC 716.3
migratory - *see* Fever, rheumatic
neuropathic (Charcôt's) 094.0 *[713.5]*
diabetic 250.6 *[713.5]*
nonsyphilitic NEC 349.9 *[713.5]*
syringomyelic 336.0 *[713.5]*
tabetic 094.0 *[713.5]*
nodosa (*see also* Osteoarthrosis) 715.9
spine 721.90
with myelopathy 721.91
nonpyogenic NEC 716.9
spine 721.90
with myelopathy 721.91
ochronotic 270.2 *[713.0]*
palindromic (*see also* Rheumatism, palindromic) 719.3
pneumococcal 711.0
postdysenteric 009.0 *[711.3]*
postrheumatic, chronic (Jaccoud's) 714.4
primary progressive 714.0
spine 720.9
proliferative 714.0
spine 720.0
psoriatic 696.0
purulent 711.0
pyogenic or pyemic 711.0
rheumatic 714.0
acute or subacute - *see* Fever, rheumatic
chronic 714.0
spine 720.9
rheumatoid (nodular) 714.0
with
splenoadenomegaly and leukopenia 714.1
visceral or systemic involvement 714.2
aortitis 714.89
carditis 714.2
heart disease 714.2
juvenile (chronic) (polyarticular) 714.30
acute 714.31
monoarticular 714.33
pauciarticular 714.32
spine 720.0
rubella 056.71
sacral, sacroiliac, sacrococcygeal (*see also* Spondylosis, sacral) 721.3
scorbutic 267
senile or senescent (*see also* Osteoarthrosis) 715.9
spine 721.90
with myelopathy 721.91
septic 711.0
serum (nontherapeutic) (therapeutic) 999.5 *[713.6]*
specified form NEC 716.8
spine 721.90
with myelopathy 721.91
atrophic 720.9
degenerative 721.90
with myelopathy 721.91
hypertrophic (with deformity) 721.90
with myelopathy 721.91
infectious or infective NEC 720.9

Arthritis, arthritic *(Continued)*
spine *(Continued)*
Marie-Strümpell 720.0
nonpyogenic 721.90
with myelopathy 721.91
pyogenic 720.9
rheumatoid 720.0
traumatic (old) 721.7
tuberculous (*see also* Tuberculosis) 015.0 *[720.81]*
staphylococcal 711.0
streptococcal 711.0
suppurative 711.0
syphilitic 094.0 *[713.5]*
congenital 090.49 *[713.5]*
syphilitica deformans (Charcôt) 094.0 *[713.5]*
temporomandibular joint 524.69
thoracic (*see also* Spondylosis, thoracic) 721.2
toxic of menopause 716.3
transient 716.4
traumatic (chronic) (old) (post) 716.1
current injury - *see* nature of injury
tuberculous (*see also* Tuberculosis, arthritis) 015.9 *[711.4]*
urethritica 099.3 *[711.1]*
urica, uratic 274.0
venereal 099.3 *[711.1]*
vertebral (*see also* Arthritis, spine) 721.90
villous 716.8
von Bechterew's 720.0
Arthrocele (*see also* Effusion, joint) 719.0
Arthrochondritis - *see* Arthritis
Arthrodesis status V45.4
Arthrodynia (*see also* Pain, joint) 719.4
psychogenic 307.89
Arthrodysplasia 755.9
Arthrofibrosis, joint (*see also* Ankylosis) 718.5
Arthrogryposis 728.3
multiplex, congenita 754.89
Arthrokatadysis 715.35
Arthrolithiasis 274.0
Arthro-onychodysplasia 756.89
Arthro-osteo-onychodysplasia 756.89
Arthropathy (*see also* Arthritis) 716.9

Note Use the following fifth-digit subclassification with categories 711-712, 716:

0 site unspecified
1 shoulder region
2 upper arm
3 forearm
4 hand
5 pelvic region and thigh
6 lower leg
7 ankle and foot
8 other specified sites
9 multiple sites

Behçet's 136.1 *[711.2]*
Charcôt's 094.0 *[713.5]*
diabetic 250.6 *[713.5]*
syringomyelic 336.0 *[713.5]*
tabetic 094.0 *[713.5]*
crystal (-induced) - *see* Arthritis, due to crystals
gouty 274.0
neurogenic, neuropathic (Charcôt's) (tabetic) 094.0 *[713.5]*
diabetic 250.6 *[713.5]*

Arthropathy *(Continued)*
neurogenic, neuropathic *(Continued)*
nonsyphilitic NEC 349.9 *[713.5]*
syringomyelic 336.0 *[713.5]*
postdysenteric NEC 009.0 *[711.3]*
postrheumatic, chronic (Jaccoud's) 714.4
psoriatic 696.0
pulmonary 731.2
specified NEC 716.8
syringomyelia 336.0 *[713.5]*
tabes dorsalis 094.0 *[713.5]*
tabetic 094.0 *[713.5]*
transient 716.4
traumatic 716.1
uric acid 274.0
Arthrophyte (*see also* Loose, body, joint) 718.1
Arthrophytis 719.80
ankle 719.87
elbow 719.82
foot 719.87
hand 719.84
hip 719.85
knee 719.86
multiple sites 719.89
pelvic region 719.85
shoulder (region) 719.81
specified site NEC 719.88
wrist 719.83
Arthropyosis (*see also* Arthritis, pyogenic) 711.0
Arthroscopic surgical procedure converted to open procedure V64.43
Arthrosis (deformans) (degenerative) (*see also* Osteoarthrosis) 715.9
Charcôt's 094.0 *[713.5]*
polyarticular 715.09
spine (*see also* Spondylosis) 721.90
Arthus phenomenon 995.21
due to
correct substance properly administered 995.21
overdose or wrong substance given or taken 977.9
specified drug - *see* Table of Drugs and Chemicals
serum 999.5
Articular - *see also* condition
disc disorder (reducing or non-reducing) 524.63
spondylolisthesis 756.12
Articulation
anterior 524.27
posterior 524.27
reverse 524.27
Artificial
device (prosthetic) - *see* Fitting, device
insemination V26.1
menopause (states) (symptoms) (syndrome) 627.4
opening status (functioning) (without complication) V44.9
anus (colostomy) V44.3
colostomy V44.3
cystostomy V44.50
appendico-vesicostomy V44.52
cutaneous-vesicostomy V44.51
specified type NEC V44.59
enterostomy V44.4
gastrostomy V44.1
ileostomy V44.2
intestinal tract NEC V44.4
jejunostomy V44.4

Artificial *(Continued)*
opening status *(Continued)*
nephrostomy V44.6
specified site NEC V44.8
tracheostomy V44.0
ureterostomy V44.6
urethrostomy V44.6
urinary tract NEC V44.6
vagina V44.7
vagina status V44.7
ARV (disease) (illness) (infection) - *see* Human immunodeficiency virus (disease) (illness) (infection)
Arytenoid - *see* condition
Asbestosis (occupational) 501
Asboe-Hansen's disease (incontinentia pigmenti) 757.33
Ascariasis (intestinal) (lung) 127.0
Ascaridiasis 127.0
Ascaridosis 127.0
Ascaris 127.0
lumbricoides (infestation) 127.0
pneumonia 127.0
Ascending - *see* condition
Aschoff's bodies (*see also* Myocarditis, rheumatic) 398.0
Ascites 789.5
abdominal NEC 789.5
cancerous (M8000/6) 197.6
cardiac 428.0
chylous (nonfilarial) 457.8
filarial (*see also* Infestation, filarial) 125.9
congenital 778.0
due to S. japonicum 120.2
fetal, causing fetopelvic disproportion 653.7
heart 428.0
joint (*see also* Effusion, joint) 719.0
malignant (M8000/6) 197.6
pseudochylous 789.5
syphilitic 095.2
tuberculous (*see also* Tuberculosis) 014.0
Ascorbic acid (vitamin C) deficiency (scurvy) 267
ASC-H (atypical squamous cells cannot exclude high grade squamous intraepithelial lesion) 795.02
ASC-US (atypical squamous cells of undetermined significance) 795.01
ASCVD (arteriosclerotic cardiovascular disease) 429.2
Aseptic - *see* condition
Asherman's syndrome 621.5
Asialia 527.7
Asiatic cholera (*see also* Cholera) 001.9
Asocial personality or trends 301.7
Asomatognosia 781.8
Aspergillosis 117.3
with pneumonia 117.3 *[484.6]*
allergic bronchopulmonary 518.6
nonsyphilitic NEC 117.3
Aspergillus (flavus) (fumigatus) (infection) (terreus) 117.3
Aspermatogenesis 606.0
Aspermia (testis) 606.0
Asphyxia, asphyxiation (by) 799.01
antenatal - *see* Distress, fetal
bedclothes 994.7
birth (*see also* Asphyxia, newborn) 768.9
bunny bag 994.7
carbon monoxide 986
caul (*see also* Asphyxia, newborn) 768.9

Asphyxia, asphyxiation *(Continued)*
cave-in 994.7
crushing - *see* Injury, internal, intrathoracic organs
constriction 994.7
crushing - *see* Injury, internal, intrathoracic organs
drowning 994.1
fetal, affecting newborn 768.9
food or foreign body (in larynx) 933.1
bronchioles 934.8
bronchus (main) 934.1
lung 934.8
nasopharynx 933.0
nose, nasal passages 932
pharynx 933.0
respiratory tract 934.9
specified part NEC 934.8
throat 933.0
trachea 934.0
gas, fumes, or vapor NEC 987.9
specified - *see* Table of Drugs and Chemicals
gravitational changes 994.7
hanging 994.7
inhalation - *see* Inhalation
intrauterine
fetal death (before onset of labor) 768.0
during labor 768.1
liveborn infant - *see* Distress, fetal, liveborn infant
local 443.0
mechanical 994.7
during birth (*see also* Distress, fetal) 768.9
mucus 933.1
bronchus (main) 934.1
larynx 933.1
lung 934.8
nasal passages 932
newborn 770.18
pharynx 933.0
respiratory tract 934.9
specified part NEC 934.8
throat 933.0
trachea 934.0
vaginal (fetus or newborn) 770.18
newborn 768.9
with neurologic involvement 768.5
blue 768.6
livida 768.6
mild or moderate 768.6
pallida 768.5
severe 768.5
white 768.5
pathological 799.01
plastic bag 994.7
postnatal (*see also* Asphyxia, newborn) 768.9
mechanical 994.7
pressure 994.7
reticularis 782.61
strangulation 994.7
submersion 994.1
traumatic NEC - *see* Injury, internal, intrathoracic organs
vomiting, vomitus - *see* Asphyxia, food or foreign body
Aspiration
acid pulmonary (syndrome) 997.3
obstetric 668.0
amniotic fluid 770.13
with respiratory symptoms 770.14
Aspiration *(Continued)*
bronchitis 507.0
clear amniotic fluid 770.13
with
pneumonia 770.14
pneumonitis 770.14
respiratory symptoms 770.14
contents of birth canal 770.17
with respiratory symptoms 770.18
fetal 770.10
blood 770.15
with
pneumonia 770.16
pneumonitis 770.16
pneumonitis 770.18
food, foreign body, or gasoline (with asphyxiation) - *see* Asphyxia, food or foreign body
meconium 770.11
with
pneumonia 770.12
pneumonitis 770.12
respiratory symptoms 770.12
below vocal cords 770.11
with respiratory symptoms 770.12
mucus 933.1
into
bronchus (main) 934.1
lung 934.8
respiratory tract 934.9
specified part NEC 934.8
trachea 934.0
newborn 770.17
vaginal (fetus or newborn) 770.17
newborn 770.10
with respiratory symptoms 770.18
blood 770.15
with
pneumonia 770.16
pneumonitis 770.16
respiratory symptoms 770.16
pneumonia 507.0
fetus or newborn 770.18
meconium 770.12
pneumonitis 507.0
fetus or newborn 770.18
meconium 770.12
obstetric 668.0
postnatal stomach contents 770.85
with
pneumonia 770.86
pneumonitis 770.86
respiratory symptoms 770.86
syndrome of newborn (massive) 770.18
meconium 770.12
vernix caseosa 770.17
Asplenia 759.0
with mesocardia 746.87
Assam fever 085.0
Assimilation, pelvis
with disproportion 653.2
affecting fetus or newborn 763.1
causing obstructed labor 660.1
affecting fetus or newborn 763.1
Assmann's focus (*see also* Tuberculosis) 011.0
Astasia (-abasia) 307.9
hysterical 300.11
Asteatosis 706.8
cutis 706.8
Astereognosis 780.99
Asterixis 781.3
in liver disease 572.8
Asteroid hyalitis 379.22
Asthenia, asthenic 780.79
cardiac (*see also* Failure, heart) 428.9
psychogenic 306.2
cardiovascular (*see also* Failure, heart) 428.9
psychogenic 306.2
heart (*see also* Failure, heart) 428.9
psychogenic 306.2
hysterical 300.11
myocardial (*see also* Failure, heart) 428.9
psychogenic 306.2
nervous 300.5
neurocirculatory 306.2
neurotic 300.5
psychogenic 300.5
psychoneurotic 300.5
psychophysiologic 300.5
reaction, psychoneurotic 300.5
senile 797
Stiller's 780.79
tropical anhidrotic 705.1
Asthenopia 368.13
accommodative 367.4
hysterical (muscular) 300.11
psychogenic 306.7
Asthenospermia 792.2
Asthma, asthmatic (bronchial) (catarrh) (spasmodic) 493.9

Note The following fifth digit subclassification is for use with codes 493.0-493.2, 493.9:

0 unspecified
1 with status asthmaticus
2 with (acute) exacerbation

with
chronic obstructive pulmonary disease (COPD) 493.2
hay fever 493.0
rhinitis, allergic 493.0
allergic 493.9
stated cause (external allergen) 493.0
atopic 493.0
cardiac (*see also* Failure, ventricular, left) 428.1
cardiobronchial (*see also* Failure, ventricular, left) 428.1
cardiorenal (*see also* Hypertension, cardiorenal) 404.90
childhood 493.0
Colliers' 500
cough variant 493.82
croup 493.9
detergent 507.8
due to
detergent 507.8
inhalation of fumes 506.3
internal immunological process 493.0
endogenous (intrinsic) 493.1
eosinophilic 518.3
exercise induced bronchospasm 493.81
exogenous (cosmetics) (dander or dust) (drugs) (dust) (feathers) (food) (hay) (platinum) (pollen) 493.0
extrinsic 493.0
grinders' 502
hay 493.0
heart (*see also* Failure, ventricular, left) 428.1
IgE 493.0

Asthma, asthmatic *(Continued)*
- infective 493.1
- intrinsic 493.1
- Kopp's 254.8
- late-onset 493.1
- meat-wrappers' 506.9
- Millar's (laryngismus stridulus) 478.75
- millstone makers' 502
- miners' 500
- Monday morning 504
- New Orleans (epidemic) 493.0
- platinum 493.0
- pneumoconiotic (occupational) NEC 505
- potters' 502
- psychogenic 316 *[493.9]*
- pulmonary eosinophilic 518.3
- red cedar 495.8
- Rostan's (*see also* Failure, ventricular, left) 428.1
- sandblasters' 502
- sequoiosis 495.8
- stonemasons' 502
- thymic 254.8
- tuberculous (*see also* Tuberculosis, pulmonary) 011.9
- Wichmann's (laryngismus stridulus) 478.75
- wood 495.8

Astigmatism (compound) (congenital) 367.20
- irregular 367.22
- regular 367.21

Astroblastoma (M9430/3)
- nose 748.1
- specified site - *see* Neoplasm, by site, malignant
- unspecified site 191.9

Astrocytoma (cystic) (M9400/3)
- anaplastic type (M9401/3)
  - specified site - *see* Neoplasm, by site, malignant
  - unspecified site 191.9
- fibrillary (M9420/3)
  - specified site - *see* Neoplasm, by site, malignant
  - unspecified site 191.9
- fibrous (M9420/3)
  - specified site - *see* Neoplasm, by site, malignant
  - unspecified site 191.9
- gemistocytic (M9411/3)
  - specified site - *see* Neoplasm, by site, malignant
  - unspecified site 191.9
- juvenile (M9421/3)
  - specified site - *see* Neoplasm, by site, malignant
  - unspecified site 191.9
- nose 748.1
- pilocytic (M9421/3)
  - specified site - *see* Neoplasm, by site, malignant
  - unspecified site 191.9
- piloid (M9421/3)
  - specified site - *see* Neoplasm, by site, malignant
  - unspecified site 191.9
- protoplasmic (M9410/3)
  - specified site - *see* Neoplasm, by site, malignant
  - unspecified site 191.9
- specified site - *see* Neoplasm, by site, malignant

Astrocytoma *(Continued)*
- subependymal (M9383/1) 237.5
  - giant cell (M9384/1) 237.5
- unspecified site 191.9

Astroglioma (M9400/3)
- nose 748.1
- specified site - *see* Neoplasm, by site, malignant
- unspecified site 191.9

Asymbolia 784.60

Asymmetrical breathing 786.09

Asymmetry - *see also* Distortion
- chest 786.9
- face 754.0
- jaw NEC 524.12
  - maxillary 524.11
- pelvis with disproportion 653.0
  - affecting fetus or newborn 763.1
  - causing obstructed labor 660.1
    - affecting fetus or newborn 763.1

Asynergia 781.3

Asynergy 781.3
- ventricular 429.89

Asystole (heart) (*see also* Arrest, cardiac) 427.5

At risk for falling V15.88

Ataxia, ataxy, ataxic 781.3
- acute 781.3
- brain 331.89
- cerebellar 334.3
  - hereditary (Marie's) 334.2
  - in
    - alcoholism 303.9 *[334.4]*
    - myxedema (*see also* Myxedema) 244.9 *[334.4]*
    - neoplastic disease NEC 239.9 *[334.4]*
- cerebral 331.89
- family, familial 334.2
  - cerebral (Marie's) 334.2
  - spinal (Friedreich's) 334.0
- Friedreich's (heredofamilial) (spinal) 334.0
- frontal lobe 781.3
- gait 781.2
  - hysterical 300.11
- general 781.3
- hereditary NEC 334.2
  - cerebellar 334.2
  - spastic 334.1
  - spinal 334.0
- heredofamilial (Marie's) 334.2
- hysterical 300.11
- locomotor (progressive) 094.0
  - diabetic 250.6 *[337.1]*
- Marie's (cerebellar) (heredofamilial) 334.2
- nonorganic origin 307.9
- partial 094.0
- postchickenpox 052.7
- progressive locomotor 094.0
- psychogenic 307.9
- Sanger-Brown's 334.2
- spastic 094.0
  - hereditary 334.1
  - syphilitic 094.0
- spinal
  - hereditary 334.0
  - progressive locomotor 094.0
- telangiectasia 334.8

Ataxia-telangiectasia 334.8

Atelectasis (absorption collapse) (complete) (compression) (massive) (partial) (postinfective) (pressure collapse) (pulmonary) (relaxation) 518.0

Atelectasis *(Continued)*
- newborn (congenital) (partial) 770.5
  - primary 770.4
- primary 770.4
- tuberculous (*see also* Tuberculosis, pulmonary) 011.9

Ateleiosis, ateliosis 253.3

Atelia - *see* Distortion

Ateliosis 253.3

Atelocardia 746.9

Atelomyelia 742.59

Athelia 757.6

Atheroembolism
- extremity
  - lower 445.02
  - upper 445.01
- kidney 445.81
- specified site NEC 445.89

Atheroma, atheromatous (*see also* Arteriosclerosis) 440.9
- aorta, aortic 440.0
  - valve (*see also* Endocarditis, aortic) 424.1
- artery - *see* Arteriosclerosis
- basilar (artery) (*see also* Occlusion, artery, basilar) 433.0
- carotid (artery) (common) (internal) (*see also* Occlusion, artery, carotid) 433.1
- cerebral (arteries) 437.0
- coronary (artery) - *see* Arteriosclerosis, coronary
- degeneration - *see* Arteriosclerosis
- heart, cardiac - *see* Arteriosclerosis, coronary
- mitral (valve) 424.0
- myocardium, myocardial - *see* Arteriosclerosis, coronary
- pulmonary valve (heart) (*see also* Endocarditis, pulmonary) 424.3
- skin 706.2
- tricuspid (heart) (valve) 424.2
- valve, valvular - *see* Endocarditis
- vertebral (artery) (*see also* Occlusion, artery, vertebral) 433.2

Atheromatosis - *see also* Arteriosclerosis
- arterial, congenital 272.8

Atherosclerosis - *see* Arteriosclerosis

Athetosis (acquired) 781.0
- bilateral 333.79 ◀▮▮
- congenital (bilateral) 333.6 ◀▮▮
- double 333.71 ◀▮▮
- unilateral 781.0

Athlete's
- foot 110.4
- heart 429.3

Athletic team examination V70.3

Athrepsia 261

Athyrea (acquired) (*see also* Hypothyroidism) 244.9
- congenital 243

Athyreosis (congenital) 243
- acquired - *see* Hypothyroidism

Athyroidism (acquired) (*see also* Hypothyroidism) 244.9
- congenital 243

Atmospheric pyrexia 992.0

Atonia, atony, atonic
- abdominal wall 728.2
- bladder (sphincter) 596.4
  - neurogenic NEC 596.54
    - with cauda equina syndrome 344.61
- capillary 448.9

- **Atonia, atony, atonic** *(Continued)*
  - cecum 564.89
    - psychogenic 306.4
  - colon 564.89
    - psychogenic 306.4
  - congenital 779.89
  - dyspepsia 536.3
    - psychogenic 306.4
  - intestine 564.89
    - psychogenic 306.4
  - stomach 536.3
    - neurotic or psychogenic 306.4
    - psychogenic 306.4
  - uterus (Revised)
    - with hemorrhage 666.1 ◀
    - without hemorrhage 669.8 ◀
    - affecting fetus or newborn 763.7
  - vesical 596.4
- **Atopy NEC** V15.09
- **Atransferrinemia, congenital** 273.8
- **Atresia, atretic** (congenital) 759.89
  - alimentary organ or tract NEC 751.8
    - lower 751.2
    - upper 750.8
  - ani, anus, anal (canal) 751.2
  - aorta 747.22
    - with hypoplasia of ascending aorta and defective development of left ventricle (with mitral valve atresia) 746.7
    - arch 747.11
    - ring 747.21
  - aortic (orifice) (valve) 746.89
    - arch 747.11
  - aqueduct of Sylvius 742.3
    - with spina bifida (*see also* Spina bifida) 741.0
  - artery NEC (*see also* Atresia, blood vessel) 747.60
    - cerebral 747.81
    - coronary 746.85
    - eye 743.58
    - pulmonary 747.3
    - umbilical 747.5
  - auditory canal (external) 744.02
  - bile, biliary duct (common) or passage 751.61
    - acquired (*see also* Obstruction, biliary) 576.2
  - bladder (neck) 753.6
  - blood vessel (peripheral) NEC 747.60
    - cerebral 747.81
    - gastrointestinal 747.61
    - lower limb 747.64
    - pulmonary artery 747.3
    - renal 747.62
    - spinal 747.82
    - upper limb 747.63
  - bronchus 748.3
  - canal, ear 744.02
  - cardiac
    - valve 746.89
      - aortic 746.89
      - mitral 746.89
      - pulmonary 746.01
      - tricuspid 746.1
  - cecum 751.2
  - cervix (acquired) 622.4
    - congenital 752.49
    - in pregnancy or childbirth 654.6
      - affecting fetus or newborn 763.89
      - causing obstructed labor 660.2
        - affecting fetus or newborn 763.1
  - choana 748.0

- **Atresia, atretic** *(Continued)*
  - colon 751.2
  - cystic duct 751.61
    - acquired 575.8
      - with obstruction (*see also* Obstruction, gallbladder) 575.2
  - digestive organs NEC 751.8
  - duodenum 751.1
  - ear canal 744.02
  - ejaculatory duct 752.89
  - epiglottis 748.3
  - esophagus 750.3
  - Eustachian tube 744.24
  - fallopian tube (acquired) 628.2
    - congenital 752.19
  - follicular cyst 620.0
  - foramen of
    - Luschka 742.3
      - with spina bifida (*see also* Spina bifida) 741.0
    - Magendie 742.3
      - with spina bifida (*see also* Spina bifida) 741.0
  - gallbladder 751.69
  - genital organ
    - external
      - female 752.49
      - male NEC 752.89
        - penis 752.69
    - internal
      - female 752.89
      - male 752.89
  - glottis 748.3
  - gullet 750.3
  - heart
    - valve NEC 746.89
      - aortic 746.89
      - mitral 746.89
      - pulmonary 746.01
      - tricuspid 746.1
  - hymen 752.42
    - acquired 623.3
    - postinfective 623.3
  - ileum 751.1
  - intestine (small) 751.1
    - large 751.2
  - iris, filtration angle (*see also* Buphthalmia) 743.20
  - jejunum 751.1
  - kidney 753.3
  - lacrimal, apparatus 743.65
    - acquired - *see* Stenosis, lacrimal
  - larynx 748.3
  - ligament, broad 752.19
  - lung 748.5
  - meatus urinarius 753.6
  - mitral valve 746.89
    - with atresia or hypoplasia of aortic orifice or valve, with hypoplasia of ascending aorta and defective development of left ventricle 746.7
  - nares (anterior) (posterior) 748.0
  - nasolacrimal duct 743.65
  - nasopharynx 748.8
  - nose, nostril 748.0
    - acquired 738.0
  - organ or site NEC - *see* Anomaly, specified type NEC
  - osseous meatus (ear) 744.03
  - oviduct (acquired) 628.2
    - congenital 752.19
  - parotid duct 750.23
    - acquired 527.8

- **Atresia, atretic** *(Continued)*
  - pulmonary (artery) 747.3
    - valve 746.01
    - vein 747.49
  - pulmonic 746.01
  - pupil 743.46
  - rectum 751.2
  - salivary duct or gland 750.23
    - acquired 527.8
  - sublingual duct 750.23
    - acquired 527.8
  - submaxillary duct or gland 750.23
    - acquired 527.8
  - trachea 748.3
  - tricuspid valve 746.1
  - ureter 753.29
  - ureteropelvic junction 753.21
  - ureterovesical orifice 753.22
  - urethra (valvular) 753.6
  - urinary tract NEC 753.29
  - uterus 752.3
    - acquired 621.8
  - vagina (acquired) 623.2
    - congenital 752.49
    - postgonococcal (old) 098.2
    - postinfectional 623.2
    - senile 623.2
  - vascular NEC (*see also* Atresia, blood vessel) 747.60
    - cerebral 747.81
  - vas deferens 752.89
  - vein NEC (*see also* Atresia, blood vessel) 747.60
    - cardiac 746.89
    - great 747.49
    - portal 747.49
    - pulmonary 747.49
  - vena cava (inferior) (superior) 747.49
  - vesicourethral orifice 753.6
  - vulva 752.49
    - acquired 624.8
- **Atrichia, atrichosis** 704.00
  - congenital (universal) 757.4
- **Atrioventricularis commune** 745.69
- **Atrophia** - *see also* Atrophy
  - alba 709.09
  - cutis 701.8
    - idiopathica progressiva 701.8
    - senilis 701.8
  - dermatological, diffuse (idiopathic) 701.8
  - flava hepatis (acuta) (subacuta) (*see also* Necrosis, liver) 570
  - gyrata of choroid and retina (central) 363.54
    - generalized 363.57
  - senilis 797
    - dermatological 701.8
  - unguium 703.8
    - congenita 757.5
- **Atrophoderma, atrophodermia** 701.9
  - diffusum (idiopathic) 701.8
  - maculatum 701.3
    - et striatum 701.3
      - due to syphilis 095.8
    - syphilitic 091.3
  - neuriticum 701.8
  - pigmentosum 757.33
  - reticulatum symmetricum faciei 701.8
  - senile 701.8
  - symmetrical 701.8
  - vermiculata 701.8

Atrophy, atrophic
adrenal (autoimmune) (capsule) (cortex) (gland) 255.4
with hypofunction 255.4
alveolar process or ridge (edentulous) 525.20
mandible 525.20
minimal 525.21
moderate 525.22
severe 525.23
maxilla 525.20
minimal 525.24
moderate 525.25
severe 525.26
appendix 543.9
Aran-Duchenne muscular 335.21
arm 728.2
arteriosclerotic - *see* Arteriosclerosis
arthritis 714.0
spine 720.9
bile duct (any) 576.8
bladder 596.8
blanche (of Milian) 701.3
bone (senile) 733.99
due to
disuse 733.7
infection 733.99
tabes dorsalis (neurogenic) 094.0
posttraumatic 733.99
brain (cortex) (progressive) 331.9
with dementia 290.10
Alzheimer's 331.0
with dementia - *see* Alzheimer's, dementia
circumscribed (Pick's) 331.11
with dementia
with behavioral disturbance 331.11 *[294.11]*
without behavioral disturbance 331.11 *[294.10]*
congenital 742.4
hereditary 331.9
senile 331.2
breast 611.4
puerperal, postpartum 676.3
buccal cavity 528.9
cardiac (brown) (senile) (*see also* Degeneration, myocardial) 429.1
cartilage (infectional) (joint) 733.99
cast, plaster of Paris 728.2
cerebellar - *see* Atrophy, brain
cerebral - *see* Atrophy, brain
cervix (endometrium) (mucosa) (myometrium) (senile) (uteri) 622.8
menopausal 627.8
Charcôt-Marie-Tooth 356.1
choroid 363.40
diffuse secondary 363.42
hereditary (*see also* Dystrophy, choroid) 363.50
gyrate
central 363.54
diffuse 363.57
generalized 363.57
senile 363.41
ciliary body 364.57
colloid, degenerative 701.3
conjunctiva (senile) 372.89
corpus cavernosum 607.89
cortical (*see also* Atrophy, brain) 331.9
Cruveilhier's 335.21
cystic duct 576.8
dacryosialadenopathy 710.2
degenerative

Atrophy, atrophic *(Continued)*
degenerative *(Continued)*
colloid 701.3
senile 701.3
Déjérine-Thomas 333.0
diffuse idiopathic, dermatological 701.8
disuse
bone 733.7
muscle 728.2
pelvic muscles and anal sphincter 618.83
Duchenne-Aran 335.21
ear 388.9
edentulous alveolar ridge 525.20
mandible 525.20
minimal 525.21
moderate 525.22
severe 525.23
maxilla 525.20
minimal 525.24
moderate 525.25
severe 525.26
emphysema, lung 492.8
endometrium (senile) 621.8
cervix 622.8
enteric 569.89
epididymis 608.3
eyeball, cause unknown 360.41
eyelid (senile) 374.50
facial (skin) 701.9
facioscapulohumeral (Landouzy-Déjérine) 359.1
fallopian tube (senile), acquired 620.3
fatty, thymus (gland) 254.8
gallbladder 575.8
gastric 537.89
gastritis (chronic) 535.1
gastrointestinal 569.89
genital organ, male 608.89
glandular 289.3
globe (phthisis bulbi) 360.41
gum (*see also* Recession, gingival) 523.20
hair 704.2
heart (brown) (senile) (*see also* Degeneration, myocardial) 429.1
hemifacial 754.0
Romberg 349.89
hydronephrosis 591
infantile 261
paralysis, acute (*see also* Poliomyelitis, with paralysis) 045.1
intestine 569.89
iris (generalized) (postinfectional) (sector shaped) 364.59
essential 364.51
progressive 364.51
sphincter 364.54
kidney (senile) (*see also* Sclerosis, renal) 587
with hypertension (*see also* Hypertension, kidney) 403.90
congenital 753.0
hydronephrotic 591
infantile 753.0
lacrimal apparatus (primary) 375.13
secondary 375.14
Landouzy-Déjérine 359.1
laryngitis, infection 476.0
larynx 478.79
Leber's optic 377.16
lip 528.5
liver (acute) (subacute) (*see also* Necrosis, liver) 570
chronic (yellow) 571.8

Atrophy, atrophic *(Continued)*
liver *(Continued)*
yellow (congenital) 570
with
abortion - *see* Abortion, by type, with specified complication NEC
ectopic pregnancy (*see also* categories 633.0-633.9) 639.8
molar pregnancy (*see also* categories 630-632) 639.8
chronic 571.8
complicating pregnancy 646.7
following
abortion 639.8
ectopic or molar pregnancy 639.8
from injection, inoculation or transfusion (onset within 8 months after administration) - *see* Hepatitis, viral
healed 571.5
obstetric 646.7
postabortal 639.8
postimmunization - *see* Hepatitis, viral
posttransfusion - *see* Hepatitis, viral
puerperal, postpartum 674.8
lung (senile) 518.89
congenital 748.69
macular (dermatological) 701.3
syphilitic, skin 091.3
striated 095.8
muscle, muscular 728.2
disuse 728.2
Duchenne-Aran 335.21
extremity (lower) (upper) 728.2
familial spinal 335.11
general 728.2
idiopathic 728.2
infantile spinal 335.0
myelopathic (progressive) 335.10
myotonic 359.2
neuritic 356.1
neuropathic (peroneal) (progressive) 356.1
peroneal 356.1
primary (idiopathic) 728.2
progressive (familial) (hereditary) (pure) 335.21
adult (spinal) 335.19
infantile (spinal) 335.0
juvenile (spinal) 335.11
spinal 335.10
adult 335.19
hereditary or familial 335.11
infantile 335.0
pseudohypertrophic 359.1
spinal (progressive) 335.10
adult 335.19
Aran-Duchenne 335.21
familial 335.11
hereditary 335.11
infantile 335.0
juvenile 335.11
syphilitic 095.6
myocardium (*see also* Degeneration, myocardial) 429.1
myometrium (senile) 621.8
cervix 622.8
myotatic 728.2
myotonia 359.2
nail 703.8
congenital 757.5

Atrophy, atrophic *(Continued)*
nasopharynx 472.2
nerve - *see also* Disorder, nerve
abducens 378.54
accessory 352.4
acoustic or auditory 388.5
cranial 352.9
first (olfactory) 352.0
second (optic) (*see also* Atrophy, optic nerve) 377.10
third (oculomotor) (partial) 378.51
total 378.52
fourth (trochlear) 378.53
fifth (trigeminal) 350.8
sixth (abducens) 378.54
seventh (facial) 351.8
eighth (auditory) 388.5
ninth (glossopharyngeal) 352.2
tenth (pneumogastric) (vagus) 352.3
eleventh (accessory) 352.4
twelfth (hypoglossal) 352.5
facial 351.8
glossopharyngeal 352.2
hypoglossal 352.5
oculomotor (partial) 378.51
total 378.52
olfactory 352.0
peripheral 355.9
pneumogastric 352.3
trigeminal 350.8
trochlear 378.53
vagus (pneumogastric) 352.3
nervous system, congenital 742.8
neuritic (*see also* Disorder, nerve) 355.9
neurogenic NEC 355.9
bone
tabetic 094.0
nutritional 261
old age 797
olivopontocerebellar 333.0
optic nerve (ascending) (descending) (infectional) (nonfamilial) (papillomacular bundle) (postretinal) (secondary NEC) (simple) 377.10
associated with retinal dystrophy 377.13
dominant hereditary 377.16
glaucomatous 377.14
hereditary (dominant) (Leber's) 377.16
Leber's (hereditary) 377.16
partial 377.15
postinflammatory 377.12
primary 377.11
syphilitic 094.84
congenital 090.49
tabes dorsalis 094.0
orbit 376.45
ovary (senile), acquired 620.3
oviduct (senile), acquired 620.3
palsy, diffuse 335.20
pancreas (duct) (senile) 577.8
papillary muscle 429.81
paralysis 355.9
parotid gland 527.0
patches skin 701.3
senile 701.8
penis 607.89
pharyngitis 472.1
pharynx 478.29
pluriglandular 258.8
polyarthritis 714.0

Atrophy, atrophic *(Continued)*
prostate 602.2
pseudohypertrophic 359.1
renal (*see also* Sclerosis, renal) 587
reticulata 701.8
retina (*see also* Degeneration, retina) 362.60
hereditary (*see also* Dystrophy, retina) 362.70
rhinitis 472.0
salivary duct or gland 527.0
scar NEC 709.2
sclerosis, lobar (of brain) 331.0
with dementia
with behavioral disturbance 331.0 *[294.11]*
without behavioral disturbance 331.0 *[294.10]*
scrotum 608.89
seminal vesicle 608.89
senile 797
degenerative, of skin 701.3
skin (patches) (senile) 701.8
spermatic cord 608.89
spinal (cord) 336.8
acute 336.8
muscular (chronic) 335.10
adult 335.19
familial 335.11
juvenile 335.10
paralysis 335.10
acute (*see also* Poliomyelitis, with paralysis) 045.1
spine (column) 733.99
spleen (senile) 289.59
spots (skin) 701.3
senile 701.8
stomach 537.89
striate and macular 701.3
syphilitic 095.8
subcutaneous 701.9
due to injection 999.9
sublingual gland 527.0
submaxillary gland 527.0
Sudeck's 733.7
suprarenal (autoimmune) (capsule) (gland) 255.4
with hypofunction 255.4
tarso-orbital fascia, congenital 743.66
testis 608.3
thenar, partial 354.0
throat 478.29
thymus (fat) 254.8
thyroid (gland) 246.8
with
cretinism 243
myxedema 244.9
congenital 243
tongue (senile) 529.8
papillae 529.4
smooth 529.4
trachea 519.19 ⬅
tunica vaginalis 608.89
turbinate 733.99
tympanic membrane (nonflaccid) 384.82
flaccid 384.81
ulcer (*see also* Ulcer, skin) 707.9
upper respiratory tract 478.9
uterus, uterine (acquired) (senile) 621.8
cervix 622.8
due to radiation (intended effect) 621.8
vagina (senile) 627.3

Atrophy, atrophic *(Continued)*
vascular 459.89
vas deferens 608.89
vertebra (senile) 733.99
vulva (primary) (senile) 624.1
Werdnig-Hoffmann 335.0
yellow (acute) (congenital) (liver) (subacute) (*see also* Necrosis, liver) 570
chronic 571.8
resulting from administration of blood, plasma, serum, or other biological substance (within 8 months of administration) - *see* Hepatitis, viral

Attack
akinetic (*see also* Epilepsy) 345.0
angina - *see* Angina
apoplectic (*see also* Disease, cerebrovascular, acute) 436
benign shuddering 333.93
bilious - *see* Vomiting
cataleptic 300.11
cerebral (*see also* Disease, cerebrovascular, acute) 436
coronary (*see also* Infarct, myocardium) 410.9
cyanotic, newborn 770.83
epileptic (*see also* Epilepsy) 345.9
epileptiform 780.39
heart (*see also* Infarct, myocardium) 410.9
hemiplegia (*see also* Disease, cerebrovascular, acute) 436
hysterical 300.11
jacksonian (*see also* Epilepsy) 345.5
myocardium, myocardial (*see also* Infarct, myocardium) 410.9
myoclonic (*see also* Epilepsy) 345.1
panic 300.01
paralysis (*see also* Disease, cerebrovascular, acute) 436
paroxysmal 780.39
psychomotor (*see also* Epilepsy) 345.4
salaam (*see also* Epilepsy) 345.6
schizophreniform (*see also* Schizophrenia) 295.4
sensory and motor 780.39
syncope 780.2
toxic, cerebral 780.39
transient ischemic (TIA) 435.9
unconsciousness 780.2
hysterical 300.11
vasomotor 780.2
vasovagal (idiopathic) (paroxysmal) 780.2

Attention to
artificial
opening (of) V55.9
digestive tract NEC V55.4
specified site NEC V55.8
urinary tract NEC V55.6
vagina V55.7
dressing ◀
wound V58.30 ◀
nonsurgical V58.30 ◀
surgical V58.31 ◀
colostomy V55.3
cystostomy V55.5
gastrostomy V55.1
ileostomy V55.2
jejunostomy V55.4
nephrostomy V55.6
surgical dressings V58.31 ⬅

Attention to *(Continued)*
sutures V58.32
tracheostomy V55.0
ureterostomy V55.6
urethrostomy V55.6
Attrition
gum (*see also* Recession, gingival) 523.20
teeth (hard tissues) 521.10
excessive 521.10
extending into
dentine 521.12
pulp 521.13
generalized 521.15
limited to enamel 521.11
localized 521.14
Atypical - *see also* condition
cells
endocervical 795.00
endometrial 795.00
glandular 795.00
distribution, vessel (congenital) (peripheral) NEC 747.60
endometrium 621.9
kidney 593.89
Atypism, cervix 622.10
Audible tinnitus (*see also* Tinnitus) 388.30
Auditory - *see* condition
Audry's syndrome (acropachyderma) 757.39
Aujeszky's disease 078.89
Aura, jacksonian (*see also* Epilepsy) 345.5
Aurantiasis, cutis 278.3
Auricle, auricular - *see* condition
Auriculotemporal syndrome 350.8
Australian
Q fever 083.0
X disease 062.4
Autism, autistic (child) (infantile) 299.0
Autodigestion 799.89
Autoerythrocyte sensitization 287.2
Autographism 708.3
Autoimmune
cold sensitivity 283.0
disease NEC 279.4
hemolytic anemia 283.0
thyroiditis 245.2
Autoinfection, septic - *see* Septicemia
Autointoxication 799.89
Automatism 348.8
epileptic (*see also* Epilepsy) 345.4
paroxysmal, idiopathic (*see also* Epilepsy) 345.4
Autonomic, autonomous
bladder 596.54
Autonomic, autonomous *(Continued)*
bladder *(Continued)*
neurogenic 596.54
with cauda equina 344.61
dysreflexia 337.3
faciocephalalgia (*see also* Neuropathy, peripheral, autonomic) 337.9
hysterical seizure 300.11
imbalance (*see also* Neuropathy, peripheral, autonomic 337.9
Autophony 388.40
Autosensitivity, erythrocyte 287.2
Autotopagnosia 780.99
Autotoxemia 799.89
Autumn - *see* condition
Avellis' syndrome 344.89
Aviators'
disease or sickness (*see also* Effect, adverse, high altitude) 993.2
ear 993.0
effort syndrome 306.2
Avitaminosis (multiple NEC) (*see also* Deficiency, vitamin) 269.2
A 264.9
B 266.9
with
beriberi 265.0
pellagra 265.2
B_1 265.1
B_2 266.0
B_6 266.1
B_{12} 266.2
C (with scurvy) 267
D 268.9
with
osteomalacia 268.2
rickets 268.0
E 269.1
G 266.0
H 269.1
K 269.0
multiple 269.2
nicotinic acid 265.2
P 269.1
Avulsion (traumatic) 879.8
blood vessel - *see* Injury, blood vessel, by site
cartilage - *see also* Dislocation, by site
knee, current (*see also* Tear, meniscus) 836.2
symphyseal (inner), complicating delivery 665.6
complicated 879.9
diaphragm - *see* Injury, internal, diaphragm
Avulsion *(Continued)*
ear - *see* Wound, open, ear
epiphysis of bone - *see* Fracture, by site
external site other than limb - *see* Wound, open, by site
eye 871.3
fingernail - *see* Wound, open, finger
fracture - *see* Fracture, by site
genital organs, external - *see* Wound, open, genital organs
head (intracranial) NEC - *see also* Injury, intracranial, with open intracranial wound
complete 874.9
external site NEC 873.8
complicated 873.9
internal organ or site - *see* Injury, internal, by site
joint - *see also* Dislocation, by site
capsule - *see* Sprain, by site
ligament - *see* Sprain, by site
limb - *see also* Amputation, traumatic, by site
skin and subcutaneous tissue - *see* Wound, open, by site
muscle - *see* Sprain, by site
nerve (root) - *see* Injury, nerve, by site
scalp - *see* Wound, open, scalp
skin and subcutaneous tissue - *see* Wound, open, by site
symphyseal cartilage (inner), complicating delivery 665.6
tendon - *see also* Sprain, by site
with open wound - *see* Wound, open, by site
toenail - *see* Wound, open, toe(s)
tooth 873.63
complicated 873.73
Awaiting organ transplant status V49.83
Awareness of heart beat 785.1
Axe grinders' disease 502
Axenfeld's anomaly or syndrome 743.44
Axilla, axillary - *see also* condition
breast 757.6
Axonotmesis - *see* Injury, nerve, by site
Ayala's disease 756.89
Ayerza's disease or syndrome (pulmonary artery sclerosis with pulmonary hypertension) 416.0
Azoospermia 606.0
Azorean disease (of the nervous system) 334.8
Azotemia 790.6
meaning uremia (*see also* Uremia) 586
Aztec ear 744.29
Azygos lobe, lung (fissure) 748.69

B

- **Baader's syndrome** (erythema multiforme exucatiuum) 695.1
- **Baastrup's syndrome** 721.5
- **Babesiasis** 088.82
- **Babesiosis** 088.82
- **Babington's disease** (familial hemorrhagic telangiectasia) 448.0
- **Babinski's syndrome** (cardiovascular syphilis) 093.89
- **Babinski-Fröhlich syndrome** (adiposogenital dystrophy) 253.8
- **Babinski-Nageotte syndrome** 344.89
- **Bacillary** - *see* condition
- **Bacilluria** 791.9
  - asymptomatic, in pregnancy or puerperium 646.5
  - tuberculous (*see also* Tuberculosis) 016.9
- **Bacillus** - *see also* Infection, bacillus
  - abortus infection 023.1
  - anthracis infection 022.9
  - coli
    - infection 041.4
      - generalized 038.42
      - intestinal 008.00
    - pyemia 038.42
    - septicemia 038.42
  - Flexner's 004.1
  - fusiformis infestation 101
  - mallei infection 024
  - Shiga's 004.0
  - suipestifer infection (*see also* Infection, Salmonella) 003.9
- **Back** - *see* condition
- **Backache** (postural) 724.5
  - psychogenic 307.89
  - sacroiliac 724.6
- **Backflow** (pyelovenous) (*see also* Disease, renal) 593.9
- **Backknee** (*see also* Genu, recurvatum) 736.5
- **Bacteremia** 790.7
  - newborn 771.83
- **Bacteria**
  - in blood (*see also* Bacteremia) 790.7
  - in urine (*see also* Bacteriuria) 791.9
- **Bacterial** - *see* condition
- **Bactericholia** (*see also* Cholecystitis, acute) 575.0
- **Bacterid, bacteride** (Andrews' pustular) 686.8
- **Bacteriuria, bacteruria** 791.9
  - with
    - urinary tract infection 599.0
  - asymptomatic 791.9
    - in pregnancy or puerperium 646.5
      - affecting fetus or newborn 760.1
- **Bad**
  - breath 784.99
  - heart - *see* Disease, heart
  - trip (*see also* Abuse, drugs, nondependent) 305.3
- **Baehr-Schiffrin disease** (thrombotic thrombocytopenic purpura) 446.6
- **Baelz's disease** (cheilitis glandularis apostematosa) 528.5
- **Baerensprung's disease** (eczema marginatum) 110.3
- **Bagassosis** (occupational) 495.1
- **Baghdad boil** 085.1
- **Bagratuni's syndrome** (temporal arteritis) 446.5
- **Baker's**
  - cyst (knee) 727.51
    - tuberculous (*see also* Tuberculosis) 015.2
  - itch 692.89
- **Bakwin-Krida syndrome** (craniometaphyseal dysplasia) 756.89
- **Balanitis** (circinata) (gangraenosa) (infectious) (vulgaris) 607.1
  - amebic 006.8
  - candidal 112.2
  - chlamydial 099.53
  - due to Ducrey's bacillus 099.0
  - erosiva circinata et gangraenosa 607.1
  - gangrenous 607.1
  - gonococcal (acute) 098.0
    - chronic or duration of 2 months or over 098.2
  - nongonococcal 607.1
  - phagedenic 607.1
  - venereal NEC 099.8
  - xerotica obliterans 607.81
- **Balanoposthitis** 607.1
  - chlamydial 099.53
  - gonococcal (acute) 098.0
    - chronic or duration of 2 months or over 098.2
  - ulcerative NEC 099.8
- **Balanorrhagia** - *see* Balanitis
- **Balantidiasis** 007.0
- **Balantidiosis** 007.0
- **Balbuties, balbutio** 307.0
- **Bald**
  - patches on scalp 704.00
  - tongue 529.4
- **Baldness** (*see also* Alopecia) 704.00
- **Balfour's disease** (chloroma) 205.3
- **Balint's syndrome** (psychic paralysis of visual fixation) 368.16
- **Balkan grippe** 083.0
- **Ball**
  - food 938
  - hair 938
- **Ballantyne** (-Runge) syndrome (postmaturity) 766.22
- **Balloon disease** (*see also* Effect, adverse, high altitude) 993.2
- **Ballooning posterior leaflet syndrome** 424.0
- **Baló's disease or concentric sclerosis** 341.1
- **Bamberger's disease** (hypertrophic pulmonary osteoarthropathy) 731.2
- **Bamberger-Marie disease** (hypertrophic pulmonary osteoarthropathy) 731.2
- **Bamboo spine** 720.0
- **Bancroft's filariasis** 125.0
- **Band(s)**
  - adhesive (*see also* Adhesions, peritoneum) 568.0
  - amniotic 658.8
    - affecting fetus or newborn 762.8
  - anomalous or congenital - *see also* Anomaly, specified type NEC
    - atrial 746.9
    - heart 746.9
    - intestine 751.4
    - omentum 751.4
    - ventricular 746.9
  - cervix 622.3
  - gallbladder (congenital) 751.69
  - intestinal (adhesive) (*see also* Adhesions, peritoneum) 568.0
    - congenital 751.4
- **Band(s)** *(Continued)*
  - obstructive (*see also* Obstruction, intestine) 560.81
  - periappendiceal (congenital) 751.4
  - peritoneal (adhesive) (*see also* Adhesions, peritoneum) 568.0
    - with intestinal obstruction 560.81
    - congenital 751.4
  - uterus 621.5
  - vagina 623.2
- **Bandl's ring** (contraction)
  - complicating delivery 661.4
    - affecting fetus or newborn 763.7
- **Bang's disease** (Brucella abortus) 023.1
- **Bangkok hemorrhagic fever** 065.4
- **Bannister's disease** 995.1
- **Bantam-Albright-Martin disease** (pseudohypoparathyroidism) 275.49
- **Banti's disease or syndrome** (with cirrhosis) (with portal hypertension) - *see* Cirrhosis, liver
- **Bar**
  - calcaneocuboid 755.67
  - calcaneonavicular 755.67
  - cubonavicular 755.67
  - prostate 600.90
    - with
      - other lower urinary tract symptoms (LUTS) 600.91
      - urinary
        - obstruction 600.91
        - retention 600.91
  - talocalcaneal 755.67
- **Baragnosis** 780.99
- **Barasheh, barashek** 266.2
- **Barcoo disease or rot** (*see also* Ulcer, skin) 707.9
- **Bard-Pic syndrome** (carcinoma, head of pancreas) 157.0
- **Bärensprung's disease** (eczema marginatum) 110.3
- **Baritosis** 503
- **Barium lung disease** 503
- **Barlow's syndrome** (meaning mitral valve prolapse) 424.0
- **Barlow** (-Möller) disease or syndrome (meaning infantile scurvy) 267
- **Barodontalgia** 993.2
- **Baron Münchausen syndrome** 301.51
- **Barosinusitis** 993.1
- **Barotitis** 993.0
- **Barotrauma** 993.2
  - odontalgia 993.2
  - otitic 993.0
  - sinus 993.1
- **Barraquer's disease or syndrome** (progressive lipodystrophy) 272.6
- **Barré-Guillain syndrome** 357.0
- **Barré-Liéou syndrome** (posterior cervical sympathetic) 723.2
- **Barrel chest** 738.3
- **Barrett's esophagus** 530.85
- **Barrett's syndrome or ulcer** (chronic peptic ulcer of esophagus) 530.85
- **Bársony-Polgár syndrome** (corkscrew esophagus) 530.5
- **Bársony-Teschendorf syndrome** (corkscrew esophagus) 530.5
- **Barth syndrome** 759.89
- **Bartholin's**
  - adenitis (*see also* Bartholinitis) 616.89
  - gland - *see* condition

Bartholinitis (suppurating) 616.89
gonococcal (acute) 098.0
chronic or duration of 2 months or over 098.2
Bartonellosis 088.0
Bartter's syndrome (secondary hyperaldosteronism with juxtaglomerular hyperplasia) 255.13
Basal - *see* condition
Basan's (hidrotic) ectodermal dysplasia 757.31
Baseball finger 842.13
Basedow's disease or syndrome (exophthalmic goiter) 242.0
Basic - *see* condition
Basilar - *see* condition
Bason's (hidrotic) ectodermal dysplasia 757.31
Basopenia 288.59
Basophilia 288.65
Basophilism (corticoadrenal) (Cushing's) (pituitary) (thymic) 255.0
Bassen-Kornzweig syndrome (abetalipoproteinemia) 272.5
Bat ear 744.29
Bateman's
disease 078.0
purpura (senile) 287.2
Bathing cramp 994.1
Bathophobia 300.23
Batten's disease, retina 330.1 [362.71]
Batten-Mayou disease 330.1 [362.71]
Batten-Steinert syndrome 359.2
Battered
adult (syndrome) 995.81
baby or child (syndrome) 995.54
spouse (syndrome) 995.81
Battey mycobacterium infection 031.0
Battledore placenta - *see* Placenta, abnormal
Battle exhaustion (*see also* Reaction, stress, acute) 308.9
Baumgarten-Cruveilhier (cirrhosis) disease, or syndrome 571.5
Bauxite
fibrosis (of lung) 503
workers' disease 503
Bayle's disease (dementia paralytica) 094.1
Bazin's disease (primary) (*see also* Tuberculosis) 017.1
Beach ear 380.12
Beaded hair (congenital) 757.4
Beals syndrome 759.82
Beard's disease (neurasthenia) 300.5
Bearn-Kunkel (-Slater) syndrome (lupoid hepatitis) 571.49
Beat
elbow 727.2
hand 727.2
knee 727.2
Beats
ectopic 427.60
escaped, heart 427.60
postoperative 997.1
premature (nodal) 427.60
atrial 427.61
auricular 427.61
postoperative 997.1
specified type NEC 427.69
supraventricular 427.61
ventricular 427.69
Beau's
disease or syndrome (*see also* Degeneration, myocardial) 429.1
Beau's *(Continued)*
lines (transverse furrows on fingernails) 703.8
Bechterew's disease (ankylosing spondylitis) 720.0
Bechterew-Strümpell-Marie syndrome (ankylosing spondylitis) 720.0
Beck's syndrome (anterior spinal artery occlusion) 433.8
Becker's
disease (idiopathic mural endomyocardial disease) 425.2
dystrophy 359.1
Beckwith (-Wiedemann) syndrome 759.89
Bedclothes, asphyxiation or suffocation by 994.7
Bed confinement status V49.84
Bednar's aphthae 528.2
Bedsore 707.00
with gangrene 707.00 *[785.4]*
Bedwetting (*see also* Enuresis) 788.36
Beer-drinkers' heart (disease) 425.5
Bee sting (with allergic or anaphylactic shock) 989.5
Begbie's disease (exophthalmic goiter) 242.0
Behavior disorder, disturbance - *see also* Disturbance, conduct
antisocial, without manifest psychiatric disorder
adolescent V71.02
adult V71.01
child V71.02
dyssocial, without manifest psychiatric disorder
adolescent V71.02
adult V71.01
child V71.02
high-risk - *see* problem
Behçet's syndrome 136.1
Behr's disease 362.50
Beigel's disease or morbus (white piedra) 111.2
Bejel 104.0
Bekhterev's (Bechterew's) disease (ankylosing spondylitis) 720.0
Bekhterev-Strümpell-Marie syndrome (ankylosing spondylitis) 720.0
Belching (*see also* Eructation) 787.3
Bell's
disease (*see also* Psychosis, affective) 296.0
mania (*see also* Psychosis, affective) 296.0
palsy, paralysis 351.0
infant 767.5
newborn 767.5
syphilitic 094.89
spasm 351.0
Bence-Jones albuminuria, albuminosuria, or proteinuria 791.0
Bends 993.3
Benedikt's syndrome (paralysis) 344.89
Benign - *see also* condition
cellular changes, cervix 795.09
prostate
hyperplasia 600.20
with
other lower urinary tract symptoms (LUTS) 600.21
urinary
obstruction 600.21
retention 600.21
neoplasm 222.2
Bennett's
disease (leukemia) 208.9
fracture (closed) 815.01
open 815.11
Benson's disease 379.22
Bent
back (hysterical) 300.11
nose 738.0
congenital 754.0
Bereavement V62.82
as adjustment reaction 309.0
Berger's paresthesia (lower limb) 782.0
Bergeron's disease (hysteroepilepsy) 300.11
Beriberi (acute) (atrophic) (chronic) (dry) (subacute) (wet) 265.0
with polyneuropathy 265.0 *[357.4]*
heart (disease) 265.0 *[425.7]*
leprosy 030.1
neuritis 265.0 *[357.4]*
Berlin's disease or edema (traumatic) 921.3
Berloque dermatitis 692.72
Bernard-Horner syndrome (*see also* Neuropathy, peripheral, autonomic) 337.9
Bernard-Sergent syndrome (acute adrenocortical insufficiency) 255.4
Bernard-Soulier disease or thrombopathy 287.1
Bernhardt's disease or paresthesia 355.1
Bernhardt-Roth disease or syndrome (paresthesia) 355.1
Bernheim's syndrome (*see also* Failure, heart) 428.0
Bertielliasis 123.8
Bertolotti's syndrome (sacralization of fifth lumbar vertebra) 756.15
Berylliosis (acute) (chronic) (lung) (occupational) 503
Besnier's
lupus pernio 135
prurigo (atopic dermatitis) (infantile eczema) 691.8
Besnier-Boeck disease or sarcoid 135
Besnier-Boeck-Schaumann disease (sarcoidosis) 135
Best's disease 362.76
Bestiality 302.1
Beta-adrenergic hyperdynamic circulatory state 429.82
Beta-aminoisobutyric aciduria 277.2
Beta-mercaptolactate-cysteine disulfiduria 270.0
Beta thalassemia (major) (minor) (mixed) 282.49
Beurmann's disease (sporotrichosis) 117.1
Bezoar 938
intestine 936
stomach 935.2
Bezold's abscess (*see also* Mastoiditis) 383.01
Bianchi's syndrome (aphasia-apraxia-alexia) 784.69
Bicornuate or bicornis uterus 752.3
in pregnancy or childbirth 654.0
with obstructed labor 660.2
affecting fetus or newborn 763.1
affecting fetus or newborn 763.89
Bicuspid aortic valve 746.4
Biedl-Bardet syndrome 759.89
Bielschowsky's disease 330.1
Bielschowsky-Jansky
amaurotic familial idiocy 330.1
disease 330.1

◀ New ⇐ Revised

- **Biemond's syndrome** (obesity, poly-dactyly, and mental retardation) 759.89
- **Biermer's anemia or disease** (pernicious anemia) 281.0
- **Biett's disease** 695.4
- **Bifid** (congenital) - *see also* Imperfect, closure
  - apex, heart 746.89
  - clitoris 752.49
  - epiglottis 748.3
  - kidney 753.3
  - nose 748.1
  - patella 755.64
  - scrotum 752.89
  - toe 755.66
  - tongue 750.13
  - ureter 753.4
  - uterus 752.3
  - uvula 749.02
    - with cleft lip (*see also* Cleft, palate, with cleft lip) 749.20
- **Biforis uterus** (suprasimplex) 752.3
- **Bifurcation** (congenital) - *see also* Imperfect, closure
  - gallbladder 751.69
  - kidney pelvis 753.3
  - renal pelvis 753.3
  - rib 756.3
  - tongue 750.13
  - trachea 748.3
  - ureter 753.4
  - urethra 753.8
  - uvula 749.02
    - with cleft lip (*see also* Cleft, palate, with cleft lip) 749.20
  - vertebra 756.19
- **Bigeminal pulse** 427.89
- **Bigeminy** 427.89
- **Big spleen syndrome** 289.4
- **Bilateral** - *see* condition
- **Bile duct** - *see* condition
- **Bile pigments in urine** 791.4
- **Bilharziasis** (*see also* Schistosomiasis) 120.9
  - chyluria 120.0
  - cutaneous 120.3
  - galacturia 120.0
  - hematochyluria 120.0
  - intestinal 120.1
  - lipemia 120.9
  - lipuria 120.0
  - Oriental 120.2
  - piarhemia 120.9
  - pulmonary 120.2
  - tropical hematuria 120.0
  - vesical 120.0
- **Biliary** - *see* condition
- **Bilious** (attack) - *see also* Vomiting
  - fever, hemoglobinuric 084.8
- **Bilirubinuria** 791.4
- **Biliuria** 791.4
- **Billroth's disease**
  - meningocele (*see also* Spina bifida) 741.9
- **Bilobate placenta** - *see* Placenta, abnormal
- **Bilocular**
  - heart 745.7
  - stomach 536.8
- **Bing-Horton syndrome** (histamine cephalgia) 346.2
- **Binswanger's disease or dementia** 290.12
- **Biörck** (-Thorson) syndrome (malignant carcinoid) 259.2
- **Biparta, bipartite** - *see also* Imperfect, closure
  - carpal scaphoid 755.59
  - patella 755.64
  - placenta - *see* Placenta, abnormal
  - vagina 752.49
- **Bird**
  - face 756.0
  - fanciers' lung or disease 495.2
- **Bird's disease** (oxaluria) 271.8
- **Birth**
  - abnormal fetus or newborn 763.9
  - accident, fetus or newborn - *see* Birth, injury
  - complications in mother - *see* Delivery, complicated
  - compression during NEC 767.9
  - defect - *see* Anomaly
  - delayed, fetus 763.9
  - difficult NEC, affecting fetus or newborn 763.9
  - dry, affecting fetus or newborn 761.1
  - forced, NEC, affecting fetus or newborn 763.89
  - forceps, affecting fetus or newborn 763.2
  - hematoma of sternomastoid 767.8
  - immature 765.1
    - extremely 765.0
  - inattention, after or at 995.52
  - induced, affecting fetus or newborn 763.89
  - infant - *see* Newborn
  - injury NEC 767.9
    - adrenal gland 767.8
    - basal ganglia 767.0
    - brachial plexus (paralysis) 767.6
    - brain (compression) (pressure) 767.0
    - cerebellum 767.0
    - cerebral hemorrhage 767.0
    - conjunctiva 767.8
    - eye 767.8
    - fracture
      - bone, any except clavicle or spine 767.3
      - clavicle 767.2
      - femur 767.3
      - humerus 767.3
      - long bone 767.3
      - radius and ulna 767.3
      - skeleton NEC 767.3
      - skull 767.3
      - spine 767.4
      - tibia and fibula 767.3
    - hematoma 767.8
      - liver (subcapsular) 767.8
      - mastoid 767.8
      - skull 767.19
      - sternomastoid 767.8
      - testes 767.8
      - vulva 767.8
    - intracranial (edema) 767.0
    - laceration
      - brain 767.0
      - by scalpel 767.8
      - peripheral nerve 767.7
    - liver 767.8
    - meninges
      - brain 767.0
      - spinal cord 767.4
    - nerves (cranial, peripheral) 767.7
      - brachial plexus 767.6
      - facial 767.5
    - paralysis 767.7

Birth *(Continued)*

- injury NEC *(Continued)*
  - paralysis *(Continued)*
    - brachial plexus 767.6
    - Erb (-Duchenne) 767.6
    - facial nerve 767.5
    - Klumpke (-Déjérine) 767.6
    - radial nerve 767.6
    - spinal (cord) (hemorrhage) (laceration) (rupture) 767.4
  - rupture
    - intracranial 767.0
    - liver 767.8
    - spinal cord 767.4
    - spleen 767.8
    - viscera 767.8
  - scalp 767.19
  - scalpel wound 767.8
  - skeleton NEC 767.3
  - specified NEC 767.8
  - spinal cord 767.4
  - spleen 767.8
  - subdural hemorrhage 767.0
  - tentorial, tear 767.0
  - testes 767.8
  - vulva 767.8
- instrumental, NEC, affecting fetus or newborn 763.2
- lack of care, after or at 995.52
- multiple
  - affected by maternal complications of pregnancy 761.5
  - healthy liveborn - *see* Newborn, multiple
- neglect, after or at 995.52
- newborn - *see* Newborn
- palsy or paralysis NEC 767.7
- precipitate, fetus or newborn 763.6
- premature (infant) 765.1
- prolonged, affecting fetus or newborn 763.9
- retarded, fetus or newborn 763.9
- shock, newborn 779.89
- strangulation or suffocation
  - due to aspiration of clear amniotic fluid 770.13
    - with respiratory symptoms 770.14
  - mechanical 767.8
- trauma NEC 767.9
- triplet
  - affected by maternal complications of pregnancy 761.5
  - healthy liveborn - *see* Newborn, multiple
- twin
  - affected by maternal complications of pregnancy 761.5
  - healthy liveborn - *see* Newborn, twin
- ventouse, affecting fetus or newborn 763.3

- **Birthmark** 757.32
- **Bisalbuminemia** 273.8
- **Biskra button** 085.1
- **Bite(s)**
  - with intact skin surface - *see* Contusion
  - animal - *see* Wound, open, by site
    - intact skin surface - *see* Contusion
  - centipede 989.5
  - chigger 133.8
  - fire ant 989.5
  - flea - *see* Injury, superficial, by site
  - human (open wound) - *see also* Wound, open, by site
    - intact skin surface - *see* Contusion

Bite(s) *(Continued)*
insect
nonvenomous - *see* Injury, superficial, by site
venomous 989.5
mad dog (death from) 071
open
anterior 524.24
posterior 524.25
poisonous 989.5
red bug 133.8
reptile 989.5
nonvenomous - *see* Wound, open, by site
snake 989.5
nonvenomous - *see* Wound, open, by site
spider (venomous) 989.5
nonvenomous - *see* Injury, superficial, by site
venomous 989.5
Biting
cheek or lip 528.9
nail 307.9
Black
death 020.9
eye NEC 921.0
hairy tongue 529.3
heel 924.20
lung disease 500
palm 923.20
Blackfan-Diamond anemia or syndrome (congenital hypoplastic anemia) 284.01
Blackhead 706.1
Blackout 780.2
Blackwater fever 084.8
Bladder - *see* condition
Blast
blindness 921.3
concussion - *see* Blast, injury
injury 869.0
with open wound into cavity 869.1
abdomen or thorax - *see* Injury, internal, by site
brain (*see also* Concussion, brain) 850.9
with skull fracture - *see* Fracture, skull
ear (acoustic nerve trauma) 951.5
with perforation, tympanic membrane - *see* Wound, open, ear, drum
lung (*see also* Injury, internal, lung) 861.20
otitic (explosive) 388.11
Blastomycosis, blastomycotic (chronic) (cutaneous) (disseminated) (lung) (pulmonary) (systemic) 116.0
Brazilian 116.1
European 117.5
keloidal 116.2
North American 116.0
primary pulmonary 116.0
South American 116.1
Bleb(s) 709.8
emphysematous (bullous) (diffuse) (lung) (ruptured) (solitary) 492.0
filtering, eye (postglaucoma) (status) V45.69
with complication 997.99
postcataract extraction (complication) 997.99
lung (ruptured) 492.0

Bleb(s) *(Continued)*
lung *(Continued)*
congenital 770.5
subpleural (emphysematous) 492.0
Bleeder (familial) (hereditary) (*see also* Defect, coagulation) 286.9
nonfamilial 286.9
Bleeding (*see also* Hemorrhage) 459.0
anal 569.3
anovulatory 628.0
atonic, following delivery 666.1
capillary 448.9
due to subinvolution 621.1
puerperal 666.2
ear 388.69
excessive, associated with menopausal onset 627.0
familial (*see also* Defect, coagulation) 286.9
following intercourse 626.7
gastrointestinal 578.9
gums 523.8
hemorrhoids - *see* Hemorrhoids, bleeding
intermenstrual
irregular 626.6
regular 626.5
intraoperative 998.11
irregular NEC 626.4
menopausal 627.0
mouth 528.9
nipple 611.79
nose 784.7
ovulation 626.5
postclimacteric 627.1
postcoital 626.7
postmenopausal 627.1
following induced menopause 627.4
postoperative 998.11
preclimacteric 627.0
puberty 626.3
excessive, with onset of menstrual periods 626.3
rectum, rectal 569.3
tendencies (*see also* Defect, coagulation) 286.9
throat 784.8
umbilical stump 772.3
umbilicus 789.9
unrelated to menstrual cycle 626.6
uterus, uterine 626.9
climacteric 627.0
dysfunctional 626.8
functional 626.8
unrelated to menstrual cycle 626.6
vagina, vaginal 623.8
functional 626.8
vicarious 625.8
Blennorrhagia, blennorrhagic - *see* Blennorrhea
Blennorrhea (acute) 098.0
adultorum 098.40
alveolaris 523.40
chronic or duration of 2 months or over 098.2
gonococcal (neonatorum) 098.40
inclusion (neonatal) (newborn) 771.6
neonatorum 098.40
Blepharelosis (*see also* Entropion) 374.00
Blepharitis (eyelid) 373.00
angularis 373.01
ciliaris 373.00
with ulcer 373.01

Blepharitis *(Continued)*
marginal 373.00
with ulcer 373.01
scrofulous (*see also* Tuberculosis) 017.3 *[373.00]*
squamous 373.02
ulcerative 373.01
Blepharochalasis 374.34
congenital 743.62
Blepharoclonus 333.81
Blepharoconjunctivitis (*see also* Conjunctivitis) 372.20
angular 372.21
contact 372.22
Blepharophimosis (eyelid) 374.46
congenital 743.62
Blepharoplegia 374.89
Blepharoptosis 374.30
congenital 743.61
Blepharopyorrhea 098.49
Blepharospasm 333.81
due to drugs 333.85
Blessig's cyst 362.62
Blighted ovum 631
Blind
bronchus (congenital) 748.3
eye - *see also* Blindness
hypertensive 360.42
hypotensive 360.41
loop syndrome (postoperative) 579.2
sac, fallopian tube (congenital) 752.19
spot, enlarged 368.42
tract or tube (congenital) NEC - *see* Atresia
Blindness (acquired) (congenital) (both eyes) 369.00
blast 921.3
with nerve injury - *see* Injury, nerve, optic
Bright's - *see* Uremia
color (congenital) 368.59
acquired 368.55
blue 368.53
green 368.52
red 368.51
total 368.54
concussion 950.9
cortical 377.75
day 368.10
acquired 368.10
congenital 368.10
hereditary 368.10
specified type NEC 368.10
due to
injury NEC 950.9
refractive error - *see* Error, refractive
eclipse (total) 363.31
emotional 300.11
hysterical 300.11
legal (both eyes) (USA definition) 369.4
with impairment of better (less impaired) eye
near-total 369.02
with
lesser eye impairment 369.02
near-total 369.04
total 369.03
profound 369.05
with
lesser eye impairment 369.05
near-total 369.07
profound 369.08
total 369.06
severe 369.21

Blindness *(Continued)*
- legal *(Continued)*
  - with impairment of better *(Continued)*
    - severe *(Continued)*
      - with
        - lesser eye impairment 369.21
          - blind 369.11
          - near-total 369.13
          - profound 369.14
          - severe 369.22
          - total 369.12
    - total
      - with lesser eye impairment
        - total 369.01
- mind 784.69
- moderate
  - both eyes 369.25
    - with impairment of lesser eye (specified as)
      - blind, not further specified 369.15
      - low vision, not further specified 369.23
      - near-total 369.17
      - profound 369.18
      - severe 369.24
      - total 369.16
  - one eye 369.74
    - with vision of other eye (specified as)
      - near-normal 369.75
      - normal 369.76
- near-total
  - both eyes 369.04
    - with impairment of lesser eye (specified as)
      - blind, not further specified 369.02
      - total 369.03
  - one eye 369.64
    - with vision of other eye (specified as)
      - near-normal 369.65
      - normal 369.66
- night 368.60
  - acquired 368.62
  - congenital (Japanese) 368.61
  - hereditary 368.61
  - specified type NEC 368.69
  - vitamin A deficiency 264.5
- nocturnal - *see* Blindness, night
- one eye 369.60
  - with low vision of other eye 369.10
- profound
  - both eyes 369.08
    - with impairment of lesser eye (specified as)
      - blind, not further specified 369.05
      - near-total 369.07
      - total 369.06
  - one eye 369.67
    - with vision of other eye (specified as)
      - near-normal 369.68
      - normal 369.69
- psychic 784.69
- severe
  - both eyes 369.22
    - with impairment of lesser eye (specified as)
      - blind, not further specified 369.11
      - low vision, not further specified 369.21

Blindness *(Continued)*
- severe *(Continued)*
  - both eyes *(Continued)*
    - with impairment of lesser eye *(Continued)*
      - near-total 369.13
      - profound 369.14
      - total 369.12
  - one eye 369.71
    - with vision of other eye (specified as)
      - near-normal 369.72
      - normal 369.73
- snow 370.24
- sun 363.31
- temporary 368.12
- total
  - both eyes 369.01
  - one eye 369.61
    - with vision of other eye (specified as)
      - near-normal 369.62
      - normal 369.63
- transient 368.12
- traumatic NEC 950.9
- word (developmental) 315.01
  - acquired 784.61
  - secondary to organic lesion 784.61

Blister - *see also* Injury, superficial, by site
- beetle dermatitis 692.89
- due to burn - *see* Burn, by site, second degree
- fever 054.9
- multiple, skin, nontraumatic 709.8

Bloating 787.3

Bloch-Siemens syndrome (incontinentia pigmenti) 757.33

Bloch-Stauffer dyshormonal dermatosis 757.33

Bloch-Sulzberger disease or syndrome (incontinentia pigmenti) (melanoblastosis) 757.33

Block
- alveolar capillary 516.3
- arborization (heart) 426.6
- arrhythmic 426.9
- atrioventricular (AV) (incomplete) (partial) 426.10
  - with
    - 2:1 atrioventricular response block 426.13
    - atrioventricular dissociation 426.0
  - first degree (incomplete) 426.11
  - second degree (Mobitz type I) 426.13
    - Mobitz (type II) 426.12
  - third degree 426.0
  - complete 426.0
    - congenital 746.86
  - congenital 746.86
  - Mobitz (incomplete)
    - type I (Wenckebach's) 426.13
    - type II 426.12
  - partial 426.13
- auriculoventricular (*see also* Block, atrioventricular) 426.10
  - complete 426.0
    - congenital 746.86
  - congenital 746.86
- bifascicular (cardiac) 426.53
- bundle branch (complete) (false) (incomplete) 426.50
  - bilateral 426.53
  - left (complete) (main stem) 426.3

Block *(Continued)*
- bundle branch *(Continued)*
  - left *(Continued)*
    - with right bundle branch block 426.53
    - anterior fascicular 426.2
      - with
        - posterior fascicular block 426.3
        - right bundle branch block 426.52
    - hemiblock 426.2
    - incomplete 426.2
      - with right bundle branch block 426.53
    - posterior fascicular 426.2
      - with
        - anterior fascicular block 426.3
        - right bundle branch block 426.51
  - right 426.4
    - with
      - left bundle branch block (incomplete) (main stem) 426.53
      - left fascicular block 426.53
        - anterior 426.52
        - posterior 426.51
  - Wilson's type 426.4
- cardiac 426.9
- conduction 426.9
  - complete 426.0
- Eustachian tube (*see also* Obstruction, Eustachian tube) 381.60
- fascicular (left anterior) (left posterior) 426.2
- foramen Magendie (acquired) 331.3
  - congenital 742.3
    - with spina bifida (*see also* Spina bifida) 741.0
- heart 426.9
  - first degree (atrioventricular) 426.11
  - second degree (atrioventricular) 426.13
  - third degree (atrioventricular) 426.0
  - bundle branch (complete) (false) (incomplete) 426.50
    - bilateral 426.53
    - left (*see also* Block, bundle branch, left) 426.3
    - right (*see also* Block, bundle branch, right) 426.4
  - complete (atrioventricular) 426.0
  - congenital 746.86
  - incomplete 426.13
  - intra-atrial 426.6
  - intraventricular NEC 426.6
  - sinoatrial 426.6
  - specified type NEC 426.6
- hepatic vein 453.0
- intraventricular (diffuse) (myofibrillar) 426.6
  - bundle branch (complete) (false) (incomplete) 426.50
    - bilateral 426.53
    - left (*see also* Block, bundle branch, left) 426.3
    - right (*see also* Block, bundle branch, right) 426.4
- kidney (*see also* Disease, renal) 593.9
  - postcystoscopic 997.5
- myocardial (*see also* Block, heart) 426.9
- nodal 426.10
- optic nerve 377.49

- **Block** *(Continued)*
  - organ or site (congenital) NEC - *see* Atresia
  - parietal 426.6
  - peri-infarction 426.6
  - portal (vein) 452
  - sinoatrial 426.6
  - sinoauricular 426.6
  - spinal cord 336.9
  - trifascicular 426.54
  - tubal 628.2
  - vein NEC 453.9
- **Blocq's disease or syndrome** (astasia-abasia) 307.9
- **Blood**
  - constituents, abnormal NEC 790.6
  - disease 289.9
    - specified NEC 289.89
  - donor V59.01
    - other blood components V59.09
    - stem cells V59.02
    - whole blood V59.01
  - dyscrasia 289.9
    - with
      - abortion - *see* Abortion, by type, with hemorrhage, delayed or excessive
      - ectopic pregnancy (*see also* categories 633.0–633.9) 639.1
      - molar pregnancy (*see also* categories 630–632) 639.1
    - fetus or newborn NEC 776.9
    - following
      - abortion 639.1
      - ectopic or molar pregnancy 639.1
    - puerperal, postpartum 666.3
  - flukes NEC (*see also* Infestation, Schistosoma) 120.9
  - in
    - feces (*see also* Melena) 578.1
      - occult 792.1
    - urine (*see also* Hematuria) 599.7
  - mole 631
  - occult 792.1
  - poisoning (*see also* Septicemia) 038.9
  - pressure
    - decreased, due to shock following injury 958.4
    - fluctuating 796.4
    - high (*see also* Hypertension) 401.9
      - incidental reading (isolated) (nonspecific), without diagnosis of hypertension 796.2
    - low (*see also* Hypotension) 458.9
      - incidental reading (isolated) (nonspecific), without diagnosis of hypotension 796.3
  - spitting (*see also* Hemoptysis) 786.3
  - staining cornea 371.12
  - transfusion
    - without reported diagnosis V58.2
    - donor V59.01
      - stem cells V59.02
    - reaction or complication - *see* Complications, transfusion
  - tumor - *see* Hematoma
  - vessel rupture - *see* Hemorrhage
  - vomiting (*see also* Hematemesis) 578.0
- **Blood-forming organ disease** 289.9
- **Bloodgood's disease** 610.1
- **Bloodshot eye** 379.93
- **Bloom** (-Machacek) (-Torre) syndrome 757.39
- **Blotch, palpebral** 372.55
- **Blount's disease** (tibia vara) 732.4
- **Blount-Barber syndrome** (tibia vara) 732.4
- **Blue**
  - baby 746.9
  - bloater 491.20
    - with
      - acute bronchitis 491.22
      - exacerbation (acute) 491.21
  - diaper syndrome 270.0
  - disease 746.9
  - dome cyst 610.0
  - drum syndrome 381.02
  - sclera 743.47
    - with fragility of bone and deafness 756.51
  - toe syndrome 445.02
- **Blueness** (*see also* Cyanosis) 782.5
- **Blurring, visual** 368.8
- **Blushing** (abnormal) (excessive) 782.62
- **BMI** (body mass index)
  - adult
    - 25.0–25.9 V85.21
    - 26.0–26.9 V85.22
    - 27.0–27.9 V85.23
    - 28.0–28.9 V85.24
    - 29.0–29.9 V85.25
    - 30.0–30.9 V85.30
    - 31.0–31.9 V85.31
    - 32.0–32.9 V85.32
    - 33.0–33.9 V85.33
    - 34.0–34.9 V85.34
    - 35.0–35.9 V85.35
    - 36.0–36.9 V85.36
    - 37.0–37.9 V85.37
    - 38.0–38.9 V85.38
    - 39.0–39.9 V85.39
    - 40.0 and over V85.4
    - between 19–24 V85.1
    - less than 19 V85.0
  - pediatric ◀
    - 5th percentile to less than 85th percentile for age V85.52 ◀
    - 85th percentile to less than 95th percentile for age V85.53 ◀
    - greater than or equal to 95th percentile for age V85.54 ◀
    - less than 5th percentile for age V85.51 ◀
- **Boarder, hospital** V65.0
  - infant V65.0
- **Bockhart's impetigo** (superficial folliculitis) 704.8
- **Bodechtel-Guttmann disease** (subacute sclerosing panencephalitis) 046.2
- **Boder-Sedgwick syndrome** (ataxia-telangiectasia) 334.8
- **Body, bodies**
  - Aschoff (*see also* Myocarditis, rheumatic) 398.0
  - asteroid, vitreous 379.22
  - choroid, colloid (degenerative) 362.57
    - hereditary 362.77
  - cytoid (retina) 362.82
  - drusen (retina) (*see also* Drusen) 362.57
    - optic disc 377.21
  - fibrin, pleura 511.0
  - foreign - *see* Foreign body
  - Hassall-Henle 371.41
  - loose
    - joint (*see also* Loose, body, joint) 718.1
      - knee 717.6
    - knee 717.6
    - sheath, tendon 727.82
  - Mallory's 034.1
  - mass index (BMI)
    - adult
      - 25.0–25.9 V85.21
      - 26.0–26.9 V85.22
      - 27.0–27.9 V85.23
      - 28.0–28.9 V85.24
      - 29.0–29.9 V85.25
      - 30.0–30.9 V85.30
      - 31.0–31.9 V85.31
      - 32.0–32.9 V85.32
      - 33.0–33.9 V85.33
      - 34.0–34.9 V85.34
      - 35.0–35.9 V85.35
      - 36.0–36.9 V85.36
      - 37.0–37.9 V85.37
      - 38.0–38.9 V85.38
      - 39.0–39.9 V85.39
      - 40.0 and over V85.4
      - between 19–24 V85.1
      - less than 19 V85.0
    - pediatric ◀
      - 5th percentile to less than 85th percentile for age V85.52 ◀
      - 85th percentile to less than 95th percentile for age V85.53 ◀
      - greater than or equal to 95th percentile for age V85.54 ◀
      - less than 5th percentile for age V85.51 ◀
  - Mooser 081.0
  - Negri 071
  - rice (joint) (*see also* Loose, body, joint) 718.1
    - knee 717.6
  - rocking 307.3
- **Boeck's**
  - disease (sarcoidosis) 135
  - lupoid (miliary) 135
  - sarcoid 135
- **Boerhaave's syndrome** (spontaneous esophageal rupture) 530.4
- **Boggy**
  - cervix 622.8
  - uterus 621.8
- **Boil** (*see also* Carbuncle) 680.9
  - abdominal wall 680.2
  - Aleppo 085.1
  - ankle 680.6
  - anus 680.5
  - arm (any part, above wrist) 680.3
  - auditory canal, external 680.0
  - axilla 680.3
  - back (any part) 680.2
  - Baghdad 085.1
  - breast 680.2
  - buttock 680.5
  - chest wall 680.2
  - corpus cavernosum 607.2
  - Delhi 085.1
  - ear (any part) 680.0
  - eyelid 373.13
  - face (any part, except eye) 680.0
  - finger (any) 680.4
  - flank 680.2
  - foot (any part) 680.7
  - forearm 680.3
  - Gafsa 085.1

◀ **New** ⬅ **Revised**

Boil *(Continued)*
genital organ, male 608.4
gluteal (region) 680.5
groin 680.2
hand (any part) 680.4
head (any part, except face) 680.8
heel 680.7
hip 680.6
knee 680.6
labia 616.4
lacrimal (*see also* Dacryocystitis) 375.30
gland (*see also* Dacryoadenitis) 375.00
passages (duct) (sac) (*see also* Dacryocystitis) 375.30
leg, any part, except foot 680.6
multiple sites 680.9
Natal 085.1
neck 680.1
nose (external) (septum) 680.0
orbit, orbital 376.01
partes posteriores 680.5
pectoral region 680.2
penis 607.2
perineum 680.2
pinna 680.0
scalp (any part) 680.8
scrotum 608.4
seminal vesicle 608.0
shoulder 680.3
skin NEC 680.9
specified site NEC 680.8
spermatic cord 608.4
temple (region) 680.0
testis 608.4
thigh 680.6
thumb 680.4
toe (any) 680.7
tropical 085.1
trunk 680.2
tunica vaginalis 608.4
umbilicus 680.2
upper arm 680.3
vas deferens 608.4
vulva 616.4
wrist 680.4
Bold hives (*see also* Urticaria) 708.9
Bolivian hemorrhagic fever 078.7
Bombé, iris 364.74
Bomford-Rhoads anemia (refractory) 238.72 (Revised)
Bone - *see* condition
Bonnevie-Ullrich syndrome 758.6
Bonnier's syndrome 386.19
Bonvale Dam fever 780.79
Bony block of joint 718.80
ankle 718.87
elbow 718.82
foot 718.87
hand 718.84
hip 718.85
knee 718.86
multiple sites 718.89
pelvic region 718.85
shoulder (region) 718.81
specified site NEC 718.88
wrist 718.83
Borderline
intellectual functioning V62.89
pelvis 653.1
with obstruction during labor 660.1
affecting fetus or newborn 763.1
psychosis (*see also* Schizophrenia) 295.5
of childhood (*see also* Psychosis, childhood) 299.8

Borderline *(Continued)*
schizophrenia (*see also* Schizophrenia) 295.5
Borna disease 062.9
Bornholm disease (epidemic pleurodynia) 074.1
Borrelia vincentii (mouth) (pharynx) (tonsils) 101
Bostock's catarrh (*see also* Fever, hay) 477.9
Boston exanthem 048
Botalli, ductus (patent) (persistent) 747.0
Bothriocephalus latus infestation 123.4
Botulism 005.1
wound - *see* Wound, open, by site, complicated (New)
Bouba (*see also* Yaws) 102.9
Bouffée délirante 298.3
Bouillaud's disease or syndrome (rheumatic heart disease) 391.9
Bourneville's disease (tuberous sclerosis) 759.5
Boutonneuse fever 082.1
Boutonniere
deformity (finger) 736.21
hand (intrinsic) 736.21
Bouveret (-Hoffmann) disease or syndrome (paroxysmal tachycardia) 427.2
Bovine heart - *see* Hypertrophy, cardiac
Bowel - *see* condition
Bowen's
dermatosis (precancerous) (M8081/2) - *see* Neoplasm, skin, in situ
disease (M8081/2) - *see* Neoplasm, skin, in situ
epithelioma (M8081/2) - *see* Neoplasm, skin, in situ
type
epidermoid carcinoma in situ (M8081/2) - *see* Neoplasm, skin, in situ
intraepidermal squamous cell carcinoma (M8081/2) - *see* Neoplasm, skin, in situ
Bowing
femur 736.89
congenital 754.42
fibula 736.89
congenital 754.43
forearm 736.09
away from midline (cubitus valgus) 736.01
toward midline (cubitus varus) 736.02
leg(s), long bones, congenital 754.44
radius 736.09
away from midline (cubitus valgus) 736.01
toward midline (cubitus varus) 736.02
tibia 736.89
congenital 754.43
Bowleg(s) 736.42
congenital 754.44
rachitic 268.1
Boyd's dysentery 004.2
Brachial - *see* condition
Brachman-de Lange syndrome (Amsterdam dwarf, mental retardation, and brachycephaly) 759.89
Brachycardia 427.89
Brachycephaly 756.0
Brachymorphism and ectopia lentis 759.89
Bradley's disease (epidemic vomiting) 078.82

Bradycardia 427.89
chronic (sinus) 427.81
newborn 779.81
nodal 427.89
postoperative 997.1
reflex 337.0
sinoatrial 427.89
with paroxysmal tachyarrhythmia or tachycardia 427.81
chronic 427.81
sinus 427.89
with paroxysmal tachyarrhythmia or tachycardia 427.81
chronic 427.81
persistent 427.81
severe 427.81
tachycardia syndrome 427.81
vagal 427.89
Bradypnea 786.09
Brailsford's disease 732.3
radial head 732.3
tarsal scaphoid 732.5
Brailsford-Morquio disease or syndrome (mucopolysaccharidosis IV) 277.5
Brain - *see also* condition
death 348.8
syndrome (acute) (chronic) (nonpsychotic) (organic) (with neurotic reaction) (with behavioral reaction) (*see also* Syndrome, brain) 310.9
with
presenile brain disease 290.10
psychosis, psychotic reaction (*see also* Psychosis, organic) 294.9
congenital (*see also* Retardation, mental) 319
Branched-chain amino-acid disease 270.3
Branchial - *see* condition
Brandt's syndrome (acrodermatitis enteropathica) 686.8
Brash (water) 787.1
Brass-founders' ague 985.8
Bravais-Jacksonian epilepsy (*see also* Epilepsy) 345.5
Braxton Hicks contractions 644.1
Braziers' disease 985.8
Brazilian
blastomycosis 116.1
leishmaniasis 085.5
BRBPR (bright red blood per rectum) 569.3
Break
cardiorenal - *see* Hypertension, cardiorenal
retina (*see also* Defect, retina) 361.30
Breakbone fever 061
Breakdown
device, implant, or graft - *see* Complications, mechanical
nervous (*see also* Disorder, mental, nonpsychotic) 300.9
perineum 674.2
Breast - *see* condition
Breast feeding difficulties 676.8
Breath
foul 784.99 (Revised)
holder, child 312.81
holding spells 786.9
shortness 786.05
Breathing
asymmetrical 786.09
bronchial 786.09
exercises V57.0
labored 786.09

ICD-9-CM B Vol. 2

Breathing *(Continued)*
- mouth 784.99
  - causing malocclusion 524.59
- periodic 786.09
  - high altitude 327.22
- tic 307.20

Breathlessness 786.09
Breda's disease (*see also* Yaws) 102.9
Breech
- delivery, affecting fetus or newborn 763.0
- extraction, affecting fetus or newborn 763.0
- presentation (buttocks) (complete) (frank) 652.2
  - with successful version 652.1
  - before labor, affecting fetus or newborn 761.7
  - during labor, affecting fetus or newborn 763.0

Breisky's disease (kraurosis vulvae) 624.0
Brennemann's syndrome (acute mesenteric lymphadenitis) 289.2
Brenner's
- tumor (benign) (M9000/0) 220
  - borderline malignancy (M9000/1) 236.2
  - malignant (M9000/3) 183.0
  - proliferating (M9000/1) 236.2

Bretonneau's disease (diphtheritic malignant angina) 032.0
Breus' mole 631
Brevicollis 756.16
Bricklayers' itch 692.89
Brickmakers' anemia 126.9
Bridge
- myocardial 746.85

Bright red blood per rectum (BRBPR) 569.3
Bright's
- blindness - *see* Uremia
- disease (*see also* Nephritis) 583.9
  - arteriosclerotic (*see also* Hypertension, kidney) 403.90

Brill's disease (recrudescent typhus) 081.1
- flea-borne 081.0
- louse-borne 081.1

Brill-Symmers disease (follicular lymphoma) (M9690/3) 202.0
Brill-Zinsser disease (recrudescent typhus) 081.1
Brinton's disease (linitis plastica) (M8142/3) 151.9
Brion-Kayser disease (*see also* Fever, paratyphoid) 002.9
Briquet's disorder or syndrome 300.81
Brissaud's
- infantilism (infantile myxedema) 244.9
- motor-verbal tic 307.23

Brissaud-Meige syndrome (infantile myxedema) 244.9
Brittle
- bones (congenital) 756.51
- nails 703.8
  - congenital 757.5

Broad - *see also* condition
- beta disease 272.2
- ligament laceration syndrome 620.6

Brock's syndrome (atelectasis due to enlarged lymph nodes) 518.0
Brocq's disease 691.8
- atopic (diffuse) neurodermatitis 691.8
- lichen simplex chronicus 698.3
- parakeratosis psoriasiformis 696.2
- parapsoriasis 696.2

Brocq-Duhring disease (dermatitis herpetiformis) 694.0
Brodie's
- abscess (localized) (chronic) (*see also* Osteomyelitis) 730.1
- disease (joint) (*see also* Osteomyelitis) 730.1

Broken
- arches 734
  - congenital 755.67
- back - *see* Fracture, vertebra, by site
- bone - *see* Fracture, by site
- compensation - *see* Disease, heart
- heart syndrome 429.83 ◀
- implant or internal device - *see* listing under Complications, mechanical
- neck - *see* Fracture, vertebra, cervical
- nose 802.0
  - open 802.1
- tooth, teeth 873.63
  - complicated 873.73

Bromhidrosis 705.89
Bromidism, bromism
- acute 967.3
  - correct substance properly administered 349.82
  - overdose or wrong substance given or taken 967.3
- chronic (*see also* Dependence) 304.1

Bromidrosiphobia 300.23
Bromidrosis 705.89
Bronchi, bronchial - *see* condition
Bronchiectasis (cylindrical) (diffuse) (fusiform) (localized) (moniliform) (postinfectious) (recurrent) (saccular) 494.0
- with acute exacerbation 494.1
- congenital 748.61
- tuberculosis (*see also* Tuberculosis) 011.5

Bronchiolectasis - *see* Bronchiectasis
Bronchiolitis (acute) (infectious) (subacute) 466.19
- with
  - bronchospasm or obstruction 466.19
  - influenza, flu, or grippe 487.1
- catarrhal (acute) (subacute) 466.19
- chemical 506.0
  - chronic 506.4
- chronic (obliterative) 491.8
- due to external agent - *see* Bronchitis, acute, due to
- fibrosa obliterans 491.8
- influenzal 487.1
- obliterans 491.8
  - with organizing pneumonia (B.O.O.P.) 516.8
  - status post lung transplant 996.84
- obliterative (chronic) (diffuse) (subacute) 491.8
  - due to fumes or vapors 506.4
- respiratory syncytial virus 466.11
- vesicular - *see* Pneumonia, broncho-

Bronchitis (diffuse) (hypostatic) (infectious) (inflammatory) (simple) 490
- with
  - emphysema - *see* Emphysema
  - influenza, flue, or grippe 487.1
  - obstruction airway, chronic 491.20

Bronchitis *(Continued)*
- with *(Continued)*
  - obstruction airway, chronic *(Continued)*
    - with
      - acute bronchitis 491.22
      - exacerbation (acute) 491.21
  - tracheitis 490
    - acute or subacute 466.0
      - with bronchospasm or obstruction 466.0
    - chronic 491.8
- acute or subacute 466.0
  - with
    - bronchospasm 466.0
    - obstruction 466.0
    - tracheitis 466.0
  - chemical (due to fumes or vapors) 506.0
  - due to
    - fumes or vapors 506.0
    - radiation 508.8
- allergic (acute) (*see also* Asthma) 493.9
- arachidic 934.1
- aspiration 507.0
  - due to fumes or vapors 506.0
- asthmatic (acute) 493.90
  - with
    - acute exacerbation 493.92
    - status asthmaticus 493.91
  - chronic 493.2
- capillary 466.19
  - with bronchospasm or obstruction 466.19
  - chronic 491.8
- caseous (*see also* Tuberculosis) 011.3
- Castellani's 104.8
- catarrhal 490
  - acute - *see* Bronchitis, acute
  - chronic 491.0
- chemical (acute) (subacute) 506.0
  - chronic 506.4
  - due to fumes or vapors (acute) (subacute) 506.0
    - chronic 506.4
- chronic 491.9
  - with
    - tracheitis (chronic) 491.8
  - asthmatic 493.2
  - catarrhal 491.0
  - chemical (due to fumes and vapors) 506.4
  - due to
    - fumes or vapors (chemical) (inhalation) 506.4
    - radiation 508.8
    - tobacco smoking 491.0
  - mucopurulent 491.1
  - obstructive 491.20
    - with
      - acute bronchitis 491.22
      - exacerbation (acute) 491.21
  - purulent 491.1
  - simple 491.0
  - specified type NEC 491.8
- croupous 466.0
  - with bronchospasm or obstruction 466.0
  - due to fumes or vapors 506.0
- emphysematous 491.20
  - with
    - acute bronchitis 491.22
    - exacerbation (acute) 491.21
- exudative 466.0

Bronchitis *(Continued)*
- fetid (chronic) (recurrent) 491.1
- fibrinous, acute or subacute 466.0
  - with bronchospasm or obstruction 466.0
- grippal 487.1
- influenzal 487.1
- membranous, acute or subacute 466.0
  - with bronchospasm or obstruction 466.0
- moulders' 502
- mucopurulent (chronic) (recurrent) 491.1
  - acute or subacute 466.0
- obliterans 491.8
- obstructive (chronic) 491.20
  - with
    - acute bronchitis 491.22
    - exacerbation (acute) 491.21
- pituitous 491.1
- plastic (inflammatory) 466.0
- pneumococcal, acute or subacute 466.0
  - with bronchospasm or obstruction 466.0
- pseudomembranous 466.0
- purulent (chronic) (recurrent) 491.1
  - acute or subacute 466.0
    - with bronchospasm or obstruction 466.0
- putrid 491.1
- scrofulous (*see also* Tuberculosis) 011.3
- senile 491.9
- septic, acute or subacute 466.0
  - with bronchospasm or obstruction 466.0
- smokers' 491.0
- spirochetal 104.8
- suffocative, acute or subacute 466.0
- summer (*see also* Asthma) 493.9
- suppurative (chronic) 491.1
  - acute or subacute 466.0
- tuberculous (*see also* Tuberculosis) 011.3
- ulcerative 491.8
  - Vincent's 101
- Vincent's 101
- viral, acute or subacute 466.0

Bronchoalveolitis 485
Bronchoaspergillosis 117.3
Bronchocele
- meaning
  - dilatation of bronchus 519.19
  - goiter 240.9

Bronchogenic carcinoma 162.9
Bronchohemisporosis 117.9
Broncholithiasis 518.89
- tuberculous (*see also* Tuberculosis) 011.3

Bronchomalacia 748.3
Bronchomoniliasis 112.89
Bronchomycosis 112.89
Bronchonocardiosis 039.1
Bronchopleuropneumonia - *see* Pneumonia, broncho-
Bronchopneumonia - *see* Pneumonia, broncho-
Bronchopneumonitis - *see* Pneumonia, broncho-
Bronchopulmonary - *see* condition
Bronchopulmonitis - *see* Pneumonia, broncho-
Bronchorrhagia 786.3
- newborn 770.3

Bronchorrhagia *(Continued)*
- tuberculous (*see also* Tuberculosis) 011.3

Bronchorrhea (chronic) (purulent) 491.0
- acute 466.0

Bronchospasm 519.11
- with
  - asthma - *see* Asthma
  - bronchiolitis, acute 466.19
    - due to respiratory syncytial virus 466.11
  - bronchitis - *see* Bronchitis
  - chronic obstructive pulmonary disease (COPD) 496
  - emphysema - *see* Emphysema
    - due to external agent - *see* Condition, respiratory, acute, due to
- acute 519.11
- exercise induced 493.81

Bronchospirochetosis 104.8
Bronchostenosis 519.19
Bronchus - *see* condition
Bronze, bronzed
- diabetes 275.0
- disease (Addison's) (skin) 255.4
  - tuberculous (*see also* Tuberculosis) 017.6

Brooke's disease or tumor (M8100/0) - *see* Neoplasm, skin, benign
Brown's tendon sheath syndrome 378.61
Brown enamel of teeth (hereditary) 520.5
Brown-Séquard's paralysis (syndrome) 344.89
Brow presentation complicating delivery 652.4
Brucella, brucellosis (infection) 023.9
- abortus 023.1
- canis 023.3
- dermatitis, skin 023.9
- melitensis 023.0
- mixed 023.8
- suis 023.2

Bruck's disease 733.99
Bruck-de Lange disease or syndrome (Amsterdam dwarf, mental retardation, and brachycephaly) 759.89
Brugada syndrome 746.89
Brug's filariasis 125.1
Brugsch's syndrome (acropachyderma) 757.39
Bruhl's disease (splenic anemia with fever) 285.8
Bruise (skin surface intact) - *see also* Contusion
- with
  - fracture - *see* Fracture, by site
  - open wound - *see* Wound, open, by site
- internal organ (abdomen, chest, or pelvis) - *see* Injury, internal, by site
- umbilical cord 663.6
  - affecting fetus or newborn 762.6

Bruit 785.9
- arterial (abdominal) (carotid) 785.9
- supraclavicular 785.9

Brushburn - *see* Injury, superficial, by site
Bruton's X-linked agammaglobulinemia 279.04
Bruxism 306.8
- sleep related 327.53

Bubbly lung syndrome 770.7
Bubo 289.3
- blennorrhagic 098.89
- chancroidal 099.0
- climatic 099.1
- due to Hemophilus ducreyi 099.0
- gonococcal 098.89
- indolent NEC 099.8
- inguinal NEC 099.8
  - chancroidal 099.0
  - climatic 099.1
  - due to H. ducreyi 099.0
- scrofulous (*see also* Tuberculosis) 017.2
- soft chancre 099.0
- suppurating 683
- syphilitic 091.0
  - congenital 090.0
- tropical 099.1
- venereal NEC 099.8
- virulent 099.0

Bubonic plague 020.0
Bubonocele - *see* Hernia, inguinal
Buccal - *see* condition
Buchanan's disease (juvenile osteochondrosis of iliac crest) 732.1
Buchem's syndrome (hyperostosis corticalis) 733.3
Buchman's disease (osteochondrosis, juvenile) 732.1
Bucket handle fracture (semilunar cartilage) (*see also* Tear, meniscus) 836.2
Budd-Chiari syndrome (hepatic vein thrombosis) 453.0
Budgerigar-fanciers' disease or lung 495.2
Büdinger-Ludloff-Läwen disease 717.89
Buerger's disease (thromboangiitis obliterans) 443.1
Bulbar - *see* condition
Bulbus cordis 745.9
- persistent (in left ventricle) 745.8

Bulging fontanels (congenital) 756.0
Bulimia 783.6
- nervosa 307.51
- nonorganic origin 307.51

Bulky uterus 621.2
Bulla(e) 709.8
- lung (emphysematous) (solitary) 492.0

Bullet wound - *see also* Wound, open, by site
- fracture - *see* Fracture, by site, open
- internal organ (abdomen, chest, or pelvis) - *see* Injury, internal, by site, with open wound
- intracranial - *see* Laceration, brain, with open wound

Bullis fever 082.8
Bullying (*see also* Disturbance, conduct) 312.0
Bundle
- branch block (complete) (false) (incomplete) 426.50
  - bilateral 426.53
  - left (*see also* Block, bundle branch, left) 426.3
    - hemiblock 426.2
  - right (*see also* Block, bundle branch, right) 426.4
- of His - *see* condition
- of Kent syndrome (anomalous atrioventricular excitation) 426.7

Bungpagga 040.81

ICD-9-CM
B
Vol. 2

◄ New ⇐ Revised

- **Bunion** 727.1
- **Bunionette** 727.1
- **Bunyamwera fever** 066.3
- **Buphthalmia, buphthalmos** (congenital) 743.20
  - associated with
    - keratoglobus, congenital 743.22
    - megalocornea 743.22
    - ocular anomalies NEC 743.22
  - isolated 743.21
  - simple 743.21
- **Bürger-Grütz disease or syndrome** (essential familial hyperlipemia) 272.3
- **Buried roots** 525.3
- **Burke's syndrome** 577.8
- **Burkitt's**
  - tumor (M9750/3) 200.2
  - type (malignant, lymphoma, lymphoblastic, or undifferentiated) (M9750/3) 200.2
- **Burn** (acid) (cathode ray) (caustic) (chemical) (electric heating appliance) (electricity) (fire) (flame) (hot liquid or object) (irradiation) (lime) (radiation) (steam) (thermal) (x-ray) 949.0

> Note Use the following fifth-digit subclassification with category 948 to indicate the percent of body surface with third degree burn:
>
> 0 less than 10 percent or unspecified
> 1 10-19 percent
> 2 20-29 percent
> 3 30-39 percent
> 4 40-49 percent
> 5 50-59 percent
> 6 60-69 percent
> 7 70-79 percent
> 8 80-89 percent
> 9 90 percent or more of body surface

  - with
    - blisters - *see* Burn, by site, second degree
    - erythema - *see* Burn, by site, first degree
    - skin loss (epidermal) - *see also* Burn, by site, second degree
      - full thickness - *see also* Burn, by site, third degree
        - with necrosis of underlying tissues - *see* Burn, by site, third degree, deep
  - first degree - *see* Burn, by site, first degree
  - second degree - *see* Burn, by site, second degree
  - third degree - *see also* Burn, by site, third degree
    - deep - *see* Burn, by site, third degree, deep
  - abdomen, abdominal (muscle) (wall) 942.03
    - with
      - trunk - *see* Burn, trunk, multiple sites
    - first degree 942.13
    - second degree 942.23
    - third degree 942.33
      - deep 942.43
        - with loss of body part 942.53

Burn *(Continued)*
  - ankle 945.03
    - with
      - lower limb(s) - *see* Burn, leg, multiple sites
    - first degree 945.13
    - second degree 945.23
    - third degree 945.33
      - deep 945.43
        - with loss of body part 945.53
  - anus - *see* Burn, trunk, specified site NEC
  - arm(s) 943.00
    - first degree 943.10
    - second degree 943.20
    - third degree 943.30
      - deep 943.40
        - with loss of body part 943.50
    - lower - *see* Burn, forearm(s)
    - multiple sites, except hand(s) or wrist(s) 943.09
      - first degree 943.19
      - second degree 943.29
      - third degree 943.39
        - deep 943.49
          - with loss of body part 943.59
    - upper 943.03
      - first degree 943.13
      - second degree 943.23
      - third degree 943.33
        - deep 943.43
          - with loss of body part 943.53
  - auditory canal (external) - *see* Burn, ear
  - auricle (ear) - *see* Burn, ear
  - axilla 943.04
    - with
      - upper limb(s), except hand(s) or wrist(s) - *see* Burn, arm(s), multiple sites
    - first degree 943.14
    - second degree 943.24
    - third degree 943.34
      - deep 943.44
        - with loss of body part 943.54
  - back 942.04
    - with
      - trunk - *see* Burn, trunk, multiple sites
    - first degree 942.14
    - second degree 942.24
    - third degree 942.34
      - deep 942.44
        - with loss of body part 942.54
  - biceps
    - brachii - *see* Burn, arm(s), upper
    - femoris - *see* Burn, thigh
  - breast(s) 942.01
    - with
      - trunk - *see* Burn, trunk, multiple sites
    - first degree 942.11
    - second degree 942.21
    - third degree 942.31
      - deep 942.41
        - with loss of body part 942.51
  - brow - *see* Burn, forehead
  - buttock(s) - *see* Burn, back
  - canthus (eye) 940.1
    - chemical 940.0
  - cervix (uteri) 947.4
  - cheek (cutaneous) 941.07
    - with
      - face or head - *see* Burn, head, multiple sites

Burn *(Continued)*
  - cheek *(Continued)*
    - first degree 941.17
    - second degree 941.27
    - third degree 941.37
      - deep 941.47
        - with loss of body part 941.57
  - chest wall (anterior) 942.02
    - with
      - trunk - *see* Burn, trunk, multiple sites
    - first degree 942.12
    - second degree 942.22
    - third degree 942.32
      - deep 942.42
        - with loss of body part 942.52
  - chin 941.04
    - with
      - face or head - *see* Burn, head, multiple sites
    - first degree 941.14
    - second degree 941.24
    - third degree 941.34
      - deep 941.44
        - with loss of body part 941.54
  - clitoris - *see* Burn, genitourinary organs, external
  - colon 947.3
  - conjunctiva (and cornea) 940.4
    - chemical
      - acid 940.3
      - alkaline 940.2
  - cornea (and conjunctiva) 940.4
    - chemical
      - acid 940.3
      - alkaline 940.2
  - costal region - *see* Burn, chest wall
  - due to ingested chemical agent - *see* Burn, internal organs
  - ear (auricle) (canal) (drum) (external) 941.01
    - with
      - face or head - *see* Burn, head, multiple sites
    - first degree 941.11
    - second degree 941.21
    - third degree 941.31
      - deep 941.41
        - with loss of a body part 941.51
  - elbow 943.02
    - with
      - hand(s) and wrist(s) - *see* Burn, multiple specified sites
      - upper limb(s), except hand(s) or wrist(s) - *see also* Burn, arm(s), multiple sites
    - first degree 943.12
    - second degree 943.22
    - third degree 943.32
      - deep 943.42
        - with loss of body part 943.52
  - electricity, electric current - *see* Burn, by site
  - entire body - *see* Burn, multiple, specified sites
  - epididymis - *see* Burn, genitourinary organs, external
  - epigastric region - *see* Burn, abdomen
  - epiglottis 947.1
  - esophagus 947.2
  - extent (percent of body surface)
    - less than 10 percent 948.0
    - 10–19 percent 948.1
    - 20–29 percent 948.2
    - 30–39 percent 948.3

Burn *(Continued)*
extent *(Continued)*
40–49 percent 948.4
50–59 percent 948.5
60–69 percent 948.6
70–79 percent 948.7
80–89 percent 948.8
90 percent or more 948.9
extremity
lower - *see* Burn, leg
upper - *see* Burn, arm(s)
eye(s) (and adnexa) (only) 940.9
with
face, head, or neck 941.02
first degree 941.12
second degree 941.22
third degree 941.32
deep 941.42
with loss of body part 941.52
other sites (classifiable to more than one category in 940–945) - *see* Burn, multiple, specified sites
resulting rupture and destruction of eyeball 940.5
specified part - *see* Burn, by site
eyeball - *see also* Burn, eye
with resulting rupture and destruction of eyeball 940.5
eyelid(s) 940.1
chemical 940.0
face - *see* Burn, head
finger (nail) (subungual) 944.01
with
hand(s) - *see* Burn, hand(s), multiple sites
other sites - *see* Burn, multiple, specified sites
thumb 944.04
first degree 944.14
second degree 944.24
third degree 944.34
deep 944.44
with loss of body part 944.54
first degree 944.11
second degree 944.21
third degree 944.31
deep 944.41
with loss of body part 944.51
multiple (digits) 944.03
with thumb - *see* Burn, finger, with thumb
first degree 944.13
second degree 944.23
third degree 944.33
deep 944.43
with loss of body part 944.53
flank - *see* Burn, abdomen
foot 945.02
with
lower limb(s) - *see* Burn, leg, multiple sites
first degree 945.12
second degree 945.22
third degree 945.32
deep 945.42
with loss of body part 945.52
forearm(s) 943.01
with
upper limb(s), except hand(s) or wrist(s) - *see* Burn, arm(s), multiple sites
first degree 943.11

Burn *(Continued)*
forearm *(Continued)*
second degree 943.21
third degree 943.31
deep 943.41
with loss of body part 943.51
forehead 941.07
with
face or head - *see* Burn, head, multiple sites
first degree 941.17
second degree 941.27
third degree 941.37
deep 941.47
with loss of body part 941.57
fourth degree - *see* Burn, by site, third degree, deep
friction - *see* Injury, superficial, by site
from swallowing caustic or corrosive substance NEC - *see* Burn, internal organs
full thickness - *see* Burn, by site, third degree
gastrointestinal tract 947.3
genitourinary organs
external 942.05
with
trunk - *see* Burn, trunk, multiple sites
first degree 942.15
second degree 942.25
third degree 942.35
deep 942.45
with loss of body part 942.55
internal 947.8
globe (eye) - *see* Burn, eyeball
groin - *see* Burn, abdomen
gum 947.0
hand(s) (phalanges) (and wrist) 944.00
first degree 944.10
second degree 944.20
third degree 944.30
deep 944.40
with loss of body part 944.50
back (dorsal surface) 944.06
first degree 944.16
second degree 944.26
third degree 944.36
deep 944.46
with loss of body part 944.56
multiple sites 944.08
first degree 944.18
second degree 944.28
third degree 944.38
deep 944.48
with loss of body part 944.58
head (and face) 941.00
eye(s) only 940.9
specified part - *see* Burn, by site
first degree 941.10
second degree 941.20
third degree 941.30
deep 941.40
with loss of body part 941.50
multiple sites 941.09
with eyes - *see* Burn, eyes, with face, head, or neck
first degree 941.19
second degree 941.29
third degree 941.39
deep 941.49
with loss of body part 941.59
heel - *see* Burn, foot

Burn *(Continued)*
hip - *see* Burn, trunk, specified site NEC
iliac region - *see* Burn, trunk, specified site NEC
infected 958.3
inhalation (*see also* Burn, internal organs) 947.9
internal organs 947.9
from caustic or corrosive substance (swallowing) NEC 947.9
specified NEC (*see also* Burn, by site) 947.8
interscapular region - *see* Burn, back
intestine (large) (small) 947.3
iris - *see* Burn, eyeball
knee 945.05
with
lower limb(s) - *see* Burn, leg, multiple sites
first degree 945.15
second degree 945.25
third degree 945.35
deep 945.45
with loss of body part 945.55
labium (majus) (minus) - *see* Burn, genitourinary organs, external
lacrimal apparatus, duct, gland, or sac 940.1
chemical 940.0
larynx 947.1
late effect - *see* Late, effects (of), burn
leg 945.00
first degree 945.10
second degree 945.20
third degree 945.30
deep 945.40
with loss of body part 945.50
lower 945.04
with other part(s) of lower limb(s) - *see* Burn, leg, multiple sites
first degree 945.14
second degree 945.24
third degree 945.34
deep 945.44
with loss of body part 945.54
multiple sites 945.09
first degree 945.19
second degree 945.29
third degree 945.39
deep 945.49
with loss of body part 945.59
upper - *see* Burn, thigh
lightning - *see* Burn, by site
limb(s)
lower (including foot or toe(s)) - *see* Burn, leg
upper (except wrist and hand) - *see* Burn, arm(s)
lip(s) 941.03
with
face or head - *see* Burn, head, multiple sites
first degree 941.13
second degree 941.23
third degree 941.33
deep 941.43
with loss of body part 941.53
lumbar region - *see* Burn, back
lung 947.1
malar region - *see* Burn, cheek
mastoid region - *see* Burn, scalp
membrane, tympanic - *see* Burn, ear
midthoracic region - *see* Burn, chest wall

ICD-9-CM B Vol. 2

Burn *(Continued)*
mouth 947.0
multiple (*see also* Burn, unspecified) 949.0
specified sites classifiable to more than one category in 940–945 946.0
first degree 946.1
second degree 946.2
third degree 946.3
deep 946.4
with loss of body part 946.5
muscle, abdominal - *see* Burn, abdomen
nasal (septum) - *see* Burn, nose
neck 941.08
with
face or head - *see* Burn, head, multiple sites
first degree 941.18
second degree 941.28
third degree 941.38
deep 941.48
with loss of body part 941.58
nose (septum) 941.05
with
face or head - *see* Burn, head, multiple sites
first degree 941.15
second degree 941.25
third degree 941.35
deep 941.45
with loss of body part 941.55
occipital region - *see* Burn, scalp
orbit region 940.1
chemical 940.0
oronasopharynx 947.0
palate 947.0
palm(s) 944.05
with
hand(s) and wrist(s) - *see* Burn, hand(s), multiple sites
first degree 944.15
second degree 944.25
third degree 944.35
deep 944.45
with loss of a body part 944.55
parietal region - *see* Burn, scalp
penis - *see* Burn, genitourinary organs, external
perineum - *see* Burn, genitourinary organs, external
periocular area 940.1
chemical 940.0
pharynx 947.0
pleura 947.1
popliteal space - *see* Burn, knee
prepuce - *see* Burn, genitourinary organs, external
pubic region - *see* Burn, genitourinary organs, external
pudenda - *see* Burn, genitourinary organs, external
rectum 947.3
sac, lacrimal 940.1
chemical 940.0
sacral region - *see* Burn, back
salivary (ducts) (glands) 947.0
scalp 941.06
with
face or neck - *see* Burn, head, multiple sites
first degree 941.16

Burn *(Continued)*
scalp *(Continued)*
second degree 941.26
third degree 941.36
deep 941.46
with loss of body part 941.56
scapular region 943.06
with
upper limb(s), except hand(s) or wrist(s) - *see* Burn, arm(s), multiple sites
first degree 943.16
second degree 943.26
third degree 943.36
deep 943.46
with loss of body part 943.56
sclera - *see* Burn, eyeball
scrotum - *see* Burn, genitourinary organs, external
septum, nasal - *see* Burn, nose
shoulder(s) 943.05
with
hand(s) and wrist(s) - *see* Burn, multiple, specified sites
upper limb(s), except hand(s) or wrist(s) - *see* Burn, arm(s), multiple sites
first degree 943.15
second degree 943.25
third degree 943.35
deep 943.45
with loss of body part 943.55
skin NEC (*see also* Burn, unspecified) 949.0
skull - *see* Burn, head
small intestine 947.3
sternal region - *see* Burn, chest wall
stomach 947.3
subconjunctival - *see* Burn, conjunctiva
subcutaneous - *see* Burn, by site, third degree
submaxillary region - *see* Burn, head
submental region - *see* Burn, chin
sun - *see* Sunburn
supraclavicular fossa - *see* Burn, neck
supraorbital - *see* Burn, forehead
temple - *see* Burn, scalp
temporal region - *see* Burn, scalp
testicle - *see* Burn, genitourinary organs, external
testis - *see* Burn, genitourinary organs, external
thigh 945.06
with
lower limb(s) - *see* Burn, leg, multiple sites
first degree 945.16
second degree 945.26
third degree 945.36
deep 945.46
with loss of body part 945.56
thorax (external) - *see* Burn, chest wall
throat 947.0
thumb(s) (nail) (subungual) 944.02
with
finger(s) - *see* Burn, finger, with other sites, thumb
hand(s) and wrist(s) - *see* Burn, hand(s), multiple sites
first degree 944.12
second degree 944.22
third degree 944.32
deep 944.42
with loss of body part 944.52

Burn *(Continued)*
toe (nail) (subungual) 945.01
with
lower limb(s) - *see* Burn, leg, multiple sites
first degree 945.11
second degree 945.21
third degree 945.31
deep 945.41
with loss of body part 945.51
tongue 947.0
tonsil 947.0
trachea 947.1
trunk 942.00
first degree 942.10
second degree 942.20
third degree 942.30
deep 942.40
with loss of body part 942.50
multiple sites 942.09
first degree 942.19
second degree 942.29
third degree 942.39
deep 942.49
with loss of body part 942.59
specified site NEC 942.09
first degree 942.19
second degree 942.29
third degree 942.39
deep 942.49
with loss of body part 942.59
tunica vaginalis - *see* Burn, genitourinary organs, external
tympanic membrane - *see* Burn, ear
tympanum - *see* Burn, ear
ultraviolet 692.82
unspecified site (multiple) 949.0
with extent of body surface involved specified
less than 10 percent 948.0
10–19 percent 948.1
20–29 percent 948.2
30–39 percent 948.3
40–49 percent 948.4
50–59 percent 948.5
60–69 percent 948.6
70–79 percent 948.7
80–89 percent 948.8
90 percent or more 948.9
first degree 949.1
second degree 949.2
third degree 949.3
deep 949.4
with loss of body part 949.5
uterus 947.4
uvula 947.0
vagina 947.4
vulva - *see* Burn, genitourinary organs, external
wrist(s) 944.07
with
hand(s) - *see* Burn, hand(s), multiple sites
first degree 944.17
second degree 944.27
third degree 944.37
deep 944.47
with loss of body part 944.57
Burnett's syndrome (milk-alkali) 275.42
Burnier's syndrome (hypophyseal dwarfism) 253.3
Burning
feet syndrome 266.2

Burning *(Continued)*
sensation (*see also* Disturbance, sensation) 782.0
tongue 529.6
Burns' disease (osteochondrosis, lower ulna) 732.3
Bursa - *see also* condition
pharynx 478.29
Bursitis NEC 727.3
Achilles tendon 726.71
adhesive 726.90
shoulder 726.0
ankle 726.79
buttock 726.5
calcaneal 726.79
collateral ligament
fibular 726.63
tibial 726.62
Duplay's 726.2
elbow 726.33
finger 726.8
foot 726.79
gonococcal 098.52
hand 726.4
hip 726.5

Bursitis NEC *(Continued)*
infrapatellar 726.69
ischiogluteal 726.5
knee 726.60
occupational NEC 727.2
olecranon 726.33
pes anserinus 726.61
pharyngeal 478.29
popliteal 727.51
prepatellar 726.65
radiohumeral 727.3
scapulohumeral 726.19
adhesive 726.0
shoulder 726.10
adhesive 726.0
subacromial 726.19
adhesive 726.0
subcoracoid 726.19
subdeltoid 726.19
adhesive 726.0
subpatellar 726.69
syphilitic 095.7
Thornwaldt's, Tornwaldt's (pharyngeal) 478.29
toe 726.79

Bursitis NEC *(Continued)*
toe 726.79
trochanteric area 726.5
wrist 726.4
Burst stitches or sutures (complication of surgery) (external) 998.32
internal 998.31
Buruli ulcer 031.1
Bury's disease (erythema elevatum diutinum) 695.89
Buschke's disease or scleredema (adultorum) 710.1
Busquet's disease (osteoperiostitis) (*see also* Osteomyelitis) 730.1
Busse-Buschke disease (cryptococcosis) 117.5
Buttock - *see* condition
Button
Biskra 085.1
Delhi 085.1
oriental 085.1
Buttonhole hand (intrinsic) 736.21
Bwamba fever (encephalitis) 066.3
Byssinosis (occupational) 504
Bywaters' syndrome 958.5

C

Cacergasia 300.9
Cachexia 799.4
cancerous - *see also* Neoplasm, by site, malignant 799.4 ◀
cardiac - *see* Disease, heart
dehydration 276.51
with
hypernatremia 276.0
hyponatremia 276.1
due to malnutrition 799.4 ⬅
exophthalmic 242.0
heart - *see* Disease, heart
hypophyseal 253.2
hypopituitary 253.2
lead 984.9
specified type of lead - *see* Table of Drugs and Chemicals
malaria 084.9
malignant - *see also* Neoplasm, by site, malignant 799.4 ◀
marsh 084.9
nervous 300.5
old age 797
pachydermic - *see* Hypothyroidism
paludal 084.9
pituitary (postpartum) 253.2
renal (*see also* Disease, renal) 593.9
saturnine 984.9
specified type of lead - *see* Table of Drugs and Chemicals
senile 797
Simmonds' (pituitary cachexia) 253.2
splenica 289.59
strumipriva (*see also* Hypothyroidism) 244.9
tuberculous NEC (*see also* Tuberculosis) 011.9
Café au lait spots 709.09
Caffey's disease or syndrome (infantile cortical hyperostosis) 756.59
Caisson disease 993.3
Caked breast (puerperal, postpartum) 676.2
Cake kidney 753.3
Calabar swelling 125.2
Calcaneal spur 726.73
Calcaneoapophysitis 732.5
Calcaneonavicular bar 755.67
Calcareous - *see* condition
Calcicosis (occupational) 502
Calciferol (vitamin D) deficiency 268.9
with
osteomalacia 268.2
rickets (*see also* Rickets) 268.0
Calcification
adrenal (capsule) (gland) 255.4
tuberculous (*see also* Tuberculosis) 017.6
aorta 440.0
artery (annular) - *see* Arteriosclerosis
auricle (ear) 380.89
bladder 596.8
due to S. hematobium 120.0
brain (cortex) - *see* Calcification, cerebral
bronchus 519.19 ⬅
bursa 727.82
cardiac (*see also* Degeneration, myocardial) 429.1
cartilage (postinfectional) 733.99
cerebral (cortex) 348.8
artery 437.0
cervix (uteri) 622.8
choroid plexus 349.2

Calcification *(Continued)*
conjunctiva 372.54
corpora cavernosa (penis) 607.89
cortex (brain) - *see* Calcification, cerebral
dental pulp (nodular) 522.2
dentinal papilla 520.4
disc, intervertebral 722.90
cervical, cervicothoracic 722.91
lumbar, lumbosacral 722.93
thoracic, thoracolumbar 722.92
fallopian tube 620.8
falx cerebri - *see* Calcification, cerebral
fascia 728.89
gallbladder 575.8
general 275.40
heart (*see also* Degeneration, myocardial) 429.1
valve - *see* Endocarditis
intervertebral cartilage or disc (postinfectional) 722.90
cervical, cervicothoracic 722.91
lumbar, lumbosacral 722.93
thoracic, thoracolumbar 722.92
intracranial - *see* Calcification, cerebral
intraspinal ligament 728.89
joint 719.80
ankle 719.87
elbow 719.82
foot 719.87
hand 719.84
hip 719.85
knee 719.86
multiple sites 719.89
pelvic region 719.85
shoulder (region) 719.81
specified site NEC 719.88
wrist 719.83
kidney 593.89
tuberculous (*see also* Tuberculosis) 016.0
larynx (senile) 478.79
lens 366.8
ligament 728.89
intraspinal 728.89
knee (medial collateral) 717.89
lung 518.89
active 518.89
postinfectional 518.89
tuberculous (*see also* Tuberculosis, pulmonary) 011.9
lymph gland or node (postinfectional) 289.3
tuberculous (*see also* Tuberculosis, lymph gland) 017.2
mammographic 793.89 ◀
massive (paraplegic) 728.10
medial (*see also* Arteriosclerosis, extremities) 440.20
meninges (cerebral) 349.2
metastatic 275.40
Mönckeberg's - *see* Arteriosclerosis
muscle 728.10
heterotopic, postoperative 728.13
myocardium, myocardial (*see also* Degeneration, myocardial) 429.1
ovary 620.8
pancreas 577.8
penis 607.89
periarticular 728.89
pericardium (*see also* Pericarditis) 423.8
pineal gland 259.8
pleura 511.0
postinfectional 518.89
tuberculous (*see also* Tuberculosis, pleura) 012.0

Calcification *(Continued)*
pulp (dental) (nodular) 522.2
renal 593.89
Rider's bone 733.99
sclera 379.16
semilunar cartilage 717.89
spleen 289.59
subcutaneous 709.3
suprarenal (capsule) (gland) 255.4
tendon (sheath) 727.82
with bursitis, synovitis, or tenosynovitis 727.82
trachea 519.19 ⬅
ureter 593.89
uterus 621.8
vitreous 379.29
Calcified - *see also* Calcification
hematoma NEC 959.9
Calcinosis (generalized) (interstitial) (tumoral) (universalis) 275.49
circumscripta 709.3
cutis 709.3
intervertebralis 275.49 *[722.90]*
Raynaud's phenomenon sclerodactylytelangiectasis (CRST) 710.1
Calciphylaxis (*see also* Calcification, by site) 275.49 ◀
Calcium
blood
high (*see also* Hypercalcemia) 275.42
low (*see also* Hypocalcemia) 275.41
deposits - *see also* Calcification, by site
in bursa 727.82
in tendon (sheath) 727.82
with bursitis, synovitis or tenosynovitis 727.82
salts or soaps in vitreous 379.22
Calciuria 791.9
Calculi - *see* Calculus
Calculosis, intrahepatic - *see* Choledocholithiasis
Calculus, calculi, calculous 592.9
ampulla of Vater - *see* Choledocholithiasis
anuria (impacted) (recurrent) 592.0
appendix 543.9
bile duct (any) - *see* Choledocholithiasis
biliary - *see* Cholelithiasis
bilirubin, multiple - *see* Cholelithiasis
bladder (encysted) (impacted) (urinary) 594.1
diverticulum 594.0
bronchus 518.89
calyx (kidney) (renal) 592.0
congenital 753.3
cholesterol (pure) (solitary) - *see* Cholelithiasis
common duct (bile) - *see* Choledocholithiasis
conjunctiva 372.54
cystic 594.1
duct - *see* Cholelithiasis
dental 523.6
subgingival 523.6
supragingival 523.6
epididymis 608.89
gallbladder - *see also* Cholelithiasis
congenital 751.69
hepatic (duct) - *see* Choledocholithiasis
intestine (impaction) (obstruction) 560.39
kidney (impacted) (multiple) (pelvis) (recurrent) (staghorn) 592.0
congenital 753.3

◀ **New** ⬅ **Revised**

Calculus, calculi, calculous *(Continued)*
lacrimal (passages) 375.57
liver (impacted) - *see* Choledocholithiasis
lung 518.89
mammographic 793.89 ◀
nephritic (impacted) (recurrent) 592.0
nose 478.19 ⬅
pancreas (duct) 577.8
parotid gland 527.5
pelvis, encysted 592.0
prostate 602.0
pulmonary 518.89
renal (impacted) (recurrent) 592.0
congenital 753.3
salivary (duct) (gland) 527.5
seminal vesicle 608.89
staghorn 592.0
Stensen's duct 527.5
sublingual duct or gland 527.5
congenital 750.26
submaxillary duct, gland, or region 527.5
suburethral 594.8
tonsil 474.8
tooth, teeth 523.6
tunica vaginalis 608.89
ureter (impacted) (recurrent) 592.1
urethra (impacted) 594.2
urinary (duct) (impacted) (passage) (tract) 592.9
lower tract NEC 594.9
specified site 594.8
vagina 623.8
vesicle (impacted) 594.1
Wharton's duct 527.5
Caliectasis 593.89
California
disease 114.0
encephalitis 062.5
Caligo cornea 371.03
Callositas, callosity (infected) 700
Callus (infected) 700
bone 726.91
excessive, following fracture - *see also* Late, effect (of), fracture
Calvé (-Perthes) disease (osteochondrosis, femoral capital) 732.1
Calvities (*see also* Alopecia) 704.00
Cameroon fever (*see also* Malaria) 084.6
Camptocormia 300.11
Camptodactyly (congenital) 755.59
Camurati-Engelmann disease (diaphyseal sclerosis) 756.59
Canal - *see* condition
Canaliculitis (lacrimal) (acute) 375.31
Actinomyces 039.8
chronic 375.41
Canavan's disease 330.0
Cancer (M8000/3) - *see also* Neoplasm, by site, malignant

Note The term "cancer" when modified by an adjective or adjectival phrase indicating a morphological type should be coded in the same manner as "carcinoma" with that adjective or phrase. Thus, "squamous-cell cancer" should be coded in the same manner as "squamous-cell carcinoma," which appears in the list under "Carcinoma."

bile duct type (M8160/3), liver 155.1
hepatocellular (M8170/3) 155.0
Cancerous (M8000/3) - *see* Neoplasm, by site, malignant
Cancerphobia 300.29
Cancrum oris 528.1
Candidiasis, candidal 112.9
with pneumonia 112.4
balanitis 112.2
congenital 771.7
disseminated 112.5
endocarditis 112.81
esophagus 112.84
intertrigo 112.3
intestine 112.85
lung 112.4
meningitis 112.83
mouth 112.0
nails 112.3
neonatal 771.7
onychia 112.3
otitis externa 112.82
otomycosis 112.82
paronychia 112.3
perionyxis 112.3
pneumonia 112.4
pneumonitis 112.4
skin 112.3
specified site NEC 112.89
systemic 112.5
urogenital site NEC 112.2
vagina 112.1
vulva 112.1
vulvovaginitis 112.1
Candidiosis - *see* Candidiasis
Candiru infection or infestation 136.8
Canities (premature) 704.3
congenital 757.4
Canker (mouth) (sore) 528.2
rash 034.1
Cannabinosis 504
Canton fever 081.9
Cap
cradle 690.11
Capillariasis 127.5
Capillary - *see* condition
Caplan's syndrome 714.81
Caplan-Colinet syndrome 714.81
Capsule - *see* condition
Capsulitis (joint) 726.90
adhesive (shoulder) 726.0
hip 726.5
knee 726.60
labyrinthine 387.8
thyroid 245.9
wrist 726.4
Caput
crepitus 756.0
medusae 456.8
succedaneum 767.19
Carapata disease 087.1
Carate - *see* Pinta
Carbohydrate-deficient glycoprotein syndrome (CDGS) 271.8
Carboxyhemoglobinemia 986
Carbuncle 680.9
abdominal wall 680.2
ankle 680.6
anus 680.5
arm (any part, above wrist) 680.3
auditory canal, external 680.0
axilla 680.3
back (any part) 680.2
breast 680.2
buttock 680.5
chest wall 680.2
Carbuncle *(Continued)*
corpus cavernosum 607.2
ear (any part) (external) 680.0
eyelid 373.13
face (any part, except eye) 680.0
finger (any) 680.4
flank 680.2
foot (any part) 680.7
forearm 680.3
genital organ (male) 608.4
gluteal (region) 680.5
groin 680.2
hand (any part) 680.4
head (any part, except face) 680.8
heel 680.7
hip 680.6
kidney (*see also* Abscess, kidney) 590.2
knee 680.6
labia 616.4
lacrimal
gland (*see also* Dacryoadenitis) 375.00
passages (duct) (sac) (*see also* Dacryocystitis) 375.30
leg, any part except foot 680.6
lower extremity, any part except foot 680.6
malignant 022.0
multiple sites 680.9
neck 680.1
nose (external) (septum) 680.0
orbit, orbital 376.01
partes posteriores 680.5
pectoral region 680.2
penis 607.2
perineum 680.2
pinna 680.0
scalp (any part) 680.8
scrotum 608.4
seminal vesicle 608.0
shoulder 680.3
skin NEC 680.9
specified site NEC 680.8
spermatic cord 608.4
temple (region) 680.0
testis 608.4
thigh 680.6
thumb 680.4
toe (any) 680.7
trunk 680.2
tunica vaginalis 608.4
umbilicus 680.2
upper arm 680.3
urethra 597.0
vas deferens 608.4
vulva 616.4
wrist 680.4
Carbunculus (*see also* Carbuncle) 680.9
Carcinoid (tumor) (M8240/1) - *see also* Neoplasm, by site, uncertain behavior
and struma ovarii (M9091/1) 236.2
argentaffin (M8241/1) - *see* Neoplasm, by site, uncertain behavior
malignant (M8241/3) - *see* Neoplasm, by site, malignant
benign (M9091/0) 220
composite (M8244/3) - *see* Neoplasm, by site, malignant
goblet cell (M8243/3) - *see* Neoplasm, by site, malignant
malignant (M8240/3) - *see* Neoplasm, by site, malignant
nonargentaffin (M8242/1) - *see also* Neoplasm, by site, uncertain behavior

ICD-9-CM C Vol. 2

Carcinoid *(Continued)*
nonargentaffin *(Continued)*
malignant (M8242/3) - *see* Neoplasm, by site, malignant
strumal (M9091/1) 236.2
syndrome (intestinal) (metastatic) 259.2
type bronchial adenoma (M8240/3) - *see* Neoplasm, lung, malignant
Carcinoidosis 259.2
Carcinoma (M8010/3) - *see also* Neoplasm, by site, malignant

Note Except where otherwise indicated, the morphological varieties of carcinoma in the list below should be coded by site as for "Neoplasm, malignant."

with
apocrine metaplasia (M8573/3)
cartilaginous (and osseous) metaplasia (M8571/3)
osseous (and cartilaginous) metaplasia (M8571/3)
productive fibrosis (M8141/3)
spindle cell metaplasia (M8572/3)
squamous metaplasia (M8570/3)
acidophil (M8280/3)
specified site - *see* Neoplasm, by site, malignant
unspecified site 194.3
acidophil-basophil, mixed (M8281/3)
specified site - *see* Neoplasm, by site, malignant
unspecified site 194.3
acinar (cell) (M8550/3)
acinic cell (M8550/3)
adenocystic (M8200/3)
adenoid
cystic (M8200/3)
squamous cell (M8075/3)
adenosquamous (M8560/3)
adnexal (skin) (M8390/3) - *see* Neoplasm, skin, malignant
adrenal cortical (M8370/3) 194.0
alveolar (M8251/3)
cell (M8250/3) - *see* Neoplasm, lung, malignant
anaplastic type (M8021/3)
apocrine (M8401/3)
breast - *see* Neoplasm, breast, malignant
specified site NEC - *see* Neoplasm, skin, malignant
unspecified site 173.9
basal cell (pigmented) (M8090/3) - *see also* Neoplasm, skin, malignant
fibro-epithelial type (M8093/3) - *see* Neoplasm, skin, malignant
morphea type (M8092/3) - *see* Neoplasm, skin, malignant
multicentric (M8091/3) - *see* Neoplasm, skin, malignant
basaloid (M8123/3)
basal-squamous cell, mixed (M8094/3) - *see* Neoplasm, skin, malignant
basophil (M8300/3)
specified site - *see* Neoplasm, by site, malignant
unspecified site 194.3
basophil-acidophil, mixed (M8281/3)
specified site - *see* Neoplasm, by site, malignant
unspecified site 194.3

Carcinoma *(Continued)*
basosquamous (M8094/3) - *see* Neoplasm, skin, malignant
bile duct type (M8160/3)
and hepatocellular, mixed (M8180/3) 155.0
liver 155.1
specified site NEC - *see* Neoplasm, by site, malignant
unspecified site 155.1
branchial or branchiogenic 146.8
bronchial or bronchogenic - *see* Neoplasm, lung, malignant
bronchiolar (terminal) (M8250/3) - *see* Neoplasm, lung, malignant
bronchiolo-alveolar (M8250/3) - *see* Neoplasm, lung, malignant
bronchogenic (epidermoid) 162.9
C cell (M8510/3)
specified site - *see* Neoplasm, by site, malignant
unspecified site 193
ceruminous (M8420/3) 173.2
chorionic (M9100/3)
specified site - *see* Neoplasm, by site, malignant
unspecified site
female 181
male 186.9
chromophobe (M8270/3)
specified site - *see* Neoplasm, by site, malignant
unspecified site 194.3
clear cell (mesonephroid type) (M8310/3)
cloacogenic (M8124/3)
specified site - *see* Neoplasm, by site, malignant
unspecified site 154.8
colloid (M8480/3)
cribriform (M8201/3)
cylindroid type (M8200/3)
diffuse type (M8145/3)
specified site - *see* Neoplasm, by site, malignant
unspecified site 151.9
duct (cell) (M8500/3)
with Paget's disease (M8541/3) - *see* Neoplasm, breast, malignant
infiltrating (M8500/3)
specified site - *see* Neoplasm, by site, malignant
unspecified site 174.9
ductal (M8500/3)
ductular, infiltrating (M8521/3)
embryonal (M9070/3)
and teratoma, mixed (M9081/3)
combined with choriocarcinoma (M9101/3) - *see* Neoplasm, by site, malignant
infantile type (M9071/3)
liver 155.0
polyembryonal type (M9072/3)
endometrioid (M8380/3)
eosinophil (M8280/3)
specified site - *see* Neoplasm, by site, malignant
unspecified site 194.3
epidermoid (M8070/3) - *see also* Carcinoma, squamous cell
and adenocarcinoma, mixed (M8560/3)
in situ, Bowen's type (M8081/2) - *see* Neoplasm, skin, in situ

Carcinoma *(Continued)*
epidermoid *(Continued)*
intradermal - *see* Neoplasm, skin, in situ
fibroepithelial type basal cell (M8093/3) - *see* Neoplasm, skin, malignant
follicular (M8330/3)
and papillary (mixed) (M8340/3) 193
moderately differentiated type (M8332/3) 193
pure follicle type (M8331/3) 193
specified site - *see* Neoplasm, by site, malignant
trabecular type (M8332/3) 193
unspecified site 193
well differentiated type (M8331/3) 193
gelatinous (M8480/3)
giant cell (M8031/3)
and spindle cell (M8030/3)
granular cell (M8320/3)
granulosa cell (M8620/3) 183.0
hepatic cell (M8170/3) 155.0
hepatocellular (M8170/3) 155.0
and bile duct, mixed (M8180/3) 155.0
hepatocholangiolitic (M8180/3) 155.0
Hürthle cell (thyroid) 193
hypernephroid (M8311/3)
in
adenomatous
polyp (M8210/3)
polyposis coli (M8220/3) 153.9
pleomorphic adenoma (M8940/3)
polypoid adenoma (M8210/3)
situ (M8010/3) - *see* Carcinoma, in situ
tubular adenoma (M8210/3)
villous adenoma (M8261/3)
infiltrating duct (M8500/3)
with Paget's disease (M8541/3) - *see* Neoplasm, breast, malignant
specified site - *see* Neoplasm, by site, malignant
unspecified site 174.9
inflammatory (M8530/3)
specified site - *see* Neoplasm, by site, malignant
unspecified site 174.9
in situ (M8010/2) - *see also* Neoplasm, by site, in situ
epidermoid (M8070/2) - *see also* Neoplasm, by site, in situ
with questionable stromal invasion (M8076/2)
specified site - *see* Neoplasm, by site, in situ
unspecified site 233.1
Bowen's type (M8081/2) - *see* Neoplasm, skin, in situ
intraductal (M8500/2)
specified site - *see* Neoplasm, by site, in situ
unspecified site 233.0
lobular (M8520/2)
specified site - *see* Neoplasm, by site, in situ
unspecified site 233.0
papillary (M8050/2) - *see* Neoplasm, by site, in situ
squamous cell (M8070/2) - *see also* Neoplasm, by site, in situ
with questionable stromal invasion (M8076/2)

Carcinoma *(Continued)*
in situ *(Continued)*
squamous cell *(Continued)*
with questionable stromal invasion *(Continued)*
specified site - *see* Neoplasm, by site, in situ
unspecified site 233.1
transitional cell (M8120/2) - *see* Neoplasm, by site, in situ
intestinal type (M8144/3)
specified site - *see* Neoplasm, by site, malignant
unspecified site 151.9
intraductal (noninfiltrating) (M8500/2)
papillary (M8503/2)
specified site - *see* Neoplasm, by site, in situ
unspecified site 233.0
specified site - *see* Neoplasm, by site, in situ
unspecified site 233.0
intraepidermal (M8070/2) - *see also* Neoplasm, skin, in situ
squamous cell, Bowen's type (M8081/2) - *see* Neoplasm, skin, in situ
intraepithelial (M8010/2) - *see also* Neoplasm, by site, in situ
squamous cell (M8072/2) - *see* Neoplasm, by site, in situ
intraosseous (M9270/3) 170.1
upper jaw (bone) 170.0
islet cell (M8150/3)
and exocrine, mixed (M8154/3)
specified site - *see* Neoplasm, by site, malignant
unspecified site 157.9
pancreas 157.4
specified site NEC - *see* Neoplasm, by site, malignant
unspecified site 157.4
juvenile, breast (M8502/3) - *see* Neoplasm, breast, malignant
Kulchitsky's cell (carcinoid tumor of intestine) 259.2
large cell (M8012/3)
squamous cell, non-keratinizing type (M8072/3)
Leydig cell (testis) (M8650/3)
specified site - *see* Neoplasm, by site, malignant
unspecified site 186.9
female 183.0
male 186.9
liver cell (M8170/3) 155.0
lobular (infiltrating) (M8520/3)
noninfiltrating (M8520/3)
specified site - *see* Neoplasm, by site, in situ
unspecified site 233.0
specified site - *see* Neoplasm, by site, malignant
unspecified site 174.9
lymphoepithelial (M8082/3)
medullary (M8510/3)
with
amyloid stroma (M8511/3)
specified site - *see* Neoplasm, by site, malignant
unspecified site 193
lymphoid stroma (M8512/3)
specified site - *see* Neoplasm, by site, malignant
unspecified site 174.9

Carcinoma *(Continued)*
mesometanephric (M9110/3)
mesonephric (M9110/3)
metastatic (M8010/6) - *see* Metastasis, cancer
metatypical (M8095/3) - *see* Neoplasm, skin, malignant
morphea type basal cell (M8092/3) - *see* Neoplasm, skin, malignant
mucinous (M8480/3)
mucin-producing (M8481/3)
mucin-secreting (M8481/3)
mucoepidermoid (M8430/3)
mucoid (M8480/3)
cell (M8300/3)
specified site - *see* Neoplasm, by site, malignant
unspecified site 194.3
mucous (M8480/3)
nonencapsulated sclerosing (M8350/3) 193
noninfiltrating
intracystic (M8504/2) - *see* Neoplasm, by site, in situ
intraductal (M8500/2)
papillary (M8503/2)
specified site - *see* Neoplasm, by site, in situ
unspecified site 233.0
specified site - *see* Neoplasm, by site, in situ
unspecified site 233.0
lobular (M8520/2)
specified site - *see* Neoplasm, by site, in situ
unspecified site 233.0
oat cell (M8042/3)
specified site - *see* Neoplasm, by site, malignant
unspecified site 162.9
odontogenic (M9270/3) 170.1
upper jaw (bone) 170.0
oncocytic (M8290/3)
oxyphilic (M8290/3)
papillary (M8050/3)
and follicular (mixed) (M8340/3) 193
epidermoid (M8052/3)
intraductal (noninfiltrating) (M8503/2)
specified site - *see* Neoplasm, by site, in situ
unspecified site 233.0
serous (M8460/3)
specified site - *see* Neoplasm, by site, malignant
surface (M8461/3)
specified site - *see* Neoplasm, by site, malignant
unspecified site 183.0
unspecified site 183.0
squamous cell (M8052/3)
transitional cell (M8130/3)
papillocystic (M8450/3)
specified site - *see* Neoplasm, by site, malignant
unspecified site 183.0
parafollicular cell (M8510/3)
specified site - *see* Neoplasm, by site, malignant
unspecified site 193
pleomorphic (M8022/3)
polygonal cell (M8034/3)
prickle cell (M8070/3)

Carcinoma *(Continued)*
pseudoglandular, squamous cell (M8075/3)
pseudomucinous (M8470/3)
specified site - *see* Neoplasm, by site, malignant
unspecified site 183.0
pseudosarcomatous (M8033/3)
regaud type (M8082/3) - *see* Neoplasm, nasopharynx, malignant
renal cell (M8312/3) 189.0
reserve cell (M8041/3)
round cell (M8041/3)
Schmincke (M8082/3) - *see* Neoplasm, nasopharynx, malignant
Schneiderian (M8121/3)
specified site - *see* Neoplasm, by site, malignant
unspecified site 160.0
scirrhous (M8141/3)
sebaceous (M8410/3) - *see* Neoplasm, skin, malignant
secondary (M8010/6) - *see* Neoplasm, by site, malignant, secondary
secretory, breast (M8502/3) - *see* Neoplasm, breast, malignant
serous (M8441/3)
papillary (M8460/3)
specified site - *see* Neoplasm, by site, malignant
unspecified site 183.0
surface, papillary (M8461/3)
specified site - *see* Neoplasm, by site, malignant
unspecified site 183.0
Sertoli cell (M8640/3)
specified site - *see* Neoplasm, by site, malignant
unspecified site 186.9
signet ring cell (M8490/3)
metastatic (M8490/6) - *see* Neoplasm, by site, secondary
simplex (M8231/3)
skin appendage (M8390/3) - *see* Neoplasm, skin, malignant
small cell (M8041/3)
fusiform cell type (M8043/3)
squamous cell, nonkeratinizing type (M8073/3)
solid (M8230/3)
with amyloid stroma (M8511/3)
specified site - *see* Neoplasm, by site, malignant
unspecified site 193
spheroidal cell (M8035/3)
spindle cell (M8032/3)
and giant cell (M8030/3)
spinous cell (M8070/3)
squamous (cell) (M8070/3)
adenoid type (M8075/3)
and adenocarcinoma, mixed (M8560/3)
intraepidermal, Bowen's type - *see* Neoplasm, skin, in situ
keratinizing type (large cell) (M8071/3)
large cell, nonkeratinizing type (M8072/3)
microinvasive (M8076/3)
specified site - *see* Neoplasm, by site, malignant
unspecified site 180.9
nonkeratinizing type (M8072/3)
papillary (M8052/3)

ICD-9-CM
C
Vol. 2

Carcinoma *(Continued)*
squamous *(Continued)*
pseudoglandular (M8075/3)
small cell, nonkeratinizing type (M8073/3)
spindle cell type (M8074/3)
verrucous (M8051/3)
superficial spreading (M8143/3)
sweat gland (M8400/3) - *see* Neoplasm, skin, malignant
theca cell (M8600/3) 183.0
thymic (M8580/3) 164.0
trabecular (M8190/3)
transitional (cell) (M8120/3)
papillary (M8130/3)
spindle cell type (M8122/3)
tubular (M8211/3)
undifferentiated type (M8020/3)
urothelial (M8120/3)
ventriculi 151.9
verrucous (epidermoid) (squamous cell) (M8051/3)
villous (M8262/3)
water-clear cell (M8322/3) 194.1
wolffian duct (M9110/3)
Carcinomaphobia 300.29
Carcinomatosis
peritonei (M8010/6) 197.6
specified site NEC (M8010/3) - *see* Neoplasm, by site, malignant
unspecified site (M8010/6) 199.0
Carcinosarcoma (M8980/3) - *see also* Neoplasm, by site, malignant
embryonal type (M8981/3) - *see* Neoplasm, by site, malignant
Cardia, cardial - *see* condition
Cardiac - *see also* condition
death - *see* Disease, heart
device
defibrillator, automatic implantable V45.02
in situ NEC V45.00
pacemaker
cardiac
fitting or adjustment V53.31
in situ V45.01
carotid sinus
fitting or adjustment V53.39
in situ V45.09
pacemaker - *see* Cardiac, device, pacemaker
tamponade 423.9
Cardialgia (*see also* Pain, precordial) 786.51
Cardiectasis - *see* Hypertrophy, cardiac
Cardiochalasia 530.81
Cardiomalacia (*see also* Degeneration, myocardial) 429.1
Cardiomegalia glycogenica diffusa 271.0
Cardiomegaly (*see also* Hypertrophy, cardiac) 429.3
congenital 746.89
glycogen 271.0
hypertensive (*see also* Hypertension, heart) 402.90
idiopathic 425.4
Cardiomyoliposis (*see also* Degeneration, myocardial) 429.1
Cardiomyopathy (congestive) (constrictive) (familial) (infiltrative) (obstructive) (restrictive) (sporadic) 425.4
alcoholic 425.5
amyloid 277.39 *[425.7]* (Revised)
Cardiomyopathy *(Continued)*
beriberi 265.0 *[425.7]*
cobalt-beer 425.5
congenital 425.3
due to
amyloidosis 277.39 *[425.7]* (Revised)
beriberi 265.0 *[425.7]*
cardiac glycogenosis 271.0 *[425.7]*
Chagas' disease 086.0
Friedreich's ataxia 334.0 *[425.8]*
hypertension - *see* Hypertension, with, heart involvement
mucopolysaccharidosis 277.5 *[425.7]*
myotonia atrophica 359.2 *[425.8]*
progressive muscular dystrophy 359.1 *[425.8]*
sarcoidosis 135 *[425.8]*
glycogen storage 271.0 *[425.7]*
hypertensive - *see* Hypertension, with, heart involvement
hypertrophic
nonobstructive 425.4
obstructive 425.1
congenital 746.84
idiopathic (concentric) 425.4
in
Chagas' disease 086.0
sarcoidosis 135 *[425.8]*
ischemic 414.8
metabolic NEC 277.9 *[425.7]*
amyloid 277.39 *[425.7]* (Revised)
thyrotoxic (*see also* Thyrotoxicosis) 242.9 *[425.7]*
thyrotoxicosis (*see also* Thyrotoxicosis) 242.9 *[425.7]*
newborn 425.4
congenital 425.3
nutritional 269.9 *[425.7]*
beriberi 265.0 *[425.7]*
obscure of Africa 425.2
peripartum 674.5
postpartum 674.5
primary 425.4
secondary 425.9
stress induced 429.83 (New)
takotsubo 429.83 (Revised)
thyrotoxic (*see also* Thyrotoxicosis) 242.9 *[425.7]*
toxic NEC 425.9
tuberculous (*see also* Tuberculosis) 017.9 *[425.8]*
Cardionephritis - *see* Hypertension, cardiorenal
Cardionephropathy - *see* Hypertension, cardiorenal
Cardionephrosis - *see* Hypertension, cardiorenal
Cardioneurosis 306.2
Cardiopathia nigra 416.0
Cardiopathy (*see also* Disease, heart) 429.9
hypertensive (*see also* Hypertension, heart) 402.90
idiopathic 425.4
mucopolysaccharidosis 277.5 *[425.7]*
Cardiopericarditis (*see also* Pericarditis) 423.9
Cardiophobia 300.29
Cardioptosis 746.87
Cardiorenal - *see* condition
Cardiorrhexis (*see also* Infarct, myocardium) 410.9
Cardiosclerosis - *see* Arteriosclerosis, coronary
Cardiosis - *see* Disease, heart
Cardiospasm (esophagus) (reflex) (stomach) 530.0
congenital 750.7
Cardiostenosis - *see* Disease, heart
Cardiosymphysis 423.1
Cardiothyrotoxicosis - *see* Hyperthyroidism
Cardiovascular - *see* condition
Carditis (acute) (bacterial) (chronic) (subacute) 429.89
Coxsackie 074.20
hypertensive (*see also* Hypertension, heart) 402.90
meningococcal 036.40
rheumatic - *see* Disease, heart, rheumatic
rheumatoid 714.2
Care (of)
child (routine) V20.1
convalescent following V66.9
chemotherapy V66.2
medical NEC V66.5
psychotherapy V66.3
radiotherapy V66.1
surgery V66.0
surgical NEC V66.0
treatment (for) V66.5
combined V66.6
fracture V66.4
mental disorder NEC V66.3
specified type NEC V66.5
end-of-life V66.7
family member (handicapped) (sick)
creating problem for family V61.49
provided away from home for holiday relief V60.5
unavailable, due to
absence (person rendering care) (sufferer) V60.4
inability (any reason) of person rendering care V60.4
holiday relief V60.5
hospice V66.7
lack of (at or after birth) (infant) (child) 995.52
adult 995.84
lactation of mother V24.1
palliative V66.7
postpartum
immediately after delivery V24.0
routine follow-up V24.2
prenatal V22.1
first pregnancy V22.0
high-risk pregnancy V23.9
specified problem NEC V23.8
terminal V66.7
unavailable, due to
absence of person rendering care V60.4
inability (any reason) of person rendering care V60.4
well baby V20.1
Caries (bone) (*see also* Tuberculosis, bone) 015.9 [730.8]
arrested 521.04
cementum 521.03
cerebrospinal (tuberculous) 015.0 *[730.88]*
dental (acute) (chronic) (incipient) (infected) 521.00
with pulp exposure 521.03
extending to
dentine 521.02
pulp 521.03

◀ New ⬅ Revised

Caries *(Continued)*
dental *(Continued)*
other specified NEC 521.09
pit and fissure 521.06
primary ◀
pit and fissure origin 521.06 ◀
root surface 521.08 ◀
smooth surface origin 521.07 ◀
root surface 521.08
smooth surface 521.07
dentin (acute) (chronic) 521.02
enamel (acute) (chronic) (incipient) 521.01
external meatus 380.89
hip (*see also* Tuberculosis) 015.1 *[730.85]*
initial 521.01
knee 015.2 *[730.86]*
labyrinth 386.8
limb NEC 015.7 *[730.88]*
mastoid (chronic) (process) 383.1
middle ear 385.89
nose 015.7 *[730.88]*
orbit 015.7 *[730.88]*
ossicle 385.24
petrous bone 383.20
sacrum (tuberculous) 015.0 *[730.88]*
spine, spinal (column) (tuberculous) 015.0 *[730.88]*
syphilitic 095.5
congenital 090.0 *[730.8]*
teeth (internal) 521.00
initial 521.01
vertebra (column) (tuberculous) 015.0 *[730.88]*
Carini's syndrome (ichthyosis congenita) 757.1
Carious teeth 521.00
Carneous mole 631
Carnosinemia 270.5
Carotid body or sinus syndrome 337.0
Carotidynia 337.0
Carotinemia (dietary) 278.3
Carotinosis (cutis) (skin) 278.3
Carpal tunnel syndrome 354.0
Carpenter's syndrome 759.89
Carpopedal spasm (*see also* Tetany) 781.7
Carpoptosis 736.05
Carrier (suspected) of
amebiasis V02.2
bacterial disease (meningococcal, staphylococcal) NEC V02.59
cholera V02.0
cystic fibrosis gene V83.81
defective gene V83.89
diphtheria V02.4
dysentery (bacillary) V02.3
amebic V02.2
Entamoeba histolytica V02.2
gastrointestinal pathogens NEC V02.3
genetic defect V83.89
gonorrhea V02.7
group B streptococcus V02.51
HAA (hepatitis Australian-antigen) V02.61
hemophilia A (asymptomatic) V83.01
symptomatic V83.02
hepatitis V02.60
Australian-antigen (HAA) V02.61
B V02.61
C V02.62
specified type NEC V02.69
serum V02.61
viral V02.60
infective organism NEC V02.9

Carrier *(Continued)*
malaria V02.9
paratyphoid V02.3
Salmonella V02.3
typhosa V02.1
serum hepatitis V02.61
Shigella V02.3
Staphylococcus NEC V02.59
Streptococcus NEC V02.52
group B V02.51
typhoid V02.1
venereal disease NEC V02.8
Carrión's disease (Bartonellosis) 088.0
Car sickness 994.6
Carter's
relapsing fever (Asiatic) 087.0
Cartilage - *see* condition
Caruncle (inflamed)
abscess, lacrimal (*see also* Dacryocystitis) 375.30
conjunctiva 372.00
acute 372.00
eyelid 373.00
labium (majus) (minus) 616.89 ⬅
lacrimal 375.30
urethra (benign) 599.3
vagina (wall) 616.89 ⬅
Cascade stomach 537.6
Caseation lymphatic gland (*see also* Tuberculosis) 017.2
Caseous
bronchitis - *see* Tuberculosis, pulmonary
meningitis 013.0
pneumonia - *see* Tuberculosis, pulmonary
Cassidy (-Scholte) syndrome (malignant carcinoid) 259.2
Castellani's bronchitis 104.8
Castleman's tumor or lymphoma (mediastinal lymph node hyperplasia) 785.6
Castration, traumatic 878.2
complicated 878.3
Casts in urine 791.7
Cat's ear 744.29
Catalepsy 300.11
catatonic (acute) (*see also* Schizophrenia) 295.2
hysterical 300.11
schizophrenic (*see also* Schizophrenia) 295.2
Cataphasia 307.0
Cataplexy (idiopathic) (*see also* Narcolepsy)
Cataract (anterior cortical) (anterior polar) (black) (capsular) (central) (cortical) (hypermature) (immature) (incipient) (mature) 366.9
anterior
and posterior axial embryonal 743.33
pyramidal 743.31
subcapsular polar
infantile, juvenile, or presenile 366.01
senile 366.13
associated with
calcinosis 275.40 *[366.42]*
craniofacial dysostosis 756.0 *[366.44]*
galactosemia 271.1 *[366.44]*
hypoparathyroidism 252.1 *[366.42]*
myotonic disorders 359.2 *[366.43]*
neovascularization 366.33
blue dot 743.39
cerulean 743.39

Cataract *(Continued)*
complicated NEC 366.30
congenital 743.30
capsular or subcapsular 743.31
cortical 743.32
nuclear 743.33
specified type NEC 743.39
total or subtotal 743.34
zonular 743.32
coronary (congenital) 743.39
acquired 366.12
cupuliform 366.14
diabetic 250.5 *[366.41]*
drug-induced 366.45
due to
chalcosis 360.24 *[366.34]*
chronic choroiditis (*see also* Choroiditis) 363.20 *[366.32]*
degenerative myopia 360.21 *[366.34]*
glaucoma (*see also* Glaucoma) 365.9 *[366.31]*
infection, intraocular NEC 366.32
inflammatory ocular disorder NEC 366.32
iridocyclitis, chronic 364.10 *[366.33]*
pigmentary retinal dystrophy 362.74 *[366.34]*
radiation 366.46
electric 366.46
glassblowers' 366.46
heat ray 366.46
heterochromic 366.33
in eye disease NEC 366.30
infantile (*see also* Cataract, juvenile) 366.00
intumescent 366.12
irradiational 366.46
juvenile 366.00
anterior subcapsular polar 366.01
combined forms 366.09
cortical 366.03
lamellar 366.03
nuclear 366.04
posterior subcapsular polar 366.02
specified NEC 366.09
zonular 366.03
lamellar 743.32
infantile juvenile, or presenile 366.03
morgagnian 366.18
myotonic 359.2 *[366.43]*
myxedema 244.9 *[366.44]*
nuclear 366.16
posterior, polar (capsular) 743.31
infantile, juvenile, or presenile 366.02
senile 366.14
presenile (*see also* Cataract, juvenile) 366.00
punctate
acquired 366.12
congenital 743.39
secondary (membrane) 366.50
obscuring vision 366.53
specified type, not obscuring vision 366.52
senile 366.10
anterior subcapsular polar 366.13
combined forms 366.19
cortical 366.15
hypermature 366.18
immature 366.12
incipient 366.12
mature 366.17
nuclear 366.16
posterior subcapsular polar 366.14

ICD-9-CM C Vol. 2

Cataract *(Continued)*
senile *(Continued)*
specified NEC 366.19
total or subtotal 366.17
snowflake 250.5 *[366.41]*
specified NEC 366.8
subtotal (senile) 366.17
congenital 743.34
sunflower 360.24 *[366.34]*
tetanic NEC 252.1 *[366.42]*
total (mature) (senile) 366.17
congenital 743.34
localized 366.21
traumatic 366.22
toxic 366.45
traumatic 366.20
partially resolved 366.23
total 366.22
zonular (perinuclear) 743.32
infantile, juvenile, or presenile 366.03
Cataracta 366.10
brunescens 366.16
cerulea 743.39
complicata 366.30
congenita 743.30
coralliformis 743.39
coronaria (congenital) 743.39
acquired 366.12
diabetic 250.5 *[366.41]*
floriformis 360.24 *[366.34]*
membranacea
accreta 366.50
congenita 743.39
nigra 366.16
Catarrh, catarrhal (inflammation) (*see also* condition) 460
acute 460
asthma, asthmatic (*see also* Asthma) 493.9
Bostock's (*see also* Fever, hay) 477.9
bowel - *see* Enteritis
bronchial 490
acute 466.0
chronic 491.0
subacute 466.0
cervix, cervical (canal) (uteri) - *see* Cervicitis
chest (*see also* Bronchitis) 490
chronic 472.0
congestion 472.0
conjunctivitis 372.03
due to syphilis 095.9
congenital 090.0
enteric - *see* Enteritis
epidemic 487.1
Eustachian 381.50
eye (acute) (vernal) 372.03
fauces (*see also* Pharyngitis) 462
febrile 460
fibrinous acute 466.0
gastroenteric - *see* Enteritis
gastrointestinal - *see* Enteritis
gingivitis 523.00
hay (*see also* Fever, hay) 477.9
infectious 460
intestinal - *see* Enteritis
larynx (*see also* Laryngitis, chronic) 476.0
liver 070.1
with hepatic coma 070.0
lung (*see also* Bronchitis) 490
acute 466.0
chronic 491.0
middle ear (chronic) - *see* Otitis media, chronic
Catarrh, catarrhal *(Continued)*
mouth 528.00
nasal (chronic) (*see also* Rhinitis) 472.0
acute 460
nasobronchial 472.2
nasopharyngeal (chronic) 472.2
acute 460
nose - *see* Catarrh, nasal
ophthalmia 372.03
pneumococcal, acute 466.0
pulmonary (*see also* Bronchitis) 490
acute 466.0
chronic 491.0
spring (eye) 372.13
suffocating (*see also* Asthma) 493.9
summer (hay) (*see also* Fever, hay) 477.9
throat 472.1
tracheitis 464.10
with obstruction 464.11
tubotympanal 381.4
acute (*see also* Otitis media, acute, nonsuppurative) 381.00
chronic 381.10
vasomotor (*see also* Fever, hay) 477.9
vesical (bladder) - *see* Cystitis
Catarrhus aestivus (*see also* Fever, hay) 477.9
Catastrophe, cerebral (*see also* Disease, cerebrovascular, acute) 436
Catatonia, catatonic (acute) 781.99
with
affective psychosis - *see* Psychosis, affective
agitation 295.2
dementia (praecox) 295.2
due to or associated with physical condition 293.89
excitation 295.2
excited type 295.2
in conditions classified elsewhere 293.89
schizophrenia 295.2
stupor 295.2
Cat-scratch - *see also* Injury, superficial
disease or fever 078.3
Cauda equina - *see also* condition
syndrome 344.60
Cauliflower ear 738.7
Caul over face 768.9
Causalgia 355.9
lower limb 355.71
upper limb 354.4
Cause
external, general effects NEC 994.9
not stated 799.9
unknown 799.9
Caustic burn - *see also* Burn, by site
from swallowing caustic or corrosive substance - *see* Burn, internal organs
Cavare's disease (familial periodic paralysis) 359.3
Cave-in, injury
crushing (severe) (*see also* Crush, by site) 869.1
suffocation 994.7
Cavernitis (penis) 607.2
lymph vessel - *see* Lymphangioma
Cavernositis 607.2
Cavernous - *see* condition
Cavitation of lung (*see also* Tuberculosis) 011.2
nontuberculous 518.89
primary, progressive 010.8
Cavity
lung - *see* Cavitation of lung
optic papilla 743.57
pulmonary - *see* Cavitation of lung
teeth 521.00
vitreous (humor) 379.21
Cavovarus foot, congenital 754.59
Cavus foot (congenital) 754.71
acquired 736.73
Cazenave's
disease (pemphigus) NEC 694.4
lupus (erythematosus) 695.4
CDGS (carbohydrate-deficient glycoprotein syndrome) 271.8
Cecitis - *see* Appendicitis
Cecocele - *see* Hernia
Cecum - *see* condition
Celiac
artery compression syndrome 447.4
disease 579.0
infantilism 579.0
Cell, cellular - *see also* condition
anterior chamber (eye) (positive aqueous ray) 364.04
Cellulitis (diffuse) (with lymphangitis) (*see also* Abscess) 682.9
abdominal wall 682.2
anaerobic (*see also* Gas gangrene) 040.0
ankle 682.6
anus 566
areola 611.0
arm (any part, above wrist) 682.3
auditory canal (external) 380.10
axilla 682.3
back (any part) 682.2
breast 611.0
postpartum 675.1
broad ligament (*see also* Disease, pelvis, inflammatory) 614.4
acute 614.3
buttock 682.5
cervical (neck region) 682.1
cervix (uteri) (*see also* Cervicitis) 616.0
cheek, external 682.0
internal 528.3
chest wall 682.2
chronic NEC 682.9
colostomy 569.61
corpus cavernosum 607.2
digit 681.9
Douglas' cul-de-sac or pouch (chronic) (*see also* Disease, pelvis, inflammatory) 614.4
acute 614.3
drainage site (following operation) 998.59
ear, external 380.10
enterostomy 569.61
erysipelar (*see also* Erysipelas) 035
esophagostomy 530.86
eyelid 373.13
face (any part, except eye) 682.0
finger (intrathecal) (periosteal) (subcutaneous) (subcuticular) 681.00
flank 682.2
foot (except toe) 682.7
forearm 682.3
gangrenous (*see also* Gangrene) 785.4
genital organ NEC
female - *see* Abscess, genital organ, female
male 608.4
glottis 478.71
gluteal (region) 682.5

- **Cellulitis** *(Continued)*
  - gonococcal NEC 098.0
  - groin 682.2
  - hand (except finger or thumb) 682.4
  - head (except face) NEC 682.8
  - heel 682.7
  - hip 682.6
  - jaw (region) 682.0
  - knee 682.6
  - labium (majus) (minus) (*see also* Vulvitis) 616.10
  - larynx 478.71
  - leg, except foot 682.6
  - lip 528.5
  - mammary gland 611.0
  - mouth (floor) 528.3
  - multiple sites NEC 682.9
  - nasopharynx 478.21
  - navel 682.2
    - newborn NEC 771.4
  - neck (region) 682.1
  - nipple 611.0
  - nose 478.19
    - external 682.0
  - orbit, orbital 376.01
  - palate (soft) 528.3
  - pectoral (region) 682.2
  - pelvis, pelvic
    - with
      - abortion - *see* Abortion, by type, with sepsis
      - ectopic pregnancy (*see also* categories 633.0–633.9) 639.0
      - molar pregnancy (*see also* categories 630–632) 639.0
    - female (*see also* Disease, pelvis, inflammatory) 614.4
      - acute 614.3
    - following
      - abortion 639.0
      - ectopic or molar pregnancy 639.0
    - male 567.21
    - puerperal, postpartum, childbirth 670
  - penis 607.2
  - perineal, perineum 682.2
  - perirectal 566
  - peritonsillar 475
  - periurethral 597.0
  - periuterine (*see also* Disease, pelvis, inflammatory) 614.4
    - acute 614.3
  - pharynx 478.21
  - phlegmonous NEC 682.9
  - rectum 566
  - retromammary 611.0
  - retroperitoneal (*see also* Peritonitis) 567.38
  - round ligament (*see also* Disease, pelvis, inflammatory) 614.4
    - acute 614.3
  - scalp (any part) 682.8
    - dissecting 704.8
  - scrotum 608.4
  - seminal vesicle 608.0
  - septic NEC 682.9
  - shoulder 682.3
  - specified sites NEC 682.8
  - spermatic cord 608.4
  - submandibular (region) (space) (triangle) 682.0
    - gland 527.3
  - submaxillary 528.3
    - gland 527.3
- **Cellulitis** *(Continued)*
  - submental (pyogenic) 682.0
    - gland 527.3
  - suppurative NEC 682.9
  - testis 608.4
  - thigh 682.6
  - thumb (intrathecal) (periosteal) (subcutaneous) (subcuticular) 681.00
  - toe (intrathecal) (periosteal) (subcutaneous) (subcuticular) 681.10
  - tonsil 475
  - trunk 682.2
  - tuberculous (primary) (*see also* Tuberculosis) 017.0
  - tunica vaginalis 608.4
  - umbilical 682.2
    - newborn NEC 771.4
  - vaccinal 999.3
  - vagina - *see* Vaginitis
  - vas deferens 608.4
  - vocal cords 478.5
  - vulva (*see also* Vulvitis) 616.10
  - wrist 682.4
- **Cementoblastoma, benign** (M9273/0) 213.1
  - upper jaw (bone) 213.0
- **Cementoma** (M9273/0) 213.1
  - gigantiform (M9276/0) 213.1
    - upper jaw (bone) 213.0
  - upper jaw (bone) 213.0
- **Cementoperiostitis** 523.40
- **Cephalgia, cephalalgia** (*see also* Headache) 784.0
  - histamine 346.2
  - nonorganic origin 307.81
  - psychogenic 307.81
  - tension 307.81
- **Cephalhematocele, cephalematocele**
  - due to birth injury 767.19
  - fetus or newborn 767.19
  - traumatic (*see also* Contusion, head) 920
- **Cephalhematoma, cephalematoma** (calcified)
  - due to birth injury 767.19
  - fetus or newborn 767.19
  - traumatic (*see also* Contusion, head) 920
- **Cephalic** - *see* condition
- **Cephalitis** - *see* Encephalitis
- **Cephalocele** 742.0
- **Cephaloma** - *see* Neoplasm, by site, malignant
- **Cephalomenia** 625.8
- **Cephalopelvic** - *see* condition
- **Cercomoniasis** 007.3
- **Cerebellitis** - *see* Encephalitis
- **Cerebellum** (cerebellar) - *see* condition
- **Cerebral** - *see* condition
- **Cerebritis** - *see* Encephalitis
- **Cerebrohepatorenal syndrome** 759.89
- **Cerebromacular degeneration** 330.1
- **Cerebromalacia** (*see also* Softening, brain) 434.9
- **Cerebrosidosis** 272.7
- **Cerebrospasticity** - *see* Palsy, cerebral
- **Cerebrospinal** - *see* condition
- **Cerebrum** - *see* condition
- **Ceroid storage disease** 272.7
- **Cerumen** (accumulation) (impacted) 380.4
- **Cervical** - *see also* condition
  - auricle 744.43
  - high risk human papillomavirus (HPV) DNA test positive 795.05
  - intraepithelial glandular neoplasia 233.1
- **Cervical** *(Continued)*
  - low risk human papillomavirus (HPV) DNA test positive 795.09
  - rib 756.2
- **Cervicalgia** 723.1
- **Cervicitis** (acute) (chronic) (nonvenereal) (subacute) (with erosion or ectropion) 616.0
  - with
    - abortion - *see* Abortion, by type, with sepsis
    - ectopic pregnancy (*see also* categories 633.0-633.9) 639.0
    - molar pregnancy (*see also* categories 630-632) 639.0
    - ulceration 616.0
  - chlamydial 099.53
  - complicating pregnancy or puerperium 646.6
    - affecting fetus or newborn 760.8
  - following
    - abortion 639.0
    - ectopic or molar pregnancy 639.0
  - gonococcal (acute) 098.15
    - chronic or duration of 2 months or more 098.35
  - senile (atrophic) 616.0
  - syphilitic 095.8
  - trichomonal 131.09
  - tuberculous (*see also* Tuberculosis) 016.7
- **Cervicoaural fistula** 744.49
- **Cervicocolpitis** (emphysematosa) (*see also* Cervicitis) 616.0
- **Cervix** - *see* condition
- **Cesarean delivery, operation or section NEC** 669.7
  - affecting fetus or newborn 763.4
  - post mortem, affecting fetus or newborn 761.6
  - previous, affecting management of pregnancy 654.2
- **Céstan's syndrome** 344.89
- **Céstan-Chenais paralysis** 344.89
- **Céstan-Raymond syndrome** 433.8
- **Cestode infestation NEC** 123.9
  - specified type NEC 123.8
- **Cestodiasis** 123.9
- **CGF** (congenital generalized fibromatosis) 759.89
- **Chabert's disease** 022.9
- **Chacaleh** 266.2
- **Chafing** 709.8
- **Chagas' disease** (*see also* Trypanosomiasis, American) 086.2
  - with heart involvement 086.0
- **Chagres fever** 084.0
- **Chalasia** (cardiac sphincter) 530.81
- **Chalazion** 373.2
- **Chalazoderma** 757.39
- **Chalcosis** 360.24
  - cornea 371.15
  - crystalline lens 360.24 *[366.34]*
  - retina 360.24
- **Chalicosis** (occupational) (pulmonum) 502
- **Chancre** (any genital site) (hard) (indurated) (infecting) (primary) (recurrent) 091.0
  - congenital 090.0
  - conjunctiva 091.2
  - Ducrey's 099.0
  - extragenital 091.2
  - eyelid 091.2
  - Hunterian 091.0
  - lip (syphilis) 091.2

- **Chancre** *(Continued)*
  - mixed 099.8
  - nipple 091.2
  - Nisbet's 099.0
  - of
    - carate 103.0
    - pinta 103.0
    - yaws 102.0
  - palate, soft 091.2
  - phagedenic 099.0
  - Ricord's 091.0
  - Rollet's (syphilitic) 091.0
  - seronegative 091.0
  - seropositive 091.0
  - simple 099.0
  - soft 099.0
    - bubo 099.0
  - urethra 091.0
  - yaws 102.0
- **Chancriform syndrome** 114.1
- **Chancroid** 099.0
  - anus 099.0
  - penis (Ducrey's bacillus) 099.0
  - perineum 099.0
  - rectum 099.0
  - scrotum 099.0
  - urethra 099.0
  - vulva 099.0
- **Chandipura fever** 066.8
- **Chandler's disease** (osteochondritis dissecans, hip) 732.7
- **Change(s) (of)** - *see also* Removal of
  - arteriosclerotic - *see* Arteriosclerosis
  - battery
    - cardiac pacemaker V53.31
  - bone 733.90
    - diabetic 250.8 *[731.8]*
    - in disease, unknown cause 733.90
  - bowel habits 787.99
  - cardiorenal (vascular) (*see also* Hypertension, cardiorenal) 404.90
  - cardiovascular - *see* Disease, cardiovascular
  - circulatory 459.9
  - cognitive or personality change of other type, nonpsychotic 310.1
  - color, teeth, tooth
    - during formation 520.8
    - extrinsic 523.6
    - intrinsic posteruptive 521.7
  - contraceptive device V25.42
  - cornea, corneal
    - degenerative NEC 371.40
    - membrane NEC 371.30
    - senile 371.41
  - coronary (*see also* Ischemia, heart) 414.9
  - degenerative
    - chamber angle (anterior) (iris) 364.56
    - ciliary body 364.57
    - spine or vertebra (*see also* Spondylosis) 721.90
  - dental pulp, regressive 522.2
  - drains V58.49
  - dressing
    - wound V58.30
      - nonsurgical V58.30
      - surgical V58.31
  - fixation device V54.89
    - external V54.89
    - internal V54.01
  - heart - *see also* Disease, heart
  - hip joint 718.95
  - hyperplastic larynx 478.79
- **Change(s) (of)** *(Continued)*
  - hypertrophic
    - nasal sinus (*see also* Sinusitis) 473.9
    - turbinate, nasal 478.0
    - upper respiratory tract 478.9
  - inflammatory - *see* Inflammation
  - joint (*see also* Derangement, joint) 718.90
    - sacroiliac 724.6
  - Kirschner wire V54.89
  - knee 717.9
  - macular, congenital 743.55
  - malignant (M----/3) - *see also* Neoplasm, by site, malignant

> Note For malignant change occurring in a neoplasm, use the appropriate M code with behavior digit/3 e.g., malignant change in uterine fibroid-M8890/3. For malignant change occurring in a nonneoplastic condition (e.g., gastric ulcer) use the M code M8000/3.

  - mental (status) NEC 780.97
    - due to or associated with physical condition - *see* Syndrome, brain
  - myocardium, myocardial - *see* Degeneration, myocardial
  - of life (*see also* Menopause) 627.2
  - pacemaker battery (cardiac) V53.31
  - peripheral nerve 355.9
  - personality (nonpsychotic) NEC 310.1
  - plaster cast V54.89
  - refractive, transient 367.81
  - regressive, dental pulp 522.2
  - retina 362.9
    - myopic (degenerative) (malignant) 360.21
    - vascular appearance 362.13
  - sacroiliac joint 724.6
  - scleral 379.19
    - degenerative 379.16
  - senile (*see also* Senility) 797
  - sensory (*see also* Disturbance, sensation) 782.0
  - skin texture 782.8
  - spinal cord 336.9
  - splint, external V54.89
  - subdermal implantable contraceptive V25.5
  - suture V58.32
  - traction device V54.89
  - trophic 355.9
    - arm NEC 354.9
    - leg NEC 355.8
    - lower extremity NEC 355.8
    - upper extremity NEC 354.9
  - vascular 459.9
  - vasomotor 443.9
  - voice 784.49
    - psychogenic 306.1
  - wound packing V58.30
    - nonsurgical V58.30
    - surgical V58.31
- **Changing sleep-work schedule, affecting sleep** 327.36
- **Changuinola fever** 066.0
- **Chapping skin** 709.8
- **Character**
  - depressive 301.12
- **Charcôt's**
  - arthropathy 094.0 *[713.5]*
  - [illegible] - *see* Cirrhosis, biliary
  - disease 094.0
    - spinal cord 094.0
- **Charcôt's** *(Continued)*
  - fever (biliary) (hepatic) (intermittent) - *see* Choledocholithiasis
  - joint (disease) 094.0 *[713.5]*
    - diabetic 250.6 *[713.5]*
    - syringomyelic 336.0 *[713.5]*
  - syndrome (intermittent claudication) 443.9
    - due to atherosclerosis 440.21
- **Charcôt-Marie-Tooth disease, paralysis, or syndrome** 356.1
- **CHARGE association** (syndrome) 759.89
- **Charleyhorse** (quadriceps) 843.8
  - muscle, except quadriceps - *see* Sprain, by site
- **Charlouis' disease** (*see also* Yaws) 102.9
- **Chauffeur's fracture** - *see* Fracture, ulna, lower end
- **Cheadle** (-Möller) (-Barlow) disease or syndrome (infantile scurvy) 267
- **Checking** (of)
  - contraceptive device (intrauterine) V25.42
  - device
    - fixation V54.89
      - external V54.89
      - internal V54.09
    - traction V54.89
  - Kirschner wire V54.89
  - plaster cast V54.89
  - splint, external V54.89
- **Checkup**
  - following treatment - *see* Examination
  - health V70.0
  - infant (not sick) V20.2
  - newborn, routine
    - initial V20.2
    - subsequent V20.2
  - pregnancy (normal) V22.1
    - first V22.0
    - high-risk pregnancy V23.9
      - specified problem NEC V23.89
- **Chédiak-Higashi** (-Steinbrinck) anomaly, disease, or syndrome (congenital gigantism of peroxidase granules) 288.2
- **Cheek** - *see also* condition
  - biting 528.9
- **Cheese itch** 133.8
- **Cheese washers' lung** 495.8
- **Cheilitis** 528.5
  - actinic (due to sun) 692.72
    - chronic NEC 692.74
      - due to radiation, except from sun 692.82
    - due to radiation, except from sun 692.82
  - acute 528.5
  - angular 528.5
  - catarrhal 528.5
  - chronic 528.5
  - exfoliative 528.5
  - gangrenous 528.5
  - glandularis apostematosa 528.5
  - granulomatosa 351.8
  - infectional 528.5
  - membranous 528.5
  - Miescher's 351.8
  - suppurative 528.5
  - ulcerative 528.5
  - vesicular 528.5
- **Cheilodynia** 528.5
- **Cheilopalatoschisis** (*see also* Cleft, palate, with cleft lip) 749.20
- **Cheilophagia** 528.9

◀ **New** ⬅ **Revised**

Cheiloschisis (*see also* Cleft, lip) 749.10
Cheilosis 528.5
with pellagra 265.2
angular 528.5
due to
dietary deficiency 266.0
vitamin deficiency 266.0
Cheiromegaly 729.89
Cheiropompholyx 705.81
Cheloid (*see also* Keloid) 701.4
Chemical burn - *see also* Burn, by site
from swallowing chemical - *see* Burn, internal organs
Chemodectoma (M8693/1) - *see* Paraganglioma, nonchromaffin
Chemoprophylaxis NEC V07.39
Chemosis, conjunctiva 372.73
Chemotherapy
convalescence V66.2
encounter (for) V58.11
maintenance V58.11
prophylactic NEC V07.39
fluoride V07.31
Cherubism 526.89
Chest - *see* condition
Cheyne-Stokes respiration (periodic) 786.04
Chiari's
disease or syndrome (hepatic vein thrombosis) 453.0
malformation
type I 348.4
type II (*see also* Spina bifida) 741.0
type III 742.0
type IV 742.2
network 746.89
Chiari-Frommel syndrome 676.6
Chicago disease (North American blastomycosis) 116.0
Chickenpox (*see also* Varicella) 052.9
exposure to V01.71
vaccination and inoculation (prophylactic) V05.4
Chiclero ulcer 085.4
Chiggers 133.8
Chignon 111.2
fetus or newborn (from vacuum extraction) 767.19
Chigoe disease 134.1
Chikungunya fever 066.3
Chilaiditi's syndrome (subphrenic displacement, colon) 751.4
Chilblains 991.5
lupus 991.5
Child
behavior causing concern V61.20
Childbed fever 670
Childbirth - *see also* Delivery
puerperal complications - *see* Puerperal
Childhood, period of rapid growth V21.0
Chill(s) 780.99
with fever 780.6
congestive 780.99
in malarial regions 084.6
septic - *see* Septicemia
urethral 599.84
Chilomastigiasis 007.8
Chin - *see* condition
Chinese dysentery 004.9
Chiropractic dislocation (*see also* Lesion, nonallopathic, by site) 739.9
Chitral fever 066.0
Chlamydia, chlamydial - *see* condition
Chloasma 709.09
cachecticorum 709.09
Chloasma *(Continued)*
eyelid 374.52
congenital 757.33
hyperthyroid 242.0
gravidarum 646.8
idiopathic 709.09
skin 709.09
symptomatic 709.09
Chloroma (M9930/3) 205.3
Chlorosis 280.9
Egyptian (*see also* Ancylostomiasis) 126.9
miners' (*see also* Ancylostomiasis) 126.9
Chlorotic anemia 280.9
Chocolate cyst (ovary) 617.1
Choked
disk or disc - *see* Papilledema
on food, phlegm, or vomitus NEC (*see also* Asphyxia, food) 933.1
phlegm 933.1
while vomiting NEC (*see also* Asphyxia, food) 933.1
Chokes (resulting from bends) 993.3
Choking sensation 784.99 ⬅
Cholangiectasis (*see also* Disease, gallbladder) 575.8
Cholangiocarcinoma (M8160/3)
and hepatocellular carcinoma, combined (M8180/3) 155.0
liver 155.1
specified site NEC - *see* Neoplasm, by site, malignant
unspecified site 155.1
Cholangiohepatitis 575.8
due to fluke infestation 121.1
Cholangiohepatoma (M8180/3) 155.0
Cholangiolitis (acute) (chronic) (extrahepatic) (gangrenous) 576.1
intrahepatic 575.8
paratyphoidal (*see also* Fever, paratyphoid) 002.9
typhoidal 002.0
Cholangioma (M8160/0) 211.5
malignant - *see* Cholangiocarcinoma
Cholangitis (acute) (ascending) (catarrhal) (chronic) (infective) (malignant) (primary) (recurrent) (sclerosing) (secondary) (stenosing) (suppurative) 576.1
chronic nonsuppurative destructive 571.6
nonsuppurative destructive (chronic) 571.6
Cholecystdocholithiasis - *see* Choledocholithiasis
Cholecystitis 575.10
with
calculus, stones in
bile duct (common) (hepatic) - *see* Choledocholithiasis
gallbladder - *see* Cholelithiasis
acute 575.0
acute and chronic 575.12
chronic 575.11
emphysematous (acute) (*see also* Cholecystitis, acute) 575.0
gangrenous (*see also* Cholecystitis, acute) 575.0
paratyphoidal, current (*see also* Fever, paratyphoid) 002.9
suppurative (*see also* Cholecystitis, acute) 575.0
typhoidal 002.0
Choledochitis (suppurative) 576.1
Choledocholith - *see* Choledocholithiasis
Choledocholithiasis 574.5

Note Use the following fifth-digit subclassification with category 574:
0 without mention of obstruction
1 with obstruction

with
cholecystitis 574.4
acute 574.3
chronic 574.4
cholelithiasis 574.9
with
cholecystitis 574.7
acute 574.6
and chronic 574.8
chronic 574.7
Cholelithiasis (impacted) (multiple) 574.2

Note Use the following fifth-digit subclassification with category 574:
0 without mention of obstruction
1 with obstruction

with
cholecystitis 574.1
acute 574.0
chronic 574.1
choledocholithiasis 574.9
with
cholecystitis 574.7
acute 574.6
and chronic 574.8
chronic cholecystitis 574.7
Cholemia (*see also* Jaundice) 782.4
familial 277.4
Gilbert's (familial nonhemolytic) 277.4
Cholemic gallstone - *see* Cholelithiasis
Choleperitoneum, choleperitonitis (*see also* Disease, gallbladder) 567.81
Cholera (algid) (Asiatic) (asphyctic) (epidemic) (gravis) (Indian) (malignant) (morbus) (pestilential) (spasmodic) 001.9
antimonial 985.4
carrier (suspected) of V02.0
classical 001.0
contact V01.0
due to
Vibrio
cholerae (Inaba, Ogawa, Hikojima serotypes) 001.0
el Tor 001.1
el Tor 001.1
exposure to V01.0
vaccination, prophylactic (against) V03.0
Cholerine (*see also* Cholera) 001.9
Cholestasis 576.8
due to total parenteral nutrition (TPN) 573.8 ◀
Cholesteatoma (ear) 385.30
attic (primary) 385.31
diffuse 385.35
external ear (canal) 380.21
marginal (middle ear) 385.32
with involvement of mastoid cavity 385.33
secondary (with middle ear involvement) 385.33
mastoid cavity 385.30
middle ear (secondary) 385.32
with involvement of mastoid cavity 385.33

ICD-9-CM C Vol. 2

Cholesteatoma *(Continued)*
postmastoidectomy cavity (recurrent) 383.32
primary 385.31
recurrent, postmastoidectomy cavity 383.32
secondary (middle ear) 385.32
with involvement of mastoid cavity 385.33
Cholesteatosis (middle ear) (*see also* Cholesteatoma) 385.30
diffuse 385.35
Cholesteremia 272.0
Cholesterin
granuloma, middle ear 385.82
in vitreous 379.22
Cholesterol
deposit
retina 362.82
vitreous 379.22
imbibition of gallbladder (*see also* Disease, gallbladder) 575.6
Cholesterolemia 272.0
essential 272.0
familial 272.0
hereditary 272.0
Cholesterosis, cholesterolosis (gallbladder) 575.6
with
cholecystitis - *see* Cholecystitis
cholelithiasis - *see* Cholelithiasis
middle ear (*see also* Cholesteatoma) 385.30
Cholocolic fistula (*see also* Fistula, gallbladder) 575.5
Choluria 791.4
Chondritis (purulent) 733.99
auricle 380.03
costal 733.6
Tietze's 733.6
patella, posttraumatic 717.7
pinna 380.03
posttraumatica patellae 717.7
tuberculous (active) (*see also* Tuberculosis) 015.9
intervertebral 015.0 *[730.88]*
Chondroangiopathia calcarea seu punctate 756.59
Chondroblastoma (M9230/0) - *see also* Neoplasm, bone, benign
malignant (M9230/3) - *see* Neoplasm, bone, malignant
Chondrocalcinosis (articular) (crystal deposition) (dihydrate) (*see also* Arthritis, due to, crystals) 275.49 [712.3]
due to
calcium pyrophosphate 275.49 *[712.2]*
dicalcium phosphate crystals 275.49 *[712.1]*
pyrophosphate crystals 275.49 *[712.2]*
Chondrodermatitis nodularis helicis 380.00
Chondrodysplasia 756.4
angiomatose 756.4
calcificans congenita 756.59
epiphysialis punctata 756.59
hereditary deforming 756.4
rhizomelic punctata 277.86
Chondrodystrophia (fetalis) 756.4
calcarea 756.4
calcificans congenita 756.59
fetalis hypoplastica 756.59
hypoplastica calcinosa 756.59
punctata 756.59
tarda 277.5
Chondrodystrophy (familial) (hypoplastic) 756.4
Chondroectodermal dysplasia 756.55
Chondrolysis 733.99
Chondroma (M9220/0) - *see also* Neoplasm, cartilage, benign
juxtacortical (M9221/0) - *see* Neoplasm, bone, benign
periosteal (M9221/0) - *see* Neoplasm, bone, benign
Chondromalacia 733.92
epiglottis (congenital) 748.3
generalized 733.92
knee 717.7
larynx (congenital) 748.3
localized, except patella 733.92
patella, patellae 717.7
systemic 733.92
tibial plateau 733.92
trachea (congenital) 748.3
Chondromatosis (M9220/1) - *see* Neoplasm, cartilage, uncertain behavior
Chondromyxosarcoma (M9220/3) - *see* Neoplasm, cartilage, malignant
Chondro-osteodysplasia (Morquio-Brailsford type) 277.5
Chondro-osteodystrophy 277.5
Chondro-osteoma (M9210/0) - *see* Neoplasm, bone, benign
Chondropathia tuberosa 733.6
Chondrosarcoma (M9220/3) - *see also* Neoplasm, cartilage, malignant
juxtacortical (M9221/3) - *see* Neoplasm, bone, malignant
mesenchymal (M9240/3) - *see* Neoplasm, connective tissue, malignant
Chordae tendineae rupture (chronic) 429.5
Chordee (nonvenereal) 607.89
congenital 752.63
gonococcal 098.2
Chorditis (fibrinous) (nodosa) (tuberosa) 478.5
Chordoma (M9370/3) - *see* Neoplasm, by site, malignant
Chorea (gravis) (minor) (spasmodic) 333.5
with
heart involvement - *see* Chorea with rheumatic heart disease
rheumatic heart disease (chronic, inactive, or quiescent) (conditions classifiable to 393–398) - *see* rheumatic heart condition involved
active or acute (conditions classifiable to 391) 392.0
acute - *see* Chorea, Sydenham's
apoplectic (*see also* Disease, cerebrovascular, acute) 436
chronic 333.4
electric 049.8
gravidarum - *see* Eclampsia, pregnancy
habit 307.22
hereditary 333.4
Huntington's 333.4
posthemiplegic 344.89
pregnancy - *see* Eclampsia, pregnancy
progressive 333.4
chronic 333.4
hereditary 333.4
rheumatic (chronic) 392.9
with heart disease or involvement - *see* Chorea, with rheumatic heart disease
senile 333.5
Sydenham's 392.9
with heart involvement - *see* Chorea, with rheumatic heart disease
Chorea *(Continued)*
Sydenham's *(Continued)*
nonrheumatic 333.5
variabilis 307.23
Choreoathetosis (paroxysmal) 333.5
Chorioadenoma (destruens) (M9100/1) 236.1
Chorioamnionitis 658.4
affecting fetus or newborn 762.7
Chorioangioma (M9120/0) 219.8
Choriocarcinoma (M9100/3)
combined with
embryonal carcinoma (M9101/3) - *see* Neoplasm, by site, malignant
teratoma (M9101/3) - *see* Neoplasm, by site, malignant
specified site - *see* Neoplasm, by site, malignant
unspecified site
female 181
male 186.9
Chorioencephalitis, lymphocytic (acute) (serous) 049.0
Chorioepithelioma (M9100/3) - *see* Choriocarcinoma
Choriomeningitis (acute) (benign) (lymphocytic) (serous) 049.0
Chorionepithelioma (M9100/3) - *see* Choriocarcinoma
Chorionitis (*see also* Scleroderma) 710.1
Chorioretinitis 363.20
disseminated 363.10
generalized 363.13
in
neurosyphilis 094.83
secondary syphilis 091.51
peripheral 363.12
posterior pole 363.11
tuberculous (*see also* Tuberculosis) 017.3 *[363.13]*
due to
histoplasmosis (*see also* Histoplasmosis) 115.92
toxoplasmosis (acquired) 130.2
congenital (active) 771.2
focal 363.00
juxtapapillary 363.01
peripheral 363.04
posterior pole NEC 363.03
juxtapapillaris, juxtapapillary 363.01
progressive myopia (degeneration) 360.21
syphilitic (secondary) 091.51
congenital (early) 090.0 *[363.13]*
late 090.5 *[363.13]*
late 095.8 *[363.13]*
tuberculous (*see also* Tuberculosis) 017.3 *[363.13]*
Choristoma - *see* Neoplasm, by site, benign
Choroid - *see* condition
Choroideremia, choroidermia (initial stage) (late stage) (partial or total atrophy) 363.55
Choroiditis (*see also* Chorioretinitis) 363.20
leprous 030.9 *[363.13]*
senile guttate 363.41
sympathetic 360.11
syphilitic (secondary) 091.51
congenital (early) 090.0 *[363.13]*
late 090.5 *[363.13]*
late 095.8 *[363.13]*
Tay's 363.41

Choroiditis *(Continued)*
tuberculous (*see also* Tuberculosis) 017.3 *[363.13]*
Choroidopathy NEC 363.9
degenerative (*see also* Degeneration, choroid) 363.40
hereditary (*see also* Dystrophy, choroid) 363.50
specified type NEC 363.8
Choroidoretinitis - *see* Chorioretinitis
Choroidosis, central serous 362.41
Choroidretinopathy, serous 362.41
Christian's syndrome (chronic histiocytosis X) 277.89
Christian-Weber disease (nodular nonsuppurative panniculitis) 729.30
Christmas disease 286.1
Chromaffinoma (M8700/0) - *see also* Neoplasm, by site, benign
malignant (M8700/3) - *see* Neoplasm, by site, malignant
Chromatopsia 368.59
Chromhidrosis, chromidrosis 705.89
Chromoblastomycosis 117.2
Chromomycosis 117.2
Chromophytosis 111.0
Chromotrichomycosis 111.8
Chronic - *see* condition
Churg-Strauss syndrome 446.4
Chyle cyst, mesentery 457.8
Chylocele (nonfilarial) 457.8
filarial (*see also* Infestation, filarial) 125.9
tunica vaginalis (nonfilarial) 608.84
filarial (*see also* Infestation, filarial) 125.9
Chylomicronemia (fasting) (with hyperprebetalipoproteinemia) 272.3
Chylopericardium (acute) 420.90
Chylothorax (nonfilarial) 457.8
filarial (*see also* Infestation, filarial) 125.9
Chylous
ascites 457.8
cyst of peritoneum 457.8
hydrocele 603.9
hydrothorax (nonfilarial) 457.8
filarial (*see also* Infestation, filarial) 125.9
Chyluria 791.1
bilharziasis 120.0
due to
Brugia (malayi) 125.1
Wuchereria (bancrofti) 125.0
malayi 125.1
filarial (*see also* Infestation, filarial) 125.9
filariasis (*see also* Infestation, filarial) 125.9
nonfilarial 791.1
Cicatricial (deformity) - *see* Cicatrix
Cicatrix (adherent) (contracted) (painful) (vicious) 709.2
adenoid 474.8
alveolar process 525.8
anus 569.49
auricle 380.89
bile duct (*see also* Disease, biliary) 576.8
bladder 596.8
bone 733.99
brain 348.8
cervix (postoperative) (postpartal) 622.3
in pregnancy or childbirth 654.6
causing obstructed labor 660.2
chorioretinal 363.30
disseminated 363.35
macular 363.32
peripheral 363.34
posterior pole NEC 363.33
Cicatrix *(Continued)*
choroid - *see* Cicatrix, chorioretinal
common duct (*see also* Disease, biliary) 576.8
congenital 757.39
conjunctiva 372.64
cornea 371.00
tuberculous (*see also* Tuberculosis) 017.3 *[371.05]*
duodenum (bulb) 537.3
esophagus 530.3
eyelid 374.46
with
ectropion - *see* Ectropion
entropion - *see* Entropion
hypopharynx 478.29
knee, semilunar cartilage 717.5
lacrimal
canaliculi 375.53
duct
acquired 375.56
neonatal 375.55
punctum 375.52
sac 375.54
larynx 478.79
limbus (cystoid) 372.64
lung 518.89
macular 363.32
disseminated 363.35
peripheral 363.34
middle ear 385.89
mouth 528.9
muscle 728.89
nasolacrimal duct
acquired 375.56
neonatal 375.55
nasopharynx 478.29
palate (soft) 528.9
penis 607.89
prostate 602.8
rectum 569.49
retina 363.30
disseminated 363.35
macular 363.32
peripheral 363.34
posterior pole NEC 363.33
semilunar cartilage - *see* Derangement, meniscus
seminal vesicle 608.89
skin 709.2
infected 686.8
postinfectional 709.2
tuberculous (*see also* Tuberculosis) 017.0
specified site NEC 709.2
throat 478.29
tongue 529.8
tonsil (and adenoid) 474.8
trachea 478.9
tuberculous NEC (*see also* Tuberculosis) 011.9
ureter 593.89
urethra 599.84
uterus 621.8
vagina 623.4
in pregnancy or childbirth 654.7
causing obstructed labor 660.2
vocal cord 478.5
wrist, constricting (annular) 709.2
CIN I [cervical intraepithelial neoplasia I] 622.11
CIN II [cervical intraepithelial neoplasia II] 622.12
CIN III [cervical intraepithelial neoplasia III] 233.1
Cinchonism
correct substance properly administered 386.9
overdose or wrong substance given or taken 961.4
Circine herpes 110.5
Circle of Willis - *see* condition
Circular - *see also* condition
hymen 752.49
Circulating anticoagulants 286.5
following childbirth 666.3
postpartum 666.3
Circulation
collateral (venous), any site 459.89
defective 459.9
congenital 747.9
lower extremity 459.89
embryonic 747.9
failure 799.89
fetus or newborn 779.89
peripheral 785.59
fetal, persistent 747.83
heart, incomplete 747.9
Circulatory system - *see* condition
Circulus senilis 371.41
Circumcision
in absence of medical indication V50.2
ritual V50.2
routine V50.2
Circumscribed - *see* condition
Circumvallata placenta - *see* Placenta, abnormal
Cirrhosis, cirrhotic 571.5
with alcoholism 571.2
alcoholic (liver) 571.2
atrophic (of liver) - *see* Cirrhosis, portal
Baumgarten-Cruveilhier 571.5
biliary (cholangiolitic) (cholangitic) (cholestatic) (extrahepatic) (hypertrophic) (intrahepatic) (nonobstructive) (obstructive) (pericholangiolitic) (posthepatic) (primary) (secondary) (xanthomatous) 571.6
due to
clonorchiasis 121.1
flukes 121.3
brain 331.9
capsular - *see* Cirrhosis, portal
cardiac 571.5
alcoholic 571.2
central (liver) - *see* Cirrhosis, liver
Charcôt's 571.6
cholangiolitic - *see* Cirrhosis, biliary
cholangitic - *see* Cirrhosis, biliary
cholestatic - *see* Cirrhosis, biliary
clitoris (hypertrophic) 624.2
coarsely nodular 571.5
congestive (liver) - *see* Cirrhosis, cardiac
Cruveilhier-Baumgarten 571.5
cryptogenic (of liver) 571.5
alcoholic 571.2
dietary (*see also* Cirrhosis, portal) 571.5
due to
bronzed diabetes 275.0
congestive hepatomegaly - *see* Cirrhosis, cardiac
cystic fibrosis 277.00
hemochromatosis 275.0
hepatolenticular degeneration 275.1
passive congestion (chronic) - *see* Cirrhosis, cardiac
Wilson's disease 275.1
xanthomatosis 272.2

ICD-9-CM
C
Vol. 2

Cirrhosis, cirrhotic *(Continued)*
extrahepatic (obstructive) - *see* Cirrhosis, biliary
fatty 571.8
alcoholic 571.0
florid 571.2
Glisson's - *see* Cirrhosis, portal
Hanot's (hypertrophic) - *see* Cirrhosis, biliary
hepatic - *see* Cirrhosis, liver
hepatolienal - *see* Cirrhosis, liver
hobnail - *see* Cirrhosis, portal
hypertrophic - *see also* Cirrhosis, liver
biliary - *see* Cirrhosis, biliary
Hanot's - *see* Cirrhosis, biliary
infectious NEC - *see* Cirrhosis, portal
insular - *see* Cirrhosis, portal
intrahepatic (obstructive) (primary) (secondary) - *see* Cirrhosis, biliary
juvenile (*see also* Cirrhosis, portal) 571.5
kidney (*see also* Sclerosis, renal) 587
Laennec's (of liver) 571.2
nonalcoholic 571.5
liver (chronic) (hepatolienal) (hypertrophic) (nodular) (splenomegalic) (unilobar) 571.5
with alcoholism 571.2
alcoholic 571.2
congenital (due to failure of obliteration of umbilical vein) 777.8
cryptogenic 571.5
alcoholic 571.2
fatty 571.8
alcoholic 571.0
macronodular 571.5
alcoholic 571.2
micronodular 571.5
alcoholic 571.2
nodular, diffuse 571.5
alcoholic 571.2
pigmentary 275.0
portal 571.5
alcoholic 571.2
postnecrotic 571.5
alcoholic 571.2
syphilitic 095.3
lung (chronic) (*see also* Fibrosis, lung) 515
macronodular (of liver) 571.5
alcoholic 571.2
malarial 084.9
metabolic NEC 571.5
micronodular (of liver) 571.5
alcoholic 571.2
monolobular - *see* Cirrhosis, portal
multilobular - *see* Cirrhosis, portal
nephritis (*see also* Sclerosis, renal) 587
nodular - *see* Cirrhosis, liver
nutritional (fatty) 571.5
obstructive (biliary) (extrahepatic) (intrahepatic) - *see* Cirrhosis, biliary
ovarian 620.8
paludal 084.9
pancreas (duct) 577.8
pericholangiolitic - *see* Cirrhosis, biliary
periportal - *see* Cirrhosis, portal
pigment, pigmentary (of liver) 275.0
portal (of liver) 571.5
alcoholic 571.2
posthepatitic (*see also* Cirrhosis, postnecrotic) 571.5
postnecrotic (of liver) 571.5
alcoholic 571.2
primary (intrahepatic) - *see* Cirrhosis, biliary

Cirrhosis, cirrhotic *(Continued)*
pulmonary (*see also* Fibrosis, lung) 515
renal (*see also* Sclerosis, renal) 587
septal (*see also* Cirrhosis, postnecrotic) 571.5
spleen 289.51
splenomegalic (of liver) - *see* Cirrhosis, liver
stasis (liver) - *see* Cirrhosis, liver
stomach 535.4
Todd's (*see also* Cirrhosis, biliary) 571.6
toxic (nodular) - *see* Cirrhosis, postnecrotic
trabecular - *see* Cirrhosis, postnecrotic
unilobar - *see* Cirrhosis, liver
vascular (of liver) - *see* Cirrhosis, liver
xanthomatous (biliary) (*see also* Cirrhosis, biliary) 571.6
due to xanthomatosis (familial) (metabolic) (primary) 272.2
Cistern, subarachnoid 793.0
Citrullinemia 270.6
Citrullinuria 270.6
Ciuffini-Pancoast tumor (M8010/3) (carcinoma, pulmonary apex) 162.3
Civatte's disease or poikiloderma 709.09
Clam diggers' itch 120.3
Clap - *see* Gonorrhea
Clark's paralysis 343.9
Clarke-Hadfield syndrome (pancreatic infantilism) 577.8
Clastothrix 704.2
Claude's syndrome 352.6
Claude Bernard-Horner syndrome (*see also* Neuropathy, peripheral, autonomic) 337.9
Claudication, intermittent 443.9
cerebral (artery) (*see also* Ischemia, cerebral, transient) 435.9
due to atherosclerosis 440.21
spinal cord (arteriosclerotic) 435.1
syphilitic 094.89
spinalis 435.1
venous (axillary) 453.8
Claudicatio venosa intermittens 453.8
Claustrophobia 300.29
Clavus (infected) 700
Clawfoot (congenital) 754.71
acquired 736.74
Clawhand (acquired) 736.06
congenital 755.59
Clawtoe (congenital) 754.71
acquired 735.5
Clay eating 307.52
Clay shovelers' fracture - *see* Fracture, vertebra, cervical
Cleansing of artificial opening (*see also* Attention to artificial opening) V55.9
Cleft (congenital) - *see also* Imperfect, closure
alveolar process 525.8
branchial (persistent) 744.41
cyst 744.42
clitoris 752.49
cricoid cartilage, posterior 748.3
facial (*see also* Cleft, lip) 749.10
lip 749.10
with cleft palate 749.20
bilateral (lip and palate) 749.24
with unilateral lip or palate 749.25
complete 749.23
incomplete 749.24
unilateral (lip and palate) 749.22
with bilateral lip or palate 749.25

Cleft *(Continued)*
lip *(Continued)*
with cleft palate *(Continued)*
unilateral *(Continued)*
complete 749.21
incomplete 749.22
bilateral 749.14
with cleft palate, unilateral 749.25
complete 749.13
incomplete 749.14
unilateral 749.12
with cleft palate, bilateral 749.25
complete 749.11
incomplete 749.12
nose 748.1
palate 749.00
with cleft lip 749.20
bilateral (lip and palate) 749.24
with unilateral lip or palate 749.25
complete 749.23
incomplete 749.24
unilateral (lip and palate) 749.22
with bilateral lip or palate 749.25
complete 749.21
incomplete 749.22
bilateral 749.04
with cleft lip, unilateral 749.25
complete 749.03
incomplete 749.04
unilateral 749.02
with cleft lip, bilateral 749.25
complete 749.01
incomplete 749.02
penis 752.69
posterior, cricoid cartilage 748.3
scrotum 752.89
sternum (congenital) 756.3
thyroid cartilage (congenital) 748.3
tongue 750.13
uvula 749.02
with cleft lip (*see also* Cleft, lip, with cleft palate) 749.20
water 366.12
Cleft hand (congenital) 755.58
Cleidocranial dysostosis 755.59
Cleidotomy, fetal 763.89
Cleptomania 312.32
Clérambault's syndrome 297.8
erotomania 302.89
Clergyman's sore throat 784.49
Click, clicking
systolic syndrome 785.2
Clifford's syndrome (postmaturity) 766.22
Climacteric (*see also* Menopause) 627.2
arthritis NEC (*see also* Arthritis, climacteric) 716.3
depression (*see also* Psychosis, affective) 296.2
disease 627.2
recurrent episode 296.3
single episode 296.2
female (symptoms) 627.2
male (symptoms) (syndrome) 608.89
melancholia (*see also* Psychosis, affective) 296.2
recurrent episode 296.3
single episode 296.2
paranoid state 297.2
paraphrenia 297.2
polyarthritis NEC 716.39
male 608.89
symptoms (female) 627.2
Clinical research investigation (control) (participant) V70.7

◀ New ⟸ Revised

- **Clinodactyly** 755.59
- **Clitoris** - *see* condition
- **Cloaca, persistent** 751.5
- **Clonorchiasis** 121.1
- **Clonorchiosis** 121.1
- **Clonorchis infection, liver** 121.1
- **Clonus** 781.0
- **Closed bite** 524.20
- **Closed surgical procedure converted to open procedure**
  - arthroscopic V64.43
  - laparoscopic V64.41
  - thoracoscopic V64.42
- **Closure**
  - artificial opening (*see also* Attention to artificial opening) V55.9
  - congenital, nose 748.0
  - cranial sutures, premature 756.0
  - defective or imperfect NEC - *see* Imperfect, closure
  - fistula, delayed - *see* Fistula
  - fontanelle, delayed 756.0
  - foramen ovale, imperfect 745.5
  - hymen 623.3
  - interauricular septum, defective 745.5
  - interventricular septum, defective 745.4
  - lacrimal duct 375.56
    - congenital 743.65
    - neonatal 375.55
  - nose (congenital) 748.0
    - acquired 738.0
  - vagina 623.2
  - valve - *see* Endocarditis
  - vulva 624.8
- **Clot** (blood)
  - artery (obstruction) (occlusion) (*see also* Embolism) 444.9
  - atrial appendage 429.89 ◄
  - bladder 596.7
  - brain (extradural or intradural) (*see also* Thrombosis, brain) 434.0
    - late effect - *see* Late effect(s) (of) cerebrovascular disease
  - circulation 444.9
  - heart (*see also* Infarct, myocardium) 410.9
    - without myocardial infarction 429.89 ◄
  - vein (*see also* Thrombosis) 453.9
- **Clotting defect NEC** (*see also* Defect, coagulation) 286.9
- **Clouded state** 780.09
  - epileptic (*see also* Epilepsy) 345.9
  - paroxysmal (idiopathic) (*see also* Epilepsy) 345.9
- **Clouding**
  - corneal graft 996.51
- **Cloudy**
  - antrum, antra 473.0
  - dialysis effluent 792.5
- **Clouston's** (hidrotic) ectodermal dysplasia 757.31
- **Clubbing of fingers** 781.5
- **Clubfinger** 736.29
  - acquired 736.29
  - congenital 754.89
- **Clubfoot** (congenital) 754.70
  - acquired 736.71
  - equinovarus 754.51
  - paralytic 736.71
- **Club hand** (congenital) 754.89
  - acquired 736.07
- **Clubnail** (acquired) 703.8
  - congenital 757.5
- **Clump kidney** 753.3
- **Clumsiness** 781.3
  - syndrome 315.4
- **Cluttering** 307.0
- **Clutton's joints** 090.5
- **Coagulation, intravascular** (diffuse) (disseminated) (*see also* Fibrinolysis) 286.6
  - newborn 776.2
- **Coagulopathy** (*see also* Defect, coagulation) 286.9
  - consumption 286.6
  - intravascular (disseminated) NEC 286.6
    - newborn 776.2
- **Coalition**
  - calcaneoscaphoid 755.67
  - calcaneus 755.67
  - tarsal 755.67
- **Coal miners'**
  - elbow 727.2
  - lung 500
- **Coal workers' lung or pneumoconiosis** 500
- **Coarctation**
  - aorta (postductal) (preductal) 747.10
  - pulmonary artery 747.3
- **Coated tongue** 529.3
- **Coats' disease** 362.12
- **Cocainism** (*see also* Dependence) 304.2
- **Coccidioidal granuloma** 114.3
- **Coccidioidomycosis** 114.9
  - with pneumonia 114.0
  - cutaneous (primary) 114.1
  - disseminated 114.3
  - extrapulmonary (primary) 114.1
  - lung 114.5
    - acute 114.0
    - chronic 114.4
    - primary 114.0
  - meninges 114.2
  - primary (pulmonary) 114.0
    - acute 114.0
  - prostate 114.3
  - pulmonary 114.5
    - acute 114.0
    - chronic 114.4
    - primary 114.0
  - specified site NEC 114.3
- **Coccidioidosis** 114.9
  - lung 114.5
    - acute 114.0
    - chronic 114.4
    - primary 114.0
  - meninges 114.2
- **Coccidiosis** (colitis) (diarrhea) (dysentery) 007.2
- **Cocciuria** 791.9
- **Coccus in urine** 791.9
- **Coccydynia** 724.79
- **Coccygodynia** 724.79
- **Coccyx** - *see* condition
- **Cochin-China**
  - diarrhea 579.1
    - anguilluliasis 127.2
  - ulcer 085.1
- **Cock's peculiar tumor** 706.2
- **Cockayne's disease or syndrome** (microcephaly and dwarfism) 759.89
- **Cockayne-Weber syndrome** (epidermolysis bullosa) 757.39
- **Cocked-up toe** 735.2
- **Codman's tumor** (benign chondroblastoma) (M9230/0) - *see* Neoplasm, bone, benign
- **Coenurosis** 123.8
- **Coffee workers' lung** 495.8
- **Cogan's syndrome** 370.52
  - congenital oculomotor apraxia 379.51
  - nonsyphilitic interstitial keratitis 370.52
- **Coiling, umbilical cord** - *see* Complications, umbilical cord
- **Coitus, painful** (female) 625.0
  - male 608.89
  - psychogenic 302.76
- **Cold** 460
  - with influenza, flu, or grippe 487.1
  - abscess - *see also* Tuberculosis, abscess
    - articular - *see* Tuberculosis, joint
  - agglutinin
    - disease (chronic) or syndrome 283.0
    - hemoglobinuria 283.0
      - paroxysmal (cold) (nocturnal) 283.2
  - allergic (*see also* Fever, hay) 477.9
  - bronchus or chest - *see* Bronchitis
    - with grippe or influenza 487.1
  - common (head) 460
    - vaccination, prophylactic (against) V04.7
  - deep 464.10
  - effects of 991.9
    - specified effect NEC 991.8
  - excessive 991.9
    - specified effect NEC 991.8
  - exhaustion from 991.8
  - exposure to 991.9
    - specified effect NEC 991.8
  - grippy 487.1
  - head 460
  - injury syndrome (newborn) 778.2
  - intolerance 780.99
  - on lung - *see* Bronchitis
  - rose 477.0
  - sensitivity, autoimmune 283.0
  - virus 460
- **Coldsore** (*see also* Herpes, simplex) 054.9
- **Colibacillosis** 041.4
  - generalized 038.42
- **Colibacilluria** 791.9
- **Colic** (recurrent) 789.0
  - abdomen 789.0
    - psychogenic 307.89
  - appendicular 543.9
  - appendix 543.9
  - bile duct - *see* Choledocholithiasis
  - biliary - *see* Cholelithiasis
  - bilious - *see* Cholelithiasis
  - common duct - *see* Choledocholithiasis
  - Devonshire NEC 984.9
    - specified type of lead - *see* Table of Drugs and Chemicals
  - flatulent 787.3
  - gallbladder or gallstone - *see* Cholelithiasis
  - gastric 536.8
  - hepatic (duct) - *see* Choledocholithiasis
  - hysterical 300.11
  - infantile 789.0
  - intestinal 789.0
  - kidney 788.0
  - lead NEC 984.9
    - specified type of lead - *see* Table of Drugs and Chemicals
  - liver (duct) - *see* Choledocholithiasis
  - mucous 564.9
    - psychogenic 316 *[564.9]*
  - nephritic 788.0
  - Painter's NEC 984.9
  - pancreas 577.8
  - psychogenic 306.4
  - renal 788.0

Colic *(Continued)*
saturnine NEC 984.9
specified type of lead - *see* Table of Drugs and Chemicals
spasmodic 789.0
ureter 788.0
urethral 599.84
due to calculus 594.2
uterus 625.8
menstrual 625.3
vermicular 543.9
virus 460
worm NEC 128.9
Colicystitis (*see also* Cystitis) 595.9
Colitis (acute) (catarrhal) (croupous) (cystica superficialis) (exudative) (hemorrhagic) (noninfectious) (phlegmonous) (presumed noninfectious) 558.9
adaptive 564.9
allergic 558.3
amebic (*see also* Amebiasis) 006.9
nondysenteric 006.2
anthrax 022.2
bacillary (*see also* Infection, Shigella) 004.9
balantidial 007.0
chronic 558.9
ulcerative (*see also* Colitis, ulcerative) 556.9
coccidial 007.2
dietetic 558.9
due to radiation 558.1
functional 558.9
gangrenous 009.0
giardial 007.1
granulomatous 555.1
gravis (*see also* Colitis, ulcerative) 556.9
infectious (*see also* Enteritis, due to, specific organism) 009.0
presumed 009.1
ischemic 557.9
acute 557.0
chronic 557.1
due to mesenteric artery insufficiency 557.1
membranous 564.9
psychogenic 316 *[564.9]*
mucous 564.9
psychogenic 316 *[564.9]*
necrotic 009.0
polyposa (*see also* Colitis, ulcerative) 556.9
protozoal NEC 007.9
pseudomembranous 008.45
pseudomucinous 564.9
regional 555.1
segmental 555.1
septic (*see also* Enteritis, due to, specific organism) 009.0
spastic 564.9
psychogenic 316 *[564.9]*
Staphylococcus 008.41
food 005.0
thromboulcerative 557.0
toxic 558.2
transmural 555.1
trichomonal 007.3
tuberculous (ulcerative) 014.8
ulcerative (chronic) (idiopathic) (nonspecific) 556.9
entero- 556.0
fulminant 557.0
ileo- 556.1
left-sided 556.5

Colitis *(Continued)*
ulcerative *(Continued)*
procto- 556.2
proctosigmoid 556.3
psychogenic 316 *[556]*
specified NEC 556.8
universal 556.6
Collagen disease NEC 710.9
nonvascular 710.9
vascular (allergic) (*see also* Angiitis, hypersensitivity) 446.20
Collagenosis (*see also* Collagen disease) 710.9
cardiovascular 425.4
mediastinal 519.3
Collapse 780.2
adrenal 255.8
cardiorenal (*see also* Hypertension, cardiorenal) 404.90
cardiorespiratory 785.51
fetus or newborn 779.85 ⬅
cardiovascular (*see also* Disease, heart) 785.51
fetus or newborn 779.85 ⬅
circulatory (peripheral) 785.59
with
abortion - *see* Abortion, by type, with shock
ectopic pregnancy (*see also* categories 633.0–633.9) 639.5
molar pregnancy (*see also* categories 630–632) 639.5
during or after labor and delivery 669.1
fetus or newborn 779.85 ⬅
following
abortion 639.5
ectopic or molar pregnancy 639.5
during or after labor and delivery 669.1
fetus or newborn 779.89
external ear canal 380.50
secondary to
inflammation 380.53
surgery 380.52
trauma 380.51
general 780.2
heart - *see* Disease, heart
heat 992.1
hysterical 300.11
labyrinth, membranous (congenital) 744.05
lung (massive) (*see also* Atelectasis) 518.0
pressure, during labor 668.0
myocardial - *see* Disease, heart
nervous (*see also* Disorder, mental, nonpsychotic) 300.9
neurocirculatory 306.2
nose 738.0
postoperative (cardiovascular) 998.0
pulmonary (*see also* Atelectasis) 518.0
fetus or newborn 770.5
partial 770.5
primary 770.4
thorax 512.8
iatrogenic 512.1
postoperative 512.1
trachea 519.19 ⬅
valvular - *see* Endocarditis
vascular (peripheral) 785.59
with
abortion - *see* Abortion, by type, with shock
ectopic pregnancy (*see also* categories 633.0–633.9) 639.5

Collapse *(Continued)*
vascular *(Continued)*
with *(Continued)*
molar pregnancy (*see also* categories 630–632) 639.5
cerebral (*see also* Disease, cerebrovascular, acute) 436
during or after labor and delivery 669.1
fetus or newborn 779.89
following
abortion 639.5
ectopic or molar pregnancy 639.5
vasomotor 785.59
vertebra 733.13
Collateral - *see also* condition
circulation (venous) 459.89
dilation, veins 459.89
Colles' fracture (closed) (reversed) (separation) 813.41
open 813.51
Collet's syndrome 352.6
Collet-Sicard syndrome 352.6
Colliculitis urethralis (*see also* Urethritis) 597.89
Colliers'
asthma 500
lung 500
phthisis (*see also* Tuberculosis) 011.4
Collodion baby (ichthyosis congenita) 757.1
Colloid milium 709.3
Coloboma NEC 743.49
choroid 743.59
fundus 743.52
iris 743.46
lens 743.36
lids 743.62
optic disc (congenital) 743.57
acquired 377.23
retina 743.56
sclera 743.47
Coloenteritis - *see* Enteritis
Colon - *see* condition
Coloptosis 569.89
Color
amblyopia NEC 368.59
acquired 368.55
blindness NEC (congenital) 368.59
acquired 368.55
Colostomy
attention to V55.3
fitting or adjustment V55.3
malfunctioning 569.62
status V44.3
Colpitis (*see also* Vaginitis) 616.10
Colpocele 618.6
Colpocystitis (*see also* Vaginitis) 616.10
Colporrhexis 665.4
Colpospasm 625.1
Column, spinal, vertebral - *see* condition
Coma 780.01
apoplectic (*see also* Disease, cerebrovascular, acute) 436
diabetic (with ketoacidosis) 250.3
hyperosmolar 250.2
eclamptic (*see also* Eclampsia) 780.39
epileptic 345.3
hepatic 572.2
hyperglycemic 250.2
hyperosmolar (diabetic) (nonketotic) 250.2
hypoglycemic 251.0
diabetic 250.3
insulin 250.3

- **Coma** *(Continued)*
  - insulin *(Continued)*
    - hyperosmolar 250.2
    - nondiabetic 251.0
    - organic hyperinsulinism 251.0
  - Kussmaul's (diabetic) 250.3
  - liver 572.2
  - newborn 779.2
  - prediabetic 250.2
  - uremic - *see* Uremia
- **Combat fatigue** (*see also* Reaction, stress, acute) 308.9
- **Combined** - *see* condition
- **Comedo** 706.1
- **Comedocarcinoma** (M8501/3) - *see also* Neoplasm, breast, malignant
  - noninfiltrating (M8501/2)
    - specified site - *see* Neoplasm, by site, in situ
    - unspecified site 233.0
- **Comedomastitis** 610.4
- **Comedones** 706.1
  - lanugo 757.4
- **Comma bacillus, carrier** (suspected) of V02.3
- **Comminuted fracture** - *see* Fracture, by site
- **Common**
  - aortopulmonary trunk 745.0
  - atrioventricular canal (defect) 745.69
  - atrium 745.69
  - cold (head) 460
    - vaccination, prophylactic (against) V04.7
  - truncus (arteriosus) 745.0
  - ventricle 745.3
- **Commotio** (current)
  - cerebri (*see also* Concussion, brain) 850.9
    - with skull fracture - *see* Fracture, skull, by site
  - retinae 921.3
  - spinalis - *see* Injury, spinal, by site
- **Commotion** (current)
  - brain (without skull fracture) (*see also* Concussion, brain) 850.9
    - with skull fracture - *see* Fracture, skull, by site
  - spinal cord - *see* Injury, spinal, by site
- **Communication**
  - abnormal - *see also* Fistula
    - between
      - base of aorta and pulmonary artery 745.0
      - left ventricle and right atrium 745.4
      - pericardial sac and pleural sac 748.8
      - pulmonary artery and pulmonary vein 747.3
    - congenital, between uterus and
      - anterior abdominal wall 752.3
      - bladder 752.3
      - intestine 752.3
      - rectum 752.3
  - left ventricular-right atrial 745.4
  - pulmonary artery-pulmonary vein 747.3
- **Compartment syndrome** - *see* Syndrome, compartment ◀
- **Compensation**
  - broken - *see* Failure, heart
  - failure - *see* Failure, heart
  - neurosis, psychoneurosis 300.11
- **Complaint** - *see also* Disease
  - bowel, functional 564.9
    - psychogenic 306.4
- **Complaint** *(Continued)*
  - intestine, functional 564.9
    - psychogenic 306.4
  - kidney (*see also* Disease, renal) 593.9
  - liver 573.9
  - miners' 500
- **Complete** - *see* condition
- **Complex**
  - cardiorenal (*see also* Hypertension, cardiorenal) 404.90
  - castration 300.9
  - Costen's 524.60
  - ego-dystonic homosexuality 302.0
  - Eisenmenger's (ventricular septal defect) 745.4
  - homosexual, ego-dystonic 302.0
  - hypersexual 302.89
  - inferiority 301.9
  - jumped process
    - spine - *see* Dislocation, vertebra
  - primary, tuberculosis (*see also* Tuberculosis) 010.0
  - Taussig-Bing (transposition, aorta and overriding pulmonary artery) 745.11
- **Complications**
  - abortion NEC - *see* categories 634–639
  - accidental puncture or laceration during a procedure 998.2
  - amputation stump (late) (surgical) 997.60
    - traumatic - *see* Amputation, traumatic
  - anastomosis (and bypass) - *see also* Complications, due to (presence of) any device, implant, or graft classified to 996.0–996.5 NEC
    - hemorrhage NEC 998.11
    - intestinal (internal) NEC 997.4
      - involving urinary tract 997.5
    - mechanical - *see* Complications, mechanical, graft
    - urinary tract (involving intestinal tract) 997.5
  - anesthesia, anesthetic NEC (*see also* Anesthesia, complication) 995.22 ◀
    - in labor and delivery 668.9
      - affecting fetus or newborn 763.5
      - cardiac 668.1
      - central nervous system 668.2
      - pulmonary 668.0
      - specified type NEC 668.8
  - aortocoronary (bypass) graft 996.03
    - atherosclerosis - *see* Arteriosclerosis, coronary
    - embolism 996.72
    - occlusion NEC 996.72
    - thrombus 996.72
  - arthroplasty (*see also* Complications, prosthetic joint) 996.49
  - artificial opening
    - cecostomy 569.60
    - colostomy 569.60
    - cystostomy 997.5
    - enterostomy 569.60
    - esophagostomy 530.87
      - infection 530.86
      - mechanical 530.87
    - gastrostomy 536.40
    - ileostomy 569.60
    - jejunostomy 569.60
    - nephrostomy 997.5
    - tracheostomy 519.00
- **Complications** *(Continued)*
  - artificial opening *(Continued)*
    - ureterostomy 997.5
    - urethrostomy 997.5
  - bariatric surgery 997.4
  - bile duct implant (prosthetic) NEC 996.79
    - infection or inflammation 996.69
    - mechanical 996.59
  - bleeding (intraoperative) (postoperative) 998.11
  - blood vessel graft 996.1
    - aortocoronary 996.03
      - atherosclerosis - *see* Arteriosclerosis, coronary
      - embolism 996.72
      - occlusion NEC 996.72
      - thrombus 996.72
    - atherosclerosis - *see* Arteriosclerosis, extremities
    - embolism 996.74
    - occlusion NEC 996.74
    - thrombus 996.74
  - bone growth stimulator NEC 996.78
    - infection or inflammation 996.67
  - bone marrow transplant 996.85
  - breast implant (prosthetic) NEC 996.79
    - infection or inflammation 996.69
    - mechanical 996.54
  - bypass - *see also* Complications, anastomosis
    - aortocoronary 996.03
      - atherosclerosis - *see* Arteriosclerosis, coronary
      - embolism 996.72
      - occlusion NEC 996.72
      - thrombus 996.72
    - carotid artery 996.1
      - atherosclerosis - *see* Arteriosclerosis, coronary
      - embolism 996.74
      - occlusion NEC 996.74
      - thrombus 996.74
  - cardiac (*see also* Disease, heart) 429.9
    - device, implant, or graft NEC 996.72
      - infection or inflammation 996.61
      - long-term effect 429.4
      - mechanical (*see also* Complications, mechanical, by type) 996.00
      - valve prosthesis 996.71
        - infection or inflammation 996.61
    - postoperative NEC 997.1
      - long-term effect 429.4
  - cardiorenal (*see also* Hypertension, cardiorenal) 404.90
  - carotid artery bypass graft 996.1
    - atherosclerosis - *see* Arteriosclerosis, coronary
    - embolism 996.74
    - occlusion NEC 996.74
    - thrombus 996.74
  - cataract fragments in eye 998.82
  - catheter device NEC - *see also* Complications, due to (presence of) any device, implant, or graft classified to 996.0-996.5 NEC
    - mechanical - *see* Complications, mechanical, catheter
  - cecostomy 569.60
  - cesarean section wound 674.3
  - chin implant (prosthetic) NEC 996.79
    - infection or inflammation 996.69
    - mechanical 996.59

Complications *(Continued)*
colostomy (enterostomy) 569.60
specified type NEC 569.69
contraceptive device, intrauterine NEC 996.76
infection 996.65
inflammation 996.65
mechanical 996.32
cord (umbilical) - *see* Complications, umbilical cord
cornea
due to
contact lens 371.82
coronary (artery) bypass (graft) NEC 996.03
atherosclerosis - *see* Arteriosclerosis, coronary
embolism 996.72
infection or inflammation 996.61
mechanical 996.03
occlusion NEC 996.72
specified type NEC 996.72
thrombus 996.72
cystostomy 997.5
delivery 669.9
procedure (instrumental) (manual) (surgical) 669.4
specified type NEC 669.8
dialysis (hemodialysis) (peritoneal) (renal) NEC 999.9
catheter NEC - *see also* Complications, due to (presence of) any device, implant, or graft classified to 996.0–996.5 NEC
infection or inflammation 996.62
peritoneal 996.68
mechanical 996.1
peritoneal 996.56
due to (presence of) any device, implant, or graft classified to 996.0–996.5 NEC 996.70
with infection or inflammation - *see* Complications, infection or inflammation, due to (presence of) any device, implant, or graft classified to 996.0–996.5 NEC
arterial NEC 996.74
coronary NEC 996.03
atherosclerosis - *see* Arteriosclerosis, coronary
embolism 996.72
occlusion NEC 996.72
specified type NEC 996.72
thrombus 996.72
renal dialysis 996.73
arteriovenous fistula or shunt NEC 996.74
bone growth stimulator 996.78
breast NEC 996.79
cardiac NEC 996.72
defibrillator 996.72
pacemaker 996.72
valve prosthesis 996.71
catheter NEC 996.79
spinal 996.75
urinary, indwelling 996.76
vascular NEC 996.74
renal dialysis 996.73
ventricular shunt 996.75
coronary (artery) bypass (graft) NEC 996.03
atherosclerosis - *see* Arteriosclerosis, coronary
embolism 996.72

Complications *(Continued)*
due to *(Continued)*
coronary *(Continued)*
occlusion NEC 996.72
thrombus 996.72
electrodes
brain 996.75
heart 996.72
esophagostomy 530.87
gastrointestinal NEC 996.79
genitourinary NEC 996.76
heart valve prosthesis NEC 996.71
infusion pump 996.74
insulin pump 996.57
internal
joint prosthesis 996.77
orthopedic NEC 996.78
specified type NEC 996.79
intrauterine contraceptive device NEC 996.76
joint prosthesis, internal NEC 996.77
mechanical - *see* Complications, mechanical
nervous system NEC 996.75
ocular lens NEC 996.79
orbital NEC 996.79
orthopedic NEC 996.78
joint, internal 996.77
renal dialysis 996.73
specified type NEC 996.79
urinary catheter, indwelling 996.76
vascular NEC 996.74
ventricular shunt 996.75
during dialysis NEC 999.9
ectopic or molar pregnancy NEC 639.9
electroshock therapy NEC 999.9
enterostomy 569.60
specified type NEC 569.69
esophagostomy 530.87
infection 530.86
mechanical 530.87
external (fixation) device with internal component(s) NEC 996.78
infection or inflammation 996.67
mechanical 996.49
extracorporeal circulation NEC 999.9
eye implant (prosthetic) NEC 996.79
infection or inflammation 996.69
mechanical
ocular lens 996.53
orbital globe 996.59
gastrointestinal, postoperative NEC (*see also* Complications, surgical procedures) 997.4
gastrostomy 536.40
specified type NEC 536.49
genitourinary device, implant, or graft NEC 996.76
infection or inflammation 996.65
urinary catheter, indwelling 996.64
mechanical (*see also* Complications, mechanical, by type) 996.30
specified NEC 996.39
graft (bypass) (patch) - *see also* Complications, due to (presence of) any device, implant, or graft classified to 996.0–996.5 NEC
bone marrow 996.85
corneal NEC 996.79
infection or inflammation 996.69
rejection or reaction 996.51
mechanical - *see* Complications, mechanical, graft

Complications *(Continued)*
graft *(Continued)*
organ (immune or nonimmune cause) (partial) (total) 996.80
bone marrow 996.85
heart 996.83
intestines 996.87
kidney 996.81
liver 996.82
lung 996.84
pancreas 996.86
specified NEC 996.89
skin NEC 996.79
infection or inflammation 996.69
rejection 996.52
artificial 996.55
decellularized allodermis 996.55
heart - *see also* Disease, heart transplant (immune or nonimmune cause) 996.83
hematoma (intraoperative) (postoperative) 998.12
hemorrhage (intraoperative) (postoperative) 998.11
hyperalimentation therapy NEC 999.9
immunization (procedure) - *see* Complications, vaccination
implant - *see also* Complications, due to (presence of) any device, implant, or graft classified to 996.0–996.5 NEC
mechanical - *see* Complications, mechanical, implant
infection and inflammation
due to (presence of) any device, implant, or graft classified to 996.0–996.5 NEC 996.60
arterial NEC 996.62
coronary 996.61
renal dialysis 996.62
arteriovenous fistula or shunt 996.62
artificial heart 996.61
bone growth stimulator 996.67
breast 996.69
cardiac 996.61
catheter NEC 996.69
peritoneal 996.68
spinal 996.63
urinary, indwelling 996.64
vascular NEC 996.62
ventricular shunt 996.63
coronary artery bypass 996.61
electrodes
brain 996.63
heart 996.61
gastrointestinal NEC 996.69
genitourinary NEC 996.65
indwelling urinary catheter 996.64
heart assist device 996.61
heart valve 996.61
infusion pump 996.62
insulin pump 996.69
intrauterine contraceptive device 996.65
joint prosthesis, internal 996.66
ocular lens 996.69
orbital (implant) 996.69
orthopedic NEC 996.67
joint, internal 996.66
specified type NEC 996.69
urinary catheter, indwelling 996.64
ventricular shunt 996.63

Complications *(Continued)*
- infusion (procedure) 999.9
  - blood - *see* Complications, transfusion
  - infection NEC 999.3
  - sepsis NEC 999.3
- inhalation therapy NEC 999.9
- injection (procedure) 999.9
  - drug reaction (*see also* Reaction, drug) 995.27 ⟸
  - infection NEC 999.3
  - sepsis NEC 999.3
  - serum (prophylactic) (therapeutic) - *see* Complications, vaccination
  - vaccine (any) - *see* Complications, vaccination
- inoculation (any) - *see* Complications, vaccination
- insulin pump 996.57
- internal device (catheter) (electronic) (fixation) (prosthetic) - *see also* Complications, due to (presence of) any device, implant, or graft classified to 996.0–996.5 NEC
  - mechanical - *see* Complications, mechanical
- intestinal transplant (immune or nonimmune cause) 996.87
- intraoperative bleeding or hemorrhage 998.11
- intrauterine contraceptive device (*see also* Complications, contraceptive device) 996.76
  - with fetal damage affecting management of pregnancy 655.8
  - infection or inflammation 996.65
- jejunostomy 569.60
- kidney transplant (immune or nonimmune cause) 996.81
- labor 669.9
  - specified condition NEC 669.8
- liver transplant (immune or nonimmune cause) 996.82
- lumbar puncture 349.0
- mechanical
  - anastomosis - *see* Complications, mechanical, graft
  - artificial heart 996.09
  - bypass - *see* Complications, mechanical, graft
  - catheter NEC 996.59
    - cardiac 996.09
    - cystostomy 996.39
    - dialysis (hemodialysis) 996.1
      - peritoneal 996.56
    - during a procedure 998.2
    - urethral, indwelling 996.31
  - colostomy 569.62
  - device NEC 996.59
    - balloon (counterpulsation), intra-aortic 996.1
    - cardiac 996.00
      - automatic implantable defibrillator 996.04
      - long-term effect 429.4
      - specified NEC 996.09
    - contraceptive, intrauterine 996.32
    - counterpulsation, intra-aortic 996.1
    - fixation, external, with internal components 996.49
    - fixation, internal (nail, rod, plate) 996.40
    - genitourinary 996.30
      - specified NEC 996.39

Complications *(Continued)*
- mechanical *(Continued)*
  - device NEC *(Continued)*
    - insulin pump 996.57
    - nervous system 996.2
    - orthopedic, internal 996.40
      - prosthetic joint (*see also* Complications, mechanical, device, orthopedic, prosthetic, joint) 996.47
    - prosthetic NEC 996.59
      - joint (*see also* Complications, prosthetic joint) 996.47
        - articular bearing surface wear 996.46
        - aseptic loosening 996.41
        - breakage 996.43
        - dislocation 996.42
        - failure 996.43
        - fracture 996.43
          - around prosthetic 996.44
          - peri-prosthetic 996.44
        - instability 996.42
        - loosening 996.41
        - peri-prosthetic osteolysis 996.45
        - subluxation 996.42
        - wear 996.46
    - umbrella, vena cava 996.1
    - vascular 996.1
  - dorsal column stimulator 996.2
  - electrode NEC 996.59
    - brain 996.2
    - cardiac 996.01
    - spinal column 996.2
  - enterostomy 569.62
  - esophagostomy 530.87
  - fistula, arteriovenous, surgically created 996.1
  - gastrostomy 536.42
  - graft NEC 996.52
    - aortic (bifurcation) 996.1
    - aortocoronary bypass 996.03
    - blood vessel NEC 996.1
    - bone 996.49
    - cardiac 996.00
    - carotid artery bypass 996.1
    - cartilage 996.49
    - corneal 996.51
    - coronary bypass 996.03
    - decellularized allodermis 996.55
    - genitourinary 996.30
      - specified NEC 996.39
    - muscle 996.49
    - nervous system 996.2
    - organ (immune or nonimmune cause) 996.80
      - heart 996.83
      - intestines 996.87
      - kidney 996.81
      - liver 996.82
      - lung 996.84
      - pancreas 996.86
      - specified NEC 996.89
    - orthopedic, internal 996.49
    - peripheral nerve 996.2
    - prosthetic NEC 996.59
    - skin 996.52
      - artificial 996.55
    - specified NEC 996.59
    - tendon 996.49
    - tissue NEC 996.52
    - tooth 996.59
    - ureter, without mention of resection 996.39
    - vascular 996.1

Complications *(Continued)*
- mechanical *(Continued)*
  - heart valve prosthesis 996.02
    - long-term effect 429.4
  - implant NEC 996.59
    - cardiac 996.00
      - automatic implantable defibrillator 996.04
      - long-term effect 429.4
      - specified NEC 996.09
    - electrode NEC 996.59
      - brain 996.2
      - cardiac 996.01
      - spinal column 996.2
    - genitourinary 996.30
    - nervous system 996.2
    - orthopedic, internal 996.49
    - prosthetic NEC 996.59
      - in
        - bile duct 996.59
        - breast 996.54
        - chin 996.59
        - eye
          - ocular lens 996.53
          - orbital globe 996.59
    - vascular 996.1
  - insulin pump 996.57
  - nonabsorbable surgical material 996.59
  - pacemaker NEC 996.59
    - brain 996.2
    - cardiac 996.01
    - nerve (phrenic) 996.2
  - patch - *see* Complications, mechanical, graft
  - prosthesis NEC 996.59
    - bile duct 996.59
    - breast 996.54
    - chin 996.59
    - ocular lens 996.53
    - reconstruction, vas deferens 996.39
  - reimplant NEC 996.59
    - extremity (*see also* Complications, reattached, extremity) 996.90
    - organ (*see also* Complications, transplant, organ, by site) 996.80
  - repair - *see* Complications, mechanical, graft
  - respirator [ventilator] V46.14
  - shunt NEC 996.59
    - arteriovenous, surgically created 996.1
    - ventricular (communicating) 996.2
  - stent NEC 996.59
  - tracheostomy 519.02
  - vas deferens reconstruction 996.39
  - ventilator [respirator] V46.14
- medical care NEC 999.9
  - cardiac NEC 997.1
  - gastrointestinal NEC 997.4
  - nervous system NEC 997.00
  - peripheral vascular NEC 997.2
  - respiratory NEC 997.3
  - urinary NEC 997.5
  - vascular
    - mesenteric artery 997.71
    - other vessels 997.79
    - peripheral vessels 997.2
    - renal artery 997.72
- nephrostomy 997.5
- nervous system
  - device, implant, or graft NEC 349.1
    - mechanical 996.2
  - postoperative NEC 997.00

Complications *(Continued)*
obstetric 669.9
procedure (instrumental) (manual) (surgical) 669.4
specified NEC 669.8
surgical wound 674.3
ocular lens implant NEC 996.79
infection or inflammation 996.69
mechanical 996.53
organ transplant - *see* Complications, transplant, organ, by site
orthopedic device, implant, or graft
internal (fixation) (nail) (plate) (rod) NEC 996.78
infection or inflammation 996.67
joint prosthesis 996.77
infection or inflammation 996.66
mechanical 996.40
pacemaker (cardiac) 996.72
infection or inflammation 996.61
mechanical 996.01
pancreas transplant (immune or nonimmune cause) 996.86
perfusion NEC 999.9
perineal repair (obstetrical) 674.3
disruption 674.2
pessary (uterus) (vagina) - *see* Complications, contraceptive device
phototherapy 990
postcystoscopic 997.5
postmastoidectomy NEC 383.30
postoperative - *see* Complications, surgical procedures
pregnancy NEC 646.9
affecting fetus or newborn 761.9
prosthetic device, internal - *see also* Complications, due to (presence of) any device, implant, or graft classified to 996.0–996.5 NEC
mechanical NEC (*see also* Complications, mechanical) 996.59
puerperium NEC (*see also* Puerperal) 674.9
puncture, spinal 349.0
pyelogram 997.5
radiation 990
radiotherapy 990
reattached
body part, except extremity 996.99
extremity (infection) (rejection) 996.90
arm(s) 996.94
digit(s) (hand) 996.93
foot 996.95
finger(s) 996.93
foot 996.95
forearm 996.91
hand 996.92
leg 996.96
lower NEC 996.96
toe(s) 996.95
upper NEC 996.94
reimplant NEC - *see also* Complications, due to (presence of) any device, implant, or graft classified to 996.0–996.5 NEC
bone marrow 996.85
extremity (*see also* Complications, reattached, extremity) 996.90
due to infection 996.90
mechanical - *see* Complications, mechanical, reimplant
organ (immune or nonimmune cause) (partial) (total) (*see also* Complications, transplant, organ, by site) 996.80

Complications *(Continued)*
renal allograft 996.81
renal dialysis - *see* Complications, dialysis
respirator [ventilator], mechanical V46.14
respiratory 519.9
device, implant, or graft NEC 996.79
infection or inflammation 996.69
mechanical 996.59
distress syndrome, adult, following trauma or surgery 518.5
insufficiency, acute, postoperative 518.5
postoperative NEC 997.3
therapy NEC 999.9
sedation during labor and delivery 668.9
affecting fetus or newborn 763.5
cardiac 668.1
central nervous system 668.2
pulmonary 668.0
specified type NEC 668.8
seroma (intraoperative) (postoperative) (noninfected) 998.13
infected 998.51
shunt - *see also* Complications, due to (presence of) any device, implant, or graft classified to 996.0–996.5 NEC
mechanical - *see* Complications, mechanical, shunt
specified body system NEC
device, implant, or graft - *see* Complications, due to (presence of) any device, implant, or graft classified to 996.0–996.5 NEC
postoperative NEC 997.99
spinal puncture or tap 349.0
stoma, external
gastrointestinal tract
colostomy 569.60
enterostomy 569.60
esophagostomy 530.87
infection 530.86
mechanical 530.87
gastrostomy 536.40
urinary tract 997.5
stomach banding 997.4
stomach stapling 997.4
surgical procedures 998.9
accidental puncture or laceration 998.2
amputation stump (late) 997.60
anastomosis - *see* Complications, anastomosis
burst stitches or sutures (external) 998.32
internal 998.31
cardiac 997.1
long-term effect following cardiac surgery 429.4
catheter device - *see* Complications, catheter device
cataract fragments in eye 998.82
cecostomy malfunction 569.62
colostomy malfunction 569.62
cystostomy malfunction 997.5
dehiscence (of incision) (external) 998.32
internal 998.31
dialysis NEC (*see also* Complications, dialysis) 999.9
disruption
anastomosis (internal) - *see* Complications, mechanical, graft

Complications *(Continued)*
surgical procedures *(Continued)*
disruption *(Continued)*
internal suture (line) 998.31
wound (external) 998.32
internal 998.31
dumping syndrome (postgastrectomy) 564.2
elephantiasis or lymphedema 997.99
postmastectomy 457.0
emphysema (surgical) 998.81
enterostomy malfunction 569.62
esophagostomy malfunction 530.87
evisceration 998.32
fistula (persistent postoperative) 998.6
foreign body inadvertently left in wound (sponge) (suture) (swab) 998.4
from nonabsorbable surgical material (Dacron) (mesh) (permanent suture) (reinforcing) (Teflon) - *see* Complications due to (presence of) any device, implant, or graft classified to 996.0–996.5 NEC
gastrointestinal NEC 997.4
gastrostomy malfunction 536.42
hematoma 998.12
hemorrhage 998.11
ileostomy malfunction 569.62
internal prosthetic device NEC (*see also* Complications, internal device) 996.70
hemolytic anemia 283.19
infection or inflammation 996.60
malfunction - *see* Complications, mechanical
mechanical complication - *see* Complications, mechanical
thrombus 996.70
jejunostomy malfunction 569.62
nervous system NEC 997.00
obstruction, internal anastomosis - *see* Complications, mechanical, graft
other body system NEC 997.99
peripheral vascular NEC 997.2
postcardiotomy syndrome 429.4
postcholecystectomy syndrome 576.0
postcommissurotomy syndrome 429.4
postgastrectomy dumping syndrome 564.2
postmastectomy lymphedema syndrome 457.0
postmastoidectomy 383.30
cholesteatoma, recurrent 383.32
cyst, mucosal 383.31
granulation 383.33
inflammation, chronic 383.33
postvagotomy syndrome 564.2
postvalvulotomy syndrome 429.4
reattached extremity (infection) (rejection) (*see also* Complications, reattached, extremity) 996.90
respiratory NEC 997.3
seroma 998.13
shock (endotoxic) (hypovolemic) (septic) 998.0
shunt, prosthetic (thrombus) - *see also* Complications, due to (presence of) any device, implant, or graft classified to 996.0–996.5 NEC
hemolytic anemia 283.19
specified complication NEC 998.89

Complications *(Continued)*
surgical procedures *(Continued)*
stitch abscess 998.59
transplant - *see* Complications, graft
ureterostomy malfunction 997.5
urethrostomy malfunction 997.5
urinary NEC 997.5
vascular
mesenteric artery 997.71
other vessels 997.79
peripheral vessels 997.2
renal artery 997.72
wound infection 998.59
therapeutic misadventure NEC 999.9
surgical treatment 998.9
tracheostomy 519.00
transfusion (blood) (lymphocytes) (plasma) NEC 999.8
acute lung injury (TRALI) 518.7 ◀
atrophy, liver, yellow, subacute (within 8 months of administration) - *see* Hepatitis, viral
bone marrow 996.85
embolism
air 999.1
thrombus 999.2
hemolysis NEC 999.8
bone marrow 996.85
hepatitis (serum) (type B) (within 8 months after administration) - *see* Hepatitis, viral
incompatibility reaction (ABO) (blood group) 999.6
Rh (factor) 999.7
infection 999.3
jaundice (serum) (within 8 months after administration) - *see* Hepatitis, viral
sepsis 999.3
shock or reaction NEC 999.8
bone marrow 996.85
subacute yellow atrophy of liver (within 8 months after administration) - *see* Hepatitis, viral
thromboembolism 999.2
transplant NEC - *see also* Complications, due to (presence of) any device, implant, or graft classified to 996.0–996.5 NEC
bone marrow 996.85
organ (immune or nonimmune cause) (partial) (total) 996.80
bone marrow 996.85
heart 996.83
intestines 996.87
kidney 996.81
liver 996.82
lung 996.84
pancreas 996.86
specified NEC 996.89
trauma NEC (early) 958.8
ultrasound therapy NEC 999.9
umbilical cord
affecting fetus or newborn 762.6
complicating delivery 663.9
affecting fetus or newborn 762.6
specified type NEC 663.8
urethral catheter NEC 996.76
infection or inflammation 996.64
mechanical 996.31
urinary, postoperative NEC 997.5
vaccination 999.9
anaphylaxis NEC 999.4
cellulitis 999.3

Complications *(Continued)*
vaccination *(Continued)*
encephalitis or encephalomyelitis 323.51 ◀
hepatitis (serum) (type B) (within 8 months after administration) - *see* Hepatitis, viral
infection (general) (local) NEC 999.3
jaundice (serum) (within 8 months after administration) - *see* Hepatitis, viral
meningitis 997.09 *[321.8]*
myelitis 323.52 ◀
protein sickness 999.5
reaction (allergic) 999.5
Herxheimer's 995.0
serum 999.5
sepsis 999.3
serum intoxication, sickness, rash, or other serum reaction NEC 999.5
shock (allergic) (anaphylactic) 999.4
subacute yellow atrophy of liver (within 8 months after administration) - *see* Hepatitis, viral
vaccinia (generalized) 999.0
localized 999.3
vascular
device, implant, or graft NEC 996.74
infection or inflammation 996.62
mechanical NEC 996.1
cardiac (*see also* Complications, mechanical, by type) 996.00
following infusion, perfusion, or transfusion 999.2
postoperative NEC 997.2
mesenteric artery 997.71
other vessels 997.79
peripheral vessels 997.2
renal artery 997.72
ventilation therapy NEC 999.9
ventilator [respirator], mechanical V46.14
Compound presentation, complicating delivery 652.8
causing obstructed labor 660.0
Compressed air disease 993.3
Compression
with injury - *see* specific injury
arm NEC 354.9
artery 447.1
celiac, syndrome 447.4
brachial plexus 353.0
brain (stem) 348.4
due to
contusion, brain - *see* Contusion, brain
injury NEC - *see also* Hemorrhage, brain, traumatic
birth - *see* Birth, injury, brain
laceration, brain - *see* Laceration, brain
osteopathic 739.0
bronchus 519.19 ◀
by cicatrix - *see* Cicatrix
cardiac 423.9
cauda equina 344.60
with neurogenic bladder 344.61
celiac (artery) (axis) 447.4
cerebral - *see* Compression, brain
cervical plexus 353.2
cord (umbilical) - *see* Compression, umbilical cord
cranial nerve 352.9
second 377.49
third (partial) 378.51
total 378.52

Compression *(Continued)*
cranial nerve *(Continued)*
fourth 378.53
fifth 350.8
sixth 378.54
seventh 351.8
divers' squeeze 993.3
duodenum (external) (*see also* Obstruction, duodenum) 537.3
during birth 767.9
esophagus 530.3
congenital, external 750.3
Eustachian tube 381.63
facies (congenital) 754.0
fracture - *see* Fracture, by site
heart - *see* Disease, heart
intestine (*see also* Obstruction, intestine) 560.9
with hernia - *see* Hernia, by site, with obstruction
laryngeal nerve, recurrent 478.79
leg NEC 355.8
lower extremity NEC 355.8
lumbosacral plexus 353.1
lung 518.89
lymphatic vessel 457.1
medulla - *see* Compression, brain
nerve NEC - *see also* Disorder, nerve
arm NEC 354.9
autonomic nervous system (*see also* Neuropathy, peripheral, autonomic) 337.9
axillary 353.0
cranial NEC 352.9
due to displacement of intervertebral disc 722.2
with myelopathy 722.70
cervical 722.0
with myelopathy 722.71
lumbar, lumbosacral 722.10
with myelopathy 722.73
thoracic, thoracolumbar 722.11
with myelopathy 722.72
iliohypogastric 355.79
ilioinguinal 355.79
leg NEC 355.8
lower extremity NEC 355.8
median (in carpal tunnel) 354.0
obturator 355.79
optic 377.49
plantar 355.6
posterior tibial (in tarsal tunnel) 355.5
root (by scar tissue) NEC 724.9
cervical NEC 723.4
lumbar NEC 724.4
lumbosacral 724.4
thoracic 724.4
saphenous 355.79
sciatic (acute) 355.0
sympathetic 337.9
traumatic - *see* Injury, nerve
ulnar 354.2
upper extremity NEC 354.9
peripheral - *see* Compression, nerve
spinal (cord) (old or nontraumatic) 336.9
by displacement of intervertebral disc - *see* Displacement, intervertebral disc
nerve
root NEC 724.9
postoperative 722.80
cervical region 722.81
lumbar region 722.83
thoracic region 722.82

Compression *(Continued)*
spinal *(Continued)*
nerve *(Continued)*
root *(Continued)*
traumatic - *see* Injury, nerve, spinal
traumatic - *see* Injury, nerve, spinal
spondylogenic 721.91
cervical 721.1
lumbar, lumbosacral 721.42
thoracic 721.41
traumatic - *see also* Injury, spinal, by site
with fracture, vertebra - *see* Fracture, vertebra, by site, with spinal cord injury
spondylogenic - *see* Compression, spinal cord, spondylogenic
subcostal nerve (syndrome) 354.8
sympathetic nerve NEC 337.9
syndrome 958.5
thorax 512.8
iatrogenic 512.1
postoperative 512.1
trachea 519.19
congenital 748.3
ulnar nerve (by scar tissue) 354.2
umbilical cord
affecting fetus or newborn 762.5
cord prolapsed 762.4
complicating delivery 663.2
cord around neck 663.1
cord prolapsed 663.0
upper extremity NEC 354.9
ureter 593.3
urethra - *see* Stricture, urethra
vein 459.2
vena cava (inferior) (superior) 459.2
vertebral NEC - *see* Compression, spinal (cord)
Compulsion, compulsive
eating 307.51
neurosis (obsessive) 300.3
personality 301.4
states (mixed) 300.3
swearing 300.3
in Gilles de la Tourette's syndrome 307.23
tics and spasms 307.22
water drinking NEC (syndrome) 307.9
Concato's disease (pericardial polyserositis) 423.2
peritoneal 568.82
pleural - *see* Pleurisy
Concavity, chest wall 738.3
Concealed
hemorrhage NEC 459.0
penis 752.65
Concentric fading 368.12
Concern (normal) about sick person in family V61.49
Concrescence (teeth) 520.2
Concretio cordis 423.1
rheumatic 393
Concretion - *see also* Calculus
appendicular 543.9
canaliculus 375.57
clitoris 624.8
conjunctiva 372.54
eyelid 374.56
intestine (impaction) (obstruction) 560.39
lacrimal (passages) 375.57
prepuce (male) 605
female (clitoris) 624.8

Concretion *(Continued)*
salivary gland (any) 527.5
seminal vesicle 608.89
stomach 537.89
tonsil 474.8
Concussion (current) 850.9
with
loss of consciousness 850.5
brief (less than one hour)
30 minutes or less 850.11
31–59 minutes 850.12
moderate (1–24 hours) 850.2
prolonged (more than 24 hours) (with complete recovery) (with return to pre-existing conscious level) 850.3
without return to pre-existing conscious level 850.4
mental confusion or disorientation (without loss of consciousness) 850.0
with loss of consciousness - *see* Concussion, with, loss of consciousness
without loss of consciousness 850.0
blast (air) (hydraulic) (immersion) (underwater) 869.0
with open wound into cavity 869.1
abdomen or thorax - *see* Injury, internal, by site
brain - *see* Concussion, brain
ear (acoustic nerve trauma) 951.5
with perforation, tympanic membrane - *see* Wound, open, ear drum
thorax - *see* Injury, internal, intrathoracic organs NEC
brain or cerebral (without skull fracture) 850.9
with
loss of consciousness 850.5
brief (less than one hour)
30 minutes or less 850.11
31–59 minutes 850.12
moderate (1–24 hours) 850.2
prolonged (more than 24 hours) (with complete recovery) (with return to pre-existing conscious level) 850.3
without return to pre-existing conscious level 850.4
mental confusion or disorientation (without loss of consciousness) 850.0
with loss of consciousness - *see* Concussion, brain, with, loss of consciousness
skull fracture - *see* Fracture, skull, by site
without loss of consciousness 850.0
cauda equina 952.4
cerebral - *see* Concussion, brain
conus medullaris (spine) 952.4
hydraulic - *see* Concussion, blast
internal organs - *see* Injury, internal, by site
labyrinth - *see* Injury, intracranial
ocular 921.3
osseous labyrinth - *see* Injury, intracranial
spinal (cord) - *see also* Injury, spinal, by site
due to
broken

Concussion *(Continued)*
spinal *(Continued)*
due to *(Continued)*
broken *(Continued)*
back - *see* Fracture, vertebra, by site, with spinal cord injury
neck - *see* Fracture, vertebra, cervical, with spinal cord injury
fracture, fracture dislocation, or compression fracture of spine or vertebra - *see* Fracture, vertebra, by site, with spinal cord injury
syndrome 310.2
underwater blast - *see* Concussion, blast
Condition - *see also* Disease
psychiatric 298.9
respiratory NEC 519.9
acute or subacute NEC 519.9
due to
external agent 508.9
specified type NEC 508.8
fumes or vapors (chemical) (inhalation) 506.3
radiation 508.0
chronic NEC 519.9
due to
external agent 508.9
specified type NEC 508.8
fumes or vapors (chemical) (inhalation) 506.4
radiation 508.1
due to
external agent 508.9
specified type NEC 508.8
fumes or vapors (chemical) inhalation 506.9
Conduct disturbance (*see also* Disturbance, conduct) 312.9
adjustment reaction 309.3
hyperkinetic 314.2
Condyloma NEC 078.10
acuminatum 078.11
gonorrheal 098.0
latum 091.3
syphilitic 091.3
congenital 090.0
venereal, syphilitic 091.3
Confinement - *see* Delivery
Conflagration - *see also* Burn, by site
asphyxia (by inhalation of smoke, gases, fumes, or vapors) 987.9
specified agent - *see* Table of Drugs and Chemicals
Conflict
family V61.9
specified circumstance NEC V61.8
interpersonal NEC V62.81
marital V61.10
involving divorce or estrangement V61.0
parent-child V61.20
partner V61.10
Confluent - *see* condition
Confusion, confused (mental) (state) (*see also* State, confusional) 298.9
acute 293.0
epileptic 293.0
postoperative 293.9
psychogenic 298.2
reactive (from emotional stress, psychological trauma) 298.2
subacute 293.1

Confusional arousals 327.41
Congelation 991.9
Congenital - *see also* condition
aortic septum 747.29
generalized fibromatosis (CGF) 759.89 ◀
intrinsic factor deficiency 281.0
malformation - *see* Anomaly
Congestion, congestive (chronic) (passive)
asphyxia, newborn 768.9
bladder 596.8
bowel 569.89
brain (*see also* Disease, cerebrovascular NEC) 437.8
malarial 084.9
breast 611.79
bronchi 519.19 ◀
bronchial tube 519.19 ◀
catarrhal 472.0
cerebral - *see* Congestion, brain
cerebrospinal - *see* Congestion, brain
chest 514
chill 780.99
malarial (*see also* Malaria) 084.6
circulatory NEC 459.9
conjunctiva 372.71
due to disturbance of circulation 459.9
duodenum 537.3
enteritis - *see* Enteritis
eye 372.71
fibrosis syndrome (pelvic) 625.5
gastroenteritis - *see* Enteritis
general 799.89
glottis 476.0
heart (*see also* Failure, heart) 428.0
hepatic 573.0
hypostatic (lung) 514
intestine 569.89
intracranial - *see* Congestion, brain
kidney 593.89
labyrinth 386.50
larynx 476.0
liver 573.0
lung 514
active or acute (*see also* Pneumonia) 486
congenital 770.0
chronic 514
hypostatic 514
idiopathic, acute 518.5
passive 514
malaria, malarial (brain) (fever) (*see also* Malaria) 084.6
medulla - *see* Congestion, brain
nasal 478.19 ◀
orbit, orbital 376.33
inflammatory (chronic) 376.10
acute 376.00
ovary 620.8
pancreas 577.8
pelvic, female 625.5
pleural 511.0
prostate (active) 602.1
pulmonary - *see* Congestion, lung
renal 593.89
retina 362.89
seminal vesicle 608.89
spinal cord 336.1
spleen 289.51
chronic 289.51
stomach 537.89
trachea 464.11
urethra 599.84

Congestion, congestive *(Continued)*
uterus 625.5
with subinvolution 621.1
viscera 799.89
Congestive - *see* Congestion
Conical
cervix 622.6
cornea 371.60
teeth 520.2
Conjoined twins 759.4
causing disproportion (fetopelvic) 653.7
Conjugal maladjustment V61.10
involving divorce or estrangement V61.0
Conjunctiva - *see* condition
Conjunctivitis (exposure) (infectious) (nondiphtheritic) (pneumococcal) (pustular) (staphylococcal) (streptococcal) NEC 372.30
actinic 370.24
acute 372.00
atopic 372.05
contagious 372.03
follicular 372.02
hemorrhagic (viral) 077.4
adenoviral (acute) 077.3
allergic (chronic) 372.14
with hay fever 372.05
anaphylactic 372.05
angular 372.03
Apollo (viral) 077.4
atopic 372.05
blennorrhagic (neonatorum) 098.40
catarrhal 372.03
chemical 372.01
allergic 372.05
meaning corrosion - *see* Burn, conjunctiva
chlamydial 077.98
due to
Chlamydia trachomatis - *see* Trachoma
paratrachoma 077.0
chronic 372.10
allergic 372.14
follicular 372.12
simple 372.11
specified type NEC 372.14
vernal 372.13
diphtheritic 032.81
due to
dust 372.05
enterovirus type 70 077.4
erythema multiforme 695.1 *[372.33]*
filariasis (*see also* Filariasis) 125.9 *[372.15]*
mucocutaneous
disease NEC 372.33
leishmaniasis 085.5 *[372.15]*
Reiter's disease 099.3 *[372.33]*
syphilis 095.8 *[372.10]*
toxoplasmosis (acquired) 130.1
congenital (active) 771.2
trachoma - *see* Trachoma
dust 372.05
eczematous 370.31
epidemic 077.1
hemorrhagic 077.4
follicular (acute) 372.02
adenoviral (acute) 077.3
chronic 372.12
glare 370.24
gonococcal (neonatorum) 098.40
granular (trachomatous) 076.1
late effect 139.1

Conjunctivitis *(Continued)*
hemorrhagic (acute) (epidemic) 077.4
herpetic (simplex) 054.43
zoster 053.21
inclusion 077.0
infantile 771.6
influenzal 372.03
Koch-Weeks 372.03
light 372.05
medicamentosa 372.05
membranous 372.04
meningococcic 036.89
Morax-Axenfeld 372.02
mucopurulent NEC 372.03
neonatal 771.6
gonococcal 098.40
Newcastle's 077.8
nodosa 360.14
of Beal 077.3
parasitic 372.15
filariasis (*see also* Filariasis) 125.9 *[372.15]*
mucocutaneous leishmaniasis 085.5 *[372.15]*
Parinaud's 372.02
petrificans 372.39
phlyctenular 370.31
pseudomembranous 372.04
diphtheritic 032.81
purulent 372.03
Reiter's 099.3 *[372.33]*
rosacea 695.3 *[372.31]*
serous 372.01
viral 077.99
simple chronic 372.11
specified NEC 372.39
sunlamp 372.04
swimming pool 077.0
trachomatous (follicular) 076.1
acute 076.0
late effect 139.1
traumatic NEC 372.39
tuberculous (*see also* Tuberculosis) 017.3 *[370.31]*
tularemic 021.3
tularensis 021.3
vernal 372.13
limbar 372.13 *[370.32]*
viral 077.99
acute hemorrhagic 077.4
specified NEC 077.8
Conjunctivochalasis 372.81
Conjunctoblepharitis - *see* Conjunctivitis
Conn (-Louis) syndrome (primary aldosteronism) 255.12
Connective tissue - *see* condition
Conradi (-Hünermann) syndrome or disease (chondrodysplasia calcificans congenita) 756.59
Consanguinity V19.7
Consecutive - *see* condition
Consolidated lung (base) - *see* Pneumonia, lobar
Constipation 564.00
atonic 564.09
drug induced
correct substance properly administered 564.09
overdose or wrong substance given or taken 977.9
specified drug - *see* Table of Drugs and Chemicals
neurogenic 564.09
other specified NEC 564.09

ICD-9-CM C Vol. 2

Constipation *(Continued)*
  outlet dysfunction 564.02
  psychogenic 306.4
  simple 564.00
  slow transit 564.01
  spastic 564.09
Constitutional - *see also* condition
  arterial hypotension (*see also* Hypotension) 458.9
  obesity 278.00
    morbid 278.01
  psychopathic state 301.9
  short stature in childhood 783.43
  state, developmental V21.9
    specified development NEC V21.8
  substandard 301.6
Constitutionally substandard 301.6
Constriction
  anomalous, meningeal bands or folds 742.8
  aortic arch (congenital) 747.10
  asphyxiation or suffocation by 994.7
  bronchus 519.19
  canal, ear (*see also* Stricture, ear canal, acquired) 380.50
  duodenum 537.3
  gallbladder (*see also* Obstruction, gallbladder) 575.2
    congenital 751.69
  intestine (*see also* Obstruction, intestine) 560.9
  larynx 478.74
    congenital 748.3
  meningeal bands or folds, anomalous 742.8
  organ or site, congenital NEC - *see* Atresia
  prepuce (congenital) 605
  pylorus 537.0
    adult hypertrophic 537.0
    congenital or infantile 750.5
    newborn 750.5
  ring (uterus) 661.4
    affecting fetus or newborn 763.7
  spastic - *see also* Spasm
    ureter 593.3
    urethra - *see* Stricture, urethra
  stomach 537.89
  ureter 593.3
  urethra - *see* Stricture, urethra
  visual field (functional) (peripheral) 368.45
Constrictive - *see* condition
Consultation V65.9
  medical - *see also* Counseling, medical
  specified reason NEC V65.8
  without complaint or sickness V65.9
    feared complaint unfounded V65.5
    specified reason NEC V65.8
Consumption - *see* Tuberculosis
Contact
  with
    AIDS virus V01.79
    anthrax V01.81
    cholera V01.0
    communicable disease V01.9
      specified type NEC V01.89
      viral NEC V01.79
    Escherichia coli (E. coli) V01.83
    German measles V01.4
    gonorrhea V01.6
    HIV V01.79
    human immunodeficiency virus V01.79
Contact *(Continued)*
  with *(Continued)*
    meningococcus V01.84
    parasitic disease NEC V01.89
    poliomyelitis V01.2
    rabies V01.5
    rubella V01.4
    SARS-associated coronavirus V01.82
    smallpox V01.3
    syphilis V01.6
    tuberculosis V01.1
    varicella V01.71
    venereal disease V01.6
    viral disease NEC V01.79
  dermatitis - *see* Dermatitis
Contamination, food (*see also* Poisoning, food) 005.9
Contraception, contraceptive
  advice NEC V25.09
    family planning V25.09
    fitting of diaphragm V25.02
    prescribing or use of
      oral contraceptive agent V25.01
      specified agent NEC V25.02
  counseling NEC V25.09
    emergency V25.03
    family planning V25.09
    fitting of diaphragm V25.02
    prescribing or use of
      oral contraceptive agent V25.01
        emergency V25.03
        postcoital V25.03
      specified agent NEC V25.02
  device (in situ) V45.59
    causing menorrhagia 996.76
    checking V25.42
    complications 996.32
    insertion V25.1
    intrauterine V45.51
    reinsertion V25.42
    removal V25.42
    subdermal V45.52
  fitting of diaphragm V25.02
  insertion
    intrauterine contraceptive device V25.1
    subdermal implantable V25.5
  maintenance V25.40
    examination V25.40
      intrauterine device V25.42
      oral contraceptive V25.41
      specified method NEC V25.49
      subdermal implantable V25.43
    intrauterine device V25.42
    oral contraceptive V25.41
    specified method NEC V25.49
    subdermal implantable V25.43
  management NEC V25.49
  prescription
    oral contraceptive agent V25.01
      emergency V25.03
      postcoital V25.03
      repeat V25.41
    specified agent NEC V25.02
      repeat V25.49
  sterilization V25.2
  surveillance V25.40
    intrauterine device V25.42
    oral contraceptive agent V25.41
    specified method NEC V25.49
    subdermal implantable V25.43
Contraction, contracture, contracted
  Achilles tendon (*see also* Short, tendon, Achilles) 727.81
Contraction, contracture, contracted *(Continued)*
  anus 564.89
  axilla 729.9
  bile duct (*see also* Disease, biliary) 576.8
  bladder 596.8
    neck or sphincter 596.0
  bowel (*see also* Obstruction, intestine) 560.9
  Braxton Hicks 644.1
  bronchus 519.19
  burn (old) - *see* Cicatrix
  cecum (*see also* Obstruction, intestine) 560.9
  cervix (*see also* Stricture, cervix) 622.4
    congenital 752.49
  cicatricial - *see* Cicatrix
  colon (*see also* Obstruction, intestine) 560.9
  conjunctiva, trachomatous, active 076.1
    late effect 139.1
  Dupuytren's 728.6
  eyelid 374.41
  eye socket (after enucleation) 372.64
  face 729.9
  fascia (lata) (postural) 728.89
    Dupuytren's 728.6
    palmar 728.6
    plantar 728.71
  finger NEC 736.29
    congenital 755.59
    joint (*see also* Contraction, joint) 718.44
  flaccid, paralytic
    joint (*see also* Contraction, joint) 718.4
    muscle 728.85
      ocular 378.50
  gallbladder (*see also* Obstruction, gallbladder) 575.2
  hamstring 728.89
    tendon 727.81
  heart valve - *see* Endocarditis
  Hicks' 644.1
  hip (*see also* Contraction, joint) 718.4
  hourglass
    bladder 596.8
      congenital 753.8
    gallbladder (*see also* Obstruction, gallbladder) 575.2
      congenital 751.69
    stomach 536.8
      congenital 750.7
      psychogenic 306.4
    uterus 661.4
      affecting fetus or newborn 763.7
  hysterical 300.11
  infantile (*see also* Epilepsy) 345.6
  internal os (*see also* Stricture, cervix) 622.4
  intestine (*see also* Obstruction, intestine) 560.9
  joint (abduction) (acquired) (adduction) (flexion) (rotation) 718.40
    ankle 718.47
    congenital NEC 755.8
      generalized or multiple 754.89
        lower limb joints 754.89
      hip (*see also* Subluxation, congenital, hip) 754.32
      lower limb (including pelvic girdle) not involving hip 754.89
      upper limb (including shoulder girdle) 755.59
    elbow 718.42

Contraction, contracture, contracted *(Continued)*
joint *(Continued)*
foot 718.47
hand 718.44
hip 718.45
hysterical 300.11
knee 718.46
multiple sites 718.49
pelvic region 718.45
shoulder (region) 718.41
specified site NEC 718.48
wrist 718.43
kidney (granular) (secondary) (*see also* Sclerosis, renal) 587
congenital 753.3
hydronephritic 591
pyelonephritic (*see also* Pyelitis, chronic) 590.00
tuberculous (*see also* Tuberculosis) 016.0
ligament 728.89
congenital 756.89
liver - *see* Cirrhosis, liver
muscle (postinfectional) (postural) NEC 728.85
congenital 756.89
sternocleidomastoid 754.1
extraocular 378.60
eye (extrinsic) (*see also* Strabismus) 378.9
paralytic (*see also* Strabismus, paralytic) 378.50
flaccid 728.85
hysterical 300.11
ischemic (Volkmann's) 958.6
paralytic 728.85
posttraumatic 958.6
psychogenic 306.0
specified as conversion reaction 300.11
myotonic 728.85
neck (*see also* Torticollis) 723.5
congenital 754.1
psychogenic 306.0
ocular muscle (*see also* Strabismus) 378.9
paralytic (*see also* Strabismus, paralytic) 378.50
organ or site, congenital NEC - *see* Atresia
outlet (pelvis) - *see* Contraction, pelvis
palmar fascia 728.6
paralytic
joint (*see also* Contraction, joint) 718.4
muscle 728.85
ocular (*see also* Strabismus, paralytic) 378.50
pelvis (acquired) (general) 738.6
affecting fetus or newborn 763.1
complicating delivery 653.1
causing obstructed labor 660.1
generally contracted 653.1
causing obstructed labor 660.1
inlet 653.2
causing obstructed labor 660.1
midpelvic 653.8
causing obstructed labor 660.1
midplane 653.8
causing obstructed labor 660.1
outlet 653.3
causing obstructed labor 660.1
plantar fascia 728.71

Contraction, contracture, contracted *(Continued)*
premature
atrial 427.61
auricular 427.61
auriculoventricular 427.61
heart (junctional) (nodal) 427.60
supraventricular 427.61
ventricular 427.69
prostate 602.8
pylorus (*see also* Pylorospasm) 537.81
rectosigmoid (*see also* Obstruction, intestine) 560.9
rectum, rectal (sphincter) 564.89
psychogenic 306.4
ring (Bandl's) 661.4
affecting fetus or newborn 763.7
scar - *see* Cicatrix
sigmoid (*see also* Obstruction, intestine) 560.9
socket, eye 372.64
spine (*see also* Curvature, spine) 737.9
stomach 536.8
hourglass 536.8
congenital 750.7
psychogenic 306.4
psychogenic 306.4
tendon (sheath) (*see also* Short, tendon) 727.81
toe 735.8
ureterovesical orifice (postinfectional) 593.3
urethra 599.84
uterus 621.8
abnormal 661.9
affecting fetus or newborn 763.7
clonic, hourglass or tetanic 661.4
affecting fetus or newborn 763.7
dyscoordinate 661.4
affecting fetus or newborn 763.7
hourglass 661.4
affecting fetus or newborn 763.7
hypotonic NEC 661.2
affecting fetus or newborn 763.7
incoordinate 661.4
affecting fetus or newborn 763.7
inefficient or poor 661.2
affecting fetus or newborn 763.7
irregular 661.2
affecting fetus or newborn 763.7
tetanic 661.4
affecting fetus or newborn 763.7
vagina (outlet) 623.2
vesical 596.8
neck or urethral orifice 596.0
visual field, generalized 368.45
Volkmann's (ischemic) 958.6
Contusion (skin surface intact) 924.9
with
crush injury - *see* Crush
dislocation - *see* Dislocation, by site
fracture - *see* Fracture, by site
internal injury - *see also* Injury, internal, by site
heart - *see* Contusion, cardiac
kidney - *see* Contusion, kidney
liver - *see* Contusion, liver
lung - *see* Contusion, lung
spleen - *see* Contusion, spleen
intracranial injury - *see* Injury, intracranial
nerve injury - *see* Injury, nerve
open wound - *see* Wound, open, by site

Contusion *(Continued)*
abdomen, abdominal (muscle) (wall) 922.2
organ(s) NEC 868.00
adnexa, eye NEC 921.9
ankle 924.21
with other parts of foot 924.20
arm 923.9
lower (with elbow) 923.10
upper 923.03
with shoulder or axillary region 923.09
auditory canal (external) (meatus) (and other part(s) of neck, scalp, or face, except eye) 920
auricle, ear (and other part(s) of neck, scalp, or face except eye) 920
axilla 923.02
with shoulder or upper arm 923.09
back 922.31
bone NEC 924.9
brain (cerebral) (membrane) (with hemorrhage) 851.8

Note Use the following fifth-digit subclassification with categories 851–854:

0 unspecified state of consciousness
1 with no loss of consciousness
2 with brief [less than one hour] loss of consciousness
3 with moderate [1-24 hours] loss of consciousness
4 with prolonged [more than 24 hours] loss of consciousness and return to pre-existing conscious level
5 with prolonged [more than 24 hours] loss of consciousness, without return to pre-existing conscious level

Use fifth-digit 5 to designate when a patient is unconscious and dies before regaining consciousness, regardless of the duration of the loss of consciousness

6 with loss of consciousness of unspecified duration
9 with concussion, unspecified

with
open intracranial wound 851.9
skull fracture - *see* Fracture, skull, by site
cerebellum 851.4
with open intracranial wound 851.5
cortex 851.0
with open intracranial wound 851.1
occipital lobe 851.4
with open intracranial wound 851.5
stem 851.4
with open intracranial wound 851.5
breast 922.0
brow (and other part(s) of neck, scalp, or face, except eye) 920
buttock 922.32
canthus 921.1
cardiac 861.01
with open wound into thorax 861.11
cauda equina (spine) 952.4
cerebellum - *see* Contusion, brain, cerebellum
cerebral - *see* Contusion, brain

ICD-9-CM C Vol. 2

Contusion *(Continued)*
cheek(s) (and other part(s) of neck, scalp, or face, except eye) 920
chest (wall) 922.1
chin (and other part(s) of neck, scalp, or face, except eye) 920
clitoris 922.4
conjunctiva 921.1
conus medullaris (spine) 952.4
cornea 921.3
corpus cavernosum 922.4
cortex (brain) (cerebral) - *see* Contusion, brain, cortex
costal region 922.1
ear (and other part(s) of neck, scalp, or face except eye) 920
elbow 923.11
with forearm 923.10
epididymis 922.4
epigastric region 922.2
eye NEC 921.9
eyeball 921.3
eyelid(s) (and periocular area) 921.1
face (and neck, or scalp, any part, except eye) 920
femoral triangle 922.2
fetus or newborn 772.6
finger(s) (nail) (subungual) 923.3
flank 922.2
foot (with ankle) (excluding toe(s)) 924.20
forearm (and elbow) 923.10
forehead (and other part(s) of neck, scalp, or face, except eye) 920
genital organs, external 922.4
globe (eye) 921.3
groin 922.2
gum(s) (and other part(s) of neck, scalp, or face, except eye) 920
hand(s) (except fingers alone) 923.20
head (any part, except eye) (and face) (and neck) 920
heart - *see* Contusion, cardiac
heel 924.20
hip 924.01
with thigh 924.00
iliac region 922.2
inguinal region 922.2
internal organs (abdomen, chest, or pelvis) NEC - *see* Injury, internal, by site
interscapular region 922.33
iris (eye) 921.3
kidney 866.01
with open wound into cavity 866.11
knee 924.11
with lower leg 924.10
labium (majus) (minus) 922.4
lacrimal apparatus, gland, or sac 921.1
larynx (and other part(s) of neck, scalp, or face, except eye) 920
late effect - *see* Late, effects (of), contusion
leg 924.5
lower (with knee) 924.10
lens 921.3
lingual (and other part(s) of neck, scalp, or face, except eye) 920
lip(s) (and other part(s) of neck, scalp, or face, except eye) 920
liver 864.01
with
laceration - *see* Laceration, liver
open wound into cavity 864.11

Contusion *(Continued)*
lower extremity 924.5
multiple sites 924.4
lumbar region 922.31
lung 861.21
with open wound into thorax 861.31
malar region (and other part(s) of neck, scalp, or face, except eye) 920
mandibular joint (and other part(s) of neck, scalp, or face, except eye) 920
mastoid region (and other part(s) of neck, scalp, or face, except eye) 920
membrane, brain - *see* Contusion, brain
midthoracic region 922.1
mouth (and other part(s) of neck, scalp, or face, except eye) 920
multiple sites (not classifiable to same three-digit category) 924.8
lower limb 924.4
trunk 922.8
upper limb 923.8
muscle NEC 924.9
myocardium - *see* Contusion, cardiac
nasal (septum) (and other part(s) of neck, scalp, or face, except eye) 920
neck (and scalp, or face, any part, except eye) 920
nerve - *see* Injury, nerve, by site
nose (and other part(s) of neck, scalp, or face, except eye) 920
occipital region (scalp) (and neck or face, except eye) 920
lobe - *see* Contusion, brain, occipital lobe
orbit (region) (tissues) 921.2
palate (soft) (and other part(s) of neck, scalp, or face, except eye) 920
parietal region (scalp) (and neck, or face, except eye) 920
lobe - *see* Contusion, brain
penis 922.4
pericardium - *see* Contusion, cardiac
perineum 922.4
periocular area 921.1
pharynx (and other part(s) of neck, scalp, or face, except eye) 920
popliteal space (*see also* Contusion, knee) 924.11
prepuce 922.4
pubic region 922.4
pudenda 922.4
pulmonary - *see* Contusion, lung
quadriceps femoralis 924.00
rib cage 922.1
sacral region 922.32
salivary ducts or glands (and other part(s) of neck, scalp, or face, except eye) 920
scalp (and neck, or face, any part, except eye) 920
scapular region 923.01
with shoulder or upper arm 923.09
sclera (eye) 921.3
scrotum 922.4
shoulder 923.00
with upper arm or axillary regions 923.09
skin NEC 924.9
skull 920

Contusion *(Continued)*
spermatic cord 922.4
spinal cord - *see also* Injury, spinal, by site
cauda equina 952.4
conus medullaris 952.4
spleen 865.01
with open wound into cavity 865.11
sternal region 922.1
stomach - *see* Injury, internal, stomach
subconjunctival 921.1
subcutaneous NEC 924.9
submaxillary region (and other part(s) of neck, scalp, or face, except eye) 920
submental region (and other part(s) of neck, scalp, or face, except eye) 920
subperiosteal NEC 924.9
supraclavicular fossa (and other part(s) of neck, scalp, or face, except eye) 920
supraorbital (and other part(s) of neck, scalp, or face, except eye) 920
temple (region) (and other part(s) of neck, scalp, or face, except eye) 920
testis 922.4
thigh (and hip) 924.00
thorax 922.1
organ - *see* Injury, internal, intrathoracic
throat (and other part(s) of neck, scalp, or face, except eye) 920
thumb(s) (nail) (subungual) 923.3
toe(s) (nail) (subungual) 924.3
tongue (and other part(s) of neck, scalp, or face, except eye) 920
trunk 922.9
multiple sites 922.8
specified site - *see* Contusion, by site
tunica vaginalis 922.4
tympanum (membrane) (and other part(s) of neck, scalp, or face, except eye) 920
upper extremity 923.9
multiple sites 923.8
uvula (and other part(s) of neck, scalp, or face, except eye) 920
vagina 922.4
vocal cord(s) (and other part(s) of neck, scalp, or face, except eye) 920
vulva 922.4
wrist 923.21
with hand(s), except finger(s) alone 923.20
Conus (any type) (congenital) 743.57
acquired 371.60
medullaris syndrome 336.8
Convalescence (following) V66.9
chemotherapy V66.2
medical NEC V66.5
psychotherapy V66.3
radiotherapy V66.1
surgery NEC V66.0
treatment (for) NEC V66.5
combined V66.6
fracture V66.4
mental disorder NEC V66.3
specified disorder NEC V66.5
Conversion
closed surgical procedure to open procedure
arthroscopic V64.43
laparoscopic V64.41
thoracoscopic V64.42

Conversion *(Continued)*
hysteria, hysterical, any type 300.11
neurosis, any 300.11
reaction, any 300.11
Converter, tuberculosis (test reaction) 795.5
Convulsions (idiopathic) 780.39
apoplectiform (*see also* Disease, cerebrovascular, acute) 436
brain 780.39
cerebral 780.39
cerebrospinal 780.39
due to trauma NEC - *see* Injury, intracranial
eclamptic (*see also* Eclampsia) 780.39
epileptic (*see also* Epilepsy) 345.9
epileptiform (*see also* Seizure, epileptiform) 780.39
epileptoid (*see also* Seizure, epileptiform) 780.39
ether
anesthetic
correct substance properly administered 780.39
overdose or wrong substance given 968.2
other specified type - *see* Table of Drugs and Chemicals
febrile (simple) 780.31
complex 780.32
generalized 780.39
hysterical 300.11
infantile 780.39
epilepsy - *see* Epilepsy
internal 780.39
jacksonian (*see also* Epilepsy) 345.5
myoclonic 333.2
newborn 779.0
paretic 094.1
pregnancy (nephritic) (uremic) - *see* Eclampsia, pregnancy
psychomotor (*see also* Epilepsy) 345.4
puerperal, postpartum - *see* Eclampsia, pregnancy
recurrent 780.39
epileptic - *see* Epilepsy
reflex 781.0
repetitive 780.39
epileptic - *see* Epilepsy
salaam (*see also* Epilepsy) 345.6
scarlatinal 034.1
spasmodic 780.39
tetanus, tetanic (*see also* Tetanus) 037
thymic 254.8
uncinate 780.39
uremic 586
Convulsive - *see also* Convulsions
disorder or state 780.39
epileptic - *see* Epilepsy
equivalent, abdominal (*see also* Epilepsy) 345.5
Cooke-Apert-Gallais syndrome (adrenogenital) 255.2
Cooley's anemia (erythroblastic) 282.49
Coolie itch 126.9
Cooper's
disease 610.1
hernia - *see* Hernia, Cooper's
Coordination disturbance 781.3
Copper wire arteries, retina 362.13
Copra itch 133.8
Coprolith 560.39
Coprophilia 302.89
Coproporphyria, hereditary 277.1
Coprostasis 560.39
with hernia - *see also* Hernia, by site, with obstruction
gangrenous - *see* Hernia, by site, with gangrene
Cor
biloculare 745.7
bovinum - *see* Hypertrophy, cardiac
bovis - *see also* Hypertrophy, cardiac
pulmonale (chronic) 416.9
acute 415.0
triatriatum, triatrium 746.82
triloculare 745.8
biatriatum 745.3
biventriculare 745.69
Corbus' disease 607.1
Cord - *see also* condition
around neck (tightly) (with compression)
affecting fetus or newborn 762.5
complicating delivery 663.1
without compression 663.3
affecting fetus or newborn 762.6
bladder NEC 344.61
tabetic 094.0
prolapse
affecting fetus or newborn 762.4
complicating delivery 663.0
Cord's angiopathy (*see also* Tuberculosis) 017.3 [362.18]
Cordis ectopia 746.87
Corditis (spermatic) 608.4
Corectopia 743.46
Cori type glycogen storage disease - *see* Disease, glycogen storage
Cork-handlers' disease or lung 495.3
Corkscrew esophagus 530.5
Corlett's pyosis (impetigo) 684
Corn (infected) 700
Cornea - *see also* condition
donor V59.5
guttata (dystrophy) 371.57
plana 743.41
Cornelia de Lange's syndrome (Amsterdam dwarf, mental retardation, and brachycephaly) 759.89
Cornual gestation or pregnancy - *see* Pregnancy, cornual
Cornu cutaneum 702.8
Coronary (artery) - *see also* condition
arising from aorta or pulmonary trunk 746.85
Corpora - *see also* condition
amylacea (prostate) 602.8
cavernosa - *see* condition
Corpulence (*see also* Obesity)
Corpus - *see* condition
Corrigan's disease - *see* Insufficiency, aortic
Corrosive burn - *see* Burn, by site
Corsican fever (*see also* Malaria) 084.6
Cortical - *see also* condition
blindness 377.75
necrosis, kidney (bilateral) 583.6
Corticoadrenal - *see* condition
Corticosexual syndrome 255.2
Coryza (acute) 460
with grippe or influenza 487.1
syphilitic 095.8
congenital (chronic) 090.0
Costen's syndrome or complex 524.60
Costiveness (*see also* Constipation) 564.00
Costochondritis 733.6
Cotard's syndrome (paranoia) 297.1
Cot death 798.0
Cotungo's disease 724.3
Cough 786.2
with hemorrhage (*see also* Hemoptysis) 786.3
affected 786.2
bronchial 786.2
with grippe or influenza 487.1
chronic 786.2
epidemic 786.2
functional 306.1
hemorrhagic 786.3
hysterical 300.11
laryngeal, spasmodic 786.2
nervous 786.2
psychogenic 306.1
smokers' 491.0
tea tasters' 112.89
Counseling NEC V65.40
without complaint or sickness V65.49
abuse victim NEC V62.89
child V61.21
partner V61.11
spouse V61.11
child abuse, maltreatment, or neglect V61.21
contraceptive NEC V25.09
device (intrauterine) V25.02
maintenance V25.40
intrauterine contraceptive device V25.42
oral contraceptive (pill) V25.41
specified type NEC V25.49
subdermal implantable V25.43
management NEC V25.9
oral contraceptive (pill) V25.01
emergency V25.03
postcoital V25.03
prescription NEC V25.02
oral contraceptive (pill) V25.01
emergency V25.03
postcoital V25.03
repeat prescription V25.41
repeat prescription V25.40
subdermal implantable V25.43
surveillance NEC V25.40
dietary V65.3
exercise V65.41
expectant mother, pediatric pre-birth visit V65.11
explanation of
investigation finding NEC V65.49
medication NEC V65.49
family planning V25.09
for nonattending third party V65.19
genetic V26.33
gonorrhea V65.45
health (advice) (education) (instruction) NEC V65.49
HIV V65.44
human immunodeficiency virus V65.44
injury prevention V65.43
insulin pump training V65.46
marital V61.10
medical (for) V65.9
boarding school resident V60.6
condition not demonstrated V65.5
feared complaint and no disease found V65.5
institutional resident V60.6
on behalf of another V65.19
person living alone V60.3

ICD-9-CM
C
Vol. 2

◀ New ◀ Revised

Counseling NEC *(Continued)*
parent-child conflict V61.20
specified problem NEC V61.29
partner abuse
perpetrator V61.12
victim V61.11
pediatric pre-birth visit for expectant mother V65.11
perpetrator of
child abuse V62.83
parental V61.22
partner abuse V61.12
spouse abuse V61.12
procreative V65.49
sex NEC V65.49
transmitted disease NEC V65.45
HIV V65.44
specified reason NEC V65.49
spousal abuse
perpetrator V61.12
victim V61.11
substance use and abuse V65.42
syphilis V65.45
victim (of)
abuse NEC V62.89
child abuse V61.21
partner abuse V61.11
spousal abuse V61.11
Coupled rhythm 427.89
Couvelaire uterus (complicating delivery) - *see* Placenta, separation
Cowper's gland - *see* condition
Cowperitis (*see also* Urethritis) 597.89
gonorrheal (acute) 098.0
chronic or duration of 2 months or over 098.2
Cowpox (abortive) 051.0
due to vaccination 999.0
eyelid 051.0 *[373.5]*
postvaccination 999.0 *[373.5]*
Coxa
plana 732.1
valga (acquired) 736.31
congenital 755.61
late effect of rickets 268.1
vara (acquired) 736.32
congenital 755.62
late effect of rickets 268.1
Coxae malum senilis 715.25
Coxalgia (nontuberculous) 719.45
tuberculous (*see also* Tuberculosis) 015.1 *[730.85]*
Coxalgic pelvis 736.30
Coxitis 716.65
Coxsackie (infection) (virus) 079.2
central nervous system NEC 048
endocarditis 074.22
enteritis 008.67
meningitis (aseptic) 047.0
myocarditis 074.23
pericarditis 074.21
pharyngitis 074.0
pleurodynia 074.1
specific disease NEC 074.8
Crabs, meaning pubic lice 132.2
Crack baby 760.75
Cracked
nipple 611.2
puerperal, postpartum 676.1
tooth 521.81
Cradle cap 690.11
Craft neurosis 300.89
Craigiasis 007.8
Cramp(s) 729.82
abdominal 789.0

Cramp(s) *(Continued)*
bathing 994.1
colic 789.0
psychogenic 306.4
due to immersion 994.1
extremity (lower) (upper) NEC 729.82
fireman 992.2
heat 992.2
hysterical 300.11
immersion 994.1
intestinal 789.0
psychogenic 306.4
linotypists' 300.89
organic 333.84
muscle (extremity) (general) 729.82
due to immersion 994.1
hysterical 300.11
occupational (hand) 300.89
organic 333.84
psychogenic 307.89
salt depletion 276.1
sleep related leg 327.52
stoker 992.2
stomach 789.0
telegraphers' 300.89
organic 333.84
typists' 300.89
organic 333.84
uterus 625.8
menstrual 625.3
writers' 333.84
organic 333.84
psychogenic 300.89
Cranial - *see* condition
Cranioclasis, fetal 763.89
Craniocleidodysostosis 755.59
Craniofenestria (skull) 756.0
Craniolacunia (skull) 756.0
Craniopagus 759.4
Craniopathy, metabolic 733.3
Craniopharyngeal - *see* condition
Craniopharyngioma (M9350/1) 237.0
Craniorachischisis (totalis) 740.1
Cranioschisis 756.0
Craniostenosis 756.0
Craniosynostosis 756.0
Craniotabes (cause unknown) 733.3
rachitic 268.1
syphilitic 090.5
Craniotomy, fetal 763.89
Cranium - *see* condition
Craw-craw 125.3
Creaking joint 719.60
ankle 719.67
elbow 719.62
foot 719.67
hand 719.64
hip 719.65
knee 719.66
multiple sites 719.69
pelvic region 719.65
shoulder (region) 719.61
specified site NEC 719.68
wrist 719.63
Creeping
eruption 126.9
palsy 335.21
paralysis 335.21
Crenated tongue 529.8
Creotoxism 005.9
Crepitus
caput 756.0
joint 719.60
ankle 719.67

Crepitus *(Continued)*
joint *(Continued)*
elbow 719.62
foot 719.67
hand 719.64
hip 719.65
knee 719.66
multiple sites 719.69
pelvic region 719.65
shoulder (region) 719.61
specified site NEC 719.68
wrist 719.63
Crescent or conus choroid, congenital 743.57
Cretin, cretinism (athyrotic) (congenital) (endemic) (metabolic) (nongoitrous) (sporadic) 243
goitrous (sporadic) 246.1
pelvis (dwarf type) (male type) 243
with disproportion (fetopelvic) 653.1
affecting fetus or newborn 763.1
causing obstructed labor 660.1
affecting fetus or newborn 763.1
pituitary 253.3
Cretinoid degeneration 243
Creutzfeldt-Jakob disease (syndrome) (new variant) 046.1
with dementia
with behavioral disturbance 046.1 *[294.11]*
without behavioral disturbance 046.1 *[294.10]*
Crib death 798.0
Cribriform hymen 752.49
Cri-du-chat syndrome 758.31
Crigler-Najjar disease or syndrome (congenital hyperbilirubinemia) 277.4
Crimean hemorrhagic fever 065.0
Criminalism 301.7
Crisis
abdomen 789.0
addisonian (acute adrenocortical insufficiency) 255.4
adrenal (cortical) 255.4
asthmatic - *see* Asthma
brain, cerebral (*see also* Disease, cerebrovascular, acute) 436
celiac 579.0
Dietl's 593.4
emotional NEC 309.29
acute reaction to stress 308.0
adjustment reaction 309.9
specific to childhood or adolescence 313.9
gastric (tabetic) 094.0
glaucomatocyclitic 364.22
heart (*see also* Failure, heart) 428.9
hypertensive - *see* Hypertension
nitritoid
correct substance properly administered 458.29
overdose or wrong substance given or taken 961.1
oculogyric 378.87
psychogenic 306.7
Pel's 094.0
psychosexual identity 302.6
rectum 094.0
renal 593.81
sickle cell 282.62
stomach (tabetic) 094.0
tabetic 094.0
thyroid (*see also* Thyrotoxicosis) 242.9
thyrotoxic (*see also* Thyrotoxicosis) 242.9

Crisis *(Continued)*
vascular - *see* Disease, cerebrovascular, acute
Crocq's disease (acrocyanosis) 443.89
Crohn's disease (*see also* Enteritis, regional) 555.9
Cronkhite-Canada syndrome 211.3
Crooked septum, nasal 470
Cross
birth (of fetus) complicating delivery 652.3
with successful version 652.1
causing obstructed labor 660.0
bite, anterior or posterior 524.27
eye (*see also* Esotropia) 378.00
Crossed ectopia of kidney 753.3
Crossfoot 754.50
Croup, croupous (acute) (angina) (catarrhal) (infective) (inflammatory) (laryngeal) (membranous) (nondiphtheritic) (pseudomembranous) 464.4
asthmatic (*see also* Asthma) 493.9
bronchial 466.0
diphtheritic (membranous) 032.3
false 478.75
spasmodic 478.75
diphtheritic 032.3
stridulous 478.75
diphtheritic 032.3
Crouzon's disease (craniofacial dysostosis) 756.0
Crowding, teeth 524.31
CRST syndrome (cutaneous systemic sclerosis) 710.1
Cruchet's disease (encephalitis lethargica) 049.8
Cruelty in children (*see also* Disturbance, conduct) 312.9
Crural ulcer (*see also* Ulcer, lower extremity) 707.10
Crush, crushed, crushing (injury) 929.9
with
fracture - *see* Fracture, by site
abdomen 926.19
internal - *see* Injury, internal, abdomen
ankle 928.21
with other parts of foot 928.20
arm 927.9
lower (and elbow) 927.10
upper 927.03
with shoulder or axillary region 927.09
axilla 927.02
with shoulder or upper arm 927.09
back 926.11
breast 926.19
buttock 926.12
cheek 925.1
chest - *see* Injury, internal, chest
ear 925.1
elbow 927.11
with forearm 927.10
face 925.1
finger(s) 927.3
with hand(s) 927.20
and wrist(s) 927.21
flank 926.19
foot, excluding toe(s) alone (with ankle) 928.20
forearm (and elbow) 927.10
genitalia, external (female) (male) 926.0
internal - *see* Injury, internal, genital organ NEC
hand, except finger(s) alone (and wrist) 927.20

Crush, crushed, crushing *(Continued)*
head - *see* Fracture, skull, by site
heel 928.20
hip 928.01
with thigh 928.00
internal organ (abdomen, chest, or pelvis) - *see* Injury, internal, by site
knee 928.11
with leg, lower 928.10
labium (majus) (minus) 926.0
larynx 925.2
late effect - *see* Late, effects (of), crushing
leg 928.9
lower 928.10
and knee 928.11
upper 928.00
limb
lower 928.9
multiple sites 928.8
upper 927.9
multiple sites 927.8
multiple sites NEC 929.0
neck 925.2
nerve - *see* Injury, nerve, by site
nose 802.0
open 802.1
penis 926.0
pharynx 925.2
scalp 925.1
scapular region 927.01
with shoulder or upper arm 927.09
scrotum 926.0
shoulder 927.00
with upper arm or axillary region 927.09
skull or cranium - *see* Fracture, skull, by site
spinal cord - *see* Injury, spinal, by site
syndrome (complication of trauma) 958.5
testis 926.0
thigh (with hip) 928.00
throat 925.2
thumb(s) (and fingers) 927.3
toe(s) 928.3
with foot 928.20
and ankle 928.21
tonsil 925.2
trunk 926.9
chest - *see* Injury, internal, intrathoracic organs NEC
internal organ - *see* Injury, internal, by site
multiple sites 926.8
specified site NEC 926.19
vulva 926.0
wrist 927.21
with hand(s), except fingers alone 927.20
Crusta lactea 690.11
Crusts 782.8
Crutch paralysis 953.4
Cruveilhier's disease 335.21
Cruveilhier-Baumgarten cirrhosis, disease, or syndrome 571.5
Cruz-Chagas disease (*see also* Trypanosomiasis) 086.2
Crying
constant, continuous
adolescent 780.95
adult 780.95
baby 780.92
child 780.95
infant 780.92
newborn 780.92

Crying *(Continued)*
excessive
adolescent 780.95
adult 780.95
baby 780.92
child 780.95
infant 780.92
newborn 780.92
Cryoglobulinemia (mixed) 273.2
Crypt (anal) (rectal) 569.49
Cryptitis (anal) (rectal) 569.49
Cryptococcosis (European) (pulmonary) (systemic) 117.5
Cryptococcus 117.5
epidermicus 117.5
neoformans, infection by 117.5
Cryptopapillitis (anus) 569.49
Cryptophthalmos (eyelid) 743.06
Cryptorchid, cryptorchism, cryptorchidism 752.51
Cryptosporidiosis 007.4
Cryptotia 744.29
Crystallopathy
calcium pyrophosphate (*see also* Arthritis) 275.49 *[712.2]*
dicalcium phosphate (*see also* Arthritis) 275.49 *[712.1]*
gouty 274.0
pyrophosphate NEC (*see also* Arthritis) 275.49 *[712.2]*
uric acid 274.0
Crystalluria 791.9
Csillag's disease (lichen sclerosus et atrophicus) 701.0
Cuban itch 050.1
Cubitus
valgus (acquired) 736.01
congenital 755.59
late effect of rickets 268.1
varus (acquired) 736.02
congenital 755.59
late effect of rickets 268.1
Cultural deprivation V62.4
Cupping of optic disc 377.14
Curling's ulcer - *see* Ulcer, duodenum
Curling esophagus 530.5
Curschmann (-Batten) (-Steinert) disease or syndrome 359.2
Curvature
organ or site, congenital NEC - *see* Distortion
penis (lateral) 752.69
Pott's (spinal) (*see also* Tuberculosis) 015.0 *[737.43]*
radius, idiopathic, progressive (congenital) 755.54
spine (acquired) (angular) (idiopathic) (incorrect) (postural) 737.9
congenital 754.2
due to or associated with
Charcôt-Marie-Tooth disease 356.1 *[737.40]*
mucopolysaccharidosis 277.5 *[737.40]*
neurofibromatosis 237.71 *[737.40]*
osteitis
deformans 731.0 *[737.40]*
fibrosa cystica 252.01 *[737.40]*
osteoporosis (*see also* Osteoporosis) 733.00 *[737.40]*
poliomyelitis (*see also* Poliomyelitis) 138 *[737.40]*
tuberculosis (Pott's curvature) (*see also* Tuberculosis) 015.0 *[737.43]*

Curvature *(Continued)*
spine *(Continued)*
kyphoscoliotic (*see also* Kyphoscoliosis) 737.30
kyphotic (*see also* Kyphosis) 737.10
late effect of rickets 268.1 *[737.40]*
Pott's 015.0 *[737.40]*
scoliotic (*see also* Scoliosis) 737.30
specified NEC 737.8
tuberculous 015.0 *[737.40]*
Cushing's
basophilism, disease, or syndrome (iatrogenic) (idiopathic) (pituitary basophilism) (pituitary dependent) 255.0
ulcer - *see* Ulcer, peptic
Cushingoid due to steroid therapy
correct substance properly administered 255.0
overdose or wrong substance given or taken 962.0
Cut (external) - *see* Wound, open, by site
Cutaneous - *see also* condition
hemorrhage 782.7
horn (cheek) (eyelid) (mouth) 702.8
larva migrans 126.9
Cutis - *see also* condition
hyperelastic 756.83
acquired 701.8
laxa 756.83
senilis 701.8
marmorata 782.61
osteosis 709.3
pendula 756.83
acquired 701.8
rhomboidalis nuchae 701.8
verticis gyrata 757.39
acquired 701.8
Cyanopathy, newborn 770.83
Cyanosis 782.5
autotoxic 289.7
common atrioventricular canal 745.69
congenital 770.83
conjunctiva 372.71
due to
endocardial cushion defect 745.60
nonclosure, foramen botalli 745.5
patent foramen botalli 745.5
persistent foramen ovale 745.5
enterogenous 289.7
fetus or newborn 770.83
ostium primum defect 745.61
paroxysmal digital 443.0
retina, retinal 362.10
Cycle
anovulatory 628.0
menstrual, irregular 626.4
Cyclencephaly 759.89
Cyclical vomiting 536.2
psychogenic 306.4
Cyclitic membrane 364.74
Cyclitis (*see also* Iridocyclitis) 364.3
acute 364.00
primary 364.01
recurrent 364.02
chronic 364.10
in
sarcoidosis 135 *[364.11]*
tuberculosis (*see also* Tuberculosis) 017.3 *[364.11]*
Fuchs' heterochromic 364.21
granulomatous 364.10
lens induced 364.23
nongranulomatous 364.00

Cyclitis *(Continued)*
posterior 363.21
primary 364.01
recurrent 364.02
secondary (noninfectious) 364.04
infectious 364.03
subacute 364.00
primary 364.01
recurrent 364.02
Cyclokeratitis - *see* Keratitis
Cyclophoria 378.44
Cyclopia, cyclops 759.89
Cycloplegia 367.51
Cyclospasm 367.53
Cyclosporiasis 007.5
Cyclothymia 301.13
Cyclothymic personality 301.13
Cyclotropia 378.33
Cyesis - *see* Pregnancy
Cylindroma (M8200/3) - *see also* Neoplasm, by site, malignant
eccrine dermal (M8200/0) - *see* Neoplasm, skin, benign
skin (M8200/0) - *see* Neoplasm, skin, benign
Cylindruria 791.7
Cyllosoma 759.89
Cynanche
diphtheritic 032.3
tonsillaris 475
Cynorexia 783.6
Cyphosis - *see* Kyphosis
Cyprus fever (*see also* Brucellosis) 023.9
Cyriax's syndrome (slipping rib) 733.99
Cyst (mucous) (retention) (serous) (simple)

Note In general, cysts are not neoplastic and are classified to the appropriate category for disease of the specified anatomical site. This generalization does not apply to certain types of cysts which are neoplastic in nature, for example, dermoid, nor does it apply to cysts of certain structures, for example, branchial cleft, which are classified as developmental anomalies.

The following listing includes some of the most frequently reported sites of cysts as well as qualifiers which indicate the type of cyst. The latter qualifiers usually are not repeated under the anatomical sites. Since the code assignment for a given site may vary depending upon the type of cyst, the coder should refer to the listings under the specified type of cyst before consideration is given to the site.

accessory, fallopian tube 752.11
adenoid (infected) 474.8
adrenal gland 255.8
congenital 759.1
air, lung 518.89
allantoic 753.7
alveolar process (jaw bone) 526.2
amnion, amniotic 658.8
anterior chamber (eye) 364.60
exudative 364.62
implantation (surgical) (traumatic) 364.61
parasitic 360.13
anterior nasopalatine 526.1
antrum 478.19 ⬅

Cyst *(Continued)*
anus 569.49
apical (periodontal) (tooth) 522.8
appendix 543.9
arachnoid, brain 348.0
arytenoid 478.79
auricle 706.2
Baker's (knee) 727.51
tuberculous (*see also* Tuberculosis) 015.2
Bartholin's gland or duct 616.2
bile duct (*see also* Disease, biliary) 576.8
bladder (multiple) (trigone) 596.8
Blessig's 362.62
blood, endocardial (*see also* Endocarditis) 424.90
blue dome 610.0
bone (local) 733.20
aneurysmal 733.22
jaw 526.2
developmental (odontogenic) 526.0
fissural 526.1
latent 526.89
solitary 733.21
unicameral 733.21
brain 348.0
congenital 742.4
hydatid (*see also* Echinococcus) 122.9
third ventricle (colloid) 742.4
branchial (cleft) 744.42
branchiogenic 744.42
breast (benign) (blue dome) (pedunculated) (solitary) (traumatic) 610.0
involution 610.4
sebaceous 610.8
broad ligament (benign) 620.8
embryonic 752.11
bronchogenic (mediastinal) (sequestration) 518.89
congenital 748.4
buccal 528.4
bulbourethral gland (Cowper's) 599.89
bursa, bursal 727.49
pharyngeal 478.26
calcifying odontogenic (M9301/0) 213.1
upper jaw (bone) 213.0
canal of Nuck (acquired) (serous) 629.1
congenital 752.41
canthus 372.75
carcinomatous (M8010/3) - *see* Neoplasm, by site, malignant
cartilage (joint) - *see* Derangement, joint
cauda equina 336.8
cavum septi pellucidi NEC 348.0
celomic (pericardium) 746.89
cerebellopontine (angle) - *see* Cyst, brain
cerebellum - *see* Cyst, brain
cerebral - *see* Cyst, brain
cervical lateral 744.42
cervix 622.8
embryonal 752.41
nabothian (gland) 616.0
chamber, anterior (eye) 364.60
exudative 364.62
implantation (surgical) (traumatic) 364.61
parasitic 360.13
chiasmal, optic NEC (*see also* Lesion, chiasmal) 377.54
chocolate (ovary) 617.1
choledochal (congenital) 751.69
acquired 576.8

Cyst *(Continued)*
choledochus 751.69
chorion 658.8
choroid plexus 348.0
chyle, mesentery 457.8
ciliary body 364.60
exudative 364.64
implantation 364.61
primary 364.63
clitoris 624.8
coccyx (*see also* Cyst, bone) 733.20
colloid
third ventricle (brain) 742.4
thyroid gland - *see* Goiter
colon 569.89
common (bile) duct (*see also* Disease, biliary) 576.8
congenital NEC 759.89
adrenal glands 759.1
epiglottis 748.3
esophagus 750.4
fallopian tube 752.11
kidney 753.10
multiple 753.19
single 753.11
larynx 748.3
liver 751.62
lung 748.4
mediastinum 748.8
ovary 752.0
oviduct 752.11
pancreas 751.7
periurethral (tissue) 753.8
prepuce NEC 752.69
penis 752.69
sublingual 750.26
submaxillary gland 750.26
thymus (gland) 759.2
tongue 750.19
ureterovesical orifice 753.4
vulva 752.41
conjunctiva 372.75
cornea 371.23
corpora quadrigemina 348.0
corpus
albicans (ovary) 620.2
luteum (ruptured) 620.1
Cowper's gland (benign) (infected) 599.89
cranial meninges 348.0
craniobuccal pouch 253.8
craniopharyngeal pouch 253.8
cystic duct (*see also* Disease, gallbladder) 575.8
Cysticercus (any site) 123.1
Dandy-Walker 742.3
with spina bifida (*see also* Spina bifida) 741.0
dental 522.8
developmental 526.0
eruption 526.0
lateral periodontal 526.0
primordial (keratocyst) 526.0
root 522.8
dentigerous 526.0
mandible 526.0
maxilla 526.0
dermoid (M9084/0) - *see also* Neoplasm, by site, benign
with malignant transformation (M9084/3) 183.0
implantation
external area or site (skin) NEC 709.8

Cyst *(Continued)*
dermoid *(Continued)*
implantation *(Continued)*
iris 364.61
skin 709.8
vagina 623.8
vulva 624.8
mouth 528.4
oral soft tissue 528.4
sacrococcygeal 685.1
with abscess 685.0
developmental of ovary, ovarian 752.0
dura (cerebral) 348.0
spinal 349.2
ear (external) 706.2
echinococcal (*see also* Echinococcus) 122.9
embryonal
cervix uteri 752.41
genitalia, female external 752.41
uterus 752.3
vagina 752.41
endometrial 621.8
ectopic 617.9
endometrium (uterus) 621.8
ectopic - *see* Endometriosis
enteric 751.5
enterogenous 751.5
epidermal (inclusion) (*see also* Cyst, skin) 706.2
epidermoid (inclusion) (*see also* Cyst, skin) 706.2
mouth 528.4
not of skin - *see* Cyst, by site
oral soft tissue 528.4
epididymis 608.89
epiglottis 478.79
epiphysis cerebri 259.8
epithelial (inclusion) (*see also* Cyst, skin) 706.2
epoophoron 752.11
eruption 526.0
esophagus 530.89
ethmoid sinus 478.19 ⇐
eye (retention) 379.8
congenital 743.03
posterior segment, congenital 743.54
eyebrow 706.2
eyelid (sebaceous) 374.84
infected 373.13
sweat glands or ducts 374.84
falciform ligament (inflammatory) 573.8
fallopian tube 620.8
female genital organs NEC 629.89 ⇐
fimbrial (congenital) 752.11
fissural (oral region) 526.1
follicle (atretic) (graafian) (ovarian) 620.0
nabothian (gland) 616.0
follicular (atretic) (ovarian) 620.0
dentigerous 526.0
frontal sinus 478.19 ⇐
gallbladder or duct 575.8
ganglion 727.43
Gartner's duct 752.41
gas, of mesentery 568.89
gingiva 523.8
gland of moll 374.84
globulomaxillary 526.1
graafian follicle 620.0
granulosal lutein 620.2
hemangiomatous (M9121/0) (*see also* Hemangioma) 228.00
hydatid (*see also* Echinococcus) 122.9
fallopian tube (Morgagni) 752.11
liver NEC 122.8

Cyst *(Continued)*
hydatid *(Continued)*
lung NEC 122.9
Morgagni 752.89
fallopian tube 752.11
specified site NEC 122.9
hymen 623.8
embryonal 752.41
hypopharynx 478.26
hypophysis, hypophyseal (duct) (recurrent) 253.8
cerebri 253.8
implantation (dermoid)
anterior chamber (eye) 364.61
external area or site (skin) NEC 709.8
iris 364.61
vagina 623.8
vulva 624.8
incisor, incisive canal 526.1
inclusion (epidermal) (epithelial) (epidermoid) (mucous) (squamous) (*see also* Cyst, skin) 706.2
not of skin - *see* Neoplasm, by site, benign
intestine (large) (small) 569.89
intracranial - *see* Cyst, brain
intraligamentous 728.89
knee 717.89
intrasellar 253.8
iris (idiopathic) 364.60
exudative 364.62
implantation (surgical) (traumatic) 364.61
miotic pupillary 364.55
parasitic 360.13
Iwanoff's 362.62
jaw (bone) (aneurysmal) (extravasation) (hemorrhagic) (traumatic) 526.2
developmental (odontogenic) 526.0
fissural 526.1
keratin 706.2
kidney (congenital) 753.10
acquired 593.2
calyceal (*see also* Hydronephrosis) 591
multiple 753.19
pyelogenic (*see also* Hydronephrosis) 591
simple 593.2
single 753.11
solitary (not congenital) 593.2
labium (majus) (minus) 624.8
sebaceous 624.8
lacrimal
apparatus 375.43
gland or sac 375.12
larynx 478.79
lens 379.39
congenital 743.39
lip (gland) 528.5
liver 573.8
congenital 751.62
hydatid (*see also* Echinococcus) 122.8
granulosis 122.0
multilocularis 122.5
lung 518.89
congenital 748.4
giant bullous 492.0
lutein 620.1
lymphangiomatous (M9173/0) 228.1
lymphoepithelial
mouth 528.4
oral soft tissue 528.4
macula 362.54

ICD-9-CM
C
Vol. 2

Cyst *(Continued)*
malignant (M8000/3) - *see* Neoplasm, by site, malignant
mammary gland (sweat gland) (*see also* Cyst, breast) 610.0
mandible 526.2
dentigerous 526.0
radicular 522.8
maxilla 526.2
dentigerous 526.0
radicular 522.8
median
anterior maxillary 526.1
palatal 526.1
mediastinum (congenital) 748.8
meibomian (gland) (retention) 373.2
infected 373.12
membrane, brain 348.0
meninges (cerebral) 348.0
spinal 349.2
meniscus knee 717.5
mesentery, mesenteric (gas) 568.89
chyle 457.8
gas 568.89
mesonephric duct 752.89
mesothelial
peritoneum 568.89
pleura (peritoneal) 568.89
milk 611.5
miotic pupillary (iris) 364.55
Morgagni (hydatid) 752.89
fallopian tube 752.11
mouth 528.4
mullerian duct 752.89
multilocular (ovary) (M8000/1) 239.5
myometrium 621.8
nabothian (follicle) (ruptured) 616.0
nasal sinus 478.19
nasoalveolar 528.4
nasolabial 528.4
nasopalatine (duct) 526.1
anterior 526.1
nasopharynx 478.26
neoplastic (M8000/1) - *see also* Neoplasm, by site, unspecified nature
benign (M8000/0) - *see* Neoplasm, by site, benign
uterus 621.8
nervous system - *see* Cyst, brain
neuroenteric 742.59
neuroepithelial ventricle 348.0
nipple 610.0
nose 478.19
skin of 706.2
odontogenic, developmental 526.0
omentum (lesser) 568.89
congenital 751.8
oral soft tissue (dermoid) (epidermoid) (lymphoepithelial) 528.4
ora serrata 361.19
orbit 376.81
ovary, ovarian (twisted) 620.2
adherent 620.2
chocolate 617.1
corpus
albicans 620.2
luteum 620.1
dermoid (M9084/0) 220
developmental 752.0
due to failure of involution NEC 620.2
endometrial 617.1
follicular (atretic) (graafian) (hemorrhagic) 620.0

Cyst *(Continued)*
ovary, ovarian *(Continued)*
hemorrhagic 620.2
in pregnancy or childbirth 654.4
affecting fetus or newborn 763.89
causing obstructed labor 660.2
affecting fetus or newborn 763.1
multilocular (M8000/1) 239.5
pseudomucinous (M8470/0) 220
retention 620.2
serous 620.2
theca lutein 620.2
tuberculous (*see also* Tuberculosis) 016.6
unspecified 620.2
oviduct 620.8
palatal papilla (jaw) 526.1
palate 526.1
fissural 526.1
median (fissural) 526.1
palatine, of papilla 526.1
pancreas, pancreatic 577.2
congenital 751.7
false 577.2
hemorrhagic 577.2
true 577.2
paranephric 593.2
paraovarian 752.11
paraphysis, cerebri 742.4
parasitic NEC 136.9
parathyroid (gland) 252.8
paratubal (fallopian) 620.8
paraurethral duct 599.89
paroophoron 752.11
parotid gland 527.6
mucous extravasation or retention 527.6
parovarian 752.11
pars planus 364.60
exudative 364.64
primary 364.63
pelvis, female
in pregnancy or childbirth 654.4
affecting fetus or newborn 763.89
causing obstructed labor 660.2
affecting fetus or newborn 763.1
penis (sebaceous) 607.89
periapical 522.8
pericardial (congenital) 746.89
acquired (secondary) 423.8
pericoronal 526.0
perineural (Tarlov's) 355.9
periodontal 522.8
lateral 526.0
peripancreatic 577.2
peripelvic (lymphatic) 593.2
peritoneum 568.89
chylous 457.8
pharynx (wall) 478.26
pilonidal (infected) (rectum) 685.1
with abscess 685.0
malignant (M9084/3) 173.5
pituitary (duct) (gland) 253.8
placenta (amniotic) - *see* Placenta, abnormal
pleura 519.8
popliteal 727.51
porencephalic 742.4
acquired 348.0
postanal (infected) 685.1
with abscess 685.0
posterior segment of eye, congenital 743.54
postmastoidectomy cavity 383.31

Cyst *(Continued)*
preauricular 744.47
prepuce 607.89
congenital 752.69
primordial (jaw) 526.0
prostate 600.3
pseudomucinous (ovary) (M8470/0) 220
pudenda (sweat glands) 624.8
pupillary, miotic 364.55
sebaceous 624.8
radicular (residual) 522.8
radiculodental 522.8
ranular 527.6
Rathke's pouch 253.8
rectum (epithelium) (mucous) 569.49
renal - *see* Cyst, kidney
residual (radicular) 522.8
retention (ovary) 620.2
retina 361.19
macular 362.54
parasitic 360.13
primary 361.13
secondary 361.14
retroperitoneal 568.89
sacrococcygeal (dermoid) 685.1
with abscess 685.0
salivary gland or duct 527.6
mucous extravasation or retention 527.6
Sampson's 617.1
sclera 379.19
scrotum (sebaceous) 706.2
sweat glands 706.2
sebaceous (duct) (gland) 706.2
breast 610.8
eyelid 374.84
genital organ NEC
female 629.89
male 608.89
scrotum 706.2
semilunar cartilage (knee) (multiple) 717.5
seminal vesicle 608.89
serous (ovary) 620.2
sinus (antral) (ethmoidal) (frontal) (maxillary) (nasal) (sphenoidal) 478.19
Skene's gland 599.89
skin (epidermal) (epidermoid, inclusion) (epithelial) (inclusion) (retention) (sebaceous) 706.2
breast 610.8
eyelid 374.84
genital organ NEC
female 629.89
male 608.89
neoplastic 216.3
scrotum 706.2
sweat gland or duct 705.89
solitary
bone 733.21
kidney 593.2
spermatic cord 608.89
sphenoid sinus 478.19
spinal meninges 349.2
spine (*see also* Cyst, bone) 733.20
spleen NEC 289.59
congenital 759.0
hydatid (*see also* Echinococcus) 122.9
spring water (pericardium) 746.89
subarachnoid 348.0
intrasellar 793.0

- **Cyst** *(Continued)*
  - subdural (cerebral) 348.0
    - spinal cord 349.2
  - sublingual gland 527.6
    - mucous extravasation or retention 527.6
  - submaxillary gland 527.6
    - mucous extravasation or retention 527.6
  - suburethral 599.89
  - suprarenal gland 255.8
  - suprasellar - *see* Cyst, brain
  - sweat gland or duct 705.89
  - sympathetic nervous system 337.9
  - synovial 727.40
    - popliteal space 727.51
  - Tarlov's 355.9
  - tarsal 373.2
  - tendon (sheath) 727.42
  - testis 608.89
  - thecalutein (ovary) 620.2
  - Thornwaldt's, Tornwaldt's 478.26
  - thymus (gland) 254.8
  - thyroglossal (duct) (infected) (persistent) 759.2
  - thyroid (gland) 246.2
    - adenomatous - *see* Goiter, nodular
    - colloid (*see also* Goiter) 240.9
  - thyrolingual duct (infected) (persistent) 759.2
  - tongue (mucous) 529.8
  - tonsil 474.8
  - tooth (dental root) 522.8
  - tubo-ovarian 620.8
    - inflammatory 614.1
  - tunica vaginalis 608.89
  - turbinate (nose) (*see also* Cyst, bone) 733.20
  - Tyson's gland (benign) (infected) 607.89
  - umbilicus 759.89
  - urachus 753.7
  - ureter 593.89
  - ureterovesical orifice 593.89
    - congenital 753.4
  - urethra 599.84
  - urethral gland (Cowper's) 599.89
  - uterine
    - ligament 620.8
      - embryonic 752.11
    - tube 620.8
  - uterus (body) (corpus) (recurrent) 621.8
    - embryonal 752.3
  - utricle (ear) 386.8
    - prostatic 599.89
  - utriculus masculinus 599.89
  - vagina, vaginal (squamous cell) (wall) 623.8
    - embryonal 752.41
    - implantation 623.8
    - inclusion 623.8
  - vallecula, vallecular 478.79
  - ventricle, neuroepithelial 348.0
  - verumontanum 599.89
  - vesical (orifice) 596.8
  - vitreous humor 379.29
  - vulva (sweat glands) 624.8
    - congenital 752.41
    - implantation 624.8
    - inclusion 624.8
    - sebaceous gland 624.8
  - vulvovaginal gland 624.8
  - wolffian 752.89
- **Cystadenocarcinoma** (M8440/3) - *see also* Neoplasm, by site, malignant
  - bile duct type (M8161/3) 155.1
  - endometrioid (M8380/3) - *see* Neoplasm, by site, malignant
  - mucinous (M8470/3)
    - papillary (M8471/3)
      - specified site - *see* Neoplasm, by site, malignant
      - unspecified site 183.0
    - specified site - *see* Neoplasm, by site, malignant
    - unspecified site 183.0
  - papillary (M8450/3)
    - mucinous (M8471/3)
      - specified site - *see* Neoplasm, by site, malignant
      - unspecified site 183.0
    - pseudomucinous (M8471/3)
      - specified site - *see* Neoplasm, by site, malignant
      - unspecified site 183.0
    - serous (M8460/3)
      - specified site - *see* Neoplasm, by site, malignant
      - unspecified site 183.0
    - specified site - *see* Neoplasm, by site, malignant
    - unspecified 183.0
  - pseudomucinous (M8470/3)
    - papillary (M8471/3)
      - specified site - *see* Neoplasm, by site, malignant
      - unspecified site 183.0
    - specified site - *see* Neoplasm, by site, malignant
    - unspecified site 183.0
  - serous (M8441/3)
    - papillary (M8460/3)
      - specified site - *see* Neoplasm, by site, malignant
      - unspecified site 183.0
    - specified site - *see* Neoplasm, by site, malignant
    - unspecified site 183.0
- **Cystadenofibroma** (M9013/0)
  - clear cell (M8313/0) - *see* Neoplasm, by site, benign
  - endometrioid (M8381/0) 220
    - borderline malignancy (M8381/1) 236.2
    - malignant (M8381/3) 183.0
  - mucinous (M9015/0)
    - specified site - *see* Neoplasm, by site, benign
    - unspecified site 220
  - serous (M9014/0)
    - specified site - *see* Neoplasm, by site, benign
    - unspecified site 220
  - specified site - *see* Neoplasm, by site, benign
  - unspecified site 220
- **Cystadenoma** (M8440/0) - *see also* Neoplasm, by site, benign
  - bile duct (M8161/0) 211.5
  - endometrioid (M8380/0) - *see also* Neoplasm, by site, benign
    - borderline malignancy (M8380/1) - *see* Neoplasm, by site, uncertain behavior
  - malignant (M8440/3) - *see* Neoplasm, by site, malignant
  - mucinous (M8470/0)
    - borderline malignancy (M8470/1)
- **Cystadenoma** *(Continued)*
  - mucinous *(Continued)*
    - borderline malignancy *(Continued)*
      - specified site - *see* Neoplasm, uncertain behavior
      - unspecified site 236.2
    - papillary (M8471/0)
      - borderline malignancy (M8471/1)
        - specified site - *see* Neoplasm, by site, uncertain behavior
        - unspecified site 236.2
      - specified site - *see* Neoplasm, by site, benign
      - unspecified site 220
    - specified site - *see* Neoplasm, by site, benign
    - unspecified site 220
  - papillary (M8450/0)
    - borderline malignancy (M8450/1)
      - specified site - *see* Neoplasm, by site, uncertain behavior
      - unspecified site 236.2
    - lymphomatosum (M8561/0) 210.2
    - mucinous (M8471/0)
      - borderline malignancy (M8471/1)
        - specified site - *see* Neoplasm, by site, uncertain behavior
        - unspecified site 236.2
      - specified site - *see* Neoplasm, by site, benign
      - unspecified site 220
    - pseudomucinous (M8471/0)
      - borderline malignancy (M8471/1)
        - specified site - *see* Neoplasm, by site, uncertain behavior
        - unspecified site 236.2
      - specified site - *see* Neoplasm, by site, benign
      - unspecified site 220
    - serous (M8460/0)
      - borderline malignancy (M8460/1)
        - specified site - *see* Neoplasm, by site, uncertain behavior
        - unspecified site 236.2
      - specified site - *see* Neoplasm, by site, benign
      - unspecified site 220
    - specified site - *see* Neoplasm, by site, benign
    - unspecified site 220
  - pseudomucinous (M8470/0)
    - borderline malignancy (M8470/1)
      - specified site - *see* Neoplasm, by site, uncertain behavior
      - unspecified site 236.2
    - papillary (M8471/0)
      - borderline malignancy (M8471/1)
        - specified site - *see* Neoplasm, by site, uncertain behavior
        - unspecified site 236.2
      - specified site - *see* Neoplasm, by site, benign
      - unspecified site 220
    - specified site - *see* Neoplasm, by site, benign
    - unspecified site 220
  - serous (M8441/0)
    - borderline malignancy (M8441/1)
      - specified site - *see* Neoplasm, by site, uncertain behavior
      - unspecified site 236.2
    - papillary (M8460/0)
      - borderline malignancy (M8460/1)
        - specified site - *see* Neoplasm, by site, uncertain behavior
        - unspecified site 236.2

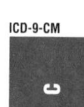

ICD-9-CM C Vol. 2

Cystadenoma *(Continued)*
serous *(Continued)*
papillary *(Continued)*
specified site - *see* Neoplasm, by site, benign
unspecified site 220
specified site - *see* Neoplasm, by site, benign
unspecified site 220
thyroid 226
Cystathioninemia 270.4
Cystathioninuria 270.4
Cystic - *see also* condition
breast, chronic 610.1
corpora lutea 620.1
degeneration, congenital
brain 742.4
kidney (*see also* Cystic, disease, kidney) 753.10
disease
breast, chronic 610.1
kidney, congenital 753.10
medullary 753.16
multiple 753.19
polycystic - *see* Polycystic, kidney
single 753.11
specified NEC 753.19
liver, congenital 751.62
lung 518.89
congenital 748.4
pancreas, congenital 751.7
semilunar cartilage 717.5
duct - *see* condition
eyeball, congenital 743.03
fibrosis (pancreas) 277.00
with
manifestations
gastrointestinal 277.03
pulmonary 277.02
specified NEC 277.09
meconium ileus 277.01
pulmonary exacerbation 277.02
hygroma (M9173/0) 228.1
kidney, congenital 753.10
medullary 753.16
multiple 753.19
polycystic - *see* Polycystic, kidney
single 753.11
specified NEC 753.19
liver, congenital 751.62
lung 518.89
congenital 748.4
mass - *see* Cyst
mastitis, chronic 610.1
ovary 620.2
pancreas, congenital 751.7
Cysticerciasis 123.1
Cysticercosis (mammary) (subretinal) 123.1
Cysticercus 123.1
cellulosae infestation 123.1
Cystinosis (malignant) 270.0
Cystinuria 270.0
Cystitis (bacillary) (colli) (diffuse) (exudative) (hemorrhagic) (purulent) (recurrent) (septic) (suppurative) (ulcerative) 595.9

Cystitis *(Continued)*
with
abortion - *see* Abortion, by type, with urinary tract infection
ectopic pregnancy (*see also* categories 633.0–633.9) 639.8
fibrosis 595.1
leukoplakia 595.1
malakoplakia 595.1
metaplasia 595.1
molar pregnancy (*see also* categories 630–632) 639.8
actinomycotic 039.8 *[595.4]*
acute 595.0
of trigone 595.3
allergic 595.89
amebic 006.8 *[595.4]*
bilharzial 120.9 *[595.4]*
blennorrhagic (acute) 098.11
chronic or duration of 2 months or more 098.31
bullous 595.89
calculous 594.1
chlamydial 099.53
chronic 595.2
interstitial 595.1
of trigone 595.3
complicating pregnancy, childbirth, or puerperium 646.6
affecting fetus or newborn 760.1
cystic(a) 595.81
diphtheritic 032.84
echinococcal
glanulosus 122.3 *[595.4]*
multilocularis 122.6 *[595.4]*
emphysematous 595.89
encysted 595.81
follicular 595.3
following
abortion 639.8
ectopic or molar pregnancy 639.8
gangrenous 595.89
glandularis 595.89
gonococcal (acute) 098.11
chronic or duration of 2 months or more 098.31
incrusted 595.89
interstitial 595.1
irradiation 595.82
irritation 595.89
malignant 595.89
monilial 112.2
of trigone 595.3
panmural 595.1
polyposa 595.89
prostatic 601.3
radiation 595.82
Reiter's (abacterial) 099.3
specified NEC 595.89
subacute 595.2
submucous 595.1
syphilitic 095.8
trichomoniasis 131.09
tuberculous (*see also* Tuberculosis) 016.1
ulcerative 595.1

Cystocele (-rectocele)
female (without uterine prolapse) 618.01
with uterine prolapse 618.4
complete 618.3
incomplete 618.2
lateral 618.02
midline 618.01
paravaginal 618.02
in pregnancy or childbirth 654.4
affecting fetus or newborn 763.89
causing obstructed labor 660.2
affecting fetus or newborn 763.1
male 596.8
Cystoid
cicatrix limbus 372.64
degeneration, macula 362.53
Cystolithiasis 594.1
Cystoma (M8440/0) - *see also* Neoplasm, by site, benign
endometrial, ovary 617.1
mucinous (M8470/0)
specified site - *see* Neoplasm, by site, benign
unspecified site 220
serous (M8441/0)
specified site - *see* Neoplasm, by site, benign
unspecified site 220
simple (ovary) 620.2
Cystoplegia 596.53
Cystoptosis 596.8
Cystopyelitis (*see also* Pyelitis) 590.80
Cystorrhagia 596.8
Cystosarcoma phyllodes (M9020/1) 238.3
benign (M9020/0) 217
malignant (M9020/3) - *see* Neoplasm, breast, malignant
Cystostomy status V44.50
with complication 997.5
appendico-vesicostomy V44.52
cutaneous-vesicostomy V44.51
specified type NEC V44.59
Cystourethritis (*see also* Urethritis) 597.89
Cystourethrocele (*see also* Cystocele)
female (without uterine prolapse) 618.09
with uterine prolapse 618.4
complete 618.3
incomplete 618.2
male 596.8
Cytomegalic inclusion disease 078.5
congenital 771.1
Cytomycosis, reticuloendothelial (*see also* Histoplasmosis, American) 115.00
Cytopenia 289.9
refractory ◀
with ◀
multilineage dysplasia (RCMD) 238.72 ◀
and ringed sideroblasts (RCMD-RS) 238.72 ◀

D

Daae (-Finsen) disease (epidemic pleurodynia) 074.1
Dabney's grip 074.1
Da Costa's syndrome (neurocirculatory asthenia) 306.2
Dacryoadenitis, dacryadenitis 375.00
acute 375.01
chronic 375.02
Dacryocystitis 375.30
acute 375.32
chronic 375.42
neonatal 771.6
phlegmonous 375.33
syphilitic 095.8
congenital 090.0
trachomatous, active 076.1
late effect 139.1
tuberculous (*see also* Tuberculosis) 017.3
Dacryocystoblenorrhea 375.42
Dacryocystocele 375.43
Dacryolith, dacryolithiasis 375.57
Dacryoma 375.43
Dacryopericystitis (acute) (subacute) 375.32
chronic 375.42
Dacryops 375.11
Dacryosialadenopathy, atrophic 710.2
Dacryostenosis 375.56
congenital 743.65
Dactylitis
bone (*see also* Osteomyelitis) 730.2
sickle-cell 282.62
Hb-C 282.64
Hb-SS 282.62
specified NEC 282.69
syphilitic 095.5
tuberculous (*see also* Tuberculosis) 015.5
Dactylolysis spontanea 136.0
Dactylosymphysis (*see also* Syndactylism) 755.10
Damage
arteriosclerotic - *see* Arteriosclerosis
brain 348.9
anoxic, hypoxic 348.1
during or resulting from a procedure 997.01
ischemic, in newborn 768.7
child NEC 343.9
due to birth injury 767.0
minimal (child) (*see also* Hyperkinesia) 314.9
newborn 767.0
cardiac - *see also* Disease, heart
cardiorenal (vascular) (*see also* Hypertension, cardiorenal) 404.90
central nervous system - *see* Damage, brain
cerebral NEC - *see* Damage, brain
coccyx, complicating delivery 665.6
coronary (*see also* Ischemia, heart) 414.9
eye, birth injury 767.8
heart - *see also* Disease, heart
valve - *see* Endocarditis
hypothalamus NEC 348.9
liver 571.9
alcoholic 571.3
myocardium (*see also* Degeneration, myocardial) 429.1
pelvic
joint or ligament, during delivery 665.6
Damage *(Continued)*
pelvic *(Continued)*
organ NEC
with
abortion - *see* Abortion, by type, with damage to pelvic organs
ectopic pregnancy (*see also* categories 633.0–633.9) 639.2
molar pregnancy (*see also* categories 630–632) 639.2
during delivery 665.5
following
abortion 639.2
ectopic or molar pregnancy 639.2
renal (*see also* Disease, renal) 593.9
skin, solar 692.79
acute 692.72
chronic 692.74
subendocardium, subendocardial (*see also* Degeneration, myocardial) 429.1
vascular 459.9
Dameshek's syndrome (erythroblastic anemia) 282.49
Dana-Putnam syndrome (subacute combined sclerosis with pernicious anemia) 281.0 *[336.2]*
Danbolt (-Closs) syndrome (acrodermatitis enteropathica) 686.8
Dandruff 690.18
Dandy fever 061
Dandy-Walker deformity or syndrome (atresia, foramen of Magendie) 742.3
with spina bifida (*see also* Spina bifida) 741.0
Dangle foot 736.79
Danielssen's disease (anesthetic leprosy) 030.1
Danlos' syndrome 756.83
Darier's disease (congenital) (keratosis follicularis) 757.39
due to vitamin A deficiency 264.8
meaning erythema annulare centrifugum 695.0
Darier-Roussy sarcoid 135
Darling's
disease (*see also* Histoplasmosis, American) 115.00
histoplasmosis (*see also* Histoplasmosis, American) 115.00
Dartre 054.9
Darwin's tubercle 744.29
Davidson's anemia (refractory) 284.9
Davies' disease 425.0
Davies-Colley syndrome (slipping rib) 733.99
Dawson's encephalitis 046.2
Day blindness (*see also* Blindness, day) 368.60
Dead
fetus
retained (in utero) 656.4
early pregnancy (death before 22 completed weeks' gestation) 632
late (death after 22 completed weeks' gestation) 656.4
syndrome 641.3
labyrinth 386.50
ovum, retained 631
Deaf and dumb NEC 389.7
Deaf mutism (acquired) (congenital) NEC 389.7
endemic 243
Deaf mutism (acquired) (congenital) NEC *(Continued)*
hysterical 300.11
syphilitic, congenital 090.0
Deafness (acquired) (complete) (congenital) (hereditary) (middle ear) (partial) 389.9
with blue sclera and fragility of bone 756.51
auditory fatigue 389.9
aviation 993.0
nerve injury 951.5
boilermakers' 951.5
central, bilateral 389.14
with conductive hearing loss 389.2
conductive (air) 389.00
with sensorineural hearing loss 389.2
combined types 389.08
external ear 389.01
inner ear 389.04
middle ear 389.03
multiple types 389.08
tympanic membrane 389.02
emotional (complete) 300.11
functional (complete) 300.11
high frequency 389.8
hysterical (complete) 300.11
injury 951.5
low frequency 389.8
mental 784.69
mixed conductive and sensorineural 389.2
nerve, bilateral 389.12
with conductive hearing loss 389.2
neural, bilateral 389.12
with conductive hearing loss 389.2
noise-induced 388.12
nerve injury 951.5
nonspeaking 389.7
perceptive 389.10
with conductive hearing loss 389.2
central, bilateral 389.14
combined types, bilateral 389.18
multiple types, bilateral 389.18
neural, bilateral 389.12
sensorineural 389.10
asymmetrical 389.16
bilateral 389.18
unilateral 389.15
sensory, bilateral 389.11
psychogenic (complete) 306.7
sensorineural (*see also* Deafness, perceptive) 389.10
asymmetrical 389.16
bilateral 389.18
unilateral 389.15
sensory, bilateral 389.11
with conductive hearing loss 389.2
specified type NEC 389.8
sudden NEC 388.2
syphilitic 094.89
transient ischemic 388.02
transmission - *see* Deafness, conductive
traumatic 951.5
word (secondary to organic lesion) 784.69
developmental 315.31
Death
after delivery (cause not stated) (sudden) 674.9
anesthetic
due to
correct substance properly administered 995.4

ICD-9-CM
D
Vol. 2

Death *(Continued)*
anesthetic *(Continued)*
due to *(Continued)*
overdose or wrong substance given 968.4
specified anesthetic - *see* Table of Drugs and Chemicals
during delivery 668.9
brain 348.8
cardiac - *see* Disease, heart
cause unknown 798.2
cot (infant) 798.0
crib (infant) 798.0
fetus, fetal (cause not stated) (intrauterine) 779.9
early, with retention (before 22 completed weeks' gestation) 632
from asphyxia or anoxia (before labor) 768.0
during labor 768.1
late, affecting management of pregnancy (after 22 completed weeks' gestation) 656.4
from pregnancy NEC 646.9
instantaneous 798.1
intrauterine (*see also* Death, fetus) 779.9
complicating pregnancy 656.4
maternal, affecting fetus or newborn 761.6
neonatal NEC 779.9
sudden (cause unknown) 798.1
during delivery 669.9
under anesthesia NEC 668.9
infant, syndrome (SIDS) 798.0
puerperal, during puerperium 674.9
unattended (cause unknown) 798.9
under anesthesia NEC
due to
correct substance properly administered 995.4
overdose or wrong substance given 968.4
specified anesthetic - *see* Table of Drugs and Chemicals
during delivery 668.9
violent 798.1
de Beurmann-Gougerot disease (sporotrichosis) 117.1
Debility (general) (infantile) (postinfectional) 799.3
with nutritional difficulty 269.9
congenital or neonatal NEC 779.9
nervous 300.5
old age 797
senile 797
Débove's disease (splenomegaly) 789.2
Decalcification
bone (*see also* Osteoporosis) 733.00
teeth 521.89 ⬅
Decapitation 874.9
fetal (to facilitate delivery) 763.89
Decapsulation, kidney 593.89
Decay
dental 521.00
senile 797
tooth, teeth 521.00
Decensus, uterus - *see* Prolapse, uterus
Deciduitis (acute)
with
abortion - *see* Abortion, by type, with sepsis
ectopic pregnancy (*see also* categories 633.0–633.9) 639.0
Deciduitis *(Continued)*
with *(Continued)*
molar pregnancy (*see also* categories 630–632) 639.0
affecting fetus or newborn 760.8
following
abortion 639.0
ectopic or molar pregnancy 639.0
in pregnancy 646.6
puerperal, postpartum 670
Deciduoma malignum (M9100/3) 181
Deciduous tooth (retained) 520.6
Decline (general) (*see also* Debility) 799.3
Decompensation
cardiac (acute) (chronic) (*see also* Disease, heart) 429.9
failure - *see* Failure, heart
cardiorenal (*see also* Hypertension, cardiorenal) 404.90
cardiovascular (*see also* Disease, cardiovascular) 429.2
heart (*see also* Disease, heart) 429.9
failure - *see* Failure, heart
hepatic 572.2
myocardial (acute) (chronic) (*see also* Disease, heart) 429.9
failure - *see* Failure, heart
respiratory 519.9
Decompression sickness 993.3
Decrease, decreased
blood
platelets (*see also* Thrombocytopenia) 287.5
pressure 796.3
due to shock following
injury 958.4
operation 998.0
white cell count 288.50 ◀
specified NEC 288.59 ◀
cardiac reserve - *see* Disease, heart
estrogen 256.39
postablative 256.2
fetal movements 655.7
fragility of erythrocytes 289.89
function
adrenal (cortex) 255.4
medulla 255.5
ovary in hypopituitarism 253.4
parenchyma of pancreas 577.8
pituitary (gland) (lobe) (anterior) 253.2
posterior (lobe) 253.8
functional activity 780.99
glucose 790.29
haptoglobin (serum) NEC 273.8
leukocytes 288.50 ◀
libido 799.81
lymphocytes 288.51 ◀
platelets (*see also* Thrombocytopenia) 287.5
pulse pressure 785.9
respiration due to shock following injury 958.4
sexual desire 799.81
tear secretion NEC 375.15
tolerance
fat 579.8
salt and water 276.9
vision NEC 369.9
white blood cell count 288.50 ◀
Decubital gangrene 707.00 *[785.4]*
Decubiti (*see also* Decubitus) 707.00
Decubitus (ulcer) 707.00
with gangrene 707.00 *[785.4]*
ankle 707.06
Decubitus *(Continued)*
back
lower 707.03
upper 707.02
buttock 707.05
elbow 707.01
head 707.09
heel 707.07
hip 707.04
other site 707.09
sacrum 707.03
shoulder blades 707.02
Deepening acetabulum 718.85
Defect, defective 759.9
3-beta-hydroxysteroid dehydrogenase 255.2
11-hydroxylase 255.2
21-hydroxylase 255.2
abdominal wall, congenital 756.70
aorticopulmonary septum 745.0
aortic septal 745.0
atrial septal (ostium secundum type) 745.5
acquired 429.71
ostium primum type 745.61
sinus venosus 745.8
atrioventricular
canal 745.69
septum 745.4
acquired 429.71
atrium secundum 745.5
acquired 429.71
auricular septal 745.5
acquired 429.71
bilirubin excretion 277.4
biosynthesis, testicular androgen 257.2
bridge 525.60 ◀
bulbar septum 745.0
butanol-insoluble iodide 246.1
chromosome - *see* Anomaly, chromosome
circulation (acquired) 459.9
congenital 747.9
newborn 747.9
clotting NEC (*see also* Defect, coagulation) 286.9
coagulation (factor) (*see also* Deficiency, coagulation factor) 286.9
with
abortion - *see* Abortion, by type, with hemorrhage
ectopic pregnancy (*see also* categories 634–638) 639.1
molar pregnancy (*see also* categories 630–632) 639.1
acquired (any) 286.7
antepartum or intrapartum 641.3
affecting fetus or newborn 762.1
causing hemorrhage of pregnancy or delivery 641.3
complicating pregnancy, childbirth, or puerperium 649.3 ◀
due to
liver disease 286.7
vitamin K deficiency 286.7
newborn, transient 776.3
postpartum 666.3
specified type NEC 286.3
conduction (heart) 426.9
bone (*see also* Deafness, conductive) 389.00
congenital, organ or site NEC - *see also* Anomaly
circulation 747.9

Defect, defective *(Continued)*
congenital, organ or site NEC *(Continued)*
Descemet's membrane 743.9
specified type NEC 743.49
diaphragm 756.6
ectodermal 757.9
esophagus 750.9
pulmonic cusps - *see* Anomaly, heart valve
respiratory system 748.9
specified type NEC 748.8
crown 525.60 ◀
cushion endocardial 745.60
dental restoration 525.60 ◀
dentin (hereditary) 520.5
Descemet's membrane (congenital) 743.9
acquired 371.30
specific type NEC 743.49
deutan 368.52
developmental - *see also* Anomaly, by site
cauda equina 742.59
left ventricle 746.9
with atresia or hypoplasia of aortic orifice or valve, with hypoplasia of ascending aorta 746.7
in hypoplastic left heart syndrome 746.7
testis 752.9
vessel 747.9
diaphragm
with elevation, eventration, or hernia - *see* Hernia, diaphragm
congenital 756.6
with elevation, eventration, or hernia 756.6
gross (with elevation, eventration, or hernia) 756.6
ectodermal, congenital 757.9
Eisenmenger's (ventricular septal defect) 745.4
endocardial cushion 745.60
specified type NEC 745.69
esophagus, congenital 750.9
extensor retinaculum 728.9
fibrin polymerization (*see also* Defect, coagulation) 286.3
filling
biliary tract 793.3
bladder 793.5
dental 525.60 ◀
gallbladder 793.3
kidney 793.5
stomach 793.4
ureter 793.5
fossa ovalis 745.5
gene, carrier (suspected) of V83.89
Gerbode 745.4
glaucomatous, without elevated tension 365.89
Hageman (factor) (*see also* Defect, coagulation) 286.3
hearing (*see also* Deafness) 389.9
high grade 317
homogentisic acid 270.2
interatrial septal 745.5
acquired 429.71
interauricular septal 745.5
acquired 429.71
interventricular septal 745.4
with pulmonary stenosis or atresia, dextraposition of aorta, and hypertrophy of right ventricle 745.2

Defect, defective *(Continued)*
interventricular septal *(Continued)*
acquired 429.71
in tetralogy of Fallot 745.2
iodide trapping 246.1
iodotyrosine dehalogenase 246.1
kynureninase 270.2
learning, specific 315.2
major osseous 731.3 ◀
mental (*see also* Retardation, mental) 319
osseous, major 731.3 ◀
osteochondral NEC 738.8
ostium
primum 745.61
secundum 745.5
pericardium 746.89
peroxidase-binding 246.1
placental blood supply - *see* Placenta, insufficiency
platelet (qualitative) 287.1
constitutional 286.4
postural, spine 737.9
protan 368.51
pulmonic cusps, congenital 746.00
renal pelvis 753.9
obstructive 753.29
specified type NEC 753.3
respiratory system, congenital 748.9
specified type NEC 748.8
retina, retinal 361.30
with detachment (*see also* Detachment, retina, with retinal defect) 361.00
multiple 361.33
with detachment 361.02
nerve fiber bundle 362.85
single 361.30
with detachment 361.01
septal (closure) (heart) NEC 745.9
acquired 429.71
atrial 745.5
specified type NEC 745.8
speech NEC 784.5
developmental 315.39
secondary to organic lesion 784.5
Taussig-Bing (transposition, aorta and overriding pulmonary artery) 745.11
teeth, wedge 521.20
thyroid hormone synthesis 246.1
tritan 368.53
ureter 753.9
obstructive 753.29
vascular (acquired) (local) 459.9
congenital (peripheral) NEC 747.60
gastrointestinal 747.61
lower limb 747.64
renal 747.62
specified NEC 747.69
spinal 747.82
upper limb 747.63
ventricular septal 745.4
with pulmonary stenosis or atresia, dextraposition of aorta, and hypertrophy of right ventricle 745.2
acquired 429.71
atrioventricular canal type 745.69
between infundibulum and anterior portion 745.4
in tetralogy of Fallot 745.2
isolated anterior 745.4
vision NEC 369.9
visual field 368.40
arcuate 368.43
heteronymous, bilateral 368.47
homonymous, bilateral 368.46

Defect, defective *(Continued)*
visual field *(Continued)*
localized NEC 368.44
nasal step 368.44
peripheral 368.44
sector 368.43
voice 784.40
wedge, teeth (abrasion) 521.20
Defeminization syndrome 255.2
Deferentitis 608.4
gonorrheal (acute) 098.14
chronic or duration of 2 months or over 098.34
Defibrination syndrome (*see also* Fibrinolysis) 286.6
Deficiency, deficient
3-beta-hydroxysteroid dehydrogenase 255.2
6-phosphogluconic dehydrogenase (anemia) 282.2
11-beta-hydroxylase 255.2
17-alpha-hydroxylase 255.2
18-hydroxysteroid dehydrogenase 255.2
20-alpha-hydroxylase 255.2
21-hydroxylase 255.2
AAT (alpha-1 antitrypsin) 273.4
abdominal muscle syndrome 756.79
accelerator globulin (Ac G) (blood) (*see also* Defect, coagulation) 286.3
AC globulin (congenital) (*see also* Defect, coagulation) 286.3
acquired 286.7
activating factor (blood) (*see also* Defect, coagulation) 286.3
adenohypophyseal 253.2
adenosine deaminase 277.2
aldolase (hereditary) 271.2
alpha-1-antitrypsin 273.4
alpha-1-trypsin inhibitor 273.4
alpha-fucosidase 271.8
alpha-lipoprotein 272.5
alpha-mannosidase 271.8
amino acid 270.9
anemia - *see* Anemia, deficiency
aneurin 265.1
with beriberi 265.0
antibody NEC 279.00
antidiuretic hormone 253.5
antihemophilic
factor (A) 286.0
B 286.1
C 286.2
globulin (AHG) NEC 286.0
antithrombin III 289.81
antitrypsin 273.4
argininosuccinate synthetase or lyase 270.6
ascorbic acid (with scurvy) 267
autoprothrombin
I (*see also* Defect, coagulation) 286.3
II 286.1
C (*see also* Defect, coagulation) 286.3
bile salt 579.8
biotin 266.2
biotinidase 277.6
bradykinase-1 277.6
brancher enzyme (amylopectinosis) 271.0
calciferol 268.9
with
osteomalacia 268.2
rickets (*see also* Rickets) 268.0
calcium 275.40
dietary 269.3
calorie, severe 261

Deficiency, deficient *(Continued)*
carbamyl phosphate synthetase 270.6
cardiac (*see also* Insufficiency, myocardial) 428.0
carnitine 277.81
due to
hemodialysis 277.83
inborn errors of metabolism 277.82
valproic acid therapy 277.83
iatrogenic 277.83
palmitoyltransferase (CPT1, CPT2) 277.85
palmityl transferase (CPT1, CPT2) 277.85
primary 277.81
secondary 277.84
carotene 264.9
Carr factor (*see also* Defect, coagulation) 286.9
central nervous system 349.9
ceruloplasmin 275.1
cevitamic acid (with scurvy) 267
choline 266.2
Christmas factor 286.1
chromium 269.3
citrin 269.1
clotting (blood) (*see also* Defect, coagulation) 286.9
coagulation factor NEC 286.9
with
abortion - *see* Abortion, by type, with hemorrhage
ectopic pregnancy (*see also* categories 634–638) 639.1
molar pregnancy (*see also* categories 630–632) 639.1
acquired (any) 286.7
antepartum or intrapartum 641.3
affecting fetus or newborn 762.1
complicating pregnancy, childbirth, or puerperium 649.3 ◀
due to
liver disease 286.7
vitamin K deficiency 286.7
newborn, transient 776.3
postpartum 666.3
specified type NEC 286.3
color vision (congenital) 368.59
acquired 368.55
combined, two or more coagulation factors (*see also* Defect, coagulation) 286.9
complement factor NEC 279.8
contact factor (*see also* Defect, coagulation) 286.3
copper NEC 275.1
corticoadrenal 255.4
craniofacial axis 756.0
cyanocobalamin (vitamin B_{12}) 266.2
debrancher enzyme (limit dextrinosis) 271.0
desmolase 255.2
diet 269.9
dihydrofolate reductase 281.2
dihydropteridine reductase 270.1
disaccharidase (intestinal) 271.3
disease NEC 269.9
ear(s) V48.8
edema 262
endocrine 259.9
enzymes, circulating NEC (*see also* Deficiency, by specific enzyme) 277.6

Deficiency, deficient *(Continued)*
ergosterol 268.9
with
osteomalacia 268.2
rickets (*see also* Rickets) 268.0
erythrocytic glutathione (anemia) 282.2
eyelid(s) V48.8
factor (*see also* Defect, coagulation) 286.9
I (congenital) (fibrinogen) 286.3
antepartum or intrapartum 641.3
affecting fetus or newborn 762.1
newborn, transient 776.3
postpartum 666.3
II (congenital) (prothrombin) 286.3
V (congenital) (labile) 286.3
VII (congenital) (stable) 286.3
VIII (congenital) (functional) 286.0
with
functional defect 286.0
vascular defect 286.4
IX (Christmas) (congenital) (functional) 286.1
X (congenital) (Stuart-Prower) 286.3
XI (congenital) (plasma thromboplastin antecedent) 286.2
XII (congenital) (Hageman) 286.3
XIII (congenital) (fibrin stabilizing) 286.3
Hageman 286.3
multiple (congenital) 286.9
acquired 286.7
fibrinase (*see also* Defect, coagulation) 286.3
fibrinogen (congenital) (*see also* Defect, coagulation) 286.3
acquired 286.6
fibrin-stabilizing factor (congenital) (*see also* Defect, coagulation) 286.3
acquired 286.7
finger - *see* Absence, finger
fletcher factor (*see also* Defect, coagulation) 286.9
fluorine 269.3
folate, anemia 281.2
folic acid (vitamin B_C) 266.2
anemia 281.2
follicle-stimulating hormone (FSH) 253.4
fructokinase 271.2
fructose-1, 6-diphosphate 271.2
fructose-1-phosphate aldolase 271.2
FSH (follicle-stimulating hormone) 253.4
fucosidase 271.8
galactokinase 271.1
galactose-1-phosphate uridyl transferase 271.1
gamma globulin in blood 279.00
glass factor (*see also* Defect, coagulation) 286.3
glucocorticoid 255.4
glucose-6-phosphatase 271.0
glucose-6-phosphate dehydrogenase anemia 282.2
glucuronyl transferase 277.4
glutathione-reductase (anemia) 282.2
glycogen synthetase 271.0
growth hormone 253.3
Hageman factor (congenital) (*see also* Defect, coagulation) 286.3
head V48.0
hemoglobin (*see also* Anemia) 285.9
hepatophosphorylase 271.0
hexose monophosphate (HMP) shunt 282.2
hGH (human growth hormone) 253.3

Deficiency, deficient *(Continued)*
HG-PRT 277.2
homogentisic acid oxidase 270.2
hormone - *see also* Deficiency, by specific hormone
anterior pituitary (isolated) (partial) NEC 253.4
growth (human) 253.3
follicle-stimulating 253.4
growth (human) (isolated) 253.3
human growth 253.3
interstitial cell-stimulating 253.4
luteinizing 253.4
melanocyte-stimulating 253.4
testicular 257.2
human growth hormone 253.3
humoral 279.00
with
hyper-IgM 279.05
autosomal recessive 279.05
X-linked 279.05
increased IgM 279.05
congenital hypogammaglobulinemia 279.04
non-sex-linked 279.06
selective immunoglobulin NEC 279.03
IgA 279.01
IgG 279.03
IgM 279.02
increased 279.05
specified NEC 279.09
hydroxylase 255.2
hypoxanthine-guanine phosphoribosyltransferase (HG-PRT) 277.2
ICSH (interstitial cell-stimulating hormone) 253.4
immunity NEC 279.3
cell-mediated 279.10
with
hyperimmunoglobulinemia 279.2
thrombocytopenia and eczema 279.12
specified NEC 279.19
combined (severe) 279.2
syndrome 279.2
common variable 279.06
humoral NEC 279.00
IgA (secretory) 279.01
IgG 279.03
IgM 279.02
immunoglobulin, selective NEC 279.03
IgA 279.01
IgG 279.03
IgM 279.02
inositol (B complex) 266.2
interferon 279.4
internal organ V47.0
interstitial cell-stimulating hormone (ICSH) 253.4
intrinsic factor (Castle's) (congenital) 281.0
intrinsic (urethral) sphincter (ISD) 599.82
invertase 271.3
iodine 269.3
iron, anemia 280.9
labile factor (congenital) (*see also* Defect, coagulation) 286.3
acquired 286.7
lacrimal fluid (acquired) 375.15
congenital 743.64
lactase 271.3
Laki-Lorand factor (*see also* Defect, coagulation) 286.3
lecithin-cholesterol acyltranferase 272.5

◀ New ⟸ Revised

Deficiency, deficient *(Continued)*
- LH (luteinizing hormone) 253.4
- limb V49.0
  - lower V49.0
    - congenital (*see also* Deficiency, lower limb, congenital) 755.30
  - upper V49.0
    - congenital (*see also* Deficiency, upper limb, congenital) 755.20
- lipocaic 577.8
- lipoid (high-density) 272.5
- lipoprotein (familial) (high-density) 272.5
- liver phosphorylase 271.0
- long chain 3-hydroxyacyl CoA dehydrogenase (LCHAD) 277.85
- long chain/very long chain acyl CoA dehydrogenase (LCAD, VLCAD) 277.85
- lower limb V49.0
  - congenital 755.30
    - with complete absence of distal elements 755.31
    - longitudinal (complete) (partial) (with distal deficiencies, incomplete) 755.32
      - with complete absence of distal elements 755.31
      - combined femoral, tibial, fibular (incomplete) 755.33
      - femoral 755.34
      - fibular 755.37
      - metatarsal(s) 755.38
      - phalange(s) 755.39
        - meaning all digits 755.31
      - tarsal(s) 755.38
      - tibia 755.36
      - tibiofibular 755.35
    - transverse 755.31
- luteinizing hormone (LH) 253.4
- lysosomal alpha-1, 4 glucosidase 271.0
- magnesium 275.2
- mannosidase 271.8
- medium chain acyl CoA dehydrogenase (MCAD) 277.85
- melanocyte-stimulating hormone (MSH) 253.4
- menadione (vitamin K) 269.0
  - newborn 776.0
- mental (familial) (hereditary) (*see also* Retardation, mental) 319
- mineral NEC 269.3
- molybdenum 269.3
- moral 301.7
- multiple, syndrome 260
- myocardial (*see also* Insufficiency, myocardial) 428.0
- myophosphorylase 271.0
- NADH (DPNH)-methemoglobin-reductase (congenital) 289.7
- NADH diaphorase or reductase (congenital) 289.7
- neck V48.1
- niacin (amide) (-tryptophan) 265.2
- nicotinamide 265.2
- nicotinic acid (amide) 265.2
- nose V48.8
- number of teeth (*see also* Anodontia) 520.0
- nutrition, nutritional 269.9
  - specified NEC 269.8
- ornithine transcarbamylase 270.6
- ovarian 256.39
- oxygen (*see also* Anoxia) 799.02
- pantothenic acid 266.2

Deficiency, deficient *(Continued)*
- parathyroid (gland) 252.1
- phenylalanine hydroxylase 270.1
- phosphoenolpyruvate carboxykinase 271.8
- phosphofructokinase 271.2
- phosphoglucomutase 271.0
- phosphohexosisomerase 271.0
- phosphomannomutase 271.8
- phosphomannose isomerase 271.8
- phosphomannosyl mutase 271.8
- phosphorylase kinase, liver 271.0
- pituitary (anterior) 253.2
  - posterior 253.5
- placenta - *see* Placenta, insufficiency
- plasma
  - cell 279.00
  - protein (paraproteinemia) (pyroglobulinemia) 273.8
    - gamma globulin 279.00
  - thromboplastin
    - antecedent (PTA) 286.2
    - component (PTC) 286.1
- platelet NEC 287.1
  - constitutional 286.4
- polyglandular 258.9
- potassium (K) 276.8
- proaccelerin (congenital) (*see also* Defect, congenital) 286.3
  - acquired 286.7
- proconvertin factor (congenital) (*see also* Defect, coagulation) 286.3
  - acquired 286.7
- prolactin 253.4
- protein 260
  - anemia 281.4
  - C 289.81
  - plasma - *see* Deficiency, plasma, protein
  - S 289.81
- prothrombin (congenital) (*see also* Defect, coagulation) 286.3
  - acquired 286.7
- Prower factor (*see also* Defect, coagulation) 286.3
- PRT 277.2
- pseudocholinesterase 289.89
- psychobiological 301.6
- PTA 286.2
- PTC 286.1
- purine nucleoside phosphorylase 277.2
- pyracin (alpha) (beta) 266.1
- pyridoxal 266.1
- pyridoxamine 266.1
- pyridoxine (derivatives) 266.1
- pyruvate carboxylase 271.8
- pyruvate dehydrogenase 271.8
- pyruvate kinase (PK) 282.3
- riboflavin (vitamin B_2) 266.0
- saccadic eye movements 379.57
- salivation 527.7
- salt 276.1
- secretion
  - ovary 256.39
  - salivary gland (any) 527.7
  - urine 788.5
- selenium 269.3
- serum
  - antitrypsin, familial 273.4
  - protein (congenital) 273.8
- short chain acyl CoA dehydrogenase (SCAD) 277.85
- smooth pursuit movements (eye) 379.58
- sodium (Na) 276.1
- SPCA (*see also* Defect, coagulation) 286.3

Deficiency, deficient *(Continued)*
- specified NEC 269.8
- stable factor (congenital) (*see also* Defect, coagulation) 286.3
  - acquired 286.7
- Stuart (-Prower) factor (*see also* Defect, coagulation) 286.3
- sucrase 271.3
- sucrase-isomaltase 271.3
- sulfite oxidase 270.0
- syndrome, multiple 260
- thiamine, thiaminic (chloride) 265.1
- thrombokinase (*see also* Defect, coagulation) 286.3
  - newborn 776.0
- thrombopoieten 287.39
- thymolymphatic 279.2
- thyroid (gland) 244.9
- tocopherol 269.1
- toe - *see* Absence, toe
- tooth bud (*see also* Anodontia) 520.0
- trunk V48.1
- UDPG-glycogen transferase 271.0
- upper limb V49.0
  - congenital 755.20
    - with complete absence of distal elements 755.21
    - longitudinal (complete) (partial) (with distal deficiencies, incomplete) 755.22
      - carpal(s) 755.28
      - combined humeral, radial, ulnar (incomplete) 755.23
      - humeral 755.24
      - metacarpal(s) 755.28
      - phalange(s) 755.29
        - meaning all digits 755.21
      - radial 755.26
      - radioulnar 755.25
      - ulnar 755.27
    - transverse (complete) (partial) 755.21
- vascular 459.9
- vasopressin 253.5
- viosterol (*see also* Deficiency, calciferol) 268.9
- vitamin (multiple) NEC 269.2
  - A 264.9
    - with
      - Bitôt's spot 264.1
        - corneal 264.2
          - with corneal ulceration 264.3
      - keratomalacia 264.4
      - keratosis, follicular 264.8
      - night blindness 264.5
      - scar of cornea, xerophthalmic 264.6
      - specified manifestation NEC 264.8
        - ocular 264.7
    - xeroderma 264.8
    - xerophthalmia 264.7
    - xerosis
      - conjunctival 264.0
        - with Bitôt's spot 264.1
      - corneal 264.2
        - with corneal ulceration 264.3
  - B (complex) NEC 266.9
    - with
      - beriberi 265.0
      - pellagra 265.2
    - specified type NEC 266.2
  - B_1 NEC 265.1
    - beriberi 265.0
  - B_2 266.0
  - B_6 266.1

ICD-9-CM
D
Vol. 2

- **Deficiency, deficient** *(Continued)*
  - vitamin *(Continued)*
    - B_{12} 266.2
    - B_C (folic acid) 266.2
    - C (ascorbic acid) (with scurvy) 267
    - D (calciferol) (ergosterol) 268.9
      - with
        - osteomalacia 268.2
        - rickets (*see also* Rickets) 268.0
    - E 269.1
    - folic acid 266.2
    - G 266.0
    - H 266.2
    - K 269.0
      - of newborn 776.0
    - nicotinic acid 265.2
    - P 269.1
    - PP 265.2
    - specified NEC 269.1
    - zinc 269.3
- **Deficient** - *see also* Deficiency
  - blink reflex 374.45
  - craniofacial axis 756.0
  - number of teeth (*see also* Anodontia) 520.0
  - secretion of urine 788.5
- **Deficit**
  - neurologic NEC 781.99
    - due to
      - cerebrovascular lesion (*see also* Disease, cerebrovascular, acute) 436
        - late effect - *see* Late effect(s) (of) cerebrovascular disease
      - transient ischemic attack 435.9
  - oxygen 799.02
- **Deflection**
  - radius 736.09
  - septum (acquired) (nasal) (nose) 470
  - spine - *see* Curvature, spine
  - turbinate (nose) 470
- **Defluvium**
  - capillorum (*see also* Alopecia) 704.00
  - ciliorum 374.55
  - unguium 703.8
- **Deformity** 738.9
  - abdomen, congenital 759.9
  - abdominal wall
    - acquired 738.8
    - congenital 756.70
    - muscle deficiency syndrome 756.79
  - acquired (unspecified site) 738.9
    - specified site NEC 738.8
  - adrenal gland (congenital) 759.1
  - alimentary tract, congenital 751.9
    - lower 751.5
    - specified type NEC 751.8
    - upper (any part, except tongue) 750.9
      - specified type NEC 750.8
      - tongue 750.10
        - specified type NEC 750.19
  - ankle (joint) (acquired) 736.70
    - abduction 718.47
    - congenital 755.69
    - contraction 718.47
    - specified NEC 736.79
  - anus (congenital) 751.5
    - acquired 569.49
  - aorta (congenital) 747.20
    - acquired 447.8
    - arch 747.21
      - acquired 447.8
    - coarctation 747.10
  - aortic
    - arch 747.21
      - acquired 447.8

- **Deformity** *(Continued)*
  - aortic *(Continued)*
    - cusp or valve (congenital) 746.9
      - acquired (*see also* Endocarditis, aortic) 424.1
    - ring 747.21
  - appendix 751.5
  - arm (acquired) 736.89
    - congenital 755.50
  - arteriovenous (congenital) (peripheral) NEC 747.60
    - gastrointestinal 747.61
    - lower limb 747.64
    - renal 747.62
    - specified NEC 747.69
    - spinal 747.82
    - upper limb 747.63
  - artery (congenital) (peripheral) NEC (*see also* Deformity, vascular) 747.60
    - acquired 447.8
    - cerebral 747.81
    - coronary (congenital) 746.85
      - acquired (*see also* Ischemia, heart) 414.9
    - retinal 743.9
    - umbilical 747.5
  - atrial septal (congenital) (heart) 745.5
  - auditory canal (congenital) (external) (*see also* Deformity, ear) 744.3
    - acquired 380.50
  - auricle
    - ear (congenital) (*see also* Deformity, ear) 744.3
      - acquired 380.32
    - heart (congenital) 746.9
  - back (acquired) - *see* Deformity, spine
  - Bartholin's duct (congenital) 750.9
  - bile duct (congenital) 751.60
    - acquired 576.8
      - with calculus, choledocholithiasis, or stones - *see* Choledocholithiasis
  - biliary duct or passage (congenital) 751.60
    - acquired 576.8
      - with calculus, choledocholithiasis, or stones - *see* Choledocholithiasis
  - bladder (neck) (sphincter) (trigone) (acquired) 596.8
    - congenital 753.9
  - bone (acquired) NEC 738.9
    - congenital 756.9
    - turbinate 738.0
  - boutonniere (finger) 736.21
  - brain (congenital) 742.9
    - acquired 348.8
    - multiple 742.4
    - reduction 742.2
    - vessel (congenital) 747.81
  - breast (acquired) 611.8
    - congenital 757.9
  - bronchus (congenital) 748.3
    - acquired 519.19 ⬅
  - bursa, congenital 756.9
  - canal of Nuck 752.9
  - canthus (congenital) 743.9
    - acquired 374.89
  - capillary (acquired) 448.9
    - congenital NEC (*see also* Deformity, vascular) 747.60
  - cardiac - *see* Deformity, heart
  - cardiovascular system (congenital) 746.9
  - caruncle, lacrimal (congenital) 743.9
    - acquired 375.69
  - cascade, stomach 537.6

- **Deformity** *(Continued)*
  - cecum (congenital) 751.5
    - acquired 569.89
  - cerebral (congenital) 742.9
    - acquired 348.8
  - cervix (acquired) (uterus) 622.8
    - congenital 752.40
  - cheek (acquired) 738.19
    - congenital 744.9
  - chest (wall) (acquired) 738.3
    - congenital 754.89
    - late effect of rickets 268.1
  - chin (acquired) 738.19
    - congenital 744.9
  - choroid (congenital) 743.9
    - acquired 363.8
    - plexus (congenital) 742.9
      - acquired 349.2
  - cicatricial - *see* Cicatrix
  - cilia (congenital) 743.9
    - acquired 374.89
  - circulatory system (congenital) 747.9
  - clavicle (acquired) 738.8
    - congenital 755.51
  - clitoris (congenital) 752.40
    - acquired 624.8
  - clubfoot - *see* Clubfoot
  - coccyx (acquired) 738.6
    - congenital 756.10
  - colon (congenital) 751.5
    - acquired 569.89
  - concha (ear) (congenital) (*see also* Deformity, ear) 744.3
    - acquired 380.32
  - congenital, organ or site not listed (*see also* Anomaly) 759.9
  - cornea (congenital) 743.9
    - acquired 371.70
  - coronary artery (congenital) 746.85
    - acquired (*see also* Ischemia, heart) 414.9
  - cranium (acquired) 738.19
    - congenital (*see also* Deformity, skull, congenital) 756.0
  - cricoid cartilage (congenital) 748.3
    - acquired 478.79
  - cystic duct (congenital) 751.60
    - acquired 575.8
  - Dandy-Walker 742.3
    - with spina bifida (*see also* Spina bifida) 741.0
  - diaphragm (congenital) 756.6
    - acquired 738.8
  - digestive organ(s) or system (congenital) NEC 751.9
    - specified type NEC 751.8
  - ductus arteriosus 747.0
  - duodenal bulb 537.89
  - duodenum (congenital) 751.5
    - acquired 537.89
  - dura (congenital) 742.9
    - brain 742.4
      - acquired 349.2
    - spinal 742.59
      - acquired 349.2
  - ear (congenital) 744.3
    - acquired 380.32
    - auricle 744.3
      - causing impairment of hearing 744.02
    - causing impairment of hearing 744.00
    - external 744.3
      - causing impairment of hearing 744.02
    - internal 744.05

- **Deformity** *(Continued)*
  - ear *(Continued)*
    - lobule 744.3
    - middle 744.03
      - ossicles 744.04
    - ossicles 744.04
  - ectodermal (congenital) NEC 757.9
    - specified type NEC 757.8
  - ejaculatory duct (congenital) 752.9
    - acquired 608.89
  - elbow (joint) (acquired) 736.00
    - congenital 755.50
    - contraction 718.42
  - endocrine gland NEC 759.2
  - epididymis (congenital) 752.9
    - acquired 608.89
    - torsion 608.24
  - epiglottis (congenital) 748.3
    - acquired 478.79
  - esophagus (congenital) 750.9
    - acquired 530.89
  - Eustachian tube (congenital) NEC 744.3
    - specified type NEC 744.24
  - extremity (acquired) 736.9
    - congenital, except reduction deformity 755.9
      - lower 755.60
      - upper 755.50
    - reduction - *see* Deformity, reduction
  - eye (congenital) 743.9
    - acquired 379.8
    - muscle 743.9
  - eyebrow (congenital) 744.89
  - eyelid (congenital) 743.9
    - acquired 374.89
    - specified type NEC 743.62
  - face (acquired) 738.19
    - congenital (any part) 744.9
      - due to intrauterine malposition and pressure 754.0
  - fallopian tube (congenital) 752.10
    - acquired 620.8
  - femur (acquired) 736.89
    - congenital 755.60
  - fetal
    - with fetopelvic disproportion 653.7
      - affecting fetus or newborn 763.1
    - causing obstructed labor 660.1
      - affecting fetus or newborn 763.1
    - known or suspected, affecting management of pregnancy 655.9
  - finger (acquired) 736.20
    - boutonniere type 736.21
    - congenital 755.50
    - flexion contracture 718.44
    - swan neck 736.22
  - flexion (joint) (acquired) 736.9
    - congenital NEC 755.9
    - hip or thigh (acquired) 736.39
      - congenital (*see also* Subluxation, congenital, hip) 754.32
  - foot (acquired) 736.70
    - cavovarus 736.75
      - congenital 754.59
    - congenital NEC 754.70
      - specified type NEC 754.79
    - valgus (acquired) 736.79
      - congenital 754.60
        - specified type NEC 754.69
    - varus (acquired) 736.79
      - congenital 754.50
        - specified type NEC 754.59
  - forearm (acquired) 736.00
    - congenital 755.50
- **Deformity** *(Continued)*
  - forehead (acquired) 738.19
    - congenital (*see also* Deformity, skull, congenital) 756.0
  - frontal bone (acquired) 738.19
    - congenital (*see also* Deformity, skull, congenital) 756.0
  - gallbladder (congenital) 751.60
    - acquired 575.8
  - gastrointestinal tract (congenital) NEC 751.9
    - acquired 569.89
    - specified type NEC 751.8
  - genitalia, genital organ(s) or system NEC
    - congenital 752.9
    - female (congenital) 752.9
      - acquired 629.89
      - external 752.40
      - internal 752.9
    - male (congenital) 752.9
      - acquired 608.89
  - globe (eye) (congenital) 743.9
    - acquired 360.89
  - gum (congenital) 750.9
    - acquired 523.9
  - gunstock 736.02
  - hand (acquired) 736.00
    - claw 736.06
    - congenital 755.50
    - minus (and plus) (intrinsic) 736.09
    - pill roller (intrinsic) 736.09
    - plus (and minus) (intrinsic) 736.09
    - swan neck (intrinsic) 736.09
  - head (acquired) 738.10
    - congenital (*see also* Deformity, skull, congenital) 756.0
    - specified NEC 738.19
  - heart (congenital) 746.9
    - auricle (congenital) 746.9
    - septum 745.9
      - auricular 745.5
      - specified type NEC 745.8
      - ventricular 745.4
    - valve (congenital) NEC 746.9
      - acquired - *see* Endocarditis
      - pulmonary (congenital) 746.00
      - specified type NEC 746.89
    - ventricle (congenital) 746.9
  - heel (acquired) 736.76
    - congenital 755.67
  - hepatic duct (congenital) 751.60
    - acquired 576.8
      - with calculus, choledocholithiasis, or stones - *see* Choledocholithiasis
  - hip (joint) (acquired) 736.30
    - congenital NEC 755.63
    - flexion 718.45
      - congenital (*see also* Subluxation, congenital, hip) 754.32
  - hourglass - *see* Contraction, hourglass
  - humerus (acquired) 736.89
    - congenital 755.50
  - hymen (congenital) 752.40
  - hypophyseal (congenital) 759.2
  - ileocecal (coil) (valve) (congenital) 751.5
    - acquired 569.89
  - ileum (intestine) (congenital) 751.5
    - acquired 569.89
  - ilium (acquired) 738.6
    - congenital 755.60
  - integument (congenital) 757.9
- **Deformity** *(Continued)*
  - intervertebral cartilage or disc (acquired) - *see also* Displacement, intervertebral disc
    - congenital 756.10
  - intestine (large) (small) (congenital) 751.5
    - acquired 569.89
  - iris (acquired) 364.75
    - congenital 743.9
    - prolapse 364.8
  - ischium (acquired) 738.6
    - congenital 755.60
  - jaw (acquired) (congenital) NEC 524.9
    - due to intrauterine malposition and pressure 754.0
  - joint (acquired) NEC 738.8
    - congenital 755.9
    - contraction (abduction) (adduction) (extension) (flexion) - *see* Contraction, joint
  - kidney(s) (calyx) (pelvis) (congenital) 753.9
    - acquired 593.89
    - vessel 747.62
      - acquired 459.9
  - Klippel-Feil (brevicollis) 756.16
  - knee (acquired) NEC 736.6
    - congenital 755.64
  - labium (majus) (minus) (congenital) 752.40
    - acquired 624.8
  - lacrimal apparatus or duct (congenital) 743.9
    - acquired 375.69
  - larynx (muscle) (congenital) 748.3
    - acquired 478.79
    - web (glottic) (subglottic) 748.2
  - leg (lower) (upper) (acquired) NEC 736.89
    - congenital 755.60
      - reduction - *see* Deformity, reduction, lower limb
  - lens (congenital) 743.9
    - acquired 379.39
  - lid (fold) (congenital) 743.9
    - acquired 374.89
  - ligament (acquired) 728.9
    - congenital 756.9
  - limb (acquired) 736.9
    - congenital, except reduction deformity 755.9
      - lower 755.60
        - reduction (*see also* Deformity, reduction, lower limb) 755.30
      - upper 755.50
        - reduction (*see also* Deformity, reduction, lower limb) 755.20
    - specified NEC 736.89
  - lip (congenital) NEC 750.9
    - acquired 528.5
    - specified type NEC 750.26
  - liver (congenital) 751.60
    - acquired 573.8
    - duct (congenital) 751.60
      - acquired 576.8
        - with calculus, choledocholithiasis, or stones - *see* Choledocholithiasis
  - lower extremity - *see* Deformity, leg
  - lumbosacral (joint) (region) (congenital) 756.10
    - acquired 738.5
  - lung (congenital) 748.60
    - acquired 518.89
    - specified type NEC 748.69

Deformity *(Continued)*
lymphatic system, congenital 759.9
Madelung's (radius) 755.54
maxilla (acquired) (congenital) 524.9
meninges or membrane (congenital) 742.9
brain 742.4
acquired 349.2
spinal (cord) 742.59
acquired 349.2
mesentery (congenital) 751.9
acquired 568.89
metacarpus (acquired) 736.00
congenital 755.50
metatarsus (acquired) 736.70
congenital 754.70
middle ear, except ossicles (congenital) 744.03
ossicles 744.04
mitral (leaflets) (valve) (congenital) 746.9
acquired - *see* Endocarditis, mitral
Ebstein's 746.89
parachute 746.5
specified type NEC 746.89
stenosis, congenital 746.5
mouth (acquired) 528.9
congenital NEC 750.9
specified type NEC 750.26
multiple, congenital NEC 759.7
specified type NEC 759.89
muscle (acquired) 728.9
congenital 756.9
specified type NEC 756.89
sternocleidomastoid (due to intrauterine malposition and pressure) 754.1
musculoskeletal system, congenital NEC 756.9
specified type NEC 756.9
nail (acquired) 703.9
congenital 757.9
nasal - *see* Deformity, nose
neck (acquired) NEC 738.2
congenital (any part) 744.9
sternocleidomastoid 754.1
nervous system (congenital) 742.9
nipple (congenital) 757.9
acquired 611.8
nose, nasal (cartilage) (acquired) 738.0
bone (turbinate) 738.0
congenital 748.1
bent 754.0
squashed 754.0
saddle 738.0
syphilitic 090.5
septum 470
congenital 748.1
sinus (wall) (congenital) 748.1
acquired 738.0
syphilitic (congenital) 090.5
late 095.8
ocular muscle (congenital) 743.9
acquired 378.60
opticociliary vessels (congenital) 743.9
orbit (congenital) (eye) 743.9
acquired NEC 376.40
associated with craniofacial deformities 376.44
due to
bone disease 376.43
surgery 376.47
trauma 376.47
organ of Corti (congenital) 744.05
ovary (congenital) 752.0
acquired 620.8

Deformity *(Continued)*
oviduct (congenital) 752.10
acquired 620.8
palate (congenital) 750.9
acquired 526.89
cleft (congenital) (*see also* Cleft, palate) 749.00
hard, acquired 526.89
soft, acquired 528.9
pancreas (congenital) 751.7
acquired 577.8
parachute, mitral valve 746.5
parathyroid (gland) 759.2
parotid (gland) (congenital) 750.9
acquired 527.8
patella (acquired) 736.6
congenital 755.64
pelvis, pelvic (acquired) (bony) 738.6
with disproportion (fetopelvic) 653.0
affecting fetus or newborn 763.1
causing obstructed labor 660.1
affecting fetus or newborn 763.1
congenital 755.60
rachitic (late effect) 268.1
penis (glans) (congenital) 752.9
acquired 607.89
pericardium (congenital) 746.9
acquired - *see* Pericarditis
pharynx (congenital) 750.9
acquired 478.29
Pierre Robin (congenital) 756.0
pinna (acquired) 380.32
congenital 744.3
pituitary (congenital) 759.2
pleural folds (congenital) 748.8
portal vein (congenital) 747.40
posture - *see* Curvature, spine
prepuce (congenital) 752.9
acquired 607.89
prostate (congenital) 752.9
acquired 602.8
pulmonary valve - *see* Endocarditis, pulmonary
pupil (congenital) 743.9
acquired 364.75
pylorus (congenital) 750.9
acquired 537.89
rachitic (acquired), healed or old 268.1
radius (acquired) 736.00
congenital 755.50
reduction - *see* Deformity, reduction, upper limb
rectovaginal septum (congenital) 752.40
acquired 623.8
rectum (congenital) 751.5
acquired 569.49
reduction (extremity) (limb) 755.4
brain 742.2
lower limb 755.30
with complete absence of distal elements 755.31
longitudinal (complete) (partial) (with distal deficiencies, incomplete) 755.32
with complete absence of distal elements 755.31
combined femoral, tibial, fibular (incomplete) 755.33
femoral 755.34
fibular 755.37
metatarsal(s) 755.38
phalange(s) 755.39
meaning all digits 755.31
tarsal(s) 755.38

Deformity *(Continued)*
reduction *(Continued)*
lower limb *(Continued)*
longitudinal *(Continued)*
tibia 755.36
tibiofibular 755.35
transverse 755.31
upper limb 755.20
with complete absence of distal elements 755.21
longitudinal (complete) (partial) (with distal deficiencies, incomplete) 755.22
with complete absence of distal elements 755.21
carpal(s) 755.28
combined humeral, radial, ulnar (incomplete) 755.23
humeral 755.24
metacarpal(s) 755.28
phalange(s) 755.29
meaning all digits 755.21
radial 755.26
radioulnar 755.25
ulnar 755.27
transverse (complete) (partial) 755.21
renal - *see* Deformity, kidney
respiratory system (congenital) 748.9
specified type NEC 748.8
rib (acquired) 738.3
congenital 756.3
cervical 756.2
rotation (joint) (acquired) 736.9
congenital 755.9
hip or thigh 736.39
congenital (*see also* Subluxation, congenital, hip) 754.32
sacroiliac joint (congenital) 755.69
acquired 738.5
sacrum (acquired) 738.5
congenital 756.10
saddle
back 737.8
nose 738.0
syphilitic 090.5
salivary gland or duct (congenital) 750.9
acquired 527.8
scapula (acquired) 736.89
congenital 755.50
scrotum (congenital) 752.9
acquired 608.89
sebaceous gland, acquired 706.8
seminal tract or duct (congenital) 752.9
acquired 608.89
septum (nasal) (acquired) 470
congenital 748.1
shoulder (joint) (acquired) 736.89
congenital 755.50
specified type NEC 755.59
contraction 718.41
sigmoid (flexure) (congenital) 751.5
acquired 569.89
sinus of Valsalva 747.29
skin (congenital) 757.9
acquired NEC 709.8
skull (acquired) 738.19
congenital 756.0
with
anencephalus 740.0
encephalocele 742.0
hydrocephalus 742.3
with spina bifida (*see also* Spina bifida) 741.0
microcephalus 742.1

Deformity *(Continued)*
  skull *(Continued)*
    congenital *(Continued)*
      due to intrauterine malposition and pressure 754.0
  soft parts, organs or tissues (of pelvis)
    in pregnancy or childbirth NEC 654.9
      affecting fetus or newborn 763.89
      causing obstructed labor 660.2
        affecting fetus or newborn 763.1
  spermatic cord (congenital) 752.9
    acquired 608.89
      torsion 608.22
        extravaginal 608.21
        intravaginal 608.22
  spinal
    column - *see* Deformity, spine
    cord (congenital) 742.9
      acquired 336.8
      vessel (congenital) 747.82
    nerve root (congenital) 742.9
      acquired 724.9
  spine (acquired) NEC 738.5
    congenital 756.10
      due to intrauterine malposition and pressure 754.2
    kyphoscoliotic (*see also* Kyphoscoliosis) 737.30
    kyphotic (*see also* Kyphosis) 737.10
    lordotic (*see also* Lordosis) 737.20
    rachitic 268.1
    scoliotic (*see also* Scoliosis) 737.30
  spleen
    acquired 289.59
    congenital 759.0
  Sprengel's (congenital) 755.52
  sternum (acquired) 738.3
    congenital 756.3
  stomach (congenital) 750.9
    acquired 537.89
  submaxillary gland (congenital) 750.9
    acquired 527.8
  swan neck (acquired)
    finger 736.22
    hand 736.09
  talipes - *see* Talipes
  teeth, tooth NEC 520.9
  testis (congenital) 752.9
    acquired 608.89
      torsion 608.20
  thigh (acquired) 736.89
    congenital 755.60
  thorax (acquired) (wall) 738.3
    congenital 754.89
    late effect of rickets 268.1
  thumb (acquired) 736.20
    congenital 755.50
  thymus (tissue) (congenital) 759.2
  thyroid (gland) (congenital) 759.2
    cartilage 748.3
      acquired 478.79
  tibia (acquired) 736.89
    congenital 755.60
    saber 090.5
  toe (acquired) 735.9
    congenital 755.66
    specified NEC 735.8
  tongue (congenital) 750.10
    acquired 529.8
  tooth, teeth NEC 520.9
  trachea (rings) (congenital) 748.3
    acquired 519.19
  transverse aortic arch (congenital) 747.21

Deformity *(Continued)*
  tricuspid (leaflets) (valve) (congenital) 746.9
    acquired - *see* Endocarditis, tricuspid
    atresia or stenosis 746.1
    specified type NEC 746.89
  trunk (acquired) 738.3
    congenital 759.9
  ulna (acquired) 736.00
    congenital 755.50
  upper extremity - *see* Deformity, arm
  urachus (congenital) 753.7
  ureter (opening) (congenital) 753.9
    acquired 593.89
  urethra (valve) (congenital) 753.9
    acquired 599.84
  urinary tract or system (congenital) 753.9
    urachus 753.7
  uterus (congenital) 752.3
    acquired 621.8
  uvula (congenital) 750.9
    acquired 528.9
  vagina (congenital) 752.40
    acquired 623.8
  valve, valvular (heart) (congenital) 746.9
    acquired - *see* Endocarditis
    pulmonary 746.00
    specified type NEC 746.89
  vascular (congenital) (peripheral) NEC 747.60
    acquired 459.9
    gastrointestinal 747.61
    lower limb 747.64
    renal 747.62
    specified site NEC 747.69
    spinal 747.82
    upper limb 747.63
  vas deferens (congenital) 752.9
    acquired 608.89
  vein (congenital) NEC (*see also* Deformity, vascular) 747.60
    brain 747.81
    coronary 746.9
    great 747.40
  vena cava (inferior) (superior) (congenital) 747.40
  vertebra - *see* Deformity, spine
  vesicourethral orifice (acquired) 596.8
    congenital NEC 753.9
      specified type NEC 753.8
  vessels of optic papilla (congenital) 743.9
  visual field (contraction) 368.45
  vitreous humor (congenital) 743.9
    acquired 379.29
  vulva (congenital) 752.40
    acquired 624.8
  wrist (joint) (acquired) 736.00
    congenital 755.50
    contraction 718.43
    valgus 736.03
      congenital 755.59
    varus 736.04
      congenital 755.59

Degeneration, degenerative
  adrenal (capsule) (gland) 255.8
    with hypofunction 255.4
    fatty 255.8
    hyaline 255.8
    infectional 255.8
    lardaceous 277.39
  amyloid (any site) (general) 277.39
  anterior cornua, spinal cord 336.8
  aorta, aortic 440.0
    fatty 447.8

Degeneration, degenerative *(Continued)*
  aorta, aortic *(Continued)*
    valve (heart) (*see also* Endocarditis, aortic) 424.1
  arteriovascular - *see* Arteriosclerosis
  artery, arterial (atheromatous) (calcareous) - *see also* Arteriosclerosis
    amyloid 277.39
    lardaceous 277.39
    medial NEC (*see also* Arteriosclerosis, extremities) 440.20
  articular cartilage NEC (*see also* Disorder, cartilage, articular) 718.0
    elbow 718.02
    knee 717.5
    patella 717.7
    shoulder 718.01
    spine (*see also* Spondylosis) 721.90
  atheromatous - *see* Arteriosclerosis
  bacony (any site) 277.39
  basal nuclei or ganglia NEC 333.0
  bone 733.90
  brachial plexus 353.0
  brain (cortical) (progressive) 331.9
    arteriosclerotic 437.0
    childhood 330.9
      specified type NEC 330.8
    congenital 742.4
    cystic 348.0
      congenital 742.4
    familial NEC 331.89
    grey matter 330.8
    heredofamilial NEC 331.89
    in
      alcoholism 303.9 *[331.7]*
      beriberi 265.0 *[331.7]*
      cerebrovascular disease 437.9 *[331.7]*
      congenital hydrocephalus 742.3 *[331.7]*
        with spina bifida (*see also* Spina bifida) 741.0 *[331.7]*
      Fabry's disease 272.7 *[330.2]*
      Gaucher's disease 272.7 *[330.2]*
      Hunter's disease or syndrome 277.5 *[330.3]*
      lipidosis
        cerebral *[330.1]*
        generalized 272.7 *[330.2]*
      mucopolysaccharidosis 277.5 *[330.3]*
      myxedema (*see also* Myxedema) 244.9 *[331.7]*
      neoplastic disease NEC (M8000/1) 239.9 *[331.7]*
      Niemann-Pick disease 272.7 *[330.2]*
      sphingolipidosis 272.7 *[330.2]*
      vitamin B_{12} deficiency 266.2 *[331.7]*
    motor centers 331.89
    senile 331.2
    specified type NEC 331.89
  breast - *see* Disease, breast
  Bruch's membrane 363.40
  bundle of His 426.50
    left 426.3
    right 426.4
  calcareous NEC 275.49
  capillaries 448.9
    amyloid 277.39
    fatty 448.9
    lardaceous 277.39
  cardiac (brown) (calcareous) (fatty) (fibrous) (hyaline) (mural) (muscular) (pigmentary) (senile) (with arteriosclerosis) (*see also* Degeneration, myocardial) 429.1

ICD-9-CM
D
Vol. 2

Degeneration, degenerative (Continued)
cardiac (Continued)
valve, valvular - see Endocarditis
cardiorenal (see also Hypertension, cardiorenal) 404.90
cardiovascular (see also Disease, cardiovascular) 429.2
renal (see also Hypertension, cardiorenal) 404.90
cartilage (joint) - see Derangement, joint
cerebellar NEC 334.9
primary (hereditary) (sporadic) 334.2
cerebral - see Degeneration, brain
cerebromacular 330.1
cerebrovascular 437.1
due to hypertension 437.2
late effect - see Late effect(s) (of) cerebrovascular disease
cervical plexus 353.2
cervix 622.8
due to radiation (intended effect) 622.8
adverse effect or misadventure 622.8
changes, spine or vertebra (see also Spondylosis) 721.90
chitinous 277.39
chorioretinal 363.40
congenital 743.53
hereditary 363.50
choroid (colloid) (drusen) 363.40
hereditary 363.50
senile 363.41
diffuse secondary 363.42
cochlear 386.8
collateral ligament (knee) (medial) 717.82
lateral 717.81
combined (spinal cord) (subacute) 266.2 [336.2]
with anemia (pernicious) 281.0 [336.2]
due to dietary deficiency 281.1 [336.2]
due to vitamin B_{12} deficiency anemia (dietary) 281.1 [336.2]
conjunctiva 372.50
amyloid 277.39 [372.50]
cornea 371.40
calcerous 371.44
familial (hereditary) (see also Dystrophy, cornea) 371.50
macular 371.55
reticular 371.54
hyaline (of old scars) 371.41
marginal (Terrien's) 371.48
mosaic (shagreen) 371.41
nodular 371.46
peripheral 371.48
senile 371.41
cortical (cerebellar) (parenchymatous) 334.2
alcoholic 303.9 [334.4]
diffuse, due to arteriopathy 437.0
corticostriatal-spinal 334.8
cretinoid 243
cruciate ligament (knee) (posterior) 717.84
anterior 717.83
cutis 709.3
amyloid 277.39
dental pulp 522.2
disc disease - see Degeneration, intervertebral disc
dorsolateral (spinal cord) - see Degeneration, combined
endocardial 424.90
extrapyramidal NEC 333.90

Degeneration, degenerative (Continued)
eye NEC 360.40
macular (see also Degeneration, macula) 362.50
congenital 362.75
hereditary 362.76
fatty (diffuse) (general) 272.8
liver 571.8
alcoholic 571.0
localized site - see Degeneration, by site, fatty
placenta - see Placenta, abnormal
globe (eye) NEC 360.40
macular - see Degeneration, macula
grey matter 330.8
heart (brown) (calcareous) (fatty) (fibrous) (hyaline) (mural) (muscular) (pigmentary) (senile) (with arteriosclerosis) (see also Degeneration, myocardial) 429.1
amyloid 277.39 [425.7]
atheromatous - see Arteriosclerosis, coronary
gouty 274.82
hypertensive (see also Hypertension, heart) 402.90
ischemic 414.9
valve, valvular - see Endocarditis
hepatolenticular (Wilson's) 275.1
hepatorenal 572.4
heredofamilial
brain NEC 331.89
spinal cord NEC 336.8
hyaline (diffuse) (generalized) 728.9
localized - see also Degeneration, by site
cornea 371.41
keratitis 371.41
hypertensive vascular - see Hypertension
infrapatellar fat pad 729.31
internal semilunar cartilage 717.3
intervertebral disc 722.6
with myelopathy 722.70
cervical, cervicothoracic 722.4
with myelopathy 722.71
lumbar, lumbosacral 722.52
with myelopathy 722.73
thoracic, thoracolumbar 722.51
with myelopathy 722.72
intestine 569.89
amyloid 277.39
lardaceous 277.39
iris (generalized) (see also Atrophy, iris) 364.59
pigmentary 364.53
pupillary margin 364.54
ischemic - see Ischemia
joint disease (see also Osteoarthrosis) 715.9
multiple sites 715.09
spine (see also Spondylosis) 721.90
kidney (see also Sclerosis, renal) 587
amyloid 277.39 [583.81]
cyst, cystic (multiple) (solitary) 593.2
congenital (see also Cystic, disease, kidney) 753.10
fatty 593.89
fibrocystic (congenital) 753.19
lardaceous 277.39 [583.81]
polycystic (congenital) 753.12
adult type (APKD) 753.13
autosomal dominant 753.13
autosomal recessive 753.14
childhood type (CPKD) 753.14
infantile type 753.14
waxy 277.39 [583.81]

Degeneration, degenerative (Continued)
Kuhnt-Junius (retina) 362.52
labyrinth, osseous 386.8
lacrimal passages, cystic 375.12
lardaceous (any site) 277.39
lateral column (posterior), spinal cord (see also Degeneration, combined) 266.2 [336.2]
lattice 362.63
lens 366.9
infantile, juvenile, or presenile 366.00
senile 366.10
lenticular (familial) (progressive) (Wilson's) (with cirrhosis of liver) 275.1
striate artery 437.0
lethal ball, prosthetic heart valve 996.02
ligament
collateral (knee) (medial) 717.82
lateral 717.81
cruciate (knee) (posterior) 717.84
anterior 717.83
liver (diffuse) 572.8
amyloid 277.39
congenital (cystic) 751.62
cystic 572.8
congenital 751.62
fatty 571.8
alcoholic 571.0
hypertrophic 572.8
lardaceous 277.39
parenchymatous, acute or subacute (see also Necrosis, liver) 570
pigmentary 572.8
toxic (acute) 573.8
waxy 277.39
lung 518.89
lymph gland 289.3
hyaline 289.3
lardaceous 277.39
macula (acquired) (senile) 362.50
atrophic 362.51
Best's 362.76
congenital 362.75
cystic 362.54
cystoid 362.53
disciform 362.52
dry 362.51
exudative 362.52
familial pseudoinflammatory 362.77
hereditary 362.76
hole 362.54
juvenile (Stargardt's) 362.75
nonexudative 362.51
pseudohole 362.54
wet 362.52
medullary - see Degeneration, brain
membranous labyrinth, congenital (causing impairment of hearing) 744.05
meniscus - see Derangement, joint
microcystoid 362.62
mitral - see Insufficiency, mitral
Mönckeberg's (see also Arteriosclerosis, extremities) 440.20
moral 301.7
motor centers, senile 331.2
mural (see also Degeneration, myocardial) 429.1
heart, cardiac (see also Degeneration, myocardial) 429.1
myocardium, myocardial (see also Degeneration, myocardial) 429.1

New   Revised

Degeneration, degenerative *(Continued)*
- muscle 728.9
  - fatty 728.9
  - fibrous 728.9
  - heart (*see also* Degeneration, myocardial) 429.1
  - hyaline 728.9
- muscular progressive 728.2
- myelin, central nervous system NEC 341.9
- myocardium, myocardial (brown) (calcareous) (fatty) (fibrous) (hyaline) (mural) (muscular) (pigmentary) (senile) (with arteriosclerosis) 429.1
  - with rheumatic fever (conditions classifiable to 390) 398.0
    - active, acute, or subacute 391.2
      - with chorea 392.0
    - inactive or quiescent (with chorea) 398.0
  - amyloid 277.39 *[425.7]*
  - congenital 746.89
  - fetus or newborn 779.89
  - gouty 274.82
  - hypertensive (*see also* Hypertension, heart) 402.90
  - ischemic 414.8
  - rheumatic (*see also* Degeneration, myocardium, with rheumatic fever) 398.0
  - syphilitic 093.82
- nasal sinus (mucosa) (*see also* Sinusitis) 473.9
  - frontal 473.1
  - maxillary 473.0
- nerve - *see* Disorder, nerve
- nervous system 349.89
  - amyloid 277.39 *[357.4]*
  - autonomic (*see also* Neuropathy, peripheral, autonomic) 337.9
  - fatty 349.89
  - peripheral autonomic NEC (*see also* Neuropathy, peripheral, autonomic) 337.9
- nipple 611.9
- nose 478.19
- oculoacousticocerebral, congenital (progressive) 743.8
- olivopontocerebellar (familial) (hereditary) 333.0
- osseous labyrinth 386.8
- ovary 620.8
  - cystic 620.2
  - microcystic 620.2
- pallidal, pigmentary (progressive) 333.0
- pancreas 577.8
  - tuberculous (*see also* Tuberculosis) 017.9
- papillary muscle 429.81
- paving stone 362.61
- penis 607.89
- peritoneum 568.89
- pigmentary (diffuse) (general)
  - localized - *see* Degeneration, by site
  - pallidal (progressive) 333.0
  - secondary 362.65
- pineal gland 259.8
- pituitary (gland) 253.8
- placenta (fatty) (fibrinoid) (fibroid) - *see* Placenta, abnormal
- popliteal fat pad 729.31
- posterolateral (spinal cord) (*see also* Degeneration, combined) 266.2 *[336.2]*
- pulmonary valve (heart) (*see also* Endocarditis, pulmonary) 424.3
- pulp (tooth) 522.2
- pupillary margin 364.54
- renal (*see also* Sclerosis, renal) 587
  - fibrocystic 753.19
  - polycystic 753.12
    - adult type (APKD) 753.13
    - autosomal dominant 753.13
    - autosomal recessive 753.14
    - childhood type (CPKD) 753.14
    - infantile type 753.14
- reticuloendothelial system 289.89
- retina (peripheral) 362.60
  - with retinal defect (*see also* Detachment, retina, with retinal defect) 361.00
  - cystic (senile) 362.50
  - cystoid 362.53
  - hereditary (*see also* Dystrophy, retina) 362.70
    - cerebroretinal 362.71
    - congenital 362.75
    - juvenile (Stargardt's) 362.75
    - macula 362.76
  - Kuhnt-Junius 362.52
  - lattice 362.63
  - macular (*see also* Degeneration, macula) 362.50
  - microcystoid 362.62
  - palisade 362.63
  - paving stone 362.61
  - pigmentary (primary) 362.74
    - secondary 362.65
  - posterior pole (*see also* Degeneration, macula) 362.50
  - secondary 362.66
  - senile 362.60
    - cystic 362.53
    - reticular 362.64
- saccule, congenital (causing impairment of hearing) 744.05
- sacculocochlear 386.8
- senile 797
  - brain 331.2
  - cardiac, heart, or myocardium (*see also* Degeneration, myocardial) 429.1
  - motor centers 331.2
  - reticule 362.64
  - retina, cystic 362.50
  - vascular - *see* Arteriosclerosis
- silicone rubber poppet (prosthetic valve) 996.02
- sinus (cystic) (*see also* Sinusitis) 473.9
  - polypoid 471.1
- skin 709.3
  - amyloid 277.39
  - colloid 709.3
- spinal (cord) 336.8
  - amyloid 277.39
  - column 733.90
  - combined (subacute) (*see also* Degeneration, combined) 266.2 *[336.2]*
    - with anemia (pernicious) 281.0 *[336.2]*
  - dorsolateral (*see also* Degeneration, combined) 266.2 *[336.2]*
  - familial NEC 336.8
  - fatty 336.8
  - funicular (*see also* Degeneration, combined) 266.2 *[336.2]*
  - heredofamilial NEC 336.8
  - posterolateral (*see also* Degeneration, combined) 266.2 *[336.2]*
  - subacute combined - *see* Degeneration, combined
  - tuberculous (*see also* Tuberculosis) 013.8
- spine 733.90
- spleen 289.59
  - amyloid 277.39
  - lardaceous 277.39
- stomach 537.89
  - lardaceous 277.39
- strionigral 333.0
- sudoriparous (cystic) 705.89
- suprarenal (capsule) (gland) 255.8
  - with hypofunction 255.4
- sweat gland 705.89
- synovial membrane (pulpy) 727.9
- tapetoretinal 362.74
  - adult or presenile form 362.50
- testis (postinfectional) 608.89
- thymus (gland) 254.8
  - fatty 254.8
  - lardaceous 277.39
- thyroid (gland) 246.8
- tricuspid (heart) (valve) - *see* Endocarditis, tricuspid
- tuberculous NEC (*see also* Tuberculosis) 011.9
- turbinate 733.90
- uterus 621.8
  - cystic 621.8
- vascular (senile) - *see also* Arteriosclerosis
  - hypertensive - *see* Hypertension
- vitreoretinal (primary) 362.73
  - secondary 362.66
- vitreous humor (with infiltration) 379.21
- wallerian NEC - *see* Disorder, nerve
- waxy (any site) 277.39
- Wilson's hepatolenticular 275.1

Deglutition
- paralysis 784.99
  - hysterical 300.11
- pneumonia 507.0

Degos' disease or syndrome 447.8

Degradation disorder, branched-chain amino-acid 270.3

Dehiscence
- anastomosis - *see* Complications, anastomosis
- cesarean wound 674.1
- episiotomy 674.2
- operation wound 998.32
  - internal 998.31
- perineal wound (postpartum) 674.2
- postoperative 998.32
  - abdomen 998.32
    - internal 998.31
  - internal 998.31
- uterine wound 674.1

Dehydration (cachexia) 276.51
- with
  - hypernatremia 276.0
  - hyponatremia 276.1
- newborn 775.5

Deiters' nucleus syndrome 386.19

Déjérine's disease 356.0

Déjérine-Klumpke paralysis 767.6

Déjérine-Roussy syndrome 338.0

Déjérine-Sottas disease or neuropathy (hypertrophic) 356.0

Déjérine-Thomas atrophy or syndrome 333.0

ICD-9-CM D Vol. 2

- **de Lange's syndrome** (Amsterdam dwarf, mental retardation, and brachycephaly) 759.89
- **Delay, delayed**
  - adaptation, cones or rods 368.63
  - any plane in pelvis
    - affecting fetus or newborn 763.1
    - complicating delivery 660.1
  - birth or delivery NEC 662.1
    - affecting fetus or newborn 763.9
    - second twin, triplet, or multiple mate 662.3
  - closure - *see also* Fistula
    - cranial suture 756.0
    - fontanel 756.0
  - coagulation NEC 790.92
  - conduction (cardiac) (ventricular) 426.9
  - delivery NEC 662.1
    - second twin, triplet, etc. 662.3
      - affecting fetus or newborn 763.89
  - development
    - in childhood 783.40
      - physiological 783.40
    - intellectual NEC 315.9
    - learning NEC 315.2
    - reading 315.00
    - sexual 259.0
    - speech 315.39
      - associated with hyperkinesis 314.1
    - spelling 315.09
  - gastric emptying 536.8
  - menarche 256.39
    - due to pituitary hypofunction 253.4
  - menstruation (cause unknown) 626.8
  - milestone in childhood 783.42
  - motility - *see* Hypomotility
  - passage of meconium (newborn) 777.1
  - primary respiration 768.9
  - puberty 259.0
  - separation of umbilical cord 779.83
  - sexual maturation, female 259.0
- **Del Castillo's syndrome** (germinal aplasia) 606.0
- **Deleage's disease** 359.89
- **Deletion syndrome**
  - 5p 758.31
  - 22q11.2 758.32
  - autosomal NEC 758.39
  - constitutional 5q deletion 758.39 ◀
- **Delhi** (boil) (button) (sore) 085.1
- **Delinquency** (juvenile) 312.9
  - group (*see also* Disturbance, conduct) 312.2
  - neurotic 312.4
- **Delirium, delirious** 780.09
  - acute (psychotic) 293.0
  - alcoholic 291.0
    - acute 291.0
    - chronic 291.1
  - alcoholicum 291.0
  - chronic (*see also* Psychosis) 293.89
    - due to or associated with physical condition - *see* Psychosis, organic
  - drug-induced 292.81
  - due to conditions classified elsewhere 293.0
  - eclamptic (*see also* Eclampsia) 780.39
  - exhaustion (*see also* Reaction, stress, acute) 308.9
  - hysterical 300.11
  - in
    - presenile dementia 290.11
    - senile dementia 290.3
  - induced by drug 292.81
  - manic, maniacal (acute) (*see also* Psychosis, affective) 296.0
    - recurrent episode 296.1
    - single episode 296.0
  - puerperal 293.9
  - senile 290.3
  - subacute (psychotic) 293.1
  - thyroid (*see also* Thyrotoxicosis) 242.9
  - traumatic - *see also* Injury, intracranial
    - with
      - lesion, spinal cord - *see* Injury, spinal, by site
      - shock, spinal - *see* Injury, spinal, by site
  - tremens (impending) 291.0
  - uremic - *see* Uremia
  - withdrawal
    - alcoholic (acute) 291.0
      - chronic 291.1
    - drug 292.0
- **Delivery**

> Note Use the following fifth-digit subclassification with categories 640–648, 651–676:
>
> 0 unspecified as to episode of care
> 1 delivered, with or without mention of antepartum condition
> 2 delivered, with mention of postpartum complication
> 3 antepartum condition or complication
> 4 postpartum condition or complication

  - breech (assisted) (buttocks) (complete) (frank) (spontaneous) 652.2
    - affecting fetus or newborn 763.0
    - extraction NEC 669.6
  - cesarean (for) 669.7
    - abnormal
      - cervix 654.6
      - pelvic organs of tissues 654.9
      - pelvis (bony) (major) NEC 653.0
      - presentation or position 652.9
        - in multiple gestation 652.6
      - size, fetus 653.5
      - soft parts (of pelvis) 654.9
      - uterus, congenital 654.0
      - vagina 654.7
      - vulva 654.8
    - abruptio placentae 641.2
    - acromion presentation 652.8
    - affecting fetus or newborn 763.4
    - anteversion, cervix or uterus 654.4
    - atony, uterus, with hemorrhage 666.1 ⬅
    - bicornis or bicornuate uterus 654.0
    - breech presentation (buttocks) (complete) (frank) 652.2
    - brow presentation 652.4
    - cephalopelvic disproportion (normally formed fetus) 653.4
    - chin presentation 652.4
    - cicatrix of cervix 654.6
    - contracted pelvis (general) 653.1
      - inlet 653.2
      - outlet 653.3
    - cord presentation or prolapse 663.0
    - cystocele 654.4
    - deformity (acquired) (congenital)
      - pelvic organs or tissues NEC 654.9
      - pelvis (bony) NEC 653.0
    - displacement, uterus NEC 654.4
    - disproportion NEC 653.9
    - distress
      - fetal 656.8
      - maternal 669.0
    - eclampsia 642.6
    - face presentation 652.4
    - failed
      - forceps 660.7
      - trial of labor NEC 660.6
      - vacuum extraction 660.7
      - ventouse 660.7
    - fetal deformity 653.7
    - fetal-maternal hemorrhage 656.0
    - fetus, fetal
      - distress 656.8
      - prematurity 656.8
    - fibroid (tumor) (uterus) 654.1
    - footling 652.8
      - with successful version 652.1
    - hemorrhage (antepartum) (intrapartum) NEC 641.9
    - hydrocephalic fetus 653.6
    - incarceration of uterus 654.3
    - incoordinate uterine action 661.4
    - inertia, uterus 661.2
      - primary 661.0
      - secondary 661.1
    - lateroversion, uterus or cervix 654.4
    - mal lie 652.9
    - malposition
      - fetus 652.9
        - in multiple gestation 652.6
      - pelvic organs or tissues NEC 654.9
      - uterus NEC or cervix 654.4
    - malpresentation NEC 652.9
      - in multiple gestation 652.6
    - maternal
      - diabetes mellitus 648.0
      - heart disease NEC 648.6
    - meconium in liquor 656.8
      - staining only 792.3
    - oblique presentation 652.3
    - oversize fetus 653.5
    - pelvic tumor NEC 654.9
    - placental insufficiency 656.5
    - placenta previa 641.0
      - with hemorrhage 641.1
    - poor dilation, cervix 661.0
    - pre-eclampsia 642.4
      - severe 642.5
    - previous
      - cesarean delivery, section 654.2
      - surgery (to)
        - cervix 654.6
        - gynecological NEC 654.9
        - rectum 654.8
        - uterus NEC 654.9
          - previous cesarean delivery, section 654.2
        - vagina 654.7
    - prolapse
      - arm or hand 652.7
      - uterus 654.4
    - prolonged labor 662.1
    - rectocele 654.4
    - retroversion, uterus or cervix 654.3

Delivery *(Continued)*
cesarean *(Continued)*
rigid
cervix 654.6
pelvic floor 654.4
perineum 654.8
vagina 654.7
vulva 654.8
sacculation, pregnant uterus 654.4
scar(s)
cervix 654.6
cesarean delivery, section 654.2
uterus NEC 654.9
due to previous cesarean delivery, section 654.2
Shirodkar suture in situ 654.5
shoulder presentation 652.8
stenosis or stricture, cervix 654.6
transverse presentation or lie 652.3
tumor, pelvic organs or tissues NEC 654.4
umbilical cord presentation or prolapse 663.0
completely normal case - *see* category 650
complicated (by) NEC 669.9
abdominal tumor, fetal 653.7
causing obstructed labor 660.1
abnormal, abnormality of
cervix 654.6
causing obstructed labor 660.2
forces of labor 661.9
formation of uterus 654.0
pelvic organs or tissues 654.9
causing obstructed labor 660.2
pelvis (bony) (major) NEC 653.0
causing obstructed labor 660.1
presentation or position NEC 652.9
causing obstructed labor 660.0
size, fetus 653.5
causing obstructed labor 660.1
soft parts (of pelvis) 654.9
causing obstructed labor 660.2
uterine contractions NEC 661.9
uterus (formation) 654.0
causing obstructed labor 660.2
vagina 654.7
causing obstructed labor 660.2
abnormally formed uterus (any type) (congenital) 654.0
causing obstructed labor 660.2
acromion presentation 652.8
causing obstructed labor 660.0
adherent placenta 667.0
with hemorrhage 666.0
adhesions, uterus (to abdominal wall) 654.4
advanced maternal age NEC 659.6
multigravida 659.6
primigravida 659.5
air embolism 673.0
amnionitis 658.4
amniotic fluid embolism 673.1
anesthetic death 668.9
annular detachment, cervix 665.3
antepartum hemorrhage - *see* Delivery, complicated, hemorrhage
anteversion, cervix or uterus 654.4
causing obstructed labor 660.2
apoplexy 674.0
placenta 641.2
arrested active phase 661.1
asymmetrical pelvis bone 653.0
causing obstructed labor 660.1

Delivery *(Continued)*
complicated (by) NEC *(Continued)*
atony, uterus, with hemorrhage (hypotonic) (inertia) 666.1 ⬅
hypertonic 661.4
Bandl's ring 661.4
Battledore placenta - *see* Placenta, abnormal
bicornis or bicornuate uterus 654.0
causing obstructed labor 660.2
birth injury to mother NEC 665.9
bleeding (*see also* Delivery, complicated, hemorrhage) 641.9
breech presentation (assisted) (buttocks) (complete) (frank) (spontaneous) 652.2
with successful version 652.1
brow presentation 652.4
cephalopelvic disproportion (normally formed fetus) 653.4
causing obstructed labor 660.1
cerebral hemorrhage 674.0
cervical dystocia 661.0
chin presentation 652.4
causing obstructed labor 660.0
cicatrix
cervix 654.6
causing obstructed labor 660.2
vagina 654.7
causing obstructed labor 660.2
coagulation defect 649.3 ◀
colporrhexis 665.4
with perineal laceration 664.0
compound presentation 652.8
causing obstructed labor 660.0
compression of cord (umbilical) 663.2
around neck 663.1
cord prolapsed 663.0
contraction, contracted pelvis 653.1
causing obstructed labor 660.1
general 653.1
causing obstructed labor 660.1
inlet 653.2
causing obstructed labor 660.1
midpelvic 653.8
causing obstructed labor 660.1
midplane 653.8
causing obstructed labor 660.1
outlet 653.3
causing obstructed labor 660.1
contraction ring 661.4
cord (umbilical) 663.9
around neck, tightly or with compression 663.1
without compression 663.3
bruising 663.6
complication NEC 663.9
specified type NEC 663.8
compression NEC 663.2
entanglement NEC 663.3
with compression 663.2
forelying 663.0
hematoma 663.6
marginal attachment 663.8
presentation 663.0
prolapse (complete) (occult) (partial) 663.0
short 663.4
specified complication NEC 663.8
thrombosis (vessels) 663.6
vascular lesion 663.6
velamentous insertion 663.8
Couvelaire uterus 641.2

Delivery *(Continued)*
complicated (by) NEC *(Continued)*
cretin pelvis (dwarf type) (male type) 653.1
causing obstructed labor 660.1
crossbirth 652.3
with successful version 652.1
causing obstructed labor 660.0
cyst (Gartner's duct) 654.7
cystocele 654.4
causing obstructed labor 660.2
death of fetus (near term) 656.4
early (before 22 completed weeks' gestation) 632
deformity (acquired) (congenital)
fetus 653.7
causing obstructed labor 660.1
pelvic organs or tissues NEC 654.9
causing obstructed labor 660.2
pelvis (bony) NEC 653.0
causing obstructed labor 660.1
delay, delayed
delivery in multiple pregnancy 662.3
due to locked mates 660.5
following rupture of membranes (spontaneous) 658.2
artificial 658.3
depressed fetal heart tones 659.7
diastasis recti 665.8
dilatation
bladder 654.4
causing obstructed labor 660.2
cervix, incomplete, poor, or slow 661.0
diseased placenta 656.7
displacement uterus NEC 654.4
causing obstructed labor 660.2
disproportion NEC 653.9
causing obstructed labor 660.1
disruptio uteri - *see* Delivery, complicated, rupture, uterus
distress
fetal 656.8
maternal 669.0
double uterus (congenital) 654.0
causing obstructed labor 660.2
dropsy amnion 657
dysfunction, uterus 661.9
hypertonic 661.4
hypotonic 661.2
primary 661.0
secondary 661.1
incoordinate 661.4
dystocia
cervical 661.0
fetal - *see* Delivery, complicated, abnormal, presentation
maternal - *see* Delivery, complicated, prolonged labor
pelvic - *see* Delivery, complicated, contraction pelvis
positional 652.8
shoulder girdle 660.4
eclampsia 642.6
ectopic kidney 654.4
causing obstructed labor 660.2
edema, cervix 654.6
causing obstructed labor 660.2
effusion, amniotic fluid 658.1
elderly multigravida 659.6
elderly primigravida 659.5
embolism (pulmonary) 673.2
air 673.0
amniotic fluid 673.1

Delivery *(Continued)*
complicated (by) NEC *(Continued)*
embolism *(Continued)*
blood-clot 673.2
cerebral 674.0
fat 673.8
pyemic 673.3
septic 673.3
entanglement, umbilical cord 663.3
with compression 663.2
around neck (with compression) 663.1
eversion, cervix or uterus 665.2
excessive
fetal growth 653.5
causing obstructed labor 660.1
size of fetus 653.5
causing obstructed labor 660.1
face presentation 652.4
causing obstructed labor 660.0
to pubes 660.3
failure, fetal head to enter pelvic brim 652.5
causing obstructed labor 660.0
female genital mutilation 660.8
fetal
acid-base balance 656.8
death (near term) NEC 656.4
early (before 22 completed weeks' gestation) 632
deformity 653.7
causing obstructed labor 660.1
distress 656.8
heart rate or rhythm 659.7
reduction of multiple fetuses reduced to single fetus 651.7
fetopelvic disproportion 653.4
causing obstructed labor 660.1
fever during labor 659.2
fibroid (tumor) (uterus) 654.1
causing obstructed labor 660.2
fibromyomata 654.1
causing obstructed labor 660.2
forelying umbilical cord 663.0
fracture of coccyx 665.6
hematoma 664.5
broad ligament 665.7
ischial spine 665.7
pelvic 665.7
perineum 664.5
soft tissues 665.7
subdural 674.0
umbilical cord 663.6
vagina 665.7
vulva or perineum 664.5
hemorrhage (uterine) (antepartum) (intrapartum) (pregnancy) 641.9
accidental 641.2
associated with
afibrinogenemia 641.3
coagulation defect 641.3
hyperfibrinolysis 641.3
hypofibrinogenemia 641.3
cerebral 674.0
due to
low-lying placenta 641.1
placenta previa 641.1
premature separation of placenta (normally implanted) 641.2
retained placenta 666.0
trauma 641.8
uterine leiomyoma 641.8
marginal sinus rupture 641.2
placenta NEC 641.9

Delivery *(Continued)*
complicated (by) NEC *(Continued)*
hemorrhage *(Continued)*
postpartum (atonic) (immediate) (within 24 hours) 666.1
with retained or trapped placenta 666.0
delayed 666.2
secondary 666.2
third stage 666.0
hourglass contraction, uterus 661.4
hydramnios 657
hydrocephalic fetus 653.6
causing obstructed labor 660.1
hydrops fetalis 653.7
causing obstructed labor 660.1
hypertension - *see* Hypertension, complicating pregnancy
hypertonic uterine dysfunction 661.4
hypotonic uterine dysfunction 661.2
impacted shoulders 660.4
incarceration, uterus 654.3
causing obstructed labor 660.2
incomplete dilation (cervix) 661.0
incoordinate uterus 661.4
indication NEC 659.9
specified type NEC 659.8
inertia, uterus 661.2
hypertonic 661.4
hypotonic 661.2
primary 661.0
secondary 661.1
infantile
genitalia 654.4
causing obstructed labor 660.2
uterus (os) 654.4
causing obstructed labor 660.2
injury (to mother) NEC 665.9
intrauterine fetal death (near term) NEC 656.4
early (before 22 completed weeks' gestation) 632
inversion, uterus 665.2
kidney, ectopic 654.4
causing obstructed labor 660.2
knot (true), umbilical cord 663.2
labor, premature (before 37 completed weeks' gestation) 644.2
laceration 664.9
anus (sphincter) 664.2
with mucosa 664.3
bladder (urinary) 665.5
bowel 665.5
central 664.4
cervix (uteri) 665.3
fourchette 664.0
hymen 664.0
labia (majora) (minora) 664.0
pelvic
floor 664.1
organ NEC 665.5
perineum, perineal 664.4
first degree 664.0
second degree 664.1
third degree 664.2
fourth degree 664.3
central 664.4
extensive NEC 664.4
muscles 664.1
skin 664.0
slight 664.0
peritoneum 665.5
periurethral tissue 665.5

Delivery *(Continued)*
complicated (by) NEC *(Continued)*
laceration *(Continued)*
rectovaginal (septum) (without perineal laceration) 665.4
with perineum 664.2
with anal or rectal mucosa 664.3
skin (perineum) 664.0
specified site or type NEC 664.8
sphincter ani 664.2
with mucosa 664.3
urethra 665.5
uterus 665.1
before labor 665.0
vagina, vaginal (deep) (high) (sulcus) (wall) (without perineal laceration) 665.4
with perineum 664.0
muscles, with perineum 664.1
vulva 664.0
lateroversion, uterus or cervix 654.4
causing obstructed labor 660.2
locked mates 660.5
low implantation of placenta - *see* Delivery, complicated, placenta, previa
mal lie 652.9
malposition
fetus NEC 652.9
causing obstructed labor 660.0
pelvic organs or tissues NEC 654.9
causing obstructed labor 660.2
placenta 641.1
without hemorrhage 641.0
uterus NEC or cervix 654.4
causing obstructed labor 660.2
malpresentation 652.9
causing obstructed labor 660.0
marginal sinus (bleeding) (rupture) 641.2
maternal hypotension syndrome 669.2
meconium in liquor 656.8
membranes, retained - *see* Delivery, complicated, placenta, retained
mentum presentation 652.4
causing obstructed labor 660.0
metrorrhagia (myopathia) - *see* Delivery, complicated, hemorrhage
metrorrhexis - *see* Delivery, complicated, rupture, uterus
multiparity (grand) 659.4
myelomeningocele, fetus 653.7
causing obstructed labor 660.1
Nägele's pelvis 653.0
causing obstructed labor 660.1
nonengagement, fetal head 652.5
causing obstructed labor 660.0
oblique presentation 652.3
causing obstructed labor 660.0
obstetric
shock 669.1
trauma NEC 665.9
obstructed labor 660.9
due to
abnormality of pelvic organs or tissues (conditions classifiable to 654.0–654.9) 660.2
deep transverse arrest 660.3
impacted shoulders 660.4
locked twins 660.5
malposition and malpresentation of fetus (conditions classifiable to 652.0–652.9) 660.0

Delivery *(Continued)*
complicated (by) NEC *(Continued)*
obstructed labor *(Continued)*
due to *(Continued)*
persistent occipitoposterior 660.3
shoulder dystocia 660.4
occult prolapse of umbilical cord 663.0
oversize fetus 653.5
causing obstructed labor 660.1
pathological retraction ring, uterus 661.4
pelvic
arrest (deep) (high) (of fetal head) (transverse) 660.3
deformity (bone) - *see also* Deformity, pelvis, with disproportion
soft tissue 654.9
causing obstructed labor 660.2
tumor NEC 654.9
causing obstructed labor 660.2
penetration, pregnant uterus by instrument 665.1
perforation - *see* Delivery, complicated, laceration
persistent
hymen 654.8
causing obstructed labor 660.2
occipitoposterior 660.3
placenta, placental
ablatio 641.2
abnormality 656.7
with hemorrhage 641.2
abruptio 641.2
accreta 667.0
with hemorrhage 666.0
adherent (without hemorrhage) 667.0
with hemorrhage 666.0
apoplexy 641.2
Battledore - *see* Placenta, abnormal
detachment (premature) 641.2
disease 656.7
hemorrhage NEC 641.9
increta (without hemorrhage) 667.0
with hemorrhage 666.0
low (implantation) 641.1
without hemorrhage 641.0
malformation 656.7
with hemorrhage 641.2
malposition 641.1
without hemorrhage 641.0
marginal sinus rupture 641.2
percreta 667.0
with hemorrhage 666.0
premature separation 641.2
previa (central) (lateral) (marginal) (partial) 641.1
without hemorrhage 641.0
retained (with hemorrhage) 666.0
without hemorrhage 667.0
rupture of marginal sinus 641.2
separation (premature) 641.2
trapped 666.0
without hemorrhage 667.0
vicious insertion 641.1
polyhydramnios 657
polyp, cervix 654.6
causing obstructed labor 660.2
precipitate labor 661.3
premature
labor (before 37 completed weeks' gestation) 644.2
rupture, membranes 658.1
delayed delivery following 658.2

Delivery *(Continued)*
complicated (by) NEC *(Continued)*
presenting umbilical cord 663.0
previous
cesarean delivery, section 654.2
surgery
cervix 654.6
causing obstructed labor 660.2
gynecological NEC 654.9
causing obstructed labor 660.2
perineum 654.8
rectum 654.8
uterus NEC 654.9
due to previous cesarean delivery, section 654.2
vagina 654.7
causing obstructed labor 660.2
vulva 654.8
primary uterine inertia 661.0
primipara, elderly or old 659.5
prolapse
arm or hand 652.7
causing obstructed labor 660.0
cord (umbilical) 663.0
fetal extremity 652.8
foot or leg 652.8
causing obstructed labor 660.0
umbilical cord (complete) (occult) (partial) 663.0
uterus 654.4
causing obstructed labor 660.2
prolonged labor 662.1
first stage 662.0
second stage 662.2
active phase 661.2
due to
cervical dystocia 661.0
contraction ring 661.4
tetanic uterus 661.4
uterine inertia 661.2
primary 661.0
secondary 661.1
latent phase 661.0
pyrexia during labor 659.2
rachitic pelvis 653.2
causing obstructed labor 660.1
rectocele 654.4
causing obstructed labor 660.2
retained membranes or portions of placenta 666.2
without hemorrhage 667.1
retarded (prolonged) birth 662.1
retention secundines (with hemorrhage) 666.2
without hemorrhage 667.1
retroversion, uterus or cervix 654.3
causing obstructed labor 660.2
rigid
cervix 654.6
causing obstructed labor 660.2
pelvic floor 654.4
causing obstructed labor 660.2
perineum or vulva 654.8
causing obstructed labor 660.2
vagina 654.7
causing obstructed labor 660.2
Robert's pelvis 653.0
causing obstructed labor 660.1
rupture - *see also* Delivery, complicated, laceration
bladder (urinary) 665.5
cervix 665.3
marginal sinus 641.2
membranes, premature 658.1

Delivery *(Continued)*
complicated (by) NEC *(Continued)*
rupture *(Continued)*
pelvic organ NEC 665.5
perineum (without mention of other laceration) - *see* Delivery, complicated, laceration, perineum
peritoneum 665.5
urethra 665.5
uterus (during labor) 665.1
before labor 665.0
sacculation, pregnant uterus 654.4
sacral teratomas, fetal 653.7
causing obstructed labor 660.1
scar(s)
cervix 654.6
causing obstructed labor 660.2
cesarean delivery, section 654.2
causing obstructed labor 660.2
perineum 654.8
causing obstructed labor 660.2
uterus NEC 654.9
causing obstructed labor 660.2
due to previous cesarean delivery, section 654.2
vagina 654.7
causing obstructed labor 660.2
vulva 654.8
causing obstructed labor 660.2
scoliotic pelvis 653.0
causing obstructed labor 660.1
secondary uterine inertia 661.1
secundines, retained - *see* Delivery, complicated, placenta, retained
separation
placenta (premature) 641.2
pubic bone 665.6
symphysis pubis 665.6
septate vagina 654.7
causing obstructed labor 660.2
shock (birth) (obstetric) (puerperal) 669.1
short cord syndrome 663.4
shoulder
girdle dystocia 660.4
presentation 652.8
causing obstructed labor 660.0
Siamese twins 653.7
causing obstructed labor 660.1
slow slope active phase 661.2
spasm
cervix 661.4
uterus 661.4
spondylolisthesis, pelvis 653.3
causing obstructed labor 660.1
spondylolysis (lumbosacral) 653.3
causing obstructed labor 660.1
spondylosis 653.0
causing obstructed labor 660.1
stenosis or stricture
cervix 654.6
causing obstructed labor 660.2
vagina 654.7
causing obstructed labor 660.2
sudden death, unknown cause 669.9
tear (pelvic organ) (*see also* Delivery, complicated, laceration) 664.9
teratomas, sacral, fetal 653.7
causing obstructed labor 660.1
tetanic uterus 661.4
tipping pelvis 653.0
causing obstructed labor 660.1

Delivery *(Continued)*
complicated (by) NEC *(Continued)*
transverse
arrest (deep) 660.3
presentation or lie 652.3
with successful version 652.1
causing obstructed labor 660.0
trauma (obstetrical) NEC 665.9
tumor
abdominal, fetal 653.7
causing obstructed labor 660.1
pelvic organs or tissues NEC 654.9
causing obstructed labor 660.2
umbilical cord (*see also* Delivery, complicated, cord) 663.9
around neck tightly, or with compression 663.1
entanglement NEC 663.3
with compression 663.2
prolapse (complete) (occult) (partial) 663.0
unstable lie 652.0
causing obstructed labor 660.0
uterine
inertia (*see also* Delivery, complicated, inertia, uterus) 661.2
spasm 661.4
vasa previa 663.5
velamentous insertion of cord 663.8
young maternal age 659.8
delayed NEC 662.1
following rupture of membranes (spontaneous) 658.2
artificial 658.3
second twin, triplet, etc. 662.3
difficult NEC 669.9
previous, affecting management of pregnancy or childbirth V23.49
specified type NEC 669.8
early onset (spontaneous) 644.2
footling 652.8
with successful version 652.1
forceps NEC 669.5
affecting fetus or newborn 763.2
missed (at or near term) 656.4
multiple gestation NEC 651.9
with fetal loss and retention of one or more fetus(es) 651.6
following (elective) fetal reduction 651.7
specified type NEC 651.8
with fetal loss and retention of one or more fetus(es) 651.6
following (elective) fetal reduction 651.7
nonviable infant 656.4
normal - *see* category 650
precipitate 661.3
affecting fetus or newborn 763.6
premature NEC (before 37 completed weeks' gestation) 644.2
previous, affecting management of pregnancy V23.41
quadruplet NEC 651.2
with fetal loss and retention of one or more fetus(es) 651.5
following (elective) fetal reduction 651.7
quintuplet NEC 651.8
with fetal loss and retention of one or more fetus(es) 651.6
following (elective) fetal reduction 651.7

Delivery *(Continued)*
sextuplet NEC 651.8
with fetal loss and retention of one or more fetus(es) 651.6
following (elective) fetal reduction 651.7
specified complication NEC 669.8
stillbirth (near term) NEC 656.4
early (before 22 completed weeks' gestation) 632
term pregnancy (live birth) NEC - *see* category 650
stillbirth NEC 656.4
threatened premature 644.2
triplets NEC 651.1
with fetal loss and retention of one or more fetus(es) 651.4
delayed delivery (one or more mates) 662.3
following (elective) fetal reduction 651.7
locked mates 660.5
twins NEC 651.0
with fetal loss and retention of one fetus 651.3
delayed delivery (one or more mates) 662.3
following (elective) fetal reduction 651.7
locked mates 660.5
uncomplicated - *see* category 650
vacuum extractor NEC 669.5
affecting fetus or newborn 763.3
ventouse NEC 669.5
affecting fetus or newborn 763.3
Dellen, cornea 371.41
Delusions (paranoid) 297.9
grandiose 297.1
parasitosis 300.29
systematized 297.1
Dementia 294.8
alcohol-induced persisting (*see also* Psychosis, alcoholic) 291.2
Alzheimer's - *see* Alzheimer's, dementia
arteriosclerotic (simple type) (uncomplicated) 290.40
with
acute confusional state 290.41
delirium 290.41
delusions 290.42
depressed mood 290.43
depressed type 290.43
paranoid type 290.42
Binswanger's 290.12
catatonic (acute) (*see also* Schizophrenia) 295.2
congenital (*see also* Retardation, mental) 319
degenerative 290.9
presenile-onset - *see* Dementia, presenile
senile-onset - *see* Dementia, senile
developmental (*see also* Schizophrenia) 295.9
dialysis 294.8
transient 293.9
drug-induced persisting (*see also* Psychosis, drug) 292.82
due to or associated with condition(s) classified elsewhere
Alzheimer's
with behavioral disturbance 331.0 *[294.11]*

Dementia *(Continued)*
due to or associated with condition(s) classified elsewhere *(Continued)*
Alzheimer's *(Continued)*
without behavioral disturbance 331.0 *[294.10]*
cerebral lipidoses
with behavioral disturbance 330.1 *[294.11]*
without behavioral disturbance 330.1 *[294.10]*
epilepsy
with behavioral disturbance 345.9 *[294.11]*
without behavioral disturbance 345.9 *[294.10]*
hepatolenticular degeneration
with behavioral disturbance 275.1 *[294.11]*
without behavioral disturbance 275.1 *[294.10]*
HIV
with behavioral disturbance 042 *[294.11]*
without behavioral disturbance 042 *[294.10]*
Huntington's chorea
with behavioral disturbance 333.4 *[294.11]*
without behavioral disturbance 333.4 *[294.10]*
Jakob-Creutzfeldt disease (new variant)
with behavioral disturbance 046.1 *[294.11]*
without behavioral disturbance 046.1 *[294.10]*
Lewy bodies
with behavioral disturbance 331.82 *[294.11]*
without behavioral disturbance 331.82 *[294.10]*
multiple sclerosis
with behavioral disturbance 340 *[294.11]*
without behavioral disturbance 340 *[294.10]*
neurosyphilis
with behavioral disturbance 094.9 *[294.11]*
without behavioral disturbance 094.9 *[294.10]*
Pelizaeus-Merzbacher disease
with behavioral disturbance 333.0 *[294.11]*
without behavioral disturbance 333.0 *[294.10]*
Parkinsonism
with behavioral disturbance 331.82 *[294.11]*
without behavioral disturbance 331.82 *[294.10]*
Pick's disease
with behavioral disturbance 331.11 *[294.11]*
without behavioral disturbance 331.11 *[294.10]*
polyarteritis nodosa
with behavioral disturbance 446.0 *[294.11]*
without behavioral disturbance 446.0 *[294.10]*
syphilis
with behavioral disturbance 094.1 *[294.11]*

Dementia *(Continued)*
due to or associated with condition(s) classified elsewhere *(Continued)*
syphilis *(Continued)*
without behavioral disturbance 094.1 *[294.10]*
Wilson's disease
with behavioral disturbance 275.1 *[294.11]*
without behavioral disturbance 275.1 *[294.10]*
frontal 331.19
with behavioral disturbance 331.19 *[294.11]*
without behavioral disturbance 331.19 *[294.10]*
frontotemporal 331.19
with behavioral disturbance 331.19 *[294.11]*
without behavioral disturbance 331.19 *[294.10]*
hebephrenic (acute) 295.1
Heller's (infantile psychosis) (*see also* Psychosis, childhood) 299.1
idiopathic 290.9
presenile-onset - *see* Dementia, presenile
senile-onset - *see* Dementia, senile
in
arteriosclerotic brain disease 290.40
senility 290.0
induced by drug 292.82
infantile, infantilia (*see also* Psychosis, childhood) 299.0
Lewy body 331.82
with behavioral disturbance 331.82 *[294.11]*
without behavioral disturbance 331.82 *[294.10]*
multi-infarct (cerebrovascular) (*see also* Dementia, arteriosclerotic) 290.40
old age 290.0
paralytica, paralytic 094.1
juvenilis 090.40
syphilitic 094.1
congenital 090.40
tabetic form 094.1
paranoid (*see also* Schizophrenia) 295.3
paraphrenic (*see also* Schizophrenia) 295.3
paretic 094.1
praecox (*see also* Schizophrenia) 295.9
presenile 290.10
with
acute confusional state 290.11
delirium 290.11
delusional features 290.12
depressive features 290.13
depressed type 290.13
paranoid type 290.12
simple type 290.10
uncomplicated 290.10
primary (acute) (*see also* Schizophrenia) 295.0
progressive, syphilitic 094.1
puerperal - *see* Psychosis, puerperal
schizophrenic (*see also* Schizophrenia) 295.9
senile 290.0
with
acute confusional state 290.3
delirium 290.3
delusional features 290.20
depressive features 290.21

Dementia *(Continued)*
senile *(Continued)*
depressed type 290.21
exhaustion 290.0
paranoid type 290.20
simple type (acute) (*see also* Schizophrenia) 295.0
simplex (acute) (*see also* Schizophrenia) 295.0
syphilitic 094.1
uremic - *see* Uremia
vascular 290.40
with
delirium 290.41
delusions 290.42
depressed mood 290.43
Demerol dependence (*see also* Dependence) 304.0
Demineralization, ankle (*see also* Osteoporosis) 733.00
Demodex folliculorum (infestation) 133.8
de Morgan's spots (senile angiomas) 448.1
Demyelinating
polyneuritis, chronic inflammatory 357.81
Demyelination, demyelinization
central nervous system 341.9
specified NEC 341.8
corpus callosum (central) 341.8
global 340
Dengue (fever) 061
sandfly 061
vaccination, prophylactic (against) V05.1
virus hemorrhagic fever 065.4
Dens
evaginatus 520.2
in dente 520.2
invaginatus 520.2
Density
increased, bone (disseminated) (generalized) (spotted) 733.99
lung (nodular) 518.89
Dental - *see also* condition
examination only V72.2
Dentia praecox 520.6
Denticles (in pulp) 522.2
Dentigerous cyst 526.0
Dentin
irregular (in pulp) 522.3
opalescent 520.5
secondary (in pulp) 522.3
sensitive 521.89
Dentinogenesis imperfecta 520.5
Dentinoma (M9271/0) 213.1
upper jaw (bone) 213.0
Dentition 520.7
abnormal 520.6
anomaly 520.6
delayed 520.6
difficult 520.7
disorder of 520.6
precocious 520.6
retarded 520.6
Denture sore (mouth) 528.9
Dependence

Note Use the following fifth-digit subclassification with category 304:

0 unspecified
1 continuous
2 episodic
3 in remission

Dependence *(Continued)*
with
withdrawal symptoms
alcohol 291.81
drug 292.0
14-hydroxy-dihydromorphinone 304.0
absinthe 304.6
acemorphan 304.0
acetanilid(e) 304.6
acetophenetidin 304.6
acetorphine 304.0
acetyldihydrocodeine 304.0
acetyldihydrocodeinone 304.0
Adalin 304.1
Afghanistan black 304.3
agrypnal 304.1
alcohol, alcoholic (ethyl) (methyl) (wood) 303.9
maternal, with suspected fetal damage affecting management of pregnancy 655.4
allobarbitone 304.1
allonal 304.1
allylisopropylacetylurea 304.1
alphaprodine (hydrochloride) 304.0
Alurate 304.1
Alvodine 304.0
amethocaine 304.6
amidone 304.0
amidopyrine 304.6
aminopyrine 304.6
amobarbital 304.1
amphetamine(s) (type) (drugs classifiable to 969.7) 304.4
amylene hydrate 304.6
amylobarbitone 304.1
amylocaine 304.6
Amytal (sodium) 304.1
analgesic (drug) NEC 304.6
synthetic with morphine-like effect 304.0
anesthetic (agent) (drug) (gas) (general) (local) NEC 304.6
Angel dust 304.6
anileridine 304.0
antipyrine 304.6
anxiolytic 304.1
aprobarbital 304.1
aprobarbitone 304.1
atropine 304.6
Avertin (bromide) 304.6
barbenyl 304.1
barbital(s) 304.1
barbitone 304.1
barbiturate(s) (compounds) (drugs classifiable to 967.0) 304.1
barbituric acid (and compounds) 304.1
benzedrine 304.4
benzylmorphine 304.0
Beta-chlor 304.1
bhang 304.3
blue velvet 304.0
Brevital 304.1
bromal (hydrate) 304.1
bromide(s) NEC 304.1
bromine compounds NEC 304.1
bromisovalum 304.1
bromoform 304.1
Bromo-seltzer 304.1
bromural 304.1
butabarbital (sodium) 304.1
butabarpal 304.1
butallylonal 304.1
butethal 304.1

ICD-9-CM
D
Vol. 2

Dependence *(Continued)*
- buthalitone (sodium) 304.1
- Butisol 304.1
- butobarbitone 304.1
- butyl chloral (hydrate) 304.1
- caffeine 304.4
- cannabis (indica) (sativa) (resin) (derivatives) (type) 304.3
- carbamazepine 304.6
- Carbrital 304.1
- carbromal 304.1
- carisoprodol 304.6
- Catha (edulis) 304.4
- chloral (betaine) (hydrate) 304.1
- chloralamide 304.1
- chloralformamide 304.1
- chloralose 304.1
- chlordiazepoxide 304.1
- Chloretone 304.1
- chlorobutanol 304.1
- chlorodyne 304.1
- chloroform 304.6
- Cliradon 304.0
- coca (leaf) and derivatives 304.2
- cocaine 304.2
  - hydrochloride 304.2
  - salt (any) 304.2
- codeine 304.0
- combination of drugs (excluding morphine or opioid type drug) NEC 304.8
  - morphine or opioid type drug with any other drug 304.7
- croton-chloral 304.1
- cyclobarbital 304.1
- cyclobarbitone 304.1
- dagga 304.3
- Delvinal 304.1
- Demerol 304.0
- desocodeine 304.0
- desomorphine 304.0
- desoxyephedrine 304.4
- DET 304.5
- dexamphetamine 304.4
- dexedrine 304.4
- dextromethorphan 304.0
- dextromoramide 304.0
- dextronorpseudoephedrine 304.4
- dextrorphan 304.0
- diacetylmorphine 304.0
- Dial 304.1
- diallylbarbituric acid 304.1
- diamorphine 304.0
- diazepam 304.1
- dibucaine 304.6
- dichloroethane 304.6
- diethyl barbituric acid 304.1
- diethylsulfone-diethylmethane 304.1
- difencloxazine 304.0
- dihydrocodeine 304.0
- dihydrocodeinone 304.0
- dihydrohydroxycodeinone 304.0
- dihydroisocodeine 304.0
- dihydromorphine 304.0
- dihydromorphinone 304.0
- dihydroxcodeinone 304.0
- Dilaudid 304.0
- dimenhydrinate 304.6
- dimethylmeperidine 304.0
- dimethyltriptamine 304.5
- Dionin 304.0
- diphenoxylate 304.6
- dipipanone 304.0
- d-lysergic acid diethylamide 304.5

Dependence *(Continued)*
- DMT 304.5
- Dolophine 304.0
- DOM 304.2
- doriden 304.1
- dormiral 304.1
- Dormison 304.1
- Dromoran 304.0
- drug NEC 304.9
  - analgesic NEC 304.6
  - combination (excluding morphine or opioid type drug) NEC 304.8
    - morphine or opioid type drug with any other drug 304.7
  - complicating pregnancy, childbirth, or puerperium 648.3
    - affecting fetus or newborn 779.5
  - hallucinogenic 304.5
  - hypnotic NEC 304.1
  - narcotic NEC 304.9
  - psychostimulant NEC 304.4
  - sedative 304.1
  - soporific NEC 304.1
  - specified type NEC 304.6
  - suspected damage to fetus affecting management of pregnancy 655.5
  - synthetic, with morphine-like effect 304.0
  - tranquilizing 304.1
- duboisine 304.6
- ectylurea 304.1
- Endocaine 304.6
- Equanil 304.1
- Eskabarb 304.1
- ethchlorvynol 304.1
- ether (ethyl) (liquid) (vapor) (vinyl) 304.6
- ethidene 304.6
- ethinamate 304.1
- ethoheptazine 304.6
- ethyl
  - alcohol 303.9
  - bromide 304.6
  - carbamate 304.6
  - chloride 304.6
  - morphine 304.0
- ethylene (gas) 304.6
  - dichloride 304.6
- ethylidene chloride 304.6
- etilfen 304.1
- etorphine 304.0
- etoval 304.1
- eucodal 304.0
- euneryl 304.1
- Evipal 304.1
- Evipan 304.1
- fentanyl 304.0
- ganja 304.3
- gardenal 304.1
- gardenpanyl 304.1
- gelsemine 304.6
- Gelsemium 304.6
- Gemonil 304.1
- glucochloral 304.1
- glue (airplane) (sniffing) 304.6
- glutethimide 304.1
- hallucinogenics 304.5
- hashish 304.3
- headache powder NEC 304.6
- Heavenly Blue 304.5
- hedonal 304.1
- hemp 304.3
- heptabarbital 304.1
- Heptalgin 304.0
- heptobarbitone 304.1

Dependence *(Continued)*
- heroin 304.0
  - salt (any) 304.0
- hexethal (sodium) 304.1
- hexobarbital 304.1
- Hycodan 304.0
- hydrocodone 304.0
- hydromorphinol 304.0
- hydromorphinone 304.0
- hydromorphone 304.0
- hydroxycodeine 304.0
- hypnotic NEC 304.1
- Indian hemp 304.3
- inhalant 304.6
- intranarcon 304.1
- Kemithal 304.1
- ketobemidone 304.0
- khat 304.4
- kif 304.3
- Lactuca (virosa) extract 304.1
- lactucarium 304.1
- laudanum 304.0
- Lebanese red 304.3
- Leritine 304.0
- lettuce opium 304.1
- Levanil 304.1
- Levo-Dromoran 304.0
- levo-iso-methadone 304.0
- levorphanol 304.0
- Librium 304.1
- Lomotil 304.6
- Lotusate 304.1
- LSD (-25) (and derivatives) 304.5
- Luminal 304.1
- lysergic acid 304.5
  - amide 304.5
- maconha 304.3
- magic mushroom 304.5
- marihuana 304.3
- MDA (methylene dioxyamphetamine) 304.4
- Mebaral 304.1
- Medinal 304.1
- Medomin 304.1
- megahallucinogenics 304.5
- meperidine 304.0
- mephobarbital 304.1
- meprobamate 304.1
- mescaline 304.5
- methadone 304.0
- methamphetamine(s) 304.4
- methaqualone 304.1
- metharbital 304.1
- methitural 304.1
- methobarbitone 304.1
- methohexital 304.1
- methopholine 304.6
- methyl
  - alcohol 303.9
  - bromide 304.6
  - morphine 304.0
  - sulfonal 304.1
- methylated spirit 303.9
- methylbutinol 304.6
- methyldihydromorphinone 304.0
- methylene
  - chloride 304.6
  - dichloride 304.6
  - dioxyamphetamine (MDA) 304.4
- methylparafynol 304.1
- methylphenidate 304.4
- methyprylone 304.1
- metopon 304.0
- Miltown 304.1

Dependence *(Continued)*
morning glory seeds 304.5,
morphinan(s) 304.0
morphine (sulfate) (sulfite) (type) (drugs classifiable to 965.00–965.09) 304.0
morphine or opioid type drug (drugs classifiable to 965.00–965.09) with any other drug 304.7
morphinol(s) 304.0
morphinon 304.0
morpholinylethylmorphine 304.0
mylomide 304.1
myristicin 304.5
narcotic (drug) NEC 304.9
nealbarbital 304.1
nealbarbitone 304.1
Nembutal 304.1
Neonal 304.1
Neraval 304.1
Neravan 304.1
neurobarb 304.1
nicotine 305.1
Nisentil 304.0
nitrous oxide 304.6
Noctec 304.1
Noludar 304.1
nonbarbiturate sedatives and tranquilizers with similar effect 304.1
noptil 304.1
normorphine 304.0
noscapine 304.0
Novocaine 304.6
Numorphan 304.0
nunol 304.1
Nupercaine 304.6
Oblivon 304.1
on
aspirator V46.0
hemodialysis V45.1
hyperbaric chamber V46.8
iron lung V46.11
machine (enabling) V46.9
specified type NEC V46.8
peritoneal dialysis V45.1
Possum (patient-operated-selector-mechanism) V46.8
renal dialysis machine V45.1
respirator [ventilator] V46.11
encounter
during
power failure V46.12
mechanical failure V46.14
for weaning V46.13
supplemental oxygen V46.2
opiate 304.0
opioids 304.0
opioid type drug 304.0
with any other drug 304.7
opium (alkaloids) (derivatives) (tincture) 304.0
ortal 304.1
Oxazepam 304.1
oxycodone 304.0
oxymorphone 304.0
Palfium 304.0
Panadol 304.6
pantopium 304.0
pantopon 304.0
papaverine 304.0
paracetamol 304.6
paracodin 304.0
paraldehyde 304.1

Dependence *(Continued)*
paregoric 304.0
Parzone 304.0
PCP (phencyclidine) 304.6
Pearly Gates 304.5
pentazocine 304.0
pentobarbital 304.1
pentobarbitone (sodium) 304.1
Pentothal 304.1
Percaine 304.6
Percodan 304.0
Perichlor 304.1
Pernocton 304.1
Pernoston 304.1
peronine 304.0
pethidine (hydrochloride) 304.0
petrichloral 304.1
peyote 304.5
Phanodorn 304.1
phenacetin 304.6
phenadoxone 304.0
phenaglycodol 304.1
phenazocine 304.0
phencyclidine 304.6
phenmetrazine 304.4
phenobal 304.1
phenobarbital 304.1
phenobarbitone 304.1
phenomorphan 304.0
phenonyl 304.1
phenoperidine 304.0
pholcodine 304.0
piminodine 304.0
Pipadone 304.0
Pitkin's solution 304.6
Placidyl 304.1
polysubstance 304.8
Pontocaine 304.6
pot 304.3
potassium bromide 304.1
Preludin 304.4
Prinadol 304.0
probarbital 304.1
procaine 304.6
propanal 304.1
propoxyphene 304.6
psilocibin 304.5
psilocin 304.5
psilocybin 304.5
psilocyline 304.5
psilocyn 304.5
psychedelic agents 304.5
psychostimulant NEC 304.4
psychotomimetic agents 304.5
pyrahexyl 304.3
Pyramidon 304.6
quinalbarbitone 304.1
racemoramide 304.0
racemorphan 304.0
Rela 304.6
scopolamine 304.6
secobarbital 304.1
seconal 304.1
sedative NEC 304.1
nonbarbiturate with barbiturate effect 304.1
Sedormid 304.1
sernyl 304.1
sodium bromide 304.1
Soma 304.6
Somnal 304.1
Somnos 304.1
Soneryl 304.1
soporific (drug) NEC 304.1

Dependence *(Continued)*
specified drug NEC 304.6
speed 304.4
spinocaine 304.6
stovaine 304.6
STP 304.5
stramonium 304.6
Sulfonal 304.1
sulfonethylmethane 304.1
sulfonmethane 304.1
Surital 304.1
synthetic drug with morphine-like effect 304.0
talbutal 304.1
tetracaine 304.6
tetrahydrocannabinol 304.3
tetronal 304.1
THC 304.3
thebacon 304.0
thebaine 304.0
thiamil 304.1
thiamylal 304.1
thiopental 304.1
tobacco 305.1
toluene, toluol 304.6
tranquilizer NEC 304.1
nonbarbiturate with barbiturate effect 304.1
tribromacetaldehyde 304.6
tribromethanol 304.6
tribromomethane 304.6
trichloroethanol 304.6
trichoroethyl phosphate 304.1
triclofos 304.1
Trional 304.1
Tuinal 304.1
Turkish green 304.3
urethan(e) 304.6
Valium 304.1
Valmid 304.1
veganin 304.0
veramon 304.1
Veronal 304.1
versidyne 304.6
vinbarbital 304.1
vinbarbitone 304.1
vinyl bitone 304.1
vitamin B_6 266.1
wine 303.9
Zactane 304.6
Dependency
passive 301.6
reactions 301.6
Depersonalization (episode, in neurotic state) (neurotic) (syndrome) 300.6
Depletion
carbohydrates 271.9
complement factor 279.8
extracellular fluid 276.52
plasma 276.52
potassium 276.8
nephropathy 588.89
salt or sodium 276.1
causing heat exhaustion or prostration 992.4
nephropathy 593.9
volume 276.50
extracellular fluid 276.52
plasma 276.52
Deposit
argentous, cornea 371.16
bone, in Boeck's sarcoid 135
calcareous, calcium - *see* Calcification

Deposit *(Continued)*
cholesterol
retina 362.82
skin 709.3
vitreous (humor) 379.22
conjunctival 372.56
cornea, corneal NEC 371.10
argentous 371.16
in
cystinosis 270.0 *[371.15]*
mucopolysaccharidosis 277.5 *[371.15]*
crystalline, vitreous (humor) 379.22
hemosiderin, in old scars of cornea 371.11
metallic, in lens 366.45
skin 709.3
teeth, tooth (betel) (black) (green) (materia alba) (orange) (soft) (tobacco) 523.6
urate, in kidney (*see also* Disease, renal) 593.9
Depraved appetite 307.52
Depression 311
acute (*see also* Psychosis, affective) 296.2
recurrent episode 296.3
single episode 296.2
agitated (*see also* Psychosis, affective) 296.2
recurrent episode 296.3
single episode 296.2
anaclitic 309.21
anxiety 300.4
arches 734
congenital 754.61
autogenous (*see also* Psychosis, affective) 296.2
recurrent episode 296.3
single episode 296.2
basal metabolic rate (BMR) 794.7
bone marrow 289.9
central nervous system 799.1
newborn 779.2
cerebral 331.9
newborn 779.2
cerebrovascular 437.8
newborn 779.2
chest wall 738.3
endogenous (*see also* Psychosis, affective) 296.2
recurrent episode 296.3
single episode 296.2
functional activity 780.99
hysterical 300.11
involutional, climacteric, or menopausal (*see also* Psychosis, affective) 296.2
recurrent episode 296.3
single episode 296.2
manic (*see also* Psychosis, affective) 296.80
medullary 348.8
newborn 779.2
mental 300.4
metatarsal heads - *see* Depression, arches
metatarsus - *see* Depression, arches
monopolar (*see also* Psychosis, affective) 296.2
recurrent episode 296.3
single episode 296.2
nervous 300.4
neurotic 300.4
nose 738.0
postpartum 648.4
psychogenic 300.4
reactive 298.0

Depression *(Continued)*
psychoneurotic 300.4
psychotic (*see also* Psychosis, affective) 296.2
reactive 298.0
recurrent episode 296.3
single episode 296.2
reactive 300.4
neurotic 300.4
psychogenic 298.0
psychoneurotic 300.4
psychotic 298.0
recurrent 296.3
respiratory center 348.8
newborn 770.89
scapula 736.89
senile 290.21
situational (acute) (brief) 309.0
prolonged 309.1
skull 754.0
sternum 738.3
visual field 368.40
Depressive reaction - *see also* Reaction, depressive
acute (transient) 309.0
with anxiety 309.28
prolonged 309.1
situational (acute) 309.0
prolonged 309.1
Deprivation
cultural V62.4
emotional V62.89
affecting
adult 995.82
infant or child 995.51
food 994.2
specific substance NEC 269.8
protein (familial) (kwashiorkor) 260
sleep V69.4
social V62.4
affecting
adult 995.82
infant or child 995.51
symptoms, syndrome
alcohol 291.81
drug 292.0
vitamins (*see also* Deficiency, vitamin) 269.2
water 994.3
de Quervain's
disease (tendon sheath) 727.04
thyroiditis (subacute granulomatous thyroiditis) 245.1
Derangement
ankle (internal) 718.97
current injury (*see also* Dislocation, ankle) 837.0
recurrent 718.37
cartilage (articular) NEC (*see also* Disorder, cartilage, articular) 718.0
knee 717.9
recurrent 718.36
recurrent 718.3
collateral ligament (knee) (medial) (tibial) 717.82
current injury 844.1
lateral (fibular) 844.0
lateral (fibular) 717.81
current injury 844.0
cruciate ligament (knee) (posterior) 717.84
anterior 717.83
current injury 844.2
current injury 844.2

Derangement *(Continued)*
elbow (internal) 718.92
current injury (*see also* Dislocation, elbow) 832.00
recurrent 718.32
gastrointestinal 536.9
heart - *see* Disease, heart
hip (joint) (internal) (old) 718.95
current injury (*see also* Dislocation, hip) 835.00
recurrent 718.35
intervertebral disc - *see* Displacement, intervertebral disc
joint (internal) 718.90
ankle 718.97
current injury - *see also* Dislocation, by site
knee, meniscus or cartilage (*see also* Tear, meniscus) 836.2
elbow 718.92
foot 718.97
hand 718.94
hip 718.95
knee 717.9
multiple sites 718.99
pelvic region 718.95
recurrent 718.30
ankle 718.37
elbow 718.32
foot 718.37
hand 718.34
hip 718.35
knee 718.36
multiple sites 718.39
pelvic region 718.35
shoulder (region) 718.31
specified site NEC 718.38
temporomandibular (old) 524.69
wrist 718.33
shoulder (region) 718.91
specified site NEC 718.98
spine NEC 724.9
temporomandibular 524.69
wrist 718.93
knee (cartilage) (internal) 717.9
current injury (*see also* Tear, meniscus) 836.2
ligament 717.89
capsular 717.85
collateral - *see* Derangement, collateral ligament
cruciate - *see* Derangement, cruciate ligament
specified NEC 717.85
recurrent 718.36
low back NEC 724.9
meniscus NEC (knee) 717.5
current injury (*see also* Tear, meniscus) 836.2
lateral 717.40
anterior horn 717.42
posterior horn 717.43
specified NEC 717.49
medial 717.3
anterior horn 717.1
posterior horn 717.2
recurrent 718.3
site other than knee - *see* Disorder, cartilage, articular
mental (*see also* Psychosis) 298.9
rotator cuff (recurrent) (tear) 726.10
current 840.4
sacroiliac (old) 724.6
current - *see* Dislocation, sacroiliac

Derangement *(Continued)*
semilunar cartilage (knee) 717.5
current injury 836.2
lateral 836.1
medial 836.0
recurrent 718.3
shoulder (internal) 718.91
current injury (*see also* Dislocation, shoulder) 831.00
recurrent 718.31
spine (recurrent) NEC 724.9
current - *see* Dislocation, spine
temporomandibular (internal) (joint) (old) 524.69
current - *see* Dislocation, jaw
Dercum's disease or syndrome (adiposis dolorosa) 272.8
Derealization (neurotic) 300.6
Dermal - *see* condition
Dermaphytid - *see* Dermatophytosis
Dermatergosis - *see* Dermatitis
Dermatitis (allergic) (contact) (occupational) (venenata) 692.9
ab igne 692.82
acneiform 692.9
actinic (due to sun) 692.70
acute 692.72
chronic NEC 692.74
other than from sun NEC 692.82
ambustionis
due to
burn or scald - *see* Burn, by site
sunburn (*see also* Sunburn) 692.71
amebic 006.6
ammonia 691.0
anaphylactoid NEC 692.9
arsenical 692.4
artefacta 698.4
psychogenic 316 *[698.4]*
asthmatic 691.8
atopic (allergic) (intrinsic) 691.8
psychogenic 316 *[691.8]*
atrophicans 701.8
diffusa 701.8
maculosa 701.3
berlock, berloque 692.72
blastomycetic 116.0
blister beetle 692.89
Brucella NEC 023.9
bullosa 694.9
striata pratensis 692.6
bullous 694.9
mucosynechial, atrophic 694.60
with ocular involvement 694.61
seasonal 694.8
calorica
due to
burn or scald - *see* Burn, by site
cold 692.89
sunburn (*see also* Sunburn) 692.71
caterpillar 692.89
cercarial 120.3
combustionis
due to
burn or scald - *see* Burn, by site
sunburn (*see also* Sunburn) 692.71
congelationis 991.5
contusiformis 695.2
diabetic 250.8
diaper 691.0
diphtheritica 032.85
due to
acetone 692.2
acids 692.4

Dermatitis *(Continued)*
due to *(Continued)*
adhesive plaster 692.4
alcohol (skin contact) (substances classifiable to 980.0–980.9) 692.4
taken internally 693.8
alkalis 692.4
allergy NEC 692.9
ammonia (household) (liquid) 692.4
animal
dander (cat) (dog) 692.84
hair (cat) (dog) 692.84
arnica 692.3
arsenic 692.4
taken internally 693.8
blister beetle 692.89
cantharides 692.3
carbon disulphide 692.2
caterpillar 692.89
caustics 692.4
cereal (ingested) 693.1
contact with skin 692.5
chemical(s) NEC 692.4
internal 693.8
irritant NEC 692.4
taken internally 693.8
chlorocompounds 692.2
coffee (ingested) 693.1
contact with skin 692.5
cold weather 692.89
cosmetics 692.81
cyclohexanes 692.2
dander, animal (cat) (dog) 692.84
deodorant 692.81
detergents 692.0
dichromate 692.4
drugs and medicinals (correct substance properly administered) (internal use) 693.0
external (in contact with skin) 692.3
wrong substance given or taken 976.9
specified substance - *see* Table of Drugs and Chemicals
wrong substance given or taken 977.9
specified substance - *see* Table of Drugs and Chemicals
dyes 692.89
hair 692.89
epidermophytosis - *see* Dermatophytosis
esters 692.2
external irritant NEC 692.9
specified agent NEC 692.89
eye shadow 692.81
fish (ingested) 693.1
contact with skin 692.5
flour (ingested) 693.1
contact with skin 692.5
food (ingested) 693.1
in contact with skin 692.5
fruit (ingested) 693.1
contact with skin 692.5
fungicides 692.3
furs 692.84
glycols 692.2
greases NEC 692.1
hair, animal (cat) (dog) 692.84
hair dyes 692.89
hot
objects and materials - *see* Burn, by site
weather or places 692.89

Dermatitis *(Continued)*
due to *(Continued)*
hydrocarbons 692.2
infrared rays, except from sun 692.82
solar NEC (*see also* Dermatitis, due to, sun) 692.70
ingested substance 693.9
drugs and medicinals (*see also* Dermatitis, due to, drugs and medicinals) 693.0
food 693.1
specified substance NEC 693.8
ingestion or injection of
chemical 693.8
drug (correct substance properly administered) 693.0
wrong substance given or taken 977.9
specified substance - *see* Table of Drugs and Chemicals
insecticides 692.4
internal agent 693.9
drugs and medicinals (*see also* Dermatitis, due to, drugs and medicinals) 693.0
food (ingested) 693.1
in contact with skin 692.5
specified agent NEC 693.8
iodine 692.3
iodoform 692.3
irradiation 692.82
jewelry 692.83
keratolytics 692.3
ketones 692.2
lacquer tree (Rhus verniciflua) 692.6
light (sun) NEC (*see also* Dermatitis, due to, sun) 692.70
other 692.82
low temperature 692.89
mascara 692.81
meat (ingested) 693.1
contact with skin 692.5
mercury, mercurials 692.3
metals 692.83
milk (ingested) 693.1
contact with skin 692.5
Neomycin 692.3
nylon 692.4
oils NEC 692.1
paint solvent 692.2
pediculocides 692.3
petroleum products (substances classifiable to 981) 692.4
phenol 692.3
photosensitiveness, photosensitivity (sun) 692.72
other light 692.82
plants NEC 692.6
plasters, medicated (any) 692.3
plastic 692.4
poison
ivy (Rhus toxicodendron) 692.6
oak (Rhus diversiloba) 692.6
plant or vine 692.6
sumac (Rhus venenata) 692.6
vine (Rhus radicans) 692.6
preservatives 692.89
primrose (primula) 692.6
primula 692.6
radiation 692.82
sun NEC (*see also* Dermatitis, due to, sun) 692.70
tanning bed 692.82
radioactive substance 692.82

Dermatitis *(Continued)*
due to *(Continued)*
radium 692.82
ragweed (Senecio jacobae) 692.6
Rhus (diversiloba) (radicans) (toxicodendron) (venenata) (verniciflua) 692.6
rubber 692.4
scabicides 692.3
Senecio jacobae 692.6
solar radiation - *see* Dermatitis, due to, sun
solvents (any) (substances classifiable to 982.0–982.8) 692.2
chlorocompound group 692.2
cyclohexane group 692.2
ester group 692.2
glycol group 692.2
hydrocarbon group 692.2
ketone group 692.2
paint 692.2
specified agent NEC 692.89
sun 692.70
acute 692.72
chronic NEC 692.74
specified NEC 692.79
sunburn (*see also* Sunburn) 692.71
sunshine NEC (*see also* Dermatitis, due to, sun) 692.70
tanning bed 692.82
tetrachlorethylene 692.2
toluene 692.2
topical medications 692.3
turpentine 692.2
ultraviolet rays, except from sun 692.82
sun NEC (*see also* Dermatitis, due to, sun) 692.70
vaccine or vaccination (correct substance properly administered) 693.0
wrong substance given or taken
bacterial vaccine 978.8
specified - *see* Table of Drugs and Chemicals
other vaccines NEC 979.9
specified - *see* Table of Drugs and Chemicals
varicose veins (*see also* Varicose, vein, inflamed or infected) 454.1
x-rays 692.82
dyshydrotic 705.81
dysmenorrheica 625.8
eczematoid NEC 692.9
infectious 690.8
eczematous NEC 692.9
epidemica 695.89
erysipelatosa 695.81
escharotica - *see* Burn, by site
exfoliativa, exfoliative 695.89
generalized 695.89
infantum 695.81
neonatorum 695.81
eyelid 373.31
allergic 373.32
contact 373.32
eczematous 373.31
herpes (zoster) 053.20
simplex 054.41
infective 373.5
due to
actinomycosis 039.3 *[373.5]*
herpes
simplex 054.41
zoster 053.20

Dermatitis *(Continued)*
eyelid *(Continued)*
infective *(Continued)*
due to *(Continued)*
impetigo 684 *[373.5]*
leprosy (*see also* Leprosy) 030.0 *[373.4]*
lupus vulgaris (tuberculous) (*see also* Tuberculosis) 017.0 *[373.4]*
mycotic dermatitis (*see also* Dermatomycosis) 111.9 *[373.5]*
vaccinia 051.0 *[373.5]*
postvaccination 999.0 *[373.5]*
yaws (*see also* Yaws) 102.9 *[373.4]*
facta, factitia 698.4
psychogenic 316 *[698.4]*
ficta 698.4
psychogenic 316 *[698.4]*
flexural 691.8
follicularis 704.8
friction 709.8
fungus 111.9
specified type NEC 111.8
gangrenosa, gangrenous (infantum) (*see also* Gangrene) 785.4
gestationis 646.8
gonococcal 098.89
gouty 274.89
harvest mite 133.8
heat 692.89
herpetiformis (bullous) (erythematous) (pustular) (vesicular) 694.0
juvenile 694.2
senile 694.5
hiemalis 692.89
hypostatic, hypostatica 454.1
with ulcer 454.2
impetiginous 684
infantile (acute) (chronic) (intertriginous) (intrinsic) (seborrheic) 690.12
infectiosa eczematoides 690.8
infectious (staphylococcal) (streptococcal) 686.9
eczematoid 690.8
infective eczematoid 690.8
Jacquet's (diaper dermatitis) 691.0
leptus 133.8
lichenified NEC 692.9
lichenoid, chronic 701.0
lichenoides purpurica pigmentosa 709.1
meadow 692.6
medicamentosa (correct substance properly administered) (internal use) (*see also* Dermatitis, due to, drugs or medicinals) 693.0
due to contact with skin 692.3
mite 133.8
multiformis 694.0
juvenile 694.2
senile 694.5
napkin 691.0
neuro 698.3
neurotica 694.0
nummular NEC 692.9
osteatosis, osteatotic 706.8
papillaris capillitii 706.1
pellagrous 265.2
perioral 695.3
perstans 696.1
photosensitivity (sun) 692.72
other light 692.82
pigmented purpuric lichenoid 709.1
polymorpha dolorosa 694.0

Dermatitis *(Continued)*
primary irritant 692.9
pruriginosa 694.0
pruritic NEC 692.9
psoriasiform nodularis 696.2
psychogenic 316
purulent 686.00
pustular contagious 051.2
pyococcal 686.00
pyocyaneus 686.09
pyogenica 686.00
radiation 692.82
repens 696.1
Ritter's (exfoliativa) 695.81
Schamberg's (progressive pigmentary dermatosis) 709.09
schistosome 120.3
seasonal bullous 694.8
seborrheic 690.10
infantile 690.12
sensitization NEC 692.9
septic (*see also* Septicemia) 686.00
gonococcal 098.89
solar, solare NEC (*see also* Dermatitis, due to, sun) 692.70
stasis 459.81
due to
postphlebitic syndrome 459.12
with ulcer 459.13
varicose veins - *see* Varicose
ulcerated or with ulcer (varicose) 454.2
sunburn (*see also* Sunburn) 692.71
suppurative 686.00
traumatic NEC 709.8
trophoneurotica 694.0
ultraviolet, except from sun 692.82
due to sun NEC (*see also* Dermatitis, due to, sun) 692.70
varicose 454.1
with ulcer 454.2
vegetans 686.8
verrucosa 117.2
xerotic 706.8
Dermatoarthritis, lipoid 272.8 [713.0]
Dermatochalasia, dermatochalasis 374.87
Dermatofibroma (lenticulare) (M8832/0) - *see also* Neoplasm, skin, benign
protuberans (M8832/1) - *see* Neoplasm, skin, uncertain behavior
Dermatofibrosarcoma (protuberans) (M8832/3) - *see* Neoplasm, skin, malignant
Dermatographia 708.3
Dermatolysis (congenital) (exfoliativa) 757.39
acquired 701.8
eyelids 374.34
palpebrarum 374.34
senile 701.8
Dermatomegaly NEC 701.8
Dermatomucomyositis 710.3
Dermatomycosis 111.9
furfuracea 111.0
specified type NEC 111.8
Dermatomyositis (acute) (chronic) 710.3
Dermatoneuritis of children 985.0
Dermatophiliasis 134.1
Dermatophytide - *see* Dermatophytosis
Dermatophytosis (Epidermophyton) (infection) (microsporum) (tinea) (Trichophyton) 110.9
beard 110.0
body 110.5
deep seated 110.6

Dermatophytosis *(Continued)*
fingernails 110.1
foot 110.4
groin 110.3
hand 110.2
nail 110.1
perianal (area) 110.3
scalp 110.0
scrotal 110.8
specified site NEC 110.8
toenails 110.1
vulva 110.8
Dermatopolyneuritis 985.0
Dermatorrhexis 756.83
acquired 701.8
Dermatosclerosis (*see also* Scleroderma) 710.1
localized 701.0
Dermatosis 709.9
Andrews' 686.8
atopic 691.8
Bowen's (M8081/2) - *see* Neoplasm, skin, in situ
bullous 694.9
specified type NEC 694.8
erythematosquamous 690.8
exfoliativa 695.89
factitial 698.4
gonococcal 098.89
herpetiformis 694.0
juvenile 694.2
senile 694.5
hysterical 300.11
linear IgA 694.8
menstrual NEC 709.8
neutrophilic, acute febrile 695.89
occupational (*see also* Dermatitis) 692.9
papulosa nigra 709.8
pigmentary NEC 709.00
progressive 709.09
Schamberg's 709.09
Siemens-Bloch 757.33
progressive pigmentary 709.09
psychogenic 316
pustular subcorneal 694.1
Schamberg's (progressive pigmentary) 709.09
senile NEC 709.3
specified NEC 702.8
Unna's (seborrheic dermatitis) 690.10
Dermographia 708.3
Dermographism 708.3
Dermoid (cyst) (M9084/0) - *see also* Neoplasm, by site, benign
with malignant transformation (M9084/3) 183.0
Dermopathy
infiltrative, with thyrotoxicosis 242.0
senile NEC 709.3
Dermophytosis - *see* Dermatophytosis
Descemet's membrane - *see* condition
Descemetocele 371.72
Descending - *see* condition
Descensus uteri (complete) (incomplete) (partial) (without vaginal wall prolapse) 618.1
with mention of vaginal wall prolapse - *see* Prolapse, uterovaginal
Desensitization to allergens V07.1
Desert
rheumatism 114.0
sore (*see also* Ulcer, skin) 707.9
Desertion (child) (newborn) 995.52
adult 995.84
Desmoid (extra-abdominal) (tumor) (M8821/1) - *see also* Neoplasm, connective tissue, uncertain behavior
abdominal (M8822/1) - *see* Neoplasm, connective tissue, uncertain behavior
Despondency 300.4
Desquamative dermatitis NEC 695.89
Destruction
articular facet (*see also* Derangement, joint) 718.9
vertebra 724.9
bone 733.90
syphilitic 095.5
joint (*see also* Derangement, joint) 718.9
sacroiliac 724.6
kidney 593.89
live fetus to facilitate birth NEC 763.89
ossicles (ear) 385.24
rectal sphincter 569.49
septum (nasal) 478.19
tuberculous NEC (*see also* Tuberculosis) 011.9
tympanic membrane 384.82
tympanum 385.89
vertebral disc - *see* Degeneration, intervertebral disc
Destructiveness (*see also* Disturbance, conduct) 312.9
adjustment reaction 309.3
Detachment
cartilage - *see also* Sprain, by site
knee - *see* Tear, meniscus
cervix, annular 622.8
complicating delivery 665.3
choroid (old) (postinfectional) (simple) (spontaneous) 363.70
hemorrhagic 363.72
serous 363.71
knee, medial meniscus (old) 717.3
current injury 836.0
ligament - *see* Sprain, by site
placenta (premature) - *see* Placenta, separation
retina (recent) 361.9
with retinal defect (rhegmatogenous) 361.00
giant tear 361.03
multiple 361.02
partial
with
giant tear 361.03
multiple defects 361.02
retinal dialysis (juvenile) 361.04
single defect 361.01
retinal dialysis (juvenile) 361.04
single 361.01
subtotal 361.05
total 361.05
delimited (old) (partial) 361.06
old
delimited 361.06
partial 361.06
total or subtotal 361.07
pigment epithelium (RPE) (serous) 362.42
exudative 362.42
hemorrhagic 362.43
rhegmatogenous (*see also* Detachment, retina, with retinal defect) 361.00
serous (without retinal defect) 361.2
specified type NEC 361.89
traction (with vitreoretinal organization) 361.81
vitreous humor 379.21
Detergent asthma 507.8
Deterioration
epileptic
with behavioral disturbance 345.9 *[294.11]*
without behavioral disturbance 345.9 *[294.10]*
heart, cardiac (*see also* Degeneration, myocardial) 429.1
mental (*see also* Psychosis) 298.9
myocardium, myocardial (*see also* Degeneration, myocardial) 429.1
senile (simple) 797
transplanted organ - *see* Complications, transplant, organ, by site
de Toni-Fanconi syndrome (cystinosis) 270.0
Deuteranomaly 368.52
Deuteranopia (anomalous trichromat) (complete) (incomplete) 368.52
Deutschländer's disease - *see* Fracture, foot
Development
abnormal, bone 756.9
arrested 783.40
bone 733.91
child 783.40
due to malnutrition (protein-calorie) 263.2
fetus or newborn 764.9
tracheal rings (congenital) 748.3
defective, congenital - *see also* Anomaly
cauda equina 742.59
left ventricle 746.9
with atresia or hypoplasia of aortic orifice or valve with hypoplasia of ascending aorta 746.7
in hypoplastic left heart syndrome 746.7
delayed (*see also* Delay, development) 783.40
arithmetical skills 315.1
language (skills) 315.31
expressive 315.31
mixed receptive-expressive 315.32
learning skill, specified NEC 315.2
mixed skills 315.5
motor coordination 315.4
reading 315.00
specified
learning skill NEC 315.2
type NEC, except learning 315.8
speech 315.39
associated with hyperkinesia 314.1
phonological 315.39
spelling 315.09
written expression 315.2
imperfect, congenital - *see also* Anomaly
heart 746.9
lungs 748.60
improper (fetus or newborn) 764.9
incomplete (fetus or newborn) 764.9
affecting management of pregnancy 656.5
bronchial tree 748.3
organ or site not listed - *see* Hypoplasia
respiratory system 748.9
sexual, precocious NEC 259.1
tardy, mental (*see also* Retardation, mental) 319
Developmental - *see* condition
Devergie's disease (pityriasis rubra pilaris) 696.4

- **Deviation**
  - conjugate (eye) 378.87
    - palsy 378.81
    - spasm, spastic 378.82
  - esophagus 530.89
  - eye, skew 378.87
  - mandible, opening and closing 524.53
  - midline (jaw) (teeth) 524.29
    - specified site NEC - *see* Malposition
  - occlusal plane 524.76
  - organ or site, congenital NEC - *see* Malposition, congenital
  - septum (acquired) (nasal) 470
    - congenital 754.0
  - sexual 302.9
    - bestiality 302.1
    - coprophilia 302.89
    - ego-dystonic
      - homosexuality 302.0
      - lesbianism 302.0
    - erotomania 302.89
      - Clérambault's 297.8
    - exhibitionism (sexual) 302.4
    - fetishism 302.81
      - transvestic 302.3
    - frotteurism 302.89
    - homosexuality, ego-dystonic 302.0
      - pedophilic 302.2
    - lesbianism, ego-dystonic 302.0
    - masochism 302.83
    - narcissism 302.89
    - necrophilia 302.89
    - nymphomania 302.89
    - pederosis 302.2
    - pedophilia 302.2
    - sadism 302.84
    - sadomasochism 302.84
    - satyriasis 302.89
    - specified type NEC 302.89
    - transvestic fetishism 302.3
    - transvestism 302.3
    - voyeurism 302.82
    - zoophilia (erotica) 302.1
  - teeth, midline 524.29
  - trachea 519.19 ◀
  - ureter (congenital) 753.4
- **Devic's disease** 341.0
- **Device**
  - cerebral ventricle (communicating) in situ V45.2
  - contraceptive - *see* Contraceptive, device
  - drainage, cerebrospinal fluid V45.2
- **Devil's**
  - grip 074.1
  - pinches (purpura simplex) 287.2
- **Devitalized tooth** 522.9
- **Devonshire colic** 984.9
  - specified type of lead - *see* Table of Drugs and Chemicals
- **Dextraposition, aorta** 747.21
  - with ventricular septal defect, pulmonary stenosis or atresia, and hypertrophy of right ventricle 745.2
  - in tetralogy of Fallot 745.2
- **Dextratransposition, aorta** 745.11
- **Dextrinosis, limit** (debrancher enzyme deficiency) 271.0
- **Dextrocardia** (corrected) (false) (isolated) (secondary) (true) 746.87
  - with
    - complete transposition of viscera 759.3
    - situs inversus 759.3
- **Dextroversion, kidney** (left) 753.3
- **Dhobie itch** 110.3
- **Diabetes, diabetic** (brittle) (congenital) (familial) (mellitus) (poorly controlled) (severe) (slight) (without complication) 250.0

> Note Use the following fifth-digit subclassification with category 250:
>
> 0 type II or unspecified type, not stated as uncontrolled
>
> Fifth-digit 0 is for use for type II patients, even if the patient requires insulin
>
> 1 type I [juvenile type], not stated as uncontrolled
>
> 2 type II or unspecified type, uncontrolled
>
> Fifth-digit 2 is for use for type II patients, even if the patient requires insulin
>
> 3 type I [juvenile type], uncontrolled

  - with
    - coma (with ketoacidosis) 250.3
      - hyperosmolar (nonketotic) 250.2
    - complication NEC 250.9
      - specified NEC 250.8
    - gangrene 250.7 *[785.4]*
    - hyperosmolarity 250.2
    - ketosis, ketoacidosis 250.1
    - osteomyelitis 250.8 *[731.8]*
    - specified manifestations NEC 250.8
  - acetonemia 250.1
  - acidosis 250.1
  - amyotrophy 250.6 *[358.1]*
  - angiopathy, peripheral 250.7 *[443.81]*
  - asymptomatic 790.29
  - autonomic neuropathy (peripheral) 250.6 *[337.1]*
  - bone change 250.8 *[731.8]*
  - bronze, bronzed 275.0
  - cataract 250.5 *[366.41]*
  - chemical 790.29
    - complicating pregnancy, childbirth, or puerperium 648.8
  - coma (with ketoacidosis) 250.3
    - hyperglycemic 250.3
    - hyperosmolar (nonketotic) 250.2
    - hypoglycemic 250.3
    - insulin 250.3
  - complicating pregnancy, childbirth, or puerperium (maternal) 648.0
    - affecting fetus or newborn 775.0
  - complication NEC 250.9
    - specified NEC 250.8
  - dorsal sclerosis 250.6 *[340]*
  - dwarfism-obesity syndrome 258.1
  - gangrene 250.7 *[785.4]*
  - gastroparesis 250.6 *[536.3]*
  - gestational 648.8
    - complicating pregnancy, childbirth, or puerperium 648.8
  - glaucoma 250.5 *[365.44]*
  - glomerulosclerosis (intercapillary) 250.4 *[581.81]*
  - glycogenosis, secondary 250.8 *[259.8]*
  - hemochromatosis 275.0
  - hyperosmolar coma 250.2
  - hyperosmolarity 250.2
  - hypertension-nephrosis syndrome 250.4 *[581.81]*

Diabetes, diabetic *(Continued)*

  - hypoglycemia 250.8
  - hypoglycemic shock 250.8
  - insipidus 253.5
    - nephrogenic 588.1
    - pituitary 253.5
    - vasopressin-resistant 588.1
  - intercapillary glomerulosclerosis 250.4 *[581.81]*
  - iritis 250.5 *[364.42]*
  - ketosis, ketoacidosis 250.1
  - Kimmelstiel (-Wilson) disease or syndrome (intercapillary glomerulosclerosis) 250.4 *[581.81]*
  - Lancereaux's (diabetes mellitus with marked emaciation) 250.8 *[261]*
  - latent (chemical) 790.29
    - complicating pregnancy, childbirth, or puerperium 648.8
  - lipoidosis 250.8 *[272.7]*
  - macular edema 250.5 *[362.07]*
  - maternal
    - with manifest disease in the infant 775.1
    - affecting fetus or newborn 775.0
  - microaneurysms, retinal 250.5 *[362.01]*
  - mononeuropathy 250.6 *[355.9]*
  - neonatal, transient 775.1
  - nephropathy 250.4 *[583.81]*
  - nephrosis (syndrome) 250.4 *[581.81]*
  - neuralgia 250.6 *[357.2]*
  - neuritis 250.6 *[357.2]*
  - neurogenic arthropathy 250.6 *[713.5]*
  - neuropathy 250.6 *[357.2]*
  - nonclinical 790.29
  - osteomyelitis 250.8 *[731.8]*
  - peripheral autonomic neuropathy 250.6 *[337.1]*
  - phosphate 275.3
  - polyneuropathy 250.6 *[357.2]*
  - renal (true) 271.4
  - retinal
    - edema 250.5 *[362.07]*
    - hemorrhage 250.5 *[362.01]*
    - microaneurysms 250.5 *[362.01]*
  - retinitis 250.5 *[362.01]*
  - retinopathy 250.5 *[362.01]*
    - background 250.5 *[362.01]*
    - nonproliferative 250.5 *[362.03]*
      - mild 250.5 *[362.04]*
      - moderate 250.5 *[362.05]*
      - severe 250.5 *[362.06]*
    - proliferative 250.5 *[362.02]*
  - steroid induced
    - correct substance properly administered 251.8
    - overdose or wrong substance given or taken 962.0
  - stress 790.29
  - subclinical 790.29
  - subliminal 790.29
  - sugar 250.0
  - ulcer (skin) 250.8 *[707.9]*
    - lower extremity 250.8 *[707.10]*
      - ankle 250.8 *[707.13]*
      - calf 250.8 *[707.12]*
      - foot 250.8 *[707.15]*
      - heel 250.8 *[707.14]*
      - knee 250.8 *[707.19]*
      - specified site NEC 250.8 *[707.19]*
      - thigh 250.8 *[707.11]*
      - toes 250.8 *[707.15]*
    - specified site NEC 250.8 *[707.8]*
  - xanthoma 250.8 *[272.2]*

◀ **New** ◀ **Revised**

Diacyclothrombopathia 287.1
Diagnosis deferred 799.9
Dialysis (intermittent) (treatment)
anterior retinal (juvenile) (with detachment) 361.04
extracorporeal V56.0
hemodialysis V56.0
status only V45.1
peritoneal V56.8
status only V45.1
renal V56.0
status only V45.1
specified type NEC V56.8
Diamond-Blackfan anemia or syndrome (congenital hypoplastic anemia) 284.01
Diamond-Gardener syndrome (autoerythrocyte sensitization) 287.2
Diaper rash 691.0
Diaphoresis (excessive) NEC (*see also* Hyperhidrosis) 780.8
Diaphragm - *see* condition
Diaphragmalgia 786.52
Diaphragmitis 519.4
Diaphyseal aclasis 756.4
Diaphysitis 733.99
Diarrhea, diarrheal (acute) (autumn) (bilious) (bloody) (catarrhal) (choleraic) (chronic) (gravis) (green) (infantile) (lienteric) (noninfectious) (presumed noninfectious) (putrefactive) (secondary) (sporadic) (summer) (symptomatic) (thermic) 787.91
achlorhydric 536.0
allergic 558.3
amebic (*see also* Amebiasis) 006.9
with abscess - *see* Abscess, amebic
acute 006.0
chronic 006.1
nondysenteric 006.2
bacillary - *see* Dysentery, bacillary
bacterial NEC 008.5
balantidial 007.0
bile salt-induced 579.8
cachectic NEC 787.91
chilomastix 007.8
choleriformis 001.1
coccidial 007.2
Cochin-China 579.1
anguilluliasis 127.2
psilosis 579.1
Dientamoeba 007.8
dietetic 787.91
due to
achylia gastrica 536.8
Aerobacter aerogenes 008.2
Bacillus coli - *see* Enteritis, E. coli
bacteria NEC 008.5
bile salts 579.8
Capillaria
hepatica 128.8
philippinensis 127.5
Clostridium perfringens (C) (F) 008.46
Enterobacter aerogenes 008.2
enterococci 008.49
Escherichia coli - *see* Enteritis, E. coli
Giardia lamblia 007.1
Heterophyes heterophyes 121.6
irritating foods 787.91
Metagonimus yokogawai 121.5
Necator americanus 126.1
Paracolobactrum arizonae 008.1

Diarrhea, diarrheal *(Continued)*
due to *(Continued)*
Paracolon bacillus NEC 008.47
Arizona 008.1
Proteus (bacillus) (mirabilis) (Morganii) 008.3
Pseudomonas aeruginosa 008.42
S. japonicum 120.2
specified organism NEC 008.8
bacterial 008.49
viral NEC 008.69
Staphylococcus 008.41
Streptococcus 008.49
anaerobic 008.46
Strongyloides stercoralis 127.2
Trichuris trichiuria 127.3
virus NEC (*see also* Enteritis, viral) 008.69
dysenteric 009.2
due to specified organism NEC 008.8
dyspeptic 787.91
endemic 009.3
due to specified organism NEC 008.8
epidemic 009.2
due to specified organism NEC 008.8
fermentative 787.91
flagellate 007.9
Flexner's (ulcerative) 004.1
functional 564.5
following gastrointestinal surgery 564.4
psychogenic 306.4
giardial 007.1
Giardia lamblia 007.1
hill 579.1
hyperperistalsis (nervous) 306.4
infectious 009.2
due to specified organism NEC 008.8
presumed 009.3
inflammatory 787.91
due to specified organism NEC 008.8
malarial (*see also* Malaria) 084.6
mite 133.8
mycotic 117.9
nervous 306.4
neurogenic 564.5
parenteral NEC 009.2
postgastrectomy 564.4
postvagotomy 564.4
prostaglandin induced 579.8
protozoal NEC 007.9
psychogenic 306.4
septic 009.2
due to specified organism NEC 008.8
specified organism NEC 008.8
bacterial 008.49
viral NEC 008.69
Staphylococcus 008.41
Streptococcus 008.49
anaerobic 008.46
toxic 558.2
travelers' 009.2
due to specified organism NEC 008.8
trichomonal 007.3
tropical 579.1
tuberculous 014.8
ulcerative (chronic) (*see also* Colitis, ulcerative) 556.9
viral (*see also* Enteritis, viral) 008.8
zymotic NEC 009.2
Diastasis
cranial bones 733.99
congenital 756.0
joint (traumatic) - *see* Dislocation, by site

Diastasis *(Continued)*
muscle 728.84
congenital 756.89
recti (abdomen) 728.84
complicating delivery 665.8
congenital 756.79
Diastema, teeth, tooth 524.30
Diastematomyelia 742.51
Diataxia, cerebral, infantile 343.0
Diathesis
allergic V15.09
bleeding (familial) 287.9
cystine (familial) 270.0
gouty 274.9
hemorrhagic (familial) 287.9
newborn NEC 776.0
oxalic 271.8
scrofulous (*see also* Tuberculosis) 017.2
spasmophilic (*see also* Tetany) 781.7
ulcer 536.9
uric acid 274.9
Diaz's disease or osteochondrosis 732.5
Dibothriocephaliasis 123.4
larval 123.5
Dibothriocephalus (infection) (infestation) (latus) 123.4
larval 123.5
Dicephalus 759.4
Dichotomy, teeth 520.2
Dichromat, dichromata (congenital) 368.59
Dichromatopsia (congenital) 368.59
Dichuchwa 104.0
Dicroceliasis 121.8
Didelphys, didelphic (*see also* Double uterus) 752.2
Didymitis (*see also* Epididymitis) 604.90
Died - *see also* Death
without
medical attention (cause unknown) 798.9
sign of disease 798.2
Dientamoeba diarrhea 007.8
Dietary
inadequacy or deficiency 269.9
surveillance and counseling V65.3
Dietl's crisis 593.4
Dieulafoy lesion (hemorrhagic)
of
duodenum 537.84
esophagus 530.82 ◄
intestine 569.86
stomach 537.84
Difficult
birth, affecting fetus or newborn 763.9
delivery NEC 669.9
Difficulty
feeding 783.3
adult 783.3
breast 676.8
child 783.3
elderly 783.3
infant 783.3
newborn 779.3
nonorganic (infant) NEC 307.59
mechanical, gastroduodenal stoma 537.89
reading 315.00
specific, spelling 315.09
swallowing (*see also* Dysphagia) 787.2
walking 719.7
Diffuse - *see* condition
Diffused ganglion 727.42
Di George's syndrome (thymic hypoplasia) 279.11
Digestive - *see* condition

Di Guglielmo's disease or syndrome (M9841/3) 207.0
Diktyoma (M9051/3) - *see* Neoplasm, by site, malignant
Dilaceration, tooth 520.4
Dilatation
anus 564.89
venule - *see* Hemorrhoids
aorta (focal) (general) (*see also* Aneurysm, aorta) 441.9
congenital 747.29
infectional 093.0
ruptured 441.5
syphilitic 093.0
appendix (cystic) 543.9
artery 447.8
bile duct (common) (cystic) (congenital) 751.69
acquired 576.8
bladder (sphincter) 596.8
congenital 753.8
in pregnancy or childbirth 654.4
causing obstructed labor 660.2
affecting fetus or newborn 763.1
blood vessel 459.89
bronchus, bronchi 494.0
with acute exacerbation 494.1
calyx (due to obstruction) 593.89
capillaries 448.9
cardiac (acute) (chronic) (*see also* Hypertrophy, cardiac) 429.3
congenital 746.89
valve NEC 746.89
pulmonary 746.09
hypertensive (*see also* Hypertension, heart) 402.90
cavum septi pellucidi 742.4
cecum 564.89
psychogenic 306.4
cervix (uteri) - *see also* Incompetency, cervix
incomplete, poor, slow
affecting fetus or newborn 763.7
complicating delivery 661.0
affecting fetus or newborn 763.7
colon 564.7
congenital 751.3
due to mechanical obstruction 560.89
psychogenic 306.4
common bile duct (congenital) 751.69
acquired 576.8
with calculus, choledocholithiasis, or stones - *see* Choledocholithiasis
cystic duct 751.69
acquired (any bile duct) 575.8
duct, mammary 610.4
duodenum 564.89
esophagus 530.89
congenital 750.4
due to
achalasia 530.0
cardiospasm 530.0
Eustachian tube, congenital 744.24
fontanel 756.0
gallbladder 575.8
congenital 751.69
gastric 536.8
acute 536.1
psychogenic 306.4
heart (acute) (chronic) (*see also* Hypertrophy, cardiac) 429.3
congenital 746.89

Dilatation *(Continued)*
heart *(Continued)*
hypertensive (*see also* Hypertension, heart) 402.90
valve - *see also* Endocarditis
congenital 746.89
ileum 564.89
psychogenic 306.4
inguinal rings - *see* Hernia, inguinal
jejunum 564.89
psychogenic 306.4
kidney (calyx) (collecting structures) (cystic) (parenchyma) (pelvis) 593.89
lacrimal passages 375.69
lymphatic vessel 457.1
mammary duct 610.4
Meckel's diverticulum (congenital) 751.0
meningeal vessels, congenital 742.8
myocardium (acute) (chronic) (*see also* Hypertrophy, cardiac) 429.3
organ or site, congenital NEC - *see* Distortion
pancreatic duct 577.8
pelvis, kidney 593.89
pericardium - *see* Pericarditis
pharynx 478.29
prostate 602.8
pulmonary
artery (idiopathic) 417.8
congenital 747.3
valve, congenital 746.09
pupil 379.43
rectum 564.89
renal 593.89
saccule vestibularis, congenital 744.05
salivary gland (duct) 527.8
sphincter ani 564.89
stomach 536.8
acute 536.1
psychogenic 306.4
submaxillary duct 527.8
trachea, congenital 748.3
ureter (idiopathic) 593.89
congenital 753.20
due to obstruction 593.5
urethra (acquired) 599.84
vasomotor 443.9
vein 459.89
ventricular, ventricle (acute) (chronic) (*see also* Hypertrophy, cardiac) 429.3
cerebral, congenital 742.4
hypertensive (*see also* Hypertension, heart) 402.90
venule 459.89
anus - *see* Hemorrhoids
vesical orifice 596.8
Dilated, dilation - *see* Dilatation
Diminished
hearing (acuity) (*see also* Deafness) 389.9
pulse pressure 785.9
vision NEC 369.9
vital capacity 794.2
Diminuta taenia 123.6
Diminution, sense or sensation (cold) (heat) (tactile) (vibratory) (*see also* Disturbance, sensation) 782.0
Dimitri-Sturge-Weber disease (encephalocutaneous angiomatosis) 759.6
Dimple
parasacral 685.1
with abscess 685.0
pilonidal 685.1
with abscess 685.0

Dimple *(Continued)*
postanal 685.1
with abscess 685.0
Dioctophyma renale (infection) (infestation) 128.8
Dipetalonemiasis 125.4
Diphallus 752.69
Diphtheria, diphtheritic (gangrenous) (hemorrhagic) 032.9
carrier (suspected) of V02.4
cutaneous 032.85
cystitis 032.84
faucial 032.0
infection of wound 032.85
inoculation (anti) (not sick) V03.5
laryngeal 032.3
myocarditis 032.82
nasal anterior 032.2
nasopharyngeal 032.1
neurological complication 032.89
peritonitis 032.83
specified site NEC 032.89
Diphyllobothriasis (intestine) 123.4
larval 123.5
Diplacusis 388.41
Diplegia (upper limbs) 344.2
brain or cerebral 437.8
congenital 343.0
facial 351.0
congenital 352.6
infantile or congenital (cerebral) (spastic) (spinal) 343.0
lower limbs 344.1
syphilitic, congenital 090.49
Diplococcus, diplococcal - *see* condition
Diplomyelia 742.59
Diplopia 368.2
refractive 368.15
Dipsomania (*see also* Alcoholism) 303.9
with psychosis (*see also* Psychosis, alcoholic) 291.9
Dipylidiasis 123.8
intestine 123.8
Direction, teeth, abnormal 524.30
Dirt-eating child 307.52
Disability
heart - *see* Disease, heart
learning NEC 315.2
special spelling 315.09
Disarticulation (*see also* Derangement, joint) 718.9
meaning
amputation
status - *see* Absence, by site
traumatic - *see* Amputation, traumatic
dislocation, traumatic or congenital - *see* Dislocation
Disaster, cerebrovascular (*see also* Disease, cerebrovascular, acute) 436
Discharge
anal NEC 787.99
breast (female) (male) 611.79
conjunctiva 372.89
continued locomotor idiopathic (*see also* Epilepsy) 345.5
diencephalic autonomic idiopathic (*see also* Epilepsy) 345.5
ear 388.60
blood 388.69
cerebrospinal fluid 388.61
excessive urine 788.42
eye 379.93
nasal 478.19 ⬅

Discharge *(Continued)*
nipple 611.79
patterned motor idiopathic (*see also* Epilepsy) 345.5
penile 788.7
postnasal - *see* Sinusitis
sinus, from mediastinum 510.0
umbilicus 789.9
urethral 788.7
bloody 599.84
vaginal 623.5
Discitis 722.90
cervical, cervicothoracic 722.91
lumbar, lumbosacral 722.93
thoracic, thoracolumbar 722.92
Discogenic syndrome - *see* Displacement, intervertebral disc
Discoid
kidney 753.3
meniscus, congenital 717.5
semilunar cartilage 717.5
Discoloration
mouth 528.9
nails 703.8
teeth 521.7
due to
drugs 521.7
metals (copper) (silver) 521.7
pulpal bleeding 521.7
during formation 520.8
extrinsic 523.6
intrinsic posteruptive 521.7
Discomfort
chest 786.59
visual 368.13
Discomycosis - *see* Actinomycosis
Discontinuity, ossicles, ossicular chain 385.23
Discrepancy
centric occlusion (Revised)
maximum intercuspation 524.55 (New)
of teeth 524.55 (New)
leg length (acquired) 736.81
congenital 755.30
uterine size-date 649.6 (Revised)
Discrimination
political V62.4
racial V62.4
religious V62.4
sex V62.4
Disease, diseased - *see also* Syndrome
Abrami's (acquired hemolytic jaundice) 283.9
absorbent system 459.89
accumulation - *see* Thesaurismosis
acid-peptic 536.8
Acosta's 993.2
Adams-Stokes (-Morgagni) (syncope with heart block) 426.9
Addison's (bronze) (primary adrenal insufficiency) 255.4
anemia (pernicious) 281.0
tuberculous (*see also* Tuberculosis) 017.6
Addison-Gull - *see* Xanthoma
adenoids (and tonsils) (chronic) 474.9
adrenal (gland) (capsule) (cortex) 255.9
hyperfunction 255.3
hypofunction 255.4
specified type NEC 255.8
ainhum (dactylolysis spontanea) 136.0
akamushi (scrub typhus) 081.2
Akureyri (epidemic neuromyasthenia) 049.8
Albarrán's (colibacilluria) 791.9

Disease, diseased *(Continued)*
Albers-Schönberg's (marble bones) 756.52
Albert's 726.71
Albright (-Martin) (-Bantam) 275.49
Alibert's (mycosis fungoides) (M9700/3) 202.1
Alibert-Bazin (M9700/3) 202.1
alimentary canal 569.9
alligator skin (ichthyosis congenita) 757.1
acquired 701.1
Almeida's (Brazilian blastomycosis) 116.1
Alpers' 330.8
alpine 993.2
altitude 993.2
alveoli, teeth 525.9
Alzheimer's - *see* Alzheimer's
amyloid (any site) 277.30 (Revised)
anarthritic rheumatoid 446.5
Anders' (adiposis tuberosa simplex) 272.8
Andersen's (glycogenosis IV) 271.0
Anderson's (angiokeratoma corporis diffusum) 272.7
Andes 993.2
Andrews' (bacterid) 686.8
angiopastic, angiospasmodic 443.9
cerebral 435.9
with transient neurologic deficit 435.9
vein 459.89
anterior
chamber 364.9
horn cell 335.9
specified type NEC 335.8
antral (chronic) 473.0
acute 461.0
anus NEC 569.49
aorta (nonsyphilitic) 447.9
syphilitic NEC 093.89
aortic (heart) (valve) (*see also* Endocarditis, aortic) 424.1
apollo 077.4
aponeurosis 726.90
appendix 543.9
aqueous (chamber) 364.9
arc-welders' lung 503
Armenian 277.31 (Revised)
Arnold-Chiari (*see also* Spina bifida) 741.0
arterial 447.9
occlusive (*see also* Occlusion, by site) 444.22
with embolus or thrombus - *see* Occlusion, by site
due to stricture or stenosis 447.1
specified type NEC 447.8
arteriocardiorenal (*see also* Hypertension, cardiorenal) 404.90
arteriolar (generalized) (obliterative) 447.90
specified type NEC 447.8
arteriorenal - *see* Hypertension, kidney
arteriosclerotic - *see also* Arteriosclerosis
cardiovascular 429.2
coronary - *see* Arteriosclerosis, coronary
heart - *see* Arteriosclerosis, coronary
vascular - *see* Arteriosclerosis
artery 447.9
cerebral 437.9
coronary - *see* Arteriosclerosis, coronary
specified type NEC 447.8
arthropod-borne NEC 088.9
specified type NEC 088.89

Disease, diseased *(Continued)*
Asboe-Hansen's (incontinentia pigmenti) 757.33
atticoantral, chronic (with posterior or superior marginal perforation of ear drum) 382.2
auditory canal, ear 380.9
Aujeszky's 078.89
auricle, ear NEC 380.30
Australian X 062.4
autoimmune NEC 279.4
hemolytic (cold type) (warm type) 283.0
parathyroid 252.1
thyroid 245.2
aviators' (*see also* Effect, adverse, high altitude) 993.2
ax(e)-grinders' 502
Ayala's 756.89
Ayerza's (pulmonary artery sclerosis with pulmonary hypertension) 416.0
Azorean (of the nervous system) 334.8
Babington's (familial hemorrhagic telangiectasia) 448.0
back bone NEC 733.90
bacterial NEC 040.89
zoonotic NEC 027.9
specified type NEC 027.8
Baehr-Schiffrin (thrombotic thrombocytopenic purpura) 446.6
Baelz's (cheilitis glandularis apostematosa) 528.5
Baerensprung's (eczema marginatum) 110.3
Balfour's (chloroma) 205.3
balloon (*see also* Effect, adverse, high altitude) 993.2
Baló's 341.1
Bamberger (-Marie) (hypertrophic pulmonary osteoarthropathy) 731.2
Bang's (Brucella abortus) 023.1
Bannister's 995.1
Banti's (with cirrhosis) (with portal hypertension) - *see* Cirrhosis, liver
Barcoo (*see also* Ulcer, skin) 707.9
barium lung 503
Barlow (-Möller) (infantile scurvy) 267
barometer makers' 985.0
Barraquer (-Simons) (progressive lipodystrophy) 272.6
basal ganglia 333.90
degenerative NEC 333.0
specified NEC 333.89
Basedow's (exophthalmic goiter) 242.0
basement membrane NEC 583.89
with
pulmonary hemorrhage (Goodpasture's syndrome) 446.21 *[583.81]*
Bateman's 078.0
purpura (senile) 287.2
Batten's 330.1 *[362.71]*
Batten-Mayou (retina) 330.1 *[362.71]*
Batten-Steinert 359.2
Battey 031.0
Baumgarten-Cruveilhier (cirrhosis of liver) 571.5
bauxite-workers' 503
Bayle's (dementia paralytica) 094.1
Bazin's (primary) (*see also* Tuberculosis) 017.1
Beard's (neurasthenia) 300.5
Beau's (*see also* Degeneration, myocardial) 429.1

ICD-9-CM
D
Vol. 2

◀ New ⬅ Revised

Disease, diseased *(Continued)*
Bechterew's (ankylosing spondylitis) 720.0
Becker's (idiopathic mural endomyocardial disease) 425.2
Begbie's (exophthalmic goiter) 242.0
Behr's 362.50
Beigel's (white piedra) 111.2
Bekhterev's (ankylosing spondylitis) 720.0
Bell's (*see also* Psychosis, affective) 296.0
Bennett's (leukemia) 208.9
Benson's 379.22
Bergeron's (hysteroepilepsy) 300.11
Berlin's 921.3
Bernard-Soulier (thrombopathy) 287.1
Bernhardt (-Roth) 355.1
beryllium 503
Besnier-Boeck (-Schaumann) (sarcoidosis) 135
Best's 362.76
Beurmann's (sporotrichosis) 117.1
Bielschowsky (-Jansky) 330.1
Biermer's (pernicious anemia) 281.0
Biett's (discoid lupus erythematosus) 695.4
bile duct (*see also* Disease, biliary) 576.9
biliary (duct) (tract) 576.9
with calculus, choledocholithiasis, or stones - *see* Choledocholithiasis
Billroth's (meningocele) (*see also* Spina bifida) 741.9
Binswanger's 290.12
Bird's (oxaluria) 271.8
bird fanciers' 495.2
black lung 500
bladder 596.9
specified NEC 596.8
bleeder's 286.0
Bloch-Sulzberger (incontinentia pigmenti) 757.33
Blocq's (astasia-abasia) 307.9
blood (-forming organs) 289.9
specified NEC 289.89
vessel 459.9
Bloodgood's 610.1
Blount's (tibia vara) 732.4
blue 746.9
Bodechtel-Guttmann (subacute sclerosing panencephalitis) 046.2
Boeck's (sarcoidosis) 135
bone 733.90
fibrocystic NEC 733.29
jaw 526.2
marrow 289.9
Paget's (osteitis deformans) 731.0
specified type NEC 733.99
von Recklinghausen's (osteitis fibrosa cystica) 252.01
Bonfils' - *see* Disease, Hodgkin's
Borna 062.9
Bornholm (epidemic pleurodynia) 074.1
Bostock's (*see also* Fever, hay) 477.9
Bouchard's (myopathic dilatation of the stomach) 536.1
Bouillaud's (rheumatic heart disease) 391.9
Bourneville (-Brissaud) (tuberous sclerosis) 759.5
Bouveret (-Hoffmann) (paroxysmal tachycardia) 427.2
bowel 569.9
functional 564.9
psychogenic 306.4

Disease, diseased *(Continued)*
Bowen's (M8081/2) - *see* Neoplasm, skin, in situ
Bozzolo's (multiple myeloma) (M9730/3) 203.0
Bradley's (epidemic vomiting) 078.82
Brailsford's 732.3
radius, head 732.3
tarsal, scaphoid 732.5
Brailsford-Morquio (mucopolysaccharidosis IV) 277.5
brain 348.9
Alzheimer's 331.0
with dementia - *see* Alzheimer's, dementia
arterial, artery 437.9
arteriosclerotic 437.0
congenital 742.9
degenerative - *see* Degeneration, brain
inflammatory - *see also* Encephalitis
late effect - *see* category 326
organic 348.9
arteriosclerotic 437.0
parasitic NEC 123.9
Pick's 331.11
with dementia
with behavioral disturbance 331.11 *[294.11]*
without behavioral disturbance 331.11 *[294.10]*
senile 331.2
braziers' 985.8
breast 611.9
cystic (chronic) 610.1
fibrocystic 610.1
inflammatory 611.0
Paget's (M8540/3) 174.0
puerperal, postpartum NEC 676.3
specified NEC 611.8
Breda's (*see also* Yaws) 102.9
Breisky's (kraurosis vulvae) 624.0
Bretonneau's (diphtheritic malignant angina) 032.0
Bright's (*see also* Nephritis) 583.9
arteriosclerotic (*see also* Hypertension, kidney) 403.90
Brill's (recrudescent typhus) 081.1
flea-borne 081.0
louse-borne 081.1
Brill-Symmers (follicular lymphoma) (M9690/3) 202.0
Brill-Zinsser (recrudescent typhus) 081.1
Brinton's (leather bottle stomach) (M8142/3) 151.9
Brion-Kayser (*see also* Fever, paratyphoid) 002.9
broad
beta 272.2
ligament, noninflammatory 620.9
specified NEC 620.8
Brocq's 691.8
meaning
atopic (diffuse) neurodermatitis 691.8
dermatitis herpetiformis 694.0
lichen simplex chronicus 698.3
parapsoriasis 696.2
prurigo 698.2
Brocq-Duhring (dermatitis herpetiformis) 694.0
Brodie's (joint) (*see also* Osteomyelitis) 730.1
bronchi 519.19
bronchopulmonary 519.19

Disease, diseased *(Continued)*
bronze (Addison's) 255.4
tuberculous (*see also* Tuberculosis) 017.6
Brown-Séquard 344.89
Bruck's 733.99
Bruck-de Lange (Amsterdam dwarf, mental retardation, and brachycephaly) 759.89
Bruhl's (splenic anemia with fever) 285.8
Bruton's (X-linked agammaglobulinemia) 279.04
buccal cavity 528.9
Buchanan's (juvenile osteochondrosis, iliac crest) 732.1
Buchman's (osteochondrosis juvenile) 732.1
Budgerigar-Fanciers' 495.2
Budinger-Ludloff-Läwen 717.89
Büerger's (thromboangiitis obliterans) 443.1
Burger-Grütz (essential familial hyperlipemia) 272.3
Burns' (lower ulna) 732.3
bursa 727.9
Bury's (erythema elevatum diutinum) 695.89
Buschke's 710.1
Busquet's (*see also* Osteomyelitis) 730.1
Busse-Buschke (cryptococcosis) 117.5
C_2 (*see also* Alcoholism) 303.9
Caffey's (infantile cortical hyperostosis) 756.59
caisson 993.3
calculous 592.9
California 114.0
Calvé (-Perthes) (osteochondrosis, femoral capital) 732.1
Camurati-Engelmann (diaphyseal sclerosis) 756.59
Canavan's 330.0
capillaries 448.9
Carapata 087.1
cardiac - *see* Disease, heart
cardiopulmonary, chronic 416.9
cardiorenal (arteriosclerotic) (hepatic) (hypertensive) (vascular) (*see also* Hypertension, cardiorenal) 404.90
cardiovascular (arteriosclerotic) 429.2
congenital 746.9
hypertensive (*see also* Hypertension, heart) 402.90
benign 402.10
malignant 402.00
renal (*see also* Hypertension, cardiorenal) 404.90
syphilitic (asymptomatic) 093.9
carotid gland 259.8
Carrión's (Bartonellosis) 088.0
cartilage NEC 733.90
specified NEC 733.99
Castellani's 104.8
cat-scratch 078.3
Cavare's (familial periodic paralysis) 359.3
Cazenave's (pemphigus) 694.4
cecum 569.9
celiac (adult) 579.0
infantile 579.0
cellular tissue NEC 709.9
central core 359.0
cerebellar, cerebellum - *see* Disease, brain
cerebral (*see also* Disease, brain) 348.9
arterial, artery 437.9
degenerative - *see* Degeneration, brain

◀ New ⬅ Revised

Disease, diseased *(Continued)*
cerebrospinal 349.9
cerebrovascular NEC 437.9
acute 436
embolic - *see* Embolism, brain
late effect - *see* Late effect(s) (of) cerebrovascular disease
puerperal, postpartum, childbirth 674.0
thrombotic - *see* Thrombosis, brain
arteriosclerotic 437.0
embolic - *see* Embolism, brain
ischemic, generalized NEC 437.1
late effect - *see* Late effect(s) (of) cerebrovascular disease
occlusive 437.1
puerperal, postpartum, childbirth 674.0
specified type NEC 437.8
thrombotic - *see* Thrombosis, brain
ceroid storage 272.7
cervix (uteri)
inflammatory 616.9
specified NEC 616.89 ◄
noninflammatory 622.9
specified NEC 622.8
Chabert's 022.9
Chagas' (*see also* Trypanosomiasis, American) 086.2
Chandler's (osteochondritis dissecans, hip) 732.7
Charcôt's (joint) 094.0 *[713.5]*
spinal cord 094.0
Charcôt-Marie-Tooth 356.1
Charlouis' (*see also* Yaws) 102.9
Cheadle (-Möller) (-Barlow) (infantile scurvy) 267
Chédiak-Steinbrinck (-Higashi) (congenital gigantism of peroxidase granules) 288.2
cheek, inner 528.9
chest 519.9
Chiari's (hepatic vein thrombosis) 453.0
Chicago (North American blastomycosis) 116.0
chignon (white piedra) 111.2
chigoe, chigo (jigger) 134.1
childhood granulomatous 288.1
Chinese liver fluke 121.1
chlamydial NEC 078.88
cholecystic (*see also* Disease, gallbladder) 575.9
choroid 363.9
degenerative (*see also* Degeneration, choroid) 363.40
hereditary (*see also* Dystrophy, choroid) 363.50
specified type NEC 363.8
Christian's (chronic histiocytosis X) 277.89
Christian-Weber (nodular nonsuppurative panniculitis) 729.30
Christmas 286.1
ciliary body 364.9
circulatory (system) NEC 459.9
chronic, maternal, affecting fetus or newborn 760.3
specified NEC 459.89
syphilitic 093.9
congenital 090.5
Civatte's (poikiloderma) 709.09
climacteric 627.2
male 608.89
coagulation factor deficiency (congenital) (*see also* Defect, coagulation) 286.9

Disease, diseased *(Continued)*
Coats' 362.12
coccidioidal pulmonary 114.5
acute 114.0
chronic 114.4
primary 114.0
residual 114.4
Cockayne's (microcephaly and dwarfism) 759.89
Cogan's 370.52
cold
agglutinin 283.0
or hemoglobinuria 283.0
paroxysmal (cold) (nocturnal) 283.2
hemagglutinin (chronic) 283.0
collagen NEC 710.9
nonvascular 710.9
specified NEC 710.8
vascular (allergic) (*see also* Angiitis, hypersensitivity) 446.20
colon 569.9
functional 564.9
congenital 751.3
ischemic 557.0
combined system (of spinal cord) 266.2 *[336.2]*
with anemia (pernicious) 281.0 *[336.2]*
compressed air 993.3
Concato's (pericardial polyserositis) 423.2
peritoneal 568.82
pleural - *see* Pleurisy
congenital NEC 799.89
conjunctiva 372.9
chlamydial 077.98
specified NEC 077.8
specified type NEC 372.89
viral 077.99
specified NEC 077.8
connective tissue, diffuse (*see also* Disease, collagen) 710.9
Conor and Bruch's (boutonneuse fever) 082.1
Conradi (-Hünermann) 756.59
Cooley's (erythroblastic anemia) 282.49
Cooper's 610.1
Corbus' 607.1
cork-handlers' 495.3
cornea (*see also* Keratopathy) 371.9
coronary (*see also* Ischemia, heart) 414.9
congenital 746.85
ostial, syphilitic 093.20
aortic 093.22
mitral 093.21
pulmonary 093.24
tricuspid 093.23
Corrigan's - *see* Insufficiency, aortic
Cotugno's 724.3
Coxsackie (virus) NEC 074.8
cranial nerve NEC 352.9
Creutzfeldt-Jakob (new variant) 046.1
with dementia
with behavioral disturbance 046.1 *[294.11]*
without behavioral disturbance 046.1 *[294.10]*
Crigler-Najjar (congenital hyperbilirubinemia) 277.4
Crocq's (acrocyanosis) 443.89
Crohn's (intestine) (*see also* Enteritis, regional) 555.9
Crouzon's (craniofacial dysostosis) 756.0
Cruchet's (encephalitis lethargica) 049.8
Cruveilhier's 335.21

Disease, diseased *(Continued)*
Cruz-Chagas (*see also* Trypanosomiasis, American) 086.2
crystal deposition (*see also* Arthritis, due to, crystals) 712.9
Csillag's (lichen sclerosus et atrophicus) 701.0
Curschmann's 359.2
Cushing's (pituitary basophilism) 255.0
cystic
breast (chronic) 610.1
kidney, congenital (*see also* Cystic, disease, kidney) 753.10
liver, congenital 751.62
lung 518.89
congenital 748.4
pancreas 577.2
congenital 751.7
renal, congenital (*see also* Cystic, disease, kidney) 753.10
semilunar cartilage 717.5
cysticercus 123.1
cystine storage (with renal sclerosis) 270.0
cytomegalic inclusion (generalized) 078.5
with
pneumonia 078.5 *[484.1]*
congenital 771.1
Daae (-Finsen) (epidemic pleurodynia) 074.1
dancing 297.8
Danielssen's (anesthetic leprosy) 030.1
Darier's (congenital) (keratosis follicularis) 757.39
erythema annulare centrifugum 695.0
vitamin A deficiency 264.8
Darling's (histoplasmosis) (*see also* Histoplasmosis, American) 115.00
Davies' 425.0
de Beurmann-Gougerot (sporotrichosis) 117.1
Débove's (splenomegaly) 789.2
deer fly (*see also* Tularemia) 021.9
deficiency 269.9
degenerative - *see also* Degeneration
disc - *see* Degeneration, intervertebral disc
Degos' 447.8
Déjérine (-Sottas) 356.0
Déleage's 359.89
demyelinating, demyelinizating (brain stem) (central nervous system) 341.9
multiple sclerosis 340
specified NEC 341.8
de Quervain's (tendon sheath) 727.04
thyroid (subacute granulomatous thyroiditis) 245.1
Dercum's (adiposis dolorosa) 272.8
Deutschländer's - *see* Fracture, foot
Devergie's (pityriasis rubra pilaris) 696.4
Devic's 341.0
diaphorase deficiency 289.7
diaphragm 519.4
diarrheal, infectious 009.2
diatomaceous earth 502
Diaz's (osteochondrosis astragalus) 732.5
digestive system 569.9
Di Guglielmo's (erythemic myelosis) (M9841/3) 207.0
Dimitri-Sturge-Weber (encephalocutaneous angiomatosis) 759.6
disc, degenerative - *see* Degeneration, intervertebral disc
discogenic (*see also* Disease, intervertebral disc) 722.90

Disease, diseased *(Continued)*
diverticular - *see* Diverticula
Down's (mongolism) 758.0
Dubini's (electric chorea) 049.8
Dubois' (thymus gland) 090.5
Duchenne's 094.0
locomotor ataxia 094.0
muscular dystrophy 359.1
paralysis 335.22
pseudohypertrophy, muscles 359.1
Duchenne-Griesinger 359.1
ductless glands 259.9
Duhring's (dermatitis herpetiformis) 694.0
Dukes (-Filatov) 057.8
duodenum NEC 537.9
specified NEC 537.89
Duplay's 726.2
Dupré's (meningism) 781.6
Dupuytren's (muscle contracture) 728.6
Durand-Nicolas-Favre (climatic bubo) 099.1
Duroziez's (congenital mitral stenosis) 746.5
Dutton's (trypanosomiasis) 086.9
Eales' 362.18
ear (chronic) (inner) NEC 388.9
middle 385.9
adhesive (*see also* Adhesions, middle ear) 385.10
specified NEC 385.89
Eberth's (typhoid fever) 002.0
Ebstein's
heart 746.2
meaning diabetes 250.4 *[581.81]*
Echinococcus (*see also* Echinococcus) 122.9
ECHO virus NEC 078.89
Economo's (encephalitis lethargica) 049.8
Eddowes' (brittle bones and blue sclera) 756.51
Edsall's 992.2
Eichstedt's (pityriasis versicolor) 111.0
Ellis-van Creveld (chondroectodermal dysplasia) 756.55
endocardium - *see* Endocarditis
endocrine glands or system NEC 259.9
specified NEC 259.8
endomyocardial, idiopathic mural 425.2
Engel-von Recklinghausen (osteitis fibrosa cystica) 252.01
Engelmann's (diaphyseal sclerosis) 756.59
English (rickets) 268.0
Engman's (infectious eczematoid dermatitis) 690.8
enteroviral, enterovirus NEC 078.89
central nervous system NEC 048
epidemic NEC 136.9
epididymis 608.9
epigastric, functional 536.9
psychogenic 306.4
Erb (-Landouzy) 359.1
Erb-Goldflam 358.00
Erichsen's (railway spine) 300.16
esophagus 530.9
functional 530.5
psychogenic 306.4
Eulenburg's (congenital paramyotonia) 359.2
Eustachian tube 381.9
Evans' (thrombocytopenic purpura) 287.32
external auditory canal 380.9
extrapyramidal NEC 333.90

Disease, diseased *(Continued)*
eye 379.90
anterior chamber 364.9
inflammatory NEC 364.3
muscle 378.9
eyeball 360.9
eyelid 374.9
eyeworm of Africa 125.2
Fabry's (angiokeratoma corporis diffusum) 272.7
facial nerve (seventh) 351.9
newborn 767.5
Fahr-Volhard (malignant nephrosclerosis) 403.00
fallopian tube, noninflammatory 620.9
specified NEC 620.8
familial periodic 277.31 ⬅
paralysis 359.3
Fanconi's (congenital pancytopenia) 284.09 ⬅
Farber's (disseminated lipogranulomatosis) 272.8
fascia 728.9
inflammatory 728.9
Fauchard's (periodontitis) 523.40 ⬅
Favre-Durand-Nicolas (climatic bubo) 099.1
Favre-Racouchot (elastoidosis cutanea nodularis) 701.8
Fede's 529.0
Feer's 985.0
Felix's (juvenile osteochondrosis, hip) 732.1
Fenwick's (gastric atrophy) 537.89
Fernels' (aortic aneurysm) 441.9
fibrocaseous, of lung (*see also* Tuberculosis, pulmonary) 011.9
fibrocystic - *see also* Fibrocystic, disease
newborn 277.01
Fiedler's (leptospiral jaundice) 100.0
fifth 057.0
Filatoff's (infectious mononucleosis) 075
Filatov's (infectious mononucleosis) 075
file-cutters' 984.9
specified type of lead - *see* Table of Drugs and Chemicals
filterable virus NEC 078.89
fish skin 757.1
acquired 701.1
Flajani (-Basedow) (exophthalmic goiter) 242.0
Flatau-Schilder 341.1
flax-dressers' 504
Fleischner's 732.3
flint 502
fluke - *see* Infestation, fluke
Følling's (phenylketonuria) 270.1
foot and mouth 078.4
foot process 581.3
Forbes' (glycogenosis III) 271.0
Fordyce's (ectopic sebaceous glands) (mouth) 750.26
Fordyce-Fox (apocrine miliaria) 705.82
Fothergill's
meaning scarlatina anginosa 034.1
neuralgia (*see also* Neuralgia, trigeminal) 350.1
Fournier's 608.83
fourth 057.8
Fox (-Fordyce) (apocrine miliaria) 705.82
Francis' (*see also* Tularemia) 021.9
Franklin's (heavy chain) 273.2
Frei's (climatic bubo) 099.1
Freiberg's (flattening metatarsal) 732.5

Disease, diseased *(Continued)*
Friedländer's (endarteritis obliterans) - *see* Arteriosclerosis
Friedreich's
combined systemic or ataxia 334.0
facial hemihypertrophy 756.0
myoclonia 333.2
Fröhlich's (adiposogenital dystrophy) 253.8
Frommel's 676.6
frontal sinus (chronic) 473.1
acute 461.1
Fuller's earth 502
fungus, fungous NEC 117.9
Gaisböck's (polycythemia hypertonica) 289.0
gallbladder 575.9
congenital 751.60
Gamna's (siderotic splenomegaly) 289.51
Gamstorp's (adynamia episodica hereditaria) 359.3
Gandy-Nanta (siderotic splenomegaly) 289.51
Gannister (occupational) 502
Garré's (*see also* Osteomyelitis) 730.1
gastric (*see also* Disease, stomach) 537.9
gastrointestinal (tract) 569.9
amyloid 277.39 ⬅
functional 536.9
psychogenic 306.4
Gaucher's (adult) (cerebroside lipidosis) (infantile) 272.7
Gayet's (superior hemorrhagic polioencephalitis) 265.1
Gee (-Herter) (-Heubner) (-Thaysen) (nontropical sprue) 579.0
generalized neoplastic (M8000/6) 199.0
genital organs NEC
female 629.9
specified NEC 629.89 ⬅
male 608.9
Gerhardt's (erythromelalgia) 443.82
Gerlier's (epidemic vertigo) 078.81
Gibert's (pityriasis rosea) 696.3
Gibney's (perispondylitis) 720.9
Gierke's (glycogenosis I) 271.0
Gilbert's (familial nonhemolytic jaundice) 277.4
Gilchrist's (North American blastomycosis) 116.0
Gilford (-Hutchinson) (progeria) 259.8
Gilles de la Tourette's (motor-verbal tic) 307.23
Giovannini's 117.9
gland (lymph) 289.9
Glanzmann's (hereditary hemorrhagic thrombasthenia) 287.1
glassblowers' 527.1
Glénard's (enteroptosis) 569.89
Glisson's (*see also* Rickets) 268.0
glomerular
membranous, idiopathic 581.1
minimal change 581.3
glycogen storage (Andersen's) (Cori types 1-7) (Forbes') (McArdle-Schmid-Pearson) (Pompe's) (types I-VII) 271.0
cardiac 271.0 *[425.7]*
generalized 271.0
glucose-6-phosphatase deficiency 271.0
heart 271.0 *[425.7]*
hepatorenal 271.0
liver and kidneys 271.0

◀ New ⬅ Revised

Disease, diseased *(Continued)*
glycogen storage *(Continued)*
myocardium 271.0 *[425.7]*
von Gierke's (glycogenosis I) 271.0
Goldflam-Erb 358.00
Goldscheider's (epidermolysis bullosa) 757.39
Goldstein's (familial hemorrhagic telangiectasia) 448.0
gonococcal NEC 098.0
Goodall's (epidemic vomiting) 078.82
Gordon's (exudative enteropathy) 579.8
Gougerot's (trisymptomatic) 709.1
Gougerot-Carteaud (confluent reticulate papillomatosis) 701.8
Gougerot-Hailey-Hailey (benign familial chronic pemphigus) 757.39
graft-versus-host (bone marrow) 996.85
due to organ transplant NEC - *see* Complications, transplant, organ
grain-handlers' 495.8
Grancher's (splenopneumonia) - *see* Pneumonia
granulomatous (childhood) (chronic) 288.1
graphite lung 503
Graves' (exophthalmic goiter) 242.0
Greenfield's 330.0
green monkey 078.89
Griesinger's (*see also* Ancylostomiasis) 126.9
grinders' 502
Grisel's 723.5
Gruby's (tinea tonsurans) 110.0
Guertin's (electric chorea) 049.8
Guillain-Barré 357.0
Guinon's (motor-verbal tic) 307.23
Gull's (thyroid atrophy with myxedema) 244.8
Gull and Sutton's - *see* Hypertension, kidney
gum NEC 523.9
Günther's (congenital erythropoietic porphyria) 277.1
gynecological 629.9
specified NEC 629.89
H 270.0
Haas' 732.3
Habermann's (acute parapsoriasis varioliformis) 696.2
Haff 985.1
Hageman (congenital factor XII deficiency) (*see also* Defect, congenital) 286.3
Haglund's (osteochondrosis os tibiale externum) 732.5
Hagner's (hypertrophic pulmonary osteoarthropathy) 731.2
Hailey-Hailey (benign familial chronic pemphigus) 757.39
hair (follicles) NEC 704.9
specified type NEC 704.8
Hallervorden-Spatz 333.0
Hallopeau's (lichen sclerosus et atrophicus) 701.0
Hamman's (spontaneous mediastinal emphysema) 518.1
hand, foot, and mouth 074.3
Hand-Schüller-Christian (chronic histiocytosis X) 277.89
Hanot's - *see* Cirrhosis, biliary
Hansen's (leprosy) 030.9
benign form 030.1
malignant form 030.0

Disease, diseased *(Continued)*
Harada's 363.22
Harley's (intermittent hemoglobinuria) 283.2
Hart's (pellagra-cerebellar ataxia-renal aminoaciduria) 270.0
Hartnup (pellagra-cerebellar ataxia-renal aminoaciduria) 270.0
Hashimoto's (struma lymphomatosa) 245.2
Hb - *see* Disease, hemoglobin
heart (organic) 429.9
with
acute pulmonary edema (*see also* Failure, ventricular, left) 428.1
hypertensive 402.91
with renal failure 404.92
benign 402.11
with renal failure 404.12
malignant 402.01
with renal failure 404.02
kidney disease - *see* Hypertension, cardiorenal
rheumatic fever (conditions classifiable to 390)
active 391.9
with chorea 392.0
inactive or quiescent (with chorea) 398.90
amyloid 277.39 *[425.7]*
aortic (valve) (*see also* Endocarditis, aortic) 424.1
arteriosclerotic or sclerotic (minimal) (senile) - *see* Arteriosclerosis, coronary
artery, arterial - *see* Arteriosclerosis, coronary
atherosclerotic - *see* Arteriosclerosis, coronary
beer drinkers' 425.5
beriberi 265.0 *[425.7]*
black 416.0
congenital NEC 746.9
cyanotic 746.9
maternal, affecting fetus or newborn 760.3
specified type NEC 746.89
congestive (*see also* Failure, heart) 428.0
coronary 414.9
cryptogenic 429.9
due to
amyloidosis 277.39 *[425.7]*
beriberi 265.0 *[425.7]*
cardiac glycogenosis 271.0 *[425.7]*
Friedreich's ataxia 334.0 *[425.8]*
gout 274.82
mucopolysaccharidosis 277.5 *[425.7]*
myotonia atrophica 359.2 *[425.8]*
progressive muscular dystrophy 359.1 *[425.8]*
sarcoidosis 135 *[425.8]*
fetal 746.9
inflammatory 746.89
fibroid (*see also* Myocarditis) 429.0
functional 427.9
postoperative 997.1
psychogenic 306.2
glycogen storage 271.0 *[425.7]*
gonococcal NEC 098.85
gouty 274.82
hypertensive (*see also* Hypertension, heart) 402.90
benign 402.10
malignant 402.00

Disease, diseased *(Continued)*
heart *(Continued)*
hyperthyroid (*see also* Hyperthyroidism) 242.9 *[425.7]*
incompletely diagnosed - *see* Disease, heart
ischemic (chronic) (*see also* Ischemia, heart) 414.9
acute (*see also* Infarct, myocardium) 410.9
without myocardial infarction 411.89
with coronary (artery) occlusion 411.81
asymptomatic 412
diagnosed on ECG or other special investigation but currently presenting no symptoms 412
kyphoscoliotic 416.1
mitral (*see also* Endocarditis, mitral) 394.9
muscular (*see also* Degeneration, myocardial) 429.1
postpartum 674.8
psychogenic (functional) 306.2
pulmonary (chronic) 416.9
acute 415.0
specified NEC 416.8
rheumatic (chronic) (inactive) (old) (quiescent) (with chorea) 398.90
active or acute 391.9
with chorea (active) (rheumatic) (Sydenham's) 392.0
specified type NEC 391.8
maternal, affecting fetus or newborn 760.3
rheumatoid - *see* Arthritis, rheumatoid
sclerotic - *see* Arteriosclerosis, coronary
senile (*see also* Myocarditis) 429.0
specified type NEC 429.89
syphilitic 093.89
aortic 093.1
aneurysm 093.0
asymptomatic 093.89
congenital 090.5
thyroid (gland) (*see also* Hyperthyroidism) 242.9 *[425.7]*
thyrotoxic (*see also* Thyrotoxicosis) 242.9 *[425.7]*
tuberculous (*see also* Tuberculosis) 017.9 *[425.8]*
valve, valvular (obstructive) (regurgitant) - *see also* Endocarditis
congenital NEC (*see also* Anomaly, heart, valve) 746.9
pulmonary 746.00
specified type NEC 746.89
vascular - *see* Disease, cardiovascular
heavy-chain (gamma G) 273.2
Heberden's 715.04
Hebra's
dermatitis exfoliativa 695.89
erythema multiforme exudativum 695.1
pityriasis
maculata et circinata 696.3
rubra 695.89
pilaris 696.4
prurigo 698.2
Heerfordt's (uveoparotitis) 135
Heidenhain's 290.10
with dementia 290.10
Heilmeyer-Schöner (M9842/3) 207.1
Heine-Medin (*see also* Poliomyelitis) 045.9

ICD-9-CM D Vol. 2

Disease, diseased *(Continued)*
Heller's (*see also* Psychosis, childhood) 299.1
Heller-Döhle (syphilitic aortitis) 093.1
hematopoietic organs 289.9
hemoglobin (Hb) 282.7
with thalassemia 282.49
abnormal (mixed) NEC 282.7
with thalassemia 282.49
AS genotype 282.5
Bart's 282.49
C (Hb-C) 282.7
with other abnormal hemoglobin NEC 282.7
elliptocytosis 282.7
Hb-S (without crisis) 282.63
with
crisis 282.64
vaso-occlusive pain 282.64
sickle-cell (without crisis) 282.63
with
crisis 282.64
vaso-occlusive pain 282.64
thalassemia 282.49
constant spring 282.7
D (Hb-D) 282.7
with other abnormal hemoglobin NEC 282.7
Hb-S (without crisis) 282.68
with crisis 282.69
sickle-cell (without crisis) 282.68
with crisis 282.69
thalassemia 282.49
E (Hb-E) 282.7
with other abnormal hemoglobin NEC 282.7
Hb-S (without crisis) 282.68
with crisis 282.69
sickle-cell (without crisis) 282.68
with crisis 282.69
thalassemia 282.49
elliptocytosis 282.7
F (Hb-F) 282.7
G (Hb-G) 282.7
H (Hb-H) 282.49
hereditary persistence, fetal (HPFH) ("Swiss variety") 282.7
high fetal gene 282.7
I thalassemia 282.49
M 289.7
S - *see also* Disease, sickle-cell, Hb-S
thalassemia (without crisis) 282.41
with
crisis 282.42
vaso-occlusive pain 282.42
spherocytosis 282.7
unstable, hemolytic 282.7
Zurich (Hb-Zurich) 282.7
hemolytic (fetus) (newborn) 773.2
autoimmune (cold type) (warm type) 283.0
due to or with
incompatibility
ABO (blood group) 773.1
blood (group) (Duffy) (Kell) (Kidd) (Lewis) (M) (S) NEC 773.2
Rh (blood group) (factor) 773.0
Rh negative mother 773.0
unstable hemoglobin 282.7
hemorrhagic 287.9
newborn 776.0
Henoch (-Schönlein) (purpura nervosa) 287.0

Disease, diseased *(Continued)*
hepatic - *see* Disease, liver
hepatolenticular 275.1
heredodegenerative NEC
brain 331.89
spinal cord 336.8
Hers' (glycogenosis VI) 271.0
Herter (-Gee) (-Heubner) (nontropical sprue) 579.0
Herxheimer's (diffuse idiopathic cutaneous atrophy) 701.8
Heubner's 094.89
Heubner-Herter (nontropical sprue) 579.0
high fetal gene or hemoglobin thalassemia 282.49
Hildenbrand's (typhus) 081.9
hip (joint) NEC 719.95
congenital 755.63
suppurative 711.05
tuberculous (*see also* Tuberculosis) 015.1 *[730.85]*
Hippel's (retinocerebral angiomatosis) 759.6
Hirschfeld's (acute diabetes mellitus) (*see also* Diabetes) 250.0
Hirschsprung's (congenital megacolon) 751.3
His (-Werner) (trench fever) 083.1
HIV 042
Hodgkin's (M9650/3) 201.9

Note Use the following fifth-digit subclassification with category 201:

0 unspecified site
1 lymph nodes of head, face, and neck
2 intrathoracic lymph nodes
3 intra-abdominal lymph nodes
4 lymph nodes of axilla and upper limb
5 lymph nodes of inguinal region and lower limb
6 intrapelvic lymph nodes
7 spleen
8 lymph nodes of multiple sites

lymphocytic
depletion (M9653/3) 201.7
diffuse fibrosis (M9654/3) 201.7
reticular type (M9655/3) 201.7
predominance (M9651/3) 201.4
lymphocytic-histiocytic predominance (M9651/3) 201.4
mixed cellularity (M9652/3) 201.6
nodular sclerosis (M9656/3) 201.5
cellular phase (M9657/3) 201.5
Hodgson's 441.9
ruptured 441.5
Hoffa (-Kastert) (liposynovitis prepatellaris) 272.8
Holla (*see also* Spherocytosis) 282.0
homozygous-Hb-S 282.61
hoof and mouth 078.4
hookworm (*see also* Ancylostomiasis) 126.9
Horton's (temporal arteritis) 446.5
host-versus-graft (immune or nonimmune cause) 996.80
bone marrow 996.85
heart 996.83
intestines 996.87
kidney 996.81
liver 996.82

Disease, diseased *(Continued)*
host-versus-graft *(Continued)*
lung 996.84
pancreas 996.86
specified NEC 996.89
HPFH (hereditary persistence of fetal hemoglobin) ("Swiss variety") 282.7
Huchard's (continued arterial hypertension) 401.9
Huguier's (uterine fibroma) 218.9
human immunodeficiency (virus) 042
hunger 251.1
Hunt's
dyssynergia cerebellaris myoclonica 334.2
herpetic geniculate ganglionitis 053.11
Huntington's 333.4
Huppert's (multiple myeloma) (M9730/3) 203.0
Hurler's (mucopolysaccharidosis I) 277.5
Hutchinson's, meaning
angioma serpiginosum 709.1
cheiropompholyx 705.81
prurigo estivalis 692.72
Hutchinson-Boeck (sarcoidosis) 135
Hutchinson-Gilford (progeria) 259.8
hyaline (diffuse) (generalized) 728.9
membrane (lung) (newborn) 769
hydatid (*see also* Echinococcus) 122.9
Hyde's (prurigo nodularis) 698.3
hyperkinetic (*see also* Hyperkinesia) 314.9
heart 429.82
hypertensive (*see also* Hypertension) 401.9
hypophysis 253.9
hyperfunction 253.1
hypofunction 253.2
Iceland (epidemic neuromyasthenia) 049.8
I cell 272.7
ill-defined 799.89
immunologic NEC 279.9
immunoproliferative 203.8
inclusion 078.5
salivary gland 078.5
infancy, early NEC 779.9
infective NEC 136.9
inguinal gland 289.9
internal semilunar cartilage, cystic 717.5
intervertebral disc 722.90
with myelopathy 722.70
cervical, cervicothoracic 722.91
with myelopathy 722.71
lumbar, lumbosacral 722.93
with myelopathy 722.73
thoracic, thoracolumbar 722.92
with myelopathy 722.72
intestine 569.9
functional 564.9
congenital 751.3
psychogenic 306.4
lardaceous 277.39 ⬅
organic 569.9
protozoal NEC 007.9
iris 364.9
iron
metabolism 275.0
storage 275.0
Isambert's (*see also* Tuberculosis, larynx) 012.3
Iselin's (osteochondrosis, fifth metatarsal) 732.5
island (scrub typhus) 081.2
itai-itai 985.5

- **Disease, diseased** *(Continued)*
  - Jadassohn's (maculopapular erythroderma) 696.2
  - Jadassohn-Pellizari's (anetoderma) 701.3
  - Jakob-Creutzfeldt (new variant) 046.1
    - with dementia
      - with behavioral disturbance 046.1 *[294.11]*
      - without behavioral disturbance 046.1 *[294.10]*
  - Jaksch (-Luzet) (pseudoleukemia infantum) 285.8
  - Janet's 300.89
  - Jansky-Bielschowsky 330.1
  - jaw NEC 526.9
    - fibrocystic 526.2
  - Jensen's 363.05
  - Jeune's (asphyxiating thoracic dystrophy) 756.4
  - jigger 134.1
  - Johnson-Stevens (erythema multiforme exudativum) 695.1
  - joint NEC 719.9
    - ankle 719.97
    - Charcôt 094.0 *[713.5]*
    - degenerative (*see also* Osteoarthrosis) 715.9
      - multiple 715.09
      - spine (*see also* Spondylosis) 721.90
    - elbow 719.92
    - foot 719.97
    - hand 719.94
    - hip 719.95
    - hypertrophic (chronic) (degenerative) (*see also* Osteoarthrosis) 715.9
      - spine (*see also* Spondylosis) 721.90
    - knee 719.96
    - Luschka 721.90
    - multiple sites 719.99
    - pelvic region 719.95
    - sacroiliac 724.6
    - shoulder (region) 719.91
    - specified site NEC 719.98
    - spine NEC 724.9
      - pseudarthrosis following fusion 733.82
      - sacroiliac 724.6
    - wrist 719.93
  - Jourdain's (acute gingivitis) 523.00
  - Jüngling's (sarcoidosis) 135
  - Kahler (-Bozzolo) (multiple myeloma) (M9730/3) 203.0
  - Kalischer's 759.6
  - Kaposi's 757.33
    - lichen ruber 697.8
      - acuminatus 696.4
      - moniliformis 697.8
  - xeroderma pigmentosum 757.33
  - Kaschin-Beck (endemic polyarthritis) 716.00
    - ankle 716.07
    - arm 716.02
      - lower (and wrist) 716.03
      - upper (and elbow) 716.02
    - foot (and ankle) 716.07
    - forearm (and wrist) 716.03
    - hand 716.04
    - leg 716.06
      - lower 716.06
      - upper 716.05
    - multiple sites 716.09
    - pelvic region (hip) (thigh) 716.05
    - shoulder region 716.01
    - specified site NEC 716.08

- **Disease, diseased** *(Continued)*
  - Katayama 120.2
  - Kawasaki 446.1
  - Kedani (scrub typhus) 081.2
  - kidney (functional) (pelvis) (*see also* Disease, renal) 593.9
    - chronic 585.9
      - requiring chronic dialysis 585.6 ◄
      - stage
        - I 585.1
        - II (mild) 585.2
        - III (moderate) 585.3
        - IV (severe) 585.4
        - V 585.5
    - cystic (congenital) 753.10
      - multiple 753.19
      - single 753.11
      - specified NEC 753.19
    - fibrocystic (congenital) 753.19
    - in gout 274.10
    - polycystic (congenital) 753.12
      - adult type (APKD) 753.13
      - autosomal dominant 753.13
      - autosomal recessive 753.14
      - childhood type (CPKD) 753.14
      - infantile type 753.14
  - Kienböck's (carpal lunate) (wrist) 732.3
  - Kimmelstiel (-Wilson) (intercapillary glomerulosclerosis) 250.4 *[581.81]*
  - Kinnier Wilson's (hepatolenticular degeneration) 275.1
  - kissing 075
  - Kleb's (*see also* Nephritis) 583.9
  - Klinger's 446.4
  - Klippel's 723.8
  - Klippel-Feil (brevicollis) 756.16
  - Knight's 911.1
  - Köbner's (epidermolysis bullosa) 757.39
  - Koenig-Wichmann (pemphigus) 694.4
  - Köhler's
    - first (osteoarthrosis juvenilis) 732.5
    - second (Freiberg's infraction, metatarsal head) 732.5
    - patellar 732.4
    - tarsal navicular (bone) (osteoarthrosis juvenilis) 732.5
  - Köhler-Freiberg (infraction, metatarsal head) 732.5
  - Köhler-Mouchet (osteoarthrosis juvenilis) 732.5
  - Köhler-Pellegrini-Stieda (calcification, knee joint) 726.62
  - Kok 759.89
  - König's (osteochondritis dissecans) 732.7
  - Korsakoff's (nonalcoholic) 294.0
    - alcoholic 291.1
  - Kostmann's (infantile genetic agranulocytosis) 288.01
  - Krabbe's 330.0
  - Kraepelin-Morel (*see also* Schizophrenia) 295.9
  - Kraft-Weber-Dimitri 759.6
  - Kufs' 330.1
  - Kugelberg-Welander 335.11
  - Kuhnt-Junius 362.52
  - Kümmell's (-Verneuil) (spondylitis) 721.7
  - Kundrat's (lymphosarcoma) 200.1
  - kuru 046.0
  - Kussmaul (-Meier) (polyarteritis nodosa) 446.0
  - Kyasanur Forest 065.2
  - Kyrle's (hyperkeratosis follicularis in cutem penetrans) 701.1

- **Disease, diseased** *(Continued)*
  - labia
    - inflammatory 616.9
      - specified NEC 616.89
    - noninflammatory 624.9
      - specified NEC 624.8
  - labyrinth, ear 386.8
  - lacrimal system (apparatus) (passages) 375.9
    - gland 375.00
    - specified NEC 375.89
  - Lafora's 333.2
  - Lagleyze-von Hippel (retinocerebral angiomatosis) 759.6
  - Lancereaux-Mathieu (leptospiral jaundice) 100.0
  - Landry's 357.0
  - Lane's 569.89
  - lardaceous (any site) 277.39
  - Larrey-Weil (leptospiral jaundice) 100.0
  - Larsen (-Johansson) (juvenile osteopathia patellae) 732.4
  - larynx 478.70
  - Lasègue's (persecution mania) 297.9
  - Leber's 377.16
  - Lederer's (acquired infectious hemolytic anemia) 283.19
  - Legg's (capital femoral osteochondrosis) 732.1
  - Legg-Calvé-Perthes (capital femoral osteochondrosis) 732.1
  - Legg-Calvé-Waldenström (femoral capital osteochondrosis) 732.1
  - Legg-Perthes (femoral capital osteochrondosis) 732.1
  - Legionnaires' 482.84
  - Leigh's 330.8
  - Leiner's (exfoliative dermatitis) 695.89
  - Leloir's (lupus erythematosus) 695.4
  - Lenegre's 426.0
  - lens (eye) 379.39
  - Leriche's (osteoporosis, posttraumatic) 733.7
  - Letterer-Siwe (acute histiocytosis X) (M9722/3) 202.5
  - Lev's (acquired complete heart block) 426.0
  - Lewandowski's (*see also* Tuberculosis) 017.0
  - Lewandowski-Lutz (epidermodysplasia verruciformis) 078.19
  - Lewy body 331.82
    - with dementia
      - with behavioral disturbance 331.82 *[294.11]*
      - without behavioral disturbance 331.82 *[294.10]*
  - Leyden's (periodic vomiting) 536.2
  - Libman-Sacks (verrucous endocarditis) 710.0 *[424.91]*
  - Lichtheim's (subacute combined sclerosis with pernicious anemia) 281.0 *[336.2]*
  - ligament 728.9
  - light chain 203.0
  - Lightwood's (renal tubular acidosis) 588.89
  - Lignac's (cystinosis) 270.0
  - Lindau's (retinocerebral angiomatosis) 759.6
  - Lindau-von Hippel (angiomatosis retinocerebellosa) 759.6
  - lip NEC 528.5

ICD-9-CM

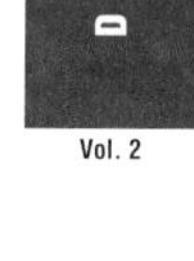

Vol. 2

◄ New   Revised

Disease, diseased *(Continued)*
lipidosis 272.7
lipoid storage NEC 272.7
Lipschütz's 616.50
Little's - *see* Palsy, cerebral
liver 573.9
alcoholic 571.3
acute 571.1
chronic 571.3
chronic 571.9
alcoholic 571.3
cystic, congenital 751.62
drug-induced 573.3
due to
chemicals 573.3
fluorinated agents 573.3
hypersensitivity drugs 573.3
isoniazids 573.3
fibrocystic (congenital) 751.62
glycogen storage 271.0
organic 573.9
polycystic (congenital) 751.62
Lobo's (keloid blastomycosis) 116.2
Lobstein's (brittle bones and blue sclera) 756.51
locomotor system 334.9
Lorain's (pituitary dwarfism) 253.3
Lou Gehrig's 335.20
Lucas-Championnière (fibrinous bronchitis) 466.0
Ludwig's (submaxillary cellulitis) 528.3
luetic - *see* Syphilis
lumbosacral region 724.6
lung NEC 518.89
black 500
congenital 748.60
cystic 518.89
congenital 748.4
fibroid (chronic) (*see also* Fibrosis, lung) 515
fluke 121.2
Oriental 121.2
in
amyloidosis 277.39 *[517.8]* (Revised)
polymyositis 710.4 *[517.8]*
sarcoidosis 135 *[517.8]*
Sjögren's syndrome 710.2 *[517.8]*
syphilis 095.1
systemic lupus erythematosus 710.0 *[517.8]*
systemic sclerosis 710.1 *[517.2]*
interstitial (chronic) 515
acute 136.3
nonspecific, chronic 496
obstructive (chronic) (COPD) 496
with
acute
bronchitis 491.22
exacerbation NEC 491.21
alveolitis, allergic (*see also* Alveolitis, allergic) 495.9
asthma (chronic) (obstructive) 493.2
bronchiectasis 494.0
with acute exacerbation 494.1
bronchitis (chronic) 491.20
with
acute bronchitis 491.22
exacerbation (acute) 491.21
decompensated 491.21 (New)
with exacerbation 491.21 (New)
emphysema NEC 492.8
diffuse (with fibrosis) 496

Disease, diseased *(Continued)*
lung NEC *(Continued)*
polycystic 518.89
asthma (chronic) (obstructive) 493.2
congenital 748.4
purulent (cavitary) 513.0
restrictive 518.89
rheumatoid 714.81
diffuse interstitial 714.81
specified NEC 518.89
Lutembacher's (atrial septal defect with mitral stenosis) 745.5
Lutz-Miescher (elastosis perforans serpiginosa) 701.1
Lutz-Splendore-de Almeida (Brazilian blastomycosis) 116.1
Lyell's (toxic epidermal necrolysis) 695.1
due to drug
correct substance properly administered 695.1
overdose or wrong substance given or taken 977.9
specific drug - *see* Table of Drugs and Chemicals
Lyme 088.81
lymphatic (gland) (system) 289.9
channel (noninfective) 457.9
vessel (noninfective) 457.9
specified NEC 457.8
lymphoproliferative (chronic) (M9970/1) 238.79 (Revised)
Machado-Joseph 334.8
Madelung's (lipomatosis) 272.8
Madura (actinomycotic) 039.9
mycotic 117.4
Magitot's 526.4
Majocchi's (purpura annularis telangiectodes) 709.1
malarial (*see also* Malaria) 084.6
Malassez's (cystic) 608.89
Malibu 919.8
infected 919.9
malignant (M8000/3) - *see also* Neoplasm, by site, malignant
previous, affecting management of pregnancy V23.89
Manson's 120.1
maple bark 495.6
maple syrup (urine) 270.3
Marburg (virus) 078.89
Marchiafava (-Bignami) 341.8
Marfan's 090.49
congenital syphilis 090.49
meaning Marfan's syndrome 759.82
Marie-Bamberger (hypertrophic pulmonary osteoarthropathy) (secondary) 731.2
primary or idiopathic (acropachyderma) 757.39
pulmonary (hypertrophic osteoarthropathy) 731.2
Marie-Strümpell (ankylosing spondylitis) 720.0
Marion's (bladder neck obstruction) 596.0
Marsh's (exophthalmic goiter) 242.0
Martin's 715.27
mast cell 757.33
systemic (M9741/3) 202.6
mastoid (*see also* Mastoiditis) 383.9
process 385.9
maternal, unrelated to pregnancy NEC, affecting fetus or newborn 760.9
Mathieu's (leptospiral jaundice) 100.0
Mauclaire's 732.3

Disease, diseased *(Continued)*
Mauriac's (erythema nodosum syphiliticum) 091.3
Maxcy's 081.0
McArdle (-Schmid-Pearson) (glycogenosis V) 271.0
mediastinum NEC 519.3
Medin's (*see also* Poliomyelitis) 045.9
Mediterranean (with hemoglobinopathy) 282.49
medullary center (idiopathic) (respiratory) 348.8
Meige's (chronic hereditary edema) 757.0
Meleda 757.39
Ménétrier's (hypertrophic gastritis) 535.2
Ménière's (active) 386.00
cochlear 386.02
cochleovestibular 386.01
inactive 386.04
in remission 386.04
vestibular 386.03
meningeal - *see* Meningitis
mental (*see also* Psychosis) 298.9
Merzbacher-Pelizaeus 330.0
mesenchymal 710.9
mesenteric embolic 557.0
metabolic NEC 277.9
metal polishers' 502
metastatic - *see* Metastasis
Mibelli's 757.39
microdrepanocytic 282.49
microvascular - *code to condition* (Revised)
Miescher's 709.3
Mikulicz's (dryness of mouth, absent or decreased lacrimation) 527.1
Milkman (-Looser) (osteomalacia with pseudofractures) 268.2
Miller's (osteomalacia) 268.2
Mills' 335.29
Milroy's (chronic hereditary edema) 757.0
Minamata 985.0
Minor's 336.1
Minot's (hemorrhagic disease, newborn) 776.0
Minot-von Willebrand-Jürgens (angiohemophilia) 286.4
Mitchell's (erythromelalgia) 443.82
mitral - *see* Endocarditis, mitral
Mljet (mal de Meleda) 757.39
Möbius', Moebius' 346.8
Möeller's 267
Möller (-Barlow) (infantile scurvy) 267
Mönckeberg's (*see also* Arteriosclerosis, extremities) 440.20
Mondor's (thrombophlebitis of breast) 451.89
Monge's 993.2
Morel-Kraepelin (*see also* Schizophrenia) 295.9
Morgagni's (syndrome) (hyperostosis frontalis interna) 733.3
Morgagni-Adams-Stokes (syncope with heart block) 426.9
Morquio (-Brailsford) (-Ullrich) (mucopolysaccharidosis IV) 277.5
Morton's (with metatarsalgia) 355.6
Morvan's 336.0
motor neuron (bulbar) (mixed type) 335.20
Mouchet's (juvenile osteochondrosis, foot) 732.5
mouth 528.9
Moyamoya 437.5

◀ New ⟸ Revised

Disease, diseased *(Continued)*
Mucha's (acute parapsoriasis varioliformis) 696.2
mu-chain 273.2
mucolipidosis (I) (II) (III) 272.7
Münchmeyer's (exostosis luxurians) 728.11
Murri's (intermittent hemoglobinuria) 283.2
muscle 359.9
inflammatory 728.9
ocular 378.9
musculoskeletal system 729.9
mushroom workers' 495.5
Myà's (congenital dilation, colon) 751.3
mycotic 117.9
myeloproliferative (chronic) (M9960/1) 238.79
myocardium, myocardial (*see also* Degeneration, myocardial) 429.1
hypertensive (*see also* Hypertension, heart) 402.90
primary (idiopathic) 425.4
myoneural 358.9
Naegeli's 287.1
nail 703.9
specified type NEC 703.8
Nairobi sheep 066.1
nasal 478.19
cavity NEC 478.19
sinus (chronic) - *see* Sinusitis
navel (newborn) NEC 779.89
delayed separation of umbilical cord 779.83
nemaline body 359.0
neoplastic, generalized (M8000/6) 199.0
nerve - *see* Disorder, nerve
nervous system (central) 349.9
autonomic, peripheral (*see also* Neuropathy, peripheral, autonomic) 337.9
congenital 742.9
inflammatory - *see* Encephalitis
parasympathetic (*see also* Neuropathy, peripheral, autonomic) 337.9
peripheral NEC 355.9
specified NEC 349.89
sympathetic (*see also* Neuropathy, peripheral, autonomic) 337.9
vegetative (*see also* Neuropathy, peripheral, autonomic) 337.9
Nettleship's (urticaria pigmentosa) 757.33
Neumann's (pemphigus vegetans) 694.4
neurologic (central) NEC (*see also* Disease, nervous system) 349.9
peripheral NEC 355.9
neuromuscular system NEC 358.9
Newcastle 077.8
Nicolas (-Durand) -Favre (climatic bubo) 099.1
Niemann-Pick (lipid histiocytosis) 272.7
nipple 611.9
Paget's (M8540/3) 174.0
Nishimoto (-Takeuchi) 437.5
nonarthropod-borne NEC 078.89
central nervous system NEC 049.9
enterovirus NEC 078.89
nonautoimmune hemolytic NEC 283.10
Nonne-Milroy-Meige (chronic hereditary edema) 757.0
Norrie's (congenital progressive oculoacousticocerebral degeneration) 743.8
nose 478.19

Disease, diseased *(Continued)*
nucleus pulposus - *see* Disease, intervertebral disc
nutritional 269.9
maternal, affecting fetus or newborn 760.4
oasthouse, urine 270.2
obliterative vascular 447.1
Odelberg's (juvenile osteochondrosis) 732.1
Oguchi's (retina) 368.61
Ohara's (*see also* Tularemia) 021.9
Ollier's (chondrodysplasia) 756.4
Opitz's (congestive splenomegaly) 289.51
Oppenheim's 358.8
Oppenheim-Urbach (necrobiosis lipoidica diabeticorum) 250.8 *[709.3]*
optic nerve NEC 377.49
orbit 376.9
specified NEC 376.89
Oriental liver fluke 121.1
Oriental lung fluke 121.2
Ormond's 593.4
Osgood's tibia (tubercle) 732.4
Osgood-Schlatter 732.4
Osler (-Vaquez) (polycythemia vera) (M9950/1) 238.4
Osler-Rendu (familial hemorrhagic telangiectasia) 448.0
osteofibrocystic 252.01
Otto's 715.35
outer ear 380.9
ovary (noninflammatory) NEC 620.9
cystic 620.2
polycystic 256.4
specified NEC 620.8
Owren's (congenital) (*see also* Defect, coagulation) 286.3
Paas' 756.59
Paget's (osteitis deformans) 731.0
with infiltrating duct carcinoma of the breast (M8541/3) - *see* Neoplasm, breast, malignant
bone 731.0
osteosarcoma in (M9184/3) - *see* Neoplasm, bone, malignant
breast (M8540/3) 174.0
extramammary (M8542/3) - *see also* Neoplasm, skin, malignant
anus 154.3
skin 173.5
malignant (M8540/3)
breast 174.0
specified site NEC (M8542/3) - *see* Neoplasm, skin, malignant
unspecified site 174.0
mammary (M8540/3) 174.0
nipple (M8540/3) 174.0
palate (soft) 528.9
Paltauf-Sternberg 201.9
pancreas 577.9
cystic 577.2
congenital 751.7
fibrocystic 277.00
Panner's 732.3
capitellum humeri 732.3
head of humerus 732.3
tarsal navicular (bone) (osteochondrosis) 732.5
panvalvular - *see* Endocarditis, mitral
parametrium 629.9
parasitic NEC 136.9
cerebral NEC 123.9
intestinal NEC 129

Disease, diseased *(Continued)*
parasitic NEC *(Continued)*
mouth 112.0
skin NEC 134.9
specified type - *see* Infestation
tongue 112.0
parathyroid (gland) 252.9
specified NEC 252.8
Parkinson's 332.0
parodontal 523.9
Parrot's (syphilitic osteochondritis) 090.0
Parry's (exophthalmic goiter) 242.0
Parson's (exophthalmic goiter) 242.0
Pavy's 593.6
Paxton's (white piedra) 111.2
Payr's (splenic flexure syndrome) 569.89
pearl-workers' (chronic osteomyelitis) (*see also* Osteomyelitis) 730.1
Pel-Ebstein - *see* Disease, Hodgkin's
Pelizaeus-Merzbacher 330.0
with dementia
with behavioral disturbance 330.0 *[294.11]*
without behavioral disturbance 330.0 *[294.10]*
Pellegrini-Stieda (calcification, knee joint) 726.62
pelvis, pelvic
female NEC 629.9
specified NEC 629.89
gonococcal (acute) 098.19
chronic or duration of 2 months or over 098.39
infection (*see also* Disease, pelvis, inflammatory) 614.9
inflammatory (female) (PID) 614.9
with
abortion - *see* Abortion, by type, with sepsis
ectopic pregnancy (*see also* categories 633.0–633.9) 639.0
molar pregnancy (*see also* categories 630–632) 639.0
acute 614.3
chronic 614.4
complicating pregnancy 646.6
affecting fetus or newborn 760.8
following
abortion 639.0
ectopic or molar pregnancy 639.0
peritonitis (acute) 614.5
chronic NEC 614.7
puerperal, postpartum, childbirth 670
specified NEC 614.8
organ, female NEC 629.9
specified NEC 629.89
peritoneum, female NEC 629.9
specified NEC 629.89
penis 607.9
inflammatory 607.2
peptic NEC 536.9
acid 536.8
periapical tissues NEC 522.9
pericardium 423.9
specified type NEC 423.8
perineum
female
inflammatory 616.9
specified NEC 616.89
noninflammatory 624.9
specified NEC 624.8
male (inflammatory) 682.2

ICD-9-CM D Vol. 2

Disease, diseased *(Continued)*
periodic (familial) (Reimann's) NEC 277.31
paralysis 359.3
periodontal NEC 523.9
specified NEC 523.8
periosteum 733.90
peripheral
arterial 443.9
autonomic nervous system (*see also* Neuropathy, autonomic) 337.9
nerve NEC (*see also* Neuropathy) 356.9
multiple - *see* Polyneuropathy
vascular 443.9
specified type NEC 443.89
peritoneum 568.9
pelvic, female 629.9
specified NEC 629.89
Perrin-Ferraton (snapping hip) 719.65
persistent mucosal (middle ear) (with posterior or superior marginal perforation of ear drum) 382.2
Perthes' (capital femoral osteochondrosis) 732.1
Petit's (*see also* Hernia, lumbar) 553.8
Peutz-Jeghers 759.6
Peyronie's 607.85
Pfeiffer's (infectious mononucleosis) 075
pharynx 478.20
Phocas' 610.1
photochromogenic (acid-fast bacilli) (pulmonary) 031.0
nonpulmonary 031.9
Pick's
brain 331.11
with dementia
with behavioral disturbance 331.11 *[294.11]*
without behavioral disturbance 331.11 *[294.10]*
cerebral atrophy 331.11
with dementia
with behavioral disturbance 331.11 *[294.11]*
without behavioral disturbance 331.11 *[294.10]*
lipid histiocytosis 272.7
liver (pericardial pseudocirrhosis of liver) 423.2
pericardium (pericardial pseudocirrhosis of liver) 423.2
polyserositis (pericardial pseudocirrhosis of liver) 423.2
Pierson's (osteochondrosis) 732.1
pigeon fanciers' or breeders' 495.2
pineal gland 259.8
pink 985.0
Pinkus' (lichen nitidus) 697.1
pinworm 127.4
pituitary (gland) 253.9
hyperfunction 253.1
hypofunction 253.2
pituitary snuff-takers' 495.8
placenta
affecting fetus or newborn 762.2
complicating pregnancy or childbirth 656.7
pleura (cavity) (*see also* Pleurisy) 511.0
Plummer's (toxic nodular goiter) 242.3
pneumatic
drill 994.9
hammer 994.9
policeman's 729.2

Disease, diseased *(Continued)*
Pollitzer's (hidradenitis suppurativa) 705.83
polycystic (congenital) 759.89
kidney or renal 753.12
adult type (APKD) 753.13
autosomal dominant 753.13
autosomal recessive 753.14
childhood type (CPKD) 753.14
infantile type 753.14
liver or hepatic 751.62
lung or pulmonary 518.89
congenital 748.4
ovary, ovaries 256.4
spleen 759.0
Pompe's (glycogenosis II) 271.0
Poncet's (tuberculous rheumatism) (*see also* Tuberculosis) 015.9
Posada-Wernicke 114.9
Potain's (pulmonary edema) 514
Pott's (*see also* Tuberculosis) 015.0 *[730.88]*
osteomyelitis 015.0 *[730.88]*
paraplegia 015.0 *[730.88]*
spinal curvature 015.0 *[737.43]*
spondylitis 015.0 *[720.81]*
Potter's 753.0
Poulet's 714.2
pregnancy NEC (*see also* Pregnancy) 646.9
Preiser's (osteoporosis) 733.09
Pringle's (tuberous sclerosis) 759.5
Profichet's 729.9
prostate 602.9
specified type NEC 602.8
protozoal NEC 136.8
intestine, intestinal NEC 007.9
pseudo-Hurler's (mucolipidosis III) 272.7
psychiatric (*see also* Psychosis) 298.9
psychotic (*see also* Psychosis) 298.9
Puente's (simple glandular cheilitis) 528.5
puerperal NEC (*see also* Puerperal) 674.9
pulmonary - *see also* Disease, lung
amyloid 277.39 *[517.8]*
artery 417.9
circulation, circulatory 417.9
specified NEC 417.8
diffuse obstructive (chronic) 496
with
acute bronchitis 491.22
asthma (chronic) (obstructive) 493.2
exacerbation NEC (acute) 491.21
heart (chronic) 416.9
specified NEC 416.8
hypertensive (vascular) 416.0
cardiovascular 416.0
obstructive diffuse (chronic) 496
with
acute bronchitis 491.22
asthma (chronic) (obstructive) 493.2
bronchitis (chronic) 491.20
with
exacerbation (acute) 491.21
acute 491.22
exacerbation NEC (acute) 491.21
decompensated 491.21
with exacerbation 491.21
valve (*see also* Endocarditis, pulmonary) 424.3
pulp (dental) NEC 522.9
pulseless 446.7
Putnam's (subacute combined sclerosis with pernicious anemia) 281.0 *[336.2]*

Disease, diseased *(Continued)*
Pyle (-Cohn) (craniometaphyseal dysplasia) 756.89
pyramidal tract 333.90
Quervain's
tendon sheath 727.04
thyroid (subacute granulomatous thyroiditis) 245.1
Quincke's - *see* Edema, angioneurotic
Quinquaud (acne decalvans) 704.09
rag sorters' 022.1
Raynaud's (paroxysmal digital cyanosis) 443.0
reactive airway - *see* Asthma
Recklinghausen's (M9540/1) 237.71
bone (osteitis fibrosa cystica) 252.01
Recklinghausen-Applebaum (hemochromatosis) 275.0
Reclus' (cystic) 610.1
rectum NEC 569.49
Refsum's (heredopathia atactica polyneuritiformis) 356.3
Reichmann's (gastrosuccorrhea) 536.8
Reimann's (periodic) 277.31
Reiter's 099.3
renal (functional) (pelvis) (*see also* Disease, kidney) 593.9
with
edema (*see also* Nephrosis) 581.9
exudative nephritis 583.89
lesion of interstitial nephritis 583.89
stated generalized cause - *see* Nephritis
acute 593.9
basement membrane NEC 583.89
with
pulmonary hemorrhage (Goodpasture's syndrome) 446.21 *[583.81]*
chronic (*see also* Disease, kidney, chronic) 585.9
complicating pregnancy or puerperium NEC 646.2
with hypertension - *see* Toxemia, of pregnancy
affecting fetus or newborn 760.1
cystic, congenital (*see also* Cystic, disease, kidney) 753.10
diabetic 250.4 *[583.81]*
due to
amyloidosis 277.39 *[583.81]*
diabetes mellitus 250.4 *[583.81]*
systemic lupus erythematosis 710.0 *[583.81]*
end-stage 585.6
exudative 583.89
fibrocystic (congenital) 753.19
gonococcal 098.19 *[583.81]*
gouty 274.10
hypertensive (*see also* Hypertension, kidney) 403.90
immune complex NEC 583.89
interstitial (diffuse) (focal) 583.89
lupus 710.0 *[583.81]*
maternal, affecting fetus or newborn 760.1
hypertensive 760.0
phosphate-losing (tubular) 588.0
polycystic (congenital) 753.12
adult type (APKD) 753.13
autosomal dominant 753.13
autosomal recessive 753.14
childhood type (CPKD) 753.14
infantile type 753.14

Disease, diseased *(Continued)*
renal *(Continued)*
specified lesion or cause NEC (*see also* Glomerulonephritis) 583.89
subacute 581.9
syphilitic 095.4
tuberculous (*see also* Tuberculosis) 016.0 *[583.81]*
tubular (*see also* Nephrosis, tubular) 584.5
Rendu-Osler-Weber (familial hemorrhagic telangiectasia) 448.0
renovascular (arteriosclerotic) (*see also* Hypertension, kidney) 403.90
respiratory (tract) 519.9
acute or subacute (upper) NEC 465.9
due to fumes or vapors 506.3
multiple sites NEC 465.8
noninfectious 478.9
streptococcal 034.0
chronic 519.9
arising in the perinatal period 770.7
due to fumes or vapors 506.4
due to
aspiration of liquids or solids 508.9
external agents NEC 508.9
specified NEC 508.8
fumes or vapors 506.9
acute or subacute NEC 506.3
chronic 506.4
fetus or newborn NEC 770.9
obstructive 496
specified type NEC 519.8
upper (acute) (infectious) NEC 465.9
multiple sites NEC 465.8
noninfectious NEC 478.9
streptococcal 034.0
retina, retinal NEC 362.9
Batten's or Batten-Mayou 330.1 *[362.71]*
degeneration 362.89
vascular lesion 362.17
rheumatic (*see also* Arthritis) 716.8
heart - *see* Disease, heart, rheumatic
rheumatoid (heart) - *see* Arthritis, rheumatoid
rickettsial NEC 083.9
specified type NEC 083.8
Riedel's (ligneous thyroiditis) 245.3
Riga (-Fede) (cachectic aphthae) 529.0
Riggs' (compound periodontitis) 523.40 ⬅
Ritter's 695.81
Rivalta's (cervicofacial actinomycosis) 039.3
Robles' (onchocerciasis) 125.3 *[360.13]*
Roger's (congenital interventricular septal defect) 745.4
Rokitansky's (*see also* Necrosis, liver) 570
Romberg's 349.89
Rosenthal's (factor XI deficiency) 286.2
Rossbach's (hyperchlorhydria) 536.8
psychogenic 306.4
Roth (-Bernhardt) 355.1
Runeberg's (progressive pernicious anemia) 281.0
Rust's (tuberculous spondylitis) (*see also* Tuberculosis) 015.0 *[720.81]*
Rustitskii's (multiple myeloma) (M9730/3) 203.0
Ruysch's (Hirschsprung's disease) 751.3
Sachs (-Tay) 330.1
sacroiliac NEC 724.6

Disease, diseased *(Continued)*
salivary gland or duct NEC 527.9
inclusion 078.5
streptococcal 034.0
virus 078.5
Sander's (paranoia) 297.1
Sandhoff's 330.1
sandworm 126.9
Savill's (epidemic exfoliative dermatitis) 695.89
Schamberg's (progressive pigmentary dermatosis) 709.09
Schaumann's (sarcoidosis) 135
Schenck's (sporotrichosis) 117.1
Scheuermann's (osteochondrosis) 732.0
Schilder (-Flatau) 341.1
Schimmelbusch's 610.1
Schlatter's tibia (tubercle) 732.4
Schlatter-Osgood 732.4
Schmorl's 722.30
cervical 722.39
lumbar, lumbosacral 722.32
specified region NEC 722.39
thoracic, thoracolumbar 722.31
Scholz's 330.0
Schönlein (-Henoch) (purpura rheumatica) 287.0
Schottmüller's (*see also* Fever, paratyphoid) 002.9
Schüller-Christian (chronic histiocytosis X) 277.89
Schultz's (agranulocytosis) 288.09 ⬅
Schwalbe-Ziehen-Oppenheimer 333.6
Schweninger-Buzzi (macular atrophy) 701.3
sclera 379.19
scrofulous (*see also* Tuberculosis) 017.2
scrotum 608.9
sebaceous glands NEC 706.9
Secretan's (posttraumatic edema) 782.3
semilunar cartilage, cystic 717.5
seminal vesicle 608.9
Senear-Usher (pemphigus erythematosus) 694.4
serum NEC 999.5
Sever's (osteochondrosis calcaneum) 732.5
Sézary's (reticulosis) (M9701/3) 202.2
Shaver's (bauxite pneumoconiosis) 503
Sheehan's (postpartum pituitary necrosis) 253.2
shimamushi (scrub typhus) 081.2
shipyard 077.1
sickle-cell 282.60
with
crisis 282.62
Hb-S disease 282.61
other abnormal hemoglobin (Hb-D) (Hb-E) (Hb-G) (Hb-J) (Hb-K) (Hb-O) (Hb-P) (high fetal gene) (without crisis) 282.68
with crisis 282.69
elliptocytosis 282.60
Hb-C (without crisis) 282.63
with
crisis 282.64
vaso-occlusive pain 282.64
Hb-S 282.61
with
crisis 282.62
Hb-C (without crisis) 282.63
with
crisis 282.64
vaso-occlusive pain 282.64

Disease, diseased *(Continued)*
sickle-cell *(Continued)*
Hb-S *(Continued)*
with *(Continued)*
other abnormal hemoglobin (Hb-D) (Hb-E) (Hb-G) (Hb-J) (Hb-K) (Hb-O) (Hb-P) (high fetal gene) (without crisis) 282.68
with crisis 282.69
spherocytosis 282.60
thalassemia (without crisis) 282.41
with
crisis 282.42
vaso-occlusive pain 282.42
Siegal-Cattan-Mamou (periodic) 277.31 ⬅
silo fillers' 506.9
Simian B 054.3
Simmonds' (pituitary cachexia) 253.2
Simons' (progressive lipodystrophy) 272.6
Sinding-Larsen (juvenile osteopathia patellae) 732.4
sinus - *see also* Sinusitis
brain 437.9
specified NEC 478.19 ⬅
Sirkari's 085.0
sixth 057.8
Sjögren (-Gougerot) 710.2
with lung involvement 710.2 *[517.8]*
Skevas-Zerfus 989.5
skin NEC 709.9
due to metabolic disorder 277.9
specified type NEC 709.8
sleeping (*see also* Narcolepsy) 347.00
meaning sleeping sickness (*see also* Trypanosomiasis) 086.5
small vessel 443.9
Smith-Strang (oasthouse urine) 270.2
Sneddon-Wilkinson (subcorneal pustular dermatosis) 694.1
South African creeping 133.8
Spencer's (epidemic vomiting) 078.82
Spielmeyer-Stock 330.1
Spielmeyer-Vogt 330.1
spine, spinal 733.90
combined system (*see also* Degeneration, combined) 266.2 *[336.2]*
with pernicious anemia 281.0 *[336.2]*
cord NEC 336.9
congenital 742.9
demyelinating NEC 341.8
joint (*see also* Disease, joint, spine) 724.9
tuberculous 015.0 *[730.8]*
spinocerebellar 334.9
specified NEC 334.8
spleen (organic) (postinfectional) 289.50
amyloid 277.39 ⬅
lardaceous 277.39 ⬅
polycystic 759.0
specified NEC 289.59
sponge divers' 989.5
Stanton's (melioidosis) 025
Stargardt's 362.75
Startle 759.89
Steinert's 359.2
Sternberg's - *see* Disease, Hodgkin's
Stevens-Johnson (erythema multiforme exudativum) 695.1
Sticker's (erythema infectiosum) 057.0
Stieda's (calcification, knee joint) 726.62
Still's (juvenile rheumatoid arthritis) 714.30

Disease, diseased *(Continued)*
Stiller's (asthenia) 780.79
Stokes' (exophthalmic goiter) 242.0
Stokes-Adams (syncope with heart block) 426.9
Stokvis (-Talma) (enterogenous cyanosis) 289.7
stomach NEC (organic) 537.9
functional 536.9
psychogenic 306.4
lardaceous 277.39 ⬅
stonemasons' 502
storage
glycogen (*see also* Disease, glycogen storage) 271.0
lipid 272.7
mucopolysaccharide 277.5
striatopallidal system 333.90
specified NEC 333.89
Strümpell-Marie (ankylosing spondylitis) 720.0
Stuart's (congenital factor X deficiency) (*see also* Defect, coagulation) 286.3
Stuart-Prower (congenital factor X deficiency) (*see also* Defect, coagulation) 286.3
Sturge (-Weber) (-Dimitri) (encephalocutaneous angiomatosis) 759.6
Stuttgart 100.89
Sudeck's 733.7
supporting structures of teeth NEC 525.9
suprarenal (gland) (capsule) 255.9
hyperfunction 255.3
hypofunction 255.4
Sutton's 709.09
Sutton and Gull's - *see* Hypertension, kidney
sweat glands NEC 705.9
specified type NEC 705.89
sweating 078.2
Sweeley-Klionsky 272.4
Swift (-Feer) 985.0
swimming pool (bacillus) 031.1
swineherd's 100.89
Sylvest's (epidemic pleurodynia) 074.1
Symmers (follicular lymphoma) (M9690/3) 202.0
sympathetic nervous system (*see also* Neuropathy, peripheral, autonomic) 337.9
synovium 727.9
syphilitic - *see* Syphilis
systemic tissue mast cell (M9741/3) 202.6
Taenzer's 757.4
Takayasu's (pulseless) 446.7
Talma's 728.85
Tangier (familial high-density lipoprotein deficiency) 272.5
Tarral-Besnier (pityriasis rubra pilaris) 696.4
Tay-Sachs 330.1
Taylor's 701.8
tear duct 375.69
teeth, tooth 525.9
hard tissues 521.9 ⬅
specified NEC 521.89 ◀
pulp NEC 522.9
tendon 727.9
inflammatory NEC 727.9
terminal vessel 443.9
testis 608.9
Thaysen-Gee (nontropical sprue) 579.0
Thomsen's 359.2

Disease, diseased *(Continued)*
Thomson's (congenital poikiloderma) 757.33
Thornwaldt's, Tornwaldt's (pharyngeal bursitis) 478.29
throat 478.20
septic 034.0
thromboembolic (*see also* Embolism) 444.9
thymus (gland) 254.9
specified NEC 254.8
thyroid (gland) NEC 246.9
heart (*see also* Hyperthyroidism) 242.9 *[425.7]*
lardaceous 277.39 ⬅
specified NEC 246.8
Tietze's 733.6
Tommaselli's
correct substance properly administered 599.7
overdose or wrong substance given or taken 961.4
tongue 529.9
tonsils, tonsillar (and adenoids) (chronic) 474.9
specified NEC 474.8
tooth, teeth 525.9
hard tissues 521.9 ⬅
specified NEC 521.89 ◀
pulp NEC 522.9
Tornwaldt's (pharyngeal bursitis) 478.29
Tourette's 307.23
trachea 519.19 ⬅
tricuspid - *see* Endocarditis, tricuspid
triglyceride-storage, type I, II, III 272.7
triple vessel - *see* Arteriosclerosis, coronary
trisymptomatic, Gougerot's 709.1
trophoblastic (*see also* Hydatidiform mole) 630
previous, affecting management of pregnancy V23.1
tsutsugamushi (scrub typhus) 081.2
tube (fallopian), noninflammatory 620.9
specified NEC 620.8
tuberculous NEC (*see also* Tuberculosis) 011.9
tubo-ovarian
inflammatory (*see also* Salpingo-oophoritis) 614.2
noninflammatory 620.9
specified NEC 620.8
tubotympanic, chronic (with anterior perforation of ear drum) 382.1
tympanum 385.9
Uhl's 746.84
umbilicus (newborn) NEC 779.89
delayed separation 779.83
Underwood's (sclerema neonatorum) 778.1
undiagnosed 799.9
Unna's (seborrheic dermatitis) 690.18
unstable hemoglobin hemolytic 282.7
Unverricht (-Lundborg) 333.2
Urbach-Oppenheim (necrobiosis lipoidica diabeticorum) 250.8 *[709.3]*
Urbach-Wiethe (lipoid proteinosis) 272.8
ureter 593.9
urethra 599.9
specified type NEC 599.84
urinary (tract) 599.9
bladder 596.9
specified NEC 596.8
maternal, affecting fetus or newborn 760.1

Disease, diseased *(Continued)*
Usher-Senear (pemphigus erythematosus) 694.4
uterus (organic) 621.9
infective (*see also* Endometritis) 615.9
inflammatory (*see also* Endometritis) 615.9
noninflammatory 621.9
specified type NEC 621.8
uveal tract
anterior 364.9
posterior 363.9
vagabonds' 132.1
vagina, vaginal
inflammatory 616.9
specified NEC 616.89 ⬅
noninflammatory 623.9
specified NEC 623.8
Valsuani's (progressive pernicious anemia, puerperal) 648.2
complicating pregnancy or puerperium 648.2
valve, valvular - *see* Endocarditis
van Bogaert-Nijssen (-Peiffer) 330.0
van Creveld-von Gierke (glycogenosis I) 271.0
van den Bergh's (enterogenous cyanosis) 289.7
van Neck's (juvenile osteochondrosis) 732.1
Vaquez (-Osler) (polycythemia vera) (M9950/1) 238.4
vascular 459.9
arteriosclerotic - *see* Arteriosclerosis
hypertensive - *see* Hypertension
obliterative 447.1
peripheral 443.9
occlusive 459.9
peripheral (occlusive) 443.9
in diabetes mellitus 250.7 *[443.81]*
specified type NEC 443.89
vas deferens 608.9
vasomotor 443.9
vasospastic 443.9
vein 459.9
venereal 099.9
chlamydial NEC 099.50
anus 099.52
bladder 099.53
cervix 099.53
epididymis 099.54
genitourinary NEC 099.55
lower 099.53
specified NEC 099.54
pelvic inflammatory disease 099.54
perihepatic 099.56
peritoneum 099.56
pharynx 099.51
rectum 099.52
specified site NEC 099.59
testis 099.54
vagina 099.53
vulva 099.53
fifth 099.1
sixth 099.1
complicating pregnancy, childbirth, or puerperium 647.2
specified nature or type NEC 099.8
chlamydial - *see* Disease, venereal, chlamydial
Verneuil's (syphilitic bursitis) 095.7
Verse's (calcinosis intervertebralis) 275.49 *[722.90]*

Disease, diseased *(Continued)*
vertebra, vertebral NEC 733.90
disc - *see* Disease, Intervertebral disc
vibration NEC 994.9
Vidal's (lichen simplex chronicus) 698.3
Vincent's (trench mouth) 101
Virchow's 733.99
virus (filterable) NEC 078.89
arbovirus NEC 066.9
arthropod-borne NEC 066.9
central nervous system NEC 049.9
specified type NEC 049.8
complicating pregnancy, childbirth, or puerperium 647.6
contact (with) V01.79
varicella V01.71
exposure to V01.79
varicella V01.71
Marburg 078.89
maternal
with fetal damage affecting management of pregnancy 655.3
nonarthropod-borne NEC 078.89
central nervous system NEC 049.9
specified NEC 049.8
vaccination, prophylactic (against) V04.89
vitreous 379.29
vocal cords NEC 478.5
Vogt's (Cecile) 333.71
Vogt-Spielmeyer 330.1
Volhard-Fahr (malignant nephrosclerosis) 403.00
Volkmann's
acquired 958.6
von Bechterew's (ankylosing spondylitis) 720.0
von Economo's (encephalitis lethargica) 049.8
von Eulenburg's (congenital paramyotonia) 359.2
von Gierke's (glycogenosis I) 271.0
von Graefe's 378.72
von Hippel's (retinocerebral angiomatosis) 759.6
von Hippel-Lindau (angiomatosis retinocerebellosa) 759.6
von Jaksch's (pseudoleukemia infantum) 285.8
von Recklinghausen's (M9540/1) 237.71
bone (osteitis fibrosa cystica) 252.01
von Recklinghausen-Applebaum (hemochromatosis) 275.0
von Willebrand (-Jürgens) (angiohemophilia) 286.4
von Zambusch's (lichen sclerosus et atrophicus) 701.0
Voorhoeve's (dyschondroplasia) 756.4
Vrolik's (osteogenesis imperfecta) 756.51
vulva
inflammatory 616.9
specified NEC 616.89
noninflammatory 624.9
specified NEC 624.8
Wagner's (colloid milium) 709.3
Waldenström's (osteochondrosis capital femoral) 732.1
Wallgren's (obstruction of splenic vein with collateral circulation) 459.89
Wardrop's (with lymphangitis) 681.9
finger 681.02
toe 681.11

Disease, diseased *(Continued)*
Wassilieff's (leptospiral jaundice) 100.0
wasting NEC 799.4
due to malnutrition 261
paralysis 335.21
Waterhouse-Friderichsen 036.3
waxy (any site) 277.39
Weber-Christian (nodular nonsuppurative panniculitis) 729.30
Wegner's (syphilitic osteochondritis) 090.0
Weil's (leptospiral jaundice) 100.0
of lung 100.0
Weir Mitchell's (erythromelalgia) 443.82
Werdnig-Hoffmann 335.0
Werlhof's (*see also* Purpura, thrombocytopenic) 287.39
Wermer's 258.0
Werner's (progeria adultorum) 259.8
Werner-His (trench fever) 083.1
Werner-Schultz (agranulocytosis) 288.09
Wernicke's (superior hemorrhagic polioencephalitis) 265.1
Wernicke-Posadas 114.9
Whipple's (intestinal lipodystrophy) 040.2
whipworm 127.3
white
blood cell 288.9
specified NEC 288.8
spot 701.0
White's (congenital) (keratosis follicularis) 757.39
Whitmore's (melioidosis) 025
Widal-Abrami (acquired hemolytic jaundice) 283.9
Wilkie's 557.1
Wilkinson-Sneddon (subcorneal pustular dermatosis) 694.1
Willis' (diabetes mellitus) (*see also* Diabetes) 250.0
Wilson's (hepatolenticular degeneration) 275.1
Wilson-Brocq (dermatitis exfoliativa) 695.89
winter vomiting 078.82
Wise's 696.2
Wohlfart-Kugelberg-Welander 335.11
Woillez's (acute idiopathic pulmonary congestion) 518.5
Wolman's (primary familial xanthomatosis) 272.7
wool-sorters' 022.1
Zagari's (xerostomia) 527.7
Zahorsky's (exanthem subitum) 057.8
Ziehen-Oppenheim 333.6
zoonotic, bacterial NEC 027.9
specified type NEC 027.8
Disfigurement (due to scar) 709.2
head V48.6
limb V49.4
neck V48.7
trunk V48.7
Disgerminoma - *see* Dysgerminoma
Disinsertion, retina 361.04
Disintegration, complete, of the body 799.89
traumatic 869.1
Disk kidney 753.3
Dislocatable hip, congenital (*see also* Dislocation, hip, congenital) 754.30

Dislocation (articulation) (closed) (displacement) (simple) (subluxation) 839.8

> Note
>
> "Closed" includes simple, complete, partial, uncomplicated, and unspecified dislocation.
>
> "Open" includes dislocation specified as infected or compound and dislocation with foreign body.
>
> "Chronic," "habitual," "old," or "recurrent" dislocations should be coded as indicated under the entry "Dislocation, recurrent"; and "pathological" as indicated under the entry "Dislocation, pathological."
>
> For late effect of dislocation see Late, effect, dislocation.

with fracture - *see* Fracture, by site
acromioclavicular (joint) (closed) 831.04
open 831.14
anatomical site (closed)
specified NEC 839.69
open 839.79
unspecified or ill-defined 839.8
open 839.9
ankle (scaphoid bone) (closed) 837.0
open 837.1
arm (closed) 839.8
open 839.9
astragalus (closed) 837.0
open 837.1
atlanto-axial (closed) 839.01
open 839.11
atlas (closed) 839.01
open 839.11
axis (closed) 839.02
open 839.12
back (closed) 839.8
open 839.9
Bell-Dally 723.8
breast bone (closed) 839.61
open 839.71
capsule, joint - *see* Dislocation, by site
carpal (bone) - *see* Dislocation, wrist
carpometacarpal (joint) (closed) 833.04
open 833.14
cartilage (joint) - *see also* Dislocation, by site
knee - *see* Tear, meniscus
cervical, cervicodorsal, or cervicothoracic (spine) (vertebra) - *see* Dislocation, vertebra, cervical
chiropractic (*see also* Lesion, nonallopathic) 739.9
chondrocostal - *see* Dislocation, costochondral
chronic - *see* Dislocation, recurrent
clavicle (closed) 831.04
open 831.14
coccyx (closed) 839.41
open 839.51
collar bone (closed) 831.04
open 831.14
compound (open) NEC 839.9
congenital NEC 755.8
hip (*see also* Dislocation, hip, congenital) 754.30
lens 743.37
rib 756.3

ICD-9-CM D Vol. 2

Dislocation *(Continued)*
congenital NEC *(Continued)*
sacroiliac 755.69
spine NEC 756.19
vertebra 756.19
coracoid (closed) 831.09
open 831.19
costal cartilage (closed) 839.69
open 839.79
costochondral (closed) 839.69
open 839.79
cricoarytenoid articulation (closed) 839.69
open 839.79
cricothyroid (cartilage) articulation (closed) 839.69
open 839.79
dorsal vertebrae (closed) 839.21
open 839.31
ear ossicle 385.23
elbow (closed) 832.00
anterior (closed) 832.01
open 832.11
congenital 754.89
divergent (closed) 832.09
open 832.19
lateral (closed) 832.04
open 832.14
medial (closed) 832.03
open 832.13
open 832.10
posterior (closed) 832.02
open 832.12
recurrent 718.32
specified type NEC 832.09
open 832.19
eye 360.81
lateral 376.36
eyeball 360.81
lateral 376.36
femur
distal end (closed) 836.50
anterior 836.52
open 836.62
lateral 836.53
open 836.63
medial 836.54
open 836.64
open 836.60
posterior 836.51
open 836.61
proximal end (closed) 835.00
anterior (pubic) 835.03
open 835.13
obturator 835.02
open 835.12
open 835.10
posterior 835.01
open 835.11
fibula
distal end (closed) 837.0
open 837.1
proximal end (closed) 836.59
open 836.69
finger(s) (phalanx) (thumb) (closed) 834.00
interphalangeal (joint) 834.02
open 834.12
metacarpal (bone), distal end 834.01
open 834.11
metacarpophalangeal (joint) 834.01
open 834.11
open 834.10
recurrent 718.34

Dislocation *(Continued)*
foot (closed) 838.00
open 838.10
recurrent 718.37
forearm (closed) 839.8
open 839.9
fracture - *see* Fracture, by site
glenoid (closed) 831.09
open 831.19
habitual - *see* Dislocation, recurrent
hand (closed) 839.8
open 839.9
hip (closed) 835.00
anterior 835.03
obturator 835.02
open 835.12
open 835.13
congenital (unilateral) 754.30
with subluxation of other hip 754.35
bilateral 754.31
developmental 718.75
open 835.10
posterior 835.01
open 835.11
recurrent 718.35
humerus (closed) 831.00
distal end (*see also* Dislocation, elbow) 832.00
open 831.10
proximal end (closed) 831.00
anterior (subclavicular) (subcoracoid) (subglenoid) (closed) 831.01
open 831.11
inferior (closed) 831.03
open 831.13
open 831.10
posterior (closed) 831.02
open 831.12
implant - *see* Complications, mechanical
incus 385.23
infracoracoid (closed) 831.01
open 831.11
innominate (pubic junction) (sacral junction) (closed) 839.69
acetabulum (*see also* Dislocation, hip) 835.00
open 839.79
interphalangeal (joint)
finger or hand (closed) 834.02
open 834.12
foot or toe (closed) 838.06
open 838.16
jaw (cartilage) (meniscus) (closed) 830.0
open 830.1
recurrent 524.69
joint NEC (closed) 839.8
developmental 718.7
open 839.9
pathological - *see* Dislocation, pathological
recurrent - *see* Dislocation, recurrent
knee (closed) 836.50
anterior 836.51
open 836.61
congenital (with genu recurvatum) 754.41
habitual 718.36
lateral 836.54
open 836.64
medial 836.53
open 836.63
old 718.36

Dislocation *(Continued)*
knee *(Continued)*
open 836.60
posterior 836.52
open 836.62
recurrent 718.36
rotatory 836.59
open 836.69
lacrimal gland 375.16
leg (closed) 839.8
open 839.9
lens (crystalline) (complete) (partial) 379.32
anterior 379.33
congenital 743.37
ocular implant 996.53
posterior 379.34
traumatic 921.3
ligament - *see* Dislocation, by site
lumbar (vertebrae) (closed) 839.20
open 839.30
lumbosacral (vertebrae) (closed) 839.20
congenital 756.19
open 839.30
mandible (closed) 830.0
open 830.1
maxilla (inferior) (closed) 830.0
open 830.1
meniscus (knee) - *see also* Tear, meniscus
other sites - *see* Dislocation, by site
metacarpal (bone)
distal end (closed) 834.01
open 834.11
proximal end (closed) 833.05
open 833.15
metacarpophalangeal (joint) (closed) 834.01
open 834.11
metatarsal (bone) (closed) 838.04
open 838.14
metatarsophalangeal (joint) (closed) 838.05
open 838.15
midcarpal (joint) (closed) 833.03
open 833.13
midtarsal (joint) (closed) 838.02
open 838.12
Monteggia's - *see* Dislocation, hip
multiple locations (except fingers only or toes only) (closed) 839.8
open 839.9
navicular (bone) foot (closed) 837.0
open 837.1
neck (*see also* Dislocation, vertebra, cervical) 839.00
Nélaton's - *see* Dislocation, ankle
nontraumatic (joint) - *see* Dislocation, pathological
nose (closed) 839.69
open 839.79
not recurrent, not current injury - *see* Dislocation, pathological
occiput from atlas (closed) 839.01
open 839.11
old - *see* Dislocation, recurrent
open (compound) NEC 839.9
ossicle, ear 385.23
paralytic (flaccid) (spastic) - *see* Dislocation, pathological
patella (closed) 836.3
congenital 755.64
open 836.4

Dislocation *(Continued)*
- pathological NEC 718.20
  - ankle 718.27
  - elbow 718.22
  - foot 718.27
  - hand 718.24
  - hip 718.25
  - knee 718.26
  - lumbosacral joint 724.6
  - multiple sites 718.29
  - pelvic region 718.25
  - sacroiliac 724.6
  - shoulder (region) 718.21
  - specified site NEC 718.28
  - spine 724.8
    - sacroiliac 724.6
  - wrist 718.23
- pelvis (closed) 839.69
  - acetabulum (*see also* Dislocation, hip) 835.00
  - open 839.79
- phalanx
  - foot or toe (closed) 838.09
    - open 838.19
  - hand or finger (*see also* Dislocation, finger) 834.00
- postpoliomyelitic - *see* Dislocation, pathological
- prosthesis, internal - *see* Complications, mechanical
- radiocarpal (joint) (closed) 833.02
  - open 833.12
- radioulnar (joint)
  - distal end (closed) 833.01
    - open 833.11
  - proximal end (*see also* Dislocation, elbow) 832.00
- radius
  - distal end (closed) 833.00
    - open 833.10
  - proximal end (closed) 832.01
    - open 832.11
- recurrent (*see also* Derangement, joint, recurrent) 718.3
  - elbow 718.32
  - hip 718.35
  - joint NEC 718.38
  - knee 718.36
  - lumbosacral (joint) 724.6
  - patella 718.36
  - sacroiliac 724.6
  - shoulder 718.31
  - temporomandibular 524.69
- rib (cartilage) (closed) 839.69
  - congenital 756.3
  - open 839.79
- sacrococcygeal (closed) 839.42
  - open 839.52
- sacroiliac (joint) (ligament) (closed) 839.42
  - congenital 755.69
  - open 839.52
  - recurrent 724.6
- sacrum (closed) 839.42
  - open 839.52
- scaphoid (bone)
  - ankle or foot (closed) 837.0
    - open 837.1
  - wrist (closed) (*see also* Dislocation, wrist) 833.00
    - open 833.10
- scapula (closed) 831.09
  - open 831.19
- semilunar cartilage, knee - *see* Tear, meniscus

Dislocation *(Continued)*
- septal cartilage (nose) (closed) 839.69
  - open 839.79
- septum (nasal) (old) 470
- sesamoid bone - *see* Dislocation, by site
- shoulder (blade) (ligament) (closed) 831.00
  - anterior (subclavicular) (subcoracoid) (subglenoid) (closed) 831.01
    - open 831.11
  - chronic 718.31
  - inferior 831.03
    - open 831.13
  - open 831.10
  - posterior (closed) 831.02
    - open 831.12
  - recurrent 718.31
- skull - *see* Injury, intracranial
- Smith's - *see* Dislocation, foot
- spine (articular process) (*see also* Dislocation, vertebra) (closed) 839.40
  - atlanto-axial (closed) 839.01
    - open 839.11
    - recurrent 723.8
  - cervical, cervicodorsal, cervicothoracic (closed) (*see also* Dislocation, vertebrae, cervical) 839.00
    - open 839.10
    - recurrent 723.8
  - coccyx 839.41
    - open 839.51
  - congenital 756.19
  - due to birth trauma 767.4
  - open 839.50
  - recurrent 724.9
  - sacroiliac 839.42
    - recurrent 724.6
  - sacrum (sacrococcygeal) (sacroiliac) 839.42
    - open 839.52
- spontaneous - *see* Dislocation, pathological
- sternoclavicular (joint) (closed) 839.61
  - open 839.71
- sternum (closed) 839.61
  - open 839.71
- subastragalar - *see* Dislocation, foot
- subglenoid (closed) 831.01
  - open 831.11
- symphysis
  - jaw (closed) 830.0
    - open 830.1
  - mandibular (closed) 830.0
    - open 830.1
  - pubis (closed) 839.69
    - open 839.79
- tarsal (bone) (joint) 838.01
  - open 838.11
- tarsometatarsal (joint) 838.03
  - open 838.13
- temporomandibular (joint) (closed) 830.0
  - open 830.1
  - recurrent 524.69
- thigh
  - distal end (*see also* Dislocation, femur, distal end) 836.50
  - proximal end (*see also* Dislocation, hip) 835.00
- thoracic (vertebrae) (closed) 839.21
  - open 839.31
- thumb(s) (*see also* Dislocation, finger) 834.00
- thyroid cartilage (closed) 839.69
  - open 839.79

Dislocation *(Continued)*
- tibia
  - distal end (closed) 837.0
    - open 837.1
  - proximal end (closed) 836.50
    - anterior 836.51
      - open 836.61
    - lateral 836.54
      - open 836.64
    - medial 836.53
      - open 836.63
    - open 836.60
    - posterior 836.52
      - open 836.62
    - rotatory 836.59
      - open 836.69
- tibiofibular
  - distal (closed) 837.0
    - open 837.1
  - superior (closed) 836.59
    - open 836.69
- toe(s) (closed) 838.09
  - open 838.19
- trachea (closed) 839.69
  - open 839.79
- ulna
  - distal end (closed) 833.09
    - open 833.19
  - proximal end - *see* Dislocation, elbow
- vertebra (articular process) (body) (closed) (traumatic) 839.40 ⬅
  - cervical, cervicodorsal or cervicothoracic (closed) 839.00
    - first (atlas) 839.01
      - open 839.11
    - second (axis) 839.02
      - open 839.12
    - third 839.03
      - open 839.13
    - fourth 839.04
      - open 839.14
    - fifth 839.05
      - open 839.15
    - sixth 839.06
      - open 839.16
    - seventh 839.07
      - open 839.17
    - congenital 756.19
    - multiple sites 839.08
      - open 839.18
    - open 839.10
  - congenital 756.19
  - dorsal 839.21
    - open 839.31
    - recurrent 724.9
  - lumbar, lumbosacral 839.20
    - open 839.30
  - non-traumatic - *see* Displacement, intervertebral disc ◀
  - open NEC 839.50
  - recurrent 724.9
  - specified region NEC 839.49
    - open 839.59
  - thoracic 839.21
    - open 839.31
- wrist (carpal bone) (scaphoid) (semilunar) (closed) 833.00
  - carpometacarpal (joint) 833.04
    - open 833.14
  - metacarpal bone, proximal end 833.05
    - open 833.15
  - midcarpal (joint) 833.03
    - open 833.13
  - open 833.10

ICD-9-CM D Vol. 2

Dislocation *(Continued)*
wrist *(Continued)*
radiocarpal (joint) 833.02
open 833.12
radioulnar (joint) 833.01
open 833.11
recurrent 718.33
specified site NEC 833.09
open 833.19
xiphoid cartilage (closed) 839.61
open 839.71
Dislodgement
artificial skin graft 996.55
decellularized allodermis graft 996.55
Disobedience, hostile (covert) (overt) (*see also* Disturbance, conduct) 312.0
Disorder - *see also* Disease
academic underachievement, childhood and adolescence 313.83
accommodation 367.51
drug-induced 367.89
toxic 367.89
adjustment (*see also* Reaction, adjustment) 309.8
with
anxiety 309.24
anxiety and depressed mood 309.28
depressed mood 309.0
disturbance of conduct 309.3
disturbance of emotions and conduct 309.4
adrenal (capsule) (cortex) (gland) 255.9
specified type NEC 255.8
adrenogenital 255.2
affective (*see also* Psychosis, affective) 296.90
atypical 296.81
aggressive, unsocialized (*see also* Disturbance, conduct) 312.0
alcohol, alcoholic (*see also* Alcohol) 291.9
allergic - *see* Allergy
amino acid (metabolic) (*see also* Disturbance, metabolism, amino acid) 270.9
albinism 270.2
alkaptonuria 270.2
argininosuccinicaciduria 270.6
beta-amino-isobutyricaciduria 277.2
cystathioninuria 270.4
cystinosis 270.0
cystinuria 270.0
glycinuria 270.0
homocystinuria 270.4
imidazole 270.5
maple syrup (urine) disease 270.3
neonatal, transitory 775.89 ⇐
oasthouse urine disease 270.2
ochronosis 270.2
phenylketonuria 270.1
phenylpyruvic oligophrenia 270.1
purine NEC 277.2
pyrimidine NEC 277.2
renal transport NEC 270.0
specified type NEC 270.8
transport NEC 270.0
renal 270.0
xanthinuria 277.2
amnestic (*see also* Amnestic syndrome) 294.8
alcohol-induced persisting 291.1
drug-induced persisting 292.83
in conditions classified elsewhere 294.0
anaerobic glycolysis with anemia 282.3

Disorder *(Continued)*
anxiety (*see also* Anxiety) 300.00
due to or associated with physical condition 293.84
arteriole 447.9
specified type NEC 447.8
artery 447.9
specified type NEC 447.8
articulation - *see* Disorder, joint
Asperger's 299.8
attachment of infancy or early childhood 313.89
attention deficit 314.00
with hyperactivity 314.01
predominantly
combined hyperactive/inattentive 314.01
hyperactive/impulsive 314.01
inattentive 314.00
residual type 314.8
autistic 299.0
autoimmune NEC 279.4
hemolytic (cold type) (warm type) 283.0
parathyroid 252.1
thyroid 245.2
avoidant, childhood or adolescence 313.21
balance
acid-base 276.9
mixed (with hypercapnia) 276.4
electrolyte 276.9
fluid 276.9
behavior NEC (*see also* Disturbance, conduct) 312.9
disruptive 312.9
bilirubin excretion 277.4
bipolar (affective) (alternating) 296.80

Note Use the following fifth-digit subclassification with categories 296.0–296.6:

0 unspecified
1 mild
2 moderate
3 severe, without mention of psychotic behavior
4 severe, specified as with psychotic behavior
5 in partial or unspecified remission
6 in full remission

atypical 296.7
specified type NEC 296.89
type I 296.7
most recent episode (or current)
depressed 296.5
hypomanic 296.4
manic 296.4
mixed 296.6
unspecified 296.7
single manic episode 296.0
type II (recurrent major depressive episodes with hypomania) 296.89
bladder 596.9
functional NEC 596.59
specified NEC 596.8
bone NEC 733.90
specified NEC 733.99
brachial plexus 353.0
branched-chain amino-acid degradation 270.3

Disorder *(Continued)*
breast 611.9
puerperal, postpartum 676.3
specified NEC 611.8
Briquet's 300.81
bursa 727.9
shoulder region 726.10
carbohydrate metabolism, congenital 271.9
cardiac, functional 427.9
postoperative 997.1
psychogenic 306.2
cardiovascular, psychogenic 306.2
cartilage NEC 733.90
articular 718.00
ankle 718.07
elbow 718.02
foot 718.07
hand 718.04
hip 718.05
knee 717.9
multiple sites 718.09
pelvic region 718.05
shoulder region 718.01
specified
site NEC 718.08
type NEC 733.99
wrist 718.03
catatonic - *see* Catatonia
central auditory processing 315.32
cervical region NEC 723.9
cervical root (nerve) NEC 353.2
congenital
glycosylation (CDG) 271.8
character NEC (*see also* Disorder, personality) 301.9
coagulation (factor) (*see also* Defect, coagulation) 286.9
factor VIII (congenital) (functional) 286.0
factor IX (congenital) (functional) 286.1
neonatal, transitory 776.3
coccyx 724.70
specified NEC 724.79
cognitive 294.9
colon 569.9
functional 564.9
congenital 751.3
communication 307.9
conduct (*see also* Disturbance, conduct) 312.9
adjustment reaction 309.3
adolescent onset type 312.82
childhood onset type 312.81
compulsive 312.30
specified type NEC 312.39
hyperkinetic 314.2
onset unspecified 312.89
socialized (type) 312.20
aggressive 312.23
unaggressive 312.21
specified NEC 312.89
conduction, heart 426.9
specified NEC 426.89
conflict
sexual orientation 302.0
convulsive (secondary) (*see also* Convulsions) 780.39
due to injury at birth 767.0
idiopathic 780.39
coordination 781.3
cornea NEC 371.89
due to contact lens 371.82

- **Disorder** *(Continued)*
  - corticosteroid metabolism NEC 255.2
  - cranial nerve - *see* Disorder, nerve, cranial
  - cyclothymic 301.13
  - degradation, branched-chain amino acid 270.3
  - delusional 297.1
  - dentition 520.6
  - depersonalization 300.6
  - depressive NEC 311
    - atypical 296.82
    - major (*see also* Psychosis, affective) 296.2
      - recurrent episode 296.3
      - single episode 296.2
  - development, specific 315.9
    - associated with hyperkinesia 314.1
    - coordination 315.4
    - language 315.31
    - learning 315.2
      - arithmetical 315.1
      - reading 315.00
    - mixed 315.5
    - motor coordination 315.4
    - specified type NEC 315.8
    - speech 315.39
  - diaphragm 519.4
  - digestive 536.9
    - fetus or newborn 777.9
      - specified NEC 777.8
    - psychogenic 306.4
  - disintegrative childhood 299.1
  - dissociative 300.15
    - identity 300.14
    - nocturnal 307.47
  - drug-related 292.9
  - dysmorphic body 300.7
  - dysthymic 300.4
  - ear 388.9
    - degenerative NEC 388.00
    - external 380.9
      - specified 380.89
    - pinna 380.30
    - specified type NEC 388.8
    - vascular NEC 388.00
  - eating NEC 307.50
  - electrolyte NEC 276.9
    - with
      - abortion - *see* Abortion, by type, with metabolic disorder
      - ectopic pregnancy (*see also* categories 633.0–633.9) 639.4
      - molar pregnancy (*see also* categories 630–632) 639.4
    - acidosis 276.2
      - metabolic 276.2
      - respiratory 276.2
    - alkalosis 276.3
      - metabolic 276.3
      - respiratory 276.3
    - following
      - abortion 639.4
      - ectopic or molar pregnancy 639.4
    - neonatal, transitory NEC 775.5
  - emancipation as adjustment reaction 309.22
  - emotional (*see also* Disorder, mental, nonpsychotic) V40.9
  - endocrine 259.9
    - specified type NEC 259.8
  - esophagus 530.9
    - functional 530.5
    - psychogenic 306.4

- **Disorder** *(Continued)*
  - explosive
    - intermittent 312.34
    - isolated 312.35
  - expressive language 315.31
  - eye 379.90
    - globe - *see* Disorder, globe
    - ill-defined NEC 379.99
    - limited duction NEC 378.63
    - specified NEC 379.8
  - eyelid 374.9
    - degenerative 374.50
    - sensory 374.44
    - specified type NEC 374.89
    - vascular 374.85
  - factitious (with combined psychological and physical signs and symptoms) (with predominantly physical signs and symptoms) 300.19
    - with predominantly psychological signs and symptoms 300.16
  - factor, coagulation (*see also* Defect, coagulation) 286.9
    - VIII (congenital) (functional) 286.0
    - IX (congenital) (functional) 286.1
  - fascia 728.9
  - fatty acid oxidation 277.85
  - feeding - *see* Feeding
  - female sexual arousal 302.72
  - fluid NEC 276.9
  - gastric (functional) 536.9
    - motility 536.8
    - psychogenic 306.4
    - secretion 536.8
  - gastrointestinal (functional) NEC 536.9
    - newborn (neonatal) 777.9
      - specified NEC 777.8
    - psychogenic 306.4
  - gender (child) 302.6
    - adolescents 302.85
    - adults (-life) 302.85
  - gender identity (childhood) 302.6
    - adolescents 302.85
    - adult-life 302.85
  - genitourinary system, psychogenic 306.50
  - globe 360.9
    - degenerative 360.20
      - specified NEC 360.29
    - specified type NEC 360.89
  - hearing - *see also* Deafness
    - conductive type (air) (*see also* Deafness, conductive) 389.00
    - mixed conductive and sensorineural 389.2
    - nerve, bilateral 389.12
    - perceptive (*see also* Deafness, perceptive) 389.10
    - sensorineural type NEC (*see also* Deafness, sensorineural) 389.10
  - heart action 427.9
    - postoperative 997.1
  - hematological, transient neonatal 776.9
    - specified type NEC 776.8
  - hematopoietic organs 289.9
  - hemorrhagic NEC 287.9
    - due to intrinsic circulating anticoagulants 286.5
    - specified type NEC 287.8
  - hemostasis (*see also* Defect, coagulation) 286.9
  - homosexual conflict 302.0

- **Disorder** *(Continued)*
  - hypomanic (chronic) 301.11
  - identity
    - childhood and adolescence 313.82
      - gender 302.6
  - immune mechanism (immunity) 279.9
    - single complement (C_1–C_9) 279.8
    - specified type NEC 279.8
  - impulse control (*see also* Disturbance, conduct, compulsive) 312.30
  - infant sialic acid storage 271.8
  - integument, fetus or newborn 778.9
    - specified type NEC 778.8
  - interactional psychotic (childhood) (*see also* Psychosis, childhood) 299.1
  - intermittent explosive 312.34
  - intervertebral disc 722.90
    - cervical, cervicothoracic 722.91
    - lumbar, lumbosacral 722.93
    - thoracic, thoracolumbar 722.92
  - intestinal 569.9
    - functional NEC 564.9
      - congenital 751.3
      - postoperative 564.4
    - psychogenic 306.4
  - introverted, of childhood and adolescence 313.22
  - iron, metabolism 275.0
  - isolated explosive 312.35
  - joint NEC 719.90
    - ankle 719.97
    - elbow 719.92
    - foot 719.97
    - hand 719.94
    - hip 719.95
    - knee 719.96
    - multiple sites 719.99
    - pelvic region 719.95
    - psychogenic 306.0
    - shoulder (region) 719.91
    - specified site NEC 719.98
    - temporomandibular 524.60
      - sounds on opening or closing 524.64
      - specified NEC 524.69
    - wrist 719.93
  - kidney 593.9
    - functional 588.9
      - specified NEC 588.89
  - labyrinth, labyrinthine 386.9
    - specified type NEC 386.8
  - lactation 676.9
  - language (developmental) (expressive) 315.31
    - mixed receptive-expressive 315.32
  - learning 315.9
  - ligament 728.9
  - ligamentous attachments, peripheral - *see also* Enthesopathy
    - spine 720.1
  - limb NEC 729.9
    - psychogenic 306.0
  - lipid
    - metabolism, congenital 272.9
    - storage 272.7
  - lipoprotein deficiency (familial) 272.5
  - low back NEC 724.9
    - psychogenic 306.0
  - lumbosacral
    - plexus 353.1
    - root (nerve) NEC 353.4
  - lymphoproliferative (chronic) NEC (M9970/1) 238.79

ICD-9-CM D Vol. 2

Disorder *(Continued)*
major depressive (*see also* Psychosis, affective) 296.2
recurrent episode 296.3
single episode 296.2
male erectile 607.84
nonorganic origin 302.72
manic (*see also* Psychosis, affective) 296.0
atypical 296.81
mathematics 315.1
meniscus NEC (*see also* Disorder, cartilage, articular) 718.0
menopausal 627.9
specified NEC 627.8
menstrual 626.9
psychogenic 306.52
specified NEC 626.8
mental (nonpsychotic) 300.9
affecting management of pregnancy, childbirth, or puerperium 648.4
drug-induced 292.9
hallucinogen persisting perception 292.89
specified type NEC 292.89
due to or associated with
alcoholism 291.9
drug consumption NEC 292.9
specified type NEC 292.89
physical condition NEC 293.9
induced by drug 292.9
specified type NEC 292.89
neurotic (*see also* Neurosis) 300.9
of infancy, childhood, or adolescence 313.9
persistent
other
due to conditions classified elsewhere 294.8
unspecified
due to conditions classified elsewhere 294.9
presenile 310.1
psychotic NEC 290.10
previous, affecting management of pregnancy V23.89
psychoneurotic (*see also* Neurosis) 300.9
psychotic (*see also* Psychosis) 298.9
brief 298.8
senile 290.20
specific, following organic brain damage 310.9
cognitive or personality change of other type 310.1
frontal lobe syndrome 310.0
postconcussional syndrome 310.2
specified type NEC 310.8
transient
in conditions classified elsewhere 293.9
metabolism NEC 277.9
with
abortion - *see* Abortion, by type, with metabolic disorder
ectopic pregnancy (*see also* categories 633.0–633.9) 639.4
molar pregnancy (*see also* categories 630–632) 639.4
alkaptonuria 270.2
amino acid (*see also* Disorder, amino acid) 270.9
specified type NEC 270.8
ammonia 270.6
arginine 270.6
argininosuccinic acid 270.6

Disorder *(Continued)*
metabolism NEC *(Continued)*
basal 794.7
bilirubin 277.4
calcium 275.40
carbohydrate 271.9
specified type NEC 271.8
cholesterol 272.9
citrulline 270.6
copper 275.1
corticosteroid 255.2
cystine storage 270.0
cystinuria 270.0
fat 272.9
fatty acid oxidation 277.85
following
abortion 639.4
ectopic or molar pregnancy 639.4
fructosemia 271.2
fructosuria 271.2
fucosidosis 271.8
galactose-1-phosphate uridyl transferase 271.1
glutamine 270.7
glycine 270.7
glycogen storage NEC 271.0
hepatorenal 271.0
hemochromatosis 275.0
in labor and delivery 669.0
iron 275.0
lactose 271.3
lipid 272.9
specified type NEC 272.8
storage 272.7
lipoprotein - *see also* Hyperlipemia deficiency (familial) 272.5
lysine 270.7
magnesium 275.2
mannosidosis 271.8
mineral 275.9
specified type NEC 275.8
mitochondrial 277.87
mucopolysaccharide 277.5
nitrogen 270.9
ornithine 270.6
oxalosis 271.8
pentosuria 271.8
phenylketonuria 270.1
phosphate 275.3
phosphorus 275.3
plasma protein 273.9
specified type NEC 273.8
porphyrin 277.1
purine 277.2
pyrimidine 277.2
serine 270.7
sodium 276.9
specified type NEC 277.89
steroid 255.2
threonine 270.7
urea cycle 270.6
xylose 271.8
micturition NEC 788.69
psychogenic 306.53
misery and unhappiness, of childhood and adolescence 313.1
mitochondrial metabolism 277.87
mitral valve 424.0
mood (*see also* Disorder, bipolar) 296.90
episodic 296.90
specified NEC 296.99
in conditions classified elsewhere 293.83

Disorder *(Continued)*
motor tic 307.20
chronic 307.22
transient (childhood) 307.21
movement NEC 333.90
hysterical 300.11
medication-induced 333.90
periodic limb 327.51
sleep related unspecified 780.58
other organic 327.59
specified type NEC 333.99
stereotypic 307.3
mucopolysaccharide 277.5
muscle 728.9
psychogenic 306.0
specified type NEC 728.3
muscular attachments, peripheral - *see also* Enthesopathy
spine 720.1
musculoskeletal system NEC 729.9
psychogenic 306.0
myeloproliferative (chronic) NEC (M9960/1) 238.79 (Revised)
myoneural 358.9
due to lead 358.2
specified type NEC 358.8
toxic 358.2
myotonic 359.2
neck region NEC 723.9
nerve 349.9
abducens NEC 378.54
accessory 352.4
acoustic 388.5
auditory 388.5
auriculotemporal 350.8
axillary 353.0
cerebral - *see* Disorder, nerve, cranial
cranial 352.9
first 352.0
second 377.49
third
partial 378.51
total 378.52
fourth 378.53
fifth 350.9
sixth 378.54
seventh NEC 351.9
eighth 388.5
ninth 352.2
tenth 352.3
eleventh 352.4
twelfth 352.5
multiple 352.6
entrapment - *see* Neuropathy, entrapment
facial 351.9
specified NEC 351.8
femoral 355.2
glossopharyngeal NEC 352.2
hypoglossal 352.5
iliohypogastric 355.79
ilioinguinal 355.79
intercostal 353.8
lateral
cutaneous of thigh 355.1
popliteal 355.3
lower limb NEC 355.8
medial, popliteal 355.4
median NEC 354.1
obturator 355.79
oculomotor
partial 378.51
total 378.52
olfactory 352.0

Disorder *(Continued)*
nerve *(Continued)*
optic 377.49
hypoplasia 377.43 ◀
ischemic 377.41
nutritional 377.33
toxic 377.34
peroneal 355.3
phrenic 354.8
plantar 355.6
pneumogastric 352.3
posterior tibial 355.5
radial 354.3
recurrent laryngeal 352.3
root 353.9
specified NEC 353.8
saphenous 355.79
sciatic NEC 355.0
specified NEC 355.9
lower limb 355.79
upper limb 354.8
spinal 355.9
sympathetic NEC 337.9
trigeminal 350.9
specified NEC 350.8
trochlear 378.53
ulnar 354.2
upper limb NEC 354.9
vagus 352.3
nervous system NEC 349.9
autonomic (peripheral) (*see also* Neuropathy, peripheral, autonomic) 337.9
cranial 352.9
parasympathetic (*see also* Neuropathy, peripheral, autonomic) 337.9
specified type NEC 349.89
sympathetic (*see also* Neuropathy, peripheral, autonomic) 337.9
vegetative (*see also* Neuropathy, peripheral, autonomic) 337.9
neurohypophysis NEC 253.6
neurological NEC 781.99
peripheral NEC 355.9
neuromuscular NEC 358.9
hereditary NEC 359.1
specified NEC 358.8
toxic 358.2
neurotic 300.9
specified type NEC 300.89
neutrophil, polymorphonuclear (functional) 288.1
nightmare 307.47
night terror 307.46
obsessive-compulsive 300.3
oppositional defiant childhood and adolescence 313.81
optic
chiasm 377.54
associated with
inflammatory disorders 377.54
neoplasm NEC 377.52
pituitary 377.51
pituitary disorders 377.51
vascular disorders 377.53
nerve 377.49
radiations 377.63
tracts 377.63
orbit 376.9
specified NEC 376.89
orgasmic
female 302.73
male 302.74

Disorder *(Continued)*
overanxious, of childhood and adolescence 313.0
oxidation, fatty acid 277.85
pancreas, internal secretion (other than diabetes mellitus) 251.9
specified type NEC 251.8
panic 300.01
with agoraphobia 300.21
papillary muscle NEC 429.81
paranoid 297.9
induced 297.3
shared 297.3
parathyroid 252.9
specified type NEC 252.8
paroxysmal, mixed 780.39
pentose phosphate pathway with anemia 282.2
periodic limb movement 327.51
peroxisomal 277.86
personality 301.9
affective 301.10
aggressive 301.3
amoral 301.7
anancastic, anankastic 301.4
antisocial 301.7
asocial 301.7
asthenic 301.6
avoidant 301.82
borderline 301.83
compulsive 301.4
cyclothymic 301.13
dependent-passive 301.6
dyssocial 301.7
emotional instability 301.59
epileptoid 301.3
explosive 301.3
following organic brain damage 310.1
histrionic 301.50
hyperthymic 301.11
hypomanic (chronic) 301.11
hypothymic 301.12
hysterical 301.50
immature 301.89
inadequate 301.6
introverted 301.21
labile 301.59
moral deficiency 301.7
narcissistic 301.81
obsessional 301.4
obsessive-compulsive 301.4
overconscientious 301.4
paranoid 301.0
passive (-dependent) 301.6
passive-aggressive 301.84
pathological NEC 301.9
pseudosocial 301.7
psychopathic 301.9
schizoid 301.20
introverted 301.21
schizotypal 301.22
schizotypal 301.22
seductive 301.59
type A 301.4
unstable 301.59
pervasive developmental 299.9
childhood-onset 299.8
specified NEC 299.8
phonological 315.39
pigmentation, choroid (congenital) 743.53
pinna 380.30
specified type NEC 380.39

Disorder *(Continued)*
pituitary, thalamic 253.9
anterior NEC 253.4
iatrogenic 253.7
postablative 253.7
specified NEC 253.8
pityriasis-like NEC 696.8
platelets (blood) 287.1
polymorphonuclear neutrophils (functional) 288.1
porphyrin metabolism 277.1
postmenopausal 627.9
specified type NEC 627.8
post-traumatic stress (PTSD) 309.81 ◀
posttraumatic stress 309.81
acute 309.81
brief 309.81
chronic 309.81
premenstrual dysphoric (PMDD) 625.4
psoriatic-like NEC 696.8
psychic, with diseases classified elsewhere 316
psychogenic NEC (*see also* condition) 300.9
allergic NEC
respiratory 306.1
anxiety 300.00
atypical 300.00
generalized 300.02
appetite 307.59
articulation, joint 306.0
asthenic 300.5
blood 306.8
cardiovascular (system) 306.2
compulsive 300.3
cutaneous 306.3
depressive 300.4
digestive (system) 306.4
dysmenorrheic 306.52
dyspneic 306.1
eczematous 306.3
endocrine (system) 306.6
eye 306.7
feeding 307.59
functional NEC 306.9
gastric 306.4
gastrointestinal (system) 306.4
genitourinary (system) 306.50
heart (function) (rhythm) 306.2
hemic 306.8
hyperventilatory 306.1
hypochondriacal 300.7
hysterical 300.10
intestinal 306.4
joint 306.0
learning 315.2
limb 306.0
lymphatic (system) 306.8
menstrual 306.52
micturition 306.53
monoplegic NEC 306.0
motor 307.9
muscle 306.0
musculoskeletal 306.0
neurocirculatory 306.2
obsessive 300.3
occupational 300.89
organ or part of body NEC 306.9
organs of special sense 306.7
paralytic NEC 306.0
phobic 300.20
physical NEC 306.9
pruritic 306.3
rectal 306.4

Disorder *(Continued)*
psychogenic NEC *(Continued)*
respiratory (system) 306.1
rheumatic 306.0
sexual (function) 302.70
specified type NEC 302.79
sexual orientation conflict 302.0
skin (allergic) (eczematous) (pruritic) 306.3
sleep 307.40
initiation or maintenance 307.41
persistent 307.42
transient 307.41
movement 780.58
sleep terror 307.46
specified type NEC 307.49
specified part of body NEC 306.8
stomach 306.4
psychomotor NEC 307.9
hysterical 300.11
psychoneurotic (*see also* Neurosis) 300.9
mixed NEC 300.89
psychophysiologic (*see also* Disorder, psychosomatic) 306.9
psychosexual identity (childhood) 302.6
adult-life 302.85
psychosomatic NEC 306.9
allergic NEC
respiratory 306.1
articulation, joint 306.0
cardiovascular (system) 306.2
cutaneous 306.3
digestive (system) 306.4
dysmenorrheic 306.52
dyspneic 306.1
endocrine (system) 306.6
eye 306.7
gastric 306.4
gastrointestinal (system) 306.4
genitourinary (system) 306.50
heart (functional) (rhythm) 306.2
hyperventilatory 306.1
intestinal 306.4
joint 306.0
limb 306.0
lymphatic (system) 306.8
menstrual 306.52
micturition 306.53
monoplegic NEC 306.0
muscle 306.0
musculoskeletal 306.0
neurocirculatory 306.2
organs of special sense 306.7
paralytic NEC 306.0
pruritic 306.3
rectal 306.4
respiratory (system) 306.1
rheumatic 306.0
sexual (function) 302.70
specified type NEC 302.79
skin 306.3
specified part of body NEC 306.8
stomach 306.4
psychotic (*see also* Psychosis) 298.9
brief 298.8
purine metabolism NEC 277.2
pyrimidine metabolism NEC 277.2
reactive attachment of infancy or early childhood 313.89
reading, developmental 315.00
reflex 796.1
REM sleep behavior 327.42
renal function, impaired 588.9
specified type NEC 588.89

Disorder *(Continued)*
renal transport NEC 588.89
respiration, respiratory NEC 519.9
due to
aspiration of liquids or solids 508.9
inhalation of fumes or vapors 506.9
psychogenic 306.1
retina 362.9
specified type NEC 362.89
rumination 307.53
sacroiliac joint NEC 724.6
sacrum 724.6
schizo-affective (*see also* Schizophrenia) 295.7
schizoid, childhood or adolescence 313.22
schizophreniform 295.4
schizotypal personality 301.22
secretion, thyrocalcitonin 246.0
seizure 345.9 (Revised)
recurrent 345.9 (Revised)
epileptic - *see* Epilepsy
sense of smell 781.1
psychogenic 306.7
separation anxiety 309.21
sexual (*see also* Deviation, sexual) 302.9
aversion 302.79
desire, hypoactive 302.71
function, psychogenic 302.70
shyness, of childhood and adolescence 313.21
single complement (C_1–C_9) 279.8
skin NEC 709.9
fetus or newborn 778.9
specified type 778.8
psychogenic (allergic) (eczematous) (pruritic) 306.3
specified type NEC 709.8
vascular 709.1
sleep 780.50
with apnea - *see* Apnea, sleep
alcohol induced 291.82
arousal 307.46
confusional 327.41
circadian rhythm 327.30
advanced sleep phase type 327.32
alcohol induced 291.82
delayed sleep phase type 327.31
drug induced 292.85
free running type 327.34
in conditions classified elsewhere 327.37
irregular sleep-wake type 327.33
jet lag type 327.35
other 327.39
shift work type 327.36
drug induced 292.85
initiation or maintenance (*see also* Insomnia) 780.52
nonorganic origin (transient) 307.41
persistent 307.42
nonorganic origin 307.40
specified type NEC 307.49
organic specified type NEC 327.8
periodic limb movement 327.51
specified NEC 780.59
wake
cycle - *see* Disorder, sleep, circadian rhythm
schedule - *see* Disorder, sleep, circadian rhythm

Disorder *(Continued)*
social, of childhood and adolescence 313.22
soft tissue 729.9
somatization 300.81
somatoform (atypical) (undifferentiated) 300.82
severe 300.81
specified type NEC 300.89
speech NEC 784.5
nonorganic origin 307.9
spine NEC 724.9
ligamentous or muscular attachments, peripheral 720.1
steroid metabolism NEC 255.2
stomach (functional) (*see also* Disorder, gastric) 536.9
psychogenic 306.4
storage, iron 275.0
stress (*see also* Reaction, stress, acute) 308.3
posttraumatic
acute 309.81
brief 309.81
chronic (motor or vocal) 309.81
substitution 300.11
suspected - *see* Observation
synovium 727.9
temperature regulation, fetus or newborn 778.4
temporomandibular joint NEC 524.60
sounds on opening or closing 524.64
specified NEC 524.69
tendon 727.9
shoulder region 726.10
thoracic root (nerve) NEC 353.3
thyrocalcitonin secretion 246.0
thyroid (gland) NEC 246.9
specified type NEC 246.8
tic 307.20
chronic (motor or vocal) 307.22
motor-verbal 307.23
organic origin 333.1
transient (of childhood) 307.21
tooth NEC 525.9
development NEC 520.9
specified type NEC 520.8
eruption 520.6
specified type NEC 525.8
Tourette's 307.23
transport, carbohydrate 271.9
specified type NEC 271.8
tubular, phosphate-losing 588.0
tympanic membrane 384.9
unaggressive, unsocialized (*see also* Disturbance, conduct) 312.1
undersocialized, unsocialized (*see also* Disturbance, conduct)
aggressive (type) 312.0
unaggressive (type) 312.1
vision, visual NEC 368.9
binocular NEC 368.30
cortex 377.73
associated with
inflammatory disorders 377.73
neoplasms 377.71
vascular disorders 377.72
pathway NEC 377.63
associated with
inflammatory disorders 377.63
neoplasms 377.61
vascular disorders 377.62

Disorder *(Continued)*
vocal tic
chronic 307.22
wakefulness (*see also* Hypersomnia) 780.54
nonorganic origin (transient) 307.43
persistent 307.44
written expression 315.2
Disorganized globe 360.29
Displacement, displaced

Note For acquired displacement of bones, cartilage, joints, tendons, due to injury, *see also* Dislocation.

Displacements at ages under one year should be considered congenital, provided there is no indication the condition was acquired after birth.

acquired traumatic of bone, cartilage, joint, tendon NEC (without fracture) (*see also* Dislocation) 839.8
with fracture - *see* Fracture, by site
adrenal gland (congenital) 759.1
alveolus and teeth, vertical 524.75
appendix, retrocecal (congenital) 751.5
auricle (congenital) 744.29
bladder (acquired) 596.8
congenital 753.8
brachial plexus (congenital) 742.8
brain stem, caudal 742.4
canaliculus lacrimalis 743.65
cardia, through esophageal hiatus 750.6
cerebellum, caudal 742.4
cervix - *see* Displacement, uterus
colon (congenital) 751.4
device, implant, or graft - *see* Complications, mechanical
epithelium
columnar of cervix 622.10
cuboidal, beyond limits of external os (uterus) 752.49
esophageal mucosa into cardia of stomach, congenital 750.4
esophagus (acquired) 530.89
congenital 750.4
eyeball (acquired) (old) 376.36
congenital 743.8
current injury 871.3
lateral 376.36
fallopian tube (acquired) 620.4
congenital 752.19
opening (congenital) 752.19
gallbladder (congenital) 751.69
gastric mucosa 750.7
into
duodenum 750.7
esophagus 750.7
Meckel's diverticulum, congenital 750.7
globe (acquired) (lateral) (old) 376.36
current injury 871.3
graft
artificial skin graft 996.55
decellularized allodermis graft 996.55
heart (congenital) 746.87
acquired 429.89
hymen (congenital) (upward) 752.49
internal prosthesis NEC - *see* Complications, mechanical

Displacement, displaced *(Continued)*
intervertebral disc (with neuritis, radiculitis, sciatica, or other pain) 722.2
with myelopathy 722.70
cervical, cervicodorsal, cervicothoracic 722.0
with myelopathy 722.71
due to major trauma - *see* Dislocation, vertebra, cervical
due to trauma - *see* Dislocation, vertebra
lumbar, lumbosacral 722.10
with myelopathy 722.73
due to major trauma - *see* Dislocation, vertebra, lumbar
thoracic, thoracolumbar 722.11
with myelopathy 722.72
due to major trauma - *see* Dislocation, vertebra, thoracic
intrauterine device 996.32
kidney (acquired) 593.0
congenital 753.3
lacrimal apparatus or duct (congenital) 743.65
macula (congenital) 743.55
Meckel's diverticulum (congenital) 751.0
nail (congenital) 757.5
acquired 703.8
opening of Wharton's duct in mouth 750.26
organ or site, congenital NEC - *see* Malposition, congenital
ovary (acquired) 620.4
congenital 752.0
free in peritoneal cavity (congenital) 752.0
into hernial sac 620.4
oviduct (acquired) 620.4
congenital 752.19
parathyroid (gland) 252.8
parotid gland (congenital) 750.26
punctum lacrimale (congenital) 743.65
sacroiliac (congenital) (joint) 755.69
current injury - *see* Dislocation, sacroiliac
old 724.6
spine (congenital) 756.19
spleen, congenital 759.0
stomach (congenital) 750.7
acquired 537.89
subglenoid (closed) 831.01
sublingual duct (congenital) 750.26
teeth, tooth 524.30
horizontal 524.33
vertical 524.34
tongue (congenital) (downward) 750.19
trachea (congenital) 748.3
ureter or ureteric opening or orifice (congenital) 753.4
uterine opening of oviducts or fallopian tubes 752.19
uterus, uterine (*see also* Malposition, uterus) 621.6
congenital 752.3
ventricular septum 746.89
with rudimentary ventricle 746.89
xyphoid bone (process) 738.3
Disproportion 653.9
affecting fetus or newborn 763.1
caused by
conjoined twins 653.7
contraction, pelvis (general) 653.1
inlet 653.2
midpelvic 653.8

Disproportion *(Continued)*
caused by *(Continued)*
contraction, pelvis *(Continued)*
midplane 653.8
outlet 653.3
fetal
ascites 653.7
hydrocephalus 653.6
hydrops 653.7
meningomyelocele 653.7
sacral teratoma 653.7
tumor 653.7
hydrocephalic fetus 653.6
pelvis, pelvic, abnormality (bony) NEC 653.0
unusually large fetus 653.5
causing obstructed labor 660.1
cephalopelvic, normally formed fetus 653.4
causing obstructed labor 660.1
fetal NEC 653.5
causing obstructed labor 660.1
fetopelvic, normally formed fetus 653.4
causing obstructed labor 660.1
mixed maternal and fetal origin, normally, formed fetus 653.4
pelvis, pelvic (bony) NEC 653.1
causing obstructed labor 660.1
specified type NEC 653.8
Disruption
cesarean wound 674.1
family V61.0
gastrointestinal anastomosis 997.4
ligament(s) - *see also* Sprain
knee
current injury - *see* Dislocation, knee
old 717.89
capsular 717.85
collateral (medial) 717.82
lateral 717.81
cruciate (posterior) 717.84
anterior 717.83
specified site NEC 717.85
marital V61.10
involving divorce or estrangement V61.0
operation wound (external) 998.32
internal 998.31
organ transplant, anastomosis site - *see* Complications, transplant, organ, by site
ossicles, ossicular chain 385.23
traumatic - *see* Fracture, skull, base
parenchyma
liver (hepatic) - *see* Laceration, liver, major
spleen - *see* Laceration, spleen, parenchyma, massive
phase-shift, of 24 hour sleep-wake cycle, unspecified 780.55
nonorganic origin 307.45
sleep-wake cycle (24 hour), unspecified 780.55
circadian rhythm 327.33
nonorganic origin 307.45
suture line (external) 998.32
internal 998.31
wound
cesarean operation 674.1
episiotomy 674.2

Disruption *(Continued)*
wound *(Continued)*
operation 998.32
cesarean 674.1
internal 998.31
perineal (obstetric) 674.2
uterine 674.1
Disruptio uteri - *see also* Rupture, uterus
complicating delivery - *see* Delivery, complicated, rupture, uterus
Dissatisfaction with
employment V62.2
school environment V62.3
Dissecting - *see* condition
Dissection
aorta 441.00
abdominal 441.02
thoracic 441.01
thoracoabdominal 441.03
artery, arterial
carotid 443.21
coronary 414.12
iliac 443.22
renal 443.23
specified NEC 443.29
vertebral 443.24
vascular 459.9
wound - *see* Wound, open, by site
Disseminated - *see* condition
Dissociated personality NEC 300.15
Dissociation
auriculoventricular or atrioventricular (any degree) (AV) 426.89
with heart block 426.0
interference 426.89
isorhythmic 426.89
rhythm
atrioventricular (AV) 426.89
interference 426.89
Dissociative
identity disorder 300.14
reaction NEC 300.15
Dissolution, vertebra (*see also* Osteoporosis) 733.00
Distention
abdomen (gaseous) 787.3
bladder 596.8
cecum 569.89
colon 569.89
gallbladder 575.8
gaseous (abdomen) 787.3
intestine 569.89
kidney 593.89
liver 573.9
seminal vesicle 608.89
stomach 536.8
acute 536.1
psychogenic 306.4
ureter 593.5
uterus 621.8
Distichia, distichiasis (eyelid) 743.63
Distoma hepaticum infestation 121.3
Distomiasis 121.9
bile passages 121.3
due to Clonorchis sinensis 121.1
hemic 120.9
hepatic (liver) 121.3
due to Clonorchis sinensis (clonorchiasis) 121.1
intestinal 121.4
liver 121.3
due to Clonorchis sinensis 121.1
lung 121.2
pulmonary 121.2
Distomolar (fourth molar) 520.1
causing crowding 524.31
Disto-occlusion (division I) (division II) 524.22
Distortion (congenital)
adrenal (gland) 759.1
ankle (joint) 755.69
anus 751.5
aorta 747.29
appendix 751.5
arm 755.59
artery (peripheral) NEC (*see also* Distortion, peripheral vascular system) 747.60
cerebral 747.81
coronary 746.85
pulmonary 747.3
retinal 743.58
umbilical 747.5
auditory canal 744.29
causing impairment of hearing 744.02
bile duct or passage 751.69
bladder 753.8
brain 742.4
bronchus 748.3
cecum 751.5
cervix (uteri) 752.49
chest (wall) 756.3
clavicle 755.51
clitoris 752.49
coccyx 756.19
colon 751.5
common duct 751.69
cornea 743.41
cricoid cartilage 748.3
cystic duct 751.69
duodenum 751.5
ear 744.29
auricle 744.29
causing impairment of hearing 744.02
causing impairment of hearing 744.09
external 744.29
causing impairment of hearing 744.02
inner 744.05
middle, except ossicles 744.03
ossicles 744.04
ossicles 744.04
endocrine (gland) NEC 759.2
epiglottis 748.3
Eustachian tube 744.24
eye 743.8
adnexa 743.69
face bone(s) 756.0
fallopian tube 752.19
femur 755.69
fibula 755.69
finger(s) 755.59
foot 755.67
gallbladder 751.69
genitalia, genital organ(s)
female 752.89
external 752.49
internal NEC 752.89
male 752.89
penis 752.69
glottis 748.3
gyri 742.4
hand bone(s) 755.59
heart (auricle) (ventricle) 746.89
valve (cusp) 746.89
hepatic duct 751.69
humerus 755.59
Distortion *(Continued)*
hymen 752.49
ileum 751.5
intestine (large) (small) 751.5
with anomalous adhesions, fixation or malrotation 751.4
jaw NEC 524.89
jejunum 751.5
kidney 753.3
knee (joint) 755.64
labium (majus) (minus) 752.49
larynx 748.3
leg 755.69
lens 743.36
liver 751.69
lumbar spine 756.19
with disproportion (fetopelvic) 653.0
affecting fetus or newborn 763.1
causing obstructed labor 660.1
lumbosacral (joint) (region) 756.19
lung (fissures) (lobe) 748.69
nerve 742.8
nose 748.1
organ
of Corti 744.05
of site not listed - *see* Anomaly, specified type NEC
ossicles, ear 744.04
ovary 752.0
oviduct 752.19
pancreas 751.7
parathyroid (gland) 759.2
patella 755.64
peripheral vascular system NEC 747.60
gastrointestinal 747.61
lower limb 747.64
renal 747.62
spinal 747.82
upper limb 747.63
pituitary (gland) 759.2
radius 755.59
rectum 751.5
rib 756.3
sacroiliac joint 755.69
sacrum 756.19
scapula 755.59
shoulder girdle 755.59
site not listed - *see* Anomaly, specified type NEC
skull bone(s) 756.0
with
anencephalus 740.0
encephalocele 742.0
hydrocephalus 742.3
with spina bifida (*see also* Spina bifida) 741.0
microcephalus 742.1
spinal cord 742.59
spine 756.19
spleen 759.0
sternum 756.3
thorax (wall) 756.3
thymus (gland) 759.2
thyroid (gland) 759.2
cartilage 748.3
tibia 755.69
toe(s) 755.66
tongue 750.19
trachea (cartilage) 748.3
ulna 755.59
ureter 753.4
causing obstruction 753.20
urethra 753.8
causing obstruction 753.6

Distortion *(Continued)*
uterus 752.3
vagina 752.49
vein (peripheral) NEC (*see also* Distortion, peripheral vascular system) 747.60
great 747.49
portal 747.49
pulmonary 747.49
vena cava (inferior) (superior) 747.49
vertebra 756.19
visual NEC 368.15
shape or size 368.14
vulva 752.49
wrist (bones) (joint) 755.59
Distress
abdomen 789.0
colon 564.9
emotional V40.9
epigastric 789.0
fetal (syndrome) 768.4
affecting management of pregnancy or childbirth 656.8
liveborn infant 768.4
first noted
before onset of labor 768.2
during labor and delivery 768.3
stillborn infant (death before onset of labor) 768.0
death during labor 768.1
gastrointestinal (functional) 536.9
psychogenic 306.4
intestinal (functional) NEC 564.9
psychogenic 306.4
intrauterine - *see* Distress, fetal
leg 729.5
maternal 669.0
mental V40.9
respiratory 786.09
acute (adult) 518.82
adult syndrome (following shock, surgery, or trauma) 518.5
specified NEC 518.82
fetus or newborn 770.89
syndrome (idiopathic) (newborn) 769
stomach 536.9
psychogenic 306.4
Distribution vessel, atypical NEC 747.60
coronary artery 746.85
spinal 747.82
Districhiasis 704.2
Disturbance - *see also* Disease
absorption NEC 579.9
calcium 269.3
carbohydrate 579.8
fat 579.8
protein 579.8
specified type NEC 579.8
vitamin (*see also* Deficiency, vitamin) 269.2
acid-base equilibrium 276.9
activity and attention, simple, with hyperkinesis 314.01
amino acid (metabolic) (*see also* Disorder, amino acid) 270.9
imidazole 270.5
maple syrup (urine) disease 270.3
transport 270.0
assimilation, food 579.9
attention, simple 314.00
with hyperactivity 314.01
auditory, nerve, except deafness 388.5

Disturbance *(Continued)*
behavior (*see also* Disturbance, conduct) 312.9
blood clotting (hypoproteinemia) (mechanism) (*see also* Defect, coagulation) 286.9
central nervous system NEC 349.9
cerebral nerve NEC 352.9
circulatory 459.9
conduct 312.9
adjustment reaction 309.3
adolescent onset type 312.82
childhood onset type 312.81

Note Use the following fifth-digit subclassification with categories 312.0–312.2:

0 unspecified
1 mild
2 moderate
3 severe

compulsive 312.30
intermittent explosive disorder 312.34
isolated explosive disorder 312.35
kleptomania 312.32
pathological gambling 312.31
pyromania 312.33
hyperkinetic 314.2
intermittent explosive 312.34
isolated explosive 312.35
mixed with emotions 312.4
socialized (type) 312.20
aggressive 312.23
unaggressive 312.21
specified type NEC 312.89
undersocialized, unsocialized
aggressive (type) 312.0
unaggressive (type) 312.1
coordination 781.3
cranial nerve NEC 352.9
deep sensibility - *see* Disturbance, sensation
digestive 536.9
psychogenic 306.4
electrolyte - *see* Imbalance, electrolyte
emotions specific to childhood or adolescence 313.9
with
academic underachievement 313.83
anxiety and fearfulness 313.0
elective mutism 313.23
identity disorder 313.82
jealousy 313.3
misery and unhappiness 313.1
oppositional defiant disorder 313.81
overanxiousness 313.0
sensitivity 313.21
shyness 313.21
social withdrawal 313.22
withdrawal reaction 313.22
involving relationship problems 313.3
mixed 313.89
specified type NEC 313.89
endocrine (gland) 259.9
neonatal, transitory 775.9
specified NEC 775.89
equilibrium 780.4
feeding (elderly) (infant) 783.3
newborn 779.3
nonorganic origin NEC 307.59
psychogenic NEC 307.59

Disturbance *(Continued)*
fructose metabolism 271.2
gait 781.2
hysterical 300.11
gastric (functional) 536.9
motility 536.8
psychogenic 306.4
secretion 536.8
gastrointestinal (functional) 536.9
psychogenic 306.4
habit, child 307.9
hearing, except deafness 388.40
heart, functional (conditions classifiable to 426, 427, 428)
due to presence of (cardiac) prosthesis 429.4
postoperative (immediate) 997.1
long-term effect of cardiac surgery 429.4
psychogenic 306.2
hormone 259.9
innervation uterus, sympathetic, parasympathetic 621.8
keratinization NEC
gingiva 523.10
lip 528.5
oral (mucosa) (soft tissue) 528.79
residual ridge mucosa
excessive 528.72
minimal 528.71
tongue 528.79
labyrinth, labyrinthine (vestibule) 386.9
learning, specific NEC 315.2
memory (*see also* Amnesia) 780.93
mild, following organic brain damage 310.8
mental (*see also* Disorder, mental) 300.9
associated with diseases classified elsewhere 316
metabolism (acquired) (congenital) (*see also* Disorder, metabolism) 277.9
with
abortion - *see* Abortion, by type, with metabolic disorder
ectopic pregnancy (*see also* categories 633.0–633.9) 639.4
molar pregnancy (*see also* categories 630–632) 639.4
amino acid (*see also* Disorder, amino acid) 270.9
aromatic NEC 270.2
branched-chain 270.3
specified type NEC 270.8
straight-chain NEC 270.7
sulfur-bearing 270.4
transport 270.0
ammonia 270.6
arginine 270.6
argininosuccinic acid 270.6
carbohydrate NEC 271.9
cholesterol 272.9
citrulline 270.6
cystathionine 270.4
fat 272.9
following
abortion 639.4
ectopic or molar pregnancy 639.4
general 277.9
carbohydrate 271.9
iron 275.0
phosphate 275.3
sodium 276.9

Disturbance *(Continued)*
metabolism *(Continued)*
glutamine 270.7
glycine 270.7
histidine 270.5
homocystine 270.4
in labor or delivery 669.0
iron 275.0
isoleucine 270.3
leucine 270.3
lipoid 272.9
specified type NEC 272.8
lysine 270.7
methionine 270.4
neonatal, transitory 775.9
specified type NEC 775.89
nitrogen 788.9
ornithine 270.6
phosphate 275.3
phosphatides 272.7
serine 270.7
sodium NEC 276.9
threonine 270.7
tryptophan 270.2
tyrosine 270.2
urea cycle 270.6
valine 270.3
motor 796.1
nervous functional 799.2
neuromuscular mechanism (eye) due to syphilis 094.84
nutritional 269.9
nail 703.8
ocular motion 378.87
psychogenic 306.7
oculogyric 378.87
psychogenic 306.7
oculomotor NEC 378.87
psychogenic 306.7
olfactory nerve 781.1
optic nerve NEC 377.49
oral epithelium, including tongue 528.79
residual ridge mucosa
excessive 528.72
minimal 528.71
personality (pattern) (trait) (*see also* Disorder, personality) 301.9
following organic brain damage 310.1
polyglandular 258.9
psychomotor 307.9
pupillary 379.49
reflex 796.1
rhythm, heart 427.9
postoperative (immediate) 997.1
long-term effect of cardiac surgery 429.4
psychogenic 306.2
salivary secretion 527.7
sensation (cold) (heat) (localization) (tactile discrimination localization) (texture) (vibratory) NEC 782.0
hysterical 300.11
skin 782.0
smell 781.1
taste 781.1
sensory (*see also* Disturbance, sensation) 782.0
innervation 782.0
situational (transient) (*see also* Reaction, adjustment) 309.9
acute 308.3

Disturbance *(Continued)*
sleep 780.50
with apnea - *see* Apnea, sleep
initiation or maintenance (*see also* Insomnia) 780.52
nonorganic origin 307.41
nonorganic origin 307.40
specified type NEC 307.49
specified NEC 780.59
nonorganic origin 307.49
wakefulness (*see also* Hypersomnia) 780.54
nonorganic origin 307.43
sociopathic 301.7
speech NEC 784.5
developmental 315.39
associated with hyperkinesis 314.1
secondary to organic lesion 784.5
stomach (functional) (*see also* Disturbance, gastric) 536.9
sympathetic (nerve) (*see also* Neuropathy, peripheral, autonomic) 337.9
temperature sense 782.0
hysterical 300.11
tooth
eruption 520.6
formation 520.4
structure, hereditary NEC 520.5
touch (*see also* Disturbance, sensation) 782.0
vascular 459.9
arteriosclerotic - *see* Arteriosclerosis
vasomotor 443.9
vasospastic 443.9
vestibular labyrinth 386.9
vision, visual NEC 368.9
psychophysical 368.16
specified NEC 368.8
subjective 368.10
voice 784.40
wakefulness (initiation or maintenance) (*see also* Hypersomnia) 780.54
nonorganic origin 307.43
Disulfiduria, beta-mercaptolactate-cysteine 270.0
Disuse atrophy, bone 733.7
Ditthomska syndrome 307.81
Diuresis 788.42
Divers'
palsy or paralysis 993.3
squeeze 993.3
Diverticula, diverticulosis, diverticulum (acute) (multiple) (perforated) (ruptured) 562.10
with diverticulitis 562.11
aorta (Kommerell's) 747.21
appendix (noninflammatory) 543.9
bladder (acquired) (sphincter) 596.3
congenital 753.8
broad ligament 620.8
bronchus (congenital) 748.3
acquired 494.0
with acute exacerbation 494.1
calyx, calyceal (kidney) 593.89
cardia (stomach) 537.1
cecum 562.10
with
diverticulitis 562.11
with hemorrhage 562.13
hemorrhage 562.12
congenital 751.5

Diverticula, diverticulosis, diverticulum *(Continued)*
colon (acquired) 562.10
with
diverticulitis 562.11
with hemorrhage 562.13
hemorrhage 562.12
congenital 751.5
duodenum 562.00
with
diverticulitis 562.01
with hemorrhage 562.03
hemorrhage 562.02
congenital 751.5
epiphrenic (esophagus) 530.6
esophagus (congenital) 750.4
acquired 530.6
epiphrenic 530.6
pulsion 530.6
traction 530.6
Zenker's 530.6
Eustachian tube 381.89
fallopian tube 620.8
gallbladder (congenital) 751.69
gastric 537.1
heart (congenital) 746.89
ileum 562.00
with
diverticulitis 562.01
with hemorrhage 562.03
hemorrhage 562.03
intestine (large) 562.10
with
diverticulitis 562.11
with hemorrhage 562.13
hemorrhage 562.12
congenital 751.5
small 562.00
with
diverticulitis 562.01
with hemorrhage 562.03
hemorrhage 562.02
congenital 751.5
jejunum 562.00
with
diverticulitis 562.01
with hemorrhage 562.03
hemorrhage 562.02
kidney (calyx) (pelvis) 593.89
with calculus 592.0
Kommerell's 747.21
laryngeal ventricle (congenital) 748.3
Meckel's (displaced) (hypertrophic) 751.0
midthoracic 530.6
organ or site, congenital NEC - *see* Distortion
pericardium (congenital) (cyst) 746.89
acquired (true) 423.8
pharyngoesophageal (pulsion) 530.6
pharynx (congenital) 750.27
pulsion (esophagus) 530.6
rectosigmoid 562.10
with
diverticulitis 562.11
with hemorrhage 562.13
hemorrhage 562.12
congenital 751.5
rectum 562.10
with
diverticulitis 562.11
with hemorrhage 562.13
hemorrhage 562.12
renal (calyces) (pelvis) 593.89
with calculus 592.0

Diverticula, diverticulosis, diverticulum *(Continued)*
Rokitansky's 530.6
seminal vesicle 608.0
sigmoid 562.10
with
diverticulitis 562.11
with hemorrhage 562.13
hemorrhage 562.12
congenital 751.5
small intestine 562.00
with
diverticulitis 562.01
with hemorrhage 562.03
hemorrhage 562.02
stomach (cardia) (juxtacardia) (juxtapyloric) (acquired) 537.1
congenital 750.7
subdiaphragmatic 530.6
trachea (congenital) 748.3
acquired 519.19
traction (esophagus) 530.6
ureter (acquired) 593.89
congenital 753.4
ureterovesical orifice 593.89
urethra (acquired) 599.2
congenital 753.8
ventricle, left (congenital) 746.89
vesical (urinary) 596.3
congenital 753.8
Zenker's (esophagus) 530.6
Diverticulitis (acute) (*see also* Diverticula) 562.11
with hemorrhage 562.13
bladder (urinary) 596.3
cecum (perforated) 562.11
with hemorrhage 562.13
colon (perforated) 562.11
with hemorrhage 562.13
duodenum 562.01
with hemorrhage 562.03
esophagus 530.6
ileum (perforated) 562.01
with hemorrhage 562.03
intestine (large) (perforated) 562.11
with hemorrhage 562.13
small 562.01
with hemorrhage 562.03
jejunum (perforated) 562.01
with hemorrhage 562.03
Meckel's (perforated) 751.0
pharyngoesophageal 530.6
rectosigmoid (perforated) 562.11
with hemorrhage 562.13
rectum 562.11
with hemorrhage 562.13
sigmoid (old) (perforated) 562.11
with hemorrhage 562.13
small intestine (perforated) 562.01
with hemorrhage 562.03
vesical (urinary) 596.3
Diverticulosis - *see* Diverticula
Division
cervix uteri 622.8
external os into two openings by frenum 752.49
external (cervical) into two openings by frenum 752.49
glans penis 752.69
hymen 752.49
labia minora (congenital) 752.49
ligament (partial or complete) (current) - *see also* Sprain, by site
with open wound - *see* Wound, open, by site

Division *(Continued)*
muscle (partial or complete) (current) - *see also* Sprain, by site
with open wound - *see* Wound, open, by site
nerve - *see* Injury, nerve, by site
penis glans 752.69
spinal cord - *see* Injury, spinal, by site
vein 459.9
traumatic - *see* Injury, vascular, by site
Divorce V61.0
Dix-Hallpike neurolabyrinthitis 386.12
Dizziness 780.4
hysterical 300.11
psychogenic 306.9
Doan-Wiseman syndrome (primary splenic neutropenia) 289.53
Dog bite - *see* Wound, open, by site
Döhle-Heller aortitis 093.1
Döhle body-panmyelopathic syndrome 288.2
Dolichocephaly, dolichocephalus 754.0
Dolichocolon 751.5
Dolichostenomelia 759.82
Donohue's syndrome (leprechaunism) 259.8
Donor
blood V59.01
other blood components V59.09
stem cells V59.02
whole blood V59.01
bone V59.2
marrow V59.3
cornea V59.5
egg (oocyte) (ovum) V59.70
over age 35 V59.73
anonymous recipient V59.73
designated recipient V59.74
under age 35 V59.71
anonymous recipient V59.71
designated recipient V59.72
heart V59.8
kidney V59.4
liver V59.6
lung V59.8
lymphocyte V59.8
organ V59.9
specified NEC V59.8
potential, examination of V70.8
skin V59.1
specified organ or tissue NEC V59.8
sperm V59.8
stem cells V59.02
tissue V59.9
specified type NEC V59.8
Donovanosis (granuloma venereum) 099.2
DOPS (diffuse obstructive pulmonary syndrome) 496
Double
albumin 273.8
aortic arch 747.21
auditory canal 744.29
auricle (heart) 746.82
bladder 753.8
external (cervical) os 752.49
kidney with double pelvis (renal) 753.3
larynx 748.3
meatus urinarius 753.8
organ or site NEC - *see* Accessory
orifice
heart valve NEC 746.89
pulmonary 746.09
outlet, right ventricle 745.11
pelvis (renal) with double ureter 753.4

Double *(Continued)*
penis 752.69
tongue 750.13
ureter (one or both sides) 753.4
with double pelvis (renal) 753.4
urethra 753.8
urinary meatus 753.8
uterus (any degree) 752.2
with doubling of cervix and vagina 752.2
in pregnancy or childbirth 654.0
affecting fetus or newborn 763.89
vagina 752.49
with doubling of cervix and uterus 752.2
vision 368.2
vocal cords 748.3
vulva 752.49
whammy (syndrome) 360.81
Douglas' pouch, cul-de-sac - *see* condition
Down's disease or syndrome (mongolism) 758.0
Down-growth, epithelial (anterior chamber) 364.61
Dracontiasis 125.7
Dracunculiasis 125.7
Dracunculosis 125.7
Drainage
abscess (spontaneous) - *see* Abscess
anomalous pulmonary veins to hepatic veins or right atrium 747.41
stump (amputation) (surgical) 997.62
suprapubic, bladder 596.8
Dream state, hysterical 300.13
Drepanocytic anemia (*see also* Disease, sickle cell) 282.60
Dresbach's syndrome (elliptocytosis) 282.1
Dreschlera (infection) 118
hawaiiensis 117.8
Dressler's syndrome (postmyocardial infarction) 411.0
Dribbling (post-void) 788.35
Drift, ulnar 736.09
Drinking (alcohol) - *see also* Alcoholism
excessive, to excess NEC (*see also* Abuse, drugs, nondependent) 305.0
bouts, periodic 305.0
continual 303.9
episodic 305.0
habitual 303.9
periodic 305.0
Drip, postnasal (chronic) 784.91
due to:
allergic rhinitis - *see* Rhinitis, allergic
common cold 460
gastroesophageal reflux - *see* Reflux, gastroesophageal
nasopharyngitis - *see* Nasopharyngitis
other known condition - *code to condition*
sinusitis - *see* Sinusitis
Drivers' license examination V70.3
Droop
Cooper's 611.8
facial 781.94
Drop
finger 736.29
foot 736.79
hematocrit (precipitous) 790.01
toe 735.8
wrist 736.05

ICD-9-CM
D
Vol. 2

Dropped
  dead 798.1
  heart beats 426.6
Dropsy, dropsical (*see also* Edema) 782.3
  abdomen 789.5
  amnion (*see also* Hydramnios) 657
  brain - *see* Hydrocephalus
  cardiac (*see also* Failure, heart) 428.0
  cardiorenal (*see also* Hypertension, cardiorenal) 404.90
  chest 511.9
  fetus or newborn 778.0
    due to isoimmunization 773.3
  gangrenous (*see also* Gangrene) 785.4
  heart (*see also* Failure, heart) 428.0
  hepatic - *see* Cirrhosis, liver
  infantile - *see* Hydrops, fetalis
  kidney (*see also* Nephrosis) 581.9
  liver - *see* Cirrhosis, liver
  lung 514
  malarial (*see also* Malaria) 084.9
  neonatorum - *see* Hydrops, fetalis
  nephritic 581.9
  newborn - *see* Hydrops, fetalis
  nutritional 269.9
  ovary 620.8
  pericardium (*see also* Pericarditis) 423.9
  renal (*see also* Nephrosis) 581.9
  uremic - *see* Uremia
Drowned, drowning 994.1
  lung 518.5
Drowsiness 780.09
Drug - *see also* condition
  addiction (*see also* Dependence) 304.9
  adverse effect NEC, correct substance properly administered 995.20
  allergy 995.27
  dependence (*see also* Dependence) 304.9
  habit (*see also* Dependence) 304.9
  hypersensitivity 995.27
  induced
    circadian rhythm sleep disorder 292.85
    hypersomnia 292.85
    insomnia 292.85
    mental disorder 292.9
      anxiety 292.89
      mood 292.84
      sexual 292.89
      sleep 292.85
      specified type 292.89
    parasomnia 292.85
    persisting
      amnestic disorder 292.83
      dementia 292.82
    psychotic disorder
      with
        delusions 292.11
        hallucinations 292.12
    sleep disorder 292.85
  intoxication 292.89
  overdose - *see* Table of Drugs and Chemicals
  poisoning - *see* Table of Drugs and Chemicals
  therapy (maintenance) status NEC
    chemotherapy, antineoplastic V58.11
    immunotherapy, antineoplastic V58.12
    long-term (current) use V58.69
      antibiotics V58.62
      anticoagulants V58.61
      anti-inflammatories, non-steroidal (NSAID) V58.64
      antiplatelets V58.63
Drug *(Continued)*
  therapy (maintenance) status NEC *(Continued)*
    long-term (current) use V58.69 *(Continued)*
      antithrombotics V58.63
      aspirin V58.66
      insulin V58.67
      steroids V58.65
  wrong substance given or taken in error - *see* Table of Drugs and Chemicals
Drunkenness (*see also* Abuse, drugs, nondependent) 305.0
  acute in alcoholism (*see also* Alcoholism) 303.0
  chronic (*see also* Alcoholism) 303.9
  pathologic 291.4
  simple (acute) 305.0
    in alcoholism 303.0
  sleep 307.47
Drusen
  optic disc or papilla 377.21
  retina (colloid) (hyaloid degeneration) 362.57
    hereditary 362.77
Drusenfieber 075
Dry, dryness - *see also* condition
  eye 375.15
    syndrome 375.15
  larynx 478.79
  mouth 527.7
  nose 478.19
  skin syndrome 701.1
  socket (teeth) 526.5
  throat 478.29
DSAP (disseminated superficial actinic porokeratosis) 692.75
Duane's retraction syndrome 378.71
Duane-Stilling-Türk syndrome (ocular retraction syndrome) 378.71
Dubin-Johnson disease or syndrome 277.4
Dubini's disease (electric chorea) 049.8
Dubois' abscess or disease 090.5
Duchenne's
  disease 094.0
    locomotor ataxia 094.0
    muscular dystrophy 359.1
    pseudohypertrophy, muscles 359.1
  paralysis 335.22
  syndrome 335.22
Duchenne-Aran myelopathic, muscular atrophy (nonprogressive) (progressive) 335.21
Duchenne-Griesinger disease 359.1
Ducrey's
  bacillus 099.0
  chancre 099.0
  disease (chancroid) 099.0
Duct, ductus - *see* condition
Duengero 061
Duhring's disease (dermatitis herpetiformis) 694.0
Dukes (-Filatov) disease 057.8
Dullness
  cardiac (decreased) (increased) 785.3
Dumb ague (*see also* Malaria) 084.6
Dumbness (*see also* Aphasia) 784.3
Dumdum fever 085.0
Dumping syndrome (postgastrectomy) 564.2
  nonsurgical 536.8
Duodenitis (nonspecific) (peptic) 535.60
  with hemorrhage 535.61
  due to
    strongyloides stercoralis 127.2
Duodenocholangitis 575.8
Duodenum, duodenal - *see* condition
Duplay's disease, periarthritis, or syndrome 726.2
Duplex - *see also* Accessory
  kidney 753.3
  placenta - *see* Placenta, abnormal
  uterus 752.2
Duplication - *see also* Accessory
  anus 751.5
  aortic arch 747.21
  appendix 751.5
  biliary duct (any) 751.69
  bladder 753.8
  cecum 751.5
    and appendix 751.5
  clitoris 752.49
  cystic duct 751.69
  digestive organs 751.8
  duodenum 751.5
  esophagus 750.4
  fallopian tube 752.19
  frontonasal process 756.0
  gallbladder 751.69
  ileum 751.5
  intestine (large) (small) 751.5
  jejunum 751.5
  kidney 753.3
  liver 751.69
  nose 748.1
  pancreas 751.7
  penis 752.69
  respiratory organs NEC 748.9
  salivary duct 750.22
  spinal cord (incomplete) 742.51
  stomach 750.7
  ureter 753.4
  vagina 752.49
  vas deferens 752.89
  vocal cords 748.3
Dupré's disease or syndrome (meningism) 781.6
Dupuytren's
  contraction 728.6
  disease (muscle contracture) 728.6
  fracture (closed) 824.4
    ankle (closed) 824.4
      open 824.5
    fibula (closed) 824.4
      open 824.5
    open 824.5
    radius (closed) 813.42
      open 813.52
  muscle contracture 728.6
Durand-Nicolas-Favre disease (climatic bubo) 099.1
Duroziez's disease (congenital mitral stenosis) 746.5
Dust
  conjunctivitis 372.05
  reticulation (occupational) 504
Dutton's
  disease (trypanosomiasis) 086.9
  relapsing fever (West African) 087.1
Dwarf, dwarfism 259.4
  with infantilism (hypophyseal) 253.3
  achondroplastic 756.4
  Amsterdam 759.89
  bird-headed 759.89
  congenital 259.4

◀ New ⬅ Revised

- **Dwarf, dwarfism** *(Continued)*
  - constitutional 259.4
  - hypophyseal 253.3
  - infantile 259.4
  - Levi type 253.3
  - Lorain-Levi (pituitary) 253.3
  - Lorain type (pituitary) 253.3
  - metatropic 756.4
  - nephrotic-glycosuric, with hypophosphatemic rickets 270.0
  - nutritional 263.2
  - ovarian 758.6
  - pancreatic 577.8
  - pituitary 253.3
  - polydystrophic 277.5
  - primordial 253.3
  - psychosocial 259.4
  - renal 588.0
    - with hypertension - *see* Hypertension, kidney
  - Russell's (uterine dwarfism and craniofacial dysostosis) 759.89
- **Dyke-Young anemia or syndrome** (acquired macrocytic hemolytic anemia) (secondary) (symptomatic) 283.9
- **Dynia abnormality** (*see also* Defect, coagulation) 286.9
- **Dysacousis** 388.40
- **Dysadrenocortism** 255.9
  - hyperfunction 255.3
  - hypofunction 255.4
- **Dysarthria** 784.5
- **Dysautonomia** (*see also* Neuropathy, peripheral, autonomic) 337.9
  - familial 742.8
- **Dysbarism** 993.3
- **Dysbasia** 719.7
  - angiosclerotica intermittens 443.9
    - due to atherosclerosis 440.21
  - hysterical 300.11
  - lordotica (progressiva) 333.6
  - nonorganic origin 307.9
  - psychogenic 307.9
- **Dysbetalipoproteinemia** (familial) 272.2
- **Dyscalculia** 315.1
- **Dyschezia** (*see also* Constipation) 564.00
- **Dyschondroplasia** (with hemangiomata) 756.4
  - Voorhoeve's 756.4
- **Dyschondrosteosis** 756.59
- **Dyschromia** 709.00
- **Dyscollagenosis** 710.9
- **Dyscoria** 743.41
- **Dyscraniopyophalangy** 759.89
- **Dyscrasia**
  - blood 289.9
    - with antepartum hemorrhage 641.3
    - fetus or newborn NEC 776.9
    - hemorrhage, subungual 287.8
    - puerperal, postpartum 666.3
  - ovary 256.8
  - plasma cell 273.9
  - pluriglandular 258.9
  - polyglandular 258.9
- **Dysdiadochokinesia** 781.3
- **Dysectasia, vesical neck** 596.8
- **Dysendocrinism** 259.9
- **Dysentery, dysenteric** (bilious) (catarrhal) (diarrhea) (epidemic) (gangrenous) (hemorrhagic) (infectious) (sporadic) (tropical) (ulcerative) 009.0
  - abscess, liver (*see also* Abscess, amebic) 006.3
- **Dysentery, dysenteric** *(Continued)*
  - amebic (*see also* Amebiasis) 006.9
    - with abscess - *see* Abscess, amebic
    - acute 006.0
    - carrier (suspected) of V02.2
    - chronic 006.1
  - arthritis (*see also* Arthritis, due to, dysentery) 009.0 *[711.3]*
    - bacillary 004.9 *[711.3]*
  - asylum 004.9
  - bacillary 004.9
    - arthritis 004.9 *[711.3]*
    - Boyd 004.2
    - Flexner 004.1
    - Schmitz (-Stutzer) 004.0
    - Shiga 004.0
    - Shigella 004.9
      - group A 004.0
      - group B 004.1
      - group C 004.2
      - group D 004.3
      - specified type NEC 004.8
    - Sonne 004.3
    - specified type NEC 004.8
  - bacterium 004.9
  - balantidial 007.0
  - Balantidium coli 007.0
  - Boyd's 004.2
  - Chilomastix 007.8
  - Chinese 004.9
  - choleriform 001.1
  - coccidial 007.2
  - Dientamoeba fragilis 007.8
  - due to specified organism NEC - *see* Enteritis, due to, by organism
  - Embadomonas 007.8
  - Endolimax nana - *see* Dysentery, amebic
  - Entamoba, entamebic - *see* Dysentery, amebic
  - Flexner's 004.1
  - Flexner-Boyd 004.2
  - giardial 007.1
  - Giardia lamblia 007.1
  - Hiss-Russell 004.1
  - lamblia 007.1
  - leishmanial 085.0
  - malarial (*see also* Malaria) 084.6
  - metazoal 127.9
  - Monilia 112.89
  - protozoal NEC 007.9
  - Russell's 004.8
  - salmonella 003.0
  - schistosomal 120.1
  - Schmitz (-Stutzer) 004.0
  - Shiga 004.0
  - Shigella NEC (*see also* Dysentery, bacillary) 004.9
    - boydii 004.2
    - dysenteriae 004.0
      - Schmitz 004.0
      - Shiga 004.0
    - flexneri 004.1
    - group A 004.0
    - group B 004.1
    - group C 004.2
    - group D 004.3
    - Schmitz 004.0
    - Shiga 004.0
    - Sonnei 004.3
  - Sonne 004.3
  - strongyloidiasis 127.2
  - trichomonal 007.3
  - tuberculous (*see also* Tuberculosis) 014.8
  - viral (*see also* Enteritis, viral) 008.8
- **Dysequilibrium** 780.4
- **Dysesthesia** 782.0
  - hysterical 300.11
- **Dysfibrinogenemia** (congenital) (*see also* Defect, coagulation) 286.3
- **Dysfunction**
  - adrenal (cortical) 255.9
    - hyperfunction 255.3
    - hypofunction 255.4
  - associated with sleep stages or arousal from sleep 780.56
    - nonorganic origin 307.47
  - bladder NEC 596.59
  - bleeding, uterus 626.8
  - brain, minimal (*see also* Hyperkinesia) 314.9
  - cerebral 348.30
  - colon 564.9
    - psychogenic 306.4
  - colostomy or enterostomy 569.62
  - cystic duct 575.8
  - diastolic 429.9
    - with heart failure - *see* Failure, heart
    - due to
      - cardiomyopathy - *see* Cardiomyopathy
      - hypertension - *see* Hypertension, heart
  - endocrine NEC 259.9
  - endometrium 621.8
  - enteric stoma 569.62
  - enterostomy 569.62
  - erectile 607.84
    - nonorganic origin 302.72
  - esophagostomy 530.87
  - Eustachian tube 381.81
  - gallbladder 575.8
  - gastrointestinal 536.9
  - gland, glandular NEC 259.9
  - heart 427.9
    - postoperative (immediate) 997.1
      - long-term effect of cardiac surgery 429.4
  - hemoglobin 289.89 (Revised)
  - hepatic 573.9
  - hepatocellular NEC 573.9
  - hypophysis 253.9
    - hyperfunction 253.1
    - hypofunction 253.2
    - posterior lobe 253.6
      - hypofunction 253.5
  - kidney (*see also* Disease, renal) 593.9
  - labyrinthine 386.50
    - specified NEC 386.58
  - liver 573.9
    - constitutional 277.4
  - minimal brain (child) (*see also* Hyperkinesia) 314.9
  - ovary, ovarian 256.9
    - hyperfunction 256.1
      - estrogen 256.0
    - hypofunction 256.39
      - postablative 256.2
    - postablative 256.2
    - specified NEC 256.8
  - papillary muscle 429.81
    - with myocardial infarction 410.8
  - parathyroid 252.8
    - hyperfunction 252.00
    - hypofunction 252.1
  - pineal gland 259.8
  - pituitary (gland) 253.9
    - hyperfunction 253.1
    - hypofunction 253.2

Dysfunction *(Continued)*
  pituitary *(Continued)*
    posterior 253.6
      hypofunction 253.5
  placental - *see* Placenta, insufficiency
  platelets (blood) 287.1
  polyglandular 258.9
    specified NEC 258.8
  psychosexual 302.70
    with
      dyspareunia (functional) (psychogenic) 302.76
      frigidity 302.72
      impotence 302.72
      inhibition
        orgasm
          female 302.73
          male 302.74
        sexual
          desire 302.71
          excitement 302.72
      premature ejaculation 302.75
      sexual aversion 302.79
      specified disorder NEC 302.79
      vaginismus 306.51
  pylorus 537.9
  rectum 564.9
    psychogenic 306.4
  segmental (*see also* Dysfunction, somatic) 739.9
  senile 797
  sexual 302.70
  sinoatrial node 427.81
  somatic 739.9
    abdomen 739.9
    acromioclavicular 739.7
    cervical 739.1
    cervicothoracic 739.1
    costochondral 739.8
    costovertebral 739.8
    extremities
      lower 739.6
      upper 739.7
    head 739.0
    hip 739.5
    lumbar, lumbosacral 739.3
    occipitocervical 739.0
    pelvic 739.5
    pubic 739.5
    rib cage 739.8
    sacral 739.4
    sacrococcygeal 739.4
    sacroiliac 739.4
    specified site NEC 739.9
    sternochondral 739.8
    sternoclavicular 739.7
    temporomandibular 739.0
    thoracic, thoracolumbar 739.2
  stomach 536.9
    psychogenic 306.4
  suprarenal 255.9
    hyperfunction 255.3
    hypofunction 255.4
  symbolic NEC 784.60
    specified type NEC 784.69
  systolic 429.9
    with heart failure - *see* Failure, heart
  temporomandibular (joint) (joint-pain-syndrome) NEC 524.60
    sounds on opening or closing 524.64
    specified NEC 524.69

Dysfunction *(Continued)*
  testicular 257.9
    hyperfunction 257.0
    hypofunction 257.2
    specified type NEC 257.8
  thymus 254.9
  thyroid 246.9
    complicating pregnancy, childbirth, or puerperium 648.1
    hyperfunction - *see* Hyperthyroidism
    hypofunction - *see* Hypothyroidism
  uterus, complicating delivery 661.9
    affecting fetus or newborn 763.7
    hypertonic 661.4
    hypotonic 661.2
      primary 661.0
      secondary 661.1
  velopharyngeal (acquired) 528.9
    congenital 750.29
  ventricular 429.9
    with congestive heart failure (*see also* Failure, heart) 428.0
    due to
      cardiomyopathy - *see* Cardiomyopathy
      hypertension - *see* Hypertension, heart
    left, reversible following sudden emotional stress 429.83 ◀
  vesicourethral NEC 596.59
  vestibular 386.50
    specified type NEC 386.58
Dysgammaglobulinemia 279.06
Dysgenesis
  gonadal (due to chromosomal anomaly) 758.6
    pure 752.7
  kidney(s) 753.0
  ovarian 758.6
  renal 753.0
  reticular 279.2
  seminiferous tubules 758.6
  tidal platelet 287.31
Dysgerminoma (M9060/3)
  specified site - *see* Neoplasm, by site, malignant
  unspecified site
    female 183.0
    male 186.9
Dysgeusia 781.1
Dysgraphia 781.3
Dyshidrosis 705.81
Dysidrosis 705.81
Dysinsulinism 251.8
Dyskaryotic cervical smear 795.09
Dyskeratosis (*see also* Keratosis) 701.1
  bullosa hereditaria 757.39
  cervix 622.10
  congenital 757.39
  follicularis 757.39
    vitamin A deficiency 264.8
  gingiva 523.8
  oral soft tissue NEC 528.79
  tongue 528.79
  uterus NEC 621.8
Dyskinesia 781.3
  biliary 575.8
  esophagus 530.5
  hysterical 300.11
  intestinal 564.89
  neuroleptic-induced tardive 333.85 ⬅
  nonorganic origin 307.9
  orofacial 333.82
    due to drugs 333.85 ◀

Dyskinesia *(Continued)*
  psychogenic 307.9
  subacute, due to drugs 333.85 ◀
  tardive (oral) 333.85 ⬅
Dyslalia 784.5
  developmental 315.39
Dyslexia 784.61
  developmental 315.02
  secondary to organic lesion 784.61
Dyslipidemia 272.4
Dysmaturity (*see also* Immaturity) 765.1
  lung 770.4
  pulmonary 770.4
Dysmenorrhea (essential) (exfoliative) (functional) (intrinsic) (membranous) (primary) (secondary) 625.3
  psychogenic 306.52
Dysmetabolic syndrome X 277.7
Dysmetria 781.3
Dysmorodystrophia mesodermalis congenita 759.82
Dysnomia 784.3
Dysorexia 783.0
  hysterical 300.11
Dysostosis
  cleidocranial, cleidocranialis 755.59
  craniofacial 756.0
  Fairbank's (idiopathic familial generalized osteophytosis) 756.50
  mandibularis 756.0
  mandibulofacial, incomplete 756.0
  multiplex 277.5
  orodigitofacial 759.89
Dyspareunia (female) 625.0
  male 608.89
  psychogenic 302.76
Dyspepsia (allergic) (congenital) (fermentative) (flatulent) (functional) (gastric) (gastrointestinal) (neurogenic) (occupational) (reflex) 536.8
  acid 536.8
  atonic 536.3
    psychogenic 306.4
  diarrhea 787.91
    psychogenic 306.4
  intestinal 564.89
    psychogenic 306.4
  nervous 306.4
  neurotic 306.4
  psychogenic 306.4
Dysphagia 787.2
  functional 300.11
  hysterical 300.11
  nervous 300.11
  psychogenic 306.4
  sideropenic 280.8
  spastica 530.5
Dysphagocytosis, congenital 288.1
Dysphasia 784.5
Dysphonia 784.49
  clericorum 784.49
  functional 300.11
  hysterical 300.11
  psychogenic 306.1
  spastica 478.79
Dyspigmentation - *see also* Pigmentation
  eyelid (acquired) 374.52
Dyspituitarism 253.9
  hyperfunction 253.1
  hypofunction 253.2
  posterior lobe 253.6

- **Dysplasia** - *see also* Anomaly
  - artery
    - fibromuscular NEC 447.8
      - carotid 447.8
      - renal 447.3
  - bladder 596.8
  - bone (fibrous) NEC 733.29
    - diaphyseal, progressive 756.59
    - jaw 526.89
    - monostotic 733.29
    - polyostotic 756.54
    - solitary 733.29
  - brain 742.9
  - bronchopulmonary, fetus or newborn 770.7
  - cervix (uteri) 622.10
    - cervical intraepithelial neoplasia I [CIN I] 622.11
    - cervical intraepithelial neoplasia II [CIN II] 622.12
    - cervical intraepithelial neoplasia III [CIN III] 233.1
    - CIN I 622.11
    - CIN II 622.12
    - CIN III 233.1
    - mild 622.11
    - moderate 622.12
    - severe 233.1
  - chondroectodermal 756.55
  - chondromatose 756.4
  - colon 211.3
  - craniocarpotarsal 759.89
  - craniometaphyseal 756.89
  - dentinal 520.5
  - diaphyseal, progressive 756.59
  - ectodermal (anhidrotic) (Bason) (Clouston's) (congenital) (Feinmesser) (hereditary) (hidrotic) (Marshall) (Robinson's) 757.31
  - epiphysealis 756.9
    - multiplex 756.56
    - punctata 756.59
  - epiphysis 756.9
    - multiple 756.56
  - epithelial
    - epiglottis 478.79
    - uterine cervix 622.10
  - erythroid NEC 289.89
  - eye (*see also* Microphthalmos) 743.10
  - familial metaphyseal 756.89
  - fibromuscular, artery NEC 447.8
    - carotid 447.8
    - renal 447.3
  - fibrous
    - bone NEC 733.29
    - diaphyseal, progressive 756.59
    - jaw 526.89
    - monostotic 733.29
    - polyostotic 756.54
    - solitary 733.29
  - high grade, focal - *see* Neoplasm, by site, benign
  - hip (congenital) 755.63
    - with dislocation (*see also* Dislocation, hip, congenital) 754.30
  - hypohidrotic ectodermal 757.31
  - joint 755.8
  - kidney 753.15
  - leg 755.69
  - linguofacialis 759.89
  - lung 748.5
  - macular 743.55
- **Dysplasia** *(Continued)*
  - mammary (benign) (gland) 610.9
    - cystic 610.1
    - specified type NEC 610.8
  - metaphyseal 756.9
    - familial 756.89
  - monostotic fibrous 733.29
  - muscle 756.89
  - myeloid NEC 289.89
  - nervous system (general) 742.9
  - neuroectodermal 759.6
  - oculoauriculovertebral 756.0
  - oculodentodigital 759.89
  - olfactogenital 253.4
  - osteo-onycho-arthro (hereditary) 756.89
  - periosteum 733.99
  - polyostotic fibrous 756.54
  - progressive diaphyseal 756.59
  - prostate 602.3
    - intraepithelial neoplasia I [PIN I] 602.3
    - intraepithelial neoplasia II [PIN II] 602.3
    - intraepithelial neoplasia III [PIN III] 233.4
  - renal 753.15
  - renofacialis 753.0
  - retinal NEC 743.56
  - retrolental 362.21
  - spinal cord 742.9
  - thymic, with immunodeficiency 279.2
  - vagina 623.0
  - vocal cord 478.5
  - vulva 624.8
    - intraepithelial neoplasia I [VIN I] 624.0 (Revised)
    - intraepithelial neoplasia II [VIN II] 624.0 (Revised)
    - intraepithelial neoplasia III [VIN III] 233.3
    - VIN I 624.0 (Revised)
    - VIN II 624.0 (Revised)
    - VIN III 233.3
- **Dyspnea** (nocturnal) (paroxysmal) 786.09
  - asthmatic (bronchial) (*see also* Asthma) 493.9
    - with bronchitis (*see also* Asthma) 493.9
      - chronic 493.2
    - cardiac (*see also* Failure, ventricular, left) 428.1
  - cardiac (*see also* Failure, ventricular, left) 428.1
  - functional 300.11
  - hyperventilation 786.01
  - hysterical 300.11
  - Monday morning 504
  - newborn 770.89
  - psychogenic 306.1
  - uremic - *see* Uremia
- **Dyspraxia** 781.3
  - syndrome 315.4
- **Dysproteinemia** 273.8
  - transient with copper deficiency 281.4
- **Dysprothrombinemia** (constitutional) (*see also* Defect, coagulation) 286.3
- **Dysreflexia, autonomic** 337.3
- **Dysrhythmia**
  - cardiac 427.9
    - postoperative (immediate) 997.1
      - long-term effect of cardiac surgery 429.4
    - specified type NEC 427.89
  - cerebral or cortical 348.30
- **Dyssecretosis, mucoserous** 710.2
- **Dyssocial reaction, without manifest psychiatric disorder**
  - adolescent V71.02
  - adult V71.01
  - child V71.02
- **Dyssomnia NEC** 780.56
  - nonorganic origin 307.47
- **Dyssplenism** 289.4
- **Dyssynergia**
  - biliary (*see also* Disease, biliary) 576.8
  - cerebellaris myoclonica 334.2
  - detrusor sphincter (bladder) 596.55
  - ventricular 429.89
- **Dystasia, hereditary areflexic** 334.3
- **Dysthymia** 300.4
- **Dysthymic disorder** 300.4
- **Dysthyroidism** 246.9
- **Dystocia** 660.9
  - affecting fetus or newborn 763.1
  - cervical 661.0
    - affecting fetus or newborn 763.7
  - contraction ring 661.4
    - affecting fetus or newborn 763.7
  - fetal 660.9
    - abnormal size 653.5
    - affecting fetus or newborn 763.1
    - deformity 653.7
  - maternal 660.9
    - affecting fetus or newborn 763.1
  - positional 660.0
    - affecting fetus or newborn 763.1
  - shoulder (girdle) 660.4
    - affecting fetus or newborn 763.1
  - uterine NEC 661.4
    - affecting fetus or newborn 763.7
- **Dystonia**
  - acute (New)
    - due to drugs 333.72 (New)
    - neuroleptic-induced acute 333.72 (New)
  - deformans progressiva 333.6
  - lenticularis 333.6
  - musculorum deformans 333.6
  - torsion (idiopathic) 333.6
    - acquired 333.79 (New)
    - fragments (of) 333.89
    - genetic 333.6 (New)
    - symptomatic 333.79 (Revised)
- **Dystonic**
  - movements 781.0
- **Dystopia kidney** 753.3
- **Dystrophy, dystrophia** 783.9
  - adiposogenital 253.8
  - asphyxiating thoracic 756.4
  - Becker's type 359.1
  - brevicollis 756.16
  - Bruch's membrane 362.77
  - cervical (sympathetic) NEC 337.0
  - chondro-osseus with punctate epiphyseal dysplasia 756.59
  - choroid (hereditary) 363.50
    - central (areolar) (partial) 363.53
      - total (gyrate) 363.54
    - circinate 363.53
    - circumpapillary (partial) 363.51
      - total 363.52
    - diffuse
      - partial 363.56
      - total 363.57
    - generalized
      - partial 363.56
      - total 363.57
    - gyrate
      - central 363.54
      - generalized 363.57

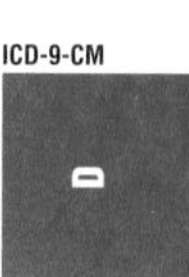

ICD-9-CM
D
Vol. 2

Dystrophy, dystrophia *(Continued)*
choroid *(Continued)*
helicoid 363.52
peripapillary - *see* Dystrophy, choroid, circumpapillary
serpiginous 363.54
cornea (hereditary) 371.50
anterior NEC 371.52
Cogan's 371.52
combined 371.57
crystalline 371.56
endothelial (Fuchs') 371.57
epithelial 371.50
juvenile 371.51
microscopic cystic 371.52
granular 371.53
lattice 371.54
macular 371.55
marginal (Terrien's) 371.48
Meesman's 371.51
microscopic cystic (epithelial) 371.52
nodular, Salzmann's 371.46
polymorphous 371.58
posterior NEC 371.58
ring-like 371.52
Salzmann's nodular 371.46
stromal NEC 371.56
dermatochondrocorneal 371.50
Duchenne's 359.1
due to malnutrition 263.9
Erb's 359.1
familial
hyperplastic periosteal 756.59
osseous 277.5
foveal 362.77
Fuchs', cornea 371.57
Gowers' muscular 359.1
hair 704.2
hereditary, progressive muscular 359.1

Dystrophy, dystrophia *(Continued)*
hypogenital, with diabetic tendency 759.81
Landouzy-Déjérine 359.1
Leyden-Möbius 359.1
mesodermalis congenita 759.82
muscular 359.1
congenital (hereditary) 359.0
myotonic 359.2
distal 359.1
Duchenne's 359.1
Erb's 359.1
fascioscapulohumeral 359.1
Gowers' 359.1
hereditary (progressive) 359.1
Landouzy-Déjérine 359.1
limb-girdle 359.1
myotonic 359.2
progressive (hereditary) 359.1
Charcôt-Marie-Tooth 356.1
pseudohypertrophic (infantile) 359.1
myocardium, myocardial (*see also* Degeneration, myocardial) 429.1
myotonic 359.2
myotonica 359.2
nail 703.8
congenital 757.5
neurovascular (traumatic) (*see also* Neuropathy, peripheral, autonomic) 337.9
nutritional 263.9
ocular 359.1
oculocerebrorenal 270.8
oculopharyngeal 359.1
ovarian 620.8
papillary (and pigmentary) 701.1
pelvicrural atrophic 359.1
pigmentary (*see also* Acanthosis) 701.2
pituitary (gland) 253.8
polyglandular 258.8

Dystrophy, dystrophia *(Continued)*
posttraumatic sympathetic - *see* Dystrophy, symphatic
progressive ophthalmoplegic 359.1
retina, retinal (hereditary) 362.70
albipunctate 362.74
Bruch's membrane 362.77
cone, progressive 362.75
hyaline 362.77
in
Bassen-Kornzweig syndrome 272.5 *[362.72]*
cerebroretinal lipidosis 330.1 *[362.71]*
Refsum's disease 356.3 *[362.72]*
systemic lipidosis 272.7 *[362.71]*
juvenile (Stargardt's) 362.75
pigmentary 362.74
pigment epithelium 362.76
progressive cone (-rod) 362.75
pseudoinflammatory foveal 362.77
rod, progressive 362.75
sensory 362.75
vitelliform 362.76
Salzmann's nodular 371.46
scapuloperoneal 359.1
skin NEC 709.9
sympathetic (posttraumatic) (reflex) 337.20
lower limb 337.22
specified site NEC 337.29
upper limb 337.21
tapetoretinal NEC 362.74
thoracic asphyxiating 756.4
unguium 703.8
congenital 757.5
vitreoretinal (primary) 362.73
secondary 362.66
vulva 624.0
Dysuria 788.1
psychogenic 306.53

E

Eagle-Barrett syndrome 756.71
Eales' disease (syndrome) 362.18
Ear - *see also* condition
ache 388.70
otogenic 388.71
referred 388.72
lop 744.29
piercing V50.3
swimmers' acute 380.12
tank 380.12
tropical 111.8 *[380.15]*
wax 380.4
Earache 388.70
otogenic 388.71
referred 388.72
Early satiety 780.94
Eaton-Lambert syndrome (*see also* Neoplasm, by site, malignant) 199.1 *[358.1]*
Eberth's disease (typhoid fever) 002.0
Ebstein's
anomaly or syndrome (downward displacement, tricuspid valve into right ventricle) 746.2
disease (diabetes) 250.4 *[581.81]*
Eccentro-osteochondrodysplasia 277.5
Ecchondroma (M9210/0) - *see* Neoplasm, bone, benign
Ecchondrosis (M9210/1) 238.0
Ecchordosis physaliphora 756.0
Ecchymosis (multiple) 459.89
conjunctiva 372.72
eye (traumatic) 921.0
eyelids (traumatic) 921.1
newborn 772.6
spontaneous 782.7
traumatic - *see* Contusion
Echinococciasis - *see* Echinococcus
Echinococcosis - *see* Echinococcus
Echinococcus (infection) 122.9
granulosus 122.4
liver 122.0
lung 122.1
orbit 122.3 *[376.13]*
specified site NEC 122.3
thyroid 122.2
liver NEC 122.8
granulosus 122.0
multilocularis 122.5
lung NEC 122.9
granulosus 122.1
multilocularis 122.6
multilocularis 122.7
liver 122.5
specified site NEC 122.6
orbit 122.9 *[376.13]*
granulosus 122.3 *[376.13]*
multilocularis 122.6 *[376.13]*
specified site NEC 122.9
granulosus 122.3
multilocularis 122.6 *[376.13]*
thyroid NEC 122.9
granulosus 122.2
multilocularis 122.6
Echinorhynchiasis 127.7
Echinostomiasis 121.8
Echolalia 784.69
ECHO virus infection NEC 079.1
Eclampsia, eclamptic (coma) (convulsions) (delirium) 780.39
female, child-bearing age NEC - *see* Eclampsia, pregnancy
gravidarum - *see* Eclampsia, pregnancy
Eclampsia, eclamptic *(Continued)*
male 780.39
not associated with pregnancy or childbirth 780.39
pregnancy, childbirth, or puerperium 642.6
with pre-existing hypertension 642.7
affecting fetus or newborn 760.0
uremic 586
Eclipse blindness (total) 363.31
Economic circumstance affecting care V60.9
specified type NEC V60.8
Economo's disease (encephalitis lethargica) 049.8
Ectasia, ectasis
aorta (*see also* Aneurysm, aorta) 441.9
ruptured 441.5
breast 610.4
capillary 448.9
cornea (marginal) (postinfectional) 371.71
duct (mammary) 610.4
kidney 593.89
mammary duct (gland) 610.4
papillary 448.9
renal 593.89
salivary gland (duct) 527.8
scar, cornea 371.71
sclera 379.11
Ecthyma 686.8
contagiosum 051.2
gangrenosum 686.09
infectiosum 051.2
Ectocardia 746.87
Ectodermal dysplasia, congenital 757.31
Ectodermosis erosiva pluriorificialis 695.1
Ectopic, ectopia (congenital) 759.89
abdominal viscera 751.8
due to defect in anterior abdominal wall 756.79
ACTH syndrome 255.0
adrenal gland 759.1
anus 751.5
auricular beats 427.61
beats 427.60
bladder 753.5
bone and cartilage in lung 748.69
brain 742.4
breast tissue 757.6
cardiac 746.87
cerebral 742.4
cordis 746.87
endometrium 617.9
gallbladder 751.69
gastric mucosa 750.7
gestation - *see* Pregnancy, ectopic
heart 746.87
hormone secretion NEC 259.3
hyperparathyroidism 259.3
kidney (crossed) (intrathoracic) (pelvis) 753.3
in pregnancy or childbirth 654.4
causing obstructed labor 660.2
lens 743.37
lentis 743.37
mole - *see* Pregnancy, ectopic
organ or site NEC - *see* Malposition, congenital
ovary 752.0
pancreas, pancreatic tissue 751.7
pregnancy - *see* Pregnancy, ectopic
pupil 364.75
renal 753.3
Ectopic, ectopia *(Continued)*
sebaceous glands of mouth 750.26
secretion
ACTH 255.0
adrenal hormone 259.3
adrenalin 259.3
adrenocorticotropin 255.0
antidiuretic hormone (ADH) 259.3
epinephrine 259.3
hormone NEC 259.3
norepinephrine 259.3
pituitary (posterior) 259.3
spleen 759.0
testis 752.51
thyroid 759.2
ureter 753.4
ventricular beats 427.69
vesicae 753.5
Ectrodactyly 755.4
finger (*see also* Absence, finger, congenital) 755.29
toe (*see also* Absence, toe, congenital) 755.39
Ectromelia 755.4
lower limb 755.30
upper limb 755.20
Ectropion 374.10
anus 569.49
cervix 622.0
with mention of cervicitis 616.0
cicatricial 374.14
congenital 743.62
eyelid 374.10
cicatricial 374.14
congenital 743.62
mechanical 374.12
paralytic 374.12
senile 374.11
spastic 374.13
iris (pigment epithelium) 364.54
lip (congenital) 750.26
acquired 528.5
mechanical 374.12
paralytic 374.12
rectum 569.49
senile 374.11
spastic 374.13
urethra 599.84
uvea 364.54
Eczema (acute) (allergic) (chronic) (erythematous) (fissum) (occupational) (rubrum) (squamous) 692.9
asteatotic 706.8
atopic 691.8
contact NEC 692.9
dermatitis NEC 692.9
due to specified cause - *see* Dermatitis, due to
dyshidrotic 705.81
external ear 380.22
flexural 691.8
gouty 274.89
herpeticum 054.0
hypertrophicum 701.8
hypostatic - *see* Varicose, vein
impetiginous 684
infantile (acute) (chronic) (due to any substance) (intertriginous) (seborrheic) 690.12
intertriginous NEC 692.9
infantile 690.12
intrinsic 691.8
lichenified NEC 692.9
marginatum 110.3
nummular 692.9

Eczema *(Continued)*
pustular 686.8
seborrheic 690.18
infantile 690.12
solare 692.72
stasis (lower extremity) 454.1
ulcerated 454.2
vaccination, vaccinatum 999.0
varicose (lower extremity) - *see* Varicose, vein
verrucosum callosum 698.3
Eczematoid, exudative 691.8
Eddowes' syndrome (brittle bones and blue sclera) 756.51
Edema, edematous 782.3
with nephritis (*see also* Nephrosis) 581.9
allergic 995.1
angioneurotic (allergic) (any site) (with urticaria) 995.1
hereditary 277.6
angiospastic 443.9
Berlin's (traumatic) 921.3
brain 348.5
due to birth injury 767.8
fetus or newborn 767.8
cardiac (*see also* Failure, heart) 428.0
cardiovascular (*see also* Failure, heart) 428.0
cerebral - *see* Edema, brain
cerebrospinal vessel - *see* Edema, brain
cervix (acute) (uteri) 622.8
puerperal, postpartum 674.8
chronic hereditary 757.0
circumscribed, acute 995.1
hereditary 277.6
complicating pregnancy (gestational) 646.1
with hypertension - *see* Toxemia, of pregnancy
conjunctiva 372.73
connective tissue 782.3
cornea 371.20
due to contact lenses 371.24
idiopathic 371.21
secondary 371.22
cystoid macular 362.53
due to
lymphatic obstruction - *see* Edema, lymphatic
salt retention 276.0
epiglottis - *see* Edema, glottis
essential, acute 995.1
hereditary 277.6
extremities, lower - *see* Edema, legs
eyelid NEC 374.82
familial, hereditary (legs) 757.0
famine 262
fetus or newborn 778.5
genital organs
female 629.89 ◄
male 608.86
gestational 646.1
with hypertension - *see* Toxemia, of pregnancy
glottis, glottic, glottides (obstructive) (passive) 478.6
allergic 995.1
hereditary 277.6
due to external agent - *see* Condition, respiratory, acute, due to specified agent
heart (*see also* Failure, heart) 428.0
newborn 779.89
heat 992.7
hereditary (legs) 757.0

Edema, edematous *(Continued)*
inanition 262
infectious 782.3
intracranial 348.5
due to injury at birth 767.8
iris 364.8
joint (*see also* Effusion, joint) 719.0
larynx (*see also* Edema, glottis) 478.6
legs 782.3
due to venous obstruction 459.2
hereditary 757.0
localized 782.3
due to venous obstruction 459.2
lower extremity 459.2
lower extremities - *see* Edema, legs
lung 514
acute 518.4
with heart disease or failure (*see also* Failure, ventricular, left) 428.1
congestive 428.0
chemical (due to fumes or vapors) 506.1
due to
external agent(s) NEC 508.9
specified NEC 508.8
fumes and vapors (chemical) (inhalation) 506.1
radiation 508.0
chemical (acute) 506.1
chronic 506.4
chronic 514
chemical (due to fumes or vapors) 506.4
due to
external agent(s) NEC 508.9
specified NEC 508.8
fumes or vapors (chemical) (inhalation) 506.4
radiation 508.1
due to
external agent 508.9
specified NEC 508.8
high altitude 993.2
near drowning 994.1
postoperative 518.4
terminal 514
lymphatic 457.1
due to mastectomy operation 457.0
macula 362.83
cystoid 362.53
diabetic 250.5 *[362.07]*
malignant (*see also* Gangrene, gas) 040.0
Milroy's 757.0
nasopharynx 478.25
neonatorum 778.5
nutritional (newborn) 262
with dyspigmentation, skin and hair 260
optic disc or nerve - *see* Papilledema
orbit 376.33
circulatory 459.89
palate (soft) (hard) 528.9
pancreas 577.8
penis 607.83
periodic 995.1
hereditary 277.6
pharynx 478.25
pitting 782.3
pulmonary - *see* Edema, lung
Quincke's 995.1
hereditary 277.6
renal (*see also* Nephrosis) 581.9
retina (localized) (macular) (peripheral) 362.83

Edema, edematous *(Continued)*
retina *(Continued)*
cystoid 362.53
diabetic 250.5 *[362.07]*
salt 276.0
scrotum 608.86
seminal vesicle 608.86
spermatic cord 608.86
spinal cord 336.1
starvation 262
stasis - *see also* Hypertension, venous 459.30
subconjunctival 372.73
subglottic (*see also* Edema, glottis) 478.6
supraglottic (*see also* Edema, glottis) 478.6
testis 608.86
toxic NEC 782.3
traumatic NEC 782.3
tunica vaginalis 608.86
vas deferens 608.86
vocal cord - *see* Edema, glottis
vulva (acute) 624.8
Edentia (complete) (partial) (*see also* Absence, tooth) 520.0
acquired (*see also* Edentulism) 525.40
due to
caries 525.13
extraction 525.10
periodontal disease 525.12
specified NEC 525.19
trauma 525.11
causing malocclusion 524.30
congenital (deficiency of tooth buds) 520.0
Edentulism 525.40
complete 525.40
class I 525.41
class II 525.42
class III 525.43
class IV 525.44
partial 525.50
class I 525.51
class II 525.52
class III 525.53
class IV 525.54
Edsall's disease 992.2
Educational handicap V62.3
Edwards' syndrome 758.2
Effect, adverse NEC
abnormal gravitational (G) forces or states 994.9
air pressure - *see* Effect, adverse, atmospheric pressure
altitude (high) - *see* Effect, adverse, high altitude
anesthetic
in labor and delivery NEC 668.9
affecting fetus or newborn 763.5
antitoxin - *see* Complications, vaccination
atmospheric pressure 993.9
due to explosion 993.4
high 993.3
low - *see* Effect, adverse, high altitude
specified effect NEC 993.8
biological, correct substance properly administered (*see also* Effect, adverse, drug) 995.20 ◄
blood (derivatives) (serum) (transfusion) - *see* Complications, transfusion
chemical substance NEC 989.9
specified - *see* Table of Drugs and Chemicals

Effect, adverse NEC *(Continued)*
cobalt, radioactive (*see also* Effect, adverse, radioactive substance) 990
cold (temperature) (weather) 991.9
chilblains 991.5
frostbite - *see* Frostbite
specified effect NEC 991.8
drugs and medicinals 995.20
correct substance properly administered 995.20
overdose or wrong substance given or taken 977.9
specified drug - *see* Table of Drugs and Chemicals
electric current (shock) 994.8
burn - *see* Burn, by site
electricity (electrocution) (shock) 994.8
burn - *see* Burn, by site
exertion (excessive) 994.5
exposure 994.9
exhaustion 994.4
external cause NEC 994.9
fallout (radioactive) NEC 990
fluoroscopy NEC 990
foodstuffs
allergic reaction (*see also* Allergy, food) 693.1
anaphylactic shock due to food NEC 995.60
noxious 988.9
specified type NEC (*see also* Poisoning, by name of noxious foodstuff) 988.8
gases, fumes, or vapors - *see* Table of Drugs and Chemicals
glue (airplane) sniffing 304.6
heat - *see* Heat
high altitude NEC 993.2
anoxia 993.2
on
ears 993.0
sinuses 993.1
polycythemia 289.0
hot weather - *see* Heat
hunger 994.2
immersion, foot 991.4
immunization - *see* Complications, vaccination
immunological agents - *see* Complications, vaccination
implantation (removable) of isotope or radium NEC 990
infrared (radiation) (rays) NEC 990
burn - *see* Burn, by site
dermatitis or eczema 692.82
infusion - *see* Complications, infusion
ingestion or injection of isotope (therapeutic) NEC 990
irradiation NEC (*see also* Effect, adverse, radiation) 990
isotope (radioactive) NEC 990
lack of care (child) (infant) (newborn) 995.52
adult 995.84
lightning 994.0
burn - *see* Burn, by site
Lirugin - *see* Complications, vaccination
medicinal substance, correct, properly administered (*see also* Effect, adverse, drugs) 995.20
mesothorium NEC 990
motion 994.6
noise, inner ear 388.10
other drug, medicinal, and biological substance 995.29

Effect, adverse NEC *(Continued)*
overheated places - *see* Heat
polonium NEC 990
psychosocial, of work environment V62.1
radiation (diagnostic) (fallout) (infrared) (natural source) (therapeutic) (tracer) (ultraviolet) (x-ray) NEC 990
with pulmonary manifestations
acute 508.0
chronic 508.1
dermatitis or eczema 692.82
due to sun NEC (*see also* Dermatitis, due to, sun) 692.70
fibrosis of lungs 508.1
maternal with suspected damage to fetus affecting management of pregnancy 655.6
pneumonitis 508.0
radioactive substance NEC 990
dermatitis or eczema 692.82
radioactivity NEC 990
radiotherapy NEC 990
dermatitis or eczema 692.82
radium NEC 990
reduced temperature 991.9
frostbite - *see* Frostbite
immersion, foot (hand) 991.4
specified effect NEC 991.8
roentgenography NEC 990
roentgenoscopy NEC 990
roentgen rays NEC 990
serum (prophylactic) (therapeutic) NEC 999.5
specified NEC 995.89
external cause NEC 994.9
strangulation 994.7
submersion 994.1
teletherapy NEC 990
thirst 994.3
transfusion - *see* Complications, transfusion
ultraviolet (radiation) (rays) NEC 990
burn - *see also* Burn, by site
from sun (*see also* Sunburn) 692.71
dermatitis or eczema 692.82
due to sun NEC (*see also* Dermatitis, due to, sun) 692.70
uranium NEC 990
vaccine (any) - *see* Complications, vaccination
weightlessness 994.9
whole blood - *see also* Complications, transfusion
overdose or wrong substance given (*see also* Table of Drugs and Chemicals) 964.7
working environment V62.1
x-rays NEC 990
dermatitis or eczema 692.82
Effect, remote
of cancer - *see* condition
Effects, late - *see* Late, effect (of)
Effluvium, telogen 704.02
Effort
intolerance 306.2
syndrome (aviators) (psychogenic) 306.2
Effusion
amniotic fluid (*see also* Rupture, membranes, premature) 658.1
brain (serous) 348.5
bronchial (*see also* Bronchitis) 490
cerebral 348.5

Effusion *(Continued)*
cerebrospinal (*see also* Meningitis) 322.9
vessel 348.5
chest - *see* Effusion, pleura
intracranial 348.5
joint 719.00
ankle 719.07
elbow 719.02
foot 719.07
hand 719.04
hip 719.05
knee 719.06
multiple sites 719.09
pelvic region 719.05
shoulder (region) 719.01
specified site NEC 719.08
wrist 719.03
meninges (*see also* Meningitis) 322.9
pericardium, pericardial (*see also* Pericarditis) 423.9
acute 420.90
peritoneal (chronic) 568.82
pleura, pleurisy, pleuritic, pleuropericardial 511.9
bacterial, nontuberculous 511.1
fetus or newborn 511.9
malignant 197.2
nontuberculous 511.9
bacterial 511.1
pneumococcal 511.1
staphylococcal 511.1
streptococcal 511.1
traumatic 862.29
with open wound 862.39
tuberculous (*see also* Tuberculosis, pleura) 012.0
primary progressive 010.1
pulmonary - *see* Effusion, pleura
spinal (*see also* Meningitis) 322.9
thorax, thoracic - *see* Effusion, pleura
Egg (oocyte) (ovum)
donor V59.70
over age 35 V59.73
anonymous recipient V59.73
designated recipient V59.74
under age 35 V59.71
anonymous recipient V59.71
designated recipient V59.72
Eggshell nails 703.8
congenital 757.5
Ego-dystonic
homosexuality 302.0
lesbianism 302.0
sexual orientation 302.0
Egyptian splenomegaly 120.1
Ehlers-Danlos syndrome 756.83
Ehrlichiosis 082.40
chaffeensis 082.41
specified type NEC 082.49
Eichstedt's disease (pityriasis versicolor) 111.0
Eisenmenger's complex or syndrome (ventricular septal defect) 745.4
Ejaculation, semen
painful 608.89
psychogenic 306.59
premature 302.75
retrograde 608.87
Ekbom syndrome (restless legs) 333.94
Ekman's syndrome (brittle bones and blue sclera) 756.51
Elastic skin 756.83
acquired 701.8
Elastofibroma (M8820/0) - *see* Neoplasm, connective tissue, benign

Elastoidosis
  cutanea nodularis 701.8
  cutis cystica et comedonica 701.8
Elastoma 757.39
  juvenile 757.39
  Miescher's (elastosis perforans serpiginosa) 701.1
Elastomyofibrosis 425.3
Elastosis 701.8
  atrophicans 701.8
  perforans serpiginosa 701.1
  reactive perforating 701.1
  senilis 701.8
  solar (actinic) 692.74
Elbow - *see* condition
Electric
  current, electricity, effects (concussion) (fatal) (nonfatal) (shock) 994.8
    burn - *see* Burn, by site
  feet (foot) syndrome 266.2
Electrocution 994.8
Electrolyte imbalance 276.9
  with
    abortion - *see* Abortion, by type, with metabolic disorder
    ectopic pregnancy (*see also* categories 633.0–633.9) 639.4
    hyperemesis gravidarum (before 22 completed weeks' gestation) 643.1
    molar pregnancy (*see also* categories 630–632) 639.4
  following
    abortion 639.4
    ectopic or molar pregnancy 639.4
Elephant man syndrome 237.71
Elephantiasis (nonfilarial) 457.1
  arabicum (*see also* Infestation, filarial) 125.9
  congenita hereditaria 757.0
  congenital (any site) 757.0
  due to
    Brugia (malayi) 125.1
    mastectomy operation 457.0
    Wuchereria (bancrofti) 125.0
      malayi 125.1
  eyelid 374.83
  filarial (*see also* Infestation, filarial) 125.9
  filariensis (*see also* Infestation, filarial) 125.9
  gingival 523.8
  glandular 457.1
  graecorum 030.9
  lymphangiectatic 457.1
  lymphatic vessel 457.1
    due to mastectomy operation 457.0
  neuromatosa 237.71
  postmastectomy 457.0
  scrotum 457.1
  streptococcal 457.1
  surgical 997.99
    postmastectomy 457.0
  telangiectodes 457.1
  vulva (nonfilarial) 624.8
Elevated - *see* Elevation
Elevation
  17-ketosteroids 791.9
  acid phosphatase 790.5
  alkaline phosphatase 790.5
  amylase 790.5
  antibody titers 795.79
  basal metabolic rate (BMR) 794.7
  blood pressure (*see also* Hypertension) 401.9

Elevation *(Continued)*
  blood pressure *(Continued)*
    reading (incidental) (isolated) (nonspecific), no diagnosis of hypertension 796.2
  body temperature (of unknown origin) (*see also* Pyrexia) 780.6
  cancer antigen 125 [CA 125] 795.82 ◀
  carcinoembryonic antigen [CEA] 795.81 ◀
  conjugate, eye 378.81
  C-reactive protein (CRP) 790.95
  CRP (C-reactive protein) 790.95
  diaphragm, congenital 756.6
  glucose
    fasting 790.21
    tolerance test 790.22
  immunoglobulin level 795.79
  indolacetic acid 791.9
  lactic acid dehydrogenase (LDH) level 790.4
  leukocytes 288.60 ◀
  lipase 790.5
  lipoprotein a level 272.8
  liver function test (LFT) 790.6
    alkaline phosphatase 790.5 ◀
    aminotransferase 790.4 ◀
    bilirubin 782.4 ◀
    hepatic enzyme NEC 790.5 ◀
    lactate dehydrogenase 790.4 ◀
  lymphocytes 288.61 ◀
  prostate specific antigen (PSA) 790.93
  renin 790.99
    in hypertension (*see also* Hypertension, renovascular) 405.91
  Rh titer 999.7
  scapula, congenital 755.52
  sedimentation rate 790.1
  SGOT 790.4
  SGPT 790.4
  transaminase 790.4
  vanillylmandelic acid 791.9
  venous pressure 459.89
  VMA 791.9
  white blood cell count 288.60 ◀
    specified NEC 288.69 ◀
Elliptocytosis (congenital) (hereditary) 282.1
  Hb-C (disease) 282.7
  hemoglobin disease 282.7
  sickle-cell (disease) 282.60
    trait 282.5
Ellis-van Creveld disease or syndrome (chondroectodermal dysplasia) 756.55
Ellison-Zollinger syndrome (gastric hypersecretion with pancreatic islet cell tumor) 251.5
Elongation, elongated (congenital) - *see also* Distortion
  bone 756.9
  cervix (uteri) 752.49
    acquired 622.6
    hypertrophic 622.6
  colon 751.5
  common bile duct 751.69
  cystic duct 751.69
  frenulum, penis 752.69
  labia minora, acquired 624.8
  ligamentum patellae 756.89
  petiolus (epiglottidis) 748.3
  styloid bone (process) 733.99
  tooth, teeth 520.2
  uvula 750.26
    acquired 528.9
Elschnig bodies or pearls 366.51

El Tor cholera 001.1
Emaciation (due to malnutrition) 261
Emancipation disorder 309.22
Embadomoniasis 007.8
Embarrassment heart, cardiac - *see* Disease, heart
Embedded tooth, teeth 520.6
  root only 525.3
Embolic - *see* condition
Embolism 444.9
  with
    abortion - *see* Abortion, by type, with embolism
    ectopic pregnancy (*see also* categories 633.0–633.9) 639.6
    molar pregnancy (*see also* categories 630–632) 639.6
  air (any site) 958.0
    with
      abortion - *see* Abortion, by type, with embolism
      ectopic pregnancy (*see also* categories 633.0–633.9) 639.6
      molar pregnancy (*see also* categories 630–632) 639.6
    due to implanted device - *see* Complications, due to (presence of) any device, implant, or graft classified to 996.0–996.5 NEC
    following
      abortion 639.6
      ectopic or molar pregnancy 639.6
      infusion, perfusion, or transfusion 999.1
    in pregnancy, childbirth, or puerperium 673.0
    traumatic 958.0
  amniotic fluid (pulmonary) 673.1
    with
      abortion - *see* Abortion, by type, with embolism
      ectopic pregnancy (*see also* categories 633.0–633.9) 639.6
      molar pregnancy (*see also* categories 630–632) 639.6
    following
      abortion 639.6
      ectopic or molar pregnancy 639.6
  aorta, aortic 444.1
    abdominal 444.0
    bifurcation 444.0
    saddle 444.0
    thoracic 444.1
  artery 444.9
    auditory, internal 433.8
    basilar (*see also* Occlusion, artery, basilar) 433.0
    bladder 444.89
    carotid (common) (internal) (*see also* Occlusion, artery, carotid) 433.1
    cerebellar (anterior inferior) (posterior inferior) (superior) 433.8
    cerebral (*see also* Embolism, brain) 434.1
    choroidal (anterior) 433.8
    communicating posterior 433.8
    coronary (*see also* Infarct, myocardium) 410.9
      without myocardial infarction 411.81
    extremity 444.22
      lower 444.22
      upper 444.21
    hypophyseal 433.8
    mesenteric (with gangrene) 557.0

◀ New   ⇐ Revised

Embolism *(Continued)*
artery *(Continued)*
ophthalmic (*see also* Occlusion, retina) 362.30
peripheral 444.22
pontine 433.8
precerebral NEC - *see* Occlusion, artery, precerebral
pulmonary - *see* Embolism, pulmonary
renal 593.81
retinal (*see also* Occlusion, retina) 362.30
specified site NEC 444.89
vertebral (*see also* Occlusion, artery, vertebral) 433.2
auditory, internal 433.8
basilar (artery) (*see also* Occlusion, artery, basilar) 433.0
birth, mother - *see* Embolism, obstetrical
blood-clot
with
abortion - *see* Abortion, by type, with embolism
ectopic pregnancy (*see also* categories 633.0–633.9) 639.6
molar pregnancy (*see also* categories 630–632) 639.6
following
abortion 639.6
ectopic or molar pregnancy 639.6
in pregnancy, childbirth, or puerperium 673.2
brain 434.1
with
abortion - *see* Abortion, by type, with embolism
ectopic pregnancy (*see also* categories 633.0–633.9) 639.6
molar pregnancy (*see also* categories 630–632) 639.6
following
abortion 639.6
ectopic or molar pregnancy 639.6
late effect - *see* Late effect(s) (of) cerebrovascular disease
puerperal, postpartum, childbirth 674.0
capillary 448.9
cardiac (*see also* Infarct, myocardium) 410.9
carotid (artery) (common) (internal) (*see also* Occlusion, artery, carotid) 433.1
cavernous sinus (venous) - *see* Embolism, intracranial venous sinus
cerebral (*see also* Embolism, brain) 434.1
cholesterol - *see* Atheroembolism
choroidal (anterior) (artery) 433.8
coronary (artery or vein) (systemic) (*see also* Infarct, myocardium) 410.9
without myocardial infarction 411.81
due to (presence of) any device, implant, or graft classifiable to 996.0–996.5 - *see* Complications, due to (presence of) any device, implant, or graft classified to 996.0–996.5 NEC
encephalomalacia (*see also* Embolism, brain) 434.1
extremities 444.22
lower 444.22
upper 444.21
eye 362.30
fat (cerebral) (pulmonary) (systemic) 958.1

Embolism *(Continued)*
fat *(Continued)*
with
abortion - *see* Abortion, by type, with embolism
ectopic pregnancy (*see also* categories 633.0–633.9) 639.6
molar pregnancy (*see also* categories 630–632) 639.6
complicating delivery or puerperium 673.8
following
abortion 639.6
ectopic or molar pregnancy 639.6
in pregnancy, childbirth, or the puerperium 673.8
femoral (artery) 444.22
vein 453.8
deep 453.41
following
abortion 639.6
ectopic or molar pregnancy 639.6
infusion, perfusion, or transfusion
air 999.1
thrombus 999.2
heart (fatty) (*see also* Infarct, myocardium) 410.9
hepatic (vein) 453.0
iliac (artery) 444.81
iliofemoral 444.81
in pregnancy, childbirth, or puerperium (pulmonary) - *see* Embolism, obstetrical
intestine (artery) (vein) (with gangrene) 557.0
intracranial (*see also* Embolism, brain) 434.1
venous sinus (any) 325
late effect - *see* category 326
nonpyogenic 437.6
in pregnancy or puerperium 671.5
kidney (artery) 593.81
lateral sinus (venous) - *see* Embolism, intracranial venous sinus
longitudinal sinus (venous) - *see* Embolism, intracranial venous sinus
lower extremity 444.22
lung (massive) - *see* Embolism, pulmonary
meninges (*see also* Embolism, brain) 434.1
mesenteric (artery) (with gangrene) 557.0
multiple NEC 444.9
obstetrical (pulmonary) 673.2
air 673.0
amniotic fluid (pulmonary) 673.1
blood-clot 673.2
cardiac 674.8
fat 673.8
heart 674.8
pyemic 673.3
septic 673.3
specified NEC 674.8
ophthalmic (*see also* Occlusion, retina) 362.30
paradoxical NEC 444.9
penis 607.82
peripheral arteries NEC 444.22
lower 444.22
upper 444.21
pituitary 253.8
popliteal (artery) 444.22
portal (vein) 452

Embolism *(Continued)*
postoperative NEC 997.2
cerebral 997.02
mesenteric artery 997.71
other vessels 997.79
peripheral vascular 997.2
pulmonary 415.11
renal artery 997.72
precerebral artery (*see also* Occlusion, artery, precerebral) 433.9
puerperal - *see* Embolism, obstetrical
pulmonary (artery) (vein) 415.19
with
abortion - *see* Abortion, by type, with embolism
ectopic pregnancy (*see also* categories 633.0–633.9) 639.6
molar pregnancy (*see also* categories 630–632) 639.6
following
abortion 639.6
ectopic or molar pregnancy 639.6
iatrogenic 415.11
in pregnancy, childbirth, or puerperium - *see* Embolism, obstetrical
postoperative 415.11
pyemic (multiple) 038.9
with
abortion - *see* Abortion, by type, with embolism
ectopic pregnancy (*see also* categories 633.0–633.9) 639.6
molar pregnancy (*see also* categories 630–632) 639.6
Aerobacter aerogenes 038.49
enteric gram-negative bacilli 038.40
Enterobacter aerogenes 038.49
Escherichia coli 038.42
following
abortion 639.6
ectopic or molar pregnancy 639.6
Hemophilus influenzae 038.41
pneumococcal 038.2
Proteus vulgaris 038.49
Pseudomonas (aeruginosa) 038.43
puerperal, postpartum, childbirth (any organism) 673.3
Serratia 038.44
specified organism NEC 038.8
staphylococcal 038.10
aureus 038.11
specified organism NEC 038.19
streptococcal 038.0
renal (artery) 593.81
vein 453.3
retina, retinal (*see also* Occlusion, retina) 362.30
saddle (aorta) 444.0
septicemic - *see* Embolism, pyemic
sinus - *see* Embolism, intracranial venous sinus
soap
with
abortion - *see* Abortion, by type, with embolism
ectopic pregnancy (*see also* categories 633.0–633.9) 639.6
molar pregnancy (*see also* categories 630–632) 639.6
following
abortion 639.6
ectopic or molar pregnancy 639.6
spinal cord (nonpyogenic) 336.1
in pregnancy or puerperium 671.5
pyogenic origin 324.1
late effect - *see* category 326

Embolism *(Continued)*
spleen, splenic (artery) 444.89
thrombus (thromboembolism) following infusion, perfusion, or transfusion 999.2
upper extremity 444.21
vein 453.9
with inflammation or phlebitis - *see* Thrombophlebitis
cerebral (*see also* Embolism, brain) 434.1
coronary (*see also* Infarct, myocardium) 410.9
without myocardial infarction 411.81
hepatic 453.0
lower extremity 453.8
deep 453.40
calf 453.42
distal (lower leg) 453.42
femoral 453.41
iliac 453.41
lower leg 453.42
peroneal 453.42
popliteal 453.41
proximal (upper leg) 453.41
thigh 453.41
tibial 453.42
mesenteric (with gangrene) 557.0
portal 452
pulmonary - *see* Embolism, pulmonary
renal 453.3
specified NEC 453.8
with inflammation or phlebitis - *see* Thrombophlebitis
vena cava (inferior) (superior) 453.2
vessels of brain (*see also* Embolism, brain) 434.1
Embolization - *see* Embolism
Embolus - *see* Embolism
Embryoma (M9080/1) - *see also* Neoplasm, by site, uncertain behavior
benign (M9080/0) - *see* Neoplasm, by site, benign
kidney (M8960/3) 189.0
liver (M8970/3) 155.0
malignant (M9080/3) - *see also* Neoplasm, by site, malignant
kidney (M8960/3) 189.0
liver (M8970/3) 155.0
testis (M9070/3) 186.9
undescended 186.0
testis (M9070/3) 186.9
undescended 186.0
Embryonic
circulation 747.9
heart 747.9
vas deferens 752.89
Embryopathia NEC 759.9
Embryotomy, fetal 763.89
Embryotoxon 743.43
interfering with vision 743.42
Emesis - *see also* Vomiting
gravidarum - *see* Hyperemesis, gravidarum
Emissions, nocturnal (semen) 608.89
Emotional
crisis - *see* Crisis, emotional
disorder (*see also* Disorder, mental) 300.9
instability (excessive) 301.3
overlay - *see* Reaction, adjustment
upset 300.9
Emotionality, pathological 301.3
Emotogenic disease (*see also* Disorder, psychogenic) 306.9
Emphysema (atrophic) (centriacinar) (centrilobular) (chronic) (diffuse) (essential) (hypertrophic) (interlobular) (lung) (obstructive) (panlobular) (paracicatricial) (paracinar) (postural) (pulmonary) (senile) (subpleural) (traction) (unilateral) (unilobular) (vesicular) 492.8
with bronchitis
chronic 491.20
with
acute bronchitis 491.22
exacerbation (acute) 491.21
bullous (giant) 492.0
cellular tissue 958.7
surgical 998.81
compensatory 518.2
congenital 770.2
conjunctiva 372.89
connective tissue 958.7
surgical 998.81
due to fumes or vapors 506.4
eye 376.89
eyelid 374.85
surgical 998.81
traumatic 958.7
fetus or newborn (interstitial) (mediastinal) (unilobular) 770.2
heart 416.9
interstitial 518.1
congenital 770.2
fetus or newborn 770.2
laminated tissue 958.7
surgical 998.81
mediastinal 518.1
fetus or newborn 770.2
newborn (interstitial) (mediastinal) (unilobular) 770.2
obstructive diffuse with fibrosis 492.8
orbit 376.89
subcutaneous 958.7
due to trauma 958.7
nontraumatic 518.1
surgical 998.81
surgical 998.81
thymus (gland) (congenital) 254.8
traumatic 958.7
tuberculous (*see also* Tuberculosis, pulmonary) 011.9
Employment examination (certification) V70.5
Empty sella (turcica) syndrome 253.8
Empyema (chest) (diaphragmatic) (double) (encapsulated) (general) (interlobar) (lung) (medial) (necessitatis) (perforating chest wall) (pleura) (pneumococcal) (residual) (sacculated) (streptococcal) (supradiaphragmatic) 510.9
with fistula 510.0
accessory sinus (chronic) (*see also* Sinusitis) 473.9
acute 510.9
with fistula 510.0
antrum (chronic) (*see also* Sinusitis, maxillary) 473.0
brain (any part) (*see also* Abscess, brain) 324.0
ethmoidal (sinus) (chronic) (*see also* Sinusitis, ethmoidal) 473.2
extradural (*see also* Abscess, extradural) 324.9
frontal (sinus) (chronic) (*see also* Sinusitis, frontal) 473.1
gallbladder (*see also* Cholecystitis, acute) 575.0
Empyema *(Continued)*
mastoid (process) (acute) (*see also* Mastoiditis, acute) 383.00
maxilla, maxillary 526.4
sinus (chronic) (*see also* Sinusitis, maxillary) 473.0
nasal sinus (chronic) (*see also* Sinusitis) 473.9
sinus (accessory) (nasal) (*see also* Sinusitis) 473.9
sphenoidal (chronic) (sinus) (*see also* Sinusitis, sphenoidal) 473.3
subarachnoid (*see also* Abscess, extradural) 324.9
subdural (*see also* Abscess, extradural) 324.9
tuberculous (*see also* Tuberculosis, pleura) 012.0
ureter (*see also* Ureteritis) 593.89
ventricular (*see also* Abscess, brain) 324.0
Enameloma 520.2
Encephalitis (bacterial) (chronic) (hemorrhagic) (idiopathic) (nonepidemic) (spurious) (subacute) 323.9
acute - *see also* Encephalitis, viral
disseminated (postinfectious) NEC 136.9 *[323.61]* ◄
postimmunization or postvaccination 323.51 ◄
inclusional 049.8
inclusion body 049.8
necrotizing 049.8
arboviral, arbovirus NEC 064
arthropod-borne (*see also* Encephalitis, viral, arthropod-borne) 064
Australian X 062.4
Bwamba fever 066.3
California (virus) 062.5
Central European 063.2
Czechoslovakian 063.2
Dawson's (inclusion body) 046.2
diffuse sclerosing 046.2
due to
actinomycosis 039.8 *[323.41]* ◄
cat-scratch disease 078.3 *[323.01]* ◄
infection classified elsewhere 136.9 *[323.41]* ◄
infectious mononucleosis 075 *[323.01]* ◄
malaria (*see also* Malaria) 084.6 *[323.2]*
Negishi virus 064
ornithosis 073.7 *[323.01]* ◄
prophylactic inoculation against smallpox 323.51 ◄
rickettsiosis (*see also* Rickettsiosis) 083.9 *[323.1]*
rubella 056.01
toxoplasmosis (acquired) 130.0
congenital (active) 771.2 *[323.41]* ◄
typhus (fever) (*see also* Typhus) 081.9 *[323.1]*
vaccination (smallpox) 323.51 ◄
Eastern equine 062.2
endemic 049.8
epidemic 049.8
equine (acute) (infectious) (viral) 062.9
eastern 062.2
Venezuelan 066.2
western 062.1
Far Eastern 063.0
following vaccination or other immunization procedure 323.51 ◄
herpes 054.3

◄ New ◄ Revised

Encephalitis *(Continued)*
- Ilheus (virus) 062.8
- inclusion body 046.2
- infectious (acute) (virus) NEC 049.8
- influenzal 487.8 *[323.41]*
  - lethargic 049.8
- Japanese (B type) 062.0
- La Crosse 062.5
- Langat 063.8
- late effect - *see* Late, effect, encephalitis
- lead 984.9 *[323.71]*
- lethargic (acute) (infectious) (influenzal) 049.8
- lethargica 049.8
- louping ill 063.1
- lupus 710.0 *[323.81]*
- lymphatica 049.0
- Mengo 049.8
- meningococcal 036.1
- mumps 072.2
- Murray Valley 062.4
- myoclonic 049.8
- Negishi virus 064
- otitic NEC 382.4 *[323.41]*
- parasitic NEC 123.9 *[323.41]*
- periaxialis (concentrica) (diffusa) 341.1
- postchickenpox 052.0
- postexanthematous NEC 057.9 *[323.62]*
- postimmunization 323.51
- postinfectious NEC 136.9 *[323.62]*
- postmeasles 055.0
- posttraumatic 323.81
- postvaccinal (smallpox) 323.51
- postvaricella 052.0
- postviral NEC 079.99 *[323.62]*
  - postexanthematous 057.9 *[323.62]*
    - specified NEC 057.8 *[323.62]*
- Powassan 063.8
- progressive subcortical (Binswanger's) 290.12
- Rasmussen 323.81
- Rio Bravo 049.8
- rubella 056.01
- Russian
  - autumnal 062.0
  - spring-summer type (taiga) 063.0
- saturnine 984.9 *[323.71]*
- Semliki Forest 062.8
- serous 048
- slow-acting virus NEC 046.8
- specified cause NEC 323.81
- St. Louis type 062.3
- subacute sclerosing 046.2
- subcorticalis chronica 290.12
- summer 062.0
- suppurative 324.0
- syphilitic 094.81
  - congenital 090.41
- tick-borne 063.9
- torula, torular 117.5 *[323.41]*
- toxic NEC 989.9 *[323.71]*
- toxoplasmic (acquired) 130.0
  - congenital (active) 771.2 *[323.41]*
- trichinosis 124 *[323.41]*
- Trypanosomiasis (*see also* Trypanosomiasis) 086.9 *[323.2]*
- tuberculous (*see also* Tuberculosis) 013.6
- type B (Japanese) 062.0
- type C 062.3
- van Bogaert's 046.2
- Venezuelan 066.2
- Vienna type 049.8
- viral, virus 049.9
  - arthropod-borne NEC 064

Encephalitis *(Continued)*
- viral, virus *(Continued)*
  - arthropod-borne NEC *(Continued)*
    - mosquito-borne 062.9
      - Australian X disease 062.4
      - California virus 062.5
      - Eastern equine 062.2
      - Ilheus virus 062.8
      - Japanese (B type) 062.0
      - Murray Valley 062.4
      - specified type NEC 062.8
      - St. Louis 062.3
      - type B 062.0
      - type C 062.3
      - Western equine 062.1
    - tick-borne 063.9
      - biundulant 063.2
      - Central European 063.2
      - Czechoslovakian 063.2
      - diphasic meningoencephalitis 063.2
      - Far Eastern 063.0
      - Langat 063.8
      - louping ill 063.1
      - Powassan 063.8
      - Russian spring-summer (taiga) 063.0
      - specified type NEC 063.8
    - vector unknown 064
  - slow acting NEC 046.8
  - specified type NEC 049.8
  - vaccination, prophylactic (against) V05.0
- von Economo's 049.8
- Western equine 062.1
- West Nile type 066.41

Encephalocele 742.0
- orbit 376.81

Encephalocystocele 742.0

Encephalomalacia (brain) (cerebellar) (cerebral) (cerebrospinal) (*see also* Softening, brain) 434.9
- due to
  - hemorrhage (*see also* Hemorrhage, brain) 431
  - recurrent spasm of artery 435.9
- embolic (cerebral) (*see also* Embolism, brain) 434.1
- subcorticalis chronicus arteriosclerotica 290.12
- thrombotic (*see also* Thrombosis, brain) 434.0

Encephalomeningitis - *see* Meningoencephalitis

Encephalomeningocele 742.0

Encephalomeningomyelitis - *see* Meningoencephalitis

Encephalomeningopathy (*see also* Meningoencephalitis) 349.9

Encephalomyelitis (chronic) (granulomatous) (hemorrhagic necrotizing, acute) (myalgic, benign) (*see also* Encephalitis) 323.9
- abortive disseminated 049.8
- acute disseminated (ADEM) (postinfectious) 136.9 *[323.61]*
  - infectious 136.9 *[323.61]*
  - noninfectious 323.81
  - postimmunization 323.51
- due to
  - cat-scratch disease 078.3 *[323.01]*
  - infectious mononucleosis 075 *[323.01]*
  - ornithosis 073.7 *[323.01]*
  - vaccination (any) 323.51

Encephalomyelitis *(Continued)*
- equine (acute) (infectious) 062.9
  - eastern 062.2
  - Venezuelan 066.2
  - western 062.1
- funicularis infectiosa 049.8
- late effect - *see* Late, effect, encephalitis
- Munch-Peterson's 049.8
- postchickenpox 052.0
- postimmunization 323.51
- postmeasles 055.0
- postvaccinal (smallpox) 323.51
- rubella 056.01
- specified cause NEC 323.81
- syphilitic 094.81
- West Nile 066.41

Encephalomyelocele 742.0

Encephalomyelomeningitis - *see* Meningoencephalitis

Encephalomyeloneuropathy 349.9

Encephalomyelopathy 349.9
- subacute necrotizing (infantile) 330.8

Encephalomyeloradiculitis (acute) 357.0

Encephalomyeloradiculoneuritis (acute) 357.0

Encephalomyeloradiculopathy 349.9

Encephalomyocarditis 074.23

Encephalopathia hyperbilirubinemica, newborn 774.7
- due to isoimmunization (conditions classifiable to 773.0–773.2) 773.4

Encephalopathy (acute) 348.30
- alcoholic 291.2
- anoxic - *see* Damage, brain, anoxic
- arteriosclerotic 437.0
  - late effect - *see* Late effect(s) (of) cerebrovascular disease
- bilirubin, newborn 774.7
  - due to isoimmunization 773.4
- congenital 742.9
- demyelinating (callosal) 341.8
- due to
  - birth injury (intracranial) 767.8
  - dialysis 294.8
    - transient 293.9
  - hyperinsulinism - *see* Hyperinsulinism
  - influenza (virus) 487.8
  - lack of vitamin (*see also* Deficiency, vitamin) 269.2
  - nicotinic acid deficiency 291.2
  - serum (nontherapeutic) (therapeutic) 999.5
  - syphilis 094.81
  - trauma (postconcussional) 310.2
    - current (*see also* Concussion, brain) 850.9
      - with skull fracture - *see* Fracture, skull, by site, with intracranial injury
  - vaccination 323.51
- hepatic 572.2
- hyperbilirubinemic, newborn 774.7
  - due to isoimmunization (conditions classifiable to 773.0–773.2) 773.4
- hypertensive 437.2
- hypoglycemic 251.2
- hypoxic - *see also* Damage, brain, anoxic
  - ischemic (HIE) 768.7
- infantile cystic necrotizing (congenital) 341.8
- lead 984.9 *[323.71]*
- leukopolio 330.0
- metabolic - *see also* Delirium 348.31
  - toxic 349.82

ICD-9-CM

E

Vol. 2

Encephalopathy *(Continued)*
  necrotizing
    hemorrhagic 323.61
    other specified type NEC 348.39
    subacute 330.8
  pellagrous 265.2
  portal-systemic 572.2
  postcontusional 310.2
  posttraumatic 310.2
  saturnine 984.9 *[323.71]*
  septic 348.31
  spongioform, subacute (viral) 046.1
  subacute
    necrotizing 330.8
    spongioform 046.1
    viral, spongioform 046.1
  subcortical progressive (Schilder) 341.1
    chronic (Binswanger's) 290.12
  toxic 349.82
    metabolic 349.82
  traumatic (postconcussional) 310.2
    current (*see also* Concussion, brain) 850.9
      with skull fracture - *see* Fracture, skull, by site, with intracranial injury
  vitamin B deficiency NEC 266.9
  Wernicke's (superior hemorrhagic polioencephalitis) 265.1
Encephalorrhagia (*see also* Hemorrhage, brain) 432.9
  healed or old V12.59
  late effect - *see* Late effect(s) (of) cerebrovascular disease
Encephalosis, posttraumatic 310.2
Enchondroma (M9220/0) - *see also* Neoplasm, bone, benign
  multiple, congenital 756.4
Enchondromatosis (cartilaginous) (congenital) (multiple) 756.4
Enchondroses, multiple (cartilaginous) (congenital) 756.4
Encopresis (*see also* Incontinence, feces) 787.6
  nonorganic origin 307.7
Encounter for - *see also* Admission for
  administrative purpose only V68.9
    referral of patient without examination or treatment V68.81
    specified purpose NEC V68.89
  chemotherapy, antineoplastic V58.11
  dialysis
    extracorporeal (renal) V56.0
    peritoneal V56.8
  end-of-life care V66.7
  hospice care V66.7
  immunotherapy, antineoplastic V58.12
  palliative care V66.7
  paternity testing V70.4
  radiotherapy V58.0
  respirator [ventilator] dependence
    during
      mechanical failure V46.14
      power failure V46.12
    for weaning V46.13
  screening mammogram NEC V76.12
    for high-risk patient V76.11
  terminal care V66.7
  weaning from respirator [ventilator] V46.13
Encystment - *see* Cyst
End-of-life care V66.7
Endamebiasis - *see* Amebiasis
Endamoeba - *see* Amebiasis
Endarteritis (bacterial, subacute) (infective) (septic) 447.6

Endarteritis *(Continued)*
  brain, cerebral or cerebrospinal 437.4
    late effect - *see* Late effect(s) (of) cerebrovascular disease
  coronary (artery) - *see* Arteriosclerosis, coronary
  deformans - *see* Arteriosclerosis
  embolic (*see also* Embolism) 444.9
  obliterans - *see also* Arteriosclerosis
    pulmonary 417.8
  pulmonary 417.8
  retina 362.18
  senile - *see* Arteriosclerosis
  syphilitic 093.89
    brain or cerebral 094.89
    congenital 090.5
    spinal 094.89
  tuberculous (*see also* Tuberculosis) 017.9
Endemic - *see* condition
Endocarditis (chronic) (indeterminate) (interstitial) (marantis) (nonbacterial thrombotic) (residual) (sclerotic) (sclerous) (senile) (valvular) 424.90
  with
    rheumatic fever (conditions classifiable to 390)
      active - *see* Endocarditis, acute, rheumatic
      inactive or quiescent (with chorea) 397.9
  acute or subacute 421.9
    rheumatic (aortic) (mitral) (pulmonary) (tricuspid) 391.1
      with chorea (acute) (rheumatic) (Sydenham's) 392.0
  aortic (heart) (nonrheumatic) (valve) 424.1
    with
      mitral (valve) disease 396.9
        active or acute 391.1
          with chorea (acute) (rheumatic) (Sydenham's) 392.0
        bacterial 421.0
      rheumatic fever (conditions classifiable to 390)
        active - *see* Endocarditis, acute, rheumatic
        inactive or quiescent (with chorea) 395.9
          with mitral disease 396.9
    acute or subacute 421.9
    arteriosclerotic 424.1
    congenital 746.89
    hypertensive 424.1
    rheumatic (chronic) (inactive) 395.9
      with mitral (valve) disease 396.9
        active or acute 391.1
          with chorea (acute) (rheumatic) (Sydenham's) 392.0
      active or acute 391.1
        with chorea (acute) (rheumatic) (Sydenham's) 392.0
    specified cause, except rheumatic 424.1
    syphilitic 093.22
  arteriosclerotic or due to arteriosclerosis 424.99
  atypical verrucous (Libman-Sacks) 710.0 *[424.91]*
  bacterial (acute) (any valve) (chronic) (subacute) 421.0
  blastomycotic 116.0 *[421.1]*
  candidal 112.81
  congenital 425.3
  constrictive 421.0
  Coxsackie 074.22

Endocarditis *(Continued)*
  due to
    blastomycosis 116.0 *[421.1]*
    candidiasis 112.81
    Coxsackie (virus) 074.22
    disseminated lupus erythematosus 710.0 *[424.91]*
    histoplasmosis (*see also* Histoplasmosis) 115.94
    hypertension (benign) 424.99
    moniliasis 112.81
    prosthetic cardiac valve 996.61
    Q fever 083.0 *[421.1]*
    serratia marcescens 421.0
    typhoid (fever) 002.0 *[421.1]*
  fetal 425.3
  gonococcal 098.84
  hypertensive 424.99
  infectious or infective (acute) (any valve) (chronic) (subacute) 421.0
  lenta (acute) (any valve) (chronic) (subacute) 421.0
  Libman-Sacks 710.0 *[424.91]*
  Loeffler's (parietal fibroplastic) 421.0
  malignant (acute) (any valve) (chronic) (subacute) 421.0
  meningococcal 036.42
  mitral (chronic) (double) (fibroid) (heart) (inactive) (valve) (with chorea) 394.9
    with
      aortic (valve) disease 396.9
        active or acute 391.1
          with chorea (acute) (rheumatic) (Sydenham's) 392.0
      rheumatic fever (conditions classifiable to 390)
        active - *see* Endocarditis, acute, rheumatic
        inactive or quiescent (with chorea) 394.9
          with aortic valve disease 396.9
    active or acute 391.1
      with chorea (acute) (rheumatic) (Sydenham's) 392.0
      bacterial 421.0
    arteriosclerotic 424.0
    congenital 746.89
    hypertensive 424.0
    nonrheumatic 424.0
      acute or subacute 421.9
    syphilitic 093.21
  monilial 112.81
  mycotic (acute) (any valve) (chronic) (subacute) 421.0
  pneumococcic (acute) (any valve) (chronic) (subacute) 421.0
  pulmonary (chronic) (heart) (valve) 424.3
    with
      rheumatic fever (conditions classifiable to 390)
        active - *see* Endocarditis, acute, rheumatic
        inactive or quiescent (with chorea) 397.1
    acute or subacute 421.9
      rheumatic 391.1
        with chorea (acute) (rheumatic) (Sydenham's) 392.0
    arteriosclerotic or due to arteriosclerosis 424.3
    congenital 746.09
    hypertensive or due to hypertension (benign) 424.3

Endocarditis *(Continued)*
pulmonary *(Continued)*
rheumatic (chronic) (inactive) (with chorea) 397.1
active or acute 391.1
with chorea (acute) (rheumatic) (Sydenham's) 392.0
syphilitic 093.24
purulent (acute) (any valve) (chronic) (subacute) 421.0
rheumatic (chronic) (inactive) (with chorea) 397.9
active or acute (aortic) (mitral) (pulmonary) (tricuspid) 391.1
with chorea (acute) (rheumatic) (Sydenham's) 392.0
septic (acute) (any valve) (chronic) (subacute) 421.0
specified cause, except rheumatic 424.99
streptococcal (acute) (any valve) (chronic) (subacute) 421.0
subacute - *see* Endocarditis, acute
suppurative (any valve) (acute) (chronic) (subacute) 421.0
syphilitic NEC 093.20
toxic (*see also* Endocarditis, acute) 421.9
tricuspid (chronic) (heart) (inactive) (rheumatic) (valve) (with chorea) 397.0
with
rheumatic fever (conditions classifiable to 390)
active - *see* Endocarditis, acute, rheumatic
inactive or quiescent (with chorea) 397.0
active or acute 391.1
with chorea (acute) (rheumatic) (Sydenham's) 392.0
arteriosclerotic 424.2
congenital 746.89
hypertensive 424.2
nonrheumatic 424.2
acute or subacute 421.9
specified cause, except rheumatic 424.2
syphilitic 093.23
tuberculous (*see also* Tuberculosis) 017.9 *[424.91]*
typhoid 002.0 *[421.1]*
ulcerative (acute) (any valve) (chronic) (subacute) 421.0
vegetative (acute) (any valve) (chronic) (subacute) 421.0
verrucous (acute) (any valve) (chronic) (subacute) NEC 710.0 *[424.91]*
nonbacterial 710.0 *[424.91]*
nonrheumatic 710.0 *[424.91]*
Endocardium, endocardial - *see also* condition
cushion defect 745.60
specified type NEC 745.69
Endocervicitis (*see also* Cervicitis) 616.0
due to
intrauterine (contraceptive) device 996.65
gonorrheal (acute) 098.15
chronic or duration of 2 months or over 098.35
hyperplastic 616.0
syphilitic 095.8
trichomonal 131.09
tuberculous (*see also* Tuberculosis) 016.7
Endocrine - *see* condition
Endocrinopathy, pluriglandular 258.9
Endodontitis 522.0
Endomastoiditis (*see also* Mastoiditis) 383.9
Endometrioma 617.9
Endometriosis 617.9
appendix 617.5
bladder 617.8
bowel 617.5
broad ligament 617.3
cervix 617.0
colon 617.5
cul-de-sac (Douglas') 617.3
exocervix 617.0
fallopian tube 617.2
female genital organ NEC 617.8
gallbladder 617.8
in scar of skin 617.6
internal 617.0
intestine 617.5
lung 617.8
myometrium 617.0
ovary 617.1
parametrium 617.3
pelvic peritoneum 617.3
peritoneal (pelvic) 617.3
rectovaginal septum 617.4
rectum 617.5
round ligament 617.3
skin 617.6
specified site NEC 617.8
stromal (M8931/1) 236.0
umbilicus 617.8
uterus 617.0
internal 617.0
vagina 617.4
vulva 617.8
Endometritis (nonspecific) (purulent) (septic) (suppurative) 615.9
with
abortion - *see* Abortion, by type, with sepsis
ectopic pregnancy (*see also* categories 633.0-633.9) 639.0
molar pregnancy (*see also* categories 630-632) 639.0
acute 615.0
blennorrhagic 098.16
acute 098.16
chronic or duration of 2 months or over 098.36
cervix, cervical (*see also* Cervicitis) 616.0
hyperplastic 616.0
chronic 615.1
complicating pregnancy 646.6
affecting fetus or newborn 760.8
decidual 615.9
following
abortion 639.0
ectopic or molar pregnancy 639.0
gonorrheal (acute) 098.16
chronic or duration of 2 months or over 098.36
hyperplastic (*see also* Hyperplasia, endometrium) 621.30
cervix 616.0
polypoid - *see* Endometritis, hyperplastic
puerperal, postpartum, childbirth 670
senile (atrophic) 615.9
subacute 615.0
tuberculous (*see also* Tuberculosis) 016.7
Endometrium - *see* condition
Endomyocardiopathy, South African 425.2
Endomyocarditis - *see* Endocarditis
Endomyofibrosis 425.0
Endomyometritis (*see also* Endometritis) 615.9
Endopericarditis - *see* Endocarditis
Endoperineuritis - *see* Disorder, nerve
Endophlebitis (*see also* Phlebitis) 451.9
leg 451.2
deep (vessels) 451.19
superficial (vessels) 451.0
portal (vein) 572.1
retina 362.18
specified site NEC 451.89
syphilitic 093.89
Endophthalmia (*see also* Endophthalmitis) 360.00
gonorrheal 098.42
Endophthalmitis (globe) (infective) (metastatic) (purulent) (subacute) 360.00
acute 360.01
bleb associated 379.63 ◀
chronic 360.03
parasitic 360.13
phacoanaphylactic 360.19
specified type NEC 360.19
sympathetic 360.11
Endosalpingioma (M9111/1) 236.2
Endosteitis - *see* Osteomyelitis
Endothelioma, bone (M9260/3) - *see* Neoplasm, bone, malignant
Endotheliosis 287.8
hemorrhagic infectional 287.8
Endotoxemia - *code to condition* ◀
Endotoxic shock 785.52
Endotrachelitis (*see also* Cervicitis) 616.0
Enema rash 692.89
Engel-von Recklinghausen disease or syndrome (osteitis fibrosa cystica) 252.01
Engelmann's disease (diaphyseal sclerosis) 756.59
English disease (*see also* Rickets) 268.0
Engman's disease (infectious eczematoid dermatitis) 690.8
Engorgement
breast 611.79
newborn 778.7
puerperal, postpartum 676.2
liver 573.9
lung 514
pulmonary 514
retina, venous 362.37
stomach 536.8
venous, retina 362.37
Enlargement, enlarged - *see also* Hypertrophy
abdomen 789.3
adenoids 474.12
and tonsils 474.10
alveolar process or ridge 525.8
apertures of diaphragm (congenital) 756.6
blind spot, visual field 368.42
gingival 523.8
heart, cardiac (*see also* Hypertrophy, cardiac) 429.3
lacrimal gland, chronic 375.03
liver (*see also* Hypertrophy, liver) 789.1
lymph gland or node 785.6
orbit 376.46
organ or site, congenital NEC - *see* Anomaly, specified type NEC
parathyroid (gland) 252.01
pituitary fossa 793.0
prostate (simple) (soft) 600.00
with ◀
other lower urinary tract symptoms (LUTS) 600.01 ◀

Enlargement, enlarged *(Continued)*
prostate *(Continued)*
with *(Continued)*
urinary
obstruction 600.01
retention 600.01
sella turcica 793.0
spleen (*see also* Splenomegaly) 789.2
congenital 759.0
thymus (congenital) (gland) 254.0
thyroid (gland) (*see also* Goiter) 240.9
tongue 529.8
tonsils 474.11
and adenoids 474.10
uterus 621.2
Enophthalmos 376.50
due to
atrophy of orbital tissue 376.51
surgery 376.52
trauma 376.52
Enostosis 526.89
Entamebiasis - *see* Amebiasis
Entamebic - *see* Amebiasis
Entanglement, umbilical cord(s) 663.3
with compression 663.2
affecting fetus or newborn 762.5
around neck with compression 663.1
twins in monoamniotic sac 663.2
Enteralgia 789.0
Enteric - *see* condition
Enteritis (acute) (catarrhal) (choleraic) (chronic) (congestive) (diarrheal) (exudative) (follicular) (hemorrhagic) (infantile) (lienteric) (noninfectious) (perforative) (phlegmonous) (presumed noninfectious) (pseudomembranous) 558.9
adaptive 564.9
aertrycke infection 003.0
allergic 558.3
amebic (*see also* Amebiasis) 006.9
with abscess - *see* Abscess, amebic
acute 006.0
with abscess - *see* Abscess, amebic
nondysenteric 006.2
chronic 006.1
with abscess - *see* Abscess, amebic
nondysenteric 006.2
nondysenteric 006.2
anaerobic (cocci) (gram-negative) (gram-positive) (mixed) NEC 008.46
bacillary NEC 004.9
bacterial NEC 008.5
specified NEC 008.49
Bacteroides (fragilis) (melaninogeniscus) (oralis) 008.46
Butyrivibrio (fibriosolvens) 008.46
Campylobacter 008.43
Candida 112.85
Chilomastix 007.8
choleriformis 001.1
chronic 558.9
ulcerative (*see also* Colitis, ulcerative) 556.9
cicatrizing (chronic) 555.0
Clostridium
botulinum 005.1
difficile 008.45
haemolyticum 008.46
novyi 008.46
perfringens (C) (F) 008.46
specified type NEC 008.46
coccidial 007.2
dietetic 558.9

Enteritis *(Continued)*
due to
achylia gastrica 536.8
adenovirus 008.62
Aerobacter aerogenes 008.2
anaerobes (*see also* Enteritis, anaerobic) 008.46
Arizona (bacillus) 008.1
astrovirus 008.66
Bacillus coli - *see* Enteritis, E. coli
bacteria NEC 008.5
specified NEC 008.49
Bacteroides (*see also* Enteritis, Bacteroides) 008.46
Butyrivibrio (fibriosolvens) 008.46
Calcivirus 008.65
Campylobacter 008.43
Clostridium - *see* Enteritis, Clostridium
Cockle agent 008.64
Coxsackie (virus) 008.67
Ditchling agent 008.64
ECHO virus 008.67
Enterobacter aerogenes 008.2
enterococci 008.49
enterovirus NEC 008.67
Escherichia coli - *see* Enteritis, E. coli
Eubacterium 008.46
Fusobacterium (nucleatum) 008.46
gram-negative bacteria NEC 008.47
anaerobic NEC 008.46
Hawaii agent 008.63
irritating foods 558.9
Klebsiella aerogenes 008.47
Marin County agent 008.66
Montgomery County agent 008.63
Norwalk-like agent 008.63
Norwalk virus 008.63
Otofuke agent 008.63
Paracolobactrum arizonae 008.1
paracolon bacillus NEC 008.47
Arizona 008.1
Paramatta agent 008.64
Peptococcus 008.46
Peptostreptococcus 008.46
Proprionibacterium 008.46
Proteus (bacillus) (mirabilis) (morganii) 008.3
Pseudomonas aeruginosa 008.42
Rotavirus 008.61
Sapporo agent 008.63
small round virus (SRV) NEC 008.64
featureless NEC 008.63
structured NEC 008.63
Snow Mountain (SM) agent 008.63
specified
bacteria NEC 008.49
organism, nonbacterial NEC 008.8
virus NEC 008.69
Staphylococcus 008.41
Streptococcus 008.49
anaerobic 008.46
Taunton agent 008.63
Torovirus 008.69
Treponema 008.46
Veillonella 008.46
virus 008.8
specified type NEC 008.69
Wollan (W) agent 008.64
Yersinia enterocolitica 008.44
dysentery - *see* Dysentery
E. coli 008.00
enterohemorrhagic 008.04
enteroinvasive 008.03
enteropathogenic 008.01
enterotoxigenic 008.02
specified type NEC 008.09

Enteritis *(Continued)*
El Tor 001.1
embadomonial 007.8
epidemic 009.0
Eubacterium 008.46
fermentative 558.9
fulminant 557.0
Fusobacterium (nucleatum) 008.46
gangrenous (*see also* Enteritis, due to, by organism) 009.0
giardial 007.1
gram-negative bacteria NEC 008.47
anaerobic NEC 008.46
infectious NEC (*see also* Enteritis, due to, by organism) 009.0
presumed 009.1
influenzal 487.8
ischemic 557.9
acute 557.0
chronic 557.1
due to mesenteric artery insufficiency 557.1
membranous 564.9
mucous 564.9
myxomembranous
necrotic (*see also* Enteritis, due to, by organism) 009.0
necroticans 005.2
necrotizing of fetus or newborn 777.5
neurogenic 564.9
newborn 777.8
necrotizing 777.5
parasitic NEC 129
paratyphoid (fever) (*see also* Fever, paratyphoid) 002.9
Peptococcus 008.46
Peptostreptococcus 008.46
Proprionibacterium 008.46
protozoal NEC 007.9
radiation 558.1
regional (of) 555.9
intestine
large (bowel, colon, or rectum) 555.1
with small intestine 555.2
small (duodenum, ileum, or jejunum) 555.0
with large intestine 555.2
Salmonella infection 003.0
salmonellosis 003.0
segmental (*see also* Enteritis, regional) 555.9
septic (*see also* Enteritis, due to, by organism) 009.0
Shigella 004.9
simple 558.9
spasmodic 564.9
spastic 564.9
staphylococcal 008.41
due to food 005.0
streptococcal 008.49
anaerobic 008.46
toxic 558.2
Treponema (denticola) (macrodentium) 008.46
trichomonal 007.3
tuberculous (*see also* Tuberculosis) 014.8
typhosa 002.0
ulcerative (chronic) (*see also* Colitis, ulcerative) 556.9
Veillonella 008.46
viral 008.8
adenovirus 008.62
enterovirus 008.67
specified virus NEC 008.69
Yersinia enterocolitica 008.44
zymotic 009.0

Enteroarticular syndrome 099.3
Enterobiasis 127.4
Enterobius vermicularis 127.4
Enterocele (*see also* Hernia) 553.9
  pelvis, pelvic (acquired) (congenital) 618.6
  vagina, vaginal (acquired) (congenital) 618.6
Enterocolitis - *see also* Enteritis
  fetus or newborn 777.8
    necrotizing 777.5
  fulminant 557.0
  granulomatous 555.2
  hemorrhagic (acute) 557.0
    chronic 557.1
  necrotizing (acute) (membranous) 557.0
  primary necrotizing 777.5
  pseudomembranous 008.45
  radiation 558.1
    newborn 777.5
  ulcerative 556.0
Enterocystoma 751.5
Enterogastritis - *see* Enteritis
Enterogenous cyanosis 289.7
Enterolith, enterolithiasis (impaction) 560.39
  with hernia - *see also* Hernia, by site, with obstruction
    gangrenous - *see* Hernia, by site, with gangrene
Enteropathy 569.9
  exudative (of Gordon) 579.8
  gluten 579.0
  hemorrhagic, terminal 557.0
  protein-losing 579.8
Enteroperitonitis (*see also* Peritonitis) 567.9
Enteroptosis 569.89
Enterorrhagia 578.9
Enterospasm 564.9
  psychogenic 306.4
Enterostenosis (*see also* Obstruction, intestine) 560.9
Enterostomy status V44.4
  with complication 569.60
Enthesopathy 726.90
  ankle and tarsus 726.70
  elbow region 726.30
    specified NEC 726.39
  hip 726.5
  knee 726.60
  peripheral NEC 726.8
  shoulder region 726.10
    adhesive 726.0
  spinal 720.1
  wrist and carpus 726.4
Entrance, air into vein - *see* Embolism, air
Entrapment, nerve - *see* Neuropathy, entrapment
Entropion (eyelid) 374.00
  cicatricial 374.04
  congenital 743.62
  late effect of trachoma (healed) 139.1
  mechanical 374.02
  paralytic 374.02
  senile 374.01
  spastic 374.03
Enucleation of eye (current) (traumatic) 871.3
Enuresis 788.30
  habit disturbance 307.6
  nocturnal 788.36
    psychogenic 307.6
  nonorganic origin 307.6
  psychogenic 307.6
Enzymopathy 277.9
Eosinopenia 288.59
Eosinophilia 288.3
  allergic 288.3
  hereditary 288.3
  idiopathic 288.3
  infiltrative 518.3
  Loeffler's 518.3
  myalgia syndrome 710.5
  pulmonary (tropical) 518.3
  secondary 288.3
  tropical 518.3
Eosinophilic - *see also* condition
  fasciitis 728.89
  granuloma (bone) 277.89
  infiltration lung 518.3
Ependymitis (acute) (cerebral) (chronic) (granular) (*see also* Meningitis) 322.9
Ependymoblastoma (M9392/3)
  specified site - *see* Neoplasm, by site, malignant
  unspecified site 191.9
Ependymoma (epithelial) (malignant) (M9391/3)
  anaplastic type (M9392/3)
    specified site - *see* Neoplasm, by site, malignant
    unspecified site 191.9
  benign (M9391/0)
    specified site - *see* Neoplasm, by site, benign
    unspecified site 225.0
  myxopapillary (M9394/1) 237.5
  papillary (M9393/1) 237.5
  specified site - *see* Neoplasm, by site, malignant
  unspecified site 191.9
Ependymopathy 349.2
  spinal cord 349.2
Ephelides, ephelis 709.09
Ephemeral fever (*see also* Pyrexia) 780.6
Epiblepharon (congenital) 743.62
Epicanthus, epicanthic fold (congenital) (eyelid) 743.63
Epicondylitis (elbow) (lateral) 726.32
  medial 726.31
Epicystitis (*see also* Cystitis) 595.9
Epidemic - *see* condition
Epidermidalization, cervix - *see* condition
Epidermidization, cervix - *see* condition
Epidermis, epidermal - *see* condition
Epidermization, cervix - *see* condition
Epidermodysplasia verruciformis 078.19
Epidermoid
  cholesteatoma - *see* Cholesteatoma
  inclusion (*see also* Cyst, skin) 706.2
Epidermolysis
  acuta (combustiformis) (toxica) 695.1
  bullosa 757.39
  necroticans combustiformis 695.1
    due to drug
      correct substance properly administered 695.1
      overdose or wrong substance given or taken 977.9
        specified drug - *see* Table of Drugs and Chemicals
Epidermophytid - *see* Dermatophytosis
Epidermophytosis (infected) - *see* Dermatophytosis
Epidermosis, ear (middle) (*see also* Cholesteatoma) 385.30
Epididymis - *see* condition
Epididymitis (nonvenereal) 604.90
  with abscess 604.0
Epididymitis *(Continued)*
  acute 604.99
  blennorrhagic (acute) 098.0
    chronic or duration of 2 months or over 098.2
  caseous (*see also* Tuberculosis) 016.4
  chlamydial 099.54
  diphtheritic 032.89 *[604.91]*
  filarial 125.9 *[604.91]*
  gonococcal (acute) 098.0
    chronic or duration of 2 months or over 098.2
  recurrent 604.99
  residual 604.99
  syphilitic 095.8 *[604.91]*
  tuberculous (*see also* Tuberculosis) 016.4
Epididymo-orchitis (*see also* Epididymitis) 604.90
  with abscess 604.0
  chlamydial 099.54
  gonococcal (acute) 098.13
    chronic or duration of 2 months or over 098.33
Epidural - *see* condition
Epigastritis (*see also* Gastritis) 535.5
Epigastrium, epigastric - *see* condition
Epigastrocele (*see also* Hernia, epigastric) 553.29
Epiglottiditis (acute) 464.30
  with obstruction 464.31
  chronic 476.1
  viral 464.30
    with obstruction 464.31
Epiglottis - *see* condition
Epiglottitis (acute) 464.30
  with obstruction 464.31
  chronic 476.1
  viral 464.30
    with obstruction 464.31
Epignathus 759.4
Epilepsia
  partialis continua (*see also* Epilepsy) 345.7
  procursiva (*see also* Epilepsy) 345.8
Epilepsy, epileptic (idiopathic) 345.9

> Note Use the following fifth-digit subclassifications with categories 345.0, 345.1, 345.4–345.9
>
> 0 without mention of intractable epilepsy
> 1 with intractable epilepsy

  abdominal 345.5
  absence (attack) 345.0
  akinetic 345.0
    psychomotor 345.4
  automatism 345.4
  autonomic diencephalic 345.5
  brain 345.9
  Bravais-Jacksonian 345.5
  cerebral 345.9
  climacteric 345.9
  clonic 345.1
  clouded state 345.9
  coma 345.3
  communicating 345.4
  complicating pregnancy, childbirth, or the puerperium 649.4
  congenital 345.9
  convulsions 345.9
  cortical (focal) (motor) 345.5
  cursive (running) 345.8
  cysticercosis 123.1

ICD-9-CM
E
Vol. 2

Epilepsy, epileptic *(Continued)*
cysticercosis *(Continued)*
deterioration with behavioral disturbance 345.9 *[294.11]*
without behavioral disturbance 345.9 *[294.10]*
due to syphilis 094.89
equivalent 345.5
fit 345.9
focal (motor) 345.5
gelastic 345.8
generalized 345.9
convulsive 345.1
flexion 345.1
nonconvulsive 345.0
grand mal (idiopathic) 345.1
Jacksonian (motor) (sensory) 345.5
Kojevnikoff's, Kojevnikov's, Kojewnikoff's 345.7
laryngeal 786.2
limbic system 345.4
localization related (focal) (partial) and epileptic syndromes ◀
with ◀
complex partial seizures 345.4 ◀
simple partial seizures 345.5 ◀
major (motor) 345.1
minor 345.0
mixed (type) 345.9
motor partial 345.5
musicogenic 345.1
myoclonus, myoclonic 345.1
progressive (familial) 333.2
nonconvulsive, generalized 345.0
parasitic NEC 123.9
partial (focalized) 345.5
with
impairment of consciousness 345.4
memory and ideational disturbances 345.4
without impairment of consciousness 345.5 ◀
abdominal type 345.5
motor type 345.5
psychomotor type 345.4
psychosensory type 345.4
secondarily generalized 345.4
sensory type 345.5
somatomotor type 345.5
somatosensory type 345.5
temporal lobe type 345.4
visceral type 345.5
visual type 345.5
peripheral 345.9
petit mal 345.0
photokinetic 345.8
progressive myoclonic (familial) 333.2
psychic equivalent 345.5
psychomotor 345.4
psychosensory 345.4
reflex 345.1
seizure 345.9
senile 345.9
sensory-induced 345.5
sleep (*see also* Narcolepsy) 347.00
somatomotor type 345.5
somatosensory 345.5
specified type NEC 345.8
status (grand mal) 345.3
focal motor 345.7
petit mal 345.2
psychomotor 345.7
temporal lobe 345.7
symptomatic 345.9
temporal lobe 345.4

Epilepsy, epileptic *(Continued)*
tonic (-clonic) 345.1
traumatic (injury unspecified) 907.0
injury specified - *see* Late, effect (of) specified injury
twilight 293.0
uncinate (gyrus) 345.4
Unverricht (-Lundborg) (familial myoclonic) 333.2
visceral 345.5
visual 345.5
Epileptiform
convulsions 780.39
seizure 780.39
Epiloia 759.5
Epimenorrhea 626.2
Epipharyngitis (*see also* Nasopharyngitis) 460
Epiphora 375.20
due to
excess lacrimation 375.21
insufficient drainage 375.22
Epiphyseal arrest 733.91
femoral head 732.2
Epiphyseolysis, epiphysiolysis (*see also* Osteochondrosis) 732.9
Epiphysitis (*see also* Osteochondrosis) 732.9
juvenile 732.6
marginal (Scheuermann's) 732.0
os calcis 732.5
syphilitic (congenital) 090.0
vertebral (Scheuermann's) 732.0
Epiplocele (*see also* Hernia) 553.9
Epiploitis (*see also* Peritonitis) 567.9
Epiplosarcomphalocele (*see also* Hernia, umbilicus) 553.1
Episcleritis 379.00
gouty 274.89 *[379.09]*
nodular 379.02
periodica fugax 379.01
angioneurotic - *see* Edema, angioneurotic
specified NEC 379.09
staphylococcal 379.00
suppurative 379.00
syphilitic 095.0
tuberculous (*see also* Tuberculosis) 017.3 *[379.09]*
Episode
brain (*see also* Disease, cerebrovascular, acute) 436
cerebral (*see also* Disease, cerebrovascular, acute) 436
depersonalization (in neurotic state) 300.6
hyporesponsive 780.09
psychotic (*see also* Psychosis) 298.9
organic, transient 293.9
schizophrenic (acute) NEC (*see also* Schizophrenia) 295.4
Epispadias
female 753.8
male 752.62
Episplenitis 289.59
Epistaxis (multiple) 784.7
hereditary 448.0
vicarious menstruation 625.8
Epithelioma (malignant) (M8011/3) - *see also* Neoplasm, by site, malignant
adenoides cysticum (M8100/0) - *see* Neoplasm, skin, benign
basal cell (M8090/3) - *see* Neoplasm, skin, malignant
benign (M8011/0) - *see* Neoplasm, by site, benign

Epithelioma *(Continued)*
Bowen's (M8081/2) - *see* Neoplasm, skin, in situ
calcifying (benign) (Malherbe's) (M8110/0) - *see* Neoplasm, skin, benign
external site - *see* Neoplasm, skin, malignant
intraepidermal, Jadassohn (M8096/0) - *see* Neoplasm, skin, benign
squamous cell (M8070/3) - *see* Neoplasm, by site, malignant
Epitheliopathy
pigment, retina 363.15
posterior multifocal placoid (acute) 363.15
Epithelium, epithelial - *see* condition
Epituberculosis (allergic) (with atelectasis) (*see also* Tuberculosis) 010.8
Eponychia 757.5
Epstein's
nephrosis or syndrome (*see also* Nephrosis) 581.9
pearl (mouth) 528.4
Epstein-Barr infection (viral) 075
chronic 780.79 *[139.8]*
Epulis (giant cell) (gingiva) 523.8
Equinia 024
Equinovarus (congenital) 754.51
acquired 736.71
Equivalent
convulsive (abdominal) (*see also* Epilepsy) 345.5
epileptic (psychic) (*see also* Epilepsy) 345.5
Erb's
disease 359.1
palsy, paralysis (birth) (brachial) (newborn) 767.6
spinal (spastic) syphilitic 094.89
pseudohypertrophic muscular dystrophy 359.1
Erb (-Duchenne) paralysis (birth injury) (newborn) 767.6
Erb-Goldflam disease or syndrome 358.00
Erdheim's syndrome (acromegalic macrospondylitis) 253.0
Erection, painful (persistent) 607.3
Ergosterol deficiency (vitamin D) 268.9
with
osteomalacia 268.2
rickets (*see also* Rickets) 268.0
Ergotism (ergotized grain) 988.2
from ergot used as drug (migraine therapy)
correct substance properly administered 349.82
overdose or wrong substance given or taken 975.0
Erichsen's disease (railway spine) 300.16
Erlacher-Blount syndrome (tibia vara) 732.4
Erosio interdigitalis blastomycetica 112.3
Erosion
arteriosclerotic plaque - *see* Arteriosclerosis, by site
artery NEC 447.2
without rupture 447.8
bone 733.99
bronchus 519.19 ⬅
cartilage (joint) 733.99
cervix (uteri) (acquired) (chronic) (congenital) 622.0
with mention of cervicitis 616.0

◀ New ⬅ Revised

Erosion *(Continued)*
cornea (recurrent) (*see also* Keratitis) 371.42
traumatic 918.1
dental (idiopathic) (occupational) 521.30
extending into
dentine 521.32
pulp 521.33
generalized 521.35
limited to enamel 521.31
localized 521.34
duodenum, postpyloric - *see* Ulcer, duodenum
esophagus 530.89
gastric 535.4
intestine 569.89
lymphatic vessel 457.8
pylorus, pyloric (ulcer) 535.4
sclera 379.16
spine, aneurysmal 094.89
spleen 289.59
stomach 535.4
teeth (idiopathic) (occupational) (*see also* Erosion, dental) 521.30
due to
medicine 521.30
persistent vomiting 521.30
urethra 599.84
uterus 621.8
vertebra 733.99
Erotomania 302.89
Clerambault's 297.8
Error
in diet 269.9
refractive 367.9
astigmatism (*see also* Astigmatism) 367.20
drug-induced 367.89
hypermetropia 367.0
hyperopia 367.0
myopia 367.1
presbyopia 367.4
toxic 367.89
Eructation 787.3
nervous 306.4
psychogenic 306.4
Eruption
creeping 126.9
drug - *see* Dermatitis, due to, drug
Hutchinson, summer 692.72
Kaposi's varicelliform 054.0
napkin (psoriasiform) 691.0
polymorphous
light (sun) 692.72
other source 692.82
psoriasiform, napkin 691.0
recalcitrant pustular 694.8
ringed 695.89
skin (*see also* Dermatitis) 782.1
creeping (meaning hookworm) 126.9
due to
chemical(s) NEC 692.4
internal use 693.8
drug - *see* Dermatitis, due to, drug
prophylactic inoculation or vaccination against disease - *see* Dermatitis, due to, vaccine
smallpox vaccination NEC - *see* Dermatitis, due to, vaccine
erysipeloid 027.1
feigned 698.4
Hutchinson, summer 692.72
Kaposi's, varicelliform 054.0
vaccinia 999.0
lichenoid, axilla 698.3
polymorphous, due to light 692.72

Eruption *(Continued)*
skin *(Continued)*
toxic NEC 695.0
vesicular 709.8
teeth, tooth
accelerated 520.6
delayed 520.6
difficult 520.6
disturbance of 520.6
in abnormal sequence 520.6
incomplete 520.6
late 520.6
natal 520.6
neonatal 520.6
obstructed 520.6
partial 520.6
persistent primary 520.6
premature 520.6
prenatal 520.6 ◀
vesicular 709.8
Erysipelas (gangrenous) (infantile) (newborn) (phlegmonous) (suppurative) 035
external ear 035 *[380.13]*
puerperal, postpartum, childbirth 670
Erysipelatoid (Rosenbach's) 027.1
Erysipeloid (Rosenbach's) 027.1
Erythema, erythematous (generalized) 695.9
ab igne - *see* Burn, by site, first degree
annulare (centrifugum) (rheumaticum) 695.0
arthriticum epidemicum 026.1
brucellum (*see also* Brucellosis) 023.9
bullosum 695.1
caloricum - *see* Burn, by site, first degree
chronicum migrans 088.81
circinatum 695.1
diaper 691.0
due to
chemical (contact) NEC 692.4
internal 693.8
drug (internal use) 693.0
contact 692.3
elevatum diutinum 695.89
endemic 265.2
epidemic, arthritic 026.1
figuratum perstans 695.0
gluteal 691.0
gyratum (perstans) (repens) 695.1
heat - *see* Burn, by site, first degree
ichthyosiforme congenitum 757.1
induratum (primary) (scrofulosorum) (*see also* Tuberculosis) 017.1
nontuberculous 695.2
infantum febrile 057.8
infectional NEC 695.9
infectiosum 057.0
inflammation NEC 695.9
intertrigo 695.89
iris 695.1
lupus (discoid) (localized) (*see also* Lupus, erythematosus) 695.4
marginatum 695.0
rheumaticum - *see* Fever, rheumatic
medicamentosum - *see* Dermatitis, due to, drug
migrans 529.1
chronicum 088.81
multiforme 695.1
bullosum 695.1
conjunctiva 695.1
exudativum (Hebra) 695.1
pemphigoides 694.5
napkin 691.0

Erythema, erythematous *(Continued)*
neonatorum 778.8
nodosum 695.2
tuberculous (*see also* Tuberculosis) 017.1
nummular, nummulare 695.1
palmar 695.0
palmaris hereditarium 695.0
pernio 991.5
perstans solare 692.72
rash, newborn 778.8
scarlatiniform (exfoliative) (recurrent) 695.0
simplex marginatum 057.8
solare (*see also* Sunburn) 692.71
streptogenes 696.5
toxic, toxicum NEC 695.0
newborn 778.8
tuberculous (primary) (*see also* Tuberculosis) 017.0
venenatum 695.0
Erythematosus - *see* condition
Erythematous - *see* condition
Erythermalgia (primary) 443.82
Erythralgia 443.82
Erythrasma 039.0
Erythredema 985.0
polyneuritica 985.0
polyneuropathy 985.0
Erythremia (acute) (M9841/3) 207.0
chronic (M9842/3) 207.1
secondary 289.0
Erythroblastopenia (acquired) 284.8
congenital 284.01 ⬅
Erythroblastophthisis 284.01 ⬅
Erythroblastosis (fetalis) (newborn) 773.2
due to
ABO
antibodies 773.1
incompatibility, maternal/fetal 773.1
isoimmunization 773.1
Rh
antibodies 773.0
incompatibility, maternal/fetal 773.0
isoimmunization 773.0
Erythrocyanosis (crurum) 443.89
Erythrocythemia - *see* Erythremia
Erythrocytopenia 285.9
Erythrocytosis (megalosplenic)
familial 289.6
oval, hereditary (*see also* Elliptocytosis) 282.1
secondary 289.0
stress 289.0
Erythroderma (*see also* Erythema) 695.9
desquamativa (in infants) 695.89
exfoliative 695.89
ichthyosiform, congenital 757.1
infantum 695.89
maculopapular 696.2
neonatorum 778.8
psoriaticum 696.1
secondary 695.9
Erythrogenesis imperfecta 284.09 ⬅
Erythroleukemia (M9840/3) 207.0
Erythromelalgia 443.82
Erythromelia 701.8
Erythropenia 285.9
Erythrophagocytosis 289.9
Erythrophobia 300.23
Erythroplakia
oral mucosa 528.79
tongue 528.79

Erythroplasia (Queyrat) (M8080/2)
specified site - *see* Neoplasm, skin, in situ
unspecified site 233.5
Erythropoiesis, idiopathic ineffective 285.0
Escaped beats, heart 427.60
postoperative 997.1
Esoenteritis - *see* Enteritis
Esophagalgia 530.89
Esophagectasis 530.89
due to cardiospasm 530.0
Esophagismus 530.5
Esophagitis (alkaline) (chemical) (chronic) (infectional) (necrotic) (peptic) (postoperative) (regurgitant) 530.10
acute 530.12
candidal 112.84
reflux 530.11
specified NEC 530.19
tuberculous (*see also* Tuberculosis) 017.8
ulcerative 530.19
Esophagocele 530.6
Esophagodynia 530.89
Esophagomalacia 530.89
Esophagoptosis 530.89
Esophagospasm 530.5
Esophagostenosis 530.3
Esophagostomiasis 127.7
Esophagostomy
complication 530.87
infection 530.86
malfunctioning 530.87
mechanical 530.87
Esophagotracheal - *see* condition
Esophagus - *see* condition
Esophoria 378.41
convergence, excess 378.84
divergence, insufficiency 378.85
Esotropia (nonaccommodative) 378.00
accommodative 378.35
alternating 378.05
with
A pattern 378.06
specified noncomitancy NEC 378.08
V pattern 378.07
X pattern 378.08
Y pattern 378.08
intermittent 378.22
intermittent 378.20
alternating 378.22
monocular 378.21
monocular 378.01
with
A pattern 378.02
specified noncomitancy NEC 378.04
V pattern 378.03
X pattern 378.04
Y pattern 378.04
intermittent 378.21
Espundia 085.5
Essential - *see* condition
Esterapenia 289.89
Esthesioneuroblastoma (M9522/3) 160.0
Esthesioneurocytoma (M9521/3) 160.0
Esthesioneuroepithelioma (M9523/3) 160.0
Esthiomene 099.1
Estivo-autumnal
fever 084.0
malaria 084.0
Estrangement V61.0
Estriasis 134.0
Ethanolaminuria 270.8
Ethanolism (*see also* Alcoholism) 303.9
Ether dependence, dependency (*see also* Dependence) 304.6
Etherism (*see also* Dependence) 304.6
Ethmoid, ethmoidal - *see* condition
Ethmoiditis (chronic) (nonpurulent) (purulent) (*see also* Sinusitis, ethmoidal) 473.2
influenzal 487.1
Woakes' 471.1
Ethylism (*see also* Alcoholism) 303.9
Eulenburg's disease (congenital paramyotonia) 359.2
Eunuchism 257.2
Eunuchoidism 257.2
hypogonadotropic 257.2
European blastomycosis 117.5
Eustachian - *see* condition
Euthyroid sick syndrome 790.94
Euthyroidism 244.9
Evaluation
fetal lung maturity 659.8
for suspected condition (*see also* Observation) V71.9
abuse V71.81
exposure
anthrax V71.82
biologic agent NEC V71.83
SARS V71.83
neglect V71.81
newborn - *see* Observation, suspected, condition, newborn
specified condition NEC V71.89
mental health V70.2
requested by authority V70.1
nursing care V63.8
social service V63.8
Evan's syndrome (thrombocytopenic purpura) 287.32
Eventration
colon into chest - *see* Hernia, diaphragm
diaphragm (congenital) 756.6
Eversion
bladder 596.8
cervix (uteri) 622.0
with mention of cervicitis 616.0
foot NEC 736.79
congenital 755.67
lacrimal punctum 375.51
punctum lacrimale (postinfectional) (senile) 375.51
ureter (meatus) 593.89
urethra (meatus) 599.84
uterus 618.1
complicating delivery 665.2
affecting fetus or newborn 763.89
puerperal, postpartum 674.8
Evidence
of malignancy
cytologic
without histologic confirmation 795.06 (Revised)
Evisceration
birth injury 767.8
bowel (congenital) - *see* Hernia, ventral
congenital (*see also* Hernia, ventral) 553.29
operative wound 998.32
traumatic NEC 869.1
eye 871.3
Evulsion - *see* Avulsion
Ewing's
angioendothelioma (M9260/3) - *see* Neoplasm, bone, malignant
Ewing's *(Continued)*
sarcoma (M9260/3) - *see* Neoplasm, bone, malignant
tumor (M9260/3) - *see* Neoplasm, bone, malignant
Exaggerated lumbosacral angle (with impinging spine) 756.12
Examination (general) (routine) (of) (for) V70.9
allergy V72.7
annual V70.0
cardiovascular preoperative V72.81
cervical Papanicolaou smear V76.2
as a part of routine gynecological examination V72.31
to confirm findings of recent normal smear following initial abnormal smear V72.32
child care (routine) V20.2
clinical research investigation (normal control patient) (participant) V70.7
dental V72.2
developmental testing (child) (infant) V20.2
donor (potential) V70.8
ear V72.19 (Revised)
eye V72.0
following
accident (motor vehicle) V71.4
alleged rape or seduction (victim or culprit) V71.5
inflicted injury (victim or culprit) NEC V71.6
rape or seduction, alleged (victim or culprit) V71.5
treatment (for) V67.9
combined V67.6
fracture V67.4
involving high-risk medication NEC V67.51
mental disorder V67.3
specified condition NEC V67.59
follow-up (routine) (following) V67.9
cancer chemotherapy V67.2
chemotherapy V67.2
disease NEC V67.59
high-risk medication NEC V67.51
injury NEC V67.59
population survey V70.6
postpartum V24.2
psychiatric V67.3
psychotherapy V67.3
radiotherapy V67.1
specified surgery NEC V67.09
surgery V67.00
vaginal pap smear V67.01
gynecological V72.31
for contraceptive maintenance V25.40
intrauterine device V25.42
pill V25.41
specified method NEC V25.49
health (of)
armed forces personnel V70.5
checkup V70.0
child, routine V20.2
defined subpopulation NEC V70.5
inhabitants of institutions V70.5
occupational V70.5
pre-employment screening V70.5
preschool children V70.5
for admission to school V70.3
prisoners V70.5
for entrance into prison V70.3
prostitutes V70.5
refugees V70.5

- **Examination** *(Continued)*
  - health *(Continued)*
    - school children V70.5
    - students V70.5
  - hearing V72.19
    - following failed hearing screening V72.11
  - infant V20.2
  - laboratory V72.6
  - lactating mother V24.1
  - medical (for) (of) V70.9
    - administrative purpose NEC V70.3
    - admission to
      - old age home V70.3
      - prison V70.3
      - school V70.3
    - adoption V70.3
    - armed forces personnel V70.5
    - at health care facility V70.0
    - camp V70.3
    - child, routine V20.2
    - clinical research investigation, (control) (normal comparison) (participant) V70.7
    - defined subpopulation NEC V70.5
    - donor (potential) V70.8
    - driving license V70.3
    - general V70.9
      - routine V70.0
      - specified reason NEC V70.8
    - immigration V70.3
    - inhabitants of institutions V70.5
    - insurance certification V70.3
    - marriage V70.3
    - medicolegal reasons V70.4
    - naturalization V70.3
    - occupational V70.5
    - population survey V70.6
    - pre-employment V70.5
    - preschool children V70.5
      - for admission to school V70.3
    - prison V70.3
    - prisoners V70.5
      - for entrance into prison V70.3
    - prostitutes V70.5
    - refugees V70.5
    - school children V70.5
    - specified reason NEC V70.8
    - sport competition V70.3
    - students V70.5
  - medicolegal reason V70.4
  - pelvic (annual) (periodic) V72.31
  - periodic (annual) (routine) V70.0
  - postpartum
    - immediately after delivery V24.0
    - routine follow-up V24.2
  - pregnancy (unconfirmed) (possible) V72.40
    - negative result V72.41
    - positive result V72.42
  - prenatal V22.1
    - first pregnancy V22.0
    - high-risk pregnancy V23.9
      - specified problem NEC V23.89
  - preoperative V72.84
    - cardiovascular V72.81
    - respiratory V72.82
    - specified NEC V72.83
  - preprocedural V72.84
    - cardiovascular V72.81
    - general physical V72.83
    - respiratory V72.82
    - specified NEC V72.83
  - psychiatric V70.2

- **Examination** *(Continued)*
  - psychiatric *(Continued)*
    - follow-up not needing further care V67.3
    - requested by authority V70.1
  - radiological NEC V72.5
  - respiratory preoperative V72.82
  - screening - *see* Screening
  - sensitization V72.7
  - skin V72.7
    - hypersensitivity V72.7
  - special V72.9
  - specified type or reason NEC V72.85
    - preoperative V72.83
      - specified NEC V72.83
  - teeth V72.2
  - vaginal Papanicolaou smear V76.47
    - following hysterectomy for malignant condition V67.01
  - victim or culprit following
    - alleged rape or seduction V71.5
    - inflicted injury NEC V71.6
  - vision V72.0
  - well baby V20.2
- **Exanthem, exanthema** (*see also* Rash) 782.1
  - Boston 048
  - epidemic, with meningitis 048
  - lichenoid psoriasiform 696.2
  - subitum 057.8
  - viral, virus NEC 057.9
    - specified type NEC 057.8
- **Excess, excessive, excessively**
  - alcohol level in blood 790.3
  - carbohydrate tissue, localized 278.1
  - carotene (dietary) 278.3
  - cold 991.9
    - specified effect NEC 991.8
  - convergence 378.84
  - crying 780.95
    - of
      - adolescent 780.95
      - adult 780.95
      - baby 780.92
      - child 780.95
      - infant (baby) 780.92
      - newborn 780.92
  - development, breast 611.1
  - diaphoresis (*see also* Hyperhidrosis) 780.8
  - distance, interarch 524.28
  - divergence 378.85
  - drinking (alcohol) NEC (*see also* Abuse, drugs, nondependent) 305.0
    - continual (*see also* Alcoholism) 303.9
    - habitual (*see also* Alcoholism) 303.9
  - eating 783.6
  - eyelid fold (congenital) 743.62
  - fat 278.02
    - in heart (*see also* Degeneration, myocardial) 429.1
    - tissue, localized 278.1
  - foreskin 605
  - gas 787.3
  - gastrin 251.5
  - glucagon 251.4
  - heat (*see also* Heat) 992.9
  - horizontal
    - overjet 524.26
    - overlap 524.26
  - interarch distance 524.28
  - intermaxillary vertical dimension 524.37
  - interocclusal distance of teeth 524.37

- **Excess, excessive, excessively** *(Continued)*
  - large
    - colon 564.7
      - congenital 751.3
    - fetus or infant 766.0
      - with obstructed labor 660.1
      - affecting management of pregnancy 656.6
      - causing disproportion 653.5
    - newborn (weight of 4500 grams or more) 766.0
    - organ or site, congenital NEC - *see* Anomaly, specified type NEC
  - lid fold (congenital) 743.62
  - long
    - colon 751.5
    - organ or site, congenital NEC - *see* Anomaly, specified type NEC
    - umbilical cord (entangled)
      - affecting fetus or newborn 762.5
      - in pregnancy or childbirth 663.3
        - with compression 663.2
  - menstruation 626.2
  - number of teeth 520.1
    - causing crowding 524.31
  - nutrients (dietary) NEC 783.6
  - potassium (K) 276.7
  - salivation (*see also* Ptyalism) 527.7
  - secretion - *see also* Hypersecretion
    - milk 676.6
    - sputum 786.4
    - sweat (*see also* Hyperhidrosis) 780.8
  - short
    - organ or site, congenital NEC - *see* Anomaly, specified type NEC
    - umbilical cord
      - affecting fetus or newborn 762.6
      - in pregnancy or childbirth 663.4
  - skin NEC 701.9
    - eyelid 743.62
      - acquired 374.30
  - sodium (Na) 276.0
  - spacing of teeth 524.32
  - sputum 786.4
  - sweating (*see also* Hyperhidrosis) 780.8
  - tearing (ducts) (eye) (*see also* Epiphora) 375.20
  - thirst 783.5
    - due to deprivation of water 994.3
  - tuberosity 524.07
  - vitamin
    - A (dietary) 278.2
      - administered as drug (chronic) (prolonged excessive intake) 278.2
        - reaction to sudden overdose 963.5
    - D (dietary) 278.4
      - administered as drug (chronic) (prolonged excessive intake) 278.4
        - reaction to sudden overdose 963.5
  - weight 278.02
    - gain 783.1
      - of pregnancy 646.1
    - loss 783.21
- **Excitability, abnormal, under minor stress** 309.29
- **Excitation**
  - catatonic (*see also* Schizophrenia) 295.2
  - psychogenic 298.1
  - reactive (from emotional stress, psychological trauma) 298.1

Excitement
manic (*see also* Psychosis, affective) 296.0
recurrent episode 296.1
single episode 296.0
mental, reactive (from emotional stress, psychological trauma) 298.1
state, reactive (from emotional stress, psychological trauma) 298.1
Excluded pupils 364.76
Excoriation (traumatic) (*see also* Injury, superficial, by site) 919.8
neurotic 698.4
Excyclophoria 378.44
Excyclotropia 378.33
Exencephalus, exencephaly 742.0
Exercise
breathing V57.0
remedial NEC V57.1
therapeutic NEC V57.1
Exfoliation, teeth due to systemic causes 525.0
Exfoliative - *see also* condition
dermatitis 695.89
Exhaustion, exhaustive (physical NEC) 780.79
battle (*see also* Reaction, stress, acute) 308.9
cardiac (*see also* Failure, heart) 428.9
delirium (*see also* Reaction, stress, acute) 308.9
due to
cold 991.8
excessive exertion 994.5
exposure 994.4
fetus or newborn 779.89
heart (*see also* Failure, heart) 428.9
heat 992.5
due to
salt depletion 992.4
water depletion 992.3
manic (*see also* Psychosis, affective) 296.0
recurrent episode 296.1
single episode 296.0
maternal, complicating delivery 669.8
affecting fetus or newborn 763.89
mental 300.5
myocardium, myocardial (*see also* Failure, heart) 428.9
nervous 300.5
old age 797
postinfectional NEC 780.79
psychogenic 300.5
psychosis (*see also* Reaction, stress, acute) 308.9
senile 797
dementia 290.0
Exhibitionism (sexual) 302.4
Exomphalos 756.79
Exophoria 378.42
convergence, insufficiency 378.83
divergence, excess 378.85
Exophthalmic
cachexia 242.0
goiter 242.0
ophthalmoplegia 242.0 *[376.22]*
Exophthalmos 376.30
congenital 743.66
constant 376.31
endocrine NEC 259.9 *[376.22]*
hyperthyroidism 242.0 *[376.21]*
intermittent NEC 376.34
malignant 242.0 *[376.21]*

Exophthalmos *(Continued)*
pulsating 376.35
endocrine NEC 259.9 *[376.22]*
thyrotoxic 242.0 *[376.21]*
Exostosis 726.91
cartilaginous (M9210/0) - *see* Neoplasm, bone, benign
congenital 756.4
ear canal, external 380.81
gonococcal 098.89
hip 726.5
intracranial 733.3
jaw (bone) 526.81
luxurians 728.11
multiple (cancellous) (congenital) (hereditary) 756.4
nasal bones 726.91
orbit, orbital 376.42
osteocartilaginous (M9210/0) - *see* Neoplasm, bone, benign
spine 721.8
with spondylosis - *see* Spondylosis
syphilitic 095.5
wrist 726.4
Exotropia 378.10
alternating 378.15
with
A pattern 378.16
specified noncomitancy NEC 378.18
V pattern 378.17
X pattern 378.18
Y pattern 378.18
intermittent 378.24
intermittent 378.20
alternating 378.24
monocular 378.23
monocular 378.11
with
A pattern 378.12
specified noncomitancy NEC 378.14
V pattern 378.13
X pattern 378.14
Y pattern 378.14
intermittent 378.23
Explanation of
investigation finding V65.4
medication V65.4
Exposure 994.9
cold 991.9
specified effect NEC 991.8
effects of 994.9
exhaustion due to 994.4
to
AIDS virus V01.79
anthrax V01.81
asbestos V15.84
body fluids (hazardous) V15.85
Escherichia coli (E. coli) V01.83
cholera V01.0
communicable disease V01.9
specified type NEC V01.89
German measles V01.4
gonorrhea V01.6
hazardous body fluids V15.85
HIV V01.79
human immunodeficiency virus V01.79
lead V15.86
meningococcus V01.84
parasitic disease V01.89
poliomyelitis V01.2

Exposure *(Continued)*
to *(Continued)*
potentially hazardous body fluids V15.85
rabies V01.5
rubella V01.4
SARS-associated coronavirus V01.82
smallpox V01.3
syphilis V01.6
tuberculosis V01.1
varicella V01.71
venereal disease V01.6
viral disease NEC V01.79
varicella V01.71
Exsanguination, fetal 772.0
Exstrophy
abdominal content 751.8
bladder (urinary) 753.5
Extensive - *see* condition
Extra - *see also* Accessory
rib 756.3
cervical 756.2
Extraction
with hook 763.89
breech NEC 669.6
affecting fetus or newborn 763.0
cataract postsurgical V45.61
manual NEC 669.8
affecting fetus or newborn 763.89
Extrasystole 427.60
atrial 427.61
postoperative 997.1
ventricular 427.69
Extrauterine gestation or pregnancy - *see* Pregnancy, ectopic
Extravasation
blood 459.0
lower extremity 459.0
chyle into mesentery 457.8
pelvicalyceal 593.4
pyelosinus 593.4
urine 788.8
from ureter 788.8
Extremity - *see* condition
Extrophy - *see* Exstrophy
Extroversion
bladder 753.5
uterus 618.1
complicating delivery 665.2
affecting fetus or newborn 763.89
postpartal (old) 618.1
Extruded tooth 524.34 ◀
Extrusion
alveolus and teeth 524.75
breast implant (prosthetic) 996.54
device, implant, or graft - *see* Complications, mechanical
eye implant (ball) (globe) 996.59
intervertebral disc - *see* Displacement, intervertebral disc
lacrimal gland 375.43
mesh (reinforcing) 996.59
ocular lens implant 996.53
prosthetic device NEC - *see* Complications, mechanical
vitreous 379.26
Exudate, pleura - *see* Effusion, pleura
Exudates, retina 362.82
Exudative - *see* condition
Eye, eyeball, eyelid - *see* condition
Eyestrain 368.13
Eyeworm disease of Africa 125.2

F

Faber's anemia or syndrome (achlorhydric anemia) 280.9
Fabry's disease (angiokeratoma corporis diffusum) 272.7
Face, facial - *see* condition
Facet of cornea 371.44
Faciocephalalgia, autonomic (*see also* Neuropathy, peripheral, autonomic) 337.9
Facioscapulohumeral myopathy 359.1
Factitious disorder, illness - *see* Illness, factitious
Factor
  deficiency - *see* Deficiency, factor
  psychic, associated with diseases classified elsewhere 316
  risk-see problem
Fahr-Volhard disease (malignant nephrosclerosis) 403.00
Failure, failed
  adenohypophyseal 253.2
  attempted abortion (legal) (*see also* Abortion, failed) 638.9
  bone marrow (anemia) 284.9
    acquired (secondary) 284.8
    congenital 284.09
    idiopathic 284.9
  cardiac (*see also* Failure, heart) 428.9
    newborn 779.89
  cardiorenal (chronic) 428.9
    hypertensive (*see also* Hypertension, cardiorenal) 404.93
  cardiorespiratory 799.1
    specified during or due to a procedure 997.1
      long-term effect of cardiac surgery 429.4
  cardiovascular (chronic) 428.9
  cerebrovascular 437.8
  cervical dilatation in labor 661.0
    affecting fetus or newborn 763.7
  circulation, circulatory 799.89
    fetus or newborn 779.89
    peripheral 785.50
  compensation - *see* Disease, heart
  congestive (*see also* Failure, heart) 428.0
  coronary (*see also* Insufficiency, coronary) 411.89
  dental restoration
    marginal integrity 525.61
    periodontal anatomical integrity 525.65
  descent of head (at term) 652.5
    affecting fetus or newborn 763.1
    in labor 660.0
      affecting fetus or newborn 763.1
  device, implant, or graft - *see* Complications, mechanical
  engagement of head NEC 652.5
    in labor 660.0
  extrarenal 788.9
  fetal head to enter pelvic brim 652.5
    affecting fetus or newborn 763.1
    in labor 660.0
      affecting fetus or newborn 763.1
  forceps NEC 660.7
    affecting fetus or newborn 763.1
  fusion (joint) (spinal) 996.49
  growth in childhood 783.43
  heart (acute) (sudden) 428.9
    with
      abortion - *see* Abortion, by type, with specified complication NEC

Failure, failed *(Continued)*
  heart *(Continued)*
    with *(Continued)*
      acute pulmonary edema (*see also* Failure, ventricular, left) 428.1
        with congestion (*see also* Failure, heart) 428.0
      decompensation (*see also* Failure, heart) 428.0
      dilation - *see* Disease, heart
      ectopic pregnancy (*see also* categories 633.0–633.9) 639.8
      molar pregnancy (*see also* categories 630–632) 639.8
    arteriosclerotic 440.9
    combined left-right sided 428.0
    combined systolic and diastolic 428.40
      acute 428.41
      acute on chronic 428.43
      chronic 428.42
    compensated (*see also* Failure, heart) 428.0
    complicating
      abortion - *see* Abortion, by type, with specified complication NEC
      delivery (cesarean) (instrumental) 669.4
      ectopic pregnancy (*see also* categories 633.0–633.9) 639.8
      molar pregnancy (*see also* categories 630–632) 639.8
      obstetric anesthesia or sedation 668.1
      surgery 997.1
    congestive (compensated) (decompensated) (*see also* Failure, heart) 428.0
      with rheumatic fever (conditions classifiable to 390)
        active 391.8
        inactive or quiescent (with chorea) 398.91
      fetus or newborn 779.89
      hypertensive (*see also* Hypertension, heart) 402.91
        with renal disease (*see also* Hypertension, cardiorenal) 404.91
          with renal failure 404.93
        benign 402.11
        malignant 402.01
      rheumatic (chronic) (inactive) (with chorea) 398.91
        active or acute 391.8
          with chorea (Sydenham's) 392.0
    decompensated (*see also* Failure, heart) 428.0
    degenerative (*see also* Degeneration, myocardial) 429.1
    diastolic 428.30
      acute 428.31
      acute on chronic 428.33
      chronic 428.32
    due to presence of (cardiac) prosthesis 429.4
    fetus or newborn 779.89
    following
      abortion 639.8
      cardiac surgery 429.4
      ectopic or molar pregnancy 639.8
    high output NEC 428.9
    hypertensive (*see also* Hypertension, heart) 402.91

Failure, failed *(Continued)*
  heart *(Continued)*
    hypertensive *(Continued)*
      with renal disease (*see also* Hypertension, cardiorenal) 404.91
        with renal failure 404.93
      benign 402.11
      malignant 402.01
    left (ventricular) (*see also* Failure, ventricular, left) 428.1
      with right-sided failure (*see also* Failure, heart) 428.0
    low output (syndrome) NEC 428.9
    organic - *see* Disease, heart
    postoperative (immediate) 997.1
      long term effect of cardiac surgery 429.4
    rheumatic (chronic) (congestive) (inactive) 398.91
    right (secondary to left heart failure, conditions classifiable to 428.1) (ventricular) (*see also* Failure, heart) 428.0
    senile 797
    specified during or due to a procedure 997.1
      long-term effect of cardiac surgery 429.4
    systolic 428.20
      acute 428.21
      acute on chronic 428.23
      chronic 428.22
    thyrotoxic (*see also* Thyrotoxicosis) 242.9 *[425.7]*
    valvular - *see* Endocarditis
  hepatic 572.8
    acute 570
    due to a procedure 997.4
  hepatorenal 572.4
  hypertensive heart (*see also* Hypertension, heart) 402.91
    benign 402.11
    malignant 402.01
  induction (of labor) 659.1
    abortion (legal) (*see also* Abortion, failed) 638.9
    affecting fetus or newborn 763.89
    by oxytocic drugs 659.1
    instrumental 659.0
    mechanical 659.0
    medical 659.1
    surgical 659.0
  initial alveolar expansion, newborn 770.4
  involution, thymus (gland) 254.8
  kidney - *see* Failure, renal
  lactation 676.4
  Leydig's cell, adult 257.2
  liver 572.8
    acute 570
  medullary 799.89
  mitral - *see* Endocarditis, mitral
  myocardium, myocardial (*see also* Failure, heart) 428.9
    chronic (*see also* Failure, heart) 428.0
    congestive (*see also* Failure, heart) 428.0
  ovarian (primary) 256.39
    iatrogenic 256.2
    postablative 256.2
    postirradiation 256.2
    postsurgical 256.2
  ovulation 628.0
  prerenal 788.9
  renal 586

ICD-9-CM F Vol. 2

Failure, failed *(Continued)*
  renal *(Continued)*
    with
      abortion - *see* Abortion, by type, with renal failure
      ectopic pregnancy (*see also* categories 633.0–633.9) 639.3
      edema (*see also* Nephrosis) 581.9
      hypertension (*see also* Hypertension, kidney) 403.91
      hypertensive heart disease (conditions classifiable to 402) 404.92
        with heart failure 404.93
        benign 404.12
          with heart failure 404.13
        malignant 404.02
          with heart failure 404.03
      molar pregnancy (*see also* categories 630–632) 639.3
      tubular necrosis (acute) 584.5
    acute 584.9
      with lesion of
        necrosis
          cortical (renal) 584.6
          medullary (renal) (papillary) 584.7
          tubular 584.5
        specified pathology NEC 584.8
    chronic 585.9
      hypertensive or with hypertension (*see also* Hypertension, kidney) 403.91
    due to a procedure 997.5
    following
      abortion 639.3
      crushing 958.5
      ectopic or molar pregnancy 639.3
      labor and delivery (acute) 669.3
    hypertensive (*see also* Hypertension, kidney) 403.91
    puerperal, postpartum 669.3
  respiration, respiratory 518.81
    acute 518.81
    acute and chronic 518.84
    center 348.8
      newborn 770.84
    chronic 518.83
    due to trauma, surgery or shock 518.5
    newborn 770.84
  rotation
    cecum 751.4
    colon 751.4
    intestine 751.4
    kidney 753.3
  segmentation - *see also* Fusion
    fingers (*see also* Syndactylism, fingers) 755.11
    toes (*see also* Syndactylism, toes) 755.13
  seminiferous tubule, adult 257.2
  senile (general) 797
    with psychosis 290.20
  testis, primary (seminal) 257.2
  to progress 661.2
    to thrive adult 783.7
    child 783.41
  transplant 996.80
    bone marrow 996.85
    organ (immune or nonimmune cause) 996.80
      bone marrow 996.85
      heart 996.83
      intestines 996.87
      kidney 996.81
      liver 996.82

Failure, failed *(Continued)*
  transplant *(Continued)*
    organ *(Continued)*
      lung 996.84
      pancreas 996.86
      specified NEC 996.89
    skin 996.52
      artificial 996.55
      decellularized allodermis 996.55
      temporary allograft or pigskin graft - *omit code*
  trial of labor NEC 660.6
    affecting fetus or newborn 763.1
  tubal ligation 998.89
  urinary 586
  vacuum extraction
    abortion - *see* Abortion, failed
    delivery NEC 660.7
      affecting fetus or newborn 763.1
  vasectomy 998.89
  ventouse NEC 660.7
    affecting fetus or newborn 763.1
  ventricular (*see also* Failure, heart) 428.9
    left 428.1
      with rheumatic fever (conditions classifiable to 390)
        active 391.8
          with chorea 392.0
        inactive or quiescent (with chorea) 398.91
      hypertensive (*see also* Hypertension, heart) 402.91
        benign 402.11
        malignant 402.01
      rheumatic (chronic) (inactive) (with chorea) 398.91
        active or acute 391.8
          with chorea 392.0
    right (*see also* Failure, heart) 428.0
  vital centers, fetus or newborn 779.89
  weight gain
    in childhood 783.41
Fainting (fit) (spell) 780.2
Falciform hymen 752.49
Fall, maternal, affecting fetus or newborn 760.5
Fallen arches 734
Falling, any organ or part - *see* Prolapse
Fallopian
    insufflation fertility testing V26.21
    following sterilization reversal V26.22
  tube - *see* condition
Fallot's
  pentalogy 745.2
  tetrad or tetralogy 745.2
  triad or trilogy 746.09
Fallout, radioactive (adverse effect) NEC 990
False - *see also* condition
  bundle branch block 426.50
  bursa 727.89
  croup 478.75
  joint 733.82
  labor (pains) 644.1
  opening, urinary, male 752.69
  passage, urethra (prostatic) 599.4
  positive
    serological test for syphilis 795.6
    Wassermann reaction 795.6
  pregnancy 300.11
Family, familial - *see also* condition
  disruption V61.0
  hemophagocytic ◀
    lymphohistiocytosis 288.4 ◀
    reticulosis 288.4 ◀

Family, familial *(Continued)*
  Li-Fraumeni (syndrome) V84.01
  planning advice V25.09
  problem V61.9
    specified circumstance NEC V61.8
  retinoblastoma (syndrome) 190.5
Famine 994.2
  edema 262
Fanconi's anemia (congenital pancytopenia) 284.09
Fanconi (-de Toni) (-Debré) syndrome (cystinosis) 270.0
Farber (-Uzman) syndrome or disease (disseminated lipogranulomatosis) 272.8
Farcin 024
Farcy 024
Farmers'
  lung 495.0
  skin 692.74
Farsightedness 367.0
Fascia - *see* condition
Fasciculation 781.0
Fasciculitis optica 377.32
Fasciitis 729.4
  eosinophilic 728.89
  necrotizing 728.86
  nodular 728.79
  perirenal 593.4
  plantar 728.71
  pseudosarcomatous 728.79
  traumatic (old) NEC 728.79
    current - *see* Sprain, by site
Fasciola hepatica infestation 121.3
Fascioliasis 121.3
Fasciolopsiasis (small intestine) 121.4
Fasciolopsis (small intestine) 121.4
Fast pulse 785.0
Fat
  embolism (cerebral) (pulmonary) (systemic) 958.1
    with
      abortion - *see* Abortion, by type, with embolism
      ectopic pregnancy (*see also* categories 633.0–633.9) 639.6
      molar pregnancy (*see also* categories 630–632) 639.6
    complicating delivery or puerperium 673.8
    following
      abortion 639.6
      ectopic or molar pregnancy 639.6
    in pregnancy, childbirth, or the puerperium 673.8
  excessive 278.02
      in heart (*see also* Degeneration, myocardial) 429.1
  general 278.02
  hernia, herniation 729.30
    eyelid 374.34
    knee 729.31
    orbit 374.34
    retro-orbital 374.34
    retropatellar 729.31
    specified site NEC 729.39
  indigestion 579.8
  in stool 792.1
  localized (pad) 278.1
    heart (*see also* Degeneration, myocardial) 429.1
    knee 729.31
    retropatellar 729.31
  necrosis - *see also* Fatty, degeneration
    breast (aseptic) (segmental) 611.3

Fat *(Continued)*
necrosis *(Continued)*
mesentery 567.82
omentum 567.82
peritoneum 567.82
pad 278.1
Fatal syncope 798.1
Fatigue 780.79
auditory deafness (*see also* Deafness) 389.9
chronic, syndrome 780.71
combat (*see also* Reaction, stress, acute) 308.9
during pregnancy 646.8
general 780.79
psychogenic 300.5
heat (transient) 992.6
muscle 729.89
myocardium (*see also* Failure, heart) 428.9
nervous 300.5
neurosis 300.5
operational 300.89
postural 729.89
posture 729.89
psychogenic (general) 300.5
senile 797
syndrome NEC 300.5
chronic 780.71
undue 780.79
voice 784.49
Fatness 278.02
Fatty - *see also* condition
apron 278.1
degeneration (diffuse) (general) NEC 272.8
localized - *see* Degeneration, by site, fatty
placenta - *see* Placenta, abnormal
heart (enlarged) (*see also* Degeneration, myocardial) 429.1
infiltration (diffuse) (general) (*see also* Degeneration, by site, fatty) 272.8
heart (enlarged) (*see also* Degeneration, myocardial) 429.1
liver 571.8
alcoholic 571.0
necrosis - *see* Degeneration, fatty
phanerosis 272.8
Fauces - *see* condition
Fauchard's disease (periodontitis) 523.40 (Revised)
Faucitis 478.29
Faulty - *see also* condition
position of teeth 524.30
Favism (anemia) 282.2
Favre-Racouchot disease (elastoidosis cutanea nodularis) 701.8
Favus 110.9
beard 110.0
capitis 110.0
corporis 110.5
eyelid 110.8
foot 110.4
hand 110.2
scalp 110.0
specified site NEC 110.8
Fear, fearfulness (complex) (reaction) 300.20
child 313.0
of
animals 300.29
closed spaces 300.29
crowds 300.29
eating in public 300.23
Fear, fearfulness *(Continued)*
of *(Continued)*
heights 300.29
open spaces 300.22
with panic attacks 300.21
public speaking 300.23
streets 300.22
with panic attacks 300.21
travel 300.22
with panic attacks 300.21
washing in public 300.23
transient 308.0
Feared complaint unfounded V65.5
Febricula (continued) (simple) (*see also* Pyrexia) 780.6
Febrile (*see also* Pyrexia) 780.6
convulsion (simple) 780.31 (Revised)
complex 780.32 (New)
seizure (simple) 780.31 (Revised)
atypical 780.32 (New)
complex 780.32 (New)
complicated 780.32 (New)
Febris (*see also* Fever) 780.6
aestiva (*see also* Fever, hay) 477.9
flava (*see also* Fever, yellow) 060.9
melitensis 023.0
pestis (*see also* Plague) 020.9
puerperalis 672
recurrens (*see also* Fever, relapsing) 087.9
pediculo vestimenti 087.0
rubra 034.1
typhoidea 002.0
typhosa 002.0
Fecal - *see* condition
Fecalith (impaction) 560.39
with hernia - *see also* Hernia, by site, with obstruction
gangrenous - *see* Hernia, by site, with gangrene
appendix 543.9
congenital 777.1
Fede's disease 529.0
Feeble-minded 317
Feeble rapid pulse due to shock following injury 958.4
Feeding
faulty (elderly) (infant) 783.3
newborn 779.3
formula check V20.2
improper (elderly) (infant) 783.3
newborn 779.3
problem (elderly) (infant) 783.3
newborn 779.3
nonorganic origin 307.59
Feer's disease 985.0
Feet - *see* condition
Feigned illness V65.2
Feil-Klippel syndrome (brevicollis) 756.16
Feinmesser's (hidrotic) ectodermal dysplasia 757.31
Felix's disease (juvenile osteochondrosis, hip) 732.1
Felon (any digit) (with lymphangitis) 681.01
herpetic 054.6
Felty's syndrome (rheumatoid arthritis with splenomegaly and leukopenia) 714.1
Feminism in boys 302.6
Feminization, testicular 259.5
with pseudohermaphroditism, male 259.5
Femoral hernia - *see* Hernia, femoral
Femora vara 736.32
Femur, femoral - *see* condition
Fenestrata placenta - *see* Placenta, abnormal
Fenestration, fenestrated - *see also* Imperfect, closure
aorta-pulmonary 745.0
aorticopulmonary 745.0
aortopulmonary 745.0
cusps, heart valve NEC 746.89
pulmonary 746.09
hymen 752.49
pulmonic cusps 746.09
Fenwick's disease 537.89
Fermentation (gastric) (gastrointestinal) (stomach) 536.8
intestine 564.89
psychogenic 306.4
psychogenic 306.4
Fernell's disease (aortic aneurysm) 441.9
Fertile eunuch syndrome 257.2
Fertility, meaning multiparity - *see* Multiparity
Fetal alcohol syndrome 760.71
Fetalis uterus 752.3
Fetid
breath 784.99 (Revised)
sweat 705.89
Fetishism 302.81
transvestic 302.3
Fetomaternal hemorrhage
affecting management of pregnancy 656.0
fetus or newborn 772.0
Fetus, fetal - *see also* condition
papyraceous 779.89
type lung tissue 770.4
Fever 780.6
with chills 780.6
in malarial regions (*see also* Malaria) 084.6
abortus NEC 023.9
aden 061
African tick-borne 087.1
American
mountain tick 066.1
spotted 082.0
and ague (*see also* Malaria) 084.6
aphthous 078.4
arbovirus hemorrhagic 065.9
Assam 085.0
Australian A or Q 083.0
Bangkok hemorrhagic 065.4
biliary, Charcôt's intermittent - *see* Choledocholithiasis
bilious, hemoglobinuric 084.8
blackwater 084.8
blister 054.9
Bonvale Dam 780.79
boutonneuse 082.1
brain 323.9
late effect - *see* category 326
breakbone 061
Bullis 082.8
Bunyamwera 066.3
Burdwan 085.0
Bwamba (encephalitis) 066.3
Cameroon (*see also* Malaria) 084.6
Canton 081.9
catarrhal (acute) 460
chronic 472.0
cat-scratch 078.3
cerebral 323.9
late effect - *see* category 326
cerebrospinal (meningococcal) (*see also* Meningitis, cerebrospinal) 036.0

Fever *(Continued)*
Chagres 084.0
Chandipura 066.8
changuinola 066.0
Charcôt's (biliary) (hepatic) (intermittent) *see* Choledocholithiasis
Chikungunya (viral) 066.3
hemorrhagic 065.4
childbed 670
Chitral 066.0
Colombo (*see also* Fever, paratyphoid) 002.9
Colorado tick (virus) 066.1
congestive
malarial (*see also* Malaria) 084.6
remittent (*see also* Malaria) 084.6
Congo virus 065.0
continued 780.6
malarial 084.0
Corsican (*see also* Malaria) 084.6
Crimean hemorrhagic 065.0
Cyprus (*see also* Brucellosis) 023.9
dandy 061
deer fly (*see also* Tularemia) 021.9
dehydration, newborn 778.4
dengue (virus) 061
hemorrhagic 065.4
desert 114.0
due to heat 992.0
Dumdum 085.0
enteric 002.0
ephemeral (of unknown origin) (*see also* Pyrexia) 780.6
epidemic, hemorrhagic of the Far East 065.0
erysipelatous (*see also* Erysipelas) 035
estivo-autumnal (malarial) 084.0
etiocholanolone 277.31 ◀
famine - *see also* Fever, relapsing
meaning typhus - *see* Typhus
Far Eastern hemorrhagic 065.0
five day 083.1
Fort Bragg 100.89
gastroenteric 002.0
gastromalarial (*see also* Malaria) 084.6
Gibraltar (*see also* Brucellosis) 023.9
glandular 075
Guama (viral) 066.3
Haverhill 026.1
hay (allergic) (with rhinitis) 477.9
with
asthma (bronchial) (*see also* Asthma) 493.0
due to
dander, animal (cat) (dog) 477.2
dust 477.8
fowl 477.8
hair, animal (cat) (dog) 477.2
pollen, any plant or tree 477.0
specified allergen other than pollen 477.8
heat (effects) 992.0
hematuric, bilious 084.8
hemoglobinuric (malarial) 084.8
bilious 084.8
hemorrhagic (arthropod-borne) NEC 065.9
with renal syndrome 078.6
arenaviral 078.7
Argentine 078.7
Bangkok 065.4
Bolivian 078.7
Central Asian 065.0
chikungunya 065.4
Crimean 065.0

Fever *(Continued)*
hemorrhagic *(Continued)*
dengue (virus) 065.4
Ebola 065.8
epidemic 078.6
of Far East 065.0
Far Eastern 065.0
Junin virus 078.7
Korean 078.6
Kyasanur forest 065.2
Machupo virus 078.7
mite-borne NEC 065.8
mosquito-borne 065.4
Omsk 065.1
Philippine 065.4
Russian (Yaroslav) 078.6
Singapore 065.4
Southeast Asia 065.4
Thailand 065.4
tick-borne NEC 065.3
hepatic (*see also* Cholecystitis) 575.8
intermittent (Charcôt's) - *see* Choledocholithiasis
herpetic (*see also* Herpes) 054.9
hyalomma tick 065.0
icterohemorrhagic 100.0
inanition 780.6
newborn 778.4
infective NEC 136.9
intermittent (bilious) (*see also* Malaria) 084.6
hepatic (Charcôt) - *see* Choledocholithiasis
of unknown origin (*see also* Pyrexia) 780.6
pernicious 084.0
iodide
correct substance properly administered 780.6
overdose or wrong substance given or taken 975.5
Japanese river 081.2
jungle yellow 060.0
Junin virus, hemorrhagic 078.7
Katayama 120.2
Kedani 081.2
Kenya 082.1
Korean hemorrhagic 078.6
Lassa 078.89
Lone Star 082.8
lung - *see* Pneumonia
Machupo virus, hemorrhagic 078.7
malaria, malarial (*see also* Malaria) 084.6
Malta (*see also* Brucellosis) 023.9
Marseilles 082.1
marsh (*see also* Malaria) 084.6
Mayaro (viral) 066.3
Mediterranean (*see also* Brucellosis) 023.9
familial 277.31 ◀
tick 082.1
meningeal - *see* Meningitis
metal fumes NEC 985.8
Meuse 083.1
Mexican - *see* Typhus, Mexican
Mianeh 087.1
miasmatic (*see also* Malaria) 084.6
miliary 078.2
milk, female 672
mill 504
mite-borne hemorrhagic 065.8
Monday 504

Fever *(Continued)*
mosquito-borne NEC 066.3
hemorrhagic NEC 065.4
mountain 066.1
meaning
Rocky Mountain spotted 082.0
undulant fever (*see also* Brucellosis) 023.9
tick (American) 066.1
Mucambo (viral) 066.3
mud 100.89
Neapolitan (*see also* Brucellosis) 023.9
neutropenic 288.00 ◀
nine-mile 083.0
nonexanthematous tick 066.1
North Asian tick-borne typhus 082.2
Omsk hemorrhagic 065.1
O'nyong nyong (viral) 066.3
Oropouche (viral) 066.3
Oroya 088.0
paludal (*see also* Malaria) 084.6
Panama 084.0
pappataci 066.0
paratyphoid 002.9
A 002.1
B (Schottmüller's) 002.2
C (Hirschfeld) 002.3
parrot 073.9
periodic 277.31 ◀
pernicious, acute 084.0
persistent (of unknown origin) (*see also* Pyrexia) 780.6
petechial 036.0
pharyngoconjunctival 077.2
adenoviral type 3 077.2
Philippine hemorrhagic 065.4
phlebotomus 066.0
Piry 066.8
Pixuna (viral) 066.3
Plasmodium ovale 084.3
pleural (*see also* Pleurisy) 511.0
pneumonic - *see* Pneumonia
polymer fume 987.8
postoperative 998.89
due to infection 998.59
pretibial 100.89
puerperal, postpartum 672
putrid - *see* Septicemia
pyemic - *see* Septicemia
Q 083.0
with pneumonia 083.0 *[484.8]*
quadrilateral 083.0
quartan (malaria) 084.2
Queensland (coastal) 083.0
seven-day 100.89
Quintan (A) 083.1
quotidian 084.0
rabbit (*see also* Tularemia) 021.9
rat-bite 026.9
due to
Spirillum minor or minus 026.0
Spirochaeta morsus muris 026.0
Streptobacillus moniliformis 026.1
recurrent - *see* Fever, relapsing
relapsing 087.9
Carter's (Asiatic) 087.0
Dutton's (West African) 087.1
Koch's 087.9
louse-borne (epidemic) 087.0
Novy's (American) 087.1
Obermeyer's (European) 087.0
spirillum NEC 087.9
tick-borne (endemic) 087.1
remittent (bilious) (congestive) (gastric) (*see also* Malaria) 084.6

Fever *(Continued)*
rheumatic (active) (acute) (chronic) (subacute) 390
with heart involvement 391.9
carditis 391.9
endocarditis (aortic) (mitral) (pulmonary) (tricuspid) 391.1
multiple sites 391.8
myocarditis 391.2
pancarditis, acute 391.8
pericarditis 391.0
specified type NEC 391.8
valvulitis 391.1
inactive or quiescent with
cardiac hypertrophy 398.99
carditis 398.90
endocarditis 397.9
aortic (valve) 395.9
with mitral (valve) disease 396.9
mitral (valve) 394.9
with aortic (valve) disease 396.9
pulmonary (valve) 397.1
tricuspid (valve) 397.0
heart conditions (classifiable to 429.3, 429.6, 429.9) 398.99
failure (congestive) (conditions classifiable to 428.0, 428.9) 398.91
left ventricular failure (conditions classifiable to 428.1) 398.91
myocardial degeneration (conditions classifiable to 429.1) 398.0
myocarditis (conditions classifiable to 429.0) 398.0
pancarditis 398.99
pericarditis 393
Rift Valley (viral) 066.3
Rocky Mountain spotted 082.0
rose 477.0
Ross river (viral) 066.3
Russian hemorrhagic 078.6
sandfly 066.0
San Joaquin (valley) 114.0
São Paulo 082.0
scarlet 034.1
septic - *see* Septicemia
seven-day 061
Japan 100.89
Queensland 100.89
shin bone 083.1
Singapore hemorrhagic 065.4
solar 061
sore 054.9
South African tick-bite 087.1
Southeast Asia hemorrhagic 065.4
spinal - *see* Meningitis
spirillary 026.0
splenic (*see also* Anthrax) 022.9
spotted (Rocky Mountain) 082.0
American 082.0
Brazilian 082.0
Colombian 082.0
meaning
cerebrospinal meningitis 036.0
typhus 082.9
spring 309.23
steroid
correct substance properly administered 780.6
overdose or wrong substance given or taken 962.0
streptobacillary 026.1

Fever *(Continued)*
subtertian 084.0
Sumatran mite 081.2
sun 061
swamp 100.89
sweating 078.2
swine 003.8
sylvatic yellow 060.0
Tahyna 062.5
tertian - *see* Malaria, tertian
Thailand hemorrhagic 065.4
thermic 992.0
three day 066.0
with Coxsackie exanthem 074.8
tick
American mountain 066.1
Colorado 066.1
Kemerovo 066.1
Mediterranean 082.1
mountain 066.1
nonexanthematous 066.1
Quaranfil 066.1
tick-bite NEC 066.1
tick-borne NEC 066.1
hemorrhagic NEC 065.3
transitory of newborn 778.4
trench 083.1
tsutsugamushi 081.2
typhogastric 002.0
typhoid (abortive) (ambulant) (any site) (hemorrhagic) (infection) (intermittent) (malignant) (rheumatic) 002.0
typhomalarial (*see also* Malaria) 084.6
typhus - *see* Typhus
undulant (*see also* Brucellosis) 023.9
unknown origin (*see also* Pyrexia) 780.6
uremic - *see* Uremia
uveoparotid 135
valley (Coccidioidomycosis) 114.0
Venezuelan equine 066.2
Volhynian 083.1
Wesselsbron (viral) 066.3
West
African 084.8
Nile (viral) 066.40
with
cranial nerve disorders 066.42
encephalitis 066.41
optic neuritis 066.42
other complications 066.49
other neurologic manifestations 066.42
polyradiculitis 066.42
Whitmore's 025
Wolhynian 083.1
worm 128.9
Yaroslav hemorrhagic 078.6
yellow 060.9
jungle 060.0
sylvatic 060.0
urban 060.1
vaccination, prophylactic (against) V04.4
Zika (viral) 066.3
Fibrillation
atrial (established) (paroxysmal) 427.31
auricular (atrial) (established) 427.31
cardiac (ventricular) 427.41
coronary (*see also* Infarct, myocardium) 410.9
heart (ventricular) 427.41
muscular 728.9
postoperative 997.1
ventricular 427.41

Fibrin
ball or bodies, pleural (sac) 511.0
chamber, anterior (eye) (gelatinous exudate) 364.04
Fibrinogenolysis (hemorrhagic) - *see* Fibrinolysis
Fibrinogenopenia (congenital) (hereditary) (*see also* Defect, coagulation) 286.3
acquired 286.6
Fibrinolysis (acquired) (hemorrhagic) (pathologic) 286.6
with
abortion - *see* Abortion, by type, with hemorrhage, delayed or excessive
ectopic pregnancy (*see also* categories 633.0–633.9) 639.1
molar pregnancy (*see also* categories 630–632) 639.1
antepartum or intrapartum 641.3
affecting fetus or newborn 762.1
following
abortion 639.1
ectopic or molar pregnancy 639.1
newborn, transient 776.2
postpartum 666.3
Fibrinopenia (hereditary) (*see also* Defect, coagulation) 286.3
acquired 286.6
Fibrinopurulent - *see* condition
Fibrinous - *see* condition
Fibroadenoma (M9010/0)
cellular intracanalicular (M9020/0) 217
giant (intracanalicular) (M9020/0) 217
intracanalicular (M9011/0)
cellular (M9020/0) 217
giant (M9020/0) 217
specified site - *see* Neoplasm, by site, benign
unspecified site 217
juvenile (M9030/0) 217
pericanicular (M9012/0)
specified site - *see* Neoplasm, by site, benign
unspecified site 217
phyllodes (M9020/0) 217
prostate 600.20
with ⇐
other lower urinary tract symptoms (LUTS) 600.21 ◀
urinary ◀
obstruction 600.21 ◀
retention 600.21 ◀
specified site - *see* Neoplasm, by site, benign
unspecified site 217
Fibroadenosis, breast (chronic) (cystic) (diffuse) (periodic) (segmental) 610.2
Fibroangioma (M9160/0) - *see also* Neoplasm, by site, benign
juvenile (M9160/0)
specified site - *see* Neoplasm, by site, benign
unspecified site 210.7
Fibrocellulitis progressiva ossificans 728.11
Fibrochondrosarcoma (M9220/3) - *see* Neoplasm, cartilage, malignant
Fibrocystic
disease 277.00
bone NEC 733.29
breast 610.1
jaw 526.2
kidney (congenital) 753.19

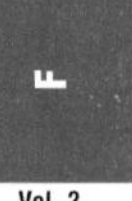

Fibrocystic *(Continued)*
  disease *(Continued)*
    liver 751.62
    lung 518.89
      congenital 748.4
    pancreas 277.00
  kidney (congenital) 753.19
Fibrodysplasia ossificans multiplex (progressiva) 728.11
Fibroelastosis (cordis) (endocardial) (endomyocardial) 425.3
Fibroid (tumor) (M8890/0) - *see also* Neoplasm, connective tissue, benign
  disease, lung (chronic) (*see also* Fibrosis, lung) 515
  heart (disease) (*see also* Myocarditis) 429.0
  induration, lung (chronic) (*see also* Fibrosis, lung) 515
  in pregnancy or childbirth 654.1
    affecting fetus or newborn 763.89
    causing obstructed labor 660.2
      affecting fetus or newborn 763.1
  liver - *see* Cirrhosis, liver
  lung (*see also* Fibrosis, lung) 515
  pneumonia (chronic) (*see also* Fibrosis, lung) 515
  uterus (M8890/0) (*see also* Leiomyoma, uterus) 218.9
Fibrolipoma (M8851/0) (*see also* Lipoma, by site) 214.9
Fibroliposarcoma (M8850/3) - *see* Neoplasm, connective tissue, malignant
Fibroma (M8810/0) - *see also* Neoplasm, connective tissue, benign
  ameloblastic (M9330/0) 213.1
    upper jaw (bone) 213.0
  bone (nonossifying) 733.99
    ossifying (M9262/0) - *see* Neoplasm, bone, benign
  cementifying (M9274/0) - *see* Neoplasm, bone, benign
  chondromyxoid (M9241/0) - *see* Neoplasm, bone, benign
  desmoplastic (M8823/1) - *see* Neoplasm, connective tissue, uncertain behavior
  facial (M8813/0) - *see* Neoplasm, connective tissue, benign
  invasive (M8821/1) - *see* Neoplasm, connective tissue, uncertain behavior
  molle (M8851/0) (*see also* Lipoma, by site) 214.9
  myxoid (M8811/0) - *see* Neoplasm, connective tissue, benign
  nasopharynx, nasopharyngeal (juvenile) (M9160/0) 210.7
  nonosteogenic (nonossifying) - *see* Dysplasia, fibrous
  odontogenic (M9321/0) 213.1
    upper jaw (bone) 213.0
  ossifying (M9262/0) - *see* Neoplasm, bone, benign
  periosteal (M8812/0) - *see* Neoplasm, bone, benign
  prostate 600.20
    with ⬅
      other lower urinary tract symptoms (LUTS) 600.21 ◀
      urinary ◀
        obstruction 600.21 ◀
        retention 600.21 ◀
  soft (M8851/0) (*see also* Lipoma, by site) 214.9

Fibromatosis 728.79 ⬅
  abdominal (M8822/1) - *see* Neoplasm, connective tissue, uncertain behavior
  aggressive (M8821/1) - *see* Neoplasm, connective tissue, uncertain behavior
  congenital generalized (CGF) 759.89 ◀
  Dupuytren's 728.6
  gingival 523.8
  plantar fascia 728.71
  proliferative 728.79
  pseudosarcomatous (proliferative) (subcutaneous) 728.79
  subcutaneous pseudosarcomatous (proliferative) 728.79
Fibromyalgia 729.1
Fibromyoma (M8890/0) - *see also* Neoplasm, connective tissue, benign
  uterus (corpus) (*see also* Leiomyoma, uterus) 218.9
    in pregnancy or childbirth 654.1
      affecting fetus or newborn 763.89
      causing obstructed labor 660.2
        affecting fetus or newborn 763.1
Fibromyositis (*see also* Myositis) 729.1
  scapulohumeral 726.2
Fibromyxolipoma (M8852/0) (*see also* Lipoma, by site) 214.9
Fibromyxoma (M8811/0) - *see* Neoplasm, connective tissue, benign
Fibromyxosarcoma (M8811/3) - *see* Neoplasm, connective tissue, malignant
Fibro-odontoma, ameloblastic (M9290/0) 213.1
  upper jaw (bone) 213.0
Fibro-osteoma (M9262/0) - *see* Neoplasm, bone, benign
Fibroplasia, retrolental 362.21
Fibropurulent - *see* condition
Fibrosarcoma (M8810/3) - *see also* Neoplasm, connective tissue, malignant
  ameloblastic (M9330/3) 170.1
    upper jaw (bone) 170.0
  congenital (M8814/3) - *see* Neoplasm, connective tissue, malignant
  fascial (M8813/3) - *see* Neoplasm, connective tissue, malignant
  infantile (M8814/3) - *see* Neoplasm, connective tissue, malignant
  odontogenic (M9330/3) 170.1
    upper jaw (bone) 170.0
  periosteal (M8812/3) - *see* Neoplasm, bone, malignant
Fibrosclerosis
  breast 610.3
  corpora cavernosa (penis) 607.89
  familial multifocal NEC 710.8
  multifocal (idiopathic) NEC 710.8
  penis (corpora cavernosa) 607.89
Fibrosis, fibrotic
  adrenal (gland) 255.8
  alveolar (diffuse) 516.3
  amnion 658.8
  anal papillae 569.49
  anus 569.49
  appendix, appendiceal, noninflammatory 543.9
  arteriocapillary - *see* Arteriosclerosis
  bauxite (of lung) 503
  biliary 576.8
    due to Clonorchis sinensis 121.1
  bladder 596.8
    interstitial 595.1

Fibrosis, fibrotic *(Continued)*
  bladder *(Continued)*
    localized submucosal 595.1
    panmural 595.1
  bone, diffuse 756.59
  breast 610.3
  capillary - *see also* Arteriosclerosis
    lung (chronic) (*see also* Fibrosis, lung) 515
  cardiac (*see also* Myocarditis) 429.0
  cervix 622.8
  chorion 658.8
  corpus cavernosum 607.89
  cystic (of pancreas) 277.00
    with
      manifestations
        gastrointestinal 277.03
        pulmonary 277.02
        specified NEC 277.09
      meconium ileus 277.01
      pulmonary exacerbation 277.02
  due to (presence of) any device, implant, or graft - *see* Complications, due to (presence of) any device, implant, or graft classified to 996.0–996.5 NEC
  ejaculatory duct 608.89
  endocardium (*see also* Endocarditis) 424.90
  endomyocardial (African) 425.0
  epididymis 608.89
  eye muscle 378.62
  graphite (of lung) 503
  heart (*see also* Myocarditis) 429.0
  hepatic - *see also* Cirrhosis, liver
    due to Clonorchis sinensis 121.1
  hepatolienal - *see* Cirrhosis, liver
  hepatosplenic - *see* Cirrhosis, liver
  infrapatellar fat pad 729.31
  interstitial pulmonary, newborn 770.7
  intrascrotal 608.89
  kidney (*see also* Sclerosis, renal) 587
  liver - *see* Cirrhosis, liver
  lung (atrophic) (capillary) (chronic) (confluent) (massive) (perialveolar) (peribronchial) 515
    with
      anthracosilicosis (occupational) 500
      anthracosis (occupational) 500
      asbestosis (occupational) 501
      bagassosis (occupational) 495.1
      bauxite 503
      berylliosis (occupational) 503
      byssinosis (occupational) 504
      calcicosis (occupational) 502
      chalicosis (occupational) 502
      dust reticulation (occupational) 504
      farmers' lung 495.0
      gannister disease (occupational) 502
      graphite 503
      pneumonoconiosis (occupational) 505
      pneumosiderosis (occupational) 503
      siderosis (occupational) 503
      silicosis (occupational) 502
      tuberculosis (*see also* Tuberculosis) 011.4
    diffuse (idiopathic) (interstitial) 516.3
    due to
      bauxite 503
      fumes or vapors (chemical) (inhalation) 506.4
      graphite 503
    following radiation 508.1

- **Fibrosis, fibrotic** *(Continued)*
  - lung *(Continued)*
    - postinflammatory 515
    - silicotic (massive) (occupational) 502
    - tuberculous (*see also* Tuberculosis) 011.4
  - lymphatic gland 289.3
  - median bar 600.90
    - with
      - other lower urinary tract symptoms (LUTS) 600.91
      - urinary
        - obstruction 600.91
        - retention 600.91
  - mediastinum (idiopathic) 519.3
  - meninges 349.2
  - muscle NEC 728.2
    - iatrogenic (from injection) 999.9
  - myocardium, myocardial (*see also* Myocarditis) 429.0
  - oral submucous 528.8
  - ovary 620.8
  - oviduct 620.8
  - pancreas 577.8
    - cystic 277.00
      - with
        - manifestations
          - gastrointestinal 277.03
          - pulmonary 277.02
          - specified NEC 277.09
        - meconium ileus 277.01
        - pulmonary exacerbation 277.02
  - penis 607.89
  - periappendiceal 543.9
  - periarticular (*see also* Ankylosis) 718.5
  - pericardium 423.1
  - perineum, in pregnancy or childbirth 654.8
    - affecting fetus or newborn 763.89
    - causing obstructed labor 660.2
      - affecting fetus or newborn 763.1
  - perineural NEC 355.9
    - foot 355.6
  - periureteral 593.89
  - placenta - *see* Placenta, abnormal
  - pleura 511.0
  - popliteal fat pad 729.31
  - preretinal 362.56
  - prostate (chronic) 600.90
    - with
      - other lower urinary tract symptoms (LUTS) 600.91
      - urinary
        - obstruction 600.91
        - retention 600.91
  - pulmonary (chronic) (*see also* Fibrosis, lung) 515
    - alveolar capillary block 516.3
    - interstitial
      - diffuse (idiopathic) 516.3
      - newborn 770.7
  - radiation - *see* Effect, adverse, radiation
  - rectal sphincter 569.49
  - retroperitoneal, idiopathic 593.4
  - sclerosing mesenteric (idiopathic) 567.82
  - scrotum 608.89
  - seminal vesicle 608.89
  - senile 797
  - skin NEC 709.2
  - spermatic cord 608.89
  - spleen 289.59
    - bilharzial (*see also* Schistosomiasis) 120.9
  - subepidermal nodular (M8832/0) - *see* Neoplasm, skin, benign
- **Fibrosis, fibrotic** *(Continued)*
  - submucous NEC 709.2
    - oral 528.8
    - tongue 528.8
  - syncytium - *see* Placenta, abnormal
  - testis 608.89
    - chronic, due to syphilis 095.8
  - thymus (gland) 254.8
  - tunica vaginalis 608.89
  - ureter 593.89
  - urethra 599.84
  - uterus (nonneoplastic) 621.8
    - bilharzial (*see also* Schistosomiasis) 120.9
    - neoplastic (*see also* Leiomyoma, uterus) 218.9
  - vagina 623.8
  - valve, heart (*see also* Endocarditis) 424.90
  - vas deferens 608.89
  - vein 459.89
    - lower extremities 459.89
  - vesical 595.1
- **Fibrositis** (periarticular) (rheumatoid) 729.0
  - humeroscapular region 726.2
  - nodular, chronic
    - Jaccoud's 714.4
    - rheumatoid 714.4
  - ossificans 728.11
  - scapulohumeral 726.2
- **Fibrothorax** 511.0
- **Fibrotic** - *see* Fibrosis
- **Fibrous** - *see* condition
- **Fibroxanthoma** (M8831/0) - *see also* Neoplasm, connective tissue, benign
  - atypical (M8831/1) - *see* Neoplasm, connective tissue, uncertain behavior
  - malignant (M8831/3) - *see* Neoplasm, connective tissue, malignant
- **Fibroxanthosarcoma** (M8831/3) - *see* Neoplasm, connective tissue, malignant
- **Fiedler's**
  - disease (leptospiral jaundice) 100.0
  - myocarditis or syndrome (acute isolated myocarditis) 422.91
- **Fiessinger-Leroy** (-Reiter) syndrome 099.3
- **Fiessinger-Rendu syndrome** (erythema muliforme exudativum) 695.1
- **Fifth disease** (eruptive) 057.0
  - venereal 099.1
- **Filaria, filarial** - *see* Infestation, filarial
- **Filariasis** (*see also* Infestation, filarial) 125.9
  - bancroftian 125.0
  - Brug's 125.1
  - due to
    - bancrofti 125.0
    - Brugia (Wuchereria) (malayi) 125.1
    - Loa loa 125.2
    - malayi 125.1
    - organism NEC 125.6
    - Wuchereria (bancrofti) 125.0
      - malayi 125.1
  - Malayan 125.1
  - ozzardi 125.5
  - specified type NEC 125.6
- **Filatoff's, Filatov's, Filatow's disease** (infectious mononucleosis) 075
- **File-cutters' disease** 984.9
  - specified type of lead - *see* Table of Drugs and Chemicals
- **Filling defect**
  - biliary tract 793.3
  - bladder 793.5
- **Filling defect** *(Continued)*
  - duodenum 793.4
  - gallbladder 793.3
  - gastrointestinal tract 793.4
  - intestine 793.4
  - kidney 793.5
  - stomach 793.4
  - ureter 793.5
- **Filtering bleb, eye** (postglaucoma) (status) V45.69
  - with complication or rupture 997.99
  - postcataract extraction (complication) 997.99
- **Fimbrial cyst** (congenital) 752.11
- **Fimbriated hymen** 752.49
- **Financial problem affecting care** V60.2
- **Findings, abnormal, without diagnosis** (examination) (laboratory test) 796.4
  - 17-ketosteroids, elevated 791.9
  - acetonuria 791.6
  - acid phosphatase 790.5
  - albumin-globulin ratio 790.99
  - albuminuria 791.0
  - alcohol in blood 790.3
  - alkaline phosphatase 790.5
  - amniotic fluid 792.3
  - amylase 790.5
  - antenatal screening 796.5
  - anthrax, positive 795.31
  - anisocytosis 790.09
  - antibody titers, elevated 795.79
  - anticardiolipin antibody 795.79
  - antigen-antibody reaction 795.79
  - antiphospholipid antibody 795.79
  - bacteriuria 791.9
  - ballistocardiogram 794.39
  - bicarbonate 276.9
  - bile in urine 791.4
  - bilirubin 277.4
  - bleeding time (prolonged) 790.92
  - blood culture, positive 790.7
  - blood gas level (arterial) 790.91
  - blood sugar level 790.29
    - high 790.29
      - fasting glucose 790.21
      - glucose tolerance test 790.22
    - low 251.2
  - C-reactive protein (CRP) 790.95
  - calcium 275.40
  - cancer antigen 125 [CA 125] 795.82
  - carbonate 276.9
  - carcinoembryonic antigen [CEA] 795.81
  - casts, urine 791.7
  - catecholamines 791.9
  - cells, urine 791.7
  - cerebrospinal fluid (color) (content) (pressure) 792.0
  - cervical
    - high risk human papillomavirus (HPV) DNA test positive 795.05
    - low risk human papillomavirus (HPV) DNA test positive 795.09
  - chloride 276.9
  - cholesterol 272.9
  - chromosome analysis 795.2
  - chyluria 791.1
  - circulation time 794.39
  - cloudy dialysis effluent 792.5
  - cloudy urine 791.9
  - coagulation study 790.92
  - cobalt, blood 790.6
  - color of urine (unusual) NEC 791.9
  - copper, blood 790.6

ICD-9-CM

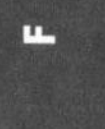

Vol. 2

Findings, abnormal, without diagnosis *(Continued)*
crystals, urine 791.9
culture, positive NEC 795.39
blood 790.7
HIV V08
human immunodeficiency virus V08
nose 795.39
skin lesion NEC 795.39
spinal fluid 792.0
sputum 795.39
stool 792.1
throat 795.39
urine 791.9
viral
human immunodeficiency V08
wound 795.39
echocardiogram 793.2
echoencephalogram 794.01
echogram NEC - *see* Findings, abnormal, structure
electrocardiogram (ECG) (EKG) 794.31
electroencephalogram (EEG) 794.02
electrolyte level, urinary 791.9
electromyogram (EMG) 794.17
ocular 794.14
electro-oculogram (EOG) 794.12
electroretinogram (ERG) 794.11
enzymes, serum NEC 790.5
fibrinogen titer coagulation study 790.92
filling defect - *see* Filling defect
function study NEC 794.9
auditory 794.15
bladder 794.9
brain 794.00
cardiac 794.30
endocrine NEC 794.6
thyroid 794.5
kidney 794.4
liver 794.8
nervous system
central 794.00
peripheral 794.19
oculomotor 794.14
pancreas 794.9
placenta 794.9
pulmonary 794.2
retina 794.11
special senses 794.19
spleen 794.9
vestibular 794.16
gallbladder, nonvisualization 793.3
glucose 790.29
elevated
fasting 790.21
tolerance test 790.22
glycosuria 791.5
heart
shadow 793.2
sounds 785.3
hematinuria 791.2
hematocrit
drop (precipitous) 790.01
elevated 282.7
low 285.9
hematologic NEC 790.99
hematuria 599.7
hemoglobin
elevated 282.7
low 285.9
hemoglobinuria 791.2
histological NEC 795.4
hormones 259.9
immunoglobulins, elevated 795.79
indolacetic acid, elevated 791.9

Findings, abnormal, without diagnosis *(Continued)*
iron 790.6
karyotype 795.2
ketonuria 791.6
lactic acid dehydrogenase (LDH) 790.4
lead 790.6 ◀
lipase 790.5
lipids NEC 272.9
lithium, blood 790.6
liver function test 790.6
lung field (coin lesion) (shadow) 793.1
magnesium, blood 790.6
mammogram 793.80
calcification 793.89 ◀
calculus 793.89 ◀
microcalcification 793.81
mediastinal shift 793.2
melanin, urine 791.9
microbiologic NEC 795.39
mineral, blood NEC 790.6
myoglobinuria 791.3
nasal swab, anthrax 795.31
neonatal screening 796.6
nitrogen derivatives, blood 790.6
nonvisualization of gallbladder 793.3
nose culture, positive 795.39
odor of urine (unusual) NEC 791.9
oxygen saturation 790.91
Papanicolaou (smear) 795.1
cervix 795.00
with
atypical squamous cells
cannot exclude high grade squamous intraepithelial lesion (ASC-H) 795.02
of undetermined significance (ASC-US) 795.01
cytologic evidence of malignancy 795.06 ◀
high grade squamous intraepithelial lesion (HGSIL) 795.04
low grade squamous intraepithelial lesion (LGSIL) 795.03
dyskaryotic 795.09
nonspecific finding NEC 795.09
other site 795.1
peritoneal fluid 792.9
phonocardiogram 794.39
phosphorus 275.3
pleural fluid 792.9
pneumoencephalogram 793.0
PO_2-oxygen ratio 790.91
poikilocytosis 790.09
potassium
deficiency 276.8
excess 276.7
PPD 795.5
prostate specific antigen (PSA) 790.93
protein, serum NEC 790.99
proteinuria 791.0
prothrombin time (prolonged) (partial) (PT) (PTT) 790.92
pyuria 791.9
radiologic (x-ray) 793.99 ⬅
abdomen 793.6
biliary tract 793.3
breast 793.89
abnormal mammogram NOS 793.80
mammographic ⬅
calcification 793.89 ◀
calculus 793.89 ◀
microcalcification 793.81 ◀
gastrointestinal tract 793.4
genitourinary organs 793.5
head 793.0

Findings, abnormal, without diagnosis *(Continued)*
radiologic *(Continued)*
image test inconclusive due to excess body fat 793.91 ◀
intrathoracic organs NEC 793.2
lung 793.1
musculoskeletal 793.7
placenta 793.99 ⬅
retroperitoneum 793.6
skin 793.99 ⬅
skull 793.0
subcutaneous tissue 793.99 ⬅
red blood cell 790.09
count 790.09
morphology 790.09
sickling 790.09
volume 790.09
saliva 792.4
scan NEC 794.9
bladder 794.9
bone 794.9
brain 794.09
kidney 794.4
liver 794.8
lung 794.2
pancreas 794.9
placental 794.9
spleen 794.9
thyroid 794.5
sedimentation rate, elevated 790.1
semen 792.2
serological (for)
human immunodeficiency virus (HIV)
inconclusive 795.71
positive V08
syphilis - *see* Findings, serology for syphilis
serology for syphilis
false positive 795.6
positive 097.1
false 795.6
follow-up of latent syphilis - *see* Syphilis, latent
only finding - *see* Syphilis, latent
serum 790.99
blood NEC 790.99
enzymes NEC 790.5
proteins 790.99
SGOT 790.4
SGPT 790.4
sickling of red blood cells 790.09
skin test, positive 795.79
tuberculin (without active tuberculosis) 795.5
sodium 790.6
deficiency 276.1
excess 276.0
spermatozoa 792.2
spinal fluid 792.0
culture, positive 792.0
sputum culture, positive 795.39
for acid-fast bacilli 795.39
stool NEC 792.1
bloody 578.1
occult 792.1
color 792.1
culture, positive 792.1
occult blood 792.1
stress test 794.39
structure, body (echogram) (thermogram) (ultrasound) (x-ray) NEC 793.99 ⬅
abdomen 793.6
breast 793.89

Findings, abnormal, without diagnosis *(Continued)*
structure, body *(Continued)*
breast *(Continued)*
abnormal mammogram NOS 793.80
mammographic
calcification 793.89
calculus 793.89
microcalcification 793.81
gastrointestinal tract 793.4
genitourinary organs 793.5
head 793.0
echogram (ultrasound) 794.01
intrathoracic organs NEC 793.2
lung 793.1
musculoskeletal 793.7
placenta 793.99
retroperitoneum 793.6
skin 793.99
subcutaneous tissue NEC 793.99
synovial fluid 792.9
thermogram - *see* Findings, abnormal, structure
throat culture, positive 795.39
thyroid (function) 794.5
metabolism (rate) 794.5
scan 794.5
uptake 794.5
total proteins 790.99
toxicology (drugs) (heavy metals) 796.0
transaminase (level) 790.4
triglycerides 272.9
tuberculin skin test (without active tuberculosis) 795.5
tumor markers NEC 795.89
ultrasound - *see also* Findings, abnormal, structure
cardiogram 793.2
uric acid, blood 790.6
urine, urinary constituents 791.9
acetone 791.6
albumin 791.0
bacteria 791.9
bile 791.4
blood 599.7
casts or cells 791.7
chyle 791.1
culture, positive 791.9
glucose 791.5
hemoglobin 791.2
ketone 791.6
protein 791.0
pus 791.9
sugar 791.5
vaginal fluid 792.9
vanillylmandelic acid, elevated 791.9
vectorcardiogram (VCG) 794.39
ventriculogram (cerebral) 793.0
VMA, elevated 791.9
Wassermann reaction
false positive 795.6
positive 097.1
follow-up of latent syphilis - *see* Syphilis, latent
only finding - *see* Syphilis, latent
white blood cell 288.9
count 288.9
elevated 288.60
low 288.50
differential 288.9
morphology 288.9
wound culture 795.39
xerography 793.89
zinc, blood 790.6

Finger - *see* condition
Fire, St. Anthony's (*see also* Erysipelas) 035
Fish
hook stomach 537.89
meal workers' lung 495.8
Fisher's syndrome 357.0
Fissure, fissured
abdominal wall (congenital) 756.79
anus, anal 565.0
congenital 751.5
buccal cavity 528.9
clitoris (congenital) 752.49
ear, lobule (congenital) 744.29
epiglottis (congenital) 748.3
larynx 478.79
congenital 748.3
lip 528.5
congenital (*see also* Cleft, lip) 749.10
nipple 611.2
puerperal, postpartum 676.1
palate (congenital) (*see also* Cleft, palate) 749.00
postanal 565.0
rectum 565.0
skin 709.8
streptococcal 686.9
spine (congenital) (*see also* Spina bifida) 741.9
sternum (congenital) 756.3
tongue (acquired) 529.5
congenital 750.13
Fistula (sinus) 686.9
abdomen (wall) 569.81
bladder 596.2
intestine 569.81
ureter 593.82
uterus 619.2
abdominorectal 569.81
abdominosigmoidal 569.81
abdominothoracic 510.0
abdominouterine 619.2
congenital 752.3
abdominovesical 596.2
accessory sinuses (*see also* Sinusitis) 473.9
actinomycotic - *see* Actinomycosis
alveolar
antrum (*see also* Sinusitis, maxillary) 473.0
process 522.7
anorectal 565.1
antrobuccal (*see also* Sinusitis, maxillary) 473.0
antrum (*see also* Sinusitis, maxillary) 473.0
anus, anal (infectional) (recurrent) 565.1
congenital 751.5
tuberculous (*see also* Tuberculosis) 014.8
aortic sinus 747.29
aortoduodenal 447.2
appendix, appendicular 543.9
arteriovenous (acquired) 447.0
brain 437.3
congenital 747.81
ruptured (*see also* Hemorrhage, subarachnoid) 430
ruptured (*see also* Hemorrhage, subarachnoid) 430
cerebral 437.3
congenital 747.81
congenital (peripheral) 747.60
brain - *see* Fistula, arteriovenous, brain, congenital

Fistula *(Continued)*
arteriovenous *(Continued)*
congenital *(Continued)*
coronary 746.85
gastrointestinal 747.61
lower limb 747.64
pulmonary 747.3
renal 747.62
specified site NEC 747.69
upper limb 747.63
coronary 414.19
congenital 746.85
heart 414.19
pulmonary (vessels) 417.0
congenital 747.3
surgically created (for dialysis) V45.1
complication NEC 996.73
atherosclerosis - *see* Arteriosclerosis, extremities
embolism 996.74
infection or inflammation 996.62
mechanical 996.1
occlusion NEC 996.74
thrombus 996.74
traumatic - *see* Injury, blood vessel, by site
artery 447.2
aural 383.81
congenital 744.49
auricle 383.81
congenital 744.49
Bartholin's gland 619.8
bile duct (*see also* Fistula, biliary) 576.4
biliary (duct) (tract) 576.4
congenital 751.69
bladder (neck) (sphincter) 596.2
into seminal vesicle 596.2
bone 733.99
brain 348.8
arteriovenous - *see* Fistula, arteriovenous, brain
branchial (cleft) 744.41
branchiogenous 744.41
breast 611.0
puerperal, postpartum 675.1
bronchial 510.0
bronchocutaneous, bronchomediastinal, bronchopleural, bronchopleuromediastinal (infective) 510.0
tuberculous (*see also* Tuberculosis) 011.3
bronchoesophageal 530.84
congenital 750.3
buccal cavity (infective) 528.3
canal, ear 380.89
carotid-cavernous
congenital 747.81
with hemorrhage 430
traumatic 900.82
with hemorrhage (*see also* Hemorrhage, brain, traumatic) 853.0
late effect 908.3
cecosigmoidal 569.81
cecum 569.81
cerebrospinal (fluid) 349.81
cervical, lateral (congenital) 744.41
cervicoaural (congenital) 744.49
cervicosigmoidal 619.1
cervicovesical 619.0
cervix 619.8
chest (wall) 510.0
cholecystocolic (*see also* Fistula, gallbladder) 575.5
cholecystocolonic (*see also* Fistula, gallbladder) 575.5

ICD-9-CM F Vol. 2

◀ New ⬅ Revised

Fistula *(Continued)*
cholecystoduodenal (*see also* Fistula, gallbladder) 575.5
cholecystoenteric (*see also* Fistula, gallbladder) 575.5
cholecystogastric (*see also* Fistula, gallbladder) 575.5
cholecystointestinal (*see also* Fistula, gallbladder) 575.5
choledochoduodenal 576.4
cholocolic (*see also* Fistula, gallbladder) 575.5
coccyx 685.1
with abscess 685.0
colon 569.81
colostomy 569.69
colovaginal (acquired) 619.1
common duct (bile duct) 576.4
congenital, NEC - *see* Anomaly, specified type NEC
cornea, causing hypotony 360.32
coronary, arteriovenous 414.19
congenital 746.85
costal region 510.0
cul-de-sac, Douglas' 619.8
cutaneous 686.9
cystic duct (*see also* Fistula, gallbladder) 575.5
congenital 751.69
dental 522.7
diaphragm 510.0
bronchovisceral 510.0
pleuroperitoneal 510.0
pulmonoperitoneal 510.0
duodenum 537.4
ear (canal) (external) 380.89
enterocolic 569.81
enterocutaneous 569.81
enteroenteric 569.81
entero-uterine 619.1
congenital 752.3
enterovaginal 619.1
congenital 752.49
enterovesical 596.1
epididymis 608.89
tuberculous (*see also* Tuberculosis) 016.4
esophagobronchial 530.89
congenital 750.3
esophagocutaneous 530.89
esophagopleurocutaneous 530.89
esophagotracheal 530.84
congenital 750.3
esophagus 530.89
congenital 750.4
ethmoid (*see also* Sinusitis, ethmoidal) 473.2
eyeball (cornea) (sclera) 360.32
eyelid 373.11
fallopian tube (external) 619.2
fecal 569.81
congenital 751.5
from periapical lesion 522.7
frontal sinus (*see also* Sinusitis, frontal) 473.1
gallbladder 575.5
with calculus, cholelithiasis, stones (*see also* Cholelithiasis) 574.2
congenital 751.69
gastric 537.4
gastrocolic 537.4
congenital 750.7
tuberculous (*see also* Tuberculosis) 014.8

Fistula *(Continued)*
gastroenterocolic 537.4
gastroesophageal 537.4
gastrojejunal 537.4
gastrojejunocolic 537.4
genital
organs
female 619.9
specified site NEC 619.8
male 608.89
tract-skin (female) 619.2
hepatopleural 510.0
hepatopulmonary 510.0
horseshoe 565.1
ileorectal 569.81
ileosigmoidal 569.81
ileostomy 569.69
ileovesical 596.1
ileum 569.81
in ano 565.1
tuberculous (*see also* Tuberculosis) 014.8
inner ear (*see also* Fistula, labyrinth) 386.40
intestine 569.81
intestinocolonic (abdominal) 569.81
intestinoureteral 593.82
intestinouterine 619.1
intestinovaginal 619.1
congenital 752.49
intestinovesical 596.1
involving female genital tract 619.9
digestive-genital 619.1
genital tract-skin 619.2
specified site NEC 619.8
urinary-genital 619.0
ischiorectal (fossa) 566
jejunostomy 569.69
jejunum 569.81
joint 719.80
ankle 719.87
elbow 719.82
foot 719.87
hand 719.84
hip 719.85
knee 719.86
multiple sites 719.89
pelvic region 719.85
shoulder (region) 719.81
specified site NEC 719.88
tuberculous - *see* Tuberculosis, joint
wrist 719.83
kidney 593.89
labium (majus) (minus) 619.8
labyrinth, labyrinthine NEC 386.40
combined sites 386.48
multiple sites 386.48
oval window 386.42
round window 386.41
semicircular canal 386.43
lacrimal, lachrymal (duct) (gland) (sac) 375.61
lacrimonasal duct 375.61
laryngotracheal 748.3
larynx 478.79
lip 528.5
congenital 750.25
lumbar, tuberculous (*see also* Tuberculosis) 015.0 *[730.8]*
lung 510.0
lymphatic (node) (vessel) 457.8
mamillary 611.0
mammary (gland) 611.0
puerperal, postpartum 675.1

Fistula *(Continued)*
mastoid (process) (region) 383.1
maxillary (*see also* Sinusitis, maxillary) 473.0
mediastinal 510.0
mediastinobronchial 510.0
mediastinocutaneous 510.0
middle ear 385.89
mouth 528.3
nasal 478.19 ⬅
sinus (*see also* Sinusitis) 473.9
nasopharynx 478.29
nipple - *see* Fistula, breast
nose 478.19 ⬅
oral (cutaneous) 528.3
maxillary (*see also* Sinusitis, maxillary) 473.0
nasal (with cleft palate) (*see also* Cleft, palate) 749.00
orbit, orbital 376.10
oro-antral (*see also* Sinusitis, maxillary) 473.0
oval window (internal ear) 386.42
oviduct (external) 619.2
palate (hard) 526.89
soft 528.9
pancreatic 577.8
pancreaticoduodenal 577.8
parotid (gland) 527.4
region 528.3
pelvoabdominointestinal 569.81
penis 607.89
perianal 565.1
pericardium (pleura) (sac) (*see also* Pericarditis) 423.8
pericecal 569.81
perineal - *see* Fistula, perineum
perineorectal 569.81
perineosigmoidal 569.81
perineo-urethroscrotal 608.89
perineum, perineal (with urethral involvement) NEC 599.1
tuberculous (*see also* Tuberculosis) 017.9
ureter 593.82
perirectal 565.1
tuberculous (*see also* Tuberculosis) 014.8
peritoneum (*see also* Peritonitis) 567.22
periurethral 599.1
pharyngo-esophageal 478.29
pharynx 478.29
branchial cleft (congenital) 744.41
pilonidal (infected) (rectum) 685.1
with abscess 685.0
pleura, pleural, pleurocutaneous, pleuroperitoneal 510.0
stomach 510.0
tuberculous (*see also* Tuberculosis) 012.0
pleuropericardial 423.8
postauricular 383.81
postoperative, persistent 998.6
preauricular (congenital) 744.46
prostate 602.8
pulmonary 510.0
arteriovenous 417.0
congenital 747.3
tuberculous (*see also* Tuberculosis, pulmonary) 011.9
pulmonoperitoneal 510.0
rectolabial 619.1
rectosigmoid (intercommunicating) 569.81

Fistula *(Continued)*
rectoureteral 593.82
rectourethral 599.1
congenital 753.8
rectouterine 619.1
congenital 752.3
rectovaginal 619.1
congenital 752.49
old, postpartal 619.1
tuberculous (*see also* Tuberculosis) 014.8
rectovesical 596.1
congenital 753.8
rectovesicovaginal 619.1
rectovulvar 619.1
congenital 752.49
rectum (to skin) 565.1
tuberculous (*see also* Tuberculosis) 014.8
renal 593.89
retroauricular 383.81
round window (internal ear) 386.41
salivary duct or gland 527.4
congenital 750.24
sclera 360.32
scrotum (urinary) 608.89
tuberculous (*see also* Tuberculosis) 016.5
semicircular canals (internal ear) 386.43
sigmoid 569.81
vesicoabdominal 596.1
sigmoidovaginal 619.1
congenital 752.49
skin 686.9
ureter 593.82
vagina 619.2
sphenoidal sinus (*see also* Sinusitis, sphenoidal) 473.3
splenocolic 289.59
stercoral 569.81
stomach 537.4
sublingual gland 527.4
congenital 750.24
submaxillary
gland 527.4
congenital 750.24
region 528.3
thoracic 510.0
duct 457.8
thoracicoabdominal 510.0
thoracicogastric 510.0
thoracicointestinal 510.0
thoracoabdominal 510.0
thoracogastric 510.0
thorax 510.0
thyroglossal duct 759.2
thyroid 246.8
trachea (congenital) (external) (internal) 748.3
tracheoesophageal 530.84
congenital 750.3
following tracheostomy 519.09
traumatic
arteriovenous (*see also* Injury, blood vessel, by site) 904.9
brain - *see* Injury, intracranial
tuberculous - *see* Tuberculosis, by site
typhoid 002.0
umbilical 759.89
umbilico-urinary 753.8
urachal, urachus 753.7
ureter (persistent) 593.82
ureteroabdominal 593.82
ureterocervical 593.82

Fistula *(Continued)*
ureterorectal 593.82
ureterosigmoido-abdominal 593.82
ureterovaginal 619.0
ureterovesical 596.2
urethra 599.1
congenital 753.8
tuberculous (*see also* Tuberculosis) 016.3
urethroperineal 599.1
urethroperineovesical 596.2
urethrorectal 599.1
congenital 753.8
urethroscrotal 608.89
urethrovaginal 619.0
urethrovesical 596.2
urethrovesicovaginal 619.0
urinary (persistent) (recurrent) 599.1
uteroabdominal (anterior wall) 619.2
congenital 752.3
uteroenteric 619.1
uterofecal 619.1
uterointestinal 619.1
congenital 752.3
uterorectal 619.1
congenital 752.3
uteroureteric 619.0
uterovaginal 619.8
uterovesical 619.0
congenital 752.3
uterus 619.8
vagina (wall) 619.8
postpartal, old 619.8
vaginocutaneous (postpartal) 619.2
vaginoileal (acquired) 619.1
vaginoperineal 619.2
vesical NEC 596.2
vesicoabdominal 596.2
vesicocervicovaginal 619.0
vesicocolic 596.1
vesicocutaneous 596.2
vesicoenteric 596.1
vesicointestinal 596.1
vesicometrorectal 619.1
vesicoperineal 596.2
vesicorectal 596.1
congenital 753.8
vesicosigmoidal 596.1
vesicosigmoidovaginal 619.1
vesicoureteral 596.2
vesicoureterovaginal 619.0
vesicourethral 596.2
vesicourethrorectal 596.1
vesicouterine 619.0
congenital 752.3
vesicovaginal 619.0
vulvorectal 619.1
congenital 752.49
Fit 780.39
apoplectic (*see also* Disease, cerebrovascular, acute) 436
late effect - *see* Late effect(s) (of) cerebrovascular disease
epileptic (*see also* Epilepsy) 345.9
fainting 780.2
hysterical 300.11
newborn 779.0
Fitting (of)
artificial
arm (complete) (partial) V52.0
breast V52.4
eye(s) V52.2
leg(s) (complete) (partial) V52.1
brain neuropacemaker V53.02
cardiac pacemaker V53.31

Fitting *(Continued)*
carotid sinus pacemaker V53.39
cerebral ventricle (communicating) shunt V53.01
colostomy belt V55.3
contact lenses V53.1
cystostomy device V53.6
defibrillator, automatic implantable cardiac V53.32
dentures V52.3
device, unspecified type V53.90
abdominal V53.5
cardiac
defibrillator, automatic implantable V53.32
pacemaker V53.31
specified NEC V53.39
cerebral ventricle (communicating) shunt V53.01
insulin pump V53.91
intrauterine contraceptive V25.1
nervous system V53.09
orthodontic V53.4
orthoptic V53.1
other device V53.99
prosthetic V52.9
breast V52.4
dental V52.3
eye V52.2
specified type NEC V52.8
special senses V53.09
substitution
auditory V53.09
nervous system V53.09
visual V53.09
urinary V53.6
diaphragm (contraceptive) V25.02
glasses (reading) V53.1
growth rod V54.02
hearing aid V53.2
ileostomy device V55.2
intestinal appliance or device NEC V53.5
intrauterine contraceptive device V25.1
neuropacemaker (brain) (peripheral nerve) (spinal cord) V53.02
orthodontic device V53.4
orthopedic (device) V53.7
brace V53.7
cast V53.7
corset V53.7
shoes V53.7
pacemaker (cardiac) V53.31
brain V53.02
carotid sinus V53.39
peripheral nerve V53.02
spinal cord V53.02
prosthesis V52.9
arm (complete) (partial) V52.0
breast V52.4
dental V52.3
eye V52.2
leg (complete) (partial) V52.1
specified type NEC V52.8
spectacles V53.1
wheelchair V53.8
Fitz's syndrome (acute hemorrhagic pancreatitis) 577.0
Fitz-Hugh and Curtis syndrome 098.86
due to:
Chlamydia trachomatis 099.56
Neisseria gonorrhoeae (gonococcal peritonitis) 098.86
Fixation
joint - *see* Ankylosis
larynx 478.79

Fixation *(Continued)*
pupil 364.76
stapes 385.22
deafness (*see also* Deafness, conductive) 389.04
uterus (acquired) - *see* Malposition, uterus
vocal cord 478.5
Flaccid - *see also* condition
foot 736.79
forearm 736.09
palate, congenital 750.26
Flail
chest 807.4
newborn 767.3
joint (paralytic) 718.80
ankle 718.87
elbow 718.82
foot 718.87
hand 718.84
hip 718.85
knee 718.86
multiple sites 718.89
pelvic region 718.85
shoulder (region) 718.81
specified site NEC 718.88
wrist 718.83
Flajani (-Basedow) syndrome or disease (exophthalmic goiter) 242.0
Flap, liver 572.8
Flare, anterior chamber (aqueous) (eye) 364.04
Flashback phenomena (drug) (hallucinogenic) 292.89
Flat
chamber (anterior) (eye) 360.34
chest, congenital 754.89
electroencephalogram (EEG) 348.8
foot (acquired) (fixed type) (painful) (postural) (spastic) 734
congenital 754.61
rocker bottom 754.61
vertical talus 754.61
rachitic 268.1
rocker bottom (congenital) 754.61
vertical talus, congenital 754.61
organ or site, congenital NEC - *see* Anomaly, specified type NEC
pelvis 738.6
with disproportion (fetopelvic) 653.2
affecting fetus or newborn 763.1
causing obstructed labor 660.1
affecting fetus or newborn 763.1
congenital 755.69
Flatau-Schilder disease 341.1
Flattening
head, femur 736.39
hip 736.39
lip (congenital) 744.89
nose (congenital) 754.0
acquired 738.0
Flatulence 787.3
Flatus 787.3
vaginalis 629.89 ◄
Flax dressers' disease 504
Flea bite - *see* Injury, superficial, by site
Fleischer (-Kayser) ring (corneal pigmentation) 275.1 [371.14]
Fleischner's disease 732.3
Fleshy mole 631
Flexibilitas cerea (*see also* Catalepsy) 300.11
Flexion
cervix - *see* Flexion, uterus ◄
contracture, joint (*see also* Contraction, joint) 718.4
deformity, joint (*see also* Contraction, joint) 736.9 ◄
hip, congenital (*see also* Subluxation, congenital, hip) 754.32
uterus (*see also* Malposition, uterus) 621.6
Flexner's
bacillus 004.1
diarrhea (ulcerative) 004.1
dysentery 004.1
Flexner-Boyd dysentery 004.2
Flexure - *see* condition
Floater, vitreous 379.24
Floating
cartilage (joint) (*see also* Disorder, cartilage, articular) 718.0
knee 717.6
gallbladder (congenital) 751.69
kidney 593.0
congenital 753.3
liver (congenital) 751.69
rib 756.3
spleen 289.59
Flooding 626.2
Floor - *see* condition
Floppy
infant NEC 781.99
valve syndrome (mitral) 424.0
Flu - *see also* Influenza
gastric NEC 008.8
Fluctuating blood pressure 796.4
Fluid
abdomen 789.5
chest (*see also* Pleurisy, with effusion) 511.9
heart (*see also* Failure, heart) 428.0
joint (*see also* Effusion, joint) 719.0
loss (acute) 276.50
with
hypernatremia 276.0
hyponatremia 276.1
lung - *see also* Edema, lung
encysted 511.8
peritoneal cavity 789.5
pleural cavity (*see also* Pleurisy, with effusion) 511.9
retention 276.6
Flukes NEC (*see also* Infestation, fluke) 121.9
blood NEC (*see also* Infestation, Schistosoma) 120.9
liver 121.3
Fluor (albus) (vaginalis) 623.5
trichomonal (Trichomonas vaginalis) 131.00
Fluorosis (dental) (chronic) 520.3
Flushing 782.62
menopausal 627.2
Flush syndrome 259.2
Flutter
atrial or auricular 427.32
heart (ventricular) 427.42
atrial 427.32
impure 427.32
postoperative 997.1
ventricular 427.42
Flux (bloody) (serosanguineous) 009.0
Focal - *see* condition
Fochier's abscess - *see* Abscess, by site
Focus, Assmann's (*see also* Tuberculosis) 011.0
Fogo selvagem 694.4
Foix-Alajouanine syndrome 336.1
Folds, anomalous - *see also* Anomaly, specified type NEC
Bowman's membrane 371.31
Descemet's membrane 371.32
epicanthic 743.63
heart 746.89
posterior segment of eye, congenital 743.54
Folie à deux 297.3
Follicle
cervix (nabothian) (ruptured) 616.0
graafian, ruptured, with hemorrhage 620.0
nabothian 616.0
Folliclis (primary) (*see also* Tuberculosis) 017.0
Follicular - *see also* condition
cyst (atretic) 620.0
Folliculitis 704.8
abscedens et suffodiens 704.8
decalvans 704.09
gonorrheal (acute) 098.0
chronic or duration of 2 months or more 098.2
keloid, keloidalis 706.1
pustular 704.8
ulerythematosa reticulata 701.8
Folliculosis, conjunctival 372.02
Følling's disease (phenylketonuria) 270.1
Follow-up (examination) (routine) (following) V67.9
cancer chemotherapy V67.2
chemotherapy V67.2
fracture V67.4
high-risk medication V67.51
injury NEC V67.59
postpartum
immediately after delivery V24.0
routine V24.2
psychiatric V67.3
psychotherapy V67.3
radiotherapy V67.1
specified condition NEC V67.59
specified surgery NEC V67.09
surgery V67.00
vaginal pap smear V67.01
treatment V67.9
combined NEC V67.6
fracture V67.4
involving high-risk medication NEC V67.51
mental disorder V67.3
specified NEC V67.59
Fong's syndrome (hereditary osteoonychodysplasia) 756.89
Food
allergy 693.1
anaphylactic shock - *see* Anaphylactic shock, due to food
asphyxia (from aspiration or inhalation) (*see also* Asphyxia, food) 933.1
choked on (*see also* Asphyxia, food) 933.1
deprivation 994.2
specified kind of food NEC 269.8
intoxication (*see also* Poisoning, food) 005.9
lack of 994.2
poisoning (*see also* Poisoning, food) 005.9
refusal or rejection NEC 307.59

Food *(Continued)*
strangulation or suffocation (*see also* Asphyxia, food) 933.1
toxemia (*see also* Poisoning, food) 005.9
Foot - *see also* condition
and mouth disease 078.4
process disease 581.3
Foramen ovale (nonclosure) (patent) (persistent) 745.5
Forbes' (glycogen storage) disease 271.0
Forbes-Albright syndrome (nonpuerperal amenorrhea and lactation associated with pituitary tumor) 253.1
Forced birth or delivery NEC 669.8
affecting fetus or newborn NEC 763.89
Forceps
delivery NEC 669.5
affecting fetus or newborn 763.2
Fordyce's disease (ectopic sebaceous glands) (mouth) 750.26
Fordyce-Fox disease (apocrine miliaria) 705.82
Forearm - *see* condition
Foreign body

Note For foreign body with open wound or other injury, see Wound, open, or the type of injury specified.

accidentally left during a procedure 998.4
anterior chamber (eye) 871.6
magnetic 871.5
retained or old 360.51
retained or old 360.61
ciliary body (eye) 871.6
magnetic 871.5
retained or old 360.52
retained or old 360.62
entering through orifice (current) (old)
accessory sinus 932
air passage (upper) 933.0
lower 934.8
alimentary canal 938
alveolar process 935.0
antrum (Highmore) 932
anus 937
appendix 936
asphyxia due to (*see also* Asphyxia, food) 933.1
auditory canal 931
auricle 931
bladder 939.0
bronchioles 934.8
bronchus (main) 934.1
buccal cavity 935.0
canthus (inner) 930.1
cecum 936
cervix (canal) uterine 939.1
coil, ileocecal 936
colon 936
conjunctiva 930.1
conjunctival sac 930.1
cornea 930.0
digestive organ or tract NEC 938
duodenum 936
ear (external) 931
esophagus 935.1
eye (external) 930.9
combined sites 930.8
intraocular - *see* Foreign body, by site
specified site NEC 930.8
eyeball 930.8
intraocular - *see* Foreign body, intraocular

Foreign body *(Continued)*
entering through orifice *(Continued)*
eyelid 930.1
retained or old 374.86
frontal sinus 932
gastrointestinal tract 938
genitourinary tract 939.9
globe 930.8
penetrating 871.6
magnetic 871.5
retained or old 360.50
retained or old 360.60
gum 935.0
Highmore's antrum 932
hypopharynx 933.0
ileocecal coil 936
ileum 936
inspiration (of) 933.1
intestine (large) (small) 936
lacrimal apparatus, duct, gland, or sac 930.2
larynx 933.1
lung 934.8
maxillary sinus 932
mouth 935.0
nasal sinus 932
nasopharynx 933.0
nose (passage) 932
nostril 932
oral cavity 935.0
palate 935.0
penis 939.3
pharynx 933.0
pyriform sinus 933.0
rectosigmoid 937
junction 937
rectum 937
respiratory tract 934.9
specified part NEC 934.8
sclera 930.1
sinus 932
accessory 932
frontal 932
maxillary 932
nasal 932
pyriform 933.0
small intestine 936
stomach (hairball) 935.2
suffocation by (*see also* Asphyxia, food) 933.1
swallowed 938
tongue 933.0
tear ducts or glands 930.2
throat 933.0
tongue 935.0
swallowed 933.0
tonsil, tonsillar 933.0
fossa 933.0
trachea 934.0
ureter 939.0
urethra 939.0
uterus (any part) 939.1
vagina 939.2
vulva 939.2
wind pipe 934.0
granuloma (old) 728.82
bone 733.99
in operative wound (inadvertently left) 998.4
due to surgical material intentionally left - *see* Complications, due to (presence of) any device, implant, or graft classified to 996.0–996.5 NEC
muscle 728.82

Foreign body *(Continued)*
granuloma *(Continued)*
skin 709.4
soft tissue NEC 709.4
subcutaneous tissue 709.4
in
bone (residual) 733.99
open wound - *see* Wound, open, by site complicated
soft tissue (residual) 729.6
inadvertently left in operation wound (causing adhesions, obstruction, or perforation) 998.4
ingestion, ingested NEC 938
inhalation or inspiration (*see also* Asphyxia, food) 933.1
internal organ, not entering through an orifice - *see* Injury, internal, by site, with open wound
intraocular (nonmagnetic) 871.6
combined sites 871.6
magnetic 871.5
retained or old 360.59
retained or old 360.69
magnetic 871.5
retained or old 360.50
retained or old 360.60
specified site NEC 871.6
magnetic 871.5
retained or old 360.59
retained or old 360.69
iris (nonmagnetic) 871.6
magnetic 871.5
retained or old 360.52
retained or old 360.62
lens (nonmagnetic) 871.6
magnetic 871.5
retained or old 360.53
retained or old 360.63
lid, eye 930.1
ocular muscle 870.4
retained or old 376.6
old or residual
bone 733.99
eyelid 374.86
middle ear 385.83
muscle 729.6
ocular 376.6
retrobulbar 376.6
skin 729.6
with granuloma 709.4
soft tissue 729.6
with granuloma 709.4
subcutaneous tissue 729.6
with granuloma 709.4
operation wound, left accidentally 998.4
orbit 870.4
retained or old 376.6
posterior wall, eye 871.6
magnetic 871.5
retained or old 360.55
retained or old 360.65
respiratory tree 934.9
specified site NEC 934.8
retained (old) (nonmagnetic) (in)
anterior chamber (eye) 360.61
magnetic 360.51
ciliary body 360.62
magnetic 360.52
eyelid 374.86
globe 360.60
magnetic 360.50
intraocular 360.60
magnetic 360.50
specified site NEC 360.69
magnetic 360.59

ICD-9-CM

Vol. 2

Foreign body *(Continued)*
retained *(Continued)*
iris 360.62
magnetic 360.52
lens 360.63
magnetic 360.53
orbit 376.6
posterior wall of globe 360.65
magnetic 360.55
retina 360.65
magnetic 360.55
retrobulbar 376.6
skin 729.6
with granuloma 709.4
soft tissue 729.6
with granuloma 709.4
subcutaneous tissue 729.6
with granuloma 709.4
vitreous 360.64
magnetic 360.54
retina 871.6
magnetic 871.5
retained or old 360.55
retained or old 360.65
superficial, without major open wound (*see also* Injury, superficial, by site) 919.6
swallowed NEC 938
vitreous (humor) 871.6
magnetic 871.5
retained or old 360.54
retained or old 360.64
Forking, aqueduct of Sylvius 742.3
with spina bifida (*see also* Spina bifida) 741.0
Formation
bone in scar tissue (skin) 709.3
connective tissue in vitreous 379.25
Elschnig pearls (postcataract extraction) 366.51
hyaline in cornea 371.49
sequestrum in bone (due to infection) (*see also* Osteomyelitis) 730.1
valve
colon, congenital 751.5
ureter (congenital) 753.29
Formication 782.0
Fort Bragg fever 100.89
Fossa - *see also* condition
pyriform - *see* condition
Foster-Kennedy syndrome 377.04
Fothergill's
disease, meaning scarlatina anginosa 034.1
neuralgia (*see also* Neuralgia, trigeminal) 350.1
Foul breath 784.99 ⬅
Found dead (cause unknown) 798.9
Foundling V20.0
Fournier's disease (idiopathic gangrene) 608.83
Fourth
cranial nerve - *see* condition
disease 057.8
molar 520.1
Foville's syndrome 344.89
Fox's
disease (apocrine miliaria) 705.82
impetigo (contagiosa) 684
Fox-Fordyce disease (apocrine miliaria) 705.82
Fracture (abduction) (adduction) (avulsion) (compression) (crush) (dislocation) (oblique) (separation) (closed) 829.0

Note For fracture of any of the following sites with fracture of other bones, *see* Fracture, multiple.

"Closed" includes the following descriptions of fractures, with or without delayed healing, unless they are specified as open or compound:

comminuted
depressed
elevated
fissured
greenstick
impacted
linear
simple
slipped epiphysis
spiral
unspecified

"Open" includes the following descriptions of fractures, with or without delayed healing:

compound
infected
missile
puncture
with foreign body

For late effect of fracture, *see* Late, effect, fracture, by site.

with
internal injuries in same region (conditions classifiable to 860–869) - *see also* Injury, internal, by site
pelvic region - *see* Fracture, pelvis
acetabulum (with visceral injury) (closed) 808.0
open 808.1
acromion (process) (closed) 811.01
open 811.11
alveolus (closed) 802.8
open 802.9
ankle (malleolus) (closed) 824.8
bimalleolar (Dupuytren's) (Pott's) 824.4
open 824.5
bone 825.21
open 825.31
lateral malleolus only (fibular) 824.2
open 824.3
medial malleolus only (tibial) 824.0
open 824.1
open 824.9
pathologic 733.16
talus 825.21
open 825.31
trimalleolar 824.6
open 824.7
antrum - *see* Fracture, skull, base
arm (closed) 818.0
and leg(s) (any bones) 828.0
open 828.1
both (any bones) (with rib(s)) (with sternum) 819.0
open 819.1
lower 813.80
open 813.90
open 818.1
upper - *see* Fracture, humerus
Fracture *(Continued)*
astragalus (closed) 825.21
open 825.31
atlas - *see* Fracture, vertebra, cervical, first
axis - *see* Fracture, vertebra, cervical, second
back - *see* Fracture, vertebra, by site
Barton's - *see* Fracture, radius, lower end
basal (skull) - *see* Fracture, skull, base
Bennett's (closed) 815.01
open 815.11
bimalleolar (closed) 824.4
open 824.5
bone (closed) NEC 829.0
birth injury NEC 767.3
open 829.1
pathological NEC (*see also* Fracture, pathologic) 733.10
stress NEC (*see also* Fracture, stress) 733.95
boot top - *see* Fracture, fibula
boxers' - *see* Fracture, metacarpal bone(s)
breast bone - *see* Fracture, sternum
bucket handle (semilunar cartilage) - *see* Tear, meniscus
bursting - *see* Fracture, phalanx, hand, distal
calcaneus (closed) 825.0
open 825.1
capitate (bone) (closed) 814.07
open 814.17
capitellum (humerus) (closed) 812.49
open 812.59
carpal bone(s) (wrist NEC) (closed) 814.00
open 814.10
specified site NEC 814.09
open 814.19
cartilage, knee (semilunar) - *see* Tear, meniscus
cervical - *see* Fracture, vertebra, cervical
chauffeur's - *see* Fracture, ulna, lower end
chisel - *see* Fracture, radius, upper end
clavicle (interligamentous part) (closed) 810.00
acromial end 810.03
open 810.13
due to birth trauma 767.2
open 810.10
shaft (middle third) 810.02
open 810.12
sternal end 810.01
open 810.11
clayshovelers' - *see* Fracture, vertebra, cervical
coccyx - *see also* Fracture, vertebra, coccyx
complicating delivery 665.6
collar bone - *see* Fracture, clavicle
Colles' (reversed) (closed) 813.41
open 813.51
comminuted - *see* Fracture, by site
compression - *see also* Fracture, by site
nontraumatic - *see* Fracture, pathologic
congenital 756.9
coracoid process (closed) 811.02
open 811.12
coronoid process (ulna) (closed) 813.02
mandible (closed) 802.23
open 802.33

Fracture *(Continued)*
  coronoid process *(Continued)*
    open 813.12
  corpus cavernosum penis 959.13
  costochondral junction - *see* Fracture, rib
  costosternal junction - *see* Fracture, rib
  cranium - *see* Fracture, skull, by site
  cricoid cartilage (closed) 807.5
    open 807.6
  cuboid (ankle) (closed) 825.23
    open 825.33
  cuneiform
    foot (closed) 825.24
      open 825.34
    wrist (closed) 814.03
      open 814.13
  dental restorative material ◀
    with loss of material 525.64 ◀
    without loss of material 525.63 ◀
  due to
    birth injury - *see* Birth injury, fracture
    gunshot - *see* Fracture, by site, open
    neoplasm - *see* Fracture, pathologic
    osteoporosis - *see* Fracture, pathologic
  Dupuytren's (ankle) (fibula) (closed) 824.4
    open 824.5
    radius 813.42
      open 813.52
  Duverney's - *see* Fracture, ilium
  elbow - *see also* Fracture, humerus, lower end
    olecranon (process) (closed) 813.01
      open 813.11
    supracondylar (closed) 812.41
      open 812.51
  ethmoid (bone) (sinus) - *see* Fracture, skull, base
  face bone(s) (closed) NEC 802.8
    with
      other bone(s) - *see* Fracture, multiple, skull
      skull - *see also* Fracture, skull
        involving other bones - *see* Fracture, multiple, skull
    open 802.9
  fatigue - *see* Fracture, march
  femur, femoral (closed) 821.00
    cervicotrochanteric 820.03
      open 820.13
    condyles, epicondyles 821.21
      open 821.31
    distal end - *see* Fracture, femur, lower end
    epiphysis (separation)
      capital 820.01
        open 820.11
      head 820.01
        open 820.11
      lower 821.22
        open 821.32
      trochanteric 820.01
        open 820.11
      upper 820.01
        open 820.11
    head 820.09
      open 820.19
    lower end or extremity (distal end) (closed) 821.20
      condyles, epicondyles 821.21
        open 821.31
      epiphysis (separation) 821.22
        open 821.32
      multiple sites 821.29
        open 821.39

Fracture *(Continued)*
  femur, femoral *(Continued)*
    lower end or extremity *(Continued)*
      open 821.30
      specified site NEC 821.29
        open 821.39
      supracondylar 821.23
        open 821.33
      T-shaped 821.21
        open 821.31
    neck (closed) 820.8
      base (cervicotrochanteric) 820.03
        open 820.13
      extracapsular 820.20
        open 820.30
      intertrochanteric (section) 820.21
        open 820.31
      intracapsular 820.00
        open 820.10
      intratrochanteric 820.21
        open 820.31
      midcervical 820.02
        open 820.12
      open 820.9
      pathologic 733.14
        specified part NEC 733.15
      specified site NEC 820.09
        open 820.19
      transcervical 820.02
        open 820.12
      transtrochanteric 820.20
        open 820.30
    open 821.10
    pathologic 733.14
      specified part NEC 733.15
    peritrochanteric (section) 820.20
      open 820.30
    shaft (lower third) (middle third) (upper third) 821.01
      open 821.11
    subcapital 820.09
      open 820.19
    subtrochanteric (region) (section) 820.22
      open 820.32
    supracondylar 821.23
      open 821.33
    transepiphyseal 820.01
      open 820.11
    trochanter (greater) (lesser) (*see also* Fracture, femur, neck, by site) 820.20
      open 820.30
    T-shaped, into knee joint 821.21
      open 821.31
    upper end 820.8
      open 820.9
  fibula (closed) 823.81
    with tibia 823.82
      open 823.92
    distal end 824.8
      open 824.9
    epiphysis
      lower 824.8
        open 824.9
      upper - *see* Fracture, fibula, upper end
    head - *see* Fracture, fibula, upper end
    involving ankle 824.2
      open 824.3
    lower end or extremity 824.8
      open 824.9
    malleolus (external) (lateral) 824.2
      open 824.3

Fracture *(Continued)*
  fibula *(Continued)*
    open NEC 823.91
    pathologic 733.16
    proximal end - *see* Fracture, fibula, upper end
    shaft 823.21
      with tibia 823.22
        open 823.32
      open 823.31
    stress 733.93
    torus 823.41
      with tibia 823.42
    upper end or extremity (epiphysis) (head) (proximal end) (styloid) 823.01
      with tibia 823.02
        open 823.12
      open 823.11
  finger(s), of one hand (closed) (*see also* Fracture, phalanx, hand) 816.00
    with
      metacarpal bone(s), of same hand 817.0
        open 817.1
      thumb of same hand 816.03
        open 816.13
    open 816.10
  foot, except toe(s) alone (closed) 825.20
    open 825.30
  forearm (closed) NEC 813.80
    lower end (distal end) (lower epiphysis) 813.40
      open 813.50
    open 813.90
    shaft 813.20
      open 813.30
    upper end (proximal end) (upper epiphysis) 813.00
      open 813.10
  fossa, anterior, middle, or posterior - *see* Fracture, skull, base
  frontal (bone) - *see also* Fracture, skull, vault
    sinus - *see* Fracture, skull, base
  Galeazzi's - *see* Fracture, radius, lower end
  glenoid (cavity) (fossa) (scapula) (closed) 811.03
    open 811.13
  Gosselin's - *see* Fracture, ankle
  greenstick - *see* Fracture, by site
  grenade-throwers' - *see* Fracture, humerus, shaft
  gutter - *see* Fracture, skull, vault
  hamate (closed) 814.08
    open 814.18
  hand, one (closed) 815.00
    carpals 814.00
      open 814.10
      specified site NEC 814.09
        open 814.19
    metacarpals 815.00
      open 815.10
    multiple, bones of one hand 817.0
      open 817.1
    open 815.10
    phalanges (*see also* Fracture, phalanx, hand) 816.00
      open 816.10
  healing
    aftercare (*see also* - Aftercare, fracture) V54.89

Fracture *(Continued)*
healing *(Continued)*
change of cast V54.89
complications - *see* condition
convalescence V66.4
removal of
cast V54.89
fixation device
external V54.89
internal V54.01
heel bone (closed) 825.0
open 825.1
hip (closed) (*see also* Fracture, femur, neck) 820.8
open 820.9
pathologic 733.14
humerus (closed) 812.20
anatomical neck 812.02
open 812.12
articular process (*see also* Fracture humerus, condyle(s)) 812.44
open 812.54
capitellum 812.49
open 812.59
condyle(s) 812.44
lateral (external) 812.42
open 812.52
medial (internal epicondyle) 812.43
open 812.53
open 812.54
distal end - *see* Fracture, humerus, lower end
epiphysis
lower (*see also* Fracture, humerus, condyle(s)) 812.44
open 812.54
upper 812.09
open 812.19
external condyle 812.42
open 812.52
great tuberosity 812.03
open 812.13
head 812.09
open 812.19
internal epicondyle 812.43
open 812.53
lesser tuberosity 812.09
open 812.19
lower end or extremity (distal end) (*see also* Fracture, humerus, by site) 812.40
multiple sites NEC 812.49
open 812.59
open 812.50
specified site NEC 812.49
open 812.59
neck 812.01
open 812.11
open 812.30
pathologic 733.11
proximal end - *see* Fracture, humerus, upper end
shaft 812.21
open 812.31
supracondylar 812.41
open 812.51
surgical neck 812.01
open 812.11
trochlea 812.49
open 812.59
T-shaped 812.44
open 812.54

Fracture *(Continued)*
humerus *(Continued)*
tuberosity - *see* Fracture, humerus, upper end
upper end or extremity (proximal end) (*see also* Fracture, humerus, by site) 812.00
open 812.10
specified site NEC 812.09
open 812.19
hyoid bone (closed) 807.5
open 807.6
hyperextension - *see* Fracture, radius, lower end
ilium (with visceral injury) (closed) 808.41
open 808.51
impaction, impacted - *see* Fracture, by site
incus - *see* Fracture, skull, base
innominate bone (with visceral injury) (closed) 808.49
open 808.59
instep, of one foot (closed) 825.20
with toe(s) of same foot 827.0
open 827.1
open 825.30
internal
ear - *see* Fracture, skull, base
semilunar cartilage, knee - *see* Tear, meniscus, medial
intertrochanteric - *see* Fracture, femur, neck, intertrochanteric
ischium (with visceral injury) (closed) 808.42
open 808.52
jaw (bone) (lower) (closed) (*see also* Fracture, mandible) 802.20
angle 802.25
open 802.35
open 802.30
upper - *see* Fracture, maxilla
knee
cap (closed) 822.0
open 822.1
cartilage (semilunar) - *see* Tear, meniscus
labyrinth (osseous) - *see* Fracture, skull, base
larynx (closed) 807.5
open 807.6
late effect - *see* Late, effects (of), fracture
Le Fort's - *see* Fracture, maxilla
leg (closed) 827.0
with rib(s) or sternum 828.0
open 828.1
both (any bones) 828.0
open 828.1
lower - *see* Fracture, tibia
open 827.1
upper - *see* Fracture, femur
limb
lower (multiple) (closed) NEC 827.0
open 827.1
upper (multiple) (closed) NEC 818.0
open 818.1
long bones, due to birth trauma - *see* Birth injury, fracture
lumbar - *see* Fracture, vertebra, lumbar
lunate bone (closed) 814.02
open 814.12
malar bone (closed) 802.4
open 802.5
Malgaigne's (closed) 808.43
open 808.53

Fracture *(Continued)*
malleolus (closed) 824.8
bimalleolar 824.4
open 824.5
lateral 824.2
and medial - *see also* Fracture, malleolus, bimalleolar
with lip of tibia - *see* Fracture, malleolus, trimalleolar
open 824.3
medial (closed) 824.0
and lateral - *see also* Fracture, malleolus, bimalleolar
with lip of tibia - *see* Fracture, malleolus, trimalleolar
open 824.1
open 824.9
trimalleolar (closed) 824.6
open 824.7
malleus - *see* Fracture, skull, base
malunion 733.81
mandible (closed) 802.20
angle 802.25
open 802.35
body 802.28
alveolar border 802.27
open 802.37
open 802.38
symphysis 802.26
open 802.36
condylar process 802.21
open 802.31
coronoid process 802.23
open 802.33
multiple sites 802.29
open 802.39
open 802.30
ramus NEC 802.24
open 802.34
subcondylar 802.22
open 802.32
manubrium - *see* Fracture, sternum
march 733.95
fibula 733.93
metatarsals 733.94
tibia 733.93
maxilla, maxillary (superior) (upper jaw) (closed) 802.4
inferior - *see* Fracture, mandible
open 802.5
meniscus, knee - *see* Tear, meniscus
metacarpus, metacarpal (bone(s)), of one hand (closed) 815.00
with phalanx, phalanges, hand (finger(s)) (thumb) of same hand 817.0
open 817.1
base 815.02
first metacarpal 815.01
open 815.11
open 815.12
thumb 815.01
open 815.11
multiple sites 815.09
open 815.19
neck 815.04
open 815.14
open 815.10
shaft 815.03
open 815.13
metatarsus, metatarsal (bone(s)), of one foot (closed) 825.25
with tarsal bone(s) 825.29
open 825.39
open 825.35

Fracture (Continued)
Monteggia's (closed) 813.03
open 813.13
Moore's - see Fracture, radius, lower end multangular bone (closed)
larger 814.05
open 814.15
smaller 814.06
open 814.16
multiple (closed) 829.0

Note Multiple fractures of sites classifiable to the same three- or four-digit category are coded to that category, except for sites classifiable to 810–818 or 820–827 in different limbs.

Multiple fractures of sites classifiable to different fourth-digit subdivisions within the same three-digit category should be dealt with according to coding rules.

Multiple fractures of sites classifiable to different three-digit categories (identifiable from the listing under "Fracture"), and of sites classifiable to 810–818 or 820–827 in different limbs should be coded according to the following list, which should be referred to in the following priority order: skull or face bones, pelvis or vertebral column, legs, arms.

arm (multiple bones in same arm except in hand alone) (sites classifiable to 810–817 with sites classifiable to a different three-digit category in 810–817 in same arm) (closed) 818.0
open 818.1
arms, both or arm(s) with rib(s) or sternum (sites classifiable to 810–818 with sites classifiable to same range of categories in other limb or to 807) (closed) 819.0
open 819.1
bones of trunk NEC (closed) 809.0
open 809.1
hand, metacarpal bone(s) with phalanx or phalanges of same hand (sites classifiable to 815 with sites classifiable to 816 in same hand) (closed) 817.0
open 817.1
leg (multiple bones in same leg) (sites classifiable to 820–826 with sites classifiable to a different three-digit category in that range in same leg) (closed) 827.0
open 827.1
legs, both or leg(s) with arm(s), rib(s), or sternum (sites classifiable to 820–827 with sites classifiable to same range of categories in other leg or to 807 or 810–819) (closed) 828.0
open 828.1
open 829.1
pelvis with other bones except skull or face bones (sites classifiable to 808 with sites classifiable to 805–807 or 810–829) (closed) 809.0
open 809.1

Fracture (Continued)
multiple (Continued)
skull, specified or unspecified bones, or face bone(s) with any other bone(s) (sites classifiable to 800–803 with sites classifiable to 805–829) (closed) 804.0

Note Use the following fifth-digit subclassification with categories 800, 801, 803, and 804:

0 unspecified state of consciousness
1 with no loss of consciousness
2 with brief [less than one hour] loss of consciousness
3 with moderate [1–24 hours] loss of consciousness
4 with prolonged [more than 24 hours] loss of consciousness and return to pre-existing conscious level
5 with prolonged [more than 24 hours] loss of consciousness, without return to pre-existing conscious level

Use fifth-digit 5 to designate when a patient is unconscious and dies before regaining consciousness, regardless of the duration of the loss of consciousness

6 with loss of consciousness of unspecified duration
9 with concussion, unspecified

with
contusion, cerebral 804.1
epidural hemorrhage 804.2
extradural hemorrhage 804.2
hemorrhage (intracranial) NEC 804.3
intracranial injury NEC 804.4
laceration, cerebral 804.1
subarachnoid hemorrhage 804.2
subdural hemorrhage 804.2
open 804.5
with
contusion, cerebral 804.6
epidural hemorrhage 804.7
extradural hemorrhage 804.7
hemorrhage (intracranial) NEC 804.8
intracranial injury NEC 804.9
laceration, cerebral 804.6
subarachnoid hemorrhage 804.7
subdural hemorrhage 804.7
vertebral column with other bones, except skull or face bones (sites classifiable to 805 or 806 with sites classifiable to 807–808 or 810–829) (closed) 809.0
open 809.1
nasal (bone(s)) (closed) 802.0
open 802.1
sinus - see Fracture, skull, base
navicular
carpal (wrist) (closed) 814.01
open 814.11
tarsal (ankle) (closed) 825.22
open 825.32
neck - see Fracture, vertebra, cervical
neural arch - see Fracture, vertebra, by site

Fracture (Continued)
nonunion 733.82
nose, nasal, (bone) (septum) (closed) 802.0
open 802.1
occiput - see Fracture, skull, base
odontoid process - see Fracture, vertebra, cervical
olecranon (process) (ulna) (closed) 813.01
open 813.11
open 829.1
orbit, orbital (bone) (region) (closed) 802.8
floor (blow-out) 802.6
open 802.7
open 802.9
roof - see Fracture, skull, base
specified part NEC 802.8
open 802.9
os
calcis (closed) 825.0
open 825.1
magnum (closed) 814.07
open 814.17
pubis (with visceral injury) (closed) 808.2
open 808.3
triquetrum (closed) 814.03
open 814.13
osseous
auditory meatus - see Fracture, skull, base
labyrinth - see Fracture, skull, base
ossicles, auditory (incus) (malleus) (stapes) - see Fracture, skull, base
osteoporotic - see Fracture, pathologic
palate (closed) 802.8
open 802.9
paratrooper - see Fracture, tibia, lower end
parietal bone - see Fracture, skull, vault
parry - see Fracture, Monteggia's
patella (closed) 822.0
open 822.1
pathologic (cause unknown) 733.10
ankle 733.16
femur (neck) 733.14
specified NEC 733.15
fibula 733.16
hip 733.14
humerus 733.11
radius (distal) 733.12
specified site NEC 733.19
tibia 733.16
ulna 733.12
vertebrae (collapse) 733.13
wrist 733.12
pedicle (of vertebral arch) - see Fracture, vertebra, by site
pelvis, pelvic (bone(s)) (with visceral injury) (closed) 808.8
multiple (with disruption of pelvic circle) 808.43
open 808.53
open 808.9
rim (closed) 808.49
open 808.59
peritrochanteric (closed) 820.20
open 820.30
phalanx, phalanges, of one
foot (closed) 826.0
with bone(s) of same lower limb 827.0
open 827.1
open 826.1

Fracture *(Continued)*
- phalanx *(Continued)*
  - hand (closed) 816.00
    - with metacarpal bone(s) of same hand 817.0
      - open 817.1
    - distal 816.02
      - open 816.12
    - middle 816.01
      - open 816.11
    - multiple sites NEC 816.03
      - open 816.13
    - open 816.10
    - proximal 816.01
      - open 816.11
- pisiform (closed) 814.04
  - open 814.14
- pond - *see* Fracture, skull, vault
- Pott's (closed) 824.4
  - open 824.5
- prosthetic device, internal - *see* Complications, mechanical
- pubis (with visceral injury) (closed) 808.2
  - open 808.3
- Quervain's (closed) 814.01
  - open 814.11
- radius (alone) (closed) 813.81
  - with ulna NEC 813.83
    - open 813.93
  - distal end - *see* Fracture, radius, lower end
  - epiphysis
    - lower - *see* Fracture, radius, lower end
    - upper - *see* Fracture, radius, upper end
  - head - *see* Fracture, radius, upper end
  - lower end or extremity (distal end) (lower epiphysis) 813.42
    - with ulna (lower end) 813.44
      - open 813.54
    - open 813.52
    - torus 813.45
  - neck - *see* Fracture, radius, upper end
  - open NEC 813.91
  - pathologic 733.12
  - proximal end - *see* Fracture, radius, upper end
  - shaft (closed) 813.21
    - with ulna (shaft) 813.23
      - open 813.33
    - open 813.31
  - upper end 813.07
    - with ulna (upper end) 813.08
      - open 813.18
    - epiphysis 813.05
      - open 813.15
    - head 813.05
      - open 813.15
    - multiple sites 813.07
      - open 813.17
    - neck 813.06
      - open 813.16
    - open 813.17
    - specified site NEC 813.07
      - open 813.17
- ramus
  - inferior or superior (with visceral injury) (closed) 808.2
    - open 808.3
  - ischium - *see* Fracture, ischium
  - mandible 802.24
    - open 802.34

Fracture *(Continued)*
- rib(s) (closed) 807.0

> Note Use the following fifth-digit subclassification with categories 807.0–807.1:
>
> 0 rib(s), unspecified
> 1 one rib
> 2 two ribs
> 3 three ribs
> 4 four ribs
> 5 five ribs
> 6 six ribs
> 7 seven ribs
> 8 eight or more ribs
> 9 multiple ribs, unspecified

  - with flail chest (open) 807.4
  - open 807.1
- root, tooth 873.63
  - complicated 873.73
- sacrum - *see* Fracture, vertebra, sacrum
- scaphoid
  - ankle (closed) 825.22
    - open 825.32
  - wrist (closed) 814.01
    - open 814.11
- scapula (closed) 811.00
  - acromial, acromion (process) 811.01
    - open 811.11
  - body 811.09
    - open 811.19
  - coracoid process 811.02
    - open 811.12
  - glenoid (cavity) (fossa) 811.03
    - open 811.13
  - neck 811.03
    - open 811.13
  - open 811.10
- semilunar
  - bone, wrist (closed) 814.02
    - open 814.12
  - cartilage (interior) (knee) - *see* Tear, meniscus
- sesamoid bone - *see* Fracture, by site
- Shepherd's (closed) 825.21
  - open 825.31
- shoulder - *see also* Fracture, humerus, upper end
  - blade - *see* Fracture, scapula
- silverfork - *see* Fracture, radius, lower end
- sinus (ethmoid) (frontal) (maxillary) (nasal) (sphenoidal) - *see* Fracture, skull, base
- Skillern's - *see* Fracture, radius, shaft
- skull (multiple NEC) (with face bones) (closed) 803.0

> Note Use the following fifth-digit subclassification with categories 800, 801, 803, and 804:
>
> 0 unspecified state of consciousness
> 1 with no loss of consciousness
> 2 with brief [less than one hour] loss of consciousness
> 3 with moderate [1-24 hours] loss of consciousness
> 4 with prolonged [more than 24 hours] loss of consciousness and return to pre-existing conscious level

Fracture *(Continued)*

> 5 with prolonged [more than 24 hours] loss of consciousness, without return to pre-existing conscious level
>
> Use fifth-digit 5 to designate when a patient is unconscious and dies before regaining consciousness, regardless of the duration of the loss of consciousness
>
> 6 with loss of consciousness of unspecified duration
> 9 with concussion, unspecified

  - with
    - contusion, cerebral 803.1
    - epidural hemorrhage 803.2
    - extradural hemorrhage 803.2
    - hemorrhage (intracranial) NEC 803.3
    - intracranial injury NEC 803.4
    - laceration, cerebral 803.1
    - other bones - *see* Fracture, multiple, skull
    - subarachnoid hemorrhage 803.2
    - subdural hemorrhage 803.2
  - base (antrum) (ethmoid bone) (fossa) (internal ear) (nasal sinus) (occiput) (sphenoid) (temporal bone) (closed) 801.0
    - with
      - contusion, cerebral 801.1
      - epidural hemorrhage 801.2
      - extradural hemorrhage 801.2
      - hemorrhage (intracranial) NEC 801.3
      - intracranial injury NEC 801.4
      - laceration, cerebral 801.1
      - subarachnoid hemorrhage 801.2
      - subdural hemorrhage 801.2
    - open 801.5
      - with
        - contusion, cerebral 801.6
        - epidural hemorrhage 801.7
        - extradural hemorrhage 801.7
        - hemorrhage (intracranial) NEC 801.8
        - intracranial injury NEC 801.9
        - laceration, cerebral 801.6
        - subarachnoid hemorrhage 801.7
        - subdural hemorrhage 801.7
  - birth injury 767.3
  - face bones - *see* Fracture, face bones
  - open 803.5
    - with
      - contusion, cerebral 803.6
      - epidural hemorrhage 803.7
      - extradural hemorrhage 803.7
      - hemorrhage (intracranial) NEC 803.8
      - intracranial injury NEC 803.9
      - laceration, cerebral 803.6
      - subarachnoid hemorrhage 803.7
      - subdural hemorrhage 803.7
  - vault (frontal bone) (parietal bone) (vertex) (closed) 800.0
    - with
      - contusion, cerebral 800.1
      - epidural hemorrhage 800.2
      - extradural hemorrhage 800.2
      - hemorrhage (intracranial) NEC 800.3

Fracture *(Continued)*
skull *(Continued)*
vault *(Continued)*
with *(Continued)*
intracranial injury NEC 800.4
laceration, cerebral 800.1
subarachnoid hemorrhage 800.2
subdural hemorrhage 800.2
open 800.5
with
contusion, cerebral 800.6
epidural hemorrhage 800.7
extradural hemorrhage 800.7
hemorrhage (intracranial) NEC 800.8
intracranial injury NEC 800.9
laceration, cerebral 800.6
subarachnoid hemorrhage 800.7
subdural hemorrhage 800.7
Smith's 813.41
open 813.51
sphenoid (bone) (sinus) - *see* Fracture, skull, base
spine - *see also* Fracture, vertebra, by site
due to birth trauma 767.4
spinous process - *see* Fracture, vertebra, by site
spontaneous - *see* Fracture, pathologic
sprinters' - *see* Fracture, ilium
stapes - *see* Fracture, skull, base
stave - *see also* Fracture, metacarpus, metacarpal bone(s)
spine - *see* Fracture, tibia, upper end
sternum (closed) 807.2
with flail chest (open) 807.4
open 807.3
Stieda's - *see* Fracture, femur, lower end
stress 733.95
fibula 733.93
metatarsals 733.94
specified site NEC 733.95
tibia 733.93
styloid process
metacarpal (closed) 815.02
open 815.12
radius - *see* Fracture, radius, lower end
temporal bone - *see* Fracture, skull, base
ulna - *see* Fracture, ulna, lower end
supracondylar, elbow 812.41
open 812.51
symphysis pubis (with visceral injury) (closed) 808.2
open 808.3
talus (ankle bone) (closed) 825.21
open 825.31
tarsus, tarsal bone(s) (with metatarsus) of one foot (closed) NEC 825.29
open 825.39
temporal bone (styloid) - *see* Fracture, skull, base
tendon - *see* Sprain, by site
thigh - *see* Fracture, femur, shaft
thumb (and finger(s)) of one hand (closed) (*see also* Fracture, phalanx, hand) 816.00
with metacarpal bone(s) of same hand 817.0
open 817.1
metacarpal(s) - *see* Fracture, metacarpus
open 816.10

Fracture *(Continued)*
thyroid cartilage (closed) 807.5
open 807.6
tibia (closed) 823.80
with fibula 823.82
open 823.92
condyles - *see* Fracture, tibia, upper end
distal end 824.8
open 824.9
epiphysis
lower 824.8
open 824.9
upper - *see* Fracture, tibia, upper end
head (involving knee joint) - *see* Fracture, tibia, upper end
intercondyloid eminence - *see* Fracture, tibia, upper end
involving ankle 824.0
open 824.1
lower end or extremity (anterior lip) (posterior lip) 824.8
open 824.9
malleolus (internal) (medial) 824.0
open 824.1
open NEC 823.90
pathologic 733.16
proximal end - *see* Fracture, tibia, upper end
shaft 823.20
with fibula 823.22
open 823.32
open 823.30
spine - *see* Fracture, tibia, upper end
stress 733.93
torus 823.40
with fibula 823.42
tuberosity - *see* Fracture, tibia, upper end
upper end or extremity (condyle) (epiphysis) (head) (spine) (proximal end) (tuberosity) 823.00
with fibula 823.02
open 823.12
open 823.10
toe(s), of one foot (closed) 826.0
with bone(s) of same lower limb 827.0
open 827.1
open 826.1
tooth (root) 873.63
complicated 873.73
torus
fibula 823.41
with tibia 823.42
radius 813.45
tibia 823.40
with fibula 823.42
trachea (closed) 807.5
open 807.6
transverse process - *see* Fracture, vertebra, by site
trapezium (closed) 814.05
open 814.15
trapezoid bone (closed) 814.06
open 814.16
trimalleolar (closed) 824.6
open 824.7
triquetral (bone) (closed) 814.03
open 814.13
trochanter (greater) (lesser) (closed) (*see also* Fracture, femur, neck, by site) 820.20

Fracture *(Continued)*
trochanter *(Continued)*
open 820.30
trunk (bones) (closed) 809.0
open 809.1
tuberosity (external) - *see* Fracture, by site
ulna (alone) (closed) 813.82
with radius NEC 813.83
open 813.93
coronoid process (closed) 813.02
open 813.12
distal end - *see* Fracture, ulna, lower end
epiphysis
lower - *see* Fracture, ulna, lower end
upper - *see* Fracture, ulna, upper, end
head - *see* Fracture, ulna, lower end
lower end (distal end) (head) (lower epiphysis) (styloid process) 813.43
with radius (lower end) 813.44
open 813.54
open 813.53
olecranon process (closed) 813.01
open 813.11
open NEC 813.92
pathologic 733.12
proximal end - *see* Fracture, ulna, upper end
shaft 813.22
with radius (shaft) 813.23
open 813.33
open 813.32
styloid process - *see* Fracture, ulna, lower end
transverse - *see* Fracture, ulna, by site
upper end (epiphysis) 813.04
with radius (upper end) 813.08
open 813.18
multiple sites 813.04
open 813.14
open 813.14
specified site NEC 813.04
open 813.14
unciform (closed) 814.08
open 814.18
vertebra, vertebral (back) (body) (column) (neural arch) (pedicle) (spine) (spinous process) (transverse process) (closed) 805.8
with
hematomyelia - *see* Fracture, vertebra, by site, with spinal cord injury
injury to
cauda equina - *see* Fracture, vertebra, sacrum, with spinal cord injury
nerve - *see* Fracture, vertebra, by site, with spinal cord injury
paralysis - *see* Fracture, vertebra, by site, with spinal cord injury
paraplegia - *see* Fracture, vertebra, by site, with spinal cord injury
quadriplegia - *see* Fracture, vertebra, by site, with spinal cord injury
spinal concussion - *see* Fracture, vertebra, by site, with spinal cord injury

Fracture *(Continued)*
  vertebra, vertebral *(Continued)*
    with *(Continued)*
      spinal cord injury (closed) NEC 806.8

> Note Use the following fifth-digit subclassification with categories 806.0–806.3:
>
> C_1–C_4 or unspecified level and D_1–D_6 (T_1–T_6) or unspecified level with:
>
> 0 unspecified spinal cord injury
> 1 complete lesion of cord
> 2 anterior cord syndrome
> 3 central cord syndrome
> 4 specified injury NEC
>
> level and D_1–D_{12} level with:
>
> 5 unspecified spinal cord injury
> 6 complete lesion of cord
> 7 anterior cord syndrome
> 8 central cord syndrome
> 9 specified injury NEC

        cervical 806.0
          open 806.1
        dorsal, dorsolumbar 806.2
          open 806.3
        open 806.9
        thoracic, thoracolumbar 806.2
          open 806.3
    atlanto-axial - *see* Fracture, vertebra, cervical
    cervical (hangman) (teardrop) (closed) 805.00
      with spinal cord injury - *see* Fracture, vertebra, with spinal cord injury, cervical
      first (atlas) 805.01
        open 805.11
      second (axis) 805.02
        open 805.12
      third 805.03
        open 805.13
      fourth 805.04
        open 805.14
      fifth 805.05
        open 805.15
      sixth 805.06
        open 805.16
      seventh 805.07
        open 805.17
      multiple sites 805.08
        open 805.18
      open 805.10
    coccyx (closed) 805.6
      with spinal cord injury (closed) 806.60
        cauda equina injury 806.62
          complete lesion 806.61
            open 806.71
          open 806.72
        open 806.70
          specified type NEC 806.69
      open 806.79
      open 805.7
    collapsed 733.13
    compression, not due to trauma 733.13
    dorsal (closed) 805.2
      with spinal cord injury - *see* Fracture, vertebra, with spinal cord injury, dorsal
      open 805.3
    dorsolumbar (closed) 805.2

Fracture *(Continued)*
    dorsolumbar *(Continued)*
      with spinal cord injury - *see* Fracture, vertebra, with spinal cord injury, dorsal
      open 805.3
    due to osteoporosis 733.13
    fetus or newborn 767.4
    lumbar (closed) 805.4
      with spinal cord injury (closed) 806.4
        open 806.5
      open 805.5
    nontraumatic 733.13
    open NEC 805.9
    pathologic (any site) 733.13
    sacrum (closed) 805.6
      with spinal cord injury 806.60
        cauda equina injury 806.62
          complete lesion 806.61
            open 806.71
          open 806.72
        open 806.70
        specified type NEC 806.69
          open 806.79
      open 805.7
    site unspecified (closed) 805.8
      with spinal cord injury (closed) 806.8
        open 806.9
      open 805.9
    stress (any site) 733.95
    thoracic (closed) 805.2
      with spinal cord injury - *see* Fracture, vertebra, with spinal cord injury, thoracic
      open 805.3
  vertex - *see* Fracture, skull, vault
  vomer (bone) 802.0
    open 802.1
  Wagstaffe's - *see* Fracture, ankle
  wrist (closed) 814.00
    open 814.10
    pathologic 733.12
  xiphoid (process) - *see* Fracture, sternum
  zygoma (zygomatic arch) (closed) 802.4
    open 802.5
Fragile X syndrome 759.83
Fragilitas
  crinium 704.2
  hair 704.2
  ossium 756.51
    with blue sclera 756.51
  unguium 703.8
    congenital 757.5
Fragility
  bone 756.51
    with deafness and blue sclera 756.51
  capillary (hereditary) 287.8
  hair 704.2
  nails 703.8
Fragmentation - *see* Fracture, by site
Frambesia, frambesial (tropica) (*see also* Yaws) 102.9
  initial lesion or ulcer 102.0
  primary 102.0
Frambeside
  gummatous 102.4
  of early yaws 102.2
Frambesioma 102.1
Franceschetti's syndrome (mandibulofacial dysostosis) 756.0
Francis' disease (*see also* Tularemia) 021.9
Frank's essential thrombocytopenia (*see also* Purpura, thrombocytopenic) 287.39

Franklin's disease (heavy chain) 273.2
Fraser's syndrome 759.89
Freckle 709.09
  malignant melanoma in (M8742/3) - *see* Melanoma
  melanotic (of Hutchinson) (M8742/2) - *see* Neoplasm, skin, in situ
Freeman-Sheldon syndrome 759.89
Freezing 991.9
  specified effect NEC 991.8
Frei's disease (climatic bubo) 099.1
Freiberg's
  disease (osteochondrosis, second metatarsal) 732.5
  infraction of metatarsal head 732.5
  osteochondrosis 732.5
Fremitus, friction, cardiac 785.3
Frenulum linguae 750.0
Frenum
  external os 752.49
  tongue 750.0
Frequency (urinary) NEC 788.41
  micturition 788.41
  nocturnal 788.43
  polyuria 788.42
  psychogenic 306.53
Frey's syndrome (auriculotemporal syndrome) 705.22
Friction
  burn (*see also* Injury, superficial, by site) 919.0
  fremitus, cardiac 785.3
  precordial 785.3
  sounds, chest 786.7
Friderichsen-Waterhouse syndrome or disease 036.3
Friedländer's
  B (bacillus) NEC (*see also* condition) 041.3
    sepsis or septicemia 038.49
  disease (endarteritis obliterans) - *see* Arteriosclerosis
Friedreich's
  ataxia 334.0
  combined systemic disease 334.0
  disease 333.2
    combined systemic 334.0
  myoclonia 333.2
  sclerosis (spinal cord) 334.0
Friedrich-Erb-Arnold syndrome (acropachyderma) 757.39
Frigidity 302.72
  psychic or psychogenic 302.72
Fröhlich's disease or syndrome (adiposogenital dystrophy) 253.8
Froin's syndrome 336.8
Frommel's disease 676.6
Frommel-Chiari syndrome 676.6
Frontal - *see also* condition
  lobe syndrome 310.0
Frostbite 991.3
  face 991.0
  foot 991.2
  hand 991.1
  specified site NEC 991.3
Frotteurism 302.89
Frozen 991.9
  pelvis 620.8
  shoulder 726.0
Fructosemia 271.2
Fructosuria (benign) (essential) 271.2
Fuchs'
  black spot (myopic) 360.21
  corneal dystrophy (endothelial) 371.57
  heterochromic cyclitis 364.21

Fucosidosis 271.8
Fugue 780.99
dissociative 300.13
hysterical (dissociative) 300.13
reaction to exceptional stress (transient) 308.1
Fukuhara syndrome 277.87
Fuller Albright's syndrome (osteitis fibrosa disseminata) 756.59
Fuller's earth disease 502
Fulminant, fulminating - *see* condition
Functional - *see* condition
Functioning
borderline intellectual V62.89
Fundus - *see also* condition
flavimaculatus 362.76
Fungemia 117.9
Fungus, fungous
cerebral 348.8
disease NEC 117.9
infection - *see* Infection, fungus
testis (*see also* Tuberculosis) 016.5 *[608.81]*
Funiculitis (acute) 608.4
chronic 608.4
endemic 608.4
gonococcal (acute) 098.14
chronic or duration of 2 months or over 098.34
tuberculous (*see also* Tuberculosis) 016.5
FUO (*see also* Pyrexia) 780.6
Funnel
breast (acquired) 738.3
congenital 754.81
late effect of rickets 268.1
chest (acquired) 738.3
congenital 754.81
late effect of rickets 268.1
pelvis (acquired) 738.6
with disproportion (fetopelvic) 653.3
affecting fetus or newborn 763.1
causing obstructed labor 660.1
affecting fetus or newborn 763.1
congenital 755.69
tuberculous (*see also* Tuberculosis) 016.9
Furfur 690.18
microsporon 111.0
Furor, paroxysmal (idiopathic) (*see also* Epilepsy) 345.8
Furriers' lung 495.8
Furrowed tongue 529.5
congenital 750.13
Furrowing nail(s) (transverse) 703.8
congenital 757.5
Furuncle 680.9
abdominal wall 680.2
ankle 680.6
anus 680.5
arm (any part, above wrist) 680.3
auditory canal, external 680.0
axilla 680.3
back (any part) 680.2
breast 680.2
buttock 680.5
chest wall 680.2
Furuncle *(Continued)*
corpus cavernosum 607.2
ear (any part) 680.0
eyelid 373.13
face (any part, except eye) 680.0
finger (any) 680.4
flank 680.2
foot (any part) 680.7
forearm 680.3
gluteal (region) 680.5
groin 680.2
hand (any part) 680.4
head (any part, except face) 680.8
heel 680.7
hip 680.6
kidney (*see also* Abscess, kidney) 590.2
knee 680.6
labium (majus) (minus) 616.4
lacrimal
gland (*see also* Dacryoadenitis) 375.00
passages (duct) (sac) (*see also* Dacryocystitis) 375.30
leg, any part except foot 680.6
malignant 022.0
multiple sites 680.9
neck 680.1
nose (external) (septum) 680.0
orbit 376.01
partes posteriores 680.5
pectoral region 680.2
penis 607.2
perineum 680.2
pinna 680.0
scalp (any part) 680.8
scrotum 608.4
seminal vesicle 608.0
shoulder 680.3
skin NEC 680.9
specified site NEC 680.8
spermatic cord 608.4
temple (region) 680.0
testis 604.90
thigh 680.6
thumb 680.4
toe (any) 680.7
trunk 680.2
tunica vaginalis 608.4
umbilicus 680.2
upper arm 680.3
vas deferens 608.4
vulva 616.4
wrist 680.4
Furunculosis (*see also* Furuncle) 680.9
external auditory meatus 680.0 *[380.13]*
Fusarium (infection) 118
Fusion, fused (congenital)
anal (with urogenital canal) 751.5
aorta and pulmonary artery 745.0
astragaloscaphoid 755.67
atria 745.5
atrium and ventricle 745.69
auditory canal 744.02
auricles, heart 745.5
binocular, with defective stereopsis 368.33
Fusion, fused *(Continued)*
bone 756.9
cervical spine - *see* Fusion, spine
choanal 748.0
commissure, mitral valve 746.5
cranial sutures, premature 756.0
cusps, heart valve NEC 746.89
mitral 746.5
tricuspid 746.89
ear ossicles 744.04
fingers (*see also* Syndactylism, fingers) 755.11
hymen 752.42
hymeno-urethral 599.89
causing obstructed labor 660.1
affecting fetus or newborn 763.1
joint (acquired) - *see also* Ankylosis
congenital 755.8
kidneys (incomplete) 753.3
labium (majus) (minus) 752.49
larynx and trachea 748.3
limb 755.8
lower 755.69
upper 755.59
lobe, lung 748.5
lumbosacral (acquired) 724.6
congenital 756.15
surgical V45.4
nares (anterior) (posterior) 748.0
nose, nasal 748.0
nostril(s) 748.0
organ or site NEC - *see* Anomaly, specified type NEC
ossicles 756.9
auditory 744.04
pulmonary valve segment 746.02
pulmonic cusps 746.02
ribs 756.3
sacroiliac (acquired) (joint) 724.6
congenital 755.69
surgical V45.4
skull, imperfect 756.0
spine (acquired) 724.9
arthrodesis status V45.4
congenital (vertebra) 756.15
postoperative status V45.4
sublingual duct with submaxillary duct at opening in mouth 750.26
talonavicular (bar) 755.67
teeth, tooth 520.2
testes 752.89
toes (*see also* Syndactylism, toes) 755.13
trachea and esophagus 750.3
twins 759.4
urethral-hymenal 599.89
vagina 752.49
valve cusps - *see* Fusion, cusps, heart valve
ventricles, heart 745.4
vertebra (arch) - *see* Fusion, spine
vulva 752.49
Fusospirillosis (mouth) (tongue) (tonsil) 101
Fussy infant (baby) 780.91

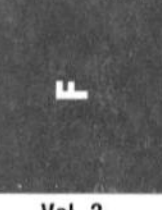

ICD-9-CM
F
Vol. 2

G

Gafsa boil 085.1
Gain, weight (abnormal) (excessive) (*see also* Weight, gain) 783.1
Gaisböck's disease or syndrome (polycythemia hypertonica) 289.0
Gait
  abnormality 781.2
    hysterical 300.11
  ataxic 781.2
    hysterical 300.11
  disturbance 781.2
    hysterical 300.11
  paralytic 781.2
  scissor 781.2
  spastic 781.2
  staggering 781.2
    hysterical 300.11
Galactocele (breast) (infected) 611.5
  puerperal, postpartum 676.8
Galactophoritis 611.0
  puerperal, postpartum 675.2
Galactorrhea 676.6
  not associated with childbirth 611.6
Galactosemia (classic) (congenital) 271.1
Galactosuria 271.1
Galacturia 791.1
  bilharziasis 120.0
Galen's vein - *see* condition
Gallbladder - *see also* condition
  acute (*see also* Disease, gallbladder) 575.0
Gall duct - *see* condition
Gallop rhythm 427.89
Gallstone (cholemic) (colic) (impacted) - *see also* Cholelithiasis
  causing intestinal obstruction 560.31
Gambling, pathological 312.31
Gammaloidosis 277.39 ⟸
Gammopathy 273.9
  macroglobulinemia 273.3
  monoclonal (benign) (essential) (idiopathic) (with lymphoplasmacytic dyscrasia) 273.1
Gamna's disease (siderotic splenomegaly) 289.51
Gampsodactylia (congenital) 754.71
Gamstorp's disease (adynamia episodica hereditaria) 359.3
Gandy-Nanta disease (siderotic splenomegaly) 289.51
Gang activity, without manifest psychiatric disorder V71.09
  adolescent V71.02
  adult V71.01
  child V71.02
Gangliocytoma (M9490/0) - *see* Neoplasm, connective tissue, benign
Ganglioglioma (M9505/1) - *see* Neoplasm, by site, uncertain behavior
Ganglion 727.43
  joint 727.41
  of yaws (early) (late) 102.6
  periosteal (*see also* Periostitis) 730.3
  tendon sheath (compound) (diffuse) 727.42
  tuberculous (*see also* Tuberculosis) 015.9
Ganglioneuroblastoma (M9490/3) - *see* Neoplasm, connective tissue, malignant
Ganglioneuroma (M9490/0) - *see also* Neoplasm, connective tissue, benign
  malignant (M9490/3) - *see* Neoplasm, connective tissue, malignant
Ganglioneuromatosis (M9491/0) - *see* Neoplasm, connective tissue, benign
Ganglionitis
  fifth nerve (*see also* Neuralgia, trigeminal) 350.1
  gasserian 350.1
  geniculate 351.1
    herpetic 053.11
    newborn 767.5
  herpes zoster 053.11
  herpetic geniculate (Hunt's syndrome) 053.11
Gangliosidosis 330.1
Gangosa 102.5
Gangrene, gangrenous (anemia) (artery) (cellulitis) (dermatitis) (dry) (infective) (moist) (pemphigus) (septic) (skin) (stasis) (ulcer) 785.4
  with
    arteriosclerosis (native artery) 440.24
      bypass graft 440.30
        autologous vein 440.31
        nonautologous biological 440.32
    diabetes (mellitus) 250.7 *[785.4]*
  abdomen (wall) 785.4
  adenitis 683
  alveolar 526.5
  angina 462
    diphtheritic 032.0
  anus 569.49
  appendices epiploicae - *see* Gangrene, mesentery
  appendix - *see* Appendicitis, acute
  arteriosclerotic - *see* Arteriosclerosis, with, gangrene
  auricle 785.4
  Bacillus welchii (*see also* Gangrene, gas) 040.0
  bile duct (*see also* Cholangitis) 576.8
  bladder 595.89
  bowel - *see* Gangrene, intestine
  cecum - *see* Gangrene, intestine
  Clostridium perfringens or welchii (*see also* Gangrene, gas) 040.0
  colon - *see* Gangrene, intestine
  connective tissue 785.4
  cornea 371.40
  corpora cavernosa (infective) 607.2
    noninfective 607.89
  cutaneous, spreading 785.4
  decubital (*see also* Decubitus) 707.00 *[785.4]*
  diabetic (any site) 250.7 *[785.4]*
  dropsical 785.4
  emphysematous (*see also* Gangrene, gas) 040.0
  epidemic (ergotized grain) 988.2
  epididymis (infectional) (*see also* Epididymitis) 604.99
  erysipelas (*see also* Erysipelas) 035
  extremity (lower) (upper) 785.4
  gallbladder or duct (*see also* Cholecystitis, acute) 575.0
  gas (bacillus) 040.0
    with
      abortion - *see* Abortion, by type, with sepsis
      ectopic pregnancy (*see also* categories 633.0–633.9) 639.0
      molar pregnancy (*see also* categories 630–632) 639.0
    following
      abortion 639.0
      ectopic or molar pregnancy 639.0
    puerperal, postpartum, childbirth 670
Gangrene, gangrenous *(Continued)*
  glossitis 529.0
  gum 523.8
  hernia - *see* Hernia, by site, with gangrene
  hospital noma 528.1
  intestine, intestinal (acute) (hemorrhagic) (massive) 557.0
    with
      hernia - *see* Hernia, by site, with gangrene
      mesenteric embolism or infarction 557.0
      obstruction (*see also* Obstruction, intestine) 560.9
  laryngitis 464.00
    with obstruction 464.01
  liver 573.8
  lung 513.0
    spirochetal 104.8
  lymphangitis 457.2
  Meleney's (cutaneous) 686.09
  mesentery 557.0
    with
      embolism or infarction 557.0
      intestinal obstruction (*see also* Obstruction, intestine) 560.9
  mouth 528.1
  noma 528.1
  orchitis 604.90
  ovary (*see also* Salpingo-oophoritis) 614.2
  pancreas 577.0
  penis (infectional) 607.2
    noninfective 607.89
  perineum 785.4
  pharynx 462
    septic 034.0
  pneumonia 513.0
  Pott's 440.24
  presenile 443.1
  pulmonary 513.0
  pulp, tooth 522.1
  quinsy 475
  Raynaud's (symmetric gangrene) 443.0 *[785.4]*
  rectum 569.49
  retropharyngeal 478.24
  rupture - *see* Hernia, by site, with gangrene
  scrotum 608.4
    noninfective 608.83
  senile 440.24
  sore throat 462
  spermatic cord 608.4
    noninfective 608.89
  spine 785.4
  spirochetal NEC 104.8
  spreading cutaneous 785.4
  stomach 537.89
  stomatitis 528.1
  symmetrical 443.0 *[785.4]*
  testis (infectional) (*see also* Orchitis) 604.99
    noninfective 608.89
  throat 462
    diphtheritic 032.0
  thyroid (gland) 246.8
  tonsillitis (acute) 463
  tooth (pulp) 522.1
  tuberculous NEC (*see also* Tuberculosis) 011.9
  tunica vaginalis 608.4
    noninfective 608.89

Gangrene, gangrenous *(Continued)*
umbilicus 785.4
uterus (*see also* Endometritis) 615.9
uvulitis 528.3
vas deferens 608.4
noninfective 608.89
vulva (*see also* Vulvitis) 616.10
Gannister disease (occupational) 502
with tuberculosis - *see* Tuberculosis, pulmonary
Ganser's syndrome, hysterical 300.16
Gardner-Diamond syndrome (autoerythrocyte sensitization) 287.2
Gargoylism 277.5
Garré's
disease (*see also* Osteomyelitis) 730.1
osteitis (sclerosing) (*see also* Osteomyelitis) 730.1
osteomyelitis (*see also* Osteomyelitis) 730.1
Garrod's pads, knuckle 728.79
Gartner's duct
cyst 752.41
persistent 752.41
Gas
asphyxia, asphyxiation, inhalation, poisoning, suffocation NEC 987.9
specified gas - *see* Table of Drugs and Chemicals
bacillus gangrene or infection - *see* Gas, gangrene
cyst, mesentery 568.89
excessive 787.3
gangrene 040.0
with
abortion - *see* Abortion, by type, with sepsis
ectopic pregnancy (*see also* categories 633.0–633.9) 639.0
molar pregnancy (*see also* categories 630–632) 639.0
following
abortion 639.0
ectopic or molar pregnancy 639.0
puerperal, postpartum, childbirth 670
on stomach 787.3
pains 787.3
Gastradenitis 535.0
Gastralgia 536.8
psychogenic 307.89
Gastrectasis, gastrectasia 536.1
psychogenic 306.4
Gastric - *see* condition
Gastrinoma (M8153/1)
malignant (M8153/3)
pancreas 157.4
specified site NEC - *see* Neoplasm, by site, malignant
unspecified site 157.4
specified site - *see* Neoplasm, by site, uncertain behavior
unspecified site 235.5
Gastritis 535.5

Note Use the following fifth-digit subclassification for category 535:

0 without mention of hemorrhage
1 with hemorrhage

acute 535.0
alcoholic 535.3
allergic 535.4
antral 535.4
atrophic 535.1
Gastritis *(Continued)*
atrophic-hyperplastic 535.1
bile-induced 535.4
catarrhal 535.0
chronic (atrophic) 535.1
cirrhotic 535.4
corrosive (acute) 535.4
dietetic 535.4
due to diet deficiency 269.9 *[535.4]*
eosinophilic 535.4
erosive 535.4
follicular 535.4
chronic 535.1
giant hypertrophic 535.2
glandular 535.4
chronic 535.1
hypertrophic (mucosa) 535.2
chronic giant 211.1
irritant 535.4
nervous 306.4
phlegmonous 535.0
psychogenic 306.4
sclerotic 535.4
spastic 536.8
subacute 535.0
superficial 535.4
suppurative 535.0
toxic 535.4
tuberculous (*see also* Tuberculosis) 017.9
Gastrocarcinoma (M8010/3) 151.9
Gastrocolic - *see* condition
Gastrocolitis - *see* Enteritis
Gastrodisciasis 121.8
Gastroduodenitis (*see also* Gastritis) 535.5
catarrhal 535.0
infectional 535.0
virus, viral 008.8
specified type NEC 008.69
Gastrodynia 536.8
Gastroenteritis (acute) (catarrhal) (congestive) (hemorrhagic) (noninfectious) (*see also* Enteritis) 558.9
aertrycke infection 003.0
allergic 558.3
chronic 558.9
ulcerative (*see also* Colitis, ulcerative) 556.9
dietetic 558.9
due to
food poisoning (*see also* Poisoning, food) 005.9
radiation 558.1
epidemic 009.0
functional 558.9
infectious (*see also* Enteritis, due to, by organism) 009.0
presumed 009.1
salmonella 003.0
septic (*see also* Enteritis, due to, by organism) 009.0
toxic 558.2
tuberculous (*see also* Tuberculosis) 014.8
ulcerative (*see also* Colitis, ulcerative) 556.9
viral NEC 008.8
specified type NEC 008.69
zymotic 009.0
Gastroenterocolitis - *see* Enteritis
Gastroenteropathy, protein-losing 579.8
Gastroenteroptosis 569.89
Gastroesophageal laceration-hemorrhage syndrome 530.7
Gastroesophagitis 530.19
Gastrohepatitis (*see also* Gastritis) 535.5
Gastrointestinal - *see* condition
Gastrojejunal - *see* condition
Gastrojejunitis (*see also* Gastritis) 535.5
Gastrojejunocolic - *see* condition
Gastroliths 537.89
Gastromalacia 537.89
Gastroparalysis 536.3
diabetic 250.6 *[536.3]*
Gastroparesis 536.3
diabetic 250.6 *[536.3]*
Gastropathy 537.9
erythematous 535.5 ◀
exudative 579.8
Gastroptosis 537.5
Gastrorrhagia 578.0
Gastrorrhea 536.8
psychogenic 306.4
Gastroschisis (congenital) 756.79
acquired 569.89
Gastrospasm (neurogenic) (reflex) 536.8
neurotic 306.4
psychogenic 306.4
Gastrostaxis 578.0
Gastrostenosis 537.89
Gastrostomy
attention to V55.1
complication 536.40
specified type 536.49
infection 536.41
malfunctioning 536.42
status V44.1
Gastrosuccorrhea (continuous) (intermittent) 536.8
neurotic 306.4
psychogenic 306.4
Gaucher's
disease (adult) (cerebroside lipidosis) (infantile) 272.7
hepatomegaly 272.7
splenomegaly (cerebroside lipidosis) 272.7
Gayet's disease (superior hemorrhagic polioencephalitis) 265.1
Gayet-Wernicke's syndrome (superior hemorrhagic polioencephalitis) 265.1
Gee (-Herter) (-Heubner) (-Thaysen) disease or syndrome (nontropical sprue) 579.0
Gélineau's syndrome (*see also* Narcolepsy) 347.00
Gemination, teeth 520.2
Gemistocytoma (M9411/3)
specified site - *see* Neoplasm, by site, malignant
unspecified site 191.9
General, generalized - *see* condition
Genetic
susceptibility to
neoplasm
malignant, of
breast V84.01
endometrium V84.04
other V84.09
ovary V84.02
prostate V84.03
other disease V84.8
Genital - *see* condition
warts 078.19
Genito-anorectal syndrome 099.1
Genitourinary system - *see* condition
Genu
congenital 755.64
extrorsum (acquired) 736.42
congenital 755.64
late effects of rickets 268.1

- **Genu** *(Continued)*
  - introrsum (acquired) 736.41
    - congenital 755.64
    - late effects of rickets 268.1
  - rachitic (old) 268.1
  - recurvatum (acquired) 736.5
    - congenital 754.40
      - with dislocation of knee 754.41
    - late effects of rickets 268.1
  - valgum (acquired) (knock-knee) 736.41
    - congenital 755.64
    - late effects of rickets 268.1
  - varum (acquired) (bowleg) 736.42
    - congenital 755.64
    - late effect of rickets 268.1
- **Geographic tongue** 529.1
- **Geophagia** 307.52
- **Geotrichosis** 117.9
  - intestine 117.9
  - lung 117.9
  - mouth 117.9
- **Gephyrophobia** 300.29
- **Gerbode defect** 745.4
- **Gerhardt's**
  - disease (erythromelalgia) 443.82
  - syndrome (vocal cord paralysis) 478.30
- **Gerlier's disease** (epidemic vertigo) 078.81
- **German measles** 056.9
  - exposure to V01.4
- **Germinoblastoma** (diffuse) (M9614/3) 202.8
  - follicular (M9692/3) 202.0
- **Germinoma** (M9064/3) - *see* Neoplasm, by site, malignant
- **Gerontoxon** 371.41
- **Gerstmann's syndrome** (finger agnosia) 784.69
- **Gestation** (period) - *see also* Pregnancy
  - ectopic NEC (*see also* Pregnancy, ectopic) 633.90
    - with intrauterine pregnancy 633.91
- **Gestational proteinuria** 646.2
  - with hypertension - *see* Toxemia, of pregnancy
- **Ghon tubercle primary infection** (*see also* Tuberculosis) 010.0
- **Ghost**
  - teeth 520.4
  - vessels, cornea 370.64
- **Ghoul hand** 102.3
- **Gianotti Crosti syndrome** 057.8
  - due to known virus - *see* Infection, virus
  - due to unknown virus 057.8
- **Giant**
  - cell
    - epulis 523.8
    - peripheral (gingiva) 523.8
    - tumor, tendon sheath 727.02
  - colon (congenital) 751.3
  - esophagus (congenital) 750.4
  - kidney 753.3
  - urticaria 995.1
    - hereditary 277.6
- **Giardia lamblia infestation** 007.1
- **Giardiasis** 007.1
- **Gibert's disease** (pityriasis rosea) 696.3
- **Gibraltar fever** - *see* Brucellosis
- **Giddiness** 780.4
  - hysterical 300.11
  - psychogenic 306.9
- **Gierke's disease** (glycogenosis I) 271.0
- **Gigantism** (cerebral) (hypophyseal) (pituitary) 253.0
- **Gilbert's disease or cholemia** (familial nonhemolytic jaundice) 277.4
- **Gilchrist's disease** (North American blastomycosis) 116.0
- **Gilford** (-Hutchinson) disease or syndrome (progeria) 259.8
- **Gilles de la Tourette's disease** (motor-verbal tic) 307.23
- **Gillespie's syndrome** (dysplasia oculodentodigitalis) 759.89
- **Gingivitis** 523.10 ⇐
  - acute 523.00 ⇐
    - necrotizing 101
    - non-plaque induced 523.01 ◀
    - plaque induced 523.00 ◀
  - catarrhal 523.00 ⇐
  - chronic 523.10 ⇐
    - non-plaque induced 523.11 ◀
  - desquamative 523.10 ⇐
  - expulsiva 523.40 ⇐
  - hyperplastic 523.10 ⇐
  - marginal, simple 523.10 ⇐
  - necrotizing, acute 101
  - non-plaque induced 523.11 ◀
  - pellagrous 265.2
  - plaque induced 523.10 ◀
  - ulcerative 523.10 ⇐
    - acute necrotizing 101
  - Vincent's 101
- **Gingivoglossitis** 529.0
- **Gingivopericementitis** 523.40 ⇐
- **Gingivosis** 523.10 ⇐
- **Gingivostomatitis** 523.10 ⇐
  - herpetic 054.2
- **Giovannini's disease** 117.9
- **GISA** (glycopeptide intermediate staphylococcus aureus) V09.8
- **Gland, glandular** - *see* condition
- **Glanders** 024
- **Glanzmann** (-Naegeli) disease or thrombasthenia 287.1
- **Glassblowers' disease** 527.1
- **Glaucoma** (capsular) (inflammatory) (noninflammatory) (primary) 365.9
  - with increased episcleral venous pressure 365.82
  - absolute 360.42
  - acute 365.22
    - narrow angle 365.22
    - secondary 365.60
  - angle closure 365.20
    - acute 365.22
    - chronic 365.23
    - intermittent 365.21
    - interval 365.21
    - residual stage 365.24
    - subacute 365.21
  - borderline 365.00
  - chronic 365.11
    - noncongestive 365.11
    - open angle 365.11
    - simple 365.11
  - closed angle - *see* Glaucoma, angle closure
  - congenital 743.20
    - associated with other eye anomalies 743.22
    - simple 743.21
  - congestive - *see* Glaucoma, narrow angle
  - corticosteroid-induced (glaucomatous stage) 365.31
    - residual stage 365.32
  - hemorrhagic 365.60
- **Glaucoma** *(Continued)*
  - hypersecretion 365.81
  - in or with
    - aniridia 743.45 *[365.42]*
    - Axenfeld's anomaly 743.44 *[365.41]*
    - concussion of globe 921.3 *[365.65]*
    - congenital syndromes NEC 759.89 *[365.44]*
    - dislocation of lens
      - anterior 379.33 *[365.59]*
      - posterior 379.34 *[365.59]*
    - disorder of lens NEC *[365.59]*
    - epithelial down-growth 364.61 *[365.64]*
    - glaucomatocyclitic crisis 364.22 *[365.62]*
    - hypermature cataract 366.18 *[365.51]*
    - hyphema 364.41 *[365.63]*
    - inflammation, ocular 365.62
    - iridocyclitis 364.3 *[365.62]*
    - iris
      - anomalies NEC 743.46 *[365.42]*
      - atrophy, essential 364.51 *[365.42]*
      - bombé 364.74 *[365.61]*
      - rubeosis 364.42 *[365.63]*
    - microcornea 743.41 *[365.43]*
    - neurofibromatosis 237.71 *[365.44]*
    - ocular
      - cysts NEC 365.64
      - disorders NEC 365.60
      - trauma 365.65
      - tumors NEC 365.64
    - postdislocation of lens
      - anterior 379.33 *[365.59]*
      - posterior 379.34 *[365.59]*
    - pseudoexfoliation of capsule 366.11 *[365.52]*
    - pupillary block or seclusion 364.74 *[365.61]*
    - recession of chamber angle 364.77 *[365.65]*
    - retinal vein occlusion 362.35 *[365.63]*
    - Rieger's anomaly or syndrome 743.44 *[365.41]*
    - rubeosis of iris 364.42 *[365.63]*
    - seclusion of pupil 364.74 *[365.61]*
    - spherophakia 743.36 *[365.59]*
    - Sturge-Weber (-Dimitri) syndrome 759.6 *[365.44]*
    - systemic syndrome NEC 365.44
    - tumor of globe 365.64
    - vascular disorders NEC 365.63
  - infantile 365.14
    - congenital 743.20
      - associated with other eye anomalies 743.22
      - simple 743.21
  - juvenile 365.14
  - low tension 365.12
  - malignant 365.83
  - narrow angle (primary) 365.20
    - acute 365.22
    - chronic 365.23
    - intermittent 365.21
    - interval 365.21
    - residual stage 365.24
    - subacute 365.21
  - newborn 743.20
    - associated with other eye anomalies 743.22
    - simple 743.21
  - noncongestive (chronic) 365.11
  - nonobstructive (chronic) 365.11
  - obstructive 365.60
    - due to lens changes 365.59
  - open angle 365.10

◀ **New** ⇐ **Revised**

- **Glaucoma** *(Continued)*
  - open angle *(Continued)*
    - with
      - borderline intraocular pressure 365.01
      - cupping of optic discs 365.01
    - primary 365.11
    - residual stage 365.15
  - phacolytic 365.51
    - with hypermature cataract 366.18 *[365.51]*
  - pigmentary 365.13
  - postinfectious 365.60
  - pseudoexfoliation 365.52
    - with pseudoexfoliation of capsule 366.11 *[365.52]*
  - secondary NEC 365.60
  - simple (chronic) 365.11
  - simplex 365.11
  - steroid responders 365.03
  - suspect 365.00
  - syphilitic 095.8
  - traumatic NEC 365.65
    - newborn 767.8
  - tuberculous (*see also* Tuberculosis) 017.3 *[365.62]*
  - wide angle (*see also* Glaucoma, open angle) 365.10
- **Glaucomatous flecks** (subcapsular) 366.31
- **Glazed tongue** 529.4
- **Gleet** 098.2
- **Glénard's disease or syndrome** (enteroptosis) 569.89
- **Glinski-Simmonds syndrome** (pituitary cachexia) 253.2
- **Glioblastoma** (multiforme) (M9440/3)
  - with sarcomatous component (M9442/3)
    - specified site - *see* Neoplasm, by site, malignant
    - unspecified site 191.9
  - giant cell (M9441/3)
    - specified site - *see* Neoplasm, by site, malignant
    - unspecified site 191.9
  - specified site - *see* Neoplasm, by site, malignant
  - unspecified site 191.9
- **Glioma** (malignant) (M9380/3)
  - astrocytic (M9400/3)
    - specified site - *see* Neoplasm, by site, malignant
    - unspecified site 191.9
  - mixed (M9382/3)
    - specified site - *see* Neoplasm, by site, malignant
    - unspecified site 191.9
  - nose 748.1
  - specified site NEC - *see* Neoplasm, by site, malignant
  - subependymal (M9383/1) 237.5
  - unspecified site 191.9
- **Gliomatosis cerebri** (M9381/3) 191.0
- **Glioneuroma** (M9505/1) - *see* Neoplasm, by site, uncertain behavior
- **Gliosarcoma** (M9380/3)
  - specified site - *see* Neoplasm, by site, malignant
  - unspecified site 191.9
- **Gliosis** (cerebral) 349.89
  - spinal 336.0
- **Glisson's**
  - cirrhosis - *see* Cirrhosis, portal
  - disease (*see also* Rickets) 268.0
- **Glissonitis** 573.3
- **Globinuria** 791.2
- **Globus** 306.4
  - hystericus 300.11
- **Glomangioma** (M8712/0) (*see also* Hemangioma) 228.00
- **Glomangiosarcoma** (M8710/3) - *see* Neoplasm, connective tissue, malignant
- **Glomerular nephritis** (*see also* Nephritis) 583.9
- **Glomerulitis** (*see also* Nephritis) 583.9
- **Glomerulonephritis** (*see also* Nephritis) 583.9
  - with
    - edema (*see also* Nephrosis) 581.9
    - lesion of
      - exudative nephritis 583.89
      - interstitial nephritis (diffuse) (focal) 583.89
      - necrotizing glomerulitis 583.4
        - acute 580.4
        - chronic 582.4
      - renal necrosis 583.9
        - cortical 583.6
        - medullary 583.7
      - specified pathology NEC 583.89
        - acute 580.89
        - chronic 582.89
    - necrosis, renal 583.9
      - cortical 583.6
      - medullary (papillary) 583.7
    - specified pathology or lesion NEC 583.89
  - acute 580.9
    - with
      - exudative nephritis 580.89
      - interstitial nephritis (diffuse) (focal) 580.89
      - necrotizing glomerulitis 580.4
    - extracapillary with epithelial crescents 580.4
    - poststreptococcal 580.0
    - proliferative (diffuse) 580.0
    - rapidly progressive 580.4
    - specified pathology NEC 580.89
  - arteriolar (*see also* Hypertension, kidney) 403.90
  - arteriosclerotic (*see also* Hypertension, kidney) 403.90
  - ascending (*see also* Pyelitis) 590.80
  - basement membrane NEC 583.89
    - with
      - pulmonary hemorrhage (Goodpasture's syndrome) 446.21 *[583.81]*
  - chronic 582.9
    - with
      - exudative nephritis 582.89
      - interstitial nephritis (diffuse) (focal) 582.89
      - necrotizing glomerulitis 582.4
      - specified pathology or lesion NEC 582.89
    - endothelial 582.2
    - extracapillary with epithelial crescents 582.4
    - hypocomplementemic persistent 582.2
    - lobular 582.2
    - membranoproliferative 582.2
    - membranous 582.1
      - and proliferative (mixed) 582.2
      - sclerosing 582.1

- **Glomerulonephritis** *(Continued)*
  - chronic *(Continued)*
    - mesangiocapillary 582.2
    - mixed membranous and proliferative 582.2
    - proliferative (diffuse) 582.0
    - rapidly progressive 582.4
    - sclerosing 582.1
  - cirrhotic - *see* Sclerosis, renal
  - desquamative - *see* Nephrosis
  - due to or associated with
    - amyloidosis 277.39 *[583.81]* ⇐
      - with nephrotic syndrome 277.39 *[581.81]* ⇐
      - chronic 277.39 *[582.81]* ⇐
    - diabetes mellitus 250.4 *[583.81]*
      - with nephrotic syndrome 250.4 *[581.81]*
    - diphtheria 032.89 *[580.81]*
    - gonococcal infection (acute) 098.19 *[583.81]*
      - chronic or duration of 2 months or over 098.39 *[583.81]*
    - infectious hepatitis 070.9 *[580.81]*
    - malaria (with nephrotic syndrome) 084.9 *[581.81]*
    - mumps 072.79 *[580.81]*
    - polyarteritis (nodosa) (with nephrotic syndrome) 446.0 *[581.81]*
    - specified pathology NEC 583.89
      - acute 580.89
      - chronic 582.89
    - streptotrichosis 039.8 *[583.81]*
    - subacute bacterial endocarditis 421.0 *[580.81]*
    - syphilis (late) 095.4
      - congenital 090.5 *[583.81]*
      - early 091.69 *[583.81]*
    - systemic lupus erythematosus 710.0 *[583.81]*
      - with nephrotic syndrome 710.0 *[581.81]*
      - chronic 710.0 *[582.81]*
    - tuberculosis (*see also* Tuberculosis) 016.0 *[583.81]*
    - typhoid fever 002.0 *[580.81]*
  - extracapillary with epithelial crescents 583.4
    - acute 580.4
    - chronic 582.4
  - exudative 583.89
    - acute 580.89
    - chronic 582.89
  - focal (*see also* Nephritis) 583.9
    - embolic 580.4
  - granular 582.89
  - granulomatous 582.89
  - hydremic (*see also* Nephrosis) 581.9
  - hypocomplementemic persistent 583.2
    - with nephrotic syndrome 581.2
    - chronic 582.2
  - immune complex NEC 583.89
  - infective (*see also* Pyelitis) 590.80
  - interstitial (diffuse) (focal) 583.89
    - with nephrotic syndrome 581.89
    - acute 580.89
    - chronic 582.89
  - latent or quiescent 582.9
  - lobular 583.2
    - with nephrotic syndrome 581.2
    - chronic 582.2
  - membranoproliferative 583.2

Glomerulonephritis *(Continued)*
membranoproliferative *(Continued)*
with nephrotic syndrome 581.2
chronic 582.2
membranous 583.1
with nephrotic syndrome 581.1
and proliferative (mixed) 583.2
with nephrotic syndrome 581.2
chronic 582.2
chronic 582.1
sclerosing 582.1
with nephrotic syndrome 581.1
mesangiocapillary 583.2
with nephrotic syndrome 581.2
chronic 582.2
minimal change 581.3
mixed membranous and proliferative 583.2
with nephrotic syndrome 581.2
chronic 582.2
necrotizing 583.4
acute 580.4
chronic 582.4
nephrotic (*see also* Nephrosis) 581.9
old - *see* Glomerulonephritis, chronic
parenchymatous 581.89
poststreptococcal 580.0
proliferative (diffuse) 583.0
with nephrotic syndrome 581.0
acute 580.0
chronic 582.0
purulent (*see also* Pyelitis) 590.80
quiescent - *see* Nephritis, chronic
rapidly progressive 583.4
acute 580.4
chronic 582.4
sclerosing membranous (chronic) 582.1
with nephrotic syndrome 581.1
septic (*see also* Pyelitis) 590.80
specified pathology or lesion NEC 583.89
with nephrotic syndrome 581.89
acute 580.89
chronic 582.89
suppurative (acute) (disseminated) (*see also* Pyelitis) 590.80
toxic - *see* Nephritis, acute
tubal, tubular - *see* Nephrosis, tubular
type II (Ellis) - *see* Nephrosis
vascular - *see* Hypertension, kidney
Glomerulosclerosis (*see also* Sclerosis, renal) 587
focal 582.1
with nephrotic syndrome 581.1
intercapillary (nodular) (with diabetes) 250.4 *[581.81]*
Glossagra 529.6
Glossalgia 529.6
Glossitis 529.0
areata exfoliativa 529.1
atrophic 529.4
benign migratory 529.1
gangrenous 529.0
Hunter's 529.4
median rhomboid 529.2
Moeller's 529.4
pellagrous 265.2
Glossocele 529.8
Glossodynia 529.6
exfoliativa 529.4
Glossoncus 529.8
Glossophytia 529.3
Glossoplegia 529.8
Glossoptosis 529.8
Glossopyrosis 529.6
Glossotrichia 529.3
Glossy skin 701.9
Glottis - *see* condition
Glottitis - *see* Glossitis
Glucagonoma (M8152/0)
malignant (M8152/3)
pancreas 157.4
specified site NEC - *see* Neoplasm, by site, malignant
unspecified site 157.4
pancreas 211.7
specified site NEC - *see* Neoplasm, by site, benign
unspecified site 211.7
Glucoglycinuria 270.7
Glue ear syndrome 381.20
Glue sniffing (airplane glue) (*see also* Dependence) 304.6
Glycinemia (with methylmalonic acidemia) 270.7
Glycinuria (renal) (with ketosis) 270.0
Glycogen
infiltration (*see also* Disease, glycogen storage) 271.0
storage disease (*see also* Disease, glycogen storage) 271.0
Glycogenosis (*see also* Disease, glycogen storage) 271.0
cardiac 271.0 *[425.7]*
Cori, types I-VII 271.0
diabetic, secondary 250.8 *[259.8]*
diffuse (with hepatic cirrhosis) 271.0
generalized 271.0
glucose-6-phosphatase deficiency 271.0
hepatophosphorylase deficiency 271.0
hepatorenal 271.0
myophosphorylase deficiency 271.0
Glycopenia 251.2
Glycopeptide
intermediate staphylococcus aureus (GISA) V09.8
resistant
enterococcus V09.8
staphylococcus aureus (GRSA) V09.8
Glycoprolinuria 270.8
Glycosuria 791.5
renal 271.4
Gnathostoma (spinigerum) (infection) (infestation) 128.1
wandering swellings from 128.1
Gnathostomiasis 128.1
Goiter (adolescent) (colloid) (diffuse) (dipping) (due to iodine deficiency) (endemic) (euthyroid) (heart) (hyperplastic) (internal) (intrathoracic) (juvenile) (mixed type) (nonendemic) (parenchymatous) (plunging) (sporadic) (subclavicular) (substernal) 240.9
with
hyperthyroidism (recurrent) (*see also* Goiter, toxic) 242.0
thyrotoxicosis (*see also* Goiter, toxic) 242.0
adenomatous (*see also* Goiter, nodular) 241.9
cancerous (M8000/3) 193
complicating pregnancy, childbirth, or puerperium 648.1
congenital 246.1
cystic (*see also* Goiter, nodular) 241.9
Goiter *(Continued)*
due to enzyme defect in synthesis of thyroid hormone (butane-insoluble iodine) (coupling) (deiodinase) (iodide trapping or organification) (iodotyrosine dehalogenase) (peroxidase) 246.1
dyshormonogenic 246.1
exophthalmic (*see also* Goiter, toxic) 242.0
familial (with deaf-mutism) 243
fibrous 245.3
lingual 759.2
lymphadenoid 245.2
malignant (M8000/3) 193
multinodular (nontoxic) 241.1
toxic or with hyperthyroidism (*see also* Goiter, toxic) 242.2
nodular (nontoxic) 241.9
with
hyperthyroidism (*see also* Goiter, toxic) 242.3
thyrotoxicosis (*see also* Goiter, toxic) 242.3
endemic 241.9
exophthalmic (diffuse) (*see also* Goiter, toxic) 242.0
multinodular (nontoxic) 241.1
sporadic 241.9
toxic (*see also* Goiter, toxic) 242.3
uninodular (nontoxic) 241.0
nontoxic (nodular) 241.9
multinodular 241.1
uninodular 241.0
pulsating (*see also* Goiter, toxic) 242.0
simple 240.0
toxic 242.0

Note Use the following fifth-digit subclassification with category 242:

0 without mention of thyrotoxic crisis or storm
1 with mention of thyrotoxic crisis or storm

adenomatous 242.3
multinodular 242.2
uninodular 242.1
multinodular 242.2
nodular 242.3
multinodular 242.2
uninodular 242.1
uninodular 242.1
uninodular (nontoxic) 241.0
toxic or with hyperthyroidism (*see also* Goiter, toxic) 242.1
Goldberg (-Maxwell) (-Morris) syndrome (testicular feminization) 259.5
Goldblatt's
hypertension 440.1
kidney 440.1
Goldenhar's syndrome (oculoauriculovertebral dysplasia) 756.0
Goldflam-Erb disease or syndrome 358.00
Goldscheider's disease (epidermolysis bullosa) 757.39
Goldstein's disease (familial hemorrhagic telangiectasia) 448.0
Golfer's elbow 726.32
Goltz-Gorlin syndrome (dermal hypoplasia) 757.39
Gonadoblastoma (M9073/1)
specified site - *see* Neoplasm, by site uncertain behavior

Gonadoblastoma *(Continued)*
unspecified site
female 236.2
male 236.4
Gonecystitis (*see also* Vesiculitis) 608.0
Gongylonemiasis 125.6
mouth 125.6
Goniosynechiae 364.73
Gonococcemia 098.89
Gonococcus, gonococcal (disease) (infection) (*see also* condition) 098.0
anus 098.7
bursa 098.52
chronic NEC 098.2
complicating pregnancy, childbirth, or puerperium 647.1
affecting fetus or newborn 760.2
conjunctiva, conjunctivitis (neonatorum) 098.40
dermatosis 098.89
endocardium 098.84
epididymo-orchitis 098.13
chronic or duration of 2 months or over 098.33
eye (newborn) 098.40
fallopian tube (chronic) 098.37
acute 098.17
genitourinary (acute) (organ) (system) (tract) (*see also* Gonorrhea) 098.0
lower 098.0
chronic 098.2
upper 098.10
chronic 098.30
heart NEC 098.85
joint 098.50
keratoderma 098.81
keratosis (blennorrhagica) 098.81
lymphatic (gland) (node) 098.89
meninges 098.82
orchitis (acute) 098.13
chronic or duration of 2 months or over 098.33
pelvis (acute) 098.19
chronic or duration of 2 months or over 098.39
pericarditis 098.83
peritonitis 098.86
pharyngitis 098.6
pharynx 098.6
proctitis 098.7
pyosalpinx (chronic) 098.37
acute 098.17
rectum 098.7
septicemia 098.89
skin 098.89
specified site NEC 098.89
synovitis 098.51
tendon sheath 098.51
throat 098.6
urethra (acute) 098.0
chronic or duration of 2 months or over 098.2
vulva (acute) 098.0
chronic or duration of 2 months or over 098.2
Gonocytoma (M9073/1)
specified site - *see* Neoplasm, by site, uncertain behavior
unspecified site
female 236.2
male 236.4
Gonorrhea 098.0
acute 098.0
Gonorrhea *(Continued)*
Bartholin's gland (acute) 098.0
chronic or duration of 2 months or over 098.2
bladder (acute) 098.11
chronic or duration of 2 months or over 098.31
carrier (suspected of) V02.7
cervix (acute) 098.15
chronic or duration of 2 months or over 098.35
chronic 098.2
complicating pregnancy, childbirth, or puerperium 647.1
affecting fetus or newborn 760.2
conjunctiva, conjunctivitis (neonatorum) 098.40
contact V01.6
Cowper's gland (acute) 098.0
chronic or duration of 2 months or over 098.2
duration of 2 months or over 098.2
exposure to V01.6
fallopian tube (chronic) 098.37
acute 098.17
genitourinary (acute) (organ) (system) (tract) 098.0
chronic 098.2
duration of 2 months or over 098.2
kidney (acute) 098.19
chronic or duration of 2 months or over 098.39
ovary (acute) 098.19
chronic or duration of 2 months or over 098.39
pelvis (acute) 098.19
chronic or duration of 2 months or over 098.39
penis (acute) 098.0
chronic or duration of 2 months or over 098.2
prostate (acute) 098.12
chronic or duration of 2 months or over 098.32
seminal vesicle (acute) 098.14
chronic or duration of 2 months or over 098.34
specified site NEC - *see* Gonococcus
spermatic cord (acute) 098.14
chronic or duration of 2 months or over 098.34
urethra (acute) 098.0
chronic or duration of 2 months or over 098.2
vagina (acute) 098.0
chronic or duration of 2 months or over 098.2
vas deferens (acute) 098.14
chronic or duration of 2 months or over 098.34
vulva (acute) 098.0
chronic or duration of 2 months or over 098.2
Goodpasture's syndrome (pneumorenal) 446.21
Good's syndrome 279.06
Gopalan's syndrome (burning feet) 266.2
Gordon's disease (exudative enteropathy) 579.8
Gorlin-Chaudhry-Moss syndrome 759.89
Gougerot's syndrome (trisymptomatic) 709.1
Gougerot-Blum syndrome (pigmented purpuric lichenoid dermatitis) 709.1
Gougerot-Carteaud disease or syndrome (confluent reticulate papillomatosis) 701.8
Gougerot-Hailey-Hailey disease (benign familial chronic pemphigus) 757.39
Gougerot (-Houwer)-Sjögren syndrome (keratoconjunctivitis sicca) 710.2
Gouley's syndrome (constrictive pericarditis) 423.2
Goundou 102.6
Gout, gouty 274.9
with specified manifestations NEC 274.89
arthritis (acute) 274.0
arthropathy 274.0
degeneration, heart 274.82
diathesis 274.9
eczema 274.89
episcleritis 274.89 *[379.09]*
external ear (tophus) 274.81
glomerulonephritis 274.10
iritis 274.89 *[364.11]*
joint 274.0
kidney 274.10
lead 984.9
specified type of lead - *see* Table of Drugs and Chemicals
nephritis 274.10
neuritis 274.89 *[357.4]*
phlebitis 274.89 *[451.9]*
rheumatic 714.0
saturnine 984.9
specified type of lead - *see* Table of Drugs and Chemicals
spondylitis 274.0
synovitis 274.0
syphilitic 095.8
tophi 274.0
ear 274.81
heart 274.82
specified site NEC 274.82
Gowers'
muscular dystrophy 359.1
syndrome (vasovagal attack) 780.2
Gowers-Paton-Kennedy syndrome 377.04
Gradenigo's syndrome 383.02
Graft-versus-host disease (bone marrow) 996.85
due to organ transplant NEC - *see* Complications, transplant, organ
Graham Steell's murmur (pulmonic regurgitation) (*see also* Endocarditis, pulmonary) 424.3
Grain-handlers' disease or lung 495.8
Grain mite (itch) 133.8
Grand
mal (idiopathic) (*see also* Epilepsy) 345.1
hysteria of Charcôt 300.11
nonrecurrent or isolated 780.39
multipara
affecting management of labor and delivery 659.4
status only (not pregnant) V61.5
Granite workers' lung 502
Granular - *see also* condition
inflammation, pharynx 472.1
kidney (contracting) (*see also* Sclerosis, renal) 587
liver - *see* Cirrhosis, liver
nephritis - *see* Nephritis
Granulation tissue, abnormal - *see also* Granuloma

ICD-9-CM
G
Vol. 2

Granulation tissue, abnormal *(Continued)*
abnormal or excessive 701.5
postmastoidectomy cavity 383.33
postoperative 701.5
skin 701.5
Granulocytopenia, granulocytopenic (primary) 288.00
malignant 288.09
Granuloma NEC 686.1
abdomen (wall) 568.89
skin (pyogenicum) 686.1
from residual foreign body 709.4
annulare 695.89
anus 569.49
apical 522.6
appendix 543.9
aural 380.23
beryllium (skin) 709.4
lung 503
bone (*see also* Osteomyelitis) 730.1
eosinophilic 277.89
from residual foreign body 733.99
canaliculus lacrimalis 375.81
cerebral 348.8
cholesterin, middle ear 385.82
coccidioidal (progressive) 114.3
lung 114.4
meninges 114.2
primary (lung) 114.0
colon 569.89
conjunctiva 372.61
dental 522.6
ear, middle (cholesterin) 385.82
with otitis media - *see* Otitis media
eosinophilic 277.89
bone 277.89
lung 277.89
oral mucosa 528.9
exuberant 701.5
eyelid 374.89
facial
lethal midline 446.3
malignant 446.3
faciale 701.8
fissuratum (gum) 523.8
foot NEC 686.1
foreign body (in soft tissue) NEC 728.82
bone 733.99
in operative wound 998.4
muscle 728.82
skin 709.4
subcutaneous tissue 709.4
fungoides 202.1
gangraenescens 446.3
giant cell (central) (jaw) (reparative) 526.3
gingiva 523.8
peripheral (gingiva) 523.8
gland (lymph) 289.3
Hodgkin's (M9661/3) 201.1
ileum 569.89
infectious NEC 136.9
inguinale (Donovan) 099.2
venereal 099.2
intestine 569.89
iridocyclitis 364.10
jaw (bone) 526.3
reparative giant cell 526.3
kidney (*see also* Infection, kidney) 590.9
lacrimal sac 375.81
larynx 478.79
lethal midline 446.3
lipid 277.89
lipoid 277.89

Granuloma NEC *(Continued)*
liver 572.8
lung (infectious) (*see also* Fibrosis, lung) 515
coccidioidal 114.4
eosinophilic 277.89
lymph gland 289.3
Majocchi's 110.6
malignant, face 446.3
mandible 526.3
mediastinum 519.3
midline 446.3
monilial 112.3
muscle 728.82
from residual foreign body 728.82
nasal sinus (*see also* Sinusitis) 473.9
operation wound 998.59
foreign body 998.4
stitch (external) 998.89
internal wound 998.89
talc 998.7
oral mucosa, eosinophilic or pyogenic 528.9
orbit, orbital 376.11
paracoccidioidal 116.1
penis, venereal 099.2
periapical 522.6
peritoneum 568.89
due to ova of helminths NEC (*see also* Helminthiasis) 128.9
postmastoidectomy cavity 383.33
postoperative - *see* Granuloma, operation wound
prostate 601.8
pudendi (ulcerating) 099.2
pudendorum (ulcerative) 099.2
pulp, internal (tooth) 521.49
pyogenic, pyogenicum (skin) 686.1
maxillary alveolar ridge 522.6
oral mucosa 528.9
rectum 569.49
reticulohistiocytic 277.89
rubrum nasi 705.89
sarcoid 135
Schistosoma 120.9
septic (skin) 686.1
silica (skin) 709.4
sinus (accessory) (infectional) (nasal) (*see also* Sinusitis) 473.9
skin (pyogenicum) 686.1
from foreign body or material 709.4
sperm 608.89
spine
syphilitic (epidural) 094.89
tuberculous (*see also* Tuberculosis) 015.0 *[730.88]*
stitch (postoperative) 998.89
internal wound 998.89
suppurative (skin) 686.1
suture (postoperative) 998.89
internal wound 998.89
swimming pool 031.1
talc 728.82
in operation wound 998.7
telangiectaticum (skin) 686.1
tracheostomy 519.09
trichophyticum 110.6
tropicum 102.4
umbilicus 686.1
newborn 771.4
urethra 599.84
uveitis 364.10
vagina 099.2
venereum 099.2

Granuloma NEC *(Continued)*
vocal cords 478.5
Wegener's (necrotizing respiratory granulomatosis) 446.4
Granulomatosis NEC 686.1
disciformis chronica et progressiva 709.3
infantiseptica 771.2
lipoid 277.89
lipophagic, intestinal 040.2
miliary 027.0
necrotizing, respiratory 446.4
progressive, septic 288.1
Wegener's (necrotizing respiratory) 446.4
Granulomatous tissue - *see* Granuloma
Granulosis rubra nasi 705.89
Graphite fibrosis (of lung) 503
Graphospasm 300.89
organic 333.84
Grating scapula 733.99
Gravel (urinary) (*see also* Calculus) 592.9
Graves' disease (exophthalmic goiter) (*see also* Goiter, toxic) 242.0
Gravis - *see* condition
Grawitz's tumor (hypernephroma) (M8312/3) 189.0
Grayness, hair (premature) 704.3
congenital 757.4
Gray or grey syndrome (chloramphenicol) (newborn) 779.4
Greenfield's disease 330.0
Green sickness 280.9
Greenstick fracture - *see* Fracture, by site
Greig's syndrome (hypertelorism) 756.0
Griesinger's disease (*see also* Ancylostomiasis) 126.9
Grinders'
asthma 502
lung 502
phthisis (*see also* Tuberculosis) 011.4
Grinding, teeth 306.8
Grip
Dabney's 074.1
devil's 074.1
Grippe, grippal - *see also* Influenza
Balkan 083.0
intestinal 487.8
summer 074.8
Grippy cold 487.1
Grisel's disease 723.5
Groin - *see* condition
Grooved
nails (transverse) 703.8
tongue 529.5
congenital 750.13
Ground itch 126.9
Growing pains, children 781.99
Growth (fungoid) (neoplastic) (new) (M8000/1) - *see also* Neoplasm, by site, unspecified nature
adenoid (vegetative) 474.12
benign (M8000/0) - *see* Neoplasm, by site, benign
fetal, poor 764.9
affecting management of pregnancy 656.5
malignant (M8000/3) - *see* Neoplasm, by site, malignant
rapid, childhood V21.0
secondary (M8000/6) - *see* Neoplasm, by site, malignant, secondary
GRSA (glycopeptide resistant staphylococcus aureus) V09.8

◀ New ⬅ Revised

Gruber's hernia - *see* Hernia, Gruber's
Gruby's disease (tinea tonsurans) 110.0
G-trisomy 758.0
Guama fever 066.3
Gubler (-Millard) paralysis or syndrome 344.89
Guérin-Stern syndrome (arthrogryposis multiplex congenita) 754.89
Guertin's disease (electric chorea) 049.8
Guillain-Barré disease or syndrome 357.0
Guinea worms (infection) (infestation) 125.7
Guinon's disease (motor-verbal tic) 307.23
Gull's disease (thyroid atrophy with myxedema) 244.8
Gull and Sutton's disease - *see* Hypertension, kidney
Gum - *see* condition
Gumboil 522.7
Gumma (syphilitic) 095.9
  artery 093.89
    cerebral or spinal 094.89
  bone 095.5
    of yaws (late) 102.6
  brain 094.89
  cauda equina 094.89
  central nervous system NEC 094.9
  ciliary body 095.8 *[364.11]*
  congenital 090.5
    testis 090.5

Gumma *(Continued)*
  eyelid 095.8 *[373.5]*
  heart 093.89
  intracranial 094.89
  iris 095.8 *[364.11]*
  kidney 095.4
  larynx 095.8
  leptomeninges 094.2
  liver 095.3
  meninges 094.2
  myocardium 093.82
  nasopharynx 095.8
  neurosyphilitic 094.9
  nose 095.8
  orbit 095.8
  palate (soft) 095.8
  penis 095.8
  pericardium 093.81
  pharynx 095.8
  pituitary 095.8
  scrofulous (*see also* Tuberculosis) 017.0
  skin 095.8
  specified site NEC 095.8
  spinal cord 094.89
  tongue 095.8
  tonsil 095.8
  trachea 095.8
  tuberculous (*see also* Tuberculosis) 017.0
  ulcerative due to yaws 102.4
  ureter 095.8

Gumma *(Continued)*
  yaws 102.4
    bone 102.6
Gunn's syndrome (jaw-winking syndrome) 742.8
Gunshot wound - *see also* Wound, open, by site
  fracture - *see* Fracture, by site, open
  internal organs (abdomen, chest, or pelvis) - *see* Injury, internal, by site, with open wound
  intracranial - *see* Laceration, brain, with open intracranial wound
Günther's disease or syndrome (congenital erythropoietic porphyria) 277.1
Gustatory hallucination 780.1
Gynandrism 752.7
Gynandroblastoma (M8632/1)
  specified site - *see* Neoplasm, by site, uncertain behavior
  unspecified site
    female 236.2
    male 236.4
Gynandromorphism 752.7
Gynatresia (congenital) 752.49
Gynecoid pelvis, male 738.6
Gynecological examination V72.31
  for contraceptive maintenance V25.40
Gynecomastia 611.1
Gynephobia 300.29
Gyrate scalp 757.39

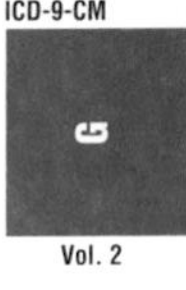

ICD-9-CM
G
Vol. 2

H

Haas' disease (osteochondrosis head of humerus) 732.3
Habermann's disease (acute parapsoriasis varioliformis) 696.2
Habit, habituation
  chorea 307.22
  disturbance, child 307.9
  drug (*see also* Dependence) 304.9
  laxative (*see also* Abuse, drugs, nondependent) 305.9
  spasm 307.20
    chronic 307.22
    transient (of childhood) 307.21
  tic 307.20
    chronic 307.22
    transient (of childhood) 307.21
  use of
    nonprescribed drugs (*see also* Abuse, drugs, nondependent) 305.9
    patent medicines (*see also* Abuse, drugs, nondependent) 305.9
  vomiting 536.2
Hadfield-Clarke syndrome (pancreatic infantilism) 577.8
Haff disease 985.1
Hag teeth, tooth 524.39
Hageman factor defect, deficiency, or disease (*see also* Defect, coagulation) 286.3
Haglund's disease (osteochondrosis os tibiale externum) 732.5
Haglund-Läwen-Fründ syndrome 717.89
Hagner's disease (hypertrophic pulmonary osteoarthropathy) 731.2
Hailey-Hailey disease (benign familial chronic pemphigus) 757.39
Hair - *see also* condition
  plucking 307.9
Hairball in stomach 935.2
Hairy black tongue 529.3
Half vertebra 756.14
Halitosis 784.99
Hallermann-Streiff syndrome 756.0
Hallervorden-Spatz disease or syndrome 333.0
Hallopeau's
  acrodermatitis (continua) 696.1
  disease (lichen sclerosis et atrophicus) 701.0
Hallucination (auditory) (gustatory) (olfactory) (tactile) 780.1
  alcohol-induced 291.3
  drug-induced 292.12
  visual 368.16
Hallucinosis 298.9
  alcohol-induced (acute) 291.3
  drug-induced 292.12
Hallus - *see* Hallux
Hallux 735.9
  malleus (acquired) 735.3
  rigidus (acquired) 735.2
    congenital 755.66
    late effects of rickets 268.1
  valgus (acquired) 735.0
    congenital 755.66
  varus (acquired) 735.1
    congenital 755.66
Halo, visual 368.15
Hamartoblastoma 759.6
Hamartoma 759.6
  epithelial (gingival), odontogenic, central, or peripheral (M9321/0) 213.1
    upper jaw (bone) 213.0
  vascular 757.32
Hamartosis, hamartoses NEC 759.6
Hamman's disease or syndrome (spontaneous mediastinal emphysema) 518.1
Hamman-Rich syndrome (diffuse interstitial pulmonary fibrosis) 516.3
Hammer toe (acquired) 735.4
  congenital 755.66
  late effects of rickets 268.1
Hand - *see* condition
Hand-Schüller-Christian disease or syndrome (chronic histiocytosis X) 277.89
Hand-foot syndrome 282.61
Hanging (asphyxia) (strangulation) (suffocation) 994.7
Hangnail (finger) (with lymphangitis) 681.02
Hangover (alcohol) (*see also* Abuse, drugs, nondependent) 305.0
Hanot's cirrhosis or disease - *see* Cirrhosis, biliary
Hanot-Chauffard (-Troisier) syndrome (bronze diabetes) 275.0
Hansen's disease (leprosy) 030.9
  benign form 030.1
  malignant form 030.0
Harada's disease or syndrome 363.22
Hard chancre 091.0
Hard firm prostate 600.10
  with
    urinary
      obstruction 600.11
      retention 600.11
Hardening
  artery - *see* Arteriosclerosis
  brain 348.8
  liver 571.8
Hare's syndrome (M8010/3) (carcinoma, pulmonary apex) 162.3
Harelip (*see also* Cleft, lip) 749.10
Harkavy's syndrome 446.0
Harlequin (fetus) 757.1
  color change syndrome 779.89
Harley's disease (intermittent hemoglobinuria) 283.2
Harris'
  lines 733.91
  syndrome (organic hyperinsulinism) 251.1
Hart's disease or syndrome (pellagra-cerebellar ataxia-renal aminoaciduria) 270.0
Hartmann's pouch (abnormal sacculation of gallbladder neck) 575.8
  of intestine V44.3
    attention to V55.3
Hartnup disease (pellagra-cerebellar ataxia-renal aminoaciduria) 270.0
Harvester lung 495.0
Hashimoto's disease or struma (struma lymphomatosa) 245.2
Hassall-Henle bodies (corneal warts) 371.41
Haut mal (*see also* Epilepsy) 345.1
Haverhill fever 026.1
Hawaiian wood rose dependence 304.5
Hawkins' keloid 701.4
Hay
  asthma (*see also* Asthma) 493.0
  fever (allergic) (with rhinitis) 477.9
    with asthma (bronchial) (*see also* Asthma) 493.0
Hay *(Continued)*
  fever *(Continued)*
    allergic, due to grass, pollen, ragweed, or tree 477.0
    conjunctivitis 372.05
    due to
      dander, animal (cat) (dog) 477.2
      dust 477.8
      fowl 477.8
      hair, animal (cat) (dog) 477.2
      pollen 477.0
      specified allergen other than pollen 477.8
Hayem-Faber syndrome (achlorhydric anemia) 280.9
Hayem-Widal syndrome (acquired hemolytic jaundice) 283.9
Haygarth's nodosities 715.04
Hazard-Crile tumor (M8350/3) 193
Hb (abnormal)
  disease - *see* Disease, hemoglobin
  trait - *see* Trait
H disease 270.0
Head - *see also* condition
  banging 307.3
Headache 784.0
  allergic 346.2
  cluster 346.2
  due to
    loss, spinal fluid 349.0
    lumbar puncture 349.0
    saddle block 349.0
  emotional 307.81
  histamine 346.2
  lumbar puncture 349.0
  menopausal 627.2
  migraine 346.9
  nonorganic origin 307.81
  postspinal 349.0
  psychogenic 307.81
  psychophysiologic 307.81
  sick 346.1
  spinal 349.0
    complicating labor and delivery 668.8
    postpartum 668.8
  spinal fluid loss 349.0
  tension 307.81
  vascular 784.0
    migraine type 346.9
  vasomotor 346.9
Health
  advice V65.4
  audit V70.0
  checkup V70.0
  education V65.4
  hazard (*see also* History of) V15.9
    falling V15.88
    specified cause NEC V15.89
  instruction V65.4
  services provided because (of)
    boarding school residence V60.6
    holiday relief for person providing home care V60.5
    inadequate
      housing V60.1
      resources V60.2
    lack of housing V60.0
    no care available in home V60.4
    person living alone V60.3
    poverty V60.3
    residence in institution V60.6
    specified cause NEC V60.8
    vacation relief for person providing home care V60.5

Healthy
donor (*see also* Donor) V59.9
infant or child
accompanying sick mother V65.0
receiving care V20.1
person
accompanying sick relative V65.0
admitted for sterilization V25.2
receiving prophylactic inoculation or vaccination (*see also* Vaccination, prophylactic) V05.9
Hearing examination V72.19
following failed hearing screening V72.11
Heart - *see* condition
Heartburn 787.1
psychogenic 306.4
Heat (effects) 992.9
apoplexy 992.0
burn - *see also* Burn, by site
from sun (*see also* Sunburn) 692.71
collapse 992.1
cramps 992.2
dermatitis or eczema 692.89
edema 992.7
erythema - *see* Burn, by site
excessive 992.9
specified effect NEC 992.8
exhaustion 992.5
anhydrotic 992.3
due to
salt (and water) depletion 992.4
water depletion 992.3
fatigue (transient) 992.6
fever 992.0
hyperpyrexia 992.0
prickly 705.1
prostration - *see* Heat, exhaustion
pyrexia 992.0
rash 705.1
specified effect NEC 992.8
stroke 992.0
sunburn (*see also* Sunburn) 692.71
syncope 992.1
Heavy-chain disease 273.2
Heavy-for-dates (fetus or infant) 766.1
4500 grams or more 766.0
exceptionally 766.0
Hebephrenia, hebephrenic (acute) (*see also* Schizophrenia) 295.1
dementia (praecox) (*see also* Schizophrenia) 295.1
schizophrenia (*see also* Schizophrenia) 295.1
Heberden's
disease or nodes 715.04
syndrome (angina pectoris) 413.9
Hebra's disease
dermatitis exfoliativa 695.89
erythema multiforme exudativum 695.1
pityriasis 695.89
maculata et circinata 696.3
rubra 695.89
pilaris 696.4
prurigo 698.2
Hebra, nose 040.1
Hedinger's syndrome (malignant carcinoid) 259.2
Heel - *see* condition
Heerfordt's disease or syndrome (uveoparotitis) 135
Hegglin's anomaly or syndrome 288.2
Heidenhain's disease 290.10
with dementia 290.10
Heilmeyer-Schoner disease (M9842/3) 207.1
Heine-Medin disease (*see also* Poliomyelitis) 045.9
Heinz-body anemia, congenital 282.7
Heller's disease or syndrome (infantile psychosis) (*see also* Psychosis, childhood) 299.1
H.E.L.L.P. 642.5
Helminthiasis (*see also* Infestation, by specific parasite) 128.9
Ancylostoma (*see also* Ancylostoma) 126.9
intestinal 127.9
mixed types (types classifiable to more than one of the categories 120.0–127.7) 127.8
specified type 127.7
mixed types (intestinal) (types classifiable to more than one of the categories 120.0–127.7) 127.8
Necator americanus 126.1
specified type NEC 128.8
Trichinella 124
Heloma 700
Hemangioblastoma (M9161/1) - *see also* Neoplasm, connective tissue, uncertain behavior
malignant (M9161/3) - *see* Neoplasm, connective tissue, malignant
Hemangioblastomatosis, cerebelloretinal 759.6
Hemangioendothelioma (M9130/1) - *see also* Neoplasm, by site, uncertain behavior
benign (M9130/0) 228.00
bone (diffuse) (M9130/3) - *see* Neoplasm, bone, malignant
malignant (M9130/3) - *see* Neoplasm, connective tissue, malignant
nervous system (M9130/0) 228.09
Hemangioendotheliosarcoma (M9130/3) - *see* Neoplasm, connective tissue, malignant
Hemangiofibroma (M9160/0) - *see* Neoplasm, by site, benign
Hemangiolipoma (M8861/0) - *see* Lipoma
Hemangioma (M9120/0) 228.00
arteriovenous (M9123/0) - *see* Hemangioma, by site
brain 228.02
capillary (M9131/0) - *see* Hemangioma, by site
cavernous (M9121/0) - *see* Hemangioma, by site
central nervous system NEC 228.09
choroid 228.09
heart 228.09
infantile (M9131/0) - *see* Hemangioma, by site
intra-abdominal structures 228.04
intracranial structures 228.02
intramuscular (M9132/0) - *see* Hemangioma, by site
iris 228.09
juvenile (M9131/0) - *see* Hemangioma, by site
malignant (M9120/3) - *see* Neoplasm, connective tissue, malignant
meninges 228.09
brain 228.02
spinal cord 228.09
Hemangioma *(Continued)*
peritoneum 228.04
placenta - *see* Placenta, abnormal
plexiform (M9131/0) - *see* Hemangioma, by site
racemose (M9123/0) - *see* Hemangioma, by site
retina 228.03
retroperitoneal tissue 228.04
sclerosing (M8832/0) - *see* Neoplasm, skin, benign
simplex (M9131/0) - *see* Hemangioma, by site
skin and subcutaneous tissue 228.01
specified site NEC 228.09
spinal cord 228.09
venous (M9122/0) - *see* Hemangioma, by site
verrucous keratotic (M9142/0) - *see* Hemangioma, by site
Hemangiomatosis (systemic) 757.32
involving single site - *see* Hemangioma
Hemangiopericytoma (M9150/1) - *see also* Neoplasm, connective tissue, uncertain behavior
benign (M9150/0) - *see* Neoplasm, connective tissue, benign
malignant (M9150/3) - *see* Neoplasm, connective tissue, malignant
Hemangiosarcoma (M9120/3) - *see* Neoplasm, connective tissue, malignant
Hemarthrosis (nontraumatic) 719.10
ankle 719.17
elbow 719.12
foot 719.17
hand 719.14
hip 719.15
knee 719.16
multiple sites 719.19
pelvic region 719.15
shoulder (region) 719.11
specified site NEC 719.18
traumatic - *see* Sprain, by site
wrist 719.13
Hematemesis 578.0
with ulcer - *see* Ulcer, by site, with hemorrhage
due to S. japonicum 120.2
Goldstein's (familial hemorrhagic telangiectasia) 448.0
newborn 772.4
due to swallowed maternal blood 777.3
Hematidrosis 705.89
Hematinuria (*see also* Hemoglobinuria) 791.2
malarial 084.8
paroxysmal 283.2
Hematite miners' lung 503
Hematobilia 576.8
Hematocele (congenital) (diffuse) (idiopathic) 608.83
broad ligament 620.7
canal of Nuck 629.0
cord, male 608.83
fallopian tube 620.8
female NEC 629.0
ischiorectal 569.89
male NEC 608.83
ovary 629.0

Hematocele *(Continued)*
pelvis, pelvic
female 629.0
with ectopic pregnancy (*see also* Pregnancy, ectopic) 633.90
with intrauterine pregnancy 633.91
male 608.83
periuterine 629.0
retrouterine 629.0
scrotum 608.83
spermatic cord (diffuse) 608.83
testis 608.84
traumatic - *see* Injury, internal, pelvis
tunica vaginalis 608.83
uterine ligament 629.0
uterus 621.4
vagina 623.6
vulva 624.5
Hematocephalus 742.4
Hematochezia (*see also* Melena) 578.1
Hematochyluria (*see also* Infestation, filarial) 125.9
Hematocolpos 626.8
Hematocornea 371.12
Hematogenous - *see* condition
Hematoma (skin surface intact) (traumatic) - *see also* Contusion

Note Hematomas are coded according to origin and the nature and site of the hematoma or the accompanying injury. Hematomas of unspecified origin are coded as injuries of the sites involved, except:

(a) hematomas of genital organs which are coded as diseases of the organ involved unless they complicate pregnancy or delivery
(b) hematomas of the eye which are coded as diseases of the eye.

For late effect of hematoma classifiable to 920–924 *see* Late, effect, contusion.

with
crush injury - *see* Crush
fracture - *see* Fracture, by site
injury of internal organs - *see also* Injury, internal, by site
kidney - *see* Hematoma, kidney, traumatic
liver - *see* Hematoma, liver, traumatic
spleen - *see* Hematoma, spleen
nerve injury - *see* Injury, nerve
open wound - *see* Wound, open, by site
skin surface intact - *see* Contusion
abdomen (wall) - *see* Contusion, abdomen
amnion 658.8
aorta, dissecting 441.00
abdominal 441.02
thoracic 441.01
thoracoabdominal 441.03
arterial (complicating trauma) 904.9
specified site - *see* Injury, blood vessel, by site
auricle (ear) 380.31

Hematoma *(Continued)*
birth injury 767.8
skull 767.19
brain (traumatic) 853.0

Note Use the following fifth-digit subclassification with categories 851–854:

0 unspecified state of consciousness
1 with no loss of consciousness
2 with brief [less than one hour] loss of consciousness
3 with moderate [1–24 hours] loss of consciousness
4 with prolonged [more than 24 hours] loss of consciousness and return to pre-existing conscious level
5 with prolonged [more than 24 hours] loss of consciousness, without return to pre-existing conscious level

Use fifth-digit 5 to designate when a patient is unconscious and dies before regaining consciousness, regardless of the duration of the loss of consciousness

6 with loss of consciousness of unspecified duration
9 with concussion, unspecified

with
cerebral
contusion - *see* Contusion, brain
laceration - *see* Laceration, brain
open intracranial wound 853.1
skull fracture - *see* Fracture, skull, by site
extradural or epidural 852.4
with open intracranial wound 852.5
fetus or newborn 767.0
nontraumatic 432.0
fetus or newborn NEC 767.0
nontraumatic (*see also* Hemorrhage, brain) 431
epidural or extradural 432.0
newborn NEC 772.8
subarachnoid, arachnoid, or meningeal (*see also* Hemorrhage, subarachnoid) 430
subdural (*see also* Hemorrhage, subdural) 432.1
subarachnoid, arachnoid, or meningeal 852.0
with open intracranial wound 852.1
fetus or newborn 772.2
nontraumatic (*see also* Hemorrhage, subarachnoid) 430
subdural 852.2
with open intracranial wound 852.3
fetus or newborn (localized) 767.0
nontraumatic (*see also* Hemorrhage, subdural) 432.1
breast (nontraumatic) 611.8
broad ligament (nontraumatic) 620.7
complicating delivery 665.7
traumatic - *see* Injury, internal, broad ligament
calcified NEC 959.9
capitis 920
due to birth injury 767.19
newborn 767.19

Hematoma *(Continued)*
cerebral - *see* Hematoma, brain
cesarean section wound 674.3
chorion - *see* Placenta, abnormal
complicating delivery (perineum) (vulva) 664.5
pelvic 665.7
vagina 665.7
corpus
cavernosum (nontraumatic) 607.82
luteum (nontraumatic) (ruptured) 620.1
dura (mater) - *see* Hematoma, brain, subdural
epididymis (nontraumatic) 608.83
epidural (traumatic) - *see also* Hematoma, brain, extradural
spinal - *see* Injury, spinal, by site
episiotomy 674.3
external ear 380.31
extradural - *see also* Hematoma, brain, extradural
fetus or newborn 767.0
nontraumatic 432.0
fetus or newborn 767.0
fallopian tube 620.8
genital organ (nontraumatic)
female NEC 629.89
male NEC 608.83
traumatic (external site) 922.4
internal - *see* Injury, internal, genital organ
graafian follicle (ruptured) 620.0
internal organs (abdomen, chest, or pelvis) - *see also* Injury, internal, by site
kidney - *see* Hematoma, kidney, traumatic
liver - *see* Hematoma, liver, traumatic
spleen - *see* Hematoma, spleen
intracranial - *see* Hematoma, brain
kidney, cystic 593.81
traumatic 866.01
with open wound into cavity 866.11
labia (nontraumatic) 624.5
lingual (and other parts of neck, scalp, or face, except eye) 920
liver (subcapsular) 573.8
birth injury 767.8
fetus or newborn 767.8
traumatic NEC 864.01
with
laceration - *see* Laceration, liver
open wound into cavity 864.11
mediastinum - *see* Injury, internal, mediastinum
meninges, meningeal (brain) - *see also* Hematoma, brain, subarachnoid
spinal - *see* Injury, spinal, by site
mesosalpinx (nontraumatic) 620.8
traumatic - *see* Injury, internal, pelvis
muscle (traumatic) - *see* Contusion, by site
nasal (septum) (and other part(s) of neck, scalp, or face, except eye) 920
obstetrical surgical wound 674.3
orbit, orbital (nontraumatic) 376.32
traumatic 921.2
ovary (corpus luteum) (nontraumatic) 620.1
traumatic - *see* Injury, internal, ovary
pelvis (female) (nontraumatic) 629.89
complicating delivery 665.7
male 608.83

Hematoma *(Continued)*
pelvis *(Continued)*
traumatic - *see also* Injury, internal, pelvis
specified organ NEC (*see also* Injury, internal, pelvis) 867.6
penis (nontraumatic) 607.82
pericranial (and neck, or face any part, except eye) 920
due to injury at birth 767.19
perineal wound (obstetrical) 674.3
complicating delivery 664.5
perirenal, cystic 593.81
pinna 380.31
placenta - *see* Placenta, abnormal
postoperative 998.12
retroperitoneal (nontraumatic) 568.81
traumatic - *see* Injury, internal, retroperitoneum
retropubic, male 568.81
scalp (and neck, or face any part, except eye) 920
fetus or newborn 767.19
scrotum (nontraumatic) 608.83
traumatic 922.4
seminal vesicle (nontraumatic) 608.83
traumatic - *see* Injury, internal, seminal, vesicle
spermatic cord - *see also* Injury, internal, spermatic cord
nontraumatic 608.83
spinal (cord) (meninges) - *see also* Injury, spinal, by site
fetus or newborn 767.4
nontraumatic 336.1
spleen 865.01
with
laceration - *see* Laceration, spleen
open wound into cavity 865.11
sternocleidomastoid, birth injury 767.8
sternomastoid, birth injury 767.8
subarachnoid - *see also* Hematoma, brain, subarachnoid
fetus or newborn 772.2
nontraumatic (*see also* Hemorrhage, subarachnoid) 430
newborn 772.2
subdural - *see also* Hematoma, brain, subdural
fetus or newborn (localized) 767.0
nontraumatic (*see also* Hemorrhage, subdural) 432.1
subperiosteal (syndrome) 267
traumatic - *see* Hematoma, by site
superficial, fetus or newborn 772.6
syncytium - *see* Placenta, abnormal
testis (nontraumatic) 608.83
birth injury 767.8
traumatic 922.4
tunica vaginalis (nontraumatic) 608.83
umbilical cord 663.6
affecting fetus or newborn 762.6
uterine ligament (nontraumatic) 620.7
traumatic - *see* Injury, internal, pelvis
uterus 621.4
traumatic - *see* Injury, internal, pelvis
vagina (nontraumatic) (ruptured) 623.6
complicating delivery 665.7
traumatic 922.4
vas deferens (nontraumatic) 608.83
traumatic - *see* Injury, internal, vas deferens
vitreous 379.23
vocal cord 920

Hematoma *(Continued)*
vulva (nontraumatic) 624.5
complicating delivery 664.5
fetus or newborn 767.8
traumatic 922.4
Hematometra 621.4
Hematomyelia 336.1
with fracture of vertebra (*see also* Fracture, vertebra, by site, with spinal cord injury) 806.8
fetus or newborn 767.4
Hematomyelitis 323.9
late effect - *see* category 326
Hematoperitoneum (*see also* Hemoperitoneum) 568.81
Hematopneumothorax (*see also* Hemothorax) 511.8
Hematopoiesis, cyclic 288.02 ◀
Hematoporphyria (acquired) (congenital) 277.1
Hematoporphyrinuria (acquired) (congenital) 277.1
Hematorachis, hematorrhachis 336.1
fetus or newborn 767.4
Hematosalpinx 620.8
with
ectopic pregnancy (*see also* categories 633.0–633.9) 639.2
molar pregnancy (*see also* categories 630–632) 639.2
infectional (*see also* Salpingo-oophoritis) 614.2
Hematospermia 608.82
Hematothorax (*see also* Hemothorax) 511.8
Hematotympanum 381.03
Hematuria (benign) (essential) (idiopathic) 599.7
due to S. hematobium 120.0
endemic 120.0
intermittent 599.7
malarial 084.8
paroxysmal 599.7
sulfonamide
correct substance properly administered 599.7
overdose or wrong substance given or taken 961.0
tropical (bilharziasis) 120.0
tuberculous (*see also* Tuberculosis) 016.9
Hematuric bilious fever 084.8
Hemeralopia 368.10
Hemiabiotrophy 799.89
Hemi-akinesia 781.8
Hemianalgesia (*see also* Disturbance, sensation) 782.0
Hemianencephaly 740.0
Hemianesthesia (*see also* Disturbance, sensation) 782.0
Hemianopia, hemianopsia (altitudinal) (homonymous) 368.46
binasal 368.47
bitemporal 368.47
heteronymous 368.47
syphilitic 095.8
Hemiasomatognosia 307.9
Hemiathetosis 781.0
Hemiatrophy 799.89
cerebellar 334.8
face 349.89
progressive 349.89
fascia 728.9
leg 728.2
tongue 529.8
Hemiballism(us) 333.5
Hemiblock (cardiac) (heart) (left) 426.2

Hemicardia 746.89
Hemicephalus, hemicephaly 740.0
Hemichorea 333.5
Hemicrania 346.9
congenital malformation 740.0
Hemidystrophy - *see* Hemiatrophy
Hemiectromelia 755.4
Hemihypalgesia (*see also* Disturbance, sensation) 782.0
Hemihypertrophy (congenital) 759.89
cranial 756.0
Hemihypesthesia (*see also* Disturbance, sensation) 782.0
Hemi-inattention 781.8
Hemimelia 755.4
lower limb 755.30
paraxial (complete) (incomplete) (intercalary) (terminal) 755.32
fibula 755.37
tibia 755.36
transverse (complete) (partial) 755.31
upper limb 755.20
paraxial (complete) (incomplete) (intercalary) (terminal) 755.22
radial 755.26
ulnar 755.27
transverse (complete) (partial) 755.21
Hemiparalysis (*see also* Hemiplegia) 342.9
Hemiparesis (*see also* Hemiplegia) 342.9
Hemiparesthesia (*see also* Disturbance, sensation) 782.0
Hemiplegia 342.9
acute (*see also* Disease, cerebrovascular, acute) 436
alternans facialis 344.89
apoplectic (*see also* Disease, cerebrovascular, acute) 436
late effect or residual
affecting
dominant side 438.21
nondominant side 438.22
unspecified side 438.20
arteriosclerotic 437.0
late effect or residual
affecting
dominant side 438.21
nondominant side 438.22
unspecified side 438.20
ascending (spinal) NEC 344.89
attack (*see also* Disease, cerebrovascular, acute) 436
brain, cerebral (current episode) 437.8
congenital 343.1
cerebral - *see* Hemiplegia, brain
congenital (cerebral) (spastic) (spinal) 343.1
conversion neurosis (hysterical) 300.11
cortical - *see* Hemiplegia, brain
due to
arteriosclerosis 437.0
late effect or residual
affecting
dominant side 438.21
nondominant side 438.22
unspecified side 438.20
cerebrovascular lesion (*see also* Disease, cerebrovascular, acute) 436
late effect
affecting
dominant side 438.21
nondominant side 438.22
unspecified side 438.20

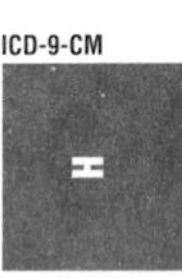

Hemiplegia *(Continued)*
  embolic (current) (*see also* Embolism, brain) 434.1
    late effect
      affecting
        dominant side 438.21
        nondominant side 438.22
        unspecified side 438.20
  flaccid 342.0
  hypertensive (current episode) 437.8
  infantile (postnatal) 343.4
  late effect
    birth injury, intracranial or spinal 343.4
    cerebrovascular lesion - *see* Late effect(s) (of) cerebrovascular disease
    viral encephalitis 139.0
  middle alternating NEC 344.89
  newborn NEC 767.0
  seizure (current episode) (*see also* Disease, cerebrovascular, acute) 436
  spastic 342.1
    congenital or infantile 343.1
  specified NEC 342.8
  thrombotic (current) (*see also* Thrombosis, brain) 434.0
    late effect - *see* Late effect(s) (of) cerebrovascular disease
Hemisection, spinal cord - *see* Fracture, vertebra, by site, with spinal cord injury
Hemispasm 781.0
  facial 781.0
Hemispatial neglect 781.8
Hemisporosis 117.9
Hemitremor 781.0
Hemivertebra 756.14
Hemobilia 576.8
Hemocholecyst 575.8
Hemochromatosis (acquired) (diabetic) (hereditary) (liver) (myocardium) (primary idiopathic) (secondary) 275.0
  with refractory anemia 238.72 ⟸
Hemodialysis V56.0
Hemoglobin - *see also* condition
  abnormal (disease) - *see* Disease, hemoglobin
  AS genotype 282.5
  fetal, hereditary persistence 282.7
  high-oxygen-affinity 289.0
  low NEC 285.9
  S (Hb-S), heterozygous 282.5
Hemoglobinemia 283.2
  due to blood transfusion NEC 999.8
    bone marrow 996.85
  paroxysmal 283.2
Hemoglobinopathy (mixed) (*see also* Disease, hemoglobin) 282.7
  with thalassemia 282.49
  sickle-cell 282.60
    with thalassemia (without crisis) 282.41
      with
        crisis 282.42
        vaso-occlusive pain 282.42
Hemoglobinuria, hemoglobinuric 791.2
  with anemia, hemolytic, acquired (chronic) NEC 283.2
  cold (agglutinin) (paroxysmal) (with Raynaud's syndrome) 283.2
  due to
    exertion 283.2
    hemolysis (from external causes) NEC 283.2
Hemoglobinuria, hemoglobinuric *(Continued)*
  exercise 283.2
  fever (malaria) 084.8
  infantile 791.2
  intermittent 283.2
  malarial 084.8
  march 283.2
  nocturnal (paroxysmal) 283.2
  paroxysmal (cold) (nocturnal) 283.2
Hemolymphangioma (M9175/0) 228.1
Hemolysis
  fetal - *see* Jaundice, fetus or newborn
  intravascular (disseminated) NEC 286.6
    with
      abortion - *see* Abortion, by type, with hemorrhage, delayed or excessive
      ectopic pregnancy (*see also* categories 633.0–633.9) 639.1
      hemorrhage of pregnancy 641.3
        affecting fetus or newborn 762.1
      molar pregnancy (*see also* categories 630–632) 639.1
    acute 283.2
    following
      abortion 639.1
      ectopic or molar pregnancy 639.1
  neonatal - *see* Jaundice, fetus or newborn
  transfusion NEC 999.8
    bone marrow 996.85
Hemolytic - *see also* condition
  anemia - *see* Anemia, hemolytic
  uremic syndrome 283.11
Hemometra 621.4
Hemopericardium (with effusion) 423.0
  newborn 772.8
  traumatic (*see also* Hemothorax, traumatic) 860.2
    with open wound into thorax 860.3
Hemoperitoneum 568.81
  infectional (*see also* Peritonitis) 567.29
  traumatic - *see* Injury, internal, peritoneum
Hemophagocytic syndrome 288.4 ◄
  infection-associated 288.4 ◄
Hemophilia (familial) (hereditary) 286.0
  A 286.0
    carrier (asymptomatic) V83.01
      symptomatic V83.02
  acquired 286.5
  B (Leyden) 286.1
  C 286.2
  calcipriva (*see also* Fibrinolysis) 286.7
  classical 286.0
  nonfamilial 286.7
  secondary 286.5
  vascular 286.4
Hemophilus influenzae NEC 041.5
  arachnoiditis (basic) (brain) (spinal) 320.0
    late effect - *see* category 326
  bronchopneumonia 482.2
  cerebral ventriculitis 320.0
    late effect - *see* category 326
  cerebrospinal inflammation 320.0
    late effect - *see* category 326
  infection NEC 041.5
  leptomeningitis 320.0
    late effect - *see* category 326
  meningitis (cerebral) (cerebrospinal) (spinal) 320.0
    late effect - *see* category 326
  meningomyelitis 320.0
    late effect - *see* category 326
Hemophilus influenzae NEC *(Continued)*
  pachymeningitis (adhesive) (fibrous) (hemorrhagic) (hypertrophic) (spinal) 320.0
    late effect - *see* category 326
  pneumonia (broncho-) 482.2
Hemophthalmos 360.43
Hemopneumothorax (*see also* Hemothorax) 511.8
  traumatic 860.4
    with open wound into thorax 860.5
Hemoptysis 786.3
  due to Paragonimus (westermani) 121.2
  newborn 770.3
  tuberculous (*see also* Tuberculosis, pulmonary) 011.9
Hemorrhage, hemorrhagic (nontraumatic) 459.0
  abdomen 459.0
  accidental (antepartum) 641.2
    affecting fetus or newborn 762.1
  adenoid 474.8
  adrenal (capsule) (gland) (medulla) 255.4
    newborn 772.5
  after labor - *see* Hemorrhage, postpartum
  alveolar
    lung, newborn 770.3
    process 525.8
  alveolus 525.8
  amputation stump (surgical) 998.11
    secondary, delayed 997.69
  anemia (chronic) 280.0
    acute 285.1
  antepartum - *see* Hemorrhage, pregnancy
  anus (sphincter) 569.3
  apoplexy (stroke) 432.9
  arachnoid - *see* Hemorrhage, subarachnoid
  artery NEC 459.0
    brain (*see also* Hemorrhage, brain) 431
    middle meningeal - *see* Hemorrhage, subarachnoid
  basilar (ganglion) (*see also* Hemorrhage, brain) 431
  bladder 596.8
  blood dyscrasia 289.9
  bowel 578.9
    newborn 772.4
  brain (miliary) (nontraumatic) 431
    with
      birth injury 767.0
    arachnoid - *see* Hemorrhage, subarachnoid
    due to
      birth injury 767.0
      rupture of aneurysm (congenital) (*see also* Hemorrhage, subarachnoid) 430
        mycotic 431
      syphilis 094.89
    epidural or extradural - *see* Hemorrhage, extradural
    fetus or newborn (anoxic) (hypoxic) (due to birth trauma) (nontraumatic) 767.0
      intraventricular 772.10
        grade I 772.11
        grade II 772.12
        grade III 772.13
        grade IV 772.14
    iatrogenic 997.02

Hemorrhage, hemorrhagic *(Continued)*
brain *(Continued)*
postoperative 997.02
puerperal, postpartum, childbirth 674.0
stem 431
subarachnoid, arachnoid, or meningeal - *see* Hemorrhage, subarachnoid
subdural - *see* Hemorrhage, subdural
traumatic NEC 853.0

Note Use the following fifth-digit subclassification with categories 851–854:

0 unspecified state of consciousness
1 with no loss of consciousness
2 with brief [less than one hour] loss of consciousness
3 with moderate [1–24 hours] loss of consciousness
4 with prolonged [more than 24 hours] loss of consciousness and return to pre-existing conscious level
5 with prolonged [more than 24 hours] loss of consciousness, without return to pre-existing conscious level

Use fifth-digit 5 to designate when a patient is unconscious and dies before regaining consciousness, regardless of the duration of the loss of consciousness

6 with loss of consciousness of unspecified duration
9 with concussion, unspecified

with
cerebral
contusion - *see* Contusion, brain
laceration - *see* Laceration, brain
open intracranial wound 853.1
skull fracture - *see* Fracture, skull, by site
extradural or epidural 852.4
with open intracranial wound 852.5
subarachnoid 852.0
with open intracranial wound 852.1
subdural 852.2
with open intracranial wound 852.3
breast 611.79
bronchial tube - *see* Hemorrhage, lung
bronchopulmonary - *see* Hemorrhage, lung
bronchus (cause unknown) (*see also* Hemorrhage, lung) 786.3
bulbar (*see also* Hemorrhage, brain) 431
bursa 727.89
capillary 448.9
primary 287.8
capsular - *see* Hemorrhage, brain
cardiovascular 429.89
cecum 578.9
cephalic (*see also* Hemorrhage, brain) 431
cerebellar (*see also* Hemorrhage, brain) 431

Hemorrhage, hemorrhagic *(Continued)*
cerebellum (*see also* Hemorrhage, brain) 431
cerebral (*see also* Hemorrhage, brain) 431
fetus or newborn (anoxic) (traumatic) 767.0
cerebromeningeal (*see also* Hemorrhage, brain) 431
cerebrospinal (*see also* Hemorrhage, brain) 431
cerebrovascular accident - *see* Hemorrhage, brain
cerebrum (*see also* Hemorrhage, brain) 431
cervix (stump) (uteri) 622.8
cesarean section wound 674.3
chamber, anterior (eye) 364.41
childbirth - *see* Hemorrhage, complicating, delivery
choroid 363.61
expulsive 363.62
ciliary body 364.41
cochlea 386.8
colon - *see* Hemorrhage, intestine
complicating
delivery 641.9
affecting fetus or newborn 762.1
associated with
afibrinogenemia 641.3
affecting fetus or newborn 763.89
coagulation defect 641.3
affecting fetus or newborn 763.89
hyperfibrinolysis 641.3
affecting fetus or newborn 763.89
hypofibrinogenemia 641.3
affecting fetus or newborn 763.89
due to
low-lying placenta 641.1
affecting fetus or newborn 762.0
placenta previa 641.1
affecting fetus or newborn 762.0
premature separation of placenta 641.2
affecting fetus or newborn 762.1
retained
placenta 666.0
secundines 666.2
trauma 641.8
affecting fetus or newborn 763.89
uterine leiomyoma 641.8
affecting fetus or newborn 763.89
surgical procedure 998.11
concealed NEC 459.0
congenital 772.9
conjunctiva 372.72
newborn 772.8
cord, newborn 772.0
slipped ligature 772.3
stump 772.3
corpus luteum (ruptured) 620.1
cortical (*see also* Hemorrhage, brain) 431
cranial 432.9
cutaneous 782.7
newborn 772.6

Hemorrhage, hemorrhagic *(Continued)*
cyst, pancreas 577.2
cystitis - *see* Cystitis
delayed
with
abortion - *see* Abortion, by type, with hemorrhage, delayed or excessive
ectopic pregnancy (*see also* categories 633.0–633.9) 639.1
molar pregnancy (*see also* categories 630–632) 639.1
following
abortion 639.1
ectopic or molar pregnancy 639.1
postpartum 666.2
diathesis (familial) 287.9
newborn 776.0
disease 287.9
newborn 776.0
specified type NEC 287.8
disorder 287.9
due to intrinsic circulating anticoagulants 286.5
specified type NEC 287.8
due to
any device, implant, or graft (presence of) classifiable to 996.0–996.5 - *see* Complications, due to (presence of) any device, implant, or graft classified to 996.0–996.5 NEC
intrinsic circulating anticoagulant 286.5
duodenum, duodenal 537.89
ulcer - *see* Ulcer, duodenum, with hemorrhage
dura mater - *see* Hemorrhage, subdural
endotracheal - *see* Hemorrhage, lung
epicranial subaponeurotic (massive) 767.11
epidural - *see* Hemorrhage, extradural
episiotomy 674.3
esophagus 530.82
varix (*see also* Varix, esophagus, bleeding) 456.0
excessive
with
abortion - *see* Abortion, by type, with hemorrhage, delayed or excessive
ectopic pregnancy (*see also* categories 633.0–633.9) 639.1
molar pregnancy (*see also* categories 630–632) 639.1
following
abortion 639.1
ectopic or molar pregnancy 639.1
external 459.0
extradural (traumatic) - *see also* Hemorrhage, brain, traumatic, extradural
birth injury 767.0
fetus or newborn (anoxic) (traumatic) 767.0
nontraumatic 432.0
eye 360.43
chamber (anterior) (aqueous) 364.41
fundus 362.81
eyelid 374.81
fallopian tube 620.8
fetomaternal 772.0
affecting management of pregnancy or puerperium 656.0

Hemorrhage, hemorrhagic *(Continued)*
fetus, fetal 772.0
from
cut end of co-twin's cord 772.0
placenta 772.0
ruptured cord 772.0
vasa previa 772.0
into
co-twin 772.0
mother's circulation 772.0
affecting management of pregnancy or puerperium 656.0
fever (*see also* Fever, hemorrhagic) 065.9
with renal syndrome 078.6
arthropod-borne NEC 065.9
Bangkok 065.4
Crimean 065.0
dengue virus 065.4
epidemic 078.6
Junin virus 078.7
Korean 078.6
Machupo virus 078.7
mite-borne 065.8
mosquito-borne 065.4
Philippine 065.4
Russian (Yaroslav) 078.6
Singapore 065.4
Southeast Asia 065.4
Thailand 065.4
tick-borne NEC 065.3
fibrinogenolysis (*see also* Fibrinolysis) 286.6
fibrinolytic (acquired) (*see also* Fibrinolysis) 286.6
fontanel 767.19
from tracheostomy stoma 519.09
fundus, eye 362.81
funis
affecting fetus or newborn 772.0
complicating delivery 663.8
gastric (*see also* Hemorrhage, stomach) 578.9
gastroenteric 578.9
newborn 772.4
gastrointestinal (tract) 578.9
newborn 772.4
genitourinary (tract) NEC 599.89
gingiva 523.8
globe 360.43
gravidarum - *see* Hemorrhage, pregnancy
gum 523.8
heart 429.89
hypopharyngeal (throat) 784.8
intermenstrual 626.6
irregular 626.6
regular 626.5
internal (organs) 459.0
capsule (*see also* Hemorrhage brain) 431
ear 386.8
newborn 772.8
intestine 578.9
congenital 772.4
newborn 772.4
into
bladder wall 596.7
bursa 727.89
corpus luysii (*see also* Hemorrhage, brain) 431
intra-abdominal 459.0
during or following surgery 998.11

Hemorrhage, hemorrhagic *(Continued)*
intra-alveolar, newborn (lung) 770.3
intracerebral (*see also* Hemorrhage, brain) 431
intracranial NEC 432.9
puerperal, postpartum, childbirth 674.0
traumatic - *see* Hemorrhage, brain, traumatic
intramedullary NEC 336.1
intraocular 360.43
intraoperative 998.11
intrapartum - *see* Hemorrhage, complicating, delivery
intrapelvic
female 629.89 (Revised)
male 459.0
intraperitoneal 459.0
intrapontine (*see also* Hemorrhage, brain) 431
intrauterine 621.4
complicating delivery - *see* Hemorrhage, complicating, delivery
in pregnancy or childbirth - *see* Hemorrhage, pregnancy
postpartum (*see also* Hemorrhage, postpartum) 666.1
intraventricular (*see also* Hemorrhage, brain) 431
fetus or newborn (anoxic) (traumatic) 772.10
grade I 772.11
grade II 772.12
grade III 772.13
grade IV 772.14
intravesical 596.7
iris (postinfectional) (postinflammatory) (toxic) 364.41
joint (nontraumatic) 719.10
ankle 719.17
elbow 719.12
foot 719.17
forearm 719.13
hand 719.14
hip 719.15
knee 719.16
lower leg 719.16
multiple sites 719.19
pelvic region 719.15
shoulder (region) 719.11
specified site NEC 719.18
thigh 719.15
upper arm 719.12
wrist 719.13
kidney 593.81
knee (joint) 719.16
labyrinth 386.8
leg NEC 459.0
lenticular striate artery (*see also* Hemorrhage, brain) 431
ligature, vessel 998.11
liver 573.8
lower extremity NEC 459.0
lung 786.3
newborn 770.3
tuberculous (*see also* Tuberculosis, pulmonary) 011.9
malaria 084.8
marginal sinus 641.2
massive subaponeurotic, birth injury 767.11
maternal, affecting fetus or newborn 762.1
mediastinum 786.3

Hemorrhage, hemorrhagic *(Continued)*
medulla (*see also* Hemorrhage, brain) 431
membrane (brain) (*see also* Hemorrhage, subarachnoid) 430
spinal cord - *see* Hemorrhage, spinal cord
meninges, meningeal (brain) (middle) (*see also* Hemorrhage, subarachnoid) 430
spinal cord - *see* Hemorrhage, spinal cord
mesentery 568.81
metritis 626.8
midbrain (*see also* Hemorrhage, brain) 431
mole 631
mouth 528.9
mucous membrane NEC 459.0
newborn 772.8
muscle 728.89
nail (subungual) 703.8
nasal turbinate 784.7
newborn 772.8
nasopharynx 478.29
navel, newborn 772.3
newborn 772.9
adrenal 772.5
alveolar (lung) 770.3
brain (anoxic) (hypoxic) (due to birth trauma) 767.0
cerebral (anoxic) (hypoxic) (due to birth trauma) 767.0
conjunctiva 772.8
cutaneous 772.6
diathesis 776.0
due to vitamin K deficiency 776.0
epicranial subaponeurotic (massive) 767.11
gastrointestinal 772.4
internal (organs) 772.8
intestines 772.4
intra-alveolar (lung) 770.3
intracranial (from any perinatal cause) 767.0
intraventricular (from any perinatal cause) 772.10
grade I 772.11
grade II 772.12
grade III 772.13
grade IV 772.14
lung 770.3
pulmonary (massive) 770.3
spinal cord, traumatic 767.4
stomach 772.4
subaponeurotic (massive) 767.11
subarachnoid (from any perinatal cause) 772.2
subconjunctival 772.8
subgaleal 767.11
umbilicus 772.0
slipped ligature 772.3
vasa previa 772.0
nipple 611.79
nose 784.7
newborn 772.8
obstetrical surgical wound 674.3
omentum 568.89
newborn 772.4
optic nerve (sheath) 377.42
orbit 376.32
ovary 620.1
oviduct 620.8
pancreas 577.8

Hemorrhage, hemorrhagic *(Continued)*
parathyroid (gland) (spontaneous) 252.8
parturition - *see* Hemorrhage, complicating, delivery
penis 607.82
pericardium, pericarditis 423.0
perineal wound (obstetrical) 674.3
peritoneum, peritoneal 459.0
peritonsillar tissue 474.8
after operation on tonsils 998.11
due to infection 475
petechial 782.7
pituitary (gland) 253.8
placenta NEC 641.9
affecting fetus or newborn 762.1
from surgical or instrumental damage 641.8
affecting fetus or newborn 762.1
previa 641.1
affecting fetus or newborn 762.0
pleura - *see* Hemorrhage, lung
polioencephalitis, superior 265.1
polymyositis - *see* Polymyositis
pons (*see also* Hemorrhage, brain) 431
pontine (*see also* Hemorrhage, brain) 431
popliteal 459.0
postcoital 626.7
postextraction (dental) 998.11
postmenopausal 627.1
postnasal 784.7
postoperative 998.11
postpartum (atonic) (following delivery of placenta) 666.1
delayed or secondary (after 24 hours) 666.2
retained placenta 666.0
third stage 666.0
pregnancy (concealed) 641.9
accidental 641.2
affecting fetus or newborn 762.1
affecting fetus or newborn 762.1
before 22 completed weeks' gestation 640.9
affecting fetus or newborn 762.1
due to
abruptio placentae 641.2
affecting fetus or newborn 762.1
afibrinogenemia or other coagulation defect (conditions classifiable to 286.0–286.9) 641.3
affecting fetus or newborn 762.1
coagulation defect 641.3
affecting fetus or newborn 762.1
hyperfibrinolysis 641.3
affecting fetus or newborn 762.1
hypofibrinogenemia 641.3
affecting fetus or newborn 762.1
leiomyoma, uterus 641.8
affecting fetus or newborn 762.1
low-lying placenta 641.1
affecting fetus or newborn 762.1
marginal sinus (rupture) 641.2
affecting fetus or newborn 762.1
placenta previa 641.1
affecting fetus or newborn 762.0
premature separation of placenta (normally implanted) 641.2
affecting fetus or newborn 762.1
threatened abortion 640.0
affecting fetus or newborn 762.1

Hemorrhage, hemorrhagic *(Continued)*
pregnancy *(Continued)*
due to *(Continued)*
trauma 641.8
affecting fetus or newborn 762.1
early (before 22 completed weeks' gestation) 640.9
affecting fetus or newborn 762.1
previous, affecting management of pregnancy or childbirth V23.49
unavoidable - *see* Hemorrhage, pregnancy, due to placenta previa
prepartum (mother) - *see* Hemorrhage, pregnancy
preretinal, cause unspecified 362.81
prostate 602.1
puerperal (*see also* Hemorrhage, postpartum) 666.1
pulmonary - *see also* Hemorrhage, lung
newborn (massive) 770.3
renal syndrome 446.21
purpura (primary) (*see also* Purpura, thrombocytopenic) 287.39
rectum (sphincter) 569.3
recurring, following initial hemorrhage at time of injury 958.2
renal 593.81
pulmonary syndrome 446.21
respiratory tract (*see also* Hemorrhage, lung) 786.3
retina, retinal (deep) (superficial) (vessels) 362.81
diabetic 250.5 *[362.01]*
due to birth injury 772.8
retrobulbar 376.89
retroperitoneal 459.0
retroplacental (*see also* Placenta, separation) 641.2
scalp 459.0
due to injury at birth 767.19
scrotum 608.83
secondary (nontraumatic) 459.0
following initial hemorrhage at time of injury 958.2
seminal vesicle 608.83
skin 782.7
newborn 772.6
spermatic cord 608.83
spinal (cord) 336.1
aneurysm (ruptured) 336.1
syphilitic 094.89
due to birth injury 767.4
fetus or newborn 767.4
spleen 289.59
spontaneous NEC 459.0
petechial 782.7
stomach 578.9
newborn 772.4
ulcer - *see* Ulcer, stomach, with hemorrhage
subaponeurotic, newborn 767.11
massive (birth injury) 767.11
subarachnoid (nontraumatic) 430
fetus or newborn (anoxic) (traumatic) 772.2
puerperal, postpartum, childbirth 674.0
traumatic - *see* Hemorrhage, brain, traumatic, subarachnoid
subconjunctival 372.72
due to birth injury 772.8
newborn 772.8
subcortical (*see also* Hemorrhage, brain) 431

Hemorrhage, hemorrhagic *(Continued)*
subcutaneous 782.7
subdiaphragmatic 459.0
subdural (nontraumatic) 432.1
due to birth injury 767.0
fetus or newborn (anoxic) (hypoxic) (due to birth trauma) 767.0
puerperal, postpartum, childbirth 674.0
spinal 336.1
traumatic - *see* Hemorrhage, brain, traumatic, subdural
subgaleal 767.11
subhyaloid 362.81
subperiosteal 733.99
subretinal 362.81
subtentorial (*see also* Hemorrhage, subdural) 432.1
subungual 703.8
due to blood dyscrasia 287.8
suprarenal (capsule) (gland) 255.4
fetus or newborn 772.5
tentorium (traumatic) - *see also* Hemorrhage, brain, traumatic
fetus or newborn 767.0
nontraumatic - *see* Hemorrhage, subdural
testis 608.83
thigh 459.0
third stage 666.0
thorax - *see* Hemorrhage, lung
throat 784.8
thrombocythemia 238.71 ⇐
thymus (gland) 254.8
thyroid (gland) 246.3
cyst 246.3
tongue 529.8
tonsil 474.8
postoperative 998.11
tooth socket (postextraction) 998.11
trachea - *see* Hemorrhage, lung
traumatic - *see also* nature of injury
brain - *see* Hemorrhage, brain, traumatic
recurring or secondary (following initial hemorrhage at time of injury) 958.2
tuberculous NEC (*see also* Tuberculosis, pulmonary) 011.9
tunica vaginalis 608.83
ulcer - *see* Ulcer, by site, with hemorrhage
umbilicus, umbilical cord 772.0
after birth, newborn 772.3
complicating delivery 663.8
affecting fetus or newborn 772.0
slipped ligature 772.3
stump 772.3
unavoidable (due to placenta previa) 641.1
affecting fetus or newborn 762.0
upper extremity 459.0
urethra (idiopathic) 599.84
uterus, uterine (abnormal) 626.9
climacteric 627.0
complicating delivery - *see* Hemorrhage, complicating, delivery
due to
intrauterine contraceptive device 996.76
perforating uterus 996.32
functional or dysfunctional 626.8
in pregnancy - *see* Hemorrhage, pregnancy

Hemorrhage, hemorrhagic *(Continued)*
uterus, uterine *(Continued)*
intermenstrual 626.6
irregular 626.6
regular 626.5
postmenopausal 627.1
postpartum (*see also* Hemorrhage, postpartum) 666.1
prepubertal 626.8
pubertal 626.3
puerperal (immediate) 666.1
vagina 623.8
vasa previa 663.5
affecting fetus or newborn 772.0
vas deferens 608.83
ventricular (*see also* Hemorrhage, brain) 431
vesical 596.8
viscera 459.0
newborn 772.8
vitreous (humor) (intraocular) 379.23
vocal cord 478.5
vulva 624.8
Hemorrhoids (anus) (rectum) (without complication) 455.6
bleeding, prolapsed, strangulated, or ulcerated NEC 455.8
external 455.5
internal 455.2
complicated NEC 455.8
complicating pregnancy and puerperium 671.8
external 455.3
with complication NEC 455.5
bleeding, prolapsed, strangulated, or ulcerated 455.5
thrombosed 455.4
internal 455.0
with complication NEC 455.2
bleeding, prolapsed, strangulated, or ulcerated 455.2
thrombosed 455.1
residual skin tag 455.9
sentinel pile 455.9
thrombosed NEC 455.7
external 455.4
internal 455.1
Hemosalpinx 620.8
Hemosiderosis 275.0
dietary 275.0
pulmonary (idiopathic) 275.0 *[516.1]*
transfusion NEC 999.8
bone marrow 996.85
Hemospermia 608.82
Hemothorax 511.8
bacterial, nontuberculous 511.1
newborn 772.8
nontuberculous 511.8
bacterial 511.1
pneumococcal 511.1
postoperative 998.11
staphylococcal 511.1
streptococcal 511.1
traumatic 860.2
with
open wound into thorax 860.3
pneumothorax 860.4
with open wound into thorax 860.5
tuberculous (*see also* Tuberculosis, pleura) 012.0
Hemotympanum 385.89
Hench-Rosenberg syndrome (palindromic arthritis) (*see also* Rheumatism, palindromic) 719.3
Henle's warts 371.41
Henoch (-Schönlein)
disease or syndrome (allergic purpura) 287.0
purpura (allergic) 287.0
Henpue, henpuye 102.6
Heparitinuria 277.5
Hepar lobatum 095.3
Hepatalgia 573.8
Hepatic - *see* also condition
flexure syndrome 569.89
Hepatitis 573.3
acute (*see also* Necrosis, liver) 570
alcoholic 571.1
infective 070.1
with hepatic coma 070.0
alcoholic 571.1
amebic - *see* Abscess, liver, amebic
anicteric (acute) - *see* Hepatitis, viral
antigen-associated (HAA) - *see* Hepatitis, viral, type B
Australian antigen (positive) - *see* Hepatitis, viral, type B
autoimmune 571.49 ◀
catarrhal (acute) 070.1
with hepatic coma 070.0
chronic 571.40
newborn 070.1
with hepatic coma 070.0
chemical 573.3
cholangiolitic 573.8
cholestatic 573.8
chronic 571.40
active 571.49
viral - *see* Hepatitis, viral
aggressive 571.49
persistent 571.41
viral - *see* Hepatitis, viral
cytomegalic inclusion virus 078.5 *[573.1]*
diffuse 573.3
"dirty needle" - *see* Hepatitis, viral
drug-induced 573.3
due to
Coxsackie 074.8 *[573.1]*
cytomegalic inclusion virus 078.5 *[573.1]*
infectious mononucleosis 075 *[573.1]*
malaria 084.9 *[573.2]*
mumps 072.71
secondary syphilis 091.62
toxoplasmosis (acquired) 130.5
congenital (active) 771.2
epidemic - *see* Hepatitis, viral, type A
fetus or newborn 774.4
fibrous (chronic) 571.49
acute 570
from injection, inoculation, or transfusion (blood) (other substance) (plasma) (serum) (onset within 8 months after administration) - *see* Hepatitis, viral
fulminant (viral) (*see also* Hepatitis, viral) 070.9
with hepatic coma 070.6
type A 070.1
with hepatic coma 070.0
type B - *see* Hepatitis, viral, type B
giant cell (neonatal) 774.4
hemorrhagic 573.8
due to adhesion with obstruction 560.81
Hepatitis *(Continued)*
history of
B V12.09
C V12.09
homologous serum - *see* Hepatitis, viral
hypertrophic (chronic) 571.49
acute 570
infectious, infective (acute) (chronic) (subacute) 070.1
with hepatic coma 070.0
inoculation - *see* Hepatitis, viral
interstitial (chronic) 571.49
acute 570
lupoid 571.49
malarial 084.9 *[573.2]*
malignant (*see also* Necrosis, liver) 570
neonatal (toxic) 774.4
newborn 774.4
parenchymatous (acute) (*see also* Necrosis, liver) 570
peliosis 573.3
persistent, chronic 571.41
plasma cell 571.49
postimmunization - *see* Hepatitis, viral
postnecrotic 571.49
posttransfusion - *see* Hepatitis, viral
recurrent 571.49
septic 573.3
serum - *see* Hepatitis, viral
carrier (suspected of) V02.61
subacute (*see also* Necrosis, liver) 570
suppurative (diffuse) 572.0
syphilitic (late) 095.3
congenital (early) 090.0 *[573.2]*
late 090.5 *[573.2]*
secondary 091.62
toxic (noninfectious) 573.3
fetus or newborn 774.4
tuberculous (*see also* Tuberculosis) 017.9
viral (acute) (anicteric) (cholangiolitic) (cholestatic) (chronic) (subacute) 070.9
with hepatic coma 070.6
AU-SH type virus - *see* Hepatitis, viral, type B
Australia antigen - *see* Hepatitis, viral, type B
B-antigen - *see* Hepatitis, viral, type B
Coxsackie 074.8 *[573.1]*
cytomegalic inclusion 078.5 *[573.1]*
IH (virus) - *see* Hepatitis, viral, type A
infectious hepatitis virus - *see* Hepatitis, viral, type A
serum hepatitis virus - *see* Hepatitis, viral, type B
SH - *see* Hepatitis, viral, type B
specified type NEC 070.59
with hepatic coma 070.49
type A 070.1
with hepatic coma 070.0
type B (acute) 070.30
with
hepatic coma 070.20
carrier status V02.61
chronic 070.32
with
hepatic coma 070.22
with hepatitis delta 070.23
hepatitis delta 070.33
with hepatic coma 070.23
with hepatitis delta 070.21
hepatitis delta 070.31
with hepatic coma 070.21

Hepatitis *(Continued)*
viral *(Continued)*
type C
acute 070.51
with hepatic coma 070.41
carrier status V02.62
chronic 070.54
with hepatic coma 070.44
in remission 070.54 ◀
unspecified 070.70
with hepatic coma 070.71
type delta (with hepatitis B carrier state) 070.52
with
active hepatitis B disease - *see* Hepatitis, viral, type B
hepatic coma 070.42
type E 070.53
with hepatic coma 070.43
vaccination and inoculation (prophylactic) V05.3
Waldenström's (lupoid hepatitis) 571.49
Hepatization, lung (acute) - *see also* Pneumonia, lobar
chronic (*see also* Fibrosis, lung) 515
Hepatoblastoma (M8970/3) 155.0
Hepatocarcinoma (M8170/3) 155.0
Hepatocholangiocarcinoma (M8180/3) 155.0
Hepatocholangioma, benign (M8180/0) 211.5
Hepatocholangitis 573.8
Hepatocystitis (*see also* Cholecystitis) 575.10
Hepatodystrophy 570
Hepatolenticular degeneration 275.1
Hepatolithiasis - *see* Choledocholithiasis
Hepatoma (malignant) (M8170/3) 155.0
benign (M8170/0) 211.5
congenital (M8970/3) 155.0
embryonal (M8970/3) 155.0
Hepatomegalia glycogenica diffusa 271.0
Hepatomegaly (*see also* Hypertrophy, liver) 789.1
congenital 751.69
syphilitic 090.0
due to Clonorchis sinensis 121.1
Gaucher's 272.7
syphilitic (congenital) 090.0
Hepatoptosis 573.8
Hepatorrhexis 573.8
Hepatosis, toxic 573.8
Hepatosplenomegaly 571.8
due to S. japonicum 120.2
hyperlipemic (Burger-Grutz type) 272.3
Herald patch 696.3
Hereditary - *see* condition
Heredodegeneration 330.9
macular 362.70
Heredopathia atactica polyneuritiformis 356.3
Heredosyphilis (*see also* Syphilis, congenital) 090.9
Hermaphroditism (true) 752.7
with specified chromosomal anomaly - *see* Anomaly, chromosomes, sex
Hernia, hernial (acquired) (recurrent) 553.9
with
gangrene (obstructed) NEC 551.9
obstruction NEC 552.9
and gangrene 551.9

Hernia, hernial *(Continued)*
abdomen (wall) - *see* Hernia, ventral
abdominal, specified site NEC 553.8
with
gangrene (obstructed) 551.8
obstruction 552.8
and gangrene 551.8
appendix 553.8
with
gangrene (obstructed) 551.8
obstruction 552.8
and gangrene 551.8
bilateral (inguinal) - *see* Hernia, inguinal
bladder (sphincter)
congenital (female) (male) 756.71
female (*see also* Cystocele, female) 618.01
male 596.8
brain 348.4
congenital 742.0
broad ligament 553.8
cartilage, vertebral - *see* Displacement, intervertebral disc
cerebral 348.4
congenital 742.0
endaural 742.0
ciliary body 364.8
traumatic 871.1
colic 553.9
with
gangrene (obstructed) 551.9
obstruction 552.9
and gangrene 551.9
colon 553.9
with
gangrene (obstructed) 551.9
obstruction 552.9
and gangrene 551.9
colostomy (stoma) 569.69
Cooper's (retroperitoneal) 553.8
with
gangrene (obstructed) 551.8
obstruction 552.8
and gangrene 551.8
crural - *see* Hernia, femoral
diaphragm, diaphragmatic 553.3
with
gangrene (obstructed) 551.3
obstruction 552.3
and gangrene 551.3
congenital 756.6
due to gross defect of diaphragm 756.6
traumatic 862.0
with open wound into cavity 862.1
direct (inguinal) - *see* Hernia, inguinal
disc, intervertebral - *see* Displacement, intervertebral disc
diverticulum, intestine 553.9
with
gangrene (obstructed) 551.9
obstruction 552.9
and gangrene 551.9
double (inguinal) - *see* Hernia, inguinal
due to adhesion with obstruction 560.81
duodenojejunal 553.8
with
gangrene (obstructed) 551.8
obstruction 552.8
and gangrene 551.8
en glissade - *see* Hernia, inguinal
enterostomy (stoma) 569.69

Hernia, hernial *(Continued)*
epigastric 553.29
with
gangrene (obstruction) 551.29
obstruction 552.29
and gangrene 551.29
recurrent 553.21
with
gangrene (obstructed) 551.21
obstruction 552.21
and gangrene 551.21
esophageal hiatus (sliding) 553.3
with
gangrene (obstructed) 551.3
obstruction 552.3
and gangrene 551.3
congenital 750.6
external (inguinal) - *see* Hernia, inguinal
fallopian tube 620.4
fascia 728.89
fat 729.30
eyelid 374.34
orbital 374.34
pad 729.30
eye, eyelid 374.34
knee 729.31
orbit 374.34
popliteal (space) 729.31
specified site NEC 729.39
femoral (unilateral) 553.00
with
gangrene (obstructed) 551.00
obstruction 552.00
with gangrene 551.00
bilateral 553.02
gangrenous (obstructed) 551.02
obstructed 552.02
with gangrene 551.02
recurrent 553.03
gangrenous (obstructed) 551.03
obstructed 552.03
with gangrene 551.03
recurrent (unilateral) 553.01
bilateral 553.03
gangrenous (obstructed) 551.03
obstructed 552.03
with gangrene 551.03
gangrenous (obstructed) 551.01
obstructed 552.01
with gangrene 551.01
foramen
Bochdalek 553.3
with
gangrene (obstructed) 551.3
obstruction 552.3
and gangrene 551.3
congenital 756.6
magnum 348.4
Morgagni, morgagnian 553.3
with
gangrene 551.3
obstruction 552.3
and gangrene 551.3
congenital 756.6
funicular (umbilical) 553.1
with
gangrene (obstructed) 551.1
obstruction 552.1
and gangrene 551.1
spermatic cord - *see* Hernia, inguinal
gangrenous - *see* Hernia, by site, with gangrene

Hernia, hernial *(Continued)*
gastrointestinal tract 553.9
with
gangrene (obstructed) 551.9
obstruction 552.9
and gangrene 551.9
gluteal - *see* Hernia, femoral
Gruber's (internal mesogastric) 553.8
with
gangrene (obstructed) 551.8
obstruction 552.8
and gangrene 551.8
Hesselbach's 553.8
with
gangrene (obstructed) 551.8
obstruction 552.8
and gangrene 551.8
hiatal (esophageal) (sliding) 553.3
with
gangrene (obstructed) 551.3
obstruction 552.3
and gangrene 551.3
congenital 750.6
incarcerated (*see also* Hernia, by site, with obstruction) 552.9
gangrenous (*see also* Hernia, by site, with gangrene) 551.9
incisional 553.21
with
gangrene (obstructed) 551.21
obstruction 552.21
and gangrene 551.21
lumbar - *see* Hernia, lumbar
recurrent 553.21
with
gangrene (obstructed) 551.21
obstruction 552.21
and gangrene 551.21
indirect (inguinal) - *see* Hernia, inguinal
infantile - *see* Hernia, inguinal
infrapatellar fat pad 729.31
inguinal (direct) (double) (encysted) (external) (funicular) (indirect) (infantile) (internal) (interstitial) (oblique) (scrotal) (sliding) 550.9

Note Use the following fifth-digit subclassification with category 550:

0 unilateral or unspecified (not specified as recurrent)
1 unilateral or unspecified, recurrent
2 bilateral (not specified as recurrent)
3 bilateral, recurrent

with
gangrene (obstructed) 550.0
obstruction 550.1
and gangrene 550.0
internal 553.8
with
gangrene (obstructed) 551.8
obstruction 552.8
and gangrene 551.8
inguinal - *see* Hernia, inguinal
interstitial 553.9
with
gangrene (obstructed) 551.9
obstruction 552.9
and gangrene 551.9
inguinal - *see* Hernia, inguinal

Hernia, hernial *(Continued)*
intervertebral cartilage or disc - *see* Displacement, intervertebral disc
intestine, intestinal 553.9
with
gangrene (obstructed) 551.9
obstruction 552.9
and gangrene 551.9
intra-abdominal 553.9
with
gangrene (obstructed) 551.9
obstruction 552.9
and gangrene 551.9
intraparietal 553.9
with
gangrene (obstructed) 551.9
obstruction 552.9
and gangrene 551.9
iris 364.8
traumatic 871.1
irreducible (*see also* Hernia, by site, with obstruction) 552.9
gangrenous (with obstruction) (*see also* Hernia, by site, with gangrene) 551.9
ischiatic 553.8
with
gangrene (obstructed) 551.8
obstruction 552.8
and gangrene 551.8
ischiorectal 553.8
with
gangrene (obstructed) 551.8
obstruction 552.8
and gangrene 551.8
lens 379.32
traumatic 871.1
linea
alba - *see* Hernia, epigastric
semilunaris - *see* Hernia, spigelian
Littre's (diverticular) 553.9
with
gangrene (obstructed) 551.9
obstruction 552.9
and gangrene 551.9
lumbar 553.8
with
gangrene (obstructed) 551.8
obstruction 552.8
and gangrene 551.8
intervertebral disc 722.10
lung (subcutaneous) 518.89
congenital 748.69
mediastinum 519.3
mesenteric (internal) 553.8
with
gangrene (obstructed) 551.8
obstruction 552.8
and gangrene 551.8
mesocolon 553.8
with
gangrene (obstructed) 551.8
obstruction 552.8
and gangrene 551.8
muscle (sheath) 728.89
nucleus pulposus - *see* Displacement, intervertebral disc
oblique (inguinal) - *see* Hernia, inguinal
obstructive (*see also* Hernia, by site, with obstruction) 552.9
gangrenous (with obstruction) (*see also* Hernia, by site, with gangrene) 551.9

Hernia, hernial *(Continued)*
obturator 553.8
with
gangrene (obstructed) 551.8
obstruction 552.8
and gangrene 551.8
omental 553.8
with
gangrene (obstructed) 551.8
obstruction 552.8
and gangrene 551.8
orbital fat (pad) 374.34
ovary 620.4
oviduct 620.4
paracolostomy (stoma) 569.69
paraduodenal 553.8
with
gangrene (obstructed) 551.8
obstruction 552.8
and gangrene 551.8
paraesophageal 553.3
with
gangrene (obstructed) 551.3
obstruction 552.3
and gangrene 551.3
congenital 750.6
parahiatal 553.3
with
gangrene (obstructed) 551.3
obstruction 552.3
and gangrene 551.3
paraumbilical 553.1
with
gangrene (obstructed) 551.1
obstruction 552.1
and gangrene 551.1
parietal 553.9
with
gangrene (obstructed) 551.9
obstruction 552.9
and gangrene 551.9
perineal 553.8
with
gangrene (obstructed) 551.8
obstruction 552.8
and gangrene 551.8
peritoneal sac, lesser 553.8
with
gangrene (obstructed) 551.8
obstruction 552.8
and gangrene 551.8
popliteal fat pad 729.31
postoperative 553.21
with
gangrene (obstructed) 551.21
obstruction 552.21
and gangrene 551.21
pregnant uterus 654.4
prevesical 596.8
properitoneal 553.8
with
gangrene (obstructed) 551.8
obstruction 552.8
and gangrene 551.8
pudendal 553.8
with
gangrene (obstructed) 551.8
obstruction 552.8
and gangrene 551.8
rectovaginal 618.6
retroperitoneal 553.8
with
gangrene (obstructed) 551.8
obstruction 552.8
and gangrene 551.8

Hernia, hernial *(Continued)*
Richter's (parietal) 553.9
with
gangrene (obstructed) 551.9
obstruction 552.9
and gangrene 551.9
Rieux's, Riex's (retrocecal) 553.8
with
gangrene (obstructed) 551.8
obstruction 552.8
and gangrene 551.8
sciatic 553.8
with
gangrene (obstructed) 551.8
obstruction 552.8
and gangrene 551.8
scrotum, scrotal - *see* Hernia, inguinal
sliding (inguinal) - *see also* Hernia, inguinal
hiatus - *see* Hernia, hiatal
spigelian 553.29
with
gangrene (obstructed) 551.29
obstruction 552.29
and gangrene 551.29
spinal (*see also* Spina bifida) 741.9
with hydrocephalus 741.0
strangulated (*see also* Hernia, by site, with obstruction) 552.9
gangrenous (with obstruction) (*see also* Hernia, by site, with gangrene) 551.9
supraumbilicus (linea alba) - *see* Hernia, epigastric
tendon 727.9
testis (nontraumatic) 550.9
meaning
scrotal hernia 550.9
symptomatic late syphilis 095.8
Treitz's (fossa) 553.8
with
gangrene (obstructed) 551.8
obstruction 552.8
and gangrene 551.8
tunica
albuginea 608.89
vaginalis 752.89
umbilicus, umbilical 553.1
with
gangrene (obstructed) 551.1
obstruction 552.1
and gangrene 551.1
ureter 593.89
with obstruction 593.4
uterus 621.8
pregnant 654.4
vaginal (posterior) 618.6
Velpeau's (femoral) (*see also* Hernia, femoral) 553.00
ventral 553.20
with
gangrene (obstructed) 551.20
obstruction 552.20
and gangrene 551.20
incisional 553.21
recurrent 553.21
with
gangrene (obstructed) 551.21
obstruction 552.21
and gangrene 551.21
vesical
congenital (female) (male) 756.71
female (*see also* Cystocele, female) 618.01
male 596.8

Hernia, hernial *(Continued)*
vitreous (into anterior chamber) 379.21
traumatic 871.1
Herniation - *see also* Hernia
brain (stem) 348.4
cerebral 348.4
gastric mucosa (into duodenal bulb) 537.89
mediastinum 519.3
nucleus pulposus - *see* Displacement, intervertebral disc
Herpangina 074.0
Herpes, herpetic 054.9
auricularis (zoster) 053.71
simplex 054.73
blepharitis (zoster) 053.20
simplex 054.41
circinate 110.5
circinatus 110.5
bullous 694.5
conjunctiva (simplex) 054.43
zoster 053.21
cornea (simplex) 054.43
disciform (simplex) 054.43
zoster 053.21
encephalitis 054.3
eye (zoster) 053.29
simplex 054.40
eyelid (zoster) 053.20
simplex 054.41
febrilis 054.9
fever 054.9
geniculate ganglionitis 053.11
genital, genitalis 054.10
specified site NEC 054.19
gestationis 646.8
gingivostomatitis 054.2
iridocyclitis (simplex) 054.44
zoster 053.22
iris (any site) 695.1
iritis (simplex) 054.44
keratitis (simplex) 054.43
dendritic 054.42
disciform 054.43
interstitial 054.43
zoster 053.21
keratoconjunctivitis (simplex) 054.43
zoster 053.21
labialis 054.9
meningococcal 036.89
lip 054.9
meningitis (simplex) 054.72
zoster 053.0
ophthalmicus (zoster) 053.20
simplex 054.40
otitis externa (zoster) 053.71
simplex 054.73
penis 054.13
perianal 054.10
pharyngitis 054.79
progenitalis 054.10
scrotum 054.19
septicemia 054.5
simplex 054.9
complicated 054.8
ophthalmic 054.40
specified NEC 054.49
specified NEC 054.79
congenital 771.2
external ear 054.73
keratitis 054.43
dendritic 054.42
meningitis 054.72
myelitis 054.74 ◄
neuritis 054.79

Herpes, herpetic *(Continued)*
simplex *(Continued)*
specified complication NEC 054.79
ophthalmic 054.49
visceral 054.71
stomatitis 054.2
tonsurans 110.0
maculosus (of Hebra) 696.3
visceral 054.71
vulva 054.12
vulvovaginitis 054.11
whitlow 054.6
zoster 053.9
auricularis 053.71
complicated 053.8
specified NEC 053.79
conjunctiva 053.21
cornea 053.21
ear 053.71
eye 053.29
geniculate 053.11
keratitis 053.21
interstitial 053.21
myelitis 053.14 ◄
neuritis 053.10
ophthalmicus(a) 053.20
oticus 053.71
otitis externa 053.71
specified complication NEC 053.79
specified site NEC 053.9
zosteriform, intermediate type 053.9
Herrick's
anemia (hemoglobin S disease) 282.61
syndrome (hemoglobin S disease) 282.61
Hers' disease (glycogenosis VI) 271.0
Herter's infantilism (nontropical sprue) 579.0
Herter (-Gee) disease or syndrome (nontropical sprue) 579.0
Herxheimer's disease (diffuse idiopathic cutaneous atrophy) 701.8
Herxheimer's reaction 995.0
Hesitancy, urinary 788.64 ◄
Hesselbach's hernia - *see* Hernia, Hesselbach's
Heterochromia (congenital) 743.46
acquired 364.53
cataract 366.33
cyclitis 364.21
hair 704.3
iritis 364.21
retained metallic foreign body 360.62
magnetic 360.52
uveitis 364.21
Heterophoria 378.40
alternating 378.45
vertical 378.43
Heterophyes, small intestine 121.6
Heterophyiasis 121.6
Heteropsia 368.8
Heterotopia, heterotopic - *see also* Malposition, congenital
cerebralis 742.4
pancreas, pancreatic 751.7
spinalis 742.59
Heterotropia 378.30
intermittent 378.20
vertical 378.31
vertical (constant) (intermittent) 378.31
Heubner's disease 094.89
Heubner-Herter disease or syndrome (nontropical sprue) 579.0
Hexadactylism 755.00
Heyd's syndrome (hepatorenal) 572.4

- **HGSIL** (high grade squamous intraepithelial lesion) 795.04
- **Hibernoma** (M8880/0) - *see* Lipoma
- **Hiccough** 786.8
  - epidemic 078.89
  - psychogenic 306.1
- **Hiccup** (*see also* Hiccough) 786.8
- **Hicks** (-Braxton) contractures 644.1
- **Hidden penis** 752.65
- **Hidradenitis** (axillaris) (suppurative) 705.83
- **Hidradenoma** (nodular) (M8400/0) - *see also* Neoplasm, skin, benign
  - clear cell (M8402/0) - *see* Neoplasm, skin, benign
  - papillary (M8405/0) - *see* Neoplasm, skin, benign
- **Hidrocystoma** (M8404/0) - *see* Neoplasm, skin, benign
- **HIE** (hypoxic-ischemic encephalopathy) 768.7 ◀
- **High**
  - A_2 anemia 282.49
  - altitude effects 993.2
    - anoxia 993.2
    - on
      - ears 993.0
      - sinuses 993.1
    - polycythemia 289.0
  - arch
    - foot 755.67
    - palate 750.26
  - artery (arterial) tension (*see also* Hypertension) 401.9
    - without diagnosis of hypertension 796.2
  - basal metabolic rate (BMR) 794.7
  - blood pressure (*see also* Hypertension) 401.9
    - incidental reading (isolated) (nonspecific), no diagnosis of hypertension 796.2
  - compliance bladder 596.4
  - diaphragm (congenital) 756.6
  - frequency deafness (congenital) (regional) 389.8
  - head at term 652.5
    - affecting fetus or newborn 763.1
  - output failure (cardiac) (*see also* Failure, heart) 428.9
  - oxygen-affinity hemoglobin 289.0
  - palate 750.26
  - risk
    - behavior - *see* problem
    - cervical, human papillomavirus (HPV) DNA test positive 795.05
    - family situation V61.9
      - specified circumstance NEC V61.8
    - individual NEC V62.89
    - infant NEC V20.1
    - patient taking drugs (prescribed) V67.51
      - nonprescribed (*see also* Abuse, drugs, nondependent) 305.9
    - pregnancy V23.9
      - inadequate prenatal care V23.7
      - specified problem NEC V23.89
  - temperature (of unknown origin) (*see also* Pyrexia) 780.6
  - thoracic rib 756.3
- **Hildenbrand's disease** (typhus) 081.9
- **Hilger's syndrome** 337.0
- **Hill diarrhea** 579.1
- **Hilliard's lupus** (*see also* Tuberculosis) 017.0
- **Hilum** - *see* condition
- **Hip** - *see* condition
- **Hippel's disease** (retinocerebral angiomatosis) 759.6
- **Hippus** 379.49
- **Hirschfeld's disease** (acute diabetes mellitus) (*see also* Diabetes) 250.0
- **Hirschsprung's disease or megacolon** (congenital) 751.3
- **Hirsuties** (*see also* Hypertrichosis) 704.1
- **Hirsutism** (*see also* Hypertrichosis) 704.1
- **Hirudiniasis** (external) (internal) 134.2
- **His-Werner disease** (trench fever) 083.1
- **Hiss-Russell dysentery** 004.1
- **Histamine cephalgia** 346.2
- **Histidinemia** 270.5
- **Histidinuria** 270.5
- **Histiocytic syndromes** 288.4 ◀
- **Histiocytoma** (M8832/0) - (*see also* Neoplasm, skin, benign)
  - fibrous (M8830/0) - (*see also* Neoplasm, skin, benign)
    - atypical (M8830/1) - *see* Neoplasm, connective tissue, uncertain behavior
    - malignant (M8830/3) - *see* Neoplasm, connective tissue, malignant
- **Histiocytosis** (acute) (chronic) (subacute) 277.89
  - acute differentiated progressive (M9722/3) 202.5
  - cholesterol 277.89
  - essential 277.89
  - lipid, lipoid (essential) 272.7
  - lipochrome (familial) 288.1
  - malignant (M9720/3) 202.3
  - X (chronic) 277.89
    - acute (progressive) (M9722/3) 202.5
- **Histoplasmosis** 115.90
  - with
    - endocarditis 115.94
    - meningitis 115.91
    - pericarditis 115.93
    - pneumonia 115.95
    - retinitis 115.92
    - specified manifestation NEC 115.99
  - African (due to Histoplasma duboisii) 115.10
    - with
      - endocarditis 115.14
      - meningitis 115.11
      - pericarditis 115.13
      - pneumonia 115.15
      - retinitis 115.12
      - specified manifestation NEC 115.19
  - American (due to Histoplasma capsulatum) 115.00
    - with
      - endocarditis 115.04
      - meningitis 115.01
      - pericarditis 115.03
      - pneumonia 115.05
      - retinitis 115.02
      - specified manifestation NEC 115.09
  - Darling's - *see* Histoplasmosis, American
  - large form (*see also* Histoplasmosis, African) 115.10
  - lung 115.05
  - small form (*see also* Histoplasmosis, American) 115.00
- **History** (personal) of
  - abuse
    - emotional V15.42
    - neglect V15.42
    - physical V15.41
    - sexual V15.41
- **History** (personal) of *(Continued)*
  - affective psychosis V11.1
  - alcoholism V11.3
    - specified as drinking problem (*see also* Abuse, drugs, nondependent) 305.0
  - allergy to
    - analgesic agent NEC V14.6
    - anesthetic NEC V14.4
    - antibiotic agent NEC V14.1
      - penicillin V14.0
    - anti-infective agent NEC V14.3
    - diathesis V15.09
    - drug V14.9
      - specified type NEC V14.8
    - eggs V15.03
    - food additives V15.05
    - insect bite V15.06
    - latex V15.07
    - medicinal agents V14.9
      - specified type NEC V14.8
    - milk products V15.02
    - narcotic agent NEC V14.5
    - nuts V15.05
      - peanuts V15.01
    - penicillin V14.0
    - radiographic dye V15.08
    - seafood V15.04
    - serum V14.7
    - specified food NEC V15.05
    - specified nonmedicinal agents NEC V15.09
    - spider bite V15.06
    - sulfa V14.2
    - sulfonamides V14.2
    - therapeutic agent NEC V15.09
    - vaccine V14.7
  - anemia V12.3
  - arthritis V13.4
  - benign neoplasm of brain V12.41
  - blood disease V12.3
  - calculi, urinary V13.01
  - cardiovascular disease V12.50
    - myocardial infarction 412
  - child abuse V15.41
  - cigarette smoking V15.82
  - circulatory system disease V12.50
    - myocardial infarction 412
  - congenital malformation V13.69
  - contraception V15.7
  - diathesis, allergic V15.09
  - digestive system disease V12.70
    - peptic ulcer V12.71
    - polyps, colonic V12.72
    - specified NEC V12.79
  - disease (of) V13.9
    - blood V12.3
    - blood-forming organs V12.3
    - cardiovascular system V12.50
    - circulatory system V12.50
    - digestive system V12.70
      - peptic ulcer V12.71
      - polyps, colonic V12.72
      - specified NEC V12.79
    - infectious V12.00
    - malaria V12.03
      - poliomyelitis V12.02
      - specified NEC V12.09
      - tuberculosis V12.01
    - parasitic V12.00
      - specified NEC V12.09
    - respiratory system V12.60
      - pneumonia V12.61
      - specified NEC V12.69

History (personal) of *(Continued)*
disease *(Continued)*
skin V13.3
specified site NEC V13.8
subcutaneous tissue V13.3
trophoblastic V13.1
affecting management of pregnancy V23.1
disorder (of) V13.9
endocrine V12.2
genital system V13.29
hematological V12.3
immunity V12.2
mental V11.9
affective type V11.1
manic-depressive V11.1
neurosis V11.2
schizophrenia V11.0
specified type NEC V11.8
metabolic V12.2
musculoskeletal NEC V13.5
nervous system V12.40
specified type NEC V12.49
obstetric V13.29
affecting management of current pregnancy V23.49
pre-term labor V23.41
pre-term labor V13.21
sense organs V12.40
specified type NEC V12.49
specified site NEC V13.8
urinary system V13.00
calculi V13.01
infection V13.02
nephrotic syndrome V13.03
specified NEC V13.09
drug use
nonprescribed (*see also* Abuse, drugs, nondependent) 305.9
patent (*see also* Abuse, drugs, nondependent) 305.9
effect NEC of external cause V15.89
embolism (pulmonary) V12.51
emotional abuse V15.42
encephalitis V12.42
endocrine disorder V12.2
extracorporeal membrane oxygenation (ECMO) V15.87
falling V15.88
family
allergy V19.6
anemia V18.2
arteriosclerosis V17.4
arthritis V17.7
asthma V17.5
blindness V19.0
blood disorder NEC V18.3
cardiovascular disease V17.4
carrier, genetic disease V18.9
cerebrovascular disease V17.1
chronic respiratory condition NEC V17.6
colonic polyps V18.51 ◀
congenital anomalies V19.5
consanguinity V19.7
coronary artery disease V17.3
cystic fibrosis V18.1
deafness V19.2
diabetes mellitus V18.0
digestive disorders V18.59 ◀
disease or disorder (of)
allergic V19.6
blood NEC V18.3
cardiovascular NEC V17.4
cerebrovascular V17.1

History (personal) of *(Continued)*
family *(Continued)*
disease or disorder *(Continued)*
colonic polyps V18.51 ◀
coronary artery V17.3
digestive V18.59 ◀
ear NEC V19.3
endocrine V18.1
eye NEC V19.1
genitourinary NEC V18.7
hypertensive V17.4
infectious V18.8
ischemic heart V17.3
kidney V18.69
polycystic V18.61
mental V17.0
metabolic V18.1
musculoskeletal NEC V17.89
osteoporosis V17.81
neurological NEC V17.2
parasitic V18.8
psychiatric condition V17.0
skin condition V19.4
ear disorder NEC V19.3
endocrine disease V18.1
epilepsy V17.2
eye disorder NEC V19.1
genetic disease carrier V18.9
genitourinary disease NEC V18.7
glomerulonephritis V18.69
gout V18.1
hay fever V17.6
hearing loss V19.2
hematopoietic neoplasia V16.7
Hodgkin's disease V16.7
Huntington's chorea V17.2
hydrocephalus V19.5
hypertension V17.4
hypospadias V13.61
infectious disease V18.8
ischemic heart disease V17.3
kidney disease V18.69
polycystic V18.61
leukemia V16.6
lymphatic malignant neoplasia NEC V16.7
malignant neoplasm (of) NEC V16.9
anorectal V16.0
anus V16.0
appendix V16.0
bladder V16.59
bone V16.8
brain V16.8
breast V16.3
male V16.8
bronchus V16.1
cecum V16.0
cervix V16.49
colon V16.0
duodenum V16.0
esophagus V16.0
eye V16.8
gallbladder V16.0
gastrointestinal tract V16.0
genital organs V16.40
hemopoietic NEC V16.7
ileum V16.0
ilium V16.8
intestine V16.0
intrathoracic organs NEC V16.2
kidney V16.51
larynx V16.2
liver V16.0
lung V16.1
lymphatic NEC V16.7

History (personal) of *(Continued)*
family *(Continued)*
malignant neoplasm (of) NEC *(Continued)*
ovary V16.41
oviduct V16.41
pancreas V16.0
penis V16.49
prostate V16.42
rectum V16.0
respiratory organs NEC V16.2
skin V16.8
specified site NEC V16.8
stomach V16.0
testis V16.43
trachea V16.1
ureter V16.59
urethra V16.59
urinary organs V16.59
uterus V16.49
vagina V16.49
vulva V16.49
mental retardation V18.4
metabolic disease NEC V18.1
mongolism V19.5
multiple myeloma V16.7
musculoskeletal disease NEC V17.89
osteoporosis V17.81
nephritis V18.69
nephrosis V18.69
osteoporosis V17.81
parasitic disease V18.8
polycystic kidney disease V18.61
psychiatric disorder V17.0
psychosis V17.0
retardation, mental V18.4
retinitis pigmentosa V19.1
schizophrenia V17.0
skin conditions V19.4
specified condition NEC V19.8
stroke (cerebrovascular) V17.1
visual loss V19.0
genital system disorder V13.29
pre-term labor V13.21
health hazard V15.9
falling V15.88
specified cause NEC V15.89
hepatitis
B V12.09
C V12.09
Hodgkin's disease V10.72
immunity disorder V12.2
infection
central nervous system V12.42
urinary (tract) V13.02
infectious disease V12.00
malaria V12.03
poliomyelitis V12.02
specified NEC V12.09
tuberculosis V12.01
injury NEC V15.5
insufficient prenatal care V23.7
irradiation V15.3
leukemia V10.60
lymphoid V10.61
monocytic V10.63
myeloid V10.62
specified type NEC V10.69
little or no prenatal care V23.7
low birth weight (*see also* Status, low birth weight) V21.30
lymphosarcoma V10.71
malaria V12.03

History (personal) of *(Continued)*
malignant neoplasm (of) V10.9
accessory sinus V10.22
adrenal V10.88
anus V10.06
bile duct V10.09
bladder V10.51
bone V10.81
brain V10.85
breast V10.3
bronchus V10.11
cervix uteri V10.41
colon V10.05
connective tissue NEC V10.89
corpus uteri V10.42
digestive system V10.00
specified part NEC V10.09
duodenum V10.09
endocrine gland NEC V10.88
epididymis V10.48
esophagus V10.03
eye V10.84
fallopian tube V10.44
female genital organ V10.40
specified site NEC V10.44
gallbladder V10.09
gastrointestinal tract V10.00
gum V10.02
hematopoietic NEC V10.79
hypopharynx V10.02
ileum V10.09
intrathoracic organs NEC V10.20
jejunum V10.09
kidney V10.52
large intestine V10.05
larynx V10.21
lip V10.02
liver V10.07
lung V10.11
lymphatic NEC V10.79
lymph glands or nodes NEC V10.79
male genital organ V10.45
specified site NEC V10.49
mediastinum V10.29
melanoma (of skin) V10.82
middle ear V10.22
mouth V10.02
specified part NEC V10.02
nasal cavities V10.22
nasopharynx V10.02
nervous system NEC V10.86
nose V10.22
oropharynx V10.02
ovary V10.43
pancreas V10.09
parathyroid V10.88
penis V10.49
pharynx V10.02
pineal V10.88
pituitary V10.88
placenta V10.44
pleura V10.29
prostate V10.46
rectosigmoid junction V10.06
rectum V10.06
renal pelvis V10.53
respiratory organs NEC V10.20
salivary gland V10.02
skin V10.83
melanoma V10.82
small intestine NEC V10.09
soft tissue NEC V10.89
specified site NEC V10.89
stomach V10.04

History (personal) of *(Continued)*
malignant neoplasm *(Continued)*
testis V10.47
thymus V10.29
thyroid V10.87
tongue V10.01
trachea V10.12
ureter V10.59
urethra V10.59
urinary organ V10.50
uterine adnexa V10.44
uterus V10.42
vagina V10.44
vulva V10.44
manic-depressive psychosis V11.1
meningitis V12.42
mental disorder V11.9
affective type V11.1
manic-depressive V11.1
neurosis V11.2
schizophrenia V11.0
specified type NEC V11.8
metabolic disorder V12.2
musculoskeletal disorder NEC V13.5
myocardial infarction 412
neglect (emotional) V15.42
nephrotic syndrome V13.03
nervous system disorder V12.40
specified type NEC V12.49
neurosis V11.2
noncompliance with medical treatment V15.81
nutritional deficiency V12.1
obstetric disorder V13.29
affecting management of current pregnancy V23.49
pre-term labor V23.21
pre-term labor V13.21
parasitic disease V12.00
specified NEC V12.09
perinatal problems V13.7
low birth weight (*see also* Status, low birth weight) V21.30
physical abuse V15.41
poisoning V15.6
poliomyelitis V12.02
polyps, colonic V12.72
poor obstetric V13.29
affecting management of current pregnancy V23.49
pre-term labor V23.21
pre-term labor V13.21
psychiatric disorder V11.9
affective type V11.1
manic-depressive V11.1
neurosis V11.2
schizophrenia V11.0
specified type NEC V11.8
psychological trauma V15.49
emotional abuse V15.42
neglect V15.42
physical abuse V15.41
rape V15.41
psychoneurosis V11.2
radiation therapy V15.3
rape V15.41
respiratory system disease V12.60
pneumonia V12.61
specified NEC V12.69
reticulosarcoma V10.71
schizophrenia V11.0
skin disease V13.3
smoking (tobacco) V15.82
subcutaneous tissue disease V13.3

History (personal) of *(Continued)*
surgery (major) to
great vessels V15.1
heart V15.1
major organs NEC V15.2
syndrome, nephrotic V13.03
thrombophlebitis V12.52
thrombosis V12.51
tobacco use V15.82
trophoblastic disease V13.1
affecting management of pregnancy V23.1
tuberculosis V12.01
ulcer, peptic V12.71
urinary system disorder V13.00
calculi V13.01
infection V13.02
nephrotic syndrome V13.03
specified NEC V13.09
HIV infection (disease) (illness) - *see* Human immunodeficiency virus (disease) (illness) (infection)
Hives (bold) (*see also* Urticaria) 708.9
Hoarseness 784.49
Hobnail liver - *see* Cirrhosis, portal
Hobo, hoboism V60.0
Hodgkin's
disease (M9650/3) 201.9
lymphocytic
depletion (M9653/3) 201.7
diffuse fibrosis (M9654/3) 201.7
reticular type (M9655/3) 201.7
predominance (M9651/3) 201.4
lymphocytic-histiocytic predominance (M9651/3) 201.4
mixed cellularity (M9652/3) 201.6
nodular sclerosis (M9656/3) 201.5
cellular phase (M9657/3) 201.5
granuloma (M9661/3) 201.1
lymphogranulomatosis (M9650/3) 201.9
lymphoma (M9650/3) 201.9
lymphosarcoma (M9650/3) 201.9
paragranuloma (M9660/3) 201.0
sarcoma (M9662/3) 201.2
Hodgson's disease (aneurysmal dilatation of aorta) 441.9
ruptured 441.5
Hodi-potsy 111.0
Hoffa (-Kastert) disease or syndrome (liposynovitis prepatellaris) 272.8
Hoffmann's syndrome 244.9 *[359.5]*
Hoffmann-Bouveret syndrome (paroxysmal tachycardia) 427.2
Hole
macula 362.54
optic disc, crater-like 377.22
retina (macula) 362.54
round 361.31
with detachment 361.01
Holla disease (*see also* Spherocytosis) 282.0
Holländer-Simons syndrome (progressive lipodystrophy) 272.6
Hollow foot (congenital) 754.71
acquired 736.73
Holmes' syndrome (visual disorientation) 368.16
Holoprosencephaly 742.2
due to
trisomy 13 758.1
trisomy 18 758.2

Holthouse's hernia - *see* Hernia, inguinal
Homesickness 309.89
Homocystinemia 270.4
Homocystinuria 270.4
Homologous serum jaundice (prophylactic) (therapeutic) - *see* Hepatitis, viral
Homosexuality - *omit code*
  ego-dystonic 302.0
  pedophilic 302.2
  problems with 302.0
Homozygous Hb-S disease 282.61
Honeycomb lung 518.89
  congenital 748.4
Hong Kong ear 117.3
HOOD (hereditary osteo-onychodysplasia) 756.89
Hooded
  clitoris 752.49
  penis 752.69
Hookworm (anemia) (disease) (infestation) - *see* Ancylostomiasis
Hoppe-Goldflam syndrome 358.00
Hordeolum (external) (eyelid) 373.11
  internal 373.12
Horn
  cutaneous 702.8
    cheek 702.8
    eyelid 702.8
    penis 702.8
  iliac 756.89
  nail 703.8
    congenital 757.5
  papillary 700
Horner's
  syndrome (*see also* Neuropathy, peripheral, autonomic) 337.9
    traumatic 954.0
  teeth 520.4
Horseshoe kidney (congenital) 753.3
Horton's
  disease (temporal arteritis) 446.5
  headache or neuralgia 346.2
Hospice care V66.7
Hospitalism (in children) NEC 309.83
Hourglass contraction, contracture
  bladder 596.8
  gallbladder 575.2
    congenital 751.69
  stomach 536.8
    congenital 750.7
    psychogenic 306.4
  uterus 661.4
    affecting fetus or newborn 763.7
Household circumstance affecting care V60.9
  specified type NEC V60.8
Housemaid's knee 727.2
Housing circumstance affecting care V60.9
  specified type NEC V60.8
Huchard's disease (continued arterial hypertension) 401.9
Hudson-Stähli lines 371.11
Huguier's disease (uterine fibroma) 218.9
Hum, venous - *omit code*
Human bite (open wound) - (*see also* Wound, open, by site)
  intact skin surface - *see* Contusion
Human immunodeficiency virus (disease) (illness) 042
  infection V08
    with symptoms, symptomatic 042
Human immunodeficiency virus-2 infection 079.53
Human immunovirus (disease) (illness) (infection) - *see* Human immunodeficiency virus (disease) (illness) (infection)
Human papillomavirus 079.4
  cervical
    high risk, DNA test positive 795.05
    low risk, DNA test positive 795.09
Human T-cell lymphotrophic virus I infection 079.51
Human T-cell lymphotrophic virus II infection 079.52
Human T-cell lymphotropic virus-III (disease) (illness) (infection) - *see* Human immunodeficiency virus (disease) (illness) (infection)
HTLV-I infection 079.51
HTLV-II infection 079.52
HTLV-III (disease) (illness) (infection) - *see* Human immunodeficiency virus (disease) (illness) (infection)
HTLV-III/LAV (disease) (illness) (infection) - *see* Human immunodeficiency virus (disease) (illness) (infection)
Humpback (acquired) 737.9
  congenital 756.19
Hunchback (acquired) 737.9
  congenital 756.19
Hunger 994.2
  air, psychogenic 306.1
  disease 251.1
Hunner's ulcer (*see also* Cystitis) 595.1
Hunt's
  neuralgia 053.11
  syndrome (herpetic geniculate ganglionitis) 053.11
    dyssynergia cerebellaris myoclonica 334.2
Hunter's glossitis 529.4
Hunter (-Hurler) syndrome (mucopolysaccharidosis II) 277.5
Hunterian chancre 091.0
Huntington's
  chorea 333.4
  disease 333.4
Huppert's disease (multiple myeloma) (M9730/3) 203.0
Hurler (-Hunter) disease or syndrome (mucopolysaccharidosis II) 277.5
Hürthle cell
  adenocarcinoma (M8290/3) 193
  adenoma (M8290/0) 226
  carcinoma (M8290/3) 193
  tumor (M8290/0) 226
Hutchinson's
  disease meaning
    angioma serpiginosum 709.1
    cheiropompholyx 705.81
    prurigo estivalis 692.72
    summer eruption, or summer prurigo 692.72
  incisors 090.5
  melanotic freckle (M8742/2) - *see also* Neoplasm, skin, in situ
    malignant melanoma in (M8742/3) - *see* Melanoma
  teeth or incisors (congenital syphilis) 090.5
Hutchinson-Boeck disease or syndrome (sarcoidosis) 135
Hutchinson-Gilford disease or syndrome (progeria) 259.8
Hyaline
  degeneration (diffuse) (generalized) 728.9
    localized - *see* Degeneration, by site
  membrane (disease) (lung) (newborn) 769
Hyalinosis cutis et mucosae 272.8
Hyalin plaque, sclera, senile 379.16
Hyalitis (asteroid) 379.22
  syphilitic 095.8
Hydatid
  cyst or tumor - *see also* Echinococcus
    fallopian tube 752.11
  mole - *see* Hydatidiform mole
  Morgagni (congenital) 752.89
    fallopian tube 752.11
Hydatidiform mole (benign) (complicating pregnancy) (delivered) (undelivered) 630
  invasive (M9100/1) 236.1
  malignant (M9100/1) 236.1
  previous, affecting management of pregnancy V23.1
Hydatidosis - *see* Echinococcus
Hyde's disease (prurigo nodularis) 698.3
Hydradenitis 705.83
Hydradenoma (M8400/0) - *see* Hidradenoma
Hydralazine lupus or syndrome
  correct substance properly administered 695.4
  overdose or wrong substance given or taken 972.6
Hydramnios 657
  affecting fetus or newborn 761.3
Hydrancephaly 742.3
  with spina bifida (*see also* Spina bifida) 741.0
Hydranencephaly 742.3
  with spina bifida (*see also* Spina bifida) 741.0
Hydrargyrism NEC 985.0
Hydrarthrosis (*see also* Effusion, joint) 719.0
  gonococcal 098.50
  intermittent (*see also* Rheumatism, palindromic) 719.3
  of yaws (early) (late) 102.6
  syphilitic 095.8
    congenital 090.5
Hydremia 285.9
Hydrencephalocele (congenital) 742.0
Hydrencephalomeningocele (congenital) 742.0
Hydroa 694.0
  aestivale 692.72
  gestationis 646.8
  herpetiformis 694.0
  pruriginosa 694.0
  vacciniforme 692.72
Hydroadenitis 705.83
Hydrocalycosis (*see also* Hydronephrosis) 591
  congenital 753.29
Hydrocalyx (*see also* Hydronephrosis) 591
Hydrocele (calcified) (chylous) (idiopathic) (infantile) (inguinal canal) (recurrent) (senile) (spermatic cord) (testis) (tunica vaginalis) 603.9
  canal of Nuck (female) 629.1
    male 603.9
  congenital 778.6
  encysted 603.0
    congenital 778.6

Hydrocele *(Continued)*
female NEC 629.89
infected 603.1
round ligament 629.89
specified type NEC 603.8
congenital 778.6
spinalis (*see also* Spina bifida) 741.9
vulva 624.8
Hydrocephalic fetus
affecting management or pregnancy 655.0
causing disproportion 653.6
with obstructed labor 660.1
affecting fetus or newborn 763.1
Hydrocephalus (acquired) (external) (internal) (malignant) (noncommunicating) (obstructive) (recurrent) 331.4
aqueduct of Sylvius stricture 742.3
with spina bifida (*see also* Spina bifida) 741.0
chronic 742.3
with spina bifida (*see also* Spina bifida) 741.0
communicating 331.3
congenital (external) (internal) 742.3
with spina bifida (*see also* Spina bifida) 741.0
due to
stricture of aqueduct of Sylvius 742.3
with spina bifida (*see also* Spina bifida) 741.0
toxoplasmosis (congenital) 771.2
fetal affecting management of pregnancy 655.0
foramen Magendie block (acquired) 331.3
congenital 742.3
with spina bifida (*see also* Spina bifida) 741.0
newborn 742.3
with spina bifida (*see also* Spina bifida) 741.0
otitic 348.2
syphilitic, congenital 090.49
tuberculous (*see also* Tuberculosis) 013.8
Hydrocolpos (congenital) 623.8
Hydrocystoma (M8404/0) - *see* Neoplasm, skin, benign
Hydroencephalocele (congenital) 742.0
Hydroencephalomeningocele (congenital) 742.0
Hydrohematopneumothorax (*see also* Hemothorax) 511.8
Hydromeningitis - *see* Meningitis
Hydromeningocele (spinal) (*see also* Spina bifida) 741.9
cranial 742.0
Hydrometra 621.8
Hydrometrocolpos 623.8
Hydromicrocephaly 742.1
Hydromphalus (congenital) (since birth) 757.39
Hydromyelia 742.53
Hydromyelocele (*see also* Spina bifida) 741.9
Hydronephrosis 591
atrophic 591
congenital 753.29
due to S. hematobium 120.0
early 591
functionless (infected) 591
infected 591
intermittent 591
Hydronephrosis *(Continued)*
primary 591
secondary 591
tuberculous (*see also* Tuberculosis) 016.0
Hydropericarditis (*see also* Pericarditis) 423.9
Hydropericardium (*see also* Pericarditis) 423.9
Hydroperitoneum 789.5
Hydrophobia 071
Hydrophthalmos (*see also* Buphthalmia) 743.20
Hydropneumohemothorax (*see also* Hemothorax) 511.8
Hydropneumopericarditis (*see also* Pericarditis) 423.9
Hydropneumopericardium (*see also* Pericarditis) 423.9
Hydropneumothorax 511.8
nontuberculous 511.8
bacterial 511.1
pneumococcal 511.1
staphylococcal 511.1
streptococcal 511.1
traumatic 860.0
with open wound into thorax 860.1
tuberculous (*see also* Tuberculosis, pleura) 012.0
Hydrops 782.3
abdominis 789.5
amnii (complicating pregnancy) (*see also* Hydramnios) 657
articulorum intermittens (*see also* Rheumatism, palindromic) 719.3
cardiac (*see also* Failure, heart) 428.0
congenital - *see* Hydrops, fetalis
endolymphatic (*see also* Disease, Meniere's) 386.00
fetal(is) or newborn 778.0
due to isoimmunization 773.3
not due to isoimmunization 778.0
gallbladder 575.3
idiopathic (fetus or newborn) 778.0
joint (*see also* Effusion, joint) 719.0
labyrinth (*see also* Disease, Meniere's) 386.00
meningeal NEC 331.4
nutritional 262
pericardium - *see* Pericarditis
pleura (*see also* Hydrothorax) 511.8
renal (*see also* Nephrosis) 581.9
spermatic cord (*see also* Hydrocele) 603.9
Hydropyonephrosis (*see also* Pyelitis) 590.80
chronic 590.00
Hydrorachis 742.53
Hydrorrhea (nasal) 478.19
gravidarum 658.1
pregnancy 658.1
Hydrosadenitis 705.83
Hydrosalpinx (fallopian tube) (follicularis) 614.1
Hydrothorax (double) (pleural) 511.8
chylous (nonfilarial) 457.8
filaria (*see also* Infestation, filarial) 125.9
nontuberculous 511.8
bacterial 511.1
pneumococcal 511.1
staphylococcal 511.1
streptococcal 511.1
traumatic 862.29
with open wound into thorax 862.39
Hydrothorax *(Continued)*
tuberculous (*see also* Tuberculosis, pleura) 012.0
Hydroureter 593.5
congenital 753.22
Hydroureteronephrosis (*see also* Hydronephrosis) 591
Hydrourethra 599.84
Hydroxykynureninuria 270.2
Hydroxyprolinemia 270.8
Hydroxyprolinuria 270.8
Hygroma (congenital) (cystic) (M9173/0) 228.1
prepatellar 727.3
subdural - *see* Hematoma, subdural
Hymen - *see* condition
Hymenolepiasis (diminuta) (infection) (infestation) (nana) 123.6
Hymenolepsis (diminuta) (infection) (infestation) (nana) 123.6
Hypalgesia (*see also* Disturbance, sensation) 782.0
Hyperabduction syndrome 447.8
Hyperacidity, gastric 536.8
psychogenic 306.4
Hyperactive, hyperactivity
basal cell, uterine cervix 622.10
bladder 596.51
bowel (syndrome) 564.9
sounds 787.5
cervix epithelial (basal) 622.10
child 314.01
colon 564.9
gastrointestinal 536.8
psychogenic 306.4
intestine 564.9
labyrinth (unilateral) 386.51
with loss of labyrinthine reactivity 386.58
bilateral 386.52
nasal mucous membrane 478.19
stomach 536.8
thyroid (gland) (*see also* Thyrotoxicosis) 242.9
Hyperacusis 388.42
Hyperadrenalism (cortical) 255.3
medullary 255.6
Hyperadrenocorticism 255.3
congenital 255.2
iatrogenic
correct substance properly administered 255.3
overdose or wrong substance given or taken 962.0
Hyperaffectivity 301.11
Hyperaldosteronism (atypical) (hyperplastic) (normoaldosteronal) (normotensive) (primary) 255.10
seconday 255.14
Hyperalgesia (*see also* Disturbance, sensation) 782.0
Hyperalimentation 783.6
carotene 278.3
specified NEC 278.8
vitamin A 278.2
vitamin D 278.4
Hyperaminoaciduria 270.9
arginine 270.6
citrulline 270.6
cystine 270.0
glycine 270.0
lysine 270.7
ornithine 270.6
renal (types I, II, III) 270.0

Hyperammonemia (congenital) 270.6
Hyperamnesia 780.99
Hyperamylasemia 790.5
Hyperaphia 782.0
Hyperazotemia 791.9
Hyperbetalipoproteinemia (acquired) (essential) (familial) (hereditary) (primary) (secondary) 272.0
  with prebetalipoproteinemia 272.2
Hyperbilirubinemia 782.4
  congenital 277.4
  constitutional 277.4
  neonatal (transient) (*see also* Jaundice, fetus or newborn) 774.6
    of prematurity 774.2
Hyperbilirubinemica encephalopathia, newborn 774.7
  due to isoimmunization 773.4
Hypercalcemia, hypercalcemic (idiopathic) 275.42
  nephropathy 588.89
Hypercalcinuria 275.40
Hypercapnia 786.09
  with mixed acid-based disorder 276.4
  fetal, affecting newborn 770.89
Hypercarotinemia 278.3
Hypercementosis 521.5
Hyperchloremia 276.9
Hyperchlorhydria 536.8
  neurotic 306.4
  psychogenic 306.4
Hypercholesterinemia - *see* Hypercholesterolemia
Hypercholesterolemia 272.0
  with hyperglyceridemia, endogenous 272.2
  essential 272.0
  familial 272.0
  hereditary 272.0
  primary 272.0
  pure 272.0
Hypercholesterolosis 272.0
Hyperchylia gastrica 536.8
  psychogenic 306.4
Hyperchylomicronemia (familial) (with hyperbetalipoproteinemia) 272.3
Hypercoagulation syndrome (primary) 289.81
  secondary 289.82
Hypercorticosteronism
  correct substance properly administered 255.3
  overdose or wrong substance given or taken 962.0
Hypercortisonism
  correct substance properly administered 255.3
  overdose or wrong substance given or taken 962.0
Hyperdynamic beta-adrenergic state or syndrome (circulatory) 429.82
Hyperekplexia 759.89
Hyperelectrolytemia 276.9
Hyperemesis 536.2
  arising during pregnancy - *see* Hyperemesis, gravidarum
  gravidarum (mild) (before 22 completed weeks' gestation) 643.0
    with
      carbohydrate depletion 643.1
      dehydration 643.1
      electrolyte imbalance 643.1
      metabolic disturbance 643.1

Hyperemesis *(Continued)*
  gravidarum *(Continued)*
    affecting fetus or newborn 761.8
    severe (with metabolic disturbance) 643.1
  psychogenic 306.4
Hyperemia (acute) 780.99
  anal mucosa 569.49
  bladder 596.7
  cerebral 437.8
  conjunctiva 372.71
  ear, internal, acute 386.30
  enteric 564.89
  eye 372.71
  eyelid (active) (passive) 374.82
  intestine 564.89
  iris 364.41
  kidney 593.81
  labyrinth 386.30
  liver (active) (passive) 573.8
  lung 514
  ovary 620.8
  passive 780.99
  pulmonary 514
  renal 593.81
  retina 362.89
  spleen 289.59
  stomach 537.89
Hyperesthesia (body surface) (*see also* Disturbance, sensation) 782.0
  larynx (reflex) 478.79
    hysterical 300.11
  pharynx (reflex) 478.29
Hyperestrinism 256.0
Hyperestrogenism 256.0
Hyperestrogenosis 256.0
Hyperexplexia 759.89
Hyperextension, joint 718.80
  ankle 718.87
  elbow 718.82
  foot 718.87
  hand 718.84
  hip 718.85
  knee 718.86
  multiple sites 718.89
  pelvic region 718.85
  shoulder (region) 718.81
  specified site NEC 718.88
  wrist 718.83
Hyperfibrinolysis - *see* Fibrinolysis
Hyperfolliculinism 256.0
Hyperfructosemia 271.2
Hyperfunction
  adrenal (cortex) 255.3
    androgenic, acquired benign 255.3
    medulla 255.6
    virilism 255.2
  corticoadrenal NEC 255.3
  labyrinth - *see* Hyperactive, labyrinth
  medulloadrenal 255.6
  ovary 256.1
    estrogen 256.0
  pancreas 577.8
  parathyroid (gland) 252.00
  pituitary (anterior) (gland) (lobe) 253.1
  testicular 257.0
Hypergammaglobulinemia 289.89
  monoclonal, benign (BMH) 273.1
  polyclonal 273.0
  Waldenström's 273.0
Hyperglobulinemia 273.8
Hyperglycemia 790.29 ⬅
  maternal
    affecting fetus or newborn 775.0
    manifest diabetes in infant 775.1

Hyperglycemia *(Continued)*
  postpancreatectomy (complete) (partial) 251.3
Hyperglyceridemia 272.1
  endogenous 272.1
  essential 272.1
  familial 272.1
  hereditary 272.1
  mixed 272.3
  pure 272.1
Hyperglycinemia 270.7
Hypergonadism
  ovarian 256.1
  testicular (infantile) (primary) 257.0
Hyperheparinemia (*see also* Circulating anticoagulants) 286.5
Hyperhidrosis, hyperidrosis 705.21
  axilla 705.21
  face 705.21
  focal (localized) 705.21
    primary 705.21
      axilla 705.21
      face 705.21
      palms 705.21
      soles 705.21
    secondary 705.22
      axilla 705.22
      face 705.22
      palms 705.22
      soles 705.22
  generalized 780.8
  palms 705.21
  psychogenic 306.3
  secondary 780.8
  soles 705.21
Hyperhistidinemia 270.5
Hyperinsulinism (ectopic) (functional) (organic) NEC 251.1
  iatrogenic 251.0
  reactive 251.2
  spontaneous 251.2
  therapeutic misadventure (from administration of insulin) 962.3
Hyperiodemia 276.9
Hyperirritability (cerebral), in newborn 779.1
Hyperkalemia 276.7
Hyperkeratosis (*see also* Keratosis) 701.1
  cervix 622.2
  congenital 757.39
  cornea 371.89
  due to yaws (early) (late) (palmar or plantar) 102.3
  eccentrica 757.39
  figurata centrifuga atrophica 757.39
  follicularis 757.39
    in cutem penetrans 701.1
  limbic (cornea) 371.89
  palmoplantaris climacterica 701.1
  pinta (carate) 103.1
  senile (with pruritus) 702.0
  tongue 528.79
  universalis congenita 757.1
  vagina 623.1
  vocal cord 478.5
  vulva 624.0
Hyperkinesia, hyperkinetic (disease) (reaction) (syndrome) 314.9
  with
    attention deficit - *see* Disorder, attention deficit
    conduct disorder 314.2
    developmental delay 314.1

Hyperkinesia, hyperkinetic *(Continued)*
with *(Continued)*
simple disturbance of activity and attention 314.01
specified manifestation NEC 314.8
heart (disease) 429.82
of childhood or adolescence NEC 314.9
Hyperlacrimation (*see also* Epiphora) 375.20
Hyperlipemia (*see also* Hyperlipidemia) 272.4
Hyperlipidemia 272.4
carbohydrate-induced 272.1
combined 272.4
endogenous 272.1
exogenous 272.3
fat-induced 272.3
group
A 272.0
B 272.1
C 272.2
D 272.3
mixed 272.2
specified type NEC 272.4
Hyperlipidosis 272.7
hereditary 272.7
Hyperlipoproteinemia (acquired) (essential) (familial) (hereditary) (primary) (secondary) 272.4
Fredrickson type
I 272.3
IIA 272.0
IIB 272.2
III 272.2
IV 272.1
V 272.3
low-density-lipoid-type (LDL) 272.0
very-low-density-lipoid-type [VLDL] 272.1
Hyperlucent lung, unilateral 492.8
Hyperluteinization 256.1
Hyperlysinemia 270.7
Hypermagnesemia 275.2
neonatal 775.5
Hypermaturity (fetus or newborn)
post-term infant 766.21
prolonged gestation infant 766.22
Hypermenorrhea 626.2
Hypermetabolism 794.7
Hypermethioninemia 270.4
Hypermetropia (congenital) 367.0
Hypermobility
cecum 564.9
coccyx 724.71
colon 564.9
psychogenic 306.4
ileum 564.89
joint (acquired) 718.80
ankle 718.87
elbow 718.82
foot 718.87
hand 718.84
hip 718.85
knee 718.86
multiple sites 718.89
pelvic region 718.85
shoulder (region) 718.81
specified site NEC 718.88
wrist 718.83
kidney, congenital 753.3
meniscus (knee) 717.5
scapula 718.81
stomach 536.8
psychogenic 306.4

Hypermobility *(Continued)*
syndrome 728.5
testis, congenital 752.52
urethral 599.81
Hypermotility
gastrointestinal 536.8
intestine 564.9
psychogenic 306.4
stomach 536.8
Hypernasality 784.49
Hypernatremia 276.0
with water depletion 276.0
Hypernephroma (M8312/3) 189.0
Hyperopia 367.0
Hyperorexia 783.6
Hyperornithinemia 270.6
Hyperosmia (*see also* Disturbance, sensation) 781.1
Hyperosmolality 276.0
Hyperosteogenesis 733.99
Hyperostosis 733.99
calvarial 733.3
cortical 733.3
infantile 756.59
frontal, internal of skull 733.3
interna frontalis 733.3
monomelic 733.99
skull 733.3
congenital 756.0
vertebral 721.8
with spondylosis - *see* Spondylosis
ankylosing 721.6
Hyperovarianism 256.1
Hyperovarism, hyperovaria 256.1
Hyperoxaluria (primary) 271.8
Hyperoxia 987.8
Hyperparathyroidism 252.00
ectopic 259.3
other 252.08
primary 252.01
secondary (of renal origin) 588.81
non-renal 252.02
tertiary 252.08
Hyperpathia (*see also* Disturbance, sensation) 782.0
psychogenic 307.80
Hyperperistalsis 787.4
psychogenic 306.4
Hyperpermeability, capillary 448.9
Hyperphagia 783.6
Hyperphenylalaninemia 270.1
Hyperphoria 378.40
alternating 378.45
Hyperphosphatemia 275.3
Hyperpiesia (*see also* Hypertension) 401.9
Hyperpiesis (*see also* Hypertension) 401.9
Hyperpigmentation - *see* Pigmentation
Hyperpinealism 259.8
Hyperpipecolatemia 270.7
Hyperpituitarism 253.1
Hyperplasia, hyperplastic
adenoids (lymphoid tissue) 474.12
and tonsils 474.10
adrenal (capsule) (cortex) (gland) 255.8
with
sexual precocity (male) 255.2
virilism, adrenal 255.2
virilization (female) 255.2
congenital 255.2
due to excess ACTH (ectopic) (pituitary) 255.0
medulla 255.8

Hyperplasia, hyperplastic *(Continued)*
alpha cells (pancreatic)
with
gastrin excess 251.5
glucagon excess 251.4
appendix (lymphoid) 543.0
artery, fibromuscular NEC 447.8
carotid 447.8
renal 447.3
bone 733.99
marrow 289.9
breast (*see also* Hypertrophy, breast) 611.1
carotid artery 447.8
cementation, cementum (teeth) (tooth) 521.5
cervical gland 785.6
cervix (uteri) 622.10
basal cell 622.10
congenital 752.49
endometrium 622.10
polypoid 622.10
chin 524.05
clitoris, congenital 752.49
dentin 521.5
endocervicitis 616.0
endometrium, endometrial (adenomatous) (atypical) (cystic) (glandular) (polypoid) (uterus) 621.30
with atypia 621.33
without atypia
complex 621.32
simple 621.31
cervix 622.10
epithelial 709.8
focal, oral, including tongue 528.79
mouth (focal) 528.79
nipple 611.8
skin 709.8
tongue (focal) 528.79
vaginal wall 623.0
erythroid 289.9
fascialis ossificans (progressiva) 728.11
fibromuscular, artery NEC 447.8
carotid 447.8
renal 447.3
genital
female 629.89 ⇐
male 608.89
gingiva 523.8
glandularis
cystica uteri 621.30
endometrium (uterus) 621.30
interstitialis uteri 621.30
granulocytic 288.69 ⇐
gum 523.8
hymen, congenital 752.49
islands of Langerhans 251.1
islet cell (pancreatic) 251.9
alpha cells
with excess
gastrin 251.5
glucagon 251.4
beta cells 251.1
juxtaglomerular (complex) (kidney) 593.89
kidney (congenital) 753.3
liver (congenital) 751.69
lymph node (gland) 785.6
lymphoid (diffuse) (nodular) 785.6
appendix 543.0
intestine 569.89
mandibular 524.02
alveolar 524.72
unilateral condylar 526.89

◀ New ⇐ Revised

Hyperplasia, hyperplastic *(Continued)*
Marchand multiple nodular (liver) - *see* Cirrhosis, postnecrotic
maxillary 524.01
alveolar 524.71
medulla, adrenal 255.8
myometrium, myometrial 621.2
nose (lymphoid) (polypoid) 478.19
oral soft tissue (inflammatory) (irritative) (mucosa) NEC 528.9
gingiva 523.8
tongue 529.8
organ or site, congenital NEC - *see* Anomaly, specified type NEC
ovary 620.8
palate, papillary 528.9
pancreatic islet cells 251.9
alpha
with excess
gastrin 251.5
glucagon 251.4
beta 251.1
parathyroid (gland) 252.01
persistent, vitreous (primary) 743.51
pharynx (lymphoid) 478.29
prostate 600.90
with
other lower urinary tract symptoms (LUTS) 600.91 ◀
urinary ◀
obstruction 600.91 ◀
retention 600.91 ◀
adenofibromatous 600.20
with
other lower urinary tract symptoms (LUTS) 600.21 ◀
urinary ◀
obstruction 600.21 ◀
retention 600.21 ◀
nodular 600.10
with
urinary ◀
obstruction 600.11 ◀
retention 600.11 ◀
renal artery (fibromuscular) 447.3
reticuloendothelial (cell) 289.9
salivary gland (any) 527.1
Schimmelbusch's 610.1
suprarenal (capsule) (gland) 255.8
thymus (gland) (persistent) 254.0
thyroid (*see also* Goiter) 240.9
primary 242.0
secondary 242.2
tonsil (lymphoid tissue) 474.11
and adenoids 474.10
urethrovaginal 599.89
uterus, uterine (myometrium) 621.2
endometrium (*see also* Hyperplasia, endometrium) 621.30
vitreous (humor), primary persistent 743.51
vulva 624.3
zygoma 738.11
Hyperpnea (*see also* Hyperventilation) 786.01
Hyperpotassemia 276.7
Hyperprebetalipoproteinemia 272.1
with chylomicronemia 272.3
familial 272.1
Hyperprolactinemia 253.1
Hyperprolinemia 270.8
Hyperproteinemia 273.8
Hyperprothrombinemia 289.89
Hyperpselaphesia 782.0
Hyperpyrexia 780.6
heat (effects of) 992.0
malarial (*see also* Malaria) 084.6
malignant, due to anesthetic 995.86
rheumatic - *see* Fever, rheumatic
unknown origin (*see also* Pyrexia) 780.6
Hyperreactor, vascular 780.2
Hyperreflexia 796.1
bladder, autonomic 596.54
with cauda equina 344.61
detrusor 344.61
Hypersalivation (*see also* Ptyalism) 527.7
Hypersarcosinemia 270.8
Hypersecretion
ACTH 255.3
androgens (ovarian) 256.1
calcitonin 246.0
corticoadrenal 255.3
cortisol 255.0
estrogen 256.0
gastric 536.8
psychogenic 306.4
gastrin 251.5
glucagon 251.4
hormone
ACTH 255.3
anterior pituitary 253.1
growth NEC 253.0
ovarian androgen 256.1
testicular 257.0
thyroid stimulating 242.8
insulin - *see* Hyperinsulinism
lacrimal glands (*see also* Epiphora) 375.20
medulloadrenal 255.6
milk 676.6
ovarian androgens 256.1
pituitary (anterior) 253.1
salivary gland (any) 527.7
testicular hormones 257.0
thyrocalcitonin 246.0
upper respiratory 478.9
Hypersegmentation, hereditary 288.2
eosinophils 288.2
neutrophil nuclei 288.2
Hypersensitive, hypersensitiveness, hypersensitivity - *see also* Allergy
angiitis 446.20
specified NEC 446.29
carotid sinus 337.0
colon 564.9
psychogenic 306.4
DNA (deoxyribonucleic acid) NEC 287.2
drug (*see also* Allergy, drug) 995.27
esophagus 530.89
insect bites - *see* Injury, superficial, by site
labyrinth 386.58
pain (*see also* Disturbance, sensation) 782.0
pneumonitis NEC 495.9
reaction (*see also* Allergy) 995.3
upper respiratory tract NEC 478.8
stomach (allergic) (nonallergic) 536.8
psychogenic 306.4
Hypersomatotropism (classic) 253.0
Hypersomnia, unspecified 780.54
with sleep apnea, unspecified 780.53
alcohol induced 291.82
drug induced 292.85
due to
medical condition classified elsewhere 327.14
mental disorder 327.15
Hypersomnia *(Continued)*
idiopathic
with long sleep time 327.11
without long sleep time 327.12
menstrual related 327.13
nonorganic origin 307.43
persistent (primary) 307.44
transient 307.43
organic 327.10
other 327.19
primary 307.44
recurrent 327.13
Hypersplenia 289.4
Hypersplenism 289.4
Hypersteatosis 706.3
Hyperstimulation, ovarian 256.1
Hypersuprarenalism 255.3
Hypersusceptibility - *see* Allergy
Hyper-TBG-nemia 246.8
Hypertelorism 756.0
orbit, orbital 376.41
Hyperthecosis, ovary 256.8
Hyperthermia (of unknown origin) (*see also* Pyrexia) 780.6
malignant (due to anesthesia) 995.86
newborn 778.4
Hyperthymergasia (*see also* Psychosis, affective) 296.0
reactive (from emotional stress, psychological trauma) 298.1
recurrent episode 296.1
single episode 296.0
Hyperthymism 254.8
Hyperthyroid (recurrent) - *see* Hyperthyroidism
Hyperthyroidism (latent) (preadult) (recurrent) (without goiter) 242.9

Note Use the following fifth-digit subclassification with category 242:
0 without mention of thyrotoxic crisis or storm
1 with mention of thyrotoxic crisis or storm

with
goiter (diffuse) 242.0
adenomatous 242.3
multinodular 242.2
uninodular 242.1
nodular 242.3
multinodular 242.2
uninodular 242.1
thyroid nodule 242.1
complicating pregnancy, childbirth, or puerperium 648.1
neonatal (transient) 775.3
Hypertonia - *see* Hypertonicity
Hypertonicity
bladder 596.51
fetus or newborn 779.89
gastrointestinal (tract) 536.8
infancy 779.89
due to electrolyte imbalance 779.89
muscle 728.85
stomach 536.8
psychogenic 306.4
uterus, uterine (contractions) 661.4
affecting fetus or newborn 763.7
Hypertony - *see* Hypertonicity
Hypertransaminemia 790.4
Hypertrichosis 704.1
congenital 757.4
eyelid 374.54

	Malignant	Benign	Unspecified
Hypertension, hypertensive (arterial) (arteriolar) (crisis) (degeneration) (disease) (essential) (fluctuating) (idiopathic) (intermittent) (labile) (low renin) (orthostatic) (paroxysmal) (primary) (systemic) (uncontrolled) (vascular)	401.0	401.1	401.9
with			
chronic kidney disease	-	-	-
stage I through stage IV, or unspecified	403.00	403.10	403.90
stage V or end stage renal disease	403.01	403.11	403.91
heart involvement (conditions classifiable to 429.0–429.3, 429.8, 429.9 due to hypertension) (*see also* Hypertension, heart)	402.00	402.10	402.90
with kidney involvement - *see* Hypertension, cardiorenal			
renal involvement (only conditions classifiable to 585, 586, 587) (excludes conditions classifiable to 584) (*see also* Hypertension, kidney)	403.00	403.10	403.90
with heart involvement - *see* Hypertension, cardiorenal			
failure (and sclerosis) (*see also* Hypertension, kidney)	403.01	403.11	403.91
sclerosis without failure (*see also* Hypertension, kidney)	403.00	403.10	403.90
accelerated (*see also* Hypertension, by type, malignant)	401.0	-	-
antepartum - *see* Hypertension, complicating pregnancy, childbirth, or the puerperium			
cardiorenal (disease)	404.00	404.10	404.90
with			
chronic kidney disease	-	-	-
stage I through stage IV, or unspecified	404.00	404.10	404.90
and heart failure	404.01	404.11	404.91
stage V or end stage renal disease	404.02	404.12	404.92
and heart failure	404.03	404.13	404.93
heart failure	404.01	404.11	404.91
and chronic kidney disease	404.02	404.12	404.92
stage I through stage IV or unspecified	404.02	404.12	404.92
stage V or end stage renal disease	404.03	404.13	404.93
cardiovascular disease (arteriosclerotic) (sclerotic)	402.00	402.10	402.90
with			
heart failure	402.01	402.11	402.91
renal involvement (conditions classifiable to 403) (*see also* Hypertension, cardiorenal)	404.00	404.10	404.90
cardiovascular renal (disease) (sclerosis) (*see also* Hypertension, cardiorenal)	404.00	404.10	404.90
cerebrovascular disease NEC	437.2	437.2	437.2
complicating pregnancy, childbirth, or the puerperium	642.2	642.0	642.9
with			
albuminuria (and edema) (mild)	-	-	642.4
severe	-	-	642.5
chronic kidney disease	642.2	642.2	642.2
and heart disease	642.2	642.2	642.2
edema (mild)	-	-	642.4
severe	-	-	642.5
heart disease	642.2	642.2	642.2
and chronic kidney disease	642.2	642.2	642.2
renal disease	642.2	642.2	642.2
and heart disease	642.2	642.2	642.2
chronic	642.2	642.0	642.0
with pre-eclampsia or eclampsia	642.7	642.7	642.7
fetus or newborn	760.0	760.0	760.0
essential	-	642.0	642.0
with pre-eclampsia or eclampsia	-	642.7	642.7
fetus or newborn	760.0	760.0	760.0
fetus or newborn	760.0	760.0	760.0
gestational	-	-	642.3
pre-existing	642.2	642.0	642.0
with pre-eclampsia or eclampsia	642.7	642.7	642.7
fetus or newborn	760.0	760.0	760.0
secondary to renal disease	642.1	642.1	642.1
with pre-eclampsia or eclampsia	642.7	642.7	642.7
fetus or newborn	760.0	760.0	760.0
transient	-	-	642.3
due to			
aldosteronism, primary	405.09	405.19	405.99
brain tumor	405.09	405.19	405.99
bulbar poliomyelitis	405.09	405.19	405.99
calculus			
kidney	405.09	405.19	405.99
ureter	405.09	405.19	405.99
coarctation, aorta	405.09	405.19	405.99
Cushing's disease	405.09	405.19	405.99
glomerulosclerosis (*see also* Hypertension, kidney)	403.00	403.10	403.90
periarteritis nodosa	405.09	405.19	405.99
pheochromocytoma	405.09	405.19	405.99
polycystic kidney(s)	405.09	405.19	405.99
polycythemia	405.09	405.19	405.99
porphyria	405.09	405.19	405.99
pyelonephritis	405.09	405.19	405.99
renal (artery)			
aneurysm	405.01	405.11	405.91
anomaly	405.01	405.11	405.91
embolism	405.01	405.11	405.91

◄ New   Revised

	Malignant	Benign	Unspecified
Hypertension, hypertensive *(Continued)*			
due to *(Continued)*			
renal *(Continued)*			
fibromuscular hyperplasia	405.01	405.11	405.91
occlusion	405.01	405.11	405.91
stenosis	405.01	405.11	405.91
thrombosis	405.01	405.11	405.91
encephalopathy	437.2	437.2	437.2
gestational (transient) NEC	-	-	642.3
Goldblatt's	440.1	440.1	440.1
heart (disease) (conditions classifiable to 429.0–429.3, 429.8, 429.9 due to hypertension)	402.00	402.10	402.90
with			
heart failure	402.01	402.11	402.91
hypertensive kidney disease (conditions classifiable to 403) (*see also* Hypertension, cardiorenal)	404.00	404.10	404.90
renal sclerosis (*see also* Hypertension, cardiorenal)	404.00	404.10	404.90
intracranial, benign	-	348.2	-
intraocular	-	-	365.04
kidney	403.00	403.10	403.90
with			
chronic kidney disease	-	-	-
stage I through stage IV, or unspecified	403.00	403.10	403.90
stage V or end stage renal disease	403.01	403.11	403.91
heart involvement (conditions classifiable to 429.0–429.3, 429.8, 429.9 due to hypertension) (*see also* Hypertension, cardiorenal)	404.00	404.10	404.90
hypertensive heart (disease) (conditions classifiable to 402) (*see also* Hypertension, cardiorenal)	404.00	404.10	404.90
renal failure (conditions classifiable to 585, 586)	403.01	403.11	403.91
lesser circulation	-	-	416.0
necrotizing	401.0	-	-
ocular	-	-	365.04
portal (due to chronic liver disease)	-	-	572.3
postoperative	-	-	997.91
psychogenic	-	-	306.2
puerperal, postpartum - *see* Hypertension, complicating pregnancy, childbirth, or the puerperium			
pulmonary (artery)	-	-	416.8
with cor pulmonale (chronic)	-	-	416.8
acute	-	-	415.0
idiopathic	-	-	416.0
primary	-	-	416.0
of newborn	-	-	747.83
secondary	-	-	416.8
renal (disease) (*see also* Hypertension, kidney)	403.00	403.10	403.90
renovascular NEC	405.01	405.11	405.91
secondary NEC	405.09	405.19	405.99
due to			
aldosteronism, primary	405.09	405.19	405.99
brain tumor	405.09	405.19	405.99
bulbar poliomyelitis	405.09	405.19	405.99
calculus			
kidney	405.09	405.19	405.99
ureter	405.09	405.19	405.99
coarctation, aorta	405.09	405.19	405.99
Cushing's disease	405.09	405.19	405.99
glomerulosclerosis (*see also* Hypertension, kidney)	403.00	403.10	403.90
periarteritis nodosa	405.09	405.19	405.99
pheochromocytoma	405.09	405.19	405.99
polycystic kidney(s)	405.09	405.19	405.99
polycythemia	405.09	405.19	405.99
porphyria	405.09	405.19	405.99
pyelonephritis	405.09	405.19	405.99
renal (artery)			
aneurysm	405.01	405.11	405.91
anomaly	405.01	405.11	405.91
embolism	405.01	405.11	405.91
fibromuscular hyperplasia	405.01	405.11	405.91
occlusion	405.01	405.11	405.91
stenosis	405.01	405.11	405.91
thrombosis	405.01	405.11	405.91
transient	-	-	796.2
of pregnancy	-	-	642.3
venous, chronic (asymptomatic) (idiopathic)	-	-	459.30
due to			
deep vein thrombosis (*see also* Syndrome, postphlebitic)	-	-	459.10
with			
complication, NEC	-	-	459.39
inflammation	-	-	459.32
with ulcer	-	-	459.33
ulcer	-	-	459.31
with inflammation	-	-	459.33

ICD-9-CM

H

Vol. 2

Hypertrichosis *(Continued)*
lanuginosa 757.4
acquired 704.1
Hypertriglyceridemia, essential 272.1
Hypertrophy, hypertrophic
adenoids (infectional) 474.12
and tonsils (faucial) (infective) (lingual) (lymphoid) 474.10
adrenal 255.8
alveolar process or ridge 525.8
anal papillae 569.49
apocrine gland 705.82
artery NEC 447.8
carotid 447.8
congenital (peripheral) NEC 747.60
gastrointestinal 747.61
lower limb 747.64
renal 747.62
specified NEC 747.69
spinal 747.82
upper limb 747.63
renal 447.3
arthritis (chronic) (*see also* Osteoarthrosis) 715.9
spine (*see also* Spondylosis) 721.90
arytenoid 478.79
asymmetrical (heart) 429.9
auricular - *see* Hypertrophy, cardiac
Bartholin's gland 624.8
bile duct 576.8
bladder (sphincter) (trigone) 596.8
blind spot, visual field 368.42
bone 733.99
brain 348.8
breast 611.1
cystic 610.1
fetus or newborn 778.7
fibrocystic 610.1
massive pubertal 611.1
puerperal, postpartum 676.3
senile (parenchymatous) 611.1
cardiac (chronic) (idiopathic) 429.3
with
rheumatic fever (conditions classifiable to 390)
active 391.8
with chorea 392.0
inactive or quiescent (with chorea) 398.99
congenital NEC 746.89
fatty (*see also* Degeneration, myocardial) 429.1
hypertensive (*see also* Hypertension, heart) 402.90
rheumatic (with chorea) 398.99
active or acute 391.8
with chorea 392.0
valve (*see also* Endocarditis) 424.90
congenital NEC 746.89
cartilage 733.99
cecum 569.89
cervix (uteri) 622.6
congenital 752.49
elongation 622.6
clitoris (cirrhotic) 624.2
congenital 752.49
colon 569.89
congenital 751.3
conjunctiva, lymphoid 372.73
cornea 371.89
corpora cavernosa 607.89
duodenum 537.89
endometrium (uterus) (*see also* Hyperplasia, endometrium) 621.30
cervix 622.6
epididymis 608.89
esophageal hiatus (congenital) 756.6

Hypertrophy, hypertrophic *(Continued)*
esophageal hiatus (*Continued*)
with hernia - *see* Hernia, diaphragm
eyelid 374.30
falx, skull 733.99
fat pad 729.30
infrapatellar 729.31
knee 729.31
orbital 374.34
popliteal 729.31
prepatellar 729.31
retropatellar 729.31
specified site NEC 729.39
foot (congenital) 755.67
frenum, frenulum (tongue) 529.8
linguae 529.8
lip 528.5
gallbladder or cystic duct 575.8
gastric mucosa 535.2
gingiva 523.8
gland, glandular (general) NEC 785.6
gum (mucous membrane) 523.8
heart (idiopathic) - *see also* Hypertrophy, cardiac
valve - *see also* Endocarditis
congenital NEC 746.89
hemifacial 754.0
hepatic - *see* Hypertrophy, liver
hiatus (esophageal) 756.6
hilus gland 785.6
hymen, congenital 752.49
ileum 569.89
infrapatellar fat pad 729.31
intestine 569.89
jejunum 569.89
kidney (compensatory) 593.1
congenital 753.3
labial frenulum 528.5
labium (majus) (minus) 624.3
lacrimal gland, chronic 375.03
ligament 728.9
spinal 724.8
linguae frenulum 529.8
lingual tonsil (infectional) 474.11
lip (frenum) 528.5
congenital 744.81
liver 789.1
acute 573.8
cirrhotic - *see* Cirrhosis, liver
congenital 751.69
fatty - *see* Fatty, liver
lymph gland 785.6
tuberculous - *see* Tuberculosis, lymph gland
mammary gland - *see* Hypertrophy, breast
maxillary frenulum 528.5
Meckel's diverticulum (congenital) 751.0
medial meniscus, acquired 717.3
median bar 600.90
with
other lower urinary tract symptoms (LUTS) 600.91
urinary
obstruction 600.91
retention 600.91
mediastinum 519.3
meibomian gland 373.2
meniscus, knee, congenital 755.64
metatarsal head 733.99
metatarsus 733.99
mouth 528.9
mucous membrane
alveolar process 523.8
nose 478.19
turbinate (nasal) 478.0

Hypertrophy, hypertrophic *(Continued)*
muscle 728.9
muscular coat, artery NEC 447.8
carotid 447.8
renal 447.3
myocardium (*see also* Hypertrophy, cardiac) 429.3
idiopathic 425.4
myometrium 621.2
nail 703.8
congenital 757.5
nasal 478.19
alae 478.19
bone 738.0
cartilage 478.19
mucous membrane (septum) 478.19
sinus (*see also* Sinusitis) 473.9
turbinate 478.0
nasopharynx, lymphoid (infectional) (tissue) (wall) 478.29
neck, uterus 622.6
nipple 611.1
normal aperture diaphragm (congenital) 756.6
nose (*see also* Hypertrophy, nasal) 478.19
orbit 376.46
organ or site, congenital NEC - *see* Anomaly, specified type NEC
osteoarthropathy (pulmonary) 731.2
ovary 620.8
palate (hard) 526.89
soft 528.9
pancreas (congenital) 751.7
papillae
anal 569.49
tongue 529.3
parathyroid (gland) 252.01
parotid gland 527.1
penis 607.89
phallus 607.89
female (clitoris) 624.2
pharyngeal tonsil 474.12
pharyngitis 472.1
pharynx 478.29
lymphoid (infectional) (tissue) (wall) 478.29
pituitary (fossa) (gland) 253.8
popliteal fat pad 729.31
preauricular (lymph) gland (Hampstead) 785.6
prepuce (congenital) 605
female 624.2
prostate (asymptomatic) (early) (recurrent) 600.90
with
other lower urinary tract symptoms (LUTS) 600.91
urinary
obstruction 600.91
retention 600.91
adenofibromatous 600.20
with
other lower urinary tract symptoms (LUTS) 600.21
urinary
obstruction 600.21
retention 600.21
benign 600.00
with
other lower urinary tract symptoms (LUTS) 600.01
urinary
obstruction 600.01
retention 600.01
congenital 752.89

Hypertrophy, hypertrophic *(Continued)*
pseudoedematous hypodermal 757.0
pseudomuscular 359.1
pylorus (muscle) (sphincter) 537.0
congenital 750.5
infantile 750.5
rectal sphincter 569.49
rectum 569.49
renal 593.1
rhinitis (turbinate) 472.0
salivary duct or gland 527.1
congenital 750.26
scaphoid (tarsal) 733.99
scar 701.4
scrotum 608.89
sella turcica 253.8
seminal vesicle 608.89
sigmoid 569.89
skin condition NEC 701.9
spermatic cord 608.89
spinal ligament 724.8
spleen - *see* Splenomegaly
spondylitis (spine) (*see also* Spondylosis) 721.90
stomach 537.89
subaortic stenosis (idiopathic) 425.1
sublingual gland 527.1
congenital 750.26
submaxillary gland 527.1
suprarenal (gland) 255.8
tendon 727.9
testis 608.89
congenital 752.89
thymic, thymus (congenital) (gland) 254.0
thyroid (gland) (*see also* Goiter) 240.9
primary 242.0
secondary 242.2
toe (congenital) 755.65
acquired 735.8
tongue 529.8
congenital 750.15
frenum 529.8
papillae (foliate) 529.3
tonsil (faucial) (infective) (lingual) (lymphoid) 474.11
with
adenoiditis 474.01
tonsillitis 474.00
and adenoiditis 474.02
and adenoids 474.10
tunica vaginalis 608.89
turbinate (mucous membrane) 478.0
ureter 593.89
urethra 599.84
uterus 621.2
puerperal, postpartum 674.8
uvula 528.9
vagina 623.8
vas deferens 608.89
vein 459.89
ventricle, ventricular (heart) (left) (right) - *see also* Hypertrophy, cardiac
congenital 746.89
due to hypertension (left) (right) (*see also* Hypertension, heart) 402.90
benign 402.10
malignant 402.00
right with ventricular septal defect, pulmonary stenosis or atresia, and dextraposition of aorta 745.2

Hypertrophy, hypertrophic *(Continued)*
verumontanum 599.89
vesical 596.8
vocal cord 478.5
vulva 624.3
stasis (nonfilarial) 624.3
Hypertropia (intermittent) (periodic) 378.31
Hypertyrosinemia 270.2
Hyperuricemia 790.6
Hypervalinemia 270.3
Hyperventilation (tetany) 786.01
hysterical 300.11
psychogenic 306.1
syndrome 306.1
Hyperviscidosis 277.00
Hyperviscosity (of serum) (syndrome) NEC 273.3
polycythemic 289.0
sclerocythemic 282.8
Hypervitaminosis (dietary) NEC 278.8
A (dietary) 278.2
D (dietary) 278.4
from excessive administration or use of vitamin preparations (chronic) 278.8
reaction to sudden overdose 963.5
vitamin A 278.2
reaction to sudden overdose 963.5
vitamin D 278.4
reaction to sudden overdose 963.5
vitamin K
correct substance properly administered 278.8
overdose or wrong substance given or taken 964.3
Hypervolemia 276.6
Hypesthesia (*see also* Disturbance, sensation) 782.0
cornea 371.81
Hyphema (anterior chamber) (ciliary body) (iris) 364.41
traumatic 921.3
Hyphemia - *see* Hyphema
Hypoacidity, gastric 536.8
psychogenic 306.4
Hypoactive labyrinth (function) - *see* Hypofunction, labyrinth
Hypoadrenalism 255.4
tuberculous (*see also* Tuberculosis) 017.6
Hypoadrenocorticism 255.4
pituitary 253.4
Hypoalbuminemia 273.8
Hypoaldosteronism 255.4 ◀
Hypoalphalipoproteinemia 272.5
Hypobarism 993.2
Hypobaropathy 993.2
Hypobetalipoproteinemia (familial) 272.5
Hypocalcemia 275.41
cow's milk 775.4
dietary 269.3
neonatal 775.4
phosphate-loading 775.4
Hypocalcification, teeth 520.4
Hypochloremia 276.9
Hypochlorhydria 536.8
neurotic 306.4
psychogenic 306.4
Hypocholesteremia 272.5
Hypochondria (reaction) 300.7
Hypochondriac 300.7
Hypochondriasis 300.7
Hypochromasia blood cells 280.9

Hypochromic anemia 280.9
due to blood loss (chronic) 280.0
acute 285.1
microcytic 280.9
Hypocoagulability (*see also* Defect, coagulation) 286.9
Hypocomplementemia 279.8
Hypocythemia (progressive) 284.9
Hypodontia (*see also* Anodontia) 520.0
Hypoeosinophilia 288.59 ⬅
Hypoesthesia (*see also* Disturbance, sensation) 782.0
cornea 371.81
tactile 782.0
Hypoestrinism 256.39
Hypoestrogenism 256.39
Hypoferremia 280.9
due to blood loss (chronic) 280.0
Hypofertility
female 628.9
male 606.1
Hypofibrinogenemia 286.3
acquired 286.6
congenital 286.3
Hypofunction
adrenal (gland) 255.4
cortex 255.4
medulla 255.5
specified NEC 255.5
cerebral 331.9
corticoadrenal NEC 255.4
intestinal 564.89
labyrinth (unilateral) 386.53
with loss of labyrinthine reactivity 386.55
bilateral 386.54
with loss of labyrinthine reactivity 386.56
Leydig cell 257.2
ovary 256.39
postablative 256.2
pituitary (anterior) (gland) (lobe) 253.2
posterior 253.5
testicular 257.2
iatrogenic 257.1
postablative 257.1
postirradiation 257.1
postsurgical 257.1
Hypogammaglobulinemia 279.00
acquired primary 279.06
non-sex-linked, congenital 279.06
sporadic 279.06
transient of infancy 279.09
Hypogenitalism (congenital) (female) (male) 752.89
penis 752.69
Hypoglycemia (spontaneous) 251.2
coma 251.0
diabetic 250.3
diabetic 250.8
due to insulin 251.0
therapeutic misadventure 962.3
familial (idiopathic) 251.2
following gastrointestinal surgery 579.3
infantile (idiopathic) 251.2
in infant of diabetic mother 775.0
leucine-induced 270.3
neonatal 775.6
reactive 251.2
specified NEC 251.1
Hypoglycemic shock 251.0
diabetic 250.8
due to insulin 251.0
functional (syndrome) 251.1

ICD-9-CM
H
Vol. 2

Hypogonadism
female 256.39
gonadotrophic (isolated) 253.4
hypogonadotropic (isolated) (with anosmia) 253.4
isolated 253.4
male 257.2
hereditary familial (Reifenstein's syndrome) 259.5
ovarian (primary) 256.39
pituitary (secondary) 253.4
testicular (primary) (secondary) 257.2
Hypohidrosis 705.0
Hypohidrotic ectodermal dysplasia 757.31
Hypoidrosis 705.0
Hypoinsulinemia, postsurgical 251.3
postpancreatectomy (complete) (partial) 251.3
Hypokalemia 276.8
Hypokinesia 780.99
Hypoleukia splenica 289.4
Hypoleukocytosis 288.50
Hypolipidemia 272.5
Hypolipoproteinemia 272.5
Hypomagnesemia 275.2
neonatal 775.4
Hypomania, hypomanic reaction (*see also* Psychosis, affective) 296.0
recurrent episode 296.1
single episode 296.0
Hypomastia (congenital) 757.6
Hypomenorrhea 626.1
Hypometabolism 783.9
Hypomotility
gastrointestinal tract 536.8
psychogenic 306.4
intestine 564.89
psychogenic 306.4
stomach 536.8
psychogenic 306.4
Hyponasality 784.49
Hyponatremia 276.1
Hypo-ovarianism 256.39
Hypo-ovarism 256.39
Hypoparathyroidism (idiopathic) (surgically induced) 252.1
neonatal 775.4
Hypopharyngitis 462
Hypophoria 378.40
Hypophosphatasia 275.3
Hypophosphatemia (acquired) (congenital) (familial) 275.3
renal 275.3
Hypophyseal, hypophysis - *see also* condition
dwarfism 253.3
gigantism 253.0
syndrome 253.8
Hypophyseothalamic syndrome 253.8
Hypopiesis - *see* Hypotension
Hypopigmentation 709.00
eyelid 374.53
Hypopinealism 259.8
Hypopituitarism (juvenile) (syndrome) 253.2
due to
hormone therapy 253.7
hypophysectomy 253.7
radiotherapy 253.7
postablative 253.7
postpartum hemorrhage 253.2
Hypoplasia, hypoplasis 759.89
adrenal (gland) 759.1
alimentary tract 751.8

Hypoplasia, hypoplasis *(Continued)*
alimentary tract *(Continued)*
lower 751.2
upper 750.8
anus, anal (canal) 751.2
aorta 747.22
aortic
arch (tubular) 747.10
orifice or valve with hypoplasia of ascending aorta and defective development of left ventricle (with mitral valve atresia) 746.7
appendix 751.2
areola 757.6
arm (*see also* Absence, arm, congenital) 755.20
artery (congenital) (peripheral) 747.60
brain 747.81
cerebral 747.81
coronary 746.85
gastrointestinal 747.61
lower limb 747.64
pulmonary 747.3
renal 747.62
retinal 743.58
specified NEC 747.69
spinal 747.82
umbilical 747.5
upper limb 747.63
auditory canal 744.29
causing impairment of hearing 744.02
biliary duct (common) or passage 751.61
bladder 753.8
bone NEC 756.9
face 756.0
malar 756.0
mandible 524.04
alveolar 524.74
marrow 284.9
acquired (secondary) 284.8
congenital 284.09
idiopathic 284.9
maxilla 524.03
alveolar 524.73
skull (*see also* Hypoplasia, skull) 756.0
brain 742.1
gyri 742.2
specified part 742.2
breast (areola) 757.6
bronchus (tree) 748.3
cardiac 746.89
valve - *see* Hypoplasia, heart, valve
vein 746.89
carpus (*see also* Absence, carpal, congenital) 755.28
cartilaginous 756.9
cecum 751.2
cementum 520.4
hereditary 520.5
cephalic 742.1
cerebellum 742.2
cervix (uteri) 752.49
chin 524.06
clavicle 755.51
coccyx 756.19
colon 751.2
corpus callosum 742.2
cricoid cartilage 748.3
dermal, focal (Goltz) 757.39
digestive organ(s) or tract NEC 751.8
lower 751.2
upper 750.8

Hypoplasia, hypoplasis *(Continued)*
ear 744.29
auricle 744.23
lobe 744.29
middle, except ossicles 744.03
ossicles 744.04
ossicles 744.04
enamel of teeth (neonatal) (postnatal) (prenatal) 520.4
hereditary 520.5
endocrine (gland) NEC 759.2
endometrium 621.8
epididymis 752.89
epiglottis 748.3
erythroid, congenital 284.01
erythropoietic, chronic acquired 284.8
esophagus 750.3
Eustachian tube 744.24
eye (*see also* Microphthalmos) 743.10
lid 743.62
face 744.89
bone(s) 756.0
fallopian tube 752.19
femur (*see also* Absence, femur, congenital) 755.34
fibula (*see also* Absence, fibula, congenital) 755.37
finger (*see also* Absence, finger, congenital) 755.29
focal dermal 757.39
foot 755.31
gallbladder 751.69
genitalia, genital organ(s)
female 752.89
external 752.49
internal NEC 752.89
in adiposogenital dystrophy 253.8
male 752.89
penis 752.69
glottis 748.3
hair 757.4
hand 755.21
heart 746.89
left (complex) (syndrome) 746.7
valve NEC 746.89
pulmonary 746.01
humerus (*see also* Absence, humerus, congenital) 755.24
hymen 752.49
intestine (small) 751.1
large 751.2
iris 743.46
jaw 524.09
kidney(s) 753.0
labium (majus) (minus) 752.49
labyrinth, membranous 744.05
lacrimal duct (apparatus) 743.65
larynx 748.3
leg (*see also* Absence, limb, congenital, lower) 755.30
limb 755.4
lower (*see also* Absence, limb, congenital, lower) 755.30
upper (*see also* Absence, limb, congenital, upper) 755.20
liver 751.69
lung (lobe) 748.5
mammary (areolar) 757.6
mandibular 524.04
alveolar 524.74
unilateral condylar 526.89
maxillary 524.03
alveolar 524.73
medullary 284.9

Hypoplasia, hypoplasis *(Continued)*
megakaryocytic 287.30
metacarpus (*see also* Absence, metacarpal, congenital) 755.28
metatarsus (*see also* Absence, metatarsal, congenital) 755.38
muscle 756.89
eye 743.69
myocardium (congenital) (Uhl's anomaly) 746.84
nail(s) 757.5
nasolacrimal duct 743.65
nervous system NEC 742.8
neural 742.8
nose, nasal 748.1
ophthalmic (*see also* Microphthalmos) 743.10
optic nerve 377.43 ◀
organ
of Corti 744.05
or site NEC - *see* Anomaly, by site
osseous meatus (ear) 744.03
ovary 752.0
oviduct 752.19
pancreas 751.7
parathyroid (gland) 759.2
parotid gland 750.26
patella 755.64
pelvis, pelvic girdle 755.69
penis 752.69
peripheral vascular system (congenital) NEC 747.60
gastrointestinal 747.61
lower limb 747.64
renal 747.62
specified NEC 747.69
spinal 747.82
upper limb 747.63
pituitary (gland) 759.2
pulmonary 748.5
arteriovenous 747.3
artery 747.3
valve 746.01
punctum lacrimale 743.65
radioulnar (*see also* Absence, radius, congenital, with ulna) 755.25
radius (*see also* Absence, radius, congenital) 755.26
rectum 751.2
respiratory system NEC 748.9
rib 756.3
sacrum 756.19
scapula 755.59
shoulder girdle 755.59
skin 757.39
skull (bone) 756.0
with
anencephalus 740.0
encephalocele 742.0
hydrocephalus 742.3
with spina bifida (*see also* Spina bifida) 741.0
microcephalus 742.1
spinal (cord) (ventral horn cell) 742.59
vessel 747.82
spine 756.19
spleen 759.0
sternum 756.3
tarsus (*see also* Absence, tarsal, congenital) 755.38
testis, testicle 752.89
thymus (gland) 279.11
thyroid (gland) 243
cartilage 748.3
tibiofibular (*see also* Absence, tibia, congenital, with fibula) 755.35

Hypoplasia, hypoplasis *(Continued)*
toe (*see also* Absence, toe, congenital) 755.39
tongue 750.16
trachea (cartilage) (rings) 748.3
Turner's (tooth) 520.4
ulna (*see also* Absence, ulna, congenital) 755.27
umbilical artery 747.5
ureter 753.29
uterus 752.3
vagina 752.49
vascular (peripheral) NEC (*see also* Hypoplasia, peripheral vascular system) 747.60
brain 747.81
vein(s) (peripheral) NEC (*see also* Hypoplasia, peripheral vascular system) 747.60
brain 747.81
cardiac 746.89
great 747.49
portal 747.49
pulmonary 747.49
vena cava (inferior) (superior) 747.49
vertebra 756.19
vulva 752.49
zonule (ciliary) 743.39
zygoma 738.12
Hypopotassemia 276.8
Hypoproaccelerinemia (*see also* Defect, coagulation) 286.3
Hypoproconvertinemia (congenital) (*see also* Defect, coagulation) 286.3
Hypoproteinemia (essential) (hypermetabolic) (idiopathic) 273.8
Hypoproteinosis 260
Hypoprothrombinemia (congenital) (hereditary) (idiopathic) (*see also* Defect, coagulation) 286.3
acquired 286.7
newborn 776.3
Hypopselaphesia 782.0
Hypopyon (anterior chamber) (eye) 364.05
iritis 364.05
ulcer (cornea) 370.04
Hypopyrexia 780.99
Hyporeflex 796.1
Hyporeninemia, extreme 790.99
in primary aldosteronism 255.10
Hyporesponsive episode 780.09
Hyposecretion
ACTH 253.4
ovary 256.39
postablative 256.2
salivary gland (any) 527.7
Hyposegmentation of neutrophils, hereditary 288.2
Hyposiderinemia 280.9
Hyposmolality 276.1
syndrome 276.1
Hyposomatotropism 253.3
Hyposomnia, unspecified (*see also* Insomnia) 780.52
with sleep apnea, unspecified 780.51 ⬅
Hypospadias (male) 752.61
female 753.8
Hypospermatogenesis 606.1
Hyposphagma 372.72
Hyposplenism 289.59
Hypostasis, pulmonary 514
Hypostatic - *see* condition

Hyposthenuria 593.89
Hyposuprarenalism 255.4
Hypo-TBG-nemia 246.8
Hypotension (arterial) (constitutional) 458.9
chronic 458.1
iatrogenic 458.29
maternal, syndrome (following labor and delivery) 669.2
of hemodialysis 458.21
orthostatic (chronic) 458.0
dysautonomic-dyskinetic syndrome 333.0
permanent idiopathic 458.1
postoperative 458.29
postural 458.0
specified type NEC 458.8
transient 796.3
Hypothermia (accidental) 991.6
anesthetic 995.89
newborn NEC 778.3
not associated with low environmental temperature 780.99
Hypothymergasia (*see also* Psychosis, affective) 296.2
recurrent episode 296.3
single episode 296.2
Hypothyroidism (acquired) 244.9
complicating pregnancy, childbirth, or puerperium 648.1
congenital 243
due to
ablation 244.1
radioactive iodine 244.1
surgical 244.0
iodine (administration) (ingestion) 244.2
radioactive 244.1
irradiation therapy 244.1
p-aminosalicylic acid (PAS) 244.3
phenylbutazone 244.3
resorcinol 244.3
specified cause NEC 244.8
surgery 244.0
goitrous (sporadic) 246.1
iatrogenic NEC 244.3
iodine 244.2
pituitary 244.8
postablative NEC 244.1
postsurgical 244.0
primary 244.9
secondary NEC 244.8
specified cause NEC 244.8
sporadic goitrous 246.1
Hypotonia, hypotonicity, hypotony 781.3
benign congenital 358.8
bladder 596.4
congenital 779.89
benign 358.8
eye 360.30
due to
fistula 360.32
ocular disorder NEC 360.33
following loss of aqueous or vitreous 360.33
primary 360.31
infantile muscular (benign) 359.0
muscle 728.9
uterus, uterine (contractions) - *see* Inertia, uterus
Hypotrichosis 704.09
congenital 757.4
lid (congenital) 757.4
acquired 374.55

Hypotrichosis *(Continued)*
postinfectional NEC 704.09
Hypotropia 378.32
Hypoventilation 786.09
congenital central alveolar syndrome 327.25
idiopathic sleep related nonobstructive alveolar 327.24
sleep related, in conditions classifiable elsewhere 327.26
Hypovitaminosis (*see also* Deficiency, vitamin) 269.2
Hypovolemia 276.52
surgical shock 998.0
traumatic (shock) 958.4
Hypoxemia (*see also* Anoxia) 799.02
Hypoxemia *(Continued)*
sleep related, in conditions classifiable elsewhere 327.26
Hypoxia (*see also* Anoxia) 799.02
cerebral 348.1
during or resulting from a procedure 997.01
newborn 770.88 ⬅
mild or moderate 768.6
severe 768.5
fetal, affecting newborn 770.88 ⬅
intrauterine - *see* Distress, fetal
myocardial (*see also* Insufficiency, coronary) 411.89
arteriosclerotic - *see* Arteriosclerosis, coronary
Hypoxia *(Continued)*
newborn 770.88 ⬅
sleep related 327.24
Hypoxic-ischemic encephalopathy (HIE) 768.7 ◀
Hypsarrhythmia (*see also* Epilepsy) 345.6
Hysteralgia, pregnant uterus 646.8
Hysteria, hysterical 300.10
anxiety 300.20
Charcôt's gland 300.11
conversion (any manifestation) 300.11
dissociative type NEC 300.15
psychosis, acute 298.1
Hysteroepilepsy 300.11
Hysterotomy, affecting fetus or newborn 763.89

◀ New ⬅ Revised

I

Iatrogenic syndrome of excess cortisol 255.0
Iceland disease (epidemic neuromyasthenia) 049.8
Ichthyosis (congenita) 757.1
  acquired 701.1
  fetalis gravior 757.1
  follicularis 757.1
  hystrix 757.39
  lamellar 757.1
  lingual 528.6
  palmaris and plantaris 757.39
  simplex 757.1
  vera 757.1
  vulgaris 757.1
Ichthyotoxism 988.0
  bacterial (*see also* Poisoning, food) 005.9
Icteroanemia, hemolytic (acquired) 283.9
  congenital (*see also* Spherocytosis) 282.0
Icterus (*see also* Jaundice) 782.4
  catarrhal - *see* Icterus, infectious
  conjunctiva 782.4
    newborn 774.6
  epidemic - *see* Icterus, infectious
  febrilis - *see* Icterus, infectious
  fetus or newborn - *see* Jaundice, fetus or newborn
  gravis (*see also* Necrosis, liver) 570
    complicating pregnancy 646.7
      affecting fetus or newborn 760.8
    fetus or newborn NEC 773.0
    obstetrical 646.7
      affecting fetus or newborn 760.8
  hematogenous (acquired) 283.9
  hemolytic (acquired) 283.9
    congenital (*see also* Spherocytosis) 282.0
  hemorrhagic (acute) 100.0
    leptospiral 100.0
    newborn 776.0
    spirochetal 100.0
  infectious 070.1
    with hepatic coma 070.0
    leptospiral 100.0
    spirochetal 100.0
  intermittens juvenilis 277.4
  malignant (*see also* Necrosis, liver) 570
  neonatorum (*see also* Jaundice, fetus or newborn) 774.6
  pernicious (*see also* Necrosis, liver) 570
  spirochetal 100.0
Ictus solaris, solis 992.0
Ideation
  suicidal V62.84
Identity disorder 313.82
  dissociative 300.14
  gender role (child) 302.6
    adult 302.85
  psychosexual (child) 302.6
    adult 302.85
Idioglossia 307.9
Idiopathic - *see* condition
Idiosyncrasy (*see also* Allergy) 995.3
  drug, medicinal substance, and biological - *see* Allergy, drug
Idiot, idiocy (congenital) 318.2
  amaurotic (Bielschowsky) (-Jansky) (family) (infantile (late)) (juvenile (late)) (Vogt-Spielmeyer) 330.1
  microcephalic 742.1
  mongolian 758.0
  oxycephalic 756.0
Id reaction (due to bacteria) 692.89
IgE asthma 493.0
Ileitis (chronic) (*see also* Enteritis) 558.9
  infectious 009.0
  noninfectious 558.9
  regional (ulcerative) 555.0
    with large intestine 555.2
  segmental 555.0
    with large intestine 555.2
  terminal (ulcerative) 555.0
    with large intestine 555.2
Ileocolitis (*see also* Enteritis) 558.9
  infectious 009.0
  regional 555.2
  ulcerative 556.1
Ileostomy status V44.2
  with complication 569.60
Ileotyphus 002.0
Ileum - *see* condition
Ileus (adynamic) (bowel) (colon) (inhibitory) (intestine) (neurogenic) (paralytic) 560.1
  arteriomesenteric duodenal 537.2
  due to gallstone (in intestine) 560.31
  duodenal, chronic 537.2
  following gastrointestinal surgery 997.4
  gallstone 560.31
  mechanical (*see also* Obstruction, intestine) 560.9
  meconium 777.1
    due to cystic fibrosis 277.01
  myxedema 564.89
  postoperative 997.4
  transitory, newborn 777.4
Iliac - *see* condition
Iliotibial band friction syndrome 728.89
Ill, louping 063.1
Illegitimacy V61.6
Illness - *see also* Disease
  factitious 300.19
    with
      combined psychological and physical signs and symptoms 300.19
      physical symptoms 300.19
      predominantly
        physical signs and symptoms 300.19
        psychological symptoms 300.16
      psychological symptoms 300.16
    chronic (with physical symptoms) 301.51
  heart - *see* Disease, heart
  manic-depressive (*see also* Psychosis, affective) 296.80
  mental (*see also* Disorder, mental) 300.9
Imbalance 781.2
  autonomic (*see also* Neuropathy, peripheral, autonomic) 337.9
  electrolyte 276.9
    with
      abortion - *see* Abortion, by type, with metabolic disorder
      ectopic pregnancy (*see also* categories 633.0–633.9) 639.4
      hyperemesis gravidarum (before 22 completed weeks' gestation) 643.1
      molar pregnancy (*see also* categories 630–632) 639.4
    following
      abortion 639.4
      ectopic or molar pregnancy 639.4
    neonatal, transitory NEC 775.5
  endocrine 259.9
Imbalance *(Continued)*
  eye muscle NEC 378.9
    heterophoria - *see* Heterophoria
  glomerulotubular NEC 593.89
  hormone 259.9
  hysterical (*see also* Hysteria) 300.10
  labyrinth NEC 386.50
  posture 729.9
  sympathetic (*see also* Neuropathy, peripheral, autonomic) 337.9
Imbecile, imbecility 318.0
  moral 301.7
  old age 290.9
  senile 290.9
  specified IQ - *see* IQ
  unspecified IQ 318.0
Imbedding, intrauterine device 996.32
Imbibition, cholesterol (gallbladder) 575.6
Imerslund (-Gräsbeck) syndrome (anemia due to familial selective vitamin B_{12} malabsorption) 281.1
Iminoacidopathy 270.8
Iminoglycinuria, familial 270.8
Immature - *see also* Immaturity
  personality 301.89
Immaturity 765.1
  extreme 765.0
  fetus or infant light-for-dates - *see* Light-for-dates
  lung, fetus or newborn 770.4
  organ or site NEC - *see* Hypoplasia
  pulmonary, fetus or newborn 770.4
  reaction 301.89
  sexual (female) (male) 259.0
Immersion 994.1
  foot 991.4
  hand 991.4
Immobile, immobility
  intestine 564.89
  joint - *see* Ankylosis
  syndrome (paraplegic) 728.3
Immunization
  ABO
    affecting management of pregnancy 656.2
      fetus or newborn 773.1
  complication - *see* Complications, vaccination
  Rh factor
    affecting management of pregnancy 656.1
      fetus or newborn 773.0
    from transfusion 999.7
Immunodeficiency 279.3
  with
    adenosine-deaminase deficiency 279.2
    defect, predominant
      B-cell 279.00
      T-cell 279.10
    hyperimmunoglobulinemia 279.2
    lymphopenia, hereditary 279.2
    thrombocytopenia and eczema 279.12
    thymic
      aplasia 279.2
      dysplasia 279.2
  autosomal recessive, Swiss-type 279.2
  common variable 279.06
  severe combined (SCID) 279.2
  to Rh factor
    affecting management of pregnancy 656.1
      fetus or newborn 773.0
  X-linked, with increased IgM 279.05

ICD-9-CM

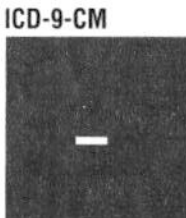

Vol. 2

Immunotherapy, prophylactic V07.2
antineoplastic V58.12
Impaction, impacted
bowel, colon, rectum 560.30
with hernia - *see also* Hernia, by site, with, obstruction
gangrenous - *see* Hernia, by site, with gangrene
by
calculus 560.39
gallstone 560.31
fecal 560.39
specified type NEC 560.39
calculus - *see* Calculus
cerumen (ear) (external) 380.4
cuspid 520.6
dental 520.6
fecal, feces 560.39
with hernia - *see also* Hernia, by site, with obstruction
gangrenous - *see* Hernia, by site, with gangrene
fracture - *see* Fracture, by site
gallbladder - *see* Cholelithiasis
gallstone(s) - *see* Cholelithiasis
in intestine (any part) 560.31
intestine(s) 560.30
with hernia - *see also* Hernia, by site, with obstruction
gangrenous - *see* Hernia, by site, with gangrene
by
calculus 560.39
gallstone 560.31
fecal 560.39
specified type NEC 560.39
intrauterine device (IUD) 996.32
molar 520.6
shoulder 660.4
affecting fetus or newborn 763.1
tooth, teeth 520.6
turbinate 733.99
Impaired, impairment (function)
arm V49.1
movement, involving
musculoskeletal system V49.1
nervous system V49.2
auditory discrimination 388.43
back V48.3
body (entire) V49.89
cognitive, mild, so stated 331.83 ◀
glucose
fasting 790.21
tolerance test (oral) 790.22
hearing (*see also* Deafness) 389.9
heart - *see* Disease, heart
kidney (*see also* Disease, renal) 593.9
disorder resulting from 588.9
specified NEC 588.89
leg V49.1
movement, involving
musculoskeletal system V49.1
nervous system V49.2
limb V49.1
movement, involving
musculoskeletal system V49.1
nervous system V49.2
liver 573.8
mastication 524.9
mild cognitive, so stated 331.83 ◀
mobility
ear ossicles NEC 385.22
incostapedial joint 385.22
malleus 385.21
myocardium, myocardial (*see also* Insufficiency, myocardial) 428.0

Impaired, impairment *(Continued)*
neuromusculoskeletal NEC V49.89
back V48.3
head V48.2
limb V49.2
neck V48.3
spine V48.3
trunk V48.3
rectal sphincter 787.99
renal (*see also* Disease, renal) 593.9
disorder resulting from 588.9
specified NEC 588.89
spine V48.3
vision NEC 369.9
both eyes NEC 369.3
moderate 369.74
both eyes 369.25
with impairment of lesser eye (specified as)
blind, not further specified 369.15
low vision, not further specified 369.23
near-total 369.17
profound 369.18
severe 369.24
total 369.16
one eye 369.74
with vision of other eye (specified as)
near-normal 369.75
normal 369.76
near-total 369.64
both eyes 369.04
with impairment of lesser eye (specified as)
blind, not further specified 369.02
total 369.03
one eye 369.64
with vision of other eye (specified as)
near-normal 369.65
normal 369.66
one eye 369.60
with low vision of other eye 369.10
profound 369.67
both eyes 369.08
with impairment of lesser eye (specified as)
blind, not further specified 369.05
near-total 369.07
total 369.06
one eye 369.67
with vision of other eye (specified as)
near-normal 369.68
normal 369.69
severe 369.71
both eyes 369.22
with impairment of lesser eye (specified as)
blind, not further specified 369.11
low vision, not further specified 369.21
near-total 369.13
profound 369.14
total 369.12
one eye 369.71
with vision of other eye (specified as)
near-normal 369.72
normal 369.73

Impaired, impairment *(Continued)*
vision NEC *(Continued)*
total
both eyes 369.01
one eye 369.61
with vision of other eye (specified as)
near-normal 369.62
normal 369.63
Impaludism - *see* Malaria
Impediment, speech NEC 784.5
psychogenic 307.9
secondary to organic lesion 784.5
Impending
cerebrovascular accident or attack 435.9
coronary syndrome 411.1
delirium tremens 291.0
myocardial infarction 411.1
Imperception, auditory (acquired) (congenital) 389.9
Imperfect
aeration, lung (newborn) 770.5
closure (congenital)
alimentary tract NEC 751.8
lower 751.5
upper 750.8
atrioventricular ostium 745.69
atrium (secundum) 745.5
primum 745.61
branchial cleft or sinus 744.41
choroid 743.59
cricoid cartilage 748.3
cusps, heart valve NEC 746.89
pulmonary 746.09
ductus
arteriosus 747.0
Botallo 747.0
ear drum 744.29
causing impairment of hearing 744.03
endocardial cushion 745.60
epiglottis 748.3
esophagus with communication to bronchus or trachea 750.3
Eustachian valve 746.89
eyelid 743.62
face, facial (*see also* Cleft, lip) 749.10
foramen
Botallo 745.5
ovale 745.5
genitalia, genital organ(s) or system
female 752.89
external 752.49
internal NEC 752.89
uterus 752.3
male 752.89
penis 752.69
glottis 748.3
heart valve (cusps) NEC 746.89
interatrial ostium or septum 745.5
interauricular ostium or septum 745.5
interventricular ostium or septum 745.4
iris 743.46
kidney 753.3
larynx 748.3
lens 743.36
lip (*see also* Cleft, lip) 749.10
nasal septum or sinus 748.1
nose 748.1
omphalomesenteric duct 751.0
optic nerve entry 743.57
organ or site NEC - *see* Anomaly, specified type, by site
ostium

Imperfect *(Continued)*
closure *(Continued)*
ostium *(Continued)*
interatrial 745.5
interauricular 745.5
interventricular 745.4
palate (*see also* Cleft, palate) 749.00
preauricular sinus 744.46
retina 743.56
roof of orbit 742.0
sclera 743.47
septum
aortic 745.0
aorticopulmonary 745.0
atrial (secundum) 745.5
primum 745.61
between aorta and pulmonary artery 745.0
heart 745.9
interatrial (secundum) 745.5
primum 745.61
interauricular (secundum) 745.5
primum 745.61
interventricular 745.4
with pulmonary stenosis or atresia, dextraposition of aorta, and hypertrophy of right ventricle 745.2
in tetralogy of Fallot 745.2
nasal 748.1
ventricular 745.4
with pulmonary stenosis or atresia, dextraposition of aorta, and hypertrophy of right ventricle 745.2
in tetralogy of Fallot 745.2
skull 756.0
with
anencephalus 740.0
encephalocele 742.0
hydrocephalus 742.3
with spina bifida (*see also* Spina bifida) 741.0
microcephalus 742.1
spine (with meningocele) (*see also* Spina bifida) 741.90
thyroid cartilage 748.3
trachea 748.3
tympanic membrane 744.29
causing impairment of hearing 744.03
uterus (with communication to bladder, intestine, or rectum) 752.3
uvula 749.02
with cleft lip (*see also* Cleft, palate, with cleft lip) 749.20
vitelline duct 751.0
development - *see* Anomaly, by site
erection 607.84
fusion - *see* Imperfect, closure
inflation lung (newborn) 770.5
intestinal canal 751.5
poise 729.9
rotation - *see* Malrotation
septum, ventricular 745.4
Imperfectly descended testis 752.51
Imperforate (congenital) - *see also* Atresia
anus 751.2
bile duct 751.61
cervix (uteri) 752.49
esophagus 750.3
hymen 752.42
intestine (small) 751.1
large 751.2
jejunum 751.1
pharynx 750.29

Imperforate *(Continued)*
rectum 751.2
salivary duct 750.23
urethra 753.6
urinary meatus 753.6
vagina 752.49
Impervious (congenital) - *see also* Atresia
anus 751.2
bile duct 751.61
esophagus 750.3
intestine (small) 751.1
large 751.5
rectum 751.2
urethra 753.6
Impetiginization of other dermatoses 684
Impetigo (any organism) (any site) (bullous) (circinate) (contagiosa) (neonatorum) (simplex) 684
Bockhart's (superficial folliculitis) 704.8
external ear 684 *[380.13]*
eyelid 684 *[373.5]*
Fox's (contagiosa) 684
furfuracea 696.5
herpetiformis 694.3
nonobstetrical 694.3
staphylococcal infection 684
ulcerative 686.8
vulgaris 684
Impingement, soft tissue between teeth 524.89
anterior 524.81
posterior 524.82
Implant, endometrial 617.9
Implantation
anomalous - *see also* Anomaly, specified type, by site
ureter 753.4
cyst
external area or site (skin) NEC 709.8
iris 364.61
vagina 623.8
vulva 624.8
dermoid (cyst)
external area or site (skin) NEC 709.8
iris 364.61
vagina 623.8
vulva 624.8
placenta, low or marginal - *see* Placenta previa
Impotence (sexual) (psychogenic) 607.84
organic origin NEC 607.84
psychogenic 302.72
Impoverished blood 285.9
Impression, basilar 756.0
Imprisonment V62.5
Improper
development, infant 764.9
Improperly tied umbilical cord (causing hemorrhage) 772.3
Impulses, obsessional 300.3
Impulsive neurosis 300.3
Inaction, kidney (*see also* Disease, renal) 593.9
Inactive - *see* condition
Inadequate, inadequacy
aesthetics of dental restoration 525.67 ◀
biologic 301.6
cardiac and renal - *see* Hypertension, cardiorenal
constitutional 301.6
development
child 783.40
fetus 764.9
affecting management of pregnancy 656.5

Inadequate, inadequacy *(Continued)*
development *(Continued)*
genitalia
after puberty NEC 259.0
congenital - *see* Hypoplasia, genitalia
lungs 748.5
organ or site NEC - *see* Hypoplasia, by site
dietary 269.9
distance, interarch 524.28
education V62.3
environment
economic problem V60.2
household condition NEC V60.1
poverty V60.2
unemployment V62.0
functional 301.6
household care, due to
family member
handicapped or ill V60.4
temporarily away from home V60.4
on vacation V60.5
technical defects in home V60.1
temporary absence from home of person rendering care V60.4
housing (heating) (space) V60.1
interarch distance 524.28
material resources V60.2
mental (*see also* Retardation, mental) 319
nervous system 799.2
personality 301.6
prenatal care in current pregnancy V23.7
pulmonary
function 786.09
newborn 770.89
ventilation, newborn 770.89
respiration 786.09
newborn 770.89
sample, Papanicolaou smear 795.08
social 301.6
Inanition 263.9
with edema 262
due to
deprivation of food 994.2
malnutrition 263.9
fever 780.6
Inappropriate secretion
ACTH 255.0
antidiuretic hormone (ADH) (excessive) 253.6
deficiency 253.5
ectopic hormone NEC 259.3
pituitary (posterior) 253.6
Inattention after or at birth 995.52
Inborn errors of metabolism - *see* Disorder, metabolism
Incarceration, incarcerated
bubonocele - *see also* Hernia, inguinal, with obstruction
gangrenous - *see* Hernia, inguinal, with gangrene
colon (by hernia) - *see also* Hernia, by site with obstruction
gangrenous - *see* Hernia, by site, with gangrene
enterocele 552.9
gangrenous 551.9
epigastrocele 552.29
gangrenous 551.29
epiplocele 552.9
gangrenous 551.9
exomphalos 552.1
gangrenous 551.1
fallopian tube 620.8

ICD-9-CM
I
Vol. 2

Incarceration, incarcerated *(Continued)*
hernia - *see also* Hernia, by site, with obstruction
gangrenous - *see* Hernia, by site, with gangrene
iris, in wound 871.1
lens, in wound 871.1
merocele (*see also* Hernia, femoral, with obstruction) 552.00
omentum (by hernia) - *see also* Hernia, by site, with obstruction
gangrenous - *see* Hernia, by site, with gangrene
omphalocele 756.79
rupture (meaning hernia) (*see also* Hernia, by site, with obstruction) 552.9
gangrenous (*see also* Hernia, by site, with gangrene) 551.9
sarcoepiplocele 552.9
gangrenous 551.9
sarcoepiplomphalocele 552.1
with gangrene 551.1
uterus 621.8
gravid 654.3
causing obstructed labor 660.2
affecting fetus or newborn 763.1
Incident, cerebrovascular (*see also* Disease, cerebrovascular, acute) 436
Incineration (entire body) (from fire, conflagration, electricity, or lightning) - *see* Burn, multiple, specified sites
Incised wound
external - *see* Wound, open, by site
internal organs (abdomen, chest, or pelvis) - *see* Injury, internal, by site, with open wound
Incision, incisional
hernia - *see* Hernia, incisional
surgical, complication - *see* Complications, surgical procedures
traumatic
external - *see* Wound, open, by site
internal organs (abdomen, chest, or pelvis) - *see* Injury, internal, by site, with open wound
Inclusion
azurophilic leukocytic 288.2
blennorrhea (neonatal) (newborn) 771.6
cyst - *see* Cyst, skin
gallbladder in liver (congenital) 751.69
Incompatibility
ABO
affecting management of pregnancy 656.2
fetus or newborn 773.1
infusion or transfusion reaction 999.6
blood (group) (Duffy) (E) (K(ell)) (Kidd) (Lewis) (M) (N) (P) (S) NEC
affecting management of pregnancy 656.2
fetus or newborn 773.2
infusion or transfusion reaction 999.6
marital V61.10
involving divorce or estrangement V61.0
Rh (blood group) (factor)
affecting management of pregnancy 656.1
fetus or newborn 773.0
infusion or transfusion reaction 999.7
Rhesus - *see* Incompatibility, Rh
Incompetency, incompetence, incompetent
annular
aortic (valve) (*see also* Insufficiency, aortic) 424.1
mitral (valve) - (*see also* Insufficiency, mitral) 424.0
pulmonary valve (heart) (*see also* Endocarditis, pulmonary) 424.3
aortic (valve) (*see also* Insufficiency, aortic) 424.1
syphilitic 093.22
cardiac (orifice) 530.0
valve - *see* Endocarditis
cervix, cervical (os) 622.5
in pregnancy 654.5
affecting fetus or newborn 761.0
contour of existing restoration of tooth ◀
with oral health 525.65 ◀
esophagogastric (junction) (sphincter) 530.0
heart valve, congenital 746.89
mitral (valve) - *see* Insufficiency, mitral
papillary muscle (heart) 429.81
pelvic fundus
pubocervical tissue 618.81
rectovaginal tissue 618.82
pulmonary valve (heart) (*see also* Endocarditis, pulmonary) 424.3
congenital 746.09
tricuspid (annular) (rheumatic) (valve) (*see also* Endocarditis, tricuspid) 397.0
valvular - *see* Endocarditis
vein, venous (saphenous) (varicose) (*see also* Varicose, vein) 454.9
velopharyngeal (closure)
acquired 528.9
congenital 750.29
Incomplete - *see also* condition
bladder emptying 788.21
expansion lungs (newborn) 770.5
gestation (liveborn) - *see* Immaturity
rotation - *see* Malrotation
Incontinence 788.30
without sensory awareness 788.34
anal sphincter 787.6
continuous leakage 788.37
feces 787.6
due to hysteria 300.11
nonorganic origin 307.7
hysterical 300.11
mixed (male) (female) (urge and stress) 788.33
overflow 788.38
paradoxical 788.39
rectal 787.6
specified NEC 788.39
stress (female) 625.6
male NEC 788.32
urethral sphincter 599.84
urge 788.31
and stress (male) (female) 788.33
urine 788.30
active 788.30
male 788.30
stress 788.32
and urge 788.33
neurogenic 788.39
nonorganic origin 307.6
stress (female) 625.6
male NEC 788.32
urge 788.31
and stress 788.33
Incontinentia pigmenti 757.33
Incoordinate
uterus (action) (contractions) 661.4
affecting fetus or newborn 763.7
Incoordination
esophageal-pharyngeal (newborn) 787.2
muscular 781.3
papillary muscle 429.81
Increase, increased
abnormal, in development 783.9
androgens (ovarian) 256.1
anticoagulants (antithrombin) (anti-VIIIa) (anti-IXa) (anti-Xa) (anti-XIa) 286.5
postpartum 666.3
cold sense (*see also* Disturbance, sensation) 782.0
estrogen 256.0
function
adrenal (cortex) 255.3
medulla 255.6
pituitary (anterior) (gland) (lobe) 253.1
posterior 253.6
heat sense (*see also* Disturbance, sensation) 782.0
intracranial pressure 781.99
injury at birth 767.8
light reflex of retina 362.13
permeability, capillary 448.9
pressure
intracranial 781.99
injury at birth 767.8
intraocular 365.00
pulsations 785.9
pulse pressure 785.9
sphericity, lens 743.36
splenic activity 289.4
venous pressure 459.89
portal 572.3
Incrustation, cornea, lead, or zinc 930.0
Incyclophoria 378.44
Incyclotropia 378.33
Indeterminate sex 752.7
India rubber skin 756.83
Indicanuria 270.2
Indigestion (bilious) (functional) 536.8
acid 536.8
catarrhal 536.8
due to decomposed food NEC 005.9
fat 579.8
nervous 306.4
psychogenic 306.4
Indirect - *see* condition
Indolent bubo NEC 099.8
Induced
abortion - *see* Abortion, induced
birth, affecting fetus or newborn 763.89
delivery - *see* Delivery
labor - *see* Delivery
Induration, indurated
brain 348.8
breast (fibrous) 611.79
puerperal, postpartum 676.3
broad ligament 620.8
chancre 091.0
anus 091.1
congenital 090.0
extragenital NEC 091.2
corpora cavernosa (penis) (plastic) 607.89
liver (chronic) 573.8
acute 573.8

Induration, indurated *(Continued)*
lung (black) (brown) (chronic) (fibroid) (*see also* Fibrosis, lung) 515
essential brown 275.0 *[516.1]*
penile 607.89
phlebitic - *see* Phlebitis
skin 782.8
stomach 537.89
Induratio penis plastica 607.89
Industrial - *see* condition
Inebriety (*see also* Abuse, drugs, nondependent) 305.0
Inefficiency
kidney (*see also* Disease, renal) 593.9
thyroid (acquired) (gland) 244.9
Inelasticity, skin 782.8
Inequality, leg (acquired) (length) 736.81
congenital 755.30
Inertia
bladder 596.4
neurogenic 596.54
with cauda equina syndrome 344.61
stomach 536.8
psychogenic 306.4
uterus, uterine 661.2
affecting fetus or newborn 763.7
primary 661.0
secondary 661.1
vesical 596.4
neurogenic 596.54
with cauda equina 344.61
Infant - *see also* condition
excessive crying of 780.92
fussy (baby) 780.91
held for adoption V68.89
newborn - *see* Newborn
post-term (gestation period over 40 completed weeks to 42 completed weeks) 766.21
prolonged gestation of (period over 42 completed weeks) 766.22
syndrome of diabetic mother 775.0
"Infant Hercules" syndrome 255.2
Infantile - *see also* condition
genitalia, genitals 259.0
in pregnancy or childbirth NEC 654.4
affecting fetus or newborn 763.89
causing obstructed labor 660.2
affecting fetus or newborn 763.1
heart 746.9
kidney 753.3
lack of care 995.52
macula degeneration 362.75
melanodontia 521.05
os, uterus (*see also* Infantile, genitalia) 259.0
pelvis 738.6
with disproportion (fetopelvic) 653.1
affecting fetus or newborn 763.1
causing obstructed labor 660.1
affecting fetus or newborn 763.1
penis 259.0
testis 257.2
uterus (*see also* Infantile, genitalia) 259.0
vulva 752.49
Infantilism 259.9
with dwarfism (hypophyseal) 253.3
Brissaud's (infantile myxedema) 244.9
celiac 579.0
Herter's (nontropical sprue) 579.0
hypophyseal 253.3
hypothalamic (with obesity) 253.8
idiopathic 259.9
Infantilism *(Continued)*
intestinal 579.0
pancreatic 577.8
pituitary 253.3
renal 588.0
sexual (with obesity) 259.0
Infants, healthy liveborn - *see* Newborn
Infarct, infarction
adrenal (capsule) (gland) 255.4
amnion 658.8
anterior (with contiguous portion of intraventricular septum) NEC (*see also* Infarct, myocardium) 410.1
appendices epiploicae 557.0
bowel 557.0
brain (stem) 434.91
embolic (*see also* Embolism, brain) 434.11
healed or old, without residuals V12.59
iatrogenic 997.02
lacunar 434.91
late effect - *see* Late effect(s) (of) cerebrovascular disease
postoperative 997.02
puerperal, postpartum, childbirth 674.0
thrombotic (*see also* Thrombosis, brain) 434.01
breast 611.8
Brewer's (kidney) 593.81
cardiac (*see also* Infarct, myocardium) 410.9
cerebellar (*see also* Infarct, brain) 434.91
embolic (*see also* Embolism, brain) 434.11
cerebral (*see also* Infarct, brain) 434.91
embolic (*see also* Embolism, brain) 434.11
thrombotic (*see also* Infarct, brain) 434.01
chorion 658.8
colon (acute) (agnogenic) (embolic) (hemorrhagic) (nonocclusive) (nonthrombotic) (occlusive) (segmental) (thrombotic) (with gangrene) 557.0
coronary artery (*see also* Infarct, myocardium) 410.9
cortical 434.91
embolic (*see also* Embolism) 444.9
fallopian tube 620.8
gallbladder 575.8
heart (*see also* Infarct, myocardium) 410.9
hepatic 573.4
hypophysis (anterior lobe) 253.8
impending (myocardium) 411.1
intestine (acute) (agnogenic) (embolic) (hemorrhagic) (nonocclusive) (nonthrombotic) (occlusive) (thrombotic) (with gangrene) 557.0
kidney 593.81
lacunar 434.91
liver 573.4
lung (embolic) (thrombotic) 415.19
with
abortion - *see* Abortion, by type, with, embolism
ectopic pregnancy (*see also* categories 633.0–633.9) 639.6
molar pregnancy (*see also* categories 630–632) 639.6
following
abortion 639.6
ectopic or molar pregnancy 639.6
Infarct, infarction *(Continued)*
lung *(Continued)*
iatrogenic 415.11
in pregnancy, childbirth, or puerperium - *see* Embolism, obstetrical
postoperative 415.11
lymph node or vessel 457.8
medullary (brain) - *see* Infarct, brain
meibomian gland (eyelid) 374.85
mesentery, mesenteric (embolic) (thrombotic) (with gangrene) 557.0
with symptoms after 8 weeks from date of infarction 414.8
non-ST elevation (NSTEMI) 410.7
ST elevation (STEMI) 410.9
anterior (wall) 410.1
anterolateral (wall) 410.0
inferior (wall) 410.4
inferolateral (wall) 410.2
inferoposterior (wall) 410.3
lateral (wall) 410.5
posterior (strictly) (true) (wall) 410.6
specified site NEC 410.8
midbrain - *see* Infarct, brain
myocardium, myocardial (acute or with a stated duration of 8 weeks or less) (with hypertension) 410.9

Note Use the following fifth-digit subclassification with category 410:

0 episode unspecified
1 initial episode
2 subsequent episode without recurrence

with symptoms after 8 weeks from date of infarction 414.8
anterior (wall) (with contiguous portion of intraventricular septum) NEC 410.1
anteroapical (with contiguous portion of intraventricular septum) 410.1
anterolateral (wall) 410.0
anteroseptal (with contiguous portion of intraventricular septum) 410.1
apical-lateral 410.5
atrial 410.8
basal-lateral 410.5
chronic (with symptoms after 8 weeks from date of infarction) 414.8
diagnosed on ECG, but presenting no symptoms 412
diaphragmatic wall (with contiguous portion of intraventricular septum) 410.4
healed or old, currently presenting no symptoms 412
high lateral 410.5
impending 411.1
inferior (wall) (with contiguous portion of intraventricular septum) 410.4
inferolateral (wall) 410.2
inferoposterior wall 410.3
lateral wall 410.5
nontransmural 410.7
papillary muscle 410.8
past (diagnosed on ECG or other special investigation, but currently presenting no symptoms) 412
with symptoms NEC 414.8
posterior (strictly) (true) (wall) 410.6
posterobasal 410.6

ICD-9-CM I Vol. 2

- **Infarct, infarction** *(Continued)*
  - with symptoms after 8 weeks from date of infarction *(Continued)*
    - posteroinferior 410.3
    - posterolateral 410.5
    - previous, currently presenting no symptoms 412
    - septal 410.8
    - specified site NEC 410.8
    - ST elevation (STEMI) 410.9
      - anterior (wall) 410.1
      - anterolateral (wall) 410.0
      - inferior (wall) 410.4
      - inferolateral (wall) 410.2
      - inferoposterior wall 410.3
      - lateral wall 410.5
      - posterior (strictly) (true) (wall) 410.6
      - specified site NEC 410.8
    - subendocardial 410.7
    - syphilitic 093.82
  - non-ST elevation myocardial infarction (NSTEMI) 410.7
  - nontransmural 410.7
  - omentum 557.0
  - ovary 620.8
  - pancreas 577.8
  - papillary muscle (*see also* Infarct, myocardium) 410.8
  - parathyroid gland 252.8
  - pituitary (gland) 253.8
  - placenta (complicating pregnancy) 656.7
    - affecting fetus or newborn 762.2
  - pontine - *see* Infarct, brain
  - posterior NEC (*see also* Infarct, myocardium) 410.6
  - prostate 602.8
  - pulmonary (artery) (hemorrhagic) (vein) 415.19
    - with
      - abortion - *see* Abortion, by type, with embolism
      - ectopic pregnancy (*see also* categories 633.0–633.9) 639.6
      - molar pregnancy (*see also* categories 630–632) 639.6
    - following
      - abortion 639.6
      - ectopic or molar pregnancy 639.6
    - iatrogenic 415.11
    - in pregnancy, childbirth, or puerperium - *see* Embolism, obstetrical
    - postoperative 415.11
  - renal 593.81
    - embolic or thrombotic 593.81
  - retina, retinal 362.84
    - with occlusion - *see* Occlusion, retina
  - spinal (acute) (cord) (embolic) (nonembolic) 336.1
  - spleen 289.59
    - embolic or thrombotic 444.89
  - subchorionic - *see* Infarct, placenta
  - subendocardial (*see also* Infarct, myocardium) 410.7
  - suprarenal (capsule) (gland) 255.4
  - syncytium - *see* Infarct, placenta
  - testis 608.83
  - thrombotic (*see also* Thrombosis) 453.9
    - artery, arterial - *see* Embolism
  - thyroid (gland) 246.3
  - ventricle (heart) (*see also* Infarct, myocardium) 410.9
- **Infecting** - *see* condition
- **Infection, infected, infective** (opportunistic) 136.9
  - with lymphangitis - *see* Lymphangitis
  - abortion - *see* Abortion, by type, with, sepsis
  - abscess (skin) - *see* Abscess, by site
  - Absidia 117.7
  - Acanthocheilonema (perstans) 125.4
    - streptocerca 125.6
  - accessory sinus (chronic) (*see also* Sinusitis) 473.9
  - Achorion - *see* Dermatophytosis
  - Acremonium falciforme 117.4
  - acromioclavicular (joint) 711.91
  - Actinobacillus
    - lignieresii 027.8
    - mallei 024
    - muris 026.1
  - Actinomadura - *see* Actinomycosis
  - Actinomyces (israelii) - *see also* Actinomycosis
    - muris-ratti 026.1
  - Actinomycetales (Actinomadura) (Actinomyces) (Nocardia) (Streptomyces) - *see* Actinomycosis
  - actinomycotic NEC (*see also* Actinomycosis) 039.9
  - adenoid (chronic) 474.01
    - acute 463
    - and tonsil (chronic) 474.02
      - acute or subacute 463
  - adenovirus NEC 079.0
    - in diseases classified elsewhere - *see* category 079
    - unspecified nature or site 079.0
  - Aerobacter aerogenes NEC 041.85
    - enteritis 008.2
  - Aerogenes capsulatus (*see also* Gangrene, gas) 040.0
  - aertrycke (*see also* Infection, Salmonella) 003.9
  - Ajellomyces dermatitidis 116.0
  - alimentary canal NEC (*see also* Enteritis, due to, by organism) 009.0
  - Allescheria boydii 117.6
  - Alternaria 118
  - alveolus, alveolar (process) (pulpal origin) 522.4
  - ameba, amebic (histolytica) (*see also* Amebiasis) 006.9
    - acute 006.0
    - chronic 006.1
    - free-living 136.2
    - hartmanni 007.8
    - specified
      - site NEC 006.8
      - type NEC 007.8
  - amniotic fluid or cavity 658.4
    - affecting fetus or newborn 762.7
  - anaerobes (cocci) (gram-negative) (gram-positive) (mixed) NEC 041.84
  - anal canal 569.49
  - Ancylostoma braziliense 126.2
  - Angiostrongylus cantonensis 128.8
  - anisakiasis 127.1
  - Anisakis larva 127.1
  - anthrax (*see also* Anthrax) 022.9
  - antrum (chronic) (*see also* Sinusitis, maxillary) 473.0
  - anus (papillae) (sphincter) 569.49
  - arbor virus NEC 066.9
  - arbovirus NEC 066.9
  - argentophil-rod 027.0
  - Ascaris lumbricoides 127.0
  - ascomycetes 117.4

Infection, infected, infective *(Continued)*
  - Aspergillus (flavus) (fumigatus) (terreus) 117.3
  - atypical
    - acid-fast (bacilli) (*see also* Mycobacterium, atypical) 031.9
    - mycobacteria (*see also* Mycobacterium, atypical) 031.9
  - auditory meatus (circumscribed) (diffuse) (external) (*see also* Otitis, externa) 380.10
  - auricle (ear) (*see also* Otitis, externa) 380.10
  - axillary gland 683
  - babesiasis 088.82
  - babesiosis 088.82
  - Bacillus NEC 041.89
    - abortus 023.1
    - anthracis (*see also* Anthrax) 022.9
    - cereus (food poisoning) 005.89
    - coli - *see* Infection, Escherichia coli
    - coliform NEC 041.85
    - Ducrey's (any location) 099.0
    - Flexner's 004.1
    - Friedländer's NEC 041.3
    - fusiformis 101
    - gas (gangrene) (*see also* Gangrene, gas) 040.0
    - mallei 024
    - melitensis 023.0
    - paratyphoid, paratyphosus 002.9
      - A 002.1
      - B 002.2
      - C 002.3
    - Schmorl's 040.3
    - Shiga 004.0
    - suipestifer (*see also* Infection, Salmonella) 003.9
    - swimming pool 031.1
    - typhosa 002.0
    - welchii (*see also* Gangrene, gas) 040.0
    - Whitmore's 025
  - bacterial NEC 041.9
    - specified NEC 041.89
      - anaerobic NEC 041.84
      - gram-negative NEC 041.85
        - anaerobic NEC 041.84
  - Bacterium
    - paratyphosum 002.9
      - A 002.1
      - B 002.2
      - C 002.3
    - typhosum 002.9
  - Bacteroides (fragilis) (melaninogenicus) (oralis) NEC 041.82
  - Balantidium coli 007.0
  - Bartholin's gland 616.89 (Revised)
  - Basidiobolus 117.7
  - Bedsonia 079.98
    - specified NEC 079.88
  - bile duct 576.1
  - bladder (*see also* Cystitis) 595.9
  - Blastomyces, blastomycotic 116.0
    - brasiliensis 116.1
    - dermatitidis 116.0
    - European 117.5
    - loboi 116.2
    - North American 116.0
    - South American 116.1
  - bleb (New)
    - postprocedural 379.60 (New)
      - stage 1 379.61 (New)
      - stage 2 379.62 (New)
      - stage 3 379.63 (New)
  - blood stream - *see* Septicemia

Infection, infected, infective *(Continued)*
bone 730.9
specified - *see* Osteomyelitis
Bordetella 033.9
bronchiseptica 033.8
parapertussis 033.1
pertussis 033.0
Borrelia
bergdorfi 088.81
vincentii (mouth) (pharynx) (tonsil) 101
brain (*see also* Encephalitis) 323.9
late effect - *see* category 326
membranes - (*see also* Meningitis) 322.9
septic 324.0
late effect - *see* category 326
meninges (*see also* Meningitis) 320.9
branchial cyst 744.42
breast 611.0
puerperal, postpartum 675.2
with nipple 675.9
specified type NEC 675.8
nonpurulent 675.2
purulent 675.1
bronchus (*see also* Bronchitis) 490
fungus NEC 117.9
Brucella 023.9
abortus 023.1
canis 023.3
melitensis 023.0
mixed 023.8
suis 023.2
Brugia (Wuchereria) malayi 125.1
bursa - *see* Bursitis
buttocks (skin) 686.9
Candida (albicans) (tropicalis) (*see also* Candidiasis) 112.9
congenital 771.7
Candiru 136.8
Capillaria
hepatica 128.8
philippinensis 127.5
cartilage 733.99
cat liver fluke 121.0
cellulitis - *see* Cellulitis, by site
Cephalosporum falciforme 117.4
Cercomonas hominis (intestinal) 007.3
cerebrospinal (*see also* Meningitis) 322.9
late effect - *see* category 326
cervical gland 683
cervix (*see also* Cervicitis) 616.0
cesarean section wound 674.3
Chilomastix (intestinal) 007.8
Chlamydia 079.98
specified NEC 079.88
Cholera (*see also* Cholera) 001.9
chorionic plate 658.8
Cladosporium
bantianum 117.8
carrionii 117.2
mansonii 111.1
trichoides 117.8
werneckii 111.1
Clonorchis (sinensis) (liver) 121.1
Clostridium (haemolyticum) (novyi) NEC 041.84
botulinum 005.1
histolyticum (*see also* Gangrene, gas) 040.0
oedematiens (*see also* Gangrene, gas) 040.0
perfringens 041.83
due to food 005.2

Infection, infected, infective *(Continued)*
Clostridium *(Continued)*
septicum (*see also* Gangrene, gas) 040.0
sordellii (*see also* Gangrene, gas) 040.0
welchii (*see also* Gangrene, gas) 040.0
due to food 005.2
Coccidioides (immitis) (*see also* Coccidioidomycosis) 114.9
coccus NEC 041.89
colon (*see also* Enteritis, due to, by organism) 009.0
bacillus - *see* Infection, Escherichia coli
colostomy or enterostomy 569.61
common duct 576.1
complicating pregnancy, childbirth, or puerperium NEC 647.9
affecting fetus or newborn 760.2
Condiobolus 117.7
congenital NEC 771.89
Candida albicans 771.7
chronic 771.2
cytomegalovirus 771.1
hepatitis, viral 771.2
herpes simplex 771.2
listeriosis 771.2
malaria 771.2
poliomyelitis 771.2
rubella 771.0
toxoplasmosis 771.2
tuberculosis 771.2
urinary (tract) 771.82
vaccinia 771.2
Conidiobolus 117.7
coronavirus 079.89
SARS-associated 079.82
corpus luteum (*see also* Salpingo-oophoritis) 614.2
Corynebacterium diphtheriae - *see* Diphtheria
Coxsackie (*see also* Coxsackie) 079.2
endocardium 074.22
heart NEC 074.20
in diseases classified elsewhere - *see* category 079
meninges 047.0
myocardium 074.23
pericardium 074.21
pharynx 074.0
specified disease NEC 074.8
unspecified nature or site 079.2
Cryptococcus neoformans 117.5
Cryptosporidia 007.4
Cunninghamella 117.7
cyst - *see* Cyst
Cysticercus cellulosae 123.1
cytomegalovirus 078.5
congenital 771.1
dental (pulpal origin) 522.4
deuteromycetes 117.4
Dicrocoelium dendriticum 121.8
Dipetalonema (perstans) 125.4
streptocerca 125.6
diphtherial - *see* Diphtheria
Diphyllobothrium (adult) (latum) (pacificum) 123.4
larval 123.5
Diplogonoporus (grandis) 123.8
Dipylidium (caninum) 123.8
Dirofilaria 125.6
dog tapeworm 123.8
Dracunculus medinensis 125.7
Dreschlera 118
hawaiiensis 117.8

Infection, infected, infective *(Continued)*
Ducrey's bacillus (any site) 099.0
due to or resulting from
device, implant, or graft (any) (presence of) - *see* Complications, infection and inflammation, due to (presence of) any device, implant, or graft classified to 996.0–996.5 NEC
injection, inoculation, infusion, transfusion, or vaccination (prophylactic) (therapeutic) 999.3
injury NEC - *see* Wound, open, by site, complicated
surgery 998.59
duodenum 535.6
ear - *see also* Otitis
external (*see also* Otitis, externa) 380.10
inner (*see also* Labyrinthitis) 386.30
middle - *see* Otitis, media
Eaton's agent NEC 041.81
Eberthella typhosa 002.0
Ebola 078.89
echinococcosis 122.9
Echinococcus (*see also* Echinococcus) 122.9
Echinostoma 121.8
ECHO virus 079.1
in diseases classified elsewhere - *see* category 079
unspecified nature or site 079.1
Ehrlichiosis 082.40
chaffeensis 082.41
specified type NEC 082.49
Endamoeba - *see* Infection, ameba
endocardium (*see also* Endocarditis) 421.0
endocervix (*see also* Cervicitis) 616.0
Entamoeba - *see* Infection, ameba
enteric (*see also* Enteritis, due to, by organism) 009.0
Enterobacter aerogenes NEC 041.85
Enterobacter sakazakii 041.85
Enterobius vermicularis 127.4
enterococcus NEC 041.04
enterovirus NEC 079.89
central nervous system NEC 048
enteritis 008.67
meningitis 047.9
Entomophthora 117.7
Epidermophyton - *see* Dermatophytosis
epidermophytosis - *see* Dermatophytosis
episiotomy 674.3
Epstein-Barr virus 075
chronic 780.79 *[139.8]*
erysipeloid 027.1
Erysipelothrix (insidiosa) (rhusiopathiae) 027.1
erythema infectiosum 057.0
Escherichia coli NEC 041.4
enteritis - *see* Enteritis, E. coli
generalized 038.42
intestinal - *see* Enteritis, E. coli
esophagostomy 530.86
ethmoidal (chronic) (sinus) (*see also* Sinusitis, ethmoidal) 473.2
Eubacterium 041.84
Eustachian tube (ear) 381.50
acute 381.51
chronic 381.52
exanthema subitum 057.8
external auditory canal (meatus) (*see also* Otitis, externa) 380.10
eye NEC 360.00

Infection, infected, infective *(Continued)*
eyelid 373.9
specified NEC 373.8
fallopian tube (*see also* Salpingo-oophoritis) 614.2
fascia 728.89
Fasciola
gigantica 121.3
hepatica 121.3
Fasciolopsis (buski) 121.4
fetus (intra-amniotic) - *see* Infection, congenital
filarial - *see* Infestation, filarial
finger (skin) 686.9
abscess (with lymphangitis) 681.00
pulp 681.01
cellulitis (with lymphangitis) 681.00
distal closed space (with lymphangitis) 681.00
nail 681.02
fungus 110.1
fish tapeworm 123.4
larval 123.5
flagellate, intestinal 007.9
fluke - *see* Infestation, fluke
focal
teeth (pulpal origin) 522.4
tonsils 474.00
and adenoids 474.02
Fonsecaea
compactum 117.2
pedrosoi 117.2
food (*see also* Poisoning, food) 005.9
foot (skin) 686.9
fungus 110.4
Francisella tularensis (*see also* Tularemia) 021.9
frontal sinus (chronic) (*see also* Sinusitis, frontal) 473.1
fungus NEC 117.9
beard 110.0
body 110.5
dematiaceous NEC 117.8
foot 110.4
groin 110.3
hand 110.2
nail 110.1
pathogenic to compromised host only 118
perianal (area) 110.3
scalp 110.0
scrotum 110.8
skin 111.9
foot 110.4
hand 110.2
toenails 110.1
trachea 117.9
Fusarium 118
Fusobacterium 041.84
gallbladder (*see also* Cholecystitis, acute) 575.0
Gardnerella vaginalis 041.89
gas bacillus (*see also* Gas, gangrene) 040.0
gastric (*see also* Gastritis) 535.5
Gastrodiscoides hominis 121.8
gastroenteric (*see also* Enteritis, due to, by organism) 009.0
gastrointestinal (*see also* Enteritis, due to, by organism) 009.0
gastrostomy 536.41
generalized NEC (*see also* Septicemia) 038.9

Infection, infected, infective *(Continued)*
genital organ or tract NEC
female 614.9
with
abortion - *see* Abortion, by type, with sepsis
ectopic pregnancy (*see also* categories 633.0–633.9) 639.0
molar pregnancy (*see also* categories 630–632) 639.0
complicating pregnancy 646.6
affecting fetus or newborn 760.8
following
abortion 639.0
ectopic or molar pregnancy 639.0
puerperal, postpartum, childbirth 670
minor or localized 646.6
affecting fetus or newborn 760.8
male 608.4
genitourinary tract NEC 599.0
Ghon tubercle, primary (*see also* Tuberculosis) 010.0
Giardia lamblia 007.1
gingival (chronic) 523.10 (Revised)
acute 523.00 (Revised)
Vincent's 101
glanders 024
Glenosporopsis amazonica 116.2
Gnathostoma spinigerum 128.1
Gongylonema 125.6
gonococcal NEC (*see also* Gonococcus) 098.0
gram-negative bacilli NEC 041.85
anaerobic 041.84
guinea worm 125.7
gum (*see also* Infection, gingival) 523.10 (Revised)
Hantavirus 079.81
heart 429.89
Helicobactor pylori 041.86
helminths NEC 128.9
intestinal 127.9
mixed (types classifiable to more than one category in 120.0–127.7) 127.8
specified type NEC 127.7
specified type NEC 128.8
Hemophilus influenzae NEC 041.5
generalized 038.41
herpes (simplex) (*see also* Herpes, simplex) 054.9
congenital 771.2
zoster (*see also* Herpes, zoster) 053.9
eye NEC 053.29
Heterophyes heterophyes 121.6
Histoplasma (*see also* Histoplasmosis) 115.90
capsulatum (*see also* Histoplasmosis, American) 115.00
duboisii (*see also* Histoplasmosis, African) 115.10
HIV V08
with symptoms, symptomatic 042
hookworm (*see also* Ancylostomiasis) 126.9
human immunodeficiency virus V08
with symptoms, symptomatic 042
human papillomavirus 079.4
hydrocele 603.1
hydronephrosis 591
Hymenolepis 123.6
hypopharynx 478.29

Infection, infected, infective *(Continued)*
inguinal glands 683
due to soft chancre 099.0
intestine, intestinal (*see also* Enteritis, due to, by organism) 009.0
intrauterine (*see also* Endometritis) 615.9
complicating delivery 646.6
Isospora belli or hominis 007.2
Japanese B encephalitis 062.0
jaw (bone) (acute) (chronic) (lower) (subacute) (upper) 526.4
joint - *see* Arthritis, infectious or infective
kidney (cortex) (hematogenous) 590.9
with
abortion - *see* Abortion, by type, with urinary tract infection
calculus 592.0
ectopic pregnancy (*see also* categories 633.0–633.9) 639.8
molar pregnancy (*see also* categories 630–632) 639.8
complicating pregnancy or puerperium 646.6
affecting fetus or newborn 760.1
following
abortion 639.8
ectopic or molar pregnancy 639.8
pelvis and ureter 590.3
Klebsiella pneumoniae NEC 041.3
knee (skin) NEC 686.9
joint - *see* Arthritis, infectious
Koch's (*see also* Tuberculosis, pulmonary) 011.9
labia (majora) (minora) (*see also* Vulvitis) 616.10
lacrimal
gland (*see also* Dacryoadenitis) 375.00
passages (duct) (sac) (*see also* Dacryocystitis) 375.30
larynx NEC 478.79
leg (skin) NEC 686.9
Leishmania (*see also* Leishmaniasis) 085.9
braziliensis 085.5
donovani 085.0
Ethiopica 085.3
furunculosa 085.1
infantum 085.0
mexicana 085.4
tropica (minor) 085.1
major 085.2
Leptosphaeria senegalensis 117.4
Leptospira (*see also* Leptospirosis) 100.9
australis 100.89
bataviae 100.89
pyrogenes 100.89
specified type NEC 100.89
leptospirochetal NEC (*see also* Leptospirosis) 100.9
Leptothrix - *see* Actinomycosis
Listeria monocytogenes (listeriosis) 027.0
congenital 771.2
liver fluke - *see* Infestation, fluke, liver
Loa loa 125.2
eyelid 125.2 *[373.6]*
Loboa loboi 116.2
local, skin (staphylococcal) (streptococcal) NEC 686.9
abscess - *see* Abscess, by site
cellulitis - *see* Cellulitis, by site
ulcer (*see also* Ulcer, skin) 707.9
Loefflerella
mallei 024
whitmori 025

Infection, infected, infective *(Continued)*
lung 518.89
atypical mycobacterium 031.0
tuberculous (*see also* Tuberculosis, pulmonary) 011.9
basilar 518.89
chronic 518.89
fungus NEC 117.9
spirochetal 104.8
virus - *see* Pneumonia, virus
lymph gland (axillary) (cervical) (inguinal) 683
mesenteric 289.2
lymphoid tissue, base of tongue or posterior pharynx, NEC 474.00
Madurella
grisea 117.4
mycetomii 117.4
major
with
abortion - *see* Abortion, by type, with sepsis
ectopic pregnancy (*see also* categories 633.0–633.9) 639.0
molar pregnancy (*see also* categories 630–632) 639.0
following
abortion 639.0
ectopic or molar pregnancy 639.0
puerperal, postpartum, childbirth 670
malarial - *see* Malaria
Malassezia furfur 111.0
Malleomyces
mallei 024
pseudomallei 025
mammary gland 611.0
puerperal, postpartum 675.2
Mansonella (ozzardi) 125.5
mastoid (suppurative) - *see* Mastoiditis
maxilla, maxillary 526.4
sinus (chronic) (*see also* Sinusitis, maxillary) 473.0
mediastinum 519.2
medina 125.7
meibomian
cyst 373.12
gland 373.12
melioidosis 025
meninges (*see also* Meningitis) 320.9
meningococcal (*see also* condition) 036.9
brain 036.1
cerebrospinal 036.0
endocardium 036.42
generalized 036.2
meninges 036.0
meningococcemia 036.2
specified site NEC 036.89
mesenteric lymph nodes or glands NEC 289.2
Metagonimus 121.5
metatarsophalangeal 711.97
microorganism resistant to drugs - *see* Resistance (to), drugs by microorganisms
Microsporidia 136.8
Microsporum, microsporic - *see* Dermatophytosis
mima polymorpha NEC 041.85
mixed flora NEC 041.89
Monilia (*see also* Candidiasis) 112.9
neonatal 771.7
monkeypox 057.8
Monosporium apiospermum 117.6
mouth (focus) NEC 528.9
parasitic 136.9

Infection, infected, infective *(Continued)*
Mucor 117.7
muscle NEC 728.89
mycelium NEC 117.9
mycetoma
actinomycotic NEC (*see also* Actinomycosis) 039.9
mycotic NEC 117.4
Mycobacterium, mycobacterial (*see also* Mycobacterium) 031.9
mycoplasma NEC 041.81
mycotic NEC 117.9
pathogenic to compromised host only 118
skin NEC 111.9
systemic 117.9
myocardium NEC 422.90
nail (chronic) (with lymphangitis) 681.9
finger 681.02
fungus 110.1
ingrowing 703.0
toe 681.11
fungus 110.1
nasal sinus (chronic) (*see also* Sinusitis) 473.9
nasopharynx (chronic) 478.29
acute 460
navel 686.9
newborn 771.4
Neisserian - *see* Gonococcus
Neotestudina rosatii 117.4
newborn, generalized 771.89
nipple 611.0
puerperal, postpartum 675.0
with breast 675.9
specified type NEC 675.8
Nocardia - *see* Actinomycosis
nose 478.19 (Revised)
nostril 478.19 (Revised)
obstetrical surgical wound 674.3
Oesophagostomum (apiostomum) 127.7
Oestrus ovis 134.0
Oidium albicans (*see also* Candidiasis) 112.9
Onchocerca (volvulus) 125.3
eye 125.3 *[360.13]*
eyelid 125.3 *[373.6]*
operation wound 998.59
Opisthorchis (felineus) (tenuicollis) (viverrini) 121.0
orbit 376.00
chronic 376.10
ovary (*see also* Salpingo-oophoritis) 614.2
Oxyuris vermicularis 127.4
pancreas 577.0
Paracoccidioides brasiliensis 116.1
Paragonimus (westermani) 121.2
parainfluenza virus 079.89
parameningococcus NEC 036.9
with meningitis 036.0
parasitic NEC 136.9
paratyphoid 002.9
type A 002.1
type B 002.2
type C 002.3
paraurethral ducts 597.89
parotid gland 527.2
Pasteurella NEC 027.2
multocida (cat-bite) (dog-bite) 027.2
pestis (*see also* Plague) 020.9
pseudotuberculosis 027.2
septica (cat-bite) (dog-bite) 027.2
tularensis (*see also* Tularemia) 021.9

Infection, infected, infective *(Continued)*
pelvic, female (*see also* Disease, pelvis, inflammatory) 614.9
penis (glans) (retention) NEC 607.2
herpetic 054.13
Peptococcus 041.84
Peptostreptococcus 041.84
periapical (pulpal origin) 522.4
peridental 523.30 (Revised)
perineal wound (obstetrical) 674.3
periodontal 523.31 (Revised)
periorbital 376.00
chronic 376.10
perirectal 569.49
perirenal (*see also* Infection, kidney) 590.9
peritoneal (*see also* Peritonitis) 567.9
periureteral 593.89
periurethral 597.89
Petriellidium boydii 117.6
pharynx 478.29
Coxsackie virus 074.0
phlegmonous 462
posterior, lymphoid 474.00
Phialophora
gougerotii 117.8
jeanselmei 117.8
verrucosa 117.2
Piedraia hortai 111.3
pinna, acute 380.11
pinta 103.9
intermediate 103.1
late 103.2
mixed 103.3
primary 103.0
pinworm 127.4
Pityrosporum furfur 111.0
pleuropneumonia-like organisms NEC (PPLO) 041.81
pneumococcal NEC 041.2
generalized (purulent) 038.2
Pneumococcus NEC 041.2
postoperative wound 998.59
posttraumatic NEC 958.3
postvaccinal 999.3
prepuce NEC 607.1
Propionibacterium 041.84
prostate (capsule) (*see also* Prostatitis) 601.9
Proteus (mirabilis) (morganii) (vulgaris) NEC 041.6
enteritis 008.3
protozoal NEC 136.8
intestinal NEC 007.9
Pseudomonas NEC 041.7
mallei 024
pneumonia 482.1
pseudomallei 025
psittacosis 073.9
puerperal, postpartum (major) 670
minor 646.6
pulmonary - *see* Infection, lung
purulent - *see* Abscess
putrid, generalized - *see* Septicemia
pyemic - *see* Septicemia
Pyrenochaeta romeroi 117.4
Q fever 083.0
rabies 071
rectum (sphincter) 569.49
renal (*see also* Infection, kidney) 590.9
pelvis and ureter 590.3
resistant to drugs - *see* Resistance (to), drugs by microorganisms
respiratory 519.8
chronic 519.8

ICD-9-CM
Vol. 2

Infection, infected, infective *(Continued)*
respiratory *(Continued)*
influenzal (acute) (upper) 487.1
lung 518.89
rhinovirus 460
syncytial virus 079.6
upper (acute) (infectious) NEC 465.9
with flu, grippe, or influenza 487.1
influenzal 487.1
multiple sites NEC 465.8
streptococcal 034.0
viral NEC 465.9
respiratory syncytial virus (RSV) 079.6
resulting from presence of shunt or other internal prosthetic device - *see* Complications, infection and inflammation, due to (presence of) any device, implant, or graft classified to 996.0–996.5 NEC
retroperitoneal 567.39
retrovirus 079.50
human immunodeficiency virus type 2 [HIV 2] 079.53
human T-cell lymphotrophic virus type I [HTLV-I] 079.51
human T-cell lymphotrophic virus type II [HTLV-II] 079.52
specified NEC 079.59
Rhinocladium 117.1
Rhinosporidium (seeberi) 117.0,
rhinovirus
in diseases classified elsewhere - *see* category 079
unspecified nature or site 079.3
Rhizopus 117.7
rickettsial 083.9
rickettsialpox 083.2
rubella (*see also* Rubella) 056.9
congenital 771.0
Saccharomyces (*see also* Candidiasis) 112.9
Saksenaea 117.7
salivary duct or gland (any) 527.2
Salmonella (aertrycke) (callinarum) (choleraesuis) (enteritidis) (suipestifer) (typhimurium) 003.9
with
arthritis 003.23
gastroenteritis 003.0
localized infection 003.20
specified type NEC 003.29
meningitis 003.21
osteomyelitis 003.24
pneumonia 003.22
septicemia 003.1
specified manifestation NEC 003.8
due to food (poisoning) (any serotype) (*see also* Poisoning, food, due to, Salmonella)
Salmonella *(Continued)*
hirschfeldii 002.3
localized 003.20
specified type NEC 003.29
paratyphi 002.9
A 002.1
B 002.2
C 002.3
schottmuelleri 002.2
specified type NEC 003.8
typhi 002.0
typhosa 002.0
saprophytic 136.8
Sarcocystis, lindemanni 136.5
SARS-associated coronavirus 079.82
scabies 133.0

Infection, infected, infective *(Continued)*
Schistosoma - *see* Infestation, Schistosoma
Schmorl's bacillus 040.3
scratch or other superficial injury - *see* Injury, superficial, by site
scrotum (acute) NEC 608.4
secondary, burn or open wound (dislocation) (fracture) 958.3
seminal vesicle (*see also* Vesiculitis) 608.0
septic
generalized - *see* Septicemia
localized, skin (*see also* Abscess) 682.9
septicemic - *see* Septicemia
seroma 998.51
Serratia (marcescens) 041.85
generalized 038.44
sheep liver fluke 121.3
Shigella 004.9
boydii 004.2
dysenteriae 004.0
Flexneri 004.1
group
A 004.0
B 004.1
C 004.2
D 004.3
Schmitz (-Stutzer) 004.0
Schmitzii 004.0
Shiga 004.0
Sonnei 004.3
specified type NEC 004.8
Sin Nombre virus 079.81
sinus (*see also* Sinusitis) 473.9
pilonidal 685.1
with abscess 685.0
skin NEC 686.9
Skene's duct or gland (*see also* Urethritis) 597.89
skin (local) (staphylococcal) (streptococcal) NEC 686.9
abscess - *see* Abscess, by site
cellulitis - *see* Cellulitis, by site
due to fungus 111.9
specified type NEC 111.8
mycotic 111.9
specified type NEC 111.8
ulcer (*see also* Ulcer, skin) 707.9
slow virus 046.9
specified condition NEC 046.8
Sparganum (mansoni) (proliferum) 123.5
spermatic cord NEC 608.4
sphenoidal (chronic) (sinus) (*see also* Sinusitis, sphenoidal) 473.3
Spherophorus necrophorus 040.3
spinal cord NEC (*see also* Encephalitis) 323.9
abscess 324.1
late effect - *see* category 326
late effect - *see* category 326
meninges - *see* Meningitis
streptococcal 320.2
Spirillum
minus or minor 026.0
morsus muris 026.0
obermeieri 087.0
spirochetal NEC 104.9
lung 104.8
specified nature or site NEC 104.8
spleen 289.59
Sporothrix schenckii 117.1
Sporotrichum (schenckii) 117.1
Sporozoa 136.8

Infection, infected, infective *(Continued)*
staphylococcal NEC 041.10
aureus 041.11
food poisoning 005.0
generalized (purulent) 038.10
aureus 038.11
specified organism NEC 038.19
pneumonia 482.40
aureus 482.41
specified type NEC 482.49
septicemia 038.10
aureus 038.11
specified organism NEC 038.19
specified NEC 041.19
steatoma 706.2
Stellantchasmus falcatus 121.6
Streptobacillus moniliformis 026.1
streptococcal NEC 041.00
generalized (purulent) 038.0
group
A 041.01
B 041.02
C 041.03
D [enterococcus] 041.04
G 041.05
pneumonia - *see* Pneumonia, streptococcal
septicemia 038.0
sore throat 034.0
specified NEC 041.09
Streptomyces - *see* Actinomycosis
streptotrichosis - *see* Actinomycosis
Strongyloides (stercoralis) 127.2
stump (amputation) (posttraumatic) (surgical) 997.62
traumatic - *see* Amputation, traumatic, by site, complicated
subcutaneous tissue, local NEC 686.9
submaxillary region 528.9
suipestifer (*see also* Infection, Salmonella) 003.9
swimming pool bacillus 031.1
syphilitic - *see* Syphilis
systemic - *see* Septicemia
Taenia - *see* Infestation, Taenia
Taeniarhynchus saginatus 123.2
tapeworm - *see* Infestation, tapeworm
tendon (sheath) 727.89
Ternidens diminutus 127.7
testis (*see also* Orchitis) 604.90
thigh (skin) 686.9
threadworm 127.4
throat 478.29
pneumococcal 462
staphylococcal 462
streptococcal 034.0
viral NEC (*see also* Pharyngitis) 462
thumb (skin) 686.9
abscess (with lymphangitis) 681.00
pulp 681.01
cellulitis (with lymphangitis) 681.00
nail 681.02
thyroglossal duct 529.8
toe (skin) 686.9
abscess (with lymphangitis) 681.10
cellulitis (with lymphangitis) 681.10
nail 681.11
fungus 110.1
tongue NEC 529.0
parasitic 112.0
tonsil (faucial) (lingual) (pharyngeal) 474.00
acute or subacute 463
and adenoid 474.02
tag 474.00

Infection, infected, infective *(Continued)*
tooth, teeth 522.4
periapical (pulpal origin) 522.4
peridental 523.30
periodontal 523.31
pulp 522.0
socket 526.5
Torula histolytica 117.5
Toxocara (cani) (cati) (felis) 128.0
Toxoplasma gondii (*see also* Toxoplasmosis) 130.9
trachea, chronic 491.8
fungus 117.9
traumatic NEC 958.3
trematode NEC 121.9
trench fever 083.1
Treponema
denticola 041.84
macrodenticum 041.84
pallidum (*see also* Syphilis) 097.9
Trichinella (spiralis) 124
Trichomonas 131.9
bladder 131.09
cervix 131.09
hominis 007.3
intestine 007.3
prostate 131.03
specified site NEC 131.8
urethra 131.02
urogenitalis 131.00
vagina 131.01
vulva 131.01
Trichophyton, trichophytid - *see* Dermatophytosis
Trichosporon (beigelii) cutaneum 111.2
Trichostrongylus 127.6
Trichuris (trichuria) 127.3
Trombicula (irritans) 133.8
Trypanosoma (*see also* Trypanosomiasis) 086.9
cruzi 086.2
tubal (*see also* Salpingo-oophoritis) 614.2
tuberculous NEC (*see also* Tuberculosis) 011.9
tubo-ovarian (*see also* Salpingo-oophoritis) 614.2
tunica vaginalis 608.4
tympanic membrane - *see* Myringitis
typhoid (abortive) (ambulant) (bacillus) 002.0
typhus 081.9
flea-borne (endemic) 081.0
louse-borne (epidemic) 080
mite-borne 081.2
recrudescent 081.1
tick-borne 082.9
African 082.1
North Asian 082.2
umbilicus (septic) 686.9
newborn NEC 771.4
ureter 593.89
urethra (*see also* Urethritis) 597.80
urinary (tract) NEC 599.0
with
abortion - *see* Abortion, by type, with urinary tract infection
ectopic pregnancy (*see also* categories 633.0–633.9) 639.8
molar pregnancy (*see also* categories 630–632) 639.8
candidal 112.2
complicating pregnancy, childbirth, or puerperium 646.6
affecting fetus or newborn 760.1
asymptomatic 646.5
affecting fetus or newborn 760.1

Infection, infected, infective *(Continued)*
urinary (tract) *(Continued)*
diplococcal (acute) 098.0
chronic 098.2
due to Trichomonas (vaginalis) 131.00
following
abortion 639.8
ectopic or molar pregnancy 639.8
gonococcal (acute) 098.0
chronic or duration of 2 months or over 098.2
newborn 771.82
trichomonal 131.00
tuberculous (*see also* Tuberculosis) 016.3
uterus, uterine (*see also* Endometritis) 615.9
utriculus masculinus NEC 597.89
vaccination 999.3
vagina (granulation tissue) (wall) (*see also* Vaginitis) 616.10
varicella 052.9
varicose veins - *see* Varicose, veins
variola 050.9
major 050.0
minor 050.1
vas deferens NEC 608.4
Veillonella 041.84
verumontanum 597.89
vesical (*see also* Cystitis) 595.9
Vibrio
cholerae 001.0
el Tor 001.1
parahaemolyticus (food poisoning) 005.4
vulnificus 041.85
Vincent's (gums) (mouth) (tonsil) 101
virus, viral 079.99
adenovirus
in diseases classified elsewhere - *see* category 079
unspecified nature or site 079.0
central nervous system NEC 049.9
enterovirus 048
meningitis 047.9
specified type NEC 047.8
slow virus 046.9
specified condition NEC 046.8
chest 519.8
conjunctivitis 077.99
specified type NEC 077.89
coronavirus 079.89
SARS-associated 079.82
Coxsackie (*see also* Infection, Coxsackie) 079.2
Ebola 065.8
ECHO
in diseases classified elsewhere - *see* category 079
unspecified nature or site 079.1
encephalitis 049.9
arthropod-borne NEC 064
tick-borne 063.9
specified type NEC 063.8
enteritis NEC (*see also* Enteritis, viral) 008.8
exanthem NEC 057.9
Hantavirus 079.81
human papilloma 079.4
in diseases classified elsewhere - *see* category 079
intestine (*see also* Enteritis, viral) 008.8
lung - *see* Pneumonia, viral
respiratory syncytial (RSV) 079.6
Retrovirus 079.50

Infection, infected, infective *(Continued)*
virus, viral *(Continued)*
rhinovirus
in diseases classified elsewhere - *see* category 079
unspecified nature or site 079.3
salivary gland disease 078.5
slow 046.9
specified condition NEC 046.8
specified type NEC 079.89
in diseases classified elsewhere - *see* category 079
unspecified nature or site 079.99
warts NEC 078.10
vulva (*see also* Vulvitis) 616.10
whipworm 127.3
Whitmore's bacillus 025
wound (local) (posttraumatic) NEC 958.3
with
dislocation - *see* Dislocation, by site, open
fracture - *see* Fracture, by site, open
open wound - *see* Wound, open, by site, complicated
postoperative 998.59
surgical 998.59
Wuchereria 125.0
bancrofti 125.0
malayi 125.1
yaws - *see* Yaws
yeast (*see also* Candidiasis) 112.9
yellow fever (*see also* Fever, yellow) 060.9
Yersinia pestis (*see also* Plague) 020.9
Zeis' gland 373.12
zoonotic bacterial NEC 027.9
Zopfia senegalensis 117.4
Infective, infectious - *see* condition
Inferiority complex 301.9
constitutional psychopathic 301.9
Infertility
female 628.9
age related 628.8
associated with
adhesions, peritubal 614.6 *[628.2]*
anomaly
cervical mucus 628.4
congenital
cervix 628.4
fallopian tube 628.2
uterus 628.3
vagina 628.4
anovulation 628.0
dysmucorrhea 628.4
endometritis, tuberculous (*see also* Tuberculosis) 016.7 *[628.3]*
Stein-Leventhal syndrome 256.4 *[628.0]*
due to
adiposogenital dystrophy 253.8 *[628.1]*
anterior pituitary disorder NEC 253.4 *[628.1]*
hyperfunction 253.1 *[628.1]*
cervical anomaly 628.4
fallopian tube anomaly 628.2
ovarian failure 256.39 *[628.0]*
Stein-Leventhal syndrome 256.4 *[628.0]*
uterine anomaly 628.3
vaginal anomaly 628.4
nonimplantation 628.3
origin
cervical 628.4
pituitary-hypothalamus NEC 253.8 *[628.1]*

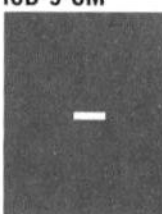
ICD-9-CM
Vol. 2

Infertility *(Continued)*
female *(Continued)*
origin *(Continued)*
anterior pituitary NEC 253.4 *[628.1]*
hyperfunction NEC 253.1 *[628.1]*
dwarfism 253.3 *[628.1]*
panhypopituitarism 253.2 *[628.1]*
specified NEC 628.8
tubal (block) (occlusion) (stenosis) 628.2
adhesions 614.6 *[628.2]*
uterine 628.3
vaginal 628.4
previous, requiring supervision of pregnancy V23.0
male 606.9
absolute 606.0
due to
azoospermia 606.0
drug therapy 606.8
extratesticular cause NEC 606.8
germinal cell
aplasia 606.0
desquamation 606.1
hypospermatogenesis 606.1
infection 606.8
obstruction, afferent ducts 606.8
oligospermia 606.1
radiation 606.8
spermatogenic arrest (complete) 606.0
incomplete 606.1
systemic disease 606.8
Infestation 134.9
Acanthocheilonema (perstans) 125.4
streptocerca 125.6
Acariasis 133.9
demodex folliculorum 133.8
sarcoptes scabiei 133.0
trombiculae 133.8
Agamofilaria streptocerca 125.6
Ancylostoma, Ankylostoma 126.9
americanum 126.1
braziliense 126.2
canium 126.8
ceylanicum 126.3
duodenale 126.0
new world 126.1
old world 126.0
Angiostrongylus cantonensis 128.8
anisakiasis 127.1
Anisakis larva 127.1
arthropod NEC 134.1
Ascaris lumbricoides 127.0
Bacillus fusiformis 101
Balantidium coli 007.0
beef tapeworm 123.2
Bothriocephalus (latus) 123.4
larval 123.5
broad tapeworm 123.4
larval 123.5
Brugia malayi 125.1
Candiru 136.8
Capillaria
hepatica 128.8
philippinensis 127.5
cat liver fluke 121.0
Cercomonas hominis (intestinal) 007.3
cestodes 123.9
specified type NEC 123.8
chigger 133.8
chigoe 134.1
Chilomastix 007.8
Clonorchis (sinensis) (liver) 121.1

Infestation *(Continued)*
coccidia 007.2
complicating pregnancy, childbirth, or puerperium 647.9
affecting fetus or newborn 760.8
Cysticercus cellulosae 123.1
Demodex folliculorum 133.8
Dermatobia (hominis) 134.0
Dibothriocephalus (latus) 123.4
larval 123.5
Dicrocoelium dendriticum 121.8
Diphyllobothrium (adult) (intestinal) (latum) (pacificum) 123.4
larval 123.5
Diplogonoporus (grandis) 123.8
Dipylidium (caninum) 123.8
Distoma hepaticum 121.3
dog tapeworm 123.8
Dracunculus medinensis 125.7
dragon worm 125.7
dwarf tapeworm 123.6
Echinococcus (*see also* Echinococcus) 122.9
Echinostoma ilocanum 121.8
Embadomonas 007.8
Endamoeba (histolytica) - *see* Infection, ameba
Entamoeba (histolytica) - *see* Infection, ameba
Enterobius vermicularis 127.4
Epidermophyton - *see* Dermatophytosis
eyeworm 125.2
Fasciola
gigantica 121.3
hepatica 121.3
Fasciolopsis (buski) (small intestine) 121.4
filarial 125.9
due to
Acanthocheilonema (perstans) 125.4
streptocerca 125.6
Brugia (Wuchereria) malayi 125.1
Dracunculus medinensis 125.7
guinea worms 125.7
Mansonella (ozzardi) 125.5
Onchocerca volvulus 125.3
eye 125.3 *[360.13]*
eyelid 125.3 *[373.6]*
Wuchereria (bancrofti) 125.0
malayi 125.1
specified type NEC 125.6
fish tapeworm 123.4
larval 123.5
fluke 121.9
blood NEC (*see also* Schistosomiasis) 120.9
cat liver 121.0
intestinal (giant) 121.4
liver (sheep) 121.3
cat 121.0
Chinese 121.1
clonorchiasis 121.1
fascioliasis 121.3
Oriental 121.1
lung (oriental) 121.2
sheep liver 121.3
fly larva 134.0
Gasterophilus (intestinalis) 134.0
Gastrodiscoides hominis 121.8
Giardia lamblia 007.1
Gnathostoma (spinigerum) 128.1
Gongylonema 125.6
guinea worm 125.7

Infestation *(Continued)*
helminth NEC 128.9
intestinal 127.9
mixed (types classifiable to more than one category in 120.0–127.7) 127.8
specified type NEC 127.7
specified type NEC 128.8
Heterophyes heterophyes (small intestine) 121.6
hookworm (*see also* Infestation, ancylostoma) 126.9
Hymenolepis (diminuta) (nana) 123.6
intestinal NEC 129
leeches (aquatic) (land) 134.2
Leishmania - *see* Leishmaniasis
lice (*see also* Infestation, pediculus) 132.9
Linguatulidae, linguatula (pentastoma) (serrata) 134.1
Loa loa 125.2
eyelid 125.2 *[373.6]*
louse (*see also* Infestation, pediculus) 132.9
body 132.1
head 132.0
pubic 132.2
maggots 134.0
Mansonella (ozzardi) 125.5
medina 125.7
Metagonimus yokogawai (small intestine) 121.5
Microfilaria streptocerca 125.3
eye 125.3 *[360.13]*
eyelid 125.3 *[373.6]*
Microsporon furfur 111.0
microsporum - *see* Dermatophytosis
mites 133.9
scabic 133.0
specified type NEC 133.8
Monilia (albicans) (*see also* Candidiasis) 112.9
vagina 112.1
vulva 112.1
mouth 112.0
Necator americanus 126.1
nematode (intestinal) 127.9
Ancylostoma (*see also* Ancylostoma) 126.9
Ascaris lumbricoides 127.0
conjunctiva NEC 128.9
Dioctophyma 128.8
Enterobius vermicularis 127.4
Gnathostoma spinigerum 128.1
Oesophagostomum (apiostomum) 127.7
Physaloptera 127.4
specified type NEC 127.7
Strongyloides stercoralis 127.2
Ternidens diminutus 127.7
Trichinella spiralis 124
Trichostrongylus 127.6
Trichuris (trichiuria) 127.3
Oesophagostomum (apiostomum) 127.7
Oestrus ovis 134.0
Onchocerca (volvulus) 125.3
eye 125.3 *[360.13]*
eyelid 125.3 *[373.6]*
Opisthorchis (felineus) (tenuicollis) (viverrini) 121.0
Oxyuris vermicularis 127.4
Paragonimus (westermani) 121.2
parasite, parasitic NEC 136.9

Infestation *(Continued)*
parasite, parasitic *(Continued)*
eyelid 134.9 *[373.6]*
intestinal 129
mouth 112.0
orbit 376.13
skin 134.9
tongue 112.0
pediculus 132.9
capitis (humanus) (any site) 132.0
corporis (humanus) (any site) 132.1
eyelid 132.0 *[373.6]*
mixed (classifiable to more than one category in 132.0–132.2) 132.3
pubis (any site) 132.2
phthirus (pubis) (any site) 132.2
with any infestation classifiable to 132.0 and 132.1 132.3
pinworm 127.4
pork tapeworm (adult) 123.0
protozoal NEC 136.8
pubic louse 132.2
rat tapeworm 123.6
red bug 133.8
roundworm (large) NEC 127.0
sand flea 134.1
saprophytic NEC 136.8
Sarcoptes scabiei 133.0
scabies 133.0
Schistosoma 120.9
bovis 120.8
cercariae 120.3
hematobium 120.0
intercalatum 120.8
japonicum 120.2
mansoni 120.1
mattheii 120.8
specified
site - *see* Schistosomiasis
type NEC 120.8
spindale 120.8
screw worms 134.0
skin NEC 134.9
Sparganum (mansoni) (proliferum) 123.5
larval 123.5
specified type NEC 134.8
Spirometra larvae 123.5
Sporozoa NEC 136.8
Stellantchasmus falcatus 121.6
Strongyloides 127.2
Strongylus (gibsoni) 127.7
Taenia 123.3
diminuta 123.6
Echinococcus (*see also* Echinococcus) 122.9
mediocanellata 123.2
nana 123.6
saginata (mediocanellata) 123.2
solium (intestinal form) 123.0
larval form 123.1
Taeniarhynchus saginatus 123.2
tapeworm 123.9
beef 123.2
broad 123.4
larval 123.5
dog 123.8
dwarf 123.6
fish 123.4
larval 123.5
pork 123.0
rat 123.6
Ternidens diminutus 127.7
Tetranychus molestissimus 133.8

Infestation *(Continued)*
threadworm 127.4
tongue 112.0
Toxocara (cani) (cati) (felis) 128.0
trematode(s) NEC 121.9
Trichina spiralis 124
Trichinella spiralis 124
Trichocephalus 127.3
Trichomonas 131.9
bladder 131.09
cervix 131.09
intestine 007.3
prostate 131.03
specified site NEC 131.8
urethra (female) (male) 131.02
urogenital 131.00
vagina 131.01
vulva 131.01
Trichophyton - *see* Dermatophytosis
Trichostrongylus instabilis 127.6
Trichuris (trichiuria) 127.3
Trombicula (irritans) 133.8
Trypanosoma - *see* Trypanosomiasis
Tunga penetrans 134.1
Uncinaria americana 126.1
whipworm 127.3
worms NEC 128.9
intestinal 127.9
Wuchereria 125.0
bancrofti 125.0
malayi 125.1
Infiltrate, infiltration
with an iron compound 275.0
amyloid (any site) (generalized) 277.39 (Revised)
calcareous (muscle) NEC 275.49
localized - *see* Degeneration, by site
calcium salt (muscle) 275.49
corneal (*see also* Edema, cornea) 371.20
eyelid 373.9
fatty (diffuse) (generalized) 272.8
localized - *see* Degeneration, by site, fatty
glycogen, glycogenic (*see also* Disease, glycogen storage) 271.0
heart, cardiac
fatty (*see also* Degeneration, myocardial) 429.1
glycogenic 271.0 *[425.7]*
inflammatory in vitreous 379.29
kidney (*see also* Disease, renal) 593.9
leukemic (M9800/3) - *see* Leukemia
liver 573.8
fatty - *see* Fatty, liver
glycogen (*see also* Disease, glycogen storage) 271.0
lung (*see also* Infiltrate, pulmonary) 518.3
eosinophilic 518.3
x-ray finding only 793.1
lymphatic (*see also* Leukemia, lymphatic) 204.9
gland, pigmentary 289.3
muscle, fatty 728.9
myelogenous (*see also* Leukemia, myeloid) 205.9
myocardium, myocardial
fatty (*see also* Degeneration, myocardial) 429.1
glycogenic 271.0 *[425.7]*
pulmonary 518.3
with
eosinophilia 518.3
pneumonia - *see* Pneumonia, by type

Infiltrate, infiltration *(Continued)*
pulmonary *(Continued)*
x-ray finding only 793.1
Ranke's primary (*see also* Tuberculosis) 010.0
skin, lymphocytic (benign) 709.8
thymus (gland) (fatty) 254.8
urine 788.8
vitreous humor 379.29
Infirmity 799.89
senile 797
Inflammation, inflamed, inflammatory (with exudation)
abducens (nerve) 378.54
accessory sinus (chronic) (*see also* Sinusitis) 473.9
adrenal (gland) 255.8
alimentary canal - *see* Enteritis
alveoli (teeth) 526.5
scorbutic 267
amnion - *see* Amnionitis
anal canal 569.49
antrum (chronic) (*see also* Sinusitis, maxillary) 473.0
anus 569.49
appendix (*see also* Appendicitis) 541
arachnoid - *see* Meningitis
areola 611.0
puerperal, postpartum 675.0
areolar tissue NEC 686.9
artery - *see* Arteritis
auditory meatus (external) (*see also* Otitis, externa) 380.10
Bartholin's gland 616.89 (Revised)
bile duct or passage 576.1
bladder (*see also* Cystitis) 595.9
bleb (New)
postprocedural 379.60 (New)
stage 1 379.61 (New)
stage 2 379.62 (New)
stage 3 379.63 (New)
bone - *see* Osteomyelitis
bowel (*see also* Enteritis) 558.9
brain (*see also* Encephalitis) 323.9
late effect - *see* category 326
membrane - *see* Meningitis
breast 611.0
puerperal, postpartum 675.2
broad ligament (*see also* Disease, pelvis, inflammatory) 614.4
acute 614.3
bronchus - *see* Bronchitis
bursa - *see* Bursitis
capsule
liver 573.3
spleen 289.59
catarrhal (*see also* Catarrh) 460
vagina 616.10
cecum (*see also* Appendicitis) 541
cerebral (*see also* Encephalitis) 323.9
late effect - *see* category 326
membrane - *see* Meningitis
cerebrospinal (*see also* Meningitis) 322.9
late effect - *see* category 326
meningococcal 036.0
tuberculous (*see also* Tuberculosis) 013.6
cervix (uteri) (*see also* Cervicitis) 616.0
chest 519.9
choroid NEC (*see also* Choroiditis) 363.20
cicatrix (tissue) - *see* Cicatrix
colon (*see also* Enteritis) 558.9
granulomatous 555.1
newborn 558.9

ICD-9-CM
Vol. 2

Inflammation, inflamed, inflammatory *(Continued)*
connective tissue (diffuse) NEC 728.9
cornea (*see also* Keratitis) 370.9
with ulcer (*see also* Ulcer, cornea) 370.00
corpora cavernosa (penis) 607.2
cranial nerve - *see* Disorder, nerve, cranial
diarrhea - *see* Diarrhea
disc (intervertebral) (space) 722.90
cervical, cervicothoracic 722.91
lumbar, lumbosacral 722.93
thoracic, thoracolumbar 722.92
Douglas' cul-de-sac or pouch (chronic) (*see also* Disease, pelvis, inflammatory) 614.4
acute 614.3
due to (presence of) any device, implant, or graft classifiable to 996.0–996.5 - *see* Complications, infection and inflammation, due to (presence of) any device, implant, or graft classified to 996.0–996.5 NEC
duodenum 535.6
dura mater - *see* Meningitis
ear - *see also* Otitis
external (*see also* Otitis, externa) 380.10
inner (*see also* Labyrinthitis) 386.30
middle - *see* Otitis media
esophagus 530.10
ethmoidal (chronic) (sinus) (*see also* Sinusitis, ethmoidal) 473.2
Eustachian tube (catarrhal) 381.50
acute 381.51
chronic 381.52
extrarectal 569.49
eye 379.99
eyelid 373.9
specified NEC 373.8
fallopian tube (*see also* Salpingo-oophoritis) 614.2
fascia 728.9
fetal membranes (acute) 658.4
affecting fetus or newborn 762.7
follicular, pharynx 472.1
frontal (chronic) (sinus) (*see also* Sinusitis, frontal) 473.1
gallbladder (*see also* Cholecystitis, acute) 575.0
gall duct (*see also* Cholecystitis) 575.10
gastrointestinal (*see also* Enteritis) 558.9
genital organ (diffuse) (internal)
female 614.9
with
abortion - *see* Abortion, by type, with sepsis
ectopic pregnancy (*see also* categories 633.0–633.9) 639.0
molar pregnancy (*see also* categories 630–632) 639.0
complicating pregnancy, childbirth, or puerperium 646.6
affecting fetus or newborn 760.8
following
abortion 639.0
ectopic or molar pregnancy 639.0
male 608.4
gland (lymph) (*see also* Lymphadenitis) 289.3
glottis (*see also* Laryngitis) 464.00
with obstruction 464.01
granular, pharynx 472.1

Inflammation, inflamed, inflammatory *(Continued)*
gum 523.10 (Revised)
heart (*see also* Carditis) 429.89
hepatic duct 576.8
hernial sac - *see* Hernia, by site
ileum (*see also* Enteritis) 558.9
terminal or regional 555.0
with large intestine 555.2
intervertebral disc 722.90
cervical, cervicothoracic 722.91
lumbar, lumbosacral 722.93
thoracic, thoracolumbar 722.92
intestine (*see also* Enteritis) 558.9
jaw (acute) (bone) (chronic) (lower) (suppurative) (upper) 526.4
jejunum - *see* Enteritis
joint NEC (*see also* Arthritis) 716.9
sacroiliac 720.2
kidney (*see also* Nephritis) 583.9
knee (joint) 716.66
tuberculous (active) (*see also* Tuberculosis) 015.2
labium (majus) (minus) (*see also* Vulvitis) 616.10
lacrimal
gland (*see also* Dacryoadenitis) 375.00
passages (duct) (sac) (*see also* Dacryocystitis) 375.30
larynx (*see also* Laryngitis) 464.00
with obstruction 464.01
diphtheritic 032.3
leg NEC 686.9
lip 528.5
liver (capsule) (*see also* Hepatitis) 573.3
acute 570
chronic 571.40
suppurative 572.0
lung (acute) (*see also* Pneumonia) 486
chronic (interstitial) 518.89
lymphatic vessel (*see also* Lymphangitis) 457.2
lymph node or gland (*see also* Lymphadenitis) 289.3
mammary gland 611.0
puerperal, postpartum 675.2
maxilla, maxillary 526.4
sinus (chronic) (*see also* Sinusitis, maxillary) 473.0
membranes of brain or spinal cord - *see* Meningitis
meninges - *see* Meningitis
mouth 528.00 (Revised)
muscle 728.9
myocardium (*see also* Myocarditis) 429.0
nasal sinus (chronic) (*see also* Sinusitis) 473.9
nasopharynx - *see* Nasopharyngitis
navel 686.9
newborn NEC 771.4
nerve NEC 729.2
nipple 611.0
puerperal, postpartum 675.0
nose 478.19 (Revised)
suppurative 472.0
oculomotor nerve 378.51
optic nerve 377.30
orbit (chronic) 376.10
acute 376.00
chronic 376.10
ovary (*see also* Salpingo-oophoritis) 614.2
oviduct (*see also* Salpingo-oophoritis) 614.2
pancreas - *see* Pancreatitis

Inflammation, inflamed, inflammatory *(Continued)*
parametrium (chronic) (*see also* Disease, pelvis, inflammatory) 614.4
acute 614.3
parotid region 686.9
gland 527.2
pelvis, female (*see also* Disease, pelvis, inflammatory) 614.9
penis (corpora cavernosa) 607.2
perianal 569.49
pericardium (*see also* Pericarditis) 423.9
perineum (female) (male) 686.9
perirectal 569.49
peritoneum (*see also* Peritonitis) 567.9
periuterine (*see also* Disease, pelvis, inflammatory) 614.9
perivesical (*see also* Cystitis) 595.9
petrous bone (*see also* Petrositis) 383.20
pharynx (*see also* Pharyngitis) 462
follicular 472.1
granular 472.1
pia mater - *see* Meningitis
pleura - *see* Pleurisy
postmastoidectomy cavity 383.30
chronic 383.33
prostate (*see also* Prostatitis) 601.9
rectosigmoid - *see* Rectosigmoiditis
rectum (*see also* Proctitis) 569.49
respiratory, upper (*see also* Infection, respiratory, upper) 465.9
chronic, due to external agent - *see* Condition, respiratory, chronic, due to, external agent
due to
fumes or vapors (chemical) (inhalation) 506.2
radiation 508.1
retina (*see also* Retinitis) 363.20
retrocecal (*see also* Appendicitis) 541
retroperitoneal (*see also* Peritonitis) 567.9
salivary duct or gland (any) (suppurative) 527.2
scorbutic, alveoli, teeth 267
scrotum 608.4
sigmoid - *see* Enteritis
sinus (*see also* Sinusitis) 473.9
Skene's duct or gland (*see also* Urethritis) 597.89
skin 686.9
spermatic cord 608.4
sphenoidal (sinus) (*see also* Sinusitis, sphenoidal) 473.3
spinal
cord (*see also* Encephalitis) 323.9
late effect - *see* category 326
membrane - *see* Meningitis
nerve - *see* Disorder, nerve
spine (*see also* Spondylitis) 720.9
spleen (capsule) 289.59
stomach - *see* Gastritis
stricture, rectum 569.49
subcutaneous tissue NEC 686.9
suprarenal (gland) 255.8
synovial (fringe) (membrane) - *see* Bursitis
tendon (sheath) NEC 726.90
testis (*see also* Orchitis) 604.90
thigh 686.9
throat (*see also* Sore throat) 462
thymus (gland) 254.8
thyroid (gland) (*see also* Thyroiditis) 245.9

Inflammation, inflamed, inflammatory *(Continued)*
tongue 529.0
tonsil - *see* Tonsillitis
trachea - *see* Tracheitis
trochlear nerve 378.53
tubal (*see also* Salpingo-oophoritis) 614.2
tuberculous NEC (*see also* Tuberculosis) 011.9
tubo-ovarian (*see also* Salpingo-oophoritis) 614.2
tunica vaginalis 608.4
tympanic membrane - *see* Myringitis
umbilicus, umbilical 686.9
newborn NEC 771.4
uterine ligament (*see also* Disease, pelvis, inflammatory) 614.4
acute 614.3
uterus (catarrhal) (*see also* Endometritis) 615.9
uveal tract (anterior) (*see also* Iridocyclitis) 364.3
posterior - *see* Chorioretinitis
sympathetic 360.11
vagina (*see also* Vaginitis) 616.10
vas deferens 608.4
vein (*see also* Phlebitis) 451.9
thrombotic 451.9
cerebral (*see also* Thrombosis, brain) 434.0
leg 451.2
deep (vessels) NEC 451.19
superficial (vessels) 451.0
lower extremity 451.2
deep (vessels) NEC 451.19
superficial (vessels) 451.0
vocal cord 478.5
vulva (*see also* Vulvitis) 616.10
Inflation, lung imperfect (newborn) 770.5
Influenza, influenzal 487.1
with
bronchitis 487.1
bronchopneumonia 487.0
cold (any type) 487.1
digestive manifestations 487.8
hemoptysis 487.1
involvement of
gastrointestinal tract 487.8
nervous system 487.8
laryngitis 487.1
manifestations NEC 487.8
respiratory 487.1
pneumonia 487.0
pharyngitis 487.1
pneumonia (any form classifiable to 480–483, 485–486) 487.0
respiratory manifestations NEC 487.1
sinusitis 487.1
sore throat 487.1
tonsillitis 487.1
tracheitis 487.1
upper respiratory infection (acute) 487.1
abdominal 487.8
Asian 487.1
bronchial 487.1
bronchopneumonia 487.0
catarrhal 487.1
epidemic 487.1
gastric 487.8
intestinal 487.8
laryngitis 487.1
maternal affecting fetus or newborn 760.2

Influenza, influenzal *(Continued)*
maternal affecting fetus or newborn *(Continued)*
manifest influenza in infant 771.2
pharyngitis 487.1
pneumonia (any form) 487.0
respiratory (upper) 487.1
stomach 487.8
vaccination, prophylactic (against) V04.81
Influenza-like disease 487.1
Infraction, Freiberg's (metatarsal head) 732.5
Infraeruption, teeth 524.34
Infusion complication, misadventure, or reaction - *see* Complication, infusion
Ingestion
chemical - *see* Table of Drugs and Chemicals
drug or medicinal substance
overdose or wrong substance given or taken 977.9
specified drug - *see* Table of Drugs and Chemicals
foreign body NEC (*see also* Foreign body) 938
Ingrowing
hair 704.8
nail (finger) (toe) (infected) 703.0
Inguinal - *see also* condition
testis 752.51
Inhalation
carbon monoxide 986
flame
mouth 947.0
lung 947.1
food or foreign body (*see also* Asphyxia, food or foreign body) 933.1
gas, fumes, or vapor (noxious) 987.9
specified agent - *see* Table of Drugs and Chemicals
liquid or vomitus (*see also* Asphyxia, food or foreign body) 933.1
lower respiratory tract NEC 934.9
meconium (fetus or newborn) 770.11
with respiratory symptoms 770.12
mucus (*see also* Asphyxia, mucus) 933.1
oil (causing suffocation) (*see also* Asphyxia, food or foreign body) 933.1
pneumonia - *see* Pneumonia, aspiration
smoke 987.9
steam 987.9
stomach contents or secretions (*see also* Asphyxia, food or foreign body) 933.1
in labor and delivery 668.0
Inhibition, inhibited
academic as adjustment reaction 309.23
orgasm
female 302.73
male 302.74
sexual
desire 302.71
excitement 302.72
work as adjustment reaction 309.23
Inhibitor, systemic lupus erythematosus (presence of) 286.5
Iniencephalus, iniencephaly 740.2
Injected eye 372.74
Injury 959.9

Note For abrasion, insect bite (nonvenomous), blister, or scratch, *see* Injury, superficial.

Injury *(Continued)*

For laceration, traumatic rupture, tear, or penetrating wound of internal organs, such as heart, lung, liver, kidney, pelvic organs, whether or not accompanied by open wound in the same region, *see* Injury, internal.

For nerve injury, *see* Injury, nerve.

For late effect of injuries classifiable to 850–854, 860–869, 900–919, 950–959, *see* Late, effect, injury, by type.

abdomen, abdominal (viscera) - *see also* Injury, internal, abdomen
muscle or wall 959.12
acoustic, resulting in deafness 951.5
adenoid 959.09
adrenal (gland) - *see* Injury, internal, adrenal
alveolar (process) 959.09
ankle (and foot) (and knee) (and leg, except thigh) 959.7
anterior chamber, eye 921.3
anus 959.19
aorta (thoracic) 901.0
abdominal 902.0
appendix - *see* Injury, internal, appendix
arm, upper (and shoulder) 959.2
artery (complicating trauma) (*see also* Injury, blood vessel, by site) 904.9
cerebral or meningeal (*see also* Hemorrhage, brain, traumatic, subarachnoid) 852.0
auditory canal (external) (meatus) 959.09
auricle, auris, ear 959.09
axilla 959.2
back 959.19
bile duct - *see* Injury, internal, bile duct
birth - *see also* Birth, injury
canal NEC, complicating delivery 665.9
bladder (sphincter) - *see* Injury, internal, bladder
blast (air) (hydraulic) (immersion) (underwater) NEC 869.0
with open wound into cavity NEC 869.1
abdomen or thorax - *see* Injury, internal, by site
brain - *see* Concussion, brain
ear (acoustic nerve trauma) 951.5
with perforation of tympanic membrane - *see* Wound, open, ear, drum
blood vessel NEC 904.9
abdomen 902.9
multiple 902.87
specified NEC 902.89
aorta (thoracic) 901.0
abdominal 902.0
arm NEC 903.9
axillary 903.00
artery 903.1
vein 903.02
azygos vein 901.89
basilic vein 903.1
brachial (artery) (vein) 903.1
bronchial 901.89
carotid artery 900.00
common 900.01
external 900.02
internal 900.03

ICD-9-CM
I
Vol. 2

Injury *(Continued)*
blood vessel *(Continued)*
celiac artery 902.20
specified branch NEC 902.24
cephalic vein (arm) 903.1
colica dextra 902.26
cystic
artery 902.24
vein 902.39
deep plantar 904.6
diffuse axonal - *see* Injury, intracranial
digital (artery) (vein) 903.5
due to accidental puncture or laceration during procedure 998.2
extremity
lower 904.8
multiple 904.7
specified NEC 904.7
upper 903.9
multiple 903.8
specified NEC 903.8
femoral
artery (superficial) 904.1
above profunda origin 904.0
common 904.0
vein 904.2
gastric
artery 902.21
vein 902.39
head 900.9
intracranial - *see* Injury, intracranial
multiple 900.82
specified NEC 900.89
hemiazygos vein 901.89
hepatic
artery 902.22
vein 902.11
hypogastric 902.59
artery 902.51
vein 902.52
ileocolic
artery 902.26
vein 902.31
iliac 902.50
artery 902.53
specified branch NEC 902.59
vein 902.54
innominate
artery 901.1
vein 901.3
intercostal (artery) (vein) 901.81
jugular vein (external) 900.81
internal 900.1
leg NEC 904.8
mammary (artery) (vein) 901.82
mesenteric
artery 902.20
inferior 902.27
specified branch NEC 902.29
superior (trunk) 902.25
branches, primary 902.26
vein 902.39
inferior 902.32
superior (and primary subdivisions) 902.31
neck 900.9
multiple 900.82
specified NEC 900.89
ovarian 902.89
artery 902.81
vein 902.82
palmar artery 903.4
pelvis 902.9
multiple 902.87
specified NEC 902.89

Injury *(Continued)*
blood vessel *(Continued)*
plantar (deep) (artery) (vein) 904.6
popliteal 904.40
artery 904.41
vein 904.42
portal 902.33
pulmonary 901.40
artery 901.41
vein 901.42
radial (artery) (vein) 903.2
renal 902.40
artery 902.41
specified NEC 902.49
vein 902.42
saphenous
artery 904.7
vein (greater) (lesser) 904.3
splenic
artery 902.23
vein 902.34
subclavian
artery 901.1
vein 901.3
suprarenal 902.49
thoracic 901.9
multiple 901.83
specified NEC 901.89
tibial 904.50
artery 904.50
anterior 904.51
posterior 904.53
vein 904.50
anterior 904.52
posterior 904.54
ulnar (artery) (vein) 903.3
uterine 902.59
artery 902.55
vein 902.56
vena cava
inferior 902.10
specified branches NEC 902.19
superior 901.2
brachial plexus 953.4
newborn 767.6
brain NEC (*see also* Injury, intracranial) 854.0
breast 959.19
broad ligament - *see* Injury, internal, broad ligament
bronchus, bronchi - *see* Injury, internal, bronchus
brow 959.09
buttock 959.19
canthus, eye 921.1
cathode ray 990
cauda equina 952.4
with fracture, vertebra - *see* Fracture, vertebra, sacrum
cavernous sinus (*see also* Injury, intracranial) 854.0
cecum - *see* Injury, internal, cecum
celiac ganglion or plexus 954.1
cerebellum (*see also* Injury, intracranial) 854.0
cervix (uteri) - *see* Injury, internal, cervix
cheek 959.09
chest - *see* Injury, internal, chest
wall 959.11
childbirth - *see also* Birth, injury
maternal NEC 665.9
chin 959.09
choroid (eye) 921.3

Injury *(Continued)*
clitoris 959.14
coccyx 959.19
complicating delivery 665.6
colon - *see* Injury, internal, colon
common duct - *see* Injury, internal, common duct
conjunctiva 921.1
superficial 918.2
cord
spermatic - *see* Injury, internal, spermatic cord
spinal - *see* Injury, spinal, by site
cornea 921.3
abrasion 918.1
due to contact lens 371.82
penetrating - *see* Injury, eyeball, penetrating
superficial 918.1
due to contact lens 371.82
cortex (cerebral) (*see also* Injury, intracranial) 854.0
visual 950.3
costal region 959.11
costochondral 959.11
cranial
bones - *see* Fracture, skull, by site
cavity (*see also* Injury, intracranial) 854.0
nerve - *see* Injury, nerve, cranial
crushing - *see* Crush
cutaneous sensory nerve
lower limb 956.4
upper limb 955.5
delivery - *see also* Birth, injury
maternal NEC 665.9
Descemet's membrane - *see* Injury, eyeball, penetrating
diaphragm - *see* Injury, internal, diaphragm
diffuse axonal - *see* Injury, intracranial
duodenum - *see* Injury, internal, duodenum
ear (auricle) (canal) (drum) (external) 959.09
elbow (and forearm) (and wrist) 959.3
epididymis 959.14
epigastric region 959.12
epiglottis 959.09
epiphyseal, current - *see* Fracture, by site
esophagus - *see* Injury, internal, esophagus
Eustachian tube 959.09
extremity (lower) (upper) NEC 959.8
eye 921.9
penetrating eyeball - *see* Injury, eyeball, penetrating
superficial 918.9
eyeball 921.3
penetrating 871.7
with
partial loss (of intraocular tissue) 871.2
prolapse or exposure (of intraocular tissue) 871.1
without prolapse 871.0
foreign body (nonmagnetic) 871.6
magnetic 871.5
superficial 918.9
eyebrow 959.09
eyelid(s) 921.1
laceration - *see* Laceration, eyelid
superficial 918.0

Injury *(Continued)*
face (and neck) 959.09
fallopian tube - *see* Injury, internal, fallopian tube
fingers(s) (nail) 959.5
flank 959.19
foot (and ankle) (and knee) (and leg, except thigh) 959.7
forceps NEC 767.9
scalp 767.19
forearm (and elbow) (and wrist) 959.3
forehead 959.09
gallbladder - *see* Injury, internal, gallbladder
gasserian ganglion 951.2
gastrointestinal tract - *see* Injury, internal, gastrointestinal tract
genital organ(s)
with
abortion - *see* Abortion, by type, with, damage to pelvic organs
ectopic pregnancy (*see also* categories 633.0–633.9) 639.2
molar pregnancy (*see also* categories 630–632) 639.2
external 959.14
fracture of corpus cavernosum penis 959.13
following
abortion 639.2
ectopic or molar pregnancy 639.2
internal - *see* Injury, internal, genital organs
obstetrical trauma NEC 665.9
affecting fetus or newborn 763.89
gland
lacrimal 921.1
laceration 870.8
parathyroid 959.09
salivary 959.09
thyroid 959.09
globe (eye) (*see also* Injury, eyeball) 921.3
grease gun - *see* Wound, open, by site, complicated
groin 959.19
gum 959.09
hand(s) (except fingers) 959.4
head NEC 959.01
with
loss of consciousness 850.5
skull fracture - *see* Fracture, skull, by site
heart - *see* Injury, internal, heart
heel 959.7
hip (and thigh) 959.6
hymen 959.14
hyperextension (cervical) (vertebra) 847.0
ileum - *see* Injury, internal, ileum
iliac region 959.19
infrared rays NEC 990
instrumental (during surgery) 998.2
birth injury - *see* Birth, injury
nonsurgical (*see also* Injury, by site) 959.9
obstetrical 665.9
affecting fetus or newborn 763.89
bladder 665.5
cervix 665.3
high vaginal 665.4
perineal NEC 664.9
urethra 665.5
uterus 665.5
internal 869.0

Injury *(Continued)*
internal *(Continued)*

Note For injury of internal organ(s) by foreign body entering through a natural orifice (e.g., inhaled, ingested, or swallowed) - *see* Foreign body, entering through orifice.

For internal injury of any of the following sites with internal injury of any other of the sites - *see* Injury, internal, multiple.

with
fracture
pelvis - *see* Fracture, pelvis
specified site, except pelvis - *see* Injury, internal, by site
open wound into cavity 869.1
abdomen, abdominal (viscera) NEC 868.00
with
fracture, pelvis - *see* Fracture, pelvis
open wound into cavity 868.10
specified site NEC 868.09
with open wound into cavity 868.19
adrenal (gland) 868.01
with open wound into cavity 868.11
aorta (thoracic) 901.0
abdominal 902.0
appendix 863.85
with open wound into cavity 863.95
bile duct 868.02
with open wound into cavity 868.12
bladder (sphincter) 867.0
with
abortion - *see* Abortion, by type, with, damage to pelvic organs
ectopic pregnancy (*see also* categories 633.0–633.9) 639.2
molar pregnancy (*see also* categories 630–632) 639.2
open wound into cavity 867.1
following
abortion 639.2
ectopic or molar pregnancy 639.2
obstetrical trauma 665.5
affecting fetus or newborn 763.89
blood vessel - *see* Injury, blood vessel, by site
broad ligament 867.6
with open wound into cavity 867.7
bronchus, bronchi 862.21
with open wound into cavity 862.31
cecum 863.89
with open wound into cavity 863.99
cervix (uteri) 867.4
with
abortion - *see* Abortion, by type, with damage to pelvic organs
ectopic pregnancy (*see also* categories 633.0–633.9) 639.2
molar pregnancy (*see also* categories 630–632) 639.2
open wound into cavity 867.5
following

Injury *(Continued)*
internal *(Continued)*
cervix *(Continued)*
following *(Continued)*
abortion 639.2
ectopic or molar pregnancy 639.2
obstetrical trauma 665.3
affecting fetus or newborn 763.89
chest (*see also* Injury, internal, intrathoracic organs) 862.8
with open wound into cavity 862.9
colon 863.40
with
open wound into cavity 863.50
rectum 863.46
with open wound into cavity 863.56
ascending (right) 863.41
with open wound into cavity 863.51
descending (left) 863.43
with open wound into cavity 863.53
multiple sites 863.46
with open wound into cavity 863.56
sigmoid 863.44
with open wound into cavity 863.54
specified site NEC 863.49
with open wound into cavity 863.59
transverse 863.42
with open wound into cavity 863.52
common duct 868.02
with open wound into cavity 868.12
complicating delivery 665.9
affecting fetus or newborn 763.89
diaphragm 862.0
with open wound into cavity 862.1
duodenum 863.21
with open wound into cavity 863.31
esophagus (intrathoracic) 862.22
with open wound into cavity 862.32
cervical region 874.4
complicated 874.5
fallopian tube 867.6
with open wound into cavity 867.7
gallbladder 868.02
with open wound into cavity 868.12
gastrointestinal tract NEC 863.80
with open wound into cavity 863.90
genital organ NEC 867.6
with open wound into cavity 867.7
heart 861.00
with open wound into thorax 861.10
ileum 863.29
with open wound into cavity 863.39
intestine NEC 863.89
with open wound into cavity 863.99
large NEC 863.40
with open wound into cavity 863.50
small NEC 863.20
with open wound into cavity 863.30

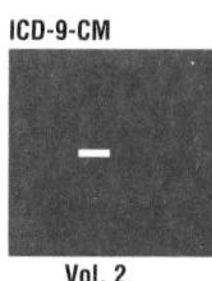

Injury *(Continued)*
internal *(Continued)*
intra-abdominal (organ) 868.00
with open wound into cavity 868.10
multiple sites 868.09
with open wound into cavity 868.19
specified site NEC 868.09
with open wound into cavity 868.19
intrathoracic organs (multiple) 862.8
with open wound into cavity 862.9
diaphragm (only) - *see* Injury, internal, diaphragm
heart (only) - *see* Injury, internal, heart
lung (only) - *see* Injury, internal, lung
specified site NEC 862.29
with open wound into cavity 862.39
intrauterine (*see also* Injury, internal, uterus) 867.4
with open wound into cavity 867.5
jejunum 863.29
with open wound into cavity 863.39
kidney (subcapsular) 866.00
with
disruption of parenchyma (complete) 866.03
with open wound into cavity 866.13
hematoma (without rupture of capsule) 866.01
with open wound into cavity 866.11
laceration 866.02
with open wound into cavity 866.12
open wound into cavity 866.10
liver 864.00
with
contusion 864.01
with open wound into cavity 864.11
hematoma 864.01
with open wound into cavity 864.11
laceration 864.05
with open wound into cavity 864.15
major (disruption of hepatic parenchyma) 864.04
with open wound into cavity 864.14
minor (capsule only) 864.02
with open wound into cavity 864.12
moderate (involving parenchyma) 864.03
with open wound into cavity 864.13
multiple 864.04
stellate 864.04
with open wound into cavity 864.14
open wound into cavity 864.10
lung 861.20
with open wound into thorax 861.30
hemopneumothorax - *see* Hemopneumothorax, traumatic

Injury *(Continued)*
internal *(Continued)*
lung *(Continued)*
hemothorax - *see* Hemothorax, traumatic
pneumohemothorax - *see* Pneumohemothorax, traumatic
pneumothorax - *see* Pneumothorax, traumatic
transfusion related, acute (TRALI) 518.7 ◀
mediastinum 862.29
with open wound into cavity 862.39
mesentery 863.89
with open wound into cavity 863.99
mesosalpinx 867.6
with open wound into cavity 867.7
multiple 869.0

Note Multiple internal injuries of sites classifiable to the same three- or four-digit category should be classified to that category.

Multiple injuries classifiable to different fourth-digit subdivisions of 861.-(heart and lung injuries) should be dealt with according to coding rules.

internal 869.0
with open wound into cavity 869.1
intra-abdominal organ (sites classifiable to 863–868)
with
intrathoracic organ(s) (sites classifiable to 861–862) 869.0
with open wound into cavity 869.1
other intra-abdominal organ(s) (sites classifiable to 863–868, except where classifiable to the same three-digit category) 868.09
with open wound into cavity 868.19
intrathoracic organ (sites classifiable to 861–862)
with
intra-abdominal organ(s) (sites classifiable to 863–868) 869.0
with open wound into cavity 869.1
other intrathoracic organs(s) (sites classifiable to 861–862, except where classifiable to the same three-digit category) 862.8
with open wound into cavity 862.9
myocardium - *see* Injury, internal, heart
ovary 867.6
with open wound into cavity 867.7
pancreas (multiple sites) 863.84
with open wound into cavity 863.94
body 863.82
with open wound into cavity 863.92
head 863.81
with open wound into cavity 863.91

Injury *(Continued)*
internal *(Continued)*
pancreas *(Continued)*
tail 863.83
with open wound into cavity 863.93
pelvis, pelvic (organs) (viscera) 867.8
with
fracture, pelvis - *see* Fracture, pelvis
open wound into cavity 867.9
specified site NEC 867.6
with open wound into cavity 867.7
peritoneum 868.03
with open wound into cavity 868.13
pleura 862.29
with open wound into cavity 862.39
prostate 867.6
with open wound into cavity 867.7
rectum 863.45
with
colon 863.46
with open wound into cavity 863.56
open wound into cavity 863.55
retroperitoneum 868.04
with open wound into cavity 868.14
round ligament 867.6
with open wound into cavity 867.7
seminal vesicle 867.6
with open wound into cavity 867.7
spermatic cord 867.6
with open wound into cavity 867.7
scrotal - *see* Wound, open, spermatic cord
spleen 865.00
with
disruption of parenchyma (massive) 865.04
with open wound into cavity 865.14
hematoma (without rupture of capsule) 865.01
with open wound into cavity 865.11
open wound into cavity 865.10
tear, capsular 865.02
with open wound into cavity 865.12
extending into parenchyma 865.03
with open wound into cavity 865.13
stomach 863.0
with open wound into cavity 863.1
suprarenal gland (multiple) 868.01
with open wound into cavity 868.11
thorax, thoracic (cavity) (organs) (multiple) (*see also* Injury, internal, intrathoracic organs) 862.8
with open wound into cavity 862.9
thymus (gland) 862.29
with open wound into cavity 862.39
trachea (intrathoracic) 862.29
with open wound into cavity 862.39
cervical region (*see also* Wound, open, trachea) 874.02
ureter 867.2
with open wound into cavity 867.3

Injury *(Continued)*
internal *(Continued)*
urethra (sphincter) 867.0
with
abortion - *see* Abortion, by type, with, damage to pelvic organs
ectopic pregnancy (*see also* categories 633.0–633.9) 639.2
molar pregnancy (*see also* categories 630–632) 639.2
open wound into cavity 867.1
following
abortion 639.2
ectopic or molar pregnancy 639.2
obstetrical trauma 665.5
affecting fetus or newborn 763.89
uterus 867.4
with
abortion - *see* Abortion, by type, with, damage to pelvic organs
ectopic pregnancy (*see also* categories 633.0–633.9) 639.2
molar pregnancy (*see also* categories 630–632) 639.2
open wound into cavity 867.5
following
abortion 639.2
ectopic or molar pregnancy 639.2
obstetrical trauma NEC 665.5
affecting fetus or newborn 763.89
vas deferens 867.6
with open wound into cavity 867.7
vesical (sphincter) 867.0
with open wound into cavity 867.1
viscera (abdominal) (*see also* Injury, internal, multiple) 868.00
with
fracture, pelvis - *see* Fracture, pelvis
open wound into cavity 868.10
thoracic NEC (*see also* Injury, internal, intrathoracic organs) 862.8
with open wound into cavity 862.9
interscapular region 959.19
intervertebral disc 959.19
intestine - *see* Injury, internal, intestine
intra-abdominal (organs) NEC - *see* Injury, internal, intra-abdominal
intracranial 854.0

Note Use the following fifth-digit subclassification with categories 851–854:

0 unspecified state of consciousness
1 with no loss of consciousness
2 with brief [less than one hour] loss of consciousness
3 with moderate [1–24 hours] loss of consciousness
4 with prolonged [more than 24 hours] loss of consciousness and return to pre-existing conscious level
5 with prolonged [more than 24 hours] loss of consciousness, without return to pre-existing conscious level

Use fifth-digit 5 to designate when a patient is unconscious and dies before regaining consciousness, regardless of the duration of the loss of consciousness

6 with loss of consciousness of unspecified duration
9 with concussion, unspecified

with
open intracranial wound 854.1
skull fracture - *see* Fracture, skull, by site
contusion 851.8
with open intracranial wound 851.9
brain stem 851.4
with open intracranial wound 851.5
cerebellum 851.4
with open intracranial wound 851.5
cortex (cerebral) 851.0
with open intracranial wound 851.2
hematoma - *see* Injury, intracranial, hemorrhage
hemorrhage 853.0
with
laceration - *see* Injury, intracranial, laceration
open intracranial wound 853.1
extradural 852.4
with open intracranial wound 852.5
subarachnoid 852.0
with open intracranial wound 852.1
subdural 852.2
with open intracranial wound 852.3
laceration 851.8
with open intracranial wound 851.9
brain stem 851.6
with open intracranial wound 851.7
cerebellum 851.6
with open intracranial wound 851.7
cortex (cerebral) 851.2
with open intracranial wound 851.3
intraocular - *see* Injury, eyeball, penetrating
intrathoracic organs (multiple) - *see* Injury, internal, intrathoracic organs
intrauterine - *see* Injury, internal, intrauterine
iris 921.3
penetrating - *see* Injury, eyeball, penetrating
jaw 959.09
jejunum - *see* Injury, internal, jejunum
joint NEC 959.9
old or residual 718.80
ankle 718.87
elbow 718.82
foot 718.87
hand 718.84
hip 718.85
knee 718.86
multiple sites 718.89

Injury *(Continued)*
joint *(Continued)*
old or residual *(Continued)*
pelvic region 718.85
shoulder (region) 718.81
specified site NEC 718.88
wrist 718.83
kidney - *see* Injury, internal, kidney
knee (and ankle) (and foot) (and leg, except thigh) 959.7
labium (majus) (minus) 959.14
labyrinth, ear 959.09
lacrimal apparatus, gland, or sac 921.1
laceration 870.8
larynx 959.09
late effect - *see* Late, effects (of), injury
leg, except thigh (and ankle) (and foot) (and knee) 959.7
upper or thigh 959.6
lens, eye 921.3
penetrating - *see* Injury, eyeball, penetrating
lid, eye - *see* Injury, eyelid
lip 959.09
liver - *see* Injury, internal, liver
lobe, parietal - *see* Injury, intracranial
lumbar (region) 959.19
plexus 953.5
lumbosacral (region) 959.19
plexus 953.5
lung - *see* Injury, internal, lung
malar region 959.09
mastoid region 959.09
maternal, during pregnancy, affecting fetus or newborn 760.5
maxilla 959.09
mediastinum - *see* Injury, internal, mediastinum
membrane
brain (*see also* Injury, intracranial) 854.0
tympanic 959.09
meningeal artery - *see* Hemorrhage, brain, traumatic, subarachnoid
meninges (cerebral) - *see* Injury, intracranial
mesenteric
artery - *see* Injury, blood vessel, mesenteric, artery
plexus, inferior 954.1
vein - *see* Injury, blood vessel, mesenteric, vein
mesentery - *see* Injury, internal, mesentery
mesosalpinx - *see* Injury, internal, mesosalpinx
middle ear 959.09
midthoracic region 959.11
mouth 959.09
multiple (sites not classifiable to the same four-digit category in 959.0–959.7) 959.8
internal 869.0
with open wound into cavity 869.1
musculocutaneous nerve 955.4
nail
finger 959.5
toe 959.7
nasal (septum) (sinus) 959.09
nasopharynx 959.09
neck (and face) 959.09
nerve 957.9
abducens 951.3
abducent 951.3

Injury *(Continued)*
nerve *(Continued)*
accessory 951.6
acoustic 951.5
ankle and foot 956.9
anterior crural, femoral 956.1
arm (*see also* Injury, nerve, upper limb) 955.9
auditory 951.5
axillary 955.0
brachial plexus 953.4
cervical sympathetic 954.0
cranial 951.9
first or olfactory 951.8
second or optic 950.0
third or oculomotor 951.0
fourth or trochlear 951.1
fifth or trigeminal 951.2
sixth or abducens 951.3
seventh or facial 951.4
eighth, acoustic, or auditory 951.5
ninth or glossopharyngeal 951.8
tenth, pneumogastric, or vagus 951.8
eleventh or accessory 951.6
twelfth or hypoglossal 951.7
newborn 767.7
cutaneous sensory
lower limb 956.4
upper limb 955.5
digital (finger) 955.6
toe 956.5
facial 951.4
newborn 767.5
femoral 956.1
finger 955.9
foot and ankle 956.9
forearm 955.9
glossopharyngeal 951.8
hand and wrist 955.9
head and neck, superficial 957.0
hypoglossal 951.7
involving several parts of body 957.8
leg (*see also* Injury, nerve, lower limb) 956.9
lower limb 956.9
multiple 956.8
specified site NEC 956.5
lumbar plexus 953.5
lumbosacral plexus 953.5
median 955.1
forearm 955.1
wrist and hand 955.1
multiple (in several parts of body) (sites not classifiable to the same three-digit category) 957.8
musculocutaneous 955.4
musculospiral 955.3
upper arm 955.3
oculomotor 951.0
olfactory 951.8
optic 950.0
pelvic girdle 956.9
multiple sites 956.8
specified site NEC 956.5
peripheral 957.9
multiple (in several regions) (sites not classifiable to the same three-digit category) 957.8
specified site NEC 957.1
peroneal 956.3
ankle and foot 956.3
lower leg 956.3

Injury *(Continued)*
nerve *(Continued)*
plantar 956.5
plexus 957.9
celiac 954.1
mesenteric, inferior 954.1
spinal 953.9
brachial 953.4
lumbosacral 953.5
multiple sites 953.8
sympathetic NEC 954.1
pneumogastric 951.8
radial 955.3
wrist and hand 955.3
sacral plexus 953.5
sciatic 956.0
thigh 956.0
shoulder girdle 955.9
multiple 955.8
specified site NEC 955.7
specified site NEC 957.1
spinal 953.9
plexus - *see* Injury, nerve, plexus, spinal
root 953.9
cervical 953.0
dorsal 953.1
lumbar 953.2
multiple sites 953.8
sacral 953.3
splanchnic 954.1
sympathetic NEC 954.1
cervical 954.0
thigh 956.9
tibial 956.5
ankle and foot 956.2
lower leg 956.5
posterior 956.2
toe 956.9
trigeminal 951.2
trochlear 951.1
trunk, excluding shoulder and pelvic girdles 954.9
specified site NEC 954.8
sympathetic NEC 954.1
ulnar 955.2
forearm 955.2
wrist (and hand) 955.2
upper limb 955.9
multiple 955.8
specified site NEC 955.7
vagus 951.8
wrist and hand 955.9
nervous system, diffuse 957.8
nose (septum) 959.09
obstetrical NEC 665.9
affecting fetus or newborn 763.89
occipital (region) (scalp) 959.09
lobe (*see also* Injury, intracranial) 854.0
optic 950.9
chiasm 950.1
cortex 950.3
nerve 950.0
pathways 950.2
orbit, orbital (region) 921.2
penetrating 870.3
with foreign body 870.4
ovary - *see* Injury, internal, ovary
paint-gun - *see* Wound, open, by site, complicated
palate (soft) 959.09
pancreas - *see* Injury, internal, pancreas

Injury *(Continued)*
parathyroid (gland) 959.09
parietal (region) (scalp) 959.09
lobe - *see* Injury, intracranial
pelvic
floor 959.19
complicating delivery 664.1
affecting fetus or newborn 763.89
joint or ligament, complicating delivery 665.6
affecting fetus or newborn 763.89
organs - *see also* Injury, internal, pelvis
with
abortion - *see* Abortion, by type, with damage to pelvic organs
ectopic pregnancy (*see also* categories 633.0–633.9) 639.2
molar pregnancy (*see also* categories 633.0–633.9) 639.2
following
abortion 639.2
ectopic or molar pregnancy 639.2
obstetrical trauma 665.5
affecting fetus or newborn 763.89
pelvis 959.19
penis 959.14
fracture of corpus cavernosum 959.13
perineum 959.14
peritoneum - *see* Injury, internal, peritoneum
periurethral tissue
with
abortion - *see* Abortion, by type, with damage to pelvic organs
ectopic pregnancy (*see also* categories 633.0–633.9) 639.2
molar pregnancy (*see also* categories 630–632) 639.2
complicating delivery 665.5
affecting fetus or newborn 763.89
following
abortion 639.2
ectopic or molar pregnancy 639.2
phalanges
foot 959.7
hand 959.5
pharynx 959.09
pleura - *see* Injury, internal, pleura
popliteal space 959.7
post-cardiac surgery (syndrome) 429.4 ◀
prepuce 959.14
prostate - *see* Injury, internal, prostate
pubic region 959.19
pudenda 959.14
radiation NEC 990
radioactive substance or radium NEC 990
rectovaginal septum 959.14
rectum - *see* Injury, internal, rectum
retina 921.3
penetrating - *see* Injury, eyeball, penetrating
retroperitoneal - *see* Injury, internal, retroperitoneum
roentgen rays NEC 990
round ligament - *see* Injury, internal, round ligament
sacral (region) 959.19
plexus 953.5
sacroiliac ligament NEC 959.19
sacrum 959.19
salivary ducts or glands 959.09

Injury *(Continued)*
- scalp 959.09
  - due to birth trauma 767.19
  - fetus or newborn 767.19
- scapular region 959.2
- sclera 921.3
  - penetrating - *see* Injury, eyeball, penetrating
  - superficial 918.2
- scrotum 959.14
- seminal vesicle - *see* Injury, internal, seminal vesicle
- shoulder (and upper arm) 959.2
- sinus
  - cavernous (*see also* Injury, intracranial) 854.0
  - nasal 959.09
- skeleton NEC, birth injury 767.3
- skin NEC 959.9
- skull - *see* Fracture, skull, by site
- soft tissue (of external sites) (severe) - *see* Wound, open, by site
- specified site NEC 959.8
- spermatic cord - *see* Injury, internal, spermatic cord
- spinal (cord) 952.9
  - with fracture, vertebra - *see* Fracture, vertebra, by site, with spinal cord injury
  - cervical (C_1–C_4) 952.00
    - with
      - anterior cord syndrome 952.02
      - central cord syndrome 952.03
      - complete lesion of cord 952.01
      - incomplete lesion NEC 952.04
      - posterior cord syndrome 952.04
    - C_5–C_7 level 952.05
      - with
        - anterior cord syndrome 952.07
        - central cord syndrome 952.08
        - complete lesion of cord 952.06
        - incomplete lesion NEC 952.09
        - posterior cord syndrome 952.09
      - specified type NEC 952.09
    - specified type NEC 952.04
  - dorsal (D_1–D_6) (T_1–T_6) (thoracic) 952.10
    - with
      - anterior cord syndrome 952.12
      - central cord syndrome 952.13
      - complete lesion of cord 952.11
      - incomplete lesion NEC 952.14
      - posterior cord syndrome 952.14
    - D_7–D_{12} level (T_7–T_{12}) 952.15
      - with
        - anterior cord syndrome 952.17
        - central cord syndrome 952.18
        - complete lesion of cord 952.16
        - incomplete lesion NEC 952.19
        - posterior cord syndrome 952.19
      - specified type NEC 952.19
    - specified type NEC 952.14
  - lumbar 952.2
  - multiple sites 952.8
  - nerve (root) NEC - *see* Injury, nerve, spinal, root
  - plexus 953.9
    - brachial 953.4
    - lumbosacral 953.5
    - multiple sites 953.8
  - sacral 952.3
  - thoracic (*see also* Injury, spinal, dorsal) 952.10

Injury *(Continued)*
- spleen - *see* Injury, internal, spleen
- stellate ganglion 954.1
- sternal region 959.11
- stomach - *see* Injury, internal, stomach
- subconjunctival 921.1
- subcutaneous 959.9
- subdural - *see* Injury, intracranial
- submaxillary region 959.09
- submental region 959.09
- subungual
  - fingers 959.5
  - toes 959.7
- superficial 919

> Note Use the following fourth-digit subdivisions with categories 910–919:
>
> 0 abrasion or friction burn without mention of infection
> 1 abrasion or friction burn, infected
> 2 blister without mention of infection
> 3 blister, infected
> 4 insect bite, nonvenomous, without mention of infection
> 5 insect bite, nonvenomous, infected
> 6 superficial foreign body (splinter) without major open wound and without mention of infection
> 7 superficial foreign body (splinter) without major open wound, infected
> 8 other and unspecified superficial injury without mention of infection
> 9 other and unspecified superficial injury, infected
>
> For late effects of superficial injury, *see* category 906.2.

  - abdomen, abdominal (muscle) (wall) (and other part(s) of trunk) 911
  - ankle (and hip, knee, leg, or thigh) 916
  - anus (and other part(s) of trunk) 911
  - arm 913
    - upper (and shoulder) 912
  - auditory canal (external) (meatus) (and other part(s) of face, neck, or scalp, except eye) 910
  - axilla (and upper arm) 912
  - back (and other part(s) of trunk) 911
  - breast (and other part(s) of trunk) 911
  - brow (and other part(s) of face, neck, or scalp, except eye) 910
  - buttock (and other part(s) of trunk) 911
  - canthus, eye 918.0
  - cheek(s) (and other part(s) of face, neck, or scalp, except eye) 910
  - chest wall (and other part(s) of trunk) 911
  - chin (and other part(s) of face, neck, or scalp, except eye) 910
  - clitoris (and other part(s) of trunk) 911
  - conjunctiva 918.2
  - cornea 918.1
    - due to contact lens 371.82

Injury *(Continued)*
- superficial *(Continued)*
  - costal region (and other part(s) of trunk) 911
  - ear(s) (auricle) (canal) (drum) (external) (and other part(s) of face, neck, or scalp, except eye) 910
  - elbow (and forearm) (and wrist) 913
  - epididymis (and other part(s) of trunk) 911
  - epigastric region (and other part(s) of trunk) 911
  - epiglottis (and other part(s) of face, neck, or scalp, except eye) 910
  - eye(s) (and adnexa) NEC 918.9
  - eyelid(s) (and periocular area) 918.0
  - face (any part(s), except eye) (and neck or scalp) 910
  - finger(s) (nail) (any) 915
  - flank (and other part(s) of trunk) 911
  - foot (phalanges) (and toe(s)) 917
  - forearm (and elbow) (and wrist) 913
  - forehead (and other part(s) of face, neck, or scalp, except eye) 910
  - globe (eye) 918.9
  - groin (and other part(s) of trunk) 911
  - gum(s) (and other part(s) of face, neck, or scalp, except eye) 910
  - hand(s) (except fingers alone) 914
  - head (and other part(s) of face, neck, or scalp, except eye) 910
  - heel (and foot or toe) 917
  - hip (and ankle, knee, leg, or thigh) 916
  - iliac region (and other part(s) of trunk) 911
  - interscapular region (and other part(s) of trunk) 911
  - iris 918.9
  - knee (and ankle, hip, leg, or thigh) 916
  - labium (majus) (minus) (and other part(s) of trunk) 911
  - lacrimal (apparatus) (gland) (sac) 918.0
  - leg (lower) (upper) (and ankle, hip, knee, or thigh) 916
  - lip(s) (and other part(s) of face, neck, or scalp, except eye) 910
  - lower extremity (except foot) 916
  - lumbar region (and other part(s) of trunk) 911
  - malar region (and other part(s) of face, neck, or scalp, except eye) 910
  - mastoid region (and other part(s) of face, neck, or scalp, except eye) 910
  - midthoracic region (and other part(s) of trunk) 911
  - mouth (and other part(s) of face, neck, or scalp, except eye) 910
  - multiple sites (not classifiable to the same three-digit category) 919
  - nasal (septum) (and other part(s) of face, neck, or scalp, except eye) 910

Injury *(Continued)*
superficial *(Continued)*
neck (and face or scalp, any part(s), except eye) 910
nose (septum) (and other part(s) of face, neck, or scalp, except eye) 910
occipital region (and other part(s) of face, neck, or scalp, except eye) 910
orbital region 918.0
palate (soft) (and other part(s) of face, neck, or scalp, except eye) 910
parietal region (and other part(s) of face, neck, or scalp, except eye) 910
penis (and other part(s) of trunk) 911
perineum (and other part(s) of trunk) 911
periocular area 918.0
pharynx (and other part(s) of face, neck, or scalp, except eye) 910
popliteal space (and ankle, hip, leg, or thigh) 916
prepuce (and other part(s) of trunk) 911
pubic region (and other part(s) of trunk) 911
pudenda (and other part(s) of trunk) 911
sacral region (and other part(s) of trunk) 911
salivary (ducts) (glands) (and other part(s) of face, neck, or scalp, except eye) 910
scalp (and other part(s) of face or neck, except eye) 910
scapular region (and upper arm) 912
sclera 918.2
scrotum (and other part(s) of trunk) 911
shoulder (and upper arm) 912
skin NEC 919
specified site(s) NEC 919
sternal region (and other part(s) of trunk) 911
subconjunctival 918.2
subcutaneous NEC 919
submaxillary region (and other part(s) of face, neck, or scalp, except eye) 910
submental region (and other part(s) of face, neck, or scalp, except eye) 910
supraclavicular fossa (and other part(s) of face, neck, or scalp, except eye) 910
supraorbital 918.0
temple (and other part(s) of face, neck, or scalp, except eye) 910
temporal region (and other part(s) of face, neck, or scalp, except eye) 910
testis (and other part(s) of trunk) 911
thigh (and ankle, hip, knee, or leg) 916
thorax, thoracic (external) (and other part(s) of trunk) 911
throat (and other part(s) of face, neck, or scalp, except eye) 910
thumb(s) (nail) 915
toe(s) (nail) (subungual) (and foot) 917
tongue (and other part(s) of face, neck, or scalp, except eye) 910

Injury *(Continued)*
superficial *(Continued)*
tooth, teeth (*see also* Abrasion, dental) 521.20
trunk (any part(s)) 911
tunica vaginalis (and other part(s) of trunk) 911
tympanum, tympanic membrane (and other part(s) of face, neck, or scalp, except eye) 910
upper extremity NEC 913
uvula (and other part(s) of face, neck, or scalp, except eye) 910
vagina (and other part(s) of trunk) 911
vulva (and other part(s) of trunk) 911
wrist (and elbow) (and forearm) 913
supraclavicular fossa 959.19
supraorbital 959.09
surgical complication (external or internal site) 998.2
symphysis pubis 959.19
complicating delivery 665.6
affecting fetus or newborn 763.89
temple 959.09
temporal region 959.09
testis 959.14
thigh (and hip) 959.6
thorax, thoracic (external) 959.11
cavity - *see* Injury, internal, thorax
internal - *see* Injury, internal, intrathoracic organs
throat 959.09
thumb(s) (nail) 959.5
thymus - *see* Injury, internal, thymus
thyroid (gland) 959.09
toe (nail) (any) 959.7
tongue 959.09
tonsil 959.09
tooth NEC 873.63
complicated 873.73
trachea - *see* Injury, internal, trachea
trunk 959.19
tunica vaginalis 959.14
tympanum, tympanic membrane 959.09
ultraviolet rays NEC 990
ureter - *see* Injury, internal, ureter
urethra (sphincter) - *see* Injury, internal, urethra
uterus - *see* Injury, internal, uterus
uvula 959.09
vagina 959.14
vascular - *see* Injury, blood vessel
vas deferens - *see* Injury, internal, vas deferens
vein (*see also* Injury, blood vessel, by site) 904.9
vena cava
inferior 902.10
superior 901.2
vesical (sphincter) - *see* Injury, internal, vesical
viscera (abdominal) - *see* Injury, internal, viscera
with fracture, pelvis - *see* Fracture, pelvis
visual 950.9
cortex 950.3
vitreous (humor) 871.2
vulva 959.14
whiplash (cervical spine) 847.0
wringer - *see* Crush, by site
wrist (and elbow) (and forearm) 959.3
x-ray NEC 990

Inoculation - *see also* Vaccination
complication or reaction - *see* Complication, vaccination
Insanity, insane (*see also* Psychosis) 298.9
adolescent (*see also* Schizophrenia) 295.9
alternating (*see also* Psychosis, affective, circular) 296.7
confusional 298.9
acute 293.0
subacute 293.1
delusional 298.9
paralysis, general 094.1
progressive 094.1
paresis, general 094.1
senile 290.20
Insect
bite - *see* Injury, superficial, by site
venomous, poisoning by 989.5
Insemination, artificial V26.1
Insensitivity
androgen 259.5
partial 259.5
Insertion
cord (umbilical) lateral or velamentous 663.8
affecting fetus or newborn 762.6
intrauterine contraceptive device V25.1
placenta, vicious - *see* Placenta, previa
subdermal implantable contraceptive V25.5
velamentous, umbilical cord 663.8
affecting fetus or newborn 762.6
Insolation 992.0
meaning sunstroke 992.0
Insomnia, unspecified 780.52
with sleep apnea, unspecified 780.51
adjustment 307.41
alcohol induced 291.82
behavioral, of childhood V69.5
drug induced 292.85
due to
medical condition classified elsewhere 327.01
mental disorder 327.02
idiopathic 307.42
nonorganic origin 307.41
persistent (primary) 307.42
transient 307.41
organic 327.00
other 327.09
paradoxical 307.42
primary 307.42
psychophysiological 307.42
subjective complaint 307.49
Inspiration
food or foreign body (*see also* Asphyxia, food or foreign body) 933.1
mucus (*see also* Asphyxia, mucus) 933.1
Inspissated bile syndrome, newborn 774.4
Instability
detrusor 596.59
emotional (excessive) 301.3
joint (posttraumatic) 718.80
ankle 718.87
elbow 718.82
foot 718.87
hand 718.84
hip 718.85
knee 718.86
lumbosacral 724.6
multiple sites 718.89
pelvic region 718.85
sacroiliac 724.6

Instability *(Continued)*
joint *(Continued)*
shoulder (region) 718.81
specified site NEC 718.88
wrist 718.83
lumbosacral 724.6
nervous 301.89
personality (emotional) 301.59
thyroid, paroxysmal 242.9
urethral 599.83
vasomotor 780.2
Insufficiency, insufficient
accommodation 367.4
adrenal (gland) (acute) (chronic) 255.4
medulla 255.5
primary 255.4
specified site NEC 255.5
adrenocortical 255.4
anterior (occlusal) guidance 524.54
anus 569.49
aortic (valve) 424.1
with
mitral (valve) disease 396.1
insufficiency, incompetence, or regurgitation 396.3
stenosis or obstruction 396.1
stenosis or obstruction 424.1
with mitral (valve) disease 396.8
congenital 746.4
rheumatic 395.1
with
mitral (valve) disease 396.1
insufficiency, incompetence, or regurgitation 396.3
stenosis or obstruction 396.1
stenosis or obstruction 395.2
with mitral (valve) disease 396.8
specified cause NEC 424.1
syphilitic 093.22
arterial 447.1
basilar artery 435.0
carotid artery 435.8
cerebral 437.1
coronary (acute or subacute) 411.89
mesenteric 557.1
peripheral 443.9
precerebral 435.9
vertebral artery 435.1
vertebrobasilar 435.3
arteriovenous 459.9
basilar artery 435.0
biliary 575.8
cardiac (*see also* Insufficiency, myocardial) 428.0
complicating surgery 997.1
due to presence of (cardiac) prosthesis 429.4
postoperative 997.1
long-term effect of cardiac surgery 429.4
specified during or due to a procedure 997.1
long-term effect of cardiac surgery 429.4
cardiorenal (*see also* Hypertension, cardiorenal) 404.90
cardiovascular (*see also* Disease, cardiovascular) 429.2
renal (*see also* Hypertension, cardiorenal) 404.90
carotid artery 435.8

Insufficiency, insufficient *(Continued)*
cerebral (vascular) 437.9
cerebrovascular 437.9
with transient focal neurological signs and symptoms 435.9
acute 437.1
with transient focal neurological signs and symptoms 435.9
circulatory NEC 459.9
fetus or newborn 779.89
convergence 378.83
coronary (acute or subacute) 411.89
chronic or with a stated duration of over 8 weeks 414.8
corticoadrenal 255.4
dietary 269.9
divergence 378.85
food 994.2
gastroesophageal 530.89
gonadal
ovary 256.39
testis 257.2
gonadotropic hormone secretion 253.4
heart - *see also* Insufficiency, myocardial
fetus or newborn 779.89
valve (*see also* Endocarditis) 424.90
congenital NEC 746.89
hepatic 573.8
idiopathic autonomic 333.0
interocclusal distance of teeth (ridge) 524.36
kidney
acute 593.9
chronic 585.9
labyrinth, labyrinthine (function) 386.53
bilateral 386.54
unilateral 386.53
lacrimal 375.15
liver 573.8
lung (acute) (*see also* Insufficiency, pulmonary) 518.82
following trauma, surgery, or shock 518.5
newborn 770.89
mental (congenital) (*see also* Retardation, mental) 319
mesenteric 557.1
mitral (valve) 424.0
with
aortic (valve) disease 396.3
insufficiency, incompetence, or regurgitation 396.3
stenosis or obstruction 396.2
obstruction or stenosis 394.2
with aortic valve disease 396.8
congenital 746.6
rheumatic 394.1
with
aortic (valve) disease 396.3
insufficiency, incompetence, or regurgitation 396.3
stenosis or obstruction 396.2
obstruction or stenosis 394.2
with aortic valve disease 396.8
active or acute 391.1
with chorea, rheumatic (Sydenham's) 392.0
specified cause, except rheumatic 424.0
muscle
heart - *see* Insufficiency, myocardial
ocular (*see also* Strabismus) 378.9

Insufficiency, insufficient *(Continued)*
myocardial, myocardium (with arteriosclerosis) 428.0
with rheumatic fever (conditions classifiable to 390)
active, acute, or subacute 391.2
with chorea 392.0
inactive or quiescent (with chorea) 398.0
congenital 746.89
due to presence of (cardiac) prosthesis 429.4
fetus or newborn 779.89
following cardiac surgery 429.4
hypertensive (*see also* Hypertension, heart) 402.91
benign 402.11
malignant 402.01
postoperative 997.1
long-term effect of cardiac surgery 429.4
rheumatic 398.0
active, acute, or subacute 391.2
with chorea (Sydenham's) 392.0
syphilitic 093.82
nourishment 994.2
organic 799.89
ovary 256.39
postablative 256.2
pancreatic 577.8
parathyroid (gland) 252.1
peripheral vascular (arterial) 443.9
pituitary (anterior) 253.2
posterior 253.5
placental - *see* Placenta, insufficiency
platelets 287.5
prenatal care in current pregnancy V23.7
progressive pluriglandular 258.9
pseudocholinesterase 289.89
pulmonary (acute) 518.82
following
shock 518.5
surgery 518.5
trauma 518.5
newborn 770.89
valve (*see also* Endocarditis, pulmonary) 424.3
congenital 746.09
pyloric 537.0
renal 593.9
acute 593.9
chronic 585.9
due to a procedure 997.5
respiratory 786.09
acute 518.82
following shock, surgery, or trauma 518.5
newborn 770.89
rotation - *see* Malrotation
suprarenal 255.4
medulla 255.5
tarso-orbital fascia, congenital 743.66
tear film 375.15
testis 257.2
thyroid (gland) (acquired) - *see also* Hypothyroidism
congenital 243
tricuspid (*see also* Endocarditis, tricuspid) 397.0
congenital 746.89
syphilitic 093.23
urethral sphincter 599.84
valve, valvular (heart) (*see also* Endocarditis) 424.90

ICD-9-CM I Vol. 2

Insufficiency, insufficient *(Continued)*
vascular 459.9
intestine NEC 557.9
mesenteric 557.1
peripheral 443.9
renal (*see also* Hypertension, kidney) 403.90
velopharyngeal
acquired 528.9
congenital 750.29
venous (peripheral) 459.81
ventricular - *see* Insufficiency, myocardial
vertebral artery 435.1
vertebrobasilar artery 435.3
weight gain during pregnancy 646.8
zinc 269.3
Insufflation
fallopian
fertility testing V26.21
following sterilization reversal V26.22
meconium 770.11
with respiratory symptoms 770.12
Insular - *see* condition
Insulinoma (M8151/0)
malignant (M8151/3)
pancreas 157.4
specified site - *see* Neoplasm, by site, malignant
unspecified site 157.4
pancreas 211.7
specified site - *see* Neoplasm, by site, benign
unspecified site 211.7
Insuloma - *see* Insulinoma
Insult
brain 437.9
acute 436
cerebral 437.9
acute 436
cerebrovascular 437.9
acute 436
vascular NEC 437.9
acute 436
Insurance examination (certification) V70.3
Intemperance (*see also* Alcoholism) 303.9
Interception of pregnancy (menstrual extraction) V25.3
Interference ◀
balancing side 524.56 ◀
non-working side 524.56 ◀
Intermenstrual
bleeding 626.6
irregular 626.6
regular 626.5
hemorrhage 626.6
irregular 626.6
regular 626.5
pain(s) 625.2
Intermittent - *see* condition
Internal - *see* condition
Interproximal wear 521.10
Interruption
aortic arch 747.11
bundle of His 426.50
fallopian tube (for sterilization) V25.2
phase-shift, sleep cycle 307.45
repeated REM-sleep 307.48
sleep
due to perceived environmental disturbances 307.48
phase-shift, of 24-hour sleep-wake cycle 307.45
repeated REM-sleep type 307.48
vas deferens (for sterilization) V25.2
Intersexuality 752.7
Interstitial - *see* condition
Intertrigo 695.89
labialis 528.5
Intervertebral disc - *see* condition
Intestine, intestinal - *see also* condition
flu 487.8
Intolerance
carbohydrate NEC 579.8
cardiovascular exercise, with pain (at rest) (with less than ordinary activity) (with ordinary activity) V47.2
cold 780.99
dissacharide (hereditary) 271.3
drug
correct substance properly administered 995.27 ⬅
wrong substance given or taken in error 977.9
specified drug - *see* Table of Drugs and Chemicals
effort 306.2
fat NEC 579.8
foods NEC 579.8
fructose (hereditary) 271.2
glucose (-galactose) (congenital) 271.3
gluten 579.0
lactose (hereditary) (infantile) 271.3
lysine (congenital) 270.7
milk NEC 579.8
protein (familial) 270.7
starch NEC 579.8
sucrose (-isomaltose) (congenital) 271.3
Intoxicated NEC (*see also* Alcoholism) 305.0
Intoxication
acid 276.2
acute
alcoholic 305.0
with alcoholism 303.0
hangover effects 305.0
caffeine 305.9
hallucinogenic (*see also* Abuse, drugs, nondependent) 305.3
alcohol (acute) 305.0
with alcoholism 303.0
hangover effects 305.0
idiosyncratic 291.4
pathological 291.4
alimentary canal 558.2
ammonia (hepatic) 572.2
caffeine 305.9
chemical - *see also* Table of Drugs and Chemicals
via placenta or breast milk 760.70
alcohol 760.71
anticonvulsants 760.77
antifungals 760.74
anti-infective agents 760.74
antimetabolics 760.78
cocaine 760.75
"crack" 760.75
hallucinogenic agents NEC 760.73
medicinal agents NEC 760.79
narcotics 760.72
obstetric anesthetic or analgesic drug 763.5
specified agent NEC 760.79
suspected, affecting management of pregnancy 655.5
cocaine, through placenta or breast milk 760.75
delirium
alcohol 291.0
drug 292.81
Intoxication *(Continued)*
drug 292.89
with delirium 292.81
correct substance properly administered (*see also* Allergy, drug) 995.27 ⬅
newborn 779.4
obstetric anesthetic or sedation 668.9
affecting fetus or newborn 763.5
overdose or wrong substance given or taken - *see* Table of Drugs and Chemicals
pathologic 292.2
specific to newborn 779.4
via placenta or breast milk 760.70
alcohol 760.71
anticonvulsants 760.77
antifungals 760.74
anti-infective agents 760.74
antimetabolics 760.78
cocaine 760.75
"crack" 760.75
hallucinogenic agents 760.73
medicinal agents NEC 760.79
narcotics 760.72
obstetric anesthetic or analgesic drug 763.5
specified agent NEC 760.79
suspected, affecting management of pregnancy 655.5
enteric - *see* Intoxication, intestinal
fetus or newborn, via placenta or breast milk 760.70
alcohol 760.71
anticonvulsants 760.77
antifungals 760.74
anti-infective agents 760.74
antimetabolics 760.78
cocaine 760.75
"crack" 760.75
hallucinogenic agents 760.73
medicinal agents NEC 760.79
narcotics 760.72
obstetric anesthetic or analgesic drug 763.5
specified agent NEC 760.79
suspected, affecting management of pregnancy 655.5
food - *see* Poisoning, food
gastrointestinal 558.2
hallucinogenic (acute) 305.3
hepatocerebral 572.2
idiosyncratic alcohol 291.4
intestinal 569.89
due to putrefaction of food 005.9
methyl alcohol (*see also* Alcoholism) 305.0
with alcoholism 303.0
pathologic 291.4
drug 292.2
potassium (K) 276.7
septic
with
abortion - *see* Abortion, by type, with sepsis
ectopic pregnancy (*see also* categories 633.0–633.9) 639.0
molar pregnancy (*see also* categories 630–632) 639.0
during labor 659.3
following
abortion 639.0
ectopic or molar pregnancy 639.0
generalized - *see* Septicemia

- **Intoxication** *(Continued)*
  - septic *(Continued)*
    - puerperal, postpartum, childbirth 670
  - serum (prophylactic) (therapeutic) 999.5
  - uremic - *see* Uremia
  - water 276.6
- **Intracranial** - *see* condition
- **Intrahepatic gallbladder** 751.69
- **Intraligamentous** - *see also* condition
  - pregnancy - *see* Pregnancy, cornual
- **Intraocular** - *see also* condition
  - sepsis 360.00
- **Intrathoracic** - *see also* condition
  - kidney 753.3
  - stomach - *see* Hernia, diaphragm
- **Intrauterine contraceptive device**
  - checking V25.42
  - insertion V25.1
  - in situ V45.51
  - management V25.42
  - prescription V25.02
    - repeat V25.42
  - reinsertion V25.42
  - removal V25.42
- **Intraventricular** - *see* condition
- **Intrinsic deformity** - *see* Deformity
- **Intruded tooth** 524.34 ◀
- **Intrusion, repetitive, of sleep** (due to environmental disturbances) (with atypical polysomnographic features) 307.48
- **Intumescent, lens** (eye) NEC 366.9
  - senile 366.12
- **Intussusception** (colon) (enteric) (intestine) (rectum) 560.0
  - appendix 543.9
  - congenital 751.5
  - fallopian tube 620.8
  - ileocecal 560.0
  - ileocolic 560.0
  - ureter (obstruction) 593.4
- **Invagination**
  - basilar 756.0
  - colon or intestine 560.0
- **Invalid** (since birth) 799.89
- **Invalidism** (chronic) 799.89
- **Inversion**
  - albumin-globulin (A-G) ratio 273.8
  - bladder 596.8
  - cecum (*see also* Intussusception) 560.0
  - cervix 622.8
  - nipple 611.79
    - congenital 757.6
    - puerperal, postpartum 676.3
  - optic papilla 743.57
  - organ or site, congenital NEC - *see* Anomaly, specified type NEC
  - sleep rhythm 327.39
    - nonorganic origin 307.45
  - testis (congenital) 752.51
  - uterus (postinfectional) (postpartal, old) 621.7
    - chronic 621.7
    - complicating delivery 665.2
      - affecting fetus or newborn 763.89
  - vagina - *see* Prolapse, vagina
- **Investigation**
  - allergens V72.7
  - clinical research (control) (normal comparison) (participant) V70.7
- **Inviability** - *see* Immaturity
- **Involuntary movement, abnormal** 781.0
- **Involution, involutional** - *see also* condition
  - breast, cystic or fibrocystic 610.1
- **Involution, involutional** *(Continued)*
  - depression (*see also* Psychosis, affective) 296.2
    - recurrent episode 296.3
    - single episode 296.2
  - melancholia (*see also* Psychosis, affective) 296.2
    - recurrent episode 296.3
    - single episode 296.2
  - ovary, senile 620.3
  - paranoid state (reaction) 297.2
  - paraphrenia (climacteric) (menopause) 297.2
  - psychosis 298.8
  - thymus failure 254.8
- **IQ**
  - under 20 318.2
  - 20–34 318.1
  - 35–49 318.0
  - 50–70 317
- **IRDS** 769
- **Irideremia** 743.45
- **Iridis rubeosis** 364.42
  - diabetic 250.5 *[364.42]*
- **Iridochoroiditis** (panuveitis) 360.12
- **Iridocyclitis NEC** 364.3
  - acute 364.00
    - primary 364.01
    - recurrent 364.02
  - chronic 364.10
    - in
      - lepromatous leprosy 030.0 *[364.11]*
      - sarcoidosis 135 *[364.11]*
      - tuberculosis (*see also* Tuberculosis) 017.3 *[364.11]*
  - due to allergy 364.04
  - endogenous 364.01
  - gonococcal 098.41
  - granulomatous 364.10
  - herpetic (simplex) 054.44
    - zoster 053.22
  - hypopyon 364.05
  - lens induced 364.23
  - nongranulomatous 364.00
  - primary 364.01
  - recurrent 364.02
  - rheumatic 364.10
  - secondary 364.04
    - infectious 364.03
    - noninfectious 364.04
  - subacute 364.00
    - primary 364.01
    - recurrent 364.02
  - sympathetic 360.11
  - syphilitic (secondary) 091.52
  - tuberculous (chronic) (*see also* Tuberculosis) 017.3 *[364.11]*
- **Iridocyclochoroiditis** (panuveitis) 360.12
- **Iridodialysis** 364.76
- **Iridodonesis** 364.8
- **Iridoplegia** (complete) (partial) (reflex) 379.49
- **Iridoschisis** 364.52
- **Iris** - *see* condition
- **Iritis** 364.3
  - acute 364.00
    - primary 364.01
    - recurrent 364.02
  - chronic 364.10
    - in
      - sarcoidosis 135 *[364.11]*
      - tuberculosis (*see also* Tuberculosis) 017.3 *[364.11]*
- **Iritis** *(Continued)*
  - diabetic 250.5 *[364.42]*
  - due to
    - allergy 364.04
    - herpes simplex 054.44
    - leprosy 030.0 *[364.11]*
  - endogenous 364.01
  - gonococcal 098.41
  - gouty 274.89 *[364.11]*
  - granulomatous 364.10
  - hypopyon 364.05
  - lens induced 364.23
  - nongranulomatous 364.00
  - papulosa 095.8 *[364.11]*
  - primary 364.01
  - recurrent 364.02
  - rheumatic 364.10
  - secondary 364.04
    - infectious 364.03
    - noninfectious 364.04
  - subacute 364.00
    - primary 364.01
    - recurrent 364.02
  - sympathetic 360.11
  - syphilitic (secondary) 091.52
    - congenital 090.0 *[364.11]*
    - late 095.8 *[364.11]*
  - tuberculous (*see also* Tuberculosis) 017.3 *[364.11]*
  - uratic 274.89 *[364.11]*
- **Iron**
  - deficiency anemia 280.9
  - metabolism disease 275.0
  - storage disease 275.0
- **Iron-miners' lung** 503
- **Irradiated enamel** (tooth, teeth) 521.89 ⟸
- **Irradiation**
  - burn - *see* Burn, by site
  - effects, adverse 990
- **Irreducible, irreducibility** - *see* condition
- **Irregular, irregularity**
  - action, heart 427.9
  - alveolar process 525.8
  - bleeding NEC 626.4
  - breathing 786.09
  - colon 569.89
  - contour of cornea 743.41
    - acquired 371.70
  - dentin in pulp 522.3
  - eye movements NEC 379.59
  - menstruation (cause unknown) 626.4
  - periods 626.4
  - prostate 602.9
  - pupil 364.75
  - respiratory 786.09
  - septum (nasal) 470
  - shape, organ or site, congenital NEC - *see* Distortion
  - sleep-wake rhythm (non-24-hour) 327.39
    - nonorganic origin 307.45
  - vertebra 733.99
- **Irritability** (nervous) 799.2
  - bladder 596.8
    - neurogenic 596.54
      - with cauda equina syndrome 344.61
  - bowel (syndrome) 564.1
  - bronchial (*see also* Bronchitis) 490
  - cerebral, newborn 779.1
  - colon 564.1
    - psychogenic 306.4
  - duodenum 564.89
  - heart (psychogenic) 306.2
  - ileum 564.89
  - jejunum 564.89

Irritability *(Continued)*
myocardium 306.2
rectum 564.89
stomach 536.9
psychogenic 306.4
sympathetic (nervous system) (*see also* Neuropathy, peripheral, autonomic) 337.9
urethra 599.84
ventricular (heart) (psychogenic) 306.2
Irritable - *see* Irritability
Irritation
anus 569.49
axillary nerve 353.0
bladder 596.8
brachial plexus 353.0
brain (traumatic) (*see also* Injury, intracranial) 854.0
nontraumatic - *see* Encephalitis
bronchial (*see also* Bronchitis) 490
cerebral (traumatic) (*see also* Injury, intracranial) 854.0
nontraumatic - *see* Encephalitis
cervical plexus 353.2
cervix (*see also* Cervicitis) 616.0
choroid, sympathetic 360.11
cranial nerve - *see* Disorder, nerve, cranial
digestive tract 536.9
psychogenic 306.4
gastric 536.9
psychogenic 306.4
gastrointestinal (tract) 536.9
functional 536.9
psychogenic 306.4
globe, sympathetic 360.11
intestinal (bowel) 564.9
labyrinth 386.50
lumbosacral plexus 353.1
meninges (traumatic) (*see also* Injury, intracranial) 854.0
nontraumatic - *see* Meningitis
myocardium 306.2
nerve - *see* Disorder, nerve
nervous 799.2
nose 478.19
penis 607.89
perineum 709.9
peripheral
autonomic nervous system (*see also* Neuropathy, peripheral, autonomic) 337.9
nerve - *see* Disorder, nerve
peritoneum (*see also* Peritonitis) 567.9
pharynx 478.29
plantar nerve 355.6
spinal (cord) (traumatic) - *see also* Injury, spinal, by site
nerve - *see also* Disorder, nerve
root NEC 724.9
traumatic - *see* Injury, nerve, spinal
nontraumatic - *see* Myelitis
stomach 536.9
psychogenic 306.4
sympathetic nerve NEC (*see also* Neuropathy, peripheral, autonomic) 337.9
ulnar nerve 354.2
vagina 623.9
Isambert's disease 012.3
Ischemia, ischemic 459.9
basilar artery (with transient neurologic deficit) 435.0
bone NEC 733.40
bowel (transient) 557.9
acute 557.0
Ischemia, ischemic *(Continued)*
bowel *(Continued)*
chronic 557.1
due to mesenteric artery insufficiency 557.1
brain - *see also* Ischemia, cerebral
recurrent focal 435.9
cardiac (*see also* Ischemia, heart) 414.9
cardiomyopathy 414.8
carotid artery (with transient neurologic deficit) 435.8
cerebral (chronic) (generalized) 437.1
arteriosclerotic 437.0
intermittent (with transient neurologic deficit) 435.9
newborn 779.2
puerperal, postpartum, childbirth 674.0
recurrent focal (with transient neurologic deficit) 435.9
transient (with transient neurologic deficit) 435.9
colon 557.9
acute 557.0
chronic 557.1
due to mesenteric artery insufficiency 557.1
coronary (chronic) (*see also* Ischemia, heart) 414.9
heart (chronic or with a stated duration of over 8 weeks) 414.9
acute or with a stated duration of 8 weeks or less (*see also* Infarct, myocardium) 410.9
without myocardial infarction 411.89
with coronary (artery) occlusion 411.81
subacute 411.89
intestine (transient) 557.9
acute 557.0
chronic 557.1
due to mesenteric artery insufficiency 557.1
kidney 593.81
labyrinth 386.50
muscles, leg 728.89
myocardium, myocardial (chronic or with a stated duration of over 8 weeks) 414.8
acute (*see also* Infarct, myocardium) 410.9
without myocardial infarction 411.89
with coronary (artery) occlusion 411.81
renal 593.81
retina, retinal 362.84
small bowel 557.9
acute 557.0
chronic 557.1
due to mesenteric artery insufficiency 557.1
spinal cord 336.1
subendocardial (*see also* Insufficiency, coronary) 411.89
vertebral artery (with transient neurologic deficit) 435.1
Ischialgia (*see also* Sciatica) 724.3
Ischiopagus 759.4
Ischium, ischial - *see* condition
Ischomenia 626.8
Ischuria 788.5
Iselin's disease or osteochondrosis 732.5
Islands of
parotid tissue in
lymph nodes 750.26
neck structures 750.26
submaxillary glands in
fascia 750.26
lymph nodes 750.26
neck muscles 750.26
Islet cell tumor, pancreas (M8150/0) 211.7
Isoimmunization NEC (*see also* Incompatibility) 656.2
fetus or newborn 773.2
ABO blood groups 773.1
rhesus (Rh) factor 773.0
Isolation V07.0
social V62.4
Isosporosis 007.2
Issue
medical certificate NEC V68.0
cause of death V68.0
fitness V68.0
incapacity V68.0
repeat prescription NEC V68.1
appliance V68.1
contraceptive V25.40
device NEC V25.49
intrauterine V25.42
specified type NEC V25.49
pill V25.41
glasses V68.1
medicinal substance V68.1
Itch (*see also* Pruritus) 698.9
bakers' 692.89
barbers' 110.0
bricklayers' 692.89
cheese 133.8
clam diggers' 120.3
coolie 126.9
copra 133.8
Cuban 050.1
dew 126.9
dhobie 110.3
eye 379.99
filarial (*see also* Infestation, filarial) 125.9
grain 133.8
grocers' 133.8
ground 126.9
harvest 133.8
jock 110.3
Malabar 110.9
beard 110.0
foot 110.4
scalp 110.0
meaning scabies 133.0
Norwegian 133.0
perianal 698.0
poultrymen's 133.8
sarcoptic 133.0
scrub 134.1
seven year V61.10
meaning scabies 133.0
straw 133.8
swimmers' 120.3
washerwoman's 692.4
water 120.3
winter 698.8
Itsenko-Cushing syndrome (pituitary basophilism) 255.0
Ivemark's syndrome (asplenia with congenital heart disease) 759.0
Ivory bones 756.52
Ixodes 134.8
Ixodiasis 134.8

J

- **Jaccoud's nodular fibrositis, chronic** (Jaccoud's syndrome) 714.4
- **Jackson's**
  - membrane 751.4
  - paralysis or syndrome 344.89
  - veil 751.4
- **Jacksonian**
  - epilepsy (*see also* Epilepsy) 345.5
  - seizures (focal) (*see also* Epilepsy) 345.5
- **Jacob's ulcer** (M8090/3) - *see* Neoplasm, skin, malignant, by site
- **Jacquet's dermatitis** (diaper dermatitis) 691.0
- **Jadassohn's**
  - blue nevus (M8780/0) - *see* Neoplasm, skin, benign
  - disease (maculopapular erythroderma) 696.2
  - intraepidermal epithelioma (M8096/0) - *see* Neoplasm, skin, benign
- **Jadassohn-Lewandowski syndrome** (pachyonychia congenita) 757.5
- **Jadassohn-Pellizari's disease** (anetoderma) 701.3
- **Jadassohn-Tièche nevus** (M8780/0) - *see* Neoplasm, skin, benign
- **Jaffe-Lichtenstein** (-Uehlinger) syndrome 252.01
- **Jahnke's syndrome** (encephalocutaneous angiomatosis) 759.6
- **Jakob-Creutzfeldt disease** (syndrome) (new variant) 046.1
  - with dementia
    - with behavioral disturbance 046.1 *[294.11]*
    - without behavioral disturbance 046.1 *[294.10]*
- **Jaksch** (-Luzet) disease or syndrome (pseudoleukemia infantum) 285.8
- **Jamaican**
  - neuropathy 349.82
  - paraplegic tropical ataxic-spastic syndrome 349.82
- **Janet's disease** (psychasthenia) 300.89
- **Janiceps** 759.4
- **Jansky-Bielschowsky amaurotic familial idiocy** 330.1
- **Japanese**
  - B-type encephalitis 062.0
  - river fever 081.2
  - seven-day fever 100.89
- **Jaundice** (yellow) 782.4
  - acholuric (familial) (splenomegalic) (*see also* Spherocytosis) 282.0
    - acquired 283.9
  - breast milk 774.39
  - catarrhal (acute) 070.1
    - with hepatic coma 070.0
    - chronic 571.9
    - epidemic - *see* Jaundice, epidemic
  - cholestatic (benign) 782.4
  - chronic idiopathic 277.4
  - epidemic (catarrhal) 070.1
    - with hepatic coma 070.0
    - leptospiral 100.0
    - spirochetal 100.0
  - febrile (acute) 070.1
    - with hepatic coma 070.0
    - leptospiral 100.0
    - spirochetal 100.0

Jaundice *(Continued)*

- fetus or newborn 774.6
  - due to or associated with
    - ABO
      - antibodies 773.1
      - incompatibility, maternal/fetal 773.1
      - isoimmunization 773.1
    - absence or deficiency of enzyme system for bilirubin conjugation (congenital) 774.39
    - blood group incompatibility NEC 773.2
    - breast milk inhibitors to conjugation 774.39
      - associated with preterm delivery 774.2
    - bruising 774.1
    - Crigler-Najjar syndrome 277.4 *[774.31]*
    - delayed conjugation 774.30
      - associated with preterm delivery 774.2
      - development 774.39
    - drugs or toxins transmitted from mother 774.1
    - G-6-PD deficiency 282.2 *[774.0]*
    - galactosemia 271.1 *[774.5]*
    - Gilbert's syndrome 277.4 *[774.31]*
    - hepatocellular damage 774.4
    - hereditary hemolytic anemia (*see also* Anemia, hemolytic) 282.9 *[774.0]*
    - hypothyroidism, congenital 243 *[774.31]*
    - incompatibility, maternal/fetal NEC 773.2
    - infection 774.1
    - inspissated bile syndrome 774.4
    - isoimmunization NEC 773.2
    - mucoviscidosis 277.01 *[774.5]*
    - obliteration of bile duct, congenital 751.61 *[774.5]*
    - polycythemia 774.1
    - preterm delivery 774.2
    - red cell defect 282.9 *[774.0]*
    - Rh
      - antibodies 773.0
      - incompatibility, maternal/fetal 773.0
      - isoimmunization 773.0
    - spherocytosis (congenital) 282.0 *[774.0]*
    - swallowed maternal blood 774.1
  - physiological NEC 774.6
- from injection, inoculation, infusion, or transfusion (blood) (plasma) (serum) (other substance) (onset within 8 months after administration) - *see* Hepatitis, viral
- Gilbert's (familial nonhemolytic) 277.4
- hematogenous 283.9
- hemolytic (acquired) 283.9
  - congenital (*see also* Spherocytosis) 282.0
- hemorrhagic (acute) 100.0
  - leptospiral 100.0
  - newborn 776.0
  - spirochetal 100.0
- hepatocellular 573.8

Jaundice *(Continued)*

- homologous (serum) - *see* Hepatitis, viral
- idiopathic, chronic 277.4
- infectious (acute) (subacute) 070.1
  - with hepatic coma 070.0
  - leptospiral 100.0
  - spirochetal 100.0
- leptospiral 100.0
- malignant (*see also* Necrosis, liver) 570
- newborn (physiological) (*see also* Jaundice, fetus or newborn) 774.6
- nonhemolytic, congenital familial (Gilbert's) 277.4
- nuclear, newborn (*see also* Kernicterus of newborn) 774.7
- obstructive NEC (*see also* Obstruction, biliary) 576.8
- postimmunization - *see* Hepatitis, viral
- posttransfusion - *see* Hepatitis, viral
- regurgitation (*see also* Obstruction, biliary) 576.8
- serum (homologous) (prophylactic) (therapeutic) - *see* Hepatitis, viral
- spirochetal (hemorrhagic) 100.0
- symptomatic 782.4
  - newborn 774.6
- **Jaw** - *see* condition
- **Jaw-blinking** 374.43
  - congenital 742.8
- **Jaw-winking phenomenon or syndrome** 742.8
- **Jealousy**
  - alcoholic 291.5
  - childhood 313.3
  - sibling 313.3
- **Jejunitis** (*see also* Enteritis) 558.9
- **Jejunostomy status** V44.4
- **Jejunum, jejunal** - *see* condition
- **Jensen's disease** 363.05
- **Jericho boil** 085.1
- **Jerks, myoclonic** 333.2
- **Jervell-Lange-Nielsen syndrome** 426.82
- **Jeune's disease or syndrome** (asphyxiating thoracic dystrophy) 756.4
- **Jigger disease** 134.1
- **Job's syndrome** (chronic granulomatous disease) 288.1
- **Jod-Basedow phenomenon** 242.8
- **Johnson-Stevens disease** (erythema multiforme exudativum) 695.1
- **Joint** - *see also* condition
  - Charcôt's 094.0 *[713.5]*
  - false 733.82
  - flail - *see* Flail, joint
  - mice - *see* Loose, body, joint, by site
  - sinus to bone 730.9
  - von Gies' 095.8
- **Jordan's anomaly or syndrome** 288.2
- **Josephs-Diamond-Blackfan anemia** (congenital hypoplastic) 284.01 ⇐
- **Joubert syndrome** 759.89
- **Jumpers' knee** 727.2
- **Jungle yellow fever** 060.0
- **Jungling's disease** (sarcoidosis) 135
- **Junin virus hemorrhagic fever** 078.7
- **Juvenile** - *see also* condition
  - delinquent 312.9
    - group (*see also* Disturbance, conduct) 312.2
    - neurotic 312.4

K

Kabuki syndrome 759.89
Kahler (-Bozzolo) disease (multiple myeloma) (M9730/3) 203.0
Kakergasia 300.9
Kakke 265.0
Kala-azar (Indian) (infantile) (Mediterranean) (Sudanese) 085.0
Kalischer's syndrome (encephalocutaneous angiomatosis) 759.6
Kallmann's syndrome (hypogonadotropic hypogonadism with anosmia) 253.4
Kanner's syndrome (autism) (*see also* Psychosis, childhood) 299.0
Kaolinosis 502
Kaposi's
disease 757.33
lichen ruber 696.4
acuminatus 696.4
moniliformis 697.8
xeroderma pigmentosum 757.33
sarcoma (M9140/3) 176.9
adipose tissue 176.1
aponeurosis 176.1
artery 176.1
blood vessel 176.1
bursa 176.1
connective tissue 176.1
external genitalia 176.8
fascia 176.1
fatty tissue 176.1
fibrous tissue 176.1
gastrointestinal tract NEC 176.3
ligament 176.1
lung 176.4
lymph
gland(s) 176.5
node(s) 176.5
lymphatic(s) NEC 176.1
muscle (skeletal) 176.1
oral cavity NEC 176.8
palate 176.2
scrotum 176.8
skin 176.0
soft tissue 176.1
specified site NEC 176.8
subcutaneous tissue 176.1
synovia 176.1
tendon (sheath) 176.1
vein 176.1
vessel 176.1
viscera NEC 176.9
vulva 176.8
varicelliform eruption 054.0
vaccinia 999.0
Kartagener's syndrome or triad (sinusitis, bronchiectasis, situs inversus) 759.3
Kasabach-Merritt syndrome (capillary hemangioma associated with thrombocytopenic purpura) 287.39
Kaschin-Beck disease (endemic polyarthritis) - *see* Disease, Kaschin-Beck
Kast's syndrome (dyschondroplasia with hemangiomas) 756.4
Katatonia- *see* Catatonia
Katayama disease or fever 120.2
Kathisophobia 781.0
Kawasaki disease 446.1
Kayser-Fleischer ring (cornea) (pseudosclerosis) 275.1 [371.14]
Kaznelson's syndrome (congenital hypoplastic anemia) 284.01 ⬅
Kearns-Sayre syndrome 277.87
Kedani fever 081.2
Kelis 701.4
Kelly (-Paterson) syndrome (sideropenic dysphagia) 280.8
Keloid, cheloid 701.4
Addison's (morphea) 701.0
cornea 371.00
Hawkins' 701.4
scar 701.4
Keloma 701.4
Kenya fever 082.1
Keratectasia 371.71
congenital 743.41
Keratinization NEC ◀
alveolar ridge mucosa ◀
excessive 528.72 ◀
minimal 528.71 ◀
Keratitis (nodular) (nonulcerative) (simple) (zonular) NEC 370.9
with ulceration (*see also* Ulcer, cornea) 370.00
actinic 370.24
arborescens 054.42
areolar 370.22
bullosa 370.8
deep - *see* Keratitis, interstitial
dendritic(a) 054.42
desiccation 370.34
diffuse interstitial 370.52
disciform(is) 054.43
varicella 052.7 *[370.44]*
epithelialis vernalis 372.13 *[370.32]*
exposure 370.34
filamentary 370.23
gonococcal (congenital) (prenatal) 098.43
herpes, herpetic (simplex) NEC 054.43
zoster 053.21
hypopyon 370.04
in
chickenpox 052.7 *[370.44]*
exanthema (*see also* Exanthem) 057.9 *[370.44]*
paravaccinia (*see also* Paravaccinia) 051.9 *[370.44]*
smallpox (*see also* Smallpox) 050.9 *[370.44]*
vernal conjunctivitis 372.13 *[370.32]*
interstitial (nonsyphilitic) 370.50
with ulcer (*see also* Ulcer, cornea) 370.00
diffuse 370.52
herpes, herpetic (simplex) 054.43
zoster 053.21
syphilitic (congenital) (hereditary) 090.3
tuberculous (*see also* Tuberculosis) 017.3 *[370.59]*
lagophthalmic 370.34
macular 370.22
neuroparalytic 370.35
neurotrophic 370.35
nummular 370.22
oyster-shuckers' 370.8
parenchymatous - *see* Keratitis, interstitial
petrificans 370.8
phlyctenular 370.31
postmeasles 055.71
punctata, punctate 370.21
leprosa 030.0 *[370.21]*
profunda 090.3
superficial (Thygeson's) 370.21
purulent 370.8
Keratitis *(Continued)*
pustuliformis profunda 090.3
rosacea 695.3 *[370.49]*
sclerosing 370.54
specified type NEC 370.8
stellate 370.22
striate 370.22
superficial 370.20
with conjunctivitis (*see also* Keratoconjunctivitis) 370.40
punctate (Thygeson's) 370.21
suppurative 370.8
syphilitic (congenital) (prenatal) 090.3
trachomatous 076.1
late effect 139.1
tuberculous (phlyctenular) (*see also* Tuberculosis) 017.3 *[370.31]*
ulcerated (*see also* Ulcer, cornea) 370.00
vesicular 370.8
welders' 370.24
xerotic (*see also* Keratomalacia) 371.45
vitamin A deficiency 264.4
Keratoacanthoma 238.2
Keratocele 371.72
Keratoconjunctivitis (*see also* Keratitis) 370.40
adenovirus type 8 077.1
epidemic 077.1
exposure 370.34
gonococcal 098.43
herpetic (simplex) 054.43
zoster 053.21
in
chickenpox 052.7 *[370.44]*
exanthema (*see also* Exanthem) 057.9 *[370.44]*
paravaccinia (*see also* Paravaccinia) 051.9 *[370.44]*
smallpox (*see also* Smallpox) 050.9 *[370.44]*
infectious 077.1
neurotrophic 370.35
phlyctenular 370.31
postmeasles 055.71
shipyard 077.1
sicca (Sjögren's syndrome) 710.2
not in Sjögren's syndrome 370.33
specified type NEC 370.49
tuberculous (phlyctenular) (*see also* Tuberculosis) 017.3 *[370.31]*
Keratoconus 371.60
acute hydrops 371.62
congenital 743.41
stable 371.61
Keratocyst (dental) 526.0
Keratoderma, keratodermia (congenital) (palmaris et plantaris) (symmetrical) 757.39
acquired 701.1
blennorrhagica 701.1
gonococcal 098.81
climacterium 701.1
eccentrica 757.39
gonorrheal 098.81
punctata 701.1
tylodes, progressive 701.1
Keratodermatocele 371.72
Keratoglobus 371.70
congenital 743.41
associated with buphthalmos 743.22
Keratohemia 371.12
Keratoiritis (*see also* Iridocyclitis) 364.3
syphilitic 090.3
tuberculous (*see also* Tuberculosis) 017.3 *[364.11]*

Keratolysis exfoliativa (congenital) 757.39
  acquired 695.89
  neonatorum 757.39
Keratoma 701.1
  congenital 757.39
  malignum congenitale 757.1
  palmaris et plantaris hereditarium 757.39
  senile 702.0
Keratomalacia 371.45
  vitamin A deficiency 264.4
Keratomegaly 743.41
Keratomycosis 111.1
  nigricans (palmaris) 111.1
Keratopathy 371.40
  band (*see also* Keratitis) 371.43
  bullous (*see also* Keratitis) 371.23
  degenerative (*see also* Degeneration, cornea) 371.40
    hereditary (*see also* Dystrophy, cornea) 371.50
  discrete colliquative 371.49
Keratoscleritis, tuberculous (*see also* Tuberculosis) 017.3 [370.31]
Keratosis 701.1
  actinic 702.0
  arsenical 692.4
  blennorrhagica 701.1
    gonococcal 098.81
  congenital (any type) 757.39
  ear (middle) (*see also* Cholesteatoma) 385.30
  female genital (external) 629.89 (Revised)
  follicular, vitamin A deficiency 264.8
  follicularis 757.39
    acquired 701.1
    congenital (acneiformis) (Siemens') 757.39
    spinulosa (decalvans) 757.39
    vitamin A deficiency 264.8
  gonococcal 098.81
  larynx, laryngeal 478.79
  male genital (external) 608.89
  middle ear (*see also* Cholesteatoma) 385.30
  nigricans 701.2
    congenital 757.39
  obturans 380.21
  oral epithelium
    residual ridge mucosa
      excessive 528.72
      minimal 528.71
  palmaris et plantaris (symmetrical) 757.39
  penile 607.89
  pharyngeus 478.29
  pilaris 757.39
    acquired 701.1
  punctata (palmaris et plantaris) 701.1
  scrotal 608.89
  seborrheic 702.19
    inflamed 702.11
  senilis 702.0
  solar 702.0
  suprafollicularis 757.39
  tonsillaris 478.29
  vagina 623.1
  vegetans 757.39
  vitamin A deficiency 264.8
Kerato-uveitis (*see also* Iridocyclitis) 364.3
Keraunoparalysis 994.0
Kerion (celsi) 110.0
Kernicterus of newborn (not due to isoimmunization) 774.7
  due to isoimmunization (conditions classifiable to 773.0–773.2) 773.4
Ketoacidosis 276.2
  diabetic 250.1
Ketonuria 791.6
  branched-chain, intermittent 270.3
Ketosis 276.2
  diabetic 250.1
Kidney - *see* condition
Kienböck's
  disease 732.3
    adult 732.8
  osteochondrosis 732.3
Kimmelstiel (-Wilson) disease or syndrome (intercapillary glomerulosclerosis) 250.4 [581.81]
Kink, kinking
  appendix 543.9
  artery 447.1
  cystic duct, congenital 751.61
  hair (acquired) 704.2
  ileum or intestine (*see also* Obstruction, intestine) 560.9
  Lane's (*see also* Obstruction, intestine) 560.9
  organ or site, congenital NEC - *see* Anomaly, specified type NEC, by site
  ureter (pelvic junction) 593.3
    congenital 753.20
  vein(s) 459.2
    caval 459.2
    peripheral 459.2
Kinnier Wilson's disease (hepatolenticular degeneration) 275.1
Kissing
  osteophytes 721.5
  spine 721.5
  vertebra 721.5
Klauder's syndrome (erythema multiforme exudativum) 695.1
Klebs' disease (*see also* Nephritis) 583.9
Klein-Waardenburg syndrome (ptosis-epicanthus) 270.2
Kleine-Levin syndrome 327.13
Kleptomania 312.32
Klinefelter's syndrome 758.7
Klinger's disease 446.4
Klippel's disease 723.8
Klippel-Feil disease or syndrome (brevicollis) 756.16
Klippel-Trenaunay syndrome 759.89
Klumpke (-Déjérine) palsy, paralysis (birth) (newborn) 767.6
Kluver-Bucy (-Terzian) syndrome 310.0
Knee - *see* condition
Knifegrinders' rot (*see also* Tuberculosis) 011.4
Knock-knee (acquired) 736.41
  congenital 755.64
Knot
  intestinal, syndrome (volvulus) 560.2
  umbilical cord (true) 663.2
    affecting fetus or newborn 762.5
Knots, surfer 919.8
  infected 919.9
Knotting (of)
  hair 704.2
  intestine 560.2
Knuckle pads (Garrod's) 728.79
Köbner's disease (epidermolysis bullosa) 757.39
Koch's
  infection (*see also* Tuberculosis, pulmonary) 011.9
  relapsing fever 087.9
Koch-Weeks conjunctivitis 372.03
Koenig-Wichman disease (pemphigus) 694.4
Köhler's disease (osteochondrosis) 732.5
  first (osteochondrosis juvenilis) 732.5
  second (Freiburg's infarction, metatarsal head) 732.5
  patellar 732.4
  tarsal navicular (bone) (osteoarthosis juvenilis) 732.5
Köhler-Mouchet disease (osteoarthrosis juvenilis) 732.5
Köhler-Pellegrini-Stieda disease or syndrome (calcification, knee joint) 726.62
Koilonychia 703.8
  congenital 757.5
Kojevnikov's, Kojewnikoff's epilepsy (*see also* Epilepsy) 345.7
König's
  disease (osteochondritis dissecans) 732.7
  syndrome 564.89
Koniophthisis (*see also* Tuberculosis) 011.4
Koplik's spots 055.9
Kopp's asthma 254.8
Korean hemorrhagic fever 078.6
Korsakoff (-Wernicke) disease, psychosis, or syndrome (nonalcoholic) 294.0
  alcoholic 291.1
Korsakov's disease - *see* Korsakoff's disease
Korsakow's disease - *see* Korsakoff's disease
Kostmann's disease or syndrome (infantile genetic agranulocytosis) 288.01 (Revised)
Krabbe's
  disease (leukodystrophy) 330.0
  syndrome
    congenital muscle hypoplasia 756.89
    cutaneocerebral angioma 759.6
Kraepelin-Morel disease (*see also* Schizophrenia) 295.9
Kraft-Weber-Dimitri disease 759.6
Kraurosis
  ani 569.49
  penis 607.0
  vagina 623.8
  vulva 624.0
Kreotoxism 005.9
Krukenberg's
  spindle 371.13
  tumor (M8490/6) 198.6
Kufs' disease 330.1
Kugelberg-Welander disease 335.11
Kuhnt-Junius degeneration or disease 362.52
Kulchitsky's cell carcinoma (carcinoid tumor of intestine) 259.2
Kummell's disease or spondylitis 721.7
Kundrat's disease (lymphosarcoma) 200.1
Kunekune - *see* Dermatophytosis
Kunkel syndrome (lupoid hepatitis) 571.49

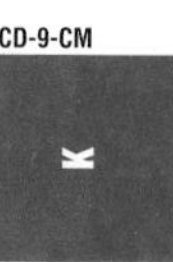

ICD-9-CM
K
Vol. 2

Kupffer cell sarcoma (M9124/3) 155.0
Kuru 046.0
Kussmaul's
  coma (diabetic) 250.3
  disease (polyarteritis nodosa) 446.0
  respiration (air hunger) 786.09
Kwashiorkor (marasmus type) 260
Kyasanur Forest disease 065.2
Kyphoscoliosis, kyphoscoliotic (acquired) (*see also* Scoliosis) 737.30
  congenital 756.19
  due to radiation 737.33
  heart (disease) 416.1
  idiopathic 737.30
    infantile
      progressive 737.32
      resolving 737.31
  late effect of rickets 268.1 *[737.43]*
  specified NEC 737.39
  thoracogenic 737.34
  tuberculous (*see also* Tuberculosis) 015.0 *[737.43]*
Kyphosis, kyphotic (acquired) (postural) 737.10
  adolescent postural 737.0
  congenital 756.19
  dorsalis juvenilis 732.0
  due to or associated with
    Charcôt-Marie-Tooth disease 356.1 *[737.41]*
    mucopolysaccharidosis 277.5 *[737.41]*
    neurofibromatosis 237.71 *[737.41]*
    osteitis
      deformans 731.0 *[737.41]*
      fibrosa cystica 252.01 *[737.41]*
    osteoporosis (*see also* Osteoporosis) 733.0 *[737.41]*
    poliomyelitis (*see also* Poliomyelitis) 138 *[737.41]*
    radiation 737.11
    tuberculosis (*see also* Tuberculosis) 015.0 *[737.41]*
  Kümmell's 721.7
  late effect of rickets 268.1 *[737.41]*
  Morquio-Brailsford type (spinal) 277.5 *[737.41]*
  pelvis 738.6
  postlaminectomy 737.12
  specified cause NEC 737.19
  syphilitic, congenital 090.5 *[737.41]*
  tuberculous (*see also* Tuberculosis) 015.0 *[737.41]*
Kyrle's disease (hyperkeratosis follicularis in cutem penetrans) 701.1

L

Labia, labium - *see* condition
Labiated hymen 752.49
Labile
blood pressure 796.2
emotions, emotionality 301.3
vasomotor system 443.9
Labioglossal paralysis 335.22
Labium leporinum (*see also* Cleft, lip) 749.10
Labor (*see also* Delivery)
with complications - *see* Delivery, complicated
abnormal NEC 661.9
affecting fetus or newborn 763.7
arrested active phase 661.1
affecting fetus or newborn 763.7
desultory 661.2
affecting fetus or newborn 763.7
dyscoordinate 661.4
affecting fetus or newborn 763.7
early onset (22–36 weeks gestation) 644.2
failed
induction 659.1
mechanical 659.0
medical 659.1
surgical 659.0
trial (vaginal delivery) 660.6
false 644.1
forced or induced, affecting fetus or newborn 763.89
hypertonic 661.4
affecting fetus or newborn 763.7
hypotonic 661.2
affecting fetus or newborn 763.7
primary 661.0
affecting fetus or newborn 763.7
secondary 661.1
affecting fetus or newborn 763.7
incoordinate 661.4
affecting fetus or newborn 763.7
irregular 661.2
affecting fetus or newborn 763.7
long - *see* Labor, prolonged
missed (at or near term) 656.4
obstructed NEC 660.9
affecting fetus or newborn 763.1
due to female genital mutilation 660.8
specified cause NEC 660.8
affecting fetus or newborn 763.1
pains, spurious 644.1
precipitate 661.3
affecting fetus or newborn 763.6
premature 644.2
threatened 644.0
prolonged or protracted 662.1
affecting fetus or newborn 763.89
first stage 662.0
affecting fetus or newborn 763.89
second stage 662.2
affecting fetus or newborn 763.89
threatened NEC 644.1
undelivered 644.1
Labored breathing (*see also* Hyperventilation) 786.09
Labyrinthitis (inner ear) (destructive) (latent) 386.30
circumscribed 386.32
diffuse 386.31
focal 386.32
purulent 386.33
serous 386.31
Labyrinthitis *(Continued)*
suppurative 386.33
syphilitic 095.8
toxic 386.34
viral 386.35
Laceration - *see also* Wound, open, by site
accidental, complicating surgery 998.2
Achilles tendon 845.09
with open wound 892.2
anus (sphincter) 879.6
with
abortion - *see* Abortion, by type, with damage to pelvic organs
ectopic pregnancy (*see also* categories 633.0–633.9) 639.2
molar pregnancy (*see also* categories 630–632) 639.2
complicated 879.7
complicating delivery 664.2
with laceration of anal or rectal mucosa 664.3
following
abortion 639.2
ectopic or molar pregnancy 639.2
nontraumatic, nonpuerperal 565.0
bladder (urinary)
with
abortion - *see* Abortion, by type, with damage to pelvic organs
ectopic pregnancy (*see also* categories 633.0–633.9) 639.2
molar pregnancy (*see also* categories 630–632) 639.2
following
abortion 639.2
ectopic or molar pregnancy 639.2
obstetrical trauma 665.5
blood vessel - *see* Injury, blood vessel, by site
bowel
with
abortion - *see* Abortion, by type, with damage to pelvic organs
ectopic pregnancy (*see also* categories 633.0–633.9) 639.2
molar pregnancy (*see also* categories 630–632) 639.2
following
abortion 639.2
ectopic or molar pregnancy 639.2
obstetrical trauma 665.5
brain (cerebral) (membrane) (with hemorrhage) 851.8

Note Use the following fifth-digit subclassification with categories 851–854:

0 unspecified state of consciousness
1 with no loss of consciousness
2 with brief [less than one hour] loss of consciousness
3 with moderate [1–24 hours] loss of consciousness
4 with prolonged [more than 24 hours] loss of consciousness and return to pre-existing conscious level
5 with prolonged [more than 24 hours] loss of consciousness, without return to pre-existing conscious level

Laceration *(Continued)*
brain *(Continued)*

Use fifth-digit 5 to designate when a patient is unconscious and dies before regaining consciousness, regardless of the duration of the loss of consciousness

6 with loss of consciousness of unspecified duration
9 with concussion, unspecified

with
open intracranial wound 851.9
skull fracture - *see* Fracture, skull, by site
cerebellum 851.6
with open intracranial wound 851.7
cortex 851.2
with open intracranial wound 851.3
during birth 767.0
stem 851.6
with open intracranial wound 851.7
broad ligament
with
abortion - *see* Abortion, by type, with damage to pelvic organs
ectopic pregnancy (*see also* categories 633.0–633.9) 639.2
molar pregnancy (*see also* categories 630–632) 639.2
following
abortion 639.2
ectopic or molar pregnancy 639.2
nontraumatic 620.6
obstetrical trauma 665.6
syndrome (nontraumatic) 620.6
capsule, joint - *see* Sprain, by site
cardiac - *see* Laceration, heart
causing eversion of cervix uteri (old) 622.0
central, complicating delivery 664.4
cerebellum - *see* Laceration, brain, cerebellum
cerebral - *see also* Laceration, brain
during birth 767.0
cervix (uteri)
with
abortion - *see* Abortion, by type, with damage to pelvic organs
ectopic pregnancy (*see also* categories 633.0–633.9) 639.2
molar pregnancy (*see also* categories 630–632) 639.2
following
abortion 639.2
ectopic or molar pregnancy 639.2
nonpuerperal, nontraumatic 622.3
obstetrical trauma (current) 665.3
old (postpartal) 622.3
traumatic - *see* Injury, internal, cervix
chordae heart 429.5
complicated 879.9
cornea - *see* Laceration, eyeball
superficial 918.1
cortex (cerebral) - *see* Laceration, brain, cortex
esophagus 530.89
eye(s) - *see* Laceration, ocular
eyeball NEC 871.4
with prolapse or exposure of intraocular tissue 871.1
penetrating - *see* Penetrating wound, eyeball

Laceration *(Continued)*
eyeball NEC *(Continued)*
specified as without prolapse of intraocular tissue 871.0
eyelid NEC 870.8
full thickness 870.1
involving lacrimal passages 870.2
skin (and periocular area) 870.0
penetrating - *see* Penetrating wound, orbit
fourchette
with
abortion - *see* Abortion, by type, with damage to pelvic organs
ectopic pregnancy (*see also* categories 633.0–633.9) 639.2
molar pregnancy (*see also* categories 630–632) 639.2
complicating delivery 664.0
following
abortion 639.2
ectopic or molar pregnancy 639.2
heart (without penetration of heart chambers) 861.02
with
open wound into thorax 861.12
penetration of heart chambers 861.03
with open wound into thorax 861.13
hernial sac - *see* Hernia, by site
internal organ (abdomen) (chest) (pelvis) NEC - *see* Injury, internal, by site
kidney (parenchyma) 866.02
with
complete disruption of parenchyma (rupture) 866.03
with open wound into cavity 866.13
open wound into cavity 866.12
labia
complicating delivery 664.0
ligament - *see also* Sprain, by site
with open wound - *see* Wound, open, by site
liver 864.05
with open wound into cavity 864.15
major (disruption of hepatic parenchyma) 864.04
with open wound into cavity 864.14
minor (capsule only) 864.02
with open wound into cavity 864.12
moderate (involving parenchyma without major disruption) 864.03
with open wound into cavity 864.13
multiple 864.04
with open wound into cavity 864.14
stellate 864.04
with open wound into cavity 864.14
lung 861.22
with open wound into thorax 861.32
meninges - *see* Laceration, brain
meniscus (knee) (*see also* Tear, meniscus) 836.2
old 717.5
site other than knee - *see also* Sprain, by site
old NEC (*see also* Disorder, cartilage, articular) 718.0

Laceration *(Continued)*
muscle - *see also* Sprain, by site
with open wound - *see* Wound, open, by site
myocardium - *see* Laceration, heart
nerve - *see* Injury, nerve, by site
ocular NEC (*see also* Laceration, eyeball) 871.4
adnexa NEC 870.8
penetrating 870.3
with foreign body 870.4
orbit (eye) 870.8
penetrating 870.3
with foreign body 870.4
pelvic
floor (muscles)
with
abortion - *see* Abortion, by type, with damage to pelvic organs
ectopic pregnancy (*see also* categories 633.0–633.9) 639.2
molar pregnancy (*see also* categories 630–632) 639.2
complicating delivery 664.1
following
abortion 639.2
ectopic or molar pregnancy 639.2
nonpuerperal 618.7
old (postpartal) 618.7
organ NEC
with
abortion - *see* Abortion, by type, with damage to pelvic organs
ectopic pregnancy (*see also* categories 633.0–633.9) 639.2
molar pregnancy (*see also* categories 630–632) 639.2
complicating delivery 665.5
affecting fetus or newborn 763.89
following
abortion 639.2
ectopic or molar pregnancy 639.2
obstetrical trauma 665.5
perineum, perineal (old) (postpartal) 618.7
with
abortion - *see* Abortion, by type, with damage to pelvic floor
ectopic pregnancy (*see also* categories 633.0–633.9) 639.2
molar pregnancy (*see also* categories 630–632) 639.2
complicating delivery 664.4
first degree 664.0
second degree 664.1
third degree 664.2
fourth degree 664.3
central 664.4
involving
anal sphincter 664.2
fourchette 664.0
hymen 664.0
labia 664.0
pelvic floor 664.1
perineal muscles 664.1
rectovaginal with septum 664.2
with anal mucosa 664.3
skin 664.0
sphincter (anal) 664.2
with anal mucosa 664.3
vagina 664.0

Laceration *(Continued)*
perineum, perineal *(Continued)*
complicating delivery *(Continued)*
involving *(Continued)*
vaginal muscles 664.1
vulva 664.0
secondary 674.2
following
abortion 639.2
ectopic or molar pregnancy 639.2
male 879.6
complicated 879.7
muscles, complicating delivery 664.1
nonpuerperal, current injury 879.6
complicated 879.7
secondary (postpartal) 674.2
peritoneum
with
abortion - *see* Abortion, by type, with damage to pelvic organs
ectopic pregnancy (*see also* categories 633.0–633.9) 639.2
molar pregnancy (*see also* categories 630–632) 639.2
following
abortion 639.2
ectopic or molar pregnancy 639.2
obstetrical trauma 665.5
periurethral tissue
with
abortion - *see* Abortion, by type, with damage to pelvic organs
ectopic pregnancy (*see also* categories 633.0–633.9) 639.2
molar pregnancy (*see also* categories 630–632) 639.2
following
abortion 639.2
ectopic or molar pregnancy 639.2
obstetrical trauma 665.5
rectovaginal (septum)
with
abortion - *see* Abortion, by type, with damage to pelvic organs
ectopic pregnancy (*see also* categories 633.0–633.9) 639.2
molar pregnancy (*see also* categories 630–632) 639.2
complicating delivery 665.4
with perineum 664.2
involving anal or rectal mucosa 664.3
following
abortion 639.2
ectopic or molar pregnancy 639.2
nonpuerperal 623.4
old (postpartal) 623.4
spinal cord (meninges) - *see also* Injury, spinal, by site
due to injury at birth 767.4
fetus or newborn 767.4
spleen 865.09
with
disruption of parenchyma (massive) 865.04
with open wound into cavity 865.14
open wound into cavity 865.19
capsule (without disruption of parenchyma) 865.02
with open wound into cavity 865.12

Laceration *(Continued)*
spleen *(Continued)*
parenchyma 865.03
with open wound into cavity 865.13
massive disruption (rupture) 865.04
with open wound into cavity 865.14
tendon 848.9
with open wound - *see* Wound, open, by site
Achilles 845.09
with open wound 892.2
lower limb NEC 844.9
with open wound NEC 894.2
upper limb NEC 840.9
with open wound NEC 884.2
tentorium cerebelli - *see* Laceration, brain, cerebellum
tongue 873.64
complicated 873.74
urethra
with
abortion - *see* Abortion, by type, with damage to pelvic organs
ectopic pregnancy (*see also* categories 633.0–633.9) 639.2
molar pregnancy (*see also* categories 630–632) 639.2
following
abortion 639.2
ectopic or molar pregnancy 639.2
nonpuerperal, nontraumatic 599.84
obstetrical trauma 665.5
uterus
with
abortion - *see* Abortion, by type, with damage to pelvic organs
ectopic pregnancy (*see also* categories 633.0–633.9) 639.2
molar pregnancy (*see also* categories 630–632) 639.2
following
abortion 639.2
ectopic or molar pregnancy 639.2
nonpuerperal, nontraumatic 621.8
obstetrical trauma NEC 665.5
old (postpartal) 621.8
vagina
with
abortion - *see* Abortion, by type, with damage to pelvic organs
ectopic pregnancy (*see also* categories 633.0–633.9) 639.2
molar pregnancy (*see also* categories 630–632) 639.2
perineal involvement, complicating delivery 664.0
complicating delivery 665.4
first degree 664.0
second degree 664.1
third degree 664.2
fourth degree 664.3
high 665.4
muscles 664.1
sulcus 665.4
wall 665.4
following
abortion 639.2
ectopic or molar pregnancy 639.2
nonpuerperal, nontraumatic 623.4
old (postpartal) 623.4
valve, heart - *see* Endocarditis

Laceration *(Continued)*
vulva
with
abortion - *see* Abortion, by type, with damage to pelvic organs
ectopic pregnancy (*see also* categories 633.0–633.9) 639.2
molar pregnancy (*see also* categories 630–632) 639.2
complicating delivery 664.0
following
abortion 639.2
ectopic or molar pregnancy 639.2
nonpuerperal, nontraumatic 624.4
old (postpartal) 624.4
Lachrymal - *see* condition
Lachrymonasal duct - *see* condition
Lack of
adequate intermaxillary vertical dimension 524.36 ◀
appetite (*see also* Anorexia) 783.0
care
in home V60.4
of adult 995.84
of infant (at or after birth) 995.52
coordination 781.3
development - *see also* Hypoplasia
physiological in childhood 783.40
education V62.3
energy 780.79
financial resources V60.2
food 994.2
in environment V60.8
growth in childhood 783.43
heating V60.1
housing (permanent) (temporary) V60.0
adequate V60.1
material resources V60.2
medical attention 799.89
memory (*see also* Amnesia) 780.93
mild, following organic brain damage 310.1
ovulation 628.0
person able to render necessary care V60.4
physical exercise V69.0
physiologic development in childhood 783.40
posterior occlusal support 524.57
prenatal care in current pregnancy V23.7
shelter V60.0
sleep V69.4
water 994.3
Lacrimal - *see* condition
Lacrimation, abnormal (*see also* Epiphora) 375.20
Lacrimonasal duct - *see* condition
Lactation, lactating (breast) (puerperal) (postpartum)
defective 676.4
disorder 676.9
specified type NEC 676.8
excessive 676.6
failed 676.4
mastitis NEC 675.2
mother (care and/or examination) V24.1
nonpuerperal 611.6
suppressed 676.5
Lacticemia 271.3
excessive 276.2
Lactosuria 271.3
Lacunar skull 756.0

Laennec's cirrhosis (alcoholic) 571.2
nonalcoholic 571.5
Lafora's disease 333.2
Lag, lid (nervous) 374.41
Lagleyze-von Hippel disease (retinocerebral angiomatosis) 759.6
Lagophthalmos (eyelid) (nervous) 374.20
cicatricial 374.23
keratitis (*see also* Keratitis) 370.34
mechanical 374.22
paralytic 374.21
La grippe - *see* Influenza
Lahore sore 085.1
Lakes, venous (cerebral) 437.8
Laki-Lorand factor deficiency (*see also* Defect, coagulation) 286.3
Lalling 307.9
Lambliasis 007.1
Lame back 724.5
Lancereaux's (diabetes, diabetes mellitus with marked emaciation) 250.8 [261]
Landouzy-Déjérine dystrophy (fascioscapulohumeral atrophy) 359.1
Landry's disease or paralysis 357.0
Landry-Guillain-Barré syndrome 357.0
Lane's
band 751.4
disease 569.89
kink (*see also* Obstruction, intestine) 560.9
Langdon Down's syndrome (mongolism) 758.0
Language abolition 784.69
Lanugo (persistent) 757.4
Laparoscopic surgical procedure converted to open procedure V64.41
Lardaceous
degeneration (any site) 277.39 ⇐
disease 277.39 ⇐
kidney 277.39 *[583.81]* ⇐
liver 277.39 ⇐
Large
baby (regardless of gestational age) 766.1
exceptionally (weight of 4500 grams or more) 766.0
of diabetic mother 775.0
ear 744.22
fetus - *see also* Oversize, fetus
causing disproportion 653.5
with obstructed labor 660.1
for dates
fetus or newborn (regardless of gestational age) 766.1
affecting management of pregnancy 656.6
exceptionally (weight of 4500 grams or more) 766.0
physiological cup 743.57
stature 783.9
waxy liver 277.39 ⇐
white kidney - *see* Nephrosis
Larsen's syndrome (flattened facies and multiple congenital dislocations) 755.8
Larsen-Johansson disease (juvenile osteopathia patellae) 732.4
Larva migrans
cutaneous NEC 126.9
ancylostoma 126.9
of Diptera in vitreous 128.0
visceral NEC 128.0
Laryngeal - *see also* condition
syncope 786.2
Laryngismus (acute) (infectious) (stridulous) 478.75
congenital 748.3
diphtheritic 032.3

Laryngitis (acute) (edematous) (fibrinous) (gangrenous) (infective) (infiltrative) (malignant) (membranous) (phlegmonous) (pneumococcal) (pseudomembranous) (septic) (subglottic) (suppurative) (ulcerative) (viral) 464.00
with
influenza, flu, or grippe 487.1
obstruction 464.01
tracheitis (*see also* Laryngotracheitis) 464.20
with obstruction 464.21
acute 464.20
with obstruction 464.21
chronic 476.1
atrophic 476.0
Borrelia vincentii 101
catarrhal 476.0
chronic 476.0
with tracheitis (chronic) 476.1
due to external agent - *see* Condition, respiratory, chronic, due to
diphtheritic (membranous) 032.3
due to external agent - *see* Inflammation, respiratory, upper, due to
H. influenzae 464.00
with obstruction 464.01
Hemophilus influenzae 464.00
with obstruction 464.01
hypertrophic 476.0
influenzal 487.1
pachydermic 478.79
sicca 476.0
spasmodic 478.75
acute 464.00
with obstruction 464.01
streptococcal 034.0
stridulous 478.75
syphilitic 095.8
congenital 090.5
tuberculous (*see also* Tuberculosis, larynx) 012.3
Vincent's 101
Laryngocele (congenital) (ventricular) 748.3
Laryngofissure 478.79
congenital 748.3
Laryngomalacia (congenital) 748.3
Laryngopharyngitis (acute) 465.0
chronic 478.9
due to external agent - *see* Condition, respiratory, chronic, due to
due to external agent - *see* Inflammation, respiratory, upper, due to
septic 034.0
Laryngoplegia (*see also* Paralysis, vocal cord) 478.30
Laryngoptosis 478.79
Laryngospasm 478.75
due to external agent - *see* Condition, respiratory, acute, due to
Laryngostenosis 478.74
congenital 748.3
Laryngotracheitis (acute) (infectional) (viral) (*see also* Laryngitis) 464.20
with obstruction 464.21
atrophic 476.1
Borrelia vincentii 101
catarrhal 476.1
chronic 476.1
due to external agent - *see* Condition, respiratory, chronic, due to
diphtheritic (membranous) 032.3

Laryngotracheitis *(Continued)*
due to external agent - *see* Inflammation, respiratory, upper, due to
H. influenzae 464.20
with obstruction 464.21
hypertrophic 476.1
influenzal 487.1
pachydermic 478.75
sicca 476.1
spasmodic 478.75
acute 464.20
with obstruction 464.21
streptococcal 034.0
stridulous 478.75
syphilitic 095.8
congenital 090.5
tuberculous (*see also* Tuberculosis, larynx) 012.3
Vincent's 101
Laryngotracheobronchitis (*see also* Bronchitis) 490
acute 466.0
chronic 491.8
viral 466.0
Laryngotracheobronchopneumonitis - *see* Pneumonia, broncho-
Larynx, laryngeal - *see* condition
Lasègue's disease (persecution mania) 297.9
Lassa fever 078.89
Lassitude (*see also* Weakness) 780.79
Late - *see also* condition
effect(s) (of) - *see also* condition
abscess
intracranial or intraspinal (conditions classifiable to 324) - *see* category 326
adverse effect of drug, medicinal or biological substance 909.5
allergic reaction 909.9
amputation
postoperative (late) 997.60
traumatic (injury classifiable to 885–887 and 895–897) 905.9
burn (injury classifiable to 948–949) 906.9
extremities NEC (injury classifiable to 943 or 945) 906.7
hand or wrist (injury classifiable to 944) 906.6
eye (injury classifiable to 940) 906.5
face, head, and neck (injury classifiable to 941) 906.5
specified site NEC (injury classifiable to 942 and 946–947) 906.8
cerebrovascular disease (conditions classifiable to 430–437) 438.9
with
alteration of sensations 438.6
aphasia 438.11
apraxia 438.81
ataxia 438.84
cognitive deficits 438.0
disturbances of vision 438.7
dysphagia 438.82
dysphasia 438.12
facial droop 438.83
facial weakness 438.83
hemiplegia/hemiparesis
affecting
dominant side 438.21
nondominant side 438.22
unspecified side 438.20

Late *(Continued)*
effect(s) *(Continued)*
cerebrovascular disease *(Continued)*
with *(Continued)*
monoplegia of lower limb
affecting
dominant side 438.41
nondominant side 438.42
unspecified side 438.40
monoplegia of upper limb
affecting
dominant side 438.31
nondominant side 438.32
unspecified side 438.30
paralytic syndrome NEC
affecting
bilateral 438.53
dominant side 438.51
nondominant side 438.52
unspecified side 438.50
speech and language deficit 438.10
specified type NEC 438.19
vertigo 438.85
specified type NEC 438.89
childbirth complication(s) 677
complication(s) of
childbirth 677
delivery 677
pregnancy 677
puerperium 677
surgical and medical care (conditions classifiable to 996–999) 909.3
trauma (conditions classifiable to 958) 908.6
contusion (injury classifiable to 920–924) 906.3
crushing (injury classifiable to 925–929) 906.4
delivery complication(s) 677
dislocation (injury classifiable to 830–839) 905.6
encephalitis or encephalomyelitis (conditions classifiable to 323) - *see* category 326
in infectious diseases 139.8
viral (conditions classifiable to 049.8, 049.9, 062–064) 139.0
external cause NEC (conditions classifiable to 995) 909.9
certain conditions classifiable to categories 991–994 909.4
foreign body in orifice (injury classifiable to 930–939) 908.5
fracture (multiple) (injury classifiable to 828–829) 905.5
extremity
lower (injury classifiable to 821–827) 905.4
neck of femur (injury classifiable to 820) 905.3
upper (injury classifiable to 810–819) 905.2
face and skull (injury classifiable to 800–804) 905.0
skull and face (injury classifiable to 800–804) 905.0
spine and trunk (injury classifiable to 805 and 807–809) 905.1
with spinal cord lesion (injury classifiable to 806) 907.2
infection
pyogenic, intracranial - *see* category 326

Late *(Continued)*
effect(s) *(Continued)*
infectious diseases (conditions classifiable to 001–136) NEC 139.8
injury (injury classifiable to 959) 908.9
blood vessel 908.3
abdomen and pelvis (injury classifiable to 902) 908.4
extremity (injury classifiable to 903–904) 908.3
head and neck (injury classifiable to 900) 908.3
intracranial (injury classifiable to 850–854) 907.0
with skull fracture 905.0
thorax (injury classifiable to 901) 908.4
internal organ NEC (injury classifiable to 867 and 869) 908.2
abdomen (injury classifiable to 863–866 and 868) 908.1
thorax (injury classifiable to 860–862) 908.0
intracranial (injury classifiable to 850–854) 907.0
with skull fracture (injury classifiable to 800–801 and 803–804) 905.0
nerve NEC (injury classifiable to 957) 907.9
cranial (injury classifiable to 950–951) 907.1
peripheral NEC (injury classifiable to 957) 907.9
lower limb and pelvic girdle (injury classifiable to 956) 907.5
upper limb and shoulder girdle (injury classifiable to 955) 907.4
roots and plexus(es), spinal (injury classifiable to 953) 907.3
trunk (injury classifiable to 954) 907.3
spinal
cord (injury classifiable to 806 and 952) 907.2
nerve root(s) and plexus(es) (injury classifiable to 953) 907.3
superficial (injury classifiable to 910–919) 906.2
tendon (tendon injury classifiable to 840–848, 880–884 with .2, and 890–894 with .2) 905.8
meningitis
bacterial (conditions classifiable to 320) - *see* category 326
unspecified cause (conditions classifiable to 322) - *see* category 326
myelitis (*see also* Late, effect(s) (of), encephalitis) - *see* category 326
parasitic diseases (conditions classifiable to 001–136 NEC) 139.8
phlebitis or thrombophlebitis of intracranial venous sinuses (conditions classifiable to 325) - *see* category 326
poisoning due to drug, medicinal, or biological substance (conditions classifiable to 960–979) 909.0
poliomyelitis, acute (conditions classifiable to 045) 138
pregnancy complication(s) 677

Late *(Continued)*
effect(s) *(Continued)*
puerperal complication(s) 677
radiation (conditions classifiable to 990) 909.2
rickets 268.1
sprain and strain without mention of tendon injury (injury classifiable to 840–848, except tendon injury) 905.7
tendon involvement 905.8
toxic effect of
drug, medicinal, or biological substance (conditions classifiable to 960–979) 909.0
nonmedical substance (conditions classifiable to 980–989) 909.1
trachoma (conditions classifiable to 076) 139.1
tuberculosis 137.0
bones and joints (conditions classifiable to 015) 137.3
central nervous system (conditions classifiable to 013) 137.1
genitourinary (conditions classifiable to 016) 137.2
pulmonary (conditions classifiable to 010–012) 137.0
specified organs NEC (conditions classifiable to 014, 017–018) 137.4
viral encephalitis (conditions classifiable to 049.8, 049.9, 062–064) 139.0
wound, open
extremity (injury classifiable to 880–884 and 890–894, except .2) 906.1
tendon (injury classifiable to 880–884 with .2 and 890–894 with .2) 905.8
head, neck, and trunk (injury classifiable to 870–879) 906.0
infant
post-term (gestation period over 40 completed weeks to 42 completed weeks) 766.21
prolonged gestation (period over 42 completed weeks) 766.22
Latent - *see* condition
Lateral - *see* condition
Laterocession - *see* Lateroversion
Lateroflexion - *see* Lateroversion
Lateroversion
cervix - *see* Lateroversion, uterus
uterus, uterine (cervix) (postinfectional) (postpartal, old) 621.6
congenital 752.3
in pregnancy or childbirth 654.4
affecting fetus or newborn 763.89
Lathyrism 988.2
Launois' syndrome (pituitary gigantism) 253.0
Launois-Bensaude's lipomatosis 272.8
Launois-Cleret syndrome (adiposogenital dystrophy) 253.8
Laurence-Moon-Biedl syndrome (obesity, polydactyly, and mental retardation) 759.89
LAV (disease) (illness) (infection) - *see* Human immunodeficiency virus (disease) (illness) (infection)
LAV/HTLV-III (disease) (illness) (infection) - *see* Human immunodeficiency virus (disease) (illness) (infection)

Lawford's syndrome (encephalocutaneous angiomatosis) 759.6
Lax, laxity - *see also* Relaxation
ligament 728.4
skin (acquired) 701.8
congenital 756.83
Laxative habit (*see also* Abuse, drugs, nondependent) 305.9
Lazy leukocyte syndrome 288.09 ◄
LCAD (long chain/very long chain acyl CoA dehydrogenase deficiency, VLCAD) 277.85
LCHAD (long chain 3-hydroxyacyl CoA dehydrogenase deficiency) 277.85
Lead - *see also* condition
exposure to V15.86
incrustation of cornea 371.15
poisoning 984.9
specified type of lead - *see* Table of Drugs and Chemicals
Lead miners' lung 503
Leakage
amniotic fluid 658.1
with delayed delivery 658.2
affecting fetus or newborn 761.1
bile from drainage tube (T tube) 997.4
blood (microscopic), fetal, into maternal circulation 656.0
affecting management of pregnancy or puerperium 656.0
device, implant, or graft - *see* Complications, mechanical
spinal fluid at lumbar puncture site 997.09
urine, continuous 788.37
Leaky heart - *see* Endocarditis
Learning defect, specific NEC (strephosymbolia) 315.2
Leather bottle stomach (M8142/3) 151.9
Leber's
congenital amaurosis 362.76
optic atrophy (hereditary) 377.16
Lederer's anemia or disease (acquired infectious hemolytic anemia) 283.19
Lederer-Brill syndrome (acquired infectious hemolytic anemia) 283.19
Leeches (aquatic) (land) 134.2
Left-sided neglect 781.8
Leg - *see* condition
Legal investigation V62.5
Legg (-Calvé)-Perthes disease or syndrome (osteochondrosis, femoral capital) 732.1
Legionnaires' disease 482.84
Leigh's disease 330.8
Leiner's disease (exfoliative dermatitis) 695.89
Leiofibromyoma (M8890/0) - *see also* Leiomyoma
uterus (cervix) (corpus) (*see also* Leiomyoma, uterus) 218.9
Leiomyoblastoma (M8891/1) - *see* Neoplasm, connective tissue, uncertain behavior
Leiomyofibroma (M8890/0) - *see also* Neoplasm, connective tissue, benign
uterus (cervix) (corpus) (*see also* Leiomyoma, uterus) 218.9
Leiomyoma (M8890/0) - *see also* Neoplasm, connective tissue, benign
bizarre (M8893/0) - *see* Neoplasm, connective tissue, benign
cellular (M8892/1) - *see* Neoplasm, connective tissue, uncertain behavior

Leiomyoma *(Continued)*
epithelioid (M8891/1) - *see* Neoplasm, connective tissue, uncertain behavior
prostate (polypoid) 600.20
with
other lower urinary tract symptoms (LUTS) 600.21
urinary
obstruction 600.21
retention 600.21
uterus (cervix) (corpus) 218.9
interstitial 218.1
intramural 218.1
submucous 218.0
subperitoneal 218.2
subserous 218.2
vascular (M8894/0) - *see* Neoplasm, connective tissue, benign
Leiomyomatosis (intravascular) (M8890/1) - *see* Neoplasm, connective tissue, uncertain behavior
Leiomyosarcoma (M8890/3) - *see also* Neoplasm, connective tissue, malignant
epithelioid (M8891/3) - *see* Neoplasm, connective tissue, malignant
Leishmaniasis 085.9
American 085.5
cutaneous 085.4
mucocutaneous 085.5
Asian desert 085.2
Brazilian 085.5
cutaneous 085.9
acute necrotizing 085.2
American 085.4
Asian desert 085.2
diffuse 085.3
dry form 085.1
Ethiopian 085.3
eyelid 085.5 *[373.6]*
late 085.1
lepromatous 085.3
recurrent 085.1
rural 085.2
ulcerating 085.1
urban 085.1
wet form 085.2
zoonotic form 085.2
dermal - *see also* Leishmaniasis, cutaneous
post kala-azar 085.0
eyelid 085.5 *[373.6]*
infantile 085.0
Mediterranean 085.0
mucocutaneous (American) 085.5
naso-oral 085.5
nasopharyngeal 085.5
Old World 085.1
tegumentaria diffusa 085.4
vaccination, prophylactic (against) V05.2
visceral (Indian) 085.0
Leishmanoid, dermal - *see also* Leishmaniasis, cutaneous
post kala-azar 085.0
Leloir's disease 695.4
Lemiere syndrome 451.89
Lenegre's disease 426.0
Lengthening, leg 736.81
Lennox-Gastaut syndrome 345.0
with tonic seizures 345.1
Lennox's syndrome (*see also* Epilepsy) 345.0
Lens - *see* condition
Lenticonus (anterior) (posterior) (congenital) 743.36
Lenticular degeneration, progressive 275.1
Lentiglobus (posterior) (congenital) 743.36
Lentigo (congenital) 709.09
juvenile 709.09
maligna (M8742/2) - *see also* Neoplasm, skin, in situ
melanoma (M8742/3) - *see* Melanoma
senile 709.09
Leonine leprosy 030.0
Leontiasis
ossium 733.3
syphilitic 095.8
congenital 090.5
Léopold-Lévi's syndrome (paroxysmal thyroid instability) 242.9
Lepore hemoglobin syndrome 282.49
Lepothrix 039.0
Lepra 030.9
Willan's 696.1
Leprechaunism 259.8
Lepromatous leprosy 030.0
Leprosy 030.9
anesthetic 030.1
beriberi 030.1
borderline (group B) (infiltrated) (neuritic) 030.3
cornea (*see also* Leprosy, by type) 030.9 *[371.89]*
dimorphous (group B) (infiltrated) (lepromatous) (neuritic) (tuberculoid) 030.3
eyelid 030.0 *[373.4]*
indeterminate (group I) (macular) (neuritic) (uncharacteristic) 030.2
leonine 030.0
lepromatous (diffuse) (infiltrated) (macular) (neuritic) (nodular) (type L) 030.0
macular (early) (neuritic) (simple) 030.2
maculoanesthetic 030.1
mixed 030.0
neuro 030.1
nodular 030.0
primary neuritic 030.3
specified type or group NEC 030.8
tubercular 030.1
tuberculoid (macular) (maculoanesthetic) (major) (minor) (neuritic) (type T) 030.1
Leptocytosis, hereditary 282.49
Leptomeningitis (chronic) (circumscribed) (hemorrhagic) (nonsuppurative) (*see also* Meningitis) 322.9
aseptic 047.9
adenovirus 049.1
Coxsackie virus 047.0
ECHO virus 047.1
enterovirus 047.9
lymphocytic choriomeningitis 049.0
epidemic 036.0
late effect - *see* category 326
meningococcal 036.0
pneumococcal 320.1
syphilitic 094.2
tuberculous (*see also* Tuberculosis, meninges) 013.0
Leptomeningopathy (*see also* Meningitis) 322.9
Leptospiral - *see* condition
Leptospirochetal - *see* condition
Leptospirosis 100.9
autumnalis 100.89
canicula 100.89
grippotyphosa 100.89
hebdomadis 100.89
icterohemorrhagica 100.0
nanukayami 100.89
pomona 100.89
Weil's disease 100.0
Leptothricosis - *see* Actinomycosis
Leptothrix infestation - *see* Actinomycosis
Leptotricosis - *see* Actinomycosis
Leptus dermatitis 133.8
Léris pleonosteosis 756.89
Léri-Weill syndrome 756.59
Leriche's syndrome (aortic bifurcation occlusion) 444.0
Lermoyez's syndrome (*see also* Disease, Ménière's) 386.00
Lesbianism - *omit code*
ego-dystonic 302.0
problems with 302.0
Lesch-Nyhan syndrome (hypoxanthine-guanine-phosphoribosyltransferase deficiency) 277.2
Lesion(s)
abducens nerve 378.54
alveolar process 525.8
anorectal 569.49
aortic (valve) - *see* Endocarditis, aortic
auditory nerve 388.5
basal ganglion 333.90
bile duct (*see also* Disease, biliary) 576.8
bladder 596.9
bone 733.90
brachial plexus 353.0
brain 348.8
congenital 742.9
vascular (*see also* Lesion, cerebrovascular) 437.9
degenerative 437.1
healed or old without residuals V12.59
hypertensive 437.2
late effect - *see* Late effect(s) (of) cerebrovascular disease
buccal 528.9
calcified - *see* Calcification
canthus 373.9
carate - *see* Pinta, lesions
cardia 537.89
cardiac - *see also* Disease, heart
congenital 746.9
valvular - *see* Endocarditis
cauda equina 344.60
with neurogenic bladder 344.61
cecum 569.89
cerebral - *see* Lesion, brain
cerebrovascular (*see also* Disease, cerebrovascular NEC) 437.9
degenerative 437.1
healed or old without residuals V12.59
hypertensive 437.2
specified type NEC 437.8
cervical root (nerve) NEC 353.2
chiasmal 377.54
associated with
inflammatory disorders 377.54
neoplasm NEC 377.52
pituitary 377.51
pituitary disorders 377.51
vascular disorders 377.53

◀ New ⬅ Revised

Lesion(s) *(Continued)*
chorda tympani 351.8
coin, lung 793.1
colon 569.89
congenital - *see* Anomaly
conjunctiva 372.9
coronary artery (*see also* Ischemia, heart) 414.9
cranial nerve 352.9
first 352.0
second 377.49
third
partial 378.51
total 378.52
fourth 378.53
fifth 350.9
sixth 378.54
seventh 351.9
eighth 388.5
ninth 352.2
tenth 352.3
eleventh 352.4
twelfth 352.5
cystic - *see* Cyst
degenerative - *see* Degeneration
dermal (skin) 709.9
Dieulafoy (hemorrhagic)
of
duodenum 537.84
intestine 569.86
stomach 537.84
duodenum 537.89
with obstruction 537.3
eyelid 373.9
gasserian ganglion 350.8
gastric 537.89
gastroduodenal 537.89
gastrointestinal 569.89
glossopharyngeal nerve 352.2
heart (organic) - *see also* Disease, heart
vascular - *see* Disease, cardiovascular
helix (ear) 709.9
high grade myelodysplastic syndrome 238.73
hyperchromic, due to pinta (carate) 103.1
hyperkeratotic (*see also* Hyperkeratosis) 701.1
hypoglossal nerve 352.5
hypopharynx 478.29
hypothalamic 253.9
ileocecal coil 569.89
ileum 569.89
iliohypogastric nerve 355.79
ilioinguinal nerve 355.79
in continuity - *see* Injury, nerve, by site
inflammatory - *see* Inflammation
intestine 569.89
intracerebral - *see* Lesion, brain
intrachiasmal (optic) (*see also* Lesion, chiasmal) 377.54
intracranial, space-occupying NEC 784.2
joint 719.90
ankle 719.97
elbow 719.92
foot 719.97
hand 719.94
hip 719.95
knee 719.96
multiple sites 719.99
pelvic region 719.95
sacroiliac (old) 724.6
shoulder (region) 719.91
specified site NEC 719.98
wrist 719.93

Lesion(s) *(Continued)*
keratotic (*see also* Keratosis) 701.1
kidney (*see also* Disease, renal) 593.9
laryngeal nerve (recurrent) 352.3
leonine 030.0
LGSIL (low grade squamous intraepithelial dysplasia 622.1
lip 528.5
liver 573.8
low grade myelodysplastic syndrome 238.72
lumbosacral
plexus 353.1
root (nerve) NEC 353.4
lung 518.89
coin 793.1
maxillary sinus 473.0
mitral - *see* Endocarditis, mitral
motor cortex 348.8
nerve (*see also* Disorder, nerve) 355.9
nervous system 349.9
congenital 742.9
nonallopathic NEC 739.9
in region (of)
abdomen 739.9
acromioclavicular 739.7
cervical, cervicothoracic 739.1
costochondral 739.8
costovertebral 739.8
extremity
lower 739.6
upper 739.7
head 739.0
hip 739.5
lower extremity 739.6
lumbar, lumbosacral 739.3
occipitocervical 739.0
pelvic 739.5
pubic 739.5
rib cage 739.8
sacral, sacrococcygeal, sacroiliac 739.4
sternochondral 739.8
sternoclavicular 739.7
thoracic, thoracolumbar 739.2
upper extremity 739.7
nose (internal) 478.19
obstructive - *see* Obstruction
obturator nerve 355.79
occlusive
artery - *see* Embolism, artery
organ or site NEC - *see* Disease, by site
osteolytic 733.90
paramacular, of retina 363.32
peptic 537.89
periodontal, due to traumatic occlusion 523.8
perirectal 569.49
peritoneum (granulomatous) 568.89
pigmented (skin) 709.00
pinta - *see* Pinta, lesions
polypoid - *see* Polyp
prechiasmal (optic) (*see also* Lesion, chiasmal) 377.54
primary - *see also* Syphilis, primary
carate 103.0
pinta 103.0
yaws 102.0
pulmonary 518.89
valve (*see also* Endocarditis, pulmonary) 424.3
pylorus 537.89
radiation NEC 990
radium NEC 990

Lesion(s) *(Continued)*
rectosigmoid 569.89
retina, retinal - *see also* Retinopathy
vascular 362.17
retroperitoneal 568.89
romanus 720.1
sacroiliac (joint) 724.6
salivary gland 527.8
benign lymphoepithelial 527.8
saphenous nerve 355.79
secondary - *see* Syphilis, secondary
sigmoid 569.89
sinus (accessory) (nasal) (*see also* Sinusitis) 473.9
skin 709.9
suppurative 686.00
SLAP (superior glenoid labrum) 840.7
space-occupying, intracranial NEC 784.2
spinal cord 336.9
congenital 742.9
traumatic (complete) (incomplete) (transverse) - *see also* Injury, spinal, by site
with
broken
back - *see* Fracture, vertebra, by site, with spinal cord injury
neck - *see* Fracture, vertebra, cervical, with spinal cord injury
fracture, vertebra - *see* Fracture, vertebra, by site, with spinal cord injury
spleen 289.50
stomach 537.89
superior glenoid labrum (SLAP) 840.7
syphilitic - *see* Syphilis
tertiary - *see* Syphilis, tertiary
thoracic root (nerve) 353.3
tonsillar fossa 474.9
tooth, teeth 525.8
white spot 521.01
traumatic NEC (*see also* nature and site of injury) 959.9
tricuspid (valve) - *see* Endocarditis, tricuspid
trigeminal nerve 350.9
ulcerated or ulcerative - *see* Ulcer
uterus NEC 621.9
vagina 623.8
vagus nerve 352.3
valvular - *see* Endocarditis
vascular 459.9
affecting central nervous system (*see also* Lesion, cerebrovascular) 437.9
following trauma (*see also* Injury, blood vessel, by site) 904.9
retina 362.17
traumatic - *see* Injury, blood vessel, by site
umbilical cord 663.6
affecting fetus or newborn 762.6
visual
cortex NEC (*see also* Disorder, visual, cortex) 377.73
pathway NEC (*see also* Disorder, visual, pathway) 377.63
warty - *see* Verruca
white spot, on teeth 521.01
x-ray NEC 990

Lethargic - *see* condition
Lethargy 780.79
Letterer-Siwe disease (acute histiocytosis X) (M9722/3) 202.5
Leucinosis 270.3
Leucocoria 360.44
Leucosarcoma (M9850/3) 207.8
Leukasmus 270.2
Leukemia, leukemic (congenital) (M9800/3) 208.9

> Note Use the following fifth-digit subclassification for categories 203–208:
>
> 0 without mention of remission
> 1 with remission

- acute NEC (M9801/3) 208.0
- aleukemic NEC (M9804/3) 208.8
  - granulocytic (M9864/3) 205.8
- basophilic (M9870/3) 205.1
- blast (cell) (M9801/3) 208.0
- blastic (M9801/3) 208.0
  - granulocytic (M9861/3) 205.0
- chronic NEC (M9803/3) 208.1
- compound (M9810/3) 207.8
- eosinophilic (M9880/3) 205.1
- giant cell (M9910/3) 207.2
- granulocytic (M9860/3) 205.9
  - acute (M9861/3) 205.0
  - aleukemic (M9864/3) 205.8
  - blastic (M9861/3) 205.0
  - chronic (M9863/3) 205.1
  - subacute (M9862/3) 205.2
  - subleukemic (M9864/3) 205.8
- hairy cell (M9940/3) 202.4
- hemoblastic (M9801/3) 208.0
- histiocytic (M9890/3) 206.9
- lymphatic (M9820/3) 204.9
  - acute (M9821/3) 204.0
  - aleukemic (M9824/3) 204.8
  - chronic (M9823/3) 204.1
  - subacute (M9822/3) 204.2
  - subleukemic (M9824/3) 204.8
- lymphoblastic (M9821/3) 204.0
- lymphocytic (M9820/3) 204.9
  - acute (M9821/3) 204.0
  - aleukemic (M9824/3) 204.8
  - chronic (M9823/3) 204.1
  - subacute (M9822/3) 204.2
  - subleukemic (M9824/3) 204.8
- lymphogenous (M9820/3) - *see* Leukemia, lymphoid
- lymphoid (M9820/3) 204.9
  - acute (M9821/3) 204.0
  - aleukemic (M9824/3) 204.8
  - blastic (M9821/3) 204.0
  - chronic (M9823/3) 204.1
  - subacute (M9822/3) 204.2
  - subleukemic (M9824/3) 204.8
- lymphosarcoma cell (M9850/3) 207.8
- mast cell (M9900/3) 207.8
- megakaryocytic (M9910/3) 207.2
- megakaryocytoid (M9910/3) 207.2
- mixed (cell) (M9810/3) 207.8
- monoblastic (M9891/3) 206.0
- monocytic (Schilling-type) (M9890/3) 206.9
  - acute (M9891/3) 206.0
  - aleukemic (M9894/3) 206.8
  - chronic (M9893/3) 206.1
  - Naegeli-type (M9863/3) 205.1
  - subacute (M9892/3) 206.2
  - subleukemic (M9894/3) 206.8

Leukemia, leukemic *(Continued)*
- monocytoid (M9890/3) 206.9
  - acute (M9891/3) 206.0
  - aleukemic (M9894/3) 206.8
  - chronic (M9893/3) 206.1
  - myelogenous (M9863/3) 205.1
  - subacute (M9892/3) 206.2
  - subleukemic (M9894/3) 206.8
- monomyelocytic (M9860/3) - *see* Leukemia, myelomonocytic
- myeloblastic (M9861/3) 205.0
- myelocytic (M9863/3) 205.1
  - acute (M9861/3) 205.0
- myelogenous (M9860/3) 205.9
  - acute (M9861/3) 205.0
  - aleukemic (M9864/3) 205.8
  - chronic (M9863/3) 205.1
  - monocytoid (M9863/3) 205.1
  - subacute (M9862/3) 205.2
  - subleukemic (M9864) 205.8
- myeloid (M9860/3) 205.9
  - acute (M9861/3) 205.0
  - aleukemic (M9864/3) 205.8
  - chronic (M9863/3) 205.1
  - subacute (M9862/3) 205.2
  - subleukemic (M9864/3) 205.8
- myelomonocytic (M9860/3) 205.9
  - acute (M9861/3) 205.0
  - chronic (M9863/3) 205.1
- Naegeli-type monocytic (M9863/3) 205.1
- neutrophilic (M9865/3) 205.1
- plasma cell (M9830/3) 203.1
- plasmacytic (M9830/3) 203.1
- prolymphocytic (M9825/3) - *see* Leukemia, lymphoid
- promyelocytic, acute (M9866/3) 205.0
- Schilling-type monocytic (M9890/3) - *see* Leukemia, monocytic
- stem cell (M9801/3) 208.0
- subacute NEC (M9802/3) 208.2
- subleukemic NEC (M9804/3) 208.8
- thrombocytic (M9910/3) 207.2
- undifferentiated (M9801/3) 208.0

Leukemoid reaction (basophilic) (lymphocytic) (monocytic) (myelocytic) (neutrophilic) 288.62
Leukoclastic vasculitis 446.29
Leukocoria 360.44
Leukocythemia - *see* Leukemia
Leukocytopenia 288.50
Leukocytosis 288.60
- basophilic 288.8
- eosinophilic 288.3
- lymphocytic 288.8
- monocytic 288.8
- neutrophilic 288.8

Leukoderma 709.09
- syphilitic 091.3
  - late 095.8

Leukodermia (*see also* Leukoderma) 709.09
Leukodystrophy (cerebral) (globoid cell) (metachromatic) (progressive) (sudanophilic) 330.0
Leukoedema, mouth or tongue 528.79
Leukoencephalitis
- acute hemorrhagic (postinfectious) NEC 136.9 *[323.61]*
  - postimmunization or postvaccinal 323.51
- subacute sclerosing 046.2
  - van Bogaert's 046.2
- van Bogaert's (sclerosing) 046.2

Leukoencephalopathy (*see also* Encephalitis) 323.9
- acute necrotizing hemorrhagic (postinfectious) 136.9 *[323.61]*
  - postimmunization or postvaccinal 323.51
- metachromatic 330.0
- multifocal (progressive) 046.3
- progressive multifocal 046.3

Leukoerythroblastosis 289.9
Leukoerythrosis 289.0
Leukokeratosis (*see also* Leukoplakia) 702.8
- mouth 528.6
- nicotina palati 528.79
- tongue 528.6

Leukokoria 360.44
Leukokraurosis vulva, vulvae 624.0
Leukolymphosarcoma (M9850/3) 207.8
Leukoma (cornea) (interfering with central vision) 371.03
- adherent 371.04

Leukomalacia, periventricular 779.7
Leukomelanopathy, hereditary 288.2
Leukonychia (punctata) (striata) 703.8
- congenital 757.5

Leukopathia
- unguium 703.8
  - congenital 757.5

Leukopenia 288.50
- basophilic 288.59
- cyclic 288.02
- eosinophilic 288.59
- familial 288.59
- malignant (*see also* Agranulocytosis) 288.09
- periodic 288.02
- transitory neonatal 776.7

Leukopenic - *see* condition
Leukoplakia 702.8
- anus 569.49
- bladder (postinfectional) 596.8
- buccal 528.6
- cervix (uteri) 622.2
- esophagus 530.83
- gingiva 528.6
- kidney (pelvis) 593.89
- larynx 478.79
- lip 528.6
- mouth 528.6
- oral soft tissue (including tongue) (mucosa) 528.6
- palate 528.6
- pelvis (kidney) 593.89
- penis (infectional) 607.0
- rectum 569.49
- syphilitic 095.8
- tongue 528.6
- tonsil 478.29
- ureter (postinfectional) 593.89
- urethra (postinfectional) 599.84
- uterus 621.8
- vagina 623.1
- vesical 596.8
- vocal cords 478.5
- vulva 624.0

Leukopolioencephalopathy 330.0
Leukorrhea (vagina) 623.5
- due to Trichomonas (vaginalis) 131.00
- trichomonal (Trichomonas vaginalis) 131.00

Leukosarcoma (M9850/3) 207.8
Leukosis (M9800/3) - *see* Leukemia
Lev's disease or syndrome (acquired complete heart block) 426.0

◀ New ⬅ Revised

Levi's syndrome (pituitary dwarfism) 253.3
Levocardia (isolated) 746.87
with situs inversus 759.3
Levulosuria 271.2
Lewandowski's disease (primary) (*see also* Tuberculosis) 017.0
Lewandowski-Lutz disease (epidermodysplasia verruciformis) 078.19
Lewy body dementia 331.82
Lewy body disease 331.82
Leyden's disease (periodic vomiting) 536.2
Leyden-Möbius dystrophy 359.1
Leydig cell
carcinoma (M8650/3)
specified site - *see* Neoplasm, by site, malignant
unspecified site
female 183.0
male 186.9
tumor (M8650/1)
benign (M8650/0)
specified site - *see* Neoplasm, by site, benign
unspecified site
female 220
male 222.0
malignant (M8650/3)
specified site - *see* Neoplasm, by site, malignant
unspecified site
female 183.0
male 186.9
specified site - *see* Neoplasm, by site, uncertain behavior
unspecified site
female 236.2
male 236.4
Leydig-Sertoli cell tumor (M8631/0)
specified site - *see* Neoplasm, by site, benign
unspecified site
female 220
male 222.0
LGSIL (low grade squamous intraepithelial lesion) 795.03
Liar, pathologic 301.7
Libman-Sacks disease or syndrome 710.0 [424.91]
Lice (infestation) 132.9
body (pediculus corporis) 132.1
crab 132.2
head (pediculus capitis) 132.0
mixed (classifiable to more than one of the categories 132.0–132.2) 132.3
pubic (pediculus pubis) 132.2
Lichen 697.9
albus 701.0
annularis 695.89
atrophicus 701.0
corneus obtusus 698.3
myxedematous 701.8
nitidus 697.1
pilaris 757.39
acquired 701.1
planopilaris 697.0
planus (acute) (chronicus) (hypertrophic) (verrucous) 697.0
morphoeicus 701.0
sclerosus (et atrophicus) 701.0
ruber 696.4
acuminatus 696.4
moniliformis 697.8
Lichen *(Continued)*
ruber *(Continued)*
obtusus corneus 698.3
of Wilson 697.0
planus 697.0
sclerosus (et atrophicus) 701.0
scrofulosus (primary) (*see also* Tuberculosis) 017.0
simplex (Vidal's) 698.3
chronicus 698.3
circumscriptus 698.3
spinulosus 757.39
mycotic 117.9
striata 697.8
urticatus 698.2
Lichenification 698.3
nodular 698.3
Lichenoides tuberculosis (primary) (*see also* Tuberculosis) 017.0
Lichtheim's disease or syndrome (subacute combined sclerosis with pernicious anemia) 281.0 [336.2]
Lien migrans 289.59
Lientery (*see also* Diarrhea) 787.91
infectious 009.2
Life circumstance problem NEC V62.89
Li-Fraumeni cancer syndrome V84.01
Ligament - *see* condition
Light-for-dates (infant) 764.0
with signs of fetal malnutrition 764.1
affecting management of pregnancy 656.5
Light-headedness 780.4
Lightning (effects) (shock) (stroke) (struck by) 994.0
burn - *see* Burn, by site
foot 266.2
Lightwood's disease or syndrome (renal tubular acidosis) 588.89
Lignac's disease (cystinosis) 270.0
Lignac (-de Toni) (-Fanconi) (-Debré) syndrome (cystinosis) 270.0
Lignac (-Fanconi) syndrome (cystinosis) 270.0
Ligneous thyroiditis 245.3
Likoff's syndrome (angina in menopausal women) 413.9
Limb - *see* condition
Limitation of joint motion (*see also* Stiffness, joint) 719.5
sacroiliac 724.6
Limit dextrinosis 271.0
Limited
cardiac reserve - *see* Disease, heart
duction, eye NEC 378.63
mandibular range of motion 524.52
Lindau's disease (retinocerebral angiomatosis) 759.6
Lindau (-von Hippel) disease (angiomatosis retinocerebellosa) 759.6
Linea corneae senilis 371.41
Lines
Beau's (transverse furrows on fingernails) 703.8
Harris' 733.91
Hudson-Stähli 371.11
Stähli's 371.11
Lingua
geographical 529.1
nigra (villosa) 529.3
plicata 529.5
congenital 750.13
tylosis 528.6
Lingual (tongue) - *see also* condition
thyroid 759.2
Linitis (gastric) 535.4
plastica (M8142/3) 151.9
Lioderma essentialis (cum melanosis et telangiectasia) 757.33
Lip - *see also* condition
biting 528.9
Lipalgia 272.8
Lipedema - *see* Edema
Lipemia (*see also* Hyperlipidemia) 272.4
retina, retinalis 272.3
Lipidosis 272.7
cephalin 272.7
cerebral (infantile) (juvenile) (late) 330.1
cerebroretinal 330.1 *[362.71]*
cerebroside 272.7
cerebrospinal 272.7
chemically induced 272.7
cholesterol 272.7
diabetic 250.8 *[272.7]*
dystopic (hereditary) 272.7
glycolipid 272.7
hepatosplenomegalic 272.3
hereditary, dystopic 272.7
sulfatide 330.0
Lipoadenoma (M8324/0 - *see* Neoplasm, by site, benign
Lipoblastoma (M8881/0) - *see* Lipoma, by site
Lipoblastomatosis (M8881/0) - *see* Lipoma, by site
Lipochondrodystrophy 277.5
Lipochrome histiocytosis (familial) 288.1
Lipodystrophia progressiva 272.6
Lipodystrophy (progressive) 272.6
insulin 272.6
intestinal 040.2
mesenteric 567.82
Lipofibroma (M8851/0) - *see* Lipoma, by site
Lipoglycoproteinosis 272.8
Lipogranuloma, sclerosing 709.8
Lipogranulomatosis (disseminated) 272.8
kidney 272.8
Lipoid - *see also* condition
histiocytosis 272.7
essential 272.7
nephrosis (*see also* Nephrosis) 581.3
proteinosis of Urbach 272.8
Lipoidemia (*see also* Hyperlipidemia) 272.4
Lipoidosis (*see also* Lipidosis) 272.7
Lipoma (M8850/0) 214.9
breast (skin) 214.1
face 214.0
fetal (M8881/0) - *see also* Lipoma, by site
fat cell (M8880/0) - *see* Lipoma, by site
infiltrating (M8856/0) - *see* Lipoma, by site
intra-abdominal 214.3
intramuscular (M8856/0) - *see* Lipoma, by site
intrathoracic 214.2
kidney 214.3
mediastinum 214.2
muscle 214.8
peritoneum 214.3
retroperitoneum 214.3
skin 214.1
face 214.0

Lipoma *(Continued)*
spermatic cord 214.4
spindle cell (M8857/0) - *see* Lipoma, by site
stomach 214.3
subcutaneous tissue 214.1
face 214.0
thymus 214.2
thyroid gland 214.2
Lipomatosis (dolorosa) 272.8
epidural 214.8
fetal (M8881/0) - *see* Lipoma, by site
Launois-Bensaude's 272.8
Lipomyohemangioma (M8860/0)
specified site - *see* Neoplasm, connective tissue, benign
unspecified site 223.0
Lipomyoma (M8860/0)
specified site - *see* Neoplasm, connective tissue, benign
unspecified site 223.0
Lipomyxoma (M8852/0) - *see* Lipoma, by site
Lipomyxosarcoma (M8852/3) - *see* Neoplasm, connective tissue, malignant
Lipophagocytosis 289.89
Lipoproteinemia (alpha) 272.4
broad-beta 272.2
floating-beta 272.2
hyper-pre-beta 272.1
Lipoproteinosis (Rossle-Urbach-Wiethe) 272.8
Liposarcoma (M8850/3) - *see also* Neoplasm, connective tissue, malignant
differentiated type (M8851/3) - *see* Neoplasm, connective tissue, malignant
embryonal (M8852/3) - *see* Neoplasm, connective tissue, malignant
mixed type (M8855/3) - *see* Neoplasm, connective tissue, malignant
myxoid (M8852/3) - *see* Neoplasm, connective tissue, malignant
pleomorphic (M8854/3) - *see* Neoplasm, connective tissue, malignant
round cell (M8853/3) - *see* Neoplasm, connective tissue, malignant
well differentiated type (M8851/3) - *see* Neoplasm, connective tissue, malignant
Liposynovitis prepatellaris 272.8
Lipping
cervix 622.0
spine (*see also* Spondylosis) 721.90
vertebra (*see also* Spondylosis) 721.90
Lip pits (mucus), congenital 750.25
Lipschütz disease or ulcer 616.50
Lipuria 791.1
bilharziasis 120.0
Liquefaction, vitreous humor 379.21
Lisping 307.9
Lissauer's paralysis 094.1
Lissencephalia, lissencephaly 742.2
Listerellose 027.0
Listeriose 027.0
Listeriosis 027.0
congenital 771.2
fetal 771.2
suspected fetal damage affecting management of pregnancy 655.4
Listlessness 780.79
Lithemia 790.6
Lithiasis - *see also* Calculus
hepatic (duct) - *see* Choledocholithiasis
urinary 592.9
Lithopedion 779.9
affecting management of pregnancy 656.8
Lithosis (occupational) 502
with tuberculosis - *see* Tuberculosis, pulmonary
Lithuria 791.9
Litigation V62.5
Little
league elbow 718.82
stroke syndrome 435.9
Little's disease - *see* Palsy, cerebral
Littre's
gland - *see* condition
hernia - *see* Hernia, Littre's
Littritis (*see also* Urethritis) 597.89
Livedo 782.61
annularis 782.61
racemose 782.61
reticularis 782.61
Live flesh 781.0
Liver - *see also* condition
donor V59.6
Livida, asphyxia
newborn 768.6
Living
alone V60.3
with handicapped person V60.4
Lloyd's syndrome 258.1
Loa loa 125.2
Loasis 125.2
Lobe, lobar - *see* condition
Lobo's disease or blastomycosis 116.2
Lobomycosis 116.2
Lobotomy syndrome 310.0
Lobstein's disease (brittle bones and blue sclera) 756.51
Lobster-claw hand 755.58
Lobulation (congenital) - *see also* Anomaly, specified type NEC, by site
kidney, fetal 753.3
liver, abnormal 751.69
spleen 759.0
Lobule, lobular - *see* condition
Local, localized - *see* condition
Locked bowel or intestine (*see also* Obstruction, intestine) 560.9
Locked-in state 344.81
Locked twins 660.5
affecting fetus or newborn 763.1
Locking
joint (*see also* Derangement, joint) 718.90
knee 717.9
Lockjaw (*see also* Tetanus) 037
Locomotor ataxia (progressive) 094.0
Löffler's
endocarditis 421.0
eosinophilia or syndrome 518.3
pneumonia 518.3
syndrome (eosinophilic pneumonitis) 518.3
Löfgren's syndrome (sarcoidosis) 135
Loiasis 125.2
eyelid 125.2 *[373.6]*
Loneliness V62.89
Lone Star fever 082.8
Long labor 662.1
affecting fetus or newborn 763.89
first stage 662.0
second stage 662.2
Longitudinal stripes or grooves, nails 703.8
congenital 757.5
Long-term (current) drug use V58.69
antibiotics V58.62
Long-term *(Continued)*
anticoagulants V58.61
anti-inflammatories, non-steroidal (NSAID) V58.64
antiplatelets/antithrombotics V58.63
aspirin V58.66
insulin V58.67
steroids V58.65
Loop
intestine (*see also* Volvulus) 560.2
intrascleral nerve 379.29
vascular on papilla (optic) 743.57
Loose - *see also* condition
body
in tendon sheath 727.82
joint 718.10
ankle 718.17
elbow 718.12
foot 718.17
hand 718.14
hip 718.15
knee 717.6
multiple sites 718.19
pelvic region 718.15
prosthetic implant - *see* Complications, mechanical
shoulder (region) 718.11
specified site NEC 718.18
wrist 718.13
cartilage (joint) (*see also* Loose, body, joint) 718.1
knee 717.6
facet (vertebral) 724.9
prosthetic implant - *see* Complications, mechanical
sesamoid, joint (*see also* Loose, body, joint) 718.1
tooth, teeth 525.8
Loosening epiphysis 732.9
Looser (-Debray)-Milkman syndrome (osteomalacia with pseudofractures) 268.2
Lop ear (deformity) 744.29
Lorain's disease or syndrome (pituitary dwarfism) 253.3
Lorain-Levi syndrome (pituitary dwarfism) 253.3
Lordosis (acquired) (postural) 737.20
congenital 754.2
due to or associated with
Charcôt-Marie-Tooth disease 356.1 *[737.42]*
mucopolysaccharidosis 277.5 *[737.42]*
neurofibromatosis 237.71 *[737.42]*
osteitis
deformans 731.0 *[737.42]*
fibrosa cystica 252.01 *[737.42]*
osteoporosis (*see also* Osteoporosis) 733.00 *[737.42]*
poliomyelitis (*see also* Poliomyelitis) 138 *[737.42]*
tuberculosis (*see also* Tuberculosis) 015.0 *[737.42]*
late effect of rickets 268.1 *[737.42]*
postlaminectomy 737.21
postsurgical NEC 737.22
rachitic 268.1 *[737.42]*
specified NEC 737.29
tuberculous (*see also* Tuberculosis) 015.0 *[737.42]*
Loss
appetite 783.0
hysterical 300.11

- **Loss** *(Continued)*
  - appetite *(Continued)*
    - nonorganic origin 307.59
    - psychogenic 307.59
  - blood - *see* Hemorrhage
  - central vision 368.41
  - consciousness 780.09
    - transient 780.2
  - control, sphincter, rectum 787.6
    - nonorganic origin 307.7
  - ear ossicle, partial 385.24
  - elasticity, skin 782.8
  - extremity or member, traumatic, current - *see* Amputation, traumatic
  - fluid (acute) 276.50
    - with
      - hypernatremia 276.0
      - hyponatremia 276.1
    - fetus or newborn 775.5
  - hair 704.00
  - hearing - *see also* Deafness
    - central, bilateral 389.14
    - conductive (air) 389.00
      - with sensorineural hearing loss 389.2
      - combined types 389.08
      - external ear 389.01
      - inner ear 389.04
      - middle ear 389.03
      - multiple types 389.08
      - tympanic membrane 389.02
    - mixed type 389.2
    - nerve, bilateral 389.12
    - neural, bilateral 389.12
    - noise-induced 388.12
    - perceptive NEC (*see also* Loss, hearing, sensorineural) 389.10
    - sensorineural 389.10
      - with conductive hearing loss 389.2
      - asymmetrical 389.16
      - central, bilateral 389.14
      - combined types, bilateral 389.18
      - multiple types, bilateral 389.18
      - neural, bilateral 389.12
      - sensory, bilateral 389.11
      - unilateral 389.15
    - sensory, bilateral 389.11
    - specified type NEC 389.8
    - sudden NEC 388.2
  - height 781.91
  - labyrinthine reactivity (unilateral) 386.55
    - bilateral 386.56
  - memory (*see also* Amnesia) 780.93
    - mild, following organic brain damage 310.1
  - mind (*see also* Psychosis) 298.9
  - occusal vertical dimension 524.37
  - organ or part - *see* Absence, by site, acquired
  - sensation 782.0
  - sense of
    - smell (*see also* Disturbance, sensation) 781.1
    - taste (*see also* Disturbance, sensation) 781.1
    - touch (*see also* Disturbance, sensation) 781.1
  - sight (acquired) (complete) (congenital) - *see* Blindness
  - spinal fluid
    - headache 349.0
- **Loss** *(Continued)*
  - substance of
    - bone (*see also* Osteoporosis) 733.00
    - cartilage 733.99
      - ear 380.32
    - vitreous (humor) 379.26
  - tooth, teeth
    - acquired 525.10
      - due to
        - caries 525.13
        - extraction 525.10
        - periodontal disease 525.12
        - specified NEC 525.19
        - trauma 525.11
  - vision, visual (*see also* Blindness) 369.9
    - both eyes (*see also* Blindness, both eyes) 369.3
    - complete (*see also* Blindness, both eyes) 369.00
    - one eye 369.8
    - sudden 368.11
    - transient 368.12
  - vitreous 379.26
  - voice (*see also* Aphonia) 784.41
  - weight (cause unknown) 783.21
- **Lou Gehrig's disease** 335.20
- **Louis-Bar syndrome** (ataxia-telangiectasia) 334.8
- **Louping ill** 063.1
- **Lousiness** - *see* Lice
- **Low**
  - back syndrome 724.2
  - basal metabolic rate (BMR) 794.7
  - birthweight 765.1
    - extreme (less than 1000 grams) 765.0
    - for gestational age 764.0
    - status (*see also* Status, low birth weight) V21.30
  - bladder compliance 596.52
  - blood pressure (*see also* Hypotension) 458.9
    - reading (incidental) (isolated) (nonspecific) 796.3
  - cardiac reserve - *see* Disease, heart
  - compliance bladder 596.52
  - frequency deafness - *see* Disorder, hearing
  - function - *see also* Hypofunction
    - kidney (*see also* Disease, renal) 593.9
    - liver 573.9
  - hemoglobin 285.9
  - implantation, placenta - *see* Placenta, previa
  - insertion, placenta - *see* Placenta, previa
  - lying
    - kidney 593.0
    - organ or site, congenital - *see* Malposition, congenital
    - placenta - *see* Placenta, previa
  - output syndrome (cardiac) (*see also* Failure, heart) 428.9
  - platelets (blood) (*see also* Thrombocytopenia) 287.5
  - reserve, kidney (*see also* Disease, renal) 593.9
  - risk
    - cervical, human papillomavirus (HPV) DNA test positive 795.09
  - salt syndrome 593.9
  - tension glaucoma 365.12
  - vision 369.9
    - both eyes 369.20
    - one eye 369.70
- **Lowe** (-Terrey-MacLachlan) syndrome (oculocerebrorenal dystrophy) 270.8
- **Lower extremity** - *see* condition
- **Lown** (-Ganong)-Levine syndrome (short P-R interval, normal QRS complex, and paroxysmal supraventricular tachycardia) 426.81
- **LSD reaction** (*see also* Abuse, drugs, nondependent) 305.3
- **L-shaped kidney** 753.3
- **Lucas-Championnière disease** (fibrinous bronchitis) 466.0
- **Lucey-Driscoll syndrome** (jaundice due to delayed conjugation) 774.30
- **Ludwig's**
  - angina 528.3
  - disease (submaxillary cellulitis) 528.3
- **Lues** (venerea), luetic - *see* Syphilis
- **Luetscher's syndrome** (dehydration) 276.51
- **Lumbago** 724.2
  - due to displacement, intervertebral disc 722.10
- **Lumbalgia** 724.2
  - due to displacement, intervertebral disc 722.10
- **Lumbar** - *see* condition
- **Lumbarization, vertebra** 756.15
- **Lumbermen's itch** 133.8
- **Lump** - *see also* Mass
  - abdominal 789.3
  - breast 611.72
  - chest 786.6
  - epigastric 789.3
  - head 784.2
  - kidney 753.3
  - liver 789.1
  - lung 786.6
  - mediastinal 786.6
  - neck 784.2
  - nose or sinus 784.2
  - pelvic 789.3
  - skin 782.2
  - substernal 786.6
  - throat 784.2
  - umbilicus 789.3
- **Lunacy** (*see also* Psychosis) 298.9
- **Lunatomalacia** 732.3
- **Lung** - *see also* condition
  - donor V59.8
  - drug addict's 417.8
  - mainliners' 417.8
  - vanishing 492.0
- **Lupoid** (miliary) of Boeck 135
- **Lupus** 710.0
  - anticoagulant 289.81
  - Cazenave's (erythematosus) 695.4
  - discoid (local) 695.4
  - disseminated 710.0
  - erythematodes (discoid) (local) 695.4
  - erythematosus (discoid) (local) 695.4
    - disseminated 710.0
    - eyelid 373.34
    - systemic 710.0
      - with
        - encephalitis 710.0 *[323.81]*
        - lung involvement 710.0 *[517.8]*
      - inhibitor (presence of) 286.5
  - exedens 017.0
  - eyelid (*see also* Tuberculosis) 017.0 *[373.4]*
  - Hilliard's 017.0

Lupus *(Continued)*
hydralazine
correct substance properly administered 695.4
overdose or wrong substance given or taken 972.6
miliaris disseminatus faciei 017.0
nephritis 710.0 *[583.81]*
acute 710.0 *[580.81]*
chronic 710.0 *[582.81]*
nontuberculous, not disseminated 695.4
pernio (Besnier) 135
tuberculous (*see also* Tuberculosis) 017.0
eyelid (*see also* Tuberculosis) 017.0 *[373.4]*
vulgaris 017.0
Luschka's joint disease 721.90
Luteinoma (M8610/0) 220
Lutembacher's disease or syndrome (atrial septal defect with mitral stenosis) 745.5
Luteoma (M8610/0) 220
Lutz-Miescher disease (elastosis perforans serpiginosa) 701.1
Lutz-Splendore-de Almeida disease (Brazilian blastomycosis) 116.1
Luxatio
bulbi due to birth injury 767.8
coxae congenita (*see also* Dislocation, hip, congenital) 754.30
erecta - *see* Dislocation, shoulder
imperfecta - *see* Sprain, by site
perinealis - *see* Dislocation, hip
Luxation - *see also* Dislocation, by site
eyeball 360.81
due to birth injury 767.8
lateral 376.36
genital organs (external) NEC - *see* Wound, open, genital organs
globe (eye) 360.81
lateral 376.36
lacrimal gland (postinfectional) 375.16
lens (old) (partial) 379.32
congenital 743.37
syphilitic 090.49 *[379.32]*
Marfan's disease 090.49
spontaneous 379.32
penis - *see* Wound, open, penis
scrotum - *see* Wound, open, scrotum
testis - *see* Wound, open, testis
L-xyloketosuria 271.8
Lycanthropy (*see also* Psychosis) 298.9
Lyell's disease or syndrome (toxic epidermal necrolysis) 695.1
due to drug
correct substance properly administered 695.1
overdose or wrong substance given or taken 977.9
specified drug - *see* Table of Drugs and Chemicals
Lyme disease 088.81
Lymph
gland or node - *see* condition
scrotum (*see also* Infestation, filarial) 125.9
Lymphadenitis 289.3
with
abortion - *see* Abortion, by type, with sepsis
ectopic pregnancy (*see also* categories 633.0–633.9) 639.0
molar pregnancy (*see also* categories 630–632) 639.0
Lymphadenitis *(Continued)*
acute 683
mesenteric 289.2
any site, except mesenteric 289.3
acute 683
chronic 289.1
mesenteric (acute) (chronic) (nonspecific) (subacute) 289.2
subacute 289.1
mesenteric 289.2
breast, puerperal, postpartum 675.2
chancroidal (congenital) 099.0
chronic 289.1
mesenteric 289.2
dermatopathic 695.89
due to
anthracosis (occupational) 500
Brugia (Wuchereria) malayi 125.1
diphtheria (toxin) 032.89
lymphogranuloma venereum 099.1
Wuchereria bancrofti 125.0
following
abortion 639.0
ectopic or molar pregnancy 639.0
generalized 289.3
gonorrheal 098.89
granulomatous 289.1
infectional 683
mesenteric (acute) (chronic) (nonspecific) (subacute) 289.2
due to Bacillus typhi 002.0
tuberculous (*see also* Tuberculosis) 014.8
mycobacterial 031.8
purulent 683
pyogenic 683
regional 078.3
septic 683
streptococcal 683
subacute, unspecified site 289.1
suppurative 683
syphilitic (early) (secondary) 091.4
late 095.8
tuberculous - *see* Tuberculosis, lymph gland
venereal 099.1
Lymphadenoid goiter 245.2
Lymphadenopathy (general) 785.6
due to toxoplasmosis (acquired) 130.7
congenital (active) 771.2
Lymphadenopathy-associated virus (disease) (illness) (infection) - *see* Human immunodeficiency virus (disease) (illness) (infection)
Lymphadenosis 785.6
acute 075
Lymphangiectasis 457.1
conjunctiva 372.89
postinfectional 457.1
scrotum 457.1
Lymphangiectatic elephantiasis, nonfilarial 457.1
Lymphangioendothelioma (M9170/0) 228.1
malignant (M9170/3) - *see* Neoplasm, connective tissue, malignant
Lymphangioma (M9170/0) 228.1
capillary (M9171/0) 228.1
cavernous (M9172/0) 228.1
cystic (M9173/0) 228.1
malignant (M9170/3) - *see* Neoplasm, connective tissue, malignant
Lymphangiomyoma (M9174/0) 228.1
Lymphangiomyomatosis (M9174/1) - *see* Neoplasm, connective tissue, uncertain behavior
Lymphangiosarcoma (M9170/3) - *see* Neoplasm, connective tissue, malignant
Lymphangitis 457.2
with
abortion - *see* Abortion, by type, with sepsis
abscess - *see* Abscess, by site
cellulitis - *see* Abscess, by site
ectopic pregnancy (*see also* categories 633.0–633.9) 639.0
molar pregnancy (*see also* categories 630–632) 639.0
acute (with abscess or cellulitis) 682.9
specified site - *see* Abscess, by site
breast, puerperal, postpartum 675.2
chancroidal 099.0
chronic (any site) 457.2
due to
Brugia (Wuchereria) malayi 125.1
Wuchereria bancrofti 125.0
following
abortion 639.0
ectopic or molar pregnancy 639.0
gangrenous 457.2
penis
acute 607.2
gonococcal (acute) 098.0
chronic or duration of 2 months or more 098.2
puerperal, postpartum, childbirth 670
strumous, tuberculous (*see also* Tuberculosis) 017.2
subacute (any site) 457.2
tuberculous - *see* Tuberculosis, lymph gland
Lymphatic (vessel) - *see* condition
Lymphatism 254.8
scrofulous (*see also* Tuberculosis) 017.2
Lymphectasia 457.1
Lymphedema (*see also* Elephantiasis) 457.1
acquired (chronic) 457.1
chronic hereditary 757.0
congenital 757.0
idiopathic hereditary 757.0
praecox 457.1
secondary 457.1
surgical NEC 997.99
postmastectomy (syndrome) 457.0
Lymph-hemangioma (M9120/0) - *see* Hemangioma, by site
Lymphoblastic - *see* condition
Lymphoblastoma (diffuse) (M9630/3) 200.1
giant follicular (M9690/3) 202.0
macrofollicular (M9690/3) 202.0
Lymphoblastosis, acute benign 075
Lymphocele 457.8
Lymphocythemia 288.51
Lymphocytic - *see also* condition
chorioencephalitis (acute) (serous) 049.0
choriomeningitis (acute) (serous) 049.0
Lymphocytoma (diffuse) (malignant) (M9620/3) 200.1
Lymphocytomatosis (M9620/3) 200.1
Lymphocytopenia 288.51
Lymphocytosis (symptomatic) 288.61
infectious (acute) 078.89
Lymphoepithelioma (M8082/3) - *see* Neoplasm, by site, malignant

- **Lymphogranuloma** (malignant) (M9650/3) 201.9
  - inguinale 099.1
  - venereal (any site) 099.1
    - with stricture of rectum 099.1
  - venereum 099.1
- **Lymphogranulomatosis** (malignant) (M9650/3) 201.9
  - benign (Boeck's sarcoid) (Schaumann's) 135
  - Hodgkin's (M9650/3) 201.9
- **Lymphohistiocytosis, familial hemophagocytic** 288.4 ◀
- **Lymphoid** - *see* condition
- **Lympholeukoblastoma** (M9850/3) 207.8
- **Lympholeukosarcoma** (M9850/3) 207.8
- **Lymphoma** (malignant) (M9590/3) 202.8

> Note Use the following fifth-digit subclassification with categories 200–202:
>
> 0 unspecified site, extranodal and solid organ sites
> 1 lymph nodes of head, face, and neck
> 2 intrathoracic lymph nodes
> 3 intra-abdominal lymph nodes
> 4 lymph nodes of axilla and upper limb
> 5 lymph nodes of inguinal region and lower limb
> 6 intrapelvic lymph nodes
> 7 spleen
> 8 lymph nodes of multiple sites

  - benign (M9590/0) - *see* Neoplasm, by site, benign
  - Burkitt's type (lymphoblastic) (undifferentiated) (M9750/3) 200.2
  - Castleman's (mediastinal lymph node hyperplasia) 785.6
  - centroblastic-centrocytic
    - diffuse (M9614/3) 202.8
    - follicular (M9692/3) 202.0
  - centroblastic type (diffuse) (M9632/3) 202.8
    - follicular (M9697/3) 202.0
  - centrocytic (M9622/3) 202.8
  - compound (M9613/3) 200.8
  - convoluted cell type (lymphoblastic) (M9602/3) 202.8
  - diffuse NEC (M9590/3) 202.8
  - follicular (giant) (M9690/3) 202.0
    - center cell (diffuse) (M9615/3) 202.8
      - cleaved (diffuse) (M9623/3) 202.8
        - follicular (M9695/3) 202.0
      - non-cleaved (diffuse) (M9633/3) 202.8
        - follicular (M9698/3) 202.0
    - centroblastic-centrocytic (M9692/3) 202.0
    - centroblastic type (M9697/3) 202.0

- **Lymphoma** *(Continued)*
  - follicular *(Continued)*
    - lymphocytic
      - intermediate differentiation (M9694/3) 202.0
      - poorly differentiated (M9696/3) 202.0
    - mixed (cell type) (lymphocytic-histiocytic) (small cell and large cell) (M9691/3) 202.0
  - germinocytic (M9622/3) 202.8
  - giant, follicular or follicle (M9690/3) 202.0
  - histiocytic (diffuse) (M9640/3) 200.0
    - nodular (M9642/3) 200.0
    - pleomorphic cell type (M9641/3) 200.0
  - Hodgkin's (M9650/3) (*see also* Disease, Hodgkin's) 201.9
  - immunoblastic (type) (M9612/3) 200.8
  - large cell (M9640/3) 200.0
    - nodular (M9642/3) 200.0
    - pleomorphic cell type (M9641/3) 200.0
  - lymphoblastic (diffuse) (M9630/3) 200.1
    - Burkitt's type (M9750/3) 200.2
    - convoluted cell type (M9602/3) 202.8
  - lymphocytic (cell type) (diffuse) (M9620/3) 200.1
    - with plasmacytoid differentiation, diffuse (M9611/3) 200.8
    - intermediate differentiation (diffuse) (M9621/3) 200.1
      - follicular (M9694/3) 202.0
      - nodular (M9694/3) 202.0
    - nodular (M9690/3) 202.0
    - poorly differentiated (diffuse) (M9630/3) 200.1
      - follicular (M9696/3) 202.0
      - nodular (M9696/3) 202.0
    - well differentiated (diffuse) (M9620/3) 200.1
      - follicular (M9693/3) 202.0
      - nodular (M9693/3) 202.0
  - lymphocytic-histiocytic, mixed (diffuse) (M9613/3) 200.8
    - follicular (M9691/3) 202.0
    - nodular (M9691/3) 202.0
  - lymphoplasmacytoid type (M9611/3) 200.8
  - lymphosarcoma type (M9610/3) 200.1
  - macrofollicular (M9690/3) 202.0
  - mixed cell type (diffuse) (M9613/3) 200.8
    - follicular (M9691/3) 202.0
    - nodular (M9691/3) 202.0
  - nodular (M9690/3) 202.0
    - histiocytic (M9642/3) 200.0
    - lymphocytic (M9690/3) 202.0
      - intermediate differentiation (M9694/3) 202.0
      - poorly differentiated (M9696/3) 202.0

- **Lymphoma** *(Continued)*
  - nodular *(Continued)*
    - mixed (cell type) (lymphocytic-histiocytic) (small cell and large cell) (M9691/3) 202.0
  - non-Hodgkin's type NEC (M9591/3) 202.8
  - reticulum cell (type) (M9640/3) 200.0
  - small cell and large cell, mixed (diffuse) (M9613/3) 200.8
    - follicular (M9691/3) 202.0
    - nodular (9691/3) 202.0
  - stem cell (type) (M9601/3) 202.8
  - T-cell 202.1
  - undifferentiated (cell type) (non-Burkitt's) (M9600/3) 202.8
    - Burkitt's type (M9750/3) 200.2
- **Lymphomatosis** (M9590/3) - *see also* Lymphoma
  - granulomatous 099.1
- **Lymphopathia**
  - venereum 099.1
  - veneris 099.1
- **Lymphopenia** 288.51 ⟸
  - familial 279.2
- **Lymphoreticulosis, benign** (of inoculation) 078.3
- **Lymphorrhea** 457.8
- **Lymphosarcoma** (M9610/3) 200.1
  - diffuse (M9610/3) 200.1
    - with plasmacytoid differentiation (M9611/3) 200.8
    - lymphoplasmacytic (M9611/3) 200.8
  - follicular (giant) (M9690/3) 202.0
    - lymphoblastic (M9696/3) 202.0
    - lymphocytic, intermediate differentiation (M9694/3) 202.0
    - mixed cell type (M9691/3) 202.0
  - giant follicular (M9690/3) 202.0
  - Hodgkin's (M9650/3) 201.9
  - immunoblastic (M9612/3) 200.8
  - lymphoblastic (diffuse) (M9630/3) 200.1
    - follicular (M9696/3) 202.0
    - nodular (M9696/3) 202.0
  - lymphocytic (diffuse) (M9620/3) 200.1
    - intermediate differentiation (diffuse) (M9621/3) 200.1
      - follicular (M9694/3) 202.0
      - nodular (M9694/3) 202.0
  - mixed cell type (diffuse) (M9613/3) 200.8
    - follicular (M9691/3) 202.0
    - nodular (M9691/3) 202.0
  - nodular (M9690/3) 202.0
    - lymphoblastic (M9696/3) 202.0
    - lymphocytic, intermediate differentiation (M9694/3) 202.0
    - mixed cell type (M9691/3) 202.0
  - prolymphocytic (M9631/3) 200.1
  - reticulum cell (M9640/3) 200.0
- **Lymphostasis** 457.8
- **Lypemania** (*see also* Melancholia) 296.2
- **Lyssa** 071

M

Macacus ear 744.29
Maceration
fetus (cause not stated) 779.9
wet feet, tropical (syndrome) 991.4
Machado-Joseph disease 334.8
Machupo virus hemorrhagic fever 078.7
Macleod's syndrome (abnormal transradiancy, one lung) 492.8
Macrocephalia, macrocephaly 756.0
Macrocheilia (congenital) 744.81
Macrochilia (congenital) 744.81
Macrocolon (congenital) 751.3
Macrocornea 743.41
associated with buphthalmos 743.22
Macrocytic - *see* condition
Macrocytosis 289.89
Macrodactylia, macrodactylism (fingers) (thumbs) 755.57
toes 755.65
Macrodontia 520.2
Macroencephaly 742.4
Macrogenia 524.05
Macrogenitosomia (female) (male) (praecox) 255.2
Macrogingivae 523.8
Macroglobulinemia (essential) (idiopathic) (monoclonal) (primary) (syndrome) (Waldenström's) 273.3
Macroglossia (congenital) 750.15
acquired 529.8
Macrognathia, macrognathism (congenital) 524.00
mandibular 524.02
alveolar 524.72
maxillary 524.01
alveolar 524.71
Macrogyria (congenital) 742.4
Macrohydrocephalus (*see also* Hydrocephalus) 331.4
Macromastia (*see also* Hypertrophy, breast) 611.1
Macrophage activation syndrome 288.4 ◀
Macropsia 368.14
Macrosigmoid 564.7
congenital 751.3
Macrospondylitis, acromegalic 253.0
Macrostomia (congenital) 744.83
Macrotia (external ear) (congenital) 744.22
Macula
cornea, corneal
congenital 743.43
interfering with vision 743.42
interfering with central vision 371.03
not interfering with central vision 371.02
degeneration (*see also* Degeneration, macula) 362.50
hereditary (*see also* Dystrophy, retina) 362.70
edema, cystoid 362.53
Maculae ceruleae 132.1
Macules and papules 709.8
Maculopathy, toxic 362.55
Madarosis 374.55
Madelung's
deformity (radius) 755.54
disease (lipomatosis) 272.8
lipomatosis 272.8
Madness (*see also* Psychosis) 298.9
myxedema (acute) 293.0
subacute 293.1
Madura
disease (actinomycotic) 039.9
mycotic 117.4
foot (actinomycotic) 039.4
mycotic 117.4
Maduromycosis (actinomycotic) 039.9
mycotic 117.4
Maffucci's syndrome (dyschondroplasia with hemangiomas) 756.4
Magenblase syndrome 306.4
Main en griffe (acquired) 736.06
congenital 755.59
Maintenance
chemotherapy regimen or treatment V58.11
dialysis regimen or treatment
extracorporeal (renal) V56.0
peritoneal V56.8
renal V56.0
drug therapy or regimen
chemotherapy, antineoplastic V58.11
immunotherapy, antineoplastic V58.12
external fixation NEC V54.89
radiotherapy V58.0
traction NEC V54.89
Majocchi's
disease (purpura annularis telangiectodes) 709.1
granuloma 110.6
Major - *see* condition
Mal
cerebral (idiopathic) (*see also* Epilepsy) 345.9
comital (*see also* Epilepsy) 345.9
de los pintos (*see also* Pinta) 103.9
de Meleda 757.39
de mer 994.6
lie - *see* Presentation, fetal
perforant (*see also* Ulcer, lower extremity) 707.15
Malabar itch 110.9
beard 110.0
foot 110.4
scalp 110.0
Malabsorption 579.9
calcium 579.8
carbohydrate 579.8
disaccharide 271.3
drug-induced 579.8
due to bacterial overgrowth 579.8
fat 579.8
folate, congenital 281.2
galactose 271.1
glucose-galactose (congenital) 271.3
intestinal 579.9
isomaltose 271.3
lactose (hereditary) 271.3
methionine 270.4
monosaccharide 271.8
postgastrectomy 579.3
postsurgical 579.3
protein 579.8
sucrose (-isomaltose) (congenital) 271.3
syndrome 579.9
postgastrectomy 579.3
postsurgical 579.3
Malacia, bone 268.2
juvenile (*see also* Rickets) 268.0
Kienböck's (juvenile) (lunate) (wrist) 732.3
adult 732.8
Malacoplakia
bladder 596.8
colon 569.89
Malacoplakia *(Continued)*
pelvis (kidney) 593.89
ureter 593.89
urethra 599.84
Malacosteon 268.2
juvenile (*see also* Rickets) 268.0
Maladaptation - *see* Maladjustment
Maladie de Roger 745.4
Maladjustment
conjugal V61.10
involving divorce or estrangement V61.0
educational V62.3
family V61.9
specified circumstance NEC V61.8
marital V61.10
involving divorce or estrangement V61.0
occupational V62.2
simple, adult (*see also* Reaction, adjustment) 309.9
situational acute (*see also* Reaction, adjustment) 309.9
social V62.4
Malaise 780.79
Malakoplakia - *see* Malacoplakia
Malaria, malarial (fever) 084.6
algid 084.9
any type, with
algid malaria 084.9
blackwater fever 084.8
fever
blackwater 084.8
hemoglobinuric (bilious) 084.8
hemoglobinuria, malarial 084.8
hepatitis 084.9 *[573.2]*
nephrosis 084.9 *[581.81]*
pernicious complication NEC 084.9
cardiac 084.9
cerebral 084.9
cardiac 084.9
carrier (suspected) of V02.9
cerebral 084.9
complicating pregnancy, childbirth, or puerperium 647.4
congenital 771.2
congestion, congestive 084.6
brain 084.9
continued 084.0
estivo-autumnal 084.0
falciparum (malignant tertian) 084.0
hematinuria 084.8
hematuria 084.8
hemoglobinuria 084.8
hemorrhagic 084.6
induced (therapeutically) 084.7
accidental - *see* Malaria, by type
liver 084.9 *[573.2]*
malariae (quartan) 084.2
malignant (tertian) 084.0
mixed infections 084.5
monkey 084.4
ovale 084.3
pernicious, acute 084.0
Plasmodium, P.
falciparum 084.0
malariae 084.2
ovale 084.3
vivax 084.1
quartan 084.2
quotidian 084.0
recurrent 084.6
induced (therapeutically) 084.7
accidental - *see* Malaria, by type

Malaria, malarial *(Continued)*
remittent 084.6
specified types NEC 084.4
spleen 084.6
subtertian 084.0
tertian (benign) 084.1
malignant 084.0
tropical 084.0
typhoid 084.6
vivax (benign tertian) 084.1
Malassez's disease (testicular cyst) 608.89
Malassimilation 579.9
Maldescent, testis 752.51
Maldevelopment - *see also* Anomaly, by site
brain 742.9
colon 751.5
hip (joint) 755.63
congenital dislocation (*see also* Dislocation, hip, congenital) 754.30
mastoid process 756.0
middle ear, except ossicles 744.03
ossicles 744.04
newborn (not malformation) 764.9
ossicles, ear 744.04
spine 756.10
toe 755.66
Male type pelvis 755.69
with disproportion (fetopelvic) 653.2
affecting fetus or newborn 763.1
causing obstructed labor 660.1
affecting fetus or newborn 763.1
Malformation (congenital) - *see also* Anomaly
bone 756.9
bursa 756.9
Chiari
type I 348.4
type II (*see also* Spina bifida) 741.0
type III 742.0
type IV 742.2
circulatory system NEC 747.9
specified type NEC 747.89
cochlea 744.05
digestive system NEC 751.9
lower 751.5
specified type NEC 751.8
upper 750.9
eye 743.9
gum 750.9
heart NEC 746.9
specified type NEC 746.89
valve 746.9
internal ear 744.05
joint NEC 755.9
specified type NEC 755.8
Mondini's (congenital) (malformation, cochlea) 744.05
muscle 756.9
nervous system (central) 742.9
pelvic organs or tissues
in pregnancy or childbirth 654.9
affecting fetus or newborn 763.89
causing obstructed labor 660.2
affecting fetus or newborn 763.1
placenta (*see also* Placenta, abnormal) 656.7
respiratory organs 748.9
specified type NEC 748.8
Rieger's 743.44
sense organs NEC 742.9
specified type NEC 742.8
skin 757.9
specified type NEC 757.8

Malformation *(Continued)*
spinal cord 742.9
teeth, tooth NEC 520.9
tendon 756.9
throat 750.9
umbilical cord (complicating delivery) 663.9
affecting fetus or newborn 762.6
umbilicus 759.9
urinary system NEC 753.9
specified type NEC 753.8
Malfunction - *see also* Dysfunction
arterial graft 996.1
cardiac pacemaker 996.01
catheter device - *see* Complications, mechanical, catheter
colostomy 569.62
valve 569.62 ◀
cystostomy 997.5
device, implant, or graft NEC - *see* Complications, mechanical
enteric stoma 569.62
enterostomy 569.62
esophagostomy 530.87
gastroenteric 536.8
gastrostomy 536.42
ileostomy ◀
valve 569.62 ◀
nephrostomy 997.5
pacemaker - *see* Complications, mechanical, pacemaker
prosthetic device, internal - *see* Complications, mechanical
tracheostomy 519.02
valve ◀
colostomy 569.62 ◀
ileostomy 569.62 ◀
vascular graft or shunt 996.1
Malgaigne's fracture (closed) 808.43
open 808.53
Malherbe's
calcifying epithelioma (M8110/0) - *see* Neoplasm, skin, benign
tumor (M8110/0) - *see* Neoplasm, skin, benign
Malibu disease 919.8
infected 919.9
Malignancy (M8000/3) - *see* Neoplasm, by site, malignant
Malignant - *see* condition
Malingerer, malingering V65.2
Mallet, finger (acquired) 736.1
congenital 755.59
late effect of rickets 268.1
Malleus 024
Mallory's bodies 034.1
Mallory-Weiss syndrome 530.7
Malnutrition (calorie) 263.9
complicating pregnancy 648.9
degree
first 263.1
second 263.0
third 262
mild 263.1
moderate 263.0
severe 261
protein-calorie 262
fetus 764.2
"light-for-dates" 764.1
following gastrointestinal surgery 579.3
intrauterine or fetal 764.2
fetus or infant "light-for-dates" 764.1

Malnutrition *(Continued)*
lack of care, or neglect (child) (infant) 995.52
adult 995.84
malignant 260
mild 263.1
moderate 263.0
protein 260
protein-calorie 263.9
severe 262
specified type NEC 263.8
severe 261
protein-calorie NEC 262
Malocclusion (teeth) 524.4
angle's class I 524.21 ◀
angle's class II 524.22 ◀
angle's class III 524.23 ◀
due to
abnormal swallowing 524.59
accessory teeth (causing crowding) 524.31
dentofacial abnormality NEC 524.89
impacted teeth (causing crowding) 520.6
missing teeth 524.30
mouth breathing 524.59
sleep postures 524.59
supernumerary teeth (causing crowding) 524.31
thumb sucking 524.59
tongue, lip, or finger habits 524.59
temporomandibular (joint) 524.69
Malposition
cardiac apex (congenital) 746.87
cervix - *see* Malposition, uterus
congenital
adrenal (gland) 759.1
alimentary tract 751.8
lower 751.5
upper 750.8
aorta 747.21
appendix 751.5
arterial trunk 747.29
artery (peripheral) NEC (*see also* Malposition, congenital, peripheral vascular system) 747.60
coronary 746.85
pulmonary 747.3
auditory canal 744.29
causing impairment of hearing 744.02
auricle (ear) 744.29
causing impairment of hearing 744.02
cervical 744.43
biliary duct or passage 751.69
bladder (mucosa) 753.8
exteriorized or extroverted 753.5
brachial plexus 742.8
brain tissue 742.4
breast 757.6
bronchus 748.3
cardiac apex 746.87
cecum 751.5
clavicle 755.51
colon 751.5
digestive organ or tract NEC 751.8
lower 751.5
upper 750.8
ear (auricle) (external) 744.29
ossicles 744.04
endocrine (gland) NEC 759.2
epiglottis 748.3

Malposition *(Continued)*
congenital *(Continued)*
Eustachian tube 744.24
eye 743.8
facial features 744.89
fallopian tube 752.19
finger(s) 755.59
supernumerary 755.01
foot 755.67
gallbladder 751.69
gastrointestinal tract 751.8
genitalia, genital organ(s) or tract
female 752.89
external 752.49
internal NEC 752.89
male 752.89
penis 752.69
scrotal transposition 752.81
glottis 748.3
hand 755.59
heart 746.87
dextrocardia 746.87
with complete transposition of viscera 759.3
hepatic duct 751.69
hip (joint) (*see also* Dislocation, hip, congenital) 754.30
intestine (large) (small) 751.5
with anomalous adhesions, fixation, or malrotation 751.4
joint NEC 755.8
kidney 753.3
larynx 748.3
limb 755.8
lower 755.69
upper 755.59
liver 751.69
lung (lobe) 748.69
nail(s) 757.5
nerve 742.8
nervous system NEC 742.8
nose, nasal (septum) 748.1
organ or site NEC - *see* Anomaly, specified type NEC, by site
ovary 752.0
pancreas 751.7
parathyroid (gland) 759.2
patella 755.64
peripheral vascular system 747.60
gastrointestinal 747.61
lower limb 747.64
renal 747.62
specified NEC 747.69
spinal 747.82
upper limb 747.63
pituitary (gland) 759.2
respiratory organ or system NEC 748.9
rib (cage) 756.3
supernumerary in cervical region 756.2
scapula 755.59
shoulder 755.59
spinal cord 742.59
spine 756.19
spleen 759.0
sternum 756.3
stomach 750.7
symphysis pubis 755.69
testis (undescended) 752.51
thymus (gland) 759.2
thyroid (gland) (tissue) 759.2
cartilage 748.3
toe(s) 755.66
supernumerary 755.02
tongue 750.19

Malposition *(Continued)*
congenital *(Continued)*
trachea 748.3
uterus 752.3
vein(s) (peripheral) NEC (*see also* Malposition, congenital, peripheral vascular system) 747.60
great 747.49
portal 747.49
pulmonary 747.49
vena cava (inferior) (superior) 747.49
device, implant, or graft - *see* Complications, mechanical
fetus NEC (*see also* Presentation, fetal) 652.9
with successful version 652.1
affecting fetus or newborn 763.1
before labor, affecting fetus or newborn 761.7
causing obstructed labor 660.0
in multiple gestation (one fetus or more) 652.6
with locking 660.5
causing obstructed labor 660.0
gallbladder (*see also* Disease, gallbladder) 575.8
gastrointestinal tract 569.89
congenital 751.8
heart (*see also* Malposition, congenital, heart) 746.87
intestine 569.89
congenital 751.5
pelvic organs or tissues
in pregnancy or childbirth 654.4
affecting fetus or newborn 763.89
causing obstructed labor 660.2
affecting fetus or newborn 763.1
placenta - *see* Placenta, previa
stomach 537.89
congenital 750.7
tooth, teeth 524.30
with impaction 520.6
uterus (acquired) (acute) (adherent) (any degree) (asymptomatic) (postinfectional) (postpartal, old) 621.6 ⬅
anteflexion or anteversion (*see also* Anteversion, uterus) 621.6
congenital 752.3
flexion 621.6
lateral (*see also* Lateroversion, uterus) 621.6
in pregnancy or childbirth 654.4
affecting fetus or newborn 763.89
causing obstructed labor 660.2
affecting fetus or newborn 763.1
inversion 621.6
lateral (flexion) (version) (*see also* Lateroversion, uterus) 621.6
lateroflexion (*see also* Lateroversion, uterus) 621.6
lateroversion (*see also* Lateroversion, uterus) 621.6
retroflexion or retroversion (*see also* Retroversion, uterus) 621.6
Malposture 729.9
Malpresentation, fetus (*see also* Presentation, fetal) 652.9
Malrotation
cecum 751.4
colon 751.4
intestine 751.4
kidney 753.3

Malta fever (*see also* Brucellosis) 023.9
Maltosuria 271.3
Maltreatment (of)
adult 995.80
emotional 995.82
multiple forms 995.85
neglect (nutritional) 995.84
physical 995.81
psychological 995.82
sexual 995.83
child 995.50
emotional 995.51
multiple forms 995.59
neglect (nutritional) 995.52
physical 995.54
shaken infant syndrome 995.55
psychological 995.51
sexual 995.53
spouse (*see also* Maltreatment, adult) 995.80
Malt workers' lung 495.4
Malum coxae senilis 715.25
Malunion, fracture 733.81
Mammillitis (*see also* Mastitis) 611.0
puerperal, postpartum 675.2
Mammitis (*see also* Mastitis) 611.0
puerperal, postpartum 675.2
Mammographic ⬅
calcification 793.89 ◀
calculus 793.89 ◀
microcalcification 793.81 ◀
Mammoplasia 611.1
Management
contraceptive V25.9
specified type NEC V25.8
procreative V26.9
specified type NEC V26.8
Mangled NEC (*see also* nature and site of injury) 959.9
Mania (monopolar) (*see also* Psychosis, affective) 296.0
alcoholic (acute) (chronic) 291.9
Bell's - *see* Mania, chronic
chronic 296.0
recurrent episode 296.1
single episode 296.0
compulsive 300.3
delirious (acute) 296.0
recurrent episode 296.1
single episode 296.0
epileptic (*see also* Epilepsy) 345.4
hysterical 300.10
inhibited 296.89
puerperal (after delivery) 296.0
recurrent episode 296.1
single episode 296.0
recurrent episode 296.1
senile 290.8
single episode 296.0
stupor 296.89
stuporous 296.89
unproductive 296.89
Manic-depressive insanity, psychosis, reaction, or syndrome (*see also* Psychosis, affective) 296.80
circular (alternating) 296.7
currently
depressed 296.5
episode unspecified 296.7
hypomanic, previously depressed 296.4
manic 296.4
mixed 296.6
depressed (type), depressive 296.2

- **Manic-depressive insanity, psychosis, reaction, or syndrome** *(Continued)*
  - depressed (type), depressive *(Continued)*
    - atypical 296.82
    - recurrent episode 296.3
    - single episode 296.2
  - hypomanic 296.0
    - recurrent episode 296.1
    - single episode 296.0
  - manic 296.0
    - atypical 296.81
    - recurrent episode 296.1
    - single episode 296.0
  - mixed NEC 296.89
  - perplexed 296.89
  - stuporous 296.89
- **Manifestations, rheumatoid**
  - lungs 714.81
  - pannus - *see* Arthritis, rheumatoid
  - subcutaneous nodules - *see* Arthritis, rheumatoid
- **Mankowsky's syndrome** (familial dysplastic osteopathy) 731.2
- **Mannoheptulosuria** 271.8
- **Mannosidosis** 271.8
- **Manson's**
  - disease (schistosomiasis) 120.1
  - pyosis (pemphigus contagiosus) 684
  - schistosomiasis 120.1
- **Mansonellosis** 125.5
- **Manual** - *see* condition
- **Maple bark disease** 495.6
- **Maple bark-strippers' lung** 495.6
- **Maple syrup** (urine) disease or syndrome 270.3
- **Marable's syndrome** (celiac artery compression) 447.4
- **Marasmus** 261
  - brain 331.9
  - due to malnutrition 261
  - intestinal 569.89
  - nutritional 261
  - senile 797
  - tuberculous NEC (*see also* Tuberculosis) 011.9
- **Marble**
  - bones 756.52
  - skin 782.61
- **Marburg disease** (virus) 078.89
- **March**
  - foot 733.94
  - hemoglobinuria 283.2
- **Marchand multiple nodular hyperplasia** (liver) 571.5
- **Marchesani** (-Weill) syndrome (brachymorphism and ectopia lentis) 759.89
- **Marchiafava** (-Bignami) disease or syndrome 341.8
- **Marchiafava-Micheli syndrome** (paroxysmal nocturnal hemoglobinuria) 283.2
- **Marcus Gunn's syndrome** (jaw-winking syndrome) 742.8
- **Marfan's**
  - congenital syphilis 090.49
  - disease 090.49
  - syndrome (arachnodactyly) 759.82
    - meaning congenital syphilis 090.49
      - with luxation of lens 090.49 *[379.32]*
- **Marginal**
  - implantation, placenta - *see* Placenta, previa
  - placenta - *see* Placenta, previa
  - sinus (hemorrhage) (rupture) 641.2
    - affecting fetus or newborn 762.1
- **Marie's**
  - cerebellar ataxia 334.2
  - syndrome (acromegaly) 253.0
- **Marie-Bamberger disease or syndrome** (hypertrophic) (pulmonary) (secondary) 731.2
  - idiopathic (acropachyderma) 757.39
  - primary (acropachyderma) 757.39
- **Marie-Charcôt-Tooth neuropathic atrophy, muscle** 356.1
- **Marie-Strümpell arthritis or disease** (ankylosing spondylitis) 720.0
- **Marihuana, marijuana**
  - abuse (*see also* Abuse, drugs, nondependent) 305.2
  - dependence (*see also* Dependence) 304.3
- **Marion's disease** (bladder neck obstruction) 596.0
- **Marital conflict** V61.10
- **Mark**
  - port wine 757.32
  - raspberry 757.32
  - strawberry 757.32
  - stretch 701.3
  - tattoo 709.09
- **Maroteaux-Lamy syndrome** (mucopolysaccharidosis VI) 277.5
- **Marriage license examination** V70.3
- **Marrow** (bone)
  - arrest 284.9
  - megakaryocytic 287.30
  - poor function 289.9
- **Marseilles fever** 082.1
- **Marsh's disease** (exophthalmic goiter) 242.0
- **Marshall's** (hidrotic) ectodermal dysplasia 757.31
- **Marsh fever** (*see also* Malaria) 084.6
- **Martin's disease** 715.27
- **Martin-Albright syndrome** (pseudohypoparathyroidism) 275.49
- **Martorell-Fabre syndrome** (pulseless disease) 446.7
- **Masculinization, female, with adrenal hyperplasia** 255.2
- **Masculinovoblastoma** (M8670/0) 220
- **Masochism** 302.83
- **Masons' lung** 502
- **Mass**
  - abdominal 789.3
  - anus 787.99
  - bone 733.90
  - breast 611.72
  - cheek 784.2
  - chest 786.6
  - cystic - *see* Cyst
  - ear 388.8
  - epigastric 789.3
  - eye 379.92
  - female genital organ 625.8
  - gum 784.2
  - head 784.2
  - intracranial 784.2
  - joint 719.60
    - ankle 719.67
    - elbow 719.62
    - foot 719.67
    - hand 719.64
    - hip 719.65
    - knee 719.66
    - multiple sites 719.69
    - pelvic region 719.65
    - shoulder (region) 719.61
    - specified site NEC 719.68
    - wrist 719.63
- **Mass** *(Continued)*
  - kidney (*see also* Disease, kidney) 593.9
  - lung 786.6
  - lymph node 785.6
  - malignant (M8000/3) - *see* Neoplasm, by site, malignant
  - mediastinal 786.6
  - mouth 784.2
  - muscle (limb) 729.89
  - neck 784.2
  - nose or sinus 784.2
  - palate 784.2
  - pelvis, pelvic 789.3
  - penis 607.89
  - perineum 625.8
  - rectum 787.99
  - scrotum 608.89
  - skin 782.2
  - specified organ NEC - *see* Disease of specified organ or site
  - splenic 789.2
  - substernal 786.6
    - thyroid (*see also* Goiter) 240.9
  - superficial (localized) 782.2
  - testes 608.89
  - throat 784.2
  - tongue 784.2
  - umbilicus 789.3
  - uterus 625.8
  - vagina 625.8
  - vulva 625.8
- **Massive** - *see* condition
- **Mastalgia** 611.71
  - psychogenic 307.89
- **Mast cell**
  - disease 757.33
    - systemic (M9741/3) 202.6
  - leukemia (M9900/3) 207.8
  - sarcoma (M9742/3) 202.6
  - tumor (M9740/1) 238.5
    - malignant (M9740/3) 202.6
- **Masters-Allen syndrome** 620.6
- **Mastitis** (acute) (adolescent) (diffuse) (interstitial) (lobular) (nonpuerperal) (nonsuppurative) (parenchymatous) (phlegmonous) (simple) (subacute) (suppurative) 611.0
  - chronic (cystic) (fibrocystic) 610.1
  - cystic 610.1
    - Schimmelbusch's type 610.1
  - fibrocystic 610.1
  - infective 611.0
  - lactational 675.2
  - lymphangitis 611.0
  - neonatal (noninfective) 778.7
    - infective 771.5
  - periductal 610.4
  - plasma cell 610.4
  - puerperal, postpartum, (interstitial) (nonpurulent) (parenchymatous) 675.2
    - purulent 675.1
    - stagnation 676.2
  - puerperalis 675.2
  - retromammary 611.0
    - puerperal, postpartum 675.1
  - submammary 611.0
    - puerperal, postpartum 675.1
- **Mastocytoma** (M9740/1) 238.5
  - malignant (M9740/3) 202.6
- **Mastocytosis** 757.33
  - malignant (M9741/3) 202.6
  - systemic (M9741/3) 202.6
- **Mastodynia** 611.71
  - psychogenic 307.89

Mastoid - *see* condition
Mastoidalgia (*see also* Otalgia) 388.70
Mastoiditis (coalescent) (hemorrhagic) (pneumococcal) (streptococcal) (suppurative) 383.9
  acute or subacute 383.00
    with
      Gradenigo's syndrome 383.02
      petrositis 383.02
      specified complication NEC 383.02
      subperiosteal abscess 383.01
  chronic (necrotic) (recurrent) 383.1
  tuberculous (*see also* Tuberculosis) 015.6
Mastopathy, mastopathia 611.9
  chronica cystica 610.1
  diffuse cystic 610.1
  estrogenic 611.8
  ovarian origin 611.8
Mastoplasia 611.1
Masturbation 307.9
Maternal condition, affecting fetus or newborn
  acute yellow atrophy of liver 760.8
  albuminuria 760.1
  anesthesia or analgesia 763.5
  blood loss 762.1
  chorioamnionitis 762.7
  circulatory disease, chronic (conditions classifiable to 390–459, 745–747) 760.3
  congenital heart disease (conditions classifiable to 745–746) 760.3
  cortical necrosis of kidney 760.1
  death 761.6
  diabetes mellitus 775.0
    manifest diabetes in the infant 775.1
  disease NEC 760.9
    circulatory system, chronic (conditions classifiable to 390–459, 745–747) 760.3
    genitourinary system (conditions classifiable to 580–599) 760.1
    respiratory (conditions classifiable to 490–519, 748) 760.3
  eclampsia 760.0
  hemorrhage NEC 762.1
  hepatitis acute, malignant, or subacute 760.8
  hyperemesis (gravidarum) 761.8
  hypertension (arising during pregnancy) (conditions classifiable to 642) 760.0
  infection
    disease classifiable to 001–136 760.2
    genital tract NEC 760.8
    urinary tract 760.1
  influenza 760.2
    manifest influenza in the infant 771.2
  injury (conditions classifiable to 800–996) 760.5
  malaria 760.2
    manifest malaria in infant or fetus 771.2
  malnutrition 760.4
  necrosis of liver 760.8
  nephritis (conditions classifiable to 580–583) 760.1
  nephrosis (conditions classifiable to 581) 760.1
  noxious substance transmitted via breast milk or placenta 760.70
    alcohol 760.71
    anticonvulsants 760.77
    antifungals 760.74
Maternal condition, affecting fetus or newborn *(Continued)*
  noxious substance transmitted via breast milk or placenta *(Continued)*
    anti-infective agents 760.74
    antimetabolics 760.78
    cocaine 760.75
    "crack" 760.75
    diethylstilbestrol [DES] 760.76
    hallucinogenic agents 760.73
    medicinal agents NEC 760.79
    narcotics 760.72
    obstetric anesthetic or analgesic drug 760.72
    specified agent NEC 760.79
  nutritional disorder (conditions classifiable to 260–269) 760.4
  operation unrelated to current delivery 760.6
  pre-eclampsia 760.0
  pyelitis or pyelonephritis, arising during pregnancy (conditions classifiable to 590) 760.1
  renal disease or failure 760.1
  respiratory disease, chronic (conditions classifiable to 490–519, 748) 760.3
  rheumatic heart disease (chronic) (conditions classifiable to 393–398) 760.3
  rubella (conditions classifiable to 056) 760.2
    manifest rubella in the infant or fetus 771.0
  surgery unrelated to current delivery 760.6
    to uterus or pelvic organs 763.89
  syphilis (conditions classifiable to 090–097) 760.2
    manifest syphilis in the infant or fetus 090.0
  thrombophlebitis 760.3
  toxemia (of pregnancy) 760.0
    pre-eclamptic 760.0
  toxoplasmosis (conditions classifiable to 130) 760.2
    manifest toxoplasmosis in the infant or fetus 771.2
  transmission of chemical substance through the placenta 760.70
    alcohol 760.71
    anticonvulsants 760.77
    antifungals 760.74
    anti-infective 760.74
    antimetabolics 760.78
    cocaine 760.75
    "crack" 760.75
    diethylstilbestrol [DES] 760.76
    hallucinogenic agents 760.73
    narcotics 760.72
    specified substance NEC 760.79
  uremia 760.1
  urinary tract conditions (conditions classifiable to 580–599) 760.1
  vomiting (pernicious) (persistent) (vicious) 761.8
Maternity - *see* Delivery
Matheiu's disease (leptospiral jaundice) 100.0
Mauclaire's disease or osteochondrosis 732.3
Maxcy's disease 081.0
Maxilla, maxillary - *see* condition
May (-Hegglin) anomaly or syndrome 288.2
Mayaro fever 066.3
Mazoplasia 610.8
MBD (minimal brain dysfunction), child (*see also* Hyperkinesia) 314.9
MCAD (medium chain acyl CoA dehydrogenase deficiency) 277.85
McArdle (-Schmid-Pearson) disease or syndrome (glycogenosis V) 271.0
McCune-Albright syndrome (osteitis fibrosa disseminata) 756.59
MCLS (mucocutaneous lymph node syndrome) 446.1
McQuarrie's syndrome (idiopathic familial hypoglycemia) 251.2
Measles (black) (hemorrhagic) (suppressed) 055.9
  with
    encephalitis 055.0
    keratitis 055.71
    keratoconjunctivitis 055.71
    otitis media 055.2
    pneumonia 055.1
  complication 055.8
    specified type NEC 055.79
  encephalitis 055.0
  French 056.9
  German 056.9
  keratitis 055.71
  keratoconjunctivitis 055.71
  liberty 056.9
  otitis media 055.2
  pneumonia 055.1
  specified complications NEC 055.79
  vaccination, prophylactic (against) V04.2
Meatitis, urethral (*see also* Urethritis) 597.89
Meat poisoning - *see* Poisoning, food
Meatus, meatal - *see* condition
Meat-wrappers' asthma 506.9
Meckel's
  diverticulitis 751.0
  diverticulum (displaced) (hypertrophic) 751.0
Meconium
  aspiration 770.11
    with
      pneumonia 770.12
      pneumonitis 770.12
      respiratory symptoms 770.12
    below vocal cords 770.11
      with respiratory symptoms 770.12
    syndrome 770.12
  delayed passage in newborn 777.1
  ileus 777.1
    due to cystic fibrosis 277.01
  in liquor 792.3
    noted during delivery 656.8
  insufflation 770.11
    with respiratory symptoms 770.12
  obstruction
    fetus or newborn 777.1
      in mucoviscidosis 277.01
  passage of 792.3
    noted during delivery 763.84
  peritonitis 777.6
  plug syndrome (newborn) NEC 777.1
  staining 779.84
Median - *see also* condition
  arcuate ligament syndrome 447.4
  bar (prostate) 600.90

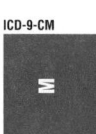

Median *(Continued)*
bar *(Continued)*
with ⬅
other lower urinary tract symptoms (LUTS) 600.91 ◀
urinary ◀
obstruction 600.91 ◀
retention 600.91 ◀
rhomboid glossitis 529.2
vesical orifice 600.90
with ⬅
other lower urinary tract symptoms (LUTS) 600.91 ◀
urinary ◀
obstruction 600.91 ◀
retention 600.91 ◀
Mediastinal shift 793.2
Mediastinitis (acute) (chronic) 519.2
actinomycotic 039.8
syphilitic 095.8
tuberculous (*see also* Tuberculosis) 012.8
Mediastinopericarditis (*see also* Pericarditis) 423.9
acute 420.90
chronic 423.8
rheumatic 393
rheumatic, chronic 393
Mediastinum, mediastinal - *see* condition
Medical services provided for - *see* Health, services provided because (of)
Medicine poisoning (by overdose) (wrong substance given or taken in error) 977.9
specified drug or substance - *see* Table of Drugs and Chemicals
Medin's disease (poliomyelitis) 045.9
Mediterranean
anemia (with other hemoglobinopathy) 282.49
disease or syndrome (hemipathic) 282.49
fever (*see also* Brucellosis) 023.9
familial 277.31 ⬅
kala-azar 085.0
leishmaniasis 085.0
tick fever 082.1
Medulla - *see* condition
Medullary
cystic kidney 753.16
sponge kidney 753.17
Medullated fibers
optic (nerve) 743.57
retina 362.85
Medulloblastoma (M9470/3)
desmoplastic (M9471/3) 191.6
specified site - *see* Neoplasm, by site, malignant
unspecified site 191.6
Medulloepithelioma (M9501/3) - *see also* Neoplasm, by site, malignant
teratoid (M9502/3) - *see* Neoplasm, by site, malignant
Medullomyoblastoma (M9472/3)
specified site - *see* Neoplasm, by site, malignant
unspecified site 191.6
Meekeren-Ehlers-Danlos syndrome 756.83
Megacaryocytic - *see* condition
Megacolon (acquired) (functional) (not Hirschsprung's disease) 564.7
aganglionic 751.3
congenital, congenitum 751.3
Hirschsprung's (disease) 751.3
psychogenic 306.4
toxic (*see also* Colitis, ulcerative) 556.9
Megaduodenum 537.3
Megaesophagus (functional) 530.0
congenital 750.4
Megakaryocytic - *see* condition
Megalencephaly 742.4
Megalerythema (epidermicum) (infectiosum) 057.0
Megalia, cutis et ossium 757.39
Megaloappendix 751.5
Megalocephalus, megalocephaly NEC 756.0
Megalocornea 743.41
associated with buphthalmos 743.22
Megalocytic anemia 281.9
Megalodactylia (fingers) (thumbs) 755.57
toes 755.65
Megaloduodenum 751.5
Megaloesophagus (functional) 530.0
congenital 750.4
Megalogastria (congenital) 750.7
Megalomania 307.9
Megalophthalmos 743.8
Megalopsia 368.14
Megalosplenia (*see also* Splenomegaly) 789.2
Megaloureter 593.89
congenital 753.22
Megarectum 569.49
Megasigmoid 564.7
congenital 751.3
Megaureter 593.89
congenital 753.22
Megrim 346.9
Meibomian
cyst 373.2
infected 373.12
gland - *see* condition
infarct (eyelid) 374.85
stye 373.11
Meibomitis 373.12
Meige
-Milroy disease (chronic hereditary edema) 757.0
syndrome (blepharospasm-oromandibular dystonia) 333.82
Melalgia, nutritional 266.2
Melancholia (*see also* Psychosis, affective) 296.90
climacteric 296.2
recurrent episode 296.3
single episode 296.2
hypochondriac 300.7
intermittent 296.2
recurrent episode 296.3
single episode 296.2
involutional 296.2
recurrent episode 296.3
single episode 296.2
menopausal 296.2
recurrent episode 296.3
single episode 296.2
puerperal 296.2
reactive (from emotional stress, psychological trauma) 298.0
recurrent 296.3
senile 290.21
stuporous 296.2
recurrent episode 296.3
single episode 296.2
Melanemia 275.0
Melanoameloblastoma (M9363/0) - *see* Neoplasm, bone, benign
Melanoblastoma (M8720/3) - *see* Melanoma
Melanoblastosis
Block-Sulzberger 757.33
cutis linearis sive systematisata 757.33
Melanocarcinoma (M8720/3) - *see* Melanoma
Melanocytoma, eyeball (M8726/0) 224.0
Melanoderma, melanodermia 709.09
Addison's (primary adrenal insufficiency) 255.4
Melanodontia, infantile 521.05
Melanodontoclasia 521.05
Melanoepithelioma (M8720/3) - *see* Melanoma
Melanoma (malignant) (M8720/3) 172.9

Note Except where otherwise indicated, the morphological varieties of melanoma in the list below should be coded by site as for "Melanoma (malignant)." Internal sites should be coded to malignant neoplasm of those sites.

abdominal wall 172.5
ala nasi 172.3
amelanotic (M8730/3) - *see* Melanoma, by site
ankle 172.7
anus, anal 154.3
canal 154.2
arm 172.6
auditory canal (external) 172.2
auricle (ear) 172.2
auricular canal (external) 172.2
axilla 172.5
axillary fold 172.5
back 172.5
balloon cell (M8722/3) - *see* Melanoma, by site
benign (M8720/0) - *see* Neoplasm, skin, benign
breast (female) (male) 172.5
brow 172.3
buttock 172.5
canthus (eye) 172.1
cheek (external) 172.3
chest wall 172.5
chin 172.3
choroid 190.6
conjunctiva 190.3
ear (external) 172.2
epithelioid cell (M8771/3) - *see also* Melanoma, by site
and spindle cell, mixed (M8775/3) - *see* Melanoma, by site
external meatus (ear) 172.2
eye 190.9
eyebrow 172.3
eyelid (lower) (upper) 172.1
face NEC 172.3
female genital organ (external) NEC 184.4
finger 172.6
flank 172.5
foot 172.7
forearm 172.6
forehead 172.3
foreskin 187.1
gluteal region 172.5
groin 172.5
hand 172.6
heel 172.7
helix 172.2
hip 172.7

Melanoma *(Continued)*
in
giant pigmented nevus (M8761/3) - *see* Melanoma, by site
Hutchinson's melanotic freckle (M8742/3) - *see* Melanoma, by site
junctional nevus (M8740/3) - *see* Melanoma, by site
precancerous melanosis (M8741/3) - *see* Melanoma, by site
interscapular region 172.5
iris 190.0
jaw 172.3
juvenile (M8770/0) - *see* Neoplasm, skin, benign
knee 172.7
labium
majus 184.1
minus 184.2
lacrimal gland 190.2
leg 172.7
lip (lower) (upper) 172.0
liver 197.7
lower limb NEC 172.7
male genital organ (external) NEC 187.9
meatus, acoustic (external) 172.2
meibomian gland 172.1
metastatic
of or from specified site - *see* Melanoma, by site
site not of skin - *see* Neoplasm, by site, malignant, secondary
to specified site - *see* Neoplasm, by site, malignant, secondary
unspecified site 172.9
nail 172.9
finger 172.6
toe 172.7
neck 172.4
nodular (M8721/3) - *see* Melanoma, by site
nose, external 172.3
orbit 190.1
penis 187.4
perianal skin 172.5
perineum 172.5
pinna 172.2
popliteal (fossa) (space) 172.7
prepuce 187.1
pubes 172.5
pudendum 184.4
retina 190.5
scalp 172.4
scrotum 187.7
septum nasal (skin) 172.3
shoulder 172.6
skin NEC 172.8
spindle cell (M8772/3) - *see also* Melanoma, by site
type A (M8773/3) 190.0
type B (M8774/3) 190.0
submammary fold 172.5
superficial spreading (M8743/3) - *see* Melanoma, by site
temple 172.3
thigh 172.7
toe 172.7
trunk NEC 172.5
umbilicus 172.5
upper limb NEC 172.6
vagina vault 184.0
vulva 184.4
Melanoplakia 528.9
Melanosarcoma (M8720/3) - *see also* Melanoma
epithelioid cell (M8771/3) - *see* Melanoma
Melanosis 709.09
addisonian (primary adrenal insufficiency) 255.4
tuberculous (*see also* Tuberculosis) 017.6
adrenal 255.4
colon 569.89
conjunctiva 372.55
congenital 743.49
corii degenerativa 757.33
cornea (presenile) (senile) 371.12
congenital 743.43
interfering with vision 743.42
prenatal 743.43
interfering with vision 743.42
eye 372.55
congenital 743.49
jute spinners' 709.09
lenticularis progressiva 757.33
liver 573.8
precancerous (M8741/2) - *see also* Neoplasm, skin, in situ
malignant melanoma in (M8741/3) - *see* Melanoma
Riehl's 709.09
sclera 379.19
congenital 743.47
suprarenal 255.4
tar 709.09
toxic 709.09
Melanuria 791.9
MELAS syndrome (mitochondrial encephalopathy, lactic acidosis and stroke-like episodes) 277.87
Melasma 709.09
adrenal (gland) 255.4
suprarenal (gland) 255.4
Melena 578.1
due to
swallowed maternal blood 777.3
ulcer - *see* Ulcer, by site, with hemorrhage
newborn 772.4
due to swallowed maternal blood 777.3
Meleney's
gangrene (cutaneous) 686.09
ulcer (chronic undermining) 686.09
Melioidosis 025
Melitensis, febris 023.0
Melitococcosis 023.0
Melkersson (-Rosenthal) syndrome 351.8
Mellitus, diabetes - *see* Diabetes
Melorheostosis (bone) (leri) 733.99
Meloschisis 744.83
Melotia 744.29
Membrana
capsularis lentis posterior 743.39
epipapillaris 743.57
Membranacea placenta - *see* Placenta, abnormal
Membranaceous uterus 621.8
Membrane, membranous - *see also* condition
folds, congenital - *see* Web
Jackson's 751.4
over face (causing asphyxia), fetus or newborn 768.9
premature rupture - *see* Rupture, membranes, premature
Membrane, membranous *(Continued)*
pupillary 364.74
persistent 743.46
retained (complicating delivery) (with hemorrhage) 666.2
without hemorrhage 667.1
secondary (eye) 366.50
unruptured (causing asphyxia) 768.9
vitreous humor 379.25
Membranitis, fetal 658.4
affecting fetus or newborn 762.7
Memory disturbance, loss or lack (*see also* Amnesia) 780.93
mild, following organic brain damage 310.1
Menadione (vitamin K) deficiency 269.0
Menarche, precocious 259.1
Mendacity, pathologic 301.7
Mende's syndrome (ptosis-epicanthus) 270.2
Mendelson's syndrome (resulting from a procedure) 997.3
obstetric 668.0
Ménétrier's disease or syndrome (hypertrophic gastritis) 535.2
Ménière's disease, syndrome, or vertigo 386.00
cochlear 386.02
cochleovestibular 386.01
inactive 386.04
in remission 386.04
vestibular 386.03
Meninges, meningeal - *see* condition
Meningioma (M9530/0) - *see also* Neoplasm, meninges, benign
angioblastic (M9535/0) - *see* Neoplasm, meninges, benign
angiomatous (M9534/0) - *see* Neoplasm, meninges, benign
endotheliomatous (M9531/0) - *see* Neoplasm, meninges, benign
fibroblastic (M9532/0) - *see* Neoplasm, meninges, benign
fibrous (M9532/0) - *see* Neoplasm, meninges, benign
hemangioblastic (M9535/0) - *see* Neoplasm, meninges, benign
hemangiopericytic (M9536/0) - *see* Neoplasm, meninges, benign
malignant (M9530/3) - *see* Neoplasm, meninges, malignant
meningiothelial (M9531/0) - *see* Neoplasm, meninges, benign
meningotheliomatous (M9531/0) - *see* Neoplasm, meninges, benign
mixed (M9537/0) - *see* Neoplasm, meninges, benign
multiple (M9530/1) 237.6
papillary (M9538/1) 237.6
psammomatous (M9533/0) - *see* Neoplasm, meninges, benign
syncytial (M9531/0) - *see* Neoplasm, meninges, benign
transitional (M9537/0) - *see* Neoplasm, meninges, benign
Meningiomatosis (diffuse) (M9530/1) 237.6
Meningism (*see also* Meningismus) 781.6
Meningismus (infectional) (pneumococcal) 781.6
due to serum or vaccine 997.09 *[321.8]*
influenzal NEC 487.8

Meningitis (basal) (basic) (basilar) (brain) (cerebral) (cervical) (congestive) (diffuse) (hemorrhagic) (infantile) (membranous) (metastatic) (nonspecific) (pontine) (progressive) (simple) (spinal) (subacute) (sympathetica) (toxic) 322.9
abacterial NEC (*see also* Meningitis, aseptic) 047.9
actinomycotic 039.8 *[320.7]*
adenoviral 049.1
Aerobacter aerogenes 320.82
anaerobes (cocci) (gram-negative) (gram-positive) (mixed) (NEC) 320.81
arbovirus NEC 066.9 *[321.2]*
specified type NEC 066.8 *[321.2]*
aseptic (acute) NEC 047.9
adenovirus 049.1
Coxsackie virus 047.0
due to
adenovirus 049.1
Coxsackie virus 047.0
echo virus 047.1
enterovirus 047.9
mumps 072.1
poliovirus (*see also* Poliomyelitis) 045.2 *[321.2]*
echo virus 047.1
herpes (simplex) virus 054.72
zoster 053.0
leptospiral 100.81
lymphocytic choriomeningitis 049.0
noninfective 322.0
Bacillus pyocyaneus 320.89
bacterial NEC 320.9
anaerobic 320.81
gram-negative 320.82
anaerobic 320.81
Bacteroides (fragilis) (oralis) (melaninogenicus) 320.81
cancerous (M8000/6) 198.4
candidal 112.83
carcinomatous (M8010/6) 198.4
caseous (*see also* Tuberculosis, meninges) 013.0
cerebrospinal (acute) (chronic) (diplococcal) (endemic) (epidemic) (fulminant) (infectious) (malignant) (meningococcal) (sporadic) 036.0
carrier (suspected) of V02.59
chronic NEC 322.2
clear cerebrospinal fluid NEC 322.0
Clostridium (haemolyticum) (novyi) NEC 320.81
coccidioidomycosis 114.2
Coxsackie virus 047.0
cryptococcal 117.5 *[321.0]*
diplococcal 036.0
gram-negative 036.0
gram-positive 320.1
Diplococcus pneumoniae 320.1
due to
actinomycosis 039.8 *[320.7]*
adenovirus 049.1
coccidiomycosis 114.2
enterovirus 047.9
specified NEC 047.8
histoplasmosis (*see also* Histoplasmosis) 115.91
listerosis 027.0 *[320.7]*
Lyme disease 088.81 *[320.7]*
moniliasis 112.83
mumps 072.1

Meningitis *(Continued)*
due to *(Continued)*
neurosyphilis 094.2
nonbacterial organisms NEC 321.8
oidiomycosis 112.83
poliovirus (*see also* Poliomyelitis) 045.2 *[321.2]*
preventive immunization, inoculation, or vaccination 997.09 *[321.8]*
sarcoidosis 135 *[321.4]*
sporotrichosis 117.1 *[321.1]*
syphilis 094.2
acute 091.81
congenital 090.42
secondary 091.81
trypanosomiasis (*see also* Trypanosomiasis) 086.9 *[321.3]*
whooping cough 033.9 *[320.7]*
E. coli 320.82
ECHO virus 047.1
endothelial-leukocytic, benign, recurrent 047.9
Enterobacter aerogenes 320.82
enteroviral 047.9
specified type NEC 047.8
enterovirus 047.9
specified NEC 047.8
eosinophilic 322.1
epidemic NEC 036.0
Escherichia coli (E. coli) 320.82
Eubacterium 320.81
fibrinopurulent NEC 320.9
specified type NEC 320.89
Friedländer (bacillus) 320.82
fungal NEC 117.9 *[321.1]*
Fusobacterium 320.81
gonococcal 098.82
gram-negative bacteria NEC 320.82
anaerobic 320.81
cocci 036.0
specified NEC 320.82
gram-negative cocci NEC 036.0
specified NEC 320.82
gram-positive cocci NEC 320.9
H. influenzae 320.0
herpes (simplex) virus 054.72
zoster 053.0
infectious NEC 320.9
influenzal 320.0
Klebsiella pneumoniae 320.82
late effect - *see* Late, effect, meningitis
leptospiral (aseptic) 100.81
Listerella (monocytogenes) 027.0 *[320.7]*
Listeria monocytogenes 027.0 *[320.7]*
lymphocytic (acute) (benign) (serous) 049.0
choriomeningitis virus 049.0
meningococcal (chronic) 036.0
Mima polymorpha 320.82
Mollaret's 047.9
monilial 112.83
mumps (virus) 072.1
mycotic NEC 117.9 *[321.1]*
Neisseria 036.0
neurosyphilis 094.2
nonbacterial NEC (*see also* Meningitis, aseptic) 047.9
nonpyogenic NEC 322.0
oidiomycosis 112.83
ossificans 349.2
Peptococcus 320.81
Peptostreptococcus 320.81
pneumococcal 320.1

Meningitis *(Continued)*
poliovirus (*see also* Poliomyelitis) 045.2 *[321.2]*
Propionibacterium 320.81
Proteus morganii 320.82
Pseudomonas (aeruginosa) (pyocyaneus) 320.82
purulent NEC 320.9
specified organism NEC 320.89
pyogenic NEC 320.9
specified organism NEC 320.89
Salmonella 003.21
septic NEC 320.9
specified organism NEC 320.89
serosa circumscripta NEC 322.0
serous NEC (*see also* Meningitis, aseptic) 047.9
lymphocytic 049.0
syndrome 348.2
Serratia (marcescens) 320.82
specified organism NEC 320.89
sporadic cerebrospinal 036.0
sporotrichosis 117.1 *[321.1]*
staphylococcal 320.3
sterile 997.09
streptococcal (acute) 320.2
suppurative 320.9
specified organism NEC 320.89
syphilitic 094.2
acute 091.81
congenital 090.42
secondary 091.81
torula 117.5 *[321.0]*
traumatic (complication of injury) 958.8
Treponema (denticola) (macrodenticum) 320.81
trypanosomiasis 086.1 *[321.3]*
tuberculous (*see also* Tuberculosis, meninges) 013.0
typhoid 002.0 *[320.7]*
Veillonella 320.81
Vibrio vulnificus 320.82
viral, virus NEC (*see also* Meningitis, aseptic) 047.9
Wallgren's (*see also* Meningitis, aseptic) 047.9
Meningocele (congenital) (spinal) (*see also* Spina bifida) 741.9
acquired (traumatic) 349.2
cerebral 742.0
cranial 742.0
Meningocerebritis - *see* Meningoencephalitis
Meningococcemia (acute) (chronic) 036.2
Meningococcus, meningococcal (*see also* condition) 036.9
adrenalitis, hemorrhagic 036.3
carditis 036.40
carrier (suspected) of V02.59
cerebrospinal fever 036.0
encephalitis 036.1
endocarditis 036.42
exposure to V01.84
infection NEC 036.9
meningitis (cerebrospinal) 036.0
myocarditis 036.43
optic neuritis 036.81
pericarditis 036.41
septicemia (chronic) 036.2
Meningoencephalitis (*see also* Encephalitis) 323.9
acute NEC 048
bacterial, purulent, pyogenic, or septic - *see* Meningitis

Meningoencephalitis *(Continued)*
chronic NEC 094.1
diffuse NEC 094.1
diphasic 063.2
due to
actinomycosis 039.8 *[320.7]*
blastomycosis NEC (*see also* Blastomycosis) 116.0 *[323.41]*
free-living amebae 136.2
Listeria monocytogenes 027.0 *[320.7]*
Lyme disease 088.81 *[320.7]*
mumps 072.2
Naegleria (amebae) (gruberi) (organisms) 136.2
rubella 056.01
sporotrichosis 117.1 *[321.1]*
toxoplasmosis (acquired) 130.0
congenital (active) 771.2 *[323.41]*
Trypanosoma 086.1 *[323.2]*
epidemic 036.0
herpes 054.3
herpetic 054.3
H. influenzae 320.0
infectious (acute) 048
influenzal 320.0
late effect - *see* category 326
Listeria monocytogenes 027.0 *[320.7]*
lymphocytic (serous) 049.0
mumps 072.2
parasitic NEC 123.9 *[323.41]*
pneumococcal 320.1
primary amebic 136.2
rubella 056.01
serous 048
lymphocytic 049.0
specific 094.2
staphylococcal 320.3
streptococcal 320.2
syphilitic 094.2
toxic NEC 989.9 *[323.71]*
due to
carbon tetrachloride 987.8 *[323.71]*
hydroxyquinoline derivatives poisoning 961.3 *[323.71]*
lead 984.9 *[323.71]*
mercury 985.0 *[323.71]*
thallium 985.8 *[323.71]*
toxoplasmosis (acquired) 130.0
trypanosomic 086.1 *[323.2]*
tuberculous (*see also* Tuberculosis, meninges) 013.0
virus NEC 048
Meningoencephalocele 742.0
syphilitic 094.89
congenital 090.49
Meningoencephalomyelitis (*see also* Meningoencephalitis) 323.9
acute NEC 048
disseminated (postinfectious) 136.9 *[323.61]*
postimmunization or postvaccination 323.51
due to
actinomycosis 039.8 *[320.7]*
torula 117.5 *[323.41]*
toxoplasma or toxoplasmosis (acquired) 130.0
congenital (active) 771.2 *[323.41]*
late effect - *see* category 326
Meningoencephalomyelopathy (*see also* Meningoencephalomyelitis) 349.9
Meningoencephalopathy (*see also* Meningoencephalitis) 348.39
Meningoencephalopoliomyelitis (*see also* Poliomyelitis, bulbar) 045.0
late effect 138
Meningomyelitis (*see also* Meningoencephalitis) 323.9
blastomycotic NEC (*see also* Blastomycosis) 116.0 *[323.41]*
due to
actinomycosis 039.8 *[320.7]*
blastomycosis (*see also* Blastomycosis) 116.0 *[323.41]*
Meningococcus 036.0
sporotrichosis 117.1 *[323.41]*
torula 117.5 *[323.41]*
late effect - *see* category 326
lethargic 049.8
meningococcal 036.0
syphilitic 094.2
tuberculous (*see also* Tuberculosis, meninges) 013.0
Meningomyelocele (*see also* Spina bifida) 741.9
syphilitic 094.89
Meningomyeloneuritis - *see* Meningoencephalitis
Meningoradiculitis - *see* Meningitis
Meningovascular - *see* condition
Meniscocytosis 282.60
Menkes' syndrome - *see* Syndrome, Menkes'
Menolipsis 626.0
Menometrorrhagia 626.2
Menopause, menopausal (symptoms) (syndrome) 627.2
arthritis (any site) NEC 716.3
artificial 627.4
bleeding 627.0
crisis 627.2
depression (*see also* Psychosis, affective) 296.2
agitated 296.2
recurrent episode 296.3
single episode 296.2
psychotic 296.2
recurrent episode 296.3
single episode 296.2
recurrent episode 296.3
single episode 296.2
melancholia (*see also* Psychosis, affective) 296.2
recurrent episode 296.3
single episode 296.2
paranoid state 297.2
paraphrenia 297.2
postsurgical 627.4
premature 256.31
postirradiation 256.2
postsurgical 256.2
psychoneurosis 627.2
psychosis NEC 298.8
surgical 627.4
toxic polyarthritis NEC 716.39
Menorrhagia (primary) 626.2
climacteric 627.0
menopausal 627.0
postclimacteric 627.1
postmenopausal 627.1
preclimacteric 627.0
premenopausal 627.0
puberty (menses retained) 626.3
Menorrhalgia 625.3
Menoschesis 626.8
Menostaxis 626.2
Menses, retention 626.8
Menstrual - *see also* Menstruation
cycle, irregular 626.4
disorders NEC 626.9
extraction V25.3
fluid, retained 626.8
molimen 625.4
period, normal V65.5
regulation V25.3
Menstruation
absent 626.0
anovulatory 628.0
delayed 626.8
difficult 625.3
disorder 626.9
psychogenic 306.52
specified NEC 626.8
during pregnancy 640.8
excessive 626.2
frequent 626.2
infrequent 626.1
irregular 626.4
latent 626.8
membranous 626.8
painful (primary) (secondary) 625.3
psychogenic 306.52
passage of clots 626.2
precocious 626.8
protracted 626.8
retained 626.8
retrograde 626.8
scanty 626.1
suppression 626.8
vicarious (nasal) 625.8
Mentagra (*see also* Sycosis) 704.8
Mental - *see also* condition
deficiency (*see also* Retardation, mental) 319
deterioration (*see also* Psychosis) 298.9
disorder (*see also* Disorder, mental) 300.9
exhaustion 300.5
insufficiency (congenital) (*see also* Retardation, mental) 319
observation without need for further medical care NEC V71.09
retardation (*see also* Retardation, mental) 319
subnormality (*see also* Retardation, mental) 319
mild 317
moderate 318.0
profound 318.2
severe 318.1
upset (*see also* Disorder, mental) 300.9
Meralgia paresthetica 355.1
Mercurial - *see* condition
Mercurialism NEC 985.0
Merergasia 300.9
Merkel cell tumor - *see* Neoplasm, by site, malignant
Merocele (*see also* Hernia, femoral) 553.00
Meromelia 755.4
lower limb 755.30
intercalary 755.32
femur 755.34
tibiofibular (complete) (incomplete) 755.33
fibula 755.37
metatarsal(s) 755.38
tarsal(s) 755.38
tibia 755.36
tibiofibular 755.35

Meromelia *(Continued)*
lower limb *(Continued)*
terminal (complete) (partial) (transverse) 755.31
longitudinal 755.32
metatarsal(s) 755.38
phalange(s) 755.39
tarsal(s) 755.38
transverse 755.31
upper limb 755.20
intercalary 755.22
carpal(s) 755.28
humeral 755.24
radioulnar (complete) (incomplete) 755.23
metacarpal(s) 755.28
phalange(s) 755.29
radial 755.26
radioulnar 755.25
ulnar 755.27
terminal (complete) (partial) (transverse) 755.21
longitudinal 755.22
carpal(s) 755.28
metacarpal(s) 755.28
phalange(s) 755.29
transverse 755.21
Merosmia 781.1
MERRF syndrome (myoclonus with epilepsy and with ragged red fibers) 277.87
Merycism - *see also* Vomiting
psychogenic 307.53
Merzbacher-Pelizaeus disease 330.0
Mesaortitis - *see* Aortitis
Mesarteritis - *see* Arteritis
Mesencephalitis (*see also* Encephalitis) 323.9
late effect - *see* category 326
Mesenchymoma (M8990/1) - *see also* Neoplasm, connective tissue, uncertain behavior
benign (M8990/0) - *see* Neoplasm, connective tissue, benign
malignant (M8990/3) - *see* Neoplasm, connective tissue, malignant
Mesenteritis
retractile 567.82
sclerosing 567.82
Mesentery, mesenteric - *see* condition
Mesiodens, mesiodentes 520.1
causing crowding 524.31
Mesio-occlusion 524.23
Mesocardia (with asplenia) 746.87
Mesocolon - *see* condition
Mesonephroma (malignant) (M9110/3) - *see also* Neoplasm, by site, malignant
benign (M9110/0) - *see* Neoplasm, by site, benign
Mesophlebitis - *see* Phlebitis
Mesostromal dysgenesis 743.51
Mesothelioma (malignant) (M9050/3) - *see also* Neoplasm, by site, malignant
benign (M9050/0) - *see* Neoplasm, by site, benign
biphasic type (M9053/3) - *see also* Neoplasm, by site, malignant
benign (M9053/0) - *see* Neoplasm, by site, benign
epithelioid (M9052/3) - *see also* Neoplasm, by site, malignant
benign (M9052/0) - *see* Neoplasm, by site, benign
fibrous (M9051/3) - *see also* Neoplasm, by site, malignant
Mesothelioma *(Continued)*
benign (M9051/0) - *see* Neoplasm, by site, benign
Metabolic syndrome 277.7
Metabolism disorder 277.9
specified type NEC 277.89
Metagonimiasis 121.5
Metagonimus infestation (small intestine) 121.5
Metal
pigmentation (skin) 709.00
polishers' disease 502
Metalliferous miners' lung 503
Metamorphopsia 368.14
Metaplasia
bone, in skin 709.3
breast 611.8
cervix - *omit code*
endometrium (squamous) 621.8
esophagus 530.85
intestinal, of gastric mucosa 537.89
kidney (pelvis) (squamous) (*see also* Disease, renal) 593.89
myelogenous 289.89
myeloid 289.89
agnogenic 238.76
megakaryocytic 238.76
spleen 289.59
squamous cell
amnion 658.8
bladder 596.8
cervix - *see* condition
trachea 519.19
tracheobronchial tree 519.19
uterus 621.8
cervix - *see* condition
Metastasis, metastatic
abscess - *see* Abscess
calcification 275.40
cancer, neoplasm, or disease
from specified site (M8000/3) - *see* Neoplasm, by site, malignant
to specified site (M8000/6) - *see* Neoplasm, by site, secondary
deposits (in) (M8000/6) - *see* Neoplasm, by site, secondary
pneumonia 038.8 *[484.8]*
spread (to) (M8000/6) - *see* Neoplasm, by site, secondary
Metatarsalgia 726.70
anterior 355.6
due to Freiberg's disease 732.5
Morton's 355.6
Metatarsus, metatarsal - *see also* condition
abductus valgus (congenital) 754.60
adductus varus (congenital) 754.53
primus varus 754.52
valgus (adductus) (congenital) 754.60
varus (abductus) (congenital) 754.53
primus 754.52
Methemoglobinemia 289.7
acquired (with sulfhemoglobinemia) 289.7
congenital 289.7
enzymatic 289.7
Hb-M disease 289.7
hereditary 289.7
toxic 289.7
Methemoglobinuria (*see also* Hemoglobinuria) 791.2
Methicillin-resistant staphylococcus aureus (MRSA) V09.0
Methioninemia 270.4
Metritis (catarrhal) (septic) (suppurative) (*see also* endometritis) 615.9
blennorrhagic 098.16
chronic or duration of 2 months or over 098.36
cervical (*see also* Cervicitis) 616.0
gonococcal 098.16
chronic or duration of 2 months or over 098.36
hemorrhagic 626.8
puerperal, postpartum, childbirth 670
tuberculous (*see also* Tuberculosis) 016.7
Metropathia hemorrhagica 626.8
Metroperitonitis (*see also* Peritonitis, pelvic, female) 614.5
Metrorrhagia 626.6
arising during pregnancy - *see* Hemorrhage, pregnancy
postpartum NEC 666.2
primary 626.6
psychogenic 306.59
puerperal 666.2
Metrorrhexis - *see* Rupture, uterus
Metrosalpingitis (*see also* Salpingo-oophoritis) 614.2
Metrostaxis 626.6
Metrovaginitis (*see also* Endometritis) 615.9
gonococcal (acute) 098.16
chronic or duration of 2 months or over 098.36
Mexican fever - *see* Typhus, Mexican
Meyenburg-Altherr-Uehlinger syndrome 733.99
Meyer-Schwickerath and Weyers syndrome (dysplasia oculodentodigitalis) 759.89
Meynert's amentia (nonalcoholic) 294.0
alcoholic 291.1
Mibelli's disease 757.39
Mice, joint (*see also* Loose, body, joint) 718.1
knee 717.6
Micheli-Rietti syndrome (thalassemia minor) 282.49
Michotte's syndrome 721.5
Micrencephalon, micrencephaly 742.1
Microalbuminuria 791.0
Microaneurysm, retina 362.14
diabetic 250.5 *[362.01]*
Microangiopathy 443.9
diabetic (peripheral) 250.7 *[443.81]*
retinal 250.5 *[362.01]*
peripheral 443.9
diabetic 250.7 *[443.81]*
retinal 362.18
diabetic 250.5 *[362.01]*
thrombotic 446.6
Moschcowitz's (thrombotic thrombocytopenic purpura) 446.6
Microcalcification, mammographic 793.81
Microcephalus, microcephalic, microcephaly 742.1
due to toxoplasmosis (congenital) 771.2
Microcheilia 744.82
Microcolon (congenital) 751.5
Microcornea (congenital) 743.41
Microcytic - *see* condition
Microdeletions NEC 758.33
Microdontia 520.2
Microdrepanocytosis (thalassemia-Hb-S disease) 282.49

Microembolism
atherothrombotic - *see* Atheroembolism
retina 362.33
Microencephalon 742.1
Microfilaria streptocerca infestation 125.3
Microgastria (congenital) 750.7
Microgenia 524.06
Microgenitalia (congenital) 752.89
penis 752.64
Microglioma (M9710/3)
specified site - *see* Neoplasm, by site, malignant
unspecified site 191.9
Microglossia (congenital) 750.16
Micrognathia, micrognathism (congenital) 524.00
mandibular 524.04
alveolar 524.74
maxillary 524.03
alveolar 524.73
Microgyria (congenital) 742.2
Microinfarct, heart (*see also* Insufficiency, coronary) 411.89
Microlithiasis, alveolar, pulmonary 516.2
Micromyelia (congenital) 742.59
Micropenis 752.64
Microphakia (congenital) 743.36
Microphthalmia (congenital) (*see also* Microphthalmos) 743.10
Microphthalmos (congenital) 743.10
associated with eye and adnexal anomalies NEC 743.12
due to toxoplasmosis (congenital) 771.2
isolated 743.11
simple 743.11
syndrome 759.89
Micropsia 368.14
Microsporidiosis 136.8
Microsporosis (*see also* Dermatophytosis) 110.9
nigra 111.1
Microsporum furfur infestation 111.0
Microstomia (congenital) 744.84
Microthelia 757.6
Microthromboembolism - *see* Embolism
Microtia (congenital) (external ear) 744.23
Microtropia 378.34
Micturition
disorder NEC 788.69
psychogenic 306.53
frequency 788.41
psychogenic 306.53
nocturnal 788.43
painful 788.1
psychogenic 306.53
Middle
ear - *see* condition
lobe (right) syndrome 518.0
Midplane - *see* condition
Miescher's disease 709.3
cheilitis 351.8
granulomatosis disciformis 709.3
Miescher-Leder syndrome or granulomatosis 709.3
Mieten's syndrome 759.89
Migraine (idiopathic) 346.9
with aura 346.0
abdominal (syndrome) 346.2
allergic (histamine) 346.2
atypical 346.1
basilar 346.2
classical 346.0
common 346.1
hemiplegic 346.8
Migraine *(Continued)*
lower-half 346.2
menstrual 625.4
ophthalmic 346.8
ophthalmoplegic 346.8
retinal 346.2
variant 346.2
Migrant, social V60.0
Migratory, migrating - *see also* condition
person V60.0
testis, congenital 752.52
Mikulicz's disease or syndrome (dryness of mouth, absent or decreased lacrimation) 527.1
Milian atrophia blanche 701.3
Miliaria (crystallina) (rubra) (tropicalis) 705.1
apocrine 705.82
Miliary - *see* condition
Milium (*see also* Cyst, sebaceous) 706.2
colloid 709.3
eyelid 374.84
Milk
crust 690.11
excess secretion 676.6
fever, female 672
poisoning 988.8
retention 676.2
sickness 988.8
spots 423.1
Milkers' nodes 051.1
Milk-leg (deep vessels) 671.4
complicating pregnancy 671.3
nonpuerperal 451.19
puerperal, postpartum, childbirth 671.4
Milkman (-Looser) disease or syndrome (osteomalacia with pseudofractures) 268.2
Milky urine (*see also* Chyluria) 791.1
Millar's asthma (laryngismus stridulus) 478.75
Millard-Gubler paralysis or syndrome 344.89
Millard-Gubler-Foville paralysis 344.89
Miller-Dieker syndrome 758.33
Miller's disease (osteomalacia) 268.2
Miller Fisher's syndrome 357.0
Milles' syndrome (encephalocutaneous angiomatosis) 759.6
Mills' disease 335.29
Millstone makers' asthma or lung 502
Milroy's disease (chronic hereditary edema) 757.0
Miners' - *see also* condition
asthma 500
elbow 727.2
knee 727.2
lung 500
nystagmus 300.89
phthisis (*see also* Tuberculosis) 011.4
tuberculosis (*see also* Tuberculosis) 011.4
Minkowski-Chauffard syndrome (*see also* Spherocytosis) 282.0
Minor - *see* condition
Minor's disease 336.1
Minot's disease (hemorrhagic disease, newborn) 776.0
Minot-von Willebrand (-Jurgens) disease or syndrome (angiohemophilia) 286.4
Minus (and plus) hand (intrinsic) 736.09
Miosis (persistent) (pupil) 379.42
Mirizzi's syndrome (hepatic duct stenosis) (*see also* Obstruction, biliary) 576.2
Mirizzi's syndrome *(Continued)*
with calculus, cholelithiasis, or stones - *see* Choledocholithiasis
Mirror writing 315.09
secondary to organic lesion 784.69
Misadventure (prophylactic) (therapeutic) (*see also* Complications) 999.9
administration of insulin 962.3
infusion - *see* Complications, infusion
local applications (of fomentations, plasters, etc.) 999.9
burn or scald - *see* Burn, by site
medical care (early) (late) NEC 999.9
adverse effect of drugs or chemicals - *see* Table of Drugs and Chemicals
burn or scald - *see* Burn, by site
radiation NEC 990
radiotherapy NEC 990
surgical procedure (early) (late) - *see* Complications, surgical procedure
transfusion - *see* Complications, transfusion
vaccination or other immunological procedure - *see* Complications, vaccination
Misanthropy 301.7
Miscarriage - *see* Abortion, spontaneous
Mischief, malicious, child (*see also* Disturbance, conduct) 312.0
Misdirection
aqueous 365.83
Mismanagement, feeding 783.3
Misplaced, misplacement
kidney (*see also* Disease, renal) 593.0
congenital 753.3
organ or site, congenital NEC - *see* Malposition, congenital
Missed
abortion 632
delivery (at or near term) 656.4
labor (at or near term) 656.4
Missing - *see also* Absence
teeth (acquired) 525.10
congenital (*see also* Anodontia) 520.0
due to
caries 525.13
extraction 525.10
periodontal disease 525.12
specified NEC 525.19
trauma 525.11
vertebrae (congenital) 756.13
Misuse of drugs NEC (*see also* Abuse, drug, nondependent) 305.9
Mitchell's disease (erythromelalgia) 443.82
Mite(s)
diarrhea 133.8
grain (itch) 133.8
hair follicle (itch) 133.8
in sputum 133.8
Mitochondrial encephalopathy, lactic acidosis and stroke-like episodes (MELAS syndrome) 277.87
Mitochondrial neurogastrointestinal encephalopathy syndrome (MNGIE) 277.87
Mitral - *see* condition
Mittelschmerz 625.2
Mixed - *see* condition
Mljet disease (mal de Meleda) 757.39
Mobile, mobility
cecum 751.4
coccyx 733.99
excessive - *see* Hypermobility

Mobile, mobility *(Continued)*
gallbladder 751.69
kidney 593.0
congenital 753.3
organ or site, congenital NEC - *see* Malposition, congenital
spleen 289.59
Mobitz heart block (atrioventricular) 426.10
type I (Wenckebach's) 426.13
type II 426.12
Möbius'
disease 346.8
syndrome
congenital oculofacial paralysis 352.6
ophthalmoplegic migraine 346.8
Moeller (-Barlow) disease (infantile scurvy) 267
glossitis 529.4
Mohr's syndrome (types I and II) 759.89
Mola destruens (M9100/1) 236.1
Molarization, premolars 520.2
Molar pregnancy 631
hydatidiform (delivered) (undelivered) 630
Mold(s) in vitreous 117.9
Molding, head (during birth) - *omit code*
Mole (pigmented) (M8720/0) - *see also* Neoplasm, skin, benign
blood 631
Breus' 631
cancerous (M8720/3) - *see* Melanoma
carneous 631
destructive (M9100/1) 236.1
ectopic - *see* Pregnancy, ectopic
fleshy 631
hemorrhagic 631
hydatid, hydatidiform (benign) (complicating pregnancy) (delivered) (undelivered) (*see also* Hydatidiform mole) 630
invasive (M9100/1) 236.1
malignant (M9100/1) 236.1
previous, affecting management of pregnancy V23.1
invasive (hydatidiform) (M9100/1) 236.1
malignant
meaning
malignant hydatidiform mole (9100/1) 236.1
melanoma (M8720/3) - *see* Melanoma
nonpigmented (M8730/0) - *see* Neoplasm, skin, benign
pregnancy NEC 631
skin (M8720/0) - *see* Neoplasm, skin, benign
tubal - *see* Pregnancy, tubal
vesicular (*see also* Hydatidiform mole) 630
Molimen, molimina (menstrual) 625.4
Mollaret's meningitis 047.9
Mollities (cerebellar) (cerebral) 437.8
ossium 268.2
Molluscum
contagiosum 078.0
epitheliale 078.0
fibrosum (M8851/0) - *see* Lipoma, by site
pendulum (M8851/0) - *see* Lipoma, by site
Mönckeberg's arteriosclerosis, degeneration, disease, or sclerosis (*see also* Arteriosclerosis, extremities) 440.20
Monday fever 504
Monday morning dyspnea or asthma 504
Mondini's malformation (cochlea) 744.05
Mondor's disease (thrombophlebitis of breast) 451.89
Mongolian, mongolianism, mongolism, mongoloid 758.0
spot 757.33
Monilethrix (congenital) 757.4
Monilia infestation - *see* Candidiasis
Moniliasis - *see also* Candidiasis
neonatal 771.7
vulvovaginitis 112.1
Monkeypox 057.8
Monoarthritis 716.60
ankle 716.67
arm 716.62
lower (and wrist) 716.63
upper (and elbow) 716.62
foot (and ankle) 716.67
forearm (and wrist) 716.63
hand 716.64
leg 716.66
lower 716.66
upper 716.65
pelvic region (hip) (thigh) 716.65
shoulder (region) 716.61
specified site NEC 716.68
Monoblastic - *see* condition
Monochromatism (cone) (rod) 368.54
Monocytic - *see* condition
Monocytopenia 288.59 ◀
Monocytosis (symptomatic) 288.63 ⬅
Monofixation syndrome 378.34
Monomania (*see also* Psychosis) 298.9
Mononeuritis 355.9
cranial nerve - *see* Disorder, nerve, cranial
femoral nerve 355.2
lateral
cutaneous nerve of thigh 355.1
popliteal nerve 355.3
lower limb 355.8
specified nerve NEC 355.79
medial popliteal nerve 355.4
median nerve 354.1
multiplex 354.5
plantar nerve 355.6
posterior tibial nerve 355.5
radial nerve 354.3
sciatic nerve 355.0
ulnar nerve 354.2
upper limb 354.9
specified nerve NEC 354.8
vestibular 388.5
Mononeuropathy (*see also* Mononeuritis) 355.9
diabetic NEC 250.6 *[355.9]*
lower limb 250.6 *[355.8]*
upper limb 250.6 *[354.9]*
iliohypogastric nerve 355.79
ilioinguinal nerve 355.79
obturator nerve 355.79
saphenous nerve 355.79
Mononucleosis, infectious 075
with hepatitis 075 *[573.1]*
Monoplegia 344.5
brain (current episode) (*see also* Paralysis, brain) 437.8
fetus or newborn 767.8
cerebral (current episode) (*see also* Paralysis, brain) 437.8
congenital or infantile (cerebral) (spastic) (spinal) 343.3
Monoplegia *(Continued)*
embolic (current) (*see also* Embolism, brain) 434.1
late effect - *see* Late effect(s) (of) cerebrovascular disease
infantile (cerebral) (spastic) (spinal) 343.3
lower limb 344.30
affecting
dominant side 344.31
nondominant side 344.32
due to late effect of cerebrovascular accident - *see* Late effect(s) (of) cerebrovascular accident
newborn 767.8
psychogenic 306.0
specified as conversion reaction 300.11
thrombotic (current) (*see also* Thrombosis, brain) 434.0
late effect - *see* Late effect(s) (of) cerebrovascular disease
transient 781.4
upper limb 344.40
affecting
dominant side 344.41
nondominant side 344.42
due to late effect of cerebrovascular accident - *see* Late effect(s) (of) cerebrovascular accident
Monorchism, monorchidism 752.89
Monteggia's fracture (closed) 813.03
open 813.13
Mood swings
brief compensatory 296.99
rebound 296.99
Moore's syndrome (*see also* Epilepsy) 345.5
Mooren's ulcer (cornea) 370.07
Mooser-Neill reaction 081.0
Mooser bodies 081.0
Moral
deficiency 301.7
imbecility 301.7
Morax-Axenfeld conjunctivitis 372.03
Morbilli (*see also* Measles) 055.9
Morbus
anglicus, anglorum 268.0
Beigel 111.2
caducus (*see also* Epilepsy) 345.9
caeruleus 746.89
celiacus 579.0
comitialis (*see also* Epilepsy) 345.9
cordis - *see also* Disease, heart
valvulorum - *see* Endocarditis
coxae 719.95
tuberculous (*see also* Tuberculosis) 015.1
hemorrhagicus neonatorum 776.0
maculosus neonatorum 772.6
renum 593.0
senilis (*see also* Osteoarthrosis) 715.9
Morel-Kraepelin disease (*see also* Schizophrenia) 295.9
Morel-Moore syndrome (hyperostosis frontalis interna) 733.3
Morel-Morgagni syndrome (hyperostosis frontalis interna) 733.3
Morgagni
cyst, organ, hydatid, or appendage 752.89
fallopian tube 752.11
disease or syndrome (hyperostosis frontalis interna) 733.3

- **Morgagni-Adams-Stokes syndrome** (syncope with heart block) 426.9
- **Morgagni-Stewart-Morel syndrome** (hyperostosis frontalis interna) 733.3
- **Moria** (*see also* Psychosis) 298.9
- **Morning sickness** 643.0
- **Moron** 317
- **Morphea** (guttate) (linear) 701.0
- **Morphine dependence** (*see also* Dependence) 304.0
- **Morphinism** (*see also* Dependence) 304.0
- **Morphinomania** (*see also* Dependence) 304.0
- **Morphoea** 701.0
- **Morquio** (-Brailsford) (-Ullrich) disease or syndrome (mucopolysaccharidosis IV) 277.5
  - kyphosis 277.5
- **Morris syndrome** (testicular feminization) 259.5
- **Morsus humanus** (open wound) - *see also* Wound, open, by site
  - skin surface intact - *see* Contusion
- **Mortification** (dry) (moist) (*see also* Gangrene) 785.4
- **Morton's**
  - disease 355.6
  - foot 355.6
  - metatarsalgia (syndrome) 355.6
  - neuralgia 355.6
  - neuroma 355.6
  - syndrome (metatarsalgia) (neuralgia) 355.6
  - toe 355.6
- **Morvan's disease** 336.0
- **Mosaicism, mosaic** (chromosomal) 758.9
  - autosomal 758.5
  - sex 758.81
- **Moschcowitz's syndrome** (thrombotic thrombocytopenic purpura) 446.6
- **Mother yaw** 102.0
- **Motion sickness** (from travel, any vehicle) (from roundabouts or swings) 994.6
- **Mottled teeth** (enamel) (endemic) (nonendemic) 520.3
- **Mottling enamel** (endemic) (nonendemic) (teeth) 520.3
- **Mouchet's disease** 732.5
- **Mould**(s) (in vitreous) 117.9
- **Moulders'**
  - bronchitis 502
  - tuberculosis (*see also* Tuberculosis) 011.4
- **Mounier-Kuhn syndrome** 748.3
  - with
    - acute exacerbation 494.1
    - bronchiectasis 494.0
      - with (acute) exacerbation 494.1
  - acquired 519.19 ⬅
    - with bronchiectasis 494.0
      - with (acute) exacerbation 494.1
- **Mountain**
  - fever - *see* Fever, mountain
  - sickness 993.2
    - with polycythemia, acquired 289.0
    - acute 289.0
  - tick fever 066.1
- **Mouse, joint** (*see also* Loose, body, joint) 718.1
  - knee 717.6
- **Mouth** - *see* condition
- **Movable**
  - coccyx 724.71
  - kidney (*see also* Disease, renal) 593.0
    - congenital 753.3
- **Movable** *(Continued)*
  - organ or site, congenital NEC - *see* Malposition, congenital
  - spleen 289.59
- **Movement**
  - abnormal (dystonic) (involuntary) 781.0
  - decreased fetal 655.7
  - paradoxical facial 374.43
- **Moya Moya disease** 437.5
- **Mozart's ear** 744.29
- **MRSA** (methicillin-resistant staphylococcus aureus) V09.0
- **Mucha's disease** (acute parapsoriasis varioliformis) 696.2
- **Mucha-Haberman syndrome** (acute parapsoriasis varioliformis) 696.2
- **Mu-chain disease** 273.2
- **Mucinosis** (cutaneous) (papular) 701.8
- **Mucocele**
  - appendix 543.9
  - buccal cavity 528.9
  - gallbladder (*see also* Disease, gallbladder) 575.3
  - lacrimal sac 375.43
  - orbit (eye) 376.81
  - salivary gland (any) 527.6
  - sinus (accessory) (nasal) 478.19 ⬅
  - turbinate (bone) (middle) (nasal) 478.19 ⬅
  - uterus 621.8
- **Mucocutaneous lymph node syndrome** (acute) (febrile) (infantile) 446.1
- **Mucoenteritis** 564.9
- **Mucolipidosis I, II, III** 272.7
- **Mucopolysaccharidosis** (types 1–6) 277.5
  - cardiopathy 277.5 *[425.7]*
- **Mucormycosis** (lung) 117.7
- **Mucositis** - *see also* Inflammation, by site 528.00 ⬅
  - cervix (ulcerative) 616.81 ◀
  - due to ◀
    - antineoplastic therapy (ulcerative) 528.01 ◀
    - other drugs (ulcerative) 528.02 ◀
    - specified NEC 528.09 ◀
  - gastrointestinal (ulcerative) 538 ◀
  - nasal (ulcerative) 478.11 ◀
  - necroticans agranulocytica (*see also* Agranulocytosis) 288.09 ⬅
  - ulcerative 528.00 ◀
  - vagina (ulcerative) 616.81 ◀
  - vulva (ulcerative) 616.81 ◀
- **Mucous** - *see also* condition
  - patches (syphilitic) 091.3
    - congenital 090.0
- **Mucoviscidosis** 277.00
  - with meconium obstruction 277.01
- **Mucus**
  - asphyxia or suffocation (*see also* Asphyxia, mucus) 933.1
    - newborn 770.18
  - in stool 792.1
  - plug (*see also* Asphyxia, mucus) 933.1
    - aspiration, of newborn 770.17
    - tracheobronchial 519.19 ⬅
      - newborn 770.18
- **Muguet** 112.0
- **Mulberry molars** 090.5
- **Mullerian mixed tumor** (M8950/3) - *see* Neoplasm, by site, malignant
- **Multicystic kidney** 753.19
- **Multilobed placenta** - *see* Placenta, abnormal
- **Multinodular prostate** 600.10
  - with ⬅
    - urinary ◀
      - obstruction 600.11 ◀
      - retention 600.11 ◀
- **Multiparity** V61.5
  - affecting
    - fetus or newborn 763.89
    - management of
      - labor and delivery 659.4
      - pregnancy V23.3
  - requiring contraceptive management (*see also* Contraception) V25.9
- **Multipartita placenta** - *see* Placenta, abnormal
- **Multiple, multiplex** - *see also* condition
  - birth
    - affecting fetus or newborn 761.5
    - healthy liveborn - *see* Newborn, multiple
  - digits (congenital) 755.00
    - fingers 755.01
    - toes 755.02
  - organ or site NEC - *see* Accessory
  - personality 300.14
  - renal arteries 747.62
- **Mumps** 072.9
  - with complication 072.8
    - specified type NEC 072.79
  - encephalitis 072.2
  - hepatitis 072.71
  - meningitis (aseptic) 072.1
  - meningoencephalitis 072.2
  - oophoritis 072.79
  - orchitis 072.0
  - pancreatitis 072.3
  - polyneuropathy 072.72
  - vaccination, prophylactic (against) V04.6
- **Mumu** (*see also* Infestation, filarial) 125.9
- **Münchausen syndrome** 301.51
- **Münchmeyer's disease or syndrome** (exostosis luxurians) 728.11
- **Mural** - *see* condition
- **Murmur** (cardiac) (heart) (nonorganic) (organic) 785.2
  - abdominal 787.5
  - aortic (valve) (*see also* Endocarditis, aortic) 424.1
  - benign - *omit code*
  - cardiorespiratory 785.2
  - diastolic - *see* condition
  - Flint (*see also* Endocarditis, aortic) 424.1
  - functional - *omit code*
  - Graham Steell (pulmonic regurgitation) (*see also* Endocarditis, pulmonary) 424.3
  - innocent - *omit code*
  - insignificant - *omit code*
  - midsystolic 785.2
  - mitral (valve) - *see* Stenosis
  - physiologic - *see* condition
  - presystolic, mitral - *see* Insufficiency, mitral
  - pulmonic (valve) (*see also* Endocarditis, pulmonary) 424.3
  - Still's (vibratory) - *omit code*
  - systolic (valvular) - *see* condition
  - tricuspid (valve) - *see* Endocarditis, tricuspid
  - undiagnosed 785.2
  - valvular - *see* condition
  - vibratory - *omit code*
- **Murri's disease** (intermittent hemoglobinuria) 283.2

Muscae volitantes 379.24
Muscle, muscular - *see* condition
Musculoneuralgia 729.1
Mushrooming hip 718.95
Mushroom workers' (pickers') lung 495.5
Mutation
factor V leiden 289.81
prothrombin gene 289.81
Mutism (*see also* Aphasia) 784.3
akinetic 784.3
deaf (acquired) (congenital) 389.7
hysterical 300.11
selective (elective) 313.23
adjustment reaction 309.83
Myà's disease (congenital dilation, colon) 751.3
Myalgia (intercostal) 729.1
eosinophilia syndrome 710.5
epidemic 074.1
cervical 078.89
psychogenic 307.89
traumatic NEC 959.9
Myasthenia 358.00
cordis - *see* Failure, heart
gravis 358.00
with exacerbation (acute) 358.01
in crisis 358.01
neonatal 775.2
pseudoparalytica 358.00
stomach 536.8
psychogenic 306.4
syndrome
in
botulism 005.1 *[358.1]*
diabetes mellitus 250.6 *[358.1]*
hypothyroidism (*see also* Hypothyroidism) 244.9 *[358.1]*
malignant neoplasm NEC 199.1 *[358.1]*
pernicious anemia 281.0 *[358.1]*
thyrotoxicosis (*see also* Thyrotoxicosis) 242.9 *[358.1]*
Myasthenic 728.87
Mycelium infection NEC 117.9
Mycetismus 988.1
Mycetoma (actinomycotic) 039.9
bone 039.8
mycotic 117.4
foot 039.4
mycotic 117.4
madurae 039.9
mycotic 117.4
maduromycotic 039.9
mycotic 117.4
mycotic 117.4
nocardial 039.9
Mycobacteriosis - *see* Mycobacterium
Mycobacterium, mycobacterial (infection) 031.9
acid-fast (bacilli) 031.9
anonymous (*see also* Mycobacterium, atypical) 031.9
atypical (acid-fast bacilli) 031.9
cutaneous 031.1
pulmonary 031.0
tuberculous (*see also* Tuberculosis, pulmonary) 011.9
specified site NEC 031.8
avium 031.0
intracellulare complex bacteremia (MAC) 031.2
balnei 031.1
Battey 031.0
cutaneous 031.1

Mycobacterium, mycobacterial *(Continued)*
disseminated 031.2
avium-intracellulare complex (DMAC) 031.2
fortuitum 031.0
intracellulare (Battey bacillus) 031.0
kakerifu 031.8
kansasii 031.0
kasongo 031.8
leprae - *see* Leprosy
luciflavum 031.0
marinum 031.1
pulmonary 031.0
tuberculous (*see also* Tuberculosis, pulmonary) 011.9
scrofulaceum 031.1
tuberculosis (human, bovine) - *see also* Tuberculosis
avian type 031.0
ulcerans 031.1
xenopi 031.0
Mycosis, mycotic 117.9
cutaneous NEC 111.9
ear 111.8 *[380.15]*
fungoides (M9700/3) 202.1
mouth 112.0
pharynx 117.9
skin NEC 111.9
stomatitis 112.0
systemic NEC 117.9
tonsil 117.9
vagina, vaginitis 112.1
Mydriasis (persistent) (pupil) 379.43
Myelatelia 742.59
Myelinoclasis, perivascular, acute (postinfectious) NEC 136.9 *[323.61]* ◄
postimmunization or postvaccinal 323.51 ◄
Myelinosis, central pontine 341.8
Myelitis (ascending) (cerebellar) (childhood) (chronic) (descending) (diffuse) (disseminated) (pressure) (progressive) (spinal cord) (subacute) (*see also* Encephalitis) 323.9 ◄
acute (transverse) 341.20 ◄
idiopathic 341.22 ◄
in conditions classified elsewhere 341.21 ◄
due to ◄
infection classified elsewhere 136.9 *[323.42]* ◄
specified cause NEC 323.82 ◄
vaccination (any) 323.52 ◄
viral diseases classified elsewhere 323.02 ◄
herpes simplex 054.74 ◄
herpes zoster 053.14 ◄
late effect - *see* category 326
optic neuritis in 341.0
postchickenpox 052.2 ◄
postimmunization 323.52 ◄
postinfectious 136.9 *[323.63]* ◄
postvaccinal 323.52 ◄
postvaricella 052.2 ◄
syphilitic (transverse) 094.89
toxic 989.9 *[323.72]* ◄
transverse 323.82 ◄
acute 341.20 ◄
idiopathic 341.22 ◄
in conditions classified elsewhere 341.21 ◄
idiopathic 341.22 ◄

Myelitis *(Continued)*
tuberculous (*see also* Tuberculosis) 013.6
virus 049.9
Myeloblastic - *see* condition
Myelocele (*see also* Spina bifida) 741.9
with hydrocephalus 741.0
Myelocystocele (*see also* Spina bifida) 741.9
Myelocytic - *see* condition
Myelocytoma 205.1
Myelodysplasia (spinal cord) 742.59
meaning myelodysplastic syndrome - *see* Syndrome, myelodysplastic
Myeloencephalitis - *see* Encephalitis
Myelofibrosis 289.83 ◄
with myeloid metaplasia 238.76 ◄
idiopathic (chronic) 238.76 ◄
megakaryocytic 238.79 ◄
primary 238.76 ◄
secondary 289.83 ◄
Myelogenous - *see* condition
Myeloid - *see* condition
Myelokathexis 288.09 ◄
Myeloleukodystrophy 330.0
Myelolipoma (M8870/0) - *see* Neoplasm, by site, benign
Myeloma (multiple) (plasma cell) (plasmacytic) (M9730/3) 203.0
monostotic (M9731/1) 238.6
solitary (M9731/1) 238.6
Myelomalacia 336.8
Myelomata, multiple (M9730/3) 203.0
Myelomatosis (M9730/3) 203.0
Myelomeningitis - *see* Meningoencephalitis
Myelomeningocele (spinal cord) (*see also* Spina bifida) 741.9
fetal, causing fetopelvic disproportion 653.7
Myelo-osteo-musculodysplasia hereditaria 756.89
Myelopathic - *see* condition
Myelopathy (spinal cord) 336.9
cervical 721.1
diabetic 250.6 *[336.3]*
drug-induced 336.8
due to or with
carbon tetrachloride 987.8 *[323.72]* ◄
degeneration or displacement, intervertebral disc 722.70
cervical, cervicothoracic 722.71
lumbar, lumbosacral 722.73
thoracic, thoracolumbar 722.72
hydroxyquinoline derivatives 961.3 *[323.72]* ◄
infection - *see* Encephalitis
intervertebral disc disorder 722.70
cervical, cervicothoracic 722.71
lumbar, lumbosacral 722.73
thoracic, thoracolumbar 722.72
lead 984.9 *[323.72]* ◄
mercury 985.0 *[323.72]* ◄
neoplastic disease (*see also* Neoplasm, by site) 239.9 *[336.3]*
pernicious anemia 281.0 *[336.3]*
spondylosis 721.91
cervical 721.1
lumbar, lumbosacral 721.42
thoracic 721.41
thallium 985.8 *[323.72]* ◄
lumbar, lumbosacral 721.42
necrotic (subacute) 336.1
radiation-induced 336.8
spondylogenic NEC 721.91

◄ New ◄ Revised

Myelopathy *(Continued)*
spondylogenic NEC *(Continued)*
cervical 721.1
lumbar, lumbosacral 721.42
thoracic 721.41
thoracic 721.41
toxic NEC 989.9 *[323.72]*
transverse (*see also* Myelitis) 323.82
vascular 336.1
Myelophthisis 284.2
Myeloproliferative disease (M9960/1) 238.79
Myeloradiculitis (*see also* Polyneuropathy) 357.0
Myeloradiculodysplasia (spinal) 742.59
Myelosarcoma (M9930/3) 205.3
Myelosclerosis 289.89
with myeloid metaplasia (M9961/1) 238.76
disseminated, of nervous system 340
megakaryocytic (M9961/1) 238.79
Myelosis (M9860/3) (*see also* Leukemia, myeloid) 205.9
acute (M9861/3) 205.0
aleukemic (M9864/3) 205.8
chronic (M9863/3) 205.1
erythremic (M9840/3) 207.0
acute (M9841/3) 207.0
megakaryocytic (M9920/3) 207.2
nonleukemic (chronic) 288.8
subacute (M9862/3) 205.2
Myesthenia - *see* Myasthenia
Myiasis (cavernous) 134.0
orbit 134.0 *[376.13]*
Myoadenoma, prostate 600.20
with
other lower urinary tract symptoms (LUTS) 600.21
urinary
obstruction 600.21
retention 600.21
Myoblastoma
granular cell (M9580/0) - *see also* Neoplasm, connective tissue, benign
malignant (M9580/3) - *see* Neoplasm, connective tissue, malignant
tongue (M9580/0) 210.1
Myocardial - *see* condition
Myocardiopathy (congestive) (constrictive) (familial) (hypertrophic nonobstructive) (idiopathic) (infiltrative) (obstructive) (primary) (restrictive) (sporadic) 425.4
alcoholic 425.5
amyloid 277.39 *[425.7]*
beriberi 265.0 *[425.7]*
cobalt-beer 425.5
due to
amyloidosis 277.39 *[425.7]*
beriberi 265.0 *[425.7]*
cardiac glycogenosis 271.0 *[425.7]*
Chagas' disease 086.0
Friedreich's ataxia 334.0 *[425.8]*
influenza 487.8 *[425.8]*
mucopolysaccharidosis 277.5 *[425.7]*
myotonia atrophica 359.2 *[425.8]*
progressive muscular dystrophy 359.1 *[425.8]*
sarcoidosis 135 *[425.8]*
glycogen storage 271.0 *[425.7]*
hypertrophic obstructive 425.1
metabolic NEC 277.9 *[425.7]*
nutritional 269.9 *[425.7]*

Myocardiopathy *(Continued)*
obscure (African) 425.2
peripartum 674.5
postpartum 674.5
secondary 425.9
thyrotoxic (*see also* Thyrotoxicosis) 242.9 *[425.7]*
toxic NEC 425.9
Myocarditis (fibroid) (interstitial) (old) (progressive) (senile) (with arteriosclerosis) 429.0
with
rheumatic fever (conditions classifiable to 390) 398.0
active (*see also* Myocarditis, acute, rheumatic) 391.2
inactive or quiescent (with chorea) 398.0
active (nonrheumatic) 422.90
rheumatic 391.2
with chorea (acute) (rheumatic) (Sydenham's) 392.0
acute or subacute (interstitial) 422.90
due to Streptococcus (beta-hemolytic) 391.2
idiopathic 422.91
rheumatic 391.2
with chorea (acute) (rheumatic) (Sydenham's) 392.0
specified type NEC 422.99
aseptic of newborn 074.23
bacterial (acute) 422.92
chagasic 086.0
chronic (interstitial) 429.0
congenital 746.89
constrictive 425.4
Coxsackie (virus) 074.23
diphtheritic 032.82
due to or in
Coxsackie (virus) 074.23
diphtheria 032.82
epidemic louse-borne typhus 080 *[422.0]*
influenza 487.8 *[422.0]*
Lyme disease 088.81 *[422.0]*
scarlet fever 034.1 *[422.0]*
toxoplasmosis (acquired) 130.3
tuberculosis (*see also* Tuberculosis) 017.9 *[422.0]*
typhoid 002.0 *[422.0]*
typhus NEC 081.9 *[422.0]*
eosinophilic 422.91
epidemic of newborn 074.23
Fiedler's (acute) (isolated) (subacute) 422.91
giant cell (acute) (subacute) 422.91
gonococcal 098.85
granulomatous (idiopathic) (isolated) (nonspecific) 422.91
hypertensive (*see also* Hypertension, heart) 402.90
idiopathic 422.91
granulomatous 422.91
infective 422.92
influenzal 487.8 *[422.0]*
isolated (diffuse) (granulomatous) 422.91
malignant 422.99
meningococcal 036.43
nonrheumatic, active 422.90
parenchymatous 422.90
pneumococcal (acute) (subacute) 422.92
rheumatic (chronic) (inactive) (with chorea) 398.0

Myocarditis *(Continued)*
rheumatic *(Continued)*
active or acute 391.2
with chorea (acute) (rheumatic) (Sydenham's) 392.0
septic 422.92
specific (giant cell) (productive) 422.91
staphylococcal (acute) (subacute) 422.92
suppurative 422.92
syphilitic (chronic) 093.82
toxic 422.93
rheumatic (*see also* Myocarditis, acute rheumatic) 391.2
tuberculous (*see also* Tuberculosis) 017.9 *[422.0]*
typhoid 002.0 *[422.0]*
valvular - *see* Endocarditis
viral, except Coxsackie 422.91
Coxsackie 074.23
of newborn (Coxsackie) 074.23
Myocardium, myocardial - *see* condition
Myocardosis (*see also* Cardiomyopathy) 425.4
Myoclonia (essential) 333.2
epileptica 333.2
Friedrich's 333.2
massive 333.2
Myoclonic
epilepsy, familial (progressive) 333.2
jerks 333.2
Myoclonus (familial essential) (multifocal) (simplex) 333.2
with epilepsy and with ragged red fibers (MERRF syndrome) 277.87
facial 351.8
massive (infantile) 333.2
pharyngeal 478.29
Myodiastasis 728.84
Myoendocarditis - *see also* Endocarditis
acute or subacute 421.9
Myoepithelioma (M8982/0) - *see* Neoplasm, by site, benign
Myofascitis (acute) 729.1
low back 724.2
Myofibroma (M8890/0) - *see also* Neoplasm, connective tissue, benign
uterus (cervix) (corpus) (*see also* Leiomyoma) 218.9
Myofibromatosis
infantile 759.89
Myofibrosis 728.2
heart (*see also* Myocarditis) 429.0
humeroscapular region 726.2
scapulohumeral 726.2
Myofibrositis (*see also* Myositis) 729.1
scapulohumeral 726.2
Myogelosis (occupational) 728.89
Myoglobinuria 791.3
Myoglobulinuria, primary 791.3
Myokymia - *see also* Myoclonus
facial 351.8
Myolipoma (M8860/0)
specified site - *see* Neoplasm, connective tissue, benign
unspecified site 223.0
Myoma (M8895/0) - *see also* Neoplasm, connective tissue, benign
cervix (stump) (uterus) (*see also* Leiomyoma) 218.9
malignant (M8895/3) - *see* Neoplasm, connective tissue, malignant
prostate 600.20

◀ New ⬅ Revised

Myoma *(Continued)*
prostate *(Continued)*
with
other lower urinary tract symptoms (LUTS) 600.21
urinary
obstruction 600.21
retention 600.21
uterus (cervix) (corpus) (*see also* Leiomyoma) 218.9
in pregnancy or childbirth 654.1
affecting fetus or newborn 763.89
causing obstructed labor 660.2
affecting fetus or newborn 763.1
Myomalacia 728.9
cordis, heart (*see also* Degeneration, myocardial) 429.1
Myometritis (*see also* Endometritis) 615.9
Myometrium - *see* condition
Myonecrosis, clostridial 040.0
Myopathy 359.9
alcoholic 359.4
amyloid 277.39 *[359.6]*
benign, congenital 359.0
central core 359.0
centronuclear 359.0
congenital (benign) 359.0
critical illness 359.81
distal 359.1
due to drugs 359.4
endocrine 259.9 *[359.5]*
specified type NEC 259.8 *[359.5]*
extraocular muscles 376.82
facioscapulohumeral 359.1
in
Addison's disease 255.4 *[359.5]*
amyloidosis 277.39 *[359.6]*
cretinism 243 *[359.5]*
Cushing's syndrome 255.0 *[359.5]*
disseminated lupus erythematosus 710.0 *[359.6]*
giant cell arteritis 446.5 *[359.6]*
hyperadrenocorticism NEC 255.3 *[359.5]*
hyperparathyroidism 252.01 *[359.5]*
hypopituitarism 253.2 *[359.5]*
hypothyroidism (*see also* Hypothyroidism) 244.9 *[359.5]*
malignant neoplasm NEC (M8000/3) 199.1 *[359.6]*
myxedema (*see also* Myxedema) 244.9 *[359.5]*
polyarteritis nodosa 446.0 *[359.6]*
rheumatoid arthritis 714.0 *[359.6]*
sarcoidosis 135 *[359.6]*

Myopathy *(Continued)*
in *(Continued)*
scleroderma 710.1 *[359.6]*
Sjögren's disease 710.2 *[359.6]*
thyrotoxicosis (*see also* Thyrotoxicosis) 242.9 *[359.5]*
inflammatory 359.89
intensive care (ICU) 359.81
limb-girdle 359.1
myotubular 359.0
necrotizing, acute 359.81
nemaline 359.0
ocular 359.1
oculopharyngeal 359.1
of critical illness 359.81
primary 359.89
progressive NEC 359.89
quadriplegic, acute 359.81
rod body 359.0
scapulohumeral 359.1
specified type NEC 359.89
toxic 359.4
Myopericarditis (*see also* Pericarditis) 423.9
Myopia (axial) (congenital) (increased curvature or refraction, nucleus of lens) 367.1
degenerative, malignant 360.21
malignant 360.21
progressive high (degenerative) 360.21
Myosarcoma (M8895/3) - *see* Neoplasm, connective tissue, malignant
Myosis (persistent) 379.42
stromal (endolymphatic) (M8931/1) 236.0
Myositis 729.1
clostridial 040.0
due to posture 729.1
epidemic 074.1
fibrosa or fibrous (chronic) 728.2
Volkmann's (complicating trauma) 958.6
infective 728.0
interstitial 728.81
multiple - *see* Polymyositis
occupational 729.1
orbital, chronic 376.12
ossificans 728.12
circumscribed 728.12
progressive 728.11
traumatic 728.12
progressive fibrosing 728.11
purulent 728.0
rheumatic 729.1
rheumatoid 729.1

Myositis *(Continued)*
suppurative 728.0
syphilitic 095.6
traumatic (old) 729.1
Myospasia impulsiva 307.23
Myotonia (acquisita) (intermittens) 728.85
atrophica 359.2
congenita 359.2
dystrophica 359.2
Myotonic pupil 379.46
Myriapodiasis 134.1
Myringitis
with otitis media - *see* Otitis media
acute 384.00
specified type NEC 384.09
bullosa hemorrhagica 384.01
bullous 384.01
chronic 384.1
Mysophobia 300.29
Mytilotoxism 988.0
Myxadenitis labialis 528.5
Myxedema (adult) (idiocy) (infantile) (juvenile) (thyroid gland) (*see also* Hypothyroidism) 244.9
circumscribed 242.9
congenital 243
cutis 701.8
localized (pretibial) 242.9
madness (acute) 293.0
subacute 293.1
papular 701.8
pituitary 244.8
postpartum 674.8
pretibial 242.9
primary 244.9
Myxochondrosarcoma (M9220/3) - *see* Neoplasm, cartilage, malignant
Myxofibroma (M8811/0) - *see also* Neoplasm, connective tissue, benign
odontogenic (M9320/0) 213.1
upper jaw (bone) 213.0
Myxofibrosarcoma (M8811/3) - *see* Neoplasm, connective tissue, malignant
Myxolipoma (M8852/0) (*see also* Lipoma, by site) 214.9
Myxoliposarcoma (M8852/3) - *see* Neoplasm, connective tissue, malignant
Myxoma (M8840/0) - *see also* Neoplasm, connective tissue, benign
odontogenic (M9320/0) 213.1
upper jaw (bone) 213.0
Myxosarcoma (M8840/3) - *see* Neoplasm, connective tissue, malignant

ICD-9-CM
M
Vol. 2

N

Naegeli's
disease (hereditary hemorrhagic thrombasthenia 287.1
leukemia, monocytic (M9863/3) 205.1
syndrome (incontinentia pigmenti) 757.33
Naffziger's syndrome 353.0
Naga sore (*see* also Ulcer, skin) 707.9
Nägele's pelvis 738.6
with disproportion (fetopelvic) 653.0
affecting fetus or newborn 763.1
causing obstructed labor 660.1
affecting fetus or newborn 763.1
Nager-de Reynier syndrome (dysostosis mandibularis) 756.0
Nail - *see* also condition
biting 307.9
patella syndrome (hereditary osteoonychodysplasia) 756.89
Nanism, nanosomia (*see* also Dwarfism) 259.4
hypophyseal 253.3
pituitary 253.3
renis, renalis 588.0
Nanukayami 100.89
Napkin rash 691.0
Narcissism 301.81
Narcolepsy 347.00
with cataplexy 347.01
in conditions classified elsewhere 347.10
with cataplexy 347.11
Narcosis
carbon dioxide (respiratory) 786.09
due to drug
correct substance properly administered 780.09
overdose or wrong substance given or taken 977.9
specified drug - *see* Table of Drugs and Chemicals
Narcotism (chronic) (*see* also Dependence) 304.9
acute
correct substance properly administered 349.82
overdose or wrong substance given or taken 967.8
specified drug - *see* Table of Drugs and Chemicals
NARP (Neuropathy, ataxia, and retinitis pigmentosa syndrome) 277.87
Narrow
anterior chamber angle 365.02
pelvis (inlet) (outlet) - *see* Contraction, pelvis
Narrowing
artery NEC 447.1
auditory, internal 433.8
basilar 433.0
with other precerebral artery 433.3
bilateral 433.3
carotid 433.1
with other precerebral artery 433.3
bilateral 433.3
cerebellar 433.8
choroidal 433.8
communicating posterior 433.8
coronary - *see also* Arteriosclerosis, coronary
congenital 746.85
due to syphilis 090.5
hypophyseal 433.8

Narrowing *(Continued)*
artery NEC *(Continued)*
pontine 433.8
precerebral NEC 433.9
multiple or bilateral 433.3
specified NEC 433.8
vertebral 433.2
with other precerebral artery 433.3
bilateral 433.3
auditory canal (external) (*see also* Stricture, ear canal, acquired) 380.50
cerebral arteries 437.0
cicatricial - *see* Cicatrix
congenital - *see* Anomaly, congenital
coronary artery - *see* Narrowing, artery, coronary
ear, middle 385.22
Eustachian tube (*see also* Obstruction, Eustachian tube) 381.60
eyelid 374.46
congenital 743.62
intervertebral disc or space NEC - *see* Degeneration, intervertebral disc
joint space, hip 719.85
larynx 478.74
lids 374.46
congenital 743.62
mesenteric artery (with gangrene) 557.0
palate 524.89
palpebral fissure 374.46
retinal artery 362.13
ureter 593.3
urethra (*see also* Stricture, urethra) 598.9
Narrowness, abnormal, eyelid 743.62
Nasal - *see* condition
Nasolacrimal - *see* condition
Nasopharyngeal - *see also* condition
bursa 478.29
pituitary gland 759.2
torticollis 723.5
Nasopharyngitis (acute) (infective) (subacute) 460
chronic 472.2
due to external agent - *see* Condition, respiratory, chronic, due to
due to external agent - *see* Condition, respiratory, due to
septic 034.0
streptococcal 034.0
suppurative (chronic) 472.2
ulcerative (chronic) 472.2
Nasopharynx, nasopharyngeal - *see* condition
Natal tooth, teeth 520.6
Nausea (*see also* Vomiting) 787.02
with vomiting 787.01
epidemic 078.82
gravidarum - *see* Hyperemesis, gravidarum
marina 994.6
Naval - *see* condition
Neapolitan fever (*see also* Brucellosis) 023.9
Nearsightedness 367.1
Near-syncope 780.2
Nebécourt's syndrome 253.3
Nebula, cornea (eye) 371.01
congenital 743.43
interfering with vision 743.42
Necator americanus infestation 126.1
Necatoriasis 126.1
Neck - *see* condition
Necrencephalus (*see also* Softening, brain) 437.8

Necrobacillosis 040.3
Necrobiosis 799.89
brain or cerebral (*see also* Softening, brain) 437.8
lipoidica 709.3
diabeticorum 250.8 *[709.3]*
Necrodermolysis 695.1
Necrolysis, toxic epidermal 695.1
due to drug
correct substance properly administered 695.1
overdose or wrong substance given or taken 977.9
specified drug - *see* Table of Drugs and Chemicals
Neuropathy, ataxia, and retinitis pigmentosa (NARP syndrome) 277.87
Necrophilia 302.89
Necrosis, necrotic
adrenal (capsule) (gland) 255.8
antrum, nasal sinus 478.19 (Revised)
aorta (hyaline) (*see also* Aneurysm, aorta) 441.9
cystic medial 441.00
abdominal 441.02
thoracic 441.01
thoracoabdominal 441.03
ruptured 441.5
arteritis 446.0
artery 447.5
aseptic, bone 733.40
femur (head) (neck) 733.42
medial condyle 733.43
humoral head 733.41
medial femoral condyle 733.43
specific site NEC 733.49
talus 733.44
avascular, bone NEC (*see also* Necrosis, aseptic, bone) 733.40
bladder (aseptic) (sphincter) 596.8
bone (*see also* Osteomyelitis) 730.1
acute 730.0
aseptic or avascular 733.40
femur (head) (neck) 733.42
medial condyle 733.43
humoral head 733.41
medial femoral condyle 733.43
specified site NEC 733.49
talus 733.44
ethmoid 478.19 (Revised)
ischemic 733.40
jaw 526.4
marrow 289.89
Paget's (osteitis deformans) 731.0
tuberculous - *see* Tuberculosis, bone
brain (softening) (*see also* Softening, brain) 437.8
breast (aseptic) (fat) (segmental) 611.3
bronchus, bronchi 519.19 (Revised)
central nervous system NEC (*see also* Softening, brain) 437.8
cerebellar (*see also* Softening, brain) 437.8
cerebral (softening) (*see also* Softening, brain) 437.8
cerebrospinal (softening) (*see also* Softening, brain) 437.8
cornea (*see also* Keratitis) 371.40
cortical, kidney 583.6
cystic medial (aorta) 441.00
abdominal 441.02
thoracic 441.01
thoracoabdominal 441.03
dental 521.09
pulp 522.1

Necrosis, necrotic *(Continued)*
due to swallowing corrosive substance - *see* Burn, by site
ear (ossicle) 385.24
esophagus 530.89
ethmoid (bone) 478.19
eyelid 374.50
fat, fatty (generalized) (*see also* Degeneration, fatty) 272.8
abdominal wall 567.82
breast (aseptic) (segmental) 611.3
intestine 569.89
localized - *see* Degeneration, by site, fatty
mesentery 567.82
omentum 567.82
pancreas 577.8
peritoneum 567.82
skin (subcutaneous) 709.3
newborn 778.1
femur (aseptic) (avascular) 733.42
head 733.42
medial condyle 733.43
neck 733.42
gallbladder (*see also* Cholecystitis, acute) 575.0
gangrenous 785.4
gastric 537.89
glottis 478.79
heart (myocardium) - *see* Infarct, myocardium
hepatic (*see also* Necrosis, liver) 570
hip (aseptic) (avascular) 733.42
intestine (acute) (hemorrhagic) (massive) 557.0
ischemic 785.4
jaw 526.4
kidney (bilateral) 583.9
acute 584.9
cortical 583.6
acute 584.6
with
abortion - *see* Abortion, by type, with renal failure
ectopic pregnancy (*see also* categories 633.0–633.9) 639.3
molar pregnancy (*see also* categories 630–632) 639.3
complicating pregnancy 646.2
affecting fetus or newborn 760.1
following labor and delivery 669.3
medullary (papillary) (*see also* Pyelitis) 590.80
in
acute renal failure 584.7
nephritis, nephropathy 583.7
papillary (*see also* Pyelitis) 590.80
in
acute renal failure 584.7
nephritis, nephropathy 583.7
tubular 584.5
with
abortion - *see* Abortion, by type, with renal failure

Necrosis, necrotic *(Continued)*
kidney *(Continued)*
tubular *(Continued)*
with *(Continued)*
ectopic pregnancy (*see also* categories 633.0–633.9) 639.3
molar pregnancy (*see also* categories 630–632) 639.3
complicating
abortion 639.3
ectopic or molar pregnancy 639.3
pregnancy 646.2
affecting fetus or newborn 760.1
following labor and delivery 669.3
traumatic 958.5
larynx 478.79
liver (acute) (congenital) (diffuse) (massive) (subacute) 570
with
abortion - *see* Abortion, by type, with specified complication NEC
ectopic pregnancy (*see also* categories 633.0–633.9) 639.8
molar pregnancy (*see also* categories 630–632) 639.8
complicating pregnancy 646.7
affecting fetus or newborn 760.8
following
abortion 639.8
ectopic or molar pregnancy 639.8
obstetrical 646.7
postabortal 639.8
puerperal, postpartum 674.8
toxic 573.3
lung 513.0
lymphatic gland 683
mammary gland 611.3
mastoid (chronic) 383.1
mesentery 557.0
fat 567.82
mitral valve - *see* Insufficiency, mitral
myocardium, myocardial - *see* Infarct, myocardium
nose (septum) 478.19
omentum 557.0
with mesenteric infarction 557.0
fat 567.82
orbit, orbital 376.10
ossicles, ear (aseptic) 385.24
ovary (*see also* Salpingo-oophoritis) 614.2
pancreas (aseptic) (duct) (fat) 577.8
acute 577.0
infective 577.0
papillary, kidney (*see also* Pyelitis) 590.80
perineum 624.8
peritoneum 557.0
with mesenteric infarction 557.0
fat 567.82
pharynx 462
in granulocytopenia 288.09
phosphorus 983.9
pituitary (gland) (postpartum) (Sheehan) 253.2

Necrosis, necrotic *(Continued)*
placenta (*see also* Placenta, abnormal) 656.7
pneumonia 513.0
pulmonary 513.0
pulp (dental) 522.1
pylorus 537.89
radiation - *see* Necrosis, by site
radium - *see* Necrosis, by site
renal - *see* Necrosis, kidney
sclera 379.19
scrotum 608.89
skin or subcutaneous tissue 709.8
due to burn - *see* Burn, by site
gangrenous 785.4
spine, spinal (column) 730.18
acute 730.18
cord 336.1
spleen 289.59
stomach 537.89
stomatitis 528.1
subcutaneous fat 709.3
fetus or newborn 778.1
subendocardial - *see* Infarct, myocardium
suprarenal (capsule) (gland) 255.8
teeth, tooth 521.09
testis 608.89
thymus (gland) 254.8
tonsil 474.8
trachea 519.19
tuberculous NEC - *see* Tuberculosis
tubular (acute) (anoxic) (toxic) 584.5
due to a procedure 997.5
umbilical cord, affecting fetus or newborn 762.6
vagina 623.8
vertebra (lumbar) 730.18
acute 730.18
tuberculous (*see also* Tuberculosis) 015.0 *[730.8]*
vesical (aseptic) (bladder) 596.8
vulva 624.8
x-ray - *see* Necrosis, by site
Necrospermia 606.0
Necrotizing angiitis 446.0
Negativism 301.7
Neglect (child) (newborn) NEC 995.52
adult 995.84
after or at birth 995.52
hemispatial 781.8
left-sided 781.8
sensory 781.8
visuospatial 781.8
Negri bodies 071
Neill-Dingwall syndrome (microcephaly and dwarfism) 759.89
Neisserian infection NEC - *see* Gonococcus
Nematodiasis NEC (*see also* Infestation, Nematode) 127.9
ancylostoma (*see also* Ancylostomiasis) 126.9
Neoformans cryptococcus infection 117.5
Neonatal - *see also* condition
adrenoleukodystrophy 277.86
teeth, tooth 520.6
Neonatorum - *see* condition

ICD-9-CM N Vol. 2

	Malignant					
	Primary	**Secondary**	**Ca in situ**	**Benign**	**Uncertain Behavior**	**Unspecified**
Neoplasm, neoplastic	199.1	199.1	234.9	229.9	238.9	239.9

Notes — 1. The list below gives the code numbers for neoplasms by anatomical site. For each site there are six possible code numbers according to whether the neoplasm in question is malignant, benign, in situ, of uncertain behavior, or of unspecified nature. The description of the neoplasm will often indicate which of the six columns is appropriate; e.g., malignant melanoma of skin, benign fibroadenoma of breast, carcinoma in situ of cervix uteri.

Where such descriptors are not present, the remainder of the Index should be consulted where guidance is given to the appropriate column for each morphological (histological) variety listed; e.g., Mesonephroma—see Neoplasm, malignant; Embryoma—see also Neoplasm, uncertain behavior; Disease, Bowen's—see Neoplasm, skin, in situ. However, the guidance in the Index can be overridden if one of the descriptors mentioned above is present; e.g., malignant adenoma of colon is coded to 153.9 and not to 211.3 as the adjective "malignant" overrides the Index entry "Adenoma - see also Neoplasm, benign."

*2. Sites marked with the sign * (e.g., face NEC*) should be classified to malignant neoplasm of skin of these sites if the variety of neoplasm is a squamous cell carcinoma or an epidermoid carcinoma and to benign neoplasm of skin of these sites if the variety of neoplasm is a papilloma (any type).*

Site	Primary	Secondary	Ca in situ	Benign	Uncertain Behavior	Unspecified
abdomen, abdominal	195.2	198.89	234.8	229.8	238.8	239.8
cavity	195.2	198.89	234.8	229.8	238.8	239.8
organ	195.2	198.89	234.8	229.8	238.8	239.8
viscera	195.2	198.89	234.8	229.8	238.8	239.8
wall	173.5	198.2	232.5	216.5	238.2	239.2
connective tissue	171.5	198.89	—	215.5	238.1	239.2
abdominopelvic	195.8	198.89	234.8	229.8	238.8	239.8
accessory sinus - *see* Neoplasm, sinus						
acoustic nerve	192.0	198.4	—	225.1	237.9	239.7
acromion (process)	170.4	198.5	—	213.4	238.0	239.2
adenoid (pharynx) (tissue)	147.1	198.89	230.0	210.7	235.1	239.0
adipose tissue (*see also* Neoplasm, connective tissue)	171.9	198.89	—	215.9	238.1	239.2
adnexa (uterine)	183.9	198.82	233.3	221.8	236.3	239.5
adrenal (cortex) (gland) (medulla)	194.0	198.7	234.8	227.0	237.2	239.7
ala nasi (external)	173.3	198.2	232.3	216.3	238.2	239.2
alimentary canal or tract NEC	159.9	197.8	230.9	211.9	235.5	239.0
alveolar	143.9	198.89	230.0	210.4	235.1	239.0
mucosa	143.9	198.89	230.0	210.4	235.1	239.0
lower	143.1	198.89	230.0	210.4	235.1	239.0
upper	143.0	198.89	230.0	210.4	235.1	239.0
ridge or process	170.1	198.5	—	213.1	238.0	239.2
carcinoma	143.9	—	—	—	—	—
lower	143.1	—	—	—	—	—
upper	143.0	—	—	—	—	—
lower	170.1	198.5	—	213.1	238.0	239.2
mucosa	143.9	198.89	230.0	210.4	235.1	239.0
lower	143.1	198.89	230.0	210.4	235.1	239.0
upper	143.0	198.89	230.0	210.4	235.1	239.0
upper	170.0	198.5	—	213.0	238.0	239.2
sulcus	145.1	198.89	230.0	210.4	235.1	239.0
alveolus	143.9	198.89	230.0	210.4	235.1	239.0
lower	143.1	198.89	230.0	210.4	235.1	239.0
upper	143.0	198.89	230.0	210.4	235.1	239.0
ampulla of Vater	156.2	197.8	230.8	211.5	235.3	239.0
ankle NEC*	195.5	198.89	232.7	229.8	238.8	239.8
anorectum, anorectal (junction)	154.8	197.5	230.7	211.4	235.2	239.0
antecubital fossa or space*	195.4	198.89	232.6	229.8	238.8	239.8
antrum (Highmore) (maxillary)	160.2	197.3	231.8	212.0	235.9	239.1
pyloric	151.2	197.8	230.2	211.1	235.2	239.0
tympanicum	160.1	197.3	231.8	212.0	235.9	239.1
anus, anal	154.3	197.5	230.6	211.4	235.5	239.0
canal	154.2	197.5	230.5	211.4	235.5	239.0
contiguous sites with rectosigmoid junction or rectum	154.8	—	—	—	—	—
margin	173.5	198.2	232.5	216.5	238.2	239.2
skin	173.5	198.2	232.5	216.5	238.2	239.2
sphincter	154.2	197.5	230.5	211.4	235.5	239.0
aorta (thoracic)	171.4	198.89	—	215.4	238.1	239.2
abdominal	171.5	198.89	—	215.5	238.1	239.2
aortic body	194.6	198.89	—	227.6	237.3	239.7
aponeurosis	171.9	198.89	—	215.9	238.1	239.2
palmar	171.2	198.89	—	215.2	238.1	239.2
plantar	171.3	198.89	—	215.3	238.1	239.2
appendix	153.5	197.5	230.3	211.3	235.2	239.0

	Malignant					
	Primary	**Secondary**	**Ca in situ**	**Benign**	**Uncertain Behavior**	**Unspecified**
Neoplasm *(Continued)*						
arachnoid (cerebral)	192.1	198.4	—	225.2	237.6	239.7
spinal	192.3	198.4	—	225.4	237.6	239.7
areola (female)	174.0	198.81	233.0	217	238.3	239.3
male	175.0	198.81	233.0	217	238.3	239.3
arm NEC*	195.4	198.89	232.6	229.8	238.8	239.8
artery - *see* Neoplasm, connective tissue						
aryepiglottic fold	148.2	198.89	230.0	210.8	235.1	239.0
hypopharyngeal aspect	148.2	198.89	230.0	210.8	235.1	239.0
laryngeal aspect	161.1	197.3	231.0	212.1	235.6	239.1
marginal zone	148.2	198.89	230.0	210.8	235.1	239.0
arytenoid (cartilage)	161.3	197.3	231.0	212.1	235.6	239.1
fold - *see* Neoplasm, aryepiglottic						
atlas	170.2	198.5	—	213.2	238.0	239.2
atrium, cardiac	164.1	198.89	—	212.7	238.8	239.8
auditory						
canal (external) (skin)	173.2	198.2	232.2	216.2	238.2	239.2
internal	160.1	197.3	231.8	212.0	235.9	239.1
nerve	192.0	198.4	—	225.1	237.9	239.7
tube	160.1	197.3	231.8	212.0	235.9	239.1
opening	147.2	198.89	230.0	210.7	235.1	239.0
auricle, ear	173.2	198.2	232.2	216.2	238.2	239.2
cartilage	171.0	198.89	—	215.0	238.1	239.2
auricular canal (external)	173.2	198.2	232.2	216.2	238.2	239.2
internal	160.1	197.3	231.8	212.0	235.9	239.1
autonomic nerve or nervous system NEC	171.9	198.89	—	215.9	238.1	239.2
axilla, axillary	195.1	198.89	234.8	229.8	238.8	239.8
fold	173.5	198.2	232.5	216.5	238.2	239.2
back NEC*	195.8	198.89	232.5	229.8	238.8	239.8
Bartholin's gland	184.1	198.82	233.3	221.2	236.3	239.5
basal ganglia	191.0	198.3	—	225.0	237.5	239.6
basis pedunculi	191.7	198.3	—	225.0	237.5	239.6
bile or biliary (tract)	156.9	197.8	230.8	211.5	235.3	239.0
canaliculi (biliferi) (intrahepatic)	155.1	197.8	230.8	211.5	235.3	239.0
canals, interlobular	155.1	197.8	230.8	211.5	235.3	239.0
contiguous sites	156.8	—	—	—	—	—
duct or passage (common) (cystic) (extrahepatic)	156.1	197.8	230.8	211.5	235.3	239.0
contiguous sites						
with gallbladder	156.8	—	—	—	—	—
interlobular	155.1	197.8	230.8	211.5	235.3	239.0
intrahepatic	155.1	197.8	230.8	211.5	235.3	239.0
and extrahepatic	156.9	197.8	230.8	211.5	235.3	239.0
bladder (urinary)	188.9	198.1	233.7	223.3	236.7	239.4
contiguous sites	188.8	—	—	—	—	—
dome	188.1	198.1	233.7	223.3	236.7	239.4
neck	188.5	198.1	233.7	223.3	236.7	239.4
orifice	188.9	198.1	233.7	223.3	236.7	239.4
ureteric	188.6	198.1	233.7	223.3	236.7	239.4
urethral	188.5	198.1	233.7	223.3	236.7	239.4
sphincter	188.8	198.1	233.7	223.3	236.7	239.4
trigone	188.0	198.1	233.7	223.3	236.7	239.4
urachus	188.7	—	233.7	223.3	236.7	239.4
wall	188.9	198.1	233.7	223.3	236.7	239.4
anterior	188.3	198.1	233.7	223.3	236.7	239.4
lateral	188.2	198.1	233.7	223.3	236.7	239.4
posterior	188.4	198.1	233.7	223.3	236.7	239.4
blood vessel - *see* Neoplasm, connective tissue						
bone (periosteum)	170.9	198.5	—	213.9	238.0	239.2

Note — Carcinomas and adenocarcinomas, of any type other than intraosseous or odontogenic, of the sites listed under "Neoplasm, bone" should be considered as constituting metastatic spread from an unspecified primary site and coded to 198.5 for morbidity coding and to 199.1 for underlying cause of death coding.

	Primary	Secondary	Ca in situ	Benign	Uncertain Behavior	Unspecified
acetabulum	170.6	198.5	—	213.6	238.0	239.2
acromion (process)	170.4	198.5	—	213.4	238.0	239.2
ankle	170.8	198.5	—	213.8	238.0	239.2
arm NEC	170.4	198.5	—	213.4	238.0	239.2

	Malignant					
	Primary	**Secondary**	**Ca in situ**	**Benign**	**Uncertain Behavior**	**Unspecified**
Neoplasm *(Continued)*						
bone *(Continued)*						
astragalus	170.8	198.5	—	213.8	238.0	239.2
atlas	170.2	198.5	—	213.2	238.0	239.2
axis	170.2	198.5	—	213.2	238.0	239.2
back NEC	170.2	198.5	—	213.2	238.0	239.2
calcaneus	170.8	198.5	—	213.8	238.0	239.2
calvarium	170.0	198.5	—	213.0	238.0	239.2
carpus (any)	170.5	198.5	—	213.5	238.0	239.2
cartilage NEC	170.9	198.5	—	213.9	238.0	239.2
clavicle	170.3	198.5	—	213.3	238.0	239.2
clivus	170.0	198.5	—	213.0	238.0	239.2
coccygeal vertebra	170.6	198.5	—	213.6	238.0	239.2
coccyx	170.6	198.5	—	213.6	238.0	239.2
costal cartilage	170.3	198.5	—	213.3	238.0	239.2
costovertebral joint	170.3	198.5	—	213.3	238.0	239.2
cranial	170.0	198.5	—	213.0	238.0	239.2
cuboid	170.8	198.5	—	213.8	238.0	239.2
cuneiform	170.9	198.5	—	213.9	238.0	239.2
ankle	170.8	198.5	—	213.8	238.0	239.2
wrist	170.5	198.5	—	213.5	238.0	239.2
digital	170.9	198.5	—	213.9	238.0	239.2
finger	170.5	198.5	—	213.5	238.0	239.2
toe	170.8	198.5	—	213.8	238.0	239.2
elbow	170.4	198.5	—	213.4	238.0	239.2
ethmoid (labyrinth)	170.0	198.5	—	213.0	238.0	239.2
face	170.0	198.5	—	213.0	238.0	239.2
lower jaw	170.1	198.5	—	213.1	238.0	239.2
femur (any part)	170.7	198.5	—	213.7	238.0	239.2
fibula (any part)	170.7	198.5	—	213.7	238.0	239.2
finger (any)	170.5	198.5	—	213.5	238.0	239.2
foot	170.8	198.5	—	213.8	238.0	239.2
forearm	170.4	198.5	—	213.4	238.0	239.2
frontal	170.0	198.5	—	213.0	238.0	239.2
hand	170.5	198.5	—	213.5	238.0	239.2
heel	170.8	198.5	—	213.8	238.0	239.2
hip	170.6	198.5	—	213.6	238.0	239.2
humerus (any part)	170.4	198.5	—	213.4	238.0	239.2
hyoid	170.0	198.5	—	213.0	238.0	239.2
ilium	170.6	198.5	—	213.6	238.0	239.2
innominate	170.6	198.5	—	213.6	238.0	239.2
intervertebral cartilage or disc	170.2	198.5	—	213.2	238.0	239.2
ischium	170.6	198.5	—	213.6	238.0	239.2
jaw (lower)	170.1	198.5	—	213.1	238.0	239.2
upper	170.0	198.5	—	213.0	238.0	239.2
knee	170.7	198.5	—	213.7	238.0	239.2
leg NEC	170.7	198.5	—	213.7	238.0	239.2
limb NEC	170.9	198.5	—	213.9	238.0	239.2
lower (long bones)	170.7	198.5	—	213.7	238.0	239.2
short bones	170.8	198.5	—	213.8	238.0	239.2
upper (long bones)	170.4	198.5	—	213.4	238.0	239.2
short bones	170.5	198.5	—	213.5	238.0	239.2
long	170.9	198.5	—	213.9	238.0	239.2
lower limbs NEC	170.7	198.5	—	213.7	238.0	239.2
upper limbs NEC	170.4	198.5	—	213.4	238.0	239.2
malar	170.0	198.5	—	213.0	238.0	239.2
mandible	170.1	198.5	—	213.1	238.0	239.2
marrow NEC	202.9	198.5	—	—	—	238.79
mastoid	170.0	198.5	—	213.0	238.0	239.2
maxilla, maxillary (superior)	170.0	198.5	—	213.0	238.0	239.2
inferior	170.1	198.5	—	213.1	238.0	239.2
metacarpus (any)	170.5	198.5	—	213.5	238.0	239.2
metatarsus (any)	170.8	198.5	—	213.8	238.0	239.2
navicular (ankle)	170.8	198.5	—	213.8	238.0	239.2
hand	170.5	198.5	—	213.5	238.0	239.2

	Malignant					
	Primary	Secondary	Ca in situ	Benign	Uncertain Behavior	Unspecified
Neoplasm *(Continued)*						
bone *(Continued)*						
nose, nasal	170.0	198.5	—	213.0	238.0	239.2
occipital	170.0	198.5	—	213.0	238.0	239.2
orbit	170.0	198.5	—	213.0	238.0	239.2
parietal	170.0	198.5	—	213.0	238.0	239.2
patella	170.8	198.5	—	213.8	238.0	239.2
pelvic	170.6	198.5	—	213.6	238.0	239.2
phalanges	170.9	198.5	—	213.9	238.0	239.2
foot	170.8	198.5	—	213.8	238.0	239.2
hand	170.5	198.5	—	213.5	238.0	239.2
pubic	170.6	198.5	—	213.6	238.0	239.2
radius (any part)	170.4	198.5	—	213.4	238.0	239.2
rib	170.3	198.5	—	213.3	238.0	239.2
sacral vertebra	170.6	198.5	—	213.6	238.0	239.2
sacrum	170.6	198.5	—	213.6	238.0	239.2
scaphoid (of hand)	170.5	198.5	—	213.5	238.0	239.2
of ankle	170.8	198.5	—	213.8	238.0	239.2
scapula (any part)	170.4	198.5	—	213.4	238.0	239.2
sella turcica	170.0	198.5	—	213.0	238.0	239.2
short	170.9	198.5	—	213.9	238.0	239.2
lower limb	170.8	198.5	—	213.8	238.0	239.2
upper limb	170.5	198.5	—	213.5	238.0	239.2
shoulder	170.4	198.5	—	213.4	238.0	239.2
skeleton, skeletal NEC	170.9	198.5	—	213.9	238.0	239.2
skull	170.0	198.5	—	213.0	238.0	239.2
sphenoid	170.0	198.5	—	213.0	238.0	239.2
spine, spinal (column)	170.2	198.5	—	213.2	238.0	239.2
coccyx	170.6	198.5	—	213.6	238.0	239.2
sacrum	170.6	198.5	—	213.6	238.0	239.2
sternum	170.3	198.5	—	213.3	238.0	239.2
tarsus (any)	170.8	198.5	—	213.8	238.0	239.2
temporal	170.0	198.5	—	213.0	238.0	239.2
thumb	170.5	198.5	—	213.5	238.0	239.2
tibia (any part)	170.7	198.5	—	213.7	238.0	239.2
toe (any)	170.8	198.5	—	213.8	238.0	239.2
trapezium	170.5	198.5	—	213.5	238.0	239.2
trapezoid	170.5	198.5	—	213.5	238.0	239.2
turbinate	170.0	198.5	—	213.0	238.0	239.2
ulna (any part)	170.4	198.5	—	213.4	238.0	239.2
unciform	170.5	198.5	—	213.5	238.0	239.2
vertebra (column)	170.2	198.5	—	213.2	238.0	239.2
coccyx	170.6	198.5	—	213.6	238.0	239.2
sacrum	170.6	198.5	—	213.6	238.0	239.2
vomer	170.0	198.5	—	213.0	238.0	239.2
wrist	170.5	198.5	—	213.5	238.0	239.2
xiphoid process	170.3	198.5	—	213.3	238.0	239.2
zygomatic	170.0	198.5	—	213.0	238.0	239.2
book-leaf (mouth)	145.8	198.89	230.0	210.4	235.1	239.0
bowel - *see* Neoplasm, intestine						
brachial plexus	171.2	198.89	—	215.2	238.1	239.2
brain NEC	191.9	198.3	—	225.0	237.5	239.6
basal ganglia	191.0	198.3	—	225.0	237.5	239.6
cerebellopontine angle	191.6	198.3	—	225.0	237.5	239.6
cerebellum NOS	191.6	198.3	—	225.0	237.5	239.6
cerebrum	191.0	198.3	—	225.0	237.5	239.6
choroid plexus	191.5	198.3	—	225.0	237.5	239.6
contiguous sites	191.8	—	—	—	—	—
corpus callosum	191.8	198.3	—	225.0	237.5	239.6
corpus striatum	191.0	198.3	—	225.0	237.5	239.6
cortex (cerebral)	191.0	198.3	—	225.0	237.5	239.6
frontal lobe	191.1	198.3	—	225.0	237.5	239.6
globus pallidus	191.0	198.3	—	225.0	237.5	239.6
hippocampus	191.2	198.3	—	225.0	237.5	239.6
hypothalamus	191.0	198.3	—	225.0	237.5	239.6

	Malignant					
	Primary	**Secondary**	**Ca in situ**	**Benign**	**Uncertain Behavior**	**Unspecified**
Neoplasm *(Continued)*						
brain NEC *(Continued)*						
internal capsule	191.0	198.3	—	225.0	237.5	239.6
medulla oblongata	191.7	198.3	—	225.0	237.5	239.6
meninges	192.1	198.4	—	225.2	237.6	239.7
midbrain	191.7	198.3	—	225.0	237.5	239.6
occipital lobe	191.4	198.3	—	225.0	237.5	239.6
parietal lobe	191.3	198.3	—	225.0	237.5	239.6
peduncle	191.7	198.3	—	225.0	237.5	239.6
pons	191.7	198.3	—	225.0	237.5	239.6
stem	191.7	198.3	—	225.0	237.5	239.6
tapetum	191.8	198.3	—	225.0	237.5	239.6
temporal lobe	191.2	198.3	—	225.0	237.5	239.6
thalamus	191.0	198.3	—	225.0	237.5	239.6
uncus	191.2	198.3	—	225.0	237.5	239.6
ventricle (floor)	191.5	198.3	—	225.0	237.5	239.6
branchial (cleft) (vestiges)	146.8	198.89	230.0	210.6	235.1	239.0
breast (connective tissue) (female) (glandular tissue) (soft parts)	174.9	198.81	233.0	217	238.3	239.3
areola	174.0	198.81	233.0	217	238.3	239.3
male	175.0	198.81	233.0	217	238.3	239.3
axillary tail	174.6	198.81	233.0	217	238.3	239.3
central portion	174.1	198.81	233.0	217	238.3	239.3
contiguous sites	174.8	—	—	—	—	—
ectopic sites	174.8	198.81	233.0	217	238.3	239.3
inner	174.8	198.81	233.0	217	238.3	239.3
lower	174.8	198.81	233.0	217	238.3	239.3
lower-inner quadrant	174.3	198.81	233.0	217	238.3	239.3
lower-outer quadrant	174.5	198.81	233.0	217	238.3	239.3
male	175.9	198.81	233.0	217	238.3	239.3
areola	175.0	198.81	233.0	217	238.3	239.3
ectopic tissue	175.9	198.81	233.0	217	238.3	239.3
nipple	175.0	198.81	233.0	217	238.3	239.3
mastectomy site (skin)	173.5	198.2	—	—	—	—
specified as breast tissue	174.8	198.81	—	—	—	—
midline	174.8	198.81	233.0	217	238.3	239.3
nipple	174.0	198.81	233.0	217	238.3	239.3
male	175.0	198.81	233.0	217	238.3	239.3
outer	174.8	198.81	233.0	217	238.3	239.3
skin	173.5	198.2	232.5	216.5	238.2	239.2
tail (axillary)	174.6	198.81	233.0	217	238.3	239.3
upper	174.8	198.81	233.0	217	238.3	239.3
upper-inner quadrant	174.2	198.81	233.0	217	238.3	239.3
upper-outer quadrant	174.4	198.81	233.0	217	238.3	239.3
broad ligament	183.3	198.82	233.3	221.0	236.3	239.5
bronchiogenic, bronchogenic (lung)	162.9	197.0	231.2	212.3	235.7	239.1
bronchiole	162.9	197.0	231.2	212.3	235.7	239.1
bronchus	162.9	197.0	231.2	212.3	235.7	239.1
carina	162.2	197.0	231.2	212.3	235.7	239.1
contiguous sites with lung or trachea	162.8	—	—	—	—	—
lower lobe of lung	162.5	197.0	231.2	212.3	235.7	239.1
main	162.2	197.0	231.2	212.3	235.7	239.1
middle lobe of lung	162.4	197.0	231.2	212.3	235.7	239.1
upper lobe of lung	162.3	197.0	231.2	212.3	235.7	239.1
brow	173.3	198.2	232.3	216.3	238.2	239.2
buccal (cavity)	145.9	198.89	230.0	210.4	235.1	239.0
commissure	145.0	198.89	230.0	210.4	235.1	239.0
groove (lower) (upper)	145.1	198.89	230.0	210.4	235.1	239.0
mucosa	145.0	198.89	230.0	210.4	235.1	239.0
sulcus (lower) (upper)	145.1	198.89	230.0	210.4	235.1	239.0
bulbourethral gland	189.3	198.1	233.9	223.81	236.99	239.5
bursa - *see* Neoplasm, connective tissue						
buttock NEC*	195.3	198.89	232.5	229.8	238.8	239.8
calf*	195.5	198.89	232.7	229.8	238.8	239.8
calvarium	170.0	198.5	—	213.0	238.0	239.2
calyx, renal	189.1	198.0	233.9	223.1	236.91	239.5

	Malignant					
	Primary	Secondary	Ca in situ	Benign	Uncertain Behavior	Unspecified
Neoplasm *(Continued)*						
canal						
anal	154.2	197.5	230.5	211.4	235.5	239.0
auditory (external)	173.2	198.2	232.2	216.2	238.2	239.2
auricular (external)	173.2	198.2	232.2	216.2	238.2	239.2
canaliculi, biliary (biliferi) (intrahepatic)	155.1	197.8	230.8	211.5	235.3	239.0
canthus (eye) (inner) (outer)	173.1	198.2	232.1	216.1	238.2	239.2
capillary - *see* Neoplasm, connective tissue						
caput coli	153.4	197.5	230.3	211.3	235.2	239.0
cardia (gastric)	151.0	197.8	230.2	211.1	235.2	239.0
cardiac orifice (stomach)	151.0	197.8	230.2	211.1	235.2	239.0
cardio-esophageal junction	151.0	197.8	230.2	211.1	235.2	239.0
cardio-esophagus	151.0	197.8	230.2	211.1	235.2	239.0
carina (bronchus) (trachea)	162.2	197.0	231.2	212.3	235.7	239.1
carotid (artery)	171.0	198.89	—	215.0	238.1	239.2
body	194.5	198.89	—	227.5	237.3	239.7
carpus (any bone)	170.5	198.5	—	213.5	238.0	239.2
cartilage (articular) (joint) NEC - *see also* Neoplasm, bone	170.9	198.5	—	213.9	238.0	239.2
arytenoid	161.3	197.3	231.0	212.1	235.6	239.1
auricular	171.0	198.89	—	215.0	238.1	239.2
bronchi	162.2	197.3	—	212.3	235.7	239.1
connective tissue - *see* Neoplasm, connective tissue						
costal	170.3	198.5	—	213.3	238.0	239.2
cricoid	161.3	197.3	231.0	212.1	235.6	239.1
cuneiform	161.3	197.3	231.0	212.1	235.6	239.1
ear (external)	171.0	198.89	—	215.0	238.1	239.2
ensiform	170.3	198.5	—	213.3	238.0	239.2
epiglottis	161.1	197.3	231.0	212.1	235.6	239.1
anterior surface	146.4	198.89	230.0	210.6	235.1	239.0
eyelid	171.0	198.89	—	215.0	238.1	239.2
intervertebral	170.2	198.5	—	213.2	238.0	239.2
larynx, laryngeal	161.3	197.3	231.0	212.1	235.6	239.1
nose, nasal	160.0	197.3	231.8	212.0	235.9	239.1
pinna	171.0	198.89	—	215.0	238.1	239.2
rib	170.3	198.5	—	213.3	238.0	239.2
semilunar (knee)	170.7	198.5	—	213.7	238.0	239.2
thyroid	161.3	197.3	231.0	212.1	235.6	239.1
trachea	162.0	197.3	231.1	212.2	235.7	239.1
cauda equina	192.2	198.3	—	225.3	237.5	239.7
cavity						
buccal	145.9	198.89	230.0	210.4	235.1	239.0
nasal	160.0	197.3	231.8	212.0	235.9	239.1
oral	145.9	198.89	230.0	210.4	235.1	239.0
peritoneal	158.9	197.6	—	211.8	235.4	239.0
tympanic	160.1	197.3	231.8	212.0	235.9	239.1
cecum	153.4	197.5	230.3	211.3	235.2	239.0
central nervous system - *see* Neoplasm, white matter	191.0	198.3	—	225.0	237.5	239.6
cerebellopontine (angle)	191.6	198.3	—	225.0	237.5	239.6
cerebellum, cerebellar	191.6	198.3	—	225.0	237.5	239.6
cerebrum, cerebral (cortex) (hemisphere) (white matter)	191.0	198.3	—	225.0	237.5	239.6
meninges	192.1	198.4	—	225.2	237.6	239.7
peduncle	191.7	198.3	—	225.0	237.5	239.6
ventricle (any)	191.5	198.3	—	225.0	237.5	239.6
cervical region	195.0	198.89	234.8	229.8	238.8	239.8
cervix (cervical) (uteri) (uterus)	180.9	198.82	233.1	219.0	236.0	239.5
canal	180.0	198.82	233.1	219.0	236.0	239.5
contiguous sites	180.8	—	—	—	—	—
endocervix (canal) (gland)	180.0	198.82	233.1	219.0	236.0	239.5
exocervix	180.1	198.82	233.1	219.0	236.0	239.5
external os	180.1	198.82	233.1	219.0	236.0	239.5
internal os	180.0	198.82	233.1	219.0	236.0	239.5
nabothian gland	180.0	198.82	233.1	219.0	236.0	239.5
squamocolumnar junction	180.8	198.82	233.1	219.0	236.0	239.5
stump	180.8	198.82	233.1	219.0	236.0	239.5

	Malignant					
	Primary	Secondary	Ca in situ	Benign	Uncertain Behavior	Unspecified
Neoplasm *(Continued)*						
cheek	195.0	198.89	234.8	229.8	238.8	239.8
external	173.3	198.2	232.3	216.3	238.2	239.2
inner aspect	145.0	198.89	230.0	210.4	235.1	239.0
internal	145.0	198.89	230.0	210.4	235.1	239.0
mucosa	145.0	198.89	230.0	210.4	235.1	239.0
chest (wall) NEC	195.1	198.89	234.8	229.8	238.8	239.8
chiasma opticum	192.0	198.4	—	225.1	237.9	239.7
chin	173.3	198.2	232.3	216.3	238.2	239.2
choana	147.3	198.89	230.0	210.7	235.1	239.0
cholangiole	155.1	197.8	230.8	211.5	235.3	239.0
choledochal duct	156.1	197.8	230.8	211.5	235.3	239.0
choroid	190.6	198.4	234.0	224.6	238.8	239.8
plexus	191.5	198.3	—	225.0	237.5	239.6
ciliary body	190.0	198.4	234.0	224.0	238.8	239.8
clavicle	170.3	198.5	—	213.3	238.0	239.2
clitoris	184.3	198.82	233.3	221.2	236.3	239.5
clivus	170.0	198.5	—	213.0	238.0	239.2
cloacogenic zone	154.8	197.5	230.7	211.4	235.5	239.0
coccygeal						
body or glomus	194.6	198.89	—	227.6	237.3	239.7
vertebra	170.6	198.5	—	213.6	238.0	239.2
coccyx	170.6	198.5	—	213.6	238.0	239.2
colon - *see also* Neoplasm, intestine, large and rectum	154.0	197.5	230.4	211.4	235.2	239.0
column, spinal - *see* Neoplasm, spine						
columnella	173.3	198.2	232.3	216.3	238.2	239.2
commissure						
labial, lip	140.6	198.89	230.0	210.4	235.1	239.0
laryngeal	161.0	197.3	231.0	212.1	235.6	239.1
common (bile) duct	156.1	197.8	230.8	211.5	235.3	239.0
concha	173.2	198.2	232.2	216.2	238.2	239.2
nose	160.0	197.3	231.8	212.0	235.9	239.1
conjunctiva	190.3	198.4	234.0	224.3	238.8	239.8
connective tissue NEC	171.9	198.89	—	215.9	238.1	239.2

Note — For neoplasms of connective tissue (blood vessel, bursa, fascia, ligament, muscle, peripheral nerves, sympathetic and parasympathetic nerves and ganglia, synovia, tendon, etc.) or of morphological types that indicate connective tissue, code according to the list under "Neoplasm, connective tissue;" for sites that do not appear in this list, code to neoplasm of that site; e.g.,

liposarcoma, shoulder 171.2
leiomyosarcoma, stomach 151.9
neurofibroma, chest wall 215.4

Morphological types that indicate connective tissue appear in their proper place in the alphabetic index with the instruction "see Neoplasm, connective tissue ...."

	Primary	Secondary	Ca in situ	Benign	Uncertain Behavior	Unspecified
abdomen	171.5	198.89	—	215.5	238.1	239.2
abdominal wall	171.5	198.89	—	215.5	238.1	239.2
ankle	171.3	198.89	—	215.3	238.1	239.2
antecubital fossa or space	171.2	198.89	—	215.2	238.1	239.2
arm	171.2	198.89	—	215.2	238.1	239.2
auricle (ear)	171.0	198.89	—	215.0	238.1	239.2
axilla	171.4	198.89	—	215.4	238.1	239.2
back	171.7	198.89	—	215.7	238.1	239.2
breast (female) (*see also* Neoplasm, breast)	174.9	198.81	233.0	217	238.3	239.3
male	175.9	198.81	233.0	217	238.3	239.3
buttock	171.6	198.89	—	215.6	238.1	239.2
calf	171.3	198.89	—	215.3	238.1	239.2
cervical region	171.0	198.89	—	215.0	238.1	239.2
cheek	171.0	198.89	—	215.0	238.1	239.2
chest (wall)	171.4	198.89	—	215.4	238.1	239.2
chin	171.0	198.89	—	215.0	238.1	239.2
contiguous sites	171.8	—	—	—	—	—
diaphragm	171.4	198.89	—	215.4	238.1	239.2
ear (external)	171.0	198.89	—	215.0	238.1	239.2
elbow	171.2	198.89	—	215.2	238.1	239.2
extrarectal	171.6	198.89	—	215.6	238.1	239.2

	Malignant					
	Primary	**Secondary**	**Ca in situ**	**Benign**	**Uncertain Behavior**	**Unspecified**
Neoplasm *(Continued)*						
connective tissue NEC *(Continued)*						
extremity	171.8	198.89	—	215.8	238.1	239.2
lower	171.3	198.89	—	215.3	238.1	239.2
upper	171.2	198.89	—	215.2	238.1	239.2
eyelid	171.0	198.89	—	215.0	238.1	239.2
face	171.0	198.89	—	215.0	238.1	239.2
finger	171.2	198.89	—	215.2	238.1	239.2
flank	171.7	198.89	—	215.7	238.1	239.2
foot	171.3	198.89	—	215.3	238.1	239.2
forearm	171.2	198.89	—	215.2	238.1	239.2
forehead	171.0	198.89	—	215.0	238.1	239.2
gastric	171.5	198.89	—	215.5	238.1	—
gastrointestinal	171.5	198.89	—	215.5	238.1	—
gluteal region	171.6	198.89	—	215.6	238.1	239.2
great vessels NEC	171.4	198.89	—	215.4	238.1	239.2
groin	171.6	198.89	—	215.6	238.1	239.2
hand	171.2	198.89	—	215.2	238.1	239.2
head	171.0	198.89	—	215.0	238.1	239.2
heel	171.3	198.89	—	215.3	238.1	239.2
hip	171.3	198.89	—	215.3	238.1	239.2
hypochondrium	171.5	198.89	—	215.5	238.1	239.2
iliopsoas muscle	171.6	198.89	—	215.5	238.1	239.2
infraclavicular region	171.4	198.89	—	215.4	238.1	239.2
inguinal (canal) (region)	171.6	198.89	—	215.6	238.1	239.2
intestine	171.5	198.89	—	215.5	238.1	—
intrathoracic	171.4	198.89	—	215.4	238.1	239.2
ischorectal fossa	171.6	198.89	—	215.6	238.1	239.2
jaw	143.9	198.89	230.0	210.4	235.1	239.0
knee	171.3	198.89	—	215.3	238.1	239.2
leg	171.3	198.89	—	215.3	238.1	239.2
limb NEC	171.9	198.89	—	215.8	238.1	239.2
lower	171.3	198.89	—	215.3	238.1	239.2
upper	171.2	198.89	—	215.2	238.1	239.2
nates	171.6	198.89	—	215.6	238.1	239.2
neck	171.0	198.89	—	215.0	238.1	239.2
orbit	190.1	198.4	234.0	224.1	238.8	239.8
pararectal	171.6	198.89	—	215.6	238.1	239.2
para-urethral	171.6	198.89	—	215.6	238.1	239.2
paravaginal	171.6	198.89	—	215.6	238.1	239.2
pelvis (floor)	171.6	198.89	—	215.6	238.1	239.2
pelvo-abdominal	171.8	198.89	—	215.8	238.1	239.2
perineum	171.6	198.89	—	215.6	238.1	239.2
perirectal (tissue)	171.6	198.89	—	215.6	238.1	239.2
periurethral (tissue)	171.6	198.89	—	215.6	238.1	239.2
popliteal fossa or space	171.3	198.89	—	215.3	238.1	239.2
presacral	171.6	198.89	—	215.6	238.1	239.2
psoas muscle	171.5	198.89	—	215.5	238.1	239.2
pterygoid fossa	171.0	198.89	—	215.0	238.1	239.2
rectovaginal septum or wall	171.6	198.89	—	215.6	238.1	239.2
rectovesical	171.6	198.89	—	215.6	238.1	239.2
retroperitoneum	158.0	197.6	—	211.8	235.4	239.0
sacrococcygeal region	171.6	198.89	—	215.6	238.1	239.2
scalp	171.0	198.89	—	215.0	238.1	239.2
scapular region	171.4	198.89	—	215.4	238.1	239.2
shoulder	171.2	198.89	—	215.2	238.1	239.2
skin (dermis) NEC	173.9	198.2	232.9	216.9	238.2	239.2
stomach	171.5	198.89	—	215.5	238.1	—
submental	171.0	198.89	—	215.0	238.1	239.2
supraclavicular region	171.0	198.89	—	215.0	238.1	239.2
temple	171.0	198.89	—	215.0	238.1	239.2
temporal region	171.0	198.89	—	215.0	238.1	239.2
thigh	171.3	198.89	—	215.3	238.1	239.2
thoracic (duct) (wall)	171.4	198.89	—	215.4	238.1	239.2
thorax	171.4	198.89	—	215.4	238.1	239.2

	Malignant					
	Primary	Secondary	Ca in situ	Benign	Uncertain Behavior	Unspecified
Neoplasm *(Continued)*						
connective tissue NEC *(Continued)*						
thumb	171.2	198.89	—	215.2	238.1	239.2
toe	171.3	198.89	—	215.3	238.1	239.2
trunk	171.7	198.89	—	215.7	238.1	239.2
umbilicus	171.5	198.89	—	215.5	238.1	239.2
vesicorectal	171.6	198.89	—	215.6	238.1	239.2
wrist	171.2	198.89	—	215.2	238.1	239.2
conus medullaris	192.2	198.3	—	225.3	237.5	239.7
cord (true) (vocal)	161.0	197.3	231.0	212.1	235.6	239.1
false	161.1	197.3	231.0	212.1	235.6	239.1
spermatic	187.6	198.82	233.6	222.8	236.6	239.5
spinal (cervical) (lumbar) (thoracic)	192.2	198.3	—	225.3	237.5	239.7
cornea (limbus)	190.4	198.4	234.0	224.4	238.8	239.8
corpus						
albicans	183.0	198.6	233.3	220	236.2	239.5
callosum, brain	191.8	198.3	—	225.0	237.5	239.6
cavernosum	187.3	198.82	233.5	222.1	236.6	239.5
gastric	151.4	197.8	230.2	211.1	235.2	239.0
penis	187.3	198.82	233.5	222.1	236.6	239.5
striatum, cerebrum	191.0	198.3	—	225.0	237.5	239.6
uteri	182.0	198.82	233.2	219.1	236.0	239.5
isthmus	182.1	198.82	233.2	219.1	236.0	239.5
cortex						
adrenal	194.0	198.7	234.8	227.0	237.2	239.7
cerebral	191.0	198.3	—	225.0	237.5	239.6
costal cartilage	170.3	198.5	—	213.3	238.0	239.2
costovertebral joint	170.3	198.5	—	213.3	238.0	239.2
Cowper's gland	189.3	198.1	233.9	223.81	236.99	239.5
cranial (fossa, any)	191.9	198.3	—	225.0	237.5	239.6
meninges	192.1	198.4	—	225.2	237.6	239.7
nerve (any)	192.0	198.4	—	225.1	237.9	239.7
craniobuccal pouch	194.3	198.89	234.8	227.3	237.0	239.7
craniopharyngeal (duct) (pouch)	194.3	198.89	234.8	227.3	237.0	239.7
cricoid	148.0	198.89	230.0	210.8	235.1	239.0
cartilage	161.3	197.3	231.0	212.1	235.6	239.1
cricopharynx	148.0	198.89	230.0	210.8	235.1	239.0
crypt of Morgagni	154.8	197.5	230.7	211.4	235.2	239.0
crystalline lens	190.0	198.4	234.0	224.0	238.8	239.8
cul-de-sac (Douglas')	158.8	197.6	—	211.8	235.4	239.0
cuneiform cartilage	161.3	197.3	231.0	212.1	235.6	239.1
cutaneous - *see* Neoplasm, skin						
cutis - *see* Neoplasm, skin						
cystic (bile) duct (common)	156.1	197.8	230.8	211.5	235.3	239.0
dermis - *see* Neoplasm, skin						
diaphragm	171.4	198.89	—	215.4	238.1	239.2
digestive organs, system, tube, or tract NEC	159.9	197.8	230.9	211.9	235.5	239.0
contiguous sites with peritoneum	159.8	—	—	—	—	—
disc, intervertebral	170.2	198.5	—	213.2	238.0	239.2
disease, generalized	199.0	199.0	234.9	229.9	238.9	199.0
disseminated	199.0	199.0	234.9	229.9	238.9	199.0
Douglas' cul-de-sac or pouch	158.8	197.6	—	211.8	235.4	239.0
duodenojejunal junction	152.8	197.4	230.7	211.2	235.2	239.0
duodenum	152.0	197.4	230.7	211.2	235.2	239.0
dura (cranial) (mater)	192.1	198.4	—	225.2	237.6	239.7
cerebral	192.1	198.4	—	225.2	237.6	239.7
spinal	192.3	198.4	—	225.4	237.6	239.7
ear (external)	173.2	198.2	232.2	216.2	238.2	239.2
auricle or auris	173.2	198.2	232.2	216.2	238.2	239.2
canal, external	173.2	198.2	232.2	216.2	238.2	239.2
cartilage	171.0	198.89	—	215.0	238.1	239.2
external meatus	173.2	198.2	232.2	216.2	238.2	239.2
inner	160.1	197.3	231.8	212.0	235.9	239.8
lobule	173.2	198.2	232.2	216.2	238.2	239.2

	Malignant					
	Primary	Secondary	Ca in situ	Benign	Uncertain Behavior	Unspecified
Neoplasm *(Continued)*						
ear *(Continued)*						
middle	160.1	197.3	231.8	212.0	235.9	239.8
contiguous sites with accessory sinuses or nasal cavities	160.8	—	—	—	—	—
skin	173.2	198.2	232.2	216.2	238.2	239.2
earlobe	173.2	198.2	232.2	216.2	238.2	239.2
ejaculatory duct	187.8	198.82	233.6	222.8	236.6	239.5
elbow NEC*	195.4	198.89	232.6	229.8	238.8	239.8
endocardium	164.1	198.89	—	212.7	238.8	239.8
endocervix (canal) (gland)	180.0	198.82	233.1	219.0	236.0	239.5
endocrine gland NEC	194.9	198.89	—	227.9	237.4	239.7
pluriglandular NEC	194.8	198.89	234.8	227.8	237.4	239.7
endometrium (gland) (stroma)	182.0	198.82	233.2	219.1	236.0	239.5
ensiform cartilage	170.3	198.5	—	213.3	238.0	239.2
enteric - *see* Neoplasm, intestine						
ependyma (brain)	191.5	198.3	—	225.0	237.5	239.6
epicardium	164.1	198.89	—	212.7	238.8	239.8
epididymis	187.5	198.82	233.6	222.3	236.6	239.5
epidural	192.9	198.4	—	225.9	237.9	239.7
epiglottis	161.1	197.3	231.0	212.1	235.6	239.1
anterior aspect or surface	146.4	198.89	230.0	210.6	235.1	239.0
cartilage	161.3	197.3	231.0	212.1	235.6	239.1
free border (margin)	146.4	198.89	230.0	210.6	235.1	239.0
junctional region	146.5	198.89	230.0	210.6	235.1	239.0
posterior (laryngeal) surface	161.1	197.3	231.0	212.1	235.6	239.1
suprahyoid portion	161.1	197.3	231.0	212.1	235.6	239.1
esophagogastric junction	151.0	197.8	230.2	211.1	235.2	239.0
esophagus	150.9	197.8	230.1	211.0	235.5	239.0
abdominal	150.2	197.8	230.1	211.0	235.5	239.0
cervical	150.0	197.8	230.1	211.0	235.5	239.0
contiguous sites	150.8	—	—	—	—	—
distal (third)	150.5	197.8	230.1	211.0	235.5	239.0
lower (third)	150.5	197.8	230.1	211.0	235.5	239.0
middle (third)	150.4	197.8	230.1	211.0	235.5	239.0
proximal (third)	150.3	197.8	230.1	211.0	235.5	239.0
specified part NEC	150.8	197.8	230.1	211.0	235.5	239.0
thoracic	150.1	197.8	230.1	211.0	235.5	239.0
upper (third)	150.3	197.8	230.1	211.0	235.5	239.0
ethmoid (sinus)	160.3	197.3	231.8	212.0	235.9	239.1
bone or labyrinth	170.0	198.5	—	213.0	238.0	239.2
Eustachian tube	160.1	197.3	231.8	212.0	235.9	239.1
exocervix	180.1	198.82	233.1	219.0	236.0	239.5
external						
meatus (ear)	173.2	198.2	232.2	216.2	238.2	239.2
os, cervix uteri	180.1	198.82	233.1	219.0	236.0	239.5
extradural	192.9	198.4	—	225.9	237.9	239.7
extrahepatic (bile) duct	156.1	197.8	230.8	211.5	235.3	239.0
contiguous sites with gallbladder	156.8	—	—	—	—	—
extraocular muscle	190.1	198.4	234.0	224.1	238.8	239.8
extrarectal	195.3	198.89	234.8	229.8	238.8	239.8
extremity*	195.8	198.89	232.8	229.8	238.8	239.8
lower*	195.5	198.89	232.7	229.8	238.8	239.8
upper*	195.4	198.89	232.6	229.8	238.8	239.8
eye NEC	190.9	198.4	234.0	224.9	238.8	239.8
contiguous sites	190.8	—	—	—	—	—
specified sites NEC	190.8	198.4	234.0	224.8	238.8	239.8
eyeball	190.0	198.4	234.0	224.0	238.8	239.8
eyebrow	173.3	198.2	232.3	216.3	238.2	239.2
eyelid (lower) (skin) (upper)	173.1	198.2	232.1	216.1	238.2	239.2
cartilage	171.0	198.89	—	215.0	238.1	239.2
face NEC*	195.0	198.89	232.3	229.8	238.8	239.8
Fallopian tube (accessory)	183.2	198.82	233.3	221.0	236.3	239.5
falx (cerebella) (cerebri)	192.1	198.4	—	225.2	237.6	239.7
fascia - *see also* Neoplasm, connective tissue						

	Malignant					
	Primary	Secondary	Ca in situ	Benign	Uncertain Behavior	Unspecified
Neoplasm *(Continued)*						
fascia *(Continued)*						
palmar	171.2	198.89	—	215.2	238.1	239.2
plantar	171.3	198.89	—	215.3	238.1	239.2
fatty tissue - *see* Neoplasm, connective tissue						
fauces, faucial NEC	146.9	198.89	230.0	210.6	235.1	239.0
pillars	146.2	198.89	230.0	210.6	235.1	239.0
tonsil	146.0	198.89	230.0	210.5	235.1	239.0
femur (any part)	170.7	198.5	—	213.7	238.0	239.2
fetal membrane	181	198.82	233.2	219.8	236.1	239.5
fibrous tissue - *see* Neoplasm, connective tissue						
fibula (any part)	170.7	198.5	—	213.7	238.0	239.2
filum terminale	192.2	198.3	—	225.3	237.5	239.7
finger NEC*	195.4	198.89	232.6	229.8	238.8	239.8
flank NEC*	195.8	198.89	232.5	229.8	238.8	239.8
follicle, nabothian	180.0	198.82	233.1	219.0	236.0	239.5
foot NEC*	195.5	198.89	232.7	229.8	238.8	239.8
forearm NEC*	195.4	198.89	232.6	229.8	238.8	239.8
forehead (skin)	173.3	198.2	232.3	216.3	238.2	239.2
foreskin	187.1	198.82	233.5	222.1	236.6	239.5
fornix						
pharyngeal	147.3	198.89	230.0	210.7	235.1	239.0
vagina	184.0	198.82	233.3	221.1	236.3	239.5
fossa (of)						
anterior (cranial)	191.9	198.3	—	225.0	237.5	239.6
cranial	191.9	198.3	—	225.0	237.5	239.6
ischiorectal	195.3	198.89	234.8	229.8	238.8	239.8
middle (cranial)	191.9	198.3	—	225.0	237.5	239.6
pituitary	194.3	198.89	234.8	227.3	237.0	239.7
posterior (cranial)	191.9	198.3	—	225.0	237.5	239.6
pterygoid	171.0	198.89	—	215.0	238.1	239.2
pyriform	148.1	198.89	230.0	210.8	235.1	239.0
Rosenmüller	147.2	198.89	230.0	210.7	235.1	239.0
tonsillar	146.1	198.89	230.0	210.6	235.1	239.0
fourchette	184.4	198.82	233.3	221.2	236.3	239.5
frenulum						
labii - *see* Neoplasm, lip, internal						
linguae	141.3	198.89	230.0	210.1	235.1	239.0
frontal						
bone	170.0	198.5	—	213.0	238.0	239.2
lobe, brain	191.1	198.3	—	225.0	237.5	239.6
meninges	192.1	198.4	—	225.2	237.6	239.7
pole	191.1	198.3	—	225.0	237.5	239.6
sinus	160.4	197.3	231.8	212.0	235.9	239.1
fundus						
stomach	151.3	197.8	230.2	211.1	235.2	239.0
uterus	182.0	198.82	233.2	219.1	236.0	239.5
gall duct (extrahepatic)	156.1	197.8	230.8	211.5	235.3	239.0
intrahepatic	155.1	197.8	230.8	211.5	235.3	239.0
gallbladder	156.0	197.8	230.8	211.5	235.3	239.0
contiguous sites with extrahepatic bile ducts	156.8	—	—	—	—	—
ganglia (*see also* Neoplasm, connective tissue)	171.9	198.89	—	215.9	238.1	239.2
basal	191.0	198.3	—	225.0	237.5	239.6
ganglion (*see also* Neoplasm, connective tissue)	171.9	198.89	—	215.9	238.1	239.2
cranial nerve	192.0	198.4	—	225.1	237.9	239.7
Gartner's duct	184.0	198.82	233.3	221.1	236.3	239.5
gastric - *see* Neoplasm, stomach						
gastrocolic	159.8	197.8	230.9	211.9	235.5	239.0
gastroesophageal junction	151.0	197.8	230.2	211.1	235.2	239.0
gastrointestinal (tract) NEC	159.9	197.8	230.9	211.9	235.5	239.0
generalized	199.0	199.0	234.9	229.9	238.9	199.0
genital organ or tract						
female NEC	184.9	198.82	233.3	221.9	236.3	239.5
contiguous sites	184.8					
specified site NEC	184.8	198.82	233.3	221.8	236.3	239.5

◀ New ⟸ Revised

	Malignant					
	Primary	Secondary	Ca in situ	Benign	Uncertain Behavior	Unspecified
Neoplasm *(Continued)*						
genital organ or tract *(Continued)*						
male NEC	187.9	198.82	233.6	222.9	236.6	239.5
contiguous sites	187.8	—	—	—	—	—
specified site NEC	187.8	198.82	233.6	222.8	236.6	239.5
genitourinary tract						
female	184.9	198.82	233.3	221.9	236.3	239.5
male	187.9	198.82	233.6	222.9	236.6	239.5
gingiva (alveolar) (marginal)	143.9	198.89	230.0	210.4	235.1	239.0
lower	143.1	198.89	230.0	210.4	235.1	239.0
mandibular	143.1	198.89	230.0	210.4	235.1	239.0
maxillary	143.0	198.89	230.0	210.4	235.1	239.0
upper	143.0	198.89	230.0	210.4	235.1	239.0
gland, glandular (lymphatic) (system) - *see also* Neoplasm, lymph gland						
endocrine NEC	194.9	198.89	—	227.9	237.4	239.7
salivary - *see* Neoplasm, salivary, gland						
glans penis	187.2	198.82	233.5	222.1	236.6	239.5
globus pallidus	191.0	198.3	—	225.0	237.5	239.6
glomus						
coccygeal	194.6	198.89	—	227.6	237.3	239.7
jugularis	194.6	198.89	—	227.6	237.3	239.7
glosso-epiglottic fold(s)	146.4	198.89	230.0	210.6	235.1	239.0
glossopalatine fold	146.2	198.89	230.0	210.6	235.1	239.0
glossopharyngeal sulcus	146.1	198.89	230.0	210.6	235.1	239.0
glottis	161.0	197.3	231.0	212.1	235.6	239.1
gluteal region*	195.3	198.89	232.5	229.8	238.8	239.8
great vessels NEC	171.4	198.89	—	215.4	238.1	239.2
groin NEC	195.3	198.89	232.5	229.8	238.8	239.8
gum	143.9	198.89	230.0	210.4	235.1	239.0
contiguous sites	143.8	—	—	—	—	—
lower	143.1	198.89	230.0	210.4	235.1	239.0
upper	143.0	198.89	230.0	210.4	235.1	239.0
hand NEC*	195.4	198.89	232.6	229.8	238.8	239.8
head NEC*	195.0	198.89	232.4	229.8	238.8	239.8
heart	164.1	198.89	—	212.7	238.8	239.8
contiguous sites with mediastinum or thymus	164.8	—	—	—	—	—
heel NEC*	195.5	198.89	232.7	229.8	238.8	239.8
helix	173.2	198.2	232.2	216.2	238.2	239.2
hematopoietic, hemopoietic tissue NEC	202.8	198.89	—	—	—	238.79 (Revised)
hemisphere, cerebral	191.0	198.3	—	225.0	237.5	239.6
hemorrhoidal zone	154.2	197.5	230.5	211.4	235.5	239.0
hepatic	155.2	197.7	230.8	211.5	235.3	239.0
duct (bile)	156.1	197.8	230.8	211.5	235.3	239.0
flexure (colon)	153.0	197.5	230.3	211.3	235.2	239.0
primary	155.0	—	—	—	—	—
hilus of lung	162.2	197.0	231.2	212.3	235.7	239.1
hip NEC*	195.5	198.89	232.7	229.8	238.8	239.8
hippocampus, brain	191.2	198.3	—	225.0	237.5	239.6
humerus (any part)	170.4	198.5	—	213.4	238.0	239.2
hymen	184.0	198.82	233.3	221.1	236.3	239.5
hypopharynx, hypopharyngeal NEC	148.9	198.89	230.0	210.8	235.1	239.0
contiguous sites	148.8	—	—	—	—	—
postcricoid region	148.0	198.89	230.0	210.8	235.1	239.0
posterior wall	148.3	198.89	230.0	210.8	235.1	239.0
pyriform fossa (sinus)	148.1	198.89	230.0	210.8	235.1	239.0
specified site NEC	148.8	198.89	230.0	210.8	235.1	239.0
wall	148.9	198.89	230.0	210.8	235.1	239.0
posterior	148.3	198.89	230.0	210.8	235.1	239.0
hypophysis	194.3	198.89	234.8	227.3	237.0	239.7
hypothalamus	191.0	198.3	—	225.0	237.5	239.6
ileocecum, ileocecal (coil) (junction) (valve)	153.4	197.5	230.3	211.3	235.2	239.0
ileum	152.2	197.4	230.7	211.2	235.2	239.0
ilium	170.6	198.5	—	213.6	238.0	239.2
immunoproliferative NEC	203.8	—	—	—	—	—
infraclavicular (region)*	195.1	198.89	232.5	229.8	238.8	239.8

	Malignant					
	Primary	Secondary	Ca in situ	Benign	Uncertain Behavior	Unspecified
Neoplasm *(Continued)*						
inguinal (region)*	195.3	198.89	232.5	229.8	238.8	239.8
insula	191.0	198.3	—	225.0	237.5	239.6
insular tissue (pancreas)	157.4	197.8	230.9	211.7	235.5	239.0
brain	191.0	198.3	—	225.0	237.5	239.6
interarytenoid fold	148.2	198.89	230.0	210.8	235.1	239.0
hypopharyngeal aspect	148.2	198.89	230.0	210.8	235.1	239.0
laryngeal aspect	161.1	197.3	231.0	212.1	235.6	239.1
marginal zone	148.2	198.89	230.0	210.8	235.1	239.0
interdental papillae	143.9	198.89	230.0	210.4	235.1	239.0
lower	143.1	198.89	230.0	210.4	235.1	239.0
upper	143.0	198.89	230.0	210.4	235.1	239.0
internal						
capsule	191.0	198.3	—	225.0	237.5	239.6
os (cervix)	180.0	198.82	233.1	219.0	236.0	239.5
intervertebral cartilage or disc	170.2	198.5	—	213.2	238.0	239.2
intestine, intestinal	159.0	197.8	230.7	211.9	235.2	239.0
large	153.9	197.5	230.3	211.3	235.2	239.0
appendix	153.5	197.5	230.3	211.3	235.2	239.0
caput coli	153.4	197.5	230.3	211.3	235.2	239.0
cecum	153.4	197.5	230.3	211.3	235.2	239.0
colon	153.9	197.5	230.3	211.3	235.2	239.0
and rectum	154.0	197.5	230.4	211.4	235.2	239.0
ascending	153.6	197.5	230.3	211.3	235.2	239.0
caput	153.4	197.5	230.3	211.3	235.2	239.0
contiguous sites	153.8	—	—	—	—	—
descending	153.2	197.5	230.3	211.3	235.2	239.0
distal	153.2	197.5	230.3	211.3	235.2	239.0
left	153.2	197.5	230.3	211.3	235.2	239.0
pelvic	153.3	197.5	230.3	211.3	235.2	239.0
right	153.6	197.5	230.3	211.3	235.2	239.0
sigmoid (flexure)	153.3	197.5	230.3	211.3	235.2	239.0
transverse	153.1	197.5	230.3	211.3	235.2	239.0
contiguous sites	153.8	—	—	—	—	—
hepatic flexure	153.0	197.5	230.3	211.3	235.2	239.0
ileocecum, ileocecal (coil) (valve)	153.4	197.5	230.3	211.3	235.2	239.0
sigmoid flexure (lower) (upper)	153.3	197.5	230.3	211.3	235.2	239.0
splenic flexure	153.7	197.5	230.3	211.3	235.2	239.0
small	152.9	197.4	230.7	211.2	235.2	239.0
contiguous sites	152.8	—	—	—	—	—
duodenum	152.0	197.4	230.7	211.2	235.2	239.0
ileum	152.2	197.4	230.7	211.2	235.2	239.0
jejunum	152.1	197.4	230.7	211.2	235.2	239.0
tract NEC	159.0	197.8	230.7	211.9	235.2	239.0
intra-abdominal	195.2	198.89	234.8	229.8	238.8	239.8
intracranial NEC	191.9	198.3	—	225.0	237.5	239.6
intrahepatic (bile) duct	155.1	197.8	230.8	211.5	235.3	239.0
intraocular	190.0	198.4	234.0	224.0	238.8	239.8
intraorbital	190.1	198.4	234.0	224.1	238.8	239.8
intrasellar	194.3	198.89	234.8	227.3	237.0	239.7
intrathoracic (cavity) (organs NEC)	195.1	198.89	234.8	229.8	238.8	239.8
contiguous sites with respiratory organs	165.8	—	—	—	—	—
iris	190.0	198.4	234.0	224.0	238.8	239.8
ischiorectal (fossa)	195.3	198.89	234.8	229.8	238.8	239.8
ischium	170.6	198.5	—	213.6	238.0	239.2
island of Reil	191.0	198.3	—	225.0	237.5	239.6
islands or islets of Langerhans	157.4	197.8	230.9	211.7	235.5	239.0
isthmus uteri	182.1	198.82	233.2	219.1	236.0	239.5
jaw	195.0	198.89	234.8	229.8	238.8	239.8
bone	170.1	198.5	—	213.1	238.0	239.2
carcinoma	143.9	—	—	—	—	—
lower	143.1	—	—	—	—	—
upper	143.0	—	—	—	—	—
lower	170.1	198.5	—	213.1	238.0	239.2
upper	170.0	198.5	—	213.0	238.0	239.2

	Malignant					
	Primary	**Secondary**	**Ca in situ**	**Benign**	**Uncertain Behavior**	**Unspecified**
Neoplasm *(Continued)*						
jaw *(Continued)*						
carcinoma (any type) (lower) (upper)	195.0	—	—	—	—	—
skin	173.3	198.2	232.3	216.3	238.2	239.2
soft tissues	143.9	198.89	230.0	210.4	235.1	239.0
lower	143.1	198.89	230.0	210.4	235.1	239.0
upper	143.0	198.89	230.0	210.4	235.1	239.0
jejunum	152.1	197.4	230.7	211.2	235.2	239.0
joint NEC (*see also* Neoplasm, bone)	170.9	198.5	—	213.9	238.0	239.2
acromioclavicular	170.4	198.5	—	213.4	238.0	239.2
bursa or synovial membrane - *see* Neoplasm, connective tissue						
costovertebral	170.3	198.5	—	213.3	238.0	239.2
sternocostal	170.3	198.5	—	213.3	238.0	239.2
temporomandibular	170.1	198.5	—	213.1	238.0	239.2
junction						
anorectal	154.8	197.5	230.7	211.4	235.5	239.0
cardioesophageal	151.0	197.8	230.2	211.1	235.2	239.0
esophagogastric	151.0	197.8	230.2	211.1	235.2	239.0
gastroesophageal	151.0	197.8	230.2	211.1	235.2	239.0
hard and soft palate	145.5	198.89	230.0	210.4	235.1	239.0
ileocecal	153.4	197.5	230.3	211.3	235.2	239.0
pelvirectal	154.0	197.5	230.4	211.4	235.2	239.0
pelviureteric	189.1	198.0	233.9	223.1	236.91	239.5
rectosigmoid	154.0	197.5	230.4	211.4	235.2	239.0
squamocolumnar, of cervix	180.8	198.82	233.1	219.0	236.0	239.5
kidney (parenchymal)	189.0	198.0	233.9	223.0	236.91	239.5
calyx	189.1	198.0	233.9	223.1	236.91	239.5
hilus	189.1	198.0	233.9	223.1	236.91	239.5
pelvis	189.1	198.0	233.9	223.1	236.91	239.5
knee NEC*	195.5	198.89	232.7	229.8	238.8	239.8
labia (skin)	184.4	198.82	233.3	221.2	236.3	239.5
majora	184.1	198.82	233.3	221.2	236.3	239.5
minora	184.2	198.82	233.3	221.2	236.3	239.5
labial - *see also* Neoplasm, lip sulcus (lower) (upper)	145.1	198.89	230.0	210.4	235.1	239.0
labium (skin)	184.4	198.82	233.3	221.2	236.3	239.5
majus	184.1	198.82	233.3	221.2	236.3	239.5
minus	184.2	198.82	233.3	221.2	236.3	239.5
lacrimal						
canaliculi	190.7	198.4	234.0	224.7	238.8	239.8
duct (nasal)	190.7	198.4	234.0	224.7	238.8	239.8
gland	190.2	198.4	234.0	224.2	238.8	239.8
punctum	190.7	198.4	234.0	224.7	238.8	239.8
sac	190.7	198.4	234.0	224.7	238.8	239.8
Langerhans, islands or islets	157.4	197.8	230.9	211.7	235.5	239.0
laryngopharynx	148.9	198.89	230.0	210.8	235.1	239.0
larynx, laryngeal NEC	161.9	197.3	231.0	212.1	235.6	239.1
aryepiglottic fold	161.1	197.3	231.0	212.1	235.6	239.1
cartilage (arytenoid) (cricoid) (cuneiform) (thyroid)	161.3	197.3	231.0	212.1	235.6	239.1
commissure (anterior) (posterior)	161.0	197.3	231.0	212.1	235.6	239.1
contiguous sites	161.8	—	—	—	—	—
extrinsic NEC	161.1	197.3	231.0	212.1	235.6	239.1
meaning hypopharynx	148.9	198.89	230.0	210.8	235.1	239.0
interarytenoid fold	161.1	197.3	231.0	212.1	235.6	239.1
intrinsic	161.0	197.3	231.0	212.1	235.6	239.1
ventricular band	161.1	197.3	231.0	212.1	235.6	239.1
leg NEC*	195.5	198.89	232.7	229.8	238.8	239.8
lens, crystalline	190.0	198.4	234.0	224.0	238.8	239.8
lid (lower) (upper)	173.1	198.2	232.1	216.1	238.2	239.2
ligament - *see also* Neoplasm, connective tissue						
broad	183.3	198.82	233.3	221.0	236.3	239.5
Mackenrodt's	183.8	198.82	233.3	221.8	236.3	239.5
non-uterine - *see* Neoplasm, connective tissue						
round	183.5	198.82	—	221.0	236.3	239.5
sacro-uterine	183.4	198.82	—	221.0	236.3	239.5
uterine	183.4	198.82	—	221.0	236.3	239.5

	Malignant					
	Primary	**Secondary**	**Ca in situ**	**Benign**	**Uncertain Behavior**	**Unspecified**
Neoplasm *(Continued)*						
ligament *(Continued)*						
utero-ovarian	183.8	198.82	233.3	221.8	236.3	239.5
uterosacral	183.4	198.82	—	221.0	236.3	239.5
limb*	195.8	198.89	232.8	229.8	238.8	239.8
lower*	195.5	198.89	232.7	229.8	238.8	239.8
upper*	195.4	198.89	232.6	229.8	238.8	239.8
limbus of cornea	190.4	198.4	234.0	224.4	238.8	239.8
lingual NEC (*see also* Neoplasm, tongue)	141.9	198.89	230.0	210.1	235.1	239.0
lingula, lung	162.3	197.0	231.2	212.3	235.7	239.1
lip (external) (lipstick area) (vermillion border)	140.9	198.89	230.0	210.0	235.1	239.0
buccal aspect - *see* Neoplasm, lip, internal						
commissure	140.6	198.89	230.0	210.4	235.1	239.0
contiguous sites	140.8	—	—	—	—	—
with oral cavity or pharynx	149.8	—	—	—	—	—
frenulum - *see* Neoplasm, lip, internal						
inner aspect - *see* Neoplasm, lip, internal						
internal (buccal) (frenulum) (mucosa) (oral)	140.5	198.89	230.0	210.0	235.1	239.0
lower	140.4	198.89	230.0	210.0	235.1	239.0
upper	140.3	198.89	230.0	210.0	235.1	239.0
lower	140.1	198.89	230.0	210.0	235.1	239.0
internal (buccal) (frenulum) (mucosa) (oral)	140.4	198.89	230.0	210.0	235.1	239.0
mucosa - *see* Neoplasm, lip, internal						
oral aspect - *see* Neoplasm, lip, internal						
skin (commissure) (lower) (upper)	173.0	198.2	232.0	216.0	238.2	239.2
upper	140.0	198.89	230.0	210.0	235.1	239.0
internal (buccal) (frenulum) (mucosa) (oral)	140.3	198.89	230.0	210.0	235.1	239.0
liver	155.2	197.7	230.8	211.5	235.3	239.0
primary	155.0	—	—	—	—	—
lobe						
azygos	162.3	197.0	231.2	212.3	235.7	239.1
frontal	191.1	198.3	—	225.0	237.5	239.6
lower	162.5	197.0	231.2	212.3	235.7	239.1
middle	162.4	197.0	231.2	212.3	235.7	239.1
occipital	191.4	198.3	—	225.0	237.5	239.6
parietal	191.3	198.3	—	225.0	237.5	239.6
temporal	191.2	198.3	—	225.0	237.5	239.6
upper	162.3	197.0	231.2	212.3	235.7	239.1
lumbosacral plexus	171.6	198.4	—	215.6	238.1	239.2
lung	162.9	197.0	231.2	212.3	235.7	239.1
azygos lobe	162.3	197.0	231.2	212.3	235.7	239.1
carina	162.2	197.0	231.2	212.3	235.7	239.1
contiguous sites with bronchus or trachea	162.8	—	—	—	—	—
hilus	162.2	197.0	231.2	212.3	235.7	239.1
lingula	162.3	197.0	231.2	212.3	235.7	239.1
lobe NEC	162.9	197.0	231.2	212.3	235.7	239.1
lower lobe	162.5	197.0	231.2	212.3	235.7	239.1
main bronchus	162.2	197.0	231.2	212.3	235.7	239.1
middle lobe	162.4	197.0	231.2	212.3	235.7	239.1
upper lobe	162.3	197.0	231.2	212.3	235.7	239.1
lymph, lymphatic channel NEC (*see also* Neoplasm, connective tissue)	171.9	198.89	—	215.9	238.1	239.2
gland (secondary)	—	196.9	—	229.0	238.8	239.8
abdominal	—	196.2	—	229.0	238.8	239.8
aortic	—	196.2	—	229.0	238.8	239.8
arm	—	196.3	—	229.0	238.8	239.8
auricular (anterior) (posterior)	—	196.0	—	229.0	238.8	239.8
axilla, axillary	—	196.3	—	229.0	238.8	239.8
brachial	—	196.3	—	229.0	238.8	239.8
bronchial	—	196.1	—	229.0	238.8	239.8
bronchopulmonary	—	196.1	—	229.0	238.8	239.8
celiac	—	196.2	—	229.0	238.8	239.8
cervical	—	196.0	—	229.0	238.8	239.8
cervicofacial	—	196.0	—	229.0	238.8	239.8
Cloquet	—	196.5	—	229.0	238.8	239.8
colic	—	196.2	—	229.0	238.8	239.8

	Malignant					
	Primary	Secondary	Ca in situ	Benign	Uncertain Behavior	Unspecified
Neoplasm *(Continued)*						
lymph, lymphatic channel NEC *(Continued)*						
gland *(Continued)*						
common duct	—	196.2	—	229.0	238.8	239.8
cubital	—	196.3	—	229.0	238.8	239.8
diaphragmatic	—	196.1	—	229.0	238.8	239.8
epigastric, inferior	—	196.6	—	229.0	238.8	239.8
epitrochlear	—	196.3	—	229.0	238.8	239.8
esophageal	—	196.1	—	229.0	238.8	239.8
face	—	196.0	—	229.0	238.8	239.8
femoral	—	196.5	—	229.0	238.8	239.8
gastric	—	196.2	—	229.0	238.8	239.8
groin	—	196.5	—	229.0	238.8	239.8
head	—	196.0	—	229.0	238.8	239.8
hepatic	—	196.2	—	229.0	238.8	239.8
hilar (pulmonary)	—	196.1	—	229.0	238.8	239.8
splenic	—	196.2	—	229.0	238.8	239.8
hypogastric	—	196.6	—	229.0	238.8	239.8
ileocolic	—	196.2	—	229.0	238.8	239.8
iliac	—	196.6	—	229.0	238.8	239.8
infraclavicular	—	196.3	—	229.0	238.8	239.8
inguina, inguinal	—	196.5	—	229.0	238.8	239.8
innominate	—	196.1	—	229.0	238.8	239.8
intercostal	—	196.1	—	229.0	238.8	239.8
intestinal	—	196.2	—	229.0	238.8	239.8
intrabdominal	—	196.2	—	229.0	238.8	239.8
intrapelvic	—	196.6	—	229.0	238.8	239.8
intrathoracic	—	196.1	—	229.0	238.8	239.9
jugular	—	196.0	—	229.0	238.8	239.8
leg	—	196.5	—	229.0	238.8	239.8
limb						
lower	—	196.5	—	229.0	238.8	239.8
upper	—	196.3	—	229.0	238.8	239.8
lower limb	—	196.5	—	229.0	238.8	238.9
lumbar	—	196.2	—	229.0	238.8	239.8
mandibular	—	196.0	—	229.0	238.8	239.8
mediastinal	—	196.1	—	229.0	238.8	239.8
mesenteric (inferior) (superior)	—	196.2	—	229.0	238.8	239.8
midcolic	—	196.2	—	229.0	238.8	239.8
multiple sites in categories 196.0–196.6	—	196.8	—	229.0	238.8	239.8
neck	—	196.0	—	229.0	238.8	239.8
obturator	—	196.6	—	229.0	238.8	239.8
occipital	—	196.0	—	229.0	238.8	239.8
pancreatic	—	196.2	—	229.0	238.8	239.8
para-aortic	—	196.2	—	229.0	238.8	239.8
paracervical	—	196.6	—	229.0	238.8	239.8
parametrial	—	196.6	—	229.0	238.8	239.8
parasternal	—	196.1	—	229.0	238.8	239.8
parotid	—	196.0	—	229.0	238.8	239.8
pectoral	—	196.3	—	229.0	238.8	239.8
pelvic	—	196.6	—	229.0	238.8	239.8
peri-aortic	—	196.2	—	229.0	238.8	239.8
peripancreatic	—	196.2	—	229.0	238.8	239.8
popliteal	—	196.5	—	229.0	238.8	239.8
porta hepatis	—	196.2	—	229.0	238.8	239.8
portal	—	196.2	—	229.0	238.8	239.8
preauricular	—	196.0	—	229.0	238.8	239.8
prelaryngeal	—	196.0	—	229.0	238.8	239.8
presymphysial	—	196.6	—	229.0	238.8	239.8
pretracheal	—	196.0	—	229.0	238.8	239.8
primary (any site) NEC	202.9	—	—	—	—	—
pulmonary (hiler)	—	196.1	—	229.0	238.8	239.8
pyloric	—	196.2	—	229.0	238.8	239.8
retroperitoneal	—	196.2	—	229.0	238.8	239.8
retropharyngeal	—	196.0	—	229.0	238.8	239.8

◀ New ⟸ Revised

	Malignant					
	Primary	**Secondary**	**Ca in situ**	**Benign**	**Uncertain Behavior**	**Unspecified**
Neoplasm *(Continued)*						
lymph, lymphatic channel NEC *(Continued)*						
gland *(Continued)*						
Rosenmüller's	—	196.5	—	229.0	238.8	239.8
sacral	—	196.6	—	229.0	238.8	239.8
scalene	—	196.0	—	229.0	238.8	239.8
site NEC	—	196.9	—	229.0	238.8	239.8
splenic (hilar)	—	196.2	—	229.0	238.8	239.8
subclavicular	—	196.3	—	229.0	238.8	239.8
subinguinal	—	196.5	—	229.0	238.8	239.8
sublingual	—	196.0	—	229.0	238.8	239.8
submandibular	—	196.0	—	229.0	238.8	239.8
submaxillary	—	196.0	—	229.0	238.8	239.8
submental	—	196.0	—	229.0	238.8	239.8
subscapular	—	196.3	—	229.0	238.8	239.8
supraclavicular	—	196.0	—	229.0	238.8	239.8
thoracic	—	196.1	—	229.0	238.8	239.8
tibial	—	196.5	—	229.0	238.8	239.8
tracheal		196.1	—	229.0	238.8	239.8
tracheobronchial	—	196.1	—	229.0	238.8	239.8
upper limb	—	196.3	—	229.0	238.8	239.8
Virchow's	—	196.0	—	229.0	238.8	239.8
node - *see also* Neoplasm, lymph gland primary NEC	202.9	—	—	—	—	—
vessel (*see also* Neoplasm, connective tissue)	171.9	198.89	—	215.9	238.1	239.2
Mackenrodt's ligament	183.8	198.82	233.3	221.8	236.3	239.5
malar region - *see* Neoplasm, cheek	170.0	198.5	—	213.0	238.0	239.2
mammary gland - *see* Neoplasm, breast						
mandible	170.1	198.5	—	213.1	238.0	239.2
alveolar						
mucosa	143.1	198.89	230.0	210.4	235.1	239.0
ridge or process	170.1	198.5	—	213.1	238.0	239.2
carcinoma	143.1	—	—	—	—	—
carcinoma	143.1	—	—	—	—	—
marrow (bone) NEC	202.9	198.5	—	—	—	238.79
mastectomy site (skin)	173.5	198.2	—	—	—	—
specified as breast tissue	174.8	198.81	—	—	—	—
mastoid (air cells) (antrum) (cavity)	160.1	197.3	231.8	212.0	235.9	239.1
bone or process	170.0	198.5	—	213.0	238.0	239.2
maxilla, maxillary (superior)	170.0	198.5	—	213.0	238.0	239.2
alveolar						
mucosa	143.0	198.89	230.0	210.4	235.1	239.0
ridge or process	170.0	198.5	—	213.0	238.0	239.2
carcinoma	143.0	—	—	—	—	—
antrum	160.2	197.3	231.8	212.0	235.9	239.1
carcinoma	143.0	—	—	—	—	—
inferior - *see* Neoplasm, mandible						
sinus	160.2	197.3	231.8	212.0	235.9	239.1
meatus						
external (ear)	173.2	198.2	232.2	216.2	238.2	239.2
Meckel's diverticulum	152.3	197.4	230.7	211.2	235.2	239.0
mediastinum, mediastinal	164.9	197.1	—	212.5	235.8	239.8
anterior	164.2	197.1	—	212.5	235.8	239.8
contiguous sites with heart and thymus	164.8	—	—	—	—	—
posterior	164.3	197.1	—	212.5	235.8	239.8
medulla						
adrenal	194.0	198.7	234.8	227.0	237.2	239.7
oblongata	191.7	198.3	—	225.0	237.5	239.6
meibomian gland	173.1	198.2	232.1	216.1	238.2	239.2
melanoma - *see* Melanoma						
meninges (brain) (cerebral) (cranial) (intracranial)	192.1	198.4	—	225.2	237.6	239.7
spinal (cord)	192.3	198.4	—	225.4	237.6	239.7
meniscus, knee joint (lateral) (medial)	170.7	198.5	—	213.7	238.0	239.2
mesentery, mesenteric	158.8	197.6	—	211.8	235.4	239.0
mesoappendix	158.8	197.6	—	211.8	235.4	239.0
mesocolon	158.8	197.6	—	211.8	235.4	239.0

	Malignant					
	Primary	Secondary	Ca in situ	Benign	Uncertain Behavior	Unspecified
Neoplasm *(Continued)*						
mesopharynx - *see* Neoplasm, oropharynx						
mesosalpinx	183.3	198.82	233.3	221.0	236.3	239.5
mesovarium	183.3	198.82	233.3	221.0	236.3	239.5
metacarpus (any bone)	170.5	198.5	—	213.5	238.0	239.2
metastatic NEC - *see also* Neoplasm, by site, secondary	—	199.1	—	—	—	—
metatarsus (any bone)	170.8	198.5	—	213.8	238.0	239.2
midbrain	191.7	198.3	—	225.0	237.5	239.6
milk duct - *see* Neoplasm, breast						
mons						
pubis	184.4	198.82	233.3	221.2	236.3	239.5
veneris	184.4	198.82	233.3	221.2	236.3	239.5
motor tract	192.9	198.4	—	225.9	237.9	239.7
brain	191.9	198.3	—	225.0	237.5	239.6
spinal	192.2	198.3	—	225.3	237.5	239.7
mouth	145.9	198.89	230.0	210.4	235.1	239.0
contiguous sites	145.8	—	—	—	—	—
floor	144.9	198.89	230.0	210.3	235.1	239.0
anterior portion	144.0	198.89	230.0	210.3	235.1	239.0
contiguous sites	144.8	—	—	—	—	—
lateral portion	144.1	198.89	230.0	210.3	235.1	239.0
roof	145.5	198.89	230.0	210.4	235.1	239.0
specified part NEC	145.8	198.89	230.0	210.4	235.1	239.0
vestibule	145.1	198.89	230.0	210.4	235.1	239.0
mucosa						
alveolar (ridge or process)	143.9	198.89	230.0	210.4	235.1	239.0
lower	143.1	198.89	230.0	210.4	235.1	239.0
upper	143.0	198.89	230.0	210.4	235.1	239.0
buccal	145.0	198.89	230.0	210.4	235.1	239.0
cheek	145.0	198.89	230.0	210.4	235.1	239.0
lip - *see* Neoplasm, lip, internal						
nasal	160.0	197.3	231.8	212.0	235.9	239.1
oral	145.0	198.89	230.0	210.4	235.1	239.0
Müllerian duct						
female	184.8	198.82	233.3	221.8	236.3	239.5
male	187.8	198.82	233.6	222.8	236.6	239.5
multiple sites NEC	199.0	199.0	234.9	229.9	238.9	199.0
muscle - *see also* Neoplasm, connective tissue extraocular	190.1	198.4	234.0	224.1	238.8	239.8
myocardium	164.1	198.89	—	212.7	238.8	239.8
myometrium	182.0	198.82	233.2	219.1	236.0	239.5
myopericardium	164.1	198.89	—	212.7	238.8	239.8
nabothian gland (follicle)	180.0	198.82	233.1	219.0	236.0	239.5
nail	173.9	198.2	232.9	216.9	238.2	239.2
finger	173.6	198.2	232.6	216.6	238.2	239.2
toe	173.7	198.2	232.7	216.7	238.2	239.2
nares, naris (anterior) (posterior)	160.0	197.3	231.8	212.0	235.9	239.1
nasal - *see* Neoplasm, nose						
nasolabial groove	173.3	198.2	232.3	216.3	238.2	239.2
nasolacrimal duct	190.7	198.4	234.0	224.7	238.8	239.8
nasopharynx, nasopharyngeal	147.9	198.89	230.0	210.7	235.1	239.0
contiguous sites	147.8	—	—	—	—	—
floor	147.3	198.89	230.0	210.7	235.1	239.0
roof	147.0	198.89	230.0	210.7	235.1	239.0
specified site NEC	147.8	198.89	230.0	210.7	235.1	239.0
wall	147.9	198.89	230.0	210.7	235.1	239.0
anterior	147.3	198.89	230.0	210.7	235.1	239.0
lateral	147.2	198.89	230.0	210.7	235.1	239.0
posterior	147.1	198.89	230.0	210.7	235.1	239.0
superior	147.0	198.89	230.0	210.7	235.1	239.0
nates	173.5	198.2	232.5	216.5	238.2	239.2
neck NEC*	195.0	198.89	234.8	229.8	238.8	239.8
nerve (autonomic) (ganglion) (parasympathetic) (peripheral) (sympathetic) - *see also* Neoplasm, connective tissue						
abducens	192.0	198.4	—	225.1	237.9	239.7
accessory (spinal)	192.0	198.4	—	225.1	237.9	239.7

	Malignant					
	Primary	Secondary	Ca in situ	Benign	Uncertain Behavior	Unspecified
Neoplasm *(Continued)*						
nerve *(Continued)*						
acoustic	192.0	198.4	—	225.1	237.9	239.7
auditory	192.0	198.4	—	225.1	237.9	239.7
brachial	171.2	198.89	—	215.2	238.1	239.2
cranial (any)	192.0	198.4	—	225.1	237.9	239.7
facial	192.0	198.4	—	225.1	237.9	239.7
femoral	171.3	198.89	—	215.3	238.1	239.2
glossopharyngeal	192.0	198.4	—	225.1	237.9	239.7
hypoglossal	192.0	198.4	—	225.1	237.9	239.7
intercostal	171.4	198.89	—	215.4	238.1	239.2
lumbar	171.7	198.89	—	215.7	238.1	239.2
median	171.2	198.89	—	215.2	238.1	239.2
obturator	171.3	198.89	—	215.3	238.1	239.2
oculomotor	192.0	198.4	—	225.1	237.9	239.7
olfactory	192.0	198.4	—	225.1	237.9	239.7
optic	192.0	198.4	—	225.1	237.9	239.7
peripheral NEC	171.9	198.89	—	215.9	238.1	239.2
radial	171.2	198.89	—	215.2	238.1	239.2
sacral	171.6	198.89	—	215.6	238.1	239.2
sciatic	171.3	198.89	—	215.3	238.1	239.2
spinal NEC	171.9	198.89	—	215.9	238.1	239.2
trigeminal	192.0	198.4	—	225.1	237.9	239.7
trochlear	192.0	198.4	—	225.1	237.9	239.7
ulnar	171.2	198.89	—	215.2	238.1	239.2
vagus	192.0	198.4	—	225.1	237.9	239.7
nervous system (central) NEC	192.9	198.4	—	225.9	237.9	239.7
autonomic NEC	171.9	198.89	—	215.9	238.1	239.2
brain - *see also* Neoplasm, brain membrane or meninges	192.1	198.4	—	225.2	237.6	239.7
contiguous sites	192.8	—	—	—	—	—
parasympathetic NEC	171.9	198.89	—	215.9	238.1	239.2
sympathetic NEC	171.9	198.89	—	215.9	238.1	239.2
nipple (female)	174.0	198.81	233.0	217	238.3	239.3
male	175.0	198.81	233.0	217	238.3	239.3
nose, nasal	195.0	198.89	234.8	229.8	238.8	239.8
ala (external)	173.3	198.2	232.3	216.3	238.2	239.2
bone	170.0	198.5	—	213.0	238.0	239.2
cartilage	160.0	197.3	231.8	212.0	235.9	239.1
cavity	160.0	197.3	231.8	212.0	235.9	239.1
contiguous sites with accessory sinuses or middle ear	160.8	—	—	—	—	—
choana	147.3	198.89	230.0	210.7	235.1	239.0
external (skin)	173.3	198.2	232.3	216.3	238.2	239.2
fossa	160.0	197.3	231.8	212.0	235.9	239.1
internal	160.0	197.3	231.8	212.0	235.9	239.1
mucosa	160.0	197.3	231.8	212.0	235.9	239.1
septum	160.0	197.3	231.8	212.0	235.9	239.1
posterior margin	147.3	198.89	230.0	210.7	235.1	239.0
sinus - *see* Neoplasm, sinus						
skin	173.3	198.2	232.3	216.3	238.2	239.2
turbinate (mucosa)	160.0	197.3	231.8	212.0	235.9	239.1
bone	170.0	198.5	—	213.0	238.0	239.2
vestibule	160.0	197.3	231.8	212.0	235.9	239.1
nostril	160.0	197.3	231.8	212.0	235.9	239.1
nucleus pulposus	170.2	198.5	—	213.2	238.0	230.2
occipital						
bone	170.0	198.5	—	213.0	238.0	239.2
lobe or pole, brain	191.4	198.3	—	225.0	237.5	239.6
odontogenic - *see* Neoplasm, jaw bone						
oesophagus - *see* Neoplasm, esophagus						
olfactory nerve or bulb	192.0	198.4	—	225.1	237.9	239.7
olive (brain)	191.7	198.3	—	225.0	237.5	239.6
omentum	158.8	197.6	—	211.8	235.4	239.0
operculum (brain)	191.0	198.3	—	225.0	237.5	239.6
optic nerve, chiasm, or tract	192.0	198.4	—	225.1	237.9	239.7

	Malignant					
	Primary	**Secondary**	**Ca in situ**	**Benign**	**Uncertain Behavior**	**Unspecified**
Neoplasm *(Continued)*						
oral (cavity)	145.9	198.89	230.0	210.4	235.1	239.0
contiguous sites with lip or pharynx	149.8	—	—	—	—	—
ill-defined	149.9	198.89	230.0	210.4	235.1	239.0
mucosa	145.9	198.89	230.0	210.4	235.1	239.0
orbit	190.1	198.4	234.0	224.1	238.8	239.8
bone	170.0	198.5	—	213.0	238.0	239.2
eye	190.1	198.4	234.0	224.1	238.8	239.8
soft parts	190.1	198.4	234.0	224.1	238.8	239.8
organ of Zuckerkandl	194.6	198.89	—	227.6	237.3	239.7
oropharynx	146.9	198.89	230.0	210.6	235.1	239.0
branchial cleft (vestige)	146.8	198.89	230.0	210.6	235.1	239.0
contiguous sites	146.8	—	—	—	—	—
junctional region	146.5	198.89	230.0	210.6	235.1	239.0
lateral wall	146.6	198.89	230.0	210.6	235.1	239.0
pillars of fauces	146.2	198.89	230.0	210.6	235.1	239.0
posterior wall	146.7	198.89	230.0	210.6	235.1	239.0
specified part NEC	146.8	198.89	230.0	210.6	235.1	239.0
vallecula	146.3	198.89	230.0	210.6	235.1	239.0
os						
external	180.1	198.82	233.1	219.0	236.0	239.5
internal	180.0	198.82	233.1	219.0	236.0	239.5
ovary	183.0	198.6	233.3	220	236.2	239.5
oviduct	183.2	198.82	233.3	221.0	236.3	239.5
palate	145.5	198.89	230.0	210.4	235.1	239.0
hard	145.2	198.89	230.0	210.4	235.1	239.0
junction of hard and soft palate	145.5	198.89	230.0	210.4	235.1	239.0
soft	145.3	198.89	230.0	210.4	235.1	239.0
nasopharyngeal surface	147.3	198.89	230.0	210.7	235.1	239.0
posterior surface	147.3	198.89	230.0	210.7	235.1	239.0
superior surface	147.3	198.89	230.0	210.7	235.1	239.0
palatoglossal arch	146.2	198.89	230.0	210.6	235.1	239.0
palatopharyngeal arch	146.2	198.89	230.0	210.6	235.1	239.0
pallium	191.0	198.3	—	225.0	237.5	239.6
palpebra	173.1	198.2	232.1	216.1	238.2	239.2
pancreas	157.9	197.8	230.9	211.6	235.5	239.0
body	157.1	197.8	230.9	211.6	235.5	239.0
contiguous sites	157.8	—	—	—	—	—
duct (of Santorini) (of Wirsung)	157.3	197.8	230.9	211.6	235.5	239.0
ectopic tissue	157.8	197.8				
head	157.0	197.8	230.9	211.6	235.5	239.0
islet cells	157.4	197.8	230.9	211.7	235.5	239.0
neck	157.8	197.8	230.9	211.6	235.5	239.0
tail	157.2	197.8	230.9	211.6	235.5	239.0
para-aortic body	194.6	198.89	—	227.6	237.3	239.7
paraganglion NEC	194.6	198.89	—	227.6	237.3	239.7
parametrium	183.4	198.82	—	221.0	236.3	239.5
paranephric	158.0	197.6	—	211.8	235.4	239.0
pararectal	195.3	198.89	—	229.8	238.8	239.8
parasagittal (region)	195.0	198.89	234.8	229.8	238.8	239.8
parasellar	192.9	198.4	—	225.9	237.9	239.7
parathyroid (gland)	194.1	198.89	234.8	227.1	237.4	239.7
paraurethral	195.3	198.89	—	229.8	238.8	239.8
gland	189.4	198.1	233.9	223.89	236.99	239.5
paravaginal	195.3	198.89	—	229.8	238.8	239.8
parenchyma, kidney	189.0	198.0	233.9	223.0	236.91	239.5
parietal						
bone	170.0	198.5	—	213.0	238.0	239.2
lobe, brain	191.3	198.3	—	225.0	237.5	239.6
paroophoron	183.3	198.82	233.3	221.0	236.3	239.5
parotid (duct) (gland)	142.0	198.89	230.0	210.2	235.0	239.0
parovarium	183.3	198.82	233.3	221.0	236.3	239.5
patella	170.8	198.5	—	213.8	238.0	239.2
peduncle, cerebral	191.7	198.3	—	225.0	237.5	239.6
pelvirectal junction	154.0	197.5	230.4	211.4	235.2	239.0

	Malignant					
	Primary	Secondary	Ca in situ	Benign	Uncertain Behavior	Unspecified
Neoplasm *(Continued)*						
pelvis, pelvic	195.3	198.89	234.8	229.8	238.8	239.8
bone	170.6	198.5	—	213.6	238.0	239.2
floor	195.3	198.89	234.8	229.8	238.8	239.8
renal	189.1	198.0	233.9	223.1	236.91	239.5
viscera	195.3	198.89	234.8	229.8	238.8	239.8
wall	195.3	198.89	234.8	229.8	238.8	239.8
pelvo-abdominal	195.8	198.89	234.8	229.8	238.8	239.8
penis	187.4	198.82	233.5	222.1	236.6	239.5
body	187.3	198.82	233.5	222.1	236.6	239.5
corpus (cavernosum)	187.3	198.82	233.5	222.1	236.6	239.5
glans	187.2	198.82	233.5	222.1	236.6	239.5
skin NEC	187.4	198.82	233.5	222.1	236.6	239.5
periadrenal (tissue)	158.0	197.6	—	211.8	235.4	239.0
perianal (skin)	173.5	198.2	232.5	216.5	238.2	239.2
pericardium	164.1	198.89	—	212.7	238.8	239.8
perinephric	158.0	197.6	—	211.8	235.4	239.0
perineum	195.3	198.89	234.8	229.8	238.8	239.8
periodontal tissue NEC	143.9	198.89	230.0	210.4	235.1	239.0
periosteum - *see* Neoplasm, bone						
peripancreatic	158.0	197.6	—	211.8	235.4	239.0
peripheral nerve NEC	171.9	198.89	—	215.9	238.1	239.2
perirectal (tissue)	195.3	198.89	—	229.8	238.8	239.8
perirenal (tissue)	158.0	197.6	—	211.8	235.4	239.0
peritoneum, peritoneal (cavity)	158.9	197.6	—	211.8	235.4	239.0
contiguous sites	158.8	—	—	—	—	—
with digestive organs	159.8	—	—	—	—	—
parietal	158.8	197.6	—	211.8	235.4	239.0
pelvic	158.8	197.6	—	211.8	235.4	239.0
specified part NEC	158.8	197.6	—	211.8	235.4	239.0
peritonsillar (tissue)	195.0	198.89	234.8	229.8	238.8	239.8
periurethral tissue	195.3	198.89	—	229.8	238.8	239.8
phalanges	170.9	198.5	—	213.9	238.0	239.2
foot	170.8	198.5	—	213.8	238.0	239.2
hand	170.5	198.5	—	213.5	238.0	239.2
pharynx, pharyngeal	149.0	198.89	230.0	210.9	235.1	239.0
bursa	147.1	198.89	230.0	210.7	235.1	239.0
fornix	147.3	198.89	230.0	210.7	235.1	239.0
recess	147.2	198.89	230.0	210.7	235.1	239.0
region	149.0	198.89	230.0	210.9	235.1	239.0
tonsil	147.1	198.89	230.0	210.7	235.1	239.0
wall (lateral) (posterior)	149.0	198.89	230.0	210.9	235.1	239.0
pia mater (cerebral) (cranial)	192.1	198.4	—	225.2	237.6	239.7
spinal	192.3	198.4	—	225.4	237.6	239.7
pillars of fauces	146.2	198.89	230.0	210.6	235.1	239.0
pineal (body) (gland)	194.4	198.89	234.8	227.4	237.1	239.7
pinna (ear) NEC	173.2	198.2	232.2	216.2	238.2	239.2
cartilage	171.0	198.89	—	215.0	238.1	239.2
piriform fossa or sinus	148.1	198.89	230.0	210.8	235.1	239.0
pituitary (body) (fossa) (gland) (lobe)	194.3	198.89	234.8	227.3	237.0	239.7
placenta	181	198.82	233.2	219.8	236.1	239.5
pleura, pleural (cavity)	163.9	197.2	—	212.4	235.8	239.1
contiguous sites	163.8	—	—	—	—	—
parietal	163.0	197.2	—	212.4	235.8	239.1
visceral	163.1	197.2	—	212.4	235.8	239.1
plexus						
brachial	171.2	198.89	—	215.2	238.1	239.2
cervical	171.0	198.89	—	215.0	238.1	239.2
choroid	191.5	198.3	—	225.0	237.5	239.6
lumbosacral	171.6	198.89	—	215.6	238.1	239.2
sacral	171.6	198.89	—	215.6	238.1	239.2
pluri-endocrine	194.8	198.89	234.8	227.8	237.4	239.7
pole						
frontal	191.1	198.3	—	225.0	237.5	239.6
occipital	191.4	198.3	—	225.0	237.5	239.6

	Malignant					
	Primary	Secondary	Ca in situ	Benign	Uncertain Behavior	Unspecified
Neoplasm *(Continued)*						
pons (varolii)	191.7	198.3	—	225.0	237.5	239.6
popliteal fossa or space*	195.5	198.89	234.8	229.8	238.8	239.8
postcricoid (region)	148.0	198.89	230.0	210.8	235.1	239.0
posterior fossa (cranial)	191.9	198.3	—	225.0	237.5	239.6
postnasal space	147.9	198.89	230.0	210.7	235.1	239.0
prepuce	187.1	198.82	233.5	222.1	236.6	239.5
prepylorus	151.1	197.8	230.2	211.1	235.2	239.0
presacral (region)	195.3	198.89	—	229.8	238.8	239.8
prostate (gland)	185	198.82	233.4	222.2	236.5	239.5
utricle	189.3	198.1	233.9	223.81	236.99	239.5
pterygoid fossa	171.0	198.89	—	215.0	238.1	239.2
pubic bone	170.6	198.5	—	213.6	238.0	239.2
pudenda, pudendum (female)	184.4	198.82	233.3	221.2	236.3	239.5
pulmonary	162.9	197.0	231.2	212.3	235.7	239.1
putamen	191.0	198.3	—	225.0	237.5	239.6
pyloric						
antrum	151.2	197.8	230.2	211.1	235.2	239.0
canal	151.1	197.8	230.2	211.1	235.2	239.0
pylorus	151.1	197.8	230.2	211.1	235.2	239.0
pyramid (brain)	191.7	198.3	—	225.0	237.5	239.6
pyriform fossa or sinus	148.1	198.89	230.0	210.8	235.1	239.0
radius (any part)	170.4	198.5	—	213.4	238.0	239.2
Rathke's pouch	194.3	198.89	234.8	227.3	237.0	239.7
rectosigmoid (colon) (junction)	154.0	197.5	230.4	211.4	235.2	239.0
contiguous sites with anus or rectum	154.8	—	—	—	—	—
rectouterine pouch	158.8	197.6	—	211.8	235.4	239.0
rectovaginal septum or wall	195.3	198.89	234.8	229.8	238.8	239.8
rectovesical septum	195.3	198.89	234.8	229.8	238.8	239.8
rectum (ampulla)	154.1	197.5	230.4	211.4	235.2	239.0
and colon	154.0	197.5	230.4	211.4	235.2	239.0
contiguous sites with anus or rectosigmoid junction	154.8	—	—	—	—	—
renal	189.0	198.0	233.9	223.0	236.91	239.5
calyx	189.1	198.0	233.9	223.1	236.91	239.5
hilus	189.1	198.0	233.9	223.1	236.91	239.5
parenchyma	189.0	198.0	233.9	223.0	236.91	239.5
pelvis	189.1	198.0	233.9	223.1	236.91	239.5
respiratory						
organs or system NEC	165.9	197.3	231.9	212.9	235.9	239.1
contiguous sites with intrathoracic organs	165.8	—	—	—	—	—
specified sites NEC	165.8	197.3	231.8	212.8	235.9	239.1
tract NEC	165.9	197.3	231.9	212.9	235.9	239.1
upper	165.0	197.3	231.9	212.9	235.9	239.1
retina	190.5	198.4	234.0	224.5	238.8	239.8
retrobulbar	190.1	198.4	—	224.1	238.8	239.8
retrocecal	158.0	197.6	—	211.8	235.4	239.0
retromolar (area) (triangle) (trigone)	145.6	198.89	230.0	210.4	235.1	239.0
retro-orbital	195.0	198.89	234.8	229.8	238.8	239.8
retroperitoneal (space) (tissue)	158.0	197.6	—	211.8	235.4	239.0
contiguous sites	158.8	—	—	—	—	—
retroperitoneum	158.0	197.6	—	211.8	235.4	239.0
contiguous sites	158.8	—	—	—	—	—
retropharyngeal	149.0	198.89	230.0	210.9	235.1	239.0
retrovesical (septum)	195.3	198.89	234.8	229.8	238.8	239.8
rhinencephalon	191.0	198.3	—	225.0	237.5	239.6
rib	170.3	198.5	—	213.3	238.0	239.2
Rosenmüller's fossa	147.2	198.89	230.0	210.7	235.1	239.0
round ligament	183.5	198.82	—	221.0	236.3	239.5
sacrococcyx, sacrococcygeal	170.6	198.5	—	213.6	238.0	239.2
region	195.3	198.89	234.8	229.8	238.8	239.8
sacrouterine ligament	183.4	198.82	—	221.0	236.3	239.5
sacrum, sacral (vertebra)	170.6	198.5	—	213.6	238.0	239.2
salivary gland or duct (major)	142.9	198.89	230.0	210.2	235.0	239.0
contiguous sites	142.8	—	—	—	—	—
minor NEC	145.9	198.89	230.0	210.4	235.1	239.0

	Malignant					
	Primary	Secondary	Ca in situ	Benign	Uncertain Behavior	Unspecified
Neoplasm *(Continued)*						
salivary gland or duct *(Continued)*						
parotid	142.0	198.89	230.0	210.2	235.0	239.0
pluriglandular	142.8	198.89	230.0	210.2	235.0	239.0
sublingual	142.2	198.89	230.0	210.2	235.0	239.0
submandibular	142.1	198.89	230.0	210.2	235.0	239.0
submaxillary	142.1	198.89	230.0	210.2	235.0	239.0
salpinx (uterine)	183.2	198.82	233.3	221.0	236.3	239.5
Santorini's duct	157.3	197.8	230.9	211.6	235.5	239.0
scalp	173.4	198.2	232.4	216.4	238.2	239.2
scapula (any part)	170.4	198.5	—	213.4	238.0	239.2
scapular region	195.1	198.89	234.8	229.8	238.8	239.8
scar NEC (*see also* Neoplasm, skin)	173.9	198.2	232.9	216.9	238.2	239.2
sciatic nerve	171.3	198.89	—	215.3	238.1	239.2
sclera	190.0	198.4	234.0	224.0	238.8	239.8
scrotum (skin)	187.7	198.82	233.6	222.4	236.6	239.5
sebaceous gland - *see* Neoplasm, skin						
sella turcica	194.3	198.89	234.8	227.3	237.0	239.7
bone	170.0	198.5	—	213.0	238.0	239.2
semilunar cartilage (knee)	170.7	198.5	—	213.7	238.0	239.2
seminal vesicle	187.8	198.82	233.6	222.8	236.6	239.5
septum						
nasal	160.0	197.3	231.8	212.0	235.9	239.1
posterior margin	147.3	198.89	230.0	210.7	235.1	239.0
rectovaginal	195.3	198.89	234.8	229.8	238.8	239.8
rectovesical	195.3	198.89	234.8	229.8	238.8	239.8
urethrovaginal	184.9	198.82	233.3	221.9	236.3	239.5
vesicovaginal	184.9	198.82	233.3	221.9	236.3	239.5
shoulder NEC*	195.4	198.89	232.6	229.8	238.8	239.8
sigmoid flexure (lower) (upper)	153.3	197.5	230.3	211.3	235.2	239.0
sinus (accessory)	160.9	197.3	231.8	212.0	235.9	239.1
bone (any)	170.0	198.5	—	213.0	238.0	239.2
contiguous sites with middle ear or nasal cavities	160.8	—	—	—	—	—
ethmoidal	160.3	197.3	231.8	212.0	235.9	239.1
frontal	160.4	197.3	231.8	212.0	235.9	239.1
maxillary	160.2	197.3	231.8	212.0	235.9	239.1
nasal, paranasal NEC	160.9	197.3	231.8	212.0	235.9	239.1
pyriform	148.1	198.89	230.0	210.8	235.1	239.0
sphenoidal	160.5	197.3	231.8	212.0	235.9	239.1
skeleton, skeletal NEC	170.9	198.5	—	213.9	238.0	239.2
Skene's gland	189.4	198.1	233.9	223.89	236.99	239.5
skin NEC	173.9	198.2	232.9	216.9	238.2	239.2
abdominal wall	173.5	198.2	232.5	216.5	238.2	239.2
ala nasi	173.3	198.2	232.3	216.3	238.2	239.2
ankle	173.7	198.2	232.7	216.7	238.2	239.2
antecubital space	173.6	198.2	232.6	216.6	238.2	239.2
anus	173.5	198.2	232.5	216.5	238.2	239.2
arm	173.6	198.2	232.6	216.6	238.2	239.2
auditory canal (external)	173.2	198.2	232.2	216.2	238.2	239.2
auricle (ear)	173.2	198.2	232.2	216.2	238.2	239.2
auricular canal (external)	173.2	198.2	232.2	216.2	238.2	239.2
axilla, axillary fold	173.5	198.2	232.5	216.5	238.2	239.2
back	173.5	198.2	232.5	216.5	238.2	239.2
breast	173.5	198.2	232.5	216.5	238.2	239.2
brow	173.3	198.2	232.3	216.3	238.2	239.2
buttock	173.5	198.2	232.5	216.5	238.2	239.2
calf	173.7	198.2	232.7	216.7	238.2	239.2
canthus (eye) (inner) (outer)	173.1	198.2	232.1	216.1	238.2	239.2
cervical region	173.4	198.2	232.4	216.4	238.2	239.2
cheek (external)	173.3	198.2	232.3	216.3	238.2	239.2
chest (wall)	173.5	198.2	232.5	216.5	238.2	239.2
chin	173.3	198.2	232.3	216.3	238.2	239.2
clavicular area	173.5	198.2	232.5	216.5	238.2	239.2
clitoris	184.3	198.82	233.3	221.2	236.3	239.5
columnella	173.3	198.2	232.3	216.3	238.2	239.2

	Malignant					
	Primary	Secondary	Ca in situ	Benign	Uncertain Behavior	Unspecified
Neoplasm *(Continued)*						
skin NEC *(Continued)*						
concha	173.2	198.2	232.2	216.2	238.2	239.2
contiguous sites	173.8	—	—	—	—	—
ear (external)	173.2	198.2	232.2	216.2	238.2	239.2
elbow	173.6	198.2	232.6	216.6	238.2	239.2
eyebrow	173.3	198.2	232.3	216.3	238.2	239.2
eyelid	173.1	198.2	232.1	216.1	238.2	239.2
face NEC	173.3	198.2	232.3	216.3	238.2	239.2
female genital organs (external)	184.4	198.82	233.3	221.2	236.3	239.5
clitoris	184.3	198.82	233.3	221.2	236.3	239.5
labium NEC	184.4	198.82	233.3	221.2	236.3	239.5
majus	184.1	198.82	233.3	221.2	236.3	239.5
minus	184.2	198.82	233.3	221.2	236.3	239.5
pudendum	184.4	198.82	233.3	221.2	236.3	239.5
vulva	184.4	198.82	233.3	221.2	236.3	239.5
finger	173.6	198.2	232.6	216.6	238.2	239.2
flank	173.5	198.2	232.5	216.5	238.2	239.2
foot	173.7	198.2	232.7	216.7	238.2	239.2
forearm	173.6	198.2	232.6	216.6	238.2	239.2
forehead	173.3	198.2	232.3	216.3	238.2	239.2
glabella	173.3	198.2	232.3	216.3	238.2	239.2
gluteal region	173.5	198.2	232.5	216.5	238.2	239.2
groin	173.5	198.2	232.5	216.5	238.2	239.2
hand	173.6	198.2	232.6	216.6	238.2	239.2
head NEC	173.4	198.2	232.4	216.4	238.2	239.2
heel	173.7	198.2	232.7	216.7	238.2	239.2
helix	173.2	198.2	232.2	216.2	238.2	239.2
hip	173.7	198.2	232.7	216.7	238.2	239.2
infraclavicular region	173.5	198.2	232.5	216.5	238.2	239.2
inguinal region	173.5	198.2	232.5	216.5	238.2	239.2
jaw	173.3	198.2	232.3	216.3	238.2	239.2
knee	173.7	198.2	232.7	216.7	238.2	239.2
labia						
majora	184.1	198.82	233.3	221.2	236.3	239.5
minora	184.2	198.82	233.3	221.2	236.3	239.5
leg	173.7	198.2	232.7	216.7	238.2	239.2
lid (lower) (upper)	173.1	198.2	232.1	216.1	238.2	239.2
limb NEC	173.9	198.2	232.9	216.9	238.2	239.5
lower	173.7	198.2	232.7	216.7	238.2	239.2
upper	173.6	198.2	232.6	216.6	238.2	239.2
lip (lower) (upper)	173.0	198.2	232.0	216.0	238.2	239.2
male genital organs	187.9	198.82	233.6	222.9	236.6	239.5
penis	187.4	198.82	233.5	222.1	236.6	239.5
prepuce	187.1	198.82	233.5	222.1	236.6	239.5
scrotum	187.7	198.82	233.6	222.4	236.6	239.5
mastectomy site	173.5	198.2	—	—	—	—
specified as breast tissue	174.8	198.81	—	—	—	—
meatus, acoustic (external)	173.2	198.2	232.2	216.2	238.2	239.2
nates	173.5	198.2	232.5	216.5	238.2	239.2
neck	173.4	198.2	232.4	216.4	238.2	239.2
nose (external)	173.3	198.2	232.3	216.3	238.2	239.2
palm	173.6	198.2	232.6	216.6	238.2	239.2
palpebra	173.1	198.2	232.1	216.1	238.2	239.2
penis NEC	187.4	198.82	233.5	222.1	236.6	239.5
perianal	173.5	198.2	232.5	216.5	238.2	239.2
perineum	173.5	198.2	232.5	216.5	238.2	239.2
pinna	173.2	198.2	232.2	216.2	238.2	239.2
plantar	173.7	198.2	232.7	216.7	238.2	239.2
popliteal fossa or space	173.7	198.2	232.7	216.7	238.2	239.2
prepuce	187.1	198.82	233.5	222.1	236.6	239.5
pubes	173.5	198.2	232.5	216.5	238.2	239.2
sacrococcygeal region	173.5	198.2	232.5	216.5	238.2	239.2
scalp	173.4	198.2	232.4	216.4	238.2	239.2
scapular region	173.5	198.2	232.5	216.5	238.2	239.2

	Malignant					
	Primary	**Secondary**	**Ca in situ**	**Benign**	**Uncertain Behavior**	**Unspecified**
Neoplasm *(Continued)*						
skin NEC *(Continued)*						
scrotum	187.7	198.82	233.6	222.4	236.6	239.5
shoulder	173.6	198.2	232.6	216.6	238.2	239.2
sole (foot)	173.7	198.2	232.7	216.7	238.2	239.2
specified sites NEC	173.8	198.2	232.8	216.8	232.8	239.2
submammary fold	173.5	198.2	232.5	216.5	238.2	239.2
supraclavicular region	173.4	198.2	232.4	216.4	238.2	239.2
temple	173.3	198.2	232.3	216.3	238.2	239.2
thigh	173.7	198.2	232.7	216.7	238.2	239.2
thoracic wall	173.5	198.2	232.5	216.5	238.2	239.2
thumb	173.6	198.2	232.6	216.6	238.2	239.2
toe	173.7	198.2	232.7	216.7	238.2	239.2
tragus	173.2	198.2	232.2	216.2	238.2	239.2
trunk	173.5	198.2	232.5	216.5	238.2	239.2
umbilicus	173.5	198.2	232.5	216.5	238.2	239.2
vulva	184.4	198.82	233.3	221.2	236.3	239.5
wrist	173.6	198.2	232.6	216.6	238.2	239.2
skull	170.0	198.5	—	213.0	238.0	239.2
soft parts or tissues - *see* Neoplasm, connective tissue						
specified site NEC	195.8	198.89	234.8	229.8	238.8	239.8
spermatic cord	187.6	198.82	233.6	222.8	236.6	239.5
sphenoid	160.5	197.3	231.8	212.0	235.9	239.1
bone	170.0	198.5	—	213.0	238.0	239.2
sinus	160.5	197.3	231.8	212.0	235.9	239.1
sphincter						
anal	154.2	197.5	230.5	211.4	235.5	239.0
of Oddi	156.1	197.8	230.8	211.5	235.3	239.0
spine, spinal (column)	170.2	198.5	—	213.2	238.0	239.2
bulb	191.7	198.3	—	225.0	237.5	239.6
coccyx	170.6	198.5	—	213.6	238.0	239.2
cord (cervical) (lumbar) (sacral) (thoracic)	192.2	198.3	—	225.3	237.5	239.7
dura mater	192.3	198.4	—	225.4	237.6	239.7
lumbosacral	170.2	198.5	—	213.2	238.0	239.2
membrane	192.3	198.4	—	225.4	237.6	239.7
meninges	192.3	198.4	—	225.4	237.6	239.7
nerve (root)	171.9	198.89	—	215.9	238.1	239.2
pia mater	192.3	198.4	—	225.4	237.6	239.7
root	171.9	198.89	—	215.9	238.1	239.2
sacrum	170.6	198.5	—	213.6	238.0	239.2
spleen, splenic NEC	159.1	197.8	230.9	211.9	235.5	239.0
flexure (colon)	153.7	197.5	230.3	211.3	235.2	239.0
stem, brain	191.7	198.3	—	225.0	237.5	239.6
Stensen's duct	142.0	198.89	230.0	210.2	235.0	239.0
sternum	170.3	198.5	—	213.3	238.0	239.2
stomach	151.9	197.8	230.2	211.1	235.2	239.0
antrum (pyloric)	151.2	197.8	230.2	211.1	235.2	239.0
body	151.4	197.8	230.2	211.1	235.2	239.0
cardia	151.0	197.8	230.2	211.1	235.2	239.0
cardiac orifice	151.0	197.8	230.2	211.1	235.2	239.0
contiguous sites	151.8	—	—	—	—	—
corpus	151.4	197.8	230.2	211.1	235.2	239.0
fundus	151.3	197.8	230.2	211.1	235.2	239.0
greater curvature NEC	151.6	197.8	230.2	211.1	235.2	239.0
lesser curvature NEC	151.5	197.8	230.2	211.1	235.2	239.0
prepylorus	151.1	197.8	230.2	211.1	235.2	239.0
pylorus	151.1	197.8	230.2	211.1	235.2	239.0
wall NEC	151.9	197.8	230.2	211.1	235.2	239.0
anterior NEC	151.8	197.8	230.2	211.1	235.2	239.0
posterior NEC	151.8	197.8	230.2	211.1	235.2	239.0
stroma, endometrial	182.0	198.82	233.2	219.1	236.0	239.5
stump, cervical	180.8	198.82	233.1	219.0	236.0	239.5
subcutaneous (nodule) (tissue) NEC - *see* Neoplasm, connective tissue						
subdural	192.1	198.4	—	225.2	237.6	239.7
subglottis, subglottic	161.2	197.3	231.0	212.1	235.6	239.1

◀ New ⬅ Revised

	Malignant					
	Primary	Secondary	Ca in situ	Benign	Uncertain Behavior	Unspecified
Neoplasm *(Continued)*						
sublingual	144.9	198.89	230.0	210.3	235.1	239.0
gland or duct	142.2	198.89	230.0	210.2	235.0	239.0
submandibular gland	142.1	198.89	230.0	210.2	235.0	239.0
submaxillary gland or duct	142.1	198.89	230.0	210.2	235.0	239.0
submental	195.0	198.89	234.8	229.8	238.8	239.8
subpleural	162.9	197.0	—	212.3	235.7	239.1
substernal	164.2	197.1	—	212.5	235.8	239.8
sudoriferous, sudoriparous gland, site unspecified	173.9	198.2	232.9	216.9	238.2	239.2
specified site - *see* Neoplasm, skin						
supraclavicular region	195.0	198.89	234.8	229.8	238.8	239.8
supraglottis	161.1	197.3	231.0	212.1	235.6	239.1
suprarenal (capsule) (cortex) (gland) (medulla)	194.0	198.7	234.8	227.0	237.2	239.7
suprasellar (region)	191.9	198.3	—	225.0	237.5	239.6
sweat gland (apocrine) (eccrine), site unspecified	173.9	198.2	232.9	216.9	238.2	239.2
specified site - *see* Neoplasm, skin						
sympathetic nerve or nervous system NEC	171.9	198.89	—	215.9	238.1	239.2
symphysis pubis	170.6	198.5	—	213.6	238.0	239.2
synovial membrane - *see* Neoplasm, connective tissue						
tapetum, brain	191.8	198.3	—	225.0	237.5	239.6
tarsus (any bone)	170.8	198.5	—	213.8	238.0	239.2
temple (skin)	173.3	198.2	232.3	216.3	238.2	239.2
temporal						
bone	170.0	198.5	—	213.0	238.0	239.2
lobe or pole	191.2	198.3	—	225.0	237.5	239.6
region	195.0	198.89	234.8	229.8	238.8	239.8
skin	173.3	198.2	232.3	216.3	238.2	239.2
tendon (sheath) - *see* Neoplasm, connective tissue						
tentorium (cerebelli)	192.1	198.4	—	225.2	237.6	239.7
testis, testes (descended) (scrotal)	186.9	198.82	233.6	222.0	236.4	239.5
ectopic	186.0	198.82	233.6	222.0	236.4	239.5
retained	186.0	198.82	233.6	222.0	236.4	239.5
undescended	186.0	198.82	233.6	222.0	236.4	239.5
thalamus	191.0	198.3	—	225.0	237.5	239.6
thigh NEC*	195.5	198.89	234.8	229.8	238.8	239.8
thorax, thoracic (cavity) (organs NEC)	195.1	198.89	234.8	229.8	238.8	239.8
duct	171.4	198.89	—	215.4	238.1	239.2
wall NEC	195.1	198.89	234.8	229.8	238.8	239.8
throat	149.0	198.89	230.0	210.9	235.1	239.0
thumb NEC*	195.4	198.89	232.6	229.8	238.8	239.8
thymus (gland)	164.0	198.89	—	212.6	235.8	239.8
contiguous sites with heart and mediastinum	164.8	—	—	—	—	—
thyroglossal duct	193	198.89	234.8	226	237.4	239.7
thyroid (gland)	193	198.89	234.8	226	237.4	239.7
cartilage	161.3	197.3	231.0	212.1	235.6	239.1
tibia (any part)	170.7	198.5	—	213.7	238.0	239.2
toe NEC*	195.5	198.89	232.7	229.8	238.8	239.8
tongue	141.9	198.89	230.0	210.1	235.1	239.0
anterior (two-thirds) NEC	141.4	198.89	230.0	210.1	235.1	239.0
dorsal surface	141.1	198.89	230.0	210.1	235.1	239.0
ventral surface	141.3	198.89	230.0	210.1	235.1	239.0
base (dorsal surface)	141.0	198.89	230.0	210.1	235.1	239.0
border (lateral)	141.2	198.89	230.0	210.1	235.1	239.0
contiguous sites	141.8	—	—	—	—	—
dorsal surface NEC	141.1	198.89	230.0	210.1	235.1	239.0
fixed part NEC	141.0	198.89	230.0	210.1	235.1	239.0
foramen cecum	141.1	198.89	230.0	210.1	235.1	239.0
frenulum linguae	141.3	198.89	230.0	210.1	235.1	239.0
junctional zone	141.5	198.89	230.0	210.1	235.1	239.0
margin (lateral)	141.2	198.89	230.0	210.1	235.1	239.0
midline NEC	141.1	198.89	230.0	210.1	235.1	239.0
mobile part NEC	141.4	198.89	230.0	210.1	235.1	239.0
posterior (third)	141.0	198.89	230.0	210.1	235.1	239.0
root	141.0	198.89	230.0	210.1	235.1	239.0

	Malignant					
	Primary	**Secondary**	**Ca in situ**	**Benign**	**Uncertain Behavior**	**Unspecified**
Neoplasm *(Continued)*						
tongue *(Continued)*						
surface (dorsal)	141.1	198.89	230.0	210.1	235.1	239.0
base	141.0	198.89	230.0	210.1	235.1	239.0
ventral	141.3	198.89	230.0	210.1	235.1	239.0
tip	141.2	198.89	230.0	210.1	235.1	239.0
tonsil	141.6	198.89	230.0	210.1	235.1	239.0
tonsil	146.0	198.89	230.0	210.5	235.1	239.0
fauces, faucial	146.0	198.89	230.0	210.5	235.1	239.0
lingual	141.6	198.89	230.0	210.1	235.1	239.0
palatine	146.0	198.89	230.0	210.5	235.1	239.0
pharyngeal	147.1	198.89	230.0	210.7	235.1	239.0
pillar (anterior) (posterior)	146.2	198.89	230.0	210.6	235.1	239.0
tonsillar fossa	146.1	198.89	230.0	210.6	235.1	239.0
tooth socket NEC	143.9	198.89	230.0	210.4	235.1	239.0
trachea (cartilage) (mucosa)	162.0	197.3	231.1	212.2	235.7	239.1
contiguous sites with bronchus or lung	162.8	—	—	—	—	—
tracheobronchial	162.8	197.3	231.1	212.2	235.7	239.1
contiguous sites with lung	162.8	—	—	—	—	—
tragus	173.2	198.2	232.2	216.2	238.2	239.2
trunk NEC*	195.8	198.89	232.5	229.8	238.8	239.8
tubo-ovarian	183.8	198.82	233.3	221.8	236.3	239.5
tunica vaginalis	187.8	198.82	233.6	222.8	236.6	239.5
turbinate (bone)	170.0	198.5	—	213.0	238.0	239.2
nasal	160.0	197.3	231.8	212.0	235.9	239.1
tympanic cavity	160.1	197.3	231.8	212.0	235.9	239.1
ulna (any part)	170.4	198.5	—	213.4	238.0	239.2
umbilicus, umbilical	173.5	198.2	232.5	216.5	238.2	239.2
uncus, brain	191.2	198.3	—	225.0	237.5	239.6
unknown site or unspecified	199.1	199.1	234.9	229.9	238.9	239.9
urachus	188.7	198.1	233.7	223.3	236.7	239.4
ureter, ureteral	189.2	198.1	233.9	223.2	236.91	239.5
orifice (bladder)	188.6	198.1	233.7	223.3	236.7	239.4
ureter-bladder (junction)	188.6	198.1	233.7	223.3	236.7	239.4
urethra, urethral (gland)	189.3	198.1	233.9	223.81	236.99	239.5
orifice, internal	188.5	198.1	233.7	223.3	236.7	239.4
urethrovaginal (septum)	184.9	198.82	233.3	221.9	236.3	239.5
urinary organ or system NEC	189.9	198.1	233.9	223.9	236.99	239.5
bladder - *see* Neoplasm, bladder						
contiguous sites	189.8	—	—	—	—	—
specified sites NEC	189.8	198.1	233.9	223.89	236.99	239.5
utero-ovarian	183.8	198.82	233.3	221.8	236.3	239.5
ligament	183.3	198.82	—	221.0	236.3	239.5
uterosacral ligament	183.4	198.82	—	221.0	236.3	239.5
uterus, uteri, uterine	179	198.82	233.2	219.9	236.0	239.5
adnexa NEC	183.9	198.82	233.3	221.8	236.3	239.5
contiguous sites	183.8	—	—	—	—	—
body	182.0	198.82	233.2	219.1	236.0	239.5
contiguous sites	182.8	—	—	—	—	—
cervix	180.9	198.82	233.1	219.0	236.0	239.5
cornu	182.0	198.82	233.2	219.1	236.0	239.5
corpus	182.0	198.82	233.2	219.1	236.0	239.5
endocervix (canal) (gland)	180.0	198.82	233.1	219.0	236.0	239.5
endometrium	182.0	198.82	233.2	219.1	236.0	239.5
exocervix	180.1	198.82	233.1	219.0	236.0	239.5
external os	180.1	198.82	233.1	219.0	236.0	239.5
fundus	182.0	198.82	233.2	219.1	236.0	239.5
internal os	180.0	198.82	233.1	219.0	236.0	239.5
isthmus	182.1	198.82	233.2	219.1	236.0	239.5
ligament	183.4	198.82	—	221.0	236.3	239.5
broad	183.3	198.82	233.3	221.0	236.3	239.5
round	183.5	198.82	—	221.0	236.3	239.5
lower segment	182.1	198.82	233.2	219.1	236.0	239.5
myometrium	182.0	198.82	233.2	219.1	236.0	239.5

	Malignant					
	Primary	Secondary	Ca in situ	Benign	Uncertain Behavior	Unspecified
Neoplasm *(Continued)*						
uterus, uteri, uterine *(Continued)*						
squamocolumnar junction	180.8	198.82	233.1	219.0	236.0	239.5
tube	183.2	198.82	233.3	221.0	236.3	239.5
utricle, prostatic	189.3	198.1	233.9	223.81	236.99	239.5
uveal tract	190.0	198.4	234.0	224.0	238.8	239.8
uvula	145.4	198.89	230.0	210.4	235.1	239.0
vagina, vaginal (fornix) (vault) (wall)	184.0	198.82	233.3	221.1	236.3	239.5
vaginovesical	184.9	198.82	233.3	221.9	236.3	239.5
septum	194.9	198.82	233.3	221.9	236.3	239.5
vallecula (epiglottis)	146.3	198.89	230.0	210.6	235.1	239.0
vascular - *see* Neoplasm, connective tissue						
vas deferens	187.6	198.82	233.6	222.8	236.6	239.5
Vater's ampulla	156.2	197.8	230.8	211.5	235.3	239.0
vein, venous - *see* Neoplasm, connective tissue						
vena cava (abdominal) (inferior)	171.5	198.89	—	215.5	238.1	239.2
superior	171.4	198.89	—	215.4	238.1	239.2
ventricle (cerebral) (floor) (fourth) (lateral) (third)	191.5	198.3	—	225.0	237.5	239.6
cardiac (left) (right)	164.1	198.89	—	212.7	238.8	239.8
ventricular band of larynx	161.1	197.3	231.0	212.1	235.6	239.1
ventriculus - *see* Neoplasm, stomach						
vermillion border - *see* Neoplasm, lip						
vermis, cerebellum	191.6	198.3	—	225.0	237.5	239.6
vertebra (column)	170.2	198.5	—	213.2	238.0	239.2
coccyx	170.6	198.5	—	213.6	238.0	239.2
sacrum	170.6	198.5	—	213.6	238.0	239.2
vesical - *see* Neoplasm, bladder						
vesicle, seminal	187.8	198.82	233.6	222.8	236.6	239.5
vesicocervical tissue	184.9	198.82	233.3	221.9	236.3	239.5
vesicorectal	195.3	198.89	234.8	229.8	238.8	239.8
vesicovaginal	184.9	198.82	233.3	221.9	236.3	239.5
septum	184.9	198.82	233.3	221.9	236.3	239.5
vessel (blood) - *see* Neoplasm, connective tissue						
vestibular gland, greater	184.1	198.82	233.3	221.2	236.3	239.5
vestibule						
mouth	145.1	198.89	230.0	210.4	235.1	239.0
nose	160.0	197.3	231.8	212.0	235.9	239.1
Virchow's gland	—	196.0	—	229.0	238.8	239.8
viscera NEC	195.8	198.89	234.8	229.8	238.8	239.8
vocal cords (true)	161.0	197.3	231.0	212.1	235.6	239.1
false	161.1	197.3	231.0	212.1	235.6	239.1
vomer	170.0	198.5	—	213.0	238.0	239.2
vulva	184.4	198.82	233.3	221.2	236.3	239.5
vulvovaginal gland	184.4	198.82	233.3	221.2	236.3	239.5
Waldeyer's ring	149.1	198.89	230.0	210.9	235.1	239.0
Wharton's duct	142.1	198.89	230.0	210.2	235.0	239.0
white matter (central) (cerebral)	191.0	198.3	—	225.0	237.5	239.6
windpipe	162.0	197.3	231.1	212.2	235.7	239.1
Wirsung's duct	157.3	197.8	230.9	211.6	235.5	239.0
wolffian (body) (duct)						
female	184.8	198.82	233.3	221.8	236.3	239.5
male	187.8	198.82	233.6	222.8	236.6	239.5
womb - *see* Neoplasm, uterus						
wrist NEC*	195.4	198.89	232.6	229.8	238.8	239.8
xiphoid process	170.3	198.5	—	213.3	238.0	239.2
Zuckerkandl's organ	194.6	198.89	—	227.6	237.3	239.7

- **Neovascularization**
  - choroid 362.16
  - ciliary body 364.42
  - cornea 370.60
    - deep 370.63
    - localized 370.61
  - iris 364.42
  - retina 362.16
  - subretinal 362.16
- **Nephralgia** 788.0
- **Nephritis, nephritic** (albuminuric) (azotemic) (congenital) (degenerative) (diffuse) (disseminated) (epithelial) (familial) (focal) (granulomatous) (hemorrhagic) (infantile) (non-suppurative, excretory) (uremic) 583.9
  - with
    - edema - *see* Nephrosis
    - lesion of
      - glomerulonephritis
        - hypocomplementemic persistent 583.2
          - with nephrotic syndrome 581.2
          - chronic 582.2
        - lobular 583.2
          - with nephrotic syndrome 581.2
          - chronic 582.2
        - membranoproliferative 583.2
          - with nephrotic syndrome 581.2
          - chronic 582.2
        - membranous 583.1
          - with nephrotic syndrome 581.1
          - chronic 582.1
        - mesangiocapillary 583.2
          - with nephrotic syndrome 581.2
          - chronic 582.2
        - mixed membranous and proliferative 583.2
          - with nephrotic syndrome 581.2
          - chronic 582.2
        - proliferative (diffuse) 583.0
          - with nephrotic syndrome 581.0
          - acute 580.0
          - chronic 582.0
        - rapidly progressive 583.4
          - acute 580.4
          - chronic 582.4
      - interstitial nephritis (diffuse) (focal) 583.89
        - with nephrotic syndrome 581.89
        - acute 580.89
        - chronic 582.89
      - necrotizing glomerulitis 583.4
        - acute 580.4
        - chronic 582.4
      - renal necrosis 583.9
        - cortical 583.6
        - medullary 583.7
      - specified pathology NEC 583.89
        - with nephrotic syndrome 581.89
        - acute 580.89
        - chronic 582.89
    - necrosis, renal 583.9
      - cortical 583.6
      - medullary (papillary) 583.7
    - nephrotic syndrome (*see also* Nephrosis) 581.9
    - papillary necrosis 583.7
    - specified pathology NEC 583.89
  - acute 580.9
    - extracapillary with epithelial crescents 580.4
    - hypertensive (*see also* Hypertension, kidney) 403.90

- **Nephritis, nephritic** *(Continued)*
  - acute *(Continued)*
    - necrotizing 580.4
    - poststreptococcal 580.0
    - proliferative (diffuse) 580.0
    - rapidly progressive 580.4
    - specified pathology NEC 580.89
  - amyloid 277.39 *[583.81]*
    - chronic 277.39 *[582.81]*
  - arteriolar (*see also* Hypertension, kidney) 403.90
  - arteriosclerotic (*see also* Hypertension, kidney) 403.90
  - ascending (*see also* Pyelitis) 590.80
  - atrophic 582.9
  - basement membrane NEC 583.89
    - with pulmonary hemorrhage (Goodpasture's syndrome) 446.21 *[583.81]*
  - calculous, calculus 592.0
  - cardiac (*see also* Hypertension, kidney) 403.90
  - cardiovascular (*see also* Hypertension, kidney) 403.90
  - chronic 582.9
    - arteriosclerotic (*see also* Hypertension, kidney) 403.90
    - hypertensive (*see also* Hypertension, kidney) 403.90
  - cirrhotic (*see also* Sclerosis, renal) 587
  - complicating pregnancy, childbirth, or puerperium 646.2
    - with hypertension 642.1
      - affecting fetus or newborn 760.0
    - affecting fetus or newborn 760.1
  - croupous 580.9
  - desquamative - *see* Nephrosis
  - due to
    - amyloidosis 277.39 *[583.81]*
      - chronic 277.39 *[582.81]*
    - arteriosclerosis (*see also* Hypertension, kidney) 403.90
    - diabetes mellitus 250.4 *[583.81]*
      - with nephrotic syndrome 250.4 *[581.81]*
    - diphtheria 032.89 *[580.81]*
    - gonococcal infection (acute) 098.19 *[583.81]*
      - chronic or duration of 2 months or over 098.39 *[583.81]*
    - gout 274.10
    - infectious hepatitis 070.9 *[580.81]*
    - mumps 072.79 *[580.81]*
    - specified kidney pathology NEC 583.89
      - acute 580.89
      - chronic 582.89
    - streptotrichosis 039.8 *[583.81]*
    - subacute bacterial endocarditis 421.0 *[580.81]*
    - systemic lupus erythematosus 710.0 *[583.81]*
      - chronic 710.0 *[582.81]*
    - typhoid fever 002.0 *[580.81]*
  - endothelial 582.2
  - end state (chronic) (terminal) NEC 585.6
  - epimembranous 581.1
  - exudative 583.89
    - with nephrotic syndrome 581.89
    - acute 580.89
    - chronic 582.89
  - gonococcal (acute) 098.19 *[583.81]*
    - chronic or duration of 2 months or over 098.39 *[583.81]*

- **Nephritis, nephritic** *(Continued)*
  - gouty 274.10
  - hereditary (Alport's syndrome) 759.89
  - hydremic - *see* Nephrosis
  - hypertensive (*see also* Hypertension, kidney) 403.90
  - hypocomplementemic persistent 583.2
    - with nephrotic syndrome 581.2
    - chronic 582.2
  - immune complex NEC 583.89
  - infective (*see also* Pyelitis) 590.80
  - interstitial (diffuse) (focal) 583.89
    - with nephrotic syndrome 581.89
    - acute 580.89
    - chronic 582.89
  - latent or quiescent - *see* Nephritis, chronic
  - lead 984.9
    - specified type of lead - *see* Table of Drugs and Chemicals
  - lobular 583.2
    - with nephrotic syndrome 581.2
    - chronic 582.2
  - lupus 710.0 *[583.81]*
    - acute 710.0 *[580.81]*
    - chronic 710.0 *[582.81]*
  - membranoproliferative 583.2
    - with nephrotic syndrome 581.2
    - chronic 582.2
  - membranous 583.1
    - with nephrotic syndrome 581.1
    - chronic 582.1
  - mesangiocapillary 583.2
    - with nephrotic syndrome 581.2
    - chronic 582.2
  - minimal change 581.3
  - mixed membranous and proliferative 583.2
    - with nephrotic syndrome 581.2
    - chronic 582.2
  - necrotic, necrotizing 583.4
    - acute 580.4
    - chronic 582.4
  - nephrotic - *see* Nephrosis
  - old - *see* Nephritis, chronic
  - parenchymatous 581.89
  - polycystic 753.12
    - adult type (APKD) 753.13
    - autosomal dominant 753.13
    - autosomal recessive 753.14
    - childhood type (CPKD) 753.14
    - infantile type 753.14
  - poststreptococcal 580.0
  - pregnancy - *see* Nephritis, complicating pregnancy
  - proliferative 583.0
    - with nephrotic syndrome 581.0
    - acute 580.0
    - chronic 582.0
  - purulent (*see also* Pyelitis) 590.80
  - rapidly progressive 583.4
    - acute 580.4
    - chronic 582.4
  - salt-losing or salt-wasting (*see also* Disease, renal) 593.9
  - saturnine 584.9
    - specified type of lead - *see* Table of Drugs and Chemicals
  - septic (*see also* Pyelitis) 590.80
  - specified pathology NEC 583.89
    - acute 580.89
    - chronic 582.89
  - staphylococcal (*see also* Pyelitis) 590.80
  - streptotrichosis 039.8 *[583.81]*

Nephritis, nephritic *(Continued)*
  subacute (*see also* Nephrosis) 581.9
  suppurative (*see also* Pyelitis) 590.80
  syphilitic (late) 095.4
    congenital 090.5 *[583.81]*
    early 091.69 *[583.81]*
  terminal (chronic) (end-stage) NEC 585.6
  toxic - *see* Nephritis, acute
  tubal, tubular - *see* Nephrosis, tubular
  tuberculous (*see also* Tuberculosis) 016.0 *[583.81]*
  type II (Ellis) - *see* Nephrosis
  vascular - *see also* Hypertension, kidney
  war 580.9
Nephroblastoma (M8960/3) 189.0
  epithelial (M8961/3) 189.0
  mesenchymal (M8962/3) 189.0
Nephrocalcinosis 275.49
Nephrocystitis, pustular (*see also* Pyelitis) 590.80
Nephrolithiasis (congenital) (pelvis) (recurrent) 592.0
  uric acid 274.11
Nephroma (M8960/3) 189.0
  mesoblastic (M8960/1) 236.9
Nephronephritis (*see also* Nephrosis) 581.9
Nephronopthisis 753.16
Nephropathy (*see also* Nephritis) 583.9
  with
    exudative nephritis 583.89
    interstitial nephritis (diffuse) (focal) 583.89
    medullary necrosis 583.7
    necrosis 583.9
      cortical 583.6
      medullary or papillary 583.7
    papillary necrosis 583.7
    specified lesion or cause NEC 583.89
  analgesic 583.89
    with medullary necrosis, acute 584.7
  arteriolar (*see also* Hypertension, kidney) 403.90
  arteriosclerotic (*see also* Hypertension, kidney) 403.90
  complicating pregnancy 646.2
  diabetic 250.4 *[583.81]*
  gouty 274.10
    specified type NEC 274.19
  hereditary amyloid 277.31 ◀
  hypercalcemic 588.89
  hypertensive (*see also* Hypertension, kidney) 403.90
  hypokalemic (vacuolar) 588.89
  IgA 583.9
  obstructive 593.89
    congenital 753.20
  phenacetin 584.7
  phosphate-losing 588.0
  potassium depletion 588.89
  proliferative (*see also* Nephritis, proliferative) 583.0
  protein-losing 588.89
  salt-losing or salt-wasting (*see also* Disease, renal) 593.9
  sickle-cell (*see also* Disease, sickle-cell) 282.60 *[583.81]*
  toxic 584.5
  vasomotor 584.5
  water-losing 588.89
Nephroptosis (*see also* Disease, renal) 593.0
  congenital (displaced) 753.3
Nephropyosis (*see also* Abscess, kidney) 590.2
Nephrorrhagia 593.81
Nephrosclerosis (arteriolar) (arteriosclerotic) (chronic) (hyaline) (*see also* Hypertension, kidney) 403.90
  gouty 274.10
  hyperplastic (arteriolar) (*see also* Hypertension, kidney) 403.90
  senile (*see also* Sclerosis, renal) 587
Nephrosis, nephrotic (Epstein's) (syndrome) 581.9
  with
    lesion of
      focal glomerulosclerosis 581.1
      glomerulonephritis
        endothelial 581.2
        hypocomplementemic persistent 581.2
        lobular 581.2
        membranoproliferative 581.2
        membranous 581.1
        mesangiocapillary 581.2
        minimal change 581.3
        mixed membranous and proliferative 581.2
        proliferative 581.0
      segmental hyalinosis 581.1
      specified pathology NEC 581.89
  acute - *see* Nephrosis, tubular
  anoxic - *see* Nephrosis, tubular
  arteriosclerotic (*see also* Hypertension, kidney) 403.90
  chemical - *see* Nephrosis, tubular
  cholemic 572.4
  complicating pregnancy, childbirth, or puerperium - *see* Nephritis, complicating pregnancy
  diabetic 250.4 *[581.81]*
  hemoglobinuric - *see* Nephrosis, tubular
  in
    amyloidosis 277.39 *[581.81]* ⟸
    diabetes mellitus 250.4 *[581.81]*
    epidemic hemorrhagic fever 078.6
    malaria 084.9 *[581.81]*
    polyarteritis 446.0 *[581.81]*
    systemic lupus erythematosus 710.0 *[581.81]*
  ischemic - *see* Nephrosis, tubular
  lipoid 581.3
  lower nephron - *see* Nephrosis, tubular
  lupoid 710.0 *[581.81]*
  lupus 710.0 *[581.81]*
  malarial 084.9 *[581.81]*
  minimal change 581.3
  necrotizing - *see* Nephrosis, tubular
  osmotic (sucrose) 588.89
  polyarteritic 446.0 *[581.81]*
  radiation 581.9
  specified lesion or cause NEC 581.89
  syphilitic 095.4
  toxic - *see* Nephrosis, tubular
  tubular (acute) 584.5
    due to a procedure 997.5
    radiation 581.9
Nephrosonephritis hemorrhagic (endemic) 078.6
Nephrostomy status V44.6
  with complication 997.5
Nerve - *see* condition
Nerves 799.2
Nervous (*see also* condition) 799.2
  breakdown 300.9
  heart 306.2
  stomach 306.4
  tension 799.2
Nervousness 799.2
Nesidioblastoma (M8150/0)
  pancreas 211.7
  specified site NEC - *see* Neoplasm, by site, benign
  unspecified site 211.7
Netherton's syndrome (ichthyosiform erythroderma) 757.1
Nettle rash 708.8
Nettleship's disease (urticaria pigmentosa) 757.33
Neumann's disease (pemphigus vegetans) 694.4
Neuralgia, neuralgic (acute) (*see also* Neuritis) 729.2
  accessory (nerve) 352.4
  acoustic (nerve) 388.5
  ankle 355.8
  anterior crural 355.8
  anus 787.99
  arm 723.4
  auditory (nerve) 388.5
  axilla 353.0
  bladder 788.1
  brachial 723.4
  brain - *see* Disorder, nerve, cranial
  broad ligament 625.9
  cerebral - *see* Disorder, nerve, cranial
  ciliary 346.2
  cranial nerve - *see also* Disorder, nerve, cranial
    fifth or trigeminal (*see also* Neuralgia, trigeminal) 350.1
  ear 388.71
    middle 352.1
  facial 351.8
  finger 354.9
  flank 355.8
  foot 355.8
  forearm 354.9
  Fothergill's (*see also* Neuralgia, trigeminal) 350.1
    postherpetic 053.12
  glossopharyngeal (nerve) 352.1
  groin 355.8
  hand 354.9
  heel 355.8
  Horton's 346.2
  Hunt's 053.11
  hypoglossal (nerve) 352.5
  iliac region 355.8
  infraorbital (*see also* Neuralgia, trigeminal) 350.1
  inguinal 355.8
  intercostal (nerve) 353.8
    postherpetic 053.19
  jaw 352.1
  kidney 788.0
  knee 355.8
  loin 355.8
  malarial (*see also* Malaria) 084.6
  mastoid 385.89
  maxilla 352.1
  median thenar 354.1
  metatarsal 355.6
  middle ear 352.1
  migrainous 346.2
  Morton's 355.6
  nerve, cranial - *see* Disorder, nerve, cranial
  nose 352.0
  occipital 723.8
  olfactory (nerve) 352.0
  ophthalmic 377.30
    postherpetic 053.19

Neuralgia, neuralgic *(Continued)*
  optic (nerve) 377.30
  penis 607.9
  perineum 355.8
  pleura 511.0
  postherpetic NEC 053.19
    geniculate ganglion 053.11
    ophthalmic 053.19
    trifacial 053.12
    trigeminal 053.12
  pubic region 355.8
  radial (nerve) 723.4
  rectum 787.99
  sacroiliac joint 724.3
  sciatic (nerve) 724.3
  scrotum 608.9
  seminal vesicle 608.9
  shoulder 354.9
  sluder's 337.0
  specified nerve NEC - *see* Disorder, nerve
  spermatic cord 608.9
  sphenopalatine (ganglion) 337.0
  subscapular (nerve) 723.4
  suprascapular (nerve) 723.4
  testis 608.89
  thenar (median) 354.1
  thigh 355.8
  tongue 352.5
  trifacial (nerve) (*see also* Neuralgia, trigeminal) 350.1
  trigeminal (nerve) 350.1
    postherpetic 053.12
  tympanic plexus 388.71
  ulnar (nerve) 723.4
  vagus (nerve) 352.3
  wrist 354.9
  writers' 300.89
    organic 333.84
Neurapraxia - *see* Injury, nerve, by site
Neurasthenia 300.5
  cardiac 306.2
  gastric 306.4
  heart 306.2
  postfebrile 780.79
  postviral 780.79
Neurilemmoma (M9560/0) - *see also* Neoplasm, connective tissue, benign
  acoustic (nerve) 225.1
  malignant (M9560/3) - *see also* Neoplasm, connective tissue, malignant
    acoustic (nerve) 192.0
Neurilemmosarcoma (M9560/3) - *see* Neoplasm, connective tissue, malignant
Neurilemoma - *see* Neurilemmoma
Neurinoma (M9560/0) - *see* Neurilemmoma
Neurinomatosis (M9560/1) - *see also* Neoplasm, connective tissue, uncertain behavior
  centralis 759.5
Neuritis (*see also* Neuralgia) 729.2
  abducens (nerve) 378.54
  accessory (nerve) 352.4
  acoustic (nerve) 388.5
    syphilitic 094.86
  alcoholic 357.5
    with psychosis 291.1
  amyloid, any site 277.39 *[357.4]* (Revised)
  anterior crural 355.8
  arising during pregnancy 646.4
  arm 723.4
  ascending 355.2
  auditory (nerve) 388.5

Neuritis *(Continued)*
  brachial (nerve) NEC 723.4
    due to displacement, intervertebral disc 722.0
  cervical 723.4
  chest (wall) 353.8
  costal region 353.8
  cranial nerve - *see also* Disorder, nerve, cranial
    first or olfactory 352.0
    second or optic 377.30
    third or oculomotor 378.52
    fourth or trochlear 378.53
    fifth or trigeminal (*see also* Neuralgia, trigeminal) 350.1
    sixth or abducens 378.54
    seventh or facial 351.8
      newborn 767.5
    eighth or acoustic 388.5
    ninth or glossopharyngeal 352.1
    tenth or vagus 352.3
    eleventh or accessory 352.4
    twelfth or hypoglossal 352.5
  Déjérine-Sottas 356.0
  diabetic 250.6 *[357.2]*
  diphtheritic 032.89 *[357.4]*
  due to
    beriberi 265.0 *[357.4]*
    displacement, prolapse, protrusion, or rupture of intervertebral disc 722.2
      cervical 722.0
      lumbar, lumbosacral 722.10
      thoracic, thoracolumbar 722.11
    herniation, nucleus pulposus 722.2
      cervical 722.0
      lumbar, lumbosacral 722.10
      thoracic, thoracolumbar 722.11
  endemic 265.0 *[357.4]*
  facial (nerve) 351.8
    newborn 767.5
  general - *see* Polyneuropathy
  geniculate ganglion 351.1
    due to herpes 053.11
  glossopharyngeal (nerve) 352.1
  gouty 274.89 *[357.4]*
  hypoglossal (nerve) 352.5
  ilioinguinal (nerve) 355.8
  in diseases classified elsewhere - *see* Polyneuropathy, in
  infectious (multiple) 357.0
  intercostal (nerve) 353.8
  interstitial hypertrophic progressive NEC 356.9
  leg 355.8
  lumbosacral NEC 724.4
  median (nerve) 354.1
    thenar 354.1
  multiple (acute) (infective) 356.9
    endemic 265.0 *[357.4]*
  multiplex endemica 265.0 *[357.4]*
  nerve root (*see also* Radiculitis) 729.2
  oculomotor (nerve) 378.52
  olfactory (nerve) 352.0
  optic (nerve) 377.30
    in myelitis 341.0
    meningococcal 036.81
  pelvic 355.8
  peripheral (nerve) - *see also* Neuropathy, peripheral
    complicating pregnancy or puerperium 646.4
    specified nerve NEC - *see* Mononeuritis

Neuritis *(Continued)*
  pneumogastric (nerve) 352.3
  postchickenpox 052.7
  postherpetic 053.19
  progressive hypertrophic interstitial NEC 356.9
  puerperal, postpartum 646.4
  radial (nerve) 723.4
  retrobulbar 377.32
    syphilitic 094.85
  rheumatic (chronic) 729.2
  sacral region 355.8
  sciatic (nerve) 724.3
    due to displacement of intervertebral disc 722.10
  serum 999.5
  specified nerve NEC - *see* Disorder, nerve
  spinal (nerve) 355.9
    root (*see also* Radiculitis) 729.2
  subscapular (nerve) 723.4
  suprascapular (nerve) 723.4
  syphilitic 095.8
  thenar (median) 354.1
  thoracic NEC 724.4
  toxic NEC 357.7
  trochlear (nerve) 378.53
  ulnar (nerve) 723.4
  vagus (nerve) 352.3
Neuroangiomatosis, encephalofacial 759.6
Neuroastrocytoma (M9505/1) - *see* Neoplasm, by site, uncertain behavior
Neuro-avitaminosis 269.2
Neuroblastoma (M9500/3)
  olfactory (M9522/3) 160.0
  specified site - *see* Neoplasm, by site, malignant
  unspecified site 194.0
Neurochorioretinitis (*see also* Chorioretinitis) 363.20
Neurocirculatory asthenia 306.2
Neurocytoma (M9506/0) - *see* Neoplasm, by site, benign
Neurodermatitis (circumscribed) (circumscripta) (local) 698.3
  atopic 691.8
  diffuse (Brocq) 691.8
  disseminated 691.8
  nodulosa 698.3
Neuroencephalomyelopathy, optic 341.0
Neuroepithelioma (M9503/3) - *see also* Neoplasm, by site, malignant
  olfactory (M9521/3) 160.0
Neurofibroma (M9540/0) - *see also* Neoplasm, connective tissue, benign
  melanotic (M9541/0) - *see* Neoplasm, connective tissue, benign
  multiple (M9540/1) 237.70
    type 1 237.71
    type 2 237.72
  plexiform (M9550/0) - *see* Neoplasm, connective tissue, benign
Neurofibromatosis (multiple) (M9540/1) 237.70
  acoustic 237.72
  malignant (M9540/3) - *see* Neoplasm, connective tissue, malignant
  type 1 237.71
  type 2 237.72
  von Recklinghausen's 237.71
Neurofibrosarcoma (M9540/3) - *see* Neoplasm, connective tissue, malignant

- **Neurogenic** - *see also* condition
  - bladder (atonic) (automatic) (autonomic) (flaccid) (hypertonic) (hypotonic) (inertia) (infranuclear) (irritable) (motor) (nonreflex) (nuclear) (paralysis) (reflex) (sensory) (spastic) (supranuclear) (uninhibited) 596.54
    - with cauda equina syndrome 344.61
  - bowel 564.81
  - heart 306.2
- **Neuroglioma** (M9505/1) - *see* Neoplasm, by site, uncertain behavior
- **Neurolabyrinthitis** (of Dix and Hallpike) 386.12
- **Neurolathyrism** 988.2
- **Neuroleprosy** 030.1
- **Neuroleptic malignant syndrome** 333.92
- **Neurolipomatosis** 272.8
- **Neuroma** (M9570/0) - *see also* Neoplasm, connective tissue, benign
  - acoustic (nerve) (M9560/0) 225.1
  - amputation (traumatic) - *see also* Injury, nerve, by site
    - surgical complication (late) 997.61
  - appendix 211.3
  - auditory nerve 225.1
  - digital 355.6
    - toe 355.6
  - interdigital (toe) 355.6
  - intermetatarsal 355.6
  - Morton's 355.6
  - multiple 237.70
    - type 1 237.71
    - type 2 237.72
  - nonneoplastic 355.9
    - arm NEC 354.9
    - leg NEC 355.8
    - lower extremity NEC 355.8
    - specified site NEC - *see* Mononeuritis, by site
    - upper extremity NEC 354.9
  - optic (nerve) 225.1
  - plantar 355.6
  - plexiform (M9550/0) - *see* Neoplasm, connective tissue, benign
  - surgical (nonneoplastic) 355.9
    - arm NEC 354.9
    - leg NEC 355.8
    - lower extremity NEC 355.8
    - upper extremity NEC 354.9
  - traumatic - *see also* Injury, nerve, by site
    - old - *see* Neuroma, nonneoplastic
- **Neuromyalgia** 729.1
- **Neuromyasthenia** (epidemic) 049.8
- **Neuromyelitis** 341.8
  - ascending 357.0
  - optica 341.0
- **Neuromyopathy NEC** 358.9
- **Neuromyositis** 729.1
- **Neuronevus** (M8725/0) - *see* Neoplasm, skin, benign
- **Neuronitis** 357.0
  - ascending (acute) 355.2
  - vestibular 386.12
- **Neuroparalytic** - *see* condition
- **Neuropathy, neuropathic** (*see also* Disorder, nerve) 355.9
  - acute motor 357.82
  - alcoholic 357.5
    - with psychosis 291.1
  - arm NEC 354.9
  - ataxia and retinitis pigmentosa (NARP syndrome) 277.87

Neuropathy, neuropathic *(Continued)*

  - autonomic (peripheral) - *see* Neuropathy, peripheral, autonomic
  - axillary nerve 353.0
  - brachial plexus 353.0
  - cervical plexus 353.2
  - chronic
    - progressive segmentally demyelinating 357.89
    - relapsing demyelinating 357.89
  - congenital sensory 356.2
  - Déjérine-Sottas 356.0
  - diabetic 250.6 *[357.2]*
  - entrapment 355.9
    - iliohypogastric nerve 355.79
    - ilioinguinal nerve 355.79
    - lateral cutaneous nerve of thigh 355.1
    - median nerve 354.0
    - obturator nerve 355.79
    - peroneal nerve 355.3
    - posterior tibial nerve 355.5
    - saphenous nerve 355.79
    - ulnar nerve 354.2
  - facial nerve 351.9
  - hereditary 356.9
    - peripheral 356.0
    - sensory (radicular) 356.2
  - hypertrophic
    - Charcôt-Marie-Tooth 356.1
    - Déjérine-Sottas 356.0
    - interstitial 356.9
    - Refsum 356.3
  - intercostal nerve 354.8
  - ischemic - *see* Disorder, nerve
  - Jamaican (ginger) 357.7
  - leg NEC 355.8
  - lower extremity NEC 355.8
  - lumbar plexus 353.1
  - median nerve 354.1
  - motor
    - acute 357.82
  - multiple (acute) (chronic) (*see also* Polyneuropathy) 356.9
  - optic 377.39
    - ischemic 377.41
    - nutritional 377.33
    - toxic 377.34
  - peripheral (nerve) (*see also* Polyneuropathy) 356.9
    - arm NEC 354.9
    - autonomic 337.9
      - amyloid 277.39 *[337.1]*
      - idiopathic 337.0
      - in
        - amyloidosis 277.39 *[337.1]*
        - diabetes (mellitus) 250.6 *[337.1]*
        - diseases classified elsewhere 337.1
        - gout 274.89 *[337.1]*
        - hyperthyroidism 242.9 *[337.1]*
    - due to
      - antitetanus serum 357.6
      - arsenic 357.7
      - drugs 357.6
      - lead 357.7
      - organophosphate compounds 357.7
      - toxic agent NEC 357.7
    - hereditary 356.0
    - idiopathic 356.9
      - progressive 356.4
      - specified type NEC 356.8
    - in diseases classified elsewhere - *see* Polyneuropathy, in
    - leg NEC 355.8

Neuropathy, neuropathic *(Continued)*

  - peripheral *(Continued)*
    - lower extremity NEC 355.8
    - upper extremity NEC 354.9
  - plantar nerves 355.6
  - progressive hypertrophic interstitial 356.9
  - radicular NEC 729.2
    - brachial 723.4
    - cervical NEC 723.4
    - hereditary sensory 356.2
    - lumbar 724.4
    - lumbosacral 724.4
    - thoracic NEC 724.4
  - sacral plexus 353.1
  - sciatic 355.0
  - spinal nerve NEC 355.9
    - root (*see also* Radiculitis) 729.2
  - toxic 357.7
  - trigeminal sensory 350.8
  - ulnar nerve 354.2
  - upper extremity NEC 354.9
  - uremic 585.9 *[357.4]*
  - vitamin B_{12} 266.2 *[357.4]*
    - with anemia (pernicious) 281.0 *[357.4]*
      - due to dietary deficiency 281.1 *[357.4]*
- **Neurophthisis** - *see also* Disorder, nerve
  - peripheral 356.9
  - diabetic 250.6 *[357.2]*
- **Neuropraxia** - *see* Injury, nerve
- **Neuroretinitis** 363.05
  - syphilitic 094.85
- **Neurosarcoma** (M9540/3) - *see* Neoplasm, connective tissue, malignant
- **Neurosclerosis** - *see* Disorder, nerve
- **Neurosis, neurotic** 300.9
  - accident 300.16
  - anancastic, anankastic 300.3
  - anxiety (state) 300.00
    - generalized 300.02
    - panic type 300.01
  - asthenic 300.5
  - bladder 306.53
  - cardiac (reflex) 306.2
  - cardiovascular 306.2
  - climacteric, unspecified type 627.2
  - colon 306.4
  - compensation 300.16
  - compulsive, compulsion 300.3
  - conversion 300.11
  - craft 300.89
  - cutaneous 306.3
  - depersonalization 300.6
  - depressive (reaction) (type) 300.4
  - endocrine 306.6
  - environmental 300.89
  - fatigue 300.5
  - functional (*see also* Disorder, psychosomatic) 306.9
  - gastric 306.4
  - gastrointestinal 306.4
  - genitourinary 306.50
  - heart 306.2
  - hypochondriacal 300.7
  - hysterical 300.10
    - conversion type 300.11
    - dissociative type 300.15
  - impulsive 300.3
  - incoordination 306.0
    - larynx 306.1
    - vocal cord 306.1
  - intestine 306.4

Neurosis, neurotic *(Continued)*
  larynx 306.1
    hysterical 300.11
    sensory 306.1
  menopause, unspecified type 627.2
  mixed NEC 300.89
  musculoskeletal 306.0
  obsessional 300.3
    phobia 300.3
  obsessive-compulsive 300.3
  occupational 300.89
  ocular 306.7
  oral 307.0
  organ (*see also* Disorder, psychosomatic) 306.9
  pharynx 306.1
  phobic 300.20
  posttraumatic (acute) (situational) 309.81
    chronic 309.81
  psychasthenic (type) 300.89
  railroad 300.16
  rectum 306.4
  respiratory 306.1
  rumination 306.4
  senile 300.89
  sexual 302.70
  situational 300.89
  specified type NEC 300.89
  state 300.9
    with depersonalization episode 300.6
  stomach 306.4
  vasomotor 306.2
  visceral 306.4
  war 300.16
Neurospongioblastosis diffusa 759.5
Neurosyphilis (arrested) (early) (inactive) (late) (latent) (recurrent) 094.9
  with ataxia (cerebellar) (locomotor) (spastic) (spinal) 094.0
  acute meningitis 094.2
  aneurysm 094.89
  arachnoid (adhesive) 094.2
  arteritis (any artery) 094.89
  asymptomatic 094.3
  congenital 090.40
  dura (mater) 094.89
  general paresis 094.1
  gumma 094.9
  hemorrhagic 094.9
  juvenile (asymptomatic) (meningeal) 090.40
  leptomeninges (aseptic) 094.2
  meningeal 094.2
  meninges (adhesive) 094.2
  meningovascular (diffuse) 094.2
  optic atrophy 094.84
  parenchymatous (degenerative) 094.1
  paresis (*see also* Paresis, general) 094.1
  paretic (*see also* Paresis, general) 094.1
  relapse 094.9
  remission in (sustained) 094.9
  serological 094.3
  specified nature or site NEC 094.89
  tabes (dorsalis) 094.0
    juvenile 090.40
  tabetic 094.0
    juvenile 090.40
  taboparesis 094.1
    juvenile 090.40
  thrombosis 094.89
  vascular 094.89
Neurotic (*see also* Neurosis) 300.9
  excoriation 698.4
    psychogenic 306.3
Neurotmesis - *see* Injury, nerve, by site
Neurotoxemia - *see* Toxemia
Neutroclusion 524.2
Neutro-occlusion 524.21
Neutropenia, neutropenic (idiopathic) (pernicious) (primary) 288.00
  chronic 288.09
    hypoplastic 288.09
  congenital (nontransient) 288.01
  cyclic 288.02
  drug induced 288.03
  due to infection 288.04
  fever 288.00
  genetic 288.01
  immune 288.09
  infantile 288.01
  malignant 288.09
  neonatal, transitory (isoimmune) (maternal transfer) 776.7
  periodic 288.02
  splenic 289.53
  splenomegaly 289.53
  toxic 288.09
Neutrophilia, hereditary giant 288.2
Nevocarcinoma (M8720/3) - *see* Melanoma
Nevus (M8720/0) - *see also* Neoplasm, skin, benign

> Note Except where otherwise indicated, varieties of nevus in the list below that are followed by a morphology code number (M----/0) should be coded by site as for "Neoplasm, skin, benign."

  acanthotic 702.8
  achromic (M8730/0)
  amelanotic (M8730/0)
  anemic, anemicus 709.09
  angiomatous (M9120/0) (*see also* Hemangioma) 228.00
  araneus 448.1
  avasculosus 709.09
  balloon cell (M8722/0)
  bathing trunk (M8761/1) 238.2
  blue (M8780/0)
    cellular (M8790/0)
    giant (M8790/0)
    Jadassohn's (M8780/0)
    malignant (M8780/3) - *see* Melanoma
  capillary (M9131/0) (*see also* Hemangioma) 228.00
  cavernous (M9121/0) (*see also* Hemangioma) 228.00
  cellular (M8720/0)
    blue (M8790/0)
  comedonicus 757.33
  compound (M8760/0)
  conjunctiva (M8720/0) 224.3
  dermal (8750/0)
    and epidermal (M8760/0)
  epithelioid cell (and spindle cell) (M8770/0)
  flammeus 757.32
    osteohypertrophic 759.89
  hairy (M8720/0)
  halo (M8723/0)
  hemangiomatous (M9120/0) (*see also* Hemangioma) 228.00
  intradermal (M8750/0)
  intraepidermal (M8740/0)
  involuting (M8724/0)
  Jadassohn's (blue) (M8780/0)

Nevus *(Continued)*
  junction, junctional (M8740/0)
    malignant melanoma in (M8740/3) - *see* Melanoma
  juvenile (M8770/0)
  lymphatic (M9170/0) 228.1
  magnocellular (M8726/0)
    specified site - *see* Neoplasm, by site, benign
    unspecified site 224.0
  malignant (M8720/3) - *see* Melanoma
  meaning hemangioma (M9120/0) (*see also* Hemangioma) 228.00
  melanotic (pigmented) (M8720/0)
  multiplex 759.5
  nonneoplastic 448.1
  nonpigmented (M8730/0)
  nonvascular (M8720/0)
  oral mucosa, white sponge 750.26
  osteohypertrophic, flammeus 759.89
  papillaris (M8720/0)
  papillomatosus (M8720/0)
  pigmented (M8720/0)
    giant (M8761/1) - *see also* Neoplasm, skin, uncertain behavior
      malignant melanoma in (M8761/3) - *see* Melanoma
    systematicus 757.33
  pilosus (M8720/0)
  port wine 757.32
  sanguineous 757.32
  sebaceous (senile) 702.8
  senile 448.1
  spider 448.1
  spindle cell (and epithelioid cell) (M8770/0)
  stellar 448.1
  strawberry 757.32
  syringocystadenomatous papilliferous (M8406/0)
  unius lateris 757.33
  Unna's 757.32
  vascular 757.32
  verrucous 757.33
  white sponge (oral mucosa) 750.26
Newborn (infant) (liveborn)
  affected by maternal abuse of drugs (gestational) (via placenta) (via breast milk) (*see also* Noxious, substances transmitted through placenta or breast milk (affecting fetus or newborn)) 760.70
  apnea 770.81
    obstructive 770.82
    specified NEC 770.82
  cardiomyopathy 425.4
    congenital 425.3
  convulsion 779.0
  electrolyte imbalance NEC (transitory) 775.5
  gestation
    24 completed weeks 765.22
    25–26 completed weeks 765.23
    27–28 completed weeks 765.24
    29–30 completed weeks 765.25
    31–32 completed weeks 765.26
    33–34 completed weeks 765.27
    35–36 completed weeks 765.28
    37 or more completed weeks 765.29
    less than 24 completed weeks 765.21
    unspecified completed weeks 765.20
  infection 771.89
    candida 771.7
    mastitis 771.5

◀ **New** **Revised**

Newborn *(Continued)*
infection *(Continued)*
specified NEC 771.89
urinary tract 771.82
mastitis 771.5
multiple NEC
born in hospital (without mention of cesarean delivery or section) V37.00
with cesarean delivery or section V37.01
born outside hospital
hospitalized V37.1
not hospitalized V37.2
mates all liveborn
born in hospital (without mention of cesarean delivery or section) V34.00
with cesarean delivery or section V34.01
born outside hospital
hospitalized V34.1
not hospitalized V34.2
mates all stillborn
born in hospital (without mention of cesarean delivery or section) V35.00
with cesarean delivery or section V35.01
born outside hospital
hospitalized V35.1
not hospitalized V35.2
mates liveborn and stillborn
born in hospital (without mention of cesarean delivery or section) V36.00
with cesarean delivery or section V36.01
born outside hospital
hospitalized V36.1
not hospitalized V36.2
omphalitis 771.4
seizure 779.0
sepsis 771.81
single
born in hospital (without mention of cesarean delivery or section) V30.00
with cesarean delivery or section V30.01
born outside hospital
hospitalized V30.1
not hospitalized V30.2
specified condition NEC 779.89
twin NEC
born in hospital (without mention of cesarean delivery or section) V33.00
with cesarean delivery or section V33.01
born outside hospital
hospitalized V33.1
not hospitalized V33.2
mate liveborn
born in hospital V31.0
born outside hospital
hospitalized V31.1
not hospitalized V31.2
mate stillborn
born in hospital V32.0
born outside hospital
hospitalized V32.1
not hospitalized V32.2

Newborn *(Continued)*
unspecified as to single or multiple birth
born in hospital (without mention of cesarean delivery or section) V39.00
with cesarean delivery or section V39.01
born outside hospital
hospitalized V39.1
not hospitalized V39.2
Newcastle's conjunctivitis or disease 077.8
Nezelof's syndrome (pure alymphocytosis) 279.13
Niacin (amide) deficiency 265.2
Nicolas-Durand-Favre disease (climatic bubo) 099.1
Nicolas-Favre disease (climatic bubo) 099.1
Nicotinic acid (amide) deficiency 265.2
Niemann-Pick disease (lipid histiocytosis) (splenomegaly) 272.7
Night
blindness (*see also* Blindness, night) 368.60
congenital 368.61
vitamin A deficiency 264.5
cramps 729.82
sweats 780.8
terrors, child 307.46
Nightmare 307.47
REM-sleep type 307.47
Nipple - *see* condition
Nisbet's chancre 099.0
Nishimoto (-Takeuchi) disease 437.5
Nitritoid crisis or reaction - *see* Crisis, nitritoid
Nitrogen retention, extrarenal 788.9
Nitrosohemoglobinemia 289.89
Njovera 104.0
No
diagnosis 799.9
disease (found) V71.9
room at the inn V65.0
Nocardiasis - *see* Nocardiosis
Nocardiosis 039.9
with pneumonia 039.1
lung 039.1
specified type NEC 039.8
Nocturia 788.43
psychogenic 306.53
Nocturnal - *see also* condition
dyspnea (paroxysmal) 786.09
emissions 608.89
enuresis 788.36
psychogenic 307.6
frequency (micturition) 788.43
psychogenic 306.53
Nodal rhythm disorder 427.89
Nodding of head 781.0
Node(s) - *see also* Nodules
Heberden's 715.04
larynx 478.79
lymph - *see* condition
milkers' 051.1
Osler's 421.0
rheumatic 729.89
Schmorl's 722.30
lumbar, lumbosacral 722.32
specified region NEC 722.39
thoracic, thoracolumbar 722.31
singers' 478.5
skin NEC 782.2

Node(s) *(Continued)*
tuberculous - *see* Tuberculosis, lymph gland
vocal cords 478.5
Nodosities, Haygarth's 715.04
Nodule(s), nodular
actinomycotic (*see also* Actinomycosis) 039.9
arthritic - *see* Arthritis, nodosa
cutaneous 782.2
Haygarth's 715.04
inflammatory - *see* Inflammation
juxta-articular 102.7
syphilitic 095.7
yaws 102.7
larynx 478.79
lung, solitary 518.89
emphysematous 492.8
milkers' 051.1
prostate 600.10
with (Revised)
urinary (New)
obstruction 600.11 (New)
retention 600.11 (New)
rheumatic 729.89
rheumatoid - *see* Arthritis rheumatoid
scrotum (inflammatory) 608.4
singers' 478.5
skin NEC 782.2
solitary, lung 518.89
emphysematous 492.8
subcutaneous 782.2
thyroid (gland) (nontoxic) (uninodular) 241.0
with
hyperthyroidism 242.1
thyrotoxicosis 242.1
toxic or with hyperthyroidism 242.1
vocal cords 478.5
Noma (gangrenous) (hospital) (infective) 528.1
auricle (*see also* Gangrene) 785.4
mouth 528.1
pudendi (*see also* Vulvitis) 616.10
vulvae (*see also* Vulvitis) 616.10
Nomadism V60.0
Non-adherence
artificial skin graft 996.55
decellularized allodermis graft 996.55
Non-autoimmune hemolytic anemia NEC 283.10
Nonclosure - *see also* Imperfect, closure
ductus
arteriosus 747.0
Botalli 747.0
Eustachian valve 746.89
foramen
Botalli 745.5
ovale 745.5
Noncompliance with medical treatment V15.81
Nondescent (congenital) - *see also* Malposition, congenital
cecum 751.4
colon 751.4
testis 752.51
Nondevelopment
brain 742.1
specified part 742.2
heart 746.89
organ or site, congenital NEC - *see* Hypoplasia

ICD-9-CM N Vol. 2

◀ New ⬅ Revised

Nonengagement
head NEC 652.5
in labor 660.1
affecting fetus or newborn 763.1
Nonexanthematous tick fever 066.1
Nonexpansion, lung (newborn) NEC 770.4
Nonfunctioning
cystic duct (*see also* Disease, gallbladder) 575.8
gallbladder (*see also* Disease, gallbladder) 575.8
kidney (*see also* Disease, renal) 593.9
labyrinth 386.58
Nonhealing
stump (surgical) 997.69
wound, surgical 998.83
Nonimplantation of ovum, causing infertility 628.3
Noninsufflation, fallopian tube 628.2
Nonne-Milroy-Meige syndrome (chronic hereditary edema) 757.0
Nonovulation 628.0
Nonpatent fallopian tube 628.2
Nonpneumatization, lung NEC 770.4
Nonreflex bladder 596.54
with cauda equina 344.61
Nonretention of food - *see* Vomiting
Nonrotation - *see* Malrotation
Nonsecretion, urine (*see also* Anuria) 788.5
newborn 753.3
Nonunion
fracture 733.82
organ or site, congenital NEC - *see* Imperfect, closure
symphysis pubis, congenital 755.69
top sacrum, congenital 756.19
Nonviability 765.0
Nonvisualization, gallbladder 793.3
Nonvitalized tooth 522.9
Non-working side interference 524.56
Normal
delivery - *see* category 650
menses V65.5
state (feared complaint unfounded) V65.5
Normoblastosis 289.89
Normocytic anemia (infectional) 285.9
due to blood loss (chronic) 280.0
acute 285.1
Norrie's disease (congenital) (progressive oculoacousticocerebral degeneration) 743.8
North American blastomycosis 116.0
Norwegian itch 133.0
Nose, nasal - *see* condition
Nosebleed 784.7
Nosomania 298.9
Nosophobia 300.29
Nostalgia 309.89
Notch of iris 743.46
Notched lip, congenital (*see also* Cleft, lip) 749.10
Notching nose, congenital (tip) 748.1
Nothnagel's
syndrome 378.52
vasomotor acroparesthesia 443.89
Novy's relapsing fever (American) 087.1
Noxious
foodstuffs, poisoning by
fish 988.0
fungi 988.1
mushrooms 988.1
plants (food) 988.2
shellfish 988.0
specified type NEC 988.8
toadstool 988.1
substances transmitted through placenta or breast milk (affecting fetus or newborn) 760.70
acetretin 760.78
alcohol 760.71
aminopterin 760.78
antiandrogens 760.79
anticonvulsant 760.77
antifungal 760.74
anti-infective agents 760.74
antimetabolic 760.78
atorvastatin 760.78
carbamazepine 760.77
cocaine 760.75
"crack" 760.75
diethylstilbestrol (DES) 760.76
divalproex sodium 760.77
endocrine disrupting chemicals 760.79
estrogens 760.79
etretinate 760.78
fluconazole 760.74
fluvastatin 760.78
hallucinogenic agents NEC 760.73
hormones 760.79
lithium 760.79
lovastatin 760.78
medicinal agents NEC 760.79
methotrexate 760.78
misoprostil 760.79
narcotics 760.72
obstetric anesthetic or analgesic 763.5
phenobarbital 760.77
phenytoin 760.77
Noxious *(Continued)*
substances transmitted through placenta or breast milk *(Continued)*
pravastatin 760.78
progestins 760.79
retinoic acid 760.78
simvastatin 760.78
solvents 760.79
specified agent NEC 760.79
statins 760.78
suspected, affecting management of pregnancy 655.5
tetracycline 760.74
thalidomide 760.79
trimethadione 760.77
valproate 760.77
valproic acid 760.77
vitamin A 760.78
Nuchal hitch (arm) 652.8
Nucleus pulposus - *see* condition
Numbness 782.0
Nuns' knee 727.2
Nursemaid's
elbow 832.0
shoulder 831.0
Nutmeg liver 573.8
Nutrition, deficient or insufficient (particular kind of food) 269.9
due to
insufficient food 994.2
lack of
care (child) (infant) 995.52
adult 995.84
food 994.2
Nyctalopia (*see also* Blindness, night) 368.60
vitamin A deficiency 264.5
Nycturia 788.43
psychogenic 306.53
Nymphomania 302.89
Nystagmus 379.50
associated with vestibular system disorders 379.54
benign paroxysmal positional 386.11
central positional 386.2
congenital 379.51
deprivation 379.53
dissociated 379.55
latent 379.52
miners' 300.89
positional
benign paroxysmal 386.11
central 386.2
specified NEC 379.56
vestibular 379.54
visual deprivation 379.53

O

Oasthouse urine disease 270.2
Obermeyer's relapsing fever (European) 087.0
Obesity (constitutional) (exogenous) (familial) (nutritional) (simple) 278.00
adrenal 255.8
complicating pregnancy, childbirth, or puerperium 649.1 ◀
due to hyperalimentation 278.00
endocrine NEC 259.9
endogenous 259.9
Fröhlich's (adiposogenital dystrophy) 253.8
glandular NEC 259.9
hypothyroid (*see also* Hypothyroidism) 244.9
morbid 278.01
of pregnancy 649.1
pituitary 253.8
severe 278.01
thyroid (*see also* Hypothyroidism) 244.9
Oblique - *see also* condition
lie before labor, affecting fetus or newborn 761.7
Obliquity, pelvis 738.6
Obliteration
abdominal aorta 446.7
appendix (lumen) 543.9
artery 447.1
ascending aorta 446.7
bile ducts 576.8
with calculus, choledocholithiasis, or stones - *see* Choledocholithiasis
congenital 751.61
jaundice from 751.61 *[774.5]*
common duct 576.8
with calculus, choledocholithiasis, or stones - *see* Choledocholithiasis
congenital 751.61
cystic duct 575.8
with calculus, choledocholithiasis, or stones - *see* Choledocholithiasis
disease, arteriolar 447.1
endometrium 621.8
eye, anterior chamber 360.34
fallopian tube 628.2
lymphatic vessel 457.1
postmastectomy 457.0
organ or site, congenital NEC - *see* Atresia
placental blood vessels - *see* Placenta, abnormal
supra-aortic branches 446.7
ureter 593.89
urethra 599.84
vein 459.9
vestibule (oral) 525.8
Observation (for) V71.9
without need for further medical care V71.9
accident NEC V71.4
at work V71.3
criminal assault V71.6
deleterious agent ingestion V71.89
disease V71.9
cardiovascular V71.7
heart V71.7
mental V71.09
specified condition NEC V71.89
foreign body ingestion V71.89
Observation *(Continued)*
growth and development variations V21.8
injuries (accidental) V71.4
inflicted NEC V71.6
during alleged rape or seduction V71.5
malignant neoplasm, suspected V71.1
postpartum
immediately after delivery V24.0
routine follow-up V24.2
pregnancy
high-risk V23.9
specified problem NEC V23.8
normal (without complication) V22.1
with nonobstetric complication V22.2
first V22.0
rape or seduction, alleged V71.5
injury during V71.5
suicide attempt, alleged V71.89
suspected (undiagnosed) (unproven)
abuse V71.81
cardiovascular disease V71.7
child or wife battering victim V71.6
concussion (cerebral) V71.6
condition NEC V71.89
infant - *see* Observation, suspected, condition, newborn
newborn V29.9
cardiovascular disease V29.8
congenital anomaly V29.8
genetic V29.3
infectious V29.0
ingestion foreign object V29.8
injury V29.8
metabolic V29.3
neoplasm V29.8
neurological V29.1
poison, poisoning V29.8
respiratory V29.2
specified NEC V29.8
exposure
anthrax V71.82
biologic agent NEC V71.83
SARS V71.83
infectious disease not requiring isolation V71.89
malignant neoplasm V71.1
mental disorder V71.09
neglect V71.81
neoplasm
benign V71.89
malignant V71.1
specified condition NEC V71.89
tuberculosis V71.2
tuberculosis, suspected V71.2
Obsession, obsessional 300.3
ideas and mental images 300.3
impulses 300.3
neurosis 300.3
phobia 300.3
psychasthenia 300.3
ruminations 300.3
state 300.3
syndrome 300.3
Obsessive-compulsive 300.3
neurosis 300.3
personality 301.4
reaction 300.3
Obstetrical trauma NEC (complicating delivery) 665.9
with
Obstetrical trauma NEC *(Continued)*
with *(Continued)*
abortion - *see* Abortion, by type, with damage to pelvic organs
ectopic pregnancy (*see also* categories 633.0-633.9) 639.2
molar pregnancy (*see also* categories 630-632) 639.2
affecting fetus or newborn 763.89
following
abortion 639.2
ectopic or molar pregnancy 639.2
Obstipation (*see also* Constipation) 564.00
psychogenic 306.4
Obstruction, obstructed, obstructive
airway NEC 519.8
with
allergic alveolitis NEC 495.9
asthma NEC (*see also* Asthma) 493.9
bronchiectasis 494.0
with acute exacerbation 494.1
bronchitis (*see also* Bronchitis, with, obstruction) 491.20
emphysema NEC 492.8
chronic 496
with
allergic alveolitis NEC 495.5
asthma NEC (*see also* Asthma) 493.2
bronchiectasis 494.0
with acute exacerbation 494.1
bronchitis (chronic) (*see also* Bronchitis, chronic, obstructive) 491.20
emphysema NEC 492.8
due to
bronchospasm 519.11
foreign body 934.9
inhalation of fumes or vapors 506.9
laryngospasm 478.75
alimentary canal (*see also* Obstruction, intestine) 560.9
ampulla of Vater 576.2
with calculus, cholelithiasis, or stones - *see* Choledocholithiasis
aortic (heart) (valve) (*see also* Stenosis, aortic) 424.1
rheumatic (*see also* Stenosis, aortic, rheumatic) 395.0
aortoiliac 444.0
aqueduct of Sylvius 331.4
congenital 742.3
with spina bifida (*see also* Spina bifida) 741.0
Arnold-Chiari (*see also* Spina bifida) 741.0
artery (*see also* Embolism, artery) 444.9
basilar (complete) (partial) (*see also* Occlusion, artery, basilar) 433.0
carotid (complete) (partial) (*see also* Occlusion, artery, carotid) 433.1
precerebral - *see* Occlusion, artery, precerebral NEC
retinal (central) (*see also* Occlusion, retina) 362.30
vertebral (complete) (partial) (*see also* Occlusion, artery, vertebral) 433.2
asthma (chronic) (with obstructive pulmonary disease) 493.2
band (intestinal) 560.81
bile duct or passage (*see also* Obstruction, biliary) 576.2
congenital 751.61
jaundice from 751.61 *[774.5]*

ICD-9-CM
O
Vol. 2

Obstruction, obstructed, obstructive *(Continued)*
biliary (duct) (tract) 576.2
with calculus 574.51
with cholecystitis (chronic) 574.41
acute 574.31
congenital 751.61
jaundice from 751.61 *[774.5]*
gallbladder 575.2
with calculus 574.21
with cholecystitis (chronic) 574.11
acute 574.01
bladder neck (acquired) 596.0
congenital 753.6
bowel (*see also* Obstruction, intestine) 560.9
bronchus 519.19
canal, ear (*see also* Stricture, ear canal, acquired) 380.50
cardia 537.89
caval veins (inferior) (superior) 459.2
cecum (*see also* Obstruction, intestine) 560.9
circulatory 459.9
colon (*see also* Obstruction, intestine) 560.9
sympathicotonic 560.89
common duct (*see also* Obstruction, biliary) 576.2
congenital 751.61
coronary (artery) (heart) - *see also* Arteriosclerosis, coronary
acute (*see also* Infarct, myocardium) 410.9
without myocardial infarction 411.81
cystic duct (*see also* Obstruction, gallbladder) 575.2
congenital 751.61
device, implant, or graft - *see* Complications, due to (presence of) any device, implant, or graft classified to 996.0–996.5 NEC
due to foreign body accidentally left in operation wound 998.4
duodenum 537.3
congenital 751.1
due to
compression NEC 537.3
cyst 537.3
intrinsic lesion or disease NEC 537.3
scarring 537.3
torsion 537.3
ulcer 532.91
volvulus 537.3
ejaculatory duct 608.89
endocardium 424.90
arteriosclerotic 424.99
specified cause, except rheumatic 424.99
esophagus 530.3
Eustachian tube (complete) (partial) 381.60
cartilaginous
extrinsic 381.63
intrinsic 381.62
due to
cholesteatoma 381.61
osseous lesion NEC 381.61
polyp 381.61
osseous 381.61

Obstruction, obstructed, obstructive *(Continued)*
fallopian tube (bilateral) 628.2
fecal 560.39
with hernia - *see also* Hernia, by site, with obstruction
gangrenous - *see* Hernia, by site, with gangrene
foramen of Monro (congenital) 742.3
with spina bifida (*see also* Spina bifida) 741.0
foreign body - *see* Foreign body
gallbladder 575.2
with calculus, cholelithiasis, or stones 574.21
with cholecystitis (chronic) 574.11
acute 574.01
congenital 751.69
jaundice from 751.69 *[774.5]*
gastric outlet 537.0
gastrointestinal (*see also* Obstruction, intestine) 560.9
glottis 478.79
hepatic 573.8
duct (*see also* Obstruction, biliary) 576.2
congenital 751.61
icterus (*see also* Obstruction, biliary) 576.8
congenital 751.61
ileocecal coil (*see also* Obstruction, intestine) 560.9
ileum (*see also* Obstruction, intestine) 560.9
iliofemoral (artery) 444.81
internal anastomosis - *see* Complications, mechanical, graft
intestine (mechanical) (neurogenic) (paroxysmal) (postinfectional) (reflex) 560.9
with
adhesions (intestinal) (peritoneal) 560.81
hernia - *see also* Hernia, by site, with obstruction
gangrenous - *see* Hernia, by site, with gangrene
adynamic (*see also* Ileus) 560.1
by gallstone 560.31
congenital or infantile (small) 751.1
large 751.2
due to
Ascaris lumbricoides 127.0
mural thickening 560.89
procedure 997.4
involving urinary tract 997.5
impaction 560.39
infantile - *see* Obstruction, intestine, congenital
newborn
due to
fecaliths 777.1
inspissated milk 777.2
meconium (plug) 777.1
in mucoviscidosis 277.01
transitory 777.4
specified cause NEC 560.89
transitory, newborn 777.4
volvulus 560.2
intracardiac ball valve prosthesis 996.02
jaundice (*see also* Obstruction, biliary) 576.8
congenital 751.61
jejunum (*see also* Obstruction, intestine) 560.9

Obstruction, obstructed, obstructive *(Continued)*
kidney 593.89
labor 660.9
affecting fetus or newborn 763.1
by
bony pelvis (conditions classifiable to 653.0–653.9) 660.1
deep transverse arrest 660.3
impacted shoulder 660.4
locked twins 660.5
malposition (fetus) (conditions classifiable to 652.0–652.9) 660.0
head during labor 660.3
persistent occipitoposterior position 660.3
soft tissue, pelvic (conditions classifiable to 654.0–654.9) 660.2
lacrimal
canaliculi 375.53
congenital 743.65
punctum 375.52
sac 375.54
lacrimonasal duct 375.56
congenital 743.65
neonatal 375.55
lacteal, with steatorrhea 579.2
laryngitis (*see also* Laryngitis) 464.01
larynx 478.79
congenital 748.3
liver 573.8
cirrhotic (*see also* Cirrhosis, liver) 571.5
lung 518.89
with
asthma - *see* Asthma
bronchitis (chronic) 491.20
emphysema NEC 492.8
airway, chronic 496
chronic NEC 496
with
asthma (chronic) (obstructive) 493.2
disease, chronic 496
with
asthma (chronic) (obstructive) 493.2
emphysematous 492.8
lymphatic 457.1
meconium
fetus or newborn 777.1
in mucoviscidosis 277.01
newborn due to fecaliths 777.1
mediastinum 519.3
mitral (rheumatic) - *see* Stenosis, mitral
nasal 478.19
duct 375.56
neonatal 375.55
sinus - *see* Sinusitis
nasolacrimal duct 375.56
congenital 743.65
neonatal 375.55
nasopharynx 478.29
nose 478.19
organ or site, congenital NEC - *see* Atresia
pancreatic duct 577.8
parotid gland 527.8
pelviureteral junction (*see also* Obstruction, ureter) 593.4
pharynx 478.29
portal (circulation) (vein) 452
prostate 600.90
with
other lower urinary tract symptoms (LUTS) 600.91

◀ New ⇐ Revised

Obstruction, obstructed, obstructive *(Continued)*
prostate *(Continued)*
with *(Continued)*
urinary ◀
obstruction 600.91 ◀
retention 600.91 ◀
valve (urinary) 596.0
pulmonary
valve (heart) (*see also* Endocarditis, pulmonary) 424.3
vein, isolated 747.49
pyemic - *see* Septicemia
pylorus (acquired) 537.0
congenital 750.5
infantile 750.5
rectosigmoid (*see also* Obstruction, intestine) 560.9
rectum 569.49
renal 593.89
respiratory 519.8
chronic 496
retinal (artery) (vein) (central) (*see also* Occlusion, retina) 362.30
salivary duct (any) 527.8
with calculus 527.5
sigmoid (*see also* Obstruction, intestine) 560.9
sinus (accessory) (nasal) (*see also* Sinusitis) 473.9
Stensen's duct 527.8
stomach 537.89
acute 536.1
congenital 750.7
submaxillary gland 527.8
with calculus 527.5
thoracic duct 457.1
thrombotic - *see* Thrombosis
tooth eruption 520.6
trachea 519.19 ⬅
tracheostomy airway 519.09
tricuspid - *see* Endocarditis, tricuspid
upper respiratory, congenital 748.8
ureter (functional) 593.4
congenital 753.20
due to calculus 592.1
ureteropelvic junction, congenital 753.21
ureterovesical junction, congenital 753.22
urethra 599.60
congenital 753.6
urinary (moderate) 599.60
organ or tract (lower) 599.60
due to
benign prostatic hypertrophy (BPH) - *see* category 600
specified NEC 599.69
due to
benign prostatic hypertrophy (BPH) - *see* category 600
prostatic valve 596.0
specified NEC 599.69
due to
benign prostatic hypertrophy (BPH) - *see* category 600
uropathy 599.60
uterus 621.8
vagina 623.2
valvular - *see* Endocarditis
vascular graft or shunt 996.1
atherosclerosis - *see* Arteriosclerosis, coronary
embolism 996.74

Obstruction, obstructed, obstructive *(Continued)*
vascular graft or shunt *(Continued)*
occlusion NEC 996.74
thrombus 996.74
vein, venous 459.2
caval (inferior) (superior) 459.2
thrombotic - *see* Thrombosis
vena cava (inferior) (superior) 459.2
ventricular shunt 996.2
vesical 596.0
vesicourethral orifice 596.0
vessel NEC 459.9
Obturator - *see* condition
Occlusal
plane deviation 524.76
wear, teeth 521.10
Occlusion
anus 569.49
congenital 751.2
infantile 751.2
aortoiliac (chronic) 444.0
aqueduct of Sylvius 331.4
congenital 742.3
with spina bifida (*see also* Spina bifida) 741.0
arteries of extremities, lower 444.22
without thrombus or embolus (*see also* Arteriosclerosis, extremities) 440.20
due to stricture or stenosis 447.1
upper 444.21
without thrombus or embolus (*see also* Arteriosclerosis, extremities) 440.20
due to stricture or stenosis 447.1
artery NEC (*see also* Embolism, artery) 444.9
auditory, internal 433.8
basilar 433.0
with other precerebral artery 433.3
bilateral 433.3
brain or cerebral (*see also* Infarct, brain) 434.9
carotid 433.1
with other precerebral artery 433.3
bilateral 433.3
cerebellar (anterior inferior) (posterior inferior) (superior) 433.8
cerebral (*see also* Infarct, brain) 434.9
choroidal (anterior) 433.8
communicating posterior 433.8
coronary (thrombotic) (*see also* Infarct, myocardium) 410.9
acute 410.9
without myocardial infarction 411.81
healed or old 412
hypophyseal 433.8
iliac 444.81
mesenteric (embolic) (thrombotic) (with gangrene) 557.0
pontine 433.8
precerebral NEC 433.9
late effect - *see* Late effect(s) (of) cerebrovascular disease
multiple or bilateral 433.3
puerperal, postpartum, childbirth 674.0
specified NEC 433.8
renal 593.81
retinal - *see* Occlusion, retina, artery
spinal 433.8
vertebral 433.2

Occlusion *(Continued)*
artery NEC *(Continued)*
vertebral *(Continued)*
with other precerebral artery 433.3
bilateral 433.3
basilar (artery) - *see* Occlusion, artery, basilar
bile duct (any) (*see also* Obstruction, biliary) 576.2
bowel (*see also* Obstruction, intestine) 560.9
brain (artery) (vascular) (*see also* Infarct, brain) 434.9
breast (duct) 611.8
carotid (artery) (common) (internal) - *see* Occlusion, artery, carotid
cerebellar (anterior inferior) (artery) (posterior inferior) (superior) 433.8
cerebral (artery) (*see also* Infarct, brain) 434.9
cerebrovascular (*see also* Infarct, brain) 434.9
diffuse 437.0
cervical canal (*see also* Stricture, cervix) 622.4
by falciparum malaria 084.0
cervix (uteri) (*see also* Stricture, cervix) 622.4
choanal 748.0
choroidal (artery) 433.8
colon (*see also* Obstruction, intestine) 560.9
communicating posterior artery 433.8
coronary (artery) (thrombotic) (*see also* Infarct, myocardium) 410.9
acute 410.9
without myocardial infarction 411.81
healed or old 412
cystic duct (*see also* Obstruction, gallbladder) 575.2
congenital 751.69
disto
division I 524.22
division II 524.22
embolic - *see* Embolism
fallopian tube 628.2
congenital 752.19
gallbladder (*see also* Obstruction, gallbladder) 575.2
congenital 751.69
jaundice from 751.69 *[744.5]*
gingiva, traumatic 523.8
hymen 623.3
congenital 752.42
hypophyseal (artery) 433.8
iliac (artery) 444.81
intestine (*see also* Obstruction, intestine) 560.9
kidney 593.89
lacrimal apparatus - *see* Stenosis, lacrimal
lung 518.89
lymph or lymphatic channel 457.1
mammary duct 611.8
mesenteric artery (embolic) (thrombotic) (with gangrene) 557.0
nose 478.19 ⬅
congenital 748.0
organ or site, congenital NEC - *see* Atresia
oviduct 628.2
congenital 752.19
periodontal, traumatic 523.8

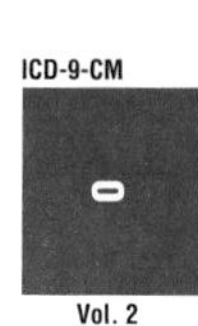
ICD-9-CM
O
Vol. 2

Occlusion *(Continued)*
peripheral arteries (lower extremity) 444.22
without thrombus or embolus (*see also* Arteriosclerosis, extremities) 440.20
due to stricture or stenosis 447.1
upper extremity 444.21
without thrombus or embolus (*see also* Arteriosclerosis, extremities) 440.20
due to stricture or stenosis 447.1
pontine (artery) 433.8
posterior lingual, of mandibular teeth 524.29
precerebral artery - *see* Occlusion, artery, precerebral NEC
puncta lacrimalia 375.52
pupil 364.74
pylorus (*see also* Stricture, pylorus) 537.0
renal artery 593.81
retina, retinal (vascular) 362.30
artery, arterial 362.30
branch 362.32
central (total) 362.31
partial 362.33
transient 362.34
tributary 362.32
vein 362.30
branch 362.36
central (total) 362.35
incipient 362.37
partial 362.37
tributary 362.36
spinal artery 433.8
stent
coronary 996.72
teeth (mandibular) (posterior lingual) 524.29
thoracic duct 457.1
tubal 628.2
ureter (complete) (partial) 593.4
congenital 753.29
urethra (*see also* Stricture, urethra) 598.9
congenital 753.6
uterus 621.8
vagina 623.2
vascular NEC 459.9
vein - *see* Thrombosis
vena cava (inferior) (superior) 453.2
ventricle (brain) NEC 331.4
vertebral (artery) - *see* Occlusion, artery, vertebral
vessel (blood) NEC 459.9
vulva 624.8
Occlusio pupillae 364.74
Occupational
problems NEC V62.2
therapy V57.21
Ochlophobia 300.29
Ochronosis (alkaptonuric) (congenital) (endogenous) 270.2
with chloasma of eyelid 270.2
Ocular muscle - *see also* condition
myopathy 359.1
torticollis 781.93
Oculoauriculovertebral dysplasia 756.0
Oculogyric
crisis or disturbance 378.87
psychogenic 306.7
Oculomotor syndrome 378.81
Oddi's sphincter spasm 576.5
Odelberg's disease (juvenile osteochondrosis) 732.1
Odontalgia 525.9
Odontoameloblastoma (M9311/0) 213.1
upper jaw (bone) 213.0
Odontoclasia 521.05
Odontoclasis 873.63
complicated 873.73
Odontodysplasia, regional 520.4
Odontogenesis imperfecta 520.5
Odontoma (M9280/0) 213.1
ameloblastic (M9311/0) 213.1
upper jaw (bone) 213.0
calcified (M9280/0) 213.1
upper jaw (bone) 213.0
complex (M9282/0) 213.1
upper jaw (bone) 213.0
compound (M9281/0) 213.1
upper jaw (bone) 213.0
fibroameloblastic (M9290/0) 213.1
upper jaw (bone) 213.0
follicular 526.0
upper jaw (bone) 213.0
Odontomyelitis (closed) (open) 522.0
Odontonecrosis 521.09
Odontorrhagia 525.8
Odontosarcoma, ameloblastic (M9290/3) 170.1
upper jaw (bone) 170.0
Odynophagia 787.2
Oesophagostomiasis 127.7
Oesophagostomum infestation 127.7
Oestriasis 134.0
Ogilvie's syndrome (sympathicotonic colon obstruction) 560.89
Oguchi's disease (retina) 368.61
Ohara's disease (*see also* Tularemia) 021.9
Oidiomycosis (*see also* Candidiasis) 112.9
Oidiomycotic meningitis 112.83
Oidium albicans infection (*see also* Candidiasis) 112.9
Old age 797
dementia (of) 290.0
Olfactory - *see* condition
Oligemia 285.9
Oligergasia (*see also* Retardation, mental) 319
Oligoamnios 658.0
affecting fetus or newborn 761.2
Oligoastrocytoma, mixed (M9382/3)
specified site - *see* Neoplasm, by site, malignant
unspecified site 191.9
Oligocythemia 285.9
Oligodendroblastoma (M9460/3)
specified site - *see* Neoplasm, by site, malignant
unspecified site 191.9
Oligodendroglioma (M9450/3)
anaplastic type (M9451/3)
specified site - *see* Neoplasm, by site, malignant
unspecified site 191.9
specified site - *see* Neoplasm, by site, malignant
unspecified site 191.9
Oligodendroma - *see* Oligodendroglioma
Oligodontia (*see also* Anodontia) 520.0
Oligoencephalon 742.1
Oligohydramnios 658.0
affecting fetus or newborn 761.2
due to premature rupture of membranes 658.1
affecting fetus or newborn 761.2
Oligohydrosis 705.0
Oligomenorrhea 626.1
Oligophrenia (*see also* Retardation, mental) 319
phenylpyruvic 270.1
Oligospermia 606.1
Oligotrichia 704.09
congenita 757.4
Oliguria 788.5
with
abortion - *see* Abortion, by type, with renal failure
ectopic pregnancy (*see also* categories 633.0–633.9) 639.3
molar pregnancy (*see also* categories 630–632) 639.3
complicating
abortion 639.3
ectopic or molar pregnancy 639.3
pregnancy 646.2
with hypertension - *see* Toxemia, of pregnancy
due to a procedure 997.5
following labor and delivery 669.3
heart or cardiac - *see* Failure, heart
puerperal, postpartum 669.3
specified due to a procedure 997.5
Ollier's disease (chondrodysplasia) 756.4
Omentitis (*see also* Peritonitis) 567.9
Omentocele (*see also* Hernia, omental) 553.8
Omentum, omental - *see* condition
Omphalitis (congenital) (newborn) 771.4
not of newborn 686.9
tetanus 771.3
Omphalocele 756.79
Omphalomesenteric duct, persistent 751.0
Omphalorrhagia, newborn 772.3
Omsk hemorrhagic fever 065.1
Onanism 307.9
Onchocerciasis 125.3
eye 125.3 *[360.13]*
Onchocercosis 125.3
Oncocytoma (M8290/0) - *see* Neoplasm, by site, benign
Ondine's curse 348.8
Oneirophrenia (*see also* Schizophrenia) 295.4
Onychauxis 703.8
congenital 757.5
Onychia (with lymphangitis) 681.9
dermatophytic 110.1
finger 681.02
toe 681.11
Onychitis (with lymphangitis) 681.9
finger 681.02
toe 681.11
Onychocryptosis 703.0
Onychodystrophy 703.8
congenital 757.5
Onychogryphosis 703.8
Onychogryposis 703.8
Onycholysis 703.8
Onychomadesis 703.8
Onychomalacia 703.8
Onychomycosis 110.1
finger 110.1
toe 110.1
Onycho-osteodysplasia 756.89
Onychophagy 307.9
Onychoptosis 703.8
Onychorrhexis 703.8
congenital 757.5

Onychoschizia 703.8
Onychotrophia (*see also* Atrophy, nail) 703.8
O'Nyong Nyong fever 066.3
Onyxis (finger) (toe) 703.0
Onyxitis (with lymphangitis) 681.9
finger 681.02
toe 681.11
Oocyte (egg) (ovum)
donor V59.70
over age 35 V59.73
anonymous recipient V59.73
designated recipient V59.74
under age 35 V59.71
anonymous recipient V59.71
designated recipient V59.72
Oophoritis (cystic) (infectional) (interstitial) (*see also* Salpingo-oophoritis) 614.2
complicating pregnancy 646.6
fetal (acute) 752.0
gonococcal (acute) 098.19
chronic or duration of 2 months or over 098.39
tuberculous (*see also* Tuberculosis) 016.6
Opacity, opacities
cornea 371.00
central 371.03
congenital 743.43
interfering with vision 743.42
degenerative (*see also* Degeneration, cornea) 371.40
hereditary (*see also* Dystrophy, cornea) 371.50
inflammatory (*see also* Keratitis) 370.9
late effect of trachoma (healed) 139.1
minor 371.01
peripheral 371.02
enamel (fluoride) (nonfluoride) (teeth) 520.3
lens (*see also* Cataract) 366.9
snowball 379.22
vitreous (humor) 379.24
congenital 743.51
Opalescent dentin (hereditary) 520.5
Open, opening
abnormal, organ or site, congenital - *see* Imperfect, closure
angle with
borderline intraocular pressure 365.01
cupping of discs 365.01
bite (anterior) (posterior) 524.29
false - *see* Imperfect, closure
margin on tooth restoration 525.61 ◀
restoration margins 525.61 ◀
wound - *see* Wound, open, by site
Operation
causing mutilation of fetus 763.89
destructive, on live fetus, to facilitate birth 763.89
for delivery, fetus or newborn 763.89
maternal, unrelated to current delivery, affecting fetus or newborn 760.6
Operational fatigue 300.89
Operative - *see* condition
Operculitis (chronic) 523.40 ⬅
acute 523.30 ⬅
Operculum, retina 361.32
with detachment 361.01
Ophiasis 704.01
Ophthalmia (*see also* Conjunctivitis) 372.30
actinic rays 370.24
allergic (acute) 372.05
chronic 372.14
Ophthalmia *(Continued)*
blennorrhagic (neonatorum) 098.40
catarrhal 372.03
diphtheritic 032.81
Egyptian 076.1
electric, electrica 370.24
gonococcal (neonatorum) 098.40
metastatic 360.11
migraine 346.8
neonatorum, newborn 771.6
gonococcal 098.40
nodosa 360.14
phlyctenular 370.31
with ulcer (*see also* Ulcer, cornea) 370.00
sympathetic 360.11
Ophthalmitis - *see* Ophthalmia
Ophthalmocele (congenital) 743.66
Ophthalmoneuromyelitis 341.0
Ophthalmopathy, infiltrative with thyrotoxicosis 242.0
Ophthalmoplegia (*see also* Strabismus) 378.9
anterior internuclear 378.86
ataxia-areflexia syndrome 357.0
bilateral 378.9
diabetic 250.5 *[378.86]*
exophthalmic 242.0 *[376.22]*
external 378.55
progressive 378.72
total 378.56
internal (complete) (total) 367.52
internuclear 378.86
migraine 346.8
painful 378.55
Parinaud's 378.81
progressive external 378.72
supranuclear, progressive 333.0
total (external) 378.56
internal 367.52
unilateral 378.9
Opisthognathism 524.00
Opisthorchiasis (felineus) (tenuicollis) (viverrini) 121.0
Opisthotonos, opisthotonus 781.0
Opitz's disease (congestive splenomegaly) 289.51
Opiumism (*see also* Dependence) 304.0
Oppenheim's disease 358.8
Oppenheim-Urbach disease or syndrome (necrobiosis lipoidica diabeticorum) 250.8 *[709.3]*
Opsoclonia 379.59
Optic nerve - *see* condition
Orbit - *see* condition
Orchioblastoma (M9071/3) 186.9
Orchitis (nonspecific) (septic) 604.90
with abscess 604.0
blennorrhagic (acute) 098.13
chronic or duration of 2 months or over 098.33
diphtheritic 032.89 *[604.91]*
filarial 125.9 *[604.91]*
gangrenous 604.99
gonococcal (acute) 098.13
chronic or duration of 2 months or over 098.33
mumps 072.0
parotidea 072.0
suppurative 604.99
syphilitic 095.8 *[604.91]*
tuberculous (*see also* Tuberculosis) 016.5 *[608.81]*
Orf 051.2
Organic - *see also* condition
heart - *see* Disease, heart
insufficiency 799.89
Oriental
bilharziasis 120.2
schistosomiasis 120.2
sore 085.1
Orientation
ego-dystonic sexual 302.0
Orifice - *see* condition
Origin, both great vessels from right ventricle 745.11
Ormond's disease or syndrome 593.4
Ornithosis 073.9
with
complication 073.8
specified NEC 073.7
pneumonia 073.0
pneumonitis (lobular) 073.0
Orodigitofacial dysostosis 759.89
Oropouche fever 066.3
Orotaciduria, oroticaciduria (congenital) (hereditary) (pyrimidine deficiency) 281.4
Oroya fever 088.0
Orthodontics V58.5
adjustment V53.4
aftercare V58.5
fitting V53.4
Orthopnea 786.02
Os, uterus - *see* condition
Osgood-Schlatter
disease 732.4
osteochondrosis 732.4
Osler's
disease (M9950/1) (polycythemia vera) 238.4
nodes 421.0
Osler-Rendu disease (familial hemorrhagic telangiectasia) 448.0
Osler-Vaquez disease (M9950/1) (polycythemia vera) 238.4
Osler-Weber-Rendu syndrome (familial hemorrhagic telangiectasia) 448.0
Osmidrosis 705.89
Osseous - *see* condition
Ossification
artery - *see* Arteriosclerosis
auricle (ear) 380.39
bronchus 519.19 ⬅
cardiac (*see also* Degeneration, myocardial) 429.1
cartilage (senile) 733.99
coronary - *see* Arteriosclerosis, coronary
diaphragm 728.10
ear 380.39
middle (*see also* Otosclerosis) 387.9
falx cerebri 349.2
fascia 728.10
fontanel
defective or delayed 756.0
premature 756.0
heart (*see also* Degeneration, myocardial) 429.1
valve - *see* Endocarditis
larynx 478.79
ligament
posterior longitudinal 724.8
cervical 723.7
meninges (cerebral) 349.2
spinal 336.8
multiple, eccentric centers 733.99
muscle 728.10
heterotopic, postoperative 728.13

ICD-9-CM

O

Vol. 2

Ossification *(Continued)*
myocardium, myocardial (*see also* Degeneration, myocardial) 429.1
penis 607.81
periarticular 728.89
sclera 379.16
tendon 727.82
trachea 519.19
tympanic membrane (*see also* Tympanosclerosis) 385.00
vitreous (humor) 360.44
Osteitis (*see also* Osteomyelitis) 730.2
acute 730.0
alveolar 526.5
chronic 730.1
condensans (ilii) 733.5
deformans (Paget's) 731.0
due to or associated with malignant neoplasm (*see also* Neoplasm, bone, malignant) 170.9 *[731.1]*
due to yaws 102.6
fibrosa NEC 733.29
cystica (generalisata) 252.01
disseminata 756.59
osteoplastica 252.01
fragilitans 756.51
Garré's (sclerosing) 730.1
infectious (acute) (subacute) 730.0
chronic or old 730.1
jaw (acute) (chronic) (lower) (neonatal) (suppurative) (upper) 526.4
parathyroid 252.01
petrous bone (*see also* Petrositis) 383.20
pubis 733.5
sclerotic, nonsuppurative 730.1
syphilitic 095.5
tuberculosa
cystica (of Jüngling) 135
multiplex cystoides 135
Osteoarthritica spondylitis (spine) (*see also* Spondylosis) 721.90
Osteoarthritis (*see also* Osteoarthrosis) 715.9
distal interphalangeal 715.9
hyperplastic 731.2
interspinalis (*see also* Spondylosis) 721.90
spine, spinal NEC (*see also* Spondylosis) 721.90
Osteoarthropathy (*see also* Osteoarthrosis) 715.9
chronic idiopathic hypertrophic 757.39
familial idiopathic 757.39
hypertrophic pulmonary 731.2
secondary 731.2
idiopathic hypertrophic 757.39
primary hypertrophic 731.2
pulmonary hypertrophic 731.2
secondary hypertrophic 731.2
Osteoarthrosis (degenerative) (hypertrophic) (rheumatoid) 715.9

Note Use the following fifth-digit subclassification with category 715:

0 site unspecified
1 shoulder region
2 upper arm
3 forearm
4 hand
5 pelvic region and thigh
6 lower leg
7 ankle and foot
8 other specified sites except spine
9 multiple sites

Osteoarthrosis *(Continued)*
deformans alkaptonurica 270.2
generalized 715.09
juvenilis (Köhler's) 732.5
localized 715.3
idiopathic 715.1
primary 715.1
secondary 715.2
multiple sites, not specified as generalized 715.89
polyarticular 715.09
spine (*see also* Spondylosis) 721.90
temporomandibular joint 524.69
Osteoblastoma (M9200/0) - *see* Neoplasm, bone, benign
Osteochondritis (*see also* Osteochondrosis) 732.9
dissecans 732.7
hip 732.7
ischiopubica 732.1
multiple 756.59
syphilitic (congenital) 090.0
Osteochondrodermodysplasia 756.59
Osteochondrodystrophy 277.5
deformans 277.5
familial 277.5
fetalis 756.4
Osteochondrolysis 732.7
Osteochondroma (M9210/0) - *see also* Neoplasm, bone, benign
multiple, congenital 756.4
Osteochondromatosis (M9210/1) 238.0
synovial 727.82
Osteochondromyxosarcoma (M9180/3) - *see* Neoplasm, bone, malignant
Osteochondropathy NEC 732.9
Osteochondrosarcoma (M9180/3) - *see* Neoplasm, bone, malignant
Osteochondrosis 732.9
acetabulum 732.1
adult spine 732.8
astragalus 732.5
Blount's 732.4
Buchanan's (juvenile osteochondrosis of iliac crest) 732.1
Buchman's (juvenile osteochondrosis) 732.1
Burns' 732.3
calcaneus 732.5
capitular epiphysis (femur) 732.1
carpal
lunate (wrist) 732.3
scaphoid 732.3
coxae juvenilis 732.1
deformans juvenilis (coxae) (hip) 732.1
Scheuermann's 732.0
spine 732.0
tibia 732.4
vertebra 732.0
Diaz's (astragalus) 732.5
dissecans (knee) (shoulder) 732.7
femoral capital epiphysis 732.1
femur (head) (juvenile) 732.1
foot (juvenile) 732.5
Freiberg's (disease) (second metatarsal) 732.5
Haas' 732.3
Haglund's (os tibiale externum) 732.5
hand (juvenile) 732.3
head of
femur 732.1
humerus (juvenile) 732.3
hip (juvenile) 732.1

Osteochondrosis *(Continued)*
humerus (juvenile) 732.3
iliac crest (juvenile) 732.1
ilium (juvenile) 732.1
ischiopubic synchondrosis 732.1
Iselin's (osteochondrosis fifth metatarsal) 732.5
juvenile, juvenilis 732.6
arm 732.3
capital femoral epiphysis 732.1
capitellum humeri 732.3
capitular epiphysis 732.1
carpal scaphoid 732.3
clavicle, sternal epiphysis 732.6
coxae 732.1
deformans 732.1
foot 732.5
hand 732.3
hip and pelvis 732.1
lower extremity, except foot 732.4
lunate, wrist 732.3
medial cuneiform bone 732.5
metatarsal (head) 732.5
metatarsophalangeal 732.5
navicular, ankle 732.5
patella 732.4
primary patellar center (of Köhler) 732.4
specified site NEC 732.6
spine 732.0
tarsal scaphoid 732.5
tibia (epiphysis) (tuberosity) 732.4
upper extremity 732.3
vertebra (body) (Calvé) 732.0
epiphyseal plates (of Scheuermann) 732.0
Kienböck's (disease) 732.3
Köhler's (disease) (navicular, ankle) 732.5
patellar 732.4
tarsal navicular 732.5
Legg-Calvé-Perthes (disease) 732.1
lower extremity (juvenile) 732.4
lunate bone 732.3
Mauclaire's 732.3
metacarpal heads (of Mauclaire) 732.3
metatarsal (fifth) (head) (second) 732.5
navicular, ankle 732.5
os calcis 732.5
Osgood-Schlatter 732.4
os tibiale externum 732.5
Panner's 732.3
patella (juvenile) 732.4
patellar center
primary (of Köhler) 732.4
secondary (of Sinding-Larsen) 732.4
pelvis (juvenile) 732.1
Pierson's 732.1
radial head (juvenile) 732.3
Scheuermann's 732.0
Sever's (calcaneum) 732.5
Sinding-Larsen (secondary patellar center) 732.4
spine (juvenile) 732.0
adult 732.8
symphysis pubis (of Pierson) (juvenile) 732.1
syphilitic (congenital) 090.0
tarsal (navicular) (scaphoid) 732.5
tibia (proximal) (tubercle) 732.4
tuberculous - *see* Tuberculosis, bone
ulna 732.3
upper extremity (juvenile) 732.3

Osteochondrosis *(Continued)*
van Neck's (juvenile osteochondrosis) 732.1
vertebral (juvenile) 732.0
adult 732.8
Osteoclastoma (M9250/1) 238.0
malignant (M9250/3) - *see* Neoplasm, bone, malignant
Osteocopic pain 733.90
Osteodynia 733.90
Osteodystrophy
azotemic 588.0
chronica deformans hypertrophica 731.0
congenital 756.50
specified type NEC 756.59
deformans 731.0
fibrosa localisata 731.0
parathyroid 252.01
renal 588.0
Osteofibroma (M9262/0) - *see* Neoplasm, bone, benign
Osteofibrosarcoma (M9182/3) - *see* Neoplasm, bone, malignant
Osteogenesis imperfecta 756.51
Osteogenic - *see* condition
Osteoma (M9180/0) - *see also* Neoplasm, bone, benign
osteoid (M9191/0) - *see also* Neoplasm, bone, benign
giant (M9200/0) - *see* Neoplasm, bone, benign
Osteomalacia 268.2
chronica deformans hypertrophica 731.0
due to vitamin D deficiency 268.2
infantile (*see also* Rickets) 268.0
juvenile (*see also* Rickets) 268.0
pelvis 268.2
vitamin D-resistant 275.3
Osteomalacic bone 268.2
Osteomalacosis 268.2
Osteomyelitis (general) (infective) (localized) (neonatal) (purulent) (pyogenic) (septic) (staphylococcal) (streptococcal) (suppurative) (with periostitis) 730.2

Note Use the following fifth-digit subclassification with category 730:

0 site unspecified
1 shoulder region
2 upper arm
3 forearm
4 hand
5 pelvic region and thigh
6 lower leg
7 ankle and foot
8 other specified sites
9 multiple sites

acute or subacute 730.0
chronic or old 730.1
due to or associated with
diabetes mellitus 250.8 *[731.8]*
tuberculosis (*see also* Tuberculosis, bone) 015.9 *[730.8]*
limb bones 015.5 *[730.8]*
specified bones NEC 015.7 *[730.8]*
spine 015.0 *[730.8]*
typhoid 002.0 *[730.8]*
Garré's 730.1
jaw (acute) (chronic) (lower) (neonatal) (suppurative) (upper) 526.4

Osteomyelitis *(Continued)*
nonsuppurating 730.1
orbital 376.03
petrous bone (*see also* Petrositis) 383.20
Salmonella 003.24
sclerosing, nonsuppurative 730.1
sicca 730.1
syphilitic 095.5
congenital 090.0 *[730.8]*
tuberculous - *see* Tuberculosis, bone
typhoid 002.0 *[730.8]*
Osteomyelofibrosis 289.89
Osteomyelosclerosis 289.89
Osteonecrosis 733.40
meaning osteomyelitis 730.1
Osteo-onycho-arthro dysplasia 756.89
Osteo-onychodysplasia, hereditary 756.89
Osteopathia
condensans disseminata 756.53
hyperostotica multiplex infantilis 756.59
hypertrophica toxica 731.2
striata 756.4
Osteopathy resulting from poliomyelitis (*see also* Poliomyelitis) 045.9 *[730.7]*
familial dysplastic 731.2
Osteopecilia 756.53
Osteopenia 733.90
Osteoperiostitis (*see also* Osteomyelitis) 730.2
ossificans toxica 731.2
toxica ossificans 731.2
Osteopetrosis (familial) 756.52
Osteophyte - *see* Exostosis
Osteophytosis - *see* Exostosis
Osteopoikilosis 756.53
Osteoporosis (generalized) 733.00
circumscripta 731.0
disuse 733.03
drug-induced 733.09
idiopathic 733.02
postmenopausal 733.01
posttraumatic 733.7
screening V82.81
senile 733.01
specified type NEC 733.09
Osteoporosis-osteomalacia syndrome 268.2
Osteopsathyrosis 756.51
Osteoradionecrosis, jaw 526.89
Osteosarcoma (M9180/3) - *see also* Neoplasm, bone, malignant
chondroblastic (M9181/3) - *see* Neoplasm, bone, malignant
fibroblastic (M9182/3) - *see* Neoplasm, bone, malignant
in Paget's disease of bone (M9184/3) - *see* Neoplasm, bone, malignant
juxtacortical (M9190/3) - *see* Neoplasm, bone malignant
parosteal (M9190/3) - *see* Neoplasm, bone, malignant
telangiectatic (M9183/3) - *see* Neoplasm, bone, malignant
Osteosclerosis 756.52
fragilis (generalisata) 756.52
Osteosclerotic anemia 289.89
Osteosis
acromegaloid 757.39
cutis 709.3
parathyroid 252.01
renal fibrocystic 588.0
Österreicher-Turner syndrome 756.89

Ostium
atrioventriculare commune 745.69
primum (arteriosum) (defect) (persistent) 745.61
secundum (arteriosum) (defect) (patent) (persistent) 745.5
Ostrum-Furst syndrome 756.59
Otalgia 388.70
otogenic 388.71
referred 388.72
Othematoma 380.31
Otitic hydrocephalus 348.2
Otitis 382.9
with effusion 381.4
purulent 382.4
secretory 381.4
serous 381.4
suppurative 382.4
acute 382.9
adhesive (*see also* Adhesions, middle ear) 385.10
chronic 382.9
with effusion 381.3
mucoid, mucous (simple) 381.20
purulent 382.3
secretory 381.3
serous 381.10
suppurative 382.3
diffuse parasitic 136.8
externa (acute) (diffuse) (hemorrhagica) 380.10
actinic 380.22
candidal 112.82
chemical 380.22
chronic 380.23
mycotic - *see* Otitis, externa, mycotic
specified type NEC 380.23
circumscribed 380.10
contact 380.22
due to
erysipelas 035 *[380.13]*
impetigo 684 *[380.13]*
seborrheic dermatitis 690.10 *[380.13]*
eczematoid 380.22
furuncular 680.0 *[380.13]*
infective 380.10
chronic 380.16
malignant 380.14
mycotic (chronic) 380.15
due to
aspergillosis 117.3 *[380.15]*
moniliasis 112.82
otomycosis 111.8 *[380.15]*
reactive 380.22
specified type NEC 380.22
tropical 111.8 *[380.15]*
insidiosa (*see also* Otosclerosis) 387.9
interna (*see also* Labyrinthitis) 386.30
media (hemorrhagic) (staphylococcal) (streptococcal) 382.9
acute 382.9
with effusion 381.00
allergic 381.04
mucoid 381.05
sanguineous 381.06
serous 381.04
catarrhal 381.00
exudative 381.00
mucoid 381.02
allergic 381.05
necrotizing 382.00
with spontaneous rupture of ear drum 382.01

ICD-9-CM O Vol. 2

- **Otitis** *(Continued)*
  - media *(Continued)*
    - acute *(Continued)*
      - necrotizing *(Continued)*
        - in
          - influenza 487.8 *[382.02]*
          - measles 055.2
          - scarlet fever 034.1 *[382.02]*
      - nonsuppurative 381.00
      - purulent 382.00
        - with spontaneous rupture of ear drum 382.01
      - sanguineous 381.03
        - allergic 381.06
      - secretory 381.01
      - seromucinous 381.02
      - serous 381.01
        - allergic 381.04
      - suppurative 382.00
        - with spontaneous rupture of ear drum 382.01
        - due to
          - influenza 487.8 *[382.02]*
          - scarlet fever 034.1 *[382.02]*
      - transudative 381.00
    - adhesive (*see also* Adhesions, middle ear) 385.10
    - allergic 381.4
      - acute 381.04
        - mucoid 381.05
        - sanguineous 381.06
        - serous 381.04
      - chronic 381.3
    - catarrhal 381.4
      - acute 381.00
      - chronic (simple) 381.10
    - chronic 382.9
      - with effusion 381.3
      - adhesive (*see also* Adhesions, middle ear) 385.10
      - allergic 381.3
      - atticoantral, suppurative (with posterior or superior marginal perforation of ear drum) 382.2
      - benign suppurative (with anterior perforation of ear drum) 382.1
      - catarrhal 381.10
      - exudative 381.3
      - mucinous 381.20
      - mucoid, mucous (simple) 381.20
      - mucosanguineous 381.29
      - nonsuppurative 381.3
      - purulent 382.3
      - secretory 381.3
      - seromucinous 381.3
      - serosanguineous 381.19
      - serous (simple) 381.10
      - suppurative 382.3
        - atticoantral (with posterior or superior marginal perforation of ear drum) 382.2
        - benign (with anterior perforation of ear drum) 382.1
        - tuberculous (*see also* Tuberculosis) 017.4
        - tubotympanic 382.1
      - transudative 381.3
    - exudative 381.4
      - acute 381.00
      - chronic 381.3
    - fibrotic (*see also* Adhesions, middle ear) 385.10
    - mucoid, mucous 381.4
      - acute 381.02
      - chronic (simple) 381.20
    - mucosanguineous, chronic 381.29
    - nonsuppurative 381.4
      - acute 381.00
      - chronic 381.3
    - postmeasles 055.2
    - purulent 382.4
      - acute 382.00
        - with spontaneous rupture of ear drum 382.01
      - chronic 382.3
    - sanguineous, acute 381.03
      - allergic 381.06
    - secretory 381.4
      - acute or subacute 381.01
      - chronic 381.3
    - seromucinous 381.4
      - acute or subacute 381.02
      - chronic 381.3
    - serosanguineous, chronic 381.19
    - serous 381.4
      - acute or subacute 381.01
      - chronic (simple) 381.10
    - subacute - *see* Otitis, media, acute
    - suppurative 382.4
      - acute 382.00
        - with spontaneous rupture of ear drum 382.01
      - chronic 382.3
        - atticoantral 382.2
        - benign 382.1
        - tuberculous (*see also* Tuberculosis) 017.4
        - tubotympanic 382.1
    - transudative 381.4
      - acute 381.00
      - chronic 381.3
    - tuberculous (*see also* Tuberculosis) 017.4
  - postmeasles 055.2
- **Otoconia** 386.8
- **Otolith syndrome** 386.19
- **Otomycosis** 111.8 *[380.15]*
  - in
    - aspergillosis 117.3 *[380.15]*
    - moniliasis 112.82
- **Otopathy** 388.9
- **Otoporosis** (*see also* Otosclerosis) 387.9
- **Otorrhagia** 388.69
  - traumatic - *see* nature of injury
- **Otorrhea** 388.60
  - blood 388.69
  - cerebrospinal (fluid) 388.61
- **Otosclerosis** (general) 387.9
  - cochlear (endosteal) 387.2
  - involving
    - otic capsule 387.2
    - oval window
      - nonobliterative 387.0
      - obliterative 387.1
    - round window 387.2
  - nonobliterative 387.0
  - obliterative 387.1
  - specified type NEC 387.8
- **Otospongiosis** (*see also* Otosclerosis) 387.9
- **Otto's disease or pelvis** 715.35
- **Outburst, aggressive** (*see also* Disturbance, conduct) 312.0
  - in children or adolescents 313.9
- **Outcome of delivery**
  - multiple birth NEC V27.9
    - all liveborn V27.5
    - all stillborn V27.7
    - some liveborn V27.6
    - unspecified V27.9
  - single V27.9
    - liveborn V27.0
    - stillborn V27.1
  - twins V27.9
    - both liveborn V27.2
    - both stillborn V27.4
    - one liveborn, one stillborn V27.3
- **Outlet** - *see also* condition
  - syndrome (thoracic) 353.0
- **Outstanding ears** (bilateral) 744.29
- **Ovalocytosis** (congenital) (hereditary) (*see also* Elliptocytosis) 282.1
- **Ovarian** - *see also* condition
  - pregnancy - *see* Pregnancy, ovarian
  - remnant syndrome 620.8
  - vein syndrome 593.4
- **Ovaritis** (cystic) (*see also* Salpingo-oophoritis) 614.2
- **Ovary, ovarian** - *see* condition
- **Overactive** - *see also* Hyperfunction
  - bladder 596.51
  - eye muscle (*see also* Strabismus) 378.9
  - hypothalamus 253.8
  - thyroid (*see also* Thyrotoxicosis) 242.9
- **Overactivity, child** 314.01
- **Overbite** (deep) (excessive) (horizontal) (vertical) 524.29
- **Overbreathing** (*see also* Hyperventilation) 786.01
- **Overconscientious personality** 301.4
- **Overdevelopment** - *see also* Hypertrophy
  - breast (female) (male) 611.1
  - nasal bones 738.0
  - prostate, congenital 752.89
- **Overdistention** - *see* Distention
- **Overdose overdosage** (drug) 977.9
  - specified drug or substance - *see* Table of Drugs and Chemicals
- **Overeating** 783.6
  - with obesity 278.00
  - nonorganic origin 307.51
- **Overexertion** (effects) (exhaustion) 994.5
- **Overexposure** (effects) 994.9
  - exhaustion 994.4
- **Overfeeding** (*see also* Overeating) 783.6
- **Overfill, endodontic** 526.62 ◀
- **Overgrowth, bone NEC** 733.99
- **Overhanging** ◀
  - tooth restoration 525.62 ◀
  - unrepairable, dental restorative materials 525.62 ◀
- **Overheated** (effects) (places) - *see* Heat
- **Overinhibited child** 313.0
- **Overjet** 524.29
  - excessive horizontal 524.26 ◀
- **Overlaid, overlying** (suffocation) 994.7
- **Overlap**
  - excessive horizontal 524.26
- **Overlapping toe** (acquired) 735.8
  - congenital (fifth toe) 755.66
- **Overload**
  - fluid 276.6
  - potassium (K) 276.7
  - sodium (Na) 276.0
- **Overnutrition** (*see also* Hyperalimentation) 783.6
- **Overproduction** - *see also* Hypersecretion
  - ACTH 255.3

Overproduction *(Continued)*
cortisol 255.0
growth hormone 253.0
thyroid-stimulating hormone (TSH) 242.8
Overriding
aorta 747.21
finger (acquired) 736.29
congenital 755.59
toe (acquired) 735.8
congenital 755.66
Oversize
fetus (weight of 4500 grams or more) 766.0
affecting management of pregnancy 656.6
causing disproportion 653.5
with obstructed labor 660.1
affecting fetus or newborn 763.1
Overstimulation, ovarian 256.1
Overstrained 780.79
heart - *see* Hypertrophy, cardiac
Overweight (*see also* Obesity) 278.02
Overwork 780.79
Oviduct - *see* condition
Ovotestis 752.7
Ovulation (cycle)
failure or lack of 628.0
pain 625.2
Ovum
blighted 631
donor V59.70
over age 35 V59.73
anonymous recipient V59.73
designated recipient V59.74
under age 35 V59.71
anonymous recipient V59.71
Ovum *(Continued)*
donor *(Continued)*
under age 35 *(Continued)*
designated recipient V59.72
dropsical 631
pathologic 631
Owren's disease or syndrome (parahemophilia) (*see also* Defect, coagulation) 286.3
Oxalosis 271.8
Oxaluria 271.8
Ox heart - *see* Hypertrophy, cardiac
OX syndrome 758.6
Oxycephaly, oxycephalic 756.0
syphilitic, congenital 090.0
Oxyuriasis 127.4
Oxyuris vermicularis (infestation) 127.4
Ozena 472.0

P

Pacemaker syndrome 429.4
Pachyderma, pachydermia 701.8
  laryngis 478.5
  laryngitis 478.79
  larynx (verrucosa) 478.79
Pachydermatitis 701.8
Pachydermatocele (congenital) 757.39
  acquired 701.8
Pachydermatosis 701.8
Pachydermoperiostitis
  secondary 731.2
Pachydermoperiostosis
  primary idiopathic 757.39
  secondary 731.2
Pachymeningitis (adhesive) (basal) (brain) (cerebral) (cervical) (chronic) (circumscribed) (external) (fibrous) (hemorrhagic) (hypertrophic) (internal) (purulent) (spinal) (suppurative) (*see also* Meningitis) 322.9
  gonococcal 098.82
Pachyonychia (congenital) 757.5
  acquired 703.8
Pachyperiosteodermia
  primary or idiopathic 757.39
  secondary 731.2
Pachyperiostosis
  primary or idiopathic 757.39
  secondary 731.2
Pacinian tumor (M9507/0) - *see* Neoplasm, skin, benign
Pads, knuckle or Garrod's 728.79
Paget's disease (osteitis deformans) 731.0
  with infiltrating duct carcinoma of the breast (M8541/3) - *see* Neoplasm, breast, malignant
  bone 731.0
    osteosarcoma in (M9184/3) - *see* Neoplasm, bone, malignant
  breast (M8540/3) 174.0
  extramammary (M8542/3) - *see also* Neoplasm, skin, malignant
    anus 154.3
    skin 173.5
  malignant (M8540/3)
    breast 174.0
    specified site NEC (M8542/3) - *see* Neoplasm, skin, malignant
    unspecified site 174.0
  mammary (M8540/3) 174.0
  necrosis of bone 731.0
  nipple (M8540/3) 174.0
  osteitis deformans 731.0
Paget-Schroetter syndrome (intermittent venous claudication) 453.8
Pain(s) 780.96 ⬅
  abdominal 789.0
  acute 338.19 ◀
    due to trauma 338.11 ◀
    postoperative 338.18 ◀
      post-thoracotomy 338.12 ◀
  adnexa (uteri) 625.9
  alimentary, due to vascular insufficiency 557.9
  anginoid (*see also* Pain, precordial) 786.51
  anus 569.42
  arch 729.5
  arm 729.5
  axillary 729.5 ◀
  back (postural) 724.5
    low 724.2
    psychogenic 307.89

Pain(s) *(Continued)*
  bile duct 576.9
  bladder 788.9
  bone 733.90
  breast 611.71
    psychogenic 307.89
  broad ligament 625.9
  cancer associated 338.3 ◀
  cartilage NEC 733.90
  cecum 789.0
  cervicobrachial 723.3
  chest (central) 786.50
    atypical 786.59
    midsternal 786.51
    musculoskeletal 786.59
    noncardiac 786.59
    substernal 786.51
    wall (anterior) 786.52
  chronic 338.29 ◀
    associated with significant psychosocial dysfunction 338.4 ◀
    due to trauma 338.21 ◀
    postoperative 338.28 ◀
      post-thoracotomy 338.22 ◀
    syndrome 338.4 ◀
  coccyx 724.79
  colon 789.0
  common duct 576.9
  coronary - *see* Angina
  costochondral 786.52
  diaphragm 786.52
  due to (presence of) any device, implant, or graft classifiable to 996.0–996.5 - *see* Complications, due to (presence of) any device, implant, or graft classified to 996.0–996.5 NEC
    malignancy (primary) (secondary) 338.3 ◀
  ear (*see also* Otalgia) 388.70
  epigastric, epigastrium 789.06
  extremity (lower) (upper) 729.5
  eye 379.91
  face, facial 784.0
    atypical 350.2
    nerve 351.8
  false (labor) 644.1
  female genital organ NEC 625.9
    psychogenic 307.89
  finger 729.5
  flank 789.0
  foot 729.5
  gallbladder 575.9
  gas (intestinal) 787.3
  gastric 536.8
  generalized 780.96 ⬅
  genital organ
    female 625.9
    male 608.9
    psychogenic 307.89
  groin 789.0
  growing 781.99
  hand 729.5
  head (*see also* Headache) 784.0
  heart (*see also* Pain, precordial) 786.51
  infraorbital (*see also* Neuralgia, trigeminal) 350.1
  intermenstrual 625.2
  jaw 526.9
  joint 719.40
    ankle 719.47
    elbow 719.42
    foot 719.47
    hand 719.44
    hip 719.45

Pain(s) *(Continued)*
  joint *(Continued)*
    knee 719.46
    multiple sites 719.49
    pelvic region 719.45
    psychogenic 307.89
    shoulder (region) 719.41
    specified site NEC 719.48
    wrist 719.43
  kidney 788.0
  labor, false or spurious 644.1
  laryngeal 784.1
  leg 729.5
  limb 729.5
  low back 724.2
  lumbar region 724.2
  mastoid (*see also* Otalgia) 388.70
  maxilla 526.9
  metacarpophalangeal (joint) 719.44
  metatarsophalangeal (joint) 719.47
  mouth 528.9
  muscle 729.1
    intercostal 786.59
  musculoskeletal (*see also* Pain, by site) 729.1 ◀
  nasal 478.19 ⬅
  nasopharynx 478.29
  neck NEC 723.1
    psychogenic 307.89
  neoplasm related (acute) (chronic) 338.3 ◀
  nerve NEC 729.2
  neuromuscular 729.1
  nose 478.19 ⬅
  ocular 379.91
  ophthalmic 379.91
  orbital region 379.91
  osteocopic 733.90
  ovary 625.9
    psychogenic 307.89
  over heart (*see also* Pain, precordial) 786.51
  ovulation 625.2
  pelvic (female) 625.9
    male NEC 789.0
      psychogenic 307.89
    psychogenic 307.89
  penis 607.9
    psychogenic 307.89
  pericardial (*see also* Pain, precordial) 786.51
  perineum
    female 625.9
    male 608.9
  pharynx 478.29
  pleura, pleural, pleuritic 786.52
  postoperative 338.18 ⬅
    acute 338.18 ◀
    chronic 338.28 ◀
  post-thoracotomy 338.12 ◀
    acute 338.12 ◀
    chronic 338.22 ◀
  preauricular 388.70
  precordial (region) 786.51
    psychogenic 307.89
  psychogenic 307.80
    cardiovascular system 307.89
    gastrointestinal system 307.89
    genitourinary system 307.89
    heart 307.89
    musculoskeletal system 307.89
    respiratory system 307.89
    skin 306.3
  radicular (spinal) (*see also* Radiculitis) 729.2

◀ **New** ⬅ **Revised**

Pain(s) *(Continued)*
  rectum 569.42
  respiration 786.52
  retrosternal 786.51
  rheumatic NEC 729.0
    muscular 729.1
  rib 786.50
  root (spinal) (*see also* Radiculitis) 729.2
  round ligament (stretch) 625.9
  sacroiliac 724.6
  sciatic 724.3
  scrotum 608.9
    psychogenic 307.89
  seminal vesicle 608.9
  sinus 478.19
  skin 782.0
  spermatic cord 608.9
  spinal root (*see also* Radiculitis) 729.2
  stomach 536.8
    psychogenic 307.89
  substernal 786.51
  temporomandibular (joint) 524.62
  temporomaxillary joint 524.62
  testis 608.9
    psychogenic 307.89
  thoracic spine 724.1
    with radicular and visceral pain 724.4
  throat 784.1
  tibia 733.90
  toe 729.5
  tongue 529.6
  tooth 525.9
  trigeminal (*see also* Neuralgia, trigeminal) 350.1
  tumor associated 338.3
  umbilicus 789.05
  ureter 788.0
  urinary (organ) (system) 788.0
  uterus 625.9
    psychogenic 307.89
  vagina 625.9
  vertebrogenic (syndrome) 724.5
  vesical 788.9
  vulva 625.9
  xiphoid 733.90
Painful - *see also* Pain
  arc syndrome 726.19
  coitus
    female 625.0
    male 608.89
    psychogenic 302.76
  ejaculation (semen) 608.89
    psychogenic 302.79
  erection 607.3
  feet syndrome 266.2
  menstruation 625.3
    psychogenic 306.52
  micturition 788.1
  ophthalmoplegia 378.55
  respiration 786.52
  scar NEC 709.2
  urination 788.1
  wire sutures 998.89
Painters' colic 984.9
  specified type of lead - *see* Table of Drugs and Chemicals
Palate - *see* condition
Palatoplegia 528.9
Palatoschisis (*see also* Cleft, palate) 749.00
Palilalia 784.69
Palindromic arthritis (*see also* Rheumatism, palindromic) 719.3
Palliative care V66.7
Pallor 782.61
  temporal, optic disc 377.15
Palmar - *see also* condition
  fascia - *see* condition
Palpable
  cecum 569.89
  kidney 593.89
  liver 573.9
  lymph nodes 785.6
  ovary 620.8
  prostate 602.9
  spleen (*see also* Splenomegaly) 789.2
  uterus 625.8
Palpitation (heart) 785.1
  psychogenic 306.2
Palsy (*see also* Paralysis) 344.9
  atrophic diffuse 335.20
  Bell's 351.0
    newborn 767.5
  birth 767.7
  brachial plexus 353.0
    fetus or newborn 767.6
  brain - *see also* Palsy, cerebral
    noncongenital or noninfantile 344.89
      late effects - *see* Late effect(s) (of) cerebrovascular disease
    syphilitic 094.89
      congenital 090.49
  bulbar (chronic) (progressive) 335.22
    pseudo NEC 335.23
    supranuclear NEC 344.89
  cerebral (congenital) (infantile) (spastic) 343.9
    athetoid 333.71
    diplegic 343.0
      late effects - *see* Late effect(s) (of) cerebrovascular disease
    hemiplegic 343.1
    monoplegic 343.3
    noncongenital or noninfantile 437.8
      late effects - *see* Late effect(s) (of) cerebrovascular disease
    paraplegic 343.0
    quadriplegic 343.2
    spastic, not congenital or infantile 344.89
    syphilitic 094.89
      congenital 090.49
    tetraplegic 343.2
  cranial nerve - *see also* Disorder, nerve, cranial
    multiple 352.6
  creeping 335.21
  divers' 993.3
  erb's (birth injury) 767.6
  facial 351.0
    newborn 767.5
  glossopharyngeal 352.2
  Klumpke (-Déjérine) 767.6
  lead 984.9
    specified type of lead - *see* Table of Drugs and Chemicals
  median nerve (tardy) 354.0
  peroneal nerve (acute) (tardy) 355.3
  progressive supranuclear 333.0
  pseudobulbar NEC 335.23
  radial nerve (acute) 354.3
  seventh nerve 351.0
    newborn 767.5
  shaking (*see also* Parkinsonism) 332.0
  spastic (cerebral) (spinal) 343.9
    hemiplegic 343.1
  specified nerve NEC - *see* Disorder, nerve
  supranuclear NEC 356.8
    progressive 333.0
  ulnar nerve (tardy) 354.2
  wasting 335.21
Paltauf-Sternberg disease 201.9
Paludism - *see* Malaria
Panama fever 084.0
Panaris (with lymphangitis) 681.9
  finger 681.02
  toe 681.11
Panaritium (with lymphangitis) 681.9
  finger 681.02
  toe 681.11
Panarteritis (nodosa) 446.0
  brain or cerebral 437.4
Pancake heart 793.2
  with cor pulmonale (chronic) 416.9
Pancarditis (acute) (chronic) 429.89
  with
    rheumatic
      fever (active) (acute) (chronic) (subacute) 391.8
        inactive or quiescent 398.99
  rheumatic, acute 391.8
    chronic or inactive 398.99
Pancoast's syndrome or tumor (carcinoma, pulmonary apex) (M8010/3) 162.3
Pancoast-Tobias syndrome (M8010/3) (carcinoma, pulmonary apex) 162.3
Pancolitis 556.6
Pancreas, pancreatic - *see* condition
Pancreatitis 577.0
  acute (edematous) (hemorrhagic) (recurrent) 577.0
  annular 577.0
  apoplectic 577.0
  calcereous 577.0
  chronic (infectious) 577.1
    recurrent 577.1
  cystic 577.2
  fibrous 577.8
  gangrenous 577.0
  hemorrhagic (acute) 577.0
  interstitial (chronic) 577.1
    acute 577.0
  malignant 577.0
  mumps 072.3
  painless 577.1
  recurrent 577.1
  relapsing 577.1
  subacute 577.0
  suppurative 577.0
  syphilitic 095.8
Pancreatolithiasis 577.8
Pancytolysis 289.9
Pancytopenia (acquired) 284.1
  with malformations 284.09
  congenital 284.09
Panencephalitis - *see also* Encephalitis
  subacute, sclerosing 046.2
Panhematopenia 284.8
  congenital 284.09
  constitutional 284.09
  splenic, primary 289.4
Panhemocytopenia 284.8
  congenital 284.09
  constitutional 284.09
Panhypogonadism 257.2
Panhypopituitarism 253.2
  prepubertal 253.3
Panic (attack) (state) 300.01
  reaction to exceptional stress (transient) 308.0
Panmyelopathy, familial constitutional 284.09
Panmyelophthisis 284.2
  acquired (secondary) 284.8
  congenital 284.2
  idiopathic 284.9

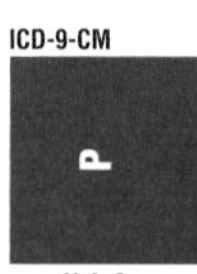
ICD-9-CM
P
Vol. 2

Panmyelosis (acute) (M9951/1) 238.79 ⬅
Panner's disease 732.3
  capitellum humeri 732.3
  head of humerus 732.3
  tarsal navicular (bone) (osteochondrosis) 732.5
Panneuritis endemica 265.0 *[357.4]*
Panniculitis 729.30
  back 724.8
  knee 729.31
  mesenteric 567.82
  neck 723.6
  nodular, nonsuppurative 729.30
  sacral 724.8
  specified site NEC 729.39
Panniculus adiposus (abdominal) 278.1
Pannus (corneal) 370.62 ⬅
  abdominal (symptomatic) 278.1 ◀
  allergic eczematous 370.62
  degenerativus 370.62
  keratic 370.62
  rheumatoid - *see* Arthritis, rheumatoid
  trachomatosus, trachomatous (active) 076.1 *[370.62]*
    late effect 139.1
Panophthalmitis 360.02
Panotitis - *see* Otitis media
Pansinusitis (chronic) (hyperplastic) (nonpurulent) (purulent) 473.8
  acute 461.8
  due to fungus NEC 117.9
  tuberculous (*see also* Tuberculosis) 012.8
Panuveitis 360.12
  sympathetic 360.11
Panvalvular disease - *see* Endocarditis, mitral
Papageienkrankheit 073.9
Papanicolaou smear
  cervix (screening test) V76.2
    as part of gynecological examination V72.31
    for suspected malignant neoplasm V76.2
      no disease found V71.1
    inadequate sample 795.08
    nonspecific abnormal finding 795.00
      with
        atypical squamous cells
          cannot exclude high grade squamous intraepithelial lesion (ASC-H) 795.02
          of undetermined significance (ASC-US) 795.01
        cytologic evidence of malignancy 795.06 ◀
        high grade squamous intraepithelial lesion (HGSIL) 795.04
        low grade squamous intraepithelial lesion (LGSIL) 795.03
      nonspecific finding NEC 795.09
      to confirm findings of recent normal smear following initial abnormal smear V72.32
      unsatisfactory 795.08
  other specified site - *see also* Screening, malignant neoplasm
    for suspected malignant neoplasm - *see also* Screening, malignant neoplasm
      no disease found V71.1
    nonspecific abnormal finding 795.1
    vagina V67.47
      following hysterectomy for malignant condition V67.01
Papilledema 377.00
  associated with
    decreased ocular pressure 377.02
    increased intracranial pressure 377.01
    retinal disorder 377.03
  choked disc 377.00
  infectional 377.00
Papillitis 377.31
  anus 569.49
  chronic lingual 529.4
  necrotizing, kidney 584.7
  optic 377.31
  rectum 569.49
  renal, necrotizing 584.7
  tongue 529.0
Papilloma (M8050/0) - *see also* Neoplasm, by site, benign

Note Except where otherwise indicated, the morphological varieties of papilloma in the list below should be coded by site as for "Neoplasm, benign".

  Acuminatum (female) (male) 078.11
  bladder (urinary) (transitional cell) (M8120/1) 236.7
    benign (M8120/0) 223.3
  choroid plexus (M9390/0) 225.0
    anaplastic type (M9390/3) 191.5
    malignant (M9390/3) 191.5
  ductal (M8503/0)
  dyskeratotic (M8052/0)
  epidermoid (M8052/0)
  hyperkeratotic (M8052/0)
  intracystic (M8504/0)
  intraductal (M8503/0)
  inverted (M8053/0)
  keratotic (M8052/0)
  parakeratotic (M8052/0)
  pinta (primary) 103.0
  renal pelvis (transitional cell) (M8120/1) 236.99
    benign (M8120/0) 223.1
  Schneiderian (M8121/0)
    specified site - *see* Neoplasm, by site, benign
    unspecified site 212.0
  serous surface (M8461/0)
    borderline malignancy (M8461/1)
      specified site - *see* Neoplasm, by site, uncertain behavior
      unspecified site 236.2
    specified site - *see* Neoplasm, by site, benign
    unspecified site 220
  squamous (cell) (M8052/0)
  transitional (cell) (M8120/0)
    bladder (urinary) (M8120/1) 236.7
    inverted type (M8121/1) - *see* Neoplasm, by site, uncertain behavior
    renal pelvis (M8120/1) 236.91
    ureter (M8120/1) 236.91
  ureter (transitional cell) (M8120/1) 236.91
    benign (M8120/0) 223.2
  urothelial (M8120/1) - *see* Neoplasm, by site, uncertain behavior
  verrucous (M8051/0)
  villous (M8261/1) - *see* Neoplasm, by site, uncertain behavior
  yaws, plantar or palmar 102.1
Papillomata, multiple, of yaws 102.1
Papillomatosis (M8060/0) - *see also* Neoplasm, by site, benign
Papillomatosis *(Continued)*
  confluent and reticulate 701.8
  cutaneous 701.8
  ductal, breast 610.1
  Gougerot-Carteaud (confluent reticulate) 701.8
  intraductal (diffuse) (M8505/0) - *see* Neoplasm, by site, benign
  subareolar duct (M8506/0) 217
Papillon-Léage and Psaume syndrome (orodigitofacial dysostosis) 759.89
Papule 709.8
  carate (primary) 103.0
  fibrous, of nose (M8724/0) 216.3
  pinta (primary) 103.0
Papulosis, malignant 447.8
Papyraceous fetus 779.89
  complicating pregnancy 646.0
Paracephalus 759.7
Parachute mitral valve 746.5
Paracoccidioidomycosis 116.1
  mucocutaneous-lymphangitic 116.1
  pulmonary 116.1
  visceral 116.1
Paracoccidiomycosis - *see* Paracoccidioidomycosis
Paracusis 388.40
Paradentosis 523.5
Paradoxical facial movements 374.43
Paraffinoma 999.9
Paraganglioma (M8680/1)
  adrenal (M8700/0) 227.0
    malignant (M8700/3) 194.0
  aortic body (M8691/1) 237.3
    malignant (M8691/3) 194.6
  carotid body (M8692/1) 237.3
    malignant (M8692/3) 194.5
  chromaffin (M8700/0) - *see also* Neoplasm, by site, benign
    malignant (M8700/3) - *see* Neoplasm, by site, malignant
  extra-adrenal (M8693/1)
    malignant (M8693/3)
      specified site - *see* Neoplasm, by site, malignant
      unspecified site 194.6
    specified site - *see* Neoplasm, by site, uncertain behavior
    unspecified site 237.3
  glomus jugulare (M8690/1) 237.3
    malignant (M8690/3) 194.6
  jugular (M8690/1) 237.3
  malignant (M8680/3)
    specified site - *see* Neoplasm, by site, malignant
    unspecified site 194.6
  nonchromaffin (M8693/1)
    malignant (M8693/3)
      specified site - *see* Neoplasm, by site, malignant
      unspecified site 194.6
    specified site - *see* Neoplasm, by site, uncertain behavior
    unspecified site 237.3
  parasympathetic (M8682/1)
    specified site - *see* Neoplasm, by site, uncertain behavior
    unspecified site 237.3
  specified site - *see* Neoplasm, by site, uncertain behavior
  sympathetic (M8681/1)
    specified site - *see* Neoplasm, by site, uncertain behavior
    unspecified site 237.3
  unspecified site 237.3

Parageusia 781.1
psychogenic 306.7
Paragonimiasis 121.2
Paragranuloma, Hodgkin's (M9660/3) 201.0
Parahemophilia (*see also* Defect, coagulation) 286.3
Parakeratosis 690.8
psoriasiformis 696.2
variegata 696.2
Paralysis, paralytic (complete) (incomplete) 344.9
with
broken
back - *see* Fracture, vertebra, by site, with spinal cord injury
neck - *see* Fracture, vertebra, cervical, with spinal cord injury
fracture, vertebra - *see* Fracture, vertebra, by site, with spinal cord injury
syphilis 094.89
abdomen and back muscles 355.9
abdominal muscles 355.9
abducens (nerve) 378.54
abductor 355.9
lower extremity 355.8
upper extremity 354.9
accessory nerve 352.4
accommodation 367.51
hysterical 300.11
acoustic nerve 388.5
agitans 332.0
arteriosclerotic 332.0
alternating 344.89
oculomotor 344.89
amyotrophic 335.20
ankle 355.8
anterior serratus 355.9
anus (sphincter) 569.49
apoplectic (current episode) (*see also* Disease, cerebrovascular, acute) 436
late effect - *see* Late effect(s) (of) cerebrovascular disease
arm 344.40
affecting
dominant side 344.41
nondominant side 344.42
both 344.2
hysterical 300.11
late effect - *see* Late effect(s) (of) cerebrovascular disease
psychogenic 306.0
transient 781.4
traumatic NEC (*see also* Injury, nerve, upper limb) 955.9
arteriosclerotic (current episode) 437.0
late effect - *see* Late effect(s) (of) cerebrovascular disease
ascending (spinal), acute 357.0
associated, nuclear 344.89
asthenic bulbar 358.00
ataxic NEC 334.9
general 094.1
athetoid 333.71
atrophic 356.9
infantile, acute (*see also* Poliomyelitis, with paralysis) 045.1
muscle NEC 355.9
progressive 335.21
spinal (acute) (*see also* Poliomyelitis, with paralysis) 045.1
attack (*see also* Disease, cerebrovascular, acute) 436

Paralysis, paralytic *(Continued)*
axillary 353.0
Babinski-Nageotte's 344.89
Bell's 351.0
newborn 767.5
Benedikt's 344.89
birth (injury) 767.7
brain 767.0
intracranial 767.0
spinal cord 767.4
bladder (sphincter) 596.53
neurogenic 596.54
with cauda equina syndrome 344.61
puerperal, postpartum, childbirth 665.5
sensory 596.54
with cauda equina 344.61
spastic 596.54
with cauda equina 344.61
bowel, colon, or intestine (*see also* Ileus) 560.1
brachial plexus 353.0
due to birth injury 767.6
newborn 767.6
brain
congenital - *see* Palsy, cerebral
current episode 437.8
diplegia 344.2
late effect - *see* Late effect(s) (of) cerebrovascular disease
hemiplegia 342.9
late effect - *see* Late effect(s) (of) cerebrovascular disease
infantile - *see* Palsy, cerebral
monoplegia - *see also* Monoplegia
late effect - *see* Late effect(s) (of) cerebrovascular disease
paraplegia 344.1
quadriplegia - *see* Quadriplegia
syphilitic, congenital 090.49
triplegia 344.89
bronchi 519.19
Brown-Séquard's 344.89
bulbar (chronic) (progressive) 335.22
infantile (*see also* Poliomyelitis, bulbar) 045.0
poliomyelitic (*see also* Poliomyelitis, bulbar) 045.0
pseudo 335.23
supranuclear 344.89
bulbospinal 358.00
cardiac (*see also* Failure, heart) 428.9
cerebral
current episode 437.8
spastic, infantile - *see* Palsy, cerebral
cerebrocerebellar 437.8
diplegic infantile 343.0
cervical
plexus 353.2
sympathetic NEC 337.0
Céstan-Chenais 344.89
Charcôt-Marie-Tooth type 356.1
childhood - *see* Palsy, cerebral
Clark's 343.9
colon (*see also* Ileus) 560.1
compressed air 993.3
compression
arm NEC 354.9
cerebral - *see* Paralysis, brain
leg NEC 355.8
lower extremity NEC 355.8
upper extremity NEC 354.9
congenital (cerebral) (spastic) (spinal) - *see* Palsy, cerebral

Paralysis, paralytic *(Continued)*
conjugate movement (of eye) 378.81
cortical (nuclear) (supranuclear) 378.81
convergence 378.83
cordis (*see also* Failure, heart) 428.9
cortical (*see also* Paralysis, brain) 437.8
cranial or cerebral nerve (*see also* Disorder, nerve, cranial) 352.9
creeping 335.21
crossed leg 344.89
crutch 953.4
deglutition 784.99
hysterical 300.11
dementia 094.1
descending (spinal) NEC 335.9
diaphragm (flaccid) 519.4
due to accidental section of phrenic nerve during procedure 998.2
digestive organs NEC 564.89
diplegic - *see* Diplegia
divergence (nuclear) 378.85
divers' 993.3
Duchenne's 335.22
due to intracranial or spinal birth injury - *see* Palsy, cerebral
embolic (current episode) (*see also* Embolism, brain) 434.1
late effect - *see* Late effect(s) (of) cerebrovascular disease
enteric (*see also* Ileus) 560.1
with hernia - *see* Hernia, by site, with obstruction
Erb's syphilitic spastic spinal 094.89
Erb (-Duchenne) (birth) (newborn) 767.6
esophagus 530.89
essential, infancy (*see also* Poliomyelitis) 045.9
extremity
lower - *see* Paralysis, leg
spastic (hereditary) 343.3
noncongenital or noninfantile 344.1
transient (cause unknown) 781.4
upper - *see* Paralysis, arm
eye muscle (extrinsic) 378.55
intrinsic 367.51
facial (nerve) 351.0
birth injury 767.5
congenital 767.5
following operation NEC 998.2
newborn 767.5
familial 359.3
periodic 359.3
spastic 334.1
fauces 478.29
finger NEC 354.9
foot NEC 355.8
gait 781.2
gastric nerve 352.3
gaze 378.81
general 094.1
ataxic 094.1
insane 094.1
juvenile 090.40
progressive 094.1
tabetic 094.1
glossopharyngeal (nerve) 352.2
glottis (*see also* Paralysis, vocal cord) 478.30
gluteal 353.4
Gubler (-Millard) 344.89
hand 354.9
hysterical 300.11
psychogenic 306.0

ICD-9-CM
P
Vol. 2

Paralysis, paralytic *(Continued)*
heart (*see also* Failure, heart) 428.9
hemifacial, progressive 349.89
hemiplegic - *see* Hemiplegia
hyperkalemic periodic (familial) 359.3
hypertensive (current episode) 437.8
hypoglossal (nerve) 352.5
hypokalemic periodic 359.3
Hyrtl's sphincter (rectum) 569.49
hysterical 300.11
ileus (*see also* Ileus) 560.1
infantile (*see also* Poliomyelitis) 045.9
atrophic acute 045.1
bulbar 045.0
cerebral - *see* Palsy, cerebral
paralytic 045.1
progressive acute 045.9
spastic - *see* Palsy, cerebral
spinal 045.9
infective (*see also* Poliomyelitis) 045.9
inferior nuclear 344.9
insane, general or progressive 094.1
internuclear 378.86
interosseous 355.9
intestine (*see also* Ileus) 560.1
intracranial (current episode) (*see also* Paralysis, brain) 437.8
due to birth injury 767.0
iris 379.49
due to diphtheria (toxin) 032.81 *[379.49]*
ischemic, Volkmann's (complicating trauma) 958.6
isolated sleep, recurrent 327.43
Jackson's 344.89
jake 357.7
Jamaica ginger (jake) 357.7
juvenile general 090.40
Klumpke (-Déjérine) (birth) (newborn) 767.6
labioglossal (laryngeal) (pharyngeal) 335.22
Landry's 357.0
laryngeal nerve (recurrent) (superior) (*see also* Paralysis, vocal cord) 478.30
larynx (*see also* Paralysis, vocal cord) 478.30
due to diphtheria (toxin) 032.3
late effect
due to
birth injury, brain or spinal (cord) - *see* Palsy, cerebral
edema, brain or cerebral - *see* Paralysis, brain
lesion
cerebrovascular - *see* Late effect(s) (of) cerebrovascular disease
spinal (cord) - *see* Paralysis, spinal
lateral 335.24
lead 984.9
specified type of lead - *see* Table of Drugs and Chemicals
left side - *see* Hemiplegia
leg 344.30
affecting
dominant side 344.31
nondominant side 344.32
both (*see also* Paraplegia) 344.1
crossed 344.89
hysterical 300.11
psychogenic 306.0
transient or transitory 781.4
traumatic NEC (*see also* Injury, nerve, lower limb) 956.9

Paralysis, paralytic *(Continued)*
levator palpebrae superioris 374.31
limb NEC 344.5
all four - *see* Quadriplegia
quadriplegia - *see* Quadriplegia
lip 528.5
Lissauer's 094.1
local 355.9
lower limb - *see also* Paralysis, leg
both (*see also* Paraplegia) 344.1
lung 518.89
newborn 770.89
median nerve 354.1
medullary (tegmental) 344.89
mesencephalic NEC 344.89
tegmental 344.89
middle alternating 344.89
Millard-Gubler-Foville 344.89
monoplegic - *see* Monoplegia
motor NEC 344.9
cerebral - *see* Paralysis, brain
spinal - *see* Paralysis, spinal
multiple
cerebral - *see* Paralysis, brain
spinal - *see* Paralysis, spinal
muscle (flaccid) 359.9
due to nerve lesion NEC 355.9
eye (extrinsic) 378.55
intrinsic 367.51
oblique 378.51
iris sphincter 364.8
ischemic (complicating trauma) (Volkmann's) 958.6
pseudohypertrophic 359.1
muscular (atrophic) 359.9
progressive 335.21
musculocutaneous nerve 354.9
musculospiral 354.9
nerve - *see also* Disorder, nerve
third or oculomotor (partial) 378.51
total 378.52
fourth or trochlear 378.53
sixth or abducens 378.54
seventh or facial 351.0
birth injury 767.5
due to
injection NEC 999.9
operation NEC 997.09
newborn 767.5
accessory 352.4
auditory 388.5
birth injury 767.7
cranial or cerebral (*see also* Disorder, nerve, cranial) 352.9
facial 351.0
birth injury 767.5
newborn 767.5
laryngeal (*see also* Paralysis, vocal cord) 478.30
newborn 767.7
phrenic 354.8
newborn 767.7
radial 354.3
birth injury 767.6
newborn 767.6
syphilitic 094.89
traumatic NEC (*see also* Injury, nerve, by site) 957.9
trigeminal 350.9
ulnar 354.2
newborn NEC 767.0
normokalemic periodic 359.3
obstetrical, newborn 767.7
ocular 378.9
oculofacial, congenital 352.6

Paralysis, paralytic *(Continued)*
oculomotor (nerve) (partial) 378.51
alternating 344.89
external bilateral 378.55
total 378.52
olfactory nerve 352.0
palate 528.9
palatopharyngolaryngeal 352.6
paratrigeminal 350.9
periodic (familial) (hyperkalemic) (hypokalemic) (normokalemic) (secondary) 359.3
peripheral
autonomic nervous system - *see* Neuropathy, peripheral, autonomic
nerve NEC 355.9
peroneal (nerve) 355.3
pharynx 478.29
phrenic nerve 354.8
plantar nerves 355.6
pneumogastric nerve 352.3
poliomyelitis (current) (*see also* Poliomyelitis, with paralysis) 045.1
bulbar 045.0
popliteal nerve 355.3
pressure (*see also* Neuropathy, entrapment) 355.9
progressive 335.21
atrophic 335.21
bulbar 335.22
general 094.1
hemifacial 349.89
infantile, acute (*see also* Poliomyelitis) 045.9
multiple 335.20
pseudobulbar 335.23
pseudohypertrophic 359.1
muscle 359.1
psychogenic 306.0
pupil, pupillary 379.49
quadriceps 355.8
quadriplegic (*see also* Quadriplegia) 344.0
radial nerve 354.3
birth injury 767.6
rectum (sphincter) 569.49
rectus muscle (eye) 378.55
recurrent
isolated sleep 327.43
laryngeal nerve (*see also* Paralysis, vocal cord) 478.30
respiratory (muscle) (system) (tract) 786.09
center NEC 344.89
fetus or newborn 770.87 (Revised)
congenital 768.9
newborn 768.9
right side - *see* Hemiplegia
Saturday night 354.3
saturnine 984.9
specified type of lead - *see* Table of Drugs and Chemicals
sciatic nerve 355.0
secondary - *see* Paralysis, late effect
seizure (cerebral) (current episode) (*see also* Disease, cerebrovascular, acute) 436
late effect - *see* Late effect(s) (of) cerebrovascular disease
senile NEC 344.9
serratus magnus 355.9
shaking (*see also* Parkinsonism) 332.0
shock (*see also* Disease, cerebrovascular, acute) 436
late effect - *see* Late effect(s) (of) cerebrovascular disease

Paralysis, paralytic *(Continued)*
shoulder 354.9
soft palate 528.9
spasmodic - *see* Paralysis, spastic
spastic 344.9
cerebral infantile - *see* Palsy, cerebral
congenital (cerebral) - *see* Palsy, cerebral
familial 334.1
hereditary 334.1
infantile 343.9
noncongenital or noninfantile, cerebral 344.9
syphilitic 094.0
spinal 094.89
sphincter, bladder (*see also* Paralysis, bladder) 596.53
spinal (cord) NEC 344.1
accessory nerve 352.4
acute (*see also* Poliomyelitis) 045.9
ascending acute 357.0
atrophic (acute) (*see also* Poliomyelitis, with paralysis) 045.1
spastic, syphilitic 094.89
congenital NEC 343.9
hemiplegic - *see* Hemiplegia
hereditary 336.8
infantile (*see also* Poliomyelitis) 045.9
late effect NEC 344.89
monoplegic - *see* Monoplegia
nerve 355.9
progressive 335.10
quadriplegic - *see* Quadriplegia
spastic NEC 343.9
traumatic - *see* Injury, spinal, by site
sternomastoid 352.4
stomach 536.3
diabetic 250.6 *[536.3]*
nerve (nondiabetic) 352.3
stroke (current episode) - *see* Infarct, brain
late effect - *see* Late effect(s) (of) cerebrovascular disease
subscapularis 354.8
superior nuclear NEC 334.9
supranuclear 356.8
sympathetic
cervical NEC 337.0
nerve NEC (*see also* Neuropathy, peripheral, autonomic) 337.9
nervous system - *see* Neuropathy, peripheral, autonomic
syndrome 344.9
specified NEC 344.89
syphilitic spastic spinal (Erb's) 094.89
tabetic general 094.1
thigh 355.8
throat 478.29
diphtheritic 032.0
muscle 478.29
thrombotic (current episode) (*see also* Thrombosis, brain) 434.0
late effect - *see* Late effect(s) (of) cerebrovascular disease
thumb NEC 354.9
tick (-bite) 989.5
Todd's (postepileptic transitory paralysis) 344.89
toe 355.6
tongue 529.8
transient
arm or leg NEC 781.4
traumatic NEC (*see also* Injury, nerve, by site) 957.9
trapezius 352.4

Paralysis, paralytic *(Continued)*
traumatic, transient NEC (*see also* Injury, nerve, by site) 957.9
trembling (*see also* Parkinsonism) 332.0
triceps brachii 354.9
trigeminal nerve 350.9
trochlear nerve 378.53
ulnar nerve 354.2
upper limb - *see also* Paralysis, arm
both (*see also* Diplegia) 344.2
uremic - *see* Uremia
uveoparotitic 135
uvula 528.9
hysterical 300.11
postdiphtheritic 032.0
vagus nerve 352.3
vasomotor NEC 337.9
velum palati 528.9
vesical (*see also* Paralysis, bladder) 596.53
vestibular nerve 388.5
visual field, psychic 368.16
vocal cord 478.30
bilateral (partial) 478.33
complete 478.34
complete (bilateral) 478.34
unilateral (partial) 478.31
complete 478.32
Volkmann's (complicating trauma) 958.6
wasting 335.21
Weber's 344.89
wrist NEC 354.9
Paramedial orifice, urethrovesical 753.8
Paramenia 626.9
Parametritis (chronic) (*see also* Disease, pelvis, inflammatory) 614.4
acute 614.3
puerperal, postpartum, childbirth 670
Parametrium, parametric - *see* condition
Paramnesia (*see also* Amnesia) 780.93
Paramolar 520.1
causing crowding 524.31
Paramyloidosis 277.30 (Revised)
Paramyoclonus multiplex 333.2
Paramyotonia 359.2
congenita 359.2
Paraneoplastic syndrome - *see* condition
Parangi (*see also* Yaws) 102.9
Paranoia 297.1
alcoholic 291.5
querulans 297.8
senile 290.20
Paranoid
dementia (*see also* Schizophrenia) 295.3
praecox (acute) 295.3
senile 290.20
personality 301.0
psychosis 297.9
alcoholic 291.5
climacteric 297.2
drug-induced 292.11
involutional 297.2
menopausal 297.2
protracted reactive 298.4
psychogenic 298.4
acute 298.3
senile 290.20
reaction (chronic) 297.9
acute 298.3
schizophrenia (acute) (*see also* Schizophrenia) 295.3
state 297.9
alcohol-induced 291.5
climacteric 297.2
drug-induced 292.11

Paranoid *(Continued)*
state *(Continued)*
due to or associated with
arteriosclerosis (cerebrovascular) 290.42
presenile brain disease 290.12
senile brain disease 290.20
involutional 297.2
menopausal 297.2
senile 290.20
simple 297.0
specified type NEC 297.8
tendencies 301.0
traits 301.0
trends 301.0
type, psychopathic personality 301.0
Paraparesis (*see also* Paralysis) 344.9
Paraphasia 784.3
Paraphilia (*see also* Deviation, sexual) 302.9
Paraphimosis (congenital) 605
chancroidal 099.0
Paraphrenia, paraphrenic (late) 297.2
climacteric 297.2
dementia (*see also* Schizophrenia) 295.3
involutional 297.2
menopausal 297.2
schizophrenia (acute) (*see also* Schizophrenia) 295.3
Paraplegia 344.1
with
broken back - *see* Fracture, vertebra, by site, with spinal cord injury
fracture, vertebra - *see* Fracture, vertebra, by site, with spinal cord injury
ataxic - *see* Degeneration, combined, spinal cord
brain (current episode) (*see also* Paralysis, brain) 437.8
cerebral (current episode) (*see also* Paralysis, brain) 437.8
congenital or infantile (cerebral) (spastic) (spinal) 343.0
cortical - *see* Paralysis, brain
familial spastic 334.1
functional (hysterical) 300.11
hysterical 300.11
infantile 343.0
late effect 344.1
Pott's (*see also* Tuberculosis) 015.0 *[730.88]*
psychogenic 306.0
spastic
Erb's spinal 094.89
hereditary 334.1
not infantile or congenital 344.1
spinal (cord)
traumatic NEC - *see* Injury, spinal, by site
syphilitic (spastic) 094.89
traumatic NEC - *see* Injury, spinal, by site
Paraproteinemia 273.2
benign (familial) 273.1
monoclonal 273.1
secondary to malignant or inflammatory disease 273.1
Parapsoriasis 696.2
en plaques 696.2
guttata 696.2
lichenoides chronica 696.2
retiformis 696.2
varioliformis (acuta) 696.2
Parascarlatina 057.8

ICD-9-CM
P
Vol. 2

Parasitic - *see also* condition
disease NEC (*see also* Infestation, parasitic) 136.9
contact V01.89
exposure to V01.89
intestinal NEC 129
skin NEC 134.9
stomatitis 112.0
sycosis 110.0
beard 110.0
scalp 110.0
twin 759.4
Parasitism NEC 136.9
intestinal NEC 129
skin NEC 134.9
specified - *see* Infestation
Parasitophobia 300.29
Parasomnia 307.47
alcohol induced 291.82
drug induced 292.85
nonorganic origin 307.47
organic 327.40
in conditions classified elsewhere 327.44
other 327.49
Paraspadias 752.69
Paraspasm facialis 351.8
Parathyroid gland - *see* condition
Parathyroiditis (autoimmune) 252.1
Parathyroprival tetany 252.1
Paratrachoma 077.0
Paratyphilitis (*see also* Appendicitis) 541
Paratyphoid (fever) - *see* Fever, paratyphoid
Paratyphus - *see* Fever, paratyphoid
Paraurethral duct 753.8
Para-urethritis 597.89
gonococcal (acute) 098.0
chronic or duration of 2 months or over 098.2
Paravaccinia NEC 051.9
milkers' node 051.1
Paravaginitis (*see also* Vaginitis) 616.10
Parencephalitis (*see also* Encephalitis) 323.9
late effect - *see* category 326
Parergasia 298.9
Paresis (*see also* Paralysis) 344.9
accommodation 367.51
bladder (spastic) (sphincter) (*see also* Paralysis, bladder) 596.53
tabetic 094.0
bowel, colon, or intestine (*see also* Ileus) 560.1
brain or cerebral - *see* Paralysis, brain
extrinsic muscle, eye 378.55
general 094.1
arrested 094.1
brain 094.1
cerebral 094.1
insane 094.1
juvenile 090.40
remission 090.49
progressive 094.1
remission (sustained) 094.1
tabetic 094.1
heart (*see also* Failure, heart) 428.9
infantile (*see also* Poliomyelitis) 045.9
insane 094.1
juvenile 090.40
late effect - *see* Paralysis, late effect
luetic (general) 094.1
peripheral progressive 356.9
pseudohypertrophic 359.1
senile NEC 344.9
stomach 536.3
diabetic 250.6 *[536.3]*

Paresis *(Continued)*
syphilitic (general) 094.1
congenital 090.40
transient, limb 781.4
vesical (sphincter) NEC 596.53
Paresthesia (*see also* Disturbance, sensation) 782.0
Berger's (paresthesia of lower limb) 782.0
Bernhardt 355.1
Magnan's 782.0
Paretic - *see* condition
Parinaud's
conjunctivitis 372.02
oculoglandular syndrome 372.02
ophthalmoplegia 378.81
syndrome (paralysis of conjugate upward gaze) 378.81
Parkes Weber and Dimitri syndrome (encephalocutaneous angiomatosis) 759.6
Parkinson's disease, syndrome, or tremor - *see* Parkinsonism
Parkinsonism (arteriosclerotic) (idiopathic) (primary) 332.0
associated with orthostatic hypotension (idiopathic) (symptomatic) 333.0
due to drugs 332.1
neuroleptic-induced 332.1
secondary 332.1
syphilitic 094.82
Parodontitis 523.4
Parodontosis 523.40 ⬅
Paronychia (with lymphangitis) 681.9
candidal (chronic) 112.3
chronic 681.9
candidal 112.3
finger 681.02
toe 681.11
finger 681.02
toe 681.11
tuberculous (primary) (*see also* Tuberculosis) 017.0
Parorexia NEC 307.52
hysterical 300.11
Parosmia 781.1
psychogenic 306.7
Parotid gland - *see* condition
Parotiditis (*see also* Parotitis) 527.2
epidemic 072.9
infectious 072.9
Parotitis 527.2
allergic 527.2
chronic 527.2
epidemic (*see also* Mumps) 072.9
infectious (*see also* Mumps) 072.9
noninfectious 527.2
nonspecific toxic 527.2
not mumps 527.2
postoperative 527.2
purulent 527.2
septic 527.2
suppurative (acute) 527.2
surgical 527.2
toxic 527.2
Paroxysmal - *see also* condition
dyspnea (nocturnal) 786.09
Parrot's disease (syphilitic osteochondritis) 090.0
Parrot fever 073.9
Parry's disease or syndrome (exophthalmic goiter) 242.0
Parry-Romberg syndrome 349.89
Parson's disease (exophthalmic goiter) 242.0

Parsonage-Aldren-Turner syndrome 353.5
Parsonage-Turner syndrome 353.5
Pars planitis 363.21
Particolored infant 757.39
Parturition - *see* Delivery
Passage
false, urethra 599.4
meconium noted during delivery 763.84
of sounds or bougies (*see also* Attention to artificial opening) V55.9
Passive - *see* condition
Pasteurella septica 027.2
Pasteurellosis (*see also* Infection, Pasteurella) 027.2
PAT (paroxysmal atrial tachycardia) 427.0
Patau's syndrome (trisomy D1) 758.1
Patch
herald 696.3
Patches
mucous (syphilitic) 091.3
congenital 090.0
smokers' (mouth) 528.6
Patellar - *see* condition
Patellofemoral syndrome 719.46
Patent - *see also* Imperfect closure
atrioventricular ostium 745.69
canal of Nuck 752.41
cervix 622.5
complicating pregnancy 654.5
affecting fetus or newborn 761.0
ductus arteriosus or Botalli 747.0
Eustachian
tube 381.7
valve 746.89
foramen
Botalli 745.5
ovale 745.5
interauricular septum 745.5
interventricular septum 745.4
omphalomesenteric duct 751.0
os (uteri) - *see* Patent, cervix
ostium secundum 745.5
urachus 753.7
vitelline duct 751.0
Paternity testing V70.4
Paterson's syndrome (sideropenic dysphagia) 280.8
Paterson (-Brown) (-Kelly) syndrome (sideropenic dysphagia) 280.8
Paterson-Kelly syndrome or web (sideropenic dysphagia) 280.8
Pathologic, pathological - *see also* condition
asphyxia 799.01
drunkenness 291.4
emotionality 301.3
fracture - *see* Fracture, pathologic
liar 301.7
personality 301.9
resorption, tooth 521.40
external 521.42
internal 521.41
specified NEC 521.49
sexuality (*see also* Deviation, sexual) 302.9
Pathology (of) - *see also* Disease ⬅
periradicular, associated with previous endodontic treatment 526.69 ◀
Patterned motor discharge, idiopathic (*see also* Epilepsy) 345.5
Patulous - *see also* Patent
anus 569.49
Eustachian tube 381.7
Pause, sinoatrial 427.81
Pavor nocturnus 307.46
Pavy's disease 593.6

- **Paxton's disease** (white piedra) 111.2
- **Payr's disease or syndrome** (splenic flexure syndrome) 569.89
- **PBA** (pseudobulbar affect) 310.8
- **Pearls**
  - Elschnig 366.51
  - enamel 520.2
- **Pearl-workers' disease** (chronic osteomyelitis) (*see also* Osteomyelitis) 730.1
- **Pectenitis** 569.49
- **Pectenosis** 569.49
- **Pectoral** - *see* condition
- **Pectus**
  - carinatum (congenital) 754.82
    - acquired 738.3
    - rachitic (*see also* Rickets) 268.0
  - excavatum (congenital) 754.81
    - acquired 738.3
    - rachitic (*see also* Rickets) 268.0
  - recurvatum (congenital) 754.81
    - acquired 738.3
- **Pedatrophia** 261
- **Pederosis** 302.2
- **Pediculosis** (infestation) 132.9
  - capitis (head louse) (any site) 132.0
  - corporis (body louse) (any site) 132.1
  - eyelid 132.0 *[373.6]*
  - mixed (classifiable to more than one category in 132.0–132.2) 132.3
  - pubis (pubic louse) (any site) 132.2
  - vestimenti 132.1
  - vulvae 132.2
- **Pediculus** (infestation) - *see* Pediculosis
- **Pedophilia** 302.2
- **Peg-shaped teeth** 520.2
- **Pel's crisis** 094.0
- **Pel-Ebstein disease** - *see* Disease, Hodgkin's
- **Pelade** 704.01
- **Pelger-Huët anomaly or syndrome** (hereditary hyposegmentation) 288.2
- **Peliosis** (rheumatica) 287.0
- **Pelizaeus-Merzbacher**
  - disease 330.0
  - sclerosis, diffuse cerebral 330.0
- **Pellagra** (alcoholic or with alcoholism) 265.2
  - with polyneuropathy 265.2 *[357.4]*
- **Pellagra-cerebellar-ataxia-renal aminoaciduria syndrome** 270.0
- **Pellegrini's disease** (calcification, knee joint) 726.62
- **Pellegrini** (-Stieda) disease or syndrome (calcification, knee joint) 726.62
- **Pellizzi's syndrome** (pineal) 259.8
- **Pelvic** - *see also* condition
  - congestion-fibrosis syndrome 625.5
  - kidney 753.3
- **Pelvioectasis** 591
- **Pelviolithiasis** 592.0
- **Pelviperitonitis**
  - female (*see also* Peritonitis, pelvic, female) 614.5
  - male (*see also* Peritonitis) 567.21
- **Pelvis, pelvic** - *see also* condition or type
  - infantile 738.6
  - Nägele's 738.6
  - obliquity 738.6
  - Robert's 755.69
- **Pemphigoid** 694.5
  - benign, mucous membrane 694.60
    - with ocular involvement 694.61
  - bullous 694.5
- **Pemphigoid** *(Continued)*
  - cicatricial 694.60
    - with ocular involvement 694.61
  - juvenile 694.2
- **Pemphigus** 694.4
  - benign 694.5
    - chronic familial 757.39
  - Brazilian 694.4
  - circinatus 694.0
  - congenital, traumatic 757.39
  - conjunctiva 694.61
  - contagiosus 684
  - erythematodes 694.4
  - erythematosus 694.4
  - foliaceus 694.4
  - frambesiodes 694.4
  - gangrenous (*see also* Gangrene) 785.4
  - malignant 694.4
  - neonatorum, newborn 684
  - ocular 694.61
  - papillaris 694.4
  - seborrheic 694.4
  - South American 694.4
  - syphilitic (congenital) 090.0
  - vegetans 694.4
  - vulgaris 694.4
  - wildfire 694.4
- **Pendred's syndrome** (familial goiter with deaf-mutism) 243
- **Pendulous**
  - abdomen 701.9
    - in pregnancy or childbirth 654.4
      - affecting fetus or newborn 763.89
  - breast 611.8
- **Penetrating wound** - *see also* Wound, open, by site
  - with internal injury - *see* Injury, internal, by site, with open wound
  - eyeball 871.7
    - with foreign body (nonmagnetic) 871.6
      - magnetic 871.5
  - ocular (*see also* Penetrating wound, eyeball) 871.7
    - adnexa 870.3
      - with foreign body 870.4
  - orbit 870.3
    - with foreign body 870.4
- **Penetration, pregnant uterus by instrument**
  - with
    - abortion - *see* Abortion, by type, with damage to pelvic organs
    - ectopic pregnancy (*see also* categories 633.0–633.9) 639.2
    - molar pregnancy (*see also* categories 630–632) 639.2
  - complication of delivery 665.1
    - affecting fetus or newborn 763.89
  - following
    - abortion 639.2
    - ectopic or molar pregnancy 639.2
- **Penfield's syndrome** (*see also* Epilepsy) 345.5
- **Penicilliosis of lung** 117.3
- **Penis** - *see* condition
- **Penitis** 607.2
- **Penta X syndrome** 758.81
- **Pentalogy** (of Fallot) 745.2
- **Pentosuria** (benign) (essential) 271.8
- **Peptic acid disease** 536.8
- **Peregrinating patient** V65.2
- **Perforated** - *see* Perforation
- **Perforation, perforative** (nontraumatic)
  - antrum (*see also* Sinusitis, maxillary) 473.0
- **Perforation, perforative** *(Continued)*
  - appendix 540.0
    - with peritoneal abscess 540.1
  - atrial septum, multiple 745.5
  - attic, ear 384.22
    - healed 384.81
  - bile duct, except cystic (*see also* Disease, biliary) 576.3
    - cystic 575.4
  - bladder (urinary) 596.6
    - with
      - abortion - *see* Abortion, by type, with damage to pelvic organs
      - ectopic pregnancy (*see also* categories 633.0–633.9) 639.2
      - molar pregnancy (*see also* categories 630–632) 639.2
    - following
      - abortion 639.2
      - ectopic or molar pregnancy 639.2
    - obstetrical trauma 665.5
  - bowel 569.83
    - with
      - abortion - *see* Abortion, by type, with damage to pelvic organs
      - ectopic pregnancy (*see also* categories 633.0–633.9) 639.2
      - molar pregnancy (*see also* categories 630–632) 639.2
    - fetus or newborn 777.6
    - following
      - abortion 639.2
      - ectopic or molar pregnancy 639.2
    - obstetrical trauma 665.5
  - broad ligament
    - with
      - abortion - *see* Abortion, by type, with damage to pelvic organs
      - ectopic pregnancy (*see also* categories 633.0–633.9) 639.2
      - molar pregnancy (*see also* categories 630–632) 639.2
    - following
      - abortion 639.2
      - ectopic or molar pregnancy 639.2
    - obstetrical trauma 665.6
  - by
    - device, implant, or graft - *see* Complications, mechanical
    - foreign body left accidentally in operation wound 998.4
    - instrument (any) during a procedure, accidental 998.2
  - cecum 540.0
    - with peritoneal abscess 540.1
  - cervix (uteri) - *see also* Injury, internal, cervix
    - with
      - abortion - *see* Abortion, by type, with damage to pelvic organs
      - ectopic pregnancy (*see also* categories 633.0–633.9) 639.2
      - molar pregnancy (*see also* categories 630–632) 639.2
    - following
      - abortion 639.2
      - ectopic or molar pregnancy 639.2
    - obstetrical trauma 665.3
  - colon 569.83
  - common duct (bile) 576.3
  - cornea (*see also* Ulcer, cornea) 370.00
    - due to ulceration 370.06
  - cystic duct 575.4
  - diverticulum (*see also* Diverticula) 562.10
    - small intestine 562.00

Perforation, perforative *(Continued)*
  duodenum, duodenal (ulcer) - *see* Ulcer, duodenum, with perforation
  ear drum - *see* Perforation, tympanum
  enteritis - *see* Enteritis
  esophagus 530.4
  ethmoidal sinus (*see also* Sinusitis, ethmoidal) 473.2
  foreign body (external site) - *see also* Wound, open, by site, complicated
    internal site, by ingested object - *see* Foreign body
  frontal sinus (*see also* Sinusitis, frontal) 473.1
  gallbladder or duct (*see also* Disease, gallbladder) 575.4
  gastric (ulcer) - *see* Ulcer, stomach, with perforation
  heart valve - *see* Endocarditis
  ileum (*see also* Perforation, intestine) 569.83
  instrumental
    external - *see* Wound, open, by site
    pregnant uterus, complicating delivery 665.9
    surgical (accidental) (blood vessel) (nerve) (organ) 998.2
  intestine 569.83
    with
      abortion - *see* Abortion, by type, with damage to pelvic organs
      ectopic pregnancy (*see also* categories 633.0–633.9) 639.2
      molar pregnancy (*see also* categories 630–632) 639.2
    fetus or newborn 777.6
    obstetrical trauma 665.5
    ulcerative NEC 569.83
  jejunum, jejunal 569.83
    ulcer - *see* Ulcer, gastrojejunal, with perforation
  mastoid (antrum) (cell) 383.89
  maxillary sinus (*see also* Sinusitis, maxillary) 473.0
  membrana tympani - *see* Perforation, tympanum
  nasal
    septum 478.19 ⇐
      congenital 748.1
      syphilitic 095.8
    sinus (*see also* Sinusitis) 473.9
      congenital 748.1
  palate (hard) 526.89
    soft 528.9
      syphilitic 095.8
    syphilitic 095.8
  palatine vault 526.89
    syphilitic 095.8
      congenital 090.5
  pelvic
    floor
      with
        abortion - *see* Abortion, by type, with damage to pelvic organs
        ectopic pregnancy (*see also* categories 633.0–633.9) 639.2
        molar pregnancy (*see also* categories 630–632) 639.2
      obstetrical trauma 664.1
    organ
      with
        abortion - *see* Abortion, by type, with damage to pelvic organs

Perforation, perforative *(Continued)*
  pelvic *(Continued)*
    organ *(Continued)*
      with *(Continued)*
        ectopic pregnancy (*see also* categories 633.0–633.9) 639.2
        molar pregnancy (*see also* categories 630–632) 639.2
      following
        abortion 639.2
        ectopic or molar pregnancy 639.2
      obstetrical trauma 665.5
  perineum - *see* Laceration, perineum
  periurethral tissue
    with
      abortion - *see* Abortion, by type, with damage to pelvic organs
      ectopic pregnancy (*see also* categories 633.0–633.9) 639.2
      molar pregnancy (*see also* categories 630–632) 639.2
  pharynx 478.29
  pylorus, pyloric (ulcer) - *see* Ulcer, stomach, with perforation
  rectum 569.49
  root canal space 526.61 ◀
  sigmoid 569.83
  sinus (accessory) (chronic) (nasal) (*see also* Sinusitis) 473.9
  sphenoidal sinus (*see also* Sinusitis, sphenoidal) 473.3
  stomach (due to ulcer) - *see* Ulcer, stomach, with perforation
  surgical (accidental) (by instrument) (blood vessel) (nerve) (organ) 998.2
  traumatic
    external - *see* Wound, open, by site
    eye (*see also* Penetrating wound, ocular) 871.7
    internal organ - *see* Injury, internal, by site
  tympanum (membrane) (persistent posttraumatic) (postinflammatory) 384.20
    with
      otitis media - *see* Otitis media
    attic 384.22
    central 384.21
    healed 384.81
    marginal NEC 384.23
    multiple 384.24
    pars flaccida 384.22
    total 384.25
    traumatic - *see* Wound, open, ear, drum
  typhoid, gastrointestinal 002.0
  ulcer - *see* Ulcer, by site, with perforation
  ureter 593.89
  urethra
    with
      abortion - *see* Abortion, by type, with damage to pelvic organs
      ectopic pregnancy (*see also* categories 633.0–633.9) 639.2
      molar pregnancy (*see also* categories 630–632) 639.2
    following
      abortion 639.2
      ectopic or molar pregnancy 639.2
    obstetrical trauma 665.5
  uterus - *see also* Injury, internal, uterus
    with
      abortion - *see* Abortion, by type, with damage to pelvic organs

Perforation, perforative *(Continued)*
  uterus *(Continued)*
    with *(Continued)*
      ectopic pregnancy (*see also* categories 633.0–633.9) 639.2
      molar pregnancy (*see also* categories 630–632) 639.2
    by intrauterine contraceptive device 996.32
    following
      abortion 639.2
      ectopic or molar pregnancy 639.2
    obstetrical trauma - *see* Injury, internal, uterus, obstetrical trauma
  uvula 528.9
    syphilitic 095.8
  vagina - *see* Laceration, vagina
  viscus NEC 799.89
    traumatic 868.00
      with open wound into cavity 868.10
Periadenitis mucosa necrotica recurrens 528.2
Periangiitis 446.0
Periantritis 535.4
Periappendicitis (acute) (*see also* Appendicitis) 541
Periarteritis (disseminated) (infectious) (necrotizing) (nodosa) 446.0
Periarthritis (joint) 726.90
  Duplay's 726.2
  gonococcal 098.50
  humeroscapularis 726.2
  scapulohumeral 726.2
  shoulder 726.2
  wrist 726.4
Periarthrosis (angioneural) - *see* Periarthritis
Peribronchitis 491.9
  tuberculous (*see also* Tuberculosis) 011.3
Pericapsulitis, adhesive (shoulder) 726.0
Pericarditis (granular) (with decompensation) (with effusion) 423.9
  with
    rheumatic fever (conditions classifiable to 390)
      active (*see also* Pericarditis, rheumatic) 391.0
      inactive or quiescent 393
  actinomycotic 039.8 *[420.0]*
  acute (nonrheumatic) 420.90
    with chorea (acute) (rheumatic) (Sydenham's) 392.0
    bacterial 420.99
    benign 420.91
    hemorrhagic 420.90
    idiopathic 420.91
    infective 420.90
    nonspecific 420.91
    rheumatic 391.0
      with chorea (acute) (rheumatic) (Sydenham's) 392.0
    sicca 420.90
    viral 420.91
  adhesive or adherent (external) (internal) 423.1
    acute - *see* Pericarditis, acute
    rheumatic (external) (internal) 393
  amebic 006.8 *[420.0]*
  bacterial (acute) (subacute) (with serous or seropurulent effusion) 420.99
  calcareous 423.2
  cholesterol (chronic) 423.8
    acute 420.90
  chronic (nonrheumatic) 423.8
    rheumatic 393

- **Pericarditis** *(Continued)*
  - constrictive 423.2
  - Coxsackie 074.21
  - due to
    - actinomycosis 039.8 *[420.0]*
    - amebiasis 006.8 *[420.0]*
    - Coxsackie (virus) 074.21
    - histoplasmosis (*see also* Histoplasmosis) 115.93
    - nocardiosis 039.8 *[420.0]*
    - tuberculosis (*see also* Tuberculosis) 017.9 *[420.0]*
  - fibrinocaseous (*see also* Tuberculosis) 017.9 *[420.0]*
  - fibrinopurulent 420.99
  - fibrinous - *see* Pericarditis, rheumatic
  - fibropurulent 420.99
  - fibrous 423.1
  - gonococcal 098.83
  - hemorrhagic 423.0
  - idiopathic (acute) 420.91
  - infective (acute) 420.90
  - meningococcal 036.41
  - neoplastic (chronic) 423.8
    - acute 420.90
  - nonspecific 420.91
  - obliterans, obliterating 423.1
  - plastic 423.1
  - pneumococcal (acute) 420.99
  - postinfarction 411.0
  - purulent (acute) 420.99
  - rheumatic (active) (acute) (with effusion) (with pneumonia) 391.0
    - with chorea (acute) (rheumatic) (Sydenham's) 392.0
    - chronic or inactive (with chorea) 393
  - septic (acute) 420.99
  - serofibrinous - *see* Pericarditis, rheumatic
  - staphylococcal (acute) 420.99
  - streptococcal (acute) 420.99
  - suppurative (acute) 420.99
  - syphilitic 093.81
  - tuberculous (acute) (chronic) (*see also* Tuberculosis) 017.9 *[420.0]*
  - uremic 585.9 *[420.0]*
  - viral (acute) 420.91
- **Pericardium, pericardial** - *see* condition
- **Pericellulitis** (*see also* Cellulitis) 682.9
- **Pericementitis** 523.40
  - acute 523.30
  - chronic (suppurative) 523.40
- **Pericholecystitis** (*see also* Cholecystitis) 575.10
- **Perichondritis**
  - auricle 380.00
    - acute 380.01
    - chronic 380.02
  - bronchus 491.9
  - ear (external) 380.00
    - acute 380.01
    - chronic 380.02
  - larynx 478.71
    - syphilitic 095.8
    - typhoid 002.0 *[478.71]*
  - nose 478.19
  - pinna 380.00
    - acute 380.01
    - chronic 380.02
  - trachea 478.9
- **Periclasia** 523.5
- **Pericolitis** 569.89
- **Pericoronitis** (chronic) 523.40
  - acute 523.30
- **Pericystitis** (*see also* Cystitis) 595.9
- **Pericytoma** (M9150/1) - *see also* Neoplasm, connective tissue, uncertain behavior
  - benign (M9150/0) - *see* Neoplasm, connective tissue, benign
  - malignant (M9150/3) - *see* Neoplasm, connective tissue, malignant
- **Peridacryocystitis, acute** 375.32
- **Peridiverticulitis** (*see also* Diverticulitis) 562.11
- **Periduodenitis** 535.6
- **Periendocarditis** (*see also* Endocarditis) 424.90
  - acute or subacute 421.9
- **Periepididymitis** (*see also* Epididymitis) 604.90
- **Perifolliculitis** (abscedens) 704.8
  - capitis, abscedens et suffodiens 704.8
  - dissecting, scalp 704.8
  - scalp 704.8
  - superficial pustular 704.8
- **Perigastritis** (acute) 535.0
- **Perigastrojejunitis** (acute) 535.0
- **Perihepatitis** (acute) 573.3
  - chlamydial 099.56
  - gonococcal 098.86
- **Peri-ileitis** (subacute) 569.89
- **Perilabyrinthitis** (acute) - *see* Labyrinthitis
- **Perimeningitis** - *see* Meningitis
- **Perimetritis** (*see also* Endometritis) 615.9
- **Perimetrosalpingitis** (*see also* Salpingo-oophoritis) 614.2
- **Perineocele** 618.05
- **Perinephric** - *see* condition
- **Perinephritic** - *see* condition
- **Perinephritis** (*see also* Infection, kidney) 590.9
  - purulent (*see also* Abscess, kidney) 590.2
- **Perineum, perineal** - *see* condition
- **Perineuritis NEC** 729.2
- **Periodic** - *see also* condition
  - disease (familial) 277.31
  - edema 995.1
    - hereditary 277.6
  - fever 277.31
  - limb movement disorder 327.51
  - paralysis (familial) 359.3
  - peritonitis 277.31
  - polyserositis 277.31
  - somnolence (*see also* Narcolepsy) 347.00
- **Periodontal**
  - cyst 522.8
  - pocket 523.8
- **Periodontitis** (chronic) (complex) (compound) (simplex) 523.40
  - acute 523.33
  - aggressive 523.30
    - generalized 523.32
    - localized 523.31
  - apical 522.6
    - acute (pulpal origin) 522.4
  - generalized 523.42
  - localized 523.41
- **Periodontoclasia** 523.5
- **Periodontosis** 523.5
- **Periods** - *see also* Menstruation
  - heavy 626.2
  - irregular 626.4
- **Perionychia** (with lymphangitis) 681.9
  - finger 681.02
  - toe 681.11
- **Perioophoritis** (*see also* Salpingo-oophoritis) 614.2
- **Periorchitis** (*see also* Orchitis) 604.90
- **Periosteum, periosteal** - *see* condition
- **Periostitis** (circumscribed) (diffuse) (infective) 730.3

> Note Use the following fifth-digit subclassification with category 730:
>
> 0 site unspecified
> 1 shoulder region
> 2 upper arm
> 3 forearm
> 4 hand
> 5 pelvic region and thigh
> 6 lower leg
> 7 ankle and foot
> 8 other specified sites
> 9 multiple sites

  - with osteomyelitis (*see also* Osteomyelitis) 730.2
    - acute or subacute 730.0
    - chronic or old 730.1
  - albuminosa, albuminosus 730.3
  - alveolar 526.5
  - alveolodental 526.5
  - dental 526.5
  - gonorrheal 098.89
  - hyperplastica, generalized 731.2
  - jaw (lower) (upper) 526.4
  - monomelic 733.99
  - orbital 376.02
  - syphilitic 095.5
    - congenital 090.0 *[730.8]*
    - secondary 091.61
  - tuberculous (*see also* Tuberculosis, bone) 015.9 *[730.8]*
  - yaws (early) (hypertrophic) (late) 102.6
- **Periostosis** (*see also* Periostitis) 730.3
  - with osteomyelitis (*see also* Osteomyelitis) 730.2
    - acute or subacute 730.0
    - chronic or old 730.1
  - hyperplastic 756.59
- **Peripartum cardiomyopathy** 674.5
- **Periphlebitis** (*see also* Phlebitis) 451.9
  - lower extremity 451.2
    - deep (vessels) 451.19
    - superficial (vessels) 451.0
  - portal 572.1
  - retina 362.18
  - superficial (vessels) 451.0
  - tuberculous (*see also* Tuberculosis) 017.9
    - retina 017.3 *[362.18]*
- **Peripneumonia** - *see* Pneumonia
- **Periproctitis** 569.49
- **Periprostatitis** (*see also* Prostatitis) 601.9
- **Perirectal** - *see* condition
- **Perirenal** - *see* condition
- **Perisalpingitis** (*see also* Salpingo-oophoritis) 614.2
- **Perisigmoiditis** 569.89
- **Perisplenitis** (infectional) 289.59
- **Perispondylitis** - *see* Spondylitis
- **Peristalsis reversed or visible** 787.4
- **Peritendinitis** (*see also* Tenosynovitis) 726.90
  - adhesive (shoulder) 726.0
- **Perithelioma** (M9150/1) - *see* Pericytoma
- **Peritoneum, peritoneal** - *see also* condition
  - equilibration test V56.32
- **Peritonitis** (acute) (adhesive) (fibrinous) (hemorrhagic) (idiopathic) (localized) (perforative) (primary) (with adhesions) (with effusion) 567.9

Peritonitis *(Continued)*
- with or following
  - abortion - *see* Abortion, by type, with sepsis
  - abscess 567.21
  - appendicitis 540.0
    - with peritoneal abscess 540.1
  - ectopic pregnancy (*see also* categories 633.0–633.9) 639.0
  - molar pregnancy (*see also* categories 630–632) 639.0
- aseptic 998.7
- bacterial 567.29
  - spontaneous 567.23
- bile, biliary 567.81
- chemical 998.7
- chlamydial 099.56
- chronic proliferative 567.89
- congenital NEC 777.6
- diaphragmatic 567.22
- diffuse NEC 567.29
- diphtheritic 032.83
- disseminated NEC 567.29
- due to
  - bile 567.81
  - foreign
    - body or object accidentally left during a procedure (instrument) (sponge) (swab) 998.4
    - substance accidentally left during a procedure (chemical) (powder) (talc) 998.7
  - talc 998.7
  - urine 567.89
- fibrinopurulent 567.29
- fibrinous 567.29
- fibrocaseous (*see also* Tuberculosis) 014.0
- fibropurulent 567.29
- general, generalized (acute) 567.21
- gonococcal 098.86
- in infective disease NEC 136.9 *[567.0]*
- meconium (newborn) 777.6
- pancreatic 577.8
- paroxysmal, benign 277.31
- pelvic
  - female (acute) 614.5
    - chronic NEC 614.7
      - with adhesions 614.6
    - puerperal, postpartum, childbirth 670
  - male (acute) 567.21
- periodic (familial) 277.31
- phlegmonous 567.29
- pneumococcal 567.1
- postabortal 639.0
- proliferative, chronic 567.89
- puerperal, postpartum, childbirth 670
- purulent 567.29
- septic 567.29
- spontaneous bacterial 567.23
- staphylococcal 567.29
- streptococcal 567.29
- subdiaphragmatic 567.29
- subphrenic 567.29
- suppurative 567.29
- syphilitic 095.2
  - congenital 090.0 *[567.0]*
- talc 998.7
- tuberculous (*see also* Tuberculosis) 014.0
- urine 567.89

Peritonsillar - *see* condition

Peritonsillitis 475

Perityphlitis (*see also* Appendicitis) 541

Periureteritis 593.89

Periurethral - *see* condition

Periurethritis (gangrenous) 597.89

Periuterine - *see* condition

Perivaginitis (*see also* Vaginitis) 616.10

Perivasculitis, retinal 362.18

Perivasitis (chronic) 608.4

Periventricular leukomalacia 779.7

Perivesiculitis (seminal) (*see also* Vesiculitis) 608.0

Perlèche 686.8
- due to
  - moniliasis 112.0
  - riboflavin deficiency 266.0

Pernicious - *see* condition

Pernio, perniosis 991.5

Persecution
- delusion 297.9
- social V62.4

Perseveration (tonic) 784.69

Persistence, persistent (congenital) 759.89
- anal membrane 751.2
- arteria stapedia 744.04
- atrioventricular canal 745.69
- bloody ejaculate 792.2
- branchial cleft 744.41
- bulbus cordis in left ventricle 745.8
- canal of Cloquet 743.51
- capsule (opaque) 743.51
- cilioretinal artery or vein 743.51
- cloaca 751.5
- communication - *see* Fistula, congenital
- convolutions
  - aortic arch 747.21
  - fallopian tube 752.19
  - oviduct 752.19
  - uterine tube 752.19
- double aortic arch 747.21
- ductus
  - arteriosus 747.0
  - Botalli 747.0
- fetal
  - circulation 747.83
  - form of cervix (uteri) 752.49
  - hemoglobin (hereditary) ("Swiss variety") 282.7
  - pulmonary hypertension 747.83
- foramen
  - Botalli 745.5
  - ovale 745.5
- Gartner's duct 752.41
- hemoglobin, fetal (hereditary) (HPFH) 282.7
- hyaloid
  - artery (generally incomplete) 743.51
  - system 743.51
- hymen (tag)
  - in pregnancy or childbirth 654.8
    - causing obstructed labor 660.2
- lanugo 757.4
- left
  - posterior cardinal vein 747.49
  - root with right arch of aorta 747.21
  - superior vena cava 747.49
- Meckel's diverticulum 751.0
- mesonephric duct 752.89
  - fallopian tube 752.11
- mucosal disease (middle ear) (with posterior or superior marginal perforation of ear drum) 382.2
- nail(s), anomalous 757.5
- occiput, anterior or posterior 660.3
  - fetus or newborn 763.1
- omphalomesenteric duct 751.0
- organ or site NEC - *see* Anomaly, specified type NEC
- ostium
  - atrioventriculare commune 745.69

Persistence, persistent *(Continued)*
- ostium *(Continued)*
  - primum 745.61
  - secundum 745.5
- ovarian rests in fallopian tube 752.19
- pancreatic tissue in intestinal tract 751.5
- primary (deciduous)
  - teeth 520.6
  - vitreous hyperplasia 743.51
- pulmonary hypertension 747.83
- pupillary membrane 743.46
  - iris 743.46
  - Rhesus (Rh) titer 999.7
- right aortic arch 747.21
- sinus
  - urogenitalis 752.89
  - venosus with imperfect incorporation in right auricle 747.49
- thymus (gland) 254.8
  - hyperplasia 254.0
- thyroglossal duct 759.2
- thyrolingual duct 759.2
- truncus arteriosus or communis 745.0
- tunica vasculosa lentis 743.39
- umbilical sinus 753.7
- urachus 753.7
- vegetative state 780.03
- vitelline duct 751.0
- wolffian duct 752.89

Person (with)
- admitted for clinical research, as participant or control subject V70.7
- awaiting admission to adequate facility elsewhere V63.2
  - undergoing social agency investigation V63.8
- concern (normal) about sick person in family V61.49
- consulting on behalf of another V65.19
  - pediatric pre-birth visit for expectant mother V65.11
- feared
  - complaint in whom no diagnosis was made V65.5
  - condition not demonstrated V65.5
- feigning illness V65.2
- healthy, accompanying sick person V65.0
- living (in)
  - alone V60.3
  - boarding school V60.6
  - residence remote from hospital or medical care facility V63.0
  - residential institution V60.6
  - without
    - adequate
      - financial resources V60.2
      - housing (heating) (space) V60.1
    - housing (permanent) (temporary) V60.0
    - material resources V60.2
    - person able to render necessary care V60.4
    - shelter V60.0
- medical services in home not available V63.1
- on waiting list V63.2
  - undergoing social agency investigation V63.8
- sick or handicapped in family V61.49
- "worried well" V65.5

Personality
- affective 301.10
- aggressive 301.3

Personality *(Continued)*
amoral 301.7
anancastic, anankastic 301.4
antisocial 301.7
asocial 301.7
asthenic 301.6
avoidant 301.82
borderline 301.83
change 310.1
compulsive 301.4
cycloid 301.13
cyclothymic 301.13
dependent 301.6
depressive (chronic) 301.12
disorder, disturbance NEC 301.9
with
antisocial disturbance 301.7
pattern disturbance NEC 301.9
sociopathic disturbance 301.7
trait disturbance 301.9
dual 300.14
dyssocial 301.7
eccentric 301.89
"haltlose" type 301.89
emotionally unstable 301.59
epileptoid 301.3
explosive 301.3
fanatic 301.0
histrionic 301.50
hyperthymic 301.11
hypomanic 301.11
hypothymic 301.12
hysterical 301.50
immature 301.89
inadequate 301.6
labile 301.59
masochistic 301.89
morally defective 301.7
multiple 300.14
narcissistic 301.81
obsessional 301.4
obsessive-compulsive 301.4
overconscientious 301.4
paranoid 301.0
passive (-dependent) 301.6
passive-aggressive 301.84
pathologic NEC 301.9
pattern defect or disturbance 301.9
pseudosocial 301.7
psychoinfantile 301.59
psychoneurotic NEC 301.89
psychopathic 301.9
with
amoral trend 301.7
antisocial trend 301.7
asocial trend 301.7
pathologic sexuality (*see also* Deviation, sexual) 302.9
mixed types 301.9
schizoid 301.20
introverted 301.21
schizotypal 301.22
with sexual deviation (*see also* Deviation, sexual) 302.9
antisocial 301.7
dyssocial 301.7
type A 301.4
unstable (emotional) 301.59
Perthes' disease (capital femoral osteochondrosis) 732.1
Pertussis (*see also* Whooping cough) 033.9
vaccination, prophylactic (against) V03.6
Peruvian wart 088.0
Perversion, perverted
appetite 307.52
hysterical 300.11
function
pineal gland 259.8
pituitary gland 253.9
anterior lobe
deficient 253.2
excessive 253.1
posterior lobe 253.6
placenta - *see* Placenta, abnormal
sense of smell or taste 781.1
psychogenic 306.7
sexual (*see also* Deviation, sexual) 302.9
Pervious, congenital - *see also* Imperfect, closure
ductus arteriosus 747.0
Pes (congenital) (*see also* Talipes) 754.70
abductus (congenital) 754.60
acquired 736.79
acquired NEC 736.79
planus 734
adductus (congenital) 754.79
acquired 736.79
cavus 754.71
acquired 736.73
planovalgus (congenital) 754.69
acquired 736.79
planus (acquired) (any degree) 734
congenital 754.61
rachitic 268.1
valgus (congenital) 754.61
acquired 736.79
varus (congenital) 754.50
acquired 736.79
Pest (*see also* Plague) 020.9
Pestis (*see also* Plague) 020.9
bubonica 020.0
fulminans 020.0
minor 020.8
pneumonica - *see* Plague, pneumonic
Petechia, petechiae 782.7
fetus or newborn 772.6
Petechial
fever 036.0
typhus 081.9
Petges-Cléjat or Petges-Clégat syndrome (poikilodermatomyositis) 710.3
Petit's
disease (*see also* Hernia, lumbar) 553.8
Petit mal (idiopathic) (*see also* Epilepsy) 345.0
status 345.2
Petrellidosis 117.6
Petrositis 383.20
acute 383.21
chronic 383.22
Peutz-Jeghers disease or syndrome 759.6
Peyronie's disease 607.85
Pfeiffer's disease 075
Phacentocele 379.32
traumatic 921.3
Phacoanaphylaxis 360.19
Phacocele (old) 379.32
traumatic 921.3
Phaehyphomycosis 117.8
Phagedena (dry) (moist) (*see also* Gangrene) 785.4
arteriosclerotic 440.24
geometric 686.09
penis 607.89
senile 440.24
sloughing 785.4
tropical (*see also* Ulcer, skin) 707.9
vulva 616.50
Phagedenic - *see also* condition
abscess - *see also* Abscess
chancroid 099.0
bubo NEC 099.8
chancre 099.0
ulcer (tropical) (*see also* Ulcer, skin) 707.9
Phagomania 307.52
Phakoma 362.89
Phantom limb (syndrome) 353.6
Pharyngeal - *see also* condition
arch remnant 744.41
pouch syndrome 279.11
Pharyngitis (acute) (catarrhal) (gangrenous) (infective) (malignant) (membranous) (phlegmonous) (pneumococcal) (pseudomembranous) (simple) (staphylococcal) (subacute) (suppurative) (ulcerative) (viral) 462
with influenza, flu, or grippe 487.1
aphthous 074.0
atrophic 472.1
chlamydial 099.51
chronic 472.1
Coxsackie virus 074.0
diphtheritic (membranous) 032.0
follicular 472.1
fusospirochetal 101
gonococcal 098.6
granular (chronic) 472.1
herpetic 054.79
hypertrophic 472.1
infectional, chronic 472.1
influenzal 487.1
lymphonodular, acute 074.8
septic 034.0
streptococcal 034.0
tuberculous (*see also* Tuberculosis) 012.8
vesicular 074.0
Pharyngoconjunctival fever 077.2
Pharyngoconjunctivitis, viral 077.2
Pharyngolaryngitis (acute) 465.0
chronic 478.9
septic 034.0
Pharyngoplegia 478.29
Pharyngotonsillitis 465.8
tuberculous 012.8
Pharyngotracheitis (acute) 465.8
chronic 478.9
Pharynx, pharyngeal - *see* condition
Phase of life problem NEC V62.89
Phenomenon
Arthus 995.21 ◄
flashback (drug) 292.89
jaw-winking 742.8
Jod-Basedow 242.8
L. E. cell 710.0
lupus erythematosus cell 710.0
Pelger-Huët (hereditary hyposegmentation) 288.2
Raynaud's (paroxysmal digital cyanosis) (secondary) 443.0
Reilly's (*see also* Neuropathy, peripheral, autonomic) 337.9
vasomotor 780.2
vasospastic 443.9
vasovagal 780.2
Wenckebach's, heart block (second degree) 426.13
Phenylketonuria (PKU) 270.1
Phenylpyruvicaciduria 270.1
Pheochromoblastoma (M8700/3)
specified site - *see* Neoplasm, by site, malignant
unspecified site 194.0

Pheochromocytoma (M8700/0)
malignant (M8700/3)
specified site - *see* Neoplasm, by site, malignant
unspecified site 194.0
specified site - *see* Neoplasm, by site, benign
unspecified site 227.0
Phimosis (congenital) 605
chancroidal 099.0
due to infection 605
Phlebectasia (*see also* Varicose, vein) 454.9
congenital NEC 747.60
esophagus (*see also* Varix, esophagus) 456.1
with hemorrhage (*see also* Varix, esophagus, bleeding) 456.0
Phlebitis (infective) (pyemic) (septic) (suppurative) 451.9
antecubital vein 451.82
arm NEC 451.84
axillary vein 451.89
basilic vein 451.82
deep 451.83
superficial 451.82
axillary vein 451.89
basilic vein 451.82
blue 451.9
brachial vein 451.83
breast, superficial 451.89
cavernous (venous) sinus - *see* Phlebitis, intracranial sinus
cephalic vein 451.82
cerebral (venous) sinus - *see* Phlebitis, intracranial sinus
chest wall, superficial 451.89
complicating pregnancy or puerperium 671.9
affecting fetus or newborn 760.3
cranial (venous) sinus - *see* Phlebitis, intracranial sinus
deep (vessels) 451.19
femoral vein 451.11
specified vessel NEC 451.19
due to implanted device - *see* Complications, due to (presence of) any device, implant, or graft classified to 996.0–996.5 NEC
during or resulting from a procedure 997.2
femoral vein (deep) (superficial) 451.11
femoropopliteal 451.19
following infusion, perfusion, or transfusion 999.2
gouty 274.89 *[451.9]*
hepatic veins 451.89
iliac vein 451.81
iliofemoral 451.11
intracranial sinus (any) (venous) 325
late effect - *see* category 326
nonpyogenic 437.6
in pregnancy or puerperium 671.5
jugular vein 451.89
lateral (venous) sinus - *see* Phlebitis, intracranial sinus
leg 451.2
deep (vessels) 451.19
specified vessel NEC 451.19
superficial (vessels) 451.0
femoral vein 451.11
longitudinal sinus - *see* Phlebitis, intracranial sinus
lower extremity 451.2
deep (vessels) 451.19
specified vessel NEC 451.19
Phlebitis *(Continued)*
lower extremity *(Continued)*
superficial (vessels) 451.0
femoral vein 451.11
migrans, migrating (superficial) 453.1
pelvic
with
abortion - *see* Abortion, by type, with sepsis
ectopic pregnancy (*see also* categories 633.0–633.9) 639.0
molar pregnancy (*see also* categories 630–632) 639.0
following
abortion 639.0
ectopic or molar pregnancy 639.0
puerperal, postpartum 671.4
popliteal vein 451.19
portal (vein) 572.1
postoperative 997.2
pregnancy 671.9
deep 671.3
specified type NEC 671.5
superficial 671.2
puerperal, postpartum, childbirth 671.9
deep 671.4
lower extremities 671.2
pelvis 671.4
specified site NEC 671.5
superficial 671.2
radial vein 451.83
retina 362.18
saphenous (great) (long) 451.0
accessory or small 451.0
sinus (meninges) - *see* Phlebitis, intracranial sinus
specified site NEC 451.89
subclavian vein 451.89
syphilitic 093.89
tibial vein 451.19
ulcer, ulcerative 451.9
leg 451.2
deep (vessels) 451.19
specified vessel NEC 451.19
superficial (vessels) 451.0
femoral vein 451.11
lower extremity 451.2
deep (vessels) 451.19
femoral vein 451.11
specified vessel NEC 451.19
superficial (vessels) 451.0
ulnar vein 451.83
umbilicus 451.89
upper extremity - *see* Phlebitis, arm
deep (veins) 451.83
brachial vein 451.83
radial vein 451.83
ulnar vein 451.83
superficial (veins) 451.82
antecubital vein 451.82
basilic vein 451.82
cephalic vein 451.82
uterus (septic) (*see also* Endometritis) 615.9
varicose (leg) (lower extremity) (*see also* Varicose, vein) 454.1
Phlebofibrosis 459.89
Phleboliths 459.89
Phlebosclerosis 459.89
Phlebothrombosis - *see* Thrombosis
Phlebotomus fever 066.0
Phlegm, choked on 933.1
Phlegmasia
alba dolens (deep vessels) 451.19
complicating pregnancy 671.3
Phlegmasia *(Continued)*
alba dolens *(Continued)*
nonpuerperal 451.19
puerperal, postpartum, childbirth 671.4
cerulea dolens 451.19
Phlegmon (*see also* Abscess) 682.9
erysipelatous (*see also* Erysipelas) 035
iliac 682.2
fossa 540.1
throat 478.29
Phlegmonous - *see* condition
Phlyctenulosis (allergic) (keratoconjunctivitis) (nontuberculous) 370.31
cornea 370.31
with ulcer (*see also* Ulcer, cornea) 370.00
tuberculous (*see also* Tuberculosis) 017.3 *[370.31]*
Phobia, phobic (reaction) 300.20
animal 300.29
isolated NEC 300.29
obsessional 300.3
simple NEC 300.29
social 300.23
specified NEC 300.29
state 300.20
Phocas' disease 610.1
Phocomelia 755.4
lower limb 755.32
complete 755.33
distal 755.35
proximal 755.34
upper limb 755.22
complete 755.23
distal 755.25
proximal 755.24
Phoria (*see also* Heterophoria) 378.40
Phosphate-losing tubular disorder 588.0
Phosphatemia 275.3
Phosphaturia 275.3
Photoallergic response 692.72
Photocoproporphyria 277.1
Photodermatitis (sun) 692.72
light other than sun 692.82
Photokeratitis 370.24
Photo-ophthalmia 370.24
Photophobia 368.13
Photopsia 368.15
Photoretinitis 363.31
Photoretinopathy 363.31
Photosensitiveness (sun) 692.72
light other than sun 692.82
Photosensitization skin (sun) 692.72
light other than sun 692.82
Phototoxic response 692.72
Phrenitis 323.9
Phrynoderma 264.8
Phthiriasis (pubis) (any site) 132.2
with any infestation classifiable to 132.0 and 132.1 132.3
Phthirus infestation - *see* Phthiriasis
Phthisis (*see also* Tuberculosis) 011.9
bulbi (infectional) 360.41
colliers' 011.4
cornea 371.05
eyeball (due to infection) 360.41
millstone makers' 011.4
miners' 011.4
potters' 011.4
sandblasters' 011.4
stonemasons' 011.4
Phycomycosis 117.7
Physalopteriasis 127.7
Physical therapy NEC V57.1
breathing exercises V57.0

Physiological cup, optic papilla
borderline, glaucoma suspect 365.00
enlarged 377.14
glaucomatous 377.14
Phytobezoar 938
intestine 936
stomach 935.2
Pian (*see also* Yaws) 102.9
Pianoma 102.1
Piarhemia, piarrhemia (*see also* Hyperlipemia) 272.4
bilharziasis 120.9
Pica 307.52
hysterical 300.11
Pick's
cerebral atrophy 331.11
with dementia
with behavioral disturbance 331.11 *[294.11]*
without behavioral disturbance 331.11 *[294.10]*
disease
brain 331.11
dementia in
with behavioral disturbance 331.11 *[294.11]*
without behavioral disturbance 331.11 *[294.10]*
lipid histiocytosis 272.7
liver (pericardial pseudocirrhosis of liver) 423.2
pericardium (pericardial pseudocirrhosis of liver) 423.2
polyserositis (pericardial pseudocirrhosis of liver) 423.2
syndrome
heart (pericardial pseudocirrhosis of liver) 423.2
liver (pericardial pseudocirrhosis of liver) 423.2
tubular adenoma (M8640/0)
specified site - *see* Neoplasm, by site, benign
unspecified site
female 220
male 222.0
Pick-Herxheimer syndrome (diffuse idiopathic cutaneous atrophy) 701.8
Pick-Niemann disease (lipid histiocytosis) 272.7
Pickwickian syndrome (cardiopulmonary obesity) 278.8
Piebaldism, classic 709.09
Piedra 111.2
beard 111.2
black 111.3
white 111.2
black 111.3
scalp 111.3
black 111.3
white 111.2
white 111.2
Pierre Marie's syndrome (pulmonary hypertrophic osteoarthropathy) 731.2
Pierre Marie-Bamberger syndrome (hypertrophic pulmonary osteoarthropathy) 731.2
Pierre Mauriac's syndrome (diabetes-dwarfism-obesity) 258.1
Pierre Robin deformity or syndrome (congenital) 756.0
Pierson's disease or osteochondrosis 732.1
Pigeon
breast or chest (acquired) 738.3
congenital 754.82
rachitic (*see also* Rickets) 268.0
Pigeon *(Continued)*
breeders' disease or lung 495.2
fanciers' disease or lung 495.2
toe 735.8
Pigmentation (abnormal) 709.00
anomalies NEC 709.00
congenital 757.33
specified NEC 709.09
conjunctiva 372.55
cornea 371.10
anterior 371.11
posterior 371.13
stromal 371.12
lids (congenital) 757.33
acquired 374.52
limbus corneae 371.10
metals 709.00
optic papilla, congenital 743.57
retina (congenital) (grouped) (nevoid) 743.53
acquired 362.74
scrotum, congenital 757.33
Piles - *see* Hemorrhoids
Pili
annulati or torti (congenital) 757.4
incarnati 704.8
Pill roller hand (intrinsic) 736.09
Pilomatrixoma (M8110/0) - *see* Neoplasm, skin, benign
Pilonidal - *see* condition
Pimple 709.8
PIN I (prostatic intraepithelial neoplasia I) 602.3
PIN II (prostatic intraepithelial neoplasia II) 602.3
PIN III (prostatic intraepithelial neoplasia III) 233.4
Pinched nerve - *see* Neuropathy, entrapment
Pineal body or gland - *see* condition
Pinealoblastoma (M9362/3) 194.4
Pinealoma (M9360/1) 237.1
malignant (M9360/3) 194.4
Pineoblastoma (M9362/3) 194.4
Pineocytoma (M9361/1) 237.1
Pinguecula 372.51
Pinhole meatus (*see also* Stricture, urethra) 598.9
Pink
disease 985.0
eye 372.03
puffer 492.8
Pinkus' disease (lichen nitidus) 697.1
Pinpoint
meatus (*see also* Stricture, urethra) 598.9
os (uteri) (*see also* Stricture, cervix) 622.4
Pinselhaare (congenital) 757.4
Pinta 103.9
cardiovascular lesions 103.2
chancre (primary) 103.0
erythematous plaques 103.1
hyperchromic lesions 103.1
hyperkeratosis 103.1
lesions 103.9
cardiovascular 103.2
hyperchromic 103.1
intermediate 103.1
late 103.2
mixed 103.3
primary 103.0
skin (achromic) (cicatricial) (dyschromic) 103.2
hyperchromic 103.1
mixed (achromic and hyperchromic) 103.3
papule (primary) 103.0
Pinta *(Continued)*
skin lesions (achromic) (cicatricial) (dyschromic) 103.2
hyperchromic 103.1
mixed (achromic and hyperchromic) 103.3
vitiligo 103.2
Pintid 103.0
Pinworms (disease) (infection) (infestation) 127.4
Piry fever 066.8
Pistol wound - *see* Gunshot wound
Pit, lip (mucus), congenital 750.25
Pitchers' elbow 718.82
Pithecoid pelvis 755.69
with disproportion (fetopelvic) 653.2
affecting fetus or newborn 763.1
causing obstructed labor 660.1
Pithiatism 300.11
Pitted - *see also* Pitting
teeth 520.4
Pitting (edema) (*see also* Edema) 782.3
lip 782.3
nail 703.8
congenital 757.5
Pituitary gland - *see* condition
Pituitary snuff-takers' disease 495.8
Pityriasis 696.5
alba 696.5
capitis 690.11
circinata (et maculata) 696.3
Hebra's (exfoliative dermatitis) 695.89
lichenoides et varioliformis 696.2
maculata (et circinata) 696.3
nigra 111.1
pilaris 757.39
acquired 701.1
Hebra's 696.4
rosea 696.3
rotunda 696.3
rubra (Hebra) 695.89
pilaris 696.4
sicca 690.18
simplex 690.18
specified type NEC 696.5
streptogenes 696.5
versicolor 111.0
scrotal 111.0
Placenta, placental
ablatio 641.2
affecting fetus or newborn 762.1
abnormal, abnormality 656.7
with hemorrhage 641.8
affecting fetus or newborn 762.1
affecting fetus or newborn 762.2
abruptio 641.2
affecting fetus or newborn 762.1
accessory lobe - *see* Placenta, abnormal
accreta (without hemorrhage) 667.0
with hemorrhage 666.0
adherent (without hemorrhage) 667.0
with hemorrhage 666.0
apoplexy - *see* Placenta, separation
battledore - *see* Placenta, abnormal
bilobate - *see* Placenta, abnormal
bipartita - *see* Placenta, abnormal
carneous mole 631
centralis - *see* Placenta, previa
circumvallata - *see* Placenta, abnormal
cyst (amniotic) - *see* Placenta, abnormal
deficiency - *see* Placenta, insufficiency
degeneration - *see* Placenta, insufficiency
detachment (partial) (premature) (with hemorrhage) 641.2
affecting fetus or newborn 762.1

ICD-9-CM
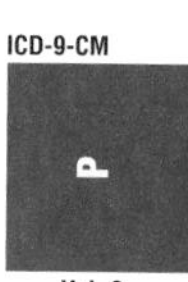
Vol. 2

- **Placenta, placental** *(Continued)*
  - dimidiata - *see* Placenta, abnormal
  - disease 656.7
    - affecting fetus or newborn 762.2
  - duplex - *see* Placenta, abnormal
  - dysfunction - *see* Placenta, insufficiency
  - fenestrata - *see* Placenta, abnormal
  - fibrosis - *see* Placenta, abnormal
  - fleshy mole 631
  - hematoma - *see* Placenta, abnormal
  - hemorrhage NEC - *see* Placenta, separation
  - hormone disturbance or malfunction - *see* Placenta, abnormal
  - hyperplasia - *see* Placenta, abnormal
  - increta (without hemorrhage) 667.0
    - with hemorrhage 666.0
  - infarction 656.7
    - affecting fetus or newborn 762.2
  - insertion, vicious - *see* Placenta, previa
  - insufficiency
    - affecting
      - fetus or newborn 762.2
      - management of pregnancy 656.5
  - lateral - *see* Placenta, previa
  - low implantation or insertion - *see* Placenta, previa
  - low-lying - *see* Placenta, previa
  - malformation - *see* Placenta, abnormal
  - malposition - *see* Placenta, previa
  - marginalis, marginata - *see* Placenta, previa
  - marginal sinus (hemorrhage) (rupture) 641.2
    - affecting fetus or newborn 762.1
  - membranacea - *see* Placenta, abnormal
  - multilobed - *see* Placenta, abnormal
  - multipartita - *see* Placenta, abnormal
  - necrosis - *see* Placenta, abnormal
  - percreta (without hemorrhage) 667.0
    - with hemorrhage 666.0
  - polyp 674.4
  - previa (central) (centralis) (complete) (lateral) (marginal) (marginalis) (partial) (partialis) (total) (with hemorrhage) 641.1
    - affecting fetus or newborn 762.0
    - noted
      - before labor, without hemorrhage (with cesarean delivery) 641.0
      - during pregnancy (without hemorrhage) 641.0
    - without hemorrhage (before labor and delivery) (during pregnancy) 641.0
  - retention (with hemorrhage) 666.0
    - fragments, complicating puerperium (delayed hemorrhage) 666.2
      - without hemorrhage 667.1
    - postpartum, puerperal 666.2
    - without hemorrhage 667.0
  - separation (normally implanted) (partial) (premature) (with hemorrhage) 641.2
    - affecting fetus or newborn 762.1
  - septuplex - *see* Placenta, abnormal
  - small - *see* Placenta, insufficiency
  - softening (premature) - *see* Placenta, abnormal
  - spuria - *see* Placenta, abnormal
  - succenturiata - *see* Placenta, abnormal
  - syphilitic 095.8
  - transfusion syndromes 762.3
  - transmission of chemical substance - *see* Absorption, chemical, through placenta
  - trapped (with hemorrhage) 666.0
    - without hemorrhage 667.0
  - trilobate - *see* Placenta, abnormal
  - tripartita - *see* Placenta, abnormal
  - triplex - *see* Placenta, abnormal
  - varicose vessel - *see* Placenta, abnormal
  - vicious insertion - *see* Placenta, previa
- **Placentitis**
  - affecting fetus or newborn 762.7
  - complicating pregnancy 658.4
- **Plagiocephaly** (skull) 754.0
- **Plague** 020.9
  - abortive 020.8
  - ambulatory 020.8
  - bubonic 020.0
  - cellulocutaneous 020.1
  - lymphatic gland 020.0
  - pneumonic 020.5
    - primary 020.3
    - secondary 020.4
  - pulmonary - *see* Plague, pneumonic
  - pulmonic - *see* Plague, pneumonic
  - septicemic 020.2
  - tonsillar 020.9
    - septicemic 020.2
  - vaccination, prophylactic (against) V03.3
- **Planning, family** V25.09
  - contraception V25.9
  - procreation V26.4
- **Plaque**
  - artery, arterial - *see* Arteriosclerosis
  - calcareous - *see* Calcification
  - Hollenhorst's (retinal) 362.33
  - tongue 528.6
- **Plasma cell myeloma** 203.0
- **Plasmacytoma, plasmocytoma** (solitary) (M9731/1) 238.6
  - benign (M9731/0) - *see* Neoplasm, by site, benign
  - malignant (M9731/3) 203.8
- **Plasmacytopenia** 288.59 ◀
- **Plasmacytosis** 288.64 ⇐
- **Plaster ulcer** (*see also* Decubitus) 707.00
- **Platybasia** 756.0
- **Platyonychia** (congenital) 757.5
  - acquired 703.8
- **Platypelloid pelvis** 738.6
  - with disproportion (fetopelvic) 653.2
    - affecting fetus or newborn 763.1
    - causing obstructed labor 660.1
      - affecting fetus or newborn 763.1
  - congenital 755.69
- **Platyspondylia** 756.19
- **Plethora** 782.62
  - newborn 776.4
- **Pleura, pleural** - *see* condition
- **Pleuralgia** 786.52
- **Pleurisy** (acute) (adhesive) (chronic) (costal) (diaphragmatic) (double) (dry) (fetid) (fibrinous) (fibrous) (interlobar) (latent) (lung) (old) (plastic) (primary) (residual) (sicca) (sterile) (subacute) (unresolved) (with adherent pleura) 511.0
  - with
    - effusion (without mention of cause) 511.9
      - bacterial, nontuberculous 511.1
      - nontuberculous NEC 511.9
        - bacterial 511.1
      - pneumococcal 511.1
      - specified type NEC 511.8
      - staphylococcal 511.1
      - streptococcal 511.1
      - tuberculous (*see also* Tuberculosis, pleura) 012.0
        - primary, progressive 010.1
    - influenza, flu, or grippe 487.1
    - tuberculosis - *see* Pleurisy, tuberculous
  - encysted 511.8
  - exudative (*see also* Pleurisy, with effusion) 511.9
    - bacterial, nontuberculous 511.1
  - fibrinopurulent 510.9
    - with fistula 510.0
  - fibropurulent 510.9
    - with fistula 510.0
  - hemorrhagic 511.8
  - influenzal 487.1
  - pneumococcal 511.0
    - with effusion 511.1
  - purulent 510.9
    - with fistula 510.0
  - septic 510.9
    - with fistula 510.0
  - serofibrinous (*see also* Pleurisy, with effusion) 511.9
    - bacterial, nontuberculous 511.1
  - seropurulent 510.9
    - with fistula 510.0
  - serous (*see also* Pleurisy, with effusion) 511.9
    - bacterial, nontuberculous 511.1
  - staphylococcal 511.0
    - with effusion 511.1
  - streptococcal 511.0
    - with effusion 511.1
  - suppurative 510.9
    - with fistula 510.0
  - traumatic (post) (current) 862.29
    - with open wound into cavity 862.39
  - tuberculous (with effusion) (*see also* Tuberculosis, pleura) 012.0
    - primary, progressive 010.1
- **Pleuritis sicca** - *see* Pleurisy
- **Pleurobronchopneumonia** (*see also* Pneumonia, broncho-) 485
- **Pleurodynia** 786.52
  - epidemic 074.1
  - viral 074.1
- **Pleurohepatitis** 573.8
- **Pleuropericarditis** (*see also* Pericarditis) 423.9
  - acute 420.90
- **Pleuropneumonia** (acute) (bilateral) (double) (septic) (*see also* Pneumonia) 486
  - chronic (*see also* Fibrosis, lung) 515
- **Pleurorrhea** (*see also* Hydrothorax) 511.8
- **Plexitis, brachial** 353.0
- **Plica**
  - knee 727.83
  - polonica 132.0
  - tonsil 474.8
- **Plicae dysphonia ventricularis** 784.49
- **Plicated tongue** 529.5
  - congenital 750.13
- **Plug**
  - bronchus NEC 519.19 ⇐
  - meconium (newborn) NEC 777.1
  - mucus - *see* Mucus, plug

◀ New ⇐ Revised

Plumbism 984.9
specified type of lead - *see* Table of Drugs and Chemicals
Plummer's disease (toxic nodular goiter) 242.3
Plummer-Vinson syndrome (sideropenic dysphagia) 280.8
Pluricarential syndrome of infancy 260
Plurideficiency syndrome of infancy 260
Plus (and minus) hand (intrinsic) 736.09
PMDD (premenstrual dysphoric disorder) 625.4
PMS 625.4
Pneumathemia - *see* Air, embolism, by type
Pneumatic drill or hammer disease 994.9
Pneumatocele (lung) 518.89
intracranial 348.8
tension 492.0
Pneumatosis
cystoides intestinalis 569.89
peritonei 568.89
pulmonum 492.8
Pneumaturia 599.84
Pneumoblastoma (M8981/3) - *see* Neoplasm, lung, malignant
Pneumocephalus 348.8
Pneumococcemia 038.2
Pneumococcus, pneumococcal - *see* condition
Pneumoconiosis (due to) (inhalation of) 505
aluminum 503
asbestos 501
bagasse 495.1
bauxite 503
beryllium 503
carbon electrode makers' 503
coal
miners' (simple) 500
workers' (simple) 500
cotton dust 504
diatomite fibrosis 502
dust NEC 504
inorganic 503
lime 502
marble 502
organic NEC 504
fumes or vapors (from silo) 506.9
Pneumoconiosis *(Continued)*
graphite 503
hard metal 503
mica 502
moldy hay 495.0
rheumatoid 714.81
silica NEC 502
and carbon 500
silicate NEC 502
talc 502
Pneumocystis carinii pneumonia 136.3
Pneumocystis jiroveci pneumonia 136.3 ◀
Pneumocystosis 136.3
with pneumonia 136.3
Pneumoenteritis 025
Pneumohemopericardium (*see also* Pericarditis) 423.9
Pneumohemothorax (*see also* Hemothorax) 511.8
traumatic 860.4
with open wound into thorax 860.5
Pneumohydropericardium (*see also* Pericarditis) 423.9
Pneumohydrothorax (*see also* Hydrothorax) 511.8

Pneumomediastinum 518.1
congenital 770.2
fetus or newborn 770.2
Pneumomycosis 117.9
Pneumonia (acute) (Alpenstich) (benign) (bilateral) (brain) (cerebral) (circumscribed) (congestive) (creeping) (delayed resolution) (double) (epidemic) (fever) (flash) (fulminant) (fungoid) (granulomatous) (hemorrhagic) (incipient) (infantile) (infectious) (infiltration) (insular) (intermittent) (latent) (lobe) (migratory) (newborn) (organized) (overwhelming) (primary) (progressive) (pseudolobar) (purulent) (resolved) (secondary) (senile) (septic) (suppurative) (terminal) (true) (unresolved) (vesicular) 486
with influenza, flu, or grippe 487.0
adenoviral 480.0
adynamic 514
alba 090.0
allergic 518.3
alveolar - *see* Pneumonia, lobar
anaerobes 482.81
anthrax 022.1 *[484.5]*
apex, apical - *see* Pneumonia, lobar
ascaris 127.0 *[484.8]*
aspiration 507.0
due to
aspiration of microorganisms
bacterial 482.9
specified type NEC 482.89
specified organism NEC 483.8
bacterial NEC 482.89
viral 480.9
specified type NEC 480.8
food (regurgitated) 507.0
gastric secretions 507.0
milk 507.0
oils, essences 507.1
solids, liquids NEC 507.8
vomitus 507.0
fetal 770.18
due to
blood 770.16
clear amniotic fluid 770.14
meconium 770.12
postnatal stomach contents 770.86
newborn 770.18
due to
blood 770.16
clear amniotic fluid 770.14
meconium 770.12
postnatal stomach contents 770.86
asthenic 514
atypical (disseminated) (focal) (primary) 486
with influenza 487.0
bacillus 482.9
specified type NEC 482.89
bacterial 482.9
specified type NEC 482.89
Bacteroides (fragilis) (oralis) (melaninogenicus) 482.81
basal, basic, basilar - *see* Pneumonia, lobar
broncho-, bronchial (confluent) (croupous) (diffuse) (disseminated) (hemorrhagic) (involving lobes) (lobar) (terminal) 485
with influenza 487.0
allergic 518.3

Pneumonia *(Continued)*
broncho- *(Continued)*
aspiration (*see also* Pneumonia, aspiration) 507.0
bacterial 482.9
specified type NEC 482.89
capillary 466.19
with bronchospasm or obstruction 466.19
chronic (*see also* Fibrosis, lung) 515
congenital (infective) 770.0
diplococcal 481
Eaton's agent 483.0
Escherichia coli (E. coli) 482.82
Friedlander's bacillus 482.0
Haemophilus influenzae 482.2
hiberno-vernal 083.0 *[484.8]*
hypostatic 514
influenzal 487.0
inhalation (*see also* Pneumonia, aspiration) 507.0
due to fumes or vapors (chemical) 506.0
Klebsiella 482.0
lipid 507.1
endogenous 516.8
Mycoplasma (pneumoniae) 483.0
ornithosis 073.0
pleuropneumonia-like organisms (PPLO) 483.0
pneumococcal 481
Proteus 482.83
Pseudomonas 482.1
specified organism NEC 483.8
bacterial NEC 482.89
staphylococcal 482.40
aureus 482.41
specified type NEC 482.49
streptococcal - *see* Pneumonia, streptococcal
typhoid 002.0 *[484.8]*
viral, virus (*see also* Pneumonia, viral) 480.9
butyrivibrio (fibriosolvens) 482.81
candida 112.4
capillary 466.19
with bronchospasm or obstruction 466.19
caseous (*see also* Tuberculosis) 011.6
catarrhal - *see* Pneumonia, broncho-
central - *see* Pneumonia, lobar
chlamydia, chlamydial 483.1
pneumoniae 483.1
psittaci 073.0
specified type NEC 483.1
trachomatis 483.1
cholesterol 516.8
chronic (*see also* Fibrosis, lung) 515
cirrhotic (chronic) (*see also* Fibrosis, lung) 515
clostridium (haemolyticum) (novyi) NEC 482.81
confluent - *see* Pneumonia, broncho-
congenital (infective) 770.0
aspiration 770.18
croupous - *see* Pneumonia, lobar
cytomegalic inclusion 078.5 *[484.1]*
deglutition (*see also* Pneumonia, aspiration) 507.0
desquamative interstitial 516.8
diffuse - *see* Pneumonia, broncho-
diplococcal, diplococcus (broncho-) (lobar) 481
disseminated (focal) - *see* Pneumonia, broncho-

ICD-9-CM
P
Vol. 2

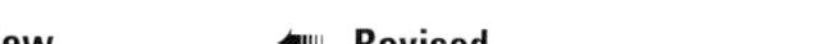

Pneumonia *(Continued)*
due to
adenovirus 480.0
anaerobes 482.81
Bacterium anitratum 482.83
Chlamydia, chlamydial 483.1
pneumoniae 483.1
psittaci 073.0
specified type NEC 483.1
trachomatis 483.1
coccidioidomycosis 114.0
Diplococcus (pneumoniae) 481
Eaton's agent 483.0
Escherichia coli (E. coli) 482.82
Friedlander's bacillus 482.0
fumes or vapors (chemical) (inhalation) 506.0
fungus NEC 117.9 *[484.7]*
coccidioidomycosis 114.0
Haemophilus influenzae (H. influenzae) 482.2
Herellea 482.83
influenza 487.0
Klebsiella pneumoniae 482.0
Mycoplasma (pneumoniae) 483.0
parainfluenza virus 480.2
pleuropneumonia-like organism (PPLO) 483.0
Pneumococcus 481
Pneumocystis carinii 136.3
Pneumocystis jiroveci 136.3 ◀
Proteus 482.83
Pseudomonas 482.1
respiratory syncytial virus 480.1
rickettsia 083.9 *[484.8]*
SARS-associated coronavirus 480.3
specified
bacteria NEC 482.89
organism NEC 483.8
virus NEC 480.8
Staphylococcus 482.40
aureus 482.41
specified type NEC 482.49
Streptococcus - *see also* Pneumonia, streptococcal
pneumoniae 481
virus (*see also* Pneumonia, viral) 480.9
SARS-associated coronavirus 480.3
Eaton's agent 483.0
embolic, embolism (*see* Embolism, pulmonary)
eosinophilic 518.3
Escherichia coli (E. coli) 482.82
eubacterium 482.81
fibrinous - *see* Pneumonia, lobar
fibroid (chronic) (*see also* Fibrosis, lung) 515
fibrous (*see also* Fibrosis, lung) 515
Friedländer's bacillus 482.0
fusobacterium (nucleatum) 482.81
gangrenous 513.0
giant cell (*see also* Pneumonia, viral) 480.9
gram-negative bacteria NEC 482.83
anaerobic 482.81
grippal 487.0
Hemophilus influenzae (bronchial) (lobar) 482.2
hypostatic (broncho-) (lobar) 514
in
actinomycosis 039.1
anthrax 022.1 *[484.5]*
aspergillosis 117.3 *[484.6]*
candidiasis 112.4
coccidioidomycosis 114.0
cytomegalic inclusion disease 078.5 *[484.1]*

Pneumonia *(Continued)*
in *(Continued)*
histoplasmosis (*see also* Histoplasmosis) 115.95
infectious disease NEC 136.9 *[484.8]*
measles 055.1
mycosis, systemic NEC 117.9 *[484.7]*
nocardiasis, nocardiosis 039.1
ornithosis 073.0
pneumocystosis 136.3
psittacosis 073.0
Q fever 083.0 *[484.8]*
salmonellosis 003.22
toxoplasmosis 130.4
tularemia 021.2
typhoid (fever) 002.0 *[484.8]*
varicella 052.1
whooping cough (*see also* Whooping cough) 033.9 *[484.3]*
infective, acquired prenatally 770.0
influenzal (broncho) (lobar) (virus) 487.0
inhalation (*see also* Pneumonia, aspiration) 507.0
fumes or vapors (chemical) 506.0
interstitial 516.8
with influenzal 487.0
acute 136.3
chronic (*see also* Fibrosis, lung) 515
desquamative 516.8
hypostatic 514
lipoid 507.1
lymphoid 516.8
plasma cell 136.3
Pseudomonas 482.1
intrauterine (infective) 770.0
aspiration 770.18
blood 770.16
clear amniotic fluid 770.14
meconium 770.12
postnatal stomach contents 770.86
Klebsiella pneumoniae 482.0
Legionnaires' 482.84
lipid, lipoid (exogenous) (interstitial) 507.1
endogenous 516.8
lobar (diplococcal) (disseminated) (double) (interstitial) (pneumococcal, any type) 481
with influenza 487.0
bacterial 482.9
specified type NEC 482.89
chronic (*see also* Fibrosis, lung) 515
Escherichia coli (E. coli) 482.82
Friedländer's bacillus 482.0
Hemophilus influenzae (H. influenzae) 482.2
hypostatic 514
influenzal 487.0
Klebsiella 482.0
ornithosis 073.0
Proteus 482.83
Pseudomonas 482.1
psittacosis 073.0
specified organism NEC 483.8
bacterial NEC 482.89
staphylococcal 482.40
aureus 482.41
specified type NEC 482.49
streptococcal - *see* Pneumonia, streptococcal
viral, virus (*see also* Pneumonia, viral) 480.9
lobular (confluent) - *see* Pneumonia, broncho-
Löffler's 518.3
massive - *see* Pneumonia, lobar

Pneumonia *(Continued)*
meconium aspiration 770.12
metastatic NEC 038.8 *[484.8]*
Mycoplasma (pneumoniae) 483.0
necrotic 513.0
nitrogen dioxide 506.9
orthostatic 514
parainfluenza virus 480.2
parenchymatous (*see also* Fibrosis, lung) 515
passive 514
patchy - *see* Pneumonia, broncho
Peptococcus 482.81
Peptostreptococcus 482.81
plasma cell 136.3
pleurolobar - *see* Pneumonia, lobar
pleuropneumonia-like organism (PPLO) 483.0
pneumococcal (broncho) (lobar) 481
Pneumocystis (carinii) (jiroveci) 136.3 ⇐
postinfectional NEC 136.9 *[484.8]*
postmeasles 055.1
postoperative 997.3
primary atypical 486
Proprionibacterium 482.81
Proteus 482.83
Pseudomonas 482.1
psittacosis 073.0
radiation 508.0
respiratory syncytial virus 480.1
resulting from a procedure 997.3
rheumatic 390 *[517.1]*
Salmonella 003.22
SARS-associated coronavirus 480.3
segmented, segmental - *see* Pneumonia, broncho-
Serratia (marcascens) 482.83
specified
bacteria NEC 482.89
organism NEC 483.8
virus NEC 480.8
spirochetal 104.8 *[484]*
staphylococcal (broncho) (lobar) 482.40
aureus 482.41
specified type NEC 482.49
static, stasis 514
streptococcal (broncho) (lobar) NEC 482.30
Group
A 482.31
B 482.32
specified NEC 482.39
pneumoniae 481
specified type NEC 482.39
Streptococcus pneumoniae 481
traumatic (complication) (early) (secondary) 958.8
tuberculous (any) (*see also* Tuberculosis) 011.6
tularemic 021.2
TWAR agent 483.1
varicella 052.1
Veillonella 482.81
viral, virus (broncho) (interstitial) (lobar) 480.9
with influenza, flu, or grippe 487.0
adenoviral 480.0
parainfluenza 480.2
respiratory syncytial 480.1
SARS-associated coronavirus 480.3
specified type NEC 480.8
white (congenital) 090.0
Pneumonic - *see* condition
Pneumonitis (acute) (primary) (*see also* Pneumonia) 486

- **Pneumonitis** *(Continued)*
  - allergic 495.9
    - specified type NEC 495.8
  - aspiration 507.0
    - due to fumes or gases 506.0
    - fetal 770.18
      - due to
        - blood 770.16
        - clear amniotic fluid 770.14
        - meconium 770.12
        - postnatal stomach contents 770.86
    - newborn 770.18
      - due to
        - blood 770.16
        - clear amniotic fluid 770.14
        - meconium 770.12
        - postnatal stomach contents 770.86
    - obstetric 668.0
  - chemical 506.0
    - due to fumes or gases 506.0
  - cholesterol 516.8
  - chronic (*see also* Fibrosis, lung) 515
  - congenital rubella 771.0
  - crack 506.0
  - due to
    - crack (cocaine) 506.0
    - fumes or vapors 506.0
    - inhalation
      - food (regurgitated), milk, vomitus 507.0
      - oils, essences 507.1
      - saliva 507.0
      - solids, liquids NEC 507.8
    - toxoplasmosis (acquired) 130.4
      - congenital (active) 771.2 *[484.8]*
  - eosinophilic 518.3
  - fetal aspiration 770.18
    - due to
      - blood 770.16
      - clear amniotic fluid 770.14
      - meconium 770.12
      - postnatal stomach contents 770.86
  - hypersensitivity 495.9
  - interstitial (chronic) (*see also* Fibrosis, lung) 515
    - lymphoid 516.8
  - lymphoid, interstitial 516.8
  - meconium aspiration 770.12
  - postanesthetic
    - correct substance properly administered 507.0
    - obstetric 668.0
    - overdose or wrong substance given 968.4
      - specified anesthetic - *see* Table of Drugs and Chemicals
  - postoperative 997.3
    - obstetric 668.0
  - radiation 508.0
  - rubella, congenital 771.0
  - "ventilation" 495.7
  - wood-dust 495.8
- **Pneumonoconiosis** - *see* Pneumoconiosis
- **Pneumoparotid** 527.8
- **Pneumopathy NEC** 518.89
  - alveolar 516.9
    - specified NEC 516.8
  - due to dust NEC 504
  - parietoalveolar 516.9
    - specified condition NEC 516.8
- **Pneumopericarditis** (*see also* Pericarditis) 423.9
  - acute 420.90
- **Pneumopericardium** - *see also* Pericarditis
  - congenital 770.2
  - fetus or newborn 770.2
  - traumatic (post) (*see also* Pneumothorax, traumatic) 860.0
    - with open wound into thorax 860.1
- **Pneumoperitoneum** 568.89
  - fetus or newborn 770.2
- **Pneumophagia** (psychogenic) 306.4
- **Pneumopleurisy, pneumopleuritis** (*see also* Pneumonia) 486
- **Pneumopyopericardium** 420.99
- **Pneumopyothorax** (*see also* Pyopneumothorax) 510.9
  - with fistula 510.0
- **Pneumorrhagia** 786.3
  - newborn 770.3
  - tuberculous (*see also* Tuberculosis, pulmonary) 011.9
- **Pneumosiderosis** (occupational) 503
- **Pneumothorax** (acute) (chronic) 512.8
  - congenital 770.2
  - due to operative injury of chest wall or lung 512.1
    - accidental puncture or laceration 512.1
  - fetus or newborn 770.2
  - iatrogenic 512.1
  - postoperative 512.1
  - spontaneous 512.8
    - fetus or newborn 770.2
    - tension 512.0
  - sucking 512.8
    - iatrogenic 512.1
    - postoperative 512.1
  - tense valvular, infectional 512.0
  - tension 512.0
    - iatrogenic 512.1
    - postoperative 512.1
    - spontaneous 512.0
  - traumatic 860.0
    - with
      - hemothorax 860.4
        - with open wound into thorax 860.5
      - open wound into thorax 860.1
  - tuberculous (*see also* Tuberculosis) 011.7
- **Pocket**(s)
  - endocardial (*see also* Endocarditis) 424.90
  - periodontal 523.8
- **Podagra** 274.9
- **Podencephalus** 759.89
- **Poikilocytosis** 790.09
- **Poikiloderma** 709.09
  - Civatte's 709.09
  - congenital 757.33
  - vasculare atrophicans 696.2
- **Poikilodermatomyositis** 710.3
- **Pointed ear** 744.29
- **Poise imperfect** 729.9
- **Poisoned** - *see* Poisoning
- **Poisoning** (acute) - *see also* Table of Drugs and Chemicals
  - Bacillus, B.
    - aertrycke (*see also* Infection, Salmonella) 003.9
    - botulinus 005.1
    - cholerae (suis) (*see also* Infection, Salmonella) 003.9
    - paratyphosus (*see also* Infection, Salmonella) 003.9
    - suipestifer (*see also* Infection, Salmonella) 003.9
  - bacterial toxins NEC 005.9
  - berries, noxious 988.2

- **Poisoning** *(Continued)*
  - blood (general) - *see* Septicemia
  - botulism 005.1
  - bread, moldy, mouldy - *see* Poisoning, food
  - damaged meat - *see* Poisoning, food
  - death-cap (Amanita phalloides) (Amanita verna) 988.1
  - decomposed food - *see* Poisoning, food
  - diseased food - *see* Poisoning, food
  - drug - *see* Table of Drugs and Chemicals
  - epidemic, fish, meat, or other food - *see* Poisoning, food
  - fava bean 282.2
  - fish (bacterial) - *see also* Poisoning, food
    - noxious 988.0
  - food (acute) (bacterial) (diseased) (infected) NEC 005.9
    - due to
      - bacillus
        - aertrycke (*see also* Poisoning, food, due to Salmonella) 003.9
        - botulinus 005.1
        - cereus 005.89
        - choleraesuis (*see also* Poisoning, food, due to Salmonella) 003.9
        - paratyphosus (*see also* Poisoning, food, due to Salmonella) 003.9
        - suipestifer (*see also* Poisoning, food, due to Salmonella) 003.9
      - Clostridium 005.3
        - botulinum 005.1
        - perfringens 005.2
        - welchii 005.2
      - Salmonella (aertrycke) (callinarum) (choleraesuis) (enteritidis) (paratyphi) (suipestifer) 003.9
        - with
          - gastroenteritis 003.0
          - localized infection(s) (*see also* Infection, Salmonella) 003.20
          - septicemia 003.1
          - specified manifestation NEC 003.8
      - specified bacterium NEC 005.89
      - Staphylococcus 005.0
      - Streptococcus 005.89
      - Vibrio parahaemolyticus 005.4
      - Vibrio vulnificus 005.81
    - noxious or naturally toxic 988.0
      - berries 988.2
      - fish 988.0
      - mushroom 988.1
      - plants NEC 988.2
  - ice cream - *see* Poisoning, food
  - ichthyotoxism (bacterial) 005.9
  - kreotoxism, food 005.9
  - malarial - *see* Malaria
  - meat - *see* Poisoning, food
  - mushroom (noxious) 988.1
  - mussel - *see also* Poisoning, food
    - noxious 988.0
  - noxious foodstuffs (*see also* Poisoning, food, noxious) 988.9
    - specified type NEC 988.8
  - plants, noxious 988.2
  - pork - *see also* Poisoning, food
    - specified NEC 988.8
    - Trichinosis 124
  - ptomaine - *see* Poisoning, food
  - putrefaction, food - *see* Poisoning, food

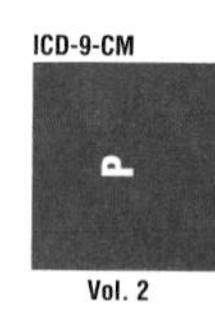

ICD-9-CM
P
Vol. 2

Poisoning *(Continued)*
radiation 508.0
Salmonella (*see also* Infection, Salmonella) 003.9
sausage - *see also* Poisoning, food
Trichinosis 124
saxitoxin 988.0
shellfish - *see also* Poisoning, food
noxious 988.0
Staphylococcus, food 005.0
toxic, from disease NEC 799.89
truffles - *see* Poisoning, food
uremic - *see* Uremia
uric acid 274.9
Poison ivy, oak, sumac or other plant dermatitis 692.6
Poker spine 720.0
Policeman's disease 729.2
Polioencephalitis (acute) (bulbar) (*see also* Poliomyelitis, bulbar) 045.0
inferior 335.22
influenzal 487.8
superior hemorrhagic (acute) (Wernicke's) 265.1
Wernicke's (superior hemorrhagic) 265.1
Polioencephalomyelitis (acute) (anterior) (bulbar) (*see also* Polioencephalitis) 045.0
Polioencephalopathy, superior hemorrhagic 265.1
with
beriberi 265.0
pellagra 265.2
Poliomeningoencephalitis - *see* Meningoencephalitis
Poliomyelitis (acute) (anterior) (epidemic) 045.9

Note Use the following fifth-digit subclassification with category 045:

0 poliovirus, unspecified type
1 poliovirus, type I
2 poliovirus, type II
3 poliovirus, type II

with
paralysis 045.1
bulbar 045.0
abortive 045.2
ascending 045.9
progressive 045.9
bulbar 045.0
cerebral 045.0
chronic 335.21
congenital 771.2
contact V01.2
deformities 138
exposure to V01.2
late effect 138
nonepidemic 045.9
nonparalytic 045.2
old with deformity 138
posterior, acute 053.19
residual 138
sequelae 138
spinal, acute 045.9
syphilitic (chronic) 094.89
vaccination, prophylactic (against) V04.0
Poliosis (eyebrow) (eyelashes) 704.3
circumscripta (congenital) 757.4
acquired 704.3
congenital 757.4
Pollakiuria 788.41
psychogenic 306.53
Pollinosis 477.0
Pollitzer's disease (hidradenitis suppurativa) 705.83
Polyadenitis (*see also* Adenitis) 289.3
malignant 020.0
Polyalgia 729.9
Polyangiitis (essential) 446.0
Polyarteritis (nodosa) (renal) 446.0
Polyarthralgia 719.49
psychogenic 306.0
Polyarthritis, polyarthropathy NEC 716.59
due to or associated with other specified conditions - *see* Arthritis, due to or associated with
endemic (*see also* Disease, Kaschin-Beck) 716.0
inflammatory 714.9
specified type NEC 714.89
juvenile (chronic) 714.30
acute 714.31
migratory - *see* Fever, rheumatic
rheumatic 714.0
fever (acute) - *see* Fever, rheumatic
Polycarential syndrome of infancy 260
Polychondritis (atrophic) (chronic) (relapsing) 733.99
Polycoria 743.46
Polycystic (congenital) (disease) 759.89
degeneration, kidney - *see* Polycystic, kidney
kidney (congenital) 753.12
adult type (APKD) 753.13
autosomal dominant 753.13
autosomal recessive 753.14
childhood type (CPKD) 753.14
infantile type 753.14
liver 751.62
lung 518.89
congenital 748.4
ovary, ovaries 256.4
spleen 759.0
Polycythemia (primary) (rubra) (vera) (M9950/1) 238.4
acquired 289.0
benign 289.0
familial 289.6
due to
donor twin 776.4
fall in plasma volume 289.0
high altitude 289.0
maternal-fetal transfusion 776.4
stress 289.0
emotional 289.0
erythropoietin 289.0
familial (benign) 289.6
Gaisböck's (hypertonica) 289.0
high altitude 289.0
hypertonica 289.0
hypoxemic 289.0
neonatorum 776.4
nephrogenous 289.0
relative 289.0
secondary 289.0
spurious 289.0
stress 289.0
Polycytosis cryptogenica 289.0
Polydactylism, polydactyly 755.00
fingers 755.01
toes 755.02
Polydipsia 783.5
Polydystrophic oligophrenia 277.5
Polyembryoma (M9072/3) - *see* Neoplasm, by site, malignant
Polygalactia 676.6
Polyglandular
deficiency 258.9
dyscrasia 258.9
Polyglandular *(Continued)*
dysfunction 258.9
syndrome 258.8
Polyhydramnios (*see also* Hydramnios) 657
Polymastia 757.6
Polymenorrhea 626.2
Polymicrogyria 742.2
Polymyalgia 725
arteritica 446.5
rheumatica 725
Polymyositis (acute) (chronic) (hemorrhagic) 710.4
with involvement of
lung 710.4 *[517.8]*
skin 710.3
ossificans (generalisata) (progressiva) 728.19
Wagner's (dermatomyositis) 710.3
Polyneuritis, polyneuritic (*see also* Polyneuropathy) 356.9
alcoholic 357.5
with psychosis 291.1
cranialis 352.6
demyelinating, chronic inflammatory 357.81
diabetic 250.6 *[357.2]*
due to lack of vitamin NEC 269.2 *[357.4]*
endemic 265.0 *[357.4]*
erythredema 985.0
febrile 357.0
hereditary ataxic 356.3
idiopathic, acute 357.0
infective (acute) 357.0
nutritional 269.9 *[357.4]*
postinfectious 357.0
Polyneuropathy (peripheral) 356.9
alcoholic 357.5
amyloid 277.39 *[357.4]* (Revised)
arsenical 357.7
critical illness 357.82
diabetic 250.6 *[357.2]*
due to
antitetanus serum 357.6
arsenic 357.7
drug or medicinal substance 357.6
correct substance properly administered 357.6
overdose or wrong substance given or taken 977.9
specified drug - *see* Table of Drugs and Chemicals
lack of vitamin NEC 269.2 *[357.4]*
lead 357.7
organophosphate compounds 357.7
pellagra 265.2 *[357.4]*
porphyria 277.1 *[357.4]*
serum 357.6
toxic agent NEC 357.7
hereditary 356.0
idiopathic 356.9
progressive 356.4
in
amyloidosis 277.39 *[357.4]* (Revised)
avitaminosis 269.2 *[357.4]*
specified NEC 269.1 *[357.4]*
beriberi 265.0 *[357.4]*
collagen vascular disease NEC 710.9 *[357.1]*
deficiency
B-complex NEC 266.2 *[357.4]*
vitamin B 266.9 *[357.4]*
vitamin B_6 266.1 *[357.4]*
diabetes 250.6 *[357.2]*

Polyneuropathy *(Continued)*
in *(Continued)*
diphtheria (*see also* Diphtheria) 032.89 *[357.4]*
disseminated lupus erythematosus 710.0 *[357.1]*
herpes zoster 053.13
hypoglycemia 251.2 *[357.4]*
malignant neoplasm (M8000/3) NEC 199.1 *[357.3]*
mumps 072.72
pellagra 265.2 *[357.4]*
polyarteritis nodosa 446.0 *[357.1]*
porphyria 277.1 *[357.4]*
rheumatoid arthritis 714.0 *[357.1]*
sarcoidosis 135 *[357.4]*
uremia 585.9 *[357.4]*
lead 357.7
nutritional 269.9 *[357.4]*
specified NEC 269.8 *[357.4]*
postherpetic 053.13
progressive 356.4
sensory (hereditary) 356.2
Polyonychia 757.5
Polyopia 368.2
refractive 368.15
Polyorchism, polyorchidism (three testes) 752.89
Polyorrhymenitis (peritoneal) (*see also* Polyserositis) 568.82
pericardial 423.2
Polyostotic fibrous dysplasia 756.54
Polyotia 744.1
Polyp, polypus

Note Polyps of organs or sites that do not appear in the list below should be coded to the residual category for diseases of the organ or site concerned.

accessory sinus 471.8
adenoid tissue 471.0
adenomatous (M8210/0) - *see also* Neoplasm, by site, benign
adenocarcinoma in (M8210/3) - *see* Neoplasm, by site, malignant
carcinoma in (M8210/3) - *see* Neoplasm, by site, malignant
multiple (M8221/0) - *see* Neoplasm, by site, benign
antrum 471.8
anus, anal (canal) (nonadenomatous) 569.0
adenomatous 211.4
Bartholin's gland 624.6
bladder (M8120/1) 236.7
broad ligament 620.8
cervix (uteri) 622.7
adenomatous 219.0
in pregnancy or childbirth 654.6
affecting fetus or newborn 763.89
causing obstructed labor 660.2
mucous 622.7
nonneoplastic 622.7
choanal 471.0
cholesterol 575.6
clitoris 624.6
colon (M8210/0) (*see also* Polyp, adenomatous) 211.3
corpus uteri 621.0
dental 522.0
ear (middle) 385.30
endometrium 621.0
ethmoidal (sinus) 471.8

Polyp, polypus *(Continued)*
fallopian tube 620.8
female genital organs NEC 624.8
frontal (sinus) 471.8
gallbladder 575.6
gingiva 523.8
gum 523.8
labia 624.6
larynx (mucous) 478.4
malignant (M8000/3) - *see* Neoplasm, by site, malignant
maxillary (sinus) 471.8
middle ear 385.30
myometrium 621.0
nares
anterior 471.9
posterior 471.0
nasal (mucous) 471.9
cavity 471.0
septum 471.9
nasopharyngeal 471.0
neoplastic (M8210/0) - *see* Neoplasm, by site, benign
nose (mucous) 471.9
oviduct 620.8
paratubal 620.8
pharynx 478.29
congenital 750.29
placenta, placental 674.4
prostate 600.20
with ⟸
other lower urinary tract symptoms (LUTS) 600.21 ◀
urinary ◀
obstruction 600.21 ◀
retention 600.21 ◀
pudenda 624.6
pulp (dental) 522.0
rectosigmoid 211.4
rectum (nonadenomatous) 569.0
adenomatous 211.4
septum (nasal) 471.9
sinus (accessory) (ethmoidal) (frontal) (maxillary) (sphenoidal) 471.8
sphenoidal (sinus) 471.8
stomach (M8210/0) 211.1
tube, fallopian 620.8
turbinate, mucous membrane 471.8
ureter 593.89
urethra 599.3
uterine
ligament 620.8
tube 620.8
uterus (body) (corpus) (mucous) 621.0
in pregnancy or childbirth 654.1
affecting fetus or newborn 763.89
causing obstructed labor 660.2
vagina 623.7
vocal cord (mucous) 478.4
vulva 624.6
Polyphagia 783.6
Polypoid - *see* condition
Polyposis - *see also* Polyp
coli (adenomatous) (M8220/0) 211.3
adenocarcinoma in (M8220/3) 153.9
carcinoma in (M8220/3) 153.9
familial (M8220/0) 211.3
intestinal (adenomatous) (M8220/0) 211.3
multiple (M8221/0) - *see* Neoplasm, by site, benign
Polyradiculitis (acute) 357.0
Polyradiculoneuropathy (acute) (segmentally demyelinating) 357.0
Polysarcia 278.00

Polyserositis (peritoneal) 568.82
due to pericarditis 423.2
paroxysmal (familial) 277.31 ⟸
pericardial 423.2
periodic (familial) 277.31 ⟸
pleural - *see* Pleurisy
recurrent 277.31 ⟸
tuberculous (*see also* Tuberculosis, polyserositis) 018.9
Polysialia 527.7
Polysplenia syndrome 759.0
Polythelia 757.6
Polytrichia (*see also* Hypertrichosis) 704.1
Polyunguia (congenital) 757.5
acquired 703.8
Polyuria 788.42
Pompe's disease (glycogenosis II) 271.0
Pompholyx 705.81
Poncet's disease (tuberculous rheumatism) (*see also* Tuberculosis) 015.9
Pond fracture - *see* Fracture, skull, vault
Ponos 085.0
Pons, pontine - *see* condition
Poor
aesthetics of existing restoration of tooth 525.67 ◀
contractions, labor 661.2
affecting fetus or newborn 763.7
fetal growth NEC 764.9
affecting management of pregnancy 656.5
incorporation
artificial skin graft 996.55
decellularized allodermis graft 996.55
obstetrical history V13.29
affecting management of current pregnancy V23.49
pre-term labor V23.41
pre-term labor V13.21
sucking reflex (newborn) 796.1
vision NEC 369.9
Poradenitis, nostras 099.1
Porencephaly (congenital) (developmental) (true) 742.4
acquired 348.0
nondevelopmental 348.0
traumatic (post) 310.2
Porocephaliasis 134.1
Porokeratosis 757.39
disseminated superficial actinic (DSAP) 692.75
Poroma, eccrine (M8402/0) - *see* Neoplasm, skin, benign
Porphyria (acute) (congenital) (constitutional) (erythropoietic) (familial) (hepatica) (idiopathic) (idiosyncratic) (intermittent) (latent) (mixed hepatic) (photosensitive) (South African genetic) (Swedish) 277.1
acquired 277.1
cutaneatarda
hereditaria 277.1
symptomatica 277.1
due to drugs
correct substance properly administered 277.1
overdose or wrong substance given or taken 977.9
specified drug - *see* Table of Drugs and Chemicals
secondary 277.1
toxic NEC 277.1
variegata 277.1
Porphyrinuria (acquired) (congenital) (secondary) 277.1

Porphyruria (acquired) (congenital) 277.1
Portal - *see* condition
Port wine nevus or mark 757.32
Posadas-Wernicke disease 114.9
Position
  fetus, abnormal (*see also* Presentation, fetal) 652.9
  teeth, faulty (*see also* Anomaly, position tooth) 524.30
Positive
  culture (nonspecific) 795.39
    AIDS virus V08
    blood 790.7
    HIV V08
    human immunodeficiency virus V08
    nose 795.39
    skin lesion NEC 795.39
    spinal fluid 792.0
    sputum 795.39
    stool 792.1
    throat 795.39
    urine 791.9
    wound 795.39
  findings, anthrax 795.31
  HIV V08
  human immunodeficiency virus (HIV) V08
  PPD 795.5
  serology
    AIDS virus V08
      inconclusive 795.71
    HIV V08
      inconclusive 795.71
    human immunodeficiency virus V08
      inconclusive 795.71
    syphilis 097.1
      with signs or symptoms - *see* Syphilis, by site and stage
      false 795.6
  skin test 795.7
    tuberculin (without active tuberculosis) 795.5
  VDRL 097.1
    with signs or symptoms - *see* Syphilis, by site and stage
    false 795.6
  Wassermann reaction 097.1
    false 795.6
Postcardiotomy syndrome 429.4
Postcaval ureter 753.4
Postcholecystectomy syndrome 576.0
Postclimacteric bleeding 627.1
Postcommissurotomy syndrome 429.4
Postconcussional syndrome 310.2
Postcontusional syndrome 310.2
Postcricoid region - *see* condition
Post-dates (pregnancy) - *see* Pregnancy
Postencephalitic - *see also* condition
  syndrome 310.8
Posterior - *see* condition
Posterolateral sclerosis (spinal cord) - *see* Degeneration, combined
Postexanthematous - *see* condition
Postfebrile - *see* condition
Postgastrectomy dumping syndrome 564.2
Posthemiplegic chorea 344.89
Posthemorrhagic anemia (chronic) 280.0
  acute 285.1
  newborn 776.5
Posthepatitis syndrome 780.79
Postherpetic neuralgia (intercostal) (syndrome) (zoster) 053.19
  geniculate ganglion 053.11
  ophthalmica 053.19
  trigeminal 053.12
Posthitis 607.1
Postimmunization complication or reaction - *see* Complications, vaccination
Postinfectious - *see* condition
Postinfluenzal syndrome 780.79
Postlaminectomy syndrome 722.80
  cervical, cervicothoracic 722.81
  kyphosis 737.12
  lumbar, lumbosacral 722.83
  thoracic, thoracolumbar 722.82
Postleukotomy syndrome 310.0
Postlobectomy syndrome 310.0
Postmastectomy lymphedema (syndrome) 457.0
Postmaturity, postmature (fetus or newborn) (gestation period over 42 completed weeks) 766.22
  affecting management of pregnancy
    post-term pregnancy 645.1
    prolonged pregnancy 645.2
  syndrome 766.22
Postmeasles - *see also* condition
  complication 055.8
    specified NEC 055.79
Postmenopausal
  endometrium (atrophic) 627.8
    suppurative (*see also* Endometritis) 615.9
  hormone replacement therapy V07.4
  status (age related) (natural) V49.81
Postnasal drip 784.91 (Revised)
Postnatal - *see* condition
Postoperative - *see also* condition
  confusion state 293.9
  psychosis 293.9
  status NEC (*see also* Status (post)) V45.89
Postpancreatectomy hyperglycemia 251.3
Postpartum - *see also* condition
  anemia 648.2
    cardiomyopathy 674.5
  observation
    immediately after delivery V24.0
    routine follow-up V24.2
Postperfusion syndrome NEC 999.8
  bone marrow 996.85
Postpoliomyelitic - *see* condition
Postsurgery status NEC (*see also* Status (post)) V45.89
Post-term (pregnancy) 645.1
  infant (gestation period over 40 completed weeks to 42 completed weeks) 766.21
Posttraumatic - *see* condition
Posttraumatic brain syndrome, nonpsychotic 310.2
Post-typhoid abscess 002.0
Post-Traumatic Stress Disorder (PTSD) 309.81 (New)
Postures, hysterical 300.11
Postvaccinal reaction or complication - *see* Complications, vaccination
Postvagotomy syndrome 564.2
Postvalvulotomy syndrome 429.4
Postvasectomy sperm count V25.8
Potain's disease (pulmonary edema) 514
Potain's syndrome (gastrectasis with dyspepsia) 536.1
Pott's
  curvature (spinal) (*see also* Tuberculosis) 015.0 *[737.43]*
  disease or paraplegia (*see also* Tuberculosis) 015.0 *[730.88]*
  fracture (closed) 824.4
    open 824.5
  gangrene 440.24
Pott's *(Continued)*
  osteomyelitis (*see also* Tuberculosis) 015.0 *[730.88]*
  spinal curvature (*see also* Tuberculosis) 015.0 *[737.43]*
  tumor, puffy (*see also* Osteomyelitis) 730.2
Potter's
  asthma 502
  disease 753.0
  facies 754.0
  lung 502
  syndrome (with renal agenesis) 753.0
Pouch
  bronchus 748.3
  Douglas' - *see* condition
  esophagus, esophageal (congenital) 750.4
    acquired 530.6
  gastric 537.1
  Hartmann's (abnormal sacculation of gallbladder neck) 575.8
    of intestine V44.3
      attention to V55.3
  pharynx, pharyngeal (congenital) 750.27
Poulet's disease 714.2
Poultrymen's itch 133.8
Poverty V60.2
Prader-Labhart-Willi-Fanconi syndrome (hypogenital dystrophy with diabetic tendency) 759.81
Prader-Willi syndrome (hypogenital dystrophy with diabetic tendency) 759.81
Preachers' voice 784.49
Pre-AIDS - *see* Human immunodeficiency virus (disease) (illness) (infection)
Preauricular appendage 744.1
Prebetalipoproteinemia (acquired) (essential) (familial) (hereditary) (primary) (secondary) 272.1
  with chylomicronemia 272.3
Precipitate labor 661.3
  affecting fetus or newborn 763.6
Preclimacteric bleeding 627.0
  menorrhagia 627.0
Precocious
  adrenarche 259.1
  menarche 259.1
  menstruation 626.8
  pubarche 259.1
  puberty NEC 259.1
  sexual development NEC 259.1
  thelarche 259.1
Precocity, sexual (constitutional) (cryptogenic) (female) (idiopathic) (male) NEC 259.1
  with adrenal hyperplasia 255.2
Precordial pain 786.51
  psychogenic 307.89
Predeciduous teeth 520.2
Prediabetes, prediabetic 790.29
  complicating pregnancy, childbirth, or puerperium 648.8
  fetus or newborn 775.89 (Revised)
Predislocation status of hip, at birth (*see also* Subluxation, congenital, hip) 754.32
Pre-eclampsia (mild) 642.4
  with pre-existing hypertension 642.7
  affecting fetus or newborn 760.0
  severe 642.5
  superimposed on pre-existing hypertensive disease 642.7
Preeruptive color change, teeth, tooth 520.8

Preexcitation 426.7
atrioventricular conduction 426.7
ventricular 426.7
Preglaucoma 365.00
Pregnancy (single) (uterine) (without sickness) V22.2

Note Use the following fifth-digit subclassification with categories 640–648, 651–676:

0 unspecified as to episode of care
1 delivered, with or without mention of antepartum condition
2 delivered, with mention of postpartum complication
3 antepartum condition or complication
4 postpartum condition or complication

abdominal (ectopic) 633.00
with intrauterine pregnancy 633.01
affecting fetus or newborn 761.4
abnormal NEC 646.9
ampullar - *see* Pregnancy, tubal
broad ligament - *see* Pregnancy, cornual
cervical - *see* Pregnancy, cornual
combined (extrauterine and intrauterine) - *see* Pregnancy, cornual
complicated (by) 646.9
abnormal, abnormality NEC 646.9
cervix 654.6
cord (umbilical) 663.9
pelvic organs or tissues NEC 654.9
pelvis (bony) 653.0
perineum or vulva 654.8
placenta, placental (vessel) 656.7
position
cervix 654.4
placenta 641.1
without hemorrhage 641.0
uterus 654.4
size, fetus 653.5
uterus (congenital) 654.0
abscess or cellulitis
bladder 646.6
genitourinary tract (conditions classifiable to 590, 595, 597, 599.0, 614.0–614.5, 614.7–614.9, 615) 646.6
kidney 646.6
urinary tract NEC 646.6
adhesion, pelvic peritoneal 648.9
air embolism 673.0
albuminuria 646.2
with hypertension - *see* Toxemia, of pregnancy
amnionitis 658.4
amniotic fluid embolism 673.1
anemia (conditions classifiable to 280–285) 648.2
appendicitis 648.9 ◀
atrophy, yellow (acute) (liver) (subacute) 646.7
bacilluria, asymptomatic 646.5
bacteriuria, asymptomatic 646.5
bariatric surgery status 649.2 ◀
bicornis or bicornuate uterus 654.0
biliary problems 646.8
bone and joint disorders (conditions classifiable to 720–724 or conditions affecting lower limbs classifiable to 711–719, 725–738) 648.7
breech presentation (buttocks) (complete) (frank) 652.2

Pregnancy *(Continued)*
complicated *(Continued)*
breech presentation *(Continued)*
with successful version 652.1
cardiovascular disease (conditions classifiable to 390–398, 410–429) 648.6
congenital (conditions classifiable to 745–747) 648.5
cerebrovascular disorders (conditions classifiable to 430–434, 436–437) 674.0
cervicitis (conditions classifiable to 616.0) 646.6
chloasma (gravidarum) 646.8
cholelithiasis 646.8
chorea (gravidarum) - *see* Eclampsia, pregnancy
coagulation defect 649.3 ◀
contraction, pelvis (general) 653.1
inlet 653.2
outlet 653.3
convulsions (eclamptic) (uremic) 642.6
with pre-existing hypertension 642.7
current disease or condition (nonobstetric)
abnormal glucose tolerance 648.8
anemia 648.2
bone and joint (lower limb) 648.7
cardiovascular 648.6
congenital 648.5
cerebrovascular 674.0
diabetic 648.0
drug dependence 648.3
female genital mutilation 648.9
genital organ or tract 646.6
gonorrheal 647.1
hypertensive 642.2
chronic kidney 642.2 ◀
renal 642.1
infectious 647.9
specified type NEC 647.8
liver 646.7
malarial 647.4
nutritional deficiency 648.9
parasitic NEC 647.8
periodontal disease 648.9
renal 646.2
hypertensive 642.1
rubella 647.5
specified condition NEC 648.9
syphilitic 647.0
thyroid 648.1
tuberculous 647.3
urinary 646.6
venereal 647.2
viral NEC 647.6
cystitis 646.6
cystocele 654.4
death of fetus (near term) 656.4
early pregnancy (before 22 completed weeks' gestation) 632
deciduitis 646.6
decreased fetal movements 655.7
diabetes (mellitus) (conditions classifiable to 250) 648.0
disorders of liver 646.7
displacement, uterus NEC 654.4
disproportion - *see* Disproportion
double uterus 654.0
drug dependence (conditions classifiable to 304) 648.3
dysplasia, cervix 654.6

Pregnancy *(Continued)*
complicated *(Continued)*
early onset of delivery (spontaneous) 644.2
eclampsia, eclamptic (coma) (convulsions) (delirium) (nephritis) (uremia) 642.6
with pre-existing hypertension 642.7
edema 646.1
with hypertension - *see* Toxemia, of pregnancy
effusion, amniotic fluid 658.1
delayed delivery following 658.2
embolism
air 673.0
amniotic fluid 673.1
blood-clot 673.2
cerebral 674.0
pulmonary NEC 673.2
pyemic 673.3
septic 673.3
emesis (gravidarum) - *see* Pregnancy, complicated, vomiting
endometritis (conditions classifiable to 615.0–615.9) 646.6
decidual 646.6
epilepsy 649.4 ◀
excessive weight gain NEC 646.1
face presentation 652.4
failure, fetal head to enter pelvic brim 652.5
false labor (pains) 644.1
fatigue 646.8
fatty metamorphosis of liver 646.7
female genital mutilation 648.9
fetal
death (near term) 656.4
early (before 22 completed weeks' gestation) 632
deformity 653.7
distress 656.8
reduction of multiple fetuses reduced to single fetus 651.7
fibroid (tumor) (uterus) 654.1
footling presentation 652.8
with successful version 652.1
gallbladder disease 646.8
gastric banding status 649.2 ◀
gastric bypass status for obesity 649.2 ◀
goiter 648.1
gonococcal infection (conditions classifiable to 098) 647.1
gonorrhea (conditions classifiable to 098) 647.1
hemorrhage 641.9
accidental 641.2
before 22 completed weeks' gestation NEC 640.9
cerebrovascular 674.0
due to
afibrinogenemia or other coagulation defect (conditions classifiable to 286.0–286.9) 641.3
leiomyoma, uterine 641.8
marginal sinus (rupture) 641.2
premature separation, placenta 641.2
trauma 641.8
early (before 22 completed weeks' gestation) 640.9
threatened abortion 640.0
unavoidable 641.1
hepatitis (acute) (malignant) (subacute) 646.7

ICD-9-CM

P

Vol. 2

- **Pregnancy** *(Continued)*
  - complicated *(Continued)*
    - hepatitis *(Continued)*
      - viral 647.6
    - herniation of uterus 654.4
    - high head at term 652.5
    - hydatidiform mole (delivered) (undelivered) 630
    - hydramnios 657
    - hydrocephalic fetus 653.6
    - hydrops amnii 657
    - hydrorrhea 658.1
    - hyperemesis (gravidarum) - *see* Hyperemesis, gravidarum
    - hypertension - *see* Hypertension, complicating pregnancy
    - hypertensive
      - chronic kidney disease 642.2 ◀
      - heart and chronic kidney disease 642.2 ◀
      - heart and renal disease 642.2
      - heart disease 642.2
      - renal disease 642.2
    - hypertensive heart and chronic kidney disease 642.2 ◀
    - hyperthyroidism 648.1
    - hypothyroidism 648.1
    - hysteralgia 646.8
    - icterus gravis 646.7
    - incarceration, uterus 654.3
    - incompetent cervix (os) 654.5
    - infection 647.9
      - amniotic fluid 658.4
      - bladder 646.6
      - genital organ (conditions classifiable to 614.0–614.5, 614.7–614.9, 615) 646.6
      - kidney (conditions classifiable to 590.0–590.9) 646.6
      - urinary (tract) 646.6
        - asymptomatic 646.5
    - infective and parasitic diseases NEC 647.8
    - inflammation
      - bladder 646.6
      - genital organ (conditions classifiable to 614.0–614.5, 614.7–614.9, 615) 646.6
      - urinary tract NEC 646.6
    - injury 648.9
      - obstetrical NEC 665.9
    - insufficient weight gain 646.8
    - intrauterine fetal death (near term) NEC 656.4
      - early (before 22 completed weeks' gestation) 632
    - malaria (conditions classifiable to 084) 647.4
    - malformation, uterus (congenital) 654.0
    - malnutrition (conditions classifiable to 260–269) 648.9
    - malposition
      - fetus - *see* Pregnancy, complicated, malpresentation
      - uterus or cervix 654.4
    - malpresentation 652.9
      - with successful version 652.1
      - in multiple gestation 652.6
      - specified type NEC 652.8
    - marginal sinus hemorrhage or rupture 641.2
    - maternal obesity syndrome 646.1
    - menstruation 640.8
    - mental disorders (conditions classifiable to 290–303, 305.0, 305.2–305.9, 306–316, 317–319) 648.4 ⬅
    - mentum presentation 652.4
    - missed
      - abortion 632
      - delivery (at or near term) 656.4
      - labor (at or near term) 656.4
    - necrosis
      - genital organ or tract (conditions classifiable to 614.0–614.5, 614.7–614.9, 615) 646.6
      - liver (conditions classifiable to 570) 646.7
      - renal, cortical 646.2
    - nephritis or nephrosis (conditions classifiable to 580–589) 646.2
      - with hypertension 642.1
    - nephropathy NEC 646.2
    - neuritis (peripheral) 646.4
    - nutritional deficiency (conditions classifiable to 260–269) 648.9
    - obesity 649.1 ◀
      - surgery status 649.2 ◀
    - oblique lie or presentation 652.3
      - with successful version 652.1
    - obstetrical trauma NEC 665.9
    - oligohydramnios NEC 658.0
    - onset of contractions before 37 weeks 644.0
    - oversize fetus 653.5
    - papyraceous fetus 646.0
    - patent cervix 654.5
    - pelvic inflammatory disease (conditions classifiable to 614.0–614.5, 614.7–614.9, 615) 646.6
    - pelvic peritoneal adhesion 648.9
    - placenta, placental
      - abnormality 656.7
      - abruptio or ablatio 641.2
      - detachment 641.2
      - disease 656.7
      - infarct 656.7
      - low implantation 641.1
        - without hemorrhage 641.0
      - malformation 656.7
      - malposition 641.1
        - without hemorrhage 641.0
      - marginal sinus hemorrhage 641.2
      - previa 641.1
        - without hemorrhage 641.0
      - separation (premature) (undelivered) 641.2
    - placentitis 658.4
    - polyhydramnios 657
    - postmaturity
      - post-term 645.1
      - prolonged 645.2
    - prediabetes 648.8
    - pre-eclampsia (mild) 642.4
      - severe 642.5
      - superimposed on pre-existing hypertensive disease 642.7
    - premature rupture of membranes 658.1
      - with delayed delivery 658.2
    - previous
      - infertility V23.0
      - nonobstetric condition V23.89
      - poor obstetrical history V23.49
      - premature delivery V23.41
      - trophoblastic disease (conditions classifiable to 630) V23.1
    - prolapse, uterus 654.4
    - proteinuria (gestational) 646.2
      - with hypertension - *see* Toxemia, of pregnancy
    - pruritus (neurogenic) 646.8
    - psychosis or psychoneurosis 648.4
    - ptyalism 646.8
    - pyelitis (conditions classifiable to 590.0–590.9) 646.6
    - renal disease or failure NEC 646.2
      - with secondary hypertension 642.1
      - hypertensive 642.2
    - retention, retained dead ovum 631
    - retroversion, uterus 654.3
    - Rh immunization, incompatibility, or sensitization 656.1
    - rubella (conditions classifiable to 056) 647.5
    - rupture
      - amnion (premature) 658.1
        - with delayed delivery 658.2
      - marginal sinus (hemorrhage) 641.2
      - membranes (premature) 658.1
        - with delayed delivery 658.2
      - uterus (before onset of labor) 665.0
    - salivation (excessive) 646.8
    - salpingo-oophoritis (conditions classifiable to 614.0–614.2) 646.6
    - septicemia (conditions classifiable to 038.0–038.9) 647.8
      - postpartum 670
      - puerperal 670
    - smoking 649.0 ◀
    - spasms, uterus (abnormal) 646.8
    - specified condition NEC 646.8
    - spotting 649.5 ◀
    - spurious labor pains 644.1
    - status post ◀
      - bariatric surgery 649.2 ◀
      - gastric banding 649.2 ◀
      - gastric bypass for obesity 649.2 ◀
      - obesity surgery 649.2 ◀
    - superfecundation 651.9
    - superfetation 651.9
    - syphilis (conditions classifiable to 090–097) 647.0
    - threatened
      - abortion 640.0
      - premature delivery 644.2
      - premature labor 644.0
    - thrombophlebitis (superficial) 671.2
      - deep 671.3
    - thrombosis 671.9
      - venous (superficial) 671.2
        - deep 671.3
    - thyroid dysfunction (conditions classifiable to 240–246) 648.1
    - thyroiditis 648.1
    - thyrotoxicosis 648.1
    - tobacco use disorder 649.0 ◀
    - torsion of uterus 654.4
    - toxemia - *see* Toxemia, of pregnancy
    - transverse lie or presentation 652.3
      - with successful version 652.1
    - trauma 648.9
      - obstetrical 665.9
    - tuberculosis (conditions classifiable to 010–018) 647.3
    - tumor
      - cervix 654.6
      - ovary 654.4
      - pelvic organs or tissue NEC 654.4
      - uterus (body) 654.1
        - cervix 654.6

Pregnancy *(Continued)*
  complicated *(Continued)*
    tumor *(Continued)*
      vagina 654.7
      vulva 654.8
    unstable lie 652.0
    uremia - *see* Pregnancy, complicated, renal disease
    urethritis 646.6
    vaginitis or vulvitis (conditions classifiable to 616.1) 646.6
    varicose
      placental vessels 656.7
      veins (legs) 671.0
        perineum 671.1
        vulva 671.1
    varicosity, labia or vulva 671.1
    venereal disease NEC (conditions classifiable to 099) 647.2
    viral disease NEC (conditions classifiable to 042, 050–055, 057–079) 647.6
    vomiting (incoercible) (pernicious) (persistent) (uncontrollable) (vicious) 643.9
      due to organic disease or other cause 643.8
      early - *see* Hyperemesis, gravidarum
      late (after 22 completed weeks gestation) 643.2
    young maternal age 659.8
  complications NEC 646.9
  cornual 633.80
    with intrauterine pregnancy 633.81
    affecting fetus or newborn 761.4
  death, maternal NEC 646.9
  delivered - *see* Delivery
  ectopic (ruptured) NEC 633.90
    with intrauterine pregnancy 633.91
    abdominal - *see* Pregnancy, abdominal
    affecting fetus or newborn 761.4
    combined (extrauterine and intrauterine) - *see* Pregnancy, cornual
    ovarian - *see* Pregnancy, ovarian
    specified type NEC 633.80
      with intrauterine pregnancy 633.81
      affecting fetus or newborn 761.4
    tubal - *see* Pregnancy, tubal
  examination, pregnancy
    negative result V72.41
    not confirmed V72.40
    positive result V72.42
  extrauterine - *see* Pregnancy, ectopic
  fallopian - *see* Pregnancy, tubal
  false 300.11
    labor (pains) 644.1
  fatigue 646.8
  illegitimate V61.6
  incidental finding V22.2
  in double uterus 654.0
  interstitial - *see* Pregnancy, cornual
  intraligamentous - *see* Pregnancy, cornual
  intramural - *see* Pregnancy, cornual
  intraperitoneal - *see* Pregnancy, abdominal
  isthmian - *see* Pregnancy, tubal
  management affected by
    abnormal, abnormality
      fetus (suspected) 655.9
        specified NEC 655.8
      placenta 656.7
    advanced maternal age NEC 659.6
      multigravida 659.6
      primigravida 659.5

Pregnancy *(Continued)*
  management affected by *(Continued)*
    antibodies (maternal)
      anti-c 656.1
      anti-d 656.1
      anti-e 656.1
      blood group (ABO) 656.2
        rh(esus) 656.1
    appendicitis 648.9 ◀
    bariatric surgery status 649.2 ◀
    coagulation defect 649.3 ◀
    elderly multigravida 659.6
    elderly primigravida 659.5
    epilepsy 649.4 ◀
    fetal (suspected)
      abnormality 655.9
        acid-base balance 656.8
        heart rate or rhythm 659.7
        specified NEC 655.8
      acidemia 656.3
      anencephaly 655.0
      bradycardia 659.7
      central nervous system malformation 655.0
      chromosomal abnormalities (conditions classifiable to 758.0–758.9) 655.1
      damage from
        drugs 655.5
          obstetric, anesthetic, or sedative 655.5
        environmental toxins 655.8
        intrauterine contraceptive device 655.8
        maternal
          alcohol addiction 655.4
          disease NEC 655.4
          drug use 655.5
          listeriosis 655.4
          rubella 655.3
          toxoplasmosis 655.4
          viral infection 655.3
        radiation 655.6
      death (near term) 656.4
        early (before 22 completed weeks' gestation) 632
      distress 656.8
      excessive growth 656.6
      growth retardation 656.5
      hereditary disease 655.2
      hydrocephalus 655.0
      intrauterine death 656.4
      poor growth 656.5
      spina bifida (with myelomeningocele) 655.0
    fetal-maternal hemorrhage 656.0
    gastric banding status 649.2 ◀
    gastric bypass status for obesity 649.2 ◀
    hereditary disease in family (possibly) affecting fetus 655.2
    incompatibility, blood groups (ABO) 656.2
      Rh(esus) 656.1
    insufficient prenatal care V23.7
    intrauterine death 656.4
    isoimmunization (ABO) 656.2
      Rh(esus) 656.1
    large-for-dates fetus 656.6
    light-for-dates fetus 656.5
    meconium in liquor 656.8
    mental disorder (conditions classifiable to 290–303, 305.0, 305.2–305.9, 306–316, 317–319) 648.4
    multiparity (grand) 659.4

Pregnancy *(Continued)*
  management affected by *(Continued)*
    obesity 649.1 ◀
      surgery status 649.2 ◀
    poor obstetric history V23.49
      pre-term labor V23.41
    postmaturity
      post-term 645.1
      prolonged 645.2
    post-term pregnancy 645.1
    possible, not (yet) confirmed V72.40
    previous
      abortion V23.2
        habitual 646.3
      cesarean delivery 654.2
      difficult delivery V23.49
      forceps delivery V23.49
      habitual abortions 646.3
      hemorrhage, antepartum or postpartum V23.49
      hydatidiform mole V23.1
      infertility V23.0
      malignancy NEC V23.89
      nonobstetrical conditions V23.89
      premature delivery V23.41
      trophoblastic disease (conditions in 630) V23.1
      vesicular mole V23.1
    prolonged pregnancy 645.2
    small-for-dates fetus 656.5
    smoking 649.0 ◀
    spotting 649.5 ◀
    tobacco use disorder 649.0 ◀
    young maternal age 659.8
  maternal death NEC 646.9
  mesometric (mural) - *see* Pregnancy, cornual
  molar 631
    hydatidiform (*see also* Hydatidiform mole) 630
      previous, affecting management of pregnancy V23.1
    previous, affecting management of pregnancy V23.49
  multiple NEC 651.9
    with fetal loss and retention of one or more fetus(es) 651.6
    affecting fetus or newborn 761.5
    following (elective) fetal reduction 651.7
    specified type NEC 651.8
      with fetal loss and retention of one or more fetus(es) 651.6
      following (elective) fetal reduction 651.7
  mural - *see* Pregnancy, cornual
  observation NEC V22.1
    first pregnancy V22.0
    high-risk V23.9
      specified problem NEC V23.89
  ovarian 633.20
    with intrauterine pregnancy 633.21
    affecting fetus or newborn 761.4
  possible, not (yet) confirmed V72.40
  postmature
    post-term 645.1
    prolonged 645.2
  post-term 645.1
  prenatal care only V22.1
    first pregnancy V22.0
    high-risk V23.9
      specified problem NEC V23.89
  prolonged 645.2
  quadruplet NEC 651.2
    with fetal loss and retention of one or more fetus(es) 651.5

ICD-9-CM
P
Vol. 2

Pregnancy *(Continued)*
quadruplet NEC *(Continued)*
affecting fetus or newborn 761.5
following (elective) fetal reduction 651.7
quintuplet NEC 651.8
with fetal loss and retention of one or more fetus(es) 651.6
affecting fetus or newborn 761.5
following (elective) fetal reduction 651.7
sextuplet NEC 651.8
with fetal loss and retention of one or more fetus(es) 651.6
affecting fetus or newborn 761.5
following (elective) fetal reduction 651.7
spurious 300.11
superfecundation NEC 651.9
with fetal loss and retention of one or more fetus(es) 651.6
following (elective) fetal reduction 651.7
superfetation NEC 651.9
with fetal loss and retention of one or more fetus(es) 651.6
following (elective) fetal reduction 651.7
supervision (of) (for) - *see also* Pregnancy, management affected
by elderly
multigravida V23.82
primigravida V23.81
high-risk V23.9
insufficient prenatal care V23.7
specified problem NEC V23.89
multiparity V23.3
normal NEC V22.1
first V22.0
poor
obstetric history V23.49
pre-term labor V23.41
reproductive history V23.5
previous
abortion V23.2
hydatidiform mole V23.1
infertility V23.0
neonatal death V23.5
stillbirth V23.5
trophoblastic disease V23.1
vesicular mole V23.1
specified problem NEC V23.89
young
multigravida V23.84
primigravida V23.83
triplet NEC 651.1
with fetal loss and retention of one or more fetus(es) 651.4
affecting fetus or newborn 761.5
following (elective) fetal reduction 651.7
tubal (with rupture) 633.10
with intrauterine pregnancy 633.11
affecting fetus or newborn 761.4
twin NEC 651.0
with fetal loss and retention of one fetus 651.3
affecting fetus or newborn 761.5
following (elective) fetal reduction 651.7
unconfirmed V72.40
undelivered (no other diagnosis) V22.2
with false labor 644.1
high-risk V23.9
specified problem NEC V23.89
unwanted NEC V61.7

Pregnant uterus - *see* condition
Preiser's disease (osteoporosis) 733.09
Prekwashiorkor 260
Preleukemia 238.75 ⬅
Preluxation of hip, congenital (*see also* Subluxation, congenital, hip) 754.32
Premature - *see also* condition
beats (nodal) 427.60
atrial 427.61
auricular 427.61
postoperative 997.1
specified type NEC 427.69
supraventricular 427.61
ventricular 427.69
birth NEC 765.1
closure
cranial suture 756.0
fontanel 756.0
foramen ovale 745.8
contractions 427.60
atrial 427.61
auricular 427.61
auriculoventricular 427.61
heart (extrasystole) 427.60
junctional 427.60
nodal 427.60
postoperative 997.1
ventricular 427.69
ejaculation 302.75
infant NEC 765.1
excessive 765.0
light-for-dates - *see* Light-for-dates
labor 644.2
threatened 644.0
lungs 770.4
menopause 256.31
puberty 259.1
rupture of membranes or amnion 658.1
affecting fetus or newborn 761.1
delayed delivery following 658.2
senility (syndrome) 259.8
separation, placenta (partial) - *see* Placenta, separation
ventricular systole 427.69
Prematurity NEC 765.1
extreme 765.0
Premenstrual syndrome 625.4
Premenstrual tension 625.4
Premolarization, cuspids 520.2
Premyeloma 273.1
Prenatal
care, normal pregnancy V22.1
first V22.0
death, cause unknown - *see* Death, fetus
screening - *see* Antenatal, screening
teeth 520.6 ◀
Prepartum - *see* condition
Preponderance, left or right ventricular 429.3
Prepuce - *see* condition
PRES (posterior reversible encephalopathy syndrome) 348.39 ◀
Presbycardia 797
hypertensive (*see also* Hypertension, heart) 402.90
Presbycusis 388.01
Presbyesophagus 530.89
Presbyophrenia 310.1
Presbyopia 367.4
Prescription of contraceptives NEC V25.02
diaphragm V25.02
oral (pill) V25.01
emergency V25.03
postcoital V25.03
repeat V25.41

Prescription of contraceptives NEC *(Continued)*
repeat V25.40
oral (pill) V25.41
Presenile - *see also* condition
aging 259.8
dementia (*see also* Dementia, presenile) 290.10
Presenility 259.8
Presentation, fetal
abnormal 652.9
with successful version 652.1
before labor, affecting fetus or newborn 761.7
causing obstructed labor 660.0
affecting fetus or newborn, any, except breech 763.1
in multiple gestation (one or more) 652.6
specified NEC 652.8
arm 652.7
causing obstructed labor 660.0
breech (buttocks) (complete) (frank) 652.2
with successful version 652.1
before labor, affecting fetus or newborn 761.7
before labor, affecting fetus or newborn 761.7
brow 652.4
causing obstructed labor 660.0
buttocks 652.2
chin 652.4
complete 652.2
compound 652.8
cord 663.0
extended head 652.4
face 652.4
to pubes 652.8
footling 652.8
frank 652.2
hand, leg, or foot NEC 652.8
incomplete 652.8
mentum 652.4
multiple gestation (one fetus or more) 652.6
oblique 652.3
with successful version 652.1
shoulder 652.8
affecting fetus or newborn 763.1
transverse 652.3
with successful version 652.1
umbilical cord 663.0
unstable 652.0
Prespondylolisthesis (congenital) (lumbosacral) 756.11
Pressure
area, skin ulcer (*see also* Decubitus) 707.00
atrophy, spine 733.99
birth, fetus or newborn NEC 767.9
brachial plexus 353.0
brain 348.4
injury at birth 767.0
cerebral - *see* Pressure, brain
chest 786.59
cone, tentorial 348.4
injury at birth 767.0
funis - *see* Compression, umbilical cord
hyposystolic (*see also* Hypotension) 458.9
increased
intracranial 781.99

Pressure *(Continued)*
increased *(Continued)*
intracranial *(Continued)*
due to
benign intracranial hypertension 348.2
hydrocephalus - *see* hydrocephalus
injury at birth 767.8
intraocular 365.00
lumbosacral plexus 353.1
mediastinum 519.3
necrosis (chronic) (skin) (*see also* Decubitus) 707.00
nerve - *see* Compression, nerve
paralysis (*see also* Neuropathy, entrapment) 355.9
sore (chronic) (*see also* Decubitus) 707.00
spinal cord 336.9
ulcer (chronic) (*see also* Decubitus) 707.00
umbilical cord - *see* Compression, umbilical cord
venous, increased 459.89
Pre-syncope 780.2
Preterm infant NEC 765.1
extreme 765.0
Priapism (penis) 607.3
Prickling sensation (*see also* Disturbance, sensation) 782.0
Prickly heat 705.1
Primary - *see* condition
Primigravida, elderly
affecting
fetus or newborn 763.89
management of pregnancy, labor, and delivery 659.5
Primipara, old
affecting
fetus or newborn 763.89
management of pregnancy, labor, and delivery 659.5
Primula dermatitis 692.6
Primus varus (bilateral) (metatarsus) 754.52
P.R.I.N.D. 436
Pringle's disease (tuberous sclerosis) 759.5
Prinzmetal's angina 413.1
Prinzmetal-Massumi syndrome (anterior chest wall) 786.52
Prizefighter ear 738.7
Problem (with) V49.9
academic V62.3
acculturation V62.4
adopted child V61.29
aged
in-law V61.3
parent V61.3
person NEC V61.8
alcoholism in family V61.41
anger reaction (*see also* Disturbance, conduct) 312.0
behavior, child 312.9
behavioral V40.9
specified NEC V40.3
betting V69.3
cardiorespiratory NEC V47.2
care of sick or handicapped person in family or household V61.49
career choice V62.2
communication V40.1
conscience regarding medical care V62.6
delinquency (juvenile) 312.9
diet, inappropriate V69.1

Problem *(Continued)*
digestive NEC V47.3
ear NEC V41.3
eating habits, inappropriate V69.1
economic V60.2
affecting care V60.9
specified type NEC V60.8
educational V62.3
enuresis, child 307.6
exercise, lack of V69.0
eye NEC V41.1
family V61.9
specified circumstance NEC V61.8
fear reaction, child 313.0
feeding (elderly) (infant) 783.3
newborn 779.3
nonorganic 307.59
fetal, affecting management of pregnancy 656.9
specified type NEC 656.8
financial V60.2
foster child V61.29
specified NEC V41.8
functional V41.9
specified type NEC V41.8
gambling V69.3
genital NEC V47.5
head V48.9
deficiency V48.0
disfigurement V48.6
mechanical V48.2
motor V48.2
movement of V48.2
sensory V48.4
specified condition NEC V48.8
hearing V41.2
high-risk sexual behavior V69.2
identity 313.82
influencing health status NEC V49.89
internal organ NEC V47.9
deficiency V47.0
mechanical or motor V47.1
interpersonal NEC V62.81
jealousy, child 313.3
learning V40.0
legal V62.5
life circumstance NEC V62.89
lifestyle V69.9
specified NEC V69.8
limb V49.9
deficiency V49.0
disfigurement V49.4
mechanical V49.1
motor V49.2
movement, involving
musculoskeletal system V49.1
nervous system V49.2
sensory V49.3
specified condition NEC V49.5
litigation V62.5
living alone V60.3
loneliness NEC V62.89
marital V61.10
involving
divorce V61.0
estrangement V61.0
psychosexual disorder 302.9
sexual function V41.7
relationship V61.10
mastication V41.6
medical care, within family V61.49
mental V40.9
specified NEC V40.2
mental hygiene, adult V40.9

Problem *(Continued)*
multiparity V61.5
nail biting, child 307.9
neck V48.9
deficiency V48.1
disfigurement V48.7
mechanical V48.3
motor V48.3
movement V48.3
sensory V48.5
specified condition NEC V48.8
neurological NEC 781.99
none (feared complaint unfounded) V65.5
occupational V62.2
parent-child V61.20
relationship V61.20
partner V61.10
relationship V61.10
personal NEC V62.89
interpersonal conflict NEC V62.81
personality (*see also* Disorder, personality) 301.9
phase of life V62.89
placenta, affecting management of pregnancy 656.9
specified type NEC 656.8
poverty V60.2
presence of sick or handicapped person in family or household V61.49
psychiatric 300.9
psychosocial V62.9
specified type NEC V62.89
relational NEC V62.81
relationship, childhood 313.3
religious or spiritual belief
other than medical care V62.89
regarding medical care V62.6
self-damaging behavior V69.8
sexual
behavior, high-risk V69.2
function NEC V41.7
sibling
relational V61.8
relationship V61.8
sight V41.0
sleep disorder, child 307.40
sleep, lack of V69.4
smell V41.5
speech V40.1
spite reaction, child (*see also* Disturbance, conduct) 312.0
spoiled child reaction (*see also* Disturbance, conduct) 312.1
swallowing V41.6
tantrum, child (*see also* Disturbance, conduct) 312.1
taste V41.5
thumb sucking, child 307.9
tic (child) 307.21
trunk V48.9
deficiency V48.1
disfigurement V48.7
mechanical V48.3
motor V48.3
movement V48.3
sensory V48.5
specified condition NEC V48.8
unemployment V62.0
urinary NEC V47.4
voice production V41.4
Procedure (surgical) not done NEC V64.3
because of
contraindication V64.1

Procedure *(Continued)*
because of *(Continued)*
patient's decision V64.2
for reasons of conscience or religion V62.6
specified reason NEC V64.3
Procidentia
anus (sphincter) 569.1
rectum (sphincter) 569.1
stomach 537.89
uteri 618.1
Proctalgia 569.42
fugax 564.6
spasmodic 564.6
psychogenic 307.89
Proctitis 569.49
amebic 006.8
chlamydial 099.52
gonococcal 098.7
granulomatous 555.1
idiopathic 556.2
with ulcerative sigmoiditis 556.3
tuberculous (*see also* Tuberculosis) 014.8
ulcerative (chronic) (nonspecific) 556.2
with ulcerative sigmoiditis 556.3
Proctocele
female (without uterine prolapse) 618.04
with uterine prolapse 618.4
complete 618.3
incomplete 618.2
male 569.49
Proctocolitis, idiopathic 556.2
with ulcerative sigmoiditis 556.3
Proctoptosis 569.1
Proctosigmoiditis 569.89
ulcerative (chronic) 556.3
Proctospasm 564.6
psychogenic 306.4
Prodromal-AIDS - *see* Human immunodeficiency virus (disease) (illness) (infection)
Profichet's disease or syndrome 729.9
Progeria (adultorum) (syndrome) 259.8
Prognathism (mandibular) (maxillary) 524.00
Progonoma (melanotic) (M9363/0) - *see* Neoplasm, by site, benign
Progressive - *see* condition
Prolapse, prolapsed
anus, anal (canal) (sphincter) 569.1
arm or hand, complicating delivery 652.7
causing obstructed labor 660.0
affecting fetus or newborn 763.1
fetus or newborn 763.1
bladder (acquired) (mucosa) (sphincter)
congenital (female) (male) 756.71
female (*see also* Cystocele, female) 618.01
male 596.8
breast implant (prosthetic) 996.54
cecostomy 569.69
cecum 569.89
cervix, cervical (hypertrophied) 618.1 ◀Revised
anterior lip, obstructing labor 660.2
affecting fetus or newborn 763.1
congenital 752.49
postpartal (old) 618.1
stump 618.84 ◀
ciliary body 871.1
colon (pedunculated) 569.89
colostomy 569.69
conjunctiva 372.73
cord - *see* Prolapse, umbilical cord

Prolapse, prolapsed *(Continued)*
disc (intervertebral) - *see* Displacement, intervertebral disc
duodenum 537.89
eye implant (orbital) 996.59
lens (ocular) 996.53
fallopian tube 620.4
fetal extremity, complicating delivery 652.8
causing obstructed labor 660.0
fetus or newborn 763.1
funis - *see* Prolapse, umbilical cord
gastric (mucosa) 537.89
genital, female 618.9
specified NEC 618.89
globe 360.81
ileostomy bud 569.69
intervertebral disc - *see* Displacement, intervertebral disc
intestine (small) 569.89
iris 364.8
traumatic 871.1
kidney (*see also* Disease, renal) 593.0
congenital 753.3
laryngeal muscles or ventricle 478.79
leg, complicating delivery 652.8
causing obstructed labor 660.0
fetus or newborn 763.1
liver 573.8
meatus urinarius 599.5
mitral valve 424.0
ocular lens implant 996.53
organ or site, congenital NEC - *see* Malposition, congenital
ovary 620.4
pelvic (floor), female 618.89
perineum, female 618.89
pregnant uterus 654.4
rectum (mucosa) (sphincter) 569.1
due to Trichuris trichiuria 127.3
spleen 289.59
stomach 537.89
umbilical cord
affecting fetus or newborn 762.4
complicating delivery 663.0
ureter 593.89
with obstruction 593.4
ureterovesical orifice 593.89
urethra (acquired) (infected) (mucosa) 599.5
congenital 753.8
uterovaginal 618.4
complete 618.3
incomplete 618.2
specified NEC 618.89
uterus (first degree) (second degree) (third degree) (complete) (without vaginal wall prolapse) 618.1
with mention of vaginal wall prolapse - *see* Prolapse, uterovaginal
congenital 752.3
in pregnancy or childbirth 654.4
affecting fetus or newborn 763.1
causing obstructed labor 660.2
affecting fetus or newborn 763.1
postpartal (old) 618.1
uveal 871.1
vagina (anterior) (posterior) (vault) (wall) (without uterine prolapse) 618.00
with uterine prolapse 618.4
complete 618.3
incomplete 618.2
paravaginal 618.02

Prolapse, prolapsed *(Continued)*
vagina *(Continued)*
posthysterectomy 618.5
specified NEC 618.09
vitreous (humor) 379.26
traumatic 871.1
womb - *see* Prolapse, uterus
Prolapsus, female 618.9
Proliferative - *see* condition
Prolinemia 270.8
Prolinuria 270.8
Prolonged, prolongation
bleeding time (*see also* Defect, coagulation) 790.92
"idiopathic" (in von Willebrand's disease) 286.4
coagulation time (*see also* Defect, coagulation) 790.92
gestation syndrome 766.22
labor 662.1
affecting fetus or newborn 763.89
first stage 662.0
second stage 662.2
PR interval 426.11
pregnancy 645.2
prothrombin time (*see also* Defect, coagulation) 790.92
QT interval 794.31
syndrome 426.82
rupture of membranes (24 hours or more prior to onset of labor) 658.2
uterine contractions in labor 661.4
affecting fetus or newborn 763.7
Prominauris 744.29
Prominence
auricle (ear) (congenital) 744.29
acquired 380.32
ischial spine or sacral promontory
with disproportion (fetopelvic) 653.3
affecting fetus or newborn 763.1
causing obstructed labor 660.1
affecting fetus or newborn 763.1
nose (congenital) 748.1
acquired 738.0
Pronation
ankle 736.79
foot 736.79
congenital 755.67
Prophylactic
administration of
antibiotics V07.39
antitoxin, any V07.2
antivenin V07.2
chemotherapeutic agent NEC V07.39
fluoride V07.31
diphtheria antitoxin V07.2
gamma globulin V07.2
immune sera (gamma globulin) V07.2
RhoGAM V07.2
tetanus antitoxin V07.2
chemotherapy NEC V07.39
fluoride V07.31
hormone replacement (postmenopausal) V07.4
immunotherapy V07.2
measure V07.9
specified type NEC V07.8
postmenopausal hormone replacement V07.4
sterilization V25.2
Proptosis (ocular) (*see also* Exophthalmos) 376.30
thyroid 242.0
Propulsion
eyeball 360.81

- **Prosecution, anxiety concerning** V62.5
- **Prostate, prostatic** - *see* condition
- **Prostatism** 600.90
  - with ⬅
    - other lower urinary tract symptoms (LUTS) 600.91 ◀
    - urinary ◀
      - obstruction 600.91 ◀
      - retention 600.91 ◀
- **Prostatitis** (congestive) (suppurative) 601.9
  - acute 601.0
  - cavitary 601.8
  - chlamydial 099.54
  - chronic 601.1
  - diverticular 601.8
  - due to Trichomonas (vaginalis) 131.03
  - fibrous 600.90
    - with ⬅
      - other lower urinary tract symptoms (LUTS) 600.91 ◀
      - urinary ◀
        - obstruction 600.91 ◀
        - retention 600.91 ◀
    - gonococcal (acute) 098.12
    - chronic or duration of 2 months or over 098.32
  - granulomatous 601.8
  - hypertrophic 600.00
    - with ⬅
      - other lower urinary tract symptoms (LUTS) 600.01 ◀
      - urinary ◀
        - obstruction 600.01 ◀
        - retention 600.01 ◀
  - specified type NEC 601.8
  - subacute 601.1
  - trichomonal 131.03
  - tuberculous (*see also* Tuberculosis) 016.5 *[601.4]*
- **Prostatocystitis** 601.3
- **Prostatorrhea** 602.8
- **Prostatoseminovesiculitis, trichomonal** 131.03
- **Prostration** 780.79
  - heat 992.5
    - anhydrotic 992.3
    - due to
      - salt (and water) depletion 992.4
      - water depletion 992.3
  - nervous 300.5
  - newborn 779.89
  - senile 797
- **Protanomaly** 368.51
- **Protanopia** (anomalous trichromat) (complete) (incomplete) 368.51
- **Protein**
  - deficiency 260
  - malnutrition 260
  - sickness (prophylactic) (therapeutic) 999.5
- **Proteinemia** 790.99
- **Proteinosis**
  - alveolar, lung or pulmonary 516.0
  - lipid 272.8
  - lipoid (of Urbach) 272.8
- **Proteinuria** (*see also* Albuminuria) 791.0
  - Bence-Jones NEC 791.0
  - gestational 646.2
    - with hypertension - *see* Toxemia, of pregnancy
  - orthostatic 593.6
  - postural 593.6
- **Proteolysis, pathologic** 286.6
- **Protocoproporphyria** 277.1
- **Protoporphyria** (erythrohepatic) (erythropoietic) 277.1
- **Protrusio acetabuli** 718.65
- **Protrusion**
  - acetabulum (into pelvis) 718.65
  - device, implant, or graft - *see* Complications, mechanical
  - ear, congenital 744.29
  - intervertebral disc - *see* Displacement, intervertebral disc
  - nucleus pulposus - *see* Displacement, intervertebral disc
- **Proud flesh** 701.5
- **Prune belly** (syndrome) 756.71
- **Prurigo** (ferox) (gravis) (Hebra's) (hebrae) (mitis) (simplex) 698.2
  - agria 698.3
  - asthma syndrome 691.8
  - Besnier's (atopic dermatitis) (infantile eczema) 691.8
  - eczematodes allergicum 691.8
  - estivalis (Hutchinson's) 692.72
  - Hutchinson's 692.72
  - nodularis 698.3
  - psychogenic 306.3
- **Pruritus, pruritic** 698.9
  - ani 698.0
    - psychogenic 306.3
  - conditions NEC 698.9
    - psychogenic 306.3
  - due to Onchocerca volvulus 125.3
  - ear 698.9
  - essential 698.9
  - genital organ(s) 698.1
    - psychogenic 306.3
  - gravidarum 646.8
  - hiemalis 698.8
  - neurogenic (any site) 306.3
  - perianal 698.0
  - psychogenic (any site) 306.3
  - scrotum 698.1
    - psychogenic 306.3
  - senile, senilis 698.8
  - trichomonas 131.9
  - vulva, vulvae 698.1
    - psychogenic 306.3
- **Psammocarcinoma** (M8140/3) - *see* Neoplasm, by site, malignant
- **Pseudarthrosis, pseudoarthrosis** (bone) 733.82
  - joint following fusion V45.4
- **Pseudoacanthosis**
  - nigricans 701.8
- **Pseudoaneurysm** - *see* Aneurysm
- **Pseudoangina** (pectoris) - *see* Angina
- **Pseudoangioma** 452
- **Pseudo-Argyll-Robertson pupil** 379.45
- **Pseudoarteriosus** 747.89
- **Pseudoarthrosis** - *see* Pseudarthrosis
- **Pseudoataxia** 799.89
- **Pseudobulbar affect (PBA)** 310.8
- **Pseudobursa** 727.89
- **Pseudocholera** 025
- **Pseudochromidrosis** 705.89
- **Pseudocirrhosis, liver, pericardial** 423.2
- **Pseudocoarctation** 747.21
- **Pseudocowpox** 051.1
- **Pseudocoxalgia** 732.1
- **Pseudocroup** 478.75
- **Pseudocyesis** 300.11
- **Pseudocyst**
  - lung 518.89
  - pancreas 577.2
  - retina 361.19
- **Pseudodementia** 300.16
- **Pseudoelephantiasis neuroarthritica** 757.0
- **Pseudoemphysema** 518.89
- **Pseudoencephalitis**
  - superior (acute) hemorrhagic 265.1
- **Pseudoerosion cervix, congenital** 752.49
- **Pseudoexfoliation, lens capsule** 366.11
- **Pseudofracture** (idiopathic) (multiple) (spontaneous) (symmetrical) 268.2
- **Pseudoglanders** 025
- **Pseudoglioma** 360.44
- **Pseudogout** - *see* Chondrocalcinosis
- **Pseudohallucination** 780.1
- **Pseudohemianesthesia** 782.0
- **Pseudohemophilia** (Bernuth's) (hereditary) (type B) 286.4
  - type A 287.8
  - vascular 287.8
- **Pseudohermaphroditism** 752.7
  - with chromosomal anomaly - *see* Anomaly, chromosomal
  - adrenal 255.2
  - female (without adrenocortical disorder) 752.7
    - with adrenocortical disorder 255.2
    - adrenal 255.2
  - male (without gonadal disorder) 752.7
    - with
      - adrenocortical disorder 255.2
      - cleft scrotum 752.7
      - feminizing testis 259.5
      - gonadal disorder 257.9
    - adrenal 255.2
- **Pseudohole, macula** 362.54
- **Pseudo-Hurler's disease** (mucolipidosis III) 272.7
- **Pseudohydrocephalus** 348.2
- **Pseudohypertrophic muscular dystrophy** (Erb's) 359.1
- **Pseudohypertrophy, muscle** 359.1
- **Pseudohypoparathyroidism** 275.49
- **Pseudoinfluenza** 487.1
- **Pseudoinsomnia** 307.49
- **Pseudoleukemia** 288.8
  - infantile 285.8
- **Pseudomembranous** - *see* condition
- **Pseudomeningocele** (cerebral) (infective) 349.2
  - postprocedural 997.01
  - spinal 349.2
- **Pseudomenstruation** 626.8
- **Pseudomucinous**
  - cyst (ovary) (M8470/0) 220
  - peritoneum 568.89
- **Pseudomyeloma** 273.1
- **Pseudomyxoma peritonei** (M8480/6) 197.6
- **Pseudoneuritis optic** (nerve) 377.24
  - papilla 377.24
    - congenital 743.57
- **Pseudoneuroma** - *see* Injury, nerve, by site
- **Pseudo-obstruction**
  - intestine (chronic) (idiopathic) (intermittent secondary) (primary) 564.89
    - acute 560.89
- **Pseudopapilledema** 377.24
- **Pseudoparalysis**
  - arm or leg 781.4
  - atonic, congenital 358.8
- **Pseudopelade** 704.09
- **Pseudophakia** V43.1
- **Pseudopolycythemia** 289.0
- **Pseudopolyposis, colon** 556.4
- **Pseudoporencephaly** 348.0

Pseudopseudohypoparathyroidism 275.49
Pseudopsychosis 300.16
Pseudopterygium 372.52
Pseudoptosis (eyelid) 374.34
Pseudorabies 078.89
Pseudoretinitis, pigmentosa 362.65
Pseudorickets 588.0
senile (Pozzi's) 731.0
Pseudorubella 057.8
Pseudoscarlatina 057.8
Pseudosclerema 778.1
Pseudosclerosis (brain)
Jakob's 046.1
of Westphal (-Strümpell) (hepatolenticular degeneration) 275.1
spastic 046.1
with dementia
with behavioral disturbance 046.1 *[294.11]*
without behavioral disturbance 046.1 *[294.10]*
Pseudoseizure 780.39
non-psychiatric 780.39
psychiatric 300.11
Pseudotabes 799.89
diabetic 250.6 *[337.1]*
Pseudotetanus (*see also* Convulsions) 780.39
Pseudotetany 781.7
hysterical 300.11
Pseudothalassemia 285.0
Pseudotrichinosis 710.3
Pseudotruncus arteriosus 747.29
Pseudotuberculosis, pasteurella (infection) 027.2
Pseudotumor
cerebri 348.2
orbit (inflammatory) 376.11
Pseudo-Turner's syndrome 759.89
Pseudoxanthoma elasticum 757.39
Psilosis (sprue) (tropical) 579.1
Monilia 112.89
nontropical 579.0
not sprue 704.00
Psittacosis 073.9
Psoitis 728.89
Psora NEC 696.1
Psoriasis 696.1
any type, except arthropathic 696.1
arthritic, arthropathic 696.0
buccal 528.6
flexural 696.1
follicularis 696.1
guttate 696.1
inverse 696.1
mouth 528.6
nummularis 696.1
psychogenic 316 *[696.1]*
punctata 696.1
pustular 696.1
rupioides 696.1
vulgaris 696.1
Psorospermiasis 136.4
Psorospermosis 136.4
follicularis (vegetans) 757.39
Psychalgia 307.80
Psychasthenia 300.89
compulsive 300.3
mixed compulsive states 300.3
obsession 300.3
Psychiatric disorder or problem NEC 300.9
Psychogenic - *see also* condition
factors associated with physical conditions 316
Psychoneurosis, psychoneurotic (*see also* Neurosis) 300.9

Psychoneurosis, psychoneurotic *(Continued)*
anxiety (state) 300.00
climacteric 627.2
compensation 300.16
compulsion 300.3
conversion hysteria 300.11
depersonalization 300.6
depressive type 300.4
dissociative hysteria 300.15
hypochondriacal 300.7
hysteria 300.10
conversion type 300.11
dissociative type 300.15
mixed NEC 300.89
neurasthenic 300.5
obsessional 300.3
obsessive-compulsive 300.3
occupational 300.89
personality NEC 301.89
phobia 300.20
senile NEC 300.89
Psychopathic - *see also* condition
constitution, posttraumatic 310.2
with psychosis 293.9
personality 301.9
amoral trends 301.7
antisocial trends 301.7
asocial trends 301.7
mixed types 301.7
state 301.9
Psychopathy, sexual (*see also* Deviation, sexual) 302.9
Psychophysiologic, psychophysiological condition - *see* Reaction, psychophysiologic
Psychose passionelle 297.8
Psychosexual identity disorder 302.6
adult-life 302.85
childhood 302.6
Psychosis 298.9
acute hysterical 298.1
affecting management of pregnancy, childbirth, or puerperium 648.4
affective (*see also* Disorder, mood) 296.90

Note Use the following fifth-digit subclassification with categories 296.0–296.6:

0 unspecified
1 mild
2 moderate
3 severe, without mention of psychotic behavior
5 in partial or unspecified remission
6 in full remission

drug-induced 292.84
due to or associated with physical condition 293.83
involutional 293.83
recurrent episode 296.3
single episode 296.2
manic-depressive 296.80
circular (alternating) 296.7
currently depressed 296.5
currently manic 296.4
depressed type 296.2
atypical 296.82
recurrent episode 296.3
single episode 296.2
manic 296.0
atypical 296.81

Psychosis *(Continued)*
affective *(Continued)*
manic-depressive *(Continued)*
manic *(Continued)*
recurrent episode 296.1
single episode 296.0
mixed type NEC 296.89
specified type NEC 296.89
senile 290.21
specified type NEC 296.99
alcoholic 291.9
with
anxiety 291.89
delirium tremens 291.0
delusions 291.5
dementia 291.2
hallucinosis 291.3
jealousy 291.5
mood disturbance 291.89
paranoia 291.5
persisting amnesia 291.1
sexual dysfunction 291.89
sleep disturbance 291.89
amnestic confabulatory 291.1
delirium tremens 291.0
hallucinosis 291.3
Korsakoff's, Korsakov's, Korsakow's 291.1
paranoid type 291.5
pathological intoxication 291.4
polyneuritic 291.1
specified type NEC 291.89
alternating (*see also* Psychosis, manic-depressive, circular) 296.7
anergastic (*see also* Psychosis, organic) 294.9
arteriosclerotic 290.40
with
acute confusional state 290.41
delirium 290.41
delusions 290.42
depressed mood 290.43
depressed type 290.43
paranoid type 290.42
simple type 290.40
uncomplicated 290.40
atypical 298.9
depressive 296.82
manic 296.81
borderline (schizophrenia) (*see also* Schizophrenia) 295.5
of childhood (*see also* Psychosis, childhood) 299.8
prepubertal 299.8
brief reactive 298.8
childhood, with origin specific to 299.9

Note Use the following fifth-digit subclassification with category 299:

0 current or active state
1 residual state

atypical 299.8
specified type NEC 299.8
circular (*see also* Psychosis, manic-depressive, circular) 296.7
climacteric (*see also* Psychosis, involutional) 298.8
confusional 298.9
acute 293.0
reactive 298.2
subacute 293.1
depressive (*see also* Psychosis, affective) 296.2
atypical 296.82
involutional 296.2

Psychosis *(Continued)*
depressive *(Continued)*
involutional *(Continued)*
with hypomania (bipolar II) 296.89
recurrent episode 296.3
single episode 296.2
psychogenic 298.0
reactive (emotional stress) (psychological trauma) 298.0
recurrent episode 296.3
with hypomania (bipolar II) 296.89
single episode 296.2
disintegrative childhood (*see also* Psychosis, childhood) 299.1
drug 292.9
with
affective syndrome 292.84
amnestic syndrome 292.83
anxiety 292.89
delirium 292.81
withdrawal 292.0
delusions 292.11
dementia 292.82
depressive state 292.84
hallucinations 292.12
hallucinosis 292.12
mood disorder 292.84
mood disturbance 292.84
organic personality syndrome NEC 292.89
sexual dysfunction 292.89
sleep disturbance 292.89
withdrawal syndrome (and delirium) 292.0
affective syndrome 292.84
delusions 292.11
hallucinatory state 292.12
hallucinosis 292.12
paranoid state 292.11
specified type NEC 292.89
withdrawal syndrome (and delirium) 292.0
due to or associated with physical condition (*see also* Psychosis, organic) 294.9
epileptic NEC 293.9
excitation (psychogenic) (reactive) 298.1
exhaustive (*see also* Reaction, stress, acute) 308.9
hypomanic (*see also* Psychosis, affective) 296.0
recurrent episode 296.1
single episode 296.0
hysterical 298.8
acute 298.1
incipient 298.8
schizophrenic (*see also* Schizophrenia) 295.5
induced 297.3
infantile (*see also* Psychosis, childhood) 299.0
infective 293.9
acute 293.0
subacute 293.1
in
conditions classified elsewhere
with
delusions 293.81
hallucinations 293.82
pregnancy, childbirth, or puerperium 648.4
interactional (childhood) (*see also* Psychosis, childhood) 299.1
involutional 298.8

Psychosis *(Continued)*
involutional *(Continued)*
depressive (*see also* Psychosis, affective) 296.2
recurrent episode 296.3
single episode 296.2
melancholic 296.2
recurrent episode 296.3
single episode 296.2
paranoid state 297.2
paraphrenia 297.2
Korsakoff's, Korakov's, Korsakow's (nonalcoholic) 294.0
alcoholic 291.1
mania (phase) (*see also* Psychosis, affective) 296.0
recurrent episode 296.1
single episode 296.0
manic (*see also* Psychosis, affective) 296.0
atypical 296.81
recurrent episode 296.1
single episode 296.0
manic-depressive 296.80
circular 296.7
currently
depressed 296.5
manic 296.4
mixed 296.6
depressive 296.2
recurrent episode 296.3
with hypomania (bipolar II) 296.89
single episode 296.2
hypomanic 296.0
recurrent episode 296.1
single episode 296.0
manic 296.0
atypical 296.81
recurrent episode 296.1
single episode 296.0
mixed NEC 296.89
perplexed 296.89
stuporous 296.89
menopausal (*see also* Psychosis, involutional) 298.8
mixed schizophrenic and affective (*see also* Schizophrenia) 295.7
multi-infarct (cerebrovascular) (*see also* Psychosis, arteriosclerotic) 290.40
organic NEC 294.9
due to or associated with
addiction
alcohol (*see also* Psychosis, alcoholic) 291.9
drug (*see also* Psychosis, drug) 292.9
alcohol intoxication, acute (*see also* Psychosis, alcoholic) 291.9
alcoholism (*see also* Psychosis, alcoholic) 291.9
arteriosclerosis (cerebral) (*see also* Psychosis, arteriosclerotic) 290.40
cerebrovascular disease
acute (psychosis) 293.0
arteriosclerotic (*see also* Psychosis, arteriosclerotic) 290.40
childbirth - *see* Psychosis, puerperal
dependence
alcohol (*see also* Psychosis, alcoholic) 291.9
drug 292.9

Psychosis *(Continued)*
organic NEC *(Continued)*
due to or associated with *(Continued)*
disease
alcoholic liver (*see also* Psychosis, alcoholic) 291.9
brain
arteriosclerotic (*see also* Psychosis, arteriosclerotic) 290.40
cerebrovascular
acute (psychosis) 293.0
arteriosclerotic (*see also* Psychosis, arteriosclerotic) 290.40
endocrine or metabolic 293.9
acute (psychosis) 293.0
subacute (psychosis) 293.1
Jakob-Creutzfeldt (new variant)
with behavioral disturbance 046.1 *[294.11]*
without behavioral disturbance 046.1 *[294.10]*
liver, alcoholic (*see also* Psychosis, alcoholic) 291.9
disorder
cerebrovascular
acute (psychosis) 293.0
endocrine or metabolic 293.9
acute (psychosis) 293.0
subacute (psychosis) 293.1
epilepsy
with behavioral disturbance 345.9 *[294.11]*
without behavioral disturbance 345.9 *[294.10]*
transient (acute) 293.0
Huntington's chorea
with behavioral disturbance 333.4 *[294.11]*
without behavioral disturbance 333.4 *[294.10]*
infection
brain 293.9
acute (psychosis) 293.0
chronic 294.8
subacute (psychosis) 293.1
intracranial NEC 293.9
acute (psychosis) 293.0
chronic 294.8
subacute (psychosis) 293.1
intoxication
alcoholic (acute) (*see also* Psychosis, alcoholic) 291.9
pathological 291.4
drug (*see also* Psychosis, drug) 292.9
ischemia
cerebrovascular (generalized) (*see also* Psychosis, arteriosclerotic) 290.40
Jakob-Creutzfeldt disease (syndrome) (new variant)
with behavioral disturbance 046.1 *[294.11]*
without behavioral disturbance 046.1 *[294.10]*
multiple sclerosis
with behavioral disturbance 340 *[294.11]*
without behavioral disturbance 340 *[294.10]*
physical condition NEC 293.9
with
delusions 293.81
hallucinations 293.82

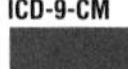
ICD-9-CM
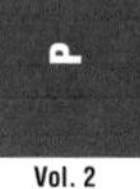
P
Vol. 2

- **Psychosis** *(Continued)*
  - organic NEC *(Continued)*
    - due to or associated with *(Continued)*
      - presenility 290.10
      - puerperium - *see* Psychosis, puerperal
      - sclerosis, multiple
        - with behavioral disturbance 340 *[294.11]*
        - without behavioral disturbance 340 *[294.10]*
      - senility 290.20
      - status epilepticus
        - with behavioral disturbance 345.3 *[294.11]*
        - without behavioral disturbance 345.3 *[294.10]*
      - trauma
        - brain (birth) (from electrical current) (surgical) 293.9
          - acute (psychosis) 293.0
          - chronic 294.8
          - subacute (psychosis) 293.1
      - unspecified physical condition 293.9
        - with
          - delusions 293.81
          - hallucinations 293.82
    - infective 293.9
      - acute (psychosis) 293.0
      - subacute 293.1
    - posttraumatic 293.9
      - acute 293.0
      - subacute 293.1
    - specified type NEC 294.8
    - transient 293.9
      - with
        - anxiety 293.84
        - delusions 293.81
        - depression 293.83
        - hallucinations 293.82
      - depressive type 293.83
      - hallucinatory type 293.82
      - paranoid type 293.81
      - specified type NEC 293.89
  - paranoic 297.1
  - paranoid (chronic) 297.9
    - alcoholic 291.5
    - chronic 297.1
    - climacteric 297.2
    - involutional 297.2
    - menopausal 297.2
    - protracted reactive 298.4
    - psychogenic 298.4
      - acute 298.3
    - schizophrenic (*see also* Schizophrenia) 295.3
    - senile 290.20
  - paroxysmal 298.9
    - senile 290.20
  - polyneuritic, alcoholic 291.1
  - postoperative 293.9
  - postpartum - *see* Psychosis, puerperal
  - prepsychotic (*see also* Schizophrenia) 295.5
  - presbyophrenic (type) 290.8
  - presenile (*see also* Dementia, presenile) 290.10
  - prison 300.16
  - psychogenic 298.8
    - depressive 298.0
    - paranoid 298.4
      - acute 298.3
  - puerperal
    - specified type - *see* categories 295–298
- **Psychosis** *(Continued)*
  - puerperal *(Continued)*
    - unspecified type 293.89
      - acute 293.0
      - chronic 293.89
      - subacute 293.1
  - reactive (emotional stress) (psychological trauma) 298.8
    - brief 298.8
    - confusion 298.2
    - depressive 298.0
    - excitation 298.1
  - schizo-affective (depressed) (excited) (*see also* Schizophrenia) 295.7
  - schizophrenia, schizophrenic (*see also* Schizophrenia) 295.9
    - borderline type 295.5
      - of childhood (*see also* Psychosis, childhood) 299.8
    - catatonic (excited) (withdrawn) 295.2
    - childhood type (*see also* Psychosis, childhood) 299.9
    - hebephrenic 295.1
    - incipient 295.5
    - latent 295.5
    - paranoid 295.3
    - prepsychotic 295.5
    - prodromal 295.5
    - pseudoneurotic 295.5
    - pseudopsychopathic 295.5
    - schizophreniform 295.4
    - simple 295.0
    - undifferentiated type 295.9
  - schizophreniform 295.4
  - senile NEC 290.20
    - with
      - delusional features 290.20
      - depressive features 290.21
    - depressed type 290.21
    - paranoid type 290.20
    - simple deterioration 290.20
    - specified type - *see* categories 295–298
  - shared 297.3
  - situational (reactive) 298.8
  - symbiotic (childhood) (*see also* Psychosis, childhood) 299.1
  - toxic (acute) 293.9
- **Psychotic** (*see also* condition) 298.9
  - episode 298.9
    - due to or associated with physical conditions (*see also* Psychosis, organic) 293.9
- **Pterygium** (eye) 372.40
  - central 372.43
  - colli 744.5
  - double 372.44
  - peripheral (stationary) 372.41
    - progressive 372.42
  - recurrent 372.45
- **Ptilosis** 374.55
- **Ptomaine** (poisoning) (*see also* Poisoning, food) 005.9
- **Ptosis** (adiposa) 374.30
  - breast 611.8
  - cecum 569.89
  - colon 569.89
  - congenital (eyelid) 743.61
    - specified site NEC - *see* Anomaly, specified type NEC
  - epicanthus syndrome 270.2
  - eyelid 374.30
    - congenital 743.61
    - mechanical 374.33
    - myogenic 374.32
    - paralytic 374.31
- **Ptosis** *(Continued)*
  - gastric 537.5
  - intestine 569.89
  - kidney (*see also* Disease, renal) 593.0
    - congenital 753.3
  - liver 573.8
  - renal (*see also* Disease, renal) 593.0
    - congenital 753.3
  - splanchnic 569.89
  - spleen 289.59
  - stomach 537.5
  - viscera 569.89
- **PTSD** (Post-Traumatic Stress Disorder) 309.81 ◀
- **Ptyalism** 527.7
  - hysterical 300.11
  - periodic 527.2
  - pregnancy 646.8
  - psychogenic 306.4
- **Ptyalolithiasis** 527.5
- **Pubalgia** 848.8
- **Pubarche, precocious** 259.1
- **Pubertas praecox** 259.1
- **Puberty** V21.1
  - abnormal 259.9
  - bleeding 626.3
  - delayed 259.0
  - precocious (constitutional) (cryptogenic) (idiopathic) NEC 259.1
    - due to
      - adrenal
        - cortical hyperfunction 255.2
        - hyperplasia 255.2
      - cortical hyperfunction 255.2
      - ovarian hyperfunction 256.1
        - estrogen 256.0
      - pineal tumor 259.8
      - testicular hyperfunction 257.0
  - premature 259.1
    - due to
      - adrenal cortical hyperfunction 255.2
      - pineal tumor 259.8
      - pituitary (anterior) hyperfunction 253.1
- **Puckering, macula** 362.56
- **Pudenda, pudendum** - *see* condition
- **Puente's disease** (simple glandular cheilitis) 528.5
- **Puerperal**
  - abscess
    - areola 675.1
    - Bartholin's gland 646.6
    - breast 675.1
    - cervix (uteri) 670
    - fallopian tube 670
    - genital organ 670
    - kidney 646.6
    - mammary 675.1
    - mesosalpinx 670
    - nabothian 646.6
    - nipple 675.0
    - ovary, ovarian 670
    - oviduct 670
    - parametric 670
    - para-uterine 670
    - pelvic 670
    - perimetric 670
    - periuterine 670
    - retro-uterine 670
    - subareolar 675.1
    - suprapelvic 670
    - tubal (ruptured) 670
    - tubo-ovarian 670

Puerperal *(Continued)*
abscess *(Continued)*
urinary tract NEC 646.6
uterine, uterus 670
vagina (wall) 646.6
vaginorectal 646.6
vulvovaginal gland 646.6
accident 674.9
adnexitis 670
afibrinogenemia, or other coagulation defect 666.3
albuminuria (acute) (subacute) 646.2
pre-eclamptic 642.4
anemia (conditions classifiable to 280–285) 648.2
anuria 669.3
apoplexy 674.0
asymptomatic bacteriuria 646.5
atrophy, breast 676.3
blood dyscrasia 666.3
caked breast 676.2
cardiomyopathy 674.5
cellulitis - *see* Puerperal, abscess
cerebrovascular disorder (conditions classifiable to 430–434, 436–437) 674.0
cervicitis (conditions classifiable to 616.0) 646.6
coagulopathy (any) 666.3
complications 674.9
specified type NEC 674.8
convulsions (eclamptic) (uremic) 642.6
with pre-existing hypertension 642.7
cracked nipple 676.1
cystitis 646.6
cystopyelitis 646.6
deciduitis (acute) 670
delirium NEC 293.9
diabetes (mellitus) (conditions classifiable to 250) 648.0
disease 674.9
breast NEC 676.3
cerebrovascular (acute) 674.0
nonobstetric NEC (*see also* Pregnancy, complicated, current disease or condition) 648.9
pelvis inflammatory 670
renal NEC 646.2
tubo-ovarian 670
Valsuani's (progressive pernicious anemia) 648.2
disorder
lactation 676.9
specified type NEC 676.8
nonobstetric NEC (*see also* Pregnancy, complicated, current disease or condition) 648.9
disruption
cesarean wound 674.1
episiotomy wound 674.2
perineal laceration wound 674.2
drug dependence (conditions classifiable to 304) 648.3
eclampsia 642.6
with pre-existing hypertension 642.7
embolism (pulmonary) 673.2
air 673.0
amniotic fluid 673.1
blood clot 673.2
brain or cerebral 674.0
cardiac 674.8
fat 673.8
intracranial sinus (venous) 671.5

Puerperal *(Continued)*
embolism *(Continued)*
pyemic 673.3
septic 673.3
spinal cord 671.5
endometritis (conditions classifiable to 615.0–615.9) 670
endophlebitis - *see* Puerperal, phlebitis
endotrachelitis 646.6
engorgement, breasts 676.2
erysipelas 670
failure
lactation 676.4
renal, acute 669.3
fever 670
meaning pyrexia (of unknown origin) 672
meaning sepsis 670
fissure, nipple 676.1
fistula
breast 675.1
mammary gland 675.1
nipple 675.0
galactophoritis 675.2
galactorrhea 676.6
gangrene
gas 670
uterus 670
gonorrhea (conditions classifiable to 098) 647.1
hematoma, subdural 674.0
hematosalpinx, infectional 670
hemiplegia, cerebral 674.0
hemorrhage 666.1
brain 674.0
bulbar 674.0
cerebellar 674.0
cerebral 674.0
cortical 674.0
delayed (after 24 hours) (uterine) 666.2
extradural 674.0
internal capsule 674.0
intracranial 674.0
intrapontine 674.0
meningeal 674.0
pontine 674.0
subarachnoid 674.0
subcortical 674.0
subdural 674.0
uterine, delayed 666.2
ventricular 674.0
hemorrhoids 671.8
hepatorenal syndrome 674.8
hypertrophy
breast 676.3
mammary gland 676.3
induration breast (fibrous) 676.3
infarction
lung - *see* Puerperal, embolism
pulmonary - *see* Puerperal, embolism
infection
Bartholin's gland 646.6
breast 675.2
with nipple 675.9
specified type NEC 675.8
cervix 646.6
endocervix 646.6
fallopian tube 670
generalized 670
genital tract (major) 670
minor or localized 646.6
kidney (bacillus coli) 646.6
mammary gland 675.2
with nipple 675.9
specified type NEC 675.8

Puerperal *(Continued)*
infection *(Continued)*
nipple 675.0
with breast 675.9
specified type NEC 675.8
ovary 670
pelvic 670
peritoneum 670
renal 646.6
tubo-ovarian 670
urinary (tract) NEC 646.6
asymptomatic 646.5
uterus, uterine 670
vagina 646.6
inflammation - *see also* Puerperal, infection
areola 675.1
Bartholin's gland 646.6
breast 675.2
broad ligament 670
cervix (uteri) 646.6
fallopian tube 670
genital organs 670
localized 646.6
mammary gland 675.2
nipple 675.0
ovary 670
oviduct 670
pelvis 670
periuterine 670
tubal 670
vagina 646.6
vein - *see* Puerperal, phlebitis
inversion, nipple 676.3
ischemia, cerebral 674.0
lymphangitis 670
breast 675.2
malaria (conditions classifiable to 084) 647.4
malnutrition 648.9
mammillitis 675.0
mammitis 675.2
mania 296.0
recurrent episode 296.1
single episode 296.0
mastitis 675.2
purulent 675.1
retromammary 675.1
submammary 675.1
melancholia 296.2
recurrent episode 296.3
single episode 296.2
mental disorder (conditions classifiable to 290–303, 305.0, 305.2–305.9, 306–316, 317–319) 648.4 (Revised)
metritis (septic) (suppurative) 670
metroperitonitis 670
metrorrhagia 666.2
metrosalpingitis 670
metrovaginitis 670
milk leg 671.4
monoplegia, cerebral 674.0
necrosis
kidney, tubular 669.3
liver (acute) (subacute) (conditions classifiable to 570) 674.8
ovary 670
renal cortex 669.3
nephritis or nephrosis (conditions classifiable to 580–589) 646.2
with hypertension 642.1
nutritional deficiency (conditions classifiable to 260–269) 648.9
occlusion, precerebral artery 674.0

ICD-9-CM P Vol. 2

Puerperal *(Continued)*
oliguria 669.3
oophoritis 670
ovaritis 670
paralysis
bladder (sphincter) 665.5
cerebral 674.0
paralytic stroke 674.0
parametritis 670
paravaginitis 646.6
pelviperitonitis 670
perimetritis 670
perimetrosalpingitis 670
perinephritis 646.6
perioophoritis 670
periphlebitis - *see* Puerperal, phlebitis
perisalpingitis 670
peritoneal infection 670
peritonitis (pelvic) 670
perivaginitis 646.6
phlebitis 671.9
deep 671.4
intracranial sinus (venous) 671.5
pelvic 671.4
specified site NEC 671.5
superficial 671.2
phlegmasia alba dolens 671.4
placental polyp 674.4
pneumonia, embolic - *see* Puerperal, embolism
prediabetes 648.8
pre-eclampsia (mild) 642.4
with pre-existing hypertension 642.7
severe 642.5
psychosis, unspecified (*see also* Psychosis, puerperal) 293.89
pyelitis 646.6
pyelocystitis 646.6
pyelohydronephrosis 646.6
pyelonephritis 646.6
pyelonephrosis 646.6
pyemia 670
pyocystitis 646.6
pyohemia 670
pyometra 670
pyonephritis 646.6
pyonephrosis 646.6
pyo-oophoritis 670
pyosalpingitis 670
pyosalpinx 670
pyrexia (of unknown origin) 672
renal
disease NEC 646.2
failure, acute 669.3
retention
decidua (fragments) (with delayed hemorrhage) 666.2
without hemorrhage 667.1
placenta (fragments) (with delayed hemorrhage) 666.2
without hemorrhage 667.1
secundines (fragments) (with delayed hemorrhage) 666.2
without hemorrhage 667.1
retracted nipple 676.0
rubella (conditions classifiable to 056) 647.5
salpingitis 670
salpingo-oophoritis 670
salpingo-ovaritis 670
salpingoperitonitis 670
sapremia 670
secondary perineal tear 674.2

Puerperal *(Continued)*
sepsis (pelvic) 670
septicemia 670
subinvolution (uterus) 674.8
sudden death (cause unknown) 674.9
suppuration - *see* Puerperal, abscess
syphilis (conditions classifiable to 090–097) 647.0
tetanus 670
thelitis 675.0
thrombocytopenia 666.3
thrombophlebitis (superficial) 671.2
deep 671.4
pelvic 671.4
specified site NEC 671.5
thrombosis (venous) - *see* Thrombosis, puerperal
thyroid dysfunction (conditions classifiable to 240–246) 648.1
toxemia (*see also* Toxemia, of pregnancy) 642.4
eclamptic 642.6
with pre-existing hypertension 642.7
pre-eclamptic (mild) 642.4
with
convulsions 642.6
pre-existing hypertension 642.7
severe 642.5
tuberculosis (conditions classifiable to 010–018) 647.3
uremia 669.3
vaginitis (conditions classifiable to 616.1) 646.6
varicose veins (legs) 671.0
vulva or perineum 671.1
vulvitis (conditions classifiable to 616.1) 646.6
vulvovaginitis (conditions classifiable to 616.1) 646.6
white leg 671.4
Pulled muscle - *see* Sprain, by site
Pulmolithiasis 518.89
Pulmonary - *see* condition
Pulmonitis (unknown etiology) 486
Pulpitis (acute) (anachoretic) (chronic) (hyperplastic) (putrescent) (suppurative) (ulcerative) 522.0
Pulpless tooth 522.9
Pulse
alternating 427.89
psychogenic 306.2
bigeminal 427.89
fast 785.0
feeble, rapid, due to shock following injury 958.4
rapid 785.0
slow 427.89
strong 785.9
trigeminal 427.89
water-hammer (*see also* Insufficiency, aortic) 424.1
weak 785.9
Pulseless disease 446.7
Pulsus
alternans or trigeminy 427.89
psychogenic 306.2
Punch drunk 310.2
Puncta lacrimalia occlusion 375.52
Punctiform hymen 752.49
Puncture (traumatic) - *see also* Wound, open, by site
accidental, complicating surgery 998.2
bladder, nontraumatic 596.6

Puncture *(Continued)*
by
device, implant, or graft - *see* Complications, mechanical
foreign body
internal organs - *see also* Injury, internal, by site
by ingested object - *see* Foreign body
left accidentally in operation wound 998.4
instrument (any) during a procedure, accidental 998.2
internal organs, abdomen, chest, or pelvis - *see* Injury, internal, by site
kidney, nontraumatic 593.89
Pupil - *see* condition
Pupillary membrane 364.74
persistent 743.46
Pupillotonia 379.46
pseudotabetic 379.46
Purpura 287.2
abdominal 287.0
allergic 287.0
anaphylactoid 287.0
annularis telangiectodes 709.1
arthritic 287.0
autoerythrocyte sensitization 287.2
autoimmune 287.0
bacterial 287.0
Bateman's (senile) 287.2
capillary fragility (hereditary) (idiopathic) 287.8
cryoglobulinemic 273.2
devil's pinches 287.2
fibrinolytic (*see also* Fibrinolysis) 286.6
fulminans, fulminous 286.6
gangrenous 287.0
hemorrhagic (*see also* Purpura, thrombocytopenic) 287.39
nodular 272.7
nonthrombocytopenic 287.0
thrombocytopenic 287.39
Henoch's (purpura nervosa) 287.0
Henoch-Schönlein (allergic) 287.0
hypergammaglobulinemic (benign primary) (Waldenström's) 273.0
idiopathic 287.31
nonthrombocytopenic 287.0
thrombocytopenic 287.31
immune thrombocytopenic 287.31
infectious 287.0
malignant 287.0
neonatorum 772.6
nervosa 287.0
newborn NEC 772.6
nonthrombocytopenic 287.2
hemorrhagic 287.0
idiopathic 287.0
nonthrombopenic 287.2
peliosis rheumatica 287.0
pigmentaria, progressiva 709.09
posttransfusion 287.4
primary 287.0
primitive 287.0
red cell membrane sensitivity 287.2
rheumatica 287.0
Schönlein (-Henoch) (allergic) 287.0
scorbutic 267
senile 287.2
simplex 287.2
symptomatica 287.0
telangiectasia annularis 709.1
thrombocytopenic (*see also* Thrombocytopenia) 287.30
congenital 287.33

Purpura *(Continued)*
thrombocytopenic *(Continued)*
essential 287.30
hereditary 287.31
idiopathic 287.31
immune 287.31
neonatal, transitory (*see also* Thrombocytopenia, neonatal transitory) 776.1
primary 287.30
puerperal, postpartum 666.3
thrombotic 446.6
thrombohemolytic (*see also* Fibrinolysis) 286.6
thrombopenic (*see also* Thrombocytopenia) 287.30
congenital 287.33
essential 287.30
thrombotic 446.6
thrombocytic 446.6
thrombocytopenic 446.6
toxic 287.0
variolosa 050.0
vascular 287.0
visceral symptoms 287.0
Werlhof's (*see also* Purpura, thrombocytopenic) 287.39
Purpuric spots 782.7
Purulent - *see* condition
Pus
absorption, general - *see* Septicemia
in
stool 792.1
urine 791.9
tube (rupture) (*see also* Salpingo-oophoritis) 614.2
Pustular rash 782.1
Pustule 686.9
malignant 022.0
nonmalignant 686.9
Putnam's disease (subacute combined sclerosis with pernicious anemia) 281.0 *[336.2]*
Putnam-Dana syndrome (subacute combined sclerosis with pernicious anemia) 281.0 *[336.2]*
Putrefaction, intestinal 569.89
Putrescent pulp (dental) 522.1
Pyarthritis - *see* Pyarthrosis
Pyarthrosis (*see also* Arthritis, pyogenic) 711.0
tuberculous - *see* Tuberculosis, joint
Pycnoepilepsy, pycnolepsy (idiopathic) (*see also* Epilepsy) 345.0
Pyelectasia 593.89
Pyelectasis 593.89
Pyelitis (congenital) (uremic) 590.80
with
abortion - *see* Abortion, by type, with specified complication NEC
contracted kidney 590.00
ectopic pregnancy (*see also* categories 633.0–633.9) 639.8
molar pregnancy (*see also* categories 630–632) 639.8
acute 590.10
with renal medullary necrosis 590.11
chronic 590.00
with
renal medullary necrosis 590.01
complicating pregnancy, childbirth, or puerperium 646.6

Pyelitis *(Continued)*
complicating pregnancy, childbirth, or puerperium *(Continued)*
affecting fetus or newborn 760.1
cystica 590.3
following
abortion 639.8
ectopic or molar pregnancy 639.8
gonococcal 098.19
chronic or duration of 2 months or over 098.39
tuberculous (*see also* Tuberculosis) 016.0 *[590.81]*
Pyelocaliectasis 593.89
Pyelocystitis (*see also* Pyelitis) 590.80
Pyelohydronephrosis 591
Pyelonephritis (*see also* Pyelitis) 590.80
acute 590.10
with renal medullary necrosis 590.11
chronic 590.00
syphilitic (late) 095.4
tuberculous (*see also* Tuberculosis) 016.0 *[590.81]*
Pyelonephrosis (*see also* Pyelitis) 590.80
chronic 590.00
Pyelophlebitis 451.89
Pyelo-ureteritis cystica 590.3
Pyemia, pyemic (purulent) (*see also* Septicemia) 038.9
abscess - *see* Abscess
arthritis (*see also* Arthritis, pyogenic) 711.0
Bacillus coli 038.42
embolism - *see* Embolism, pyemic
fever 038.9
infection 038.9
joint (*see also* Arthritis, pyogenic) 711.0
liver 572.1
meningococcal 036.2
newborn 771.81
phlebitis - *see* Phlebitis
pneumococcal 038.2
portal 572.1
postvaccinal 999.3
specified organism NEC 038.8
staphylococcal 038.10
aureus 038.11
specified organism NEC 038.19
streptococcal 038.0
tuberculous - *see* Tuberculosis, miliary
Pygopagus 759.4
Pykno-epilepsy, pyknolepsy (idiopathic) (*see also* Epilepsy) 345.0
Pyle (-Cohn) disease (craniometaphyseal dysplasia) 756.89
Pylephlebitis (suppurative) 572.1
Pylethrombophlebitis 572.1
Pylethrombosis 572.1
Pyloritis (*see also* Gastritis) 535.5
Pylorospasm (reflex) 537.81
congenital or infantile 750.5
neurotic 306.4
newborn 750.5
psychogenic 306.4
Pylorus, pyloric - *see* condition
Pyoarthrosis - *see* Pyarthrosis
Pyocele
mastoid 383.00
sinus (accessory) (nasal) (*see also* Sinusitis) 473.9
turbinate (bone) 473.9
urethra (*see also* Urethritis) 597.0
Pyococcal dermatitis 686.00

Pyococcide, skin 686.00
Pyocolpos (*see also* Vaginitis) 616.10
Pyocyaneus dermatitis 686.09
Pyocystitis (*see also* Cystitis) 595.9
Pyoderma, pyodermia 686.00
gangrenosum 686.01
specified type NEC 686.09
vegetans 686.8
Pyodermatitis 686.00
vegetans 686.8
Pyogenic - *see* condition
Pyohemia - *see* Septicemia
Pyohydronephrosis (*see also* Pyelitis) 590.80
Pyometra 615.9
Pyometritis (*see also* Endometritis) 615.9
Pyometrium (*see also* Endometritis) 615.9
Pyomyositis 728.0
ossificans 728.19
tropical (bungpagga) 040.81
Pyonephritis (*see also* Pyelitis) 590.80
chronic 590.00
Pyonephrosis (congenital) (*see also* Pyelitis) 590.80
acute 590.10
Pyo-oophoritis (*see also* Salpingo-oophoritis) 614.2
Pyo-ovarium (*see also* Salpingo-oophoritis) 614.2
Pyopericarditis 420.99
Pyopericardium 420.99
Pyophlebitis - *see* Phlebitis
Pyopneumopericardium 420.99
Pyopneumothorax (infectional) 510.9
with fistula 510.0
subdiaphragmatic (*see also* Peritonitis) 567.29
subphrenic (*see also* Peritonitis) 567.29
tuberculous (*see also* Tuberculosis, pleura) 012.0
Pyorrhea (alveolar) (alveolaris) 523.40 ⇐
degenerative 523.5
Pyosalpingitis (*see also* Salpingo-oophoritis) 614.2
Pyosalpinx (*see also* Salpingo-oophoritis) 614.2
Pyosepticemia - *see* Septicemia
Pyosis
Corlett's (impetigo) 684
Manson's (pemphigus contagiosus) 684
Pyothorax 510.9
with fistula 510.0
tuberculous (*see also* Tuberculosis, pleura) 012.0
Pyoureter 593.89
tuberculous (*see also* Tuberculosis) 016.2
Pyramidopallidonigral syndrome 332.0
Pyrexia (of unknown origin) (P.U.O.) 780.6
atmospheric 992.0
during labor 659.2
environmentally-induced newborn 778.4
heat 992.0
newborn, environmentally-induced 778.4
puerperal 672
Pyroglobulinemia 273.8
Pyromania 312.33
Pyrosis 787.1
Pyrroloporphyria 277.1
Pyuria (bacterial) 791.9

Q

Q fever 083.0
with pneumonia 083.0 *[484.8]*
Quadricuspid aortic valve 746.89
Quadrilateral fever 083.0
Quadriparesis - *see* Quadriplegia
meaning muscle weakness 728.87
Quadriplegia 344.00
with fracture, vertebra (process) - *see* Fracture, vertebra, cervical, with spinal cord injury
brain (current episode) 437.8
C_1–C_4
complete 344.01
incomplete 344.02
C_5–C_7
complete 344.03
incomplete 344.04
cerebral (current episode) 437.8
congenital or infantile (cerebral) (spastic) (spinal) 343.2
cortical 437.8
embolic (current episode) (*see also* Embolism, brain) 434.1
infantile (cerebral) (spastic) (spinal) 343.2

Quadriplegia *(Continued)*
newborn NEC 767.0
specified NEC 344.09
thrombotic (current episode) (*see also* Thrombosis, brain) 434.0
traumatic - *see* Injury, spinal, cervical
Quadruplet
affected by maternal complications of pregnancy 761.5
healthy liveborn - *see* Newborn, multiple
pregnancy (complicating delivery) NEC 651.8
with fetal loss and retention of one or more fetus(es) 651.5
following (elective) fetal reduction 651.7
Quarrelsomeness 301.3
Quartan
fever 084.2
malaria (fever) 084.2
Queensland fever 083.0
coastal 083.0
seven-day 100.89
Quervain's disease 727.04
thyroid (subacute granulomatous thyroiditis) 245.1

Queyrat's erythroplasia (M8080/2)
specified site - *see* Neoplasm, skin, in situ
unspecified site 233.5
Quincke's disease or edema - *see* Edema, angioneurotic
Quinquaud's disease (acne decalvans) 704.09
Quinsy (gangrenous) 475
Quintan fever 083.1
Quintuplet
affected by maternal complications of pregnancy 761.5
healthy liveborn - *see* Newborn, multiple
pregnancy (complicating delivery) NEC 651.2
with fetal loss and retention of one or more fetus(es) 651.6
following (elective) fetal reduction 651.7
Quotidian
fever 084.0
malaria (fever) 084.0

R

Rabbia 071
Rabbit fever (*see also* Tularemia) 021.9
Rabies 071
contact V01.5
exposure to V01.5
inoculation V04.5
reaction - *see* Complications, vaccination
vaccination, prophylactic (against) V04.5
Rachischisis (*see also* Spina bifida) 741.9
Rachitic - *see also* condition
deformities of spine 268.1
pelvis 268.1
with disproportion (fetopelvic) 653.2
affecting fetus or newborn 763.1
causing obstructed labor 660.1
affecting fetus or newborn 763.1
Rachitis, rachitism - *see also* Rickets
acute 268.0
fetalis 756.4
renalis 588.0
tarda 268.0
Racket nail 757.5
Radial nerve - *see* condition
Radiation effects or sickness - *see also* Effect, adverse, radiation
cataract 366.46
dermatitis 692.82
sunburn (*see also* Sunburn) 692.71
Radiculitis (pressure) (vertebrogenic) 729.2
accessory nerve 723.4
anterior crural 724.4
arm 723.4
brachial 723.4
cervical NEC 723.4
due to displacement of intervertebral disc - *see* Neuritis, due to, displacement intervertebral disc
leg 724.4
lumbar NEC 724.4
lumbosacral 724.4
rheumatic 729.2
syphilitic 094.89
thoracic (with visceral pain) 724.4
Radiculomyelitis 357.0
toxic, due to
Clostridium tetani 037
Corynebacterium diphtheriae 032.89
Radiculopathy (*see also* Radiculitis) 729.2
Radioactive substances, adverse effect - *see* Effect, adverse, radioactive substance
Radiodermal burns (acute) (chronic) (occupational) - *see* Burn, by site
Radiodermatitis 692.82
Radionecrosis - *see* Effect, adverse, radiation
Radiotherapy session V58.0
Radium, adverse effect - *see* Effect, adverse, radioactive substance
Raeder-Harbitz syndrome (pulseless disease) 446.7
Rage (*see also* Disturbance, conduct) 312.0
meaning rabies 071
Rag sorters' disease 022.1
Raillietiniasis 123.8
Railroad neurosis 300.16
Railway spine 300.16
Raised - *see* Elevation
Raiva 071
Rake teeth, tooth 524.39
Rales 786.7
Ramifying renal pelvis 753.3
Ramsay Hunt syndrome (herpetic geniculate ganglionitis) 053.11
meaning dyssynergia cerebellaris myoclonica 334.2
Ranke's primary infiltration (*see also* Tuberculosis) 010.0
Ranula 527.6
congenital 750.26
Rape
adult 995.83
alleged, observation or examination V71.5
child 995.53
Rapid
feeble pulse, due to shock, following injury 958.4
heart (beat) 785.0
psychogenic 306.2
respiration 786.06
psychogenic 306.1
second stage (delivery) 661.3
affecting fetus or newborn 763.6
time-zone change syndrome 327.35
Rarefaction, bone 733.99
Rash 782.1
canker 034.1
diaper 691.0
drug (internal use) 693.0
contact 692.3
ECHO 9 virus 078.89
enema 692.89
food (*see also* Allergy, food) 693.1
heat 705.1
napkin 691.0
nettle 708.8
pustular 782.1
rose 782.1
epidemic 056.9
of infants 057.8
scarlet 034.1
serum (prophylactic) (therapeutic) 999.5
toxic 782.1
wandering tongue 529.1
Rasmussen's aneurysm (*see also* Tuberculosis) 011.2
Rat-bite fever 026.9
due to Streptobacillus moniliformis 026.1
spirochetal (morsus muris) 026.0
Rathke's pouch tumor (M9350/1) 237.0
Raymond (-Céstan) syndrome 433.8
Raynaud's
disease or syndrome (paroxysmal digital cyanosis) 443.0
gangrene (symmetric) 443.0 *[785.4]*
phenomenon (paroxysmal digital cyanosis) (secondary) 443.0
RDS 769
Reaction
acute situational maladjustment (*see also* Reaction, adjustment) 309.9
adaptation (*see also* Reaction, adjustment) 309.9
adjustment 309.9
with
anxious mood 309.24
with depressed mood 309.28
conduct disturbance 309.3
Reaction *(Continued)*
adjustment *(Continued)*
with *(Continued)*
conduct disturbance *(Continued)*
combined with disturbance of emotions 309.4
depressed mood 309.0
brief 309.0
with anxious mood 309.28
prolonged 309.1
elective mutism 309.83
mixed emotions and conduct 309.4
mutism, elective 309.83
physical symptoms 309.82
predominant disturbance (of)
conduct 309.3
emotions NEC 309.29
mixed 309.28
mixed, emotions and conduct 309.4
specified type NEC 309.89
specific academic or work inhibition 309.23
withdrawal 309.83
depressive 309.0
with conduct disturbance 309.4
brief 309.0
prolonged 309.1
specified type NEC 309.89
adverse food NEC 995.7
affective (*see also* Psychosis, affective) 296.90
specified type NEC 296.99
aggressive 301.3
unsocialized (*see also* Disturbance, conduct) 312.0
allergic (*see also* Allergy) 995.3
drug, medicinal substance, and biological - *see* Allergy, drug
food - *see* Allergy, food
serum 999.5
anaphylactic - *see* Shock, anaphylactic
anesthesia - *see* Anesthesia, complication
anger 312.0
antisocial 301.7
antitoxin (prophylactic) (therapeutic) - *see* Complications, vaccination
anxiety 300.00
Arthus 995.21 ◀
asthenic 300.5
compulsive 300.3
conversion (anesthetic) (autonomic) (hyperkinetic) (mixed paralytic) (paresthetic) 300.11
deoxyribonuclease (DNA) (DNase) hypersensitivity NEC 287.2
depressive 300.4
acute 309.0
affective (*see also* Psychosis, affective) 296.2
recurrent episode 296.3
single episode 296.2
brief 309.0
manic (*see also* Psychosis, affective) 296.80
neurotic 300.4
psychoneurotic 300.4
psychotic 298.0
dissociative 300.15
drug NEC (*see also* Table of Drugs and Chemicals) 995.20 ◀
allergic - *see also* Allergy, drug 995.27 ◀

ICD-9-CM R Vol. 2

Reaction *(Continued)*
drug NEC *(Continued)*
correct substance properly administered 995.20 ⬅
obstetric anesthetic or analgesic NEC 668.9
affecting fetus or newborn 763.5
specified drug - *see* Table of Drugs and Chemicals
overdose or poisoning 977.9
specified drug - *see* Table of Drugs and Chemicals
specific to newborn 779.4
transmitted via placenta or breast milk - *see* Absorption, drug, through placenta
withdrawal NEC 292.0
infant of dependent mother 779.5
wrong substance given or taken in error 977.9
specified drug - *see* Table of Drugs and Chemicals
dyssocial 301.7
dystonic, acute, due to drugs 333.72 ◀
erysipeloid 027.1
fear 300.20
child 313.0
fluid loss, cerebrospinal 349.0
food - *see also* Allergy, food
adverse NEC 995.7
anaphylactic shock - *see* Anaphylactic shock, due to, food
foreign
body NEC 728.82
in operative wound (inadvertently left) 998.4
due to surgical material intentionally left - *see* Complications, due to (presence of) any device, implant, or graft classified to 996.0–996.5 NEC
substance accidentally left during a procedure (chemical) (powder) (talc) 998.7
body or object (instrument) (sponge) (swab) 998.4
graft-versus-host (GVH) 996.85
grief (acute) (brief) 309.0
prolonged 309.1
gross stress (*see also* Reaction, stress, acute) 308.9
group delinquent (*see also* Disturbance, conduct) 312.2
Herxheimer's 995.0
hyperkinetic (*see also* Hyperkinesia) 314.9
hypochondriacal 300.7
hypoglycemic, due to insulin 251.0
therapeutic misadventure 962.3
hypomanic (*see also* Psychosis, affective) 296.0
recurrent episode 296.1
single episode 296.0
hysterical 300.10
conversion type 300.11
dissociative 300.15
id (bacterial cause) 692.89
immaturity NEC 301.89
aggressive 301.3
emotional instability 301.59
immunization - *see* Complications, vaccination

Reaction *(Continued)*
incompatibility
blood group (ABO) (infusion) (transfusion) 999.6
Rh (factor) (infusion) (transfusion) 999.7
inflammatory - *see* Infection
infusion - *see* Complications, infusion
inoculation (immune serum) - *see* Complications, vaccination
insulin 995.23 ⬅
involutional
paranoid 297.2
psychotic (*see also* Psychosis, affective, depressive) 296.2
leukemoid (basophilic) (lymphocytic) (monocytic) (myelocytic) (neutrophilic) 288.62 ⬅
LSD (*see also* Abuse, drugs, nondependent) 305.3
lumbar puncture 349.0
manic-depressive (*see also* Psychosis, affective) 296.80
depressed 296.2
recurrent episode 296.3
single episode 296.2
hypomanic 296.0
neurasthenic 300.5
neurogenic (*see also* Neurosis) 300.9
neurotic NEC 300.9
neurotic-depressive 300.4
nitritoid - *see* Crisis, nitritoid
obsessive compulsive 300.3
organic 293.9
acute 293.0
subacute 293.1
overanxious, child or adolescent 313.0
paranoid (chronic) 297.9
acute 298.3
climacteric 297.2
involutional 297.2
menopausal 297.2
senile 290.20
simple 297.0
passive
aggressive 301.84
dependency 301.6
personality (*see also* Disorder, personality) 301.9
phobic 300.20
postradiation - *see* Effect, adverse, radiation
psychogenic NEC 300.9
psychoneurotic (*see also* Neurosis) 300.9
anxiety 300.00
compulsive 300.3
conversion 300.11
depersonalization 300.6
depressive 300.4
dissociative 300.15
hypochondriacal 300.7
hysterical 300.10
conversion type 300.11
dissociative type 300.15
neurasthenic 300.5
obsessive 300.3
obsessive-compulsive 300.3
phobic 300.20
tension state 300.9
psychophysiologic NEC (*see also* Disorder, psychosomatic) 306.9
cardiovascular 306.2

Reaction *(Continued)*
psychophysiologic NEC *(Continued)*
digestive 306.4
endocrine 306.6
gastrointestinal 306.4
genitourinary 306.50
heart 306.2
hemic 306.8
intestinal (large) (small) 306.4
laryngeal 306.1
lymphatic 306.8
musculoskeletal 306.0
pharyngeal 306.1
respiratory 306.1
skin 306.3
special sense organs 306.7
psychosomatic (*see also* Disorder, psychosomatic) 306.9
psychotic (*see also* Psychosis) 298.9
depressive 298.0
due to or associated with physical condition (*see also* Psychosis, organic) 293.9
involutional (*see also* Psychosis, affective) 296.2
recurrent episode 296.3
single episode 296.2
pupillary (myotonic) (tonic) 379.46
radiation - *see* Effect, adverse, radiation
runaway - *see also* Disturbance, conduct
socialized 312.2
undersocialized, unsocialized 312.1
scarlet fever toxin - *see* Complications, vaccination
schizophrenic (*see also* Schizophrenia) 295.9
latent 295.5
serological for syphilis - *see* Serology for syphilis
serum (prophylactic) (therapeutic) 999.5
immediate 999.4
situational (*see also* Reaction, adjustment) 309.9
acute, to stress 308.3
adjustment (*see also* Reaction, adjustment) 309.9
somatization (*see also* Disorder, psychosomatic) 306.9
spinal puncture 349.0
spite, child (*see also* Disturbance, conduct) 312.0
stress, acute 308.9
with predominant disturbance (of)
consciousness 308.1
emotions 308.0
mixed 308.4
psychomotor 308.2
bone or cartilage - *see* fracture stress
specified type NEC 308.3
surgical procedure - *see* Complications, surgical procedure
tetanus antitoxin - *see* Complications, vaccination
toxin-antitoxin - *see* Complications, vaccination
transfusion (blood) (bone marrow) (lymphocytes) (allergic) - *see* Complications, transfusion
tuberculin skin test, nonspecific (without active tuberculosis) 795.5
positive (without active tuberculosis) 795.5
ultraviolet - *see* Effect, adverse, ultraviolet

Reaction *(Continued)*
undersocialized, unsocialized - *see also* Disturbance, conduct
aggressive (type) 312.0
unaggressive (type) 312.1
vaccination (any) - *see* Complications, vaccination
white graft (skin) 996.52
withdrawing, child or adolescent 313.22
x-ray - *see* Effect, adverse, x-rays
Reactive depression (*see also* Reaction, depressive) 300.4
neurotic 300.4
psychoneurotic 300.4
psychotic 298.0
Rebound tenderness 789.6
Recalcitrant patient V15.81
Recanalization, thrombus - *see* Thrombosis
Recession, receding
chamber angle (eye) 364.77
chin 524.06
gingival (post-infective) (postoperative) 523.20
generalized 523.25
localized 523.24
minimal 523.21
moderate 523.22
severe 523.23
Recklinghausen's disease (M9540/1) 237.71
bones (osteitis fibrosa cystica) 252.01
Recklinghausen-Applebaum disease (hemochromatosis) 275.0
Reclus' disease (cystic) 610.1
Recrudescent typhus (fever) 081.1
Recruitment, auditory 388.44
Rectalgia 569.42
Rectitis 569.49
Rectocele
female (without uterine prolapse) 618.04
with uterine prolapse 618.4
complete 618.3
incomplete 618.2
in pregnancy or childbirth 654.4
causing obstructed labor 660.2
affecting fetus or newborn 763.1
male 569.49
vagina, vaginal (outlet) 618.04
Rectosigmoiditis 569.89
ulcerative (chronic) 556.3
Rectosigmoid junction - *see* condition
Rectourethral - *see* condition
Rectovaginal - *see* condition
Rectovesical - *see* condition
Rectum, rectal - *see* condition
Recurrent - *see* condition
Red bugs 133.8
Red cedar asthma 495.8
Redness
conjunctiva 379.93
eye 379.93
nose 478.19
Reduced ventilatory or vital capacity 794.2
Reduction
function
kidney (*see also* Disease, renal) 593.9
liver 573.8
ventilatory capacity 794.2
vital capacity 794.2
Redundant, redundancy
abdomen 701.9

Redundant, redundancy *(Continued)*
anus 751.5
cardia 537.89
clitoris 624.2
colon (congenital) 751.5
foreskin (congenital) 605
intestine 751.5
labia 624.3
organ or site, congenital NEC - *see* Accessory
panniculus (abdominal) 278.1
prepuce (congenital) 605
pylorus 537.89
rectum 751.5
scrotum 608.89
sigmoid 751.5
skin (of face) 701.9
eyelids 374.30
stomach 537.89
uvula 528.9
vagina 623.8
Reduplication - *see* Duplication
Referral
adoption (agency) V68.89
nursing care V63.8
patient without examination or treatment V68.81
social services V63.8
Reflex - *see also* condition
blink, deficient 374.45
hyperactive gag 478.29
neurogenic bladder NEC 596.54
atonic 596.54
with cauda equina syndrome 344.61
vasoconstriction 443.9
vasovagal 780.2
Reflux
esophageal 530.81
with esophagitis 530.11
esophagitis 530.11
gastroesophageal 530.81
mitral - *see* Insufficiency, mitral
ureteral - *see* Reflux, vesicoureteral
vesicoureteral 593.70
with
reflux nephropathy 593.73
bilateral 593.72
unilateral 593.71
Reformed gallbladder 576.0
Reforming, artificial openings (*see also* Attention to, artificial, opening) V55.9
Refractive error (*see also* Error, refractive) 367.9
Refsum's disease or syndrome (heredopathia atactica polyneuritiformis) 356.3
Refusal of
food 307.59
hysterical 300.11
treatment because of, due to
patient's decision NEC V64.2
reason of conscience or religion V62.6
Regaud
tumor (M8082/3) - *see* Neoplasm, nasopharynx, malignant
type carcinoma (M8082/3) - *see* Neoplasm, nasopharynx, malignant
Regional - *see* condition
Regulation feeding (elderly) (infant) 783.3
newborn 779.3

Regurgitated
food, choked on 933.1
stomach contents, choked on 933.1
Regurgitation
aortic (valve) (*see also* Insufficiency, aortic) 424.1
congenital 746.4
syphilitic 093.22
food - *see also* Vomiting
with reswallowing - *see* Rumination
newborn 779.3
gastric contents - *see* Vomiting
heart - *see* Endocarditis
mitral (valve) - *see also* Insufficiency, mitral
congenital 746.6
myocardial - *see* Endocarditis
pulmonary (heart) (valve) (*see also* Endocarditis, pulmonary) 424.3
stomach - *see* Vomiting
tricuspid - *see* Endocarditis, tricuspid
valve, valvular - *see* Endocarditis
vesicoureteral - *see* Reflux, vesicoureteral
Rehabilitation V57.9
multiple types V57.89
occupational V57.21
specified type NEC V57.89
speech V57.3
vocational V57.22
Reichmann's disease or syndrome (gastrosuccorrhea) 536.8
Reifenstein's syndrome (hereditary familial hypogonadism, male) 259.5
Reilly's syndrome or phenomenon (*see also* Neuropathy, peripheral, autonomic) 337.9
Reimann's periodic disease 277.31
Reinsertion, contraceptive device V25.42
Reiter's disease, syndrome, or urethritis 099.3 *[711.1]*
Rejection
food, hysterical 300.11
transplant 996.80
bone marrow 996.85
corneal 996.51
organ (immune or nonimmune cause) 996.80
bone marrow 996.85
heart 996.83
intestines 996.87
kidney 996.81
liver 996.82
lung 996.84
pancreas 996.86
specified NEC 996.89
skin 996.52
artificial 996.55
decellularized allodermis 996.55
Relapsing fever 087.9
Carter's (Asiatic) 087.0
Dutton's (West African) 087.1
Koch's 087.9
louse-borne (epidemic) 087.0
Novy's (American) 087.1
Obermeyer's (European) 087.0
Spirillum 087.9
tick-borne (endemic) 087.1
Relaxation
anus (sphincter) 569.49
due to hysteria 300.11
arch (foot) 734
congenital 754.61
back ligaments 728.4

Relaxation *(Continued)*
bladder (sphincter) 596.59
cardio-esophageal 530.89
cervix (*see also* Incompetency, cervix) 622.5
diaphragm 519.4
inguinal rings - *see* Hernia, inguinal
joint (capsule) (ligament) (paralytic) (*see also* Derangement, joint) 718.90
congenital 755.8
lumbosacral joint 724.6
pelvic floor 618.89
pelvis 618.89
perineum 618.89
posture 729.9
rectum (sphincter) 569.49
sacroiliac (joint) 724.6
scrotum 608.89
urethra (sphincter) 599.84
uterus (outlet) 618.89
vagina (outlet) 618.89
vesical 596.59
Remains
canal of Cloquet 743.51
capsule (opaque) 743.51
Remittent fever (malarial) 084.6
Remnant
canal of Cloquet 743.51
capsule (opaque) 743.51
cervix, cervical stump (acquired) (postoperative) 622.8
cystic duct, postcholecystectomy 576.0
fingernail 703.8
congenital 757.5
meniscus, knee 717.5
thyroglossal duct 759.2
tonsil 474.8
infected 474.00
urachus 753.7
Remote effect of cancer - *see* condition
Removal (of)
catheter (urinary) (indwelling) V53.6
from artificial opening - *see* Attention to, artificial, opening
non-vascular V58.82
vascular V58.81
cerebral ventricle (communicating) shunt V53.01
device - *see also* Fitting (of)
contraceptive V25.42
fixation
external V54.89
internal V54.01
traction V54.89
drains V58.49 ◀
dressing ⬅
wound V58.30 ◀
nonsurgical V58.30 ◀
surgical V58.31 ◀
ileostomy V55.2
Kirschner wire V54.89
non-vascular catheter V58.82
pin V54.01
plaster cast V54.89
plate (fracture) V54.01
rod V54.01
screw V54.01
splint, external V54.89
staples V58.32 ◀
subdermal implantable contraceptive V25.43
sutures V58.32 ⬅

Removal (of) *(Continued)*
traction device, external V54.89
vascular catheter V58.81
wound packing V58.30 ◀
nonsurgical V58.30 ◀
surgical V58.31 ◀
Ren
arcuatus 753.3
mobile, mobilis (*see also* Disease, renal) 593.0
congenital 753.3
unguliformis 753.3
Renal - *see also* condition
glomerulohyalinosis-diabetic syndrome 250.4 *[581.81]*
Rendu-Osler-Weber disease or syndrome (familial hemorrhagic telangiectasia) 448.0
Reninoma (M8361/1) 236.91
Rénon-Delille syndrome 253.8
Repair
pelvic floor, previous, in pregnancy or childbirth 654.4
affecting fetus or newborn 763.89
scarred tissue V51
Replacement by artificial or mechanical device or prosthesis of (*see also* Fitting (of))
artificial skin V43.83
bladder V43.5
blood vessel V43.4
breast V43.82
eye globe V43.0
heart
with
assist device V43.21
fully implantable artificial heart V43.22
valve V43.3
intestine V43.89
joint V43.60
ankle V43.66
elbow V43.62
finger V43.69
hip (partial) (total) V43.64
knee V43.65
shoulder V43.61
specified NEC V43.69
wrist V43.63
kidney V43.89
larynx V43.81
lens V43.1
limb(s) V43.7
liver V43.89
lung V43.89
organ NEC V43.89
pancreas V43.89
skin (artificial) V43.83
tissue NEC V43.89
Reprogramming
cardiac pacemaker V53.31
Request for expert evidence V68.2
Reserve, decreased or low
cardiac - *see* Disease, heart
kidney (*see also* Disease, renal) 593.9
Residual - *see also* condition
bladder 596.8
foreign body - *see* Retention, foreign body
state, schizophrenic (*see also* Schizophrenia) 295.6
urine 788.69

Resistance, resistant (to)
activated protein C 289.81

Note Use the following subclassification for categories V09.5, V09.7, V09.8, V09.9:

0 without mention of resistance to multiple drugs
1 with resistance to multiple drugs
V09.5 quinolones and fluoroquinolones
V09.7 antimycobacterial agents
V09.8 specified drugs NEC
V09.9 unspecified drugs
9 multiple sites

drugs by microorganisms V09.90
amikacin V09.4
aminoglycosides V09.4
amodiaquine V09.5
amoxicillin V09.0
ampicillin V09.0
antimycobacterial agents V09.7
azithromycin V09.2
azlocillin V09.0
aztreonam V09.1
B-lactam antibiotics V09.1
bacampicillin V09.0
bacitracin V09.8
benznidazole V09.8
capreomycin V09.7
carbenicillin V09.0
cefaclor V09.1
cefadroxil V09.1
cefamandole V09.1
cefatetan V09.1
cefazolin V09.1
cefixime V09.1
cefonicid V09.1
cefoperazone V09.1
ceforanide V09.1
cefotaxime V09.1
cefoxitin V09.1
ceftazidine V09.1
ceftizoxime V09.1
ceftriaxone V09.1
cefuroxime V09.1
cephalexin V09.1
cephaloglycin V09.1
cephaloridine V09.1
cephalosporins V09.1
cephalothin V09.1
cephapirin V09.1
cephradine V09.1
chloramphenicol V09.8
chloraquine V09.5
chlorguanide V09.8
chlorproguanil V09.8
chlortetracycline V09.3
cinoxacin V09.5
ciprofloxacin V09.5
clarithromycin V09.2
clindamycin V09.8
clioquinol V09.5
clofazimine V09.7
cloxacillin V09.0
cyclacillin V09.0
cycloserine V09.7
dapsone [Dz] V09.7
demeclocycline V09.3
dicloxacillin V09.0
doxycycline V09.3
enoxacin V09.5
erythromycin V09.2

◀ New ⬅ Revised

Resistance, resistant *(Continued)*
drugs by microorganisms *(Continued)*
ethambutol [Emb] V09.7
ethionamide [Eta] V09.7
fluoroquinolones NEC V09.5
gentamicin V09.4
halofantrine V09.8
imipenem V09.1
iodoquinol V09.5
isoniazid [INH] V09.7
kanamycin V09.4
macrolides V09.2
mafenide V09.6
MDRO (multiple drug resistant organisms) NOS V09.91
mefloquine V09.8
melarsoprol V09.8
methicillin V09.0
methacycline V09.3
methenamine V09.8
metronidazole V09.8
mezlocillin V09.0
minocycline V09.3
multiple drug resistant organisms NOS V09.91
nafcillin V09.0
nalidixic acid V09.5
natamycin V09.2
neomycin V09.4
netilmicin V09.4
nimorazole V09.8
nitrofurantoin V09.8
norfloxacin V09.5
nystatin V09.2
ofloxacin V09.5
oleandomycin V09.2
oxacillin V09.0
oxytetracycline V09.3
para-amino salicyclic acid [PAS] V09.7
paromomycin V09.4
penicillin (G) (V) (Vk) V09.0
penicillins V09.0
pentamidine V09.8
piperacillin V09.0
primaquine V09.5
proguanil V09.8
pyrazinamide [Pza] V09.7
pyrimethamine/sulfalene V09.8
pyrimethamine/sulfodoxine V09.8
quinacrine V09.5
quinidine V09.8
quinine V09.8
quinolones V09.5
rifabutin V09.7
rifampin [Rif] V09.7
rifamycin V09.7
rolitetracycline V09.3
specified drugs NEC V09.8
spectinomycin V09.8
spiramycin V09.2
streptomycin [Sm] V09.4
sulfacetamide V09.6
sulfacytine V09.6
sulfadiazine V09.6
sulfadoxine V09.6
sulfamethoxazole V09.6
sulfapyridine V09.6
sulfasalizine V09.6
sulfasoxazone V09.6
sulfonamides V09.6
sulfoxone V09.7
tetracycline V09.3
tetracyclines V09.3

Resistance, resistant *(Continued)*
drugs by microorganisms *(Continued)*
thiamphenicol V09.8
ticarcillin V09.0
tinidazole V09.8
tobramycin V09.4
triamphenicol V09.8
trimethoprim V09.8
vancomycin V09.8
insulin 277.7
thyroid hormone 246.8 ◀
Resorption
biliary 576.8
purulent or putrid (*see also* Cholecystitis) 576.8
dental (roots) 521.40
alveoli 525.8
pathological
external 521.42
internal 521.41
specified NEC 521.49
septic - *see* Septicemia
teeth (roots) 521.40
pathological
external 521.42
internal 521.41
specified NEC 521.49
Respiration
asymmetrical 786.09
bronchial 786.09
Cheyne-Stokes (periodic respiration) 786.04
decreased, due to shock following injury 958.4
disorder of 786.00
psychogenic 306.1
specified NEC 786.09
failure 518.81
acute 518.81
acute and chronic 518.84
chronic 518.83
newborn 770.84
insufficiency 786.09
acute 518.82
newborn NEC 770.89
Kussmaul (air hunger) 786.09
painful 786.52
periodic 786.09
high altitude 327.22
poor 786.09
newborn NEC 770.89
sighing 786.7
psychogenic 306.1
wheezing 786.07
Respiratory - *see also* condition
distress 786.09
acute 518.82
fetus or newborn NEC 770.89
syndrome (newborn) 769
adult (following shock, surgery, or trauma) 518.5
specified NEC 518.82
failure 518.81
acute 518.81
acute and chronic 518.84
chronic 518.83
Respiratory syncytial virus (RSV) 079.6
bronchiolitis 466.11
pneumonia 480.1
vaccination, prophylactic (against) V04.82
Response
photoallergic 692.72
phototoxic 692.72

Rest, rests
mesonephric duct 752.89
fallopian tube 752.11
ovarian, in fallopian tubes 752.19
wolffian duct 752.89
Restless legs syndrome (RLS) 333.94 ⬅
Restlessness 799.2
Restoration of organ continuity from previous sterilization (tuboplasty) (vasoplasty) V26.0
Restriction of housing space V60.1
Restzustand, schizophrenic (*see also* Schizophrenia) 295.6
Retained - *see* Retention
Retardation
development, developmental, specific (*see also* Disorder, development, specific) 315.9
learning, specific 315.2
arithmetical 315.1
language (skills) 315.31
expressive 315.31
mixed receptive-expressive 315.32
mathematics 315.1
reading 315.00
phonological 315.39
written expression 315.2
motor 315.4
endochondral bone growth 733.91
growth (physical) in childhood 783.43
due to malnutrition 263.2
fetal (intrauterine) 764.9
affecting management of pregnancy 656.5
intrauterine growth 764.9
affecting management of pregnancy 656.5
mental 319
borderline V62.89
mild, IQ 50–70 317
moderate, IQ 35–49 318.0
profound, IQ under 20 318.2
severe, IQ 20–34 318.1
motor, specific 315.4
physical 783.43
child 783.43
due to malnutrition 263.2
fetus (intrauterine) 764.9
affecting management of pregnancy 656.5
psychomotor NEC 307.9
reading 315.00
Retching - *see* Vomiting
Retention, retained
bladder (*see also* Retention, urine) 788.20
psychogenic 306.53
carbon dioxide 276.2
cyst - *see* Cyst
dead
fetus (after 22 completed weeks' gestation) 656.4
early fetal death (before 22 completed weeks' gestation) 632
ovum 631
decidua (following delivery) (fragments) (with hemorrhage) 666.2
without hemorrhage 667.1
deciduous tooth 520.6
dental root 525.3
fecal (*see also* Constipation) 564.00
fluid 276.6

ICD-9-CM
R
Vol. 2

Retention, retained *(Continued)*
foreign body - *see also* Foreign body, retained
bone 733.99
current trauma - *see* Foreign body, by site or type
middle ear 385.83
muscle 729.6
soft tissue NEC 729.6
gastric 536.8
membranes (following delivery) (with hemorrhage) 666.2
with abortion - *see* Abortion, by type
without hemorrhage 667.1
menses 626.8
milk (puerperal) 676.2
nitrogen, extrarenal 788.9
placenta (total) (with hemorrhage) 666.0
with abortion - *see* Abortion, by type
portions or fragments 666.2
without hemorrhage 667.1
without hemorrhage 667.0
products of conception
early pregnancy (fetal death before 22 completed weeks' gestation) 632
following
abortion - *see* Abortion, by type
delivery 666.2
with hemorrhage 666.2
without hemorrhage 667.1
secundines (following delivery) (with hemorrhage) 666.2
with abortion - *see* Abortion, by type
complicating puerperium (delayed hemorrhage) 666.2
without hemorrhage 667.1
smegma, clitoris 624.8
urine NEC 788.20
bladder, incomplete emptying 788.21
due to
benign prostatic hypertrophy (BPH) - *see* category 600
due to
benign prostatic hypertrophy (BPH) - *see* category 600
psychogenic 306.53
specified NEC 788.29
water (in tissue) (*see also* Edema) 782.3
Reticulation, dust (occupational) 504
Reticulocytosis NEC 790.99
Reticuloendotheliosis
acute infantile (M9722/3) 202.5
leukemic (M9940/3) 202.4
malignant (M9720/3) 202.3
nonlipid (M9722/3) 202.5
Reticulohistiocytoma (giant cell) 277.89
Reticulohistiocytosis, multicentric 272.8
Reticulolymphosarcoma (diffuse) (M9613/3) 200.8
follicular (M9691/3) 202.0
nodular (M9691/3) 202.0
Reticulosarcoma (M9640/3) 200.0
nodular (M9642/3) 200.0
pleomorphic cell type (M9641/3) 200.0
Reticulosis (skin)
acute of infancy (M9722/3) 202.5
familial hemophagocytic 288.4 ◀
histiocytic medullary (M9721/3) 202.3
lipomelanotic 695.89
malignant (M9720/3) 202.3
Sezary's (M9701/3) 202.2
Retina, retinal - *see* condition

Retinitis (*see also* Chorioretinitis) 363.20
albuminurica 585.9 *[363.10]*
arteriosclerotic 440.8 *[362.13]*
central angiospastic 362.41
Coat's 362.12
diabetic 250.5 *[362.01]*
disciformis 362.52
disseminated 363.10
metastatic 363.14
neurosyphilitic 094.83
pigment epitheliopathy 363.15
exudative 362.12
focal 363.00
in histoplasmosis 115.92
capsulatum 115.02
duboisii 115.12
juxtapapillary 363.05
macular 363.06
paramacular 363.06
peripheral 363.08
posterior pole NEC 363.07
gravidarum 646.8
hemorrhagica externa 362.12
juxtapapillary (Jensen's) 363.05
luetic - *see* Retinitis, syphilitic
metastatic 363.14
pigmentosa 362.74
proliferans 362.29
proliferating 362.29
punctata albescens 362.76
renal 585.9 *[363.13]*
syphilitic (secondary) 091.51
congenital 090.0 *[363.13]*
early 091.51
late 095.8 *[363.13]*
syphilitica, central, recurrent 095.8 *[363.13]*
tuberculous (*see also* Tuberculosis) 017.3 *[363.13]*
Retinoblastoma (M9510/3) 190.5
differentiated type (M9511/3) 190.5
undifferentiated type (M9512/3) 190.5
Retinochoroiditis (*see also* Chorioretinitis) 363.20
central angiospastic 362.41
disseminated 363.10
metastatic 363.14
neurosyphilitic 094.83
pigment epitheliopathy 363.15
syphilitic 094.83
due to toxoplasmosis (acquired) (focal) 130.2
focal 363.00
in histoplasmosis 115.92
capsulatum 115.02
duboisii 115.12
juxtapapillary (Jensen's) 363.05
macular 363.06
paramacular 363.06
peripheral 363.08
posterior pole NEC 363.07
juxtapapillaris 363.05
syphilitic (disseminated) 094.83
Retinopathy (background) 362.10
arteriosclerotic 440.8 *[362.13]*
atherosclerotic 440.8 *[362.13]*
central serous 362.41
circinate 362.10
Coat's 362.12
diabetic 250.5 *[362.01]*
nonproliferative 250.5 *[362.03]*
mild 250.5 *[362.04]*
moderate 250.5 *[362.05]*
severe 250.5 *[362.06]*
proliferative 250.5 *[362.02]*

Retinopathy *(Continued)*
exudative 362.12
hypertensive 362.11
nonproliferative
diabetic 250.5 *[362.03]*
mild 250.5 *[362.04]*
moderate 250.5 *[362.05]*
severe 250.5 *[362.06]*
of prematurity 362.21
pigmentary, congenital 362.74
proliferative 362.29
diabetic 250.5 *[362.02]*
sickle-cell 282.60 *[362.29]*
solar 363.31
Retinoschisis 361.10
bullous 361.12
congenital 743.56
flat 361.11
juvenile 362.73
Retractile testis 752.52
Retraction
cervix - *see* Retraction, uterus ⬅
drum (membrane) 384.82
eyelid 374.41
finger 736.29
head 781.0
lid 374.41
lung 518.89
mediastinum 519.3
nipple 611.79
congenital 757.6
puerperal, postpartum 676.0
palmar fascia 728.6
pleura (*see also* Pleurisy) 511.0
ring, uterus (Bandl's) (pathological) 661.4
affecting fetus or newborn 763.7
sternum (congenital) 756.3
acquired 738.3
during respiration 786.9
substernal 738.3
supraclavicular 738.8
syndrome (Duane's) 378.71
uterus 621.6 ⬅
valve (heart) - *see* Endocarditis
Retrobulbar - *see* condition
Retrocaval ureter 753.4
Retrocecal - *see also* condition
appendix (congenital) 751.5
Retrocession - *see* Retroversion
Retrodisplacement - *see* Retroversion
Retroflection, retroflexion - *see* Retroversion
Retrognathia, retrognathism (mandibular) (maxillary) 524.10
Retrograde
ejaculation 608.87
menstruation 626.8
Retroiliac ureter 753.4
Retroperineal - *see* condition
Retroperitoneal - *see* condition
Retroperitonitis 567.39 ⬅
Retropharyngeal - *see* condition
Retroplacental - *see* condition
Retroposition - *see* Retroversion
Retrosternal thyroid (congenital) 759.2
Retroversion, retroverted
cervix - *see* Retroversion, uterus ⬅
female NEC (*see also* Retroversion, uterus) 621.6
iris 364.70
testis (congenital) 752.51
uterus, uterine (acquired) (acute) (adherent) (any degree) (asymptomatic) (cervix) (postinfectional) (postpartal, old) 621.6

Retroversion, retroverted *(Continued)*
uterus, uterine *(Continued)*
congenital 752.3
in pregnancy or childbirth 654.3
affecting fetus or newborn 763.89
causing obstructed labor 660.2
affecting fetus or newborn 763.1
Retrusion, premaxilla (developmental) 524.04
Rett's syndrome 330.8
Reverse, reversed
peristalsis 787.4
Reye's syndrome 331.81
Reye-Sheehan syndrome (postpartum pituitary necrosis) 253.2
Rh (factor)
hemolytic disease 773.0
incompatibility, immunization, or sensitization
affecting management of pregnancy 656.1
fetus or newborn 773.0
transfusion reaction 999.7
negative mother, affecting fetus or newborn 773.0
titer elevated 999.7
transfusion reaction 999.7
Rhabdomyolysis (idiopathic) 728.88
Rhabdomyoma (M8900/0) - *see also* Neoplasm, connective tissue, benign
adult (M8904/0) - *see* Neoplasm, connective tissue, benign
fetal (M8903/0) - *see* Neoplasm, connective tissue, benign
glycogenic (M8904/0) - *see* Neoplasm, connective tissue, benign
Rhabdomyosarcoma (M8900/3) - *see also* Neoplasm, connective tissue, malignant
alveolar (M8920/3) - *see* Neoplasm, connective tissue, malignant
embryonal (M8910/3) - *see* Neoplasm, connective tissue, malignant
mixed type (M8902/3) - *see* Neoplasm, connective tissue, malignant
pleomorphic (M8901/3) - *see* Neoplasm, connective tissue, malignant
Rhabdosarcoma (M8900/3) - *see* Rhabdomyosarcoma
Rhesus (factor) (Rh) incompatibility - *see* Rh, incompatibility
Rheumaticosis - *see* Rheumatism
Rheumatism, rheumatic (acute NEC) 729.0
adherent pericardium 393
arthritis
acute or subacute - *see* Fever, rheumatic
chronic 714.0
spine 720.0
articular (chronic) NEC (*see also* Arthritis) 716.9
acute or subacute - *see* Fever, rheumatic
back 724.9
blennorrhagic 098.59
carditis - *see* Disease, heart, rheumatic
cerebral - *see* Fever, rheumatic
chorea (acute) - *see* Chorea, rheumatic
chronic NEC 729.0
coronary arteritis 391.9
chronic 398.99
degeneration, myocardium (*see also* Degeneration, myocardium, with rheumatic fever) 398.0

Rheumatism, rheumatic *(Continued)*
desert 114.0
febrile - *see* Fever, rheumatic
fever - *see* Fever, rheumatic
gonococcal 098.59
gout 274.0
heart
disease (*see also* Disease, heart, rheumatic) 398.90
failure (chronic) (congestive) (inactive) 398.91
hemopericardium - *see* Rheumatic, pericarditis
hydropericardium - *see* Rheumatic, pericarditis
inflammatory (acute) (chronic) (subacute) - *see* Fever, rheumatic
intercostal 729.0
meaning Tietze's disease 733.6
joint (chronic) NEC (*see also* Arthritis) 716.9
acute - *see* Fever, rheumatic
mediastinopericarditis - *see* Rheumatic, pericarditis
muscular 729.0
myocardial degeneration (*see also* Degeneration, myocardium, with rheumatic fever) 398.0
myocarditis (chronic) (inactive) (with chorea) 398.0
active or acute 391.2
with chorea (acute) (rheumatic) (Sydenham's) 392.0
myositis 729.1
neck 724.9
neuralgic 729.0
neuritis (acute) (chronic) 729.2
neuromuscular 729.0
nodose - *see* Arthritis, nodosa
nonarticular 729.0
palindromic 719.30
ankle 719.37
elbow 719.32
foot 719.37
hand 719.34
hip 719.35
knee 719.36
multiple sites 719.39
pelvic region 719.35
shoulder (region) 719.31
specified site NEC 719.38
wrist 719.33
pancarditis, acute 391.8
with chorea (acute) (rheumatic) (Sydenham's) 392.0
chronic or inactive 398.99
pericarditis (active) (acute) (with effusion) (with pneumonia) 391.0
with chorea (acute) (rheumatic) (Sydenham's) 392.0
chronic or inactive 393
pericardium - *see* Rheumatic, pericarditis
pleuropericarditis - *see* Rheumatic, pericarditis
pneumonia 390 *[517.1]*
pneumonitis 390 *[517.1]*
pneumopericarditis - *see* Rheumatic, pericarditis
polyarthritis
acute or subacute - *see* Fever, rheumatic
chronic 714.0
polyarticular NEC (*see also* Arthritis) 716.9

Rheumatism, rheumatic *(Continued)*
psychogenic 306.0
radiculitis 729.2
sciatic 724.3
septic - *see* Fever, rheumatic
spine 724.9
subacute NEC 729.0
torticollis 723.5
tuberculous NEC (*see also* Tuberculosis) 015.9
typhoid fever 002.0
Rheumatoid - *see also* condition
lungs 714.81
Rhinitis (atrophic) (catarrhal) (chronic) (croupous) (fibrinous) (hyperplastic) (hypertrophic) (membranous) (purulent) (suppurative) (ulcerative) 472.0
with
hay fever (*see also* Fever, hay) 477.9
with asthma (bronchial) 493.0
sore throat - *see* Nasopharyngitis
acute 460
allergic (nonseasonal) (seasonal) (*see also* Fever, hay) 477.9
with asthma (*see also* Asthma) 493.0
due to food 477.1
granulomatous 472.0
infective 460
obstructive 472.0
pneumococcal 460
syphilitic 095.8
congenital 090.0
tuberculous (*see also* Tuberculosis) 012.8
vasomotor (*see also* Fever, hay) 477.9
Rhinoantritis (chronic) 473.0
acute 461.0
Rhinodacryolith 375.57
Rhinolalia (aperta) (clausa) (open) 784.49
Rhinolith 478.19 ⇐
nasal sinus (*see also* Sinusitis) 473.9
Rhinomegaly 478.19 ⇐
Rhinopharyngitis (acute) (subacute) (*see also* Nasopharyngitis) 460
chronic 472.2
destructive ulcerating 102.5
mutilans 102.5
Rhinophyma 695.3
Rhinorrhea 478.19 ⇐
cerebrospinal (fluid) 349.81
paroxysmal (*see also* Fever, hay) 477.9
spasmodic (*see also* Fever, hay) 477.9
Rhinosalpingitis 381.50
acute 381.51
chronic 381.52
Rhinoscleroma 040.1
Rhinosporidiosis 117.0
Rhinovirus infection 079.3
Rhizomelic chrondrodysplasia punctata 277.86
Rhizomelique, pseudopolyarthritic 446.5
Rhoads and Bomford anemia (refractory) 238.72 ⇐
Rhus
diversiloba dermatitis 692.6
radicans dermatitis 692.6
toxicodendron dermatitis 692.6
venenata dermatitis 692.6
verniciflua dermatitis 692.6
Rhythm
atrioventricular nodal 427.89
disorder 427.9
coronary sinus 427.89
ectopic 427.89
nodal 427.89

Rhythm *(Continued)*
escape 427.89
heart, abnormal 427.9
fetus or newborn - *see* Abnormal, heart rate
idioventricular 426.89
accelerated 427.89
nodal 427.89
sleep, inversion 327.39
nonorganic origin 307.45
Rhytidosis facialis 701.8
Rib - *see also* condition
cervical 756.2
Riboflavin deficiency 266.0
Rice bodies (*see also* Loose, body, joint) 718.1
knee 717.6
Richter's hernia - *see* Hernia, Richter's
Ricinism 988.2
Rickets (active) (acute) (adolescent) (adult) (chest wall) (congenital) (current) (infantile) (intestinal) 268.0
celiac 579.0
fetal 756.4
hemorrhagic 267
hypophosphatemic with nephrotic-glycosuric dwarfism 270.0
kidney 588.0
late effect 268.1
renal 588.0
scurvy 267
vitamin D-resistant 275.3
Rickettsial disease 083.9
specified type NEC 083.8
Rickettsialpox 083.2
Rickettsiosis NEC 083.9
specified type NEC 083.8
tick-borne 082.9
specified type NEC 082.8
vesicular 083.2
Ricord's chancre 091.0
Riddoch's syndrome (visual disorientation) 368.16
Rider's
bone 733.99
chancre 091.0
Ridge, alveolus - *see also* condition
edentulous
atrophy 525.20
mandible 525.20
minimal 525.21
moderate 525.22
severe 525.23
maxilla 525.20
minimal 525.24
moderate 525.25
severe 525.26
flabby 525.20
Ridged ear 744.29
Riedel's
disease (ligneous thyroiditis) 245.3
lobe, liver 751.69
struma (ligneous thyroiditis) 245.3
thyroiditis (ligneous) 245.3
Rieger's anomaly or syndrome (mesodermal dysgenesis, anterior ocular segment) 743.44
Riehl's melanosis 709.09
Rietti-Greppi-Micheli anemia or syndrome 282.49
Rieux's hernia - *see* Hernia, Rieux's
Rift Valley fever 066.3
Riga's disease (cachectic aphthae) 529.0
Riga-Fede disease (cachectic aphthae) 529.0
Riggs' disease (compound periodontitis) 523.40
Right middle lobe syndrome 518.0
Rigid, rigidity - *see also* condition
abdominal 789.4
articular, multiple congenital 754.89
back 724.8
cervix uteri
in pregnancy or childbirth 654.6
affecting fetus or newborn 763.89
causing obstructed labor 660.2
affecting fetus or newborn 763.1
hymen (acquired) (congenital) 623.3
nuchal 781.6
pelvic floor
in pregnancy or childbirth 654.4
affecting fetus or newborn 763.89
causing obstructed labor 660.2
affecting fetus or newborn 763.1
perineum or vulva
in pregnancy or childbirth 654.8
affecting fetus or newborn 763.89
causing obstructed labor 660.2
affecting fetus or newborn 763.1
spine 724.8
vagina
in pregnancy or childbirth 654.7
affecting fetus or newborn 763.89
causing obstructed labor 660.2
affecting fetus or newborn 763.1
Rigors 780.99
Riley-Day syndrome (familial dysautonomia) 742.8
Ring(s)
aorta 747.21
Bandl's, complicating delivery 661.4
affecting fetus or newborn 763.7
contraction, complicating delivery 661.4
affecting fetus or newborn 763.7
esophageal (congenital) 750.3
Fleischer (-Kayser) (cornea) 275.1 *[371.14]*
hymenal, tight (acquired) (congenital) 623.3
Kayser-Fleischer (cornea) 275.1 *[371.14]*
retraction, uterus, pathological 661.4
affecting fetus or newborn 763.7
Schatzki's (esophagus) (congenital) (lower) 750.3
acquired 530.3
Soemmering's 366.51
trachea, abnormal 748.3
vascular (congenital) 747.21
Vossius' 921.3
late effect 366.21
Ringed hair (congenital) 757.4
Ringing in the ear (*see also* Tinnitus) 388.30
Ringworm 110.9
beard 110.0
body 110.5
burmese 110.9
corporeal 110.5
foot 110.4
groin 110.3
hand 110.2
honeycomb 110.0
nails 110.1
perianal (area) 110.3
scalp 110.0
specified site NEC 110.8
Tokelau 110.5
Rise, venous pressure 459.89
Risk
factor - *see* Problem
falling V15.88
suicidal 300.9
Ritter's disease (dermatitis exfoliativa neonatorum) 695.81
Rivalry, sibling 313.3
Rivalta's disease (cervicofacial actinomycosis) 039.3
River blindness 125.3 *[360.13]*
Robert's pelvis 755.69
with disproportion (fetopelvic) 653.0
affecting fetus or newborn 763.1
causing obstructed labor 660.1
affecting fetus or newborn 763.1
Robin's syndrome 756.0
Robinson's (hidrotic) ectodermal dysplasia 757.31
Robles' disease (onchocerciasis) 125.3 *[360.13]*
Rochalimaea - *see* Rickettsial disease
Rocky Mountain fever (spotted) 082.0
Rodent ulcer (M8090/3) - *see also* Neoplasm, skin, malignant
cornea 370.07
Roentgen ray, adverse effect - *see* Effect, adverse, x-ray
Roetheln 056.9
Roger's disease (congenital interventricular septal defect) 745.4
Rokitansky's
disease (*see also* Necrosis, liver) 570
tumor 620.2
Rokitansky-Aschoff sinuses (mucosal outpouching of gallbladder) (*see also* Disease, gallbladder) 575.8
Rokitansky-Kuster-Hauser syndrome (congenital absence vagina) 752.49
Rollet's chancre (syphilitic) 091.0
Rolling of head 781.0
Romano-Ward syndrome (prolonged QT interval syndrome) 426.82
Romanus lesion 720.1
Romberg's disease or syndrome 349.89
Roof, mouth - *see* condition
Rosacea 695.3
acne 695.3
keratitis 695.3 *[370.49]*
Rosary, rachitic 268.0
Rose
cold 477.0
fever 477.0
rash 782.1
epidemic 056.9
of infants 057.8
Rosen-Castleman-Liebow syndrome (pulmonary proteinosis) 516.0
Rosenbach's erysipelatoid or erysipeloid 027.1
Rosenthal's disease (factor XI deficiency) 286.2
Roseola 057.8
infantum, infantilis 057.8
Rossbach's disease (hyperchlorhydria) 536.8
psychogenic 306.4
Rossle-Urbach-Wiethe lipoproteinosis 272.8
Ross river fever 066.3
Rostan's asthma (cardiac) (*see also* Failure, ventricular, left) 428.1
Rot
Barcoo (*see also* Ulcer, skin) 707.9
knife-grinders' (*see also* Tuberculosis) 011.4

◀ New ⬅ Revised

Rot-Bernhardt disease 355.1
Rotation
anomalous, incomplete or insufficient - *see* Malrotation
cecum (congenital) 751.4
colon (congenital) 751.4
manual, affecting fetus or newborn 763.89
spine, incomplete or insufficient 737.8
tooth, teeth 524.35
vertebra, incomplete or insufficient 737.8
Röteln 056.9
Roth's disease or meralgia 355.1
Roth-Bernhardt disease or syndrome 355.1
Rothmund (-Thomson) syndrome 757.33
Rotor's disease or syndrome (idiopathic hyperbilirubinemia) 277.4
Rotundum ulcus - *see* Ulcer, stomach
Round
back (with wedging of vertebrae) 737.10
late effect of rickets 268.1
hole, retina 361.31
with detachment 361.01
ulcer (stomach) - *see* Ulcer, stomach
worms (infestation) (large) NEC 127.0
Roussy-Lévy syndrome 334.3
Routine postpartum follow-up V24.2
Roy (-Jutras) syndrome (acropachyderma) 757.39
Rubella (German measles) 056.9
complicating pregnancy, childbirth, or puerperium 647.5
complication 056.8
neurological 056.00
encephalomyelitis 056.01
specified type NEC 056.09
specified type NEC 056.79
congenital 771.0
contact V01.4
exposure to V01.4
maternal
with suspected fetal damage affecting management of pregnancy 655.3
affecting fetus or newborn 760.2
manifest rubella in infant 771.0
specified complications NEC 056.79
vaccination, prophylactic (against) V04.3
Rubeola (measles) (*see also* Measles) 055.9
complicated 055.8
meaning rubella (*see also* Rubella) 056.9
scarlatinosis 057.8
Rubeosis iridis 364.42
diabetica 250.5 *[364.42]*
Rubinstein-Taybi's syndrome (brachydactylia, short stature and mental retardation) 759.89
Rud's syndrome (mental deficiency, epilepsy, and infantilism) 759.89
Rudimentary (congenital) - *see also* Agenesis
arm 755.22
bone 756.9
cervix uteri 752.49
eye (*see also* Microphthalmos) 743.10
fallopian tube 752.19
leg 755.32
lobule of ear 744.21
patella 755.64
respiratory organs in thoracopagus 759.4
tracheal bronchus 748.3

Rudimentary *(Continued)*
uterine horn 752.3
uterus 752.3
in male 752.7
solid or with cavity 752.3
vagina 752.49
Ruiter-Pompen (-Wyers) syndrome (angiokeratoma corporis diffusum) 272.7
Ruled out condition (*see also* Observation, suspected) V71.9
Rumination - *see also* Vomiting
disorder 307.53
neurotic 300.3
obsessional 300.3
psychogenic 307.53
Runaway reaction - *see also* Disturbance, conduct
socialized 312.2
undersocialized, unsocialized 312.1
Runeberg's disease (progressive pernicious anemia) 281.0
Runge's syndrome (postmaturity) 766.22
Rupia 091.3
congenital 090.0
tertiary 095.9
Rupture, ruptured 553.9
abdominal viscera NEC 799.89
obstetrical trauma 665.5
abscess (spontaneous) - *see* Abscess, by site
amnion - *see* Rupture, membranes
aneurysm - *see* Aneurysm
anus (sphincter) - *see* Laceration, anus
aorta, aortic 441.5
abdominal 441.3
arch 441.1
ascending 441.1
descending 441.5
abdominal 441.3
thoracic 441.1
syphilitic 093.0
thoracoabdominal 441.6
thorax, thoracic 441.1
transverse 441.1
traumatic (thoracic) 901.0
abdominal 902.0
valve or cusp (*see also* Endocarditis, aortic) 424.1
appendix (with peritonitis) 540.0
with peritoneal abscess 540.1
traumatic - *see* Injury, internal, gastrointestinal tract
arteriovenous fistula, brain (congenital) 430
artery 447.2
brain (*see also* Hemorrhage, brain) 431
coronary (*see also* Infarct, myocardium) 410.9
heart (*see also* Infarct, myocardium) 410.9
pulmonary 417.8
traumatic (complication) (*see also* Injury, blood vessel, by site) 904.9
bile duct, except cystic (*see also* Disease, biliary) 576.3
cystic 575.4
traumatic - *see* Injury, internal, intra-abdominal
bladder (sphincter) 596.6
with
abortion - *see* Abortion, by type, with damage to pelvic organs
ectopic pregnancy (*see also* categories 633.0–633.9) 639.2

Rupture, ruptured *(Continued)*
bladder *(Continued)*
with *(Continued)*
molar pregnancy (*see also* categories 630–632) 639.2
following
abortion 639.2
ectopic or molar pregnancy 639.2
nontraumatic 596.6
obstetrical trauma 665.5
spontaneous 596.6
traumatic - *see* Injury, internal, bladder
blood vessel (*see also* Hemorrhage) 459.0
brain (*see also* Hemorrhage, brain) 431
heart (*see also* Infarct, myocardium) 410.9
traumatic (complication) (*see also* Injury, blood vessel, by site) 904.9
bone - *see* Fracture, by site
bowel 569.89
traumatic - *see* Injury, internal, intestine
Bowman's membrane 371.31
brain
aneurysm (congenital) (*see also* Hemorrhage, subarachnoid) 430
late effect - *see* Late effect(s) (of) cerebrovascular disease
syphilitic 094.87
hemorrhagic (*see also* Hemorrhage, brain) 431
injury at birth 767.0
syphilitic 094.89
capillaries 448.9
cardiac (*see also* Infarct, myocardium) 410.9
cartilage (articular) (current) - *see also* Sprain, by site
knee - *see* Tear, meniscus
semilunar - *see* Tear, meniscus
cecum (with peritonitis) 540.0
with peritoneal abscess 540.1
traumatic 863.89
with open wound into cavity 863.99
cerebral aneurysm (congenital) (*see also* Hemorrhage, subarachnoid) 430
late effect - *see* Late effect(s) (of) cerebrovascular disease
cervix (uteri)
with
abortion - *see* Abortion, by type, with damage to pelvic organs
ectopic pregnancy (*see also* categories 633.0–633.9) 639.2
molar pregnancy (*see also* categories 630–632) 639.2
following
abortion 639.2
ectopic or molar pregnancy 639.2
obstetrical trauma 665.3
traumatic - *see* Injury, internal, cervix
chordae tendineae 429.5
choroid (direct) (indirect) (traumatic) 363.63
circle of Willis (*see also* Hemorrhage, subarachnoid) 430
late effect - *see* Late effect(s) (of) cerebrovascular disease
colon 569.89
traumatic - *see* Injury, internal, colon
cornea (traumatic) - *see also* Rupture, eye

Rupture, ruptured *(Continued)*
cornea *(Continued)*
due to ulcer 370.00
coronary (artery) (thrombotic) (*see also* Infarct, myocardium) 410.9
corpus luteum (infected) (ovary) 620.1
cyst - *see* Cyst
cystic duct (*see also* Disease, gallbladder) 575.4
Descemet's membrane 371.33
traumatic - *see* Rupture, eye
diaphragm - *see also* Hernia, diaphragm
traumatic - *see* Injury, internal, diaphragm
diverticulum
bladder 596.3
intestine (large) (*see also* Diverticula) 562.10
small 562.00
duodenal stump 537.89
duodenum (ulcer) - *see* Ulcer, duodenum, with perforation
ear drum (*see also* Perforation, tympanum) 384.20
with otitis media - *see* Otitis media
traumatic - *see* Wound, open, ear
esophagus 530.4
traumatic 862.22
with open wound into cavity 862.32
cervical region - *see* Wound, open, esophagus
eye (without prolapse of intraocular tissue) 871.0
with
exposure of intraocular tissue 871.1
partial loss of intraocular tissue 871.2
prolapse of intraocular tissue 871.1
due to burn 940.5
fallopian tube 620.8
due to pregnancy - *see* Pregnancy, tubal
traumatic - *see* Injury, internal, fallopian tube
fontanel 767.3
free wall (ventricle) (*see also* Infarct, myocardium) 410.9
gallbladder or duct (*see also* Disease, gallbladder) 575.4
traumatic - *see* Injury, internal, gallbladder
gastric (*see also* Rupture, stomach) 537.89
vessel 459.0
globe (eye) (traumatic) - *see* Rupture, eye
graafian follicle (hematoma) 620.0
heart (auricle) (ventricle) (*see also* Infarct, myocardium) 410.9
infectional 422.90
traumatic - *see* Rupture, myocardium, traumatic
hymen 623.8
internal
organ, traumatic - *see also* Injury, internal, by site
heart - *see* Rupture, myocardium, traumatic
kidney - *see* Rupture, kidney
liver - *see* Rupture, liver
spleen - *see* Rupture, spleen, traumatic
semilunar cartilage - *see* Tear, meniscus

Rupture, ruptured *(Continued)*
intervertebral disc - *see* Displacement, intervertebral disc
traumatic (current) - *see* Dislocation, vertebra
intestine 569.89
traumatic - *see* Injury, internal, intestine
intracranial, birth injury 767.0
iris 364.76
traumatic - *see* Rupture, eye
joint capsule - *see* Sprain, by site
kidney (traumatic) 866.03
with open wound into cavity 866.13
due to birth injury 767.8
nontraumatic 593.89
lacrimal apparatus (traumatic) 870.2
lens (traumatic) 366.20
ligament - *see also* Sprain, by site
with open wound - *see* Wound, open, by site
old (*see also* Disorder, cartilage, articular) 718.0
liver (traumatic) 864.04
with open wound into cavity 864.14
due to birth injury 767.8
nontraumatic 573.8
lymphatic (node) (vessel) 457.8
marginal sinus (placental) (with hemorrhage) 641.2
affecting fetus or newborn 762.1
meaning hernia - *see* Hernia
membrana tympani (*see also* Perforation, tympanum) 384.20
with otitis media - *see* Otitis media
traumatic - *see* Wound, open, ear
membranes (spontaneous)
artificial
delayed delivery following 658.3
affecting fetus or newborn 761.1
fetus or newborn 761.1
delayed delivery following 658.2
affecting fetus or newborn 761.1
premature (less than 24 hours prior to onset of labor) 658.1
affecting fetus or newborn 761.1
delayed delivery following 658.2
affecting fetus or newborn 761.1
meningeal artery (*see also* Hemorrhage, subarachnoid) 430
late effect - *see* Late effect(s) (of) cerebrovascular disease
meniscus (knee) - *see also* Tear, meniscus
old (*see also* Derangement, meniscus) 717.5
site other than knee - *see* Disorder, cartilage, articular
site other than knee - *see* Sprain, by site
mesentery 568.89
traumatic - *see* Injury, internal, mesentery
mitral - *see* Insufficiency, mitral
muscle (traumatic) NEC - *see also* Sprain, by site
with open wound - *see* Wound, open, by site
nontraumatic 728.83
musculotendinous cuff (nontraumatic) (shoulder) 840.4
mycotic aneurysm, causing cerebral hemorrhage (*see also* Hemorrhage, subarachnoid) 430
late effect - *see* Late effect(s) (of) cerebrovascular disease

Rupture, ruptured *(Continued)*
myocardium, myocardial (*see also* Infarct, myocardium) 410.9
traumatic 861.03
with open wound into thorax 861.13
nontraumatic (meaning hernia) (*see also* Hernia, by site) 553.9
obstructed (*see also* Hernia, by site, with obstruction) 552.9
gangrenous (*see also* Hernia, by site, with gangrene) 551.9
operation wound 998.32
internal 998.31
ovary, ovarian 620.8
corpus luteum 620.1
follicle (graafian) 620.0
oviduct 620.8
due to pregnancy - *see* Pregnancy, tubal
pancreas 577.8
traumatic - *see* Injury, internal, pancreas
papillary muscle (ventricular) 429.6
pelvic
floor, complicating delivery 664.1
organ NEC - *see* Injury, pelvic, organs
penis (traumatic) - *see* Wound, open, penis
perineum 624.8
during delivery (*see also* Laceration, perineum, complicating delivery) 664.4
pharynx (nontraumatic) (spontaneous) 478.29
pregnant uterus (before onset of labor) 665.0
prostate (traumatic) - *see* Injury, internal, prostate
pulmonary
artery 417.8
valve (heart) (*see also* Endocarditis, pulmonary) 424.3
vein 417.8
vessel 417.8
pupil, sphincter 364.75
pus tube (*see also* Salpingo-oophoritis) 614.2
pyosalpinx (*see also* Salpingo-oophoritis) 614.2
rectum 569.49
traumatic - *see* Injury, internal, rectum
retina, retinal (traumatic) (without detachment) 361.30
with detachment (*see also* Detachment, retina, with retinal defect) 361.00
rotator cuff (capsule) (traumatic) 840.4
nontraumatic, complete 727.61
sclera 871.0
semilunar cartilage, knee (*see also* Tear, meniscus) 836.2
old (*see also* Derangement, meniscus) 717.5
septum (cardiac) 410.8
sigmoid 569.89
traumatic - *see* Injury, internal, colon, sigmoid
sinus of Valsalva 747.29
spinal cord - *see also* Injury, spinal, by site
due to injury at birth 767.4
fetus or newborn 767.4
syphilitic 094.89

Rupture, ruptured *(Continued)*
spinal cord *(Continued)*
traumatic - *see also* Injury, spinal, by site
with fracture - *see* Fracture, vertebra, by site, with spinal cord injury
spleen 289.59
congenital 767.8
due to injury at birth 767.8
malarial 084.9
nontraumatic 289.59
spontaneous 289.59
traumatic 865.04
with open wound into cavity 865.14
splenic vein 459.0
stomach 537.89
due to injury at birth 767.8
traumatic - *see* Injury, internal, stomach
ulcer - *see* Ulcer, stomach, with perforation
synovium 727.50
specified site NEC 727.59
tendon (traumatic) - *see also* Sprain, by site
with open wound - *see* Wound, open, by site
Achilles 845.09
nontraumatic 727.67
ankle 845.09
nontraumatic 727.68
biceps (long bead) 840.8
nontraumatic 727.62
foot 845.10
interphalangeal (joint) 845.13
metatarsophalangeal (joint) 845.12
nontraumatic 727.68
specified site NEC 845.19
tarsometatarsal (joint) 845.11
hand 842.10
carpometacarpal (joint) 842.11
interphalangeal (joint) 842.13
metacarpophalangeal (joint) 842.12
nontraumatic 727.63
extensors 727.63
flexors 727.64
specified site NEC 842.19
nontraumatic 727.60
specified site NEC 727.69
patellar 844.8
nontraumatic 727.66
rotator cuff (capsule) 840.4
nontraumatic, complete 727.61
wrist 842.00
carpal (joint) 842.01
nontraumatic 727.63

Rupture, ruptured *(Continued)*
tendon *(Continued)*
wrist *(Continued)*
nontraumatic *(Continued)*
extensors 727.63
flexors 727.64
radiocarpal (joint) (ligament) 842.02
radioulnar (joint), distal 842.09
specified site NEC 842.09
testis (traumatic) 878.2
complicated 878.3
due to syphilis 095.8
thoracic duct 457.8
tonsil 474.8
traumatic
with open wound - *see* Wound, open, by site
aorta - *see* Rupture, aorta, traumatic
ear drum - *see* Wound, open, ear, drum
external site - *see* Wound, open, by site
eye 871.2
globe (eye) - *see* Wound, open, eyeball
internal organ (abdomen, chest, or pelvis) - *see also* Injury, internal, by site
heart - *see* Rupture, myocardium, traumatic
kidney - *see* Rupture, kidney
liver - *see* Rupture, liver
spleen - *see* Rupture, spleen, traumatic
ligament, muscle, or tendon - *see also* Sprain, by site
with open wound - *see* Wound, open, by site
meaning hernia - *see* Hernia
tricuspid (heart) (valve) - *see* Endocarditis, tricuspid
tube, tubal 620.8
abscess (*see also* Salpingo-oophoritis) 614.2
due to pregnancy - *see* Pregnancy, tubal
tympanum, tympanic (membrane) (*see also* Perforation, tympanum) 384.20
with otitis media - *see* Otitis media
traumatic - *see* Wound, open, ear, drum
umbilical cord 663.8
fetus or newborn 772.0
ureter (traumatic) (*see also* Injury, internal, ureter) 867.2
nontraumatic 593.89

Rupture, ruptured *(Continued)*
urethra 599.84
with
abortion - *see* Abortion, by type, with damage to pelvic organs
ectopic pregnancy (*see also* categories 633.0–633.9) 639.2
molar pregnancy (*see also* categories 630–632) 639.2
following
abortion 639.2
ectopic or molar pregnancy 639.2
obstetrical trauma 665.5
traumatic - *see* Injury, internal urethra
uterosacral ligament 620.8
uterus (traumatic) - *see also* Injury, internal, uterus
affecting fetus or newborn 763.89
during labor 665.1
nonpuerperal, nontraumatic 621.8
nontraumatic 621.8
pregnant (during labor) 665.1
before labor 665.0
vagina 878.6
complicated 878.7
complicating delivery - *see* Laceration, vagina, complicating delivery
valve, valvular (heart) - *see* Endocarditis
varicose vein - *see* Varicose, vein
varix - *see* Varix
vena cava 459.0
ventricle (free wall) (left) (*see also* Infarct, myocardium) 410.9
vesical (urinary) 596.6
traumatic - *see* Injury, internal, bladder
vessel (blood) 459.0
pulmonary 417.8
viscus 799.89
vulva 878.4
complicated 878.5
complicating delivery 664.0
Russell's dwarf (uterine dwarfism and craniofacial dysostosis) 759.89
Russell's dysentery 004.8
Russell (-Silver) syndrome (congenital hemihypertrophy and short stature) 759.89
Russian spring-summer type encephalitis 063.0
Rust's disease (tuberculous spondylitis) 015.0 *[720.81]*
Rustitskii's disease (multiple myeloma) (M9730/3) 203.0
Ruysch's disease (Hirschsprung's disease) 751.3
Rytand-Lipsitch syndrome (complete atrioventricular block) 426.0

S

Saber
- shin 090.5
- tibia 090.5

Sac, lacrimal - *see* condition
Saccharomyces infection (*see also* Candidiasis) 112.9
Saccharopinuria 270.7
Saccular - *see* condition
Sacculation
- aorta (nonsyphilitic) (*see also* Aneurysm, aorta) 441.9
  - ruptured 441.5
  - syphilitic 093.0
- bladder 596.3
- colon 569.89
- intralaryngeal (congenital) (ventricular) 748.3
- larynx (congenital) (ventricular) 748.3
- organ or site, congenital - *see* Distortion
- pregnant uterus, complicating delivery 654.4
  - affecting fetus or newborn 763.1
    - causing obstructed labor 660.2
      - affecting fetus or newborn 763.1
- rectosigmoid 569.89
- sigmoid 569.89
- ureter 593.89
- urethra 599.2
- vesical 596.3

Sachs (-Tay) disease (amaurotic familial idiocy) 330.1
Sacks-Libman disease 710.0 [424.91]
Sacralgia 724.6
Sacralization
- fifth lumbar vertebra 756.15
- incomplete (vertebra) 756.15

Sacrodynia 724.6
Sacroiliac joint - *see* condition
Sacroiliitis NEC 720.2
Sacrum - *see* condition
Saddle
- back 737.8
- embolus, aorta 444.0
- nose 738.0
  - congenital 754.0
  - due to syphilis 090.5

Sadism (sexual) 302.84
Saemisch's ulcer 370.04
Saenger's syndrome 379.46
Sago spleen 277.39 ⬅
Sailors' skin 692.74
Saint
- Anthony's fire (*see also* Erysipelas) 035
- Guy's dance - *see* Chorea
- Louis-type encephalitis 062.3
- triad (*see also* Hernia, diaphragm) 553.3
- Vitus' dance - *see* Chorea

Salicylism
- correct substance properly administered 535.4
- overdose or wrong substance given or taken 965.1

Salivary duct or gland - *see also* condition
- virus disease 078.5

Salivation (excessive) (*see also* Ptyalism) 527.7
Salmonella (aertrycke) (choleraesuis) (enteritidis) (gallinarum) (suipestifer) (typhimurium) (*see also* Infection, Salmonella) 003.9
- arthritis 003.23
- carrier (suspected) of V02.3
- meningitis 003.21

Salmonella *(Continued)*
- osteomyelitis 003.24
- pneumonia 003.22
- septicemia 003.1
- typhosa 002.0
  - carrier (suspected) of V02.1

Salmonellosis 003.0
- with pneumonia 003.22

Salpingitis (catarrhal) (fallopian tube) (nodular) (pseudofollicular) (purulent) (septic) (*see also* Salpingo-oophoritis) 614.2
- ear 381.50
  - acute 381.51
  - chronic 381.52
- Eustachian (tube) 381.50
  - acute 381.51
  - chronic 381.52
- follicularis 614.1
- gonococcal (chronic) 098.37
  - acute 098.17
- interstitial, chronic 614.1
- isthmica nodosa 614.1
- old - *see* Salpingo-oophoritis, chronic
- puerperal, postpartum, childbirth 670
- specific (chronic) 098.37
  - acute 098.17
- tuberculous (acute) (chronic) (*see also* Tuberculosis) 016.6
- venereal (chronic) 098.37
  - acute 098.17

Salpingocele 620.4
Salpingo-oophoritis (catarrhal) (purulent) (ruptured) (septic) (suppurative) 614.2
- acute 614.0
  - with
    - abortion - *see* Abortion, by type, with sepsis
    - ectopic pregnancy (*see also* categories 633.0–633.9) 639.0
    - molar pregnancy (*see also* categories 630–632) 639.0
  - following
    - abortion 639.0
    - ectopic or molar pregnancy 639.0
  - gonococcal 098.17
  - puerperal, postpartum, childbirth 670
  - tuberculous (*see also* Tuberculosis) 016.6
- chronic 614.1
  - gonococcal 098.37
  - tuberculous (*see also* Tuberculosis) 016.6
- complicating pregnancy 646.6
  - affecting fetus or newborn 760.8
- gonococcal (chronic) 098.37
  - acute 098.17
- old - *see* Salpingo-oophoritis, chronic
- puerperal 670
- specific - *see* Salpingo-oophoritis, gonococcal
- subacute (*see also* Salpingo-oophoritis, acute) 614.0
- tuberculous (acute) (chronic) (*see also* Tuberculosis) 016.6
- venereal - *see* Salpingo-oophoritis, gonococcal

Salpingo-ovaritis (*see also* Salpingo-oophoritis) 614.2
Salpingoperitonitis (*see also* Salpingo-oophoritis) 614.2
Salt-losing
- nephritis (*see also* Disease, renal) 593.9
- syndrome (*see also* Disease, renal) 593.9

Salt-rheum (*see also* Eczema) 692.9
Salzmann's nodular dystrophy 371.46
Sampson's cyst or tumor 617.1
Sandblasters'
- asthma 502
- lung 502

Sander's disease (paranoia) 297.1
Sandfly fever 066.0
Sandhoff's disease 330.1
Sanfilippo's syndrome (mucopolysaccharidosis III) 277.5
Sanger-Brown's ataxia 334.2
San Joaquin Valley fever 114.0
Sao Paulo fever or typhus 082.0
Saponification, mesenteric 567.89
Sapremia - *see* Septicemia
Sarcocele (benign)
- syphilitic 095.8
  - congenital 090.5

Sarcoepiplocele (*see also* Hernia) 553.9
Sarcoepiplomphalocele (*see also* Hernia, umbilicus) 553.1
Sarcoid (any site) 135
- with lung involvement 135 *[517.8]*
- Boeck's 135
- Darier-Roussy 135
- Spiegler-Fendt 686.8

Sarcoidosis 135
- cardiac 135 *[425.8]*
- lung 135 *[517.8]*

Sarcoma (M8800/3) - *see also* Neoplasm, connective tissue, malignant
- alveolar soft part (M9581/3) - *see* Neoplasm, connective tissue, malignant
- ameloblastic (M9330/3) 170.1
  - upper jaw (bone) 170.0
- botryoid (M8910/3) - *see* Neoplasm, connective tissue, malignant
- botryoides (M8910/3) - *see* Neoplasm, connective tissue, malignant
- cerebellar (M9480/3) 191.6
  - circumscribed (arachnoidal) (M9471/3) 191.6
- circumscribed (arachnoidal) cerebellar (M9471/3) 191.6
- clear cell, of tendons and aponeuroses (M9044/3) - *see* Neoplasm, connective tissue, malignant
- embryonal (M8991/3) - *see* Neoplasm, connective tissue, malignant
- endometrial (stromal) (M8930/3) 182.0
  - isthmus 182.1
- endothelial (M9130/3) - *see also* Neoplasm, connective tissue, malignant
  - bone (M9260/3) - *see* Neoplasm, bone, malignant
- epithelioid cell (M8804/3) - *see* Neoplasm, connective tissue, malignant
- Ewing's (M9260/3) - *see* Neoplasm, bone, malignant
- follicular dendritic cell 202.9
- germinoblastic (diffuse) (M9632/3) 202.8
  - follicular (M9697/3) 202.0
- giant cell (M8802/3) - *see also* Neoplasm, connective tissue, malignant
  - bone (M9250/3) - *see* Neoplasm, bone, malignant
- glomoid (M8710/3) - *see* Neoplasm, connective tissue, malignant
- granulocytic (M9930/3) 205.3
- hemangioendothelial (M9130/3) - *see* Neoplasm, connective tissue, malignant
- hemorrhagic, multiple (M9140/3) - *see* Kaposi's, sarcoma

Sarcoma *(Continued)*
Hodgkin's (M9662/3) 201.2
immunoblastic (M9612/3) 200.8
interdigitating dendritic cell 202.9
Kaposi's (M9140/3) - *see* Kaposi's, sarcoma
Kupffer cell (M9124/3) 155.0
Langerhans cell 202.9
leptomeningeal (M9530/3) - *see* Neoplasm, meninges, malignant
lymphangioendothelial (M9170/3) - *see* Neoplasm, connective tissue, malignant
lymphoblastic (M9630/3) 200.1
lymphocytic (M9620/3) 200.1
mast cell (M9740/3) 202.6
melanotic (M8720/3) - *see* Melanoma
meningeal (M9530/3) - *see* Neoplasm, meninges, malignant
meningothelial (M9530/3) - *see* Neoplasm, meninges, malignant
mesenchymal (M8800/3) - *see also* Neoplasm, connective tissue, malignant
mixed (M8990/3) - *see* Neoplasm, connective tissue, malignant
mesothelial (M9050/3) - *see* Neoplasm, by site, malignant
monstrocellular (M9481/3)
specified site - *see* Neoplasm, by site, malignant
unspecified site 191.9
myeloid (M9930/3) 205.3
neurogenic (M9540/3) - *see* Neoplasm, connective tissue, malignant
odontogenic (M9270/3) 170.1
upper jaw (bone) 170.0
osteoblastic (M9180/3) - *see* Neoplasm, bone, malignant
osteogenic (M9180/3) - *see also* Neoplasm, bone, malignant
juxtacortical (M9190/3) - *see* Neoplasm, bone, malignant
periosteal (M9190/3) - *see* Neoplasm, bone, malignant
periosteal (M8812/3) - *see also* Neoplasm, bone, malignant
osteogenic (M9190/3) - *see* Neoplasm, bone, malignant
plasma cell (M9731/3) 203.8
pleomorphic cell (M8802/3) - *see* Neoplasm, connective tissue, malignant
reticuloendothelial (M9720/3) 202.3
reticulum cell (M9640/3) 200.0
nodular (M9642/3) 200.0
pleomorphic cell type (M9641/3) 200.0
round cell (M8803/3) - *see* Neoplasm, connective tissue, malignant
small cell (M8803/3) - *see* Neoplasm, connective tissue, malignant
spindle cell (M8801/3) - *see* Neoplasm, connective tissue, malignant
stromal (endometrial) (M8930/3) 182.0
isthmus 182.1
synovial (M9040/3) - *see also* Neoplasm, connective tissue, malignant
biphasic type (M9043/3) - *see* Neoplasm, connective tissue, malignant
epithelioid cell type (M9042/3) - *see* Neoplasm, connective tissue, malignant
spindle cell type (M9041/3) - *see* Neoplasm, connective tissue, malignant

Sarcomatosis
meningeal (M9539/3) - *see* Neoplasm, meninges, malignant
specified site NEC (M8800/3) - *see* Neoplasm, connective tissue, malignant
unspecified site (M8800/6) 171.9
Sarcosinemia 270.8
Sarcosporidiosis 136.5
Satiety, early 780.94
Saturnine - *see* condition
Saturnism 984.9
specified type of lead - *see* Table of Drugs and Chemicals
Satyriasis 302.89
Sauriasis - *see* Ichthyosis
Sauriderma 757.39
Sauriosis - *see* Ichthyosis
Savill's disease (epidemic exfoliative dermatitis) 695.89
SBE (subacute bacterial endocarditis) 421.0
Scabies (any site) 133.0
Scabs 782.8
Scaglietti-Dagnini syndrome (acromegalic macrospondylitis) 253.0
Scald, scalded - *see also* Burn, by site
skin syndrome 695.1
Scalenus anticus (anterior) syndrome 353.0
Scales 782.8
Scalp - *see* condition
Scaphocephaly 756.0
Scaphoiditis, tarsal 732.5
Scapulalgia 733.90
Scapulohumeral myopathy 359.1
Scar, scarring (*see also* Cicatrix) 709.2
adherent 709.2
atrophic 709.2
cervix
in pregnancy or childbirth 654.6
affecting fetus or newborn 763.89
causing obstructed labor 660.2
affecting fetus or newborn 763.1
cheloid 701.4
chorioretinal 363.30
disseminated 363.35
macular 363.32
peripheral 363.34
posterior pole NEC 363.33
choroid (*see also* Scar, chorioretinal) 363.30
compression, pericardial 423.9
congenital 757.39
conjunctiva 372.64
cornea 371.00
xerophthalmic 264.6
due to previous cesarean delivery, complicating pregnancy or childbirth 654.2
affecting fetus or newborn 763.89
duodenal (bulb) (cap) 537.3
hypertrophic 701.4
keloid 701.4
labia 624.4
lung (base) 518.89
macula 363.32
disseminated 363.35
peripheral 363.34
muscle 728.89
myocardium, myocardial 412
painful 709.2
papillary muscle 429.81
posterior pole NEC 363.33
macular - *see* Scar, macula

Scar, scarring *(Continued)*
postnecrotic (hepatic) (liver) 571.9
psychic V15.49
retina (*see also* Scar, chorioretinal) 363.30
trachea 478.9
uterus 621.8
in pregnancy or childbirth NEC 654.9
affecting fetus or newborn 763.89
from previous cesarean delivery 654.2
vulva 624.4
Scarabiasis 134.1
Scarlatina 034.1
anginosa 034.1
maligna 034.1
myocarditis, acute 034.1 *[422.0]*
old (*see also* Myocarditis) 429.0
otitis media 034.1 *[382.02]*
ulcerosa 034.1
Scarlatinella 057.8
Scarlet fever (albuminuria) (angina) (convulsions) (lesions of lid) (rash) 034.1
Schamberg's disease, dermatitis, or dermatosis (progressive pigmentary dermatosis) 709.09
Schatzki's ring (esophagus) (lower) (congenital) 750.3
acquired 530.3
Schaufenster krankheit 413.9
Schaumann's
benign lymphogranulomatosis 135
disease (sarcoidosis) 135
syndrome (sarcoidosis) 135
Scheie's syndrome (mucopolysaccharidosis IS) 277.5
Schenck's disease (sporotrichosis) 117.1
Scheuermann's disease or osteochondrosis 732.0
Scheuthauer-Marie-Sainton syndrome (cleidocranialis dysostosis) 755.59
Schilder (-Flatau) disease 341.1
Schilling-type monocytic leukemia (M9890/3) 206.9
Schimmelbusch's disease, cystic mastitis, or hyperplasia 610.1
Schirmer's syndrome (encephalocutaneous angiomatosis) 759.6
Schistocelia 756.79
Schistoglossia 750.13
Schistosoma infestation - *see* Infestation, Schistosoma
Schistosomiasis 120.9
Asiatic 120.2
bladder 120.0
chestermani 120.8
colon 120.1
cutaneous 120.3
due to
S. hematobium 120.0
S. japonicum 120.2
S. mansoni 120.1
S. mattheii 120.8
eastern 120.2
genitourinary tract 120.0
intestinal 120.1
lung 120.2
Manson's (intestinal) 120.1
Oriental 120.2
pulmonary 120.2
specified type NEC 120.8
vesical 120.0
Schizencephaly 742.4
Schizo-affective psychosis (*see also* Schizophrenia) 295.7
Schizodontia 520.2

ICD-9-CM
S
Vol. 2

Schizoid personality 301.20
introverted 301.21
schizotypal 301.22
Schizophrenia, schizophrenic (reaction) 295.9

Note Use the following fifth-digit subclassification with category 295:
0 unspecified
1 subchronic
2 chronic
3 subchronic with acute exacerbation
4 chronic with acute exacerbation
5 in remission

acute (attack) NEC 295.8
episode 295.4
atypical form 295.8
borderline 295.5
catalepsy 295.2
catatonic (type) (acute) (excited) (withdrawn) 295.2
childhood (type) (*see also* Psychosis, childhood) 299.9
chronic NEC 295.6
coenesthesiopathic 295.8
cyclic (type) 295.7
disorganized (type) 295.1
flexibilitas cerea 295.2
hebephrenic (type) (acute) 295.1
incipient 295.5
latent 295.5
paranoid (type) (acute) 295.3
paraphrenic (acute) 295.3
prepsychotic 295.5
primary (acute) 295.0
prodromal 295.5
pseudoneurotic 295.5
pseudopsychopathic 295.5
reaction 295.9
residual type (state) 295.6
restzustand 295.6
schizo-affective (type) (depressed) (excited) 295.7
schizophreniform type 295.4
simple (type) (acute) 295.0
simplex (acute) 295.0
specified type NEC 295.8
syndrome of childhood NEC (*see also* Psychosis, childhood) 299.9
undifferentiated type 295.9
acute 295.8
chronic 295.6
Schizothymia 301.20
introverted 301.21
schizotypal 301.22
Schlafkrankheit 086.5
Schlatter's tibia (osteochondrosis) 732.4
Schlatter-Osgood disease (osteochondrosis, tibial tubercle) 732.4
Schloffer's tumor (*see also* Peritonitis) 567.29
Schmidt's syndrome
sphallo-pharyngo-laryngeal hemiplegia 352.6
thyroid-adrenocortical insufficiency 258.1
vagoaccessory 352.6
Schmincke
carcinoma (M8082/3) - *see* Neoplasm, nasopharynx, malignant
tumor (M8082/3) - *see* Neoplasm, nasopharynx, malignant
Schmitz (-Stutzer) dysentery 004.0
Schmorl's disease or nodes 722.30
lumbar, lumbosacral 722.32
specified region NEC 722.39
thoracic, thoracolumbar 722.31
Schneider's syndrome 047.9
Schneiderian
carcinoma (M8121/3)
specified site - *see* Neoplasm, by site, malignant
unspecified site 160.0
papilloma (M8121/0)
specified site - *see* Neoplasm, by site, benign
unspecified site 212.0
Schnitzler syndrome 273.1
Schoffer's tumor (*see also* Peritonitis) 567.29
Scholte's syndrome (malignant carcinoid) 259.2
Scholz's disease 330.0
Scholz (-Bielschowsky-Henneberg) syndrome 330.0
Schönlein (-Henoch) disease (primary) (purpura) (rheumatic) 287.0
School examination V70.3
Schottmüller's disease (*see also* Fever, paratyphoid) 002.9
Schroeder's syndrome (endocrine-hypertensive) 255.3
Schüller-Christian disease or syndrome (chronic histiocytosis X) 277.89
Schultz's disease or syndrome (agranulocytosis) 288.09
Schultze's acroparesthesia, simple 443.89
Schwalbe-Ziehen-Oppenheimer disease 333.6
Schwannoma (M9560/0) - *see also* Neoplasm, connective tissue, benign
malignant (M9560/3) - *see* Neoplasm, connective tissue, malignant
Schwartz (-Jampel) syndrome 756.89
Schwartz-Bartter syndrome (inappropriate secretion of antidiuretic hormone) 253.6
Schweninger-Buzzi disease (macular atrophy) 701.3
Sciatic - *see* condition
Sciatica (infectional) 724.3
due to
displacement of intervertebral disc 722.10
herniation, nucleus pulposus 722.10
wallet 724.3
Scimitar syndrome (anomalous venous drainage, right lung to inferior vena cava) 747.49
Sclera - *see* condition
Sclerectasia 379.11
Scleredema
adultorum 710.1
Buschke's 710.1
newborn 778.1
Sclerema
adiposum (newborn) 778.1
adultorum 710.1
edematosum (newborn) 778.1
neonatorum 778.1
newborn 778.1
Scleriasis - *see* Scleroderma
Scleritis 379.00
with corneal involvement 379.05
anterior (annular) (localized) 379.03
brawny 379.06
granulomatous 379.09
posterior 379.07
Scleritis *(Continued)*
specified NEC 379.09
suppurative 379.09
syphilitic 095.0
tuberculous (nodular) (*see also* Tuberculosis) 017.3 *[379.09]*
Sclerochoroiditis (*see also* Scleritis) 379.00
Scleroconjunctivitis (*see also* Scleritis) 379.00
Sclerocystic ovary (syndrome) 256.4
Sclerodactylia 701.0
Scleroderma, sclerodermia (acrosclerotic) (diffuse) (generalized) (progressive) (pulmonary) 710.1
circumscribed 701.0
linear 701.0
localized (linear) 701.0
newborn 778.1
Sclerokeratitis 379.05
meaning sclerosing keratitis 370.54
tuberculous (*see also* Tuberculosis) 017.3 *[379.09]*
Scleroma, trachea 040.1
Scleromalacia
multiple 731.0
perforans 379.04
Scleromyxedema 701.8
Scleroperikeratitis 379.05
Sclerose en plaques 340
Sclerosis, sclerotic
adrenal (gland) 255.8
Alzheimer's 331.0
with dementia - *see* Alzheimer's, dementia
amyotrophic (lateral) 335.20
annularis fibrosi
aortic 424.1
mitral 424.0
aorta, aortic 440.0
valve (*see also* Endocarditis, aortic) 424.1
artery, arterial, arteriolar, arteriovascular - *see* Arteriosclerosis
ascending multiple 340
Baló's (concentric) 341.1
basilar - *see* Sclerosis, brain
bone (localized) NEC 733.99
brain (general) (lobular) 341.9
Alzheimer's - *see* Alzheimer's, dementia
artery, arterial 437.0
atrophic lobar 331.0
with dementia
with behavioral disturbance 331.0 *[294.11]*
without behavioral disturbance 331.0 *[294.10]*
diffuse 341.1
familial (chronic) (infantile) 330.0
infantile (chronic) (familial) 330.0
Pelizaeus-Merzbacher type 330.0
disseminated 340
hereditary 334.2
infantile (degenerative) (diffuse) 330.0
insular 340
Krabbe's 330.0
miliary 340
multiple 340
Pelizaeus-Merzbacher 330.0
progressive familial 330.0
senile 437.0
tuberous 759.5
bulbar, progressive 340

Sclerosis, sclerotic *(Continued)*
bundle of His 426.50
left 426.3
right 426.4
cardiac - *see* Arteriosclerosis, coronary
cardiorenal (*see also* Hypertension, cardiorenal) 404.90
cardiovascular (*see also* Disease, cardiovascular) 429.2
renal (*see also* Hypertension, cardiorenal) 404.90
centrolobar, familial 330.0
cerebellar - *see* Sclerosis, brain
cerebral - *see* Sclerosis, brain
cerebrospinal 340
disseminated 340
multiple 340
cerebrovascular 437.0
choroid 363.40
diffuse 363.56
combined (spinal cord) - *see also* Degeneration, combined
multiple 340
concentric, Baló's 341.1
cornea 370.54
coronary (artery) - *see* Arteriosclerosis, coronary
corpus cavernosum
female 624.8
male 607.89
Dewitzky's
aortic 424.1
mitral 424.0
diffuse NEC 341.1
disease, heart - *see* Arteriosclerosis, coronary
disseminated 340
dorsal 340
dorsolateral (spinal cord) - *see* Degeneration, combined
endometrium 621.8
extrapyramidal 333.90
eye, nuclear (senile) 366.16
Friedreich's (spinal cord) 334.0
funicular (spermatic cord) 608.89
gastritis 535.4
general (vascular) - *see* Arteriosclerosis
gland (lymphatic) 457.8
hepatic 571.9
hereditary
cerebellar 334.2
spinal 334.0
idiopathic cortical (Garré's) (*see also* Osteomyelitis) 730.1
ilium, piriform 733.5
insular 340
pancreas 251.8
Islands of Langerhans 251.8
kidney - *see* Sclerosis, renal
larynx 478.79
lateral 335.24
amyotrophic 335.20
descending 335.24
primary 335.24
spinal 335.24
liver 571.9
lobar, atrophic (of brain) 331.0
with dementia
with behavioral disturbance 331.0 *[294.11]*
without behavioral disturbance 331.0 *[294.10]*
lung (*see also* Fibrosis, lung) 515
mastoid 383.1
mitral - *see* Endocarditis, mitral

Sclerosis, sclerotic *(Continued)*
Mönckeberg's (medial) (*see also* Arteriosclerosis, extremities) 440.20
multiple (brain stem) (cerebral) (generalized) (spinal cord) 340
myocardium, myocardial - *see* Arteriosclerosis, coronary
nuclear (senile), eye 366.16
ovary 620.8
pancreas 577.8
penis 607.89
peripheral arteries (*see also* Arteriosclerosis, extremities) 440.20
plaques 340
pluriglandular 258.8
polyglandular 258.8
posterior (spinal cord) (syphilitic) 094.0
posterolateral (spinal cord) - *see* Degeneration, combined
prepuce 607.89
primary lateral 335.24
progressive systemic 710.1
pulmonary (*see also* Fibrosis, lung) 515
artery 416.0
valve (heart) (*see also* Endocarditis, pulmonary) 424.3
renal 587
with
cystine storage disease 270.0
hypertension (*see also* Hypertension, kidney) 403.90
hypertensive heart disease (conditions classifiable to 402) (*see also* Hypertension, cardiorenal) 404.90
arteriolar (hyaline) (*see also* Hypertension, kidney) 403.90
hyperplastic (*see also* Hypertension, kidney) 403.90
retina (senile) (vascular) 362.17
rheumatic
aortic valve 395.9
mitral valve 394.9
Schilder's 341.1
senile - *see* Arteriosclerosis
spinal (cord) (general) (progressive) (transverse) 336.8
ascending 357.0
combined - *see also* Degeneration, combined
multiple 340
syphilitic 094.89
disseminated 340
dorsolateral - *see* Degeneration, combined
hereditary (Friedreich's) (mixed form) 334.0
lateral (amyotrophic) 335.24
multiple 340
posterior (syphilitic) 094.0
stomach 537.89
subendocardial, congenital 425.3
systemic (progressive) 710.1
with lung involvement 710.1 *[517.2]*
tricuspid (heart) (valve) - *see* Endocarditis, tricuspid
tuberous (brain) 759.5
tympanic membrane (*see also* Tympanosclerosis) 385.00
valve, valvular (heart) - *see* Endocarditis
vascular - *see* Arteriosclerosis
vein 459.89
Sclerotenonitis 379.07

Sclerotitis (*see also* Scleritis) 379.00
syphilitic 095.0
tuberculous (*see also* Tuberculosis) 017.3 *[379.09]*
Scoliosis (acquired) (postural) 737.30
congenital 754.2
due to or associated with
Charcôt-Marie-Tooth disease 356.1 *[737.43]*
mucopolysaccharidosis 277.5 *[737.43]*
neurofibromatosis 237.71 *[737.43]*
osteitis
deformans 731.0 *[737.43]*
fibrosa cystica 252.01 *[737.43]*
osteoporosis (*see also* Osteoporosis) 733.00 *[737.43]*
poliomyelitis 138 *[737.43]*
radiation 737.33
tuberculosis (*see also* Tuberculosis) 015.0 *[737.43]*
idiopathic 737.30
infantile
progressive 737.32
resolving 737.31
paralytic 737.39
rachitic 268.1
sciatic 724.3
specified NEC 737.39
thoracogenic 737.34
tuberculous (*see also* Tuberculosis) 015.0 *[737.43]*
Scoliotic pelvis 738.6
with disproportion (fetopelvic) 653.0
affecting fetus or newborn 763.1
causing obstructed labor 660.1
affecting fetus or newborn 763.1
Scorbutus, scorbutic 267
anemia 281.8
Scotoma (ring) 368.44
arcuate 368.43
Bjerrum 368.43
blind spot area 368.42
central 368.41
centrocecal 368.41
paracecal 368.42
paracentral 368.41
scintillating 368.12
Seidel 368.43
Scratch - *see* Injury, superficial, by site
Screening (for) V82.9
alcoholism V79.1
anemia, deficiency NEC V78.1
iron V78.0
anomaly, congenital V82.89
antenatal, of mother V28.9 ⇐
alphafetoprotein levels, raised V28.1
based on amniocentesis V28.2
chromosomal anomalies V28.0
raised alphafetoprotein levels V28.1
fetal growth retardation using ultrasonics V28.4
genetic V82.79 ◄
disease carrier status V82.71 ◄
isoimmunization V28.5
malformations using ultrasonics V28.3
raised alphafetoprotein levels V28.1
specified condition NEC V28.8
Streptococcus B V28.6
arterial hypertension V81.1
arthropod-borne viral disease NEC V73.5
asymptomatic bacteriuria V81.5
bacterial
conjunctivitis V74.4
disease V74.9
specified condition NEC V74.8

Screening *(Continued)*
bacteriuria, asymptomatic V81.5
blood disorder NEC V78.9
specified type NEC V78.8
bronchitis, chronic V81.3
brucellosis V74.8
cancer - *see* Screening, malignant neoplasm
cardiovascular disease NEC V81.2
cataract V80.2
Chagas' disease V75.3
chemical poisoning V82.5
cholera V74.0
cholesterol level V77.91
chromosomal
anomalies
by amniocentesis, antenatal V28.0
maternal postnatal V82.4
athletes V70.3
condition
cardiovascular NEC V81.2
eye NEC V80.2
genitourinary NEC V81.6
neurological V80.0
respiratory NEC V81.4
skin V82.0
specified NEC V82.89
congenital
anomaly V82.89
eye V80.2
dislocation of hip V82.3
eye condition or disease V80.2
conjunctivitis, bacterial V74.4
contamination NEC (*see also* Poisoning) V82.5
coronary artery disease V81.0
cystic fibrosis V77.6
deficiency anemia NEC V78.1
iron V78.0
dengue fever V73.5
depression V79.0
developmental handicap V79.9
in early childhood V79.3
specified type NEC V79.8
diabetes mellitus V77.1
diphtheria V74.3
disease or disorder V82.9
bacterial V74.9
specified NEC V74.8
blood V78.9
specified type NEC V78.8
blood-forming organ V78.9
specified type NEC V78.8
cardiovascular NEC V81.2
hypertensive V81.1
ischemic V81.0
Chagas' V75.3
chlamydial V73.98
specified NEC V73.88
ear NEC V80.3
endocrine NEC V77.99
eye NEC V80.2
genitourinary NEC V81.6
heart NEC V81.2
hypertensive V81.1
ischemic V81.0
immunity NEC V77.99
infectious NEC V75.9
lipoid NEC V77.91
mental V79.9
specified type NEC V79.8
metabolic NEC V77.99
inborn NEC V77.7
neurological V80.0

Screening *(Continued)*
disease or disorder *(Continued)*
nutritional NEC V77.99
rheumatic NEC V82.2
rickettsial V75.0
sickle-cell V78.2
trait V78.2
specified type NEC V82.89
thyroid V77.0
vascular NEC V81.2
ischemic V81.0
venereal V74.5
viral V73.99
arthropod-borne NEC V73.5
specified type NEC V73.89
dislocation of hip, congenital V82.3
drugs in athletes V70.3
emphysema (chronic) V81.3
encephalitis, viral (mosquito- or tick-borne) V73.5
endocrine disorder NEC V77.99
eye disorder NEC V80.2
congenital V80.2
fever
dengue V73.5
hemorrhagic V73.5
yellow V73.4
filariasis V75.6
galactosemia V77.4
genitourinary condition NEC V81.6
glaucoma V80.1
gonorrhea V74.5
gout V77.5
Hansen's disease V74.2
heart disease NEC V81.2
hypertensive V81.1
ischemic V81.0
heavy metal poisoning V82.5
helminthiasis, intestinal V75.7
hematopoietic malignancy V76.89
hemoglobinopathies NEC V78.3
hemorrhagic fever V73.5
Hodgkin's disease V76.89
hormones in athletes V70.3
hypercholesterolemia V77.91
hyperlipidemia V77.91
hypertension V81.1
immunity disorder NEC V77.99
inborn errors of metabolism NEC V77.7
infection
bacterial V74.9
specified type NEC V74.8
mycotic V75.4
parasitic NEC V75.8
infectious disease V75.9
specified type NEC V75.8
ingestion of radioactive substance V82.5
intestinal helminthiasis V75.7
iron deficiency anemia V78.0
ischemic heart disease V81.0
lead poisoning V82.5
leishmaniasis V75.2
leprosy V74.2
leptospirosis V74.8
leukemia V76.89
lipoid disorder NEC V77.91
lymphoma V76.89
malaria V75.1
malignant neoplasm (of) V76.9
bladder V76.3
blood V76.89
breast V76.10
mammogram NEC V76.12
for high-risk patient V76.11
specified type NEC V76.19
cervix V76.2

Screening *(Continued)*
malignant neoplasm (of) *(Continued)*
colon V76.51
colorectal V76.51
hematopoietic system V76.89
intestine V76.50
colon V76.51
small V76.52
lung V76.0
lymph (glands) V76.89
nervous system V76.81
oral cavity V76.42
other specified neoplasm NEC V76.89
ovary V76.46
prostate V76.44
rectum V76.41
respiratory organs V76.0
skin V76.43
specified sites NEC V76.49
testis V76.45
vagina V76.47
following hysterectomy for malignant condition V67.01
malnutrition V77.2
mammogram NEC V76.12
for high-risk patient V76.11
maternal postnatal chromosomal anomalies V82.4
measles V73.2
mental
disorder V79.9
specified type NEC V79.8
retardation V79.2
metabolic disorder NEC V77.99
metabolic errors, inborn V77.7
mucoviscidosis V77.6
multiphasic V82.6
mycosis V75.4
mycotic infection V75.4
nephropathy V81.5
neurological condition V80.0
nutritional disorder NEC V77.99
obesity V77.8
osteoporosis V82.81
parasitic infection NEC V75.8
phenylketonuria V77.3
plague V74.8
poisoning
chemical NEC V82.5
contaminated water supply V82.5
heavy metal V82.5
poliomyelitis V73.0
postnatal chromosomal anomalies
maternal V82.4
prenatal - *see* Screening, antenatal
pulmonary tuberculosis V74.1
radiation exposure V82.5
renal disease V81.5
respiratory condition NEC V81.4
rheumatic disorder NEC V82.2
rheumatoid arthritis V82.1
rickettsial disease V75.0
rubella V73.3
schistosomiasis V75.5
senile macular lesions of eye V80.2
sickle-cell anemia, disease, or trait V78.2
skin condition V82.0
sleeping sickness V75.3
smallpox V73.1
special V82.9
specified condition NEC V82.89
specified type NEC V82.89
spirochetal disease V74.9
specified type NEC V74.8
stimulants in athletes V70.3

Screening *(Continued)*
- syphilis V74.5
- tetanus V74.8
- thyroid disorder V77.0
- trachoma V73.6
- trypanosomiasis V75.3
- tuberculosis, pulmonary V74.1
- venereal disease V74.5
- viral encephalitis
  - mosquito-borne V73.5
  - tick-borne V73.5
- whooping cough V74.8
- worms, intestinal V75.7
- yaws V74.6
- yellow fever V73.4

Scrofula (*see also* Tuberculosis) 017.2
Scrofulide (primary) (*see also* Tuberculosis) 017.0
Scrofuloderma, scrofulodermia (any site) (primary) (*see also* Tuberculosis) 017.0
Scrofulosis (universal) (*see also* Tuberculosis) 017.2
Scrofulosis lichen (primary) (*see also* Tuberculosis) 017.0
Scrofulous - *see* condition
Scrotal tongue 529.5
- congenital 750.13

Scrotum - *see* condition
Scurvy (gum) (infantile) (rickets) (scorbutic) 267
Sea-blue histiocyte syndrome 272.7
Seabright-Bantam syndrome (pseudohypoparathyroidism) 275.49
Seasickness 994.6
Seatworm 127.4
Sebaceous
- cyst (*see also* Cyst, sebaceous) 706.2
- gland disease NEC 706.9

Sebocystomatosis 706.2
Seborrhea, seborrheic 706.3
- adiposa 706.3
- capitis 690.11
- congestiva 695.4
- corporis 706.3
- dermatitis 690.10
  - infantile 690.12
- diathesis in infants 695.89
- eczema 690.18
  - infantile 690.12
- keratosis 702.19
  - inflamed 702.11
- nigricans 759.89
- sicca 690.18
- wart 702.19
  - inflamed 702.11

Seckel's syndrome 759.89
Seclusion pupil 364.74
Seclusiveness, child 313.22
Secondary - *see also* condition
- neoplasm - *see* Neoplasm, by site, malignant, secondary

Secretan's disease or syndrome (posttraumatic edema) 782.3
Secretion
- antidiuretic hormone, inappropriate (syndrome) 253.6
- catecholamine, by pheochromocytoma 255.6
- hormone
  - antidiuretic, inappropriate (syndrome) 253.6
  - by
    - carcinoid tumor 259.2
    - pheochromocytoma 255.6
  - ectopic NEC 259.3

Secretion *(Continued)*
- urinary
  - excessive 788.42
  - suppression 788.5

Section
- cesarean
  - affecting fetus or newborn 763.4
  - post mortem, affecting fetus or newborn 761.6
  - previous, in pregnancy or childbirth 654.2
    - affecting fetus or newborn 763.89
- nerve, traumatic - *see* Injury, nerve, by site

Seeligmann's syndrome (ichthyosis congenita) 757.1
Segmentation, incomplete (congenital) - *see also* Fusion
- bone NEC 756.9
- lumbosacral (joint) 756.15
- vertebra 756.15
  - lumbosacral 756.15

Seizure 780.39
- akinetic (idiopathic) (*see also* Epilepsy) 345.0
  - psychomotor 345.4
- apoplexy, apoplectic (*see also* Disease, cerebrovascular, acute) 436
- atonic (*see also* Epilepsy) 345.0
- autonomic 300.11
- brain or cerebral (*see also* Disease, cerebrovascular, acute) 436
- convulsive (*see also* Convulsions) 780.39
- cortical (focal) (motor) (*see also* Epilepsy) 345.5
- epilepsy, epileptic (cryptogenic) (*see also* Epilepsy) 345.9
- epileptiform, epileptoid 780.39
  - focal (*see also* Epilepsy) 345.5
- febrile (simple) 780.31 ⇐ Revised
  - with status epilepticus 345.3
  - atypical 780.32 ◀ New
  - complex 780.32 ◀ New
  - complicated 780.32 ◀ New
- heart - *see* Disease, heart
- hysterical 300.11
- Jacksonian (focal) (*see also* Epilepsy) 345.5
  - motor type 345.5
  - sensory type 345.5
- newborn 779.0
- paralysis (*see also* Disease, cerebrovascular, acute) 436
- recurrent 345.9 ⇐ Revised
  - epileptic - *see* Epilepsy
- repetitive 780.39
  - epileptic - *see* Epilepsy
- salaam (*see also* Epilepsy) 345.6
- uncinate (*see also* Epilepsy) 345.4

Self-mutilation 300.9
Semicoma 780.09
Semiconsciousness 780.09
Seminal
- vesicle - *see* condition
- vesiculitis (*see also* Vesiculitis) 608.0

Seminoma (M9061/3)
- anaplastic type (M9062/3)
  - specified site - *see* Neoplasm, by site, malignant
  - unspecified site 186.9
- specified site - *see* Neoplasm, by site, malignant
- spermatocytic (M9063/3)
  - specified site - *see* Neoplasm, by site, malignant
  - unspecified site 186.9
- unspecified site 186.9

Semliki Forest encephalitis 062.8
Senear-Usher disease or syndrome (pemphigus erythematosus) 694.4
Senecio jacobae dermatitis 692.6
Senectus 797
Senescence 797
Senile (*see also* condition) 797
- cervix (atrophic) 622.8
- degenerative atrophy, skin 701.3
- endometrium (atrophic) 621.8
- fallopian tube (atrophic) 620.3
- heart (failure) 797
- lung 492.8
- ovary (atrophic) 620.3
- syndrome 259.8
- vagina, vaginitis (atrophic) 627.3
- wart 702.0

Senility 797
- with
  - acute confusional state 290.3
  - delirium 290.3
  - mental changes 290.9
  - psychosis NEC (*see also* Psychosis, senile) 290.20
- premature (syndrome) 259.8

Sensation
- burning (*see also* Disturbance, sensation) 782.0
  - tongue 529.6
- choking 784.99 ⇐ Revised
- loss of (*see also* Disturbance, sensation) 782.0
- prickling (*see also* Disturbance, sensation) 782.0
- tingling (*see also* Disturbance, sensation) 782.0

Sense loss (touch) (*see also* Disturbance, sensation) 782.0
- smell 781.1
- taste 781.1

Sensibility disturbance NEC (cortical) (deep) (vibratory) (*see also* Disturbance, sensation) 782.0
Sensitive dentine 521.89 ⇐ Revised
Sensitiver Beziehungswahn 297.8
Sensitivity, sensitization - *see also* Allergy
- autoerythrocyte 287.2
- carotid sinus 337.0
- child (excessive) 313.21
- cold, autoimmune 283.0
- methemoglobin 289.7
- suxamethonium 289.89
- tuberculin, without clinical or radiological symptoms 795.5

Sensory
- extinction 781.8
- neglect 781.8

Separation
- acromioclavicular - *see* Dislocation, acromioclavicular
- anxiety, abnormal 309.21
- apophysis, traumatic - *see* Fracture, by site
- choroid 363.70
  - hemorrhagic 363.72
  - serous 363.71
- costochondral (simple) (traumatic) - *see* Dislocation, costochondral
- delayed
  - umbilical cord 779.83
- epiphysis, epiphyseal
  - nontraumatic 732.9
    - upper femoral 732.2
  - traumatic - *see* Fracture, by site
- fracture - *see* Fracture, by site

Separation *(Continued)*
infundibulum cardiac from right ventricle by a partition 746.83
joint (current) (traumatic) - *see* Dislocation, by site
placenta (normally implanted) - *see* Placenta, separation
pubic bone, obstetrical trauma 665.6
retina, retinal (*see also* Detachment, retina) 361.9
layers 362.40
sensory (*see also* Retinoschisis) 361.10
pigment epithelium (exudative) 362.42
hemorrhagic 362.43
sternoclavicular (traumatic) - *see* Dislocation, sternoclavicular
symphysis pubis, obstetrical trauma 665.6
tracheal ring, incomplete (congenital) 748.3
Sepsis (generalized) 995.91
with
abortion - *see* Abortion, by type, with sepsis
acute organ dysfunction 995.92 ◀
ectopic pregnancy (*see also* categories 633.0–633.9) 639.0
molar pregnancy (*see also* categories 630–632) 639.0
multiple organ dysfunction (MOD) 995.92 ◀
buccal 528.3
complicating labor 659.3
dental (pulpal origin) 522.4
female genital organ NEC 614.9
fetus (intrauterine) 771.81
following
abortion 639.0
ectopic or molar pregnancy 639.0
infusion, perfusion, or transfusion 999.3
Friedländer's 038.49
intraocular 360.00
localized
in operation wound 998.59
skin (*see also* Abscess) 682.9
malleus 024
nadir 038.9
newborn (organism unspecified) NEC 771.81
oral 528.3
puerperal, postpartum, childbirth (pelvic) 670
resulting from infusion, injection, transfusion, or vaccination 999.3
severe 995.92
skin, localized (*see also* Abscess) 682.9
umbilical (newborn) (organism unspecified) 771.89
tetanus 771.3
urinary 599.0
meaning sepsis 995.91
meaning urinary tract infection 599.0
Septate - *see also* Septum
Septic - *see also* condition
adenoids 474.01
and tonsils 474.02
arm (with lymphangitis) 682.3
embolus - *see* Embolism
finger (with lymphangitis) 681.00
foot (with lymphangitis) 682.7
gallbladder (*see also* Cholecystitis) 575.8
hand (with lymphangitis) 682.4

Septic *(Continued)*
joint (*see also* Arthritis, septic) 711.0
kidney (*see also* Infection, kidney) 590.9
leg (with lymphangitis) 682.6
mouth 528.3
nail 681.9
finger 681.02
toe 681.11
shock (endotoxic) 785.52 sore (*see also* Abscess) 682.9
throat 034.0
milk-borne 034.0
streptococcal 034.0
spleen (acute) 289.59
teeth (pulpal origin) 522.4
throat 034.0
thrombus - *see* Thrombosis
toe (with lymphangitis) 681.10
tonsils 474.00
and adenoids 474.02
umbilical cord (newborn) (organism unspecified) 771.89
uterus (*see also* Endometritis) 615.9
Septicemia, septicemic (generalized) (suppurative) 038.9
with
abortion - *see* Abortion, by type, with sepsis
ectopic pregnancy (*see also* categories 633.0–633.9) 639.0
molar pregnancy (*see also* categories 630–632) 639.0
Aerobacter aerogenes 038.49
anaerobic 038.3
anthrax 022.3
Bacillus coli 038.42
Bacteroides 038.3
Clostridium 038.3
complicating labor 659.3
cryptogenic 038.9
enteric gram-negative bacilli 038.40
Enterobacter aerogenes 038.49
Erysipelothrix (insidiosa) (rhusiopathiae) 027.1
Escherichia coli 038.42
following
abortion 639.0
ectopic or molar pregnancy 639.0
infusion, injection, transfusion, or vaccination 999.3
Friedländer's (bacillus) 038.49
gangrenous 038.9
gonococcal 098.89
gram-negative (organism) 038.40
anaerobic 038.3
Hemophilus influenzae 038.41
herpes (simplex) 054.5
herpetic 054.5
Listeria monocytogenes 027.0
meningeal - *see* Meningitis
meningococcal (chronic) (fulminating) 036.2
navel, newborn (organism unspecified) 771.89
newborn (organism unspecified) 771.81
plague 020.2
pneumococcal 038.2
postabortal 639.0
postoperative 998.59
Proteus vulgaris 038.49
Pseudomonas (aeruginosa) 038.43
puerperal, postpartum 670
Salmonella (aertrycke) (callinarum) (choleraesuis) (enteritidis) (suipestifer) 003.1
Serratia 038.44

Septicemia, septicemic *(Continued)*
Shigella (*see also* Dysentery, bacillary) 004.9
specified organism NEC 038.8
staphylococcal 038.10
aureus 038.11
specified organism NEC 038.19
streptococcal (anaerobic) 038.0
Streptococcus pneumoniae 038.2
suipestifer 003.1
umbilicus, newborn (organism unspecified) 771.89
viral 079.99
Yersinia enterocolitica 038.49
Septum, septate (congenital) - *see also* Anomaly, specified type NEC
anal 751.2
aqueduct of Sylvius 742.3
with spina bifida (*see also* Spina bifida) 741.0
hymen 752.49
uterus (*see also* Double, uterus) 752.2
vagina 752.49
in pregnancy or childbirth 654.7
affecting fetus or newborn 763.89
causing obstructed labor 660.2
affecting fetus or newborn 763.1
Sequestration
lung (congenital) (extralobar) (intralobar) 748.5
orbit 376.10
pulmonary artery (congenital) 747.3
splenic 289.52
Sequestrum
bone (*see also* Osteomyelitis) 730.1
jaw 526.4
dental 525.8
jaw bone 526.4
sinus (accessory) (nasal) (*see also* Sinusitis) 473.9
maxillary 473.0
Sequoiosis asthma 495.8
Serology for syphilis
doubtful
with signs or symptoms - *see* Syphilis, by site and stage
follow-up of latent syphilis - *see* Syphilis, latent
false positive 795.6
negative, with signs or symptoms - *see* Syphilis, by site and stage
positive 097.1
with signs or symptoms - *see* Syphilis, by site and stage
false 795.6
follow-up of latent syphilis - *see* Syphilis, latent
only finding - *see* Syphilis, latent
reactivated 097.1
Seroma - (postoperative) (non-infected) 998.13
infected 998.51
Seropurulent - *see* condition
Serositis, multiple 569.89
pericardial 423.2
peritoneal 568.82
pleural - *see* Pleurisy
Serotonin syndrome 333.99
Serous - *see* condition
Sertoli cell
adenoma (M8640/0)
specified site - *see* Neoplasm, by site, benign
unspecified site
female 220
male 222.0

Sertoli cell *(Continued)*
carcinoma (M8640/3)
specified site - *see* Neoplasm, by site, malignant
unspecified site 186.9
syndrome (germinal aplasia) 606.0
tumor (M8640/0)
with lipid storage (M8641/0)
specified site - *see* Neoplasm, by site, benign
unspecified site
female 220
male 222.0
specified site - *see* Neoplasm, by site, benign
unspecified site
female 220
male 222.0
Sertoli-Leydig cell tumor (M8631/0)
specified site - *see* Neoplasm, by site, benign
unspecified site
female 220
male 222.0
Serum
allergy, allergic reaction 999.5
shock 999.4
arthritis 999.5 *[713.6]*
complication or reaction NEC 999.5
disease NEC 999.5
hepatitis 070.3
intoxication 999.5
jaundice (homologous) - *see* Hepatitis, viral, type B
neuritis 999.5
poisoning NEC 999.5
rash NEC 999.5
reaction NEC 999.5
sickness NEC 999.5
Sesamoiditis 733.99
Seven-day fever 061
of
Japan 100.89
Queensland 100.89
Sever's disease or osteochondrosis (calcaneum) 732.5
Sex chromosome mosaics 758.81
Sextuplet
affected by maternal complication of pregnancy 761.5
healthy liveborn - *see* Newborn, multiple
pregnancy (complicating delivery) NEC 651.8
with fetal loss and retention of one or more fetus(es) 651.6
following (elective) fetal reduction 651.7
Sexual
anesthesia 302.72
deviation (*see also* Deviation, sexual) 302.9
disorder (*see also* Deviation, sexual) 302.9
frigidity (female) 302.72
function, disorder of (psychogenic) 302.70
specified type NEC 302.79
immaturity (female) (male) 259.0
impotence 607.84
organic origin NEC 607.84
psychogenic 302.72
precocity (constitutional) (cryptogenic) (female) (idiopathic) (male) NEC 259.1
with adrenal hyperplasia 255.2
Sexual *(Continued)*
sadism 302.84
Sexuality, pathological (*see also* Deviation, sexual) 302.9
Sézary's disease, reticulosis, or syndrome (M9701/3) 202.2
Shadow, lung 793.1
Shaken infant syndrome 995.55
Shaking
head (tremor) 781.0
palsy or paralysis (*see also* Parkinsonism) 332.0
Shallowness, acetabulum 736.39
Shaver's disease or syndrome (bauxite pneumoconiosis) 503
Shearing
artificial skin graft 996.55
decellularized allodermis graft 996.55
Sheath (tendon) - *see* condition
Shedding
nail 703.8
teeth, premature, primary (deciduous) 520.6
Sheehan's disease or syndrome (postpartum pituitary necrosis) 253.2
Shelf, rectal 569.49
Shell
shock (current) (*see also* Reaction, stress, acute) 308.9
lasting state 300.16
teeth 520.5
Shield kidney 753.3
Shift, mediastinal 793.2
Shifting
pacemaker 427.89
sleep-work schedule (affecting sleep) 327.36
Shiga's
bacillus 004.0
dysentery 004.0
Shigella (dysentery) (*see also* Dysentery, bacillary) 004.9
carrier (suspected) of V02.3
Shigellosis (*see also* Dysentery, bacillary) 004.9
Shingles (*see also* Herpes, zoster) 053.9
eye NEC 053.29
Shin splints 844.9
Shipyard eye or disease 077.1
Shirodkar suture, in pregnancy 654.5
Shock 785.50
with
abortion - *see* Abortion, by type, with shock
ectopic pregnancy (*see also* categories 633.0–633.9) 639.5
molar pregnancy (*see also* categories 630–632) 639.5
allergic - *see* Shock, anaphylactic
anaclitic 309.21
anaphylactic 995.0
chemical - *see* Table of Drugs and Chemicals
correct medicinal substance properly administered 995.0
drug or medicinal substance
correct substance properly administered 995.0
overdose or wrong substance given or taken 977.9
specified drug - *see* Table of Drugs and Chemicals
following sting(s) 989.5
food - *see* Anaphylactic shock, due to, food
Shock *(Continued)*
anaphylactic *(Continued)*
immunization 999.4
serum 999.4
anaphylactoid - *see* Shock, anaphylactic
anesthetic
correct substance properly administered 995.4
overdose or wrong substance given 968.4
specified anesthetic - *see* Table of Drugs and Chemicals
birth, fetus or newborn NEC 779.89
cardiogenic 785.51
chemical substance - *see* Table of Drugs and Chemicals
circulatory 785.59
complicating
abortion - *see* Abortion, by type, with shock
ectopic pregnancy - *see also* categories 633.0–633.9) 639.5
labor and delivery 669.1
molar pregnancy (*see also* categories 630–632) 639.5
culture 309.29
due to
drug 995.0
correct substance properly administered 995.0
overdose or wrong substance given or taken 977.9
specified drug - *see* Table of Drugs and Chemicals
food - *see* Anaphylactic shock, due to, food
during labor and delivery 669.1
electric 994.8
endotoxic 785.52
due to surgical procedure 998.0
following
abortion 639.5
ectopic or molar pregnancy 639.5
injury (immediate) (delayed) 958.4
labor and delivery 669.1
gram-negative 785.52
hematogenic 785.59
hemorrhagic
due to
disease 785.59
surgery (intraoperative) (postoperative) 998.0
trauma 958.4
hypovolemic NEC 785.59
surgical 998.0
traumatic 958.4
insulin 251.0
therapeutic misadventure 962.3
kidney 584.5
traumatic (following crushing) 958.5
lightning 994.0
lung 518.5
nervous (*see also* Reaction, stress, acute) 308.9
obstetric 669.1
with
abortion - *see* Abortion, by type, with shock
ectopic pregnancy (*see also* categories 633.0–633.9) 639.5
molar pregnancy (*see also* categories 630–632) 639.5
following
abortion 639.5
ectopic or molar pregnancy 639.5

Shock *(Continued)*
paralysis, paralytic (*see also* Disease, cerebrovascular, acute) 436
late effect - *see* Late effect(s) (of) cerebrovascular disease
pleural (surgical) 998.0
due to trauma 958.4
postoperative 998.0
with
abortion - *see* Abortion, by type, with shock
ectopic pregnancy (*see also* categories 633.0–633.9) 639.5
molar pregnancy (*see also* categories 630–632) 639.5
following
abortion 639.5
ectopic or molar pregnancy 639.5
psychic (*see also* Reaction, stress, acute) 308.9
past history (of) V15.49
psychogenic (*see also* Reaction, stress, acute) 308.9
septic 785.52
with
abortion - *see* Abortion, by type, with shock
ectopic pregnancy (*see also* categories 633.0–633.9) 639.5
molar pregnancy (*see also* categories 630–632) 639.5
due to
surgical procedure 998.0
transfusion NEC 999.8
bone marrow 996.85
following
abortion 639.5
ectopic or molar pregnancy 639.5
surgical procedure 998.0
transfusion NEC 999.8
bone marrow 996.85
spinal - *see also* Injury, spinal, by site
with spinal bone injury - *see* Fracture, vertebra, by site, with spinal cord injury
surgical 998.0
therapeutic misadventure NEC (*see also* Complications) 998.89
thyroxin 962.7
toxic 040.82
transfusion - *see* Complications, transfusion
traumatic (immediate) (delayed) 958.4
Shoemakers' chest 738.3
Short, shortening, shortness
Achilles tendon (acquired) 727.81
arm 736.89
congenital 755.20
back 737.9
bowel syndrome 579.3
breath 786.05
chain acyl CoA dehydrogenase deficiency (SCAD) 277.85
common bile duct, congenital 751.69
cord (umbilical) 663.4
affecting fetus or newborn 762.6
cystic duct, congenital 751.69
esophagus (congenital) 750.4
femur (acquired) 736.81
congenital 755.34
frenulum linguae 750.0
frenum, lingual 750.0
hamstrings 727.81
hip (acquired) 736.39
congenital 755.63
Short, shortening, shortness *(Continued)*
leg (acquired) 736.81
congenital 755.30
metatarsus (congenital) 754.79
acquired 736.79
organ or site, congenital NEC - *see* Distortion
palate (congenital) 750.26
P-R interval syndrome 426.81
radius (acquired) 736.09
congenital 755.26
round ligament 629.89 ⬅
sleeper 307.49
stature, constitutional (hereditary) 783.43
tendon 727.81
Achilles (acquired) 727.81
congenital 754.79
congenital 756.89
thigh (acquired) 736.81
congenital 755.34
tibialis anticus 727.81
umbilical cord 663.4
affecting fetus or newborn 762.6
urethra 599.84
uvula (congenital) 750.26
vagina 623.8
Shortsightedness 367.1
Shoshin (acute fulminating beriberi) 265.0
Shoulder - *see* condition
Shovel-shaped incisors 520.2
Shower, thromboembolic - *see* Embolism
Shunt (status)
aortocoronary bypass V45.81
arterial-venous (dialysis) V45.1
arteriovenous, pulmonary (acquired) 417.0
congenital 747.3
traumatic (complication) 901.40
cerebral ventricle (communicating) in situ V45.2
coronary artery bypass V45.81
surgical, prosthetic, with complications - *see* Complications, shunt
vascular NEC V45.89
Shutdown
renal 586
with
abortion - *see* Abortion, by type, with renal failure
ectopic pregnancy (*see also* categories 633.0–633.9) 639.3
molar pregnancy (*see also* categories 630–632) 639.3
complicating
abortion 639.3
ectopic or molar pregnancy 639.3
following labor and delivery 669.3
Shwachman's syndrome 288.02 ⬅
Shy-Drager syndrome (orthostatic hypotension with multisystem degeneration) 333.0
Sialadenitis (any gland) (chronic) (suppurative) 527.2
epidemic - *see* Mumps
Sialadenosis, periodic 527.2
Sialaporia 527.7
Sialectasia 527.8
Sialitis 527.2
Sialoadenitis (*see also* Sialadenitis) 527.2
Sialoangitis 527.2
Sialodochitis (fibrinosa) 527.2
Sialodocholithiasis 527.5
Sialolithiasis 527.5
Sialorrhea (*see also* Ptyalism) 527.7
periodic 527.2
Sialosis 527.8
rheumatic 710.2
Siamese twin 759.4
Sicard's syndrome 352.6
Sicca syndrome (keratoconjunctivitis) 710.2
Sick 799.9
cilia syndrome 759.89
or handicapped person in family V61.49
Sickle-cell
anemia (*see also* Disease, sickle-cell) 282.60
disease (*see also* Disease, sickle-cell) 282.60
hemoglobin
C disease (without crisis) 282.63
with
crisis 282.64
vaso-occlusive pain 282.64
D disease (without crisis) 282.68
with crisis 282.69
E disease (without crisis) 282.68
with crisis 282.69
thalassemia (without crisis) 282.41
with
crisis 282.42
vaso-occlusive pain 282.42
trait 282.5
Sicklemia (*see also* Disease, sickle-cell) 282.60
trait 282.5
Sickness
air (travel) 994.6
airplane 994.6
alpine 993.2
altitude 993.2
Andes 993.2
aviators' 993.2
balloon 993.2
car 994.6
compressed air 993.3
decompression 993.3
green 280.9
harvest 100.89
milk 988.8
morning 643.0
motion 994.6
mountain 993.2
acute 289.0
protein (*see also* Complications, vaccination) 999.5
radiation NEC 990
roundabout (motion) 994.6
sea 994.6
serum NEC 999.5
sleeping (African) 086.5
by Trypanosoma 086.5
gambiense 086.3
rhodesiense 086.4
Gambian 086.3
late effect 139.8
Rhodesian 086.4
sweating 078.2
swing (motion) 994.6
train (railway) (travel) 994.6
travel (any vehicle) 994.6
Sick sinus syndrome 427.81
Sideropenia (*see also* Anemia, iron deficiency) 280.9
Siderosis (lung) (occupational) 503
cornea 371.15
eye (bulbi) (vitreous) 360.23
lens 360.23
Siegal-Cattan-Mamou disease (periodic) 277.31 ⬅

Siemens' syndrome
ectodermal dysplasia 757.31
keratosis follicularis spinulosa (decalvans) 757.39
Sighing respiration 786.7
Sigmoid
flexure - *see* condition
kidney 753.3
Sigmoiditis - *see* Enteritis
Silfverskiöld's syndrome 756.50
Silicosis, silicotic (complicated) (occupational) (simple) 502
fibrosis, lung (confluent) (massive) (occupational) 502
non-nodular 503
pulmonum 502
Silicotuberculosis (*see also* Tuberculosis) 011.4
Silo fillers' disease 506.9
Silver's syndrome (congenital hemihypertrophy and short stature) 759.89
Silver wire arteries, retina 362.13
Silvestroni-Bianco syndrome (thalassemia minima) 282.49
Simian crease 757.2
Simmonds' cachexia or disease (pituitary cachexia) 253.2
Simons' disease or syndrome (progressive lipodystrophy) 272.6
Simple, simplex - *see* condition
Sinding-Larsen disease (juvenile osteopathia patellae) 732.4
Singapore hemorrhagic fever 065.4
Singers' node or nodule 478.5
Single
atrium 745.69
coronary artery 746.85
umbilical artery 747.5
ventricle 745.3
Singultus 786.8
epidemicus 078.89
Sinus - *see also* Fistula
abdominal 569.81
arrest 426.6
arrhythmia 427.89
bradycardia 427.89
chronic 427.81
branchial cleft (external) (internal) 744.41
coccygeal (infected) 685.1
with abscess 685.0
dental 522.7
dermal (congenital) 685.1
with abscess 685.0
draining - *see* Fistula
infected, skin NEC 686.9
marginal, rupture or bleeding 641.2
affecting fetus or newborn 762.1
pause 426.6
pericranii 742.0
pilonidal (infected) (rectum) 685.1
with abscess 685.0
preauricular 744.46
rectovaginal 619.1
sacrococcygeal (dermoid) (infected) 685.1
with abscess 685.0
skin
infected NEC 686.9
noninfected- *see* Ulcer, skin
tachycardia 427.89
tarsi syndrome 726.79
testis 608.89
tract (postinfectional) - *see* Fistula
urachus 753.7
Sinuses, Rokitansky-Aschoff (*see also* Disease, gallbladder) 575.8
Sinusitis (accessory) (chronic) (hyperplastic) (nasal) (nonpurulent) (purulent) 473.9
with influenza, flu, or grippe 487.1
acute 461.9
ethmoidal 461.2
frontal 461.1
maxillary 461.0
specified type NEC 461.8
sphenoidal 461.3
allergic (*see also* Fever, hay) 477.9
antrum - *see* Sinusitis, maxillary
due to
fungus, any sinus 117.9
high altitude 993.1
ethmoidal 473.2
acute 461.2
frontal 473.1
acute 461.1
influenzal 478.19 (Revised)
maxillary 473.0
acute 461.0
specified site NEC 473.8
sphenoidal 473.3
acute 461.3
syphilitic, any sinus 095.8
tuberculous, any sinus (*see also* Tuberculosis) 012.8
Sinusitis-bronchiectasis-situs inversus (syndrome) (triad) 759.3
Sipple's syndrome (medullary thyroid carcinoma-pheochromocytoma) 193
Sirenomelia 759.89
Siriasis 992.0
Sirkari's disease 085.0
SIRS systemic inflammatory response syndrome 995.90
due to
infectious process 995.91
with acute organ dysfunction 995.92 (Revised)
non-infectious process 995.93
with acute organ dysfunction 995.94 (Revised)
Siti 104.0
Sitophobia 300.29
Situation, psychiatric 300.9
Situational
disturbance (transient) (*see also* Reaction, adjustment) 309.9
acute 308.3
maladjustment, acute (*see also* Reaction, adjustment) 309.9
reaction (*see also* Reaction, adjustment) 309.9
acute 308.3
Situs inversus or transversus 759.3
abdominalis 759.3
thoracis 759.3
Sixth disease 057.8
Sjögren (-Gougerot) syndrome or disease (keratoconjunctivitis sicca) 710.2
with lung involvement 710.2 *[517.8]*
Sjögren-Larsson syndrome (ichthyosis congenita) 757.1
Skeletal - *see* condition
Skene's gland - *see* condition
Skenitis (*see also* Urethritis) 597.89
gonorrheal (acute) 098.0
chronic or duration of 2 months or over 098.2
Skerljevo 104.0
Skevas-Zerfus disease 989.5
Skin - *see also* condition
donor V59.1
hidebound 710.9
SLAP lesion (superior glenoid labrum) 840.7
Slate-dressers' lung 502
Slate-miners' lung 502
Sleep
deprivation V69.4
disorder 780.50
with apnea - *see* Apnea, sleep
child 307.40
movement, unspecified 780.58
nonorganic origin 307.40
specified type NEC 307.49
disturbance 780.50
with apnea - *see* Apnea, sleep
nonorganic origin 307.40
specified type NEC 307.49
drunkenness 307.47
movement disorder, unspecified 780.58
paroxysmal (*see also* Narcolepsy) 347.00
related movement disorder, unspecified 780.58
rhythm inversion 327.39
nonorganic origin 307.45
walking 307.46
hysterical 300.13
Sleeping sickness 086.5
late effect 139.8
Sleeplessness (*see also* Insomnia) 780.52
menopausal 627.2
nonorganic origin 307.41
Slipped, slipping
epiphysis (postinfectional) 732.9
traumatic (old) 732.9
current - *see* Fracture, by site
upper femoral (nontraumatic) 732.2
intervertebral disc - *see* Displacement, intervertebral disc
ligature, umbilical 772.3
patella 717.89
rib 733.99
sacroiliac joint 724.6
tendon 727.9
ulnar nerve, nontraumatic 354.2
vertebra NEC (*see also* Spondylolisthesis) 756.12
Slocumb's syndrome 255.3
Sloughing (multiple) (skin) 686.9
abscess - *see* Abscess, by site
appendix 543.9
bladder 596.8
fascia 728.9
graft - *see* Complications, graft
phagedena (*see also* Gangrene) 785.4
reattached extremity (*see also* Complications, reattached extremity) 996.90
rectum 569.49
scrotum 608.89
tendon 727.9
transplanted organ (*see also* Rejection, transplant, organ, by site) 996.80
ulcer (*see also* Ulcer, skin) 707.9
Slow
feeding newborn 779.3
fetal, growth NEC 764.9
affecting management of pregnancy 656.5
Slowing
heart 427.89
urinary stream 788.62
Sluder's neuralgia or syndrome 337.0
Slurred, slurring, speech 784.5

ICD-9-CM
S
Vol. 2

- **Small, smallness**
  - cardia reserve - *see* Disease, heart
  - for dates
    - fetus or newborn 764.0
      - with malnutrition 764.1
      - affecting management of pregnancy 656.5
  - infant, term 764.0
    - with malnutrition 764.1
    - affecting management of pregnancy 656.5
  - introitus, vagina 623.3
  - kidney, unknown cause 589.9
    - bilateral 589.1
    - unilateral 589.0
  - ovary 620.8
  - pelvis
    - with disproportion (fetopelvic) 653.1
      - affecting fetus or newborn 763.1
    - causing obstructed labor 660.1
      - affecting fetus or newborn 763.1
  - placenta - *see* Placenta, insufficiency
  - uterus 621.8
  - white kidney 582.9
- **Small-for-dates** (*see also* Light-for-dates) 764.0
  - affecting management of pregnancy 656.5
- **Smallpox** 050.9
  - contact V01.3
  - exposure to V01.3
  - hemorrhagic (pustular) 050.0
  - malignant 050.0
  - modified 050.2
  - vaccination
    - complications - *see* Complications, vaccination
    - prophylactic (against) V04.1
- **Smith's fracture** (separation) (closed) 813.41
  - open 813.51
- **Smith-Lemli-Opitz syndrome** (cerebrohepatorenal syndrome) 759.89
- **Smith-Magenis syndrome** 758.33
- **Smith-Strang disease** (oasthouse urine) 270.2
- **Smokers'**
  - bronchitis 491.0
  - cough 491.0
  - syndrome (*see also* Abuse, drugs, nondependent) 305.1
  - throat 472.1
  - tongue 528.6
- **Smoking complicating pregnancy, childbirth, or the puerperium** 649.0 ◄
- **Smothering spells** 786.09
- **Snaggle teeth, tooth** 524.39
- **Snapping**
  - finger 727.05
  - hip 719.65
  - jaw 524.69
    - temporomandibular joint sounds on opening or closing 524.64
  - knee 717.9
  - thumb 727.05
- **Sneddon-Wilkinson disease or syndrome** (subcorneal pustular dermatosis) 694.1
- **Sneezing** 784.99
  - intractable 478.19
- **Sniffing**
  - cocaine (*see also* Dependence) 304.2
  - ether (*see also* Dependence) 304.6
  - glue (airplane) (*see also* Dependence) 304.6
- **Snoring** 786.09
- **Snow blindness** 370.24
- **Snuffles** (nonsyphilitic) 460
  - syphilitic (infant) 090.0
- **Social migrant** V60.0
- **Sodoku** 026.0
- **Soemmering's ring** 366.51
- **Soft** - *see also* condition
  - enlarged prostate 600.00
    - with
      - other lower urinary tract symptoms (LUTS) 600.01 ◄
      - urinary ◄
        - obstruction 600.01 ◄
        - retention 600.01 ◄
  - nails 703.8
- **Softening**
  - bone 268.2
  - brain (necrotic) (progressive) 434.9
    - arteriosclerotic 437.0
    - congenital 742.4
    - embolic (*see also* Embolism, brain) 434.1
    - hemorrhagic (*see also* Hemorrhage, brain) 431
    - occlusive 434.9
    - thrombotic (*see also* Thrombosis, brain) 434.0
  - cartilage 733.92
  - cerebellar - *see* Softening, brain
  - cerebral - *see* Softening, brain
  - cerebrospinal - *see* Softening, brain
  - myocardial, heart (*see also* Degeneration, myocardial) 429.1
  - nails 703.8
  - spinal cord 336.8
  - stomach 537.89
- **Solar fever** 061
- **Soldier's**
  - heart 306.2
  - patches 423.1
- **Solitary**
  - cyst
    - bone 733.21
    - kidney 593.2
  - kidney (congenital) 753.0
  - tubercle, brain (*see also* Tuberculosis, brain) 013.2
  - ulcer, bladder 596.8
- **Somatization reaction, somatic reaction** (*see also* Disorder, psychosomatic) 306.9
  - disorder 300.81
- **Somatoform disorder** 300.82
  - atypical 300.82
  - severe 300.81
  - undifferentiated 300.82
- **Somnambulism** 307.46
  - hysterical 300.13
- **Somnolence** 780.09
  - nonorganic origin 307.43
  - periodic 349.89
- **Sonne dysentery** 004.3
- **Soor** 112.0
- **Sore**
  - Delhi 085.1
  - desert (*see also* Ulcer, skin) 707.9
  - eye 379.99
  - Lahore 085.1
  - mouth 528.9
    - canker 528.2
    - due to dentures 528.9
  - muscle 729.1
  - Naga (*see also* Ulcer, skin) 707.9
  - oriental 085.1

Sore *(Continued)*
  - pressure (*see also* Decubitus) 707.00
    - with gangrene (*see also* Decubitus) 707.00 *[785.4]*
  - skin NEC 709.9
  - soft 099.0
  - throat 462
    - with influenza, flu, or grippe 487.1
    - acute 462
    - chronic 472.1
    - clergyman's 784.49
    - Coxsackie (virus) 074.0
    - diphtheritic 032.0
    - epidemic 034.0
    - gangrenous 462
    - herpetic 054.79
    - influenzal 487.1
    - malignant 462
    - purulent 462
    - putrid 462
    - septic 034.0
    - streptococcal (ulcerative) 034.0
    - ulcerated 462
    - viral NEC 462
      - Coxsackie 074.0
  - tropical (*see also* Ulcer, skin) 707.9
  - veldt (*see also* Ulcer, skin) 707.9
- **Sotos' syndrome** (cerebral gigantism) 253.0
- **Sounds**
  - friction, pleural 786.7
  - succussion, chest 786.7
  - temporomandibular joint
    - on opening or closing 524.64
- **South African cardiomyopathy syndrome** 425.2
- **South American**
  - blastomycosis 116.1
  - trypanosomiasis - *see* Trypanosomiasis
- **Southeast Asian hemorrhagic fever** 065.4
- **Spacing, teeth, abnormal** 524.30
  - excessive 524.32
- **Spade-like hand** (congenital) 754.89
- **Spading nail** 703.8
  - congenital 757.5
- **Spanemia** 285.9
- **Spanish collar** 605
- **Sparganosis** 123.5
- **Spasm, spastic, spasticity** (*see also* condition) 781.0
  - accommodation 367.53
  - ampulla of Vater (*see also* Disease, gallbladder) 576.8
  - anus, ani (sphincter) (reflex) 564.6
    - psychogenic 306.4
  - artery NEC 443.9
    - basilar 435.0
    - carotid 435.8
    - cerebral 435.9
      - specified artery NEC 435.8
    - retinal (*see also* Occlusion, retinal, artery) 362.30
    - vertebral 435.1
    - vertebrobasilar 435.3
  - Bell's 351.0
  - bladder (sphincter, external or internal) 596.8
  - bowel 564.9
    - psychogenic 306.4
  - bronchus, bronchiole 519.11
  - cardia 530.0
  - cardiac - *see* Angina
  - carpopedal (*see also* Tetany) 781.7
  - cecum 564.9
    - psychogenic 306.4

Spasm, spastic, spasticity *(Continued)*
cerebral (arteries) (vascular) 435.9
specified artery NEC 435.8
cerebrovascular 435.9
cervix, complicating delivery 661.4
affecting fetus or newborn 763.7
ciliary body (of accommodation) 367.53
colon 564.1
psychogenic 306.4
common duct (*see also* Disease, biliary) 576.8
compulsive 307.22
conjugate 378.82
convergence 378.84
coronary (artery) - *see* Angina
diaphragm (reflex) 786.8
psychogenic 306.1
duodenum, duodenal (bulb) 564.89
esophagus (diffuse) 530.5
psychogenic 306.4
facial 351.8
fallopian tube 620.8
gait 781.2
gastrointestinal (tract) 536.8
psychogenic 306.4
glottis 478.75
hysterical 300.11
psychogenic 306.1
specified as conversion reaction 300.11
reflex through recurrent laryngeal nerve 478.75
habit 307.20
chronic 307.22
transient (of childhood) 307.21
heart - *see* Angina
hourglass - *see* Contraction, hourglass
hysterical 300.11
infantile (*see also* Epilepsy) 345.6
internal oblique, eye 378.51
intestinal 564.9
psychogenic 306.4
larynx, laryngeal 478.75
hysterical 300.11
psychogenic 306.1
specified as conversion reaction 300.11
levator palpebrae superioris 333.81
lightning (*see also* Epilepsy) 345.6
mobile 781.0
muscle 728.85
back 724.8
psychogenic 306.0
nerve, trigeminal 350.1
nervous 306.0
nodding 307.3
infantile (*see also* Epilepsy) 345.6
occupational 300.89
oculogyric 378.87
ophthalmic artery 362.30
orbicularis 781.0
perineal 625.8
peroneo-extensor (*see also* Flat, foot) 734
pharynx (reflex) 478.29
hysterical 300.11
psychogenic 306.1
specified as conversion reaction 300.11
pregnant uterus, complicating delivery 661.4
psychogenic 306.0
pylorus 537.81
adult hypertrophic 537.0
congenital or infantile 750.5
psychogenic 306.4

Spasm, spastic, spasticity *(Continued)*
rectum (sphincter) 564.6
psychogenic 306.4
retinal artery NEC (*see also* Occlusion, retina, artery) 362.30
sacroiliac 724.6
salaam (infantile) (*see also* Epilepsy) 345.6
saltatory 781.0
sigmoid 564.9
psychogenic 306.4
sphincter of Oddi (*see also* Disease, gallbladder) 576.5
stomach 536.8
neurotic 306.4
throat 478.29
hysterical 300.11
psychogenic 306.1
specified as conversion reaction 300.11
tic 307.20
chronic 307.22
transient (of childhood) 307.21
tongue 529.8
torsion 333.6
trigeminal nerve 350.1
postherpetic 053.12
ureter 593.89
urethra (sphincter) 599.84
uterus 625.8
complicating labor 661.4
affecting fetus or newborn 763.7
vagina 625.1
psychogenic 306.51
vascular NEC 443.9
vasomotor NEC 443.9
vein NEC 459.89
vesical (sphincter, external or internal) 596.8
viscera 789.0
Spasmodic - *see* condition
Spasmophilia (*see also* Tetany) 781.7
Spasmus nutans 307.3
Spastic - *see also* Spasm
child 343.9
Spasticity - *see also* Spasm
cerebral, child 343.9
Speakers' throat 784.49
Specific, specified - *see* condition
Speech
defect, disorder, disturbance, impediment NEC 784.5
psychogenic 307.9
therapy V57.3
Spells 780.39
breath-holding 786.9
Spencer's disease (epidemic vomiting) 078.82
Spens' syndrome (syncope with heart block) 426.9
Spermatic cord - *see* condition
Spermatocele 608.1
congenital 752.89
Spermatocystitis 608.4
Spermatocytoma (M9063/3)
specified site - *see* Neoplasm, by site, malignant
unspecified site 186.9
Spermatorrhea 608.89
Sperm counts
fertility testing V26.21
following sterilization reversal V26.22
postvasectomy V25.8
Sphacelus (*see also* Gangrene) 785.4
Sphenoidal - *see* condition

Sphenoiditis (chronic) (*see also* Sinusitis, sphenoidal) 473.3
Sphenopalatine ganglion neuralgia 337.0
Sphericity, increased, lens 743.36
Spherocytosis (congenital) (familial) (hereditary) 282.0
hemoglobin disease 282.7
sickle-cell (disease) 282.60
Spherophakia 743.36
Sphincter - *see* condition
Sphincteritis, sphincter of Oddi (*see also* Cholecystitis) 576.8
Sphingolipidosis 272.7
Sphingolipodystrophy 272.7
Sphingomyelinosis 272.7
Spicule tooth 520.2
Spider
finger 755.59
nevus 448.1
vascular 448.1
Spiegler-Fendt sarcoid 686.8
Spielmeyer-Stock disease 330.1
Spielmeyer-Vogt disease 330.1
Spina bifida (aperta) 741.9

Note Use the following fifth-digit subclassification with category 741:

0 unspecified region
1 cervical region
2 dorsal [thoracic] region
3 lumbar region

with hydrocephalus 741.0
fetal (suspected), affecting management of pregnancy 655.0
occulta 756.17
Spindle, Krukenberg's 371.13
Spine, spinal - *see* condition
Spiradenoma (eccrine) (M8403/0) - *see* Neoplasm, skin, benign
Spirillosis NEC (*see also* Fever, relapsing) 087.9
Spirillum minus 026.0
Spirillum obermeieri infection 087.0
Spirochetal - *see* condition
Spirochetosis 104.9
arthritic, arthritica 104.9 *[711.8]*
bronchopulmonary 104.8
icterohemorrhagica 100.0
lung 104.8
Spitting blood (*see also* Hemoptysis) 786.3
Splanchnomegaly 569.89
Splanchnoptosis 569.89
Spleen, splenic - *see also* condition
agenesis 759.0
flexure syndrome 569.89
neutropenia syndrome 289.53 (Revised)
sequestration syndrome 289.52
Splenectasis (*see also* Splenomegaly) 789.2
Splenitis (interstitial) (malignant) (nonspecific) 289.59
malarial (*see also* Malaria) 084.6
tuberculous (*see also* Tuberculosis) 017.7
Splenocele 289.59
Splenomegalia - *see* Splenomegaly
Splenomegalic - *see* condition
Splenomegaly 789.2
Bengal 789.2
cirrhotic 289.51
congenital 759.0
congestive, chronic 289.51
cryptogenic 789.2
Egyptian 120.1
Gaucher's (cerebroside lipidosis) 272.7
idiopathic 789.2

ICD-9-CM
S
Vol. 2

Splenomegaly *(Continued)*
malarial (*see also* Malaria) 084.6
neutropenic 289.53 ⇐ Revised
Niemann-Pick (lipid histiocytosis) 272.7
siderotic 289.51
syphilitic 095.8
congenital 090.0
tropical (Bengal) (idiopathic) 789.2
Splenopathy 289.50
Splenopneumonia - *see* Pneumonia
Splenoptosis 289.59
Splinter - *see* Injury, superficial, by site
Split, splitting
heart sounds 427.89
lip, congenital (*see also* Cleft, lip) 749.10
nails 703.8
urinary stream 788.61
Spoiled child reaction (*see also* Disturbance, conduct) 312.1
Spondylarthritis (*see also* Spondylosis) 721.90
Spondylarthrosis (*see also* Spondylosis) 721.90
Spondylitis 720.9
ankylopoietica 720.0
ankylosing (chronic) 720.0
atrophic 720.9
ligamentous 720.9
chronic (traumatic) (*see also* Spondylosis) 721.90
deformans (chronic) (*see also* Spondylosis) 721.90
gonococcal 098.53
gouty 274.0
hypertrophic (*see also* Spondylosis) 721.90
infectious NEC 720.9
juvenile (adolescent) 720.0
Kummell's 721.7
Marie-Strümpell (ankylosing) 720.0
muscularis 720.9
ossificans ligamentosa 721.6
osteoarthritica (*see also* Spondylosis) 721.90
posttraumatic 721.7
proliferative 720.0
rheumatoid 720.0
rhizomelica 720.0
sacroiliac NEC 720.2
senescent (*see also* Spondylosis) 721.90
senile (*see also* Spondylosis) 721.90
static (*see also* Spondylosis) 721.90
traumatic (chronic) (*see also* Spondylosis) 721.90
tuberculous (*see also* Tuberculosis) 015.0 *[720.81]*
typhosa 002.0 *[720.81]*
Spondyloarthrosis (*see also* Spondylosis) 721.90
Spondylolisthesis (congenital) (lumbosacral) 756.12
with disproportion (fetopelvic) 653.3
affecting fetus or newborn 763.1
causing obstructed labor 660.1
affecting fetus or newborn 763.1
acquired 738.4
degenerative 738.4
traumatic 738.4
acute (lumbar) - *see* Fracture, vertebra, lumbar
site other than lumbosacral - *see* Fracture, vertebra, by site
Spondylolysis (congenital) 756.11
acquired 738.4
cervical 756.19
Spondylolysis *(Continued)*
lumbosacral region 756.11
with disproportion (fetopelvic) 653.3
affecting fetus or newborn 763.1
causing obstructed labor 660.1
affecting fetus or newborn 763.1
Spondylopathy
inflammatory 720.9
specified type NEC 720.89
traumatic 721.7
Spondylose rhizomelique 720.0
Spondylosis 721.90
with
disproportion 653.3
affecting fetus or newborn 763.1
causing obstructed labor 660.1
affecting fetus or newborn 763.1
myelopathy NEC 721.91
cervical, cervicodorsal 721.0
with myelopathy 721.1
inflammatory 720.9
lumbar, lumbosacral 721.3
with myelopathy 721.42
sacral 721.3
with myelopathy 721.42
thoracic 721.2
with myelopathy 721.41
traumatic 721.7
Sponge
divers' disease 989.5
inadvertently left in operation wound 998.4
kidney (medullary) 753.17
Spongioblastoma (M9422/3)
multiforme (M9440/3)
specified site - *see* Neoplasm, by site, malignant
unspecified site 191.9
polare (M9423/3)
specified site - *see* Neoplasm, by site, malignant
unspecified site 191.9
primitive polar (M9443/3)
specified site - *see* Neoplasm, by site, malignant
unspecified site 191.9
specified site - *see* Neoplasm, by site, malignant
unspecified site 191.9
Spongiocytoma (M9400/3)
specified site - *see* Neoplasm, by site, malignant
unspecified site 191.9
Spongioneuroblastoma (M9504/3) - *see* Neoplasm, by site, malignant
Spontaneous - *see also* condition
fracture - *see* Fracture, pathologic
Spoon nail 703.8
congenital 757.5
Sporadic - *see* condition
Sporotrichosis (bones) (cutaneous) (disseminated) (epidermal) (lymphatic) (lymphocutaneous) (mucous membranes) (pulmonary) (skeletal) (visceral) 117.1
Sporotrichum schenckii infection 117.1
Spots, spotting
atrophic (skin) 701.3
Bitôt's (in the young child) 264.1
café au lait 709.09
cayenne pepper 448.1
complicating pregnancy 649.5 ◀ New
cotton wool (retina) 362.83
de Morgan's (senile angiomas) 448.1
Spots, spotting *(Continued)*
Fúchs' black (myopic) 360.21
intermenstrual
irregular 626.6
regular 626.5
interpalpebral 372.53
Koplik's 055.9
liver 709.09
Mongolian (pigmented) 757.33
of pregnancy 641.9
purpuric 782.7
ruby 448.1
Spotted fever - *see* Fever, spotted
Sprain, strain (joint) (ligament) (muscle) (tendon) 848.9
abdominal wall (muscle) 848.8
Achilles tendon 845.09
acromioclavicular 840.0
ankle 845.00
and foot 845.00
anterior longitudinal, cervical 847.0
arm 840.9
upper 840.9
and shoulder 840.9
astragalus 845.00
atlanto-axial 847.0
atlanto-occipital 847.0
atlas 847.0
axis 847.0
back (*see also* Sprain, spine) 847.9
breast bone 848.40
broad ligaments - *see* Injury, internal, broad ligament
calcaneofibular 845.02
carpal 842.01
carpometacarpal 842.11
cartilage
costal, without mention of injury to sternum 848.3
involving sternum 848.42
ear 848.8
knee 844.9
with current tear (*see also* Tear, meniscus) 836.2
semilunar (knee) 844.8
with current tear (*see also* Tear, meniscus) 836.2
septal, nose 848.0
thyroid region 848.2
xiphoid 848.49
cervical, cervicodorsal, cervicothoracic 847.0
chondrocostal, without mention of injury to sternum 848.3
involving sternum 848.42
chondrosternal 848.42
chronic (joint) - *see* Derangement, joint
clavicle 840.9
coccyx 847.4
collar bone 840.9
collateral, knee (medial) (tibial) 844.1
lateral (fibular) 844.0
recurrent or old 717.89
lateral 717.81
medial 717.82
coracoacromial 840.8
coracoclavicular 840.1
coracohumeral 840.2
coracoid (process) 840.9
coronary, knee 844.8
costal cartilage, without mention of injury to sternum 848.3
involving sternum 848.42
cricoarytenoid articulation 848.2
cricothyroid articulation 848.2

Sprain, strain *(Continued)*
cruciate
knee 844.2
old 717.89
anterior 717.83
posterior 717.84
deltoid
ankle 845.01
shoulder 840.8
dorsal (spine) 847.1
ear cartilage 848.8
elbow 841.9
and forearm 841.9
specified site NEC 841.8
femur (proximal end) 843.9
distal end 844.9
fibula (proximal end) 844.9
distal end 845.00
fibulocalcaneal 845.02
finger(s) 842.10
foot 845.10
and ankle 845.00
forearm 841.9
and elbow 841.9
specified site NEC 841.8
glenoid (shoulder) (*see also* SLAP lesion) 840.8
hand 842.10
hip 843.9
and thigh 843.9
humerus (proximal end) 840.9
distal end 841.9
iliofemoral 843.0
infraspinatus 840.3
innominate
acetabulum 843.9
pubic junction 848.5
sacral junction 846.1
internal
collateral, ankle 845.01
semilunar cartilage 844.8
with current tear (*see also* Tear, meniscus) 836.2
old 717.5
interphalangeal
finger 842.13
toe 845.13
ischiocapsular 843.1
jaw (cartilage) (meniscus) 848.1
old 524.69
knee 844.9
and leg 844.9
old 717.5
collateral
lateral 717.81
medial 717.82
cruciate
anterior 717.83
posterior 717.84
late effect - *see* Late, effects (of), sprain
lateral collateral, knee 844.0
old 717.81
leg 844.9
and knee 844.9
ligamentum teres femoris 843.8
low back 846.9
lumbar (spine) 847.2
lumbosacral 846.0
chronic or old 724.6
mandible 848.1
old 524.69
maxilla 848.1
medial collateral, knee 844.1
old 717.82
meniscus

Sprain, strain *(Continued)*
meniscus *(Continued)*
jaw 848.1
old 524.69
knee 844.8
with current tear (*see also* Tear, meniscus) 836.2
old 717.5
mandible 848.1
old 524.69
specified site NEC 848.8
metacarpal 842.10
distal 842.12
proximal 842.11
metacarpophalangeal 842.12
metatarsal 845.10
metatarsophalangeal 845.12
midcarpal 842.19
midtarsal 845.19
multiple sites, except fingers alone or toes alone 848.8
neck 847.0
nose (septal cartilage) 848.0
occiput from atlas 847.0
old - *see* Derangement, joint
orbicular, hip 843.8
patella(r) 844.8
old 717.89
pelvis 848.5
phalanx
finger 842.10
toe 845.10
radiocarpal 842.02
radiohumeral 841.2
radioulnar 841.9
distal 842.09
radius, radial (proximal end) 841.9
and ulna 841.9
distal 842.09
collateral 841.0
distal end 842.00
recurrent - *see* Sprain, by site
rib (cage), without mention of injury to sternum 848.3
involving sternum 848.42
rotator cuff (capsule) 840.4
round ligament - *see also* Injury, internal, round ligament
femur 843.8
sacral (spine) 847.3
sacrococcygeal 847.3
sacroiliac (region) 846.9
chronic or old 724.6
ligament 846.1
specified site NEC 846.8
sacrospinatus 846.2
sacrospinous 846.2
sacrotuberous 846.3
scaphoid bone, ankle 845.00
scapula(r) 840.9
semilunar cartilage (knee) 844.8
with current tear (*see also* Tear, meniscus) 836.2
old 717.5
septal cartilage (nose) 848.0
shoulder 840.9
and arm, upper 840.9
blade 840.9
specified site NEC 848.8
spine 847.9
cervical 847.0
coccyx 847.4
dorsal 847.1
lumbar 847.2
lumbosacral 846.0
chronic or old 724.6

Sprain, strain *(Continued)*
spine *(Continued)*
sacral 847.3
sacroiliac (*see also* Sprain, sacroiliac) 846.9
chronic or old 724.6
thoracic 847.1
sternoclavicular 848.41
sternum 848.40
subglenoid (*see also* SLAP lesion) 840.8
subscapularis 840.5
supraspinatus 840.6
symphysis
jaw 848.1
old 524.69
mandibular 848.1
old 524.69
pubis 848.5
talofibular 845.09
tarsal 845.10
tarsometatarsal 845.11
temporomandibular 848.1
old 524.69
teres
ligamentum femoris 843.8
major or minor 840.8
thigh (proximal end) 843.9
and hip 843.9
distal end 844.9
thoracic (spine) 847.1
thorax 848.8
thumb 842.10
thyroid cartilage or region 848.2
tibia (proximal end) 844.9
distal end 845.00
tibiofibular
distal 845.03
superior 844.3
toe(s) 845.10
trachea 848.8
trapezoid 840.8
ulna, ulnar (proximal end) 841.9
collateral 841.1
distal end 842.00
ulnohumeral 841.3
vertebrae (*see also* Sprain, spine) 847.9
cervical, cervicodorsal, cervicothoracic 847.0
wrist (cuneiform) (scaphoid) (semilunar) 842.00
xiphoid cartilage 848.49
Sprengel's deformity (congenital) 755.52
Spring fever 309.23
Sprue 579.1
celiac 579.0
idiopathic 579.0
meaning thrush 112.0
nontropical 579.0
tropical 579.1
Spur - *see also* Exostosis
bone 726.91
calcaneal 726.73
calcaneal 726.73
iliac crest 726.5
nose (septum) 478.19 ◄
bone 726.91
septal 478.19 ◄
Spuria placenta - *see* Placenta, abnormal
Spurway's syndrome (brittle bones and blue sclera) 756.51
Sputum, abnormal (amount) (color) (excessive) (odor) (purulent) 786.4
bloody 786.3
Squamous - *see also* condition
cell metaplasia

Squamous *(Continued)*
cell metaplasia *(Continued)*
bladder 596.8
cervix - *see* condition
epithelium in
cervical canal (congenital) 752.49
uterine mucosa (congenital) 752.3
metaplasia
bladder 596.8
cervix - *see* condition
Squashed nose 738.0
congenital 754.0
Squeeze, divers' 993.3
Squint (*see also* Strabismus) 378.9
accommodative (*see also* Esotropia) 378.00
concomitant (*see also* Heterotropia) 378.30
Stab - *see also* Wound, open, by site
internal organs - *see* Injury, internal, by site, with open wound
Staggering gait 781.2
hysterical 300.11
Staghorn calculus 592.0
Stähl's
ear 744.29
pigment line (cornea) 371.11
Stähli's pigment lines (cornea) 371.11
Stain, staining
meconium 779.84
port wine 757.32
tooth, teeth (hard tissues) 521.7
due to
accretions 523.6
deposits (betel) (black) (green) (materia alba) (orange) (tobacco) 523.6
metals (copper) (silver) 521.7
nicotine 523.6
pulpal bleeding 521.7
tobacco 523.6
Stammering 307.0
Standstill
atrial 426.6
auricular 426.6
cardiac (*see also* Arrest, cardiac) 427.5
sinoatrial 426.6
sinus 426.6
ventricular (*see also* Arrest, cardiac) 427.5
Stannosis 503
Stanton's disease (melioidosis) 025
Staphylitis (acute) (catarrhal) (chronic) (gangrenous) (membranous) (suppurative) (ulcerative) 528.3
Staphylococcemia 038.10
aureus 038.11
specified organism NEC 038.19
Staphylococcus, staphylococcal - *see* condition
Staphyloderma (skin) 686.00
Staphyloma 379.11
anterior, localized 379.14
ciliary 379.11
cornea 371.73
equatorial 379.13
posterior 379.12
posticum 379.12
ring 379.15
sclera NEC 379.11
Starch eating 307.52
Stargardt's disease 362.75
Starvation (inanition) (due to lack of food) 994.2
edema 262
voluntary NEC 307.1

Stasis
bile (duct) (*see also* Disease, biliary) 576.8
bronchus (*see also* Bronchitis) 490
cardiac (*see also* Failure, heart) 428.0
cecum 564.89
colon 564.89
dermatitis (*see also* Varix, with stasis dermatitis) 454.1
duodenal 536.8
eczema (*see also* Varix, with stasis dermatitis) 454.1
edema (*see also* Hypertension, venous) 459.30
foot 991.4
gastric 536.3
ileocecal coil 564.89
ileum 564.89
intestinal 564.89
jejunum 564.89
kidney 586
liver 571.9
cirrhotic - *see* Cirrhosis, liver
lymphatic 457.8
pneumonia 514
portal 571.9
pulmonary 514
rectal 564.89
renal 586
tubular 584.5
stomach 536.3
ulcer
with varicose veins 454.0
without varicose veins 459.81
urine NEC (*see also* Retention, urine) 788.20
venous 459.81
State
affective and paranoid, mixed, organic psychotic 294.8
agitated 307.9
acute reaction to stress 308.2
anxiety (neurotic) (*see also* Anxiety) 300.00
specified type NEC 300.09
apprehension (*see also* Anxiety) 300.00
specified type NEC 300.09
climacteric, female 627.2
following induced menopause 627.4
clouded
epileptic (*see also* Epilepsy) 345.9
paroxysmal (idiopathic) (*see also* Epilepsy) 345.9
compulsive (mixed) (with obsession) 300.3
confusional 298.9
acute 293.0
with
arteriosclerotic dementia 290.41
presenile brain disease 290.11
senility 290.3
alcoholic 291.0
drug-induced 292.81
epileptic 293.0
postoperative 293.9
reactive (emotional stress) (psychological trauma) 298.2
subacute 293.1
constitutional psychopathic 301.9
convulsive (*see also* Convulsions) 780.39
depressive NEC 311
induced by drug 292.84
neurotic 300.4
dissociative 300.15
hallucinatory 780.1

State *(Continued)*
hallucinatory *(Continued)*
induced by drug 292.12
hypercoagulable (primary) 289.81
secondary 289.82
hyperdynamic beta-adrenergic circulatory 429.82
locked-in 344.81
menopausal 627.2
artificial 627.4
following induced menopause 627.4
neurotic NEC 300.9
with depersonalization episode 300.6
obsessional 300.3
oneiroid (*see also* Schizophrenia) 295.4
panic 300.01
paranoid 297.9
alcohol-induced 291.5
arteriosclerotic 290.42
climacteric 297.2
drug-induced 292.11
in
presenile brain disease 290.12
senile brain disease 290.20
involutional 297.2
menopausal 297.2
senile 290.20
simple 297.0
postleukotomy 310.0
pregnant (*see also* Pregnancy) V22.2
psychogenic, twilight 298.2
psychotic, organic (*see also* Psychosis, organic) 294.9
mixed paranoid and affective 294.8
senile or presenile NEC 290.9
transient NEC 293.9
with
anxiety 293.84
delusions 293.81
depression 293.83
hallucinations 293.82
residual schizophrenic (*see also* Schizophrenia) 295.6
tension (*see also* Anxiety) 300.9
transient organic psychotic 293.9
anxiety type 293.84
depressive type 293.83
hallucinatory type 293.83
paranoid type 293.81
specified type NEC 293.89
twilight
epileptic 293.0
psychogenic 298.2
vegetative (persistent) 780.03
Status (post)
absence
epileptic (*see also* Epilepsy) 345.2
of organ, acquired (postsurgical) - *see* Absence, by site, acquired
anastomosis of intestine (for bypass) V45.3
anginosus 413.9
angioplasty, percutaneous transluminal coronary V45.82
ankle prosthesis V43.66
aortocoronary bypass or shunt V45.81
arthrodesis V45.4
artificially induced condition NEC V45.89
artificial opening (of) V44.9
gastrointestinal tract NEC V44.4
specified site NEC V44.8
urinary tract NEC V44.6
vagina V44.7
aspirator V46.0

Status (post) *(Continued)*
- asthmaticus (*see also* Asthma) 493.9
- awaiting organ transplant V49.83
- bariatric surgery V45.86 ◀
  - complicating pregnancy, childbirth, or the puerperium 649.2 ◀
- bed confinement V49.84
- breast implant removal V45.83
- cardiac
  - device (in situ) V45.00
    - carotid sinus V45.09
      - fitting or adjustment V53.39
    - defibrillator, automatic implantable V45.02
    - pacemaker V45.01
      - fitting or adjustment V53.31
- carotid sinus stimulator V45.09
- cataract extraction V45.61
- chemotherapy V66.2
  - current V58.69
- circumcision, female 629.20
- clitorectomy (female genital mutilation type I) 629.21
  - with excision of labia minora (female genital mutilation type II) 629.22
- colostomy V44.3
- contraceptive device V45.59
  - intrauterine V45.51
  - subdermal V45.52
- convulsivus idiopathicus (*see also* Epilepsy) 345.3
- coronary artery bypass or shunt V45.81
- cutting ◀
  - female genital 629.20 ◀
    - specified NEC 629.29 ◀
    - type I 629.21 ◀
    - type II 629.22 ◀
    - type III 629.23 ◀
    - type IV 629.29 ◀
- cystostomy V44.50
  - appendico-vesicostomy V44.52
  - cutaneous-vesicostomy V44.51
  - specified type NEC V44.59
- defibrillator, automatic implantable cardiac V45.02
- dental crowns V45.84
- dental fillings V45.84
- dental restoration V45.84
- dental sealant V49.82
- dialysis (hemo) (peritoneal) V45.1
- donor V59.9
- drug therapy or regimen V67.59
  - high-risk medication NEC V67.51
- elbow prosthesis V43.62
- enterostomy V44.4
- epileptic, epilepticus (absence) (grand mal) (*see also* Epilepsy) 345.3
  - focal motor 345.7
  - partial 345.7
  - petit mal 345.2
  - psychomotor 345.7
  - temporal lobe 345.7
- estrogen receptor ◀
  - negative [ER-] V86.1 ◀
  - positive [ER+] V86.0 ◀
- eye (adnexa) surgery V45.69
- female genital ⬅
  - cutting 629.20 ◀
    - specified NEC 629.29 ◀
    - type I 629.21 ◀
    - type II 629.22 ◀
    - type III 629.23 ◀
    - type IV 629.29 ◀
  - mutilation 629.20 ◀
    - type IV 629.29 ◀

Status (post) *(Continued)*
- female genital *(Continued)*
    - type I 629.21
    - type II 629.22
    - type III 629.23
- filtering bleb (eye) (postglaucoma) V45.69
  - with rupture or complication 997.99
  - postcataract extraction (complication) 997.99
- finger joint prosthesis V43.69
- gastric ◀
  - banding V45.86 ◀
    - complicating pregnancy, childbirth, or the puerperium 649.2 ◀
  - bypass for obesity V45.86 ◀
    - complicating pregnancy, childbirth, or the puerperium 649.2 ◀
- gastrostomy V44.1
- grand mal 345.3
- heart valve prosthesis V43.3
- hemodialysis V45.1
- hip prosthesis (joint) (partial) (total) V43.64
- ileostomy V44.2
- infibulation (female genital mutilation type III) 629.23
- insulin pump V45.85
- intestinal bypass V45.3
- intrauterine contraceptive device V45.51
- jejunostomy V44.4
- knee joint prosthesis V43.65
- lacunaris 437.8
- lacunosis 437.8
- low birth weight V21.30
  - less than 500 grams V21.31
  - 500–999 grams V21.32
  - 1000–1499 grams V21.33
  - 1500–1999 grams V21.34
  - 2000–2500 grams V21.35
- lymphaticus 254.8
- malignant neoplasm, ablated or excised - *see* History, malignant neoplasm
- marmoratus 333.79 ⬅
- mutilation, female 629.20
  - type I 629.21
  - type II 629.22
  - type III 629.23
  - type IV 629.29 ◀
- nephrostomy V44.6
- neuropacemaker NEC V45.89
  - brain V45.89
  - carotid sinus V45.09
  - neurologic NEC V45.89
- obesity surgery V45.86 ◀
  - complicating pregnancy, childbirth, or the puerperium 649.2 ◀
- organ replacement
  - by artificial or mechanical device or prosthesis of
    - artery V43.4
    - artificial skin V43.83
    - bladder V43.5
    - blood vessel V43.4
    - breast V43.82
    - eye globe V43.0
    - heart
      - assist device V43.21
      - fully implantable artificial heart V43.22
      - valve V43.3
    - intestine V43.89
    - joint V43.60

Status (post) *(Continued)*
- organ replacement *(Continued)*
  - by artificial or mechanical device or eye globe V43.0 *(Continued)*
    - joint V43.60 *(Continued)*
      - ankle V43.66
      - elbow V43.62
      - finger V43.69
      - hip (partial) (total) V43.64
      - knee V43.65
      - shoulder V43.61
      - specified NEC V43.69
      - wrist V43.63
    - kidney V43.89
    - larynx V43.81
    - lens V43.1
    - limb(s) V43.7
    - liver V43.89
    - lung V43.89
    - organ NEC V43.89
    - pancreas V43.89
    - skin (artificial) V43.83
    - tissue NEC V43.89
    - vein V43.4
  - by organ transplant (heterologous) (homologous) - *see* Status, transplant
- pacemaker
  - brain V45.89
  - cardiac V45.01
  - carotid sinus V45.09
  - neurologic NEC V45.89
  - specified site NEC V45.89
- percutaneous transluminal coronary angioplasty V45.82
- peritoneal dialysis V45.1
- petit mal 345.2
- postcommotio cerebri 310.2
- postmenopausal (age related) (natural) V49.81
- postoperative NEC V45.89
- postpartum NEC V24.2
  - care immediately following delivery V24.0
  - routine follow-up V24.2
- postsurgical NEC V45.89
- renal dialysis V45.1
- respirator [ventilator] V46.11
  - encounter
    - during
      - mechanical failure V46.14
      - power failure V46.12
    - for weaning V46.13
- reversed jejunal transposition (for bypass) V45.3
- shoulder prosthesis V43.61
- shunt
  - aortocoronary bypass V45.81
  - arteriovenous (for dialysis) V45.1
  - cerebrospinal fluid V45.2
  - vascular NEC V45.89
    - aortocoronary (bypass) V45.81
  - ventricular (communicating) (for drainage) V45.2
- sterilization
  - tubal ligation V26.51
  - vasectomy V26.52
- subdermal contraceptive device V45.52
- thymicolymphaticus 254.8
- thymicus 254.8
- thymolymphaticus 254.8
- tooth extraction 525.10
- tracheostomy V44.0
- transplant
  - blood vessel V42.89

Status (post) *(Continued)*
transplant *(Continued)*
bone V42.4
marrow V42.81
cornea V42.5
heart V42.1
valve V42.2
intestine V42.84
kidney V42.0
liver V42.7
lung V42.6
organ V42.9
specified site NEC V42.89
pancreas V42.83
peripheral stem cells V42.82
skin V42.3
stem cells, peripheral V42.82
tissue V42.9
specified type NEC V42.89
vessel, blood V42.89
tubal ligation V26.51
ureterostomy V44.6
urethrostomy V44.6
vagina, artificial V44.7
vascular shunt NEC V45.89
aortocoronary (bypass) V45.81
vasectomy V26.52
ventilator [respirator] V46.11
encounter
during
mechanical failure V46.14
power failure V46.12
for weaning V46.13
wrist prosthesis V43.63
Stave fracture - *see* Fracture, metacarpus, metacarpal bone(s)
Steal
subclavian artery 435.2
vertebral artery 435.1
Stealing, solitary, child problem (*see also* Disturbance, conduct) 312.1
Steam burn - *see* Burn, by site
Steatocystoma multiplex 706.2
Steatoma (infected) 706.2
eyelid (cystic) 374.84
infected 373.13
Steatorrhea (chronic) 579.8
with lacteal obstruction 579.2
idiopathic 579.0
adult 579.0
infantile 579.0
pancreatic 579.4
primary 579.0
secondary 579.8
specified cause NEC 579.8
tropical 579.1
Steatosis 272.8
heart (*see also* Degeneration, myocardial) 429.1
kidney 593.89
liver 571.8
Steele-Richardson (-Olszewski) syndrome 333.0
Stein's syndrome (polycystic ovary) 256.4
Stein-Leventhal syndrome (polycystic ovary) 256.4
Steinbrocker's syndrome (*see also* Neuropathy, peripheral, autonomic) 337.9
Steinert's disease 359.2
STEMI (ST elevation myocardial infarction) (*see also* - Infarct, myocardium, ST elevation) 410.9 ◀
Stenocardia (*see also* Angina) 413.9
Stenocephaly 756.0
Stenosis (cicatricial) - *see also* Stricture
ampulla of Vater 576.2
with calculus, cholelithiasis, or stones - *see* Choledocholithiasis
anus, anal (canal) (sphincter) 569.2
congenital 751.2
aorta (ascending) 747.22
arch 747.10
arteriosclerotic 440.0
calcified 440.0
aortic (valve) 424.1
with
mitral (valve)
insufficiency or incompetence 396.2
stenosis or obstruction 396.0
atypical 396.0
congenital 746.3
rheumatic 395.0
with
insufficiency, incompetency or regurgitation 395.2
with mitral (valve) disease 396.8
mitral (valve)
disease (stenosis) 396.0
insufficiency or incompetence 396.2
stenosis or obstruction 396.0
specified cause, except rheumatic 424.1
syphilitic 093.22
aqueduct of Sylvius (congenital) 742.3
with spina bifida (*see also* Spina bifida) 741.0
acquired 331.4
artery NEC 447.1
basilar - *see* Narrowing, artery, basilar
carotid (common) (internal) - *see* Narrowing, artery, carotid
celiac 447.4
cerebral 437.0
due to
embolism (*see also* Embolism, brain) 434.1
thrombus (*see also* Thrombosis, brain) 434.0
precerebral - *see* Narrowing, artery, precerebral
pulmonary (congenital) 747.3
acquired 417.8
renal 440.1
vertebral - *see* Narrowing, artery, vertebral
bile duct or biliary passage (*see also* Obstruction, biliary) 576.2
congenital 751.61
bladder neck (acquired) 596.0
congenital 753.6
brain 348.8
bronchus 519.19 ⬅
syphilitic 095.8
cardia (stomach) 537.89
congenital 750.7
cardiovascular (*see also* Disease, cardiovascular) 429.2
carotid artery - *see* Narrowing, artery, carotid
cervix, cervical (canal) 622.4
congenital 752.49
in pregnancy or childbirth 654.6
affecting fetus or newborn 763.89
causing obstructed labor 660.2
affecting fetus or newborn 763.1
Stenosis *(Continued)*
colon (*see also* Obstruction, intestine) 560.9
congenital 751.2
colostomy 569.62
common bile duct (*see also* Obstruction, biliary) 576.2
congenital 751.61
coronary (artery) - *see* Arteriosclerosis, coronary
cystic duct (*see also* Obstruction, gallbladder) 575.2
congenital 751.61
due to (presence of) any device, implant, or graft classifiable to 996.0–996.5 - *see* Complications, due to (presence of) any device, implant, or graft classified to 996.0–996.5 NEC
duodenum 537.3
congenital 751.1
ejaculatory duct NEC 608.89
endocervical os - *see* Stenosis, cervix
enterostomy 569.62
esophagostomy 530.87
esophagus 530.3
congenital 750.3
syphilitic 095.8
congenital 090.5
external ear canal 380.50
secondary to
inflammation 380.53
surgery 380.52
trauma 380.51
gallbladder (*see also* Obstruction, gallbladder) 575.2
glottis 478.74
heart valve (acquired) - *see also* Endocarditis
congenital NEC 746.89
aortic 746.3
mitral 746.5
pulmonary 746.02
tricuspid 746.1
hepatic duct (*see also* Obstruction, biliary) 576.2
hymen 623.3
hypertrophic subaortic (idiopathic) 425.1
infundibulum cardiac 746.83
intestine (*see also* Obstruction, intestine) 560.9
congenital (small) 751.1
large 751.2
lacrimal
canaliculi 375.53
duct 375.56
congenital 743.65
punctum 375.52
congenital 743.65
sac 375.54
congenital 743.65
lacrimonasal duct 375.56
congenital 743.65
neonatal 375.55
larynx 478.74
congenital 748.3
syphilitic 095.8
congenital 090.5
mitral (valve) (chronic) (inactive) 394.0
with
aortic (valve)
disease (insufficiency) 396.1
insufficiency or incompetence 396.1
stenosis or obstruction 396.0

Steroid *(Continued)*
mitral *(Continued)*
with *(Continued)*
incompetency, insufficiency or regurgitation 394.2
with aortic valve disease 396.8
active or acute 391.1
with chorea (acute) (rheumatic) (Sydenham's) 392.0
congenital 746.5
specified cause, except rheumatic 424.0
syphilitic 093.21
myocardium, myocardial (*see also* Degeneration, myocardial) 429.1
hypertrophic subaortic (idiopathic) 425.1
nares (anterior) (posterior) 478.19
congenital 748.0
nasal duct 375.56
congenital 743.65
nasolacrimal duct 375.56
congenital 743.65
neonatal 375.55
organ or site, congenital NEC - *see* Atresia
papilla of Vater 576.2
with calculus, cholelithiasis, or stones - *see* Choledocholithiasis
pulmonary (artery) (congenital) 747.3
with ventricular septal defect, dextraposition of aorta and hypertrophy of right ventricle 745.2
acquired 417.8
infundibular 746.83
in tetralogy of Fallot 745.2
subvalvular 746.83
valve (*see also* Endocarditis, pulmonary) 424.3
congenital 746.02
vein 747.49
acquired 417.8
vessel NEC 417.8
pulmonic (congenital) 746.02
infundibular 746.83
subvalvular 746.83
pylorus (hypertrophic) 537.0
adult 537.0
congenital 750.5
infantile 750.5
rectum (sphincter) (*see also* Stricture, rectum) 569.2
renal artery 440.1
salivary duct (any) 527.8
sphincter of Oddi (*see also* Obstruction, biliary) 576.2
spinal 724.00
cervical 723.0
lumbar, lumbosacral 724.02
nerve (root) NEC 724.9
specified region NEC 724.09
thoracic, thoracolumbar 724.01
stomach, hourglass 537.6
subaortic 746.81
hypertrophic (idiopathic) 425.1
supra (valvular)-aortic 747.22
trachea 519.19
congenital 748.3
syphilitic 095.8
tuberculous (*see also* Tuberculosis) 012.8
tracheostomy 519.02
tricuspid (valve) (*see also* Endocarditis, tricuspid) 397.0
congenital 746.1
nonrheumatic 424.2

Stenosis *(Continued)*
tubal 628.2
ureter (*see also* Stricture, ureter) 593.3
congenital 753.29
urethra (*see also* Stricture, urethra) 598.9
vagina 623.2
congenital 752.49
in pregnancy or childbirth 654.7
affecting fetus or newborn 763.89
causing obstructed labor 660.2
affecting fetus or newborn 763.1
valve (cardiac) (heart) (*see also* Endocarditis) 424.90
congenital NEC 746.89
aortic 746.3
mitral 746.5
pulmonary 746.02
tricuspid 746.1
urethra 753.6
valvular (*see also* Endocarditis) 424.90
congenital NEC 746.89
urethra 753.6
vascular graft or shunt 996.1
atherosclerosis - *see* Arteriosclerosis, extremities
embolism 996.74
occlusion NEC 996.74
thrombus 996.74
vena cava (inferior) (superior) 459.2
congenital 747.49
ventricular shunt 996.2
vulva 624.8
Stercolith (*see also* Fecalith) 560.39
appendix 543.9
Stercoraceous, stercoral ulcer 569.82
anus or rectum 569.41
Stereopsis, defective
with fusion 368.33
without fusion 368.32
Stereotypies NEC 307.3
Sterility
female - *see* Infertility, female
male (*see also* Infertility, male) 606.9
Sterilization, admission for V25.2
status
tubal ligation V26.51
vasectomy V26.52
Sternalgia (*see also* Angina) 413.9
Sternopagus 759.4
Sternum bifidum 756.3
Sternutation 784.99
Steroid
effects (adverse) (iatrogenic)
cushingoid
correct substance properly administered 255.0
overdose or wrong substance given or taken 962.0
diabetes
correct substance properly administered 251.8
overdose or wrong substance given or taken 962.0
due to
correct substance properly administered 255.8
overdose or wrong substance given or taken 962.0
fever
correct substance properly administered 780.6
overdose or wrong substance given or taken 962.0

Steroid *(Continued)*
effects *(Continued)*
withdrawal
correct substance properly administered 255.4
overdose or wrong substance given or taken 962.0
responder 365.03
Stevens-Johnson disease or syndrome (erythema multiforme exudativum) 695.1
Stewart-Morel syndrome (hyperostosis frontalis interna) 733.3
Sticker's disease (erythema infectiosum) 057.0
Stickler syndrome 759.89
Sticky eye 372.03
Stieda's disease (calcification, knee joint) 726.62
Stiff
back 724.8
neck (*see also* Torticollis) 723.5
Stiff-baby 759.89
Stiff-man syndrome 333.91
Stiffness, joint NEC 719.50
ankle 719.57
back 724.8
elbow 719.52
finger 719.54
hip 719.55
knee 719.56
multiple sites 719.59
sacroiliac 724.6
shoulder 719.51
specified site NEC 719.58
spine 724.9
surgical fusion V45.4
wrist 719.53
Stigmata, congenital syphilis 090.5
Still's disease or syndrome 714.30
Still-Felty syndrome (rheumatoid arthritis with splenomegaly and leukopenia) 714.1
Stillbirth, stillborn NEC 779.9
Stiller's disease (asthenia) 780.79
Stilling-Türk-Duane syndrome (ocular retraction syndrome) 378.71
Stimulation, ovary 256.1
Sting (animal) (bee) (fish) (insect) (jellyfish) (Portuguese man-o-war) (wasp) (venomous) 989.5
anaphylactic shock or reaction 989.5
plant 692.6
Stippled epiphyses 756.59
Stitch
abscess 998.59
burst (in external operation wound) 998.32
internal 998.31
in back 724.5
Stojano's (subcostal) syndrome 098.86
Stokes' disease (exophthalmic goiter) 242.0
Stokes-Adams syndrome (syncope with heart block) 426.9
Stokvis' (-Talma) disease (enterogenous cyanosis) 289.7
Stomach - *see* condition
Stoma malfunction
colostomy 569.62
cystostomy 997.5
enterostomy 569.62
esophagostomy 530.87
gastrostomy 536.42
ileostomy 569.62

Stoma malfunction *(Continued)*
- nephrostomy 997.5
- tracheostomy 519.02
- ureterostomy 997.5

Stomatitis 528.00 ⬅
- angular 528.5
  - due to dietary or vitamin deficiency 266.0
- aphthous 528.2
- candidal 112.0
- catarrhal 528.00 ⬅
- denture 528.9
- diphtheritic (membranous) 032.0
- due to
  - dietary deficiency 266.0
  - thrush 112.0
  - vitamin deficiency 266.0
- epidemic 078.4
- epizootic 078.4
- follicular 528.00 ⬅
- gangrenous 528.1
- herpetic 054.2
- herpetiformis 528.2
- malignant 528.00 ⬅
- membranous acute 528.00 ⬅
- monilial 112.0
- mycotic 112.0
- necrotic 528.1
  - ulcerative 101
- necrotizing ulcerative 101
- parasitic 112.0
- septic 528.00 ⬅
- specified NEC 528.09 ◀
- spirochetal 101
- suppurative (acute) 528.00 ⬅
- ulcerative 528.00 ⬅
  - necrotizing 101
- ulceromembranous 101
- vesicular 528.00 ⬅
  - with exanthem 074.3
- Vincent's 101

Stomatocytosis 282.8

Stomatomycosis 112.0

Stomatorrhagia 528.9

Stone(s) - *see also* Calculus
- bladder 594.1
  - diverticulum 594.0
- cystine 270.0
- heart syndrome (*see also* Failure, ventricular, left) 428.1
- kidney 592.0
- prostate 602.0
- pulp (dental) 522.2
- renal 592.0
- salivary duct or gland (any) 527.5
- ureter 592.1
- urethra (impacted) 594.2
- urinary (duct) (impacted) (passage) 592.9
  - bladder 594.1
    - diverticulum 594.0
  - lower tract NEC 594.9
  - specified site 594.8
- xanthine 277.2

Stonecutters' lung 502
- tuberculous (*see also* Tuberculosis) 011.4

Stonemasons'
- asthma, disease, or lung 502
  - tuberculous (*see also* Tuberculosis) 011.4
- phthisis (*see also* Tuberculosis) 011.4

Stoppage
- bowel (*see also* Obstruction, intestine) 560.9
- heart (*see also* Arrest, cardiac) 427.5
- intestine (*see also* Obstruction, intestine) 560.9
- urine NEC (*see also* Retention, urine) 788.20

Storm, thyroid (apathetic) (*see also* Thyrotoxicosis) 242.9

Strabismus (alternating) (congenital) (nonparalytic) 378.9
- concomitant (*see also* Heterotropia) 378.30
  - convergent (*see also* Esotropia) 378.00
  - divergent (*see also* Exotropia) 378.10
- convergent (*see also* Esotropia) 378.00
- divergent (*see also* Exotropia) 378.10
- due to adhesions, scars - *see* Strabismus, mechanical
- in neuromuscular disorder NEC 378.73
  - intermittent 378.20
    - vertical 378.31
- latent 378.40
  - convergent (esophoria) 378.41
  - divergent (exophoria) 378.42
  - vertical 378.43
- mechanical 378.60
  - due to
    - Brown's tendon sheath syndrome 378.61
    - specified musculofascial disorder NEC 378.62
- paralytic 378.50
  - third or oculomotor nerve (partial) 378.51
    - total 378.52
  - fourth or trochlear nerve 378.53
  - sixth or abducens nerve 378.54
- specified type NEC 378.73
- vertical (hypertropia) 378.31

Strain - *see also* Sprain, by site
- eye NEC 368.13
- heart - *see* Disease, heart
- meaning gonorrhea - *see* Gonorrhea
- on urination 788.65 ◀
- physical NEC V62.89
- postural 729.9
- psychological NEC V62.89

Strands
- conjunctiva 372.62
- vitreous humor 379.25

Strangulation, strangulated 994.7
- appendix 543.9
- asphyxiation or suffocation by 994.7
- bladder neck 596.0
- bowel - *see* Strangulation, intestine
- colon - *see* Strangulation, intestine
- cord (umbilical) - *see* Compression, umbilical cord
- due to birth injury 767.8
- food or foreign body (*see also* Asphyxia, food) 933.1
- hemorrhoids 455.8
  - external 455.5
  - internal 455.2
- hernia - *see also* Hernia, by site, with obstruction
  - gangrenous - *see* Hernia, by site, with gangrene
- intestine (large) (small) 560.2
  - with hernia - *see also* Hernia, by site, with obstruction
    - gangrenous - *see* Hernia, by site, with gangrene
  - congenital (small) 751.1
    - large 751.2
- mesentery 560.2
- mucus (*see also* Asphyxia, mucus) 933.1
  - newborn 770.18
- omentum 560.2
- organ or site, congenital NEC - *see* Atresia
- ovary 620.8
  - due to hernia 620.4
- penis 607.89
  - foreign body 939.3
- rupture (*see also* Hernia, by site, with obstruction) 552.9
  - gangrenous (*see also* Hernia, by site, with gangrene) 551.9
- stomach, due to hernia (*see also* Hernia, by site, with obstruction) 552.9
  - with gangrene (*see also* Hernia, by site, with gangrene) 551.9
- umbilical cord - *see* Compression, umbilical cord
- vesicourethral orifice 596.0

Strangury 788.1

Strawberry
- gallbladder (*see also* Disease, gallbladder) 575.6
- mark 757.32
- tongue (red) (white) 529.3

Straw itch 133.8

Streak, ovarian 752.0

Strephosymbolia 315.01
- secondary to organic lesion 784.69

Streptobacillary fever 026.1

Streptobacillus moniliformis 026.1

Streptococcemia 038.0

Streptococcicosis - *see* Infection, streptococcal

Streptococcus, streptococcal - *see* condition

Streptoderma 686.00

Streptomycosis - *see* Actinomycosis

Streptothricosis - *see* Actinomycosis

Streptothrix - *see* Actinomycosis

Streptotrichosis - *see* Actinomycosis

Stress
- fracture - *see* Fracture, stress
- polycythemia 289.0
- reaction (gross) (*see also* Reaction, stress, acute) 308.9

Stretching, nerve - *see* Injury, nerve, by site

Striae (albicantes) (atrophicae) (cutis distensae) (distensae) 701.3

Striations of nails 703.8

Stricture (*see also* Stenosis) 799.89
- ampulla of Vater 576.2
  - with calculus, cholelithiasis, or stones - *see* Choledocholithiasis
- anus (sphincter) 569.2
  - congenital 751.2
  - infantile 751.2
- aorta (ascending) 747.22
  - arch 747.10
  - arteriosclerotic 440.0
  - calcified 440.0
- aortic (valve) (*see also* Stenosis, aortic) 424.1
  - congenital 746.3
- aqueduct of Sylvius (congenital) 742.3
  - with spina bifida (*see also* Spina bifida) 741.0
  - acquired 331.4
- artery 447.1
  - basilar - *see* Narrowing, artery, basilar
  - carotid (common) (internal) - *see* Narrowing, artery, carotid
  - celiac 447.4

- **Stricture** *(Continued)*
  - artery *(Continued)*
    - cerebral 437.0
      - congenital 747.81
      - due to
        - embolism (*see also* Embolism, brain) 434.1
        - thrombus (*see also* Thrombosis, brain) 434.0
    - congenital (peripheral) 747.60
      - cerebral 747.81
      - coronary 746.85
      - gastrointestinal 747.61
      - lower limb 747.64
      - renal 747.62
      - retinal 743.58
      - specified NEC 747.69
      - spinal 747.82
      - umbilical 747.5
      - upper limb 747.63
    - coronary - *see* Arteriosclerosis, coronary
      - congenital 746.85
    - precerebral - *see* Narrowing, artery, precerebral NEC
    - pulmonary (congenital) 747.3
      - acquired 417.8
    - renal 440.1
    - vertebral - *see* Narrowing, artery, vertebral
  - auditory canal (congenital) (external) 744.02
    - acquired (*see also* Stricture, ear canal, acquired) 380.50
  - bile duct or passage (any) (postoperative) (*see also* Obstruction, biliary) 576.2
    - congenital 751.61
  - bladder 596.8
    - congenital 753.6
    - neck 596.0
      - congenital 753.6
  - bowel (*see also* Obstruction, intestine) 560.9
  - brain 348.8
  - bronchus 519.19
    - syphilitic 095.8
  - cardia (stomach) 537.89
    - congenital 750.7
  - cardiac - *see also* Disease, heart orifice (stomach) 537.89
  - cardiovascular (*see also* Disease, cardiovascular) 429.2
  - carotid artery - *see* Narrowing, artery, carotid
  - cecum (*see also* Obstruction, intestine) 560.9
  - cervix, cervical (canal) 622.4
    - congenital 752.49
    - in pregnancy or childbirth 654.6
      - affecting fetus or newborn 763.89
      - causing obstructed labor 660.2
        - affecting fetus or newborn 763.1
  - colon (*see also* Obstruction, intestine) 560.9
    - congenital 751.2
  - colostomy 569.62
  - common bile duct (*see also* Obstruction, biliary) 576.2
    - congenital 751.61
  - coronary (artery) - *see* Arteriosclerosis, coronary
    - congenital 746.85
  - cystic duct (*see also* Obstruction, gallbladder) 575.2
    - congenital 751.61

- **Stricture** *(Continued)*
  - cystostomy 997.5
  - digestive organs NEC, congenital 751.8
  - duodenum 537.3
    - congenital 751.1
  - ear canal (external) (congenital) 744.02
    - acquired 380.50
      - secondary to
        - inflammation 380.53
        - surgery 380.52
        - trauma 380.51
  - ejaculatory duct 608.85
  - enterostomy 569.62
  - esophagostomy 530.87
  - esophagus (corrosive) (peptic) 530.3
    - congenital 750.3
    - syphilitic 095.8
      - congenital 090.5
  - Eustachian tube (*see also* Obstruction, Eustachian tube) 381.60
    - congenital 744.24
  - fallopian tube 628.2
    - gonococcal (chronic) 098.37
      - acute 098.17
    - tuberculous (*see also* Tuberculosis) 016.6
  - gallbladder (*see also* Obstruction, gallbladder) 575.2
    - congenital 751.69
  - glottis 478.74
  - heart - *see also* Disease, heart
    - congenital NEC 746.89
    - valve - *see also* Endocarditis
      - congenital NEC 746.89
        - aortic 746.3
        - mitral 746.5
        - pulmonary 746.02
        - tricuspid 746.1
  - hepatic duct (*see also* Obstruction, biliary) 576.2
  - hourglass, of stomach 537.6
  - hymen 623.3
  - hypopharynx 478.29
  - intestine (*see also* Obstruction, intestine) 560.9
    - congenital (small) 751.1
      - large 751.2
    - ischemic 557.1
  - lacrimal
    - canaliculi 375.53
      - congenital 743.65
    - punctum 375.52
      - congenital 743.65
    - sac 375.54
      - congenital 743.65
  - lacrimonasal duct 375.56
    - congenital 743.65
    - neonatal 375.55
  - larynx 478.79
    - congenital 748.3
    - syphilitic 095.8
      - congenital 090.5
  - lung 518.89
  - meatus
    - ear (congenital) 744.02
      - acquired (*see also* Stricture, ear canal, acquired) 380.50
    - osseous (congenital) (ear) 744.03
      - acquired (*see also* Stricture, ear canal, acquired) 380.50
    - urinarius (*see also* Stricture, urethra) 598.9
      - congenital 753.6
  - mitral (valve) (*see also* Stenosis, mitral) 394.0

- **Stricture** *(Continued)*
  - mitral *(Continued)*
    - congenital 746.5
    - specified cause, except rheumatic 424.0
  - myocardium, myocardial (*see also* Degeneration, myocardial) 429.1
    - hypertrophic subaortic (idiopathic) 425.1
  - nares (anterior) (posterior) 478.19
    - congenital 748.0
  - nasal duct 375.56
    - congenital 743.65
    - neonatal 375.55
  - nasolacrimal duct 375.56
    - congenital 743.65
    - neonatal 375.55
  - nasopharynx 478.29
    - syphilitic 095.8
  - nephrostomy 997.5
  - nose 478.19
    - congenital 748.0
  - nostril (anterior) (posterior) 478.19
    - congenital 748.0
  - organ or site, congenital NEC - *see* Atresia
  - osseous meatus (congenital) (ear) 744.03
    - acquired (*see also* Stricture, ear canal, acquired) 380.50
  - os uteri (*see also* Stricture, cervix) 622.4
  - oviduct - *see* Stricture, fallopian tube
  - pelviureteric junction 593.3
  - pharynx (dilation) 478.29
  - prostate 602.8
  - pulmonary, pulmonic
    - artery (congenital) 747.3
      - acquired 417.8
      - noncongenital 417.8
    - infundibulum (congenital) 746.83
    - valve (*see also* Endocarditis, pulmonary) 424.3
      - congenital 746.02
    - vein (congenital) 747.49
      - acquired 417.8
    - vessel NEC 417.8
  - punctum lacrimale 375.52
    - congenital 743.65
  - pylorus (hypertrophic) 537.0
    - adult 537.0
    - congenital 750.5
    - infantile 750.5
  - rectosigmoid 569.89
  - rectum (sphincter) 569.2
    - congenital 751.2
    - due to
      - chemical burn 947.3
      - irradiation 569.2
      - lymphogranuloma venereum 099.1
    - gonococcal 098.7
    - inflammatory 099.1
    - syphilitic 095.8
    - tuberculous (*see also* Tuberculosis) 014.8
  - renal artery 440.1
  - salivary duct or gland (any) 527.8
  - sigmoid (flexure) (*see also* Obstruction, intestine) 560.9
  - spermatic cord 608.85
  - stoma (following) (of)
    - colostomy 569.62
    - cystostomy 997.5
    - enterostomy 569.62
    - esophagostomy 530.87
    - gastrostomy 536.42
    - ileostomy 569.62

ICD-9-CM

S

Vol. 2

Stricture *(Continued)*
stoma *(Continued)*
nephrostomy 997.5
tracheostomy 519.02
ureterostomy 997.5
stomach 537.89
congenital 750.7
hourglass 537.6
subaortic 746.81
hypertrophic (acquired) (idiopathic) 425.1
subglottic 478.74
syphilitic NEC 095.8
tendon (sheath) 727.81
trachea 519.19
congenital 748.3
syphilitic 095.8
tuberculous (*see also* Tuberculosis) 012.8
tracheostomy 519.02
tricuspid (valve) (*see also* Endocarditis, tricuspid) 397.0
congenital 746.1
nonrheumatic 424.2
tunica vaginalis 608.85
ureter (postoperative) 593.3
congenital 753.29
tuberculous (*see also* Tuberculosis) 016.2
ureteropelvic junction 593.3
congenital 753.21
ureterovesical orifice 593.3
congenital 753.22
urethra (anterior) (meatal) (organic) (posterior) (spasmodic) 598.9
associated with schistosomiasis (*see also* Schistosomiasis) 120.9 *[598.01]*
congenital (valvular) 753.6
due to
infection 598.00
syphilis 095.8 *[598.01]*
trauma 598.1
gonococcal 098.2 *[598.01]*
gonorrheal 098.2 *[598.01]*
infective 598.00
late effect of injury 598.1
postcatheterization 598.2
postobstetric 598.1
postoperative 598.2
specified cause NEC 598.8
syphilitic 095.8 *[598.01]*
traumatic 598.1
valvular, congenital 753.6
urinary meatus (*see also* Stricture, urethra) 598.9
congenital 753.6
uterus, uterine 621.5
os (external) (internal) - *see* Stricture, cervix
vagina (outlet) 623.2
congenital 752.49
valve (cardiac) (heart) (*see also* Endocarditis) 424.90
congenital (cardiac) (heart) NEC 746.89
aortic 746.3
mitral 746.5
pulmonary 746.02
tricuspid 746.1
urethra 753.6
valvular (*see also* Endocarditis) 424.90
vascular graft or shunt 996.1
atherosclerosis - *see* Arteriosclerosis, extremities
embolism 996.74

Stricture *(Continued)*
vascular graft or shunt *(Continued)*
occlusion NEC 996.74
thrombus 996.74
vas deferens 608.85
congenital 752.89
vein 459.2
vena cava (inferior) (superior) NEC 459.2
congenital 747.49
ventricular shunt 996.2
vesicourethral orifice 596.0
congenital 753.6
vulva (acquired) 624.8
Stridor 786.1
congenital (larynx) 748.3
Stridulous - *see* condition
Strippling of nails 703.8
Stroke 434.91
apoplectic (*see also* Disease, cerebrovascular, acute) 436
brain - *see* Infarct, brain
embolic 434.11
epileptic - *see* Epilepsy
healed or old V12.59
heart - *see* Disease, heart
heat 992.0
hemorrhagic - *see* Hemorrhage, brain
iatrogenic 997.02
in evolution 435.9
ischemic 434.91
late effect - *see* Late effect(s) (of) cerebrovascular disease
lightning 994.0
paralytic - *see* Infarct, brain
postoperative 997.02
progressive 435.9
thrombotic 434.01
Stromatosis, endometrial (M8931/1) 236.0
Strong pulse 785.9
Strongyloides stercoralis infestation 127.2
Strongyloidiasis 127.2
Strongyloidosis 127.2
Strongylus (gibsoni) infestation 127.7
Strophulus (newborn) 779.89
pruriginosus 698.2
Struck by lighting 994.0
Struma (*see also* Goiter) 240.9
fibrosa 245.3
Hashimoto (struma lymphomatosa) 245.2
lymphomatosa 245.2
nodosa (simplex) 241.9
endemic 241.9
multinodular 241.1
sporadic 241.9
toxic or with hyperthyroidism 242.3
multinodular 242.2
uninodular 242.1
toxicosa 242.3
multinodular 242.2
uninodular 242.1
uninodular 241.0
ovarii (M9090/0) 220
and carcinoid (M9091/1) 236.2
malignant (M9090/3) 183.0
Riedel's (ligneous thyroiditis) 245.3
scrofulous (*see also* Tuberculosis) 017.2
tuberculous (*see also* Tuberculosis) 017.2
abscess 017.2
adenitis 017.2
lymphangitis 017.2
ulcer 017.2
Strumipriva cachexia (*see also* Hypothyroidism) 244.9

Strümpell-Marie disease or spine (ankylosing spondylitis) 720.0
Strümpell-Westphal pseudosclerosis (hepatolenticular degeneration) 275.1
Stuart's disease (congenital factor X deficiency) (*see also* Defect, coagulation) 286.3
Stuart-Prower factor deficiency (congenital factor X deficiency) (*see also* Defect, coagulation) 286.3
Students' elbow 727.2
Stuffy nose 478.19
Stump - *see also* Amputation
cervix, cervical (healed) 622.8
Stupor 780.09
catatonic (*see also* Schizophrenia) 295.2
circular (*see also* Psychosis, manic-depressive, circular) 296.7
manic 296.89
manic-depressive (*see also* Psychosis, affective) 296.89
mental (anergic) (delusional) 298.9
psychogenic 298.8
reaction to exceptional stress (transient) 308.2
traumatic NEC - *see also* Injury, intracranial
with spinal (cord)
lesion - *see* Injury, spinal, by site
shock - *see* Injury, spinal, by site
Sturge (-Weber) (-Dimitri) disease or syndrome (encephalocutaneous angiomatosis) 759.6
Sturge-Kalischer-Weber syndrome (encephalocutaneous angiomatosis) 759.6
Stuttering 307.0
Sty, stye 373.11
external 373.11
internal 373.12
meibomian 373.12
Subacidity, gastric 536.8
psychogenic 306.4
Subacute - *see* condition
Subarachnoid - *see* condition
Subclavian steal syndrome 435.2
Subcortical - *see* condition
Subcostal syndrome 098.86
nerve compression 354.8
Subcutaneous, subcuticular - *see* condition
Subdelirium 293.1
Subdural - *see* condition
Subendocardium - *see* condition
Subependymoma (M9383/1) 237.5
Suberosis 495.3
Subglossitis - *see* Glossitis
Subhemophilia 286.0
Subinvolution (uterus) 621.1
breast (postlactational) (postpartum) 611.8
chronic 621.1
puerperal, postpartum 674.8
Sublingual - *see* condition
Sublinguitis 527.2
Subluxation - *see also* Dislocation, by site
congenital NEC - *see also* Malposition, congenital
hip (unilateral) 754.32
with dislocation of other hip 754.35
bilateral 754.33
joint
lower limb 755.69
shoulder 755.59
upper limb 755.59

Subluxation *(Continued)*
congenital NEC *(Continued)*
lower limb (joint) 755.69
shoulder (joint) 755.59
upper limb (joint) 755.59
lens 379.32
anterior 379.33
posterior 379.34
rotary, cervical region of spine - *see* Fracture, vertebra, cervical
Submaxillary - *see* condition
Submersion (fatal) (nonfatal) 994.1
Submissiveness (undue), in child 313.0
Submucous - *see* condition
Subnormal, subnormality
accommodation (*see also* Disorder, accommodation) 367.9
mental (*see also* Retardation, mental) 319
mild 317
moderate 318.0
profound 318.2
severe 318.1
temperature (accidental) 991.6
not associated with low environmental temperature 780.99
Subphrenic - *see* condition
Subscapular nerve - *see* condition
Subseptus uterus 752.3
Subsiding appendicitis 542
Substernal thyroid (*see also* Goiter) 240.9
congenital 759.2
Substitution disorder 300.11
Subtentorial - *see* condition
Subtertian
fever 084.0
malaria (fever) 084.0
Subthyroidism (acquired) (*see also* Hypothyroidism) 244.9
congenital 243
Succenturiata placenta - *see* Placenta, abnormal
Succussion sounds, chest 786.7
Sucking thumb, child 307.9
Sudamen 705.1
Sudamina 705.1
Sudanese kala-azar 085.0
Sudden
death, cause unknown (less than 24 hours) 798.1
during childbirth 669.9
infant 798.0
puerperal, postpartum 674.9
hearing loss NEC 388.2
heart failure (*see also* Failure, heart) 428.9
infant death syndrome 798.0
Sudeck's atrophy, disease, or syndrome 733.7
SUDS (Sudden unexplained death) 798.2
Suffocation (*see also* Asphyxia) 799.01
by
bed clothes 994.7
bunny bag 994.7
cave-in 994.7
constriction 994.7
drowning 994.1
inhalation
food or foreign body (*see also* Asphyxia, food or foreign body) 933.1
oil or gasoline (*see also* Asphyxia, food or foreign body) 933.1
overlying 994.7
plastic bag 994.7

Suffocation *(Continued)*
by *(Continued)*
pressure 994.7
strangulation 994.7
during birth 768.1
mechanical 994.7
Sugar
blood
high 790.29
low 251.2
in urine 791.5
Suicide, suicidal (attempted)
by poisoning - *see* Table of Drugs and Chemicals
ideation V62.84
risk 300.9
tendencies 300.9
trauma NEC (*see also* nature and site of injury) 959.9
Suipestifer infection (*see also* Infection, Salmonella) 003.9
Sulfatidosis 330.0
Sulfhemoglobinemia, sulphemoglobinemia (acquired) (congenital) 289.7
Sumatran mite fever 081.2
Summer - *see* condition
Sunburn 692.71
dermatitis 692.71
due to
other ultraviolet radiation 692.82
tanning bed 692.82
first degree 692.71
second degree 692.76
third degree 692.77
Sunken
acetabulum 718.85
fontanels 756.0
Sunstroke 992.0
Superfecundation
with fetal loss and retention of one or more fetus(es) 651.6
following (elective) fetal reduction 651.7
Superfetation 651.9
with fetal loss and retention of one or more fetus(es) 651.6
following (elective) fetal reduction 651.7
Superinvolution uterus 621.8
Supernumerary (congenital)
aortic cusps 746.89
auditory ossicles 744.04
bone 756.9
breast 757.6
carpal bones 755.56
cusps, heart valve NEC 746.89
mitral 746.5
pulmonary 746.09
digit(s) 755.00
finger 755.01
toe 755.02
ear (lobule) 744.1
fallopian tube 752.19
finger 755.01
hymen 752.49
kidney 753.3
lacrimal glands 743.64
lacrimonasal duct 743.65
lobule (ear) 744.1
mitral cusps 746.5
muscle 756.82
nipples 757.6
organ or site NEC - *see* Accessory
ossicles, auditory 744.04
ovary 752.0
oviduct 752.19
pulmonic cusps 746.09

Supernumerary *(Continued)*
rib 756.3
cervical or first 756.2
syndrome 756.2
roots (of teeth) 520.2
spinal vertebra 756.19
spleen 759.0
tarsal bones 755.67
teeth 520.1
causing crowding 524.31
testis 752.89
thumb 755.01
toe 755.02
uterus 752.2
vagina 752.49
vertebra 756.19
Supervision (of)
contraceptive method previously prescribed V25.40
intrauterine device V25.42
oral contraceptive (pill) V25.41
specified type NEC V25.49
subdermal implantable contraceptive V25.43
dietary (for) V65.3
allergy (food) V65.3
colitis V65.3
diabetes mellitus V65.3
food allergy intolerance V65.3
gastritis V65.3
hypercholesterolemia V65.3
hypoglycemia V65.3
intolerance (food) V65.3
obesity V65.3
specified NEC V65.3
lactation V24.1
pregnancy - *see* Pregnancy, supervision of
Supplemental teeth 520.1
causing crowding 524.31
Suppression
binocular vision 368.31
lactation 676.5
menstruation 626.8
ovarian secretion 256.39
renal 586
urinary secretion 788.5
urine 788.5
Suppuration, suppurative - *see also* condition
accessory sinus (chronic) (*see also* Sinusitis) 473.9
adrenal gland 255.8
antrum (chronic) (*see also* Sinusitis, maxillary) 473.0
bladder (*see also* Cystitis) 595.89
bowel 569.89
brain 324.0
late effect 326
breast 611.0
puerperal, postpartum 675.1
dental periosteum 526.5
diffuse (skin) 686.00
ear (middle) (*see also* Otitis media) 382.4
external (*see also* Otitis, externa) 380.10
internal 386.33
ethmoidal (sinus) (chronic) (*see also* Sinusitis, ethmoidal) 473.2
fallopian tube (*see also* Salpingo-oophoritis) 614.2
frontal (sinus) (chronic) (*see also* Sinusitis, frontal) 473.1
gallbladder (*see also* Cholecystitis, acute) 575.0
gum 523.30

ICD-9-CM S Vol. 2

Suppuration, suppurative *(Continued)*
hernial sac - *see* Hernia, by site
intestine 569.89
joint (*see also* Arthritis, suppurative) 711.0
labyrinthine 386.33
lung 513.0
mammary gland 611.0
puerperal, postpartum 675.1
maxilla, maxillary 526.4
sinus (chronic) (*see also* Sinusitis, maxillary) 473.0
muscle 728.0
nasal sinus (chronic) (*see also* Sinusitis) 473.9
pancreas 577.0
parotid gland 527.2
pelvis, pelvic
female (*see also* Disease, pelvis, inflammatory) 614.4
acute 614.3
male (*see also* Peritonitis) 567.21
pericranial (*see also* Osteomyelitis) 730.2
salivary duct or gland (any) 527.2
sinus (nasal) (*see also* Sinusitis) 473.9
sphenoidal (sinus) (chronic) (*see also* Sinusitis, sphenoidal) 473.3
thymus (gland) 254.1
thyroid (gland) 245.0
tonsil 474.8
uterus (*see also* Endometritis) 615.9
vagina 616.10
wound - *see also* Wound, open, by site, complicated
dislocation - *see* Dislocation, by site, compound
fracture - *see* Fracture, by site, open
scratch or other superficial injury - *see* Injury, superficial, by site
Supraeruption, teeth 524.34
Supraglottitis 464.50
with obstruction 464.51
Suprapubic drainage 596.8
Suprarenal (gland) - *see* condition
Suprascapular nerve - *see* condition
Suprasellar - *see* condition
Supraspinatus syndrome 726.10
Surfer knots 919.8
infected 919.9
Surgery
cosmetic NEC V50.1
following healed injury or operation V51
hair transplant V50.0
elective V50.9
breast augmentation or reduction V50.1
circumcision, ritual or routine (in absence of medical indication) V50.2
cosmetic NEC V50.1
ear piercing V50.3
face-lift V50.1
following healed injury or operation V51
hair transplant V50.0
not done because of
contraindication V64.1
patient's decision V64.2
specified reason NEC V64.3
plastic
breast augmentation or reduction V50.1
cosmetic V50.1
face-lift V50.1

Surgery *(Continued)*
plastic *(Continued)*
following healed injury or operation V51
repair of scarred tissue (following healed injury or operation) V51
specified type NEC V50.8
previous, in pregnancy or childbirth
cervix 654.6
affecting fetus or newborn 763.89
causing obstructed labor 660.2
affecting fetus or newborn 763.1
pelvic soft tissues NEC 654.9
affecting fetus or newborn 763.89
causing obstructed labor 660.2
affecting fetus or newborn 763.1
perineum or vulva 654.8
uterus NEC 654.9
affecting fetus or newborn 763.89
causing obstructed labor 660.2
affecting fetus or newborn 763.1
from previous cesarean delivery 654.2
vagina 654.7
Surgical
abortion - *see* Abortion, legal
emphysema 998.81
kidney (*see also* Pyelitis) 590.80
operation NEC 799.9
procedures, complication or misadventure - *see* Complications, surgical procedure
shock 998.0
Susceptibility
genetic
to
neoplasm
maglignant, of
breast V84.01
endometrium V84.04
other V84.09
ovary V84.02
prostate V84.03
other disease V84.8
Suspected condition, ruled out (*see also* Observation, suspected) V71.9
specified condition NEC V71.89
Suspended uterus, in pregnancy or childbirth 654.4
affecting fetus or newborn 763.89
causing obstructed labor 660.2
affecting fetus or newborn 763.1
Sutton's disease 709.09
Sutton and Gull's disease (arteriolar nephrosclerosis) (*see also* Hypertension, kidney) 403.90
Suture
burst (in external operation wound) 998.32
internal 998.31
inadvertently left in operation wound 998.4
removal V58.32 (Revised)
shirodkar, in pregnancy (with or without cervical incompetence) 654.5
Swab inadvertently left in operation wound 998.4
Swallowed, swallowing
difficulty (*see also* Dysphagia) 787.2
foreign body NEC (*see also* Foreign body) 938
Swamp fever 100.89
Swan neck hand (intrinsic) 736.09
Sweat(s), sweating
disease or sickness 078.2

Sweat(s), sweating *(Continued)*
excessive (*see also* Hyperhidrosis) 780.8
fetid 705.89
fever 078.2
gland disease 705.9
specified type NEC 705.89
miliary 078.2
night 780.8
Sweeley-Klionsky disease (angiokeratoma corporis diffusum) 272.7
Sweet's syndrome (acute febrile neutrophilic dermatosis) 695.89
Swelling
abdominal (not referable to specific organ) 789.3
adrenal gland, cloudy 255.8
ankle 719.07
anus 787.99
arm 729.81
breast 611.72
Calabar 125.2
cervical gland 785.6
cheek 784.2
chest 786.6
ear 388.8
epigastric 789.3
extremity (lower) (upper) 729.81
eye 379.92
female genital organ 625.8
finger 729.81
foot 729.81
glands 785.6
gum 784.2
hand 729.81
head 784.2
inflammatory - *see* Inflammation
joint (*see also* Effusion, joint) 719.0
tuberculous - *see* Tuberculosis, joint
kidney, cloudy 593.89
leg 729.81
limb 729.81
liver 573.8
lung 786.6
lymph nodes 785.6
mediastinal 786.6
mouth 784.2
muscle (limb) 729.81
neck 784.2
nose or sinus 784.2
palate 784.2
pelvis 789.3
penis 607.83
perineum 625.8
rectum 787.99
scrotum 608.86
skin 782.2
splenic (*see also* Splenomegaly) 789.2
substernal 786.6
superficial, localized (skin) 782.2
testicle 608.86
throat 784.2
toe 729.81
tongue 784.2
tubular (*see also* Disease, renal) 593.9
umbilicus 789.3
uterus 625.8
vagina 625.8
vulva 625.8
wandering, due to Gnathostoma (spinigerum) 128.1
white - *see* Tuberculosis, arthritis
Swift's disease 985.0
Swimmers'
ear (acute) 380.12
itch 120.3

Swimming in the head 780.4
Swollen - *see also* Swelling
glands 785.6
Swyer-James syndrome (unilateral hyperlucent lung) 492.8
Swyer's syndrome (XY pure gonadal dysgenesis) 752.7
Sycosis 704.8
barbae (not parasitic) 704.8
contagiosa 110.0
lupoid 704.8
mycotic 110.0
parasitic 110.0
vulgaris 704.8
Sydenham's chorea - *see* Chorea, Sydenham's
Sylvatic yellow fever 060.0
Sylvest's disease (epidemic pleurodynia) 074.1
Symblepharon 372.63
congenital 743.62
Symonds' syndrome 348.2
Sympathetic - *see* condition
Sympatheticotonia (*see also* Neuropathy, peripheral, autonomic) 337.9
Sympathicoblastoma (M9500/3)
specified site - *see* Neoplasm, by site, malignant
unspecified site 194.0
Sympathicogonioma (M9500/3) - *see* Sympathicoblastoma
Sympathoblastoma (M9500/3) - *see* Sympathicoblastoma
Sympathogonioma (M9500/3) - *see* Sympathicoblastoma
Symphalangy (*see also* Syndactylism) 755.10
Symptoms, specified (general) NEC 780.99
abdomen NEC 789.9
bone NEC 733.90
breast NEC 611.79
cardiac NEC 785.9
cardiovascular NEC 785.9
chest NEC 786.9
development NEC 783.9
digestive system NEC 787.99
eye NEC 379.99
gastrointestinal tract NEC 787.99
genital organs NEC
female 625.9
male 608.9
head and neck NEC 784.99 ⬅
heart NEC 785.9
joint NEC 719.60
ankle 719.67
elbow 719.62
foot 719.67
hand 719.64
hip 719.65
knee 719.66
multiple sites 719.69
pelvic region 719.65
shoulder (region) 719.61
specified site NEC 719.68
wrist 719.63
larynx NEC 784.99 ⬅
limbs NEC 729.89
lymphatic system NEC 785.9
menopausal 627.2
metabolism NEC 783.9
mouth NEC 528.9
muscle NEC 728.9
musculoskeletal NEC 781.99
limbs NEC 729.89

Symptoms, specified *(Continued)*
nervous system NEC 781.99
neurotic NEC 300.9
nutrition, metabolism, and development NEC 783.9
pelvis NEC 789.9
female 625.9
peritoneum NEC 789.9
respiratory system NEC 786.9
skin and integument NEC 782.9
subcutaneous tissue NEC 782.9
throat NEC 784.99 ⬅
tonsil NEC 784.99 ⬅
urinary system NEC 788.9
vascular NEC 785.9
Sympus 759.89
Synarthrosis 719.80
ankle 719.87
elbow 719.82
foot 719.87
hand 719.84
hip 719.85
knee 719.86
multiple sites 719.89
pelvic region 719.85
shoulder (region) 719.81
specified site NEC 719.88
wrist 719.83
Syncephalus 759.4
Synchondrosis 756.9
abnormal (congenital) 756.9
ischiopubic (van Neck's) 732.1
Synchysis (senile) (vitreous humor) 379.21
scintillans 379.22
Syncope (near) (pre-) 780.2
anginosa 413.9
bradycardia 427.89
cardiac 780.2
carotid sinus 337.0
complicating delivery 669.2
due to lumbar puncture 349.0
fatal 798.1
heart 780.2
heat 992.1
laryngeal 786.2
tussive 786.2
vasoconstriction 780.2
vasodepressor 780.2
vasomotor 780.2
vasovagal 780.2
Syncytial infarct - *see* Placenta, abnormal
Syndactylism, syndactyly (multiple sites) 755.10
fingers (without fusion of bone) 755.11
with fusion of bone 755.12
toes (without fusion of bone) 755.13
with fusion of bone 755.14
Syndrome - *see also* Disease
5q minus 238.74 ◀
abdominal
acute 789.0
migraine 346.2
muscle deficiency 756.79
Abercrombie's (amyloid degeneration) 277.39 ⬅
abnormal innervation 374.43
abstinence
alcohol 291.81
drug 292.0
Abt-Letterer-Siwe (acute histiocytosis X) (M9722/3) 202.5
Achard-Thiers (adrenogenital) 255.2

Syndrome *(Continued)*
acid pulmonary aspiration 997.3
obstetric (Mendelson's) 668.0
acquired immune deficiency 042
acquired immunodeficiency 042
acrocephalosyndactylism 755.55
acute abdominal 789.0
acute chest 517.3
acute coronary 411.1
Adair-Dighton (brittle bones and blue sclera, deafness) 756.51
Adams-Stokes (-Morgagni) (syncope with heart block) 426.9
Addisonian 255.4
Adie (-Holmes) (pupil) 379.46
adiposogenital 253.8
adrenal
hemorrhage 036.3
meningococcic 036.3
adrenocortical 255.3
adrenogenital (acquired) (congenital) 255.2
feminizing 255.2
iatrogenic 760.79
virilism (acquired) (congenital) 255.2
affective organic NEC 293.89
drug-induced 292.84
afferent loop NEC 537.89
African macroglobulinemia 273.3
Ahumada-Del Castillo (nonpuerperal galactorrhea and amenorrhea) 253.1
air blast concussion - *see* Injury, internal, by site
Alagille 759.89
Albright (-Martin) (pseudohypoparathyroidism) 275.49
Albright-McCune-Sternberg (osteitis fibrosa disseminata) 756.59
alcohol withdrawal 291.81
Alder's (leukocyte granulation anomaly) 288.2
Aldrich (-Wiskott) (eczema-thrombocytopenia) 279.12
Alibert-Bazin (mycosis fungoides) (M9700/3) 202.1
Alice in Wonderland 293.89
Allen-Masters 620.6
Alligator baby (ichthyosis congenita) 757.1
Alport's (hereditary hematuria-nephropathy-deafness) 759.89
Alvarez (transient cerebral ischemia) 435.9
alveolar capillary block 516.3
Alzheimer's 331.0
with dementia - *see* Alzheimer's, dementia
amnestic (confabulatory) 294.0
alcohol-induced persisting 291.1
drug-induced 292.83
posttraumatic 294.0
amotivational 292.89
amyostatic 275.1
amyotrophic lateral sclerosis 335.20
androgen insensitivity 259.5
Angelman 759.89
angina (*see also* Angina) 413.9
ankyloglossia superior 750.0
anterior
chest wall 786.52
compartment (tibial) 958.8
spinal artery 433.8
compression 721.1
tibial (compartment) 958.8

ICD-9-CM
S
Vol. 2

Syndrome *(Continued)*
antibody deficiency 279.00
agammaglobulinemic 279.00
congenital 279.04
hypogammaglobulinemic 279.00
anticardiolipin antibody 795.79
antimongolism 758.39
antiphospholipid antibody 795.79
Anton (-Babinski) (hemiasomatognosia) 307.9
anxiety (*see also* Anxiety) 300.00
organic 293.84
aortic
arch 446.7
bifurcation (occlusion) 444.0
ring 747.21
Apert's (acrocephalosyndactyly) 755.55
Apert-Gallais (adrenogenital) 255.2
aphasia-apraxia-alexia 784.69
apical ballooning 429.83 ⬅
"approximate answers" 300.16
arcuate ligament (-celiac axis) 447.4
arcus aortae 446.7
arc welders' 370.24
argentaffin, argentaffinoma 259.2
Argonz-Del Castillo (nonpuerperal galactorrhea and amenorrhea) 253.1
Argyll Robertson's (syphilitic) 094.89
nonsyphilitic 379.45
Armenian 277.31 ◀
arm-shoulder (*see also* Neuropathy, peripheral, autonomic) 337.9
Arnold-Chiari (*see also* Spina bifida) 741.0
type I 348.4
type II 741.0
type III 742.0
type IV 742.2
Arrillaga-Ayerza (pulmonary artery sclerosis with pulmonary hypertension) 416.0
arteriomesenteric duodenum occlusion 537.89
arteriovenous steal 996.73
arteritis, young female (obliterative brachiocephalic) 446.7
aseptic meningitis - *see* Meningitis, aseptic
Asherman's 621.5
Asperger's 299.8
asphyctic (*see also* Anxiety) 300.00
aspiration, of newborn, massive 770.18
meconium 770.12
ataxia-telangiectasia 334.8
Audry's (acropachyderma) 757.39
auriculotemporal 350.8
autosomal - *see also* Abnormal, autosomes NEC
deletion 758.39
5p 758.31
22g11.2 758.32
Avellis' 344.89
Axenfeld's 743.44
Ayerza (-Arrillaga) (pulmonary artery sclerosis with pulmonary hypertension) 416.0
Baader's (erythema multiforme exudativum) 695.1
Baastrup's 721.5
Babinski (-Vaquez) (cardiovascular syphilis) 093.89
Babinski-Fröhlich (adiposogenital dystrophy) 253.8
Babinski-Nageotte 344.89
Bagratuni's (temporal arteritis) 446.5

Syndrome *(Continued)*
Bakwin-Krida (craniometaphyseal dysplasia) 756.89
Balint's (psychic paralysis of visual disorientation) 368.16
Ballantyne (-Runge) (postmaturity) 766.22
ballooning posterior leaflet 424.0
Banti's - *see* Cirrhosis, liver
Bard-Pic's (carcinoma, head of pancreas) 157.0
Bardet-Biedl (obesity, polydactyly, and mental retardation) 759.89
Barlow's (mitral valve prolapse) 424.0
Barlow (-Möller) (infantile scurvy) 267
Baron Munchausen's 301.51
Barré-Guillain 357.0
Barré-Liéou (posterior cervical sympathetic) 723.2
Barrett's (chronic peptic ulcer of esophagus) 530.85
Bársony-Pólgar (corkscrew esophagus) 530.5
Bársony-Teschendorf (corkscrew esophagus) 530.5
Barth 759.89
Bartter's (secondary hyperaldosteronism with juxtaglomerular hyperplasia) 255.13
Basedow's (exophthalmic goiter) 242.0
basilar artery 435.0
basofrontal 377.04
Bassen-Kornzweig (abetalipoproteinemia) 272.5
Batten-Steinert 359.2
battered
adult 995.81
baby or child 995.54
spouse 995.81
Baumgarten-Cruveilhier (cirrhosis of liver) 571.5
Beals 759.82
Bearn-Kunkel (-Slater) (lupoid hepatitis) 571.49
Beau's (*see also* Degeneration, myocardial) 429.1
Bechterew-Strümpell-Marie (ankylosing spondylitis) 720.0
Beck's (anterior spinal artery occlusion) 433.8
Beckwith (-Wiedemann) 759.89
Behçet's 136.1
Bekhterev-Strümpell-Marie (ankylosing spondylitis) 720.0
Benedikt's 344.89
Béquez César (-Steinbrinck-Chédiak-Higashi) (congenital gigantism of peroxidase granules) 288.2
Bernard-Horner (*see also* Neuropathy, peripheral, autonomic) 337.9
Bernard-Sergent (acute adrenocortical insufficiency) 255.4
Bernhardt-Roth 355.1
Bernheim's (*see also* Failure, heart) 428.0
Bertolotti's (sacralization of fifth lumbar vertebra) 756.15
Besnier-Boeck-Schaumann (sarcoidosis) 135
Bianchi's (aphasia-apraxia-alexia syndrome) 784.69
Biedl-Bardet (obesity, polydactyly, and mental retardation) 759.89
Biemond's (obesity, polydactyly, and mental retardation) 759.89
big spleen 289.4

Syndrome *(Continued)*
bilateral polycystic ovarian 256.4
Bing-Horton's 346.2
Biörck (-Thorson) (malignant carcinoid) 259.2
Blackfan-Diamond (congenital hypoplastic anemia) 284.01 ⬅
black lung 500
black widow spider bite 989.5
bladder neck (*see also* Incontinence, urine) 788.30
blast (concussion) - *see* Blast, injury
blind loop (postoperative) 579.2
Block-Siemens (incontinentia pigmenti) 757.33
Bloch-Sulzberger (incontinentia pigmenti) 757.33
Bloom (-Machacek) (-Torre) 757.39
Blount-Barber (tibia vara) 732.4
blue
bloater 491.20
with
acute bronchitis 491.22
exacerbation (acute) 491.21
diaper 270.0
drum 381.02
sclera 756.51
toe 445.02
Boder-Sedgwick (ataxia-telangiectasia) 334.8
Boerhaave's (spontaneous esophageal rupture) 530.4
Bonnevie-Ullrich 758.6
Bonnier's 386.19
Borjeson-Forssman-Lehmann 759.89 ◀
Bouillaud's (rheumatic heart disease) 391.9
Bourneville (-Pringle) (tuberous sclerosis) 759.5
Bouveret (-Hoffmann) (paroxysmal tachycardia) 427.2
brachial plexus 353.0
Brachman-de Lange (Amsterdam dwarf, mental retardation, and brachycephaly) 759.89
bradycardia-tachycardia 427.81
Brailsford-Morquio (dystrophy) (mucopolysaccharidosis IV) 277.5
brain (acute) (chronic) (nonpsychotic) (organic) (with behavioral reaction) (with neurotic reaction) 310.9
with
presenile brain disease (*see also* Dementia, presenile) 290.10
psychosis, psychotic reaction (*see also* Psychosis, organic) 294.9
chronic alcoholic 291.2
congenital (*see also* Retardation, mental) 319
postcontusional 310.2
posttraumatic
nonpsychotic 310.2
psychotic 293.9
acute 293.0
chronic (*see also* Psychosis, organic) 294.8
subacute 293.1
psycho-organic (*see also* Syndrome, psycho-organic) 310.9
psychotic (*see also* Psychosis, organic) 294.9
senile (*see also* Dementia, senile) 290.0
branchial arch 744.41
Brandt's (acrodermatitis enteropathica) 686.8

◀ New ⬅ Revised

Syndrome *(Continued)*
Brennemann's 289.2
Briquet's 300.81
Brissaud-Meige (infantile myxedema) 244.9
broad ligament laceration 620.6
Brock's (atelectasis due to enlarged lymph nodes) 518.0
broken heart 429.83 ◀
Brown's tendon sheath 378.61
Brown-Séquard 344.89
brown spot 756.59
Brugada 746.89
Brugsch's (acropachyderma) 757.39
bubbly lung 770.7
Buchem's (hyperostosis corticalis) 733.3
Budd-Chiari (hepatic vein thrombosis) 453.0
Büdinger-Ludloff-Läwen 717.89
bulbar 335.22
lateral (*see also* Disease, cerebrovascular, acute) 436
Bullis fever 082.8
bundle of Kent (anomalous atrioventricular excitation) 426.7
Burger-Grutz (essential familial hyperlipemia) 272.3
Burke's (pancreatic insufficiency and chronic neutropenia) 577.8
Burnett's (milk-alkali) 275.42
Burnier's (hypophyseal dwarfism) 253.3
burning feet 266.2
Bywaters' 958.5
Caffey's (infantile cortical hyperostosis) 756.59
Calvé-Legg-Perthes (osteochrondrosis, femoral capital) 732.1
Caplan (-Colinet) syndrome 714.81
capsular thrombosis (*see also* Thrombosis, brain) 434.0
carbohydrate-deficient glycoprotein (CDGS) 271.8
carcinogenic thrombophlebitis 453.1
carcinoid 259.2
cardiac asthma (*see also* Failure, ventricular, left) 428.1
cardiacos negros 416.0
cardiopulmonary obesity 278.8
cardiorenal (*see also* Hypertension, cardiorenal) 404.90
cardiorespiratory distress (idiopathic), newborn 769
cardiovascular renal (*see also* Hypertension, cardiorenal) 404.90
cardiovasorenal 272.7
Carini's (ichthyosis congenita) 757.1
carotid
artery (internal) 435.8
body or sinus 337.0
carpal tunnel 354.0
Carpenter's 759.89
Cassidy (-Scholte) (malignant carcinoid) 259.2
cat-cry 758.31
cauda equina 344.60
causalgia 355.9
lower limb 355.71
upper limb 354.4
cavernous sinus 437.6
celiac 579.0
artery compression 447.4
axis 447.4
central pain 338.0 ◀
cerebellomedullary malformation (*see also* Spina bifida) 741.0

Syndrome *(Continued)*
cerebral gigantism 253.0
cerebrohepatorenal 759.89
cervical (root) (spine) NEC 723.8
disc 722.71
posterior, sympathetic 723.2
rib 353.0
sympathetic paralysis 337.0
traumatic (acute) NEC 847.0
cervicobrachial (diffuse) 723.3
cervicocranial 723.2
cervicodorsal outlet 353.2
Céstan's 344.89
Céstan (-Raymond) 433.8
Céstan-Chenais 344.89
chancriform 114.1
Charcôt's (intermittent claudication) 443.9
angina cruris 443.9
due to atherosclerosis 440.21
Charcôt-Marie-Tooth 356.1
Charcôt-Weiss-Baker 337.0
CHARGE association 759.89
Cheadle (-Möller) (-Barlow) (infantile scurvy) 267
Chédiak-Higashi (-Steinbrinck) (congenital gigantism of peroxidase granules) 288.2
chest wall 786.52
Chiari's (hepatic vein thrombosis) 453.0
Chiari-Frommel 676.6
chiasmatic 368.41
Chilaiditi's (subphrenic displacement, colon) 751.4
chondroectodermal dysplasia 756.55
chorea-athetosis-agitans 275.1
Christian's (chronic histiocytosis X) 277.89
chromosome 4 short arm deletion 758.39
chronic pain 338.4 ◀
Churg-Strauss 446.4
Clarke-Hadfield (pancreatic infantilism) 577.8
Claude's 352.6
Claude Bernard-Horner (*see also* Neuropathy, peripheral, autonomic) 337.9
Clérambault's
automatism 348.8
erotomania 297.8
Clifford's (postmaturity) 766.22
climacteric 627.2
Clouston's (hidrotic ectodermal dysplasia) 757.31
clumsiness 315.4
Cockayne's (microencephaly and dwarfism) 759.89
Cockayne-Weber (epidermolysis bullosa) 757.39
Coffin-Lowry 759.89
Cogan's (nonsyphilitic interstitial keratitis) 370.52
cold injury (newborn) 778.2
Collet (-Sicard) 352.6
combined immunity deficiency 279.2
compartment(al) (anterior) (deep) (posterior) 958.8 ⇐
nontraumatic ⇐
abdomen 729.73 ◀
arm 729.71 ◀
buttock 729.72 ◀
fingers 729.71 ◀
foot 729.72 ◀
forearm 729.71 ◀

Syndrome *(Continued)*
compartment(al) *(Continued)*
nontraumatic *(Continued)*
hand 729.71 ◀
hip 729.72 ◀
leg 729.72 ◀
lower extremity 729.72 ◀
shoulder 729.71 ◀
specified site NEC 729.79 ◀
thigh 729.72 ◀
toes 729.72 ◀
upper extremity 729.71 ◀
wrist 729.71 ◀
traumatic 958.90 ◀
abdomen 958.93 ◀
arm 958.91 ◀
buttock 958.92 ◀
fingers 958.91 ◀
foot 958.92 ◀
forearm 958.91 ◀
hand 958.91 ◀
hip 958.92 ◀
leg 958.92 ◀
lower extremity 958.92 ◀
shoulder 958.91 ◀
specified site NEC 958.99 ◀
thigh 958.92 ◀
tibial 958.92 ◀
toes 958.92 ◀
upper extremity 958.91 ◀
wrist 958.91 ◀
compression 958.5
cauda equina 344.60
with neurogenic bladder 344.61
concussion 310.2
congenital
affecting more than one system 759.7
specified type NEC 759.89
congenital central alveolar hypoventilation 327.25
facial diplegia 352.6
muscular hypertrophy-cerebral 759.89
congestion-fibrosis (pelvic) 625.5
conjunctivourethrosynovial 099.3
Conn (-Louis) (primary aldosteronism) 255.12
Conradi (-Hünermann) (chondrodysplasia calcificans congenita) 756.59
conus medullaris 336.8
Cooke-Apert-Gallais (adrenogenital) 255.2
Cornelia de Lange's (Amsterdam dwarf, mental retardation, and brachycephaly) 759.8
coronary insufficiency or intermediate 411.1
cor pulmonale 416.9
corticosexual 255.2
Costen's (complex) 524.60
costochondral junction 733.6
costoclavicular 353.0
costovertebral 253.0
Cotard's (paranoia) 297.1
Cowden 759.6
craniovertebral 723.2
Creutzfeldt-Jakob (new variant) 046.1
with dementia
with behavioral disturbance 046.1 *[294.11]*
without behavioral disturbance 046.1 *[294.10]*
crib death 798.0
cricopharyngeal 787.2
cri-du-chat 758.31

Syndrome *(Continued)*
- Crigler-Najjar (congenital hyperbilirubinemia) 277.4
- crocodile tears 351.8
- Cronkhite-Canada 211.3
- croup 464.4
- CRST (cutaneous systemic sclerosis) 710.1
- crush 958.5
- crushed lung (*see also* Injury, internal, lung) 861.20
- Cruveilhier-Baumgarten (cirrhosis of liver) 571.5
- cubital tunnel 354.2
- Cuiffini-Pancoast (M8010/3) (carcinoma, pulmonary apex) 162.3
- Curschmann (-Batten) (-Steinert) 359.2
- Cushing's (iatrogenic) (idiopathic) (pituitary basophilism) (pituitary-dependent) 255.0
  - overdose or wrong substance given or taken 962.0
- Cyriax's (slipping rib) 733.99
- cystic duct stump 576.0
- Da Costa's (neurocirculatory asthenia) 306.2
- Dameshek's (erythroblastic anemia) 282.49
- Dana-Putnam (subacute combined sclerosis with pernicious anemia) 281.0 *[336.2]*
- Danbolt (-Closs) (acrodermatitis enteropathica) 686.8
- Dandy-Walker (atresia, foramen of Magendie) 742.3
  - with spina bifida (*see also* Spina bifida) 741.0
- Danlos' 756.83
- Davies-Colley (slipping rib) 733.99
- dead fetus 641.3
- defeminization 255.2
- defibrination (*see also* Fibrinolysis) 286.6
- Degos' 447.8
- Deiters' nucleus 386.19
- Déjérine-Roussy 338.0 ⬅ Revised
- Déjérine-Thomas 333.0
- de Lange's (Amsterdam dwarf, mental retardation, and brachycephaly) (Cornelia) 759.89
- Del Castillo's (germinal aplasia) 606.0
- deletion chromosomes 758.39
- delusional
  - induced by drug 292.11
- dementia-aphonia, of childhood (*see also* Psychosis, childhood) 299.1
- demyelinating NEC 341.9
- denial visual hallucination 307.9
- depersonalization 300.6
- Dercum's (adiposis dolorosa) 272.8
- de Toni-Fanconi (-Debré) (cystinosis) 270.0
- diabetes-dwarfism-obesity (juvenile) 258.1
- diabetes mellitus-hypertension-nephrosis 250.4 *[581.81]*
- diabetes mellitus in newborn infant 775.1
- diabetes-nephrosis 250.4 *[581.81]*
- diabetic amyotrophy 250.6 *[358.1]*
- Diamond-Blackfan (congenital hypoplastic anemia) 284.01 ⬅ Revised
- Diamond-Gardner (autoerythrocyte sensitization) 287.2

Syndrome *(Continued)*
- DIC (diffuse or disseminated intravascular coagulopathy) (*see also* Fibrinolysis) 286.6
- diencephalohypophyseal NEC 253.8
- diffuse cervicobrachial 723.3
- diffuse obstructive pulmonary 496
- DiGeorge's (thymic hypoplasia) 279.11
- Dighton's 756.51
- Di Guglielmo's (erythremic myelosis) (M9841/3) 207.0
- disequilibrium 276.9
- disseminated platelet thrombosis 446.6
- Ditthomska 307.81
- Doan-Wiseman (primary splenic neutropenia) 289.53 ⬅ Revised
- Döhle body-panmyelopathic 288.2
- Donohue's (leprechaunism) 259.8
- dorsolateral medullary (*see also* Disease, cerebrovascular, acute) 436
- double athetosis 333.71 ◀ New
- double whammy 360.81
- Down's (mongolism) 758.0
- Dresbach's (elliptocytosis) 282.1
- Dressler's (postmyocardial infarction) 411.0
  - hemoglobinuria 283.2
  - postcardiotomy 429.4 ◀ New
- drug withdrawal, infant, of dependent mother 779.5
- dry skin 701.1
  - eye 375.15
- DSAP (disseminated superficial actinic porokeratosis) 692.75
- Duane's (retraction) 378.71
- Duane-Stilling-Türk (ocular retraction syndrome) 378.71
- Dubin-Johnson (constitutional hyperbilirubinemia) 277.4
- Dubin-Sprinz (constitutional hyperbilirubinemia) 277.4
- Duchenne's 335.22
- due to abnormality
  - autosomal NEC (*see also* Abnormal, autosomes NEC) 758.5
    - 13 758.1
    - 18 758.2
    - 21 or 22 758.0
    - D_1 758.1
    - E_3 758.2
    - G 758.0
  - chromosomal 758.89
    - sex 758.81
- dumping 564.2
  - nonsurgical 536.8
- Duplay's 726.2
- Dupré's (meningism) 781.6
- Dyke-Young (acquired macrocytic hemolytic anemia) 283.9
- dyspraxia 315.4
- dystocia, dystrophia 654.9
- Eagle-Barret 756.71
- Eales' 362.18
- Eaton-Lambert (*see also* Neoplasm, by site, malignant) 199.1 *[358.1]*
- Ebstein's (downward displacement, tricuspid valve into right ventricle) 746.2
- ectopic ACTH secretion 255.0
- eczema-thrombocytopenia 279.12
- Eddowes' (brittle bones and blue sclera) 756.51
- Edwards' 758.2
- efferent loop 537.89
- effort (aviators') (psychogenic) 306.2

Syndrome *(Continued)*
- Ehlers-Danlos 756.83
- Eisenmenger's (ventricular septal defect) 745.4
- Ekbom's (restless legs) 333.94 ⬅ Revised
- Ekman's (brittle bones and blue sclera) 756.51
- electric feet 266.2
- Elephant man 237.71
- Ellison-Zollinger (gastric hypersecretion with pancreatic islet cell tumor) 251.5
- Ellis-van Creveld (chondroectodermal dysplasia) 756.55
- embryonic fixation 270.2
- empty sella (turcica) 253.8
- endocrine-hypertensive 255.3
- Engel-von Recklinghausen (osteitis fibrosa cystica) 252.01
- enteroarticular 099.3
- entrapment - *see* Neuropathy, entrapment
- eosinophilia myalgia 710.5
- epidemic vomiting 078.82
- Epstein's - *see* Nephrosis
- Erb (-Oppenheim)-Goldflam 358.00
- Erdheim's (acromegalic macrospondylitis) 253.0
- Erlacher-Blount (tibia vara) 732.4
- erythrocyte fragmentation 283.19
- euthyroid sick 790.94
- Evans' (thrombocytopenic purpura) 287.32
- excess cortisol, iatrogenic 255.0
- exhaustion 300.5
- extrapyramidal 333.90
- eyelid-malar-mandible 756.0
- eye retraction 378.71
- Faber's (achlorhydric anemia) 280.9
- Fabry (-Anderson) (angiokeratoma corporis diffusum) 272.7
- facet 724.8
- Fallot's 745.2
- falx (*see also* Hemorrhage, brain) 431
- familial eczema-thrombocytopenia 279.12
- Fanconi's (anemia) (congenital pancytopenia) 284.09 ⬅ Revised
- Fanconi (-de Toni) (-Debré) (cystinosis) 270.0
- Farber (-Uzman) (disseminated lipogranulomatosis) 272.8
- fatigue NEC 300.5
  - chronic 780.71
- faulty bowel habit (idiopathic megacolon) 564.7
- FDH (focal dermal hypoplasia) 757.39
- fecal reservoir 560.39
- Feil-Klippel (brevicollis) 756.16
- Felty's (rheumatoid arthritis with splenomegaly and leukopenia) 714.1
- fertile eunuch 257.2
- fetal alcohol 760.71
  - late effect 760.71
- fibrillation-flutter 427.32
- fibrositis (periarticular) 729.0
- Fiedler's (acute isolated myocarditis) 422.91
- Fiessinger-Leroy (-Reiter) 099.3
- Fiessinger-Rendu (erythema multiforme exudativum) 695.1
- first arch 756.0
- fish odor 270.8 ◀ New
- Fisher's 357.0

Syndrome *(Continued)*
- Fitz's (acute hemorrhagic pancreatitis) 577.0
- Fitz-Hugh and Curtis 098.86
  - due to:
    - Chlamydia trachomatis 099.56
    - Neisseria gonorrhoeae (gonococcal peritonitis) 098.86
- Flajani (-Basedow) (exophthalmic goiter) 242.0
- floppy
  - infant 781.99
  - valve (mitral) 424.0
- flush 259.2
- Foix-Alajouanine 336.1
- Fong's (hereditary osteo-onychodysplasia) 756.89
- foramen magnum 348.4
- Forbes-Albright (nonpuerperal amenorrhea and lactation associated with pituitary tumor) 253.1
- Foster-Kennedy 377.04
- Foville's (peduncular) 344.89
- fragile X 759.83
- Franceschetti's (mandibulofacial dysostosis) 756.0
- Fraser's 759.89
- Freeman-Sheldon 759.89
- Frey's (auriculotemporal) 705.22
- Friderichsen-Waterhouse 036.3
- Friedrich-Erb-Arnold (acropachyderma) 757.39
- Fröhlich's (adiposogenital dystrophy) 253.8
- Froin's 336.8
- Frommel-Chiari 676.6
- frontal lobe 310.0
- Fukuhara 277.87
- Fuller Albright's (osteitis fibrosa disseminata) 756.59
- functional
  - bowel 564.9
  - prepubertal castrate 752.89
- Gaisbock's (polycythemia hypertonica) 289.0
- ganglion (basal, brain) 333.90
  - geniculi 351.1
- Ganser's, hysterical 300.16
- Gardner-Diamond (autoerythrocyte sensitization) 287.2
- gastroesophageal junction 530.0
- gastroesophageal laceration-hemorrhage 530.7
- gastrojejunal loop obstruction 537.89
- Gayet-Wernicke's (superior hemorrhagic polioencephalitis) 265.1
- Gee-Herter-Heubner (nontropical sprue) 579.0
- Gélineau's (*see also* Narcolepsy) 347.00
- genito-anorectal 099.1
- Gerhardt's (vocal cord paralysis) 478.30
- Gerstmann's (finger agnosia) 784.69
- Gianotti Crosti 057.8
  - due to known virus - *see* Infection, virus
  - due to unknown virus 057.8
- Gilbert's 277.4
- Gilford (-Hutchinson) (progeria) 259.8
- Gilles de la Tourette's 307.23
- Gillespie's (dysplasia oculodentodigitalis) 759.89
- Glénard's (enteroptosis) 569.89
- Glinski-Simmonds (pituitary cachexia) 253.2
- glucuronyl transferase 277.4

Syndrome *(Continued)*
- glue ear 381.20
- Goldberg (-Maxwell) (-Morris) (testicular feminization) 259.5
- Goldenhar's (oculoauriculovertebral dysplasia) 756.0
- Goldflam-Erb 358.00
- Goltz-Gorlin (dermal hypoplasia) 757.39
- Goodpasture's (pneumorenal) 446.21
- Good's 279.06
- Gopalan's (burning feet) 266.2
- Gorlin-Chaudhry-Moss 759.89
- Gougerot (-Houwer)-Sjögren (keratoconjunctivitis sicca) 710.2
- Gougerot-Blum (pigmented purpuric lichenoid dermatitis) 709.1
- Gougerot-Carteaud (confluent reticulate papillomatosis) 701.8
- Gouley's (constrictive pericarditis) 423.2
- Gowers' (vasovagal attack) 780.2
- Gowers-Paton-Kennedy 377.04
- Gradenigo's 383.02
- Gray or grey (chloramphenicol) (newborn) 779.4
- Greig's (hypertelorism) 756.0
- Gubler-Millard 344.89
- Guérin-Stern (arthrogryposis multiplex congenita) 754.89
- Guillain-Barré (-Strohl) 357.0
- Gunn's (jaw-winking syndrome) 742.8
- Gunther's (congenital erythropoietic porphyria) 277.1
- gustatory sweating 350.8
- H_3O 759.81
- Hadfield-Clarke (pancreatic infantilism) 577.8
- Haglund-Läwen-Fründ 717.89
- hair tourniquet - *see also* Injury, superficial, by site
  - finger 915.8
    - infected 915.9
  - penis 911.8
    - infected 911.9
  - toe 917.8
    - infected 917.9
- hairless women 257.8
- Hallermann-Strieff 756.0
- Hallervorden-Spatz 333.0
- Hamman's (spontaneous mediastinal emphysema) 518.1
- Hamman-Rich (diffuse interstitial pulmonary fibrosis) 516.3
- Hand-Schüller-Christian (chronic histiocytosis X) 277.89
- hand-foot 282.61
- Hanot-Chauffard (-Troisier) (bronze diabetes) 275.0
- Harada's 363.22
- Hare's (M8010/3) (carcinoma, pulmonary apex) 162.3
- Harkavy's 446.0
- harlequin color change 779.89
- Harris' (organic hyperinsulinism) 251.1
- Hart's (pellagra-cerebellar ataxia-renal aminoaciduria) 270.0
- Hayem-Faber (achlorhydric anemia) 280.9
- Hayem-Widal (acquired hemolytic jaundice) 283.9
- Heberden's (angina pectoris) 413.9
- Hedinger's (malignant carcinoid) 259.2
- Hegglin's 288.2

Syndrome *(Continued)*
- Heller's (infantile psychosis) (*see also* Psychosis, childhood) 299.1
- H.E.L.L.P. 642.5
- hemolytic-uremic (adult) (child) 283.11
- hemophagocytic 288.4 ◀
  - infection-associated 288.4 ◀
- Hench-Rosenberg (palindromic arthritis) (*see also* Rheumatism, palindromic) 719.3
- Henoch-Schönlein (allergic purpura) 287.0
- hepatic flexure 569.89
- hepatorenal 572.4
  - due to a procedure 997.4
  - following delivery 674.8
- hepatourologic 572.4
- Herrick's (hemoglobin S disease) 282.61
- Herter (-Gee) (nontropical sprue) 579.0
- Heubner-Herter (nontropical sprue) 579.0
- Heyd's (hepatorenal) 572.4
- HHHO 759.81
- high grade myelodysplastic 238.73 ◀
  - with 5q deletion 238.73 ◀
- Hilger's 337.0
- histiocytic 288.4 ◀
- Hoffa (-Kastert) (liposynovitis prepatellaris) 272.8
- Hoffmann's 244.9 *[359.5]*
- Hoffmann-Bouveret (paroxysmal tachycardia) 427.2
- Hoffmann-Werdnig 335.0
- Holländer-Simons (progressive lipodystrophy) 272.6
- Holmes' (visual disorientation) 368.16
- Holmes-Adie 379.46
- Hoppe-Goldflam 358.00
- Horner's (*see also* Neuropathy, peripheral, autonomic) 337.9
  - traumatic - *see* Injury, nerve, cervical sympathetic
- hospital addiction 301.51
- Hunt's (herpetic geniculate ganglionitis) 053.11
  - dyssynergia cerebellaris myoclonica 334.2
- Hunter (-Hurler) (mucopolysaccharidosis II) 277.5
- hunterian glossitis 529.4
- Hurler (-Hunter) (mucopolysaccharidosis II) 277.5
- Hutchinson's incisors or teeth 090.5
- Hutchinson-Boeck (sarcoidosis) 135
- Hutchinson-Gilford (progeria) 259.8
- hydralazine
  - correct substance properly administered 695.4
  - overdose or wrong substance given or taken 972.6
- hydraulic concussion (abdomen) (*see also* Injury, internal, abdomen) 868.00
- hyperabduction 447.8
- hyperactive bowel 564.9
- hyperaldosteronism with hypokalemic alkalosis (Bartter's) 255.13
- hypercalcemic 275.42
- hypercoagulation NEC 289.89
- hypereosinophilic (idiopathic) 288.3
- hyperkalemic 276.7
- hyperkinetic - *see also* Hyperkinesia, heart 429.82
- hyperlipemia-hemolytic anemia-icterus 571.1

ICD-9-CM S Vol. 2

Syndrome *(Continued)*
hypermobility 728.5
hypernatremia 276.0
hyperosmolarity 276.0
hypersomnia-bulimia 349.89
hypersplenic 289.4
hypersympathetic (*see also* Neuropathy, peripheral, autonomic) 337.9
hypertransfusion, newborn 776.4
hyperventilation, psychogenic 306.1
hyperviscosity (of serum) NEC 273.3
polycythemic 289.0
sclerothymic 282.8
hypoglycemic (familial) (neonatal) 251.2
functional 251.1
hypokalemic 276.8
hypophyseal 253.8
hypophyseothalamic 253.8
hypopituitarism 253.2
hypoplastic left heart 746.7
hypopotassemia 276.8
hyposmolality 276.1
hypotension, maternal 669.2
hypotonia-hypomentia-hypogonadism-obesity 759.81
ICF (intravascular coagulation-fibrinolysis) (*see also* Fibrinolysis) 286.6
idiopathic cardiorespiratory distress, newborn 769
idiopathic nephrotic (infantile) 581.9
iliotibial band 728.89
Imerslund (-Gräsbeck) (anemia due to familial selective vitamin B_{12} malabsorption) 281.1
immobility (paraplegic) 728.3
immunity deficiency, combined 279.2
impending coronary 411.1
impingement
shoulder 726.2
vertebral bodies 724.4
inappropriate secretion of antidiuretic hormone (ADH) 253.6
incomplete
mandibulofacial 756.0
infant
death, sudden (SIDS) 798.0
Hercules 255.2
of diabetic mother 775.0
shaken 995.55
infantilism 253.3
inferior vena cava 459.2
influenza-like 487.1
inspissated bile, newborn 774.4
insufficient sleep 307.44
intermediate coronary (artery) 411.1
internal carotid artery (*see also* Occlusion, artery, carotid) 433.1
interspinous ligament 724.8
intestinal
carcinoid 259.2
gas 787.3
knot 560.2
intravascular
coagulation-fibrinolysis (ICF) (*see also* Fibrinolysis) 286.6
coagulopathy (*see also* Fibrinolysis) 286.6
inverted Marfan's 759.89
IRDS (idiopathic respiratory distress, newborn) 769
irritable
bowel 564.1
heart 306.2
weakness 300.5

Syndrome *(Continued)*
ischemic bowel (transient) 557.9
chronic 557.1
due to mesenteric artery insufficiency 557.1
Itsenko-Cushing (pituitary basophilism) 255.0
IVC (intravascular coagulopathy) (*see also* Fibrinolysis) 286.6
Ivemark's (asplenia with congenital heart disease) 759.0
Jaccoud's 714.4
Jackson's 344.89
Jadassohn-Lewandowski (pachyonychia congenita) 757.5
Jaffe-Lichtenstein (-Uehlinger) 252.01
Jahnke's (encephalocutaneous angiomatosis) 759.6
Jakob-Creutzfeldt (new variant) 046.1
with dementia
with behavioral disturbance 046.1 *[294.11]*
without behavioral disturbance 046.1 *[294.10]*
Jaksch's (pseudoleukemia infantum) 285.8
Jaksch-Hayem (-Luzet) (pseudoleukemia infantum) 285.8
jaw-winking 742.8
jejunal 564.2
Jervell-Lange-Nielsen 426.82
jet lag 327.35
Jeune's (asphyxiating thoracic dystrophy of newborn) 756.4
Job's (chronic granulomatous disease) 288.1
Jordan's 288.2
Joseph-Diamond-Blackfan (congenital hypoplastic anemia) 284.01 (Revised)
Joubert 759.89
jugular foramen 352.6
Kabuki 759.89
Kahler's (multiple myeloma) (M9730/3) 203.0
Kalischer's (encephalocutaneous angiomatosis) 759.6
Kallmann's (hypogonadotropic hypogonadism with anosmia) 253.4
Kanner's (autism) (*see also* Psychosis, childhood) 299.0
Kartagener's (sinusitis, bronchiectasis, situs inversus) 759.3
Kasabach-Merritt (capillary hemangioma associated with thrombocytopenic purpura) 287.39
Kast's (dyschondroplasia with hemangiomas) 756.4
Kaznelson's (congenital hypoplastic anemia) 284.01 (Revised)
Kearns-Sayre 277.87
Kelly's (sideropenic dysphagia) 280.8
Kimmelstiel-Wilson (intercapillary glomerulosclerosis) 250.4 *[581.81]*
Klauder's (erythema multiforme exudativum) 695.1
Klein-Waardenburg (ptosis-epicanthus) 270.2
Kleine-Levin 327.13
Klinefelter's 758.7
Klippel-Feil (brevicollis) 756.16
Klippel-Trenaunay 759.89
Klumpke (-Déjérine) (injury to brachial plexus at birth) 767.6
Klüver-Bucy (-Terzian) 310.0

Syndrome *(Continued)*
Köhler-Pelligrini-Stieda (calcification, knee joint) 726.62
König's 564.89
Korsakoff's (nonalcoholic) 294.0
alcoholic 291.1
Korsakoff (-Wernicke) (nonalcoholic) 294.0
alcoholic 291.1
Kostmann's (infantile genetic agranulocytosis) 288.01 (Revised)
Krabbe's
congenital muscle hypoplasia 756.89
cutaneocerebral angioma 759.6
Kunkel (lupoid hepatitis) 571.49
labyrinthine 386.50
laceration, broad ligament 620.6
Langdon Down (mongolism) 758.0
Larsen's (flattened facies and multiple congenital dislocations) 755.8
lateral
cutaneous nerve of thigh 355.1
medullary (*see also* Disease, cerebrovascular, acute) 436
Launois' (pituitary gigantism) 253.0
Launois-Cléret (adiposogenital dystrophy) 253.8
Laurence-Moon (-Bardet)-Biedl (obesity, polydactyly, and mental retardation) 759.89
Lawford's (encephalocutaneous angiomatosis) 759.6
lazy
leukocyte 288.09 (Revised)
posture 728.3
Lederer-Brill (acquired infectious hemolytic anemia) 283.19
Legg-Calvé-Perthes (osteochondrosis capital femoral) 732.1
Lemierre 451.89
Lennox's (*see also* Epilepsy) 345.0
Lennox-Gastaut 345.0
with tonic seizures 345.1
lenticular 275.1
Leopold-Levi's (paroxysmal thyroid instability) 242.9
Lepore hemoglobin 282.49
Léri-Weill 756.59
Leriche's (aortic bifurcation occlusion) 444.0
Lermoyez's (*see also* Disease, Ménière's) 386.00
Lesch-Nyhan (hypoxanthine-guanine-phosphoribosyltransferase deficiency) 277.2
Lev's (acquired complete heart block) 426.0
Levi's (pituitary dwarfism) 253.3
Lévy-Roussy 334.3
Lichtheim's (subacute combined sclerosis with pernicious anemia) 281.0 *[336.2]*
Li-Fraumeni V84.01
Lightwood's (renal tubular acidosis) 588.89
Lignac (-de Toni) (-Fanconi) (-Debré) (cystinosis) 270.0
Likoff's (angina in menopausal women) 413.9
liver-kidney 572.4
Lloyd's 258.1
lobotomy 310.0
Löffler's (eosinophilic pneumonitis) 518.3
Löfgren's (sarcoidosis) 135
long arm 18 or 21 deletion 758.39

Syndrome *(Continued)*
- Looser (-Debray)-Milkman (osteomalacia with pseudofractures) 268.2
- Lorain-Levi (pituitary dwarfism) 253.3
- Louis-Bar (ataxia-telangiectasia) 334.8
- low
  - atmospheric pressure 993.2
  - back 724.2
    - psychogenic 306.0
  - output (cardiac) (*see also* Failure, heart) 428.9
- Lowe's (oculocerebrorenal dystrophy) 270.8
- Lowe-Terrey-MacLachlan (oculocerebrorenal dystrophy) 270.8
- lower radicular, newborn 767.4
- Lown (-Ganong)-Levine (short P-R internal, normal QRS complex, and supraventricular tachycardia) 426.81
- Lucey-Driscoll (jaundice due to delayed conjugation) 774.30
- Luetscher's (dehydration) 276.51
- lumbar vertebral 724.4
- Lutembacher's (atrial septal defect with mitral stenosis) 745.5
- Lyell's (toxic epidermal necrolysis) 695.1
  - due to drug
    - correct substance properly administered 695.1
    - overdose or wrong substance given or taken 977.9
      - specified drug - *see* Table of Drugs and Chemicals
- MacLeod's 492.8
- macrogenitosomia praecox 259.8
- macroglobulinemia 273.3
- macrophage activation 288.4 ◀
- Maffucci's (dyschondroplasia with hemangiomas) 756.4
- Magenblase 306.4
- magnesium-deficiency 781.7
- Mal de Debarquement 780.4
- malabsorption 579.9
  - postsurgical 579.3
  - spinal fluid 331.3
- malignant carcinoid 259.2
- Mallory-Weiss 530.7
- mandibulofacial dysostosis 756.0
- manic-depressive (*see also* Psychosis, affective) 296.80
- Mankowsky's (familial dysplastic osteopathy) 731.2
- maple syrup (urine) 270.3
- Marable's (celiac artery compression) 447.4
- Marchesani (-Weill) (brachymorphism and ectopia lentis) 759.89
- Marchiafava-Bignami 341.8
- Marchiafava-Micheli (paroxysmal nocturnal hemoglobinuria) 283.2
- Marcus Gunn's (jaw-winking syndrome) 742.8
- Marfan's (arachnodactyly) 759.82
  - meaning congenital syphilis 090.49
    - with luxation of lens 090.49 *[379.32]*
- Marie's (acromegaly) 253.0
  - primary or idiopathic (acropachyderma) 757.39
  - secondary (hypertrophic pulmonary osteoarthropathy) 731.2
- Markus-Adie 379.46
- Maroteaux-Lamy (mucopolysaccharidosis VI) 277.5

Syndrome *(Continued)*
- Martin's 715.27
- Martin-Albright (pseudohypoparathyroidism) 275.49
- Martorell-Fabré (pulseless disease) 446.7
- massive aspiration of newborn 770.18
- Masters-Allen 620.6
- mastocytosis 757.33
- maternal hypotension 669.2
- maternal obesity 646.1
- May (-Hegglin) 288.2
- McArdle (-Schmid) (-Pearson) (glycogenosis V) 271.0
- McCune-Albright (osteitis fibrosa disseminata) 756.59
- McQuarrie's (idiopathic familial hypoglycemia) 251.2
- meconium
  - aspiration 770.12
  - plug (newborn) NEC 777.1
- median arcuate ligament 447.4
- mediastinal fibrosis 519.3
- Meekeren-Ehlers-Danlos 756.83
- Meige (blepharospasm-oromandibular dystonia) 333.82
  - -Milroy (chronic hereditary edema) 757.0
- MELAS (mitochondrial encephalopathy, lactic acidosis and stroke-like episodes) 277.87
- Melkersson (-Rosenthal) 351.8
- Mende's (ptosis-epicanthus) 270.2
- Mendelson's (resulting from a procedure) 997.3
  - during labor 668.0
  - obstetric 668.0
- Ménétrier's (hypertrophic gastritis) 535.2
- Ménière's (*see also* Disease, Ménière's) 386.00
- meningo-eruptive 047.1
- Menkes' 759.89
  - glutamic acid 759.89
  - maple syrup (urine) disease 270.3
- menopause 627.2
  - postartificial 627.4
- menstruation 625.4
- MERRF (myoclonus with epilepsy and with ragged red fibers) 277.87
- mesenteric
  - artery, superior 557.1
  - vascular insufficiency (with gangrene) 557.1
- metabolic 277.7
- metastatic carcinoid 259.2
- Meyenburg-Altherr-Uehlinger 733.99
- Meyer-Schwickerath and Weyers (dysplasia oculodentodigitalis) 759.89
- Micheli-Rietti (thalassemia minor) 282.49
- Michotte's 721.5
- micrognathia-glossoptosis 756.0
- microphthalmos (congenital) 759.89
- midbrain 348.8
- middle
  - lobe (lung) (right) 518.0
  - radicular 353.0
- Miescher's
  - familial acanthosis nigricans 701.2
  - granulomatosis disciformis 709.3
- Mieten's 759.89
- migraine 346.0
- Mikity-Wilson (pulmonary dysmaturity) 770.7

Syndrome *(Continued)*
- Mikulicz's (dryness of mouth, absent or decreased lacrimation) 527.1
- milk alkali (milk drinkers') 275.42
- Milkman (-Looser) (osteomalacia with pseudofractures) 268.2
- Millard-Gubler 344.89
- Miller Fisher's 357.0
- Miller-Dieker 758.33
- Milles' (encephalocutaneous angiomatosis) 759.6
- Minkowski-Chauffard (*see also* Spherocytosis) 282.0
- Mirizzi's (hepatic duct stenosis) 576.2
  - with calculus, cholelithiasis, or stones - *see* Choledocholithiasis
- mitochondrial neurogastrointestinal encephalopathy (MNGIE) 277.87
- mitral
  - click (-murmur) 785.2
  - valve prolapse 424.0
- MNGIE (mitochondrial neurogastrointestinal encephalopathy) 277.87
- Möbius'
  - congenital oculofacial paralysis 352.6
  - ophthalmoplegic migraine 346.8
- Mohr's (types I and II) 759.89
- monofixation 378.34
- Moore's (*see also* Epilepsy) 345.5
- Morel-Moore (hyperostosis frontalis interna) 733.3
- Morel-Morgagni (hyperostosis frontalis interna) 733.3
- Morgagni (-Stewart-Morel) (hyperostosis frontalis interna) 733.3
- Morgagni-Adams-Stokes (syncope with heart block) 426.9
- Morquio (-Brailsford) (-Ullrich) (mucopolysaccharidosis IV) 277.5
- Morris (testicular feminization) 259.5
- Morton's (foot) (metatarsalgia) (metatarsal neuralgia) (neuralgia) (neuroma) (toe) 355.6
- Moschcowitz (-Singer-Symmers) (thrombotic thrombocytopenic purpura) 446.6
- Mounier-Kuhn 748.3
  - with
    - acute exacerbation 494.1
    - bronchiectasis 494.0
      - with (acute) exacerbation 494.1
  - acquired 519.19 ⬅
    - with bronchiectasis 494.0
      - with (acute) exacerbation 494.1
- Mucha-Haberman (acute parapsoriasis varioliformis) 696.2
- mucocutaneous lymph node (acute) (febrile) (infantile) (MCLS) 446.1
- multiple
  - deficiency 260
  - operations 301.51
- Munchausen's 301.51
- Munchmeyer's (exostosis luxurians) 728.11
- Murchison-Sanderson - *see* Disease, Hodgkin's
- myasthenic - *see* Myasthenia, syndrome
- myelodysplastic 238.75 ⬅
  - with 5q deletion 238.74 ◀
  - high grade with 5q deletion 238.73 ◀
- myeloproliferative (chronic) (M9960/1) 238.79 ⬅
- myofascial pain NEC 729.1
- Naffziger's 353.0

Syndrome *(Continued)*
Nager-de Reynier (dysostosis mandibularis) 756.0
nail-patella (hereditary osteo-onychodysplasia) 756.89
NARP (neuropathy, ataxia, and retinitis pigmentosa) 277.87
Nebécourt's 253.3
Neill Dingwall (microencephaly and dwarfism) 759.89
nephrotic (*see also* Nephrosis) 581.9
diabetic 250.4 *[581.81]*
Netherton's (ichthyosiform erythroderma) 757.1
neurocutaneous 759.6
neuroleptic malignant 333.92
Nezelof's (pure alymphocytosis) 279.13
Niemann-Pick (lipid histiocytosis) 272.7
Nonne-Milroy-Meige (chronic hereditary edema) 757.0
nonsense 300.16
Noonan's 759.89
Nothnagel's
ophthalmoplegia-cerebellar ataxia 378.52
vasomotor acroparesthesia 443.89
nucleus ambiguous-hypoglossal 352.6
OAV (oculoauriculovertebral dysplasia) 756.0
obsessional 300.3
oculocutaneous 364.24
oculomotor 378.81
oculourethroarticular 099.3
Ogilvie's (sympathicotonic colon obstruction) 560.89
ophthalmoplegia-cerebellar ataxia 378.52
Oppenheim-Urbach (necrobiosis lipoidica diabeticorum) 250.8 *[709.3]*
oral-facial-digital 759.89
organic
affective NEC 293.83
drug-induced 292.84
anxiety 293.84
delusional 293.81
alcohol-induced 291.5
drug-induced 292.11
due to or associated with
arteriosclerosis 290.42
presenile brain disease 290.12
senility 290.20
depressive 293.83
drug-induced 292.84
due to or associated with
arteriosclerosis 290.43
presenile brain disease 290.13
senile brain disease 290.21
hallucinosis 293.82
drug-induced 292.84
organic affective 293.83
induced by drug 292.84
organic personality 310.1
induced by drug 292.89
Ormond's 593.4
orodigitofacial 759.89
orthostatic hypotensive-dysautonomic-dyskinetic 333.0
Osler-Weber-Rendu (familial hemorrhagic telangiectasia) 448.0
osteodermopathic hyperostosis 757.39
osteoporosis-osteomalacia 268.2
Österreicher-Turner (hereditary osteo-onychodysplasia) 756.89

Syndrome *(Continued)*
Ostrum-Furst 756.59
otolith 386.19
otopalatodigital 759.89
outlet (thoracic) 353.0
ovarian remnant 620.8
ovarian vein 593.4
Owren's (*see also* Defect, coagulation) 286.3
OX 758.6
pacemaker 429.4
Paget-Schroetter (intermittent venous claudication) 453.8
pain - *see also* Pain (Revised)
central 338.0 (New)
chronic 338.4 (New)
myelopathic 338.0 (New)
thalamic (hyperesthetic) 338.0 (New)
painful
apicocostal vertebral (M8010/3) 162.3
arc 726.19
bruising 287.2
feet 266.2
Pancoast's (carcinoma, pulmonary apex) (M8010/3) 162.3
panhypopituitary (postpartum) 253.2
papillary muscle 429.81
with myocardial infarction 410.8
Papillon-Léage and Psaume (orodigitofacial dysostosis) 759.89
paraneoplastic- *see* condition
parobiotic (transfusion)
donor (twin) 772.0
recipient (twin) 776.4
paralysis agitans 332.0
paralytic 344.9
specified type NEC 344.89
paraneoplastic - *see* Condition
Parinaud's (paralysis of conjugate upward gaze) 378.81
oculoglandular 372.02
Parkes Weber and Dimitri (encephalocutaneous angiomatosis) 759.6
Parkinson's (*see also* Parkinsonism) 332.0
parkinsonian (*see also* Parkinsonism) 332.0
Parry's (exophthalmic goiter) 242.0
Parry-Romberg 349.89
Parsonage-Aldren-Turner 353.5
Parsonage-Turner 353.5
Patau's (trisomy D_1) 758.1
patellofemoral 719.46
Paterson (-Brown) (-Kelly) (sideropenic dysphagia) 280.8
Payr's (splenic flexure syndrome) 569.89
pectoral girdle 447.8
pectoralis minor 447.8
Pelger-Huët (hereditary hyposegmentation) 288.2
Pellagra-cerebellar ataxia-renal aminoaciduria 270.0
Pellegrini-Stieda 726.62
pellagroid 265.2
Pellizzi's (pineal) 259.8
pelvic congestion (-fibrosis) 625.5
Pendred's (familial goiter with deaf-mutism) 243
Penfield's (*see also* Epilepsy) 345.5
Penta X 758.81
peptic ulcer - *see* Ulcer, peptic 533.9
perabduction 447.8
periodic 277.31 (Revised)
periurethral fibrosis 593.4
persistent fetal circulation 747.83

Syndrome *(Continued)*
Petges-Cléjat (poikilodermatomyositis) 710.3
Peutz-Jeghers 759.6
Pfeiffer (acrocephalosyndactyly) 755.55
phantom limb 353.6
pharyngeal pouch 279.11
Pick's (pericardial pseudocirrhosis of liver) 423.2
heart 423.2
liver 423.2
Pick-Herxheimer (diffuse idiopathic cutaneous atrophy) 701.8
Pickwickian (cardiopulmonary obesity) 278.8
PIE (pulmonary infiltration with eosinophilia 518.3
Pierre Marie-Bamberger (hypertrophic pulmonary osteoarthropathy) 731.2
Pierre Mauriac's (diabetes-dwarfism-obesity) 258.1
Pierre Robin 756.0
pigment dispersion, iris 364.53
pineal 259.8
pink puffer 492.8
pituitary 253.0
placental
dysfunction 762.2
insufficiency 762.2
transfusion 762.3
plantar fascia 728.71
plica knee 727.83
Plummer-Vinson (sideropenic dysphagia) 280.8
pluricarential of infancy 260
plurideficiency of infancy 260
pluriglandular (compensatory) 258.8
polycarential of infancy 260
polyglandular 258.8
polysplenia 759.0
pontine 433.8
popliteal
artery entrapment 447.8
web 756.89
postartificial menopause 627.4
postcardiac injury (New)
postcardiotomy 429.4 (New)
postmyocardial infarction 411.0 (New)
postcardiotomy 429.4
postcholecystectomy 576.0
postcommissurotomy 429.4
postconcussional 310.2
postcontusional 310.2
postencephalitic 310.8
posterior
cervical sympathetic 723.2
fossa compression 348.4
inferior cerebellar artery (*see also* Disease, cerebrovascular, acute) 436
reversible encephalopathy (PRES) 348.39 (New)
postgastrectomy (dumping) 564.2
post-gastric surgery 564.2
posthepatitis 780.79
posttherpetic (neuralgia) (zoster) 053.19
geniculate ganglion 053.11
ophthalmica 053.19
postimmunization - *see* Complications, vaccination
postinfarction 411.0
postinfluenza (asthenia) 780.79
postirradiation 990
postlaminectomy 722.80
cervical, cervicothoracic 722.81

◀ New ⟸ Revised

Syndrome *(Continued)*
postlaminectomy *(Continued)*
lumbar, lumbosacral 722.83
thoracic, thoracolumbar 722.82
postleukotomy 310.0
postlobotomy 310.0
postmastectomy lymphedema 457.0
postmature (of newborn) 766.22
postmyocardial infarction 411.0
postoperative NEC 998.9
blind loop 579.2
postpartum panhypopituitary 253.2
postperfusion NEC 999.8
bone marrow 996.85
postpericardiotomy 429.4
postphlebitic (asymptomatic) 459.10
with
complications NEC 459.19
inflammation 459.12
and ulcer 459.13
stasis dermatitis 459.12
with ulcer 459.13
ulcer 459.11
with inflammation 459.13
postpolio (myelitis) 138
postvagotomy 564.2
postvalvulotomy 429.4
postviral (asthenia) NEC 780.79
Potain's (gastrectasis with dyspepsia) 536.1
potassium intoxication 276.7
Potter's 753.0
Prader (-Labhart)-Willi (-Fanconi) 759.81
preinfarction 411.1
preleukemic 238.75 (Revised)
premature senility 259.8
premenstrual 625.4
premenstrual tension 625.4
pre-ulcer 536.9
Prinzmetal-Massumi (anterior chest wall syndrome) 786.52
Profichet's 729.9
progeria 259.8
progressive pallidal degeneration 333.0
prolonged gestation 766.22
Proteus (dermal hypoplasia) 757.39
prune belly 756.71
prurigo-asthma 691.8
pseudocarpal tunnel (sublimis) 354.0
pseudohermaphroditism-virilism-hirsutism 255.2
pseudoparalytica 358.00
pseudo-Turner's 759.89
psycho-organic 293.9
acute 293.0
anxiety type 293.84
depressive type 293.83
hallucinatory type 293.82
nonpsychotic severity 310.1
specified focal (partial) NEC 310.8
paranoid type 293.81
specified type NEC 293.89
subacute 293.1
pterygolymphangiectasia 758.6
ptosis-epicanthus 270.2
pulmonary
arteriosclerosis 416.0
hypoperfusion (idiopathic) 769
renal (hemorrhagic) 446.21
pulseless 446.7
Putnam-Dana (subacute combined sclerosis with pernicious anemia) 281.0 *[336.2]*
pyloroduodenal 537.89

Syndrome *(Continued)*
pyramidopallidonigral 332.0
pyriformis 355.0
QT interval prolongation 426.82
radicular NEC 729.2
lower limbs 724.4
upper limbs 723.4
newborn 767.4
Raeder-Harbitz (pulseless disease) 446.7
Ramsay Hunt's
dyssynergia cerebellaris myoclonica 334.2
herpetic geniculate ganglionitis 053.11
rapid time-zone change 327.35
Raymond (-Céstan) 433.8
Raynaud's (paroxysmal digital cyanosis) 443.0
RDS (respiratory distress syndrome, newborn) 769
Refsum's (heredopathia atactica polyneuritiformis) 356.3
Reichmann's (gastrosuccorrhea) 536.8
Reifenstein's (hereditary familial hypogonadism, male) 259.5
Reilly's (*see also* Neuropathy, peripheral, autonomic 337.9
Reiter's 099.3
renal glomerulohyalinosis-diabetic 250.4 *[581.81]*
Rendu-Osler-Weber (familial hemorrhagic telangiectasia) 448.0
renofacial (congenital biliary fibroangiomatosis) 753.0
Rénon-Delille 253.8
respiratory distress (idiopathic) (newborn) 769
adult (following shock, surgery, or trauma) 518.5
specified NEC 518.82
type II 770.6 (New)
restless legs (RLS) 333.94 (Revised)
retinoblastoma (familial) 190.5
retraction (Duane's) 378.71
retroperitoneal fibrosis 593.4
retroviral seroconversion (acute) V08 (New)
Rett's 330.8
Reye's 331.81
Reye-Sheehan (postpartum pituitary necrosis) 253.2
Riddoch's (visual disorientation) 368.16
Ridley's (*see also* Failure, ventricular, left) 428.1
Rieger's (mesodermal dysgenesis, anterior ocular segment) 743.44
Rietti-Greppi-Micheli (thalassemia minor) 282.49
right ventricular obstruction - *see* Failure, heart
Riley-Day (familial dysautonomia) 742.8
Robin's 756.0
Rokitansky-Kuster-Hauser (congenital absence, vagina) 752.49
Romano-Ward (prolonged QT interval syndrome) 426.82
Romberg's 349.89
Rosen-Castleman-Liebow (pulmonary proteinosis) 516.0
rotator cuff, shoulder 726.10
Roth's 355.1
Rothmund's (congenital poikiloderma) 757.33
Rotor's (idiopathic hyperbilirubinemia) 277.4
Roussy-Lévy 334.3
Roy (-Jutras) (acropachyderma) 757.39

Syndrome *(Continued)*
rubella (congenital) 771.0
Rubinstein-Taybi's (brachydactylia, short stature, and mental retardation) 759.89
Rud's (mental deficiency, epilepsy, and infantilism) 759.89
Ruiter-Pompen (-Wyers) (angiokeratoma corporis diffusum) 272.7
Runge's (postmaturity) 766.22
Russell (-Silver) (congenital hemihypertrophy and short stature) 759.89
Rytand-Lipsitch (complete atrioventricular block) 426.0
sacralization-scoliosis-sciatica 756.15
sacroiliac 724.6
Saenger's 379.46
salt
depletion (*see also* Disease, renal) 593.9
due to heat NEC 992.8
causing heat exhaustion or prostration 992.4
low (*see also* Disease, renal) 593.9
salt-losing (*see also* Disease, renal) 593.9
Sanfilippo's (mucopolysaccharidosis III) 277.5
Scaglietti-Dagnini (acromegalic macrospondylitis) 253.0
scalded skin 695.1
scalenus anticus (anterior) 353.0
scapulocostal 354.8
scapuloperoneal 359.1
scapulovertebral 723.4
Schaumann's (sarcoidosis) 135
Scheie's (mucopolysaccharidosis IS) 277.5
Scheuthauer-Marie-Sainton (cleidocranialis dysostosis) 755.59
Schirmer's (encephalocutaneous angiomatosis) 759.6
schizophrenic, of childhood NEC (*see also* Psychosis, childhood) 299.9
Schmidt's
sphallo-pharyngo-laryngeal hemiplegia 352.6
thyroid-adrenocortical insufficiency 258.1
vagoaccessory 352.6
Schneider's 047.9
Schnitzler 273.1
Scholte's (malignant carcinoid) 259.2
Scholz (-Bielschowsky-Henneberg) 330.0
Schroeder's (endocrine-hypertensive) 255.3
Schüller-Christian (chronic histiocytosis X) 277.89
Schultz's (agranulocytosis) 288.09 (Revised)
Schwachman's 288.02 (Revised)
Schwartz (-Jampel) 756.89
Schwartz-Bartter (inappropriate secretion of antidiuretic hormone) 253.6
scimitar (anomalous venous drainage, right lung to inferior vena cava) 747.49
sclerocystic ovary 256.4
sea-blue histiocyte 272.7
Seabright-Bantam (pseudohypoparathyroidism) 275.49
Seckel's 759.89
Secretan's (posttraumatic edema) 782.3
secretoinhibitor (keratoconjunctivitis sicca) 710.2

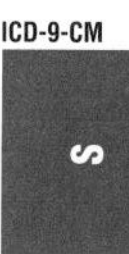
ICD-9-CM
S
Vol. 2

Syndrome *(Continued)*
  Seeligmann's (ichthyosis congenita) 757.1
  Senear-Usher (pemphigus erythematosus) 694.4
  senilism 259.8
  seroconversion, retroviral (acute) V08 ◄
  serotonin 333.99
  serous meningitis 348.2
  Sertoli cell (germinal aplasia) 606.0
  sex chromosome mosaic 758.81
  Sézary's (reticulosis) (M9701/3) 202.2
  shaken infant 995.55
  Shaver's (bauxite pneumoconiosis) 503
  Sheehan's (postpartum pituitary necrosis) 253.2
  shock (traumatic) 958.4
    kidney 584.5
      following crush injury 958.5
    lung 518.5
    neurogenic 308.9
    psychic 308.9
  short
    bowel 579.3
    P-R interval 426.81
  shoulder-arm (*see also* Neuropathy, peripheral, autonomic) 337.9
  shoulder-girdle 723.4
  shoulder-hand (*see also* Neuropathy, peripheral, autonomic) 337.9
  Shwachman's 288.0
  Shy-Drager (orthostatic hypotension with multisystem degeneration) 333.0
  Sicard's 352.6
  sicca (keratoconjunctivitis) 710.2
  sick
    cell 276.1
    cilia 759.89
    sinus 427.81
  sideropenic 280.8
  Siemens'
    ectodermal dysplasia 757.31
    keratosis follicularis spinulosa (decalvans) 757.39
  Silfverskiöld's (osteochondrodystrophy, extremities) 756.50
  Silver's (congenital hemihypertrophy and short stature) 759.89
  Silvestroni-Bianco (thalassemia minima) 282.49
  Simons' (progressive lipodystrophy) 272.6
  sinus tarsi 726.79
  sinusitis-bronchiectasis-situs inversus 759.3
  Sipple's (medullary thyroid carcinoma-pheochromocytoma) 193
  Sjögren (-Gougerot) (keratoconjunctivitis sicca) 710.2
    with lung involvement 710.2 *[517.8]*
  Sjögren-Larsson (ichthyosis congenita) 757.1
  Slocumb's 255.3
  Sluder's 337.0
  Smith-Lemli-Opitz (cerebrohepatorenal syndrome) 759.89
  Smith-Magenis 758.33
  smokers' 305.1
  Sneddon-Wilkinson (subcorneal pustular dermatosis) 694.1
  Sotos' (cerebral gigantism) 253.0
  South African cardiomyopathy 425.2
  spasmodic
    upward movement, eye(s) 378.82
    winking 307.20

Syndrome *(Continued)*
  Spens' (syncope with heart block) 426.9
  spherophakia-brachymorphia 759.89
  spinal cord injury - *see also* Injury, spinal, by site
    with fracture, vertebra - *see* Fracture, vertebra, by site, with spinal cord injury
    cervical - *see* Injury, spinal, cervical
    fluid malabsorption (acquired) 331.3
  splenic
    agenesis 759.0
    flexure 569.89
    neutropenia 289.53 ⟸
    sequestration 289.52
  Spurway's (brittle bones and blue sclera) 756.51
  staphylococcal scalded skin 695.1
  Stein's (polycystic ovary) 256.4
  Stein-Leventhal (polycystic ovary) 256.4
  Steinbrocker's (*see also* Neuropathy, peripheral, autonomic) 337.9
  Stevens-Johnson (erythema multiforme exudativum) 695.1
  Stewart-Morel (hyperostosis frontalis interna) 733.3
  Stickler 759.89
  stiff-baby 759.89
  stiff-man 333.91
  Still's (juvenile rheumatoid arthritis) 714.30
  Still-Felty (rheumatoid arthritis with splenomegaly and leukopenia) 714.1
  Stilling-Türk-Duane (ocular retraction syndrome) 378.71
  Stojano's (subcostal) 098.86
  Stokes (-Adams) (syncope with heart block) 426.9
  Stokvis-Talma (enterogenous cyanosis) 289.7
  stone heart (*see also* Failure, ventricular, left) 428.1
  straight-back 756.19
  stroke (*see also* Disease, cerebrovascular, acute) 436
    little 435.9
  Sturge-Kalischer-Weber (encephalotrigeminal angiomatosis) 759.6
  Sturge-Weber (-Dimitri) (encephalocutaneous angiomatosis) 759.6
  subclavian-carotid obstruction (chronic) 446.7
  subclavian steal 435.2
  subcoracoid-pectoralis minor 447.8
  subcostal 098.86
    nerve compression 354.8
  subperiosteal hematoma 267
  subphrenic interposition 751.4
  sudden infant death (SIDS) 798.0
  Sudeck's 733.7
  Sudeck-Leriche 733.7
  superior
    cerebellar artery (*see also* Disease, cerebrovascular, acute) 436
    mesenteric artery 557.1
    pulmonary sulcus (tumor) (M8010/3) 162.3
    vena cava 459.2
  suprarenal cortical 255.3
  supraspinatus 726.10
  swallowed blood 777.3
  sweat retention 705.1

Syndrome *(Continued)*
  Sweet's (acute febrile neutrophilic dermatosis) 695.89
  Swyer-James (unilateral hyperlucent lung) 492.8
  Swyer's (XY pure gonadal dysgenesis) 752.7
  Symonds' 348.2
  sympathetic
    cervical paralysis 337.0
    pelvic 625.5
  syndactylic oxycephaly 755.55
  syphilitic-cardiovascular 093.89
  systemic
    fibrosclerosing 710.8
    inflammatory response (SIRS) 995.90
      due to infectious process 995.91
        with acute organ dysfunction 995.92 ⟸
      non-infectious process 995.93
        with acute organ dysfunction 995.94 ⟸
  systolic click (-murmur) 785.2
  Tabagism 305.1
  tachycardia-bradycardia 427.81
  Takayasu (-Onishi) (pulseless disease) 446.7
  Takotsubo 429.83 ◄
  Tapia's 352.6
  tarsal tunnel 355.5
  Taussig-Bing (transposition, aorta and overriding pulmonary artery) 745.11
  Taybi's (otopalatodigital) 759.89
  Taylor's 625.5
  teething 520.7
  tegmental 344.89
  telangiectasis-pigmentation-cataract 757.33
  temporal 383.02
    lobectomy behavior 310.0
  temporomandibular joint-pain-dysfunction [TMJ] NEC 524.60
    specified NEC 524.69
  Terry's 362.21
  testicular feminization 259.5
  testis, nonvirilizing 257.8
  tethered (spinal) cord 742.59
  thalamic 338.0 ⟸
  Thibierge-Weissenbach (cutaneous systemic sclerosis) 710.1
  Thiele 724.6
  thoracic outlet (compression) 353.0
  thoracogenous rheumatic (hypertrophic pulmonary osteoarthropathy) 731.2
  Thorn's (*see also* Disease, renal) 593.9
  Thorson-Biörck (malignant carcinoid) 259.2
  thrombopenia-hemangioma 287.39
  thyroid-adrenocortical insufficiency 258.1
  Tietze's 733.6
  time-zone (rapid) 327.35
  Tobias' (carcinoma, pulmonary apex) (M8010/3) 162.3
  toilet seat 926.0
  Tolosa-Hunt 378.55
  Toni-Fanconi (cystinosis) 270.0
  Touraine's (hereditary osteo-onychodysplasia) 756.89
  Touraine-Solente-Golé (acropachyderma) 757.39
  toxic
    oil 710.5
    shock 040.82

Syndrome *(Continued)*
transfusion
fetal-maternal 772.0
twin
donor (infant) 772.0
recipient (infant) 776.4
transient left ventricular apical ballooning 429.83 ◀
Treacher Collins' (incomplete mandibulofacial dysostosis) 756.0
trigeminal plate 259.8
triplex X female 758.81
trisomy NEC 758.5
13 or D_1 758.1
16–18 or E 758.2
18 or E_3 758.2
20 758.5
21 or G (mongolism) 758.0
22 or G (mongolism) 758.0
G 758.0
Troisier-Hanot-Chauffard (bronze diabetes) 275.0
tropical wet feet 991.4
Trousseau's (thrombophlebitis migrans visceral cancer) 453.1
Türk's (ocular retraction syndrome) 378.71
Turner's 758.6
Turner-Varny 758.6
twin-to-twin transfusion 762.3
recipient twin 776.4
Uehlinger's (acropachyderma) 757.39
Ullrich (-Bonnevie) (-Turner) 758.6
Ullrich-Feichtiger 759.89
underwater blast injury (abdominal) (*see also* Injury, internal, abdomen) 868.00
universal joint, cervix 620.6
Unverricht (-Lundborg) 333.2
Unverricht-Wagner (dermatomyositis) 710.3
upward gaze 378.81
Urbach-Oppenheim (necrobiosis lipoidica diabeticorum) 250.8 *[709.3]*
Urbach-Wiethe (lipoid proteinosis) 272.8
uremia, chronic 585.9
urethral 597.81
urethro-oculoarticular 099.3
urethro-oculosynovial 099.3
urohepatic 572.4
uveocutaneous 364.24
uveomeningeal, uveomeningitis 363.22
vagohypoglossal 352.6
vagovagal 780.2
van Buchem's (hyperostosis corticalis) 733.3
van der Hoeve's (brittle bones and blue sclera, deafness) 756.51
van der Hoeve-Halbertsma-Waardenburg (ptosis-epicanthus) 270.2
van der Hoeve-Waardenburg-Gualdi (ptosis-epicanthus) 270.2
vanishing twin 651.33
van Neck-Odelberg (juvenile osteochondrosis) 732.1
vascular splanchnic 557.0
vasomotor 443.9
vasovagal 780.2
VATER 759.89
Velo-cardio-facial 758.32
vena cava (inferior) (superior) (obstruction) 459.2
Verbiest's (claudicatio intermittens spinalis) 435.1

Syndrome *(Continued)*
Vernet's 352.6
vertebral
artery 435.1
compression 721.1
lumbar 724.4
steal 435.1
vertebrogenic (pain) 724.5
vertiginous NEC 386.9
video display tube 723.8
Villaret's 352.6
Vinson-Plummer (sideropenic dysphagia) 280.8
virilizing adrenocortical hyperplasia, congenital 255.2
virus, viral 079.99
visceral larval migrans 128.0
visual disorientation 368.16
vitamin B_6 deficiency 266.1
vitreous touch 997.99
Vogt's (corpus striatum) 333.71 ⬅
Vogt-Koyanagi 364.24
Volkmann's 958.6
von Bechterew-Strümpell (ankylosing spondylitis) 720.0
von Graefe's 378.72
von Hippel-Lindau (angiomatosis retinocerebellosa) 759.6
von Schroetter's (intermittent venous claudication) 453.8
von Willebrand (-Jürgens) (angiohemophilia) 286.4
Waardenburg-Klein (ptosis epicanthus) 270.2
Wagner (-Unverricht) (dermatomyositis) 710.3
Waldenström's (macroglobulinemia) 273.3
Waldenström-Kjellberg (sideropenic dysphagia) 280.8
Wallenberg's (posterior inferior cerebellar artery) (*see also* Disease, cerebrovascular, acute) 436
Waterhouse (-Friderichsen) 036.3
water retention 276.6
Weber's 344.89
Weber-Christian (nodular nonsuppurative panniculitis) 729.30
Weber-Cockayne (epidermolysis bullosa) 757.39
Weber-Dimitri (encephalocutaneous angiomatosis) 759.6
Weber-Gubler 344.89
Weber-Leyden 344.89
Weber-Osler (familial hemorrhagic telangiectasia) 448.0
Wegener's (necrotizing respiratory granulomatosis) 446.4
Weill-Marchesani (brachymorphism and ectopia lentis) 759.89
Weingarten's (tropical eosinophilia) 518.3
Weiss-Baker (carotid sinus syncope) 337.0
Weissenbach-Thibierge (cutaneous systemic sclerosis) 710.1
Werdnig-Hoffmann 335.0
Werlhof-Wichmann (*see also* Purpura, thrombocytopenic) 287.39
Wermer's (polyendocrine adenomatosis) 258.0
Werner's (progeria adultorum) 259.8
Wernicke's (nonalcoholic) (superior hemorrhagic polioencephalitis) 265.1

Syndrome *(Continued)*
Wernicke-Korsakoff (nonalcoholic) 294.0
alcoholic 291.1
Westphal-Strümpell (hepatolenticular degeneration) 275.1
wet
brain (alcoholic) 303.9
feet (maceration) (tropical) 991.4
lung
adult 518.5
newborn 770.6
whiplash 847.0
Whipple's (intestinal lipodystrophy) 040.2
"whistling face" (craniocarpotarsal dystrophy) 759.89
Widal (-Abrami) (acquired hemolytic jaundice) 283.9
Wilkie's 557.1
Wilkinson-Sneddon (subcorneal pustular dermatosis) 694.1
Willan-Plumbe (psoriasis) 696.1
Willebrand (-Jürgens) (angiohemophilia) 286.4
Willi-Prader (hypogenital dystrophy with diabetic tendency) 759.81
Wilson's (hepatolenticular degeneration) 275.1
Wilson-Mikity 770.7
Wiskott-Aldrich (eczema-thrombocytopenia) 279.12
withdrawal
alcohol 291.81
drug 292.0
infant of dependent mother 779.5
Woakes' (ethmoiditis) 471.1
Wolff-Parkinson-White (anomalous atrioventricular excitation) 426.7
Wright's (hyperabduction) 447.8
X
cardiac 413.9
dysmetabolic 277.7
xiphoidalgia 733.99
XO 758.6
XXX 758.81
XXXXY 758.81
XXY 758.7
yellow vernix (placental dysfunction) 762.2
Zahorsky's 074.0
Zellweger 277.86
Zieve's (jaundice, hyperlipemia and hemolytic anemia) 571.1
Zollinger-Ellison (gastric hypersecretion with pancreatic islet cell tumor) 251.5
Zuelzer-Ogden (nutritional megaloblastic anemia) 281.2
Synechia (iris) (pupil) 364.70
anterior 364.72
peripheral 364.73
intrauterine (traumatic) 621.5
posterior 364.71
vulvae, congenital 752.49
Synesthesia (*see also* Disturbance, sensation) 782.0
Synodontia 520.2
Synophthalmus 759.89
Synorchidism 752.89
Synorchism 752.89
Synostosis (congenital) 756.59
astragaloscaphoid 755.67
radioulnar 755.53
talonavicular (bar) 755.67
tarsal 755.67

Synovial - *see* condition
Synovioma (M9040/3) - *see also* Neoplasm, connective tissue, malignant
benign (M9040/0) - *see* Neoplasm, connective tissue, benign
Synoviosarcoma (M9040/3) - *see* Neoplasm, connective tissue, malignant
Synovitis 727.00
chronic crepitant, wrist 727.2
due to crystals - *see* Arthritis, due to crystals
gonococcal 098.51
gouty 274.0
syphilitic 095.7
congenital 090.0
traumatic, current - *see* Sprain, by site
tuberculous - *see* Tuberculosis, synovitis
villonodular 719.20
ankle 719.27
elbow 719.22
foot 719.27
hand 719.24
hip 719.25
knee 719.26
multiple sites 719.29
pelvic region 719.25
shoulder (region) 719.21
specified site NEC 719.28
wrist 719.23
Syphilide 091.3
congenital 090.0
newborn 090.0
tubercular 095.8
congenital 090.0
Syphilis, syphilitic (acquired) 097.9
with lung involvement 095.1
abdomen (late) 095.2
acoustic nerve 094.86
adenopathy (secondary) 091.4
adrenal (gland) 095.8
with cortical hypofunction 095.8
age under 2 years NEC (*see also* Syphilis, congenital) 090.9
acquired 097.9
alopecia (secondary) 091.82
anemia 095.8
aneurysm (artery) (ruptured) 093.89
aorta 093.0
central nervous system 094.89
congenital 090.5
anus 095.8
primary 091.1
secondary 091.3
aorta, aortic (arch) (abdominal) (insufficiency) (pulmonary) (regurgitation) (stenosis) (thoracic) 093.89
aneurysm 093.0
arachnoid (adhesive) 094.2
artery 093.89
cerebral 094.89
spinal 094.89
arthropathy (neurogenic) (tabetic) 094.0 *[713.5]*
asymptomatic - *see* Syphilis, latent
ataxia, locomotor (progressive) 094.0
atrophoderma maculatum 091.3
auricular fibrillation 093.89
Bell's palsy 094.89
bladder 095.8
bone 095.5
secondary 091.61
brain 094.89
breast 095.8
bronchus 095.8

Syphilis, syphilitic *(Continued)*
bubo 091.0
bulbar palsy 094.89
bursa (late) 095.7
cardiac decompensation 093.89
cardiovascular (early) (late) (primary) (secondary) (tertiary) 093.9
specified type and site NEC 093.89
causing death under 2 years of age (*see also* Syphilis, congenital) 090.9
stated to be acquired NEC 097.9
central nervous system (any site) (early) (late) (latent) (primary) (recurrent) (relapse) (secondary) (tertiary) 094.9
with
ataxia 094.0
paralysis, general 094.1
juvenile 090.40
paresis (general) 094.1
juvenile 090.40
tabes (dorsalis) 094.0
juvenile 090.40
taboparesis 094.1
juvenile 090.40
aneurysm (ruptured) 094.87
congenital 090.40
juvenile 090.40
remission in (sustained) 094.9
serology doubtful, negative, or positive 094.9
specified nature or site NEC 094.89
vascular 094.89
cerebral 094.89
meningovascular 094.2
nerves 094.89
sclerosis 094.89
thrombosis 094.89
cerebrospinal 094.89
tabetic 094.0
cerebrovascular 094.89
cervix 095.8
chancre (multiple) 091.0
extragenital 091.2
Rollet's 091.2
Charcôt's joint 094.0 *[713.5]*
choked disc 094.89 *[377.00]*
chorioretinitis 091.51
congenital 090.0 *[363.13]*
late 094.83
choroiditis 091.51
congenital 090.0 *[363.13]*
late 094.83
prenatal 090.0 *[363.13]*
choroidoretinitis (secondary) 091.51
congenital 090.0 *[363.13]*
late 094.83
ciliary body (secondary) 091.52
late 095.8 *[364.11]*
colon (late) 095.8
combined sclerosis 094.89
complicating pregnancy, childbirth, or puerperium 647.0
affecting fetus or newborn 760.2
condyloma (latum) 091.3
congenital 090.9
with
encephalitis 090.41
paresis (general) 090.40
tabes (dorsalis) 090.40
taboparesis 090.40
chorioretinitis, choroiditis 090.0 *[363.13]*
early or less than 2 years after birth NEC 090.2

Syphilis, syphilitic *(Continued)*
congenital *(Continued)*
early or less than 2 years after birth NEC *(Continued)*
with manifestations 090.0
latent (without manifestations) 090.1
negative spinal fluid test 090.1
serology, positive 090.1
symptomatic 090.0
interstitial keratitis 090.3
juvenile neurosyphilis 090.40
late or 2 years or more after birth NEC 090.7
chorioretinitis, choroiditis 090.5 *[363.13]*
interstitial keratitis 090.3
juvenile neurosyphilis NEC 090.40
latent (without manifestations) 090.6
negative spinal fluid test 090.6
serology, positive 090.6
symptomatic or with manifestations NEC 090.5
interstitial keratitis 090.3
conjugal 097.9
tabes 094.0
conjunctiva 095.8 *[372.10]*
contact V01.6
cord, bladder 094.0
cornea, late 095.8 *[370.59]*
coronary (artery) 093.89
sclerosis 093.89
coryza 095.8
congenital 090.0
cranial nerve 094.89
cutaneous - *see* Syphilis, skin
dacryocystitis 095.8
degeneration, spinal cord 094.89
d'emblée 095.8
dementia 094.1
paralytica 094.1
juvenilis 090.40
destruction of bone 095.5
dilatation, aorta 093.0
due to blood transfusion 097.9
dura mater 094.89
ear 095.8
inner 095.8
nerve (eighth) 094.86
neurorecurrence 094.86
early NEC 091.0
cardiovascular 093.9
central nervous system 094.9
paresis 094.1
tabes 094.0
latent (without manifestations) (less than 2 years after infection) 092.9
negative spinal fluid test 092.9
serological relapse following treatment 092.0
serology positive 092.9
paresis 094.1
relapse (treated, untreated) 091.7
skin 091.3
symptomatic NEC 091.89
extragenital chancre 091.2
primary, except extragenital chancre 091.0
secondary (*see also* Syphilis, secondary) 091.3
relapse (treated, untreated) 091.7
tabes 094.0
ulcer 091.3
eighth nerve 094.86

Syphilis, syphilitic *(Continued)*
endemic, nonvenereal 104.0
endocarditis 093.20
aortic 093.22
mitral 093.21
pulmonary 093.24
tricuspid 093.23
epididymis (late) 095.8
epiglottis 095.8
epiphysitis (congenital) 090.0
esophagus 095.8
Eustachian tube 095.8
exposure to V01.6
eye 095.8 *[363.13]*
neuromuscular mechanism 094.85
eyelid 095.8 *[373.5]*
with gumma 095.8 *[373.5]*
ptosis 094.89
fallopian tube 095.8
fracture 095.5
gallbladder (late) 095.8
gastric 095.8
crisis 094.0
polyposis 095.8
general 097.9
paralysis 094.1
juvenile 090.40
genital (primary) 091.0
glaucoma 095.8
gumma (late) NEC 095.9
cardiovascular system 093.9
central nervous system 094.9
congenital 090.5
heart or artery 093.89
heart 093.89
block 093.89
decompensation 093.89
disease 093.89
failure 093.89
valve (*see also* Syphilis, endocarditis) 093.20
hemianesthesia 094.89
hemianopsia 095.8
hemiparesis 094.89
hemiplegia 094.89
hepatic artery 093.89
hepatitis 095.3
hepatomegaly 095.3
congenital 090.0
hereditaria tarda (*see also* Syphilis, congenital, late) 090.7
hereditary (*see also* Syphilis, congenital) 090.9
interstitial keratitis 090.3
Hutchinson's teeth 090.5
hyalitis 095.8
inactive - *see* Syphilis, latent
infantum NEC (*see also* Syphilis, congenital) 090.9
inherited - *see* Syphilis, congenital
internal ear 095.8
intestine (late) 095.8
iris, iritis (secondary) 091.52
late 095.8 *[364.11]*
joint (late) 095.8
keratitis (congenital) (early) (interstitial) (late) (parenchymatous) (punctata profunda) 090.3
kidney 095.4
lacrimal apparatus 095.8
laryngeal paralysis 095.8
larynx 095.8
late 097.0
cardiovascular 093.9
central nervous system 094.9

Syphilis, syphilitic *(Continued)*
late *(Continued)*
latent or 2 years or more after infection (without manifestation) 096
negative spinal fluid test 096
serology positive 096
paresis 094.1
specified site NEC 095.8
symptomatic or with symptoms 095.9
tabes 094.0
latent 097.1
central nervous system 094.9
date of infection unspecified 097.1
early or less than 2 years after infection 092.9
late or 2 years or more after infection 096
serology
doubtful
follow-up of latent syphilis 097.1
central nervous system 094.9
date of infection unspecified 097.1
early or less than 2 years after infection 092.9
late or 2 years or more after infection 096
positive, only finding 097.1
date of infection unspecified 097.1
early or less than 2 years after infection 097.1
late or 2 years or more after infection 097.1
lens 095.8
leukoderma 091.3
late 095.8
lienis 095.8
lip 091.3
chancre 091.2
late 095.8
primary 091.2
Lissauer's paralysis 094.1
liver 095.3
secondary 091.62
locomotor ataxia 094.0
lung 095.1
lymphadenitis (secondary) 091.4
lymph gland (early) (secondary) 091.4
late 095.8
macular atrophy of skin 091.3
striated 095.8
maternal, affecting fetus or newborn 760.2
manifest syphilis in newborn - *see* Syphilis, congenital
mediastinum (late) 095.8
meninges (adhesive) (basilar) (brain) (spinal cord) 094.2
meningitis 094.2
acute 091.81
congenital 090.42
meningoencephalitis 094.2
meningovascular 094.2
congenital 090.49
mesarteritis 093.89
brain 094.89
spine 094.89
middle ear 095.8
mitral stenosis 093.21
monoplegia 094.89
mouth (secondary) 091.3
late 095.8
mucocutaneous 091.3
late 095.8

Syphilis, syphilitic *(Continued)*
mucous
membrane 091.3
late 095.8
patches 091.3
congenital 090.0
mulberry molars 090.5
muscle 095.6
myocardium 093.82
myositis 095.6
nasal sinus 095.8
neonatorum NEC (*see also* Syphilis, congenital) 090.9
nerve palsy (any cranial nerve) 094.89
nervous system, central 094.9
neuritis 095.8
acoustic nerve 094.86
neurorecidive of retina 094.83
neuroretinitis 094.85
newborn (*see also* Syphilis, congenital) 090.9
nodular superficial 095.8
nonvenereal, endemic 104.0
nose 095.8
saddle back deformity 090.5
septum 095.8
perforated 095.8
occlusive arterial disease 093.89
ophthalmic 095.8 *[363.13]*
ophthalmoplegia 094.89
optic nerve (atrophy) (neuritis) (papilla) 094.84
orbit (late) 095.8
orchitis 095.8
organic 097.9
osseous (late) 095.5
osteochondritis (congenital) 090.0
osteoporosis 095.5
ovary 095.8
oviduct 095.8
palate 095.8
gumma 095.8
perforated 090.5
pancreas (late) 095.8
pancreatitis 095.8
paralysis 094.89
general 094.1
juvenile 090.40
paraplegia 094.89
paresis (general) 094.1
juvenile 090.40
paresthesia 094.89
Parkinson's disease or syndrome 094.82
paroxysmal tachycardia 093.89
pemphigus (congenital) 090.0
penis 091.0
chancre 091.0
late 095.8
pericardium 093.81
perichondritis, larynx 095.8
periosteum 095.5
congenital 090.0
early 091.61
secondary 091.61
peripheral nerve 095.8
petrous bone (late) 095.5
pharynx 095.8
secondary 091.3
pituitary (gland) 095.8
placenta 095.8
pleura (late) 095.8
pneumonia, white 090.0
pontine (lesion) 094.89
portal vein 093.89
primary NEC 091.2

Syphilis, syphilitic *(Continued)*
primary *(Continued)*
anal 091.1
and secondary (*see also* Syphilis, secondary) 091.9
cardiovascular 093.9
central nervous system 094.9
extragenital chancre NEC 091.2
fingers 091.2
genital 091.0
lip 091.2
specified site NEC 091.2
tonsils 091.2
prostate 095.8
psychosis (intracranial gumma) 094.89
ptosis (eyelid) 094.89
pulmonary (late) 095.1
artery 093.89
pulmonum 095.1
pyelonephritis 095.4
recently acquired, symptomatic NEC 091.89
rectum 095.8
respiratory tract 095.8
retina
late 094.83
neurorecidive 094.83
retrobulbar neuritis 094.85
salpingitis 095.8
sclera (late) 095.0
sclerosis
cerebral 094.89
coronary 093.89
multiple 094.89
subacute 094.89
scotoma (central) 095.8
scrotum 095.8
secondary (and primary) 091.9
adenopathy 091.4
anus 091.3
bone 091.61
cardiovascular 093.9
central nervous system 094.9
chorioretinitis, choroiditis 091.51
hepatitis 091.62
liver 091.62
lymphadenitis 091.4
meningitis, acute 091.81
mouth 091.3
mucous membranes 091.3
periosteum 091.61
periostitis 091.61
pharynx 091.3
relapse (treated) (untreated) 091.7
skin 091.3
specified form NEC 091.89
tonsil 091.3
ulcer 091.3
viscera 091.69
vulva 091.3
seminal vesicle (late) 095.8
seronegative
with signs or symptoms - *see* Syphilis, by site and stage

Syphilis, syphilitic *(Continued)*
seropositive
with signs or symptoms - *see* Syphilis, by site or stage
follow-up of latent syphilis - *see* Syphilis, latent
only finding - *see* Syphilis, latent
seventh nerve (paralysis) 094.89
sinus 095.8
sinusitis 095.8
skeletal system 095.5
skin (early) (secondary) (with ulceration) 091.3
late or tertiary 095.8
small intestine 095.8
spastic spinal paralysis 094.0
spermatic cord (late) 095.8
spinal (cord) 094.89
with
paresis 094.1
tabes 094.0
spleen 095.8
splenomegaly 095.8
spondylitis 095.5
staphyloma 095.8
stigmata (congenital) 090.5
stomach 095.8
synovium (late) 095.7
tabes dorsalis (early) (late) 094.0
juvenile 090.40
tabetic type 094.0
juvenile 090.40
taboparesis 094.1
juvenile 090.40
tachycardia 093.89
tendon (late) 095.7
tertiary 097.0
with symptoms 095.8
cardiovascular 093.9
central nervous system 094.9
multiple NEC 095.8
specified site NEC 095.8
testis 095.8
thorax 095.8
throat 095.8
thymus (gland) 095.8
thyroid (late) 095.8
tongue 095.8
tonsil (lingual) 095.8
primary 091.2
secondary 091.3
trachea 095.8
tricuspid valve 093.23
tumor, brain 094.89
tunica vaginalis (late) 095.8
ulcer (any site) (early) (secondary) 091.3
late 095.9
perforating 095.9
foot 094.0
urethra (stricture) 095.8
urogenital 095.8
uterus 095.8
uveal tract (secondary) 091.50
late 095.8 *[363.13]*

Syphilis, syphilitic *(Continued)*
uveitis (secondary) 091.50
late 095.8 *[363.13]*
uvula (late) 095.8
perforated 095.8
vagina 091.0
late 095.8
valvulitis NEC 093.20
vascular 093.89
brain or cerebral 094.89
vein 093.89
cerebral 094.89
ventriculi 095.8
vesicae urinariae 095.8
viscera (abdominal) 095.2
secondary 091.69
vitreous (hemorrhage) (opacities) 095.8
vulva 091.0
late 095.8
secondary 091.3
Syphiloma 095.9
cardiovascular system 093.9
central nervous system 094.9
circulatory system 093.9
congenital 090.5
Syphilophobia 300.29
Syringadenoma (M8400/0) - *see also* Neoplasm, skin, benign
papillary (M8406/0) - *see* Neoplasm, skin, benign
Syringobulbia 336.0
Syringocarcinoma (M8400/3) - *see* Neoplasm, skin, malignant
Syringocystadenoma (M8400/0) - *see also* Neoplasm, skin, benign
papillary (M8406/0) - *see* Neoplasm, skin, benign
Syringocystoma (M8407/0) - *see* Neoplasm, skin, benign
Syringoma (M8407/0) - *see also* Neoplasm, skin, benign
chondroid (M8940/0) - *see* Neoplasm, by site, benign
Syringomyelia 336.0
Syringomyelitis 323.9
late effect - *see* category 326
Syringomyelocele (*see also* Spina bifida) 741.9
Syringopontia 336.0
System, systemic - *see also* condition
disease, combined - *see* Degeneration, combined
fibrosclerosing syndrome 710.8
inflammatory response syndrome (SIRS) 995.90
due to
infectious process 995.91
with acute organ dysfunction 995.92 ⇐
non-infectious process 995.93
with acute organ dysfunction 995.94 ⇐
lupus erythematosus 710.0
inhibitor 286.5

T

Tab - *see* Tag
Tabacism 989.84
Tabacosis 989.84
Tabardillo 080
  flea-borne 081.0
  louse-borne 080
Tabes, tabetic
  with
    central nervous system syphilis 094.0
    Charcôt's joint 094.0 *[713.5]*
    cord bladder 094.0
    crisis, viscera (any) 094.0
    paralysis, general 094.1
    paresis (general) 094.1
    perforating ulcer 094.0
  arthropathy 094.0 *[713.5]*
  bladder 094.0
  bone 094.0
  cerebrospinal 094.0
  congenital 090.40
  conjugal 094.0
  dorsalis 094.0
    neurosyphilis 094.0
  early 094.0
  juvenile 090.40
  latent 094.0
  mesenterica (*see also* Tuberculosis) 014.8
  paralysis insane, general 094.1
  peripheral (nonsyphilitic) 799.89
  spasmodic 094.0
    not dorsal or dorsalis 343.9
  syphilis (cerebrospinal) 094.0
Taboparalysis 094.1
Taboparesis (remission) 094.1
  with
    Charcôt's joint 094.1 *[713.5]*
    cord bladder 094.1
    perforating ulcer 094.1
  juvenile 090.40
Tache noir 923.20 ◀
Tachyalimentation 579.3
Tachyarrhythmia, tachyrhythmia - *see also* Tachycardia
  paroxysmal with sinus bradycardia 427.81
Tachycardia 785.0
  atrial 427.89
  auricular 427.89
  AV nodal re-entry (re-entrant) 427.89
  newborn 779.82
  nodal 427.89
    nonparoxysmal atrioventricular 426.89
  nonparoxysmal atrioventricular (nodal) 426.89
  paroxysmal 427.2
    with sinus bradycardia 427.81
    atrial (PAT) 427.0
      psychogenic 316 *[427.0]*
    atrioventricular (AV) 427.0
      psychogenic 316 *[427.0]*
    essential 427.2
    junctional 427.0
    nodal 427.0
    psychogenic 316 *[427.2]*
      atrial 316 *[427.0]*
      supraventricular 316 *[427.0]*
      ventricular 316 *[427.1]*
    supraventricular 427.0
      psychogenic 316 *[427.0]*
    ventricular 427.1
      psychogenic 316 *[427.1]*

Tachycardia *(Continued)*
  postoperative 997.1
  psychogenic 306.2
  sick sinus 427.81
  sinoauricular 427.89
  sinus 427.89
  supraventricular 427.89
  ventricular (paroxysmal) 427.1
    psychogenic 316 *[427.1]*
Tachygastria 536.8 ◀
Tachypnea 786.06
  hysterical 300.11
  newborn (idiopathic) (transitory) 770.6
  psychogenic 306.1
  transitory, of newborn 770.6
Taenia (infection) (infestation) (*see also* Infestation, taenia) 123.3
  diminuta 123.6
  echinococcal infestation (*see also* Echinococcus) 122.9
  nana 123.6
  saginata infestation 123.2
  solium (intestinal form) 123.0
    larval form 123.1
Taeniasis (intestine) (*see also* Infestation, taenia) 123.3
  saginata 123.2
  solium 123.0
Taenzer's disease 757.4
Tag (hypertrophied skin) (infected) 701.9
  adenoid 474.8
  anus 455.9
  endocardial (*see also* Endocarditis) 424.90
  hemorrhoidal 455.9
  hymen 623.8
  perineal 624.8
  preauricular 744.1
  rectum 455.9
  sentinel 455.9
  skin 701.9
    accessory 757.39
    anus 455.9
    congenital 757.39
    preauricular 744.1
    rectum 455.9
  tonsil 474.8
  urethra, urethral 599.84
  vulva 624.8
Tahyna fever 062.5
Takayasu (-Onishi) disease or syndrome (pulseless disease) 446.7
Takotsubo syndrome 429.83 ◀
Talc granuloma 728.82
  in operation wound 998.7
Talcosis 502
Talipes (congenital) 754.70
  acquired NEC 736.79
    planus 734
  asymmetric 754.79
    acquired 736.79
  calcaneovalgus 754.62
    acquired 736.76
  calcaneovarus 754.59
    acquired 736.76
  calcaneus 754.79
    acquired 736.76
  cavovarus 754.59
    acquired 736.75
  cavus 754.71
    acquired 736.73
  equinovalgus 754.69
    acquired 736.72
  equinovarus 754.51
    acquired 736.71

Talipes *(Continued)*
  equinus 754.79
    acquired, NEC 736.72
  percavus 754.71
    acquired 736.73
  planovalgus 754.69
    acquired 736.79
  planus (acquired) (any degree) 734
    congenital 754.61
    due to rickets 268.1
  valgus 754.60
    acquired 736.79
  varus 754.50
    acquired 736.79
Talma's disease 728.85
Talon noir 924.20 ◀
  hand 923.20 ◀
  heel 924.20 ◀
  toe 924.3 ◀
Tamponade heart (Rose's) (*see also* Pericarditis) 423.9
Tanapox 078.89
Tangier disease (familial high-density lipoprotein deficiency) 272.5
Tank ear 380.12
Tantrum (childhood) (*see also* Disturbance, conduct) 312.1
Tapeworm (infection) (infestation) (*see also* Infestation, tapeworm) 123.9
Tapia's syndrome 352.6
Tarantism 297.8
Target-oval cell anemia 282.49
Tarlov's cyst 355.9
Tarral-Besnier disease (pityriasis rubra pilaris) 696.4
Tarsalgia 729.2
Tarsal tunnel syndrome 355.5
Tarsitis (eyelid) 373.00
  syphilitic 095.8 *[373.00]*
  tuberculous (*see also* Tuberculosis) 017.0 *[373.4]*
Tartar (teeth) 523.6
Tattoo (mark) 709.09
Taurodontism 520.2
Taussig-Bing defect, heart, or syndrome (transposition, aorta and overriding pulmonary artery) 745.11
Tay's choroiditis 363.41
Tay-Sachs
  amaurotic familial idiocy 330.1
  disease 330.1
Taybi's syndrome (otopalatodigital) 759.89
Taylor's
  disease (diffuse idiopathic cutaneous atrophy) 701.8
  syndrome 625.5
Tear, torn (traumatic) - *see also* Wound, open, by site
  anus, anal (sphincter) 863.89
    with open wound in cavity 863.99
    complicating delivery 664.2
      with mucosa 664.3
    nontraumatic, nonpuerperal 565.0
  articular cartilage, old (*see also* Disorder, cartilage, articular) 718.0
  bladder
    with
      abortion - *see* Abortion, by type, with damage to pelvic organs
      ectopic pregnancy (*see also* categories 633.0–633.9) 639.2
      molar pregnancy (*see also* categories 630–632) 639.2

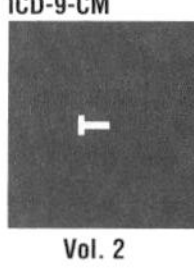
T

- **Tear, torn** *(Continued)*
  - bladder *(Continued)*
    - following
      - abortion 639.2
      - ectopic or molar pregnancy 639.2
    - obstetrical trauma 665.5
  - bowel
    - with
      - abortion - *see* Abortion, by type, with damage to pelvic organs
      - ectopic pregnancy (*see also* categories 633.0–633.9) 639.2
      - molar pregnancy (*see also* categories 630–632) 639.2
    - following
      - abortion 639.2
      - ectopic or molar pregnancy 639.2
    - obstetrical trauma 665.5
  - broad ligament
    - with
      - abortion - *see* Abortion, by type, with damage to pelvic organs
      - ectopic pregnancy (*see also* categories 633.0–633.9) 639.2
      - molar pregnancy (*see also* categories 630–632) 639.2
    - following
      - abortion 639.2
      - ectopic or molar pregnancy 639.2
    - obstetrical trauma 665.6
  - bucket handle (knee) (meniscus) - *see* Tear, meniscus
  - capsule
    - joint - *see* Sprain, by site
    - spleen - *see* Laceration, spleen, capsule
  - cartilage - *see also* Sprain, by site
    - articular, old (*see also* Disorder, cartilage, articular) 718.0
    - knee - *see* Tear, meniscus
    - semilunar (knee) (current injury) - *see* Tear, meniscus
  - cervix
    - with
      - abortion - *see* Abortion, by type, with damage to pelvic organs
      - ectopic pregnancy (*see also* categories 633.0–633.9) 639.2
      - molar pregnancy (*see also* categories 630–632) 639.2
    - following
      - abortion 639.2
      - ectopic or molar pregnancy 639.2
    - obstetrical trauma (current) 665.3
    - old 622.3
  - internal organ (abdomen, chest, or pelvis) - *see* Injury, internal, by site
  - ligament - *see also* Sprain, by site
    - with open wound - *see* Wound, open, by site
  - meniscus (knee) (current injury) 836.2
    - bucket handle 836.0
      - old 717.0
    - lateral 836.1
      - anterior horn 836.1
        - old 717.42
      - bucket handle 836.1
        - old 717.41
      - old 717.40
      - posterior horn 836.1
        - old 717.43
      - specified site NEC 836.1
        - old 717.49

- **Tear, torn** *(Continued)*
  - meniscus *(Continued)*
    - medial 836.0
      - anterior horn 836.0
        - old 717.1
      - bucket handle 836.0
        - old 717.0
      - old 717.3
      - posterior horn 836.0
        - old 717.2
    - old NEC 717.5
    - site other than knee - *see* Sprain, by site
  - muscle - *see also* Sprain, by site
    - with open wound - *see* Wound, open, by site
  - pelvic
    - floor, complicating delivery 664.1
    - organ NEC
      - with
        - abortion - *see* Abortion, by type, with damage to pelvic organs
        - ectopic pregnancy (*see also* categories 633.0–633.9) 639.2
        - molar pregnancy (*see also* categories 630–632) 639.2
      - following
        - abortion 639.2
        - ectopic or molar pregnancy 639.2
      - obstetrical trauma 665.5
  - perineum - *see also* Laceration, perineum
    - obstetrical trauma 665.5
  - periurethral tissue
    - with
      - abortion - *see* Abortion, by type, with damage to pelvic organs
      - ectopic pregnancy (*see also* categories 633.0–633.9) 639.2
      - molar pregnancy (*see also* categories 630–632) 639.2
    - following
      - abortion 639.2
      - ectopic or molar pregnancy 639.2
    - obstetrical trauma 665.5
  - rectovaginal septum - *see* Laceration, rectovaginal septum
  - retina, retinal (recent) (with detachment) 361.00
    - without detachment 361.30
    - dialysis (juvenile) (with detachment) 361.04
    - giant (with detachment) 361.03
    - horseshoe (without detachment) 361.32
    - multiple (with detachment) 361.02
      - without detachment 361.33
    - old
      - delimited (partial) 361.06
      - partial 361.06
      - total or subtotal 361.07
    - partial (without detachment)
      - giant 361.03
      - multiple defects 361.02
      - old (delimited) 361.06
      - single defect 361.01
    - round hole (without detachment) 361.31
    - single defect (with detachment) 361.01
    - total or subtotal (recent) 361.05
      - old 361.07
  - rotator cuff (traumatic) 840.4
    - current injury 840.4
    - degenerative 726.10
    - nontraumatic 727.61

- **Tear, torn** *(Continued)*
  - semilunar cartilage, knee (*see also* Tear, meniscus) 836.2
    - old 717.5
  - tendon - *see also* Sprain, by site
    - with open wound - *see* Wound, open, by site
  - tentorial, at birth 767.0
  - umbilical cord
    - affecting fetus or newborn 772.0
    - complicating delivery 663.8
  - urethra
    - with
      - abortion - *see* Abortion, by type, with damage to pelvic organs
      - ectopic pregnancy (*see also* categories 633.0–663.9) 639.2
      - molar pregnancy (*see also* categories 630–632) 639.2
    - following
      - abortion 639.2
      - ectopic or molar pregnancy 639.2
    - obstetrical trauma 665.5
  - uterus - *see* Injury, internal, uterus
  - vagina - *see* Laceration, vagina
  - vessel, from catheter 998.2
  - vulva, complicating delivery 664.0
- **Tear stone** 375.57
- **Teeth, tooth** - *see also* condition
  - grinding 306.8
  - prenatal 520.6 ◀
- **Teething** 520.7
  - syndrome 520.7
- **Tegmental syndrome** 344.89
- **Telangiectasia, telangiectasis** (verrucous) 448.9
  - ataxic (cerebellar) 334.8
  - familial 448.0
  - hemorrhagic, hereditary (congenital) (senile) 448.0
  - hereditary hemorrhagic 448.0
  - retina 362.15
  - spider 448.1
- **Telecanthus** (congenital) 743.63
- **Telescoped bowel or intestine** (*see also* Intussusception) 560.0
- **Teletherapy, adverse effect** NEC 990
- **Telogen effluvium** 704.02
- **Temperature**
  - body, high (of unknown origin) (*see also* Pyrexia) 780.6
  - cold, trauma from 991.9
    - newborn 778.2
    - specified effect NEC 991.8
  - high
    - body (of unknown origin) (*see also* Pyrexia) 780.6
    - trauma from - *see* Heat
- **Temper tantrum** (childhood) (*see also* Disturbance, conduct) 312.1
- **Temple** - *see* condition
- **Temporal** - *see also* condition
  - lobe syndrome 310.0
- **Temporomandibular joint-pain-dysfunction syndrome** 524.60
- **Temporosphenoidal** - *see* condition
- **Tendency**
  - bleeding (*see also* Defect, coagulation) 286.9
  - homosexual, ego-dystonic 302.0
  - paranoid 301.0
  - suicide 300.9

Tenderness
abdominal (generalized) (localized) 789.6
rebound 789.6
skin 782.0
Tendinitis, tendonitis (*see also* Tenosynovitis) 726.90
Achilles 726.71
adhesive 726.90
shoulder 726.0
calcific 727.82
shoulder 726.11
gluteal 726.5
patellar 726.64
peroneal 726.79
pes anserinus 726.61
psoas 726.5
tibialis (anterior) (posterior) 726.72
trochanteric 726.5
Tendon - *see* condition
Tendosynovitis - *see* Tenosynovitis
Tendovaginitis - *see* Tenosynovitis
Tenesmus 787.99
rectal 787.99
vesical 788.9
Tenia - *see* Taenia
Teniasis - *see* Taeniasis
Tennis elbow 726.32
Tenonitis - *see also* Tenosynovitis
eye (capsule) 376.04
Tenontosynovitis - *see* Tenosynovitis
Tenontothecitis - *see* Tenosynovitis
Tenophyte 727.9
Tenosynovitis 727.00
adhesive 726.90
shoulder 726.0
ankle 727.06
bicipital (calcifying) 726.12
buttock 727.09
due to crystals - *see* Arthritis, due to crystals
elbow 727.09
finger 727.05
foot 727.06
gonococcal 098.51
hand 727.05
hip 727.09
knee 727.09
radial styloid 727.04
shoulder 726.10
adhesive 726.0
spine 720.1
supraspinatus 726.10
toe 727.06
tuberculous - *see* Tuberculosis, tenosynovitis
wrist 727.05
Tenovaginitis - *see* Tenosynovitis
Tension
arterial, high (*see also* Hypertension) 401.9
without diagnosis of hypertension 796.2
headache 307.81
intraocular (elevated) 365.00
nervous 799.2
ocular (elevated) 365.00
pneumothorax 512.0
iatrogenic 512.1
postoperative 512.1
spontaneous 512.0
premenstrual 625.4
state 300.9
Tentorium - *see* condition

Teratencephalus 759.89
Teratism 759.7
Teratoblastoma (malignant) (M9080/3) - *see* Neoplasm, by site, malignant
Teratocarcinoma (M9081/3) - *see also* Neoplasm, by site, malignant
liver 155.0
Teratoma (solid) (M9080/1) - *see also* Neoplasm, by site, uncertain behavior
adult (cystic) (M9080/0) - *see* Neoplasm, by site, benign
and embryonal carcinoma, mixed (M9081/3) - *see* Neoplasm, by site, malignant
benign (M9080/0) - *see* Neoplasm, by site, benign
combined with choriocarcinoma (M9101/3) - *see* Neoplasm, by site, malignant
cystic (adult) (M9080/0) - *see* Neoplasm, by site, benign
differentiated type (M9080/0) - *see* Neoplasm, by site, benign
embryonal (M9080/3) - *see also* Neoplasm, by site, malignant
liver 155.0
fetal
sacral, causing fetopelvic disproportion 653.7
immature (M9080/3) - *see* Neoplasm, by site, malignant
liver (M9080/3) 155.0
adult, benign, cystic, differentiated type, or mature (M9080/0) 211.5
malignant (M9080/3) - *see also* Neoplasm, by site, malignant
anaplastic type (M9082/3) - *see* Neoplasm, by site, malignant
intermediate type (M9083/3) - *see* Neoplasm, by site, malignant
liver (M9080/3) 155.0
trophoblastic (M9102/3)
specified site - *see* Neoplasm, by site, malignant
unspecified site 186.9
undifferentiated type (M9082/3) - *see* Neoplasm, by site, malignant
mature (M9080/0) - *see* Neoplasm, by site, benign
ovary (M9080/0) 220
embryonal, immature, or malignant (M9080/3) 183.0
suprasellar (M9080/3) - *see* Neoplasm, by site, malignant
testis (M9080/3) 186.9
adult, benign, cystic, differentiated type or mature (M9080/0) 222.0
undescended 186.0
Terminal care V66.7
Termination
anomalous - *see also* Malposition, congenital
portal vein 747.49
right pulmonary vein 747.42
pregnancy (legal) (therapeutic) (*see* Abortion, legal) 635.9
fetus NEC 779.6
illegal (*see also* Abortion, illegal) 636.9
Ternidens diminutus infestation 127.7
Terrors, night (child) 307.46
Terry's syndrome 362.21
Tertiary - *see* condition
Tessellated fundus, retina (tigroid) 362.89

Test(s)
adequacy
hemodialysis V56.31
peritoneal dialysis V56.32
AIDS virus V72.6
allergen V72.7
bacterial disease NEC (*see also* Screening, by name of disease) V74.9
basal metabolic rate V72.6
blood-alcohol V70.4
blood-drug V70.4
for therapeutic drug monitoring V58.83
blood typing V72.86
Rh typing V72.86 ◀
developmental, infant or child V20.2
Dick V74.8
fertility V26.21
genetic ⬅
female V26.32 ◀
for genetic disease carrier status ⬅
female V26.31 ◀
male V26.34 ◀
male V26.39 ◀
hearing V72.19 ⬅
following failed hearing screening V72.11 ◀
HIV V72.6
human immunodeficiency virus V72.6
Kveim V82.89
laboratory V72.6
for medicolegal reason V70.4
male partner of habitual aborter V26.35 ◀
Mantoux (for tuberculosis) V74.1
mycotic organism V75.4
parasitic agent NEC V75.8
paternity V70.4
peritoneal equilibration V56.32
pregnancy
positive result V72.42
first pregnancy V72.42
negative result V72.41
unconfirmed V72.40
preoperative V72.84
cardiovascular V72.81
respiratory V72.82
specified NEC V72.83
procreative management NEC V26.29
genetic disease carrier status ◀
female V26.31 ◀
male V26.34 ◀
Rh typing V72.86 ◀
sarcoidosis V82.89
Schick V74.3
Schultz-Charlton V74.8
skin, diagnostic
allergy V72.7
bacterial agent NEC (*see also* Screening, by name of disease) V74.9
Dick V74.8
hypersensitivity V72.7
Kveim V82.89
Mantoux V74.1
mycotic organism V75.4
parasitic agent NEC V75.8
sarcoidosis V82.89
Schick V74.3
Schultz-Charlton V74.8
st()tuberculin V74.1
specified type NEC V72.85
tuberculin V74.1
vision V72.0

ICD-9-CM
T
Vol. 2

Test(s) *(Continued)*
Wassermann
positive (*see also* Serology for syphilis, positive) 097.1
false 795.6
Testicle, testicular, testis - *see also* condition
feminization (syndrome) 259.5
Tetanus, tetanic (cephalic) (convulsions) 037
with
abortion - *see* Abortion, by type, with sepsis
ectopic pregnancy (*see also* categories 633.0–633.9) 639.0
molar pregnancy (*see* categories 630–632) 639.0
following
abortion 639.0
ectopic or molar pregnancy 639.0
Tetanus, tetanic *(Continued)*
inoculation V03.7
reaction (due to serum) - *see* Complications, vaccination
neonatorum 771.3
puerperal, postpartum, childbirth 670
Tetany, tetanic 781.7
alkalosis 276.3
associated with rickets 268.0
convulsions 781.7
hysterical 300.11
functional (hysterical) 300.11
hyperkinetic 781.7
hysterical 300.11
hyperpnea 786.01
hysterical 300.11
psychogenic 306.1
hyperventilation 786.01
hysterical 300.11
psychogenic 306.1
hypocalcemic, neonatal 775.4
hysterical 300.11
neonatal 775.4
parathyroid (gland) 252.1
parathyroprival 252.1
postoperative 252.1
postthyroidectomy 252.1
pseudotetany 781.7
hysterical 300.11
psychogenic 306.1
specified as conversion reaction 300.11
Tetralogy of Fallot 745.2
Tetraplegia - *see* Quadriplegia
Thailand hemorrhagic fever 065.4
Thalassanemia 282.49
Thalassemia (alpha) (beta) (disease) (Hb-C) (Hb-D) (Hb-E) (Hb-H) (Hb-I) (high fetal gene) (high fetal hemoglobin) (intermedia) (major) (minima) (minor) (mixed) (trait) (with other hemoglobinopathy) 282.49
Hb-S (without crisis) 282.41
with
crisis 282.42
vaso-occlusive pain 282.42
sickle-cell (without crisis) 282.41
with
crisis 282.42
vaso-occlusive pain 282.42
Thalassemic variants 282.49
Thaysen-Gee disease (nontropical sprue) 579.0
Thecoma (M8600/0) 220
malignant (M8600/3) 183.0
Thelarche, precocious 259.1
Thelitis 611.0
puerperal, postpartum 675.0
Therapeutic - *see* condition
Therapy V57.9
blood transfusion, without reported diagnosis V58.2
breathing V57.0
chemotherapy, antineoplastic V58.11
fluoride V07.31
prophylactic NEC V07.39
dialysis (intermittent) (treatment)
extracorporeal V56.0
peritoneal V56.8
renal V56.0
specified type NEC V56.8
exercise NEC V57.1
breathing V57.0
extracorporeal dialysis (renal) V56.0
fluoride prophylaxis V07.31
Therapy *(Continued)*
hemodialysis V56.0
hormone replacement (postmenopausal) V07.4
immunotherapy antineoplastic V58.12
long term oxygen therapy V46.2
occupational V57.21
orthoptic V57.4
orthotic V57.81
peritoneal dialysis V56.8
physical NEC V57.1
postmenopausal hormone replacement V07.4
radiation V58.0
speech V57.3
vocational V57.22
Thermalgesia 782.0
Thermalgia 782.0
Thermanalgesia 782.0
Thermanesthesia 782.0
Thermic - *see* condition
Thermography (abnormal) 793.99 ⇐
breast 793.89
Thermoplegia 992.0
Thesaurismosis
amyloid 277.39 ⇐
bilirubin 277.4
calcium 275.40
cystine 270.0
glycogen (*see also* Disease, glycogen storage) 271.0
kerasin 272.7
lipoid 272.7
melanin 255.4
phosphatide 272.7
urate 274.9
Thiaminic deficiency 265.1
with beriberi 265.0
Thibierge-Weissenbach syndrome (cutaneous systemic sclerosis) 710.1
Thickened endometrium 793.5
Thickening
bone 733.99
extremity 733.99
breast 611.79
hymen 623.3
larynx 478.79
nail 703.8
congenital 757.5
periosteal 733.99
pleura (*see also* Pleurisy) 511.0
skin 782.8
subepiglottic 478.79
tongue 529.8
valve, heart - *see* Endocarditis
Thiele syndrome 724.6
Thigh - *see* condition
Thinning vertebra (*see also* Osteoporosis) 733.00
Thirst, excessive 783.5
due to deprivation of water 994.3
Thomsen's disease 359.2
Thomson's disease (congenital poikiloderma) 757.33
Thoracic - *see also* condition
kidney 753.3
outlet syndrome 353.0
stomach - *see* Hernia, diaphragm
Thoracogastroschisis (congenital) 759.89
Thoracopagus 759.4
Thoracoschisis 756.3
Thoracoscopic surgical procedure converted to open procedure V64.42
Thorax - *see* condition
Thorn's syndrome (*see also* Disease, renal) 593.9
Thornwaldt's, Tornwaldt's
bursitis (pharyngeal) 478.29
cyst 478.26
disease (pharyngeal bursitis) 478.29
Thorson-Biörck syndrome (malignant carcinoid) 259.2
Threadworm (infection) (infestation) 127.4
Threatened
abortion or miscarriage 640.0
with subsequent abortion (*see also* Abortion, spontaneous) 634.9
affecting fetus 762.1
labor 644.1
affecting fetus or newborn 761.8
premature 644.0
miscarriage 640.0
affecting fetus 762.1
premature
delivery 644.2
affecting fetus or newborn 761.8
labor 644.0
before 22 completed weeks of gestation 640.0
Three-day fever 066.0
Threshers' lung 495.0
Thrix annulata (congenital) 757.4
Throat - *see* condition
Thrombasthenia (Glanzmann's) (hemorrhagic) (hereditary) 287.1
Thromboangiitis 443.1
obliterans (general) 443.1
cerebral 437.1
vessels
brain 437.1
spinal cord 437.1
Thromboarteritis - *see* Arteritis
Thromboasthenia (Glanzmann's) (hemorrhagic) (hereditary) 287.1
Thrombocytasthenia (Glanzmann's) 287.1
Thrombocythemia (primary) (M9962/1) 238.71 ⇐
essential 238.71 ◀
hemorrhagic 238.71 ◀
idiopathic (hemorrhagic) (M9962/1) 238.71 ⇐
Thrombocytopathy (dystrophic) (granulopenic) 287.1
Thrombocytopenia, thrombocytopenic 287.5
with
absent radii (TAR) syndrome 287.33
giant hemangioma 287.39
amegakaryocytic, congenital 287.33

- **Thrombocytopenia, thrombocytopenic** *(Continued)*
  - congenital 287.33
  - cyclic 287.39
  - dilutional 287.4
  - due to
    - drugs 287.4
    - extracorporeal circulation of blood 287.4
    - massive blood transfusion 287.4
    - platelet alloimmunization 287.4
  - essential 287.30
  - hereditary 287.33
  - Kasabach-Merritt 287.39
  - neonatal, transitory 776.1
    - due to
      - exchange transfusion 776.1
      - idiopathic maternal thrombocytopenia 776.1
      - isoimmunization 776.1
  - primary 287.30
  - puerperal, postpartum 666.3
  - purpura (*see also* Purpura, thrombocytopenic) 287.30
    - thrombotic 446.6
  - secondary 287.4
  - sex-linked 287.39
- **Thrombocytosis** 238.71 (Revised)
  - essential 238.71 ◀
  - primary 238.71 ◀
- **Thromboembolism** - *see* Embolism
- **Thrombopathy** (Bernard-Soulier) 287.1
  - constitutional 286.4
  - Willebrand-Jürgens (angiohemophilia) 286.4
- **Thrombopenia** (*see also* Thrombocytopenia) 287.5
- **Thrombophlebitis** 451.9
  - antecubital vein 451.82
  - antepartum (superficial) 671.2
    - affecting fetus or newborn 760.3
    - deep 671.3
  - arm 451.89
    - deep 451.83
    - superficial 451.82
  - breast, superficial 451.89
  - cavernous (venous) sinus - *see* Thrombophlebitis, intracranial venous sinus
  - cephalic vein 451.82
  - cerebral (sinus) (vein) 325
    - late effect - *see* category 326
    - nonpyogenic 437.6
      - in pregnancy or puerperium 671.5
      - late effect - *see* Late effect(s) (of) cerebrovascular disease
  - due to implanted device - *see* Complications, due to (presence of) any device, implant, or graft classified to 996.0–996.5 NEC
  - during or resulting from a procedure NEC 997.2
  - femoral 451.11
  - femoropopliteal 451.19
  - following infusion, perfusion, or transfusion 999.2
  - hepatic (vein) 451.89
  - idiopathic, recurrent 453.1
  - iliac vein 451.81
  - iliofemoral 451.11
  - intracranial venous sinus (any) 325
    - late effect - *see* category 326
    - nonpyogenic 437.6
      - in pregnancy or puerperium 671.5
      - late effect - *see* Late effect(s) (of) cerebrovascular disease
- **Thrombophlebitis** *(Continued)*
  - jugular vein 451.89
  - lateral (venous) sinus - *see* Thrombophlebitis, intracranial venous sinus
  - leg 451.2
    - deep (vessels) 451.19
      - femoral vein 451.11
      - specified vessel NEC 451.19
    - superficial (vessels) 451.0
      - femoral vein 451.11
  - longitudinal (venous) sinus - *see* Thrombophlebitis, intracranial venous sinus
  - lower extremity 451.2
    - deep (vessels) 451.19
      - femoral vein 451.11
      - specified vessel NEC 451.19
    - superficial (vessels) 451.0
  - migrans, migrating 453.1
  - pelvic
    - with
      - abortion - *see* Abortion, by type, with sepsis
      - ectopic pregnancy (*see also* categories 633.0–633.9) 639.0
      - molar pregnancy (*see also* categories 630–632) 639.0
    - following
      - abortion 639.0
      - ectopic or molar pregnancy 639.0
    - puerperal 671.4
  - popliteal vein 451.19
  - portal (vein) 572.1
  - postoperative 997.2
  - pregnancy (superficial) 671.2
    - affecting fetus or newborn 760.3
    - deep 671.3
  - puerperal, postpartum, childbirth (extremities) (superficial) 671.2
    - deep 671.4
    - pelvic 671.4
    - specified site NEC 671.5
  - radial vein 451.82
  - saphenous (greater) (lesser) 451.0
  - sinus (intracranial) - *see* Thrombophlebitis, intracranial venous sinus
  - specified site NEC 451.89
  - tibial vein 451.19
- **Thrombosis, thrombotic** (marantic) (multiple) (progressive) (septic) (vein) (vessel) 453.9
  - with childbirth or during the puerperium - *see* Thrombosis, puerperal, postpartum
  - without endocarditis 429.89 ◀
  - antepartum - *see* Thrombosis, pregnancy
  - aorta, aortic 444.1
    - abdominal 444.0
    - bifurcation 444.0
    - saddle 444.0
    - terminal 444.0
    - thoracic 444.1
    - valve - *see* Endocarditis, aortic
  - apoplexy (*see also* Thrombosis, brain) 434.0
    - late effect - *see* Late effect(s) (of) cerebrovascular disease
  - appendix, septic - *see* Appendicitis, acute
  - arteriolar-capillary platelet, disseminated 446.6
  - artery, arteries (postinfectional) 444.9
    - auditory, internal 433.8
- **Thrombosis, thrombotic** *(Continued)*
  - artery, arteries *(Continued)*
    - basilar (*see also* Occlusion, artery, basilar) 433.0
    - carotid (common) (internal) (*see also* Occlusion, artery, carotid) 433.1
      - with other precerebral artery 433.3
    - cerebellar (anterior inferior) (posterior inferior) (superior) 433.8
    - cerebral (*see also* Thrombosis, brain) 434.0
    - choroidal (anterior) 433.8
    - communicating posterior 433.8
    - coronary (*see also* Infarct, myocardium) 410.9
      - without myocardial infarction 411.81
      - due to syphilis 093.89
      - healed or specified as old 412
    - extremities 444.22
      - lower 444.22
      - upper 444.21
    - femoral 444.22
    - hepatic 444.89
    - hypophyseal 433.8
    - meningeal, anterior or posterior 433.8
    - mesenteric (with gangrene) 557.0
    - ophthalmic (*see also* Occlusion, retina) 362.30
    - pontine 433.8
    - popliteal 444.22
    - precerebral - *see* Occlusion, artery, precerebral NEC
    - pulmonary 415.19
      - iatrogenic 415.11
      - postoperative 415.11
    - renal 593.81
    - retinal (*see also* Occlusion, retina) 362.30
    - specified site NEC 444.89
    - spinal, anterior or posterior 433.8
    - traumatic (complication) (early) (*see also* Injury, blood vessel, by site) 904.9
    - vertebral (*see also* Occlusion, artery, vertebral) 433.2
      - with other precerebral artery 433.3
  - atrial (endocardial) 424.90
    - due to syphilis 093.89
  - auricular (*see also* Infarct, myocardium) 410.9
  - axillary (vein) 453.8
  - basilar (artery) (*see also* Occlusion, artery, basilar) 433.0
  - bland NEC 453.9
  - brain (artery) (stem) 434.0
    - due to syphilis 094.89
    - iatrogenic 997.02
    - late effect - *see* Late effect(s) (of) cerebrovascular disease
    - postoperative 997.02
    - puerperal, postpartum, childbirth 674.0
    - sinus (*see also* Thrombosis, intracranial venous sinus) 325
  - capillary 448.9
    - arteriolar, generalized 446.6
  - cardiac (*see also* Infarct, myocardium) 410.9
    - due to syphilis 093.89
    - healed or specified as old 412
    - valve - *see* Endocarditis
  - carotid (artery) (common) (internal) (*see also* Occlusion, artery, carotid) 433.1
    - with other precerebral artery 433.3

ICD-9-CM
T
Vol. 2

Thrombosis, thrombotic *(Continued)*
cavernous sinus (venous) - *see* Thrombosis, intracranial venous sinus
cerebellar artery (anterior inferior) (posterior inferior) (superior) 433.8
late effect - *see* Late effect(s) (of) cerebrovascular disease
cerebral (arteries) (*see also* Thrombosis, brain) 434.0
late effect - *see* Late effect(s) (of) cerebrovascular disease
coronary (artery) (*see also* Infarct, myocardium) 410.9
without myocardial infarction 411.81
due to syphilis 093.89
healed or specified as old 412
corpus cavernosum 607.82
cortical (*see also* Thrombosis, brain) 434.0
due to (presence of) any device, implant, or graft classifiable to 996.0–996.5 - *see* Complications, due to (presence of) any device, implant, or graft classified to 996.0–996.5 NEC
effort 453.8
endocardial - *see* Infarct, myocardium
eye (*see also* Occlusion, retina) 362.30
femoral (vein) 453.8
with inflammation or phlebitis 451.11
artery 444.22
deep 453.41
genital organ, male 608.83
heart (chamber) (*see also* Infarct, myocardium) 410.9
hepatic (vein) 453.0
artery 444.89
infectional or septic 572.1
iliac (vein) 453.8
with inflammation or phlebitis 451.81
artery (common) (external) (internal) 444.81
inflammation, vein - *see* Thrombophlebitis
internal carotid artery (*see also* Occlusion, artery, carotid) 433.1
with other precerebral artery 433.3
intestine (with gangrene) 557.0
intracranial (*see also* Thrombosis, brain) 434.0
venous sinus (any) 325
nonpyogenic origin 437.6
in pregnancy or puerperium 671.5
intramural (*see also* Infarct, myocardium) 410.9
without
cardiac condition 429.89
coronary artery disease 429.89
myocardial infarction 429.89
healed or specified as old 412
jugular (bulb) 453.8
kidney 593.81
artery 593.81
lateral sinus (venous) - *see* Thrombosis, intracranial venous sinus
leg 453.8
with inflammation or phlebitis - *see* Thrombophlebitis
deep (vessels) 453.40
lower (distal) 453.42
upper (proximal) 453.41
superficial (vessels) 453.8

Thrombosis, thrombotic *(Continued)*
liver (venous) 453.0
artery 444.89
infectional or septic 572.1
portal vein 452
longitudinal sinus (venous) - *see* Thrombosis, intracranial venous sinus
lower extremity 453.8
deep vessels 453.40
calf 453.42
distal (lower leg) 453.42
femoral 453.41
iliac 453.41
lower leg 453.42
peroneal 453.42
popliteal 453.41
proximal (upper leg) 453.41
thigh 453.41
tibial 453.42
lung 415.19
iatrogenic 415.11
postoperative 415.11
marantic, dural sinus 437.6
meninges (brain) (*see also* Thrombosis, brain) 434.0
mesenteric (artery) (with gangrene) 557.0
vein (inferior) (superior) 557.0
mitral - *see* Insufficiency, mitral
mural (heart chamber) (*see also* Infarct, myocardium) 410.9
without
without
cardiac condition 429.89
coronary artery disease 429.89
myocardial infarction 429.89
due to syphilis 093.89
following myocardial infarction 429.79
healed or specified as old 412
omentum (with gangrene) 557.0
ophthalmic (artery) (*see also* Occlusion, retina) 362.30
pampiniform plexus (male) 608.83
female 620.8
parietal (*see also* Infarct, myocardium) 410.9
penis, penile 607.82
peripheral arteries 444.22
lower 444.22
upper 444.21
platelet 446.6
portal 452
due to syphilis 093.89
infectional or septic 572.1
precerebral artery - *see also* Occlusion, artery, precerebral NEC
pregnancy 671.9
deep (vein) 671.3
superficial (vein) 671.2
puerperal, postpartum, childbirth 671.9
brain (artery) 674.0
venous 671.5
cardiac 674.8
cerebral (artery) 674.0
venous 671.5
deep (vein) 671.4
intracranial sinus (nonpyogenic) (venous) 671.5
pelvic 671.4
pulmonary (artery) 673.2
specified site NEC 671.5
superficial 671.2

Thrombosis, thrombotic *(Continued)*
pulmonary (artery) (vein) 415.19
iatrogenic 415.11
postoperative 415.11
renal (artery) 593.81
vein 453.3
resulting from presence of shunt or other internal prosthetic device - *see* Complications, due to (presence of) any device, implant, or graft classifiable to 996.0–996.5 NEC
retina, retinal (artery) 362.30
arterial branch 362.32
central 362.31
partial 362.33
vein
central 362.35
tributary (branch) 362.36
scrotum 608.83
seminal vesicle 608.83
sigmoid (venous) sinus (*see* Thrombosis, intracranial venous sinus) 325
silent NEC 453.9
sinus, intracranial (venous) (any) (*see also* Thrombosis, intracranial venous sinus) 325
softening, brain (*see also* Thrombosis, brain) 434.0
specified site NEC 453.8
spermatic cord 608.83
spinal cord 336.1
due to syphilis 094.89
in pregnancy or puerperium 671.5
pyogenic origin 324.1
late effect - *see* category 326
spleen, splenic 289.59
artery 444.89
testis 608.83
traumatic (complication) (early) (*see also* Injury, blood vessel, by site) 904.9
tricuspid - *see* Endocarditis, tricuspid
tumor - *see* Neoplasm, by site
tunica vaginalis 608.83
umbilical cord (vessels) 663.6
affecting fetus or newborn 762.6
vas deferens 608.83
vein
deep 453.40
lower extremity - *see* Thrombosis, lower extremity
vena cava (inferior) (superior) 453.2
Thrombus - *see* Thrombosis
Thrush 112.0
newborn 771.7
Thumb - *see also* condition
gamekeeper's 842.12
sucking (child problem) 307.9
Thygeson's superficial punctate keratitis 370.21
Thymergasia (*see also* Psychosis, affective) 296.80
Thymitis 254.8
Thymoma (benign) (M8580/0) 212.6
malignant (M8580/3) 164.0
Thymus, thymic (gland) - *see* condition
Thyrocele (*see also* Goiter) 240.9
Thyroglossal - *see also* condition
cyst 759.2
duct, persistent 759.2
Thyroid (body) (gland) - *see also* condition
hormone resistance 246.8 ◀
lingual 759.2
Thyroiditis 245.9
acute (pyogenic) (suppurative) 245.0
nonsuppurative 245.0

Thyroiditis *(Continued)*
autoimmune 245.2
chronic (nonspecific) (sclerosing) 245.8
fibrous 245.3
lymphadenoid 245.2
lymphocytic 245.2
lymphoid 245.2
complicating pregnancy, childbirth, or puerperium 648.1
de Quervain's (subacute granulomatous) 245.1
fibrous (chronic) 245.3
giant (cell) (follicular) 245.1
granulomatous (de Quervain's) (subacute) 245.1
Hashimoto's (struma lymphomatosa) 245.2
iatrogenic 245.4
invasive (fibrous) 245.3
ligneous 245.3
lymphocytic (chronic) 245.2
lymphoid 245.2
lymphomatous 245.2
pseudotuberculous 245.1
pyogenic 245.0
radiation 245.4
Riedel's (ligneous) 245.3
subacute 245.1
suppurative 245.0
tuberculous (*see also* Tuberculosis) 017.5
viral 245.1
woody 245.3
Thyrolingual duct, persistent 759.2
Thyromegaly 240.9
Thyrotoxic
crisis or storm (*see also* Thyrotoxicosis) 242.9
heart failure (*see also* Thyrotoxicosis) 242.9 *[425.7]*
Thyrotoxicosis 242.9

Note Use the following fifth-digit subclassification with category 242:

0 without mention of thyrotoxic crisis or storm
1 with mention of thyrotoxic crisis or storm

with
goiter (diffuse) 242.0
adenomatous 242.3
multinodular 242.2
uninodular 242.1
nodular 242.3
multinodular 242.2
uninodular 242.1
infiltrative
dermopathy 242.0
ophthalmopathy 242.0
thyroid acropachy 242.0
complicating pregnancy, childbirth, or puerperium 648.1
due to
ectopic thyroid nodule 242.4
ingestion of (excessive) thyroid material 242.8
specified cause NEC 242.8
factitia 242.8
heart 242.9 *[425.7]*
neonatal (transient) 775.3
TIA (transient ischemic attack) 435.9
with transient neurologic deficit 435.9
late effect - *see* Late effect(s) (of) cerebrovascular disease
Tibia vara 732.4
Tic 307.20
breathing 307.20
child problem 307.21
compulsive 307.22
convulsive 307.20
degenerative (generalized) (localized) 333.3
facial 351.8
douloureux (*see also* Neuralgia, trigeminal) 350.1
atypical 350.2
habit 307.20
chronic (motor or vocal) 307.22
transient (of childhood) 307.21
lid 307.20
transient (of childhood) 307.21
motor-verbal 307.23
occupational 300.89
orbicularis 307.20
transient (of childhood) 307.21
organic origin 333.3
postchoreic - *see* Chorea
psychogenic 307.20
compulsive 307.22
salaam 781.0
spasm 307.20
chronic (motor or vocal) 307.22
transient (of childhood) 307.21
Tick (-borne) fever NEC 066.1
American mountain 066.1
Colorado 066.1
hemorrhagic NEC 065.3
Crimean 065.0
Kyasanur Forest 065.2
Omsk 065.1
Tick *(Continued)*
mountain 066.1
nonexanthematous 066.1
Tick-bite fever NEC 066.1
African 087.1
Colorado (virus) 066.1
Rocky Mountain 082.0
Tick paralysis 989.5
Tics and spasms, compulsive 307.22
Tietze's disease or syndrome 733.6
Tight, tightness
anus 564.89
chest 786.59
fascia (lata) 728.9
foreskin (congenital) 605
hymen 623.3
introitus (acquired) (congenital) 623.3
rectal sphincter 564.89
tendon 727.81
Achilles (heel) 727.81
urethral sphincter 598.9
Tilting vertebra 737.9
Timidity, child 313.21
Tinea (intersecta) (tarsi) 110.9
amiantacea 110.0
asbestina 110.0
barbae 110.0
beard 110.0
black dot 110.0
blanca 111.2
capitis 110.0
corporis 110.5
cruris 110.3
decalvans 704.09
flava 111.0
foot 110.4
furfuracea 111.0
imbricata (Tokelau) 110.5
Tinea *(Continued)*
lepothrix 039.0
manuum 110.2
microsporic (*see also* Dermatophytosis) 110.9
nigra 111.1
nodosa 111.2
pedis 110.4
scalp 110.0
specified site NEC 110.8
sycosis 110.0
tonsurans 110.0
trichophytic (*see also* Dermatophytosis) 110.9
unguium 110.1
versicolor 111.0
Tingling sensation (*see also* Disturbance, sensation) 782.0
Tin-miners' lung 503
Tinnitus (aurium) 388.30
audible 388.32
objective 388.32
subjective 388.31
Tipped, teeth 524.33 ◀
Tipping
pelvis 738.6
with disproportion (fetopelvic) 653.0
affecting fetus or newborn 763.1
causing obstructed labor 660.1
affecting fetus or newborn 763.1
teeth 524.33
Tiredness 780.79
Tissue - *see* condition
Tobacco
abuse (affecting health) NEC (*see also* Abuse, drugs, nondependent) 305.1
heart 989.84
use disorder complicating pregnancy, childbirth, or the puerperium 649.0 ◀
Tobias' syndrome (carcinoma, pulmonary apex) (M8010/3) 162.3
Tocopherol deficiency 269.1
Todd's
cirrhosis - *see* Cirrhosis, biliary
paralysis (postepileptic transitory paralysis) 344.89
Toe - *see* condition
Toilet, artificial opening (*see also* Attention to, artificial, opening) V55.9
Tokelau ringworm 110.5
Tollwut 071
Tolosa-Hunt syndrome 378.55
Tommaselli's disease
correct substance properly administered 599.7
overdose or wrong substance given or taken 961.4
Tongue - *see also* condition
worms 134.1
Tongue tie 750.0
Toni-Fanconi syndrome (cystinosis) 270.0
Tonic pupil 379.46
Tonsil - *see* condition
Tonsillitis (acute) (catarrhal) (croupous) (follicular) (gangrenous) (infective) (lacunar) (lingual) (malignant) (membranous) (phlegmonous) (pneumococcal) (pseudomembranous) (purulent) (septic) (staphylococcal) (subacute) (suppurative) (toxic) (ulcerative) (vesicular) (viral) 463
with influenza, flu, or grippe 487.1
chronic 474.00
diphtheritic (membranous) 032.0

Tonsillitis *(Continued)*
  hypertrophic 474.00
  influenzal 487.1
  parenchymatous 475
  streptococcal 034.0
  tuberculous (*see also* Tuberculosis) 012.8
  Vincent's 101
Tonsillopharyngitis 465.8
Tooth, teeth - *see* condition
Toothache 525.9
Topagnosis 782.0
Tophi (gouty) 274.0
  ear 274.81
  heart 274.82
  specified site NEC 274.82
Torn - *see* Tear, torn
Tornwaldt's bursitis (disease) (pharyngeal bursitis) 478.29
  cyst 478.26
Torpid liver 573.9
Torsion
  accessory tube 620.5
  adnexa (female) 620.5
  aorta (congenital) 747.29
    acquired 447.1
  appendix ⬅
    epididymis 608.24 ◀
    testis 608.23 ◀
  bile duct 576.8
    with calculus, choledocholithiasis or stones - *see* Choledocholithiasis
    congenital 751.69
  bowel, colon, or intestine 560.2
  cervix - *see* Malposition, uterus ⬅
  duodenum 537.3
  dystonia - *see* Dystonia, torsion
  epididymis 608.24 ⬅
    appendix 608.24 ⬅
  fallopian tube 620.5
  gallbladder (*see also* Disease, gallbladder) 575.8
    congenital 751.69
Torsion *(Continued)*
  gastric 537.89
  hydatid of Morgagni (female) 620.5
  kidney (pedicle) 593.89
  Meckel's diverticulum (congenital) 751.0
  mesentery 560.2
  omentum 560.2
  organ or site, congenital NEC - *see* Anomaly, specified type NEC
  ovary (pedicle) 620.5
    congenital 752.0
  oviduct 620.5
  penis 607.89
    congenital 752.69
  renal 593.89
  spasm - *see* Dystonia, torsion
  spermatic cord 608.22 ⬅
    extravaginal 608.21 ◀
    intravaginal 608.22 ◀
  spleen 289.59
  testicle, testis 608.20 ⬅
    appendix 608.23 ◀
  tibia 736.89
  umbilical cord - *see* Compression, umbilical cord
  uterus (*see also* Malposition, uterus) 621.6
Torticollis (intermittent) (spastic) 723.5
  congenital 754.1
    sternomastoid 754.1
  due to birth injury 767.8
Torticollis *(Continued)*
  hysterical 300.11
  ocular 781.93
  psychogenic 306.0
    specified as conversion reaction 300.11
  rheumatic 723.5
  rheumatoid 714.0
  spasmodic 333.83
  traumatic, current NEC 847.0
Tortuous
  artery 447.1
  fallopian tube 752.19
  organ or site, congenital NEC - *see* Distortion
  renal vessel (congenital) 747.62
  retina vessel (congenital) 743.58
    acquired 362.17
  ureter 593.4
  urethra 599.84
  vein - *see* Varicose, vein
Torula, torular (infection) 117.5
  histolytica 117.5
  lung 117.5
Torulosis 117.5
Torus
  fracture
    fibula 823.41
      with tibia 823.42
    radius 813.45
    tibia 823.40
      with fibula 823.42
  mandibularis 526.81
  palatinus 526.81
Touch, vitreous 997.99
Touraine's syndrome (hereditary osteo-onychodysplasia) 756.89
Touraine-Solente-Golé syndrome (acropachyderma) 757.39
Tourette's disease (motor-verbal tic) 307.23
Tower skull 756.0
  with exophthalmos 756.0
Toxemia 799.89
  with
    abortion - *see* Abortion, by type, with toxemia
  bacterial - *see* Septicemia
  biliary (*see also* Disease, biliary) 576.8
  burn - *see* Burn, by site
  congenital NEC 779.89
  eclamptic 642.6
    with pre-existing hypertension 642.7
  erysipelatous (*see also* Erysipelas) 035
  fatigue 799.89
  fetus or newborn NEC 779.89
  food (*see also* Poisoning, food) 005.9
  gastric 537.89
  gastrointestinal 558.2
  intestinal 558.2
  kidney (*see also* Disease, renal) 593.9
  lung 518.89
  malarial NEC (*see also* Malaria) 084.6
  maternal (of pregnancy), affecting fetus or newborn 760.0
  myocardial - *see* Myocarditis, toxic
  of pregnancy (mild) (pre-eclamptic) 642.4
    with
      convulsions 642.6
      pre-existing hypertension 642.7
    affecting fetus or newborn 760.0
    severe 642.5
Toxemia *(Continued)*
  pre-eclamptic - *see* Toxemia, of pregnancy
  puerperal, postpartum - *see* Toxemia, of pregnancy
  pulmonary 518.89
  renal (*see also* Disease, renal) 593.9
  septic (*see also* Septicemia) 038.9
  small intestine 558.2
  staphylococcal 038.10
    aureus 038.11
    due to food 005.0
    specified organism NEC 038.19
  stasis 799.89
  stomach 537.89
  uremic (*see also* Uremia) 586
  urinary 586
Toxemica cerebropathia psychica (nonalcoholic) 294.0
  alcoholic 291.1
Toxic (poisoning) - *see also* condition
  from drug or poison - *see* Table of Drugs and Chemicals
  oil syndrome 710.5
  shock syndrome 040.82
  thyroid (gland) (*see also* Thyrotoxicosis) 242.9
Toxicemia - *see* Toxemia
Toxicity
  dilantin
    asymptomatic 796.0
    symptomatic -*see* Table of Drugs and Chemicals
  drug
    asymptomatic 796.0
    symptomatic - *see* Table of Drugs and Chemicals
  fava bean 282.2
  from drug or poison
    asymptomatic 796.0
    symptomatic - *see* Table of Drugs and Chemicals
Toxicosis (*see also* Toxemia) 799.89
  capillary, hemorrhagic 287.0
Toxinfection 799.89
  gastrointestinal 558.2
Toxocariasis 128.0
Toxoplasma infection, generalized 130.9
Toxoplasmosis (acquired) 130.9
  with pneumonia 130.4
  congenital, active 771.2
  disseminated (multisystemic) 130.8
  maternal
    with suspected damage to fetus affecting management of pregnancy 655.4
    affecting fetus or newborn 760.2
      manifest toxoplasmosis in fetus or newborn 771.2
  multiple sites 130.8
  multisystemic disseminated 130.8
  specified site NEC 130.7
Trabeculation, bladder 596.8
Trachea - *see* condition
Tracheitis (acute) (catarrhal) (infantile) (membranous) (plastic) (pneumococcal) (septic) (suppurative) (viral) 464.10
  with
    bronchitis 490
      acute or subacute 466.0
      chronic 491.8
      tuberculosis - *see* Tuberculosis, pulmonary

◀ New ⬅ Revised

Tracheitis *(Continued)*
with *(Continued)*
laryngitis (acute) 464.20
with obstruction 464.21
chronic 476.1
tuberculous (*see also* Tuberculosis, larynx) 012.3
obstruction 464.11
chronic 491.8
with
bronchitis (chronic) 491.8
laryngitis (chronic) 476.1
due to external agent - *see* Condition, respiratory, chronic, due to
diphtheritic (membranous) 032.3
due to external agent - *see* Inflammation, respiratory, upper, due to
edematous 464.11
influenzal 487.1
streptococcal 034.0
syphilitic 095.8
tuberculous (*see also* Tuberculosis) 012.8
Trachelitis (nonvenereal) (*see also* Cervicitis) 616.0
trichomonal 131.09
Tracheobronchial - *see* condition
Tracheobronchitis (*see also* Bronchitis) 490
acute or subacute 466.0
with bronchospasm or obstruction 466.0
chronic 491.8
influenzal 487.1
senile 491.8
Tracheobronchomegaly (congenital) 748.3
with bronchiectasis 494.0
with (acute) exacerbation 494.1
acquired 519.19
with bronchiectasis 494.0
with (acute) exacerbation 494.1
Tracheobronchopneumonitis - *see* Pneumonia, broncho
Tracheocele (external) (internal) 519.19
congenital 748.3
Tracheomalacia 519.19
congenital 748.3
Tracheopharyngitis (acute) 465.8
chronic 478.9
due to external agent - *see* Condition, respiratory, chronic, due to
due to external agent - *see* Inflammation, respiratory, upper, due to
Tracheostenosis 519.19
congenital 748.3
Tracheostomy
attention to V55.0
complication 519.00
granuloma 519.09
hemorrhage 519.09
infection 519.01
malfunctioning 519.02
obstruction 519.09
sepsis 519.01
status V44.0
stenosis 519.02
Trachoma, trachomatous 076.9
active (stage) 076.1
contraction of conjunctiva 076.1
dubium 076.0
healed or late effect 139.1
initial (stage) 076.0
Türck's (chronic catarrhal laryngitis) 476.0
Trachyphonia 784.49
Training
insulin pump V65.46
orthoptic V57.4
orthotic V57.81
Train sickness 994.6
Trait
hemoglobin
abnormal NEC 282.7
with thalassemia 282.49
C (*see also* Disease, hemoglobin, C) 282.7
with elliptocytosis 282.7
S (Hb-S) 282.5
Lepore 282.49
with other abnormal hemoglobin NEC 282.49
paranoid 301.0
sickle-cell 282.5
with
elliptocytosis 282.5
spherocytosis 282.5
Traits, paranoid 301.0
Tramp V60.0
Trance 780.09
hysterical 300.13
Transaminasemia 790.4
Transfusion, blood
donor V59.01
stem cells V59.02
incompatible 999.6
reaction or complication - *see* Complications, transfusion
related acute lung injury (TRALI) 518.7
syndrome
fetomaternal 772.0
twin-to-twin
blood loss (donor twin) 772.0
recipient twin 776.4
without reported diagnosis V58.2
Transient - *see also* condition
alteration of awareness 780.02
blindness 368.12
deafness (ischemic) 388.02
global amnesia 437.7
person (homeless) NEC V60.0
Transitional, lumbosacral joint of vertebra 756.19
Translocation
autosomes NEC 758.5
13–15 758.1
16–18 758.2
21 or 22 758.0
balanced in normal individual 758.4
D_1 758.1
E_3 758.2
G 758.0
balanced autosomal in normal individual 758.4
chromosomes NEC 758.89
Down's syndrome 758.0
Translucency, iris 364.53
Transmission of chemical substances through the placenta (affecting fetus or newborn) 760.70
alcohol 760.71
anticonvulsants 760.77
antifungals 760.74
anti-infective agents 760.74
antimetabolics 760.78
cocaine 760.75
"crack" 760.75
diethylstilbestrol [DES] 760.76
Transmission of chemical substances through the placenta *(Continued)*
hallucinogenic agents 760.73
medicinal agents NEC 760.79
narcotics 760.72
obstetric anesthetic or analgesic drug 763.5
specified agent NEC 760.79
suspected, affecting management of pregnancy 655.5
Transplant (ed)
bone V42.4
marrow V42.81
complication - *see also* Complications, due to (presence of) any device, implant, or graft classified to 996.0–996.5 NEC
bone marrow 996.85
corneal graft NEC 996.79
infection or inflammation 996.69
reaction 996.51
rejection 996.51
organ (failure) (immune or nonimmune cause) (infection) (rejection) 996.80
bone marrow 996.85
heart 996.83
intestines 996.87
kidney 996.81
liver 996.82
lung 996.84
pancreas 996.86
specified NEC 996.89
skin NEC 996.79
infection or inflammation 996.69
rejection 996.52
artificial 996.55
decellularized allodermis 996.55
cornea V42.5
hair V50.0
heart V42.1
valve V42.2
intestine V42.84
kidney V42.0
liver V42.7
lung V42.6
organ V42.9
specified NEC V42.89
pancreas V42.83
peripheral stem cells V42.82
skin V42.3
stem cells, peripheral V42.82
tissue V42.9
specified NEC V42.89
Transplants, ovarian, endometrial 617.1
Transposed - *see* Transposition
Transposition (congenital) - *see also* Malposition, congenital
abdominal viscera 759.3
aorta (dextra) 745.11
appendix 751.5
arterial trunk 745.10
colon 751.5
great vessels (complete) 745.10
both originating from right ventricle 745.11
corrected 745.12
double outlet right ventricle 745.11
incomplete 745.11
partial 745.11
specified type NEC 745.19
heart 746.87
with complete transposition of viscera 759.3

Transposition *(Continued)*
intestine (large) (small) 751.5
pulmonary veins 747.49
reversed jejunal (for bypass) (status) V45.3
scrotal 752.81
stomach 750.7
with general transposition of viscera 759.3
teeth, tooth 524.30
vessels (complete) 745.10
partial 745.11
viscera (abdominal) (thoracic) 759.3
Trans-sexualism 302.50
with
asexual history 302.51
heterosexual history 302.53
homosexual history 302.52
Transverse - *see also* condition
arrest (deep), in labor 660.3
affecting fetus or newborn 763.1
lie 652.3
before labor, affecting fetus or newborn 761.7
causing obstructed labor 660.0
affecting fetus or newborn 763.1
during labor, affecting fetus or newborn 763.1
Transvestism, transvestitism (transvestic fetishism) 302.3
Trapped placenta (with hemorrhage) 666.0
without hemorrhage 667.0
Trauma, traumatism (*see also* Injury, by site) 959.9
birth - *see* Birth, injury NEC
causing hemorrhage of pregnancy or delivery 641.8
complicating
abortion - *see* Abortion, by type, with damage to pelvic organs
ectopic pregnancy (*see also* categories 633.0–633.9) 639.2
molar pregnancy (*see also* categories 630–632) 639.2
during delivery NEC 665.9
following
abortion 639.2
ectopic or molar pregnancy 639.2
maternal, during pregnancy, affecting fetus or newborn 760.5
neuroma - *see* Injury, nerve, by site
previous major, affecting management of pregnancy, childbirth, or puerperium V23.8
psychic (current) - *see also* Reaction, adjustment
previous (history) V15.49
psychologic, previous (affecting health) V15.49
transient paralysis - *see* Injury, nerve, by site
Traumatic - *see* condition
Treacher Collins' syndrome (incomplete facial dysostosis) 756.0
Treitz's hernia - *see* Hernia, Treitz's
Trematode infestation NEC 121.9
Trematodiasis NEC 121.9
Trembles 988.8
Trembling paralysis (*see also* Parkinsonism) 332.0
Tremor 781.0
essential (benign) 333.1
familial 333.1
flapping (liver) 572.8
Tremor *(Continued)*
hereditary 333.1
hysterical 300.11
intention 333.1
medication-induced postural 333.1
mercurial 985.0
muscle 728.85
Parkinson's (*see also* Parkinsonism) 332.0
psychogenic 306.0
specified as conversion reaction 300.11
senilis 797
specified type NEC 333.1
Trench
fever 083.1
foot 991.4
mouth 101
nephritis - *see* Nephritis, acute
Treponema pallidum infection (*see also* Syphilis) 097.9
Treponematosis 102.9
due to
T. pallidum - *see* Syphilis
T. pertenue (yaws) (*see also* Yaws) 102.9
Triad
Kartagener's 759.3
Reiter's (complete) (incomplete) 099.3
Saint's (*see also* Hernia, diaphragm) 553.3
Trichiasis 704.2
cicatricial 704.2
eyelid 374.05
with entropion (*see also* Entropion) 374.00
Trichinella spiralis (infection) (infestation) 124
Trichinelliasis 124
Trichinellosis 124
Trichiniasis 124
Trichinosis 124
Trichobezoar 938
intestine 936
stomach 935.2
Trichocephaliasis 127.3
Trichocephalosis 127.3
Trichocephalus infestation 127.3
Trichoclasis 704.2
Trichoepithelioma (M8100/0) - *see also* Neoplasm, skin, benign
breast 217
genital organ NEC - *see* Neoplasm, by site, benign
malignant (M8100/3) - *see* Neoplasm, skin, malignant
Trichofolliculoma (M8101/0) - *see* Neoplasm, skin, benign
Tricholemmoma (M8102/0) - *see* Neoplasm, skin, benign
Trichomatosis 704.2
Trichomoniasis 131.9
bladder 131.09
cervix 131.09
intestinal 007.3
prostate 131.03
seminal vesicle 131.09
specified site NEC 131.8
urethra 131.02
urogenitalis 131.00
vagina 131.01
vulva 131.01
vulvovaginal 131.01
Trichomycosis 039.0
axillaris 039.0
nodosa 111.2
nodularis 111.2
rubra 039.0
Trichonocardiosis (axillaris) (palmellina) 039.0
Trichonodosis 704.2
Trichophytid, trichophyton infection (*see also* Dermatophytosis) 110.9
Trichophytide - *see* Dermatophytosis
Trichophytobezoar 938
intestine 936
stomach 935.2
Trichophytosis - *see* Dermatophytosis
Trichoptilosis 704.2
Trichorrhexis (nodosa) 704.2
Trichosporosis nodosa 111.2
Trichostasis spinulosa (congenital) 757.4
Trichostrongyliasis (small intestine) 127.6
Trichostrongylosis 127.6
Trichostrongylus (instabilis) infection 127.6
Trichotillomania 312.39
Trichromat, anomalous (congenital) 368.59
Trichromatopsia, anomalous (congenital) 368.59
Trichuriasis 127.3
Trichuris trichiura (any site) (infection) (infestation) 127.3
Tricuspid (valve) - *see* condition
Trifid - *see also* Accessory
kidney (pelvis) 753.3
tongue 750.13
Trigeminal neuralgia (*see also* Neuralgia, trigeminal) 350.1
Trigeminoencephaloangiomatosis 759.6
Trigeminy 427.89
postoperative 997.1
Trigger finger (acquired) 727.03
congenital 756.89
Trigonitis (bladder) (chronic) (pseudomembranous) 595.3
tuberculous (*see also* Tuberculosis) 016.1
Trigonocephaly 756.0
Trihexosidosis 272.7
Trilobate placenta - *see* Placenta, abnormal
Trilocular heart 745.8
Trimethylaminuria 270.8 ◀
Tripartita placenta - *see* Placenta, abnormal
Triple - *see also* Accessory
kidneys 753.3
uteri 752.2
X female 758.81
Triplegia 344.89
congenital or infantile 343.8
Triplet
affected by maternal complications of pregnancy 761.5
healthy liveborn - *see* Newborn, multiple
pregnancy (complicating delivery) NEC 651.1
with fetal loss and retention of one or more fetus(es) 651.4
following (elective) fetal reduction 651.7
Triplex placenta - *see* Placenta, abnormal
Triplication - *see* Accessory

Trismus 781.0
neonatorum 771.3
newborn 771.3
Trisomy (syndrome) NEC 758.5
13 (partial) 758.1
16–18 758.2
18 (partial) 758.2
21 (partial) 758.0
22 758.0
autosomes NEC 758.5
D_1 758.1
E_3 758.2
G (group) 758.0
group D_1 758.1
group E 758.2
group G 758.0
Tritanomaly 368.53
Tritanopia 368.53
Troisier-Hanot-Chauffard syndrome (bronze diabetes) 275.0
Trombidiosis 133.8
Trophedema (hereditary) 757.0
congenital 757.0
Trophoblastic disease (*see also* Hydatidiform mole) 630
previous, affecting management of pregnancy V23.1
Tropholymphedema 757.0
Trophoneurosis NEC 356.9
arm NEC 354.9
disseminated 710.1
facial 349.89
leg NEC 355.8
lower extremity NEC 355.8
upper extremity NEC 354.9
Tropical - *see also* condition
maceration feet (syndrome) 991.4
wet foot (syndrome) 991.4
Trouble - *see also* Disease
bowel 569.9
heart - *see* Disease, heart
intestine 569.9
kidney (*see also* Disease, renal) 593.9
nervous 799.2
sinus (*see also* Sinusitis) 473.9
Trousseau's syndrome (thrombophlebitis migrans) 453.1
Truancy, childhood - *see also* Disturbance, conduct
socialized 312.2
undersocialized, unsocialized 312.1
Truncus
arteriosus (persistent) 745.0
common 745.0
communis 745.0
Trunk - *see* condition
Trychophytide - *see* Dermatophytosis
Trypanosoma infestation - *see* Trypanosomiasis
Trypanosomiasis 086.9
with meningoencephalitis 086.9 [323.2]
African 086.5
due to Trypanosoma 086.5
gambiense 086.3
rhodesiense 086.4
American 086.2
with
heart involvement 086.0
other organ involvement 086.1
without mention of organ involvement 086.2
Brazilian - *see* Trypanosomiasis, American
Chagas' - *see* Trypanosomiasis, American

Trypanosomiasis *(Continued)*
due to Trypanosoma
cruzi - *see* Trypanosomiasis, American
gambiense 086.3
rhodesiense 086.4
gambiensis, Gambian 086.3
North American - *see* Trypanosomiasis, American
rhodesiensis, Rhodesian 086.4
South American - *see* Trypanosomiasis, American
T-shaped incisors 520.2
Tsutsugamushi fever 081.2
Tube, tubal, tubular - *see also* condition
ligation, admission for V25.2
Tubercle - *see also* Tuberculosis
brain, solitary 013.2
Darwin's 744.29
epithelioid noncaseating 135
Ghon, primary infection 010.0
Tuberculid, tuberculide (indurating) (lichenoid) (miliary) (papulonecrotic) (primary) (skin) (subcutaneous) (*see also* Tuberculosis) 017.0
Tuberculoma - *see also* Tuberculosis
brain (any part) 013.2
meninges (cerebral) (spinal) 013.1
spinal cord 013.4
Tuberculosis, tubercular, tuberculous (calcification) (calcified) (caseous) (chromogenic acid-fast bacilli) (congenital) (degeneration) (disease) (fibrocaseous) (fistula) (gangrene) (interstitial) (isolated circumscribed lesions) (necrosis) (parenchymatous) (ulcerative) 011.9

Note Use the following fifth-digit subclassification with categories 010–018:

0 unspecified
1 bacteriological or histological examination not done
2 bacteriological or histological examination unknown (at present)
3 tubercle bacilli found (in sputum) by microscopy
4 tubercle bacilli not found (in sputum) by microscopy, but found by bacterial culture
5 tubercle bacilli not found by bacteriological examination, but tuberculosis confirmed histologically
6 tubercle bacilli not found by bacteriological or histological examination, but tuberculosis confirmed by other methods [inoculation of animals]

For tuberculous conditions specified as late effects or sequelae, *see* category 137.

abdomen 014.8
lymph gland 014.8
abscess 011.9
arm 017.9
bone (*see also* Osteomyelitis, due to, tuberculosis) 015.9 *[730.8]*
hip 015.1 *[730.85]*
knee 015.2 *[730.86]*
sacrum 015.0 *[730.88]*
specified site NEC 015.7 *[730.88]*

Tuberculosis, tubercular, tuberculous *(Continued)*
abscess *(Continued)*
bone *(Continued)*
spinal 015.0 *[730.88]*
vertebra 015.0 *[730.88]*
brain 013.3
breast 017.9
Cowper's gland 016.5
dura (mater) 013.8
brain 013.3
spinal cord 013.5
epidural 013.8
brain 013.3
spinal cord 013.5
frontal sinus - *see* Tuberculosis, sinus
genital organs NEC 016.9
female 016.7
male 016.5
genitourinary NEC 016.9
gland (lymphatic) - *see* Tuberculosis, lymph gland
hip 015.1
iliopsoas 015.0 *[730.88]*
intestine 014.8
ischiorectal 014.8
joint 015.9
hip 015.1
knee 015.2
specified joint NEC 015.8
vertebral 015.0 *[730.88]*
kidney 016.0 *[590.81]*
knee 015.2
lumbar 015.0 *[730.88]*
lung 011.2
primary, progressive 010.8
meninges (cerebral) (spinal) 013.0
pelvic 016.9
female 016.7
male 016.5
perianal 014.8
fistula 014.8
perinephritic 016.0 *[590.81]*
perineum 017.9
perirectal 014.8
psoas 015.0 *[730.88]*
rectum 014.8
retropharyngeal 012.8
sacrum 015.0 *[730.88]*
scrofulous 017.2
scrotum 016.5
skin 017.0
primary 017.0
spinal cord 013.5
spine or vertebra (column) 015.0 *[730.88]*
strumous 017.2
subdiaphragmatic 014.8
testis 016.5
thigh 017.9
urinary 016.3
kidney 016.0 *[590.81]*
uterus 016.7
accessory sinus - *see* Tuberculosis, sinus
Addison's disease 017.6
adenitis (*see also* Tuberculosis, lymph gland) 017.2
adenoids 012.8
adenopathy (*see also* Tuberculosis, lymph gland) 017.2
tracheobronchial 012.1
primary progressive 010.8
adherent pericardium 017.9 *[420.0]*
adnexa (uteri) 016.7

Tuberculosis, tubercular, tuberculous *(Continued)*
adrenal (capsule) (gland) 017.6
air passage NEC 012.8
alimentary canal 014.8
anemia 017.9
ankle (joint) 015.8
bone 015.5 *[730.87]*
anus 014.8
apex (*see also* Tuberculosis, pulmonary) 011.9
apical (*see also* Tuberculosis, pulmonary) 011.9
appendicitis 014.8
appendix 014.8
arachnoid 013.0
artery 017.9
arthritis (chronic) (synovial) 015.9 *[711.40]*
ankle 015.8 *[730.87]*
hip 015.1 *[711.45]*
knee 015.2 *[711.46]*
specified site NEC 015.8 *[711.48]*
spine or vertebra (column) 015.0 *[720.81]*
wrist 015.8 *[730.83]*
articular - *see* Tuberculosis, joint
ascites 014.0
asthma (*see also* Tuberculosis, pulmonary) 011.9
axilla, axillary 017.2
gland 017.2
bilateral (*see also* Tuberculosis, pulmonary) 011.9
bladder 016.1
bone (*see also* Osteomyelitis, due to, tuberculosis) 015.9 *[730.8]*
hip 015.1 *[730.85]*
knee 015.2 *[730.86]*
limb NEC 015.5 *[730.88]*
sacrum 015.0 *[730.88]*
specified site NEC 015.7 *[730.88]*
spinal or vertebral column 015.0 *[730.88]*
bowel 014.8
miliary 018.9
brain 013.2
breast 017.9
broad ligament 016.7
bronchi, bronchial, bronchus 011.3
ectasia, ectasis 011.5
fistula 011.3
primary, progressive 010.8
gland 012.1
primary, progressive 010.8
isolated 012.2
lymph gland or node 012.1
primary, progressive 010.8
bronchiectasis 011.5
bronchitis 011.3
bronchopleural 012.0
bronchopneumonia, bronchopneumonic 011.6
bronchorrhagia 011.3
bronchotracheal 011.3
isolated 012.2
bronchus - *see* Tuberculosis, bronchi
bronze disease (Addison's) 017.6
buccal cavity 017.9
bulbourethral gland 016.5
bursa (*see also* Tuberculosis, joint) 015.9
cachexia NEC (*see also* Tuberculosis, pulmonary) 011.9

Tuberculosis, tubercular, tuberculous *(Continued)*
cardiomyopathy 017.9 *[425.8]*
caries (*see also* Tuberculosis, bone) 015.9 *[730.8]*
cartilage (*see also* Tuberculosis, bone) 015.9 *[730.8]*
intervertebral 015.0 *[730.88]*
catarrhal (*see also* Tuberculosis, pulmonary) 011.9
cecum 014.8
cellular tissue (primary) 017.0
cellulitis (primary) 017.0
central nervous system 013.9
specified site NEC 013.8
cerebellum (current) 013.2
cerebral (current) 013.2
meninges 013.0
cerebrospinal 013.6
meninges 013.0
cerebrum (current) 013.2
cervical 017.2
gland 017.2
lymph nodes 017.2
cervicitis (uteri) 016.7
cervix 016.7
chest (*see also* Tuberculosis, pulmonary) 011.9
childhood type or first infection 010.0
choroid 017.3 *[363.13]*
choroiditis 017.3 *[363.13]*
ciliary body 017.3 *[364.11]*
colitis 014.8
colliers' 011.4
colliquativa (primary) 017.0
colon 014.8
ulceration 014.8
complex, primary 010.0
complicating pregnancy, childbirth, or puerperium 647.3
affecting fetus or newborn 760.2
congenital 771.2
conjunctiva 017.3 *[370.31]*
connective tissue 017.9
bone - *see* Tuberculosis, bone
contact V01.1
converter (tuberculin skin test) (without disease) 795.5
cornea (ulcer) 017.3 *[370.31]*
Cowper's gland 016.5
coxae 015.1 *[730.85]*
coxalgia 015.1 *[730.85]*
cul-de-sac of Douglas 014.8
curvature, spine 015.0 *[737.40]*
cutis (colliquativa) (primary) 017.0
cyst, ovary 016.6
cystitis 016.1
dacryocystitis 017.3 *[375.32]*
dactylitis 015.5
diarrhea 014.8
diffuse (*see also* Tuberculosis, miliary) 018.9
lung - *see* Tuberculosis, pulmonary
meninges 013.0
digestive tract 014.8
disseminated (*see also* Tuberculosis, miliary) 018.9
meninges 013.0
duodenum 014.8
dura (mater) 013.9
abscess 013.8
cerebral 013.3
spinal 013.5
dysentery 014.8

Tuberculosis, tubercular, tuberculous *(Continued)*
ear (inner) (middle) 017.4
bone 015.6
external (primary) 017.0
skin (primary) 017.0
elbow 015.8
emphysema - *see* Tuberculosis, pulmonary
empyema 012.0
encephalitis 013.6
endarteritis 017.9
endocarditis (any valve) 017.9 *[424.91]*
endocardium (any valve) 017.9 *[424.91]*
endocrine glands NEC 017.9
endometrium 016.7
enteric, enterica 014.8
enteritis 014.8
enterocolitis 014.8
epididymis 016.4
epididymitis 016.4
epidural abscess 013.8
brain 013.3
spinal cord 013.5
epiglottis 012.3
episcleritis 017.3 *[379.00]*
erythema (induratum) (nodosum) (primary) 017.1
esophagus 017.8
Eustachian tube 017.4
exposure to V01.1
exudative 012.0
primary, progressive 010.1
eye 017.3
glaucoma 017.3 *[365.62]*
eyelid (primary) 017.0
lupus 017.0 *[373.4]*
fallopian tube 016.6
fascia 017.9
fauces 012.8
finger 017.9
first infection 010.0
fistula, perirectal 014.8
Florida 011.6
foot 017.9
funnel pelvis 137.3
gallbladder 017.9
galloping (*see also* Tuberculosis, pulmonary) 011.9
ganglionic 015.9
gastritis 017.9
gastrocolic fistula 014.8
gastroenteritis 014.8
gastrointestinal tract 014.8
general, generalized 018.9
acute 018.0
chronic 018.8
genital organs NEC 016.9
female 016.7
male 016.5
genitourinary NEC 016.9
genu 015.2
glandulae suprarenalis 017.6
glandular, general 017.2
glottis 012.3
grinders' 011.4
groin 017.2
gum 017.9
hand 017.9
heart 017.9 *[425.8]*
hematogenous - *see* Tuberculosis, miliary
hemoptysis (*see also* Tuberculosis, pulmonary) 011.9
hemorrhage NEC (*see also* Tuberculosis, pulmonary) 011.9

Tuberculosis, tubercular, tuberculous *(Continued)*
hemothorax 012.0
hepatitis 017.9
hilar lymph nodes 012.1
primary, progressive 010.8
hip (disease) (joint) 015.1
bone 015.1 *[730.85]*
hydrocephalus 013.8
hydropneumothorax 012.0
hydrothorax 012.0
hypoadrenalism 017.6
hypopharynx 012.8
ileocecal (hyperplastic) 014.8
ileocolitis 014.8
ileum 014.8
iliac spine (superior) 015.0 *[730.88]*
incipient NEC (*see also* Tuberculosis, pulmonary) 011.9
indurativa (primary) 017.1
infantile 010.0
infection NEC 011.9
without clinical manifestation 010.0
infraclavicular gland 017.2
inguinal gland 017.2
inguinalis 017.2
intestine (any part) 014.8
iris 017.3 *[364.11]*
iritis 017.3 *[364.11]*
ischiorectal 014.8
jaw 015.7 *[730.88]*
jejunum 014.8
joint 015.9
hip 015.1
knee 015.2
specified site NEC 015.8
vertebral 015.0 *[730.88]*
keratitis 017.3 *[370.31]*
interstitial 017.3 *[370.59]*
keratoconjunctivitis 017.3 *[370.31]*
kidney 016.0
knee (joint) 015.2
kyphoscoliosis 015.0 *[737.43]*
kyphosis 015.0 *[737.41]*
lacrimal apparatus, gland 017.3
laryngitis 012.3
larynx 012.3
leptomeninges, leptomeningitis (cerebral) (spinal) 013.0
lichenoides (primary) 017.0
linguae 017.9
lip 017.9
liver 017.9
lordosis 015.0 *[737.42]*
lung - *see* Tuberculosis, pulmonary
luposa 017.0
eyelid 017.0 *[373.4]*
lymphadenitis - *see* Tuberculosis, lymph gland
lymphangitis - *see* Tuberculosis, lymph gland
lymphatic (gland) (vessel) - *see* Tuberculosis, lymph gland
lymph gland or node (peripheral) 017.2
abdomen 014.8
bronchial 012.1
primary, progressive 010.8
cervical 017.2
hilar 012.1
primary, progressive 010.8
intrathoracic 012.1
primary, progressive 010.8
mediastinal 012.1
primary, progressive 010.8

Tuberculosis, tubercular, tuberculous *(Continued)*
lymph gland or node *(Continued)*
mesenteric 014.8
peripheral 017.2
retroperitoneal 014.8
tracheobronchial 012.1
primary, progressive 010.8
malignant NEC (*see also* Tuberculosis, pulmonary) 011.9
mammary gland 017.9
marasmus NEC (*see also* Tuberculosis, pulmonary) 011.9
mastoiditis 015.6
maternal, affecting fetus or newborn 760.2
mediastinal (lymph) gland or node 012.1
primary, progressive 010.8
mediastinitis 012.8
primary, progressive 010.8
mediastinopericarditis 017.9 *[420.0]*
mediastinum 012.8
primary, progressive 010.8
medulla 013.9
brain 013.2
spinal cord 013.4
melanosis, Addisonian 017.6
membrane, brain 013.0
meninges (cerebral) (spinal) 013.0
meningitis (basilar) (brain) (cerebral) (cerebrospinal) (spinal) 013.0
meningoencephalitis 013.0
mesentery, mesenteric 014.8
lymph gland or node 014.8
miliary (any site) 018.9
acute 018.0
chronic 018.8
specified type NEC 018.8
millstone makers' 011.4
miners' 011.4
moulders' 011.4
mouth 017.9
multiple 018.9
acute 018.0
chronic 018.8
muscle 017.9
myelitis 013.6
myocarditis 017.9 *[422.0]*
myocardium 017.9 *[422.0]*
nasal (passage) (sinus) 012.8
nasopharynx 012.8
neck gland 017.2
nephritis 016.0 *[583.81]*
nerve 017.9
nose (septum) 012.8
ocular 017.3
old NEC 137.0
without residuals V12.01
omentum 014.8
oophoritis (acute) (chronic) 016.6
optic 017.3 *[377.39]*
nerve trunk 017.3 *[377.39]*
papilla, papillae 017.3 *[377.39]*
orbit 017.3
orchitis 016.5 *[608.81]*
organ, specified NEC 017.9
orificialis (primary) 017.0
osseous (*see also* Tuberculosis, bone) 015.9 *[730.8]*
osteitis (*see also* Tuberculosis, bone) 015.9 *[730.8]*
osteomyelitis (*see also* Tuberculosis, bone) 015.9 *[730.8]*
otitis (media) 017.4

Tuberculosis, tubercular, tuberculous *(Continued)*
ovaritis (acute) (chronic) 016.6
ovary (acute) (chronic) 016.6
oviducts (acute) (chronic) 016.6
pachymeningitis 013.0
palate (soft) 017.9
pancreas 017.9
papulonecrotic (primary) 017.0
parathyroid glands 017.9
paronychia (primary) 017.0
parotid gland or region 017.9
pelvic organ NEC 016.9
female 016.7
male 016.5
pelvis (bony) 015.7 *[730.85]*
penis 016.5
peribronchitis 011.3
pericarditis 017.9 *[420.0]*
pericardium 017.9 *[420.0]*
perichondritis, larynx 012.3
perineum 017.9
periostitis (*see also* Tuberculosis, bone) 015.9 *[730.8]*
periphlebitis 017.9
eye vessel 017.3 *[362.18]*
retina 017.3 *[362.18]*
perirectal fistula 014.8
peritoneal gland 014.8
peritoneum 014.0
peritonitis 014.0
pernicious NEC (*see also* Tuberculosis, pulmonary) 011.9
pharyngitis 012.8
pharynx 012.8
phlyctenulosis (conjunctiva) 017.3 *[370.31]*
phthisis NEC (*see also* Tuberculosis, pulmonary) 011.9
pituitary gland 017.9
placenta 016.7
pleura, pleural, pleurisy, pleuritis (fibrinous) (obliterative) (purulent) (simple plastic) (with effusion) 012.0
primary, progressive 010.1
pneumonia, pneumonic 011.6
pneumothorax 011.7
polyserositis 018.9
acute 018.0
chronic 018.8
potters' 011.4
prepuce 016.5
primary 010.9
complex 010.0
complicated 010.8
with pleurisy or effusion 010.1
progressive 010.8
with pleurisy or effusion 010.1
skin 017.0
proctitis 014.8
prostate 016.5 *[601.4]*
prostatitis 016.5 *[601.4]*
pulmonaris (*see also* Tuberculosis, pulmonary) 011.9
pulmonary (artery) (incipient) (malignant) (multiple round foci) (pernicious) (reinfection stage) 011.9
cavitated or with cavitation 011.2
primary, progressive 010.8
childhood type or first infection 010.0
chromogenic acid-fast bacilli 795.39
fibrosis or fibrotic 011.4
infiltrative 011.0
primary, progressive 010.9

Tuberculosis, tubercular, tuberculous *(Continued)*
pulmonary *(Continued)*
nodular 011.1
specified NEC 011.8
sputum positive only 795.39
status following surgical collapse of lung NEC 011.9
pyelitis 016.0 *[590.81]*
pyelonephritis 016.0 *[590.81]*
pyemia - *see* Tuberculosis, miliary
pyonephrosis 016.0
pyopneumothorax 012.0
pyothorax 012.0
rectum (with abscess) 014.8
fistula 014.8
reinfection stage (*see also* Tuberculosis, pulmonary) 011.9
renal 016.0
renes 016.0
reproductive organ 016.7
respiratory NEC (*see also* Tuberculosis, pulmonary) 011.9
specified site NEC 012.8
retina 017.3 *[363.13]*
retroperitoneal (lymph gland or node) 014.8
gland 014.8
retropharyngeal abscess 012.8
rheumatism 015.9
rhinitis 012.8
sacroiliac (joint) 015.8
sacrum 015.0 *[730.88]*
salivary gland 017.9
salpingitis (acute) (chronic) 016.6
sandblasters' 011.4
sclera 017.3 *[379.09]*
scoliosis 015.0 *[737.43]*
scrofulous 017.2
scrotum 016.5
seminal tract or vesicle 016.5 *[608.81]*
senile NEC (*see also* Tuberculosis, pulmonary) 011.9
septic NEC (*see also* Tuberculosis, miliary) 018.9
shoulder 015.8
blade 015.7 *[730.8]*
sigmoid 014.8
sinus (accessory) (nasal) 012.8
bone 015.7 *[730.88]*
epididymis 016.4
skeletal NEC (*see also* Osteomyelitis, due to tuberculosis) 015.9 *[730.8]*
skin (any site) (primary) 017.0
small intestine 014.8
soft palate 017.9
spermatic cord 016.5
spinal
column 015.0 *[730.88]*
cord 013.4
disease 015.0 *[730.88]*
medulla 013.4
membrane 013.0
meninges 013.0
spine 015.0 *[730.88]*
spleen 017.7
splenitis 017.7
spondylitis 015.0 *[720.81]*
spontaneous pneumothorax - *see* Tuberculosis, pulmonary
sternoclavicular joint 015.8
stomach 017.9
stonemasons' 011.4
struma 017.2

Tuberculosis, tubercular, tuberculous *(Continued)*
subcutaneous tissue (cellular) (primary) 017.0
subcutis (primary) 017.0
subdeltoid bursa 017.9
submaxillary 017.9
region 017.9
supraclavicular gland 017.2
suprarenal (capsule) (gland) 017.6
swelling, joint (*see also* Tuberculosis, joint) 015.9
symphysis pubis 015.7 *[730.88]*
synovitis 015.9 *[727.01]*
hip 015.1 *[727.01]*
knee 015.2 *[727.01]*
specified site NEC 015.8 *[727.01]*
spine or vertebra 015.0 *[727.01]*
systemic - *see* Tuberculosis, miliary
tarsitis (eyelid) 017.0 *[373.4]*
ankle (bone) 015.5 *[730.87]*
tendon (sheath) - *see* Tuberculosis, tenosynovitis
tenosynovitis 015.9 *[727.01]*
hip 015.1 *[727.01]*
knee 015.2 *[727.01]*
specified site NEC 015.8 *[727.01]*
spine or vertebra 015.0 *[727.01]*
testis 016.5 *[608.81]*
throat 012.8
thymus gland 017.9
thyroid gland 017.5
toe 017.9
tongue 017.9
tonsil (lingual) 012.8
tonsillitis 012.8
trachea, tracheal 012.8
gland 012.1
primary, progressive 010.8
isolated 012.2
tracheobronchial 011.3
glandular 012.1
primary, progressive 010.8
isolated 012.2
lymph gland or node 012.1
primary, progressive 010.8
tubal 016.6
tunica vaginalis 016.5
typhlitis 014.8
ulcer (primary) (skin) 017.0
bowel or intestine 014.8
specified site NEC - *see* Tuberculosis, by site
unspecified site - *see* Tuberculosis, pulmonary
ureter 016.2
urethra, urethral 016.3
urinary organ or tract 016.3
kidney 016.0
uterus 016.7
uveal tract 017.3 *[363.13]*
uvula 017.9
vaccination, prophylactic (against) V03.2
vagina 016.7
vas deferens 016.5
vein 017.9
verruca (primary) 017.0
verrucosa (cutis) (primary) 017.0
vertebra (column) 015.0 *[730.88]*
vesiculitis 016.5 *[608.81]*
viscera NEC 014.8
vulva 016.7 *[616.51]*
wrist (joint) 015.8
bone 015.5 *[730.83]*

Tuberculum
auriculae 744.29
occlusal 520.2
paramolare 520.2
Tuberosity ◀
jaw, excessive 524.07 ◀
maxillary, entire 524.07 ◀
Tuberous sclerosis (brain) 759.5
Tubo-ovarian - *see* condition
Tuboplasty, after previous sterilization V26.0
Tubotympanitis 381.10
Tularemia 021.9
with
conjunctivitis 021.3
pneumonia 021.2
bronchopneumonic 021.2
conjunctivitis 021.3
cryptogenic 021.1
disseminated 021.8
enteric 021.1
generalized 021.8
glandular 021.8
intestinal 021.1
oculoglandular 021.3
ophthalmic 021.3
pneumonia 021.2
pulmonary 021.2
specified NEC 021.8
typhoidal 021.1
ulceroglandular 021.0
vaccination, prophylactic (against) V03.4
Tularensis conjunctivitis 021.3
Tumefaction - *see also* Swelling
liver (*see also* Hypertrophy, liver) 789.1
Tumor (M8000/1) - *see also* Neoplasm, by site, unspecified nature
Abrikosov's (M9580/0) - *see also* Neoplasm, connective tissue, benign
malignant (M9580/3) - *see* Neoplasm, connective tissue, malignant
acinar cell (M8550/1) - *see* Neoplasm, by site, uncertain behavior
acinic cell (M8550/1) - *see* Neoplasm, by site, uncertain behavior
adenomatoid (M9054/0) - *see also* Neoplasm, by site, benign
odontogenic (M9300/0) 213.1
upper jaw (bone) 213.0
adnexal (skin) (M8390/0) - *see* Neoplasm, skin, benign
adrenal
cortical (benign) (M8370/0) 227.0
malignant (M8370/3) 194.0
rest (M8671/0) - *see* Neoplasm, by site, benign
alpha cell (M8152/0)
malignant (M8152/3)
pancreas 157.4
specified site NEC - *see* Neoplasm, by site, malignant
unspecified site 157.4
pancreas 211.7
specified site NEC - *see* Neoplasm, by site, benign
unspecified site 211.7
aneurysmal (*see also* Aneurysm) 442.9
aortic body (M8691/1) 237.3
malignant (M8691/3) 194.6
argentaffin (M8241/1) - *see* Neoplasm, by site, uncertain behavior
basal cell (M8090/1) - *see also* Neoplasm, skin, uncertain behavior

Tumor *(Continued)*
benign (M8000/0) - *see* Neoplasm, by site, benign
beta cell (M8151/0)
malignant (M8151/3)
pancreas 157.4
specified site - *see* Neoplasm, by site, malignant
unspecified site 157.4
pancreas 211.7
specified site NEC - *see* Neoplasm, by site, benign
unspecified site 211.7
blood - *see* Hematoma
Brenner (M9000/0) 220
borderline malignancy (M9000/1) 236.2
malignant (M9000/3) 183.0
proliferating (M9000/1) 236.2
Brooke's (M8100/0) - *see* Neoplasm, skin, benign
brown fat (M8880/0) - *see* Lipoma, by site
Burkitt's (M9750/3) 200.2
calcifying epithelial odontogenic (M9340/0) 213.1
upper jaw (bone) 213.0
carcinoid (M8240/1) - *see* Carcinoid
carotid body (M8692/1) 237.3
malignant (M8692/3) 194.5
Castleman's (mediastinal lymph node hyperplasia) 785.6
cells (M8001/1) - *see also* Neoplasm, by site, unspecified nature
benign (M8001/0) - *see* Neoplasm, by site, benign
malignant (M8001/3) - *see* Neoplasm, by site, malignant
uncertain whether benign or malignant (M8001/1) - *see* Neoplasm, by site, uncertain nature
cervix
in pregnancy or childbirth 654.6
affecting fetus or newborn 763.89
causing obstructed labor 660.2
affecting fetus or newborn 763.1
chondromatous giant cell (M9230/0) - *see* Neoplasm, bone, benign
chromaffin (M8700/0) - *see also* Neoplasm, by site, benign
malignant (M8700/3) - *see* Neoplasm, by site, malignant
Cock's peculiar 706.2
Codman's (benign chondroblastoma) (M9230/0) - *see* Neoplasm, bone, benign
dentigerous, mixed (M9282/0) 213.1
upper jaw (bone) 213.0
dermoid (M9084/0) - *see* Neoplasm, by site, benign
with malignant transformation (M9084/3) 183.0
desmoid (extra-abdominal) (M8821/1) - *see also* Neoplasm, connective tissue, uncertain behavior
abdominal (M8822/1) - *see* Neoplasm, connective tissue, uncertain behavior
embryonal (mixed) (M9080/1) - *see also* Neoplasm, by site, uncertain behavior
liver (M9080/3) 155.0

Tumor *(Continued)*
endodermal sinus (M9071/3)
specified site - *see* Neoplasm, by site, malignant
unspecified site
female 183.0
male 186.9
epithelial
benign (M8010/0) - *see* Neoplasm, by site, benign
malignant (M8010/3) - *see* Neoplasm, by site, malignant
Ewing's (M9260/3) - *see* Neoplasm, bone, malignant
fatty - *see* Lipoma
fetal, causing disproportion 653.7
causing obstructed labor 660.1
fibroid (M8890/0) - *see* Leiomyoma
G cell (M8153/1)
malignant (M8153/3)
pancreas 157.4
specified site NEC - *see* Neoplasm, by site, malignant
unspecified site 157.4
specified site - *see* Neoplasm, by site, uncertain behavior
unspecified site 235.5
giant cell (type) (M8003/1) - *see also* Neoplasm, by site, unspecified nature
bone (M9250/1) 238.0
malignant (M9250/3) - *see* Neoplasm, bone, malignant
chondromatous (M9230/0) - *see* Neoplasm, bone, benign
malignant (M8003/3) - *see* Neoplasm, by site, malignant
peripheral (gingiva) 523.8
soft parts (M9251/1) - *see also* Neoplasm, connective tissue, uncertain behavior
malignant (M9251/3) - *see* Neoplasm, connective tissue, malignant
tendon sheath 727.02
glomus (M8711/0) - *see also* Hemangioma, by site
jugulare (M8690/1) 237.3
malignant (M8690/3) 194.6
gonadal stromal (M8590/1) - *see* Neoplasm, by site, uncertain behavior
granular cell (M9580/0) - *see also* Neoplasm, connective tissue, benign
malignant (M9580/3) - *see* Neoplasm, connective tissue, malignant
granulosa cell (M8620/1) 236.2
malignant (M8620/3) 183.0
granulosa cell-theca cell (M8621/1) 236.2
malignant (M8621/3) 183.0
Grawitz's (hypernephroma) (M8312/3) 189.0
hazard-crile (M8350/3) 193
hemorrhoidal - *see* Hemorrhoids
hilar cell (M8660/0) 220
Hürthle cell (benign) (M8290/0) 226
malignant (M8290/3) 193
hydatid (*see also* Echinococcus) 122.9
hypernephroid (M8311/1) - *see also* Neoplasm, by site, uncertain behavior
interstitial cell (M8650/1) - *see also* Neoplasm, by site, uncertain behavior

Tumor *(Continued)*
interstitial cell *(Continued)*
benign (M8650/0) - *see* Neoplasm, by site, benign
malignant (M8650/3) - *see* Neoplasm, by site, malignant
islet cell (M8150/0)
malignant (M8150/3)
pancreas 157.4
specified site - *see* Neoplasm, by site, malignant
unspecified site 157.4
pancreas 211.7
specified site NEC - *see* Neoplasm, by site, benign
unspecified site 211.7
juxtaglomerular (M8361/1) 236.91
Krukenberg's (M8490/6) 198.6
Leydig cell (M8650/1)
benign (M8650/0)
specified site - *see* Neoplasm, by site, benign
unspecified site
female 220
male 222.0
malignant (M8650/3)
specified site - *see* Neoplasm, by site, malignant
unspecified site
female 183.0
male 186.9
specified site - *see* Neoplasm, by site, uncertain behavior
unspecified site
female 236.2
male 236.4
lipid cell, ovary (M8670/0) 220
lipoid cell, ovary (M8670/0) 220
lymphomatous, benign (M9590/0) - *see also* Neoplasm, by site, benign
Malherbe's (M8110/0) - *see* Neoplasm, skin, benign
malignant (M8000/3) - *see also* Neoplasm, by site, malignant
fusiform cell (type) (M8004/3) - *see* Neoplasm, by site, malignant
giant cell (type) (M8003/3) - *see* Neoplasm, by site, malignant
mixed NEC (M8940/3) - *see* Neoplasm, by site, malignant
small cell (type) (M8002/3) - *see* Neoplasm, by site, malignant
spindle cell (type) (M8004/3) - *see* Neoplasm, by site, malignant
mast cell (M9740/1) 238.5
malignant (M9740/3) 202.6
melanotic, neuroectodermal (M9363/0) - *see* Neoplasm, by site, benign
Merkel cell - *see* Neoplasm, by site, malignant
mesenchymal
malignant (M8800/3) - *see* Neoplasm, connective tissue, malignant
mixed (M8990/1) - *see* Neoplasm, connective tissue, uncertain behavior
mesodermal, mixed (M8951/3) - *see also* Neoplasm, by site, malignant
liver 155.0
mesonephric (M9110/1) - *see also* Neoplasm, by site, uncertain behavior
malignant (M9110/3) - *see* Neoplasm, by site, malignant

Tumor *(Continued)*
metastatic
from specified site (M8000/3) - *see* Neoplasm, by site, malignant
to specified site (M8000/6) - *see* Neoplasm, by site, malignant, secondary
mixed NEC (M8940/0) - *see also* Neoplasm, by site, benign
malignant (M8940/3) - *see* Neoplasm, by site, malignant
mucocarcinoid, malignant (M8243/3) - *see* Neoplasm, by site, malignant
mucoepidermoid (M8430/1) - *see* Neoplasm, by site, uncertain behavior
Mullerian, mixed (M8950/3) - *see* Neoplasm, by site, malignant
myoepithelial (M8982/0) - *see* Neoplasm, by site, benign
neurogenic olfactory (M9520/3) 160.0
nonencapsulated sclerosing (M8350/3) 193
odontogenic (M9270/1) 238.0
adenomatoid (M9300/0) 213.1
upper jaw (bone) 213.0
benign (M9270/0) 213.1
upper jaw (bone) 213.0
calcifying epithelial (M9340/0) 213.1
upper jaw (bone) 213.0
malignant (M9270/3) 170.1
upper jaw (bone) 170.0
squamous (M9312/0) 213.1
upper jaw (bone) 213.0
ovarian stromal (M8590/1) 236.2
ovary
in pregnancy or childbirth 654.4
affecting fetus or newborn 763.89
causing obstructed labor 660.2
affecting fetus or newborn 763.1
pacinian (M9507/0) - *see* Neoplasm, skin, benign
Pancoast's (M8010/3) 162.3
papillary - *see* Papilloma
pelvic, in pregnancy or childbirth 654.9
affecting fetus or newborn 763.89
causing obstructed labor 660.2
affecting fetus or newborn 763.1
phantom 300.11
plasma cell (M9731/1) 238.6
benign (M9731/0) - *see* Neoplasm, by site, benign
malignant (M9731/3) 203.8
polyvesicular vitelline (M9071/3)
specified site - *see* Neoplasm, by site, malignant
unspecified site
female 183.0
male 186.9
Pott's puffy (*see also* Osteomyelitis) 730.2
Rathke's pouch (M9350/1) 237.0
Regaud's (M8082/3) - *see* Neoplasm, nasopharynx, malignant
rete cell (M8140/0) 222.0
retinal anlage (M9363/0) - *see* Neoplasm, by site, benign
Rokitansky's 620.2
salivary gland type, mixed (M8940/0) - *see also* Neoplasm, by site, benign
malignant (M8940/3) - *see* Neoplasm, by site, malignant
Sampson's 617.1
Schloffer's (*see also* Peritonitis) 567.29

Tumor *(Continued)*
Schmincke's (M8082/3) - *see* Neoplasm, nasopharynx, malignant
sebaceous (*see also* Cyst, sebaceous) 706.2
secondary (M8000/6) - *see* Neoplasm, by site, secondary
Sertoli cell (M8640/0)
with lipid storage (M8641/0)
specified site - *see* Neoplasm, by site, benign
unspecified site
female 220
male 222.0
specified site - *see* Neoplasm, by site, benign
unspecified site
female 220
male 222.0
Sertoli-Leydig cell (M8631/0)
specified site - *see* Neoplasm, by site, benign
unspecified site
female 220
male 222.0
sex cord (-stromal) (M8590/1) - *see* Neoplasm, by site, uncertain behavior
skin appendage (M8390/0) - *see* Neoplasm, skin, benign
soft tissue
benign (M8800/0) - *see* Neoplasm, connective tissue, benign
malignant (M8800/3) - *see* Neoplasm, connective tissue, malignant
sternomastoid 754.1
stromal
abdomen ◀
benign 215.5 ◀
malignant 171.5 ◀
uncertain behavior 238.1 ◀
digestive system 238.1 ◀
benign 215.5 ◀
malignant 171.5 ◀
uncertain behavior 238.1 ◀
gastric 238.1
benign 215.5
malignant 171.5
uncertain behavior 238.1
gastrointestinal 238.1
benign 215.5
malignant 171.5
uncertain behavior 238.1
intestine (small) (large) 238.1 ⬅
benign 215.5
malignant 171.5
uncertain behavior 238.1
stomach 238.1
benign 215.5
malignant 171.5
uncertain behavior 238.1
superior sulcus (lung) (pulmonary) (syndrome) (M8010/3) 162.3
suprasulcus (M8010/3) 162.3
sweat gland (M8400/1) - *see also* Neoplasm, skin, uncertain behavior
benign (M8400/0) - *see* Neoplasm, skin, benign
malignant (M8400/3) - *see* Neoplasm, skin, malignant
syphilitic brain 094.89
congenital 090.49
testicular stromal (M8590/1) 236.4
theca cell (M8600/0) 220
theca cell-granulosa cell (M8621/1) 236.2

Tumor *(Continued)*
theca-lutein (M8610/0) 220
turban (M8200/0) 216.4
uterus
in pregnancy or childbirth 654.1
affecting fetus or newborn 763.89
causing obstructed labor 660.2
affecting fetus or newborn 763.1
vagina
in pregnancy or childbirth 654.7
affecting fetus or newborn 763.89
causing obstructed labor 660.2
affecting fetus or newborn 763.1
varicose (*see also* Varicose, vein) 454.9
von Recklinghausen's (M9540/1) 237.71
vulva
in pregnancy or childbirth 654.8
affecting fetus or newborn 763.89
causing obstructed labor 660.2
affecting fetus or newborn 763.1
Warthin's (salivary gland) (M8561/0) 210.2
white - *see also* Tuberculosis, arthritis
White-Darier 757.39
Wilms' (nephroblastoma) (M8960/3) 189.0
yolk sac (M9071/3)
specified site - *see* Neoplasm, by site, malignant
unspecified site
female 183.0
male 186.9
Tumorlet (M8040/1) - *see* Neoplasm, by site, uncertain behavior
Tungiasis 134.1
Tunica vasculosa lentis 743.39
Tunnel vision 368.45
Turban tumor (M8200/0) 216.4
Türck's trachoma (chronic catarrhal laryngitis) 476.0
Türk's syndrome (ocular retraction syndrome) 378.71
Turner's
hypoplasia (tooth) 520.4
syndrome 758.6
tooth 520.4
Turner-Kieser syndrome (hereditary osteo-onychodysplasia) 756.89
Turner-Varny syndrome 758.6
Turricephaly 756.0
Tussis convulsiva (*see also* Whooping cough) 033.9
Twin
affected by maternal complications of pregnancy 761.5
conjoined 759.4
healthy liveborn - *see* Newborn, twin
pregnancy (complicating delivery) NEC 651.0
with fetal loss and retention of one fetus 651.3
following (elective) fetal reduction 651.7
Twinning, teeth 520.2
Twist, twisted
bowel, colon, or intestine 560.2
hair (congenital) 757.4
mesentery 560.2
omentum 560.2
organ or site, congenital NEC - *see* Anomaly, specified type NEC
ovarian pedicle 620.5
congenital 752.0
umbilical cord - *see* Compression, umbilical cord

Twitch 781.0
Tylosis 700
buccalis 528.6
gingiva 523.8
linguae 528.6
palmaris et plantaris 757.39
Tympanism 787.3
Tympanites (abdominal) (intestine) 787.3
Tympanitis - *see* Myringitis
Tympanosclerosis 385.00
involving
combined sites NEC 385.09
with tympanic membrane 385.03
tympanic membrane 385.01
with ossicles 385.02
and middle ear 385.03
Tympanum - *see* condition
Tympany
abdomen 787.3
chest 786.7
Typhlitis (*see also* Appendicitis) 541
Typhoenteritis 002.0
Typhogastric fever 002.0
Typhoid (abortive) (ambulant) (any site) (fever) (hemorrhagic) (infection) (intermittent) (malignant) (rheumatic) 002.0
with pneumonia 002.0 *[484.8]*
abdominal 002.0
carrier (suspected) of V02.1
cholecystitis (current) 002.0
clinical (Widal and blood test negative) 002.0
Typhoid *(Continued)*
endocarditis 002.0 *[421.1]*
inoculation reaction - *see* Complications, vaccination
meningitis 002.0 *[320.7]*
mesenteric lymph nodes 002.0
myocarditis 002.0 *[422.0]*
osteomyelitis (*see also* Osteomyelitis, due to, typhoid) 002.0 *[730.8]*
perichondritis, larynx 002.0 *[478.71]*
pneumonia 002.0 *[484.8]*
spine 002.0 *[720.81]*
ulcer (perforating) 002.0
vaccination, prophylactic (against) V03.1
Widal negative 002.0
Typhomalaria (fever) (*see also* Malaria) 084.6
Typhomania 002.0
Typhoperitonitis 002.0
Typhus (fever) 081.9
abdominal, abdominalis 002.0
African tick 082.1
amarillic (*see also* Fever, yellow) 060.9
brain 081.9
cerebral 081.9
classical 080
endemic (flea-borne) 081.0
epidemic (louse-borne) 080
exanthematic NEC 080
exanthematicus SAI 080
brillii SAI 081.1
mexicanus SAI 081.0
Typhus *(Continued)*
exanthematicus SAI *(Continued)*
pediculo vestimenti causa 080
typhus murinus 081.0
flea-borne 081.0
Indian tick 082.1
Kenya tick 082.1
louse-borne 080
Mexican 081.0
flea-borne 081.0
louse-borne 080
tabardillo 080
mite-borne 081.2
murine 081.0
North Asian tick-borne 082.2
petechial 081.9
Queensland tick 082.3
rat 081.0
recrudescent 081.1
recurrent (*see also* Fever, relapsing) 087.9
São Paulo 082.0
scrub (China) (India) (Malaya) (New Guinea) 081.2
shop (of Malaya) 081.0
Siberian tick 082.2
tick-borne NEC 082.9
tropical 081.2
vaccination, prophylactic (against) V05.8
Tyrosinemia 270.2
neonatal 775.89 ⬅
Tyrosinosis (Medes) (Sakai) 270.2
Tyrosinuria 270.2
Tyrosyluria 270.2

ICD-9-CM
T
Vol. 2

U

Uehlinger's syndrome (acropachyderma) 757.39
Uhl's anomaly or disease (hypoplasia of myocardium, right ventricle) 746.84
Ulcer, ulcerated, ulcerating, ulceration, ulcerative 707.9
with gangrene 707.9 *[785.4]*
abdomen (wall) (*see also* Ulcer, skin) 707.8
ala, nose 478.19
alveolar process 526.5
amebic (intestine) 006.9
skin 006.6
anastomotic - *see* Ulcer, gastrojejunal
anorectal 569.41
antral - *see* Ulcer, stomach
anus (sphincter) (solitary) 569.41
varicose - *see* Varicose, ulcer, anus
aorta - *see* Aneurysm
aphthous (oral) (recurrent) 528.2
genital organ(s)
female 616.89
male 608.89
mouth 528.2
arm (*see also* Ulcer, skin) 707.8
arteriosclerotic plaque - *see* Arteriosclerosis, by site
artery NEC 447.2
without rupture 447.8
atrophic NEC - *see* Ulcer, skin
Barrett's (chronic peptic ulcer of esophagus) 530.85
bile duct 576.8
bladder (solitary) (sphincter) 596.8
bilharzial (*see also* Schistosomiasis) 120.9 *[595.4]*
submucosal (*see also* Cystitis) 595.1
tuberculous (*see also* Tuberculosis) 016.1
bleeding NEC - *see* Ulcer, peptic, with hemorrhage
bone 730.9
bowel (*see also* Ulcer, intestine) 569.82
breast 611.0
bronchitis 491.8
bronchus 519.19
buccal (cavity) (traumatic) 528.9
burn (acute) - *see* Ulcer, duodenum
Buruli 031.1
buttock (*see also* Ulcer, skin) 707.8
decubitus (*see also* Ulcer, decubitus) 707.00
cancerous (M8000/3) - *see* Neoplasm, by site, malignant
cardia - *see* Ulcer, stomach
cardio-esophageal (peptic) 530.20
with bleeding 530.21
cecum (*see also* Ulcer, intestine) 569.82
cervix (uteri) (trophic) 622.0
with mention of cervicitis 616.0
chancroidal 099.0
chest (wall) (*see also* Ulcer, skin) 707.8
Chiclero 085.4
chin (pyogenic) (*see also* Ulcer, skin) 707.8
chronic (cause unknown) - *see also* Ulcer, skin
penis 607.89
Cochin-China 085.1
colitis - *see* Colitis, ulcerative
colon (*see also* Ulcer, intestine) 569.82
conjunctiva (acute) (postinfectional) 372.00

Ulcer, ulcerated, ulcerating, ulceration, ulcerative *(Continued)*
cornea (infectional) 370.00
with perforation 370.06
annular 370.02
catarrhal 370.01
central 370.03
dendritic 054.42
marginal 370.01
mycotic 370.05
phlyctenular, tuberculous (*see also* Tuberculosis) 017.3 *[370.31]*
ring 370.02
rodent 370.07
serpent, serpiginous 370.04
superficial marginal 370.01
tuberculous (*see also* Tuberculosis) 017.3 *[370.31]*
corpus cavernosum (chronic) 607.89
crural - *see* Ulcer, lower extremity
Curling's - *see* Ulcer, duodenum
Cushing's - *see* Ulcer, peptic
cystitis (interstitial) 595.1
decubitus (unspecified site) 707.00
with gangrene 707.00 *[785.4]*
ankle 707.06
back
lower 707.03
upper 707.02
buttock 707.05
elbow 707.01
head 707.09
heel 707.07
hip 707.04
other site 707.09
sacrum 707.03
shoulder blades 707.02
dendritic 054.42
diabetes, diabetic (mellitus) 250.8 *[707.9]*
lower limb 250.8 *[707.10]*
ankle 250.8 *[707.13]*
calf 250.8 *[707.12]*
foot 250.8 *[707.15]*
heel 250.8 *[707.14]*
knee 250.8 *[707.19]*
specified site NEC 250.8 *[707.19]*
thigh 250.8 *[707.11]*
toes 250.8 *[707.15]*
specified site NEC 250.8 *[707.8]*
Dieulafoy - *see* Lesion, Dieulafoy
due to
infection NEC - *see* Ulcer, skin
radiation, radium - *see* Ulcer, by site
trophic disturbance (any region) - *see* Ulcer, skin
x-ray - *see* Ulcer, by site
duodenum, duodenal (eroded) (peptic) 532.9

> Note Use the following fifth-digit subclassification with categories 531–534:
>
> 0 without mention of obstruction
> 1 with obstruction

with
hemorrhage (chronic) 532.4
and perforation 532.6
perforation (chronic) 532.5
and hemorrhage 532.6
acute 532.3
with
hemorrhage 532.0
and perforation 532.2

Ulcer, ulcerated, ulcerating, ulceration, ulcerative *(Continued)*
duodenum, duodenal *(Continued)*
acute *(Continued)*
with *(Continued)*
perforation 532.1
and hemorrhage 532.2
bleeding (recurrent) - *see* Ulcer, duodenum, with hemorrhage
chronic 532.7
with
hemorrhage 532.4
and perforation 532.6
perforation 532.5
and hemorrhage 532.6
penetrating - *see* Ulcer, duodenum, with perforation
perforating - *see* Ulcer, duodenum, with perforation
dysenteric NEC 009.0
elusive 595.1
endocarditis (any valve) (acute) (chronic) (subacute) 421.0
enteritis - *see* Colitis, ulcerative
enterocolitis 556.0
epiglottis 478.79
esophagus (peptic) 530.20
with bleeding 530.21
due to ingestion
aspirin 530.20
chemicals 530.20
medicinal agents 530.20
fungal 530.20
infectional 530.20
varicose (*see also* Varix, esophagus) 456.1
bleeding (*see also* Varix, esophagus, bleeding) 456.0
eye NEC 360.00
dendritic 054.42
eyelid (region) 373.01
face (*see also* Ulcer, skin) 707.8
fauces 478.29
Fenwick (-Hunner) (solitary) (*see also* Cystitis) 595.1
fistulous NEC - *see* Ulcer, skin
foot (indolent) (*see also* Ulcer, lower extremity) 707.15
perforating 707.15
leprous 030.1
syphilitic 094.0
trophic 707.15
varicose 454.0
inflamed or infected 454.2
frambesial, initial or primary 102.0
gallbladder or duct 575.8
gall duct 576.8
gangrenous (*see also* Gangrene) 785.4
gastric - *see* Ulcer, stomach
gastrocolic - *see* Ulcer, gastrojejunal
gastroduodenal - *see* Ulcer, peptic
gastroesophageal - *see* Ulcer, stomach
gastrohepatic - *see* Ulcer, stomach
gastrointestinal - *see* Ulcer, gastrojejunal
gastrojejunal (eroded) (peptic) 534.9

> Note Use the following fifth-digit subclassification with categories 531–534:
>
> 0 without mention of obstruction
> 1 with obstruction

with
hemorrhage (chronic) 534.4
and perforation 534.6

Ulcer, ulcerated, ulcerating, ulceration, ulcerative *(Continued)*
gastrojejunal *(Continued)*
with *(Continued)*
perforation 534.5
and hemorrhage 534.6
acute 534.3
with
hemorrhage 534.0
and perforation 534.2
perforation 534.1
and hemorrhage 534.2
bleeding (recurrent) - *see* Ulcer, gastrojejunal, with hemorrhage
chronic 534.7
with
hemorrhage 534.4
and perforation 534.6
perforation 534.5
and hemorrhage 534.6
penetrating - *see* Ulcer, gastrojejunal, with perforation
perforating - *see* Ulcer, gastrojejunal, with perforation
gastrojejunocolic - *see* Ulcer, gastrojejunal
genital organ
female 629.89 ⇐
male 608.89
gingiva 523.8
gingivitis 523.10 ⇐
glottis 478.79
granuloma of pudenda 099.2
groin (*see also* Ulcer, skin) 707.8
gum 523.8
gumma, due to yaws 102.4
hand (*see also* Ulcer, skin) 707.8
hard palate 528.9
heel (*see also* Ulcer, lower extremity) 707.14
decubitus (*see also* Ulcer, decubitus) 707.07
hemorrhoids 455.8
external 455.5
internal 455.2
hip (*see also* Ulcer, skin) 707.8
decubitus (*see also* Ulcer, decubitus) 707.04
Hunner's 595.1
hypopharynx 478.29
hypopyon (chronic) (subacute) 370.04
hypostaticum - *see* Ulcer, varicose
ileocolitis 556.1
ileum (*see also* Ulcer, intestine) 569.82
intestine, intestinal 569.82
with perforation 569.83
amebic 006.9
duodenal - *see* Ulcer, duodenum
granulocytopenic (with hemorrhage) 288.09 ⇐
marginal 569.82
perforating 569.83
small, primary 569.82
stercoraceous 569.82
stercoral 569.82
tuberculous (*see also* Tuberculosis) 014.8
typhoid (fever) 002.0
varicose 456.8
ischemic 707.9
lower extremity (*see also* Ulcer, lower extremity) 707.10
ankle 707.13
calf 707.12

Ulcer, ulcerated, ulcerating, ulceration, ulcerative *(Continued)*
ischemic *(Continued)*
lower extremity *(Continued)*
foot 707.15
heel 707.14
knee 707.19
specified site NEC 707.19
thigh 707.11
toes 707.15
jejunum, jejunal - *see* Ulcer, gastrojejunal
keratitis (*see also* Ulcer, cornea) 370.00
knee - *see* Ulcer, lower extremity
labium (majus) (minus) 616.50
laryngitis (*see also* Laryngitis) 464.00
with obstruction 464.01
larynx (aphthous) (contact) 478.79
diphtheritic 032.3
leg - *see* Ulcer, lower extremity
lip 528.5
Lipschütz's 616.50
lower extremity (atrophic) (chronic) (neurogenic) (perforating) (pyogenic) (trophic) (tropical) 707.10
with gangrene (*see also* Ulcer, lower extremity) 707.10 *[785.4]*
ankle 707.13
arteriosclerotic 440.23
with gangrene 440.24
calf 707.12
decubitus 707.00
with gangrene 707.00 *[785.4]*
ankle 707.06
buttock 707.05
heel 707.07
hip 707.04
foot 707.15
heel 707.14
knee 707.19
specified site NEC 707.19
thigh 707.11
toes 707.15
varicose 454.0
inflamed or infected 454.2
luetic - *see* Ulcer, syphilitic
lung 518.89
tuberculous (*see also* Tuberculosis) 011.2
malignant (M8000/3) - *see* Neoplasm, by site, malignant
marginal NEC - *see* Ulcer, gastrojejunal
meatus (urinarius) 597.89
Meckel's diverticulum 751.0
Meleney's (chronic undermining) 686.09
Mooren's (cornea) 370.07
mouth (traumatic) 528.9
mycobacterial (skin) 031.1
nasopharynx 478.29
navel cord (newborn) 771.4
neck (*see also* Ulcer, skin) 707.8
uterus 622.0
neurogenic NEC - *see* Ulcer, skin
nose, nasal (infectional) (passage) 478.19 ⇐
septum 478.19 ⇐
varicose 456.8
skin - *see* Ulcer, skin
spirochetal NEC 104.8
oral mucosa (traumatic) 528.9
palate (soft) 528.9
penetrating NEC - *see* Ulcer, peptic, with perforation
penis (chronic) 607.89

Ulcer, ulcerated, ulcerating, ulceration, ulcerative *(Continued)*
peptic (site unspecified) 533.9

> Note Use the following fifth-digit subclassification with categories 531–534:
>
> 0 without mention of obstruction
> 1 with obstruction

with
hemorrhage 533.4
and perforation 533.6
perforation (chronic) 533.5
and hemorrhage 533.6
acute 533.3
with
hemorrhage 533.0
and perforation 533.2
perforation 533.1
and hemorrhage 533.2
bleeding (recurrent) - *see* Ulcer, peptic, with hemorrhage
chronic 533.7
with
hemorrhage 533.4
and perforation 533.6
perforation 533.5
and hemorrhage 533.6
penetrating - *see* Ulcer, peptic, with perforation
perforating NEC (*see also* Ulcer, peptic, with perforation) 533.5
skin 707.9
perineum (*see also* Ulcer, skin) 707.8
peritonsillar 474.8
phagedenic (tropical) NEC - *see* Ulcer, skin
pharynx 478.29
phlebitis - *see* Phlebitis
plaster (*see also* Ulcer, decubitus) 707.00
popliteal space - *see* Ulcer, lower extremity
postpyloric - *see* Ulcer, duodenum
prepuce 607.89
prepyloric - *see* Ulcer, stomach
pressure (*see also* Ulcer, decubitus) 707.00
primary of intestine 569.82
with perforation 569.83
proctitis 556.2
with ulcerative sigmoiditis 556.3
prostate 601.8
pseudopeptic - *see* Ulcer, peptic
pyloric - *see* Ulcer, stomach
rectosigmoid 569.82
with perforation 569.83
rectum (sphincter) (solitary) 569.41
stercoraceous, stercoral 569.41
varicose - *see* Varicose, ulcer, anus
retina (*see also* Chorioretinitis) 363.20
rodent (M8090/3) - *see also* Neoplasm, skin, malignant
cornea 370.07
round - *see* Ulcer, stomach
sacrum (region) (*see also* Ulcer, skin) 707.8
Saemisch's 370.04
scalp (*see also* Ulcer, skin) 707.8
sclera 379.09
scrofulous (*see also* Tuberculosis) 017.2
scrotum 608.89
tuberculous (*see also* Tuberculosis) 016.5
varicose 456.4

ICD-9-CM

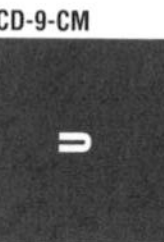

Vol. 2

Ulcer, ulcerated, ulcerating, ulceration, ulcerative *(Continued)*
seminal vesicle 608.89
sigmoid 569.82
with perforation 569.83
skin (atrophic) (chronic) (neurogenic) (non-healing) (perforating) (pyogenic) (trophic) 707.9
with gangrene 707.9 *[785.4]*
amebic 006.6
decubitus (*see also* Ulcer, decubitus) 707.00
with gangrene 707.00 *[785.4]*
in granulocytopenia 288.09
lower extremity (*see also* Ulcer, lower extremity) 707.10
with gangrene 707.10 *[785.4]*
ankle 707.13
arteriosclerotic 440.24
arteriosclerotic 440.23
with gangrene 440.24
calf 707.12
foot 707.15
heel 707.14
knee 707.19
specified site NEC 707.19
thigh 707.11
toes 707.15
mycobacterial 031.1
syphilitic (early) (secondary) 091.3
tuberculous (primary) (*see also* Tuberculosis) 017.0
varicose - *see* Ulcer, varicose
sloughing NEC - *see* Ulcer, skin
soft palate 528.9
solitary, anus or rectum (sphincter) 569.41
sore throat 462
streptococcal 034.0
spermatic cord 608.89
spine (tuberculous) 015.0 *[730.88]*
stasis (leg) (venous) 454.0
with varicose veins 454.0
without varicose veins 459.81
inflamed or infected 454.2
stercoral, stercoraceous 569.82
with perforation 569.83
anus or rectum 569.41
stoma, stomal - *see* Ulcer, gastrojejunal
stomach (eroded) (peptic) (round) 531.9

Note Use the following fifth-digit subclassification with categories 531–534:

0 without mention of obstruction
1 with obstruction

with
hemorrhage 531.4
and perforation 531.6
perforation (chronic) 531.5
and hemorrhage 531.6
acute 531.3
with
hemorrhage 531.0
and perforation 531.2
perforation 531.1
and hemorrhage 531.2
bleeding (recurrent) - *see* Ulcer, stomach, with hemorrhage
chronic 531.7
with
hemorrhage 531.4
and perforation 531.6

Ulcer, ulcerated, ulcerating, ulceration, ulcerative *(Continued)*
stomach *(Continued)*
chronic *(Continued)*
with *(Continued)*
perforation 531.5
and hemorrhage 531.6
penetrating - *see* Ulcer, stomach, with perforation
perforating - *see* Ulcer, stomach, with perforation
stomatitis 528.00
stress - *see* Ulcer, peptic
strumous (tuberculous) (*see also* Tuberculosis) 017.2
submental (*see also* Ulcer, skin) 707.8
submucosal, bladder 595.1
syphilitic (any site) (early) (secondary) 091.3
late 095.9
perforating 095.9
foot 094.0
testis 608.89
thigh - *see* Ulcer, lower extremity
throat 478.29
diphtheritic 032.0
toe - *see* Ulcer, lower extremity
tongue (traumatic) 529.0
tonsil 474.8
diphtheritic 032.0
trachea 519.19
trophic - *see* Ulcer, skin
tropical NEC (*see also* Ulcer, skin) 707.9
tuberculous - *see* Tuberculosis, ulcer
tunica vaginalis 608.89
turbinate 730.9
typhoid (fever) 002.0
perforating 002.0
umbilicus (newborn) 771.4
unspecified site NEC - *see* Ulcer, skin
urethra (meatus) (*see also* Urethritis) 597.89
uterus 621.8
cervix 622.0
with mention of cervicitis 616.0
neck 622.0
with mention of cervicitis 616.0
vagina 616.89
valve, heart 421.0
varicose (lower extremity, any part) 454.0
anus - *see* Varicose, ulcer, anus
broad ligament 456.5
esophagus (*see also* Varix, esophagus) 456.1
bleeding (*see also* Varix, esophagus, bleeding) 456.0
inflamed or infected 454.2
nasal septum 456.8
perineum 456.6
rectum - *see* Varicose, ulcer, anus
scrotum 456.4
specified site NEC 456.8
sublingual 456.3
vulva 456.6
vas deferens 608.89
vesical (*see also* Ulcer, bladder) 596.8
vulva (acute) (infectional) 616.50
Behçet's syndrome 136.1 *[616.51]*
herpetic 054.12
tuberculous 016.7 *[616.51]*
vulvobuccal, recurring 616.50
x-ray - *see* Ulcer, by site
yaws 102.4
Ulcerosa scarlatina 034.1

Ulcus - *see also* Ulcer
cutis tuberculosum (*see also* Tuberculosis) 017.0
duodeni - *see* Ulcer, duodenum
durum 091.0
extragenital 091.2
gastrojejunale - *see* Ulcer, gastrojejunal
hypostaticum - *see* Ulcer, varicose
molle (cutis) (skin) 099.0
serpens corneae (pneumococcal) 370.04
ventriculi - *see* Ulcer, stomach
Ulegyria 742.4
Ulerythema
acneiforma 701.8
centrifugum 695.4
ophryogenes 757.4
Ullrich (-Bonnevie) (-Turner) syndrome 758.6
Ullrich-Feichtiger syndrome 759.89
Ulnar - *see* condition
Ulorrhagia 523.8
Ulorrhea 523.8
Umbilicus, umbilical - *see also* condition
cord necrosis, affecting fetus or newborn 762.6
Unacceptable
existing dental restoration
contours 525.65
morphology 525.65
Unavailability of medical facilities (at) V63.9
due to
investigation by social service agency V63.8
lack of services at home V63.1
remoteness from facility V63.0
waiting list V63.2
home V63.1
outpatient clinic V63.0
specified reason NEC V63.8
Uncinaria americana infestation 126.1
Uncinariasis (*see also* Ancylostomiasis) 126.9
Unconscious, unconsciousness 780.09
Underdevelopment - *see also* Undeveloped
sexual 259.0
Underfill, endodontic 526.63
Undernourishment 269.9
Undernutrition 269.9
Under observation - *see* Observation
Underweight 783.22
for gestational age - *see* Light-for-dates
Underwood's disease (sclerema neonatorum) 778.1
Undescended - *see also* Malposition, congenital
cecum 751.4
colon 751.4
testis 752.51
Undetermined diagnosis or cause 799.9
Undeveloped, undevelopment - *see also* Hypoplasia
brain (congenital) 742.1
cerebral (congenital) 742.1
fetus or newborn 764.9
heart 746.89
lung 748.5
testis 257.2
uterus 259.0
Undiagnosed (disease) 799.9
Undulant fever (*see also* Brucellosis) 023.9
Unemployment, anxiety concerning V62.0

Unequal leg (acquired) (length) 736.81
congenital 755.30
Unerupted teeth, tooth 520.6
Unextracted dental root 525.3
Unguis incarnatus 703.0
Unicornis uterus 752.3
Unicorporeus uterus 752.3
Uniformis uterus 752.3
Unilateral - *see also* condition
development, breast 611.8
organ or site, congenital NEC - *see* Agenesis
vagina 752.49
Unilateralis uterus 752.3
Unilocular heart 745.8
Uninhibited bladder 596.54
with cauda equina syndrome 344.61
neurogenic (*see also* Neurogenic, bladder) 596.54
Union, abnormal - *see also* Fusion
divided tendon 727.89
larynx and trachea 748.3
Universal
joint, cervix 620.6
mesentery 751.4
Unknown
cause of death 799.9
diagnosis 799.9
Unna's disease (seborrheic dermatitis) 690.10
Unresponsiveness, adrenocorticotropin (ACTH) 255.4
Unsatisfactory ⬅
restoration, tooth (existing) 525.60 ◀
specified NEC 525.69 ◀
smear 795.08 ◀
Unsoundness of mind (*see also* Psychosis) 298.9
Unspecified cause of death 799.9
Unstable
back NEC 724.9
colon 569.89
joint - *see* Instability, joint
lie 652.0
affecting fetus or newborn (before labor) 761.7
causing obstructed labor 660.0
affecting fetus or newborn 763.1
lumbosacral joint (congenital) 756.19
acquired 724.6
sacroiliac 724.6
spine NEC 724.9
Untruthfulness, child problem (*see also* Disturbance, conduct) 312.0
Unverricht (-Lundborg) disease, syndrome, or epilepsy 333.2
Unverricht-Wagner syndrome (dermatomyositis) 710.3
Upper respiratory - *see* condition
Upset
gastric 536.8
psychogenic 306.4
gastrointestinal 536.8
psychogenic 306.4
virus (*see also* Enteritis, viral) 008.8
intestinal (large) (small) 564.9
psychogenic 306.4
menstruation 626.9
mental 300.9
stomach 536.8
psychogenic 306.4
Urachus - *see also* condition
patent 753.7
persistent 753.7
Uratic arthritis 274.0
Urbach's lipoid proteinosis 272.8
Urbach-Oppenheim disease or syndrome (necrobiosis lipoidica diabeticorum) 250.8 [709.3]
Urbach-Wiethe disease or syndrome (lipoid proteinosis) 272.8
Urban yellow fever 060.1
Urea, blood, high - *see* Uremia
Uremia, uremic (absorption) (amaurosis) (amblyopia) (aphasia) (apoplexy) (coma) (delirium) (dementia) (dropsy) (dyspnea) (fever) (intoxication) (mania) (paralysis) (poisoning) (toxemia) (vomiting) 586
with
abortion - *see* Abortion, by type, with renal failure
ectopic pregnancy (*see also* categories 633.0–633.9) 639.3
hypertension (*see also* Hypertension, kidney) 403.91
molar pregnancy (*see also* categories 630–632) 639.3
chronic 585.9
complicating
abortion 639.3
ectopic or molar pregnancy 639.3
hypertension (*see also* Hypertension, kidney) 403.91
labor and delivery 669.3
congenital 779.89
extrarenal 788.9
hypertensive (chronic) (*see also* Hypertension, kidney) 403.91
maternal NEC, affecting fetus or newborn 760.1
neuropathy 585.9 *[357.4]*
pericarditis 585.9 *[420.0]*
prerenal 788.9
pyelitic (*see also* Pyelitis) 590.80
Ureter, ureteral - *see* condition
Ureteralgia 788.0
Ureterectasis 593.89
Ureteritis 593.89
cystica 590.3
due to calculus 592.1
gonococcal (acute) 098.19
chronic or duration of 2 months or over 098.39
nonspecific 593.89
Ureterocele (acquired) 593.89
congenital 753.23
Ureterolith 592.1
Ureterolithiasis 592.1
Ureterostomy status V44.6
with complication 997.5
Urethra, urethral - *see* condition
Urethralgia 788.9
Urethritis (abacterial) (acute) (allergic) (anterior) (chronic) (nonvenereal) (posterior) (recurrent) (simple) (subacute) (ulcerative) (undifferentiated) 597.80
diplococcal (acute) 098.0
chronic or duration of 2 months or over 098.2
due to Trichomonas (vaginalis) 131.02
gonococcal (acute) 098.0
chronic or duration of 2 months or over 098.2
nongonococcal (sexually transmitted) 099.40
Chlamydia trachomatis 099.41
Urethritis *(Continued)*
nongonococcal *(Continued)*
Reiter's 099.3
specified organism NEC 099.49
nonspecific (sexually transmitted) (*see also* Urethritis, nongonococcal) 099.40
not sexually transmitted 597.80
Reiter's 099.3
trichomonal or due to Trichomonas (vaginalis) 131.02
tuberculous (*see also* Tuberculosis) 016.3
venereal NEC (*see also* Urethritis, nongonococcal) 099.40
Urethrocele
female 618.03
with uterine prolapse 618.4
complete 618.3
incomplete 618.2
male 599.5
Urethrolithiasis 594.2
Urethro-oculoarticular syndrome 099.3
Urethro-oculosynovial syndrome 099.3
Urethrorectal - *see* condition
Urethrorrhagia 599.84
Urethrorrhea 788.7
Urethrostomy status V44.6
with complication 997.5
Urethrotrigonitis 595.3
Urethrovaginal - *see* condition
Urhidrosis, uridrosis 705.89
Uric acid
diathesis 274.9
in blood 790.6
Uricacidemia 790.6
Uricemia 790.6
Uricosuria 791.9
Urination
frequent 788.41
painful 788.1
urgency 788.63
Urine, urinary - *see also* condition
abnormality NEC 788.69
blood in (*see also* Hematuria) 599.7
discharge, excessive 788.42
enuresis 788.30
nonorganic origin 307.6
extravasation 788.8
frequency 788.41
hesitancy 788.64 ◀
incontinence 788.30
active 788.30
female 788.30
stress 625.6
and urge 788.33
male 788.30
stress 788.32
and urge 788.33
mixed (stress and urge) 788.33
neurogenic 788.39
nonorganic origin 307.6
overflow 788.38
stress (female) 625.6
male NEC 788.32
intermittent stream 788.61
pus in 791.9
retention or stasis NEC 788.20
bladder, incomplete emptying 788.21
psychogenic 306.53
specified NEC 788.29
secretion
deficient 788.5
excessive 788.42
frequency 788.41

◀ New ⬅ Revised

Urine, urinary *(Continued)*
- strain 788.65 ◀
- stream
  - intermittent 788.61
  - slowing 788.62
  - splitting 788.61
  - weak 788.62
- urgency 788.63

Urinemia - *see* Uremia
Urinoma NEC 599.9
- bladder 596.8
- kidney 593.89
- renal 593.89
- ureter 593.89
- urethra 599.84

Uroarthritis, infectious 099.3
Urodialysis 788.5
Urolithiasis 592.9
Uronephrosis 593.89
Uropathy 599.9
- obstructive 599.60

Urosepsis 599.0
- meaning sepsis 995.91
- meaning urinary tract infection 599.0

Urticaria 708.9
- with angioneurotic edema 995.1
  - hereditary 277.6
- allergic 708.0
- cholinergic 708.5
- chronic 708.8
- cold, familial 708.2
- dermatographic 708.3
- due to
  - cold or heat 708.2
  - drugs 708.0
  - food 708.0
  - inhalants 708.0
  - plants 708.8
  - serum 999.5
- factitial 708.3
- giant 995.1

Urticaria *(Continued)*
- giant *(Continued)*
  - hereditary 277.6
- gigantea 995.1
  - hereditary 277.6
- idiopathic 708.1
- larynx 995.1
  - hereditary 277.6
- neonatorum 778.8
- nonallergic 708.1
- papulosa (Hebra) 698.2
- perstans hemorrhagica 757.39
- pigmentosa 757.33
- recurrent periodic 708.8
- serum 999.5
- solare 692.72
- specified type NEC 708.8
- thermal (cold) (heat) 708.2
- vibratory 708.4

Urticarioides acarodermatitis 133.9
Use of
- nonprescribed drugs (*see also* Abuse, drugs, nondependent) 305.9
- patent medicines (*see also* Abuse, drugs, nondependent) 305.9

Usher-Senear disease (pemphigus erythematosus) 694.4
Uta 085.5
Uterine size-date discrepancy 649.6 ⬅
Uteromegaly 621.2
Uterovaginal - *see* condition
Uterovesical - *see* condition
Uterus - *see* condition
Utriculitis (utriculus prostaticus) 597.89
Uveal - *see* condition
Uveitis (anterior) (*see also* Iridocyclitis) 364.3
- acute or subacute 364.00
  - due to or associated with
    - gonococcal infection 098.41
    - herpes (simplex) 054.44

Uveitis *(Continued)*
- acute or subacute *(Continued)*
  - due to or associated with *(Continued)*
    - zoster 053.22
  - primary 364.01
  - recurrent 364.02
  - secondary (noninfectious) 364.04
    - infectious 364.03
- allergic 360.11
- chronic 364.10
  - due to or associated with
    - sarcoidosis 135 *[364.11]*
    - tuberculosis (*see also* Tuberculosis) 017.3 *[364.11]*
- due to
  - operation 360.11
  - toxoplasmosis (acquired) 130.2
    - congenital (active) 771.2
- granulomatous 364.10
- heterochromic 364.21
- lens-induced 364.23
- nongranulomatous 364.00
- posterior 363.20
  - disseminated - *see* Chorioretinitis, disseminated
  - focal - *see* Chorioretinitis, focal
- recurrent 364.02
- sympathetic 360.11
- syphilitic (secondary) 091.50
  - congenital 090.0 *[363.13]*
  - late 095.8 *[363.13]*
- tuberculous (*see also* Tuberculosis) 017.3 *[364.11]*

Uveoencephalitis 363.22
Uveokeratitis (*see also* Iridocyclitis) 364.3
Uveoparotid fever 135
Uveoparotitis 135
Uvula - *see* condition
Uvulitis (acute) (catarrhal) (chronic) (gangrenous) (membranous) (suppurative) (ulcerative) 528.3

V

Vaccination
complication or reaction - *see* Complications, vaccination
not carried out V64.00
because of
acute illness V64.01
allergy to vaccine or component V64.04
caregiver refusal V64.05
chronic illness V64.02
immune compromised state V64.03
patient had disease being vaccinated against V64.08
patient refusal V64.06
reason NEC V64.09
religious reasons V64.07
prophylactic (against) V05.9
arthropod-borne viral
disease NEC V05.1
encephalitis V05.0
chicken pox V05.4
cholera (alone) V03.0
with typhoid-paratyphoid (cholera + TAB) V06.0
common cold V04.7
diphtheria (alone) V03.5
with
poliomyelitis (DTP + polio) V06.3
tetanus V06.5
pertussis combined [DTP] [DTaP] V06.1
typhoid-paratyphoid (DTP + TAB) V06.2
disease (single) NEC V05.9
bacterial NEC V03.9
specified type NEC V03.89
combination NEC V06.9
specified type NEC V06.8
specified type NEC V05.8
encephalitis, viral, arthropod-borne V05.0
Haemophilus influenzae, type B [Hib] V03.81
hepatitis, viral V05.3
influenza V04.81
with
Streptococcus pneumoniae [pneumococcus] V06.6
leishmaniasis V05.2
measles (alone) V04.2
with mumps-rubella (MMR) V06.4
mumps (alone) V04.6
with measles and rubella (MMR) V06.4
pertussis alone V03.6
plague V03.3
poliomyelitis V04.0
with diphtheria-tetanus-pertussis (DTP + polio) V06.3
rabies V04.5
respiratory syncytial virus (RSV) V04.82
rubella (alone) V04.3
with measles and mumps (MMR) V06.4
smallpox V04.1
Streptococcus pneumoniae [pneumococcus] V03.82
with
influenza V06.6

Vaccination *(Continued)*
prophylactic *(Continued)*
tetanus toxoid (alone) V03.7
with diphtheria [Td] [DT] V06.5
with
pertussis (DTP) (DTaP) V06.1
with poliomyelitis (DTP + polio) V06.3
tuberculosis (BCG) V03.2
tularemia V03.4
typhoid-paratyphoid (TAB) (alone) V03.1
with diphtheria-tetanus-pertussis (TAB + DTP) V06.2
varicella V05.4
viral
disease NEC V04.89
encephalitis, arthropod-borne V05.0
hepatitis V05.3
yellow fever V04.4
Vaccinia (generalized) 999.0
congenital 771.2
conjunctiva 999.3
eyelids 999.0 *[373.5]*
localized 999.3
nose 999.3
not from vaccination 051.0
eyelid 051.0 *[373.5]*
sine vaccinatione 051.0
without vaccination 051.0
Vacuum
extraction of fetus or newborn 763.3
in sinus (accessory) (nasal) (*see also* Sinusitis) 473.9
Vagabond V60.0
Vagabondage V60.0
Vagabonds' disease 132.1
Vagina, vaginal - *see* condition
Vaginalitis (tunica) 608.4
Vaginismus (reflex) 625.1
functional 306.51
hysterical 300.11
psychogenic 306.51
Vaginitis (acute) (chronic) (circumscribed) (diffuse) (emphysematous) (Haemophilus vaginalis) (nonspecific) (nonvenereal) (ulcerative) 616.10
with
abortion - *see* Abortion, by type, with sepsis
ectopic pregnancy (*see also* categories 633.0–633.9) 639.0
molar pregnancy (*see also* categories 630–632) 639.0
adhesive, congenital 752.49
atrophic, postmenopausal 627.3
bacterial 616.10
blennorrhagic (acute) 098.0
chronic or duration of 2 months or over 098.2
candidal 112.1
chlamydial 099.53
complicating pregnancy or puerperium 646.6
affecting fetus or newborn 760.8
congenital (adhesive) 752.49
due to
C. albicans 112.1
Trichomonas (vaginalis) 131.01
following
abortion 639.0
ectopic or molar pregnancy 639.0

Vaginitis *(Continued)*
gonococcal (acute) 098.0
chronic or duration of 2 months or over 098.2
granuloma 099.2
Monilia 112.1
mycotic 112.1
pinworm 127.4 *[616.11]*
postirradiation 616.10
postmenopausal atrophic 627.3
senile (atrophic) 627.3
syphilitic (early) 091.0
late 095.8
trichomonal 131.01
tuberculous (*see also* Tuberculosis) 016.7
venereal NEC 099.8
Vaginosis - *see* Vaginitis
Vagotonia 352.3
Vagrancy V60.0
Vallecula - *see* condition
Valley fever 114.0
Valsuani's disease (progressive pernicious anemia, puerperal) 648.2
Valve, valvular (formation) - *see also* condition
cerebral ventricle (communicating) in situ V45.2
cervix, internal os 752.49
colon 751.5
congenital NEC - *see* Atresia
formation, congenital, NEC - *see* Atresia
heart defect - *see* Anomaly, heart, valve
ureter 753.29
pelvic junction 753.21
vesical orifice 753.22
urethra 753.6
Valvulitis (chronic) (*see also* Endocarditis) 424.90
rheumatic (chronic) (inactive) (with chorea) 397.9
active or acute (aortic) (mitral) (pulmonary) (tricuspid) 391.1
syphilitic NEC 093.20
aortic 093.22
mitral 093.21
pulmonary 093.24
tricuspid 093.23
Valvulopathy - *see* Endocarditis
van Bogaert's leukoencephalitis (sclerosing) (subacute) 046.2
van Bogaert-Nijssen (-Peiffer) disease 330.0
van Buchem's syndrome (hyperostosis corticalis) 733.3
Vancomycin (glycopeptide)
intermediate staphylococcus aureus (VISA/GISA) V09.8
resistant
enterococcus (VRE) V09.8
staphylococcus aureus (VRSA/GRSA) V09.8
van Creveld-von Gierke disease (glycogenosis I) 271.0
van den Bergh's disease (enterogenous cyanosis) 289.7
van der Hoeve's syndrome (brittle bones and blue sclera, deafness) 756.51
van der Hoeve-Halbertsma-Waardenburg syndrome (ptosis-epicanthus) 270.2
van der Hoeve-Waardenburg-Gualdi syndrome (ptosis-epicanthus) 270.2
Vanillism 692.89
Vanishing lung 492.0

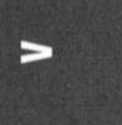

Vanishing twin 651.33
van Neck (-Odelberg) disease or syndrome (juvenile osteochondrosis) 732.1
Vapor asphyxia or suffocation NEC 987.9
specified agent - *see* Table of Drugs and Chemicals
Vaquez's disease (M9950/1) 238.4
Vaquez-Osler disease (polycythemia vera) (M9950/1) 238.4
Variance, lethal ball, prosthetic heart valve 996.02
Variants, thalassemic 282.49
Variations in hair color 704.3
Varicella 052.9
with
complication 052.8
specified NEC 052.7
pneumonia 052.1
exposure to V01.71
vaccination and inoculation (against) (prophylactic) V05.4
Varices - *see* Varix
Varicocele (scrotum) (thrombosed) 456.4
ovary 456.5
perineum 456.6
spermatic cord (ulcerated) 456.4
Varicose
aneurysm (ruptured) (*see also* Aneurysm) 442.9
dermatitis (lower extremity) - *see* Varicose, vein, inflamed or infected
eczema - *see* Varicose, vein
phlebitis - *see* Varicose, vein, inflamed or infected
placental vessel - *see* Placenta, abnormal
tumor - *see* Varicose, vein
ulcer (lower extremity, any part) 454.0
anus 455.8
external 455.5
internal 455.2
esophagus (*see also* Varix, esophagus) 456.1
bleeding (*see also* Varix, esophagus, bleeding) 456.0
inflamed or infected 454.2
nasal septum 456.8
perineum 456.6
rectum - *see* Varicose, ulcer, anus
scrotum 456.4
specified site NEC 456.8
vein (lower extremity) (ruptured) (*see also* Varix) 454.9
with
complications NEC 454.8
edema 454.8
inflammation or infection 454.1
ulcerated 454.2
pain 454.8
stasis dermatitis 454.1
with ulcer 454.2
swelling 454.8
ulcer 454.0
inflamed or infected 454.2
anus - *see* Hemorrhoids
broad ligament 456.5
congenital (peripheral) 747.60
gastrointestinal 747.61
lower limb 747.64
renal 747.62
specified NEC 747.69
upper limb 747.63

Varicose *(Continued)*
vein *(Continued)*
esophagus (ulcerated (*see also* Varix, esophagus) 456.1
bleeding (*see also* Varix, esophagus, bleeding) 456.0
inflamed or infected 454.1
with ulcer 454.2
in pregnancy or puerperium 671.0
vulva or perineum 671.1
nasal septum (with ulcer) 456.8
pelvis 456.5
perineum 456.6
in pregnancy, childbirth, or puerperium 671.1
rectum - *see* Hemorrhoids
scrotum (ulcerated) 456.4
specified site NEC 456.8
sublingual 456.3
ulcerated 454.0
inflamed or infected 454.2
umbilical cord, affecting fetus or newborn 762.6
urethra 456.8
vulva 456.6
in pregnancy, childbirth, or puerperium 671.1
vessel - *see also* Varix
placenta - *see* Placenta, abnormal
Varicosis, varicosities, varicosity (*see also* Varix) 454.9
Variola 050.9
hemorrhagic (pustular) 050.0
major 050.0
minor 050.1
modified 050.2
Varioloid 050.2
Variolosa, purpura 050.0
Varix (lower extremity) (ruptured) 454.9
with
complications NEC 454.8
edema 454.8
inflammation or infection 454.1
with ulcer 454.2
pain 454.8
stasis dermatitis 454.1
with ulcer 454.2
swelling 454.8
ulcer 454.0
with inflammation or infection 454.2
aneurysmal (*see also* Aneurysm) 442.9
anus - *see* Hemorrhoids
arteriovenous (congenital) (peripheral) NEC 747.60
gastrointestinal 747.61
lower limb 747.64
renal 747.62
specified NEC 747.69
spinal 747.82
upper limb 747.63
bladder 456.5
broad ligament 456.5
congenital (peripheral) 747.60
esophagus (ulcerated) 456.1
bleeding 456.0
in
cirrhosis of liver 571.5 *[456.20]*
portal hypertension 572.3 *[456.20]*
congenital 747.69
in
cirrhosis of liver 571.5 *[456.21]*
with bleeding 571.5 *[456.20]*

Varix *(Continued)*
esophagus *(Continued)*
in *(Continued)*
portal hypertension 572.3 *[456.21]*
with bleeding 572.3 *[456.20]*
gastric 456.8
inflamed or infected 454.1
ulcerated 454.2
in pregnancy or puerperium 671.0
perineum 671.1
vulva 671.1
labia (majora) 456.6
orbit 456.8
congenital 747.69
ovary 456.5
papillary 448.1
pelvis 456.5
perineum 456.6
in pregnancy or puerperium 671.1
pharynx 456.8
placenta - *see* Placenta, abnormal
prostate 456.8
rectum - *see* Hemorrhoids
renal papilla 456.8
retina 362.17
scrotum (ulcerated) 456.4
sigmoid colon 456.8
specified site NEC 456.8
spinal (cord) (vessels) 456.8
spleen, splenic (vein) (with phlebolith) 456.8
sublingual 456.3
ulcerated 454.0
inflamed or infected 454.2
umbilical cord, affecting fetus or newborn 762.6
uterine ligament 456.5
vocal cord 456.8
vulva 456.6
in pregnancy, childbirth, or puerperium 671.1
Vasa previa 663.5
affecting fetus or newborn 762.6
hemorrhage from, affecting fetus or newborn 772.0
Vascular - *see also* condition
loop on papilla (optic) 743.57
sheathing, retina 362.13
spasm 443.9
spider 448.1
Vascularity, pulmonary, congenital 747.3
Vascularization
choroid 362.16
cornea 370.60
deep 370.63
localized 370.61
retina 362.16
subretinal 362.16
Vasculitis 447.6
allergic 287.0
cryoglobulinemic 273.2
disseminated 447.6
kidney 447.8
leukocytoclastic 446.29
nodular 695.2
retinal 362.18
rheumatic - *see* Fever, rheumatic
Vasculopathy
cardiac allograft 996.83
Vas deferens - *see* condition
Vas deferentitis 608.4
Vasectomy, admission for V25.2
Vasitis 608.4
nodosa 608.4

Vasitis *(Continued)*
scrotum 608.4
spermatic cord 608.4
testis 608.4
tuberculous (*see also* Tuberculosis) 016.5
tunica vaginalis 608.4
vas deferens 608.4
Vasodilation 443.9
Vasomotor - *see* condition
Vasoplasty, after previous sterilization V26.0
Vasoplegia, splanchnic (*see also* Neuropathy, peripheral, autonomic) 337.9
Vasospasm 443.9
cerebral (artery) 435.9
with transient neurologic deficit 435.9
coronary 413.1
nerve
arm NEC 354.9
autonomic 337.9
brachial plexus 353.0
cervical plexus 353.2
leg NEC 355.8
lower extremity NEC 355.8
peripheral NEC 335.9
spinal NEC 355.9
sympathetic 337.9
upper extremity NEC 354.9
peripheral NEC 443.9
retina (artery) (*see also* Occlusion, retinal, artery) 362.30
Vasospastic - *see* condition
Vasovagal attack (paroxysmal) 780.2
psychogenic 306.2
Vater's ampulla - *see* condition
VATER syndrome 759.89
Vegetation, vegetative
adenoid (nasal fossa) 474.2
consciousness (persistent) 780.03
endocarditis (acute) (any valve) (chronic) (subacute) 421.0
heart (mycotic) (valve) 421.0
state (persistent) 780.03
Veil
Jackson's 751.4
over face (causing asphyxia) 768.9
Vein, venous - *see* condition
Veldt sore (*see also* Ulcer, skin) 707.9
Velo-cardio-facial syndrome 758.32
Velpeau's hernia - *see* Hernia, femoral
Venereal
balanitis NEC 099.8
bubo 099.1
disease 099.9
specified nature or type NEC 099.8
granuloma inguinale 099.2
lymphogranuloma (Durand-Nicolas-Favre), any site 099.1
salpingitis 098.37
urethritis (*see also* Urethritis, nongonococcal) 099.40
vaginitis NEC 099.8
warts 078.19
Vengefulness, in child (*see also* Disturbance, conduct) 312.0
Venofibrosis 459.89
Venom, venomous
bite or sting (animal or insect) 989.5
poisoning 989.5
Venous - *see* condition
Ventouse delivery NEC 669.5
affecting fetus or newborn 763.3
Ventral - *see* condition
Ventricle, ventricular - *see also* condition
escape 427.69
standstill (*see also* Arrest, cardiac) 427.5
Ventriculitis, cerebral (*see also* Meningitis) 322.9
Ventriculostomy status V45.2
Verbiest's syndrome (claudicatio intermittens spinalis) 435.1
Vernet's syndrome 352.6
Verneuil's disease (syphilitic bursitis) 095.7
Verruca (filiformis) 078.10
acuminata (any site) 078.11
necrogenica (primary) (*see also* Tuberculosis) 017.0
peruana 088.0
peruviana 088.0
plana (juvenilis) 078.19
plantaris 078.19
seborrheica 702.19
inflamed 702.11
senilis 702.0
tuberculosa (primary) (*see also* Tuberculosis) 017.0
venereal 078.19
viral NEC 078.10
Verrucosities (*see also* Verruca) 078.10
Verrucous endocarditis (acute) (any valve) (chronic) (subacute) 710.0 *[424.91]*
nonbacterial 710.0 *[424.91]*
Verruga
peruana 088.0
peruviana 088.0
Verse's disease (calcinosis intervertebralis) 275.49 [722.90]
Version
before labor, affecting fetus or newborn 761.7
cephalic (correcting previous malposition) 652.1
affecting fetus or newborn 763.1
cervix - *see* Version, uterus
uterus (postinfectional) (postpartal, old) (*see also* Malposition, uterus) 621.6
forward - *see* Anteversion, uterus
lateral - *see* Lateroversion, uterus
Vertebra, vertebral - *see* condition
Vertigo 780.4
auditory 386.19
aural 386.19
benign paroxysmal positional 386.11
central origin 386.2
cerebral 386.2
Dix and Hallpike (epidemic) 386.12
endemic paralytic 078.81
epidemic 078.81
Dix and Hallpike 386.12
Gerlier's 078.81
Pedersen's 386.12
vestibular neuronitis 386.12
epileptic - *see* Epilepsy
Gerlier's (epidemic) 078.81
hysterical 300.11
labyrinthine 386.10
laryngeal 786.2
malignant positional 386.2
Ménière's (*see also* Disease, Ménière's) 386.00
menopausal 627.2
otogenic 386.19
paralytic 078.81
paroxysmal positional, benign 386.11
Pedersen's (epidemic) 386.12
Vertigo *(Continued)*
peripheral 386.10
specified type NEC 386.19
positional
benign paroxysmal 386.11
malignant 386.2
Verumontanitis (chronic) (*see also* Urethritis) 597.89
Vesania (*see also* Psychosis) 298.9
Vesical - *see* condition
Vesicle
cutaneous 709.8
seminal - *see* condition
skin 709.8
Vesicocolic - *see* condition
Vesicoperineal - *see* condition
Vesicorectal - *see* condition
Vesicourethrorectal - *see* condition
Vesicovaginal - *see* condition
Vesicular - *see* condition
Vesiculitis (seminal) 608.0
amebic 006.8
gonorrheal (acute) 098.14
chronic or duration of 2 months or over 098.34
trichomonal 131.09
tuberculous (*see also* Tuberculosis) 016.5 *[608.81]*
Vestibulitis (ear) (*see also* Labyrinthitis) 386.30
nose (external) 478.19
vulvar 616.10
Vestibulopathy, acute peripheral (recurrent) 386.12
Vestige, vestigial - *see also* Persistence
branchial 744.41
structures in vitreous 743.51
Vibriosis NEC 027.9
Vidal's disease (lichen simplex chronicus) 698.3
Video display tube syndrome 723.8
Vienna-type encephalitis 049.8
Villaret's syndrome 352.6
Villous - *see* condition
VIN I (vulvar intraepithelial neoplasia I) 624.0
VIN II (vulvar intraepithelial neoplasia II) 624.0
VIN III (vulvar intraepithelial neoplasia III) 233.3
Vincent's
angina 101
bronchitis 101
disease 101
gingivitis 101
infection (any site) 101
laryngitis 101
stomatitis 101
tonsillitis 101
Vinson-Plummer syndrome (sideropenic dysphagia) 280.8
Viosterol deficiency (*see also* Deficiency, calciferol) 268.9
Virchow's disease 733.99
Viremia 790.8
Virilism (adrenal) (female) NEC 255.2
with
3-beta-hydroxysteroid dehydrogenase defect 255.2
11-hydroxylase defect 255.2
21-hydroxylase defect 255.2
adrenal
hyperplasia 255.2
insufficiency (congenital) 255.2
cortical hyperfunction 255.2

Virilization (female) (suprarenal) (*see also* Virilism) 255.2
isosexual 256.4
Virulent bubo 099.0
Virus, viral - *see also* condition
infection NEC (*see also* Infection, viral) 079.99
septicemia 079.99
VISA (vancomycin intermediate staphylococcus aureus) V09.8
Viscera, visceral - *see* condition
Visceroptosis 569.89
Visible peristalsis 787.4
Vision, visual
binocular, suppression 368.31
blurred, blurring 368.8
hysterical 300.11
defect, defective (*see also* Impaired, vision) 369.9
disorientation (syndrome) 368.16
disturbance NEC (*see also* Disturbance, vision) 368.9
hysterical 300.11
examination V72.0
field, limitation 368.40
fusion, with defective stereopsis 368.33
hallucinations 368.16
halos 368.16
loss 369.9
both eyes (*see also* Blindness, both eyes) 369.3
complete (*see also* Blindness, both eyes) 369.00
one eye 369.8
sudden 368.16
low (both eyes) 369.20
one eye (other eye normal) (*see also* Impaired, vision) 369.70
blindness, other eye 369.10
perception, simultaneous without fusion 368.32
tunnel 368.45
Vitality, lack or want of 780.79
newborn 779.89
Vitamin deficiency NEC (*see also* Deficiency, vitamin) 269.2
Vitelline duct, persistent 751.0
Vitiligo 709.01
due to pinta (carate) 103.2
eyelid 374.53
vulva 624.8
Vitium cordis - *see* Disease, heart
Vitreous - *see also* condition
touch syndrome 997.99
VLCAD (long chain/very long chain acyl CoA dehydrogenase deficiency, LCAD) 277.85
Vocal cord - *see* condition
Vocational rehabilitation V57.22
Vogt's (Cecile) disease or syndrome 333.7
Vogt-Koyanagi syndrome 364.24
Vogt-Spielmeyer disease (amaurotic familial idiocy) 330.1
Voice
change (*see also* Dysphonia) 784.49
loss (*see also* Aphonia) 784.41
Volhard-Fahr disease (malignant nephrosclerosis) 403.00
Volhynian fever 083.1
Volkmann's ischemic contracture or paralysis (complicating trauma) 958.6
Voluntary starvation 307.1
Volvulus (bowel) (colon) (intestine) 560.2
with
hernia - *see also* Hernia, by site, with obstruction
gangrenous - *see* Hernia, by site, with gangrene
perforation 560.2
congenital 751.5
duodenum 537.3
fallopian tube 620.5
oviduct 620.5
stomach (due to absence of gastrocolic ligament) 537.89
Vomiting 787.03
with nausea 787.01
allergic 535.4
asphyxia 933.1
bilious (cause unknown) 787.0
following gastrointestinal surgery 564.3
blood (*see also* Hematemesis) 578.0
causing asphyxia, choking, or suffocation (*see also* Asphyxia, food) 933.1
cyclical 536.2
psychogenic 306.4
epidemic 078.82
fecal matter 569.89
following gastrointestinal surgery 564.3
functional 536.8
psychogenic 306.4
habit 536.2
hysterical 300.11
nervous 306.4
neurotic 306.4
newborn 779.3
of or complicating pregnancy 643.9
due to
organic disease 643.8
specific cause NEC 643.8
early - *see* Hyperemesis, gravidarum
late (after 22 completed weeks of gestation) 643.2
pernicious or persistent 536.2
complicating pregnancy - *see* Hyperemesis, gravidarum
psychogenic 306.4
physiological 787.0
psychic 306.4
psychogenic 307.54
stercoral 569.89
uncontrollable 536.2
psychogenic 306.4
uremic - *see* Uremia
winter 078.82
von Bechterew (-Strümpell) disease or syndrome (ankylosing spondylitis) 720.0
von Bezold's abscess 383.01
von Economo's disease (encephalitis lethargica) 049.8
von Eulenburg's disease (congenital paramyotonia) 359.2
von Gierke's disease (glycogenosis I) 271.0
von Gies' joint 095.8
von Graefe's disease or syndrome 378.72
von Hippel (-Lindau) disease or syndrome (retinocerebral angiomatosis) 759.6
von Jaksch's anemia or disease (pseudoleukemia infantum) 285.8
von Recklinghausen's
disease or syndrome (nerves) (skin) (M9540/1) 237.71
bones (osteitis fibrosa cystica) 252.01
tumor (M9540/1) 237.71
von Recklinghausen-Applebaum disease (hemochromatosis) 275.0
von Schroetter's syndrome (intermittent venous claudication) 453.8
von Willebrand (-Jürgens) (-Minot) disease or syndrome (angiohemophilia) 286.4
von Zambusch's disease (lichen sclerosus et atrophicus) 701.0
Voorhoeve's disease or dyschondroplasia 756.4
Vossius' ring 921.3
late effect 366.21
Voyeurism 302.82
VRE (vancomycin resistant enterococcus) V09.8
Vrolik's disease (osteogenesis imperfecta) 756.51
VRSA (vancomycin resistant staphylococcus aureus) V09.8
Vulva - *see* condition
Vulvismus 625.1
Vulvitis (acute) (allergic) (aphthous) (chronic) (gangrenous) (hypertrophic) (intertriginous) 616.10
with
abortion - *see* Abortion, by type, with sepsis
ectopic pregnancy (*see also* categories 633.0–633.9) 639.0
molar pregnancy (*see also* categories 630–632) 639.0
adhesive, congenital 752.49
blennorrhagic (acute) 098.0
chronic or duration of 2 months or over 098.2
chlamydial 099.53
complicating pregnancy or puerperium 646.6
due to Ducrey's bacillus 099.0
following
abortion 639.0
ectopic or molar pregnancy 639.0
gonococcal (acute) 098.0
chronic or duration of 2 months or over 098.2
herpetic 054.11
leukoplakic 624.0
monilial 112.1
puerperal, postpartum, childbirth 646.6
syphilitic (early) 091.0
late 095.8
trichomonal 131.01
Vulvodynia 625.9
Vulvorectal - *see* condition
Vulvovaginitis (*see also* Vulvitis) 616.10
amebic 006.8
chlamydial 099.53
gonococcal (acute) 098.0
chronic or duration of 2 months or over 098.2
herpetic 054.11
monilial 112.1
trichomonal (Trichomonas vaginalis) 131.01

◀ New ⇐ Revised

W

Waardenburg's syndrome 756.89
meaning ptosis-epicanthus 270.2
Waardenburg-Klein syndrome (ptosis-epicanthus) 270.2
Wagner's disease (colloid milium) 709.3
Wagner (-Unverricht) syndrome (dermatomyositis) 710.3
Waiting list, person on V63.2
undergoing social agency investigation V63.8
Wakefulness disorder (*see also* Hypersomnia) 780.54
nonorganic origin 307.43
Waldenström's
disease (osteochondrosis, capital femoral) 732.1
hepatitis (lupoid hepatitis) 571.49
hypergammaglobulinemia 273.0
macroglobulinemia 273.3
purpura, hypergammaglobulinemic 273.0
syndrome (macroglobulinemia) 273.3
Waldenström-Kjellberg syndrome (sideropenic dysphagia) 280.8
Walking
difficulty 719.7
psychogenic 307.9
sleep 307.46
hysterical 300.13
Wall, abdominal - *see* condition
Wallenberg's syndrome (posterior inferior cerebellar artery) (*see also* Disease, cerebrovascular, acute) 436
Wallgren's
disease (obstruction of splenic vein with collateral circulation) 459.89
meningitis (*see also* Meningitis, aseptic) 047.9
Wandering
acetabulum 736.39
gallbladder 751.69
kidney, congenital 753.3
organ or site, congenital NEC - *see* Malposition, congenital
pacemaker (atrial) (heart) 427.89
spleen 289.59
Wardrop's disease (with lymphangitis) 681.9
finger 681.02
toe 681.11
War neurosis 300.16
Wart (common) (digitate) (filiform) (infectious) (viral) 078.10
external genital organs (venereal) 078.19
fig 078.19
Hassall-Henle's (of cornea) 371.41
Henle's (of cornea) 371.41
juvenile 078.19
moist 078.10
Peruvian 088.0
plantar 078.19
prosector (*see also* Tuberculosis) 017.0
seborrheic 702.19
inflamed 702.11
senile 702.0
specified NEC 078.19
syphilitic 091.3
tuberculous (*see also* Tuberculosis) 017.0
venereal (female) (male) 078.19
Warthin's tumor (salivary gland) (M8561/0) 210.2
Washerwoman's itch 692.4
Wassilieff's disease (leptospiral jaundice) 100.0
Wasting
disease 799.4
due to malnutrition 261
extreme (due to malnutrition) 261
muscular NEC 728.2
palsy, paralysis 335.21
pelvic muscle 618.83
Water
clefts 366.12
deprivation of 994.3
in joint (*see also* Effusion, joint) 719.0
intoxication 276.6
itch 120.3
lack of 994.3
loading 276.6
on
brain - *see* Hydrocephalus
chest 511.8
poisoning 276.6
Waterbrash 787.1
Water-hammer pulse (*see also* Insufficiency, aortic) 424.1
Waterhouse (-Friderichsen) disease or syndrome 036.3
Water-losing nephritis 588.89
Wax in ear 380.4
Waxy
degeneration, any site 277.39 (Revised)
disease 277.39 (Revised)
kidney 277.39 *[583.81]* (Revised)
liver (large) 277.39 (Revised)
spleen 277.39 (Revised)
Weak, weakness (generalized) 780.79
arches (acquired) 734
congenital 754.61
bladder sphincter 596.59
congenital 779.89
eye muscle - *see* Strabismus
facial 781.94
foot (double) - *see* Weak, arches
heart, cardiac (*see also* Failure, heart) 428.9
congenital 746.9
mind 317
muscle (generalized) 728.87
myocardium (*see also* Failure, heart) 428.9
newborn 779.89
pelvic fundus
pubocervical tissue 618.81
rectovaginal tissue 618.82
pulse 785.9
senile 797
urinary stream 788.62
valvular - *see* Endocarditis
Wear, worn, tooth, teeth (approximal) (hard tissues) (interproximal) (occlusal) - *see also* Attrition, teeth 521.10
Weather, weathered
effects of
cold NEC 991.9
specified effect NEC 991.8
hot (*see also* Heat) 992.9
skin 692.74
Web, webbed (congenital) - *see also* Anomaly, specified type NEC
canthus 743.63
digits (*see also* Syndactylism) 755.10
duodenal 751.5
esophagus 750.3
fingers (*see also* Syndactylism, fingers) 755.11
Web, webbed *(Continued)*
larynx (glottic) (subglottic) 748.2
neck (pterygium colli) 744.5
Paterson-Kelly (sideropenic dysphagia) 280.8
popliteal syndrome 756.89
toes (*see also* Syndactylism, toes) 755.13
Weber's paralysis or syndrome 344.89
Weber-Christian disease or syndrome (nodular nonsuppurative panniculitis) 729.30
Weber-Cockayne syndrome (epidermolysis bullosa) 757.39
Weber-Dimitri syndrome 759.6
Weber-Gubler syndrome 344.89
Weber-Leyden syndrome 344.89
Weber-Osler syndrome (familial hemorrhagic telangiectasia) 448.0
Wedge-shaped or wedging vertebra (*see also* Osteoporosis) 733.00
Wegener's granulomatosis or syndrome 446.4
Wegner's disease (syphilitic osteochondritis) 090.0
Weight
gain (abnormal) (excessive) 783.1
during pregnancy 646.1
insufficient 646.8
less than 1000 grams at birth 765.0
loss (cause unknown) 783.21
Weightlessness 994.9
Weil's disease (leptospiral jaundice) 100.0
Weill-Marchesani syndrome (brachymorphism and ectopia lentis) 759.89
Weingarten's syndrome (tropical eosinophilia) 518.3
Weir Mitchell's disease (erythromelalgia) 443.82
Weiss-Baker syndrome (carotid sinus syncope) 337.0
Weissenbach-Thibierge syndrome (cutaneous systemic sclerosis) 710.1
Wen (*see also* Cyst, sebaceous) 706.2
Wenckebach's phenomenon, heart block (second degree) 426.13
Werdnig-Hoffmann syndrome (muscular atrophy) 335.0
Werlhof's disease (*see also* Purpura, thrombocytopenic) 287.39
Werlhof-Wichmann syndrome (*see also* Purpura, thrombocytopenic) 287.39
Wermer's syndrome or disease (polyendocrine adenomatosis) 258.0
Werner's disease or syndrome (progeria adultorum) 259.8
Werner-His disease (trench fever) 083.1
Werner-Schultz disease (agranulocytosis) 288.09 (Revised)
Wernicke's encephalopathy, disease, or syndrome (superior hemorrhagic polioencephalitis) 265.1
Wernicke-Korsakoff syndrome or psychosis (nonalcoholic) 294.0
alcoholic 291.1
Wernicke-Posadas disease (*see also* Coccidioidomycosis) 114.9
Wesselsbron fever 066.3
West African fever 084.8
West Nile
encephalitis 066.41
encephalomyelitis 066.41
fever 066.40
with
cranial nerve disorders 066.42

West Nile *(Continued)*
fever *(Continued)*
with *(Continued)*
encephalitis 066.41
optic neuritis 066.42
other complications 066.49
other neurologic manifestations 066.42
polyradiculitis 066.42
virus 066.40
Westphal-Strümpell syndrome (hepatolenticular degeneration) 275.1
Wet
brain (alcoholic) (*see also* Alcoholism) 303.9
feet, tropical (syndrome) (maceration) 991.4
lung (syndrome)
adult 518.5
newborn 770.6
Wharton's duct - *see* condition
Wheal 709.8
Wheezing 786.07
Whiplash injury or syndrome 847.0
Whipple's disease or syndrome (intestinal lipodystrophy) 040.2
Whipworm 127.3
"Whistling face" syndrome (craniocarpotarsal dystrophy) 759.89
White - *see also* condition
kidney
large - *see* Nephrosis
small 582.9
leg, puerperal, postpartum, childbirth 671.4
nonpuerperal 451.19
mouth 112.0
patches of mouth 528.6
sponge nevus of oral mucosa 750.26
spot lesions, teeth 521.01
White's disease (congenital) (keratosis follicularis) 757.39
Whitehead 706.2
Whitlow (with lymphangitis) 681.01
herpetic 054.6
Whitmore's disease or fever (melioidosis) 025
Whooping cough 033.9
with pneumonia 033.9 *[484.3]*
due to
Bordetella
bronchoseptica 033.8
with pneumonia 033.8 *[484.3]*
parapertussis 033.1
with pneumonia 033.1 *[484.3]*
pertussis 033.0
with pneumonia 033.0 *[484.3]*
specified organism NEC 033.8
with pneumonia 033.8 *[484.3]*
vaccination, prophylactic (against) V03.6
Wichmann's asthma (laryngismus stridulus) 478.75
Widal (-Abrami) syndrome (acquired hemolytic jaundice) 283.9
Widening aorta (*see also* Aneurysm, aorta) 441.9
ruptured 441.5
Wilkie's disease or syndrome 557.1
Wilkinson-Sneddon disease or syndrome (subcorneal pustular dermatosis) 694.1
Willan's lepra 696.1
Willan-Plumbe syndrome (psoriasis) 696.1
Willebrand (-Jürgens) syndrome or thrombopathy (angiohemophilia) 286.4
Willi-Prader syndrome (hypogenital dystrophy with diabetic tendency) 759.81
Willis' disease (diabetes mellitus) (*see also* Diabetes) 250.0
Wilms' tumor or neoplasm (nephroblastoma) (M8960/3) 189.0
Wilson's
disease or syndrome (hepatolenticular degeneration) 275.1
hepatolenticular degeneration 275.1
lichen ruber 697.0
Wilson-Brocq disease (dermatitis exfoliativa) 695.89
Wilson-Mikity syndrome 770.7
Window - *see also* Imperfect, closure aorticopulmonary 745.0
Winged scapula 736.89
Winter - *see also* condition
vomiting disease 078.82
Wise's disease 696.2
Wiskott-Aldrich syndrome (eczema-thrombocytopenia) 279.12
Withdrawal symptoms, syndrome
alcohol 291.81
delirium (acute) 291.0
chronic 291.1
newborn 760.71
drug or narcotic 292.0
newborn, infant of dependent mother 779.5
steroid NEC
correct substance properly administered 255.4
overdose or wrong substance given or taken 962.0
Withdrawing reaction, child or adolescent 313.22
Witts' anemia (achlorhydric anemia) 280.9
Witzelsucht 301.9
Woakes' syndrome (ethmoiditis) 471.1
Wohlfart-Kugelberg-Welander disease 335.11
Woillez's disease (acute idiopathic pulmonary congestion) 518.5
Wolff-Parkinson-White syndrome (anomalous atrioventricular excitation) 426.7
Wolhynian fever 083.1
Wolman's disease (primary familial xanthomatosis) 272.7
Wood asthma 495.8
Woolly, wooly hair (congenital) (nevus) 757.4
Wool-sorters' disease 022.1
Word
blindness (congenital) (developmental) 315.01
secondary to organic lesion 784.61
deafness (secondary to organic lesion) 784.69
developmental 315.31
Worm(s) (colic) (fever) (infection) (infestation) (*see also* Infestation) 128.9
guinea 125.7
in intestine NEC 127.9
Worm-eaten soles 102.3
Worn out (*see also* Exhaustion) 780.79
"Worried well" V65.5
Wound, open (by cutting or piercing instrument) (by firearms) (cut) (dissection) (incised) (laceration) (penetration) (perforating) (puncture) (with initial hemorrhage, not internal) 879.8

> Note For fracture with open wound, see Fracture.
>
> For laceration, traumatic rupture, tear, or penetrating wound of internal organs, such as heart, lung, liver, kidney, pelvic organs, etc., whether or not accompanied by open wound or fracture in the same region, see Injury, internal. For contused wound, see Contusion. For crush injury, see Crush. For abrasion, insect bite (nonvenomous), blister, or scratch, see Injury, superficial.
>
> Complicated includes wounds with:
>
> delayed healing
> delayed treatment
> foreign body
> primary infection
>
> For late effect of open wound, see Late, effect, wound, open, by site.

abdomen, abdominal (external) (muscle) 879.2
complicated 879.3
wall (anterior) 879.2
complicated 879.3
lateral 879.4
complicated 879.5
alveolar (process) 873.62
complicated 873.72
ankle 891.0
with tendon involvement 891.2
complicated 891.1
anterior chamber, eye (*see also* Wound, open, intraocular) 871.9
anus 879.6
complicated 879.7
arm 884.0
with tendon involvement 884.2
complicated 884.1
forearm 881.00
with tendon involvement 881.20
complicated 881.10
multiple sites - *see* Wound, open, multiple, upper limb
upper 880.03
with tendon involvement 880.23
complicated 880.13
multiple sites (with axillary or shoulder regions) 880.09
with tendon involvement 880.29
complicated 880.19
artery - *see* Injury, blood vessel, by site
auditory
canal (external) (meatus) 872.02
complicated 872.12
ossicles (incus) (malleus) (stapes) 872.62
complicated 872.72
auricle, ear 872.01
complicated 872.11
axilla 880.02
with tendon involvement 880.22
complicated 880.12
with tendon involvement 880.29
involving other sites of upper arm 880.09
complicated 880.19

Wound, open *(Continued)*
- back 876.0
  - complicated 876.1
- bladder - *see* Injury, internal, bladder
- blood vessel - *see* Injury, blood vessel, by site
- brain - *see* Injury, intracranial, with open intracranial wound
- breast 879.0
  - complicated 879.1
- brow 873.42
  - complicated 873.52
- buccal mucosa 873.61
  - complicated 873.71
- buttock 877.0
  - complicated 877.1
- calf 891.0
  - with tendon involvement 891.2
  - complicated 891.1
- canaliculus lacrimalis 870.8
  - with laceration of eyelid 870.2
- canthus, eye 870.8
  - laceration - *see* Laceration, eyelid
- cavernous sinus - *see* Injury, intracranial
- cerebellum - *see* Injury, intracranial
- cervical esophagus 874.4
  - complicated 874.5
- cervix - *see* Injury, internal, cervix
- cheek(s) (external) 873.41
  - complicated 873.51
  - internal 873.61
    - complicated 873.71
- chest (wall) (external) 875.0
  - complicated 875.1
- chin 873.44
  - complicated 873.54
- choroid 363.63
- ciliary body (eye) (*see also* Wound, open, intraocular) 871.9
- clitoris 878.8
  - complicated 878.9
- cochlea 872.64
  - complicated 872.74
- complicated 879.9
- conjunctiva - *see* Wound, open, intraocular
- cornea (nonpenetrating) (*see also* Wound, open, intraocular) 871.9
- costal region 875.0
  - complicated 875.1
- Descemet's membrane (*see also* Wound, open, intraocular) 871.9
- digit(s)
  - foot 893.0
    - with tendon involvement 893.2
    - complicated 893.1
  - hand 883.0
    - with tendon involvement 883.2
    - complicated 883.1
- drumhead, ear 872.61
  - complicated 872.71
- ear 872.8
  - canal 872.02
    - complicated 872.12
  - complicated 872.9
  - drum 872.61
    - complicated 872.71
  - external 872.00
    - complicated 872.10
  - multiple sites 872.69
    - complicated 872.79
  - ossicles (incus) (malleus) (stapes) 872.62
    - complicated 872.72

Wound, open *(Continued)*
- ear *(Continued)*
  - specified part NEC 872.69
    - complicated 872.79
- elbow 881.01
  - with tendon involvement 881.21
  - complicated 881.11
- epididymis 878.2
  - complicated 878.3
- epigastric region 879.2
  - complicated 879.3
- epiglottis 874.01
  - complicated 874.11
- esophagus (cervical) 874.4
  - complicated 874.5
  - thoracic - *see* Injury, internal, esophagus
- Eustachian tube 872.63
  - complicated 872.73
- extremity
  - lower (multiple) NEC 894.0
    - with tendon involvement 894.2
    - complicated 894.1
  - upper (multiple) NEC 884.0
    - with tendon involvement 884.2
    - complicated 884.1
- eye(s) (globe) - *see* Wound, open, intraocular
- eyeball NEC 871.9
  - laceration (*see also* Laceration, eyeball) 871.4
  - penetrating (*see also* Penetrating wound, eyeball) 871.7
- eyebrow 873.42
  - complicated 873.52
- eyelid NEC 870.8
  - laceration - *see* Laceration, eyelid
- face 873.40
  - complicated 873.50
  - multiple sites 873.49
    - complicated 873.59
  - specified part NEC 873.49
    - complicated 873.59
- fallopian tube - *see* Injury, internal, fallopian tube
- finger(s) (nail) (subungual) 883.0
  - with tendon involvement 883.2
  - complicated 883.1
- flank 879.4
  - complicated 879.5
- foot (any part, except toe(s) alone) 892.0
  - with tendon involvement 892.2
  - complicated 892.1
- forearm 881.00
  - with tendon involvement 881.20
  - complicated 881.10
- forehead 873.42
  - complicated 873.52
- genital organs (external) NEC 878.8
  - complicated 878.9
  - internal - *see* Injury, internal, by site
- globe (eye) (*see also* Wound, open, eyeball) 871.9
- groin 879.4
  - complicated 879.5
- gum(s) 873.62
  - complicated 873.72
- hand (except finger(s) alone) 882.0
  - with tendon involvement 882.2
  - complicated 882.1
- head NEC 873.8
  - with intracranial injury - *see* Injury, intracranial

Wound, open *(Continued)*
- head NEC *(Continued)*
  - with *(Continued)*
    - due to or associated with skull fracture - *see* Fracture, skull
  - complicated 873.9
  - scalp - *see* Wound, open, scalp
- heel 892.0
  - with tendon involvement 892.2
  - complicated 892.1
- high-velocity (grease gun) - *see* Wound, open, complicated, by site
- hip 890.0
  - with tendon involvement 890.2
  - complicated 890.1
- hymen 878.6
  - complicated 878.7
- hypochondrium 879.4
  - complicated 879.5
- hypogastric region 879.2
  - complicated 879.3
- iliac (region) 879.4
  - complicated 879.5
- incidental to
  - dislocation - *see* Dislocation, open, by site
  - fracture - *see* Fracture, open, by site
  - intracranial injury - *see* Injury, intracranial, with open intracranial wound
  - nerve injury - *see* Injury, nerve, by site
- inguinal region 879.4
  - complicated 879.5
- instep 892.0
  - with tendon involvement 892.2
  - complicated 892.1
- interscapular region 876.0
  - complicated 876.1
- intracranial - *see* Injury, intracranial, with open intracranial wound
- intraocular 871.9
  - with
    - partial loss (of intraocular tissue) 871.2
    - prolapse or exposure (of intraocular tissue) 871.1
  - laceration (*see also* Laceration, eyeball) 871.4
  - penetrating 871.7
    - with foreign body (nonmagnetic) 871.6
      - magnetic 871.5
  - without prolapse (of intraocular tissue) 871.0
- iris (*see also* Wound, open, eyeball) 871.9
- jaw (fracture not involved) 873.44
  - with fracture - *see* Fracture, jaw
  - complicated 873.54
- knee 891.0
  - with tendon involvement 891.2
  - complicated 891.1
- labium (majus) (minus) 878.4
  - complicated 878.5
- lacrimal apparatus, gland, or sac 870.8
  - with laceration of eyelid 870.2
- larynx 874.01
  - with trachea 874.00
    - complicated 874.10
  - complicated 874.11
- leg (multiple) 891.0
  - with tendon involvement 891.2
  - complicated 891.1

Wound, open *(Continued)*
leg *(Continued)*
lower 891.0
with tendon involvement 891.2
complicated 891.1
thigh 890.0
with tendon involvement 890.2
complicated 890.1
upper 890.0
with tendon involvement 890.2
complicated 890.1
lens (eye) (alone) (*see also* Cataract, traumatic) 366.20
with involvement of other eye structures - *see* Wound, open, eyeball
limb
lower (multiple) NEC 894.0
with tendon involvement 894.2
complicated 894.1
upper (multiple) NEC 884.0
with tendon involvement 884.2
complicated 884.1
lip 873.43
complicated 873.53
loin 876.0
complicated 876.1
lumbar region 876.0
complicated 876.1
malar region 873.41
complicated 873.51
mastoid region 873.49
complicated 873.59
mediastinum - *see* Injury, internal, mediastinum
midthoracic region 875.0
complicated 875.1
mouth 873.60
complicated 873.70
floor 873.64
complicated 873.74
multiple sites 873.69
complicated 873.79
specified site NEC 873.69
complicated 873.79
multiple, unspecified site(s) 879.8

Note Multiple open wounds of sites classifiable to the same four-digit category should be classified to that category unless they are in different limbs.

Multiple open wounds of sites classifiable to different four-digit categories, or to different limbs, should be coded separately.

complicated 879.9
lower limb(s) (one or both) (sites classifiable to more than one three-digit category in 890–893) 894.0
with tendon involvement 894.2
complicated 894.1
upper limb(s) (one or both) (sites classifiable to more than one three-digit category in 880–883) 884.0
with tendon involvement 884.2
complicated 884.1
muscle - *see* Sprain, by site
nail
finger(s) 883.0
complicated 883.1
thumb 883.0
complicated 883.1

Wound, open *(Continued)*
nail *(Continued)*
toe(s) 893.0
complicated 893.1
nape (neck) 874.8
complicated 874.9
specified part NEC 874.8
complicated 874.9
nasal - *see also* Wound, open, nose
cavity 873.22
complicated 873.32
septum 873.21
complicated 873.31
sinuses 873.23
complicated 873.33
nasopharynx 873.22
complicated 873.32
neck 874.8
complicated 874.9
nape 874.8
complicated 874.9
specified part NEC 874.8
complicated 874.9
nerve - *see* Injury, nerve, by site
non-healing surgical 998.83
nose 873.20
complicated 873.30
multiple sites 873.29
complicated 873.39
septum 873.21
complicated 873.31
sinuses 873.23
complicated 873.33
occipital region - *see* Wound, open, scalp
ocular NEC 871.9
adnexa 870.9
specified region NEC 870.8
laceration (*see also* Laceration, ocular) 871.4
muscle (extraocular) 870.3
with foreign body 870.4
eyelid 870.1
intraocular - *see* Wound, open, eyeball
penetrating (*see also* Penetrating wound, ocular) 871.7
orbit 870.8
penetrating 870.3
with foreign body 870.4
orbital region 870.9
ovary - *see* Injury, internal, pelvic organs
palate 873.65
complicated 873.75
palm 882.0
with tendon involvement 882.2
complicated 882.1
parathyroid (gland) 874.2
complicated 874.3
parietal region - *see* Wound, open, scalp
pelvic floor or region 879.6
complicated 879.7
penis 878.0
complicated 878.1
perineum 879.6
complicated 879.7
periocular area 870.8
laceration of skin 870.0
pharynx 874.4
complicated 874.5
pinna 872.01
complicated 872.11
popliteal space 891.0
with tendon involvement 891.2
complicated 891.1

Wound, open *(Continued)*
prepuce 878.0
complicated 878.1
pubic region 879.2
complicated 879.3
pudenda 878.8
complicated 878.9
rectovaginal septum 878.8
complicated 878.9
sacral region 877.0
complicated 877.1
sacroiliac region 877.0
complicated 877.1
salivary (ducts) (glands) 873.69
complicated 873.79
scalp 873.0
complicated 873.1
scalpel, fetus or newborn 767.8
scapular region 880.01
with tendon involvement 880.21
complicated 880.11
involving other sites of upper arm 880.09
with tendon involvement 880.29
complicated 880.19
sclera (*see also* Wound, open, intraocular) 871.9
scrotum 878.2
complicated 878.3
seminal vesicle - *see* Injury, internal, pelvic organs
shin 891.0
with tendon involvement 891.2
complicated 891.1
shoulder 880.00
with tendon involvement 880.20
complicated 880.10
involving other sites of upper arm 880.09
with tendon involvement 880.29
complicated 880.19
skin NEC 879.8
complicated 879.9
skull - *see also* Injury, intracranial, with open intracranial wound
with skull fracture - *see* Fracture, skull
spermatic cord (scrotal) 878.2
complicated 878.3
pelvic region - *see* Injury, internal, spermatic cord
spinal cord - *see* Injury, spinal
sternal region 875.0
complicated 875.1
subconjunctival - *see* Wound, open, intraocular
subcutaneous NEC 879.8
complicated 879.9
submaxillary region 873.44
complicated 873.54
submental region 873.44
complicated 873.54
subungual
finger(s) (thumb) - *see* Wound, open, finger
toe(s) - *see* Wound, open, toe
supraclavicular region 874.8
complicated 874.9
supraorbital 873.42
complicated 873.52
surgical, non-healing 998.83
temple 873.49
complicated 873.59
temporal region 873.49
complicated 873.59

Wound, open *(Continued)*
testis 878.2
complicated 878.3
thigh 890.0
with tendon involvement 890.2
complicated 890.1
thorax, thoracic (external) 875.0
complicated 875.1
throat 874.8
complicated 874.9
thumb (nail) (subungual) 883.0
with tendon involvement 883.2
complicated 883.1
thyroid (gland) 874.2
complicated 874.3
toe(s) (nail) (subungual) 893.0
with tendon involvement 893.2
complicated 893.1
tongue 873.64
complicated 873.74
tonsil - *see* Wound, open, neck
trachea (cervical region) 874.02
with larynx 874.00
complicated 874.10
complicated 874.12

Wound, open *(Continued)*
trachea *(Continued)*
intrathoracic - *see* Injury, internal, trachea
trunk (multiple) NEC 879.6
complicated 879.7
specified site NEC 879.6
complicated 879.7
tunica vaginalis 878.2
complicated 878.3
tympanic membrane 872.61
complicated 872.71
tympanum 872.61
complicated 872.71
umbilical region 879.2
complicated 879.3
ureter - *see* Injury, internal, ureter
urethra - *see* Injury, internal, urethra
uterus - *see* Injury, internal, uterus
uvula 873.69
complicated 873.79
vagina 878.6
complicated 878.7
vas deferens - *see* Injury, internal, vas deferens
vitreous (humor) 871.2

Wound, open *(Continued)*
vulva 878.4
complicated 878.5
wrist 881.02
with tendon involvement 881.22
complicated 881.12
Wright's syndrome (hyperabduction) 447.8
pneumonia 390 *[517.1]*
Wringer injury - *see* Crush injury, by site
Wrinkling of skin 701.8
Wrist - *see also* condition
drop (acquired) 736.05
Wrong drug (given in error) NEC 977.9
specified drug or substance - *see* Table of Drugs and Chemicals
Wry neck - *see also* Torticollis
congenital 754.1
Wuchereria infestation 125.0
bancrofti 125.0
Brugia malayi 125.1
malayi 125.1
Wuchereriasis 125.0
Wuchereriosis 125.0
Wuchernde struma langhans (M8332/3) 193

X

Xanthelasma 272.2
- eyelid 272.2 *[374.51]*
- palpebrarum 272.2 *[374.51]*

Xanthelasmatosis (essential) 272.2
Xanthelasmoidea 757.33
Xanthine stones 277.2
Xanthinuria 277.2
Xanthofibroma (M8831/0) - *see* Neoplasm, connective tissue, benign
Xanthoma(s), xanthomatosis 272.2
- with
  - hyperlipoproteinemia
    - type I 272.3
    - type III 272.2
    - type IV 272.1
    - type V 272.3
- bone 272.7
- craniohypophyseal 277.89
- cutaneotendinous 272.7
- diabeticorum 250.8 *[272.2]*
- disseminatum 272.7
- eruptive 272.2
- eyelid 272.2 *[374.51]*
- familial 272.7
- hereditary 272.7
- hypercholesterinemic 272.0
- hypercholesterolemic 272.0
- hyperlipemic 272.4
- hyperlipidemic 272.4
- infantile 272.7
- joint 272.7
- juvenile 272.7
- multiple 272.7
- multiplex 272.7
- primary familial 272.7
- tendon (sheath) 272.7
- tuberosum 272.2
- tuberous 272.2
- tubo-eruptive 272.2

Xanthosis 709.09
- surgical 998.81

Xenophobia 300.29
Xeroderma (congenital) 757.39
- acquired 701.1
  - eyelid 373.33
- eyelid 373.33
- pigmentosum 757.33
- vitamin A deficiency 264.8

Xerophthalmia 372.53
- vitamin A deficiency 264.7

Xerosis
- conjunctiva 372.53
  - with Bitôt's spot 372.53
    - vitamin A deficiency 264.1
  - vitamin A deficiency 264.0
- cornea 371.40
  - with corneal ulceration 370.00
    - vitamin A deficiency 264.3
  - vitamin A deficiency 264.2
- cutis 706.8
- skin 706.8

Xerostomia 527.7
Xiphodynia 733.90
Xiphoidalgia 733.90
Xiphoiditis 733.99
Xiphopagus 759.4
XO syndrome 758.6
X-ray
- effects, adverse, NEC 990
- of chest
  - for suspected tuberculosis V71.2
  - routine V72.5

XXX syndrome 758.81
XXXXY syndrome 758.81
XXY syndrome 758.7
Xyloketosuria 271.8
Xylosuria 271.8
Xylulosuria 271.8
XYY syndrome 758.81

Y

Yawning 786.09
psychogenic 306.1
Yaws 102.9
bone or joint lesions 102.6
butter 102.1
chancre 102.0
cutaneous, less than five years after infection 102.2
early (cutaneous) (macular) (maculopapular) (micropapular) (papular) 102.2
frambeside 102.2
skin lesions NEC 102.2
eyelid 102.9 *[373.4]*
ganglion 102.6
gangosis, gangosa 102.5
gumma, gummata 102.4
bone 102.6
gummatous
frambeside 102.4
osteitis 102.6
periostitis 102.6
hydrarthrosis 102.6
hyperkeratosis (early) (late) (palmar) (plantar) 102.3
initial lesions 102.0
joint lesions 102.6
Yaws *(Continued)*
juxta-articular nodules 102.7
late nodular (ulcerated) 102.4
latent (without clinical manifestations) (with positive serology) 102.8
mother 102.0
mucosal 102.7
multiple papillomata 102.1
nodular, late (ulcerated) 102.4
osteitis 102.6
papilloma, papillomata (palmar) (plantar) 102.1
periostitis (hypertrophic) 102.6
ulcers 102.4
wet crab 102.1
Yeast infection (*see also* Candidiasis) 112.9
Yellow
atrophy (liver) 570
chronic 571.8
resulting from administration of blood, plasma, serum, or other biological substance (within 8 months of administration) - *see* Hepatitis, viral
fever - *see* Fever, yellow
jack (*see also* Fever, yellow) 060.9
jaundice (*see also* Jaundice) 782.4
Yersinia septica 027.8

Z

Zagari's disease (xerostomia) 527.7
Zahorsky's disease (exanthema subitum) 057.8
syndrome (herpangina) 074.0
Zellweger syndrome 277.86
Zenker's diverticulum (esophagus) 530.6
Ziehen-Oppenheim disease 333.6
Zieve's syndrome (jaundice, hyperlipemia, and hemolytic anemia) 571.1
Zika fever 066.3
Zollinger-Ellison syndrome (gastric hypersecretion with pancreatic islet cell tumor) 251.5
Zona (*see also* Herpes, zoster) 053.9
Zoophilia (erotica) 302.1
Zoophobia 300.29
Zoster (herpes) (*see also* Herpes, zoster) 053.9
Zuelzer (-Ogden) anemia or syndrome (nutritional megaloblastic anemia) 281.2
Zygodactyly (*see also* Syndactylism) 755.10
Zygomycosis 117.7
Zymotic - *see* condition

SECTION II TABLE OF DRUGS AND CHEMICALS

ALPHABETIC INDEX TO POISONING AND EXTERNAL CAUSES OF ADVERSE EFFECTS OF DRUGS AND OTHER CHEMICAL SUBSTANCES

This table contains a classification of drugs and other chemical substances to identify poisoning states and external causes of adverse effects.

Each of the listed substances in the table is assigned a code according to the poisoning classification (960–989). These codes are used when there is a statement of poisoning, overdose, wrong substance given or taken, or intoxication.

The table also contains a listing of external causes of adverse effects. An adverse effect is a pathologic manifestation due to ingestion or exposure to drugs or other chemical substances (e.g., dermatitis, hypersensitivity reaction, aspirin gastritis). The adverse effect is to be identified by the appropriate code found in Section I, Index to Diseases and Injuries. An external cause code can then be used to identify the circumstances involved. The table headings pertaining to external causes are defined below:

Accidental poisoning (E850–E869)-accidental overdose of drug, wrong substance given or taken, drug taken inadvertently, accidents in the usage of drugs and biologicals in medical and surgical procedures, and to show external causes of poisonings classifiable to 980–989.

Therapeutic use (E930–E949)-a correct substance properly administered in therapeutic or prophylactic dosage as the external cause of adverse effects.

Suicide attempt (E950–E952)-instances in which self-inflicted injuries or poisonings are involved.

Assault (E961–E962)-injury or poisoning inflicted by another person with the intent to injure or kill.

Undetermined (E980–E982)-to be used when the intent of the poisoning or injury cannot be determined whether it was intentional or accidental.

The American Hospital Formulary Service (AHFS) list numbers are included in the table to help classify new drugs not identified in the table by name. The AHFS list numbers are keyed to the continually revised AHFS (American Hospital Formulary Service, 2 vol. Washington, D.C.: American Society of Hospital Pharmacists, 1959-). These listings are found in the table under the main term **Drug.**

Excluded from the table are radium and other radioactive substances. The classification of adverse effects and complications pertaining to these substances will be found in Index to Diseases and Injuries, and Index to External Causes of Injuries.

Although certain substances are indexed with one or more subentries, the majority are listed according to one use or state. It is recognized that many substances may be used in various ways, in medicine and in industry, and may cause adverse effects whatever the state of the agent (solid, liquid, or fumes arising from a liquid). In cases in which the reported data indicate a use or state not in the table, or which is clearly different from the one listed, an attempt should be made to classify the substance in the form which most nearly expresses the reported facts.

Substance	Poisoning	External Cause (E-Code) Accident	Therapeutic Use	Suicide Attempt	Assault	Undetermined
1-propanol	980.3	E860.4	—	E950.9	E962.1	E980.9
2-propanol	980.2	E860.3	—	E950.9	E962.1	E980.9
2,4-D (dichlorophenoxyacetic acid)	989.4	E863.5	—	E950.6	E962.1	E980.7
2,4-toluene diisocyanate	983.0	E864.0	—	E950.7	E962.1	E980.6
2,4,5-T (trichlorophenoxyacetic acid)	989.2	E863.5	—	E950.6	E962.1	E980.7
14-hydroxydihydromorphinone	965.09	E850.2	E935.2	E950.0	E962.0	E980.0
ABOB	961.7	E857	E931.7	E950.4	E962.0	E980.4
Abrus (seed)	988.2	E865.3	—	E950.9	E962.1	E980.9
Absinthe	980.0	E860.1	—	E950.9	E962.1	E980.9
beverage	980.0	E860.0	—	E950.9	E962.1	E980.9
Acenocoumarin, acenocoumarol	964.2	E858.2	E934.2	E950.4	E962.0	E980.4
Acepromazine	969.1	E853.0	E939.1	E950.3	E962.0	E980.3
Acetal	982.8	E862.4	—	E950.9	E962.1	E980.9
Acetaldehyde (vapor)	987.8	E869.8	—	E952.8	E962.2	E982.8
liquid	989.89	E866.8	—	E950.9	E962.1	E980.9
Acetaminophen	965.4	E850.4	E935.4	E950.0	E962.0	E980.0
Acetaminosalol	965.1	E850.3	E935.3	E950.0	E962.0	E980.0
Acetanilid(e)	965.4	E850.4	E935.4	E950.0	E962.0	E980.0
Acetarsol, acetarsone	961.1	E857	E931.1	E950.4	E962.0	E980.4
Acetazolamide	974.2	E858.5	E944.2	E950.4	E962.0	E980.4
Acetic	—	—	—	—	—	—
acid	983.1	E864.1	—	E950.7	E962.1	E980.6
with sodium acetate (ointment)	976.3	E858.7	E946.3	E950.4	E962.0	E980.4
irrigating solution	974.5	E858.5	E944.5	E950.4	E962.0	E980.4
lotion	976.2	E858.7	E946.2	E950.4	E962.0	E980.4
anhydride	983.1	E864.1	—	E950.7	E962.1	E980.6
ether (vapor)	982.8	E862.4	—	E950.9	E962.1	E980.9
Acetohexamide	962.3	E858.0	E932.3	E950.4	E962.0	E980.4
Acetomenaphthone	964.3	E858.2	E934.3	E950.4	E962.0	E980.4
Acetomorphine	965.01	E850.0	E935.0	E950.0	E962.0	E980.0
Acetone (oils) (vapor)	982.8	E862.4	—	E950.9	E962.1	E980.9
Acetophenazine (maleate)	969.1	E853.0	E939.1	E950.3	E962.0	E980.3
Acetophenetidin	965.4	E850.4	E935.4	E950.0	E962.0	E980.0
Acetophenone	982.0	E862.4	—	E950.9	E962.1	E980.9
Acetorphine	965.09	E850.2	E935.2	E950.0	E962.0	E980.0
Acetosulfone (sodium)	961.8	E857	E931.8	E950.4	E962.0	E980.4
Acetrizoate (sodium)	977.8	E858.8	E947.8	E950.4	E962.0	E980.4
Acetylcarbromal	967.3	E852.2	E937.3	E950.2	E962.0	E980.2
Acetylcholine (chloride)	971.0	E855.3	E941.0	E950.4	E962.0	E980.4
Acetylcysteine	975.5	E858.6	E945.5	E950.4	E962.0	E980.4
Acetyldigitoxin	972.1	E858.3	E942.1	E950.4	E962.0	E980.4
Acetyldihydrocodeine	965.09	E850.2	E935.2	E950.0	E962.0	E980.0
Acetyldihydrocodeinone	965.09	E850.2	E935.2	E950.0	E962.0	E980.0
Acetylene (gas) (industrial)	987.1	E868.1	—	E951.8	E962.2	E981.8
incomplete combustion of - *see* Carbon monoxide, fuel, utility	—	—	—	—	—	—
tetrachloride (vapor)	982.3	E862.4	—	E950.9	E962.1	E980.9
Acetyliodosalicylic acid	965.1	E850.3	E935.3	E950.0	E962.0	E980.0
Acetylphenylhydrazine	965.8	E850.8	E935.8	E950.0	E962.0	E980.0
Acetylsalicylic acid	965.1	E850.3	E935.3	E950.0	E962.0	E980.0
Achromycin	960.4	E856	E930.4	E950.4	E962.0	E980.4
ophthalmic preparation	976.5	E858.7	E946.5	E950.4	E962.0	E980.4
topical NEC	976.0	E858.7	E946.0	E950.4	E962.0	E980.4
Acidifying agents	963.2	E858.1	E933.2	E950.4	E962.0	E980.4
Acids (corrosive) NEC	983.1	E864.1	—	E950.7	E962.1	E980.6
Aconite (wild)	988.2	E865.4	—	E950.9	E962.1	E980.9
Aconitine (liniment)	976.8	E858.7	E946.8	E950.4	E962.0	E980.4
Aconitum ferox	988.2	E865.4	—	E950.9	E962.1	E980.9
Acridine	983.0	E864.0	—	E950.7	E962.1	E980.6
vapor	987.8	E869.8	—	E952.8	E962.2	E982.8
Acriflavine	961.9	E857	E931.9	E950.4	E962.0	E980.4
Acrisorcin	976.0	E858.7	E946.0	E950.4	E962.0	E980.4

Substance	Poisoning	External Cause (E-Code)				
		Accident	Therapeutic Use	Suicide Attempt	Assault	Undetermined
Acrolein (gas)	987.8	E869.8	—	E952.8	E962.2	E982.8
liquid	989.89	E866.8	—	E950.9	E962.1	E980.9
Actaea spicata	988.2	E865.4	—	E950.9	E962.1	E980.9
Acterol	961.5	E857	E931.5	E950.4	E962.0	E980.4
ACTH	962.4	E858.0	E932.4	E950.4	E962.0	E980.4
Acthar	962.4	E858.0	E932.4	E950.4	E962.0	E980.4
Actinomycin (C) (D)	960.7	E856	E930.7	E950.4	E962.0	E980.4
Adalin (acetyl)	967.3	E852.2	E937.3	E950.2	E962.0	E980.2
Adenosine (phosphate)	977.8	E858.8	E947.8	E950.4	E962.0	E980.4
Adhesives	989.89	E866.6	—	E950.9	E962.1	E980.9
ADH	962.5	E858.0	E932.5	E950.4	E962.0	E980.4
Adicillin	960.0	E856	E930.0	E950.4	E962.0	E980.4
Adiphenine	975.1	E855.6	E945.1	E950.4	E962.0	E980.4
Adjunct, pharmaceutical	977.4	E858.8	E947.4	E950.4	E962.0	E980.4
Adrenal (extract, cortex or medulla) (glucocorticoids) (hormones) (mineralocorticoids)	962.0	E858.0	E932.0	E950.4	E962.0	E980.4
ENT agent	976.6	E858.7	E946.6	E950.4	E962.0	E980.4
ophthalmic preparation	976.5	E858.7	E946.5	E950.4	E962.0	E980.4
topical NEC	976.0	E858.7	E946.0	E950.4	E962.0	E980.4
Adrenalin	971.2	E855.5	E941.2	E950.4	E962.0	E980.4
Adrenergic blocking agents	971.3	E855.6	E941.3	E950.4	E962.0	E980.4
Adrenergics	971.2	E855.5	E941.2	E950.4	E962.0	E980.4
Adrenochrome (derivatives)	972.8	E858.3	E942.8	E950.4	E962.0	E980.4
Adrenocorticotropic hormone	962.4	E858.0	E932.4	E950.4	E962.0	E980.4
Adrenocorticotropin	962.4	E858.0	E932.4	E950.4	E962.0	E980.4
Adriamycin	960.7	E856	E930.7	E950.4	E962.0	E980.4
Aerosol spray - *see* Sprays	—	—	—	—	—	—
Aerosporin	960.8	E856	E930.8	E950.4	E962.0	E980.4
ENT agent	976.6	E858.7	E946.6	E950.4	E962.0	E980.4
ophthalmic preparation	976.5	E858.7	E946.5	E950.4	E962.0	E980.4
topical NEC	976.0	E858.7	E946.0	E950.4	E962.0	E980.4
Aethusa cynapium	988.2	E865.4	—	E950.9	E962.1	E980.9
Afghanistan black	969.6	E854.1	E939.6	E950.3	E962.0	E980.3
Aflatoxin	989.7	E865.9	—	E950.9	E962.1	E980.9
African boxwood	988.2	E865.4	—	E950.9	E962.1	E980.9
Agar (-agar)	973.3	E858.4	E943.3	E950.4	E962.0	E980.4
Agricultural agent NEC	989.89	E863.9	—	E950.6	E962.1	E980.7
Agrypnal	967.0	E851	E937.0	E950.1	E962.0	E980.1
Air contaminant(s), source or type not specified	—	—	—	—	—	—
specified type - *see* specific substance	987.9	E869.9	—	E952.9	E962.2	E982.9
Akee	988.2	E865.4	—	E950.9	E962.1	E980.9
Akrinol	976.0	E858.7	E946.0	E950.4	E962.0	E980.4
Alantolactone	961.6	E857	E931.6	E950.4	E962.0	E980.4
Albamycin	960.8	E856	E930.8	E950.4	E962.0	E980.4
Albumin (normal human serum)	964.7	E858.2	E934.7	E950.4	E962.0	E980.4
Albuterol	975.7	E858.6	E945.7	E950.4	E962.0	E980.4
Alcohol	980.9	E860.9	—	E950.9	E962.1	E980.9
absolute	980.0	E860.1	—	E950.9	E962.1	E980.9
beverage	980.0	E860.0	E947.8	E950.9	E962.1	E980.9
amyl	980.3	E860.4	—	E950.9	E962.1	E980.9
antifreeze	980.1	E860.2	—	E950.9	E962.1	E980.9
butyl	980.3	E860.4	—	E950.9	E962.1	E980.9
dehydrated	980.0	E860.1	—	E950.9	E862.1	E980.9
beverage	980.0	E860.0	E947.8	E950.9	E962.1	E980.9
denatured	980.0	E860.1	—	E950.9	E962.1	E980.9
deterrents	977.3	E858.8	E947.3	E950.4	E962.0	E980.4
diagnostic (gastric function)	977.8	E858.8	E947.8	E950.4	E962.0	E980.4
ethyl	980.0	E860.1	—	E950.9	E962.1	E980.9
beverage	980.0	E860.0	E947.8	E950.9	E962.1	E980.9
grain	980.0	E860.1	—	E950.9	E962.1	E980.9
beverage	980.0	E860.0	E947.8	E950.9	E962.1	E980.9

◀ New ⇐ Revised

Substance	Poisoning	External Cause (E-Code) Accident	Therapeutic Use	Suicide Attempt	Assault	Undetermined
Alcohol *(Continued)*						
industrial	980.9	E860.9	—	E950.9	E962.1	E980.9
isopropyl	980.2	E860.3	—	E950.9	E962.1	E980.9
methyl	980.1	E860.2	—	E950.9	E962.1	E980.9
preparation for consumption	980.0	E860.0	E947.8	E950.9	E962.1	E980.9
propyl	980.3	E860.4	—	E950.9	E962.1	E980.9
secondary	980.2	E860.3	—	E950.9	E962.1	E980.9
radiator	980.1	E860.2	—	E950.9	E962.1	E980.9
rubbing	980.2	E860.3	—	E950.9	E962.1	E980.9
specified type NEC	980.8	E860.8	—	E950.9	E962.1	E980.9
surgical	980.9	E860.9	—	E950.9	E962.1	E980.9
vapor (from any type of alcohol)	987.8	E869.8	—	E952.8	E962.2	E982.8
wood	980.1	E860.2	—	E950.9	E962.1	E980.9
Alcuronium chloride	975.2	E858.6	E945.2	E950.4	E962.0	E980.4
Aldactone	974.4	E858.5	E944.4	E950.4	E962.0	E980.4
Aldicarb	989.3	E863.2	—	E950.6	E962.1	E980.7
Aldomet	972.6	E858.3	E942.6	E950.4	E962.0	E980.4
Aldosterone	962.0	E858.0	E932.0	E950.4	E962.0	E980.4
Aldrin (dust)	989.2	E863.0	—	E950.6	E962.1	E980.7
Aleve - *see* Naproxen	—	—	—	—	—	—
Algeldrate	973.0	E858.4	E943.0	E950.4	E962.0	E980.4
Alidase	963.4	E858.1	E933.4	E950.4	E962.0	E980.4
Aliphatic thiocyanates	989.0	E866.8	—	E950.9	E962.1	E980.9
Alkaline antiseptic solution (aromatic)	976.6	E858.7	E946.6	E950.4	E962.0	E980.4
Alkalinizing agents (medicinal)	963.3	E858.1	E933.3	E950.4	E962.0	E980.4
Alkalis, caustic	983.2	E864.2	—	E950.7	E962.1	E980.6
Alkalizing agents (medicinal)	963.3	E858.1	E933.3	E950.4	E962.0	E980.4
Alka-seltzer	965.1	E850.3	E935.3	E950.0	E962.0	E980.0
Alkavervir	972.6	E858.3	E942.6	E950.4	E962.0	E980.4
Allegron	969.0	E854.0	E939.0	E950.3	E962.0	E980.3
Allobarbital, allobarbitone	967.0	E851	E937.0	E950.1	E962.0	E980.1
Allopurinol	974.7	E858.5	E944.7	E950.4	E962.0	E980.4
Allylestrenol	962.2	E858.0	E932.2	E950.4	E962.0	E980.4
Allylisopropylacetylurea	967.8	E852.8	E937.8	E950.2	E962.0	E980.2
Allylisopropylmalonylurea	967.0	E851	E937.0	E950.1	E962.0	E980.1
Allyltribromide	967.3	E852.2	E937.3	E950.2	E962.0	E980.2
Aloe, aloes, aloin	973.1	E858.4	E943.1	E950.4	E962.0	E980.4
Alosetron	973.8	E858.4	E943.8	E950.4	E962.0	E980.4
Aloxidone	966.0	E855.0	E936.0	E950.4	E962.0	E980.4
Aloxiprin	965.1	E850.3	E935.3	E950.0	E962.0	E980.0
Alpha amylase	963.4	E858.1	E933.4	E950.4	E962.0	E980.4
Alphaprodine (hydrochloride)	965.09	E850.2	E935.2	E950.0	E962.0	E980.0
Alpha tocopherol	963.5	E858.1	E933.5	E950.4	E962.0	E980.4
Alseroxylon	972.6	E858.3	E942.6	E950.4	E962.0	E980.4
Alum (ammonium) (potassium)	983.2	E864.2	—	E950.7	E962.1	E980.6
medicinal (astringent) NEC	976.2	E858.7	E946.2	E950.4	E962.0	E980.4
Aluminium, aluminum (gel) (hydroxide)	973.0	E858.4	E943.0	E950.4	E962.0	E980.4
acetate solution	976.2	E858.7	E946.2	E950.4	E962.0	E980.4
aspirin	965.1	E850.3	E935.3	E950.0	E962.0	E980.0
carbonate	973.0	E858.4	E943.0	E950.4	E962.0	E980.4
glycinate	973.0	E858.4	E943.0	E950.4	E962.0	E980.4
nicotinate	972.2	E858.3	E942.2	E950.4	E962.0	E980.4
ointment (surgical) (topical)	976.3	E858.7	E946.3	E950.4	E962.0	E980.4
phosphate	973.0	E858.4	E943.0	E950.4	E962.0	E980.4
subacetate	976.2	E858.7	E946.2	E950.4	E962.0	E980.4
topical NEC	976.3	E858.7	E946.3	E950.4	E962.0	E980.4
Alurate	967.0	E851	E937.0	E950.1	E962.0	E980.1
Alverine (citrate)	975.1	E858.6	E945.1	E950.4	E962.0	E980.4
Alvodine	965.09	E850.2	E935.2	E950.0	E962.0	E980.0
Amanita phalloides	988.1	E865.5	—	E950.9	E962.1	E980.9
Amantadine (hydrochloride)	966.4	E855.0	E936.4	E950.4	E962.0	E980.4

Substance	Poisoning	External Cause (E-Code)				
		Accident	Therapeutic Use	Suicide Attempt	Assault	Undetermined
Ambazone	961.9	E857	E931.9	E950.4	E962.0	E980.4
Ambenonium	971.0	E855.3	E941.0	E950.4	E962.0	E980.4
Ambutonium bromide	971.1	E855.4	E941.1	E950.4	E962.0	E990.4
Ametazole	977.8	E858.8	E947.8	E950.4	E962.0	E980.4
Amethocaine (infiltration) (topical)	968.5	E855.2	E938.5	E950.4	E962.0	E980.4
nerve block (peripheral) (plexus)	968.6	E855.2	E938.6	E950.4	E962.0	E980.4
spinal	968.7	E855.2	E938.7	E950.4	E962.0	E980.4
Amethopterin	963.1	E858.1	E933.1	E950.4	E962.0	E980.4
Amfepramone	977.0	E858.8	E947.0	E950.4	E962.0	E980.4
Amidone	965.02	E850.1	E935.1	E950.0	E962.0	E980.0
Amidopyrine	965.5	E850.5	E935.5	E950.0	E962.0	E980.0
Aminacrine	976.0	E858.7	E946.0	E950.4	E962.0	E980.4
Aminitrozole	961.5	E857	E931.5	E950.4	E962.0	E980.4
Aminoacetic acid	974.5	E858.5	E944.5	E950.4	E962.0	E980.4
Amino acids	974.5	E858.5	E944.5	E950.4	E962.0	E980.4
Aminocaproic acid	964.4	E858.2	E934.4	E950.4	E962.0	E980.4
Aminoethylisothiourium	963.8	E858.1	E933.8	E950.4	E962.0	E980.4
Aminoglutethimide	966.3	E855.0	E936.3	E950.4	E962.0	E980.4
Aminometradine	974.3	E858.5	E944.3	E950.4	E962.0	E980.4
Aminopentamide	971.1	E855.4	E941.1	E950.4	E962.0	E980.4
Aminophenazone	965.5	E850.5	E935.5	E950.0	E962.0	E980.0
Aminophenol	983.0	E864.0	—	E950.7	E962.1	E980.6
Aminophenylpyridone	969.5	E853.8	E939.5	E950.3	E962.0	E980.3
Aminophylline	975.7	E858.6	E945.7	E950.4	E962.0	E980.4
Aminopterin	963.1	E858.1	E933.1	E950.4	E962.0	E980.4
Aminopyrine	965.5	E850.5	E935.5	E950.0	E962.0	E980.0
Aminosalicylic acid	961.8	E857	E931.8	E950.4	E962.0	E980.4
Amiphenazole	970.1	E854.3	E940.1	E950.4	E962.0	E980.4
Amiquinsin	972.6	E858.3	E942.6	E950.4	E962.0	E980.4
Amisometradine	974.3	E858.5	E944.3	E950.4	E962.0	E980.4
Amitriptyline	969.0	E854.0	E939.0	E950.3	E962.0	E980.3
Ammonia (fumes) (gas) (vapor)	987.8	E869.8	—	E952.8	E962.2	E982.8
liquid (household) NEC	983.2	E861.4	—	E950.7	E962.1	E980.6
spirit, aromatic	970.8	E854.3	E940.8	E950.4	E962.0	E980.4
Ammoniated mercury	976.0	E858.7	E946.0	E950.4	E962.0	E980.4
Ammonium	—	—	—	—	—	—
carbonate	983.2	E864.2	—	E950.7	E962.1	E980.6
chloride (acidifying agent)	963.2	E858.1	E933.2	E950.4	E962.0	E980.4
expectorant	975.5	E858.6	E945.5	E950.4	E962.0	E980.4
compounds (household) NEC	983.2	E861.4	—	E950.7	E962.1	E980.6
fumes (any usage)	987.8	E869.8	—	E952.8	E962.2	E982.8
industrial	983.2	E864.2	—	E950.7	E962.1	E980.6
ichthosulfonate	976.4	E858.7	E946.4	E950.4	E962.0	E980.4
mandelate	961.9	E857	E931.9	E950.4	E962.0	E980.4
Amobarbital	967.0	E851	E937.0	E950.1	E962.0	E980.1
Amodiaquin(e)	961.4	E857	E931.4	E950.4	E962.0	E980.4
Amopyroquin(e)	961.4	E857	E931.4	E950.4	E962.0	E980.4
Amphenidone	969.5	E853.8	E939.5	E950.3	E962.0	E980.3
Amphetamine	969.7	E854.2	E939.7	E950.3	E962.0	E980.3
Amphomycin	960.8	E856	E930.8	E950.4	E962.0	E980.4
Amphotericin B	960.1	E856	E930.1	E950.4	E962.0	E980.4
topical	976.0	E858.7	E946.0	E950.4	E962.0	E980.4
Ampicillin	960.0	E856	E930.0	E950.4	E962.0	E980.4
Amprotropine	971.1	E855.4	E941.1	E950.4	E962.0	E980.4
Amygdalin	977.8	E858.8	E947.8	E950.4	E962.0	E980.4
Amyl	—	—	—	—	—	—
acetate (vapor)	982.8	E862.4	—	E950.9	E962.1	E980.9
alcohol	980.3	E860.4	—	E950.9	E962.1	E980.9
nitrite (medicinal)	972.4	E858.3	E942.4	E950.4	E962.0	E980.4
Amylase (alpha)	963.4	E858.1	E933.4	E950.4	E962.0	E980.4
Amylene hydrate	980.8	E860.8	—	E950.9	E962.1	E980.9

Substance	Poisoning	External Cause (E-Code)				
		Accident	Therapeutic Use	Suicide Attempt	Assault	Undetermined
Amylobarbitone	967.0	E851	E937.0	E950.1	E962.0	E980.1
Amylocaine	968.9	E855.2	E938.9	E950.4	E962.0	E980.4
infiltration (subcutaneous)	968.5	E855.2	E938.5	E950.4	E962.0	E980.4
nerve block (peripheral) (plexus)	968.6	E855.2	E938.6	E950.4	E962.0	E980.4
spinal	968.7	E855.2	E938.7	E950.4	E962.0	E980.4
topical (surface)	968.5	E855.2	E938.5	E950.4	E962.0	E980.4
Amytal (sodium)	967.0	E851	E937.0	E950.1	E962.0	E980.1
Analeptics	970.0	E854.3	E940.0	E950.4	E962.0	E980.4
Analgesics	965.9	E850.9	E935.9	E950.0	E962.0	E980.0
aromatic NEC	965.4	E850.4	E935.4	E950.0	E962.0	E980.0
non-narcotic NEC	965.7	E850.7	E935.7	E950.0	E962.0	E980.0
specified NEC	965.8	E850.8	E935.8	E950.0	E962.0	E980.0
Anamirta cocculus	988.2	E865.3	—	E950.9	E962.1	E980.9
Ancillin	960.0	E856	E930.0	E950.4	E962.0	E980.4
Androgens (anabolic congeners)	962.1	E858.0	E932.1	E950.4	E962.0	E980.4
Androstalone	962.1	E858.0	E932.1	E950.4	E962.0	E980.4
Androsterone	962.1	E858.0	E932.1	E950.4	E962.0	E980.4
Anemone pulsatilla	988.2	E865.4	—	E950.9	E962.1	E980.9
Anesthesia, anesthetic (general) NEC	968.4	E855.1	E938.4	E950.4	E962.0	E980.4
block (nerve) (plexus)	968.6	E855.2	E938.6	E950.4	E962.0	E980.4
gaseous NEC	968.2	E855.1	E938.2	E950.4	E962.0	E980.4
halogenated hydrocarbon derivatives NEC	968.2	E855.1	E938.2	E950.4	E962.0	E980.4
infiltration (intradermal) (subcutaneous) (submucosal)	968.5	E855.2	E938.5	E950.4	E962.0	E980.4
intravenous	968.3	E855.1	E938.3	E950.4	E962.0	E980.4
local NEC	968.9	E855.2	E938.9	E950.4	E962.0	E980.4
nerve blocking (peripheral) (plexus)	968.6	E855.2	E938.6	E950.4	E962.0	E980.4
rectal NEC	968.3	E855.1	E938.3	E950.4	E962.0	E980.4
spinal	968.7	E855.2	E938.7	E950.4	E962.0	E980.4
surface	968.5	E855.2	E938.5	E950.4	E962.0	E980.4
topical	968.5	E855.2	E938.5	E950.4	E962.0	E980.4
Aneurine	963.5	E858.1	E933.5	E950.4	E962.0	E980.4
Angio-Conray	977.8	E858.8	E947.8	E950.4	E962.0	E980.4
Angiotensin	971.2	E855.5	E941.2	E950.4	E962.0	E980.4
Anhydrohydroxyprogesterone	962.2	E858.0	E932.2	E950.4	E962.0	E980.4
Anhydron	974.3	E858.5	E944.3	E950.4	E962.0	E980.4
Anileridine	965.09	E850.2	E935.2	E950.0	E962.0	E980.0
Aniline (dye) (liquid)	983.0	E864.0	—	E950.7	E962.1	E980.6
analgesic	965.4	E850.4	E935.4	E950.0	E962.0	E980.0
derivatives, therapeutic NEC	965.4	E850.4	E935.4	E950.0	E962.0	E980.0
vapor	987.8	E869.8	—	E952.8	E962.2	E982.8
Aniscoropine	971.1	E855.4	E941.1	E950.4	E962.0	E980.4
Anisindione	964.2	E858.2	E934.2	E950.4	E962.0	E980.4
Anorexic agents	977.0	E858.8	E947.0	E950.4	E962.0	E980.4
Ant (bite) (sting)	989.5	E905.5	—	E950.9	E962.1	E980.9
Antabuse	977.3	E858.8	E947.3	E950.4	E962.0	E980.4
Antacids	973.0	E858.4	E943.0	E950.4	E962.0	E980.4
Antazoline	963.0	E858.1	E933.0	E950.4	E962.0	E980.4
Anthelmintics	961.6	E857	E931.6	E950.4	E962.0	E980.4
Anthralin	976.4	E858.7	E946.4	E950.4	E962.0	E980.4
Anthramycin	960.7	E856	E930.7	E950.4	E962.0	E980.4
Antiadrenergics	971.3	E855.6	E941.3	E950.4	E962.0	E980.4
Antiallergic agents	963.0	E858.1	E933.0	E950.4	E962.0	E980.4
Antianemic agents NEC	964.1	E858.2	E934.1	E950.4	E962.0	E980.4
Antiaris toxicaria	988.2	E865.4	—	E950.9	E962.1	E980.9
Antiarteriosclerotic agents	972.2	E858.3	E942.2	E950.4	E962.0	E980.4
Antiasthmatics	975.7	E858.6	E945.7	E950.4	E962.0	E980.4
Antibiotics	960.9	E856	E930.9	E950.4	E962.0	E980.4
antifungal	960.1	E856	E930.1	E950.4	E962.0	E980.4
antimycobacterial	960.6	E856	E930.6	E950.4	E962.0	E980.4
antineoplastic	960.7	E856	E930.7	E950.4	E962.0	E980.4
cephalosporin (group)	960.5	E856	E930.5	E950.4	E962.0	E980.4

Substance	Poisoning	External Cause (E-Code)				
		Accident	Therapeutic Use	Suicide Attempt	Assault	Undetermined
Antibiotics *(Continued)*						
chloramphenicol (group)	960.2	E856	E930.2	E950.4	E962.0	E980.4
macrolides	960.3	E856	E930.3	E950.4	E962.0	E980.4
specified NEC	960.8	E856	E930.8	E950.4	E962.0	E980.4
tetracycline (group)	960.4	E856	E930.4	E950.4	E962.0	E980.4
Anticancer agents NEC	963.1	E858.1	E933.1	E950.4	E962.0	E980.4
antibiotics	960.7	E856	E930.7	E950.4	E962.0	E980.4
Anticholinergics	971.1	E855.4	E941.1	E950.4	E962.0	E980.4
Anticholinesterase (organophosphorus) (reversible)	971.0	E855.3	E941.0	E950.4	E962.0	E980.4
Anticoagulants	964.2	E858.2	E934.2	E950.4	E962.0	E980.4
antagonists	964.5	E858.2	E934.5	E950.4	E962.0	E980.4
Anti-common cold agents NEC	975.6	E858.6	E945.6	E950.4	E962.0	E980.4
Anticonvulsants NEC	966.3	E855.0	E936.3	E950.4	E962.0	E980.4
Antidepressants	969.0	E854.0	E939.0	E950.3	E962.0	E980.3
Antidiabetic agents	962.3	E858.0	E932.3	E950.4	E962.0	E980.4
Antidiarrheal agents	973.5	E858.4	E943.5	E950.4	E962.0	E980.4
Antidiuretic hormone	962.5	E858.0	E932.5	E950.4	E962.0	E980.4
Antidotes NEC	977.2	E858.8	E947.2	E950.4	E962.0	E980.4
Antiemetic agents	963.0	E858.1	E933.0	E950.4	E962.0	E980.4
Antiepilepsy agent NEC	966.3	E855.0	E936.3	E950.4	E962.0	E980.4
Antifertility pills	962.2	E858.0	E932.2	E950.4	E962.0	E980.4
Antiflatulents	973.8	E858.4	E943.8	E950.4	E962.0	E980.4
Antifreeze	989.89	E866.8	—	E950.9	E962.1	E980.9
alcohol	980.1	E860.2	—	E950.9	E962.1	E980.9
ethylene glycol	982.8	E862.4	—	E950.9	E962.1	E980.9
Antifungals (nonmedicinal) (sprays)	989.4	E863.6	—	E950.6	E962.1	E980.7
medicinal NEC	961.9	E857	E931.9	E950.4	E962.0	E980.4
antibiotic	960.1	E856	E930.1	E950.4	E962.0	E980.4
topical	976.0	E858.7	E946.0	E950.4	E962.0	E980.4
Antigastric secretion agents	973.0	E858.4	E943.0	E950.4	E962.0	E980.4
Antihelmintics	961.6	E857	E931.6	E950.4	E962.0	E980.4
Antihemophilic factor (human)	964.7	E858.2	E934.7	E950.4	E962.0	E980.4
Antihistamine	963.0	E858.1	E933.0	E950.4	E962.0	E980.4
Antihypertensive agents NEC	972.6	E858.3	E942.6	E950.4	E962.0	E980.4
Anti-infectives NEC	961.9	E857	E931.9	E950.4	E962.0	E980.4
antibiotics	960.9	E856	E930.9	E950.4	E962.0	E980.4
specified NEC	960.8	E856	E930.8	E950.4	E962.0	E980.4
anthelmintic	961.6	E857	E931.6	E950.4	E962.0	E980.4
antimalarial	961.4	E857	E931.4	E950.4	E962.0	E980.4
antimycobacterial NEC	961.8	E857	E931.8	E950.4	E962.0	E980.4
antibiotics	960.6	E856	E930.6	E950.4	E962.0	E980.4
antiprotozoal NEC	961.5	E857	E931.5	E950.4	E962.0	E980.4
blood	961.4	E857	E931.4	E950.4	E962.0	E980.4
antiviral	961.7	E857	E931.7	E950.4	E962.0	E980.4
arsenical	961.1	E857	E931.1	E950.4	E962.0	E980.4
ENT agents	976.6	E858.7	E946.6	E950.4	E962.0	E980.4
heavy metals NEC	961.2	E857	E931.2	E950.4	E962.0	E980.4
local	976.0	E858.7	E946.0	E950.4	E962.0	E980.4
ophthalmic preparation	976.5	E858.7	E946.5	E950.4	E962.0	E980.4
topical NEC	976.0	E858.7	E946.0	E950.4	E962.0	E980.4
Anti-inflammatory agents (topical)	976.0	E858.7	E946.0	E950.4	E962.0	E980.4
Antiknock (tetraethyl lead)	984.1	E862.1	—	E950.9	E962.1	E980.9
Antilipemics	972.2	E858.3	E942.2	E950.4	E962.0	E980.4
Antimalarials	961.4	E857	E931.4	E950.4	E962.0	E980.4
Antimony (compounds) (vapor) NEC	985.4	E866.2	—	E950.9	E962.1	E980.9
anti-infectives	961.2	E857	E931.2	E950.4	E962.0	E980.4
pesticides (vapor)	985.4	E863.4	—	E950.6	E962.2	E980.7
potassium tartrate	961.2	E857	E931.2	E950.4	E962.0	E980.4
tartrated	961.2	E857	E931.2	E950.4	E962.0	E980.4
Antimuscarinic agents	971.1	E855.4	E941.1	E950.4	E962.0	E980.4
Antimycobacterials NEC	961.8	E857	E931.8	E950.4	E962.0	E980.4
antibiotics	960.6	E856	E930.6	E950.4	E962.0	E980.4

Substance	Poisoning	External Cause (E-Code)				
		Accident	Therapeutic Use	Suicide Attempt	Assault	Undetermined
Antineoplastic agents	963.1	E858.1	E933.1	E950.4	E962.0	E980.4
antibiotics	960.7	E856	E930.7	E950.4	E962.0	E980.4
Anti-Parkinsonism agents	966.4	E855.0	E936.4	E950.4	E962.0	E980.4
Antiphlogistics	965.69	E850.6	E935.6	E950.0	E962.0	E980.0
Antiprotozoals NEC	961.5	E857	E931.5	E950.4	E962.0	E980.4
blood	961.4	E857	E931.4	E950.4	E962.0	E980.4
Antipruritics (local)	976.1	E858.7	E946.1	E950.4	E962.0	E980.4
Antipsychotic agents NEC	969.3	E853.8	E939.3	E950.3	E962.0	E980.3
Antipyretics	965.9	E850.9	E935.9	E950.0	E962.0	E980.0
specified NEC	965.8	E850.8	E935.8	E950.0	E962.0	E980.0
Antipyrine	965.5	E850.5	E935.5	E950.0	E962.0	E980.0
Antirabies serum (equine)	979.9	E858.8	E949.9	E950.4	E962.0	E980.4
Antirheumatics	965.69	E850.6	E935.6	E950.0	E962.0	E980.0
Antiseborrheics	976.4	E858.7	E946.4	E950.4	E962.0	E980.4
Antiseptics (external) (medicinal)	976.0	E858.7	E946.0	E950.4	E962.0	E980.4
Antistine	963.0	E858.1	E933.0	E950.4	E962.0	E980.4
Antithyroid agents	962.8	E858.0	E932.8	E950.4	E962.0	E980.4
Antitoxin, any	979.9	E858.8	E949.9	E950.4	E962.0	E980.4
Antituberculars	961.8	E857	E931.8	E950.4	E962.0	E980.4
antibiotics	960.6	E856	E930.6	E950.4	E962.0	E980.4
Antitussives	975.4	E858.6	E945.4	E950.4	E962.0	E980.4
Antivaricose agents (sclerosing)	972.7	E858.3	E942.7	E950.4	E962.0	E980.4
Antivenin (crotaline) (spider-bite)	979.9	E858.8	E949.9	E950.4	E962.0	E980.4
Antivert	963.0	E858.1	E933.0	E950.4	E962.0	E980.4
Antivirals NEC	961.7	E857	E931.7	E950.4	E962.0	E980.4
Ant poisons - *see* Pesticides	—	—	—	—	—	—
Antrol	989.4	E863.4	—	E950.6	E962.1	E980.7
fungicide	989.4	E863.6	—	E950.6	E962.1	E980.7
Apomorphine hydrochloride (emetic)	973.6	E858.4	E943.6	E950.4	E962.0	E980.4
Appetite depressants, central	977.0	E858.8	E947.0	E950.4	E962.0	E980.4
Apresoline	972.6	E858.3	E942.6	E950.4	E962.0	E980.4
Aprobarbital, aprobarbitone	967.0	E851	E937.0	E950.1	E962.0	E980.1
Apronalide	967.8	E852.8	E937.8	E950.2	E962.0	E980.2
Aqua fortis	983.1	E864.1	—	E950.7	E962.1	E980.6
Arachis oil (topical)	976.3	E858.7	E946.3	E950.4	E962.0	E980.4
cathartic	973.2	E858.4	E943.2	E950.4	E962.0	E980.4
Aralen	961.4	E857	E931.4	E950.4	E962.0	E980.4
Arginine salts	974.5	E858.5	E944.5	E950.4	E962.0	E980.4
Argyrol	976.0	E858.7	E946.0	E950.4	E962.0	E980.4
ENT agent	976.6	E858.7	E946.6	E950.4	E962.0	E980.4
ophthalmic preparation	976.5	E858.7	E946.5	E950.4	E962.0	E980.4
Aristocort	962.0	E858.0	E932.0	E950.4	E962.0	E980.4
ENT agent	976.6	E858.7	E946.6	E950.4	E962.0	E980.4
ophthalmic preparation	976.5	E858.7	E946.5	E950.4	E962.0	E980.4
topical NEC	976.0	E858.7	E946.0	E950.4	E962.0	E980.4
Aromatics, corrosive	983.0	E864.0	—	E950.7	E962.1	E980.6
disinfectants	983.0	E861.4	—	E950.7	E962.1	E980.6
Arsenate of lead (insecticide)	985.1	E863.4	—	E950.8	E962.1	E980.8
herbicide	985.1	E863.5	—	E950.8	E962.1	E980.8
Arsenic, arsenicals (compounds) (dust) (fumes) (vapor) NEC	985.1	E866.3	—	E950.8	E962.1	E980.8
anti-infectives	961.1	E857	E931.1	E950.4	E962.0	E980.4
pesticide (dust) (fumes)	985.1	E863.4	—	E950.8	E962.1	E980.8
Arsine (gas)	985.1	E866.3	—	E950.8	E962.1	E980.8
Arsphenamine (silver)	961.1	E857	E931.1	E950.4	E962.0	E980.4
Arsthinol	961.1	E857	E931.1	E950.4	E962.0	E980.4
Artane	971.1	E855.4	E941.1	E950.4	E962.0	E980.4
Arthropod (venomous) NEC	989.5	E905.5	—	E950.9	E962.1	E980.9
Asbestos	989.81	E866.8	—	E950.9	E962.1	E980.9
Ascaridole	961.6	E857	E931.6	E950.4	E962.0	E980.4
Ascorbic acid	963.5	E858.1	E933.5	E950.4	E962.0	E980.4
Asiaticoside	976.0	E858.7	E946.0	E950.4	E962.0	E980.4

Substance	Poisoning	External Cause (E-Code) Accident	Therapeutic Use	Suicide Attempt	Assault	Undetermined
Aspidium (oleoresin)	961.6	E857	E931.6	E950.4	E962.0	E980.4
Aspirin	965.1	E850.3	E935.3	E950.0	E962.0	E980.0
Astringents (local)	976.2	E858.7	E946.2	E950.4	E962.0	E980.4
Atabrine	961.3	E857	E931.3	E950.4	E962.0	E980.4
Ataractics	969.5	E853.8	E939.5	E950.3	E962.0	E980.3
Atonia drug, intestinal	973.3	E858.4	E943.3	E950.4	E962.0	E980.4
Atophan	974.7	E858.5	E944.7	E950.4	E962.0	E980.4
Atropine	971.1	E855.4	E941.1	E950.4	E962.0	E980.4
Attapulgite	973.5	E858.4	E943.5	E950.4	E962.0	E980.4
Attenuvax	979.4	E858.8	E949.4	E950.4	E962.0	E980.4
Aureomycin	960.4	E856	E930.4	E950.4	E962.0	E980.4
ophthalmic preparation	976.5	E858.7	E946.5	E950.4	E962.0	E980.4
topical NEC	976.0	E858.7	E946.0	E950.4	E962.0	E980.4
Aurothioglucose	965.69	E850.6	E935.6	E950.0	E962.0	E980.0
Aurothioglycanide	965.69	E850.6	E935.6	E950.0	E962.0	E980.0
Aurothiomalate	965.69	E850.6	E935.6	E950.0	E962.0	E980.0
Automobile fuel	981	E862.1	—	E950.9	E962.1	E980.9
Autonomic nervous system agents NEC	971.9	E855.9	E941.9	E950.4	E962.0	E980.4
Avlosulfon	961.8	E857	E931.8	E950.4	E962.0	E980.4
Avomine	967.8	E852.8	E937.8	E950.2	E962.0	E980.2
Azacyclonol	969.5	E853.8	E939.5	E950.3	E962.0	E980.3
Azapetine	971.3	E855.6	E941.3	E950.4	E962.0	E980.4
Azaribine	963.1	E858.1	E933.1	E950.4	E962.0	E980.4
Azaserine	960.7	E856	E930.7	E950.4	E962.0	E980.4
Azathioprine	963.1	E858.1	E933.1	E950.4	E962.0	E980.4
Azosulfamide	961.0	E857	E931.0	E950.4	E962.0	E980.4
Azulfidine	961.0	E857	E931.0	E950.4	E962.0	E980.4
Azuresin	977.8	E858.8	E947.8	E950.4	E962.0	E980.4
Bacimycin	976.0	E858.7	E946.0	E950.4	E962.0	E980.4
ophthalmic preparation	976.5	E858.7	E946.5	E950.4	E962.0	E980.4
Bacitracin	960.8	E856	E930.8	E950.4	E962.0	E980.4
ENT agent	976.6	E858.7	E946.6	E950.4	E962.0	E980.4
ophthalmic preparation	976.5	E858.7	E946.5	E950.4	E962.0	E980.4
topical NEC	976.0	E858.7	E946.0	E950.4	E962.0	E980.4
Baking soda	963.3	E858.1	E933.3	E950.4	E962.0	E980.4
BAL	963.8	E858.1	E933.8	E950.4	E962.0	E980.4
Bamethan (sulfate)	972.5	E858.3	E942.5	E950.4	E962.0	E980.4
Bamipine	963.0	E858.1	E933.0	E950.4	E962.0	E980.4
Baneberry	988.2	E865.4	—	E950.9	E962.1	E980.9
Banewort	988.2	E865.4	—	E950.9	E962.1	E980.9
Barbenyl	967.0	E851	E937.0	E950.1	E962.0	E980.1
Barbital, barbitone	967.0	E851	E937.0	E950.1	E962.0	E980.1
Barbiturates, barbituric acid	967.0	E851	E937.0	E950.1	E962.0	E980.1
anesthetic (intravenous)	968.3	E855.1	E938.3	E950.4	E962.0	E980.4
Barium (carbonate) (chloride) (sulfate)	985.8	E866.4	—	E950.9	E962.1	E980.9
diagnostic agent	977.8	E858.8	E947.8	E950.4	E962.0	E980.4
pesticide	985.8	E863.4	—	E950.6	E962.1	E980.7
rodenticide	985.8	E863.7	—	E950.6	E962.1	E980.7
Barrier cream	976.3	E858.7	E946.3	E950.4	E962.0	E980.4
Battery acid or fluid	983.1	E864.1	—	E950.7	E962.1	E980.6
Bay rum	980.8	E860.8	—	E950.9	E962.1	E980.9
BCG vaccine	978.0	E858.8	E948.0	E950.4	E962.0	E980.4
Bearsfoot	988.2	E865.4	—	E950.9	E962.1	E980.9
Beclamide	966.3	E855.0	E936.3	E950.4	E962.0	E980.4
Bee (sting) (venom)	989.5	E905.3	—	E950.9	E962.1	E980.9
Belladonna (alkaloids)	971.1	E855.4	E941.1	E950.4	E962.0	E980.4
Bemegride	970.0	E854.3	E940.0	E950.4	E962.0	E980.4
Benactyzine	969.8	E855.8	E939.8	E950.3	E962.0	E980.3
Benadryl	963.0	E858.1	E933.0	E950.4	E962.0	E980.4
Bendrofluazide	974.3	E858.5	E944.3	E950.4	E962.0	E980.4
Bendroflumethiazide	974.3	E858.5	E944.3	E950.4	E962.0	E980.4

Substance	Poisoning	External Cause (E-Code) Accident	Therapeutic Use	Suicide Attempt	Assault	Undetermined
Benemid	974.7	E858.5	E944.7	E950.4	E962.0	E980.4
Benethamine penicillin G	960.0	E856	E930.0	E950.4	E962.0	E980.4
Benisone	976.0	E858.7	E946.0	E950.4	E962.0	E980.4
Benoquin	976.8	E858.7	E946.8	E950.4	E962.0	E980.4
Benoxinate	968.5	E855.2	E938.5	E950.4	E962.0	E980.4
Bentonite	976.3	E858.7	E946.3	E950.4	E962.0	E980.4
Benzalkonium (chloride)	976.0	E858.7	E946.0	E950.4	E962.0	E980.4
ophthalmic preparation	976.5	E858.7	E946.5	E950.4	E962.0	E980.4
Benzamidosalicylate (calcium)	961.8	E857	E931.8	E950.4	E962.0	E980.4
Benzathine penicillin	960.0	E856	E930.0	E950.4	E962.0	E980.4
Benzcarbimine	963.1	E858.1	E933.1	E950.4	E962.0	E980.4
Benzedrex	971.2	E855.5	E941.2	E950.4	E962.0	E980.4
Benzedrine (amphetamine)	969.7	E854.2	E939.7	E950.3	E962.0	E980.3
Benzene (acetyl) (dimethyl) (methyl) (solvent) (vapor)	982.0	E862.4	—	E950.9	E962.1	E980.9
hexachloride (gamma) (insecticide) (vapor)	989.2	E863.0	—	E950.6	E962.1	E980.7
Benzethonium	976.0	E858.7	E946.0	E950.4	E962.0	E980.4
Benzhexol (chloride)	966.4	E855.0	E936.4	E950.4	E962.0	E980.4
Benzilonium	971.1	E855.4	E941.1	E950.4	E962.0	E980.4
Benzin(e) - *see* Ligroin	—	—	—	—	—	—
Benziodarone	972.4	E858.3	E942.4	E950.4	E962.0	E980.4
Benzocaine	968.5	E855.2	E938.5	E950.4	E962.0	E980.4
Benzodiapin	969.4	E853.2	E939.4	E950.3	E962.0	E980.3
Benzodiazepines (tranquilizers) NEC	969.4	E853.2	E939.4	E950.3	E962.0	E980.3
Benzoic acid (with salicylic acid) (anti-infective)	976.0	E858.7	E946.0	E950.4	E962.0	E980.4
Benzoin	976.3	E858.7	E946.3	E950.4	E962.0	E980.4
Benzol (vapor)	982.0	E862.4	—	E950.9	E962.1	E980.9
Benzomorphan	965.09	E850.2	E935.2	E950.0	E962.0	E980.0
Benzonatate	975.4	E858.6	E945.4	E950.4	E962.0	E980.4
Benzothiadiazides	974.3	E858.5	E944.3	E950.4	E962.0	E980.4
Benzoylpas	961.8	E857	E931.8	E950.4	E962.0	E980.4
Benzperidol	969.5	E853.8	E939.5	E950.3	E962.0	E980.3
Benzphetamine	977.0	E858.8	E947.0	E950.4	E962.0	E980.4
Benzpyrinium	971.0	E855.3	E941.0	E950.4	E962.0	E980.4
Benzquinamide	963.0	E858.1	E933.0	E950.4	E962.0	E980.4
Benzthiazide	974.3	E858.5	E944.3	E950.4	E962.0	E980.4
Benztropine	971.1	E855.4	E941.1	E950.4	E962.0	E980.4
Benzyl	—	—	—	—	—	—
acetate	982.8	E862.4	—	E950.9	E962.1	E980.9
benzoate (anti-infective)	976.0	E858.7	E946.0	E950.4	E962.0	E980.4
morphine	965.09	E850.2	E935.2	E950.0	E962.0	E980.0
penicillin	960.0	E856	E930.0	E950.4	E962.0	E980.4
Bephenium	—	—	—	—	—	—
hydroxynapthoate	961.6	E857	E931.6	E950.4	E962.0	E980.4
Bergamot oil	989.89	E866.8	—	E950.9	E962.1	E980.9
Berries, poisonous	988.2	E865.3	—	E950.9	E962.1	E980.9
Beryllium (compounds) (fumes)	985.3	E866.4	—	E950.9	E962.1	E980.9
Beta-carotene	976.3	E858.7	E946.3	E950.4	E962.0	E980.4
Beta-Chlor	967.1	E852.0	E937.1	E950.2	E962.0	E980.2
Betamethasone	962.0	E858.0	E932.0	E950.4	E962.0	E980.4
topical	976.0	E858.7	E946.0	E950.4	E962.0	E980.4
Betazole	977.8	E858.8	E947.8	E950.4	E962.0	E980.4
Bethanechol	971.0	E855.3	E941.0	E950.4	E962.0	E980.4
Bethanidine	972.6	E858.3	E942.6	E950.4	E962.0	E980.4
Betula oil	976.3	E858.7	E946.3	E950.4	E962.0	E980.4
Bhang	969.6	E854.1	E939.6	E950.3	E962.0	E980.3
Bialamicol	961.5	E857	E931.5	E950.4	E962.0	E980.4
Bichloride of mercury - *see* Mercury, chloride	—	—	—	—	—	—
Bichromates (calcium) (crystals) (potassium) (sodium)	983.9	E864.3	—	E950.7	E962.1	E980.6
fumes	987.8	E869.8	—	E952.8	E962.2	E982.8
Biguanide derivatives, oral	962.3	E858.0	E932.3	E950.4	E962.0	E980.4
Biligrafin	977.8	E858.8	E947.8	E950.4	E962.0	E980.4

Substance	Poisoning	External Cause (E-Code)				
		Accident	Therapeutic Use	Suicide Attempt	Assault	Undetermined
Bilopaque	977.8	E858.8	E947.8	E950.4	E962.0	E980.4
Bioflavonoids	972.8	E858.3	E942.8	E950.4	E962.0	E980.4
Biological substance NEC	979.9	E858.8	E949.9	E950.4	E962.0	E980.4
Biperiden	966.4	E855.0	E936.4	E950.4	E962.0	E980.4
Bisacodyl	973.1	E858.4	E943.1	E950.4	E962.0	E980.4
Bishydroxycoumarin	964.2	E858.2	E934.2	E950.4	E962.0	E980.4
Bismarsen	961.1	E857	E931.1	E950.4	E962.0	E980.4
Bismuth (compounds) NEC	985.8	E866.4	—	E950.9	E962.1	E980.9
anti-infectives	961.2	E857	E931.2	E950.4	E962.0	E980.4
subcarbonate	973.5	E858.4	E943.5	E950.4	E962.0	E980.4
sulfarsphenamine	961.1	E857	E931.1	E950.4	E962.0	E980.4
Bithionol	961.6	E857	E931.6	E950.4	E962.0	E980.4
Bitter almond oil	989.0	E866.8	—	E950.9	E962.1	E980.9
Bittersweet	988.2	E865.4	—	E950.9	E962.1	E930.9
Black	—	—	—	—	—	—
flag	989.4	E863.4	—	E950.6	E962.1	E980.7
henbane	988.2	E865.4	—	E950.9	E962.1	E980.9
leaf (40)	989.4	E863.4	—	E950.6	E962.1	E980.7
widow spider (bite)	989.5	E905.1	—	E950.9	E962.1	E980.9
antivenin	979.9	E858.8	E949.9	E950.4	E962.0	E980.4
Blast furnace gas (carbon monoxide from)	986	E868.8	—	E952.1	E962.2	E982.1
Bleach NEC	983.9	E864.3	—	E950.7	E962.1	E980.6
Bleaching solutions	983.9	E864.3	—	E950.7	E962.1	E980.6
Bleomycin (sulfate)	960.7	E856	E930.7	E950.4	E962.0	E980.4
Blockain	968.9	E855.2	E938.9	E950.4	E962.0	E980.4
infiltration (subcutaneous)	968.5	E855.2	E938.5	E950.4	E962.0	E980.4
nerve block (peripheral) (plexus)	968.6	E855.2	E938.6	E950.4	E962.0	E980.4
topical (surface)	968.5	E855.2	E938.5	E950.4	E962.0	E980.4
Blood (derivatives) (natural) (plasma) (whole)	964.7	E858.2	E934.7	E950.4	E962.0	E980.4
affecting agent	964.9	E858.2	E934.9	E950.4	E962.0	E980.4
specified NEC	964.8	E858.2	E934.8	E950.4	E962.0	E980.4
substitute (macromolecular)	964.8	E858.2	E934.8	E950.4	E962.0	E980.4
Blue velvet	965.09	E850.2	E935.2	E950.0	E962.0	E980.0
Bone meal	989.89	E866.5	—	E950.9	E962.1	E980.9
Bonine	963.0	E858.1	E933.0	E950.4	E962.0	E980.4
Boracic acid	976.0	E858.7	E946.0	E950.4	E962.0	E980.4
ENT agent	976.6	E858.7	E946.6	E950.4	E962.0	E980.4
ophthalmic preparation	976.5	E858.7	E946.5	E950.4	E962.0	E980.4
Borate (cleanser) (sodium)	989.6	E861.3	—	E950.9	E962.1	E980.9
Borax (cleanser)	989.6	E861.3	—	E950.9	E962.1	E980.9
Boric acid	976.0	E858.7	E946.0	E950.4	E962.0	E980.4
ENT agent	976.6	E858.7	E946.6	E950.4	E962.0	E980.4
ophthalmic preparation	976.5	E858.7	E946.5	E950.4	E962.0	E980.4
Boron hydride NEC	989.89	E866.8	—	E950.9	E962.1	E980.9
fumes or gas	987.8	E869.8	—	E952.8	E962.2	E982.8
Botox	975.3	E858.6	E945.3	E950.4	E962.0	E980.4
Brake fluid vapor	987.8	E869.8	—	E952.8	E962.2	E982.8
Brass (compounds) (fumes)	985.8	E866.4	—	E950.9	E962.1	E980.9
Brasso	981	E861.3	—	E950.9	E962.1	E980.9
Bretylium (tosylate)	972.6	E858.3	E942.6	E950.4	E962.0	E980.4
Brevital (sodium)	968.3	E855.1	E938.3	E950.4	E962.0	E980.4
British antilewisite	963.8	E858.1	E933.8	E950.4	E962.0	E980.4
Bromal (hydrate)	967.3	E852.2	E937.3	E950.2	E962.0	E980.2
Bromelains	963.4	E858.1	E933.4	E950.4	E962.0	E980.4
Bromides NEC	967.3	E852.2	E937.3	E950.2	E962.0	E980.2
Bromine (vapor)	987.8	E869.8	—	E952.8	E962.2	E982.8
compounds (medicinal)	967.3	E852.2	E937.3	E950.2	E962.0	E980.2
Bromisovalum	967.3	E852.2	E937.3	E950.2	E962.0	E980.2
Bromobenzyl cyanide	987.5	E869.3	—	E952.8	E962.2	E982.8
Bromodiphenhydramine	963.0	E858.1	E933.0	E950.4	E962.0	E980.4
Bromoform	967.3	E852.2	E937.3	E950.2	E962.0	E980.2

◀ New ⬅ Revised

Substance	Poisoning	External Cause (E-Code)				
		Accident	Therapeutic Use	Suicide Attempt	Assault	Undetermined
Bromophenol blue reagent	977.8	E858.8	E947.8	E950.4	E962.0	E980.4
Bromosalicylhydroxamic acid	961.8	E857	E931.8	E950.4	E962.0	E980.4
Bromo-seltzer	965.4	E850.4	E935.4	E950.0	E962.0	E980.0
Brompheniramine	963.0	E858.1	E933.0	E950.4	E962.0	E980.4
Bromural	967.3	E852.2	E937.3	E950.2	E962.0	E980.2
Brown spider (bite) (venom)	989.5	E905.1	—	E950.9	E962.1	E980.9
Brucia	988.2	E865.3	—	E950.9	E962.1	E980.9
Brucine	989.1	E863.7	—	E950.6	E962.1	E980.7
Brunswick green - *see* Copper	—	—	—	—	—	—
Bruten - *see* Ibuprofen	—	—	—	—	—	—
Bryonia (alba) (dioica)	988.2	E865.4	—	E950.9	E962.1	E980.9
Buclizine	969.5	E853.8	E939.5	E950.3	E962.0	E980.3
Bufferin	965.1	E850.3	E935.3	E950.0	E962.0	E980.0
Bufotenine	969.6	E854.1	E939.6	E950.3	E962.0	E980.3
Buphenine	971.2	E855.5	E941.2	E950.4	E962.0	E980.4
Bupivacaine	968.9	E855.2	E938.9	E950.4	E962.0	E980.4
infiltration (subcutaneous)	968.5	E855.2	E938.5	E950.4	E962.0	E980.4
nerve block (peripheral) (plexus)	968.6	E855.2	E938.6	E950.4	E962.0	E980.4
Busulfan	963.1	E858.1	E933.1	E950.4	E962.0	E980.4
Butabarbital (sodium)	967.0	E851	E937.0	E950.1	E962.0	E980.1
Butabarbitone	967.0	E851	E937.0	E950.1	E962.0	E980.1
Butabarpal	967.0	E851	E937.0	E950.1	E962.0	E980.1
Butacaine	968.5	E855.2	E938.5	E950.4	E962.0	E980.4
Butallylonal	967.0	E851	E937.0	E950.1	E962.0	E980.1
Butane (distributed in mobile container)	987.0	E868.0	—	E951.1	E962.2	E981.1
distributed through pipes	987.0	E867	—	E951.0	E962.2	E981.0
incomplete combustion of - *see* Carbon monoxide, butane	—	—	—	—	—	—
Butanol	980.3	E860.4	—	E950.9	E962.1	E980.9
Butanone	982.8	E862.4	—	E950.9	E962.1	E980.9
Butaperazine	969.1	E853.0	E939.1	E950.3	E962.0	E980.3
Butazolidin	965.5	E850.5	E935.5	E950.0	E962.0	E980.0
Butethal	967.0	E851	E937.0	E950.1	E962.0	E980.1
Butethamate	971.1	E855.4	E941.1	E950.4	E962.0	E980.4
Buthalitone (sodium)	968.3	E855.1	E938.3	E950.4	E962.0	E980.4
Butisol (sodium)	967.0	E851	E937.0	E950.1	E962.0	E980.1
Butobarbital, butobarbitone	967.0	E851	E937.0	E950.1	E962.0	E980.1
Butriptyline	969.0	E854.0	E939.0	E950.3	E962.0	E980.3
Buttercups	988.2	E865.4	—	E950.9	E962.1	E980.9
Butter of antimony - *see* Antimony	—	—	—	—	—	—
Butyl	—	—	—	—	—	—
acetate (secondary)	982.8	E862.4	—	E950.9	E962.1	E980.9
alcohol	980.3	E860.4	—	E950.9	E962.1	E980.9
carbinol	980.8	E860.8	—	E950.9	E962.1	E980.9
carbitol	982.8	E862.4	—	E950.9	E962.1	E980.9
cellosolve	982.8	E862.4	—	E950.9	E962.1	E980.9
chloral (hydrate)	967.1	E852.0	E937.1	E950.2	E962.0	E980.2
formate	982.8	E862.4	—	E950.9	E962.1	E980.9
scopolammonium bromide	971.1	E855.4	E941.1	E950.4	E962.0	E980.4
Butyn	968.5	E855.2	E938.5	E950.4	E962.0	E980.4
Butyrophenone (-based tranquilizers)	969.2	E853.1	E939.2	E950.3	E962.0	E980.3
Cacodyl, cacodylic acid - *see* Arsenic	—	—	—	—	—	—
Cactinomycin	960.7	E856	E930.7	E950.4	E962.0	E980.4
Cade oil	976.4	E858.7	E946.4	E950.4	E962.0	E980.4
Cadmium (chloride) (compounds) (dust) (fumes) (oxide)	985.5	E866.4	—	E950.9	E962.1	E980.9
sulfide (medicinal) NEC	976.4	E858.7	E946.4	E950.4	E962.0	E980.4
Caffeine	969.7	E854.2	E939.7	E950.3	E962.0	E980.3
Calabar bean	988.2	E865.4	—	E950.9	E962.1	E980.9
Caladium seguinium	988.2	E865.4	—	E950.9	E962.1	E980.9
Calamine (liniment) (lotion)	976.3	E858.7	E946.3	E950.4	E962.0	E980.4
Calciferol	963.5	E858.1	E933.5	E950.4	E962.0	E980.4
Calcium (salts) NEC	974.5	E858.5	E944.5	E950.4	E962.0	E980.4
acetylsalicylate	965.1	E850.3	E935.3	E950.0	E962.0	E980.0

Substance	Poisoning	External Cause (E-Code) Accident	Therapeutic Use	Suicide Attempt	Assault	Undetermined
Calcium *(Continued)*						
benzamidosalicylate	961.8	E857	E931.8	E950.4	E962.0	E980.4
carbaspirin	965.1	E850.3	E935.3	E950.0	E962.0	E980.0
carbimide (citrated)	977.3	E858.8	E947.3	E950.4	E962.0	E980.4
carbonate (antacid)	973.0	E858.4	E943.0	E950.4	E962.0	E980.4
cyanide (citrated)	977.3	E858.8	E947.3	E950.4	E962.0	E980.4
dioctyl sulfosuccinate	973.2	E858.4	E943.2	E950.4	E962.0	E980.4
disodium edathamil	963.8	E858.1	E933.8	E950.4	E962.0	E980.4
disodium edetate	963.8	E858.1	E933.8	E950.4	E962.0	E980.4
EDTA	963.8	E858.1	E933.8	E950.4	E962.0	E980.4
hydrate, hydroxide	983.2	E864.2	—	E950.7	E962.1	E980.6
mandelate	961.9	E857	E931.9	E950.4	E962.0	E980.4
oxide	983.2	E864.2	—	E950.7	E962.1	E980.6
Calomel - *see* Mercury, chloride	—	—	—	—	—	—
Caloric agents NEC	974.5	E858.5	E944.5	E950.4	E962.0	E980.4
Calusterone	963.1	E858.1	E933.1	E950.4	E962.0	E980.4
Camoquin	961.4	E857	E931.4	E950.4	E962.0	E980.4
Camphor (oil)	976.1	E858.7	E946.1	E950.4	E962.0	E980.4
Candeptin	976.0	E858.7	E946.0	E950.4	E962.0	E980.4
Candicidin	976.0	E858.7	E946.0	E950.4	E962.0	E980.4
Cannabinols	969.6	E854.1	E939.6	E950.3	E962.0	E980.3
Cannabis (derivatives) (indica) (sativa)	969.6	E854.1	E939.6	E950.3	E962.0	E980.3
Canned heat	980.1	E860.2	—	E950.9	E962.1	E980.9
Cantharides, cantharidin, cantharis	976.8	E858.7	E946.8	E950.4	E962.0	E980.4
Capillary agents	972.8	E858.3	E942.8	E950.4	E962.0	E980.4
Capreomycin	960.6	E856	E930.6	E950.4	E962.0	E980.4
Captodiame, captodiamine	969.5	E853.8	E939.5	E950.3	E962.0	E980.3
Caramiphen (hydrochloride)	971.1	E855.4	E941.1	E950.4	E962.0	E980.4
Carbachol	971.0	E855.3	E941.0	E950.4	E962.0	E980.4
Carbacrylamine resins	974.5	E858.5	E944.5	E950.4	E962.0	E980.4
Carbamate (sedative)	967.8	E852.8	E937.8	E950.2	E962.0	E980.2
herbicide	989.3	E863.5	—	E950.6	E962.1	E980.7
insecticide	989.3	E863.2	—	E950.6	E962.1	E980.7
Carbamazepine	966.3	E855.0	E936.3	E950.4	E962.0	E980.4
Carbamic esters	967.8	E852.8	E937.8	E950.2	E962.0	E980.2
Carbamide	974.4	E858.5	E944.4	E950.4	E962.0	E980.4
topical	976.8	E858.7	E946.8	E950.4	E962.0	E980.4
Carbamylcholine chloride	971.0	E855.3	E941.0	E950.4	E962.0	E980.4
Carbarsone	961.1	E857	E931.1	E950.4	E962.0	E980.4
Carbaryl	989.3	E863.2	—	E950.6	E962.1	E980.7
Carbaspirin	965.1	E850.3	E935.3	E950.0	E962.0	E980.0
Carbazochrome	972.8	E858.3	E942.8	E950.4	E962.0	E980.4
Carbenicillin	960.0	E856	E930.0	E950.4	E962.0	E980.4
Carbenoxolone	973.8	E858.4	E943.8	E950.4	E962.0	E980.4
Carbetapentane	975.4	E858.6	E945.4	E950.4	E962.0	E980.4
Carbimazole	962.8	E858.0	E932.8	E950.4	E962.0	E980.4
Carbinol	980.1	E860.2	—	E950.9	E962.1	E980.9
Carbinoxamine	963.0	E858.1	E933.0	E950.4	E962.0	E980.4
Carbitol	982.8	E862.4	—	E950.9	E962.1	E980.9
Carbocaine	968.9	E855.2	E938.9	E950.4	E962.0	E980.4
infiltration (subcutaneous)	968.5	E855.2	E938.5	E950.4	E962.0	E980.4
nerve block (peripheral) (plexus)	968.6	E855.2	E938.6	E950.4	E962.0	E980.4
topical (surface)	968.5	E855.2	E938.5	E950.4	E962.0	E980.4
Carbol-fuchsin solution	976.0	E858.7	E946.0	E950.4	E962.0	E980.4
Carbolic acid (*see also* Phenol)	983.0	E864.0	—	E950.7	E962.1	E980.6
Carbomycin	960.8	E856	E930.8	E950.4	E962.0	E980.4
Carbon	—	—	—	—	—	—
bisulfide (liquid) (vapor)	982.2	E862.4	—	E950.9	E962.1	E980.9
dioxide (gas)	987.8	E869.8	—	E952.8	E962.2	E982.8
disulfide (liquid) (vapor)	982.2	E862.4	—	E950.9	E962.1	E980.9
monoxide (from incomplete combustion of) (in) NEC	986	E868.9	—	E952.1	E962.2	E982.1
blast furnace gas	986	E868.8	—	E952.1	E962.2	E982.1

◀ New ⟸ Revised

Substance	Poisoning	External Cause (E-Code)				
		Accident	Therapeutic Use	Suicide Attempt	Assault	Undetermined
Carbon *(Continued)*						
monoxide *(Continued)*						
butane (distributed in mobile container)	986	E868.0	—	E951.1	E962.2	E981.1
distributed through pipes	986	E867	—	E951.0	E962.2	E981.0
charcoal fumes	986	E868.3	—	E952.1	E962.2	E982.1
coal						
gas (piped)	986	E867	—	E951.0	E962.2	E981.0
solid (in domestic stoves, fireplaces)	986	E868.3	—	E952.1	E962.2	E982.1
coke (in domestic stoves, fireplaces)	986	E868.3	—	E952.1	E962.2	E982.1
exhaust gas (motor) not in transit	986	E868.2	—	E952.0	E962.2	E982.0
combustion engine, any not in watercraft	986	E868.2	—	E952.0	E962.2	E982.0
farm tractor, not in transit	986	E868.2	—	E952.0	E962.2	E982.0
gas engine	986	E868.2	—	E952.0	E962.2	E982.0
motor pump	986	E868.2	—	E952.0	E962.2	E982.0
motor vehicle, not in transit	986	E868.2	—	E952.0	E962.2	E982.0
fuel (in domestic use)	986	E868.3	—	E952.1	E962.2	E982.1
gas (piped)	986	E867	—	E951.0	E962.2	E981.0
in mobile container	986	E868.0	—	E951.1	E962.2	E981.1
utility	986	E868.1	—	E951.8	E962.2	E981.1
in mobile container	986	E868.0	—	E951.1	E962.2	E981.1
piped (natural)	986	E867	—	E951.0	E962.2	E981.0
illuminating gas	986	E868.1	—	E951.8	E962.2	E981.8
industrial fuels or gases, any	986	E868.8	—	E952.1	E962.2	E982.1
kerosene (in domestic stoves, fireplaces)	986	E868.3	—	E952.1	E962.2	E982.1
kiln gas or vapor	986	E868.8	—	E952.1	E962.2	E982.1
motor exhaust gas, not in transit	986	E868.2	—	E952.0	E962.2	E982.0
piped gas (manufactured) (natural)	986	E867	—	E951.0	E962.2	E981.0
producer gas	986	E868.8	—	E952.1	E962.2	E982.1
propane (distributed in mobile container)	986	E868.0	—	E951.1	E962.2	E981.1
distributed through pipes	986	E867	—	E951.0	E962.2	E981.0
specified source NEC	986	E868.8	—	E952.1	E962.2	E982.1
stove gas	986	E868.1	—	E951.8	E962.2	E981.8
piped	986	E867	—	E951.0	E962.2	E981.0
utility gas	986	E868.1	—	E951.8	E962.2	E981.8
piped	986	E867	—	E951.0	E962.2	E981.0
water gas	986	E868.1	—	E951.8	E962.2	E981.8
wood (in domestic stoves, fireplaces)	986	E868.3	—	E952.1	E962.2	E982.1
tetrachloride (vapor) NEC	987.8	E869.8	—	E952.8	E962.2	E982.8
liquid (cleansing agent) NEC	982.1	E861.3	—	E950.9	E962.1	E980.9
solvent	982.1	E862.4	—	E950.9	E962.1	E980.9
Carbonic acid (gas)	987.8	E869.8	—	E952.8	E962.2	E982.8
anhydrase inhibitors	974.2	E858.5	E944.2	E950.4	E962.0	E980.4
Carbowax	976.3	E858.7	E946.3	E950.4	E962.0	E980.4
Carbrital	967.0	E851	E937.0	E950.1	E962.0	E980.1
Carbromal (derivatives)	967.3	E852.2	E937.3	E950.2	E962.0	E980.2
Cardiac	—	—	—	—	—	—
depressants	972.0	E858.3	E942.0	E950.4	E962.0	E980.4
rhythm regulators	972.0	E858.3	E942.0	E950.4	E962.0	E980.4
Cardiografin	977.8	E858.8	E947.8	E950.4	E962.0	E980.4
Cardio-green	977.8	E858.8	E947.8	E950.4	E962.0	E980.4
Cardiotonic glycosides	972.1	E858.3	E942.1	E950.4	E962.0	E980.4
Cardiovascular agents NEC	972.9	E858.3	E942.9	E950.4	E962.0	E980.4
Cardrase	974.2	E858.5	E944.2	E950.4	E962.0	E980.4
Carfusin	976.0	E858.7	E946.0	E950.4	E962.0	E980.4
Carisoprodol	968.0	E855.1	E938.0	E950.4	E962.0	E980.4
Carmustine	963.1	E858.1	E933.1	E950.4	E962.0	E980.4
Carotene	963.5	E858.1	E933.5	E950.4	E962.0	E980.4
Carphenazine (maleate)	969.1	E853.0	E939.1	E950.3	E962.0	E980.3
Carter's Little Pills	973.1	E858.4	E943.1	E950.4	E962.0	E980.4
Cascara (sagrada)	973.1	E858.4	E943.1	E950.4	E962.0	E980.4
Cassava	988.2	E865.4	—	E950.9	E962.1	E980.9
Castellani's paint	976.0	E858.7	E946.0	E950.4	E962.0	E980.4

Substance	Poisoning	External Cause (E-Code)				
		Accident	Therapeutic Use	Suicide Attempt	Assault	Undetermined
Castor	—	—	—	—	—	—
bean	988.2	E865.3	—	E950.9	E962.1	E980.9
oil	973.1	E858.4	E943.1	E950.4	E962.0	E980.4
Caterpillar (sting)	989.5	E905.5	—	E950.9	E962.1	E980.9
Catha (edulis)	970.8	E854.3	E940.8	E950.4	E962.0	E980.4
Cathartics NEC	973.3	E858.4	E943.3	E950.4	E962.0	E980.4
contact	973.1	E858.4	E943.1	E950.4	E962.0	E980.4
emollient	973.2	E858.4	E943.2	E950.4	E962.0	E980.4
intestinal irritants	973.1	E858.4	E943.1	E950.4	E962.0	E980.4
saline	973.3	E858.4	E943.3	E950.4	E962.0	E980.4
Cathomycin	960.8	E856	E930.8	E950.4	E962.0	E980.4
Caustic(s)	983.9	E864.4	—	E950.7	E962.1	E980.6
alkali	983.2	E864.2	—	E950.7	E962.1	E980.6
hydroxide	983.2	E864.2	—	E950.7	E962.1	E980.6
potash	983.2	E864.2	—	E950.7	E962.1	E980.6
soda	983.2	E864.2	—	E950.7	E962.1	E980.6
specified NEC	983.9	E864.3	—	E950.7	E962.1	E980.6
Ceepryn	976.0	E858.7	E946.0	E950.4	E962.0	E980.4
ENT agent	976.6	E858.7	E946.6	E950.4	E962.0	E980.4
lozenges	976.6	E858.7	E946.6	E950.4	E962.0	E980.4
Celestone	962.0	E858.0	E932.0	E950.4	E962.0	E980.4
topical	976.0	E858.7	E946.0	E950.4	E962.0	E980.4
Cellosolve	982.8	E862.4	—	E950.9	E962.1	E980.9
Cell stimulants and proliferants	976.8	E858.7	E946.8	E950.4	E962.0	E980.4
Cellulose derivatives, cathartic	973.3	E858.4	E943.3	E950.4	E962.0	E980.4
nitrates (topical)	976.3	E858.7	E946.3	E950.4	E962.0	E980.4
Centipede (bite)	989.5	E905.4	—	E950.9	E962.1	E980.9
Central nervous system	—	—	—	—	—	—
depressants	968.4	E855.1	E938.4	E950.4	E962.0	E980.4
anesthetic (general) NEC	968.4	E855.1	E938.4	E950.4	E962.0	E980.4
gases NEC	968.2	E855.1	E938.2	E950.4	E962.0	E980.4
intravenous	968.3	E855.1	E938.3	E950.4	E962.0	E980.4
barbiturates	967.0	E851	E937.0	E950.1	E962.0	E980.1
bromides	967.3	E852.2	E937.3	E950.2	E962.0	E980.2
cannabis sativa	969.6	E854.1	E939.6	E950.3	E962.0	E980.3
chloral hydrate	967.1	E852.0	E937.1	E950.2	E962.0	E980.2
hallucinogenics	969.6	E854.1	E939.6	E950.3	E962.0	E980.3
hypnotics	967.9	E852.9	E937.9	E950.2	E962.0	E980.2
specified NEC	967.8	E852.8	E937.8	E950.2	E962.0	E980.2
muscle relaxants	968.0	E855.1	E938.0	E950.4	E962.0	E980.4
paraldehyde	967.2	E852.1	E937.2	E950.2	E962.0	E980.2
sedatives	967.9	E852.9	E937.9	E950.2	E962.0	E980.2
mixed NEC	967.6	E852.5	E937.6	E950.2	E962.0	E980.2
specified NEC	967.8	E852.8	E937.8	E950.2	E962.0	E980.2
muscle-tone depressants	968.0	E855.1	E938.0	E950.4	E962.0	E980.4
stimulants	970.9	E854.3	E940.9	E950.4	E962.0	E980.4
amphetamines	969.7	E854.2	E939.7	E950.3	E962.0	E980.3
analeptics	970.0	E854.3	E940.0	E950.4	E962.0	E980.4
antidepressants	969.0	E854.0	E939.0	E950.3	E962.0	E980.3
opiate antagonists	970.1	E854.3	E940.0	E950.4	E962.0	E980.4
specified NEC	970.8	E854.3	E940.8	E950.4	E962.0	E980.4
Cephalexin	960.5	E856	E930.5	E950.4	E962.0	E980.4
Cephaloglycin	960.5	E856	E930.5	E950.4	E962.0	E980.4
Cephaloridine	960.5	E856	E930.5	E950.4	E962.0	E980.4
Cephalosporins NEC	960.5	E856	E930.5	E950.4	E962.0	E980.4
N (adicillin)	960.0	E856	E930.0	E950.4	E962.0	E980.4
Cephalothin (sodium)	960.5	E856	E930.5	E950.4	E962.0	E980.4
Cerbera (odallam)	988.2	E865.4	—	E950.9	E962.1	E980.9
Cerberin	972.1	E858.3	E942.1	E950.4	E962.0	E980.4
Cerebral stimulants	970.9	E854.3	E940.9	E950.4	E962.0	E980.4
psychotherapeutic	969.7	E854.2	E939.7	E950.3	E962.0	E980.3
specified NEC	970.8	E854.3	E940.8	E950.4	E962.0	E980.4

Substance	Poisoning	External Cause (E-Code) Accident	Therapeutic Use	Suicide Attempt	Assault	Undetermined
Cetalkonium (chloride)	976.0	E858.7	E946.0	E950.4	E962.0	E980.4
Cetoxime	963.0	E858.1	E933.0	E950.4	E962.0	E980.4
Cetrimide	976.2	E858.7	E946.2	E950.4	E962.0	E980.4
Cetylpyridinium	976.0	E858.7	E946.0	E950.4	E962.0	E980.4
ENT agent	976.6	E858.7	E946.6	E950.4	E962.0	E980.4
lozenges	976.6	E858.7	E946.6	E950.4	E962.0	E980.4
Cevadilla - *see* Sabadilla	—	—	—	—	—	—
Cevitamic acid	963.5	E858.1	E933.5	E950.4	E962.0	E980.4
Chalk, precipitated	973.0	E858.4	E943.0	E950.4	E962.0	E980.4
Charcoal	—	—	—	—	—	—
fumes (carbon monoxide)	986	E868.3	—	E952.1	E962.2	E982.1
industrial	986	E868.8	—	E952.1	E962.2	E982.1
medicinal (activated)	973.0	E858.4	E943.0	E950.4	E962.0	E980.4
Chelating agents NEC	977.2	E858.8	E947.2	E950.4	E962.0	E980.4
Chelidonium majus	988.2	E865.4	—	E950.9	E962.1	E980.9
Chemical substance	989.9	E866.9	—	E950.9	E962.1	E980.9
specified NEC	989.89	E866.8	—	E950.9	E962.1	E980.9
Chemotherapy, antineoplastic	963.1	E858.1	E933.1	E950.4	E962.0	E980.4
Chenopodium (oil)	961.6	E857	E931.6	E950.4	E962.0	E980.4
Cherry laurel	988.2	E865.4	—	E950.9	E962.1	E980.9
Chiniofon	961.3	E857	E931.3	E950.4	E962.0	E980.4
Chlophedianol	975.4	E858.6	E945.4	E950.4	E962.0	E980.4
Chloral (betaine) (formamide) (hydrate)	967.1	E852.0	E937.1	E950.2	E962.0	E980.2
Chloralamide	967.1	E852.0	E937.1	E950.2	E962.0	E980.2
Chlorambucil	963.1	E858.1	E933.1	E950.4	E962.0	E980.4
Chloramphenicol	960.2	E856	E930.2	E950.4	E962.0	E980.4
ENT agent	976.6	E858.7	E946.6	E950.4	E962.0	E980.4
ophthalmic preparation	976.5	E858.7	E946.5	E950.4	E962.0	E980.4
topical NEC	976.0	E858.7	E946.0	E950.4	E962.0	E980.4
Chlorate(s) (potassium) (sodium) NEC	983.9	E864.3	—	E950.7	E962.1	E980.6
herbicides	989.4	E863.5	—	E950.6	E962.1	E980.7
Chlorcyclizine	963.0	E858.1	E933.0	E950.4	E962.0	E980.4
Chlordan(e) (dust)	989.2	E863.0	—	E950.6	E962.1	E980.7
Chlordantoin	976.0	E858.7	E946.0	E950.4	E962.0	E980.4
Chlordiazepoxide	969.4	E853.2	E939.4	E950.3	E962.0	E980.3
Chloresium	976.8	E858.7	E946.8	E950.4	E962.0	E980.4
Chlorethiazol	967.1	E852.0	E937.1	E950.2	E962.0	E980.2
Chlorethyl - *see* Ethyl, chloride	—	—	—	—	—	—
Chloretone	967.1	E852.0	E937.1	E950.2	E962.0	E980.2
Chlorex	982.3	E862.4	—	E950.9	E962.1	E980.9
Chlorhexadol	967.1	E852.0	E937.1	E950.2	E962.0	E980.2
Chlorhexidine (hydrochloride)	976.0	E858.7	E946.0	E950.4	E962.0	E980.4
Chlorhydroxyquinolin	976.0	E858.7	E946.0	E950.4	E962.0	E980.4
Chloride of lime (bleach)	983.9	E864.3	—	E950.7	E962.1	E980.6
Chlorinated	—	—	—	—	—	—
camphene	989.2	E863.0	—	E950.6	E962.1	E980.7
diphenyl	989.89	E866.8	—	E950.9	E962.1	E980.9
hydrocarbons NEC	989.2	E863.0	—	E950.6	E962.1	E980.7
solvent	982.3	E862.4	—	E950.9	E962.1	E980.9
lime (bleach)	983.9	E864.3	—	E950.7	E962.1	E980.6
naphthalene - *see* Naphthalene	—	—	—	—	—	—
pesticides NEC	989.2	E863.0	—	E950.6	E962.1	E980.7
soda - *see* Sodium, hypochlorite	—	—	—	—	—	—
Chlorine (fumes) (gas)	987.6	E869.8	—	E952.8	E962.2	E982.8
bleach	983.9	E864.3	—	E950.7	E962.1	E980.6
compounds NEC	983.9	E864.3	—	E950.7	E962.1	E980.6
disinfectant	983.9	E861.4	—	E950.7	E962.1	E980.6
releasing agents NEC	983.9	E864.3	—	E950.7	E962.1	E980.6
Chlorisondamine	972.3	E858.3	E942.3	E950.4	E962.0	E980.4
Chlormadinone	962.2	E858.0	E932.2	E950.4	E962.0	E980.4
Chlormerodrin	974.0	E858.5	E944.0	E950.4	E962.0	E980.4

Substance	Poisoning	External Cause (E-Code) Accident	Therapeutic Use	Suicide Attempt	Assault	Undetermined
Chlormethiazole	967.1	E852.0	E937.1	E950.2	E962.0	E980.2
Chlormethylenecycline	960.4	E856	E930.4	E950.4	E962.0	E980.4
Chlormezanone	969.5	E853.8	E939.5	E950.3	E962.0	E980.3
Chloroacetophenone	987.5	E869.3	—	E952.8	E962.2	E982.8
Chloroaniline	983.0	E864.0	—	E950.7	E962.1	E980.6
Chlorobenzene, chlorobenzol	982.0	E862.4	—	E950.9	E962.1	E980.9
Chlorobutanol	967.1	E852.0	E937.1	E950.2	E962.0	E980.2
Chlorodinitrobenzene	983.0	E864.0	—	E950.7	E962.1	E980.6
dust or vapor	987.8	E869.8	—	E952.8	E962.2	E982.8
Chloroethane - *see* Ethyl, chloride	—	—	—	—	—	—
Chloroform (fumes) (vapor)	987.8	E869.8	—	E952.8	E962.2	E982.8
anesthetic (gas)	968.2	E855.1	E938.2	E950.4	E962.0	E980.4
liquid NEC	968.4	E855.1	E938.4	E950.4	E962.0	E980.4
solvent	982.3	E862.4	—	E950.9	E962.1	E980.9
Chloroguanide	961.4	E857	E931.4	E950.4	E962.0	E980.4
Chloromycetin	960.2	E856	E930.2	E950.4	E962.0	E980.4
ENT agent	976.6	E858.7	E946.6	E950.4	E962.0	E980.4
ophthalmic preparation	976.5	E858.7	E946.5	E950.4	E962.0	E980.4
otic solution	976.6	E858.7	E946.6	E950.4	E962.0	E980.4
topical NEC	976.0	E858.7	E946.0	E950.4	E962.0	E980.4
Chloronitrobenzene	983.0	E864.0	—	E950.7	E962.1	E980.6
dust or vapor	987.8	E869.8	—	E952.8	E962.2	E982.8
Chlorophenol	983.0	E864.0	—	E950.7	E962.1	E980.6
Chlorophenothane	989.2	E863.0	—	E950.6	E962.1	E980.7
Chlorophyll (derivatives)	976.8	E858.7	E946.8	E950.4	E962.0	E980.4
Chloropicrin (fumes)	987.8	E869.8	—	E952.8	E962.2	E982.8
fumigant	989.4	E863.8	—	E950.6	E962.1	E980.7
fungicide	989.4	E863.6	—	E950.6	E962.1	E980.7
pesticide (fumes)	989.4	E863.4	—	E950.6	E962.1	E980.7
Chloroprocaine	968.9	E855.2	E938.9	E950.4	E962.0	E980.4
infiltration (subcutaneous)	968.5	E855.2	E938.5	E950.4	E962.0	E980.4
nerve block (peripheral) (plexus)	968.6	E855.2	E938.6	E950.4	E962.0	E980.4
Chloroptic	976.5	E858.7	E946.5	E950.4	E962.0	E980.4
Chloropurine	963.1	E858.1	E933.1	E950.4	E962.0	E980.4
Chloroquine (hydrochloride) (phosphate)	961.4	E857	E931.4	E950.4	E962.0	E980.4
Chlorothen	963.0	E858.1	E933.0	E950.4	E962.0	E980.4
Chlorothiazide	974.3	E858.5	E944.3	E950.4	E962.0	E980.4
Chlorotrianisene	962.2	E858.0	E932.2	E950.4	E962.0	E980.4
Chlorovinyldichloroarsine	985.1	E866.3	—	E950.8	E962.1	E980.8
Chloroxylenol	976.0	E858.7	E946.0	E950.4	E962.0	E980.4
Chlorphenesin (carbamate)	968.0	E855.1	E938.0	E950.4	E962.0	E980.4
topical (antifungal)	976.0	E858.7	E946.0	E950.4	E962.0	E980.4
Chlorpheniramine	963.0	E858.1	E933.0	E950.4	E962.0	E980.4
Chlorphenoxamine	966.4	E855.0	E936.4	E950.4	E962.0	E980.4
Chlorphentermine	977.0	E858.8	E947.0	E950.4	E962.0	E980.4
Chlorproguanil	961.4	E857	E931.4	E950.4	E962.0	E980.4
Chlorpromazine	969.1	E853.0	E939.1	E950.3	E962.0	E980.3
Chlorpropamide	962.3	E858.0	E932.3	E950.4	E962.0	E980.4
Chlorprothixene	969.3	E853.8	E939.3	E950.3	E962.0	E980.3
Chlorquinaldol	976.0	E858.7	E946.0	E950.4	E962.0	E980.4
Chlortetracycline	960.4	E856	E930.4	E950.4	E962.0	E980.4
Chlorthalidone	974.4	E858.5	E944.4	E950.4	E962.0	E980.4
Chlortrianisene	962.2	E858.0	E932.2	E950.4	E962.0	E980.4
Chlor-Trimeton	963.0	E858.1	E933.0	E950.4	E962.0	E980.4
Chlorzoxazone	968.0	E855.1	E938.0	E950.4	E962.0	E980.4
Choke damp	987.8	E869.8	—	E952.8	E962.2	E982.8
Cholebrine	977.8	E858.8	E947.8	E950.4	E962.0	E980.4
Cholera vaccine	978.2	E858.8	E948.2	E950.4	E962.0	E980.4
Cholesterol-lowering agents	972.2	E858.3	E942.2	E950.4	E962.0	E980.4
Cholestyramine (resin)	972.2	E858.3	E942.2	E950.4	E962.0	E980.4
Cholic acid	973.4	E858.4	E943.4	E950.4	E962.0	E980.4

Substance	Poisoning	External Cause (E-Code) Accident	Therapeutic Use	Suicide Attempt	Assault	Undetermined
Choline	—	—	—	—	—	—
dihydrogen citrate	977.1	E858.8	E947.1	E950.4	E962.0	E980.4
salicylate	965.1	E850.3	E935.3	E950.0	E962.0	E980.0
theophyllinate	974.1	E858.5	E944.1	E950.4	E962.0	E980.4
Cholinergics	971.0	E855.3	E941.0	E950.4	E962.0	E980.4
Chholografin	977.8	E858.8	E947.8	E950.4	E962.0	E980.4
Chorionic gonadotropin	962.4	E858.0	E932.4	E950.4	E962.0	E980.4
Chromates	983.9	E864.3	—	E950.7	E962.1	E980.6
dust or mist	987.8	E869.8	—	E952.8	E962.2	E982.8
lead	984.0	E866.0	—	E950.9	E962.1	E980.9
paint	984.0	E861.5	—	E950.9	E962.1	E980.9
Chromic acid	983.9	E864.3	—	E950.7	E962.1	E980.6
dust or mist	987.8	E869.8	—	E952.8	E962.2	E982.8
Chromium	985.6	E866.4	—	E950.9	E962.1	E980.9
compounds - *see* Chromates	—	—	—	—	—	—
Chromonar	972.4	E858.3	E942.4	E950.4	E962.0	E980.4
Chromyl chloride	983.9	E864.3	—	E950.7	E962.1	E980.6
Chrysarobin (ointment)	976.4	E858.7	E946.4	E950.4	E962.0	E980.4
Chrysazin	973.1	E858.4	E943.1	E950.4	E962.0	E980.4
Chymar	963.4	E858.1	E933.4	E950.4	E962.0	E980.4
ophthalmic preparation	976.5	E858.7	E946.5	E950.4	E962.0	E980.4
Chymotrypsin	963.4	E858.1	E933.4	E950.4	E962.0	E980.4
ophthalmic preparation	976.5	E858.7	E946.5	E950.4	E962.0	E980.4
Cicuta maculata or virosa	988.2	E865.4	—	E950.9	E962.1	E980.9
Cigarette lighter fluid	981	E862.1	—	E950.9	E962.1	E980.9
Cinchocaine (spinal)	968.7	E855.2	E938.7	E950.4	E962.0	E980.4
topical (surface)	968.5	E855.2	E938.5	E950.4	E962.0	E980.4
Cinchona	961.4	E857	E931.4	E950.4	E962.0	E980.4
Cinchonine alkaloids	961.4	E857	E931.4	E950.4	E962.0	E980.4
Cinchophen	974.7	E858.5	E944.7	E950.4	E962.0	E980.4
Cinnarizine	963.0	E858.1	E933.0	E950.4	E962.0	E980.4
Citanest	968.9	E855.2	E938.9	E950.4	E962.0	E980.4
infiltration (subcutaneous)	968.5	E855.2	E938.5	E950.4	E962.0	E980.4
nerve block (peripheral) (plexus)	968.6	E855.2	E938.6	E950.4	E962.0	E980.4
Citric acid	989.89	E866.8	—	E950.9	E962.1	E980.9
Citrovorum factor	964.1	E858.2	E934.1	E950.4	E962.0	E980.4
Claviceps purpurea	988.2	E865.4	—	E950.9	E962.1	E980.9
Cleaner, cleansing agent NEC	989.89	E861.3	—	E950.9	E962.1	E980.9
of paint or varnish	982.8	E862.9	—	E950.9	E962.1	E980.9
Clematis vitalba	988.2	E865.4	—	E950.9	E962.1	E980.9
Clemizole	963.0	E858.1	E933.0	E950.4	E962.0	E980.4
penicillin	960.0	E856	E930.0	E950.4	E962.0	E980.4
Clidinium	971.1	E855.4	E941.1	E950.4	E962.0	E980.4
Clindamycin	960.8	E856	E930.8	E950.4	E962.0	E980.4
Cliradon	965.09	E850.2	E935.2	E950.0	E962.0	E980.0
Clocortolone	962.0	E858.0	E932.0	E950.4	E962.0	E980.4
Clofedanol	975.4	E858.6	E945.4	E950.4	E962.0	E980.4
Clofibrate	972.2	E858.3	E942.2	E950.4	E962.0	E980.4
Clomethiazole	967.1	E852.0	E937.1	E950.2	E962.0	E980.2
Clomiphene	977.8	E858.8	E947.8	E950.4	E962.0	E980.4
Clonazepam	969.4	E853.2	E939.4	E950.3	E962.0	E980.3
Clonidine	972.6	E858.3	E942.6	E950.4	E962.0	E980.4
Clopamide	974.3	E858.5	E944.3	E950.4	E962.0	E980.4
Clorazepate	969.4	E853.2	E939.4	E950.3	E962.0	E980.3
Clorexolone	974.4	E858.5	E944.4	E950.4	E962.0	E980.4
Clorox (bleach)	983.9	E864.3	—	E950.7	E962.1	E980.6
Clortermine	977.0	E858.8	E947.0	E950.4	E962.0	E980.4
Clotrimazole	976.0	E858.7	E946.0	E950.4	E962.0	E980.4
Cloxacillin	960.0	E856	E930.0	E950.4	E962.0	E980.4
Coagulants NEC	964.5	E858.2	E934.5	E950.4	E962.0	E980.4
Coal (carbon monoxide from) - *see also* Carbon, monoxide, coal	—	—	—	—	—	—
oil - *see* Kerosene	—	—	—	—	—	—

Substance	Poisoning	External Cause (E-Code)				
		Accident	Therapeutic Use	Suicide Attempt	Assault	Undetermined
Coal *(Continued)*						
tar NEC	983.0	E864.0	—	E950.7	E962.1	E980.6
fumes	987.8	E869.8	—	E952.8	E962.2	E982.8
medicinal (ointment)	976.4	E858.7	E946.4	E950.4	E962.0	E980.4
analgesics NEC	965.5	E850.5	E935.5	E950.0	E962.0	E980.0
naphtha (solvent)	981	E862.0	—	E950.9	E962.1	E980.9
Cobalt (fumes) (industrial)	985.8	E866.4	—	E950.9	E962.1	E980.9
Cobra (venom)	989.5	E905.0	—	E950.9	E962.1	E980.9
Coca (leaf)	970.8	E854.3	E940.8	E950.4	E962.0	E980.4
Cocaine (hydrochloride) (salt)	970.8	E854.3	E940.8	E950.4	E962.0	E980.4
topical anesthetic	968.5	E855.2	E938.5	E950.4	E962.0	E980.4
Coccidioidin	977.8	E858.8	E947.8	E950.4	E962.0	E980.4
Cocculus indicus	988.2	E865.3	—	E950.9	E962.1	E980.9
Cochineal	989.89	E866.8	—	E950.9	E962.1	E980.9
medicinal products	977.4	E858.8	E947.4	E950.4	E962.0	E980.4
Codeine	965.09	E850.2	E935.2	E950.0	E962.0	E980.0
Coffee	989.89	E866.8	—	E950.9	E962.1	E980.9
Cogentin	971.1	E855.4	E941.1	E950.4	E962.0	E980.4
Coke fumes or gas (carbon monoxide)	986	E868.3	—	E952.1	E962.2	E982.1
industrial use	986	E868.8	—	E952.1	E962.2	E982.1
Colace	973.2	E858.4	E943.2	E950.4	E962.0	E980.4
Colchicine	974.7	E858.5	E944.7	E950.4	E962.0	E980.4
Colchicum	988.2	E865.3	—	E950.9	E962.1	E980.9
Cold cream	976.3	E858.7	E946.3	E950.4	E962.0	E980.4
Colestipol	972.2	E858.3	E942.2	E950.4	E962.0	E980.4
Colistimethate	960.8	E856	E930.8	E950.4	E962.0	E980.4
Colistin	960.8	E856	E930.8	E950.4	E962.0	E980.4
Collagen	977.8	E866.8	E947.8	E950.9	E962.1	E980.9
Collagenase	976.8	E858.7	E946.8	E950.4	E962.0	E980.4
Collodion (flexible)	976.3	E858.7	E946.3	E950.4	E962.0	E980.4
Colocynth	973.1	E858.4	E943.1	E950.4	E962.0	E980.4
Coloring matter - *see* Dye(s)	—	—	—	—	—	—
Combustion gas - *see* Carbon, monoxide	—	—	—	—	—	—
Compazine	969.1	E853.0	E939.1	E950.3	E962.0	E980.3
Compound	—	—	—	—	—	—
42 (warfarin)	989.4	E863.7	—	E950.6	E962.1	E980.7
269 (endrin)	989.2	E863.0	—	E950.6	E962.1	E980.7
497 (dieldrin)	989.2	E863.0	—	E950.6	E962.1	E980.7
1080 (sodium fluoroacetate)	989.4	E863.7	—	E950.6	E962.1	E980.7
3422 (parathion)	989.3	E863.1	—	E950.6	E962.1	E980.7
3911 (phorate)	989.3	E863.1	—	E950.6	E962.1	E980.7
3956 (toxaphene)	989.2	E863.0	—	E950.6	E962.1	E980.7
4049 (malathion)	989.3	E863.1	—	E950.6	E962.1	E980.7
4124 (dicapthon)	989.4	E863.4	—	E950.6	E962.1	E980.7
E (cortisone)	962.0	E858.0	E932.0	E950.4	E962.0	E980.4
F (hydrocortisone)	962.0	E858.0	E932.0	E950.4	E962.0	E980.4
Congo red	977.8	E858.8	E947.8	E950.4	E962.0	E980.4
Coniine, conine	965.7	E850.7	E935.7	E950.0	E962.0	E980.0
Conium (maculatum)	988.2	E865.4	—	E950.9	E962.1	E980.9
Conjugated estrogens (equine)	962.2	E858.0	E932.2	E950.4	E962.0	E980.4
Contac	975.6	E858.6	E945.6	E950.4	E962.0	E980.4
Contact lens solution	976.5	E858.7	E946.5	E950.4	E962.0	E980.4
Contraceptives (oral)	962.2	E858.0	E932.2	E950.4	E962.0	E980.4
vaginal	976.8	E858.7	E946.8	E950.4	E962.0	E980.4
Contrast media (roentgenographic)	977.8	E858.8	E947.8	E950.4	E962.0	E980.4
Convallaria majalis	988.2	E865.4	—	E950.9	E962.1	E980.9
Copper (dust) (fumes) (salts) NEC	985.8	E866.4	—	E950.9	E962.1	E980.9
arsenate, arsenite	985.1	E866.3	—	E950.8	E962.1	E980.8
insecticide	985.1	E863.4	—	E950.8	E962.1	E980.8
emetic	973.6	E858.4	E943.6	E950.4	E962.0	E980.4
fungicide	985.8	E863.6	—	E950.6	E962.1	E980.7

Substance	Poisoning	External Cause (E-Code)				
		Accident	Therapeutic Use	Suicide Attempt	Assault	Undetermined
Copper *(Continued)*						
insecticide	985.8	E863.4	—	E950.6	E962.1	E980.7
oleate	976.0	E858.7	E946.0	E950.4	E962.0	E980.4
sulfate	983.9	E864.3	—	E950.7	E962.1	E980.6
fungicide	983.9	E863.6	—	E950.7	E962.1	E980.6
cupric	973.6	E858.4	E943.6	E950.4	E962.0	E980.4
cuprous	983.9	E864.3	—	E950.7	E962.1	E980.6
Copperhead snake (bite) (venom)	989.5	E905.0	—	E950.9	E962.1	E980.9
Coral (sting)	989.5	E905.6	—	E950.9	E962.1	E980.9
snake (bite) (venom)	989.5	E905.0	—	E950.9	E962.1	E980.9
Cordran	976.0	E858.7	E946.0	E950.4	E962.0	E980.4
Corn cures	976.4	E858.7	E946.4	E950.4	E962.0	E980.4
Cornhusker's lotion	976.3	E858.7	E946.3	E950.4	E962.0	E980.4
Corn starch	976.3	E858.7	E946.3	E950.4	E962.0	E980.4
Corrosive	983.9	E864.4	—	E950.7	E962.1	E980.6
acids NEC	983.1	E864.1	—	E950.7	E962.1	E980.6
aromatics	983.0	E864.0	—	E950.7	E962.1	E980.6
disinfectant	983.0	E861.4	—	E950.7	E962.1	E980.6
fumes NEC	987.9	E869.9	—	E952.9	E962.2	E982.9
specified NEC	983.9	E864.3	—	E950.7	E962.1	E980.6
sublimate - *see* Mercury, chloride	—	—	—	—	—	—
Cortate	962.0	E858.0	E932.0	E950.4	E962.0	E980.4
Cort-Dome	962.0	E858.0	E932.0	E950.4	E962.0	E980.4
ENT agent	976.6	E858.7	E946.6	E950.4	E962.0	E980.4
ophthalmic preparation	976.5	E858.7	E946.5	E950.4	E962.0	E980.4
topical NEC	976.0	E858.7	E946.0	E950.4	E962.0	E980.4
Cortef	962.0	E858.0	E932.0	E950.4	E962.0	E980.4
ENT agent	976.6	E858.7	E946.6	E950.4	E962.0	E980.4
ophthalmic preparation	976.5	E858.7	E946.5	E950.4	E962.0	E980.4
topical NEC	976.0	E858.7	E946.0	E950.4	E962.0	E980.4
Corticosteroids (fluorinated)	962.0	E858.0	E932.0	E950.4	E962.0	E980.4
ENT agent	976.6	E858.7	E946.6	E950.4	E962.0	E980.4
ophthalmic preparation	976.5	E858.7	E946.5	E950.4	E962.0	E980.4
topical NEC	976.0	E858.7	E946.0	E950.4	E962.0	E980.4
Corticotropin	962.4	E858.0	E932.4	E950.4	E962.0	E980.4
Cortisol	962.0	E858.0	E932.0	E950.4	E962.0	E980.4
ENT agent	976.6	E858.7	E946.6	E950.4	E962.0	E980.4
ophthalmic preparation	976.5	E858.7	E946.5	E950.4	E962.0	E980.4
topical NEC	976.0	E858.7	E946.0	E950.4	E962.0	E980.4
Cortisone derivatives (acetate)	962.0	E858.0	E932.0	E950.4	E962.0	E980.4
ENT agent	976.6	E858.7	E946.6	E950.4	E962.0	E980.4
ophthalmic preparation	976.5	E858.7	E946.5	E950.4	E962.0	E980.4
topical NEC	976.0	E858.7	E946.0	E950.4	E962.0	E980.4
Cortogen	962.0	E858.0	E932.0	E950.4	E962.0	E980.4
ENT agent	976.6	E858.7	E946.6	E950.4	E962.0	E980.4
ophthalmic preparation	976.5	E858.7	E946.5	E950.4	E962.0	E980.4
Cortone	962.0	E858.0	E932.0	E950.4	E962.0	E980.4
ENT agent	976.6	E858.7	E946.6	E950.4	E962.0	E980.4
ophthalmic preparation	976.5	E858.7	E946.5	E950.4	E962.0	E980.4
Cortril	962.0	E858.0	E932.0	E950.4	E962.0	E980.4
ENT agent	976.6	E858.7	E946.6	E950.4	E962.0	E980.4
ophthalmic preparation	976.5	E858.7	E946.5	E950.4	E962.0	E980.4
topical NEC	976.0	E858.7	E946.0	E950.4	E962.0	E980.4
Cosmetics	989.89	E866.7	—	E950.9	E962.1	E980.9
Cosyntropin	977.8	E858.8	E947.8	E950.4	E962.0	E980.4
Cotarnine	964.5	E858.2	E934.5	E950.4	E962.0	E980.4
Cottonseed oil	976.3	E858.7	E946.3	E950.4	E962.0	E980.4
Cough mixtures (antitussives)	975.4	E858.6	E945.4	E950.4	E962.0	E980.4
containing opiates	965.09	E850.2	E935.2	E950.0	E962.0	E980.0
expectorants	975.5	E858.6	E945.5	E950.4	E962.0	E980.4
Coumadin	964.2	E858.2	E934.2	E950.4	E962.0	E980.4
rodenticide	989.4	E863.7	—	E950.6	E962.1	E980.7

Substance	Poisoning	External Cause (E-Code) Accident	Therapeutic Use	Suicide Attempt	Assault	Undetermined
Coumarin	964.2	E858.2	E934.2	E950.4	E962.0	E980.4
Coumetarol	964.2	E858.2	E934.2	E950.4	E962.0	E980.4
Cowbane	988.2	E865.4	—	E950.9	E962.1	E980.9
Cozyme	963.5	E858.1	E933.5	E950.4	E962.0	E980.4
Crack	970.8	E854.3	E940.8	E950.4	E962.0	E980.4
Creolin	983.0	E864.0	—	E950.7	E962.1	E980.6
disinfectant	983.0	E861.4	—	E950.7	E962.1	E980.6
Creosol (compound)	983.0	E864.0	—	E950.7	E962.1	E980.6
Creosote (beechwood) (coal tar)	983.0	E864.0	—	E950.7	E962.1	E980.6
medicinal (expectorant)	975.5	E858.6	E945.5	E950.4	E962.0	E980.4
syrup	975.5	E858.6	E945.5	E950.4	E962.0	E980.4
Cresol	983.0	E864.0	—	E950.7	E962.1	E980.6
disinfectant	983.0	E861.4	—	E950.7	E962.1	E980.6
Cresylic acid	983.0	E864.0	—	E950.7	E962.1	E980.6
Cropropamide	965.7	E850.7	E935.7	E950.0	E962.0	E980.0
with crotethamide	970.0	E854.3	E940.0	E950.4	E962.0	E980.4
Crotamiton	976.0	E858.7	E946.0	E950.4	E962.0	E980.4
Crotethamide	965.7	E850.7	E935.7	E950.0	E962.0	E980.0
with cropropamide	970.0	E854.3	E940.0	E950.4	E962.0	E980.4
Croton (oil)	973.1	E858.4	E943.1	E950.4	E962.0	E980.4
chloral	967.1	E852.0	E937.1	E950.2	E962.0	E980.2
Crude oil	981	E862.1	—	E950.9	E962.1	E980.9
Cryogenine	965.8	E850.8	E935.8	E950.0	E962.0	E980.0
Cryolite (pesticide)	989.4	E863.4	—	E950.6	E962.1	E980.7
Cryptenamine	972.6	E858.3	E942.6	E950.4	E962.0	E980.4
Crystal violet	976.0	E858.7	E946.0	E950.4	E962.0	E980.4
Cuckoopint	988.2	E865.4	—	E950.9	E962.1	E980.9
Cumetharol	964.2	E858.2	E934.2	E950.4	E962.0	E980.4
Cupric sulfate	973.6	E858.4	E943.6	E950.4	E962.0	E980.4
Cuprous sulfate	983.9	E864.3	—	E950.7	E962.1	E980.6
Curare, curarine	975.2	E858.6	E945.2	E950.4	E962.0	E980.4
Cyanic acid - *see* Cyanide(s)	—	—	—	—	—	—
Cyanide(s) (compounds) (hydrogen) (potassium) (sodium) NEC	989.0	E866.8	—	E950.9	E962.1	E980.9
dust or gas (inhalation) NEC	987.7	E869.8	—	E952.8	E962.2	E982.8
fumigant	989.0	E863.8	—	E950.6	E962.1	E980.7
mercuric - *see* Mercury	—	—	—	—	—	—
pesticide (dust) (fumes)	989.0	E863.4	—	E950.6	E962.1	E980.7
Cyanocobalamin	964.1	E858.2	E934.1	E950.4	E962.0	E980.4
Cyanogen (chloride) (gas)	—	—	—	—	—	—
NEC	987.8	E869.8	—	E952.8	E962.2	E982.8
Cyclaine	968.5	E855.2	E938.5	E950.4	E962.0	E980.4
Cyclamen europaeum	988.2	E865.4	—	E950.9	E962.1	E980.9
Cyclandelate	972.5	E858.3	E942.5	E950.4	E962.0	E980.4
Cyclazocine	965.09	E850.2	E935.2	E950.0	E962.0	E980.0
Cyclizine	963.0	E858.1	E933.0	E950.4	E962.0	E980.4
Cyclobarbital, cyclobarbitone	967.0	E851	E937.0	E950.1	E962.0	E980.1
Cycloguanil	961.4	E857	E931.4	E950.4	E962.0	E980.4
Cyclohexane	982.0	E862.4	—	E950.9	E962.1	E980.9
Cyclohexanol	980.8	E860.8	—	E950.9	E962.1	E980.9
Cyclohexanone	982.8	E862.4	—	E950.9	E962.1	E980.9
Cyclomethycaine	968.5	E855.2	E938.5	E950.4	E962.0	E980.4
Cyclopentamine	971.2	E855.5	E941.2	E950.4	E962.0	E980.4
Cyclopenthiazide	974.3	E858.5	E944.3	E950.4	E962.0	E980.4
Cyclopentolate	971.1	E855.4	E941.1	E950.4	E962.0	E980.4
Cyclophosphamide	963.1	E858.1	E933.1	E950.4	E962.0	E980.4
Cyclopropane	968.2	E855.1	E938.2	E950.4	E962.0	E980.4
Cycloserine	960.6	E856	E930.6	E950.4	E962.0	E980.4
Cyclothiazide	974.3	E858.5	E944.3	E950.4	E962.0	E980.4
Cycrimine	966.4	E855.0	E936.4	E950.4	E962.0	E980.4
Cymarin	972.1	E858.3	E942.1	E950.4	E962.0	E980.4
Cyproheptadine	963.0	E858.1	E933.0	E950.4	E962.0	E980.4

Substance	Poisoning	External Cause (E-Code)				
		Accident	Therapeutic Use	Suicide Attempt	Assault	Undetermined
Cyprolidol	969.0	E854.0	E939.0	E950.3	E962.0	E980.3
Cytarabine	963.1	E858.1	E933.1	E950.4	E962.0	E980.4
Cytisus	—	—	—	—	—	—
laburnum	988.2	E865.4	—	E950.9	E962.1	E980.9
scoparius	988.2	E865.4	—	E950.9	E962.1	E980.9
Cytomel	962.7	E858.0	E932.7	E950.4	E962.0	E980.4
Cytosine (antineoplastic)	963.1	E858.1	E933.1	E950.4	E962.0	E980.4
Cytoxan	963.1	E858.1	E933.1	E950.4	E962.0	E980.4
Dacarbazine	963.1	E858.1	E933.1	E950.4	E962.0	E980.4
Dactinomycin	960.7	E856	E930.7	E950.4	E962.0	E980.4
DADPS	961.8	E857	E931.8	E950.4	E962.0	E980.4
Dakin's solution (external)	976.0	E858.7	E946.0	E950.4	E962.0	E980.4
Dalmane	969.4	E853.2	E939.4	E950.3	E962.0	E980.3
DAM	977.2	E858.8	E947.2	E950.4	E962.0	E980.4
Danilone	964.2	E858.2	E934.2	E950.4	E962.0	E980.4
Danthron	973.1	E858.4	E943.1	E950.4	E962.0	E980.4
Dantrolene	975.2	E858.6	E945.2	E950.4	E962.0	E980.4
Daphne (gnidium) (mezereum)	988.2	E865.4	—	E950.9	E962.1	E980.9
berry	988.2	E865.3	—	E950.9	E962.1	E980.9
Dapsone	961.8	E857	E931.8	E950.4	E962.0	E980.4
Daraprim	961.4	E857	E931.4	E950.4	E962.0	E980.4
Darnel	988.2	E865.3	—	E950.9	E962.1	E980.9
Darvon	965.8	E850.8	E935.8	E950.0	E962.0	E980.0
Daunorubicin	960.7	E856	E930.7	E950.4	E962.0	E980.4
DBI	962.3	E858.0	E932.3	E950.4	E962.0	E980.4
D-Con (rodenticide)	989.4	E863.7	—	E950.6	E962.1	E980.7
DDS	961.8	E857	E931.8	E950.4	E962.0	E980.4
DDT	989.2	E863.0	—	E950.6	E962.1	E980.7
Deadly nightshade	988.2	E865.4	—	E950.9	E962.1	E980.9
berry	988.2	E865.3	—	E950.9	E962.1	E980.9
Deanol	969.7	E854.2	E939.7	E950.3	E962.0	E980.3
Debrisoquine	972.6	E858.3	E942.6	E950.4	E962.0	E980.4
Decaborane	989.89	E866.8	—	E950.9	E962.1	E980.9
fumes	987.8	E869.8	—	E952.8	E962.2	E982.8
Decadron	962.0	E858.0	E932.0	E950.4	E962.0	E980.4
ENT agent	976.6	E858.7	E946.6	E950.4	E962.0	E980.4
ophthalmic preparation	976.5	E858.7	E946.5	E950.4	E962.0	E980.4
topical NEC	976.0	E858.7	E946.0	E950.4	E962.0	E980.4
Decahydronaphthalene	982.0	E862.4	—	E950.9	E962.1	E980.9
Decalin	982.0	E862.4	—	E950.9	E962.1	E980.9
Decamethonium	975.2	E858.6	E945.2	E950.4	E962.0	E980.4
Decholin	973.4	E858.4	E943.4	E950.4	E962.0	E980.4
sodium (diagnostic)	977.8	E858.8	E947.8	E950.4	E962.0	E980.4
Declomycin	960.4	E856	E930.4	E950.4	E962.0	E980.4
Deferoxamine	963.8	E858.1	E933.8	E950.4	E962.0	E980.4
Dehydrocholic acid	973.4	E858.4	E943.4	E950.4	E962.0	E980.4
DeKalin	982.0	E862.4	—	E950.9	E962.1	E980.9
Delalutin	962.2	E858.0	E932.2	E950.4	E962.0	E980.4
Delphinium	988.2	E865.3	—	E950.9	E962.1	E980.9
Deltasone	962.0	E858.0	E932.0	E950.4	E962.0	E980.4
Deltra	962.0	E858.0	E932.0	E950.4	E962.0	E980.4
Delvinal	967.0	E851	E937.0	E950.1	E962.0	E980.1
Demecarium (bromide)	971.0	E855.3	E941.0	E950.4	E962.0	E980.4
Demeclocycline	960.4	E856	E930.4	E950.4	E962.0	E980.4
Demecolcine	963.1	E858.1	E933.1	E950.4	E962.0	E980.4
Demelanizing agents	976.8	E858.7	E946.8	E950.4	E962.0	E980.4
Demerol	965.09	E850.2	E935.2	E950.0	E962.0	E980.0
Demethylchlortetracycline	960.4	E856	E930.4	E950.4	E962.0	E980.4
Demethyltetracycline	960.4	E856	E930.4	E950.4	E962.0	E980.4
Demeton	989.3	E863.1	—	E950.6	E962.1	E980.7
Demulcents	976.3	E858.7	E946.3	E950.4	E962.0	E980.4

Substance	Poisoning	External Cause (E-Code)				
		Accident	Therapeutic Use	Suicide Attempt	Assault	Undetermined
Demulen	962.2	E858.0	E932.2	E950.4	E962.0	E980.4
Denatured alcohol	980.0	E860.1	—	E950.9	E962.1	E980.9
Dendrid	976.5	E858.7	E946.5	E950.4	E962.0	E980.4
Dental agents, topical	976.7	E858.7	E946.7	E950.4	E962.0	E980.4
Deodorant spray (feminine hygiene)	976.8	E858.7	E946.8	E950.4	E962.0	E980.4
Deoxyribonuclease	963.4	E858.1	E933.4	E950.4	E962.0	E980.4
Depressants	—	—	—	—	—	—
appetite, central	977.0	E858.8	E947.0	E950.4	E962.0	E980.4
cardiac	972.0	E858.3	E942.0	E950.4	E962.0	E980.4
central nervous system (anesthetic)	968.4	E855.1	E938.4	E950.4	E962.0	E980.4
psychotherapeutic	969.5	E853.9	E939.5	E950.3	E962.0	E980.3
Dequalinium	976.0	E858.7	E946.0	E950.4	E962.0	E980.4
Dermolate	976.2	E858.7	E946.2	E950.4	E962.0	E980.4
DES	962.2	E858.0	E932.2	E950.4	E962.0	E980.4
Desenex	976.0	E858.7	E946.0	E950.4	E962.0	E980.4
Deserpidine	972.6	E858.3	E942.6	E950.4	E962.0	E980.4
Desipramine	969.0	E854.0	E939.0	E950.3	E962.0	E980.3
Deslanoside	972.1	E858.3	E942.1	E950.4	E962.0	E980.4
Desocodeine	965.09	E850.2	E935.2	E950.0	E962.0	E980.0
Desomorphine	965.09	E850.2	E935.2	E950.0	E962.0	E980.0
Desonide	976.0	E858.7	E946.0	E950.4	E962.0	E980.4
Desoxycorticosterone derivatives	962.0	E858.0	E932.0	E950.4	E962.0	E980.4
Desoxyephedrine	969.7	E854.2	E939.7	E950.3	E962.0	E980.3
DET	969.6	E854.1	E939.6	E950.3	E962.0	E980.3
Detergents (ingested) (synthetic)	989.6	E861.0	—	E950.9	E962.1	E980.9
external medication	976.2	E858.7	E946.2	E950.4	E962.0	E980.4
Deterrent, alcohol	977.3	E858.8	E947.3	E950.4	E962.0	E980.4
Detrothyronine	962.7	E858.0	E932.7	E950.4	E962.0	E980.4
Dettol (external medication)	976.0	E858.7	E946.0	E950.4	E962.0	E980.4
Dexamethasone	962.0	E858.0	E932.0	E950.4	E962.0	E980.4
ENT agent	976.6	E858.7	E946.6	E950.4	E962.0	E980.4
ophthalmic preparation	976.5	E858.7	E946.5	E950.4	E962.0	E980.4
topical NEC	976.0	E858.7	E946.0	E950.4	E962.0	E980.4
Dexamphetamine	969.7	E854.2	E939.7	E950.3	E962.0	E980.3
Dexedrine	969.7	E854.2	E939.7	E950.3	E962.0	E980.3
Dexpanthenol	963.5	E858.1	E933.5	E950.4	E962.0	E980.4
Dextran	964.8	E858.2	E934.8	E950.4	E962.0	E980.4
Dextriferron	964.0	E858.2	E934.0	E950.4	E962.0	E980.4
Dextroamphetamine	969.7	E854.2	E939.7	E950.3	E962.0	E980.3
Dextro calcium pantothenate	963.5	E858.1	E933.5	E950.4	E962.0	E980.4
Dextromethorphan	975.4	E858.6	E945.4	E950.4	E962.0	E980.4
Dextromoramide	965.09	E850.2	E935.2	E950.0	E962.0	E980.0
Dextro pantothenyl alcohol	963.5	E858.1	E933.5	E950.4	E962.0	E980.4
topical	976.8	E858.7	E946.8	E950.4	E962.0	E980.4
Dextropropoxyphene (hydrochloride)	965.8	E850.8	E935.8	E950.0	E962.0	E980.0
Dextrorphan	965.09	E850.2	E935.2	E950.0	E962.0	E980.0
Dextrose NEC	974.5	E858.5	E944.5	E950.4	E962.0	E980.4
Dextrothyroxine	962.7	E858.0	E932.7	E950.4	E962.0	E980.4
DFP	971.0	E855.3	E941.0	E950.4	E962.0	E980.4
DHE-45	972.9	E858.3	E942.9	E950.4	E962.0	E980.4
Diabinese	962.3	E858.0	E932.3	E950.4	E962.0	E980.4
Diacetyl monoxime	977.2	E858.8	E947.2	E950.4	E962.0	E980.4
Diacetylmorphine	965.01	E850.0	E935.0	E950.0	E962.0	E980.0
Diagnostic agents	977.8	E858.8	E947.8	E950.4	E962.0	E980.4
Dial (soap)	976.2	E858.7	E946.2	E950.4	E962.0	E980.4
sedative	967.0	E851	E937.0	E950.1	E962.0	E980.1
Diallylbarbituric acid	967.0	E851	E937.0	E950.1	E962.0	E980.1
Diaminodiphenyisulfone	961.8	E857	E931.8	E950.4	E962.0	E980.4
Diamorphine	965.01	E850.0	E935.0	E950.0	E962.0	E980.0
Diamox	974.2	E858.5	E944.2	E950.4	E962.0	E980.4
Diamthazole	976.0	E858.7	E946.0	E950.4	E962.0	E980.4

◀ New ⟸ Revised

Substance	Poisoning	External Cause (E-Code) Accident	Therapeutic Use	Suicide Attempt	Assault	Undetermined
Diaphenyisulfone	961.8	E857	E931.8	E950.4	E962.0	E980.4
Diasone (sodium)	961.8	E857	E931.8	E950.4	E962.0	E980.4
Diazepam	969.4	E853.2	E939.4	E950.3	E962.0	E980.3
Diazinon	989.3	E863.1	—	E950.6	E962.1	E980.7
Diazomethane (gas)	987.8	E869.8	—	E952.8	E962.2	E982.8
Diazoxide	972.5	E858.3	E942.5	E950.4	E962.0	E980.4
Dibenamine	971.3	E855.6	E941.3	E950.4	E962.0	E980.4
Dibenzheptropine	963.0	E858.1	E933.0	E950.4	E962.0	E980.4
Dibenzyline	971.3	E855.6	E941.3	E950.4	E962.0	E980.4
Diborane (gas)	987.8	E869.8	—	E952.8	E962.2	E982.8
Dibromomannitol	963.1	E858.1	E933.1	E950.4	E962.0	E980.4
Dibucaine (spinal)	968.7	E855.2	E938.7	E950.4	E962.0	E980.4
topical (surface)	968.5	E855.2	E938.5	E950.4	E962.0	E980.4
Dibunate sodium	975.4	E858.6	E945.4	E950.4	E962.0	E980.4
Dibutoline	971.1	E855.4	E941.1	E950.4	E962.0	E980.4
Dicapthon	989.4	E863.4	—	E950.6	E962.1	E980.7
Dichloralphenazone	967.1	E852.0	E937.1	E950.2	E962.0	E980.2
Dichlorodifluoromethane	987.4	E869.2	—	E952.8	E962.2	E982.8
Dichloroethane	982.3	E862.4	—	E950.9	E962.1	E980.9
Dichloroethylene	982.3	E862.4	—	E950.9	E962.1	E980.9
Dichloroethyl sulfide	987.8	E869.8	—	E952.8	E962.2	E982.8
Dichlorohydrin	982.3	E862.4	—	E950.9	E962.1	E980.9
Dichloromethane (solvent) (vapor)	982.3	E862.4	—	E950.9	E962.1	E980.9
Dichlorophen(e)	961.6	E857	E931.6	E950.4	E962.0	E980.4
Dichlorphenamide	974.2	E858.5	E944.2	E950.4	E962.0	E980.4
Dichlorvos	989.3	E863.1	—	E950.6	E962.1	E980.7
Diclofenac sodium	965.69	E850.6	E935.6	E950.0	E962.0	E980.0
Dicoumarin, dicumarol	964.2	E858.2	E934.2	E950.4	E962.0	E980.4
Dicyanogen (gas)	987.8	E869.8	—	E952.8	E962.2	E982.8
Dicyclomine	971.1	E855.4	E941.1	E950.4	E962.0	E980.4
Dieldrin (vapor)	989.2	E863.0	—	E950.6	E962.1	E980.7
Dienestrol	962.2	E858.0	E932.2	E950.4	E962.0	E980.4
Dietetics	977.0	E858.8	E947.0	E950.4	E962.0	E980.4
Diethazine	966.4	E855.0	E936.4	E950.4	E962.0	E980.4
Diethyl	—	—	—	—	—	—
barbituric acid	967.0	E851	E937.0	E950.1	E962.0	E980.1
carbamazine	961.6	E857	E931.6	E950.4	E962.0	E980.4
carbinol	980.8	E860.8	—	E950.9	E962.1	E980.9
carbonate	982.8	E862.4	—	E950.9	E962.1	E980.9
ether (vapor) - *see* Ether(s)	—	—	—	—	—	—
propion	977.0	E858.8	E947.0	E950.4	E962.0	E980.4
stilbestrol	962.2	E858.0	E932.2	E950.4	E962.0	E980.4
Diethylene	—	—	—	—	—	—
dioxide	982.8	E862.4	—	E950.9	E962.1	E980.9
glycol (monoacetate) (monoethyl ether)	982.8	E862.4	—	E950.9	E962.1	E980.9
Diethylsulfone-diethylmethane	967.8	E852.8	E937.8	E950.2	E962.0	E980.2
Difencloxazine	965.09	E850.2	E935.2	E950.0	E962.0	E980.0
Diffusin	963.4	E858.1	E933.4	E950.4	E962.0	E980.4
Diflos	971.0	E855.3	E941.0	E950.4	E962.0	E980.4
Digestants	973.4	E858.4	E943.4	E950.4	E962.0	E980.4
Digitalin(e)	972.1	E858.3	E942.1	E950.4	E962.0	E980.4
Digitalis glycosides	972.1	E858.3	E942.1	E950.4	E962.0	E980.4
Digitoxin	972.1	E858.3	E942.1	E950.4	E962.0	E980.4
Digoxin	972.1	E858.3	E942.1	E950.4	E962.0	E980.4
Dihydrocodeine	965.09	E850.2	E935.2	E950.0	E962.0	E980.0
Dihydrocodeinone	965.09	E850.2	E935.2	E950.0	E962.0	E980.0
Dihydroergocristine	972.9	E858.3	E942.9	E950.4	E962.0	E980.4
Dihydroergotamine	972.9	E858.3	E942.9	E950.4	E962.0	E980.4
Dihydroergotoxine	972.9	E858.3	E942.9	E950.4	E962.0	E980.4
Dihydrohydroxycodeinone	965.09	E850.2	E935.2	E950.0	E962.0	E980.0
Dihydrohydroxymorphinone	965.09	E850.2	E935.2	E950.0	E962.0	E980.0

Substance	Poisoning	External Cause (E-Code) Accident	Therapeutic Use	Suicide Attempt	Assault	Undetermined
Dihydroisocodeine	965.09	E850.2	E935.2	E950.0	E962.0	E980.0
Dihydromorphine	965.09	E850.2	E935.2	E950.0	E962.0	E980.0
Dihydromorphinone	965.09	E850.2	E935.2	E950.0	E962.0	E980.0
Dihydrostreptomycin	960.6	E856	E930.6	E950.4	E962.0	E980.4
Dihydrotachysterol	962.6	E858.0	E932.6	E950.4	E962.0	E980.4
Dihydroxyanthraquinone	973.1	E858.4	E943.1	E950.4	E962.0	E980.4
Dihydroxycodeinone	965.09	E850.2	E935.2	E950.0	E962.0	E980.0
Diiodohydroxyquin	961.3	E857	E931.3	E950.4	E962.0	E980.4
topical	976.0	E858.7	E946.0	E950.4	E962.0	E980.4
Diiodohydroxyquinoline	961.3	E857	E931.3	E950.4	E962.0	E980.4
Dilantin	966.1	E855.0	E936.1	E950.4	E962.0	E980.4
Dilaudid	965.09	E850.2	E935.2	E950.0	E962.0	E980.0
Diloxanide	961.5	E857	E931.5	E950.4	E962.0	E980.4
Dimefline	970.0	E854.3	E940.0	E950.4	E962.0	E980.4
Dimenhydrinate	963.0	E858.1	E933.0	E950.4	E962.0	E980.4
Dimercaprol	963.8	E858.1	E933.8	E950.4	E962.0	E980.4
Dimercaptopropanol	963.8	E858.1	E933.8	E950.4	E962.0	E980.4
Dimetane	963.0	E858.1	E933.0	E950.4	E962.0	E980.4
Dimethicone	976.3	E858.7	E946.3	E950.4	E962.0	E980.4
Dimethindene	963.0	E858.1	E933.0	E950.4	E962.0	E980.4
Dimethisoquin	968.5	E855.2	E938.5	E950.4	E962.0	E980.4
Dimethisterone	962.2	E858.0	E932.2	E950.4	E962.0	E980.4
Dimethoxanate	975.4	E858.6	E945.4	E950.4	E962.0	E980.4
Dimethyl	—	—	—	—	—	—
arsine, arsinic acid - *see* Arsenic	—	—	—	—	—	—
carbinol	980.2	E860.3	—	E950.9	E962.1	E980.9
diguanide	962.3	E858.0	E932.3	E950.4	E962.0	E980.4
ketone	982.8	E862.4	—	E950.9	E962.1	E980.9
vapor	987.8	E869.8	—	E952.8	E962.2	E982.8
meperidine	965.09	E850.2	E935.2	E950.0	E962.0	E980.0
parathion	989.3	E863.1	—	E950.6	E962.1	E980.7
polysiloxane	973.8	E858.4	E943.8	E950.4	E962.0	E980.4
sulfate (fumes)	987.8	E869.8	—	E952.8	E962.2	E982.8
liquid	983.9	E864.3	—	E950.7	E962.1	E980.6
sulfoxide NEC	982.8	E862.4	—	E950.9	E962.1	E980.9
medicinal	976.4	E858.7	E946.4	E950.4	E962.0	E980.4
triptamine	969.6	E854.1	E939.6	E950.3	E962.0	E980.3
tubocurarine	975.2	E858.6	E945.2	E950.4	E962.0	E980.4
Dindevan	964.2	E858.2	E934.2	E950.4	E962.0	E980.4
Dinitro (-ortho-) cresol (herbicide) (spray)	989.4	E863.5	—	E950.6	E962.1	E980.7
insecticide	989.4	E863.4	—	E950.6	E962.1	E980.7
Dinitrobenzene	983.0	E864.0	—	E950.7	E962.1	E980.6
vapor	987.8	E869.8	—	E952.8	E962.2	E982.8
Dinitro-orthocresol (herbicide)	989.4	E863.5	—	E950.6	E962.1	E980.7
insecticide	989.4	E863.4	—	E950.6	E962.1	E980.7
Dinitrophenol (herbicide) (spray)	989.4	E863.5	—	E950.6	E962.1	E980.7
insecticide	989.4	E863.4	—	E950.6	E962.1	E980.7
Dinoprost	975.0	E858.6	E945.0	E950.4	E962.0	E980.4
Dioctyl sulfosuccinate (calcium) (sodium)	973.2	E858.4	E943.2	E950.4	E962.0	E980.4
Diodoquin	961.3	E857	E931.3	E950.4	E962.0	E980.4
Dione derivatives NEC	966.3	E855.0	E936.3	E950.4	E962.0	E980.4
Dionin	965.09	E850.2	E935.2	E950.0	E962.0	E980.0
Dioxane	982.8	E862.4	—	E950.9	E962.1	E980.9
Dioxin - *see* herbicide	—	—	—	—	—	—
Dioxyline	972.5	E858.3	E942.5	E950.4	E962.0	E980.4
Dipentene	982.8	E862.4	—	E950.9	E962.1	E980.9
Diphemanil	971.1	E855.4	E941.1	E950.4	E962.0	E980.4
Diphenadione	964.2	E858.2	E934.2	E950.4	E962.0	E980.4
Diphenhydramine	963.0	E858.1	E933.0	E950.4	E962.0	E980.4
Diphenidol	963.0	E858.1	E933.0	E950.4	E962.0	E980.4
Diphenoxylate	973.5	E858.4	E943.5	E950.4	E962.0	E980.4

Substance	Poisoning	External Cause (E-Code)				
		Accident	Therapeutic Use	Suicide Attempt	Assault	Undetermined
Diphenylchlorarsine	985.1	E866.3	—	E950.8	E962.1	E980.8
Diphenylhydantoin (sodium)	966.1	E855.0	E936.1	E950.4	E962.0	E980.4
Diphenylpyraline	963.0	E858.1	E933.0	E950.4	E962.0	E980.4
Diphtheria	—	—	—	—	—	—
antitoxin	979.9	E858.8	E949.9	E950.4	E962.0	E980.4
toxoid	978.5	E858.8	E948.5	E950.4	E962.0	E980.4
with tetanus toxoid	978.9	E858.8	E948.9	E950.4	E962.0	E980.4
with pertussis component	978.6	E858.8	E948.6	E950.4	E962.0	E980.4
vaccine	978.5	E858.8	E948.5	E950.4	E962.0	E980.4
Dipipanone	965.09	E850.2	E935.2	E950.0	E962.0	E980.0
Diplovax	979.5	E858.8	E949.5	E950.4	E962.0	E980.4
Diprophylline	975.1	E858.6	E945.1	E950.4	E962.0	E980.4
Dipyridamole	972.4	E858.3	E942.4	E950.4	E962.0	E980.4
Dipyrone	965.5	E850.5	E935.5	E950.0	E962.0	E980.0
Diquat	989.4	E863.5	—	E950.6	E962.1	E980.7
Disinfectant NEC	983.9	E861.4	—	E950.7	E962.1	E980.6
alkaline	983.2	E861.4	—	E950.7	E962.1	E980.6
aromatic	983.0	E861.4	—	E950.7	E962.1	E980.6
Disipal	966.4	E855.0	E936.4	E950.4	E962.0	E980.4
Disodium edetate	963.8	E858.1	E933.8	E950.4	E962.0	E980.4
Disulfamide	974.4	E858.5	E944.4	E950.4	E962.0	E980.4
Disulfanilamide	961.0	E857	E931.0	E950.4	E962.0	E980.4
Disulfiram	977.3	E858.8	E947.3	E950.4	E962.0	E980.4
Dithiazanine	961.6	E857	E931.6	E950.4	E962.0	E980.4
Dithioglycerol	963.8	E858.1	E933.8	E950.4	E962.0	E980.4
Dithranol	976.4	E858.7	E946.4	E950.4	E962.0	E980.4
Diucardin	974.3	E858.5	E944.3	E950.4	E962.0	E980.4
Diupres	974.3	E858.5	E944.3	E950.4	E962.0	E980.4
Diuretics NEC	974.4	E858.5	E944.4	E950.4	E962.0	E980.4
carbonic acid anhydrase inhibitors	974.2	E858.5	E944.2	E950.4	E962.0	E980.4
mercurial	974.0	E858.5	E944.0	E950.4	E962.0	E980.4
osmotic	974.4	E858.5	E944.4	E950.4	E962.0	E980.4
purine derivatives	974.1	E858.5	E944.1	E950.4	E962.0	E980.4
saluretic	974.3	E858.5	E944.3	E950.4	E962.0	E980.4
Diuril	974.3	E858.5	E944.3	E950.4	E962.0	E980.4
Divinyl ether	968.2	E855.1	E938.2	E950.4	E962.0	E980.4
D-lysergic acid diethylamide	969.6	E854.1	E939.6	E950.3	E962.0	E980.3
DMCT	960.4	E856	E930.4	E950.4	E962.0	E980.4
DMSO	982.8	E862.4	—	E950.9	E962.1	E980.9
DMT	969.6	E854.1	E939.6	E950.3	E962.0	E980.3
DNOC	989.4	E863.5	—	E950.6	E962.1	E980.7
DOCA	962.0	E858.0	E932.0	E950.4	E962.0	E980.4
Dolophine	965.02	E850.1	E935.1	E950.0	E962.0	E980.0
Doloxene	965.8	E850.8	E935.8	E950.0	E962.0	E980.0
DOM	969.6	E854.1	E939.6	E950.3	E962.0	E980.3
Domestic gas - *see* Gas, utility	—	—	—	—	—	—
Domiphen (bromide) (lozenges)	976.6	E858.7	E946.6	E950.4	E962.0	E980.4
Dopa (levo)	966.4	E855.0	E936.4	E950.4	E962.0	E980.4
Dopamine	971.2	E855.5	E941.2	E950.4	E962.0	E980.4
Doriden	967.5	E852.4	E937.5	E950.2	E962.0	E980.2
Dormiral	967.0	E851	E937.0	E950.1	E962.0	E980.1
Dormison	967.8	E852.8	E937.8	E950.2	E962.0	E980.2
Dornase	963.4	E858.1	E933.4	E950.4	E962.0	E980.4
Dorsacaine	968.5	E855.2	E938.5	E950.4	E962.0	E980.4
Dothiepin hydrochloride	969.0	E854.0	E939.0	E950.3	E962.0	E980.3
Doxapram	970.0	E854.3	E940.0	E950.4	E962.0	E980.4
Doxepin	969.0	E854.0	E939.0	E950.3	E962.0	E980.3
Doxorubicin	960.7	E856	E930.7	E950.4	E962.0	E980.4
Doxycycline	960.4	E856	E930.4	E950.4	E962.0	E980.4
Doxylamine	963.0	E858.1	E933.0	E950.4	E962.0	E980.4
Dramamine	963.0	E858.1	E933.0	E950.4	E962.0	E980.4

Substance	Poisoning	External Cause (E-Code) Accident	Therapeutic Use	Suicide Attempt	Assault	Undetermined
Drano (drain cleaner)	983.2	E864.2	—	E950.7	E962.1	E980.6
Dromoran	965.09	E850.2	E935.2	E950.0	E962.0	E980.0
Dromostanolone	962.1	E858.0	E932.1	E950.4	E962.0	E980.4
Droperidol	969.2	E853.1	E939.2	E950.3	E962.0	E980.3
Drotrecogin alfa	964.2	E858.2	E934.2	E950.4	E962.0	E980.4
Drug	977.9	E858.9	E947.9	E950.5	E962.0	E980.5
specified NEC	977.8	E858.8	E947.8	E950.4	E962.0	E980.4
AHFS List	—	—	—	—	—	—
4:00 antihistamine drugs	963.0	E858.1	E933.0	E950.4	E962.0	E980.4
8:04 amebacides	961.5	E857	E931.5	E950.4	E962.0	E980.4
arsenical anti-infectives	961.1	E857	E931.1	E950.4	E962.0	E980.4
quinoline derivatives	961.3	E857	E931.3	E950.4	E962.0	E980.4
8:08 anthelmintics	961.6	E857	E931.6	E950.4	E962.0	E980.4
quinoline derivatives	961.3	E857	E931.3	E950.4	E962.0	E980.4
8:12.04 antifungal antibiotics	960.1	E856	E930.1	E950.4	E962.0	E980.4
8:12.06 cephalosporins	960.5	E856	E930.5	E950.4	E962.0	E980.4
8:12.08 chloramphenicol	960.2	E856	E930.2	E950.4	E962.0	E980.4
8:12.12 erythromycins	960.3	E856	E930.3	E950.4	E962.0	E980.4
8:12.16 penicillins	960.0	E856	E930.0	E950.4	E962.0	E980.4
8:12.20 streptomycins	960.6	E856	E930.6	E950.4	E962.0	E980.4
8:12.24 tetracyclines	960.4	E856	E930.4	E950.4	E962.0	E980.4
8:12.28 other antibiotics	960.8	E856	E930.8	E950.4	E962.0	E980.4
antimycobacterial	960.6	E856	E930.6	E950.4	E962.0	E980.4
macrolides	960.3	E856	E930.3	E950.4	E962.0	E980.4
8:16 antituberculars	961.8	E857	E931.8	E950.4	E962.0	E980.4
antibiotics	960.6	E856	E930.6	E950.4	E962.0	E980.4
8:18 antivirals	961.7	E857	E931.7	E950.4	E962.0	E980.4
8:20 plasmodicides (antimalarials)	961.4	E857	E931.4	E950.4	E962.0	E980.4
8:24 sulfonamides	961.0	E857	E931.0	E950.4	E962.0	E980.4
8:26 sulfones	961.8	E857	E931.8	E950.4	E962.0	E980.4
8:28 treponemicides	961.2	E857	E931.2	E950.4	E962.0	E980.4
8:32 trichomonacides	961.5	E857	E931.5	E950.4	E962.0	E980.4
quinoline derivatives	961.3	E857	E931.3	E950.4	E962.0	E980.4
nitrofuran derivatives	961.9	E857	E931.9	E950.4	E962.0	E980.4
8:36 urinary germicides	961.9	E857	E931.9	E950.4	E962.0	E980.4
quinoline derivatives	961.3	E857	E931.3	E950.4	E962.0	E980.4
8:40 other anti-infectives	961.9	E857	E931.9	E950.4	E962.0	E980.4
10:00 antineoplastic agents	963.1	E858.1	E933.1	E950.4	E962.0	E980.4
antibiotics	960.7	E856	E930.7	E950.4	E962.0	E980.4
progestogens	962.2	E858.0	E932.2	E950.4	E962.0	E980.4
12:04 parasympathomimetic (cholinergic) agents	971.0	E855.3	E941.0	E950.4	E962.0	E980.4
12:08 parasympatholytic (cholinergic-blocking) agents	971.1	E855.4	E941.1	E950.4	E962.0	E980.4
12:12 sympathomimetic (adrenergic) agents	971.2	E855.5	E941.2	E950.4	E962.0	E980.4
12:16 sympatholytic (adrenergic-blocking) agents	971.3	E855.6	E941.3	E950.4	E962.0	E980.4
12:20 skeletal muscle relaxants	—	—	—	—	—	—
central nervous system muscle-tone depressants	968.0	E855.1	E938.0	E950.4	E962.0	E980.4
myoneural blocking agents	975.2	E858.6	E945.2	E950.4	E962.0	E980.4
16:00 blood derivatives	964.7	E858.2	E934.7	E950.4	E962.0	E980.4
20:04 antianemia drugs	964.1	E858.2	E934.1	E950.4	E962.0	E980.4
20:04.04 iron preparations	964.0	E858.2	E934.0	E950.4	E962.0	E980.4
20:04.08 liver and stomach preparations	964.1	E858.2	E934.1	E950.4	E962.0	E980.4
20:12.04 anticoagulants	964.2	E858.2	E934.2	E950.4	E962.0	E980.4
20:12.08 antiheparin agents	964.5	E858.2	E934.5	E950.4	E962.0	E980.4
20:12.12 coagulants	964.5	E858.2	E934.5	E950.4	E962.0	E980.4
20:12.16 hemostatics NEC	964.5	E858.2	E934.5	E950.4	E962.0	E980.4
capillary active drugs	972.8	E858.3	E942.8	E950.4	E962.0	E980.4
24:04 cardiac drugs	972.9	E858.3	E942.9	E950.4	E962.0	E980.4
cardiotonic agents	972.1	E858.3	E942.1	E950.4	E962.0	E980.4
rhythm regulators	972.0	E858.3	E942.0	E950.4	E962.0	E980.4
24:06 antilipemic agents	972.2	E858.3	E942.2	E950.4	E962.0	E980.4
thyroid derivatives	962.7	E858.0	E932.7	E950.4	E962.0	E980.4

Substance	Poisoning	External Cause (E-Code)				
		Accident	Therapeutic Use	Suicide Attempt	Assault	Undetermined
Drug *(Continued)*						
24:08 hypotensive agents	972.6	E858.3	E942.6	E950.4	E962.0	E980.4
adrenergic blocking agents	971.3	E855.6	E941.3	E950.4	E962.0	E980.4
ganglion blocking agents	972.3	E858.3	E942.3	E950.4	E962.0	E980.4
vasodilators	972.5	E858.3	E942.5	E950.4	E962.0	E980.4
24:12 vasodilating agents NEC	972.5	E858.3	E942.5	E950.4	E962.0	E980.4
coronary	972.4	E858.3	E942.4	E950.4	E962.0	E980.4
nicotinic acid derivatives	972.2	E858.3	E942.2	E950.4	E962.0	E980.4
24:16 sclerosing agents	972.7	E858.3	E942.7	E950.4	E962.0	E980.4
28:04 general anesthetics	968.4	E855.1	E938.4	E950.4	E962.0	E980.4
gaseous anesthetics	968.2	E855.1	E938.2	E950.4	E962.0	E980.4
halothane	968.1	E855.1	E938.1	E950.4	E962.0	E980.4
intravenous anesthetics	968.3	E855.1	E938.3	E950.4	E962.0	E980.4
28:08 analgesics and antipyretics	965.9	E850.9	E935.9	E950.0	E962.0	E980.0
antirheumatics	965.69	E850.6	E935.6	E950.0	E962.0	E980.0
aromatic analgesics	965.4	E850.4	E935.4	E950.0	E962.0	E980.0
non-narcotic NEC	965.7	E850.7	E935.7	E950.0	E962.0	E980.0
opium alkaloids	965.00	E850.2	E935.2	E950.0	E962.0	E980.0
heroin	965.01	E850.0	E935.0	E950.0	E962.0	E980.0
methadone	965.02	E850.1	E935.1	E950.0	E962.0	E980.0
specified type NEC	965.09	E850.2	E935.2	E950.0	E962.0	E980.0
pyrazole derivatives	965.5	E850.5	E935.5	E950.0	E962.0	E980.0
salicylates	965.1	E850.3	E935.3	E950.0	E962.0	E980.0
specified NEC	965.8	E850.8	E935.8	E950.0	E962.0	E980.0
28:10 narcotic antagonists	970.1	E854.3	E940.1	E950.4	E962.0	E980.4
28:12 anticonvulsants	966.3	E855.0	E936.3	E950.4	E962.0	E980.4
barbiturates	967.0	E851	E937.0	E950.1	E962.0	E980.1
benzodiazepine-based tranquilizers	969.4	E853.4	E939.4	E950.3	E962.0	E980.3
bromides	967.3	E852.2	E937.3	E950.2	E962.0	E980.2
hydantoin derivatives	966.1	E855.0	E936.1	E950.4	E962.0	E980.4
oxazolidine (derivatives)	966.0	E855.0	E936.0	E950.4	E962.0	E980.4
succinimides	966.2	E855.0	E936.2	E950.4	E962.0	E980.4
28:16.04 antidepressants	969.0	E854.0	E939.0	E950.3	E962.0	E980.3
28:16.08 tranquilizers	969.5	E853.9	E939.5	E950.3	E962.0	E980.3
benzodiazepine-based	969.4	E853.2	E939.4	E950.3	E962.0	E980.3
butyrophenone-based	969.2	E853.1	E939.2	E950.3	E962.0	E980.3
major NEC	969.3	E853.8	E939.3	E950.3	E962.0	E980.3
phenothiazine-based	969.1	E853.0	E939.1	E950.3	E962.0	E980.3
28:16.12 other psychotherapeutic agents	969.8	E855.8	E939.8	E950.3	E962.0	E980.3
28:20 respiratory and cerebral stimulants	970.9	E854.3	E940.9	E950.4	E962.0	E980.4
analeptics	970.0	E854.3	E940.0	E950.4	E962.0	E980.4
anorexigenic agents	977.0	E858.8	E947.0	E950.4	E962.0	E980.4
psychostimulants	969.7	E854.2	E939.7	E950.3	E962.0	E980.3
specified NEC	970.8	E854.3	E940.8	E950.4	E962.0	E980.4
28:24 sedatives and hypnotics	967.9	E852.9	E937.9	E950.2	E962.0	E980.2
barbiturates	967.0	E851	E937.0	E950.1	E962.0	E980.1
benzodiazepine-based tranquilizers	969.4	E853.2	E939.4	E950.3	E962.0	E980.3
chloral hydrate (group)	967.1	E852.0	E937.1	E950.2	E962.0	E980.2
glutethimide group	967.5	E852.4	E937.5	E950.2	E962.0	E980.2
intravenous anesthetics	968.3	E855.1	E938.3	E950.4	E962.0	E980.4
methaqualone (compounds)	967.4	E852.3	E937.4	E950.2	E962.0	E980.2
paraldehyde	967.2	E852.1	E937.2	E950.2	E962.0	E980.2
phenothiazine-based tranquilizers	969.1	E853.0	E939.1	E950.3	E962.0	E980.3
specified NEC	967.8	E852.8	E937.8	E950.2	E962.0	E980.2
thiobarbiturates	968.3	E855.1	E938.3	E950.4	E962.0	E980.4
tranquilizer NEC	969.5	E853.9	E939.5	E950.3	E962.0	E980.3
36:04 to 36:88 diagnostic agents	977.8	E858.8	E947.8	E950.4	E962.0	E980.4
40:00 electrolyte, caloric, and water balance agents NEC	974.5	E858.5	E944.5	E950.4	E962.0	E980.4
40:04 acidifying agents	963.2	E858.1	E933.2	E950.4	E962.0	E980.4
40:08 alkalinizing agents	963.3	E858.1	E933.3	E950.4	E962.0	E980.4
40:10 ammonia detoxicants	974.5	E858.5	E944.5	E950.4	E962.0	E980.4

Substance	Poisoning	External Cause (E-Code) Accident	Therapeutic Use	Suicide Attempt	Assault	Undetermined
Drug *(Continued)*						
40:12 replacement solutions	974.5	E858.5	E944.5	E950.4	E962.0	E980.4
plasma expanders	964.8	E858.2	E934.8	E950.4	E962.0	E980.4
40:16 sodium-removing resins	974.5	E858.5	E944.5	E950.4	E962.0	E980.4
40:18 potassium-removing resins	974.5	E858.5	E944.5	E950.4	E962.0	E980.4
40:20 caloric agents	974.5	E858.5	E944.5	E950.4	E962.0	E980.4
40:24 salt and sugar substitutes	974.5	E858.5	E944.5	E950.4	E962.0	E980.4
40:28 diuretics NEC	974.4	E858.5	E944.4	E950.4	E962.0	E980.4
carbonic acid anhydrase inhibitors	974.2	E858.5	E944.2	E950.4	E962.0	E980.4
mercurials	974.0	E858.5	E944.0	E950.4	E962.0	E980.4
purine derivatives	974.1	E858.5	E944.1	E950.4	E962.0	E980.4
saluretics	974.3	E858.5	E944.3	E950.4	E962.0	E980.4
thiazides	974.3	E858.5	E944.3	E950.4	E962.0	E980.4
40:36 irrigating solutions	974.5	E858.5	E944.5	E950.4	E962.0	E980.4
40:40 uricosuric agents	974.7	E858.5	E944.7	E950.4	E962.0	E980.4
44:00 enzymes	963.4	E858.1	E933.4	E950.4	E962.0	E980.4
fibrinolysis-affecting agents	964.4	E858.2	E934.4	E950.4	E962.0	E980.4
gastric agents	973.4	E858.4	E943.4	E950.4	E962.0	E980.4
48:00 expectorants and cough preparations	—	—	—	—	—	—
antihistamine agents	963.0	E858.1	E933.0	E950.4	E962.0	E980.4
antitussives	975.4	E858.6	E945.4	E950.4	E962.0	E980.4
codeine derivatives	965.09	E850.2	E935.2	E950.0	E962.0	E980.0
expectorants	975.5	E858.6	E945.5	E950.4	E962.0	E980.4
narcotic agents NEC	965.09	E850.2	E935.2	E950.0	E962.0	E980.0
52:04 anti-infectives (EENT)	—	—	—	—	—	—
ENT agent	976.6	E858.7	E946.6	E950.4	E962.0	E980.4
ophthalmic preparation	976.5	E858.7	E946.5	E950.4	E962.0	E980.4
52:04.04 antibiotics (EENT)	—	—	—	—	—	—
ENT agent	976.6	E858.7	E946.6	E950.4	E962.0	E980.4
ophthalmic preparation	976.5	E858.7	E946.5	E950.4	E962.0	E980.4
52:04.06 antivirals (EENT)	—	—	—	—	—	—
ENT agent	976.6	E858.7	E946.6	E950.4	E962.0	E980.4
ophthalmic preparation	976.5	E858.7	E946.5	E950.4	E962.0	E980.4
2:04.08 sulfonamides (EENT)	—	—	—	—	—	—
ENT agent	976.6	E858.7	E946.6	E950.4	E962.0	E980.4
ophthalmic preparation	976.5	E858.7	E946.5	E950.4	E962.0	E980.4
52:04.12 miscellaneous anti-infectives (EENT)	—	—	—	—	—	—
ENT agent	976.6	E858.7	E946.6	E950.4	E962.0	E980.4
ophthalmic preparation	976.5	E858.7	E946.5	E950.4	E962.0	E980.4
52:08 anti-inflammatory agents (EENT)	—	—	—	—	—	—
ENT agent	976.6	E858.7	E946.6	E950.4	E962.0	E980.4
ophthalmic preparation	976.5	E858.7	E946.5	E950.4	E962.0	E980.4
52:10 carbonic anhydrase inhibitors	974.2	E858.5	E944.2	E950.4	E962.0	E980.4
52:12 contact lens solutions	976.5	E858.7	E946.5	E950.4	E962.0	E980.4
52:16 local anesthetics (EENT)	968.5	E855.2	E938.5	E950.4	E962.0	E980.4
52:20 miotics	971.0	E855.3	E941.0	E950.4	E962.0	E980.4
52:24 mydriatics	—	—	—	—	—	—
adrenergics	971.2	E855.5	E941.2	E950.4	E962.0	E980.4
anticholinergics	971.1	E855.4	E941.1	E950.4	E962.0	E980.4
antimuscarinics	971.1	E855.4	E941.1	E950.4	E962.0	E980.4
parasympatholytics	971.1	E855.4	E941.1	E950.4	E962.0	E980.4
spasmolytics	971.1	E855.4	E941.1	E950.4	E962.0	E980.4
sympathomimetics	971.2	E855.5	E941.2	E950.4	E962.0	E980.4
52:28 mouth washes and gargles	976.6	E858.7	E946.6	E950.4	E962.0	E980.4
52:32 vasoconstrictors (EENT)	971.2	E855.5	E941.2	E950.4	E962.0	E980.4
52:36 unclassified agents (EENT)	—	—	—	—	—	—
ENT agent	976.6	E858.7	E946.6	E950.4	E962.0	E980.4
ophthalmic preparation	976.5	E858.7	E946.5	E950.4	E962.0	E980.4
56:04 antacids and adsorbents	973.0	E858.4	E943.0	E950.4	E962.0	E980.4
56:08 antidiarrhea agents	973.5	E858.4	E943.5	E950.4	E962.0	E980.4
56:10 antiflatulents	973.8	E858.4	E943.8	E950.4	E962.0	E980.4

◀ New ⬅ Revised

Substance	Poisoning	External Cause (E-Code)				
		Accident	Therapeutic Use	Suicide Attempt	Assault	Undetermined
Drug *(Continued)*						
56:12 cathartics NEC	973.3	E858.4	E943.3	E950.4	E962.0	E980.4
emollients	973.2	E858.4	E943.2	E950.4	E962.0	E980.4
irritants	973.1	E858.4	E943.1	E950.4	E962.0	E980.4
56:16 digestants	973.4	E858.4	E943.4	E950.4	E962.0	E980.4
56:20 emetics and antiemetics	—	—	—	—	—	—
antiemetics	963.0	E858.1	E933.0	E950.4	E962.0	E980.4
emetics	973.6	E858.4	E943.6	E950.4	E962.0	E980.4
56:24 lipotropic agents	977.1	E858.8	E947.1	E950.4	E962.0	E980.4
56:40 miscellaneous G.I. drugs	973.8	E858.4	E943.8	E950.4	E962.0	E980.4
60:00 gold compounds	965.69	E850.6	E935.6	E950.0	E962.0	E980.0
64:00 heavy metal antagonists	963.8	E858.1	E933.8	E950.4	E962.0	E980.4
68:04 adrenals	962.0	E858.0	E932.0	E950.4	E962.0	E980.4
68:08 androgens	962.1	E858.0	E932.1	E950.4	E962.0	E980.4
68:12 contraceptives, oral	962.2	E858.0	E932.2	E950.4	E962.0	E980.4
68:16 estrogens	962.2	E858.0	E932.2	E950.4	E962.0	E980.4
68:18 gonadotropins	962.4	E858.0	E932.4	E950.4	E962.0	E980.4
68:20 insulins and antidiabetic agents	962.3	E858.0	E932.3	E950.4	E962.0	E980.4
68:20.08 insulins	962.3	E858.0	E932.3	E950.4	E962.0	E980.4
68:24 parathyroid	962.6	E858.0	E932.6	E950.4	E962.0	E980.4
68:28 pituitary (posterior)	962.5	E858.0	E932.5	E950.4	E962.0	E980.4
anterior	962.4	E858.0	E932.4	E950.4	E962.0	E980.4
68:32 progestogens	962.2	E858.0	E932.2	E950.4	E962.0	E980.4
68:34 other corpus luteum hormones NEC	962.2	E858.0	E932.2	E950.4	E962.0	E980.4
68:36 thyroid and antithyroid	—	—	—	—	—	—
antithyroid	962.8	E858.0	E932.8	E950.4	E962.0	E980.4
thyroid (derivatives)	962.7	E858.0	E932.7	E950.4	E962.0	E980.4
72:00 local anesthetics NEC	968.9	E855.2	E938.9	E950.4	E962.0	E980.4
topical (surface)	968.5	E855.2	E938.5	E950.4	E962.0	E980.4
infiltration (intradermal) (subcutaneous) (submucosal)	968.5	E855.2	E938.5	E950.4	E962.0	E980.4
nerve blocking (peripheral) (plexus) (regional)	968.6	E855.2	E938.6	E950.4	E962.0	E980.4
spinal	968.7	E855.2	E938.7	E950.4	E962.0	E980.4
76:00 oxytocics	975.0	E858.6	E945.0	E950.4	E962.0	E980.4
78:00 radioactive agents	990	—	—	—	—	—
80:04 serums NEC	979.9	E858.8	E949.9	E950.4	E962.0	E980.4
immune gamma globulin (human)	964.6	E858.2	E934.6	E950.4	E962.0	E980.4
80:08 toxoids NEC	978.8	E858.8	E948.8	E950.4	E962.0	E980.4
diphtheria	978.5	E858.8	E948.5	E950.4	E962.0	E980.4
and tetanus	978.9	E858.8	E948.9	E950.4	E962.0	E980.4
with pertussis component	978.6	E858.8	E948.6	E950.4	E962.0	E980.4
tetanus	978.4	E858.8	E948.4	E950.4	E962.0	E980.4
and diphtheria	978.9	E858.8	E948.9	E950.4	E962.0	E980.4
with pertussis component	978.6	E858.8	E948.6	E950.4	E962.0	E980.4
80:12 vaccines	979.9	E858.8	E949.9	E950.4	E962.0	E980.4
bacterial NEC	978.8	E858.8	E948.8	E950.4	E962.0	E980.4
with	—	—	—	—	—	—
other bacterial components	978.9	E858.8	E948.9	E950.4	E962.0	E980.4
pertussis component	978.6	E858.8	E948.6	E950.4	E962.0	E980.4
viral and rickettsial components	979.7	E858.8	E949.7	E950.4	E962.0	E980.4
rickettsial NEC	979.6	E858.8	E949.6	E950.4	E962.0	E980.4
with	—	—	—	—	—	—
bacterial component	979.7	E858.8	E949.7	E950.4	E962.0	E980.4
pertussis component	978.6	E858.8	E948.6	E950.4	E962.0	E980.4
viral component	979.7	E858.8	E949.7	E950.4	E962.0	E980.4
viral NEC	979.6	E858.8	E949.6	E950.4	E962.0	E980.4
with	—	—	—	—	—	—
bacterial component	979.7	E858.8	E949.7	E950.4	E962.0	E980.4
pertussis component	978.6	E858.8	E948.6	E950.4	E962.0	E980.4
rickettsial component	979.7	E858.8	E949.7	E950.4	E962.0	E980.4
84:04.04 antibiotics (skin and mucous membrane)	976.0	E858.7	E946.0	E950.4	E962.0	E980.4
84:04.08 fungicides (skin and mucous membrane)	976.0	E858.7	E946.0	E950.4	E962.0	E980.4
84:04.12 scabicides and pediculicides (skin and mucous membrane)	976.0	E858.7	E946.0	E950.4	E962.0	E980.4

Substance	Poisoning	External Cause (E-Code): Accident	Therapeutic Use	Suicide Attempt	Assault	Undetermined
Drug *(Continued)*						
84:04.16 miscellaneous local anti-infectives (skin and mucous membrane)	976.0	E858.7	E946.0	E950.4	E962.0	E980.4
84:06 anti-inflammatory agents (skin and mucous membrane)	976.0	E858.7	E946.0	E950.4	E962.0	E980.4
84:08 antipruritics and local anesthetics	—	—	—	—	—	—
antipruritics	976.1	E858.7	E946.1	E950.4	E962.0	E980.4
local anesthetics	968.5	E855.2	E938.5	E950.4	E962.0	E980.4
84:12 astringents	976.2	E858.7	E946.2	E950.4	E962.0	E980.4
84:16 cell stimulants and proliferants	976.8	E858.7	E946.8	E950.4	E962.0	E980.4
84:20 detergents	976.2	E858.7	E946.2	E950.4	E962.0	E980.4
84:24 emollients, demulcents, and protectants	976.3	E858.7	E946.3	E950.4	E962.0	E980.4
84:28 keratolytic agents	976.4	E858.7	E946.4	E950.4	E962.0	E980.4
84:32 keratoplastic agents	976.4	E858.7	E946.4	E950.4	E962.0	E980.4
84:36 miscellaneous agents (skin and mucous membrane)	976.8	E858.7	E946.8	E950.4	E962.0	E980.4
86:00 spasmolytic agents	975.1	E858.6	E945.1	E950.4	E962.0	E980.4
antiasthmatics	975.7	E858.6	E945.7	E950.4	E962.0	E980.4
papaverine	972.5	E858.3	E942.5	E950.4	E962.0	E980.4
theophylline	974.1	E858.5	E944.1	E950.4	E962.0	E980.4
88:04 vitamin A	963.5	E858.1	E933.5	E950.4	E962.0	E980.4
88:08 vitamin B complex	963.5	E858.1	E933.5	E950.4	E962.0	E980.4
hematopoietic vitamin	964.1	E858.2	E934.1	E950.4	E962.0	E980.4
nicotinic acid derivatives	972.2	E858.3	E942.2	E950.4	E962.0	E980.4
88:12 vitamin C	963.5	E858.1	E933.5	E950.4	E962.0	E980.4
88:16 vitamin D	963.5	E858.1	E933.5	E950.4	E962.0	E980.4
88:20 vitamin E	963.5	E858.1	E933.5	E950.4	E962.0	E980.4
88:24 vitamin K activity	964.3	E858.2	E934.3	E950.4	E962.0	E980.4
88:28 multivitamin preparations	963.5	E858.1	E933.5	E950.4	E962.0	E980.4
92:00 unclassified therapeutic agents	977.8	E858.8	E947.8	E950.4	E962.0	E980.4
Duboisine	971.1	E855.4	E941.1	E950.4	E962.0	E980.4
Dulcolax	973.1	E858.4	E943.1	E950.4	E962.0	E980.4
Duponol (C) (EP)	976.2	E858.7	E946.2	E950.4	E962.0	E980.4
Durabolin	962.1	E858.0	E932.1	E950.4	E962.0	E980.4
Dyclone	968.5	E855.2	E938.5	E950.4	E962.0	E980.4
Dyclonine	968.5	E855.2	E938.5	E950.4	E962.0	E980.4
Dydrogesterone	962.2	E858.0	E932.2	E950.4	E962.0	E980.4
Dyes NEC	989.89	E866.8	—	E950.9	E962.1	E980.9
diagnostic agents	977.8	E858.8	E947.8	E950.4	E962.0	E980.4
pharmaceutical NEC	977.4	E858.8	E947.4	E950.4	E962.0	E980.4
Dyflos	971.0	E855.3	E941.0	E950.4	E962.0	E980.4
Dymelor	962.3	E858.0	E932.3	E950.4	E962.0	E980.4
Dynamite	989.89	E866.8	—	E950.9	E962.1	E980.9
fumes	987.8	E869.8	—	E952.8	E962.2	E982.8
Dyphylline	975.1	E858.6	E945.1	E950.4	E962.0	E980.4
Ear preparations	976.6	E858.7	E946.6	E950.4	E962.0	E980.4
Echothiopate, ecothiopate	971.0	E855.3	E941.0	E950.4	E962.0	E980.4
Ecstasy	969.7	E854.2	E939.7	E950.3	E962.0	E980.3
Ectylurea	967.8	E852.8	E937.8	E950.2	E962.0	E980.2
Edathamil disodium	963.8	E858.1	E933.8	E950.4	E962.0	E980.4
Edecrin	974.4	E858.5	E944.4	E950.4	E962.0	E980.4
Edetate, disodium (calcium)	963.8	E858.1	E933.8	E950.4	E962.0	E980.4
Edrophonium	971.0	E855.3	E941.0	E950.4	E962.0	E980.4
Elase	976.8	E858.7	E946.8	E950.4	E962.0	E980.4
Elaterium	973.1	E858.4	E943.1	E950.4	E962.0	E980.4
Elder	988.2	E865.4	—	E950.9	E962.1	E980.9
berry (unripe)	988.2	E865.3	—	E950.9	E962.1	E980.9
Electrolytes NEC	974.5	E858.5	E944.5	E950.4	E962.0	E980.4
Electrolytic agent NEC	974.5	E858.5	E944.5	E950.4	E962.0	E980.4
Embramine	963.0	E858.1	E933.0	E950.4	E962.0	E980.4
Emetics	973.6	E858.4	E943.6	E950.4	E962.0	E980.4
Emetine (hydrochloride)	961.5	E857	E931.5	E950.4	E962.0	E980.4
Emollients	976.3	E858.7	E946.3	E950.4	E962.0	E980.4
Emylcamate	969.5	E853.8	E939.5	E950.3	E962.0	E980.3
Encyprate	969.0	E854.0	E939.0	E950.3	E962.0	E980.3

Substance	Poisoning	External Cause (E-Code)				
		Accident	Therapeutic Use	Suicide Attempt	Assault	Undetermined
Endocaine	968.5	E855.2	E938.5	E950.4	E962.0	E980.4
Endrin	989.2	E863.0	—	E950.6	E962.1	E980.7
Enflurane	968.2	E855.1	E938.2	E950.4	E962.0	E980.4
Enovid	962.2	E858.0	E932.2	E950.4	E962.0	E980.4
ENT preparations (anti-infectives)	976.6	E858.7	E946.6	E950.4	E962.0	E980.4
Enzodase	963.4	E858.1	E933.4	E950.4	E962.0	E980.4
Enzymes NEC	963.4	E858.1	E933.4	E950.4	E962.0	E980.4
Epanutin	966.1	E855.0	E936.1	E950.4	E962.0	E980.4
Ephedra (tincture)	971.2	E855.5	E941.2	E950.4	E962.0	E980.4
Ephedrine	971.2	E855.5	E941.2	E950.4	E962.0	E980.4
Epiestriol	962.2	E858.0	E932.2	E950.4	E962.0	E980.4
Epilim - *see* Sodium valproate	—	—	—	—	—	—
Epinephrine	971.2	E855.5	E941.2	E950.4	E962.0	E980.4
Epsom salt	973.3	E858.4	E943.3	E950.4	E962.0	E980.4
Equanil	969.5	E853.8	E939.5	E950.3	E962.0	E980.3
Equisetum (diuretic)	974.4	E858.5	E944.4	E950.4	E962.0	E980.4
Ergometrine	975.0	E858.6	E945.0	E950.4	E962.0	E980.4
Ergonovine	975.0	E858.6	E945.0	E950.4	E962.0	E980.4
Ergot NEC	988.2	E865.4	—	E950.9	E962.1	E980.9
medicinal (alkaloids)	975.0	E858.6	E945.0	E950.4	E962.0	E980.4
Ergotamine (tartrate) (for migraine) NEC	972.9	E858.3	E942.9	E950.4	E962.0	E980.4
Ergotrate	975.0	E858.6	E945.0	E950.4	E962.0	E980.4
Erythrityl tetranitrate	972.4	E858.3	E942.4	E950.4	E962.0	E980.4
Erythrol tetranitrate	972.4	E858.3	E942.4	E950.4	E962.0	E980.4
Erythromycin	960.3	E856	E930.3	E950.4	E962.0	E980.4
ophthalmic preparation	976.5	E858.7	E946.5	E950.4	E962.0	E980.4
topical NEC	976.0	E858.7	E946.0	E950.4	E962.0	E980.4
Eserine	971.0	E855.3	E941.0	E950.4	E962.0	E980.4
Eskabarb	967.0	E851	E937.0	E950.1	E962.0	E980.1
Eskalith	969.8	E855.8	E939.8	E950.3	E962.0	E980.3
Estradiol (cypionate) (dipropionate) (valerate)	962.2	E858.0	E932.2	E950.4	E962.0	E980.4
Estriol	962.2	E858.0	E932.2	E950.4	E962.0	E980.4
Estrogens (with progestogens)	962.2	E858.0	E932.2	E950.4	E962.0	E980.4
Estrone	962.2	E858.0	E932.2	E950.4	E962.0	E980.4
Etafedrine	971.2	E855.5	E941.2	E950.4	E962.0	E980.4
Ethacrynate sodium	974.4	E858.5	E944.4	E950.4	E962.0	E980.4
Ethacrynic acid	974.4	E858.5	E944.4	E950.4	E962.0	E980.4
Ethambutol	961.8	E857	E931.8	E950.4	E962.0	E980.4
Ethamide	974.2	E858.5	E944.2	E950.4	E962.0	E980.4
Ethamivan	970.0	E854.3	E940.0	E950.4	E962.0	E980.4
Ethamsylate	964.5	E858.2	E934.5	E950.4	E962.0	E980.4
Ethanol	980.0	E860.1	—	E950.9	E962.1	E980.9
beverage	980.0	E860.0	—	E950.9	E962.1	E980.9
Ethchlorvynol	967.8	E852.8	E937.8	E950.2	E962.0	E980.2
Ethebenecid	974.7	E858.5	E944.7	E950.4	E962.0	E980.4
Ether(s) (diethyl) (ethyl) (vapor)	987.8	E869.8	—	E952.8	E962.2	E982.8
anesthetic	968.2	E855.1	E938.2	E950.4	E962.0	E980.4
petroleum - *see* Ligroin solvent	982.8	E862.4	—	E950.9	E962.1	E980.9
Ethidine chloride (vapor)	987.8	E869.8	—	E952.8	E962.2	E982.8
liquid (solvent)	982.3	E862.4	—	E950.9	E962.1	E980.9
Ethinamate	967.8	E852.8	E937.8	E950.2	E962.0	E980.2
Ethinylestradiol	962.2	E858.0	E932.2	E950.4	E962.0	E980.4
Ethionamide	961.8	E857	E931.8	E950.4	E962.0	E980.4
Ethisterone	962.2	E858.0	E932.2	E950.4	E962.0	E980.4
Ethobral	967.0	E851	E937.0	E950.1	E962.0	E980.1
Ethocaine (infiltration) (topical)	968.5	E855.2	E938.5	E950.4	E962.0	E980.4
nerve block (peripheral) (plexus)	968.6	E855.2	E938.6	E950.4	E962.0	E980.4
spinal	968.7	E855.2	E938.7	E950.4	E962.0	E980.4
Ethoheptazine (citrate)	965.7	E850.7	E935.7	E950.0	E962.0	E980.0
Ethopropazine	966.4	E855.0	E936.4	E950.4	E962.0	E980.4
Ethosuximide	966.2	E855.0	E936.2	E950.4	E962.0	E980.4
Ethotoin	966.1	E855.0	E936.1	E950.4	E962.0	E980.4

Substance	Poisoning	External Cause (E-Code)				
		Accident	Therapeutic Use	Suicide Attempt	Assault	Undetermined
Ethoxazene	961.9	E857	E931.9	E950.4	E962.0	E980.4
Ethoxzolamide	974.2	E858.5	E944.2	E950.4	E962.0	E980.4
Ethyl	—	—	—	—	—	—
acetate (vapor)	982.8	E862.4	—	E950.9	E962.1	E980.9
alcohol	980.0	E860.1	—	E950.9	E962.1	E980.9
beverage	980.0	E860.0	—	E950.9	E962.1	E980.9
aldehyde (vapor)	987.8	E869.8	—	E952.8	E962.2	E982.8
liquid	989.89	E866.8	—	E950.9	E962.1	E980.9
aminobenzoate	968.5	E855.2	E938.5	E950.4	E962.0	E980.4
biscoumacetate	964.2	E858.2	E934.2	E950.4	E962.0	E980.4
bromide (anesthetic)	968.2	E855.1	E938.2	E950.4	E962.0	E980.4
carbamate (antineoplastic)	963.1	E858.1	E933.1	E950.4	E962.0	E980.4
carbinol	980.3	E860.4	—	E950.9	E962.1	E980.9
chaulmoograte	961.8	E857	E931.8	E950.4	E962.0	E980.4
chloride (vapor)	987.8	E869.8	—	E952.8	E962.2	E982.8
anesthetic (local)	968.5	E855.2	E938.5	E950.4	E962.0	E980.4
inhaled	968.2	E855.1	E938.2	E950.4	E962.0	E980.4
solvent	982.3	E862.4	—	E950.9	E962.1	E980.9
estranol	962.1	E858.0	E932.1	E950.4	E962.0	E980.4
ether - *see* Ether(s)	—	—	—	—	—	—
formate (solvent) NEC	982.8	E862.4	—	E950.9	E962.1	E980.9
iodoacetate	987.5	E869.3	—	E952.8	E962.2	E982.8
lactate (solvent) NEC	982.8	E862.4	—	E950.9	E962.1	E980.9
methylcarbinol	980.8	E860.8	—	E950.9	E962.1	E980.9
morphine	965.09	E850.2	E935.2	E950.0	E962.0	E980.0
Ethylene (gas)	987.1	E869.8	—	E952.8	E962.2	E982.8
anesthetic (general)	968.2	E855.1	E938.2	E950.4	E962.0	E980.4
chlorohydrin (vapor)	982.3	E862.4	—	E950.9	E962.1	E980.9
dichloride (vapor)	982.3	E862.4	—	E950.9	E962.1	E980.9
glycol(s) (any) (vapor)	982.8	E862.4	—	E950.9	E962.1	E980.9
Ethylidene	—	—	—	—	—	—
chloride NEC	982.3	E862.4	—	E950.9	E962.1	E980.9
diethyl ether	982.8	E862.4	—	E950.9	E962.1	E980.9
Ethynodiol	962.2	E858.0	E932.2	E950.4	E962.0	E980.4
Etidocaine	968.9	E855.2	E938.9	E950.4	E962.0	E980.4
infiltration (subcutaneous)	968.5	E855.2	E938.5	E950.4	E962.0	E980.4
nerve (peripheral) (plexus)	968.6	E855.2	E938.6	E950.4	E962.0	E980.4
Etilfen	967.0	E851	E937.0	E950.1	E962.0	E980.1
Etomide	965.7	E850.7	E935.7	E950.0	E962.0	E980.0
Etorphine	965.09	E850.2	E935.2	E950.0	E962.0	E980.0
Etoval	967.0	E851	E937.0	E950.1	E962.0	E980.1
Etryptamine	969.0	E854.0	E939.0	E950.3	E962.0	E980.3
Eucaine	968.5	E855.2	E938.5	E950.4	E962.0	E980.4
Eucalyptus (oil) NEC	975.5	E858.6	E945.5	E950.4	E962.0	E980.4
Eucatropine	971.1	E855.4	E941.1	E950.4	E962.0	E980.4
Eucodal	965.09	E850.2	E935.2	E950.0	E962.0	E980.0
Euneryl	967.0	E851	E937.0	E950.1	E962.0	E980.1
Euphthalmine	971.1	E855.4	E941.1	E950.4	E962.0	E980.4
Eurax	976.0	E858.7	E946.0	E950.4	E962.0	E980.4
Euresol	976.4	E858.7	E946.4	E950.4	E962.0	E980.4
Euthroid	962.7	E858.0	E932.7	E950.4	E962.0	E980.4
Evans blue	977.8	E858.8	E947.8	E950.4	E962.0	E980.4
Evipal	967.0	E851	E937.0	E950.1	E962.0	E980.1
sodium	968.3	E855.1	E938.3	E950.4	E962.0	E980.4
Evipan	967.0	E851	E937.0	E950.1	E962.0	E980.1
sodium	968.3	E855.1	E938.3	E950.4	E962.0	E980.4
Exalgin	965.4	E850.4	E935.4	E950.0	E962.0	E980.0
Excipients, pharmaceutical	977.4	E858.8	E947.4	E950.4	E962.0	E980.4
Exhaust gas - *see* Carbon, monoxide	—	—	—	—	—	—
Ex-Lax (phenolphthalein)	973.1	E858.4	E943.1	E950.4	E962.0	E980.4
Expectorants	975.5	E858.6	E945.5	E950.4	E962.0	E980.4

◀ New ⟸ Revised

Substance	Poisoning	External Cause (E-Code)				
		Accident	Therapeutic Use	Suicide Attempt	Assault	Undetermined
External medications (skin) (mucous membrane)	976.9	E858.7	E946.9	E950.4	E962.0	E980.4
dental agent	976.7	E858.7	E946.7	E950.4	E962.0	E980.4
ENT agent	976.6	E858.7	E946.6	E950.4	E962.0	E980.4
ophthalmic preparation	976.5	E858.7	E946.5	E950.4	E962.0	E980.4
specified NEC	976.8	E858.7	E946.8	E950.4	E962.0	E980.4
Eye agents (anti-infective)	976.5	E858.7	E946.5	E950.4	E962.0	E980.4
Factor IX complex (human)	964.5	E858.2	E934.5	E950.4	E962.0	E980.4
Fecal softeners	973.2	E858.4	E943.2	E950.4	E962.0	E980.4
Fenbutrazate	977.0	E858.8	E947.0	E950.4	E962.0	E980.4
Fencamfamin	970.8	E854.3	E940.8	E950.4	E962.0	E980.4
Fenfluramine	977.0	E858.8	E947.0	E950.4	E962.0	E980.4
Fenoprofen	965.61	E850.6	E935.6	E950.0	E962.0	E980.0
Fentanyl	965.09	E850.2	E935.2	E950.0	E962.0	E980.0
Fentazin	969.1	E853.0	E939.1	E930.3	E962.0	E980.3
Fenticlor, fentichlor	976.0	E858.7	E946.0	E950.4	E962.0	E980.4
Fer de lance (bite) (venom)	989.5	E905.0	—	E950.9	E962.1	E980.9
Ferric - *see* Iron	—	—	—	—	—	—
Ferrocholinate	964.0	E858.2	E934.0	E950.4	E962.0	E980.4
Ferrous fumerate, gluconate, lactate, salt NEC, sulfate (medicinal)	964.0	E858.2	E934.0	E950.4	E962.0	E980.4
Ferrum - *see* Iron	—	—	—	—	—	—
Fertilizers NEC	989.89	E866.5	—	E950.9	E962.1	E980.4
with herbicide mixture	989.4	E863.5	—	E950.6	E962.1	E980.7
Fibrinogen (human)	964.7	E858.2	E934.7	E950.4	E962.0	E980.4
Fibrinolysin	964.4	E858.2	E934.4	E950.4	E962.0	E980.4
Fibrinolysis-affecting agents	964.4	E858.2	E934.4	E950.4	E962.0	E980.4
Filix mas	961.6	E857	E931.6	E950.4	E962.0	E980.4
Fiorinal	965.1	E850.3	E935.3	E950.0	E962.0	E980.0
Fire damp	987.1	E869.8	—	E952.8	E962.2	E982.8
Fish, nonbacterial or noxious	988.0	E865.2	—	E950.9	E962.1	E980.9
shell	988.0	E865.1	—	E950.9	E962.1	E980.9
Flagyl	961.5	E857	E931.5	E950.4	E962.0	E980.4
Flavoxate	975.1	E858.6	E945.1	E950.4	E962.0	E980.4
Flaxedil	975.2	E858.6	E945.2	E950.4	E962.0	E980.4
Flaxseed (medicinal)	976.3	E858.7	E946.3	E950.4	E962.0	E980.4
Florantyrone	973.4	E858.4	E943.4	E950.4	E962.0	E980.4
Floraquin	961.3	E857	E931.3	E950.4	E962.0	E980.4
Florinef	962.0	E858.0	E932.0	E950.4	E962.0	E980.4
ENT agent	976.6	E858.7	E946.6	E950.4	E962.0	E980.4
ophthalmic preparation	976.5	E858.7	E946.5	E950.4	E962.0	E980.4
topical NEC	976.0	E858.7	E946.0	E950.4	E962.0	E980.4
Flowers of sulfur	976.4	E858.7	E946.4	E950.4	E962.0	E980.4
Floxuridine	963.1	E858.1	E933.1	E950.4	E962.0	E980.4
Flucytosine	961.9	E857	E931.9	E950.4	E962.0	E980.4
Fludrocortisone	962.0	E858.0	E932.0	E950.4	E962.0	E980.4
ENT agent	976.6	E858.7	E946.6	E950.4	E962.0	E980.4
ophthalmic preparation	976.5	E858.7	E946.5	E950.4	E962.0	E980.4
topical NEC	976.0	E858.7	E946.0	E950.4	E962.0	E980.4
Flumethasone	976.0	E858.7	E946.0	E950.4	E962.0	E980.4
Flumethiazide	974.3	E858.5	E944.3	E950.4	E962.0	E980.4
Flumidin	961.7	E857	E931.7	E950.4	E962.0	E980.4
Flunitrazepam	969.4	E853.2	E939.4	E950.3	E962.0	E980.3
Fluocinolone	976.0	E858.7	E946.0	E950.4	E962.0	E980.4
Fluocortolone	962.0	E858.0	E932.0	E950.4	E962.0	E980.4
Fluohydrocortisone	962.0	E858.0	E932.0	E950.4	E962.0	E980.4
ENT agent	976.6	E858.7	E946.6	E950.4	E962.0	E980.4
ophthalmic preparation	976.5	E858.7	E946.5	E950.4	E962.0	E980.4
topical NEC	976.0	E858.7	E946.0	E950.4	E962.0	E980.4
Fluonid	976.0	E858.7	E946.0	E950.4	E962.0	E980.4
Fluopromazine	969.1	E853.0	E939.1	E950.3	E962.0	E980.3
Fluoracetate	989.4	E863.7	—	E950.6	E962.1	E980.7
Fluorescein (sodium)	977.8	E858.8	E947.8	E950.4	E962.0	E980.4

Substance	Poisoning	External Cause (E-Code) Accident	Therapeutic Use	Suicide Attempt	Assault	Undetermined
Fluoride(s) (pesticides) (sodium) NEC	989.4	E863.4	—	E950.6	E962.1	E980.7
hydrogen - *see* Hydrofluoric acid	—	—	—	—	—	—
medicinal	976.7	E858.7	E946.7	E950.4	E962.0	E980.4
not pesticide NEC	983.9	E864.4	—	E950.7	E962.1	E980.6
stannous	976.7	E858.7	E946.7	E950.4	E962.0	E980.4
Fluorinated corticosteroids	962.0	E858.0	E932.0	E950.4	E962.0	E980.4
Fluorine (compounds) (gas)	987.8	E869.8	—	E952.8	E962.2	E982.8
salt - *see* Fluoride(s)	—	—	—	—	—	—
Fluoristan	976.7	E858.7	E946.7	E950.4	E962.0	E980.4
Fluoroacetate	989.4	E863.7	—	E950.6	E962.1	E980.7
Fluorodeoxyuridine	963.1	E858.1	E933.1	E950.4	E962.0	E980.4
Fluorometholone (topical) NEC	976.0	E858.7	E946.0	E950.4	E962.0	E980.4
ophthalmic preparation	976.5	E858.7	E946.5	E950.4	E962.0	E980.4
Fluorouracil	963.1	E858.1	E933.1	E950.4	E962.0	E980.4
Fluothane	968.1	E855.1	E938.1	E950.4	E962.0	E980.4
Fluoxetine hydrochloride	969.0	E854.0	E939.0	E950.3	E962.0	E980.3
Fluoxymesterone	962.1	E858.0	E932.1	E950.4	E962.0	E980.4
Fluphenazine	969.1	E853.0	E939.1	E950.3	E962.0	E980.3
Fluprednisolone	962.0	E858.0	E932.0	E950.4	E962.0	E980.4
Flurandrenolide	976.0	E858.7	E946.0	E950.4	E962.0	E980.4
Flurazepam (hydrochloride)	969.4	E853.2	E939.4	E950.3	E962.0	E980.3
Flurbiprofen	965.61	E850.6	E935.6	E950.0	E962.0	E980.0
Flurobate	976.0	E858.7	E946.0	E950.4	E962.0	E980.4
Flurothyl	969.8	E855.8	E939.8	E950.3	E962.0	E980.3
Fluroxene	968.2	E855.1	E938.2	E950.4	E962.0	E980.4
Folacin	964.1	E858.2	E934.1	E950.4	E962.0	E980.4
Folic acid	964.1	E858.2	E934.1	E950.4	E962.0	E980.4
Follicle stimulating hormone	962.4	E858.0	E932.4	E950.4	E962.0	E980.4
Food, foodstuffs, nonbacterial or noxious	988.9	E865.9	—	E950.9	E962.1	E980.9
berries, seeds	988.2	E865.3	—	E950.9	E962.1	E980.9
fish	988.0	E865.2	—	E950.9	E962.1	E980.9
mushrooms	988.1	E865.5	—	E950.9	E962.1	E980.9
plants	988.2	E865.9	—	E950.9	E962.1	E980.9
specified type NEC	988.2	E865.4	—	E950.9	E962.1	E980.9
shellfish	988.0	E865.1	—	E950.9	E962.1	E980.9
specified NEC	988.8	E865.8	—	E950.9	E962.1	E980.9
Fool's parsley	988.2	E865.4	—	E950.9	E962.1	E980.9
Formaldehyde (solution)	989.89	E861.4	—	E950.9	E962.1	E980.9
fungicide	989.4	E863.6	—	E950.6	E962.1	E980.7
gas or vapor	987.8	E869.8	—	E952.8	E962.2	E982.8
Formalin	989.89	E861.4	—	E950.9	E962.1	E980.9
fungicide	989.4	E863.6	—	E950.6	E962.1	E980.7
vapor	987.8	E869.8	—	E952.8	E962.2	E982.8
Formic acid	983.1	E864.1	—	E950.7	E962.1	E980.6
vapor	987.8	E869.8	—	E952.8	E962.2	E982.8
Fowler's solution	985.1	E866.3	—	E950.8	E962.1	E980.8
Foxglove	988.2	E865.4	—	E950.9	E962.1	E980.9
Fox green	977.8	E858.8	E947.8	E950.4	E962.0	E980.4
Framycetin	960.8	E856	E930.8	E950.4	E962.0	E980.4
Frangula (extract)	973.1	E858.4	E943.1	E950.4	E962.0	E980.4
Frei antigen	977.8	E858.8	E947.8	E950.4	E962.0	E980.4
Freons	987.4	E869.2	—	E952.8	E962.2	E982.8
Fructose	974.5	E858.5	E944.5	E950.4	E962.0	E980.4
Frusemide	974.4	E858.5	E944.4	E950.4	E962.0	E980.4
FSH	962.4	E858.0	E932.4	E950.4	E962.0	E980.4
Fuel	—	—	—	—	—	—
automobile	981	E862.1	—	E950.9	E962.1	E980.9
exhaust gas, not in transit	986	E868.2	—	E952.0	E962.2	E982.0
vapor NEC	987.1	E869.8	—	E952.8	E962.2	E982.8
gas (domestic use) - *see also* Carbon, monoxide, fuel	—	—	—	—	—	—
utility	987.1	E868.1	—	E951.8	E962.2	E981.8
incomplete combustion of - *see* Carbon, monoxide, fuel, utility	—	—	—	—	—	—

Substance	Poisoning	External Cause (E-Code) Accident	Therapeutic Use	Suicide Attempt	Assault	Undetermined
Fuel *(Continued)*						
gas *(Continued)*						
utility *(Continued)*						
in mobile container	987.0	E868.0	—	E951.1	E962.2	E981.1
piped (natural)	987.1	E867	—	E951.0	E962.2	E981.0
industrial, incomplete combustion	986	E868.3	—	E952.1	E962.2	E982.1
Fugillin	960.8	E856	E930.8	E950.4	E962.0	E980.4
Fulminate of mercury	985.0	E866.1	—	E950.9	E962.1	E980.9
Fulvicin	960.1	E856	E930.1	E950.4	E962.0	E980.4
Fumadil	960.8	E856	E930.8	E950.4	E962.0	E980.4
Fumagillin	960.8	E856	E930.8	E950.4	E962.0	E980.4
Fumes (from)	987.9	E869.9	—	E952.9	E962.2	E982.9
carbon monoxide - *see* Carbon, monoxide	—	—	—	—	—	—
charcoal (domestic use)	986	E868.3	—	E952.1	E962.2	E982.1
chloroform - *see* Chloroform						
coke (in domestic stoves, fireplaces)	986	E868.3	—	E952.1	E962.2	E982.1
corrosive NEC	987.8	E869.8	—	E952.8	E962.2	E982.8
ether - *see* Ether(s)						
freons	987.4	E869.2	—	E952.8	E962.2	E982.8
hydrocarbons	987.1	E869.8	—	E952.8	E962.2	E982.8
petroleum (liquefied)	987.0	E868.0	—	E951.1	E962.2	E981.1
distributed through pipes (pure or mixed with air)	987.0	E867	—	E951.0	E962.2	E981.0
lead - *see* Lead	—	—	—	—	—	—
metals - *see* specified metal	—	—	—	—	—	—
nitrogen dioxide	987.2	E869.0	—	E952.8	E962.2	E982.8
pesticides - *see* Pesticides	—	—	—	—	—	—
petroleum (liquefied)	987.0	E868.0	—	E951.1	E962.2	E981.1
distributed through pipes (pure or mixed with air)	987.0	E867	—	E951.0	E962.2	E981.0
polyester	987.8	E869.8	—	E952.8	E962.2	E982.8
specified source, other (*see also* substance specified)	987.8	E869.8	—	E952.8	E962.2	E982.8
sulfur dioxide	987.3	E869.1	—	E952.8	E962.2	E982.8
Fumigants	989.4	E863.8	—	E950.6	E962.1	E980.7
Fungi, noxious, used as food	988.1	E865.5	—	E950.9	E962.1	E980.9
Fungicides (*see also* Antifungals)	989.4	E863.6	—	E950.6	E962.1	E980.7
Fungizone	960.1	E856	E930.1	E950.4	E962.0	E980.4
topical	976.0	E858.7	E946.0	E950.4	E962.0	E980.4
Furacin	976.0	E858.7	E946.0	E950.4	E962.0	E980.4
Furadantin	961.9	E857	E931.9	E950.4	E962.0	E980.4
Furazolidone	961.9	E857	E931.9	E950.4	E962.0	E980.4
Furnace (coal burning) (domestic), gas from	986	E868.3	—	E952.1	E962.2	E982.1
industrial	986	E868.8	—	E952.1	E962.2	E982.1
Furniture polish	989.89	E861.2	—	E950.9	E962.1	E980.9
Furosemide	974.4	E858.5	E944.4	E950.4	E962.0	E980.4
Furoxone	961.9	E857	E931.9	E950.4	E962.0	E980.4
Fusel oil (amyl) (butyl) (propyl)	980.3	E860.4	—	E950.9	E962.1	E980.9
Fusidic acid	960.8	E856	E930.8	E950.4	E962.0	E980.4
Gallamine	975.2	E858.6	E945.2	E950.4	E962.0	E980.4
Gallotannic acid	976.2	E858.7	E946.2	E950.4	E962.0	E980.4
Gamboge	973.1	E858.4	E943.1	E950.4	E962.0	E980.4
Gamimune	964.6	E858.2	E934.6	E950.4	E962.0	E980.4
Gamma-benzene hexachloride (vapor)	989.2	E863.0	—	E950.6	E962.1	E980.7
Gamma globulin	964.6	E858.2	E934.6	E950.4	E962.0	E980.4
Gamma hydroxy butyrate (GHB)	968.4	E855.1	E938.4	E950.4	E962.0	E980.4
Gamulin	964.6	E858.2	E934.6	E950.4	E962.0	E980.4
Ganglionic blocking agents	972.3	E858.3	E942.3	E950.4	E962.0	E980.4
Ganja	969.6	E854.1	E939.6	E950.3	E962.0	E980.3
Garamycin	960.8	E856	E930.8	E950.4	E962.0	E980.4
ophthalmic preparation	976.5	E858.7	E946.5	E950.4	E962.0	E980.4
topical NEC	976.0	E858.7	E946.0	E950.4	E962.0	E980.4
Gardenal	967.0	E851	E937.0	E950.1	E962.0	E980.1
Gardepanyl	967.0	E851	E937.0	E950.1	E962.0	E980.1

		External Cause (E-Code)				
Substance	**Poisoning**	**Accident**	**Therapeutic Use**	**Suicide Attempt**	**Assault**	**Undetermined**
Gas	987.9	E869.9	—	E952.9	E962.2	E982.9
acetylene	987.1	E868.1	—	E951.8	E962.2	E981.8
incomplete combustion of - *see* Carbon, monoxide, fuel, utility	—	—	—	—	—	—
air contaminants, source or type not specified	987.9	E869.9	—	E952.9	E962.2	E982.9
anesthetic (general) NEC	968.2	E855.1	E938.2	E950.4	E962.0	E980.4
blast furnace	986	E868.8	—	E952.1	E962.2	E982.1
butane - *see* Butane	—	—	—	—	—	—
carbon monoxide - *see* Carbon, monoxide, chlorine	987.6	E869.8	—	E952.8	E962.2	E982.8
coal - *see* Carbon, monoxide, coal	—	—	—	—	—	—
cyanide	987.7	E869.8	—	E952.8	E962.2	E982.8
dicyanogen	987.8	E869.8	—	E952.8	E962.2	E982.8
domestic - *see* Gas, utility	—	—	—	—	—	—
exhaust - *see* Carbon, monoxide, exhaust gas	—	—	—	—	—	—
from wood- or coal-burning stove or fireplace	986	E868.3	—	E952.1	E962.2	E982.1
fuel (domestic use) - *see also* Carbon, monoxide, fuel	—	—	—	—	—	—
industrial use	986	E868.8	—	E952.1	E962.2	E982.1
utility	987.1	E868.1	—	E951.8	E962.2	E981.8
incomplete combustion of - *see* Carbon, monoxide, fuel, utility	—	—	—	—	—	—
in mobile container	987.0	E868.0	—	E951.1	E962.2	E981.1
piped (natural)	987.1	E867	—	E951.0	E962.2	E981.0
garage	986	E868.2	—	E952.0	E962.2	E982.0
hydrocarbon NEC	987.1	E869.8	—	E952.8	E962.2	E982.8
incomplete combustion of - *see* Carbon, monoxide, fuel, utility	—	—	—	—	—	—
liquefied (mobile container)	987.0	E868.0	—	E951.1	E962.2	E981.1
piped	987.0	E867	—	E951.0	E962.2	E981.0
hydrocyanic acid	987.7	E869.8	—	E952.8	E962.2	E982.8
illuminating - *see* Gas, utility	—	—	—	—	—	—
incomplete combustion, any - *see* Carbon, monoxide	—	—	—	—	—	—
kiln	986	E868.8	—	E952.1	E962.2	E982.1
lacrimogenic	987.5	E869.3	—	E952.8	E962.2	E982.8
marsh	987.1	E869.8	—	E952.8	E962.2	E982.8
motor exhaust, not in transit	986	E868.8	—	E952.1	E962.2	E982.1
mustard - *see* Mustard, gas	—	—	—	—	—	—
natural	987.1	E867	—	E951.0	E962.2	E981.0
nerve (war)	987.9	E869.9	—	E952.9	E962.2	E982.9
oils	981	E862.1	—	E950.9	E962.1	E980.9
petroleum (liquefied) (distributed in mobile containers)	987.0	E868.0	—	E951.1	E962.2	E981.1
piped (pure or mixed with air)	987.0	E867	—	E951.1	E962.2	E981.1
piped (manufactured) (natural) NEC	987.1	E867	—	E951.0	E962.2	E981.0
producer	986	E868.8	—	E952.1	E962.2	E982.1
propane - *see* Propane	—	—	—	—	—	—
refrigerant (freon)	987.4	E869.2	—	E952.8	E962.2	E982.8
not freon	987.9	E869.9	—	E952.9	E962.2	E982.9
sewer	987.8	E869.8	—	E952.8	E962.2	E982.8
specified source NEC (*see also* substance specified)	987.8	E869.8	—	E952.8	E962.2	E982.8
stove - *see* Gas, utility	—	—	—	—	—	—
tear	987.5	E869.3	—	E952.8	E962.2	E982.8
utility (for cooking, heating, or lighting) (piped) NEC	987.1	E868.1	—	E951.8	E962.2	E981.8
incomplete combustion of - *see* Carbon, monoxide, fuel, utilty	—	—	—	—	—	—
in mobile container	987.0	E868.0	—	E951.1	E962.2	E981.1
piped (natural)	987.1	E867	—	E951.0	E962.2	E981.0
water	987.1	E868.1	—	E951.8	E962.2	E981.8
incomplete combustion of - *see* Carbon, monoxide, fuel, utility	—	—	—	—	—	—
Gaseous substance - *see* Gas	—	—	—	—	—	—
Gasoline, gasolene	981	E862.1	—	E950.9	E962.1	E980.9
vapor	987.1	E869.8	—	E952.8	E962.2	E982.8
Gastric enzymes	973.4	E858.4	E943.4	E950.4	E962.0	E980.4
Gastrografin	977.8	E858.8	E947.8	E950.4	E962.0	E980.4
Gastrointestinal agents	973.9	E858.4	E943.9	E950.4	E962.0	E980.4
specified NEC	973.8	E858.4	E943.8	E950.4	E962.0	E980.4
Gaultheria procumbens	988.2	E865.4	—	E950.9	E962.1	E980.9

◀ New ⟸ Revised

Substance	Poisoning	External Cause (E-Code)				
		Accident	Therapeutic Use	Suicide Attempt	Assault	Undetermined
Gelatin (intravenous)	964.8	E858.2	E934.8	E950.4	E962.0	E980.4
absorbable (sponge)	964.5	E858.2	E934.5	E950.4	E962.0	E980.4
Gelfilm	976.8	E858.7	E946.8	E950.4	E962.0	E980.4
Gelfoam	964.5	E858.2	E934.5	E950.4	E962.0	E980.4
Gelsemine	970.8	E854.3	E940.8	E950.4	E962.0	E980.4
Gelsemium (sempervirens)	988.2	E865.4	—	E950.9	E962.1	E980.9
Gemonil	967.0	E851	E937.0	E950.1	E962.0	E980.1
Gentamicin	960.8	E856	E930.8	E950.4	E962.0	E980.4
ophthalmic preparation	976.5	E858.7	E946.5	E950.4	E962.0	E980.4
topical NEC	976.0	E858.7	E946.0	E950.4	E962.0	E980.4
Gentian violet	976.0	E858.7	E946.0	E950.4	E962.0	E980.4
Gexane	976.0	E858.7	E946.0	E950.4	E962.0	E980.4
Gila monster (venom)	989.5	E905.0	—	E950.9	E962.1	E980.9
Ginger, Jamaica	989.89	E866.8	—	E950.9	E962.1	E980.9
Gitalin	972.1	E858.3	E942.1	E950.4	E962.0	E980.4
Gitoxin	972.1	E858.3	E942.1	E950.4	E962.0	E980.4
Glandular extract (medicinal) NEC	977.9	E858.9	E947.9	E950.5	E962.0	E980.5
Glaucarubin	961.5	E857	E931.5	E950.4	E962.0	E980.4
Globin zinc insulin	962.3	E858.0	E932.3	E950.4	E962.0	E980.4
Glucagon	962.3	E858.0	E932.3	E950.4	E962.0	E980.4
Glucochloral	967.1	E852.0	E937.1	E950.2	E962.0	E980.2
Glucocorticoids	962.0	E858.0	E932.0	E950.4	E962.0	E980.4
Glucose	974.5	E858.5	E944.5	E950.4	E962.0	E980.4
oxidase reagent	977.8	E858.8	E947.8	E950.4	E962.0	E980.4
Glucosulfone sodium	961.8	E857	E931.8	E950.4	E962.0	E980.4
Glue(s)	989.89	E866.6	—	E950.9	E962.1	E980.9
Glutamic acid (hydrochloride)	973.4	E858.4	E943.4	E950.4	E962.0	E980.4
Glutaraldehyde	989.89	E861.4	—	E950.9	E962.1	E980.9
Glutathione	963.8	E858.1	E933.8	E950.4	E962.0	E980.4
Glutethimide (group)	967.5	E852.4	E937.5	E950.2	E962.0	E980.2
Glycerin (lotion)	976.3	E858.7	E946.3	E950.4	E962.0	E980.4
Glycerol (topical)	976.3	E858.7	E946.3	E950.4	E962.0	E980.4
Glyceryl	—	—	—	—	—	—
guaiacolate	975.5	E858.6	E945.5	E950.4	E962.0	E980.4
triacetate (topical)	976.0	E858.7	E946.0	E950.4	E962.0	E980.4
trinitrate	972.4	E858.3	E942.4	E950.4	E962.0	E980.4
Glycine	974.5	E858.5	E944.5	E950.4	E962.0	E980.4
Glycobiarsol	961.1	E857	E931.1	E950.4	E962.0	E980.4
Glycols (ether)	982.8	E862.4	—	E950.9	E962.1	E980.9
Glycopyrrolate	971.1	E855.4	E941.1	E950.4	E962.0	E980.4
Glymidine	962.3	E858.0	E932.3	E950.4	E962.0	E980.4
Gold (compounds) (salts)	965.69	E850.6	E935.6	E950.0	E962.0	E980.0
Golden sulfide of antimony	985.4	E866.2	—	E950.9	E962.1	E980.9
Goldylocks	988.2	E865.4	—	E950.9	E962.1	E980.9
Gonadal tissue extract	962.9	E858.0	E932.9	E950.4	E962.0	E980.4
female	962.2	E858.0	E932.2	E950.4	E962.0	E980.4
male	962.1	E858.0	E932.1	E950.4	E962.0	E980.4
Gonadotropin	962.4	E858.0	E932.4	E950.4	E962.0	E980.4
Grain alcohol	980.0	E860.1	—	E950.9	E962.1	E980.9
beverage	980.0	E860.0	—	E950.9	E962.1	E980.9
Gramicidin	960.8	E856	E930.8	E950.4	E962.0	E980.4
Gratiola officinalis	988.2	E865.4	—	E950.9	E962.1	E980.9
Grease	989.89	E866.8	—	E950.9	E962.1	E980.9
Green hellebore	988.2	E865.4	—	E950.9	E962.1	E980.9
Green soap	976.2	E858.7	E946.2	E950.4	E962.0	E980.4
Grifulvin	960.1	E856	E930.1	E950.4	E962.0	E980.4
Griseofulvin	960.1	E856	E930.1	E950.4	E962.0	E980.4
Growth hormone	962.4	E858.0	E932.4	E950.4	E962.0	E980.4
Guaiacol	975.5	E858.6	E945.5	E950.4	E962.0	E980.4
Giuaiac reagent	977.8	E858.8	E947.8	E950.4	E962.0	E980.4
Guaifenesin	975.5	E858.6	E945.5	E950.4	E962.0	E980.4
Guaiphenesin	975.5	E858.6	E945.5	E950.4	E962.0	E980.4

Substance	Poisoning	External Cause (E-Code)				
		Accident	Therapeutic Use	Suicide Attempt	Assault	Undetermined
Guanatol	961.4	E857	E931.4	E950.4	E962.0	E980.4
Guanethidine	972.6	E858.3	E942.6	E950.4	E962.0	E980.4
Guano	989.89	E866.5	—	E950.9	E962.1	E980.9
Guanochlor	972.6	E858.3	E942.6	E950.4	E962.0	E980.4
Guanoctine	972.6	E858.3	E942.6	E950.4	E962.0	E980.4
Guanoxan	972.6	E858.3	E942.6	E950.4	E962.0	E980.4
Hair treatment agent NEC	976.4	E858.7	E946.4	E950.4	E962.0	E980.4
Halcinonide	976.0	E858.7	E946.0	E950.4	E962.0	E980.4
Halethazole	976.0	E858.7	E946.0	E950.4	E962.0	E980.4
Hallucinogens	969.6	E854.1	E939.6	E950.3	E962.0	E980.3
Haloperidol	969.2	E853.1	E939.2	E950.3	E962.0	E980.3
Haloprogin	976.0	E858.7	E946.0	E950.4	E962.0	E980.4
Halotex	976.0	E858.7	E946.0	E950.4	E962.0	E980.4
Halothane	968.1	E855.1	E938.1	E950.4	E962.0	E980.4
Halquinols	976.0	E858.7	E946.0	E950.4	E962.0	E980.4
Harmonyl	972.6	E858.3	E942.6	E950.4	E962.0	E980.4
Hartmann's solution	974.5	E858.5	E944.5	E950.4	E962.0	E980.4
Hashish	969.6	E854.1	E939.6	E950.3	E962.0	E980.3
Hawaiian wood rose seeds	969.6	E854.1	E939.6	E950.3	E962.0	E980.3
Headache cures, drugs, powders NEC	977.9	E858.9	E947.9	E950.5	E962.0	E980.9
Heavenly Blue (morning glory)	969.6	E854.1	E939.6	E950.3	E962.0	E980.3
Heavy metal antagonists	963.8	E858.1	E933.8	E950.4	E962.0	E980.4
anti-infectives	961.2	E857	E931.2	E950.4	E962.0	E980.4
Hedaquinium	976.0	E858.7	E946.0	E950.4	E962.0	E980.4
Hedge hyssop	988.2	E865.4	—	E950.9	E962.1	E980.9
Heet	976.8	E858.7	E946.8	E950.4	E962.0	E980.4
Helenin	961.6	E857	E931.6	E950.4	E962.0	E980.4
Hellebore (black) (green) (white)	988.2	E865.4	—	E950.9	E962.1	E980.9
Hemlock	988.2	E865.4	—	E950.9	E962.1	E980.9
Hemostatics	964.5	E858.2	E934.5	E950.4	E962.0	E980.4
capillary active drugs	972.8	E858.3	E942.8	E950.4	E962.0	E980.4
Henbane	988.2	E865.4	—	E950.9	E962.1	E980.9
Heparin (sodium)	964.2	E858.2	E934.2	E950.4	E962.0	E980.4
Heptabarbital, heptabarbitone	967.0	E851	E937.0	E950.1	E962.0	E980.1
Heptachlor	989.2	E863.0	—	E950.6	E962.1	E980.7
Heptalgin	965.09	E850.2	E935.2	E950.0	E962.0	E980.0
Herbicides	989.4	E863.5	—	E950.6	E962.1	E980.7
Heroin	965.01	E850.0	E935.0	E950.0	E962.0	E980.0
Herplex	976.5	E858.7	E946.5	E950.4	E962.0	E980.4
HES	964.8	E858.2	E934.8	E950.4	E962.0	E980.4
Hetastarch	964.8	E858.2	E934.8	E950.4	E962.0	E980.7
Hexachlorocyclohexane	989.2	E863.0	—	E950.6	E962.1	E980.7
Hexachlorophene	976.2	E858.7	E946.2	E950.4	E962.0	E980.4
Hexadimethrine (bromide)	964.5	E858.2	E934.5	E950.4	E962.0	E980.4
Hexafluorenium	975.2	E858.6	E945.2	E950.4	E962.0	E980.4
Hexa-germ	976.2	E858.7	E946.2	E950.4	E962.0	E980.4
Hexahydrophenol	980.8	E860.8	—	E950.9	E962.1	E980.9
Hexalen	980.8	E860.8	—	E950.9	E962.1	E980.9
Hexamethonium	972.3	E858.3	E942.3	E950.4	E962.0	E980.4
Hexamethylenamine	961.9	E857	E931.9	E950.4	E962.0	E980.4
Hexamine	961.9	E857	E931.9	E950.4	E962.0	E980.4
Hexanone	982.8	E862.4	—	E950.9	E962.1	E980.9
Hexapropymate	967.8	E852.8	E937.8	E950.2	E962.0	E980.2
Hexestrol	962.2	E858.0	E932.2	E950.4	E962.0	E980.4
Hexethal (sodium)	967.0	E851	E937.0	E950.1	E962.0	E980.1
Hexetidine	976.0	E858.7	E946.0	E950.4	E962.0	E980.4
Hexobarbital, hexobarbitone	967.0	E851	E937.0	E950.1	E962.0	E980.1
sodium (anesthetic)	968.3	E855.1	E938.3	E950.4	E962.0	E980.4
soluble	968.3	E855.1	E938.3	E950.4	E962.0	E980.4
Hexocyclium	971.1	E855.4	E941.1	E950.4	E962.0	E980.4
Hexoestrol	962.2	E858.0	E932.2	E950.4	E962.0	E980.4
Hexone	982.8	E862.4	—	E950.9	E962.1	E980.9

◀ New ⟸ Revised

Substance	Poisoning	External Cause (E-Code)				
		Accident	Therapeutic Use	Suicide Attempt	Assault	Undetermined
Hexylcaine	968.5	E855.2	E938.5	E950.4	E962.0	E980.4
Hexylresorcinol	961.6	E857	E931.6	E950.4	E962.0	E980.4
Hinkle's pills	973.1	E858.4	E943.1	E950.4	E962.0	E980.4
Histalog	977.8	E858.8	E947.8	E950.4	E962.0	E980.4
Histamine (phosphate)	972.5	E858.3	E942.5	E950.4	E962.0	E980.4
Histoplasmin	977.8	E858.8	E947.8	E950.4	E962.0	E980.4
Holly berries	988.2	E865.3	—	E950.9	E962.1	E980.9
Homatropine	971.1	E855.4	E941.1	E950.4	E962.0	E980.4
Homo-tet	964.6	E858.2	E934.6	E950.4	E962.0	E980.4
Hormones (synthetic substitute) NEC	962.9	E858.0	E932.9	E950.4	E962.0	E980.4
adrenal cortical steroids	962.0	E858.0	E932.0	E950.4	E962.0	E980.4
antidiabetic agents	962.3	E858.0	E932.3	E950.4	E962.0	E980.4
follicle stimulating	962.4	E858.0	E932.4	E950.4	E962.0	E980.4
gonadotropic	962.4	E858.0	E932.4	E950.4	E962.0	E980.4
growth	962.4	E858.0	E932.4	E950.4	E962.0	E980.4
ovarian (substitutes)	962.2	E858.0	E932.2	E950.4	E962.0	E980.4
parathyroid (derivatives)	962.6	E858.0	E932.6	E950.4	E962.0	E980.4
pituitary (posterior)	962.5	E858.0	E932.5	E950.4	E962.0	E980.4
anterior	962.4	E858.0	E932.4	E950.4	E962.0	E980.4
thyroid (derivative)	962.7	E858.0	E932.7	E950.4	E962.0	E980.4
Hornet (sting)	989.5	E905.3	—	E950.9	E962.1	E980.9
Horticulture agent NEC	989.4	E863.9	—	E950.6	E962.1	E980.7
Hyaluronidase	963.4	E858.1	E933.4	E950.4	E962.0	E980.4
Hyazyme	963.4	E858.1	E933.4	E950.4	E962.0	E980.4
Hycodan	965.09	E850.2	E935.2	E950.0	E962.0	E980.0
Hydantoin derivatives	966.1	E855.0	E936.1	E950.4	E962.0	E980.4
Hydeltra	962.0	E858.0	E932.0	E950.4	E962.0	E980.4
Hydergine	971.3	E855.6	E941.3	E950.4	E962.0	E980.4
Hydrabamine penicillin	960.0	E856	E930.0	E950.4	E962.0	E980.4
Hydralazine, hydrallazine	972.6	E858.3	E942.6	E950.4	E962.0	E980.4
Hydrargaphen	976.0	E858.7	E946.0	E950.4	E962.0	E980.4
Hydrazine	983.9	E864.3	—	E950.7	E962.1	E980.6
Hydriodic acid	975.5	E858.6	E945.5	E950.4	E962.0	E980.4
Hydrocarbon gas	987.1	E869.8	—	E952.8	E962.2	E982.8
incomplete combustion of - *see* Carbon, monoxide, fuel, utility	—	—	—	—	—	—
liquefied (mobile container)	987.0	E868.0	—	E951.1	E962.2	E981.1
piped (natural)	987.0	E867	—	E951.0	E962.2	E981.0
Hydrochloric acid (liquid)	983.1	E864.1	—	E950.7	E962.1	E980.6
medicinal	973.4	E858.4	E943.4	E950.4	E962.0	E980.4
vapor	987.8	E869.8	—	E952.8	E962.2	E982.8
Hydrochlorothiazide	974.3	E858.5	E944.3	E950.4	E962.0	E980.4
Hydrocodone	965.09	E850.2	E935.2	E950.0	E962.0	E980.0
Hydrocortisone	962.0	E858.0	E932.0	E950.4	E962.0	E980.4
ENT agent	976.6	E858.7	E946.6	E950.4	E962.0	E980.4
ophthalmic preparation	976.5	E858.7	E946.5	E950.4	E962.0	E980.4
topical NEC	976.0	E858.7	E946.0	E950.4	E962.0	E980.4
Hydrocortone	962.0	E858.0	E932.0	E950.4	E962.0	E980.4
ENT agent	976.6	E858.7	E946.6	E950.4	E962.0	E980.4
ophthalmic preparation	976.5	E858.7	E946.5	E950.4	E962.0	E980.4
topical NEC	976.0	E858.7	E946.0	E950.4	E962.0	E980.4
Hydrocyanic acid - *see* Cyanide(s)	—	—	—	—	—	—
Hydroflumethiazide	974.3	E858.5	E944.3	E950.4	E962.0	E980.4
Hydrofluoric acid (liquid)	983.1	E864.1	—	E950.7	E962.1	E980.6
vapor	987.8	E869.8	—	E952.8	E962.2	E982.8
Hydrogen	987.8	E869.8	—	E952.8	E962.2	E982.8
arsenide	985.1	E866.3	—	E950.8	E962.1	E980.8
arseniurated	985.1	E866.3	—	E950.8	E962.1	E980.8
cyanide (salts)	989.0	E866.8	—	E950.9	E962.1	E980.9
gas	987.7	E869.8	—	E952.8	E962.2	E982.8
fluoride (liquid)	983.1	E864.1	—	E950.7	E962.1	E980.6
vapor	987.8	E869.8	—	E952.8	E962.2	E982.8
peroxide (solution)	976.6	E858.7	E946.6	E950.4	E962.0	E980.4

Substance	Poisoning	External Cause (E-Code) Accident	Therapeutic Use	Suicide Attempt	Assault	Undetermined
Hydrogen *(Continued)*						
phosphorated	987.8	E869.8	—	E952.8	E962.2	E982.8
sulfide (gas)	987.8	E869.8	—	E952.8	E962.2	E982.8
arseniurated	985.1	E866.3	—	E950.8	E962.1	E980.8
sulfureted	987.8	E869.8	—	E952.8	E962.2	E982.8
Hydromorphinol	965.09	E850.2	E935.2	E950.0	E962.0	E980.0
Hydromorphinone	965.09	E850.2	E935.2	E950.0	E962.0	E980.0
Hydromorphone	965.09	E850.2	E935.2	E950.0	E962.0	E980.0
Hydromox	974.3	E858.5	E944.3	E950.4	E962.0	E980.4
Hydrophilic lotion	976.3	E858.7	E946.3	E950.4	E962.0	E980.4
Hydroquinone	983.0	E864.0	—	E950.7	E962.1	E980.6
vapor	987.8	E869.8	—	E952.8	E962.2	E982.8
Hydrosulfuric acid (gas)	987.8	E869.8	—	E952.8	E962.2	E982.8
Hydrous wool fat (lotion)	976.3	E858.7	E946.3	E950.4	E962.0	E980.4
Hydroxide, caustic	983.2	E864.2	—	E950.7	E962.1	E980.6
Hydroxocobalamin	964.1	E858.2	E934.1	E950.4	E962.0	E980.4
Hydroxyamphetamine	971.2	E855.5	E941.2	E950.4	E962.0	E980.4
Hydroxychloroquine	961.4	E857	E931.4	E950.4	E962.0	E980.4
Hydroxydihydrocodeinone	965.09	E850.2	E935.2	E950.0	E962.0	E980.0
Hydroxyethyl starch	964.8	E858.2	E934.8	E950.4	E962.0	E980.4
Hydroxyphenamate	969.5	E853.8	E939.5	E950.3	E962.0	E980.3
Hydroxyphenylbutazone	965.5	E850.5	E935.5	E950.0	E962.0	E980.0
Hydroxyprogesterone	962.2	E858.0	E932.2	E950.4	E962.0	E980.4
Hydroxyquinoline derivatives	961.3	E857	E931.3	E950.4	E962.0	E980.4
Hydroxystilbamidine	961.5	E857	E931.5	E950.4	E962.0	E980.4
Hydroxyurea	963.1	E858.1	E933.1	E950.4	E962.0	E980.4
Hydroxyzine	969.5	E853.8	E939.5	E950.3	E962.0	E980.3
Hyoscine (hydrobromide)	971.1	E855.4	E941.1	E950.4	E962.0	E980.4
Hyoscyamine	971.1	E855.4	E941.1	E950.4	E962.0	E980.4
Hyoscyamus (albus) (niger)	988.2	E865.4	—	E950.9	E962.1	E980.9
Hypaque	977.8	E858.8	E947.8	E950.4	E962.0	E980.4
Hypertussis	964.6	E858.2	E934.6	E950.4	E962.0	E980.4
Hypnotics NEC	967.9	E852.9	E937.9	E950.2	E962.0	E980.2
Hypochlorites - *see* Sodium, hypochlorite	—	—	—	—	—	—
Hypotensive agents NEC	972.6	E858.3	E942.6	E950.4	E962.0	E980.4
Ibufenac	965.69	E850.6	E935.6	E950.0	E962.0	E980.0
Ibuprofen	965.61	E850.6	E935.6	E950.0	E962.0	E980.0
ICG	977.8	E858.8	E947.8	E950.4	E962.0	E980.4
Ichthammol	976.4	E858.7	E946.4	E950.4	E962.0	E980.4
Ichthyol	976.4	E858.7	E946.4	E950.4	E962.0	E980.4
Idoxuridine	976.5	E858.7	E946.5	E950.4	E962.0	E980.4
IDU	976.5	E858.7	E946.5	E950.4	E962.0	E980.4
Iletin	962.3	E858.0	E932.3	E950.4	E962.0	E980.4
Ilex	988.2	E865.4	—	E950.9	E962.1	E980.9
Illuminating gas - *see* Gas, utility	—	—	—	—	—	—
Ilopan	963.5	E858.1	E933.5	E950.4	E962.0	E980.4
Ilotycin	960.3	E856	E930.3	E950.4	E962.0	E980.4
ophthalmic preparation	976.5	E858.7	E946.5	E950.4	E962.0	E980.4
topical NEC	976.0	E858.7	E946.0	E950.4	E962.0	E980.4
Imipramine	969.0	E854.0	E939.0	E950.3	E962.0	E980.3
Immu-G	964.6	E858.2	E934.6	E950.4	E962.0	E980.4
Immuglobin	964.6	E858.2	E934.6	E950.4	E962.0	E980.4
Immune serum globulin	964.6	E858.2	E934.6	E950.4	E962.0	E980.4
Immunosuppressive agents	963.1	E858.1	E933.1	E950.4	E962.0	E980.4
Immu-tetanus	964.6	E858.2	E934.6	E950.4	E962.0	E980.4
Indandione (derivatives)	964.2	E858.2	E934.2	E950.4	E962.0	E980.4
Inderal	972.0	E858.3	E942.0	E950.4	E962.0	E980.4
Indian	—	—	—	—	—	—
hemp	969.6	E854.1	E939.6	E950.3	E962.0	E980.3
tobacco	988.2	E865.4	—	E950.9	E962.1	E980.9
Indigo carmine	977.8	E858.8	E947.8	E950.4	E962.0	E980.4
Indocin	965.69	E850.6	E935.6	E950.0	E962.0	E980.0

Substance	Poisoning	External Cause (E-Code) Accident	Therapeutic Use	Suicide Attempt	Assault	Undetermined
Indocyanine green	977.8	E858.8	E947.8	E950.4	E962.0	E980.4
Indomethacin	965.69	E850.6	E935.6	E950.0	E962.0	E980.0
Industrial	—	—	—	—	—	—
alcohol	980.9	E860.9	—	E950.9	E962.1	E980.9
fumes	987.8	E869.8	—	E952.8	E962.2	E982.8
solvents (fumes) (vapors)	982.8	E862.9	—	E950.9	E962.1	E980.9
Influenza vaccine	979.6	E858.8	E949.6	E950.4	E962.0	E982.8
Ingested substances NEC	989.9	E866.9	—	E950.9	E962.1	E980.9
INH (isoniazid)	961.8	E857	E931.8	E950.4	E962.0	E980.4
Inhalation, gas (noxious) - *see* Gas	—	—	—	—	—	—
Ink	989.89	E866.8	—	E950.9	E962.1	E980.9
Innovar	967.6	E852.5	E937.6	E950.2	E962.0	E980.2
Inositol niacinate	972.2	E858.3	E942.2	E950.4	E962.0	E980.4
Inproquone	963.1	E858.1	E933.1	E950.4	E962.0	E980.4
Insect (sting), venomous	989.5	E905.5	—	E950.9	E962.1	E980.9
Insecticides (*see also* Pesticides)	989.4	E863.4	—	E950.6	E962.1	E980.7
chlorinated	989.2	E863.0	—	E950.6	E962.1	E980.7
mixtures	989.4	E863.3	—	E950.6	E962.1	E980.7
organochlorine (compounds)	989.2	E863.0	—	E950.6	E962.1	E980.7
organophosphorus (compounds)	989.3	E863.1	—	E950.6	E962.1	E980.7
Insular tissue extract	962.3	E858.0	E932.3	E950.4	E962.0	E980.4
Insulin (amorphous) (globin) (isophane) (Lente) (NPH) (Protamine) (Semilente) (Ultralente) (zinc)	962.3	E858.0	E932.3	E950.4	E962.0	E980.4
Intranarcon	968.3	E855.1	E938.3	E950.4	E962.0	E980.4
Inulin	977.8	E858.8	E947.8	E950.4	E962.0	E980.4
Invert sugar	974.5	E858.5	E944.5	E950.4	E962.0	E980.4
Inza - see Naproxen	—	—	—	—	—	—
Iodide NEC (*see also* Iodine)	976.0	E858.7	E946.0	E950.4	E962.0	E980.4
mercury (ointment)	976.0	E858.7	E946.0	E950.4	E962.0	E980.4
methylate	976.0	E858.7	E946.0	E950.4	E962.0	E980.4
potassium (expectorant) NEC	975.5	E858.6	E945.5	E950.4	E962.0	E980.4
Iodinated glycerol	975.5	E858.6	E945.5	E950.4	E962.0	E980.4
Iodine (antiseptic, external) (tincture) NEC	976.0	E858.7	E946.0	E950.4	E962.0	E980.4
diagnostic	977.8	E858.8	E947.8	E950.4	E962.0	E980.4
for thyroid conditions (antithyroid)	962.8	E858.0	E932.8	E950.4	E962.0	E980.4
vapor	987.8	E869.8	—	E952.8	E962.2	E982.8
Iodized oil	977.8	E858.8	E947.8	E950.4	E962.0	E980.4
Iodobismitol	961.2	E857	E931.2	E950.4	E962.0	E980.4
Iodochlorhydroxyquin	961.3	E857	E931.3	E950.4	E962.0	E980.4
topical	976.0	E858.7	E946.0	E950.4	E962.0	E980.4
Iodoform	976.0	E858.7	E946.0	E950.4	E962.0	E980.4
Iodopanoic acid	977.8	E858.8	E947.8	E950.4	E962.0	E980.4
Iodophthalein	977.8	E858.8	E947.8	E950.4	E962.0	E980.4
Ion exchange resins	974.5	E858.5	E944.5	E950.4	E962.0	E980.4
Iopanoic acid	977.8	E858.8	E947.8	E950.4	E962.0	E980.4
Iophendylate	977.8	E858.8	E947.8	E950.4	E962.0	E980.4
Iothiouracil	962.8	E858.0	E932.8	E950.4	E962.0	E980.4
Ipecac	973.6	E858.4	E943.6	E950.4	E962.0	E980.4
Ipecacuanha	973.6	E858.4	E943.6	E950.4	E962.0	E980.4
Ipodate	977.8	E858.8	E947.8	E950.4	E962.0	E980.4
Ipral	967.0	E851	E937.0	E950.1	E962.0	E980.1
Ipratropium	975.1	E858.6	E945.1	E950.4	E962.0	E980.4
Iproniazid	969.0	E854.0	E939.0	E950.3	E962.0	E980.3
Iron (compounds) (medicinal) (preparations)	964.0	E858.2	E934.0	E950.4	E962.0	E980.4
dextran	964.0	E858.2	E934.0	E950.4	E962.0	E980.4
nonmedicinal (dust) (fumes) NEC	985.8	E866.4	—	E950.9	E962.1	E980.9
Irritant drug	977.9	E858.9	E947.9	E950.5	E962.0	E980.5
Ismelin	972.6	E858.3	E942.6	E950.4	E962.0	E980.4
Isoamyl nitrite	972.4	E858.3	E942.4	E950.4	E962.0	E980.4
Isobutyl acetate	982.8	E862.4	—	E950.9	E962.1	E980.9
Isocarboxazid	969.0	E854.0	E939.0	E950.3	E962.0	E980.3
Isoephedrine	971.2	E855.5	E941.2	E950.4	E962.0	E980.4

Substance	Poisoning	External Cause (E-Code)				
		Accident	Therapeutic Use	Suicide Attempt	Assault	Undetermined
Isoetharine	971.2	E855.5	E941.2	E950.4	E962.0	E980.4
Isofluorophate	971.0	E855.3	E941.0	E950.4	E962.0	E980.4
Isoniazid (INH)	961.8	E857	E931.8	E950.4	E962.0	E980.4
Isopentaquine	961.4	E857	E931.4	E950.4	E962.0	E980.4
Isophane insulin	962.3	E858.0	E932.3	E950.4	E962.0	E980.4
Isopregnenone	962.2	E858.0	E932.2	E950.4	E962.0	E980.4
Isoprenaline	971.2	E855.5	E941.2	E950.4	E962.0	E980.4
Isopropamide	971.1	E855.4	E941.1	E950.4	E962.0	E980.4
Isopropanol	980.2	E860.3	—	E950.9	E962.1	E980.9
topical (germicide)	976.0	E858.7	E946.0	E950.4	E962.0	E980.4
Isopropyl	—	—	—	—	—	—
acetate	982.8	E862.4	—	E950.9	E962.1	E980.9
alcohol	980.2	E860.3	—	E950.9	E962.1	E980.9
topical (germicide)	976.0	E858.7	E946.0	E950.4	E962.0	E980.4
ether	982.8	E862.4	—	E950.9	E962.1	E980.9
Isoproterenol	971.2	E855.5	E941.2	E950.4	E962.0	E980.4
Isosorbide dinitrate	972.4	E858.3	E942.4	E950.4	E962.0	E980.4
Isothipendyl	963.0	E858.1	E933.0	E950.4	E962.0	E980.4
Isoxazolyl penicillin	960.0	E856	E930.0	E950.4	E962.0	E980.4
Isoxsuprine hydrochloride	972.5	E858.3	E942.5	E950.4	E962.0	E980.4
I-thyroxine sodium	962.7	E858.0	E932.7	E950.4	E962.0	E980.4
Jaborandi (pilocarpus) (extract)	971.0	E855.3	E941.0	E950.4	E962.0	E980.4
Jalap	973.1	E858.4	E943.1	E950.4	E962.0	E980.4
Jamaica	—	—	—	—	—	—
dogwood (bark)	965.7	E850.7	E935.7	E950.0	E962.0	E980.0
ginger	989.89	E866.8	—	E950.9	E962.1	E980.9
Jatropha	988.2	E865.4	—	E950.9	E962.1	E980.9
curcas	988.2	E865.3	—	E950.9	E962.1	E980.9
Jectofer	964.0	E858.2	E934.0	E950.4	E962.0	E980.4
Jellyfish (sting)	989.5	E905.6	—	E950.9	E962.1	E980.9
Jequirity (bean)	988.2	E865.3	—	E950.9	E962.1	E980.9
Jimson weed	988.2	E865.4	—	E950.9	E962.1	E980.9
seeds	988.2	E865.3	—	E950.9	E962.1	E980.9
Juniper tar (oil) (ointment)	976.4	E858.7	E946.4	E950.4	E962.0	E980.4
Kallikrein	972.5	E858.3	E942.5	E950.4	E962.0	E980.4
Kanamycin	960.6	E856	E930.6	E950.4	E962.0	E980.4
Kantrex	960.6	E856	E930.6	E950.4	E962.0	E980.4
Kaolin	973.5	E858.4	E943.5	E950.4	E962.0	E980.4
Karaya (gum)	973.3	E858.4	E943.3	E950.4	E962.0	E980.4
Kemithal	968.3	E855.1	E938.3	E950.4	E962.0	E980.4
Kenacort	962.0	E858.0	E932.0	E950.4	E962.0	E980.4
Keratolytics	976.4	E858.7	E946.4	E950.4	E962.0	E980.4
Keratoplastics	976.4	E858.7	E946.4	E950.4	E962.0	E980.4
Kerosene, kerosine (fuel) (solvent) NEC	981	E862.1	—	E950.9	E962.1	E980.9
insecticide	981	E863.4	—	E950.6	E962.1	E980.7
vapor	987.1	E869.8	—	E952.8	E962.2	E982.8
Ketamine	968.3	E855.1	E938.3	E950.4	E962.0	E980.4
Ketobemidone	965.09	E850.2	E935.2	E950.0	E962.0	E980.0
Ketols	982.8	E862.4	—	E950.9	E962.1	E980.9
Ketone oils	982.8	E862.4	—	E950.9	E962.1	E980.9
Ketoprofen	965.61	E850.6	E935.6	E950.0	E962.0	E980.0
Kiln gas or vapor (carbon monoxide)	986	E868.8	—	E952.1	E962.2	E982.1
Konsyl	973.3	E858.4	E943.3	E950.4	E962.0	E980.4
Kosam seed	988.2	E865.3	—	E950.9	E962.1	E980.9
Krait (venom)	989.5	E905.0	—	E950.9	E962.1	E980.9
Kwell (insecticide)	989.2	E863.0	—	E950.6	E962.1	E980.7
anti-infective (topical)	976.0	E858.7	E946.0	E950.4	E962.0	E980.4
Laburnum (flowers) (seeds)	988.2	E865.3	—	E950.9	E962.1	E980.9
leaves	988.2	E865.4	—	E950.9	E962.1	E980.9
Lacquers	989.89	E861.6	—	E950.9	E962.1	E980.9
Lacrimogenic gas	987.5	E869.3	—	E952.8	E962.2	E982.8
Lactic acid	983.1	E864.1	—	E950.7	E962.1	E980.6

Substance	Poisoning	Accident	Therapeutic Use	Suicide Attempt	Assault	Undetermined
		External Cause (E-Code)				
Lactobacillus acidophilus	973.5	E858.4	E943.5	E950.4	E962.0	E980.4
Lactoflavin	963.5	E858.1	E933.5	E950.4	E962.0	E980.4
Lactuca (virosa) (extract)	967.8	E852.8	E937.8	E950.2	E962.0	E980.2
Lactucarium	967.8	E852.8	E937.8	E950.2	E962.0	E980.2
Laevulose	974.5	E858.5	E944.5	E950.4	E962.0	E980.4
Lanatoside (C)	972.1	E858.3	E942.1	E950.4	E962.0	E980.4
Lanolin (lotion)	976.3	E858.7	E946.3	E950.4	E962.0	E980.4
Largactil	969.1	E853.0	E939.1	E950.3	E962.0	E980.3
Larkspur	988.2	E865.3	—	E950.9	E962.1	E980.9
Laroxyl	969.0	E854.0	E939.0	E950.3	E962.0	E980.3
Lasix	974.4	E858.5	E944.4	E950.4	E962.0	E980.4
Latex	989.82	E866.8	—	E950.9	E962.1	E980.9
Lathyrus (seed)	988.2	E865.3	—	E950.9	E962.1	E980.9
Laudanum	965.09	E850.2	E935.2	E950.0	E962.0	E980.0
Laudexium	975.2	E858.6	E945.2	E950.4	E962.0	E980.4
Laurel, black or cherry	988.2	E865.4	—	E950.9	E962.1	E980.9
Laurolinium	976.0	E858.7	E946.0	E950.4	E962.0	E980.4
Lauryl sulfoacetate	976.2	E858.7	E946.2	E950.4	E962.0	E980.4
Laxatives NEC	973.3	E858.4	E943.3	E950.4	E962.0	E980.4
emollient	973.2	E858.4	E943.2	E950.4	E962.0	E980.4
L-dopa	966.4	E855.0	E936.4	E950.4	E962.0	E980.4
L-Tryptophan - *see* amino acid	—	—	—	—	—	—
Lead (dust) (fumes) (vapor) NEC	984.9	E866.0	—	E950.9	E962.1	E980.9
acetate (dust)	984.1	E866.0	—	E950.9	E962.1	E980.9
anti-infectives	961.2	E857	E931.2	E950.4	E962.0	E980.4
antiknock compound (tetra-ethyl)	984.1	E862.1	—	E950.9	E962.1	E980.9
arsenate, arsenite (dust) (insecticide) (vapor)	985.1	E863.4	—	E950.8	E962.1	E980.8
herbicide	985.1	E863.5	—	E950.8	E962.1	E980.8
carbonate	984.0	E866.0	—	E950.9	E962.1	E980.9
paint	984.0	E861.5	—	E950.9	E962.1	E980.9
chromate	984.0	E866.0	—	E950.9	E962.1	E980.9
paint	984.0	E861.5	—	E950.9	E962.1	E980.9
dioxide	984.0	E866.0	—	E950.9	E962.1	E980.9
inorganic (compound)	984.0	E866.0	—	E950.9	E962.1	E980.9
paint	984.0	E861.5	—	E950.9	E962.1	E980.9
iodide	984.0	E866.0	—	E950.9	E962.1	E980.9
pigment (paint)	984.0	E861.5	—	E950.9	E962.1	E980.9
monoxide (dust)	984.0	E866.0	—	E950.9	E962.1	E980.9
paint	984.0	E861.5	—	E950.9	E962.1	E980.9
organic	984.1	E866.0	—	E950.9	E962.1	E980.9
oxide	984.0	E866.0	—	E950.9	E962.1	E980.9
paint	984.0	E861.5	—	E950.9	E962.1	E980.9
paint	984.0	E861.5	—	E950.9	E962.1	E980.9
salts	984.0	E866.0	—	E950.9	E962.1	E980.9
specified compound NEC	984.8	E866.0	—	E950.9	E962.1	E980.9
tetra-ethyl	984.1	E862.1	—	E950.9	E962.1	E980.9
Lebanese red	969.6	E854.1	E939.6	E950.3	E962.0	E980.3
Lente Iletin (insulin)	962.3	E858.0	E932.3	E950.4	E962.0	E980.4
Leptazol	970.0	E854.3	E940.0	E950.4	E962.0	E980.4
Leritine	965.09	E850.2	E935.2	E950.0	E962.0	E980.0
Letter	962.7	E858.0	E932.7	E950.4	E962.0	E980.4
Lettuce opium	967.8	E852.8	E937.8	E950.2	E962.0	E980.2
Leucovorin (factor)	964.1	E858.2	E934.1	E950.4	E962.0	E980.4
Leukeran	963.1	E858.1	E933.1	E950.4	E962.0	E980.4
Levalbuterol	975.7	E858.6	E945.7	E950.4	E962.0	E980.4
Levallorphan	970.1	E854.3	E940.1	E950.4	E962.0	E980.4
Levanil	967.8	E852.8	E937.8	E950.2	E962.0	E980.2
Levarterenol	971.2	E855.5	E941.2	E950.4	E962.0	E980.4
Levodopa	966.4	E855.0	E936.4	E950.4	E962.0	E980.4
Levo-dromoran	965.09	E850.2	E935.2	E950.0	E962.0	E980.0
Levoid	962.7	E858.0	E932.7	E950.4	E962.0	E980.4
Levo-iso-methadone	965.02	E850.1	E935.1	E950.0	E962.0	E980.0

Substance	Poisoning	External Cause (E-Code)				
		Accident	Therapeutic Use	Suicide Attempt	Assault	Undetermined
Levomepromazine	967.8	E852.8	E937.8	E950.2	E962.0	E980.2
Levoprome	967.8	E852.8	E937.8	E950.2	E962.0	E980.2
Levopropoxyphene	975.4	E858.6	E945.4	E950.4	E962.0	E980.4
Levorphan, levophanol	965.09	E850.2	E935.2	E950.0	E962.0	E980.0
Levothyroxine (sodium)	962.7	E858.0	E932.7	E950.4	E962.0	E980.4
Levsin	971.1	E855.4	E941.1	E950.4	E962.0	E980.4
Levulose	974.5	E858.5	E944.5	E950.4	E962.0	E980.4
Lewisite (gas)	985.1	E866.3	—	E950.8	E962.1	E980.8
Librium	969.4	E853.2	E939.4	E950.3	E962.0	E980.3
Lidex	976.0	E858.7	E946.0	E950.4	E962.0	E980.4
Lidocaine (infiltration) (topical)	968.5	E855.2	E938.5	E950.4	E962.0	E980.4
nerve block (peripheral) (plexus)	968.6	E855.2	E938.6	E950.4	E962.0	E980.4
spinal	968.7	E855.2	E938.7	E950.4	E962.0	E980.4
Lighter fluid	981	E862.1	—	E950.9	E962.1	E980.9
Lignocaine (infiltration) (topical)	968.5	E855.2	E938.5	E950.4	E962.0	E980.4
nerve block (peripheral) (plexus)	968.6	E855.2	E938.6	E950.4	E962.0	E980.4
spinal	968.7	E855.2	E938.7	E950.4	E962.0	E980.4
Ligroin(e) (solvent)	981	E862.0	—	E950.9	E962.1	E980.9
vapor	987.1	E869.8	—	E952.8	E962.2	E982.8
Ligustrum vulgare	988.2	E865.3	—	E950.9	E962.1	E980.9
Lily of the valley	988.2	E865.4	—	E950.9	E962.1	E980.9
Lime (chloride)	983.2	E864.2	—	E950.7	E962.1	E980.6
solution, sulferated	976.4	E858.7	E946.4	E950.4	E962.0	E980.4
Limonene	982.8	E862.4	—	E950.9	E962.1	E980.9
Lincomycin	960.8	E856	E930.8	E950.4	E962.0	E980.4
Lindane (insecticide) (vapor)	989.2	E863.0	—	E950.6	E962.1	E980.7
anti-infective (topical)	976.0	E858.7	E946.0	E950.4	E962.0	E980.4
Liniments NEC	976.9	E858.7	E946.9	E950.4	E962.0	E980.4
Linoleic acid	972.2	E858.3	E942.2	E950.4	E962.0	E980.4
Liothyronine	962.7	E858.0	E932.7	E950.4	E962.0	E980.4
Liotrix	962.7	E858.0	E932.7	E950.4	E962.0	E980.4
Lipancreatin	973.4	E858.4	E943.4	E950.4	E962.0	E980.4
Lipo-Lutin	962.2	E858.0	E932.2	E950.4	E962.0	E980.4
Lipotropic agents	977.1	E858.8	E947.1	E950.4	E962.0	E980.4
Liquefied petroleum gases	987.0	E868.0	—	E951.1	E962.2	E981.1
piped (pure or mixed with air)	987.0	E867	—	E951.0	E962.2	E981.0
Liquid petrolatum	973.2	E858.4	E943.2	E950.4	E962.0	E980.4
substance	989.9	E866.9	—	E950.9	E962.1	E980.9
specified NEC	989.89	E866.8	—	E950.9	E962.1	E980.9
Lirugen	979.4	E858.8	E949.4	E950.4	E962.0	E980.4
Lithane	969.8	E855.8	E939.8	E950.3	E962.0	E980.3
Lithium	985.8	E866.4	—	E950.9	E962.1	E980.9
carbonate	969.8	E855.8	E939.8	E950.3	E962.0	E980.3
Lithonate	969.8	E855.8	E939.8	E950.3	E962.0	E980.3
Liver (extract) (injection) (preparations)	964.1	E858.2	E934.1	E950.4	E962.0	E980.4
Lizard (bite) (venom)	989.5	E905.0	—	E950.9	E962.1	E980.9
LMD	964.8	E858.2	E934.8	E950.4	E962.0	E980.4
Lobelia	988.2	E865.4	—	E950.9	E962.1	E980.9
Lobeline	970.0	E854.3	E940.0	E950.4	E962.0	E980.4
Locorten	976.0	E858.7	E946.0	E950.4	E962.0	E980.4
Lolium temulentum	988.2	E865.3	—	E950.9	E962.1	E980.9
Lomotil	973.5	E858.4	E943.5	E950.4	E962.0	E980.4
Lomustine	963.1	E858.1	E933.1	E950.4	E962.0	E980.4
Lophophora williamsii	969.6	E854.1	E939.6	E950.3	E962.0	E980.3
Lorazepam	969.4	E853.2	E939.4	E950.3	E962.0	E980.3
Lotions NEC	976.9	E858.7	E946.9	E950.4	E962.0	E980.4
Lotronex	973.8	E858.4	E943.8	E950.4	E962.0	E980.4
Lotusate	967.0	E851	E937.0	E950.1	E962.0	E980.1
Lowila	976.2	E858.7	E946.2	E950.4	E962.0	E980.4
Loxapine	969.3	E853.8	E939.3	E950.3	E962.0	E980.3
Lozenges (throat)	976.6	E858.7	E946.6	E950.4	E962.0	E980.4

◀ New ⬅ Revised

Substance	Poisoning	External Cause (E-Code)				
		Accident	Therapeutic Use	Suicide Attempt	Assault	Undetermined
LSD (25)	969.6	E854.1	E939.6	E950.3	E962.0	E980.3
Lubricating oil NEC	981	E862.2	—	E950.9	E962.1	E980.9
Lucanthone	961.6	E857	E931.6	E950.4	E962.0	E980.4
Luminal	967.0	E851	E937.0	E950.1	E962.0	E980.1
Lung irritant (gas) NEC	987.9	E869.9	—	E952.9	E962.2	E982.9
Lutocylol	962.2	E858.0	E932.2	E950.4	E962.0	E980.4
Lutromone	962.2	E858.0	E932.2	E950.4	E962.0	E980.4
Lututrin	975.0	E858.6	E945.0	E950.4	E962.0	E980.4
Lye (concentrated)	983.2	E864.2	—	E950.7	E962.1	E980.6
Lygranum (skin test)	977.8	E858.8	E947.8	E950.4	E962.0	E980.4
Lymecycline	960.4	E856	E930.4	E950.4	E962.0	E980.4
Lymphogranuloma venereum antigen	977.8	E858.8	E947.8	E950.4	E962.0	E980.4
Lynestrenol	962.2	E858.0	E932.2	E950.4	E962.0	E980.4
Lyovac Sodium Edecrin	974.4	E858.5	E944.4	E950.4	E962.0	E980.4
Lypressin	962.5	E858.0	E932.5	E950.4	E962.0	E980.4
Lysergic acid (amide) (diethylamide)	969.6	E854.1	E939.6	E950.3	E962.0	E980.3
Lysergide	969.6	E854.1	E939.6	E950.3	E962.0	E980.3
Lysine vasopressin	962.5	E858.0	E932.5	E950.4	E962.0	E980.4
Lysol	983.0	E864.0	—	E950.7	E962.1	E980.6
Lytta (vitatta)	976.8	E858.7	E946.8	E950.4	E962.0	E980.4
Mace	987.5	E869.3	—	E952.8	E962.2	E982.8
Macrolides (antibiotics)	960.3	E856	E930.3	E950.4	E962.0	E980.4
Mafenide	976.0	E858.7	E946.0	E950.4	E962.0	E980.4
Magaldrate	973.0	E858.4	E943.0	E950.4	E962.0	E980.4
Magic mushroom	969.6	E854.1	E939.6	E950.3	E962.0	E980.3
Magnamycin	960.8	E856	E930.8	E950.4	E962.0	E980.4
Magnesia magma	973.0	E858.4	E943.0	E950.4	E962.0	E980.4
Magnesium (compounds) (fumes) NEC	985.8	E866.4	—	E950.9	E962.1	E980.9
antacid	973.0	E858.4	E943.0	E950.4	E962.0	E980.4
carbonate	973.0	E858.4	E943.0	E950.4	E962.0	E980.4
cathartic	973.3	E858.4	E943.3	E950.4	E962.0	E980.4
citrate	973.3	E858.4	E943.3	E950.4	E962.0	E980.4
hydroxide	973.0	E858.4	E943.0	E950.4	E962.0	E980.4
oxide	973.0	E858.4	E943.0	E950.4	E962.0	E980.4
sulfate (oral)	973.3	E858.4	E943.3	E950.4	E962.0	E980.4
intravenous	966.3	E855.0	E936.3	E950.4	E962.0	E980.4
trisilicate	973.0	E858.4	E943.0	E950.4	E962.0	E980.4
Malathion (insecticide)	989.3	E863.1	—	E950.6	E962.1	E980.7
Male fern (oleoresin)	961.6	E857	E931.6	E950.4	E962.0	E980.4
Mandelic acid	961.9	E857	E931.9	E950.4	E962.0	E980.4
Manganese compounds (fumes) NEC	985.2	E866.4	—	E950.9	E962.1	E980.9
Mannitol (diuretic) (medicinal) NEC	974.4	E858.5	E944.4	E950.4	E962.0	E980.4
hexanitrate	972.4	E858.3	E942.4	E950.4	E962.0	E980.4
mustard	963.1	E858.1	E933.1	E950.4	E962.0	E980.4
Mannomustine	963.1	E858.1	E933.1	E950.4	E962.0	E980.4
MAO inhibitors	969.0	E854.0	E939.0	E950.3	E962.0	E980.3
Mapharsen	961.1	E857	E931.1	E950.4	E962.0	E980.4
Marcaine	968.9	E855.2	E938.9	E950.4	E962.0	E980.4
infiltration (subcutaneous)	968.5	E855.2	E938.5	E950.4	E962.0	E980.4
nerve block (peripheral) (plexus)	968.6	E855.2	E938.6	E950.4	E962.0	E980.4
Marezine	963.0	E858.1	E933.0	E950.4	E962.0	E980.4
Marihuana, marijuana (derivatives)	969.6	E854.1	E939.6	E950.3	E962.0	E980.3
Marine animals or plants (sting)	989.5	E905.6	—	E950.9	E962.1	E980.9
Marplan	969.0	E854.0	E939.0	E950.3	E962.0	E980.3
Marsh gas	987.1	E869.8	—	E952.8	E962.2	E982.8
Marsilid	969.0	E854.0	E939.0	E950.3	E962.0	E980.3
Matulane	963.1	E858.1	E933.1	E950.4	E962.0	E980.4
Mazindol	977.0	E858.8	E947.0	E950.4	E962.0	E980.4
MDMA	969.7	E854.2	E939.7	E950.3	E962.0	E980.3
Meadow saffron	988.2	E865.3	—	E950.9	E962.1	E980.9
Measles vaccine	979.4	E858.8	E949.4	E950.4	E962.0	E980.4

Substance	Poisoning	External Cause (E-Code) Accident	Therapeutic Use	Suicide Attempt	Assault	Undetermined
Meat, noxious or nonbacterial	988.8	E865.0	—	E950.9	E962.1	E980.9
Mebanazine	969.0	E854.0	E939.0	E950.3	E962.0	E980.3
Mebaral	967.0	E851	E937.0	E950.1	E962.0	E980.1
Mebendazole	961.6	E857	E931.6	E950.4	E962.0	E980.4
Mebeverine	975.1	E858.6	E945.1	E950.4	E962.0	E980.4
Mebhydroline	963.0	E858.1	E933.0	E950.4	E962.0	E980.4
Mebrophenhydramine	963.0	E858.1	E933.0	E950.4	E962.0	E980.4
Mebutamate	969.5	E853.8	E939.5	E950.3	E962.0	E980.3
Mecamylamine (chloride)	972.3	E858.3	E942.3	E950.4	E962.0	E980.4
Mechlorethamine hydrochloride	963.1	E858.1	E933.1	E950.4	E962.0	E980.4
Meclizene (hydrochloride)	963.0	E858.1	E933.0	E950.4	E962.0	E980.4
Meclofenoxate	970.0	E854.3	E940.0	E950.4	E962.0	E980.4
Meclozine (hydrochloride)	963.0	E858.1	E933.0	E950.4	E962.0	E980.4
Medazepam	969.4	E853.2	E939.4	E950.3	E962.0	E980.3
Medicine, medicinal substance	977.9	E858.9	E947.9	E950.5	E962.0	E980.5
specified NEC	977.8	E858.8	E947.8	E950.4	E962.0	E980.4
Medinal	967.0	E851	E937.0	E950.1	E962.0	E980.1
Medomin	967.0	E851	E937.0	E950.1	E962.0	E980.1
Medroxyprogesterone	962.2	E858.0	E932.2	E950.4	E962.0	E980.4
Medrysone	976.5	E858.7	E946.5	E950.4	E962.0	E980.4
Mefenamic acid	965.7	E850.7	E935.7	E950.0	E962.0	E980.0
Megahallucinogen	969.6	E854.1	E939.6	E950.3	E962.0	E980.3
Megestrol	962.2	E858.0	E932.2	E950.4	E962.0	E980.4
Meglumine	977.8	E858.8	E947.8	E950.4	E962.0	E980.4
Meladinin	976.3	E858.7	E946.3	E950.4	E962.0	E980.4
Melanizing agents	976.3	E858.7	E946.3	E950.4	E962.0	E980.4
Melarsoprol	961.1	E857	E931.1	E950.4	E962.0	E980.4
Melia azedarach	988.2	E865.3	—	E950.9	E962.1	E980.9
Mellaril	969.1	E853.0	E939.1	E950.3	E962.0	E980.3
Meloxine	976.3	E858.7	E946.3	E950.4	E962.0	E980.4
Melphalan	963.1	E858.1	E933.1	E950.4	E962.0	E980.4
Menadiol sodium diphosphate	964.3	E858.2	E934.3	E950.4	E962.0	E980.4
Menadione (sodium bisulfite)	964.3	E858.2	E934.3	E950.4	E962.0	E980.4
Menaphthone	964.3	E858.2	E934.3	E950.4	E962.0	E980.4
Meningococcal vaccine	978.8	E858.8	E948.8	E950.4	E962.0	E980.4
Menningovax-C	978.8	E858.8	E948.8	E950.4	E962.0	E980.4
Menotropins	962.4	E858.0	E932.4	E950.4	E962.0	E980.4
Menthol NEC	976.1	E858.7	E946.1	E950.4	E962.0	E980.4
Mepacrine	961.3	E857	E931.3	E950.4	E962.0	E980.4
Meparfynol	967.8	E852.8	E937.8	E950.2	E962.0	E980.2
Mepazine	969.1	E853.0	E939.1	E950.3	E962.0	E980.3
Mepenzolate	971.1	E855.4	E941.1	E950.4	E962.0	E980.4
Meperidine	965.09	E850.2	E935.2	E950.0	E962.0	E980.0
Mephenamin(e)	966.4	E855.0	E936.4	E950.4	E962.0	E980.4
Mephenesin (carbamate)	968.0	E855.1	E938.0	E950.4	E962.0	E980.4
Mephenoxalone	969.5	E853.8	E939.5	E950.3	E962.0	E980.3
Mephentermine	971.2	E855.5	E941.2	E950.4	E962.0	E980.4
Mephenytoin	966.1	E855.0	E936.1	E950.4	E962.0	E980.4
Mephobarbital	967.0	E851	E937.0	E950.1	E962.0	E980.1
Mepiperphenidol	971.1	E855.4	E941.1	E950.4	E962.0	E980.4
Mepivacaine	968.9	E855.2	E938.9	E950.4	E962.0	E980.4
infiltration (subcutaneous)	968.5	E855.2	E938.5	E950.4	E962.0	E980.4
nerve block (peripheral) (plexus)	968.6	E855.2	E938.6	E950.4	E962.0	E980.4
topical (surface)	968.5	E855.2	E938.5	E950.4	E962.0	E980.4
Meprednisone	962.0	E858.0	E932.0	E950.4	E962.0	E980.4
Meprobam	969.5	E853.8	E939.5	E950.3	E962.0	E980.3
Meprobamate	969.5	E853.8	E939.5	E950.3	E962.0	E980.3
Mepyramine (maleate)	963.0	E858.1	E933.0	E950.4	E962.0	E980.4
Meralluride	974.0	E858.5	E944.0	E950.4	E962.0	E980.4
Merbaphen	974.0	E858.5	E944.0	E950.4	E962.0	E980.4
Merbromin	976.0	E858.7	E946.0	E950.4	E962.0	E980.4

Substance	Poisoning	External Cause (E-Code) Accident	Therapeutic Use	Suicide Attempt	Assault	Undetermined
Mercaptomerin	974.0	E858.5	E944.0	E950.4	E962.0	E980.4
Mercaptopurine	963.1	E858.1	E933.1	E950.4	E962.0	E980.4
Mercumatilin	974.0	E858.5	E944.0	E950.4	E962.0	E980.4
Mercuramide	974.0	E858.5	E944.0	E950.4	E962.0	E980.4
Mercuranin	976.0	E858.7	E946.0	E950.4	E962.0	E980.4
Mercurochrome	976.0	E858.7	E946.0	E950.4	E962.0	E980.4
Mercury, mercuric, mercurous (compounds) (cyanide) (fumes) (nonmedicinal) (vapor) NEC	985.0	E866.1	—	E950.9	E962.1	E980.9
ammoniated	976.0	E858.7	E946.0	E950.4	E962.0	E980.4
anti-infective	961.2	E857	E931.2	E950.4	E962.0	E980.4
topical	976.0	E858.7	E946.0	E950.4	E962.0	E980.4
chloride (antiseptic) NEC	976.0	E858.7	E946.0	E950.4	E962.0	E980.4
fungicide	985.0	E863.6	—	E950.6	E962.1	E980.7
diuretic compounds	974.0	E858.5	E944.0	E950.4	E962.0	E980.4
fungicide	985.0	E863.6	—	E950.6	E962.1	E980.7
organic (fungicide)	985.0	E863.6	—	E950.6	E962.1	E980.7
Merethoxylline	974.0	E858.5	E944.0	E950.4	E962.0	E980.4
Mersalyl	974.0	E858.5	E944.0	E950.4	E962.0	E980.4
Merthiolate (topical)	976.0	E858.7	E946.0	E950.4	E962.0	E980.4
ophthalmic preparation	976.5	E858.7	E946.5	E950.4	E962.0	E980.4
Meruvax	979.4	E858.8	E949.4	E950.4	E962.0	E980.4
Mescal buttons	969.6	E854.1	E939.6	E950.3	E962.0	E980.3
Mescaline (salts)	969.6	E854.1	E939.6	E950.3	E962.0	E980.3
Mesoridazine besylate	969.1	E853.0	E939.1	E950.3	E962.0	E980.3
Mestanolone	962.1	E858.0	E932.1	E950.4	E962.0	E980.4
Mestranol	962.2	E858.0	E932.2	E950.4	E962.0	E980.4
Metactesylacetate	976.0	E858.7	E946.0	E950.4	E962.0	E980.4
Metaldehyde (snail killer) NEC	989.4	E863.4	—	E950.6	E962.1	E980.7
Metals (heavy) (nonmedicinal) NEC	985.9	E866.4	—	E950.9	E962.1	E980.9
dust, fumes, or vapor NEC	985.9	E866.4	—	E950.9	E962.1	E980.9
light NEC	985.9	E866.4	—	E950.9	E962.1	E980.9
dust, fumes, or vapor NEC	985.9	E866.4	—	E950.9	E962.1	E980.9
pesticides (dust) (vapor)	985.9	E863.4	—	E950.6	E962.1	E980.7
Metamucil	973.3	E858.4	E943.3	E950.4	E962.0	E980.4
Metaphen	976.0	E858.7	E946.0	E950.4	E962.0	E980.4
Metaproterenol	975.1	E858.6	E945.1	E950.4	E962.0	E980.4
Metaraminol	972.8	E858.3	E942.8	E950.4	E962.0	E980.4
Metaxalone	968.0	E855.1	E938.0	E950.4	E962.0	E980.4
Metformin	962.3	E858.0	E932.3	E950.4	E962.0	E980.4
Methacycline	960.4	E856	E930.4	E950.4	E962.0	E980.4
Methadone	965.02	E850.1	E935.1	E950.0	E962.0	E980.0
Methallenestril	962.2	E858.0	E932.2	E950.4	E962.0	E980.4
Methamphetamine	969.7	E854.2	E939.7	E950.3	E962.0	E980.3
Methandienone	962.1	E858.0	E932.1	E950.4	E962.0	E980.4
Methandriol	962.1	E858.0	E932.1	E950.4	E962.0	E980.4
Methandrostenolone	962.1	E858.0	E932.1	E950.4	E962.0	E980.4
Methane gas	987.1	E869.8	—	E952.8	E962.2	E982.8
Methanol	980.1	E860.2	—	E950.9	E962.1	E980.9
vapor	987.8	E869.8	—	E952.8	E962.2	E982.8
Methantheline	971.1	E855.4	E941.1	E950.4	E962.0	E980.4
Methaphenilene	963.0	E858.1	E933.0	E950.4	E962.0	E980.4
Methapyrilene	963.0	E858.1	E933.0	E950.4	E962.0	E980.4
Methaqualone (compounds)	967.4	E852.3	E937.4	E950.2	E962.0	E980.2
Metharbital, metharbitone	967.0	E851	E937.0	E950.1	E962.0	E980.1
Methazolamide	974.2	E858.5	E944.2	E950.4	E962.0	E980.4
Methdilazine	963.0	E858.1	E933.0	E950.4	E962.0	E980.4
Methedrine	969.7	E854.2	E939.7	E950.3	E962.0	E980.3
Methenamine (mandelate)	961.9	E857	E931.9	E950.4	E962.0	E980.4
Methenolone	962.1	E858.0	E932.1	E950.4	E962.0	E980.4
Methergine	975.0	E858.6	E945.0	E950.4	E962.0	E980.4
Methiacil	962.8	E858.0	E932.8	E950.4	E962.0	E980.4

Substance	Poisoning	External Cause (E-Code) Accident	Therapeutic Use	Suicide Attempt	Assault	Undetermined
Methicillin (sodium)	960.0	E856	E930.0	E950.4	E962.0	E980.4
Methimazole	962.8	E858.0	E932.8	E950.4	E962.0	E980.4
Methionine	977.1	E858.8	E947.1	E950.4	E962.0	E980.4
Methisazone	961.7	E857	E931.7	E950.4	E962.0	E980.4
Methitural	967.0	E851	E937.0	E950.1	E962.0	E980.1
Methixene	971.1	E855.4	E941.1	E950.4	E962.0	E980.4
Methobarbital, methobarbitone	967.0	E851	E937.0	E950.1	E962.0	E980.1
Methocarbamol	968.0	E855.1	E938.0	E950.4	E962.0	E980.4
Methohexital, methohexitone (sodium)	968.3	E855.1	E938.3	E950.4	E962.0	E980.4
Methoin	966.1	E855.0	E936.1	E950.4	E962.0	E980.4
Methopholine	965.7	E850.7	E935.7	E950.0	E962.0	E980.0
Methorate	975.4	E858.6	E945.4	E950.4	E962.0	E980.4
Methoserpidine	972.6	E858.3	E942.6	E950.4	E962.0	E980.4
Methotrexate	963.1	E858.1	E933.1	E950.4	E962.0	E980.4
Methotrimeprazine	967.8	E852.8	E937.8	E950.2	E962.0	E980.2
Methoxa-Dome	976.3	E858.7	E946.3	E950.4	E962.0	E980.4
Methoxamine	971.2	E855.5	E941.2	E950.4	E962.0	E980.4
Methoxsalen	976.3	E858.7	E946.3	E950.4	E962.0	E980.4
Methoxybenzyl penicillin	960.0	E856	E930.0	E950.4	E962.0	E980.4
Methoxychlor	989.2	E863.0	—	E950.6	E962.1	E980.7
Methoxyflurane	968.2	E855.1	E938.2	E950.4	E962.0	E980.4
Methoxyphenamine	971.2	E855.5	E941.2	E950.4	E962.0	E980.4
Methoxypromazine	969.1	E853.0	E939.1	E950.3	E962.0	E980.3
Methoxypsoralen	976.3	E858.7	E946.3	E950.4	E962.0	E980.4
Methscopolamine (bromide)	971.1	E855.4	E941.1	E950.4	E962.0	E980.4
Methsuximide	966.2	E855.0	E936.2	E950.4	E962.0	E980.4
Methyclothiazide	974.3	E858.5	E944.3	E950.4	E962.0	E980.4
Methyl	—	—	—	—	—	—
acetate	982.8	E862.4	—	E950.9	E962.1	E980.9
acetone II	982.8	E862.4	—	E950.9	E962.1	E980.9
alcohol	980.1	E860.2	—	E950.9	E962.1	E980.9
amphetamine	969.7	E854.2	E939.7	E950.3	E962.0	E980.3
androstanolone	962.1	E858.0	E932.1	E950.4	E962.0	E980.4
atropine	971.1	E855.4	E941.1	E950.4	E962.0	E980.4
benzene	982.0	E862.4	—	E950.9	E962.1	E980.9
bromide (gas)	987.8	E869.8	—	E952.8	E962.2	E982.8
fumigant	987.8	E863.8	—	E950.6	E962.2	E980.7
butanol	980.8	E860.8	—	E950.9	E962.1	E980.9
carbinol	980.1	E860.2	—	E950.9	E962.1	E980.9
cellosolve	982.8	E862.4	—	E950.9	E962.1	E980.9
cellulose	973.3	E858.4	E943.3	E950.4	E961.0	E980.4
chloride (gas)	987.8	E869.8	—	E952.8	E962.2	E982.8
cyclohexane	982.8	E862.4	—	E950.9	E962.1	E980.9
cyclohexanone	982.8	E862.4	—	E950.9	E962.1	E980.9
dihydromorphinone	965.09	E850.2	E935.2	E950.0	E962.0	E980.0
ergometrine	975.0	E858.6	E945.0	E950.4	E962.0	E980.4
ergonovine	975.0	E858.6	E945.0	E950.4	E962.0	E980.4
ethyl ketone	982.8	E862.4	—	E950.9	E962.1	E980.9
hydrazine	983.9	E864.3	—	E950.7	E962.1	E980.6
isobutyl ketone	982.8	E862.4	—	E950.9	E962.1	E980.9
morphine NEC	965.09	E850.2	E935.2	E950.0	E962.0	E980.0
parafynol	967.8	E852.8	E937.8	E950.2	E962.0	E980.2
parathion	989.3	E863.1	—	E950.6	E962.1	E980.7
pentynol NEC	967.8	E852.8	E937.8	E950.2	E962.0	E980.2
peridol	969.2	E853.1	E939.2	E950.3	E962.0	E980.3
phenidate	969.7	E854.2	E939.7	E950.3	E962.0	E980.3
prednisolone	962.0	E858.0	E932.0	E950.4	E962.0	E980.4
ENT agent	976.6	E858.7	E946.6	E950.4	E962.0	E980.4
ophthalmic preparation	976.5	E858.7	E946.5	E950.4	E962.0	E980.4
topical NEC	976.0	E858.7	E946.0	E950.4	E962.0	E980.4
propylcarbinol	980.8	E860.8	—	E950.9	E962.1	E980.9

Substance	Poisoning	Accident	Therapeutic Use	Suicide Attempt	Assault	Undetermined
		External Cause (E-Code)				
Methyl *(Continued)*						
rosaniline NEC	976.0	E858.7	E946.0	E950.4	E962.0	E980.4
salicylate NEC	976.3	E858.7	E946.3	E950.4	E962.0	E980.4
sulfate (fumes)	987.8	E869.8	—	E952.8	E962.2	E982.8
liquid	983.9	E864.3	—	E950.7	E962.1	E980.6
sulfonal	967.8	E852.8	E937.8	E950.2	E962.0	E980.2
testosterone	962.1	E858.0	E932.1	E950.4	E962.0	E980.4
thiouracil	962.8	E858.0	E932.8	E950.4	E962.0	E980.4
Methylated spirit	980.0	E860.1	—	E950.9	E962.1	E980.9
Methyldopa	972.6	E858.3	E942.6	E950.4	E962.0	E980.4
Methylene blue	961.9	E857	E931.9	E950.4	E962.0	E980.4
chloride or dichloride (solvent) NEC	982.3	E862.4	—	E950.9	E962.1	E980.9
Methylhexabital	967.0	E851	E937.0	E950.1	E962.0	E980.1
Methylparaben (ophthalmic)	976.5	E858.7	E946.5	E950.4	E962.0	E980.4
Methyprylon	967.5	E852.4	E937.5	E950.2	E962.0	E980.2
Methysergide	971.3	E855.6	E941.3	E950.4	E962.0	E980.4
Metoclopramide	963.0	E858.1	E933.0	E950.4	E962.0	E980.4
Metofoline	965.7	E850.7	E935.7	E950.0	E962.0	E980.0
Metopon	965.09	E850.2	E935.2	E950.0	E962.0	E980.0
Metronidazole	961.5	E857	E931.5	E950.4	E962.0	E980.4
Metycaine	968.9	E855.2	E938.9	E950.4	E962.0	E980.4
infiltration (subcutaneous)	968.5	E855.2	E938.5	E950.4	E962.0	E980.4
nerve block (peripheral) (plexus)	968.6	E855.2	E938.6	E950.4	E962.0	E980.4
topical (surface)	968.5	E855.2	E938.5	E950.4	E962.0	E980.4
Metyrapone	977.8	E858.8	E947.8	E950.4	E962.0	E980.4
Mevinphos	989.3	E863.1	—	E950.6	E962.1	E980.7
Mezereon (berries)	988.2	E865.3	—	E950.9	E962.1	E980.9
Micatin	976.0	E858.7	E946.0	E950.4	E962.0	E980.4
Miconazole	976.0	E858.7	E946.0	E950.4	E962.0	E980.4
Midol	965.1	E850.3	E935.3	E950.0	E962.0	E980.0
Mifepristone	962.9	E858.0	E932.9	E950.4	E962.0	E980.4
Milk of magnesia	973.0	E858.4	E943.0	E950.4	E962.0	E980.4
Millipede (tropical) (venomous)	989.5	E905.4	—	E950.9	E962.1	E980.9
Miltown	969.5	E853.8	E939.5	E950.3	E962.0	E980.3
Mineral	—	—	—	—	—	—
oil (medicinal)	973.2	E858.4	E943.2	E950.4	E962.0	E980.4
nonmedicinal	981	E862.1	—	E950.9	E962.1	E980.9
topical	976.3	E858.7	E946.3	E950.4	E962.0	E980.4
salts NEC	974.6	E858.5	E944.6	E950.4	E962.0	E980.4
spirits	981	E862.0	—	E950.9	E962.1	E980.9
Minocycline	960.4	E856	E930.4	E950.4	E962.0	E980.4
Mithramycin (antineoplastic)	960.7	E856	E930.7	E950.4	E962.0	E980.4
Mitobronitol	963.1	E858.1	E933.1	E950.4	E962.0	E980.4
Mitomycin (antineoplastic)	960.7	E856	E930.7	E950.4	E962.0	E980.4
Mitotane	963.1	E858.1	E933.1	E950.4	E962.0	E980.4
Moderil	972.6	E858.3	E942.6	E950.4	E962.0	E980.4
Mogadon - *see* Nitrazepam	—	—	—	—	—	—
Molindone	969.3	E853.8	E939.3	E950.3	E962.0	E980.3
Monistat	976.0	E858.7	E946.0	E950.4	E962.0	E980.4
Monkshood	988.2	E865.4	—	E950.9	E962.1	E980.9
Monoamine oxidase inhibitors	969.0	E854.0	E939.0	E950.3	E962.0	E980.3
Monochlorobenzene	982.0	E862.4	—	E950.9	E962.1	E980.9
Monosodium glutamate	989.89	E866.8	—	E950.9	E962.1	E980.9
Monoxide, carbon - *see* Carbon, monoxide	—	—	—	—	—	—
Moperone	969.2	E853.1	E939.2	E950.3	E962.0	E980.3
Morning glory seeds	969.6	E854.1	E939.6	E950.3	E962.0	E980.3
Moroxydine (hydrochloride)	961.7	E857	E931.7	E950.4	E962.0	E980.4
Morphazinamide	961.8	E857	E931.8	E950.4	E962.0	E980.4
Morphinans	965.09	E850.2	E935.2	E950.0	E962.0	E980.0
Morphine NEC	965.09	E850.2	E935.2	E950.0	E962.0	E980.0
antagonists	970.1	E854.3	E940.1	E950.4	E962.0	E980.4

Substance	Poisoning	External Cause (E-Code) Accident	Therapeutic Use	Suicide Attempt	Assault	Undetermined
Morpholinylethyl morphine	965.09	E850.2	E935.2	E950.0	E962.0	E980.0
Morrhuate sodium	972.7	E858.3	E942.7	E950.4	E962.0	E980.4
Moth balls (*see also* Pesticides)	989.4	E863.4	—	E950.6	E962.1	E980.7
naphthalene	983.0	E863.4	—	E950.7	E962.1	E980.6
Motor exhaust gas - *see* Carbon, monoxide, exhaust gas	—	—	—	—	—	—
Mouth wash	976.6	E858.7	E946.6	E950.4	E962.0	E980.4
Mucolytic agent	975.5	E858.6	E945.5	E950.4	E962.0	E980.4
Mucomyst	975.5	E858.6	E945.5	E950.4	E962.0	E980.4
Mucous membrane agents (external)	976.9	E858.7	E946.9	E950.4	E962.0	E980.4
specified NEC	976.8	E858.7	E946.8	E950.4	E962.0	E980.4
Mumps	—	—	—	—	—	—
immune globulin (human)	964.6	E858.2	E934.6	E950.4	E962.0	E980.4
skin test antigen	977.8	E858.8	E947.8	E950.4	E962.0	E980.4
vaccine	979.6	E858.8	E949.6	E950.4	E962.0	E980.4
Mumpsvax	979.6	E858.8	E949.6	E950.4	E962.0	E980.4
Muriatic acid - *see* Hydrochloric acid	—	—	—	—	—	—
Muscarine	971.0	E855.3	E941.0	E950.4	E962.0	E980.4
Muscle affecting agents NEC	975.3	E858.6	E945.3	E950.4	E962.0	E980.4
oxytocic	975.0	E858.6	E945.0	E950.4	E962.0	E980.4
relaxants	975.3	E858.6	E945.3	E950.4	E962.0	E980.4
central nervous system	968.0	E855.1	E938.0	E950.4	E962.0	E980.4
skeletal	975.2	E858.6	E945.2	E950.4	E962.0	E980.4
smooth	975.1	E858.6	E945.1	E950.4	E962.0	E980.4
Mushrooms, noxious	988.1	E865.5	—	E950.9	E962.1	E980.9
Mussel, noxious	988.0	E865.1	—	E950.9	E962.1	E980.9
Mustard (emetic)	973.6	E858.4	E943.6	E950.4	E962.0	E980.4
gas	987.8	E869.8	—	E952.8	E962.2	E982.8
nitrogen	963.1	E858.1	E933.1	E950.4	E962.0	E980.4
Mustine	963.1	E858.1	E933.1	E950.4	E962.0	E980.4
M-vac	979.4	E858.8	E949.4	E950.4	E962.0	E980.4
Mycifradin	960.8	E856	E930.8	E950.4	E962.0	E980.4
topical	976.0	E858.7	E946.0	E950.4	E962.0	E980.4
Mycitracin	960.8	E856	E930.8	E950.4	E962.0	E980.4
ophthalmic preparation	976.5	E858.7	E946.5	E950.4	E962.0	E980.4
Mycostatin	960.1	E856	E930.1	E950.4	E962.0	E980.4
topical	976.0	E858.7	E946.0	E950.4	E962.0	E980.4
Mydriacyl	971.1	E855.4	E941.1	E950.4	E962.0	E980.4
Myelobromal	963.1	E858.1	E933.1	E950.4	E962.0	E980.4
Myleran	963.1	E858.1	E933.1	E950.4	E962.0	E980.4
Myochrysin(e)	965.69	E850.6	E935.6	E950.0	E962.0	E980.0
Myoneural blocking agents	975.2	E858.6	E945.2	E950.4	E962.0	E980.4
Myristica fragrans	988.2	E865.3	—	E950.9	E962.1	E980.9
Myristicin	988.2	E865.3	—	E950.9	E962.1	E980.9
Mysoline	966.3	E855.0	E936.3	E950.4	E962.0	E980.4
Nafcillin (sodium)	960.0	E856	E930.0	E950.4	E962.0	E980.4
Nail polish remover	982.8	E862.4	—	E950.9	E962.1	E980.9
Nalidixic acid	961.9	E857	E931.9	E950.4	E962.0	E980.4
Nalorphine	970.1	E854.3	E940.1	E950.4	E962.0	E980.4
Naloxone	970.1	E854.3	E940.1	E950.4	E962.0	E980.4
Nandrolone (decanoate) (phenpropionate)	962.1	E858.0	E932.1	E950.4	E962.0	E980.4
Naphazoline	971.2	E855.5	E941.2	E950.4	E962.0	E980.4
Naphtha (painter's) (petroleum)	981	E862.0	—	E950.9	E962.1	E980.9
solvent	981	E862.0	—	E950.9	E962.1	E980.9
vapor	987.1	E869.8	—	E952.8	E962.2	E982.8
Naphthalene (chlorinated)	983.0	E864.0	—	E950.7	E962.1	E980.6
insecticide or moth repellent	983.0	E863.4	—	E950.7	E962.1	E980.6
vapor	987.8	E869.8	—	E952.8	E962.2	E982.8
Naphthol	983.0	E864.0	—	E950.7	E962.1	E980.6
Naphthylamine	983.0	E864.0	—	E950.7	E962.1	E980.6
Naprosyn - *see* Naproxen	—	—	—	—	—	—
Naproxen	965.61	E850.6	E935.6	E950.0	E962.0	E980.0

Substance	Poisoning	External Cause (E-Code)				
		Accident	Therapeutic Use	Suicide Attempt	Assault	Undetermined
Narcotic (drug)	967.9	E852.9	E937.9	E950.2	E962.0	E980.2
analgesic NEC	965.8	E850.8	E935.8	E950.0	E962.0	E980.0
antagonist	970.1	E854.3	E940.1	E950.4	E962.0	E980.4
specified NEC	967.8	E852.8	E937.8	E950.2	E962.0	E980.2
Narcotine	975.4	E858.6	E945.4	E950.4	E962.0	E980.4
Nardil	969.0	E854.0	E939.0	E950.3	E962.0	E980.3
Natrium cyanide - *see* Cyanide(s)	—	—	—	—	—	—
Natural	—	—	—	—	—	—
blood (product)	964.7	E858.2	E934.7	E950.4	E962.0	E980.4
gas (piped)	987.1	E867	—	E951.0	E962.2	E981.0
incomplete combustion	986	E867	—	E951.0	E962.2	E981.0
Nealbarbital, nealbarbitone	967.0	E851	E937.0	E950.1	E962.0	E980.1
Nectadon	975.4	E858.6	E945.4	E950.4	E962.0	E980.4
Nematocyst (sting)	989.5	E905.6	—	E950.9	E962.1	E980.9
Nembutal	967.0	E851	E937.0	E950.1	E962.0	E980.1
Neoarsphenamine	961.1	E857	E931.1	E950.4	E962.0	E980.4
Neocinchophen	974.7	E858.5	E944.7	E950.4	E962.0	E980.4
Neomycin	960.8	E856	E930.8	E950.4	E962.0	E980.4
ENT agent	976.6	E858.7	E946.6	E950.4	E962.0	E980.4
ophthalmic preparation	976.5	E858.7	E946.5	E950.4	E962.0	E980.4
topical NEC	976.0	E858.7	E946.0	E950.4	E962.0	E980.4
Neonal	967.0	E851	E937.0	E950.1	E962.0	E980.1
Neoprontosil	961.0	E857	E931.0	E950.4	E962.0	E980.4
Neosalvarsan	961.1	E857	E931.1	E950.4	E962.0	E980.4
Neosilversalvarsan	961.1	E857	E931.1	E950.4	E962.0	E980.4
Neosporin	960.8	E856	E930.8	E950.4	E962.0	E980.4
ENT agent	976.6	E858.7	E946.6	E950.4	E962.0	E980.4
ophthalmic preparation	976.5	E858.7	E946.5	E950.4	E962.0	E980.4
topical NEC	976.0	E858.7	E946.0	E950.4	E962.0	E980.4
Neostigmine	971.0	E855.3	E941.0	E950.4	E962.0	E980.4
Neraval	967.0	E851	E937.0	E950.1	E962.0	E980.1
Neravan	967.0	E851	E937.0	E950.1	E962.0	E980.1
Nerium oleander	988.2	E865.4	—	E950.9	E962.1	E980.9
Nerve gases (war)	987.9	E869.9	—	E952.9	E962.2	E982.9
Nesacaine	968.9	E855.2	E938.9	E950.4	E962.0	E980.4
infiltration (subcutaneous)	968.5	E855.2	E938.5	E950.4	E962.0	E980.4
nerve block (peripheral) (plexus)	968.6	E855.2	E938.6	E950.4	E962.0	E980.4
Neurobarb	967.0	E851	E937.0	E950.1	E962.0	E980.1
Neuroleptics NEC	969.3	E853.8	E939.3	E950.3	E962.0	E980.3
Neuroprotective agent	977.8	E858.8	E947.8	E950.4	E962.0	E980.4
Neutral spirits	980.0	E860.1	—	E950.9	E962.1	E980.9
beverage	980.0	E860.0	—	E950.9	E962.1	E980.9
Niacin, niacinamide	972.2	E858.3	E942.2	E950.4	E962.0	E980.4
Nialamide	969.0	E854.0	E939.0	E950.3	E962.0	E980.3
Nickle (carbonyl) (compounds) (fumes) (tetracarbonyl) (vapor)	985.8	E866.4	—	E950.9	E962.1	E980.9
Niclosamide	961.6	E857	E931.6	E950.4	E962.0	E980.4
Nicomorphine	965.09	E850.2	E935.2	E950.0	E962.0	E980.0
Nicotinamide	972.2	E858.3	E942.2	E950.4	E962.0	E980.4
Nicotine (insecticide) (spray) (sulfate) NEC	989.4	E863.4	—	E950.6	E962.1	E980.7
not insecticide	989.89	E866.8	—	E950.9	E962.1	E980.9
Nicotinic acid (derivatives)	972.2	E858.3	E942.2	E950.4	E962.0	E980.4
Nicotinyl alcohol	972.2	E858.3	E942.2	E950.4	E962.0	E980.4
Nicoumalone	964.2	E858.2	E934.2	E950.4	E962.0	E980.4
Nifenazone	965.5	E850.5	E935.5	E950.0	E962.0	E980.0
Nifuraldezone	961.9	E857	E931.9	E950.4	E962.0	E980.4
Nightshade (deadly)	988.2	E865.4	—	E950.9	E962.1	E980.9
Nikethamide	970.0	E854.3	E940.0	E950.4	E962.0	E980.4
Nilstat	960.1	E856	E930.1	E950.4	E962.0	E980.4
topical	976.0	E858.7	E946.0	E950.4	E962.0	E980.4
Nimodipine	977.8	E858.8	E947.8	E950.4	E962.0	E980.4
Niridazole	961.6	E857	E931.6	E950.4	E962.0	E980.4

Substance	Poisoning	External Cause (E-Code) Accident	Therapeutic Use	Suicide Attempt	Assault	Undetermined
Nisentil	965.09	E850.2	E935.2	E950.0	E962.0	E980.0
Nitrates	972.4	E858.3	E942.4	E950.4	E962.0	E980.4
Nitrazepam	969.4	E853.2	E939.4	E950.3	E962.0	E980.3
Nitric	—	—	—	—	—	—
acid (liquid)	983.1	E864.1	—	E950.7	E962.1	E980.6
vapor	987.8	E869.8	—	E952.8	E962.2	E982.8
oxide (gas)	987.2	E869.0	—	E952.8	E962.2	E982.8
Nitrite, amyl (medicinal) (vapor)	972.4	E858.3	E942.4	E950.4	E962.0	E980.4
Nitroaniline	983.0	E864.0	—	E950.7	E962.1	E980.6
vapor	987.8	E869.8	—	E952.8	E962.2	E982.8
Nitrobenzene, nitrobenzol	983.0	E864.0	—	E950.7	E962.1	E980.6
vapor	987.8	E869.8	—	E952.8	E962.2	E982.8
Nitrocellulose	976.3	E858.7	E946.3	E950.4	E962.0	E980.4
Nitrofuran derivatives	961.9	E857	E931.9	E950.4	E962.0	E980.4
Nitrofurantoin	961.9	E857	E931.9	E950.4	E962.0	E980.4
Nitrofurazone	976.0	E858.7	E946.0	E950.4	E962.0	E980.4
Nitrogen (dioxide) (gas) (oxide)	987.2	E869.0	—	E952.8	E962.2	E982.8
mustard (antineoplastic)	963.1	E858.1	E933.1	E950.4	E962.0	E980.4
Nitroglycerin, nitroglycerol (medicinal)	972.4	E858.3	E942.4	E950.4	E962.0	E980.4
nonmedicinal	989.89	E866.8	—	E950.9	E962.1	E980.9
fumes	987.8	E869.8	—	E952.8	E962.2	E982.8
Nitrohydrochloric acid	983.1	E864.1	—	E950.7	E962.1	E980.6
Nitromersol	976.0	E858.7	E946.0	E950.4	E962.0	E980.4
Nitronaphthalene	983.0	E864.0	—	E950.7	E962.2	E980.6
Nitrophenol	983.0	E864.0	—	E950.7	E962.2	E980.6
Nitrothiazol	961.6	E857	E931.6	E950.4	E962.0	E980.4
Nitrotoluene, nitrotoluol	983.0	E864.0	—	E950.7	E962.1	E980.6
vapor	987.8	E869.8	—	E952.8	E962.2	E982.8
Nitrous	968.2	E855.1	E938.2	E950.4	E962.0	E980.4
acid (liquid)	983.1	E864.1	—	E950.7	E962.1	E980.6
fumes	987.2	E869.0	—	E952.8	E962.2	E982.8
oxide (anesthetic) NEC	968.2	E855.1	E938.2	E950.4	E962.0	E980.4
Nitrozone	976.0	E858.7	E946.0	E950.4	E962.0	E980.4
Noctec	967.1	E852.0	E937.1	E950.2	E962.0	E980.2
Noludar	967.5	E852.4	E937.5	E950.2	E962.0	E980.2
Noptil	967.0	E851	E937.0	E950.1	E962.0	E980.1
Noradrenalin	971.2	E855.5	E941.2	E950.4	E962.0	E980.4
Noramidopyrine	965.5	E850.5	E935.5	E950.0	E962.0	E980.0
Norepinephrine	971.2	E855.5	E941.2	E950.4	E962.0	E980.4
Norethandrolone	962.1	E858.0	E932.1	E950.4	E962.0	E980.4
Norethindrone	962.2	E858.0	E932.2	E950.4	E962.0	E980.4
Norethisterone	962.2	E858.0	E932.2	E950.4	E962.0	E980.4
Norethynodrel	962.2	E858.0	E932.2	E950.4	E962.0	E980.4
Norlestrin	962.2	E858.0	E932.2	E950.4	E962.0	E980.4
Norlutin	962.2	E858.0	E932.2	E950.4	E962.0	E980.4
Normison - *see* Benzodiazepines	—	—	—	—	—	—
Normorphine	965.09	E850.2	E935.2	E950.0	E962.0	E980.0
Nortriptyline	969.0	E854.0	E939.0	E950.3	E962.0	E980.3
Noscapine	975.4	E858.6	E945.4	E950.4	E962.0	E980.4
Nose preparations	976.6	E858.7	E946.6	E950.4	E962.0	E980.4
Novobiocin	960.8	E856	E930.8	E950.4	E962.0	E980.4
Novocain (infiltration) (topical)	968.5	E855.2	E938.5	E950.4	E962.0	E980.4
nerve block (peripheral) (plexus)	968.6	E855.2	E938.6	E950.4	E962.0	E980.4
spinal	968.7	E855.2	E938.7	E950.4	E962.0	E980.4
Noxythiolin	961.9	E857	E931.9	E950.4	E962.0	E980.4
NPH Iletin (insulin)	962.3	E858.0	E932.3	E950.4	E962.0	E980.4
Numorphan	965.09	E850.2	E935.2	E950.0	E962.0	E980.0
Nunol	967.0	E851	E937.0	E950.1	E962.0	E980.1
Nupercaine (spinal anesthetic)	968.7	E855.2	E938.7	E950.4	E962.0	E980.4
topical (surface)	968.5	E855.2	E938.5	E950.4	E962.0	E980.4
Nutmeg oil (liniment)	976.3	E858.7	E946.3	E950.4	E962.0	E980.4

Substance	Poisoning	External Cause (E-Code)				
		Accident	Therapeutic Use	Suicide Attempt	Assault	Undetermined
Nux vomica	989.1	E863.7	—	E950.6	E962.1	E980.7
Nydrazid	961.8	E857	E931.8	E950.4	E962.0	E980.4
Nylidrin	971.2	E855.5	E941.2	E950.4	E962.0	E980.4
Nystatin	960.1	E856	E930.1	E950.4	E962.0	E980.4
topical	976.0	E858.7	E946.0	E950.4	E962.0	E980.4
Nytol	963.0	E858.1	E933.0	E950.4	E962.0	E980.4
Oblivion	967.8	E852.8	E937.8	E950.2	E962.0	E980.2
Octyl nitrite	972.4	E858.3	E942.4	E950.4	E962.0	E980.4
Oestradiol (cypionate) (dipropionate) (valerate)	962.2	E858.0	E932.2	E950.4	E962.0	E980.4
Oestriol	962.2	E858.0	E932.2	E950.4	E962.0	E980.4
Oestrone	962.2	E858.0	E932.2	E950.4	E962.0	E980.4
Oil (of) NEC	989.89	E866.8	—	E950.9	E962.1	E980.9
bitter almond	989.0	E866.8	—	E950.9	E962.1	E980.9
camphor	976.1	E858.7	E946.1	E950.4	E962.0	E980.4
colors	989.89	E861.6	—	E950.9	E962.1	E980.9
fumes	987.8	E869.8	—	E952.8	E962.2	E982.8
lubricating	981	E862.2	—	E950.9	E962.1	E980.9
specified source, other - *see* substance specified	—	—	—	—	—	—
vitriol (liquid)	983.1	E864.1	—	E950.7	E962.1	E980.6
fumes	987.8	E869.8	—	E952.8	E962.2	E982.8
wintergreen (bitter) NEC	976.3	E858.7	E946.3	E950.4	E962.0	E980.4
Ointments NEC	976.9	E858.7	E946.9	E950.4	E962.0	E980.4
Oleander	988.2	E865.4	—	E950.9	E962.1	E980.9
Oleandomycin	960.3	E856	E930.3	E950.4	E962.0	E980.4
Oleovitamin A	963.5	E858.1	E933.5	E950.4	E962.0	E980.4
Oleum ricini	973.1	E858.4	E943.1	E950.4	E962.0	E980.4
Olive oil (medicinal) NEC	973.2	E858.4	E943.2	E950.4	E962.0	E980.4
OMPA	989.3	E863.1	—	E950.6	E962.1	E980.7
Oncovin	963.1	E858.1	E933.1	E950.4	E962.0	E980.4
Ophthaine	968.5	E855.2	E938.5	E950.4	E962.0	E980.4
Ophthetic	968.5	E855.2	E938.5	E950.4	E962.0	E980.4
Opiates, opioids, opium NEC	965.00	E850.2	E935.2	E950.0	E962.0	E980.0
antagonists	970.1	E854.3	E940.1	E950.4	E962.0	E980.4
Oracon	962.2	E858.0	E932.2	E950.4	E962.0	E980.4
Oragrafin	977.8	E858.8	E947.8	E950.4	E962.0	E980.4
Oral contraceptives	962.2	E858.0	E932.2	E950.4	E962.0	E980.4
Orciprenaline	975.1	E858.6	E945.1	E950.4	E962.0	E980.4
Organidin	975.5	E858.6	E945.5	E950.4	E962.0	E980.4
Organophosphates	989.3	E863.1	—	E950.6	E962.1	E980.7
Orimune	979.5	E858.8	E949.5	E950.4	E962.0	E980.4
Orinase	962.3	E858.0	E932.3	E950.4	E962.0	E980.4
Orphenadrine	966.4	E855.0	E936.4	E950.4	E962.0	E980.4
Ortal (sodium)	967.0	E851	E937.0	E950.1	E962.0	E980.1
Orthoboric acid	976.0	E858.7	E946.0	E950.4	E962.0	E980.4
ENT agent	976.6	E858.7	E946.6	E950.4	E962.0	E980.4
ophthalmic preparation	976.5	E858.7	E946.5	E950.4	E962.0	E980.4
Orthocaine	968.5	E855.2	E938.5	E950.4	E962.0	E980.4
Ortho-Novum	962.2	E858.0	E932.2	E950.4	E962.0	E980.4
Orthotolidine (reagent)	977.8	E858.8	E947.8	E950.4	E962.0	E980.4
Osmic acid (liquid)	983.1	E864.1	—	E950.7	E962.1	E980.6
fumes	987.8	E869.8	—	E952.8	E962.2	E982.8
Osmotic diuretics	974.4	E858.5	E944.4	E950.4	E962.0	E980.4
Ouabain	972.1	E858.3	E942.1	E950.4	E962.0	E980.4
Ovarian hormones (synthetic substitutes)	962.2	E858.0	E932.2	E950.4	E962.0	E980.4
Ovral	962.2	E858.0	E932.2	E950.4	E962.0	E980.4
Ovulation suppressants	962.2	E858.0	E932.2	E950.4	E962.0	E980.4
Ovulen	962.2	E858.0	E932.2	E950.4	E962.0	E980.4
Oxacillin (sodium)	960.0	E856	E930.0	E950.4	E962.0	E980.4
Oxalic acid	983.1	E864.1	—	E950.7	E962.1	E980.6
Oxanamide	969.5	E853.8	E939.5	E950.3	E962.0	E980.3
Oxandrolone	962.1	E858.0	E932.1	E950.4	E962.0	E980.4

Substance	Poisoning	External Cause (E-Code) Accident	Therapeutic Use	Suicide Attempt	Assault	Undetermined
Oxaprozin	965.61	E850.6	E935.6	E950.0	E962.0	E980.0
Oxazepam	969.4	E853.2	E939.4	E950.3	E962.0	E980.3
Oxazolidine derivatives	966.0	E855.0	E936.0	E950.4	E962.0	E980.4
Ox bile extract	973.4	E858.4	E943.4	E950.4	E962.0	E980.4
Oxedrine	971.2	E855.5	E941.2	E950.4	E962.0	E980.4
Oxeladin	975.4	E858.6	E945.4	E950.4	E962.0	E980.4
Oxethazaine NEC	968.5	E855.2	E938.5	E950.4	E962.0	E980.4
Oxidizing agents NEC	983.9	E864.3	—	E950.7	E962.1	E980.6
Oxolinic acid	961.3	E857	E931.3	E950.4	E962.0	E980.4
Oxophenarsine	961.1	E857	E931.1	E950.4	E962.0	E980.4
Oxsoralen	976.3	E858.7	E946.3	E950.4	E962.0	E980.4
Oxtriphylline	976.7	E858.6	E945.7	E950.4	E962.0	E980.4
Oxybuprocaine	968.5	E855.2	E938.5	E950.4	E962.0	E980.4
Oxybutynin	975.1	E858.6	E945.1	E950.4	E962.0	E980.4
Oxycodone	965.09	E850.2	E935.2	E950.0	E962.0	E980.0
Oxygen	987.8	E869.8	—	E952.8	E962.2	E982.8
Oxylone	976.0	E858.7	E946.0	E950.4	E962.0	E980.4
ophthalmic preparation	976.5	E858.7	E946.5	E950.4	E962.0	E980.4
Oxymesterone	962.1	E858.0	E932.1	E950.4	E962.0	E980.4
Oxymetazoline	971.2	E855.5	E941.2	E950.4	E962.0	E980.4
Oxymetholone	962.1	E858.0	E932.1	E950.4	E962.0	E980.4
Oxymorphone	965.09	E850.2	E935.2	E950.0	E962.0	E980.0
Oxypertine	969.0	E854.0	E939.0	E950.3	E962.0	E980.3
Oxyphenbutazone	965.5	E850.5	E935.5	E950.0	E962.0	E980.0
Oxyphencyclimine	971.1	E855.4	E941.1	E950.4	E962.0	E980.4
Oxyphenisatin	973.1	E858.4	E943.1	E950.4	E962.0	E980.4
Oxyphenonium	971.1	E855.4	E941.1	E950.4	E962.0	E980.4
Oxyquinoline	961.3	E857	E931.3	E950.4	E962.0	E980.4
Oxytetracycline	960.4	E856	E930.4	E950.4	E962.0	E980.4
Oxytocics	975.0	E858.6	E945.0	E950.4	E962.0	E980.4
Oxytocin	975.0	E858.6	E945.0	E950.4	E962.0	E980.4
Ozone	987.8	E869.8	—	E952.8	E962.2	E982.8
PABA	976.3	E858.7	E946.3	E950.4	E962.0	E980.4
Packed red cells	964.7	E858.2	E934.7	E950.4	E962.0	E980.4
Paint NEC	989.89	E861.6	—	E950.9	E962.1	E980.9
cleaner	982.8	E862.9	—	E950.9	E962.1	E980.9
fumes NEC	987.8	E869.8	—	E952.8	E962.1	E982.8
lead (fumes)	984.0	E861.5	—	E950.9	E962.1	E980.9
solvent NEC	982.8	E862.9	—	E950.9	E962.1	E980.9
stripper	982.8	E862.9	—	E950.9	E962.1	E980.9
Palfium	965.09	E850.2	E935.2	E950.0	E962.0	E980.0
Palivizumab	979.9	E858.8	E949.6	E950.4	E962.0	E980.4
Paludrine	961.4	E857	E931.4	E950.4	E962.0	E980.4
PAM	977.2	E855.8	E947.2	E950.4	E962.0	E980.4
Pamaquine (napthoate)	961.4	E857	E931.4	E950.4	E962.0	E980.4
Pamprin	965.1	E850.3	E935.3	E950.0	E962.0	E980.0
Panadol	965.4	E850.4	E935.4	E950.0	E962.0	E980.0
Pancreatic dornase (mucolytic)	963.4	E858.1	E933.4	E950.4	E962.0	E980.4
Pancreatin	973.4	E858.4	E943.4	E950.4	E962.0	E980.4
Pancrelipase	973.4	E858.4	E943.4	E950.4	E962.0	E980.4
Pangamic acid	963.5	E858.1	E933.5	E950.4	E962.0	E980.4
Panthenol	963.5	E858.1	E933.5	E950.4	E962.0	E980.4
topical	976.8	E858.7	E946.8	E950.4	E962.0	E980.4
Pantopaque	977.8	E858.8	E947.8	E950.4	E962.0	E980.4
Pantopon	965.00	E850.2	E935.2	E950.0	E962.0	E980.0
Pantothenic acid	963.5	E858.1	E933.5	E950.4	E962.0	E980.4
Panwarfin	964.2	E858.2	E934.2	E950.4	E962.0	E980.4
Papain	973.4	E858.4	E943.4	E950.4	E962.0	E980.4
Papaverine	972.5	E858.3	E942.5	E950.4	E962.0	E980.4
Para-aminobenzoic acid	976.3	E858.7	E946.3	E950.4	E962.0	E980.4
Para-aminophenol derivatives	965.4	E850.4	E935.4	E950.0	E962.0	E980.0

◀ New ⟸ Revised

Substance	Poisoning	External Cause (E-Code) Accident	Therapeutic Use	Suicide Attempt	Assault	Undetermined
Para-aminosalicylic acid (derivatives)	961.8	E857	E931.8	E950.4	E962.0	E980.4
Paracetaldehyde (medicinal)	967.2	E852.1	E937.2	E950.2	E962.0	E980.2
Paracetamol	965.4	E850.4	E935.4	E950.0	E962.0	E980.0
Paracodin	965.09	E850.2	E935.2	E950.0	E962.0	E980.0
Paradione	966.0	E855.0	E936.0	E950.4	E962.0	E980.4
Paraffin(s) (wax)	981	E862.3	—	E950.9	E962.1	E980.9
liquid (medicinal)	973.2	E858.4	E943.2	E950.4	E962.0	E980.4
nonmedicinal (oil)	981	E962.1	—	E950.9	E962.1	E980.9
Paraldehyde (medicinal)	967.2	E852.1	E937.2	E950.2	E962.0	E980.2
Paramethadione	966.0	E855.0	E936.0	E950.4	E962.0	E980.4
Paramethasone	962.0	E858.0	E932.0	E950.4	E962.0	E980.4
Paraquat	989.4	E863.5	—	E950.6	E962.1	E980.7
Parasympatholytics	971.1	E855.4	E941.1	E950.4	E962.0	E980.4
Parasympathomimetics	971.0	E855.3	E941.0	E950.4	E962.0	E980.4
Parathion	989.3	E863.1	—	E950.6	E962.1	E980.7
Parathormone	962.6	E858.0	E932.6	E950.4	E962.0	E980.4
Parathyroid (derivatives)	962.6	E858.0	E932.6	E950.4	E962.0	E980.4
Paratyphoid vaccine	978.1	E858.8	E948.1	E950.4	E962.0	E980.4
Paredrine	971.2	E855.5	E941.2	E950.4	E962.0	E980.4
Paregoric	965.00	E850.2	E935.2	E950.0	E962.0	E980.0
Pargyline	972.3	E858.3	E942.3	E950.4	E962.0	E980.4
Paris green	985.1	E866.3	—	E950.8	E962.1	E980.8
insecticide	985.1	E863.4	—	E950.8	E962.1	E980.8
Parnate	969.0	E854.0	E939.0	E950.3	E962.0	E980.3
Paromomycin	960.8	E856	E930.8	E950.4	E962.0	E980.4
Paroxypropione	963.1	E858.1	E933.1	E950.4	E962.0	E980.4
Parzone	965.09	E850.2	E935.2	E950.0	E962.0	E980.0
PAS	961.8	E857	E931.8	E950.4	E962.0	E980.4
PCBs	981	E862.3	—	E950.9	E962.1	E980.9
PCP (pentachlorophenol)	989.4	E863.6	—	E950.6	E962.1	E980.7
herbicide	989.4	E863.5	—	E950.6	E962.1	E980.7
insecticide	989.4	E863.4	—	E950.6	E962.1	E980.7
phencyclidine	968.3	E855.1	E938.3	E950.4	E962.0	E980.4
Peach kernel oil (emulsion)	973.2	E858.4	E943.2	E950.4	E962.0	E980.4
Peanut oil (emulsion) NEC	973.2	E858.4	E943.2	E950.4	E962.0	E980.4
topical	976.3	E858.7	E946.3	E950.4	E962.0	E980.4
Pearly Gates (morning glory seeds)	969.6	E854.1	E939.6	E950.3	E962.0	E980.3
Pecazine	969.1	E853.0	E939.1	E950.3	E962.0	E980.3
Pecilocin	960.1	E856	E930.1	E950.4	E962.0	E980.4
Pectin (with kaolin) NEC	973.5	E858.4	E943.5	E950.4	E962.0	E980.4
Pelletierine tannate	961.6	E857	E931.6	E950.4	E962.0	E980.4
Pemoline	969.7	E854.2	E939.7	E950.3	E962.0	E980.3
Pempidine	972.3	E858.3	E942.3	E950.4	E962.0	E980.4
Penamecillin	960.0	E856	E930.0	E950.4	E962.0	E980.4
Penethamate hydriodide	960.0	E856	E930.0	E950.4	E962.0	E980.4
Penicillamine	963.8	E858.1	E933.8	E950.4	E962.0	E980.4
Penicillin (any type)	960.0	E856	E930.0	E950.4	E962.0	E980.4
Penicillinase	963.4	E858.1	E933.4	E950.4	E962.0	E980.4
Pentachlorophenol (fungicide)	989.4	E863.6	—	E950.6	E962.1	E980.7
herbicide	989.4	E863.5	—	E950.6	E962.1	E980.7
insecticide	989.4	E863.4	—	E950.6	E962.1	E980.7
Pentaerythritol	972.4	E858.3	E942.4	E950.4	E962.0	E980.4
chloral	967.1	E852.0	E937.1	E950.2	E962.0	E980.2
tetranitrate NEC	972.4	E858.3	E942.4	E950.4	E962.0	E980.4
Pentagastrin	977.8	E858.8	E947.8	E950.4	E962.0	E980.4
Pentalin	982.3	E862.4	—	E950.9	E962.1	E980.9
Pentamethonium (bromide)	972.3	E858.3	E942.3	E950.4	E962.0	E980.4
Pentamidine	961.5	E857	E931.5	E950.4	E962.0	E980.4
Pentanol	980.8	E860.8	—	E950.9	E962.1	E980.9
Pentaquine	961.4	E857	E931.4	E950.4	E962.0	E980.4
Pentazocine	965.8	E850.8	E935.8	E950.0	E962.0	E980.0

Substance	Poisoning	External Cause (E-Code)				
		Accident	Therapeutic Use	Suicide Attempt	Assault	Undetermined
Penthienate	971.1	E855.4	E941.1	E950.4	E962.0	E980.4
Pentobarbital, pentobarbitone (sodium)	967.0	E851	E937.0	E950.1	E962.0	E980.1
Pentolinium (tartrate)	972.3	E858.3	E942.3	E950.4	E962.0	E980.4
Pentothal	968.3	E855.1	E938.3	E950.4	E962.0	E980.4
Pentylenetetrazol	970.0	E854.3	E940.0	E950.4	E962.0	E980.4
Pentylsalicylamide	961.8	E857	E931.8	E950.4	E962.0	E980.4
Pepsin	973.4	E858.4	E943.4	E950.4	E962.0	E980.4
Peptavlon	977.8	E858.8	E947.8	E950.4	E962.0	E980.4
Percaine (spinal)	968.7	E855.2	E938.7	E950.4	E962.0	E980.4
topical (surface)	968.5	E855.2	E938.5	E950.4	E962.0	E980.4
Perchloroethylene (vapor)	982.3	E862.4	—	E950.9	E962.1	E980.9
medicinal	961.6	E857	E931.6	E950.4	E962.0	E980.4
Percodan	965.09	E850.2	E935.2	E950.0	E962.0	E980.0
Percogesic	965.09	E850.2	E935.2	E950.0	E962.0	E980.0
Percorten	962.0	E858.0	E932.0	E950.4	E962.0	E980.4
Pergonal	962.4	E858.0	E932.4	E950.4	E962.0	E980.4
Perhexiline	972.4	E858.3	E942.4	E950.4	E962.0	E980.4
Periactin	963.0	E858.1	E933.0	E950.4	E962.0	E980.4
Periclor	967.1	E852.0	E937.1	E950.2	E962.0	E980.2
Pericyazine	969.1	E853.0	E939.1	E950.3	E962.0	E980.3
Peritrate	972.4	E858.3	E942.4	E950.4	E962.0	E980.4
Permanganates NEC	983.9	E864.3	—	E950.7	E962.1	E980.6
potassium (topical)	976.0	E858.7	E946.0	E950.4	E962.0	E980.4
Pernocton	967.0	E851	E937.0	E950.1	E962.0	E980.1
Pernoston	967.0	E851	E937.0	E950.1	E962.0	E980.1
Peronin(e)	965.09	E850.2	E935.2	E950.0	E962.0	E980.0
Perphenazine	969.1	E853.0	E939.1	E950.3	E962.0	E980.3
Pertofrane	969.0	E854	E939.0	E950.3	E962.0	E980.3
Pertussis	—	—	—	—	—	—
immune serum (human)	964.6	E858.2	E934.6	E950.4	E962.0	E980.4
vaccine (with diphtheria toxoid) (with tetanus toxoid)	978.6	E858.8	E948.6	E950.4	E962.0	E980.4
Peruvian balsam	976.8	E858.7	E946.8	E950.4	E962.0	E980.4
Pesticides (dust) (fumes) (vapor)	989.4	E863.4	—	E950.6	E962.1	E980.7
arsenic	985.1	E863.4	—	E950.8	E962.1	E980.8
chlorinated	989.2	E863.0	—	E950.6	E962.1	E980.7
cyanide	989.0	E863.4	—	E950.6	E962.1	E980.7
kerosene	981	E863.4	—	E950.6	E962.1	E980.7
mixture (of compounds)	989.4	E863.3	—	E950.6	E962.1	E980.7
naphthalene	983.0	E863.4	—	E950.7	E962.1	E980.6
organochlorine (compounds)	989.2	E863.0	—	E950.6	E962.1	E980.7
petroleum (distillate) (products) NEC	981	E863.4	—	E950.6	E962.1	E980.7
specified ingredient NEC	989.4	E863.4	—	E950.6	E962.1	E980.7
strychnine	989.1	E863.4	—	E950.6	E962.1	E980.7
thallium	985.8	E863.7	—	E950.6	E962.1	E980.7
Pethidine (hydrochloride)	965.09	E850.2	E935.2	E950.0	E962.0	E980.0
Petrichloral	967.1	E852.0	E937.1	E950.2	E962.0	E980.2
Petrol	981	E862.1	—	E950.9	E962.1	E980.9
vapor	987.1	E869.8	—	E952.8	E962.2	E982.8
Petrolatum (jelly) (ointment)	976.3	E858.7	E946.3	E950.4	E962.0	E980.4
hydrophilic	976.3	E858.7	E946.3	E950.4	E962.0	E980.4
liquid	973.2	E858.4	E943.2	E950.4	E962.0	E980.4
topical	976.3	E858.7	E946.3	E950.4	E962.0	E980.4
nonmedicinal	981	E862.1	—	E950.9	E962.1	E980.9
Petroleum (cleaners) (fuels) (products) NEC	981	E862.1	—	E950.9	E962.1	E980.9
benzin(e) - *see* Ligroin	—	—	—	—	—	—
ether - *see* Ligroin	—	—	—	—	—	—
jelly - *see* Petrolatum	—	—	—	—	—	—
aphtha - *see* Ligroin	—	—	—	—	—	—
pesticide	981	E863.4	—	E950.6	E962.1	E980.7
solids	981	E862.3	—	E950.9	E962.1	E980.9
solvents	981	E862.0	—	E950.9	E962.1	E980.9
vapor	987.1	E869.8	—	E952.8	E962.2	E982.8

Substance	Poisoning	External Cause (E-Code)				
		Accident	Therapeutic Use	Suicide Attempt	Assault	Undetermined
Peyote	969.6	E854.1	E939.6	E950.3	E962.0	E980.3
Phanodorm, phanodorn	967.0	E851	E937.0	E950.1	E962.0	E980.1
Phanquinone, phanquone	961.5	E857	E931.5	E950.4	E962.0	E980.4
Pharmaceutical excipient or adjunct	977.4	E858.8	E947.4	E950.4	E962.0	E980.4
Phenacemide	966.3	E855.0	E936.3	E950.4	E962.0	E980.4
Phenacetin	965.4	E850.4	E935.4	E950.0	E962.0	E980.0
Phenadoxone	965.09	E850.2	E935.2	E950.0	E962.0	E980.0
Phenaglycodol	969.5	E853.8	E939.5	E950.3	E962.0	E980.3
Phenantoin	966.1	E855.0	E936.1	E950.4	E962.0	E980.4
Phenaphthazine reagent	977.8	E858.8	E947.8	E950.4	E962.0	E980.4
Phenazocine	965.09	E850.2	E935.2	E950.0	E962.0	E980.0
Phenazone	965.5	E850.5	E935.5	E950.0	E962.0	E980.0
Phenazopyridine	976.1	E858.7	E946.1	E950.4	E962.0	E980.4
Phenbenicillin	960.0	E856	E930.0	E950.4	E962.0	E980.4
Phenbutrazate	977.0	E858.8	E947.0	E950.4	E962.0	E980.4
Phencyclidine	968.3	E855.1	E938.3	E950.4	E962.0	E980.4
Phendimetrazine	977.0	E858.8	E947.0	E950.4	E962.0	E980.4
Phenelzine	969.0	E854.0	E939.0	E950.3	E962.0	E980.3
Phenergan	967.8	E852.8	E937.8	E950.2	E962.0	E980.2
Phenethicillin (potassium)	960.0	E856	E930.0	E950.4	E962.0	E980.4
Phenetsal	965.1	E850.3	E935.3	E950.0	E962.0	E980.0
Pheneturide	966.3	E855.0	E936.3	E950.4	E962.0	E980.4
Phenformin	962.3	E858.0	E932.3	E950.4	E962.0	E980.4
Phenglutarimide	971.1	E855.4	E941.1	E950.4	E962.0	E980.4
Phenicarbazide	965.8	E850.8	E935.8	E950.0	E962.0	E980.0
Phenindamine (tartrate)	963.0	E858.1	E933.0	E950.4	E962.0	E980.4
Phenindione	964.2	E858.2	E934.2	E950.4	E962.0	E980.4
Pheniprazine	969.0	E854.0	E939.0	E950.3	E962.0	E980.3
Pheniramine (maleate)	963.0	E858.1	E933.0	E950.4	E962.0	E980.4
Phenmetrazine	977.0	E858.8	E947.0	E950.4	E962.0	E980.4
Phenobal	967.0	E851	E937.0	E950.1	E962.0	E980.1
Phenobarbital	967.0	E851	E937.0	E950.1	E962.0	E980.1
Phenobarbitone	967.0	E851	E937.0	E950.1	E962.0	E980.1
Phenoctide	976.0	E858.7	E946.0	E950.4	E962.0	E980.4
Phenol (derivatives) NEC	983.0	E864.0	—	E950.7	E962.1	E980.6
disinfectant	983.0	E864.0	—	E950.7	E962.1	E980.6
pesticide	989.4	E863.4	—	E950.6	E962.1	E980.7
red	977.8	E858.8	E947.8	E950.4	E962.0	E980.4
Phenolphthalein	973.1	E858.4	E943.1	E950.4	E962.0	E980.4
Phenolsulfonphthalein	977.8	E858.8	E947.8	E950.4	E962.0	E980.4
Phenomorphan	965.09	E850.2	E935.2	E950.0	E962.0	E980.0
Phenonyl	967.0	E851	E937.0	E950.1	E962.0	E980.1
Phenoperidine	965.09	E850.2	E935.2	E950.0	E962.0	E980.0
Phenoquin	974.7	E858.5	E944.7	E950.4	E962.0	E980.4
Phenothiazines (tranquilizers) NEC	969.1	E853.0	E939.1	E950.3	E962.0	E980.3
insecticide	989.3	E863.4	—	E950.6	E962.1	E980.7
Phenoxybenzamine	971.3	E855.6	E941.3	E950.4	E962.0	E980.4
Phenoxymethyl penicillin	960.0	E856	E930.0	E950.4	E962.0	E980.4
Phenprocoumon	964.2	E858.2	E934.2	E950.4	E962.0	E980.4
Phensuximide	966.2	E855.0	E936.2	E950.4	E962.0	E980.4
Phentermine	977.0	E858.8	E947.0	E950.4	E962.0	E980.4
Phentolamine	971.3	E855.6	E941.3	E950.4	E962.0	E980.4
Phenyl	—	—	—	—	—	—
butazone	965.5	E850.5	E935.5	E950.0	E962.0	E980.0
enediamine	983.0	E864.0	—	E950.7	E962.1	E980.6
hydrazine	983.0	E864.0	—	E950.7	E962.1	E980.6
antineoplastic	963.1	E858.1	E933.1	E950.4	E962.0	E980.4
mercuric compounds - *see* Mercury	—	—	—	—	—	—
salicylate	976.3	E858.7	E946.3	E950.4	E962.0	E980.4
Phenylephrine	971.2	E855.5	E941.2	E950.4	E962.0	E980.4
Phenylethylbiguanide	962.3	E858.0	E932.3	E950.4	E962.0	E980.4
Phenylpropanolamine	971.2	E855.5	E941.2	E950.4	E962.0	E980.4

Substance	Poisoning	External Cause (E-Code) Accident	Therapeutic Use	Suicide Attempt	Assault	Undetermined
Phenylsulfthion	989.3	E863.1	—	E950.6	E962.1	E980.7
Phenyramidol, phenyramidon	965.7	E850.7	E935.7	E950.0	E962.0	E980.0
Phenytoin	966.1	E855.0	E936.1	E950.4	E962.0	E980.4
pHisoHex	976.2	E858.7	E946.2	E950.4	E962.0	E980.4
Pholcodine	965.09	E850.2	E935.2	E950.0	E962.0	E980.0
Phorate	989.3	E863.1	—	E950.6	E962.1	E980.7
Phosdrin	989.3	E863.1	—	E950.6	E962.1	E980.7
Phosgene (gas)	987.8	E869.8	—	E952.8	E962.2	E982.8
Phosphate (tricresyl)	989.89	E866.8	—	E950.9	E962.1	E980.9
organic	989.3	E863.1	—	E950.6	E962.1	E980.7
solvent	982.8	E862.4	—	E950.9	E962.1	E980.9
Phosphine	987.8	E869.8	—	E952.8	E962.2	E982.8
fumigant	987.8	E863.8	—	E950.6	E962.2	E980.7
Phospholine	971.0	E855.3	E941.0	E950.4	E962.0	E980.4
Phosphoric acid	983.1	E864.1	—	E950.7	E962.1	E980.6
Phosphorus (compounds) NEC	983.9	E864.3	—	E950.7	E962.1	E980.6
rodenticide	983.9	E863.7	—	E950.7	E962.1	E980.6
Phthalimidoglutarimide	967.8	E852.8	E937.8	E950.2	E962.0	E980.2
Phthalylsulfathiazole	961.0	E857	E931.0	E950.4	E962.0	E980.4
Phylloquinone	964.3	E858.2	E934.3	E950.4	E962.0	E980.4
Physeptone	965.02	E850.1	E935.1	E950.0	E962.0	E980.0
Physostigma venenosum	988.2	E865.4	—	E950.9	E962.1	E980.9
Physostigmine	971.0	E855.3	E941.0	E950.4	E962.0	E980.4
Phytolacca decandra	988.2	E865.4	—	E950.9	E962.1	E980.9
Phytomenadione	964.3	E858.2	E934.3	E950.4	E962.0	E980.4
Phytonadione	964.3	E858.2	E934.3	E950.4	E962.0	E980.4
Picric (acid)	983.0	E864.0	—	E950.7	E962.1	E980.6
Picrotoxin	970.0	E854.3	E940.0	E950.4	E962.0	E980.4
Pilocarpine	971.0	E855.3	E941.0	E950.4	E962.0	E980.4
Pilocarpus (jaborandi) extract	971.0	E855.3	E941.0	E950.4	E962.0	E980.4
Pimaricin	960.1	E856	E930.1	E950.4	E962.0	E980.4
Piminodine	965.09	E850.2	E935.2	E950.0	E962.0	E980.0
Pine oil, pinesol (disinfectant)	983.9	E861.4	—	E950.7	E962.1	E980.6
Pinkroot	961.6	E857	E931.6	E950.4	E962.0	E980.4
Pipadone	965.09	E850.2	E935.2	E950.0	E962.0	E980.0
Pipamazine	963.0	E858.1	E933.0	E950.4	E962.0	E980.4
Pipazethate	975.4	E858.6	E945.4	E950.4	E962.0	E980.4
Pipenzolate	971.1	E855.4	E941.1	E950.4	E962.0	E980.4
Piperacetazine	969.1	E853.0	E939.1	E950.3	E962.0	E980.3
Piperazine NEC	961.6	E857	E931.6	E950.4	E962.0	E980.4
estrone sulfate	962.2	E858.0	E932.2	E950.4	E962.0	E980.4
Piper cubeba	988.2	E865.4	—	E950.9	E962.1	E980.9
Piperidione	975.4	E858.6	E945.4	E950.4	E962.0	E980.4
Piperidolate	971.1	E855.4	E941.1	E950.4	E962.0	E980.4
Piperocaine	968.9	E855.2	E938.9	E950.4	E962.0	E980.4
infiltration (subcutaneous)	968.5	E855.2	E938.5	E950.4	E962.0	E980.4
nerve block (peripheral) (plexus)	968.6	E855.2	E938.6	E950.4	E962.0	E980.4
topical (surface)	968.5	E855.2	E938.5	E950.4	E962.0	E980.4
Pipobroman	963.1	E858.1	E933.1	E950.4	E962.0	E980.4
Pipradrol	970.8	E854.3	E940.8	E950.4	E962.0	E980.4
Piscidia (bark) (erythrina)	965.7	E850.7	E935.7	E950.0	E962.0	E980.0
Pitch	983.0	E864.0	—	E950.7	E962.1	E980.6
Pitkin's solution	968.7	E855.2	E938.7	E950.4	E962.0	E980.4
Pitocin	975.0	E858.6	E945.0	E950.4	E962.0	E980.4
Pitressin (tannate)	962.5	E858.0	E932.5	E950.4	E962.0	E980.4
Pituitary extracts (posterior)	962.5	E858.0	E932.5	E950.4	E962.0	E980.4
anterior	962.4	E858.0	E932.4	E950.4	E962.0	E980.4
Pituitrin	962.5	E858.0	E932.5	E950.4	E962.0	E980.4
Placental extract	962.9	E858.0	E932.9	E950.4	E962.0	E980.4
Placidyl	967.8	E852.8	E937.8	E950.2	E962.0	E980.2
Plague vaccine	978.3	E858.8	E948.3	E950.4	E962.0	E980.4

Substance	Poisoning	External Cause (E-Code)				
		Accident	Therapeutic Use	Suicide Attempt	Assault	Undetermined
Plant foods or fertilizers NEC	989.89	E866.5	—	E950.9	E962.1	E980.9
mixed with herbicides	989.4	E863.5	—	E950.6	E962.1	E930.7
Plants, noxious, used as food	988.2	E865.9	—	E950.9	E962.1	E980.9
berries and seeds	988.2	E865.3	—	E950.9	E962.1	E980.9
specified type NEC	988.2	E865.4	—	E950.9	E962.1	E980.9
Plasma (blood)	964.7	E858.2	E934.7	E950.4	E962.0	E980.4
expanders	964.8	E858.2	E934.8	E950.4	E962.0	E980.4
Plasmanate	964.7	E858.2	E934.7	E950.4	E962.0	E980.4
Plegicil	969.1	E853.0	E939.1	E950.3	E962.0	E980.3
Podophyllin	976.4	E858.7	E946.4	E950.4	E962.0	E980.4
Podophyllum resin	976.4	E858.7	E946.4	E950.4	E962.0	E980.4
Poison NEC	989.9	E866.9	—	E950.9	E962.1	E980.9
Poisonous berries	988.2	E865.3	—	E950.9	E962.1	E980.9
Pokeweed (any part)	988.2	E865.4	—	E950.9	E962.1	E980.9
Poldine	971.1	E855.4	E941.1	E950.4	E962.0	E980.4
Poliomyelitis vaccine	979.5	E858.8	E949.5	E950.4	E962.0	E980.4
Poliovirus vaccine	979.5	E858.8	E949.5	E950.4	E962.0	E980.4
Polish (car) (floor) (furniture) (metal) (silver)	989.89	E861.2	—	E950.9	E962.1	E980.9
abrasive	989.89	E861.3	—	E950.9	E962.1	E980.9
porcelain	989.89	E861.3	—	E950.9	E962.1	E980.9
Poloxalkol	973.2	E858.4	E943.2	E950.4	E962.0	E980.4
Polyaminostyrene resins	974.5	E858.5	E944.5	E950.4	E962.0	E980.4
Polychlorinated biphenyl - *see* PCBs	—	—	—	—	—	—
Polycycline	960.4	E856	E930.4	E950.4	E962.0	E980.4
Polyester resin hardener	982.8	E862.4	—	E950.9	E962.1	E980.9
fumes	987.8	E869.8	—	E952.8	E962.2	E982.8
Polyestradiol (phosphate)	962.2	E858.0	E932.2	E950.4	E962.0	E980.4
Polyethanolamine alkyl sulfate	976.2	E858.7	E946.2	E950.4	E962.0	E980.4
Polyethylene glycol	976.3	E858.7	E946.3	E950.4	E962.0	E980.4
Polyferose	964.0	E858.2	E934.0	E950.4	E962.0	E980.4
Polymyxin B	960.8	E856	E930.8	E950.4	E962.0	E980.4
ENT agent	976.6	E858.7	E946.6	E950.4	E962.0	E980.4
ophthalmic preparation	976.5	E858.7	E946.5	E950.4	E962.0	E980.4
topical NEC	976.0	E858.7	E946.0	E950.4	E962.0	E980.4
Polynoxylin(e)	976.0	E858.7	E946.0	E950.4	E962.0	E980.4
Polyoxymethyleneurea	976.0	E858.7	E946.0	E950.4	E962.0	E980.4
Polytetrafluoroethylene (inhaled)	987.8	E869.8	—	E952.8	E962.2	E982.8
Polythiazide	974.3	E858.5	E944.3	E950.4	E962.0	E980.4
Polyvinylpyrrolidone	964.8	E858.2	E934.8	E950.4	E962.0	E980.4
Pontocaine (hydrochloride) (infiltration) (topical)	968.5	E855.2	E938.5	E950.4	E962.0	E980.4
nerve block (peripheral) (plexus)	968.6	E855.2	E938.6	E950.4	E962.0	E980.4
spinal	968.7	E855.2	E938.7	E950.4	E962.0	E980.4
Pot	969.6	E854.1	E939.6	E950.3	E962.0	E980.3
Potash (caustic)	983.2	E864.2	—	E950.7	E962.1	E980.6
Potassic saline injection (lactated)	974.5	E858.5	E944.5	E950.4	E962.0	E980.4
Potassium (salts) NEC	974.5	E858.5	E944.5	E950.4	E962.0	E980.4
aminosalicylate	961.8	E857	E931.8	E950.4	E962.0	E980.4
arsenite (solution)	985.1	E866.3	—	E950.8	E962.1	E980.8
bichromate	983.9	E864.3	—	E950.7	E962.1	E980.6
bisulfate	983.9	E864.3	—	E950.7	E962.1	E980.6
bromide (medicinal) NEC	967.3	E852.2	E937.3	E950.2	E962.0	E980.2
carbonate	983.2	E864.2	—	E950.7	E962.1	E980.6
chlorate NEC	983.9	E864.3	—	E950.7	E962.1	E980.6
cyanide - *see* Cyanide	—	—	—	—	—	—
hydroxide	983.2	E864.2	—	E950.7	E962.1	E980.6
iodide (expectorant) NEC	975.5	E858.6	E945.5	E950.4	E962.0	E980.4
nitrate	989.89	E866.8	—	E950.9	E962.1	E980.9
oxalate	983.9	E864.3	—	E950.7	E962.1	E980.6
perchlorate NEC	977.8	E858.8	E947.8	E950.4	E962.0	E980.4
antithyroid	962.8	E858.0	E932.8	E950.4	E962.0	E980.4
permanganate	976.0	E858.7	E946.0	E950.4	E962.0	E980.4
nonmedicinal	983.9	E864.3	—	E950.7	E962.1	E980.6

Substance	Poisoning	External Cause (E-Code)				
		Accident	Therapeutic Use	Suicide Attempt	Assault	Undetermined
Povidone-iodine (anti-infective) NEC	976.0	E858.7	E946.0	E950.4	E962.0	E980.4
Practolol	972.0	E858.3	E942.0	E950.4	E962.0	E980.4
Pralidoxime (chloride)	977.2	E858.8	E947.2	E950.4	E962.0	E980.4
Pramoxine	968.5	E855.2	E938.5	E950.4	E962.0	E980.4
Prazosin	972.6	E858.3	E942.6	E950.4	E962.0	E980.4
Prednisolone	962.0	E858.0	E932.0	E950.4	E962.0	E980.4
ENT agent	976.6	E858.7	E946.6	E950.4	E962.0	E980.4
ophthalmic preparation	976.5	E858.7	E946.5	E950.4	E962.0	E980.4
topical NEC	976.0	E858.7	E946.0	E950.4	E962.0	E980.4
Prednisone	962.0	E858.0	E932.0	E950.4	E962.0	E980.4
Pregnanediol	962.2	E858.0	E932.2	E950.4	E962.0	E990.4
Pregneninolone	962.2	E858.0	E932.2	E950.4	E962.0	E980.4
Preludin	977.0	E858.8	E947.0	E950.4	E962.0	E980.4
Premarin	962.2	E858.0	E932.2	E950.4	E962.0	E980.4
Prenylamine	972.4	E858.3	E942.4	E950.4	E962.0	E980.4
Preparation H	976.8	E858.7	E946.8	E950.4	E962.0	E980.4
Preservatives	989.89	E866.8	—	E950.9	E962.1	E980.9
Pride of China	988.2	E865.3	—	E950.9	E962.1	E980.9
Prilocaine	968.9	E855.2	E938.9	E950.4	E962.0	E980.4
infiltration (subcutaneous)	968.5	E855.2	E938.5	E950.4	E962.0	E980.4
nerve block (peripheral) (plexus)	968.6	E855.2	E938.6	E950.4	E962.0	E980.4
Primaquine	961.4	E857	E931.4	E950.4	E962.0	E980.4
Primidone	966.3	E855.0	E936.3	E950.4	E962.0	E980.4
Primula (veris)	988.2	E865.4	—	E950.9	E962.1	E980.9
Prinodol	965.09	E850.2	E935.2	E950.0	E962.0	E980.0
Priscol, Priscoline	971.3	E855.6	E941.3	E950.4	E962.0	E980.4
Privet	988.2	E865.4	—	E950.9	E962.1	E980.9
Privine	971.2	E855.5	E941.2	E950.4	E962.0	E980.4
Pro-Banthine	971.1	E855.4	E941.1	E950.4	E962.0	E980.4
Probarbital	967.0	E851	E937.0	E950.1	E962.0	E980.1
Probenecid	974.7	E858.5	E944.7	E950.4	E962.0	E990.4
Procainamide (hydrochloride)	972.0	E858.3	E942.0	E950.4	E962.0	E980.4
Procaine (hydrochloride) (infiltration) (topical)	968.5	E855.2	E938.5	E950.4	E962.0	E980.4
nerve block (periphreal) (plexus)	968.6	E855.2	E938.6	E950.4	E962.0	E980.4
penicillin G	960.0	E856	E930.0	E950.4	E962.0	E980.4
spinal	968.7	E855.2	E938.7	E950.4	E962.0	E980.4
Procalmidol	969.5	E853.8	E939.5	E950.3	E962.0	E980.3
Procarbazine	963.1	E858.1	E933.1	E950.4	E962.0	E980.4
Prochlorperazine	969.1	E853.0	E939.1	E950.3	E962.0	E980.3
Procyclidine	966.4	E855.0	E936.4	E950.4	E962.0	E980.4
Producer gas	986	E868.8	—	E952.1	E962.2	E982.1
Profenamine	966.4	E855.0	E936.4	E950.4	E962.0	E980.4
Profenil	975.1	E858.6	E945.1	E950.4	E962.0	E980.4
Progesterones	962.2	E858.0	E932.2	E950.4	E962.0	E980.4
Progestin	962.2	E858.0	E932.2	E950.4	E962.0	E980.4
Progestogens (with estrogens)	962.2	E858.0	E932.2	E950.4	E962.0	E980.4
Progestone	962.2	E858.0	E932.2	E950.4	E962.0	E980.4
Proguanil	961.4	E857	E931.4	E950.4	E962.0	E980.4
Prolactin	962.4	E858.0	E932.4	E950.4	E962.0	E980.4
Proloid	962.7	E858.0	E932.7	E950.4	E962.0	E980.4
Proluton	962.2	E858.0	E932.2	E950.4	E962.0	E980.4
Promacetin	961.8	E857	E931.8	E950.4	E962.0	E980.4
Promazine	969.1	E853.0	E939.1	E950.3	E962.0	E980.3
Promedrol	965.09	E850.2	E935.2	E950.0	E962.0	E980.0
Promethazine	967.8	E852.8	E937.8	E950.2	E962.0	E980.2
Promine	961.8	E857	E931.8	E950.4	E962.0	E980.4
Pronestyl (hydrochloride)	972.0	E858.3	E942.0	E950.4	E962.0	E980.4
Pronetalol, pronethalol	972.0	E858.3	E942.0	E950.4	E962.0	E980.4
Prontosil	961.0	E857	E931.0	E950.4	E962.0	E980.4
Propamidine isethionate	961.5	E857	E931.5	E950.4	E962.0	E980.4
Propanal (medicinal)	967.8	E852.8	E937.8	E950.2	E962.0	E980.2

◀ New ⟵ Revised

Substance	Poisoning	External Cause (E-Code)				
		Accident	Therapeutic Use	Suicide Attempt	Assault	Undetermined
Propane (gas) (distributed in mobile container)	987.0	E868.0	—	E951.1	E962.2	E981.1
distributed through pipes	987.0	E867	—	E951.0	E962.2	E981.0
incomplete combustion of - *see* Carbon monoxide, Propane	—	—	—	—	—	—
Propanidid	968.3	E855.1	E938.3	E950.4	E962.0	E980.4
Propanol	980.3	E860.4	—	E950.9	E962.1	E980.9
Propantheline	971.1	E855.4	E941.1	E950.4	E962.0	E980.4
Proparacaine	968.5	E855.2	E938.5	E950.4	E962.0	E980.4
Propatyl nitrate	972.4	E858.3	E942.4	E950.4	E962.0	E980.4
Propicillin	960.0	E856	E930.0	E950.4	E962.0	E980.4
Propiolactone (vapor)	987.8	E869.8	—	E952.8	E962.2	E982.8
Propiomazine	967.8	E852.8	E937.8	E950.2	E962.0	E980.2
Propionaldehyde (medicinal)	967.8	E852.8	E937.8	E950.2	E962.0	E980.2
Propionate compound	976.0	E858.7	E946.0	E950.4	E962.0	E980.4
Propion gel	976.0	E858.7	E946.0	E950.4	E962.0	E980.4
Propitocaine	968.9	E855.2	E938.9	E950.4	E962.0	E980.4
infiltration (subcutaneous)	968.5	E855.2	E938.5	E950.4	E962.0	E980.4
nerve block (peripheral) (plexus)	968.6	E855.2	E938.6	E950.4	E962.0	E980.4
Propoxur	989.3	E863.2	—	E950.6	E962.1	E980.7
Propoxycaine	968.9	E855.2	E938.9	E950.4	E962.0	E980.4
infiltration (subcutaneous)	968.5	E855.2	E938.5	E950.4	E962.0	E980.4
nerve block (peripheral) (plexus)	968.6	E855.2	E938.6	E950.4	E962.0	E980.4
topical (surface)	968.5	E855.2	E938.5	E950.4	E962.0	E980.4
Propoxyphene (hydrochloride)	965.8	E850.8	E935.8	E950.0	E962.0	E980.0
Propranolol	972.0	E858.3	E942.0	E950.4	E962.0	E980.4
Propyl	—	—	—	—	—	—
alcohol	980.3	E860.4	—	E950.9	E962.1	E980.9
carbinol	980.3	E860.4	—	E950.9	E962.1	E980.9
hexadrine	971.2	E855.5	E941.2	E950.4	E962.0	E980.4
iodone	977.8	E858.8	E947.8	E950.4	E962.0	E980.4
thiouracil	962.8	E858.0	E932.8	E950.4	E962.0	E980.4
Propylene	987.1	E869.8	—	E952.8	E962.2	E982.8
Propylparaben (ophthalmic)	976.5	E858.7	E946.5	E950.4	E962.0	E980.4
Proscillaridin	972.1	E858.3	E942.1	E950.4	E962.0	E980.4
Prostaglandins	975.0	E858.6	E945.0	E950.4	E962.0	E980.4
Prostigmin	971.0	E855.3	E941.0	E950.4	E962.0	E980.4
Protamine (sulfate)	964.5	E858.2	E934.5	E950.4	E962.0	E980.4
zinc insulin	962.3	E858.0	E932.3	E950.4	E962.0	E980.4
Protectants (topical)	976.3	E858.7	E946.3	E950.4	E962.0	E980.4
Protein hydrolysate	974.5	E858.5	E944.5	E950.4	E962.0	E980.4
Prothiaden - *see* Dothiepin hydrochloride	—	—	—	—	—	—
Prothionamide	961.8	E857	E931.8	E950.4	E962.0	E980.4
Prothipendyl	969.5	E853.8	E939.5	E950.3	E962.0	E980.3
Protokylol	971.2	E855.5	E941.2	E950.4	E962.0	E980.4
Protopam	977.2	E858.8	E947.2	E950.4	E962.0	E980.4
Protoveratrine(s) (A) (B)	972.6	E858.3	E942.6	E950.4	E962.0	E980.4
Protriptyline	969.0	E854.0	E939.0	E950.3	E962.0	E980.3
Provera	962.2	E858.0	E932.2	E950.4	E962.0	E980.4
Provitamin A	963.5	E858.1	E933.5	E950.4	E962.0	E980.4
Proxymetacaine	968.5	E855.2	E938.5	E950.4	E962.0	E980.4
Proxyphylline	975.1	E858.6	E945.1	E950.4	E962.0	E980.4
Prozac - *see* Fluoxetine hydrochloride	—	—	—	—	—	—
Prunus	—	—	—	—	—	—
laurocerasus	988.2	E865.4	—	E950.9	E962.1	E980.9
virginiana	988.2	E865.4	—	E950.9	E962.1	E980.9
Prussic acid	989.0	E866.8	—	E950.9	E962.1	E980.9
vapor	987.7	E869.8	—	E952.8	E962.2	E982.8
Pseudoephedrine	971.2	E855.5	E941.2	E950.4	E962.0	E980.4
Psilocin	969.6	E854.1	E939.6	E950.3	E962.0	E980.3
Psilocybin	969.6	E854.1	E939.6	E950.3	E962.0	E980.3
PSP	977.8	E858.8	E947.8	E950.4	E962.0	E980.4
Psychedelic agents	969.6	E854.1	E939.6	E950.3	E962.0	E980.3

Substance	Poisoning	External Cause (E-Code) Accident	Therapeutic Use	Suicide Attempt	Assault	Undetermined
Psychodysleptics	969.6	E854.1	E939.6	E950.3	E962.0	E980.3
Psychostimulants	969.7	E854.2	E939.7	E950.3	E962.0	E980.3
Psychotherapeutic agents	969.9	E855.9	E939.9	E950.3	E962.0	E980.3
antidepressants	969.0	E854.0	E939.0	E950.3	E962.0	E980.3
specified NEC	969.8	E855.8	E939.8	E950.3	E962.0	E980.3
tranquilizers NEC	969.5	E853.9	E939.5	E950.3	E962.0	E980.3
Psychotomimetic agents	969.6	E854.1	E939.6	E950.3	E962.0	E980.3
Psychotropic agents	969.9	E854.8	E939.9	E950.3	E962.0	E980.3
specified NEC	969.8	E854.8	E939.8	E950.3	E962.0	E980.3
Psyllium	973.3	E858.4	E943.3	E950.4	E962.0	E980.4
Pteroylglutamic acid	964.1	E858.2	E934.1	E950.4	E962.0	E980.4
Pteroyltriglutamate	963.1	E858.1	E933.1	E950.4	E962.0	E980.4
PTFE	987.8	E869.8	—	E952.8	E962.2	E982.8
Pulsatilla	988.2	E865.4	—	E950.9	E962.1	E980.9
Purex (bleach)	983.9	E864.3	—	E950.7	E962.1	E980.6
Purine diuretics	974.1	E858.5	E944.1	E950.4	E962.0	E980.4
Purinethol	963.1	E858.1	E933.1	E950.4	E962.0	E980.4
PVP	964.8	E858.2	E934.8	E950.4	E962.0	E980.4
Pyrabital	965.7	E850.7	E935.7	E950.0	E962.0	E980.0
Pyramidon	965.5	E850.5	E935.5	E950.0	E962.0	E980.0
Pyrantel (pamoate)	961.6	E857	E931.6	E950.4	E962.0	E980.4
Pyrathiazine	963.0	E858.1	E933.0	E950.4	E962.0	E980.4
Pyrazinamide	961.8	E857	E931.8	E950.4	E962.0	E980.4
Pyrazinoic acid (amide)	961.8	E857	E931.8	E950.4	E962.0	E980.4
Pyrazole (derivatives)	965.5	E850.5	E935.5	E950.0	E962.0	E980.0
Pyrazolone (analgesics)	965.5	E850.5	E935.5	E950.0	E962.0	E980.0
Pyrethrins, pyrethrum	989.4	E863.4	—	E950.6	E962.1	E980.7
Pyribenzamine	963.0	E858.1	E933.0	E950.4	E962.0	E980.4
Pyridine (liquid) (vapor)	982.0	E862.4	—	E950.9	E962.1	E980.9
aldoxime chloride	977.2	E858.8	E947.2	E950.4	E962.0	E980.4
Pyridium	976.1	E858.7	E946.1	E950.4	E962.0	E980.4
Pyridostigmine	971.0	E855.3	E941.0	E950.4	E962.0	E980.4
Pyridoxine	963.5	E858.1	E933.5	E950.4	E962.0	E980.4
Pyrilamine	963.0	E858.1	E933.0	E950.4	E962.0	E980.4
Pyrimethamine	961.4	E857	E931.4	E950.4	E962.0	E980.4
Pyrogallic acid	983.0	E864.0	—	E950.7	E962.1	E980.6
Pyroxylin	976.3	E858.7	E946.3	E950.4	E962.0	E980.4
Pyrrobutamine	963.0	E858.1	E933.0	E950.4	E962.0	E980.4
Pyrrocitine	968.5	E855.2	E938.5	E950.4	E962.0	E980.4
Pyrvinium (pamoate)	961.6	E857	E931.6	E950.4	E962.0	E980.4
PZI	962.3	E858.0	E932.3	E950.4	E962.0	E980.4
Quaalude	967.4	E852.3	E937.4	E950.2	E962.0	E980.2
Quaternary ammonium derivatives	971.1	E855.4	E941.1	E950.4	E962.0	E980.4
Quicklime	983.2	E864.2	—	E950.7	E962.1	E980.6
Quinacrine	961.3	E857	E931.3	E950.4	E962.0	E980.4
Quinaglute	972.0	E858.3	E942.0	E950.4	E962.0	E980.4
Quinalbarbitone	967.0	E851	E937.0	E950.1	E962.0	E980.1
Quinestradiol	962.2	E858.0	E932.2	E950.4	E962.0	E980.4
Quinethazone	974.3	E858.5	E944.3	E950.4	E962.0	E980.4
Quinidine (gluconate) (polygalacturonate) (salts) (sulfate)	972.0	E858.3	E942.0	E950.4	E962.0	E980.4
Quinine	961.4	E857	E931.4	E950.4	E962.0	E980.4
Quiniobine	961.3	E857	E931.3	E950.4	E962.0	E980.4
Quinolines	961.3	E857	E931.3	E950.4	E962.0	E980.4
Quotane	968.5	E855.2	E938.5	E950.4	E962.0	E980.4
Rabies	—	—	—	—	—	—
immune globulin (human)	964.6	E858.2	E934.6	E950.4	E962.0	E980.4
vaccine	979.1	E858.8	E949.1	E950.4	E962.0	E980.4
Racemoramide	965.09	E850.2	E935.2	E950.0	E962.0	E980.0
Racemorphan	965.09	E850.2	E935.2	E950.0	E962.0	E980.0
Radiator alcohol	980.1	E860.2	—	E950.9	E962.1	E980.9
Radio-opaque (drugs) (materials)	977.8	E858.8	E947.8	E950.4	E962.0	E980.4

◀ New ⟸ Revised

Substance	Poisoning	External Cause (E-Code)				
		Accident	Therapeutic Use	Suicide Attempt	Assault	Undetermined
Ranunculus	988.2	E865.4	—	E950.9	E962.1	E980.9
Rat poison	989.4	E863.7	—	E950.6	E962.1	E980.7
Rattlesnake (venom)	989.5	E905.0	—	E950.9	E962.1	E980.9
Raudixin	972.6	E858.3	E942.6	E950.4	E962.0	E980.4
Rautensin	972.6	E858.3	E942.6	E950.4	E962.0	E980.4
Rautina	972.6	E858.3	E942.6	E950.4	E962.0	E980.4
Rautotal	972.6	E858.3	E942.6	E950.4	E962.0	E980.4
Rauwiloid	972.6	E858.3	E942.6	E950.4	E962.0	E980.4
Rauwoldin	972.6	E858.3	E942.6	E950.4	E962.0	E980.4
Rauwolfia (alkaloids)	972.6	E858.3	E942.6	E950.4	E962.0	E980.4
Realgar	985.1	E866.3	—	E950.8	E962.1	E980.8
Red cells, packed	964.7	E858.2	E934.7	E950.4	E962.0	E980.4
Reducing agents, industrial NEC	983.9	E864.3	—	E950.7	E962.1	E980.6
Refrigerant gas (freon)	987.4	E869.2	—	E952.8	E962.2	E982.8
not freon	987.9	E869.9	—	E952.9	E962.2	E982.9
Regroton	974.4	E858.5	E944.4	E950.4	E962.0	E980.4
Rela	968.0	E855.1	E938.0	E950.4	E962.0	E980.4
Relaxants, skeletal muscle (autonomic)	975.2	E858.6	E945.2	E950.4	E962.0	E980.4
central nervous system	968.0	E855.1	E938.0	E950.4	E962.0	E980.4
Renese	974.3	E858.5	E944.3	E950.4	E962.0	E980.4
Renografin	977.8	E858.8	E947.8	E950.4	E962.0	E980.4
Replacement solutions	974.5	E858.5	E944.5	E950.4	E962.0	E980.4
Rescinnamine	972.6	E858.3	E942.6	E950.4	E962.0	E980.4
Reserpine	972.6	E858.3	E942.6	E950.4	E962.0	E980.4
Resorcin, resorcinol	976.4	E858.7	E946.4	E950.4	E962.0	E980.4
Respaire	975.5	E858.6	E945.5	E950.4	E962.0	E980.4
Respiratory agents NEC	975.8	E858.6	E945.8	E950.4	E962.0	E980.4
Retinoic acid	976.8	E858.7	E946.8	E950.4	E962.0	E980.4
Retinol	963.5	E858.1	E933.5	E950.4	E962.0	E980.4
Rh (D) immune globulin (human)	964.6	E858.2	E934.6	E950.4	E962.0	E980.4
Rhodine	965.1	E850.3	E935.3	E950.0	E962.0	E980.0
RhoGAM	964.6	E858.2	E934.6	E950.4	E962.0	E980.4
Riboflavin	963.5	E858.1	E933.5	E950.4	E962.0	E980.4
Ricin	989.89	E866.8	—	E950.9	E962.1	E980.9
Ricinus communis	988.2	E865.3	—	E950.9	E962.1	E980.9
Rickettsial vaccine NEC	979.6	E858.8	E949.6	E950.4	E962.0	E980.4
with viral and bacterial vaccine	979.7	E858.8	E949.7	E950.4	E962.0	E980.4
Rifampin	960.6	E856	E930.6	E950.4	E962.0	E980.4
Rimifon	961.8	E857	E931.8	E950.4	E962.0	E980.4
Ringer's injection (lactated)	974.5	E858.5	E944.5	E950.4	E962.0	E980.4
Ristocetin	960.8	E856	E930.8	E950.4	E962.0	E980.4
Ritalin	969.7	E854.2	E939.7	E950.3	E962.0	E980.3
Roach killers - *see* Pesticides	—	—	—	—	—	—
Rocky Mountain spotted fever vaccine	979.6	E858.8	E949.6	E950.4	E962.0	E980.4
Rodenticides	989.4	E863.7	—	E950.6	E962.1	E980.7
Rohypnol	969.4	E853.2	E939.4	E950.3	E962.0	E980.3
Rolaids	973.0	E858.4	E943.0	E950.4	E962.0	E980.4
Rolitetracycline	960.4	E856	E930.4	E950.4	E962.0	E980.4
Romilar	975.4	E858.6	E945.4	E950.4	E962.0	E980.4
Rose water ointment	976.3	E858.7	E946.3	E950.4	E962.0	E980.4
Rotenone	989.4	E863.7	—	E950.6	E962.1	E980.7
Rotoxamine	963.0	E858.1	E933.0	E950.4	E962.0	E980.4
Rough-on-rats	989.4	E863.7	—	E950.6	E962.1	E980.7
RU486	962.9	E858.0	E932.9	E950.4	E962.0	E980.4
Rubbing alcohol	980.2	E860.3	—	E950.9	E962.1	E980.9
Rubella virus vaccine	979.4	E858.8	E949.4	E950.4	E962.0	E980.4
Rubelogen	979.4	E858.8	E949.4	E950.4	E962.0	E980.4
Rubeovax	979.4	E858.8	E949.4	E950.4	E962.0	E980.4
Rubidomycin	960.7	E856	E930.7	E950.4	E962.0	E980.4
Rue	988.2	E865.4	—	E950.9	E962.1	E980.9
Ruta	988.2	E865.4	—	E950.9	E962.1	E980.9

Substance	Poisoning	External Cause (E-Code)				
		Accident	Therapeutic Use	Suicide Attempt	Assault	Undetermined
Sabadilla (medicinal)	976.0	E858.7	E946.0	E950.4	E962.0	E980.4
pesticide	989.4	E863.4	—	E950.6	E962.1	E980.7
Sabin oral vaccine	979.5	E858.8	E949.5	E950.4	E962.0	E980.4
Saccharated iron oxide	964.0	E858.2	E934.0	E950.4	E962.0	E980.4
Saccharin	974.5	E858.5	E944.5	E950.4	E962.0	E980.4
Safflower oil	972.2	E858.3	E942.2	E950.4	E962.0	E980.4
Salbutamol sulfate	975.7	E858.6	E945.7	E950.4	E962.0	E980.4
Salicylamide	965.1	E850.3	E935.3	E950.0	E962.0	E980.0
Salicylate(s)	965.1	E850.3	E935.3	E950.0	E962.0	E980.0
methyl	976.3	E858.7	E946.3	E950.4	E962.0	E980.4
theobromine calcium	974.1	E858.5	E944.1	E950.4	E962.0	E980.4
Salicylazosulfapyridine	961.0	E857	E931.0	E950.4	E962.0	E980.4
Salicylhydroxamic acid	976.0	E858.7	E946.0	E950.4	E962.0	E980.4
Salicylic acid (keratolytic) NEC	976.4	E858.7	E946.4	E950.4	E962.0	E980.4
congeners	965.1	E850.3	E935.3	E950.0	E962.0	E980.0
salts	965.1	E850.3	E935.3	E950.0	E962.0	E980.0
Saliniazid	961.8	E857	E931.8	E950.4	E962.0	E980.4
Salol	976.3	E858.7	E946.3	E950.4	E962.0	E980.4
Salt (substitute) NEC	974.5	E858.5	E944.5	E950.4	E962.0	E980.4
Saluretics	974.3	E858.5	E944.3	E950.4	E962.0	E980.4
Saluron	974.3	E858.5	E944.3	E950.4	E962.0	E980.4
Salvarsan 606 (neosilver) (silver)	961.1	E857	E931.1	E950.4	E962.0	E980.4
Sambucus canadensis	988.2	E865.4	—	E950.9	E962.1	E980.9
berry	988.2	E865.3	—	E950.9	E962.1	E980.9
Sandril	972.6	E858.3	E942.6	E950.4	E962.0	E980.4
Sanguinaria canadensis	988.2	E865.4	—	E950.9	E962.1	E980.9
Saniflush (cleaner)	983.9	E861.3	—	E950.7	E962.1	E980.6
Santonin	961.6	E857	E931.6	E950.4	E962.0	E980.4
Santyl	976.8	E858.7	E946.8	E950.4	E962.0	E980.4
Sarkomycin	960.7	E856	E930.7	E950.4	E962.0	E980.4
Saroten	969.0	E854.0	E939.0	E950.3	E962.0	E980.3
Saturnine - *see* Lead	—	—	—	—	—	—
Savin (oil)	976.4	E858.7	E946.4	E950.4	E962.0	E980.4
Scammony	973.1	E858.4	E943.1	E950.4	E962.0	E980.4
Scarlet red	976.8	E858.7	E946.8	E950.4	E962.0	E980.4
Scheele's green	985.1	E866.3	—	E950.8	E962.1	E980.8
insecticide	985.1	E863.4	—	E950.8	E962.1	E980.8
Schradan	989.3	E863.1	—	E950.6	E962.1	E980.7
Schweinfurt(h) green	985.1	E866.3	—	E950.8	E962.1	E980.8
insecticide	985.1	E863.4	—	E950.8	E962.1	E980.8
Scilla - *see* Squill	—	—	—	—	—	—
Sclerosing agents	972.7	E858.3	E942.7	E950.4	E962.0	E980.4
Scopolamine	971.1	E855.4	E941.1	E950.4	E962.0	E980.4
Scouring powder	989.89	E861.3	—	E950.9	E962.1	E980.9
Sea	—	—	—	—	—	—
anemone (sting)	989.5	E905.6	—	E950.9	E962.1	E980.9
cucumber (sting)	989.5	E905.6	—	E950.9	E962.1	E980.9
snake (bite) (venom)	989.5	E905.0	—	E950.9	E962.1	E980.9
urchin spine (puncture)	989.5	E905.6	—	E950.9	E962.1	E980.9
Secbutabarbital	967.0	E851	E937.0	E950.1	E962.0	E980.1
Secbutabarbitone	967.0	E851	E937.0	E950.1	E962.0	E980.1
Secobarbital	967.0	E851	E937.0	E950.1	E962.0	E980.1
Seconal	967.0	E851	E937.0	E950.1	E962.0	E980.1
Secretin	977.8	E858.8	E947.8	E950.4	E962.0	E980.4
Sedatives, nonbarbiturate	967.9	E852.9	E937.9	E950.2	E962.0	E980.2
specified NEC	967.8	E852.8	E937.8	E950.2	E962.0	E980.2
Sedormid	967.8	E852.8	E937.8	E950.2	E962.0	E980.2
Seed (plant)	988.2	E865.3	—	E950.9	E962.1	E980.9
disinfectant or dressing	989.89	E866.5	—	E950.9	E962.1	E980.9
Selenium (fumes) NEC	985.8	E866.4	—	E950.9	E962.1	E980.9
disulfide or sulfide	976.4	E858.7	E946.4	E950.4	E962.0	E980.4
Selsun	976.4	E858.7	E946.4	E950.4	E962.0	E980.4

Substance	Poisoning	External Cause (E-Code) Accident	Therapeutic Use	Suicide Attempt	Assault	Undetermined
Senna	973.1	E858.4	E943.1	E950.4	E962.0	E980.4
Septisol	976.2	E858.7	E946.2	E950.4	E962.0	E980.4
Serax	969.4	E853.2	E939.4	E950.3	E962.0	E980.3
Serenesil	967.8	E852.8	E937.8	E950.2	E962.0	E980.2
Serenium (hydrochloride)	961.9	E857	E931.9	E950.4	E962.0	E980.4
Serepax - *see* Oxazepam	—	—	—	—	—	—
Sernyl	968.3	E855.1	E938.3	E950.4	E962.0	E980.4
Serotonin	977.8	E858.8	E947.8	E950.4	E962.0	E980.4
Serpasil	972.6	E858.3	E942.6	E950.4	E962.0	E980.4
Sewer gas	987.8	E869.8	—	E952.8	E962.2	E982.8
Shampoo	989.6	E861.0	—	E950.9	E962.1	E980.9
Shellfish, nonbacterial or noxious	988.0	E865.1	—	E950.9	E962.1	E980.9
Silicones NEC	989.83	E866.8	E947.8	E950.9	E962.1	E980.9
Silvadene	976.0	E858.7	E946.0	E950.4	E962.0	E980.4
Silver (compound) (medicinal) NEC	976.0	E858.7	E946.0	E950.4	E962.0	E980.4
anti-infectives	976.0	E858.7	E946.0	E950.4	E962.0	E980.4
arsphenamine	961.1	E857	E931.1	E950.4	E962.0	E980.4
nitrate	976.0	E858.7	E946.0	E950.4	E962.0	E980.4
ophthalmic preparation	976.5	E858.7	E946.5	E950.4	E962.0	E980.4
toughened (keratolytic)	976.4	E858.7	E946.4	E950.4	E962.0	E980.4
nonmedicinal (dust)	985.8	E866.4	—	E950.9	E962.1	E980.9
protein (mild) (strong)	976.0	E858.7	E946.0	E950.4	E962.0	E980.4
salvarsan	961.1	E857	E931.1	E950.4	E962.0	E980.4
Simethicone	973.8	E858.4	E943.8	E950.4	E962.0	E980.4
Sinequan	969.0	E854.0	E939.0	E950.3	E962.0	E980.3
Singoserp	972.6	E858.3	E942.6	E950.4	E962.0	E980.4
Sintrom	964.2	E858.2	E934.2	E950.4	E962.0	E980.4
Sitosterols	972.2	E858.3	E942.2	E950.4	E962.0	E980.4
Skeletal muscle relaxants	975.2	E858.6	E945.2	E950.4	E962.0	E980.4
Skin	—	—	—	—	—	—
agents (external)	976.9	E858.7	E946.9	E950.4	E962.0	E980.4
specified NEC	976.8	E858.7	E946.8	E950.4	E962.0	E980.4
test antigen	977.8	E858.8	E947.8	E950.4	E962.0	E980.4
Sleep-eze	963.0	E858.1	E933.0	E950.4	E962.0	E980.4
Sleeping draught (drug) (pill) (tablet)	967.9	E852.9	E937.9	E950.2	E962.0	E980.2
Smallpox vaccine	979.0	E858.8	E949.0	E950.4	E962.0	E980.4
Smelter fumes NEC	985.9	E866.4	—	E950.9	E962.1	E980.9
Smog	987.3	E869.1	—	E952.8	E962.2	E982.8
Smoke NEC	987.9	E869.9	—	E952.9	E962.2	E982.9
Smooth muscle relaxant	975.1	E858.6	E945.1	E950.4	E962.0	E980.4
Snail killer	989.4	E863.4	—	E950.6	E962.1	E980.7
Snake (bite) (venom)	989.5	E905.0	—	E950.9	E962.1	E980.9
Snuff	989.89	E866.8	—	E950.9	E962.1	E980.9
Soap (powder) (product)	989.6	E861.1	—	E950.9	E962.1	E980.9
medicinal, soft	976.2	E858.7	E946.2	E950.4	E962.0	E980.4
Soda (caustic)	983.2	E864.2	—	E950.7	E962.1	E980.6
bicarb	963.3	E858.1	E933.3	E950.4	E962.0	E980.4
chlorinated - *see* Sodium, hypochlorite	—	—	—	—	—	—
Sodium	—	—	—	—	—	—
acetosulfone	961.8	E857	E931.8	E950.4	E962.0	E980.4
acetrizoate	977.8	E858.8	E947.8	E950.4	E962.0	E980.4
amytal	967.0	E851	E937.0	E950.1	E962.0	E980.1
arsenate - *see* Arsenic	—	—	—	—	—	—
bicarbonate	963.3	E858.1	E933.3	E950.4	E962.0	E980.4
bichromate	983.9	E864.3	—	E950.7	E962.1	E980.6
biphosphate	963.2	E858.1	E933.2	E950.4	E962.0	E980.4
bisulfate	983.9	E864.3	—	E950.7	E962.1	E980.6
borate (cleanser)	989.6	E861.3	—	E950.9	E962.1	E980.9
bromide NEC	967.3	E852.2	E937.3	E950.2	E962.0	E980.2
cacodylate (nonmedicinal) NEC	978.8	E858.8	E948.8	E950.4	E962.0	E980.4
anti-infective	961.1	E857	E931.1	E950.4	E962.0	E980.4
herbicide	989.4	E863.5	—	E950.6	E962.1	E980.7

Substance	Poisoning	Accident	Therapeutic Use	Suicide Attempt	Assault	Undetermined
		External Cause (E-Code)				
Sodium *(Continued)*						
calcium edetate	963.8	E858.1	E933.8	E950.4	E962.0	E980.4
carbonate NEC	983.2	E864.2	—	E950.7	E962.1	E980.6
chlorate NEC	983.9	E864.3	—	E950.7	E962.1	E980.6
herbicide	983.9	E863.5	—	E950.7	E962.1	E980.6
chloride NEC	974.5	E858.5	E944.5	E950.4	E962.0	E980.4
chromate	983.9	E864.3	—	E950.7	E962.1	E980.6
citrate	963.3	E858.1	E933.3	E950.4	E962.0	E980.4
cyanide - *see* Cyanide(s)	—	—	—	—	—	—
cyclamate	974.5	E858.5	E944.5	E950.4	E962.0	E980.4
diatrizoate	977.8	E858.8	E947.8	E950.4	E962.0	E980.4
dibunate	975.4	E858.6	E945.4	E950.4	E962.0	E980.4
dioctyl sulfosuccinate	973.2	E858.4	E943.2	E950.4	E962.0	E980.4
edetate	963.8	E858.1	E933.8	E950.4	E962.0	E980.4
ethacrynate	974.4	E858.5	E944.4	E950.4	E962.0	E980.4
fluoracetate (dust) (rodenticide)	989.4	E863.7	—	E950.6	E962.1	E980.7
fluoride - *see* Fluoride(s)	—	—	—	—	—	—
free salt	974.5	E858.5	E944.5	E950.4	E962.0	E980.4
glucosulfone	961.8	E857	E931.8	E950.4	E962.0	E980.4
hydroxide	983.2	E864.2	—	E950.7	E962.1	E980.6
hypochlorite (bleach) NEC	983.9	E864.3	—	E950.7	E962.1	E980.6
disinfectant	983.9	E861.4	—	E950.7	E962.1	E980.6
medicinal (anti-infective) (external)	976.0	E858.7	E946.0	E950.4	E962.0	E980.4
vapor	987.8	E869.8	—	E952.8	E962.2	E982.8
hyposulfite	976.0	E858.7	E946.0	E950.4	E962.0	E980.4
indigotindisulfonate	977.8	E858.8	E947.8	E950.4	E962.0	E980.4
iodide	977.8	E858.8	E947.8	E950.4	E962.0	E980.4
iothalamate	977.8	E858.8	E947.8	E950.4	E962.0	E980.4
iron edetate	964.0	E858.2	E934.0	E950.4	E962.0	E980.4
lactate	963.3	E858.1	E933.3	E950.4	E962.0	E980.4
lauryl sulfate	976.2	E858.7	E946.2	E950.4	E962.0	E980.4
L-triiodothyronine	962.7	E858.0	E932.7	E950.4	E962.0	E980.4
metrizoate	977.8	E858.8	E947.8	E950.4	E962.0	E980.4
monofluoracetate (dust) (rodenticide)	989.4	E863.7	—	E950.6	E962.1	E980.7
morrhuate	972.7	E858.3	E942.7	E950.4	E962.0	E980.4
nafcillin	960.0	E856	E930.0	E950.4	E962.0	E980.4
nitrate (oxidizing agent)	983.9	E864.3	—	E950.7	E962.1	E980.6
nitrite (medicinal)	972.4	E858.3	E942.4	E950.4	E962.0	E980.4
nitroferricyanide	972.6	E858.3	E942.6	E950.4	E962.0	E980.4
nitroprusside	972.6	E858.3	E942.6	E950.4	E962.0	E980.4
para-aminohippurate	977.8	E858.8	E947.8	E950.4	E962.0	E980.4
perborate (nonmedicinal) NEC	989.89	E866.8	—	E950.9	E962.1	E980.9
medicinal	976.6	E858.7	E946.6	E950.4	E962.0	E980.4
soap	989.6	E861.1	—	E950.9	E962.1	E980.9
percarbonate - *see* Sodium, perborate	—	—	—	—	—	—
phosphate	973.3	E858.4	E943.3	E950.4	E962.0	E980.4
polystyrene sulfonate	974.5	E858.5	E944.5	E950.4	E962.0	E980.4
propionate	976.0	E858.7	E946.0	E950.4	E962.0	E980.4
psylliate	972.7	E858.3	E942.7	E950.4	E962.0	E980.4
removing resins	974.5	E858.5	E944.5	E950.4	E962.0	E980.4
salicylate	965.1	E850.3	E935.3	E950.0	E962.0	E980.0
sulfate	973.3	E858.4	E943.3	E950.4	E962.0	E980.4
sulfoxone	961.8	E857	E931.8	E950.4	E962.0	E980.4
tetradecyl sulfate	972.7	E858.3	E942.7	E950.4	E962.0	E980.4
thiopental	968.3	E855.1	E938.3	E950.4	E962.0	E980.4
thiosalicylate	965.1	E850.3	E935.3	E950.0	E962.0	E980.0
thiosulfate	976.0	E858.7	E946.0	E950.4	E962.0	E980.4
tolbutamide	977.8	E858.8	E947.8	E950.4	E962.0	E980.4
tyropanoate	977.8	E858.8	E947.8	E950.4	E962.0	E980.4
valproate	966.3	E855.0	E936.3	E950.4	E962.0	E980.4
Solanine	977.8	E858.8	E947.8	E950.4	E962.0	E980.4

Substance	Poisoning	External Cause (E-Code)				
		Accident	Therapeutic Use	Suicide Attempt	Assault	Undetermined
Solanum dulcamara	988.2	E865.4	—	E950.9	E962.1	E980.9
Solapsone	961.8	E857	E931.8	E950.4	E962.0	E980.4
Solasulfone	961.8	E857	E931.8	E950.4	E962.0	E980.4
Soldering fluid	983.1	E864.1	—	E950.7	E962.1	E980.6
Solid substance	989.9	E866.9	—	E950.9	E962.1	E980.9
specified NEC	989.9	E866.8	—	E950.9	E962.1	E980.9
Solvents, industrial	982.8	E862.9	—	E950.9	E962.1	E980.9
naphtha	981	E862.0	—	E950.9	E962.1	E980.9
petroleum	981	E862.0	—	E950.9	E962.1	E980.9
specified NEC	982.8	E862.4	—	E950.9	E962.1	E980.9
Soma	968.0	E855.1	E938.0	E950.4	E962.0	E980.4
Somatotropin	962.4	E858.0	E932.4	E950.4	E962.0	E980.4
Sominex	963.0	E858.1	E933.0	E950.4	E962.0	E980.4
Somnos	967.1	E852.0	E937.1	E950.2	E962.0	E980.2
Somonal	967.0	E851	E937.0	E950.1	E962.0	E980.1
Soneryl	967.0	E851	E937.0	E950.1	E962.0	E980.1
Soothing syrup	977.9	E858.9	E947.9	E950.5	E962.0	E980.5
Sopor	967.4	E852.3	E937.4	E950.2	E962.0	E980.2
Soporific drug	967.9	E852.9	E937.9	E950.2	E962.0	E980.2
specified type NEC	967.8	E852.8	E937.8	E950.2	E962.0	E980.2
Sorbitol NEC	977.4	E858.8	E947.4	E950.4	E962.0	E980.4
Sotradecol	972.7	E858.3	E942.7	E950.4	E962.0	E980.4
Spacoline	975.1	E858.6	E945.1	E950.4	E962.0	E980.4
Spanish fly	976.8	E858.7	E946.8	E950.4	E962.0	E980.4
Sparine	969.1	E853.0	E939.1	E950.3	E962.0	E980.3
Sparteine	975.0	E858.6	E945.0	E950.4	E962.0	E980.4
Spasmolytics	975.1	E858.6	E945.1	E950.4	E962.0	E980.4
anticholinergics	971.1	E855.4	E941.1	E950.4	E962.0	E980.4
Spectinomycin	960.8	E856	E930.8	E950.4	E962.0	E980.4
Speed	969.7	E854.2	E939.7	E950.3	E962.0	E980.3
Spermicides	976.8	E858.7	E946.8	E950.4	E962.0	E980.4
Spider (bite) (venom)	989.5	E905.1	—	E950.9	E962.1	E980.9
antivenin	979.9	E858.8	E949.9	E950.4	E962.0	E980.4
Spigelia (root)	961.6	E857	E931.6	E950.4	E962.0	E980.4
Spiperone	969.2	E853.1	E939.2	E950.3	E962.0	E980.3
Spiramycin	960.3	E856	E930.3	E950.4	E962.0	E980.4
Spirilene	969.5	E853.8	E939.5	E950.3	E962.0	E980.3
Spirit(s) (neutral) NEC	980.0	E860.1	—	E950.9	E962.1	E980.9
beverage	980.0	E860.0	—	E950.9	E962.1	E980.9
industrial	980.9	E860.9	—	E950.9	E962.1	E980.9
mineral	981	E862.0	—	E950.9	E962.1	E980.9
of salt - *see* Hydrochloric acid	—	—	—	—	—	—
surgical	980.9	E860.9	—	E950.9	E962.1	E980.9
Spironolactone	974.4	E858.5	E944.4	E950.4	E962.0	E980.4
Sponge, absorbable (gelatin)	964.5	E858.2	E934.5	E950.4	E962.0	E980.4
Sporostacin	976.0	E858.7	E946.0	E950.4	E962.0	E980.4
Sprays (aerosol)	989.89	E866.8	—	E950.9	E962.1	E980.9
cosmetic	989.89	E866.7	—	E950.9	E962.1	E980.9
medicinal NEC	977.9	E858.9	E947.9	E950.5	E962.0	E980.5
pesticides - *see* Pesticides	—	—	—	—	—	—
specified content - *see* substance specified	—	—	—	—	—	—
Spurge flax	988.2	E865.4	—	E950.9	E962.1	E980.9
Spurges	988.2	E865.4	—	E950.9	E962.1	E980.9
Squill (expectorant) NEC	975.5	E858.6	E945.5	E950.4	E962.0	E980.4
rat poison	989.4	E863.7	—	E950.6	E962.1	E980.7
Squirting cucumber (cathartic)	973.1	E858.4	E943.1	E950.4	E962.0	E980.4
Stains	989.89	E866.8	—	E950.9	E962.1	E980.9
Stannous - *see also* Tin fluoride	976.7	E858.7	E946.7	E950.4	E962.0	E980.4
Stanolone	962.1	E858.0	E932.1	E950.4	E962.0	E980.4
Stanozolol	962.1	E858.0	E932.1	E950.4	E962.0	E980.4
Staphisagria or stavesacre (pediculicide)	976.0	E858.7	E946.0	E950.4	E962.0	E980.4

Substance	Poisoning	External Cause (E-Code) Accident	Therapeutic Use	Suicide Attempt	Assault	Undetermined
Stelazine	969.1	E853.0	E939.1	E950.3	E962.0	E980.3
Stemetil	969.1	E853.0	E939.1	E950.3	E962.0	E980.3
Sterculia (cathartic) (gum)	973.3	E858.4	E943.3	E950.4	E962.0	E980.4
Sternutator gas	987.8	E869.8	—	E952.8	E962.2	E982.8
Steroids NEC	962.0	E858.0	E932.0	E950.4	E962.0	E980.4
ENT agent	976.6	E858.7	E946.6	E950.4	E962.0	E980.4
ophthalmic preparation	976.5	E858.7	E946.5	E950.4	E962.0	E980.4
topical NEC	976.0	E858.7	E946.0	E950.4	E962.0	E980.4
Stibine	985.8	E866.4	—	E950.9	E962.1	E980.9
Stibophen	961.2	E857	E931.2	E950.4	E962.0	E980.4
Stilbamide, stilbamidine	961.5	E857	E931.5	E950.4	E962.0	E980.4
Stilbestrol	962.2	E858.0	E932.2	E950.4	E962.0	E980.4
Stimulants (central nervous system)	970.9	E854.3	E940.9	E950.4	E962.0	E980.4
analeptics	970.0	E854.3	E940.0	E950.4	E962.0	E980.4
opiate antagonist	970.1	E854.3	E940.1	E950.4	E962.0	E980.4
psychotherapeutic NEC	969.0	E854.0	E939.0	E950.3	E962.0	E980.3
specified NEC	970.8	E854.3	E940.8	E950.4	E962.0	E980.4
Storage batteries (acid) (cells)	983.1	E864.1	—	E950.7	E962.1	E980.6
Stovaine	968.9	E855.2	E938.9	E950.4	E962.0	E980.4
infiltration (subcutaneous)	968.5	E855.2	E938.5	E950.4	E962.0	E980.4
nerve block (peripheral) (plexus)	968.6	E855.2	E938.6	E950.4	E962.0	E980.4
spinal	968.7	E855.2	E938.7	E950.4	E962.0	E980.4
topical (surface)	968.5	E855.2	E938.5	E950.4	E962.0	E980.4
Stovarsal	961.1	E857	E931.1	E950.4	E962.0	E980.4
Stove gas - *see* Gas, utility	—	—	—	—	—	—
Stoxil	976.5	E858.7	E946.5	E950.4	E962.0	E980.4
STP	969.6	E854.1	E939.6	E950.3	E962.0	E980.3
Stramonium (medicinal) NEC	971.1	E855.4	E941.1	E950.4	E962.0	E980.4
natural state	988.2	E865.4	—	E950.9	E962.1	E980.9
Streptodornase	964.4	E858.2	E934.4	E950.4	E962.0	E980.4
Streptoduocin	960.6	E856	E930.6	E950.4	E962.0	E980.4
Streptokinase	964.4	E858.2	E934.4	E950.4	E962.0	E980.4
Streptomycin	960.6	E856	E930.6	E950.4	E962.0	E980.4
Streptozocin	960.7	E856	E930.7	E950.4	E962.0	E980.4
Stripper (paint) (solvent)	982.8	E862.9	—	E950.9	E962.1	E980.9
Strobane	989.2	E863.0	—	E950.6	E962.1	E980.7
Strophanthin	972.1	E858.3	E942.1	E950.4	E962.0	E980.4
Strophanthus hispidus or kombe	988.2	E865.4	—	E950.9	E962.1	E980.9
Strychnine (rodenticide) (salts)	989.1	E863.7	—	E950.6	E962.1	E980.7
medicinal NEC	970.8	E854.3	E940.8	E950.4	E962.0	E980.4
Strychnos (ignatii) - *see* Strychnine	—	—	—	—	—	—
Styramate	968.0	E855.1	E938.0	E950.4	E962.0	E980.4
Styrene	983.0	E864.0	—	E950.7	E962.1	E980.6
Succinimide (anticonvulsant)	966.2	E855.0	E936.2	E950.4	E962.0	E980.4
mercuric - *see* Mercury	—	—	—	—	—	—
Succinylcholine	975.2	E858.6	E945.2	E950.4	E962.0	E980.4
Succinylsulfathiazole	961.0	E857	E931.0	E950.4	E962.0	E980.4
Sucrose	974.5	E858.5	E944.5	E950.4	E962.0	E980.4
Sulfacetamide	961.0	E857	E931.0	E950.4	E962.0	E980.4
ophthalmic preparation	976.5	E858.7	E946.5	E950.4	E962.0	E980.4
Sulfachlorpyridazine	961.0	E857	E931.0	E950.4	E962.0	E980.4
Sulfacytine	961.0	E857	E931.0	E950.4	E962.0	E980.4
Sulfadiazine	961.0	E857	E931.0	E950.4	E962.0	E980.4
silver (topical)	976.0	E858.7	E946.0	E950.4	E962.0	E980.4
Sulfadimethoxine	961.0	E857	E931.0	E950.4	E962.0	E980.4
Sulfadimidine	961.0	E857	E931.0	E950.4	E962.0	E980.4
Sulfaethidole	961.0	E857	E931.0	E950.4	E962.0	E980.4
Sulfafurazole	961.0	E857	E931.0	E950.4	E962.0	E980.4
Sulfaguanidine	961.0	E857	E931.0	E950.4	E962.0	E980.4
Sulfamerazine	961.0	E857	E931.0	E950.4	E962.0	E980.4
Sulfameter	961.0	E857	E931.0	E950.4	E962.0	E980.4

◀ New ⟸ Revised

Substance	Poisoning	External Cause (E-Code) Accident	Therapeutic Use	Suicide Attempt	Assault	Undetermined
Sulfamethizole	961.0	E857	E931.0	E950.4	E962.0	E980.4
Sulfamethoxazole	961.0	E857	E931.0	E950.4	E962.0	E980.4
Sulfamethoxydiazine	961.0	E857	E931.0	E950.4	E962.0	E980.4
Sulfamethoxypyridazine	961.0	E857	E931.0	E950.4	E962.0	E980.4
Sulfamethylthiazole	961.0	E857	E931.0	E950.4	E962.0	E980.4
Sulfamylon	976.0	E858.7	E946.0	E950.4	E962.0	E980.4
Sulfan blue (diagnostic dye)	977.8	E858.8	E947.8	E950.4	E962.0	E980.4
Sulfanilamide	961.0	E857	E931.0	E950.4	E962.0	E980.4
Sulfanilylguanidine	961.0	E857	E931.0	E950.4	E962.0	E980.4
Sulfaphenazole	961.0	E857	E931.0	E950.4	E962.0	E980.4
Sulfaphenylthiazole	961.0	E857	E931.0	E950.4	E962.0	E980.4
Sulfaproxyline	961.0	E857	E931.0	E950.4	E962.0	E980.4
Sulfapyridine	961.0	E857	E931.0	E950.4	E962.0	E980.4
Sulfapyrimidine	961.0	E857	E931.0	E950.4	E962.0	E980.4
Sulfarsphenamine	961.1	E857	E931.1	E950.4	E962.0	E980.4
Sulfasalazine	961.0	E857	E931.0	E950.4	E962.0	E980.4
Sulfasomizole	961.0	E857	E931.0	E950.4	E962.0	E980.4
Sulfasuxidine	961.0	E857	E931.0	E950.4	E962.0	E980.4
Sulfinpyrazone	974.7	E858.5	E944.7	E950.4	E962.0	E980.4
Sulfisoxazole	961.0	E857	E931.0	E950.4	E962.0	E980.4
ophthalmic preparation	976.5	E858.7	E946.5	E950.4	E962.0	E980.4
Sulfomyxin	960.8	E856	E930.8	E950.4	E962.0	E980.4
Sulfonal	967.8	E852.8	E937.8	E950.2	E962.0	E980.2
Sulfonamides (mixtures)	961.0	E857	E931.0	E950.4	E962.0	E980.4
Sulfones	961.8	E857	E931.8	E950.4	E962.0	E980.4
Sulfonethylmethane	967.8	E852.8	E937.8	E950.2	E962.0	E980.2
Sulfonmethane	967.8	E852.8	E937.8	E950.2	E962.0	E980.2
Sulfonphthal, sulfonphthol	977.8	E858.8	E947.8	E950.4	E962.0	E980.4
Sulfonylurea derivatives, oral	962.3	E858.0	E932.3	E950.4	E962.0	E980.4
Sulfoxone	961.8	E857	E931.8	E950.4	E962.0	E980.4
Sulfur, sulfureted, sulfuric, sulfurous, sulfuryl (compounds) NEC	989.89	E866.8	—	E950.9	E962.1	E980.9
acid	983.1	E864.1	—	E950.7	E962.1	E980.6
dioxide	987.3	E869.1	—	E952.8	E962.2	E982.8
ether - *see* Ether(s)	—	—	—	—	—	—
hydrogen	987.8	E869.8	—	E952.8	E962.2	E982.8
medicinal (keratolytic) (ointment) NEC	976.4	E858.7	E946.4	E950.4	E962.0	E980.4
pesticide (vapor)	989.4	E863.4	—	E950.6	E962.1	E980.7
vapor NEC	987.8	E869.8	—	E952.8	E962.2	E982.8
Sulkowitch's reagent	977.8	E858.8	E947.8	E950.4	E962.0	E980.4
Sulph - *see also* Sulf-	—	—	—	—	—	—
Sulphadione	961.8	E857	E931.8	E950.4	E962.0	E980.4
Sulthiame, sultiame	966.3	E855.0	E936.3	E950.4	E962.0	E980.4
Superinone	975.5	E858.6	E945.5	E950.4	E962.0	E980.4
Suramin	961.5	E857	E931.5	E950.4	E962.0	E980.4
Surfacaine	968.5	E855.2	E938.5	E950.4	E962.0	E980.4
Surital	968.3	E855.1	E938.3	E950.4	E962.0	E980.4
Sutilains	976.8	E858.7	E946.8	E950.4	E962.0	E980.4
Suxamethonium (bromide) (chloride) (iodide)	975.2	E858.6	E945.2	E950.4	E962.0	E980.4
Suxethonium (bromide)	975.2	E858.6	E945.2	E950.4	E962.0	E980.4
Sweet oil (birch)	976.3	E858.7	E946.3	E950.4	E962.0	E980.4
Sym-dichloroethyl ether	982.3	E862.4	—	E950.9	E962.1	E980.9
Sympatholytics	971.3	E855.6	E941.3	E950.4	E962.0	E980.4
Sympathomimetics	971.2	E855.5	E941.2	E950.4	E962.0	E980.4
Synagis	979.6	E858.8	E949.6	E950.4	E962.0	E980.4
Synalar	976.0	E858.7	E946.0	E950.4	E962.0	E980.4
Synthroid	962.7	E858.0	E932.7	E950.4	E962.0	E980.4
Syntocinon	975.0	E858.6	E945.0	E950.4	E962.0	E950.4
Syrosingopine	972.6	E858.3	E942.6	E950.4	E962.0	E980.4
Systemic agents (primarily)	963.9	E858.1	E933.9	E950.4	E962.0	E980.4
specified NEC	963.8	E858.1	E933.8	E950.4	E962.0	E980.4
Tablets (*see also* specified substance)	977.9	E858.9	E947.9	E950.5	E962.0	E980.5

Substance	Poisoning	External Cause (E-Code) Accident	Therapeutic Use	Suicide Attempt	Assault	Undetermined
Tace	962.2	E858.0	E932.2	E950.4	E962.0	E980.4
Tacrine	971.0	E855.3	E941.0	E950.4	E962.0	E980.4
Talbutal	967.0	E851	E937.0	E950.1	E962.0	E980.1
Talc	976.3	E858.7	E946.3	E950.4	E962.0	E980.4
Talcum	976.3	E858.7	E946.3	E950.4	E962.0	E980.4
Tandearil, tanderil	965.5	E850.5	E935.5	E950.0	E962.0	E980.0
Tannic acid	983.1	E864.1	—	E950.7	E962.1	E980.6
medicinal (astringent)	976.2	E858.7	E946.2	E950.4	E962.0	E980.4
Tannin - *see* Tannic acid	—	—	—	—	—	—
Tansy	988.2	E865.4	—	E950.9	E962.1	E980.9
TAO	960.3	E856	E930.3	E950.4	E962.0	E980.4
Tapazole	962.8	E858.0	E932.8	E950.4	E962.0	E980.4
Tar NEC	983.0	E864.0	—	E950.7	E962.1	E980.6
camphor - *see* Naphthalene	—	—	—	—	—	—
fumes	987.8	E869.8	—	E952.8	E962.2	E982.8
Taractan	969.3	E853.8	E939.3	E950.3	E962.0	E980.3
Tarantula (venomous)	989.5	E905.1	—	E950.9	E962.1	E980.9
Tartar emetic (anti-infective)	961.2	E857	E931.2	E950.4	E962.0	E980.4
Tartaric acid	983.1	E864.1	—	E950.7	E962.1	E980.6
Tartrated antimony (anti-infective)	961.2	E857	E931.2	E950.4	E962.0	E980.4
TCA - *see* Trichloroacetic acid	—	—	—	—	—	—
TDI	983.0	E864.0	—	E950.7	E962.1	E980.6
vapor	987.8	E869.8	—	E952.8	E962.2	E982.8
Tear gas	987.5	E869.3	—	E952.8	E962.2	E982.8
Teclothiazide	974.3	E858.5	E944.3	E950.4	E962.0	E980.4
Tegretol	966.3	E855.0	E936.3	E950.4	E962.0	E980.4
Telepaque	977.8	E858.8	E947.8	E950.4	E962.0	E980.4
Tellurium	985.8	E866.4	—	E950.9	E962.1	E980.9
fumes	985.8	E866.4	—	E950.9	E962.1	E980.9
TEM	963.1	E858.1	E933.1	E950.4	E962.0	E980.4
Temazepam - *see* Benzodiazepines	—	—	—	—	—	—
TEPA	963.1	E858.1	E933.1	E950.4	E962.0	E980.4
TEPP	989.3	E863.1	—	E950.6	E962.1	E980.7
Terbutaline	971.2	E855.5	E941.2	E950.4	E962.0	E980.4
Teroxalene	961.6	E857	E931.6	E950.4	E962.0	E980.4
Terpin hydrate	975.5	E858.6	E945.5	E950.4	E962.0	E980.4
Terramycin	960.4	E856	E930.4	E950.4	E962.0	E980.4
Tessalon	975.4	E858.6	E945.4	E950.4	E962.0	E980.4
Testosterone	962.1	E858.0	E932.1	E950.4	E962.0	E980.4
Tetanus (vaccine)	978.4	E858.8	E948.4	E950.4	E962.0	E980.4
antitoxin	979.9	E858.8	E949.9	E950.4	E962.0	E980.4
immune globulin (human)	964.6	E858.2	E934.6	E950.4	E962.0	E980.4
toxoid	978.4	E858.8	E948.4	E950.4	E962.0	E980.4
with diphtheria toxoid	978.9	E858.8	E948.9	E950.4	E962.0	E980.4
with pertussis	978.6	E858.8	E948.6	E950.4	E962.0	E980.4
Tetrabenazine	969.5	E853.8	E939.5	E950.3	E962.0	E980.3
Tetracaine (infiltration) (topical)	968.5	E855.2	E938.5	E950.4	E962.0	E980.4
nerve block (peripheral) (plexus)	968.6	E855.2	E938.6	E950.4	E962.0	E980.4
spinal	968.7	E855.2	E938.7	E950.4	E962.0	E980.4
Tetrachlorethylene - *see* Tetrachloroethylene	—	—	—	—	—	—
Tetrachlormethiazide	974.3	E858.5	E944.3	E950.4	E962.0	E980.4
Tetrachloroethane (liquid) (vapor)	982.3	E862.4	—	E950.9	E962.1	E980.9
paint or varnish	982.3	E861.6	—	E950.9	E962.1	E980.9
Tetrachloroethylene (liquid) (vapor)	982.3	E862.4	—	E950.9	E962.1	E980.9
medicinal	961.6	E857	E931.6	E950.4	E962.0	E980.4
Tetrachloromethane - *see* Carbon, tetrachloride	—	—	—	—	—	—
Tetracycline	960.4	E856	E930.4	E950.4	E962.0	E980.4
ophthalmic preparation	976.5	E858.7	E946.5	E950.4	E962.0	E980.4
topical NEC	976.0	E858.7	E946.0	E950.4	E962.0	E980.4
Tetraethylammonium chloride	972.3	E858.3	E942.3	E950.4	E962.0	E980.4
Tetraethyl lead (antiknock compound)	984.1	E862.1	—	E950.9	E962.1	E980.9

◀ New ⬅ Revised

Substance	Poisoning	External Cause (E-Code) Accident	Therapeutic Use	Suicide Attempt	Assault	Undetermined
Tetraethyl pyrophosphate	989.3	E863.1	—	E950.6	E962.1	E980.7
Tetraethylthiuram disulfide	977.3	E858.8	E947.3	E950.4	E962.0	E980.4
Tetrahydroaminoacridine	971.0	E855.3	E941.0	E950.4	E962.0	E980.4
Tetrahydrocannabinol	969.6	E854.1	E939.6	E950.3	E962.0	E980.3
Tetrahydronaphthalene	982.0	E862.4	—	E950.9	E962.1	E980.9
Tetrahydrozoline	971.2	E855.5	E941.2	E950.4	E962.0	E980.4
Tetralin	982.0	E862.4	—	E950.9	E962.1	E980.9
Tetramethylthiuram (disulfide) NEC	989.4	E863.6	—	E950.6	E962.1	E980.7
medicinal	976.2	E858.7	E946.2	E950.4	E962.0	E980.4
Tetronal	967.8	E852.8	E937.8	E950.2	E962.0	E980.2
Tetryl	983.0	E864.0	—	E950.7	E962.1	E980.6
Thalidomide	967.8	E852.8	E937.8	E950.2	E962.0	E980.2
Thallium (compounds) (dust) NEC	985.8	E866.4	—	E950.9	E962.1	E980.9
pesticide (rodenticide)	985.8	E863.7	—	E950.6	E962.1	E980.7
THC	969.6	E854.1	E939.6	E950.3	E962.0	E980.3
Thebacon	965.09	E850.2	E935.2	E950.0	E962.0	E980.0
Thebaine	965.09	E850.2	E935.2	E950.0	E962.0	E980.0
Theobromine (calcium salicylate)	974.1	E858.5	E944.1	E950.4	E962.0	E980.4
Theophylline (diuretic)	974.1	E858.5	E944.1	E950.4	E962.0	E980.4
ethylenediamine	975.7	E858.6	E945.7	E950.4	E962.0	E980.4
Thiabendazole	961.6	E857	E931.6	E950.4	E962.0	E980.4
Thialbarbital, thialbarbitone	968.3	E855.1	E938.3	E950.4	E962.0	E980.4
Thiamine	963.5	E858.1	E933.5	E950.4	E962.0	E980.4
Thiamylal (sodium)	968.3	E855.1	E938.3	E950.4	E962.0	E980.4
Thiazesim	969.0	E854.0	E939.0	E950.3	E962.0	E980.3
Thiazides (diuretics)	974.3	E858.5	E944.3	E950.4	E962.0	E980.4
Thiethylperazine	963.0	E858.1	E933.0	E950.4	E962.0	E980.4
Thimerosal (topical)	976.0	E858.7	E946.0	E950.4	E962.0	E980.4
ophthalmic preparation	976.5	E858.7	E946.5	E950.4	E962.0	E980.4
Thioacetazone	961.8	E857	E931.8	E950.4	E962.0	E980.4
Thiobarbiturates	968.3	E855.1	E938.3	E950.4	E962.0	E980.4
Thiobismol	961.2	E857	E931.2	E950.4	E962.0	E980.4
Thiocarbamide	962.8	E858.0	E932.8	E950.4	E962.0	E980.4
Thiocarbarsone	961.1	E857	E931.1	E950.4	E962.0	E980.4
Thiocarlide	961.8	E857	E931.8	E950.4	E962.0	E980.4
Thioguanine	963.1	E858.1	E933.1	E950.4	E962.0	E980.4
Thiomercaptomerin	974.0	E858.5	E944.0	E950.4	E962.0	E980.4
Thiomerin	974.0	E858.5	E944.0	E950.4	E962.0	E980.4
Thiopental, thiopentone (sodium)	968.3	E855.1	E938.3	E950.4	E962.0	E980.4
Thiopropazate	969.1	E853.0	E939.1	E950.3	E962.0	E980.3
Thioproperazine	969.1	E853.0	E939.1	E950.3	E962.0	E980.3
Thioridazine	969.1	E853.0	E939.1	E950.3	E962.0	E980.3
Thio-TEPA, thiotepa	963.1	E858.1	E933.1	E950.4	E962.0	E980.4
Thiothixene	969.3	E853.8	E939.3	E950.3	E962.0	E980.3
Thiouracil	962.8	E858.0	E932.8	E950.4	E962.0	E980.4
Thiourea	962.8	E858.0	E932.8	E950.4	E962.0	E980.4
Thiphenamil	971.1	E855.4	E941.1	E950.4	E962.0	E980.4
Thiram NEC	989.4	E863.	—	E950.6	E962.1	E980.7
medicinal	976.2	E858.7	E946.2	E950.4	E962.0	E980.4
Thonzylamine	963.0	E858.1	E933.0	E950.4	E962.0	E980.4
Thorazine	969.1	E853.0	E939.1	E950.3	E962.0	E980.3
Thornapple	988.2	E865.4	—	E950.9	E962.1	E980.9
Throat preparation (lozenges) NEC	976.6	E858.7	E946.6	E950.4	E962.0	E980.4
Thrombin	964.5	E858.2	E934.5	E950.4	E962.0	E980.4
Thrombolysin	964.4	E858.2	E934.4	E950.4	E962.0	E980.4
Thymol	983.0	E864.0	—	E950.7	E962.1	E980.6
Thymus extract	962.9	E858.0	E932.9	E950.4	E962.0	E980.4
Thyroglobulin	962.7	E858.0	E932.7	E950.4	E962.0	E980.4
Thyroid (derivatives) (extract)	962.7	E858.0	E932.7	E950.4	E962.0	E980.4
Thyrolar	962.7	E858.0	E932.7	E950.4	E962.0	E980.4
Thyrotrophin, thyrotropin	977.8	E858.8	E947.8	E950.4	E962.0	E980.4

Substance	Poisoning	External Cause (E-Code) Accident	Therapeutic Use	Suicide Attempt	Assault	Undetermined
Thyroxin(e)	962.7	E858.0	E932.7	E950.4	E962.0	E980.4
Tigan	963.0	E858.1	E933.0	E950.4	E962.0	E980.4
Tigloidine	968.0	E855.1	E938.0	E950.4	E962.0	E980.4
Tin (chloride) (dust) (oxide) NEC	985.8	E866.4	—	E950.9	E962.1	E980.9
anti-infectives	961.2	E857	E931.2	E950.4	E962.0	E980.4
Tinactin	976.0	E858.7	E946.0	E950.4	E962.0	E980.4
Tincture, iodine - *see* Iodine	—	—	—	—	—	—
Tindal	969.1	E853.0	E939.1	E950.3	E962.0	E980.3
Titanium (compounds) (vapor)	985.8	E866.4	—	E950.9	E962.1	E980.9
ointment	976.3	E858.7	E946.3	E950.4	E962.0	E980.4
Titroid	962.7	E858.0	E932.7	E950.4	E962.0	E980.4
TMTD - *see* Tetramethylthiuram disulfide	—	—	—	—	—	—
TNT	989.89	E866.8	—	E950.9	E962.1	E980.9
fumes	987.8	E869.8	—	E952.8	E962.2	E982.8
Toadstool	988.1	E865.5	—	E950.9	E962.1	E980.9
Tobacco NEC	989.84	E866.8	—	E950.9	E962.1	E980.9
Indian	988.2	E865.4	—	E950.9	E962.1	E980.9
smoke, second-hand	987.8	E869.4	—	—	—	—
Tocopherol	963.5	E858.1	E933.5	E950.4	E962.0	E980.4
Tocosamine	975.0	E858.6	E945.0	E950.4	E962.0	E980.4
Tofranil	969.0	E854.0	E939.0	E950.3	E962.0	E980.3
Toilet deodorizer	989.89	E866.8	—	E950.9	E962.1	E980.9
Tolazamide	962.3	E858.0	E932.3	E950.4	E962.0	E980.4
Tolazoline	971.3	E855.6	E941.3	E950.4	E962.0	E980.4
Tolbutamide	962.3	E858.0	E932.3	E950.4	E962.0	E980.4
sodium	977.8	E858.8	E947.8	E950.4	E962.0	E980.4
Tolmetin	965.69	E856.0	E935.6	E950.0	E962.0	E980.0
Tolnaftate	976.0	E858.7	E946.0	E950.4	E962.0	E980.4
Tolpropamine	976.1	E858.7	E946.1	E950.4	E962.0	E980.4
Tolserol	968.0	E855.1	E938.0	E950.4	E962.0	E980.4
Toluene (liquid) (vapor)	982.0	E862.4	—	E950.9	E962.1	E980.9
diisocyanate	983.0	E864.0	—	E950.7	E962.1	E980.6
Toluidine	983.0	E864.0	—	E950.7	E962.1	E980.6
vapor	987.8	E869.8	—	E952.8	E962.2	E982.8
Toluol (liquid) (vapor)	982.0	E862.4	—	E950.9	E962.1	E980.9
Tolylene-2,4-diisocyanate	983.0	E864.0	—	E950.7	E962.1	E980.6
Tonics, cardiac	972.1	E858.3	E942.1	E950.4	E962.0	E980.4
Toxaphene (dust) (spray)	989.2	E863.0	—	E950.6	E962.1	E980.7
Toxoids NEC	978.8	E858.8	E948.8	E950.4	E962.0	E980.4
Tractor fuel NEC	981	E862.1	—	E950.9	E962.1	E980.9
Tragacanth	973.3	E858.4	E943.3	E950.4	E962.0	E980.4
Tramazoline	971.2	E855.5	E941.2	E950.4	E962.0	E980.4
Tranquilizers	969.5	E853.9	E939.5	E950.3	E962.0	E980.3
benzodiazepine-based	969.4	E853.2	E939.4	E950.3	E962.0	E980.3
butyrophenone-based	969.2	E853.1	E939.2	E950.3	E962.0	E980.3
major NEC	969.3	E853.8	E939.3	E950.3	E962.0	E980.3
phenothiazine-based	969.1	E853.0	E939.1	E950.3	E962.0	E980.3
specified NEC	969.5	E853.8	E939.5	E950.3	E962.0	E980.3
Trantoin	961.9	E857	E931.9	E950.4	E962.0	E980.4
Tranxene	969.4	E853.2	E939.4	E950.3	E962.0	E980.3
Tranylcypromine (sulfate)	969.0	E854.0	E939.0	E950.3	E962.0	E980.3
Trasentine	975.1	E858.6	E945.1	E950.4	E962.0	E980.4
Travert	974.5	E858.5	E944.5	E950.4	E962.0	E980.4
Trecator	961.8	E857	E931.8	E950.4	E962.0	E980.4
Tretinoin	976.8	E858.7	E946.8	E950.4	E962.0	E980.4
Triacetin	976.0	E858.7	E946.0	E950.4	E962.0	E980.4
Triacetyloleandomycin	960.3	E856	E930.3	E950.4	E962.0	E980.4
Triamcinolone	962.0	E858.0	E932.0	E950.4	E962.0	E980.4
ENT agent	976.6	E858.7	E946.6	E950.4	E962.0	E980.4
ophthalmic preparation	976.5	E858.7	E946.5	E950.4	E962.0	E980.4
topical NEC	976.0	E858.7	E946.0	E950.4	E962.0	E980.4
Triamterene	974.4	E858.5	E944.4	E950.4	E962.0	E980.4

Substance	Poisoning	External Cause (E-Code)				
		Accident	Therapeutic Use	Suicide Attempt	Assault	Undetermined
Triaziquone	963.1	E858.1	E933.1	E950.4	E962.0	E980.4
Tribromacetaldehyde	967.3	E852.2	E937.3	E950.2	E962.0	E980.2
Tribromoethanol	968.2	E855.1	E938.2	E950.4	E962.0	E980.4
Tribromomethane	967.3	E852.2	E937.3	E950.2	E962.0	E980.2
Trichlorethane	982.3	E862.4	—	E950.9	E962.1	E980.9
Trichlormethiazide	974.3	E858.5	E944.3	E950.4	E962.0	E980.4
Trichloroacetic acid	983.1	E864.1	—	E950.7	E962.1	E980.6
medicinal (keratolytic)	976.4	E858.7	E946.4	E950.4	E962.0	E980.4
Trichloroethanol	967.1	E852.0	E937.1	E950.2	E962.0	E980.2
Trichloroethylene (liquid) (vapor)	982.3	E862.4	—	E950.9	E962.1	E980.9
anesthetic (gas)	968.2	E855.1	E938.2	E950.4	E962.0	E980.4
Trichloroethyl phosphate	967.1	E852.0	E937.1	E950.2	E962.0	E980.2
Trichlorofluoromethane NEC	987.4	E869.2	—	E952.8	E962.2	E982.8
Trichlorotriethylamine	963.1	E858.1	E933.1	E950.4	E962.0	E980.4
Trichomonacides NEC	961.5	E857	E931.5	E950.4	E962.0	E980.4
Trichomycin	960.1	E856	E930.1	E950.4	E962.0	E980.4
Triclofos	967.1	E852.0	E937.1	E950.2	E962.0	E980.2
Tricresyl phosphate	989.89	E866.8	—	E950.9	E962.1	E980.9
solvent	982.8	E862.4	—	E950.9	E962.1	E980.9
Tricyclamol	966.4	E855.0	E936.4	E950.4	E962.0	E980.4
Tridesilon	976.0	E858.7	E946.0	E950.4	E962.0	E980.4
Tridihexethyl	971.1	E855.4	E941.1	E950.4	E962.0	E980.4
Tridione	966.0	E855.0	E936.0	E950.4	E962.0	E980.4
Triethanolamine NEC	983.2	E864.2	—	E950.7	E962.1	E980.6
detergent	983.2	E861.0	—	E950.7	E962.1	E980.6
trinitrate	972.4	E858.3	E942.4	E950.4	E962.0	E980.4
Triethanomelamine	963.1	E858.1	E933.1	E950.4	E962.0	E980.4
Triethylene melamine	963.1	E858.1	E933.1	E950.4	E962.0	E980.4
Triethylenephosphoramide	963.1	E858.1	E933.1	E950.4	E962.0	E980.4
Triethylenethiophosphoramide	963.1	E858.1	E933.1	E950.4	E962.0	E980.4
Trifluoperazine	969.1	E853.0	E939.1	E950.3	E962.0	E980.3
Trifluperidol	969.2	E853.1	E939.2	E950.3	E962.0	E980.3
Triflupromazine	969.1	E853.0	E939.1	E950.3	E962.0	E980.3
Trihexyphenidyl	971.1	E855.4	E941.1	E950.4	E962.0	E980.4
Triiodothyronine	962.7	E858.0	E932.7	E950.4	E962.0	E980.4
Trilene	968.2	E855.1	E938.2	E950.4	E962.0	E980.4
Trimeprazine	963.0	E858.1	E933.0	E950.4	E962.0	E980.4
Trimetazidine	972.4	E858.3	E942.4	E950.4	E962.0	E980.4
Trimethadione	966.0	E855.0	E936.0	E950.4	E962.0	E980.4
Trimethaphan	972.3	E858.3	E942.3	E950.4	E962.0	E980.4
Trimethidinium	972.3	E858.3	E942.3	E950.4	E962.0	E980.4
Trimethobenzamide	963.0	E858.1	E933.0	E950.4	E962.0	E980.4
Trimethylcarbinol	980.8	E860.8	—	E950.9	E962.1	E980.9
Trimethylpsoralen	976.3	E858.7	E946.3	E950.4	E962.0	E980.4
Trimeton	963.0	E858.1	E933.0	E950.4	E962.0	E980.4
Trimipramine	969.0	E854.0	E939.0	E950.3	E962.0	E980.3
Trimustine	963.1	E858.1	E933.1	E950.4	E962.0	E980.4
Trinitrin	972.4	E858.3	E942.4	E950.4	E962.0	E980.4
Trinitrophenol	983.0	E864.0	—	E950.7	E962.1	E980.6
Trinitrotoluene	989.89	E866.8	—	E950.9	E962.1	E980.9
fumes	987.8	E869.8	—	E952.8	E962.2	E982.8
Trional	967.8	E852.8	E937.8	E950.2	E962.0	E980.2
Trioxide of arsenic - *see* Arsenic	—	—	—	—	—	—
Trioxsalen	976.3	E858.7	E946.3	E950.4	E962.0	E980.4
Tripelennamine	963.0	E858.1	E933.0	E950.4	E962.0	E980.4
Triperidol	969.2	E853.1	E939.2	E950.3	E962.0	E980.3
Triprolidine	963.0	E858.1	E933.0	E950.4	E962.0	E980.4
Trisoralen	976.3	E858.7	E946.3	E950.4	E962.0	E980.4
Troleandomycin	960.3	E856	E930.3	E950.4	E962.0	E980.4
Trolnitrate (phosphate)	972.4	E858.3	E942.4	E950.4	E962.0	E980.4
Trometamol	963.3	E858.1	E933.3	E950.4	E962.0	E980.4
Tromethamine	963.3	E858.1	E933.3	E950.4	E962.0	E980.4

Substance	Poisoning	External Cause (E-Code) Accident	Therapeutic Use	Suicide Attempt	Assault	Undetermined
Tronothane	968.5	E855.2	E938.5	E950.4	E962.0	E980.4
Tropicamide	971.1	E855.4	E941.1	E950.4	E962.0	E980.4
Troxidone	966.0	E855.0	E936.0	E950.4	E962.0	E980.4
Tryparsamide	961.1	E857	E931.1	E950.4	E962.0	E980.4
Trypsin	963.4	E858.1	E933.4	E950.4	E962.0	E980.4
Tryptizol	969.0	E854.0	E939.0	E950.3	E962.0	E980.3
Tuaminoheptane	971.2	E855.5	E941.2	E950.4	E962.0	E980.4
Tuberculin (old)	977.8	E858.8	E947.8	E950.4	E962.0	E980.4
Tubocurare	975.2	E858.6	E945.2	E950.4	E962.0	E980.4
Tubocurarine	975.2	E858.6	E945.2	E950.4	E962.0	E980.4
Turkish green	969.6	E854.1	E939.6	E950.3	E962.0	E980.3
Turpentine (spirits of) (liquid) (vapor)	982.8	E862.4	—	E950.9	E962.1	E980.9
Tybamate	969.5	E853.8	E939.5	E950.3	E962.0	E980.3
Tyloxapol	975.5	E858.6	E945.5	E950.4	E962.0	E980.4
Tymazoline	971.2	E855.5	E941.2	E950.4	E962.0	E980.4
Typhoid vaccine	978.1	E858.8	E948.1	E950.4	E962.0	E980.4
Typhus vaccine	979.2	E858.8	E949.2	E950.4	E962.0	E980.4
Tyrothricin	976.0	E858.7	E946.0	E950.4	E962.0	E980.4
ENT agent	976.6	E858.7	E946.6	E950.4	E962.0	E980.4
ophthalmic preparation	976.5	E858.7	E946.5	E950.4	E962.0	E980.4
Undecenoic acid	976.0	E858.7	E946.0	E950.4	E962.0	E980.4
Undecylenic acid	976.0	E858.7	E946.0	E950.4	E962.0	E980.4
Unna's boot	976.3	E858.7	E946.3	E950.4	E962.0	E980.4
Uracil mustard	963.1	E858.1	E933.1	E950.4	E962.0	E980.4
Uramustine	963.1	E858.1	E933.1	E950.4	E962.0	E980.4
Urari	975.2	E858.6	E945.2	E950.4	E962.0	E980.4
Urea	974.4	E858.5	E944.4	E950.4	E962.0	E980.4
topical	976.8	E858.7	E946.8	E950.4	E962.0	E980.4
Urethan(e) (antineoplastic)	963.1	E858.1	E933.1	E950.4	E962.0	E980.4
Urginea (maritima) (scilla) - *see* Squill	—	—	—	—	—	—
Uric acid metabolism agents NEC	974.7	E858.5	E944.7	E950.4	E962.0	E980.4
Urokinase	964.4	E858.2	E934.4	E950.4	E962.0	E980.4
Urokon	977.8	E858.8	E947.8	E950.4	E962.0	E980.4
Urotropin	961.9	E857	E931.9	E950.4	E962.0	E980.4
Urtica	988.2	E865.4	—	E950.9	E962.1	E980.9
Utility gas - *see* Gas, utility	—	—	—	—	—	—
Vaccine NEC	979.9	E858.8	E949.9	E950.4	E962.0	E980.4
bacterial NEC	978.8	E858.8	E948.8	E950.4	E962.0	E980.4
with	—	—	—	—	—	—
other bacterial component	978.9	E858.8	E948.9	E950.4	E962.0	E980.4
pertussis component	978.6	E858.8	E948.6	E950.4	E962.0	E980.4
viral-rickettsial component	979.7	E858.8	E949.7	E950.4	E962.0	E980.4
mixed NEC	978.9	E858.8	E948.9	E950.4	E962.0	E980.4
BCG	978.0	E858.8	E948.0	E950.4	E962.0	E980.4
cholera	978.2	E858.8	E948.2	E950.4	E962.0	E980.4
diphtheria	978.5	E858.8	E948.5	E950.4	E962.0	E980.4
influenza	979.6	E858.8	E949.6	E950.4	E962.0	E980.4
measles	979.4	E858.8	E949.4	E950.4	E962.0	E980.4
meningococcal	978.8	E858.8	E948.8	E950.4	E962.0	E980.4
mumps	979.6	E858.8	E949.6	E950.4	E962.0	E980.4
paratyphoid	978.1	E858.8	E948.1	E950.4	E962.0	E980.4
pertussis (with diphtheria toxoid) (with tetanus toxoid)	978.6	E858.8	E948.6	E950.4	E962.0	E980.4
plague	978.3	E858.8	E948.3	E950.4	E962.0	E980.4
poliomyelitis	979.5	E858.8	E949.5	E950.4	E962.0	E980.4
poliovirus	979.5	E858.8	E949.5	E950.4	E962.0	E980.4
rabies	979.1	E858.8	E949.1	E950.4	E962.0	E980.4
respiratory syncytial virus	979.6	E858.8	E949.6	E950.4	E962.0	E980.4
rickettsial NEC	979.6	E858.8	E949.6	E950.4	E962.0	E980.4
with	—	—	—	—	—	—
bacterial component	979.7	E858.8	E949.7	E950.4	E962.0	E980.4
pertussis component	978.6	E858.8	E948.6	E950.4	E962.0	E980.4
viral component	979.7	E858.8	E949.7	E950.4	E962.0	E980.4

◀ New ⟸ Revised

Substance	Poisoning	External Cause (E-Code)				
		Accident	Therapeutic Use	Suicide Attempt	Assault	Undetermined
Vaccine NEC *(Continued)*						
Rocky Mountain spotted fever	979.6	E858.8	E949.6	E950.4	E962.0	E980.4
rotavirus	979.6	E858.8	E949.6	E950.4	E962.0	E980.4
rubella virus	979.4	E858.8	E949.4	E950.4	E962.0	E980.4
sabin oral	979.5	E858.8	E949.5	E950.4	E962.0	E980.4
smallpox	979.0	E858.8	E949.0	E950.4	E962.0	E980.4
tetanus	978.4	E858.8	E948.4	E950.4	E962.0	E980.4
typhoid	978.1	E858.8	E948.1	E950.4	E962.0	E980.4
typhus	979.2	E858.8	E949.2	E950.4	E962.0	E980.4
viral NEC	979.6	E858.8	E949.6	E950.4	E962.0	E980.4
with	—	—	—	—	—	—
bacterial component	979.7	E858.8	E949.7	E950.4	E962.0	E980.4
pertussis component	978.6	E858.8	E948.6	E950.4	E962.0	E980.4
rickettsial component	979.7	E858.8	E949.7	E950.4	E962.0	E980.4
yellow fever	979.3	E858.8	E949.3	E950.4	E962.0	E980.4
Vaccinia immune globulin (human)	964.6	E858.2	E934.6	E950.4	E962.0	E980.4
Vaginal contraceptives	976.8	E858.7	E946.8	E950.4	E962.0	E980.4
Valethamate	971.1	E855.4	E941.1	E950.4	E962.0	E980.4
Valisone	976.0	E858.7	E946.0	E950.4	E962.0	E980.4
Valium	969.4	E853.2	E939.4	E950.3	E962.0	E980.3
Valmid	967.8	E852.8	E937.8	E950.2	E962.0	E980.2
Vanadium	985.8	E866.4	—	E950.9	E962.1	E980.9
Vancomycin	960.8	E856	E930.8	E950.4	E962.0	E980.4
Vapor (*see also* Gas)	987.9	E869.9	—	E952.9	E962.2	E982.9
kiln (carbon monoxide)	986	E868.8	—	E952.1	E962.2	E982.1
lead - *see* Lead	—	—	—	—	—	—
specified source NEC - (*see also* specific substance)	987.8	E869.8	—	E952.8	E962.2	E982.8
Varidase	964.4	E858.2	E934.4	E950.4	E962.0	E980.4
Varnish	989.89	E861.6	—	E950.9	E962.1	E980.9
cleaner	982.8	E862.9	—	E950.9	E962.1	E980.9
Vaseline	976.3	E858.7	E946.3	E950.4	E962.0	E980.4
Vasodilan	972.5	E858.3	E942.5	E950.4	E962.0	E980.4
Vasodilators NEC	972.5	E858.3	E942.5	E950.4	E962.0	E980.4
coronary	972.4	E858.3	E942.4	E950.4	E962.0	E980.4
Vasopressin	962.5	E858.0	E932.5	E950.4	E962.0	E980.4
Vasopressor drugs	962.5	E858.0	E932.5	E950.4	E962.0	E980.4
Venom, venomous (bite) (sting)	989.5	E905.9	—	E950.9	E962.1	E980.9
arthropod NEC	989.5	E905.5	—	E950.9	E962.1	E980.9
bee	989.5	E905.3	—	E950.9	E962.1	E980.9
centipede	989.5	E905.4	—	E950.9	E962.1	E980.9
hornet	989.5	E905.3	—	E950.9	E962.1	E980.9
lizard	989.5	E905.0	—	E950.9	E962.1	E980.9
marine animals or plants	989.5	E905.6	—	E950.9	E962.1	E980.9
millipede (tropical)	989.5	E905.4	—	E950.9	E962.1	E980.9
plant NEC	989.5	E905.7	—	E950.9	E962.1	E980.9
marine	989.5	E905.6	—	E950.9	E962.1	E980.9
scorpion	989.5	E905.2	—	E950.9	E962.1	E980.9
snake	989.5	E905.0	—	E950.9	E962.1	E980.9
specified NEC	989.5	E905.8	—	E950.9	E962.1	E980.9
spider	989.5	E905.1	—	E950.9	E962.1	E980.9
wasp	989.5	E905.3	—	E950.9	E962.1	E980.9
Ventolin - *see* Salbutamol sulfate	—	—	—	—	—	—
Veramon	967.0	E851	E937.0	E950.1	E962.0	E980.1
Veratrum	—	—	—	—	—	—
album	988.2	E865.4	—	E950.9	E962.1	E980.9
alkaloids	972.6	E858.3	E942.6	E950.4	E962.0	E980.4
viride	988.2	E865.4	—	E950.9	E962.1	E980.9
Verdigris (*see also* Copper)	985.8	E866.4	—	E950.9	E962.1	E980.9
Veronal	967.0	E851	E937.0	E950.1	E962.0	E980.1
Veroxil	961.6	E857	E931.6	E950.4	E962.0	E980.4
Versidyne	965.7	E850.7	E935.7	E950.0	E962.0	E980.0

Substance	Poisoning	External Cause (E-Code)				
		Accident	Therapeutic Use	Suicide Attempt	Assault	Undetermined
Viagra	972.5	E858.3	E942.5	E950.4	E962.0	E980.4
Vienna	—	—	—	—	—	—
green	985.1	E866.3	—	E950.8	E962.1	E980.8
insecticide	985.1	E863.4	—	E950.6	E962.1	E980.7
red	989.89	E866.8	—	E950.9	E962.1	E980.9
pharmaceutical dye	977.4	E858.8	E947.4	E950.4	E962.0	E980.4
Vinbarbital, vinbarbitone	967.0	E851	E937.0	E950.1	E962.0	E980.1
Vinblastine	963.1	E858.1	E933.1	E950.4	E962.0	E980.4
Vincristine	963.1	E858.1	E933.1	E950.4	E962.0	E980.4
Vinesthene, vinethene	968.2	E855.1	E938.2	E950.4	E962.0	E980.4
Vinyl	—	—	—	—	—	—
bital	967.0	E851	E937.0	E950.1	E962.0	E980.1
ether	968.2	E855.1	E938.2	E950.4	E962.0	E980.4
Vioform	961.3	E857	E931.3	E950.4	E962.0	E980.4
topical	976.0	E858.7	E946.0	E950.4	E962.0	E980.4
Viomycin	960.6	E856	E930.6	E950.4	E962.0	E980.4
Viosterol	963.5	E858.1	E933.5	E950.4	E962.0	E980.4
Viper (venom)	989.5	E905.0	—	E950.9	E962.1	E980.9
Viprynium (embonate)	961.6	E857	E931.6	E950.4	E962.0	E980.4
Virugon	961.7	E857	E931.7	E950.4	E962.0	E980.4
Visine	976.5	E858.7	E946.5	E950.4	E962.0	E980.4
Vitamins NEC	963.5	E858.1	E933.5	E950.4	E962.0	E980.4
B_{12}	964.1	E858.2	E934.1	E950.4	E962.0	E980.4
hematopoietic	964.1	E858.2	E934.1	E950.4	E962.0	E980.4
K	964.3	E858.2	E934.3	E950.4	E962.0	E980.4
Vleminckx's solution	976.4	E858.7	E946.4	E950.4	E962.0	E980.4
Voltaren - *see* Diclofenac sodium	—	—	—	—	—	—
Warfarin (potassium) (sodium)	964.2	E858.2	E934.2	E950.4	E962.0	E980.4
rodenticide	989.4	E863.7	—	E950.6	E962.1	E980.7
Wasp (sting)	989.5	E905.3	—	E950.9	E962.1	E980.9
Water	—	—	—	—	—	—
balance agents NEC	974.5	E858.5	E944.5	E950.4	E962.0	E980.4
gas	987.1	E868.1	—	E951.8	E962.2	E981.8
incomplete combustion of - *see* Carbon, monoxide, fuel, utility	—	—	—	—	—	—
hemlock	988.2	E865.4	—	E950.9	E962.1	E980.9
moccasin (venom)	989.5	E905.0	—	E950.9	E962.1	E980.9
Wax (paraffin) (petroleum)	981	E862.3	—	E950.9	E962.1	E980.9
automobile	989.89	E861.2	—	E950.9	E962.1	E980.9
floor	981	E862.0	—	E950.9	E962.1	E980.9
Weed killers NEC	989.4	E863.5	—	E950.6	E962.1	E980.7
Welldorm	967.1	E852.0	E937.1	E950.2	E962.0	E980.2
White	—	—	—	—	—	—
arsenic - *see* Arsenic	—	—	—	—	—	—
hellebore	988.2	E865.4	—	E950.9	E962.1	E980.9
lotion (keratolytic)	976.4	E858.7	E946.4	E950.4	E962.0	E980.4
spirit	981	E862.0	—	E950.9	E962.1	E980.9
Whitewashes	989.89	E861.6	—	E950.9	E962.1	E980.9
Whole blood	964.7	E858.2	E934.7	E950.4	E962.0	E980.4
Wild	—	—	—	—	—	—
black cherry	988.2	E865.4	—	E950.9	E962.1	E980.9
poisonous plants NEC	988.2	E865.4	—	E950.9	E962.1	E980.9
Window cleaning fluid	989.89	E861.3	—	E950.9	E962.1	E980.9
Wintergreen (oil)	976.3	E858.7	E946.3	E950.4	E962.0	E980.4
Witch hazel	976.2	E858.7	E946.2	E950.4	E962.0	E980.4
Wood	—	—	—	—	—	—
alcohol	980.1	E860.2	—	E950.9	E962.1	E980.9
spirit	980.1	E860.2	—	E950.9	E962.1	E980.9
Woorali	975.2	E858.6	E945.2	E950.4	E962.0	E980.4
Wormseed, American	961.6	E857	E931.6	E950.4	E962.0	E980.4
Xanthine diuretics	974.1	E858.5	E944.1	E950.4	E962.0	E980.4
Xanthocillin	960.0	E856	E930.0	E950.4	E962.0	E980.4

Substance	Poisoning	Accident	Therapeutic Use	Suicide Attempt	Assault	Undetermined
	External Cause (E-Code)					
Xanthotoxin	976.3	E858.7	E946.3	E950.4	E962.0	E980.4
Xigris	964.2	E858.2	E934.2	E950.4	E962.0	E980.4
Xylene (liquid) (vapor)	982.0	E862.4	—	E950.9	E962.1	E980.9
Xylocaine (infiltration) (topical)	968.5	E855.2	E938.5	E950.4	E962.0	E980.4
nerve block (peripheral) (plexus)	968.6	E855.2	E938.6	E950.4	E962.0	E980.4
spinal	968.7	E855.2	E938.7	E950.4	E962.0	E980.4
Xylol (liquid) (vapor)	982.0	E862.4	—	E950.9	E962.1	E980.9
Xylometazoline	971.2	E855.5	E941.2	E950.4	E962.0	E980.4
Yellow	—	—	—	—	—	—
fever vaccine	979.3	E858.8	E949.3	E950.4	E962.0	E980.4
jasmine	988.2	E865.4	—	E950.9	E962.1	E980.9
Yew	988.2	E865.4	—	E950.9	E962.1	E980.9
Zactane	965.7	E850.7	E935.7	E950.0	E962.0	E980.0
Zaroxolyn	974.3	E858.5	E944.3	E950.4	E962.0	E980.4
Zephiran (topical)	976.0	E858.7	E946.0	E950.4	E962.0	E980.4
ophthalmic preparation	976.5	E858.7	E946.5	E950.4	E962.0	E980.4
Zerone	980.1	E860.2	—	E950.9	E962.1	E980.9
Zinc (compounds) (fumes) (salts) (vapor) NEC	985.8	E866.4	—	E950.9	E962.1	E980.9
anti-infectives	976.0	E858.7	E946.0	E950.4	E962.0	E980.4
antivaricose	972.7	E858.3	E942.7	E950.4	E962.0	E980.4
bacitracin	976.0	E858.7	E946.0	E950.4	E962.0	E980.4
chloride	976.2	E858.7	E946.2	E950.4	E962.0	E980.4
gelatin	976.3	E858.7	E946.3	E950.4	E962.0	E980.4
oxide	976.3	E858.7	E946.3	E950.4	E962.0	E980.4
peroxide	976.0	E858.7	E946.0	E950.4	E962.0	E980.4
pesticides	985.8	E863.4	—	E950.6	E962.1	E980.7
phosphide (rodenticide)	985.8	E863.7	—	E950.6	E962.1	E980.7
stearate	976.3	E858.7	E946.3	E950.4	E962.0	E980.4
sulfate (antivaricose)	972.7	E858.3	E942.7	E950.4	E962.0	E980.4
ENT agent	976.6	E858.7	E946.6	E950.4	E962.0	E980.4
ophthalmic solution	976.5	E858.7	E946.5	E950.4	E962.0	E980.4
topical NEC	976.0	E858.7	E946.0	E950.4	E962.0	E980.4
undecylenate	976.0	E858.7	E946.0	E950.4	E962.0	E980.4
Zovant	964.2	E858.2	E934.2	E950.4	E962.0	E980.4
Zoxazolamine	968.0	E855.1	E938.0	E950.4	E962.0	E980.4
Zygadenus (venenosus)	988.2	E865.4	—	E950.9	E962.1	E980.9

SECTION III

INDEX TO EXTERNAL CAUSES OF INJURY (E CODE)

This section contains the index to the codes which classify environmental events, circumstances, and other conditions as the cause of injury and other adverse effects. Where a code from the section Supplementary Classification of External Causes of Injury and Poisoning (E800–E998) is applicable, it is intended that the E code shall be used in addition to a code from the main body of the classification, Chapters 1 to 17.

The alphabetic index to the E codes is organized by main terms which describe the accident, circumstance, event, or specific agent which caused the injury or other adverse effect.

Note Transport accidents (E800–E848) include accidents involving:

aircraft and spacecraft (E840–E845)
watercraft (E830–E838)
motor vehicle (E810–E825)
railway (E800–E807)
other road vehicles (E826–E829)

For definitions and examples related to transport accidents - see Supplementary Classification of External Causes of Injury and Poisoning (E800–E999).

The fourth-digit subdivisions for use with categories E800–E848 to identify the injured person are found at the end of this section.

For identifying the place in which an accident or poisoning occurred (circumstances classifiable to categories E850–E869 and E880–E928) - see the listing in this section under "Accident, occurring."

See the Table of Drugs and Chemicals (Section 2 of this volume) for identifying the specific agent involved in drug overdose or a wrong substance given or taken in error, and for intoxication or poisoning by a drug or other chemical substance.

The specific adverse effect, reaction, or localized toxic effect of a correct drug or substance properly administered in therapeutic or prophylactic dosage should be classified according to the nature of the adverse effect (e.g., allergy, dermatitis, tachycardia) listed in Section I of this volume.

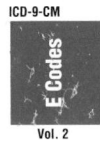
ICD-9-CM
E Codes
Vol. 2

A

Abandonment
- causing exposure to weather conditions - *see* Exposure
- child, with intent to injure or kill E968.4
- helpless person, infant, newborn E904.0
  - with intent to injure or kill E968.4

Abortion, criminal, injury to child E968.8

Abuse (alleged) (suspected)
- adult
  - by
    - child E967.4
    - ex-partner E967.3
    - ex-spouse E967.3
    - father E967.0
    - grandchild E967.7
    - grandparent E967.6
    - mother E967.2
    - non-related caregiver E967.8
    - other relative E967.7
    - other specified person E967.1
    - partner E967.3
    - sibling E967.5
    - spouse E967.3
    - stepfather E967.0
    - stepmother E967.2
    - unspecified person E967.9
- child
  - by
    - boyfriend of parent or guardian E967.0
    - child E967.4
    - father E967.0
    - female partner of parent or guardian E967.2
    - girlfriend of parent or guardian E967.2
    - grandchild E967.7
    - grandparent E967.6
    - male partner of parent or guardian E967.0
    - mother E967.2
    - non-related caregiver E967.8
    - other relative E967.7
    - other specified person(s) E967.1
    - sibling E967.5
    - stepfather E967.0
    - stepmother E967.2
    - unspecified person E967.9

Accident (to) E928.9
- aircraft (in transit) (powered) E841
  - at landing, take-off E840
  - due to, caused by cataclysm - *see* categories E908, E909
  - late effect of E929.1
  - unpowered (*see also* Collision, aircraft, unpowered) E842
  - while alighting, boarding E843
- amphibious vehicle
  - on
    - land - *see* Accident, motor vehicle
    - water - *see* Accident, watercraft
- animal, ridden NEC E828
- animal-drawn vehicle NEC E827
- balloon (*see also* Collision, aircraft, unpowered) E842
- caused by, due to
  - abrasive wheel (metalworking) E919.3
  - animal NEC E906.9
    - being ridden (in sport or transport) E828
  - avalanche NEC E909.2

Accident *(Continued)*
- caused by, due to *(Continued)*
  - band saw E919.4
  - bench saw E919.4
  - bore, earth-drilling or mining (land) (seabed) E919.1
  - bulldozer E919.7
  - cataclysmic
    - earth surface movement or eruption E909.9
    - storm E908.9
  - chain
    - hoist E919.2
      - agricultural operations E919.0
      - mining operations E919.1
    - saw E920.1
  - circular saw E919.4
  - cold (excessive) (*see also* Cold, exposure to) E901.9
  - combine E919.0
    - conflagration - *see* Conflagration
  - corrosive liquid, substance NEC E924.1
  - cotton gin E919.8
  - crane E919.2
    - agricultural operations E919.0
    - mining operations E919.1
  - cutting or piercing instrument (*see also* Cut) E920.9
  - dairy equipment E919.8
  - derrick E919.2
    - agricultural operations E919.0
    - mining operations E919.1
  - drill E920.1
    - earth (land) (seabed) E919.1
    - hand (powered) E920.1
      - not powered E920.4
    - metalworking E919.3
    - woodworking E919.4
  - earth(-)
    - drilling machine E919.1
    - moving machine E919.7
    - scraping machine E919.7
  - electric
    - current (*see also* Electric shock) E925.9
    - motor - *see also* Accident, machine, by type of machine
      - current (of) - *see* Electric shock
  - elevator (building) (grain) E919.2
    - agricultural operations E919.0
    - mining operations E919.1
  - environmental factors NEC E928.9
  - excavating machine E919.7
  - explosive material (*see also* Explosion) E923.9
  - farm machine E919.0
  - fire, flames - *see also* Fire
    - conflagration - *see* Conflagration
  - firearm missile - *see* Shooting
  - forging (metalworking) machine E919.3
  - forklift (truck) E919.2
    - agricultural operations E919.0
    - mining operations E919.1
  - gas turbine E919.5
  - harvester E919.0
  - hay derrick, mower, or rake E919.0
  - heat (excessive) (*see also* Heat) E900.9
  - hoist (*see also* Accident, caused by, due to, lift) E919.2
    - chain - *see* Accident, caused by, due to, chain
    - shaft E919.1

Accident *(Continued)*
- caused by, due to *(Continued)*
  - hot
    - liquid E924.0
      - caustic or corrosive E924.1
    - object (not producing fire or flames) E924.8
    - substance E924.9
      - caustic or corrosive E924.1
      - liquid (metal) NEC E924.0
      - specified type NEC E924.8
  - human bite E928.3
  - ignition - *see* Ignition E919.4
  - internal combustion engine E919.5
  - landslide NEC E909.2
  - lathe (metalworking) E919.3
    - turnings E920.8
    - woodworking E919.4
  - lift, lifting (appliances) E919.2
    - agricultural operations E919.0
    - mining operations E919.1
    - shaft E919.1
  - lightning NEC E907
  - machine, machinery - *see also* Accident, machine
    - drilling, metal E919.3
    - manufacturing, for manufacture of steam
      - beverages E919.8
      - clothing E919.8
      - foodstuffs E919.8
      - paper E919.8
      - textiles E919.8
    - milling, metal E919.3
    - moulding E919.4
    - power press, metal E919.3
    - printing E919.8
    - rolling mill, metal E919.3
    - sawing, metal E919.3
    - specified type NEC E919.8
    - spinning E919.8
    - weaving E919.8
  - natural factor NEC E928.9
  - overhead plane E919.4
  - plane E920.4
    - overhead E919.4
  - powered
    - hand tool NEC E920.1
    - saw E919.4
      - hand E920.1
  - printing machine E919.8
  - pulley (block) E919.2
    - agricultural operations E919.0
    - mining operations E919.1
    - transmission E919.6
  - radial saw E919.4
  - radiation - *see* Radiation
  - reaper E919.0
  - road scraper E919.7
    - when in transport under its own power - *see* categories E810–E825
  - roller coaster E919.8
  - sander E919.4
  - saw E920.4
    - band E919.4
    - bench E919.4
    - chain E920.1
    - circular E919.4
    - hand E920.4
      - powered E920.1
    - powered, except hand E919.4
    - radial E919.4
  - sawing machine, metal E919.3

Accident *(Continued)*
caused by, due to *(Continued)*
shaft
hoist E919.1
lift E919.1
transmission E919.6
shears E920.4
hand E920.4
powered E920.1
mechanical E919.3
shovel E920.4
steam E919.7
spinning machine E919.8
steam - *see also* Burning, steam
engine E919.5
shovel E919.7
thresher E919.0
thunderbolt NEC E907
tractor E919.0
when in transport under its own power - *see* categories E810–E825
transmission belt, cable, chain, gear, pinion, pulley, shaft E919.6
turbine (gas) (water driven) E919.5
under-cutter E919.1
weaving machine E919.8
winch E919.2
agricultural operations E919.0
mining operations E919.1
diving E883.0
with insufficient air supply E913.2
glider (hang) (*see also* Collision, aircraft, unpowered) E842
hovercraft
on
land - *see* Accident, motor vehicle
water - *see* Accident, watercraft
ice yacht (*see also* Accident, vehicle NEC) E848
in
medical, surgical procedure
as, or due to misadventure - *see* Misadventure
causing an abnormal reaction or later complication without mention of misadventure - *see* Reaction, abnormal
kite carrying a person (*see also* Collision, involving aircraft, unpowered) E842
land yacht (*see also* Accident, vehicle NEC) E848
late effect of - *see* Late effect
launching pad E845
machine, machinery (*see also* Accident, caused by, due to, by specific type of machine) E919.9
agricultural including animal-powered premises E919.0
earth-drilling E919.1
earth moving or scraping E919.7
excavating E919.7
involving transport under own power on highway or transport vehicle - *see* categories E810-E825, E840-E845
lifting (appliances) E919.2
metalworking E919.3
mining E919.1
prime movers, except electric motors E919.5
electric motors - *see* Accident, machine, by specific type of machine

Accident *(Continued)*
machine, machinery *(Continued)*
recreational E919.8
specified type NEC E919.8
transmission E919.6
watercraft (deck) (engine room) (galley) (laundry) (loading) E836
woodworking or forming E919.4
motor vehicle (on public highway) (traffic) E819
due to cataclysm - *see* categories E908, E909
involving
collision (*see also* Collision, motor vehicle) E812
nontraffic, not on public highway - *see* categories E820–E825
not involving collision - *see* categories E816–E819
nonmotor vehicle NEC E829
nonroad - *see* Accident, vehicle NEC
road, except pedal cycle, animal-drawn vehicle, or animal being ridden E829
nonroad vehicle NEC - *see* Accident, vehicle NEC
not elsewhere classifiable involving
cable car (not on rails) E847
on rails E829
coal car in mine E846
hand truck - *see* Accident, vehicle NEC
logging car E846
sled(ge), meaning snow or ice vehicle E848
tram, mine or quarry E846
truck
mine or quarry E846
self-propelled, industrial E846
station baggage E846
tub, mine or quarry E846
vehicle NEC E848
snow and ice E848
used only on industrial premises E846
wheelbarrow E848
occurring (at) (in)
apartment E849.0
baseball field, diamond E849.4
construction site, any E849.3
dock E849.8
yard E849.3
dormitory E849.7
factory (building) (premises) E849.3
farm E849.1
buildings E849.1
house E849.0
football field E849.4
forest E849.8
garage (place of work) E849.3
private (home) E849.0
gravel pit E849.2
gymnasium E849.4
highway E849.5
home (private) (residential) E849.0
institutional E849.7
hospital E849.7
hotel E849.6
house (private) (residential) E849.0
movie E849.6
public E849.6
institution, residential E849.7
jail E849.7
mine E849.2

Accident *(Continued)*
occurring *(Continued)*
motel E849.6
movie house E849.6
office (building) E849.6
orphanage E849.7
park (public) E849.4
mobile home E849.8
trailer E849.8
parking lot or place E849.8
place
industrial NEC E849.3
parking E849.8
public E849.6
specified place NEC E849.5
recreational NEC E849.4
sport NEC E849.4
playground (park) (school) E849.4
prison E849.6
public building NEC E849.6
quarry E849.2
railway
line NEC E849.8
yard E849.3
residence
home (private) E849.0
resort (beach) (lake) (mountain) (seashore) (vacation) E849.4
restaurant E849.6
sand pit E849.2
school (building) (private) (public) (state) E849.6
reform E849.7
riding E849.4
seashore E849.8
resort E849.4
shop (place of work) E849.3
commercial E849.6
skating rink E849.4
sports palace E849.4
stadium E849.4
store E849.6
street E849.5
swimming pool (public) E849.4
private home or garden E849.0
tennis court E849.4 public
theatre, theater E849.6
trailer court E849.8
tunnel E849.8
under construction E849.2
warehouse E849.3
yard
dock E849.3
industrial E849.3
private (home) E849.0
railway E849.3
off-road type motor vehicle (not on public highway) NEC E821
on public highway - *see* categories E810–E819
pedal cycle E826
railway E807
due to cataclysm - *see* categories E908, E909
involving
avalanche E909.2
burning by engine, locomotive, train (*see also* Explosion, railway engine) E803
collision (*see also* collision, railway) E800
derailment (*see also* Derailment, railway) E802
explosion (*see also* Explosion, railway engine) E803

Accident *(Continued)*
railway *(Continued)*
involving *(Continued)*
fall (*see also* Fall, from, railway rolling stock) E804
fire (*see also* Explosion, railway engine) E803
hitting by, being struck by
object falling in, on, from, rolling stock, train, vehicle E806
rolling stock, train, vehicle E805
overturning, railway rolling stock, train, vehicle (*see also* Derailment, railway) E802
running off rails, railway (*see also* Derailment, railway) E802
specified circumstances NEC E806
train or vehicle hit by
avalanche E909.2
falling object (earth, rock, tree) E806
due to cataclysm - *see* categories E908, E909
landslide E909.2
roller skate E885.1
scooter (nonmotorized) E885.0
skateboard E885.2
ski(ing) E885.3
jump E884.9
lift or tow (with chair or gondola) E847
snow vehicle, motor driven (not on public highway) E820
on public highway - *see* categories E810–E819
snowboard E885.4
spacecraft E845
specified cause NEC E928.8
street car E829
traffic NEC E819
vehicle NEC (with pedestrian) E848
battery powered
airport passenger vehicle E846
truck (baggage) (mail) E846
powered commercial or industrial (with other vehicle or object within commercial or industrial premises) E846
watercraft E838
with
drowning or submersion resulting from
accident other than to watercraft E832
accident to watercraft E830
injury, except drowning or submersion, resulting from
accident other than to watercraft - *see* categories E833–E838
accident to watercraft E831
due to, caused by cataclysm - *see* categories E908, E909
machinery E836
Acid throwing E961
Acosta syndrome E902.0
Aeroneurosis E902.1
Aero-otitis media - *see* Effects of, air pressure
Aerosinusitis - *see* Effects of, air pressure
After-effect, late - *see* Late effect
Air
blast
in
terrorism E979.2
war operations E993
Air *(Continued)*
embolism (traumatic) NEC E928.9
in
infusion or transfusion E874.1
perfusion E874.2
sickness E903
Alpine sickness E902.0
Altitude sickness - *see* Effects of, air pressure
Anaphylactic shock, anaphylaxis (*see also* Table of Drugs and Chemicals) E947.9
due to bite or sting (venomous) - *see* Bite, venomous
Andes disease E902.0
Apoplexy
heat - *see* Heat
Arachnidism E905.1
Arson E968.0
Asphyxia, asphyxiation
by
chemical
in
terrorism E979.7
war operations E997.2
explosion - *see* Explosion
food (bone) (regurgitated food) (seed) E911
foreign object, except food E912
fumes
in
terrorism (chemical weapons) E979.7
war operations E997.2
gas - *see also* Table of Drugs and Chemicals
in
terrorism E979.7
war operations E997.2
legal
execution E978
intervention (tear) E972
tear E972
mechanical means (*see also* Suffocation) E913.9
from
conflagration - *see* Conflagration
fire - *see also* Fire E899
in
terrorism E979.3
war operations E990.9
ignition - *see* Ignition
Aspiration
foreign body - *see* Foreign body, aspiration
mucus, not of newborn (with asphyxia, obstruction respiratory passage, suffocation) E912
phlegm (with asphyxia, obstruction respiratory passage, suffocation) E912
vomitus (with asphyxia, obstruction respiratory passage, suffocation) (*see also* Foreign body, aspiration, food) E911
Assassination (attempt) (*see also* Assault) E968.9
Assault (homicidal) (by) (in) E968.9
acid E961
swallowed E962.1
air gun E968.6
BB gun E968.6
bite NEC E968.8
of human being E968.7
Assault *(Continued)*
bomb ((placed in) car or house) E965.8
antipersonnel E965.5
letter E965.7
petrol E965.6
brawl (hand) (fists) (foot) E960.0
burning, burns (by fire) E968.0
acid E961
swallowed E962.1
caustic, corrosive substance E961
swallowed E962.1
chemical from swallowing caustic, corrosive substance NEC E962.1
hot liquid E968.3
scalding E968.3
vitriol E961
swallowed E962.1
caustic, corrosive substance E961
swallowed E962.1
cut, any part of body E966
dagger E966
drowning E964
explosives E965.9
bomb (*see also* Assault, bomb) E965.8
dynamite E965.8
fight (hand) (fists) (foot) E960.0
with weapon E968.9
blunt or thrown E968.2
cutting or piercing E966
firearm - *see* Shooting, homicide
fire E968.0
firearm(s) - *see* Shooting, homicide
garrotting E963
gunshot (wound) - *see* Shooting, homicide
hanging E963
injury NEC E968.9
knife E966
late effect of E969
ligature E963
poisoning E962.9
drugs or medicinals E962.0
gas(es) or vapors, except drugs and medicinals E962.2
solid or liquid substances, except drugs and medicinals E962.1
puncture, any part of body E966
pushing
before moving object, train, vehicle E968.5
from high place E968.1
rape E960.1
scalding E968.3
shooting - *see* Shooting, homicide
sodomy E960.1
stab, any part of body E966
strangulation E963
submersion E964
suffocation E963
transport vehicle E968.5
violence NEC E968.9
vitriol E961
swallowed E962.1
weapon E968.9
blunt or thrown E968.2
cutting or piercing E966
firearm - *see* Shooting, homicide
wound E968.9
cutting E966
gunshot - *see* Shooting, homicide
knife E966
piercing E966
puncture E966
stab E966

Attack by animal NEC E906.9
Avalanche E909.2
falling on or hitting
motor vehicle (in motion) (on public highway) E909.2
railway train E909.2
Aviators' disease E902.1

B

Barotitis, barodontalgia, barosinusitis, barotrauma (otitic) (sinus) - *see* Effects of, air pressure
Battered
baby or child (syndrome) - *see* Abuse, child; category E967
person other than baby or child - *see* Assault
Bayonet wound (*see also* Cut, by bayonet) E920.3
in
legal intervention E974
terrorism E979.8
war operations E995
Bean in nose E912
Bed set on fire NEC E898.0
Beheading (by guillotine)
homicide E966
legal execution E978
Bending, injury in E927
Bends E902.0
Bite
animal NEC E906.5
other specified (except arthropod) E906.3
venomous NEC E905.9
arthropod (nonvenomous) NEC E906.4
venomous - *see* Sting
black widow spider E905.1
cat E906.3
centipede E905.4
cobra E905.0
copperhead snake E905.0
coral snake E905.0
dog E906.0
fer de lance E905.0
gila monster E905.0
human being
accidental E928.3
assault E968.7
insect (nonvenomous) E906.4
venomous - *see* Sting
krait E905.0
late effect of - *see* Late effect
lizard E906.2
venomous E905.0
mamba E905.0
marine animal
nonvenomous E906.3
snake E906.2
venomous E905.6
snake E905.0
millipede E906.4
venomous E905.4
moray eel E906.3
rat E906.1
rattlesnake E905.0
rodent, except rat E906.3
serpent - *see* Bite, snake
shark E906.3
snake (venomous) E905.0
nonvenomous E906.2
sea E905.0
Bite *(Continued)*
spider E905.1
nonvenomous E906.4
tarantula (venomous) E905.1
venomous NEC E905.9
by specific animal - *see* category E905
viper E905.0
water moccasin E905.0
Blast (air)
in
terrorism E979.2
from nuclear explosion E979.5
underwater E979.0
war operations E993
from nuclear explosion E996
underwater E992
Blizzard E908.3
Blow E928.9
by law-enforcing agent, police (on duty) E975
with blunt object (baton) (nightstick) (stave) (truncheon) E973
Blowing up (*see also* Explosion) E923.9
Brawl (hand) (fists) (foot) E960.0
Breakage (accidental)
cable of cable car not on rails E847
ladder (causing fall) E881.0
part (any) of
animal-drawn vehicle E827
ladder (causing fall) E881.0
motor vehicle
in motion (on public highway) E818
not on public highway E825
nonmotor road vehicle, except animal-drawn vehicle or pedal cycle E829
off-road type motor vehicle (not on public highway) NEC E821
on public highway E818
pedal cycle E826
scaffolding (causing fall) E881.1
snow vehicle, motor-driven (not on public highway) E820
on public highway E818
vehicle NEC - *see* Accident, vehicle
Broken
glass,
fall on E888.0
injury by E920.8
power line (causing electric shock) E925.1
Bumping against, into (accidentally)
object (moving) E917.9
caused by crowd E917.1
with subsequent fall E917.6
furniture E917.3
with subsequent fall E917.7
in
running water E917.2
sports E917.0
with subsequent fall E917.5
stationary E917.4
with subsequent fall E917.8
person(s) E917.9
with fall E886.9
in sports E886.0
as, or caused by, a crowd E917.1
with subsequent fall E917.6
in sports E917.0
with fall E886.0
Burning, burns (accidental) (by) (from) (on) E899
acid (any kind) E924.1
swallowed - *see* Table of Drugs and Chemicals
Burning, burns *(Continued)*
bedclothes (*see also* Fire, specified NEC) E898.0
blowlamp (*see also* Fire, specified NEC) E898.1
blowtorch (*see also* Fire, specified NEC) E898.1
boat, ship, watercraft - *see* categories E830, E831, E837
bonfire (controlled) E897
uncontrolled E892
candle (*see also* Fire, specified NEC) E898.1
caustic liquid, substance E924.1
swallowed - *see* Table of Drugs and Chemicals
chemical E924.1
from swallowing caustic, corrosive substance - *see* Table of Drugs and Chemicals
in
terrorism E979.7
war operations E997.2
cigar(s) or cigarette(s) (*see also* Fire, specified NEC) E898.1
clothes, clothing, nightdress - *see* Ignition, clothes
with conflagration - *see* Conflagration
conflagration - *see* Conflagration
corrosive liquid, substance E924.1
swallowed - *see* Table of Drugs and Chemicals
electric current (*see also* Electric shock) E925.9
fire, flames (*see also* Fire) E899
flare, Verey pistol E922.8
heat
from appliance (electrical) E924.8
in local application, or packing during medical or surgical procedure E873.5
homicide (attempt) (*see also* Assault, burning) E968.0
hot
liquid E924.0
caustic or corrosive E924.1
object (not producing fire or flames) E924.8
substance E924.9
caustic or corrosive E924.1
liquid (metal) NEC E924.0
specified type NEC E924.8
tap water E924.2
ignition - *see also* Ignition
clothes, clothing, nightdress - *see also* Ignition, clothes
with conflagration - *see* Conflagration
highly inflammable material (benzine) (fat) (gasoline) (kerosene) (paraffin) (petrol) E894
inflicted by other person
stated as
homicidal, intentional (*see also* Assault, burning) E968.0
undetermined whether accidental or intentional (*see also* Burn, stated as undetermined whether accidental or intentional) E988.1
internal, from swallowed caustic, corrosive liquid, substance - *see* Table of Drugs and Chemicals

Burning, burns *(Continued)*
in
terrorism E979.3
from nuclear explosion E979.5
petrol bomb E979.3
war operations (from fire-producing device or conventional weapon) E990.9
from nuclear explosion E996
petrol bomb E990.0
lamp (*see also* Fire, specified NEC) E898.1
late effect of NEC E929.4
lighter (cigar) (cigarette) (*see also* Fire, specified NEC) E898.1
lightning E907
liquid (boiling) (hot) (molten) E924.0
caustic, corrosive (external) E924.1
swallowed - *see* Table of Drugs and Chemicals
local application of externally applied substance in medical or surgical care E873.5
machinery - *see* Accident, machine
matches (*see also* Fire, specified NEC) E898.1
medicament, externally applied E873.5
metal, molten E924.0
object (hot) E924.8
producing fire or flames - *see* Fire
oven (electric) (gas) E924.8
pipe (smoking) (*see also* Fire, specified NEC) E898.1
radiation - *see* Radiation
railway engine, locomotive, train (*see also* Explosion, railway engine) E803
self-inflicted (unspecified whether accidental or intentional) E988.1
caustic or corrosive substance NEC E988.7
stated as intentional, purposeful E958.1
caustic or corrosive substance NEC E958.7
stated as undetermined whether accidental or intentional E988.1
caustic or corrosive substance NEC E988.7
steam E924.0
pipe E924.8
substance (hot) E924.9
boiling or molten E924.0
caustic, corrosive (external) E924.1
swallowed - *see* Table of Drugs and Chemicals
suicidal (attempt) NEC E958.1
caustic substance E958.7
late effect of E959
tanning bed E926.2
therapeutic misadventure
overdose of radiation E873.2
torch, welding (*see also* Fire, specified NEC) E898.1
trash fire (*see also* Burning, bonfire) E897
vapor E924.0
vitriol E924.1
x-rays E926.3
in medical, surgical procedure - *see* Misadventure, failure, in dosage, radiation operations
Butted by animal E906.8

C

Cachexia, lead or saturnine E866.0
from pesticide NEC (*see also* Table of Drugs and Chemicals) E863.4
Caisson disease E902.2
Capital punishment (any means) E978
Car sickness E903
Casualty (not due to war) NEC E928.9
terrorism E979.8
war (*see also* War operations) E995
Cat
bite E906.3
scratch E906.8
Cataclysmic (any injury)
earth surface movement or eruption E909.9
specified type NEC E909.8
storm or flood resulting from storm E908.9
specified type NEC E909.8
Catching fire - *see* Ignition
Caught
between
objects (moving) (stationary and moving) E918
and machinery - *see* Accident, machine
by cable car, not on rails E847
in
machinery (moving parts of) - *see* Accident, machine
object E918
Cave-in (causing asphyxia, suffocation (by pressure)) (*see also* Suffocation, due to, cave-in) E913.3
with injury other than asphyxia or suffocation E916
with asphyxia or suffocation (*see also* Suffocation, due to, cave-in) E913.3
struck or crushed by E916
with asphyxia or suffocation (*see also* Suffocation, due to, cave-in) E913.3
Change(s) in air pressure - *see also* Effects of, air pressure
sudden, in aircraft (ascent) (descent) (causing aeroneurosis or aviators' disease) E902.1
Chilblains E901.0
due to manmade conditions E901.1
Choking (on) (any object except food or vomitus) E912
apple E911
bone E911
food, any type (regurgitated) E911
mucus or phlegm E912
seed E911
Civil insurrection - *see* War operations
Cloudburst E908.8
Cold, exposure to (accidental) (excessive) (extreme) (place) E901.9
causing chilblains or immersion foot E901.0
due to
manmade conditions E901.1
specified cause NEC E901.8
weather (conditions) E901.0
late effect of NEC E929.5
self-inflicted (undetermined whether accidental or intentional) E988.3
suicidal E958.3
suicide E958.3
Colic, lead, painters', or saturnine - *see* category E866
Collapse
building E916
burning (uncontrolled fire) E891.8
in terrorism E979.3
private E890.8
dam E909.3
due to heat - *see* Heat
machinery - *see* Accident, machine or vehicle
man-made structure E909.3
postoperative NEC E878.9
structure
burning (uncontrolled fire NEC) E891.8
in terrorism E979.3
Collision (accidental)

Note In the case of collisions between different types of vehicles, persons, and objects, priority in classification is in the following order:

Aircraft
Watercraft
Motor vehicle
Railway vehicle
Pedal cycle
Animal-drawn vehicle
Animal being ridden
Streetcar or other nonmotor road vehicle
Other vehicle
Pedestrian or person using pedestrian conveyance
Object (except where falling from or set in motion by vehicle, etc. listed above)

In the listing below, the combinations are listed only under the vehicle, etc., having priority. For definitions, *see* Supplementary Classification of External Causes of Injury and Poisoning (E800–E999).

aircraft (with object or vehicle) (fixed)- entrance (on (movable) (moving)) E841
with
person (while landing, taking off) vehicle off the (without accident to aircraft) E844
powered (in transit) (with unpowered aircraft) E841
while landing, taking off E840
unpowered E842
while landing, taking off E840
animal being ridden (in sport or transport) E828
and
animal (being ridden) (herded) (unattended) E828
nonmotor road vehicle, except pedal cycle or animal-drawn vehicle E828
object (fallen) (fixed) (movable) (moving) not falling from or set in motion by vehicle of higher priority E828
pedestrian (conveyance or vehicle) E828

Collision *(Continued)*
animal-drawn vehicle E827
and
animal (being ridden) (herded) (unattended) E827
nonmotor road vehicle, except pedal cycle E827
object (fallen) (fixed) (movable) (moving) not falling from or set in motion by vehicle of higher priority E827
pedestrian (conveyance or vehicle) E827
streetcar E827
motor vehicle (on public highway) (traffic accident) E812
after leaving, running off, public highway (without antecedent collision) (without re-entry) E816
with antecedent collision on public highway - *see* categories E810–E815
with re-entrance collision with another motor vehicle E811
and
abutment (bridge) (overpass) E815
animal (herded) (unattended) E815
carrying person, property E813
animal-drawn vehicle E813
another motor vehicle (abandoned) (disabled) (parked) (stalled) (stopped) E812
with, involving re-entrance (on same roadway) (across median strip) E811
any object, person, or vehicle off the public highway resulting from a noncollision motor vehicle nontraffic accident E816
avalanche, fallen or not moving E815
falling E909.2
boundary fence E815
culvert E815
fallen
stone E815
tree E815
guard post or guard rail E815
inter-highway divider E815
landslide, fallen or not moving E815
moving E909.2
machinery (road) E815
nonmotor road vehicle NEC E813
object (any object, person, or vehicle off the public highway resulting from a noncollision motor vehicle nontraffic accident) E815
off, normally not on, public highway resulting from a noncollision motor vehicle traffic accident E816
pedal cycle E813
pedestrian (conveyance) E814
person (using pedestrian conveyance) E814
post or pole (lamp) (light) (signal) (telephone) (utility) E815
railway rolling stock, train, vehicle E810
safety island E815

Collision *(Continued)*
motor vehicle *(Continued)*
and *(Continued)*
street car E813
traffic signal, sign, or marker (temporary) E815
tree E815
tricycle E813
wall or cut made for road E815
due to cataclysm - *see* categories E908, E909
not on public highway, nontraffic accident E822
and
animal (carrying person, property) (herded) (unattended) E822
animal-drawn vehicle E822
another motor vehicle (moving), except off-road motor vehicle E822
stationary E823
avalanche, fallen, not moving NEC E823
moving E909.2
landslide, fallen, not moving E823
moving E909.2
nonmotor vehicle (moving) E822
stationary E823
object (fallen) ((normally) (fixed)) (movable but not in motion) (stationary) E823
moving, except when falling from, set in motion by, aircraft or cataclysm E822
pedal cycle (moving) E822
stationary E823
pedestrian (conveyance) E822
person (using pedestrian conveyance) E822
railway rolling stock, train, vehicle (moving) E822
stationary E823
road vehicle (any) (moving) E822
stationary E823
tricycle (moving) E822
stationary E823
off-road type motor vehicle (not on public highway) E821
and
animal (being ridden) (-drawn vehicle) E821
another off-road motor vehicle, except snow vehicle E821
other motor vehicle, not on public highway E821
other object or vehicle NEC, fixed or movable, not set in motion by aircraft, motor vehicle on highway, or snow vehicle, motor-driven E821
pedal cycle E821
pedestrian (conveyance) E821
railway train E821
on public highway - *see* Collision, motor vehicle
pedal cycle E826
and
animal (carrying person, property) (herded) (unherded) E826
animal-drawn vehicle E826
another pedal cycle E826
nonmotor road vehicle E826

Collision *(Continued)*
pedal cycle *(Continued)*
and *(Continued)*
object (fallen) (fixed) (movable) (moving) not falling from or set in motion by aircraft, motor vehicle, or railway train NEC E826
pedestrian (conveyance) E826
person (using pedestrian conveyance) E826
street car E826
pedestrian(s) (conveyance) E917.9
with fall E886.9
in sports E886.0
and
crowd, human stampede E917.1
with subsequent fall E917.6
furniture E917.3
with subsequent fall E917.7
machinery - *see* Accident, machine
object (fallen) (moving) not falling from or set in motion by any vehicle classifiable to E800–E848, E917.9
caused by a crowd E917.1
with subsequent fall E917.6
furniture E917.3
with subsequent fall E917.7
in
running water E917.2
with drowning or submersion - *see* Submersion
sports E917.0
with subsequent fall E917.5
stationary E917.4
with subsequent fall E917.8
vehicle, nonmotor, nonroad E848
in
running water E917.2
with drowning or submersion - *see* Submersion
sports E917.0
with fall E886.0
person(s) (using pedestrian conveyance) (*see also* Collision, pedestrian) E917.9
railway (rolling stock) (train) (vehicle) (with (subsequent) derailment, explosion, fall or fire) E800
with antecedent derailment E802
and
animal (carrying person) (herded) (unattended) E801
another railway train or vehicle E800
buffers E801
fallen tree on railway E801
farm machinery, nonmotor (in transport) (stationary) E801
gates E801
nonmotor vehicle E801
object (fallen) (fixed) (movable) (movable) (moving) not falling from, set in motion by, aircraft or motor vehicle NEC E801
pedal cycle E801
pedestrian (conveyance) E805
person (using pedestrian conveyance) E805
platform E801
rock on railway E801
street car E801

Collision *(Continued)*
snow vehicle, motor-driven (not on public highway) E820
and
animal (being ridden) (-drawn vehicle) E820
another off-road motor vehicle E820
other motor vehicle, not on public highway E820
other object or vehicle NEC, fixed or movable, not set in motion by aircraft or motor vehicle on highway E820
pedal cycle E820
pedestrian (conveyance) E820
railway train E820
on public highway - *see* Collision, motor vehicle
street car(s) E829
and
animal, herded, not being ridden, unattended E829
nonmotor road vehicle NEC E829
object (fallen) (fixed) (movable) (moving) not falling from or set in motion by aircraft, animal-drawn vehicle, animal being ridden, motor vehicle, pedal cycle, or railway train E829
pedestrian (conveyance) E829
person (using pedestrian conveyance) E829
vehicle
animal-drawn - *see* Collision, animal-drawn vehicle
motor - *see* Collision, motor vehicle
nonmotor
nonroad E848
and
another nonmotor, nonroad vehicle E848
object (fallen) (fixed) (movable) (moving) not falling from or set in motion by aircraft, animal-drawn vehicle, animal being ridden, motor vehicle, nonmotor road vehicle, pedal cycle, railway train, or streetcar E848
road, except animal being ridden, animal-drawn vehicle, or pedal cycle E829
and
animal, herded, not being ridden, unattended E829
another nonmotor road vehicle, except animal being ridden, animal-drawn vehicle, or pedal cycle E829
object (fallen) (fixed) (movable) (moving) not falling from or set in motion by, aircraft, animal-drawn vehicle, animal being ridden, motor vehicle, pedal cycle, or railway train E829
pedestrian (conveyance) E829
person (using pedestrian conveyance) E829
vehicle, nonmotor, nonroad E829

Collision *(Continued)*
watercraft E838
and
person swimming or water skiing E838
causing
drowning, submersion E830
injury except drowning, submersion E831
Combustion, spontaneous - *see* Ignition
Complication of medical or surgical procedure or treatment
as an abnormal reaction - *see* Reaction, abnormal
delayed, without mention of misadventure - *see* Reaction, abnormal
due to misadventure - *see* Misadventure
Compression
divers' squeeze E902.2
trachea by
food E911
foreign body, except food E912
Conflagration
building or structure, except private dwelling (barn) (church) (convalescent or residential home) (factory) (farm outbuilding) (hospital) (hotel) or (institution (educational) (dormitory) (residential)) (school) (shop) (store) (theatre) E891.9
with or causing (injury due to)
accident or injury NEC E891.9
specified circumstance NEC E891.8
burns, burning E891.3
carbon monoxide E891.2
fumes E891.2
polyvinylchloride (PVC) or similar material E891.1
smoke E891.2
causing explosion E891.0
in terrorism E979.3
not in building or structure E892
private dwelling (apartment) (boarding house) (camping place) (caravan) (farmhouse) (home (private)) (house) (lodging house) (private garage) (rooming house) (tenement) E890.9
with or causing (injury due to) accident or injury NEC E890.9
specified circumstance NEC E890.8
burns, burning E890.3
carbon monoxide E890.2
fumes E890.2
polyvinylchloride (PVC) or similar material E890.1
smoke E890.2
causing explosion E890.0
Constriction, external
caused by
hair E928.4
other object E928.5
Contact with
dry ice E901.1
liquid air, hydrogen, nitrogen E901.1
Cramp(s)
Heat - *see* Heat
swimmers (*see also* category E910) E910.2
not in recreation or sport E910.3
Cranking (car) (truck) (bus) (engine) injury by E917.9

Crash
aircraft (in transit) (powered) E841
at landing, take-off E840
in
terrorism E979.1
war operations E994
on runway NEC E840
stated as
homicidal E968.8
suicidal E958.6
undetermined whether accidental or intentional E988.6
unpowered E842
glider E842
motor vehicle - *see also* Accident, motor vehicle
homicidal E968.5
suicidal E958.5
undetermined whether accidental or intentional E988.5
Crushed (accidentally) E928.9
between
boat(s), ship(s), watercraft (and dock or pier) (without accident to watercraft) E838
after accident to, or collision, watercraft E831
objects (moving) (stationary and moving) E918
by
avalanche NEC E909.2
boat, ship, watercraft after accident to, collision, watercraft E831
cave-in E916
with asphyxiation or suffocation (*see also* Suffocation, due to, cave-in) E913.3
crowd, human stampede E917.1
falling
aircraft (*see also* Accident, aircraft) E841
in
terrorism E979.1
war operations E994
earth, material E916
with asphyxiation or suffocation (*see also* Suffocation, due to, cave-in) E913.3
object E916
on ship, watercraft E838
while loading, unloading watercraft E838
landslide NEC E909.2
lifeboat after abandoning ship E831
machinery - *see* Accident, machine
railway rolling stock, train, vehicle (part of) E805
street car E829
vehicle NEC - *see* Accident, vehicle NEC
in
machinery - *see* Accident, machine
object E918
transport accident - *see* categories E800–E848
late effect of NEC E929.9
Cut, cutting (any part of body) (accidental) E920.9
by
arrow E920.8
axe E920.4
bayonet (*see also* Bayonet wound) E920.3
blender E920.2

Cut, cutting *(Continued)*
by *(Continued)*
broken glass E920.8
following fall E888.0
can opener E920.4
powered E920.2
chisel E920.4
circular saw E919.4
cutting or piercing instrument - *see also* category E920
following fall E888.0
late effect of E929.8
dagger E920.3
dart E920.8
drill - *see* Accident, caused by drill
edge of stiff paper E920.8
electric
beater E920.2
fan E920.2
knife E920.2
mixer E920.2
fork E920.4
garden fork E920.4
hand saw or tool (not powered) E920.4
powered E920.1
hedge clipper E920.4
powered E920.1
hoe E920.4
ice pick E920.4
knife E920.3
electric E920.2
lathe turnings E920.8
lawn mower E920.4
powered E920.0
riding E919.8
machine - *see* Accident, machine
meat
grinder E919.8
slicer E919.8
nails E920.8
needle E920.4
hypodermic E920.5
object, edged, pointed, sharp - *see* category E920
following fall E888.0
paper cutter E920.4
piercing instrument - *see also* category E920
late effect of E929.8
pitchfork E920.4
powered
can opener E920.2
garden cultivator E920.1
riding E919.8
hand saw E920.1
hand tool NEC E920.1
hedge clipper E920.1
household appliance or implement E920.2
lawn mower (hand) E920.0
riding E919.8
rivet gun E920.1
staple gun E920.1
rake E920.4
saw
circular E919.4
hand E920.4
scissors E920.4
screwdriver E920.4
sewing machine (electric) (powered) E920.2
not powered E920.4
shears E920.4

Cut, cutting *(Continued)*
by *(Continued)*
shovel E920.4
spade E920.4
splinters E920.8
sword E920.3
tin can lid E920.8
wood slivers E920.8
homicide (attempt) E966
inflicted by other person
stated as
intentional, homicidal E966
undetermined whether accidental or intentional E986
late effect of NEC E929.8
legal
execution E978
intervention E974
self-inflicted (unspecified whether accidental or intentional) E986
stated as intentional, purposeful E956
stated as undetermined whether accidental or intentional E986
suicidal (attempt) E956
terrorism E979.8
war operations E995
Cyclone E908.1

D

Death due to injury occurring one year or more previous - *see* Late effect
Decapitation (accidental circumstances) NEC E928.9
homicidal E966
legal execution (by guillotine) E978
Deprivation - *see also* Privation action E913.3
homicidal intent E968.4
Derailment (accidental)
railway (rolling stock) (train) (vehicle) (with subsequent collision) E802
with
collision (antecedent) (*see also* Collision, railway) E800
explosion (subsequent) (without antecedent collision) E802
antecedent collision E803
fall (without collision (antecedent)) E802
fire (without collision (antecedent)) E802
street car E829
Descent
parachute (voluntary) (without accident to aircraft) E844
due to accident to aircraft - *see* categories E840–E842
Desertion
child, with intent to injure or kill E968.4
helpless person, infant, newborn E904.0
with intent to injure or kill E968.4
Destitution - *see* Privation
Disability, late effect or sequela of injury - *see* Late effect
Disease
Andes E902.0
aviators' E902.1
caisson E902.2
range E902.0
Divers' disease, palsy, paralysis, squeeze E902.0
Dog bite E906.0
Dragged by
cable car (not on rails) E847
on rails E829
motor vehicle (on highway) E814
not on highway, nontraffic accident E825
street car E829
Drinking poison (accidental) - *see* Table of Drugs and Chemicals
Drowning - *see* Submersion
Dust in eye E914

E

Earth falling (on) (with asphyxia or suffocation (by pressure)) (*see also* Suffocation, due to, cave-in) E913.3
as, or due to, a cataclysm (involving any transport vehicle) - *see* categories E908, E909
not due to cataclysmic action E913.3
motor vehicle (in motion) (on public highway) E818
not on public highway E825
nonmotor road vehicle NEC E829
pedal cycle E826
railway rolling stock, train, vehicle E806
street car E829
struck or crushed by E916
with asphyxiation or suffocation E913.3
with injury other than asphyxia, suffocation E916
Earthquake (any injury) E909.0
Effect(s) (adverse) of
air pressure E902.9
at high altitude E902.9
in aircraft E902.1
residence or prolonged visit (causing conditions classifiable to E902.0) E902.0
due to
diving E902.2
specified cause NEC E902.8
in aircraft E902.1
cold, excessive (exposure to) (*see also* Cold, exposure to) E901.9
heat (excessive) (*see also* Heat) E900.9
hot
place - *see* Heat
weather E900.0
insulation - *see* Heat
late - *see* Late effect of
motion E903
nuclear explosion or weapon
in
terrorism E979.5
war operations (blast) (fireball) (heat) (radiation) (direct) (secondary) E996
radiation - *see* Radiation
terrorism, secondary E979.9
travel E903
Electric shock, electrocution (accidental) (from exposed wire, faulty appliance, high voltage cable, live rail, open socket) (by) (in) E925.9
appliance or wiring
domestic E925.0
factory E925.2
farm (building) E925.8
house E925.0

Electric shock, electrocution *(Continued)*
appliance or wiring *(Continued)*
home E925.0
industrial (conductor) (control apparatus) (transformer) E925.2
outdoors E925.8
public building E925.8
residential institution E925.8
school E925.8
specified place NEC E925.8
caused by other person
stated as
intentional, homicidal E968.8
undetermined whether accidental or intentional E988.4
electric power generating plant, distribution station E925.1
homicidal (attempt) E968.8
legal execution E978
lightning E907
machinery E925.9
domestic E925.0
factory E925.2
farm E925.8
home E925.0
misadventure in medical or surgical procedure
in electroshock therapy E873.4
self-inflicted (undetermined whether accidental or intentional) E988.4
stated as intentional E958.4
stated as undetermined whether accidental or intentional E988.4
suicidal (attempt) E958.4
transmission line E925.1
Electrocution - *see* Electric shock
Embolism E921.1
air (traumatic) NEC - *see* Air, embolism
Encephalitis
lead or saturnine E866.0
from pesticide NEC E863.4
Entanglement
in
bedclothes, causing suffocation E913.0
wheel of pedal cycle E826
Entry of foreign body, material, any - *see* Foreign body
Execution, legal (any method) E978
Exhaustion
cold - *see* Cold, exposure to
due to excessive exertion E927
heat - *see* Heat
Explosion (accidental) (in) (of) (on) E923.9
acetylene E923.2
aerosol can E921.8
aircraft (in transit) (powered) E841
at landing, take-off E840
in
terrorism E979.1
war operations E994
unpowered E842
air tank (compressed) (in machinery) E921.1
anesthetic gas in operating theatre E923.2
automobile tire NEC E921.8
causing transport accident - *see* categories E810-E825
blasting (cap) (materials) E923.1
boiler (machinery), not on transport vehicle E921.0
steamship - *see* Explosion, water craft

Explosion *(Continued)*
bomb E923.8
in
terrorism E979.2
war operations E993
after cessation of hostilities E998
atom, hydrogen, or nuclear E996
injury by fragments from E991.9
antipersonnel bomb E991.3
butane E923.2
caused by
other person
stated as
intentional, homicidal - *see* Assault, explosive
undetermined whether accidental or homicidal E985.5
coal gas E923.2
detonator E923.1
dynamite E923.1
explosive (material) NEC E923.9
gas(es) E923.2
missile E923.8
in
terrorism E979.2
war operations E993
injury by fragments from E991.9
antipersonnel bomb E991.3
used in blasting operations E923.1
fire-damp E923.2
fireworks E923.0
gas E923.2
cylinder (in machinery) E921.1
pressure tank (in machinery) E921.1
gasoline (fumes) (tank) not in moving motor vehicle E923.2
grain store (military) (munitions) E923.8
grenade E923.8
in
terrorism E979.2
war operations E993
injury by fragments from E991.9
homicide (attempt) - *see* Assault, explosive
hot water heater, tank (in machinery) E921.0
in mine (of explosive gases) NEC E923.2
late effect of NEC E929.8
machinery - *see also* Accident, machine
pressure vessel - *see* Explosion, pressure vessel
methane E923.2
missile E923.8
in
terrorism E979.2
war operations E993
injury by fragments from E991.9
motor vehicle (part of)
in motion (on public highway) E818
not on public highway E825
munitions (dump) (factory) E923.8
in
terrorism E979.2
war operations E993
of mine E923.8
in
terrorism
at sea or in harbor E979.0
land E979.2
marine E979.0
war operations
after cessation of hostilities E998

Explosion *(Continued)*
of mine *(Continued)*
in *(Continued)*
war operations *(Continued)*
at sea or in harbor E992
land E993
after cessation of hostilities E998
injured by fragments from E991.9
marine E992
own weapons
in
terrorism (*see also* Suicide) E979.2
war operations E993
injured by fragments from E991.9
antipersonnel bomb E991.3
pressure
cooker E921.8
gas tank (in machinery) E921.1
vessel (in machinery) E921.9
on transport vehicle - *see* categories E800-E848
specified type NEC E921.8
propane E923.2
railway engine, locomotive, train (boiler) (with subsequent collision, derailment, fall) E803
with
collision (antecedent) (*see also* Collision, railway) E800
derailment (antecedent) E802
fire (without antecedent collision or derailment) E803
secondary fire resulting from - *see* Fire
self-inflicted (unspecified whether accidental or intentional) E985.5
stated as intentional, purposeful E955.5
shell (artillery) E923.8
in
terrorism E979.2
war operations E993
injury by fragments from E991.9
stated as undetermined whether caused accidentally or purposely inflicted E985.5
steam or water lines (in machinery) E921.0
suicide (attempted) E955.5
torpedo E923.8
in
terrorism E979.0
war operations E992
transport accident - *see* categories E800–E848
war operations - *see* War operations, explosion
watercraft (boiler) E837
causing drowning, submersion (after jumping from watercraft) E830
Exposure (conditions) (rain) (weather) (wind) E904.3
with homicidal intent E968.4
excessive E904.3
cold (*see also* Cold, exposure to) E901.9
self-inflicted - *see* Cold, exposure to, self-inflicted
heat (*see also* Heat) E900.9
helpless person, infant, newborn due to abandonment or neglect E904.0
noise E928.1

ICD-9-CM
E Codes
Vol. 2

Exposure *(Continued)*
prolonged in deep-freeze unit or refrigerator E901.1
radiation - *see* Radiation
resulting from transport accident - *see* categories E800–E848
smoke from, due to
fire - *see* Fire
tobacco, second-hand E869.4
vibration E928.2

F

Fall, falling (accidental) E888.9
building E916
burning E891.8
private E890.8
down
escalator E880.0
ladder E881.0
in boat, ship, watercraft E833
staircase E880.9
stairs, steps - *see* Fall, from, stairs
earth (with asphyxia or suffocation (by pressure)) (*see also* Earth, falling) E913.3
from, off
aircraft (at landing, take-off) (in transit) (while alighting, boarding) E843
resulting from accident to aircraft - *see* categories E840–E842
animal (in sport or transport) E828
animal-drawn vehicle E827
balcony E882
bed E884.4
bicycle E826
boat, ship, watercraft (into water) E832
after accident to, collision, fire on E830
and subsequently struck by (part of) boat E831
and subsequently struck by (part of) while alighting, boat E838
burning, crushed, sinking E830
and subsequently struck by (part of) boat E831
bridge E882
building E882
burning (uncontrolled fire) E891.8
in terrorism E979.3
private E890.8
bunk in boat, ship, watercraft E834
due to accident to watercraft E831
cable car (not on rails) E847
on rails E829
car - *see* Fall from motor vehicle
chair E884.2
cliff E884.1
commode E884.6
curb (sidewalk) E880.1
elevation aboard ship E834
due to accident to ship E831
embankment E884.9
escalator E880.0
fire escape E882
flagpole E882
furniture NEC E884.5
gangplank (into water) (*see also* Fall, from, boat) E832
to deck, dock E834
hammock on ship E834
due to accident to watercraft E831
haystack E884.9

Fall, falling *(Continued)*
from, off *(Continued)*
high place NEC E884.9
stated as undetermined whether accidental or intentional - *see* Jumping, from, high place
horse (in sport or transport) E828
in-line skates E885.1
ladder E881.0
in boat, ship, watercraft E833
due to accident to watercraft E831
machinery - *see also* Accident, machine
not in operation E884.9
motor vehicle (in motion) (on public highway) E818
not on public highway E825
stationary, except while alighting, boarding, entering, leaving E884.9
while alighting, boarding, entering, leaving E824
stationary, except while alighting, boarding, entering, leaving E884.9
while alighting, boarding, entering, leaving, except off-road type motor vehicle E817
off-road type - *see* Fall, from, off-road type motor vehicle
nonmotor road vehicle (while alighting, boarding) NEC E829
stationary, except while alighting, boarding, entering, leaving E884.9
off-road type motor vehicle (not on public highway) NEC E821
on public highway E818
while alighting, boarding, entering, leaving E817
snow vehicle - *see* Fall from snow vehicle, motor-driven
one
deck to another on ship E834
due to accident to ship E831
level to another NEC E884.9
boat, ship, or watercraft E834
due to accident to watercraft E831
pedal cycle E826
playground equipment E884.0
railway rolling stock, train, vehicle (while alighting, boarding) E804
with
collision (*see also* Collision, railway) E800
derailment (*see also* Derailment, railway) E802
explosion (*see also* Explosion, railway engine) E803
rigging (aboard ship) E834
due to accident to watercraft E831
roller skates E885.1
scaffolding E881.1
scooter (nonmotorized) E885.0
sidewalk (curb) E880.1
moving E885.9
skateboard E885.2
skis E885.3
snow vehicle, motor-driven (not on public highway) E820
on public highway E818
while alighting, boarding, entering, leaving E817

Fall, falling *(Continued)*
from, off *(Continued)*
snowboard E885.4
stairs, steps E880.9
boat, ship, watercraft E833
due to accident to watercraft E831
motor bus, motor vehicle - *see* Fall, from, motor vehicle, while alighting, boarding
street car E829
stationary vehicle NEC E884.9
stepladder E881.0
street car (while boarding, alighting) E829
stationary, except while boarding or alighting E884.9
structure NEC E882
burning (uncontrolled fire) E891.8
in terrorism E979.3
table E884.9
toilet E884.6
tower E882
tree E884.9
turret E882
vehicle NEC - *see also* Accident, vehicle NEC
stationary E884.9
viaduct E882
wall E882
wheelchair E884.3
window E882
in, on
aircraft (at landing, take-off) (in transit) E843
resulting from accident to aircraft - *see* categories E840–E842
boat, ship, watercraft E835
due to accident to watercraft E831
one level to another NEC E834
on ladder, stairs E833
cutting or piercing instrument machine E888.0
deck (of boat, ship, watercraft) E835
due to accident to watercraft E831
escalator E880.0
gangplank E835
glass, broken E888.0
knife E888.0
ladder E881.0
in boat, ship, watercraft E833
due to accident to watercraft E831
object
edged, pointed or sharp E888.0
other E888.1
pitchfork E888.0
railway rolling stock, train, vehicle (while alighting, boarding) E804
with
collision (*see also* Collision, railway) E800
derailment (*see also* Derailment, railway) E802
explosion (*see also* Explosion, railway engine) E803
scaffolding E881.1
scissors E888.0
staircase, stairs, steps (*see also* Fall, from, stairs) E880.9
street car E829
water transport (*see also* Fall, in, boat) E835

Fall, falling *(Continued)*
into
cavity E883.9
dock E883.9
from boat, ship, watercraft (*see also* Fall, from, boat) E832
hold (of ship) E834
due to accident to watercraft E831
hole E883.9
manhole E883.2
moving part of machinery - *see* Accident, machine
opening in surface NEC E883.9
pit E883.9
quarry E883.9
shaft E883.9
storm drain E883.2
tank E883.9
water (with drowning or submersion) E910.9
well E883.1
late effect of NEC E929.3
object (*see also* Hit by, object, falling) E916
other E888.8
over
animal E885.9
cliff E884.1
embankment E884.9
small object E885.9
overboard (*see also* Fall, from, boat) E832
resulting in striking against object E888.1
sharp E888.0
rock E916
same level NEC E888.9
aircraft (any kind) E843
resulting from accident to aircraft - *see* categories E840–E842
boat, ship, watercraft E835
due to accident to, collision, watercraft E831
from
collision, pushing, shoving, by or with other person(s) E886.9
as, or caused by, a crowd E917.6
in sports E886.0
in-line skates E885.1
roller skates E885.1
scooter (nonmotorized) E885.0
skateboard E885.2
skis E885.3
slipping, stumbling, tripping E885.9
snowboard E885.4
snowslide E916
as avalanche E909.2
stone E916
through
hatch (on ship) E834
due to accident to watercraft E831
roof E882
window E882
timber E916
while alighting from, boarding, entering, leaving
aircraft (any kind) E843
motor bus, motor vehicle - *see* Fall, from, motor vehicle, while alighting, boarding
nonmotor road vehicle NEC E829
railway train E804
street car E829

Fallen on by
animal (horse) (not being ridden) E906.8
being ridden (in sport or transport) E828
Fell or jumped from high place, so stated - *see* Jumping, from, high place
Felo-de-se (*see also* Suicide) E958.9
Fever
heat - *see* Heat
thermic - *see* Heat
Fight (hand) (fist) (foot) (*see also* Assault, fight) E960.0
Fire (accidental) (caused by great heat from appliance (electrical), hot object, or hot substance) (secondary, resulting from explosion) E899
conflagration - *see* Conflagration
controlled, normal (in brazier, fireplace, furnace, or stove) (charcoal) (coal) (coke) (electric) (gas) (wood)
bonfire E897
brazier, not in building or structure E897
in building or structure, except private dwelling (barn) (church) (convalescent or residential home) (factory) (farm outbuilding) (hospital) (hotel) (institution (educational) (dormitory) (residential)) (private garage) (school) (shop) (store) (theatre) E896
in private dwelling (apartment) (boarding house) (camping place) (caravan) (farmhouse) (home (private)) (house) (lodging house) (rooming house) (tenement) E895
not in building or structure E897
trash E897
forest (uncontrolled) E892
grass (uncontrolled) E892
hay (uncontrolled) E892
homicide (attempt) E968.0
late effect of E969
in, of, on, starting in E892
aircraft (in transit) (powered) E841
at landing, take-off E840
stationary E892
unpowered (balloon) (glider) E842
balloon E842
boat, ship, watercraft - *see* categories E830, E831, E837
building or structure, except private dwelling (barn) (church) (convalescent or residential home) (factory) (farm outbuilding) (hospital) (hotel) (institution) (educational) (dormitory) (residential)) (school) (shop) (store) (theatre) (*see also* Conflagration, building or structure, except private dwelling) E891.9
forest (uncontrolled) E892
glider E842
grass (uncontrolled) E892
hay (uncontrolled) E892
lumber (uncontrolled) E892
machinery - *see* Accident, machine
mine (uncontrolled) E892
motor vehicle (in motion) (on public highway) E818
not on public highway E825
stationary E892

Fire *(Continued)*
in, of, on, starting in *(Continued)*
prairie (uncontrolled) E892
private dwelling (apartment) (boarding house) (camping place) (caravan) (farmhouse) (home (private)) (house) (lodging house) (private garage) (rooming house) (tenement) (*see also* Conflagration, private dwelling) E890.9
railway rolling stock, train, vehicle (*see also* Explosion, railway engine) E803
stationary E892
room NEC E898.1
street car (in motion) E829
stationary E892
terrorism (by fire-producing device) E979.3
fittings or furniture (burning buildings) (uncontrolled fire) E979.3
from nuclear explosion E979.5
transport vehicle, stationary NEC E892
tunnel (uncontrolled) E892
war operations (by fire-producing device or conventional weapon) E990.9
from nuclear explosion E996
petrol bomb E990.0
late effect of NEC E929.4
lumber (uncontrolled) E892
mine (uncontrolled) E892
prairie (uncontrolled) E892
self-inflicted (unspecified whether accidental or intentional) E988.1
stated as intentional, purposeful E958.1
specified NEC E898.1
with
conflagration - *see* Conflagration
ignition (of)
clothing - *see* Ignition, clothes
highly inflammable material (benzine) (fat) (gasoline) (kerosene) (paraffin) (petrol) E894
started by other person
stated as
with intent to injure or kill E968.0
undetermined whether or not with intent to injure or kill E988.1
suicide (attempted) E958.1
late effect of E959
tunnel (uncontrolled) E892
Fireball effects from nuclear explosion
in
terrorism E979.5
war operations E996
Fireworks (explosion) E923.0
Flash burns from explosion (*see also* Explosion) E923.9
Flood (any injury) (resulting from storm) E908.2
caused by collapse of dam or manmade structure E909.3
Forced landing (aircraft) E840
Foreign body, object or material (entrance into (accidental))
air passage (causing injury) E915
with asphyxia, obstruction, suffocation E912
food or vomitus E911

Foreign body, object or material *(Continued)*
air passage *(Continued)*
nose (with asphyxia, obstruction, suffocation) E912
causing injury without asphyxia, obstruction, suffocation E915
alimentary canal (causing injury) (with obstruction) E915
with asphyxia, obstruction respiratory passage, suffocation E912
food E911
mouth E915
with asphyxia, obstruction, suffocation E912
food E911
pharynx E915
with asphyxia, obstruction, suffocation E912
food E911
aspiration (with asphyxia, obstruction respiratory passage, suffocation) E912
causing injury without asphyxia, obstruction respiratory passage, suffocation E915
food (regurgitated) (vomited) E911
causing injury without asphyxia, obstruction respiratory passage, suffocation E915
mucus (not of newborn) E912
phlegm E912
bladder (causing injury or obstruction) E915
bronchus, bronchi - *see* Foreign body, air passages
conjunctival sac E914
digestive system - *see* Foreign body, alimentary canal
ear (causing injury or obstruction) E915
esophagus (causing injury or obstruction) (*see also* Foreign body, alimentary canal) E915
eye (any part) E914
eyelid E914
hairball (stomach) (with obstruction) E915
ingestion - *see* Foreign body, alimentary canal
inhalation - *see* Foreign body, aspiration
intestine (causing injury or obstruction) E915
iris E914
lacrimal apparatus E914
larynx - *see* Foreign body, air passage
late effect of NEC E929.8
lung - *see* Foreign body, air passage
mouth - *see* Foreign body, alimentary canal, mouth
nasal passage - *see* Foreign body, air passage, nose
nose - *see* Foreign body, air passage, nose
ocular muscle E914
operation wound (left in) - *see* Misadventure, foreign object
orbit E914
pharynx - *see* Foreign body, alimentary canal, pharynx
rectum (causing injury or obstruction) E915
stomach (hairball) (causing injury or obstruction) E915
tear ducts or glands E914

Foreign body, object or material *(Continued)*
trachea - *see* Foreign body, air passage
urethra (causing injury or obstruction) E915
vagina (causing injury or obstruction) E915
Found dead, injured
from exposure (to) - *see* Exposure
on
public highway E819
railway right of way E807
Fracture (circumstances unknown or unspecified) E887
due to specified external means - *see* manner of accident
late effect of NEC E929.3
occurring in water transport NEC E835
Freezing - *see* Cold, exposure to
Frostbite E901.0
due to manmade conditions E901.1
Frozen - *see* Cold, exposure to

G

Garrotting, homicidal (attempted) E963
Gored E906.8
Gunshot wound (*see also* Shooting) E922.9

H

Hailstones, injury by E904.3
Hairball (stomach) (with obstruction) E915
Hanged himself (*see also* Hanging, self-inflicted) E983.0
Hang gliding E842
Hanging (accidental) E913.8
caused by other person
in accidental circumstances E913.8
stated as
intentional, homicidal E963
undetermined whether accidental or intentional E983.0
homicide (attempt) E963
in bed or cradle E913.0
legal execution E978
self-inflicted (unspecified whether accidental or intentional) E983.0
in accidental circumstances E913.8
stated as intentional, purposeful E953.0
stated as undetermined whether accidental or intentional E983.0
suicidal (attempt) E953.0
Heat (apoplexy) (collapse) (cramps) (effects of) (excessive) (exhaustion) (fever) (prostration) (stroke) E900.9
due to
manmade conditions (as listed in E900.1, except boat, ship, watercraft) E900.1
weather (conditions) E900.0
from
electric heating apparatus causing burning E924.8
nuclear explosion
in
terrorism E979.5
war operations E996
generated in, boiler, engine, evaporator, fire room of boat, ship, watercraft E838

Heat *(Continued)*
inappropriate in local application or packing in medical or surgical procedure E873.5
late effect of NEC E989
Hemorrhage
delayed following medical or surgical treatment without mention of misadventure - *see* Reaction, abnormal
during medical or surgical treatment as misadventure - *see* Misadventure, cut
High
altitude, effects E902.9
level of radioactivity, effects - *see* Radiation
pressure effects - *see also* Effects of, air pressure
from rapid descent in water (causing caisson or divers' disease, palsy, or paralysis) E902.2
temperature, effects - *see* Heat
Hit, hitting (accidental) by
aircraft (propeller) (without accident to aircraft) E844
unpowered E842
avalanche E909.2
being thrown against object in or part of
motor vehicle (in motion) (on public highway) E818
not on public highway E825
nonmotor road vehicle NEC E829
street car E829
boat, ship, watercraft
after fall from watercraft E838
damaged, involved in accident E831
while swimming, water skiing E838
bullet (*see also* Shooting) E922.9
from air gun E922.4
in
terrorism E979.4
war operations E991.2
rubber E991.0
flare, Verey pistol (*see also* Shooting) E922.8
hailstones E904.3
landslide E909.2
law-enforcing agent (on duty) E975
with blunt object (baton) (night stick) (stave) (truncheon) E973
machine - *see* Accident, machine
missile
firearm (*see also* Shooting) E922.9
in
terrorism - *see* Terrorism, missile
war operations - *see* War operations, missile
motor vehicle (on public highway) (traffic accident) E814
not on public highway, nontraffic accident E822
nonmotor road vehicle NEC E829
object
falling E916
from, in, on
aircraft E844
due to accident to aircraft - *see* categories E840–E842
unpowered E842
boat, ship, watercraft E838
due to accident to watercraft E831

Hit, hitting *(Continued)*
object *(Continued)*
falling *(Continued)*
from, in, on *(Continued)*
building E916
burning E891.8
in terrorism E979.3
private E890.8
cataclysmic
earth surface movement or eruption E909.9
storm E908.9
cave-in E916
with asphyxiation or suffocation (*see also* Suffocation, due to, cave-in) E913.3
earthquake E909.0
motor vehicle (in motion) (on public highway) E818
not on public highway E825
stationary E916
nonmotor road vehicle NEC E829
pedal cycle E826
railway rolling stock, train, vehicle E806
street car E829
structure, burning NEC E891.8
vehicle, stationary E916
moving NEC - *see* Striking against, object
projected NEC - *see* Striking against, object
set in motion by
compressed air or gas, spring, striking, throwing - *see* Striking against, object
explosion - *see* Explosion
thrown into, on, or towards
motor vehicle (in motion) (on public highway) E818
not on public highway E825
nonmotor road vehicle NEC E829
pedal cycle E826
street car E829
off-road type motor vehicle (not on public highway) E821
on public highway E814
other person(s) E917.9
with blunt or thrown object E917.9
in sports E917.0
with subsequent fall E917.5
intentionally, homicidal E968.2
as, or caused by, a crowd E917.1
with subsequent fall E917.6
in sports E917.0
pedal cycle E826
police (on duty) E975
with blunt object (baton) (nightstick) (stave) (truncheon) E973
railway, rolling stock, train, vehicle (part of) E805
shot - *see* Shooting
snow vehicle, motor-driven (not on public highway) E820
on public highway E814
street car E829
vehicle NEC - *see* Accident, vehicle NEC
Homicide, homicidal (attempt) (justifiable) (*see also* Assault) E968.9
Hot
liquid, object, substance, accident caused by - *see also* Accident, caused by, hot, by type of substance
late effect of E929.8
Hot *(Continued)*
place, effects - *see* Heat
weather, effects E900.0
Humidity, causing problem E904.3
Hunger E904.1
resulting from
abandonment or neglect E904.0
transport accident - *see* categories E800–E848
Hurricane (any injury) E908.0
Hypobarism, hypobaropathy - *see* Effects of, air pressure
Hypothermia - *see* Cold, exposure to

I

Ictus
caloris - *see* Heat
solaris E900.0
Ignition (accidental)
anesthetic gas in operating theatre E923.2
bedclothes
with
conflagration - *see* Conflagration
ignition (of)
clothing - *see* Ignition, clothes
highly inflammable material obstruction (benzine) (fat) (gasoline) (kerosene) (paraffin) (petrol) E894
benzine E894
clothes, clothing (from controlled fire) (in building) E893.9
with conflagration - *see* Conflagration
from
bonfire E893.2
highly inflammable material E894
sources or material as listed in E893.8
trash fire E893.2
uncontrolled fire - *see* Conflagration
in
private dwelling E893.0
specified building or structure, except of private dwelling E893.1
not in building or structure E893.2
explosive material - *see* Explosion
fat E894
gasoline E894
kerosene E894
material
explosive - *see* Explosion
highly inflammable E894
with conflagration - *see* Conflagration
with explosion E923.2
nightdress - *see* Ignition, clothes
paraffin E894
petrol E894
Immersion - *see* Submersion
Implantation of quills of porcupine E906.8
Inanition (from) E904.9
hunger - *see* Lack of, food
resulting from homicidal intent E968.4
thirst - *see* Lack of, water
Inattention after, at birth E904.0
homicidal, infanticidal intent E968.4
Infanticide (*see also* Assault)
Ingestion
foreign body (causing injury) (with obstruction) - *see* Foreign body, alimentary canal
poisonous substance NEC - *see* Table of Drugs and Chemicals
Inhalation
excessively cold substance, manmade E901.1
foreign body - *see* Foreign body, aspiration
liquid air, hydrogen, nitrogen E901.1
mucus, not of newborn (with asphyxia, obstruction respiratory passage, suffocation) E912
phlegm (with asphyxia, obstruction respiratory passage, suffocation) E912
poisonous gas - *see* Table of Drugs and Chemicals
smoke from, due to
fire - *see* Fire
tobacco, second-hand E869.4
vomitus (with asphyxia, obstruction respiratory passage, suffocation) E911
Injury, injured (accidental(ly)) NEC E928.9
by, caused by, from
air rifle (B-B gun) E922.4
animal (not being ridden) NEC E906.9
being ridden (in sport or transport) E828
assault (*see also* Assault) E968.9
avalanche E909.2
bayonet (*see also* Bayonet wound) E920.3
being thrown against some part of, or object in
motor vehicle (in motion) (on public highway) E818
not on public highway E825
nonmotor road vehicle NEC E829
off-road motor vehicle NEC E821
railway train E806
snow vehicle, motor-driven E820
street car E829
bending E927
bite, human E928.3
broken glass E920.8
bullet - *see* Shooting
cave-in (*see also* Suffocation, due to, cave-in) E913.3
earth surface movement or eruption E909.9
storm E908.9
without asphyxiation or suffocation E916
cloudburst E908.8
cutting or piercing instrument (*see also* Cut) E920.9
cyclone E908.1
earth surface movement or eruption E909.9
earthquake E909.0
electric current (*see also* Electric shock) E925.9
explosion (*see also* Explosion) E923.9
fire - *see* Fire
flare, Verey pistol E922.8
flood E908.2
foreign body - *see* Foreign body
hailstones E904.3

ICD-9-CM
E Codes
Vol. 2

Injury, injured *(Continued)*
by, caused by, from *(Continued)*
hurricane E908.0
landslide E909.2
law-enforcing agent, police, in course of legal intervention - *see* Legal intervention
lightning E907
live rail or live wire - *see* Electric shock
machinery - *see also* Accident, machine aircraft, without accident to aircraft E844
boat, ship, watercraft (deck) (engine room) (galley) (laundry) (loading) E836
missile
explosive E923.8
firearm - *see* Shooting
in
terrorism - *see* Terrorism, missile
war operations - *see* War operations, missile
moving part of motor vehicle (in motion) (on public highway) E818
not on public highway, nontraffic accident E825
while alighting, boarding, entering, leaving - *see* Fall, from, motor vehicle, while alighting, boarding
nail E920.8
needle (sewing) E920.4
hypodermic E920.5
noise E928.1
object
fallen on
motor vehicle (in motion) (on public highway) E818
not on public highway E825
falling - *see* Hit by, object, falling
paintball gun E922.5
radiation - *see* Radiation
railway rolling stock, train, vehicle (part of) E805
door or window E806
rotating propeller, aircraft E844
rough landing of off-road type motor vehicle (after leaving ground or rough terrain) E821
snow vehicle E820
saber (*see also* Wound, saber) E920.3
shot - *see* Shooting
sound waves E928.1
splinter or sliver, wood E920.8
straining E927
street car (door) E829
suicide (attempt) E958.9
sword E920.3
terrorism - *see* Terrorism
third rail - *see* Electric shock
thunderbolt E907
tidal wave E909.4
caused by storm E908.0
tornado E908.1
torrential rain E908.2
twisting E927
vehicle NEC - *see* Accident, vehicle NEC
vibration E928.2
volcanic eruption E909.1
weapon burst, in war operations E993
weightlessness (in spacecraft, real or simulated) E928.0
wood splinter or sliver E920.8

Injury, injured *(Continued)*
due to
civil insurrection - *see* War operations
occurring after cessation of hostilities E998
terrorism - *see* Terrorism
war operations - *see* War operations
occurring after cessation of hostilities E998
homicidal (*see also* Assault) E968.9
in, on
civil insurrection - *see* War operations
fight E960.0
parachute descent (voluntary) (without accident to aircraft) E844
with accident to aircraft - *see* categories E840-E842
public highway E819
railway right of way E807
terrorism - *see* Terrorism
war operations - *see* War operations
inflicted (by)
in course of arrest (attempted), suppression of disturbance, maintenance of order, by law enforcing agents - *see* Legal intervention
law-enforcing agent (on duty) - *see* Legal intervention
other person
stated as
accidental E928.9
homicidal, intentional - *see* Assault
undetermined whether accidental or intentional - *see* Injury, stated as undetermined
police (on duty) - *see* Legal intervention
late effect of E929.9
purposely (inflicted) by other person(s) - *see* Assault
self-inflicted (unspecified whether accidental or intentional) E988.9
stated as
accidental E928.9
intentionally, purposely E958.9
specified cause NEC E928.8
stated as
undetermined whether accidentally or purposely inflicted (by) E988.9
cut (any part of body) E986
cutting or piercing instrument (classifiable to E920) E986
drowning E984
explosive(s) (missile) E985.5
falling from high place E987.9
manmade structure, except residential E987.1
natural site E987.2
residential premises E987.0
hanging E983.0
knife E986
late effect of E989
puncture (any part of body) E986
shooting - *see* Shooting, stated as undetermined whether accidental or intentional
specified means NEC E988.8
stab (any part of body) E986
strangulation - *see* Suffocation, stated as undetermined whether accidental or intentional
submersion E984

Injury, injured *(Continued)*
stated as *(Continued)*
suffocation - *see* Suffocation, stated as undetermined whether accidental or intentional
to child due to criminal abortion E968.8
Insufficient nourishment - *see also* Lack of, food
homicidal intent E968.4
Insulation, effects - *see* Heat
Interruption of respiration by
food lodged in esophagus E911
foreign body, except food, in esophagus E912
Intervention, legal - *see* Legal intervention
Intoxication, drug or poison - *see* Table of Drugs and Chemicals
Irradiation - *see* Radiation

J

Jammed (accidentally)
between objects (moving) (stationary and moving) E918
in object E918
Jumped or fell from high place, so stated - *see* Jumping, from, high place, stated as
in undetermined circumstances
Jumping
before train, vehicle or other moving object (unspecified whether accidental or intentional) E988.0
stated as
intentional, purposeful E958.0
suicidal (attempt) E958.0
from
aircraft
by parachute (voluntarily) (without accident to aircraft) E844
due to accident to aircraft - *see* categories E840–E842
boat, ship, watercraft (into water)
after accident to, fire on, watercraft E830
and subsequently struck by (part of) boat E831
burning, crushed, sinking E830
and subsequently struck by (part of) boat E831
voluntarily, without accident (to boat) with injury other than drowning or submersion E883.0
building *see also* Jumping, from, high place
burning (uncontrolled fire) E891.8
in terrorism E979.3
private E890.8
cable car (not on rails) E847
on rails E829
high place
in accidental circumstances or in sport - *see* categories E880–E884
stated as
with intent to injure self E957.9
man-made structures NEC E957.1
natural sites E957.2
residential premises E957.0

Jumping *(Continued)*
from *(Continued)*
high place *(Continued)*
stated as *(Continued)*
in undetermined circumstances E987.9
man-made structures NEC E987.1
natural sites E987.2
residential premises E987.0
suicidal (attempt) E957.9
man-made structures NEC E957.1
natural sites E957.1
residential premises E957.0
motor vehicle (in motion) (on public highway) - *see* Fall, from, motor vehicle
nonmotor road vehicle NEC E829
street car E829
structure - *see also* Jumping, from high places
burning NEC (uncontrolled fire) E891.8
in terrorism E979.3
into water
with injury other than drowning or submersion E883.0
drowning or submersion - *see* Submersion
from, off, watercraft - *see* Jumping, from, boat
Justifiable homicide - *see* Assault

K

Kicked by
animal E906.8
person(s) (accidentally) E917.9
with intent to injure or kill E960.0
as, or caused by a crowd E917.1
with subsequent fall E917.6
in fight E960.0
in sports E917.0
with subsequent fall E917.5
Kicking against
object (moving) E917.9
in sports E917.0
with subsequent fall E917.5
stationary E917.4
with subsequent fall E917.8
person - *see* Striking against, person
Killed, killing (accidentally) NEC (*see also* Injury) E928.9
in
action - *see* War operations
brawl, fight (hand) (fists) (foot) E960.0
by weapon - *see also* Assault
cutting, piercing E966
firearm - *see* Shooting, homicide
self
stated as
accident E928.9
suicide - *see* Suicide
unspecified whether accidental or suicidal E988.9
Knocked down (accidentally) (by) NEC E928.9
animal (not being ridden) E906.8
being ridden (in sport or transport) E828
blast from explosion (*see also* Explosion) E923.9

Knocked down *(Continued)*
crowd, human stampede E917.6
late effect of - *see* Late effect
person (accidentally) E917.9
in brawl, fight E960.0
in sports E917.5
transport vehicle - *see* vehicle involved under Hit by
while boxing E917.5

L

Laceration NEC E928.9
Lack of
air (refrigerator or closed place), suffocation by E913.2
care (helpless person) (infant) (newborn) E904.0
homicidal intent E968.4
food except as result of transport accident E904.1
helpless person, infant, newborn due to abandonment or neglect E904.0
water except as result of transport accident E904.2
helpless person, infant, newborn due to abandonment or neglect E904.0
Landslide E909.2
falling on, hitting
motor vehicle (any) (in motion) (on or off public highway) E909.2
railway rolling stock, train, vehicle E909.2
Late effect of
accident NEC (accident classifiable to E928.9) E929.9
specified NEC (accident classifiable to E910–E928.8) E929.8
assault E969
fall, accidental (accident classifiable to E880–E888) E929.3
fire, accident caused by (accident classifiable to E890–E899) E929.4
homicide, attempt (any means) E969
injury due to terrorism E999.1
injury undetermined whether accidentally or purposely inflicted (injury classifiable to E980–E988) E989
legal intervention (injury classifiable to E970–E976) E977
medical or surgical procedure, test or therapy
as, or resulting in, or from
abnormal or delayed reaction or complication - *see* Reaction, abnormal
misadventure - *see* Misadventure
motor vehicle accident (accident classifiable to E810–E825) E929.0
natural or environmental factor, accident due to (accident classifiable to E900–E909) E929.5
poisoning, accidental (accident classifiable to E850–E858, E860–E869) E929.2
suicide, attempt (any means) E959
transport accident NEC (accident classifiable to E800–E807, E826–E838, E840–E848) E929.1
war operations, injury due to (injury classifiable to E990–E998) E999.0

Launching pad accident E845
Legal
execution, any method E978
intervention (by) (injury from) E976
baton E973
bayonet E974
blow E975
blunt object (baton) (nightstick) (stave) (truncheon) E973
cutting or piercing instrument E974
dynamite E971
execution, any method E973
explosive(s) (shell) E971
firearm(s) E970
gas (asphyxiation) (poisoning) (tear) E972
grenade E971
late effect of E977
machine gun E970
manhandling E975
mortar bomb E971
nightstick E973
revolver E970
rifle E970
specified means NEC E975
stabbing E974
stave E973
truncheon E973
Lifting, injury in E927
Lightning (shock) (stroke) (struck by) E907
Liquid (noncorrosive) in eye E914
corrosive E924.1
Loss of control
motor vehicle (on public highway) (without antecedent collision) E816
with
antecedent collision on public highway - *see* Collision, motor vehicle
involving any object, person or vehicle not on public highway E816
on public highway - *see* Collision, motor vehicle
not on public highway, nontraffic accident E825
with antecedent collision - *see* Collision, motor vehicle, not on public highway
off-road type motor vehicle (not on public highway) E821
on public highway - *see* Loss of control, motor vehicle
snow vehicle, motor-driven (not on public highway) E820
on public highway - *see* Loss of control, motor vehicle
Lost at sea E832
with accident to watercraft E830
in war operations E995
Low
pressure, effects - *see* Effects of, air pressure
temperature, effects - *see* Cold exposure to
Lying before train, vehicle or other moving object (unspecified whether accidental or intentional) E988.0
stated as intentional, purposeful, suicidal (attempt) E958.0
Lynching (*see also* Assault) E968.9

M

Malfunction, atomic power plant in water transport E838
Mangled (accidentally) NEC E928.9
Manhandling (in brawl, fight) E960.0
legal intervention E975
Manslaughter (nonaccidental) - *see* Assault
Marble in nose E912
Mauled by animal E906.8
Medical procedure, complication of
delayed or as an abnormal reaction without mention of misadventure - *see* Reaction, abnormal
due to or as a result of misadventure - *see* Misadventure
Melting of fittings and furniture in burning
in terrorism E979.3
Minamata disease E865.2
Misadventure(s) to patient(s) during surgical or medical care E876.9
contaminated blood, fluid, drug or biological substance (presence of agents and toxins as listed in E875) E875.9
administered (by) NEC E875.9
infusion E875.0
injection E875.1
specified means NEC E875.2
transfusion E875.0
vaccination E875.1
cut, cutting, puncture, perforation or hemorrhage (accidental) (inadvertent) (inappropriate) (during) E870.9
aspiration of fluid or tissue (by puncture or catheterization, except heart) E870.5
biopsy E870.8
needle (aspirating) E870.5
blood sampling E870.5
catheterization E870.5
heart E870.6
dialysis (kidney) E870.2
endoscopic examination E870.4
enema E870.7
infusion E870.1
injection E870.3
lumbar puncture E870.5
needle biopsy E870.5
paracentesis, abdominal E870.5
perfusion E870.2
specified procedure NEC E870.8
surgical operation E870.0
thoracentesis E870.5
transfusion E870.1
vaccination E870.3
excessive amount of blood or other fluid during transfusion or infusion E873.0
failure
in dosage E873.9
electroshock therapy E873.4
inappropriate temperature (too hot or too cold) in local application and packing E873.5
infusion
excessive amount of fluid E873.0
incorrect dilution of fluid E873.1
insulin-shock therapy E873.4
nonadministration of necessary drug or medicinal E873.6

Misadventure(s) to patient(s) during surgical or medical care *(Continued)*
failure *(Continued)*
in dosage *(Continued)*
overdose - *see also* Overdose
radiation, in therapy E873.2
radiation
inadvertent exposure of patient (receiving radiation for test or therapy) E873.3
not receiving radiation for test or therapy - *see* Radiation
overdose E873.2
specified procedure NEC E873.8
transfusion
excessive amount of blood E873.0
mechanical, of instrument or apparatus (during procedure) E874.9
aspiration of fluid or tissue (by puncture or catheterization, except of heart) E874.4
biopsy E874.8
needle (aspirating) E874.4
blood sampling E874.4
catheterization E874.4
heart E874.5
dialysis (kidney) E874.2
endoscopic examination E874.3
enema E874.8
infusion E874.1
injection E874.8
lumbar puncture E874.4
needle biopsy E874.4
paracentesis, abdominal E874.4
perfusion E874.2
specified procedure NEC E874.8
surgical operation E874.0
thoracentesis E874.4
transfusion E874.1
vaccination E874.8
sterile precautions (during procedure) E872.9
aspiration of fluid or tissue (by puncture or catheterization, except heart) E872.5
biopsy E872.8
needle (aspirating) E872.5
blood sampling E872.5
catheterization E872.5
heart E872.6
dialysis (kidney) E872.2
endoscopic examination E872.4
enema E872.8
infusion E872.1
injection E872.3
lumbar puncture E872.5
needle biopsy E872.5
paracentesis, abdominal E872.5
perfusion E872.2
removal of catheter or packing E872.8
specified procedure NEC E872.8
surgical operation E872.0
thoracentesis E872.5
transfusion E872.1
vaccination E872.3
suture or ligature during surgical procedure E876.2
to introduce or to remove tube or instrument E876.4
foreign object left in body - *see* Misadventure, foreign object

Misadventure(s) to patient(s) during surgical or medical care *(Continued)*
foreign object left in body (during procedure) E871.9
aspiration of fluid or tissue (by puncture or catheterization, except heart) E871.5
biopsy E871.8
needle (aspirating) E871.5
blood sampling E871.5
catheterization E871.5
heart E871.6
dialysis (kidney) E871.2
endoscopic examination E871.4
enema E871.8
infusion E871.1
injection E871.3
lumbar puncture E871.5
needle biopsy E871.5
paracentesis, abdominal E871.5
perfusion E871.2
removal of catheter or packing E871.7
specified procedure NEC E871.8
surgical operation E871.0
thoracentesis E871.5
transfusion E871.1
vaccination E871.3
hemorrhage - *see* Misadventure, cut
inadvertent exposure of patient to radiation (being received for test or therapy) E873.3
inappropriate
operation performed E876.5
temperature (too hot or too cold) in local application or packing E873.5
infusion - *see also* Misadventure, by specific type, infusion
excessive amount of fluid E873.0
incorrect dilution of fluid E873.1
wrong fluid E876.1
mismatched blood in transfusion E876.0
nonadministration of necessary drug or medicinal E873.6
overdose - *see also* Overdose
radiation, in therapy E873.2
perforation - *see* Misadventure, cut
performance of inappropriate operation E876.5
puncture - *see* Misadventure, cut
specified type NEC E876.8
failure
suture or ligature during surgical operation E876.2
to introduce or to remove tube or instrument E876.4
foreign object left in body E871.9
infusion of wrong fluid E876.1
performance of inappropriate operation E876.5
transfusion of mismatched blood E876.0
wrong
fluid in infusion E876.1
placement of endotracheal tube during anesthetic procedure E876.3
transfusion - *see also* Misadventure, by specific type, transfusion
excessive amount of blood E873.0
mismatched blood E876.0
wrong
drug given in error - *see* Table of Drugs and Chemicals

Misadventure(s) to patient(s) during surgical or medical care *(Continued)*
wrong *(Continued)*
fluid in infusion E876.1
placement of endotracheal tube during anesthetic procedure E876.3
Motion (effects) E903
sickness E903
Mountain sickness E902.0
Mucus aspiration or inhalation, not of newborn (with asphyxia, obstruction respiratory passage, suffocation) E912
Mudslide of cataclysmic nature E909.2
Murder (attempt) (*see also* Assault) E968.9

N

Nail, injury by E920.8
Needlestick (sewing needle) E920.4
hypodermic E920.5
Neglect - *see also* Privation
criminal E968.4
homicidal intent E968.4
Noise (causing injury) (pollution) E928.1

O

Object
falling
from, in, on, hitting
aircraft E844
due to accident to aircraft - *see* categories E840–E842
machinery - *see also* Accident, machine
not in operation E916
motor vehicle (in motion) (on public highway) E818
not on public highway E825
stationary E916
nonmotor road vehicle NEC E829
pedal cycle E826
person E916
railway rolling stock, train, vehicle E806
street car E829
watercraft E838
due to accident to watercraft E831
set in motion by
accidental explosion of pressure vessel - *see* category E921
firearm - *see* category E922
machine(ry) - *see* Accident, machine
transport vehicle - *see* categories E800–E848
thrown from, in, on, towards
aircraft E844
cable car (not on rails) E847
on rails E829
motor vehicle (in motion) (on public highway) E818
not on public highway E825
nonmotor road vehicle NEC E829
pedal cycle E826
street car E829
vehicle NEC - *see* Accident, vehicle NEC
Obstruction
air passages, larynx, respiratory passages
by
external means NEC - *see* Suffocation
food, any type (regurgitated) (vomited) E911
material or object, except food E912
mucus E912
phlegm E912
vomitus E911
digestive tract, except mouth or pharynx
by
food, any type E915
foreign body (any) E915
esophagus
food E911
foreign body, except food E912
without asphyxia or obstruction of respiratory passage E915
mouth or pharynx
by
food, any type E911
material or object, except food E912
respiration - *see* Obstruction, air passages
Oil in eye E914
Overdose
anesthetic (drug) - *see* Table of Drugs and Chemicals
drug - *see* Table of Drugs and Chemicals
Overexertion (lifting) (pulling) (pushing) E927
Overexposure (accidental) (to)
cold (*see also* Cold, exposure to) E901.9
due to manmade conditions E901.1
heat (*see also* Heat) E900.9
radiation - *see* Radiation
radioactivity - *see* Radiation
sun, except sunburn E900.0
weather - *see* Exposure
wind - *see* Exposure
Overheated (*see also* Heat) E900.9
Overlaid E913.0
Overturning (accidental)
animal-drawn vehicle E827
boat, ship, watercraft
causing
drowning, submersion E830
injury except drowning, submersion E831
machinery - *see* Accident, machine
motor vehicle (*see also* Loss of control, motor vehicle) E816
with antecedent collision on public highway - *see* Collision, motor vehicle
not on public highway, nontraffic accident E825
with antecedent collision - *see* Collision, motor vehicle, not on public highway
nonmotor road vehicle NEC E829
off-road type motor vehicle - *see* Loss of control, off-road type motor vehicle
pedal cycle E826
railway rolling stock, train, vehicle (*see also* Derailment, railway) E802
street car E829
vehicle NEC - *see* Accident, vehicle NEC

P

Palsy, divers' E902.2
Parachuting (voluntary) (without accident to aircraft) E844
due to accident to aircraft - *see* categories E840–E842
Paralysis
divers' E902.2
lead or saturnine E866.0
from pesticide NEC E863.4
Pecked by bird E906.8
Phlegm aspiration or inhalation (with asphyxia, obstruction respiratory passage, suffocation) E912
Piercing (*see also* Cut) E920.9
Pinched
between objects (moving) (stationary and moving) E918
in object E918
Pinned under
machine(ry) - *see* Accident, machine
Place of occurrence of accident - *see* Accident (to), occurring (at) (in)
Plumbism E866.0
from insecticide NEC E863.4
Poisoning (accidental) (by) - *see also* Table of Drugs and Chemicals
carbon monoxide
generated by
aircraft in transit E844
motor vehicle
in motion (on public highway) E818
not on public highway E825
watercraft (in transit) (not in transit) E838
caused by injection of poisons or toxins into or through skin by plant thorns, spines, or other mechanism E905.7
marine or sea plants E905.6
fumes or smoke due to
conflagration - *see* Conflagration
explosion or fire - *see* Fire
ignition - *see* Ignition
gas
in legal intervention E972
legal execution, by E978
on watercraft E838
used as anesthetic - *see* Table of Drugs and Chemicals
in
terrorism (chemical weapons) E979.7
war operations E997.2
late effect of - *see* Late effect
legal
execution E978
intervention
by gas E972
Pressure, external, causing asphyxia, suffocation (*see also* Suffocation) E913.9
Privation E904.9
food (*see also* Lack of, food) E904.1
helpless person, infant, newborn due to abandonment or neglect E904.0
late effect of NEC E929.5
resulting from transport accident - *see* categories E800–E848
water (*see also* Lack of, water) E904.2
Projected objects, striking against or struck by - *see* Striking against, object

ICD-9-CM
E Codes
Vol. 2

Prolonged stay in
high altitude (causing conditions as listed in E902.0) E902.0
weightless environment E928.0
Prostration
heat - *see* Heat
Pulling, injury in E927
Puncture, puncturing (*see also* Cut) E920.9
by
plant thorns or spines E920.8
toxic reaction E905.7
marine or sea plants E905.6
sea-urchin spine E905.6
Pushing (injury in) (overexertion) E927
by other person(s) (accidental) E917.9
as, or caused by, a crowd, human stampede E917.1
with subsequent fall E917.6
before moving vehicle or object
stated as
intentional, homicidal E968.8
undetermined whether accidental or intentional E988.8
from
high place
in accidental circumstances - *see* categories E880–E884
stated as
intentional, homicidal E968.1
undetermined whether accidental or intentional E987.9
man-made structure, except residential E987.1
natural site E987.2
residential E987.0
motor vehicle (*see also* Fall, from, motor vehicle) E818
stated as
intentional, homicidal E968.5
undetermined whether accidental or intentional E988.8
in sports E917.0
with fall E886.0
with fall E886.9
in sports E886.0

R

Radiation (exposure to) E926.9
abnormal reaction to medical test or therapy E879.2
arc lamps E926.2
atomic power plant (malfunction) NEC E926.9
in water transport E838
electromagnetic, ionizing E926.3
gamma rays E926.3
in
terrorism (from or following nuclear explosion) (direct) (secondary) E979.5
laser E979.8
war operations (from or following nuclear explosion) (direct) (secondary) E996
laser(s) E997.0
water transport E838
inadvertent exposure of patient (receiving test or therapy) E873.3
infrared (heaters and lamps) E926.1
excessive heat E900.1
Radiation *(Continued)*
ionized, ionizing (particles, artificially accelerated) E926.8
electromagnetic E926.3
isotopes, radioactive - *see* Radiation, radioactive isotopes
laser(s) E926.4
in
terrorism E979.8
war operations E997.0
misadventure in medical care - *see* Misadventure, failure, in dosage, radiation
late effect of NEC E929.8
excessive heat from - *see* Heat
light sources (visible) (ultraviolet) E926.2
misadventure in medical or surgical procedure - *see* Misadventure, failure, in dosage, radiation
overdose (in medical or surgical pacemaker procedure) E873.2
radar E926.0
radioactive isotopes E926.5
atomic power plant malfunction E926.5
in water transport E838
misadventure in medical or surgical treatment - *see* Misadventure, failure, in dosage, radiation
radiobiologicals - *see* Radiation, radioactive isotopes
radiofrequency E926.0
radiopharmaceuticals - *see* Radiation, radioactive isotopes
radium NEC E926.9
sun E926.2
excessive heat from E900.0
tanning bed E926.2
welding arc or torch E926.2
excessive heat from E900.1
x-rays (hard) (soft) E926.3
misadventure in medical or surgical treatment - *see* Misadventure, failure, in dosage, radiation
Rape E960.1
Reaction, abnormal, to or following (medical or surgical procedure) E879.9
amputation (of limbs) E878.5
anastomosis (arteriovenous) (blood vessel) (gastrojejunal) (skin) (tendon) (natural, artificial material, tissue) E878.2
external stoma, creation of E878.3
aspiration (of fluid) E879.4
tissue E879.8
biopsy E879.8
blood
sampling E879.7
transfusion
procedure E879.8
bypass - *see* Reaction, abnormal, anastomosis
catheterization
cardiac E879.0
urinary E879.6
colostomy E878.3
cystostomy E878.3
dialysis (kidney) E879.1
drugs or biologicals - *see* Table of Drugs and Chemicals
duodenostomy E878.3
electroshock therapy E879.3
formation of external stoma E878.3
Reaction, abnormal, to or following *(Continued)*
gastrostomy E878.3
graft - *see* Reaction, abnormal, anastomosis
hypothermia E879.8
implant, implantation (of)
artificial
internal device (cardiac pacemaker) (electrodes in brain) (heart valve prosthesis) (orthopedic) E878.1
material or tissue (for anastomosis or bypass) E878.2
with creation of external stoma E878.3
natural tissues (for anastomosis or bypass) E878.2
as transplantion - *see* Reaction, abnormal, transplant
with creation of external stoma E878.3
infusion
procedure E879.8
injection
procedure E879.8
insertion of gastric or duodenal sound E879.5
insulin-shock therapy E879.3
lumbar puncture E879.4
perfusion E879.1
procedures other than surgical operation (*see also* Reaction, abnormal, by specific type of procedure) E879.9
specified procedure NEC E879.8
radiological procedure or therapy E879.2
removal of organ (partial) (total) NEC E878.6
with
anastomosis, bypass or graft E878.2
formation of external stoma E878.3
implant of artificial internal device E878.1
transplant(ation)
partial organ E878.4
whole organ E878.0
sampling
blood E879.7
fluid NEC E879.4
tissue E879.8
shock therapy E879.3
surgical operation (*see also* Reaction, abnormal, by specified type of operation) E878.9
restorative NEC E878.4
with
anastomosis, bypass or graft E878.2
formation of external stoma E878.3
implant(ation) - *see* Reaction, abnormal, implant
transplantation - *see* Reaction, abnormal, transplant
specified operation NEC E878.8
thoracentesis E879.4
transfusion
procedure E879.8
transplant, transplantation (heart) (kidney) (liver) E878.0
partial organ E878.4
ureterostomy E878.3
vaccination E879.8

Reduction in
atmospheric pressure - *see also* Effects of, air pressure
while surfacing from
deep water diving causing caisson or divers' disease, palsy or paralysis E902.2
underground E902.8
Residual (effect) - *see* Late effect
Rock falling on or hitting (accidentally)
motor vehicle (in motion) (on public highway) E818
not on public highway E825
nonmotor road vehicle NEC E829
pedal cycle E826
person E916
railway rolling stock, train, vehicle E806
Running off, away
animal (being ridden) (in sport or transport) E828
not being ridden E906.8
animal-drawn vehicle E827
rails, railway (*see also* Derailment) E802
roadway
motor vehicle (without antecedent collision) E816
nontraffic accident E825
with antecedent collision - *see* Collision, motor vehicle, not on public highway
with
antecedent collision - *see* Collision, motor vehicle
subsequent collision
involving any object, person or vehicle not on public highway E816
on public highway E811
nonmotor road vehicle NEC E829
pedal cycle E826
Run over (accidentally) (by)
animal (not being ridden) E906.8
being ridden (in sport or transport) E828
animal-drawn vehicle E827
machinery - *see* Accident, machine
motor vehicle (on public highway) - *see* Hit by, motor vehicle
nonmotor road vehicle NEC E829
railway train E805
street car E829
vehicle NEC E848

S

Saturnism E866.0
from insecticide NEC E863.4
Scald, scalding (accidental) (by) (from) (in) E924.0
acid - *see* Scald, caustic
boiling tap water E924.2
caustic or corrosive liquid, substance E924.1
swallowed - *see* Table of Drugs and Chemicals
homicide (attempt) - *see* Assault, burning
inflicted by other person
stated as
intentional or homicidal E968.3
undetermined whether accidental or intentional E988.2
late effect of NEC E929.8
Scald, scalding *(Continued)*
liquid (boiling) (hot) E924.0
local application of externally applied substance in medical or surgical care E873.5
molten metal E924.0
self-inflicted (unspecified whether accidental or intentional) E988.2
stated as intentional, purposeful E958.2
stated as undetermined whether accidental or intentional E988.2
steam E924.0
tap water (boiling) E924.2
transport accident - *see* categories E800–E848
vapor E924.0
Scratch, cat E906.8
Sea
sickness E903
Self-mutilation - *see* Suicide
Sequelae (of)
in
terrorism E999.1
war operations E999.0
Shock
anaphylactic (*see also* Table of Drugs and Chemicals) E947.9
due to
bite (venomous) - *see* Bite, venomous NEC
sting - *see* Sting
electric (*see also* Electric shock) E925.9
from electric appliance or current (*see also* Electric shock) E925.9
Shooting, shot (accidental(ly)) E922.9
air gun E922.4
BB gun E922.4
hand gun (pistol) (revolver) E922.0
himself (*see also* Shooting, self-inflicted) E985.4
hand gun (pistol) (revolver) E985.0
military firearm, except hand gun E985.3
hand gun (pistol) (revolver) E985.0
rifle (hunting) E985.2
military E985.3
shotgun (automatic) E985.1
specified firearm NEC E985.4
Verey pistol E985.4
homicide (attempt) E965.4
air gun E968.6
BB gun E968.6
hand gun (pistol) (revolver) E965.0
military firearm, except hand gun E965.3
hand gun (pistol) (revolver) E965.0
paintball gun E965.4
rifle (hunting) E965.2
military E965.3
shotgun (automatic) E965.1
specified firearm NEC E965.4
Verey pistol E965.4
inflicted by other person
in accidental circumstances E922.9
hand gun (pistol) (revolver) E922.0
military firearm, except hand gun E922.3
hand gun (pistol) (revolver) E922.0
rifle (hunting) E922.2
military E922.3
shotgun (automatic) E922.1
Shooting, shot *(Continued)*
inflicted by other person *(Continued)*
in accidental circumstances *(Continued)*
specified firearm NEC E922.8
Verey pistol E922.8
stated as
intentional, homicidal E965.4
hand gun (pistol) (revolver) E965
military firearm, except hand gun E965.3
hand gun (pistol) (revolver) E965.0
paintball gun E965.4
rifle (hunting) E965.2
military E965.3
shotgun (automatic) E965.1
specified firearm E965.4
Verey pistol E965.4
undetermined whether accidental or intentional E985.4
air gun E985.6
BB gun E985.6
hand gun (pistol) (revolver) E985.0
military firearm, except hand gun E985.3
hand gun (pistol) (revolver) E985.0
paintball gun E985.7
rifle (hunting) E985.2
shotgun (automatic) E985.1
specified firearm NEC E985.4
Verey pistol E985.4
in
terrorism - *see* Terrorism, shooting
war operations - *see* War operations, shooting
legal
execution E978
intervention E970
military firearm, except hand gun E922.3
hand gun (pistol) (revolver) E922.0
paintball gun E922.5
rifle (hunting) E922.2
military E922.3
self-inflicted (unspecified whether accidental or intentional) E985.4
air gun E985.6
BB gun E985.6
hand gun (pistol) (revolver) E985.0
military firearm, except hand gun E985.3
hand gun (pistol) (revolver) E985.0
paintball gun E985.7
rifle (hunting) E985.2
military E985.3
shotgun (automatic) E985.1
specified firearm NEC E985.4
stated as
accidental E922.9
hand gun (pistol) (revolver) E922.0
military firearm, except hand gun E922.3
hand gun (pistol) (revolver) E922.0
paintball gun 922.5
rifle (hunting) E922.2
military E922.3
shotgun (automatic) E922.1
specified firearm NEC E922.8
Verey pistol E922.8

Shooting, shot *(Continued)*
self-inflicted *(Continued)*
stated as *(Continued)*
intentional, purposeful E955.4
hand gun (pistol) (revolver) E955.0
military firearm, except hand gun E955.3
hand gun (pistol) (revolver) E955.0
paintball gun E955.7
rifle (hunting) E955.2
military E955.3
shotgun (automatic) E955.1
specified firearm NEC E955.4
Verey pistol E955.4
shotgun (automatic) E922.1
specified firearm NEC E922.8
stated as undetermined whether accidental or intentional E985.4
hand gun (pistol) (revolver) E985.0
military firearm, except hand gun E985.3
hand gun (pistol) (revolver) E985.0
paintball gun E985.7
rifle (hunting) E985.2
military E985.3
shotgun (automatic) E985.1
specified firearm NEC E985.4
Verey pistol E985.4
suicidal (attempt) E955.4
air gun E985.6
BB gun E985.6
hand gun (pistol) (revolver) E955.0
military firearm, except hand gun E955.3
hand gun (pistol) (revolver) E955.0
paintball gun E955.7
rifle (hunting) E955.2
military E955.3
shotgun (automatic) E955.1
specified firearm NEC E955.4
Verey pistol E955.4
Verey pistol E922.8
Shoving (accidentally) by other person (*see also* Pushing by other person) E917.9
Sickness
air E903
alpine E902.0
car E903
motion E903
mountain E902.0
sea E903
travel E903
Sinking (accidental)
boat, ship, watercraft (causing drowning, submersion) E830
causing injury except drowning, submersion E831
Siriasis E900.0
Skydiving E844
Slashed wrists (*see also* Cut, self-inflicted) E986
Slipping (accidental)
on
deck (of boat, ship, watercraft) (icy) (oily) (wet) E835
ice E885.9
ladder of ship E833
due to accident to watercraft E831
mud E885.9
oil E885.9
snow E885.9
Slipping *(Continued)*
on *(Continued)*
stairs of ship E833
due to accident to watercraft E831
surface
slippery E885.9
wet E885.9
Sliver, wood, injury by E920.8
Smothering, smothered (*see also* Suffocation) E913.9
Smouldering building or structure in terrorism E979.3
Sodomy (assault) E960.1
Solid substance in eye (any part) or adnexa E914
Sound waves (causing injury) E928.1
Splinter, injury by E920.8
Stab, stabbing E966
accidental - *see* Cut
Starvation E904.1
helpless person, infant, newborn - *see* Lack of food
homicidal intent E968.4
late effect of NEC E929.5
resulting from accident connected with transport - *see* categories E800–E848
Stepped on
by
animal (not being ridden) E906.8
being ridden (in sport or transport) E828
crowd E917.1
person E917.9
in sports E917.0
in sports E917.0
Stepping on
object (moving) E917.9
in sports E917.0
with subsequent fall E917.5
stationary E917.4
with subsequent fall E917.8
person E917.9
as, or caused by a crowd E917.1
with subsequent fall E917.6
in sports E917.0
Sting E905.9
ant E905.5
bee E905.3
caterpillar E905.5
coral E905.6
hornet E905.3
insect NEC E905.5
jelly fish E905.6
marine animal or plant E905.6
nematocysts E905.6
scorpion E905.2
sea anemone E905.6
sea cucumber E905.6
wasp E905.3
yellow jacket E905.3
Storm E908.9
specified type NEC E908.8
Straining, injury in E927
Strangling - *see* Suffocation
Strangulation - *see* Suffocation
Strenuous movements (in recreational or other activities) E927
Striking against
bottom (when jumping or diving into water) E883.0
object (moving) E917.9
caused by crowd E917.1
with subsequent fall E917.6
Striking against *(Continued)*
object *(Continued)*
furniture E917.3
with subsequent fall E917.7
in
running water E917.2
with drowning or submersion - *see* Submersion
sports E917.0
with subsequent fall E917.5
stationary E917.4
with subsequent fall E917.8
person(s) E917.9
with fall E886.9
in sports E886.0
as, or caused by, a crowd E917.1
with subsequent fall E917.6
in sports E917.0
with fall E886.0
Stroke
heat - *see* Heat
lightning E907
Struck by - *see also* Hit by
bullet
in
terrorism E979.4
war operations E991.2
rubber E991.0
lightning E907
missile
in terrorism - *see* Terrorism, missile
object
falling
from, in, on
building
burning (uncontrolled fire)
in terrorism E979.3
thunderbolt E907
Stumbling over animal, carpet, curb, rug or (small) object (with fall) E885.9
without fall - *see* Striking against, object
Submersion (accidental) E910.8
boat, ship, watercraft (causing drowning, submersion) E830
causing injury except drowning, submersion E831
by other person
in accidental circumstances - *see* category E910
intentional, homicidal E964
stated as undetermined whether accidental or intentional E984
due to
accident
machinery - *see* Accident, machine
to boat, ship, watercraft E830
transport - *see* categories E800-E848
avalanche E909.2
cataclysmic
earth surface movement or eruption E909.9
storm E908.9
cloudburst E908.8
cyclone E908.1
fall
from
boat, ship, watercraft (not involved in accident) E832
burning, crushed E830
involved in accident, collision E830
gangplank (into water) E832
overboard NEC E832

Submersion *(Continued)*
due to *(Continued)*
flood E908.2
hurricane E908.0
jumping into water E910.8
from boat, ship, watercraft
burning, crushed, sinking E830
involved in accident, collision E830
not involved in accident, for swim E910.2
in recreational activity (without diving equipment) E910.2
with or using diving equipment E910.1
to rescue another person E910.3
homicide (attempt) E964
in
bathtub E910.4
specified activity, not sport, transport or recreational E910.3
sport or recreational activity (without diving equipment) E910.2
with or using diving equipment E910.1
water skiing E910.0
swimming pool NEC E910.8
terrorism E979.8
war operations E995
water transport E832
due to accident to boat, ship, watercraft E830
landslide E909.2
overturning boat, ship, watercraft E909.2
sinking boat, ship, watercraft E909.2
submersion boat, ship, watercraft E909.2
tidal wave E909.4
caused by storm E908.0
torrential rain E908.2
late effect of NEC E929.8
quenching tank E910.8
self-inflicted (unspecified whether accidental or intentional) E984
in accidental circumstances - *see* category E910
stated as intentional, purposeful E954
stated as undetermined whether accidental or intentional E984
suicidal (attempted) E954
while
attempting rescue of another person E910.3
engaged in
marine salvage E910.3
underwater construction or repairs E910.3
fishing, not from boat E910.2
hunting, not from boat E910.2
ice skating E910.2
pearl diving E910.3
placing fishing nets E910.3
playing in water E910.2
scuba diving E910.1
nonrecreational E910.3
skin diving E910.1
snorkel diving E910.2
spear fishing underwater E910.1
surfboarding E910.2
swimming (swimming pool) E910.2
wading (in water) E910.2
water skiing E910.0

Sucked
into
jet (aircraft) E844

Suffocation (accidental) (by external means) (by pressure) (mechanical) E913.9
caused by other person
in accidental circumstances - *see* category E913
stated as
intentional, homicidal E963
undetermined whether accidental or intentional E983.9
by, in
hanging E983.0
plastic bag E983.1
specified means NEC E983.8
due to, by
avalanche E909.2
bedclothes E913.0
bib E913.0
blanket E913.0
cave-in E913.3
caused by cataclysmic earth surface movement or eruption E909.9
conflagration - *see* Conflagration
explosion - *see* Explosion
falling earth, other substance E913.3
fire - *see* Fire
food, any type (ingestion) (inhalation) (regurgitated) (vomited) E911
foreign body, except food (ingestion) (inhalation) E912
ignition - *see* Ignition
landslide E909.2
machine(ry) - *see* Accident, machine
material object except food entering by nose or mouth, ingested, inhaled E912
mucus (aspiration) (inhalation), not of newborn E912
phlegm (aspiration) (inhalation) E912
pillow E913.0
plastic bag - *see* Suffocation, in, plastic bag
sheet (plastic) E913.0
specified means NEC E913.8
vomitus (aspiration) (inhalation) E911
homicidal (attempt) E963
in
airtight enclosed place E913.2
baby carriage E913.0
bed E913.0
closed place E913.2
cot, cradle E913.0
perambulator E913.0
plastic bag (in accidental circumstances) E913.1
homicidal, purposely inflicted by other person E963
self-inflicted (unspecified whether accidental or intentional) E983.1
in accidental circumstances E913.1
intentional, suicidal E953.1
stated as undetermined whether accidentally or purposely inflicted E983.1
suicidal, purposely self-inflicted E953.1
refrigerator E913.2

Suffocation *(Continued)*
self-inflicted - *see also* Suffocation, stated as undetermined whether accidental or intentional E953.9
in accidental circumstances - *see* category E913
stated as intentional, purposeful - *see* Suicide, suffocation
stated as undetermined whether accidental or intentional E983.9
by, in
hanging E983.0
plastic bag E983.1
specified means NEC E983.8
suicidal - *see* Suicide, suffocation

Suicide, suicidal (attempted) (by) E958.9
burning, burns E958.1
caustic substance E958.7
poisoning E950.7
swallowed E950.7
cold, extreme E958.3
cut (any part of body) E956
cutting or piercing instrument (classifiable to E920) E956
drowning E954
electrocution E958.4
explosive(s) (classifiable to E923) E955.5
fire E958.1
firearm (classifiable to E922) - *see* Shooting, suicidal
hanging E953.0
jumping
before moving object, train, vehicle E958.0
from high place - *see* Jumping, from, high place, stated as, suicidal
knife E956
late effect of E959
motor vehicle, crashing of E958.5
poisoning - *see* Table of Drugs and Chemicals
puncture (any part of body) E956
scald E958.2
shooting - *see* Shooting, suicidal
specified means NEC E958.8
stab (any part of body) E956
strangulation - *see* Suicide, suffocation
submersion E954
suffocation E953.9
by, in
hanging E953.0
plastic bag E953.1
specified means NEC E953.8
wound NEC E958.9

Sunburn E926.2

Sunstroke E900.0

Supersonic waves (causing injury) E928.1

Surgical procedure, complication of
delayed or as an abnormal reaction without mention of misadventure, *see* Reaction, abnormal
due to or as a result of misadventure - *see* Misadventure

Swallowed, swallowing
foreign body - *see* Foreign body, alimentary canal
poison - *see* Table of Drugs and Chemicals
substance
caustic - *see* Table of Drugs and Chemicals
corrosive - *see* Table of Drugs and Chemicals

Swallowed, swallowing *(Continued)*
substance *(Continued)*
poisonous - *see* Table of Drugs and Chemicals
Swimmers' cramp (*see also* category E910) E910.2
not in recreation or sport E910.3
Syndrome, battered
baby or child - *see* Abuse, child
wife - *see* Assault

T

Tackle in sport E886.0
Terrorism (injury) (by) (in) E979.8
air blast E979.2
aircraft burned, destroyed, exploded, shot down E979.1
used as a weapon E979.1
anthrax E979.6
asphyxia from
chemical (weapons) E979.7
fire, conflagration (caused by fire-producing device) E979.3
from nuclear explosion E979.5
gas or fumes E979.7
bayonet E979.8
biological agents E979.6
blast (air) (effects) E979.2
from nuclear explosion E979.5
underwater E979.0
bomb (antipersonnel) (mortar) (explosion) (fragments) E979.2
bullet(s) (from carbine, machine gun, pistol, rifle, shotgun) E979.4
burn from
chemical E979.7
fire, conflagration (caused by fire-producing device) E979.3
from nuclear explosion E979.5
gas E979.7
burning aircraft E979.1
chemical E979.7
cholera E979.6
conflagration E979.3
crushed by falling aircraft E979.1
depth-charge E979.0
destruction of aircraft E979.1
disability, as sequelae one year or more after injury E999.1
drowning E979.8
effect
of nuclear weapon (direct) (secondary) E979.5
secondary NEC E979.9
sequelae E999.1
explosion (artillery shell) (breech-block) (cannon block) E979.2
aircraft E979.1
bomb (antipersonnel) (mortar) E979.2
nuclear (atom) (hydrogen) E979.5
depth-charge E979.0
grenade E979.2
injury by fragments from E979.2
land-mine E979.2
marine weapon E979.0
mine (land) E979.2
at sea or in harbor E979.0
marine E979.0
missile (explosive) NEC E979.2
munitions (dump) (factory) E979.2
nuclear (weapon) E979.5
other direct or secondary effects of E979.5

Terrorism *(Continued)*
explosion *(Continued)*
sea-based artillery shell E979.0
torpedo E979.0
exposure to ionizing radiation from nuclear explosion E979.5
falling aircraft E979.1
fire or fire-producing device E979.3
firearms E979.4
fireball effects from nuclear explosion E979.5
fragments from artillery shell, bomb NEC, grenade, guided missile, land-mine, rocket, shell, shrapnel E979.2
gas or fumes E979.7
grenade (explosion) (fragments) E979.2
guided missile (explosion) (fragments) E979.2
nuclear E979.5
heat from nuclear explosion E979.5
hot substances E979.3
hydrogen cyanide E979.7
land-mine (explosion) (fragments) E979.2
laser(s) E979.8
late effect of E999.1
lewisite E979.9
lung irritant (chemical) (fumes) (gas) E979.7
marine mine E979.0
mine E979.2
at sea E979.0
in harbor E979.0
land (explosion) (fragments) E979.2
marine E979.0
missile (explosion) (fragments) (guided) E979.2
marine E979.0
nuclear E979.5
mortar bomb (explosion) (fragments) (guided) E979.2
mustard gas E979.7
nerve gas E979.7
nuclear weapons E979.5
pellets (shotgun) E979.4
petrol bomb E979.3
piercing object E979.8
phosgene E979.7
poisoning (chemical) (fumes) (gas) E979.7
radiation, ionizing from nuclear explosion E979.5
rocket (explosion) (fragments) E979.2
saber, sabre E979.8
sarin E979.7
screening smoke E979.7
sequelae effect (of) E999.1
shell (aircraft) (artillery) (cannon) (land-based) (explosion) (fragments) E979.2
sea-based E979.0
shooting E979.4
bullet(s) E979.4
pellet(s) (rifle) (shotgun) E979.4
shrapnel E979.2
smallpox E979.7
stabbing object(s) E979.8
submersion E979.8
torpedo E979.0
underwater blast E979.0
vesicant (chemical) (fumes) (gas) E979.7
weapon burst E979.2
Thermic fever E900.9
Thermoplegia E900.9
Thirst - *see also* Lack of water
resulting from accident connected with transport - *see* categories E800–E848
Thrown (accidentally)
against object in or part of vehicle
by motion of vehicle
aircraft E844
boat, ship, watercraft E838
motor vehicle (on public highway) E818
not on public highway E825
off-road type (not on public highway) E821
on public highway E818
snow vehicle E820
on public highway E818
nonmotor road vehicle NEC E829
railway rolling stock, train, vehicle E806
street car E829
from
animal (being ridden) (in sport or transport) E828
high place, homicide (attempt) E968.1
machinery - *see* Accident, machine
vehicle NEC - *see* Accident, vehicle NEC
off - *see* Thrown, from
overboard (by motion of boat, ship, watercraft) E832
by accident to boat, ship, watercraft E830
Thunderbolt NEC E907
Tidal wave (any injury) E909.4
caused by storm E908.0
Took
overdose of drug - *see* Table of Drugs and Chemicals
poison - *see* Table of Drugs and Chemicals
Tornado (any injury) E908.1
Torrential rain (any injury) E908.2
Traffic accident NEC E819
Trampled by animal E906.8
being ridden (in sport or transport) E828
Trapped (accidentally)
between
objects (moving) (stationary and moving) E918
by
door of
elevator E918
motor vehicle (on public highway) (while alighting, boarding) - *see* Fall, from, motor vehicle, while alighting
railway train (underground) E806
street car E829
subway train E806
in object E918
Travel (effects) E903
sickness E903
Tree
falling on or hitting E916
motor vehicle (in motion) (on public highway) E818
not on public highway E825
nonmotor road vehicle NEC E829
pedal cycle E826
person E916
railway rolling stock, train, vehicle E806
street car E829

Trench foot E901.0
Tripping over animal, carpet, curb, rug, or small object (with fall) E885.9
  without fall - *see* Striking against, object
Tsunami E909.4
Twisting, Injury in E927

V

Violence, nonaccidental (*see also* Assault) E968.9
Volcanic eruption (any injury) E909.1
Vomitus in air passages (with asphyxia, obstruction or suffocation) E911

W

War operations (during hostilities) (injury) (by) (in) E995
  after cessation of hostilities, injury due to E998
  air blast E993
  aircraft burned, destroyed, exploded, shot down E991.9
  asphyxia from
    chemical E997.2
    fire, conflagration (caused by fire-producing device or conventional weapon) E990.9
      from nuclear explosion E996
      petrol bomb E990.0
    fumes E997.2
    gas E997.2
  battle wound NEC E995
  bayonet E995
  biological warfare agents E997.1
  blast (air) (effects) E993
    from nuclear explosion E996
    underwater E992
  bomb (mortar) (explosion) E993
    after cessation of hostilities E998
    fragments, injury by E991.9
      antipersonnel E991.3
  bullet(s) (from carbine, machine gun, pistol, rifle, shotgun) E991.2
    rubber E991.0
  burn from
    chemical E997.2
    fire, conflagration (caused by fire-producing device or conventional weapon) E990.9
      from nuclear explosion E996
      petrol bomb E990.0
    gas E997.2
  burning aircraft E994
  chemical E997.2
  chlorine E997.2
  conventional warfare, specified form NEC E995
  crushing by falling aircraft E994
  depth charge E992
  destruction of aircraft E994
  disability as sequela one year or more after injury E999.0
  drowning E995

War operations *(Continued)*
  effect (direct) (secondary) of nuclear weapon E996
  explosion (artillery shell) (breech block) (cannon shell) E993
    after cessation of hostilities of bomb, mine placed in war E998
    aircraft E994
    bomb (mortar) E993
      atom E996
      hydrogen E996
      injury by fragments from E991.9
        antipersonnel E991.3
      nuclear E996
    depth charge E992
    injury by fragments from E991.9
      antipersonnel E991.3
    marine weapon E992
    mine
      at sea or in harbor E992
      land E993
        injury by fragments from E991.9
      marine E992
    munitions (accidental) (being used in war) (dump) (factory) E993
    nuclear (weapon) E996
    own weapons (accidental) E993
      injury by fragments from E991.9
        antipersonnel E991.3
    sea-based artillery shell E992
    torpedo E992
  exposure to ionizing radiation from nuclear explosion E996
  falling aircraft E994
  fire or fire-producing device E990.9
    petrol bomb E990.0
  fireball effects from nuclear explosion E996
  fragments from
    antipersonnel bomb E991.3
    artillery shell, bomb NEC, grenade, guided missile, land mine, rocket, shell, shrapnel E991.9
  fumes E997.2
  gas E997.2
  grenade (explosion) E993
    fragments, injury by E991.9
  guided missile (explosion) E993
    fragments, injury by E991.9
    nuclear E996
  heat from nuclear explosion E996
  injury due to, but occurring after cessation of hostilities E998
  lacrimator (gas) (chemical) E997.2
  land mine (explosion) E993
    after cessation of hostilities E998
    fragments, injury by E991.9
  laser(s) E997.0
  late effect of E999.0
  lewisite E997.2
  lung irritant (chemical) (fumes) (gas) E997.2
  marine mine E992
  mine
    after cessation of hostilities E998
    at sea E992
    in harbor E992

War operations *(Continued)*
  mine *(Continued)*
    land (explosion) E993
      fragments, injury by E991.9
    marine E992
  missile (guided) (explosion) E993
    fragments, injury by E991.9
    marine E992
    nuclear E996
  mortar bomb (explosion) E993
    fragments, injury by E991.9
  mustard gas E997.2
  nerve gas E997.2
  phosgene E997.2
  poisoning (chemical) (fumes) (gas) E997.2
  radiation, ionizing from nuclear explosion E996
  rocket (explosion) E993
    fragments, injury by E991.9
  saber, sabre E995
  screening smoke E997.8
  shell (aircraft) (artillery) (cannon) (land based) (explosion) E993
    fragments, injury by E991.9
    sea-based E992
  shooting E991.2
    after cessation of hostilities E998
    bullet(s) E991.2
      rubber E991.0
    pellet(s) (rifle) E991.1
    shrapnel E991.9
    submersion E995
    torpedo E992
    unconventional warfare, except by nuclear weapon E997.9
    biological (warfare) E997.1
    gas, fumes, chemicals E997.2
    laser(s) E997.0
    specified type NEC E997.8
  underwater blast E992
  vesicant (chemical) (fumes) (gas) E997.2
  weapon burst E993
Washed
  away by flood - *see* Flood
  away by tidal wave - *see* Tidal wave
  off road by storm (transport vehicle) E908.9
  overboard E832
Weather exposure - *see also* Exposure
  cold E901.0
  hot E900.0
Weightlessness (causing injury) (effects of) (in spacecraft, real or simulated) E928.0
Wound (accidental) NEC (*see also* Injury) E928.9
  battle (*see also* War operations) E995
  bayonet E920.3
    in
      legal intervention E974
      war operations E995
  gunshot - *see* Shooting
  incised - *see* Cut
  saber, sabre E920.3
    in war operations E995

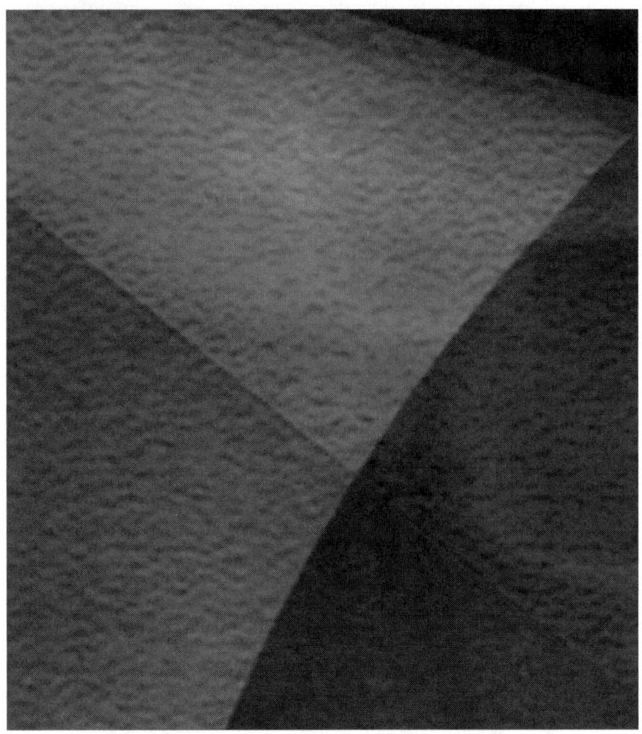

PART III

Diseases: Tabular List Volume 1

1. INFECTIOUS AND PARASITIC DISEASES (001–139)

Note: Categories for "late effects" of infectious and parasitic diseases are to be found at 137–139.

Includes: diseases generally recognized as communicable or transmissible as well as a few diseases of unknown but possibly infectious origin

Excludes *acute respiratory infections (460–466)*
carrier or suspected carrier of infectious organism (V02.0–V02.9)
certain localized infections
influenza (487.0–487.8)

INTESTINAL INFECTIOUS DISEASES (001–009)

Excludes *helminthiases (120.0–129)*
Diseases or infestations caused by parasitic worms

● 001 Cholera
- **001.0 Due to Vibrio cholerae**
- **001.1 Due to Vibrio cholerae el tor**
- ❑ **001.9 Cholera, unspecified**

● 002 Typhoid and paratyphoid fevers
- **002.0 Typhoid fever**
  Typhoid (fever) (infection) [any site]
- **002.1 Paratyphoid fever A**
- **002.2 Paratyphoid fever B**
- **002.3 Paratyphoid fever C**
- ❑ **002.9 Paratyphoid fever, unspecified**

Item 1-1 Salmonella is a bacterium that lives in the intestines of fowl and mammals and can spread to humans through improper food preparation and cooking. The most frequent clinical manifestation of a salmonella infection is food poisoning. Patients with immunocompromised systems in chronic, ill health are more likely to have the infection invade their bloodstream with life-threatening results. For example, patients with sickle cell disease are more prone to salmonella osteomyelitis than others.

● 003 Other salmonella infections

Includes: infection or food poisoning by Salmonella [any serotype]

- **003.0 Salmonella gastroenteritis**
  Salmonellosis
- **003.1 Salmonella septicemia**
- ● **003.2 Localized salmonella infections**
  - ❑ **003.20 Localized salmonella infection, unspecified**
    Specified in the documentation as localized, but unspecified as to type
  - **003.21 Salmonella meningitis**
    Specified as localized in the meninges
  - **003.22 Salmonella pneumonia**
    Specified as localized in the lungs
  - **003.23 Salmonella arthritis**
    Specified as localized in the joints
  - **003.24 Salmonella osteomyelitis**
    Specified as localized in bone
  - ❑ **003.29 Other**
    Specified as localized (because it is still under localized heading) but does not assign into any of the above codes
- ❑ **003.8 Other specified salmonella infections**
  Any specified salmonella infection which does NOT assign into any of the above codes (not specified as localized)
- ❑ **003.9 Salmonella infection, unspecified**
  Unspecified in the documentation as to specific type of salmonella

● 004 Shigellosis

Includes: bacillary dysentery

- **004.0 Shigella dysenteriae**
  Infection by group A Shigella (Schmitz) (Shiga)
- **004.1 Shigella flexneri**
  Infection by group B Shigella

004.2 **Shigella boydii**
Infection by group C Shigella

004.3 **Shigella sonnei**
Infection by group D Shigella

❏004.8 **Other specified shigella infections**

❏004.9 **Shigellosis, unspecified**

● 005 **Other food poisoning (bacterial)**

Excludes *salmonella infections (003.0–003.9)*
toxic effect of:
food contaminants (989.7)
noxious foodstuffs (988.0–988.9)

005.0 **Staphylococcal food poisoning**
Staphylococcal toxemia specified as due to food

005.1 **Botulism**
Food poisoning due to Clostridium botulinum

005.2 **Food poisoning due to Clostridium perfringens [C. welchii]**
Enteritis necroticans

005.3 **Food poisoning due to other Clostridia**

005.4 **Food poisoning due to Vibrio parahaemolyticus**

● 005.8 **Other bacterial food poisoning**

Excludes *salmonella food poisoning (003.0–003.9)*

005.81 **Food poisoning due to Vibrio vulnificus**

❏005.89 **Other bacterial food poisoning**
Food poisoning due to Bacillus cereus

❏005.9 **Food poisoning, unspecified**

● 006 **Amebiasis**

Includes: infection due to Entamoeba histolytica

Excludes *amebiasis due to organisms other than Entamoeba histolytica (007.8)*

006.0 **Acute amebic dysentery without mention of abscess**
Acute amebiasis

006.1 **Chronic intestinal amebiasis without mention of abscess**
Chronic:
amebiasis
amebic dysentery

006.2 **Amebic nondysenteric colitis**

006.3 **Amebic liver abscess**
Hepatic amebiasis

006.4 **Amebic lung abscess**
Amebic abscess of lung (and liver)

006.5 **Amebic brain abscess**
Amebic abscess of brain (and liver) (and lung)

006.6 **Amebic skin ulceration**
Cutaneous amebiasis

❏006.8 **Amebic infection of other sites**
Amebic:
appendicitis
balanitis
Ameboma

Excludes *specific infections by free-living amebae (136.2)*

❏006.9 **Amebiasis, unspecified**
Amebiasis NOS

● 007 **Other protozoal intestinal diseases**

Includes: protozoal:
colitis
diarrhea
dysentery

007.0 **Balantidiasis**
Infection by Balantidium coli

007.1 **Giardiasis**
Infection by Giardia lamblia
Lambliasis

007.2 **Coccidiosis**
Infection by Isospora belli and Isospora hominis
Isosporiasis

007.3 **Intestinal trichomoniasis**

007.4 **Cryptosporidiosis**

007.5 **Cyclosporiasis**

❏007.8 **Other specified protozoal intestinal diseases**
Amebiasis due to organisms other than Entamoeba histolytica

❏007.9 **Unspecified protozoal intestinal disease**
Flagellate diarrhea
Protozoal dysentery NOS

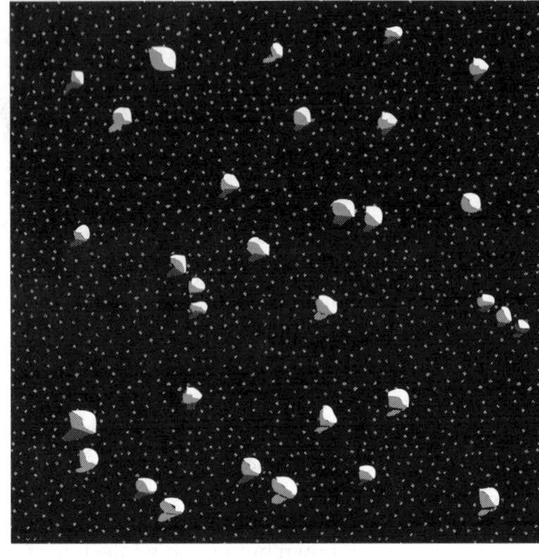

Figure 1–1 *E. coli* particles.

Item 1–2 ***Escherichia coli [E. coli]*** **is a gram-negative bacterium found in the intestinal tracts of humans and animals and is usually nonpathogenic. Pathogenic strains can cause diarrhea or pyogenic (pus-producing) infections.**

● 008 **Intestinal infections due to other organisms**

Includes: any condition classifiable to 009.0–009.3 with mention of the responsible organisms

Excludes *food poisoning by these organisms (005.0–005.9)*

● 008.0 **Escherichia coli [E. coli]**

❏008.00 **E. coli, unspecified**
E. coli enteritis NOS

008.01 **Enteropathogenic E. coli**

008.02 **Enterotoxigenic E. coli**

008.03 **Enteroinvasive E. coli**

008.04 **Enterohemorrhagic E. coli**

❏008.09 **Other intestinal E. coli infections**

008.1 **Arizona group of paracolon bacilli**

008.2 **Aerobacter aerogenes**
Enterobacter aerogenes

008.3 **Proteus (mirabilis) (morganii)**

● 008.4 **Other specified bacteria**

008.41 **Staphylococcus**
Staphylococcal enterocolitis

008.42 **Pseudomonas**

008.43 **Campylobacter**

008.44 **Yersinia enterocolitica**

008.45 Clostridium difficile
Pseudomembranous colitis

❑**008.46 Other anaerobes**
Anaerobic enteritis NOS
Bacteroides (fragilis)
Gram-negative anaerobes

❑**008.47 Other gram-negative bacteria**
Gram-negative enteritis NOS

Excludes *gram-negative anaerobes (008.46)*

❑**008.49 Other**

❑**008.5 Bacterial enteritis, unspecified**

● **008.6 Enteritis due to specified virus**

008.61 Rotavirus

008.62 Adenovirus

008.63 Norwalk virus
Norwalk-like agent

❑**008.64 Other small round viruses [SRVs]**
Small round virus NOS

008.65 Calcivirus

008.66 Astrovirus

008.67 Enterovirus NEC
Coxsackie virus
Echovirus

Excludes *poliovirus (045.0–045.9)*

❑**008.69 Other viral enteritis**
Torovirus

❑**008.8 Other organism, not elsewhere classified**
Viral:
enteritis NOS
gastroenteritis

Excludes *influenza with involvement of gastrointestinal tract (487.8)*

● **009 Ill-defined intestinal infections**

Excludes *diarrheal disease or intestinal infection due to specified organism (001.0–008.8)*
diarrhea following gastrointestinal surgery (564.4)
intestinal malabsorption (579.0–579.9)
ischemic enteritis (557.0–557.9)
other noninfectious gastroenteritis and colitis (558.1–558.9)
regional enteritis (555.0–555.9)
ulcerative colitis (556)

009.0 Infectious colitis, enteritis, and gastroenteritis
Colitis (septic)
Dysentery:
NOS
catarrhal
hemorrhagic
Enteritis (septic)
Gastroenteritis (septic)

009.1 Colitis, enteritis, and gastroenteritis of presumed infectious origin

Excludes *colitis NOS (558.9)*
enteritis NOS (558.9)
gastroenteritis NOS (558.9)

009.2 Infectious diarrhea
Diarrhea:
dysenteric
epidemic
Infectious diarrheal disease NOS

009.3 Diarrhea of presumed infectious origin

Excludes *diarrhea NOS (787.91)*

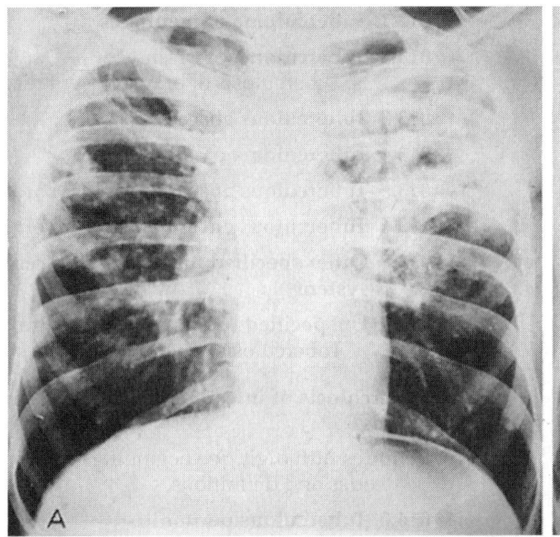
A

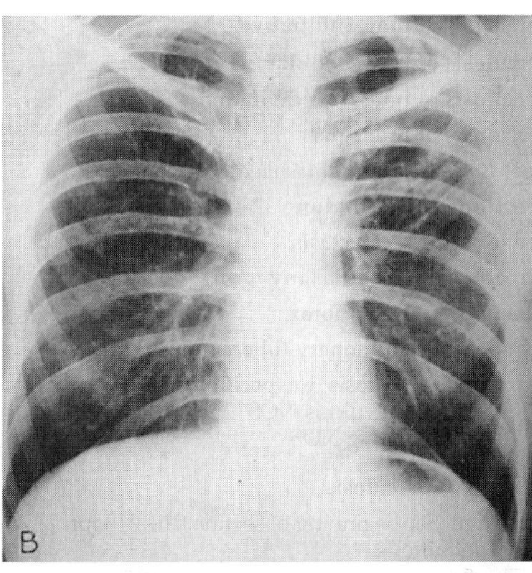
B

Figure 1–2 Far advanced bilateral pulmonary tuberculosis before and after 8 months of treatment with streptomycin, PAS, and isoniazid. (From Hinshaw HC, Garland LH: Diseases of the Chest, 2nd ed. Philadelphia, WB Saunders, 1963, p. 538.)

Item 1-3 Tuberculosis is caused by the ***Mycobacterium tuberculosis*** organism. The first tuberculosis infection is called the **primary infection.** A **Ghon** lesion is the **initial lesion.** A **secondary lesion** occurs when the tubercle bacilli are carried to other areas.

TUBERCULOSIS (010–018)

Includes: infection by Mycobacterium tuberculosis (human) (bovine)

Excludes *congenital tuberculosis (771.2)*
late effects of tuberculosis (137.0–137.4)

The following fifth-digit subclassification is for use with categories 010–018:

❑ 0 **unspecified**
1 **bacteriological or histological examination not done**
2 **bacteriological or histological examination unknown (at present)**
3 **tubercle bacilli found (in sputum) by microscopy**
4 **tubercle bacilli not found (in sputum) by microscopy, but found by bacterial culture**
5 **tubercle bacilli not found by bacteriological examination, but tuberculosis confirmed histologically**
6 **tubercle bacilli not found by bacteriological or histological examination, but tuberculosis confirmed by other methods [inoculation of animals]**

● **010 Primary tuberculous infection**

Requires fifth digit. See beginning of section 010–018 for codes and definitions.

● **010.0 Primary tuberculous infection**

Excludes *nonspecific reaction to tuberculin skin test without active tuberculosis (795.5)*
positive PPD (795.5)
positive tuberculin skin test without active tuberculosis (795.5)

● **010.1 Tuberculous pleurisy in primary progressive tuberculosis**

● ❑ **010.8 Other primary progressive tuberculosis**

Excludes *tuberculous erythema nodosum (017.1)*

● ❑ **010.9 Primary tuberculous infection, unspecified**

● **011 Pulmonary tuberculosis**

Requires fifth digit. See beginning of section 010–018 for codes and definitions.

Use additional code to identify any associated silicosis (502)

● **011.0 Tuberculosis of lung, infiltrative**

● **011.1 Tuberculosis of lung, nodular**

● **011.2 Tuberculosis of lung with cavitation**

● **011.3 Tuberculosis of bronchus**

Excludes *isolated bronchial tuberculosis (012.2)*

● **011.4 Tuberculous fibrosis of lung**

● **011.5 Tuberculous bronchiectasis**

● **011.6 Tuberculous pneumonia [any form]**

● **011.7 Tuberculous pneumothorax**

● ❑ **011.8 Other specified pulmonary tuberculosis**

● ❑ **011.9 Pulmonary tuberculosis, unspecified**
Respiratory tuberculosis NOS
Tuberculosis of lung NOS

● **012 Other respiratory tuberculosis**

Requires fifth digit. See beginning of section 010–018 for codes and definitions.

Excludes *respiratory tuberculosis, unspecified (011.9)*

● **012.0 Tuberculous pleurisy**
Tuberculosis of pleura
Tuberculous empyema
Tuberculous hydrothorax

Excludes *pleurisy with effusion without mention of cause (511.9)*
tuberculous pleurisy in primary progressive tuberculosis (010.1)

● **012.1 Tuberculosis of intrathoracic lymph nodes**
Tuberculosis of lymph nodes:
hilar
mediastinal
tracheobronchial
Tuberculous tracheobronchial adenopathy

Excludes *that specified as primary (010.0–010.9)*

● **012.2 Isolated tracheal or bronchial tuberculosis**

● **012.3 Tuberculous laryngitis**
Tuberculosis of glottis

● ❑ **012.8 Other specified respiratory tuberculosis**
Tuberculosis of:
mediastinum
nasopharynx
nose (septum)
sinus [any nasal]

Item 1-4 Although it primarily affects the lungs, the bacteria ***Mycobacterium tuberculosis*** can travel from the pulmonary circulation to virtually any organ in the body, much as a cancer metastasizes to a secondary site. If the immune system becomes compromised by age or disease, what would otherwise be a self-limiting primary tuberculosis in the lungs will develop in other organs. These are known as extrapulmonary sites. The bones and kidneys are two of the most common extrapulmonary sites of tuberculosis.

● **013 Tuberculosis of meninges and central nervous system**

Requires fifth digit. See beginning of section 010–018 for codes and definitions.

● **013.0 Tuberculous meningitis**
Tuberculosis of meninges (cerebral) (spinal)
Tuberculous:
leptomeningitis
meningoencephalitis

Excludes *tuberculoma of meninges (013.1)*

● **013.1 Tuberculoma of meninges**

● **013.2 Tuberculoma of brain**
Tuberculosis of brain (current disease)

● **013.3 Tuberculous abscess of brain**

● **013.4 Tuberculoma of spinal cord**

● **013.5 Tuberculous abscess of spinal cord**

● **013.6 Tuberculous encephalitis or myelitis**

● ❑ **013.8 Other specified tuberculosis of central nervous system**

● ❑ **013.9 Unspecified tuberculosis of central nervous system**
Tuberculosis of central nervous system NOS

● **014 Tuberculosis of intestines, peritoneum, and mesenteric glands**

Requires fifth digit. See beginning of section 010–018 for codes and definitions.

● **014.0 Tuberculous peritonitis**
Tuberculous ascites

014.8 Other
Tuberculosis (of):
anus
intestine (large) (small)
mesenteric glands
rectum
retroperitoneal (lymph nodes)
Tuberculous enteritis

015 Tuberculosis of bones and joints

Requires fifth digit. See beginning of section 010–018 for codes and definitions.

Use additional code to identify manifestation, as:
tuberculous:
arthropathy (711.4)
necrosis of bone (730.8)
osteitis (730.8)
osteomyelitis (730.8)
synovitis (727.01)
tenosynovitis (727.01)

015.0 Vertebral colum
Pott's disease
Use additional code to identify manifestation, as:
curvature of spine [Pott's] (737.4)
kyphosis (737.4)
spondylitis (720.81)

015.1 Hip

015.2 Knee

015.5 Limb bones
Tuberculous dactylitis

015.6 Mastoid
Tuberculous mastoiditis

015.7 Other specified bone

015.8 Other specified joint

015.9 Tuberculosis of unspecified bones and joints

016 Tuberculosis of genitourinary system

Requires fifth digit. See beginning of section 010–018 for codes and definitions.

016.0 Kidney
Renal tuberculosis

Use additional code to identify manifestation, as:
tuberculous:
nephropathy (583.81)
pyelitis (590.81)
pyelonephritis (590.81)

016.1 Bladder

016.2 Ureter

016.3 Other urinary organs

016.4 Epididymis

016.5 Other male genital organs
Use additional code to identify manifestation, as:
tuberculosis of:
prostate (601.4)
seminal vesicle (608.81)
testis (608.81)

016.6 Tuberculous oophoritis and salpingitis

016.7 Other female genital organs
Tuberculous:
cervicitis
endometritis

016.9 Genitourinary tuberculosis, unspecified

017 Tuberculosis of other organs

Requires fifth digit. See beginning of section 010–018 for codes and definitions.

017.0 Skin and subcutaneous cellular tissue

Lupus:	Tuberculosis:
exedens	colliquativa
vulgaris	cutis
Scrofuloderma	lichenoides
	papulonecrotica
	verrucosa cutis

Excludes *lupus erythematosus (695.4)*
disseminated (710.0)
lupus NOS (710.0)
nonspecific reaction to tuberculin skin test without active tuberculosis (795.5)
positive PPD (795.5)
positive tuberculin skin test without active tuberculosis (795.5)

017.1 Erythema nodosum with hypersensitivity reaction in tuberculosis
Bazin's disease
Erythema:
induratum
nodosum, tuberculous
Tuberculosis indurativa

Excludes *erythema nodosum NOS (695.2)*

017.2 Peripheral lymph nodes
Scrofula
Scrofulous abscess
Tuberculous adenitis

Excludes *tuberculosis of lymph nodes:*
bronchial and mediastinal (012.1)
mesenteric and retroperitoneal (014.8)
tuberculous tracheobronchial adenopathy (012.1)

017.3 Eye
Use additional code to identify manifestation, as:
tuberculous:
episcleritis (379.09)
interstitial keratitis (370.59)
iridocyclitis, chronic (364.11)
keratoconjunctivitis (phlyctenular) (370.31)

017.4 Ear
Tuberculosis of ear
Tuberculous otitis media

Excludes *tuberculous mastoiditis (015.6)*

017.5 Thyroid gland

017.6 Adrenal glands
Addison's disease, tuberculous

017.7 Spleen

017.8 Esophagus

017.9 Other specified organs
Use additional code to identify manifestation, as:
tuberculosis of:
endocardium [any valve] (424.91)
myocardium (422.0)
pericardium (420.0)

Item 1-5 Miliary tuberculosis can be a life-threatening condition. If a tuberculous lesion enters a blood vessel, immense dissemination of tuberculous organisms can occur if the immune system is too weak to fight it off. High-risk populations—children under 4 years of age and the elderly or immunocompromised—are particularly prone to this type of infection. The lesions will have a millet seed-like appearance on chest x-ray. Bronchial washings and biopsy may also aid in diagnosis.

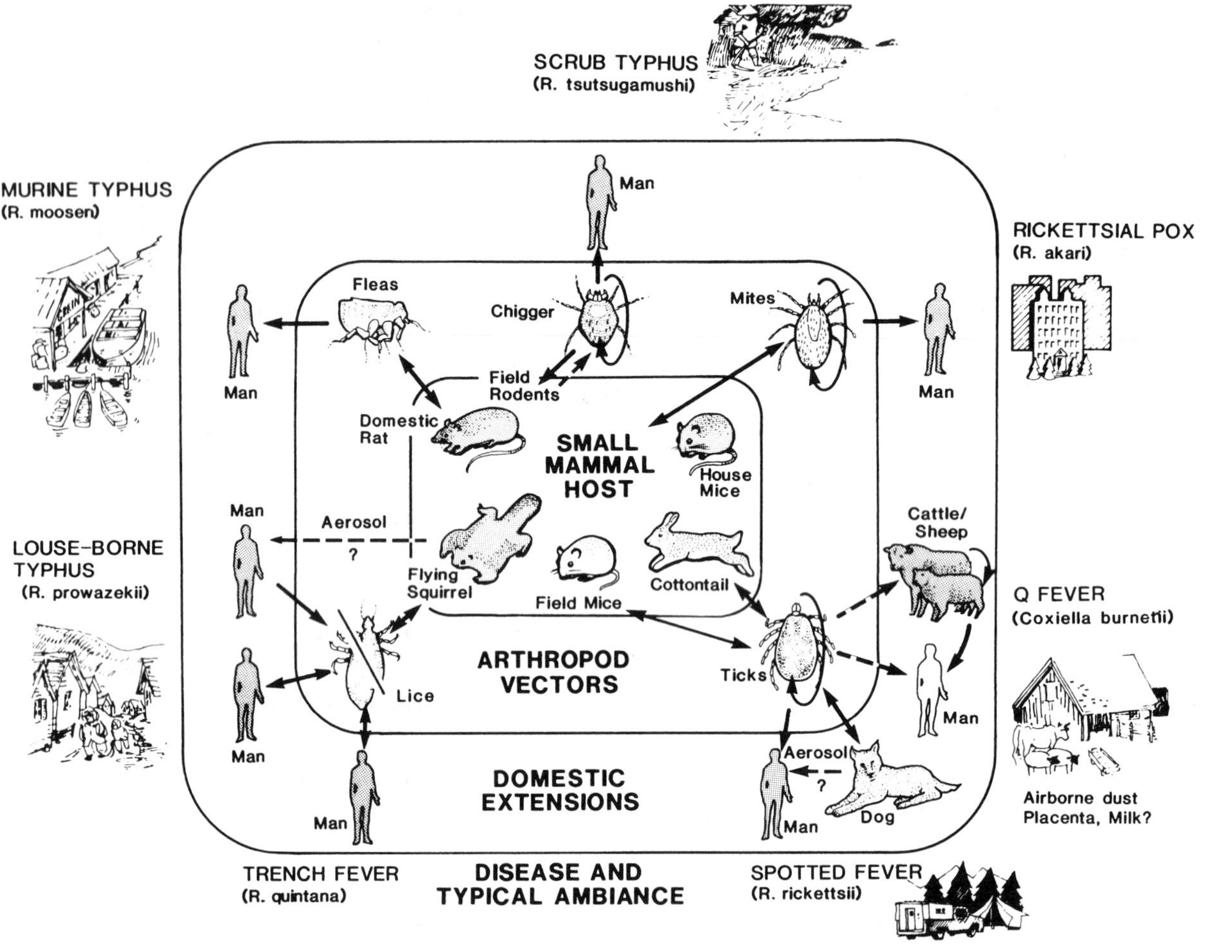

SCRUB TYPHUS
(R. tsutsugamushi)
MURINE TYPHUS
(R. moosen)
RICKETTSIAL POX
(R. akari)
LOUSE-BORNE TYPHUS
(R. prowazekii)
Q FEVER
(Coxiella burnetii)
Airborne dust
Placenta, Milk?
TRENCH FEVER
(R. quintana)
DISEASE AND TYPICAL AMBIANCE
SPOTTED FEVER
(R. rickettsii)
Man
Fleas
Chigger
Mites
Field Rodents
Domestic Rat
SMALL MAMMAL HOST
House Mice
Aerosol
?
Flying Squirrel
Field Mice
Cottontail
Cattle/ Sheep
ARTHROPOD VECTORS
Lice
Ticks
DOMESTIC EXTENSIONS
Aerosol
Dog

Figure 1–3 Schematic summary of some major interactions between rickettsial organisms and their small animal hosts and arthropod vectors, the participation of domestic animals, and examples of the typical ambiance under which each rickettsial infection is contacted by humans. (From Strickland GT: Hunter's Tropical Medicine, 7th ed. Philadelphia, WB Saunders, 1991, p. 261. Courtesy of Dr. J. K. Frenkel, University of Kansas Medical Center, Kansas City, KS.)

● **018 Miliary tuberculosis**

Requires fifth digit. See beginning of section 010–018 for codes and definitions.

Includes: tuberculosis:
- disseminated
- generalized
- miliary, whether of a single specified site, multiple sites, or unspecified site
- polyserositis

● **018.0 Acute miliary tuberculosis**

● ❑ **018.8 Other specified miliary tuberculosis**

● ❑ **018.9 Miliary tuberculosis, unspecified**

ZOONOTIC BACTERIAL DISEASES (020–027)

● **020 Plague**

Includes: infection by Yersinia [Pasteurella] pestis

020.0 Bubonic

020.1 Cellulocutaneous

020.2 Septicemic

020.3 Primary pneumonic

020.4 Secondary pneumonic

❑ **020.5 Pneumonic, unspecified**

❑ **020.8 Other specified types of plague**
- Abortive plague
- Ambulatory plague
- Pestis minor

❑ **020.9 Plague, unspecified**

● **021 Tularemia**

Includes: deerfly fever
- infection by Francisella [Pasteurella] tularensis
- rabbit fever

021.0 Ulceroglandular tularemia

021.1 Enteric tularemia

Tularemia:
- cryptogenic
- intestinal
- typhoidal

021.2 Pulmonary tularemia

Bronchopneumonic tularemia

021.3 Oculoglandular tularemia

❑ **021.8 Other specified tularemia**

Tularemia:
- generalized or disseminated
- glandular

❑ **021.9 Unspecified tularemia**

● **022 Anthrax**

022.0 Cutaneous anthrax
Malignant pustule

022.1 Pulmonary anthrax
Respiratory anthrax
Wool-sorters' disease

022.2 Gastrointestinal anthrax

022.3 Anthrax septicemia

❑ **022.8 Other specified manifestations of anthrax**

❑ **022.9 Anthrax, unspecified**

● **023 Brucellosis**

Includes: fever:
Malta
Mediterranean
undulant

023.0 Brucella melitensis

023.1 Brucella abortus

023.2 Brucella suis

023.3 Brucella canis

❑ **023.8 Other brucellosis**
Infection by more than one organism

❑ **023.9 Brucellosis, unspecified**

024 Glanders
Infection by:
Actinobacillus mallei
Malleomyces mallei
Pseudomonas mallei
Farcy
Malleus

025 Melioidosis
Infection by:
Malleomyces pseudomallei
Pseudomonas pseudomallei
Whitmore's bacillus
Pseudoglanders

● **026 Rat-bite fever**

026.0 Spirillary fever
Rat-bite fever due to Spirillum minor [S. minus]
Sodoku

026.1 Streptobacillary fever
Epidemic arthritic erythema
Haverhill fever
Rat-bite fever due to Streptobacillus moniliformis

❑ **026.9 Unspecified rat-bite fever**

● **027 Other zoonotic bacterial diseases**

027.0 Listeriosis
Infection by Listeria monocytogenes
Septicemia by Listeria monocytogenes

Use additional code to identify manifestations, as meningitis (320.7)

Excludes *congenital listeriosis (771.2)*

027.1 Erysipelothrix infection
Erysipeloid (of Rosenbach)
Infection by Erysipelothrix insidiosa [E. rhusiopathiae]
Septicemia by Erysipelothrix insidiosa [E. rhusiopathiae]

027.2 Pasteurellosis
Pasteurella pseudotuberculosis infection by Pasteurella multocida [P. septica]
Mesenteric adenitis by Pasteurella multocida [P. septica]
Septic infection (cat bite) (dog bite) by Pasteurella multocida [P. septica]

Excludes *infection by:*
Francisella [Pasteurella] tularensis (021.0–021.9)
Yersinia [Pasteurella] pestis (020.0–020.9)

❑ **027.8 Other specified zoonotic bacterial diseases**

❑ **027.9 Unspecified zoonotic bacterial disease**

OTHER BACTERIAL DISEASES (030–041)

Excludes *bacterial venereal diseases (098.0–099.9)*
bartonellosis (088.0)

● **030 Leprosy**

Includes: Hansen's disease
infection by Mycobacterium leprae

030.0 Lepromatous [type L]
Lepromatous leprosy (macular) (diffuse) (infiltrated) (nodular) (neuritic)

030.1 Tuberculoid [type T]
Tuberculoid leprosy (macular) (maculoanesthetic) (major) (minor) (neuritic)

030.2 Indeterminate [group I]
Indeterminate [uncharacteristic] leprosy (macular) (neuritic)

030.3 Borderline [group B]
Borderline or dimorphous leprosy (infiltrated) (neuritic)

❑ **030.8 Other specified leprosy**

❑ **030.9 Leprosy, unspecified**

● **031 Diseases due to other mycobacteria**

031.0 Pulmonary
Battey disease
Infection by Mycobacterium:
avium
intracellulare [Battey bacillus]
kansasii

031.1 Cutaneous
Buruli ulcer
Infection by Mycobacterium:
marinum [M. balnei]
ulcerans

031.2 Disseminated
Disseminated mycobacterium avium-intracellulare complex (DMAC)
Mycobacterium avium-intracellulare complex (MAC) bacteremia

❑ **031.8 Other specified mycobacterial diseases**

❑ **031.9 Unspecified diseases due to mycobacteria**
Atypical mycobacterium infection NOS

● **032 Diphtheria**

Includes: infection by Corynebacterium diphtheriae

032.0 Faucial diphtheria
Membranous angina, diphtheritic

032.1 Nasopharyngeal diphtheria

032.2 Anterior nasal diphtheria

032.3 Laryngeal diphtheria
Laryngotracheitis, diphtheritic

● 032.8 **Other specified diphtheria**

032.81 **Conjunctival diphtheria**
Pseudomembranous diphtheritic conjunctivitis

032.82 **Diphtheritic myocarditis**

032.83 **Diphtheritic peritonitis**

032.84 **Diphtheritic cystitis**

032.85 **Cutaneous diphtheria**

❑ 032.89 **Other**

❑ 032.9 **Diphtheria, unspecified**

● 033 **Whooping cough**

Includes: pertussis
Use additional code to identify any associated pneumonia (484.3)

033.0 **Bordetella pertussis [B. pertussis]**

033.1 **Bordetella parapertussis [B. parapertussis]**

❑ 033.8 **Whooping cough due to other specified organism**
Bordetella bronchiseptica [B. bronchiseptica]

❑ 033.9 **Whooping cough, unspecified organism**

Item 1-6 034.0 is the common "strep throat" (sore throat with strep infection). It is grouped in the same three-digit category with scarlet fever. If a patient has both scarlet fever and the strep throat, you would use both codes. "Streptococcal" must be indicated on the laboratory report to use 034.0; otherwise use 462 for "sore throat" (pharyngitis).

● 034 **Streptococcal sore throat and scarlet fever**

034.0 **Streptococcal sore throat**

Septic:	Streptococcal:
angina	angina
sore throat	laryngitis
	pharyngitis
	tonsillitis

034.1 **Scarlet fever**
Scarlatina

Excludes *parascarlatina (057.8)*

035 **Erysipelas**

Excludes *postpartum or puerperal erysipelas (670)*

● 036 **Meningococcal infection**

036.0 **Meningococcal meningitis**
Cerebrospinal fever (meningococcal)
Meningitis:
cerebrospinal
epidemic

036.1 **Meningococcal encephalitis**

036.2 **Meningococcemia**
Meningococcal septicemia

036.3 **Waterhouse-Friderichsen syndrome, meningococcal**
Meningococcal hemorrhagic adrenalitis
Meningococcic adrenal syndrome
Waterhouse-Friderichsen syndrome NOS

● 036.4 **Meningococcal carditis**

❑ 036.40 **Meningococcal carditis, unspecified**

036.41 **Meningococcal pericarditis**

036.42 **Meningococcal endocarditis**

036.43 **Meningococcal myocarditis**

● 036.8 **Other specified meningococcal infections**

036.81 **Meningococcal optic neuritis**

036.82 **Meningococcal arthropathy**

❑ 036.89 **Other**

❑ 036.9 **Meningococcal infection, unspecified**
Meningococcal infection NOS

037 **Tetanus**

Excludes *tetanus:*
complicating:
abortion (634–638 with .0, 639.0)
ectopic or molar pregnancy (639.0)
neonatorum (771.3)
puerperal (670)

● 038 **Septicemia**

Note: Use additional code for systemic inflammatory response syndrome (SIRS) (995.91–995.92).

Excludes *bacteremia (790.7)*
septicemia (sepsis) of newborn (771.81)

038.0 **Streptococcal septicemia**

● 038.1 **Staphylococcal septicemia**

❑ 038.10 **Staphylococcal septicemia, unspecified**

038.11 **Staphylococcus aureus septicemia**

❑ 038.19 **Other staphylococcal septicemia**

038.2 **Pneumococcal septicemia [Streptococcus pneumoniae septicemia]**

038.3 **Septicemia due to anaerobes**
Septicemia due to Bacteroides

Excludes *gas gangrene (040.0)*
that due to anaerobic streptococci (038.0)

● 038.4 **Septicemia due to other gram-negative organisms**

❑ 038.40 **Gram-negative organism, unspecified**
Gram-negative septicemia NOS

038.41 **Hemophilus influenzae [H. influenzae]**

038.42 **Escherichia coli [E. coli]**

038.43 **Pseudomonas**

038.44 **Serratia**

❑ 038.49 **Other**

❑ 038.8 **Other specified septicemias**

Excludes *septicemia (due to):*
anthrax (022.3)
gonococcal (098.89)
herpetic (054.5)
meningococcal (036.2)
septicemic plague (020.2)

❑ 038.9 **Unspecified septicemia**
Septicemia NOS

Excludes *bacteremia NOS (790.7)*

● 039 **Actinomycotic infections**

Includes: actinomycotic mycetoma
infection by Actinomycetales, such as species of Actinomyces, Actinomadura, Nocardia, Streptomyces
maduromycosis (actinomycotic)
schizomycetoma (actinomycotic)

039.0 **Cutaneous**
Erythrasma
Trichomycosis axillaris

039.1 **Pulmonary**
Thoracic actinomycosis

039.2 **Abdominal**

039.3 **Cervicofacial**

039.4 **Madura foot**

Excludes *madura foot due to mycotic infection (117.4)*

❑039.8 **Of other specified sites**

❑039.9 **Of unspecified site**
Actinomycosis NOS
Maduromycosis NOS
Nocardiosis NOS

Item 1-7 Gas gangrene is a necrotizing subcutaneous infection that will cause tissue death. Patients with poor circulation (e.g., diabetes, peripheral nephropathy) will have low oxygen content in their tissues (hypoxia), which makes the Clostridium bacteria flourish. Gas gangrene often occurs at the site of a surgical wound or trauma. Treatment can include debridement, amputation, and/or hyperbaric oxygen treatments.

● 040 **Other bacterial diseases**

Excludes *bacteremia NOS (790.7)*
bacterial infection NOS (041.9)

040.0 **Gas gangrene**
Gas bacillus infection or gangrene
Infection by Clostridium:
histolyticum
oedematiens
perfringens [welchii]
septicum
sordellii
Malignant edema
Myonecrosis, clostridial
Myositis, clostridial

040.1 **Rhinoscleroma**

040.2 **Whipple's disease**
Intestinal lipodystrophy

040.3 **Necrobacillosis**

● 040.8 **Other specified bacterial diseases**

040.81 **Tropical pyomyositis**

040.82 **Toxic shock syndrome**
Use additional code to identify the organism

❑040.89 **Other**

● 041 **Bacterial infection in conditions classified elsewhere and of unspecified site**

Note: This category is provided to be used as an additional code to identify the bacterial agent in diseases classified elsewhere. This category will also be used to classify bacterial infections of unspecified nature or site.

Excludes *bacteremia NOS (790.7)*
septicemia (038.0–038.9)

● 041.0 **Streptococcus**

❑041.00 **Streptococcus, unspecified**
Specified in documentation as streptococcus, but unspecified as to Group

041.01 **Group A**
Specified as Group A

041.02 **Group B**
Specified as Group B

041.03 **Group C**
Specified as Group C

041.04 **Group D [Enterococcus]**
Specified as Group D

041.05 **Group G**
Specified as Group G

❑041.09 **Other Streptococcus**
Streptococcus that is documented but not specified as Group A, B, C, D, or G

● 041.1 **Staphylococcus**

❑041.10 **Staphylococcus, unspecified**

041.11 **Staphylococcus aureus**

❑041.19 **Other Staphylococcus**

041.2 **Pneumococcus**

041.3 **Friedländer's bacillus**
Infection by Klebsiella pneumoniae

041.4 **Escherichia coli [E. coli]**

041.5 **Hemophilus influenzae [H. influenzae]**

041.6 **Proteus (mirabilis) (morganii)**

041.7 **Pseudomonas**

● 041.8 **Other specified bacterial infections**

041.81 **Mycoplasma**
Eaton's agent
Pleuropneumonia-like organisms [PPLO]

041.82 **Bacteroides fragilis**

041.83 **Clostridium perfringens**

❑041.84 **Other anaerobes**
Gram-negative anaerobes

Excludes *Helicobacter pylori (041.86)*

041.85 **Other gram-negative organisms**
Aerobacter aerogenes
Gram-negative bacteria NOS
Mima polymorpha
Serratia

Excludes *gram-negative anaerobes (041.84)*

041.86 **Helicobacter pylori (H. pylori)**

❑041.89 **Other specified bacteria**

❑041.9 **Bacterial infection, unspecified**

Item 1-8 AIDS (acquired immune deficiency syndrome) is caused by HIV (human immunodeficiency virus). HIV affects certain white blood cells (T-4 lymphocytes) and destroys the ability of the cells to fight infections, making patients susceptible to a host of infectious diseases, e.g., *Pneumocystis carinii* pneumonia (PCP), Kaposi's sarcoma, and lymphoma. AIDS-related complex (ARC) is an early stage of AIDS in which tests for HIV are positive but the symptoms are mild.

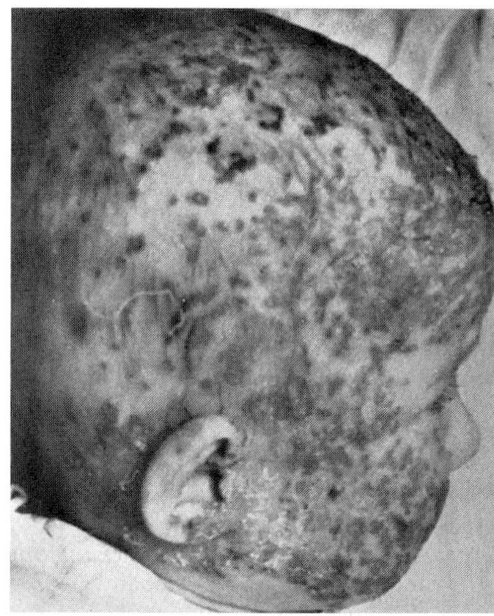

Figure 1–4 Vesicular, pustular, scabby, and necrotic lesions in Kaposi's sarcoma. (From Debre R, Celers J: Clinical Virology—The Evaluation and Management of Human Viral Infections. Philadelphia, WB Saunders, 1970, p. 460. Copyright Medicales Flammarion [Paris, France].)

ICD-9-CM 001-099 Vol. 1

HUMAN IMMUNODEFICIENCY VIRUS (HIV) INFECTION (042)

042 Human immunodeficiency virus [HIV] disease
Acquired immune deficiency syndrome
Acquired immunodeficiency syndrome
AIDS
AIDS-like syndrome
AIDS-related complex
ARC
HIV infection, symptomatic

Use additional code(s) to identify all manifestations of HIV

Use additional code to identify HIV-2 infection (079.53)

Excludes *asymptomatic HIV infection status (V08)*
exposure to HIV virus (V01.79)
nonspecific serologic evidence of HIV (795.71)

POLIOMYELITIS AND OTHER NON-ARTHROPOD-BORNE VIRAL DISEASES OF CENTRAL NERVOUS SYSTEM (045–049)

● **045 Acute poliomyelitis**
Excludes *late effects of acute poliomyelitis (138)*

The following fifth-digit subclassification is for use with category 045:
❑ **0 poliovirus, unspecified type**
1 poliovirus type I
2 poliovirus type II
3 poliovirus type III

● **045.0 Acute paralytic poliomyelitis specified as bulbar**
Infantile paralysis (acute) specified as bulbar
Poliomyelitis (acute) (anterior) specified as bulbar
Polioencephalitis (acute) (bulbar)
Polioencephalomyelitis (acute) (anterior) (bulbar)

● ❑ **045.1 Acute poliomyelitis with other paralysis**
Paralysis:
acute atrophic, spinal
infantile, paralytic
Poliomyelitis (acute) with paralysis except bulbar
anterior with paralysis except bulbar
epidemic with paralysis except bulbar

● **045.2 Acute nonparalytic poliomyelitis**
Poliomyelitis (acute) specified as nonparalytic
anterior specified as nonparalytic
epidemic specified as nonparalytic

● ❑ **045.9 Acute poliomyelitis, unspecified**
Infantile paralysis unspecified whether paralytic or nonparalytic
Poliomyelitis (acute) unspecified whether paralytic or nonparalytic
anterior unspecified whether paralytic or nonparalytic
epidemic unspecified whether paralytic or nonparalytic

● **046 Slow virus infection of central nervous system**

046.0 Kuru

046.1 Jakob-Creutzfeldt disease *JCD*
Subacute spongiform encephalopathy

046.2 Subacute sclerosing panencephalitis
Dawson's inclusion body encephalitis
Van Bogaert's sclerosing leukoencephalitis

046.3 Progressive multifocal leukoencephalopathy
Multifocal leukoencephalopathy NOS

❑ **046.8 Other specified slow virus infection of central nervous system**

❑ **046.9 Unspecified slow virus infection of central nervous system**

● **047 Meningitis due to enterovirus**
Includes: meningitis:
abacterial
aseptic
viral

Excludes *meningitis due to:*
adenovirus (049.1)
arthropod-borne virus (060.0–066.9)
leptospira (100.81)
virus of:
herpes simplex (054.72)
herpes zoster (053.0)
lymphocytic choriomeningitis (049.0)
mumps (072.1)
poliomyelitis (045.0–045.9)
any other infection specifically classified elsewhere

047.0 Coxsackie virus

047.1 ECHO virus
Meningo-eruptive syndrome

❑ **047.8 Other specified viral meningitis**

❑ **047.9 Unspecified viral meningitis**
Viral meningitis NOS

❑ **048 Other enterovirus diseases of central nervous system**
Boston exanthem

● **049 Other non-arthropod-borne viral diseases of central nervous system**
Excludes *late effects of viral encephalitis (139.0)*

049.0 Lymphocytic choriomeningitis
Lymphocytic:
meningitis (serous) (benign)
meningoencephalitis (serous) (benign)

049.1 Meningitis due to adenovirus

❑ **049.8 Other specified non-arthropod-borne viral diseases of central nervous system**
Encephalitis:
acute:
inclusion body
necrotizing
epidemic
lethargica
Rio Bravo
von Economo's disease

❑ **049.9 Unspecified non-arthropod-borne viral diseases of central nervous system**
Viral encephalitis NOS

VIRAL DISEASES ACCOMPANIED BY EXANTHEM (050–057)

Excludes *arthropod-borne viral diseases (060.0–066.9)*
Boston exanthem (048)

● **050 Smallpox**

050.0 Variola major
Hemorrhagic (pustular) smallpox
Malignant smallpox
Purpura variolosa

050.1 Alastrim
Variola minor

050.2 Modified smallpox
Varioloid

❑ **050.9 Smallpox, unspecified**

● **051 Cowpox and paravaccinia**

051.0 Cowpox
Vaccinia not from vaccination
Excludes *vaccinia (generalized) (from vaccination) (999.0)*

051.1 **Pseudocowpox**
Milkers' node

051.2 **Contagious pustular dermatitis**
Ecthyma contagiosum
Orf

❑051.9 **Paravaccinia, unspecified**

● 052 Chickenpox

052.0 **Postvaricella encephalitis**
Postchickenpox encephalitis

052.1 **Varicella (hemorrhagic) pneumonitis**

052.2 **Postvaricella myelitis** ◀
Postchickenpox myelitis ◀

❑052.7 **With other specified complications**

❑052.8 **With unspecified complication**

052.9 **Varicella without mention of complication**
Chickenpox NOS
Varicella NOS

● 053 Herpes zoster

Includes: shingles
zona

053.0 **With meningitis**

● 053.1 **With other nervous system complications**

❑053.10 **With unspecified nervous system complication**

053.11 **Geniculate herpes zoster**
Herpetic geniculate ganglionitis

053.12 **Postherpetic trigeminal neuralgia**

053.13 **Postherpetic polyneuropathy**

053.14 **Herpes zoster myelitis** ◀

❑053.19 **Other**

● 053.2 **With ophthalmic complications**

053.20 **Herpes zoster dermatitis of eyelid**
Herpes zoster ophthalmicus

053.21 **Herpes zoster keratoconjunctivitis**

053.22 **Herpes zoster iridocyclitis**

❑053.29 **Other**

Item 1-9 Herpes is a viral disease for which there is no cure. There are two types of the herpes simplex virus: Type I causes cold sores or fever blisters and Type II causes genital herpes. The virus can be spread from a sore on the lips to the genitals or from the genitals to the lips.

● 053.7 **With other specified complications**

053.71 **Otitis externa due to herpes zoster**

❑053.79 **Other**

❑053.8 **With unspecified complication**

053.9 **Herpes zoster without mention of complication**
Herpes zoster NOS

● 054 Herpes simplex

Excludes *congenital herpes simplex (771.2)*

054.0 **Eczema herpeticum**
Kaposi's varicelliform eruption

● 054.1 **Genital herpes**

❑054.10 **Genital herpes, unspecified**
Herpes progenitalis

054.11 **Herpetic vulvovaginitis**

054.12 **Herpetic ulceration of vulva**

054.13 **Herpetic infection of penis**

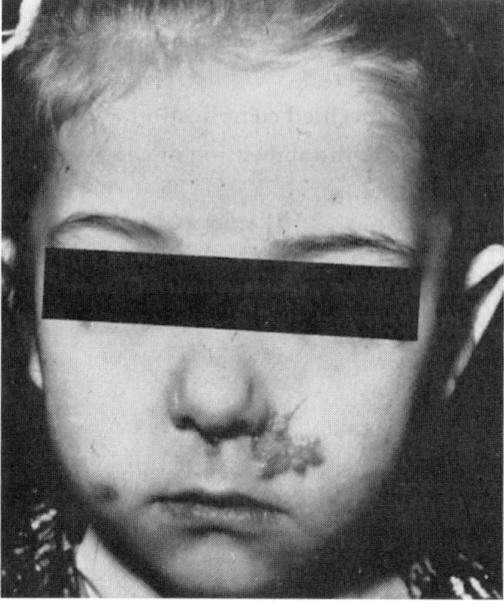

Figure 1-5 Grouped outbursts of herpes vesicles on the face. (From Debre R, Celers J: Clinical Virology—The Evaluation and Management of Human Viral Infections. Philadelphia, WB Saunders, 1970, p. 460. Copyright Medicales Flammarion [Paris, France].)

❑054.19 **Other**

054.2 **Herpetic gingivostomatitis**

054.3 **Herpetic meningoencephalitis**
Herpes encephalitis   Simian B disease

● 054.4 **With ophthalmic complications**

❑054.40 **With unspecified ophthalmic complication**

054.41 **Herpes simplex dermatitis of eyelid**

054.42 **Dendritic keratitis**

054.43 **Herpes simplex disciform keratitis**

054.44 **Herpes simplex iridocyclitis**

❑054.49 **Other**

054.5 **Herpetic septicemia**

054.6 **Herpetic whitlow**
Herpetic felon

● 054.7 **With other specified complications**

054.71 **Visceral herpes simplex**

054.72 **Herpes simplex meningitis**

054.73 **Herpes simplex otitis externa**

054.74 **Herpes simplex myelitis** ◀

❑054.79 **Other**

❑054.8 **With unspecified complication**

054.9 **Herpes simplex without mention of complication**

Item 1-10 Rubeola (055) and rubella (056) are medical terms for two different strains of measles. The MMR (measles, mumps, and rubella) vaccination is an attempt to eradicate these childhood diseases.

● 055 Measles

Includes: morbilli
rubeola

055.0 **Postmeasles encephalitis**

055.1 **Postmeasles pneumonia**

055.2 **Postmeasles otitis media**

● 055.7 **With other specified complications**

055.71 **Measles keratoconjunctivitis**
Measles keratitis

❑055.79 **Other**

❑055.8 **With unspecified complication**

055.9 **Measles without mention of complication**

Item 1-11 Rubeola (055) and **rubella** (056) are medical terms for two different strains of measles. The MMR (measles, mumps, and rubella) vaccination is an attempt to eradicate these childhood diseases.

● 056 **Rubella**

Includes: German measles

Excludes *congenital rubella (771.0)*

● 056.0 **With neurological complications**

❑056.00 **With unspecified neurological complication**

056.01 **Encephalomyelitis due to rubella**
Encephalitis due to rubella
Meningoencephalitis due to rubella

❑056.09 **Other**

● 056.7 **With other specified complications**

056.71 **Arthritis due to rubella**

❑056.79 **Other**

❑056.8 **With unspecified complications**

056.9 **Rubella without mention of complication**

● 057 **Other viral exanthemata**

057.0 **Erythema infectiosum [fifth disease]**

❑057.8 **Other specified viral exanthemata**
Dukes (-Filatow) disease
Exanthema subitum [sixth disease]
Fourth disease
Parascarlatina
Pseudoscarlatina
Roseola infantum

❑057.9 **Viral exanthem, unspecified**

ARTHROPOD-BORNE VIRAL DISEASES (060–066)

Use additional code to identify any associated meningitis (321.2)

Excludes *late effects of viral encephalitis (139.0)*

● 060 **Yellow fever**

060.0 **Sylvatic**
Yellow fever:
jungle
sylvan

060.1 **Urban**

❑060.9 **Yellow fever, unspecified**

061 **Dengue**
Breakbone fever

Excludes *hemorrhagic fever caused by dengue virus (065.4)*

● 062 **Mosquito-borne viral encephalitis**

062.0 **Japanese encephalitis**
Japanese B encephalitis

062.1 **Western equine encephalitis**

062.2 **Eastern equine encephalitis**

Excludes *Venezuelan equine encephalitis (066.2)*

062.3 **St. Louis encephalitis**

062.4 **Australian encephalitis**
Australian arboencephalitis
Australian X disease
Murray Valley encephalitis

062.5 **California virus encephalitis**
Encephalitis:
California
La Crosse
Encephalitis:
Tahyna fever

❑062.8 **Other specified mosquito-borne viral encephalitis**
Encephalitis by Ilheus virus

Excludes *West Nile virus (066.40–066.49)*

❑062.9 **Mosquito-borne viral encephalitis, unspecified**

● 063 **Tick-borne viral encephalitis**

Includes: diphasic meningoencephalitis

063.0 **Russian spring-summer [taiga] encephalitis**

063.1 **Louping ill**

063.2 **Central European encephalitis**

❑063.8 **Other specified tick-borne viral encephalitis**
Langat encephalitis
Powassan encephalitis

❑063.9 **Tick-borne viral encephalitis, unspecified**

064 **Viral encephalitis transmitted by other and unspecified arthropods**
Arthropod-borne viral encephalitis, vector unknown
Negishi virus encephalitis

Excludes *viral encephalitis NOS (049.9)*

● 065 **Arthropod-borne hemorrhagic fever**

065.0 **Crimean hemorrhagic fever [CHF Congo virus]**
Central Asian hemorrhagic fever

065.1 **Omsk hemorrhagic fever**

065.2 **Kyasanur Forest disease**

❑065.3 **Other tick-borne hemorrhagic fever**

065.4 **Mosquito-borne hemorrhagic fever**
Chikungunya hemorrhagic fever
Dengue hemorrhagic fever

Excludes *Chikungunya fever (066.3)*
dengue (061)
yellow fever (060.0–060.9)

❑065.8 **Other specified arthropod-borne hemorrhagic fever**
Mite-borne hemorrhagic fever

❑065.9 **Arthropod-borne hemorrhagic fever, unspecified**
Arbovirus hemorrhagic fever NOS

● 066 **Other arthropod-borne viral diseases**

066.0 **Phlebotomus fever**
Changuinola fever
Sandfly fever

066.1 **Tick-borne fever**
Nairobi sheep disease
Tick fever:
American mountain
Colorado
Kemerovo
Quaranfil

066.2 **Venezuelan equine fever**
Venezuelan equine encephalitis

❑066.3 **Other mosquito-borne fever**
Fever (viral):
Bunyamwera
Bwamba
Chikungunya
Guama
Mayaro
Mucambo
O' Nyong-Nyong
Fever (viral):
Oropouche
Pixuna
Rift valley
Ross river
Wesselsbron
Zika

Excludes *dengue (061)*
yellow fever (060.0–060.9)

● 066.4 **West Nile fever**

❑066.40 **West Nile fever, unspecified**
West Nile fever NOS
West Nile fever without complications
West Nile virus NOS

066.41 **West Nile fever with encephalitis**
West Nile encephalitis
West Nile encephalomyelitis

066.42 **West Nile fever with other neurologic manifestation**
Use additional code to specify the neurologic manifestation

066.49 **West Nile fever with other complications**
Use additional code to specify the other conditions

❑066.8 **Other specified arthropod-borne viral diseases**
Chandipura fever
Piry fever

❑066.9 **Arthropod-borne viral disease, unspecified**
Arbovirus infection NOS

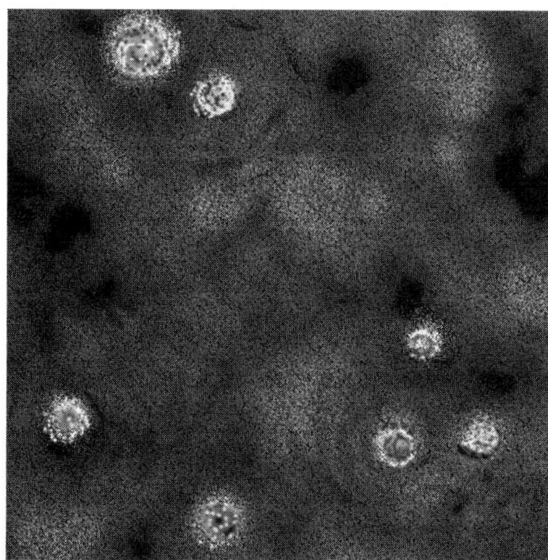

Figure 1–6 Hepatitis B virions (Dane particles).

Item 1–12 Hepatitis A (HAV) was formerly called epidemic, infectious, short-incubation, or acute catarrhal jaundice hepatitis. The primary transmission mode is the oral–fecal route.

Item 1–13 Hepatitis B (HBV) was formerly called long-incubation period, serum, or homologous serum hepatitis. Transmission modes are through body fluids and from mother to neonate.

Item 1–14 Hepatitis C, caused by the hepatitis C virus, is primarily transfusion associated.

Item 1–15 Hepatitis D, also called delta hepatitis, is caused by the hepatitis D virus in patients formerly or currently infected with hepatitis B.

Item 1–16 Hepatitis E is also called enterically transmitted non-A, non-B hepatitis. The primary transmission mode is the oral–fecal route, usually through contaminated water.

OTHER DISEASES DUE TO VIRUSES AND CHLAMYDIAE (070–079)

● 070 **Viral hepatitis**

Includes: viral hepatitis (acute) (chronic)

Excludes *cytomegalic inclusion virus hepatitis (078.5)*

The following fifth-digit subclassification is for use with categories 070.2 and 070.3:

❑ 0 **acute or unspecified, without mention of hepatitis delta**
❑ 1 **acute or unspecified, with hepatitis delta**
2 **chronic, without mention of hepatitis delta**
3 **chronic, with hepatitis delta**

070.0 **Viral hepatitis A with hepatic coma**

070.1 **Viral hepatitis A without mention of hepatic coma**
Infectious hepatitis

● 070.2 **Viral hepatitis B with hepatic coma**

● 070.3 **Viral hepatitis B without mention of hepatic coma**
Serum hepatitis

● 070.4 **Other specified viral hepatitis with hepatic coma**

❑070.41 **Acute hepatitis C with hepatic coma**

070.42 **Hepatitis delta without mention of active hepatitis B disease with hepatic coma**
Hepatitis delta with hepatitis B carrier state

070.43 **Hepatitis E with hepatic coma**

070.44 **Chronic hepatitis C with hepatic coma**

❑070.49 **Other specified viral hepatitis with hepatic coma**

● 070.5 **Other specified viral hepatitis without mention of hepatic coma**

❑070.51 **Acute hepatitis C without mention of hepatic coma**

070.52 **Hepatitis delta without mention of active hepatitis B disease or hepatic coma**

070.53 **Hepatitis E without mention of hepatic coma**

070.54 **Chronic hepatitis C without mention of hepatic coma**

❑070.59 **Other specified viral hepatitis without mention of hepatic coma**

❑070.6 **Unspecified viral hepatitis with hepatic coma**

Excludes *unspecified viral hepatitis C with hepatic coma (070.71)*

● 070.7 **Unspecified viral hepatitis C**

❑070.70 **Unspecified viral hepatitis C without hepatic coma**
Unspecified viral hepatitis C NOS

❑070.71 **Unspecified viral hepatitis C with hepatic coma**

❑070.9 **Unspecified viral hepatitis without mention of hepatic coma**
Viral hepatitis NOS

Excludes *unspecified viral hepatitis C without hepatic coma (070.70)*

071 **Rabies**
Hydrophobia
Lyssa

● 072 **Mumps**

072.0 **Mumps orchitis**

072.1 **Mumps meningitis**

072.2 **Mumps encephalitis**
Mumps meningoencephalitis

072.3 **Mumps pancreatitis**

● 072.7 **Mumps with other specified complications**

072.71 **Mumps hepatitis**

072.72 **Mumps polyneuropathy**

❑072.79 **Other**

❑072.8 **Mumps with unspecified complication**

❑072.9 **Mumps without mention of complication**
Epidemic parotitis
Infectious parotitis

● 073 **Ornithosis**

Includes: parrot fever
psittacosis

073.0 **With pneumonia**
Lobular pneumonitis due to ornithosis

❑073.7 **With other specified complications**

❑073.8 **With unspecified complication**

❑073.9 **Ornithosis, unspecified**

● 074 **Specific diseases due to Coxsackie virus**

Excludes *Coxsackie virus:*
infection NOS (079.2)
meningitis (047.0)

074.0 **Herpangina**
Vesicular pharyngitis

074.1 **Epidemic pleurodynia**
Bornholm disease
Devil's grip
Epidemic:
myalgia
myositis

● 074.2 **Coxsackie carditis**

❑074.20 **Coxsackie carditis, unspecified**

074.21 **Coxsackie pericarditis**

074.22 **Coxsackie endocarditis**

074.23 **Coxsackie myocarditis**
Aseptic myocarditis of newborn

074.3 **Hand, foot, and mouth disease**
Vesicular stomatitis and exanthem

Note: Check your documentation—this code is HAND, foot, and mouth disease. Code 078.4 is foot and mouth disease only.

❑074.8 **Other specified diseases due to Coxsackie virus**
Acute lymphonodular pharyngitis

075 **Infectious mononucleosis**
Glandular fever
Monocytic angina
Pfeiffer's disease

● 076 **Trachoma**

Excludes *late effect of trachoma (139.1)*

076.0 **Initial stage**
Trachoma dubium

076.1 **Active stage**
Granular conjunctivitis (trachomatous)
Trachomatous:
follicular conjunctivitis
pannus

❑076.9 **Trachoma, unspecified**
Trachoma NOS

● 077 **Other diseases of conjunctiva due to viruses and Chlamydiae**

Excludes *ophthalmic complications of viral diseases classified elsewhere*

077.0 **Inclusion conjunctivitis**
Paratrachoma
Swimming pool conjunctivitis

Excludes *inclusion blennorrhea (neonatal) (771.6)*

077.1 **Epidemic keratoconjunctivitis**
Shipyard eye

077.2 **Pharyngoconjunctival fever**
Viral pharyngoconjunctivitis

❑077.3 **Other adenoviral conjunctivitis**
Acute adenoviral follicular conjunctivitis

077.4 **Epidemic hemorrhagic conjunctivitis**
Apollo:
conjunctivitis
disease
Conjunctivitis due to enterovirus type 70
Hemorrhagic conjunctivitis (acute) (epidemic)

❑077.8 **Other viral conjunctivitis**
Newcastle conjunctivitis

● 077.9 **Unspecified diseases of conjunctiva due to viruses and Chlamydiae**

❑077.98 **Due to Chlamydiae**

❑077.99 **Due to viruses**
Viral conjunctivitis NOS

● 078 **Other diseases due to viruses and Chlamydiae**

Excludes *viral infection NOS (079.0–079.9)*
viremia NOS (790.8)

078.0 **Molluscum contagiosum**

● 078.1 **Viral warts**
Viral warts due to human papillomavirus

❑078.10 **Viral warts, unspecified**
Condyloma NOS
Verruca NOS:
NOS
Vulgaris
Warts (infectious)

078.11 **Condyloma acuminatum**

❑078.19 **Other specified viral warts**
Genital warts NOS
Verruca
plana
plantaris

078.2 **Sweating fever**
Miliary fever
Sweating disease

078.3 **Cat-scratch disease**
Benign lymphoreticulosis (of inoculation)
Cat-scratch fever

078.4 **Foot and mouth disease**
Aphthous fever
Epizootic:
aphthae
stomatitis

Check your documentation. Code 074.3 is for HAND, foot, and mouth disease.

078.5 **Cytomegaloviral disease**
Cytomegalic inclusion disease
Salivary gland virus disease

Use additional code to identify manifestation, as:
cytomegalic inclusion virus:
hepatitis (573.1)
pneumonia (484.1)

Excludes *congenital cytomegalovirus infection (771.1)*

078.6 **Hemorrhagic nephrosonephritis**
Hemorrhagic fever:
epidemic
Korean
Russian with renal syndrome

078.7 Arenaviral hemorrhagic fever
Hemorrhagic fever:
Argentine
Bolivian
Junin virus
Machupo virus

● **078.8 Other specified diseases due to viruses and Chlamydiae**
Excludes *epidemic diarrhea (009.2)*
lymphogranuloma venereum (099.1)

078.81 Epidemic vertigo

078.82 Epidemic vomiting syndrome
Winter vomiting disease

❑ **078.88 Other specified diseases due to Chlamydiae**

❑ **078.89 Other specified diseases due to viruses**
Epidemic cervical myalgia
Marburg disease
Tanapox

Item 1-17 Retrovirus develops by copying its RNA, genetic materials, into the DNA, which then produces new virus particles. It is from the Retroviridae virus family. **Human T-cell lymphotropic virus, Type I (HTLV-I)** is also called human T-cell leukemia virus, Type I, and is a retrovirus thought to cause T-cell leukemia/lymphoma. **Human T-cell lymphotropic virus, Type II (HTLV-II),** is also called human T-cell leukemia virus, Type II, and is a retrovirus associated with hematologic disorders. **HIV-2** is one of the serotypes of HIV and is usually confined to West Africa, whereas HIV-1 is found worldwide.

● **079 Viral and chlamydial infection in conditions classified elsewhere and of unspecified site**
Note: This category is provided to be used as an additional code to identify the viral agent in diseases classifiable elsewhere. This category will also be used to classify virus infection of unspecified nature or site.

079.0 Adenovirus

079.1 ECHO virus

079.2 Coxsackie virus

079.3 Rhinovirus

079.4 Human papillomavirus

● **079.5 Retrovirus**
Excludes *human immunodeficiency virus, type 1 [HIV-1] (042)*
human T-cell lymphotropic virus, type III [HTLV-III] (042)
lymphadenopathy-associated virus [LAV] (042)

❑ **079.50 Retrovirus, unspecified**

079.51 Human T-cell lymphotropic virus, type I [HTLV-I]

079.52 Human T-cell lymphotropic virus, type II [HTLV-II]

079.53 Human immunodeficiency virus, type 2 [HIV-2]

❑ **079.59 Other specified retrovirus**

079.6 Respiratory syncytial virus (RSV)

● **079.8 Other specified viral and chlamydial infections**

079.81 Hantavirus

079.82 SARS-associated coronavirus

❑ **079.88 Other specified chlamydial infection**

❑ **079.89 Other specified viral infection**

● **079.9 Unspecified viral and chlamydial infections**
Excludes *viremia NOS (790.8)*

❑ **079.98 Unspecified chlamydial infection**
Chlamydial infection NOS

❑ **079.99 Unspecified viral infection**
Viral infection NOS

Item 1-18 Rickettsioses are diseases spread from ticks, lice, fleas, or mites to humans. See Figure 1-3. **Typhus** is spread to humans chiefly by the fleas of rats. **Endemic** identifies a disease as being present in low numbers of humans at all times, whereas, **epidemic** identifies a disease as being present in high numbers of humans at a specific time. Morbidity (death) is higher in epidemic diseases.
Brill's disease, also known as **Brill-Zinsser disease,** is spread from human to human by body lice and also from the lice of flying squirrels. **Scrub typhus** is spread in the same ways as Brill's disease.
Malaria is spread to humans by mosquitos.

RICKETTSIOSES AND OTHER ARTHROPOD-BORNE DISEASES (080–088)

Excludes *arthropod-borne viral diseases (060.0–066.9)*

080 Louse-borne [epidemic] typhus
Typhus (fever):
classical
epidemic
exanthematic NOS
louse-borne

● **081 Other typhus**

081.0 Murine [endemic] typhus
Typhus (fever):
endemic
flea-borne

081.1 Brill's disease
Brill-Zinsser disease
Recrudescent typhus (fever)

081.2 Scrub typhus
Japanese river fever
Kedani fever
Mite-borne typhus
Tsutsugamushi

❑ **081.9 Typhus, unspecified**
Typhus (fever) NOS

● **082 Tick-borne rickettsioses**

082.0 Spotted fevers
Rocky mountain spotted fever
São Paulo fever

082.1 Boutonneuse fever
African tick typhus
India tick typhus
Kenya tick typhus
Marseilles fever
Mediterranean tick fever

082.2 North Asian tick fever
Siberian tick typhus

082.3 Queensland tick typhus

● **082.4 Ehrlichiosis**

❑ **082.40 Ehrlichiosis, unspecified**

082.41 Ehrlichiosis chafeensis (E. chafeensis)

❑ **082.49 Other ehrlichiosis**

❑ **082.8 Other specified tick-borne rickettsioses**
Lone star fever

❑ **082.9 Tick-borne rickettsiosis, unspecified**
Tick-borne typhus NOS

● 083 **Other rickettsioses**

083.0 **Q fever**

083.1 **Trench fever**
Quintan fever
Wolhynian fever

083.2 **Rickettsialpox**
Vesicular rickettsiosis

❑083.8 **Other specified rickettsioses**

❑083.9 **Rickettsiosis, unspecified**

● 084 **Malaria**

Note: Subcategories 084.0–084.6 exclude the listed conditions with mention of pernicious complications (084.8–084.9).

Excludes *congenital malaria (771.2)*

084.0 **Falciparum malaria [malignant tertian]**
Malaria (fever):
by Plasmodium falciparum
subtertian

084.1 **Vivax malaria [benign tertian]**
Malaria (fever) by Plasmodium vivax

084.2 **Quartan malaria**
Malaria (fever) by Plasmodium malariae
Malariae malaria

084.3 **Ovale malaria**
Malaria (fever) by Plasmodium ovale

❑084.4 **Other malaria**
Monkey malaria

084.5 **Mixed malaria**
Malaria (fever) by more than one parasite

❑084.6 **Malaria, unspecified**
Malaria (fever) NOS

084.7 **Induced malaria**
Therapeutically induced malaria

Excludes *accidental infection from syringe, blood transfusion, etc. (084.0–084.6, above, according to parasite species)*
transmission from mother to child during delivery (771.2)

084.8 **Blackwater fever**
Hemoglobinuric:
fever (bilious)
malaria
Malarial hemoglobinuria

❑084.9 **Other pernicious complications of malaria**
Algid malaria
Cerebral malaria

Use additional code to identify complication, as:
malarial:
hepatitis (573.2)
nephrosis (581.81)

● 085 **Leishmaniasis**

085.0 **Visceral [kala-azar]**
Dumdum fever
Infection by Leishmania:
donovani
infantum
Leishmaniasis:
dermal, post-kala-azar
Mediterranean
visceral (Indian)

085.1 **Cutaneous, urban**
Aleppo boil
Baghdad boil
Delhi boil
Infection by Leishmania tropica (minor)
Leishmaniasis, cutaneous:
dry form
late
recurrent
ulcerating
Oriental sore

085.2 **Cutaneous, Asian desert**
Infection by Leishmania tropica major
Leishmaniasis, cutaneous:
acute necrotizing
rural
wet form
zoonotic form

085.3 **Cutaneous, Ethiopian**
Infection by Leishmania ethiopica
Leishmaniasis, cutaneous:
diffuse
lepromatous

085.4 **Cutaneous, American**
Chiclero ulcer
Infection by Leishmania mexicana
Leishmaniasis tegumentaria diffusa

085.5 **Mucocutaneous (American)**
Espundia
Infection by Leishmania braziliensis
Uta

❑085.9 **Leishmaniasis, unspecified**

● 086 **Trypanosomiasis**

Use additional code to identify manifestations, as:
trypanosomiasis:
encephalitis (323.2)
meningitis (321.3)

086.0 **Chagas' disease with heart involvement**
American trypanosomiasis with heart involvement
Infection by Trypanosoma cruzi with heart involvement
Any condition classifiable to 086.2 with heart involvement

086.1 **Chagas' disease with other organ involvement**
American trypanosomiasis with involvement of organ other than heart
Infection by Trypanosoma cruzi with involvement of organ other than heart
Any condition classifiable to 086.2 with involvement of organ other than heart

086.2 **Chagas' disease without mention of organ involvement**
American trypanosomiasis
Infection by Trypanosoma cruzi

086.3 **Gambian trypanosomiasis**
Gambian sleeping sickness
Infection by Trypanosoma gambiense

086.4 **Rhodesian trypanosomiasis**
Infection by Trypanosoma rhodesiense
Rhodesian sleeping sickness

❑086.5 **African trypanosomiasis, unspecified**
Sleeping sickness NOS

❑086.9 **Trypanosomiasis, unspecified**

● 087 **Relapsing fever**

Includes: recurrent fever

087.0 **Louse-borne**

087.1 **Tick-borne**

❑087.9 **Relapsing fever, unspecified**

● 088 **Other arthropod-borne diseases**

088.0 **Bartonellosis**
Carrión's disease
Oroya fever
Verruga peruana

● ❑ 088.8 **Other specified arthropod-borne diseases**

088.81 **Lyme disease**
Erythema chronicum migrans

088.82 **Babesiosis**
Babesiasis

❑ 088.89 **Other**

❑ 088.9 **Arthropod-borne disease, unspecified**

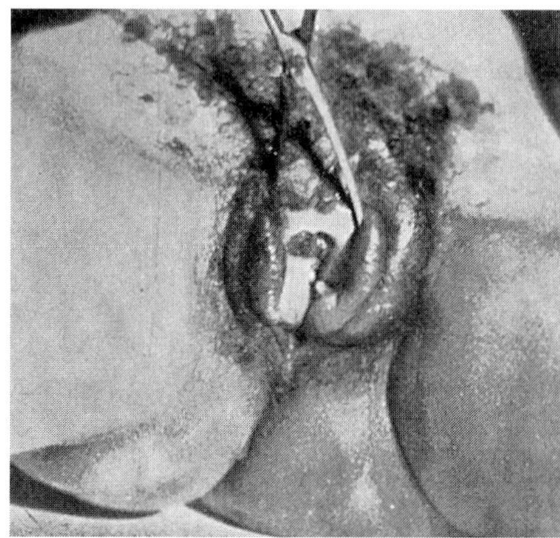

Figure 1–7 Chancre. (From Delp MH, Manning RT: Major Physical Diagnosis, 8th ed. Philadelphia, WB Saunders, 1975, p. 613.)

Item 1–19 Syphilis, also known as lues, is the most serious of the venereal diseases caused by *Treponema pallidum.* The primary stage is characterized by an ulceration known as chancre, which usually appears on the genitals but can also develop on the anus, lips, tonsils, breasts, or fingers.
The secondary stage is characterized by a rash that can affect any area of the body. Latent syphilis is divided into early, which is diagnosed within two years of infection, and late, which is diagnosed two years or more after infection. Congenital syphilis is also labeled early or late based on the time of diagnosis.

SYPHILIS AND OTHER VENEREAL DISEASES (090–099)

Excludes *nonvenereal endemic syphilis (104.0)*
urogenital trichomoniasis (131.0)

● 090 **Congenital syphilis**

090.0 **Early congenital syphilis, symptomatic**
Congenital syphilitic:
choroiditis
coryza (chronic)
hepatomegaly
mucous patches
periostitis
splenomegaly
Syphilitic (congenital):
epiphysitis
osteochondritis
pemphigus
Any congenital syphilitic condition specified as early or manifesting less than two years after birth

090.1 **Early congenital syphilis, latent**
Congenital syphilis without clinical manifestations, with positive serological reaction and negative spinal fluid test, less than two years after birth

❑ 090.2 **Early congenital syphilis, unspecified**
Congenital syphilis NOS, less than two years after birth

090.3 **Syphilitic interstitial keratitis**
Syphilitic keratitis:
parenchymatous
punctata profunda

Excludes *interstitial keratitis NOS (370.50)*

● 090.4 **Juvenile neurosyphilis**
Use additional code to identify any associated mental disorder

❑ 090.40 **Juvenile neurosyphilis, unspecified**
Congenital neurosyphilis
Dementia paralytica juvenilis
Juvenile:
general paresis
tabes
taboparesis

090.41 **Congenital syphilitic encephalitis**

090.42 **Congenital syphilitic meningitis**

❑ 090.49 **Other**

❑ 090.5 **Other late congenital syphilis, symptomatic**
Gumma due to congenital syphilis
Hutchinson's teeth
Syphilitic saddle nose
Any congenital syphilitic condition specified as late or manifesting two years or more after birth

090.6 **Late congenital syphilis, latent**
Congenital syphilis without clinical manifestations, with positive serological reaction and negative spinal fluid test, two years or more after birth

❑ 090.7 **Late congenital syphilis, unspecified**
Congenital syphilis NOS, two years or more after birth

❑ 090.9 **Congenital syphilis, unspecified**

● 091 **Early syphilis, symptomatic**

Excludes *early cardiovascular syphilis (093.0–093.9)*
early neurosyphilis (094.0–094.9)

091.0 **Genital syphilis (primary)**
Genital chancre

091.1 **Primary anal syphilis**

❑ 091.2 **Other primary syphilis**
Primary syphilis of:
breast
fingers
lip
tonsils

091.3 **Secondary syphilis of skin or mucous membranes**
Condyloma latum
Secondary syphilis of:
anus
mouth
pharynx
skin
tonsils
vulva

091.4 **Adenopathy due to secondary syphilis**
Syphilitic adenopathy (secondary)
Syphilitic lymphadenitis (secondary)

Item 1-20 Notice the placement of this combination code in with the Infectious and Parasitic Disease codes (syphilis). This uveitis does not appear in the eye code section because it is a manifestation of the underlying disease of syphilis.

● 091.5 **Uveitis due to secondary syphilis**

❑ 091.50 **Syphilitic uveitis, unspecified**

091.51 **Syphilitic chorioretinitis (secondary)**

091.52 **Syphilitic iridocyclitis (secondary)**

● 091.6 **Secondary syphilis of viscera and bone**

091.61 **Secondary syphilitic periostitis**

091.62 **Secondary syphilitic hepatitis**
Secondary syphilis of liver

❑ 091.69 **Other viscera**

091.7 **Secondary syphilis, relapse**
Secondary syphilis, relapse (treated) (untreated)

● 091.8 **Other forms of secondary syphilis**

091.81 **Acute syphilitic meningitis (secondary)**

091.82 **Syphilitic alopecia**

❑ 091.89 **Other**

❑ 091.9 **Unspecified secondary syphilis**

● 092 Early syphilis, latent

Includes: syphilis (acquired) without clinical manifestations, with positive serological reaction and negative spinal fluid test, less than two years after infection

092.0 **Early syphilis, latent, serological relapse after treatment**

❑ 092.9 **Early syphilis, latent, unspecified**

● 093 Cardiovascular syphilis

093.0 **Aneurysm of aorta, specified as syphilitic**
Dilatation of aorta, specified as syphilitic

093.1 **Syphilitic aortitis**

● 093.2 **Syphilitic endocarditis**

❑ 093.20 **Valve, unspecified**
Syphilitic ostial coronary disease

093.21 **Mitral valve**

093.22 **Aortic valve**
Syphilitic aortic incompetence or stenosis

093.23 **Tricuspid valve**

093.24 **Pulmonary valve**

● 093.8 **Other specified cardiovascular syphilis**

093.81 **Syphilitic pericarditis**

093.82 **Syphilitic myocarditis**

❑ 093.89 **Other**

❑ 093.9 **Cardiovascular syphilis, unspecified**

● 094 Neurosyphilis

Use additional code to identify any associated mental disorder

094.0 **Tabes dorsalis**
Locomotor ataxia (progressive)
Posterior spinal sclerosis (syphilitic)
Tabetic neurosyphilis

Use additional code to identify manifestation, as:
neurogenic arthropathy [Charcot's joint disease] (713.5)

094.1 **General paresis**
Dementia paralytica
General paralysis (of the insane) (progressive)
Paretic neurosyphilis
Taboparesis

094.2 **Syphilitic meningitis**
Meningovascular syphilis

Excludes *acute syphilitic meningitis (secondary) (091.81)*

094.3 **Asymptomatic neurosyphilis**

● 094.8 **Other specified neurosyphilis**

094.81 **Syphilitic encephalitis**

094.82 **Syphilitic Parkinsonism**

094.83 **Syphilitic disseminated retinochoroiditis**

094.84 **Syphilitic optic atrophy**

094.85 **Syphilitic retrobulbar neuritis**

094.86 **Syphilitic acoustic neuritis**

094.87 **Syphilitic ruptured cerebral aneurysm**

❑ 094.89 **Other**

❑ 094.9 **Neurosyphilis, unspecified**
Gumma (syphilitic) of central nervous system NOS
Syphilis (early) (late) of central nervous system NOS
Syphiloma of central nervous system NOS

● 095 Other forms of late syphilis, with symptoms

Includes: gumma (syphilitic)
tertiary, or unspecified stage

095.0 **Syphilitic episcleritis**

095.1 **Syphilis of lung**

095.2 **Syphilitic peritonitis**

095.3 **Syphilis of liver**

095.4 **Syphilis of kidney**

095.5 **Syphilis of bone**

095.6 **Syphilis of muscle**
Syphilitic myositis

095.7 **Syphilis of synovium, tendon, and bursa**
Syphilitic:
bursitis
synovitis

❑ 095.8 **Other specified forms of late symptomatic syphilis**

Excludes *cardiovascular syphilis (093.0–093.9)*
neurosyphilis (094.0–094.9)

❑ 095.9 **Late symptomatic syphilis, unspecified**

096 Late syphilis, latent
Syphilis (acquired) without clinical manifestations, with positive serological reaction and negative spinal fluid test, two years or more after infection

● 097 Other and unspecified syphilis

❑ 097.0 **Late syphilis, unspecified**

❑ 097.1 **Latent syphilis, unspecified**
Positive serological reaction for syphilis

❑ 097.9 **Syphilis, unspecified**
Syphilis (acquired) NOS

Excludes *syphilis NOS causing death under two years of age (090.9)*

● 098 Gonococcal infections

098.0 **Acute, of lower genitourinary tract**
Gonococcal:
Bartholinitis (acute)
urethritis (acute)
vulvovaginitis (acute)
Gonorrhea (acute):
NOS
genitourinary (tract) NOS

● 098.1 **Acute, of upper genitourinary tract**

❑ 098.10 **Gonococcal infection (acute) of upper genitourinary tract, site unspecified**

098.11 Gonococcal cystitis (acute)
Gonorrhea (acute) of bladder

098.12 Gonococcal prostatitis (acute)

098.13 Gonococcal epididymo-orchitis (acute)
Gonococcal orchitis (acute)

098.14 Gonococcal seminal vesiculitis (acute)
Gonorrhea (acute) of seminal vesicle

098.15 Gonococcal cervicitis (acute)
Gonorrhea (acute) of cervix

098.16 Gonococcal endometritis (acute)
Gonorrhea (acute) of uterus

098.17 Gonococcal salpingitis, specified as acute

❑**098.19 Other**

098.2 Chronic, of lower genitourinary tract
Gonococcal specified as chronic or with duration of two months or more:
Bartholinitis specified as chronic or with duration of two months or more
urethritis specified as chronic or with duration of two months or more
vulvovaginitis specified as chronic or with duration of two months or more
Gonorrhea specified as chronic or with duration of two months or more:
NOS specified as chronic or with duration of two months or more
genitourinary (tract) specified as chronic or with duration of two months or more
Any condition classifiable to 098.0 specified as chronic or with duration of two months or more

● **098.3 Chronic, of upper genitourinary tract**
Any condition classifiable to 098.1 stated as chronic or with a duration of two months or more

❑**098.30 Chronic gonococcal infection of upper genitourinary tract, site unspecified**

098.31 Gonococcal cystitis, chronic
Any condition classifiable to 098.11, specified as chronic
Gonorrhea of bladder, chronic

098.32 Gonococcal prostatitis, chronic
Any condition classifiable to 098.12, specified as chronic

098.33 Gonococcal epididymo-orchitis, chronic
Any condition classifiable to 098.13, specified as chronic
Chronic gonococcal orchitis

098.34 Gonococcal seminal vesiculitis, chronic
Any condition classifiable to 098.14, specified as chronic
Gonorrhea of seminal vesicle, chronic

098.35 Gonococcal cervicitis, chronic
Any condition classifiable to 098.15, specified as chronic
Gonorrhea of cervix, chronic

098.36 Gonococcal endometritis, chronic
Any condition classifiable to 098.16, specified as chronic

098.37 Gonococcal salpingitis (chronic)

❑**098.39 Other**

● **098.4 Gonococcal infection of eye**

098.40 Gonococcal conjunctivitis (neonatorum)
Gonococcal ophthalmia (neonatorum)

098.41 Gonococcal iridocyclitis

098.42 Gonococcal endophthalmia

098.43 Gonococcal keratitis

❑**098.49 Other**

● **098.5 Gonococcal infection of joint**

098.50 Gonococcal arthritis
Gonococcal infection of joint NOS

098.51 Gonococcal synovitis and tenosynovitis

098.52 Gonococcal bursitis

098.53 Gonococcal spondylitis

❑**098.59 Other**
Gonococcal rheumatism

098.6 Gonococcal infection of pharynx

098.7 Gonococcal infection of anus and rectum
Gonococcal proctitis

● **098.8 Gonococcal infection of other specified sites**

098.81 Gonococcal keratosis (blennorrhagica)

098.82 Gonococcal meningitis

098.83 Gonococcal pericarditis

098.84 Gonococcal endocarditis

❑**098.85 Other gonococcal heart disease**

098.86 Gonococcal peritonitis

❑**098.89 Other**
Gonococcemia

● **099 Other venereal diseases**

099.0 Chancroid
Bubo (inguinal):
chancroidal
due to Hemophilus ducreyi
Chancre:
Ducrey's simple soft
Ulcus molle (cutis) (skin)

099.1 Lymphogranuloma venereum
Climatic or tropical bubo
(Durand-) Nicolas-Favre disease
Esthiomene
Lymphogranuloma inguinale

099.2 Granuloma inguinale
Donovanosis
Granuloma pudendi (ulcerating)
Granuloma venereum
Pudendal ulcer

099.3 Reiter's disease
Reiter's syndrome

Use additional code for associated:
arthropathy (711.1)
conjunctivitis (372.33)

● **099.4 Other nongonococcal urethritis [NGU]**

❑**099.40 Unspecified**
Nonspecific urethritis

099.41 Chlamydia trachomatis

❑**099.49 Other specified organism**

● **099.5 Other venereal diseases due to Chlamydia trachomatis**

Excludes *Chlamydia trachomatis infection of conjunctiva (076.0–076.9, 077.0, 077.9)*
Lymphogranuloma venereum (099.1)

❑**099.50 Unspecified site**

099.51 Pharynx

099.52 Anus and rectum

ICD-9-CM 001 - 099 Vol. 1

099.53 **Lower genitourinary sites**

Excludes *urethra (099.41)*

Use additional code to specify site of infection, such as:
bladder (595.4)
cervix (616.0)
vagina and vulva (616.11)

❑099.54 **Other genitourinary sites**

Use additional code to specify site of infection, such as:
pelvic inflammatory disease NOS (614.9)
testis and epididymis (604.91)

❑099.55 **Unspecified genitourinary site**

099.56 **Peritoneum**
Perihepatitis

❑099.59 **Other specified site**

❑099.8 **Other specified venereal diseases**

❑099.9 **Venereal disease, unspecified**

OTHER SPIROCHETAL DISEASES (100–104)

● 100 **Leptospirosis**

100.0 **Leptospirosis icterohemorrhagica**
Leptospiral or spirochetal jaundice (hemorrhagic)
Weil's disease

● 100.8 **Other specified leptospiral infections**

100.81 **Leptospiral meningitis (aseptic)**

❑100.89 **Other**
Fever:
Fort Bragg
pretibial
swamp
Infection by Leptospira:
australis
bataviae
pyrogenes

❑100.9 **Leptospirosis, unspecified**

101 **Vincent's angina**
Acute necrotizing ulcerative:
gingivitis
stomatitis
Fusospirochetal pharyngitis
Spirochetal stomatitis
Trench mouth
Vincent's:
gingivitis
infection [any site]

● 102 **Yaws**

Includes: frambesia
pian

102.0 **Initial lesions**
Chancre of yaws
Frambesia, initial or primary
Initial frambesial ulcer
Mother yaw

102.1 **Multiple papillomata and wet crab yaws**
Butter yaws
Frambesioma
Pianoma
Plantar or palmar papilloma of yaws

❑102.2 **Other early skin lesions**
Cutaneous yaws, less than five years after infection
Early yaws (cutaneous) (macular) (papular) (maculopapular) (micropapular)
Frambeside of early yaws

102.3 **Hyperkeratosis**
Ghoul hand
Hyperkeratosis, palmar or plantar (early) (late) due to yaws
Worm-eaten soles

102.4 **Gummata and ulcers**
Nodular late yaws (ulcerated)
Gummatous frambeside

102.5 **Gangosa**
Rhinopharyngitis mutilans

102.6 **Bone and joint lesions**
Goundou of yaws (late)
Gumma, bone of yaws (late)
Gummatous osteitis or periostitis of yaws (late)
Hydrarthrosis of yaws (early) (late)
Osteitis of yaws (early) (late)
Periostitis (hypertrophic) of yaws (early) (late)

❑102.7 **Other manifestations**
Juxta-articular nodules of yaws
Mucosal yaws

102.8 **Latent yaws**
Yaws without clinical manifestations, with positive serology

❑102.9 **Yaws, unspecified**

● 103 **Pinta**

103.0 **Primary lesions**
Chancre (primary) of pinta [carate]
Papule (primary) of pinta [carate]
Pintid of pinta [carate]

103.1 **Intermediate lesions**
Erythematous plaques of pinta [carate]
Hyperchromic lesions of pinta [carate]
Hyperkeratosis of pinta [carate]

103.2 **Late lesions**
Cardiovascular lesions of pinta [carate]
Skin lesions of pinta [carate]:
achromic of pinta [carate]
cicatricial of pinta [carate]
dyschromic of pinta [carate]
Vitiligo of pinta [carate]

103.3 **Mixed lesions**
Achromic and hyperchromic skin lesions of pinta [carate]

❑103.9 **Pinta, unspecified**

● 104 **Other spirochetal infection**

104.0 **Nonvenereal endemic syphilis**
Bejel
Njovera

❑104.8 **Other specified spirochetal infections**

Excludes *relapsing fever (087.0–087.9)*
syphilis (090.0–097.9)

❑104.9 **Spirochetal infection, unspecified**

MYCOSES (110–118)

Use additional code to identify manifestation, as:
arthropathy (711.6)
meningitis (321.0–321.1)
otitis externa (380.15)

Excludes *infection by Actinomycetales, such as species of Actinomyces, Actinomadura, Nocardia, Streptomyces (039.0–039.9)*

● 110 **Dermatophytosis**

Includes: infection by species of Epidermophyton, Microsporum, and Trichophyton
tinea, any type except those in 111

110.0 **Of scalp and beard**
Kerion
Sycosis, mycotic
Trichophytic tinea [black dot tinea], scalp

110.1 **Of nail**
Dermatophytic onychia
Onychomycosis
Tinea unguium

110.2 **Of hand**
Tinea manuum

110.3 **Of groin and perianal area**
Dhobie itch
Eczema marginatum
Tinea cruris

110.4 **Of foot**
Athlete's foot
Tinea pedis

110.5 **Of the body**
Herpes circinatus
Tinea imbricata [Tokelau]

110.6 **Deep seated dermatophytosis**
Granuloma trichophyticum
Majocchi's granuloma

❑110.8 **Of other specified sites**

❑110.9 **Of unspecified site**
Favus NOS
Microsporic tinea NOS
Ringworm NOS

● 111 **Dermatomycosis, other and unspecified**

111.0 **Pityriasis versicolor**
Infection by Malassezia [Pityrosporum] furfur
Tinea flava
Tinea versicolor

111.1 **Tinea nigra**
Infection by Cladosporium species
Keratomycosis nigricans
Microsporosis nigra
Pityriasis nigra
Tinea palmaris nigra

111.2 **Tinea blanca**
Infection by Trichosporon (beigelii) cutaneum
White piedra

111.3 **Black piedra**
Infection by Piedraia hortai

❑111.8 **Other specified dermatomycoses**

❑111.9 **Dermatomycosis, unspecified**

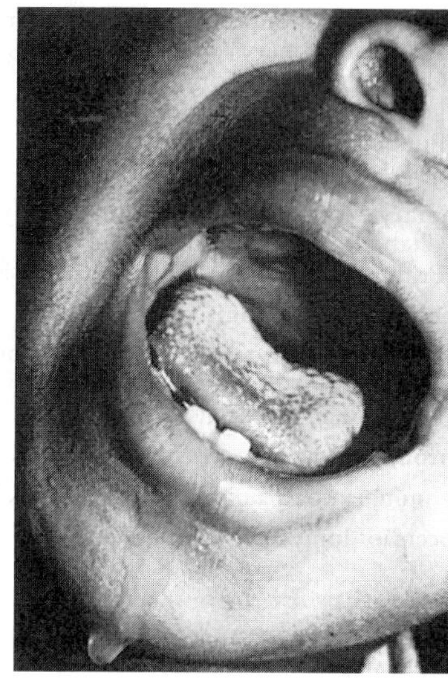

Figure 1–8 Oral candidiasis, also called thrush. (From Rippon JW: Medical Mycology, 3rd ed. Philadelphia, WB Saunders, 1988, p. 542.)

ICD-9-CM 100-199 Vol. 1

Item 1–21 Candidiasis, also called oidiomycosis or moniliasis, is a fungal infection. It most often appears on moist cutaneous areas of the body, but can also be responsible for a variety of systemic infections such as endocarditis, meningitis, arthritis, and myositis.

● 112 **Candidiasis**

Includes: infection by Candida species
moniliasis

Excludes *neonatal monilial infection (771.7)*

112.0 **Of mouth**
Thrush (oral)

112.1 **Of vulva and vagina**
Candidal vulvovaginitis
Monilial vulvovaginitis

❑112.2 **Of other urogenital sites**
Candidal balanitis

112.3 **Of skin and nails**
Candidal intertrigo
Candidal onychia
Candidal perionyxis [paronychia]

112.4 **Of lung**
Candidal pneumonia

112.5 **Disseminated**
Systemic candidiasis

● 112.8 **Of other specified sites**

112.81 **Candidal endocarditis**

112.82 **Candidal otitis externa**
Otomycosis in moniliasis

112.83 **Candidal meningitis**

112.84 **Candidal esophagitis**

112.85 **Candidal enteritis**

112.89 **Other**

❑112.9 **Of unspecified site**

● 114 **Coccidioidomycosis**

Includes: infection by Coccidioides (immitis)
Posada-Wernicke disease

114.0 Primary coccidioidomycosis (pulmonary)
Acute pulmonary coccidioidomycosis
Coccidioidomycotic pneumonitis
Desert rheumatism
Pulmonary coccidioidomycosis
San Joaquin Valley fever

114.1 Primary extrapulmonary coccidioidomycosis
Chancriform syndrome
Primary cutaneous coccidioidomycosis

114.2 Coccidioidal meningitis

❑ **114.3 Other forms of progressive coccidioidomycosis**
Coccidioidal granuloma
Disseminated coccidioidomycosis

114.4 Chronic pulmonary coccidioidomycosis

❑ **114.5 Pulmonary coccidioidomycosis, unspecified**

❑ **114.9 Coccidioidomycosis, unspecified**

Item 1-22 Bird and bat droppings that fall into the soil give rise to a fungus that can spread airborne spores. When inhaled into the lungs, these spores divide and multiply into lesions. Histoplasmosis capsulatum takes three forms: primary (lodged in the lungs only), chronic (resembles TB), and disseminated (infection has moved to other organs). This is an opportunistic infection in immunosuppressed patients.

● **115 Histoplasmosis**
The following fifth-digit subclassification is for use with category 115:
0 without mention of manifestation
1 meningitis
2 retinitis
3 pericarditis
4 endocarditis
5 pneumonia
❑ **9 other**

● **115.0 Infection by Histoplasma capsulatum**
American histoplasmosis
Darling's disease
Reticuloendothelial cytomycosis
Small form histoplasmosis

● **115.1 Infection by Histoplasma duboisii**
African histoplasmosis
Large form histoplasmosis

● ❑ **115.9 Histoplasmosis, unspecified**
Histoplasmosis NOS

● **116 Blastomycotic infection**

116.0 Blastomycosis
Blastomycotic dermatitis
Chicago disease
Cutaneous blastomycosis
Disseminated blastomycosis
Gilchrist's disease
Infection by Blastomyces [Ajellomyces] dermatitidis
North American blastomycosis
Primary pulmonary blastomycosis

116.1 Paracoccidioidomycosis
Brazilian blastomycosis
Infection by Paracoccidioides [Blastomyces] brasiliensis
Lutz-Splendore-Almeida disease
Mucocutaneous-lymphangitic paracoccidioidomycosis
Pulmonary paracoccidioidomycosis
South American blastomycosis
Visceral paracoccidioidomycosis

116.2 Lobomycosis
Infections by Loboa [Blastomyces] loboi
Keloidal blastomycosis
Lobo's disease

● **117 Other mycoses**

117.0 Rhinosporidiosis
Infection by Rhinosporidium seeberi

117.1 Sporotrichosis
Cutaneous sporotrichosis
Disseminated sporotrichosis
Infection by Sporothrix [Sporotrichum] schenckii
Lymphocutaneous sporotrichosis
Pulmonary sporotrichosis
Sporotrichosis of the bones

117.2 Chromoblastomycosis
Chromomycosis
Infection by Cladosporidium carrionii, Fonsecaea compactum, Fonsecaea pedrosoi, Phialophora verrucosa

117.3 Aspergillosis
Infection by Aspergillus species, mainly A. fumigatus, A. flavus group, A. terreus group

117.4 Mycotic mycetomas
Infection by various genera and species of Ascomycetes and Deuteromycetes, such as Acremonium [Cephalosporium] falciforme, Neotestudina rosatii, Madurella grisea, Madurella mycetomii, Pyrenochaeta romeroi, Zopfia [Leptosphaeria] senegalensis
Madura foot, mycotic
Maduromycosis, mycotic

Excludes *actinomycotic mycetomas (039.0–039.9)*

117.5 Cryptococcosis
Busse-Buschke's disease
European cryptococcosis
Infection by Cryptococcus neoformans
Pulmonary cryptococcosis
Systemic cryptococcosis
Torula

117.6 Allescheriosis [Petriellidosis]
Infections by Allescheria [Petriellidium] boydii [Monosporium apiospermum]

Excludes *mycotic mycetoma (117.4)*

117.7 Zygomycosis [Phycomycosis or Mucormycosis]
Infection by species of Absidia, Basidiobolus, Conidiobolus, Cunninghamella, Entomophthora, Mucor, Rhizopus, Saksenaea

117.8 Infection by dematiacious fungi [Phaehyphomycosis]
Infection by dematiacious fungi, such as Cladosporium trichoides [bantianum], Dreschlera hawaiiensis, Phialophora gougerotii, Phialophora jeanselmi

❑ **117.9 Other and unspecified mycoses**

118 Opportunistic mycoses
Infection of skin, subcutaneous tissues, and/or organs by a wide variety of fungi generally considered to be pathogenic to compromised hosts only (e.g., infection by species of Alternaria, Dreschlera, Fusarium)

HELMINTHIASES (120–129)

● **120 Schistosomiasis [bilharziasis]**

120.0 Schistosoma haematobium
Vesical schistosomiasis NOS

120.1 Schistosoma mansoni
Intestinal schistosomiasis NOS

120.2 Schistosoma japonicum
Asiatic schistosomiasis NOS
Katayama disease or fever

120.3 Cutaneous
Cercarial dermatitis
Infection by cercariae of Schistosoma
Schistosome dermatitis
Swimmers' itch

❑**120.8 Other specified schistosomiasis**
Infection by Schistosoma:
bovis
intercalatum
mattheii
spindale
Schistosomiasis chestermani

❑**120.9 Schistosomiasis, unspecified**
Blood flukes NOS
Hemic distomiasis

● **121 Other trematode infections**

121.0 Opisthorchiasis
Infection by:
cat liver fluke
Opisthorchis (felineus) (tenuicollis) (viverrini)

121.1 Clonorchiasis
Biliary cirrhosis due to clonorchiasis
Chinese liver fluke disease
Hepatic distomiasis due to Clonorchis sinensis
Oriental liver fluke disease

121.2 Paragonimiasis
Infection by Paragonimus
Lung fluke disease (oriental)
Pulmonary distomiasis

121.3 Fascioliasis
Infection by Fasciola:
gigantica
hepatica
Liver flukes NOS
Sheep liver fluke infection

121.4 Fasciolopsiasis
Infection by Fasciolopsis (buski)
Intestinal distomiasis

121.5 Metagonimiasis
Infection by Metagonimus yokogawai

121.6 Heterophyiasis
Infection by:
Heterophyes heterophyes
Stellantchasmus falcatus

❑**121.8 Other specified trematode infections**
Infection by:
Dicrocoelium dendriticum
Echinostoma ilocanum
Gastrodiscoides hominis

❑**121.9 Trematode infection, unspecified**
Distomiasis NOS
Fluke disease NOS

● **122 Echinococcosis**

Includes: echinococciasis
hydatid disease
hydatidosis

122.0 Echinococcus granulosus infection of liver

122.1 Echinococcus granulosus infection of lung

122.2 Echinococcus granulosus infection of thyroid

❑**122.3 Echinococcus granulosus infection, other**

❑**122.4 Echinococcus granulosus infection, unspecified**

122.5 Echinococcus multilocularis infection of liver

❑**122.6 Echinococcus multilocularis infection, other**

❑**122.7 Echinococcus multilocularis infection, unspecified**

❑**122.8 Echinococcosis, unspecified, of liver**

❑**122.9 Echinococcosis, other and unspecified**

● **123 Other cestode infection**

123.0 Taenia solium infection, intestinal form
Pork tapeworm (adult) (infection)

123.1 Cysticercosis
Cysticerciasis
Infection by Cysticercus cellulosae [larval form of Taenia solium]

123.2 Taenia saginata infection
Beef tapeworm (infection)
Infection by Taeniarhynchus saginatus

❑**123.3 Taeniasis, unspecified**

123.4 Diphyllobothriasis, intestinal
Diphyllobothrium (adult) (latum) (pacificum) infection
Fish tapeworm (infection)

123.5 Sparganosis [larval diphyllobothriasis]
Infection by:
Diphyllobothrium larvae
Sparganum (mansoni) (proliferum)
Spirometra larvae

123.6 Hymenolepiasis
Dwarf tapeworm (infection)
Hymenolepis (diminuta) (nana) infection
Rat tapeworm (infection)

❑**123.8 Other specified cestode infection**
Diplogonoporus (grandis) infection
Dipylidium (caninum) infection
Dog tapeworm (infection)

❑**123.9 Cestode infection, unspecified**
Tapeworm (infection) NOS

124 Trichinosis
Trichinella spiralis infection
Trichinellosis
Trichiniasis

● **125 Filarial infection and dracontiasis**

125.0 Bancroftian filariasis
Chyluria due to Wuchereria bancrofti
Elephantiasis due to Wuchereria bancrofti
Infection due to Wuchereria bancrofti
Lymphadenitis due to Wuchereria bancrofti
Lymphangitis due to Wuchereria bancrofti
Wuchereriasis

125.1 Malayan filariasis
Brugia filariasis due to Brugia [Wuchereria] malayi
Chyluria due to Brugia [Wuchereria] malayi
Elephantiasis due to Brugia [Wuchereria] malayi
Infection due to Brugia [Wuchereria] malayi
Lymphadenitis due to Brugia [Wuchereria] malayi
Lymphangitis due to Brugia [Wuchereria] malayi

125.2 Loiasis
Eyeworm disease of Africa
Loa loa infection

125.3 Onchocerciasis
Onchocerca volvulus infection
Onchocercosis

125.4 Dipetalonemiasis
Infection by:
Acanthocheilonema perstans
Dipetalonema perstans

125.5 Mansonella ozzardi infection
Filariasis ozzardi

❑**125.6 Other specified filariasis**
Dirofilaria infection
Infection by:
Acanthocheilonema streptocerca
Dipetalonema streptocerca

125.7 Dracontiasis
Guinea-worm infection
Infection by Dracunculus medinensis

❑**125.9 Unspecified filariasis**

● 126 **Ancylostomiasis and necatoriasis**
Includes: cutaneous larva migrans due to Ancylostoma
hookworm (disease) (infection)
uncinariasis

126.0 **Ancylostoma duodenale**

126.1 **Necator americanus**

126.2 **Ancylostoma braziliense**

126.3 **Ancylostoma ceylanicum**

❑126.8 **Other specified Ancylostoma**

❑126.9 **Ancylostomiasis and necatoriasis, unspecified**
Creeping eruption NOS
Cutaneous larva migrans NOS

● 127 **Other intestinal helminthiases**

127.0 **Ascariasis**
Ascaridiasis
Infection by Ascaris lumbricoides
Roundworm infection

127.1 **Anisakiasis**
Infection by Anisakis larva

127.2 **Strongyloidiasis**
Infection by Strongyloides stercoralis
Excludes *trichostrongyliasis (127.6)*

127.3 **Trichuriasis**
Infection by Trichuris trichiuria
Trichocephaliasis
Whipworm (disease) (infection)

127.4 **Enterobiasis**
Infection by Enterobius vermicularis
Oxyuriasis
Oxyuris vermicularis infection
Pinworm (disease) (infection)
Threadworm infection

127.5 **Capillariasis**
Infection by Capillaria philippinensis
Excludes *infection by Capillaria hepatica (128.8)*

127.6 **Trichostrongyliasis**
Infection by Trichostrongylus species

❑127.7 **Other specified intestinal helminthiasis**
Infection by:
Oesophagostomum apiostomum and related species
Ternidens diminutus
Other specified intestinal helminth
Physalopteriasis

127.8 **Mixed intestinal helminthiasis**
Infection by intestinal helminths classified to more than one of the categories 120.0–127.7
Mixed helminthiasis NOS

❑127.9 **Intestinal helminthiasis, unspecified**

● 128 **Other and unspecified helminthiases**

128.0 **Toxocariasis**
Larva migrans visceralis
Toxocara (canis) (cati) infection
Visceral larva migrans syndrome

128.1 **Gnathostomiasis**
Infection by Gnathostoma spinigerum and related species

❑128.8 **Other specified helminthiasis**
Infection by:
Angiostrongylus cantonensis
Capillaria hepatica
Other specified helminth

❑128.9 **Helminth infection, unspecified**
Helminthiasis NOS
Worms NOS

❑129 **Intestinal parasitism, unspecified**

Item 1-23 Toxoplasmosis is caused by the protozoa Toxoplasma gondii, of which the house cat can be a host. Human infection occurs when contact is made with materials containing the pathogen, such as feces or contaminated soil.
Infection can also occur with ingestion of lamb, goat, and pork meat, especially when the meat contains infected cysts.

OTHER INFECTIOUS AND PARASITIC DISEASES (130–136)

● 130 **Toxoplasmosis**
Includes: infection by toxoplasma gondii
toxoplasmosis (acquired)
Excludes *congenital toxoplasmosis (771.2)*

130.0 **Meningoencephalitis due to toxoplasmosis**
Encephalitis due to acquired toxoplasmosis

130.1 **Conjunctivitis due to toxoplasmosis**

130.2 **Chorioretinitis due to toxoplasmosis**
Focal retinochoroiditis due to acquired toxoplasmosis

130.3 **Myocarditis due to toxoplasmosis**

130.4 **Pneumonitis due to toxoplasmosis**

130.5 **Hepatitis due to toxoplasmosis**

❑130.7 **Toxoplasmosis of other specified sites**

130.8 **Multisystemic disseminated toxoplasmosis**
Toxoplasmosis of multiple sites

❑130.9 **Toxoplasmosis, unspecified**

● 131 **Trichomoniasis**
Includes: infection due to Trichomonas (vaginalis)

● 131.0 **Urogenital trichomoniasis**

❑131.00 **Urogenital trichomoniasis, unspecified**
Fluor (vaginalis) trichomonal or due to Trichomonas (vaginalis)
Leukorrhea (vaginalis) trichomonal or due to Trichomonas (vaginalis)

131.01 **Trichomonal vulvovaginitis**
Vaginitis, trichomonal or due to Trichomonas (vaginalis)

131.02 **Trichomonal urethritis**

131.03 **Trichomonal prostatitis**

❑131.09 **Other**

❑131.8 **Other specified sites**
Excludes *intestinal (007.3)*

❑131.9 **Trichomoniasis, unspecified**

● 132 **Pediculosis and Phthirus infestation**

132.0 **Pediculus capitis [head louse]**

132.1 **Pediculus corporis [body louse]**

132.2 **Phthirus pubis [pubic louse]**
Pediculus pubis

132.3 **Mixed infestation**
Infestation classifiable to more than one of the categories 132.0–132.2

❑132.9 **Pediculosis, unspecified**

● 133 **Acariasis**

133.0 **Scabies**
Infestation by Sarcoptes scabiei
Norwegian scabies
Sarcoptic itch

❑133.8 **Other acariasis**
Chiggers
Infestation by:
Demodex folliculorum
Trombicula

❑133.9 **Acariasis, unspecified**
Infestation by mites NOS

● 134 **Other infestation**

134.0 **Myiasis**
Infestation by:
Dermatobia (hominis)
fly larvae
Gasterophilus (intestinalis)
maggots
Oestrus ovis

❑134.1 **Other arthropod infestation**
Infestation by:
chigoe
sand flea
Tunga penetrans
Jigger disease
Scarabiasis
Tungiasis

134.2 **Hirudiniasis**
Hirudiniasis (external) (internal)
Leeches (aquatic) (land)

❑134.8 **Other specified infestations**

❑134.9 **Infestation, unspecified**
Infestation (skin) NOS
Skin parasites NOS

135 **Sarcoidosis**
Besnier-Boeck-Schaumann disease
Lupoid (miliary) of Boeck
Lupus pernio (Besnier)
Lymphogranulomatosis, benign (Schaumann's)
Sarcoid (any site):
NOS
Boeck
Darier-Roussy
Uveoparotid fever

● 136 **Other and unspecified infectious and parasitic diseases**

136.0 **Ainhum**
Dactylolysis spontanea

136.1 **Behçet's syndrome**

136.2 **Specific infections by free-living amebae**
Meningoencephalitis due to Naegleria

136.3 **Pneumocystosis**
Pneumonia due to Pneumocystis carinii
Pneumonia due to Pneumocystis jiroveci ◀

136.4 **Psorospermiasis**

136.5 **Sarcosporidiosis**
Infection by Sarcocystis lindemanni

❑136.8 **Other specified infectious and parasitic diseases**
Candiru infestation

❑136.9 **Unspecified infectious and parasitic diseases**
Infectious disease NOS
Parasitic disease NOS

LATE EFFECTS OF INFECTIOUS AND PARASITIC DISEASES (137–139)

Item 1-24 Before you use this late code, check your documentation. The original problem (tuberculosis, TB) that is causing the current late effect (necrosis) must have been attributable to categories 010–018. A patient who originally had TB of a joint (015.2X) now has a late effect (137.3), which is necrosis of bone (730.8). Because there is no active TB, 015.2X is not coded but serves as an authorization to use the late effect code. Remember to code the manifestation of the late effect, which is the current problem (necrosis).

● 137 **Late effects of tuberculosis**

Note: This category is to be used to indicate conditions classifiable to 010–018 as the cause of late effects, which are themselves classified elsewhere. The "late effects" include those specified as such, as sequelae, or as due to old or inactive tuberculosis, without evidence of active disease.

❑137.0 **Late effects of respiratory or unspecified tuberculosis**

❑137.1 **Late effects of central nervous system tuberculosis**

❑137.2 **Late effects of genitourinary tuberculosis**

❑137.3 **Late effects of tuberculosis of bones and joints**

❑137.4 **Late effects of tuberculosis of other specified organs**

138 **Late effects of acute poliomyelitis**

Note: This category is to be used to indicate conditions classifiable to 045 as the cause of late effects, which are themselves classified elsewhere. The "late effects" include conditions specified as such, or as sequelae, or as due to old or inactive poliomyelitis, without evidence of active disease.

● ❑139 **Late effects of other infectious and parasitic diseases**

Note: This category is to be used to indicate conditions classifiable to categories 001–009, 020–041, 046–136 as the cause of late effects, which are themselves classified elsewhere. The "late effects" include conditions specified as such; they also include sequelae of diseases classifiable to the above categories if there is evidence that the disease itself is no longer present.

139.0 **Late effects of viral encephalitis**
Late effects of conditions classifiable to 049.8–049.9, 062–064

❑139.1 **Late effects of trachoma**
Late effects of conditions classifiable to 076

❑139.8 **Late effects of other and unspecified infectious and parasitic diseases**

Item 2-1 Neoplasm: Neo = new, plasm = growth, development, formation. This new growth (mass, tumor) can be malignant or benign, which is confirmed only by the pathology report. Do not assign a code to a neoplasm until you check the pathology report. Certain CPT codes will specify benign or malignant lesion, so be certain the diagnosis code supports the procedure code.

2. NEOPLASMS (140–239)

1. Content:
   This chapter contains the following broad groups:
   - 140–195 Malignant neoplasms, stated or presumed to be primary, of specified sites, except of lymphatic and hematopoietic tissue
   - 196–198 Malignant neoplasms, stated or presumed to be secondary, of specified sites
   - 199 Malignant neoplasms, without specification of site
   - 200–208 Malignant neoplasms, stated or presumed to be primary, of lymphatic and hematopoietic tissue
   - 210–229 Benign neoplasms
   - 230–234 Carcinoma in situ
   - 235–238 Neoplasms of uncertain behavior [see Note, at beginning of section 235–238]
   - 239 Neoplasms of unspecified nature
2. Functional activity
   All neoplasms are classified in this chapter, whether or not functionally active. An additional code from Chapter 3 may be used to identify such functional activity associated with any neoplasm, e.g.:
   catecholamine-producing malignant pheochromocytoma of adrenal:
   code 194.0, additional code 255.6
   basophil adenoma of pituitary with Cushing's syndrome:
   code 227.3, additional code 255.0
3. Morphology [Histology]
   For those wishing to identify the histological type of neoplasms, a comprehensive coded nomenclature, which comprises the morphology rubrics of the ICD-Oncology, is given after the E-code chapter.
4. Malignant neoplasms overlapping site boundaries
   Categories 140–195 are for the classification of primary malignant neoplasms according to their point of origin. A malignant neoplasm that overlaps two or more subcategories within a three-digit rubric and whose point of origin cannot be determined should be classified to the subcategory .8 "Other." For example, "carcinoma involving tip and ventral surface of tongue" should be assigned to 141.8.

   On the other hand, "carcinoma of tip of tongue, extending to involve the ventral surface" should be coded to 141.2, as the point of origin, the tip, is known. Three subcategories (149.8, 159.8, 165.8) have been provided for malignant neoplasms that overlap the boundaries of three-digit rubrics within certain systems. Overlapping malignant neoplasms that cannot be classified as indicated above should be assigned to the appropriate subdivision of category 195 (Malignant neoplasm of other and ill-defined sites).

MALIGNANT NEOPLASM OF LIP, ORAL CAVITY, AND PHARYNX (140–149)

Excludes *carcinoma in situ (230.0)*

● **140 Malignant neoplasm of lip**

Excludes *skin of lip (173.0)*

140.0 Upper lip, vermilion border
Upper lip:
NOS
external
Upper lip:
lipstick area

140.1 Lower lip, vermilion border
Lower lip:
NOS
external
Lower lip:
lipstick area

140.3 Upper lip, inner aspect
Upper lip:
buccal aspect
frenulum
Upper lip:
mucosa
oral aspect

140.4 Lower lip, inner aspect
Lower lip:
buccal aspect
frenulum
Lower lip:
mucosa
oral aspect

❑ **140.5 Lip, unspecified, inner aspect**
Lip, not specified whether upper or lower:
buccal aspect
frenulum
mucosa
oral aspect

140.6 Commissure of lip
Labial commissure

❑ **140.8 Other sites of lip**
Malignant neoplasm of contiguous or overlapping sites of lip whose point of origin cannot be determined

❑ **140.9 Lip, unspecified, vermilion border**
Lip, not specified as upper or lower:
NOS
external
lipstick area

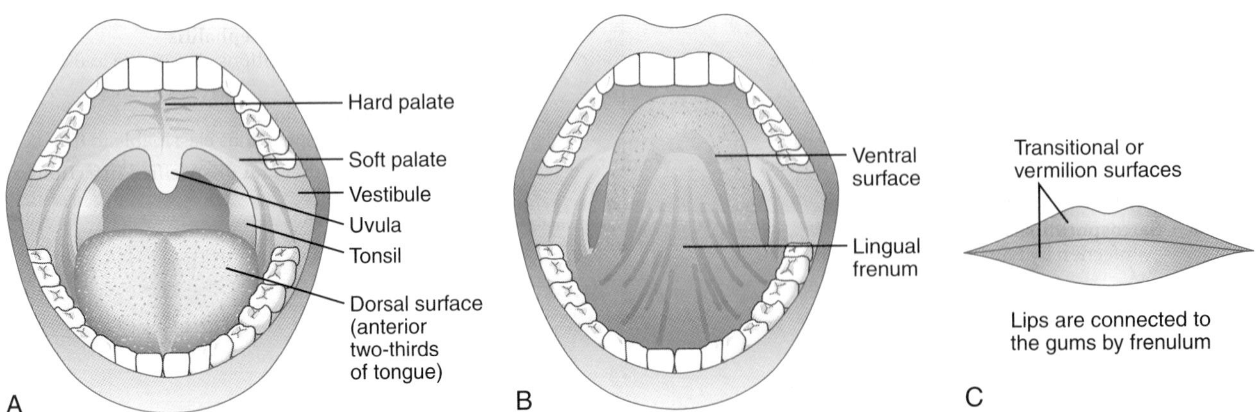
Hard palate
Soft palate
Vestibule
Uvula
Tonsil
Dorsal surface (anterior two-thirds of tongue)
A
Ventral surface
Lingual frenum
B
Transitional or vermilion surfaces
Lips are connected to the gums by frenulum
C

Figure 2-1 Anatomical structures of the mouth and lips. **A.** Dorsal surface. **B.** Ventral surface. **C.** Transitional or vermilion borders. Lips are connected to the gums by frenulum.

● **141 Malignant neoplasm of tongue**

141.0 Base of tongue
Dorsal surface of base of tongue
Fixed part of tongue NOS

141.1 Dorsal surface of tongue
Anterior two-thirds of tongue, dorsal surface
Dorsal tongue NOS
Midline of tongue

Excludes *dorsal surface of base of tongue (141.0)*

141.2 Tip and lateral border of tongue

141.3 Ventral surface of tongue
Anterior two-thirds of tongue, ventral surface
Frenulum linguae

❑**141.4 Anterior two-thirds of tongue, part unspecified**
Mobile part of tongue NOS

141.5 Junctional zone
Border of tongue at junction of fixed and mobile parts at insertion of anterior tonsillar pillar

141.6 Lingual tonsil

❑**141.8 Other sites of tongue**
Malignant neoplasm of contiguous or overlapping sites of tongue whose point of origin cannot be determined

❑**141.9 Tongue, unspecified**
Tongue NOS

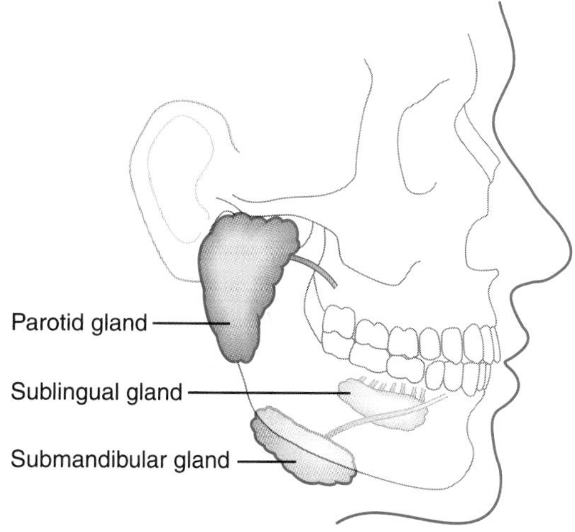
Parotid gland
Sublingual gland
Submandibular gland

Figure 2–2 Major salivary glands.

● **142 Malignant neoplasm of major salivary glands**

Includes: salivary ducts

Excludes *malignant neoplasm of minor salivary glands:*
NOS (145.9)
buccal mucosa (145.0)
soft palate (145.3)
tongue (141.0–141.9)
tonsil, palatine (146.0)

142.0 Parotid gland

142.1 Submandibular gland
Submaxillary gland

142.2 Sublingual gland

❑**142.8 Other major salivary glands**
Malignant neoplasm of contiguous or overlapping sites of salivary glands and ducts whose point of origin cannot be determined

❑**142.9 Salivary gland, unspecified**
Salivary gland (major) NOS

● **143 Malignant neoplasm of gum**

Includes: alveolar (ridge) mucosa
gingiva (alveolar) (marginal)
interdental papillae

Excludes *malignant odontogenic neoplasms (170.0–170.1)*

143.0 Upper gum

143.1 Lower gum

❑**143.8 Other sites of gum**
Malignant neoplasm of contiguous or overlapping sites of gum whose point of origin cannot be determined

❑**143.9 Gum, unspecified**

● **144 Malignant neoplasm of floor of mouth**

144.0 Anterior portion
Anterior to the premolar-canine junction

144.1 Lateral portion

❑**144.8 Other sites of floor of mouth**
Malignant neoplasm of contiguous or overlapping sites of floor of mouth whose point of origin cannot be determined

❑**144.9 Floor of mouth, part unspecified**

● **145 Malignant neoplasm of other and unspecified parts of mouth**

Excludes *mucosa of lips (140.0–140.9)*

145.0 Cheek mucosa
Buccal mucosa
Cheek, inner aspect

145.1 Vestibule of mouth
Buccal sulcus (upper) (lower)
Labial sulcus (upper) (lower)

145.2 Hard palate

145.3 Soft palate

Excludes *nasopharyngeal [posterior] [superior] surface of soft palate (147.3)*

145.4 Uvula

❑**145.5 Palate, unspecified**
Junction of hard and soft palate
Roof of mouth

145.6 Retromolar area

❑**145.8 Other specified parts of mouth**
Malignant neoplasm of contiguous or overlapping sites of mouth whose point of origin cannot be determined

❑**145.9 Mouth, unspecified**
Buccal cavity NOS
Minor salivary gland, unspecified site
Oral cavity NOS

● **146 Malignant neoplasm of oropharynx**

146.0 Tonsil

Tonsil:	Tonsil:
NOS	palatine
faucial	

Excludes *lingual tonsil (141.6)*
pharyngeal tonsil (147.1)

146.1 Tonsillar fossa

146.2 Tonsillar pillars (anterior) (posterior)
Faucial pillar
Glossopalatine fold
Palatoglossal arch
Palatopharyngeal arch

146.3 Vallecula
Anterior and medial surface of the pharyngoepiglottic fold

146.4 Anterior aspect of epiglottis
Epiglottis, free border [margin]
Glossoepiglottic fold(s)

Excludes *epiglottis:*
NOS (161.1)
suprahyoid portion (161.1)

146.5 Junctional region
Junction of the free margin of the epiglottis, the aryepiglottic fold, and the pharyngoepiglottic fold

146.6 Lateral wall of oropharynx

146.7 Posterior wall of oropharynx

❑**146.8 Other specified sites of oropharynx**
Branchial cleft
Malignant neoplasm of contiguous or overlapping sites of oropharynx whose point of origin cannot be determined

❑**146.9 Oropharynx, unspecified**

● **147 Malignant neoplasm of nasopharynx**

147.0 Superior wall
Roof of nasopharynx

147.1 Posterior wall
Adenoid
Pharyngeal tonsil

147.2 Lateral wall
Fossa of Rosenmüller
Pharyngeal recess
Opening of auditory tube

147.3 Anterior wall
Floor of nasopharynx
Nasopharyngeal [posterior] [superior] surface of soft palate
Posterior margin of nasal septum and choanae

❑**147.8 Other specified sites of nasopharynx**
Malignant neoplasm of contiguous or overlapping sites of nasopharynx whose point of origin cannot be determined

❑**147.9 Nasopharynx, unspecified**
Nasopharyngeal wall NOS

● **148 Malignant neoplasm of hypopharynx**

148.0 Postcricoid region

148.1 Pyriform sinus
Pyriform fossa

148.2 Aryepiglottic fold, hypopharyngeal aspect
Aryepiglottic fold or interarytenoid fold:
NOS
marginal zone

Excludes *aryepiglottic fold or interarytenoid fold, laryngeal aspect (161.1)*

148.3 Posterior hypopharyngeal wall

❑**148.8 Other specified sites of hypopharynx**
Malignant neoplasm of contiguous or overlapping sites of hypopharynx whose point of origin cannot be determined

❑**148.9 Hypopharynx, unspecified**
Hypopharyngeal wall NOS
Hypopharynx NOS

● **149 Malignant neoplasm of other and ill-defined sites within the lip, oral cavity, and pharynx**

❑**149.0 Pharynx, unspecified**

149.1 Waldeyer's ring

❑**149.8 Other**
Malignant neoplasms of lip, oral cavity, and pharynx whose point of origin cannot be assigned to any one of the categories 140–148

Excludes *"book leaf" neoplasm [ventral surface of tongue and floor of mouth] (145.8)*

❑**149.9 Ill-defined**

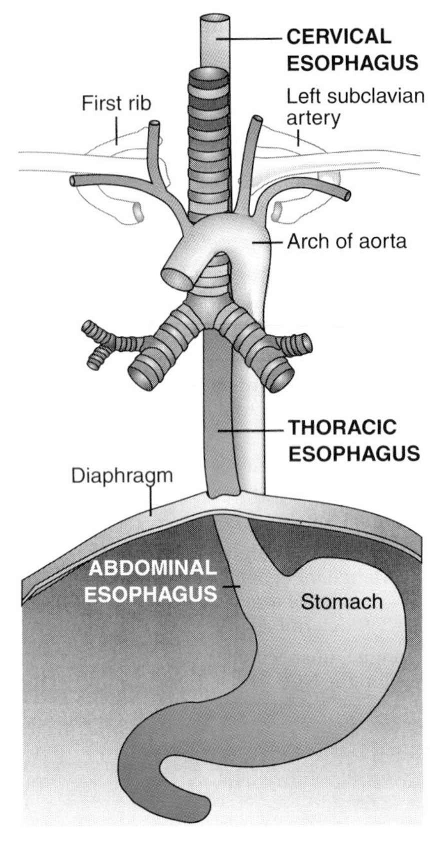
CERVICAL ESOPHAGUS
First rib
Left subclavian artery
Arch of aorta
THORACIC ESOPHAGUS
Diaphragm
ABDOMINAL ESOPHAGUS
Stomach

Figure 2–3 The esophagus is the muscular tube that connects the pharynx and the stomach. The 10 inch (25 cm) long esophagus is divided into three parts: **cervical, thoracic,** and **abdominal.**

MALIGNANT NEOPLASM OF DIGESTIVE ORGANS AND PERITONEUM (150–159)

Excludes *carcinoma in situ (230.1–230.9)*

● **150 Malignant neoplasm of esophagus**

150.0 Cervical esophagus

150.1 Thoracic esophagus

150.2 Abdominal esophagus

Excludes *adenocarcinoma (151.0)*
cardioesophageal junction (151.0)

150.3 Upper third of esophagus
Proximal third of esophagus

150.4 Middle third of esophagus

150.5 Lower third of esophagus
Distal third of esophagus

Excludes *adenocarcinoma (151.0)*
cardioesophageal junction (151.0)

❑**150.8 Other specified part**
Malignant neoplasm of contiguous or overlapping sites of esophagus whose point of origin cannot be determined

❑**150.9 Esophagus, unspecified**

Item 2–2 The esophagus enters the stomach through the **cardiac orifice,** also called the **cardioesophageal junction.** The **cardia** is adjacent to the cardiac orifice. The stomach widens into the **greater** and **lesser curvatures.** The **pyloric antrum** precedes the **pylorus,** which connects to the duodenum.

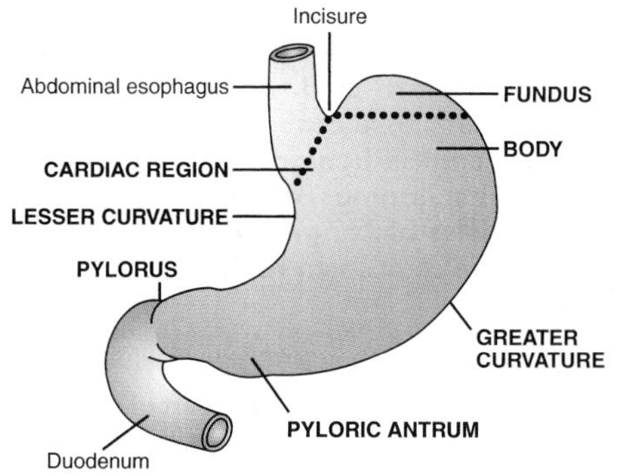
Incisure
Abdominal esophagus
FUNDUS
BODY
CARDIAC REGION
LESSER CURVATURE
PYLORUS
GREATER CURVATURE
PYLORIC ANTRUM
Duodenum

Figure 2–4 Parts of the stomach.

● **151 Malignant neoplasm of stomach**

Excludes *malignant stromal tumor of stomach (171.5)* ◀

151.0 Cardia
Cardiac orifice
Cardioesophageal junction

Excludes *squamous cell carcinoma (150.2, 150.5)*

151.1 Pylorus
Prepylorus
Pyloric canal

151.2 Pyloric antrum
Antrum of stomach NOS

151.3 Fundus of stomach

151.4 Body of stomach

❑ **151.5 Lesser curvature, unspecified**
Lesser curvature, not classifiable to 151.1–151.4

❑ **151.6 Greater curvature, unspecified**
Greater curvature, not classifiable to 151.0–151.4

❑ **151.8 Other specified sites of stomach**
Anterior wall, not classifiable to 151.0–151.4
Posterior wall, not classifiable to 151.0–151.4
Malignant neoplasm of contiguous or overlapping sites of stomach whose point of origin cannot be determined

❑ **151.9 Stomach, unspecified**
Carcinoma ventriculi
Gastric cancer

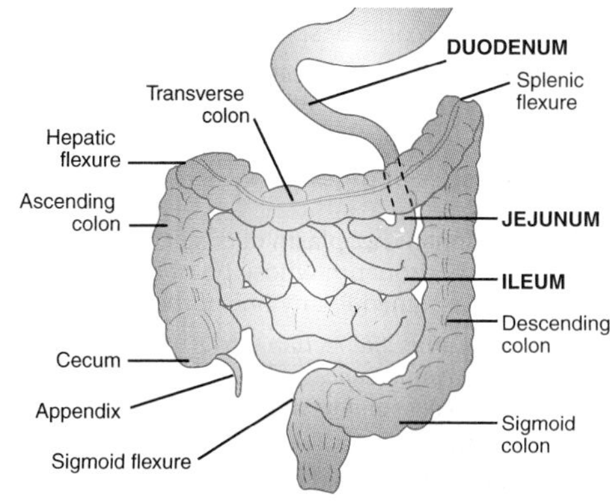
DUODENUM
Transverse colon
Splenic flexure
Hepatic flexure
Ascending colon
JEJUNUM
ILEUM
Descending colon
Cecum
Appendix
Sigmoid colon
Sigmoid flexure

Figure 2–5 Small intestine and colon.

● **152 Malignant neoplasm of small intestine, including duodenum**

Excludes *malignant stromal tumor of small intestine (171.5)* ◀

152.0 Duodenum

152.1 Jejunum

152.2 Ileum

Excludes *ileocecal valve (153.4)*

152.3 Meckel's diverticulum

❑ **152.8 Other specified sites of small intestine**
Duodenojejunal junction
Malignant neoplasm of contiguous or overlapping sites of small intestine whose point of origin cannot be determined

❑ **152.9 Small intestine, unspecified**

● **153 Malignant neoplasm of colon**

153.0 Hepatic flexure
A flexure is a bending in a structure or organ. Note the three flexures illustrated in Figure 2–5. Hepatic = liver, sigmoid = colon, splenic = spleen.

153.1 Transverse colon

153.2 Descending colon
Left colon

153.3 Sigmoid colon
Sigmoid (flexure)

Excludes *rectosigmoid junction (154.0)*

A flexure is a bending in a structure or organ. Note the three flexures illustrated in Figure 2–5. Hepatic = liver, sigmoid = colon, splenic = spleen.

153.4 Cecum
Ileocecal valve

153.5 Appendix

153.6 Ascending colon
Right colon

153.7 Splenic flexure
A flexure is a bending in a structure or organ. Note the three flexures illustrated in Figure 2–5. Hepatic = liver, sigmoid = colon, splenic = spleen.

❑ **153.8 Other specified sites of large intestine**
Malignant neoplasm of contiguous or overlapping sites of colon whose point of origin cannot be determined

Excludes *ileocecal valve (153.4)*
rectosigmoid junction (154.0)

❑ **153.9 Colon, unspecified**
Large intestine NOS

● **154 Malignant neoplasm of rectum, rectosigmoid junction, and anus**

154.0 Rectosigmoid junction
Colon with rectum
Rectosigmoid (colon)

154.1 Rectum
Rectal ampulla

154.2 Anal canal
Anal sphincter

Excludes *skin of anus (172.5, 173.5)*

❑ **154.3 Anus, unspecified**

Excludes *anus:*
margin (172.5, 173.5)
skin (172.5, 173.5)
perianal skin (172.5, 173.5)

❑154.8 **Other**
Anorectum
Cloacogenic zone
Malignant neoplasm of contiguous or overlapping sites of rectum, rectosigmoid junction, and anus whose point of origin cannot be determined

● 155 **Malignant neoplasm of liver and intrahepatic bile ducts**

155.0 **Liver, primary**
Carcinoma:
liver, specified as primary
hepatocellular
liver cell
Hepatoblastoma

155.1 **Intrahepatic bile ducts**
Canaliculi biliferi
Interlobular:
bile ducts
biliary canals
Intrahepatic:
biliary passages
canaliculi
gall duct

Excludes *hepatic duct (156.1)*

❑155.2 **Liver, not specified as primary or secondary**

● 156 **Malignant neoplasm of gallbladder and extrahepatic bile ducts**

156.0 **Gallbladder**

156.1 **Extrahepatic bile ducts**
Biliary duct or passage NOS
Common bile duct
Cystic duct
Hepatic duct
Sphincter of Oddi

156.2 **Ampulla of Vater**

❑156.8 **Other specified sites of gallbladder and extrahepatic bile ducts**
Malignant neoplasm of contiguous or overlapping sites of gallbladder and extrahepatic bile ducts whose point of origin cannot be determined

❑156.9 **Biliary tract, part unspecified**
Malignant neoplasm involving both intrahepatic and extrahepatic bile ducts

● 157 **Malignant neoplasm of pancreas**

157.0 **Head of pancreas**

157.1 **Body of pancreas**

157.2 **Tail of pancreas**

157.3 **Pancreatic duct**
Duct of:
Santorini
Wirsung

Item 2-3 Islet cells in the pancreas make and secrete hormones that regulate the body's production of insulin, glucagon, and stomach acid. Breakdown of the insulin-producing cells can cause diabetes mellitus.
Islet cell tumors can be benign or malignant and include glucagonomas, insulinomas, and gastrinomas. Also called Islet cell tumor, Islet of Langerhans tumor, and neuroendocrine tumor. The neoplasm table must be consulted for the correct code.

157.4 **Islets of Langerhans**
Islets of Langerhans, any part of pancreas

Use additional code to identify any functional activity

❑157.8 **Other specified sites of pancreas**
Ectopic pancreatic tissue
Malignant neoplasm of contiguous or overlapping sites of pancreas whose point of origin cannot be determined

❑157.9 **Pancreas, part unspecified**

● 158 **Malignant neoplasm of retroperitoneum and peritoneum**

158.0 **Retroperitoneum**
Periadrenal tissue
Perinephric tissue
Perirenal tissue
Retrocecal tissue

❑158.8 **Specified parts of peritoneum**
Cul-de-sac (of Douglas)
Mesentery
Mesocolon
Omentum
Peritoneum:
parietal
pelvic
Rectouterine pouch
Malignant neoplasm of contiguous or overlapping sites of retroperitoneum and peritoneum whose point of origin cannot be determined

❑158.9 **Peritoneum, unspecified**

● 159 **Malignant neoplasm of other and ill-defined sites within the digestive organs and peritoneum**

❑159.0 **Intestinal tract, part unspecified**
Intestine NOS

❑159.1 **Spleen, not elsewhere classified**
Angiosarcoma of spleen
Fibrosarcoma of spleen

Excludes *Hodgkin's disease (201.0–201.9)*
lymphosarcoma (200.1)
reticulosarcoma (200.0)

❑159.8 **Other sites of digestive system and intra-abdominal organs**
Malignant neoplasm of digestive organs and peritoneum whose point of origin cannot be assigned to any one of the categories 150–158

Excludes *anus and rectum (154.8)*
cardioesophageal junction (151.0)
colon and rectum (154.0)

❑159.9 **Ill-defined**
Alimentary canal or tract NOS
Gastrointestinal tract NOS

Excludes *abdominal NOS (195.2)*
intra-abdominal NOS (195.2)

MALIGNANT NEOPLASM OF RESPIRATORY AND INTRATHORACIC ORGANS (160–165)

Excludes *carcinoma in situ (231.0–231.9)*

● **160 Malignant neoplasm of nasal cavities, middle ear, and accessory sinuses**

160.0 Nasal cavities
Cartilage of nose
Conchae, nasal
Internal nose
Septum of nose
Vestibule of nose

Excludes *nasal bone (170.0)*
nose NOS (195.0)
olfactory bulb (192.0)
posterior margin of septum and choanae (147.3)
skin of nose (172.3, 173.3)
turbinates (170.0)

160.1 Auditory tube, middle ear, and mastoid air cells
Antrum tympanicum
Eustachian tube
Tympanic cavity

Excludes *auditory canal (external) (172.2, 173.2)*
bone of ear (meatus) (170.0)
cartilage of ear (171.0)
ear (external) (skin) (172.2, 173.2)

160.2 Maxillary sinus
Antrum (Highmore) (maxillary)

160.3 Ethmoidal sinus

160.4 Frontal sinus

160.5 Sphenoidal sinus

❑ **160.8 Other**
Malignant neoplasm of contiguous or overlapping sites of nasal cavities, middle ear, and accessory sinuses whose point of origin cannot be determined

❑ **160.9 Accessory sinus, unspecified**

● **161 Malignant neoplasm of larynx**

161.0 Glottis
Intrinsic larynx
Laryngeal commissure (anterior) (posterior)
True vocal cord
The true vocal cords ("lower vocal folds") produce vocalization when air from the lungs passes between them. Check your documentation. Code 161.1 is for malignant neoplasm of the false vocal cords.
Vocal cord NOS

161.1 Supraglottis
Aryepiglottic fold or interarytenoid fold, laryngeal aspect
Epiglottis (suprahyoid portion) NOS
Extrinsic larynx
False vocal cords
The false vocal cords ("upper vocal folds") are not involved in vocalization. Check your documentation. Code 161.0 is for true vocal cords.
Posterior (laryngeal) surface of epiglottis
Ventricular bands

Excludes *anterior aspect of epiglottis (146.4)*
aryepiglottic fold or interarytenoid fold:
NOS (148.2)
hypopharyngeal aspect (148.2)
marginal zone (148.2)

161.2 Subglottis

161.3 Laryngeal cartilages
Cartilage:
arytenoid
cricoid
cuneiform
thyroid

❑ **161.8 Other specified sites of larynx**
Malignant neoplasm of contiguous or overlapping sites of larynx whose point of origin cannot be determined

❑ **161.9 Larynx, unspecified**

● **162 Malignant neoplasm of trachea, bronchus, and lung**

162.0 Trachea
Cartilage of trachea
Mucosa of trachea

162.2 Main bronchus
Carina
Hilus of lung

162.3 Upper lobe, bronchus or lung

162.4 Middle lobe, bronchus or lung

162.5 Lower lobe, bronchus or lung

❑ **162.8 Other parts of bronchus or lung**
Malignant neoplasm of contiguous or overlapping sites of bronchus or lung whose point of origin cannot be determined

❑ **162.9 Bronchus and lung, unspecified**

The pleura is a serous membrane that lines the thoracic cavity (parietal) and covers the lungs (visceral).

● **163 Malignant neoplasm of pleura**

163.0 Parietal pleura

163.1 Visceral pleura

❑ **163.8 Other specified sites of pleura**
Malignant neoplasm of contiguous or overlapping sites of pleura whose point of origin cannot be determined

❑ **163.9 Pleura, unspecified**

● **164 Malignant neoplasm of thymus, heart, and mediastinum**

164.0 Thymus

164.1 Heart
Endocardium
Epicardium
Myocardium
Pericardium

Excludes *great vessels (171.4)*

164.2 Anterior mediastinum

164.3 Posterior mediastinum

❑ **164.8 Other**
Malignant neoplasm of contiguous or overlapping sites of thymus, heart, and mediastinum whose point of origin cannot be determined

❑ **164.9 Mediastinum, part unspecified**

● **165 Malignant neoplasm of other and ill-defined sites within the respiratory system and intrathoracic organs**

❑ **165.0 Upper respiratory tract, part unspecified**

❑ **165.8 Other**
Malignant neoplasm of respiratory and intrathoracic organs whose point of origin cannot be assigned to any one of the categories 160–164

❑ **165.9 Ill-defined sites within the respiratory system**
Respiratory tract NOS

Excludes *intrathoracic NOS (195.1)*
thoracic NOS (195.1)

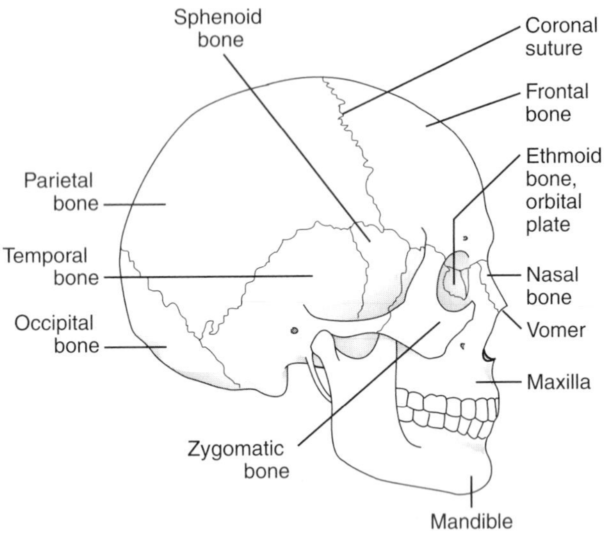

Sphenoid bone
Coronal suture
Frontal bone
Ethmoid bone, orbital plate
Parietal bone
Temporal bone
Nasal bone
Occipital bone
Vomer
Maxilla
Zygomatic bone
Mandible

Figure 2–6 Bones of the skull and face.

MALIGNANT NEOPLASM OF BONE, CONNECTIVE TISSUE, SKIN, AND BREAST (170–176)

Excludes *carcinoma in situ:*
breast (233.0)
skin (232.0–232.9)

● **170 Malignant neoplasm of bone and articular cartilage**

Includes: cartilage (articular) (joint)
periosteum

Excludes *bone marrow NOS (202.9)*
cartilage:
ear (171.0)
eyelid (171.0)
larynx (161.3)
nose (160.0)
synovia (171.0–171.9)

170.0 Bones of skull and face, except mandible

Bone:
ethmoid
frontal
malar
nasal
occipital
orbital
parietal

Bone:
sphenoid
temporal
zygomatic
Maxilla (superior)
Turbinate
Upper jaw bone
Vomer

Excludes *carcinoma, any type except intraosseous or odontogenic:*
maxilla, maxillary (sinus) (160.2)
upper jaw bone (143.0)
jaw bone (lower) (170.1)

170.1 Mandible

Inferior maxilla
Jaw bone NOS
Lower jaw bone

Excludes *carcinoma, any type except intraosseous or odontogenic:*
jaw bone NOS (143.9)
lower (143.1)
upper jaw bone (170.0)

170.2 Vertebral column, excluding sacrum and coccyx

Spinal column
Spine
Vertebra

Excludes *sacrum and coccyx (170.6)*

170.3 Ribs, sternum, and clavicle

Costal cartilage
Costovertebral joint
Xiphoid process

170.4 Scapula and long bones of upper limb

Acromion
Bones NOS of upper limb
Humerus
Radius
Ulna

170.5 Short bones of upper limb

Carpal
Cuneiform, wrist
Metacarpal
Navicular, of hand
Phalanges of hand
Pisiform
Scaphoid (of hand)
Semilunar or lunate
Trapezium
Trapezoid
Unciform

170.6 Pelvic bones, sacrum, and coccyx

Coccygeal vertebra
Ilium
Ischium
Pubic bone
Sacral vertebra

170.7 Long bones of lower limb

Bones NOS of lower limb
Femur
Fibula
Tibia

170.8 Short bones of lower limb

Astragalus [talus]
Calcaneus
Cuboid
Cuneiform, ankle
Metatarsal
Navicular (of ankle)
Patella
Phalanges of foot
Tarsal

❑ **170.9 Bone and articular cartilage, site unspecified**

● **171 Malignant neoplasm of connective and other soft tissue**

Includes: blood vessel
bursa
fascia
fat
ligament, except uterine
malignant stromal tumors ◀
muscle
peripheral, sympathetic, and parasympathetic nerves and ganglia
synovia
tendon (sheath)

Excludes *cartilage (of):*
articular (170.0–170.9)
larynx (161.3)
nose (160.0)
connective tissue:
breast (174.0–175.9)
internal organs (except stromal tumors)—code to malignant neoplasm of the site [e.g., leiomyosarcoma of stomach, 151.9] ⬅
heart (164.1)
uterine ligament (183.4)

171.0 Head, face, and neck

Cartilage of:
ear
eyelid

171.2 Upper limb, including shoulder

Arm
Finger
Forearm
Hand

171.3 Lower limb, including hip

Foot
Leg
Popliteal space
Popliteal space = popliteal cavity, popliteal fossa. Depression in the posterior aspect of the knee (behind the knee).
Thigh
Toe

171.4 Thorax
Axilla
Diaphragm
Great vessels

Excludes *heart (164.1)*
mediastinum (164.2–164.9)
thymus (164.0)

171.5 Abdomen
Abdominal wall
Hypochondrium

Excludes *peritoneum (158.8)*
retroperitoneum (158.0)

171.6 Pelvis
Buttock
Groin
Inguinal region
Perineum

Excludes *pelvic peritoneum (158.8)*
retroperitoneum (158.0)
uterine ligament, any (183.3–183.5)

❑**171.7 Trunk, unspecified**
Back NOS
Flank NOS

❑**171.8 Other specified sites of connective and other soft tissue**
Malignant neoplasm of contiguous or overlapping sites of connective tissue whose point of origin cannot be determined

❑**171.9 Connective and other soft tissue, site unspecified**

● **172 Malignant melanoma of skin**

Includes: melanocarcinoma
melanoma (skin) NOS

Excludes *skin of genital organs (184.0–184.9, 187.1–187.9)*
sites other than skin - code to malignant neoplasm of the site

172.0 Lip

Excludes *vermilion border of lip (140.0–140.1, 140.9)*

172.1 Eyelid, including canthus

172.2 Ear and external auditory canal
Auricle (ear)
Auricular canal, external
External [acoustic] meatus
Pinna

❑**172.3 Other and unspecified parts of face**
Cheek (external)
Chin
Eyebrow
Forehead
Nose, external
Temple

172.4 Scalp and neck

172.5 Trunk, except scrotum
Axilla
Breast
Buttock
Groin
Perianal skin
Perineum
Umbilicus

Excludes *anal canal (154.2)*
anus NOS (154.3)
scrotum (187.7)

172.6 Upper limb, including shoulder
Arm
Finger
Forearm
Hand

172.7 Lower limb, including hip
Ankle
Foot
Heel
Knee
Leg
Popliteal area
Thigh
Toe

❑**172.8 Other specified sites of skin**
Malignant melanoma of contiguous or overlapping sites of skin whose point of origin cannot be determined

❑**172.9 Melanoma of skin, site unspecified**

● **173 Other malignant neoplasm of skin**

Includes: malignant neoplasm of:
sebaceous glands
sudoriferous, sudoriparous glands
sweat glands

Excludes *Kaposi's sarcoma (176.0–176.9)*
malignant melanoma of skin (172.0–172.9)
skin of genital organs (184.0–184.9, 187.1–187.9)

173.0 Skin of lip

Excludes *vermilion border of lip (140.0–140.1, 140.9)*

173.1 Eyelid, including canthus

Excludes *cartilage of eyelid (171.0)*

173.2 Skin of ear and external auditory canal
Auricle (ear)
Auricular canal, external
External meatus
Pinna

Excludes *cartilage of ear (171.0)*

❑**173.3 Skin of other and unspecified parts of face**
Cheek, external
Chin
Eyebrow
Forehead
Nose, external
Temple

173.4 Scalp and skin of neck

173.5 Skin of trunk, except scrotum
Axillary fold
Perianal skin
Skin of:
abdominal wall
anus
back
breast
buttock
chest wall
groin
perineum
umbilicus

Excludes *anal canal (154.2)*
anus NOS (154.3)
skin of scrotum (187.7)

173.6 Skin of upper limb, including shoulder
Arm
Finger
Forearm
Hand

173.7 Skin of lower limb, including hip
Ankle
Foot
Heel
Knee
Leg
Popliteal area
Thigh
Toe

❑**173.8 Other specified sites of skin**
Malignant neoplasm of contiguous or overlapping sites of skin whose point of origin cannot be determined

❑**173.9 Skin, site unspecified**

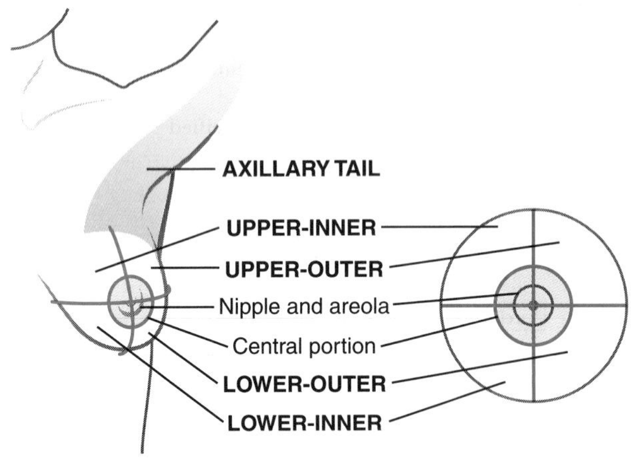
AXILLARY TAIL
UPPER-INNER
UPPER-OUTER
Nipple and areola
Central portion
LOWER-OUTER
LOWER-INNER

Figure 2–7 Female breast quadrants and axillary tail.

● 174 **Malignant neoplasm of female breast**

Includes: breast (female)
connective tissue
soft parts
Paget's disease of:
breast
nipple

Use additional code to identify estrogen receptor status (V86.0, V86.1) ◀

Excludes *skin of breast (172.5, 173.5)*

174.0 **Nipple and areola**

174.1 **Central portion**

174.2 **Upper-inner quadrant**

174.3 **Lower-inner quadrant**

174.4 **Upper-outer quadrant**

174.5 **Lower-outer quadrant**

174.6 **Axillary tail**

❑ 174.8 **Other specified sites of female breast**
Ectopic sites
Inner breast
Lower breast
Malignant neoplasm of contiguous or overlapping sites of breast whose point of origin cannot be determined
Midline of breast
Outer breast
Upper breast

❑ 174.9 **Breast (female), unspecified**

● 175 **Malignant neoplasm of male breast**

Use additional code to identify estrogen receptor status (V86.0, V86.1) ◀

Excludes *skin of breast (172.5, 173.5)*

175.0 **Nipple and areola**

❑ 175.9 **Other and unspecified sites of male breast**
Ectopic breast tissue, male

Item 2-4 Kaposi's sarcoma is a cancer that begins in blood vessels and can affect tissues under the skin or the mucous membranes before it spreads to other organs. Patients who have had organ transplants or patients with AIDS are at high risk for this malignancy.

● 176 **Kaposi's sarcoma**

176.0 **Skin**

176.1 **Soft tissue**
Blood vessel
Connective tissue
Fascia
Ligament
Lymphatic(s) NEC
Muscle

Excludes *lymph glands and nodes (176.5)*

176.2 **Palate**

176.3 **Gastrointestinal sites**

176.4 **Lung**

176.5 **Lymph nodes**

❑ 176.8 **Other specified sites**

Includes: Oral cavity NEC

❑ 176.9 **Unspecified**
Viscera NOS

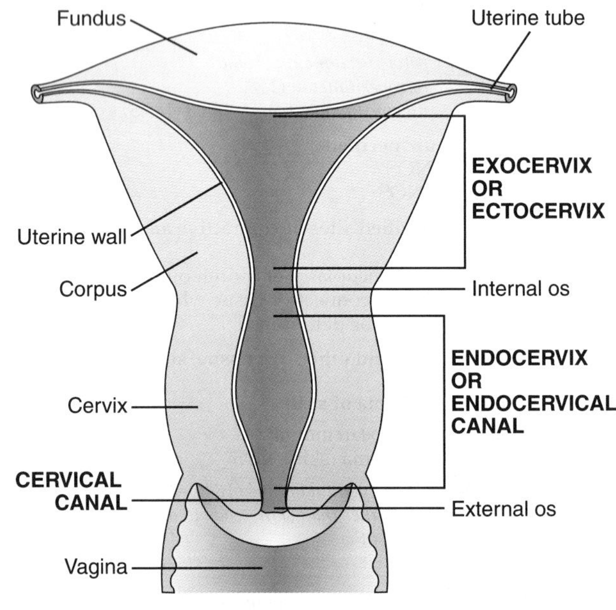
Fundus
Uterine tube
EXOCERVIX
OR
ECTOCERVIX
Uterine wall
Corpus
Internal os
ENDOCERVIX
OR
ENDOCERVICAL
CANAL
Cervix
CERVICAL
CANAL
External os
Vagina

Figure 2–8 Cervix uteri.

MALIGNANT NEOPLASM OF GENITOURINARY ORGANS (179–189)

Excludes *carcinoma in situ (233.1–233.9)*

❑ 179 **Malignant neoplasm of uterus, part unspecified**

● 180 **Malignant neoplasm of cervix uteri**

Includes: invasive malignancy [carcinoma]

Excludes *carcinoma in situ (233.1)*

180.0 **Endocervix**
Cervical canal NOS
Endocervical canal
Endocervical gland

180.1 **Exocervix**

❑ 180.8 **Other specified sites of cervix**
Cervical stump
Squamocolumnar junction of cervix
Malignant neoplasm of contiguous or overlapping sites of cervix uteri whose point of origin cannot be determined

❑ 180.9 **Cervix uteri, unspecified**

181 Malignant neoplasm of placenta
Choriocarcinoma NOS
Chorioepithelioma NOS
Excludes *chorioadenoma (destruens) (236.1)*
hydatidiform mole (630)
malignant (236.1)
invasive mole (236.1)
male choriocarcinoma NOS (186.0–186.9)

● **182 Malignant neoplasm of body of uterus**
Excludes *carcinoma in situ (233.2)*

182.0 Corpus uteri, except isthmus
Cornu
Endometrium
Fundus
Myometrium

182.1 Isthmus
Lower uterine segment

❑ **182.8 Other specified sites of body of uterus**
Malignant neoplasm of contiguous or overlapping sites of body of uterus whose point of origin cannot be determined
Excludes *uterus NOS (179)*

● **183 Malignant neoplasm of ovary and other uterine adnexa**
Excludes *Douglas' cul-de-sac (158.8)*

183.0 Ovary
Use additional code to identify any functional activity

183.2 Fallopian tube
Oviduct
Uterine tube

183.3 Broad ligament
Mesovarium
Parovarian region

183.4 Parametrium
Uterine ligament NOS
Uterosacral ligament

183.5 Round ligament

❑ **183.8 Other specified sites of uterine adnexa**
Tubo-ovarian
Utero-ovarian
Malignant neoplasm of contiguous or overlapping sites of ovary and other uterine adnexa whose point of origin cannot be determined

❑ **183.9 Uterine adnexa, unspecified**

● **184 Malignant neoplasm of other and unspecified female genital organs**
Excludes *carcinoma in situ (233.3)*

184.0 Vagina
Gartner's duct
Vaginal vault

184.1 Labia majora
Greater vestibular [Bartholin's] gland

184.2 Labia minora

184.3 Clitoris

❑ **184.4 Vulva, unspecified**
External female genitalia NOS
Pudendum

❑ **184.8 Other specified sites of female genital organs**
Malignant neoplasm of contiguous or overlapping sites of female genital organs whose point of origin cannot be determined

❑ **184.9 Female genital organ, site unspecified**
Female genitourinary tract NOS

185 Malignant neoplasm of prostate
Excludes *seminal vesicles (187.8)*

● **186 Malignant neoplasm of testis**
Use additional code to identify any functional activity

186.0 Undescended testis
Ectopic testis
Retained testis

❑ **186.9 Other and unspecified testis**
Testis:
NOS
descended
Testis:
scrotal

● **187 Malignant neoplasm of penis and other male genital organs**

187.1 Prepuce
Foreskin

187.2 Glans penis

187.3 Body of penis
Corpus cavernosum

❑ **187.4 Penis, part unspecified**
Skin of penis NOS

187.5 Epididymis

187.6 Spermatic cord
Vas deferens

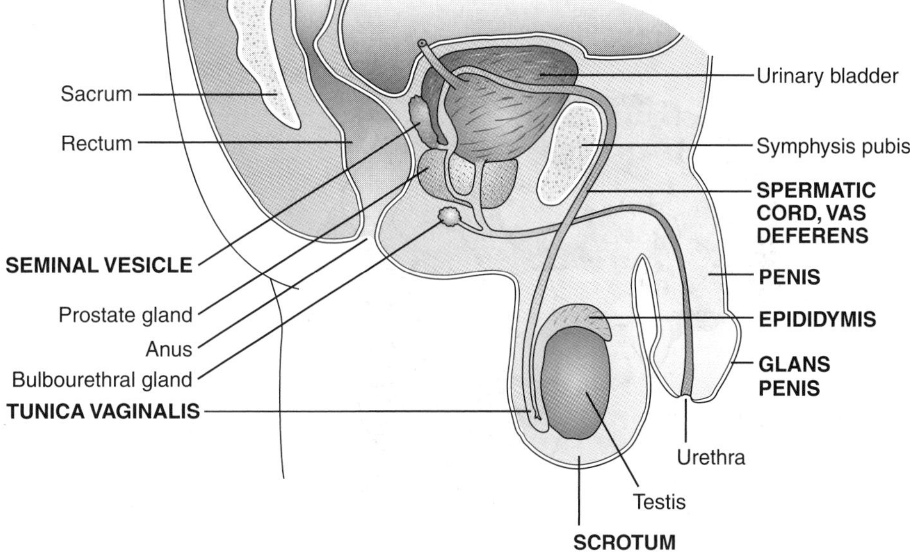

Sacrum
Rectum
SEMINAL VESICLE
Prostate gland
Anus
Bulbourethral gland
TUNICA VAGINALIS
Urinary bladder
Symphysis pubis
SPERMATIC CORD, VAS DEFERENS
PENIS
EPIDIDYMIS
GLANS PENIS
Urethra
Testis
SCROTUM

Figure 2–9 Penis and other male genital organs.

187.7 **Scrotum**
Skin of scrotum

❑187.8 **Other specified sites of male genital organs**
Seminal vesicle
Tunica vaginalis
Malignant neoplasm of contiguous or overlapping sites of penis and other male genital organs whose point of origin cannot be determined

❑187.9 **Male genital organ, site unspecified**
Male genital organ or tract NOS

● 188 **Malignant neoplasm of bladder**

Excludes *carcinoma in situ (233.7)*

188.0 **Trigone of urinary bladder**

188.1 **Dome of urinary bladder**

188.2 **Lateral wall of urinary bladder**

188.3 **Anterior wall of urinary bladder**

188.4 **Posterior wall of urinary bladder**

188.5 **Bladder neck**
Internal urethral orifice

188.6 **Ureteric orifice**

188.7 **Urachus**

❑188.8 **Other specified sites of bladder**
Malignant neoplasm of contiguous or overlapping sites of bladder whose point of origin cannot be determined

❑188.9 **Bladder, part unspecified**
Bladder wall NOS

● 189 **Malignant neoplasm of kidney and other and unspecified urinary organs**

189.0 **Kidney, except pelvis**
Kidney NOS
Kidney parenchyma

189.1 **Renal pelvis**
Renal calyces
Ureteropelvic junction

189.2 **Ureter**

Excludes *ureteric orifice of bladder (188.6)*

189.3 **Urethra**

Excludes *urethral orifice of bladder (188.5)*

189.4 **Paraurethral glands**

❑189.8 **Other specified sites of urinary organs**
Malignant neoplasm of contiguous or overlapping sites of kidney and other urinary organs whose point of origin cannot be determined

❑189.9 **Urinary organ, site unspecified**
Urinary system NOS

MALIGNANT NEOPLASM OF OTHER AND UNSPECIFIED SITES (190–199)

Excludes *carcinoma in situ (234.0–234.9)*

● 190 **Malignant neoplasm of eye**

Excludes *carcinoma in situ (234.0)*
eyelid (skin) (172.1, 173.1)
cartilage (171.0)
optic nerve (192.0)
orbital bone (170.0)

190.0 **Eyeball, except conjunctiva, cornea, retina, and choroid**

Note the use of "except" in this code.

Ciliary body
Crystalline lens
Iris
Sclera
Uveal tract

190.1 **Orbit**
Connective tissue of orbit
Extraocular muscle
Retrobulbar

Excludes *bone of orbit (170.0)*

190.2 **Lacrimal gland**

190.3 **Conjunctiva**

190.4 **Cornea**

190.5 **Retina**

190.6 **Choroid**

190.7 **Lacrimal duct**
Lacrimal sac
Nasolacrimal duct

❑190.8 **Other specified sites of eye**
Malignant neoplasm of contiguous or overlapping sites of eye whose point of origin cannot be determined

❑190.9 **Eye, part unspecified**

● 191 **Malignant neoplasm of brain**

Excludes *cranial nerves (192.0)*
retrobulbar area (190.1)

191.0 **Cerebrum, except lobes and ventricles**
Basal ganglia
Cerebral cortex
Corpus striatum
Globus pallidus
Hypothalamus
Thalamus

191.1 **Frontal lobe**

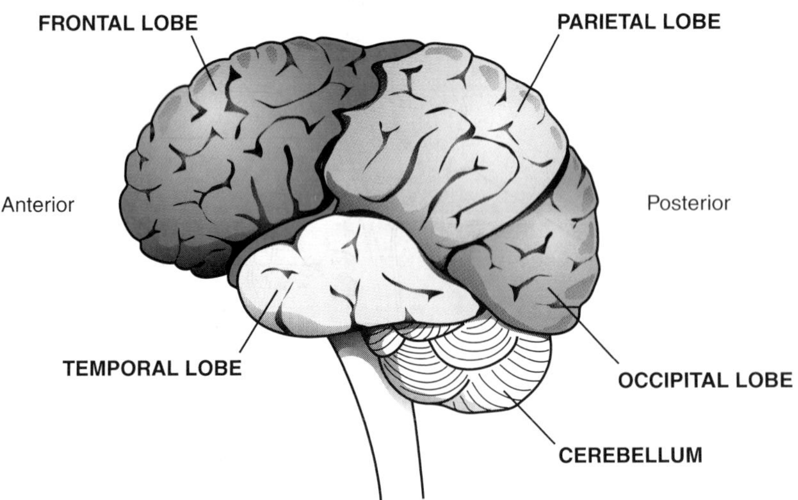
FRONTAL LOBE
PARIETAL LOBE
Anterior
Posterior
TEMPORAL LOBE
OCCIPITAL LOBE
CEREBELLUM

Figure 2–10 The brain.

191.2 Temporal lobe
Hippocampus
Uncus

191.3 Parietal lobe

191.4 Occipital lobe

191.5 Ventricles
Choroid plexus
Floor of ventricle

191.6 Cerebellum NOS
Cerebellopontine angle

191.7 Brain stem
Cerebral peduncle
Medulla oblongata
Midbrain
Pons

❑ **191.8 Other parts of brain**
Corpus callosum
Tapetum
Malignant neoplasm of contiguous or overlapping sites of brain whose point of origin cannot be determined

❑ **191.9 Brain, unspecified**
Cranial fossa NOS

● **192 Malignant neoplasm of other and unspecified parts of nervous system**

Excludes *peripheral, sympathetic, and parasympathetic nerves and ganglia (171.0–171.9)*

192.0 Cranial nerves
Olfactory bulb

192.1 Cerebral meninges
Dura (mater)
Falx (cerebelli) (cerebri)
Meninges NOS
Tentorium

192.2 Spinal cord
Cauda equina

192.3 Spinal meninges

❑ **192.8 Other specified sites of nervous system**
Malignant neoplasm of contiguous or overlapping sites of other parts of nervous system whose point of origin cannot be determined

❑ **192.9 Nervous system, part unspecified**
Nervous system (central) NOS

Excludes *meninges NOS (192.1)*

193 Malignant neoplasm of thyroid gland
Sipple's syndrome
Thyroglossal duct

Use additional code to identify any functional activity

● **194 Malignant neoplasm of other endocrine glands and related structures**

Use additional code to identify any functional activity

Excludes *islets of Langerhans (157.4)*
ovary (183.0)
testis (186.0–186.9)
thymus (164.0)

194.0 Adrenal gland
Adrenal cortex
Adrenal medulla
Suprarenal gland

194.1 Parathyroid gland

194.3 Pituitary gland and craniopharyngeal duct
Craniobuccal pouch
Hypophysis
Rathke's pouch
Sella turcica

194.4 Pineal gland

194.5 Carotid body

194.6 Aortic body and other paraganglia
Coccygeal body
Glomus jugulare
Para-aortic body

❑ **194.8 Other**
Pluriglandular involvement NOS

Note: If the sites of multiple involvements are known, they should be coded separately.

❑ **194.9 Endocrine gland, site unspecified**

● **195 Malignant neoplasm of other and ill-defined sites**

Includes: malignant neoplasms of contiguous sites, not elsewhere classified, whose point of origin cannot be determined

Excludes *malignant neoplasm:*
lymphatic and hematopoietic tissue (200.0–208.9)
secondary sites (196.0–198.8)
unspecified site (199.0–199.1)

195.0 Head, face, and neck
Cheek NOS
Jaw NOS
Nose NOS
Supraclavicular region NOS

195.1 Thorax
Axilla
Chest (wall) NOS
Intrathoracic NOS

195.2 Abdomen
Intra-abdominal NOS

195.3 Pelvis
Groin
Inguinal region NOS
Presacral region
Sacrococcygeal region
Sites overlapping systems within pelvis, as:
rectovaginal (septum)
rectovesical (septum)

195.4 Upper limb

195.5 Lower limb

❑ **195.8 Other specified sites**
Back NOS
Flank NOS
Trunk NOS

● **196 Secondary and unspecified malignant neoplasm of lymph nodes**

Excludes *any malignant neoplasm of lymph nodes, specified as primary (200.0–202.9)*
Hodgkin's disease (201.0–201.9)
lymphosarcoma (200.1)
reticulosarcoma (200.0)
other forms of lymphoma (202.0–202.9)

196.0 Lymph nodes of head, face, and neck
Cervical
Cervicofacial
Scalene
Supraclavicular

196.1 Intrathoracic lymph nodes
Bronchopulmonary
Intercostal
Mediastinal
Tracheobronchial

196.2 Intra-abdominal lymph nodes
Intestinal
Mesenteric
Retroperitoneal

196.3 Lymph nodes of axilla and upper limb
Brachial
Epitrochlear
Infraclavicular
Pectoral

196.5 Lymph nodes of inguinal region and lower limb
Femoral
Groin
Popliteal
Tibial

196.6 Intrapelvic lymph nodes
Hypogastric
Iliac
Obturator
Parametrial

❑**196.8 Lymph nodes of multiple sites**

❑**196.9 Site unspecified**
Lymph nodes NOS

● **197 Secondary malignant neoplasm of respiratory and digestive systems**

Excludes *lymph node metastasis (196.0–196.9)*

197.0 Lung
Bronchus

197.1 Mediastinum

197.2 Pleura

❑**197.3 Other respiratory organs**
Trachea

197.4 Small intestine, including duodenum

197.5 Large intestine and rectum

197.6 Retroperitoneum and peritoneum

197.7 Liver, specified as secondary

❑**197.8 Other digestive organs and spleen**

● **198 Secondary malignant neoplasm of other specified sites**

Excludes *lymph node metastasis (196.0–196.9)*

198.0 Kidney

❑**198.1 Other urinary organs**

198.2 Skin
Skin of breast

198.3 Brain and spinal cord

❑**198.4 Other parts of nervous system**
Meninges (cerebral) (spinal)

198.5 Bone and bone marrow

198.6 Ovary

198.7 Adrenal gland
Suprarenal gland

● **198.8 Other specified sites**

198.81 Breast

Excludes *skin of breast (198.2)*

198.82 Genital organs

❑**198.89 Other**

Excludes *retroperitoneal lymph nodes (196.2)*

● **199 Malignant neoplasm without specification of site**

199.0 Disseminated
Carcinomatosis unspecified site (primary) (secondary)
Generalized:
cancer unspecified site (primary) (secondary)
malignancy unspecified site (primary) (secondary)
Multiple cancer unspecified site (primary) (secondary)

❑**199.1 Other**
Cancer unspecified site (primary) (secondary)
Carcinoma unspecified site (primary) (secondary)
Malignancy unspecified site (primary) (secondary)

MALIGNANT NEOPLASM OF LYMPHATIC AND HEMATOPOIETIC TISSUE (200–208)

Excludes *secondary neoplasm of:*
bone marrow (198.5)
spleen (197.8)
secondary and unspecified neoplasm of lymph nodes (196.0–196.9)

The following fifth-digit subclassification is for use with categories 200–202:
❑ 0 **unspecified site, extranodal and solid organ sites**
1 **lymph nodes of head, face, and neck**
2 **intrathoracic lymph nodes**
3 **intra-abdominal lymph nodes**
4 **lymph nodes of axilla and upper limb**
5 **lymph nodes of inguinal region and lower limb**
6 **intrapelvic lymph nodes**
7 **spleen**
8 **lymph nodes of multiple sites**

● **200 Lymphosarcoma and reticulosarcoma**

Requires fifth digit. See note before section 200 for codes and definitions.

● **200.0 Reticulosarcoma**
Lymphoma (malignant):
histiocytic (diffuse):
nodular
pleomorphic cell type
reticulum cell type
Reticulum cell sarcoma:
NOS
pleomorphic cell type

● **200.1 Lymphosarcoma**
Lymphoblastoma (diffuse)
Lymphoma (malignant):
lymphoblastic (diffuse)
lymphocytic (cell type) (diffuse)
lymphosarcoma type
Lymphosarcoma:
NOS
diffuse NOS
lymphoblastic (diffuse)
lymphocytic (diffuse)
prolymphocytic

Excludes *lymphosarcoma:*
follicular or nodular (202.0)
mixed cell type (200.8)
lymphosarcoma cell leukemia (207.8)

● **200.2 Burkitt's tumor or lymphoma**
Malignant lymphoma, Burkitt's type

● ❑**200.8 Other named variants**
Lymphoma (malignant):
lymphoplasmacytoid type
mixed lymphocytic-histiocytic (diffuse)
Lymphosarcoma, mixed cell type (diffuse)
Reticulolymphosarcoma (diffuse)

● **201 Hodgkin's disease**

Requires fifth digit. See note before section 200 for codes and definitions.

● **201.0 Hodgkin's paragranuloma**

● **201.1 Hodgkin's granuloma**

● **201.2 Hodgkin's sarcoma**

● **201.4 Lymphocytic-histiocytic predominance**

● **201.5 Nodular sclerosis**
Hodgkin's disease, nodular sclerosis:
NOS
cellular phase

● **201.6 Mixed cellularity**

● **201.7 Lymphocytic depletion**
Hodgkin's disease, lymphocytic depletion:
NOS
diffuse fibrosis
reticular type

● ❑ **201.9 Hodgkin's disease, unspecified**
Hodgkin's:
disease NOS
lymphoma NOS
Malignant:
lymphogranuloma
lymphogranulomatosis

● **202 Other malignant neoplasms of lymphoid and histiocytic tissue**

Requires fifth digit. See note before section 200 for codes and definitions.

● **202.0 Nodular lymphoma** (Revised)
Brill-Symmers disease
Lymphoma:
follicular (giant)
lymphocytic, nodular
Lymphosarcoma:
follicular (giant)
nodular

● **202.1 Mycosis fungoides**

● **202.2 Sézary's disease**

● **202.3 Malignant histiocytosis**
Histiocytic medullary reticulosis
Malignant:
reticuloendotheliosis
reticulosis

● **202.4 Leukemic reticuloendotheliosis**
Hairy-cell leukemia

● **202.5 Letterer-Siwe disease**
Acute:
differentiated progressive histiocytosis
histiocytosis X (progressive)
infantile reticuloendotheliosis
reticulosis of infancy

Excludes *Hand-Schüller-Christian disease (277.89)*
histiocytosis (acute) (chronic) (277.89)
histiocytosis X (chronic) (277.89)

● **202.6 Malignant mast cell tumors**
Malignant:
mastocytoma
mastocytosis
Mast cell sarcoma
Systemic tissue mast cell disease

Excludes *mast cell leukemia (207.8)*

● ❑ **202.8 Other lymphomas**
Lymphoma (malignant):
NOS
diffuse

Excludes *benign lymphoma (229.0)*

● ❑ **202.9 Other and unspecified malignant neoplasms of lymphoid and histiocytic tissue**
Follicular dendritic cell sarcoma
Interdigitating dendritic cell sarcoma
Langerhans cell sarcoma
Malignant neoplasm of bone marrow NOS

● **203 Multiple myeloma and immunoproliferative neoplasms**

The following fifth-digit subclassification is for use with category 203:
0 without mention of remission
1 in remission

● **203.0 Multiple myeloma**
Kahler's disease
Myelomatosis

Excludes *solitary myeloma (238.6)*

● **203.1 Plasma cell leukemia**
Plasmacytic leukemia

● ❑ **203.8 Other immunoproliferative neoplasms**

● **204 Lymphoid leukemia**

Includes: leukemia:
lymphatic
lymphoblastic
leukemia:
lymphocytic
lymphogenous

The following fifth-digit subclassification is for use with category 204:
0 without mention of remission
1 in remission

● **204.0 Acute**

Excludes *acute exacerbation of chronic lymphoid leukemia (204.1)*

● **204.1 Chronic**

● **204.2 Subacute**

● ❑ **204.8 Other lymphoid leukemia**
Aleukemic leukemia:
lymphatic
lymphocytic
lymphoid

● ❑ **204.9 Unspecified lymphoid leukemia**

● **205 Myeloid leukemia**

Includes: leukemia:
granulocytic
myeloblastic
myelocytic
myelogenous
leukemia:
myelomonocytic
myelosclerotic
myelosis

The following fifth-digit subclassification is for use with category 205:
0 without mention of remission
1 in remission

● **205.0 Acute**
Acute promyelocytic leukemia

Excludes *acute exacerbation of chronic myeloid leukemia (205.1)*

● **205.1 Chronic**
Eosinophilic leukemia
Neutrophilic leukemia

● **205.2 Subacute**

● **205.3 Myeloid sarcoma**
Chloroma
Granulocytic sarcoma

● ❑ **205.8 Other myeloid leukemia**
Aleukemic leukemia:
granulocytic
myelogenous
myeloid
Aleukemic myelosis

● ❑ **205.9 Unspecified myeloid leukemia**

●206 **Monocytic leukemia**
Includes: leukemia:
histiocytic
monoblastic
monocytoid

The following fifth-digit subclassification is for use with category 206:
0 **without mention of remission**
1 **in remission**

●206.0 **Acute**
Excludes *acute exacerbation of chronic monocytic leukemia (206.1)*

●206.1 **Chronic**

●206.2 **Subacute**

●❑206.8 **Other monocytic leukemia**
Aleukemic:
monocytic leukemia
monocytoid leukemia

●❑206.9 **Unspecified monocytic leukemia**

●207 **Other specified leukemia**
Excludes *leukemic reticuloendotheliosis (202.4)*
plasma cell leukemia (203.1)

The following fifth-digit subclassification is for use with category 207:
0 **without mention of remission**
1 **in remission**

●207.0 **Acute erythremia and erythroleukemia**
Acute erythremic myelosis
Di Guglielmo's disease
Erythremic myelosis

●207.1 **Chronic erythremia**
Heilmeyer-Schöner disease

●207.2 **Megakaryocytic leukemia**
Megakaryocytic myelosis
Thrombocytic leukemia

●❑207.8 **Other specified leukemia**
Lymphosarcoma cell leukemia

●208 **Leukemia of unspecified cell type**
The following fifth-digit subclassification is for use with category 208:
0 **without mention of remission**
1 **in remission**

●❑208.0 **Acute**
Acute leukemia NOS
Blast cell leukemia
Stem cell leukemia
Excludes *acute exacerbation of chronic unspecified leukemia (208.1)*

●❑208.1 **Chronic**
Chronic leukemia NOS

●❑208.2 **Subacute**
Subacute leukemia NOS

●❑208.8 **Other leukemia of unspecified cell type**

●❑208.9 **Unspecified leukemia**
Leukemia NOS

BENIGN NEOPLASMS (210–229)

●210 **Benign neoplasm of lip, oral cavity, and pharynx**
Excludes *cyst (of):*
jaw (526.0–526.2, 526.89)
oral soft tissue (528.4)
radicular (522.8)

210.0 **Lip**
Frenulum labii
Lip (inner aspect) (mucosa) (vermilion border)
Excludes *labial commissure (210.4)*
skin of lip (216.0)

210.1 **Tongue**
Lingual tonsil

210.2 **Major salivary glands**
Gland:
parotid
sublingual
submandibular
Excludes *benign neoplasms of minor salivary glands:*
NOS (210.4)
buccal mucosa (210.4)
lips (210.0)
palate (hard) (soft) (210.4)
tongue (210.1)
tonsil, palatine (210.5)

210.3 **Floor of mouth**

❑210.4 **Other and unspecified parts of mouth**
Gingiva
Gum (upper) (lower)
Labial commissure
Oral cavity NOS
Oral mucosa
Palate (hard) (soft)
Uvula
Excludes *benign odontogenic neoplasms of bone (213.0–213.1)*
developmental odontogenic cysts (526.0)
mucosa of lips (210.0)
nasopharyngeal [posterior] [superior] surface of soft palate (210.7)

210.5 **Tonsil**
Tonsil (faucial) (palatine)
Excludes *lingual tonsil (210.1)*
pharyngeal tonsil (210.7)
tonsillar:
fossa (210.6)
pillars (210.6)

❑210.6 **Other parts of oropharynx**
Branchial cleft or vestiges
Epiglottis, anterior aspect
Fauces NOS
Mesopharynx NOS
Tonsillar:
fossa
pillars
Vallecula
Excludes *epiglottis:*
NOS (212.1)
suprahyoid portion (212.1)

210.7 **Nasopharynx**
Adenoid tissue
Lymphadenoid tissue
Pharyngeal tonsil
Posterior nasal septum

210.8 **Hypopharynx**
Arytenoid fold
Laryngopharynx
Postcricoid region
Pyriform fossa

❑210.9 **Pharynx, unspecified**
Throat NOS

● 211 Benign neoplasm of other parts of digestive system

Excludes *benign stromal tumors of digestive system (215.5)* ◀

211.0 Esophagus

211.1 Stomach
Body of stomach
Cardia of stomach
Fundus of stomach
Cardiac orifice
Pylorus

211.2 Duodenum, jejunum, and ileum
Small intestine NOS

Excludes *ampulla of Vater (211.5)*
ileocecal valve (211.3)

211.3 Colon
Appendix
Cecum
Ileocecal valve
Large intestine NOS

Excludes *rectosigmoid junction (211.4)*

211.4 Rectum and anal canal
Anal canal or sphincter
Anus NOS
Rectosigmoid junction

Excludes *anus:*
margin (216.5)
skin (216.5)
perianal skin (216.5)

211.5 Liver and biliary passages
Ampulla of Vater
Common bile duct
Cystic duct
Gallbladder
Hepatic duct
Sphincter of Oddi

211.6 Pancreas, except islets of Langerhans

211.7 Islets of Langerhans
Islet cell tumor

Use additional code to identify any functional activity

211.8 Retroperitoneum and peritoneum
Mesentery
Mesocolon
Omentum
Retroperitoneal tissue

❑ **211.9 Other and unspecified site**
Alimentary tract NOS
Digestive system NOS
Gastrointestinal tract NOS
Intestinal tract NOS
Intestine NOS
Spleen, not elsewhere classified

● 212 Benign neoplasm of respiratory and intrathoracic organs

212.0 Nasal cavities, middle ear, and accessory sinuses
Cartilage of nose
Eustachian tube
Nares
Septum of nose
Sinus:
ethmoidal
frontal
Sinus:
maxillary
sphenoidal

Excludes *auditory canal (external) (216.2)*
bone of:
ear (213.0)
nose [turbinates] (213.0)
cartilage of ear (215.0)
ear (external) (skin) (216.2)
nose NOS (229.8)
skin (216.3)
olfactory bulb (225.1)
polyp of:
accessory sinus (471.8)
ear (385.30–385.35)
nasal cavity (471.0)
posterior margin of septum and choanae (210.7)

212.1 Larynx
Cartilage:
arytenoid
cricoid
cuneiform
thyroid
Epiglottis (suprahyoid portion) NOS
Glottis
Vocal cords (false) (true)

Excludes *epiglottis, anterior aspect (210.6)*
polyp of vocal cord or larynx (478.4)

212.2 Trachea

212.3 Bronchus and lung
Carina
Hilus of lung

212.4 Pleura

212.5 Mediastinum

212.6 Thymus

212.7 Heart

Excludes *great vessels (215.4)*

❑ **212.8 Other specified sites**

❑ **212.9 Site unspecified**
Respiratory organ NOS
Upper respiratory tract NOS

Excludes *intrathoracic NOS (229.8)*
thoracic NOS (229.8)

● 213 Benign neoplasm of bone and articular cartilage

Includes: cartilage (articular) (joint)
periosteum

Excludes *cartilage of:*
ear (215.0)
eyelid (215.0)
larynx (212.1)
nose (212.0)
exostosis NOS (726.91)
synovia (215.0–215.9)

213.0 Bones of skull and face

Excludes *lower jaw bone (213.1)*

213.1 Lower jaw bone

213.2 Vertebral column, excluding sacrum and coccyx

213.3 Ribs, sternum, and clavicle

213.4 Scapula and long bones of upper limb

213.5 Short bones of upper limb

213.6 Pelvic bones, sacrum, and coccyx

213.7 Long bones of lower limb

213.8 Short bones of lower limb

❑ **213.9 Bone and articular cartilage, site unspecified**

● 214 Lipoma

Includes: angiolipoma
fibrolipoma
hibernoma
lipoma (fetal) (infiltrating) (intramuscular)
myelolipoma
myxolipoma

214.0 Skin and subcutaneous tissue of face

❑ **214.1 Other skin and subcutaneous tissue**

214.2 Intrathoracic organs

214.3 Intra-abdominal organs

214.4 Spermatic cord

❑ **214.8 Other specified sites**

❑ **214.9 Lipoma, unspecified site**

● **215 Other benign neoplasm of connective and other soft tissue**

Includes: blood vessel
bursa
fascia
ligament
muscle
peripheral, sympathetic, and parasympathetic nerves and ganglia
synovia
tendon (sheath)

Excludes *cartilage:*
articular (213.0–213.9)
larynx (212.1)
nose (212.0)
connective tissue of:
breast (217)
internal organ, except lipoma and hemangioma - code to benign neoplasm of the site
lipoma (214.0–214.9)

215.0 Head, face, and neck

215.2 Upper limb, including shoulder

215.3 Lower limb, including hip

215.4 Thorax

Excludes *heart (212.7)*
mediastinum (212.5)
thymus (212.6)

215.5 Abdomen
Abdominal wall
Benign stromal tumors of abdomen ◀
Hypochondrium

215.6 Pelvis
Buttock
Groin
Inguinal region
Perineum

Excludes *uterine:*
leiomyoma (218.0–218.9)
ligament, any (221.0)

❑**215.7 Trunk, unspecified**
Back NOS
Flank NOS

❑**215.8 Other specified sites**

❑**215.9 Site unspecified**

● **216 Benign neoplasm of skin**

Includes: blue nevus
dermatofibroma
hydrocystoma
pigmented nevus
syringoadenoma
syringoma

Excludes *skin of genital organs (221.0–222.9)*

216.0 Skin of lip

Excludes *vermilion border of lip (210.0)*

216.1 Eyelid, including canthus

Excludes *cartilage of eyelid (215.0)*

216.2 Ear and external auditory canal
Auricle (ear)
Auricular canal, external
External meatus
Pinna

Excludes *cartilage of ear (215.0)*

❑**216.3 Skin of other and unspecified parts of face**
Cheek, external
Eyebrow
Nose, external
Temple

216.4 Scalp and skin of neck

216.5 Skin of trunk, except scrotum
Axillary fold
Perianal skin
Skin of:
abdominal wall
anus
back
breast
buttock
Skin of:
chest wall
groin
perineum
Umbilicus

Excludes *anal canal (211.4)*
anus NOS (211.4)
skin of scrotum (222.4)

216.6 Skin of upper limb, including shoulder

216.7 Skin of lower limb, including hip

❑**216.8 Other specified sites of skin**

❑**216.9 Skin, site unspecified**

217 Benign neoplasm of breast

Note no gender difference for this code.

Breast (male) (female)
connective tissue
glandular tissue
soft parts

Excludes *adenofibrosis (610.2)*
benign cyst of breast (610.0)
fibrocystic disease (610.1)
skin of breast (216.5)

● **218 Uterine leiomyoma**

Includes: fibroid (bleeding) (uterine)
uterine:
fibromyoma
myoma

218.0 Submucous leiomyoma of uterus

218.1 Intramural leiomyoma of uterus
Interstitial leiomyoma of uterus

218.2 Subserous leiomyoma of uterus
Subperitoneal leiomyoma of uterus

❑**218.9 Leiomyoma of uterus, unspecified**

● **219 Other benign neoplasm of uterus**

219.0 Cervix uteri

219.1 Corpus uteri
Endometrium
Fundus
Myometrium

❑**219.8 Other specified parts of uterus**

❑**219.9 Uterus, part unspecified**

220 Benign neoplasm of ovary

Use additional code to identify any functional activity (256.0–256.1)

Excludes *cyst:*
corpus albicans (620.2)
corpus luteum (620.1)
endometrial (617.1)
follicular (atretic) (620.0)
graafian follicle (620.0)
ovarian NOS (620.2)
retention (620.2)

Item 2-5 Teratoma: terat = monster, oma = mass, tumor. Alternate terms: dermoid cyst of the ovary, ovarian teratoma. Teratomas arise from germ cells (ovaries in female and testes in male) and can be benign or malignant. Teratomas have been known to contain hair, nails, and teeth, giving them a bizarre ("monster") appearance.

● **221 Benign neoplasm of other female genital organs**

Includes: adenomatous polyp
benign teratoma

Excludes *cyst:*
epoophoron (752.11)
fimbrial (752.11)
Gartner's duct (752.11)
parovarian (752.11)

221.0 Fallopian tube and uterine ligaments
Oviduct
Parametrium
Uterine ligament (broad) (round) (uterosacral)
Uterine tube

221.1 Vagina

221.2 Vulva
Clitoris
External female genitalia NOS
Greater vestibular [Bartholin's] gland
Labia (majora) (minora)
Pudendum

Excludes *Bartholin's (duct) (gland) cyst (616.2)*

❑ **221.8 Other specified sites of female genital organs**

❑ **221.9 Female genital organ, site unspecified**
Female genitourinary tract NOS

● **222 Benign neoplasm of male genital organs**

222.0 Testis

Use additional code to identify any functional activity

222.1 Penis
Corpus cavernosum
Glans penis
Prepuce

222.2 Prostate

Excludes *adenomatous hyperplasia of prostate (600.20–600.21)*
prostatic:
adenoma (600.20–600.21)
enlargement (600.00–600.01)
hypertrophy (600.00–600.01)

222.3 Epididymis

222.4 Scrotum
Skin of scrotum

❑ **222.8 Other specified sites of male genital organs**
Seminal vesicle
Spermatic cord

❑ **222.9 Male genital organ, site unspecified**
Male genitourinary tract NOS

● **223 Benign neoplasm of kidney and other urinary organs**

223.0 Kidney, except pelvis
Kidney NOS

Excludes *renal:*
calyces (223.1)
pelvis (223.1)

223.1 Renal pelvis

223.2 Ureter

Excludes *ureteric orifice of bladder (223.3)*

223.3 Bladder

● **223.8 Other specified sites of urinary organs**

223.81 Urethra

Excludes *urethral orifice of bladder (223.3)*

❑ **223.89 Other**
Paraurethral glands

❑ **223.9 Urinary organ, site unspecified**
Urinary system NOS

● **224 Benign neoplasm of eye**

Excludes *cartilage of eyelid (215.0)*
eyelid (skin) (216.1)
optic nerve (225.1)
orbital bone (213.0)

224.0 Eyeball, except conjunctiva, cornea, retina, and choroid
Ciliary body
Iris
Sclera
Uveal tract

224.1 Orbit

Excludes *bone of orbit (213.0)*

224.2 Lacrimal gland

224.3 Conjunctiva

224.4 Cornea

224.5 Retina

Excludes *hemangioma of retina (228.03)*

224.6 Choroid

224.7 Lacrimal duct
Lacrimal sac
Nasolacrimal duct

❑ **224.8 Other specified parts of eye**

❑ **224.9 Eye, part unspecified**

● **225 Benign neoplasm of brain and other parts of nervous system**

Excludes *hemangioma (228.02)*
neurofibromatosis (237.7)
peripheral, sympathetic, and parasympathetic nerves and ganglia (215.0–215.9)
retrobulbar (224.1)

225.0 Brain

225.1 Cranial nerves

225.2 Cerebral meninges
Meninges NOS
Meningioma (cerebral)

225.3 Spinal cord
Cauda equina

225.4 Spinal meninges
Spinal meningioma

❑ **225.8 Other specified sites of nervous system**

❑ **225.9 Nervous system, part unspecified**
Nervous system (central) NOS

Excludes *meninges NOS (225.2)*

226 Benign neoplasm of thyroid glands

Use additional code to identify any functional activity

● **227 Benign neoplasm of other endocrine glands and related structures**

Use additional code to identify any functional activity

Excludes *ovary (220)*
pancreas (211.6)
testis (222.0)

227.0 Adrenal gland
Suprarenal gland

227.1 Parathyroid gland

227.3 Pituitary gland and craniopharyngeal duct (pouch)
Craniobuccal pouch
Hypophysis
Rathke's pouch
Sella turcica

227.4 Pineal gland
Pineal body

227.5 Carotid body

227.6 **Aortic body and other paraganglia**
Coccygeal body
Glomus jugulare
Para-aortic body

❑227.8 **Other**

❑227.9 **Endocrine gland, site unspecified**

● 228 **Hemangioma and lymphangioma, any site**

Includes: angioma (benign) (cavernous) (congenital) NOS
cavernous nevus
glomus tumor
hemangioma (benign) (congenital)

Excludes *benign neoplasm of spleen, except hemangioma and lymphangioma (211.9)*
glomus jugulare (227.6)
nevus:
NOS (216.0–216.9)
blue or pigmented (216.0–216.9)
vascular (757.32)

● 228.0 **Hemangioma, any site**

❑228.00 **Of unspecified site**

228.01 **Of skin and subcutaneous tissue**

228.02 **Of intracranial structures**

228.03 **Of retina**

228.04 **Of intra-abdominal structures**
Peritoneum
Retroperitoneal tissue

❑228.09 **Of other sites**
Systemic angiomatosis

228.1 **Lymphangioma, any site**
Congenital lymphangioma
Lymphatic nevus

● 229 **Benign neoplasm of other and unspecified sites**

229.0 **Lymph nodes**

Excludes *lymphangioma (228.1)*

❑229.8 **Other specified sites**
Intrathoracic NOS
Thoracic NOS

❑229.9 **Site unspecified**

CARCINOMA IN SITU (230–234)

Includes: Bowen's disease
erythroplasia
Queyrat's erythroplasia

Excludes *leukoplakia - see Alphabetic Index*

● 230 **Carcinoma in situ of digestive organs**

230.0 **Lip, oral cavity, and pharynx**
Gingiva
Hypopharynx
Mouth [any part]
Nasopharynx
Oropharynx
Salivary gland or duct
Tongue

Excludes *aryepiglottic fold or interarytenoid fold, laryngeal aspect (231.0)*
epiglottis:
NOS (231.0)
suprahyoid portion (231.0)
skin of lip (232.0)

230.1 **Esophagus**

230.2 **Stomach**
Body of stomach
Cardia of stomach
Fundus of stomach
Cardiac orifice
Pylorus

230.3 **Colon**
Appendix
Cecum
Ileocecal valve
Large intestine NOS

Excludes *rectosigmoid junction (230.4)*

230.4 **Rectum**
Rectosigmoid junction

230.5 **Anal canal**
Anal sphincter

❑230.6 **Anus, unspecified**

Excludes *anus:*
margin (232.5)
skin (232.5)
perianal skin (232.5)

❑230.7 **Other and unspecified parts of intestine**
Duodenum
Ileum
Jejunum
Small intestine NOS

Excludes *ampulla of Vater (230.8)*

230.8 **Liver and biliary system**
Ampulla of Vater
Common bile duct
Cystic duct
Gallbladder
Hepatic duct
Sphincter of Oddi

❑230.9 **Other and unspecified digestive organs**
Digestive organ NOS
Gastrointestinal tract NOS
Pancreas
Spleen

● 231 **Carcinoma in situ of respiratory system**

231.0 **Larynx**
Cartilage:
arytenoid
cricoid
cuneiform
thyroid
Epiglottis:
NOS
posterior surface
suprahyoid portion
Vocal cords (false) (true)

Excludes *aryepiglottic fold or interarytenoid fold:*
NOS (230.0)
hypopharyngeal aspect (230.0)
marginal zone (230.0)

231.1 **Trachea**

231.2 **Bronchus and lung**
Carina
Hilus of lung

❑231.8 **Other specified parts of respiratory system**
Accessory sinuses
Middle ear
Nasal cavities
Pleura

Excludes *ear (external) (skin) (232.2)*
nose NOS (234.8)
skin (232.3)

❑231.9 **Respiratory system, part unspecified**
Respiratory organ NOS

● 232 **Carcinoma in situ of skin**

Includes: pigment cells

232.0 **Skin of lip**

Excludes *vermilion border of lip (230.0)*

232.1 **Eyelid, including canthus**

232.2 **Ear and external auditory canal**

❑232.3 **Skin of other and unspecified parts of face**

232.4 **Scalp and skin of neck**

232.5 **Skin of trunk, except scrotum**

Anus, margin
Axillary fold
Perianal skin
Skin of:
abdominal wall
anus
back
Skin of:
breast
buttock
chest wall
groin
perineum
Umbilicus

Excludes *anal canal (230.5)*
anus NOS (230.6)
skin of genital organs (233.3, 233.5–233.6)

232.6 **Skin of upper limb, including shoulder**

232.7 **Skin of lower limb, including hip**

❑232.8 **Other specified sites of skin**

❑232.9 **Skin, site unspecified**

● 233 **Carcinoma in situ of breast and genitourinary system**

This category incorporates specific male and female genitourinary designations (233.0–233.6), while codes 233.7 and 233.9 apply to either male or female organs.

233.0 **Breast**

Excludes *Paget's disease (174.0–174.9)*
skin of breast (232.5)

233.1 **Cervix uteri**

Cervical intraepithelial glandular neoplasia ◀
Cervical intraepithelial neoplasia III [CIN III]
Severe dysplasia of cervix

Excludes *cervical intraepithelial neoplasia II [CIN II] (622.12)*
cytologic evidence of malignancy without histologic confirmation (795.06)
high grade squamous intraepithelial lesion (HGSIL) (795.04)
moderate dysplasia of cervix (622.12)

❑233.2 **Other and unspecified parts of uterus**

❑233.3 **Other and unspecified female genital organs**

233.4 **Prostate**

233.5 **Penis**

❑233.6 **Other and unspecified male genital organs**

233.7 **Bladder**

❑233.9 **Other and unspecified urinary organs**

● 234 **Carcinoma in situ of other and unspecified sites**

234.0 **Eye**

Excludes *cartilage of eyelid (234.8)*
eyelid (skin) (232.1)
optic nerve (234.8)
orbital bone (234.8)

❑234.8 **Other specified sites**

Endocrine gland [any]

❑234.9 **Site unspecified**

Carcinoma in situ NOS

NEOPLASMS OF UNCERTAIN BEHAVIOR (235–238)

Note: Categories 235–238 classify by site certain histomorphologically well-defined neoplasms, the subsequent behavior of which cannot be predicted from the present appearance.

● 235 **Neoplasm of uncertain behavior of digestive and respiratory systems**

Excludes *stromal tumors of uncertain behavior of digestive system (238.1)* ◀

235.0 **Major salivary glands**

Gland:
parotid
sublingual
submandibular

Excludes *minor salivary glands (235.1)*

235.1 **Lip, oral cavity, and pharynx**

Gingiva
Hypopharynx
Minor salivary glands
Mouth
Nasopharynx
Oropharynx
Tongue

Excludes *aryepiglottic fold or interarytenoid fold, laryngeal aspect (235.6)*
epiglottis:
NOS (235.6)
suprahyoid portion (235.6)
skin of lip (238.2)

235.2 **Stomach, intestines, and rectum**

235.3 **Liver and biliary passages**

Ampulla of Vater
Bile ducts [any]
Gallbladder
Liver

235.4 **Retroperitoneum and peritoneum**

❑235.5 **Other and unspecified digestive organs**

Anal:
canal
sphincter
Anus NOS
Esophagus
Pancreas
Spleen

Excludes *anus:*
margin (238.2)
skin (238.2)
perianal skin (238.2)

235.6 **Larynx**

Excludes *aryepiglottic fold or interarytenoid fold:*
NOS (235.1)
hypopharyngeal aspect (235.1)
marginal zone (235.1)

235.7 **Trachea, bronchus, and lung**

235.8 **Pleura, thymus, and mediastinum**

❑235.9 **Other and unspecified respiratory organs**

Accessory sinuses
Middle ear
Nasal cavities
Respiratory organ NOS

Excludes *ear (external) (skin) (238.2)*
nose (238.8)
skin (238.2)

● 236 **Neoplasm of uncertain behavior of genitourinary organs**

236.0 **Uterus**

236.1 **Placenta**

Chorioadenoma (destruens)
Invasive mole
Malignant hydatid(iform) mole

236.2 **Ovary**

Use additional code to identify any functional activity

❑236.3 **Other and unspecified female genital organs**

236.4 **Testis**

Use additional code to identify any functional activity

236.5 **Prostate**

❑236.6 **Other and unspecified male genital organs**

236.7 **Bladder**

● 236.9 **Other and unspecified urinary organs**

❑236.90 **Urinary organ, unspecified**

236.91 Kidney and ureter

❑236.99 Other

● 237 **Neoplasm of uncertain behavior of endocrine glands and nervous system**

237.0 **Pituitary gland and craniopharyngeal duct**

Use additional code to identify any functional activity

237.1 **Pineal gland**

237.2 **Adrenal gland**

Suprarenal gland

Use additional code to identify any functional activity

The adrenal glands are actually a pair of glands, as one is situated on top of or above each kidney ("suprarenal").

237.3 **Paraganglia**

Aortic body
Carotid body
Coccygeal body
Glomus jugulare

❑237.4 **Other and unspecified endocrine glands**

Parathyroid gland
Thyroid gland

237.5 **Brain and spinal cord**

237.6 **Meninges**

Meninges:
NOS
cerebral
spinal

● 237.7 **Neurofibromatosis**

von Recklinghausen's disease

❑237.70 **Neurofibromatosis, unspecified**

237.71 **Neurofibromatosis, type 1 [von Recklinghausen's disease]**

237.72 **Neurofibromatosis, type 2 [acoustic neurofibromatosis]**

❑237.9 **Other and unspecified parts of nervous system**

Cranial nerves

Excludes *peripheral, sympathetic, and parasympathetic nerves and ganglia (238.1)*

● 238 **Neoplasm of uncertain behavior of other and unspecified sites and tissues**

238.0 **Bone and articular cartilage**

Excludes *cartilage:*
ear (238.1)
eyelid (238.1)
larynx (235.6)
nose (235.9)
synovia (238.1)

❑238.1 **Connective and other soft tissue**

Peripheral, sympathetic, and parasympathetic nerves and ganglia
Stromal tumors of digestive system ◄

Excludes *cartilage (of):*
articular (238.0)
larynx (235.6)
nose (235.9)
connective tissue of breast (238.3)

238.2 **Skin**

Excludes *anus NOS (235.5)*
skin of genital organs (236.3, 236.6)
vermilion border of lip (235.1)

238.3 **Breast**

Excludes *skin of breast (238.2)*

238.4 **Polycythemia vera**

Primary polycythemia. Secondary polycythemia is 289.0. Check your documentation. Polycythemia is caused by too many red blood cells, which increase the thickness of blood (viscosity). This can cause engorgement of the spleen (splenomegaly) with extra RBCs and potential clot formation.

238.5 **Histiocytic and mast cells**

Mast cell tumor NOS
Mastocytoma NOS

238.6 **Plasma cells**

Plasmacytoma NOS
Solitary myeloma

● 238.7 **Other lymphatic and hematopoietic tissues** ⬅

Excludes *acute myelogenous leukemia (205.0)* ◄
chronic myelomonocytic leukemia (205.1) ◄
myelofibrosis (289.83) ⬅
myelosclerosis NOS (289.89)
myelosis:
NOS (205.9)
megakaryocytic (207.2)

238.71 **Essential thrombocythemia** ◄

Essential hemorrhagic thrombocythemia ◄
Essential thrombocytosis ◄
Idiopathic (hemorrhagic) thrombocythemia ◄
Primary thrombocytosis ◄

238.72 **Low grade myelodysplastic syndrome lesions** ◄

Refractory anemia (RA) ◄
Refractory anemia with ringed sideroblasts (RARS) ◄
Refractory cytopenia with multilineage dysplasia (RCMD) ◄
Refractory cytopenia with multilineage dysplasia and ringed sideroblasts (RCMD-RS) ◄

238.73 **High grade myelodysplastic syndrome lesions** ◄

Refractory anemia with excess blasts-1 (RAEB-1) ◄
Refractory anemia with excess blasts-2 (RAEB-2) ◄

238.74 **Myelodysplastic syndrome with 5q deletion** ◄

5q minus syndrome NOS ◄

Excludes *constitutional 5q deletion (758.39)* ◄
high grade myelodysplastic syndrome with 5q deletion (238.73) ◄

238.75 **Myelodysplastic syndrome, unspecified** ◄

238.76 **Myelofibrosis with myeloid metaplasia** ◄

Agnogenic myeloid metaplasia ◄
Idiopathic myelofibrosis (chronic) ◄
Myelosclerosis with myeloid metaplasia ◄
Primary myelofibrosis ◄

Excludes *myelofibrosis NOS (289.83)* ◄
myelophthisic anemia (284.2) ◄
myelophthisis (284.2) ◄
secondary myelofibrosis (289.83) ◄

❑238.79 **Other lymphatic and hematopoietic tissues** ◄

Lymphoproliferative disease (chronic) NOS ◄
Megakaryocytic myelosclerosis ◄
Myeloproliferative disease (chronic) NOS ◄
Panmyelosis (acute) ◄

❑238.8 **Other specified sites**

Eye
Heart

Excludes *eyelid (skin) (238.2)*
cartilage (238.1)

❑238.9 **Site unspecified**

NEOPLASMS OF UNSPECIFIED NATURE (239)

● **239 Neoplasms of unspecified nature**

Note: Category 239 classifies by site neoplasms of unspecified morphology and behavior. The term "mass," unless otherwise stated, is not to be regarded as a neoplastic growth.

Includes: "growth" NOS
neoplasm NOS
new growth NOS
tumor NOS

❑ **239.0 Digestive system**

Excludes *anus:*
margin (239.2)
skin (239.2)
perianal skin (239.2)

❑ **239.1 Respiratory system**

❑ **239.2 Bone, soft tissue, and skin**

Excludes *anal canal (239.0)*
anus NOS (239.0)
bone marrow (202.9)
cartilage:
larynx (239.1)
nose (239.1)
connective tissue of breast (239.3)
skin of genital organs (239.5)
vermilion border of lip (239.0)

❑ **239.3 Breast**

Excludes *skin of breast (239.2)*

❑ **239.4 Bladder**

❑ **239.5 Other genitourinary organs**

❑ **239.6 Brain**

Excludes *cerebral meninges (239.7)*
cranial nerves (239.7)

❑ **239.7 Endocrine glands and other parts of nervous system**

Excludes *peripheral, sympathetic, and parasympathetic nerves and ganglia (239.2)*

❑ **239.8 Other specified sites**

Excludes *eyelid (skin) (239.2)*
cartilage (239.2)
great vessels (239.2)
optic nerve (239.7)

❑ **239.9 Site unspecified**

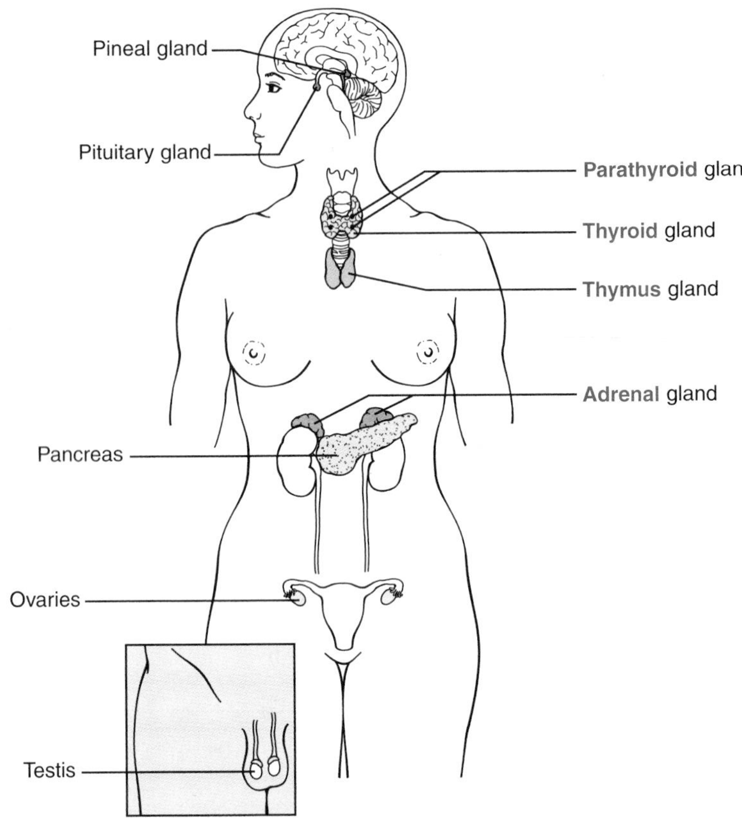
Pineal gland
Pituitary gland
Parathyroid gland
Thyroid gland
Thymus gland
Adrenal gland
Pancreas
Ovaries
Testis

Figure 3–1 The endocrine system. (From Buck CJ: Step-by-Step Medical Coding, 2005 ed. Philadelphia, WB Saunders, 2005.)

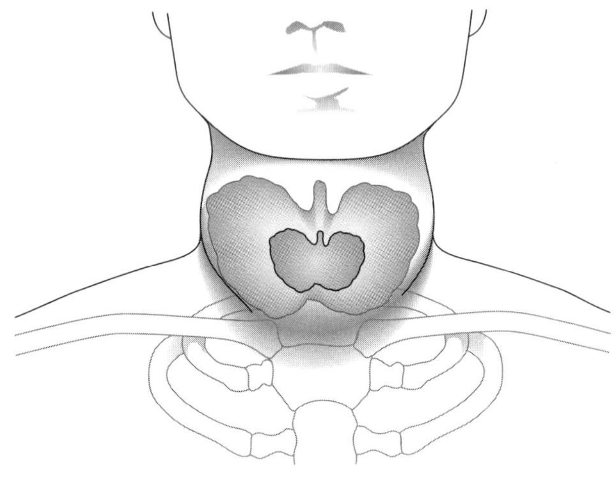

Figure 3–2 **Goiter** is an enlargement of the thyroid gland.

Item 3–1 Simple indicates no nodules are present. The most common type of goiter is a diffuse colloidal, also called a nontoxic or endemic goiter. Goiters classifiable to 240.0 or 240.9 are those goiters without mention of nodules.

3. ENDOCRINE, NUTRITIONAL AND METABOLIC DISEASES, AND IMMUNITY DISORDERS (240–279)

Excludes *endocrine and metabolic disturbances specific to the fetus and newborn (775.0–775.9)*

Note: All neoplasms, whether functionally active or not, are classified in Chapter 2. Codes in Chapter 3 (i.e., 242.8, 246.0, 251–253, 255–259) may be used to identify such functional activity associated with any neoplasm, or by ectopic endocrine tissue.

DISORDERS OF THYROID GLAND (240–246)

● **240 Simple and unspecified goiter**

240.0 Goiter, specified as simple
Any condition classifiable to 240.9, specified as simple

❑ **240.9 Goiter, unspecified**
Enlargement of thyroid
Goiter or struma:
NOS
diffuse colloid
endemic
Goiter or struma:
hyperplastic
nontoxic (diffuse)
parenchymatous
sporadic

Excludes *congenital (dyshormonogenic) goiter (246.1)*

● **241 Nontoxic nodular goiter**

Excludes *adenoma of thyroid (226)*
cystadenoma of thyroid (226)

241.0 Nontoxic uninodular goiter
Thyroid nodule
Uninodular goiter (nontoxic)

241.1 Nontoxic multinodular goiter
Multinodular goiter (nontoxic)

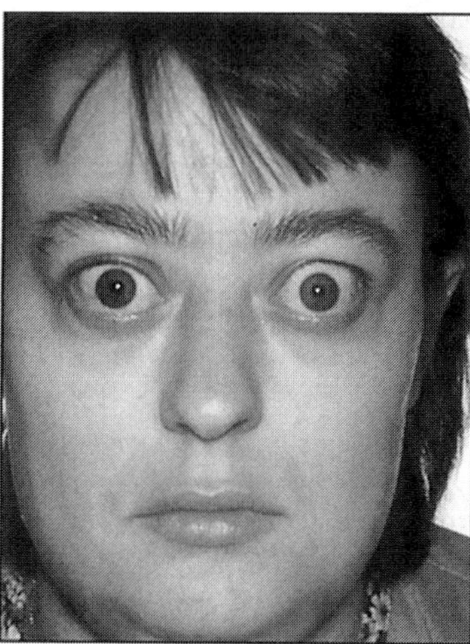

Figure 3–3 The characteristic protruding eyeballs **(exophthalmos)** of the patient with **Graves' disease.** (From Mir MA: Atlas of Clinical Diagnosis. Philadelphia, WB Saunders, 1995, p. 14.)

❑241.9 **Unspecified nontoxic nodular goiter**
Adenomatous goiter
Nodular goiter (nontoxic) NOS
Struma nodosa (simplex)

Item 3-2 Thyrotoxicosis is a condition caused by excessive amounts of the thyroid hormone thyroxine. The condition is also called hyperthyroidism. Graves' disease is associated with hyperthyroidism (known as Basedow's disease in Europe).

● 242 **Thyrotoxicosis with or without goiter**
Excludes *neonatal thyrotoxicosis (775.3)*
The following fifth-digit subclassification is for use with category 242:
0 **without mention of thyrotoxic crisis or storm**
1 **with mention of thyrotoxic crisis or storm**

● 242.0 **Toxic diffuse goiter**
Basedow's disease
Exophthalmic or toxic goiter NOS
Graves' disease
Primary thyroid hyperplasia

● 242.1 **Toxic uninodular goiter**
Thyroid nodule, toxic or with hyperthyroidism
Uninodular goiter, toxic or with hyperthyroidism

● 242.2 **Toxic multinodular goiter**
Secondary thyroid hyperplasia

● ❑242.3 **Toxic nodular goiter, unspecified**
Adenomatous goiter, toxic or with hyperthyroidism
Nodular goiter, toxic or with hyperthyroidism
Struma nodosa, toxic or with hyperthyroidism
Any condition classifiable to 241.9 specified as toxic or with hyperthyroidism

● 242.4 **Thyrotoxicosis from ectopic thyroid nodule**

● ❑242.8 **Thyrotoxicosis of other specified origin**
Overproduction of thyroid-stimulating hormone [TSH]
Thyrotoxicosis:
factitia from ingestion of excessive thyroid material
Use additional E code to identify cause, if drug-induced

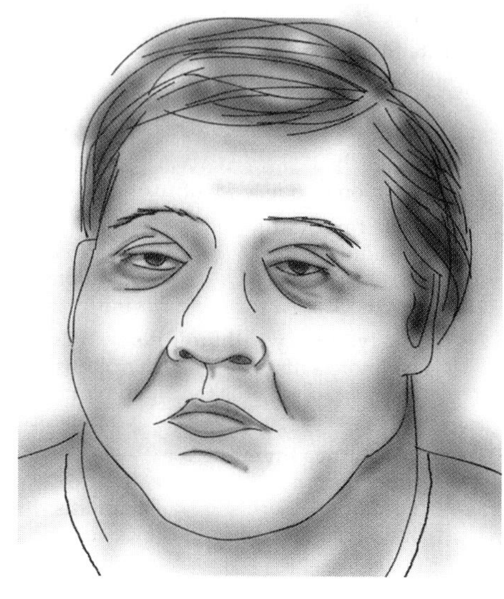

Figure 3–4 Myxedema is severe hypothyroidism.

● ❑242.9 **Thyrotoxicosis without mention of goiter or other cause**
Hyperthyroidism NOS
Thyrotoxicosis NOS
Thyrotoxicosis is also listed under "thyroid storm" in the Index.

ICD-9-CM 200-299 Vol. 1

Item 3-3 Hypothyroidism is a condition in which there are insufficient levels of thyroxine.
Cretinism is congenital hypothyroidism, which can result in mental and physical retardation.

243 **Congenital hypothyroidism**
Congenital thyroid insufficiency
Cretinism (athyrotic) (endemic)
Use additional code to identify associated mental retardation
Excludes *congenital (dyshormonogenic) goiter (246.1)*

● 244 **Acquired hypothyroidism**
Includes: athyroidism (acquired)
hypothyroidism (acquired)
myxedema (adult) (juvenile)
thyroid (gland) insufficiency (acquired)

244.0 **Postsurgical hypothyroidism**

❑244.1 **Other postablative hypothyroidism**
Hypothyroidism following therapy, such as irradiation

244.2 **Iodine hypothyroidism**
Hypothyroidism resulting from administration or ingestion of iodide
Use additional E code to identify drug

❑244.3 **Other iatrogenic hypothyroidism**
Hypothyroidism resulting from:
P-aminosalicylic acid [PAS]
Phenylbutazone
Resorcinol
Iatrogenic hypothyroidism NOS
Use additional E code to identify drug

❑244.8 **Other specified acquired hypothyroidism**
Secondary hypothyroidism NEC

❑244.9 **Unspecified hypothyroidism**
Hypothyroidism, primary or NOS
Myxedema, primary or NOS

● 245 **Thyroiditis**

245.0 **Acute thyroiditis**
Abscess of thyroid
Thyroiditis:
nonsuppurative, acute
pyogenic
Thyroiditis:
suppurative
Use additional code to identify organism

245.1 **Subacute thyroiditis**
Thyroiditis:
de Quervain's
giant cell
Thyroiditis:
granulomatous
viral

245.2 **Chronic lymphocytic thyroiditis**
Hashimoto's disease
Struma lymphomatosa
Thyroiditis:
autoimmune
lymphocytic (chronic)

245.3 **Chronic fibrous thyroiditis**
Struma fibrosa
Thyroiditis:
invasive (fibrous)
ligneous
Thyroiditis:
Riedel's

245.4 **Iatrogenic thyroiditis**
Use additional E to identify cause

❑245.8 **Other and unspecified chronic thyroiditis**
Chronic thyroiditis:
NOS
nonspecific

❑245.9 **Thyroiditis, unspecified**
Thyroiditis NOS

● 246 **Other disorders of thyroid**

246.0 **Disorders of thyrocalcitonin secretion**
Hypersecretion of calcitonin or thyrocalcitonin

246.1 **Dyshormonogenic goiter**
Congenital (dyshormonogenic) goiter
Goiter due to enzyme defect in synthesis of thyroid hormone
Goitrous cretinism (sporadic)

246.2 **Cyst of thyroid**
Excludes *cystadenoma of thyroid (226)*

246.3 **Hemorrhage and infarction of thyroid**

❑246.8 **Other specified disorders of thyroid**
Abnormality of thyroid-binding globulin
Atrophy of thyroid
Hyper-TBG-nemia
Hypo-TBG-nemia

❑246.9 **Unspecified disorder of thyroid**

DISEASES OF OTHER ENDOCRINE GLANDS (250–259)

● 250 **Diabetes mellitus**
Excludes *gestational diabetes (648.8)*
hyperglycemia NOS (790.6)
neonatal diabetes mellitus (775.1)
nonclinical diabetes (790.29)

The following fifth-digit subclassification is for use with category 250:
0 **type II or unspecified type, not stated as uncontrolled**
Fifth-digit 0 is for use for type II patients, even if the patient requires insulin
Use additional code, if applicable, for associated long-term (current) insulin use V58.67
1 **type I [juvenile type], not stated as uncontrolled**
2 **type II or unspecified type, uncontrolled**
Fifth-digit 2 is for use for type II patients, even if the patient requires insulin
Use additional code, if applicable, for associated long-term (current) insulin use V58.67
3 **type I [juvenile type], uncontrolled**

● 250.0 **Diabetes mellitus without mention of complication**
Diabetes mellitus without mention of complication or manifestation classifiable to 250.1–250.9
Diabetes (mellitus) NOS

● 250.1 **Diabetes with ketoacidosis**
Diabetic:
acidosis without mention of coma
ketosis without mention of coma

● 250.2 **Diabetes with hyperosmolarity**
Hyperosmolar (nonketotic) coma

● 250.3 **Diabetes with other coma**
Diabetic coma (with ketoacidosis)
Diabetic hypoglycemic coma
Insulin coma NOS
Excludes *diabetes with hyperosmolar coma (250.2)*

● 250.4 **Diabetes with renal manifestations**
Use additional code to identify manifestation, as:
chronic kidney disease (585.1–585.9) diabetic:
nephropathy NOS (583.81)
nephrosis (581.81)
intercapillary glomerulosclerosis (581.81)
Kimmelstiel-Wilson syndrome (581.81)

● 250.5 **Diabetes with ophthalmic manifestations**
Use additional code to identify manifestation, as:
diabetic:
blindness (369.00–369.9)
cataract (366.41)
glaucoma (365.44)
macular edema (362.07)
retinal edema (362.07)
retinopathy (362.01–362.07)

● 250.6 **Diabetes with neurological manifestations**
Use additional code to identify manifestation, as:
diabetic:
amyotrophy (358.1)
gastroparalysis (536.3)
gastroparesis (536.3)
mononeuropathy (354.0–355.9)
neurogenic arthropathy (713.5)
peripheral autonomic neuropathy (337.1)
polyneuropathy (357.2)

● 250.7 **Diabetes with peripheral circulatory disorders**
Use additional code to identify manifestation, as:
diabetic:
gangrene (785.4)
peripheral angiopathy (443.81)

● ❑250.8 **Diabetes with other specified manifestations**
Diabetic hypoglycemia
Hypoglycemic shock
Use additional code to identify manifestation, as:
any associated ulceration (707.10–707.9)
diabetic bone changes (731.8)
Use additional E code to identify cause, if drug-induced

● ❑250.9 **Diabetes with unspecified complication**

● 251 **Other disorders of pancreatic internal secretion**

251.0 **Hypoglycemic coma**
Iatrogenic hyperinsulinism
Non-diabetic insulin coma
Use additional E code to identify cause, if drug-induced
Excludes *hypoglycemic coma in diabetes mellitus (250.3)*

❑251.1 **Other specified hypoglycemia**
Hyperinsulinism:
NOS
ectopic
functional
Hyperplasia of pancreatic islet beta cells NOS
Use additional E code to identify cause, if drug-induced
Excludes *hypoglycemia in diabetes mellitus (250.8)*
hypoglycemia in infant of diabetic mother (775.0)
hypoglycemic coma (251.0)
neonatal hypoglycemia (775.6)

❑251.2 **Hypoglycemia, unspecified**
Hypoglycemia:
NOS
reactive
spontaneous
Excludes *hypoglycemia:*
with coma (251.0)
in diabetes mellitus (250.8)
leucine-induced (270.3)

251.3 **Postsurgical hypoinsulinemia**
Hypoinsulinemia following complete or partial pancreatectomy
Postpancreatectomy hyperglycemia

251.4 **Abnormality of secretion of glucagon**
Hyperplasia of pancreatic islet alpha cells with glucagon excess

251.5 **Abnormality of secretion of gastrin**
Hyperplasia of pancreatic alpha cells with gastrin excess
Zollinger-Ellison syndrome

❑251.8 **Other specified disorders of pancreatic internal secretion**

❑251.9 **Unspecified disorder of pancreatic internal secretion**
Islet cell hyperplasia NOS

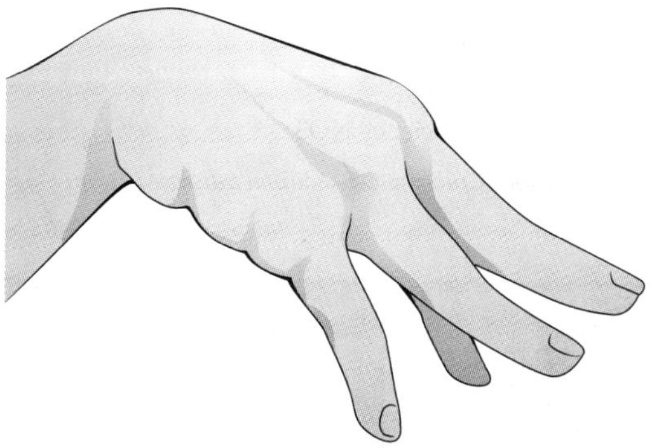

Figure 3–5 Tetany caused by hypoparathyroidism.

Item 3–4 Hyperparathyroidism is an overactive parathyroid gland that secretes excessive parathormone, causing increased levels of circulating calcium. This results in a loss of calcium in the bone.
Hypoparathyroidism is an underactive parathyroid gland that results in decreased levels of circulating calcium. The primary manifestation is tetany, a continuous muscle spasm.

● 252 **Disorders of parathyroid gland**

● 252.0 **Hyperparathyroidism**
Excludes *ectopic hyperparathyroidism (259.3)*

❑252.00 **Hyperparathyroidism, unspecified**

252.01 **Primary hyperparathyroidism**
Hyperplasia of parathyroid

252.02 **Secondary hyperparathyroidism, non-renal**
Excludes *secondary hyperparathyroidism (of renal origin) (588.81)*

252.08 **Other hyperparathyroidism**
Tertiary hyperparathyroidism

252.1 **Hypoparathyroidism**
Parathyroiditis (autoimmune)
Tetany:
parathyroid
parathyroprival
Excludes *pseudohypoparathyroidism (275.49)*
pseudopseudohypoparathyroidism (275.49)
tetany NOS (781.7)
transitory neonatal hypoparathyroidism (775.4)

❑252.8 **Other specified disorders of parathyroid gland**
Cyst of parathyroid gland
Hemorrhage of parathyroid gland

❑252.9 **Unspecified disorder of parathyroid gland**

● 253 **Disorders of the pituitary gland and its hypothalamic control**
Includes: the listed conditions whether the disorder is in the pituitary or the hypothalamus
Excludes *Cushing's syndrome (255.0)*

253.0 **Acromegaly and gigantism**
Overproduction of growth hormone

❑253.1 **Other and unspecified anterior pituitary hyperfunction**
Forbes-Albright syndrome
Excludes *overproduction of:*
ACTH (255.3)
thyroid-stimulating hormone [TSH] (242.8)

253.2 **Panhypopituitarism**
Cachexia, pituitary
Necrosis of pituitary (postpartum)
Pituitary insufficiency NOS
Sheehan's syndrome
Simmonds' disease
Excludes *iatrogenic hypopituitarism (253.7)*

253.3 **Pituitary dwarfism**
Isolated deficiency of (human) growth hormone [HGH]
Lorain-Levi dwarfism

❑253.4 **Other anterior pituitary disorders**
Isolated or partial deficiency of an anterior pituitary hormone, other than growth hormone
Prolactin deficiency

253.5 **Diabetes insipidus**
Vasopressin deficiency
Excludes *nephrogenic diabetes insipidus (588.1)*

❑253.6 **Other disorders of neurohypophysis**
Syndrome of inappropriate secretion of antidiuretic hormone [ADH]
Excludes *ectopic antidiuretic hormone secretion (259.3)*

253.7 **Iatrogenic pituitary disorders**
Hypopituitarism:
hormone-induced
hypophysectomy-induced
postablative
radiotherapy-induced
Use additional E code to identify cause

❑253.8 **Other disorders of the pituitary and other syndromes of diencephalohypophyseal origin**
Abscess of pituitary
Adiposogenital dystrophy
Cyst of Rathke's pouch
Fröhlich's syndrome
Excludes *craniopharyngioma (237.0)*

ICD-9-CM 200-299 Vol. 1

❑253.9 **Unspecified**
Dyspituitarism

● 254 **Diseases of thymus gland**

Excludes *aplasia or dysplasia with immunodeficiency (279.2)*
hypoplasia with immunodeficiency (279.2)
myasthenia gravis (358.00–358.01)

254.0 **Persistent hyperplasia of thymus**
Hypertrophy of thymus

254.1 **Abscess of thymus**

❑254.8 **Other specified diseases of thymus gland**
Atrophy of thymus
Cyst of thymus

Excludes *thymoma (212.6)*

❑254.9 **Unspecified disease of thymus gland**

Item 3-5 Hyperadrenalism is overactivity of the adrenal cortex, which secretes a variety of hormones. Excessive glucocorticoid hormone results in hyperglycemia (Cushing's syndrome), and excessive aldosterone results in Conn's syndrome. Adrenogenital syndrome is the result of excessive secretion of androgens, male hormones, which stimulates premature sexual development. Hypoadrenalism, Addison's disease, is a condition in which the adrenal glands atrophy.

● 255 **Disorders of adrenal glands**

Includes: the listed conditions whether the basic disorder is in the adrenals or is pituitary-induced

255.0 **Cushing's syndrome**
Adrenal hyperplasia due to excess ACTH
Cushing's syndrome:
NOS
iatrogenic
idiopathic
pituitary-dependent
Ectopic ACTH syndrome
Iatrogenic syndrome of excess cortisol
Overproduction of cortisol

Use additional E code to identify cause, if drug-induced

Excludes *congenital adrenal hyperplasia (255.2)*

● 255.1 **Hyperaldosteronism**

255.10 **Hyperaldosteronism, unspecified** ⇐
Aldosteronism NOS
Primary aldosteronism, unspecified ◀

Excludes *Conn's syndrome (255.12)*

255.11 **Glucocorticoid-remediable aldosteronism**
Familial aldosteronism type I

Excludes *Conn's syndrome (255.12)*

255.12 **Conn's syndrome**

255.13 **Bartter's syndrome**

❑255.14 **Other secondary aldosteronism**

255.2 **Adrenogenital disorders**
Achard-Thiers syndrome
Adrenogenital syndromes, virilizing or feminizing, whether acquired or associated with congenital adrenal hyperplasia consequent on inborn enzyme defects in hormone synthesis
Congenital adrenal hyperplasia
Female adrenal pseudohermaphroditism
Male:
macrogenitosomia praecox
sexual precocity with adrenal hyperplasia
Virilization (female) (suprarenal)

Excludes *adrenal hyperplasia due to excess ACTH (255.0)*
isosexual virilization (256.4)

❑255.3 **Other corticoadrenal overactivity**
Acquired benign adrenal androgenic overactivity
Overproduction of ACTH

255.4 **Corticoadrenal insufficiency**
Addisonian crisis
Addison's disease NOS
Adrenal:
atrophy (autoimmune)
calcification
crisis
hemorrhage
infarction
insufficiency NOS

Excludes *tuberculous Addison's disease (017.6)*

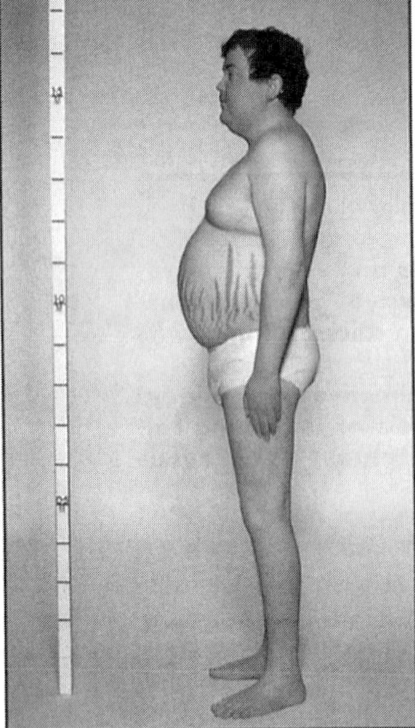

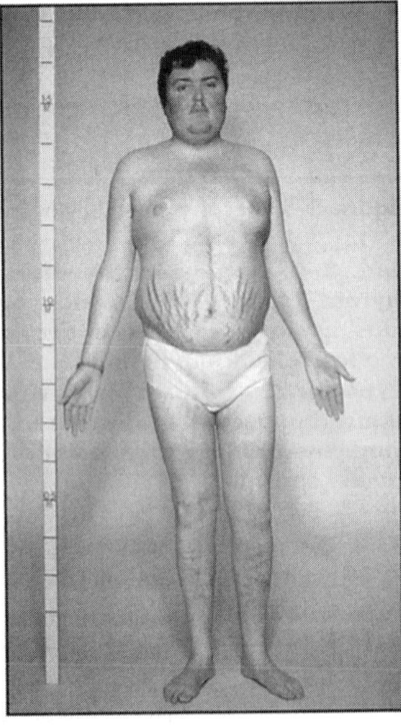

Figure 3–6 Cushing's syndrome, showing characteristic purple striae and abdominal obesity. (From Mir MA: Atlas of Clinical Diagnosis. Philadelphia, WB Saunders, 1995, p. 10.)

❑255.5 **Other adrenal hypofunction**
Adrenal medullary insufficiency

Excludes *Waterhouse-Friderichsen syndrome (meningococcal) (036.3)*

255.6 **Medulloadrenal hyperfunction**
Catecholamine secretion by pheochromocytoma

❑255.8 **Other specified disorders of adrenal glands**
Abnormality of cortisol-binding globulin

❑255.9 **Unspecified disorder of adrenal glands**

● 256 **Ovarian dysfunction**

256.0 **Hyperestrogenism**

❑256.1 **Other ovarian hyperfunction**
Hypersecretion of ovarian androgens

256.2 **Postablative ovarian failure**
Ovarian failure:
iatrogenic
postirradiation
postsurgical

Use additional code for states associated with artificial menopause (627.4)

Excludes *acquired absence of ovary (V45.77)*
asymptomatic age-related (natural) postmenopausal status (V49.81)

● 256.3 **Other ovarian failure**

Excludes *asymptomatic age-related (natural) postmenopausal status (V49.81)*

Use additional code for states associated with natural menopause (627.4)

256.31 **Premature menopause**

❑256.39 **Other ovarian failure**
Delayed menarche
Ovarian hypofunction
Primary ovarian failure NOS

256.4 **Polycystic ovaries**
Isosexual virilization Stein-Leventhal syndrome

❑256.8 **Other ovarian dysfunction**

❑256.9 **Unspecified ovarian dysfunction**

● 257 **Testicular dysfunction**

257.0 **Testicular hyperfunction**
Hypersecretion of testicular hormones

257.1 **Postablative testicular hypofunction**
Testicular hypofunction:
iatrogenic
postirradiation
postsurgical

❑257.2 **Other testicular hypofunction**
Defective biosynthesis of testicular androgen
Eunuchoidism:
NOS
hypogonadotropic
Failure:
Leydig's cell, adult
seminiferous tubule, adult
Testicular hypogonadism

Excludes *azoospermia (606.0)*

❑257.8 **Other testicular dysfunction**

Excludes *androgen insensitivity syndrome (259.5)*

❑257.9 **Unspecified testicular dysfunction**

● 258 **Polyglandular dysfunction and related disorders**

258.0 **Polyglandular activity in multiple endocrine adenomatosis**
Wermer's syndrome

❑258.1 **Other combinations of endocrine dysfunction**
Lloyd's syndrome
Schmidt's syndrome

❑258.8 **Other specified polyglandular dysfunction**

❑258.9 **Polyglandular dysfunction, unspecified**

● 259 **Other endocrine disorders**

259.0 **Delay in sexual development and puberty, not elsewhere classified**
Delayed puberty

259.1 **Precocious sexual development and puberty, not elsewhere classified**
Sexual precocity:
NOS
constitutional
cryptogenic
idiopathic

259.2 **Carcinoid syndrome**
Hormone secretion by carcinoid tumors

259.3 **Ectopic hormone secretion, not elsewhere classified**
Ectopic:
antidiuretic hormone secretion [ADH]
hyperparathyroidism

Excludes *ectopic ACTH syndrome (255.0)*

259.4 **Dwarfism, not elsewhere classified**
Dwarfism:
NOS
constitutional

Excludes *dwarfism:*
achondroplastic (756.4)
intrauterine (759.7)
nutritional (263.2)
pituitary (253.3)
renal (588.0)
progeria (259.8)

259.5 **Androgen insensitivity syndrome**
Partial androgen insensitivity
Reifenstein syndrome

❑259.8 **Other specified endocrine disorders**
Pineal gland dysfunction
Progeria
Werner's syndrome

❑259.9 **Unspecified endocrine disorder**
Disturbance:
endocrine NOS
hormone NOS
Infantilism NOS

NUTRITIONAL DEFICIENCIES (260–269)

Excludes *deficiency anemias (280.0–281.9)*

260 **Kwashiorkor**
Nutritional edema with dyspigmentation of skin and hair

261 **Nutritional marasmus**
Nutritional atrophy
Severe calorie deficiency
Severe malnutrition NOS

❑262 **Other severe protein-calorie malnutrition**
Nutritional edema without mention of dyspigmentation of skin and hair

● 263 **Other and unspecified protein-calorie malnutrition**

263.0 **Malnutrition of moderate degree**

263.1 **Malnutrition of mild degree**

263.2 **Arrested development following protein-calorie malnutrition**
Nutritional dwarfism
Physical retardation due to malnutrition

❑263.8 **Other protein-calorie malnutrition**

❑263.9 **Unspecified protein-calorie malnutrition**
Dystrophy due to malnutrition
Malnutrition (calorie) NOS
Excludes *nutritional deficiency NOS (269.9)*

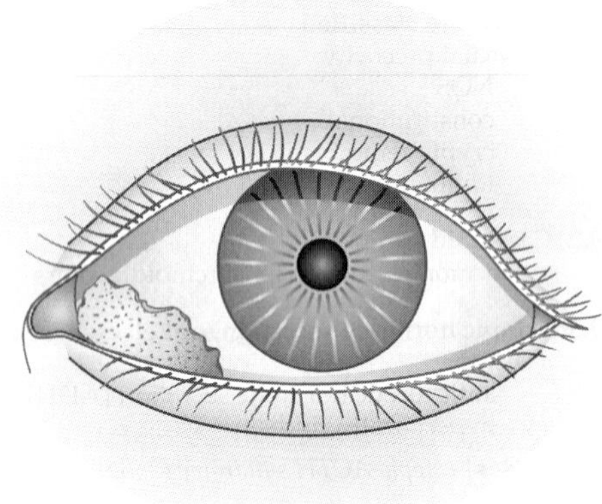

Figure 3–7 Bitot's spot on the conjunctiva.

Item 3-6 Bitot's spot is a gray, foamy erosion on the conjunctiva, usually associated with vitamin A deficiency. The disease may progress to keratomalacia, which can result in eventual prolapse of the iris and loss of the lens.

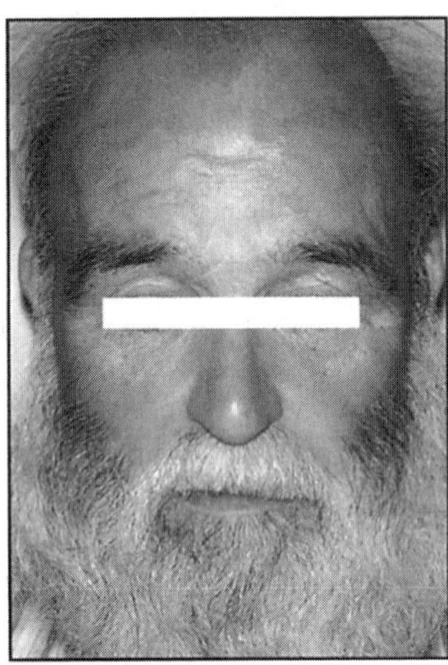

Figure 3–8 In chronic **pellagra,** the skin changes include thickening, scaling, pigmentation, and hyperkeratinization. (From Mir MA: Atlas of Clinical Diagnosis. Philadelphia, WB Saunders, 1995, p. 57.)

Item 3-7 Pellagra is associated with a deficiency of niacin and its precursor, tryptophan. Characteristics of the condition include dermatitis on exposed skin surfaces. Beriberi is associated with thiamine deficiency.

● 264 **Vitamin A deficiency**

264.0 **With conjunctival xerosis**

264.1 **With conjunctival xerosis and Bitot's spot**
Bitot's spot in the young child

264.2 **With corneal xerosis**

264.3 **With corneal ulceration and xerosis**

264.4 **With keratomalacia**

264.5 **With night blindness**

264.6 **With xerophthalmic scars of cornea**

❑264.7 **Other ocular manifestations of vitamin A deficiency**
Xerophthalmia due to vitamin A deficiency

❑264.8 **Other manifestations of vitamin A deficiency**
Follicular keratosis due to vitamin A deficiency
Xeroderma due to vitamin A deficiency

❑264.9 **Unspecified vitamin A deficiency**
Hypovitaminosis A NOS

● 265 **Thiamine and niacin deficiency states**

265.0 **Beriberi**

❑265.1 **Other and unspecified manifestations of thiamine deficiency**
Other vitamin B_1 deficiency states

265.2 **Pellagra**
Deficiency:
niacin (-tryptophan)
nicotinamide
nicotinic acid
vitamin PP
Pellagra (alcoholic)

● 266 **Deficiency of B-complex components**

266.0 **Ariboflavinosis**
Riboflavin [vitamin B_2] deficiency

266.1 **Vitamin B_6 deficiency**
Deficiency:
pyridoxal
pyridoxamine
pyridoxine
Vitamin B_6 deficiency syndrome
Excludes *vitamin B_6-responsive sideroblastic anemia (285.0)*

❑266.2 **Other B-complex deficiencies**
Deficiency:
cyanocobalamin
folic acid
vitamin B_{12}
Excludes *combined system disease with anemia (281.0–281.1)*
deficiency anemias (281.0–281.9)
subacute degeneration of spinal cord with anemia (281.0–281.1)

❑266.9 **Unspecified vitamin B deficiency**

267 **Ascorbic acid deficiency**
Deficiency of vitamin C
Scurvy
Excludes *scorbutic anemia (281.8)*

● 268 **Vitamin D deficiency**
Excludes *vitamin D-resistant:*
osteomalacia (275.3)
rickets (275.3)

268.0 **Rickets, active**
Excludes *celiac rickets (579.0)*
renal rickets (588.0)

❑268.1 **Rickets, late effect**
Any condition specified as due to rickets and stated to be a late effect or sequela of rickets
Use additional code to identify the nature of late effect

❑268.2 **Osteomalacia, unspecified**

❑268.9 **Unspecified vitamin D deficiency**
Avitaminosis D

● 269 **Other nutritional deficiencies**

269.0 **Deficiency of vitamin K**
Excludes *deficiency of coagulation factor due to vitamin K deficiency (286.7)*
vitamin K deficiency of newborn (776.0)

❑269.1 **Deficiency of other vitamins**
Deficiency:
vitamin E
vitamin P

❑269.2 **Unspecified vitamin deficiency**
Multiple vitamin deficiency NOS

269.3 **Mineral deficiency, not elsewhere classified**
Deficiency:
calcium, dietary
iodine
Excludes *deficiency:*
calcium NOS (275.40)
potassium (276.8)
sodium (276.1)

❑269.8 **Other nutritional deficiency**
Excludes *adult failure to thrive (783.7)*
failure to thrive in childhood (783.41)
feeding problems (783.3)
newborn (779.3)

❑269.9 **Unspecified nutritional deficiency**

OTHER METABOLIC AND IMMUNITY DISORDERS (270–279)

Use additional code to identify any associated mental retardation

● 270 **Disorders of amino-acid transport and metabolism**
Excludes *abnormal findings without manifest disease (790.0–796.9)*
disorders of purine and pyrimidine metabolism (277.1–277.2)
gout (274.0–274.9)

270.0 **Disturbances of amino-acid transport**
Cystinosis
Cystinuria
Fanconi (-de Toni) (-Debré) syndrome
Glycinuria (renal)
Hartnup disease

270.1 **Phenylketonuria [PKU]**
Hyperphenylalaninemia

❑270.2 **Other disturbances of aromatic amino-acid metabolism**
Albinism
Alkaptonuria
Alkaptonuric ochronosis
Disturbances of metabolism of tyrosine and tryptophan
Homogentisic acid defects
Hydroxykynureninuria
Hypertyrosinemia
Indicanuria
Kynureninase defects
Oasthouse urine disease
Ochronosis
Tyrosinosis
Tyrosinuria
Waardenburg syndrome
Excludes *vitamin B_6-deficiency syndrome (266.1)*

270.3 **Disturbances of branched-chain amino-acid metabolism**
Disturbances of metabolism of leucine, isoleucine, and valine
Hypervalinemia
Intermittent branched-chain ketonuria
Leucine-induced hypoglycemia
Leucinosis
Maple syrup urine disease

270.4 **Disturbances of sulphur-bearing amino-acid metabolism**
Cystathioninemia
Cystathioninuria
Disturbances of metabolism of methionine, homocystine, and cystathionine
Homocystinuria
Hypermethioninemia
Methioninemia

270.5 **Disturbances of histidine metabolism**
Carnosinemia
Histidinemia
Hyperhistidinemia
Imidazole aminoaciduria

270.6 **Disorders of urea cycle metabolism**
Argininosuccinic aciduria
Citrullinemia
Disorders of metabolism of ornithine, citrulline, argininosuccinic acid, arginine, and ammonia
Hyperammonemia
Hyperornithinemia

❑270.7 **Other disturbances of straight-chain amino-acid metabolism**
Glucoglycinuria
Glycinemia (with methylmalonic acidemia)
Hyperglycinemia
Hyperlysinemia
Pipecolic acidemia
Saccharopinuria
Other disturbances of metabolism of glycine, threonine, serine, glutamine, and lysine

Item 3-8 Any term ending with "emia" will be a blood condition. Any term ending with "uria" will have to do with urine. A term ending with "opathy" is a disease condition. Check for laboratory work.

❑270.8 **Other specified disorders of amino-acid metabolism**
Alaninemia
Ethanolaminuria
Glycoprolinuria
Hydroxyprolinemia
Hyperprolinemia
Iminoacidopathy
Prolinemia
Prolinuria
Sarcosinemia

❑270.9 **Unspecified disorder of amino-acid metabolism**

● **271 Disorders of carbohydrate transport and metabolism**

Excludes *abnormality of secretion of glucagon (251.4)*
diabetes mellitus (250.0–250.9)
hypoglycemia NOS (251.2)
mucopolysaccharidosis (277.5)

271.0 Glycogenosis
Amylopectinosis
Glucose-6-phosphatase deficiency
Glycogen storage disease
McArdle's disease
Pompe's disease
von Gierke's disease

271.1 Galactosemia
Galactose-1-phosphate uridyl transferase deficiency
Galactosuria

271.2 Hereditary fructose intolerance
Essential benign fructosuria
Fructosemia

271.3 Intestinal disaccharidase deficiencies and disaccharide malabsorption
Intolerance or malabsorption (congenital) (of):
glucose-galactose
lactose
sucrose-isomaltose

271.4 Renal glycosuria
Renal diabetes

❑**271.8 Other specified disorders of carbohydrate transport and metabolism**
Essential benign pentosuria
Fucosidosis
Glycolic aciduria
Hyperoxaluria (primary)
Mannosidosis
Oxalosis
Xylosuria
Xylulosuria

❑**271.9 Unspecified disorder of carbohydrate transport and metabolism**

● **272 Disorders of lipoid metabolism**

Excludes *localized cerebral lipidoses (330.1)*

272.0 Pure hypercholesterolemia
Familial hypercholesterolemia
Fredrickson Type IIa hyperlipoproteinemia
Hyperbetalipoproteinemia
Hyperlipidemia, Group A
Low-density-lipoid-type [LDL] hyperlipoproteinemia

272.1 Pure hyperglyceridemia
Endogenous hyperglyceridemia
Fredrickson Type IV hyperlipoproteinemia
Hyperlipidemia, Group B
Hyperprebetalipoproteinemia
Hypertriglyceridemia, essential
Very-low-density-lipoid-type [VLDL] hyperlipoproteinemia

272.2 Mixed hyperlipidemia
Broad- or floating-betalipoproteinemia
Fredrickson Type IIb or III hyperlipoproteinemia
Hypercholesterolemia with endogenous hyperglyceridemia
Hyperbetalipoproteinemia with prebetalipoproteinemia
Tubo-eruptive xanthoma
Xanthoma tuberosum

272.3 Hyperchylomicronemia
Bürger-Grütz syndrome
Fredrickson type I or V hyperlipoproteinemia
Hyperlipidemia, Group D
Mixed hyperglyceridemia

❑**272.4 Other and unspecified hyperlipidemia**
Alpha-lipoproteinemia
Combined hyperlipidemia
Hyperlipidemia NOS
Hyperlipoproteinemia NOS

272.5 Lipoprotein deficiencies
Abetalipoproteinemia
Bassen-Kornzweig syndrome
High-density lipoid deficiency
Hypoalphalipoproteinemia
Hypobetalipoproteinemia (familial)

272.6 Lipodystrophy
Barraquer-Simons disease
Progressive lipodystrophy

Use additional E code to identify cause, if iatrogenic

Excludes *intestinal lipodystrophy (040.2)*

272.7 Lipidoses
Chemically induced lipidosis
Disease:
Anderson's
Fabry's
Gaucher's
I cell [mucolipidosis I]
lipoid storage NOS
Niemann-Pick
pseudo-Hurler's or mucolipidosis III
triglyceride storage, Type I or II
Wolman's or triglyceride storage, Type III
Mucolipidosis II
Primary familial xanthomatosis

Excludes *cerebral lipidoses (330.1)*
Tay-Sachs disease (330.1)

❑**272.8 Other disorders of lipoid metabolism**
Hoffa's disease or liposynovitis prepatellaris
Launois-Bensaude's lipomatosis
Lipoid dermatoarthritis

❑**272.9 Unspecified disorder of lipoid metabolism**

● **273 Disorders of plasma protein metabolism**

Excludes *agammaglobulinemia and hypogammaglobulinemia (279.0–279.2)*
coagulation defects (286.0–286.9)
hereditary hemolytic anemias (282.0–282.9)

273.0 Polyclonal hypergammaglobulinemia
Hypergammaglobulinemic purpura:
benign primary
Waldenström's

273.1 Monoclonal paraproteinemia
Benign monoclonal hypergammaglobulinemia [BMH]
Monoclonal gammopathy:
NOS
associated with lymphoplasmacytic dyscrasias
benign
Paraproteinemia:
benign (familial)
secondary to malignant or inflammatory disease

❑**273.2 Other paraproteinemias**
Cryoglobulinemic:
purpura
vasculitis
Mixed cryoglobulinemia

273.3 Macroglobulinemia
Macroglobulinemia (idiopathic) (primary)
Waldenström's macroglobulinemia

273.4 Alpha-1-antitrypsin deficiency
AAT deficiency

❑273.8 **Other disorders of plasma protein metabolism**
Abnormality of transport protein
Bisalbuminemia

❑273.9 **Unspecified disorder of plasma protein metabolism**

● 274 **Gout**
Excludes *lead gout (984.0–984.9)*

274.0 **Gouty arthropathy**

● 274.1 **Gouty nephropathy**

❑274.10 **Gouty nephropathy, unspecified**

274.11 **Uric acid nephrolithiasis**

❑274.19 **Other**

● 274.8 **Gout with other specified manifestations**

274.81 **Gouty tophi of ear**

❑274.82 **Gouty tophi of other sites**
Gouty tophi of heart

❑274.89 **Other**
Use additional code to identify manifestations, as:
gouty:
iritis (364.11)
neuritis (357.4)

❑274.9 **Gout, unspecified**

● 275 **Disorders of mineral metabolism**
Excludes *abnormal findings without manifest disease (790.0–796.9)*

275.0 **Disorders of iron metabolism**
Bronzed diabetes
Hemochromatosis
Pigmentary cirrhosis (of liver)
Excludes *anemia:*
iron deficiency (280.0–280.9)
sideroblastic (285.0)

275.1 **Disorders of copper metabolism**
Hepatolenticular degeneration
Wilson's disease

275.2 **Disorders of magnesium metabolism**
Hypermagnesemia
Hypomagnesemia

275.3 **Disorders of phosphorus metabolism**
Familial hypophosphatemia
Hypophosphatasia
Vitamin D-resistant:
osteomalacia
rickets

● 275.4 **Disorders of calcium metabolism**
Excludes *parathyroid disorders (252.00–252.9)*
vitamin D deficiency (268.0–268.9)

❑275.40 **Unspecified disorder of calcium metabolism**

275.41 **Hypocalcemia**

275.42 **Hypercalcemia**

❑275.49 **Other disorders of calcium metabolism**
Nephrocalcinosis
Pseudohypoparathyroidism
Pseudopseudohypoparathyroidism

❑275.8 **Other specified disorders of mineral metabolism**

❑275.9 **Unspecified disorder of mineral metabolism**

● 276 **Disorders of fluid, electrolyte, and acid-base balance**
Excludes *diabetes insipidus (253.5)*
familial periodic paralysis (359.3)

276.0 **Hyperosmolality and/or hypernatremia**
Sodium [Na] excess
Sodium [Na] overload

276.1 **Hyposmolality and/or hyponatremia**
Sodium [Na] deficiency

276.2 **Acidosis**
Acidosis:
NOS
lactic
metabolic
respiratory
Excludes *diabetic acidosis (250.1)*

276.3 **Alkalosis**
Alkalosis:
NOS
metabolic
respiratory

276.4 **Mixed acid-base balance disorder**
Hypercapnia with mixed acid-base disorder

Item 3-9 Circulating fluid volume in the body is regulated by the vascular system, the brain, and the kidneys. Too much (fluid overload) or too little fluid volume (volume depletion) will affect blood pressure. Severe cases of vomiting, diarrhea, bleeding, and burns (fluid loss through exposed burn surface area) can contribute to fluid loss. Internal body environment must maintain a precise balance (homeostasis) between too much fluid and too little fluid.

● 276.5 **Volume depletion**
Excludes *hypovolemic shock:*
postoperative (998.0)
traumatic (958.4)

❑276.50 **Volume depletion, unspecified**

276.51 **Dehydration**

276.52 **Hypovolemia**
Depletion of volume of plasma

276.6 **Fluid overload**
Fluid retention
Excludes *ascites (789.5)*
localized edema (782.3)

276.7 **Hyperpotassemia**
Hyperkalemia
Potassium [K]:
excess
intoxication
Potassium [K]:
overload

276.8 **Hypopotassemia**
Hypokalemia
Potassium [K] deficiency

❑276.9 **Electrolyte and fluid disorders not elsewhere classified**
Electrolyte imbalance
Hyperchloremia
Hypochloremia
Excludes *electrolyte imbalance:*
associated with hyperemesis gravidarum (643.1)
complicating labor and delivery (669.0)
following abortion and ectopic or molar pregnancy (634–638 with .4, 639.4)

● 277 **Other and unspecified disorders of metabolism**

● 277.0 **Cystic fibrosis**
Fibrocystic disease of the pancreas
Mucoviscidosis

277.00 **Without mention of meconium ileus**
Cystic fibrosis NOS

277.01 **With meconium ileus**
Meconium:
ileus (of newborn)
obstruction of intestine in mucoviscidosis

277.02 **With pulmonary manifestations**
Cystic fibrosis with pulmonary exacerbation
Use additional code to identify any infectious organism present, such as:
pseudomonas (041.7)

277.03 **With gastrointestinal manifestations**

Excludes *with meconium ileus (277.01)*

❑277.09 **With other manifestations**

277.1 **Disorders of porphyrin metabolism**
Hematoporphyria
Hematoporphyrinuria
Hereditary coproporphyria
Porphyria
Porphyrinuria
Protocoproporphyria
Protoporphyria
Pyrroloporphyria

❑277.2 **Other disorders of purine and pyrimidine metabolism**
Hypoxanthine-guanine-phosphoribosyltransferase deficiency [HG-PRT deficiency]
Lesch-Nyhan syndrome
Xanthinuria

Excludes *gout (274.0–274.9)*
orotic aciduric anemia (281.4)

● 277.3 **Amyloidosis** ⬅ (Revised)
❑277.30 **Amyloidosis, unspecified** ◀
Amyloidosis NOS ◀

277.31 **Familial Mediterranean fever** ◀
Benign paroxysmal peritonitis ◀
Hereditary amyloid nephropathy ◀
Periodic familial polyserositis ◀
Recurrent polyserositis ◀

❑277.39 **Other amyloidosis** ◀
Hereditary cardiac amyloidosis ◀
Inherited systemic amyloidosis ◀
Neuropathic (Portuguese) (Swiss) amyloidosis ◀
Secondary amyloidosis ◀

277.4 **Disorders of bilirubin excretion**
Hyperbilirubinemia:
congenital
constitutional
Syndrome:
Crigler-Najjar
Dubin-Johnson
Gilbert's
Rotor's

Excludes *hyperbilirubinemias specific to the perinatal period (774.0–774.7)*

277.5 **Mucopolysaccharidosis**
Gargoylism
Hunter's syndrome
Hurler's syndrome
Lipochondrodystrophy
Maroteaux-Lamy syndrome
Morquio-Brailsford disease
Osteochondrodystrophy
Sanfilippo's syndrome
Scheie's syndrome

❑277.6 **Other deficiencies of circulating enzymes**
Hereditary angioedema

277.7 **Dysmetabolic syndrome X**
Use additional code for associated manifestation, such as:
cardiovascular disease (414.00–414.07)
obesity (278.00–278.01)

● 277.8 **Other specified disorders of metabolism**
277.81 **Primary carnitine deficiency**

277.82 **Carnitine deficiency due to inborn errors of metabolism**

277.83 **Iatrogenic carnitine deficiency**
Carnitine deficiency due to:
hemodialysis
valproic acid therapy

277.84 **Other secondary carnitine deficiency**

277.85 **Disorders of fatty acid oxidation**
Carnitine palmitoyltransferase deficiencies (CPT1, CPT2)
Glutaric aciduria type II (type IIA, IIB, IIC)
Long chain 3-hydroxyacyl CoA dehydrogenase deficiency (LCHAD)
Long chain/very long chain acyl CoA dehydrogenase deficiency (LCAD, VLCAD)
Medium chain acyl CoA dehydrogenase deficiency (MCAD)
Short chain acyl CoA dehydrogenase deficiency (SCAD)

Excludes *primary carnitine deficiency (277.81)*

277.86 **Paroxysmal disorders**
Adrenomyeloneuropathy
Neonatal adrenoleukodystrophy
Rhizomelic chondrodysplasia punctata
X-linked adrenoleukodystrophy
Zellweger syndrome

Excludes *infantile Refsum disease (356.3)*

277.87 **Disorders of mitochondrial metabolism**
Kearns-Sayre syndrome
Mitochondrial Encephalopathy, Lactic Acidosis and Stroke-like episodes (MELAS syndrome)
Mitochondrial Neurogastrointestinal Encephalopathy syndrome (MNGIE)
Myoclonus with Epilepsy and with Ragged Red Fibers (MERRF syndrome)
Neuropathy, Ataxia and Retinitis Pigmentosa (NARP syndrome)
Use additional code for associated conditions

Excludes *disorders of pyruvate metabolism (271.8)*
Leber's optic atrophy (377.16)
Leigh's subacute necrotizing encephalopathy (330.8)
Reye's syndrome (331.81)

❑277.89 **Other specified disorders of metabolism**
Hand-Schüller-Christian disease
Histiocytosis (acute) (chronic)
Histiocytosis X (chronic)

Excludes *histiocytosis:*
acute differentiated progressive (202.5)
X, acute (progressive) (202.5)

❑277.9 **Unspecified disorder of metabolism**
Enzymopathy NOS

● 278 **Overweight, obesity, and other hyperalimentation**

Excludes *hyperalimentation NOS (783.6)*
poisoning by vitamins NOS (963.5)
polyphagia (783.6)

● 278.0 **Overweight and obesity**
Use additional code to identify Body Mass Index (BMI), if known (V85.0–V85.54) ⬅ (Revised)

Excludes *adiposogenital dystrophy (253.8)*
obesity of endocrine origin NOS (259.9)

❑278.00 **Obesity, unspecified**
Obesity NOS

278.01 **Morbid obesity**
Severe obesity

278.02 **Overweight**

278.1 Localized adiposity
Fat pad

278.2 Hypervitaminosis A

278.3 Hypercarotinemia

278.4 Hypervitaminosis D

❑ **278.8 Other hyperalimentation**

● **279 Disorders involving the immune mechanism**

● **279.0 Deficiency of humoral immunity**

❑ **279.00 Hypogammaglobulinemia, unspecified**
Agammaglobulinemia NOS

279.01 Selective IgA immunodeficiency

279.02 Selective IgM immunodeficiency

❑ **279.03 Other selective immunoglobulin deficiencies**
Selective deficiency of IgG

279.04 Congenital hypogammaglobulinemia
Agammaglobulinemia:
- Bruton's type
- X-linked

279.05 Immunodeficiency with increased IgM
Immunodeficiency with hyper-IgM:
- autosomal recessive
- X-linked

279.06 Common variable immunodeficiency
Dysgammaglobulinemia (acquired) (congenital) (primary)
Hypogammaglobulinemia:
- acquired primary
- congenital non-sex-linked
- sporadic

❑ **279.09 Other**
Transient hypogammaglobulinemia of infancy

● **279.1 Deficiency of cell-mediated immunity**

❑ **279.10 Immunodeficiency with predominant T-cell defect, unspecified**

279.11 DiGeorge's syndrome
Pharyngeal pouch syndrome
Thymic hypoplasia

279.12 Wiskott-Aldrich syndrome

279.13 Nezelof's syndrome
Cellular immunodeficiency with abnormal immunoglobulin deficiency

❑ **279.19 Other**

Excludes *ataxia-telangiectasia (334.8)*

279.2 Combined immunity deficiency
Agammaglobulinemia:
- autosomal recessive
- Swiss-type
- X-linked recessive

Severe combined immunodeficiency [SCID]
Thymic:
- alymphoplasia
- aplasia or dysplasia with immunodeficiency

Excludes *thymic hypoplasia (279.11)*

❑ **279.3 Unspecified immunity deficiency**

❑ **279.4 Autoimmune disease, not elsewhere classified**
Autoimmune disease NOS

Excludes *transplant failure or rejection (996.80–996.89)*

❑ **279.8 Other specified disorders involving the immune mechanism**
Single complement [C_1-C_9] deficiency or dysfunction

❑ **279.9 Unspecified disorder of immune mechanism**

ICD-9-CM 200-299 Vol. 1

4. DISEASES OF THE BLOOD AND BLOOD-FORMING ORGANS (280–289)

Excludes *anemia complicating pregnancy or the puerperium (648.2)*

● 280 Iron deficiency anemias

Includes: anemia:
- asiderotic
- hypochromic-microcytic
- sideropenic

Excludes *familial microcytic anemia (282.49)*

280.0 Secondary to blood loss (chronic)
Normocytic anemia due to blood loss

Excludes *acute posthemorrhagic anemia (285.1)*

280.1 Secondary to inadequate dietary iron intake

❑280.8 Other specified iron deficiency anemias
Paterson-Kelly syndrome
Plummer-Vinson syndrome
Sideropenic dysphagia

❑280.9 Iron deficiency anemia, unspecified
Anemia:
- achlorhydric
- chlorotic
- idiopathic hypochromic
- iron [Fe] deficiency NOS

● 281 Other deficiency anemias

281.0 Pernicious anemia
Anemia:
- Addison's
- Biermer's
- congenital pernicious

Congenital intrinsic factor [Castle's] deficiency

Excludes *combined system disease without mention of anemia (266.2)*
subacute degeneration of spinal cord without mention of anemia (266.2)

❑281.1 Other vitamin B_{12} deficiency anemia
Anemia:
- vegan's
- vitamin B_{12} deficiency (dietary)
- due to selective vitamin B_{12} malabsorption with proteinuria

Syndrome:
- Imerslund's
- Imerslund-Gräsbeck

Excludes *combined system disease without mention of anemia (266.2)*
subacute degeneration of spinal cord without mention of anemia (266.2)

281.2 Folate-deficiency anemia
Congenital folate malabsorption
Folate or folic acid deficiency anemia:
- NOS
- dietary
- drug-induced

Goat's milk anemia
Nutritional megaloblastic anemia (of infancy)

Use additional E code to identify drug

❑281.3 Other specified megaloblastic anemias, not elsewhere classified
Combined B_{12} and folate-deficiency anemia

281.4 Protein-deficiency anemia
Amino-acid-deficiency anemia

❑281.8 Anemia associated with other specified nutritional deficiency
Scorbutic anemia

❑281.9 Unspecified deficiency anemia
Anemia:
- dimorphic
- macrocytic
- megaloblastic NOS
- nutritional NOS
- simple chronic

● 282 Hereditary hemolytic anemias

282.0 Hereditary spherocytosis
Acholuric (familial) jaundice
Congenital hemolytic anemia (spherocytic)
Congenital spherocytosis
Minkowski-Chauffard syndrome
Spherocytosis (familial)

Excludes *hemolytic anemia of newborn (773.0–773.5)*

282.1 Hereditary elliptocytosis
Elliptocytosis (congenital)
Ovalocytosis (congenital) (hereditary)

282.2 Anemias due to disorders of glutathione metabolism
Anemia:
- 6-phosphogluconic dehydrogenase deficiency
- enzyme deficiency, drug-induced
- erythrocytic glutathione deficiency
- glucose-6-phosphate dehydrogenase [G-6-PD] deficiency
- glutathione-reductase deficiency
- hemolytic nonspherocytic (hereditary), type I

Disorder of pentose phosphate pathway
Favism

❑282.3 Other hemolytic anemias due to enzyme deficiency
Anemia:
- hemolytic nonspherocytic (hereditary), type II
- hexokinase deficiency
- pyruvate kinase [PK] deficiency
- triosephosphate isomerase deficiency

● 282.4 Thalassemias

Excludes *sickle-cell:*
disease (282.60–282.69)
trait (282.5)

282.41 Sickle-cell thalassemia without crisis
Sickle-cell thalassemia NOS
Thalassemia Hb-S disease without crisis

A sickle-cell "crisis" is precipitated when the abnormally crescent-shaped red blood cells form clots and interrupt blood flow to major organs, causing severe pain and organ damage.

282.42 Sickle-cell thalassemia with crisis
Sickle-cell thalassemia with vasco-occlusive pain
Thalassemia Hb-S disease with crisis

Use additional code for types of crisis, such as:
- acute chest syndrome (517.3)
- splenic sequestration (289.52)

Splenic sequestration (to set apart) occurs when sickled red blood cells become entrapped in the spleen, causing splenomegaly (enlargement) and decreased circulating blood volume. Transfusions can be given to replace blood volume, or removal of the spleen (splenectomy) may be the treatment of choice. Splenic sequestration has its own code, 289.52, but code sickle-cell crisis first if it applies.

❑282.49 **Other thalassemia**
Cooley's anemia
Hb-Bart's disease
Hereditary leptocytosis
Mediterranean anemia (with other hemoglobinopathy)
Microdrepanocytosis
Thalassemia (alpha) (beta) (intermedia) (major) (minima) (minor) (mixed) (trait) (with other hemoglobinopathy)
Thalassemia NOS

282.5 Sickle-cell trait
Hb-AS genotype
Hemoglobin S [Hb-S] trait
Heterozygous:
hemoglobin S
Hb-S

Excludes *that with other hemoglobinopathy (282.60–282.69)*
that with thalassemia (282.49)

● **282.6 Sickle-cell disease**
Sickle-cell anemia

Excludes *sickle-cell thalassemia (282.41–282.42)*
sickle-cell trait (282.5)

❑282.60 **Sickle-cell disease, unspecified**
Sickle-cell anemia NOS

282.61 Hb-SS disease without crisis

282.62 Hb-SS disease with crisis
Hb-SS disease with vaso-occlusive pain
Sickle-cell crisis NOS

Use additional code for types of crisis, such as:
acute chest syndrome (517.3)
splenic sequestration (289.52)

282.63 Sickle-cell/Hb-C disease without crisis
Hb-S/Hb-C disease without crisis

282.64 Sickle-cell/Hb-C disease with crisis
Hb-S/Hb-C disease with crisis
Sickle-cell/Hb-C disease with vaso-occlusive pain

Use additional code for types of crisis, such as:
acute chest syndrome (517.3)
splenic sequestration (289.52)

282.68 Other sickle-cell disease without crisis
Hb-S/Hb-D disease without crisis
Hb-S/Hb-E disease without crisis
Sickle-cell/Hb-D disease without crisis
Sickle-cell/Hb-E disease without crisis

❑282.69 **Other sickle-cell disease with crisis**
Hb-S/Hb-D disease with crisis
Hb-S/Hb-E disease with crisis
Other sickle-cell disease with vaso-occlusive pain
Sickle-cell/Hb-D disease with crisis
Sickle-cell/Hb-E disease with crisis

Use additional code for types of crisis, such as:
acute chest syndrome (517.3)
splenic sequestration (289.52)

❑282.7 **Other hemoglobinopathies**
Abnormal hemoglobin NOS
Congenital Heinz-body anemia
Disease:
hemoglobin C [Hb-C]
hemoglobin D [Hb-D]
hemoglobin E [Hb-E]
hemoglobin Zurich [Hb-Zurich]
Hemoglobinopathy NOS
Hereditary persistence of fetal hemoglobin [HPFH]
Unstable hemoglobin hemolytic disease

Excludes *familial polycythemia (289.6)*
hemoglobin M [Hb-M] disease (289.7)
high-oxygen-affinity hemoglobin (289.0)

❑282.8 **Other specified hereditary hemolytic anemias**
Stomatocytosis

❑282.9 **Hereditary hemolytic anemia, unspecified**
Hereditary hemolytic anemia NOS

● **283 Acquired hemolytic anemias**

283.0 Autoimmune hemolytic anemias
Autoimmune hemolytic disease (cold type) (warm type)
Chronic cold hemagglutinin disease
Cold agglutinin disease or hemoglobinuria
Hemolytic anemia:
cold type (secondary) (symptomatic)
drug-induced
warm type (secondary) (symptomatic)

Use additional E code to identify cause, if drug-induced

Excludes *Evans'syndrome (287.32)*
hemolytic disease of newborn (773.0–773.5)

● **283.1 Non-autoimmune hemolytic anemias**

❑283.10 **Non-autoimmune hemolytic anemia, unspecified**

283.11 Hemolytic-uremic syndrome

❑283.19 **Other non-autoimmune hemolytic anemias**
Hemolytic anemia:
mechanical
microangiopathic
toxic

Use additional E code to identify cause

283.2 Hemoglobinuria due to hemolysis from external causes
Acute intravascular hemolysis
Hemoglobinuria:
from exertion
march
paroxysmal (cold) (nocturnal)
due to other hemolysis
Marchiafava-Micheli syndrome

Use additional E code to identify cause

❑283.9 **Acquired hemolytic anemia, unspecified**
Acquired hemolytic anemia NOS
Chronic idiopathic hemolytic anemia

● **284 Aplastic anemia and other bone marrow failure syndromes** ⇐

● **284.0 Constitutional aplastic anemia** ⇐

Marked deficiency of all the blood elements: red blood cells (erythrocytes), white blood cells (leukocytes), and platelets (thrombocytes). Check laboratory results.

284.01 Constitutional red blood cell aplasia ◀
Aplasia, (pure) red cell: ◀
congenital ◀
of infants ◀
primary ◀
Blackfan-Diamond syndrome ◀
Familial hypoplastic anemia ◀

ICD-9-CM 200-299 Vol. 1

❑284.09 **Other constitutional aplastic anemia** ◀
Fanconi's anemia ◀
Pancytopenia with malformations ◀

284.1 Pancytopenia ◀

Excludes *pancytopenia (due to) (with):* ◀
aplastic anemia NOS (284.9) ◀
bone marrow infiltration (284.2) ◀
constitutional red blood cell aplasia (284.01) ◀
drug induced (284.8) ◀
hairy cell leukemia (202.4) ◀
human immunodeficiency virus disease (042) ◀
leukoerythroblastic anemia (284.2) ◀
malformations (284.09) ◀
myelodysplastic syndromes (238.72–238.75) ◀
myeloproliferative disease (238.79) ◀
other constitutional aplastic anemia (284.09) ◀

● *284.2 Myelophthisis* ◀
Leukoerythroblastic anemia ◀
Myelophthisic anemia ◀

Code first the underlying disorder, such as: ◀
malignant neoplasm of breast (174.0–174.9, 175.0–175.9) ◀
tuberculosis (015.0–015.9) ◀

Excludes *idiopathic myelofibrosis (238.76)* ◀
myelofibrosis NOS (289.83) ◀
myelofibrosis with myeloid metaplasia (238.76) ◀
primary myelofibrosis (238.76) ◀
secondary myelofibrosis (289.83) ◀

❑284.8 **Other specified aplastic anemias** (Revised)
Aplastic anemia (due to):
chronic systemic disease
drugs
infection
radiation
toxic (paralytic)
Red cell aplasia (acquired) (adult) (pure) (with thymoma)

Use additional E code to identify cause

❑284.9 **Aplastic anemia, unspecified**
Anemia:
aplastic (idiopathic) NOS
aregenerative
hypoplastic NOS
nonregenerative
Medullary hypoplasia

Excludes *refractory anemia (238.72)* (Revised)

● **285 Other and unspecified anemias**

285.0 Sideroblastic anemia
Anemia:
hypochromic with iron loading
sideroachrestic
sideroblastic
acquired
congenital
hereditary
primary
secondary (drug-induced) (due to disease)
sex-linked hypochromic
vitamin B_6-responsive
Pyridoxine-responsive (hypochromic) anemia

Use additional E code to identify cause, if drug-induced

Excludes *refractory sideroblastic anemia (238.72)* (Revised)

285.1 Acute posthemorrhagic anemia
Anemia due to acute blood loss

Excludes *anemia due to chronic blood loss (280.0)*
blood loss anemia NOS (280.0)

● **285.2 Anemia of chronic disease** (Revised)
Anemia in chronic illness ◀

285.21 Anemia in chronic kidney disease
Anemia in end stage renal disease
Erythropoietin-resistant anemia (EPO resistant anemia)

285.22 Anemia in neoplastic disease

285.29 Anemia of other chronic disease (Revised)
Anemia in other chronic illness ◀

❑285.8 **Other specified anemias** (Revised)
Anemia:
dyserythropoietic (congenital)
dyshematopoietic (congenital)
von Jaksch's
Infantile pseudoleukemia

❑285.9 **Anemia, unspecified**
Anemia:
NOS
essential
normocytic, not due to blood loss
profound
progressive
secondary
Oligocythemia

Excludes *anemia (due to):*
blood loss:
acute (285.1)
chronic or unspecified (280.0)
iron deficiency (280.0–280.9)

● **286 Coagulation defects**

286.0 Congenital factor VIII disorder
Antihemophilic globulin [AHG] deficiency
Factor VIII (functional) deficiency
Hemophilia:
NOS
A
classical
familial
hereditary
Subhemophilia

Excludes *factor VIII deficiency with vascular defect (286.4)*

286.1 Congenital factor IX disorder
Christmas disease
Deficiency:
factor IX (functional)
plasma thromboplastin component [PTC]
Hemophilia B

286.2 Congenital factor XI deficiency
Hemophilia C
Plasma thromboplastin antecedent [PTA] deficiency
Rosenthal's disease

❑286.3 **Congenital deficiency of other clotting factors**
Congenital afibrinogenemia
Deficiency:
AC globulin factor:
I [fibrinogen]
II [prothrombin]
V [labile]
VII [stable]
X [Stuart-Prower]
XII [Hageman]
XIII [fibrin stabilizing]
Laki-Lorand factor
proaccelerin
Disease:
Owren's
Stuart-Prower
Dysfibrinogenemia (congenital)
Dysprothrombinemia (constitutional)
Hypoproconvertinemia
Hypoprothrombinemia (hereditary)
Parahemophilia

286.4 von Willebrand's disease
Angiohemophilia (A) (B)
Constitutional thrombopathy
Factor VIII deficiency with vascular defect
Pseudohemophilia type B
Vascular hemophilia
von Willebrand's (-Jürgens') disease

Excludes *factor VIII deficiency:*
NOS (286.0)
with functional defect (286.0)
hereditary capillary fragility (287.8)

286.5 Hemorrhagic disorder due to intrinsic circulating anticoagulants
Antithrombinemia
Antithromboplastinemia
Antithromboplastinogenemia
Hyperheparinemia
Increase in:
anti-VIIIa
anti-IXa
anti-Xa
anti-XIa
antithrombin
Secondary hemophilia
Systemic lupus erythematosus [SLE] inhibitor

286.6 Defibrination syndrome
Afibrinogenemia, acquired
Consumption coagulopathy
Diffuse or disseminated intravascular coagulation [DIC syndrome]
Fibrinolytic hemorrhage, acquired
Hemorrhagic fibrinogenolysis
Pathologic fibrinolysis
Purpura:
fibrinolytic
fulminans

Excludes *that complicating:*
abortion (634–638 with .1, 639.1)
pregnancy or the puerperium (641.3, 666.3)
disseminated intravascular coagulation in newborn (776.2)

286.7 Acquired coagulation factor deficiency
Deficiency of coagulation factor due to:
liver disease
vitamin K deficiency
Hypoprothrombinemia, acquired

Excludes *vitamin K deficiency of newborn (776.0)*

Use additional E code to identify cause, if drug-induced

❑**286.9 Other and unspecified coagulation defects**
Defective coagulation NOS
Deficiency, coagulation factor NOS
Delay, coagulation
Disorder:
coagulation
hemostasis

Excludes *abnormal coagulation profile (790.92)*
hemorrhagic disease of newborn (776.0)
that complicating:
abortion (634–638 with .1, 639.1)
pregnancy or the puerperium (641.3, 666.3)

● **287 Purpura and other hemorrhagic conditions**

Excludes *hemorrhagic thrombocythemia (238.79)* ⬅
purpura fulminans (286.6)

287.0 Allergic purpura
Peliosis rheumatica
Purpura:
anaphylactoid
autoimmune
Henoch's
nonthrombocytopenic:
hemorrhagic
idiopathic
rheumatica
Schönlein-Henoch
vascular
Vasculitis, allergic

Excludes *hemorrhagic purpura (287.39)*
purpura annularis telangiectodes (709.1)

287.1 Qualitative platelet defects
Thrombasthenia (hemorrhagic) (hereditary)
Thrombocytasthenia
Thrombocytopathy (dystrophic)
Thrombopathy (Bernard-Soulier)

Excludes *von Willebrand's disease (286.4)*

❑**287.2 Other nonthrombocytopenic purpuras**
Purpura:
NOS
senile
simplex

● **287.3 Primary thrombocytopenia**

Excludes *thrombotic thrombocytopenic purpura (446.6)*
transient thrombocytopenia of newborn (776.1)

Thrombo = clot forming, cyto = cell, penia = deficiency of: deficiency of platelets.

❑**287.30 Primary thrombocytopenia, unspecified**
Megakaryocytic hypoplasia

287.31 Immune thrombocytopenic purpura
Idiopathic thrombocytopenic purpura
Tidal platelet dysgenesis

287.32 Evans' syndrome

287.33 Congenital and hereditary thrombocytopenic purpura
Congenital and hereditary thrombocytopenia
Thrombocytopenia with absent radii (TAR) syndrome

Excludes *Wiskott-Aldrich syndrome (279.12)*

287.39 Other primary thrombocytopenia

287.4 Secondary thrombocytopenia
Posttransfusion purpura
Thrombocytopenia (due to):
dilutional
drugs
extracorporeal circulation of blood
massive blood transfusion
platelet alloimmunization

Use additional E code to identify cause

Excludes *transient thrombocytopenia of newborn (776.1)*

❑**287.5 Thrombocytopenia, unspecified**

❑**287.8 Other specified hemorrhagic conditions**
Capillary fragility (hereditary)
Vascular pseudohemophilia

❑**287.9 Unspecified hemorrhagic conditions**
Hemorrhagic diathesis (familial)

● **288 Diseases of white blood cells**

Excludes *leukemia (204.0–208.9)*

● **288.0 Neutropenia** ⬅
Decreased Absolute Neutrophil Count (ANC) ◀

Use additional code for any associated fever (780.6) ◀

Excludes *neutropenic splenomegaly (289.53)* ◀
transitory neonatal neutropenia (776.7)

❑288.00 **Neutropenia, unspecified** ◀

288.01 **Congenital neutropenia** ◀
Congenital agranulocytosis ◀
Infantile genetic agranulocytosis ◀
Kostmann's syndrome ◀

288.02 **Cyclic neutropenia** ◀
Cyclic hematopoiesis ◀
Periodic neutropenia ◀

288.03 **Drug induced neutropenia** ◀
Use additional E code to identify drug ◀

288.04 **Neutropenia due to infection** ◀

❑288.09 **Other neutropenia** ◀
Agranulocytosis ◀
Neutropenia: ◀
immune ◀
toxic ◀

288.1 **Functional disorders of polymorphonuclear neutrophils**
Chronic (childhood) granulomatous disease
Congenital dysphagocytosis
Job's syndrome
Lipochrome histiocytosis (familial)
Progressive septic granulomatosis

288.2 **Genetic anomalies of leukocytes**
Anomaly (granulation) (granulocyte) or syndrome:
Alder's (-Reilly)
Chédiak-Steinbrinck (-Higashi)
Jordan's
May-Hegglin
Pelger-Huet
Hereditary:
hypersegmentation
hyposegmentation
leukomelanopathy

288.3 **Eosinophilia**
Eosinophilia
allergic
hereditary
idiopathic
secondary
Eosinophilic leukocytosis

Excludes *Löffler's syndrome (518.3)*
pulmonary eosinophilia (518.3)

288.4 **Hemophagocytic syndromes** ◀
Familial hemophagocytic lymphohistiocytosis ◀
Familial hemophagocytic reticulosis ◀
Hemophagocytic syndrome, infection-associated ◀
Histiocytic syndromes ◀
Macrophage activation syndrome ◀

● 288.5 **Decreased white blood cell count category** ◀

Excludes *neutropenia (288.01–288.09)* ◀

❑288.50 **Leukocytopenia, unspecified** ◀
Decreased leukocytes, unspecified ◀
Decreased white blood cell count, unspecified ◀
Leukopenia NOS ◀

288.51 **Lymphocytopenia** ◀
Decreased lymphocytes ◀

❑288.59 **Other decreased white blood cell count** ◀
Basophilic leukopenia ◀
Eosinophilic leukopenia ◀
Monocytopenia ◀
Plasmacytopenia ◀

● 288.6 **Elevated white blood cell count category** ◀

Excludes *eosinophilia (288.3)* ◀

❑288.60 **Leukocytosis, unspecified** ◀
Elevated leukocytes, unspecified ◀
Elevated white blood cell count, unspecified ◀

288.61 **Lymphocytosis (symptomatic)** ◀
Elevated lymphocytes ◀

288.62 **Leukemoid reaction** ◀
Basophilic leukemoid reaction ◀
Lymphocytic leukemoid reaction ◀
Monocytic leukemoid reaction ◀
Myelocytic leukemoid reaction ◀
Neutrophilic leukemoid reaction ◀

288.63 **Monocytosis (symptomatic)** ◀

Excludes *infectious mononucleosis (075)* ◀

288.64 **Plasmacytosis** ◀

288.65 **Basophilia** ◀

❑288.69 **Other elevated white blood cell count** ◀

❑288.8 **Other specified disease of white blood cells** ⬅

Excludes *decreased white blood cell counts (288.50–288.59)* ◀
elevated white blood cell counts (288.60–288.69) ◀
immunity disorders (279.0–279.9)

❑288.9 **Unspecified disease of white blood cells**

● 289 **Other diseases of blood and blood-forming organs**

289.0 **Polycythemia, secondary**

See 238.4 for primary polycythemia (= polycythemia vera)

High-oxygen-affinity hemoglobin
Polycythemia:
acquired
benign
due to:
fall in plasma volume
high altitude
emotional
erythropoietin
hypoxemic
nephrogenous
relative
spurious
stress

Excludes *polycythemia:*
neonatal (776.4)
primary (238.4)
vera (238.4)

289.1 **Chronic lymphadenitis**
Chronic:
adenitis any lymph node, except mesenteric
lymphadenitis any lymph node, except mesenteric

Excludes *acute lymphadenitis (683)*
mesenteric (289.2)
enlarged glands NOS (785.6)

❑289.2 **Nonspecific mesenteric lymphadenitis**
Mesenteric lymphadenitis (acute) (chronic)

❑289.3 **Lymphadenitis, unspecified, except mesenteric**

289.4 **Hypersplenism**
"Big spleen" syndrome
Dyssplenism
Hypersplenia

Excludes *primary splenic neutropenia (289.53)* ⬅

● 289.5 **Other diseases of spleen**

❑289.50 **Disease of spleen, unspecified**

289.51 **Chronic congestive splenomegaly**

● 289.52 *Splenic sequestration*

Code first sickle-cell disease in crisis (282.42, 282.62, 282.64, 282.69)

289.53 Neutropenic splenomegaly ◀

❑ **289.59 Other**

Lien migrans
Perisplenitis
Splenic:
abscess
atrophy
cyst
Splenic:
fibrosis
infarction
rupture, nontraumatic
Splenitis
Wandering spleen

Excludes *bilharzial splenic fibrosis (120.0–120.9)*
hepatolienal fibrosis (571.5)
splenomegaly NOS (789.2)

289.6 Familial polycythemia

Familial:
benign polycythemia
erythrocytosis

289.7 Methemoglobinemia

Congenital NADH [DPNH]-methemoglobin-reductase deficiency
Hemoglobin M [Hb-M] disease
Methemoglobinemia:
NOS
acquired (with sulfhemoglobinemia)
hereditary
toxic
Stokvis' disease
Sulfhemoglobinemia

Use additional E code to identify cause

● **289.8 Other specified diseases of blood and blood-forming organs**

289.81 Primary hypercoagulable state

Activated protein C resistance
Antithrombin III deficiency
Factor V Leiden mutation
Lupus anticoagulant
Protein C deficiency
Protein S deficiency
Prothrombin gene mutation

289.82 Secondary hypercoagulable state

● 289.83 *Myelofibrosis* ◀

Myelofibrosis NOS ◀
Secondary myelofibrosis ◀

Code first the underlying disorder, such as: ◀
malignant neoplasm of breast (174.0–174.9, 175.0–175.9) ◀

Excludes *idiopathic myelofibrosis (238.76)* ◀
leukoerythroblastic anemia (284.2) ◀
myelofibrosis with myeloid metaplasia (238.76) ◀
myelophthisic anemia (284.2) ◀
myelophthisis (284.2) ◀
primary myelofibrosis (238.76) ◀

❑ **289.89 Other specified disease of blood and blood-forming organs** ⬅

Hypergammaglobulinemia
Pseudocholinesterase deficiency

❑ **289.9 Unspecified diseases of blood and blood-forming organs**

Blood dyscrasia NOS
Erythroid hyperplasia

5. MENTAL DISORDERS (290–319)

In the International Classification of Diseases, 9th Revision (ICD-9), the corresponding Chapter V, Mental Disorders, includes a glossary that defines the contents of each category. The introduction to Chapter V in ICD-9 indicates that the glossary is included so psychiatrists can make the diagnosis based on the descriptions provided rather than from the category titles. Lay coders are instructed to code whatever diagnosis the physician records.

Chapter 5, Mental Disorders, in ICD-9-CM uses the standard classification format with inclusion and exclusion terms, omitting the glossary as part of the main text.

The mental disorders section of ICD-9-CM has been expanded to incorporate additional psychiatric disorders not listed in ICD-9. The glossary from ICD-9 does not contain all these terms. It now appears in Appendix B, which also contains descriptions and definitions for the terms added in ICD-9-CM. Some of these were provided by the American Psychiatric Association's Task Force on Nomenclature and Statistics, which is preparing the Diagnostic and Statistical Manual, Third Edition (DSM-III), and others from A Psychiatric Glossary.

The American Psychiatric Association provided invaluable assistance in modifying Chapter 5 of ICD-9-CM to incorporate detail useful to American clinicians and gave permission to use material from the aforementioned sources.

1. Manual of the International Statistical Classification of Diseases, Injuries, and Causes of Death, 9th Revision, World Health Organization, Geneva, Switzerland, 1975.
2. American Psychiatric Association, Task Force on Nomenclature and Statistics, Robert L. Spitzer, M.D., Chairman.
3. A Psychiatric Glossary, Fourth Edition, American Psychiatric Association, Washington, D.C., 1975.

PSYCHOSES (290–299)

Excludes *mental retardation (317–319)*

ORGANIC PSYCHOTIC CONDITIONS (290–294)

Includes: psychotic organic brain syndrome

Excludes *nonpsychotic syndromes of organic etiology (310.0–310.9)*
psychoses classifiable to 295–298 and without impairment of orientation, comprehension, calculation, learning capacity, and judgment, but associated with physical disease, injury, or condition affecting the brain [e.g., following childbirth] (295.0–298.8)

● **290 Dementias**

Code first the associated neurological condition

Excludes *dementia due to alcohol (291.0–291.2)*
dementia due to drugs (292.82)
dementia not classified as senile, presenile, or arteriosclerotic (294.10–294.11)
psychoses classifiable to 295–298 occurring in the senium without dementia or delirium (295.0–298.8)
senility with mental changes of nonpsychotic severity (310.1)
transient organic psychotic conditions (293.0–293.9)

290.0 Senile dementia, uncomplicated
Senile dementia:
NOS
simple type

Excludes *mild memory disturbances, not amounting to dementia, associated with senile brain disease (310.1)*
senile dementia with:
delirium or confusion (290.3)
delusional [paranoid] features (290.20)
depressive features (290.21)

● **290.1 Presenile dementia**
Brain syndrome with presenile brain disease

Excludes *arteriosclerotic dementia (290.40–290.43)*
dementia associated with other cerebral conditions (294.10–294.11)

290.10 Presenile dementia, uncomplicated
Presenile dementia:
NOS
simple type

290.11 Presenile dementia with delirium
Presenile dementia with acute confusional state

290.12 Presenile dementia with delusional features
Presenile dementia, paranoid type

290.13 Presenile dementia with depressive features
Presenile dementia, depressed type

● **290.2 Senile dementia with delusional or depressive features**

Excludes *senile dementia:*
NOS (290.0)
with delirium and/or confusion (290.3)

290.20 Senile dementia with delusional features
Senile dementia, paranoid type
Senile psychosis NOS

290.21 Senile dementia with depressive features

290.3 Senile dementia with delirium
Senile dementia with acute confusional state

Excludes *senile:*
dementia NOS (290.0)
psychosis NOS (290.20)

● **290.4 Vascular dementia**
Multi-infarct dementia or psychosis

Use additional code to identify cerebral atherosclerosis (437.0)

Excludes *suspected cases with no clear evidence of arteriosclerosis (290.9)*

290.40 Vascular dementia, uncomplicated
Arteriosclerotic dementia:
NOS
simple type

290.41 Vascular dementia with delirium
Arteriosclerotic dementia with acute confusional state

290.42 Vascular dementia with delusions
Arteriosclerotic dementia, paranoid type

290.43 Vascular dementia with depressed mood
Arteriosclerotic dementia, depressed type

❑ **290.8 Other specified senile psychotic conditions**
Presbyophrenic psychosis

❑ **290.9 Unspecified senile psychotic condition**

● **291 Alcohol-induced mental disorders**

Excludes *alcoholism without psychosis (303.0–303.9)*

291.0 Alcohol withdrawal delirium
Alcoholic delirium
Delirium tremens

Excludes *alcohol withdrawal (291.81)*

291.1 Alcohol-induced persisting amnestic disorder
Alcoholic polyneuritic psychosis
Korsakoff's psychosis, alcoholic
Wernicke-Korsakoff syndrome (alcoholic)

❑ **291.2 Alcohol-induced persisting dementia**
Alcoholic dementia NOS
Alcoholism associated with dementia NOS
Chronic alcoholic brain syndrome

291.3 Alcohol-induced psychotic disorder with hallucinations
Alcoholic:
hallucinosis (acute)
psychosis with hallucinosis

Excludes *alcohol withdrawal with delirium (291.0)*
schizophrenia (295.0–295.9) and paranoid states (297.0–297.9) taking the form of chronic hallucinosis with clear consciousness in an alcoholic

291.4 Idiosyncratic alcohol intoxication
Pathologic:
alcohol intoxication
drunkenness

Excludes *acute alcohol intoxication (305.0)*
in alcoholism (303.0)
simple drunkenness (305.0)

291.5 Alcoholic-induced psychotic disorder with delusions
Alcoholic:
paranoia
psychosis, paranoid type

Excludes *nonalcoholic paranoid states (297.0–297.9)*
schizophrenia, paranoid type (295.3)

● **291.8 Other specified alcohol-induced mental disorders**

291.81 Alcohol withdrawal
Alcohol:
abstinence syndrome or symptoms
withdrawal syndrome or symptoms

Excludes *alcohol withdrawal:*
delirium (291.0)
hallucinosis (291.3)
delirium tremens (291.0)

❑ **291.82 Alcohol induced sleep disorders**
Alcohol induced circadian rhythm sleep disorders
Alcohol induced hypersomnia
Alcohol induced insomnia
Alcohol induced parasomnia

❑ **291.89 Other**
Alcohol-induced anxiety disorder
Alcohol-induced mood disorder
Alcohol-induced sexual dysfunction

❑ **291.9 Unspecified alcohol-induced mental disorders**
Alcohol-related disorder NOS
Alcoholic:
mania NOS
psychosis NOS
Alcoholism (chronic) with psychosis

● **292 Drug-induced mental disorders**

Includes: organic brain syndrome associated with consumption of drugs

Use additional code for any associated drug dependence (304.0–304.9)

Use E code to identify drug

292.0 Drug withdrawal
Drug:
abstinence syndrome or symptoms
withdrawal syndrome or symptoms

● **292.1 Drug-induced psychotic disorders**

292.11 Drug-induced psychotic disorder with delusions
Paranoid state induced by drugs

292.12 Drug-induced psychotic disorder with hallucinations
Hallucinatory state induced by drugs

Excludes *states following LSD or other hallucinogens, lasting only a few days or less ["bad trips"] (305.3)*

292.2 Pathological drug intoxication
Drug reaction: resulting in brief psychotic states
NOS
idiosyncratic
pathologic

Excludes *expected brief psychotic reactions to hallucinogens ["bad trips"] (305.3)*
physiological side-effects of drugs (e.g., dystonias)

● **292.8 Other specified drug-induced mental disorders**

292.81 Drug-induced delirium

292.82 Drug-induced persisting dementia

292.83 Drug-induced persisting amnestic disorder

292.84 Drug-induced mood disorder
Depressive state induced by drugs

292.85 Drug induced sleep disorders
Drug induced circadian rhythm sleep disorder
Drug induced hypersomnia
Drug induced insomnia
Drug induced parasomnia

❑ **292.89 Other**
Drug-induced anxiety disorder
Drug-induced organic personality syndrome
Drug-induced sexual dysfunction
Drug intoxication

❑ **292.9 Unspecified drug-induced mental disorder**
Drug-related disorder NOS
Organic psychosis NOS due to or associated with drugs

ICD-9-CM 200-299 Vol. 1

● **293 Transient mental disorders due to conditions classified elsewhere**

Includes: transient organic mental disorders not associated with alcohol or drugs

Code first the associated physical or neurological condition

Excludes *confusional state or delirium superimposed on senile dementia (290.3)*
dementia due to:
alcohol (291.0–291.9)
arteriosclerosis (290.40–290.43)
drugs (292.82)
senility (290.0)

● ***293.0 Delirium due to conditions classified elsewhere***
Acute:
confusional state
infective psychosis
organic reaction
posttraumatic organic psychosis
psycho-organic syndrome
Acute psychosis associated with endocrine, metabolic, or cerebrovascular disorder
Epileptic:
confusional state
twilight state

● ***293.1 Subacute delirium***
Subacute:
confusional state
infective psychosis
organic reaction
posttraumatic organic psychosis
psycho-organic syndrome
psychosis associated with endocrine or metabolic disorder

● **293.8 Other specified transient mental disorders due to conditions classified elsewhere**

● ***293.81 Psychotic disorder with delusions in conditions classified elsewhere***
Transient organic psychotic condition, paranoid type

● *293.82 Psychotic disorder with hallucinations in conditions classified elsewhere*
Transient organic psychotic condition, hallucinatory type

● *293.83 Mood disorder in conditions classified elsewhere*
Transient organic psychotic condition, depressive type

● *293.84 Anxiety disorder in conditions classified elsewhere*

● ❑*293.89 Other*
Catatonic disorder in conditions classified elsewhere

● ❑*293.9 Unspecified transient mental disorder in conditions classified elsewhere*
Organic psychosis:
infective NOS
posttraumatic NOS
transient NOS
Psycho-organic syndrome

● **294 Persistent mental disorders due to conditions classified elsewhere**

Includes: organic psychotic brain syndromes (chronic), not elsewhere classified

● *294.0 Amnestic disorder in conditions classified elsewhere*
Korsakoff's psychosis or syndrome (nonalcoholic)

Code first underlying condition

Excludes *alcoholic:*
amnestic syndrome (291.1)
Korsakoff's psychosis (291.1)

● **294.1 Dementia in conditions classified elsewhere**
Code first any underlying physical condition as:
dementia in:
Alzheimer's disease (331.0)
Cerebral lipidoses (330.1)
Dementia of the Alzheimer's type
Dementia with Lewy bodies (331.82)
Dementia with Parkinsonism (331.82)
Epilepsy (345.0–345.9)
Frontal dementia (331.19)
Frontotemporal dementia (331.19)
General paresis [syphilis] (094.1)
Hepatolenticular degeneration (275.1)
Huntington's chorea (333.4)
Jakob-Creutzfeldt disease (046.1)
Multiple sclerosis (340)
Pick's disease of the brain (331.11)
Polyarteritis nodosa (446.0)
Syphilis (094.1)

Excludes *dementia:*
arteriosclerotic (290.40–290.43)
presenile (290.10–290.13)
senile (290.0)
epileptic psychosis NOS (294.8)

● *294.10 Dementia in conditions classified elsewhere without behavioral disturbance*
Dementia in conditions classified elsewhere NOS

● *294.11 Dementia in conditions classified elsewhere with behavioral disturbance*
Aggressive behavior
Combative behavior
Violent behavior
Wandering off

❑**294.8 Other persistent mental disorders due to conditions classified elsewhere**
Amnestic disorder NOS
Dementia NOS
Epileptic psychosis NOS
Mixed paranoid and affective organic psychotic states

Use additional code for associated epilepsy (345.0–345.9)

Excludes *mild memory disturbances, not amounting to dementia (310.1)*

❑**294.9 Unspecified persistent mental disorders due to conditions classified elsewhere**
Cognitive disorder NOS
Organic psychosis (chronic)

OTHER PSYCHOSES (295–299)

Use additional code to identify any associated physical disease, injury, or condition affecting the brain with psychoses classifiable to 295–298

● **295 Schizophrenic disorders**

Includes: schizophrenia of the types described in 295.0–295.9 occurring in children

Excludes *childhood type schizophrenia (299.9)*
infantile autism (299.0)

The following fifth-digit subclassification is for use with category 295:
❑ **0 unspecified**
1 subchronic
2 chronic
3 subchronic with acute exacerbation
4 chronic with acute exacerbation
5 in remission

● **295.0 Simple type**
Schizophrenia simplex

Excludes *latent schizophrenia (295.5)*

● **295.1 Disorganized type**
Hebephrenia
Hebephrenic type schizophrenia

● **295.2 Catatonic type**
Catatonic (schizophrenia):
agitation
excitation
excited type
stupor
withdrawn type
Schizophrenic:
catalepsy
catatonia
flexibilitas cerea

● **295.3 Paranoid type**
Paraphrenic schizophrenia

Excludes *involutional paranoid state (297.2)*
paranoia (297.1)
paraphrenia (297.2)

● **295.4 Schizophreniform disorder**
Oneirophrenia
Schizophreniform:
attack
psychosis, confusional type

Excludes *acute forms of schizophrenia of:*
catatonic type (295.2)
hebephrenic type (295.1)
paranoid type (295.3)
simple type (295.0)
undifferentiated type (295.8)

● **295.5 Latent schizophrenia**
Latent schizophrenic reaction
Schizophrenia: borderline, incipient, prepsychotic
Schizophrenia: prodromal, pseudoneurotic, pseudopsychopathic
Excludes *schizoid personality (301.20–301.22)*

● **295.6 Residual type**
Chronic undifferentiated schizophrenia
Restzustand (schizophrenic)
Schizophrenic residual state

● **295.7 Schizoaffective disorder**
Cyclic schizophrenia
Mixed schizophrenic and affective psychosis
Schizo-affective psychosis
Schizophreniform psychosis, affective type

● ❑ **295.8 Other specified types of schizophrenia**
Acute (undifferentiated) schizophrenia
Atypical schizophrenia
Cenesthopathic schizophrenia
Excludes *infantile autism (299.0)*

● ❑ **295.9 Unspecified schizophrenia**
Schizophrenia: NOS, mixed NOS
Schizophrenia: undifferentiated type, undifferentiated NOS
Schizophrenic reaction NOS
Schizophreniform psychosis NOS

● 296 Episodic mood disorders

Includes: episodic affective disorders

Excludes *neurotic depression (300.4)*
reactive depressive psychosis (298.0)
reactive excitation (298.1)

The following fifth-digit subclassification is for use with categories 296.0–296.6:

❑ **0 unspecified**
1 mild
2 moderate
3 severe, without mention of psychotic behavior
4 severe, specified as with psychotic behavior
5 in partial or unspecified remission
6 in full remission

● **296.0 Bipolar I disorder, single manic episode**
Hypomania (mild) NOS single episode or unspecified
Hypomanic psychosis single episode or unspecified
Mania (monopolar) NOS single episode or unspecified
Manic-depressive psychosis or reaction, single episode or unspecified:
hypomanic, single episode or unspecified
manic, single episode or unspecified
Excludes *circular type, if there was a previous attack of depression (296.4)*

● **296.1 Manic disorder, recurrent episode**
Any condition classifiable to 296.0, stated to be recurrent
Excludes *circular type, if there was a previous attack of depression (296.4)*

● **296.2 Major depressive disorder, single episode**
Depressive psychosis, single episode or unspecified
Endogenous depression, single episode or unspecified
Involutional melancholia, single episode or unspecified
Manic-depressive psychosis or reaction, depressed type, single episode or unspecified
Monopolar depression, single episode or unspecified
Psychotic depression, single episode or unspecified
Excludes *circular type, if previous attack was of manic type (296.5)*
depression NOS (311)
reactive depression (neurotic) (300.4)
psychotic (298.0)

● **296.3 Major depressive disorder, recurrent episode**
Any condition classifiable to 296.2, stated to be recurrent
Excludes *circular type, if previous attack was of manic type (296.5)*
depression NOS (311)
reactive depression (neurotic) (300.4)
psychotic (298.0)

● **296.4 Bipolar I disorder, most recent episode (or current) manic**
Bipolar disorder, now manic
Manic-depressive psychosis, circular type but currently manic
Excludes *brief compensatory or rebound mood swings (296.99)*

● **296.5 Bipolar I disorder, most recent episode (or current) depressed**
Bipolar disorder, now depressed
Manic-depressive psychosis, circular type but currently depressed
Excludes *brief compensatory or rebound mood swings (296.99)*

● **296.6 Bipolar I disorder, most recent episode (or current) mixed**
Manic-depressive psychosis, circular type, mixed

❑ **296.7 Bipolar I disorder, most recent episode (or current) unspecified**
Atypical bipolar affective disorder NOS
Manic-depressive psychosis, circular type, current condition not specified as either manic or depressive

● **296.8 Other and unspecified bipolar disorders**

❑ **296.80 Bipolar disorder, unspecified**
Bipolar disorder NOS
Manic-depressive:
reaction NOS
syndrome NOS

296.81 Atypical manic disorder

296.82 Atypical depressive disorder

❑ **296.89 Other**
Bipolar II disorder
Manic-depressive psychosis, mixed type

● **296.9 Other and unspecified episodic mood disorder**
Excludes *psychogenic affective psychoses (298.0–298.8)*

❑ **296.90 Unspecified episodic mood disorder**
Affective psychosis NOS
Melancholia NOS
Mood disorder NOS

❑ **296.99 Other specified episodic mood disorder**
Mood swings:
brief compensatory
rebound

● 297 Delusional disorders

Includes: paranoid disorders

Excludes *acute paranoid reaction (298.3)*
alcoholic jealousy or paranoid state (291.5)
paranoid schizophrenia (295.3)

297.0 Paranoid state, simple

297.1 Delusional disorder
Chronic paranoid psychosis
Sander's disease
Systematized delusions
Excludes *paranoid personality disorder (301.0)*

297.2 Paraphrenia
Involutional paranoid state
Late paraphrenia
Paraphrenia (involutional)

ICD-9-CM 200–299 Vol. 1

297.3 Shared psychotic disorder
Folie à deux
Induced psychosis or paranoid disorder

❑**297.8 Other specified paranoid states**
Paranoia querulans
Sensitiver Beziehungswahn

Excludes *acute paranoid reaction or state (298.3)*
senile paranoid state (290.20)

❑**297.9 Unspecified paranoid state**
Paranoid:
disorder NOS
psychosis NOS
reaction NOS
state NOS

● **298 Other nonorganic psychoses**

Includes: psychotic conditions due to or provoked by:
emotional stress
environmental factors as major part of etiology

298.0 Depressive type psychosis
Psychogenic depressive psychosis
Psychotic reactive depression
Reactive depressive psychosis

Excludes *manic-depressive psychosis, depressed type (296.2–296.3)*
neurotic depression (300.4)
reactive depression NOS (300.4)

298.1 Excitative type psychosis
Acute hysterical psychosis
Psychogenic excitation
Reactive excitation

Excludes *manic-depressive psychosis, manic type (296.0–296.1)*

298.2 Reactive confusion
Psychogenic confusion
Psychogenic twilight state

Excludes *acute confusional state (293.0)*

298.3 Acute paranoid reaction
Acute psychogenic paranoid psychosis
Bouffée délirante

Excludes *paranoid states (297.0–297.9)*

298.4 Psychogenic paranoid psychosis
Protracted reactive paranoid psychosis

❑**298.8 Other and unspecified reactive psychosis**
Brief psychotic disorder
Brief reactive psychosis NOS
Hysterical psychosis
Psychogenic psychosis NOS
Psychogenic stupor

Excludes *acute hysterical psychosis (298.1)*

❑**298.9 Unspecified psychosis**
Atypical psychosis
Psychosis NOS
Psychotic disorder NOS

● **299 Pervasive developmental disorders**

Excludes *adult type psychoses occurring in childhood, as:*
affective disorders (296.0–296.9)
manic-depressive disorders (296.0–296.9)
schizophrenia (295.0–295.9)

The following fifth-digit subclassification is for use with category 299:
0 current or active state
1 residual state

● **299.0 Autistic disorder**
Childhood autism
Infantile psychosis
Kanner's syndrome

Excludes *disintegrative psychosis (299.1)*
Heller's syndrome (299.1)
schizophrenic syndrome of childhood (299.9)

● **299.1 Childhood disintegrative disorder**
Heller's syndrome

Use additional code to identify any associated neurological disorder

Excludes *infantile autism (299.0)*
schizophrenic syndrome of childhood (299.9)

● ❑**299.8 Other specified pervasive developmental disorders**
Asperger's disorder
Atypical childhood psychosis
Borderline psychosis of childhood

Excludes *simple stereotypes without psychotic disturbance (307.3)*

● ❑**299.9 Unspecified pervasive developmental disorder**
Child psychosis NOS
Pervasive developmental disorder NOS
Schizophrenia, childhood type NOS
Schizophrenic syndrome of childhood NOS

Excludes *schizophrenia of adult type occurring in childhood (295.0–295.9)*

NEUROTIC DISORDERS, PERSONALITY DISORDERS, AND OTHER NONPSYCHOTIC MENTAL DISORDERS (300–316)

● **300 Anxiety, dissociative, and somatoform disorders**

● **300.0 Anxiety states**

Excludes *anxiety in:*
acute stress reaction (308.0)
transient adjustment reaction (309.24)
neurasthenia (300.5)
psychophysiological disorders (306.0–306.9)
separation anxiety (309.21)

❑**300.00 Anxiety state, unspecified**
Anxiety:
neurosis
reaction
state (neurotic)
Atypical anxiety disorder

300.01 Panic disorder without agoraphobia
Panic:
attack
state

Excludes *panic disorder with agoraphobia (300.21)*

300.02 Generalized anxiety disorder

❑**300.09 Other**

300.1 Dissociative, conversion, and factitious disorders

Excludes *adjustment reaction (309.0–309.9)*
anorexia nervosa (307.1)
gross stress reaction (308.0–308.9)
hysterical personality (301.50–301.59)
psychophysiologic disorders (306.0–306.9)

❑**300.10 Hysteria, unspecified**

300.11 Conversion disorder
Astasia-abasia, hysterical
Conversion hysteria or reaction
Hysterical:
blindness
deafness
paralysis

300.12 Dissociative amnesia
Hysterical amnesia

300.13 Dissociative fugue
Hysterical fugue

300.14 Dissociative identity disorder

❑**300.15 Dissociative disorder or reaction, unspecified**

300.16 Factitious disorder with predominantly psychological signs and symptoms
Compensation neurosis
Ganser's syndrome, hysterical

❑**300.19 Other and unspecified factitious illness**
Factitious disorder (with combined psychological and physical signs and symptoms) (with predominantly physical signs and symptoms)
NOS

Excludes *multiple operations or hospital addiction syndrome (301.51)*

● **300.2 Phobic disorders**

Excludes *anxiety state not associated with a specific situation or object (300.00–300.09)*
obsessional phobias (300.3)

❑**300.20 Phobia, unspecified**
Anxiety-hysteria NOS
Phobia NOS

300.21 Agoraphobia with panic disorder
Fear of:
open spaces with panic attacks
streets with panic attacks
travel with panic attacks
Panic disorder with agoraphobia

Excludes *agoraphobia without panic disorder (300.22)*
panic disorder without agoraphobia (300.01)

300.22 Agoraphobia without mention of panic attacks
Any condition classifiable to 300.21 without mention of panic attacks

300.23 Social phobia
Fear of:
eating in public
public speaking
washing in public

❑**300.29 Other isolated or specific phobias**
Acrophobia
Animal phobias
Claustrophobia
Fear of crowds

300.3 Obsessive-compulsive disorders *OCD*
Anancastic neurosis
Compulsive neurosis
Obsessional phobia [any]

Excludes *obsessive-compulsive symptoms occurring in:*
endogenous depression (296.2–296.3)
organic states (e.g., encephalitis)
schizophrenia (295.0–295.9)

300.4 Dysthymic disorder
Anxiety depression
Depression with anxiety
Depressive reaction
Neurotic depressive state
Reactive depression

Excludes *adjustment reaction with depressive symptoms (309.0–309.1)*
depression NOS (311)
manic-depressive psychosis, depressed type (296.2–296.3)
reactive depressive psychosis (298.0)

300.5 Neurasthenia
Fatigue neurosis
Nervous debility
Psychogenic:
asthenia
general fatigue

Use additional code to identify any associated physical disorder

Excludes *anxiety state (300.00–300.09)*
neurotic depression (300.4)
psychophysiological disorders (306.0–306.9)
specific nonpsychotic mental disorders following organic brain damage (310.0–310.9)

300.6 Depersonalization disorder
Derealization (neurotic)
Neurotic state with depersonalization episode

Excludes *depersonalization associated with:*
anxiety (300.00–300.09)
depression (300.4)
manic-depressive disorder or psychosis (296.0–296.9)
schizophrenia (295.0–295.9)

300.7 Hypochondriasis
Body dysmorphic disorder

Excludes *hypochondriasis in:*
hysteria (300.10–300.19)
manic-depressive psychosis, depressed type (296.2–296.3)
neurasthenia (300.5)
obsessional disorder (300.3)
schizophrenia (295.0–295.9)

● **300.8 Somatoform disorders**

300.81 Somatization disorder
Briquet's disorder
Severe somatoform disorder

300.82 Undifferentiated somatoform disorder
Atypical somatoform disorder
Somatoform disorder NOS

❑**300.89 Other somatoform disorders**
Occupational neurosis, including writers' cramp
Psychasthenia
Psychasthenic neurosis

❑**300.9 Unspecified nonpsychotic mental disorder**
Psychoneurosis NOS

● **301 Personality disorders**

Includes: character neurosis

Use additional code to identify any associated neurosis or psychosis, or physical condition

Excludes *nonpsychotic personality disorder associated with organic brain syndromes (310.0–310.9)*

301.0 Paranoid personality disorder
Fanatic personality
Paranoid personality (disorder)
Paranoid traits

Excludes *acute paranoid reaction (298.3)*
alcoholic paranoia (291.5)
paranoid schizophrenia (295.3)
paranoid states (297.0–297.9)

● **301.1 Affective personality disorder**

Excludes *affective psychotic disorders (296.0–296.9)*
neurasthenia (300.5)
neurotic depression (300.4)

301.10 Affective personality disorder, unspecified

301.11 Chronic hypomanic personality disorder
Chronic hypomanic disorder
Hypomanic personality

301.12 Chronic depressive personality disorder
Chronic depressive disorder
Depressive character or personality

301.13 Cyclothymic disorder
Cycloid personality
Cyclothymia
Cyclothymic personality

● **301.2 Schizoid personality disorder**
Excludes *schizophrenia (295.0–295.9)*

❑ **301.20 Schizoid personality disorder, unspecified**

301.21 Introverted personality

301.22 Schizotypal personality disorder

301.3 Explosive personality disorder
Aggressive:
personality
reaction
Aggressiveness
Emotional instability (excessive)
Pathological emotionality
Quarrelsomeness
Excludes *dyssocial personality (301.7)*
hysterical neurosis (300.10–300.19)

301.4 Obsessive-compulsive personality disorder
Anancastic personality
Obsessional personality
Excludes *obsessive-compulsive disorder (300.3)*
phobic state (300.20–300.29)

● **301.5 Histrionic personality disorder**
Excludes *hysterical neurosis (300.10–300.19)*

❑ **301.50 Histrionic personality disorder, unspecified**
Hysterical personality NOS

301.51 Chronic factitious illness with physical symptoms
Hospital addiction syndrome
Multiple operations syndrome
Munchausen syndrome

❑ **301.59 Other histrionic personality disorder**
Personality:
emotionally unstable
labile
Personality:
psychoinfantile

301.6 Dependent personality disorder
Asthenic personality
Inadequate personality
Passive personality
Excludes *neurasthenia (300.5)*
passive-aggressive personality (301.84)

301.7 Antisocial personality disorder
Amoral personality
Asocial personality
Dyssocial personality
Personality disorder with predominantly sociopathic or asocial manifestation
Excludes *disturbance of conduct without specifiable personality disorder (312.0–312.9)*
explosive personality (301.3)

● **301.8 Other personality disorders**

301.81 Narcissistic personality disorder

301.82 Avoidant personality disorder

301.83 Borderline personality disorder

301.84 Passive-aggressive personality

❑ **301.89 Other**
Personality:
eccentric
"haltlose" type
immature
Personality:
masochistic
psychoneurotic
Excludes *psychoinfantile personality (301.59)*

❑ **301.9 Unspecified personality disorder**
Pathological personality NOS
Personality disorder NOS
Psychopathic:
constitutional state
personality (disorder)

● **302 Sexual and gender identity disorders**
Excludes *sexual disorder manifest in:*
organic brain syndrome (290.0–294.9, 310.0–310.9)
psychosis (295.0–298.9)

302.0 Ego-dystonic sexual orientation
Ego-dystonic lesbianism
Sexual orientation conflict disorder
Excludes *homosexual pedophilia (302.2)*

302.1 Zoophilia
Bestiality

302.2 Pedophilia

302.3 Transvestic fetishism
Excludes *trans-sexualism (302.5)*

302.4 Exhibitionism

● **302.5 Trans-sexualism**
Excludes *transvestism (302.3)*

❑ **302.50 With unspecified sexual history**

302.51 With asexual history

302.52 With homosexual history

302.53 With heterosexual history

302.6 Gender identity disorder in children
Feminism in boys
Gender identity disorder NOS
Excludes *gender identity disorder in adult (302.85)*
trans-sexualism (302.50–302.53)
transvestism (302.3)

● **302.7 Psychosexual dysfunction**
Excludes *impotence of organic origin (607.84)*
normal transient symptoms from ruptured hymen
transient or occasional failures of erection due to fatigue, anxiety, alcohol, or drugs

❑ **302.70 Psychosexual dysfunction, unspecified**
Sexual dysfunction NOS

302.71 Hypoactive sexual desire disorder
Excludes *decreased sexual desire NOS (799.81)*

302.72 With inhibited sexual excitement
Female sexual arousal disorder
Male erectile disorder

302.73 Female orgasmic disorder

302.74 Male orgasmic disorder

302.75 Premature ejaculation

302.76 Dyspareunia, psychogenic

❑ **302.79 With other specified psychosexual dysfunctions**
Sexual aversion disorder

● **302.8 Other specified psychosexual disorders**

302.81 Fetishism

302.82 Voyeurism

302.83 Sexual masochism

302.84 Sexual sadism

302.85 Gender identity disorder in adolescents or adults
Excludes *gender identity disorder NOS (302.6)*
gender identity disorder in children (302.6)

❑302.89 Other
Frotteurism
Nymphomania
Satyriasis

❑302.9 **Unspecified psychosexual disorder**
Paraphilia NOS
Pathologic sexuality NOS
Sexual deviation NOS
Sexual disorder NOS

● 303 **Alcohol dependence syndrome**

Use additional code to identify any associated condition, as:
alcoholic psychoses (291.0–291.9)
drug dependence (304.0–304.9)
physical complications of alcohol, such as:
cerebral degeneration (331.7)
cirrhosis of liver (571.2)
epilepsy (345.0–345.9)
gastritis (535.3)
hepatitis (571.1)
liver damage NOS (571.3)

Excludes *drunkenness NOS (305.0)*

The following fifth-digit subclassification is for use with category 303:
❑ 0 **unspecified**
1 **continuous**
2 **episodic**
3 **in remission**

● 303.0 **Acute alcoholic intoxication**
Acute drunkenness in alcoholism

● ❑303.9 **Other and unspecified alcohol dependence**
Chronic alcoholism
Dipsomania

● 304 **Drug dependence**

Excludes *nondependent abuse of drugs (305.1–305.9)*

The following fifth-digit subclassification is for use with category 304:
❑ 0 **unspecified**
1 **continuous**
2 **episodic**
3 **in remission**

● 304.0 **Opioid type dependence**
Heroin
Meperidine
Methadone
Morphine
Opium
Opium alkaloids and their derivatives
Synthetics with morphine-like effects

● 304.1 **Sedative, hypnotic, or anxiolytic dependence**
Barbiturates
Nonbarbiturate sedatives and tranquilizers with a similar effect:
chlordiazepoxide
diazepam
glutethimide
meprobamate
methaqualone

● 304.2 **Cocaine dependence**
Coca leaves and derivatives

● 304.3 **Cannabis dependence**
Hashish
Hemp
Marihuana

● 304.4 **Amphetamine and other psychostimulant dependence**
Methylphenidate
Phenmetrazine

● 304.5 **Hallucinogen dependence**
Dimethyltryptamine [DMT]
Lysergic acid diethylamide [LSD] and derivatives
Mescaline
Psilocybin

● ❑304.6 **Other specified drug dependence**
Absinthe addiction
Glue sniffing
Inhalant dependence
Phencyclidine dependence

Excludes *tobacco dependence (305.1)*

● 304.7 **Combinations of opioid type drug with any other**

● 304.8 **Combinations of drug dependence excluding opioid type drug**

● ❑304.9 **Unspecified drug dependence**
Drug addiction NOS
Drug dependence NOS

● 305 **Nondependent abuse of drugs**

Note: Includes cases where a person, for whom no other diagnosis is possible, has come under medical care because of the maladaptive effect of a drug on which he is not dependent and that he has taken on his own initiative to the detriment of his health or social functioning.

Excludes *alcohol dependence syndrome (303.0–303.9)*
drug dependence (304.0–304.9)
drug withdrawal syndrome (292.0)
poisoning by drugs or medicinal substances (960.0–979.9)

The following fifth-digit subclassification is for use with codes 305.0, 305.2–305.9:
❑ 0 **unspecified**
1 **continuous**
2 **episodic**
3 **in remission**

● 305.0 **Alcohol abuse**
Drunkenness NOS
Excessive drinking of alcohol NOS
"Hangover" (alcohol)
Inebriety NOS

Excludes *acute alcohol intoxication in alcoholism (303.0)*
alcoholic psychoses (291.0–291.9)

● 305.1 **Tobacco use disorder**
Tobacco dependence

Excludes *history of tobacco use (V15.82)*
smoking complicating pregnancy (649.0) ◀
tobacco use disorder complicating pregnancy (649.0) ◀

● 305.2 **Cannabis abuse**

● 305.3 **Hallucinogen abuse**
Acute intoxication from hallucinogens ["bad trips"]
LSD reaction

● 305.4 **Sedative, hypnotic, or anxiolytic abuse**

● 305.5 **Opioid abuse**

● 305.6 **Cocaine abuse**

● 305.7 **Amphetamine or related acting sympathomimetic abuse**

● 305.8 **Antidepressant type abuse**

305.9 Other, mixed, or unspecified drug abuse
Caffeine intoxication
Inhalant abuse
"Laxative habit"
Misuse of drugs NOS
Nonprescribed use of drugs or patent medicinals
Phencyclidine abuse

306 Physiological malfunction arising from mental factors

Includes: psychogenic:
physical symptoms not involving tissue damage
physiological manifestations not involving tissue damage

Excludes *hysteria (300.11–300.19)*
physical symptoms secondary to a psychiatric disorder classified elsewhere
psychic factors associated with physical conditions involving tissue damage classified elsewhere (316)
specific nonpsychotic mental disorders following organic brain damage (310.0–310.9)

306.0 Musculoskeletal
Psychogenic paralysis
Psychogenic torticollis

Excludes *Gilles de la Tourette's syndrome (307.23)*
paralysis as hysterical or conversion reaction (300.11)
tics (307.20–307.22)

306.1 Respiratory
Psychogenic:
air hunger
cough
hiccough
hyperventilation
yawning

Excludes *psychogenic asthma (316 and 493.9)*

306.2 Cardiovascular
Cardiac neurosis
Cardiovascular neurosis
Neurocirculatory asthenia
Psychogenic cardiovascular disorder

Excludes *psychogenic paroxysmal tachycardia (316 and 427.2)*

306.3 Skin
Psychogenic pruritus

Excludes *psychogenic:*
alopecia (316 and 704.00)
dermatitis (316 and 692.9)
eczema (316 and 691.8 or 692.9)
urticaria (316 and 708.0–708.9)

306.4 Gastrointestinal
Aerophagy
Cyclical vomiting, psychogenic
Diarrhea, psychogenic
Nervous gastritis
Psychogenic dyspepsia

Excludes *cyclical vomiting NOS (536.2)*
globus hystericus (300.11)
mucous colitis (316 and 564.9)
psychogenic:
cardiospasm (316 and 530.0)
duodenal ulcer (316 and 532.0–532.9)
gastric ulcer (316 and 531.0–531.9)
peptic ulcer NOS (316 and 533.0–533.9)
vomiting NOS (307.54)

306.5 Genitourinary

Excludes *enuresis, psychogenic (307.6)*
frigidity (302.72)
impotence (302.72)
psychogenic dyspareunia (302.76)

306.50 Psychogenic genitourinary malfunction, unspecified

306.51 Psychogenic vaginismus
Functional vaginismus

306.52 Psychogenic dysmenorrhea

306.53 Psychogenic dysuria

306.59 Other

306.6 Endocrine

306.7 Organs of special sense

Excludes *hysterical blindness or deafness (300.11)*
psychophysical visual disturbances (368.16)

306.8 Other specified psychophysiological malfunction
Bruxism
Teeth grinding

306.9 Unspecified psychophysiological malfunction
Psychophysiologic disorder NOS
Psychosomatic disorder NOS

307 Special symptoms or syndromes, not elsewhere classified

Note: This category is intended for use if the psychopathology is manifested by a single specific symptom or group of symptoms which are not part of an organic illness or other mental disorder classifiable elsewhere.

Excludes *those due to mental disorders classified elsewhere*
those of organic origin

307.0 Stuttering

Excludes *dysphasia (784.5)*
lisping or lalling (307.9)
retarded development of speech (315.31–315.39)

307.1 Anorexia nervosa

Excludes *eating disturbance NOS (307.50)*
feeding problem (783.3)
of nonorganic origin (307.59)
loss of appetite (783.0)
of nonorganic origin (307.59)

307.2 Tics

Excludes *nail-biting or thumb-sucking (307.9)*
stereotypes occurring in isolation (307.3)
tics of organic origin (333.3)

307.20 Tic disorder, unspecified
Tic disorder NOS

307.21 Transient tic disorder

307.22 Chronic motor or vocal tic disorder

307.23 Tourette's disorder
Motor-verbal tic disorder

307.3 Stereotypic movement disorder
Body-rocking
Head banging
Spasmus nutans
Stereotypes NOS

Excludes *tics (307.20–307.23)*
of organic origin (333.3)

307.4 Specific disorders of sleep of nonorganic origin

Excludes *narcolepsy (347.00–347.11)*
organic hypersomnia (327.10–327.19)
organic insomnia (327.00–327.09)
those of unspecified cause (780.50–780.59)

307.40 Nonorganic sleep disorder, unspecified

307.41 Transient disorder of initiating or maintaining sleep
Adjustment insomnia
Hyposomnia associated with acute or intermittent emotional reactions or conflicts
Insomnia associated with acute or intermittent emotional reactions or conflicts
Sleeplessness associated with acute or intermittent emotional reactions or conflicts

307.42 Persistent disorder of initiating or maintaining sleep
Hyposomnia, insomnia, or sleeplessness associated with:
anxiety
conditioned arousal
depression (major) (minor)
psychosis
Idiopathic insomnia
Paradoxical insomnia
Primary insomnia
Psychophysiological insomnia

307.43 Transient disorder of initiating or maintaining wakefulness
Hypersomnia associated with acute or intermittent emotional reactions or conflicts

307.44 Persistent disorder of initiating or maintaining wakefulness
Hypersomnia associated with depression (major) (minor)
Insufficient sleep syndrome
Primary hypersomnia

Excludes *sleep deprivation (V69.4)*

307.45 Circadian rhythm sleep disorder of nonorganic origin

307.46 Sleep arousal disorder
Night terror disorder
Night terrors
Sleep terror disorder
Sleepwalking
Somnambulism

❑**307.47 Other dysfunctions of sleep stages or arousal from sleep**
Nightmare disorder
Nightmares:
NOS
REM-sleep type
Sleep drunkenness

307.48 Repetitive intrusions of sleep
Repetitive intrusions of sleep with:
atypical polysomnographic features
environmental disturbances
repeated REM-sleep interruptions

❑**307.49 Other**
"Short-sleeper"
Subjective insomnia complaint

● **307.5 Other and unspecified disorders of eating**

Excludes *anorexia:*
nervosa (307.1)
of unspecified cause (783.0)
overeating, of unspecified cause (783.6)
vomiting:
NOS (787.0)
cyclical (536.2)
psychogenic (306.4)

❑**307.50 Eating disorder, unspecified**
Eating disorder NOS

307.51 Bulimia nervosa
Overeating of nonorganic origin

307.52 Pica
Perverted appetite of nonorganic origin
Craving and eating substances such as paint, clay, or dirt to replace a nutritional deficit in the body. Can also be a symptom of mental illness.

307.53 Rumination disorder
Regurgitation, of nonorganic origin, of food with reswallowing

Excludes *obsessional rumination (300.3)*

307.54 Psychogenic vomiting

❑**307.59 Other**
Feeding disorder of infancy or early childhood of nonorganic origin
Infantile feeding disturbances of nonorganic origin
Loss of appetite of nonorganic origin

Item 5-1 Enuresis: Bed wetting by children at night. Causes can be either psychological or medical (diabetes, urinary tract infections, or abnormalities).
Encopresis: Overflow incontinence of bowels sometimes resulting from chronic constipation or fecal impaction. Check your documentation for additional diagnoses.

307.6 Enuresis
Enuresis (primary) (secondary) of nonorganic origin

Excludes *enuresis of unspecified cause (788.3)*

307.7 Encopresis
Encopresis (continuous) (discontinuous) of nonorganic origin

Excludes *encopresis of unspecified cause (787.6)*

ICD-9-CM 300-399 Vol. 1

● **307.8 Pain disorders related to psychological factors**

❑**307.80 Psychogenic pain, site unspecified**

307.81 Tension headache

Excludes *headache:*
NOS (784.0)
migraine (346.0–346.9)

❑**307.89 Other**
Code first to type or site of pain (Revised)

Excludes *pain disorder exclusively attributed to psychological factors (307.80)*
psychogenic pain (307.80)

❑**307.9 Other and unspecified special symptoms or syndromes, not elsewhere classified**
Communication disorder NOS
Hair plucking
Lalling
Lisping
Masturbation
Nail-biting
Thumb-sucking

● **308 Acute reaction to stress**

Includes: catastrophic stress
combat fatigue
gross stress reaction (acute)
transient disorders in response to exceptional physical or mental stress which usually subside within hours or days

Excludes *adjustment reaction or disorder (309.0–309.9)*
chronic stress reaction (309.1–309.9)

308.0 Predominant disturbance of emotions
Anxiety as acute reaction to exceptional [gross] stress
Emotional crisis as acute reaction to exceptional [gross] stress
Panic state as acute reaction to exceptional [gross] stress

308.1 Predominant disturbance of consciousness
Fugues as acute reaction to exceptional [gross] stress

308.2 Predominant psychomotor disturbance
Agitation states as acute reaction to exceptional [gross] stress
Stupor as acute reaction to exceptional [gross] stress

❑ **308.3 Other acute reactions to stress**
Acute situational disturbance
Acute stress disorder

Excludes *prolonged posttraumatic emotional disturbance (309.81)*

308.4 Mixed disorders as reaction to stress

❑ **308.9 Unspecified acute reaction to stress**

● **309 Adjustment reaction**

Includes: adjustment disorders
reaction (adjustment) to chronic stress

Excludes *acute reaction to major stress (308.0–308.9)*
neurotic disorders (300.0–300.9)

309.0 Adjustment disorder with depressed mood
Grief reaction

Excludes *affective psychoses (296.0–296.9)*
neurotic depression (300.4)
prolonged depressive reaction (309.1)
psychogenic depressive psychosis (298.0)

309.1 Prolonged depressive reaction

Excludes *affective psychoses (296.0–296.9)*
brief depressive reaction (309.0)
neurotic depression (300.4)
psychogenic depressive psychosis (298.0)

● **309.2 With predominant disturbance of other emotions**

309.21 Separation anxiety disorder

309.22 Emancipation disorder of adolescence and early adult life

309.23 Specific academic or work inhibition

309.24 Adjustment disorder with anxiety

309.28 Adjustment disorder with mixed anxiety and depressed mood
Adjustment reaction with anxiety and depression

❑ **309.29 Other**
Culture shock

309.3 Adjustment disorder with disturbance of conduct
Conduct disturbance as adjustment reaction
Destructiveness as adjustment reaction

Excludes *destructiveness in child (312.9)*
disturbance of conduct NOS (312.9)
dyssocial behavior without manifest psychiatric disorder (V71.01–V71.02)
personality disorder with predominantly sociopathic or asocial manifestations (301.7)

309.4 Adjustment disorder with mixed disturbance of emotions and conduct

● **309.8 Other specified adjustment reactions**

309.81 Posttraumatic stress disorder
Chronic posttraumatic stress disorder
Concentration camp syndrome
Post-Traumatic Stress Disorder (PTSD) ◀
Posttraumatic stress disorder NOS

Excludes *acute stress disorder (308.3)*
posttraumatic brain syndrome:
nonpsychotic (310.2)
psychotic (293.0–293.9)

309.82 Adjustment reaction with physical symptoms

309.83 Adjustment reaction with withdrawal
Elective mutism as adjustment reaction
Hospitalism (in children) NOS

❑ **309.89 Other**

❑ **309.9 Unspecified adjustment reaction**
Adaptation reaction NOS
Adjustment reaction NOS

● **310 Specific nonpsychotic mental disorders due to brain damage**

Excludes *neuroses, personality disorders, or other nonpsychotic conditions occurring in a form similar to that seen with functional disorders but in association with a physical condition (300.0–300.9, 301.0–301.9)*

310.0 Frontal lobe syndrome
Lobotomy syndrome
Postleucotomy syndrome [state]

Excludes *postcontusion syndrome (310.2)*

310.1 Personality change due to conditions classified elsewhere
Cognitive or personality change of other type, of nonpsychotic severity
Organic psychosyndrome of nonpsychotic severity
Presbyophrenia NOS
Senility with mental changes of nonpsychotic severity

Excludes *memory loss of unknown cause (780.93)*

310.2 Postconcussion syndrome
Postcontusion syndrome or encephalopathy
Posttraumatic brain syndrome, nonpsychotic
Status postcommotio cerebri

Excludes *any organic psychotic conditions following head injury (293.0–294.0)*
frontal lobe syndrome (310.0)
postencephalitic syndrome (310.8)

❑ **310.8 Other specified nonpsychotic mental disorders following organic brain damage**
Mild memory disturbance
Postencephalitic syndrome
Other focal (partial) organic psychosyndromes

❑ **310.9 Unspecified nonpsychotic mental disorder following organic brain damage**

311 Depressive disorder, not elsewhere classified
Depressive disorder NOS
Depressive state NOS
Depression NOS
Excludes *acute reaction to major stress with depressive symptoms (308.0)*
affective personality disorder (301.10–301.13)
affective psychoses (296.0–296.9)
brief depressive reaction (309.0)
depressive states associated with stressful events (309.0–309.1)
disturbance of emotions specific to childhood and adolescence, with misery and unhappiness (313.1)
mixed adjustment reaction with depressive symptoms (309.4)
neurotic depression (300.4)
prolonged depressive adjustment reaction (309.1)
psychogenic depressive psychosis (298.0)

● **312 Disturbance of conduct, not elsewhere classified**
Excludes *adjustment reaction with disturbance of conduct (309.3)*
drug dependence (304.0–304.9)
dyssocial behavior without manifest psychiatric disorder (V71.01–V71.02)
personality disorder with predominantly sociopathic or asocial manifestations (301.7)
sexual deviations (302.0–302.9)

The following fifth-digit subclassification is for use with categories 312.0–312.2:
❑ **0 unspecified**
1 mild
2 moderate
3 severe

● **312.0 Undersocialized conduct disorder, aggressive type**
Aggressive outburst
Anger reaction
Unsocialized aggressive disorder

● **312.1 Undersocialized conduct disorder, unaggressive type**
Childhood truancy, unsocialized
Solitary stealing
Tantrums

● **312.2 Socialized conduct disorder**
Childhood truancy, socialized
Group delinquency
Excludes *gang activity without manifest psychiatric disorder (V71.01)*

● **312.3 Disorders of impulse control, not elsewhere classified**
❑**312.30 Impulse control disorder, unspecified**
312.31 Pathological gambling
312.32 Kleptomania *(Stealing)*
312.33 Pyromania *(Setting fires)*
312.34 Intermittent explosive disorder
312.35 Isolated explosive disorder
❑**312.39 Other**
Trichotillomania
Pulling or twisting hair until it falls out

312.4 Mixed disturbance of conduct and emotions
Neurotic delinquency
Excludes *compulsive conduct disorder (312.3)*

● **312.8 Other specified disturbances of conduct, not elsewhere classified**
312.81 Conduct disorder, childhood onset type
312.82 Conduct disorder, adolescent onset type
❑**312.89 Other conduct disorder**
Conduct disorder of unspecified onset

❑**312.9 Unspecified disturbance of conduct**
Delinquency (juvenile)
Disruptive behavior disorder NOS

● **313 Disturbance of emotions specific to childhood and adolescence**
Excludes *adjustment reaction (309.0–309.9)*
emotional disorder of neurotic type (300.0–300.9)
masturbation, nail-biting, thumb-sucking, and other isolated symptoms (307.0–307.9)

313.0 Overanxious disorder
Anxiety and fearfulness of childhood and adolescence
Overanxious disorder of childhood and adolescence
Excludes *abnormal separation anxiety (309.21)*
anxiety states (300.00–300.09)
hospitalism in children (309.83)
phobic state (300.20–300.29)

313.1 Misery and unhappiness disorder
Excludes *depressive neurosis (300.4)*

● **313.2 Sensitivity, shyness, and social withdrawal disorder**
Excludes *infantile autism (299.0)*
schizoid personality (301.20–301.22)
schizophrenia (295.0–295.9)

313.21 Shyness disorder of childhood
Sensitivity reaction of childhood or adolescence

313.22 Introverted disorder of childhood
Social withdrawal of childhood or adolescence
Withdrawal reaction of childhood or adolescence

313.23 Selective mutism
Excludes *elective mutism as adjustment reaction (309.83)*

313.3 Relationship problems
Sibling jealousy
Excludes *relationship problems associated with aggression, destruction, or other forms of conduct disturbance (312.0–312.9)*

● **313.8 Other or mixed emotional disturbances of childhood or adolescence**
313.81 Oppositional defiant disorder
313.82 Identity disorder
Identity problem
313.83 Academic underachievement disorder
❑**313.89 Other**
Reactive attachment disorder of infancy or early childhood

❑**313.9 Unspecified emotional disturbance of childhood or adolescence**
Mental disorder of infancy, childhood, or adolescence NOS

● **314 Hyperkinetic syndrome of childhood**
Excludes *hyperkinesis as symptom of underlying disorder - code the underlying disorder*

● **314.0 Attention deficit disorder** *ADD*
Adult
Child

314.00 Without mention of hyperactivity
Predominantly inattentive type

314.01 **With hyperactivity**
Attention deficit disorder with hyperactivity = ADHD
Combined type
Overactivity NOS
Predominantly hyperactive/impulsive type
Simple disturbance of attention with overactivity

314.1 **Hyperkinesis with developmental delay**
Developmental disorder of hyperkinesis

Use additional code to identify any associated neurological disorder

314.2 **Hyperkinetic conduct disorder**
Hyperkinetic conduct disorder without developmental delay

Excludes *hyperkinesis with significant delays in specific skills (314.1)*

❑314.8 **Other specified manifestations of hyperkinetic syndrome**

❑314.9 **Unspecified hyperkinetic syndrome**
Hyperkinetic reaction of childhood or adolescence NOS
Hyperkinetic syndrome NOS

● 315 **Specific delays in development**

Excludes *that due to a neurological disorder (320.0–389.9)*

● 315.0 **Specific reading disorder**

❑315.00 **Reading disorder, unspecified**

315.01 **Alexia**

315.02 **Developmental dyslexia**

❑315.09 **Other**
Specific spelling difficulty

315.1 **Mathematics disorder**
Dyscalculia

❑315.2 **Other specific learning difficulties**
Disorder of written expression

Excludes *specific arithmetical disorder (315.1)*
specific reading disorder (315.00–315.09)

● 315.3 **Developmental speech or language disorder**

315.31 **Expressive language disorder**
Developmental aphasia
Word deafness

Excludes *acquired aphasia (784.3)*
elective mutism (309.83, 313.0, 313.23)

315.32 **Mixed receptive-expressive language disorder**

❑315.39 **Other**
Developmental articulation disorder
Dyslalia
Phonological disorder

Excludes *lisping and lalling (307.9)*
stammering and stuttering (307.0)

315.4 **Developmental coordination disorder**
Clumsiness syndrome
Dyspraxia syndrome
Specific motor development disorder

315.5 **Mixed development disorder**

❑315.8 **Other specified delays in development**

❑315.9 **Unspecified delay in development**
Developmental disorder NOS
Learning disorder NOS

316 **Psychic factors associated with diseases classified elsewhere**
Psychologic factors in physical conditions classified elsewhere

Use additional code to identify the associated physical condition, as:
psychogenic:
asthma (493.9)
dermatitis (692.9)
duodenal ulcer (532.0–532.9)
eczema (691.8, 692.9)
gastric ulcer (531.0–531.9)
mucous colitis (564.9)
paroxysmal tachycardia (427.2)
ulcerative colitis (556)
urticaria (708.0–708.9)
psychosocial dwarfism (259.4)

Excludes *physical symptoms and physiological malfunctions, not involving tissue damage, of mental origin (306.0–306.9)*

MENTAL RETARDATION (317–319)

Use additional code(s) to identify any associated psychiatric or physical condition(s)

317 **Mild mental retardation**
High-grade defect
IQ 50–70
Mild mental subnormality

● 318 **Other specified mental retardation**

318.0 **Moderate mental retardation**
IQ 35–49
Moderate mental subnormality

318.1 **Severe mental retardation**
IQ 20–34
Severe mental subnormality

318.2 **Profound mental retardation**
IQ under 20
Profound mental subnormality

❑319 **Unspecified mental retardation**
Mental deficiency NOS
Mental subnormality NOS

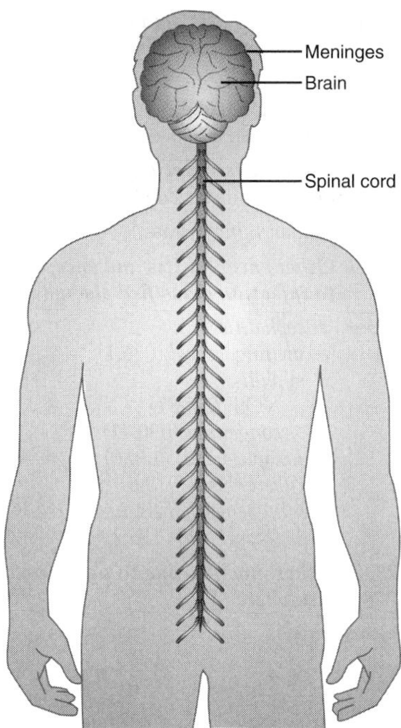
Meninges
Brain
Spinal cord

Figure 6–1 The brain and spinal cord make up the central nervous system.

Item 6–1 The two major classifications of the nervous system are the peripheral nervous system and the central nervous system (CNS). The central nervous system contains the brain and the spinal cord. Encephalitis is the swelling of the brain. Meningitis is swelling of the covering of the brain, the meninges. Types and causes of brain infections are:

Type	Cause
purulent	bacterial
aseptic/abacterial	viral
chronic meningitis	mycobacterial and fungal

6. DISEASES OF THE NERVOUS SYSTEM AND SENSE ORGANS (320–389)

INFLAMMATORY DISEASES OF THE CENTRAL NERVOUS SYSTEM (320–326)

● **320 Bacterial meningitis**

Includes: arachnoiditis bacterial
leptomeningitis bacterial
meningitis bacterial
meningoencephalitis bacterial
meningomyelitis bacterial
pachymeningitis bacterial

320.0 Haemophilus meningitis
Meningitis due to Haemophilus influenzae [H. influenzae]

320.1 Pneumococcal meningitis

320.2 Streptococcal meningitis

320.3 Staphylococcal meningitis

● *320.7 Meningitis in other bacterial diseases classified elsewhere*

Code first underlying disease as:
actinomycosis (039.8)
listeriosis (027.0)
typhoid fever (002.0)
whooping cough (033.0–033.9)

Excludes *meningitis (in):*
epidemic (036.0)
gonococcal (098.82)
meningococcal (036.0)
salmonellosis (003.21)
syphilis:
NOS (094.2)
congenital (090.42)
meningovascular (094.2)
secondary (091.81)
tuberculosis (013.0)

● **320.8 Meningitis due to other specified bacteria**

320.81 Anaerobic meningitis
Bacteroides (fragilis)
Gram-negative anaerobes

320.82 Meningitis due to gram-negative bacteria, not elsewhere classified
Aerobacter aerogenes
Escherichia coli [E. coli]
Friedlander bacillus
Klebsiella pneumoniae
Proteus morganii
Pseudomonas

Excludes *gram-negative anaerobes (320.81)*

❑ **320.89 Meningitis due to other specified bacteria**
Bacillus pyocyaneus

❑ **320.9 Meningitis due to unspecified bacterium**
Meningitis:
bacterial NOS
purulent NOS
pyogenic NOS
suppurative NOS

ICD-9-CM 300-399 Vol. 1

● **321 Meningitis due to other organisms**

Includes: arachnoiditis due to organisms other than bacteria
leptomeningitis due to organisms other than bacteria
meningitis due to organisms other than bacteria
pachymeningitis due to organisms other than bacteria

● *321.0 Cryptococcal meningitis*

Code first underlying disease (117.5)

● ❑ *321.1 Meningitis in other fungal diseases*

Code first underlying disease (110.0–118)

Excludes *meningitis in:*
candidiasis (112.83)
coccidioidomycosis (114.2)
histoplasmosis (115.01, 115.11, 115.91)

● *321.2 Meningitis due to viruses not elsewhere classified*

Code first underlying disease, as:
meningitis due to arbovirus (060.0–066.9)

Excludes *meningitis (due to):*
abacterial (047.0–047.9)
adenovirus (049.1)
aseptic NOS (047.9)
Coxsackie (virus) (047.0)
ECHO virus (047.1)
enterovirus (047.0–047.9)
herpes simplex virus (054.72)
herpes zoster virus (053.0)
lymphocytic choriomeningitis virus (049.0)
mumps (072.1)
viral NOS (047.9)
meningo-eruptive syndrome (047.1)

● ***321.3 Meningitis due to trypanosomiasis***
Code first underlying disease (086.0–086.9)

● ***321.4 Meningitis in sarcoidosis***
Code first underlying disease (135)

● ❑***321.8 Meningitis due to other nonbacterial organisms classified elsewhere***
Code first underlying disease
Excludes *leptospiral meningitis (100.81)*

● **322 Meningitis of unspecified cause**
Includes: arachnoiditis with no organism specified as cause
leptomeningitis with no organism specified as cause
meningitis with no organism specified as cause
pachymeningitis with no organism specified as cause

322.0 Nonpyogenic meningitis
Meningitis with clear cerebrospinal fluid

322.1 Eosinophilic meningitis

322.2 Chronic meningitis

❑**322.9 Meningitis, unspecified**

● **323 Encephalitis, myelitis, and encephalomyelitis**
Includes: acute disseminated encephalomyelitis
meningoencephalitis, except bacterial
meningomyelitis, except bacterial
myelitis: (Revised)
ascending
transverse
Excludes *acute transverse myelitis NOS (341.20)* ◀
acute transverse myelitis in conditions classified elsewhere (341.21) ◀
bacterial:
meningoencephalitis (320.0–320.9)
meningomyelitis (320.0–320.9)
idiopathic transverse myelitis (341.22) ◀

● ***323.0 Encephalitis, myelitis, and encephalomyelitis in viral diseases classified elsewhere*** (Revised)
Code first underlying disease, as:
cat-scratch disease (078.3)
infectious mononucleosis (075)
ornithosis (073.7)

● ***323.01 Encephalitis and encephalomyelitis in viral diseases classified elsewhere*** ◀
Excludes *encephalitis (in):* ◀
arthropod-borne viral (062.0–064) ◀
herpes simplex (054.3) ◀
mumps (072.2) ◀
other viral diseases of central nervous system (049.8–049.9) ◀
poliomyelitis (045.0–045.9) ◀
rubella (056.01) ◀
slow virus infections of central nervous system (046.0–046.9) ◀
viral NOS (049.9) ◀
West Nile (066.41) ◀

● ***323.02 Myelitis in viral diseases classified elsewhere*** ◀
Excludes *myelitis (in):* ◀
herpes simplex (054.74) ◀
herpes zoster (053.14) ◀
poliomyelitis (045.0–045.9) ◀
rubella (056.01) ◀
other viral diseases of central nervous system (049.8–049.9) ◀

● ***323.1 Encephalitis, myelitis, and encephalomyelitis in rickettsial diseases classified elsewhere*** (Revised)
Code first underlying disease (080–083.9)

● ***323.2 Encephalitis, myelitis, and encephalomyelitis in protozoal diseases classified elsewhere*** (Revised)
Code first underlying disease, as:
malaria (084.0–084.9)
trypanosomiasis (086.0–086.9)

● ***323.4 Other encephalitis, myelitis, and encephalomyelitis due to infection classified elsewhere*** (Revised)
Code first underlying disease

● ***323.41 Other encephalitis and encephalomyelitis due to infection classified elsewhere*** ◀
Excludes *encephalitis (in):* ◀
meningococcal (036.1) ◀
syphilis: ◀
NOS (094.81) ◀
congenital (090.41) ◀
toxoplasmosis (130.0) ◀
tuberculosis (013.6) ◀
meningoencephalitis due to free-living ameba [Naegleria] (136.2) ◀

● ***323.42 Other myelitis due to infection classified elsewhere*** ◀
Excludes *myelitis (in):* ◀
syphilis (094.89) ◀
tuberculosis (013.6) ◀

● **323.5 Encephalitis, myelitis, and encephalomyelitis following immunization procedures** (Revised)
Use additional E code to identify vaccine

323.51 Encephalitis and encephalomyelitis following immunization procedures ◀
Encephalitis postimmunization or postvaccinal ◀
Encephalomyelitis postimmunization or postvaccinal ◀

323.52 Myelitis following immunization procedures ◀
Myelitis postimmunization or postvaccinal ◀

● ***323.6 Postinfectious encephalitis, myelitis, and encephalomyelitis*** (Revised)
Code first underlying disease

● ***323.61 Infectious acute disseminated encephalomyelitis (ADEM)*** ◀
Acute necrotizing hemorrhagic encephalopathy ◀
Excludes *noninfectious acute disseminated encephalomyelitis (ADEM) (323.81)* ◀

● ***323.62 Other postinfectious encephalitis and encephalomyelitis*** ◀
Excludes *encephalitis:* ◀
postchickenpox (052.0) ◀
postmeasles (055.0) ◀

● ***323.63 Postinfectious myelitis*** ◀
Excludes *postchickenpox myelitis (052.2)* ◀
herpes simplex myelitis (054.74) ◀
herpes zoster myelitis (053.14) ◀

● ***323.7 Toxic encephalitis, myelitis, and encephalomyelitis*** (Revised)
Code first underlying cause, as:
carbon tetrachloride (982.1)
hydroxyquinoline derivatives (961.3)
lead (984.0–984.9)
mercury (985.0)
thallium (985.8)

● ***323.71 Toxic encephalitis and encephalomyelitis*** ◀

● ***323.71 Toxic myelitis*** ◀

● **323.8 Other causes of encephalitis, myelitis, and encephalomyelitis** (Revised)

❑323.81 **Other causes of encephalitis and encephalomyelitis** ◄
Noninfectious acute disseminated encephalomyelitis (ADEM) ◄

❑323.82 **Other causes of myelitis** ◄
Transverse myelitis NOS ◄

❑323.9 **Unspecified cause of encephalitis, myelitis, and encephalomyelitis** ⇐

● 324 **Intracranial and intraspinal abscess**

324.0 **Intracranial abscess**
Abscess (embolic):
cerebellar
cerebral
Abscess (embolic) of brain [any part]:
epidural
extradural
otogenic
subdural

Excludes *tuberculous (013.3)*

324.1 **Intraspinal abscess**
Abscess (embolic) of spinal cord [any part]:
epidural
extradural
subdural

Excludes *tuberculous (013.5)*

❑324.9 **Of unspecified site**
Extradural or subdural abscess NOS

325 **Phlebitis and thrombophlebitis of intracranial venous sinuses**
Embolism of cavernous, lateral, or other intracranial or unspecified intracranial venous sinus
Endophlebitis of cavernous, lateral, or other intracranial or unspecified intracranial venous sinus
Phlebitis, septic or suppurative of cavernous, lateral, or other intracranial or unspecified intracranial venous sinus
Thrombophlebitis of cavernous, lateral, or other intracranial or unspecified intracranial venous sinus
Thrombosis of cavernous, lateral, or other intracranial or unspecified intracranial venous sinus

Excludes *that specified as:*
complicating pregnancy, childbirth, or the puerperium (671.5)
of nonpyogenic origin (437.6)

❑326 **Late effects of intracranial abscess or pyogenic infection**
Note: This category is to be used to indicate conditions whose primary classification is to 320–325 [excluding 320.7, 321.0–321.8, 323.01–323.42, 323.6–323.7] ⇐ as the cause of late effects, themselves classifiable elsewhere. The "late effects" include conditions specified as such, or as sequelae, which may occur at any time after the resolution of the causal condition.

Use additional code to identify condition, as:
hydrocephalus (331.4)
paralysis (342.0–342.9, 344.0–344.9)

ORGANIC SLEEP DISORDERS (327) ◄

● 327 **Organic sleep disorders**

● 327.0 **Organic disorders of initiating and maintaining sleep [Organic insomnia]**

Excludes *insomnia NOS (780.52)*
insomnia not due to a substance or known physiological condition (307.41–307.42)
insomnia with sleep apnea NOS (780.51)

❑327.00 **Organic insomnia, unspecified**

● 327.01 ***Insomnia due to medical condition classified elsewhere***
Code first underlying condition

Excludes *insomnia due to mental disorder (327.02)*

● 327.02 ***Insomnia due to mental disorder***
Code first mental disorder

Excludes *alcohol induced insomnia (291.82)*
drug induced insomnia (292.85)

❑327.09 **Other organic insomnia**

● 327.1 **Organic disorder of excessive somnolence [Organic hypersomnia]**

Excludes *hypersomnia NOS (780.54)*
hypersomnia not due to a substance or known physiological condition (307.43–307.44)
hypersomnia with sleep apnea NOS (780.53)

❑327.10 **Organic hypersomnia, unspecified**

327.11 **Idiopathic hypersomnia with long sleep time**

327.12 **Idiopathic hypersomnia without long sleep time**

327.13 **Recurrent hypersomnia**
Kleine-Levin syndrome
Menstrual related hypersomnia

● 327.14 ***Hypersomnia due to medical condition classified elsewhere***
Code first underlying condition

Excludes *hypersomnia due to mental disorder (327.15)*

● 327.15 ***Hypersomnia due to mental disorder***
Code first mental disorder

Excludes *alcohol induced insomnia (291.82)*
drug induced insomnia (292.85)

❑327.19 **Other organic hypersomnia**

● 327.2 **Organic sleep apnea**

Excludes *Cheyne-Stokes breathing (786.04)*
hypersomnia with sleep apnea NOS (780.53)
insomnia with sleep apnea NOS (780.51)
sleep apnea in newborn (770.81–770.82)
sleep apnea NOS (780.57)

❑327.20 **Organic sleep apnea, unspecified**

327.21 **Primary central sleep apnea**

327.22 **High altitude periodic breathing**

327.23 **Obstructive sleep apnea (adult) (pediatric)**

327.24 **Idiopathic sleep related nonobstructive alveolar hypoventilation**
Sleep related hypoxia

327.25 **Congenital central alveolar hypoventilation syndrome**

● 327.26 ***Sleep related hypoventilation/hypoxemia in conditions classifiable elsewhere***
Code first underlying condition

● 327.27 ***Central sleep apnea in conditions classified elsewhere***
Code first underlying condition

❑327.29 **Other organic sleep apnea**

● **327.3 Circadian rhythm sleep disorder**
Organic disorder of sleep wake cycle
Organic disorder of sleep wake schedule
Excludes *alcohol induced circadian rhythm sleep disorder (291.82)*
circadian rhythm sleep disorder of nonorganic origin (307.45)
disruption of 24 hour sleep wake cycle NOS (780.55)
drug induced circadian rhythm sleep disorder (292.85)

❑ **327.30 Circadian rhythm sleep disorder, unspecified**

327.31 Circadian rhythm sleep disorder, delayed sleep phase type

327.32 Circadian rhythm sleep disorder, advanced sleep phase type

327.33 Circadian rhythm sleep disorder, irregular sleep-wake type

327.34 Circadian rhythm sleep disorder, free-running type

327.35 Circadian rhythm sleep disorder, jet lag type

327.36 Circadian rhythm sleep disorder, shift work type

● ***327.37 Circadian rhythm sleep disorder in conditions classified elsewhere***
Code first underlying condition

❑ **327.39 Other circadian rhythm sleep disorder**

● **327.4 Organic parasomnia**
Excludes *alcohol induced parasomnia (291.82)*
drug induced parasomnia (292.85)
parasomnia not due to a known physiological conditions (307.47)

❑ **327.40 Organic parasomnia, unspecified**

327.41 Confusional arousals

327.42 REM sleep behavior disorder

327.43 Recurrent isolated sleep paralysis

● ***327.44 Parasomnia in conditions classified elsewhere***
Code first underlying condition

❑ **327.49 Other organic parasomnia**

● **327.5 Organic sleep related movement disorders**
Excludes *restless legs syndrome (333.94)* ⇐
sleep related movement disorder NOS (780.58)

327.51 Periodic limb movement disorder
Periodic limb movement sleep disorder

327.52 Sleep related leg cramps

327.53 Sleep related bruxism

❑ **327.59 Other organic sleep related movement disorders**

327.8 Other organic sleep disorders

Item 6-2 Leukodystrophy is characterized by degeneration and/or failure of the myelin formation of the central nervous system and sometimes of the peripheral nervous system. The disease is inherited and progressive.

HEREDITARY AND DEGENERATIVE DISEASES OF THE CENTRAL NERVOUS SYSTEM (330–337)

Excludes *hepatolenticular degeneration (275.1)*
multiple sclerosis (340)
other demyelinating diseases of central nervous system (341.0–341.9)

● **330 Cerebral degenerations usually manifest in childhood**
Use additional code to identify associated mental retardation

330.0 Leukodystrophy
Krabbe's disease
Leukodystrophy:
NOS
globoid cell
metachromatic
sudanophilic
Pelizaeus-Merzbacher disease
Sulfatide lipidosis

330.1 Cerebral lipidoses
Amaurotic (familial) idiocy
Disease:
Batten
Jansky-Bielschowsky
Kufs'
Spielmeyer-Vogt
Tay-Sachs
Gangliosidosis

● ***330.2 Cerebral degeneration in generalized lipidoses***
Code first underlying disease, as:
Fabry's disease (272.7)
Gaucher's disease (272.7)
Niemann-Pick disease (272.7)
sphingolipidosis (272.7)

● ❑ ***330.3 Cerebral degeneration of childhood in other diseases classified elsewhere***
Code first underlying disease, as:
Hunter's disease (277.5)
mucopolysaccharidosis (277.5)

❑ **330.8 Other specified cerebral degenerations in childhood**
Alpers' disease or gray-matter degeneration
Infantile necrotizing encephalomyelopathy
Leigh's disease
Subacute necrotizing encephalopathy or encephalomyelopathy

❑ **330.9 Unspecified cerebral degeneration in childhood**

Item 6-3 Pick's disease is the atrophy of the frontal and temporal lobes, causing dementia; Alzheimer's is characterized by a more diffuse cerebral atrophy.

● **331 Other cerebral degenerations**

331.0 Alzheimer's disease

● **331.1 Frontotemporal dementia**
Use additional code for associated behavioral disturbances (294.10–294.11)

331.11 Pick's disease

331.19 Other frontotemporal dementia
Frontal dementia

331.2 Senile degeneration of brain
Excludes *senility NOS (797)*

331.3 Communicating hydrocephalus
Excludes *congenital hydrocephalus (741.0, 742.3)*

331.4 Obstructive hydrocephalus
Acquired hydrocephalus NOS
Excludes *congenital hydrocephalus (741.0, 742.3)*

● ***331.7 Cerebral degeneration in diseases classified elsewhere***
Code first underlying disease, as:
alcoholism (303.0–303.9)
beriberi (265.0)
cerebrovascular disease (430–438)
congenital hydrocephalus (741.0, 742.3)
neoplastic disease (140.0–239.9)
myxedema (244.0–244.9)
vitamin B_{12} deficiency (266.2)
Excludes *cerebral degeneration in:*
Jakob-Creutzfeldt disease (046.1)
progressive multifocal leukoencephalopathy (046.3)
subacute spongiform encephalopathy (046.1)

● **331.8 Other cerebral degeneration**
331.81 Reye's syndrome
331.82 Dementia with Lewy bodies
Dementia with Parkinsonism
Lewy body dementia
Lewy body disease
Use additional code for associated behavioral disturbances (294.10–294.11)
331.83 Mild cognitive impairment, so stated ◀
Excludes *altered mental status (780.97)* ◀
cerebral degeneration (331.0–331.9) ◀
change in mental status (780.97) ◀
cognitive deficits following (late effects of) cerebral hemorrhage or infarction (438.0) ◀
cognitive impairment due to intracranial or head injury (850–854, 959.01) ◀
cognitive impairment due to late effect of intracranial injury (907.0) ◀
dementia (290.0–290.43, 294.8) ◀
mild memory disturbance (310.8) ◀
neurologic neglect syndrome (781.8) ◀
personality change, nonpsychotic (310.1) ◀
❑ **331.89 Other**
Cerebral ataxia

❑ **331.9 Cerebral degeneration, unspecified**

● **332 Parkinson's disease**
Excludes *dementia with Parkinsonism (331.82)*
332.0 Paralysis agitans
Parkinsonism or Parkinson's disease:
NOS
idiopathic
primary
332.1 Secondary Parkinsonism
Neuroleptic-induced Parkinsonism
Parkinsonism due to drugs
Use additional E code to identify drug, if drug-induced
Excludes *Parkinsonism (in):*
Huntington's disease (333.4)
progressive supranuclear palsy (333.0)
Shy-Drager syndrome (333.0)
syphilitic (094.82)

● **333 Other extrapyramidal disease and abnormal movement disorders**
Includes: other forms of extrapyramidal, basal ganglia, or striatopallidal disease
Excludes *abnormal movements of head NOS (781.0)*
sleep related movement disorders (327.51–327.59)

❑ **333.0 Other degenerative diseases of the basal ganglia**
Atrophy or degeneration:
olivopontocerebellar [Déjérine-Thomas syndrome]
pigmentary pallidal [Hallervorden-Spatz disease]
striatonigral
Parkinsonian syndrome associated with:
idiopathic orthostatic hypotension
symptomatic orthostatic hypotension
Progressive supranuclear ophthalmoplegia
Shy-Drager syndrome

❑ **333.1 Essential and other specified forms of tremor**
Benign essential tremor
Familial tremor
Medication-induced postural tremor
Use additional E code to identify drug, if drug-induced
Excludes *tremor NOS (781.0)*

333.2 Myoclonus
Familial essential myoclonus
Progressive myoclonic epilepsy
Unverricht-Lundborg disease
Use additional E code to identify drug, if drug-induced

333.3 Tics of organic origin
Excludes *Gilles de la Tourette's syndrome (307.23)*
habit spasm (307.22)
tic NOS (307.20)
Use additional E code to identify drug, if drug-induced

Item 6-4 Huntington's disease is characterized by ceaseless, jerky movements and progressive cognitive and behavioral deterioration.

ICD-9-CM 300-399 Vol. 1

333.4 Huntington's chorea

❑ **333.5 Other choreas**
Hemiballism(us)
Paroxysmal choreo-athetosis
Excludes *Sydenham's or rheumatic chorea (392.0–392.9)*
Use additional E code to identify drug, if drug-induced

333.6 Genetic torsion dystonia (Revised)
Dystonia:
deformans progressiva
musculorum deformans
(Schwalbe-) Ziehen-Oppenheim disease

● **333.7 Acquired torsion dystonia** (Revised)
333.71 Athetoid cerebral palsy ◀
Double athetosis (syndrome) ◀
Vogt's disease ◀
Excludes *infantile cerebral palsy (343.0–343.9)* ◀
333.72 Acute dystonia due to drugs ◀
Acute dystonic reaction due to drugs ◀
Neuroleptic induced acute dystonia ◀
Use additional E code to identify drug ◀
Excludes *blepharospasm due to drugs (333.85)* ◀
orofacial dyskinesia due to drugs (333.85) ◀
secondary Parkinsonism (332.1) ◀
subacute dyskinesia due to drugs (333.85) ◀
tardive dyskinesia (333.85) ◀
❑ **333.79 Other acquired torsion dystonia** ◀

● **333.8 Fragments of torsion dystonia**
Use additional E code to identify drug, if drug-induced

333.81 **Blepharospasm**

Excludes *blepharospasm due to drugs (333.85)* ◀

333.82 **Orofacial dyskinesia** ⇐

Excludes *orofacial dyskinesia due to drugs (333.85)* ◀

333.83 **Spasmodic torticollis**

Excludes *torticollis:*
NOS (723.5)
hysterical (300.11)
psychogenic (306.0)

333.84 **Organic writers' cramp**

Excludes *psychogenic (300.89)*

333.85 **Subacute dyskinesia due to drugs** ◀
Blepharospasm due to drugs ◀
Orofacial dyskinesia due to drugs ◀
Tardive dyskinesia ◀

Use additional E code to identify drug ◀

Excludes *acute dystonia due to drugs (333.72)* ◀
acute dystonic reaction due to drugs (333.72) ◀
secondary Parkinsonism (332.1) ◀

❑333.89 **Other**

● 333.9 **Other and unspecified extrapyramidal diseases and abnormal movement disorders**

❑333.90 **Unspecified extrapyramidal disease and abnormal movement disorder**
Medication-induced movement disorders NOS

Use additional E code to identify drug, if drug-induced

333.91 **Stiff-man syndrome**

333.92 **Neuroleptic malignant syndrome**

Use additional E code to identify drug

Excludes *neuroleptic induced Parkinsonism (332.1)* ◀

333.93 **Benign shuddering attacks**

333.94 **Restless legs syndrome (RLS)** ◀

❑333.99 **Other** ⇐
Neuroleptic-induced acute akathisia
Also listed in the Index as Restless leg syndrome (RLS)

Use additional E code to identify drug, if drug-induced

● 334 **Spinocerebellar disease**

Excludes *olivopontocerebellar degeneration (333.0)*
peroneal muscular atrophy (356.1)

334.0 **Friedreich's ataxia**

334.1 **Hereditary spastic paraplegia**

334.2 **Primary cerebellar degeneration**
Cerebellar ataxia:
Marie's
Sanger-Brown
Dyssynergia cerebellaris myoclonica
Primary cerebellar degeneration:
NOS
hereditary
sporadic

❑334.3 **Other cerebellar ataxia**
Cerebellar ataxia NOS

Use additional E code to identify drug, if drug-induced

●334.4 ***Cerebellar ataxia in diseases classified elsewhere***

Code first underlying disease, as:
alcoholism (303.0–303.9)
myxedema (244.0–244.9)
neoplastic disease (140.0–239.9)

❑334.8 **Other spinocerebellar diseases**
Ataxia-telangiectasia [Louis-Bar syndrome]
Corticostriatal-spinal degeneration

❑334.9 **Spinocerebellar disease, unspecified**

● 335 **Anterior horn cell disease**

335.0 **Werdnig-Hoffmann disease**
Infantile spinal muscular atrophy
Progressive muscular atrophy of infancy

● 335.1 **Spinal muscular atrophy**

❑335.10 **Spinal muscular atrophy, unspecified**

335.11 **Kugelberg-Welander disease**
Spinal muscular atrophy:
familial
juvenile

❑335.19 **Other**
Adult spinal muscular atrophy

● 335.2 **Motor neuron disease**

335.20 **Amyotrophic lateral sclerosis**
Also listed in the Index as Lou Gehrig's disease (ALS)
Motor neuron disease (bulbar) (mixed type)

335.21 **Progressive muscular atrophy**
Duchenne-Aran muscular atrophy
Progressive muscular atrophy (pure)

335.22 **Progressive bulbar palsy**

335.23 **Pseudobulbar palsy**

335.24 **Primary lateral sclerosis**

❑335.29 **Other**

❑335.8 **Other anterior horn cell diseases**

❑335.9 **Anterior horn cell disease, unspecified**

● 336 **Other diseases of spinal cord**

336.0 **Syringomyelia and syringobulbia**

336.1 **Vascular myelopathies**
Acute infarction of spinal cord (embolic) (nonembolic)
Arterial thrombosis of spinal cord
Edema of spinal cord
Hematomyelia
Subacute necrotic myelopathy

● 336.2 ***Subacute combined degeneration of spinal cord in diseases classified elsewhere***

Code first underlying disease, as:
pernicious anemia (281.0)
other vitamin B_{12} deficiency anemia (281.1)
vitamin B_{12} deficiency (266.2)

● 336.3 ***Myelopathy in other diseases classified elsewhere***

Code first underlying disease, as:
myelopathy in neoplastic disease (140.0–239.9)

Excludes *myelopathy in:*
intervertebral disc disorder (722.70–722.73)
spondylosis (721.1, 721.41–721.42, 721.91)

❑336.8 **Other myelopathy**
Myelopathy:
drug-induced
radiation-induced

Use additional E code to identify cause

❑336.9 **Unspecified disease of spinal cord**
Cord compression NOS
Myelopathy NOS
Excludes *myelitis (323.02, 323.1, 323.2, 323.42, 323.52, 323.63, 323.72, 323.82, 323.9)*
spinal (canal) stenosis (723.0, 724.00–724.09)

● 337 **Disorders of the autonomic nervous system**
Includes: disorders of peripheral autonomic, sympathetic, parasympathetic, or vegetative system
Excludes *familial dysautonomia [Riley-Day syndrome] (742.8)*

337.0 **Idiopathic peripheral autonomic neuropathy**
Carotid sinus syncope or syndrome
Cervical sympathetic dystrophy or paralysis

● 337.1 ***Peripheral autonomic neuropathy in disorders classified elsewhere***
Code first underlying disease, as:
amyloidosis (277.30–277.39)
diabetes (250.6)

● 337.2 **Reflex sympathetic dystrophy**
❑337.20 **Reflex sympathetic dystrophy, unspecified**
337.21 **Reflex sympathetic dystrophy of the upper limb**
337.22 **Reflex sympathetic dystrophy of the lower limb**
❑337.29 **Reflex sympathetic dystrophy of other specified site**

337.3 **Autonomic dysreflexia**
Use additional code to identify the cause, such as:
decubitus ulcer (707.00–707.09)
fecal impaction (560.39)
urinary tract infection (599.0)

❑337.9 **Unspecified disorder of autonomic nervous system**

PAIN (338)

● 338 **Pain, not elsewhere classified**
Use additional code to identify:
pain associated with psychological factors (307.89)
Excludes *generalized pain (780.96)*
localized pain, unspecified type – code to pain by site
pain disorder exclusively attributed to psychological factors (307.80)

338.0 **Central pain syndrome**
Déjérine-Roussy syndrome
Myelopathic pain syndrome
Thalamic pain syndrome (hyperesthetic)

● 338.1 **Acute pain**
338.11 **Acute pain due to trauma**
338.12 **Acute post-thoracotomy pain**
Post-thoracotomy pain NOS
❑338.18 **Other acute postoperative pain**
Postoperative pain NOS
❑338.19 **Other acute pain**
Excludes *neoplasm related acute pain (338.3)*

● 338.2 **Chronic pain**
Excludes *causalgia (355.9)*
lower limb (355.71)
upper limb (354.4)
chronic pain syndrome (338.4)
myofascial pain syndrome (729.1)
neoplasm related chronic pain (338.3)
reflex sympathetic dystrophy (337.20–337.29)
338.21 **Chronic pain due to trauma**
338.22 **Chronic post-thoracotomy pain**
❑338.28 **Other chronic postoperative pain**
❑338.29 **Other chronic pain**

338.3 **Neoplasm related pain (acute) (chronic)**
Cancer associated pain
Pain due to malignancy (primary) (secondary)
Tumor associated pain

338.4 **Chronic pain syndrome**
Chronic pain associated with significant psychosocial dysfunction

OTHER DISORDERS OF THE CENTRAL NERVOUS SYSTEM (340–349)

340 **Multiple sclerosis**
Disseminated or multiple sclerosis:
NOS
brain stem
cord
generalized

● 341 **Other demyelinating diseases of central nervous system**
341.0 **Neuromyelitis optica**
341.1 **Schilder's disease**
Balo's concentric sclerosis
Encephalitis periaxialis:
concentrica [Balo's]
diffusa [Schilder's]

● 341.2 **Acute (transverse) myelitis**
Excludes *acute (transverse) myelitis (in) (due to):*
following immunization procedures (323.52)
infection classified elsewhere (323.42)
postinfectious (323.63)
protozoal diseases classified elsewhere (323.2)
rickettsial diseases classified elsewhere (323.1)
toxic (323.72)
viral diseases classified elsewhere (323.02)
transverse myelitis NOS (323.82)
341.20 **Acute (transverse) myelitis NOS**
● 341.21 ***Acute (transverse) myelitis in conditions classified elsewhere***
Code first underlying condition
341.22 **Idiopathic transverse myelitis**

❑341.8 **Other demyelinating diseases of central nervous system**
Central demyelination of corpus callosum
Central pontine myelinosis
Marchiafava (-Bignami) disease

❑341.9 **Demyelinating disease of central nervous system, unspecified**

ICD-9-CM 300-399 Vol. 1

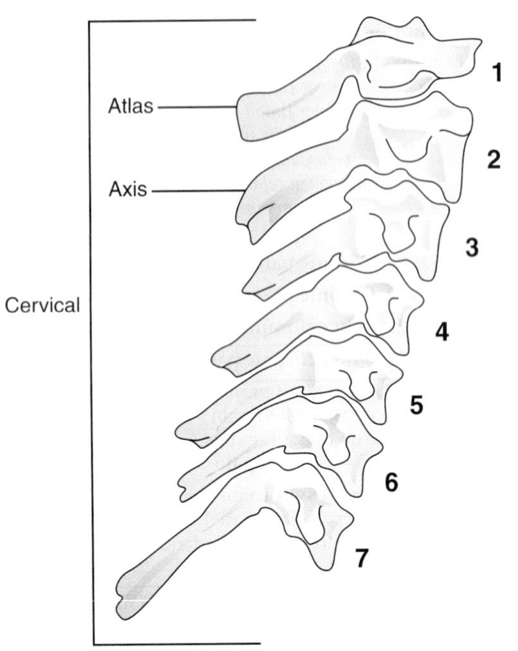
Atlas
Axis
Cervical
1
2
3
4
5
6
7

Figure 6–2 Cervical vertebrae.

Item 6–5 Hemiplegia is complete paralysis of one side of the body—arm, leg, and trunk. Hemiparesis is a generalized weakness or incomplete paralysis of one side of the body. If most activities (eating, writing) are performed with the right hand, the right is the dominant side, and the left is the nondominant side. Quadriplegia, also called tetraplegia, is the complete paralysis of all four limbs. Quadriparesis is the incomplete paralysis of all four limbs. Nerve damage in C1–C4 is associated with lower limb paralysis and C5–C7 damage is associated with upper limb paralysis. Diplegia is the paralysis of the upper limbs. Monoplegia is the complete paralysis of one limb. There are separate codes for upper (344.4x) and lower (344.3x) limb. Dominant, nondominant, or unspecified side becomes the fifth digit. Dominant side (right/left) is the side that a person leads with for movement, such as in writing and sports.
Cauda equina syndrome is due to pressure on the roots of the spinal nerves and causes paresthesia (abnormal sensations).

● **342 Hemiplegia and hemiparesis**

Note: This category is to be used when hemiplegia (complete) (incomplete) is reported without further specification, or is stated to be old or long-standing but of unspecified cause. The category is also for use in multiple coding to identify these types of hemiplegia resulting from any cause.

Excludes *congenital (343.1)*
hemiplegia due to late effect of cerebrovascular accident (438.20–438.22)
infantile NOS (343.4)

The following fifth digits are for use with codes 342.0–342.9
❑ **0 affecting unspecified side**
1 affecting dominant side
2 affecting nondominant side

● **342.0 Flaccid hemiplegia**

● **342.1 Spastic hemiplegia**

● ❑ **342.8 Other specified hemiplegia**

● ❑ **342.9 Hemiplegia, unspecified**

● **343 Infantile cerebral palsy**

Includes: cerebral:
palsy NOS
spastic infantile paralysis
congenital spastic paralysis (cerebral)
Little's disease
paralysis (spastic) due to birth injury:
intracranial
spinal

Excludes *athetoid cerebral palsy (333.71)* ◀
hereditary cerebral paralysis, such as:
hereditary spastic paraplegia (334.1)
Vogt's disease (333.71) ⬅
spastic paralysis specified as noncongenital or noninfantile (344.0–344.9)

343.0 Diplegic
Congenital diplegia
Congenital paraplegia

343.1 Hemiplegic
Congenital hemiplegia

Excludes *infantile hemiplegia NOS (343.4)*

343.2 Quadriplegic
Tetraplegic

343.3 Monoplegic

343.4 Infantile hemiplegia
Infantile hemiplegia (postnatal) NOS

❑ **343.8 Other specified infantile cerebral palsy**

❑ **343.9 Infantile cerebral palsy, unspecified**
Cerebral palsy NOS

● **344 Other paralytic syndromes**

Note: This category is to be used when the listed conditions are reported without further specification or are stated to be old or long-standing but of unspecified cause. The category is also for use in multiple coding to identify these conditions resulting from any cause.

Includes: paralysis (complete) (incomplete), except as classifiable to 342 and 343

Excludes *congenital or infantile cerebral palsy (343.0–343.9)*
hemiplegia (342.0–342.9)
congenital or infantile (343.1, 343.4)

● **344.0 Quadriplegia and quadriparesis**

❑ **344.00 Quadriplegia, unspecified**

344.01 C_1-C_4, complete

344.02 C_1-C_4, incomplete

344.03 C_5-C_7, complete

344.04 C_5-C_7, incomplete

❑ **344.09 Other**

344.1 Paraplegia
Paralysis of both lower limbs
Paraplegia (lower)

344.2 Diplegia of upper limbs
Diplegia (upper)
Paralysis of both upper limbs

● **344.3 Monoplegia of lower limb**
Paralysis of lower limb

Excludes *Monoplegia of lower limb due to late effect of cerebrovascular accident (438.40–438.42)*

❑ **344.30 Affecting unspecified side**

344.31 Affecting dominant side

344.32 Affecting nondominant side

● **344.4 Monoplegia of upper limb**
Paralysis of upper limb

Excludes *monoplegia of upper limb due to late effect of cerebrovascular accident (438.30–438.32)*

❑ **344.40 Affecting unspecified side**

344.41 Affecting dominant side

344.42 Affecting nondominant side

❑ **344.5 Unspecified monoplegia**

● **344.6 Cauda equina syndrome**

344.60 Without mention of neurogenic bladder

344.61 With neurogenic bladder
Acontractile bladder
Autonomic hyperreflexia of bladder
Cord bladder
Detrusor hyperreflexia

● **344.8 Other specified paralytic syndromes**

344.81 Locked-in state

❑ **344.89 Other specified paralytic syndrome**

❑ **344.9 Paralysis, unspecified**

● **345 Epilepsy and recurrent seizures** (Revised)

The following fifth-digit subclassification is for use with categories 345.0, .1, .4–.9:
- **0 without mention of intractable epilepsy**
- **1 with intractable epilepsy**

Excludes *progressive myoclonic epilepsy (333.2)*

● **345.0 Generalized nonconvulsive epilepsy**
Absences:
- atonic
- typical

Minor epilepsy
Petit mal
Pykno-epilepsy
Seizures:
- akinetic
- atonic

● **345.1 Generalized convulsive epilepsy**
Epileptic seizures:
- clonic
- myoclonic
- tonic

Epileptic seizures:
- tonic-clonic

Grand mal
Major epilepsy

Excludes *convulsions:*
- *NOS (780.39)* (Revised)
- *infantile (780.39)* (Revised)
- *newborn (779.0)*

infantile spasms (345.6)

345.2 Petit mal status
Epileptic absence status
Petit mal seizures can be referred to as "absence seizures."

345.3 Grand mal status
Status epilepticus NOS
Grand mal seizures can be referred to as "tonic-clonic seizures."

Excludes *epilepsia partialis continua (345.7) status:*
- *psychomotor (345.7)*
- *temporal lobe (345.7)*

● **345.4 Localization-related (focal) (partial) epilepsy and epileptic syndromes with complex partial seizures** (Revised)
Epilepsy:
- limbic system
- partial:
  - secondarily generalized
  - with impairment of consciousness (New)
  - with memory and ideational disturbances
- psychomotor
- psychosensory
- temporal lobe

Epileptic automatism

● **345.5 Localization-related (focal) (partial) epilepsy and epileptic syndromes with simple partial seizures** (Revised)
Epilepsy:
- Bravais-Jacksonian NOS
- focal (motor) NOS
- Jacksonian NOS
- motor partial
- partial NOS
  - without impairment of consciousness (New)
- sensory-induced
- somatomotor
- somatosensory
- visceral
- visual

● **345.6 Infantile spasms**
Hypsarrhythmia
Lightning spasms
Salaam attacks

Excludes *salaam tic (781.0)*

● **345.7 Epilepsia partialis continua**
Kojevnikov's epilepsy

● ❑ **345.8 Other forms of epilepsy and recurrent seizures** (Revised)
Epilepsy:
- cursive [running]
- gelastic

● ❑ **345.9 Epilepsy, unspecified**
Epileptic convulsions, fits, or seizures NOS
Recurrent seizures NOS (New)
Seizure disorder NOS (New)

Excludes *convulsion (convulsive) disorder (780.39)* (New)
convulsive seizure or fit NOS (780.39) (Revised)
recurrent convulsions (780.39) (New)

● **346 Migraine**

The following fifth-digit subclassification is for use with category 346:
- **0 without mention of intractable migraine**
- **1 with intractable migraine, so stated**

Intractable migraine: Not easily cured or managed; relentless pain from a migraine

● **346.0 Classical migraine**
Migraine preceded or accompanied by transient focal neurological phenomena
Migraine with aura

● **346.1 Common migraine**
Atypical migraine
Sick headache

● 346.2 **Variants of migraine**
Cluster headache
Histamine cephalgia
Horton's neuralgia
Migraine:
abdominal
basilar
lower half
retinal
Neuralgia:
ciliary
migrainous

● ❑ 346.8 **Other forms of migraine**
Migraine:
hemiplegic
ophthalmoplegic

● ❑ 346.9 **Migraine, unspecified**

● 347 **Cataplexy and narcolepsy**

● 347.0 **Narcolepsy**

347.00 **Without cataplexy**
Narcolepsy NOS

347.01 **With cataplexy**

● *347.1* ***Narcolepsy in conditions classified elsewhere***

Code first underlying condition

● *347.10* ***Without cataplexy***

● *347.11* ***With cataplexy***

● 348 **Other conditions of brain**

348.0 **Cerebral cysts**
Arachnoid cyst
Porencephalic cyst
Porencephaly, acquired
Pseudoporencephaly

Excludes *porencephaly (congenital) (724.4)*

Anoxic brain damage: Brain permanently damaged by lack of oxygen perfusion through brain tissues. This is the result of the problem; use an additional E code to identify the cause.

348.1 **Anoxic brain damage**

Excludes *that occurring in:*
abortion (634–638 with .7, 639.8)
ectopic or molar pregnancy (639.8)
labor or delivery (668.2, 669.4)
that of newborn (767.0, 768.0–768.9, 772.1–772.2)

Use additional E code to identify cause

348.2 **Benign intracranial hypertension**
Pseudotumor cerebri

Excludes *hypertensive encephalopathy (437.2)*

● 348.3 **Encephalopathy, not elsewhere classified**

❑ 348.30 **Encephalopathy, unspecified**

348.31 **Metabolic encephalopathy**
Septic encephalopathy

Excludes *toxic metabolic encephalopathy (349.82)* ◀

❑ 348.39 **Other encephalopathy**

Excludes *encephalopathy:*
alcoholic (291.2)
hepatic encephalopathy (572.2)
hypertensive (437.2)
toxic encephalopathy (349.82)

348.4 **Compression of brain**
Compression brain (stem)
Herniation brain (stem)
Posterior fossa compression syndrome

348.5 **Cerebral edema**

❑ 348.8 **Other conditions of brain**
Cerebral:
calcification
Cerebral:
fungus

❑ 348.9 **Unspecified condition of brain**

● 349 **Other and unspecified disorders of the nervous system**

349.0 **Reaction to spinal or lumbar puncture**
Headache following lumbar puncture
Cerebral spinal fluid (CSF) maintains a specific level of pressure inside the brain and spinal cord. If this pressure does not return to normal after a spinal or lumbar puncture, a headache will result.

349.1 **Nervous system complications from surgically implanted device**

Excludes *immediate postoperative complications (997.00–997.09)*
mechanical complications of nervous system device (996.2)

❑ 349.2 **Disorders of meninges, not elsewhere classified**
Adhesions, meningeal (cerebral) (spinal)
Cyst, spinal meninges
Meningocele, acquired
Pseudomeningocele, acquired

● 349.8 **Other specified disorders of nervous system**

349.81 **Cerebrospinal fluid rhinorrhea**

Excludes *cerebrospinal fluid otorrhea (388.61)*

349.82 **Toxic encephalopathy**
Toxic metabolic encephalopathy ◀

Use additional E code to identify cause

❑ 349.89 **Other**

❑ 349.9 **Unspecified disorders of nervous system**
Disorder of nervous system (central) NOS

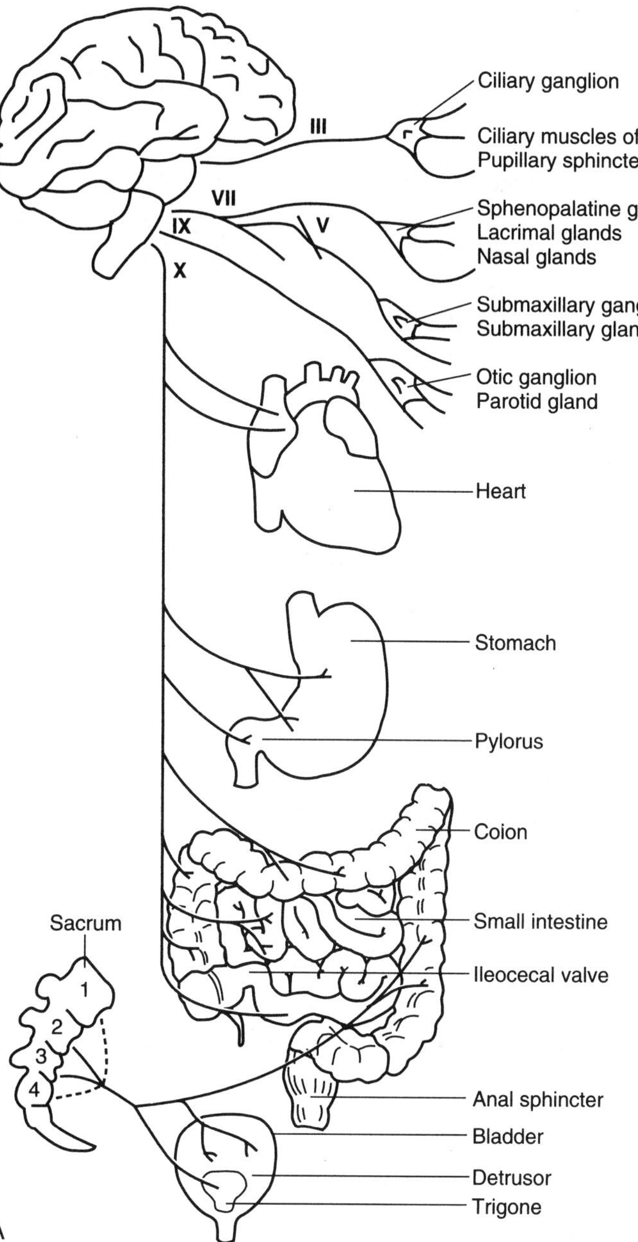
Ciliary ganglion
III
Ciliary muscles of eye
Pupillary sphincter
VII
IX
V
Sphenopalatine ganglion
Lacrimal glands
Nasal glands
X
Submaxillary ganglion
Submaxillary gland
Otic ganglion
Parotid gland
Heart
Stomach
Pylorus
Colon
Small intestine
Sacrum
Ileocecal valve
1
2
3
4
Anal sphincter
Bladder
Detrusor
Trigone

Figure 6–3 A. Parasympathetic nervous system. A

Item 6–6 The peripheral nervous system consists of 31 pairs of spinal nerves, 12 pairs of cranial nerves, and the autonomic nerves, which are divided into the parasympathetic and sympathetic nerves. The cranial nerves are: olfactory (I), optic (II), oculomotor (III), trochlear (IV), trigeminal (V), abducens (VI), facial (VII), vestibulocochlear (VIII), glossopharyngeal (IX), vagus (X), accessory (XI), and hypoglossal (XII).

DISORDERS OF THE PERIPHERAL NERVOUS SYSTEM (350–359)

Excludes *diseases of:*
acoustic [8th] nerve (388.5)
oculomotor [3rd, 4th, 6th] nerves (378.0–378.9)
optic [2nd] nerve (377.0–377.9)
peripheral autonomic nerves (337.0–337.9)
neuralgia NOS or "rheumatic" (729.2)
neuritis NOS or "rheumatic" (729.2)
radiculitis NOS or "rheumatic" (729.2)
peripheral neuritis in pregnancy (646.4)

● **350 Trigeminal nerve disorders**

Includes: disorders of 5th cranial nerve

350.1 Trigeminal neuralgia
Tic douloureux
Trifacial neuralgia
Trigeminal neuralgia NOS

Excludes *postherpetic (053.12)*

350.2 Atypical face pain

❑ **350.8 Other specified trigeminal nerve disorders**

❑ **350.9 Trigeminal nerve disorder, unspecified**

● **351 Facial nerve disorders**

Includes: disorders of 7th cranial nerve

Excludes *that in newborn (767.5)*

351.0 Bell's palsy
Facial palsy

ICD-9-CM 300-399 Vol. 1

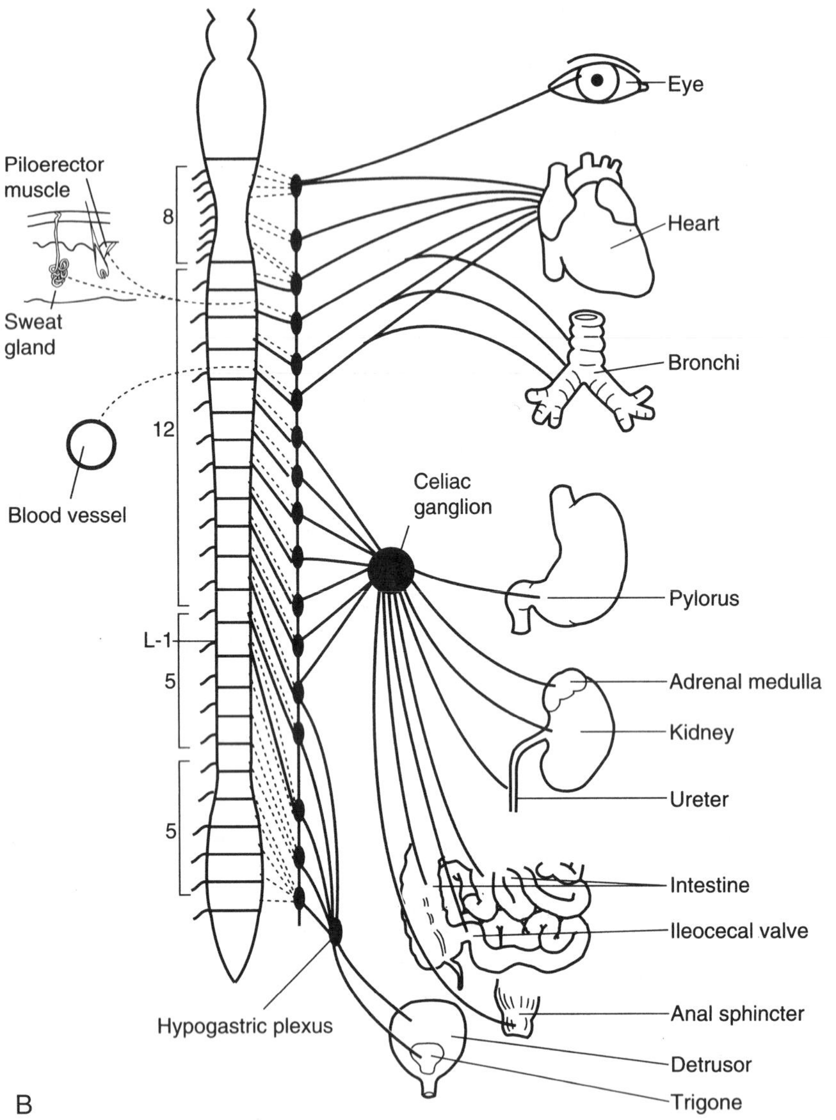

Eye
Piloerector muscle
8
Heart
Sweat gland
Bronchi
12
Blood vessel
Celiac ganglion
Pylorus
L-1
5
Adrenal medulla
Kidney
Ureter
5
Intestine
Ileocecal valve
Anal sphincter
Hypogastric plexus
Detrusor
Trigone
B

Figure 6–3 B. Sympathetic nervous system. (From Buck CJ: Step-by-Step Medical Coding, 2nd ed. Philadelphia, WB Saunders, 1998, pp 186 and 187.)

351.1 Geniculate ganglionitis
Geniculate ganglionitis NOS

Excludes *herpetic (053.11)*

❑**351.8 Other facial nerve disorders**
Facial myokymia
Melkersson's syndrome

❑**351.9 Facial nerve disorder, unspecified**

● **352 Disorders of other cranial nerves**

352.0 Disorders of olfactory [1st] nerve

352.1 Glossopharyngeal neuralgia

❑**352.2 Other disorders of glossopharyngeal [9th] nerve**

352.3 Disorders of pneumogastric [10th] nerve
Disorders of vagal nerve

Excludes *paralysis of vocal cords or larynx (478.30–478.34)*

352.4 Disorders of accessory [11th] nerve

352.5 Disorders of hypoglossal [12th] nerve

352.6 Multiple cranial nerve palsies
Collet-Sicard syndrome
Polyneuritis cranialis

❑**352.9 Unspecified disorder of cranial nerves**

● **353 Nerve root and plexus disorders**

Excludes *conditions due to:*
intervertebral disc disorders (722.0–722.9)
spondylosis (720.0–721.9)
vertebrogenic disorders (723.0–724.9)

353.0 Brachial plexus lesions
Cervical rib syndrome
Costoclavicular syndrome
Scalenus anticus syndrome
Thoracic outlet syndrome

Excludes *brachial neuritis or radiculitis NOS (723.4)*
that in newborn (767.6)

353.1 Lumbosacral plexus lesions

353.2 Cervical root lesions, not elsewhere classified

353.3 Thoracic root lesions, not elsewhere classified

353.4 Lumbosacral root lesions, not elsewhere classified

353.5 Neuralgic amyotrophy
Parsonage-Aldren-Turner syndrome

Phantom limb syndrome: Patients with amputated limbs feel sensations (cramping, itching) in a limb that no longer exists. Phantom limb pain is perceived by the patient to be coming from the missing limb and can be bearable to intolerable. There is no separate code for phantom limb pain, and the pain can be part of the syndrome.

353.6 Phantom limb (syndrome)

❑**353.8 Other nerve root and plexus disorders**

❑**353.9 Unspecified nerve root and plexus disorder**

● **354 Mononeuritis of upper limb and mononeuritis multiplex**

354.0 Carpal tunnel syndrome *CTS*
Median nerve entrapment
Partial thenar atrophy

❑**354.1 Other lesion of median nerve**
Median nerve neuritis

354.2 Lesion of ulnar nerve
Cubital tunnel syndrome
Tardy ulnar nerve palsy

354.3 Lesion of radial nerve
Acute radial nerve palsy

354.4 Causalgia of upper limb
Excludes *causalgia:*
NOS (355.9)
lower limb (355.71)

354.5 Mononeuritis multiplex
Combinations of single conditions classifiable to 354 or 355

❑**354.8 Other mononeuritis of upper limb**

❑**354.9 Mononeuritis of upper limb, unspecified**

● **355 Mononeuritis of lower limb**

355.0 Lesion of sciatic nerve
Excludes *sciatica NOS (724.3)*

355.1 Meralgia paresthetica
Lateral cutaneous femoral nerve of thigh compression or syndrome

❑**355.2 Other lesion of femoral nerve**

355.3 Lesion of lateral popliteal nerve
Lesion of common peroneal nerve

355.4 Lesion of medial popliteal nerve

355.5 Tarsal tunnel syndrome

355.6 Lesion of plantar nerve
Morton's metatarsalgia, neuralgia, or neuroma

● **355.7 Other mononeuritis of lower limb**

355.71 Causalgia of lower limb
Excludes *causalgia:*
NOS (355.9)
upper limb (354.4)

❑**355.79 Other mononeuritis of lower limb**

❑**355.8 Mononeuritis of lower limb, unspecified**

❑**355.9 Mononeuritis of unspecified site**
Causalgia NOS
Excludes *causalgia:*
lower limb (355.71)
upper limb (354.4)

● **356 Hereditary and idiopathic peripheral neuropathy**

356.0 Hereditary peripheral neuropathy
Déjérine-Sottas disease

356.1 Peroneal muscular atrophy
Charcot-Marie-Tooth disease
Neuropathic muscular atrophy

356.2 Hereditary sensory neuropathy

356.3 Refsum's disease
Heredopathia atactica polyneuritiformis

356.4 Idiopathic progressive polyneuropathy

❑**356.8 Other specified idiopathic peripheral neuropathy**
Supranuclear paralysis

❑**356.9 Unspecified**

● **357 Inflammatory and toxic neuropathy**

357.0 Acute infective polyneuritis
Guillain-Barre syndrome
Postinfectious polyneuritis

●***357.1 Polyneuropathy in collagen vascular disease***
Code first underlying disease, as:
disseminated lupus erythematosus (710.0)
polyarteritis nodosa (446.0)
rheumatoid arthritis (714.0)

●***357.2 Polyneuropathy in diabetes***
Code first underlying disease (250.6)

●***357.3 Polyneuropathy in malignant disease***
Code first underlying disease (140.0–208.9)

● ❑***357.4 Polyneuropathy in other diseases classified elsewhere***
Code first underlying disease, as:
amyloidosis (277.30–277.39) ⬅
beriberi (265.0)
chronic uremia (585.9) ◀
deficiency of B vitamins (266.0–266.9)
diphtheria (032.0–032.9)
hypoglycemia (251.2)
pellagra (265.2)
porphyria (277.1)
sarcoidosis (135)
uremia NOS (586) ⬅
Excludes *polyneuropathy in:*
herpes zoster (053.13)
mumps (072.72)

ICD-9-CM 300-399 Vol. 1

357.5 Alcoholic polyneuropathy

357.6 Polyneuropathy due to drugs
Use additional E code to identify drug

❑**357.7 Polyneuropathy due to other toxic agents**
Use additional E code to identify toxic agent

● ❑**357.8 Other**

357.81 Chronic inflammatory demyelinating polyneuritis

357.82 Critical illness polyneuropathy
Acute motor neuropathy

❑**357.89 Other inflammatory and toxic neuropathy**

❑**357.9 Unspecified**

● **358 Myoneural disorders**

● **358.0 Myasthenia gravis**

❑**358.00 Myasthenia gravis without (acute) exacerbation**
Myasthenia gravis NOS

❑**358.01 Myasthenia gravis with acute exacerbation**
Myasthenia gravis in crisis

●***358.1 Myasthenic syndromes in diseases classified elsewhere***
Amyotrophy from stated cause classified elsewhere
Eaton-Lambert syndrome from stated cause classified elsewhere
Code first underlying disease, as:
botulism (005.1)
diabetes mellitus (250.6)
hypothyroidism (244.0–244.9)
malignant neoplasm (140.0–208.9)
pernicious anemia (281.0)
thyrotoxicosis (242.0–242.9)

358.2 Toxic myoneural disorders

Use additional E code to identify toxic agent

358.8 Other specified myoneural disorders

358.9 Myoneural disorders, unspecified

● **359 Muscular dystrophies and other myopathies**

Excludes *idiopathic polymyositis (710.4)*

359.0 Congenital hereditary muscular dystrophy

Benign congenital myopathy
Central core disease
Centronuclear myopathy
Myotubular myopathy
Nemaline body disease

Excludes *arthrogryposis multiplex congenita (754.89)*

359.1 Hereditary progressive muscular dystrophy

Muscular dystrophy:
- NOS
- distal
- Duchenne
- Erb's
- fascioscapulohumeral
- Gower's
- Landouzy-Déjérine
- limb-girdle
- ocular
- oculopharyngeal

359.2 Myotonic disorders

Dystrophia myotonica
Eulenburg's disease
Myotonia congenita
Paramyotonia congenita
Steinert's disease
Thomsen's disease

359.3 Familial periodic paralysis

Hypokalemic familial periodic paralysis

359.4 Toxic myopathy

Use additional E code to identify toxic agent

● *359.5* ***Myopathy in endocrine diseases classified elsewhere***

Code first underlying disease, as:
Addison's disease (255.4)
Cushing's syndrome (255.0)
hypopituitarism (253.2)
myxedema (244.0–244.9)
thyrotoxicosis (242.0–242.9)

● *359.6* ***Symptomatic inflammatory myopathy in diseases classified elsewhere***

Code first underlying disease, as:
amyloidosis (277.30–277.39) ⬅
disseminated lupus erythematosus (710.0)
malignant neoplasm (140.0–208.9)
polyarteritis nodosa (446.0)
rheumatoid arthritis (714.0)
sarcoidosis (135)
scleroderma (710.1)
Sjögren's disease (710.2)

● ❑ **359.8 Other myopathies**

359.81 Critical illness myopathy

Acute necrotizing myopathy
Acute quadriplegic myopathy
Intensive care (ICU) myopathy
Myopathy of critical illness

❑ **359.89 Other myopathies**

❑ **359.9 Myopathy, unspecified**

DISORDERS OF THE EYE AND ADNEXA (360–379)

● **360 Disorders of the globe**

Includes: disorders affecting multiple structures of eye

● **360.0 Purulent endophthalmitis**

Excludes *bleb associated endophthalmitis (379.63)* ◀

❑ **360.00 Purulent endophthalmitis, unspecified**

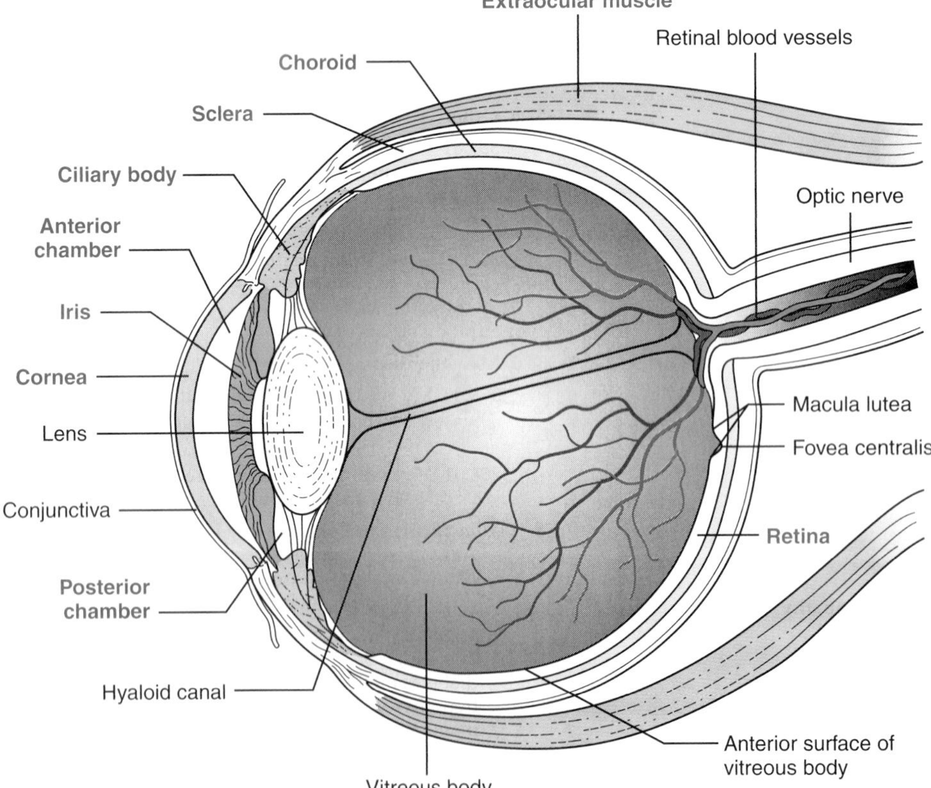
Extraocular muscle
Retinal blood vessels
Choroid
Sclera
Ciliary body
Optic nerve
Anterior chamber
Iris
Cornea
Macula lutea
Lens
Fovea centralis
Conjunctiva
Retina
Posterior chamber
Hyaloid canal
Anterior surface of vitreous body
Vitreous body

Figure 6–4 Eye and ocular adnexa. (From Buck CJ: Step-by-Step Medical Coding, 2005 ed. Philadelphia, WB Saunders, 2005.)

360.01 **Acute endophthalmitis**

360.02 **Panophthalmitis**

360.03 **Chronic endophthalmitis**

360.04 **Vitreous abscess**

● **360.1 Other endophthalmitis**

Excludes *bleb associated endophthalmitis (379.63)* ◄

360.11 **Sympathetic uveitis**

360.12 **Panuveitis**

360.13 **Parasitic endophthalmitis NOS**

360.14 **Ophthalmia nodosa**

❑360.19 **Other**
Phacoanaphylactic endophthalmitis

● **360.2 Degenerative disorders of globe**

❑360.20 **Degenerative disorder of globe, unspecified**

360.21 **Progressive high (degenerative) myopia**
Malignant myopia

360.23 **Siderosis**

❑360.24 **Other metallosis**
Chalcosis

❑360.29 **Other**

Excludes *xerophthalmia (264.7)*

● **360.3 Hypotony of eye**

❑360.30 **Hypotony, unspecified**

360.31 **Primary hypotony**

360.32 **Ocular fistula causing hypotony**

❑360.33 **Hypotony associated with other ocular disorders**

360.34 **Flat anterior chamber**

● **360.4 Degenerated conditions of globe**

❑360.40 **Degenerated globe or eye, unspecified**

360.41 **Blind hypotensive eye**
Atrophy of globe
Phthisis bulbi

360.42 **Blind hypertensive eye**
Absolute glaucoma

360.43 **Hemophthalmos, except current injury**

Excludes *traumatic (871.0–871.9, 921.0–921.9)*

360.44 **Leucocoria**

● **360.5 Retained (old) intraocular foreign body, magnetic**

Excludes *current penetrating injury with magnetic foreign body (871.5)*
retained (old) foreign body of orbit (376.6)

❑360.50 **Foreign body, magnetic, intraocular, unspecified**

360.51 **Foreign body, magnetic, in anterior chamber**

360.52 **Foreign body, magnetic, in iris or ciliary body**

360.53 **Foreign body, magnetic, in lens**

360.54 **Foreign body, magnetic, in vitreous**

360.55 **Foreign body, magnetic, in posterior wall**

❑360.59 **Foreign body, magnetic, in other or multiple sites**

● **360.6 Retained (old) intraocular foreign body, nonmagnetic**
Retained (old) foreign body:
NOS
nonmagnetic

Excludes *current penetrating injury with (nonmagnetic) foreign body (871.6)*
retained (old) foreign body in orbit (376.6)

❑360.60 **Foreign body, intraocular, unspecified**

360.61 **Foreign body in anterior chamber**

360.62 **Foreign body in iris or ciliary body**

360.63 **Foreign body in lens**

360.64 **Foreign body in vitreous**

360.65 **Foreign body in posterior wall**

❑360.69 **Foreign body in other or multiple sites**

● **360.8 Other disorders of globe**

360.81 **Luxation of globe**

❑360.89 **Other**

❑**360.9 Unspecified disorder of globe**

● **361 Retinal detachments and defects**

● **361.0 Retinal detachment with retinal defect**
Rhegmatogenous retinal detachment

Excludes *detachment of retinal pigment epithelium (362.42–362.43)*
retinal detachment (serous) (without defect) (361.2)

❑361.00 **Retinal detachment with retinal defect, unspecified**

361.01 **Recent detachment, partial, with single defect**

361.02 **Recent detachment, partial, with multiple defects**

361.03 **Recent detachment, partial, with giant tear**

361.04 **Recent detachment, partial, with retinal dialysis**
Dialysis (juvenile) of retina (with detachment)

361.05 **Recent detachment, total or subtotal**

361.06 **Old detachment, partial**
Delimited old retinal detachment

361.07 **Old detachment, total or subtotal**

● **361.1 Retinoschisis and retinal cysts**

Excludes *juvenile retinoschisis (362.73)*
microcystoid degeneration of retina (362.62)
parasitic cyst of retina (360.13)

❑361.10 **Retinoschisis, unspecified**

361.11 **Flat retinoschisis**

361.12 **Bullous retinoschisis**

361.13 **Primary retinal cysts**

361.14 **Secondary retinal cysts**

❑361.19 **Other**
Pseudocyst of retina

361.2 Serous retinal detachment
Retinal detachment without retinal defect

Excludes *central serous retinopathy (362.41)*
retinal pigment epithelium detachment (362.42–362.43)

● **361.3 Retinal defects without detachment**

Excludes *chorioretinal scars after surgery for detachment (363.30–363.35)*
peripheral retinal degeneration without defect (362.60–362.66)

❑361.30 **Retinal defect, unspecified**
Retinal break(s) NOS

361.31 **Round hole of retina without detachment**

361.32 **Horseshoe tear of retina without detachment**
Operculum of retina without mention of detachment

❑361.33 **Multiple defects of retina without detachment**

●361.8 **Other forms of retinal detachment**

361.81 **Traction detachment of retina**
Traction detachment with vitreoretinal organization

❑361.89 **Other**

❑361.9 **Unspecified retinal detachment**

●362 **Other retinal disorders**

Excludes *chorioretinal scars (363.30–363.35)*
chorioretinitis (363.0–363.2)

●362.0 ***Diabetic retinopathy***

Code first diabetes (250.5)

● 362.01 ***Background diabetic retinopathy***
Diabetic retinal microaneurysms
Diabetic retinopathy NOS

● 362.02 ***Proliferative diabetic retinopathy***

● 362.03 ***Nonproliferative diabetic retinopathy NOS***

● 362.04 ***Mild nonproliferative diabetic retinopathy***

● 362.05 ***Moderate nonproliferative diabetic retinopathy***

● 362.06 ***Severe nonproliferative diabetic retinopathy***

● 362.07 ***Diabetic macular edema***
Diabetic retinal edema

Note: Code 362.07 must be used with a code for diabetic retinopathy (362.01–362.06)

●362.1 **Other background retinopathy and retinal vascular changes**

❑362.10 **Background retinopathy, unspecified**

362.11 **Hypertensive retinopathy**

362.12 **Exudative retinopathy**
Coats' syndrome

362.13 **Changes in vascular appearance**
Vascular sheathing of retina

Use additional code for any associated atherosclerosis (440.8)

362.14 **Retinal microaneurysms NOS**

362.15 **Retinal telangiectasia**

362.16 **Retinal neovascularization NOS**
Neovascularization:
choroidal
subretinal

❑362.17 **Other intraretinal microvascular abnormalities**
Retinal varices

362.18 **Retinal vasculitis**
Eales' disease
Retinal:
arteritis
endarteritis
perivasculitis
phlebitis

●362.2 **Other proliferative retinopathy**

362.21 **Retrolental fibroplasia**

❑362.29 **Other nondiabetic proliferative retinopathy**

●362.3 **Retinal vascular occlusion**

❑362.30 **Retinal vascular occlusion, unspecified**

362.31 **Central retinal artery occlusion**

362.32 **Arterial branch occlusion**

362.33 **Partial arterial occlusion**
Hollenhorst plaque
Retinal microembolism

362.34 **Transient arterial occlusion**
Amaurosis fugax

362.35 **Central retinal vein occlusion**

362.36 **Venous tributary (branch) occlusion**

362.37 **Venous engorgement**
Occlusion:
of retinal vein
incipient of retinal vein
partial of retinal vein

●362.4 **Separation of retinal layers**

Excludes *retinal detachment (serous) (361.2)*
rhegmatogenous (361.00–361.07)

❑362.40 **Retinal layer separation, unspecified**

362.41 **Central serous retinopathy**

362.42 **Serous detachment of retinal pigment epithelium**
Exudative detachment of retinal pigment epithelium

362.43 **Hemorrhagic detachment of retinal pigment epithelium**

●362.5 **Degeneration of macula and posterior pole**

Excludes *degeneration of optic disc (377.21–377.24)*
hereditary retinal degeneration [dystrophy] (362.70–362.77)

❑362.50 **Macular degeneration (senile), unspecified**

362.51 **Nonexudative senile macular degeneration**
Senile macular degeneration:
atrophic
dry

362.52 **Exudative senile macular degeneration**
Kuhnt-Junius degeneration
Senile macular degeneration:
disciform
wet

362.53 **Cystoid macular degeneration**
Cystoid macular edema

362.54 **Macular cyst, hole, or pseudohole**

362.55 **Toxic maculopathy**

Use additional E code to identify drug, if drug induced

362.56 **Macular puckering**
Preretinal fibrosis

362.57 **Drusen (degenerative)**

●362.6 **Peripheral retinal degenerations**

Excludes *hereditary retinal degeneration [dystrophy] (362.70–362.77)*
retinal degeneration with retinal defect (361.00–361.07)

❑362.60 **Peripheral retinal degeneration, unspecified**

362.61 **Paving stone degeneration**

362.62 **Microcystoid degeneration**
Blessig's cysts
Iwanoff's cysts

362.63 **Lattice degeneration**
Palisade degeneration of retina

362.64 **Senile reticular degeneration**

362.65 **Secondary pigmentary degeneration**
Pseudoretinitis pigmentosa

362.66 **Secondary vitreoretinal degenerations**

●362.7 **Hereditary retinal dystrophies**

❑362.70 **Hereditary retinal dystrophy, unspecified**

● 362.71 ***Retinal dystrophy in systemic or cerebroretinal lipidoses***
Code first underlying disease, as:
cerebroretinal lipidoses (330.1)
systemic lipidoses (272.7)

● ❑362.72 ***Retinal dystrophy in other systemic disorders and syndromes***
Code first underlying disease, as:
Bassen-Kornzweig syndrome (272.5)
Refsum's disease (356.3)

362.73 **Vitreoretinal dystrophies**
Juvenile retinoschisis

362.74 **Pigmentary retinal dystrophy**
Retinal dystrophy, albipunctate
Retinitis pigmentosa

❑362.75 **Other dystrophies primarily involving the sensory retina**
Progressive cone (-rod) dystrophy
Stargardt's disease

362.76 **Dystrophies primarily involving the retinal pigment epithelium**
Fundus flavimaculatus
Vitelliform dystrophy

362.77 **Dystrophies primarily involving Bruch's membrane**
Dystrophy:
hyaline
pseudoinflammatory foveal
Hereditary drusen

362.8 Other retinal disorders
Excludes *chorioretinal inflammations (363.0–363.2)*
chorioretinal scars (363.30–363.35)

362.81 **Retinal hemorrhage**
Hemorrhage:
preretinal
retinal (deep) (superficial)
subretinal

362.82 **Retinal exudates and deposits**

362.83 **Retinal edema**
Retinal:
cotton wool spots
edema (localized) (macular) (peripheral)

362.84 **Retinal ischemia**

362.85 **Retinal nerve fiber bundle defects**

❑362.89 **Other retinal disorders**

❑362.9 **Unspecified retinal disorder**

363 **Chorioretinal inflammations, scars, and other disorders of choroid**

363.0 **Focal chorioretinitis and focal retinochoroiditis**
Excludes *focal chorioretinitis or retinochoroiditis in:*
histoplasmosis (115.02, 115.12, 115.92)
toxoplasmosis (130.2)
congenital infection (771.2)

❑363.00 **Focal chorioretinitis, unspecified**
Focal:
choroiditis or chorioretinitis NOS
retinitis or retinochoroiditis NOS

363.01 **Focal choroiditis and chorioretinitis, juxtapapillary**

❑363.03 **Focal choroiditis and chorioretinitis of other posterior pole**

363.04 **Focal choroiditis and chorioretinitis, peripheral**

363.05 **Focal retinitis and retinochoroiditis, juxtapapillary**
Neuroretinitis

363.06 **Focal retinitis and retinochoroiditis, macular or paramacular**

❑363.07 **Focal retinitis and retinochoroiditis of other posterior pole**

363.08 **Focal retinitis and retinochoroiditis, peripheral**

363.1 **Disseminated chorioretinitis and disseminated retinochoroiditis**
Excludes *disseminated choroiditis or chorioretinitis in secondary syphilis (091.51)*
neurosyphilitic disseminated retinitis or retinochoroiditis (094.83)
retinal (peri)vasculitis (362.18)

❑363.10 **Disseminated chorioretinitis, unspecified**
Disseminated:
choroiditis or chorioretinitis NOS
retinitis or retinochoroiditis NOS

363.11 **Disseminated choroiditis and chorioretinitis, posterior pole**

363.12 **Disseminated choroiditis and chorioretinitis, peripheral**

363.13 **Disseminated choroiditis and chorioretinitis, generalized**
Code first any underlying disease, as:
tuberculosis (017.3)

363.14 **Disseminated retinitis and retinochoroiditis, metastatic**

363.15 **Disseminated retinitis and retinochoroiditis, pigment epitheliopathy**
Acute posterior multifocal placoid pigment epitheliopathy

363.2 **Other and unspecified forms of chorioretinitis and retinochoroiditis**
Excludes *panophthalmitis (360.02)*
sympathetic uveitis (360.11)
uveitis NOS (364.3)

❑363.20 **Chorioretinitis, unspecified**
Choroiditis NOS
Retinitis NOS
Uveitis, posterior NOS

363.21 **Pars planitis**
Posterior cyclitis

363.22 **Harada's disease**

363.3 **Chorioretinal scars**
Scar (postinflammatory) (postsurgical) (post-traumatic):
choroid
retina

❑363.30 **Chorioretinal scar, unspecified**

363.31 **Solar retinopathy**

❑363.32 **Other macular scars**

❑363.33 **Other scars of posterior pole**

363.34 **Peripheral scars**

363.35 **Disseminated scars**

363.4 **Choroidal degenerations**

❑363.40 **Choroidal degeneration, unspecified**
Choroidal sclerosis NOS

363.41 **Senile atrophy of choroid**

363.42 **Diffuse secondary atrophy of choroid**

363.43 **Angioid streaks of choroid**

363.5 **Hereditary choroidal dystrophies**
Hereditary choroidal atrophy:
partial [choriocapillaris]
total [all vessels]

❑363.50 **Hereditary choroidal dystrophy or atrophy, unspecified**

363.51 **Circumpapillary dystrophy of choroid, partial**

363.52 **Circumpapillary dystrophy of choroid, total**
Helicoid dystrophy of choroid

363.53 **Central dystrophy of choroid, partial**
Dystrophy, choroidal:
central areolar
circinate

363.54 **Central choroidal atrophy, total**
Dystrophy, choroidal:
central gyrate
serpiginous

363.55 **Choroideremia**

❑363.56 **Other diffuse or generalized dystrophy, partial**
Diffuse choroidal sclerosis

❑363.57 **Other diffuse or generalized dystrophy, total**
Generalized gyrate atrophy, choroid

● 363.6 **Choroidal hemorrhage and rupture**

❑363.61 **Choroidal hemorrhage, unspecified**

363.62 **Expulsive choroidal hemorrhage**

363.63 **Choroidal rupture**

● 363.7 **Choroidal detachment**

❑363.70 **Choroidal detachment, unspecified**

363.71 **Serous choroidal detachment**

363.72 **Hemorrhagic choroidal detachment**

❑363.8 **Other disorders of choroid**

❑363.9 **Unspecified disorder of choroid**

● 364 **Disorders of iris and ciliary body**

● 364.0 **Acute and subacute iridocyclitis**
Anterior uveitis, acute, subacute
Cyclitis, acute, subacute
Iridocyclitis, acute, subacute
Iritis, acute, subacute

Excludes *gonococcal (098.41)*
herpes simplex (054.44)
herpes zoster (053.22)

❑364.00 **Acute and subacute iridocyclitis, unspecified**

364.01 **Primary iridocyclitis**

364.02 **Recurrent iridocyclitis**

364.03 **Secondary iridocyclitis, infectious**

364.04 **Secondary iridocyclitis, noninfectious**
Aqueous:
cells
fibrin
flare

364.05 **Hypopyon**

● 364.1 **Chronic iridocyclitis**

Excludes *posterior cyclitis (363.21)*

❑364.10 **Chronic iridocyclitis, unspecified**

● 364.11 ***Chronic iridocyclitis in diseases classified elsewhere***

Code first underlying disease, as:
sarcoidosis (135)
tuberculosis (017.3)

Excludes *syphilitic iridocyclitis (091.52)*

● 364.2 **Certain types of iridocyclitis**

Excludes *posterior cyclitis (363.21)*
sympathetic uveitis (360.11)

364.21 **Fuchs' heterochromic cyclitis**

364.22 **Glaucomatocyclitic crises**

364.23 **Lens-induced iridocyclitis**

364.24 **Vogt-Koyanagi syndrome**

❑364.3 **Unspecified iridocyclitis**
Uveitis NOS

● 364.4 **Vascular disorders of iris and ciliary body**

364.41 **Hyphema**
Hemorrhage of iris or ciliary body

364.42 **Rubeosis iridis**
Neovascularization of iris or ciliary body

● 364.5 **Degenerations of iris and ciliary body**

364.51 **Essential or progressive iris atrophy**

364.52 **Iridoschisis**

364.53 **Pigmentary iris degeneration**
Acquired heterochromia of iris
Pigment dispersion syndrome of iris
Translucency of iris

364.54 **Degeneration of pupillary margin**
Atrophy of sphincter of iris
Ectropion of pigment epithelium of iris

364.55 **Miotic cysts of pupillary margin**

364.56 **Degenerative changes of chamber angle**

364.57 **Degenerative changes of ciliary body**

❑364.59 **Other iris atrophy**
Iris atrophy (generalized) (sector shaped)

● 364.6 **Cysts of iris, ciliary body, and anterior chamber**

Excludes *miotic pupillary cyst (364.55)*
parasitic cyst (360.13)

364.60 **Idiopathic cysts**

364.61 **Implantation cysts**
Epithelial down-growth, anterior chamber
Implantation cysts (surgical) (traumatic)

364.62 **Exudative cysts of iris or anterior chamber**

364.63 **Primary cyst of pars plana**

364.64 **Exudative cyst of pars plana**

● 364.7 **Adhesions and disruptions of iris and ciliary body**

Excludes *flat anterior chamber (360.34)*

❑364.70 **Adhesions of iris, unspecified**
Synechiae (iris) NOS

364.71 **Posterior synechiae**

364.72 **Anterior synechiae**

364.73 **Goniosynechiae**
Peripheral anterior synechiae

364.74 **Pupillary membranes**
Iris bombé
Pupillary:
occlusion
seclusion

364.75 **Pupillary abnormalities**
Deformed pupil
Ectopic pupil
Rupture of sphincter, pupil

364.76 **Iridodialysis**

364.77 **Recession of chamber angle**

❑364.8 **Other disorders of iris and ciliary body**
Prolapse of iris NOS

Excludes *prolapse of iris in recent wound (871.1)*

❑364.9 **Unspecified disorder of iris and ciliary body**

● 365 **Glaucoma**

Excludes *blind hypertensive eye [absolute glaucoma] (360.42)*
congenital glaucoma (743.20–743.22)

● 365.0 **Borderline glaucoma [glaucoma suspect]**

❑365.00 **Preglaucoma, unspecified**

365.01 **Open angle with borderline findings**
Open angle with:
borderline intraocular pressure
cupping of optic discs

365.02 **Anatomical narrow angle**

365.03 **Steroid responders**

❑365.04 **Ocular hypertension**

● 365.1 **Open-angle glaucoma**

❑365.10 **Open-angle glaucoma, unspecified**
Wide-angle glaucoma NOS

365.11 **Primary open angle glaucoma**
Chronic simple glaucoma

365.12 **Low tension glaucoma**

365.13 **Pigmentary glaucoma**

365.14 **Glaucoma of childhood**
Infantile or juvenile glaucoma

365.15 **Residual stage of open angle glaucoma**

● 365.2 **Primary angle-closure glaucoma**

❑365.20 **Primary angle-closure glaucoma, unspecified**

365.21 **Intermittent angle-closure glaucoma**
Angle-closure glaucoma:
interval
subacute

365.22 **Acute angle-closure glaucoma**

365.23 **Chronic angle-closure glaucoma**

365.24 **Residual stage of angle-closure glaucoma**

● 365.3 **Corticosteroid-induced glaucoma**

365.31 **Glaucomatous stage**

365.32 **Residual stage**

● 365.4 **Glaucoma associated with congenital anomalies, dystrophies, and systemic syndromes**

● *365.41* ***Glaucoma associated with chamber angle anomalies***

Code first associated disorder, as:
Axenfeld's anomaly (743.44)
Rieger's anomaly or syndrome (743.44)

● *365.42* ***Glaucoma associated with anomalies of iris***

Code first associated disorder, as:
aniridia (743.45)
essential iris atrophy (364.51)

● ❑*365.43* ***Glaucoma associated with other anterior segment anomalies***

Code first associated disorder, as:
microcornea (743.41)

● *365.44* ***Glaucoma associated with systemic syndromes***

Code first associated disease, as:
neurofibromatosis (237.7)
Sturge-Weber (-Dimitri) syndrome (759.6)

● 365.5 **Glaucoma associated with disorders of the lens**

365.51 **Phacolytic glaucoma**

Use additional code for associated
hypermature cataract (366.18)

365.52 **Pseudoexfoliation glaucoma**

Use additional code for associated
pseudoexfoliation of capsule (366.11)

❑365.59 **Glaucoma associated with other lens disorders**

Use additional code for associated disorder, as:
dislocation of lens (379.33–379.34)
spherophakia (743.36)

● 365.6 **Glaucoma associated with other ocular disorders**

❑365.60 **Glaucoma associated with unspecified ocular disorder**

365.61 **Glaucoma associated with pupillary block**

Use additional code for associated disorder, as:
seclusion of pupil [iris bombé] (364.74)

365.62 **Glaucoma associated with ocular inflammations**

Use additional code for associated disorder, as:
glaucomatocyclitic crises (364.22)
iridocyclitis (364.0–364.3)

365.63 **Glaucoma associated with vascular disorders**

Use additional code for associated disorder, as:
central retinal vein occlusion (362.35)
hyphema (364.41)

365.64 **Glaucoma associated with tumors or cysts**

Use additional code for associated disorder, as:
benign neoplasm (224.0–224.9)
epithelial down-growth (364.61)
malignant neoplasm (190.0–190.9)

365.65 **Glaucoma associated with ocular trauma**

Use additional code for associated condition, as:
contusion of globe (921.3)
recession of chamber angle (364.77)

● 365.8 **Other specified forms of glaucoma**

365.81 **Hypersecretion glaucoma**

365.82 **Glaucoma with increased episcleral venous pressure**

365.83 **Aqueous misdirection**
Malignant glaucoma

❑365.89 **Other specified glaucoma**

❑365.9 **Unspecified glaucoma**

● 366 Cataract

Excludes *congenital cataract (743.30–743.34)*

● 366.0 **Infantile, juvenile, and presenile cataract**

❑366.00 **Nonsenile cataract, unspecified**

366.01 **Anterior subcapsular polar cataract**

366.02 **Posterior subcapsular polar cataract**

366.03 **Cortical, lamellar, or zonular cataract**

366.04 **Nuclear cataract**

❑366.09 **Other and combined forms of nonsenile cataract**

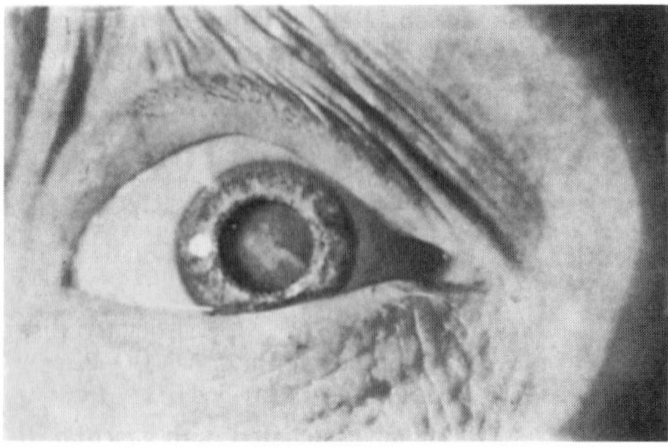

Figure 6–5 Mature cataract with gray fissures. (From Pau H: Differential Diagnosis of Eye Diseases. Philadelphia, WB Saunders, 1978, p 240. Copyright Georg Thieme Verlag [Stuttgart, Germany].)

Item 6–7 Senile cataracts are linked to the aging process. The most common area for the formation of a cataract is the cortical area of the lens. **Polar cataracts** can be either anterior or posterior. **Anterior polar cataracts** are more common and are small, white, capsular cataracts located on the anterior portion of the lens.
Total cataracts, also called **complete** or **mature,** cause an opacity of all fibers of the lens.
Hypermature describes a mature cataract with a swollen, milky cortex that covers the entire lens.
Immature, also called **incipient,** cataracts have a clear cortex and are only slightly opaque.

● **366.1 Senile cataract**

❑ **366.10 Senile cataract, unspecified**

366.11 Pseudoexfoliation of lens capsule

366.12 Incipient cataract
Cataract:
coronary
immature NOS
punctate
Water clefts

366.13 Anterior subcapsular polar senile cataract

366.14 Posterior subcapsular polar senile cataract

366.15 Cortical senile cataract

366.16 Nuclear sclerosis
Cataracta brunescens
Nuclear cataract

366.17 Total or mature cataract

366.18 Hypermature cataract
Morgagni cataract

❑ **366.19 Other and combined forms of senile cataract**

● **366.2 Traumatic cataract**

❑ **366.20 Traumatic cataract, unspecified**

366.21 Localized traumatic opacities
Vossius' ring

366.22 Total traumatic cataract

366.23 Partially resolved traumatic cataract

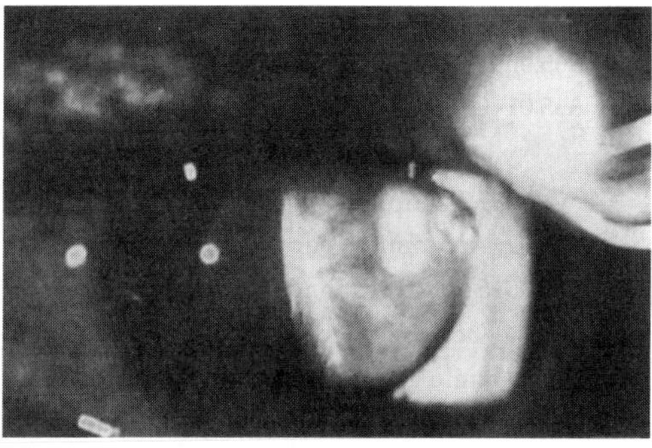

Figure 6–6 Perforation rosette of the lens; feathery opacities along suture lines beneath the posterior capsule. (From Pau H: Differential Diagnosis of Eye Diseases. Philadelphia, WB Saunders, 1978, p 250. Copyright Georg Thieme Verlag [Stuttgart, Germany].)

Item 6–8 **Vossius' ring** is the result of contusion-type traumatic injury and results in a ring of iris pigment pressed onto the anterior lens capsule.

● **366.3 Cataract secondary to ocular disorders**

❑ **366.30 Cataracta complicata, unspecified**

● ***366.31 Glaucomatous flecks (subcapsular)***
Code first underlying glaucoma (365.0–365.9)

● ***366.32 Cataract in inflammatory disorders***
Code first underlying condition, as:
chronic choroiditis (363.0–363.2)

● ***366.33 Cataract with neovascularization***
Code first underlying condition, as:
chronic iridocyclitis (364.10)

● ***366.34 Cataract in degenerative disorders***
Sunflower cataract
Code first underlying condition, as:
chalcosis (360.24)
degenerative myopia (360.21)
pigmentary retinal dystrophy (362.74)

● **366.4 Cataract associated with other disorders**

● ***366.41 Diabetic cataract***
Code first diabetes (250.5)

● ***366.42 Tetanic cataract***
Code first underlying disease, as:
calcinosis (275.40)
hypoparathyroidism (252.1)

● ***366.43 Myotonic cataract***
Code first underlying disorder (359.2)

● ❑ ***366.44 Cataract associated with other syndromes***
Code first underlying condition, as:
craniofacial dysostosis (756.0)
galactosemia (271.1)

366.45 Toxic cataract
Drug-induced cataract
Use additional E code to identify drug or other toxic substance

❑ **366.46 Cataract associated with radiation and other physical influences**
Use additional E code to identify cause

● **366.5 After-cataract**

❑ **366.50 After-cataract, unspecified**
Secondary cataract NOS

366.51 Soemmering's ring

❑366.52 **Other after-cataract, not obscuring vision**

366.53 **After-cataract, obscuring vision**

❑366.8 **Other cataract**
Calcification of lens

❑366.9 **Unspecified cataract**

● 367 **Disorders of refraction and accommodation**

367.0 **Hypermetropia**
Far-sightedness
Hyperopia

367.1 **Myopia**
Near-sightedness

● 367.2 **Astigmatism**

❑367.20 **Astigmatism, unspecified**

367.21 **Regular astigmatism**

367.22 **Irregular astigmatism**

● 367.3 **Anisometropia and aniseikonia**

367.31 **Anisometropia**

367.32 **Aniseikonia**

367.4 **Presbyopia**

● 367.5 **Disorders of accommodation**

367.51 **Paresis of accommodation**
Cycloplegia

367.52 **Total or complete internal ophthalmoplegia**

367.53 **Spasm of accommodation**

● 367.8 **Other disorders of refraction and accommodation**

367.81 **Transient refractive change**

❑367.89 **Other**
Drug-induced disorders of refraction and accommodation
Toxic disorders of refraction and accommodation

❑367.9 **Unspecified disorder of refraction and accommodation**

● 368 **Visual disturbances**

Excludes *electrophysiological disturbances (794.11–794.14)*

● 368.0 **Amblyopia ex anopsia**

❑368.00 **Amblyopia, unspecified**

368.01 **Strabismic amblyopia**
Suppression amblyopia

368.02 **Deprivation amblyopia**

368.03 **Refractive amblyopia**

● 368.1 **Subjective visual disturbances**

❑368.10 **Subjective visual disturbance, unspecified**

368.11 **Sudden visual loss**

368.12 **Transient visual loss**
Concentric fading
Scintillating scotoma

368.13 **Visual discomfort**
Asthenopia
Eye strain
Photophobia

368.14 **Visual distortions of shape and size**
Macropsia
Metamorphopsia
Micropsia

❑368.15 **Other visual distortions and entoptic phenomena**
Photopsia
Refractive:
diplopia
polyopia
Visual halos

368.16 **Psychophysical visual disturbances**
Visual:
agnosia
disorientation syndrome
hallucinations

368.2 **Diplopia**
Double vision

● 368.3 **Other disorders of binocular vision**

❑368.30 **Binocular vision disorder, unspecified**

368.31 **Suppression of binocular vision**

368.32 **Simultaneous visual perception without fusion**

368.33 **Fusion with defective stereopsis**

368.34 **Abnormal retinal correspondence**

● 368.4 **Visual field defects**

❑368.40 **Visual field defect, unspecified**

368.41 **Scotoma involving central area**
Scotoma:
central
centrocecal
paracentral

368.42 **Scotoma of blind spot area**
Enlarged:
angioscotoma
blind spot
Paracecal scotoma

368.43 **Sector or arcuate defects**
Scotoma:
arcuate
Bjerrum
Seidel

❑368.44 **Other localized visual field defect**
Scotoma:
NOS
ring
Visual field defect:
nasal step
peripheral

368.45 **Generalized contraction or constriction**

368.46 **Homonymous bilateral field defects**
Hemianopsia (altitudinal) (homonymous)
Quadrant anopia

368.47 **Heteronymous bilateral field defects**
Hemianopsia:
binasal
bitemporal

● 368.5 **Color vision deficiencies**
Color blindness

368.51 **Protan defect**
Protanomaly
Protanopia

368.52 **Deutan defect**
Deuteranomaly
Deuteranopia

368.53 **Tritan defect**
Tritanomaly
Tritanopia

368.54 **Achromatopsia**
Monochromatism (cone) (rod)

368.55 **Acquired color vision deficiencies**

❑368.59 **Other color vision deficiencies**

● 368.6 **Night blindness**
Nyctalopia

❑368.60 **Night blindness, unspecified**

368.61 **Congenital night blindness**
Hereditary night blindness
Oguchi's disease

368.62 **Acquired night blindness**

Excludes *that due to vitamin A deficiency (264.5)*

368.63 **Abnormal dark adaptation curve**
Abnormal threshold of cones or rods
Delayed adaptation of cones or rods

❑368.69 **Other night blindness**

❑368.8 **Other specified visual disturbances**
Blurred vision NOS

❑368.9 **Unspecified visual disturbance**

Classification		**Levels of Visual Impairment**	**Additional Descriptors Which May Be Encountered**
"Legal"	***WHO***	***Visual Acuity and/or Visual Field Limitation (Whichever Is Worse)***	
	(Near-) normal vision	Range of Normal Vision 20/10 20/13 20/16 20/20 20/25 2.0 1.6 1.25 1.0 0.8	
		Near-Normal Vision 20/30 20/40 20/50 20/60 0.7 0.6 0.5 0.4 0.3	
	Low vision	Moderate Visual Impairment 20/70 20/80 20/100 20/125 20/160 0.25 0.20 0.16 0.12	Moderate low vision
		Severe Visual Impairment 20/200 20/250 20/320 20/400 0.10 0.08 0.06 0.05 Visual field: 20 degrees or less	Severe low vision, "Legal" blindness
Legal Blindness (U.S.A.) both eyes	Blindness (WHO) one or both eyes	Profound Visual Impairment 20/500 20/630 20/800 20/1000 0.04 0.03 0.025 0.02 Count fingers at: less than 3 m (10 ft) Visual field: 10 degrees or less	Profound low vision, Moderate blindness
		Near-Total Visual Impairment Visual acuity: less than 0.02 (20/1000) Count fingers: 1 m (3 ft) or less Hand movements: 5 m (15 ft) or less Light projection, light perception Visual field: 5 degrees or less	Severe blindness, Near-total blindness
		Total Visual Impairment No light perception (NLP)	Total blindness

Visual acuity refers to best achievable acuity with correction.
Non-listed Snellen fractions may be classified by converting to the nearest decimal equivalent, e.g., 10/200 = 0.05, 6/30 = 0.20.
CF (count fingers) without designation of distance, may be classified to profound impairment.
HM (hand motion) without designation of distance, may be classified to near-total impairment.
Visual field measurements refer to the largest field diameter for a 1/100 white test object.

● 369 **Blindness and low vision**

Excludes *correctable impaired vision due to refractive errors (367.0–367.9)*

Note: Visual impairment refers to a functional limitation of the eye (e.g., limited visual acuity or visual field). It should be distinguished from visual disability, indicating a limitation of the abilities of the individual (e.g., limited reading skills, vocational skills), and from visual handicap, indicating a limitation of personal and socioeconomic independence (e.g., limited mobility, limited employability).

The levels of impairment defined in the table after 369.9 are based on the recommendations of the WHO Study Group on Prevention of Blindness (Geneva, November 6–10, 1972; WHO Technical Report Series 518), and of the International Council of Ophthalmology (1976).

Note that definitions of blindness vary in different settings.

For international reporting, WHO defines blindness as profound impairment. This definition can be applied to blindness of one eye (369.1, 369.6) and to blindness of the individual (369.0).

For determination of benefits in the U.S.A., the definition of legal blindness as severe impairment is often used. This definition applies to blindness of the individual only.

● 369.0 **Profound impairment, both eyes**

❑369.00 **Impairment level not further specified**
Blindness:
NOS according to WHO definition
both eyes

❑369.01 **Better eye: total impairment; lesser eye: total impairment**

❑369.02 **Better eye: near-total impairment; lesser eye: not further specified**

❑369.03 **Better eye: near-total impairment; lesser eye: total impairment**

❑369.04 **Better eye: near-total impairment; lesser eye: near-total impairment**

❑369.05 **Better eye: profound impairment; lesser eye: not further specified**

❑369.06 **Better eye: profound impairment; lesser eye: total impairment**

❑369.07 **Better eye: profound impairment; lesser eye: near-total impairment**

❑369.08 **Better eye: profound impairment; lesser eye: profound impairment**

● 369.1 **Moderate or severe impairment, better eye, profound impairment, lesser eye**

❑369.10 **Impairment level not further specified**
Blindness, one eye, low vision, other eye

❑369.11 **Better eye: severe impairment; lesser eye: blind, not further specified**

369.12 **Better eye: severe impairment; lesser eye: total impairment**

369.13 **Better eye: severe impairment; lesser eye: near-total impairment**

369.14 **Better eye: severe impairment; lesser eye: profound impairment**

❑369.15 **Better eye: moderate impairment; lesser eye: blind, not further specified**

369.16 **Better eye: moderate impairment; lesser eye: total impairment**

369.17 **Better eye: moderate impairment; lesser eye: near-total impairment**

369.18 **Better eye: moderate impairment; lesser eye: profound impairment**

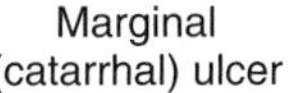
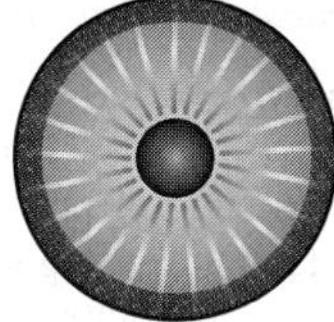
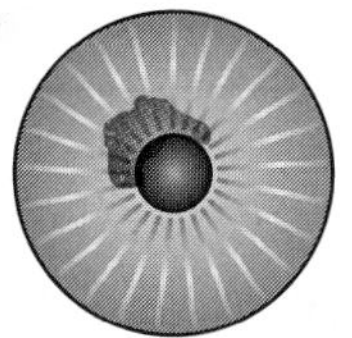
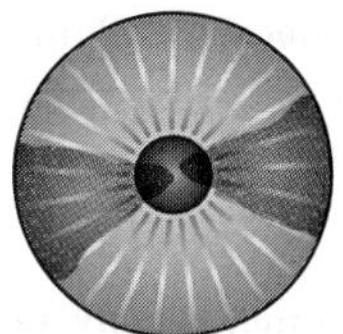
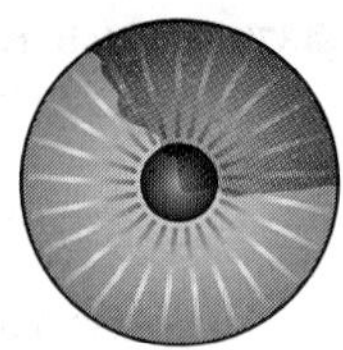
Marginal (catarrhal) ulcer
Ring ulcer
Central corneal ulcer
Rosacea ulcer
Mooren's (rodent) ulcer

Figure 6–7 Corneal ulcers: marginal, ring, central corneal, rosacea, and Mooren's.

● **369.2 Moderate or severe impairment, both eyes**

❑ **369.20 Impairment level not further specified**
Low vision, both eyes NOS

❑ **369.21 Better eye: severe impairment; lesser eye: not further specified**

369.22 Better eye: severe impairment; lesser eye: severe impairment

❑ **369.23 Better eye: moderate impairment; lesser eye: not further specified**

369.24 Better eye: moderate impairment; lesser eye: severe impairment

369.25 Better eye: moderate impairment; lesser eye: moderate impairment

369.3 Unqualified visual loss, both eyes

Excludes *blindness NOS:*
legal [U.S.A. definition] (369.4)
WHO definition (369.00)

369.4 Legal blindness, as defined in U.S.A.
Blindness NOS according to U.S.A. definition

Excludes *legal blindness with specification of impairment level (369.01–369.08, 369.11–369.14, 369.21–369.22)*

● **369.6 Profound impairment, one eye**

❑ **369.60 Impairment level not further specified**
Blindness, one eye

❑ **369.61 One eye: total impairment; other eye: not specified**

369.62 One eye: total impairment; other eye: near-normal vision

369.63 One eye: total impairment; other eye: normal vision

❑ **369.64 One eye: near-total impairment; other eye: not specified**

369.65 One eye: near-total impairment; other eye: near-normal vision

369.66 One eye: near-total impairment; other eye: normal vision

❑ **369.67 One eye: profound impairment; other eye: not specified**

369.68 One eye: profound impairment; other eye: near-normal vision

369.69 One eye: profound impairment; other eye: normal vision

● **369.7 Moderate or severe impairment, one eye**

❑ **369.70 Impairment level not further specified**
Low vision, one eye

❑ **369.71 One eye: severe impairment; other eye: not specified**

369.72 One eye: severe impairment; other eye: near-normal vision

369.73 One eye: severe impairment; other eye: normal vision

❑ **369.74 One eye: moderate impairment; other eye: not specified**

369.75 One eye: moderate impairment; other eye: near-normal vision

369.76 One eye: moderate impairment; other eye: normal vision

369.8 Unqualified visual loss, one eye

❑ **369.9 Unspecified visual loss**

Item 6-9 An infected ulcer is usually called a **serpiginous** or **hypopyon** ulcer which is a pus sac in the anterior chamber of the eye.
Marginal ulcers are usually asymptomatic, not primary, and are often superficial and simple. More severe marginal ulcers spread to form a ring ulcer. **Ring** ulcers can extend around the entire corneal periphery.
Central corneal ulcers develop when there is an abrasion to the epithelium and an infection develops in the eroded area.
The **pyocyaneal** ulcer is the most serious corneal infection, which, if left untreated, can lead to loss of the eye.

● **370.0 Corneal ulcer**

Excludes *that due to vitamin A deficiency (264.3)*

❑ **370.00 Corneal ulcer, unspecified**

370.01 Marginal corneal ulcer

370.02 Ring corneal ulcer

370.03 Central corneal ulcer

370.04 Hypopyon ulcer
Serpiginous ulcer

370.05 Mycotic corneal ulcer

370.06 Perforated corneal ulcer

370.07 Mooren's ulcer

● **370.2 Superficial keratitis without conjunctivitis**

Excludes *dendritic [herpes simplex] keratitis (054.42)*

❑ **370.20 Superficial keratitis, unspecified**

370.21 Punctate keratitis
Thygeson's superficial punctate keratitis

370.22 Macular keratitis
Keratitis:
areolar
nummular
stellate
striate

370.23 Filamentary keratitis

370.24 Photokeratitis
Snow blindness
Welders' keratitis

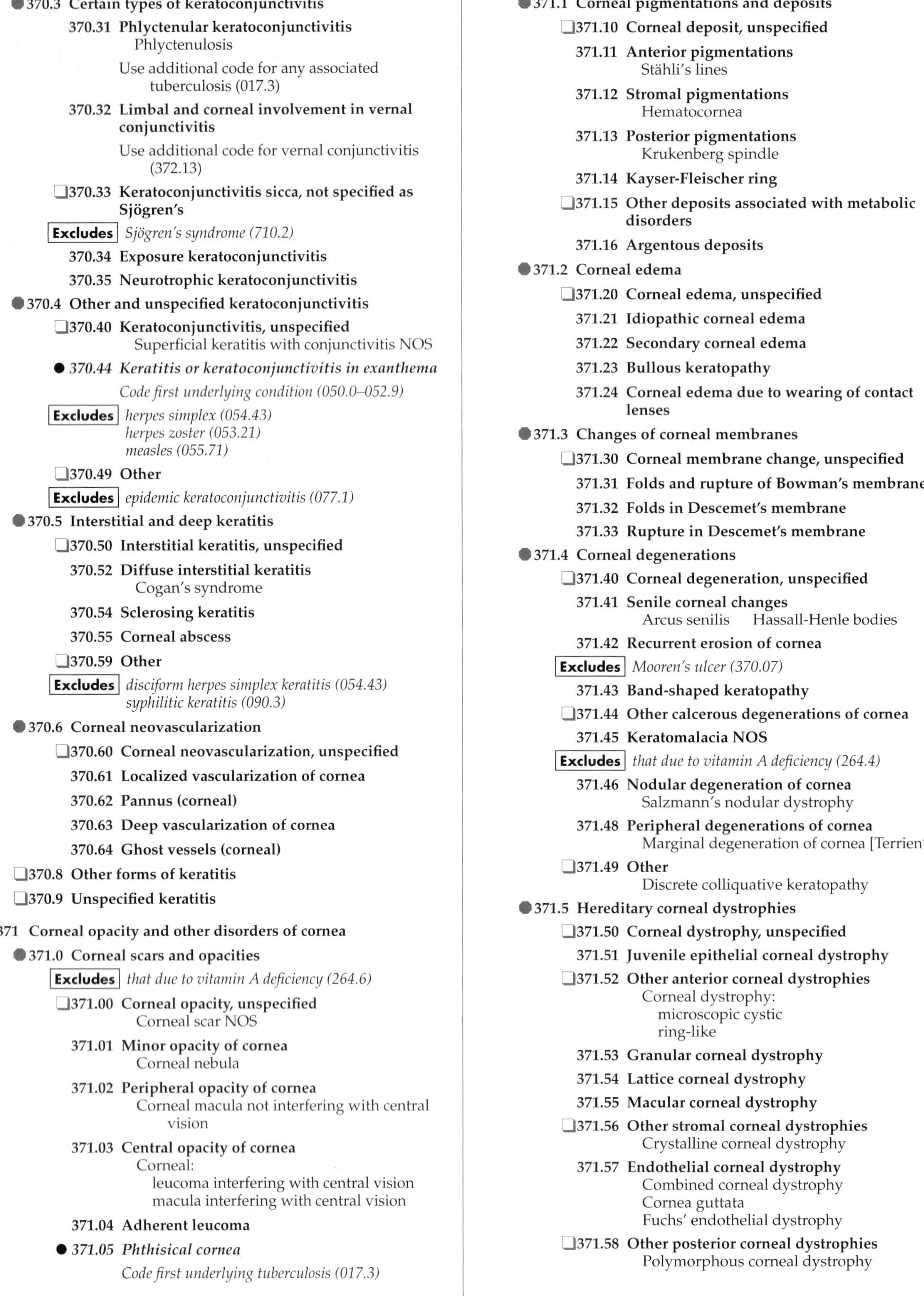

● 370.3 Certain types of keratoconjunctivitis

370.31 **Phlyctenular keratoconjunctivitis**
Phlyctenulosis

Use additional code for any associated tuberculosis (017.3)

370.32 **Limbal and corneal involvement in vernal conjunctivitis**

Use additional code for vernal conjunctivitis (372.13)

❑ 370.33 **Keratoconjunctivitis sicca, not specified as Sjögren's**

Excludes *Sjögren's syndrome (710.2)*

370.34 **Exposure keratoconjunctivitis**

370.35 **Neurotrophic keratoconjunctivitis**

● 370.4 Other and unspecified keratoconjunctivitis

❑ 370.40 **Keratoconjunctivitis, unspecified**
Superficial keratitis with conjunctivitis NOS

● *370.44 Keratitis or keratoconjunctivitis in exanthema*

Code first underlying condition (050.0–052.9)

Excludes *herpes simplex (054.43)*
herpes zoster (053.21)
measles (055.71)

❑ 370.49 **Other**

Excludes *epidemic keratoconjunctivitis (077.1)*

● 370.5 Interstitial and deep keratitis

❑ 370.50 **Interstitial keratitis, unspecified**

370.52 **Diffuse interstitial keratitis**
Cogan's syndrome

370.54 **Sclerosing keratitis**

370.55 **Corneal abscess**

❑ 370.59 **Other**

Excludes *disciform herpes simplex keratitis (054.43)*
syphilitic keratitis (090.3)

● 370.6 Corneal neovascularization

❑ 370.60 **Corneal neovascularization, unspecified**

370.61 **Localized vascularization of cornea**

370.62 **Pannus (corneal)**

370.63 **Deep vascularization of cornea**

370.64 **Ghost vessels (corneal)**

❑ 370.8 Other forms of keratitis

❑ 370.9 Unspecified keratitis

● 371 Corneal opacity and other disorders of cornea

● 371.0 Corneal scars and opacities

Excludes *that due to vitamin A deficiency (264.6)*

❑ 371.00 **Corneal opacity, unspecified**
Corneal scar NOS

371.01 **Minor opacity of cornea**
Corneal nebula

371.02 **Peripheral opacity of cornea**
Corneal macula not interfering with central vision

371.03 **Central opacity of cornea**
Corneal:
leucoma interfering with central vision
macula interfering with central vision

371.04 **Adherent leucoma**

● *371.05 Phthisical cornea*

Code first underlying tuberculosis (017.3)

● 371.1 Corneal pigmentations and deposits

❑ 371.10 **Corneal deposit, unspecified**

371.11 **Anterior pigmentations**
Stähli's lines

371.12 **Stromal pigmentations**
Hematocornea

371.13 **Posterior pigmentations**
Krukenberg spindle

371.14 **Kayser-Fleischer ring**

❑ 371.15 **Other deposits associated with metabolic disorders**

371.16 **Argentous deposits**

● 371.2 Corneal edema

❑ 371.20 **Corneal edema, unspecified**

371.21 **Idiopathic corneal edema**

371.22 **Secondary corneal edema**

371.23 **Bullous keratopathy**

371.24 **Corneal edema due to wearing of contact lenses**

● 371.3 Changes of corneal membranes

❑ 371.30 **Corneal membrane change, unspecified**

371.31 **Folds and rupture of Bowman's membrane**

371.32 **Folds in Descemet's membrane**

371.33 **Rupture in Descemet's membrane**

● 371.4 Corneal degenerations

❑ 371.40 **Corneal degeneration, unspecified**

371.41 **Senile corneal changes**
Arcus senilis   Hassall-Henle bodies

371.42 **Recurrent erosion of cornea**

Excludes *Mooren's ulcer (370.07)*

371.43 **Band-shaped keratopathy**

❑ 371.44 **Other calcerous degenerations of cornea**

371.45 **Keratomalacia NOS**

Excludes *that due to vitamin A deficiency (264.4)*

371.46 **Nodular degeneration of cornea**
Salzmann's nodular dystrophy

371.48 **Peripheral degenerations of cornea**
Marginal degeneration of cornea [Terrien's]

❑ 371.49 **Other**
Discrete colliquative keratopathy

● 371.5 Hereditary corneal dystrophies

❑ 371.50 **Corneal dystrophy, unspecified**

371.51 **Juvenile epithelial corneal dystrophy**

❑ 371.52 **Other anterior corneal dystrophies**
Corneal dystrophy:
microscopic cystic
ring-like

371.53 **Granular corneal dystrophy**

371.54 **Lattice corneal dystrophy**

371.55 **Macular corneal dystrophy**

❑ 371.56 **Other stromal corneal dystrophies**
Crystalline corneal dystrophy

371.57 **Endothelial corneal dystrophy**
Combined corneal dystrophy
Cornea guttata
Fuchs' endothelial dystrophy

❑ 371.58 **Other posterior corneal dystrophies**
Polymorphous corneal dystrophy

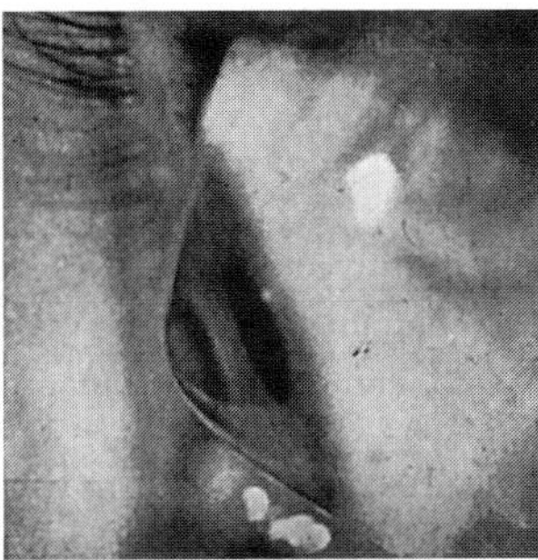

Figure 6–8 Keratoconus. (From Adler FH: Textbook of Ophthalmology, 7th ed. Philadelphia, WB Saunders, 1962, p 223.)

Item 6–10 Keratoconus is corneal degeneration that begins in childhood and gradually forms a cone at the apex of the eye even though the intraocular pressure is normal. The apex of the cornea becomes increasingly thin and can rupture, resulting in scarring.

● 371.6 Keratoconus
- ❑ 371.60 Keratoconus, unspecified
- 371.61 Keratoconus, stable condition
- 371.62 Keratoconus, acute hydrops

● 371.7 Other corneal deformities
- ❑ 371.70 Corneal deformity, unspecified
- 371.71 Corneal ectasia
- 371.72 Descemetocele
- 371.73 Corneal staphyloma

● ❑ 371.8 Other corneal disorders
- 371.81 Corneal anesthesia and hypoesthesia
- 371.82 Corneal disorder due to contact lens

Excludes *corneal edema due to contact lens (371.24)*
- ❑ 371.89 Other

❑ 371.9 Unspecified corneal disorder

● 372 Disorders of conjunctiva

Excludes *keratoconjunctivitis (370.3–370.4)*

● 372.0 Acute conjunctivitis
- ❑ 372.00 Acute conjunctivitis, unspecified
- 372.01 Serous conjunctivitis, except viral

Excludes *viral conjunctivitis NOS (077.9)*
- 372.02 Acute follicular conjunctivitis
  Conjunctival folliculosis NOS

Excludes *conjunctivitis:*
adenoviral (acute follicular) (077.3)
epidemic hemorrhagic (077.4)
inclusion (077.0)
Newcastle (077.8)
epidemic keratoconjunctivitis (077.1)
pharyngoconjunctival fever (077.2)
- ❑ 372.03 Other mucopurulent conjunctivitis
  Catarrhal conjunctivitis

Excludes *blennorrhea neonatorum (gonococcal) (098.40)*
neonatal conjunctivitis (771.6)
ophthalmia neonatorum NOS (771.6)
- 372.04 Pseudomembranous conjunctivitis
  Membranous conjunctivitis

Excludes *diphtheritic conjunctivitis (032.81)*
- 372.05 Acute atopic conjunctivitis

● 372.1 Chronic conjunctivitis
- ❑ 372.10 Chronic conjunctivitis, unspecified
- 372.11 Simple chronic conjunctivitis
- 372.12 Chronic follicular conjunctivitis
- 372.13 Vernal conjunctivitis
- ❑ 372.14 Other chronic allergic conjunctivitis
- ● *372.15 Parasitic conjunctivitis*
  Code first underlying disease, as:
  filariasis (125.0–125.9)
  mucocutaneous leishmaniasis (085.5)

● 372.2 Blepharoconjunctivitis
- ❑ 372.20 Blepharoconjunctivitis, unspecified
- 372.21 Angular blepharoconjunctivitis
- 372.22 Contact blepharoconjunctivitis

● 372.3 Other and unspecified conjunctivitis
- ❑ 372.30 Conjunctivitis, unspecified
- ● *372.31 Rosacea conjunctivitis*
  Code first underlying rosacea dermatitis (695.3)
- ● *372.33 Conjunctivitis in mucocutaneous disease*
  Code first underlying disease, as:
  erythema multiforme (695.1)
  Reiter's disease (099.3)

Excludes *ocular pemphigoid (694.61)*
- ❑ 372.39 Other

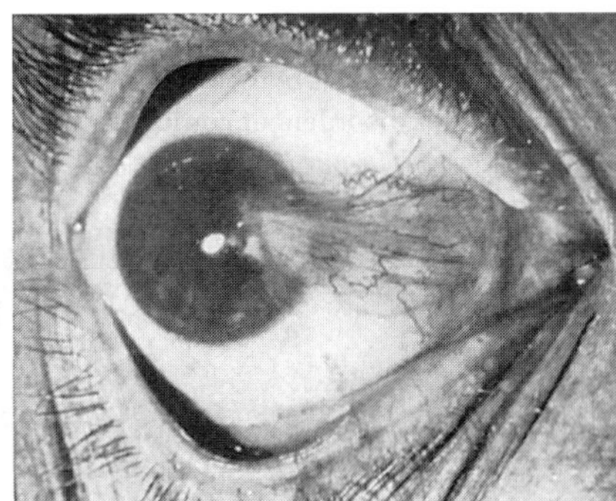

Figure 6–9 Pterygium. (From Adler FH: Textbook of Ophthalmology, 7th ed. Philadelphia, WB Saunders, 1962, p 194.)

Item 6–11 Pterygium is Greek for batlike. The condition is characterized by a membrane that extends from the limbus to the center of the cornea and resembles a wing.

● 372.4 Pterygium

Excludes *pseudopterygium (372.52)*
- ❑ 372.40 Pterygium, unspecified
- 372.41 Peripheral pterygium, stationary
- 372.42 Peripheral pterygium, progressive
- 372.43 Central pterygium
- 372.44 Double pterygium
- 372.45 Recurrent pterygium

● 372.5 Conjunctival degenerations and deposits
- ❑ 372.50 Conjunctival degeneration, unspecified

ICD-9-CM 300-399 Vol. 1

372.51 **Pinguecula**

372.52 **Pseudopterygium**

372.53 **Conjunctival xerosis**

Excludes *conjunctival xerosis due to vitamin A deficiency (264.0, 264.1, 264.7)*

372.54 **Conjunctival concretions**

372.55 **Conjunctival pigmentations**
Conjunctival argyrosis

372.56 **Conjunctival deposits**

● 372.6 **Conjunctival scars**

372.61 **Granuloma of conjunctiva**

372.62 **Localized adhesions and strands of conjunctiva**

372.63 **Symblepharon**
Extensive adhesions of conjunctiva

372.64 **Scarring of conjunctiva**
Contraction of eye socket (after enucleation)

● 372.7 **Conjunctival vascular disorders and cysts**

372.71 **Hyperemia of conjunctiva**

372.72 **Conjunctival hemorrhage**
Hyposphagma
Subconjunctival hemorrhage

372.73 **Conjunctival edema**
Chemosis of conjunctiva
Subconjunctival edema

372.74 **Vascular abnormalities of conjunctiva**
Aneurysm(ata) of conjunctiva

372.75 **Conjunctival cysts**

● ❑ 372.8 **Other disorders of conjunctiva**

372.81 **Conjunctivochalasis**

❑ 372.89 **Other disorders of conjunctivitis**

❑ 372.9 **Unspecified disorder of conjunctiva**

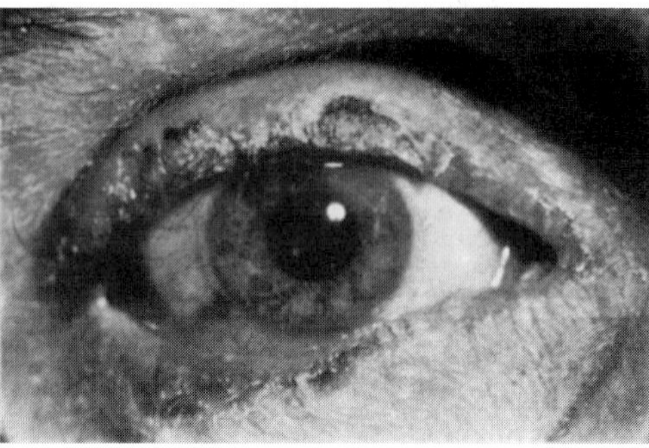

Figure 6–10 Ulcerating blepharitis caused by a staphylococcal infection. (From Pau H: Differential Diagnosis of Eye Diseases. Philadelphia, WB Saunders, 1978, p 106. Copyright Georg Thieme Verlag [Stuttgart, Germany].)

Item 6–12 Blepharitis is a common condition in which the lid is swollen and yellow scaling and conjunctivitis develop. Usually the hair on the scalp and brow is involved.

Item 6–13 Hordeolum is the inflammation of the sebaceous gland of the eyelid.

● 373 **Inflammation of eyelids**

● 373.0 **Blepharitis**

Excludes *blepharoconjunctivitis (372.20–372.22)*

❑ 373.00 **Blepharitis, unspecified**

373.01 **Ulcerative blepharitis**

372.02 **Squamous blepharitis**

● 373.1 **Hordeolum and other deep inflammation of eyelid**

373.11 **Hordeolum externum**
Hordeolum NOS
Stye

373.12 **Hordeolum internum**
Infection of meibomian gland

373.13 **Abscess of eyelid**
Furuncle of eyelid

373.2 **Chalazion**
Meibomian (gland) cyst

Excludes *infected meibomian gland (373.12)*

● 373.3 **Noninfectious dermatoses of eyelid**

373.31 **Eczematous dermatitis of eyelid**

373.32 **Contact and allergic dermatitis of eyelid**

373.33 **Xeroderma of eyelid**

373.34 **Discoid lupus erythematosus of eyelid**

● *373.4* ***Infective dermatitis of eyelid of types resulting in deformity***

Code first underlying disease, as:
leprosy (030.0–030.9)
lupus vulgaris (tuberculous) (017.0)
yaws (102.0–102.9)

● ❑ *373.5* ***Other infective dermatitis of eyelid***

Code first underlying disease, as:
actinomycosis (039.3)
impetigo (684)
mycotic dermatitis (110.0–111.9)
vaccinia (051.0)
postvaccination (999.0)

Excludes *herpes:*
simplex (054.41)
zoster (053.20)

● *373.6* ***Parasitic infestation of eyelid***

Code first underlying disease, as:
leishmaniasis (085.0–085.9)
loiasis (125.2)
onchocerciasis (125.3)
pediculosis (132.0)

❑ 373.8 **Other inflammations of eyelids**

❑ 373.9 **Unspecified inflammation of eyelid**

A

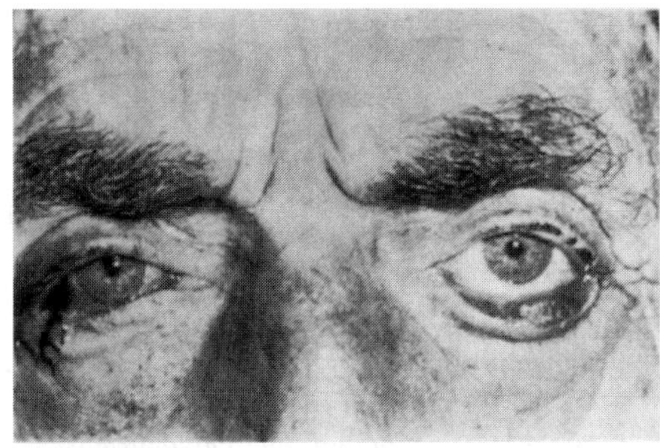

B

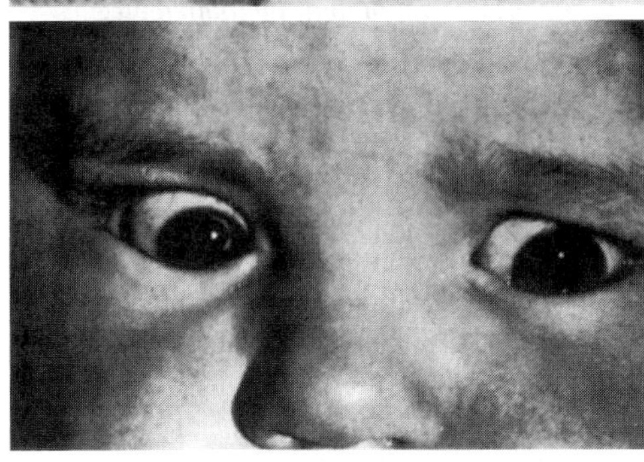

Figure 6–11 **A.** A 72-year-old male with senile ectropion. **B.** Entropion in a 6-month-old male infant. (From Pau H: Differential Diagnosis of Eye Diseases. Philadelphia, WB Saunders, 1978, p 90. Copyright Georg Thieme Verlag [Stuttgart, Germany].)

● **374 Other disorders of eyelids**

● **374.0 Entropion and trichiasis of eyelid**

❑ **374.00 Entropion, unspecified**

374.01 Senile entropion

374.02 Mechanical entropion

374.03 Spastic entropion

374.04 Cicatricial entropion

374.05 Trichiasis without entropion

● **374.1 Ectropion**

❑ **374.10 Ectropion, unspecified**

374.11 Senile ectropion

374.12 Mechanical ectropion

374.13 Spastic ectropion

374.14 Cicatricial ectropion

● **374.2 Lagophthalmos**

❑ **374.20 Lagophthalmos, unspecified**

374.21 Paralytic lagophthalmos

374.22 Mechanical lagophthalmos

374.23 Cicatricial lagophthalmos

● **374.3 Ptosis of eyelid**

Falling forward, drooping, sagging of a body part

❑ **374.30 Ptosis of eyelid, unspecified**

374.31 Paralytic ptosis

374.32 Myogenic ptosis

374.33 Mechanical ptosis

374.34 Blepharochalasis
Pseudoptosis

● **374.4 Other disorders affecting eyelid function**

Excludes *blepharoclonus (333.81)*
blepharospasm (333.81)
facial nerve palsy (351.0)
third nerve palsy or paralysis (378.51–378.52)
tic (psychogenic) (307.20–307.23)
organic (333.3)

374.41 Lid retraction or lag

374.43 Abnormal innervation syndrome
Jaw-blinking
Paradoxical facial movements

374.44 Sensory disorders

❑ **374.45 Other sensorimotor disorders**
Deficient blink reflex

374.46 Blepharophimosis
Ankyloblepharon

● **374.5 Degenerative disorders of eyelid and periocular area**

❑ **374.50 Degenerative disorder of eyelid, unspecified**

● ***374.51 Xanthelasma***
Xanthoma (planum) (tuberosum) of eyelid
Code first underlying condition (272.0–272.9)

374.52 Hyperpigmentation of eyelid
Chloasma
Dyspigmentation

374.53 Hypopigmentation of eyelid
Vitiligo of eyelid

374.54 Hypertrichosis of eyelid

374.55 Hypotrichosis of eyelid
Madarosis of eyelid

❑ **374.56 Other degenerative disorders of skin affecting eyelid**

● **374.8 Other disorders of eyelid**

374.81 Hemorrhage of eyelid

Excludes *black eye (921.0)*

374.82 Edema of eyelid
Hyperemia of eyelid

374.83 Elephantiasis of eyelid

374.84 Cysts of eyelids
Sebaceous cyst of eyelid

374.85 Vascular anomalies of eyelid

374.86 Retained foreign body of eyelid

374.87 Dermatochalasis

❑ **374.89 Other disorders of eyelid**

❑ **374.9 Unspecified disorder of eyelid**

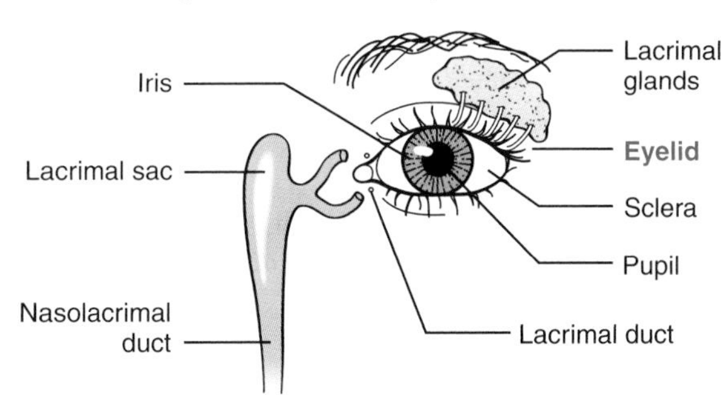
Iris
Lacrimal glands
Eyelid
Lacrimal sac
Sclera
Pupil
Nasolacrimal duct
Lacrimal duct

Figure 6–12 Lacrimal apparatus. (From Buck CJ: Step-by-Step Medical Coding, 3rd ed. Philadelphia, WB Saunders, 2000, p 205.)

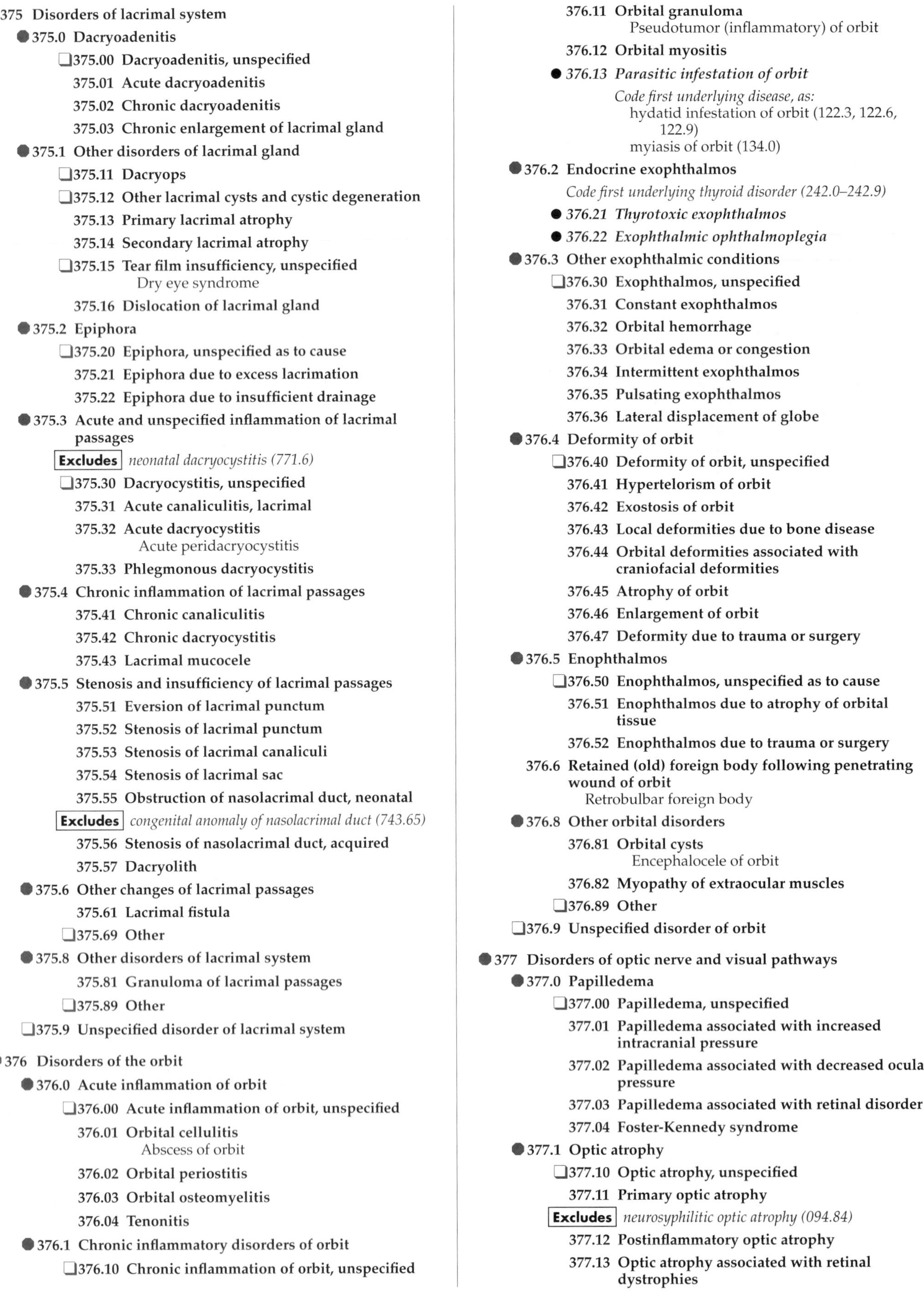

375 Disorders of lacrimal system

375.0 Dacryoadenitis

375.00 Dacryoadenitis, unspecified

375.01 Acute dacryoadenitis

375.02 Chronic dacryoadenitis

375.03 Chronic enlargement of lacrimal gland

375.1 Other disorders of lacrimal gland

375.11 Dacryops

375.12 Other lacrimal cysts and cystic degeneration

375.13 Primary lacrimal atrophy

375.14 Secondary lacrimal atrophy

375.15 Tear film insufficiency, unspecified
Dry eye syndrome

375.16 Dislocation of lacrimal gland

375.2 Epiphora

375.20 Epiphora, unspecified as to cause

375.21 Epiphora due to excess lacrimation

375.22 Epiphora due to insufficient drainage

375.3 Acute and unspecified inflammation of lacrimal passages

Excludes *neonatal dacryocystitis (771.6)*

375.30 Dacryocystitis, unspecified

375.31 Acute canaliculitis, lacrimal

375.32 Acute dacryocystitis
Acute peridacryocystitis

375.33 Phlegmonous dacryocystitis

375.4 Chronic inflammation of lacrimal passages

375.41 Chronic canaliculitis

375.42 Chronic dacryocystitis

375.43 Lacrimal mucocele

375.5 Stenosis and insufficiency of lacrimal passages

375.51 Eversion of lacrimal punctum

375.52 Stenosis of lacrimal punctum

375.53 Stenosis of lacrimal canaliculi

375.54 Stenosis of lacrimal sac

375.55 Obstruction of nasolacrimal duct, neonatal

Excludes *congenital anomaly of nasolacrimal duct (743.65)*

375.56 Stenosis of nasolacrimal duct, acquired

375.57 Dacryolith

375.6 Other changes of lacrimal passages

375.61 Lacrimal fistula

375.69 Other

375.8 Other disorders of lacrimal system

375.81 Granuloma of lacrimal passages

375.89 Other

375.9 Unspecified disorder of lacrimal system

376 Disorders of the orbit

376.0 Acute inflammation of orbit

376.00 Acute inflammation of orbit, unspecified

376.01 Orbital cellulitis
Abscess of orbit

376.02 Orbital periostitis

376.03 Orbital osteomyelitis

376.04 Tenonitis

376.1 Chronic inflammatory disorders of orbit

376.10 Chronic inflammation of orbit, unspecified

376.11 Orbital granuloma
Pseudotumor (inflammatory) of orbit

376.12 Orbital myositis

376.13 Parasitic infestation of orbit

Code first underlying disease, as:
hydatid infestation of orbit (122.3, 122.6, 122.9)
myiasis of orbit (134.0)

376.2 Endocrine exophthalmos

Code first underlying thyroid disorder (242.0–242.9)

376.21 Thyrotoxic exophthalmos

376.22 Exophthalmic ophthalmoplegia

376.3 Other exophthalmic conditions

376.30 Exophthalmos, unspecified

376.31 Constant exophthalmos

376.32 Orbital hemorrhage

376.33 Orbital edema or congestion

376.34 Intermittent exophthalmos

376.35 Pulsating exophthalmos

376.36 Lateral displacement of globe

376.4 Deformity of orbit

376.40 Deformity of orbit, unspecified

376.41 Hypertelorism of orbit

376.42 Exostosis of orbit

376.43 Local deformities due to bone disease

376.44 Orbital deformities associated with craniofacial deformities

376.45 Atrophy of orbit

376.46 Enlargement of orbit

376.47 Deformity due to trauma or surgery

376.5 Enophthalmos

376.50 Enophthalmos, unspecified as to cause

376.51 Enophthalmos due to atrophy of orbital tissue

376.52 Enophthalmos due to trauma or surgery

376.6 Retained (old) foreign body following penetrating wound of orbit
Retrobulbar foreign body

376.8 Other orbital disorders

376.81 Orbital cysts
Encephalocele of orbit

376.82 Myopathy of extraocular muscles

376.89 Other

376.9 Unspecified disorder of orbit

377 Disorders of optic nerve and visual pathways

377.0 Papilledema

377.00 Papilledema, unspecified

377.01 Papilledema associated with increased intracranial pressure

377.02 Papilledema associated with decreased ocular pressure

377.03 Papilledema associated with retinal disorder

377.04 Foster-Kennedy syndrome

377.1 Optic atrophy

377.10 Optic atrophy, unspecified

377.11 Primary optic atrophy

Excludes *neurosyphilitic optic atrophy (094.84)*

377.12 Postinflammatory optic atrophy

377.13 Optic atrophy associated with retinal dystrophies

377.14 **Glaucomatous atrophy [cupping] of optic disc**

377.15 **Partial optic atrophy**
Temporal pallor of optic disc

377.16 **Hereditary optic atrophy**
Optic atrophy:
dominant hereditary
Leber's

● 377.2 **Other disorders of optic disc**

377.21 **Drusen of optic disc**

377.22 **Crater-like holes of optic disc**

377.23 **Coloboma of optic disc**

377.24 **Pseudopapilledema**

● 377.3 **Optic neuritis**

Excludes *meningococcal optic neuritis (036.81)*

❑ 377.30 **Optic neuritis, unspecified**

377.31 **Optic papillitis**

377.32 **Retrobulbar neuritis (acute)**

Excludes *syphilitic retrobulbar neuritis (094.85)*

377.33 **Nutritional optic neuropathy**

377.34 **Toxic optic neuropathy**
Toxic amblyopia

❑ 377.39 **Other**

Excludes *ischemic optic neuropathy (377.41)*

● 377.4 **Other disorders of optic nerve**

377.41 **Ischemic optic neuropathy**

377.42 **Hemorrhage in optic nerve sheaths**

377.43 **Optic nerve hypoplasia** ◀

❑ 377.49 **Other**
Compression of optic nerve

● 377.5 **Disorders of optic chiasm**

377.51 **Associated with pituitary neoplasms and disorders**

❑ 377.52 **Associated with other neoplasms**

377.53 **Associated with vascular disorders**

377.54 **Associated with inflammatory disorders**

● 377.6 **Disorders of other visual pathways**

377.61 **Associated with neoplasms**

377.62 **Associated with vascular disorders**

377.63 **Associated with inflammatory disorders**

● 377.7 **Disorders of visual cortex**

Excludes *visual:*
agnosia (368.16)
hallucinations (368.16)
halos (368.15)

377.71 **Associated with neoplasms**

377.72 **Associated with vascular disorders**

377.73 **Associated with inflammatory disorders**

377.75 **Cortical blindness**

❑ 377.9 **Unspecified disorder of optic nerve and visual pathways**

● 378 **Strabismus and other disorders of binocular eye movements**

Excludes *nystagmus and other irregular eye movements (379.50–379.59)*

● 378.0 **Esotropia**
Convergent concomitant strabismus

Excludes *intermittent esotropia (378.20–378.22)*

❑ 378.00 **Esotropia, unspecified**

378.01 **Monocular esotropia**

378.02 **Monocular esotropia with A pattern**

378.03 **Monocular esotropia with V pattern**

❑ 378.04 **Monocular esotropia with other noncomitancies**
Monocular esotropia with X or Y pattern

378.05 **Alternating esotropia**

378.06 **Alternating esotropia with A pattern**

378.07 **Alternating esotropia with V pattern**

❑ 378.08 **Alternating esotropia with other noncomitancies**
Alternating esotropia with X or Y pattern

● 378.1 **Exotropia**
Divergent concomitant strabismus

Excludes *intermittent exotropia (378.20, 378.23–378.24)*

❑ 378.10 **Exotropia, unspecified**

378.11 **Monocular exotropia**

378.12 **Monocular exotropia with A pattern**

378.13 **Monocular exotropia with V pattern**

❑ 378.14 **Monocular exotropia with other noncomitancies**
Monocular exotropia with X or Y pattern

378.15 **Alternating exotropia**

378.16 **Alternating exotropia with A pattern**

378.17 **Alternating exotropia with V pattern**

❑ 378.18 **Alternating exotropia with other noncomitancies**
Alternating exotropia with X or Y pattern

● 378.2 **Intermittent heterotropia**

Excludes *vertical heterotropia (intermittent) (378.31)*

❑ 378.20 **Intermittent heterotropia, unspecified**
Intermittent:
esotropia NOS
exotropia NOS

378.21 **Intermittent esotropia, monocular**

378.22 **Intermittent esotropia, alternating**

378.23 **Intermittent exotropia, monocular**

378.24 **Intermittent exotropia, alternating**

● 378.3 **Other and unspecified heterotropia**

❑ 378.30 **Heterotropia, unspecified**

378.31 **Hypertropia**
Vertical heterotropia (constant) (intermittent)

378.32 **Hypotropia**

378.33 **Cyclotropia**

378.34 **Monofixation syndrome**
Microtropia

378.35 **Accommodative component in esotropia**

● 378.4 **Heterophoria**

❑ 378.40 **Heterophoria, unspecified**

378.41 **Esophoria**

378.42 **Exophoria**

378.43 **Vertical heterophoria**

378.44 **Cyclophoria**

378.45 **Alternating hyperphoria**

● 378.5 **Paralytic strabismus**

❑ 378.50 **Paralytic strabismus, unspecified**

378.51 **Third or oculomotor nerve palsy, partial**

378.52 **Third or oculomotor nerve palsy, total**

378.53 **Fourth or trochlear nerve palsy**

378.54 **Sixth or abducens nerve palsy**

378.55 **External ophthalmoplegia**

378.56 **Total ophthalmoplegia**

● 378.6 **Mechanical strabismus**

❑ 378.60 **Mechanical strabismus, unspecified**

378.61 **Brown's (tendon) sheath syndrome**

❑ 378.62 **Mechanical strabismus from other musculofascial disorders**

❑ 378.63 **Limited duction associated with other conditions**

● 378.7 **Other specified strabismus**

378.71 **Duane's syndrome**

378.72 **Progressive external ophthalmoplegia**

❑ 378.73 **Strabismus in other neuromuscular disorders**

● 378.8 **Other disorders of binocular eye movements**

Excludes *nystagmus (379.50–379.56)*

378.81 **Palsy of conjugate gaze**

378.82 **Spasm of conjugate gaze**

378.83 **Convergence insufficiency or palsy**

378.84 **Convergence excess or spasm**

378.85 **Anomalies of divergence**

378.86 **Internuclear ophthalmoplegia**

❑ 378.87 **Other dissociated deviation of eye movements**
Skew deviation

❑ 378.9 **Unspecified disorder of eye movements**
Ophthalmoplegia NOS
Strabismus NOS

● 379 **Other disorders of eye**

● 379.0 **Scleritis and episcleritis**

Excludes *syphilitic episcleritis (095.0)*

❑ 379.00 **Scleritis, unspecified**
Episcleritis NOS

379.01 **Episcleritis periodica fugax**

379.02 **Nodular episcleritis**

379.03 **Anterior scleritis**

379.04 **Scleromalacia perforans**

379.05 **Scleritis with corneal involvement**
Scleroperikeratitis

379.06 **Brawny scleritis**

379.07 **Posterior scleritis**
Sclerotenonitis

❑ 379.09 **Other**
Scleral abscess

● 379.1 **Other disorders of sclera**

Excludes *blue sclera (743.47)*

379.11 **Scleral ectasia**
Scleral staphyloma NOS

379.12 **Staphyloma posticum**

379.13 **Equatorial staphyloma**

379.14 **Anterior staphyloma, localized**

379.15 **Ring staphyloma**

❑ 379.16 **Other degenerative disorders of sclera**

❑ 379.19 **Other**

● 379.2 **Disorders of vitreous body**

379.21 **Vitreous degeneration**
Vitreous:
cavitation
detachment
liquefaction

379.22 **Crystalline deposits in vitreous**
Asteroid hyalitis
Synchysis scintillans

379.23 **Vitreous hemorrhage**

❑ 379.24 **Other vitreous opacities**
Vitreous floaters

Small clumps of cells that float in the eye vitreous, appearing as black specks or dots in the field of vision. Floaters are more common in the aging eye. Although usually harmless, a sudden increase in floaters may be a sign of retinal detachment.

379.25 **Vitreous membranes and strands**

379.26 **Vitreous prolapse**

❑ 379.29 **Other disorders of vitreous**

Excludes *vitreous abscess (360.04)*

● 379.3 **Aphakia and other disorders of lens**

Excludes *after-cataract (366.50–366.53)*

379.31 **Aphakia**

Excludes *cataract extraction status (V45.61)*

379.32 **Subluxation of lens**

379.33 **Anterior dislocation of lens**

379.34 **Posterior dislocation of lens**

❑ 379.39 **Other disorders of lens**

● 379.4 **Anomalies of pupillary function**

❑ 379.40 **Abnormal pupillary function, unspecified**

379.41 **Anisocoria**

379.42 **Miosis (persistent), not due to miotics**

379.43 **Mydriasis (persistent), not due to mydriatics**

379.45 **Argyll Robertson pupil, atypical**
Argyll Robertson phenomenon or pupil, nonsyphilitic

Excludes *Argyll Robertson pupil (syphilitic) (094.89)*

379.46 **Tonic pupillary reaction**
Adie's pupil or syndrome

❑ 379.49 **Other**
Hippus
Pupillary paralysis

● 379.5 **Nystagmus and other irregular eye movements**

❑ 379.50 **Nystagmus, unspecified**

379.51 **Congenital nystagmus**

379.52 **Latent nystagmus**

379.53 **Visual deprivation nystagmus**

379.54 **Nystagmus associated with disorders of the vestibular system**

379.55 **Dissociated nystagmus**

❑ 379.56 **Other forms of nystagmus**

379.57 **Deficiencies of saccadic eye movements**
Abnormal optokinetic response

379.58 **Deficiencies of smooth pursuit movements**

❑ 379.59 **Other irregularities of eye movements**
Opsoclonus

● 379.6 **Inflammation (infection) of postprocedural bleb** ◀
Postprocedural blebitis ◀

379.60 **Inflammation (infection) of postprocedural bleb, unspecified** ◀

379.61 **Inflammation (infection) of postprocedural bleb, stage 1** ◀

379.62 Inflammation (infection) of postprocedural bleb, stage 2 ◀

379.63 Inflammation (infection) of postprocedural bleb, stage 3 ◀

Bleb associated endophthalmitis ◀

❑ **379.8 Other specified disorders of eye and adnexa**

● **379.9 Unspecified disorder of eye and adnexa**

❑ **379.90 Disorder of eye, unspecified**

379.91 Pain in or around eye

379.92 Swelling or mass of eye

379.93 Redness or discharge of eye

❑ **379.99 Other ill-defined disorders of eye**

Excludes *blurred vision NOS (368.8)*

DISEASES OF THE EAR AND MASTOID PROCESS (380–389)

● **380 Disorders of external ear**

● **380.0 Perichondritis and chondritis of pinna**

Chondritis of auricle
Perichondritis of auricle

❑ **380.00 Perichondritis of pinna, unspecified**

380.01 Acute perichondritis of pinna

380.02 Chronic perichondritis of pinna

380.03 Chondritis of pinna

● **380.1 Infective otitis externa**

❑ **380.10 Infective otitis externa, unspecified**

Otitis externa (acute):
- NOS
- circumscribed
- diffuse
- hemorrhagica
- infective NOS

380.11 Acute infection of pinna

Excludes *furuncular otitis externa (680.0)*

380.12 Acute swimmers' ear

Beach ear
Tank ear

● ❑ ***380.13 Other acute infections of external ear***

Code first underlying disease, as:
- erysipelas (035)
- impetigo (684)
- seborrheic dermatitis (690.10–690.18)

Excludes *herpes simplex (054.73)*
herpes zoster (053.71)

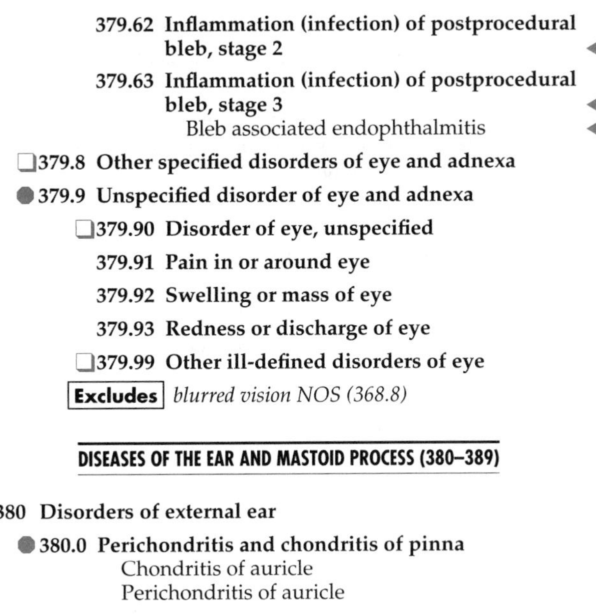
External ear
Auricle or pinna
External acoustic meatus
Middle ear
Incus
Malleus
Stapes
Tympanic membrane
Oval window
Eustachian tube
Internal ear
Vestibular nerve
Facial nerve
Cochlear nerve
Cochlea

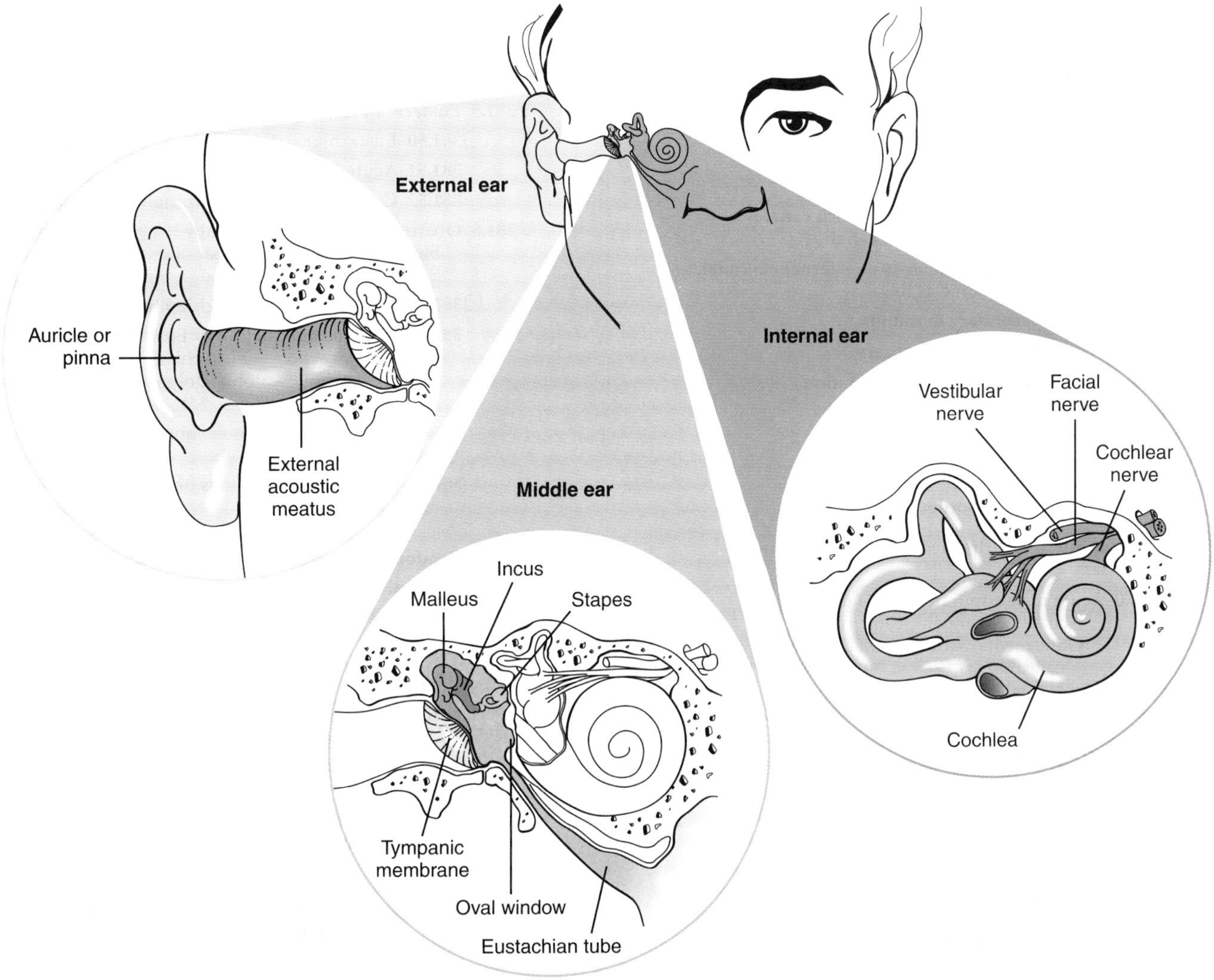

Figure 6–13 Auditory system. (From Buck CJ: Step-by-Step Medical Coding, 2005 ed. Philadelphia, WB Saunders, 2005.)

380.14 Malignant otitis externa

● *380.15 Chronic mycotic otitis externa*

Code first underlying disease, as:
aspergillosis (117.3)
otomycosis NOS (111.9)

Excludes *candidal otitis externa (112.82)*

❑380.16 **Other chronic infective otitis externa**
Chronic infective otitis externa NOS

● **380.2 Other otitis externa**

380.21 Cholesteatoma of external ear
Keratosis obturans of external ear (canal)

Excludes *cholesteatoma NOS (385.30–385.35)*
postmastoidectomy (383.32)

❑380.22 **Other acute otitis externa**
Acute otitis externa:
actinic
chemical
contact
eczematoid
reactive

❑380.23 **Other chronic otitis externa**
Chronic otitis externa NOS

● **380.3 Noninfectious disorders of pinna**

❑380.30 **Disorder of pinna, unspecified**

380.31 Hematoma of auricle or pinna

380.32 Acquired deformities of auricle or pinna

Excludes *cauliflower ear (738.7)*

❑380.39 **Other**

Excludes *gouty tophi of ear (274.81)*

380.4 Impacted cerumen
Wax in ear

● **380.5 Acquired stenosis of external ear canal**
Collapse of external ear canal

❑380.50 **Acquired stenosis of external ear canal, unspecified as to cause**

380.51 Secondary to trauma

380.52 Secondary to surgery

380.53 Secondary to inflammation

● **380.8 Other disorders of external ear**

380.81 Exostosis of external ear canal

❑380.89 **Other**

❑380.9 **Unspecified disorder of external ear**

● **381 Nonsuppurative otitis media and Eustachian tube disorders**

● **381.0 Acute nonsuppurative otitis media**
Acute tubotympanic catarrh
Otitis media, acute or subacute:
catarrhal
exudative
transudative
with effusion

Excludes *otitic barotrauma (993.0)*

❑381.00 **Acute nonsuppurative otitis media, unspecified**

381.01 Acute serous otitis media
Acute or subacute secretory otitis media

381.02 Acute mucoid otitis media
Acute or subacute seromucinous otitis media
Blue drum syndrome

381.03 Acute sanguinous otitis media

381.04 Acute allergic serous otitis media

381.05 Acute allergic mucoid otitis media

381.06 Acute allergic sanguinous otitis media

● **381.1 Chronic serous otitis media**
Chronic tubotympanic catarrh

381.10 Chronic serous otitis media, simple or unspecified

❑381.19 **Other**
Serosanguinous chronic otitis media

● **381.2 Chronic mucoid otitis media**
Glue ear

Excludes *adhesive middle ear disease (385.10–385.19)*

381.20 Chronic mucoid otitis media, simple or unspecified

❑381.29 **Other**
Mucosanguinous chronic otitis media

❑381.3 **Other and unspecified chronic nonsuppurative otitis media**
Otitis media, chronic:
allergic
exudative
secretory
Otitis media, chronic:
seromucinous
transudative
with effusion

❑381.4 **Nonsuppurative otitis media, not specified as acute or chronic**
Otitis media:
allergic
catarrhal
exudative
mucoid
secretory
Otitis media:
seromucinous
serous
transudative
with effusion

● **381.5 Eustachian salpingitis**

❑381.50 **Eustachian salpingitis, unspecified**

381.51 Acute Eustachian salpingitis

381.52 Chronic Eustachian salpingitis

● **381.6 Obstruction of Eustachian tube**
Stenosis of Eustachian tube
Stricture of Eustachian tube

❑381.60 **Obstruction of Eustachian tube, unspecified**

381.61 Osseous obstruction of Eustachian tube
Obstruction of Eustachian tube from cholesteatoma, polyp, or other osseous lesion

381.62 Intrinsic cartilaginous obstruction of Eustachian tube

381.63 Extrinsic cartilaginous obstruction of Eustachian tube
Compression of Eustachian tube

381.7 Patulous Eustachian tube

● **381.8 Other disorders of Eustachian tube**

381.81 Dysfunction of Eustachian tube

❑381.89 **Other**

❑381.9 **Unspecified Eustachian tube disorder**

● **382 Suppurative and unspecified otitis media**

● **382.0 Acute suppurative otitis media**

Suppurative: Discharging pus

Otitis media, acute:
necrotizing NOS
purulent

Purulent: Pus-filled

382.00 Acute suppurative otitis media without spontaneous rupture of ear drum

382.01 Acute suppurative otitis media with spontaneous rupture of ear drum

● ❑382.02 ***Acute suppurative otitis media in diseases classified elsewhere***
Code first underlying disease, as:
influenza (487.8)
scarlet fever (034.1)

Excludes *postmeasles otitis (055.2)*

382.1 Chronic tubotympanic suppurative otitis media
Benign chronic suppurative otitis media (with anterior perforation of ear drum)
Chronic tubotympanic disease (with anterior perforation of ear drum)

382.2 Chronic atticoantral suppurative otitis media
Chronic atticoantral disease (with posterior or superior marginal perforation of ear drum)
Persistent mucosal disease (with posterior or superior marginal perforation of ear drum)

❑**382.3 Unspecified chronic suppurative otitis media**
Chronic purulent otitis media

Excludes *tuberculous otitis media (017.4)*

❑**382.4 Unspecified suppurative otitis media**
Purulent otitis media NOS

❑**382.9 Unspecified otitis media**
Otitis media:
NOS
acute NOS
chronic NOS

● **383 Mastoiditis and related conditions**

● **383.0 Acute mastoiditis**
Abscess of mastoid
Empyema of mastoid

383.00 Acute mastoiditis without complications

383.01 Subperiosteal abscess of mastoid

❑**383.02 Acute mastoiditis with other complications**
Gradenigo's syndrome

383.1 Chronic mastoiditis
Caries of mastoid
Fistula of mastoid

Excludes *tuberculous mastoiditis (015.6)*

● **383.2 Petrositis**
Coalescing osteitis of petrous bone
Inflammation of petrous bone
Osteomyelitis of petrous bone

❑**383.20 Petrositis, unspecified**

383.21 Acute petrositis

383.22 Chronic petrositis

● **383.3 Complications following mastoidectomy**

❑**383.30 Postmastoidectomy complication, unspecified**

383.31 Mucosal cyst of postmastoidectomy cavity

383.32 Recurrent cholesteatoma of postmastoidectomy cavity

383.33 Granulations of postmastoidectomy cavity
Chronic inflammation of postmastoidectomy cavity

● **383.8 Other disorders of mastoid**

383.81 Postauricular fistula

❑**383.89 Other**

❑**383.9 Unspecified mastoiditis**

● **384 Other disorders of tympanic membrane**

● **384.0 Acute myringitis without mention of otitis media**

❑**384.00 Acute myringitis, unspecified**
Acute tympanitis NOS

384.01 Bullous myringitis
Myringitis bullosa hemorrhagica

❑**384.09 Other**

384.1 Chronic myringitis without mention of otitis media
Chronic tympanitis

● **384.2 Perforation of tympanic membrane**
Perforation of ear drum:
NOS
persistent posttraumatic
postinflammatory

Excludes *otitis media with perforation of tympanic membrane (382.00–382.9)*
traumatic perforation [current injury] (872.61)

❑**384.20 Perforation of tympanic membrane, unspecified**

384.21 Central perforation of tympanic membrane

384.22 Attic perforation of tympanic membrane
Pars flaccida

❑**384.23 Other marginal perforation of tympanic membrane**

384.24 Multiple perforations of tympanic membrane

384.25 Total perforation of tympanic membrane

● **384.8 Other specified disorders of tympanic membrane**

384.81 Atrophic flaccid tympanic membrane
Healed perforation of ear drum

384.82 Atrophic nonflaccid tympanic membrane

❑**384.9 Unspecified disorder of tympanic membrane**

● **385 Other disorders of middle ear and mastoid**

Excludes *mastoiditis (383.0–383.9)*

● **385.0 Tympanosclerosis**

❑**385.00 Tympanosclerosis, unspecified as to involvement**

385.01 Tympanosclerosis involving tympanic membrane only

385.02 Tympanosclerosis involving tympanic membrane and ear ossicles

385.03 Tympanosclerosis involving tympanic membrane, ear ossicles, and middle ear

❑**385.09 Tympanosclerosis involving other combination of structures**

● **385.1 Adhesive middle ear disease**
Adhesive otitis
Otitis media:
chronic adhesive
Otitis media:
fibrotic

Excludes *glue ear (381.20–381.29)*

❑**385.10 Adhesive middle ear disease, unspecified as to involvement**

385.11 Adhesions of drum head to incus

385.12 Adhesions of drum head to stapes

385.13 Adhesions of drum head to promontorium

❑**385.19 Other adhesions and combinations**

● **385.2 Other acquired abnormality of ear ossicles**

385.21 Impaired mobility of malleus
Ankylosis of malleus

❑**385.22 Impaired mobility of other ear ossicles**
Ankylosis of ear ossicles, except malleus

385.23 Discontinuity or dislocation of ear ossicles

385.24 Partial loss or necrosis of ear ossicles

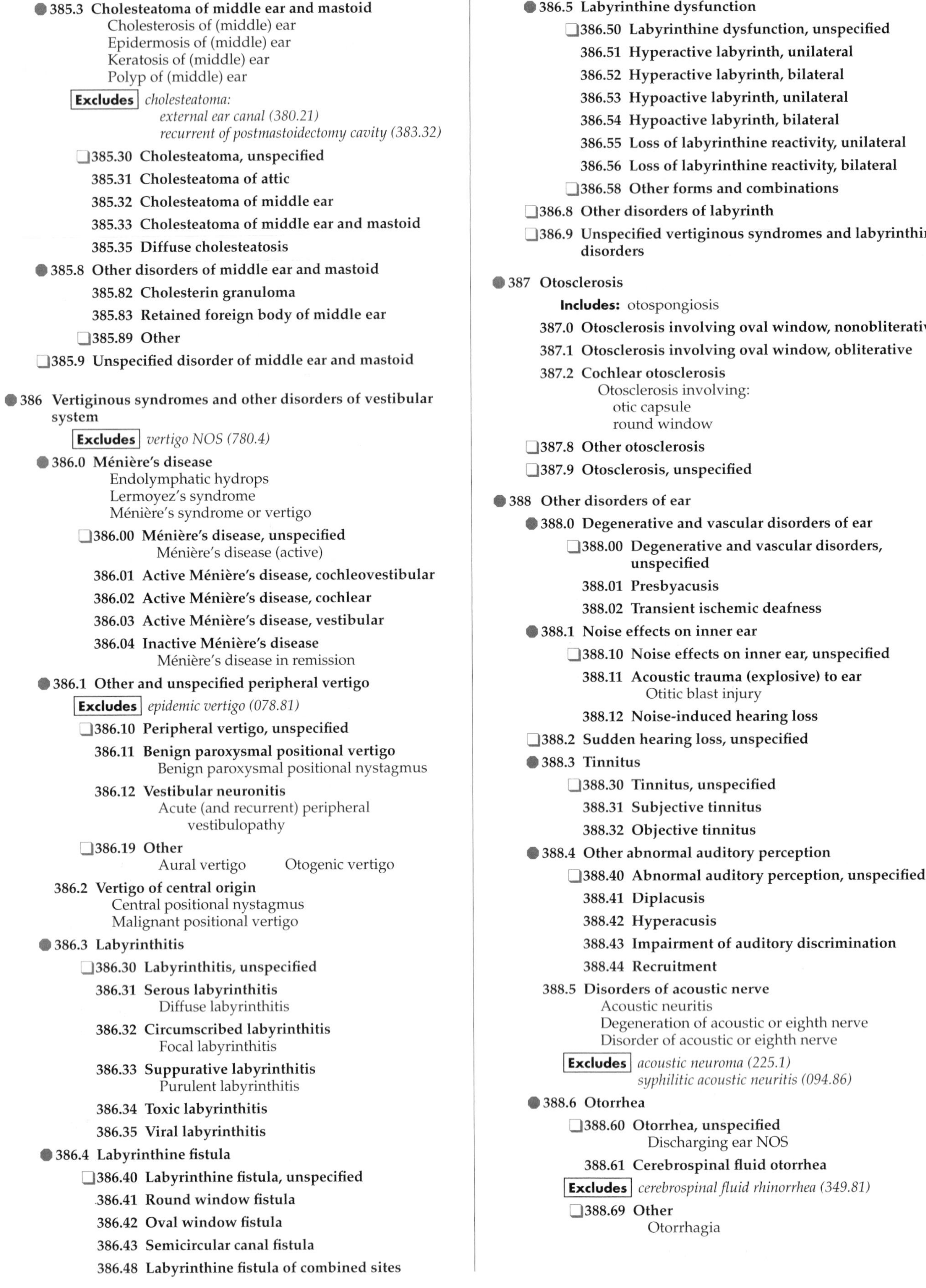

● **385.3 Cholesteatoma of middle ear and mastoid**
Cholesterosis of (middle) ear
Epidermosis of (middle) ear
Keratosis of (middle) ear
Polyp of (middle) ear

Excludes *cholesteatoma:*
external ear canal (380.21)
recurrent of postmastoidectomy cavity (383.32)

❑ **385.30 Cholesteatoma, unspecified**

385.31 Cholesteatoma of attic

385.32 Cholesteatoma of middle ear

385.33 Cholesteatoma of middle ear and mastoid

385.35 Diffuse cholesteatosis

● **385.8 Other disorders of middle ear and mastoid**

385.82 Cholesterin granuloma

385.83 Retained foreign body of middle ear

❑ **385.89 Other**

❑ **385.9 Unspecified disorder of middle ear and mastoid**

● **386 Vertiginous syndromes and other disorders of vestibular system**

Excludes *vertigo NOS (780.4)*

● **386.0 Ménière's disease**
Endolymphatic hydrops
Lermoyez's syndrome
Ménière's syndrome or vertigo

❑ **386.00 Ménière's disease, unspecified**
Ménière's disease (active)

386.01 Active Ménière's disease, cochleovestibular

386.02 Active Ménière's disease, cochlear

386.03 Active Ménière's disease, vestibular

386.04 Inactive Ménière's disease
Ménière's disease in remission

● **386.1 Other and unspecified peripheral vertigo**

Excludes *epidemic vertigo (078.81)*

❑ **386.10 Peripheral vertigo, unspecified**

386.11 Benign paroxysmal positional vertigo
Benign paroxysmal positional nystagmus

386.12 Vestibular neuronitis
Acute (and recurrent) peripheral vestibulopathy

❑ **386.19 Other**
Aural vertigo Otogenic vertigo

386.2 Vertigo of central origin
Central positional nystagmus
Malignant positional vertigo

● **386.3 Labyrinthitis**

❑ **386.30 Labyrinthitis, unspecified**

386.31 Serous labyrinthitis
Diffuse labyrinthitis

386.32 Circumscribed labyrinthitis
Focal labyrinthitis

386.33 Suppurative labyrinthitis
Purulent labyrinthitis

386.34 Toxic labyrinthitis

386.35 Viral labyrinthitis

● **386.4 Labyrinthine fistula**

❑ **386.40 Labyrinthine fistula, unspecified**

386.41 Round window fistula

386.42 Oval window fistula

386.43 Semicircular canal fistula

386.48 Labyrinthine fistula of combined sites

● **386.5 Labyrinthine dysfunction**

❑ **386.50 Labyrinthine dysfunction, unspecified**

386.51 Hyperactive labyrinth, unilateral

386.52 Hyperactive labyrinth, bilateral

386.53 Hypoactive labyrinth, unilateral

386.54 Hypoactive labyrinth, bilateral

386.55 Loss of labyrinthine reactivity, unilateral

386.56 Loss of labyrinthine reactivity, bilateral

❑ **386.58 Other forms and combinations**

❑ **386.8 Other disorders of labyrinth**

❑ **386.9 Unspecified vertiginous syndromes and labyrinthine disorders**

● **387 Otosclerosis**

Includes: otospongiosis

387.0 Otosclerosis involving oval window, nonobliterative

387.1 Otosclerosis involving oval window, obliterative

387.2 Cochlear otosclerosis
Otosclerosis involving:
otic capsule
round window

❑ **387.8 Other otosclerosis**

❑ **387.9 Otosclerosis, unspecified**

● **388 Other disorders of ear**

● **388.0 Degenerative and vascular disorders of ear**

❑ **388.00 Degenerative and vascular disorders, unspecified**

388.01 Presbyacusis

388.02 Transient ischemic deafness

● **388.1 Noise effects on inner ear**

❑ **388.10 Noise effects on inner ear, unspecified**

388.11 Acoustic trauma (explosive) to ear
Otitic blast injury

388.12 Noise-induced hearing loss

❑ **388.2 Sudden hearing loss, unspecified**

● **388.3 Tinnitus**

❑ **388.30 Tinnitus, unspecified**

388.31 Subjective tinnitus

388.32 Objective tinnitus

● **388.4 Other abnormal auditory perception**

❑ **388.40 Abnormal auditory perception, unspecified**

388.41 Diplacusis

388.42 Hyperacusis

388.43 Impairment of auditory discrimination

388.44 Recruitment

388.5 Disorders of acoustic nerve
Acoustic neuritis
Degeneration of acoustic or eighth nerve
Disorder of acoustic or eighth nerve

Excludes *acoustic neuroma (225.1)*
syphilitic acoustic neuritis (094.86)

● **388.6 Otorrhea**

❑ **388.60 Otorrhea, unspecified**
Discharging ear NOS

388.61 Cerebrospinal fluid otorrhea

Excludes *cerebrospinal fluid rhinorrhea (349.81)*

❑ **388.69 Other**
Otorrhagia

● 388.7 **Otalgia**

❑ 388.70 **Otalgia, unspecified**
Earache NOS

388.71 **Otogenic pain**

388.72 **Referred pain**

Pain from a diseased area of the body that is not felt directly in that area, but in another part of the body. Throat pain may often be referred pain in the ear.

❑ 388.8 **Other disorders of ear**

❑ 388.9 **Unspecified disorder of ear**

● 389 **Hearing loss**

● 389.0 **Conductive hearing loss**
Conductive deafness

❑ 389.00 **Conductive hearing loss, unspecified**

389.01 **Conductive hearing loss, external ear**

389.02 **Conductive hearing loss, tympanic membrane**

389.03 **Conductive hearing loss, middle ear**

389.04 **Conductive hearing loss, inner ear**

389.08 **Conductive hearing loss of combined types**

● 389.1 **Sensorineural hearing loss**
Perceptive hearing loss or deafness

Excludes *abnormal auditory perception (388.40–388.44)*
psychogenic deafness (306.7)

❑ 389.10 **Sensorineural hearing loss, unspecified**

389.11 **Sensory hearing loss, bilateral** (Revised)

389.12 **Neural hearing loss, bilateral** (Revised)

389.14 **Central hearing loss, bilateral** (Revised)

389.15 **Sensorineural hearing loss, unilateral** ◀

389.16 **Sensorineural hearing loss, asymmetrical** ◀

389.18 **Sensorineural hearing loss of combined types, bilateral** (Revised)

389.2 **Mixed conductive and sensorineural hearing loss**
Deafness or hearing loss of type classifiable to 389.0 with type classifiable to 389.1

389.7 **Deaf mutism, not elsewhere classifiable**
Deaf, nonspeaking

❑ 389.8 **Other specified forms of hearing loss**

❑ 389.9 **Unspecified hearing loss**
Deafness NOS

ICD-9-CM 300-399 Vol. 1

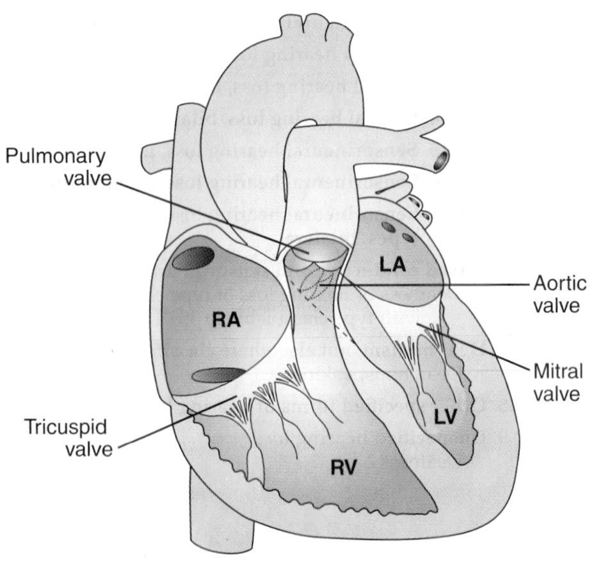
Pulmonary valve
LA
RA
Aortic valve
Mitral valve
Tricuspid valve
LV
RV

Figure 7–1 Cardiovascular valves.

Item 7–1 Rheumatic fever is the inflammation of the valve(s) of the heart, usually the mitral or aortic, which leads to valve damage. Rheumatic heart inflammations are usually pericarditis (heart), endocarditis (heart cavity), or myocarditis (heart muscle).

Item 7–2 Rheumatic chorea, also called Sydenham's, juvenile, minor, simple, or St. Vitus' dance, is a condition linked with rheumatic fever and is characterized by ceaseless, jerky movements.

7. DISEASES OF THE CIRCULATORY SYSTEM (390–459)

ACUTE RHEUMATIC FEVER (390–392)

390 Rheumatic fever without mention of heart involvement
Arthritis, rheumatic, acute or subacute
Rheumatic fever (active) (acute)
Rheumatism, articular, acute or subacute
Excludes *that with heart involvement (391.0–391.9)*

● **391 Rheumatic fever with heart involvement**
Excludes *chronic heart diseases of rheumatic origin (393.0–398.9) unless rheumatic fever is also present or there is evidence of recrudescence or activity of the rheumatic process*

391.0 Acute rheumatic pericarditis
Rheumatic:
fever (active) (acute) with pericarditis
pericarditis (acute)
Any condition classifiable to 390 with pericarditis
Excludes *that not specified as rheumatic (420.0–420.9)*

391.1 Acute rheumatic endocarditis
Rheumatic:
endocarditis, acute
fever (active) (acute) with endocarditis or valvulitis
valvulitis, acute
Any condition classifiable to 390 with endocarditis or valvulitis

391.2 Acute rheumatic myocarditis
Rheumatic fever (active) (acute) with myocarditis
Any condition classifiable to 390 with myocarditis

❑ **391.8 Other acute rheumatic heart disease**
Rheumatic:
fever (active) (acute) with other or multiple types of heart involvement
pancarditis, acute
Any condition classifiable to 390 with other or multiple types of heart involvement

❑ **391.9 Acute rheumatic heart disease, unspecified**
Rheumatic:
carditis, acute
fever (active) (acute) with unspecified type of heart involvement
heart disease, active or acute
Any condition classifiable to 390 with unspecified type of heart involvement

● **392 Rheumatic chorea**
Includes: Sydenham's chorea
Excludes *chorea:*
NOS (333.5)
Huntington's (333.4)

392.0 With heart involvement
Rheumatic chorea with heart involvement of any type classifiable to 391

392.9 Without mention of heart involvement

CHRONIC RHEUMATIC HEART DISEASE (393–398)

393 Chronic rheumatic pericarditis
Adherent pericardium, rheumatic
Chronic rheumatic:
mediastinopericarditis
myopericarditis
Excludes *pericarditis NOS or not specified as rheumatic (423.0–423.9)*

Item 7–3 Mitral stenosis is the narrowing of the mitral valve. Mitral insufficiency is the improper closure of the mitral valve. These conditions lead to enlargement (hypertrophy) of the left atrium.

● **394 Diseases of mitral valve**
Excludes *that with aortic valve involvement (396.0–396.9)*

394.0 Mitral stenosis
Mitral (valve):
obstruction (rheumatic)
stenosis NOS

394.1 Rheumatic mitral insufficiency
Rheumatic mitral:
incompetence
regurgitation
Excludes *that not specified as rheumatic (424.0)*

394.2 Mitral stenosis with insufficiency
Mitral stenosis with incompetence or regurgitation

❑ **394.9 Other and unspecified mitral valve diseases**
Mitral (valve):
disease (chronic)
failure

Item 7–4 Aortic stenosis is the narrowing of the aortic valve. Aortic insufficiency is the improper closure of the aortic valve. These conditions lead to enlargement (hypertrophy) of the left ventricle.

● 395 Diseases of aortic valve

Excludes *that not specified as rheumatic (424.1)*
that with mitral valve involvement (396.0–396.9)

395.0 Rheumatic aortic stenosis
Rheumatic aortic (valve) obstruction

395.1 Rheumatic aortic insufficiency
Rheumatic aortic:
incompetence
regurgitation

395.2 Rheumatic aortic stenosis with insufficiency
Rheumatic aortic stenosis with incompetence or regurgitation

❑ 395.9 Other and unspecified rheumatic aortic diseases
Rheumatic aortic (valve) disease

Item 7-5 Mitral and aortic valve stenosis is the narrowing of these valves, which leads to enlargement (hypertrophy) of the left atrium and left ventricle.
Mitral and aortic insufficiency is the improper closure of the mitral and aortic valves, which leads to enlargement (hypertrophy) of the left atrium and left ventricle.

● 396 Diseases of mitral and aortic valves

Includes: involvement of both mitral and aortic valves, whether specified as rheumatic or not

396.0 Mitral valve stenosis and aortic valve stenosis
Atypical aortic (valve) stenosis
Mitral and aortic (valve) obstruction (rheumatic)

396.1 Mitral valve stenosis and aortic valve insufficiency

396.2 Mitral valve insufficiency and aortic valve stenosis

396.3 Mitral valve insufficiency and aortic valve insufficiency
Mitral and aortic (valve):
incompetence
regurgitation

396.8 Multiple involvement of mitral and aortic valves
Stenosis and insufficiency of mitral or aortic valve with stenosis or insufficiency, or both, of the other valve

❑ 396.9 Mitral and aortic valve diseases, unspecified

● 397 Diseases of other endocardial structures

397.0 Diseases of tricuspid valve
Tricuspid (valve) (rheumatic):
disease
insufficiency
obstruction
regurgitation
stenosis

397.1 Rheumatic diseases of pulmonary valve

Excludes *that not specified as rheumatic (424.3)*

❑ 397.9 Rheumatic diseases of endocardium, valve unspecified
Rheumatic:
endocarditis (chronic)
valvulitis (chronic)

Excludes *that not specified as rheumatic (424.90–424.99)*

● 398 Other rheumatic heart disease

398.0 Rheumatic myocarditis
Rheumatic degeneration of myocardium

Excludes *myocarditis not specified as rheumatic (429.0)*

● 398.9 Other and unspecified rheumatic heart diseases

❑ 398.90 Rheumatic heart disease, unspecified
Rheumatic:
carditis
heart disease NOS

Excludes *carditis not specified as rheumatic (429.89)*
heart disease NOS not specified as rheumatic (429.9)

398.91 Rheumatic heart failure (congestive)
Rheumatic left ventricular failure

❑ 398.99 Other

Item 7-6 Hypertension is caused by high arterial blood pressure in the arteries. **Essential, primary,** or **idiopathic** hypertension occurs without identifiable organic cause.
Secondary hypertension is that which has an organic cause. **Malignant** hypertension is severely elevated blood pressure. **Benign** hypertension is mildly elevated blood pressure.

HYPERTENSIVE DISEASE (401–405)

Excludes *that complicating pregnancy, childbirth, or the puerperium (642.0–642.9)*
that involving coronary vessels (410.00–414.9)

● 401 Essential hypertension

Includes: high blood pressure
hyperpiesia
hyperpiesis
hypertension (arterial) (essential) (primary) (systemic)
hypertensive vascular:
degeneration
disease

Excludes *elevated blood pressure without diagnosis of hypertension (796.2)*
pulmonary hypertension (416.0–416.9)
that involving vessels of:
brain (430–438)
eye (362.11)

401.0 Malignant

401.1 Benign

❑ 401.9 Unspecified

● 402 Hypertensive heart disease

Includes: hypertensive:
cardiomegaly
cardiopathy
cardiovascular disease
heart (disease) (failure)
any condition classifiable to 429.0–429.3, 429.8, 429.9 due to hypertension

Use additional code to specify type of heart failure (428.0–428.43), if known

● 402.0 Malignant

402.00 Without heart failure

❑ 402.01 With heart failure

● 402.1 Benign

402.10 Without heart failure

402.11 With heart failure

● **402.9 Unspecified**

❑ **402.90 Without heart failure**

❑ **402.91 With heart failure**

● **403 Hypertensive chronic kidney disease**

Includes: arteriolar nephritis
arteriosclerosis of:
kidney
renal arterioles
arteriosclerotic nephritis (chronic) (interstitial)
hypertensive:
nephropathy
renal failure
uremia (chronic)
nephrosclerosis
renal sclerosis with hypertension
any condition classifiable to 585, 586, or 587 with any condition classifiable to 401

Excludes *acute renal failure (584.5–584.9)*
renal disease stated as not due to hypertension
renovascular hypertension (405.0–405.9 with fifth-digit 1)

The following fifth-digit subclassification is for use with category 403:

0 **with chronic kidney disease stage I through stage IV, or unspecified**
Use additional code to identify the stage of chronic kidney disease (585.1–585.4, 585.9) ◀

1 **with chronic kidney disease stage V or end stage renal disease**
Use additional code to identify the stage of chronic kidney disease (585.5, 585.6) ◀

● **403.0 Malignant**

● **403.1 Benign**

● ❑ **403.9 Unspecified**

● **404 Hypertensive heart and chronic kidney disease**

Includes: disease:
cardiorenal
cardiovascular renal
any condition classifiable to 402 with any condition classifiable to 403

Use additional code to specify type of heart failure (428.0–428.43), if known

The following fifth-digit subclassification is for use with category 404:

0 **without heart failure and with chronic kidney disease stage I through stage IV, or unspecified**
Use additional code to identify the stage of chronic kidney disease (585.1–585.4, 585.9) ◀

1 **with heart failure and with chronic kidney disease stage I through IV, or unspecified**
Use additional code to identify the stage of chronic kidney disease (585.1–585.4, 585.9) ◀

2 **without heart failure and with chronic kidney disease stage V or end stage renal disease**
Use additional code to identify the stage of chronic kidney disease (585.5, 585.6) ◀

3 **with heart failure and chronic kidney disease stage V or end stage renal disease**
Use additional code to identify the stage of chronic kidney disease (585.5, 585.6) ◀

● **404.0 Malignant**

● **404.1 Benign**

● ❑ **404.9 Unspecified**

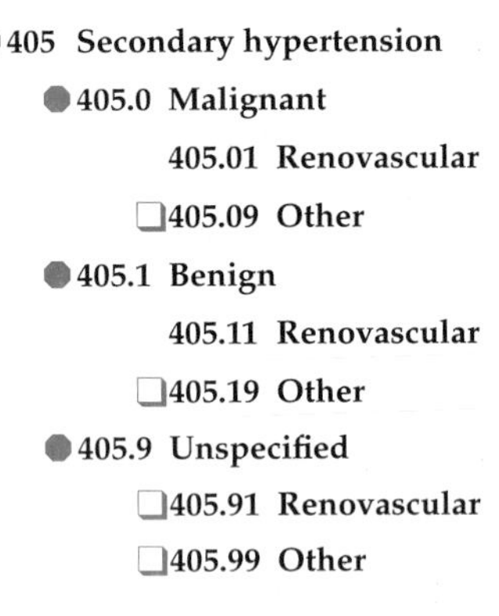

● **405 Secondary hypertension**

● **405.0 Malignant**

405.01 Renovascular

❑ **405.09 Other**

● **405.1 Benign**

405.11 Renovascular

❑ **405.19 Other**

● **405.9 Unspecified**

❑ **405.91 Renovascular**

❑ **405.99 Other**

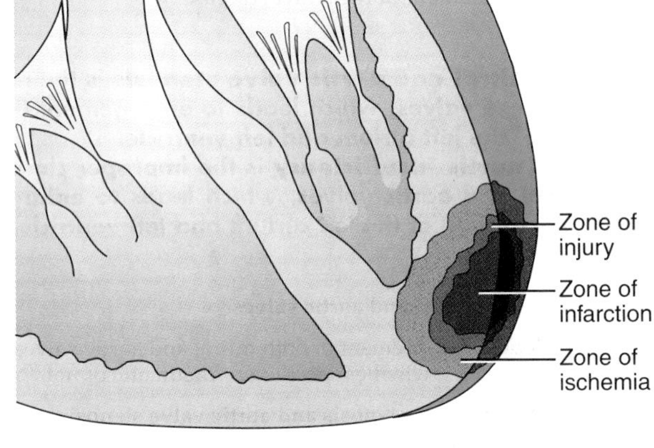
Zone of injury
Zone of infarction
Zone of ischemia

Figure 7–2 Myocardial infarction.

Item 7–7 Myocardial infarction is a sudden decrease in the coronary artery blood flow that results in death of the heart muscle. Classifications are based on the affected heart tissue.

ISCHEMIC HEART DISEASE (410–414)

Includes: that with mention of hypertension

Use additional code to identify presence of hypertension (401.0–405.9)

● **410 Acute myocardial infarction**

Includes: cardiac infarction
coronary (artery):
embolism
occlusion
rupture
thrombosis
infarction of heart, myocardium, or ventricle
rupture of heart, myocardium, or ventricle
ST elevation (STEMI) and non-ST elevation (NSTEMI) myocardial infarction
any condition classifiable to 414.1–414.9 specified as acute or with a stated duration of 8 weeks or less

The following fifth-digit subclassification is for use with category 410:

❑ 0 **episode of care unspecified**
Use when the source document does not contain sufficient information for the assignment of fifth-digit 1 or 2.

1 **initial episode of care**
Use fifth-digit 1 to designate the first episode of care (regardless of facility site) for a newly diagnosed myocardial infarction. The fifth-digit 1 is assigned regardless of the number of times a patient may be transferred during the initial episode of care.

2 **subsequent episode of care**
Use fifth-digit 2 to designate an episode of care following the initial episode when the patient is admitted for further observation, evaluation, or treatment for a myocardial infarction that has received initial treatment, but is still less than 8 weeks old.

● **410.0 Of anterolateral wall**
ST elevation myocardial infarction (STEMI) of anterolateral wall

● ❑ **410.1 Of other anterior wall**
Infarction:
anterior (wall) NOS (with contiguous portion of intraventricular septum)
anteroapical (with contiguous portion of intraventricular septum)
anteroseptal (with contiguous portion of intraventricular septum)
ST elevation myocardial infarction (STEMI) of other anterior wall

● **410.2 Of inferolateral wall**
ST elevation myocardial infarction (STEMI) of inferolateral wall

● **410.3 Of inferoposterior wall**
ST elevation myocardial infarction (STEMI) of inferoposterior wall

● ❑ **410.4 Of other inferior wall**
Infarction:
diaphragmatic wall NOS (with contiguous portion of intraventricular septum)
inferior (wall) NOS (with contiguous portion of intraventricular septum)
ST elevation myocardial infarction (STEMI) of other inferior wall

● ❑ **410.5 Of other lateral wall**
Infarction:
apical-lateral
basal-lateral
high lateral
posterolateral
ST elevation myocardial infarction (STEMI) of other lateral wall

● **410.6 True posterior wall infarction**
Infarction:
posterobasal
strictly posterior
ST elevation myocardial infarction (STEMI) of true posterior wall

● **410.7 Subendocardial infarction**
Nontransmural infarction
Non-ST elevation myocardial infarction (NSTEMI)

● ❑ **410.8 Of other specified sites**
Infarction of:
atrium
papillary muscle
septum alone
ST elevation myocardial infarction (STEMI) of other specified sites

● ❑ **410.9 Unspecified site**
Acute myocardial infarction NOS
Coronary occlusion NOS
Myocardial infarction NOS

● **411 Other acute and subacute forms of ischemic heart disease**

411.0 Postmyocardial infarction syndrome
Dressler's syndrome

411.1 Intermediate coronary syndrome
Impending infarction
Preinfarction angina
Preinfarction syndrome
Unstable angina

Excludes *angina (pectoris) (413.9)*
decubitus (413.0)

● **411.8 Other**

411.81 Acute coronary occlusion without myocardial infarction
Acute coronary (artery):
embolism without or not resulting in myocardial infarction
obstruction without or not resulting in myocardial infarction
occlusion without or not resulting in myocardial infarction
thrombosis without or not resulting in myocardial infarction

Excludes *obstruction without infarction due to atherosclerosis (414.00–414.07)*
occlusion without infarction due to atherosclerosis (414.00–414.07)

❑ **411.89 Other**
Coronary insufficiency (acute)
Subendocardial ischemia

Item 7-8 "Old" (healed) myocardial infarction: Code 412 cannot be used if the patient is experiencing current ischemic heart disease symptoms. Recent infarctions still under care cannot be coded to 412. This code is only assigned if infarction has some impact on the current episode of care—essentially, it is a history of (H/O) a past, healed MI. (There is no V code for this status/post MI.)

ICD-9-CM 400-499 Vol. 1

412 Old myocardial infarction
Healed myocardial infarction
Past myocardial infarction diagnosed on ECG [EKG] or other special investigation, but currently presenting no symptoms

● **413 Angina pectoris**

413.0 Angina decubitus
Nocturnal angina

413.1 Prinzmetal angina
Variant angina pectoris

❑ **413.9 Other and unspecified angina pectoris**
Angina:
NOS
cardiac
of effort
Anginal syndrome
Status anginosus
Stenocardia
Syncope anginosa

Excludes *preinfarction angina (411.1)*

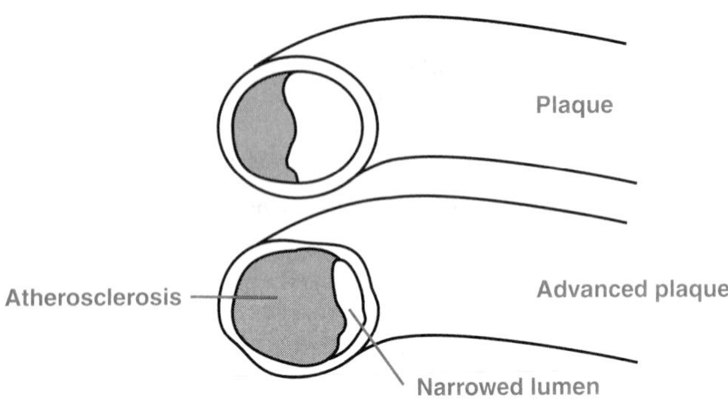
Plaque
Atherosclerosis
Advanced plaque
Narrowed lumen

Figure 7–3 Atherosclerosis. (From Buck CJ: Step-by-Step Medical Coding, 2005 ed. Philadelphia, WB Saunders, 2005.)

Item 7–9 Classification is based on the location of the atherosclerosis. **"Of native coronary artery"** indicates the atherosclerosis is within an original heart artery. **"Of autologous vein bypass graft"** indicates that the atherosclerosis is within a vein graft that was taken from within the patient. **"Of nonautologous biological bypass graft"** indicates the atherosclerosis is within a vessel grafted from other than the patient. **"Of artery bypass graft"** indicates the atherosclerosis is within an artery that was grafted from within the patient.

● **414 Other forms of chronic ischemic heart disease**

Excludes *arteriosclerotic cardiovascular disease [ASCVD] (429.2)*
cardiovascular:
arteriosclerosis or sclerosis (429.2)
degeneration or disease (429.2)

● **414.0 Coronary atherosclerosis**

Arteriosclerotic heart disease [ASHD]
Atherosclerotic heart disease
Coronary (artery):
arteriosclerosis
arteritis or endarteritis
atheroma
sclerosis
stricture

Excludes *embolism of graft (996.72)*
occlusion NOS of graft (996.72)
thrombus of graft (996.72)

❑ **414.00 Of unspecified type of vessel, native or graft**

414.01 Of native coronary artery

414.02 Of autologous biological bypass graft

414.03 Of nonautologous biological bypass graft

414.04 Of artery bypass graft
Internal mammary artery

414.05 Of unspecified type of bypass graft
Bypass graft NOS

414.06 Of native coronary artery of transplanted heart

414.07 Of bypass graft (artery) (vein) of transplanted heart

● **414.1 Aneurysm and dissection of heart**

414.10 Aneurysm of heart (wall)
Aneurysm (arteriovenous):
mural
ventricular

414.11 Aneurysm of coronary vessels
Aneurysm (arteriovenous) of coronary vessels

414.12 Dissection of coronary artery

❑ **414.19 Other aneurysm of heart**
Arteriovenous fistula, acquired, of heart

❑ **414.8 Other specified forms of chronic ischemic heart disease**
Chronic coronary insufficiency
Ischemia, myocardial (chronic)
Any condition classifiable to 410 specified as chronic, or presenting with symptoms after 8 weeks from date of infarction

Excludes *coronary insufficiency (acute) (411.89)*

❑ **414.9 Chronic ischemic heart disease, unspecified**
Ischemic heart disease NOS

DISEASES OF PULMONARY CIRCULATION (415–417)

● **415 Acute pulmonary heart disease**

415.0 Acute cor pulmonale

Excludes *cor pulmonale NOS (416.9)*

● **415.1 Pulmonary embolism and infarction**
Pulmonary (artery) (vein):
apoplexy
embolism
infarction (hemorrhagic)
thrombosis

Excludes *that complicating:*
abortion (634–638 with .6, 639.6)
ectopic or molar pregnancy (639.6)
pregnancy, childbirth, or the puerperium (673.0–673.8)

415.11 Iatrogenic pulmonary embolism and infarction

❑ **415.19 Other**

● **416 Chronic pulmonary heart disease**

416.0 Primary pulmonary hypertension
Idiopathic pulmonary arteriosclerosis
Pulmonary hypertension (essential) (idiopathic) (primary)

416.1 Kyphoscoliotic heart disease

❑ **416.8 Other chronic pulmonary heart diseases**
Pulmonary hypertension, secondary

❑ **416.9 Chronic pulmonary heart disease, unspecified**
Chronic cardiopulmonary disease
Cor pulmonale (chronic) NOS

● **417 Other diseases of pulmonary circulation**

417.0 Arteriovenous fistula of pulmonary vessels

Excludes *congenital arteriovenous fistula (747.3)*

417.1 Aneurysm of pulmonary artery

Excludes *congenital aneurysm (747.3)*

❑ **417.8 Other specified diseases of pulmonary circulation**
Pulmonary:
arteritis
endarteritis
Rupture of pulmonary vessel
Stricture of pulmonary vessel

❑ **417.9 Unspecified disease of pulmonary circulation**

OTHER FORMS OF HEART DISEASE (420–429)

● **420 Acute pericarditis**

Includes: acute:
mediastinopericarditis
myopericarditis
pericardial effusion
pleuropericarditis
pneumopericarditis

Excludes *acute rheumatic pericarditis (391.0)*
postmyocardial infarction syndrome [Dressler's] (411.0)

● ❑ ***420.0 Acute pericarditis in diseases classified elsewhere***

Code first underlying disease, as:
actinomycosis (039.8)
amebiasis (006.8)
chronic uremia (585.9) ◀
nocardiosis (039.8)
tuberculosis (017.9)
uremia NOS (586) ⬅

Excludes *pericarditis (acute) (in):*
Coxsackie (virus) (074.21)
gonococcal (098.83)
histoplasmosis (115.0–115.9 with fifth-digit 3)
meningococcal infection (036.41)
syphilitic (093.81)

● **420.9 Other and unspecified acute pericarditis**

❑ **420.90 Acute pericarditis, unspecified**
Pericarditis (acute):
NOS
infective NOS
sicca

420.91 Acute idiopathic pericarditis
Pericarditis, acute:
benign
nonspecific
viral

❑ **420.99 Other**
Pericarditis (acute):
pneumococcal
purulent
staphylococcal
streptococcal
suppurative
Pneumopyopericardium
Pyopericardium

Excludes *pericarditis in diseases classified elsewhere (420.0)*

● **421 Acute and subacute endocarditis**

421.0 Acute and subacute bacterial endocarditis
Endocarditis (acute) (chronic) (subacute):
bacterial
infective NOS
lenta
malignant
purulent
septic
ulcerative
vegetative
Infective aneurysm
Subacute bacterial endocarditis [SBE]

Use additional code, if desired, to identify infectious organism [e.g., Streptococcus 041.0, Staphylococcus 041.1]

● ❑ ***421.1 Acute and subacute infective endocarditis in diseases classified elsewhere***

Code first underlying disease, as:
blastomycosis (116.0)
Q fever (083.0)
typhoid (fever) (002.0)

Excludes *endocarditis (in):*
Coxsackie (virus) (074.22)
gonococcal (098.84)
histoplasmosis (115.0–115.9 with fifth-digit 4)
meningococcal infection (036.42)
monilial (112.81)

❑ **421.9 Acute endocarditis, unspecified**
Endocarditis, acute or subacute
Myoendocarditis, acute or subacute
Periendocarditis, acute or subacute

Excludes *acute rheumatic endocarditis (391.1)*

● **422 Acute myocarditis**

Excludes *acute rheumatic myocarditis (391.2)*

● ❑ ***422.0 Acute myocarditis in diseases classified elsewhere***

Code first underlying disease, as:
myocarditis (acute):
influenzal (487.8)
tuberculous (017.9)

Excludes *myocarditis (acute) (due to):*
aseptic, of newborn (074.23)
Coxsackie (virus) (074.23)
diphtheritic (032.82)
meningococcal infection (036.43)
syphilitic (093.82)
toxoplasmosis (130.3)

● **422.9 Other and unspecified acute myocarditis**

❑ **422.90 Acute myocarditis, unspecified**
Acute or subacute (interstitial) myocarditis

422.91 Idiopathic myocarditis
Myocarditis (acute or subacute):
Fiedler's
giant cell
isolated (diffuse) (granulomatous)
nonspecific granulomatous

422.92 Septic myocarditis
Myocarditis, acute or subacute:
pneumococcal
staphylococcal

Use additional code to identify infectious organism [e.g., Staphylococcus 041.1]

Excludes *myocarditis, acute or subacute:*
in bacterial diseases classified elsewhere (422.0)
streptococcal (391.2)

422.93 Toxic myocarditis

❑ **422.99 Other**

● **423 Other diseases of pericardium**

Excludes *that specified as rheumatic (393)*

423.0 Hemopericardium

423.1 Adhesive pericarditis
Adherent pericardium
Fibrosis of pericardium
Milk spots
Pericarditis:
adhesive
obliterative
Soldiers' patches

423.2 Constrictive pericarditis
Concato's disease
Pick's disease of heart (and liver)

❑423.8 **Other specified diseases of pericardium**
Calcification of pericardium
Fistula of pericardium

❑423.9 **Unspecified disease of pericardium**

● 424 **Other diseases of endocardium**

Excludes *bacterial endocarditis (421.0–421.9)*
rheumatic endocarditis (391.1, 394.0–397.9)
syphilitic endocarditis (093.20–093.24)

424.0 **Mitral valve disorders**
Mitral (valve):
incompetence NOS of specified cause, except rheumatic
insufficiency NOS of specified cause, except rheumatic
regurgitation NOS of specified cause, except rheumatic

Excludes *mitral (valve):*
disease (394.9)
failure (394.9)
stenosis (394.0)
the listed conditions:
specified as rheumatic (394.1)
unspecified as to cause but with mention of:
diseases of aortic valve (396.0–396.9)
mitral stenosis or obstruction (394.2)

424.1 **Aortic valve disorders**
Aortic (valve):
incompetence NOS of specified cause, except rheumatic
insufficiency NOS of specified cause, except rheumatic
regurgitation NOS of specified cause, except rheumatic
stenosis NOS of specified cause, except rheumatic

Excludes *hypertrophic subaortic stenosis (425.1)*
that specified as rheumatic (395.0–395.9)
that of unspecified cause but with mention of diseases of mitral valve (396.0–396.9)

424.2 **Tricuspid valve disorders, specified as nonrheumatic**
Tricuspid valve:
incompetence of specified cause, except rheumatic
insufficiency of specified cause, except rheumatic
regurgitation of specified cause, except rheumatic
stenosis of specified cause, except rheumatic

Excludes *rheumatic or of unspecified cause (397.0)*

424.3 **Pulmonary valve disorders**
Pulmonic:
incompetence NOS
insufficiency NOS
regurgitation NOS
stenosis NOS

Excludes *that specified as rheumatic (397.1)*

● 424.9 **Endocarditis, valve unspecified**

❑424.90 **Endocarditis, valve unspecified, unspecified cause**
Endocarditis (chronic):
NOS
nonbacterial thrombotic
Valvular:
incompetence of unspecified valve, unspecified cause
insufficiency of unspecified valve, unspecified cause
regurgitation of unspecified valve, unspecified cause
stenosis of unspecified valve, unspecified cause
Valvulitis (chronic)

● ❑*424.91* ***Endocarditis in diseases classified elsewhere***
Code first underlying disease, as:
atypical verrucous endocarditis [Libman-Sacks] (710.0)
disseminated lupus erythematosus (710.0)
tuberculosis (017.9)

Excludes *syphilitic (093.20–093.24)*

❑424.99 **Other**
Any condition classifiable to 424.90 with specified cause, except rheumatic

Excludes *endocardial fibroelastosis (425.3)*
that specified as rheumatic (397.9)

● 425 **Cardiomyopathy**

Includes: myocardiopathy

425.0 **Endomyocardial fibrosis**

425.1 **Hypertrophic obstructive cardiomyopathy**
Hypertrophic subaortic stenosis (idiopathic)

425.2 **Obscure cardiomyopathy of Africa**
Becker's disease
Idiopathic mural endomyocardial disease

425.3 **Endocardial fibroelastosis**
Elastomyofibrosis

❑425.4 **Other primary cardiomyopathies**
Cardiomyopathy:
NOS
congestive
constrictive
familial
hypertrophic
idiopathic
nonobstructive
obstructive
restrictive
Cardiovascular collagenosis

425.5 **Alcoholic cardiomyopathy**

● *425.7* ***Nutritional and metabolic cardiomyopathy***
Code first underlying disease, as:
amyloidosis (277.30–277.39) ◀
beriberi (265.0)
cardiac glycogenosis (271.0)
mucopolysaccharidosis (277.5)
thyrotoxicosis (242.0–242.9)

Excludes *gouty tophi of heart (274.82)*

● ❑*425.8* ***Cardiomyopathy in other diseases classified elsewhere***
Code first underlying disease, as:
Friedreich's ataxia (334.0)
myotonia atrophica (359.2)
progressive muscular dystrophy (359.1)
sarcoidosis (135)

Excludes *cardiomyopathy in Chagas' disease (086.0)*

❑425.9 **Secondary cardiomyopathy, unspecified**

● 426 **Conduction disorders**

426.0 **Atrioventricular block, complete**
Third degree atrioventricular block

● 426.1 **Atrioventricular block, other and unspecified**

❑426.10 **Atrioventricular block, unspecified**
Atrioventricular [AV] block (incomplete) (partial)

426.11 **First degree atrioventricular block**
Incomplete atrioventricular block, first degree
Prolonged P-R interval NOS

426.12 Mobitz (type) II atrioventricular block
Incomplete atrioventricular block:
Mobitz (type) II
second degree, Mobitz (type) II

❑**426.13 Other second degree atrioventricular block**
Incomplete atrioventricular block:
Mobitz (type) I [Wenckebach's]
second degree:
NOS
Mobitz (type) I
with 2:1 atrioventricular response [block]
Wenckebach's phenomenon

426.2 Left bundle branch hemiblock
Block:
left anterior fascicular
left posterior fascicular

❑**426.3 Other left bundle branch block**
Left bundle branch block:
NOS
anterior fascicular with posterior fascicular
complete
main stem

426.4 Right bundle branch block

● **426.5 Bundle branch block, other and unspecified**

❑**426.50 Bundle branch block, unspecified**

426.51 Right bundle branch block and left posterior fascicular block

426.52 Right bundle branch block and left anterior fascicular block

❑**426.53 Other bilateral bundle branch block**
Bifascicular block NOS
Bilateral bundle branch block NOS
Right bundle branch with left bundle branch block (incomplete) (main stem)

426.54 Trifascicular block

❑**426.6 Other heart block**
Intraventricular block:
NOS
diffuse
myofibrillar
Sinoatrial block
Sinoauricular block

426.7 Anomalous atrioventricular excitation
Atrioventricular conduction:
accelerated
accessory
pre-excitation
Ventricular pre-excitation
Wolff-Parkinson-White syndrome

● **426.8 Other specified conduction disorders**

426.81 Lown-Ganong-Levine syndrome
Syndrome of short P-R interval, normal QRS complexes, and supraventricular tachycardias

426.82 Long QT syndrome

❑**426.89 Other**
Dissociation:
atrioventricular [AV]
interference
isorhythmic
Nonparoxysmal AV nodal tachycardia

❑**426.9 Conduction disorder, unspecified**
Heart block NOS
Stokes-Adams syndrome

● **427 Cardiac dysrhythmias**

Excludes *that complicating:*
abortion (634–638 with .7, 639.8)
ectopic or molar pregnancy (639.8)
labor or delivery (668.1, 669.4)

427.0 Paroxysmal supraventricular tachycardia
Paroxysmal tachycardia:
atrial [PAT]
atrioventricular [AV]
junctional
nodal

427.1 Paroxysmal ventricular tachycardia
Ventricular tachycardia (paroxysmal)

❑**427.2 Paroxysmal tachycardia, unspecified**
Bouveret-Hoffmann syndrome
Paroxysmal tachycardia:
NOS
essential

● **427.3 Atrial fibrillation and flutter**

427.31 Atrial fibrillation

Most common abnormal heart rhythm (arrhythmia) presenting as irregular, rapid beating (tachycardia) of the heart's upper chamber. This occurs as a result of a malfunction of the heart's electrical system.

427.32 Atrial flutter

Rapid contractions of the upper heart chamber, but regular, rather than irregular, beats.

● **427.4 Ventricular fibrillation and flutter**

427.41 Ventricular fibrillation

427.42 Ventricular flutter

❑**427.5 Cardiac arrest**
Cardiorespiratory arrest

● **427.6 Premature beats**

❑**427.60 Premature beats, unspecified**
Ectopic beats
Extrasystoles
Extrasystolic arrhythmia
Premature contractions or systoles NOS

427.61 Supraventricular premature beats
Atrial premature beats, contractions, or systoles

❑**427.69 Other**
Ventricular premature beats, contractions, or systoles

● **427.8 Other specified cardiac dysrhythmias**

427.81 Sinoatrial node dysfunction
Sinus bradycardia:
persistent
severe
Syndrome:
sick sinus
tachycardia-bradycardia

Excludes *sinus bradycardia NOS (427.89)*

❑**427.89 Other**
Rhythm disorder:
coronary sinus
ectopic
nodal
Wandering (atrial) pacemaker

Excludes *carotid sinus syncope (337.0)*
neonatal bradycardia (779.81)
neonatal tachycardia (779.82)
reflex bradycardia (337.0)
tachycardia NOS (785.0)

❑**427.9 Cardiac dysrhythmia, unspecified**
Arrhythmia (cardiac) NOS

ICD-9-CM 400-499 Vol. 1

● **428 Heart failure**

Excludes *rheumatic (398.91)*
that complicating:
abortion (634–638 with .7, 639.8)
ectopic or molar pregnancy (639.8)
labor or delivery (668.1, 669.4)

Code, if applicable, heart failure due to hypertension first (402.0–402.9, with fifth-digit 1 or 404.0–404.9 with fifth-digit 1 or 3)

❑ **428.0 Congestive heart failure, unspecified**
Congestive heart disease
Right heart failure (secondary to left heart failure)

Excludes *fluid overload NOS (276.6)*

428.1 Left heart failure
Acute edema of lung with heart disease NOS or heart failure
Acute pulmonary edema with heart disease NOS or heart failure
Cardiac asthma
Left ventricular failure

● **428.2 Systolic heart failure**

Excludes *combined systolic and diastolic heart failure (428.40–428.43)*

❑ **428.20 Unspecified**

428.21 Acute

Presenting a short and relatively severe episode

428.22 Chronic

Long-lasting, presenting over time

428.23 Acute on chronic

Combination code. What is usually a chronic condition now has an acute exacerbation (to make more severe). Because two conditions are now present, the combination code reports both.

● **428.3 Diastolic heart failure**

Excludes *combined systolic and diastolic heart failure (428.40–428.43)*

❑ **428.30 Unspecified**

428.31 Acute

428.32 Chronic

428.33 Acute on chronic

● **428.4 Combined systolic and diastolic heart failure**

❑ **428.40 Unspecified**

428.41 Acute

428.42 Chronic

428.43 Acute on chronic

❑ **428.9 Heart failure, unspecified**
Cardiac failure NOS
Heart failure NOS
Myocardial failure NOS
Weak heart

● **429 Ill-defined descriptions and complications of heart disease**

❑ **429.0 Myocarditis, unspecified**
Myocarditis (with mention of arteriosclerosis):
NOS (with mention of arteriosclerosis)
chronic (interstitial) (with mention of arteriosclerosis)
fibroid (with mention of arteriosclerosis)
senile (with mention of arteriosclerosis)

Use additional code to identify presence of arteriosclerosis

Excludes *acute or subacute (422.0–422.9)*
rheumatic (398.0)
acute (391.2)
that due to hypertension (402.0–402.9)

429.1 Myocardial degeneration
Degeneration of heart or myocardium (with mention of arteriosclerosis):
fatty (with mention of arteriosclerosis)
mural (with mention of arteriosclerosis)
muscular (with mention of arteriosclerosis)
Myocardial (with mention of arteriosclerosis):
degeneration (with mention of arteriosclerosis)
disease (with mention of arteriosclerosis)

Use additional code to identify presence of arteriosclerosis

Excludes *that due to hypertension (402.0–402.9)*

❑ **429.2 Cardiovascular disease, unspecified**
Arteriosclerotic cardiovascular disease [ASCVD]
Cardiovascular arteriosclerosis
Cardiovascular:
degeneration (with mention of arteriosclerosis)
disease (with mention of arteriosclerosis)
sclerosis (with mention of arteriosclerosis)

Use additional code to identify presence of arteriosclerosis

Excludes *that due to hypertension (402.0–402.9)*

429.3 Cardiomegaly
Cardiac:
dilatation
hypertrophy
Ventricular dilatation

Excludes *that due to hypertension (402.0–402.9)*

429.4 Functional disturbances following cardiac surgery
Cardiac insufficiency following cardiac surgery or due to prosthesis
Heart failure following cardiac surgery or due to prosthesis
Postcardiotomy syndrome
Postvalvulotomy syndrome

Excludes *cardiac failure in the immediate postoperative period (997.1)*

429.5 Rupture of chordae tendineae

429.6 Rupture of papillary muscle

● **429.7 Certain sequelae of myocardial infarction, not elsewhere classified**

Use additional code to identify the associated myocardial infarction:
with onset of 8 weeks or less (410.00–410.92)
with onset of more than 8 weeks (414.8)

Excludes *congenital defects of heart (745, 746)*
coronary aneurysm (414.11)
disorders of papillary muscle (429.6, 429.81)
postmyocardial infarction syndrome (411.0)
rupture of chordae tendineae (429.5)

429.71 Acquired cardiac septal defect

Excludes *acute septal infarction (410.00–410.92)*

❑ **429.79 Other**
Mural thrombus (atrial) (ventricular) acquired, following myocardial infarction

● **429.8 Other ill-defined heart diseases**

❑ **429.81 Other disorders of papillary muscle**
Papillary muscle:
atrophy
degeneration
dysfunction
incompetence
incoordination
scarring

429.82 Hyperkinetic heart disease

429.83 **Takotsubo syndrome** ◀
Broken heart syndrome ◀
Reversible left ventricular dysfunction following sudden emotional stress ◀
Stress induced cardiomyopathy ◀
Transient left ventricular apical ballooning syndrome ◀

❑429.89 **Other**
Carditis

Excludes *that due to hypertension (402.0–402.9)*

❑429.9 **Heart disease, unspecified**
Heart disease (organic) NOS
Morbus cordis NOS

Excludes *that due to hypertension (402.0–402.9)*

CEREBROVASCULAR DISEASE (430–438)

Includes: with mention of hypertension (conditions classifiable to 401–405)

Use additional code to identify presence of hypertension

Excludes *any condition classifiable to 430–434, 436, 437 occurring during pregnancy, childbirth, or the puerperium, or specified as puerperal (674.0)*
iatrogenic cerebrovascular infarction or hemorrhage (997.02)

430 **Subarachnoid hemorrhage**
Meningeal hemorrhage
Ruptured:
berry aneurysm
(congenital) cerebral aneurysm NOS

Excludes *syphilitic ruptured cerebral aneurysm (094.87)*

431 **Intracerebral hemorrhage**
Hemorrhage (of):
basilar
bulbar
cerebellar
cerebral
cerebromeningeal
cortical
internal capsule
intrapontine
pontine
subcortical
ventricular
Rupture of blood vessel in brain

● 432 **Other and unspecified intracranial hemorrhage**

432.0 **Nontraumatic extradural hemorrhage**
Nontraumatic epidural hemorrhage

432.1 **Subdural hemorrhage**
Subdural hematoma, nontraumatic

❑432.9 **Unspecified intracranial hemorrhage**
Intracranial hemorrhage NOS

● 433 **Occlusion and stenosis of precerebral arteries**

The following fifth-digit subclassification is for use with category 433:
0 **without mention of cerebral infarction**
1 **with cerebral infarction**

Includes: embolism of basilar, carotid, and vertebral arteries
narrowing of basilar, carotid, and vertebral arteries
obstruction of basilar, carotid, and vertebral arteries
thrombosis of basilar, carotid, and vertebral arteries

Excludes *insufficiency NOS of precerebral arteries (435.0–435.9)*

● 433.0 **Basilar artery**

● 433.1 **Carotid artery**

● 433.2 **Vertebral artery**

● 433.3 **Multiple and bilateral**

● ❑433.8 **Other specified precerebral artery**

● ❑433.9 **Unspecified precerebral artery**
Precerebral artery NOS

● 434 **Occlusion of cerebral arteries**

The following fifth-digit subclassification is for use with category 434:
0 **without mention of cerebral infarction**
1 **with cerebral infarction**

● 434.0 **Cerebral thrombosis**
Thrombosis of cerebral arteries

● 434.1 **Cerebral embolism**

● ❑434.9 **Cerebral artery occlusion, unspecified**

● 435 **Transient cerebral ischemia**

Includes: cerebrovascular insufficiency (acute) with transient focal neurological signs and symptoms
insufficiency of basilar, carotid, and vertebral arteries
spasm of cerebral arteries

Excludes *acute cerebrovascular insufficiency NOS (437.1)*
that due to any condition classifiable to 433 (433.0–433.9)

435.0 **Basilar artery syndrome**

435.1 **Vertebral artery syndrome**

435.2 **Subclavian steal syndrome**

435.3 **Vertebrobasilar artery syndrome**

❑435.8 **Other specified transient cerebral ischemias**

❑435.9 **Unspecified transient cerebral ischemia**
Impending cerebrovascular accident
Intermittent cerebral ischemia
Transient ischemic attack [TIA]

436 **Acute, but ill-defined, cerebrovascular disease**
Apoplexy, apoplectic:
NOS
attack
cerebral
seizure
Cerebral seizure

Excludes *any condition classifiable to categories 430–435*
cerebrovascular accident (434.91)
CVA (ischemic) (434.91)
embolic (434.11)
hemorrhagic (430, 431, 432.0–432.9)
thrombotic (434.01)
postoperative cerebrovascular accident (997.02)
stroke (ischemic) (434.91)
embolic (434.11)
hemorrhagic (430, 431, 432.0–432.9)
thrombotic (434.01)

● 437 **Other and ill-defined cerebrovascular disease**

437.0 **Cerebral atherosclerosis**
Atheroma of cerebral arteries
Cerebral arteriosclerosis

❑437.1 **Other generalized ischemic cerebrovascular disease**
Acute cerebrovascular insufficiency NOS
Cerebral ischemia (chronic)

437.2 **Hypertensive encephalopathy**

ICD-9-CM 400-499 Vol. 1

437.3 **Cerebral aneurysm, nonruptured**
Internal carotid artery, intracranial portion
Internal carotid artery NOS

Excludes *congenital cerebral aneurysm, nonruptured (747.81)*
internal carotid artery, extracranial portion (442.81)

437.4 **Cerebral arteritis**

437.5 **Moyamoya disease**

437.6 **Nonpyogenic thrombosis of intracranial venous sinus**

Excludes *pyogenic (325)*

437.7 **Transient global amnesia**

❑437.8 **Other**

❑437.9 **Unspecified**
Cerebrovascular disease or lesion NOS

● 438 **Late effects of cerebrovascular disease**

Note: This category is to be used to indicate conditions in 430–437 as the cause of late effects. The "late effects" include conditions specified as such, or as sequelae, which may occur at any time after the onset of the causal condition.

438.0 **Cognitive deficits**

● 438.1 **Speech and language deficits**

❑438.10 **Speech and language deficit, unspecified**

438.11 **Aphasia**

438.12 **Dysphasia**

❑438.19 **Other speech and language deficits**

● 438.2 **Hemiplegia/hemiparesis**

❑438.20 **Hemiplegia affecting unspecified side**

438.21 **Hemiplegia affecting dominant side**

438.22 **Hemiplegia affecting nondominant side**

● 438.3 **Monoplegia of upper limb**

❑438.30 **Monoplegia of upper limb affecting unspecified side**

438.31 **Monoplegia of upper limb affecting dominant side**

438.32 **Monoplegia of upper limb affecting nondominant side**

● 438.4 **Monoplegia of lower limb**

❑438.40 **Monoplegia of lower limb affecting unspecified side**

438.41 **Monoplegia of lower limb affecting dominant side**

438.42 **Monoplegia of lower limb affecting nondominant side**

● 438.5 **Other paralytic syndrome**

Use additional code to identify type of paralytic syndrome, such as:
locked-in state (344.81)
quadriplegia (344.00–344.09)

Excludes *late effects of cerebrovascular accident with:*
hemiplegia/hemiparesis (438.20–438.22)
monoplegia of lower limb (438.40–438.42)
monoplegia of upper limb (438.40–438.42)

❑438.50 **Other paralytic syndrome affecting unspecified side**

438.51 **Other paralytic syndrome affecting dominant side**

438.52 **Other paralytic syndrome affecting nondominant side**

438.53 **Other paralytic syndrome, bilateral**

438.6 **Alterations of sensations**

Use additional code to identify the altered sensation

438.7 **Disturbances of vision**

Use additional code to identify the visual disturbance

● 438.8 **Other late effects of cerebrovascular disease**

438.81 **Apraxia**

438.82 **Dysphagia**

438.83 **Facial weakness**
Facial droop

438.84 **Ataxia**

438.85 **Vertigo**

❑438.89 **Other late effects of cerebrovascular disease**

❑438.9 **Unspecified late effects of cerebrovascular disease**
Use additional code to identify the late effect

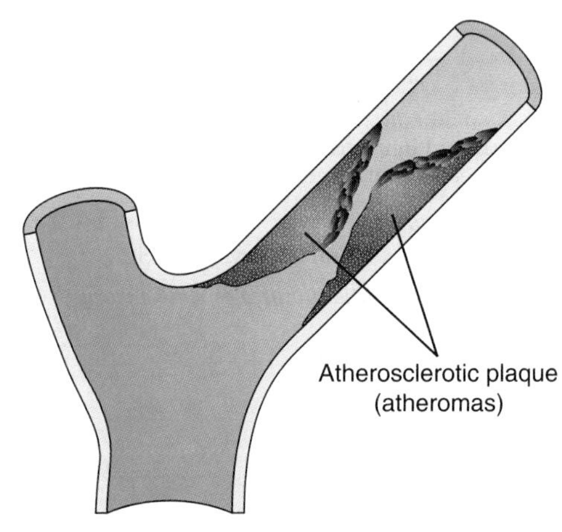
Atherosclerotic plaque
(atheromas)

Figure 7–4 Atherosclerotic plaque.

Item 7–10 Classification is based on the location of the atherosclerosis.

DISEASES OF ARTERIES, ARTERIOLES, AND CAPILLARIES (440–448)

● 440 **Atherosclerosis**

Includes: arteriolosclerosis
arteriosclerosis (obliterans) (senile)
arteriosclerotic vascular disease
atheroma
degeneration:
arterial
arteriovascular
vascular
endarteritis deformans or obliterans
senile:
arteritis
endarteritis

Excludes *atheroembolism (445.01–445.89)*
atherosclerosis of bypass graft of the extremities (440.30–440.32)

440.0 **Of aorta**

440.1 **Of renal artery**

Excludes *atherosclerosis of renal arterioles (403.00–403.91)*

● **440.2 Of native arteries of the extremities**

Excludes *atherosclerosis of bypass graft of the extremities (440.30–440.32)*

❑**440.20 Atherosclerosis of the extremities, unspecified**

440.21 Atherosclerosis of the extremities with intermittent claudication

440.22 Atherosclerosis of the extremities with rest pain

Any condition classifiable to 440.21

440.23 Atherosclerosis of the extremities with ulceration

Any condition classifiable to 440.21–440.22

Use additional code for any associated ulceration (707.10–707.9)

440.24 Atherosclerosis of the extremities with gangrene

Any condition classifiable to 440.21, 440.22, and 440.23 with ischemic gangrene 785.4

Use additional code for any associated ulceration (707.10–707.9) ◀

Excludes *gas gangrene (040.0)*

❑**440.29 Other**

● **440.3 Of bypass graft of the extremities**

Excludes *atherosclerosis of native artery of the extremity (440.21–440.24)*
embolism [occlusion NOS] [thrombus] of graft (996.74)

❑**440.30 Of unspecified graft**

440.31 Of autologous vein bypass graft

440.32 Of nonautologous vein bypass graft

❑**440.8 Of other specified arteries**

Excludes *basilar (433.0)*
carotid (433.1)
cerebral (437.0)
coronary (414.00–414.07)
mesenteric (557.1)
precerebral (433.0–433.9)
pulmonary (416.0)
vertebral (433.2)

❑**440.9 Generalized and unspecified atherosclerosis**

Arteriosclerotic vascular disease NOS

Excludes *arteriosclerotic cardiovascular disease [ASCVD] (429.2)*

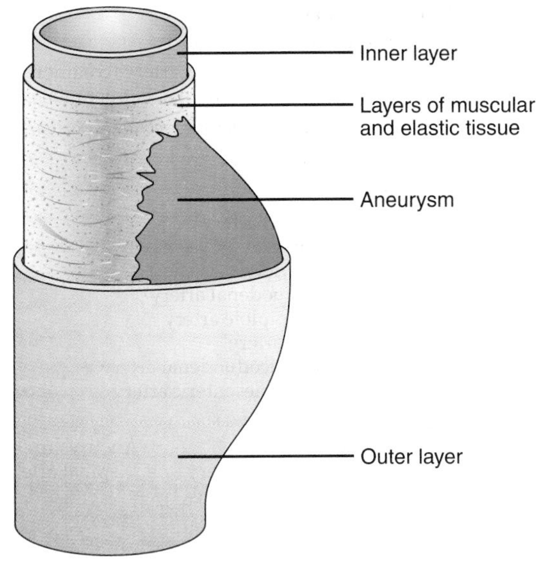

Inner layer
Layers of muscular and elastic tissue
Aneurysm
Outer layer

Figure 7–5 An aneurysm is an enclosed swelling on the wall of the vessel.

Item 7–11 Rupture is the tearing of the aneurysm.

● **441 Aortic aneurysm and dissection**

Excludes *syphilitic aortic aneurysm (093.0)*
traumatic aortic aneurysm (901.0, 902.0)

● **441.0 Dissection of aorta**

❑**441.00 Unspecified site**

441.01 Thoracic

441.02 Abdominal

441.03 Thoracoabdominal

441.1 Thoracic aneurysm, ruptured

441.2 Thoracic aneurysm without mention of rupture

441.3 Abdominal aneurysm, ruptured

441.4 Abdominal aneurysm without mention of rupture

❑**441.5 Aortic aneurysm of unspecified site, ruptured**

Rupture of aorta NOS

441.6 Thoracoabdominal aneurysm, ruptured

441.7 Thoracoabdominal aneurysm, without mention of rupture

❑**441.9 Aortic aneurysm of unspecified site without mention of rupture**

Aneurysm
Dilatation of aorta
Hyaline necrosis of aorta

● **442 Other aneurysm**

Includes: aneurysm (ruptured) (cirsoid) (false) (varicose)
aneurysmal varix

Excludes *arteriovenous aneurysm or fistula:*
acquired (447.0)
congenital (747.60–747.69)
traumatic (900.0–904.9)

442.0 Of artery of upper extremity

442.1 Of renal artery

442.2 Of iliac artery

442.3 Of artery of lower extremity

Aneurysm:
femoral artery
popliteal artery

ICD-9-CM 400-499 Vol. 1

● **442.8 Of other specified artery**

442.81 Artery of neck
Aneurysm of carotid artery (common) (external) (internal, extracranial portion)

Excludes *internal carotid artery, intracranial portion (437.3)*

442.82 Subclavian artery

442.83 Splenic artery

❑ **442.84 Other visceral artery**
Aneurysm:
celiac artery
gastroduodenal artery
gastroepiploic artery
hepatic artery
pancreaticoduodenal artery
superior mesenteric artery

❑ **442.89 Other**
Aneurysm:
mediastinal artery
Aneurysm:
spinal artery

Excludes *cerebral (nonruptured) (437.3)*
congenital (747.81)
ruptured (430)
coronary (414.11)
heart (414.10)
pulmonary (417.1)

❑ **442.9 Of unspecified site**

● **443 Other peripheral vascular disease**

443.0 Raynaud's syndrome
Raynaud's:
disease
phenomenon (secondary)

Use additional code to identify gangrene (785.4)

443.1 Thromboangiitis obliterans [Buerger's disease]
Presenile gangrene

● **443.2 Other arterial dissection**

Excludes *dissection of aorta (441.00–441.03)*
dissection of coronary arteries (414.12)

443.21 Dissection of carotid artery

443.22 Dissection of iliac artery

443.23 Dissection of renal artery

443.24 Dissection of vertebral artery

❑ **443.29 Dissection of other artery**

● **443.8 Other specified peripheral vascular diseases**

● ***443.81 Peripheral angiopathy in diseases classified elsewhere***

Code first underlying disease, as:
diabetes mellitus (250.7)

443.82 Erythromelalgia

❑ **443.89 Other**
Acrocyanosis
Acroparesthesia:
simple [Schultze's type]
vasomotor [Nothnagel's type]
Erythrocyanosis

Excludes *chilblains (991.5)*
frostbite (991.0–991.3)
immersion foot (991.4)

❑ **443.9 Peripheral vascular disease, unspecified**
Intermittent claudication NOS
Peripheral:
angiopathy NOS
vascular disease NOS
Spasm of artery

Excludes *atherosclerosis of the arteries of the extremities (440.20–440.22)*
spasm of cerebral artery (435.0–435.9)

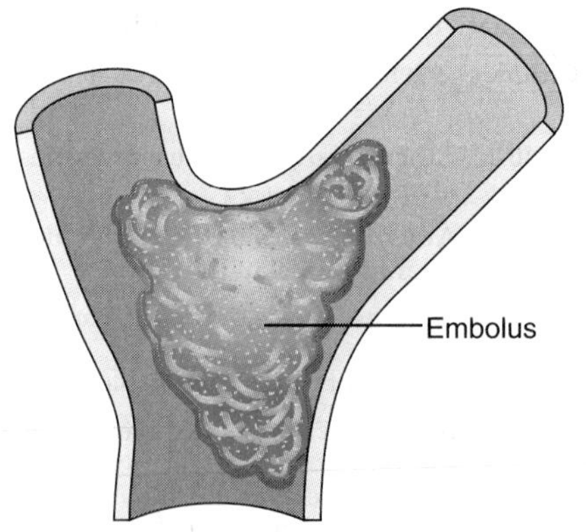
Embolus

Figure 7–6 An arterial embolism.

Item 7–12 An embolus is a mass of undissolved matter present in the blood that is transported by the blood current. A thrombus is a blood clot that occludes or shuts off a vessel. When a thrombus is dislodged, it becomes an embolus.

● **444 Arterial embolism and thrombosis**

Includes: infarction:
embolic
thrombotic
occlusion

Excludes *that complicating:*
abortion (634–638 with .6, 639.6)
atheroembolism (445.01–445.89)
ectopic or molar pregnancy (639.6)
pregnancy, childbirth, or the puerperium (673.0–673.8)

444.0 Of abdominal aorta
Aortic bifurcation syndrome
Aortoiliac obstruction
Leriche's syndrome
Saddle embolus

444.1 Of thoracic aorta
Embolism or thrombosis of aorta (thoracic)

● **444.2 Of arteries of the extremities**

444.21 Upper extremity

444.22 Lower extremity
Arterial embolism or thrombosis:
femoral
popliteal
peripheral NOS

Excludes *iliofemoral (444.81)*

● **444.8 Of other specified artery**

444.81 Iliac artery

❑ **444.89 Other**

Excludes *basilar (433.0)*
carotid (433.1)
cerebral (434.0–434.9)
coronary (410.00–410.92)
mesenteric (557.0)
ophthalmic (362.30–362.34)
precerebral (433.0–433.9)
pulmonary (415.19)
renal (593.81)
retinal (362.30–362.34)
vertebral (433.2)

❑ **444.9 Of unspecified artery**

● 445 Atheroembolism

Includes: atherothrombotic microembolism
cholesterol embolism

● 445.0 Of extremities

445.01 Upper extremity

445.02 Lower extremity

● 445.8 Of other sites

445.81 Kidney

Use additional code for any associated acute renal failure or chronic kidney disease (584, 585)

❑ 445.89 Other site

● 446 Polyarteritis nodosa and allied conditions

446.0 Polyarteritis nodosa
Disseminated necrotizing periarteritis
Necrotizing angiitis
Panarteritis (nodosa)
Periarteritis (nodosa)

446.1 Acute febrile mucocutaneous lymph node syndrome [MCLS]
Kawasaki disease

● 446.2 Hypersensitivity angiitis

Excludes *antiglomerular basement membrane disease without pulmonary hemorrhage (583.89)*

❑ 446.20 Hypersensitivity angiitis, unspecified

446.21 Goodpasture's syndrome
Antiglomerular basement membrane antibody-mediated nephritis with pulmonary hemorrhage

Use additional code to identify renal disease (583.81)

❑ 446.29 Other specified hypersensitivity angiitis

446.3 Lethal midline granuloma
Malignant granuloma of face

446.4 Wegener's granulomatosis
Necrotizing respiratory granulomatosis
Wegener's syndrome

446.5 Giant cell arteritis
Cranial arteritis
Horton's disease
Temporal arteritis

446.6 Thrombotic microangiopathy
Moschcowitz's syndrome
Thrombotic thrombocytopenic purpura

446.7 Takayasu's disease
Aortic arch arteritis
Pulseless disease

● 447 Other disorders of arteries and arterioles

447.0 Arteriovenous fistula, acquired
Arteriovenous aneurysm, acquired

Excludes *cerebrovascular (437.3)*
coronary (414.19)
pulmonary (417.0)
surgically created arteriovenous shunt or fistula:
complication (996.1, 996.61–996.62)
status or presence (V45.1)
traumatic (900.0–904.9)

447.1 Stricture of artery

447.2 Rupture of artery
Erosion of artery
Fistula, except arteriovenous, of artery
Ulcer of artery

Excludes *traumatic rupture of artery (900.0–904.9)*

447.3 Hyperplasia of renal artery
Fibromuscular hyperplasia of renal artery

447.4 Celiac artery compression syndrome
Celiac axis syndrome
Marable's syndrome

447.5 Necrosis of artery

❑ 447.6 Arteritis, unspecified
Aortitis NOS
Endarteritis NOS

Excludes *arteritis, endarteritis:*
aortic arch (446.7)
cerebral (437.4)
coronary (414.00–414.07)
deformans (440.0–440.9)
obliterans (440.0–440.9)
pulmonary (417.8)
senile (440.0–440.9)
polyarteritis NOS (446.0)
syphilitic aortitis (093.1)

❑ 447.8 Other specified disorders of arteries and arterioles
Fibromuscular hyperplasia of arteries, except renal

❑ 447.9 Unspecified disorders of arteries and arterioles

● 448 Disease of capillaries

448.0 Hereditary hemorrhagic telangiectasia
Rendu-Osler-Weber disease

448.1 Nevus, non-neoplastic
Nevus:
araneus
senile
spider
stellar

Excludes *neoplastic (216.0–216.9)*
port wine (757.32)
strawberry (757.32)

❑ 448.9 Other and unspecified capillary diseases
Capillary:
hemorrhage
hyperpermeability
thrombosis

Excludes *capillary fragility (hereditary) (287.8)*

DISEASES OF VEINS AND LYMPHATICS, AND OTHER DISEASES OF CIRCULATORY SYSTEM (451–459)

● 451 Phlebitis and thrombophlebitis

Includes: endophlebitis
inflammation, vein
periphlebitis
suppurative phlebitis

Use additional E code to identify drug, if drug-induced

Excludes *that complicating:*
abortion (634–638 with .7, 639.8)
ectopic or molar pregnancy (639.8)
pregnancy, childbirth, or the puerperium (671.0–671.9)
that due to or following:
implant or catheter device (996.61–996.62)
infusion, perfusion, or transfusion (999.2)

451.0 Of superficial vessels of lower extremities
Saphenous vein (greater) (lesser)

● 451.1 Of deep vessels of lower extremities

451.11 Femoral vein (deep) (superficial)

❑ 451.19 Other
Femoropopliteal vein
Popliteal vein
Tibial vein

❑ 451.2 Of lower extremities, unspecified

● 451.8 **Of other sites**

Excludes *intracranial venous sinus (325)*
nonpyogenic (437.6)
portal (vein) (572.1)

451.81 **Iliac vein**

451.82 **Of superficial veins of upper extremities**
Antecubital vein
Basilic vein
Cephalic vein

451.83 **Of deep veins of upper extremities**
Brachial vein
Radial vein
Ulnar vein

❑ 451.84 **Of upper extremities, unspecified**

❑ 451.89 **Other**
Axillary vein
Jugular vein
Subclavian vein
Thrombophlebitis of breast (Mondor's disease)

❑ 451.9 **Of unspecified site**

452 **Portal vein thrombosis**
Portal (vein) obstruction

Excludes *hepatic vein thrombosis (453.0)*
phlebitis of portal vein (572.1)

● 453 **Other venous embolism and thrombosis**

Excludes *that complicating:*
abortion (634–638 with .7, 639.8)
ectopic or molar pregnancy (639.8)
pregnancy, childbirth, or the puerperium (671.0–671.9)
that with inflammation, phlebitis, and thrombophlebitis (451.0–451.9)

453.0 **Budd-Chiari syndrome**
Hepatic vein thrombosis

453.1 **Thrombophlebitis migrans**

453.2 **Of vena cava**

453.3 **Of renal vein**

● 453.4 **Venous embolism and thrombosis of deep vessels of lower extremity**

❑ 453.40 **Venous embolism and thrombosis of unspecified deep vessels of lower extremity**
Deep vein thrombosis NOS
DVT NOS

453.41 **Venous embolism and thrombosis of deep vessels of proximal lower extremity**
Femoral
Iliac
Popliteal
Thigh
Upper leg NOS

453.42 **Venous embolism and thrombosis of deep vessels of distal lower extremity**
Calf
Lower leg NOS
Peroneal
Tibial

❑ 453.8 **Of other specified veins**

Excludes *cerebral (434.0–434.9)*
coronary (410.00–410.92)
intracranial venous sinus (325)
nonpyogenic (437.6)
mesenteric (557.0)
portal (452)
precerebral (433.0–433.9)
pulmonary (415.19)

❑ 453.9 **Of unspecified site**
Embolism of vein
Thrombosis (vein)

Item 7-13 Varicose/Varicosities (varix = singular, varices = plural): Enlarged, engorged, tortuous, twisted vascular vessels (veins, arteries, lymphatics). As such, the condition can present in various parts of the body, although the most familiar locations are the lower extremities. Varicosities of the anus and rectum are called hemorrhoids. There are additional codes for esophageal, sublingual (under the tongue), scrotal, pelvic, vulval, and nasal varices as well.

● 454 **Varicose veins of lower extremities**

Excludes *that complicating pregnancy, childbirth, or the puerperium (671.0)*

454.0 **With ulcer**
Varicose ulcer (lower extremity, any part)
Varicose veins with ulcer of lower extremity [any part] or of unspecified site
Any condition classifiable to 454.9 with ulcer or specified as ulcerated

454.1 **With inflammation**
Stasis dermatitis
Varicose veins with inflammation of lower extremity [any part] or of unspecified site
Any condition classifiable to 454.9 with inflammation or specified as inflamed

454.2 **With ulcer and inflammation**
Varicose veins with ulcer and inflammation of lower extremity [any part] or of unspecified site
Any condition classifiable to 454.9 with ulcer and inflammation

❑ 454.8 **With other complications**
Edema
Pain
Swelling

454.9 **Asymptomatic varicose veins**
Phlebectasia of lower extremity [any part] or of unspecified site
Varicose veins NOS
Varicose veins of lower extremity [any part] or of unspecified site
Varix of lower extremity [any part] or of unspecified site

● 455 **Hemorrhoids**

Includes: hemorrhoids (anus) (rectum)
piles
varicose veins, anus or rectum

Excludes *that complicating pregnancy, childbirth, or the puerperium (671.8)*

455.0 **Internal hemorrhoids without mention of complication**

455.1 **Internal thrombosed hemorrhoids**

❑ 455.2 **Internal hemorrhoids with other complication**
Internal hemorrhoids:
bleeding
prolapsed
strangulated
ulcerated

455.3 **External hemorrhoids without mention of complication**

455.4 **External thrombosed hemorrhoids**

❑455.5 **External hemorrhoids with other complication**
External hemorrhoids:
bleeding
prolapsed
strangulated
ulcerated

❑455.6 **Unspecified hemorrhoids without mention of complication**
Hemorrhoids NOS

❑455.7 **Unspecified thrombosed hemorrhoids**
Thrombosed hemorrhoids, unspecified whether internal or external

❑455.8 **Unspecified hemorrhoids with other complication**
Hemorrhoids, unspecified whether internal or external:
bleeding
prolapsed
strangulated
ulcerated

455.9 **Residual hemorrhoidal skin tags**
Skin tags, anus or rectum

● 456 **Varicose veins of other sites**

456.0 **Esophageal varices with bleeding**

456.1 **Esophageal varices without mention of bleeding**

● 456.2 **Esophageal varices in diseases classified elsewhere**

Code first underlying disease, as:
cirrhosis of liver (571.0–571.9)
portal hypertension (572.3)

● *456.20 With bleeding*

● *456.21 Without mention of bleeding*

456.3 **Sublingual varices**

456.4 **Scrotal varices**
Varicocele

456.5 **Pelvic varices**
Varices of broad ligament

456.6 **Vulval varices**
Varices of perineum

Excludes *that complicating pregnancy, childbirth, or the puerperium (671.1)*

❑456.8 **Varices of other sites**
Varicose veins of nasal septum (with ulcer)

Excludes *placental varices (656.7)*
retinal varices (362.17)
varicose ulcer of unspecified site (454.0)
varicose veins of unspecified site (454.9)

● 457 **Noninfectious disorders of lymphatic channels**

457.0 **Postmastectomy lymphedema syndrome**
Elephantiasis due to mastectomy
Obliteration of lymphatic vessel due to mastectomy

❑457.1 **Other lymphedema**
Elephantiasis (nonfilarial) NOS
Lymphangiectasis
Lymphedema:
acquired (chronic)
praecox
secondary
Obliteration, lymphatic vessel

Excludes *elephantiasis (nonfilarial):*
congenital (757.0)
eyelid (374.83)
vulva (624.8)

457.2 **Lymphangitis**
Lymphangitis:
NOS
chronic
subacute

Excludes *acute lymphangitis (682.0–682.9)*

❑457.8 **Other noninfectious disorders of lymphatic channels**
Chylocele (nonfilarial)
Chylous:
ascites
cyst
Lymph node or vessel:
fistula
infarction
rupture

Excludes *chylocele:*
filarial (125.0–125.9)
tunica vaginalis (nonfilarial) (608.84)

❑457.9 **Unspecified noninfectious disorder of lymphatic channels**

● 458 **Hypotension**

Includes: hypopiesis

Excludes *cardiovascular collapse (785.50)*
maternal hypotension syndrome (669.2)
shock (785.50–785.59)
Shy-Drager syndrome (333.0)

458.0 **Orthostatic hypotension**
Hypotension:
orthostatic (chronic)
postural
Relates to the patient's postural position. Moving from a sitting or reclining position to a standing position precipitates a sudden drop in blood pressure (hypotension).

458.1 **Chronic hypotension**
Permanent idiopathic hypotension

458.2 **Iatrogenic hypotension**

458.21 **Hypotension of hemodialysis**
Intra-dialytic hypotension

458.29 **Other iatrogenic hypotension**
Postoperative hypotension

❑458.8 **Other specified hypotension**

❑458.9 **Hypotension, unspecified**
Hypotension (arterial) NOS

● 459 **Other disorders of circulatory system**

❑459.0 **Hemorrhage, unspecified**
Rupture of blood vessel NOS
Spontaneous hemorrhage NEC

Excludes *hemorrhage:*
gastrointestinal NOS (578.9)
in newborn NOS (772.9)
secondary or recurrent following trauma (958.2)
traumatic rupture of blood vessel (900.0–904.9)

● 459.1 **Postphlebitic syndrome**
Chronic venous hypertension due to deep vein thrombosis

Excludes *chronic venous hypertension without deep vein thrombosis (459.30–459.39)*

459.10 **Postphlebitic syndrome without complications**
Asymptomatic postphlebitic syndrome
Postphlebitic syndrome NOS

459.11 **Postphlebitic syndrome with ulcer**

459.12 **Postphlebitic syndrome with inflammation**

459.13 Postphlebitic syndrome with ulcer and inflammation

❑**459.19 Postphlebitic syndrome with other complication**

459.2 Compression of vein
Stricture of vein
Vena cava syndrome (inferior) (superior)

●**459.3 Chronic venous hypertension (idiopathic)**
Stasis edema

Excludes *chronic venous hypertension due to deep vein thrombosis (459.10–459.19)*
varicose veins (454.0–454.9)

459.30 Chronic venous hypertension without complications
Asymptomatic chronic venous hypertension
Chronic venous hypertension NOS

459.31 Chronic venous hypertension with ulcer

459.32 Chronic venous hypertension with inflammation

459.33 Chronic venous hypertension with ulcer and inflammation

❑**459.39 Chronic venous hypertension with other complication**

●**459.8 Other specified disorders of circulatory system**

❑**459.81 Venous (peripheral) insufficiency, unspecified**
Chronic venous insufficiency NOS

Use additional code for any associated ulceration (707.10–707.9)

❑**459.89 Other**
Collateral circulation (venous), any site
Phlebosclerosis
Venofibrosis

❑**459.9 Unspecified circulatory system disorder**

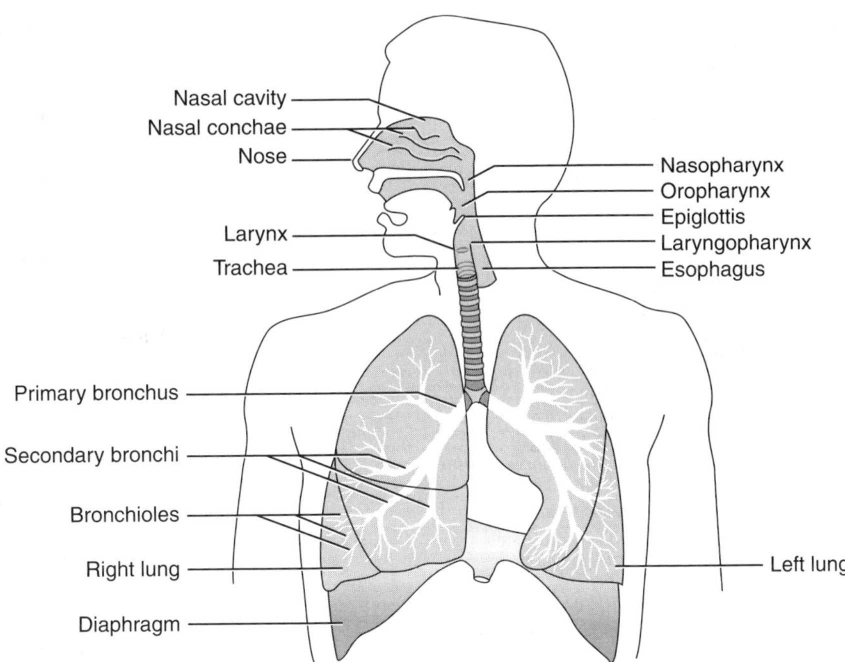
Nasal cavity
Nasal conchae
Nose
Larynx
Trachea
Nasopharynx
Oropharynx
Epiglottis
Laryngopharynx
Esophagus
Primary bronchus
Secondary bronchi
Bronchioles
Right lung
Diaphragm
Left lung

Figure 8–1 Respiratory system. (From Buck CJ: Step-by-Step Medical Coding, 2005 ed. Philadelphia, WB Saunders, 2005.)

8. DISEASES OF THE RESPIRATORY SYSTEM (460–519)

Use additional code to identify infectious organism

ACUTE RESPIRATORY INFECTIONS (460–466)

Excludes *pneumonia and influenza (480.0–487.8)*

460 Acute nasopharyngitis [common cold]
Coryza (acute)
Nasal catarrh, acute
Nasopharyngitis:
NOS
acute
infective NOS
Rhinitis:
acute
infective

Excludes *nasopharyngitis, chronic (472.2)*
pharyngitis:
acute or unspecified (462)
chronic (472.1)
rhinitis:
allergic (477.0–477.9)
chronic or unspecified (472.0)
sore throat:
acute or unspecified (462)
chronic (472.1)

461 Acute sinusitis

Includes: abscess, acute, of sinus (accessory) (nasal)
empyema, acute, of sinus (accessory) (nasal)
infection, acute, of sinus (accessory) (nasal)
inflammation, acute, of sinus (accessory) (nasal)
suppuration, acute, of sinus (accessory) (nasal)

Excludes *chronic or unspecified sinusitis (473.0–473.9)*

461.0 Maxillary
Acute antritis

461.1 Frontal

461.2 Ethmoidal

461.3 Sphenoidal

461.8 Other acute sinusitis
Acute pansinusitis

461.9 Acute sinusitis, unspecified
Acute sinusitis NOS

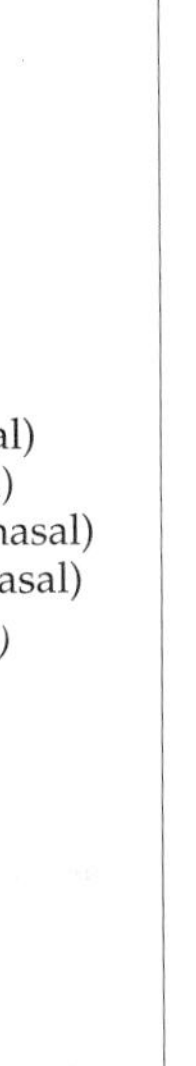

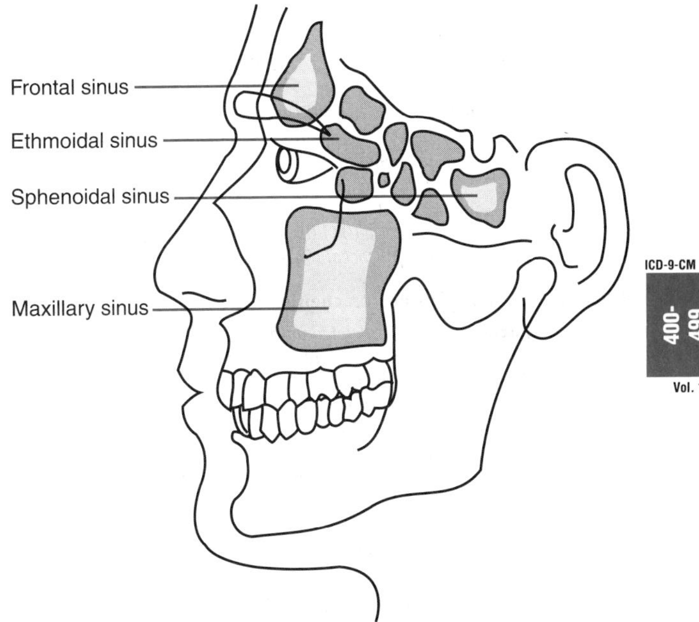
Frontal sinus
Ethmoidal sinus
Sphenoidal sinus
Maxillary sinus

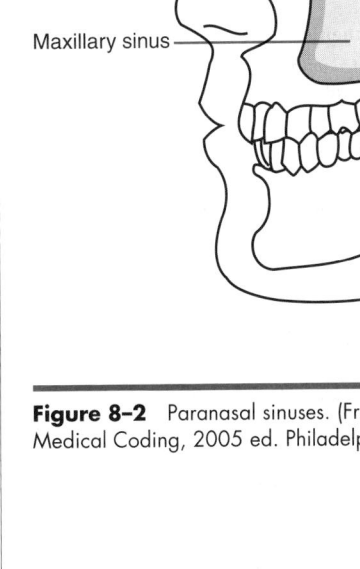

Figure 8–2 Paranasal sinuses. (From Buck CJ: Step-by-Step Medical Coding, 2005 ed. Philadelphia, WB Saunders, 2005.)

462 Acute pharyngitis
Acute sore throat NOS
Pharyngitis (acute):
NOS
gangrenous
infective
phlegmonous
pneumococcal
staphylococcal
suppurative
ulcerative
Sore throat (viral) NOS
Viral pharyngitis

Excludes *abscess:*
peritonsillar [quinsy] (475)
pharyngeal NOS (478.29)
retropharyngeal (478.24)
chronic pharyngitis (472.1)
infectious mononucleosis (075)
that specified as (due to):
Coxsackie (virus) (074.0)
gonococcus (098.6)
herpes simplex (054.79)
influenza (487.1)
septic (034.0)
streptococcal (034.0)

463 Acute tonsillitis
Tonsillitis (acute):
NOS
follicular
gangrenous
infective
pneumococcal
Tonsillitis (acute):
septic
staphylococcal
suppurative
ulcerative
viral

Excludes *chronic tonsillitis (474.0)*
hypertrophy of tonsils (474.1)
peritonsillar abscess [quinsy] (475)
sore throat:
acute or NOS (462)
septic (034.0)
streptococcal tonsillitis (034.0)

● **464 Acute laryngitis and tracheitis**

Excludes *that associated with influenza (487.1)*
that due to Streptococcus (034.0)

● **464.0 Acute laryngitis**
Laryngitis (acute):
NOS
edematous
Hemophilus influenzae [H. influenzae]
pneumococcal
septic
suppurative
ulcerative

Excludes *chronic laryngitis (476.0–476.1)*
influenzal laryngitis (487.1)

464.00 Without mention of obstruction

464.01 With obstruction

● **464.1 Acute tracheitis**
Tracheitis (acute):
NOS
catarrhal
Tracheitis (acute):
viral

Excludes *chronic tracheitis (491.8)*

464.10 Without mention of obstruction

464.11 With obstruction

● **464.2 Acute laryngotracheitis**
Laryngotracheitis (acute)
Tracheitis (acute) with laryngitis (acute)

Excludes *chronic laryngotracheitis (476.1)*

464.20 Without mention of obstruction

464.21 With obstruction

● **464.3 Acute epiglottitis**
Viral epiglottitis

Excludes *epiglottitis, chronic (476.1)*

464.30 Without mention of obstruction

464.31 With obstruction

464.4 Croup
Croup syndrome

● **464.5 Supraglottitis, unspecified**

464.50 Without mention of obstruction

464.51 With obstruction

● **465 Acute upper respiratory infections of multiple or unspecified sites**

Excludes *upper respiratory infection due to:*
influenza (487.1)
Streptococcus (034.0)

465.0 Acute laryngopharyngitis

❑ **465.8 Other multiple sites**
Multiple URI

❑ **465.9 Unspecified site**
Acute URI NOS
Upper respiratory infection (acute)

● **466 Acute bronchitis and bronchiolitis**

Includes: that with:
bronchospasm
obstruction

466.0 Acute bronchitis
Bronchitis, acute or subacute:
fibrinous
membranous
pneumococcal
purulent
Bronchitis, acute or subacute:
septic
viral
with tracheitis
Croupous bronchitis
Tracheobronchitis, acute

Excludes *acute bronchitis with chronic obstructive pulmonary disease (491.22)*

● **466.1 Acute bronchiolitis**
Bronchiolitis (acute)
Capillary pneumonia

466.11 Acute bronchiolitis due to respiratory syncytial virus (RSV)

❑ **466.19 Acute bronchiolitis due to other infectious organisms**
Use additional code to identify organism

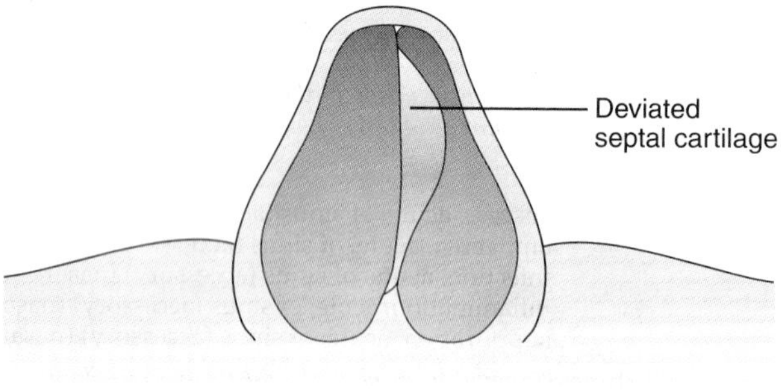

Deviated
septal cartilage

Figure 8–3 Deviated nasal septum.

Item 8–1 A deviated nasal septum is the displacement of the septal cartilage that separates the nares. This displacement causes obstructed air flow through the nasal passages. A child can be born with this displacement (congenital), or the condition may be acquired through trauma, such as a sports injury. Septoplasty is surgical repair of this condition.

OTHER DISEASES OF THE UPPER RESPIRATORY TRACT (470–478)

470 Deviated nasal septum
Deflected septum (nasal) (acquired)
Excludes *congenital (754.0)*

● **471 Nasal polyps**
Excludes *adenomatous polyps (212.0)*

471.0 Polyp of nasal cavity
Polyp:
choanal
nasopharyngeal

471.1 Polypoid sinus degeneration
Woakes' syndrome or ethmoiditis

❑ **471.8 Other polyp of sinus**
Polyp of sinus:
accessory
ethmoidal
maxillary
sphenoidal

❑ **471.9 Unspecified nasal polyp**
Nasal polyp NOS

● **472 Chronic pharyngitis and nasopharyngitis**

472.0 Chronic rhinitis
Ozena
Rhinitis:
NOS
atrophic
granulomatous
hypertrophic
Rhinitis:
obstructive
purulent
ulcerative
Excludes *allergic rhinitis (477.0–477.9)*

472.1 Chronic pharyngitis
Chronic sore throat
Pharyngitis:
atrophic
granular (chronic)
Pharyngitis:
hypertrophic

472.2 Chronic nasopharyngitis
Excludes *acute or unspecified nasopharyngitis (460)*

● **473 Chronic sinusitis**
Includes: abscess (chronic) of sinus (accessory) (nasal)
empyema (chronic) of sinus (accessory) (nasal)
infection (chronic) of sinus (accessory) (nasal)
suppuration (chronic) of sinus (accessory) (nasal)
Excludes *acute sinusitis (461.0–461.9)*

473.0 Maxillary
Antritis (chronic)

473.1 Frontal

473.2 Ethmoidal
Excludes *Woakes' ethmoiditis (471.1)*

473.3 Sphenoidal

❑ **473.8 Other chronic sinusitis**
Pansinusitis (chronic)

❑ **473.9 Unspecified sinusitis (chronic)**
Sinusitis (chronic) NOS

● **474 Chronic disease of tonsils and adenoids**

● **474.0 Chronic tonsillitis and adenoiditis**
Excludes *acute or unspecified tonsillitis (463)*

474.00 Chronic tonsillitis

474.01 Chronic adenoiditis

474.02 Chronic tonsillitis and adenoiditis

● **474.1 Hypertrophy of tonsils and adenoids**
Enlargement of tonsils or adenoids
Hyperplasia of tonsils or adenoids
Hypertrophy of tonsils or adenoids
Excludes *that with:*
adenoiditis (474.01)
adenoiditis and tonsillitis (474.02)
tonsillitis (474.00)

474.10 Tonsils with adenoids

474.11 Tonsils alone

474.12 Adenoids alone

474.2 Adenoid vegetations

❑ **474.8 Other chronic disease of tonsils and adenoids**
Amygdalolith
Calculus, tonsil
Cicatrix of tonsil (and adenoid)
Tonsillar tag
Ulcer, tonsil

❑ **474.9 Unspecified chronic disease of tonsils and adenoids**
Disease (chronic) of tonsils (and adenoids)

475 Peritonsillar abscess
Abscess of tonsil
Peritonsillar cellulitis
Quinsy
Excludes *tonsillitis:*
acute or NOS (463)
chronic (474.0)

● **476 Chronic laryngitis and laryngotracheitis**

476.0 Chronic laryngitis
Laryngitis:
catarrhal
hypertrophic
Laryngitis:
sicca

476.1 Chronic laryngotracheitis
Laryngitis, chronic, with tracheitis (chronic)
Tracheitis, chronic, with laryngitis
Excludes *chronic tracheitis (491.8)*
laryngitis and tracheitis, acute or unspecified (464.00–464.51)

● **477 Allergic rhinitis**
Includes: allergic rhinitis (nonseasonal) (seasonal)
hay fever
spasmodic rhinorrhea
Excludes *allergic rhinitis with asthma (bronchial) (493.0)*

477.0 Due to pollen
Pollinosis

477.1 Due to food

477.2 Due to animal (cat) (dog) hair and dander

❑ **477.8 Due to other allergen**

❑ **477.9 Cause unspecified**

● **478 Other diseases of upper respiratory tract**

478.0 Hypertrophy of nasal turbinates

● **478.1 Other diseases of nasal cavity and sinuses** ⇐
Excludes *varicose ulcer of nasal septum (456.8)*

478.11 Nasal mucositis (ulcerative) ◀

Use additional E code to identify adverse effects of therapy, such as: ◀
antineoplastic and immunosuppressive drugs (E930.7, E933.1) ◀
radiation therapy (E879.2) ◀

❑ **478.19 Other diseases of nasal cavity and sinuses** ◀
Abscess of nose (septum) ◀
Cyst or mucocele of sinus (nasal) ◀
Necrosis of nose (septum) ◀
Rhinolith ◀
Ulcer of nose (septum) ◀

ICD-9-CM 400-499 Vol. 1

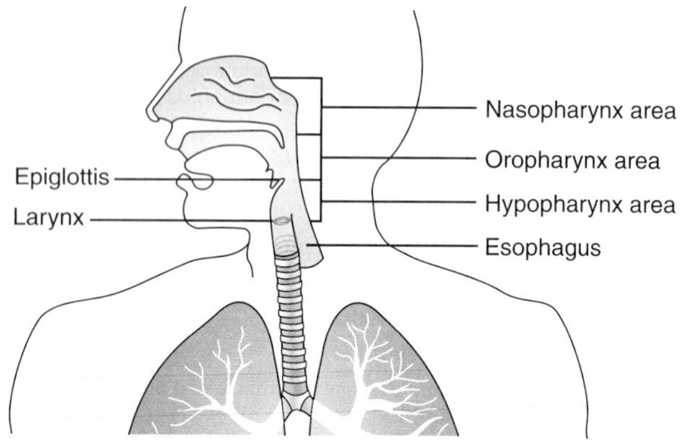
Nasopharynx area
Oropharynx area
Hypopharynx area
Esophagus
Epiglottis
Larynx

Figure 8–4 The pharynx.

Item 8–2 The **pharynx** is the passage for both food and air between the mouth and the esophagus and is divided into three areas: nasopharynx, oropharynx, and hypopharynx. The hypopharynx branches into the esophagus and the voice box.

● **478.2 Other diseases of pharynx, not elsewhere classified**

❑ **478.20 Unspecified disease of pharynx**

478.21 Cellulitis of pharynx or nasopharynx

478.22 Parapharyngeal abscess

478.24 Retropharyngeal abscess

478.25 Edema of pharynx or nasopharynx

478.26 Cyst of pharynx or nasopharynx

❑ **478.29 Other**
Abscess of pharynx or nasopharynx

Excludes *ulcerative pharyngitis (462)*

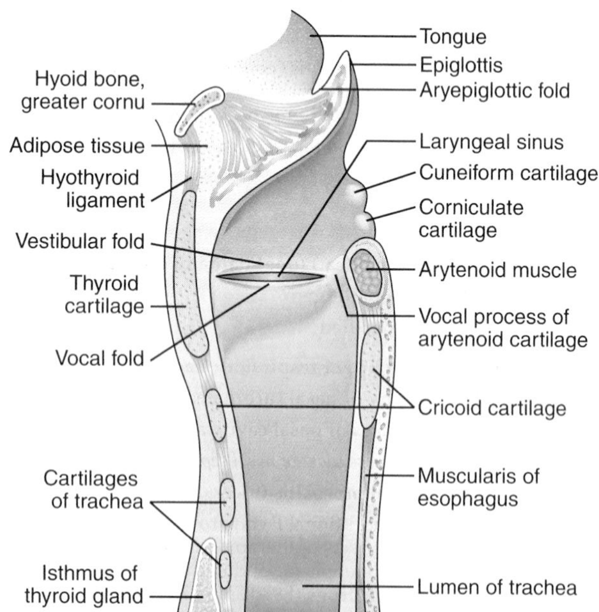
Tongue
Epiglottis
Aryepiglottic fold
Hyoid bone, greater cornu
Adipose tissue
Hyothyroid ligament
Laryngeal sinus
Cuneiform cartilage
Corniculate cartilage
Vestibular fold
Arytenoid muscle
Thyroid cartilage
Vocal process of arytenoid cartilage
Vocal fold
Cricoid cartilage
Cartilages of trachea
Muscularis of esophagus
Isthmus of thyroid gland
Lumen of trachea

Figure 8–5 Coronal section of the larynx.

Item 8–3 The **larynx** extends from the tongue to the trachea and is divided into an upper and lower portion separated by folds. The framework of the larynx is cartilage composed of the single cricoid, thyroid, and epiglottic cartilages, and the paired arytenoid, cuneiform, and corniculate cartilages.

● **478.3 Paralysis of vocal cords or larynx**

❑ **478.30 Paralysis, unspecified**
Laryngoplegia
Paralysis of glottis

478.31 Unilateral, partial

478.32 Unilateral, complete

478.33 Bilateral, partial

478.34 Bilateral, complete

478.4 Polyp of vocal cord or larynx

Excludes *adenomatous polyps (212.1)*

❑ **478.5 Other diseases of vocal cords**
Abscess of vocal cords
Cellulitis of vocal cords
Granuloma of vocal cords
Leukoplakia of vocal cords
Chorditis (fibrinous) (nodosa) (tuberosa)
Singers' nodes

478.6 Edema of larynx
Edema (of):
glottis
subglottic
supraglottic

● **478.7 Other diseases of larynx, not elsewhere classified**

❑ **478.70 Unspecified disease of larynx**

478.71 Cellulitis and perichondritis of larynx

478.74 Stenosis of larynx

478.75 Laryngeal spasm
Laryngismus (stridulus)

❑ **478.79 Other**
Abscess of larynx
Necrosis of larynx
Obstruction of larynx
Pachyderma of larynx
Ulcer of larynx

Excludes *ulcerative laryngitis (464.00–464.01)*

❑ **478.8 Upper respiratory tract hypersensitivity reaction, site unspecified**

Excludes *hypersensitivity reaction of lower respiratory tract, as:*
extrinsic allergic alveolitis (495.0–495.9)
pneumoconiosis (500–505)

❑ **478.9 Other and unspecified diseases of upper respiratory tract**
Abscess of trachea
Cicatrix of trachea

PNEUMONIA AND INFLUENZA (480–487)

Excludes *pneumonia:*
allergic or eosinophilic (518.3)
aspiration:
NOS
newborn (770.18)
solids and liquids (507.0–507.8)
congenital (770.0)
lipoid (507.1)
passive (514)
rheumatic (390)

● 480 **Viral pneumonia**

480.0 **Pneumonia due to adenovirus**

480.1 **Pneumonia due to respiratory syncytial virus**

480.2 **Pneumonia due to parainfluenza virus**

480.3 **Pneumonia due to SARS-associated coronavirus**

❑ 480.8 **Pneumonia due to other virus not elsewhere classified**

Excludes *congenital rubella pneumonitis (771.0)*
influenza with pneumonia, any form (487.0)
pneumonia complicating viral diseases classified elsewhere (484.1–484.8)

❑ 480.9 **Viral pneumonia, unspecified**

481 **Pneumococcal pneumonia [Streptococcus pneumoniae pneumonia]**
Lobar pneumonia, organism unspecified

● 482 **Other bacterial pneumonia**

482.0 **Pneumonia due to Klebsiella pneumoniae**

482.1 **Pneumonia due to Pseudomonas**

482.2 **Pneumonia due to Haemophilus influenzae [H. influenzae]**

● 482.3 **Pneumonia due to Streptococcus**

Excludes *Streptococcus pneumoniae pneumonia (481)*

❑ 482.30 **Streptococcus, unspecified**

482.31 **Group A**

482.32 **Group B**

❑ 482.39 **Other Streptococcus**

● 482.4 **Pneumonia due to Staphylococcus**

❑ 482.40 **Pneumonia due to *Staphylococcus*, unspecified**

482.41 **Pneumonia due to *Staphylococcus aureus***

❑ 482.49 **Other *Staphylococcus* pneumonia**

● 482.8 **Pneumonia due to other specified bacteria**

Excludes *pneumonia complicating infectious disease classified elsewhere (484.1–484.8)*

482.81 **Anaerobes**
Bacteroides (melaninogenicus)
Gram-negative anaerobes

482.82 **Escherichia coli [E. coli]**

❑ 482.83 **Other gram-negative bacteria**
Gram-negative pneumonia NOS
Proteus
Serratia marcescens

Excludes *gram-negative anaerobes (482.81)*
Legionnaires' disease (482.84)

482.84 **Legionnaires' disease**

❑ 482.89 **Other specified bacteria**

❑ 482.9 **Bacterial pneumonia unspecified**

● 483 **Pneumonia due to other specified organism**

483.0 **Mycoplasma pneumoniae**
Eaton's agent
Pleuropneumonia-like organisms [PPLO]

483.1 **Chlamydia**

❑ 483.8 **Other specified organism**

● 484 **Pneumonia in infectious diseases classified elsewhere**

Excludes *influenza with pneumonia, any form (487.0)*

● 484.1 ***Pneumonia in cytomegalic inclusion disease***

Code first underlying disease, as: (078.5)

● 484.3 ***Pneumonia in whooping cough***

Code first underlying disease, as: (033.0–033.9)

● 484.5 ***Pneumonia in anthrax***

Code first underlying disease (022.1)

● 484.6 ***Pneumonia in aspergillosis***

Code first underlying disease (117.3)

● ❑ 484.7 ***Pneumonia in other systemic mycoses***

Code first underlying disease

Excludes *pneumonia in:*
candidiasis (112.4)
coccidioidomycosis (114.0)
histoplasmosis (115.0–115.9 with fifth-digit 5)

● ❑ 484.8 ***Pneumonia in other infectious diseases classified elsewhere***

Code first underlying disease, as:
Q fever (083.0)
typhoid fever (002.0)

Excludes *pneumonia in:*
actinomycosis (039.1)
measles (055.1)
nocardiosis (039.1)
ornithosis (073.0)
Pneumocystis carinii (136.3)
salmonellosis (003.22)
toxoplasmosis (130.4)
tuberculosis (011.6)
tularemia (021.2)
varicella (052.1)

❑ 485 **Bronchopneumonia, organism unspecified**

Bronchopneumonia:	Pneumonia:
hemorrhagic	lobular
terminal	segmental

Pleurobronchopneumonia

Excludes *bronchiolitis (acute) (466.11–466.19)*
chronic (491.8)
lipoid pneumonia (507.1)

❑ 486 **Pneumonia, organism unspecified**

Excludes *hypostatic or passive pneumonia (514)*
influenza with pneumonia, any form (487.0)
inhalation or aspiration pneumonia due to foreign materials (507.0–507.8)
pneumonitis due to fumes and vapors (506.0)

● 487 **Influenza**

Excludes *Hemophilus influenzae [H. influenzae]:*
infection NOS (041.5)
laryngitis (464.00–464.01)
meningitis (320.0)

487.0 **With pneumonia**
Influenza with pneumonia, any form
Influenzal:
bronchopneumonia
pneumonia

Use additional code to identify the type of pneumonia (480.0–480.9, 481, 482.0–482.9, 483.0–483.8, 485)

❑ 487.1 **With other respiratory manifestations**
Influenza NOS
Influenzal:
laryngitis
pharyngitis
respiratory infection (upper) (acute)

❑ 487.8 **With other manifestations**
Encephalopathy due to influenza
Influenza with involvement of gastrointestinal tract

Excludes *"intestinal flu" [viral gastroenteritis] (008.8)*

CHRONIC OBSTRUCTIVE PULMONARY DISEASE AND ALLIED CONDITIONS (490–496)

Item 8-4 Chronic bronchitis is usually defined as being present in any patient who has persistent cough with sputum production for at least three months in at least two consecutive years. **Simple chronic bronchitis** is marked by a productive cough but no pathological airflow obstruction. **Chronic obstructive pulmonary disease (COPD)** is a group of conditions—bronchitis, emphysema, asthma, bronchiectasis, allergic alveolitis—marked by dyspnea. **Catarrhal** bronchitis is an acute form of bronchitis marked by profuse mucus and pus production (**mucopurulent** discharge). **Croupous** bronchitis, also known as pseudomembranous, fibrinous, plastic, exudative, or membranous, is marked by a violent cough and dyspnea.

❑**490 Bronchitis, not specified as acute or chronic**
Bronchitis NOS:
catarrhal
with tracheitis NOS
Tracheobronchitis NOS
Excludes *bronchitis:*
allergic NOS (493.9)
asthmatic NOS (493.9)
due to fumes and vapors (506.0)

●**491 Chronic bronchitis**
Excludes *chronic obstructive asthma (493.2)*

491.0 Simple chronic bronchitis
Catarrhal bronchitis, chronic
Smokers' cough

491.1 Mucopurulent chronic bronchitis
Bronchitis (chronic) (recurrent):
fetid
mucopurulent
purulent

●**491.2 Obstructive chronic bronchitis**
Bronchitis:
emphysematous
obstructive (chronic) (diffuse)
Bronchitis with:
chronic airway obstruction
emphysema
Excludes *asthmatic bronchitis (acute) (NOS) 493.9*
chronic obstructive asthma 493.2

491.20 Without exacerbation
Emphysema with chronic bronchitis

491.21 With (acute) exacerbation
Acute exacerbation of chronic obstructive pulmonary disease [COPD]
Decompensated chronic obstructive pulmonary disease [COPD]
Decompensated chronic obstructive pulmonary disease [COPD] with exacerbation
Excludes *chronic obstructive asthma with acute exacerbation (493.22)*

491.22 With acute bronchitis

❑**491.8 Other chronic bronchitis**
Chronic:
tracheitis
tracheobronchitis

❑**491.9 Unspecified chronic bronchitis**

●**492 Emphysema**

492.0 Emphysematous bleb
Giant bullous emphysema
Ruptured emphysematous bleb
Tension pneumatocele
Vanishing lung

❑**492.8 Other emphysema**
Emphysema (lung or pulmonary):
NOS
centriacinar
centrilobular
obstructive
panacinar
panlobular
unilateral
vesicular
MacLeod's syndrome
Swyer-James syndrome
Unilateral hyperlucent lung
Excludes *emphysema:*
with chronic bronchitis (491.20–491.22)
compensatory (518.2)
due to fumes and vapors (506.4)
interstitial (518.1)
newborn (770.2)
mediastinal (518.1)
surgical (subcutaneous) (998.81)
traumatic (958.7)

Item 8-5 Asthma is a bronchial condition marked by airway obstruction, hyper-responsiveness, and inflammation. **Extrinsic** asthma, also known as allergic asthma, is characterized by the same symptoms that occur with exposure to allergens and is divided into the following types: **atopic, occupational, and allergic bronchopulmonary aspergillosis. Intrinsic** asthma occurs in patients who have no history of allergy or sensitivities to allergens and is divided into the following types: **nonreaginic and pharmacologic. Status asthmaticus** is the most severe form of asthma attack and can last for days or weeks.

●**493 Asthma**
The following fifth-digit subclassification is for use with category 493.0–493.2, 493.9:
0 unspecified
1 with status asthmaticus
2 with (acute) exacerbation
Excludes *wheezing NOS (786.07)*

●**493.0 Extrinsic asthma**
Asthma:
allergic with stated cause
atopic
childhood
hay
platinum
Hay fever with asthma
Excludes *asthma:*
allergic NOS (493.9)
detergent (507.8)
miners' (500)
wood (495.8)

●**493.1 Intrinsic asthma**
Late-onset asthma

●**493.2 Chronic obstructive asthma**
Asthma with chronic obstructive pulmonary disease (COPD)
Chronic asthmatic bronchitis
Excludes *acute bronchitis (466.0)*
chronic obstructive bronchitis (491.20–491.22)

●**493.8 Other forms of asthma**
493.81 Exercise induced bronchospasm
493.82 Cough variant asthma

●❑**493.9 Asthma, unspecified**
Asthma (bronchial) (allergic NOS)
Bronchitis:
allergic
asthmatic

● **494 Bronchiectasis**
Bronchiectasis (fusiform) (postinfectious) (recurrent)
Bronchiolectasis
Excludes *congenital (748.61)*
tuberculous bronchiectasis (current disease) (011.5)

494.0 Bronchiectasis without acute exacerbation

494.1 Bronchiectasis with acute exacerbation

● **495 Extrinsic allergic alveolitis**
Includes: allergic alveolitis and pneumonitis due to inhaled organic dust particles of fungal, thermophilic actinomycete, or other origin

495.0 Farmers' lung

495.1 Bagassosis

495.2 Bird-fanciers' lung
Budgerigar-fanciers' disease or lung
Pigeon-fanciers' disease or lung

495.3 Suberosis
Cork-handlers' disease or lung

495.4 Malt workers' lung
Alveolitis due to Aspergillus clavatus

495.5 Mushroom workers' lung

495.6 Maple bark-strippers' lung
Alveolitis due to Cryptostroma corticale

495.7 "Ventilation" pneumonitis
Allergic alveolitis due to fungal, thermophilic actinomycete, and other organisms growing in ventilation [air conditioning] systems

❑ **495.8 Other specified allergic alveolitis and pneumonitis**
Cheese-washers' lung
Coffee workers' lung
Fish-meal workers' lung
Furriers' lung
Grain-handlers' disease or lung
Pituitary snuff-takers' disease
Sequoiosis or red-cedar asthma
Wood asthma

❑ **495.9 Unspecified allergic alveolitis and pneumonitis**
Alveolitis, allergic (extrinsic)
Hypersensitivity pneumonitis

❑ **496 Chronic airway obstruction, not elsewhere classified**
Chronic:
nonspecific lung disease
obstructive lung disease
obstructive pulmonary disease [COPD] NOS

Note: This code is not to be used with any code from categories 491–493.

Excludes *chronic obstructive lung disease [COPD] specified (as) (with):*
allergic alveolitis (495.0–495.9)
asthma (493.2)
bronchiectasis (494.0–494.1)
bronchitis (491.20–491.22)
with emphysema (491.20–491.22)
decompensated (491.21) ◀
emphysema (492.0–492.8)

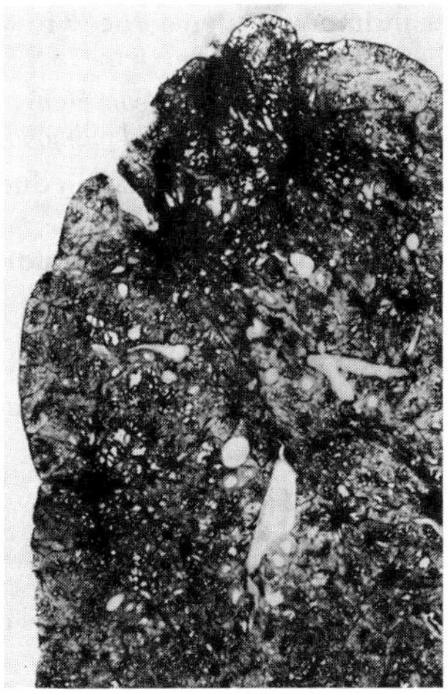

Figure 8–6 Progressive massive fibrosis superimposed on coalworkers' pneumoconiosis. The large, blackened scars are located principally in the upper lobe. Note extensions of scars into surrounding parenchyma and retraction of adjacent pleura. (From Cotran R, Kumar V, Collins T: Robbins Pathologic Basis of Disease, 6th ed. Philadelphia, WB Saunders, 1999, p 730. Courtesy of Dr. Warner Laquer, Dr. Jerome Kleinerman, and the National Institute of Occupational Safety and Health, Morgantown, WV.)

Item 8–6 Pneumoconiosis refers to a lung condition resulting from exposure to inorganic or organic airborne particles, such as coal dust or moldy hay, as well as chemical fumes and vapors, such as insecticides. In this condition, the lungs retain the airborne particles.

PNEUMOCONIOSES AND OTHER LUNG DISEASES DUE TO EXTERNAL AGENTS (500–508)

500 Coal workers' pneumoconiosis
Anthracosilicosis
Anthracosis
Black lung disease
Coal workers' lung
Miners' asthma

501 Asbestosis

❑ **502 Pneumoconiosis due to other silica or silicates**
Pneumoconiosis due to talc
Silicotic fibrosis (massive) of lung
Silicosis (simple) (complicated)

❑ **503 Pneumoconiosis due to other inorganic dust**
Aluminosis (of lung)
Bauxite fibrosis (of lung)
Berylliosis
Graphite fibrosis (of lung)
Siderosis
Stannosis

❑ **504 Pneumonopathy due to inhalation of other dust**
Byssinosis
Cannabinosis
Flax-dressers' disease
Excludes *allergic alveolitis (495.0–495.9)*
asbestosis (501)
bagassosis (495.1)
farmers' lung (495.0)

❑ **505 Pneumoconiosis, unspecified**

● **506 Respiratory conditions due to chemical fumes and vapors**
Use additional E code to identify cause

506.0 Bronchitis and pneumonitis due to fumes and vapors
Chemical bronchitis (acute)

ICD-9-CM 500-599 Vol. 1

506.1 Acute pulmonary edema due to fumes and vapors
Chemical pulmonary edema (acute)

Excludes *acute pulmonary edema NOS (518.4)*
chronic or unspecified pulmonary edema (514)

506.2 Upper respiratory inflammation due to fumes and vapors

❑**506.3 Other acute and subacute respiratory conditions due to fumes and vapors**

506.4 Chronic respiratory conditions due to fumes and vapors
Emphysema (diffuse) (chronic) due to inhalation of chemical fumes and vapors
Obliterative bronchiolitis (chronic) (subacute) due to inhalation of chemical fumes and vapors
Pulmonary fibrosis (chronic) due to inhalation of chemical fumes and vapors

❑**506.9 Unspecified respiratory conditions due to fumes and vapors**
Silo-fillers' disease

● **507 Pneumonitis due to solids and liquids**

Excludes *fetal aspiration pneumonitis (770.18)*

507.0 Due to inhalation of food or vomitus
Aspiration pneumonia (due to):
NOS
food (regurgitated)
gastric secretions
milk
saliva
vomitus

507.1 Due to inhalation of oils and essences
Lipoid pneumonia (exogenous)

Excludes *endogenous lipoid pneumonia (516.8)*

❑**507.8 Due to other solids and liquids**
Detergent asthma

● **508 Respiratory conditions due to other and unspecified external agents**

Use additional E code to identify cause

508.0 Acute pulmonary manifestations due to radiation
Radiation pneumonitis

508.1 Chronic and other pulmonary manifestations due to radiation
Fibrosis of lung following radiation

❑**508.8 Respiratory conditions due to other specified external agents**

❑**508.9 Respiratory conditions due to unspecified external agent**

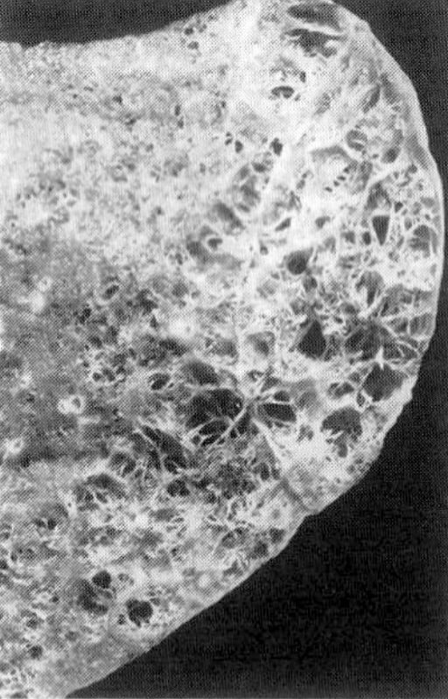

Figure 8–7 The apex of a lung (to the right) in a heavy cigarette smoker with severe emphysema (enlargement and distortion of the airspaces). (From Cotran R, Kumar V, Robbins S: Robbins Pathologic Basis of Disease. Philadelphia, WB Saunders, 1994, p 381.)

Item 8–7 Empyema is a condition in which pus accumulates in a body cavity. Empyema with fistula occurs when the pus passes from one cavity to another organ or structure.

OTHER DISEASES OF RESPIRATORY SYSTEM (510–519)

● **510 Empyema**

Use additional code to identify infectious organism (041.0–041.9)

Excludes *abscess of lung (513.0)*

510.0 With fistula
Fistula:
bronchocutaneous
bronchopleural
hepatopleural
mediastinal
pleural
thoracic
Any condition classifiable to 510.9 with fistula

510.9 Without mention of fistula
Abscess:
pleura
thorax
Empyema (chest) (lung) (pleura)
Fibrinopurulent pleurisy
Pleurisy:
purulent
septic
seropurulent
suppurative
Pyopneumothorax
Pyothorax

● **511 Pleurisy**

Excludes *malignant pleural effusion (197.2)*
pleurisy with mention of tuberculosis, current disease (012.0)

511.0 Without mention of effusion or current tuberculosis
Adhesion, lung or pleura
Calcification of pleura
Pleurisy (acute) (sterile):
diaphragmatic
fibrinous
interlobar
Pleurisy:
NOS
pneumococcal
staphylococcal
streptococcal
Thickening of pleura

❑**511.1 With effusion, with mention of a bacterial cause other than tuberculosis**
Pleurisy with effusion (exudative) (serous):
pneumococcal
staphylococcal
streptococcal
other specified nontuberculous bacterial cause

❑**511.8 Other specified forms of effusion, except tuberculous**
Encysted pleurisy
Hemopneumothorax
Hemothorax
Hydropneumothorax
Hydrothorax

Excludes *traumatic (860.2–860.5, 862.29, 862.39)*

❑**511.9 Unspecified pleural effusion**
Pleural effusion NOS
Pleurisy:
exudative
serofibrinous
serous
with effusion NOS

● **512 Pneumothorax**

512.0 Spontaneous tension pneumothorax

512.1 Iatrogenic pneumothorax
Postoperative pneumothorax

❑**512.8 Other spontaneous pneumothorax**
Pneumothorax:
NOS
acute
chronic

Excludes *pneumothorax:*
congenital (770.2)
traumatic (860.0–860.1, 860.4–860.5)
tuberculous, current disease (011.7)

● **513 Abscess of lung and mediastinum**

513.0 Abscess of lung
Abscess (multiple) of lung
Gangrenous or necrotic pneumonia
Pulmonary gangrene or necrosis

513.1 Abscess of mediastinum

514 Pulmonary congestion and hypostasis
Hypostatic:
bronchopneumonia
pneumonia
Passive pneumonia
Pulmonary congestion (chronic) (passive)
Pulmonary edema:
NOS
chronic

Excludes *acute pulmonary edema:*
NOS (518.4)
with mention of heart disease or failure (428.1)
hypostatic pneumonia due to or specified as a specific type of pneumonia—code to the type of pneumonia (480.0–480.9, 481, 482.0–482.49, 483.0–483.8, 485, 486, 487.0) ◀

515 Postinflammatory pulmonary fibrosis
Cirrhosis of lung chronic or unspecified
Fibrosis of lung (atrophic) (confluent) (massive) (perialveolar) (peribronchial) chronic or unspecified
Induration of lung chronic or unspecified

● **516 Other alveolar and parietoalveolar pneumonopathy**

516.0 Pulmonary alveolar proteinosis

● ***516.1 Idiopathic pulmonary hemosiderosis***
Essential brown induration of lung

Code first underlying disease (275.0)

516.2 Pulmonary alveolar microlithiasis

516.3 Idiopathic fibrosing alveolitis
Alveolar capillary block
Diffuse (idiopathic) (interstitial) pulmonary fibrosis
Hamman-Rich syndrome

❑**516.8 Other specified alveolar and parietoalveolar pneumonopathies**
Endogenous lipoid pneumonia
Interstitial pneumonia (desquamative) (lymphoid)

Excludes *lipoid pneumonia, exogenous or unspecified (507.1)*

❑**516.9 Unspecified alveolar and parietoalveolar pneumonopathy**

● **517 Lung involvement in conditions classified elsewhere**

Excludes *rheumatoid lung (714.81)*

● ***517.1 Rheumatic pneumonia***

Code first underlying disease (390)

● ***517.2 Lung involvement in systemic sclerosis***

Code first underlying disease (710.1)

● ***517.3 Acute chest syndrome***

Code first sickle-cell disease in crisis (282.42, 282.62, 282.64, 282.69)

● ❑***517.8 Lung involvement in other diseases classified elsewhere***

Code first underlying disease, as:
amyloidosis (277.30–277.39) ⬅
polymyositis (710.4)
sarcoidosis (135)
Sjögren's disease (710.2)
systemic lupus erythematosus (710.0)

Excludes *syphilis (095.1)*

● **518 Other diseases of lung**

518.0 Pulmonary collapse
Atelectasis
Collapse of lung
Middle lobe syndrome

Excludes *atelectasis:*
congenital (partial) (770.5)
primary (770.4)
tuberculous, current disease (011.8)

518.1 Interstitial emphysema
Mediastinal emphysema

Excludes *surgical (subcutaneous) emphysema (998.81)*
that in fetus or newborn (770.2)
traumatic emphysema (958.7)

518.2 Compensatory emphysema

518.3 Pulmonary eosinophilia
Eosinophilic asthma
Löffler's syndrome
Pneumonia:
allergic
eosinophilic
Tropical eosinophilia

❑**518.4 Acute edema of lung, unspecified**
Acute pulmonary edema NOS
Pulmonary edema, postoperative

Excludes *pulmonary edema:*
acute, with mention of heart disease or failure (428.1)
chronic or unspecified (514)
due to external agents (506.0–508.9)

518.5 Pulmonary insufficiency following trauma and surgery
Adult respiratory distress syndrome
Pulmonary insufficiency following:
shock
surgery
trauma
Shock lung

Excludes *adult respiratory distress syndrome associated with other conditions (518.82)*
pneumonia:
aspiration (507.0)
hypostatic (514)
respiratory failure in other conditions (518.81, 518.83–518.84)

518.6 Allergic bronchopulmonary aspergillosis

518.7 Transfusion related acute lung injury (TRALI) ◀

● **518.8 Other diseases of lung**

518.81 Acute respiratory failure
Respiratory failure NOS

Excludes *acute and chronic respiratory failure (518.84)*
acute respiratory distress (518.82)
chronic respiratory failure (518.83)
respiratory arrest (799.1)
respiratory failure, newborn (770.84)

❑518.82 **Other pulmonary insufficiency, not elsewhere classified**
Acute respiratory distress
Acute respiratory insufficiency
Adult respiratory distress syndrome NEC

Excludes *adult respiratory distress syndrome associated with trauma or surgery (518.5)*
pulmonary insufficiency following trauma or surgery (518.5)
respiratory distress:
NOS (786.09)
newborn (770.89)
syndrome, newborn (769)
shock lung (518.5)

518.83 **Chronic respiratory failure**

518.84 **Acute and chronic respiratory failure**
Acute on chronic respiratory failure

❑518.89 **Other diseases of lung, not elsewhere classified**
Broncholithiasis
Calcification of lung
Lung disease NOS
Pulmolithiasis

● 519 **Other diseases of respiratory system**

● 519.0 **Tracheostomy complications**

❑519.00 **Tracheostomy complication, unspecified**

519.01 **Infection of tracheostomy**

Use additional code to identify type of infection, such as:
abscess or cellulitis of neck (682.1)
septicemia (038.0–038.9)

Use additional code to identify organism (041.00–041.9)

519.02 **Mechanical complication of tracheostomy**
Tracheal stenosis due to tracheostomy

519.09 **Other tracheostomy complications**
Hemorrhage due to tracheostomy
Tracheoesophageal fistula due to tracheostomy

● 519.1 **Other diseases of trachea and bronchus, not elsewhere classified** ⬅

519.11 **Acute bronchospasm** ◀
Bronchospasm NOS ◀

Excludes *acute bronchitis with bronchospasm (466.0)* ◀
asthma (493.00–493.92) ◀
exercise induced bronchospasm (493.81) ◀

❑519.19 **Other diseases of trachea and bronchus** ◀
Calcification of bronchus or trachea ◀
Stenosis of bronchus or trachea ◀
Ulcer of bronchus or trachea ◀

519.2 **Mediastinitis**

❑519.3 **Other diseases of mediastinum, not elsewhere classified**
Fibrosis of mediastinum
Hernia of mediastinum
Retraction of mediastinum

519.4 **Disorders of diaphragm**
Diaphragmitis
Paralysis of diaphragm
Relaxation of diaphragm

Excludes *congenital defect of diaphragm (756.6)*
diaphragmatic hernia (551–553 with .3)
congenital (756.6)

❑519.8 **Other diseases of respiratory system, not elsewhere classified**

❑519.9 **Unspecified disease of respiratory system**
Respiratory disease (chronic) NOS

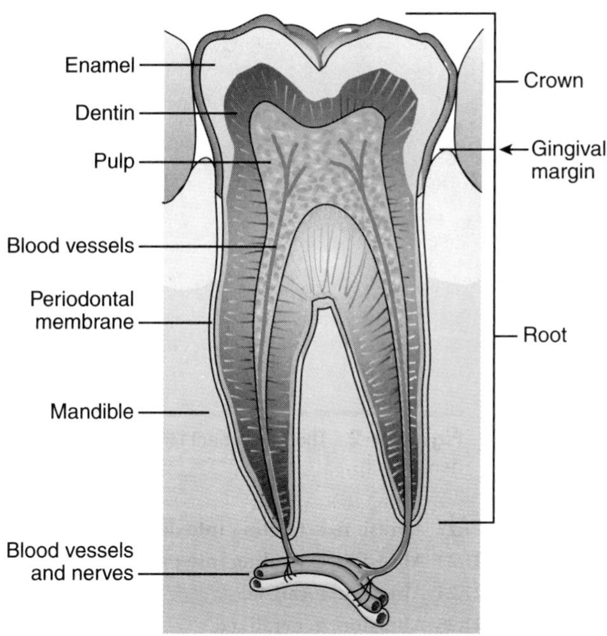
Enamel
Dentin
Pulp
Blood vessels
Periodontal membrane
Mandible
Blood vessels and nerves
Crown
Gingival margin
Root

Figure 9–1 Anatomy of a tooth.

Item 9–1 **Anodontia** is the congenital absence of teeth. **Hypodontia** is partial anodontia. **Oligodontia** is the congenital absence of some teeth, whereas **supernumerary** is having more teeth than the normal number. **Mesiodens** are small extra teeth that often appear in pairs, although single small teeth are not uncommon.

9. DISEASES OF THE DIGESTIVE SYSTEM (520–579)

DISEASES OF ORAL CAVITY, SALIVARY GLANDS, AND JAWS (520–529)

● **520 Disorders of tooth development and eruption**

520.0 Anodontia
Absence of teeth (complete) (congenital) (partial)
Hypodontia
Oligodontia

Excludes *acquired absence of teeth (525.10–525.19)*

520.1 Supernumerary teeth
Distomolar
Fourth molar
Mesiodens
Paramolar
Supplemental teeth

Excludes *supernumerary roots (520.2)*

520.2 Abnormalities of size and form
Concrescence of teeth
Fusion of teeth
Gemination of teeth
Dens evaginatus
Dens in dente
Dens invaginatus
Enamel pearls
Macrodontia
Microdontia
Peg-shaped [conical] teeth
Supernumerary roots
Taurodontism
Tuberculum paramolare

Excludes *that due to congenital syphilis (090.5)*
tuberculum Carabelli, which is regarded as a normal variation

520.3 Mottled teeth
Dental fluorosis
Mottling of enamel
Nonfluoride enamel opacities

520.4 Disturbances of tooth formation
Aplasia and hypoplasia of cementum
Dilaceration of tooth
Enamel hypoplasia (neonatal) (postnatal) (prenatal)
Horner's teeth
Hypocalcification of teeth
Regional odontodysplasia
Turner's tooth

Excludes *Hutchinson's teeth and mulberry molars in congenital syphilis (090.5)*
mottled teeth (520.3)

520.5 Hereditary disturbances in tooth structure, not elsewhere classified
Amelogenesis imperfecta
Dentinogenesis imperfecta
Odontogenesis imperfecta
Dentinal dysplasia
Shell teeth

520.6 Disturbances in tooth eruption
Teeth:
- embedded
- impacted
- natal
- neonatal
- prenatal
- primary [deciduous]:
  - persistent
  - shedding, premature

Tooth eruption:
- late
- obstructed
- premature

Excludes *exfoliation of teeth (attributable to disease of surrounding tissues) (525.0–525.19)*

520.7 Teething syndrome

❑ **520.8 Other specified disorders of tooth development and eruption**
Color changes during tooth formation
Pre-eruptive color changes

Excludes *posteruptive color changes (521.7)*

❑ **520.9 Unspecified disorder of tooth development and eruption**

ICD-9-CM 500-599 Vol. 1

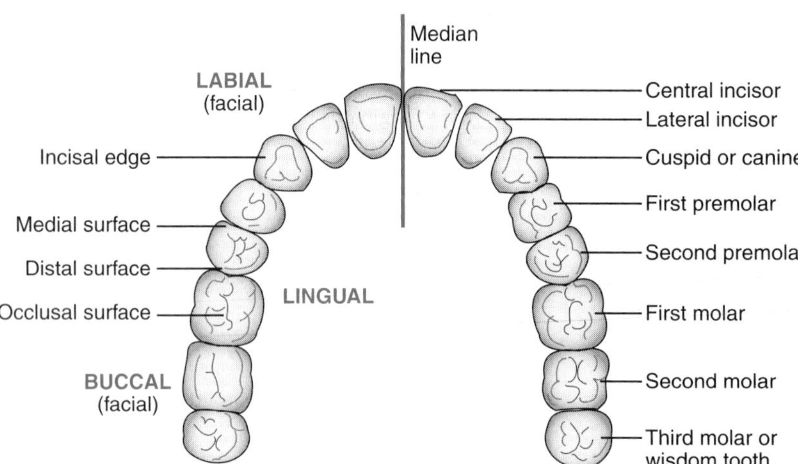
Median line
LABIAL (facial)
Incisal edge
Medial surface
Distal surface
Occlusal surface
LINGUAL
BUCCAL (facial)
Central incisor
Lateral incisor
Cuspid or canine
First premolar
Second premolar
First molar
Second molar
Third molar or wisdom tooth

Figure 9–2 The permanent teeth within the dental arch.

Item 9-2 Each dental arch (jaw) normally contains 16 teeth. Tooth decay or dental caries is a disease of the enamel, dentin, and cementum of the tooth and can result in a cavity.

● **521 Diseases of hard tissues of teeth**

● **521.0 Dental caries**

❑ **521.00 Dental caries, unspecified**

521.01 Dental caries limited to enamel
Initial caries
White spot lesion

521.02 Dental caries extending into dentin

521.03 Dental caries extending into pulp

521.04 Arrested dental caries

521.05 Odontoclasia
Infantile melanodontia
Melanodontoclasia

Excludes *internal and external resorption of teeth (521.40–521.49)*

521.06 Dental caries pit and fissure
Primary dental caries, pit and fissure origin ◀

521.07 Dental caries of smooth surface
Primary dental caries, smooth surface origin ◀

521.08 Dental caries of root surface
Primary dental caries, root surface ◀

❑ **521.09 Other dental caries**

● **521.1 Excessive attrition (approximal wear) (occlusal wear)**

❑ **521.10 Excessive attrition, unspecified**

521.11 Excessive attrition, limited to enamel

521.12 Excessive attrition, extending into dentine

521.13 Excessive attrition, extending into pulp

521.14 Excessive attrition, localized

521.15 Excessive attrition, generalized

● **521.2 Abrasion**
Abrasion of teeth:
dentifrice
habitual
occupational
ritual
traditional
Wedge defect NOS of teeth

❑ **521.20 Abrasion, unspecified**

521.21 Abrasion, limited to enamel

521.22 Abrasion, extending into dentine

521.23 Abrasion, extending into pulp

521.24 Abrasion, localized

521.25 Abrasion, generalized

● **521.3 Erosion**
Erosion of teeth:
NOS
due to:
medicine
persistent vomiting
idiopathic
occupational

❑ **521.30 Erosion, unspecified**

521.31 Erosion, limited to enamel

521.32 Erosion, extending into dentine

521.33 Erosion, extending into pulp

521.34 Erosion, localized

521.35 Erosion, generalized

● **521.4 Pathological resorption**

❑ **521.40 Pathological resorption, unspecified**

521.41 Pathological resorption, internal

521.42 Pathological resorption, external

❑ **521.49 Other pathological resorption**
Internal granuloma of pulp

521.5 Hypercementosis
Cementation hyperplasia

521.6 Ankylosis of teeth

521.7 Intrinsic posteruptive color changes
Staining [discoloration] of teeth:
NOS
due to:
drugs
metals
pulpal bleeding

Excludes *accretions [deposits] on teeth (523.6)*
extrinsic color changes (523.6)
pre-eruptive color changes (520.8)

● **521.8 Other specified diseases of hard tissues of teeth** ⬅

521.81 Cracked tooth ◀

Excludes *asymptomatic craze lines in enamel – omit code* ◀
broken tooth due to trauma (873.63, 873.73) ◀
fractured tooth due to trauma (873.63, 873.73) ◀

❑521.89 **Other specified diseases of hard tissues of teeth** ◀
Irradiated enamel ◀
Sensitive dentin ◀

❑521.9 **Unspecified disease of hard tissues of teeth**

● 522 **Diseases of pulp and periapical tissues**

522.0 **Pulpitis**
Pulpal:
abscess
polyp
Pulpitis:
acute
chronic (hyperplastic) (ulcerative)
suppurative

522.1 **Necrosis of the pulp**
Pulp gangrene

522.2 **Pulp degeneration**
Denticles
Pulp stones
Pulp calcifications

522.3 **Abnormal hard tissue formation in pulp**
Secondary or irregular dentin

522.4 **Acute apical periodontitis of pulpal origin**

522.5 **Periapical abscess without sinus**
Abscess:
dental
dentoalveolar

Excludes *periapical abscess with sinus (522.7)*

522.6 **Chronic apical periodontitis**
Apical or periapical granuloma
Apical periodontitis NOS

522.7 **Periapical abscess with sinus**
Fistula:
alveolar process
dental

522.8 **Radicular cyst**
Cyst:
apical (periodontal)
periapical
radiculodental
residual radicular

Excludes *lateral developmental or lateral periodontal cyst (526.0)*

❑522.9 **Other and unspecified diseases of pulp and periapical tissues**

Item 9-3 Acute gingivitis, also known as orilitis or ulitis, is the short-term, severe inflammation of the gums (gingiva) caused by bacteria. **Chronic gingivitis** is persistent inflammation of the gums. When the gingivitis moves into the periodontium it is called periodontitis, also known as paradentitis.

● 523 **Gingival and periodontal diseases**

● 523.0 **Acute gingivitis** ⬅

Excludes *acute necrotizing ulcerative gingivitis (101)*
herpetic gingivostomatitis (054.2)

523.00 **Acute gingivitis, plaque induced** ◀
Acute gingivitis NOS ◀

523.01 **Acute gingivitis, non-plaque induced** ◀

● 523.1 **Chronic gingivitis** ⬅
Gingivitis (chronic):
desquamative
hyperplastic
simple marginal
ulcerative

Excludes *herpetic gingivostomatitis (054.2)*

523.10 **Chronic gingivitis, plaque induced** ◀
Chronic gingivitis NOS ◀
Gingivitis NOS ◀

523.11 **Chronic gingivitis, non-plaque induced** ◀

● 523.2 **Gingival recession**
Gingival recession (postinfective) (postoperative)

❑523.20 **Gingival recession, unspecified**

523.21 **Gingival recession, minimal**

523.22 **Gingival recession, moderate**

523.23 **Gingival recession, severe**

523.24 **Gingival recession, localized**

523.25 **Gingival recession, generalized**

● 523.3 **Aggressive and acute periodontitis** ⬅
Acute:
pericementitis
pericoronitis

Excludes *acute apical periodontitis (522.4)*
periapical abscess (522.5, 522.7)

❑523.30 **Aggressive periodontitis, unspecified** ◀

523.31 **Aggressive periodontitis, localized** ◀
Periodontal abscess ◀

523.32 **Aggressive periodontitis, generalized** ◀

523.33 **Acute periodontitis** ◀

● 523.4 **Chronic periodontitis** ⬅
Chronic pericoronitis
Pericementitis (chronic)
Periodontitis:
NOS
complex
simplex

Excludes *chronic apical periodontitis (522.6)*

❑523.40 **Chronic periodontitis, unspecified** ◀

523.41 **Chronic periodontitis, localized** ◀

523.42 **Chronic periodontitis, generalized** ◀

523.5 **Periodontosis**

523.6 **Accretions on teeth**
Dental calculus:
subgingival
supragingival
Deposits on teeth:
betel
materia alba
soft
tartar
tobacco
Extrinsic discoloration of teeth

Excludes *intrinsic discoloration of teeth (521.7)*

❑523.8 **Other specified periodontal diseases**
Giant cell:
epulis
peripheral granuloma
Gingival:
cysts
enlargement NOS
fibromatosis
Gingival polyp
Periodontal lesions due to traumatic occlusion
Peripheral giant cell granuloma

Excludes *leukoplakia of gingiva (528.6)*

❑523.9 **Unspecified gingival and periodontal disease**

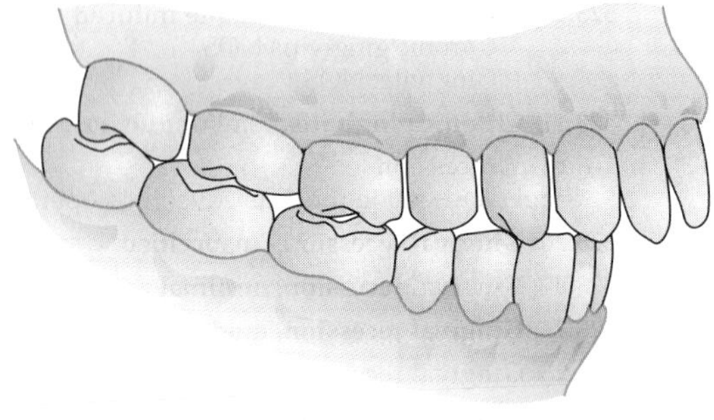

Figure 9–3 Dentofacial malocclusion.

Item 9–4 Hyperplasia is a condition of overdevelopment, whereas hypoplasia is a condition of underdevelopment. Macrogenia is overdevelopment of the chin, whereas microgenia is underdevelopment of the chin.

● **524 Dentofacial anomalies, including malocclusion**

● **524.0 Major anomalies of jaw size**

Excludes *hemifacial atrophy or hypertrophy (754.0)*
unilateral condylar hyperplasia or hypoplasia of mandible

❑ **524.00 Unspecified anomaly**

524.01 Maxillary hyperplasia

524.02 Mandibular hyperplasia

524.03 Maxillary hypoplasia

524.04 Mandibular hypoplasia

524.05 Macrogenia

524.06 Microgenia

524.07 Excessive tuberosity of jaw
Entire maxillary tuberosity ◀

❑ **524.09 Other specified anomaly**

● **524.1 Anomalies of relationship of jaw to cranial base**

❑ **524.10 Unspecified anomaly**
Prognathism Retrognathism

524.11 Maxillary asymmetry

❑ **524.12 Other jaw asymmetry**

❑ **524.19 Other specified anomaly**

● **524.2 Anomalies of dental arch relationship**
Anomaly of dental arch ◀

Excludes *hemifacial atrophy or hypertrophy (754.0)*
soft tissue impingement (524.81–524.82)
unilateral condylar hyperplasia or hypoplasia of mandible (526.89)

❑ **524.20 Unspecified anomaly of dental arch relationship**

524.21 Malocclusion, Angle's class I ⬅
Neutro-occlusion

524.22 Malocclusion, Angle's class II ⬅
Disto-occlusion Division I
Disto-occlusion Division II

524.23 Malocclusion, Angle's class III ⬅
Mesio-occlusion

524.24 Open anterior occlusal relationship
Anterior open bite ◀

524.25 Open posterior occlusal relationship
Posterior open bite ◀

524.26 Excessive horizontal overlap
Excessive horizontal overjet ◀

524.27 Reverse articulation
Anterior articulation
Crossbite ◀
Posterior articulation

524.28 Anomalies of interarch distance
Excessive interarch distance
Inadequate interarch distance

524.29 Other anomalies of dental arch relationship
Other anomalies of dental arch ◀

● **524.3 Anomalies of tooth position of fully erupted teeth**

Excludes *impacted or embedded teeth with abnormal position of such teeth or adjacent teeth (520.6)*

❑ **524.30 Unspecified anomaly of tooth position**
Diastema of teeth NOS
Displacement of teeth NOS
Transposition of teeth NOS

524.31 Crowding of teeth

524.32 Excessive spacing of teeth

524.33 Horizontal displacement of teeth
Tipped teeth ◀
Tipping of teeth

524.34 Vertical displacement of teeth
Extruded tooth ◀
Infraeruption of teeth
Intruded tooth ◀
Supraeruption of teeth

524.35 Rotation of tooth/teeth ⬅

524.36 Insufficient interocclusal distance of teeth (ridge)
Lack of adequate intermaxillary vertical dimension ◀

524.37 Excessive interocclusal distance of teeth
Excessive intermaxillary vertical dimension ◀
Loss of occlusal vertical dimension

524.39 Other anomalies of tooth position

❑ **524.4 Malocclusion, unspecified**

● **524.5 Dentofacial functional abnormalities**

❑ **524.50 Dentofacial functional abnormality, unspecified**

524.51 Abnormal jaw closure

524.52 Limited mandibular range of motion

524.53 Deviation in opening and closing of the mandible

524.54 Insufficient anterior guidance
Insufficient anterior occlusal guidance ◀

524.55 Centric occlusion maximum intercuspation discrepancy
Centric occlusion of teeth discrepancy ◀

524.56 Non-working side interference
Balancing side interference ◀

524.57 Lack of posterior occlusal support

❑ **524.59 Other dentofacial functional abnormalities**
Abnormal swallowing
Mouth breathing
Sleep postures
Tongue, lip, or finger habits

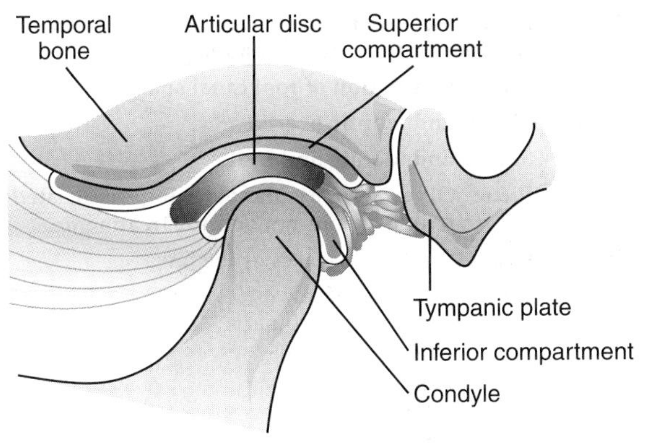
Temporal bone
Articular disc
Superior compartment
Tympanic plate
Inferior compartment
Condyle

Figure 9–4 Temporomandibular joint.

Item 9-5 Dysfunction of the temporomandibular joint is termed temporomandibular joint (TMJ) syndrome and is characterized by pain and tenderness/spasm of the muscles of mastication, joint noise, and in the later stages, limited mandibular movement.

● **524.6 Temporomandibular joint disorders**

Excludes *current temporomandibular joint:*
dislocation (830.0–830.1)
strain (848.1)

❑ **524.60 Temporomandibular joint disorders, unspecified**
Temporomandibular joint-pain-dysfunction syndrome [TMJ]

524.61 Adhesions and ankylosis (bony or fibrous)

524.62 Arthralgia of temporomandibular joint

524.63 Articular disc disorder (reducing or nonreducing)

524.64 Temporomandibular joint sounds on opening and/or closing the jaw

❑ **524.69 Other specified temporomandibular joint disorders**

● **524.7 Dental alveolar anomalies**

❑ **524.70 Unspecified alveolar anomaly**

524.71 Alveolar maxillary hyperplasia

524.72 Alveolar mandibular hyperplasia

524.73 Alveolar maxillary hypoplasia

524.74 Alveolar mandibular hypoplasia

524.75 Vertical displacement of alveolus and teeth
Extrusion of alveolus and teeth

524.76 Occlusal plane deviation

❑ **524.79 Other specified alveolar anomaly**

● **524.8 Other specified dentofacial anomalies**

524.81 Anterior soft tissue impingement

524.82 Posterior soft tissue impingement

❑ **524.89 Other specified dentofacial anomalies**

❑ **524.9 Unspecified dentofacial anomalies**

● **525 Other diseases and conditions of the teeth and supporting structures**

525.0 Exfoliation of teeth due to systemic causes

● *525.1 Loss of teeth due to trauma, extraction, or periodontal disease*

Code first class of edentulism (525.40–525.44, 525.50–525.54)

● ❑ *525.10 Acquired absence of teeth, unspecified*
Tooth extraction status, NOS

● *525.11 Loss of teeth due to trauma*

● *525.12 Loss of teeth due to periodontal disease*

● *525.13 Loss of teeth due to caries*

● ❑ *525.19 Other loss of teeth*

● **525.2 Atrophy of edentulous alveolar ridge**

❑ **525.20 Unspecified atrophy of edentulous alveolar ridge**
Atrophy of the mandible NOS
Atrophy of the maxilla NOS

525.21 Minimal atrophy of the mandible

525.22 Moderate atrophy of the mandible

525.23 Severe atrophy of the mandible

525.24 Minimal atrophy of the maxilla

525.25 Moderate atrophy of the maxilla

525.26 Severe atrophy of the maxilla

525.3 Retained dental root

● **525.4 Complete edentulism**

Use additional code to identify cause of edentulism (525.10–525.19)

❑ **525.40 Complete edentulism, unspecified**
Edentulism NOS

525.41 Complete edentulism, class I

525.42 Complete edentulism, class II

525.43 Complete edentulism, class III

525.44 Complete edentulism, class IV

● **525.5 Partial edentulism**

Use additional code to identify cause of edentulism (525.10–525.19)

❑ **525.50 Partial edentulism, unspecified**

525.51 Partial edentulism, class I

525.52 Partial edentulism, class II

525.53 Partial edentulism, class III

525.54 Partial edentulism, class IV

● **525.6 Unsatisfactory restoration of tooth** ◀
Defective bridge, crown, fillings ◀
Defective dental restoration ◀

Excludes *dental restoration status (V45.84)* ◀
unsatisfactory endodontic treatment (526.61–526.69) ◀

❑ **525.60 Unspecified unsatisfactory restoration of tooth** ◀
Unspecified defective dental restoration ◀

525.61 Open restoration margins ◀
Dental restoration failure of marginal integrity ◀
Open margin on tooth restoration ◀

525.62 Unrepairable overhanging of dental restorative materials ◀
Overhanging of tooth restoration ◀

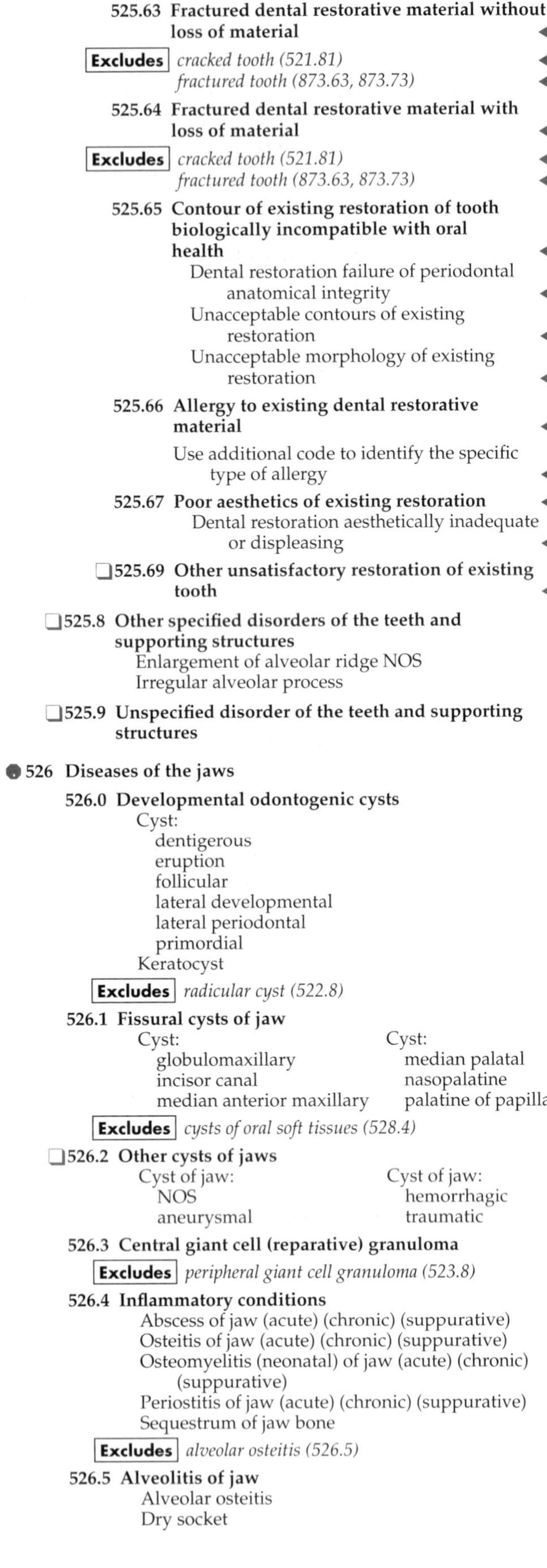

525.63 **Fractured dental restorative material without loss of material** ◀

Excludes *cracked tooth (521.81)* ◀
fractured tooth (873.63, 873.73) ◀

525.64 **Fractured dental restorative material with loss of material** ◀

Excludes *cracked tooth (521.81)* ◀
fractured tooth (873.63, 873.73) ◀

525.65 **Contour of existing restoration of tooth biologically incompatible with oral health** ◀
Dental restoration failure of periodontal anatomical integrity ◀
Unacceptable contours of existing restoration ◀
Unacceptable morphology of existing restoration ◀

525.66 **Allergy to existing dental restorative material** ◀
Use additional code to identify the specific type of allergy ◀

525.67 **Poor aesthetics of existing restoration** ◀
Dental restoration aesthetically inadequate or displeasing ◀

❑525.69 **Other unsatisfactory restoration of existing tooth** ◀

❑525.8 **Other specified disorders of the teeth and supporting structures**
Enlargement of alveolar ridge NOS
Irregular alveolar process

❑525.9 **Unspecified disorder of the teeth and supporting structures**

● 526 **Diseases of the jaws**

526.0 **Developmental odontogenic cysts**
Cyst:
dentigerous
eruption
follicular
lateral developmental
lateral periodontal
primordial
Keratocyst

Excludes *radicular cyst (522.8)*

526.1 **Fissural cysts of jaw**
Cyst:
globulomaxillary
incisor canal
median anterior maxillary
Cyst:
median palatal
nasopalatine
palatine of papilla

Excludes *cysts of oral soft tissues (528.4)*

❑526.2 **Other cysts of jaws**
Cyst of jaw:
NOS
aneurysmal
Cyst of jaw:
hemorrhagic
traumatic

526.3 **Central giant cell (reparative) granuloma**

Excludes *peripheral giant cell granuloma (523.8)*

526.4 **Inflammatory conditions**
Abscess of jaw (acute) (chronic) (suppurative)
Osteitis of jaw (acute) (chronic) (suppurative)
Osteomyelitis (neonatal) of jaw (acute) (chronic) (suppurative)
Periostitis of jaw (acute) (chronic) (suppurative)
Sequestrum of jaw bone

Excludes *alveolar osteitis (526.5)*

526.5 **Alveolitis of jaw**
Alveolar osteitis
Dry socket

● 526.6 **Periradicular pathology associated with previous category endodontic treatment** ◀

526.61 **Perforation of root canal space** ◀

526.62 **Endodontic overfill** ◀

526.63 **Endodontic underfill** ◀

❑526.69 **Other periradicular pathology associated with previous endodontic treatment** ◀

● 526.8 **Other specified diseases of the jaws**

526.81 **Exostosis of jaw**
Torus mandibularis
Torus palatinus

❑526.89 **Other**
Cherubism
Fibrous dysplasia of jaw(s)
Latent bone cyst of jaw(s)
Osteoradionecrosis of jaw(s)
Unilateral condylar hyperplasia or hypoplasia of mandible

❑526.9 **Unspecified disease of the jaws**

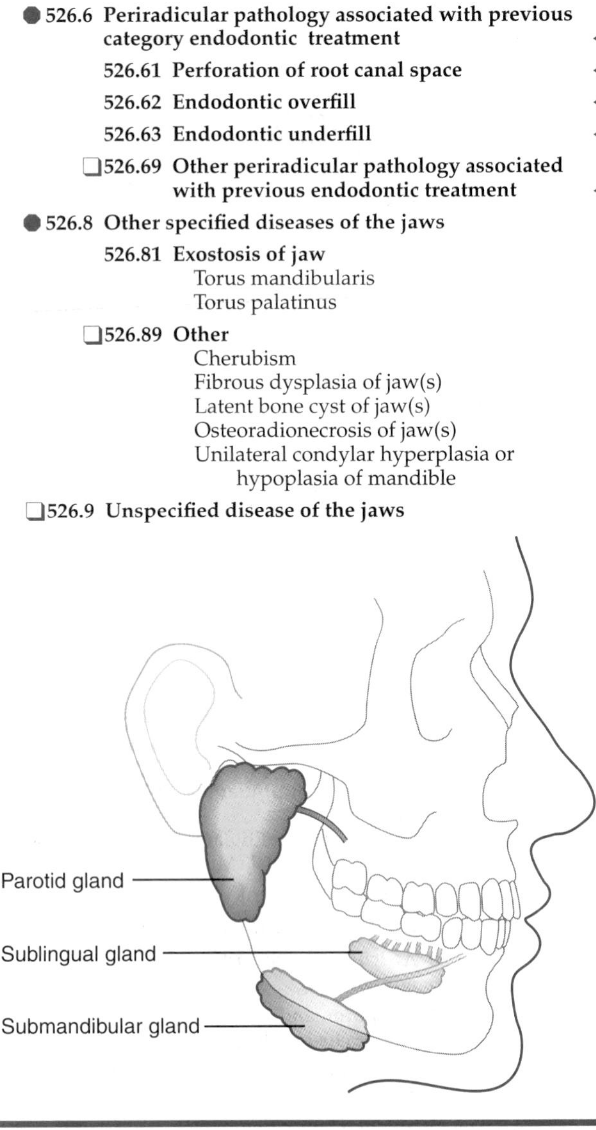
Parotid gland
Sublingual gland
Submandibular gland

Figure 9–5 Major salivary glands.

Item 9-6 Atrophy is wasting away of a tissue or organ, whereas hypertrophy is overdevelopment or enlargement of a tissue or organ. Sialoadenitis is salivary gland inflammation. Parotitis is the inflammation of the parotid gland. In the epidemic form, parotitis is also known as mumps.
Sialolithiasis is the formation of calculus within a salivary gland. Mucocele is a polyp composed of mucus.

● 527 **Diseases of the salivary glands**

527.0 **Atrophy**

527.1 **Hypertrophy**

527.2 **Sialoadenitis**
Parotitis:
NOS
allergic
toxic
Sialoangitis
Sialodochitis

Excludes *epidemic or infectious parotitis (072.0–072.9)*
uveoparotid fever (135)

527.3 **Abscess**

527.4 **Fistula**

Excludes *congenital fistula of salivary gland (750.24)*

527.5 **Sialolithiasis**
Calculus of salivary gland or duct
Stone of salivary gland or duct
Sialodocholithiasis

527.6 **Mucocele**
Mucous:
extravasation cyst of salivary gland
retention cyst of salivary gland
Ranula

527.7 **Disturbance of salivary secretion**
Hyposecretion
Ptyalism
Sialorrhea
Xerostomia

❑527.8 **Other specified diseases of the salivary glands**
Benign lymphoepithelial lesion of salivary gland
Sialectasia
Sialosis
Stenosis of salivary duct
Stricture of salivary duct

❑527.9 **Unspecified disease of the salivary glands**

Item 9-7 Stomatitis is the inflammation of the oral mucosa. Cancrum oris, also known as noma or gangrenous stomatitis, begins as an ulcer of the gingiva and results in a progressive gangrenous process.

● 528 **Diseases of the oral soft tissues, excluding lesions specific for gingiva and tongue**

● 528.0 **Stomatitis and mucositis (ulcerative)** (Revised)

Excludes *stomatitis:*
acute necrotizing ulcerative (101)
aphthous (528.2)
cellulitis and abscess of mouth (528.3) ◀
diphtheritic stomatitis (032.0) ◀
epizootic stomatitis (78.4) ◀
gangrenous (528.1)
gingivitis (523.0–523.1) ◀
herpetic (054.2)
oral thrush (112.0) ◀
Stevens-Johnson syndrome (695.1) ◀
Vincent's (101)

❑528.00 **Stomatitis and mucositis, unspecified** ◀
Mucositis NOS ◀
Ulcerative mucositis NOS ◀
Ulcerative stomatitis NOS ◀
Vesicular stomatitis NOS ◀

528.01 **Mucositis (ulcerative) due to antineoplastic therapy** ◀
Use additional E code to identify adverse effects of therapy, such as: ◀
antineoplastic and immunosuppressive drugs (E930.7, E933.1) ◀
radiation therapy (E879.2) ◀

528.02 **Mucositis (ulcerative) due to other drugs** ◀
Use additional E code to identify drug ◀

❑528.09 **Other stomatitis and mucositis (ulcerative)** ◀

528.1 **Cancrum oris**
Gangrenous stomatitis
Noma

528.2 **Oral aphthae**
Aphthous stomatitis
Canker sore
Periadenitis mucosa necrotica recurrens
Recurrent aphthous ulcer
Stomatitis herpetiformis

Excludes *herpetic stomatitis (054.2)*

528.3 **Cellulitis and abscess**
Cellulitis of mouth (floor)
Ludwig's angina
Oral fistula

Excludes *abscess of tongue (529.0)*
cellulitis or abscess of lip (528.5)
fistula (of):
dental (522.7)
lip (528.5)
gingivitis (523.00–523.11) (Revised)

528.4 **Cysts**
Dermoid cyst of mouth
Epidermoid cyst of mouth
Epstein's pearl of mouth
Lymphoepithelial cyst of mouth
Nasoalveolar cyst of mouth
Nasolabial cyst of mouth

Excludes *cyst:*
gingiva (523.8)
tongue (529.8)

528.5 **Diseases of lips**
Abscess of lip(s)
Cellulitis of lip(s)
Fistula of lip(s)
Hypertrophy of lip(s)
Cheilitis:
NOS
angular
Cheilodynia
Cheilosis

Excludes *actinic cheilitis (692.79)*
congenital fistula of lip (750.25)
leukoplakia of lips (528.6)

528.6 **Leukoplakia of oral mucosa, including tongue**
Leukokeratosis of oral mucosa
Leukoplakia of:
gingiva
lips
tongue

Excludes *carcinoma in situ (230.0, 232.0)*
leukokeratosis nicotina palati (528.79)

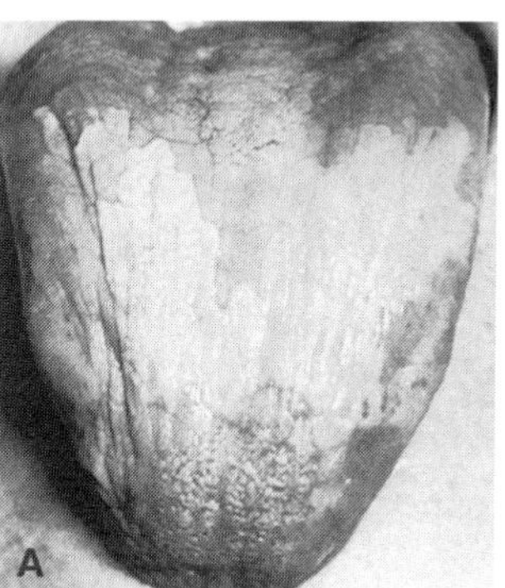
A
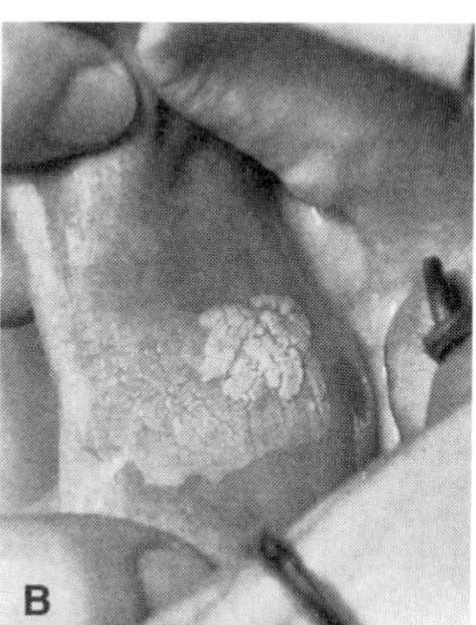
B

Figure 9-6 **A.** Lingual leukoplakia. **B.** Buccal leukoplakia. (From Pindborg JJ: In Jones JH, Mason DK (eds): Oral Manifestations of Systemic Disease. Philadelphia, WB Saunders, 1980, p 322.)

● 528.7 **Other disturbances of oral epithelium, including tongue**

Excludes *carcinoma in situ (230.0, 232.0)*
leukokeratosis NOS (702)

528.71 **Minimal keratinized residual ridge mucosa**
Minimal keratinization of alveolar ridge mucosa ◀

528.72 **Excessive keratinized residual ridge mucosa**
Excessive keratinization of alveolar ridge mucosa ◀

ICD-9-CM 500-599 Vol. 1

❑528.79 **Other disturbances of oral epithelium, including tongue**
Erythroplakia of mouth or tongue
Focal epithelial hyperplasia of mouth or tongue
Leukoedema of mouth or tongue
Leukokeratosis nicotina palate
Other oral epithelium disturbances ◀

528.8 **Oral submucosal fibrosis, including of tongue**

❑528.9 **Other and unspecified diseases of the oral soft tissues**
Cheek and lip biting
Denture sore mouth
Denture stomatitis
Melanoplakia
Papillary hyperplasia of palate
Eosinophilic granuloma of oral mucosa
Irritative hyperplasia of oral mucosa
Pyogenic granuloma of oral mucosa
Ulcer (traumatic) of oral mucosa

● 529 **Diseases and other conditions of the tongue**

529.0 **Glossitis**
Abscess of tongue
Ulceration (traumatic) of tongue

Excludes *glossitis:*
benign migratory (529.1)
Hunter's (529.4)
median rhomboid (529.2)
Moeller's (529.4)

529.1 **Geographic tongue**
Benign migratory glossitis
Glossitis areata exfoliativa

529.2 **Median rhomboid glossitis**

529.3 **Hypertrophy of tongue papillae**
Black hairy tongue
Coated tongue
Hypertrophy of foliate papillae
Lingua villosa nigra

529.4 **Atrophy of tongue papillae**
Bald tongue
Glazed tongue
Glossitis:
Hunter's
Moeller's
Glossodynia exfoliativa
Smooth atrophic tongue

529.5 **Plicated tongue**
Fissured tongue
Furrowed tongue
Scrotal tongue

Excludes *fissure of tongue, congenital (750.13)*

529.6 **Glossodynia**
Glossopyrosis
Painful tongue

Excludes *glossodynia exfoliativa (529.4)*

❑529.8 **Other specified conditions of the tongue**
Atrophy (of) tongue
Crenated (of) tongue
Enlargement (of) tongue
Hypertrophy (of) tongue
Glossocele
Glossoptosis

Excludes *erythroplasia of tongue (528.79)*
leukoplakia of tongue (528.6)
macroglossia (congenital) (750.15)
microglossia (congenital) (750.16)
oral submucosal fibrosis (528.8)

❑529.9 **Unspecified condition of the tongue**

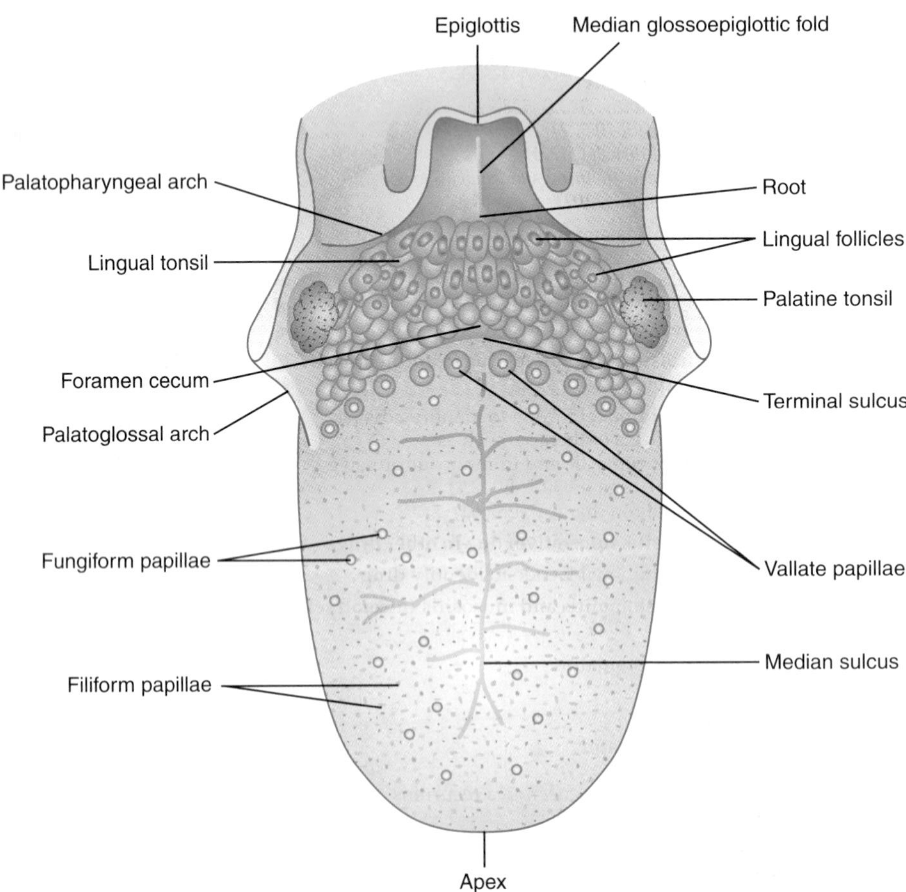
Epiglottis
Median glossoepiglottic fold
Palatopharyngeal arch
Root
Lingual follicles
Lingual tonsil
Palatine tonsil
Foramen cecum
Terminal sulcus
Palatoglossal arch
Fungiform papillae
Vallate papillae
Median sulcus
Filiform papillae
Apex

Figure 9–7 Structure of the tongue.

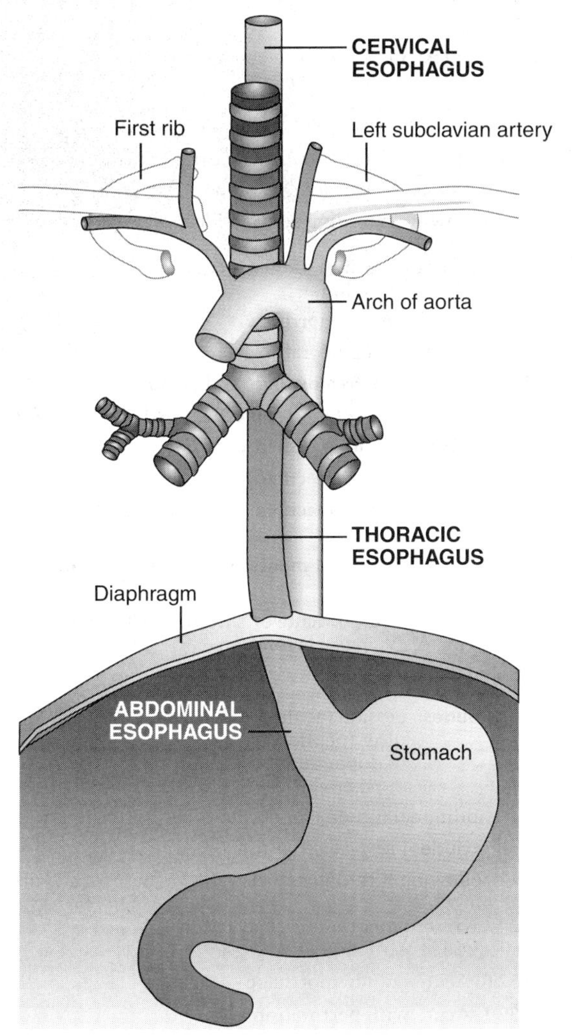
CERVICAL ESOPHAGUS
First rib
Left subclavian artery
Arch of aorta
THORACIC ESOPHAGUS
Diaphragm
ABDOMINAL ESOPHAGUS
Stomach

Figure 9–8 The esophagus is the muscular tube that connects the pharynx and the stomach. The 10 inch (25 cm) long esophagus is divided into three parts: **cervical, thoracic,** and **abdominal.**

Item 9–8 Achalasia is a condition in which the smooth muscle fibers of the esophagus do not relax. Most frequently, this condition occurs at the esophagogastric sphincter. Cardiospasm, also known as megaesophagus, is achalasia of the thoracic esophagus.

Item 9–9 Dyskinesia is difficulty in moving, and diverticulum is a sac or pouch.

DISEASES OF ESOPHAGUS, STOMACH, AND DUODENUM (530–538)

● **530 Diseases of esophagus**

Excludes *esophageal varices (456.0–456.2)*

530.0 Achalasia and cardiospasm
Achalasia (of cardia)
Aperistalsis of esophagus
Megaesophagus

Excludes *congenital cardiospasm (750.7)*

● **530.1 Esophagitis**
Abscess of esophagus
Esophagitis:
NOS
chemical
peptic
Esophagitis:
postoperative
regurgitant

Use additional E code to identify cause, if induced by chemical

Excludes *tuberculous esophagitis (017.8)*

❑ **530.10 Esophagitis, unspecified**

530.11 Reflux esophagitis

530.12 Acute esophagitis

❑ **530.19 Other esophagitis**

● **530.2 Ulcer of esophagus**
Ulcer of esophagus
fungal
peptic
Ulcer of esophagus due to ingestion of:
aspirin
medicines
chemicals

Use additional E code to identify cause, if induced by chemical or drug

530.20 Ulcer of esophagus without bleeding
Ulcer of esophagus NOS

530.21 Ulcer of esophagus with bleeding

Excludes *bleeding esophageal varices (456.0, 456.20)*

530.3 Stricture and stenosis of esophagus
Compression of esophagus
Obstruction of esophagus

Excludes *congenital stricture of esophagus (750.3)*

530.4 Perforation of esophagus
Rupture of esophagus

Excludes *traumatic perforation of esophagus (862.22, 862.32, 874.4–874.5)*

530.5 Dyskinesia of esophagus
Corkscrew esophagus
Curling esophagus
Esophagospasm
Spasm of esophagus

Excludes *cardiospasm (530.0)*

530.6 Diverticulum of esophagus, acquired
Diverticulum, acquired:
epiphrenic
pharyngoesophageal
pulsion
subdiaphragmatic
traction
Zenker's (hypopharyngeal)
Esophageal pouch, acquired
Esophagocele, acquired

Excludes *congenital diverticulum of esophagus (750.4)*

530.7 Gastroesophageal laceration-hemorrhage syndrome
Mallory-Weiss syndrome

● **530.8 Other specified disorders of esophagus**

530.81 Esophageal reflux
Gastroesophageal reflux

Excludes *reflux esophagitis (530.11)*

530.82 Esophageal hemorrhage

Excludes *hemorrhage due to esophageal varices (456.0–456.2)*

530.83 Esophageal leukoplakia

530.84 Tracheoesophageal fistula

Excludes *congenital tracheoesophageal fistula (750.3)*

530.85 Barrett's esophagus

ICD-9-CM 500-599 Vol. 1

530.86 **Infection of esophagostomy**
Use additional code to specify infection

530.87 **Mechanical complication of esophagostomy**
Malfunction of esophagostomy

❑530.89 **Other**
Excludes *Paterson-Kelly syndrome (280.8)*

❑530.9 **Unspecified disorder of esophagus**

Item 9-10 Esophageal reflux is the return flow of the contents of the stomach to the esophagus. **Gastroesophageal reflux** is the return flow of the contents of the stomach and duodenum to the esophagus. **Esophageal leukoplakia** are white areas on the mucous membrane of the esophagus for which no specific cause can be identified.

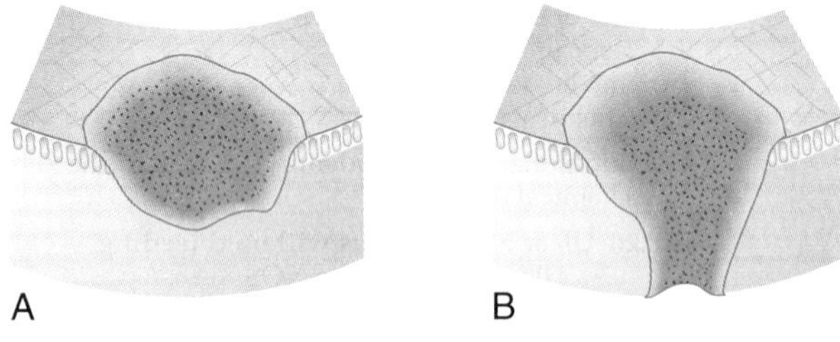
A
B

Figure 9–9 **A.** Ulcer. **B.** Perforated ulcer.

Item 9-11 Gastric ulcers are lesions of the stomach that result in the death of the tissue and a defect of the surface. **Perforated ulcers** are those in which the lesion penetrates the gastric wall, leaving a hole. **Peptic ulcers** are lesions of the stomach or the duodenum. **Peptic** refers to the gastric juice, pepsin.

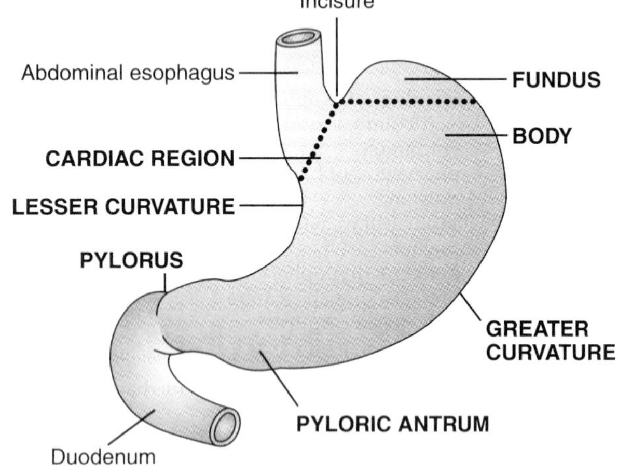
Incisure
Abdominal esophagus
FUNDUS
BODY
CARDIAC REGION
LESSER CURVATURE
PYLORUS
GREATER CURVATURE
PYLORIC ANTRUM
Duodenum

Figure 9–10 Parts of the stomach.

● **531 Gastric ulcer**

Includes: ulcer (peptic):
prepyloric
pylorus
stomach

Use additional E code to identify drug, if drug-induced

Excludes *peptic ulcer NOS (533.0–533.9)*

The following fifth-digit subclassification is for use with category 531:
0 **without mention of obstruction**
1 **with obstruction**

● 531.0 **Acute with hemorrhage**

● 531.1 **Acute with perforation**

● 531.2 **Acute with hemorrhage and perforation**

● 531.3 **Acute without mention of hemorrhage or perforation**

● 531.4 **Chronic or unspecified with hemorrhage**

● 531.5 **Chronic or unspecified with perforation**

● 531.6 **Chronic or unspecified with hemorrhage and perforation**

● 531.7 **Chronic without mention of hemorrhage or perforation**

● ❑531.9 **Unspecified as acute or chronic, without mention of hemorrhage or perforation**

● **532 Duodenal ulcer**

Includes: erosion (acute) of duodenum
ulcer (peptic):
duodenum
postpyloric

Use additional E code to identify drug, if drug-induced

Excludes *peptic ulcer NOS (533.0–533.9)*

The following fifth-digit subclassification is for use with category 532:
0 **without mention of obstruction**
1 **with obstruction**

● 532.0 **Acute with hemorrhage**

● 532.1 **Acute with perforation**

● 532.2 **Acute with hemorrhage and perforation**

● 532.3 **Acute without mention of hemorrhage or perforation**

● 532.4 **Chronic or unspecified with hemorrhage**

● 532.5 **Chronic or unspecified with perforation**

● 532.6 **Chronic or unspecified with hemorrhage and perforation**

● 532.7 **Chronic without mention of hemorrhage or perforation**

● ❑532.9 **Unspecified as acute or chronic, without mention of hemorrhage or perforation**

● **533 Peptic ulcer, site unspecified**

Includes: gastroduodenal ulcer NOS
peptic ulcer NOS
stress ulcer NOS

Use additional E code to identify drug, if drug-induced

Excludes *peptic ulcer:*
duodenal (532.0–532.9)
gastric (531.0–531.9)

The following fifth-digit subclassification is for use with category 533:
0 **without mention of obstruction**
1 **with obstruction**

● 533.0 **Acute with hemorrhage**

● 533.1 **Acute with perforation**

● 533.2 **Acute with hemorrhage and perforation**

● 533.3 **Acute without mention of hemorrhage and perforation**

● 533.4 **Chronic or unspecified with hemorrhage**

● 533.5 **Chronic or unspecified with perforation**

● 533.6 **Chronic or unspecified with hemorrhage and perforation**

● 533.7 **Chronic without mention of hemorrhage or perforation**

● ☐ 533.9 **Unspecified as acute or chronic, without mention of hemorrhage or perforation**

● 534 **Gastrojejunal ulcer**

Includes: ulcer (peptic) or erosion:
anastomotic
gastrocolic
gastrointestinal
gastrojejunal
jejunal
marginal
stomal

Excludes *primary ulcer of small intestine (569.82)*

The following fifth-digit subclassification is for use with category 534:
0 **without mention of obstruction**
1 **with obstruction**

● 534.0 **Acute with hemorrhage**

● 534.1 **Acute with perforation**

● 534.2 **Acute with hemorrhage and perforation**

● 534.3 **Acute without mention of hemorrhage or perforation**

● 534.4 **Chronic or unspecified with hemorrhage**

● 534.5 **Chronic or unspecified with perforation**

● 534.6 **Chronic or unspecified with hemorrhage and perforation**

● 534.7 **Chronic without mention of hemorrhage or perforation**

● ☐ 534.9 **Unspecified as acute or chronic, without mention of hemorrhage or perforation**

Item 9-12 Gastritis is a severe inflammation of the stomach. Atrophic gastritis is a chronic inflammation of the stomach that results in destruction of the cells of the mucosa of the stomach.

● 535 **Gastritis and duodenitis**

The following fifth-digit subclassification is for use with category 535:
0 **without mention of hemorrhage**
1 **with hemorrhage**

● 535.0 **Acute gastritis**

● 535.1 **Atrophic gastritis**
Gastritis:
atrophic-hyperplastic
chronic (atrophic)

● 535.2 **Gastric mucosal hypertrophy**
Hypertrophic gastritis

● 535.3 **Alcoholic gastritis**

● ☐ 535.4 **Other specified gastritis**
Gastritis:
allergic
bile induced
irritant
superficial
toxic

● ☐ 535.5 **Unspecified gastritis and gastroduodenitis**

● 535.6 **Duodenitis**

Item 9-13 Achlorhydria, also known as gastric anacidity, is the absence of gastric acid. Gastroparesis is paralysis of the stomach.

● 536 **Disorders of function of stomach**

Excludes *functional disorders of stomach specified as psychogenic (306.4)*

536.0 **Achlorhydria**

536.1 **Acute dilatation of stomach**
Acute distention of stomach

536.2 **Persistent vomiting**
Habit vomiting
Persistent vomiting [not of pregnancy]
Uncontrollable vomiting

Excludes *excessive vomiting in pregnancy (643.0–643.9)*
vomiting NOS (787.0)

536.3 **Gastroparesis**
Gastroparalysis

● 536.4 **Gastrostomy complications**

☐ 536.40 **Gastrostomy complication, unspecified**

536.41 **Infection of gastrostomy**

Use additional code to identify type of infection, such as:
abscess or cellulitis of abdomen (682.2)
septicemia (038.0–038.9)

Use additional code to identify organism (041.00–041.9)

536.42 **Mechanical complication of gastrostomy**

☐ 536.49 **Other gastrostomy complications**

☐ 536.8 **Dyspepsia and other specified disorders of function of stomach**
Achylia gastrica
Hourglass contraction of stomach
Hyperacidity
Hyperchlorhydria
Hypochlorhydria
Indigestion
Tachygastria ◄

Excludes *achlorhydria (536.0)*
heartburn (787.1)

☐ 536.9 **Unspecified functional disorder of stomach**
Functional gastrointestinal:
disorder
disturbance
irritation

● 537 **Other disorders of stomach and duodenum**

537.0 **Acquired hypertrophic pyloric stenosis**
Constriction of pylorus, acquired or adult
Obstruction of pylorus, acquired or adult
Stricture of pylorus, acquired or adult

Excludes *congenital or infantile pyloric stenosis (750.5)*

537.1 **Gastric diverticulum**

Excludes *congenital diverticulum of stomach (750.7)*

537.2 **Chronic duodenal ileus**

☐ 537.3 **Other obstruction of duodenum**
Cicatrix of duodenum
Stenosis of duodenum
Stricture of duodenum
Volvulus of duodenum

Excludes *congenital obstruction of duodenum (751.1)*

537.4 **Fistula of stomach or duodenum**
Gastrocolic fistula
Gastrojejunocolic fistula

537.5 **Gastroptosis**

537.6 **Hourglass stricture or stenosis of stomach**
Cascade stomach

Excludes *congenital hourglass stomach (750.7)*
hourglass contraction of stomach (536.8)

● 537.8 **Other specified disorders of stomach and duodenum**

537.81 **Pylorospasm**

Excludes *congenital pylorospasm (750.5)*

537.82 **Angiodysplasia of stomach and duodenum without mention of hemorrhage**

537.83 **Angiodysplasia of stomach and duodenum with hemorrhage**

537.84 **Dieulafoy lesion (hemorrhagic) of stomach and duodenum**

❑537.89 **Other**
Gastric or duodenal:
prolapse
rupture
Intestinal metaplasia of gastric mucosa
Passive congestion of stomach

Excludes *diverticula of duodenum (562.00–562.01)*
gastrointestinal hemorrhage (578.0–578.9)

❑537.9 **Unspecified disorder of stomach and duodenum**

538 **Gastrointestinal mucositis (ulcerative)** ◀

Use additional E code to identify adverse effects of therapy, such as: ◀
antineoplastic and immunosuppressive drugs (E930.7, E933.1) ◀
radiation therapy (E879.2) ◀

Excludes *mucositis (ulcerative) of mouth and oral soft tissue (528.00–528.09)* ◀

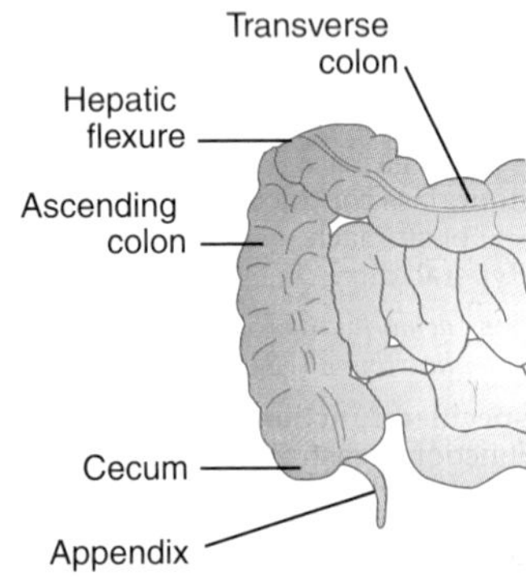
Transverse colon
Hepatic flexure
Ascending colon
Cecum
Appendix

Figure 9–11 Acute appendicitis is the inflammation of the appendix, usually associated with obstruction. Most often this is a disease of adolescents and young adults.

APPENDICITIS (540–543)

● 540 **Acute appendicitis**

540.0 **With generalized peritonitis**
Appendicitis (acute) with: perforation, peritonitis (generalized), rupture:
fulminating
gangrenous
obstructive
Cecitis (acute) with: perforation, peritonitis (generalized), rupture
Rupture of appendix

Excludes *acute appendicitis with peritoneal abscess (540.1)*

540.1 **With peritoneal abscess**
Abscess of appendix
With generalized peritonitis

540.9 **Without mention of peritonitis**
Acute:
appendicitis without mention of perforation, peritonitis, or rupture:
fulminating
gangrenous
inflamed
obstructive
cecitis without mention of perforation, peritonitis, or rupture

❑541 **Appendicitis, unqualified**

❑542 **Other appendicitis**
Appendicitis:
chronic
recurrent
relapsing
subacute

Excludes *hyperplasia (lymphoid) of appendix (543.0)*

● 543 **Other diseases of appendix**

543.0 **Hyperplasia of appendix (lymphoid)**

❑543.9 **Other and unspecified diseases of appendix**
Appendicular or appendiceal:
colic
concretion
fistula
Diverticulum of appendix
Fecalith of appendix
Intussusception of appendix
Mucocele of appendix
Stercolith of appendix

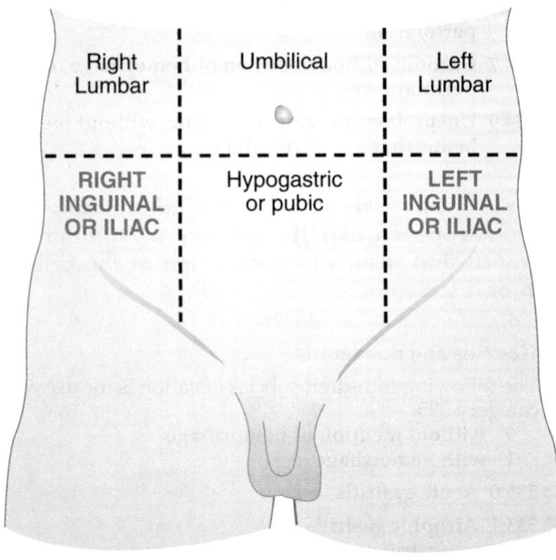
Right Lumbar
Umbilical
Left Lumbar
RIGHT INGUINAL OR ILIAC
Hypogastric or pubic
LEFT INGUINAL OR ILIAC

Figure 9–12 Inguinal hernias are those that are located in the inguinal or iliac areas of the abdomen.

Item 9–14 Hernias of the groin are the most common type, accounting for 80 percent of all hernias. There are two major types of inguinal hernias: indirect (oblique) and direct. **Indirect inguinal hernias** result when the intestines emerge through the abdominal wall in an indirect fashion through the inguinal canal. **Direct inguinal hernias** penetrate through the abdominal wall in a direct fashion.
Femoral hernias occur at the femoral ring where the femoral vessels enter the thigh.
Classification is based on location of the hernia and whether there is obstruction or gangrene.

HERNIA OF ABDOMINAL CAVITY (550–553)

Includes: hernia:
acquired
congenital, except diaphragmatic or hiatal

● **550 Inguinal hernia**

Includes: bubonocele
inguinal hernia (direct) (double) (indirect) (oblique) (sliding)
scrotal hernia

The following fifth-digit subclassification is for use with category 550:

❑ **0 unilateral or unspecified (not specified as recurrent)**
Unilateral NOS
1 unilateral or unspecified, recurrent
2 bilateral (not specified as recurrent)
Bilateral NOS
3 bilateral, recurrent

● **550.0 Inguinal hernia, with gangrene**
Inguinal hernia with gangrene (and obstruction)

● **550.1 Inguinal hernia, with obstruction, without mention of gangrene**
Inguinal hernia with mention of incarceration, irreducibility, or strangulation

● **550.9 Inguinal hernia, without mention of obstruction or gangrene**
Inguinal hernia NOS

● **551 Other hernia of abdominal cavity, with gangrene**

Includes: that with gangrene (and obstruction)

● **551.0 Femoral hernia with gangrene**

❑ **551.00 Unilateral or unspecified (not specified as recurrent)**
Femoral hernia NOS with gangrene

551.01 Unilateral or unspecified, recurrent

551.02 Bilateral (not specified as recurrent)

551.03 Bilateral, recurrent

551.1 Umbilical hernia with gangrene
Parumbilical hernia specified as gangrenous

● **551.2 Ventral hernia with gangrene**

❑ **551.20 Ventral, unspecified, with gangrene**

551.21 Incisional, with gangrene
Hernia:
postoperative specified as gangrenous
recurrent, ventral specified as gangrenous

❑ **551.29 Other**
Epigastric hernia specified as gangrenous

551.3 Diaphragmatic hernia with gangrene
Hernia:
hiatal (esophageal) (sliding) specified as gangrenous
paraesophageal specified as gangrenous
Thoracic stomach specified as gangrenous

Excludes *congenital diaphragmatic hernia (756.6)*

❑ **551.8 Hernia of other specified sites, with gangrene**
Any condition classifiable to 553.8 if specified as gangrenous

❑ **551.9 Hernia of unspecified site, with gangrene**
Any condition classifiable to 553.9 if specified as gangrenous

● **552 Other hernia of abdominal cavity, with obstruction, but without mention of gangrene**

Excludes *that with mention of gangrene (551.0–551.9)*

● **552.0 Femoral hernia with obstruction**
Femoral hernia specified as incarcerated, irreducible, strangulated, or causing obstruction

❑ **552.00 Unilateral or unspecified (not specified as recurrent)**

552.01 Unilateral or unspecified, recurrent

552.02 Bilateral (not specified as recurrent)

552.03 Bilateral, recurrent

552.1 Umbilical hernia with obstruction
Parumbilical hernia specified as incarcerated, irreducible, strangulated, or causing obstruction

● **552.2 Ventral hernia with obstruction**
Ventral hernia specified as incarcerated, irreducible, strangulated, or causing obstruction

❑ **552.20 Ventral, unspecified, with obstruction**

552.21 Incisional, with obstruction
Hernia:
postoperative specified as incarcerated, irreducible, strangulated, or causing obstruction
recurrent, ventral specified as incarcerated, irreducible, strangulated, or causing obstruction

❑ **552.29 Other**
Epigastric hernia specified as incarcerated, irreducible, strangulated, or causing obstruction

552.3 Diaphragmatic hernia with obstruction
Hernia:
hiatal (esophageal) (sliding) specified as incarcerated, irreducible, strangulated, or causing obstruction
paraesophageal specified as incarcerated, irreducible, strangulated, or causing obstruction
Thoracic stomach specified as incarcerated, irreducible, strangulated, or causing obstruction

Excludes *congenital diaphragmatic hernia (756.6)*

❑ **552.8 Hernia of other specified sites, with obstruction**
Any condition classifiable to 553.8 if specified as incarcerated, irreducible, strangulated, or causing obstruction

Excludes *hernia due to adhesion with obstruction (560.81)*

❑ **552.9 Hernia of unspecified site, with obstruction**
Any condition classifiable to 553.9 if specified as incarcerated, irreducible, strangulated, or causing obstruction

● **553 Other hernia of abdominal cavity without mention of obstruction or gangrene**

Excludes *the listed conditions with mention of:*
gangrene (and obstruction) (551.0–551.9)
obstruction (552.0–552.9)

● **553.0 Femoral hernia**

❑ **553.00 Unilateral or unspecified (not specified as recurrent)**
Femoral hernia NOS

553.01 Unilateral or unspecified, recurrent

553.02 Bilateral (not specified as recurrent)

553.03 Bilateral, recurrent

553.1 Umbilical hernia
Parumbilical hernia

● **553.2 Ventral hernia**

❑ **553.20 Ventral, unspecified**

553.21 Incisional
Hernia:
postoperative
recurrent, ventral

❑ **553.29 Other**
Hernia:
epigastric
spigelian

553.3 Diaphragmatic hernia
Hernia:
hiatal (esophageal) (sliding)
paraesophageal
Thoracic stomach

Excludes *congenital:*
diaphragmatic hernia (756.6)
hiatal hernia (750.6)
esophagocele (530.6)

❑553.8 **Hernia of other specified sites**
Hernia:
ischiatic
ischiorectal
lumbar
obturator
pudendal
retroperitoneal
sciatic
Other abdominal hernia of specified site

Excludes *vaginal enterocele (618.6)*

❑553.9 **Hernia of unspecified site**
Enterocele
Epiplocele
Hernia:
NOS
interstitial
intestinal
intra-abdominal
Rupture (nontraumatic)
Sarcoepiplocele

NONINFECTIOUS ENTERITIS AND COLITIS (555–558)

● 555 **Regional enteritis**

Includes: Crohn's disease
Granulomatous enteritis

Excludes *ulcerative colitis (556)*

555.0 **Small intestine**
Ileitis:
regional
segmental
terminal
Regional enteritis or Crohn's disease of:
duodenum
ileum
jejunum

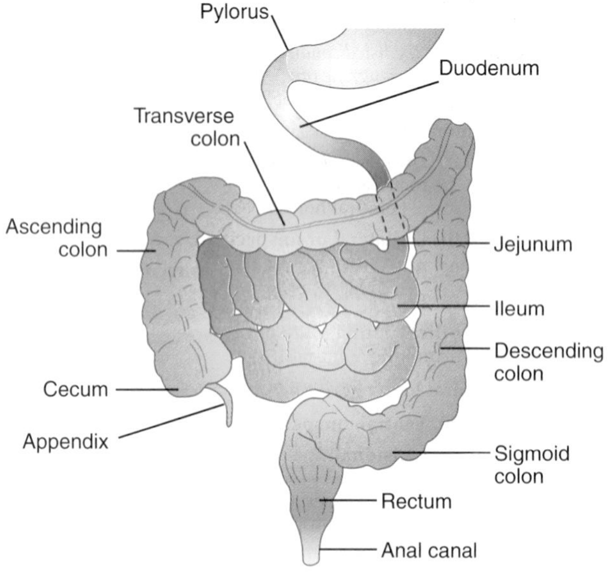
Pylorus
Duodenum
Transverse colon
Ascending colon
Jejunum
Ileum
Descending colon
Cecum
Appendix
Sigmoid colon
Rectum
Anal canal

Figure 9–13 Small and large intestines.

Item 9-15 Crohn's disease, also known as regional enteritis, is a chronic inflammatory disease of the intestines. Classification is based on location in the small (duodenum, ileum, jejunum) or large (cecum, colon, rectum, anal canal) intestine.

555.1 **Large intestine**
Colitis:
granulomatous
regional
transmural
Regional enteritis or Crohn's disease of:
colon
large bowel
rectum

555.2 **Small intestine with large intestine**
Regional ileocolitis

❑555.9 **Unspecified site**
Crohn's disease NOS
Regional enteritis NOS

● 556 **Ulcerative colitis**

556.0 **Ulcerative (chronic) enterocolitis**

556.1 **Ulcerative (chronic) ileocolitis**

556.2 **Ulcerative (chronic) proctitis**

Item 9-16 Ulcerative colitis attacks the colonic mucosa and forms abscesses. The disease involves the intestines. Classification is based on the location:
enterocolitis: large and small intestine
ileocolitis: ileum and colon
proctitis: rectum
proctosigmoiditis: sigmoid colon and rectum

556.3 **Ulcerative (chronic) proctosigmoiditis**

556.4 **Pseudopolyposis of colon**

556.5 **Left-sided ulcerative (chronic) colitis**

556.6 **Universal ulcerative (chronic) colitis**
Pancolitis

❑556.8 **Other ulcerative colitis**

❑556.9 **Ulcerative colitis, unspecified**
Ulcerative enteritis NOS

● 557 **Vascular insufficiency of intestine**

Excludes *necrotizing enterocolitis of the newborn (777.5)*

557.0 **Acute vascular insufficiency of intestine**
Acute:
hemorrhagic enterocolitis
ischemic colitis, enteritis, or enterocolitis
massive necrosis of intestine
Bowel infarction
Embolism of mesenteric artery
Fulminant enterocolitis
Hemorrhagic necrosis of intestine
Infarction of appendices epiploicae
Intestinal gangrene
Intestinal infarction (acute) (agnogenic) (hemorrhagic) (nonocclusive)
Mesenteric infarction (embolic) (thrombotic)
Necrosis of intestine
Terminal hemorrhagic enteropathy
Thrombosis of mesenteric artery

557.1 **Chronic vascular insufficiency of intestine**
Angina, abdominal
Chronic ischemic colitis, enteritis, or enterocolitis
Ischemic stricture of intestine
Mesenteric:
angina
artery syndrome (superior)
vascular insufficiency

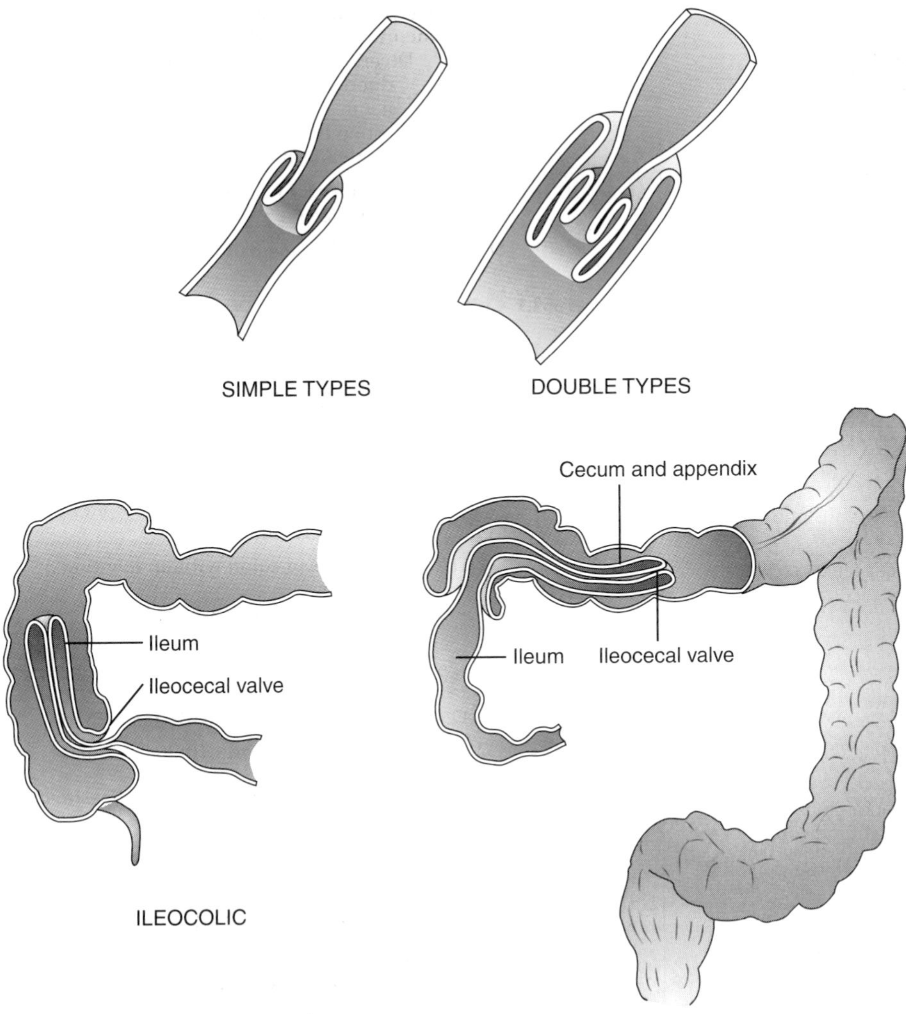
SIMPLE TYPES
DOUBLE TYPES
Cecum and appendix
Ileum
Ileocecal valve
Ileum
Ileocecal valve
ILEOCOLIC
ILEOCECAL

Figure 9–14 Types of intussusception.

❑557.9 **Unspecified vascular insufficiency of intestine**
Alimentary pain due to vascular insufficiency
Ischemic colitis, enteritis, or enterocolitis NOS

● 558 **Other and unspecified noninfectious gastroenteritis and colitis**

Excludes *infectious:*
colitis, enteritis, or gastroenteritis (009.0–009.1)
diarrhea (009.2–009.3)

558.1 **Gastroenteritis and colitis due to radiation**
Radiation enterocolitis

558.2 **Toxic gastroenteritis and colitis**
Use additional E code to identify cause

558.3 **Allergic gastroenteritis and colitis**
Use additional code to identify type of food allergy (V15.01–V15.05)

❑558.9 **Other and unspecified noninfectious gastroenteritis and colitis**
Colitis, NOS, dietetic, or noninfectious
Enteritis, NOS, dietetic, or noninfectious
Gastroenteritis, NOS, dietetic, or noninfectious
Ileitis, NOS, dietetic, or noninfectious
Jejunitis, NOS, dietetic, or noninfectious
Sigmoiditis, NOS, dietetic, or noninfectious

Item 9–17 Intussusception is the prolapse of a part of the intestine into another adjacent part of the intestine. Intussusception may be enteric (ileoileal, jejunoileal, jejunojejunal), colic (colocolic), or intracolic (ileocecal, ileocolic).

Item 9–18 Volvulus is the twisting of a segment of the intestine, resulting in obstruction.

OTHER DISEASES OF INTESTINES AND PERITONEUM (560–569)

● 560 **Intestinal obstruction without mention of hernia**

Excludes *duodenum (537.2–537.3)*
inguinal hernia with obstruction (550.1)
intestinal obstruction complicating hernia (552.0–552.9)
mesenteric:
embolism (557.0)
infarction (557.0)
thrombosis (557.0)
neonatal intestinal obstruction (277.01, 777.1–777.2, 777.4)

560.0 Intussusception
Intussusception (colon) (intestine) (rectum)
Invagination of intestine or colon

Excludes *intussusception of appendix (543.9)*

560.1 Paralytic ileus
Adynamic ileus
Ileus (of intestine) (of bowel) (of colon)
Paralysis of intestine or colon

Excludes *gallstone ileus (560.31)*

560.2 Volvulus
Knotting of intestine, bowel, or colon
Strangulation of intestine, bowel, or colon
Torsion of intestine, bowel, or colon
Twist of intestine, bowel, or colon

● **560.3 Impaction of intestine**

❑ **560.30 Impaction of intestine, unspecified**
Impaction of colon

560.31 Gallstone ileus
Obstruction of intestine by gallstone

❑ **560.39 Other**
Concretion of intestine
Enterolith
Fecal impaction

● **560.8 Other specified intestinal obstruction**

560.81 Intestinal or peritoneal adhesions with obstruction (postoperative) (postinfection)

Excludes *adhesions without obstruction (568.0)*

❑ **560.89 Other**
Acute pseudo-obstruction of intestine
Mural thickening causing obstruction

Excludes *ischemic stricture of intestine (557.1)*

❑ **560.9 Unspecified intestinal obstruction**
Enterostenosis
Obstruction of intestine or colon
Occlusion of intestine or colon
Stenosis of intestine or colon
Stricture of intestine or colon

Excludes *congenital stricture or stenosis of intestine (751.1–751.2)*

Item 9-19 Diverticula of the intestines are acquired herniations of the mucosa. Diverticulum (singular): Pocket or pouch that bulges outward through a weak spot (herniation) in the colon. Diverticula (plural). Diverticulosis is the condition of having diverticula. Diverticulitis is inflammation of these pouches or herniations.
Classification is based on location (small intestine or colon) and whether it occurs with or without hemorrhage.

● **562 Diverticula of intestine**

Use additional code to identify any associated:
peritonitis (567.0–567.9)

Excludes *congenital diverticulum of colon (751.5)*
diverticulum of appendix (543.9)
Meckel's diverticulum (751.0)

● **562.0 Small intestine**

562.00 Diverticulosis of small intestine (without mention of hemorrhage)
Diverticulosis:
duodenum without mention of diverticulitis
ileum without mention of diverticulitis
jejunum without mention of diverticulitis

562.01 Diverticulitis of small intestine (without mention of hemorrhage)
Diverticulitis (with diverticulosis):
duodenum
ileum
jejunum
small intestine

562.02 Diverticulosis of small intestine with hemorrhage

562.03 Diverticulitis of small intestine with hemorrhage

● **562.1 Colon**

562.10 Diverticulosis of colon (without mention of hemorrhage)
Diverticulosis without mention of diverticulitis:
NOS
intestine (large) without mention of diverticulitis
Diverticular disease (colon) without mention of diverticulitis

562.11 Diverticulitis of colon without mention of hemorrhage
Diverticulitis (with diverticulosis):
NOS
colon
intestine (large)

562.12 Diverticulosis of colon with hemorrhage

562.13 Diverticulitis of colon with hemorrhage

● **564 Functional digestive disorders, not elsewhere classified**

Excludes *functional disorders of stomach (536.0–536.9)*
those specified as psychogenic (306.4)

● **564.0 Constipation**

❑ **564.00 Constipation, unspecified**

564.01 Slow transit constipation

564.02 Outlet dysfunction constipation

❑ **564.09 Other constipation**

564.1 Irritable bowel syndrome
Irritable colon

564.2 Postgastric surgery syndromes
Dumping syndrome
Jejunal syndrome
Postgastrectomy syndrome
Postvagotomy syndrome

Excludes *malnutrition following gastrointestinal surgery (579.3)*
postgastrojejunostomy ulcer (534.0–534.9)

564.3 Vomiting following gastrointestinal surgery
Vomiting (bilious) following gastrointestinal surgery

❑ **564.4 Other postoperative functional disorders**
Diarrhea following gastrointestinal surgery

Excludes *colostomy and enterostomy complications (569.60–569.69)*

564.5 Functional diarrhea

Excludes *diarrhea:*
NOS (787.91)
psychogenic (306.4)

564.6 Anal spasm
Proctalgia fugax

564.7 Megacolon, other than Hirschsprung's
Dilatation of colon

Excludes *megacolon:*
congenital [Hirschsprung's] (751.3)
toxic (556)

● 564.8 **Other specified functional disorders of intestine**

Excludes *malabsorption (579.0–579.9)*

564.81 **Neurogenic bowel**

❑ 564.89 **Other functional disorders of intestine**
Atony of colon

❑ 564.9 **Unspecified functional disorder of intestine**

Item 9-20 A fissure is a groove in the surface, whereas a **fistula** is an abnormal passage.

● 565 **Anal fissure and fistula**

565.0 **Anal fissure**
Tear of anus, nontraumatic

Excludes *traumatic (863.89, 863.99)*

565.1 **Anal fistula**
Fistula:
anorectal
rectal
rectum to skin

Excludes *fistula of rectum to internal organs - see Alphabetic Index*
ischiorectal fistula (566)
rectovaginal fistula (619.1)

566 **Abscess of anal and rectal regions**
Abscess:
ischiorectal
perianal
perirectal
Cellulitis:
anal
perirectal
rectal
Ischiorectal fistula

● 567 **Peritonitis and retroperitoneal infections**

Excludes *peritonitis:*
benign paroxysmal (277.31) (Revised)
pelvic, female (614.5, 614.7)
periodic familial (277.31) (Revised)
puerperal (670)
with or following:
abortion (634–638 with .0, 639.0)
appendicitis (540.0–540.1)
ectopic or molar pregnancy (639.0)

● 567.0 ***Peritonitis in infectious diseases classified elsewhere***

Code first underlying disease

Excludes *peritonitis:*
gonococcal (098.86)
syphilitic (095.2)
tuberculous (014.0)

567.1 **Pneumococcal peritonitis**

● 567.2 **Other suppurative peritonitis**

567.21 **Peritonitis (acute) generalized**
Pelvic peritonitis, male

567.22 **Peritoneal abscess**

Abscess (of):	Abscess (of):
abdominopelvic	retrocecal
mesenteric	subdiaphragmatic
omentum	subhepatic
peritoneum	subphrenic

567.23 **Spontaneous bacterial peritonitis**

Excludes *bacterial peritonitis NOS (567.29)* (New)

❑ 567.29 **Other suppurative peritonitis**
Subphrenic peritonitis

● 567.3 **Retroperitoneal infections**

567.31 **Psoas muscle abscess**

❑ 567.38 **Other retroperitoneal abscess**

❑ 567.39 **Other retroperitoneal infections**

● 567.8 **Other specified peritonitis**

567.81 **Choleperitonitis**
Peritonitis due to bile

567.82 **Sclerosing mesenteritis**
Fat necrosis of peritoneum
(Idiopathic) sclerosing mesenteric fibrosis
Mesenteric lipodystrophy
Mesenteric panniculitis
Retractile mesenteritis

❑ 567.89 **Other specified peritonitis**
Chronic proliferative peritonitis
Mesenteric saponification
Peritonitis due to urine

❑ 567.9 **Unspecified peritonitis**

Peritonitis:	Peritonitis:
NOS	of unspecified cause

● 568 **Other disorders of peritoneum**

568.0 **Peritoneal adhesions (postoperative) (postinfection)**

Adhesions (of):	Adhesions (of):
abdominal (wall)	mesenteric
diaphragm	omentum
intestine	stomach
male pelvis	

Adhesive bands

Excludes *adhesions:*
pelvic, female (614.6)
with obstruction:
duodenum (537.3)
intestine (560.81)

● 568.8 **Other specified disorders of peritoneum**

568.81 **Hemoperitoneum (nontraumatic)**

568.82 **Peritoneal effusion (chronic)**

Excludes *ascites NOS (789.5)*

❑ 568.89 **Other**
Peritoneal:

cyst	granuloma

❑ 568.9 **Unspecified disorder of peritoneum**

● 569 **Other disorders of intestine**

569.0 **Anal and rectal polyp**
Anal and rectal polyp NOS

Excludes *adenomatous anal and rectal polyp (211.4)*

569.1 **Rectal prolapse**

Procidentia:	Prolapse:
anus (sphincter)	anal canal
rectum (sphincter)	rectal mucosa

Proctoptosis

Excludes *prolapsed hemorrhoids (455.2, 455.5)*

569.2 **Stenosis of rectum and anus**
Stricture of anus (sphincter)

569.3 **Hemorrhage of rectum and anus**

Excludes *gastrointestinal bleeding NOS (578.9)*
melena (578.1)

● 569.4 **Other specified disorders of rectum and anus**

569.41 **Ulcer of anus and rectum**
Solitary ulcer of anus (sphincter) or rectum (sphincter)
Stercoral ulcer of anus (sphincter) or rectum (sphincter)

569.42 **Anal or rectal pain**

❑569.49 **Other**
Granuloma of rectum (sphincter)
Rupture of rectum (sphincter)
Hypertrophy of anal papillae
Proctitis NOS

Excludes *fistula of rectum to:*
internal organs - see Alphabetic Index
skin (565.1)
hemorrhoids (455.0–455.9)
incontinence of sphincter ani (787.6)

569.5 **Abscess of intestine**

Excludes *appendiceal abscess (540.1)*

● 569.6 **Colostomy and enterostomy complications**

❑569.60 **Colostomy and enterostomy complication, unspecified**

569.61 **Infection of colostomy and enterostomy**
Use additional code to identify organism (041.00–041.9)
Use additional code to specify type of infection, such as:
abscess or cellulitis of abdomen (682.2)
septicemia (038.0–038.9)

569.62 **Mechanical complication of colostomy and enterostomy**
Malfunction of colostomy and enterostomy

❑569.69 **Other complication**
Fistula
Hernia
Prolapse

● 569.8 **Other specified disorders of intestine**

569.81 **Fistula of intestine, excluding rectum and anus**
Fistula:
abdominal wall
enterocolic
enteroenteric
ileorectal

Excludes *fistula of intestine to internal organs - see Alphabetic Index*
persistent postoperative fistula (998.6)

569.82 **Ulceration of intestine**
Primary ulcer of intestine
Ulceration of colon

Excludes *that with perforation (569.83)*

569.83 **Perforation of intestine**

569.84 **Angiodysplasia of intestine (without mention of hemorrhage)**

569.85 **Angiodysplasia of intestine with hemorrhage**

569.86 **Dieulafoy lesion (hemorrhagic) of intestine**

❑569.89 **Other**
Enteroptosis
Granuloma of intestine
Prolapse of intestine
Pericolitis
Perisigmoiditis
Visceroptosis

Excludes *gangrene of intestine, mesentery, or omentum (557.0)*
hemorrhage of intestine NOS (578.9)
obstruction of intestine (560.0–560.9)

❑569.9 **Unspecified disorder of intestine**

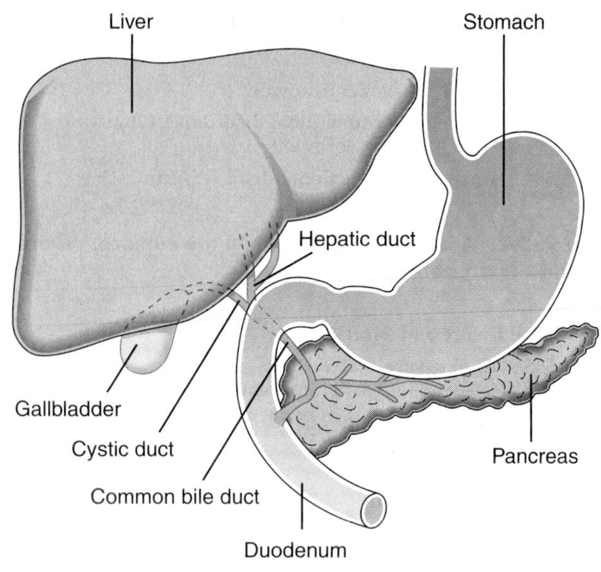

Liver
Stomach
Hepatic duct
Gallbladder
Cystic duct
Common bile duct
Pancreas
Duodenum

Figure 9–15 Liver and bile ducts.

Item 9–21 Cirrhosis is the progressive fibrosis of the liver resulting in loss of liver function. The main causes of cirrhosis of the liver are alcohol abuse, chronic hepatitis (inflammation of the liver), biliary disease, and excessive amounts of iron. **Alcoholic cirrhosis of the liver** is also called portal, Laënnec's, or fatty nutritional cirrhosis.

OTHER DISEASES OF DIGESTIVE SYSTEM (570–579)

570 **Acute and subacute necrosis of liver**
Acute hepatic failure
Acute or subacute hepatitis, not specified as infective
Necrosis of liver (acute) (diffuse) (massive) (subacute)
Parenchymatous degeneration of liver
Yellow atrophy (liver) (acute) (subacute)

Excludes *icterus gravis of newborn (773.0–773.2)*
serum hepatitis (070.2–070.3)
that with:
abortion (634–638 with .7, 639.8)
ectopic or molar pregnancy (639.8)
pregnancy, childbirth, or the puerperium (646.7)
viral hepatitis (070.0–070.9)

● 571 **Chronic liver disease and cirrhosis**

571.0 **Alcoholic fatty liver**

571.1 **Acute alcoholic hepatitis**
Acute alcoholic liver disease

571.2 **Alcoholic cirrhosis of liver**
Florid cirrhosis
Laënnec's cirrhosis (alcoholic)

❑571.3 **Alcoholic liver damage, unspecified**

● 571.4 **Chronic hepatitis**

Excludes *viral hepatitis (acute) (chronic) (070.0–070.9)*

❑571.40 **Chronic hepatitis, unspecified**

571.41 **Chronic persistent hepatitis**

❑571.49 **Other**
Chronic hepatitis:
active
aggressive
Recurrent hepatitis

571.5 Cirrhosis of liver without mention of alcohol
Cirrhosis of liver:
NOS
cryptogenic
macronodular
Cirrhosis of liver:
micronodular
posthepatitic
postnecrotic
Healed yellow atrophy (liver)
Portal cirrhosis

571.6 Biliary cirrhosis
Chronic nonsuppurative destructive cholangitis
Cirrhosis:
cholangitic
cholestatic

❑ **571.8 Other chronic nonalcoholic liver disease**
Chronic yellow atrophy (liver)
Fatty liver, without mention of alcohol

❑ **571.9 Unspecified chronic liver disease without mention of alcohol**

● **572 Liver abscess and sequelae of chronic liver disease**

572.0 Abscess of liver
Excludes *amebic liver abscess (006.3)*

572.1 Portal pyemia
Phlebitis of portal vein
Portal thrombophlebitis
Pylephlebitis
Pylethrombophlebitis

572.2 Hepatic coma
Hepatic encephalopathy
Hepatocerebral intoxication
Portal-systemic encephalopathy

572.3 Portal hypertension

572.4 Hepatorenal syndrome
Excludes *that following delivery (674.8)*

❑ **572.8 Other sequelae of chronic liver disease**

● **573 Other disorders of liver**
Excludes *amyloid or lardaceous degeneration of liver (277.39)* ◀
congenital cystic disease of liver (751.62)
glycogen infiltration of liver (271.0)
hepatomegaly NOS (789.1)
portal vein obstruction (452)

573.0 Chronic passive congestion of liver

● ***573.1 Hepatitis in viral diseases classified elsewhere***
Code first underlying disease, as:
Coxsackie virus disease (074.8)
cytomegalic inclusion virus disease (078.5)
infectious mononucleosis (075)
Excludes *hepatitis (in):*
mumps (072.71)
viral (070.0–070.9)
yellow fever (060.0–060.9)

● ❑ ***573.2 Hepatitis in other infectious diseases classified elsewhere***
Code first underlying disease, as:
malaria (084.9)
Excludes *hepatitis in:*
late syphilis (095.3)
secondary syphilis (091.62)
toxoplasmosis (130.5)

❑ **573.3 Hepatitis, unspecified**
Toxic (noninfectious) hepatitis
Use additional E code to identify cause

573.4 Hepatic infarction

❑ **573.8 Other specified disorders of liver**
Hepatoptosis

❑ **573.9 Unspecified disorder of liver**

● **574 Cholelithiasis**
The following fifth-digit subclassification is for use with category 574:
0 **without mention of obstruction**
1 **with obstruction**

● **574.0 Calculus of gallbladder with acute cholecystitis**
Biliary calculus with acute cholecystitis
Calculus of cystic duct with acute cholecystitis
Cholelithiasis with acute cholecystitis
Any condition classifiable to 574.2 with acute cholecystitis

● ❑ **574.1 Calculus of gallbladder with other cholecystitis**
Biliary calculus with cholecystitis
Calculus of cystic duct with cholecystitis
Cholelithiasis with cholecystitis
Cholecystitis with cholelithiasis NOS
Any condition classifiable to 574.2 with cholecystitis (chronic)

● **574.2 Calculus of gallbladder without mention of cholecystitis**
Biliary:
calculus NOS
colic NOS
Calculus of cystic duct
Cholelithiasis NOS
Colic (recurrent) of gallbladder
Gallstone (impacted)

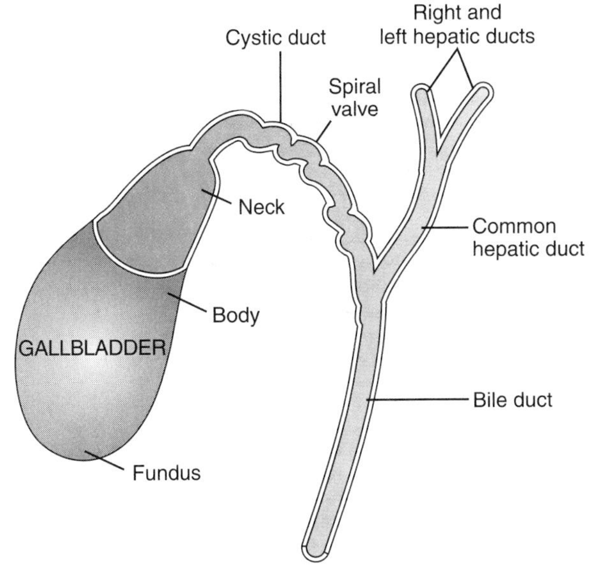
Cystic duct
Right and left hepatic ducts
Spiral valve
Neck
Common hepatic duct
Body
GALLBLADDER
Bile duct
Fundus

Figure 9–16 Gallbladder and bile ducts.

● **574.3 Calculus of bile duct with acute cholecystitis**
Calculus of bile duct [any] with acute cholecystitis
Choledocholithiasis with acute cholecystitis
Any condition classifiable to 574.5 with acute cholecystitis

● ❑ **574.4 Calculus of bile duct with other cholecystitis**
Calculus of bile duct [any] with cholecystitis (chronic)
Choledocholithiasis with cholecystitis (chronic)
Any condition classifiable to 574.5 with cholecystitis (chronic)

● **574.5 Calculus of bile duct without mention of cholecystitis**
Calculus of:
bile duct [any]
common duct
hepatic duct
Choledocholithiasis
Hepatic:
colic (recurrent)
lithiasis

● **574.6 Calculus of gallbladder and bile duct with acute cholecystitis**
Any condition classifiable to 574.0 and 574.3

● **574.7 Calculus of gallbladder and bile duct with other cholecystitis**
Any condition classifiable to 574.1 and 574.4

● **574.8 Calculus of gallbladder and bile duct with acute and chronic cholecystitis**
Any condition classifiable to 574.6 and 574.7

● **574.9 Calculus of gallbladder and bile duct without cholecystitis**
Any condition classifiable to 574.2 and 574.5

● **575 Other disorders of gallbladder**

575.0 Acute cholecystitis
Abscess of gallbladder without mention of calculus
Angiocholecystitis without mention of calculus
Cholecystitis without mention of calculus:
emphysematous (acute)
gangrenous
suppurative
Empyema of gallbladder without mention of calculus
Gangrene of gallbladder without mention of calculus

Excludes *that with:*
acute and chronic cholecystitis (575.12)
choledocholithiasis (574.3)
choledocholithiasis and cholelithiasis (574.6)
cholelithiasis (574.0)

● **575.1 Other cholecystitis**
Cholecystitis without mention of calculus:
NOS without mention of calculus
chronic without mention of calculus

Excludes *that with:*
choledocholithiasis (574.4)
choledocholithiasis and cholelithiasis (574.8)
cholelithiasis (574.1)

❑ **575.10 Cholecystitis, unspecified**
Cholecystitis NOS

575.11 Chronic cholecystitis

575.12 Acute and chronic cholecystitis

575.2 Obstruction of gallbladder
Occlusion of cystic duct or gallbladder without mention of calculus
Stenosis of cystic duct or gallbladder without mention of calculus
Stricture of cystic duct or gallbladder without mention of calculus

Excludes *that with calculus (574.0–574.2 with fifth digit 1)*

575.3 Hydrops of gallbladder
Mucocele of gallbladder

575.4 Perforation of gallbladder
Rupture of cystic duct or gallbladder

575.5 Fistula of gallbladder
Fistula:
cholecystoduodenal
Fistula:
cholecystoenteric

575.6 Cholesterolosis of gallbladder
Strawberry gallbladder

❑ **575.8 Other specified disorders of gallbladder**
Adhesions (of) cystic duct gallbladder
Atrophy (of) cystic duct gallbladder
Cyst (of) cystic duct gallbladder
Hypertrophy (of) cystic duct gallbladder
Nonfunctioning (of) cystic duct gallbladder
Ulcer (of) cystic duct gallbladder
Biliary dyskinesia

Excludes *Hartmann's pouch of intestine (V44.3)*
nonvisualization of gallbladder (793.3)

❑ **575.9 Unspecified disorder of gallbladder**

● **576 Other disorders of biliary tract**

Excludes *that involving the:*
cystic duct (575.0–575.9)
gallbladder (575.0–575.9)

576.0 Postcholecystectomy syndrome

576.1 Cholangitis
Cholangitis:
NOS
acute
ascending
chronic
primary
Cholangitis:
recurrent
sclerosing
secondary
stenosing
suppurative

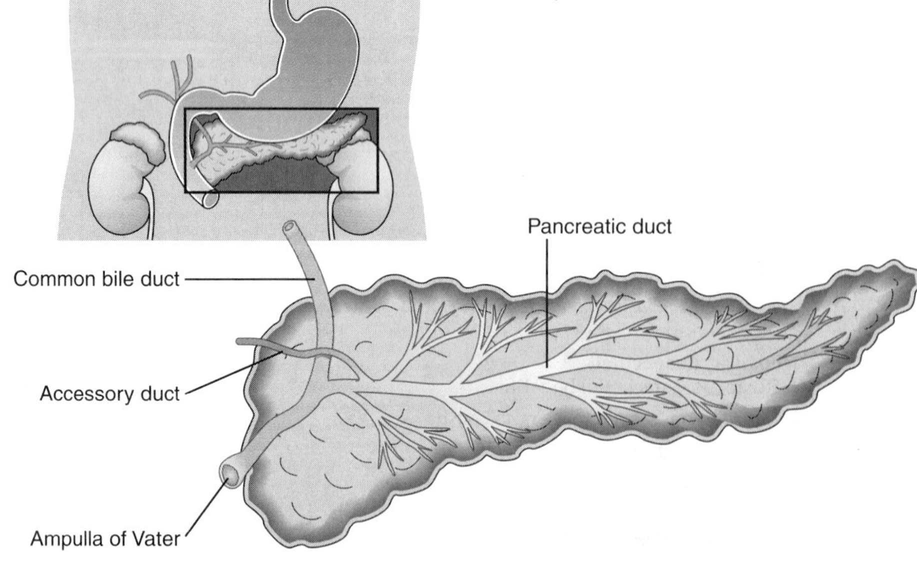

Pancreatic duct
Common bile duct
Accessory duct
Ampulla of Vater

Figure 9–17 Pancreas.

576.2 Obstruction of bile duct
Occlusion of bile duct, except cystic duct, without mention of calculus
Stenosis of bile duct, except cystic duct, without mention of calculus
Stricture of bile duct, except cystic duct, without mention of calculus
Excludes *congenital (751.61)*
that with calculus (574.3–574.5 with fifth-digit 1)

576.3 Perforation of bile duct
Rupture of bile duct, except cystic duct

576.4 Fistula of bile duct
Choledochoduodenal fistula

576.5 Spasm of sphincter of Oddi

❑ **576.8 Other specified disorders of biliary tract**
Adhesions of bile duct [any]
Atrophy of bile duct [any]
Cyst of bile duct [any]
Hypertrophy of bile duct [any]
Stasis of bile duct [any]
Ulcer of bile duct [any]
Excludes *congenital choledochal cyst (751.69)*

❑ **576.9 Unspecified disorder of biliary tract**

● **577 Diseases of pancreas**

577.0 Acute pancreatitis
Abscess of pancreas
Necrosis of pancreas:
acute
infective
Pancreatitis:
NOS
acute (recurrent)
apoplectic
hemorrhagic
subacute
suppurative
Excludes *mumps pancreatitis (072.3)*

577.1 Chronic pancreatitis
Chronic pancreatitis:
NOS
infectious
interstitial
Pancreatitis:
painless
recurrent
relapsing

577.2 Cyst and pseudocyst of pancreas

❑ **577.8 Other specified diseases of pancreas**
Atrophy of pancreas
Calculus of pancreas
Cirrhosis of pancreas
Fibrosis of pancreas
Pancreatic:
infantilism
necrosis:
NOS
aseptic
fat
Pancreatolithiasis
Excludes *fibrocystic disease of pancreas (277.00–277.09)*
islet cell tumor of pancreas (211.7)
pancreatic steatorrhea (579.4)

❑ **577.9 Unspecified disease of pancreas**

● **578 Gastrointestinal hemorrhage**
Excludes *that with mention of:*
angiodysplasia of stomach and duodenum (537.83)
angiodysplasia of intestine (569.85)
diverticulitis, intestine:
large (562.13)
small (562.03)
diverticulosis, intestine:
large (562.12)
small (562.02)
gastritis and duodenitis (535.0–535.6)
ulcer:
duodenal, gastric, gastrojejunal, or peptic (531.00–534.91)

578.0 Hematemesis
Vomiting of blood

578.1 Blood in stool
Melena
Excludes *melena of the newborn (772.4, 777.3)*
occult blood (792.1)

❑ **578.9 Hemorrhage of gastrointestinal tract, unspecified**
Gastric hemorrhage
Intestinal hemorrhage

● **579 Intestinal malabsorption**

579.0 Celiac disease
Celiac:
crisis
infantilism
rickets
Gee (-Herter) disease
Gluten enteropathy
Idiopathic steatorrhea
Nontropical sprue

579.1 Tropical sprue
Sprue:
NOS
tropical
Tropical steatorrhea

579.2 Blind loop syndrome
Postoperative blind loop syndrome

❑ **579.3 Other and unspecified postsurgical nonabsorption**
Hypoglycemia following gastrointestinal surgery
Malnutrition following gastrointestinal surgery

579.4 Pancreatic steatorrhea

❑ **579.8 Other specified intestinal malabsorption**
Enteropathy:
exudative
protein-losing
Steatorrhea (chronic)

❑ **579.9 Unspecified intestinal malabsorption**
Malabsorption syndrome NOS

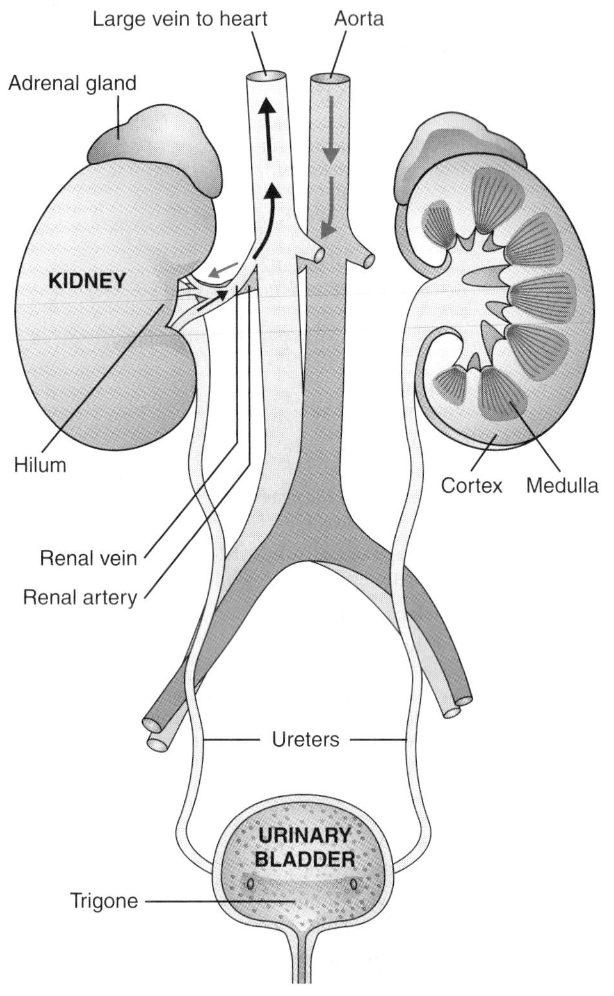
Large vein to heart
Aorta
Adrenal gland
KIDNEY
Hilum
Cortex
Medulla
Renal vein
Renal artery
Ureters
URINARY BLADDER
Trigone

Figure 10–1 Kidneys within the urinary system.

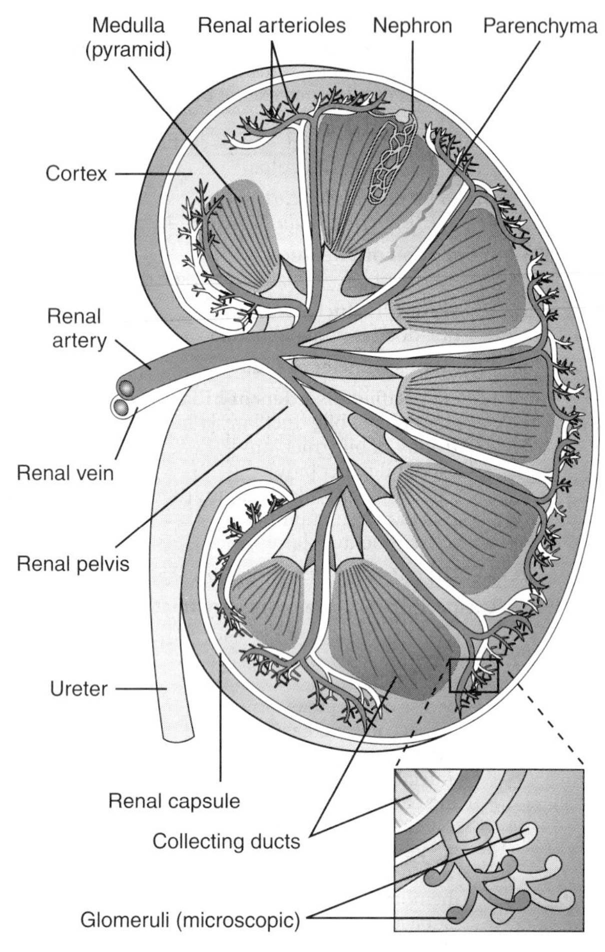
Medulla (pyramid)
Renal arterioles
Nephron
Parenchyma
Cortex
Renal artery
Renal vein
Renal pelvis
Ureter
Renal capsule
Collecting ducts
Glomeruli (microscopic)

Figure 10–2 Kidney.

Item 10-1 Glomerulonephritis is nephritis accompanied by inflammation of the glomeruli of the kidney, resulting in the degeneration of the glomeruli and the nephrons. **Acute glomerulonephritis** primarily affects children and young adults and is usually a result of a streptococcal infection.
Proliferative glomerulonephritis is the acute form of the disease resulting from a streptococcal infection.
Rapidly progressive glomerulonephritis, also known as **crescentic** or **malignant glomerulonephritis,** is the acute form of the disease, which leads quickly to rapid and progressive decline in renal function.

10. DISEASES OF THE GENITOURINARY SYSTEM (580–629)

NEPHRITIS, NEPHROTIC SYNDROME, AND NEPHROSIS (580–589)

Excludes *hypertensive chronic kidney disease (403.00–403.91, 404.00–404.93)*

● 580 **Acute glomerulonephritis**

Includes: acute nephritis

580.0 **With lesion of proliferative glomerulonephritis**
Acute (diffuse) proliferative glomerulonephritis
Acute poststreptococcal glomerulonephritis

580.4 **With lesion of rapidly progressive glomerulonephritis**
Acute nephritis with lesion of necrotizing glomerulitis

● 580.8 **With other specified pathological lesion in kidney**

● *580.81 Acute glomerulonephritis in diseases classified elsewhere*

Code first underlying disease, as:
infectious hepatitis (070.0–070.9)
mumps (072.79)
subacute bacterial endocarditis (421.0)
typhoid fever (002.0)

❑ 580.89 **Other**
Glomerulonephritis, acute, with lesion of:
exudative nephritis
interstitial (diffuse) (focal) nephritis

❑ 580.9 **Acute glomerulonephritis with unspecified pathological lesion in kidney**
Glomerulonephritis: specified as acute
NOS specified as acute
hemorrhagic specified as acute
Nephritis specified as acute
Nephropathy specified as acute

Item 10-2 Nephrotic syndrome (NS) is marked by massive proteinuria (protein in the urine) and water retention. Patients with NS are particularly vulnerable to staphylococcal and pneumococcal infections.
NS with lesion of proliferative glomerulonephritis results from a streptococcal infection.
NS with lesion of membranous glomerulonephritis results in thickening of the capillary walls.
NS with lesion of minimal change glomerulonephritis is usually a benign disorder that occurs mostly in children and requires electron microscopy to verify changes in the glomeruli.

● 581 Nephrotic syndrome

581.0 With lesion of proliferative glomerulonephritis

581.1 With lesion of membranous glomerulonephritis
Epimembranous nephritis
Idiopathic membranous glomerular disease
Nephrotic syndrome with lesion of:
focal glomerulosclerosis
sclerosing membranous glomerulonephritis
segmental hyalinosis

581.2 With lesion of membranoproliferative glomerulonephritis
Nephrotic syndrome with lesion (of):
endothelial glomerulonephritis
hypocomplementemic glomerulonephritis persistent glomerulonephritis
lobular glomerulonephritis
mesangiocapillary glomerulonephritis
mixed membranous and proliferative glomerulonephritis

581.3 With lesion of minimal change glomerulonephritis
Foot process disease
Lipoid nephrosis
Minimal change:
glomerular disease
glomerulitis
nephrotic syndrome

● 581.8 With other specified pathological lesion in kidney

● *581.81 Nephrotic syndrome in diseases classified elsewhere*

Code first underlying disease, as:
amyloidosis (277.30–277.39) ◄
diabetes mellitus (250.4)
malaria (084.9)
polyarteritis (446.0)
systemic lupus erythematosus (710.0)

Excludes *nephrosis in epidemic hemorrhagic fever (078.6)*

❑ 581.89 Other
Glomerulonephritis with edema and lesion of:
exudative nephritis
interstitial (diffuse) (focal) nephritis

❑ 581.9 Nephrotic syndrome with unspecified pathological lesion in kidney
Glomerulonephritis with edema NOS
Nephritis:
nephrotic NOS
with edema NOS
Nephrosis NOS
Renal disease with edema NOS

Item 10-3 Chronic glomerulonephritis (GN) persists over a period of years, with remissions and exacerbation.
Chronic GN with lesion of proliferative glomerulonephritis results from a streptococcal infection.
Chronic GN with lesion of membranous glomerulonephritis, also known as membranous nephropathy, is characterized by deposits along the epithelial side of the basement membrane.
Chronic GN with lesion of membranoproliferative glomerulonephritis (MPGN) is a group of disorders characterized by alterations in the basement membranes of the kidney and the glomerular cells.
Chronic GN with lesion of rapidly progressive glomerulonephritis is characterized by necrosis, endothelial proliferation, and mesangial proliferation. The condition is marked by rapid and progressive decline in renal function.

● 582 Chronic glomerulonephritis

Includes: chronic nephritis

582.0 With lesion of proliferative glomerulonephritis
Chronic (diffuse) proliferative glomerulonephritis

582.1 With lesion of membranous glomerulonephritis
Chronic glomerulonephritis:
membranous
sclerosing
Focal glomerulosclerosis
Segmental hyalinosis

582.2 With lesion of membranoproliferative glomerulonephritis
Chronic glomerulonephritis:
endothelial
hypocomplementemic persistent
lobular
membranoproliferative
mesangiocapillary
mixed membranous and proliferative

582.4 With lesion of rapidly progressive glomerulonephritis
Chronic nephritis with lesion of necrotizing glomerulitis

● 582.8 With other specified pathological lesion in kidney

● *582.81 Chronic glomerulonephritis in diseases classified elsewhere*

Code first underlying disease, as:
amyloidosis (277.30–277.39) ◄
systemic lupus erythematosus (710.0)

❑ 582.89 Other
Chronic glomerulonephritis with lesion of:
exudative nephritis
interstitial (diffuse) (focal) nephritis

❑ 582.9 Chronic glomerulonephritis with unspecified pathological lesion in kidney
Glomerulonephritis: specified as chronic
NOS specified as chronic
hemorrhagic specified as chronic
Nephritis specified as chronic
Nephropathy specified as chronic

Item 10-4 Nephritis (inflammation) or **nephropathy** (disease) **with lesion of proliferative glomerulonephritis** results from a streptococcal infection.
Nephritis (inflammation) or **nephropathy** (disease) **with lesion of membranous glomerulonephritis** is characterized by deposits along the epithelial side of the basement membrane.
Nephritis (inflammation) or **nephropathy** (disease) **with lesion of membranoproliferative glomerulonephritis** is characterized by alterations in the basement membranes of the kidney and the glomerular cells.
Nephritis (inflammation) or **nephropathy** (disease) **with lesion of rapidly progressive glomerulonephritis** is characterized by rapid and progressive decline in renal function.
Nephritis (inflammation) or **nephropathy** (disease) **with lesion of renal cortical necrosis** is characterized by death of the cortical tissues.
Nephritis (inflammation) or **nephropathy** (disease) **with lesion of renal medullary necrosis** is characterized by death of the tissues that collect urine.

● **583 Nephritis and nephropathy, not specified as acute or chronic**

Includes: "renal disease" so stated, not specified as acute or chronic but with stated pathology or cause

583.0 With lesion of proliferative glomerulonephritis
Proliferative:
glomerulonephritis (diffuse) NOS
nephritis NOS
nephropathy NOS

583.1 With lesion of membranous glomerulonephritis
Membranous:
glomerulonephritis NOS
nephritis NOS
Membranous nephropathy NOS

583.2 With lesion of membranoproliferative glomerulonephritis
Membranoproliferative:
glomerulonephritis NOS
nephritis NOS
nephropathy NOS
Nephritis NOS, with lesion of:
hypocomplementemic persistent glomerulonephritis
lobular glomerulonephritis
mesangiocapillary glomerulonephritis
mixed membranous and proliferative glomerulonephritis

583.4 With lesion of rapidly progressive glomerulonephritis
Necrotizing or rapidly progressive:
glomerulitis NOS
glomerulonephritis NOS
nephritis NOS
nephropathy NOS
Nephritis, unspecified, with lesion of necrotizing glomerulitis

583.6 With lesion of renal cortical necrosis
Nephritis NOS with (renal) cortical necrosis
Nephropathy NOS with (renal) cortical necrosis
Renal cortical necrosis NOS

583.7 With lesion of renal medullary necrosis
Nephritis NOS with (renal) medullary [papillary] necrosis
Nephropathy NOS with (renal) medullary [papillary] necrosis

● **583.8 With other specified pathological lesion in kidney**

● *583.81 **Nephritis and nephropathy, not specified as acute or chronic, in diseases classified elsewhere***

Code first underlying disease, as:
amyloidosis (277.30–277.39) ⬅
diabetes mellitus (250.4)
gonococcal infection (098.19)
Goodpasture's syndrome (446.21)
systemic lupus erythematosus (710.0)
tuberculosis (016.0)

Excludes *gouty nephropathy (274.10)*
syphilitic nephritis (095.4)

❑ **583.89 Other**
Glomerulitis with lesion of:
exudative nephritis
interstitial nephritis
Glomerulonephritis with lesion of:
exudative nephritis
interstitial nephritis
Nephritis with lesion of:
exudative nephritis
interstitial nephritis
Nephropathy with lesion of:
exudative nephritis
interstitial nephritis
Renal disease with lesion of:
exudative nephritis
interstitial nephritis

❑ **583.9 With unspecified pathological lesion in kidney**
Glomerulitis NOS
Glomerulonephritis NOS
Nephritis NOS
Nephropathy NOS

Excludes *nephropathy complicating pregnancy, labor, or the puerperium (642.0–642.9, 646.2)*
renal disease NOS with no stated cause (593.9)

Item 10-5 Decreased blood flow is the usual cause of **acute renal failure** that offers a good prognosis for recovery. **Chronic renal failure** is usually the result of long-standing kidney disease and is a very serious condition that generally results in death.

● **584 Acute renal failure**

Excludes *following labor and delivery (669.3)*
posttraumatic (958.5)
that complicating:
abortion (634–638 with .3, 639.3)
ectopic or molar pregnancy (639.3)

584.5 With lesion of tubular necrosis
Lower nephron nephrosis
Renal failure with (acute) tubular necrosis
Tubular necrosis:
NOS
acute

584.6 With lesion of renal cortical necrosis

584.7 With lesion of renal medullary [papillary] necrosis
Necrotizing renal papillitis

❑ **584.8 With other specified pathological lesion in kidney**

❑ **584.9 Acute renal failure, unspecified**

● **585 Chronic kidney disease (CKD)** ⇐
Chronic uremia
Code first hypertensive chronic kidney disease, if applicable, (403.00–403.91, 404.00–404.94) ◀
Use additional code to identify kidney transplant status, if applicable (V42.0)
Use additional code to identify manifestation as:
uremic:
neuropathy (357.4)
pericarditis (420.0)

585.1 Chronic kidney disease, Stage I

585.2 Chronic kidney disease, Stage II (mild)

585.3 Chronic kidney disease, Stage III (moderate)

585.4 Chronic kidney disease, Stage IV (severe)

585.5 Chronic kidney disease, Stage V
Excludes *chronic kidney disease, stage V requiring chronic dialysis (585.6)* ◀

585.6 End stage renal disease
Chronic kidney disease requiring chronic dialysis ◀

585.9 Chronic kidney disease, unspecified
Chronic renal disease
Chronic renal failure NOS
Chronic renal insufficiency

❑ **586 Renal failure, unspecified**
Uremia NOS
Excludes *following labor and delivery (669.3)*
posttraumatic renal failure (958.5)
that complicating:
abortion (634–638 with .3, 639.3)
ectopic or molar pregnancy (639.3)
uremia:
extrarenal (788.9)
prerenal (788.9)
with any condition classifiable to 401 (403.0–403.9 with fifth-digit 1)

❑ **587 Renal sclerosis, unspecified**
Atrophy of kidney
Contracted kidney
Renal:
cirrhosis
fibrosis
Excludes *nephrosclerosis (arteriolar) (arteriosclerotic) (403.00–403.92)*
with hypertension (403.00–403.92)

● **588 Disorders resulting from impaired renal function**

588.0 Renal osteodystrophy
Azotemic osteodystrophy
Phosphate-losing tubular disorders
Renal:
dwarfism
infantilism
rickets

588.1 Nephrogenic diabetes insipidus
Excludes *diabetes insipidus NOS (253.5)*

● **588.8 Other specified disorders resulting from impaired renal function**
Excludes *secondary hypertension (405.0–405.9)*

588.81 Secondary hyperparathyroidism (of renal origin)
Secondary hyperparathyroidism NOS

588.89 Other specified disorders resulting from impaired renal function
Hypokalemic nephropathy

❑ **588.9 Unspecified disorder resulting from impaired renal function**

● **589 Small kidney of unknown cause**

589.0 Unilateral small kidney

589.1 Bilateral small kidneys

❑ **589.9 Small kidney, unspecified**

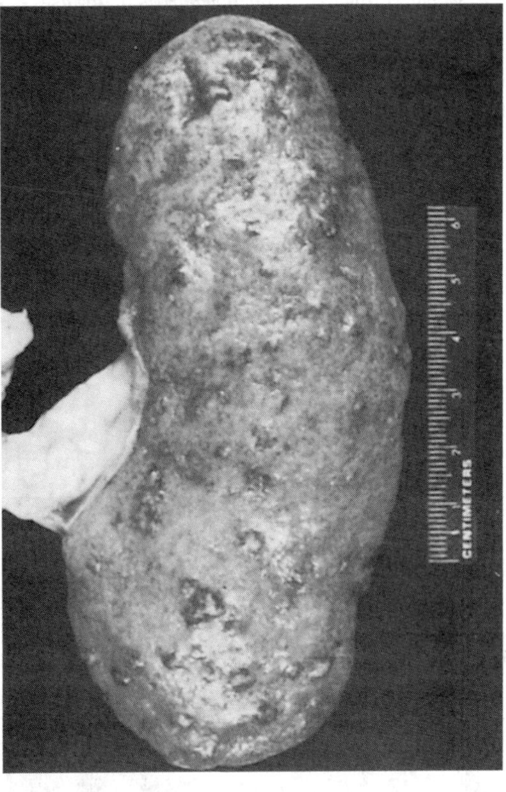
CENTIMETERS

Figure 10–3 Acute pyelonephritis. Cortical surface is dotted with abscesses. (From Cotran R, Kumar V, Robbins S: Robbins Pathologic Basis of Disease. Philadelphia, WB Saunders, 1994, p 969.)

OTHER DISEASES OF URINARY SYSTEM (590–599)

● **590 Infections of kidney**
Use additional code to identify organism, such as Escherichia coli [E. coli] (041.4)

● **590.0 Chronic pyelonephritis**
Chronic pyelitis
Chronic pyonephrosis
Code, if applicable, any causal condition first

590.00 Without lesion of renal medullary necrosis

590.01 With lesion of renal medullary necrosis

● **590.1 Acute pyelonephritis**
Acute pyelitis
Acute pyonephrosis

590.10 Without lesion of renal medullary necrosis

590.11 With lesion of renal medullary necrosis

590.2 Renal and perinephric abscess
Abscess:
kidney
nephritic
perirenal
Carbuncle of kidney

590.3 Pyeloureteritis cystica
Infection of renal pelvis and ureter
Ureteritis cystica

● **590.8 Other pyelonephritis or pyonephrosis, not specified as acute or chronic**

❑ **590.80 Pyelonephritis, unspecified**
Pyelitis NOS
Pyelonephritis NOS

● ***590.81 Pyelitis or pyelonephritis in diseases classified elsewhere***
Code first underlying disease, as:
tuberculosis (016.0)

❑ **590.9 Infection of kidney, unspecified**
Excludes *urinary tract infection NOS (599.0)*

591 Hydronephrosis
Hydrocalycosis
Hydronephrosis
Hydroureteronephrosis
Excludes *congenital hydronephrosis (753.29)*
hydroureter (593.5)

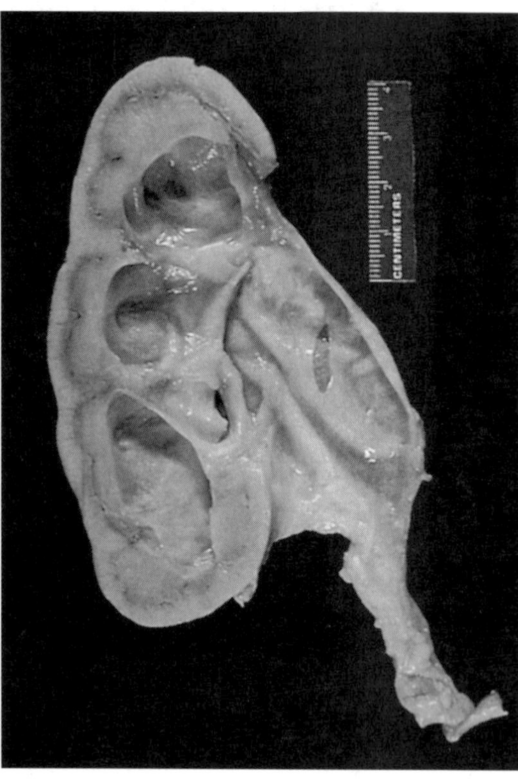
CENTIMETERS

Figure 10–4 Hydronephrosis of the kidney, with marked dilatation of pelvis and calyces and thinning of renal parenchyma. (From Cotran R, Kumar V, Collins T: Robbins Pathologic Basis of Disease, 6th ed. Philadelphia, WB Saunders, 1999, p 989.)

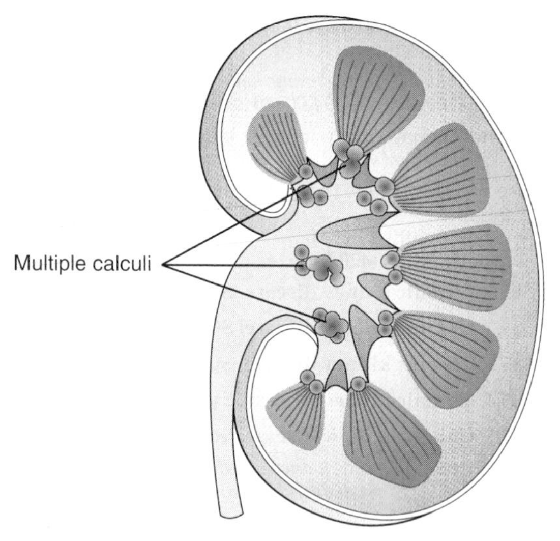
Multiple calculi

Figure 10–5 Multiple urinary calculi.

● **592 Calculus of kidney and ureter**
Excludes *nephrocalcinosis (275.49)*

592.0 Calculus of kidney
Nephrolithiasis NOS
Renal calculus or stone
Staghorn calculus
Stone in kidney
Excludes *uric acid nephrolithiasis (274.11)*

592.1 Calculus of ureter
Ureteric stone
Ureterolithiasis

❑ **592.9 Urinary calculus, unspecified**

● **593 Other disorders of kidney and ureter**

593.0 Nephroptosis
Floating kidney
Mobile kidney

593.1 Hypertrophy of kidney

593.2 Cyst of kidney, acquired
Cyst (multiple) (solitary) of kidney, not congenital
Peripelvic (lymphatic) cyst
Excludes *calyceal or pyelogenic cyst of kidney (591)*
congenital cyst of kidney (753.1)
polycystic (disease of) kidney (753.1)

593.3 Stricture or kinking of ureter
Angulation of ureter (postoperative)
Constriction of ureter (postoperative)
Stricture of pelviureteric junction

❑ **593.4 Other ureteric obstruction**
Idiopathic retroperitoneal fibrosis
Occlusion NOS of ureter
Excludes *that due to calculus (592.1)*

593.5 Hydroureter
Excludes *congenital hydroureter (753.22)*
hydroureteronephrosis (591)

593.6 Postural proteinuria
Benign postural proteinuria
Orthostatic proteinuria
Excludes *proteinuria NOS (791.0)*

Item 10-6 Vesicoureteral reflux occurs when urine flows from the bladder back into the ureters, often resulting in urinary tract infection.

● **593.7 Vesicoureteral reflux**

❑ **593.70 Unspecified or without reflux nephropathy**

593.71 With reflux nephropathy, unilateral

593.72 With reflux nephropathy, bilateral

❑ **593.73 With reflux nephropathy NOS**

● **593.8 Other specified disorders of kidney and ureter**

593.81 Vascular disorders of kidney
Renal (artery):
embolism
hemorrhage
thrombosis
Renal infarction

593.82 Ureteral fistula
Intestinoureteral fistula

Excludes *fistula between ureter and female genital tract (619.0)*

❑ **593.89 Other**
Adhesions, kidney or ureter
Periureteritis
Polyp of ureter
Pyelectasia
Ureterocele

Excludes *tuberculosis of ureter (016.2)*
ureteritis cystica (590.3)

❑ **593.9 Unspecified disorder of kidney and ureter**
Acute renal disease
Acute renal insufficiency
Renal disease NOS
Salt-losing nephritis or syndrome

Excludes *chronic renal insufficiency (585.9)*
cystic kidney disease (753.1)
nephropathy, so stated (583.0–583.9)
renal disease:
arising in pregnancy or the puerperium (642.1–642.2, 642.4–642.7, 646.2)
not specified as acute or chronic, but with stated pathology or cause (583.0–583.9)

● **594 Calculus of lower urinary tract**

594.0 Calculus in diverticulum of bladder

❑ **594.1 Other calculus in bladder**
Urinary bladder stone

Excludes *staghorn calculus (592.0)*

594.2 Calculus in urethra

❑ **594.8 Other lower urinary tract calculus**

❑ **594.9 Calculus of lower urinary tract, unspecified**

Excludes *calculus of urinary tract NOS (592.9)*

● **595 Cystitis**

Excludes *prostatocystitis (601.3)*

Use additional code to identify organism, such as Escherichia coli [E. coli] (041.4)

595.0 Acute cystitis

Excludes *trigonitis (595.3)*

595.1 Chronic interstitial cystitis
Hunner's ulcer
Panmural fibrosis of bladder
Submucous cystitis

❑ **595.2 Other chronic cystitis**
Chronic cystitis NOS
Subacute cystitis

Excludes *trigonitis (595.3)*

595.3 Trigonitis
Follicular cystitis
Trigonitis (acute) (chronic)
Urethrotrigonitis

● *595.4 Cystitis in diseases classified elsewhere*

Code first underlying disease, as:
actinomycosis (039.8)
amebiasis (006.8)
bilharziasis (120.0–120.9)
Echinococcus infestation (122.3, 122.6)

Excludes *cystitis:*
diphtheritic (032.84)
gonococcal (098.11, 098.31)
monilial (112.2)
trichomonal (131.09)
tuberculous (016.1)

● **595.8 Other specified types of cystitis**

595.81 Cystitis cystica

595.82 Irradiation cystitis

Use additional E code to identify cause

❑ **595.89 Other**
Abscess of bladder
Cystitis:
bullous
emphysematous
glandularis

❑ **595.9 Cystitis, unspecified**

Item 10-7 Intestinovesical fistula is a passage between the bladder and the intestine. **Diverticulum of the bladder** is the formation of a sac from a herniation of the wall of the bladder through a deviation. **Atony of the bladder** is diminished tone of the bladder muscle.

● **596 Other disorders of bladder**

Use additional code to identify urinary incontinence (625.6, 788.30–788.39)

596.0 Bladder neck obstruction
Contracture (acquired) of bladder neck or vesicourethral orifice
Obstruction (acquired) of bladder neck or vesicourethral orifice
Stenosis (acquired) of bladder neck or vesicourethral orifice

Excludes *congenital (753.6)*

596.1 Intestinovesical fistula
Fistula:
enterovesical
vesicocolic
Fistula:
vesicoenteric
vesicorectal

596.2 Vesical fistula, not elsewhere classified
Fistula:
bladder NOS
urethrovesical
Fistula:
vesicocutaneous
vesicoperineal

Excludes *fistula between bladder and female genital tract (619.0)*

596.3 Diverticulum of bladder
Diverticulitis of bladder
Diverticulum (acquired) (false) of bladder

Excludes *that with calculus in diverticulum of bladder (594.0)*

596.4 Atony of bladder
High compliance bladder
Hypotonicity of bladder
Inertia of bladder

Excludes *neurogenic bladder (596.54)*

● **596.5 Other functional disorders of bladder**

Excludes *cauda equina syndrome with neurogenic bladder (344.61)*

596.51 Hypertonicity of bladder
Hyperactivity
Overactive bladder

596.52 Low bladder compliance

596.53 Paralysis of bladder

596.54 Neurogenic bladder NOS

596.55 Detrusor sphincter dyssynergia

❑ **596.59 Other functional disorder of bladder**
Detrusor instability

596.6 Rupture of bladder, nontraumatic

596.7 Hemorrhage into bladder wall
Hyperemia of bladder

Excludes *acute hemorrhagic cystitis (595.0)*

❑ **596.8 Other specified disorders of bladder**
Calcified
Contracted
Hemorrhage
Hypertrophy

Excludes *cystocele, female (618.01–618.02, 618.09, 618.2–618.4)*
hernia or prolapse of bladder, female (618.01–618.02, 618.09, 618.2–618.4)

❑ **596.9 Unspecified disorder of bladder**

● **597 Urethritis, not sexually transmitted, and urethral syndrome**

Excludes *nonspecific urethritis, so stated (099.4)*

597.0 Urethral abscess
Abscess of:
bulbourethral gland
Cowper's gland
Littré's gland
Abscess:
periurethral
urethral (gland)
Periurethral cellulitis

Excludes *urethral caruncle (599.3)*

● **597.8 Other urethritis**

❑ **597.80 Urethritis, unspecified**

597.81 Urethral syndrome NOS

❑ **597.89 Other**
Adenitis, Skene's glands
Cowperitis
Meatitis, urethral
Ulcer, urethra (meatus)
Verumontanitis

Excludes *trichomonal (131.02)*

● **598 Urethral stricture**

Includes: pinhole meatus
stricture of urinary meatus

Use additional code to identify urinary incontinence (625.6, 788.30–788.39)

Excludes *congenital stricture of urethra and urinary meatus (753.6)*

● **598.0 Urethral stricture due to infection**

❑ **598.00 Due to unspecified infection**

● ***598.01 Due to infective diseases classified elsewhere***

Code first underlying disease, as:
gonococcal infection (098.2)
schistosomiasis (120.0–120.9)
syphilis (095.8)

598.1 Traumatic urethral stricture
Stricture of urethra:
late effect of injury
postobstetric

Excludes *postoperative following surgery on genitourinary tract (598.2)*

598.2 Postoperative urethral stricture
Postcatheterization stricture of urethra

❑ **598.8 Other specified causes of urethral stricture**

❑ **598.9 Urethral stricture, unspecified**

● **599 Other disorders of urethra and urinary tract**

❑ **599.0 Urinary tract infection, site not specified**

Excludes *Candidiasis of urinary tract (112.2)*
urinary tract infection of newborn (771.82)

Use additional code to identify organism, such as Escherichia coli [E. coli] (041.4)

599.1 Urethral fistula
Fistula:
urethroperineal
urethrorectal
Urinary fistula NOS

Excludes *fistula:*
urethroscrotal (608.89)
urethrovaginal (619.0)
urethrovesicovaginal (619.0)

599.2 Urethral diverticulum

599.3 Urethral caruncle
Polyp of urethra

599.4 Urethral false passage

599.5 Prolapsed urethral mucosa
Prolapse of urethra
Urethrocele

Excludes *urethrocele, female (618.03, 618.09, 618.2–618.4)*

● **599.6 Urinary obstruction** ⇐

Use additional code to identify urinary incontinence (625.6, 788.30–788.39)

Excludes *obstructive nephropathy NOS (593.89)*

❑ **599.60 Urinary obstruction, unspecified**
Obstructive uropathy NOS
Urinary (tract) obstruction NOS

❑ **599.69 Urinary obstruction, not elsewhere classified**

Code, if applicable, any causal condition first, such as: ◀
hyperplasia of prostate (600.0–600.9 with fifth-digit 1) ◀

599.7 Hematuria
Hematuria (benign) (essential)

Excludes *hemoglobinuria (791.2)*

● **599.8 Other specified disorders of urethra and urinary tract**

Use additional code to identify urinary incontinence (625.6, 788.30–788.39)

Excludes *symptoms and other conditions classifiable to 788.0–788.2, 788.4–788.9, 791.0–791.9*

599.81 Urethral hypermobility

599.82 Intrinsic (urethral) sphincter deficiency [ISD]

599.83 Urethral instability

❑ **599.84 Other specified disorders of urethra**
Rupture of urethra (nontraumatic)
Urethral:
cyst
granuloma

❑ **599.89 Other specified disorders of urinary tract**

❑ **599.9 Unspecified disorder of urethra and urinary tract**

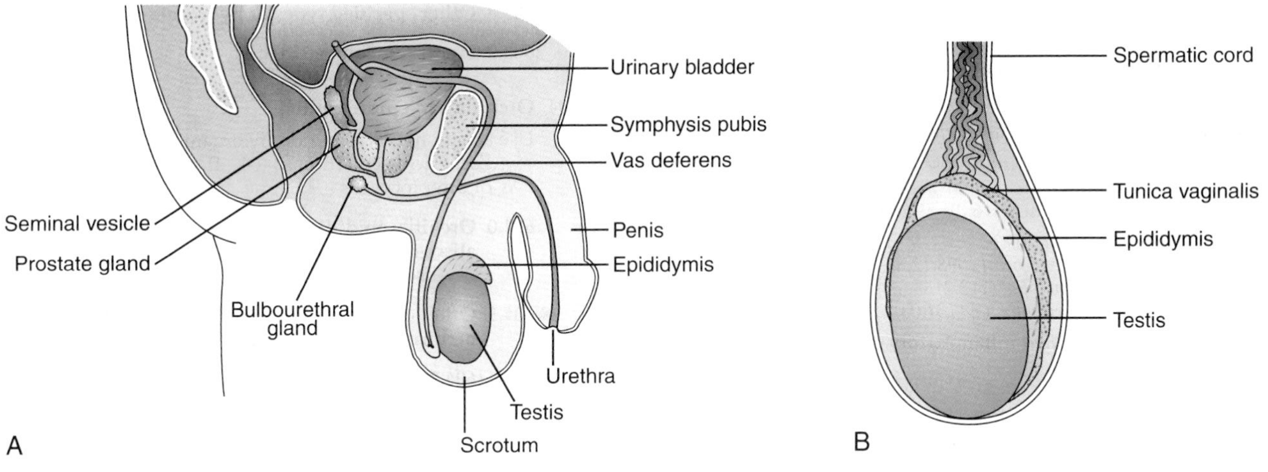
Urinary bladder
Symphysis pubis
Vas deferens
Seminal vesicle
Prostate gland
Penis
Epididymis
Bulbourethral gland
Urethra
Testis
Scrotum
A
Spermatic cord
Tunica vaginalis
Epididymis
Testis
B

Figure 10–6 **A.** Male genital system. **B.** Testis.

DISEASES OF MALE GENITAL ORGANS (600–608)

● **600 Hyperplasia of prostate**
Includes: enlarged prostate ◀

● **600.0 Hypertrophy (benign) of prostate**
Benign prostatic hypertrophy
Enlargement of prostate
Smooth enlarged prostate
Soft enlarged prostate

600.00 Hypertropy (benign) of prostate without urinary obstruction and other lower urinary tract symptoms (LUTS) ⬅
Hypertrophy (benign) of prostate NOS

600.01 Hypertrophy (benign) of prostate with urinary obstruction and other lower urinary tract symptoms (LUTS) ⬅
Hypertrophy (benign) of prostate with urinary retention

Use additional code to identify symptoms: ◀
incomplete bladder emptying (788.21) ◀
nocturia (788.43) ◀
straining on urination (788.65) ◀
urinary frequency (788.41) ◀
urinary hesitancy (788.64) ◀
urinary incontinence (788.30–788.39) ◀
urinary obstruction (599.69) ◀
urinary retention (788.20) ◀
urinary urgency (788.63) ◀
weak urinary stream (788.62) ◀

● **600.1 Nodular prostate**
Hard, firm prostate
Multinodular prostate
Excludes *malignant neoplasm of prostate (185)*

600.10 Nodular prostate without urinary obstruction
Nodular prostate NOS

600.11 Nodular prostate with urinary obstruction
Nodular prostate with urinary retention

● **600.2 Benign localized hyperplasia of prostate**
Adenofibromatous hypertrophy of prostate
Adenoma of prostate
Fibroadenoma of prostate
Fibroma of prostate
Myoma of prostate
Polyp of prostate
Excludes *benign neoplasms of prostate (222.2)*
hypertrophy of prostate (600.00–600.01)
malignant neoplasm of prostate (185)

600.20 Benign localized hyperplasia of prostate without urinary obstruction and other lower urinary tract symptoms (LUTS) ⬅
Benign localized hyperplasia of prostate NOS

600.21 Benign localized hyperplasia of prostate with urinary obstruction and other lower urinary tract symptoms (LUTS) ⬅
Benign localized hyperplasia of prostate with urinary retention

Use additional code to identify symptoms: ◀
incomplete bladder emptying (788.21) ◀
nocturia (788.43) ◀
straining on urination (788.65) ◀
urinary frequency (788.41) ◀
urinary hesitancy (788.64) ◀
urinary incontinence (788.30–788.39) ◀
urinary obstruction (599.69) ◀
urinary retention (788.20) ◀
urinary urgency (788.63) ◀
weak urinary stream (788.62) ◀

600.3 Cyst of prostate

● **600.9 Hyperplasia of prostate, unspecified**
Median bar
Prostatic obstruction NOS

❑ **600.90 Hyperplasia of prostate, unspecified, without urinary obstruction and other lower urinary tract symptoms (LUTS)** ⬅
Hyperplasia of prostate NOS

❑ **600.91 Hyperplasia of prostate, unspecified, with urinary obstruction and other lower urinary tract symptoms (LUTS)** ⬅
Hyperplasia of prostate, unspecified, with urinary retention

Use additional code to identify symptoms: ◀
incomplete bladder emptying (788.21) ◀
nocturia (788.43) ◀
straining on urination (788.65) ◀
urinary frequency (788.41) ◀
urinary hesitancy (788.64) ◀
urinary incontinence (788.30–788.39) ◀
urinary obstruction (599.69) ◀
urinary retention (788.20) ◀
urinary urgency (788.63) ◀
weak urinary stream (788.62) ◀

● **601 Inflammatory diseases of prostate**
Use additional code to identify organism, such as Staphylococcus (041.1), or Streptococcus (041.0)

601.0 **Acute prostatitis**

601.1 **Chronic prostatitis**

601.2 **Abscess of prostate**

601.3 **Prostatocystitis**

● *601.4 **Prostatitis in diseases classified elsewhere***

Code first underlying disease, as:
actinomycosis (039.8) syphilis (095.8)
blastomycosis (116.0) tuberculosis (016.5)

Excludes *prostatitis:*
gonococcal (098.12, 098.32)
monilial (112.2)
trichomonal (131.03)

❑601.8 **Other specified inflammatory diseases of prostate**
Prostatitis:
cavitary
diverticular
granulomatous

❑601.9 **Prostatitis, unspecified**
Prostatitis NOS

● 602 **Other disorders of prostate**

602.0 **Calculus of prostate**
Prostatic stone

602.1 **Congestion or hemorrhage of prostate**

602.2 **Atrophy of prostate**

602.3 **Dysplasia of prostate**
Prostatic intraepithelial neoplasia I (PIN I)
Prostatic intraepithelial neoplasia II (PIN II)

Excludes *Prostatic intraepithelial neoplasia III (PIN III) (233.4)*

❑602.8 **Other specified disorders of prostate**
Fistula of prostate
Infarction of prostate
Stricture of prostate
Periprostatic adhesions

❑602.9 **Unspecified disorder of prostate**

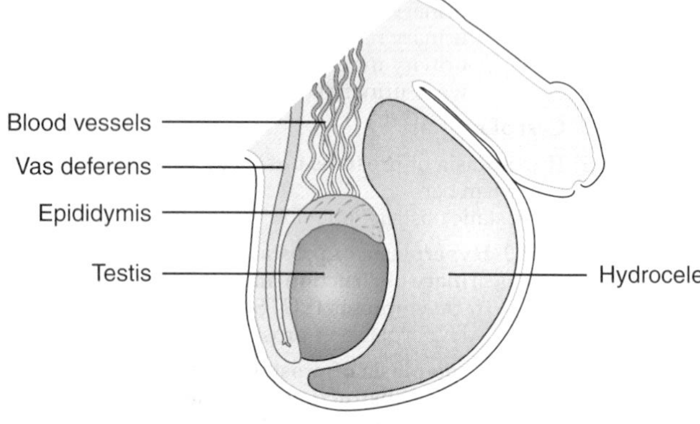

Blood vessels
Vas deferens
Epididymis
Testis
Hydrocele

Figure 10–7 Hydrocele.

Item 10–8 Hydrocele is a sac of fluid in the testes membrane.

● 603 **Hydrocele**

Includes: hydrocele of spermatic cord, testis, or tunica vaginalis

Excludes *congenital (778.6)*

603.0 **Encysted hydrocele**

603.1 **Infected hydrocele**
Use additional code to identify organism

❑603.8 **Other specified types of hydrocele**

❑603.9 **Hydrocele, unspecified**

● 604 **Orchitis and epididymitis**

Use additional code to identify organism, such as Escherichia coli [E. coli] (041.4), Staphylococcus (041.1), or Streptococcus (041.0)

604.0 **Orchitis, epididymitis, and epididymo-orchitis, with abscess**
Abscess of epididymis or testis

● 604.9 **Other orchitis, epididymitis, and epididymo-orchitis, without mention of abscess**

❑604.90 **Orchitis and epididymitis, unspecified**

● *604.91 **Orchitis and epididymitis in diseases classified elsewhere***

Code first underlying disease, as:
diphtheria (032.89)
filariasis (125.0–125.9)
syphilis (095.8)

Excludes *orchitis:*
gonococcal (098.13, 098.33)
mumps (072.0)
tuberculous (016.5)
tuberculous epididymitis (016.4)

❑604.99 **Other**

605 **Redundant prepuce and phimosis**
Adherent prepuce
Paraphimosis
Phimosis (congenital)
Tight foreskin

● 606 **Infertility, male**

606.0 **Azoospermia**
Absolute infertility
Infertility due to:
germinal (cell) aplasia
spermatogenic arrest (complete)

606.1 **Oligospermia**
Infertility due to:
germinal cell desquamation
hypospermatogenesis
incomplete spermatogenic arrest

606.8 **Infertility due to extratesticular causes**
Infertility due to:
drug therapy
infection
obstruction of efferent ducts
radiation
systemic disease

❑606.9 **Male infertility, unspecified**

● 607 **Disorders of penis**

Excludes *phimosis (605)*

607.0 **Leukoplakia of penis**
Kraurosis of penis

Excludes *carcinoma in situ of penis (233.5)*
erythroplasia of Queyrat (233.5)

607.1 **Balanoposthitis**
Balanitis

Use additional code to identify organism

❑607.2 **Other inflammatory disorders of penis**
Abscess of corpus cavernosum or penis
Boil of corpus cavernosum or penis
Carbuncle of corpus cavernosum or penis
Cellulitis of corpus cavernosum or penis
Cavernitis (penis)

Use additional code to identify organism

Excludes *herpetic infection (054.13)*

607.3 **Priapism**
Painful erection

● 607.8 **Other specified disorders of penis**

607.81 **Balanitis xerotica obliterans**
Induratio penis plastica

607.82 **Vascular disorders of penis**
Embolism of corpus cavernosum or penis
Hematoma (nontraumatic) of corpus cavernosum or penis
Hemorrhage of corpus cavernosum or penis
Thrombosis of corpus cavernosum or penis

607.83 **Edema of penis**

607.84 **Impotence of organic origin**

Excludes *nonorganic (302.72)*

607.85 **Peyronie's disease**

❑607.89 **Other**
Atrophy of corpus cavernosum or penis
Fibrosis of corpus cavernosum or penis
Hypertrophy of corpus cavernosum or penis
Ulcer (chronic) of corpus cavernosum or penis

❑607.9 **Unspecified disorder of penis**

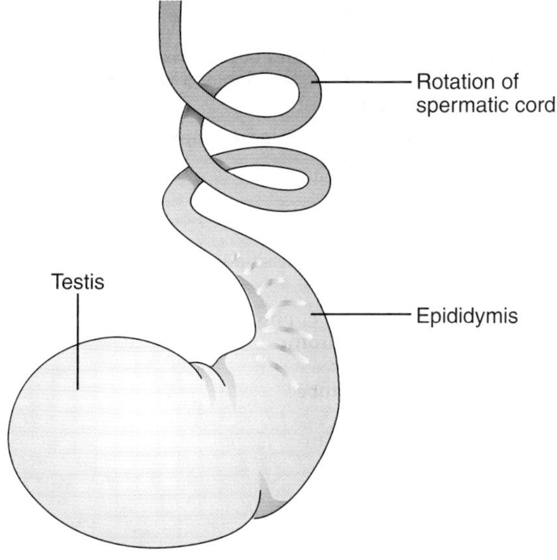
Rotation of
spermatic cord
Testis
Epididymis

Figure 10–8 Torsion of testis.

Item 10–9 Rotation of the spermatic cord causes strangulation and infarction of the testis by cutting off blood circulation to the area.

● 608 **Other disorders of male genital organs**

608.0 **Seminal vesiculitis**
Abscess of seminal vesicle
Cellulitis of seminal vesicle
Vesiculitis (seminal)

Use additional code to identify organism

Excludes *gonococcal infection (098.14, 098.34)*

608.1 **Spermatocele**

● 608.2 **Torsion of testis** ⇐

❑608.20 **Torsion of testis, unspecified** ◀

608.21 **Extravaginal torsion of spermatic cord** ◀

608.22 **Intravaginal torsion of spermatic cord** ◀

608.23 **Torsion of appendix testis** ◀

608.24 **Torsion of appendix epididymis** ◀

608.3 **Atrophy of testis**

❑608.4 **Other inflammatory disorders of male genital organs**
Abscess of scrotum, spermatic cord, testis [except abscess], tunica vaginalis, or vas deferens
Boil of scrotum, spermatic cord, testis [except abscess], tunica vaginalis, or vas deferens
Carbuncle of scrotum, spermatic cord, testis [except abscess], tunica vaginalis, or vas deferens
Cellulitis of scrotum, spermatic cord, testis [except abscess], tunica vaginalis, or vas deferens
Vasitis

Use additional code to identify organism

Excludes *abscess of testis (604.0)*

● 608.8 **Other specified disorders of male genital organs**

● 608.81 ***Disorders of male genital organs in diseases classified elsewhere***

Code first underlying disease, as:
filariasis (125.0–125.9)
tuberculosis (016.5)

608.82 **Hematospermia**

608.83 **Vascular disorders**
Hematoma (nontraumatic) of seminal vesicle, spermatic cord, testis, scrotum, tunica vaginalis, or vas deferens
Hemorrhage of seminal vesicle, spermatic cord, testis, scrotum, tunica vaginalis, or vas deferens
Thrombosis of seminal vesicle, spermatic cord, testis, scrotum, tunica vaginalis, or vas deferens
Hematocele NOS, male

608.84 **Chylocele of tunica vaginalis**

608.85 **Stricture**
Stricture of:
spermatic cord
tunica vaginalis
Stricture of:
vas deferens

608.86 **Edema**

608.87 **Retrograde ejaculation**

❑608.89 **Other**
Atrophy of seminal vesicle, spermatic cord, testis, scrotum, tunica vaginalis, or vas deferens
Fibrosis of seminal vesicle, spermatic cord, testis, scrotum, tunica vaginalis, or vas deferens
Hypertrophy of seminal vesicle, spermatic cord, testis, scrotum, tunica vaginalis, or vas deferens
Ulcer of seminal vesicle, spermatic cord, testis, scrotum, tunica vaginalis, or vas deferens

Excludes *atrophy of testis (608.3)*

❑608.9 **Unspecified disorder of male genital organs**

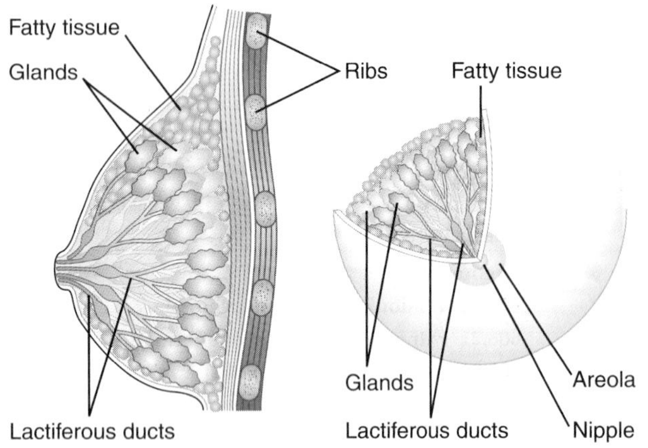
Fatty tissue
Glands
Ribs
Fatty tissue
Glands
Areola
Lactiferous ducts
Lactiferous ducts
Nipple

Figure 10–9 Breast.

DISORDERS OF BREAST (610–611)

● **610 Benign mammary dysplasias**

610.0 Solitary cyst of breast
Cyst (solitary) of breast

610.1 Diffuse cystic mastopathy
Chronic cystic mastitis
Cystic breast
Fibrocystic disease of breast

610.2 Fibroadenosis of breast
Fibroadenosis of breast:
NOS
chronic
cystic
Fibroadenosis of breast:
diffuse
periodic
segmental

610.3 Fibrosclerosis of breast

610.4 Mammary duct ectasia
Comedomastitis
Duct ectasia
Mastitis:
periductal
plasma cell

❑ **610.8 Other specified benign mammary dysplasias**
Mazoplasia
Sebaceous cyst of breast

❑ **610.9 Benign mammary dysplasia, unspecified**

● **611 Other disorders of breast**

Excludes *that associated with lactation or the puerperium (675.0–676.9)*

611.0 Inflammatory disease of breast
Abscess (acute) (chronic) (nonpuerperal) of:
areola
breast
Mammillary fistula
Mastitis (acute) (subacute) (nonpuerperal):
NOS
infective
retromammary
submammary

Excludes *carbuncle of breast (680.2)*
chronic cystic mastitis (610.1)
neonatal infective mastitis (771.5)
thrombophlebitis of breast [Mondor's disease] (451.89)

611.1 Hypertrophy of breast
Gynecomastia
Hypertrophy of breast:
NOS
massive pubertal

611.2 Fissure of nipple

611.3 Fat necrosis of breast
Fat necrosis (segmental) of breast

611.4 Atrophy of breast

611.5 Galactocele

611.6 Galactorrhea not associated with childbirth

● **611.7 Signs and symptoms in breast**

611.71 Mastodynia
Pain in breast

611.72 Lump or mass in breast

❑ **611.79 Other**
Induration of breast
Inversion of nipple
Nipple discharge
Retraction of nipple

❑ **611.8 Other specified disorders of breast**
Hematoma (nontraumatic) of breast
Infarction of breast
Occlusion of breast duct
Subinvolution of breast (postlactational) (postpartum)

❑ **611.9 Unspecified breast disorder**

INFLAMMATORY DISEASE OF FEMALE PELVIC ORGANS (614–616)

Use additional code to identify organism, such as Staphylococcus (041.1), or Streptococcus (041.0)

Excludes *that associated with pregnancy, abortion, childbirth, or the puerperium (630–676.9)*

● **614 Inflammatory disease of ovary, fallopian tube, pelvic cellular tissue, and peritoneum**

Excludes *endometritis (615.0–615.9)*
major infection following delivery (670)
that complicating:
abortion (634–638 with .0, 639.0)
ectopic or molar pregnancy (639.0)
pregnancy or labor (646.6)

614.0 Acute salpingitis and oophoritis
Any condition classifiable to 614.2, specified as acute or subacute

614.1 Chronic salpingitis and oophoritis
Hydrosalpinx
Salpingitis:
follicularis
isthmica nodosa
Any condition classifiable to 614.2, specified as chronic

❑ **614.2 Salpingitis and oophoritis not specified as acute, subacute, or chronic**
Abscess (of):
fallopian tube
ovary
tubo-ovarian
Oophoritis
Perioophoritis
Perisalpingitis
Pyosalpinx
Salpingitis
Salpingo-oophoritis
Tubo-ovarian inflammatory disease

Excludes *gonococcal infection (chronic) (098.37)*
acute (098.17)
tuberculous (016.6)

614.3 Acute parametritis and pelvic cellulitis
Acute inflammatory pelvic disease
Any condition classifiable to 614.4, specified as acute

614.4 Chronic or unspecified parametritis and pelvic cellulitis
Abscess (of):
broad ligament chronic or NOS
parametrium chronic or NOS
pelvis, female chronic or NOS
pouch of Douglas chronic or NOS
Chronic inflammatory pelvic disease
Pelvic cellulitis, female

Excludes *tuberculous (016.7)*

614.5 Acute or unspecified pelvic peritonitis, female

614.6 Pelvic peritoneal adhesions, female (postoperative) (postinfection)
Adhesions:
peritubal
tubo-ovarian

Use additional code to identify any associated infertility (628.2)

❑**614.7 Other chronic pelvic peritonitis, female**

Excludes *tuberculous (016.7)*

❑**614.8 Other specified inflammatory disease of female pelvic organs and tissues**

❑**614.9 Unspecified inflammatory disease of female pelvic organs and tissues**
Pelvic infection or inflammation, female NOS
Pelvic inflammatory disease [PID]

● **615 Inflammatory diseases of uterus, except cervix**

Excludes *following delivery (670)*
hyperplastic endometritis (621.30–621.33)
that complicating:
abortion (634–638 with .0, 639.0)
ectopic or molar pregnancy (639.0)
pregnancy or labor (646.6)

615.0 Acute
Any condition classifiable to 615.9, specified as acute or subacute

615.1 Chronic
Any condition classifiable to 615.9, specified as chronic

❑**615.9 Unspecified inflammatory disease of uterus**
Endometritis
Endomyometritis
Metritis
Myometritis
Perimetritis
Pyometra
Uterine abscess

● **616 Inflammatory disease of cervix, vagina, and vulva**

Excludes *that complicating:*
abortion (634–638 with .0, 639.0)
ectopic or molar pregnancy (639.0)
pregnancy, childbirth, or the puerperium (646.6)

616.0 Cervicitis and endocervicitis
Cervicitis with or without mention of erosion or ectropion
Endocervicitis with or without mention of erosion or ectropion
Nabothian (gland) cyst or follicle

Excludes *erosion or ectropion without mention of cervicitis (622.0)*

● **616.1 Vaginitis and vulvovaginitis**

❑**616.10 Vaginitis and vulvovaginitis, unspecified**
Vaginitis:
NOS
postirradiation
Vulvitis NOS
Vulvovaginitis NOS

Use additional code to identify organism, such as Escherichia coli [E. coli] (041.4), Staphylococcus (041.1), or Streptococcus (041.0)

Excludes *noninfective leukorrhea (623.5)*
postmenopausal or senile vaginitis (627.3)

● ***616.11 Vaginitis and vulvovaginitis in diseases classified elsewhere***

Code first underlying disease, as:
pinworm vaginitis (127.4)

Excludes *herpetic vulvovaginitis (054.11)*
monilial vulvovaginitis (112.1)
trichomonal vaginitis or vulvovaginitis (131.01)

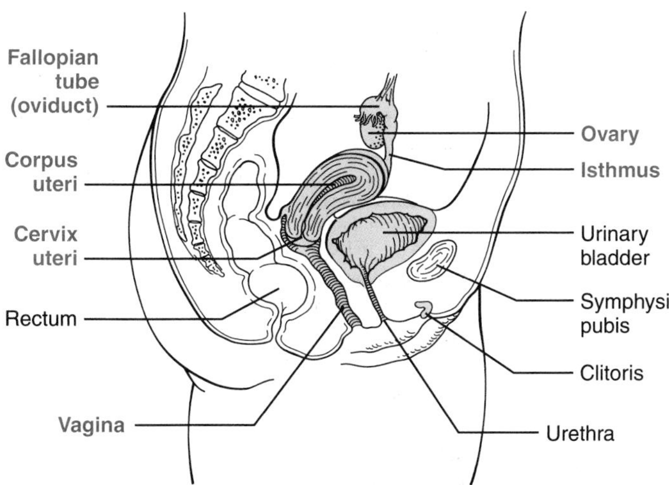
Fallopian tube (oviduct)
Corpus uteri
Cervix uteri
Rectum
Vagina
Ovary
Isthmus
Urinary bladder
Symphysis pubis
Clitoris
Urethra
A

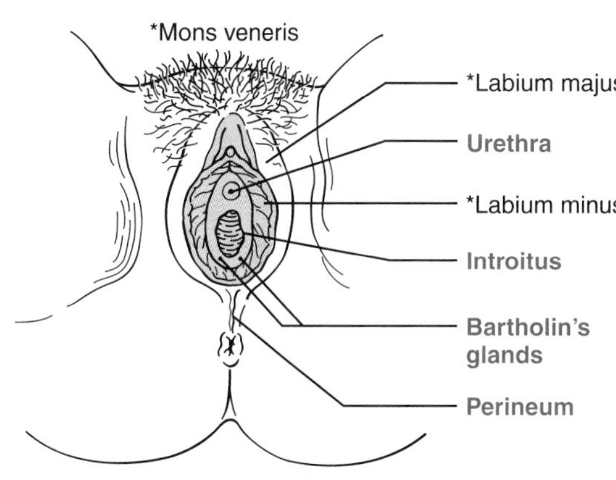
*Mons veneris
*Labium majus
Urethra
*Labium minus
Introitus
Bartholin's glands
Perineum
B
*The three parts of the vulva

Figure 10–10 A. Female genital system. **B.** External female genital system. (From Buck CJ: Step-by-Step Medical Coding, 2005 ed. Philadelphia, WB Saunders, 2005.)

616.2 **Cyst of Bartholin's gland**
Bartholin's duct cyst

616.3 **Abscess of Bartholin's gland**
Vulvovaginal gland abscess

❑616.4 **Other abscess of vulva**
Abscess of vulva
Carbuncle of vulva
Furuncle of vulva

● 616.5 **Ulceration of vulva**

616.50 **Ulceration of vulva, unspecified**
Ulcer NOS of vulva

● 616.51 ***Ulceration of vulva in diseases classified elsewhere***
Code first underlying disease, as:
Behçet's syndrome (136.1)
tuberculosis (016.7)

Excludes *vulvar ulcer (in):*
gonococcal (098.0)
herpes simplex (054.12)
syphilitic (091.0)

● 616.8 **Other specified inflammatory diseases of cervix, vagina, and vulva** ⇐

Excludes *noninflammatory disorders of:*
cervix (622.0–622.9)
vagina (623.0–623.9)
vulva (624.0–624.9)

616.81 **Mucositis (ulcerative) of cervix, vagina, and vulva** ◀
Use additional E code to identify adverse effects of therapy, such as: ◀
antineoplastic and immunosuppressive drugs (E930.7, E933.1) ◀
radiation therapy (E879.2) ◀

❑616.89 **Other inflammatory disease of cervix, vagina and vulva** ◀
Caruncle, vagina or labium ◀
Ulcer, vagina ◀

❑616.9 **Unspecified inflammatory disease of cervix, vagina, and vulva**

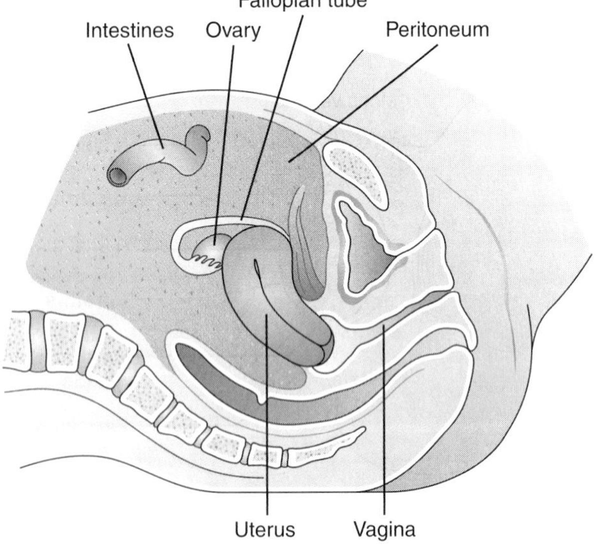
Fallopian tube
Intestines
Ovary
Peritoneum
Uterus
Vagina

Figure 10–11 Sites of potential endometrial implants.

Item 10–10 Endometriosis is a condition for which no clear cause has been identified. Endometrial tissue is expelled from the uterus into the body and can implant onto a variety of organs. Classification is based on the site of implant of the endometrial tissue.

OTHER DISORDERS OF FEMALE GENITAL TRACT (617–629)

● 617 **Endometriosis**

617.0 **Endometriosis of uterus**
Adenomyosis
Endometriosis:
cervix
internal
myometrium

Excludes *stromal endometriosis (236.0)*

617.1 **Endometriosis of ovary**
Chocolate cyst of ovary
Endometrial cystoma of ovary

617.2 **Endometriosis of fallopian tube**

617.3 **Endometriosis of pelvic peritoneum**
Endometriosis:
broad ligament
cul-de-sac (Douglas')
parametrium
round ligament

617.4 **Endometriosis of rectovaginal septum and vagina**

617.5 **Endometriosis of intestine**
Endometriosis:
appendix
colon
rectum

617.6 **Endometriosis in scar of skin**

❑617.8 **Endometriosis of other specified sites**
Endometriosis:
bladder
lung
umbilicus
vulva

❑617.9 **Endometriosis, site unspecified**

● 618 **Genital prolapse**
Use additional code to identify urinary incontinence (625.6, 788.31, 788.33–788.39)

Excludes *that complicating pregnancy, labor, or delivery (654.4)*

● 618.0 **Prolapse of vaginal walls without mention of uterine prolapse**

Excludes *that with uterine prolapse (618.2–618.4)*
enterocele (618.6)
vaginal vault prolapse following hysterectomy (618.5)

❑618.00 **Unspecified prolapse of vaginal walls**
Vaginal prolapse NOS

618.01 **Cystocele, midline**
Cystocele NOS

618.02 **Cystocele, lateral**
Paravaginal

618.03 **Urethrocele**

618.04 **Rectocele**
Proctocele

618.05 **Perineocele**

❑618.09 **Other prolapse of vaginal walls without mention of uterine prolapse**
Cystourethrocele

618.1 Uterine prolapse without mention of vaginal wall prolapse
Descensus uteri
Uterine prolapse:
NOS
complete
first degree
second degree
third degree
Excludes *that with mention of cystocele, urethrocele, or rectocele (618.2–618.4)*

618.2 Uterovaginal prolapse, incomplete

618.3 Uterovaginal prolapse, complete

❑ **618.4 Uterovaginal prolapse, unspecified**

618.5 Prolapse of vaginal vault after hysterectomy

618.6 Vaginal enterocele, congenital or acquired
Pelvic enterocele, congenital or acquired

618.7 Old laceration of muscles of pelvic floor

● **618.8 Other specified genital prolapse**

618.81 Incompetence or weakening of pubocervical tissue

618.82 Incompetence or weakening of rectovaginal tissue

618.83 Pelvic muscle wasting
Disuse atrophy of pelvic muscles and anal sphincter

618.84 Cervical stump prolapse ◀

❑ **618.89 Other specified genital prolapse**

❑ **618.9 Unspecified genital prolapse**

● **619 Fistula involving female genital tract**
Excludes *vesicorectal and intestinovesical fistula (596.1)*

619.0 Urinary-genital tract fistula, female
Fistula:
cervicovesical
ureterovaginal
urethrovaginal
urethrovesicovaginal
uteroureteric
uterovesical
vesicocervicovaginal
vesicovaginal

619.1 Digestive-genital tract fistula, female
Fistula:
intestinouterine
intestinovaginal
rectovaginal
Fistula:
rectovulval
sigmoidovaginal
uterorectal

619.2 Genital tract-skin fistula, female
Fistula:
uterus to abdominal wall
vaginoperineal

❑ **619.8 Other specified fistulas involving female genital tract**
Fistula:
cervix
cul-de-sac (Douglas')
uterus
vagina

❑ **619.9 Unspecified fistula involving female genital tract**

● **620 Noninflammatory disorders of ovary, fallopian tube, and broad ligament**
Excludes *hydrosalpinx (614.1)*

620.0 Follicular cyst of ovary
Cyst of graafian follicle

620.1 Corpus luteum cyst or hematoma
Corpus luteum hemorrhage or rupture
Lutein cyst

❑ **620.2 Other and unspecified ovarian cyst**
Cyst of ovary:
NOS
corpus albicans
retention NOS
serous
theca-lutein
Simple cystoma of ovary
Excludes *cystadenoma (benign) (serous) (220)*
developmental cysts (752.0)
neoplastic cysts (220)
polycystic ovaries (256.4)
Stein-Leventhal syndrome (256.4)

620.3 Acquired atrophy of ovary and fallopian tube
Senile involution of ovary

620.4 Prolapse or hernia of ovary and fallopian tube
Displacement of ovary and fallopian tube
Salpingocele

620.5 Torsion of ovary, ovarian pedicle, or fallopian tube
Torsion:
accessory tube
hydatid of Morgagni

620.6 Broad ligament laceration syndrome
Masters-Allen syndrome

620.7 Hematoma of broad ligament
Hematocele, broad ligament

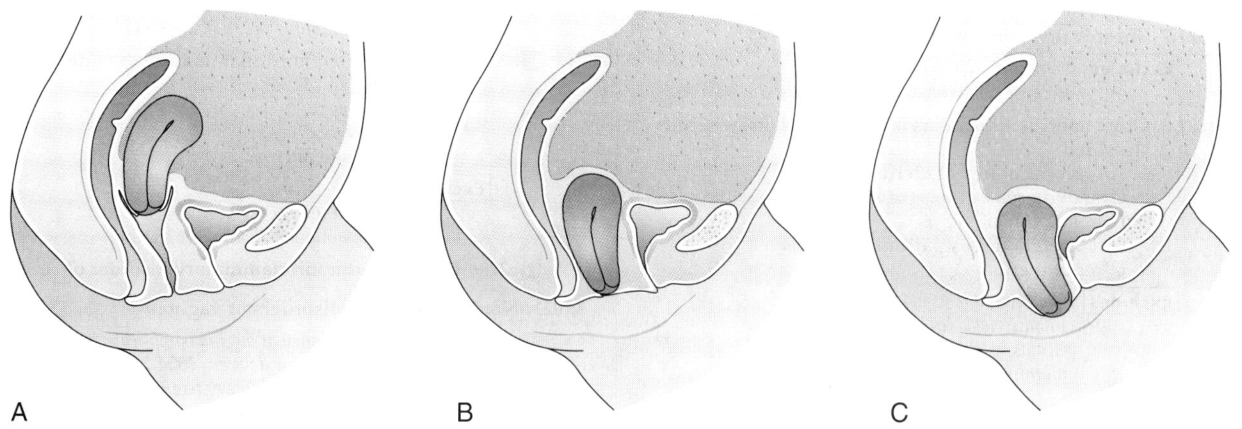
A
B
C

Figure 10–12 Three stages of uterine prolapse. **A.** Uterus is prolapsed. **B.** Vagina and uterus are prolapsed (incomplete uterovaginal prolapse). **C.** Vagina and uterus are completely prolapsed and are exposed through the external genitalia (complete uterovaginal prolapse).

❑620.8 **Other noninflammatory disorders of ovary, fallopian tube, and broad ligament**
Cyst of broad ligament or fallopian tube
Polyp of broad ligament or fallopian tube
Infarction of ovary or fallopian tube
Rupture of ovary or fallopian tube
Hematosalpinx of ovary or fallopian tube

Excludes *hematosalpinx in ectopic pregnancy (639.2)*
peritubal adhesions (614.6)
torsion of ovary, ovarian pedicle, or fallopian tube (620.5)

❑620.9 **Unspecified noninflammatory disorder of ovary, fallopian tube, and broad ligament**

● 621 **Disorders of uterus, not elsewhere classified**

621.0 **Polyp of corpus uteri**
Polyp:
endometrium
uterus NOS

Excludes *cervical polyp NOS (622.7)*

621.1 **Chronic subinvolution of uterus**

Excludes *puerperal (674.8)*

621.2 **Hypertrophy of uterus**
Bulky or enlarged uterus

Excludes *puerperal (674.8)*

● 621.3 **Endometrial hyperplasia**
Hyperplasia (adenomatous) (cystic) (glandular) of endometrium
Hyperplastic endometritis

❑621.30 **Endometrial hyperplasia, unspecified**
Endometrial hyperplasia NOS

621.31 **Simple endometrial hyperplasia without atypia**

621.32 **Complex endometrial hyperplasia without atypia**

621.33 **Endometrial hyperplasia with atypia**

621.4 **Hematometra**
Hemometra

Excludes *that in congenital anomaly (752.2–752.3)*

621.5 **Intrauterine synechiae**
Adhesions of uterus
Band(s) of uterus

621.6 **Malposition of uterus**
Anteversion of uterus
Retroflexion of uterus
Retroversion of uterus

Excludes *malposition complicating pregnancy, labor, or delivery (654.3–654.4)*
prolapse of uterus (618.1–618.4)

621.7 **Chronic inversion of uterus**

Excludes *current obstetrical trauma (665.2)*
prolapse of uterus (618.1–618.4)

❑621.8 **Other specified disorders of uterus, not elsewhere classified**
Atrophy, acquired of uterus
Cyst of uterus
Fibrosis NOS of uterus
Old laceration (postpartum) of uterus
Ulcer of uterus

Excludes *bilharzial fibrosis (120.0–120.9)*
endometriosis (617.0)
fistulas (619.0–619.8)
inflammatory diseases (615.0–615.9)

❑621.9 **Unspecified disorder of uterus**

● 622 **Noninflammatory disorders of cervix**

Excludes *abnormality of cervix complicating pregnancy, labor, or delivery (654.5–654.6)*
fistula (619.0–619.8)

622.0 **Erosion and ectropion of cervix**
Eversion of cervix
Ulcer of cervix

Excludes *that in chronic cervicitis (616.0)*

● 622.1 **Dysplasia of cervix (uteri)**

Excludes *abnormal results from cervical cytologic examination*
carcinoma in situ of cervix (233.1)
cervical intraepithelial neoplasia III [CIN III] (233.1)
without histologic confirmation (795.00–795.09)

❑622.10 **Dysplasia of cervix, unspecified**
Anaplasia of cervix
Cervical atypism
Cervical dysplasia NOS

622.11 **Mild dysplasia of cervix**
Cervical intraepithelial neoplasia I [CIN I]

622.12 **Moderate dysplasia of cervix**
Cervical intraepithelial neoplasia II [CIN II]

Excludes *carcinoma in situ of cervix (233.1)*
cervical intraepithelial neoplasia III [CIN III] (233.1)
severe dysplasia (233.1)

622.2 **Leukoplakia of cervix (uteri)**

Excludes *carcinoma in situ of cervix (233.1)*

622.3 **Old laceration of cervix**
Adhesions of cervix
Band(s) of cervix
Cicatrix (postpartum) of cervix

Excludes *current obstetrical trauma (665.3)*

622.4 **Stricture and stenosis of cervix**
Atresia (acquired) of cervix
Contracture of cervix
Occlusion of cervix
Pinpoint os uteri

Excludes *congenital (752.49)*
that complicating labor (654.6)

622.5 **Incompetence of cervix**

Excludes *complicating pregnancy (654.5)*
that affecting fetus or newborn (761.0)

622.6 **Hypertrophic elongation of cervix**

622.7 **Mucous polyp of cervix**
Polyp NOS of cervix

Excludes *adenomatous polyp of cervix (219.0)*

❑622.8 **Other specified noninflammatory disorders of cervix**
Atrophy (senile) of cervix
Cyst of cervix
Fibrosis of cervix
Hemorrhage of cervix

Excludes *endometriosis (617.0)*
fistula (619.0–619.8)
inflammatory diseases (616.0)

❑622.9 **Unspecified noninflammatory disorder of cervix**

● 623 **Noninflammatory disorders of vagina**

Excludes *abnormality of vagina complicating pregnancy, labor, or delivery (654.7)*
congenital absence of vagina (752.49)
congenital diaphragm or bands (752.49)
fistulas involving vagina (619.0–619.8)

623.0 Dysplasia of vagina

Excludes *carcinoma in situ of vagina (233.3)*

623.1 Leukoplakia of vagina

623.2 Stricture or atresia of vagina

Adhesions (postoperative) (postradiation) of vagina
Occlusion of vagina
Stenosis, vagina

Use additional E code to identify any external cause

Excludes *congenital atresia or stricture (752.49)*

623.3 Tight hymenal ring

Rigid hymen acquired or congenital
Tight hymenal ring acquired or congenital
Tight introitus acquired or congenital

Excludes *imperforate hymen (752.42)*

623.4 Old vaginal laceration

Excludes *old laceration involving muscles of pelvic floor (618.7)*

623.5 Leukorrhea, not specified as infective

Leukorrhea NOS of vagina
Vaginal discharge NOS

Excludes *trichomonal (131.00)*

623.6 Vaginal hematoma

Excludes *current obstetrical trauma (665.7)*

623.7 Polyp of vagina

❑ **623.8 Other specified noninflammatory disorders of vagina**

Cyst of vagina
Hemorrhage of vagina

❑ **623.9 Unspecified noninflammatory disorder of vagina**

● **624 Noninflammatory disorders of vulva and perineum**

Excludes *abnormality of vulva and perineum complicating pregnancy, labor, or delivery (654.8)*
condyloma acuminatum (078.1)
fistulas involving:
perineum - see Alphabetic Index
vulva (619.0–619.8)
vulval varices (456.6)
vulvar involvement in skin conditions (690–709.9)

624.0 Dystrophy of vulva

Kraurosis of vulva
Leukoplakia of vulva

Excludes *carcinoma in situ of vulva (233.3)*

624.1 Atrophy of vulva

624.2 Hypertrophy of clitoris

Excludes *that in endocrine disorders (255.2, 256.1)*

624.3 Hypertrophy of labia

Hypertrophy of vulva NOS

624.4 Old laceration or scarring of vulva

624.5 Hematoma of vulva

Excludes *that complicating delivery (664.5)*

624.6 Polyp of labia and vulva

❑ **624.8 Other specified noninflammatory disorders of vulva and perineum**

Cyst of vulva
Edema of vulva
Stricture of vulva

❑ **624.9 Unspecified noninflammatory disorder of vulva and perineum**

● **625 Pain and other symptoms associated with female genital organs**

625.0 Dyspareunia

Excludes *psychogenic dyspareunia (302.76)*

625.1 Vaginismus

Colpospasm
Vulvismus

Excludes *psychogenic vaginismus (306.51)*

625.2 Mittelschmerz

Intermenstrual pain
Ovulation pain

625.3 Dysmenorrhea

Painful menstruation

Excludes *psychogenic dysmenorrhea (306.52)*

625.4 Premenstrual tension syndrome

Menstrual:
migraine
molimen
Premenstrual dysphoric disorder
Premenstrual syndrome
Premenstrual tension NOS

625.5 Pelvic congestion syndrome

Congestion-fibrosis syndrome
Taylor's syndrome

625.6 Stress incontinence, female

Excludes *mixed incontinence (788.33)*
stress incontinence, male (788.32)

❑ **625.8 Other specified symptoms associated with female genital organs**

❑ **625.9 Unspecified symptoms associated with female genital organs**

● **626 Disorders of menstruation and other abnormal bleeding from female genital tract**

Excludes *menopausal and premenopausal bleeding (627.0)*
pain and other symptoms associated with menstrual cycle (625.2–625.4)
postmenopausal bleeding (627.1)

626.0 Absence of menstruation

Amenorrhea (primary) (secondary)

626.1 Scanty or infrequent menstruation

Hypomenorrhea
Oligomenorrhea

626.2 Excessive or frequent menstruation

Heavy periods
Menometrorrhagia
Menorrhagia
Polymenorrhea

Excludes *premenopausal (627.0)*
that in puberty (626.3)

626.3 Puberty bleeding

Excessive bleeding associated with onset of menstrual periods
Pubertal menorrhagia

626.4 Irregular menstrual cycle

Irregular:
bleeding NOS
menstruation
periods

626.5 Ovulation bleeding

Regular intermenstrual bleeding

626.6 Metrorrhagia

Bleeding unrelated to menstrual cycle
Irregular intermenstrual bleeding

626.7 Postcoital bleeding

❑ **626.8 Other**

Dysfunctional or functional uterine hemorrhage NOS
Menstruation:
retained
suppression of

❑ **626.9 Unspecified**

● 627 **Menopausal and postmenopausal disorders**

Excludes *asymptomatic age-related (natural) postmenopausal status (V49.81)*

627.0 **Premenopausal menorrhagia**
Excessive bleeding associated with onset of menopause
Menorrhagia: climacteric, menopausal, preclimacteric

627.1 **Postmenopausal bleeding**

627.2 **Symptomatic or female climacteric states**
Symptoms, such as flushing, sleeplessness, headache, lack of concentration, associated with the menopause

627.3 **Postmenopausal atrophic vaginitis**
Senile (atrophic) vaginitis

627.4 **Symptomatic states associated with artificial menopause**
Postartificial menopause syndromes
Any condition classifiable to 627.1, 627.2, or 627.3 which follows induced menopause

❑627.8 **Other specified menopausal and postmenopausal disorders**

Excludes *premature menopause NOS (256.31)*

❑627.9 **Unspecified menopausal and postmenopausal disorder**

● 628 **Infertility, female**

Includes: primary and secondary sterility

628.0 **Associated with anovulation**
Anovulatory cycle

Use additional code for any associated Stein-Leventhal syndrome (256.4)

● 628.1 ***Of pituitary-hypothalamic origin***

Code first underlying disease, as:
adiposogenital dystrophy (253.8)
anterior pituitary disorder (253.0–253.4)

628.2 **Of tubal origin**
Infertility associated with congenital anomaly of tube
Tubal: block, occlusion, stenosis

Use additional code for any associated peritubal adhesions (614.6)

628.3 **Of uterine origin**
Infertility associated with congenital anomaly of uterus
Nonimplantation

Use additional code for any associated tuberculous endometritis (016.7)

628.4 **Of cervical or vaginal origin**
Infertility associated with:
anomaly or cervical mucus
congenital structural anomaly
dysmucorrhea

❑628.8 **Of other specified origin**

❑628.9 **Of unspecified origin**

● 629 **Other disorders of female genital organs**

629.0 **Hematocele, female, not elsewhere classified**

Excludes *hematocele or hematoma:*
broad ligament (620.7)
fallopian tube (620.8)
that associated with ectopic pregnancy (633.00–633.91)
uterus (621.4)
vagina (623.6)
vulva (624.5)

629.1 **Hydrocele, canal of Nuck**
Cyst of canal of Nuck (acquired)

Excludes *congenital (752.41)*

● 629.2 **Female genital multilation status**
Female circumcision status
Female genital cutting ◀

❑629.20 **Female genital mutilation status, unspecified**
Female genital cutting status, unspecified ◀
Female genital mutilation status NOS

629.21 **Female genital mutilation Type I status**
Clitorectomy status
Female genital cutting Type I status ◀

629.22 **Female genital mutilation Type II status**
Clitorectomy with excision of labia minora status
Female genital cutting Type II status ◀

629.23 **Female genital mutilation Type III status**
Female genital cutting Type III status ◀
Infibulation status

❑629.29 **Other female genital mutilation status** ◀
Female genital cutting Type IV status ◀
Female genital mutilation Type IV status ◀
Other female genital cutting status ◀

● 629.8 **Other specified disorders of female genital organs**

629.81 **Habitual aborter without current pregnancy** ◀

Excludes *habitual aborter with current pregnancy (646.3)* ◀

❑629.89 **Other specified disorders of female genital organs** ◀

❑629.9 **Unspecified disorder of female genital organs** ⬅

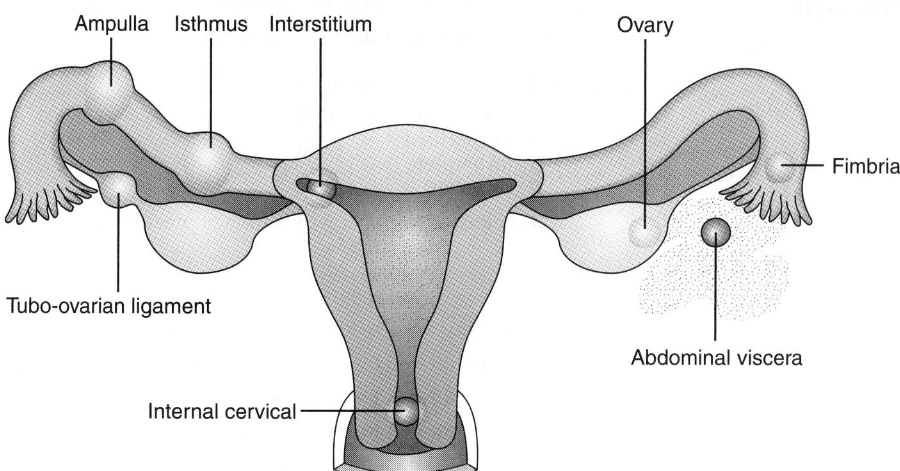
Ampulla
Isthmus
Interstitium
Ovary
Fimbria
Tubo-ovarian ligament
Abdominal viscera
Internal cervical

Figure 11–1 Implantation sites of ectopic pregnancy.

Item 11-1 A hydatidiform mole is a benign tumor of the placenta. The tumor secretes a hormone, chorionic gonadotropic hormone (CGH), that indicates a positive pregnancy test.

Item 11-2 Ectopic pregnancy most often occurs in the fallopian tube. Pregnancy outside the uterus may end in a life-threatening rupture.

11. COMPLICATIONS OF PREGNANCY, CHILDBIRTH, AND THE PUERPERIUM (630–677)

ECTOPIC AND MOLAR PREGNANCY (630–633)

Use additional code from category 639 to identify any complications

630 Hydatidiform mole
Trophoblastic disease NOS
Vesicular mole
Excludes *chorioadenoma (destruens) (236.1)*
chorioepithelioma (181)
malignant hydatidiform mole (236.1)

❑ **631 Other abnormal product of conception**
Blighted ovum
Mole:
NOS
carneous
fleshy
stone

632 Missed abortion
Early fetal death before completion of 22 weeks' gestation with retention of dead fetus
Retained products of conception, not following spontaneous or induced abortion or delivery
Excludes *failed induced abortion (638.0–638.9)*
fetal death (intrauterine) (late) (656.4)
missed delivery (656.4)
that with abnormal product of conception (630, 631)

● **633 Ectopic pregnancy**
Includes: ruptured ectopic pregnancy

● **633.0 Abdominal pregnancy**
Intraperitoneal pregnancy

633.00 Abdominal pregnancy without intrauterine pregnancy

633.01 Abdominal pregnancy with intrauterine pregnancy

● **633.1 Tubal pregnancy**
Fallopian pregnancy
Rupture of (fallopian) tube due to pregnancy
Tubal abortion

633.10 Tubal pregnancy without intrauterine pregnancy

633.11 Tubal pregnancy with intrauterine pregnancy

● **633.2 Ovarian pregnancy**

633.20 Ovarian pregnancy without intrauterine pregnancy

633.21 Ovarian pregnancy with intrauterine pregnancy

● ❑ **633.8 Other ectopic pregnancy**
Pregnancy:
cervical
combined
cornual
intraligamentous
mesometric
mural

633.80 Other ectopic pregnancy without intrauterine pregnancy

633.81 Other ectopic pregnancy with intrauterine pregnancy

● **633.9 Unspecified ectopic pregnancy**

❑ **633.90 Unspecified ectopic pregnancy without intrauterine pregnancy**

❑ **633.91 Unspecified ectopic pregnancy with intrauterine pregnancy**

OTHER PREGNANCY WITH ABORTIVE OUTCOME (634–639)

The following fourth digit subdivisions are for use with categories 634–638:

.0 Complicated by genital tract and pelvic infection
Endometritis
Salpingo-oophoritis
Sepsis NOS
Septicemia NOS
Any condition classifiable to 639.0, with condition classifiable to 634–638

Excludes *urinary tract infection (634–638 with .7)*

.1 Complicated by delayed or excessive hemorrhage
Afibrinogenemia
Defibrination syndrome
Intravascular hemolysis
Any condition classifiable to 639.1, with condition classifiable to 634–638

.2 Complicated by damage to pelvic organs and tissues
Laceration, perforation, or tear of:
bladder
uterus
Any condition classifiable to 639.2, with condition classifiable to 634–638

.3 Complicated by renal failure
Oliguria
Uremia
Any condition classifiable to 639.3, with condition classifiable to 634–638

.4 Complicated by metabolic disorder
Electrolyte imbalance with conditions classifiable to 634–638

.5 Complicated by shock
Circulatory collapse
Shock (postoperative) (septic)
Any condition classifiable to 639.5, with condition classifiable to 634–638

.6 Complicated by embolism
Embolism:
NOS
amniotic fluid
pulmonary
Any condition classifiable to 639.6, with condition classifiable to 634–638

❑ **.7 With other specified complications**
Cardiac arrest or failure
Urinary tract infection
Any condition classifiable to 639.8, with condition classifiable to 634–638

❑ **.8 With unspecified complications**
.9 Without mention of complication

● **634 Spontaneous abortion**
Requires fifth digit to identify stage:
❑ **0 unspecified**
1 incomplete
2 complete

Includes: miscarriage
spontaneous abortion

● **634.0 Complicated by genital tract and pelvic infection**
● **634.1 Complicated by delayed or excessive hemorrhage**
● **634.2 Complicated by damage to pelvic organs or tissues**
● **634.3 Complicated by renal failure**
● **634.4 Complicated by metabolic disorder**
● **634.5 Complicated by shock**
● **634.6 Complicated by embolism**
● ❑ **634.7 With other specified complications**
● ❑ **634.8 With unspecified complication**
● **634.9 Without mention of complication**

● **635 Legally induced abortion**
Requires fifth digit to identify stage:
❑ **0 unspecified**
1 incomplete
2 complete

Includes: abortion or termination of pregnancy:
elective
legal
therapeutic

Excludes *menstrual extraction or regulation (V25.3)*

● **635.0 Complicated by genital tract and pelvic infection**
● **635.1 Complicated by delayed or excessive hemorrhage**
● **635.2 Complicated by damage to pelvic organs or tissues**
● **635.3 Complicated by renal failure**
● **635.4 Complicated by metabolic disorder**
● **635.5 Complicated by shock**
● **635.6 Complicated by embolism**
● ❑ **635.7 With other specified complications**
● ❑ **635.8 With unspecified complication**
● **635.9 Without mention of complication**

● **636 Illegally induced abortion**
Requires fifth digit to identify stage:
❑ **0 unspecified**
1 incomplete
2 complete

Includes: abortion:
criminal
illegal
self-induced

● **636.0 Complicated by genital tract and pelvic infection**
● **636.1 Complicated by delayed or excessive hemorrhage**
● **636.2 Complicated by damage to pelvic organs or tissues**
● **636.3 Complicated by renal failure**
● **636.4 Complicated by metabolic disorder**
● **636.5 Complicated by shock**
● **636.6 Complicated by embolism**
● ❑ **636.7 With other specified complications**
● ❑ **636.8 With unspecified complication**
● **636.9 Without mention of complication**

● **637 Unspecified abortion**
Requires following fifth digit to identify stage:
❑ **0 unspecified**
1 incomplete
2 complete

Includes: abortion NOS
retained products of conception following abortion, not classifiable elsewhere

● ❑ **637.0 Complicated by genital tract and pelvic infection**
● ❑ **637.1 Complicated by delayed or excessive hemorrhage**
● ❑ **637.2 Complicated by damage to pelvic organs or tissues**
● ❑ **637.3 Complicated by renal failure**
● ❑ **637.4 Complicated by metabolic disorder**
● ❑ **637.5 Complicated by shock**
● ❑ **637.6 Complicated by embolism**

637.7 With other specified complications

637.8 With unspecified complication

637.9 Without mention of complication

638 Failed attempted abortion

Includes: failure of attempted induction of (legal) abortion

Excludes *incomplete abortion (634.0–637.9)*

638.0 Complicated by genital tract and pelvic infection

638.1 Complicated by delayed or excessive hemorrhage

638.2 Complicated by damage to pelvic organs or tissues

638.3 Complicated by renal failure

638.4 Complicated by metabolic disorder

638.5 Complicated by shock

638.6 Complicated by embolism

638.7 With other specified complications

638.8 With unspecified complication

638.9 Without mention of complication

639 Complications following abortion and ectopic and molar pregnancies

Note: This category is provided for use when it is required to classify separately the complications classifiable to the fourth digit level in categories 634–638; for example:
a) when the complication itself was responsible for an episode of medical care, the abortion, ectopic or molar pregnancy itself having been dealt with at a previous episode
b) when these conditions are immediate complications of ectopic or molar pregnancies classifiable to 630–633 where they cannot be identified at fourth digit level.

639.0 Genital tract and pelvic infection
Endometritis following conditions classifiable to 630–638
Parametritis following conditions classifiable to 630–638
Pelvic peritonitis following conditions classifiable to 630–638
Salpingitis following conditions classifiable to 630–638
Salpingo-oophoritis following conditions classifiable to 630–638
Sepsis NOS following conditions classifiable to 630–638
Septicemia NOS following conditions classifiable to 630–638

Excludes *urinary tract infection (639.8)*

639.1 Delayed or excessive hemorrhage
Afibrinogenemia following conditions classifiable to 630–638
Defibrination syndrome following conditions classifiable to 630–638
Intravascular hemolysis following conditions classifiable to 630–638

639.2 Damage to pelvic organs and tissues
Laceration, perforation, or tear of:
bladder following conditions classifiable to 630–638
bowel following conditions classifiable to 630–638
broad ligament following conditions classifiable to 630–638
cervix following conditions classifiable to 630–638
periurethral tissue following conditions classifiable to 630–638
uterus following conditions classifiable to 630–638
vagina following conditions classifiable to 630–638

639.3 Renal failure
Oliguria following conditions classifiable to 630–638
Renal:
failure (acute) following conditions classifiable to 630–638
shutdown following conditions classifiable to 630–638
tubular necrosis following conditions classifiable to 630–638
Uremia following conditions classifiable to 630–638

639.4 Metabolic disorders
Electrolyte imbalance following conditions classifiable to 630–638

639.5 Shock
Circulatory collapse following conditions classifiable to 630–638
Shock (postoperative) (septic) following conditions classifiable to 630–638

639.6 Embolism
Embolism:
NOS following conditions classifiable to 630–638
air following conditions classifiable to 630–638
amniotic fluid following conditions classifiable to 630–638
blood-clot following conditions classifiable to 630–638
fat following conditions classifiable to 630–638
pulmonary following conditions classifiable to 630–638
pyemic following conditions classifiable to 630–638
septic following conditions classifiable to 630–638
septic following conditions classifiable to 630–638
soap following conditions classifiable to 630–638

639.8 Other specified complications following abortion or ectopic and molar pregnancy
Acute yellow atrophy or necrosis of liver following conditions classifiable to 630–638
Cardiac arrest or failure following conditions classifiable to 630–638
Cerebral anoxia following conditions classifiable to 630–638
Urinary tract infection following conditions classifiable to 630–638

639.9 Unspecified complication following abortion or ectopic and molar pregnancy
Complication(s) not further specified following conditions classifiable to 630–638

ICD-9-CM 600–699 Vol. 1

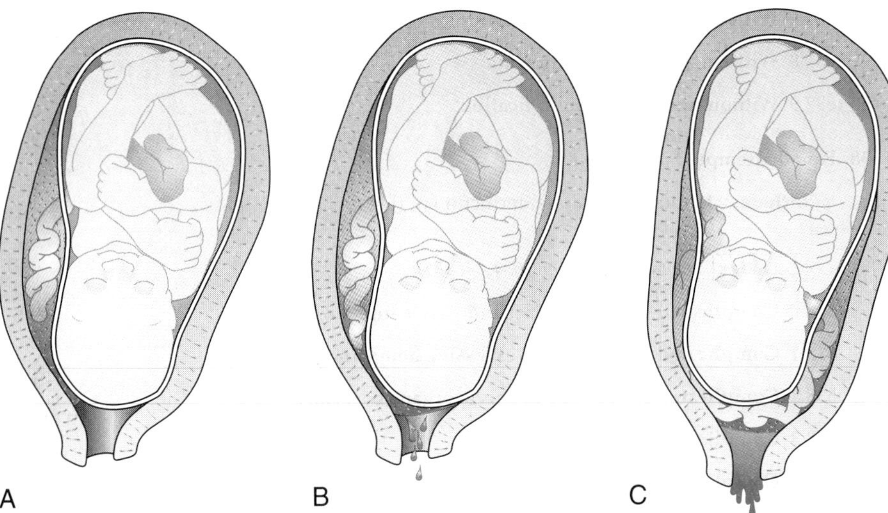
A
B
C

Figure 11–2 A. Marginal placenta previa. **B.** Partial placenta previa. **C.** Total placenta previa.

COMPLICATIONS MAINLY RELATED TO PREGNANCY (640–649)

Includes: the listed conditions even if they arose or were present during labor, delivery, or the puerperium

The following fifth-digit subclassification is for use with categories 640–649 to denote the current episode of care:

- ❑ 0 **unspecified as to episode of care or not applicable**
- 1 **delivered, with or without mention of antepartum condition**
  - Antepartum condition with delivery
  - Delivery NOS (with mention of antepartum complication during current episode of care)
  - Intrapartum
    - obstetric condition (with mention of antepartum complication during current episode of care)
  - Pregnancy, delivered (with mention of antepartum complication during current episode of care)
- 2 **delivered, with mention of postpartum complication**
  - Delivery with mention of puerperal complication during current episode of care
- 3 **antepartum condition or complication**
  - Antepartum obstetric condition, not delivered during the current episode of care
- 4 **postpartum condition or complication**
  - Postpartum or puerperal obstetric condition or complication following delivery that occurred:
    - during previous episode of care
    - outside hospital, with subsequent admission for observation or care

● **640 Hemorrhage in early pregnancy**

Requires fifth digit; valid digits are in [brackets] under each code. See beginning of section 640–648 for definitions.

Includes: hemorrhage before completion of 22 weeks' gestation

● **640.0 Threatened abortion**
[0,1,3]

● ❑ **640.8 Other specified hemorrhage in early pregnancy**
[0,1,3]

● ❑ **640.9 Unspecified hemorrhage in early pregnancy**
[0,1,3]

● **641 Antepartum hemorrhage, abruptio placentae, and placenta previa**

Requires fifth digit; valid digits are in [brackets] under each code. See beginning of section 640–648 for definitions.

● **641.0 Placenta previa without hemorrhage**
[0,1,3] Low implantation of placenta without hemorrhage
Placenta previa noted:
- during pregnancy without hemorrhage
- before labor (and delivered by cesarean delivery) without hemorrhage

● **641.1 Hemorrhage from placenta previa**
[0,1,3] Low-lying placenta NOS or with hemorrhage (intrapartum)
Placenta previa:
- incomplete NOS or with hemorrhage (intrapartum)
- marginal NOS or with hemorrhage (intrapartum)
- partial NOS or with hemorrhage (intrapartum)
- total NOS or with hemorrhage (intrapartum)

Excludes *hemorrhage from vasa previa (663.5)*

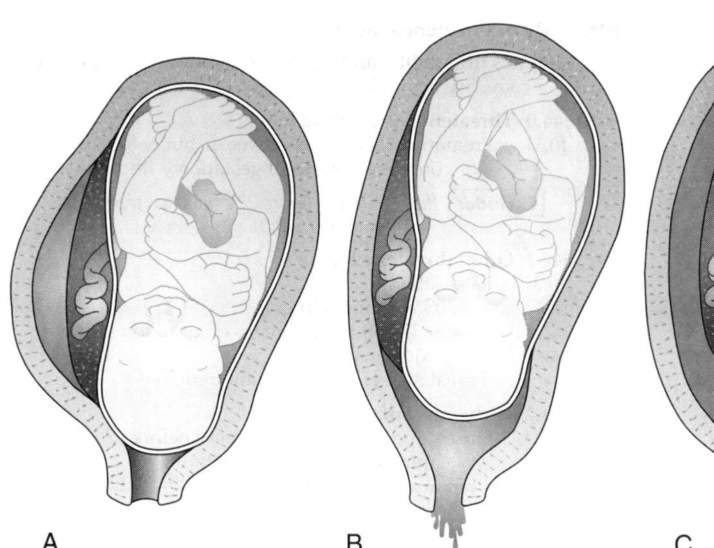
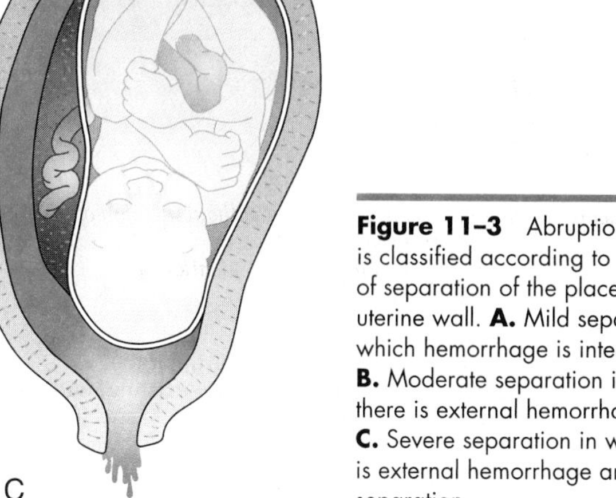
A
B
C

Figure 11-3 Abruptio placentae is classified according to the grade of separation of the placenta from the uterine wall. **A.** Mild separation in which hemorrhage is internal. **B.** Moderate separation in which there is external hemorrhage. **C.** Severe separation in which there is external hemorrhage and extreme separation.

Item 11-3 Placenta previa is a condition in which the opening of the cervix is obstructed by the displaced placenta. The three types, marginal, partial, and total, are varying degrees of placenta displacement.

● **641.2 Premature separation of placenta**
[0,1,3] Ablatio placentae
Abruptio placentae
Accidental antepartum hemorrhage
Couvelaire uterus
Detachment of placenta (premature)
Premature separation of normally implanted placenta

● **641.3 Antepartum hemorrhage associated with coagulation defects**
[0,1,3] Antepartum or intrapartum hemorrhage associated with:
afibrinogenemia
hyperfibrinolysis
hypofibrinogenemia

Excludes *coagulation defects not associated with antepartum hemorrhage (649.3)* ◀

● ❑ **641.8 Other antepartum hemorrhage**
[0,1,3] Antepartum or intrapartum hemorrhage associated with:
trauma
uterine leiomyoma

● ❑ **641.9 Unspecified antepartum hemorrhage**
[0,1,3] Hemorrhage:
antepartum NOS
intrapartum NOS
of pregnancy NOS

● **642 Hypertension complicating pregnancy, childbirth, and the puerperium**

Requires fifth digit; valid digits are in [brackets] under each code. See beginning of section 640–648 for definitions.

● **642.0 Benign essential hypertension complicating pregnancy, childbirth, and the puerperium**
[0–4] Hypertension:
benign essential specified as complicating, or as a reason for obstetric care during pregnancy, childbirth, or the puerperium
chronic NOS specified as complicating, or as a reason for obstetric care during pregnancy, childbirth, or the puerperium
essential specified as complicating, or as a reason for obstetric care during pregnancy, childbirth, or the puerperium
pre-existing NOS specified as complicating, or as a reason for obstetric care during pregnancy, childbirth, or the puerperium

● **642.1 Hypertension secondary to renal disease, complicating pregnancy, childbirth, and the puerperium**
[0–4] Hypertension secondary to renal disease, specified as complicating, or as a reason for obstetric care during pregnancy, childbirth, or the puerperium

● **642.2 Other pre-existing hypertension complicating pregnancy, childbirth, and the puerperium**
[0–4] Hypertensive:
chronic kidney disease specified as complicating, or as a reason for obstetric care during pregnancy, childbirth, or the puerperium ⟸
heart and chronic kidney disease specified as complicating, or as a reason for obstetric care during pregnancy, childbirth, or the puerperium ⟸
heart disease specified as complicating, or as a reason for obstetric care during pregnancy, childbirth, or the puerperium
Malignant hypertension specified as complicating, or as a reason for obstetric care during pregnancy, childbirth, or the puerperium

● **642.3 Transient hypertension of pregnancy**
[0–4] Gestational hypertension
Transient hypertension, so described, in pregnancy, childbirth, or the puerperium

642.4 Mild or unspecified pre-eclampsia
[0–4] Hypertension in pregnancy, childbirth, or the puerperium, not specified as pre-existing, with either albuminuria or edema, or both; mild or unspecified
Pre-eclampsia:
NOS
mild
Toxemia (pre-eclamptic):
NOS
mild

Excludes *albuminuria in pregnancy, without mention of hypertension (646.2)*
edema in pregnancy, without mention of hypertension (646.1)

642.5 Severe pre-eclampsia
[0–4] Hypertension in pregnancy, childbirth, or the puerperium, not specified as pre-existing, with either albuminuria or edema, or both; specified as severe
Pre-eclampsia, severe
Toxemia (pre-eclamptic), severe

642.6 Eclampsia
[0–4] Toxemia:
eclamptic
with convulsions

642.7 Pre-eclampsia or eclampsia superimposed on pre-existing hypertension
[0–4] Conditions classifiable to 642.4–642.6, with conditions classifiable to 642.0–642.2

642.9 Unspecified hypertension complicating pregnancy, childbirth, or the puerperium
[0–4] Hypertension NOS, without mention of albuminuria or edema, complicating pregnancy, childbirth, or the puerperium

643 Excessive vomiting in pregnancy

Requires fifth digit; valid digits are in [brackets] under each code. See beginning of section 640–648 for definitions.

Includes: hyperemesis arising during pregnancy
hyperemesis gravidarum
vomiting:
persistent arising during pregnancy
vicious arising during pregnancy

643.0 Mild hyperemesis gravidarum
[0,1,3] Hyperemesis gravidarum, mild or unspecified, starting before the end of the 22nd week of gestation

643.1 Hyperemesis gravidarum with metabolic disturbance
[0,1,3] Hyperemesis gravidarum, starting before the end of the 22nd week of gestation, with metabolic disturbance, such as:
carbohydrate depletion
dehydration
electrolyte imbalance

643.2 Late vomiting of pregnancy
[0,1,3] Excessive vomiting starting after 22 completed weeks of gestation

643.8 Other vomiting complicating pregnancy
[0,1,3] Vomiting due to organic disease or other cause, specified as complicating pregnancy, or as a reason for obstetric care during pregnancy
Use additional code to specify cause

643.9 Unspecified vomiting of pregnancy
[0,1,3] Vomiting as a reason for care during pregnancy, length of gestation unspecified

644 Early or threatened labor

Requires fifth digit; valid digits are in [brackets] under each code. See beginning of section 640–648 for definitions.

644.0 Threatened premature labor
[0,3] Premature labor after 22 weeks, but before 37 completed weeks of gestation without delivery

Excludes *that occurring before 22 completed weeks of gestation (640.0)*

644.1 Other threatened labor
[0,3] False labor:
NOS without delivery
after 37 completed weeks of gestation without delivery
Threatened labor NOS without delivery

644.2 Early onset of delivery
[0–1] Onset (spontaneous) of delivery before 37 completed weeks of gestation
Premature labor with onset of delivery before 37 completed weeks of gestation

645 Late pregnancy

Requires fifth digit; valid digits are in [brackets] under each code. See beginning of section 640–648 for definitions.

645.1 Post term pregnancy
[0,1,3] Pregnancy over 40 completed weeks to 42 completed weeks gestation

645.2 Prolonged pregnancy
[0,1,3] Pregnancy which has advanced beyond 42 completed weeks of gestation

646 Other complications of pregnancy, not elsewhere classified

Use additional code(s) to further specify complication

Requires fifth digit; valid digits are in [brackets] under each code. See beginning of section 640–648 for definitions.

646.0 Papyraceous fetus
[0,1,3]

646.1 Edema or excessive weight gain in pregnancy, without mention of hypertension
[0–4] Gestational edema
Maternal obesity syndrome

Excludes *that with mention of hypertension (642.0–642.9)*

646.2 Unspecified renal disease in pregnancy, without mention of hypertension
[0–4] Albuminuria in pregnancy or the puerperium, without mention of hypertension
Nephropathy NOS in pregnancy or the puerperium, without mention of hypertension
Renal disease NOS in pregnancy or the puerperium, without mention of hypertension
Uremia in pregnancy or the puerperium, without mention of hypertension
Gestational proteinuria in pregnancy or the puerperium, without mention of hypertension

Excludes *that with mention of hypertension (642.0–642.9)*

646.3 Habitual aborter
[0–1,3]

Excludes *with current abortion (634.0–634.9)*
without current pregnancy (629.9)

646.4 Peripheral neuritis in pregnancy
[0–4]

646.5 Asymptomatic bacteriuria in pregnancy
[0–4]

● **646.6 Infections of genitourinary tract in pregnancy**
[0–4] Conditions classifiable to 590, 595, 597, 599.0, 616 complicating pregnancy, childbirth, or the puerperium
Conditions classifiable to 614.0–614.5, 614.7–614.9, 615

Excludes *major puerperal infection (670)*

● **646.7 Liver disorders in pregnancy**
[0,1,3] Acute yellow atrophy of liver (obstetric) (true) of pregnancy
Icterus gravis of pregnancy
Necrosis of liver of pregnancy

Excludes *hepatorenal syndrome following delivery (674.8)*
viral hepatitis (647.6)

● ❑ **646.8 Other specified complications of pregnancy**
[0–4] Fatigue during pregnancy
Herpes gestationis
Insufficient weight gain of pregnancy

● ❑ **646.9 Unspecified complication of pregnancy**
[0,1,3]

● **647 Infectious and parasitic conditions in the mother classifiable elsewhere, but complicating pregnancy, childbirth, or the puerperium**

Use additional code(s) to further specify complication

Requires fifth digit; valid digits are in [brackets] under each code. See beginning of section 640–648 for definitions.

Includes: the listed conditions when complicating the pregnant state, aggravated by the pregnancy, or when a main reason for obstetric care

Excludes *those conditions in the mother known or suspected to have affected the fetus (655.0–655.9)*

● **647.0 Syphilis**
[0–4] Conditions classifiable to 090–097

● **647.1 Gonorrhea**
[0–4] Conditions classifiable to 098

● ❑ **647.2 Other venereal diseases**
[0–4] Conditions classifiable to 099

● **647.3 Tuberculosis**
[0–4] Conditions classifiable to 010–018

● **647.4 Malaria**
[0–4] Conditions classifiable to 084

● **647.5 Rubella**
[0–4] Conditions classifiable to 056

● ❑ **647.6 Other viral diseases**
[0–4] Conditions classifiable to 042 and 050–079, except 056

● ❑ **647.8 Other specified infectious and parasitic diseases**
[0–4]

● ❑ **647.9 Unspecified infection or infestation**
[0–4]

● **648 Other current conditions in the mother classifiable elsewhere, but complicating pregnancy, childbirth, or the puerperium**

Use additional code(s) to identify the condition

Requires fifth digit; valid digits are in [brackets] under each code. See beginning of section 640–648 for definitions.

Includes: the listed conditions when complicating the pregnant state, aggravated by the pregnancy, or when a main reason for obstetric care

Excludes *those conditions in the mother known or suspected to have affected the fetus (655.0–665.9)*

● **648.0 Diabetes mellitus**
[0–4] Conditions classifiable to 250

Excludes *gestational diabetes (648.8)*

● **648.1 Thyroid dysfunction**
[0–4] Conditions classifiable to 240–246

● **648.2 Anemia**
[0–4] Conditions classifiable to 280–285

● **648.3 Drug dependence**
[0–4] Conditions classifiable to 304

● **648.4 Mental disorders**
[0–4] Conditions classifiable to 290–303, 305.0, 305.2–305.9, 306–316, 317–319

● **648.5 Congenital cardiovascular disorders**
[0–4] Conditions classifiable to 745–747

● ❑ **648.6 Other cardiovascular diseases**
[0–4] Conditions classifiable to 390–398, 410–429

Excludes *cerebrovascular disorders in the puerperium (674.0)*
peripartum cardiomyopathy (674.5)
venous complications (671.0–671.9)

● **648.7 Bone and joint disorders of back, pelvis, and lower**
[0–4] **limbs**
Conditions classifiable to 720–724, and those classifiable to 711–719 or 725–738, specified as affecting the lower limbs

● **648.8 Abnormal glucose tolerance**
[0–4] Conditions classifiable to 790.21–790.29
Gestational diabetes

Use additional code, if applicable, for associated long-term (current) insulin use (V58.67)

● ❑ **648.9 Other current conditions classifiable elsewhere**
[0–4] Conditions classifiable to 440–459
Nutritional deficiencies [conditions classifiable to 260–269]

● **649 Other conditions or status of the mother complicating pregnancy, childbirth, or the puerperium** ◀

649.0 Tobacco use disorder complicating pregnancy,
[0–4] **childbirth, or the puerperium** ◀
Smoking complicating pregnancy, childbirth, or the puerperium ◀

649.1 Obesity complicating pregnancy, childbirth, or the
[0–4] **puerperium** ◀

Use additional code to identify the obesity (278.00, 278.01) ◀

649.2 Bariatric surgery status complicating pregnancy,
[0–4] **childbirth, or the puerperium** ◀
Gastric banding status complicating pregnancy, childbirth, or the puerperium ◀
Gastric bypass status for obesity complicating pregnancy, childbirth, or the puerperium ◀
Obesity surgery status complicating pregnancy, childbirth, or the puerperium ◀

649.3 Coagulation defects complicating pregnancy,
[0–4] **childbirth, or the puerperium** ◀
Conditions classifiable to 286 ◀

Use additional code to identify the specific coagulation defect (286.0–286.9) ◀

Excludes *coagulation defects causing antepartum hemorrhage (641.3)* ◀
postpartum coagulation defects (666.3) ◀

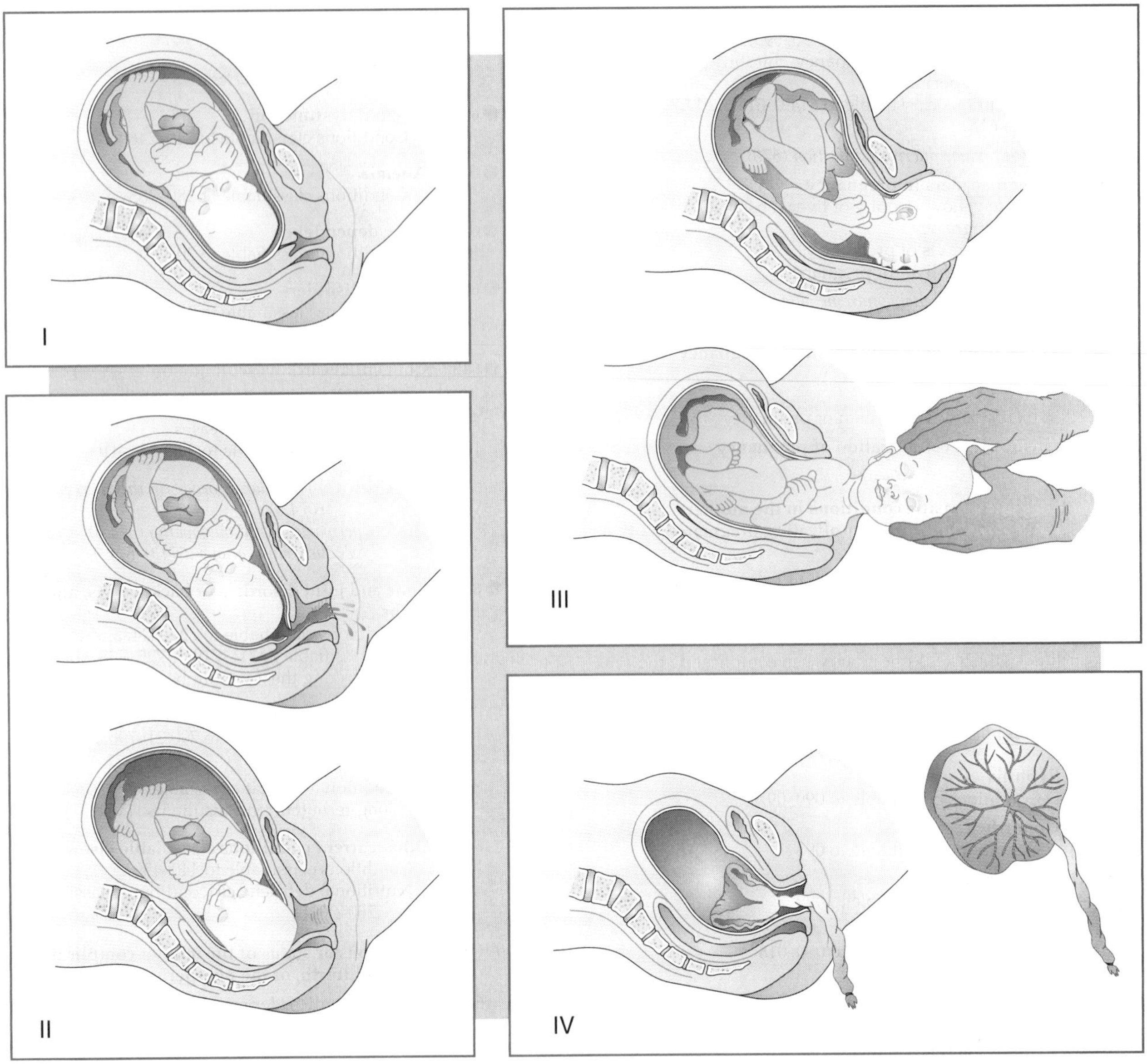

Figure 11–4 The four stages of normal delivery: **I.** Lightening, which occurs 2 to 4 weeks before birth, at which time the fetus turns with head toward the vagina. **II.** Regular contractions begin, the amniotic sac ruptures, and dilation is complete. **III.** Delivery of the head and rotation. **IV.** Recovery of the mother to full homeostasis.

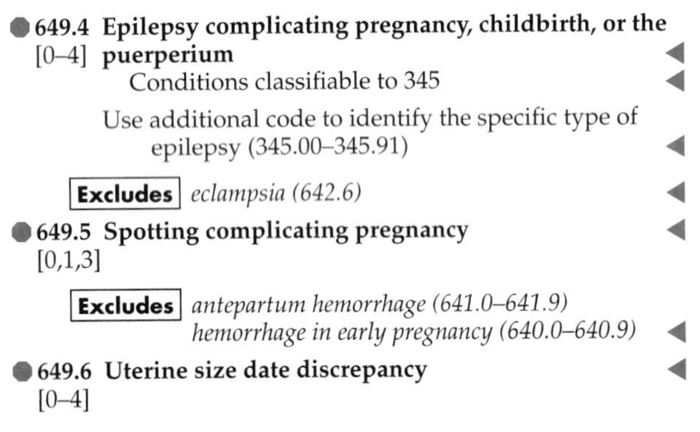

● **649.4 Epilepsy complicating pregnancy, childbirth, or the**
[0–4] **puerperium** ◀
Conditions classifiable to 345 ◀

Use additional code to identify the specific type of epilepsy (345.00–345.91) ◀

Excludes *eclampsia (642.6)* ◀

● **649.5 Spotting complicating pregnancy** ◀
[0,1,3]

Excludes *antepartum hemorrhage (641.0–641.9)*
hemorrhage in early pregnancy (640.0–640.9) ◀

● **649.6 Uterine size date discrepancy** ◀
[0–4]

NORMAL DELIVERY, AND OTHER INDICATIONS FOR CARE IN PREGNANCY, LABOR, AND DELIVERY (650–659)

The following fifth-digit subclassification is for use with categories 651–659 to denote the current episode of care:

❑ **0 unspecified as to episode of care or not applicable**
1 delivered, with or without mention of antepartum condition
2 delivered, with mention of postpartum complication
3 antepartum condition or complication
4 postpartum condition or complication

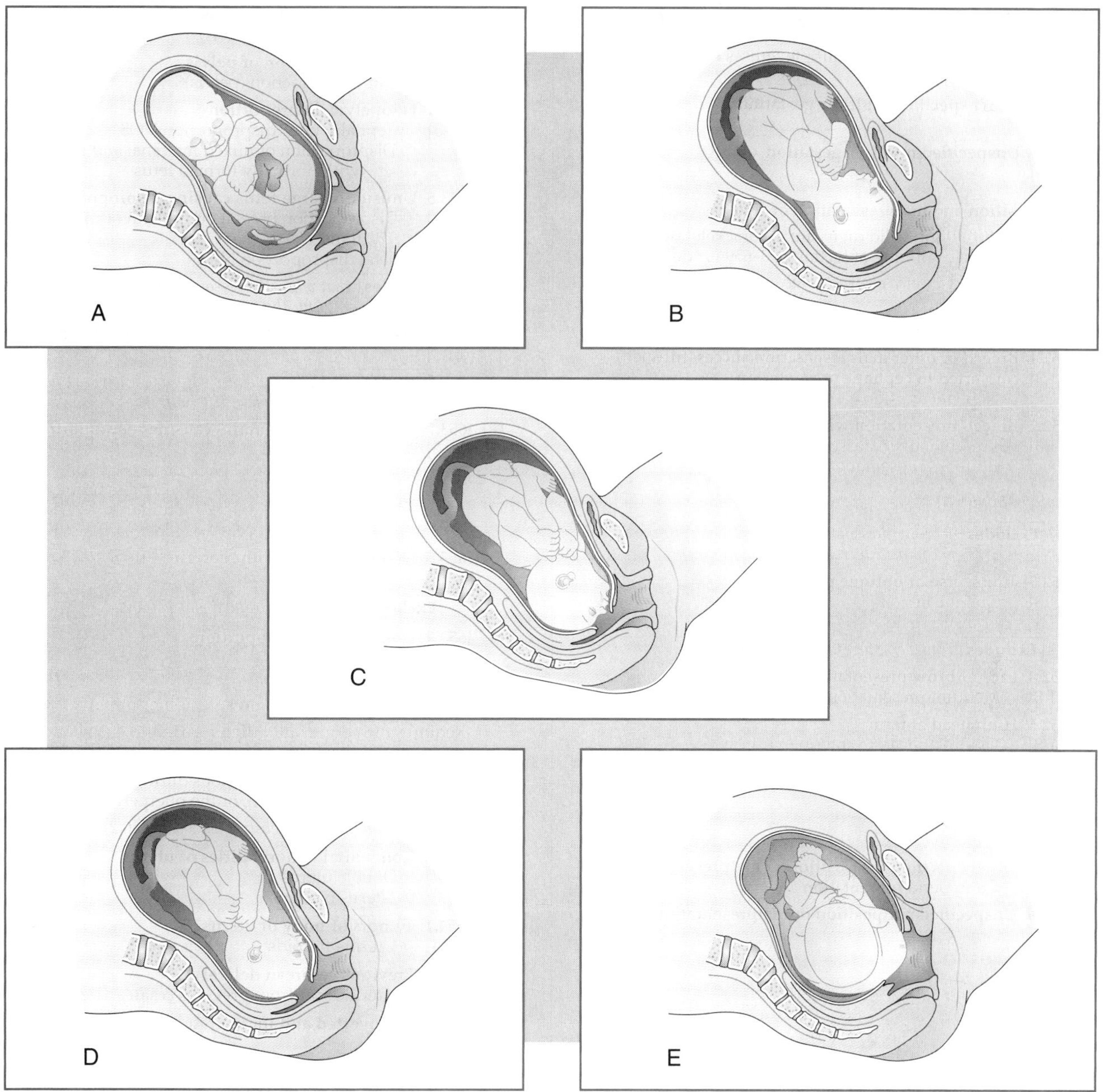
A
B
C
D
E

Figure 11–5 Five types of malposition and malpresentation of the fetus: **A.** Breech. **B.** Vertex. **C.** Face. **D.** Brow. **E.** Shoulder.

650 **Normal delivery**

Delivery requiring minimal or no assistance, with or without episiotomy, without fetal manipulation [e.g., rotation version] or instrumentation [forceps] of a spontaneous, cephalic, vaginal, full-term, single, live-born infant. This code is for use as a single diagnosis code and is not to be used with any other code in the range 630–676.

Use additional code to indicate outcome of delivery (V27.0)

Excludes *breech delivery (assisted) (spontaneous) NOS (652.2)*
delivery by vacuum extractor, forceps, cesarean section, or breech extraction, without specified complication (669.5–669.7)

● 651 **Multiple gestation**

Requires fifth digit; valid digits are in [brackets] under each code. See beginning of section 650–659 for definitions.

● 651.0 **Twin pregnancy**
[0,1,3]

● 651.1 **Triplet pregnancy**
[0,1,3]

● 651.2 **Quadruplet pregnancy**
[0,1,3]

● 651.3 **Twin pregnancy with fetal loss and retention of one fetus**
[0,1,3]

● 651.4 **Triplet pregnancy with fetal loss and retention of one or more fetus(es)**
[0,1,3]

● 651.5 **Quadruplet pregnancy with fetal loss and retention of one or more fetus(es)**
[0,1,3]

● ❑ 651.6 **Other multiple pregnancy with fetal loss and retention of one or more fetus(es)**
[0,1,3]

ICD-9-CM 600-669 Vol. 1

● 651.7 **Multiple gestation following (elective) fetal reduction**
[0,1,3]
Fetal reduction of multiple fetuses reduced to single fetus

● ❑ 651.8 **Other specified multiple gestation**
[0,1,3]

● ❑ 651.9 **Unspecified multiple gestation**
[0,1,3]

● 652 **Malposition and malpresentation of fetus**

Requires fifth digit; valid digits are in [brackets] under each code. See beginning of section 650–659 for definitions.

Code first any associated obstructed labor (660.0)

● 652.0 **Unstable lie**
[0,1,3]

● 652.1 **Breech or other malpresentation successfully converted to cephalic presentation**
[0,1,3]
Cephalic version NOS

● 652.2 **Breech presentation without mention of version**
[0,1,3]
Breech delivery (assisted) (spontaneous) NOS
Buttocks presentation
Complete breech
Frank breech

Excludes *footling presentation (652.8)*
incomplete breech (652.8)

● 652.3 **Transverse or oblique presentation**
[0,1,3]
Oblique lie
Transverse lie

Excludes *transverse arrest of fetal head (660.3)*

● 652.4 **Face or brow presentation**
[0,1,3]
Mentum presentation

● 652.5 **High head at term**
[0,1,3]
Failure of head to enter pelvic brim

● 652.6 **Multiple gestation with malpresentation of one fetus or more**
[0,1,3]

● 652.7 **Prolapsed arm**
[0,1,3]

● ❑ 652.8 **Other specified malposition or malpresentation**
[0,1,3]
Compound presentation

● ❑ 652.9 **Unspecified malposition or malpresentation**
[0,1,3]

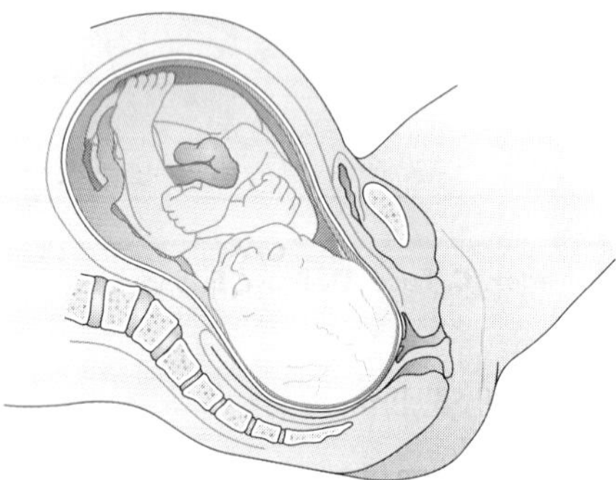

Figure 11–6 Hydrocephalic fetus causing disproportion.

● 653 **Disproportion**

Requires fifth digit; valid digits are in [brackets] under each code. See beginning of section 650–659 for definitions.

Code first any associated obstructed labor (660.1)

● 653.0 **Major abnormality of bony pelvis, not further specified**
[0,1,3]
Pelvic deformity NOS

● 653.1 **Generally contracted pelvis**
[0,1,3]
Contracted pelvis NOS

● 653.2 **Inlet contraction of pelvis**
[0,1,3]
Inlet contraction (pelvis)

● 653.3 **Outlet contraction of pelvis**
[0,1,3]
Outlet contraction (pelvis)

● 653.4 **Fetopelvic disproportion**
[0,1,3]
Cephalopelvic disproportion NOS
Disproportion of mixed maternal and fetal origin, with normally formed fetus

● 653.5 **Unusually large fetus causing disproportion**
[0,1,3]
Disproportion of fetal origin with normally formed fetus
Fetal disproportion NOS

Excludes *that when the reason for medical care was concern for the fetus (656.6)*

● 653.6 **Hydrocephalic fetus causing disproportion**
[0,1,3]

Excludes *that when the reason for medical care was concern for the fetus (655.0)*

● ❑ 653.7 **Other fetal abnormality causing disproportion**
[0,1,3]
Conjoined twins
Fetal:
ascites
hydrops
myelomeningocele
Fetal:
sacral teratoma
tumor

● ❑ 653.8 **Disproportion of other origin**
[0,1,3]

Excludes *shoulder (girdle) dystocia (660.4)*

● ❑ 653.9 **Unspecified disproportion**
[0,1,3]

● 654 **Abnormality of organs and soft tissues of pelvis**

Requires fifth digit; valid digits are in [brackets] under each code. See beginning of section 650–659 for definitions.

Includes: the listed conditions during pregnancy, childbirth, or the puerperium

Code first any associated obstructed labor (660.2)

● 654.0 **Congenital abnormalities of uterus**
[0–4]
Double uterus
Uterus bicornis

● 654.1 **Tumors of body of uterus**
[0–4]
Uterine fibroids

● 654.2 **Previous cesarean delivery**
[0,1,3]
Uterine scar from previous cesarean delivery

● 654.3 **Retroverted and incarcerated gravid uterus**
[0–4]

● ❑ 654.4 **Other abnormalities in shape or position of gravid uterus and of neighboring structures**
[0–4]
Cystocele
Pelvic floor repair
Pendulous abdomen
Prolapse of gravid uterus
Rectocele
Rigid pelvic floor

● 654.5 **Cervical incompetence**
[0–4]
Presence of Shirodkar suture with or without mention of cervical incompetence

● ❑ 654.6 **Other congenital or acquired abnormality of cervix**
[0–4]
Cicatricial cervix
Polyp of cervix
Previous surgery to cervix
Rigid cervix (uteri)
Stenosis or stricture of cervix
Tumor of cervix

● 654.7 **Congenital or acquired abnormality of vagina**
[0–4]
Previous surgery to vagina
Septate vagina
Stenosis of vagina (acquired) (congenital)
Stricture of vagina
Tumor of vagina

● **654.8 Congenital or acquired abnormality of vulva**
[0–4] Fibrosis of perineum
Persistent hymen
Previous surgery to perineum or vulva
Rigid perineum
Tumor of vulva

Excludes *varicose veins of vulva (671.1)*

● ❑ **654.9 Other and unspecified**
[0–4] Uterine scar NEC

● **655 Known or suspected fetal abnormality affecting management of mother**

Requires fifth digit; valid digits are in [brackets] under each code. See beginning of section 650–659 for definitions.

Includes: the listed conditions in the fetus as a reason for observation or obstetrical care of the mother, or for termination of pregnancy

● **655.0 Central nervous system malformation in fetus**
[0,1,3] Fetal or suspected fetal:
anencephaly
hydrocephalus
spina bifida (with myelomeningocele)

● **655.1 Chromosomal abnormality in fetus**
[0,1,3]

● **655.2 Hereditary disease in family possibly affecting fetus**
[0,1,3]

● **655.3 Suspected damage to fetus from viral disease in the mother**
[0,1,3]
Suspected damage to fetus from maternal rubella

● ❑ **655.4 Suspected damage to fetus from other disease in the mother**
[0,1,3]
Suspected damage to fetus from maternal:
alcohol addiction
listeriosis
toxoplasmosis

● **655.5 Suspected damage to fetus from drugs**
[0,1,3]

● **655.6 Suspected damage to fetus from radiation**
[0,1,3]

● **655.7 Decreased fetal movements**
[0,1,3]

● ❑ **655.8 Other known or suspected fetal abnormality, not elsewhere classified**
[0,1,3]
Suspected damage to fetus from:
environmental toxins
intrauterine contraceptive device

● ❑ **655.9 Unspecified**
[0,1,3]

● **656 Other fetal and placental problems affecting management of mother**

Requires fifth digit; valid digits are in [brackets] under each code. See beginning of section 650–659 for definitions.

● **656.0 Fetal-maternal hemorrhage**
[0,1,3] Leakage (microscopic) of fetal blood into maternal circulation

● **656.1 Rhesus isoimmunization**
[0,1,3] Anti-D [Rh] antibodies
Rh incompatibility

● ❑ **656.2 Isoimmunization from other and unspecified blood-group incompatibility**
[0,1,3]
ABO isoimmunization

● **656.3 Fetal distress**
[0,1,3] Fetal metabolic acidemia

Excludes *abnormal fetal acid-base balance (656.8)*
abnormality in fetal heart rate or rhythm (659.7)
fetal bradycardia (659.7)
fetal tachycardia (659.7)
meconium in liquor (656.8)

● **656.4 Intrauterine death**
[0,1,3] Fetal death:
NOS
after completion of 22 weeks' gestation
late
Missed delivery

Excludes *missed abortion (632)*

● **656.5 Poor fetal growth**
[0,1,3] "Light-for-dates"
"Placental insufficiency"
"Small-for-dates"

● **656.6 Excessive fetal growth**
[0,1,3] "Large-for-dates"

● ❑ **656.7 Other placental conditions**
[0,1,3] Abnormal placenta
Placental infarct

Excludes *placental polyp (674.4)*
placentitis (658.4)

● ❑ **656.8 Other specified fetal and placental problems**
[0,1,3] Abnormal acid-base balance
Intrauterine acidosis
Lithopedian
Meconium in liquor

● ❑ **656.9 Unspecified fetal and placental problem**
[0,1,3]

● **657 Polyhydramnios**
[0,1,3] Hydramnios

Requires fifth digit; valid digits are in [brackets] under each code. See beginning of section 650–659 for definitions.

Use 0 as fourth digit for category 657

● **658 Other problems associated with amniotic cavity and membranes**

Requires fifth digit; valid digits are in [brackets] under each code. See beginning of section 650–659 for definitions.

Excludes *amniotic fluid embolism (673.1)*

● **658.0 Oligohydramnios**
[0,1,3] Oligohydramnios without mention of rupture of membranes

● **658.1 Premature rupture of membranes**
[0,1,3] Rupture of amniotic sac less than 24 hours prior to the onset of labor

● **658.2 Delayed delivery after spontaneous or unspecified rupture of membranes**
[0,1,3]
Prolonged rupture of membranes NOS
Rupture of amniotic sac 24 hours or more prior to the onset of labor

● **658.3 Delayed delivery after artificial rupture of membranes**
[0,1,3]

● **658.4 Infection of amniotic cavity**
[0,1,3] Amnionitis
Chorioamnionitis
Membranitis
Placentitis

● ❑ **658.8 Other**
[0,1,3] Amnion nodosum
Amniotic cyst

● ❑ **658.9 Unspecified**
[0,1,3]

ICD-9-CM
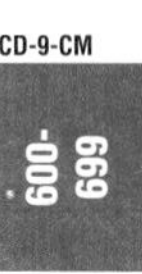
600-699
Vol. 1

659 Other indications for care or intervention related to labor and delivery, not elsewhere classified

Requires fifth digit; valid digits are in [brackets] under each code. See beginning of section 650–659 for definitions.

659.0 Failed mechanical induction
[0,1,3] Failure of induction of labor by surgical or other instrumental methods

659.1 Failed medical or unspecified induction
[0,1,3] Failed induction NOS
Failure of induction of labor by medical methods, such as oxytocic drugs

659.2 Maternal pyrexia during labor, unspecified
[0,1,3]

659.3 Generalized infection during labor
[0,1,3] Septicemia during labor

659.4 Grand multiparity
[0,1,3]

Excludes *supervision only, in pregnancy (V23.3)*
without current pregnancy (V61.5)

659.5 Elderly primigravida
[0,1,3] First pregnancy in a woman who will be 35 years of age or older at expected date of delivery

Excludes *supervision only, in pregnancy (V23.81)*

659.6 Elderly multigravida
[0,1,3] Second or more pregnancy in a woman who will be 35 years of age or older at expected date of delivery

Excludes *elderly primigravida (659.5)*
supervision only, in pregnancy (V23.82)

659.7 Abnormality in fetal heart rate or rhythm
[0,1,3] Depressed fetal heart tones
Fetal:
bradycardia
tachycardia
Fetal heart rate decelerations
Non-reassuring fetal heart rate or rhythm

659.8 Other specified indications for care or intervention
[0,1,3] **related to labor and delivery**
Pregnancy in a female less than 16 years of age at expected date of delivery
Very young maternal age

659.9 Unspecified indication for care or intervention
[0,1,3] **related to labor and delivery**

COMPLICATIONS OCCURRING MAINLY IN THE COURSE OF LABOR AND DELIVERY (660–669)

The following fifth-digit subclassification is for use with categories 660–669 to denote the current episode of care:

0 **unspecified as to episode of care or not applicable**
1 **delivered, with or without mention of antepartum condition**
2 **delivered, with mention of postpartum complication**
3 **antepartum condition or complication**
4 **postpartum condition or complication**

660 Obstructed labor

Requires fifth digit; valid digits are in [brackets] under each code. See beginning of section 660–669 for definitions.

660.0 Obstruction caused by malposition of fetus at onset
[0,1,3] **of labor**
Any condition classifiable to 652, causing obstruction during labor
Use additional code from 652.0–652.9 to identify condition

660.1 Obstruction by bony pelvis
[0,1,3] Any condition classifiable to 653, causing obstruction during labor
Use additional code from 653.0–653.9 to identify condition

660.2 Obstruction by abnormal pelvic soft tissues
[0,1,3] Prolapse of anterior lip of cervix
Any condition classifiable to 654, causing obstruction during labor
Use additional code from 654.0–654.9 to identify condition

660.3 Deep transverse arrest and persistent occipito-
[0,1,3] **posterior position**

660.4 Shoulder (girdle) dystocia
[0,1,3] Impacted shoulders

660.5 Locked twins
[0,1,3]

660.6 Failed trial of labor, unspecified
[0,1,3] Failed trial of labor, without mention of condition or suspected condition

660.7 Failed forceps or vacuum extractor, unspecified
[0,1,3] Application of ventouse or forceps, without mention of condition

660.8 Other causes of obstructed labor
[0,1,3] Use additional code to identify condition

660.9 Unspecified obstructed labor
[0,1,3] Dystocia:
NOS
fetal NOS
maternal NOS

661 Abnormality of forces of labor

Requires fifth digit; valid digits are in [brackets] under each code. See beginning of section 660–669 for definitions.

661.0 Primary uterine inertia
[0,1,3] Failure of cervical dilation
Hypotonic uterine dysfunction, primary
Prolonged latent phase of labor

661.1 Secondary uterine inertia
[0,1,3] Arrested active phase of labor
Hypotonic uterine dysfunction, secondary

661.2 Other and unspecified uterine inertia
[0,1,3] Desultory labor
Irregular labor
Poor contractions
Slow slope active phase of labor

661.3 Precipitate labor
[0,1,3]

661.4 Hypertonic, incoordinate, or prolonged uterine
[0,1,3] **contractions**
Cervical spasm
Contraction ring (dystocia)
Dyscoordinate labor
Hourglass contraction of uterus
Hypertonic uterine dysfunction
Incoordinate uterine action
Retraction ring (Bandl's) (pathological)
Tetanic contractions
Uterine dystocia NOS
Uterine spasm

661.9 Unspecified abnormality of labor
[0,1,3]

662 Long labor

Requires fifth digit; valid digits are in [brackets] under each code. See beginning of section 660–669 for definitions.

662.0 Prolonged first stage
[0,1,3]

662.1 Prolonged labor, unspecified
[0,1,3]

662.2 Prolonged second stage
[0,1,3]

662.3 Delayed delivery of second twin, triplet, etc.
[0,1,3]

663 Umbilical cord complications

Requires fifth digit; valid digits are in [brackets] under each code. See beginning of section 660–669 for definitions.

663.0 Prolapse of cord
[0,1,3] Presentation of cord

663.1 Cord around neck, with compression
[0,1,3] Cord tightly around neck

663.2 Other and unspecified cord entanglement, with compression
[0,1,3] Entanglement of cords of twins in mono-amniotic sac
Knot in cord (with compression)

663.3 Other and unspecified cord entanglement, without mention of compression
[0,1,3]

663.4 Short cord
[0,1,3]

663.5 Vasa previa
[0,1,3]

663.6 Vascular lesions of cord
[0,1,3] Bruising of cord
Hematoma of cord
Thrombosis of vessels of cord

663.8 Other umbilical cord complications
[0,1,3] Velamentous insertion of umbilical cord

663.9 Unspecified umbilical cord complication
[0,1,3]

664 Trauma to perineum and vulva during delivery

Requires fifth digit; valid digits are in [brackets] under each code. See beginning of section 660–669 for definitions.

Includes: damage from instruments
that from extension of episiotomy

664.0 First-degree perineal laceration
[0,1,4] Perineal laceration, rupture, or tear involving:
fourchette
hymen
labia
skin
vagina
vulva

664.1 Second-degree perineal laceration
[0,1,4] Perineal laceration, rupture, or tear (following episiotomy) involving:
pelvic floor
perineal muscles
vaginal muscles

Excludes *that involving anal sphincter (664.2)*

664.2 Third-degree perineal laceration
[0,1,4] Perineal laceration, rupture, or tear (following episiotomy) involving:
anal sphincter
rectovaginal septum
sphincter NOS

Excludes *that with anal or rectal mucosal laceration (664.3)*

664.3 Fourth-degree perineal laceration
[0,1,4] Perineal laceration, rupture, or tear as classifiable to 664.2 and involving also:
anal mucosa
rectal mucosa

664.4 Unspecified perineal laceration
[0,1,4] Central laceration

664.5 Vulval and perineal hematoma
[0,1,4]

664.8 Other specified trauma to perineum and vulva
[0,1,4]

664.9 Unspecified trauma to perineum and vulva
[0,1,4]

665 Other obstetrical trauma

Requires fifth digit; valid digits are in [brackets] under each code. See beginning of section 660–669 for definitions.

Includes: damage from instruments

665.0 Rupture of uterus before onset of labor
[0,1,3]

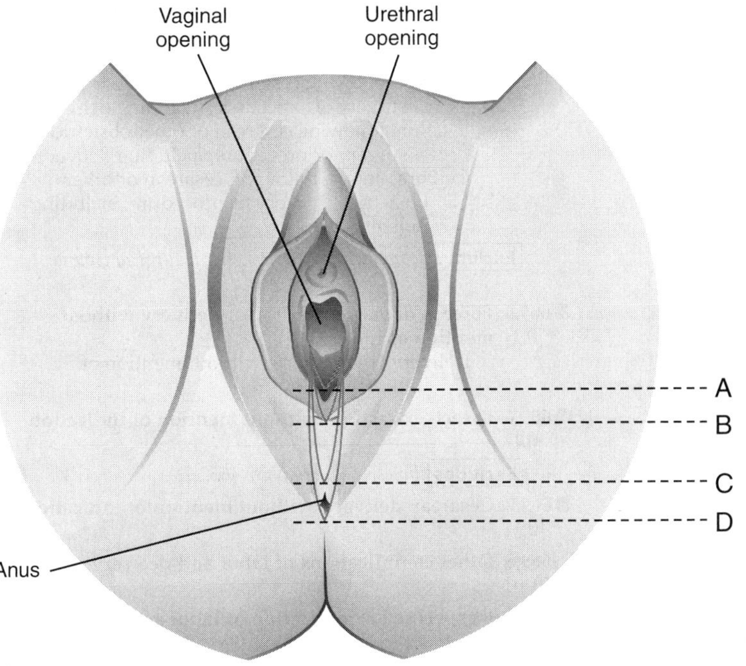

Vaginal opening
Urethral opening
A
B
C
D
Anus

Figure 11-7 Perineal lacerations: **A.** First-degree is laceration of superficial tissues. **B.** Second-degree is limited to the pelvic floor and may involve the perineal or vaginal muscles. **C.** Third-degree involves the anal sphincter. **D.** Fourth-degree involves anal or rectal mucosa.

ICD-9-CM 600-669 Vol. 1

665.1 Rupture of uterus during labor
[0,1] Rupture of uterus NOS

665.2 Inversion of uterus
[0,2,4]

665.3 Laceration of cervix
[0,1,4]

665.4 High vaginal laceration
[0,1,4] Laceration of vaginal wall or sulcus without mention of perineal laceration

665.5 Other injury to pelvic organs
[0,1,4] Injury to:
bladder
urethra

665.6 Damage to pelvic joints and ligaments
[0,1,4] Avulsion of inner symphyseal cartilage
Damage to coccyx
Separation of symphysis (pubis)

665.7 Pelvic hematoma
[0–2,4] Hematoma of vagina

665.8 Other specified obstetrical trauma
[0–4]

665.9 Unspecified obstetrical trauma
[0–4]

666 Postpartum hemorrhage

Requires fifth digit; valid digits are in [brackets] under each code. See beginning of section 660–669 for definitions.

666.0 Third-stage hemorrhage
[0,2,4] Hemorrhage associated with retained, trapped, or adherent placenta
Retained placenta NOS

666.1 Other immediate postpartum hemorrhage
[0,2,4] Atony of uterus with hemorrhage
Hemorrhage within the first 24 hours following delivery of placenta
Postpartum hemorrhage (atonic) NOS

Excludes *atony of uterus without hemorrhage (669.8)*

666.2 Delayed and secondary postpartum hemorrhage
[0,2,4] Hemorrhage:
after the first 24 hours following delivery
associated with retained portions of placenta or membranes
Postpartum hemorrhage specified as delayed or secondary
Retained products of conception NOS, following delivery

666.3 Postpartum coagulation defects
[0,2,4] Postpartum:
afibrinogenemia
fibrinolysis

667 Retained placenta without hemorrhage

Requires fifth digit; valid digits are in [brackets] under each code. See beginning of section 660–669 for definitions.

667.0 Retained placenta without hemorrhage
[0,2,4] Placenta accreta without hemorrhage
Retained placenta:
NOS without hemorrhage
total without hemorrhage

667.1 Retained portions of placenta or membranes, without hemorrhage
[0,2,4] Retained products of conception following delivery, without hemorrhage

668 Complications of the administration of anesthetic or other sedation in labor and delivery

Use additional code(s) to further specify complication

Requires fifth digit; valid digits are in [brackets] under each code. See beginning of section 660–669 for definitions.

Includes: complications arising from the administration of a general or local anesthetic, analgesic, or other sedation in labor and delivery

Excludes *reaction to spinal or lumbar puncture (349.0)*
spinal headache (349.0)

668.0 Pulmonary complications
[0–4] Inhalation [aspiration] of stomach contents or secretions following anesthesia or other sedation in labor or delivery
Mendelson's syndrome following anesthesia or other sedation in labor or delivery
Pressure collapse of lung following anesthesia or other sedation in labor or delivery

668.1 Cardiac complications
[0–4] Cardiac arrest or failure following anesthesia or other sedation in labor and delivery

668.2 Central nervous system complications
[0–4] Cerebral anoxia following anesthesia or other sedation in labor and delivery

668.8 Other complications of anesthesia or other sedation in labor and delivery
[0–4]

668.9 Unspecified complication of anesthesia and other sedation
[0–4]

669 Other complications of labor and delivery, not elsewhere classified

Requires fifth digit; valid digits are in [brackets] under each code. See beginning of section 660–669 for definitions.

669.0 Maternal distress
[0–4] Metabolic disturbance in labor and delivery

669.1 Shock during or following labor and delivery
[0–4] Obstetric shock

669.2 Maternal hypotension syndrome
[0–4]

669.3 Acute renal failure following labor and delivery
[0,2,4]

669.4 Other complications of obstetrical surgery and procedures
[0–4] Cardiac:
arrest following cesarean or other obstetrical surgery or procedure, including delivery NOS
failure following cesarean or other obstetrical surgery or procedure, including delivery NOS
Cerebral anoxia following cesarean or other obstetrical surgery or procedure, including delivery NOS

Excludes *complications of obstetrical surgical wounds (674.1–674.3)*

669.5 Forceps or vacuum extractor delivery without mention of indication
[0,1] Delivery by ventouse, without mention of indication

669.6 Breech extraction, without mention of indication
[0,1]

Excludes *breech delivery NOS (652.2)*

669.7 Cesarean delivery, without mention of indication
[0,1]

669.8 Other complications of labor and delivery
[0–4]

669.9 Unspecified complication of labor and delivery
[0–4]

COMPLICATIONS OF THE PUERPERIUM (670–677)

Note: Categories 671 and 673–676 include the listed conditions even if they occur during pregnancy or childbirth.

The following fifth-digit subclassification is for use with categories 670–676 to denote the current episode of care:

❑ **0 unspecified as to episode of care or not applicable**
1 delivered, with or without mention of antepartum condition
2 delivered, with mention of postpartum complication
3 antepartum condition or complication
4 postpartum condition or complication

● **670 Major puerperal infection**
[0,2,4]

Requires fifth digit; valid digits are in [brackets] under each code. See beginning of section 670–676 for definitions.

Use 0 as fourth digit for category 670

Puerperal:
endometritis
fever (septic)
pelvic:
cellulitis
sepsis

Puerperal:
peritonitis
pyemia
salpingitis
septicemia

Excludes *infection following abortion (639.0)*
minor genital tract infection following delivery (646.6)
puerperal fever NOS (672)
puerperal pyrexia NOS (672)
puerperal pyrexia of unknown origin (672)
urinary tract infection following delivery (646.6)

● **671 Venous complications in pregnancy and the puerperium**

Requires fifth digit; valid digits are in [brackets] under each code. See beginning of section 670–676 for definitions.

● **671.0 Varicose veins of legs**
[0–4] Varicose veins NOS

● **671.1 Varicose veins of vulva and perineum**
[0–4]

● **671.2 Superficial thrombophlebitis**
[0–4] Thrombophlebitis (superficial)

● **671.3 Deep phlebothrombosis, antepartum**
[0,1,3] Deep-vein thrombosis, antepartum

● **671.4 Deep phlebothrombosis, postpartum**
[0,2,4] Deep-vein thrombosis, postpartum
Pelvic thrombophlebitis, postpartum
Phlegmasia alba dolens (puerperal)

● ❑**671.5 Other phlebitis and thrombosis**
[0–4] Cerebral venous thrombosis
Thrombosis of intracranial venous sinus

● ❑**671.8 Other venous complications**
[0–4] Hemorrhoids

● ❑**671.9 Unspecified venous complication**
[0–4] Phlebitis NOS
Thrombosis NOS

● **672 Pyrexia of unknown origin during the puerperium**
[0,2,4] Postpartum fever NOS
Puerperal fever NOS
Puerperal pyrexia NOS

Requires fifth digit; valid digits are in [brackets] under each code. See beginning of section 670–676 for definitions.

Use 0 as fourth digit for category 672

● **673 Obstetrical pulmonary embolism**

Requires fifth digit; valid digits are in [brackets] under each code. See beginning of section 670–676 for definitions.

Includes: pulmonary emboli in pregnancy, childbirth, or the puerperium, or specified as puerperal

Excludes *embolism following abortion (639.6)*

● **673.0 Obstetrical air embolism**
[0–4]

● **673.1 Amniotic fluid embolism**
[0–4]

● **673.2 Obstetrical blood-clot embolism**
[0–4] Puerperal pulmonary embolism NOS

● **673.3 Obstetrical pyemic and septic embolism**
[0–4]

● ❑**673.8 Other pulmonary embolism**
[0–4] Fat embolism

● **674 Other and unspecified complications of the puerperium, not elsewhere classified**

Requires fifth digit; valid digits are in [brackets] under each code. See beginning of section 670–676 for definitions.

● **674.0 Cerebrovascular disorders in the puerperium**
[0–4] Any condition classifiable to 430–434, 436–437 occurring during pregnancy, childbirth, or the puerperium, or specified as puerperal

Excludes *intracranial venous sinus thrombosis (671.5)*

● **674.1 Disruption of cesarean wound**
[0,2,4] Dehiscence or disruption of uterine wound

Excludes *uterine rupture before onset of labor (665.0)*
uterine rupture during labor (665.1)

● **674.2 Disruption of perineal wound**
[0,2,4] Breakdown of perineum
Disruption of wound of:
episiotomy
perineal laceration
Secondary perineal tear

● ❑**674.3 Other complications of obstetrical surgical wounds**
[0,2,4] Hematoma of cesarean section or perineal wound
Hemorrhage of cesarean section or perineal wound
Infection of cesarean section or perineal wound

Excludes *damage from instruments in delivery (664.0–665.9)*

● **674.4 Placental polyp**
[0,2,4]

674.5 Peripartum cardiomyopathy
[0–4] Postpartum cardiomyopathy

● ❑**674.8 Other**
[0,2,4] Hepatorenal syndrome, following delivery
Postpartum:
subinvolution of uterus
uterine hypertrophy

● ❑**674.9 Unspecified**
[0,2,4] Sudden death of unknown cause during the puerperium

● **675 Infections of the breast and nipple associated with childbirth**

Requires fifth digit; valid digits are in [brackets] under each code. See beginning of section 670–676 for definitions.

Includes: the listed conditions during pregnancy, childbirth, or the puerperium

● **675.0 Infections of nipple**
[0–4] Abscess of nipple

675.1 Abscess of breast
[0–4] Abscess:
mammary
subareolar
submammary
Mastitis:
purulent
retromammary
submammary

675.2 Nonpurulent mastitis
[0–4] Lymphangitis of breast
Mastitis:
NOS
interstitial
parenchymatous

675.8 Other specified infections of the breast and nipple
[0–4]

675.9 Unspecified infection of the breast and nipple
[0–4]

676 Other disorders of the breast associated with childbirth and disorders of lactation

Requires fifth digit; valid digits are in [brackets] under each code. See beginning of section 670–676 for definitions.

Includes: the listed conditions during pregnancy, the puerperium, or lactation

676.0 Retracted nipple
[0–4]

676.1 Cracked nipple
[0–4] Fissure of nipple

676.2 Engorgement of breasts
[0–4]

676.3 Other and unspecified disorder of breast
[0–4]

676.4 Failure of lactation
[0–4] Agalactia

676.5 Suppressed lactation
[0–4]

676.6 Galactorrhea
[0–4]

Excludes *galactorrhea not associated with childbirth (611.6)*

676.8 Other disorders of lactation
[0–4] Galactocele

676.9 Unspecified disorder of lactation
[0–4]

677 Late effect of complication of pregnancy, childbirth, and the puerperium

Note: This category is to be used to indicate conditions in 632–648.9 and 651–676.9 as the cause of the late effect, themselves classifiable elsewhere. The "late effects " include conditions specified as such, or as sequelae, which may occur at any time after the puerperium.

Code first any sequelae

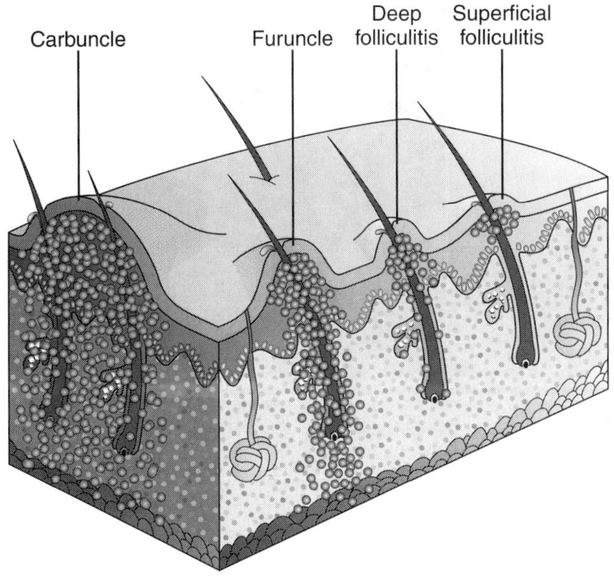
Carbuncle
Furuncle
Deep folliculitis
Superficial folliculitis

Figure 12–1 Furuncle, also known as a boil, is a staphylococcal infection. The organism enters the body through a hair follicle and so furuncles usually appear in hairy areas of the body. A cluster of furuncles is known as a carbuncle and involves infection into the deep subcutaneous fascia. These usually appear on the back and neck.

12. DISEASES OF THE SKIN AND SUBCUTANEOUS TISSUE (680–709)

INFECTIONS OF SKIN AND SUBCUTANEOUS TISSUE (680–686)

Excludes *certain infections of skin classified under "Infectious and Parasitic Diseases," such as:*
erysipelas (035)
erysipeloid of Rosenbach (027.1)
herpes:
simplex (054.0–054.9)
zoster (053.0–053.9)
molluscum contagiosum (078.0)
viral warts (078.1)

● **680 Carbuncle and furuncle**
Includes: boil
furunculosis

680.0 Face
Ear [any part]
Face [any part, except eye]
Nose (septum)
Temple (region)
Excludes *eyelid (373.13)*
lacrimal apparatus (375.31)
orbit (376.01)

680.1 Neck

680.2 Trunk
Abdominal wall
Back [any part, except buttocks]
Breast
Chest wall
Flank
Groin
Pectoral region
Perineum
Umbilicus
Excludes *buttocks (680.5)*
external genital organs:
female (616.4)
male (607.2, 608.4)

680.3 Upper arm and forearm
Arm [any part, except hand]
Axilla
Shoulder

680.4 Hand
Finger [any]
Thumb
Wrist

680.5 Buttock
Anus
Gluteal region

680.6 Leg, except foot
Ankle
Hip
Knee
Thigh

680.7 Foot
Heel
Toe

❑ **680.8 Other specified sites**
Head [any part, except face]
Scalp
Excludes *external genital organs:*
female (616.4)
male (607.2, 608.4)

❑ **680.9 Unspecified site**
Boil NOS
Carbuncle NOS
Furuncle NOS

● **681 Cellulitis and abscess of finger and toe**
Includes: that with lymphangitis
Use additional code to identify organism, such as Staphylococcus (041.1)

● **681.0 Finger**

681.00 Cellulitis and abscess, unspecified

681.01 Felon
Pulp abscess
Whitlow
Excludes *herpetic whitlow (054.6)*

681.02 Onychia and paronychia of finger
Panaritium of finger
Perionychia of finger

● **681.1 Toe**

❑ **681.10 Cellulitis and abscess, unspecified**

681.11 Onychia and paronychia of toe
Panaritium of toe
Perionychia of toe

❑ **681.9 Cellulitis and abscess of unspecified digit**
Infection of nail NOS

● **682 Other cellulitis and abscess**
Includes: abscess (acute) (with lymphangitis) except of finger or toe
cellulitis (diffuse) (with lymphangitis) except of finger or toe
lymphangitis, acute (with lymphangitis) except of finger or toe
Use additional code to identify organism, such as Staphylococcus (041.1)
Excludes *lymphangitis (chronic) (subacute) (457.2)*

682.0 Face
Cheek, external
Chin
Forehead
Nose, external
Submandibular
Temple (region)
Excludes *ear [any part] (380.10–380.16)*
eyelid (373.13)
lacrimal apparatus (375.31)
lip (528.5)
mouth (528.3)
nose (internal) (478.1)
orbit (376.01)

682.1 **Neck**

682.2 **Trunk**
Abdominal wall
Back [any part, except buttocks]
Chest wall
Flank
Groin
Pectoral region
Perineum
Umbilicus, except newborn

Excludes *anal and rectal regions (566)*
breast:
NOS (611.0)
puerperal (675.1)
external genital organs:
female (616.3–616.4)
male (604.0, 607.2, 608.4)
umbilicus, newborn (771.4)

682.3 **Upper arm and forearm**
Arm [any part, except hand]
Axilla
Shoulder

Excludes *hand (682.4)*

682.4 **Hand, except finger and thumb**
Wrist

Excludes *fingers and thumb (681.00–681.02)*

682.5 **Buttock**
Gluteal region

Excludes *anal and rectal regions (566)*

682.6 **Leg, except foot**
Ankle
Hip
Knee
Thigh

682.7 **Foot, except toes**
Heel

Excludes *toe (681.10–681.11)*

❑682.8 **Other specified sites**
Head [except face]
Scalp

Excludes *face (682.0)*

❑682.9 **Unspecified site**
Abscess NOS
Cellulitis NOS
Lymphangitis, acute NOS

Excludes *lymphangitis NOS (457.2)*

683 **Acute lymphadenitis**
Abscess (acute) lymph gland or node, except mesenteric
Adenitis, acute lymph gland or node, except mesenteric
Lymphadenitis, acute lymph gland or node, except mesenteric

Use additional code to identify organism such as Staphylococcus (041.1)

Excludes *enlarged glands NOS (785.6)*
lymphadenitis:
chronic or subacute, except mesenteric (289.1)
mesenteric (acute) (chronic) (subacute) (289.2)
unspecified (289.3)

684 **Impetigo**
Impetiginization of other dermatoses
Impetigo (contagiosa) [any site] [any organism]:
bullous
circinate
neonatorum
simplex
Pemphigus neonatorum

Excludes *impetigo herpetiformis (694.3)*

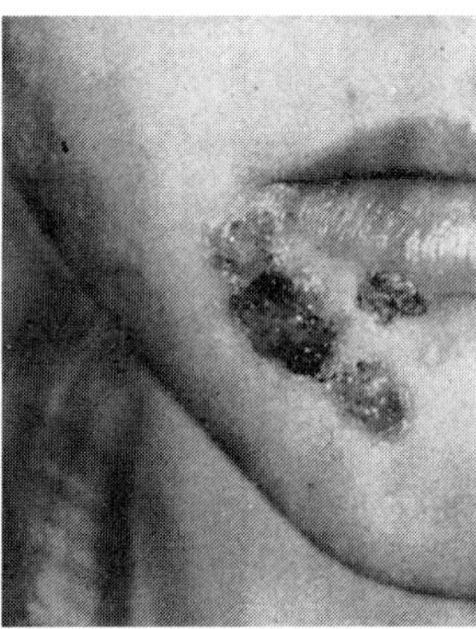

Figure 12–2 Impetigo is a contagious, superficial skin infection caused by *Staphylococcus aureus*. It appears most frequently in infants. (From Lewis GM, Wheeler CE, Jr: Practical Dermatology, 3rd ed. Philadelphia, WB Saunders, 1967, p 234, Plate 79B.)

Item 12–1 Pilonidal cyst, also called a coccygeal cyst, is the result of a disorder called pilonidal disease. The cyst usually contains hair and pus.

● 685 **Pilonidal cyst**

Includes: fistula, coccygeal or pilonidal
sinus, coccygeal or pilonidal

685.0 **With abscess**

685.1 **Without mention of abscess**

● 686 **Other local infections of skin and subcutaneous tissue**

Use additional code to identify any infectious organism (041.0–041.8)

● 686.0 **Pyoderma**
Dermatitis:
purulent
septic
suppurative

❑686.00 **Pyoderma, unspecified**

686.01 **Pyoderma gangrenosum**

❑686.09 **Other pyoderma**

686.1 **Pyogenic granuloma**
Granuloma:
septic
suppurative
telangiectaticum

Excludes *pyogenic granuloma of oral mucosa (528.9)*

❑686.8 **Other specified local infections of skin and subcutaneous tissue**
Bacterid (pustular)
Dermatitis vegetans
Ecthyma
Perlèche

Excludes *dermatitis infectiosa eczematoides (690.8)*
panniculitis (729.30–729.39)

❑686.9 **Unspecified local infection of skin and subcutaneous tissue**
Fistula of skin NOS
Skin infection NOS

Excludes *fistula to skin from internal organs—see Alphabetic Index*

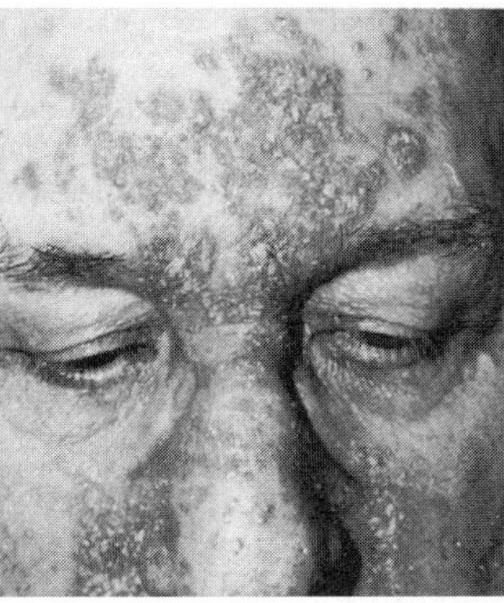

Figure 12–3 Severe seborrheic dermatitis. (From Arnold HL, Odom RB, James WD: Andrews' Diseases of the Skin, Clinical Dermatology, 8th ed. Philadelphia, WB Saunders, 1990, p 195.)

Item 12–2 Seborrheic dermatitis is characterized by greasy, scaly, red patches and is associated with oily skin and scalp.

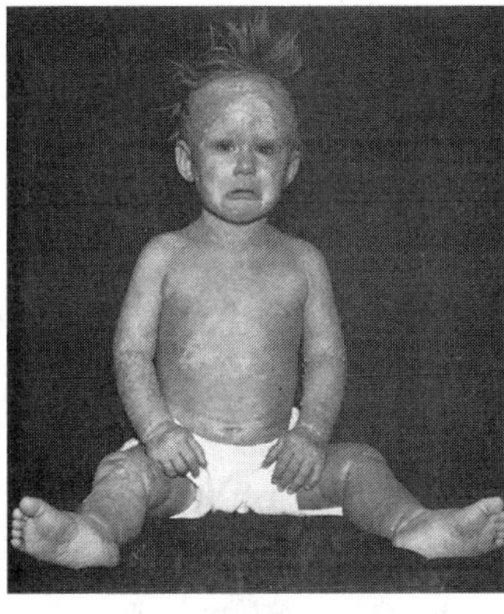

Figure 12–4 Atopic dermatitis. (From Moschella SL, Hurley HJ: Dermatology, 2nd ed. Philadelphia, WB Saunders, 1985, p 336.)

Item 12–3 Atopic dermatitis, also known as atopic eczema, infantile eczema, disseminated neurodermatitis, flexural eczema, and *prurigo diathesique* (Besnier), is characterized by intense itching and is often hereditary.

OTHER INFLAMMATORY CONDITIONS OF SKIN AND SUBCUTANEOUS TISSUE (690–698)

Excludes *panniculitis (729.30–729.39)*

● **690 Erythematosquamous dermatosis**

Excludes *eczematous dermatitis of eyelid (373.31)*
parakeratosis variegata (696.2)
psoriasis (696.0–696.1)
seborrheic keratosis (702.11–702.19)

● **690.1 Seborrheic dermatitis**

❑ **690.10 Seborrheic dermatitis, unspecified**
Seborrheic dermatitis NOS

690.11 Seborrhea capitis
Cradle cap

690.12 Seborrheic infantile dermatitis

❑ **690.18 Other seborrheic dermatitis**

❑ **690.8 Other erythematosquamous dermatosis**

● **691 Atopic dermatitis and related conditions**

691.0 Diaper or napkin rash
Ammonia dermatitis
Diaper or napkin:
- dermatitis
- erythema
- rash

Psoriasiform napkin eruption

❑ **691.8 Other atopic dermatitis and related conditions**
Atopic dermatitis
Besnier's prurigo
Eczema:
- atopic
- flexural
- intrinsic (allergic)

Neurodermatitis:
- atopic
- diffuse (of Brocq)

● **692 Contact dermatitis and other eczema**

Includes: dermatitis:
- NOS
- contact
- occupational
- venenata

eczema (acute) (chronic):
- NOS
- allergic
- erythematous
- occupational

Excludes *allergy NOS (995.3)*
contact dermatitis of eyelids (373.32)
dermatitis due to substances taken internally (693.0–693.9)
eczema of external ear (380.22)
perioral dermatitis (695.3)
urticarial reactions (708.0–708.9, 995.1)

692.0 Due to detergents

692.1 Due to oils and greases

692.2 Due to solvents
Dermatitis due to solvents of:
- chlorocompound group
- cyclohexane group
- ester group
- glycol group
- hydrocarbon group
- ketone group

692.3 Due to drugs and medicines in contact with skin
Dermatitis (allergic) (contact) due to:
- arnica
- fungicides
- iodine
- keratolytics
- mercurials
- neomycin
- pediculocides
- phenols
- scabicides
- any drug applied to skin

Dermatitis medicamentosa due to drug applied to skin

Use additional E code to identify drug

Excludes *allergy NOS due to drugs (995.27)* ◄
dermatitis due to ingested drugs (693.0)
dermatitis medicamentosa NOS (693.0)

❑ **692.4 Due to other chemical products**

Dermatitis due to:	Dermatitis due to:
acids	insecticide
adhesive plaster	nylon
alkalis	plastic
caustics	rubber
dichromate	

692.5 Due to food in contact with skin
Dermatitis, contact, due to:
cereals
fish
flour
fruit
meat
milk

Excludes *dermatitis due to:*
dyes (692.89)
ingested foods (693.1)
preservatives (692.89)

692.6 Due to plants [except food]
Dermatitis due to:
lacquer tree [Rhus verniciflua]
poison:
ivy [Rhus toxicodendron]
oak [Rhus diversiloba]
sumac [Rhus venenata]
vine [Rhus radicans]
primrose [Primula]
ragweed [Senecio jacobae]
other plants in contact with the skin

Excludes *allergy NOS due to pollen (477.0)*
nettle rash (708.8)

● **692.7 Due to solar radiation**

Excludes *sunburn due to other ultraviolet radiation exposure (692.82)*

❑ **692.70 Unspecified dermatitis due to sun**

692.71 Sunburn
First degree sunburn
Sunburn NOS

692.72 Acute dermatitis due to solar radiation
Berloque dermatitis
Photoallergic response
Phototoxic response
Polymorphous light eruption
Acute solar skin damage NOS

Excludes *sunburn (692.71, 692.76–692.77)*

Use additional E code to identify drug, if drug induced

692.73 Actinic reticuloid and actinic granuloma

❑ **692.74 Other chronic dermatitis due to solar radiation**
Chronic solar skin damage NOS
Solar elastosis

Excludes *actinic [solar] keratosis (702.0)*

692.75 Disseminated superficial actinic porokeratosis (DSAP)

692.76 Sunburn of second degree

692.77 Sunburn of third degree

❑ **692.79 Other dermatitis due to solar radiation**
Hydroa aestivale
Photodermatitis (due to sun)
Photosensitiveness (due to sun)
Solar skin damage NOS

● **692.8 Due to other specified agents**

692.81 Dermatitis due to cosmetics

❑ **692.82 Dermatitis due to other radiation**
Infrared rays
Light, except from sun
Radiation NOS
Tanning bed
Ultraviolet rays, except from sun
X-rays

Excludes *that due to solar radiation (692.70–692.79)*

692.83 Dermatitis due to metals
Jewelry

692.84 Due to animal (cat) (dog) dander
Due to animal (cat) (dog) hair

❑ **692.89 Other**
Dermatitis due to:
cold weather
dyes
hot weather
preservatives

Excludes *allergy (NOS) (rhinitis) due to animal hair or dander (477.2)*
allergy to dust (477.8)
sunburn (692.71, 692.76–692.77)

❑ **692.9 Unspecified cause**
Dermatitis:
NOS
contact NOS
venenata NOS
Eczema NOS

● **693 Dermatitis due to substances taken internally**

Excludes *adverse effect NOS of drugs and medicines (995.20)* ⇐
allergy NOS (995.3)
contact dermatitis (692.0–692.9)
urticarial reactions (708.0–708.9, 995.1)

693.0 Due to drugs and medicines
Dermatitis medicamentosa NOS

Use additional E code to identify drug

Excludes *that due to drugs in contact with skin (692.3)*

693.1 Due to food

❑ **693.8 Due to other specified substances taken internally**

❑ **693.9 Due to unspecified substance taken internally**

Excludes *dermatitis NOS (692.9)*

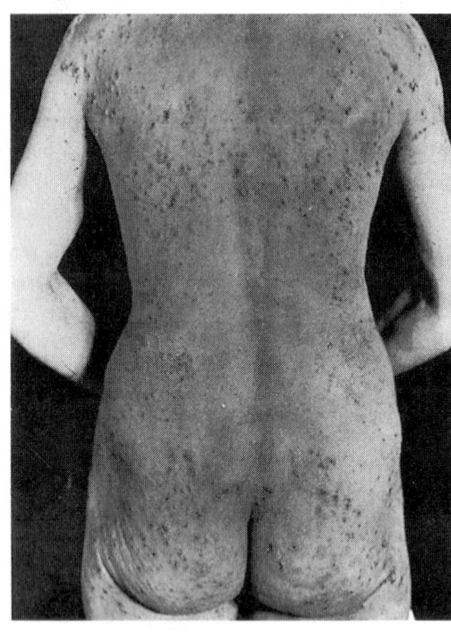

Figure 12–5 Dermatitis herpetiformis. (From Arnold HL, Odom RB, James WD: Andrews' Diseases of the Skin, Clinical Dermatology, 8th ed. Philadelphia, WB Saunders, 1990, p 553.)

Item 12–4 Dermatitis herpetiformis, also known as Duhring's disease, is a systemic disease characterized by small blisters (3 to 5 mm) and occasionally large bullae (+5 mm).

● **694 Bullous dermatoses**

694.0 Dermatitis herpetiformis
Dermatosis herpetiformis
Duhring's disease
Hydroa herpetiformis

Excludes *herpes gestationis (646.8)*
dermatitis herpetiformis:
juvenile (694.2)
senile (694.5)

694.1 Subcorneal pustular dermatosis
Sneddon-Wilkinson disease or syndrome

694.2 Juvenile dermatitis herpetiformis
Juvenile pemphigoid

694.3 Impetigo herpetiformis

694.4 Pemphigus
Pemphigus:
NOS
erythematosus
foliaceus
malignant
vegetans
vulgaris

Excludes *pemphigus neonatorum (684)*

694.5 Pemphigoid
Benign pemphigus NOS
Bullous pemphigoid
Herpes circinatus bullosus
Senile dermatitis herpetiformis

● **694.6 Benign mucous membrane pemphigoid**
Cicatricial pemphigoid
Mucosynechial atrophic bullous dermatitis

694.60 Without mention of ocular involvement

694.61 With ocular involvement
Ocular pemphigus

❑ **694.8 Other specified bullous dermatoses**

Excludes *herpes gestationis (646.8)*

❑ **694.9 Unspecified bullous dermatoses**

● **695 Erythematous conditions**

695.0 Toxic erythema
Erythema venenatum

695.1 Erythema multiforme
Erythema iris
Herpes iris
Lyell's syndrome
Scalded skin syndrome
Stevens-Johnson syndrome
Toxic epidermal necrolysis

695.2 Erythema nodosum

Excludes *tuberculous erythema nodosum (017.1)*

695.3 Rosacea
Acne:
erythematosa
rosacea
Perioral dermatitis
Rhinophyma

695.4 Lupus erythematosus
Lupus:
erythematodes (discoid)
erythematosus (discoid), not disseminated

Excludes *lupus (vulgaris) NOS (017.0)*
systemic [disseminated] lupus erythematosus (710.0)

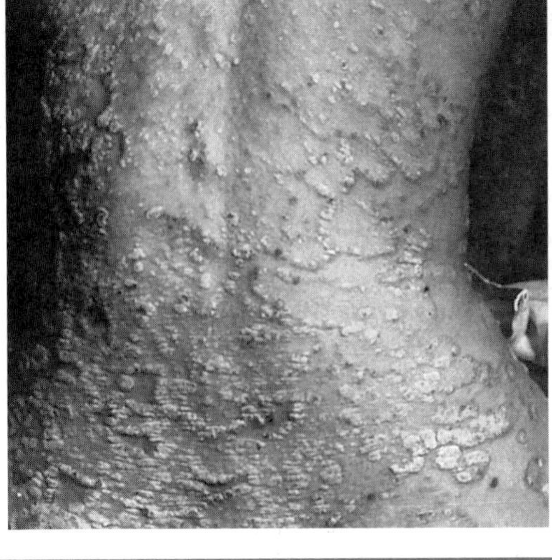

Figure 12–6 Psoriasis. (From Moschella SL, Hurley HJ: Dermatology, 2nd ed. Philadelphia, WB Saunders, 1985, p 512.)

Item 12-5 Psoriasis is a chronic, recurrent inflammatory skin disease characterized by small patches covered with thick silvery scales. **Parapsoriasis** is a treatment-resistant erythroderma. **Pityriasis rosea** is characterized by a herald patch that is a single large lesion and that usually appears on the trunk and is followed by scattered, smaller lesions.

● **695.8 Other specified erythematous conditions**

695.81 Ritter's disease
Dermatitis exfoliativa neonatorum

❑ **695.89 Other**
Erythema intertrigo
Intertrigo
Pityriasis rubra (Hebra)

Excludes *mycotic intertrigo (111.0–111.9)*

❑ **695.9 Unspecified erythematous condition**
Erythema NOS
Erythroderma (secondary)

● **696 Psoriasis and similar disorders**

696.0 Psoriatic arthropathy

❑ **696.1 Other psoriasis**
Acrodermatitis continua
Dermatitis repens
Psoriasis:
NOS
any type, except arthropathic

Excludes *psoriatic arthropathy (696.0)*

696.2 Parapsoriasis
Parakeratosis variegata
Parapsoriasis lichenoides chronica
Pityriasis lichenoides et varioliformis

696.3 Pityriasis rosea
Pityriasis circinata (et maculata)

696.4 Pityriasis rubra pilaris
Devergie's disease
Lichen ruber acuminatus

Excludes *pityriasis rubra (Hebra) (695.89)*

❑696.5 **Other and unspecified pityriasis**
Pityriasis:
NOS
alba
streptogenes
Excludes *pityriasis:*
simplex (690.18)
versicolor (111.0)

❑696.8 **Other**

● 697 **Lichen**
Excludes *lichen:*
obtusus corneus (698.3)
pilaris (congenital) (757.39)
ruber acuminatus (696.4)
sclerosus et atrophicus (701.0)
scrofulosus (017.0)
simplex chronicus (698.3)
spinulosus (congenital) (757.39)
urticatus (698.2)

697.0 **Lichen planus**
Lichen:
planopilaris
ruber planus

697.1 **Lichen nitidus**
Pinkus' disease

❑697.8 **Other lichen, not elsewhere classified**
Lichen:
ruber moniliforme
striata

❑697.9 **Lichen, unspecified**

● 698 **Pruritus and related conditions**
Excludes *pruritus specified as psychogenic (306.3)*

698.0 **Pruritus ani**
Perianal itch

698.1 **Pruritus of genital organs**

698.2 **Prurigo**
Lichen urticatus
Prurigo:
NOS
Hebra's
mitis
simplex
Urticaria papulosa (Hebra)
Excludes *prurigo nodularis (698.3)*

698.3 **Lichenification and lichen simplex chronicus**
Hyde's disease
Neurodermatitis (circumscripta) (local)
Prurigo nodularis
Excludes *neurodermatitis, diffuse (of Brocq) (691.8)*

698.4 **Dermatitis factitia [artefacta]**
Dermatitis ficta
Neurotic excoriation

Use additional code to identify any associated mental disorder

❑698.8 **Other specified pruritic conditions**
Pruritus:
hiemalis
senilis
Winter itch

❑698.9 **Unspecified pruritic disorder**
Itch NOS
Pruritus NOS

Item 12-6 Keratoderma is characterized by firm horny papules that have a cobblestone appearance. **Keratoderma climactericum,** also known as endocrine keratoderma, is hyperkeratosis located on the palms and soles.

OTHER DISEASES OF SKIN AND SUBCUTANEOUS TISSUE (700–709)

Excludes *conditions confined to eyelids (373.0–374.9)*
congenital conditions of skin, hair, and nails (757.0–757.9)

700 **Corns and callosities**
Callus
Clavus

● 701 **Other hypertrophic and atrophic conditions of skin**
Excludes *dermatomyositis (710.3)*
hereditary edema of legs (757.0)
scleroderma (generalized) (710.1)

701.0 **Circumscribed scleroderma**
Addison's keloid
Dermatosclerosis, localized
Lichen sclerosus et atrophicus
Morphea
Scleroderma, circumscribed or localized

701.1 **Keratoderma, acquired**
Acquired:
ichthyosis
keratoderma palmaris et plantaris
Elastosis perforans serpiginosa
Hyperkeratosis:
NOS
follicularis in cutem penetrans
palmoplantaris climacterica
Keratoderma:
climactericum
tylodes, progressive
Keratosis (blennorrhagica)
Excludes *Darier's disease [keratosis follicularis] (congenital) (757.39)*
keratosis:
arsenical (692.4)
gonococcal (098.81)

701.2 **Acquired acanthosis nigricans**
Keratosis nigricans

701.3 **Striae atrophicae**
Atrophic spots of skin
Atrophoderma maculatum
Atrophy blanche (of Milian)
Degenerative colloid atrophy
Senile degenerative atrophy
Striae distensae

701.4 **Keloid scar**
Cheloid
Hypertrophic scar
Keloid

❑701.5 **Other abnormal granulation tissue**
Excessive granulation

❑701.8 **Other specified hypertrophic and atrophic conditions of skin**
Acrodermatitis atrophicans chronica
Atrophia cutis senilis
Atrophoderma neuriticum
Confluent and reticulate papillomatosis
Cutis laxa senilis
Elastosis senilis
Folliculitis ulerythematosa reticulata
Gougerot-Carteaud syndrome or disease

❑701.9 **Unspecified hypertrophic and atrophic conditions of skin**
Atrophoderma

● 702 **Other dermatoses**
Excludes *carcinoma in situ (232.0–232.9)*

702.0 **Actinic keratosis**

● 702.1 **Seborrheic keratosis**

702.11 **Inflamed seborrheic keratosis**

❑ 702.19 **Other seborrheic keratosis**
Seborrheic keratosis NOS

❑ 702.8 **Other specified dermatoses**

● 703 **Diseases of nail**

Excludes *congenital anomalies (757.5)*
onychia and paronychia (681.02, 681.11)

703.0 **Ingrowing nail**
Ingrowing nail with infection
Unguis incarnatus

Excludes *infection, nail NOS (681.9)*

❑ 703.8 **Other specified diseases of nail**
Dystrophia unguium
Hypertrophy of nail
Koilonychia
Leukonychia (punctata) (striata)
Onychauxis
Onychogryposis
Onycholysis

❑ 703.9 **Unspecified disease of nail**

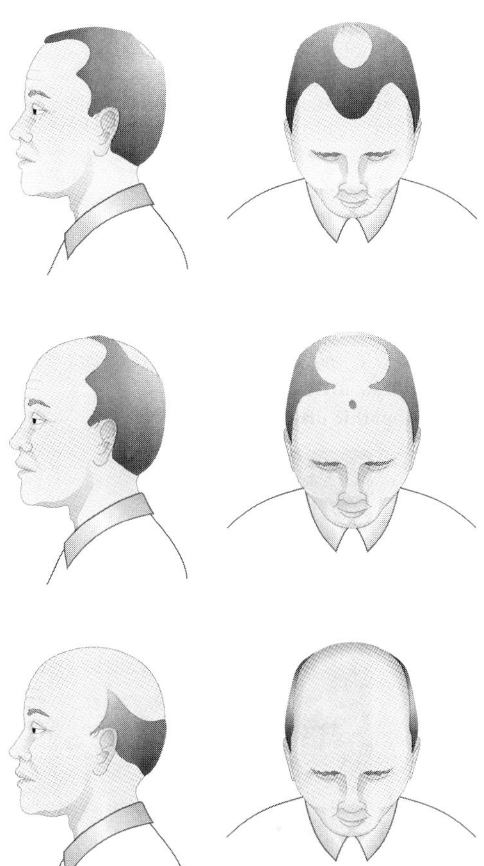

Figure 12-7 Male pattern alopecia.

Item 12-7 Alopecia is lack of hair and takes many forms. The most common is male pattern alopecia, also known as **androgenetic alopecia. Telogen effluvium** is early and excessive loss of hair resulting from a trauma to the hair (fever, drugs, surgery, etc.).

● 704 **Diseases of hair and hair follicles**

Excludes *congenital anomalies (757.4)*

● 704.0 **Alopecia**

Excludes *madarosis (374.55)*
syphilitic alopecia (091.82)

❑ 704.00 **Alopecia, unspecified**
Baldness
Loss of hair

704.01 **Alopecia areata**
Ophiasis

704.02 **Telogen effluvium**

❑ 704.09 **Other**
Folliculitis decalvans
Hypotrichosis:
NOS
postinfectional NOS
Pseudopelade

Item 12-8 Hirsutism is excessive growth of hair.

704.1 **Hirsutism**
Hypertrichosis:
NOS
lanuginosa, acquired
Polytrichia

Excludes *hypertrichosis of eyelid (374.54)*

704.2 **Abnormalities of the hair**
Atrophic hair
Clastothrix
Fragilitas crinium
Trichiasis:
NOS
cicatrical
Trichorrhexis (nodosa)

Excludes *trichiasis of eyelid (374.05)*

704.3 **Variations in hair color**
Canities (premature)
Grayness, hair (premature)
Heterochromia of hair
Poliosis:
NOS
circumscripta, acquired

❑ 704.8 **Other specified diseases of hair and hair follicles**
Folliculitis:
NOS
abscedens et suffodiens
pustular
Perifolliculitis:
NOS
capitis abscedens et suffodiens
scalp
Sycosis:
NOS
barbae [not parasitic]
lupoid
vulgaris

❑ 704.9 **Unspecified disease of hair and hair follicles**

● 705 **Disorders of sweat glands**

705.0 **Anhidrosis**
Hypohidrosis
Oligohidrosis

705.1 **Prickly heat**
Heat rash
Miliaria rubra (tropicalis)
Sudamina

● 705.2 **Focal hyperhidrosis**

Excludes *generalized (secondary) hyperhidrosis (780.8)*

705.21 **Primary focal hyperhidrosis**
Focal hyperhidrosis NOS
Hyperhidrosis NOS
Hyperhidrosis of:
axilla
face
palms
soles

705.22 **Secondary focal hyperhidrosis**
Frey's syndrome

● 705.8 **Other specified disorders of sweat glands**

705.81 **Dyshidrosis**
Cheiropompholyx
Pompholyx

705.82 **Fox-Fordyce disease**

705.83 **Hidradenitis**
Hidradenitis suppurativa

❑705.89 **Other**
Bromhidrosis
Chromhidrosis
Granulosis rubra nasi
Urhidrosis

Excludes *hidrocystoma (216.0–216.9)*
generalized hyperhidrosis (780.8)

❑705.9 **Unspecified disorder of sweat glands**
Disorder of sweat glands NOS

● 706 **Diseases of sebaceous glands**

706.0 **Acne varioliformis**
Acne:
frontalis
necrotica

❑706.1 **Other acne**
Acne:
NOS
conglobata
cystic
pustular
vulgaris
Blackhead
Comedo

Excludes *acne rosacea (695.3)*

706.2 **Sebaceous cyst**
Atheroma, skin
Keratin cyst
Wen

706.3 **Seborrhea**

Excludes *seborrhea:*
capitis (690.11)
sicca (690.18)
seborrheic:
dermatitis (690.10)
keratosis (702.11–702.19)

❑706.8 **Other specified diseases of sebaceous glands**
Asteatosis (cutis)
Xerosis cutis

❑706.9 **Unspecified disease of sebaceous glands**

● 707 **Chronic ulcer of skin**

Includes: non-infected sinus of skin
non-healing ulcer

Excludes *specific infections classified under "Infectious and Parasitic Diseases" (001.0–136.9)*
varicose ulcer (454.0, 454.2)

● 707.0 **Decubitus ulcer**
Bed sore
Decubitus ulcer [any site]
Plaster ulcer
Pressure ulcer

❑707.00 **Unspecified site**

707.01 **Elbow**

707.02 **Upper back**
Shoulder blades

707.03 **Lower back**
Sacrum

707.04 **Hip**

707.05 **Buttock**

707.06 **Ankle**

707.07 **Heel**

707.09 **Other site**
Head

● 707.1 **Ulcer of lower limbs, except decubitus**
Ulcer, chronic, of lower limb:
neurogenic of lower limb
trophic of lower limb

Code if applicable, any causal condition first:
atherosclerosis of the extremities with ulceration (440.23)
chronic venous hypertension with ulcer (459.31)
chronic venous hypertension with ulcer and inflammation (459.33)
diabetes mellitus (250.80–250.83)
postphlebitic syndrome with ulcer (459.11)
postphlebitic syndrome with ulcer and inflammation (459.13)

❑707.10 **Ulcer of lower limb, unspecified**

707.11 **Ulcer of thigh**

707.12 **Ulcer of calf**

707.13 **Ulcer of ankle**

707.14 **Ulcer of heel and midfoot**
Plantar surface of midfoot

707.15 **Ulcer of other part of foot**
Toes

707.19 **Ulcer of other part of lower limb**

❑707.8 **Chronic ulcer of other specified sites**
Ulcer, chronic, of other specified sites:
neurogenic of other specified sites
trophic of other specified sites

❑707.9 **Chronic ulcer of unspecified site**
Chronic ulcer NOS
Trophic ulcer NOS
Tropical ulcer NOS
Ulcer of skin NOS

● 708 **Urticaria**

Excludes *edema:*
angioneurotic (995.1)
Quincke's (995.1)
hereditary angioedema (277.6)
urticaria:
giant (995.1)
papulosa (Hebra) (698.2)
pigmentosa (juvenile) (congenital) (757.33)

708.0 **Allergic urticaria**

708.1 **Idiopathic urticaria**

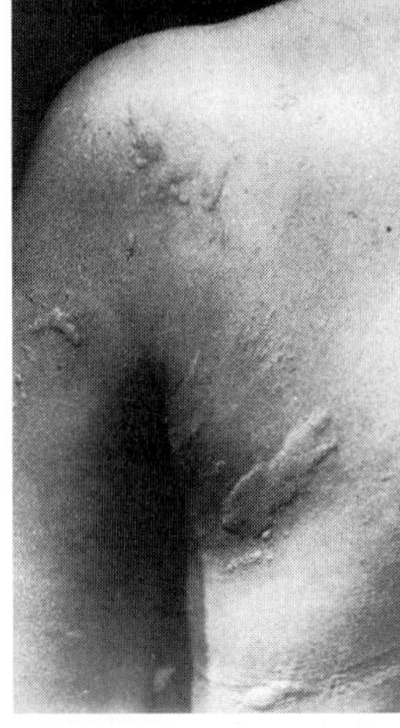

Figure 12–8 Urticaria, or hives. (From Arnold HL, Odom RB, James WD: Andrews' Diseases of the Skin, Clinical Dermatology, 8th ed. Philadelphia, WB Saunders, 1990, p 148.)

Item 12–9 Urticaria is a vascular reaction in which wheals surrounded by a red halo appear and cause severe itching. The causes of urticaria or hives are extensive and varied (e.g., food, heat, cold, drugs, stress, infections).

708.2 Urticaria due to cold and heat
Thermal urticaria

708.3 Dermatographic urticaria
Dermatographia
Factitial urticaria

708.4 Vibratory urticaria

708.5 Cholinergic urticaria

❑ **708.8 Other specified urticaria**
Nettle rash
Urticaria:
chronic
recurrent periodic

❑ **708.9 Urticaria, unspecified**
Hives NOS

● **709 Other disorders of skin and subcutaneous tissue**

● **709.0 Dyschromia**

Excludes *albinism (270.2)*
pigmented nevus (216.0–216.9)
that of eyelid (374.52–374.53)

❑ **709.00 Dyschromia, unspecified**

709.01 Vitiligo

❑ **709.09 Other**

709.1 Vascular disorders of skin
Angioma serpiginosum
Purpura (primary) annularis telangiectodes

709.2 Scar conditions and fibrosis of skin
Adherent scar (skin)
Cicatrix
Disfigurement (due to scar)
Fibrosis, skin NOS
Scar NOS

Excludes *keloid scar (701.4)*

709.3 Degenerative skin disorders
Calcinosis:
circumscripta
cutis
Colloid milium
Degeneration, skin
Deposits, skin
Senile dermatosis NOS
Subcutaneous calcification

709.4 Foreign body granuloma of skin and subcutaneous tissue

Excludes *residual foreign body without granuloma of skin and subcutaneous tissue (729.6)*
that of muscle (728.82)

❑ **709.8 Other specified disorders of skin**
Epithelial hyperplasia
Menstrual dermatosis
Vesicular eruption

❑ **709.9 Unspecified disorder of skin and subcutaneous tissue**
Dermatosis NOS

13. DISEASES OF THE MUSCULOSKELETAL SYSTEM AND CONNECTIVE TISSUE (710–739)

The following fifth-digit subclassification is for use with categories 711–712, 715–716, 718–719, and 730:

❑ **0 site unspecified**
1 shoulder region
Acromioclavicular joint(s)
Clavicle
Glenohumeral joint(s)
Scapula
Sternoclavicular joint(s)
2 upper arm
Elbow joint
Humerus
3 forearm
Radius
Ulna
Wrist joint
4 hand
Carpus
Metacarpus
Phalanges [fingers]
5 pelvic region and thigh
Buttock
Femur
Hip (joint)
6 lower leg
Fibula
Knee joint
Patella
Tibia
7 ankle and foot
Ankle joint
Digits [toes]
Metatarsus
Phalanges, foot
Tarsus
Other joints in foot
❑ **8 other specified sites**
Head
Neck
Ribs
Skull
Trunk
Vertebral column
❑ **9 multiple sites**

ARTHROPATHIES AND RELATED DISORDERS (710–719)

Excludes *disorders of spine (720.0–724.9)*

● **710 Diffuse diseases of connective tissue**

Includes: all collagen diseases whose effects are not mainly confined to a single system

Excludes *those affecting mainly the cardiovascular system, i.e., polyarteritis nodosa and allied conditions (446.0–446.7)*

710.0 Systemic lupus erythematosus
Disseminated lupus erythematosus
Libman-Sacks disease

Use additional code to identify manifestation, as:
endocarditis (424.91)
nephritis (583.81)
chronic (582.81)
nephrotic syndrome (581.81)

Excludes *lupus erythematosus (discoid) NOS (695.4)*

710.1 Systemic sclerosis
Acrosclerosis
CRST syndrome
Progressive systemic sclerosis
Scleroderma

Use additional code to identify manifestations, as:
lung involvement (517.2)
myopathy (359.6)

Excludes *circumscribed scleroderma (701.0)*

710.2 Sicca syndrome
Keratoconjunctivitis sicca
Sjögren's disease

710.3 Dermatomyositis
Poikilodermatomyositis
Polymyositis with skin involvement

710.4 Polymyositis

710.5 Eosinophilia myalgia syndrome
Toxic oil syndrome

Use additional E code to identify drug, if drug induced

❑ **710.8 Other specified diffuse diseases of connective tissue**
Multifocal fibrosclerosis (idiopathic) NEC
Systemic fibrosclerosing syndrome

❑ **710.9 Unspecified diffuse connective tissue disease**
Collagen disease NOS

● **711 Arthropathy associated with infections**

Includes: arthritis associated with conditions classifiable below
arthropathy associated with conditions classifiable below
polyarthritis associated with conditions classifiable below
polyarthropathy associated with conditions classifiable below

Excludes *rheumatic fever (390)*

The following fifth-digit subclassification is for use with category 711; valid digits are in [brackets] under each code. See list at beginning of chapter for definitions:

❑ **0 site unspecified**
1 shoulder region
2 upper arm
3 forearm
4 hand
5 pelvic region and thigh
6 lower leg
7 ankle and foot
❑ **8 other specified sites**
❑ **9 multiple sites**

● **711.0 Pyogenic arthritis**
[0–9] Arthritis or polyarthritis (due to):
coliform [*Escherichia coli*]
Hemophilus influenzae [H. influenzae]
pneumococcal
Pseudomonas
staphylococcal
streptococcal
Pyarthrosis

Use additional code to identify infectious organism (041.0–041.8)

●● ***711.1 Arthropathy associated with Reiter's disease and nonspecific urethritis***
[0–9]

Code first underlying disease, as:
nonspecific urethritis (099.4)
Reiter's disease (099.3)

●● ***711.2 Arthropathy in Behçet's syndrome***
[0–9] *Code first underlying disease (136.1)*

● ● *711.3 Postdysentericarthropathy*
[0–9] *Code first underlying disease, as:*
dysentery (009.0)
enteritis, infectious (008.0–009.3)
paratyphoid fever (002.1–002.9)
typhoid fever (002.0)

Excludes *salmonella arthritis (003.23)*

● ● ❑ *711.4 Arthropathy associated with other bacterial diseases*
[0–9] *Code first underlying disease, as:*
diseases classifiable to 010–040, 090–099, except as in 711.1, 711.3, and 713.5
leprosy (030.0–030.9)
tuberculosis (015.0–015.9)

Excludes *gonococcal arthritis (098.50)*
meningococcal arthritis (036.82)

● ● ❑ *711.5 Arthropathy associated with other viral diseases*
[0–9] *Code first underlying disease, as:*
diseases classifiable to 045–049, 050–079, 480, 487
O'nyong-nyong (066.3)

Excludes *that due to rubella (056.71)*

● ● *711.6 Arthropathy associated with mycoses*
[0–9] *Code first underlying disease (110.0–118)*

● ● *711.7 Arthropathy associated with helminthiasis*
[0–9] *Code first underlying disease, as:*
filariasis (125.0–125.9)

● ● ❑ *711.8 Arthropathy associated with other infectious and*
[0–9] *parasitic diseases*
Code first underlying disease, as:
diseases classifiable to 080–088, 100–104, 130–136

Excludes *arthropathy associated with sarcoidosis (713.7)*

● ❑ **711.9 Unspecified infective arthritis**
[0–9] Infective arthritis or polyarthritis (acute) (chronic) (subacute) NOS

● **712 Crystal arthropathies**

Includes: crystal-induced arthritis and synovitis

Excludes *gouty arthropathy (274.0)*

The following fifth-digit subclassification is for use with category 712; valid digits are in [brackets] under each code. See list at beginning of chapter for definitions:
❑ **0 site unspecified**
1 shoulder region
2 upper arm
3 forearm
4 hand
5 pelvic region and thigh
6 lower leg
7 ankle and foot
❑ **8 other specified sites**
❑ **9 multiple sites**

● ● *712.1 Chondrocalcinosis due to dicalcium phosphate*
[0–9] *crystals*
Chondrocalcinosis due to dicalcium phosphate crystals (with other crystals)
Code first underlying disease (275.49)

● ● *712.2 Chondrocalcinosis due to pyrophosphate crystals*
[0–9] *Code first underlying disease (275.49)*

● ● ❑ *712.3 Chondrocalcinosis, unspecified*
[0–9] *Code first underlying disease (275.49)*

● ❑ **712.8 Other specified crystal arthropathies**
[0–9]

● ❑ **712.9 Unspecified crystal arthropathy**
[0–9]

● **713 Arthropathy associated with other disorders classified elsewhere**

Includes: arthritis associated with conditions classifiable below
arthropathy associated with conditions classifiable below
polyarthritis associated with conditions classifiable below
polyarthropathy associated with conditions classifiable below

● ❑ *713.0 Arthropathy associated with other endocrine and metabolic disorders*
Code first underlying disease, as:
acromegaly (253.0)
hemochromatosis (275.0)
hyperparathyroidism (252.00–252.08)
hypogammaglobulinemia (279.00–279.09)
hypothyroidism (243–244.9)
lipoid metabolism disorder (272.0–272.9)
ochronosis (270.2)

Excludes *arthropathy associated with:*
amyloidosis (713.7)
crystal deposition disorders, except gout (712.1–712.9)
diabetic neuropathy (713.5)
gouty arthropathy (274.0)

● *713.1 Arthropathy associated with gastrointestinal conditions other than infections*
Code first underlying disease, as:
regional enteritis (555.0–555.9)
ulcerative colitis (556)

● *713.2 Arthropathy associated with hematological disorders*
Code first underlying disease, as:
hemoglobinopathy (282.4–282.7)
hemophilia (286.0–286.2)
leukemia (204.0–208.9)
malignant reticulosis (202.3)
multiple myelomatosis (203.0)

Excludes *arthropathy associated with Henoch-Schönlein purpura (713.6)*

● *713.3 Arthropathy associated with dermatological disorders*
Code first underlying disease, as:
erythema multiforme (695.1)
erythema nodosum (695.2)

Excludes *psoriatic arthropathy (696.0)*

● *713.4 Arthropathy associated with respiratory disorders*
Code first underlying disease, as:
diseases classifiable to 490–519

Excludes *arthropathy associated with respiratory infections (711.0, 711.4–711.8)*

● *713.5 Arthropathy associated with neurological disorders*
Charcot's arthropathy associated with diseases classifiable elsewhere
Neuropathic arthritis associated with diseases classifiable elsewhere
Code first underlying disease, as:
neuropathic joint disease [Charcot's joints]:
NOS (094.0)
diabetic (250.6)
syringomyelic (336.0)
tabetic [syphilitic] (094.0)

● 713.6 *Arthropathy associated with hypersensitivity reaction*

Code first underlying disease, as:
Henoch (-Schönlein) purpura (287.0)
serum sickness (999.5)

Excludes *allergic arthritis NOS (716.2)*

● ❑713.7 *Other general diseases with articular involvement*

Code first underlying disease, as:
amyloidosis (277.30–277.39)
familial Mediterranean fever (277.31)
sarcoidosis (135)

● ❑713.8 *Arthropathy associated with other conditions classifiable elsewhere*

Code first underlying disease, as:
conditions classifiable elsewhere except as in 711.1–711.8, 712, and 713.0–713.7

● **714 Rheumatoid arthritis and other inflammatory polyarthropathies**

Excludes *rheumatic fever (390)*
rheumatoid arthritis of spine NOS (720.0)

714.0 Rheumatoid arthritis
Arthritis or polyarthritis:
atrophic
rheumatic (chronic)

Use additional code to identify manifestation, as:
myopathy (359.6)
polyneuropathy (357.1)

Excludes *juvenile rheumatoid arthritis NOS (714.30)*

714.1 Felty's syndrome
Rheumatoid arthritis with splenoadenomegaly and leukopenia

❑**714.2 Other rheumatoid arthritis with visceral or systemic involvement**
Rheumatoid carditis

● **714.3 Juvenile chronic polyarthritis**

❑**714.30 Polyarticular juvenile rheumatoid arthritis, chronic or unspecified**
Juvenile rheumatoid arthritis NOS
Still's disease

714.31 Polyarticular juvenile rheumatoid arthritis, acute

714.32 Pauciarticular juvenile rheumatoid arthritis

714.33 Monoarticular juvenile rheumatoid arthritis

714.4 Chronic postrheumatic arthropathy
Chronic rheumatoid nodular fibrositis
Jaccoud's syndrome

● **714.8 Other specified inflammatory polyarthropathies**

714.81 Rheumatoid lung
Caplan's syndrome
Diffuse interstitial rheumatoid disease of lung
Fibrosing alveolitis, rheumatoid

❑**714.89 Other**

❑**714.9 Unspecified inflammatory polyarthropathy**
Inflammatory polyarthropathy or polyarthritis NOS

Excludes *polyarthropathy NOS (716.5)*

● **715 Osteoarthrosis and allied disorders**

Note: Localized, in the subcategories below, includes bilateral involvement of the same site.

Includes: arthritis or polyarthritis:
degenerative
hypertrophic
degenerative joint disease
osteoarthritis

Excludes *Marie-Strümpell spondylitis (720.0)*
osteoarthrosis [osteoarthritis] of spine (721.0–721.9)

The following fifth-digit subclassification is for use with category 715; valid digits are in [brackets] under each code. See list at beginning of chapter for definitions:
❑ **0 site unspecified**
1 shoulder region
2 upper arm
3 forearm
4 hand
5 pelvic region and thigh
6 lower leg
7 ankle and foot
❑ **8 other specified sites**
❑ **9 multiple sites**

● **715.0 Osteoarthrosis, generalized**
[0,4,9] Degenerative joint disease, involving multiple joints
Primary generalized hypertrophic osteoarthrosis

● **715.1 Osteoarthrosis, localized, primary**
[0–8] Localized osteoarthropathy, idiopathic

● **715.2 Osteoarthrosis, localized, secondary**
[0–8] Coxae malum senilis

● ❑**715.3 Osteoarthrosis, localized, not specified whether**
[0–8] **primary or secondary**
Otto's pelvis

● ❑**715.8 Osteoarthrosis involving, or with mention of more**
[0,9] **than one site, but not specified as generalized**

● ❑**715.9 Osteoarthrosis, unspecified whether generalized or**
[0–8] **localized**

● **716 Other and unspecified arthropathies**

Excludes *cricoarytenoid arthropathy (478.79)*

The following fifth-digit subclassification is for use with category 716; valid digits are in [brackets] under each code. See list at beginning of chapter for definitions:
❑ **0 site unspecified**
1 shoulder region
2 upper arm
3 forearm
4 hand
5 pelvic region and thigh
6 lower leg
7 ankle and foot
❑ **8 other specified sites**
❑ **9 multiple sites**

● **716.0 Kaschin-Beck disease**
[0–9] Endemic polyarthritis

● **716.1 Traumatic arthropathy**
[0–9]

● **716.2 Allergic arthritis**
[0–9]

Excludes *arthritis associated with Henoch-Schönlein purpura or serum sickness (713.6)*

● **716.3 Climacteric arthritis**
[0–9] Menopausal arthritis

● **716.4 Transient arthropathy**
[0–9]

Excludes *palindromic rheumatism (719.3)*

716.5 Unspecified polyarthropathy or polyarthritis
[0–9]

716.6 Unspecified monoarthritis
[0–8] Coxitis

716.8 Other specified arthropathy
[0–9]

716.9 Arthropathy, unspecified
[0–9] Arthritis (acute) (chronic) (subacute)
Arthropathy (acute) (chronic) (subacute)
Articular rheumatism (chronic)
Inflammation of joint NOS

717 Internal derangement of knee

Includes: degeneration of articular cartilage or meniscus of knee
rupture, old of articular cartilage or meniscus of knee
tear, old of articular cartilage or meniscus of knee

Excludes *acute derangement of knee (836.0–836.6)*
ankylosis (718.5)
contracture (718.4)
current injury (836.0–836.6)
deformity (736.4–736.6)
recurrent dislocation (718.3)

717.0 Old bucket handle tear of medial meniscus
Old bucket handle tear of unspecified cartilage

717.1 Derangement of anterior horn of medial meniscus

717.2 Derangement of posterior horn of medial meniscus

717.3 Other and unspecified derangement of medial meniscus
Degeneration of internal semilunar cartilage

717.4 Derangement of lateral meniscus

717.40 Derangement of lateral meniscus, unspecified

717.41 Bucket handle tear of lateral meniscus

717.42 Derangement of anterior horn of lateral meniscus

717.43 Derangement of posterior horn of lateral meniscus

717.49 Other

717.5 Derangement of meniscus, not elsewhere classified
Congenital discoid meniscus
Cyst of semilunar cartilage
Derangement of semilunar cartilage NOS

717.6 Loose body in knee
Joint mice, knee
Rice bodies, knee (joint)

717.7 Chondromalacia of patella
Chondromalacia patellae
Degeneration [softening] of articular cartilage of patella

717.8 Other internal derangement of knee

717.81 Old disruption of lateral collateral ligament

717.82 Old disruption of medial collateral ligament

717.83 Old disruption of anterior cruciate ligament

717.84 Old disruption of posterior cruciate ligament

717.85 Old disruption of other ligaments of knee
Capsular ligament of knee

717.89 Other
Old disruption of ligaments of knee NOS

717.9 Unspecified internal derangement of knee
Derangement NOS of knee

718 Other derangement of joint

Excludes *current injury (830.0–848.9)*
jaw (524.60–524.69)

The following fifth-digit subclassification is for use with category 718; valid digits are in [brackets] under each code. See list at beginning of chapter for definitions:

- **0 site unspecified**
- **1 shoulder region**
- **2 upper arm**
- **3 forearm**
- **4 hand**
- **5 pelvic region and thigh**
- **6 lower leg**
- **7 ankle and foot**
- **8 other specified sites**
- **9 multiple sites**

718.0 Articular cartilage disorder
[0–5,7–9] Meniscus:
disorder
rupture, old
tear, old
Old rupture of ligament(s) of joint NOS

Excludes *articular cartilage disorder:*
in ochronosis (270.2)
knee (717.0–717.9)
chondrocalcinosis (275.40)
metastatic calcification (275.40)

718.1 Loose body in joint
[0–5,7–9] Joint mice

Excludes *knee (717.6)*

718.2 Pathological dislocation
[0–9] Dislocation or displacement of joint, not recurrent and not current

718.3 Recurrent dislocation of joint
[0–9]

718.4 Contracture of joint
[0–9]

718.5 Ankylosis of joint
[0–9] Ankylosis of joint (fibrous) (osseous)

Excludes *spine (724.9)*
stiffness of joint without mention of ankylosis (719.5)

718.6 Unspecified intrapelvic protrusion of acetabulum
[0,5] Protrusio acetabuli, unspecified

718.7 Developmental dislocation of joint
[0–9]

Excludes *congenital dislocation of joint (754.0–755.8)*
traumatic dislocation of joint (830–839)

718.8 Other joint derangement, not elsewhere classified
[0–9] Flail joint (paralytic)
Instability of joint

Excludes *deformities classifiable to 736 (736.0–736.9)*

718.9 Unspecified derangement of joint
[0–5,7–9]

Excludes *knee (717.9)*

ICD-9-CM 700-799 Vol. 1

719 Other and unspecified disorders of joint

Excludes *jaw (524.60–524.69)*

The following fifth-digit subclassification is for use with codes 719.0–719.6, 719.8–719.9; valid digits are in [brackets] under each code. See list at beginning of chapter for definitions:

- **0 site unspecified**
- **1 shoulder region**
- **2 upper arm**
- **3 forearm**
- **4 hand**
- **5 pelvic region and thigh**
- **6 lower leg**
- **7 ankle and foot**
- **8 other specified sites**
- **9 multiple sites**

719.0 Effusion of joint
[0–9] Hydrarthrosis
Swelling of joint, with or without pain

Excludes *intermittent hydrarthrosis (719.3)*

719.1 Hemarthrosis
[0–9]

Excludes *current injury (840.0–848.9)*

719.2 Villonodular synovitis
[0–9]

719.3 Palindromic rheumatism
[0–9] Hench-Rosenberg syndrome
Intermittent hydrarthrosis

719.4 Pain in joint
[0–9] Arthralgia

719.5 Stiffness of joint, not elsewhere classified
[0–9]

719.6 Other symptoms referable to joint
[0–9] Joint crepitus
Snapping hip

719.7 Difficulty in walking

Excludes *abnormality of gait (781.2)*

719.8 Other specified disorders of joint
[0–9] Calcification of joint
Fistula of joint

Excludes *temporomandibular joint-pain-dysfunction syndrome [Costen's syndrome] (524.60)*

719.9 Unspecified disorder of joint
[0–9]

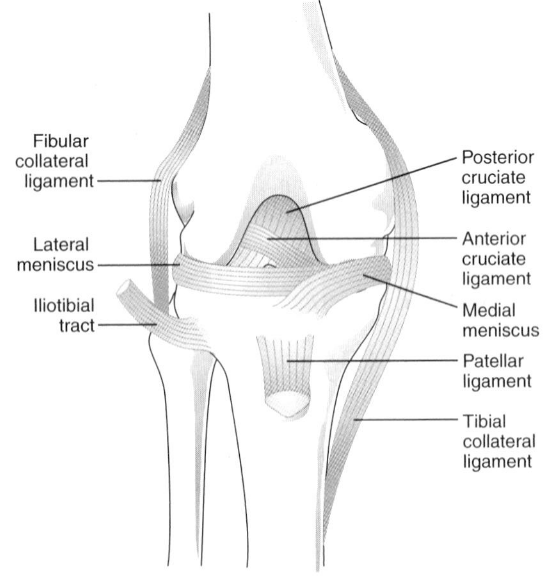
Fibular collateral ligament
Lateral meniscus
Iliotibial tract
Posterior cruciate ligament
Anterior cruciate ligament
Medial meniscus
Patellar ligament
Tibial collateral ligament

Figure 13–1 Anterior aspect of the right knee joint.

DORSOPATHIES (720–724)

Excludes *curvature of spine (737.0–737.9)*
osteochondrosis of spine (juvenile) (732.0) adult (732.8)

720 Ankylosing spondylitis and other inflammatory spondylopathies

720.0 Ankylosing spondylitis
Rheumatoid arthritis of spine NOS
Spondylitis:
Marie-Strümpell
rheumatoid

720.1 Spinal enthesopathy
Disorder of peripheral ligamentous or muscular attachments of spine
Romanus lesion

720.2 Sacroiliitis, not elsewhere classified
Inflammation of sacroiliac joint NOS

720.8 Other inflammatory spondylopathies

720.81 Inflammatory spondylopathies in diseases classified elsewhere
Code first underlying disease, as:
tuberculosis (015.0)

720.89 Other

720.9 Unspecified inflammatory spondylopathy
Spondylitis NOS

721 Spondylosis and allied disorders

721.0 Cervical spondylosis without myelopathy
Cervical or cervicodorsal:
arthritis
osteoarthritis
spondylarthritis

721.1 Cervical spondylosis with myelopathy
Anterior spinal artery compression syndrome
Spondylogenic compression of cervical spinal cord
Vertebral artery compression syndrome

721.2 Thoracic spondylosis without myelopathy
Thoracic:
arthritis
osteoarthritis
spondylarthritis

721.3 Lumbosacral spondylosis without myelopathy
Lumbar or lumbosacral:
arthritis
osteoarthritis
spondylarthritis

721.4 Thoracic or lumbar spondylosis with myelopathy

721.41 Thoracic region
Spondylogenic compression of thoracic spinal cord

721.42 Lumbar region
Spondylogenic compression of lumbar spinal cord

721.5 Kissing spine
Baastrup's syndrome

721.6 Ankylosing vertebral hyperostosis

721.7 Traumatic spondylopathy
Kümmell's disease or spondylitis

721.8 Other allied disorders of spine

721.9 Spondylosis of unspecified site

721.90 Without mention of myelopathy
Spinal:
arthritis (deformans) (degenerative) (hypertrophic)
osteoarthritis NOS
Spondylarthrosis NOS

721.91 With myelopathy
Spondylogenic compression of spinal cord NOS

722 Intervertebral disc disorders

722.0 Displacement of cervical intervertebral disc without myelopathy
Neuritis (brachial) or radiculitis due to displacement or rupture of cervical intervertebral disc
Any condition classifiable to 722.2 of the cervical or cervicothoracic intervertebral disc

722.1 Displacement of thoracic or lumbar intervertebral disc without myelopathy

722.10 Lumbar intervertebral disc without myelopathy
Lumbago or sciatica due to displacement of intervertebral disc
Neuritis or radiculitis due to displacement or rupture of lumbar intervertebral disc
Any condition classifiable to 722.2 of the lumbar or lumbosacral intervertebral disc

722.11 Thoracic intervertebral disc without myelopathy
Any condition classifiable to 722.2 of thoracic intervertebral disc

722.2 Displacement of intervertebral disc, site unspecified, without myelopathy
Discogenic syndrome NOS
Herniation of nucleus pulposus NOS
Intervertebral disc NOS:
extrusion
prolapse
protrusion
rupture
Neuritis or radiculitis due to displacement or rupture of intervertebral disc

722.3 Schmorl's nodes

722.30 Unspecified region

722.31 Thoracic region

722.32 Lumbar region

722.39 Other

722.4 Degeneration of cervical intervertebral disc
Degeneration of cervicothoracic intervertebral disc

722.5 Degeneration of thoracic or lumbar intervertebral disc

722.51 Thoracic or thoracolumbar intervertebral disc

722.52 Lumbar or lumbosacral intervertebral disc

722.6 Degeneration of intervertebral disc, site unspecified
Degenerative disc disease NOS
Narrowing of intervertebral disc or space NOS

722.7 Intervertebral disc disorder with myelopathy

722.70 Unspecified region

722.71 Cervical region

722.72 Thoracic region

722.73 Lumbar region

722.8 Postlaminectomy syndrome

722.80 Unspecified region

722.81 Cervical region

722.82 Thoracic region

722.83 Lumbar region

722.9 Other and unspecified disc disorder
Calcification of intervertebral cartilage or disc
Discitis

722.90 Unspecified region

722.91 Cervical region

722.92 Thoracic region

722.93 Lumbar region

723 Other disorders of cervical region

Excludes *conditions due to:*
intervertebral disc disorders (722.0–722.9)
spondylosis (721.0–721.9)

723.0 Spinal stenosis of cervical region

723.1 Cervicalgia
Pain in neck

723.2 Cervicocranial syndrome
Barré-Liéou syndrome
Posterior cervical sympathetic syndrome

723.3 Cervicobrachial syndrome (diffuse)

723.4 Brachia neuritis or radiculitis NOS
Cervical radiculitis
Radicular syndrome of upper limbs

723.5 Torticollis, unspecified
Contracture of neck

Excludes *congenital (754.1)*
due to birth injury (767.8)
hysterical (300.11)
ocular torticollis (781.93)
psychogenic (306.0)
spasmodic (333.83)
traumatic, current (847.0)

723.6 Panniculitis specified as affecting neck

723.7 Ossification of posterior longitudinal ligament in cervical region

723.8 Other syndromes affecting cervical region
Cervical syndrome NEC
Klippel's disease
Occipital neuralgia

723.9 Unspecified musculoskeletal disorders and symptoms referable to neck
Cervical (region) disorder NOS

724 Other and unspecified disorders of back

Excludes *collapsed vertebra (code to cause, e.g., osteoporosis, 733.00–733.09)*
conditions due to:
intervertebral disc disorders (722.0–722.9)
spondylosis (721.0–721.9)

724.0 Spinal stenosis, other than cervical

724.00 Spinal stenosis, unspecified region

724.01 Thoracic region

724.02 Lumbar region

724.09 Other

724.1 Pain in thoracic spine

724.2 Lumbago
Low back pain
Low back syndrome
Lumbalgia

724.3 Sciatica
Neuralgia or neuritis of sciatic nerve

Excludes *specified lesion of sciatic nerve (355.0)*

724.4 Thoracic or lumbosacral neuritis or radiculitis, unspecified
Radicular syndrome of lower limbs

724.5 Backache, unspecified
Vertebrogenic (pain) syndrome NOS

724.6 Disorders of sacrum
Ankylosis, lumbosacral or sacroiliac (joint)
Instability, lumbosacral or sacroiliac (joint)

724.7 Disorders of coccyx

724.70 Unspecified disorder of coccyx

724.71 Hypermobility of coccyx

724.79 Other
Coccygodynia

724.8 Other symptoms referable to back
Ossification of posterior longitudinal ligament NOS
Panniculitis specified as sacral or affecting back

724.9 Other unspecified back disorders
Ankylosis of spine NOS
Compression of spinal nerve root NEC
Spinal disorder NOS

Excludes *sacroiliitis (720.2)*

Item 13-1 Polymyalgia rheumatica is a syndrome characterized by aching and morning stiffness and is related to aging and hereditary predisposition.

RHEUMATISM, EXCLUDING THE BACK (725–729)

Includes: disorders of muscles and tendons and their attachments, and of other soft tissues

725 **Polymyalgia rheumatica**

● 726 **Peripheral enthesopathies and allied syndromes**

Note: Enthesopathies are disorders of peripheral ligamentous or muscular attachments.

Excludes *spinal enthesopathy (720.1)*

726.0 **Adhesive capsulitis of shoulder**

● 726.1 **Rotator cuff syndrome of shoulder and allied disorders**

❑ 726.10 **Disorders of bursae and tendons in shoulder region, unspecified**
Rotator cuff syndrome NOS
Supraspinatus syndrome NOS

726.11 **Calcifying tendinitis of shoulder**

726.12 **Bicipital tenosynovitis**

❑ 726.19 **Other specified disorders**

Excludes *complete rupture of rotator cuff, nontraumatic (727.61)*

❑ 726.2 **Other affections of shoulder region, not elsewhere classified**
Periarthritis of shoulder
Scapulohumeral fibrositis

● 726.3 **Enthesopathy of elbow region**

❑ 726.30 **Enthesopathy of elbow, unspecified**

726.31 **Medial epicondylitis**

726.32 **Lateral epicondylitis**
Epicondylitis NOS
Golfers' elbow
Tennis elbow

726.33 **Olecranon bursitis**
Bursitis of elbow

❑ 726.39 **Other**

726.4 **Enthesopathy of wrist and carpus**
Bursitis of hand or wrist
Periarthritis of wrist

726.5 **Enthesopathy of hip region**
Bursitis of hip
Gluteal tendinitis
Iliac crest spur
Psoas tendinitis
Trochanteric tendinitis

● 726.6 **Enthesopathy of knee**

❑ 726.60 **Enthesopathy of knee, unspecified**
Bursitis of knee NOS

726.61 **Pes anserinus tendinitis or bursitis**

726.62 **Tibial collateral ligament bursitis**
Pellegrini-Stieda syndrome

726.63 **Fibular collateral ligament bursitis**

726.64 **Patellar tendinitis**

726.65 **Prepatellar bursitis**

❑ 726.69 **Other**
Bursitis:
infrapatellar
subpatellar

● 726.7 **Enthesopathy of ankle and tarsus**

❑ 726.70 **Enthesopathy of ankle and tarsus, unspecified**
Metatarsalgia NOS

Excludes *Morton's metatarsalgia (355.6)*

726.71 **Achilles bursitis or tendinitis**

726.72 **Tibialis tendinitis**
Tibialis (anterior) (posterior) tendinitis

726.73 **Calcaneal spur**

❑ 726.79 **Other**
Peroneal tendinitis

❑ 726.8 **Other peripheral enthesopathies**

● 726.9 **Unspecified enthesopathy**

❑ 726.90 **Enthesopathy of unspecified site**
Capsulitis NOS
Periarthritis NOS
Tendinitis NOS

❑ 726.91 **Exostosis of unspecified site**
Bone spur NOS

● 727 **Other disorders of synovium, tendon, and bursa**

● 727.0 **Synovitis and tenosynovitis**

❑ 727.00 **Synovitis and tenosynovitis, unspecified**
Synovitis NOS
Tenosynovitis NOS

● 727.01 ***Synovitis and tenosynovitis in diseases classified elsewhere***

Code first underlying disease, as:
tuberculosis (015.0–015.9)

Excludes *crystal-induced (275.49)* *gonococcal (098.51)* *gouty (274.0)* *syphilitic (095.7)*

727.02 **Giant cell tumor of tendon sheath**

727.03 **Trigger finger (acquired)**

727.04 **Radial styloid tenosynovitis**
de Quervain's disease

❑ 727.05 **Other tenosynovitis of hand and wrist**

727.06 **Tenosynovitis of foot and ankle**

❑ 727.09 **Other**

727.1 **Bunion**

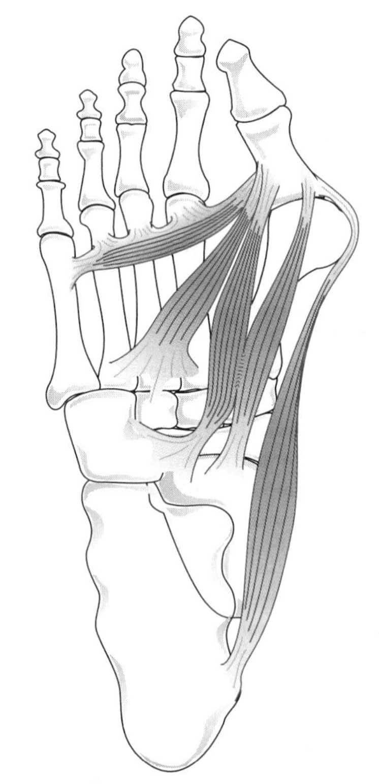

Figure 13–2 Hallux valgus or bunion.

Item 13-2 Hallux valgus, or bunion, is a bursa usually found along the medial aspect of the big toe. It is most often attributed to heredity or poorly fitted shoes.

❑727.2 **Specific bursitides often of occupational origin**
Beat:
elbow
hand
knee
Chronic crepitant synovitis of wrist
Miners':
elbow
knee

❑727.3 **Other bursitis**
Bursitis NOS
Excludes *bursitis:*
gonococcal (098.52)
subacromial (726.19)
subcoracoid (726.19)
subdeltoid (726.19)
syphilitic (095.7)
"frozen shoulder" (726.0)

● 727.4 **Ganglion and cyst of synovium, tendon, and bursa**

❑727.40 **Synovial cyst, unspecified**
Excludes *that of popliteal space (727.51)*

727.41 **Ganglion of joint**

727.42 **Ganglion of tendon sheath**

❑727.43 **Ganglion, unspecified**

❑727.49 **Other**
Cyst of bursa

● 727.5 **Rupture of synovium**

❑727.50 **Rupture of synovium, unspecified**

727.51 **Synovial cyst of popliteal space**
Baker's cyst (knee)

❑727.59 **Other**

● 727.6 **Rupture of tendon, nontraumatic**

❑727.60 **Nontraumatic rupture of unspecified tendon**

727.61 **Complete rupture of rotator cuff**

727.62 **Tendons of biceps (long head)**

727.63 **Extensor tendons of hand and wrist**

727.64 **Flexor tendons of hand and wrist**

727.65 **Quadriceps tendon**

727.66 **Patellar tendon**

727.67 **Achilles tendon**

❑727.68 **Other tendons of foot and ankle**

❑727.69 **Other**

● 727.8 **Other disorders of synovium, tendon, and bursa**

727.81 **Contracture of tendon (sheath)**
Short Achilles tendon (acquired)

727.82 **Calcium deposits in tendon and bursa**
Calcification of tendon NOS
Calcific tendinitis NOS
Excludes *peripheral ligamentous or muscular attachments (726.0–726.9)*

727.83 **Plica syndrome**
Plica knee

❑727.89 **Other**
Abscess of bursa or tendon
Excludes *xanthomatosis localized to tendons (272.7)*

❑727.9 **Unspecified disorder of synovium, tendon, and bursa**

● 728 **Disorders of muscle, ligament, and fascia**
Excludes *enthesopathies (726.0–726.9)*
muscular dystrophies (359.0–359.1)
myoneural disorders (358.00–358.9)
myopathies (359.2–359.9)
old disruption of ligaments of knee (717.81–717.89)

728.0 **Infective myositis**
Myositis:
purulent
suppurative
Excludes *myositis:*
epidemic (074.1)
interstitial (728.81)
syphilitic (095.6)
tropical (040.81)

● 728.1 **Muscular calcification and ossification**

❑728.10 **Calcification and ossification, unspecified**
Massive calcification (paraplegic)

728.11 **Progressive myositis ossificans**

728.12 **Traumatic myositis ossificans**
Myositis ossificans (circumscripta)

728.13 **Postoperative heterotopic calcification**

❑728.19 **Other**
Polymyositis ossificans

728.2 **Muscular wasting and disuse atrophy, not elsewhere classified**
Amyotrophia NOS
Myofibrosis
Excludes *neuralgic amyotrophy (353.5)*
pelvic muscle wasting and disuse atrophy (618.83)
progressive muscular atrophy (335.0–335.9)

❑728.3 **Other specific muscle disorders**
Arthrogryposis
Immobility syndrome (paraplegic)
Excludes *arthrogryposis multiplex congenita (754.89)*
stiff-man syndrome (333.91)

728.4 **Laxity of ligament**

728.5 **Hypermobility syndrome**

728.6 **Contracture of palmar fascia**
Dupuytren's contracture

● 728.7 **Other fibromatoses**

728.71 **Plantar fascial fibromatosis**
Contracture of plantar fascia
Plantar fasciitis (traumatic)

❑728.79 **Other**
Garrod's or knuckle pads
Nodular fasciitis
Pseudosarcomatous fibromatosis (proliferative) (subcutaneous)

● 728.8 **Other disorders of muscle, ligament, and fascia**

728.81 **Interstitial myositis**

728.82 **Foreign body granuloma of muscle**
Talc granuloma of muscle

728.83 **Rupture of muscle, nontraumatic**

728.84 **Diastasis of muscle**
Diastasis recti (abdomen)
Excludes *diastasis recti complicating pregnancy, labor, and delivery (665.8)*

728.85 **Spasm of muscle**

728.86 **Necrotizing fasciitis**
Use additional code to identify:
infectious organism (041.00–041.89)
gangrene (785.4), if applicable

728.87 **Muscle weakness (generalized)**
Excludes *generalized weakness (780.79)*

728.88 **Rhabdomyolysis**

❑728.89 **Other**
Eosinophilic fasciitis
Use additional E code to identify drug, if drug induced

❑728.9 **Unspecified disorder of muscle, ligament, and fascia**

● 729 **Other disorders of soft tissues**

Excludes *acroparesthesia (443.89)*
carpal tunnel syndrome (354.0)
disorders of the back (720.0–724.9)
entrapment syndromes (354.0–355.9)
palindromic rheumatism (719.3)
periarthritis (726.0–726.9)
psychogenic rheumatism (306.0)

❑729.0 **Rheumatism, unspecified, and fibrositis**

❑729.1 **Myalgia and myositis, unspecified**
Fibromyositis NOS

❑729.2 **Neuralgia, neuritis, and radiculitis, unspecified**

Excludes *brachia radiculitis (723.4)*
cervical radiculitis (723.4)
lumbosacral radiculitis (724.4)
mononeuritis (354.0–355.9)
radiculitis due to intervertebral disc involvement (722.0–722.2, 722.7)
sciatica (724.3)

Item 13-3 Panniculitis is an inflammation of the adipose tissue of the heel pad.

● 729.3 **Panniculitis, unspecified**

❑729.30 **Panniculitis, unspecified site**
Weber-Christian disease

729.31 **Hypertrophy of fat pad, knee**
Hypertrophy of infrapatellar fat pad

❑729.39 **Other site**

Excludes *panniculitis specified as (affecting):*
back (724.8)
neck (723.6)
sacral (724.8)

❑729.4 **Fasciitis, unspecified**

Excludes *necrotizing fasciitis (728.86)*
nodular fasciitis (728.79)

729.5 **Pain in limb**

729.6 **Residual foreign body in soft tissue**

Excludes *foreign body granuloma:*
muscle (728.82)
skin and subcutaneous tissue (709.4)

● 729.7 **Nontraumatic compartment syndrome** ◀

Excludes *compartment syndrome NOS (958.90)* ◀
traumatic compartment syndrome (958.90–958.99) ◀

729.71 **Nontraumatic compartment syndrome of upper extremity** ◀
Nontraumatic compartment syndrome of shoulder, arm, forearm, wrist, hand, and fingers ◀

729.72 **Nontraumatic compartment syndrome of lower extremity** ◀
Nontraumatic compartment syndrome of hip, buttock, thigh, leg, foot, and toes ◀

729.73 **Nontraumatic compartment syndrome of abdomen** ◀

❑729.79 **Nontraumatic compartment syndrome of other sites** ◀

● 729.8 **Other musculoskeletal symptoms referable to limbs**

729.81 **Swelling of limb**

729.82 **Cramp**

❑729.89 **Other**

Excludes *abnormality of gait (781.2)*
tetany (781.7)
transient paralysis of limb (781.4)

❑729.9 **Other and unspecified disorders of soft tissue**
Polyalgia

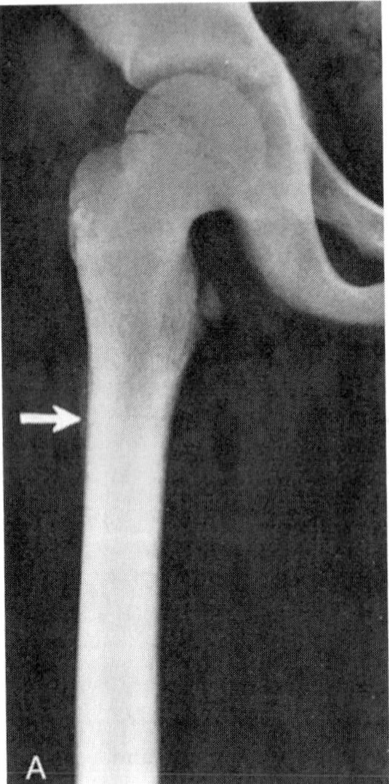
A

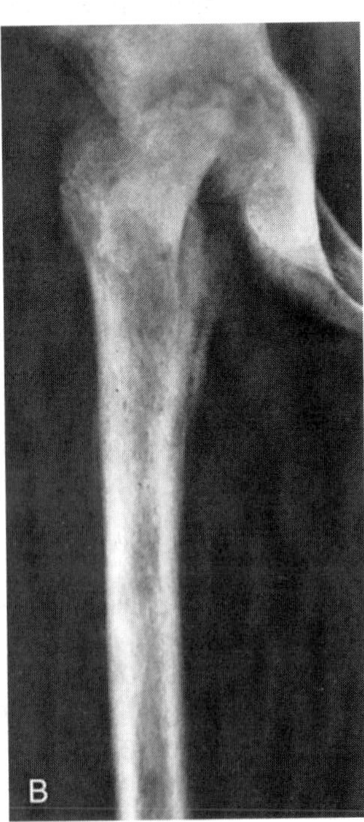
B

Figure 13–3 Suppurative osteomyelitis. The initial radiograph **(A)** shows only minimal periosteal reaction along the lateral aspect of the proximal femur *(arrow)*. Eight months after onset **(B)** there is gross destruction of the joint and the proximal femur. (From Aegerter E, Kirkpatrick J Jr: Orthopedic Diseases, 4th ed. Philadelphia, WB Saunders, 1975, p 257.)

Item 13-4 Osteomyelitis is an inflammation of the bone. Acute osteomyelitis is a rapidly destructive, pus-producing infection capable of causing severe bone destruction. Chronic osteomyelitis can remain long after the initial acute episode has passed and may lead to a recurrence of the acute phase. Brodie's abscess is an encapsulated focal abscess that must be surgically drained.

OSTEOPATHIES, CHONDROPATHIES, AND ACQUIRED MUSCULOSKELETAL DEFORMITIES (730–739)

● 730 **Osteomyelitis, periostitis, and other infections involving bone**

Excludes *jaw (526.4–526.5)*
petrous bone (383.2)

Use additional code to identify organism, such as Staphylococcus (041.1)

The following fifth-digit subclassification is for use with category 730; valid digits are in [brackets] under each code. See list at beginning of chapter for definitions:

❑ 0 **site unspecified**
1 **shoulder region**
2 **upper arm**
3 **forearm**
4 **hand**
5 **pelvic region and thigh**
6 **lower leg**
7 **ankle and foot**
❑ 8 **other specified sites**
❑ 9 **multiple sites**

● 730.0 **Acute osteomyelitis**
[0–9] Abscess of any bone except accessory sinus, jaw, or mastoid
Acute or subacute osteomyelitis, with or without mention of periostitis

Use additional code to identify major osseous defect, if applicable (731.3) ◀

● 730.1 **Chronic osteomyelitis**
[0–9] Brodie's abscess
Chronic or old osteomyelitis, with or without mention of periostitis
Sequestrum
Sclerosing osteomyelitis of Garré

Excludes *aseptic necrosis of bone (733.40–733.49)*

Use additional code to identify major osseous defect, if applicable (731.3) ◀

● ❑730.2 **Unspecified osteomyelitis**
[0–9] Osteitis or osteomyelitis NOS, with or without mention of periostitis

Use additional code to identify major osseous defect, if applicable (731.3) ◀

● 730.3 **Periostitis without mention of osteomyelitis**
[0–9] Abscess of periosteum, without mention of osteomyelitis
Periostosis, without mention of osteomyelitis

Excludes *that in secondary syphilis (091.61)*

● ● 730.7 ***Osteopathy resulting from poliomyelitis***
[0–9] *Code first underlying disease* (045.0–045.9)

● ● ❑730.8 ***Other infections involving bone in disease classified elsewhere***
[0–9]

Code first underlying disease, as:
tuberculosis (015.0–015.9)
typhoid fever (002.0)

Excludes *syphilitis of bone NOS (095.5)*

● ❑730.9 **Unspecified infection of bone**
[0–9]

● 731 **Osteitis deformans and osteopathies associated with other disorders classified elsewhere**

731.0 **Osteitis deformans without mention of bone tumor**
Paget's disease of bone

● 731.1 ***Osteitis deformans in diseases classified elsewhere***
Code first underlying disease, as:
malignant neoplasm of bone (170.0–170.9)

731.2 **Hypertrophic pulmonary osteoarthropathy**
Bamberger-Marie disease

731.3 ***Major osseous defects*** ◀
Code first underlying disease, if known, such as: ◀
aseptic necrosis (733.40–733.49) ◀
malignant neoplasm of bone (170.0–170.9) ◀
osteomyelitis (730.00–730.29) ◀
osteoporosis (733.00–733.09) ◀
peri-prosthetic osteolysis (996.45) ◀

●❑731.8 ***Other bone involvement in diseases classified elsewhere***
Code first underlying disease, as:
diabetes mellitus (250.8)

Use additional code to specify bone condition, such as:
acute osteomyelitis (730.00–730.09)

● 732 **Osteochondropathies**

732.0 **Juvenile osteochondrosis of spine**
Juvenile osteochondrosis (of):
marginal or vertebral ephiphysis (of Scheuermann) spine NOS
Vertebral epiphysitis

Excludes *adolescent postural kyphosis (737.0)*

732.1 **Juvenile osteochondrosis of hip and pelvis**
Coxa plana
Ischiopubic synchondrosis (of van Neck)
Osteochondrosis (juvenile) of:
acetabulum
head of femur (of Legg-Calvé-Perthes)
iliac crest (of Buchanan)
symphysis pubis (of Pierson)
Pseudocoxalgia

732.2 **Nontraumatic slipped upper femoral epiphysis**
Slipped upper femoral epiphysis NOS

732.3 **Juvenile osteochondrosis of upper extremity**
Osteochondrosis (juvenile) of:
capitulum of humerus (of Panner)
carpal lunate (of Kienbock)
hand NOS
head of humerus (of Haas)
heads of metacarpals (of Mauclaire)
lower ulna (of Burns)
radial head (of Brailsford)
upper extremity NOS

732.4 **Juvenile osteochondrosis of lower extremity, excluding foot**
Osteochondrosis (juvenile) of:
lower extremity NOS
primary patellar center (of Köhler)
proximal tibia (of Blount)
secondary patellar center (of Sinding-Larsen)
tibial tubercle (of Osgood-Schlatter)
Tibia vara

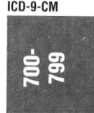

732.5 **Juvenile osteochondrosis of foot**
Calcaneal apophysitis
Epiphysitis, os calcis
Osteochondrosis (juvenile) of:
astragalus (of Diaz)
calcaneum (of Sever)
foot NOS
metatarsal:
second (of Freiberg)
fifth (of Iselin)
os tibiale externum (of Haglund)
tarsal navicular (of Köhler)

❑732.6 **Other juvenile osteochondrosis**
Apophysitis specified as juvenile, of other site, or site NOS
Epiphysitis specified as juvenile, of other site, or site NOS
Osteochondritis specified as juvenile, of other site, or site NOS
Osteochondrosis specified as juvenile, of other site, or site NOS

732.7 **Osteochondritis dissecans**

❑732.8 **Other specified forms of osteochondropathy**
Adult osteochondrosis of spine

❑732.9 **Unspecified osteochondropathy**
Apophysitis
NOS
not specified as adult or juvenile, of unspecified site
Epiphysitis
NOS
not specified as adult or juvenile, of unspecified site
Osteochondritis
NOS
not specified as adult or juvenile, of unspecified site
Osteochondrosis
NOS
not specified as adult or juvenile, of unspecified site

● 733 **Other disorders of bone and cartilage**

Excludes *bone spur (726.91)*
cartilage of, or loose body in, joint (717.0–717.9, 718.0–718.9)
giant cell granuloma of jaw (526.3)
osteitis fibrosa cystica generalisata (252.01)
osteomalacia (268.2)
polyostotic fibrous dysplasia of bone (756.54)
prognathism, retrognathism (524.1)
xanthomatosis localized to bone (272.7)

● 733.0 **Osteoporosis**
Use additional code to identify major osseous defect, if applicable (731.3) ◀

❑733.00 **Osteoporosis, unspecified**
Wedging of vertebra NOS

733.01 **Senile osteoporosis**
Postmenopausal osteoporosis

733.02 **Idiopathic osteoporosis**

733.03 **Disuse osteoporosis**

❑733.09 **Other**
Drug-induced osteoporosis
Use additional E code to identify drug

● 733.1 **Pathologic fracture**
Spontaneous fracture

Excludes *stress fracture (733.93–733.95)*
traumatic fractures (800–829)

❑733.10 **Pathologic fracture, unspecified site**

733.11 **Pathologic fracture of humerus**

733.12 **Pathologic fracture of distal radius and ulna**
Wrist NOS

733.13 **Pathologic fracture of vertebrae**
Collapse of vertebra NOS

733.14 **Pathologic fracture of neck of femur**
Femur NOS
Hip NOS

❑733.15 **Pathologic fracture of other specified part of femur**

733.16 **Pathologic fracture of tibia and fibula**
Ankle NOS

❑733.19 **Pathologic fracture of other specified site**

● 733.2 **Cyst of bone**

❑733.20 **Cyst of bone (localized), unspecified**

733.21 **Solitary bone cyst**
Unicameral bone cyst

733.22 **Aneurysmal bone cyst**

❑733.29 **Other**
Fibrous dysplasia (monostotic)

Excludes *cyst of jaw (526.0–526.2, 526.89)*
osteitis fibrosa cystica (252.01)
polyostotic fibrous dysplasia of bone (756.54)

733.3 **Hyperostosis of skull**
Hyperostosis interna frontalis
Leontiasis ossium

● 733.4 **Aseptic necrosis of bone**
Use additional code to identify major osseous defect, if applicable (731.3) ◀

Excludes *osteochondropathies (732.0–732.9)*

❑733.40 **Aseptic necrosis of bone, site unspecified**

733.41 **Head of humerus**

733.42 **Head and neck of femur**
Femur NOS

Excludes *Legg-Calvé-Perthes disease (732.1)*

733.43 **Medial femoral condyle**

733.44 **Talus**

❑733.49 **Other**

733.5 **Osteitis condensans**
Piriform sclerosis of ilium

733.6 **Tietze's disease**
Costochondral junction syndrome
Costochondritis

733.7 **Algoneurodystrophy**
Disuse atrophy of bone
Sudeck's atrophy

● 733.8 **Malunion and nonunion of fracture**

733.81 **Malunion of fracture**

733.82 **Nonunion of fracture**
Pseudoarthrosis (bone)

● 733.9 **Other and unspecified disorders of bone and cartilage**

❑733.90 **Disorder of bone and cartilage, unspecified**

733.91 **Arrest of bone development or growth**
Epiphyseal arrest

733.92 **Chondromalacia**
Chondromalacia:
NOS
localized, except patella
systemic
tibial plateau

Excludes *chondromalacia of patella (717.7)*

733.93 Stress fracture of tibia or fibula
Stress reaction of tibia or fibula

733.94 Stress fracture of the metatarsals
Stress reaction of metatarsals

❑ **733.95 Stress fracture of other bone**
Stress reaction of other bone

❑ **733.99 Other**
Diaphysitis
Hypertrophy of bone
Relapsing polychondritis

734 Flat foot
Pes planus (acquired)
Talipes planus (acquired)

Excludes *congenital (754.61)*
rigid flat foot (754.61)
spastic (everted) flat foot (754.61)

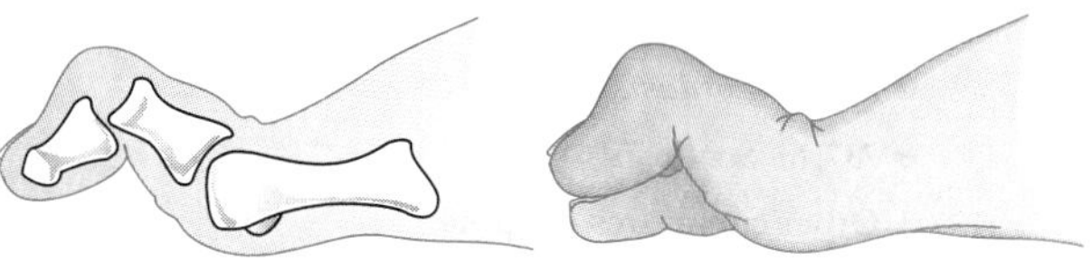

Figure 13–4 Claw toe.

Item 13–5 Claw toe is caused by a contraction of the flexor tendon producing a flexion deformity characterized by hyperextension of the big toe.

● **735 Acquired deformities of toe**

Excludes *congenital (754.60–754.69, 755.65–755.66)*

735.0 Hallux valgus (acquired)

735.1 Hallux varus (acquired)

735.2 Hallux rigidus

735.3 Hallux malleus

❑ **735.4 Other hammer toe (acquired)**

735.5 Claw toe (acquired)

❑ **735.8 Other acquired deformities of toe**

❑ **735.9 Unspecified acquired deformity of toe**

● **736 Other acquired deformities of limbs**

Excludes *congenital (754.3–755.9)*

● **736.0 Acquired deformities of forearm, excluding fingers**

❑ **736.00 Unspecified deformity**
Deformity of elbow, forearm, hand, or wrist (acquired) NOS

736.01 Cubitus valgus (acquired)

736.02 Cubitus varus (acquired)

736.03 Valgus deformity of wrist (acquired)

736.04 Varus deformity of wrist (acquired)

736.05 Wrist drop (acquired)

736.06 Claw hand (acquired)

736.07 Club hand (acquired)

❑ **736.09 Other**

736.1 Mallet finger

● **736.2 Other acquired deformities of finger**

❑ **736.20 Unspecified deformity**
Deformity of finger (acquired) NOS

736.21 Boutonniere deformity

736.22 Swan-neck deformity

❑ **736.29 Other**

Excludes *trigger finger (727.03)*

● **736.3 Acquired deformities of hip**

❑ **736.30 Unspecified deformity**
Deformity of hip (acquired) NOS

736.31 Coxa valga (acquired)

736.32 Coxa vara (acquired)

❑ **736.39 Other**

● **736.4 Genu valgum or varum (acquired)**

736.41 Genu valgum (acquired)

736.42 Genu varum (acquired)

736.5 Genu recurvatum (acquired)

❑ **736.6 Other acquired deformities of knee**
Deformity of knee (acquired) NOS

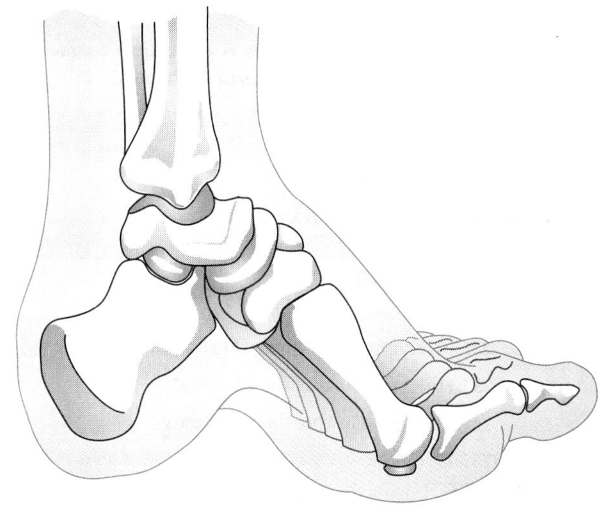

Figure 13–5 Pes cavovarus, meaning "foot with high arch."

Item 13–6 Equinus foot is a term referring to the hoof of a horse. The deformity is usually congenital or spastic.

● **736.7 Other acquired deformities of ankle and foot**

Excludes *deformities of toe (acquired) (735.0–735.9)*
pes planus (acquired) (734)

❑ **736.70 Unspecified deformity of ankle and foot, acquired**

ICD-9-CM 700-799 Vol. 1

736.71 **Acquired equinovarus deformity**
Clubfoot, acquired

Excludes *clubfoot not specified as acquired (754.5–754.7)*

736.72 **Equinus deformity of foot, acquired**

736.73 **Cavus deformity of foot**

Excludes *that with claw foot (736.74)*

736.74 **Claw foot, acquired**

736.75 **Cavovarus deformity of foot, acquired**

❑736.76 **Other calcaneus deformity**

❑736.79 **Other**
Acquired:
pes not elsewhere classified
talipes not elsewhere classified

● 736.8 **Acquired deformities of other parts of limbs**

736.81 **Unequal leg length (acquired)**

❑736.89 **Other**
Deformity (acquired):
arm or leg, not elsewhere classified
shoulder

❑736.9 **Acquired deformity of limb, site unspecified**

Item 13-7 Kyphosis is an abnormal curvature of the spine. **Senile kyphosis** is a result of disc degeneration causing ossification (turning to bone). **Adolescent** or **juvenile kyphosis** is also known as **Scheuermann's disease,** a condition in which the discs of the lower thoracic spine herniate, causing the disc space to narrow and the spine to tilt forward. This condition is attributed to poor posture.

Item 13-8 Spondylolisthesis is a condition caused by the slipping forward of one disc over another.

● 737 **Curvature of spine**

Excludes *congenital (754.2)*

737.0 **Adolescent postural kyphosis**

Excludes *osteochondrosis of spine (juvenile) (732.0)*
adult (732.8)

● ❑737.1 **Kyphosis (acquired)**

737.10 **Kyphosis (acquired) (postural)**

737.11 **Kyphosis due to radiation**

737.12 **Kyphosis, postlaminectomy**

❑737.19 **Other**

Excludes *that associated with conditions classifiable elsewhere (737.41)*

● 737.2 **Lordosis (acquired)**

737.20 **Lordosis (acquired) (postural)**

737.21 **Lordosis, postlaminectomy**

737.22 **Other postsurgical lordosis**

❑737.29 **Other**

Excludes *that associated with conditions classifiable elsewhere (737.42)*

● 737.3 **Kyphoscoliosis and scoliosis**

737.30 **Scoliosis [and kyphoscoliosis], idiopathic**

737.31 **Resolving infantile idiopathic scoliosis**

737.32 **Progressive infantile idiopathic scoliosis**

737.33 **Scoliosis due to radiation**

737.34 **Thoracogenic scoliosis**

❑737.39 **Other**

Excludes *that associated with conditions classifiable elsewhere (737.43)*
that in kyphoscoliotic heart disease (416.1)

● 737.4 ***Curvature of spine associated with other conditions***

Code first associated condition, as:
Charcot-Marie-Tooth disease (356.1)
mucopolysaccharidosis (277.5)
neurofibromatosis (237.7)
osteitis deformans (731.0)
osteitis fibrosa cystica (252.01)
osteoporosis (733.00–733.09)
poliomyelitis (138)
tuberculosis [Pott's curvature] (015.0)

● ❑*737.40* ***Curvature of spine, unspecified***

● *737.41* ***Kyphosis***

● *737.42* ***Lordosis***

● *737.43* ***Scoliosis***

❑737.8 **Other curvatures of spine**

❑737.9 **Unspecified curvature of spine**
Curvature of spine (acquired) (idiopathic) NOS
Hunchback, acquired

Excludes *deformity of spine NOS (738.5)*

● 738 **Other acquired deformity**

Excludes *congenital (754.0–756.9, 758.0–759.9)*
dentofacial anomalies (524.0–524.9)

738.0 **Acquired deformity of nose**
Deformity of nose (acquired)
Overdevelopment of nasal bones

Excludes *deflected or deviated nasal septum (470)*

● 738.1 **Other acquired deformity of head**

❑738.10 **Unspecified deformity**

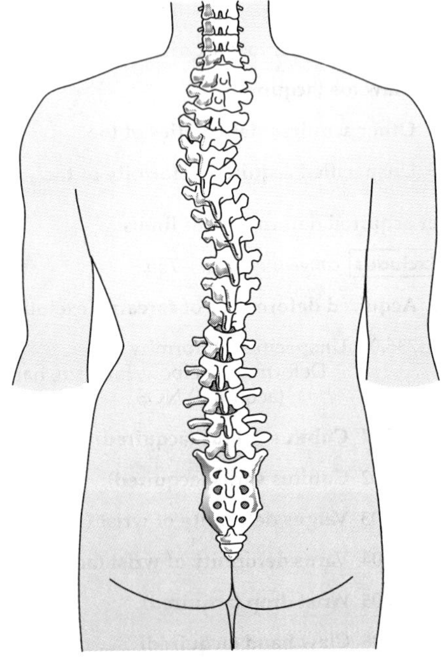

Figure 13-6 Scoliosis is a lateral curvature of the spine.

738.11 **Zygomatic hyperplasia**

738.12 **Zygomatic hypoplasia**

❑738.19 **Other specified deformity**

738.2 **Acquired deformity of neck**

738.3 **Acquired deformity of chest and rib**
Deformity:
chest (acquired)
rib (acquired)
Pectus:
carinatum, acquired
excavatum, acquired

738.4 **Acquired spondylolisthesis**
Degenerative spondylolisthesis
Spondylolysis, acquired

Excludes *congenital (756.12)*

❑738.5 **Other acquired deformity of back or spine**
Deformity of spine NOS

Excludes *curvature of spine (737.0–737.9)*

738.6 **Acquired deformity of pelvis**
Pelvic obliquity

Excludes *intrapelvic protrusion of acetabulum (718.6)*
that in relation to labor and delivery (653.0–653.4, 653.8–653.9)

738.7 **Cauliflower ear**

❑738.8 **Acquired deformity of other specified site**
Deformity of clavicle

❑738.9 **Acquired deformity of unspecified site**

● 739 **Nonallopathic lesions, not elsewhere classified**
Includes: segmental dysfunction
somatic dysfunction

739.0 **Head region**
Occipitocervical region

739.1 **Cervical region**
Cervicothoracic region

739.2 **Thoracic region**
Thoracolumbar region

739.3 **Lumbar region**
Lumbosacral region

739.4 **Sacral region**
Sacrococcygeal region
Sacroiliac region

739.5 **Pelvic region**
Hip region
Pubic region

739.6 **Lower extremities**

739.7 **Upper extremities**
Acromioclavicular region
Sternoclavicular region

739.8 **Rib cage**
Costochondral region
Costovertebral region
Sternochondral region

739.9 **Abdomen and other**

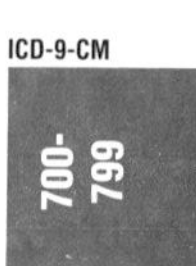
700-
799

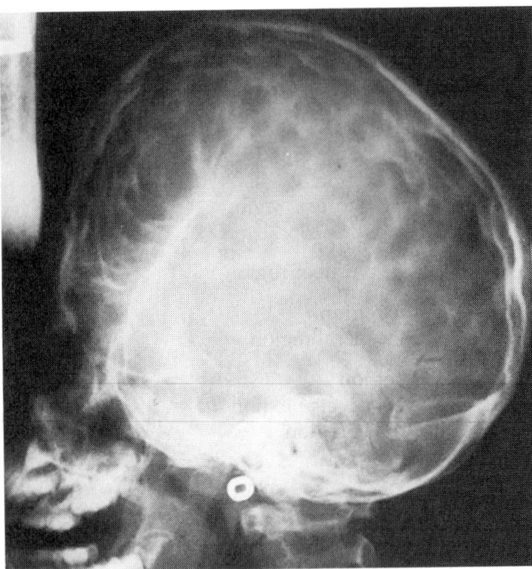

Figure 14–1 Generalized craniosynostosis in a 4-year-old girl without symptoms or signs of increased intracranial pressure. The child was referred for medical evaluation because of abnormal facial characteristics, features similar to those of her mother and aunt. Her fronto-occipital head circumference was found to be 47 cm. (From Bell WE, McCormick WF: Increased Intracranial Pressure in Children, 2nd ed. Philadelphia, WB Saunders, 1978, p 116.)

Item 14–1 Anencephalus is a congenital deformity of the cranial vault. Craniosynostosis, also known as craniostenosis and stenocephaly, signifies any form of congenital deformity of the skull that results from the premature closing of the sutures of the skull. Iniencephaly is a deformity in which the head and neck are flexed backward to a great extent and the head is very large in comparison to the shortened body.

14. CONGENITAL ANOMALIES (740–759)

● **740 Anencephalus and similar anomalies**

740.0 Anencephalus
- Acrania
- Amyelencephalus
- Hemianencephaly
- Hemicephaly

740.1 Craniorachischisis

740.2 Iniencephaly

Item 14–2 Spina bifida is a midline spinal defect in which one or more vertebrae fail to fuse, leaving an opening in the vertebral canal. When the defect is not visible, it is called spina bifida occulta, and when it is visible, it is called spina bifida cystica.

● **741 Spina bifida**

Excludes *spina bifida occulta (756.17)*

The following fifth-digit subclassification is for use with category 741:
- ❑ 0 **unspecified region**
- 1 **cervical region**
- 2 **dorsal (thoracic) region**
- 3 **lumbar region**

● **741.0 With hydrocephalus**
- Arnold-Chiari syndrome, type II
- Any condition classifiable to 741.9 with any condition classifiable to 742.3
- Chiari malformation, type II

● **741.9 Without mention of hydrocephalus**
- Hydromeningocele (spinal)
- Hydromyelocele
- Meningocele (spinal)
- Meningomyelocele
- Myelocele
- Myelocystocele
- Rachischisis
- Spina bifida (aperta)
- Syringomyelocele

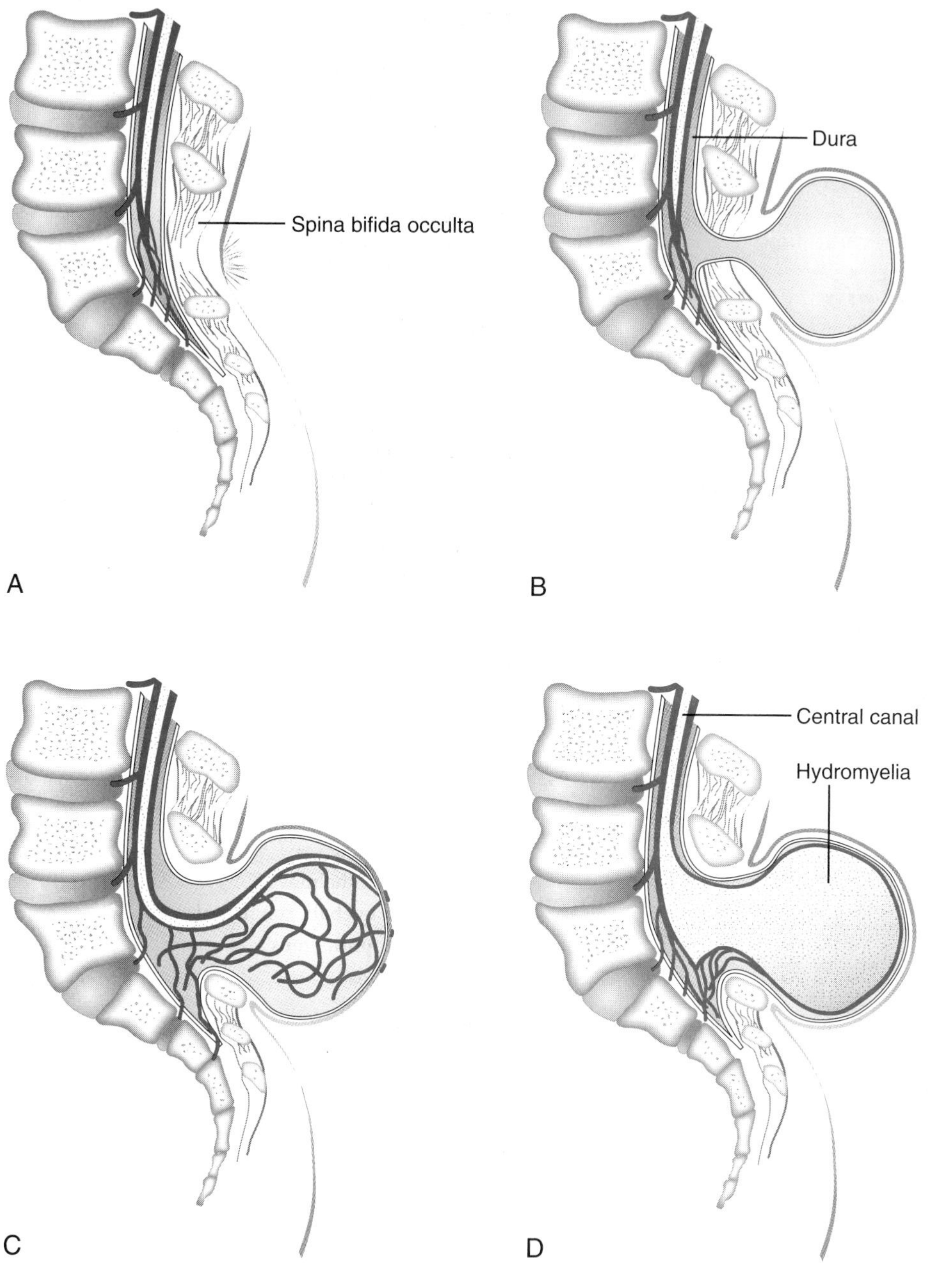

Spina bifida occulta

A

Dura

B

C

Central canal

Hydromyelia

D

Figure 14–2 **A.** Spina bifida occulta. **B.** Meningocele. **C.** Myelomeningocele. **D.** Myelocystocele (syringomyelocele) or hydromyelia.

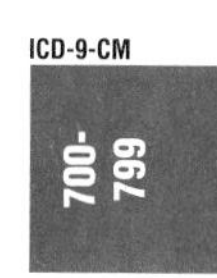
ICD-9-CM
700-
799
Vol. 1

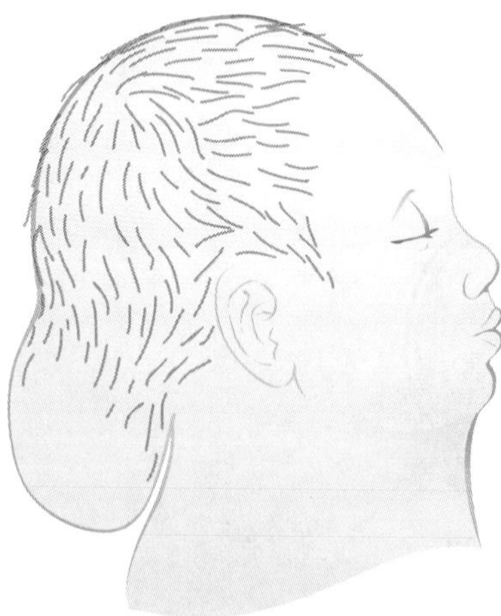

Figure 14–3 Encephalocele is a protrusion of the brain through an opening in the skull.

● 742 **Other congenital anomalies of nervous system**

Excludes *congenital central alveolar hypoventilation syndrome (327.25)*

742.0 **Encephalocele**
Encephalocystocele
Encephalomyelocele
Hydroencephalocele
Hydromeningocele, cranial
Meningocele, cerebral
Meningoencephalocele

742.1 **Microcephalus**
Hydromicrocephaly
Micrencephaly

742.2 **Reduction deformities of brain**
Absence of part of brain
Agenesis of part of brain
Agyria
Aplasia of part of brain
Arhinencephaly
Holoprosencephaly
Hypoplasia of part of brain
Microgyria

742.3 **Congenital hydrocephalus**
Aqueduct of Sylvius:
anomaly
obstruction, congenital
stenosis
Atresia of foramina of Magendie and Luschka
Hydrocephalus in newborn

Excludes *hydrocephalus:*
acquired (331.3–331.4)
due to congenital toxoplasmosis (771.2)
with any condition classifiable to 741.9 (741.0)

❑742.4 **Other specified anomalies of brain**
Congenital cerebral cyst
Macroencephaly
Macrogyria
Megalencephaly
Multiple anomalies of brain NOS
Porencephaly
Ulegyria

● 742.5 **Other specified anomalies of spinal cord**

742.51 **Diastematomyelia**

742.53 **Hydromyelia**
Hydrorhachis

❑742.59 **Other**
Amyelia
Atelomyelia
Congenital anomaly of spinal meninges
Defective development of cauda equina
Hypoplasia of spinal cord
Myelatelia
Myelodysplasia

❑742.8 **Other specified anomalies of nervous system**
Agenesis of nerve
Displacement of brachial plexus
Familial dysautonomia
Jaw-winking syndrome
Marcus-Gunn syndrome
Riley-Day syndrome

Excludes *neurofibromatosis (237.7)*

❑742.9 **Unspecified anomaly of brain, spinal cord, and nervous system**
Anomaly of brain, nervous system, and spinal cord
Congenital, of brain, nervous system, and spinal cord:
disease of brain, nervous system, and spinal cord
lesion of brain, nervous system, and spinal cord
Deformity of brain, nervous system, and spinal cord

Item 14–3 Anophthalmia is the absence of the eye and the optic pit. Microphthalmia is the partial absence of the eye and optic pit.

● 743 **Congenital anomalies of eye**

● 743.0 **Anophthalmos**

❑743.00 **Clinical anophthalmos, unspecified**
Agenesis
Congenital absence of eye
Anophthalmos NOS

743.03 **Cystic eyeball, congenital**

743.06 **Cryptophthalmos**

● 743.1 **Microphthalmos**
Dysplasia of eye
Hypoplasia of eye
Rudimentary eye

❑743.10 **Microphthalmos, unspecified**

743.11 **Simple microphthalmos**

❑743.12 **Microphthalmos associated with other anomalies of eye and adnexa**

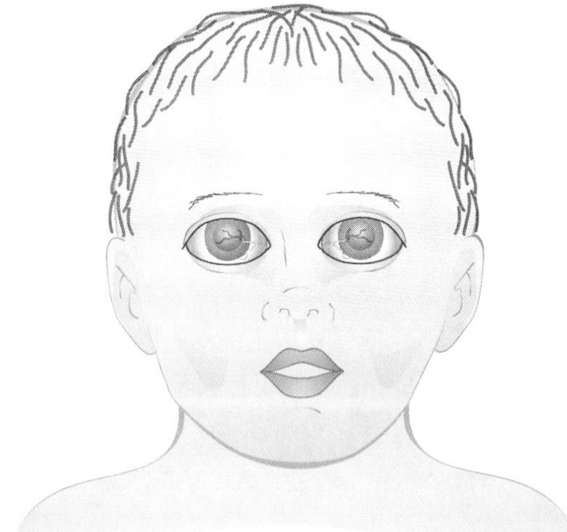

Figure 14–4 Bilateral congenital hydrophthalmia, in which the eyes are very large in comparison to the other facial features.

● **743.2 Buphthalmos**
Glaucoma:
congenital
newborn
Hydrophthalmos

Excludes *glaucoma of childhood (365.14)*
traumatic glaucoma due to birth injury (767.8)

❑ **743.20 Buphthalmos, unspecified**

743.21 Simple buphthalmos

❑ **743.22 Buphthalmos associated with other ocular anomalies**
Keratoglobus, congenital, associated with buphthalmos
Megalocornea associated with buphthalmos

● **743.3 Congenital cataract and lens anomalies**

Excludes *infantile cataract (366.00–366.09)*

❑ **743.30 Congenital cataract, unspecified**

743.31 Capsular and subcapsular cataract

743.32 Cortical and zonular cataract

743.33 Nuclear cataract

743.34 Total and subtotal cataract, congenital

743.35 Congenital aphakia
Congenital absence of lens

743.36 Anomalies of lens shape
Microphakia
Spherophakia

743.37 Congenital ectopic lens

❑ **743.39 Other**

● **743.4 Coloboma and other anomalies of anterior segment**

743.41 Anomalies of corneal size and shape
Microcornea

Excludes *that associated with buphthalmos (743.22)*

743.42 Corneal opacities, interfering with vision, congenital

❑ **743.43 Other corneal opacities, congenital**

❑ **743.44 Specified anomalies of anterior chamber, chamber angle, and related structures**
Anomaly:
Axenfeld's
Peters'
Rieger's

743.45 Aniridia

❑ **743.46 Other specified anomalies of iris and ciliary body**
Anisocoria, congenital
Atresia of pupil
Coloboma of iris
Corectopia

❑ **743.47 Specified anomalies of sclera**

❑ **743.48 Multiple and combined anomalies of anterior segment**

❑ **743.49 Other**

● **743.5 Congenital anomalies of posterior segment**

743.51 Vitreous anomalies
Congenital vitreous opacity

743.52 Fundus coloboma

743.53 Chorioretinal degeneration, congenital

743.54 Congenital folds and cysts of posterior segment

743.55 Congenital macular changes

❑ **743.56 Other retinal changes, congenital**

❑ **743.57 Specified anomalies of optic disc**
Coloboma of optic disc (congenital)

743.58 Vascular anomalies
Congenital retinal aneurysm

❑ **743.59 Other**

● **743.6 Congenital anomalies of eyelids, lacrimal system, and orbit**

743.61 Congenital ptosis

743.62 Congenital deformities of eyelids
Ablepharon
Absence of eyelid
Accessory eyelid
Congenital:
ectropion
entropion

❑ **743.63 Other specified congenital anomalies of eyelid**
Absence, agenesis, of cilia

❑ **743.64 Specified congenital anomalies of lacrimal gland**

❑ **743.65 Specified congenital anomalies of lacrimal passages**
Absence, agenesis, of:
lacrimal apparatus
punctum lacrimale
Accessory lacrimal canal

❑ **743.66 Specified congenital anomalies of orbit**

❑ **743.69 Other**
Accessory eye muscles

❑ **743.8 Other specified anomalies of eye**

Excludes *congenital nystagmus (379.51)*
ocular albinism (270.2)
optic nerve hypoplasia (377.43) ◄
retinitis pigmentosa (362.74)

❑ **743.9 Unspecified anomaly of eye**
Congenital:
anomaly NOS of eye [any part]
deformity NOS of eye [any part]

● **744 Congenital anomalies of ear, face, and neck**

Excludes *anomaly of:*
cervical spine (754.2, 756.10–756.19)
larynx (748.2–748.3)
nose (748.0–748.1)
parathyroid gland (759.2)
thyroid gland (759.2)
cleft lip (749.10–749.25)

● ❑ **744.0 Anomalies of ear causing impairment of hearing**

Excludes *congenital deafness without mention of cause (380.0–389.9)*

❑ **744.00 Unspecified anomaly of ear with impairment of hearing**

744.01 Absence of external ear
Absence of:
auditory canal (external)
auricle (ear) (with stenosis or atresia of auditory canal)

❑ **744.02 Other anomalies of external ear with impairment of hearing**
Atresia or stricture of auditory canal (external)

744.03 Anomaly of middle ear, except ossicles
Atresia or stricture of osseous meatus (ear)

744.04 Anomalies of ear ossicles
Fusion of ear ossicles

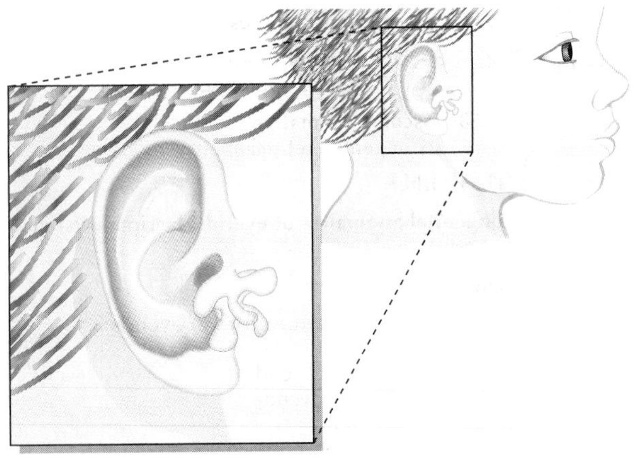

Figure 14–5 Multiple auricular appendage.

744.05 **Anomalies of inner ear**
Congenital anomaly of:
membranous labyrinth
organ of Corti

❑744.09 **Other**
Absence of ear, congenital

744.1 **Accessory auricle**
Accessory tragus
Polyotia
Preauricular appendage
Supernumerary:
ear
lobule

● 744.2 **Other specified anomalies of ear**

Excludes *that with impairment of hearing (744.00–744.09)*

744.21 **Absence of ear lobe, congenital**

744.22 **Macrotia**

744.23 **Microtia**

❑744.24 **Specified anomalies of Eustachian tube**
Absence of Eustachian tube

❑744.29 **Other**
Bat ear
Darwin's tubercle
Ridge ear
Prominence of auricle
Pointed ear

Excludes *preauricular sinus (744.46)*

❑744.3 **Unspecified anomaly of ear**
Congenital:
anomaly NOS of ear, NEC
deformity NOS of ear, NEC

● 744.4 **Branchial cleft cyst or fistula; preauricular sinus**

744.41 **Branchial cleft sinus or fistula**
Branchial:
sinus (external) (internal)
vestige

744.42 **Branchial cleft cyst**

744.43 **Cervical auricle**

744.46 **Preauricular sinus or fistula**

744.47 **Preauricular cyst**

❑744.49 **Other**
Fistula (of):
auricle, congenital
cervicoaural

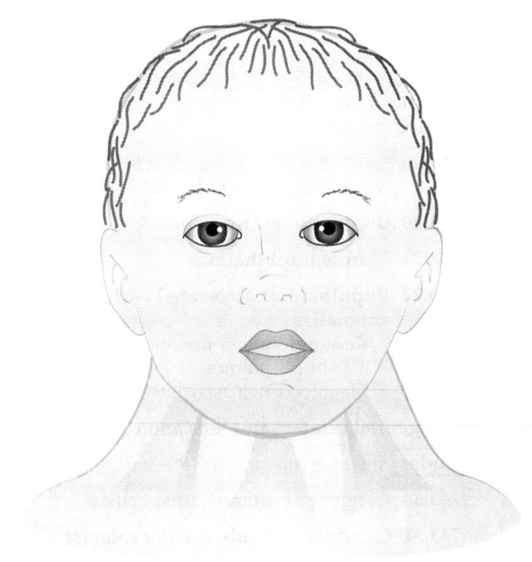

Figure 14–6 Webbing of the neck.

744.5 **Webbing of neck**
Pterygium colli

● 744.8 **Other specified anomalies of face and neck**

744.81 **Macrocheilia**
Hypertrophy of lip, congenital

744.82 **Microcheilia**

744.83 **Macrostomia**

744.84 **Microstomia**

❑744.89 **Other**

Excludes *congenital fistula of lip (750.25)*
musculoskeletal anomalies (754.0–754.1, 756.0)

❑744.9 **Unspecified anomalies of face and neck**
Congenital:
anomaly NOS of face [any part] or neck [any part]
deformity NOS of face [any part] or neck [any part]

● 745 **Bulbus cordis anomalies and anomalies of cardiac septal closure**

745.0 **Common truncus**
Absent septum between aorta and pulmonary artery
Communication (abnormal) between aorta and pulmonary artery
Aortic septal defect
Common aortopulmonary trunk
Persistent truncus arteriosus

● 745.1 **Transposition of great vessels**

745.10 **Complete transposition of great vessels**
Transposition of great vessels:
NOS
classical

745.11 **Double outlet right ventricle**
Dextrotransposition of aorta
Incomplete transposition of great vessels
Origin of both great vessels from right ventricle
Taussig-Bing syndrome or defect

745.12 **Corrected transposition of great vessels**

❑745.19 **Other**

745.2 Tetralogy of Fallot
Fallot's pentalogy
Ventricular septal defect with pulmonary stenosis or atresia, dextroposition of aorta, and hypertrophy of right ventricle

Excludes *Fallot's triad (746.09)*

745.3 Common ventricle
Cor triloculare biatriatum
Single ventricle

745.4 Ventricular septal defect
Eisenmenger's defect or complex
Gerbode defect
Interventricular septal defect
Left ventricular-right atrial communication
Roger's disease

Excludes *common atrioventricular canal type (745.69)*
single ventricle (745.3)

745.5 Ostium secundum type atrial septal defect
Defect:
atrium secundum
fossa ovalis
Patent or persistent:
foramen ovale
ostium secundum
Lutembacher's syndrome

● **745.6 Endocardial cushion defects**

❑ **745.60 Endocardial cushion defect, unspecified type**

745.61 Ostium primum defect
Persistent ostium primum

❑ **745.69 Other**
Absence of atrial septum
Atrioventricular canal type ventricular septal defect
Common atrioventricular canal
Common atrium

745.7 Cor biloculare
Absence of atrial and ventricular septa

❑ **745.8 Other**

❑ **745.9 Unspecified defect of septal closure**
Septal defect NOS

● **746 Other congenital anomalies of heart**

Excludes *endocardial fibroelastosis (425.3)*

● **746.0 Anomalies of pulmonary valve**

Excludes *infundibular or subvalvular pulmonic stenosis (746.83)*
tetralogy of Fallot (745.2)

❑ **746.00 Pulmonary valve anomaly, unspecified**

746.01 Atresia, congenital
Congenital absence of pulmonary valve

746.02 Stenosis, congenital

❑ **746.09 Other**
Congenital insufficiency of pulmonary valve
Fallot's triad or trilogy

746.1 Tricuspid atresia and stenosis, congenital
Absence of tricuspid valve

746.2 Ebstein's anomaly

746.3 Congenital stenosis of aortic valve
Congenital aortic stenosis

Excludes *congenital:*
subaortic stenosis (746.81)
supravalvular aortic stenosis (747.22)

746.4 Congenital insufficiency of aortic valve
Bicuspid aortic valve
Congenital aortic insufficiency

746.5 Congenital mitral stenosis
Fused commissure of mitral valve
Parachute deformity of mitral valve
Supernumerary cusps of mitral valve

746.6 Congenital mitral insufficiency

746.7 Hypoplastic left heart syndrome
Atresia, or marked hypoplasia, of aortic orifice or valve, with hypoplasia of ascending aorta and defective development of left ventricle (with mitral valve atresia)

● **746.8 Other specified anomalies of heart**

746.81 Subaortic stenosis

746.82 Cor triatriatum

746.83 Infundibular pulmonic stenosis
Subvalvular pulmonic stenosis

746.84 Obstructive anomalies of heart, NEC
Uhl's disease

746.85 Coronary artery anomaly
Anomalous origin or communication of coronary artery
Arteriovenous malformation of coronary artery
Coronary artery:
absence
arising from aorta or pulmonary trunk
single

746.86 Congenital heart block
Complete or incomplete atrioventricular [AV] block

746.87 Malposition of heart and cardiac apex
Abdominal heart
Dextrocardia
Ectopia cordis
Levocardia (isolated)
Mesocardia

Excludes *dextrocardia with complete transposition of viscera (759.3)*

❑ **746.89 Other**
Atresia of cardiac vein
Hypoplasia of cardiac vein
Congenital:
cardiomegaly
diverticulum, left ventricle
pericardial defect

❑ **746.9 Unspecified anomaly of heart**
Congenital:
anomaly of heart NOS
heart disease NOS

● **747 Other congenital anomalies of circulatory system**

747.0 Patent ductus arteriosus
Patent ductus Botalli
Persistent ductus arteriosus

● **747.1 Coarctation of aorta**

747.10 Coarctation of aorta (preductal) (postductal)
Hypoplasia of aortic arch

747.11 Interruption of aortic arch

● **747.2 Other anomalies of aorta**

❑ **747.20 Anomaly of aorta, unspecified**

747.21 Anomalies of aortic arch
Anomalous origin, right subclavian artery
Dextroposition of aorta
Double aortic arch
Kommerell's diverticulum
Overriding aorta
Persistent:
convolutions, aortic arch
right aortic arch
Vascular ring

Excludes *hypoplasia of aortic arch (747.10)*

747.22 Atresia and stenosis of aorta
Absence of aorta
Aplasia of aorta
Hypoplasia of aorta
Stricture of aorta
Supra (valvular)-aortic stenosis

Excludes *congenital aortic (valvular) stenosis or stricture, so stated (746.3)*
hypoplasia of aorta in hypoplastic left heart syndrome (746.7)

❑**747.29 Other**
Aneurysm of sinus of Valsalva
Congenital:
aneurysm of aorta
Congenital:
dilation of aorta

747.3 Anomalies of pulmonary artery
Agenesis of pulmonary artery
Anomaly of pulmonary artery
Atresia of pulmonary artery
Coarctation of pulmonary artery
Hypoplasia of pulmonary artery
Stenosis of pulmonary artery
Pulmonary arteriovenous aneurysm

● **747.4 Anomalies of great veins**

❑**747.40 Anomaly of great veins, unspecified**
Anomaly NOS of:
pulmonary veins
Anomaly NOS of:
vena cava

747.41 Total anomalous pulmonary venous connection
Total anomalous pulmonary venous return [TAPVR]:
subdiaphragmatic
supradiaphragmatic

747.42 Partial anomalous pulmonary venous connection
Partial anomalous pulmonary venous return

❑**747.49 Other anomalies of great veins**
Absence of vena cava (inferior) (superior)
Congenital stenosis of vena cava (inferior) (superior)
Persistent:
left posterior cardinal vein
left superior vena cava
Scimitar syndrome
Transposition of pulmonary veins NOS

747.5 Absence or hypoplasia of umbilical artery
Single umbilical artery

● **747.6 Other anomalies of peripheral vascular system**
Absence of artery or vein, NEC
Anomaly of artery or vein, NEC
Atresia of artery or vein, NEC
Arteriovenous aneurysm (peripheral)
Arteriovenous malformation of the peripheral vascular system
Congenital:
aneurysm (peripheral)
phlebectasia
Congenital:
stricture, artery
varix
Multiple renal arteries

Excludes *anomalies of:*
cerebral vessels (747.81)
pulmonary artery (747.3)
congenital retinal aneurysm (743.58)
hemangioma (228.00–228.09)
lymphangioma (228.1)

❑**747.60 Anomaly of the peripheral vascular system, unspecified site**

747.61 Gastrointestinal vessel anomaly

747.62 Renal vessel anomaly

747.63 Upper limb vessel anomaly

747.64 Lower limb vessel anomaly

❑**747.69 Anomalies of other specified sites of peripheral vascular system**

● **747.8 Other specified anomalies of circulatory system**

747.81 Anomalies of cerebrovascular system
Arteriovenous malformation of brain
Cerebral arteriovenous aneurysm, congenital
Congenital anomalies of cerebral vessels

Excludes *ruptured cerebral (arteriovenous) aneurysm (430)*

747.82 Spinal vessel anomaly
Arteriovenous malformation of spinal vessel

747.83 Persistent fetal circulation
Persistent pulmonary hypertension
Primary pulmonary hypertension of newborn

❑**747.89 Other**
Aneurysm, congenital, specified site not elsewhere classified

Excludes *congenital aneurysm:*
coronary (746.85)
peripheral (747.6)
congenital aneurysm:
pulmonary (747.3)
retinal (743.58)

❑**747.9 Unspecified anomaly of circulatory system**

● **748 Congenital anomalies of respiratory system**

Excludes *congenital central alveolar hypoventilation syndrome (327.25)*
congenital defect of diaphragm (756.6)

748.0 Choanal atresia
Atresia of nares (anterior) (posterior)
Congenital stenosis of nares (anterior) (posterior)

❑**748.1 Other anomalies of nose**
Absent nose
Accessory nose
Cleft nose
Deformity of wall of nasal sinus
Congenital:
deformity of nose
notching of tip of nose
perforation of wall of nasal sinus

Excludes *congenital deviation of nasal septum (754.0)*

748.2 Web of larynx
Web of larynx:
NOS
glottic
Web of larynx:
subglottic

❑**748.3 Other anomalies of larynx, trachea, and bronchus**
Absence or agenesis of:
bronchus
larynx
trachea
Anomaly (of):
cricoid cartilage
epiglottis
Anomaly (of):
thyroid cartilage
tracheal cartilage
Atresia (of):
epiglottis
glottis
Atresia (of):
larynx
trachea
Cleft thyroid, cartilage, congenital
Congenital:
dilation, trachea
stenosis:
larynx
trachea
tracheocele
Diverticulum:
bronchus
trachea
Fissure of epiglottis
Laryngocele
Posterior cleft of cricoid cartilage (congenital)
Rudimentary tracheal bronchus
Stridor, laryngeal, congenital

748.4 Congenital cystic lung
Disease, lung:
cystic, congenital
polycystic, congenital
Honeycomb lung, congenital
Excludes *acquired or unspecified cystic lung (518.89)*

748.5 Agenesis, hypoplasia, and dysplasia of lung
Absence of lung (fissures) (lobe)
Aplasia of lung
Hypoplasia of lung (lobe)
Sequestration of lung

● **748.6 Other anomalies of lung**

❑ **748.60 Anomaly of lung, unspecified**

748.61 Congenital bronchiectasis

❑ **748.69 Other**
Accessory lung (lobe)
Azygos lobe (fissure), lung

❑ **748.8 Other specified anomalies of respiratory system**
Abnormal communication between pericardial and pleural sacs
Anomaly, pleural folds
Atresia of nasopharynx
Congenital cyst of mediastinum

❑ **748.9 Unspecified anomaly of respiratory system**
Anomaly of respiratory system NOS

● **749 Cleft palate and cleft lip**

● **749.0 Cleft palate**

❑ **749.00 Cleft palate, unspecified**

749.01 Unilateral, complete

749.02 Unilateral, incomplete
Cleft uvula

749.03 Bilateral, complete

749.04 Bilateral, incomplete

● **749.1 Cleft lip**
Cheiloschisis
Congenital fissure of lip
Harelip
Labium leporinum

❑ **749.10 Cleft lip, unspecified**

749.11 Unilateral, complete

749.12 Unilateral, incomplete

749.13 Bilateral, complete

749.14 Bilateral, incomplete

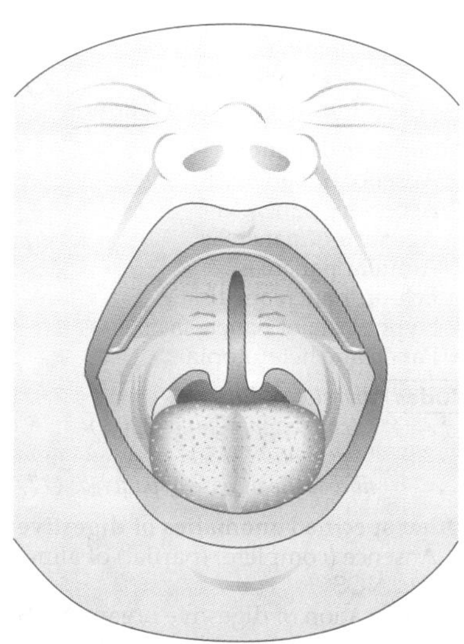

Figure 14–7 Cleft palate.

● **749.2 Cleft palate with cleft lip**
Cheilopalatoschisis

❑ **749.20 Cleft palate with cleft lip, unspecified**

749.21 Unilateral, complete

749.22 Unilateral, incomplete

749.23 Bilateral, complete

749.24 Bilateral, incomplete

❑ **749.25 Other combinations**

● **750 Other congenital anomalies of upper alimentary tract**
Excludes *dentofacial anomalies (524.0–524.9)*

750.0 Tongue tie
Ankyloglossia

● **750.1 Other anomalies of tongue**

❑ **750.10 Anomaly of tongue, unspecified**

750.11 Aglossia

750.12 Congenital adhesions of tongue

750.13 Fissure of tongue
Bifid tongue
Double tongue

750.15 Macroglossia
Congenital hypertrophy of tongue

750.16 Microglossia
Hypoplasia of tongue

❑ **750.19 Other**

● **750.2 Other specified anomalies of mouth and pharynx**

750.21 Absence of salivary gland

750.22 Accessory salivary gland

750.23 Atresia, salivary gland
Imperforate salivary duct

750.24 Congenital fistula of salivary gland

750.25 Congenital fistula of lip
Congenital (mucus) lip pits

❑ **750.26 Other specified anomalies of mouth**
Absence of uvula

750.27 Diverticulum of pharynx
Pharyngeal pouch

❑ **750.29 Other specified anomalies of pharynx**
Imperforate pharynx

750.3 Tracheoesophageal fistula, esophageal atresia and stenosis
Absent esophagus
Atresia of esophagus
Congenital:
esophageal ring
stenosis of esophagus
stricture of esophagus
Congenital fistula:
esophagobronchial
esophagotracheal
Imperforate esophagus
Webbed esophagus

❑ **750.4 Other specified anomalies of esophagus**
Dilatation, congenital, of esophagus
Displacement, congenital, of esophagus
Diverticulum of esophagus
Duplication of esophagus
Esophageal pouch
Giant esophagus
Excludes *congenital hiatus hernia (750.6)*

750.5 Congenital hypertrophic pyloric stenosis
Congenital or infantile:
constriction of pylorus
hypertrophy of pylorus
spasm of pylorus
stenosis of pylorus
stricture of pylorus

750.6 Congenital hiatus hernia
Displacement of cardia through esophageal hiatus

Excludes *congenital diaphragmatic hernia (756.6)*

❑ **750.7 Other specified anomalies of stomach**
Congenital:
cardiospasm
hourglass stomach
Displacement of stomach
Diverticulum of stomach, congenital
Duplication of stomach
Megalogastria
Microgastria
Transposition of stomach

❑ **750.8 Other specified anomalies of upper alimentary tract**

❑ **750.9 Unspecified anomaly of upper alimentary tract**
Congenital:
anomaly NOS of upper alimentary tract [any part, except tongue]
deformity NOS of upper alimentary tract [any part, except tongue]

● **751 Other congenital anomalies of digestive system**

751.0 Meckel's diverticulum
Meckel's diverticulum (displaced) (hypertrophic)
Persistent:
omphalomesenteric duct
vitelline duct

751.1 Atresia and stenosis of small intestine
Atresia of:
duodenum
ileum
intestine NOS
Congenital:
absence of small intestine or intestine NOS
obstruction of small intestine or intestine NOS
stenosis of small intestine or intestine NOS
stricture of small intestine or intestine NOS
Imperforate jejunum

751.2 Atresia and stenosis of large intestine, rectum, and anal canal
Absence:
anus (congenital)
appendix, congenital
large instestine, congenital
rectum
Atresia of:
anus
colon
rectum
Congenital or infantile:
obstruction of large intestine
occlusion of anus
stricture of anus
Imperforate:
anus
rectum
Stricture of rectum, congenital

❑ **751.3 Hirschsprung's disease and other congenital functional disorders of colon**
Aganglionosis
Congenital dilation of colon
Congenital megacolon
Macrocolon

751.4 Anomalies of intestinal fixation
Congenital adhesions:
omental, anomalous
peritoneal
Jackson's membrane
Malrotation of colon
Rotation of cecum or colon:
failure of
incomplete
insufficient
Universal mesentery

❑ **751.5 Other anomalies of intestine**
Congenital diverticulum, colon
Dolichocolon
Duplication of:
anus
appendix
cecum
intestine
Ectopic anus
Megaloappendix
Megaloduodenum
Microcolon
Persistent cloaca
Transposition of:
appendix
colon
intestine

● **751.6 Anomalies of gallbladder, bile ducts, and liver**

❑ **751.60 Unspecified anomaly of gallbladder, bile ducts, and liver**

751.61 Biliary atresia
Congenital:
absence of bile duct (common) or passage
hypoplasia of bile duct (common) or passage
obstruction of bile duct (common) or passage
stricture of bile duct (common) or passage

751.62 Congenital cystic disease of liver
Congenital polycystic disease of liver
Fibrocystic disease of liver

❑ **751.69 Other anomalies of gallbladder, bile ducts, and liver**
Absence of:
gallbladder, congenital
liver (lobe)
Accessory:
hepatic ducts
liver
Congenital:
choledochal cyst
hepatomegaly
Duplication of:
biliary duct
cystic duct
Floating:
gallbladder
Intrahepatic gallbladder
Duplication of:
gallbladder
liver
Floating:
liver

751.7 Anomalies of pancreas
Absence of pancreas
Accessory pancreas
Agenesis of pancreas
Annular pancreas
Ectopic pancreatic tissue
Hypoplasia of pancreas
Pancreatic heterotopia

Excludes *diabetes mellitus:*
congenital (250.0–250.9)
neonatal (775.1)
fibrocystic disease of pancreas (277.00–277.09)

❑ **751.8 Other specified anomalies of digestive system**
Absence (complete) (partial) of alimentary tract NOS
Duplication of digestive organs NOS
Malposition, congenital, of digestive organs NOS

Excludes *congenital diaphragmatic hernia (756.6)*
congenital hiatus hernia (750.6)

❑751.9 **Unspecified anomaly of digestive system**
Congenital:
anomaly NOS of digestive system NOS
deformity NOS of digestive system NOS

● 752 **Congenital anomalies of genital organs**

Excludes *syndromes associated with anomalies in the number and form of chromosomes (758.0–758.9)*
testicular feminization syndrome (259.5)

752.0 **Anomalies of ovaries**
Absence, congenital, of ovary
Accessory ovary
Ectopic ovary
Streak of ovary

● 752.1 **Anomalies of fallopian tubes and broad ligaments**

❑752.10 **Unspecified anomaly of fallopian tubes and broad ligaments**

752.11 **Embryonic cyst of fallopian tubes and broad ligaments**
Cyst:
epoöphoron
fimbrial
parovarian

❑752.19 **Other**
Absence of fallopian tube or broad ligament
Accessory fallopian tube or broad ligament
Atresia of fallopian tube or broad ligament

752.2 **Doubling of uterus**
Didelphic uterus
Doubling of uterus [any degree] (associated with doubling of cervix and vagina)

❑752.3 **Other anomalies of uterus**
Absence, congenital, of uterus
Agenesis of uterus
Aplasia of uterus
Bicornuate uterus
Uterus unicornis
Uterus with only one functioning horn

● 752.4 **Anomalies of cervix, vagina, and external female genitalia**

❑752.40 **Unspecified anomaly of cervix, vagina, and external female genitalia**

752.41 **Embryonic cyst of cervix, vagina, and external female genitalia**
Cyst of:
canal of Nuck, congenital
Gartner's duct
vagina, embryonal
vulva, congenital

752.42 **Imperforate hymen**

❑752.49 **Other anomalies of cervix, vagina, and external female genitalia**
Absence of cervix, clitoris, vagina, or vulva
Agenesis of cervix, clitoris, vagina, or vulva
Congenital stenosis or stricture of:
cervical canal
vagina

Excludes *double vagina associated with total duplication (752.2)*

● 752.5 **Undescended and retractile testicle**

752.51 **Undescended testis**
Cryptorchism
Ectopic testis

752.52 **Retractile testis**

Item 14-4 Testes form in the abdomen of the male and only descend into the scrotum during normal embryonic development. "Ectopic" testes are out of their normal place or "retained" (left behind) in the abdomen. Crypto (hidden) orchism (testicle) is a major risk factor for testicular cancer.

● 752.6 **Hypospadias and epispadias and other penile anomalies**

752.61 **Hypospadias**

752.62 **Epispadias**
Anaspadias

752.63 **Congenital chordee**

752.64 **Micropenis**

752.65 **Hidden penis**

❑752.69 **Other penile anomalies**

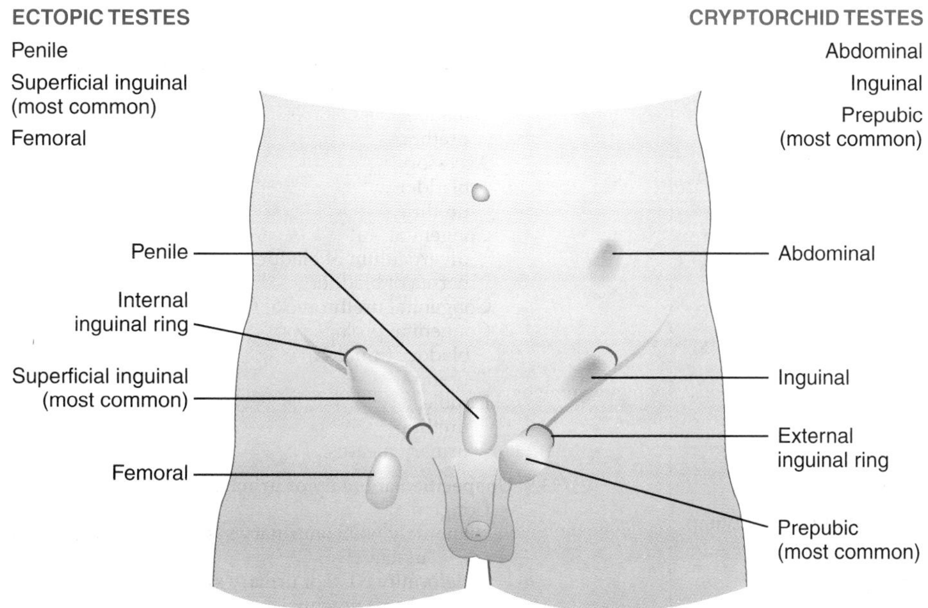
ECTOPIC TESTES
Penile
Superficial inguinal (most common)
Femoral
CRYPTORCHID TESTES
Abdominal
Inguinal
Prepubic (most common)
Penile
Internal inguinal ring
Superficial inguinal (most common)
Femoral
Abdominal
Inguinal
External inguinal ring
Prepubic (most common)

Figure 14-8 Undescended testes and the positions of the testes in various types of cryptorchidism or abnormal paths of descent.

ICD-9-CM 700-799 Vol. 1

752.7 Indeterminate sex and pseudohermaphroditism
Gynandrism
Hermaphroditism
Ovotestis
Pseudohermaphroditism (male) (female)
Pure gonadal dysgenesis

Excludes *pseudohermaphroditism:*
female, with adrenocortical disorder (255.2)
male, with gonadal disorder (257.8)
with specified chromosomal anomaly (758.0–758.9)
testicular feminization syndrome (259.5)

● **752.8 Other specified anomalies of genital organs**

Excludes *congenital hydrocele (778.6)*
penile anomalies (752.61–752.69)
phimosis or paraphimosis (605)

752.81 Scrotal transposition

❑ **752.89 Other specified anomalies of genital organs**
Absence of:
prostate
spermatic cord
vas deferens
Anorchism
Aplasia (congenital) of:
prostate
round ligament
testicle
Atresia of:
ejaculatory duct
vas deferens
Fusion of testes
Hypoplasia of testis
Monorchism
Polyorchism

❑ **752.9 Unspecified anomaly of genital organs**
Congenital:
anomaly NOS of genital organ, NEC
deformity NOS of genital organ, NEC

● **753 Congenital anomalies of urinary system**

753.0 Renal agenesis and dysgenesis
Atrophy of kidney:
congenital
infantile
Congenital absence of kidney(s)
Hypoplasia of kidney(s)

● **753.1 Cystic kidney disease**

Excludes *acquired cyst of kidney (593.2)*

❑ **753.10 Cystic kidney disease, unspecified**

753.11 Congenital single renal cyst

❑ **753.12 Polycystic kidney, unspecified type**
PKD (polycystic kidney disease)

753.13 Polycystic kidney, autosomal dominant

753.14 Polycystic kidney, autosomal recessive

753.15 Renal dysplasia

753.16 Medullary cystic kidney
Nephronophthisis

753.17 Medullary sponge kidney

❑ **753.19 Other specified cystic kidney disease**
Multicystic kidney

● **753.2 Obstructive defects of renal pelvis and ureter**

❑ **753.20 Unspecified obstructive defect of renal pelvis and ureter**

753.21 Congenital obstruction of ureteropelvic junction

753.22 Congenital obstruction of ureterovesical junction
Adynamic ureter
Congenital hydroureter

753.23 Congenital ureterocele

❑ **753.29 Other**

❑ **753.3 Other specified anomalies of kidney**
Accessory kidney
Congenital:
calculus of kidney
displaced kidney
Discoid kidney
Double kidney with double pelvis
Ectopic kidney
Fusion of kidneys
Giant kidney
Horseshoe kidney
Hyperplasia of kidney
Lobulation of kidney
Malrotation of kidney
Trifid kidney (pelvis)

❑ **753.4 Other specified anomalies of ureter**
Absent ureter
Accessory ureter
Deviaton of ureter
Displaced ureteric orifice
Double ureter
Ectopic ureter
Implantation, anomalous, of ureter

753.5 Exstrophy of urinary bladder
Ectopia vesicae
Extroversion of bladder

753.6 Atresia and stenosis of urethra and bladder neck
Congenital obstruction:
bladder neck
urethra
Congenital stricture of:
urethra (valvular)
urinary meatus
vesicourethral orifice
Imperforate urinary meatus
Impervious urethra
Urethral valve formation

753.7 Anomalies of urachus
Cyst (of) urachus
Fistula (of) urachus
Patent (of) urachus
Persistent umbilical sinus

❑ **753.8 Other specified anomalies of bladder and urethra**
Absence, congenital, of:
bladder
urethra
Accessory:
bladder
urethra
Congenital:
diverticulum of bladder
hernia of bladder
Congenital urethrorectal fistula
Congenital prolapse of:
bladder (mucosa)
urethra
Double:
urethra
urinary meatus

❑ **753.9 Unspecified anomaly of urinary system**
Congenital:
anomaly NOS of urinary system [any part, except urachus]
deformity NOS of urinary system [any part, except urachus]

754 Certain congenital musculoskeletal deformities

Includes: nonteratogenic deformities which are considered to be due to intrauterine malposition and pressure

754.0 Of skull, face, and jaw
Asymmetry of face
Compression facies
Depressions in skull
Deviation of nasal septum, congenital
Dolichocephaly
Plagiocephaly
Potter's facies
Squashed or bent nose, congenital

Excludes *dentofacial anomalies (524.0–524.9)*
syphilitic saddle nose (090.5)

754.1 Of sternocleidomastoid muscle
Congenital sternomastoid torticollis
Congenital wryneck
Contracture of sternocleidomastoid (muscle)
Sternomastoid tumor

754.2 Of spine
Congenital postural:
lordosis
scoliosis

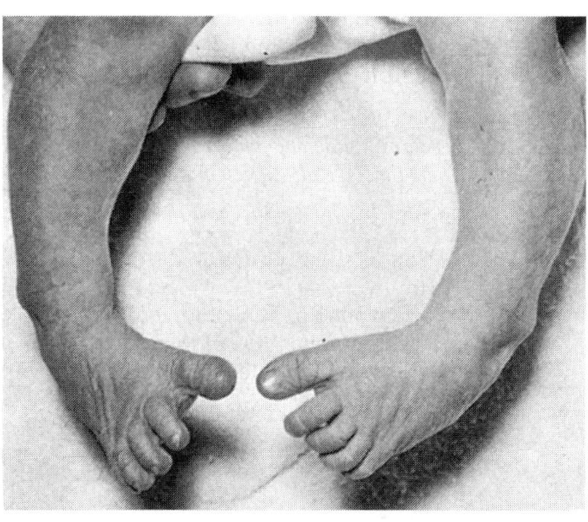

Figure 14–9 Mild to moderate inbowing of the lower leg. (From Jones KL: Smith's Recognizable Patterns of Human Malformation, 4th ed. Philadelphia, WB Saunders, 1988, p 671.)

754.3 Congenital dislocation of hip

754.30 Congenital dislocation of hip, unilateral
Congenital dislocation of hip NOS

754.31 Congenital dislocation of hip, bilateral

754.32 Congenital subluxation of hip, unilateral
Congenital flexion deformity, hip or thigh
Predislocation status of hip at birth
Preluxation of hip, congenital

754.33 Congenital subluxation of hip, bilateral

754.35 Congenital dislocation of one hip with subluxation of other hip

754.4 Congenital genu recurvatum and bowing of long bones of leg

754.40 Genu recurvatum

754.41 Congenital dislocation of knee (with genu recurvatum)

754.42 Congenital bowing of femur

754.43 Congenital bowing of tibia and fibula

754.44 Congenital bowing of unspecified long bones of leg

754.5 Varus deformities of feet

Excludes *acquired (736.71, 736.75, 736.79)*

754.50 Talipes varus
Congenital varus deformity of foot, unspecified
Pes varus

754.51 Talipes equinovarus
Equinovarus (congenital)

754.52 Metatarsus primus varus

754.53 Metatarsus varus

754.59 Other
Talipes calcaneovarus

754.6 Valgus deformities of feet

Excludes *valgus deformity of foot (acquired) (736.79)*

754.60 Talipes valgus
Congenital valgus deformity of foot, unspecified

754.61 Congenital pes planus
Congenital rocker bottom flat foot
Flat foot, congenital

Excludes *pes planus (acquired) (734)*

754.62 Talipes calcaneovalgus

754.69 Other
Talipes:
equinovalgus
planovalgus

754.7 Other deformities of feet

Excludes *acquired (736.70–736.79)*

754.70 Talipes, unspecified
Congenital deformity of foot NOS

754.71 Talipes cavus
Cavus foot (congenital)

754.79 Other
Asymmetric talipes
Talipes:
calcaneus
equinus

754.8 Other specified nonteratogenic anomalies

754.81 Pectus excavatum
Congenital funnel chest

754.82 Pectus carinatum
Congenital pigeon chest [breast]

754.89 Other
Club hand (congenital)
Congenital:
deformity of chest wall
dislocation of elbow
Generalized flexion contractures of lower limb joints, congenital
Spade-like hand (congenital)

755 Other congenital anomalies of limbs

Excludes *those deformities classifiable to 754.0–754.8*

755.0 Polydactyly

755.00 Polydactyly, unspecified digits
Supernumerary digits

755.01 Of fingers
Accessory fingers

755.02 Of toes
Accessory toes

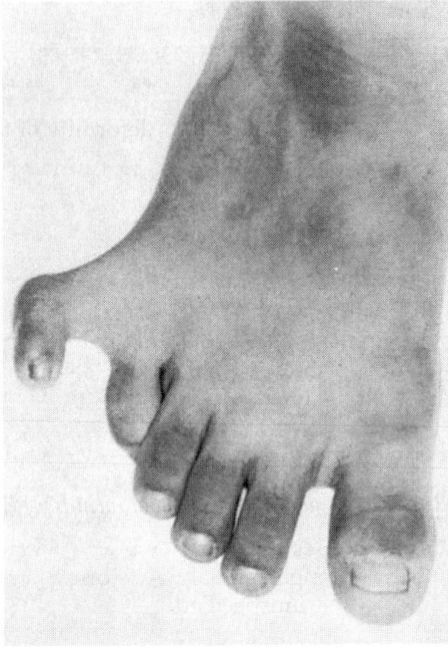

Figure 14–10 Polydactyly. (From Tachdjian MO: Pediatric Orthopedics, 2nd ed, Vol 4. Philadelphia, WB Saunders, 1990, p 2644.)

● **755.1 Syndactyly**
Symphalangy
Webbing of digits

❑ **755.10 Of multiple and unspecified sites**

755.11 Of fingers without fusion of bone

755.12 Of fingers with fusion of bone

755.13 Of toes without fusion of bone

755.14 Of toes with fusion of bone

● **755.2 Reduction deformities of upper limb**

❑ **755.20 Unspecified reduction deformity of upper limb**
Ectromelia NOS of upper limb
Hemimelia NOS of upper limb
Shortening of arm, congenital

755.21 Transverse deficiency of upper limb
Amelia of upper limb
Congenital absence of:
fingers, all (complete or partial)
forearm, including hand and fingers
upper limb, complete
Congenital amputation of upper limb
Transverse hemimelia of upper limb

755.22 Longitudinal deficiency of upper limb, NEC
Phocomelia NOS of upper limb
Rudimentary arm

755.23 Longitudinal deficiency, combined, involving humerus, radius, and ulna (complete or incomplete)
Congenital absence of arm and forearm (complete or incomplete) with or without metacarpal deficiency and/or phalangeal deficiency, incomplete
Phocomelia, complete, of upper limb

755.24 Longitudinal deficiency, humeral, complete or partial (with or without distal deficiencies, incomplete)
Congenital absence of humerus (with or without absence of some [but not all] distal elements)
Proximal phocomelia of upper limb

755.25 Longitudinal deficiency, radioulnar, complete or partial (with or without distal deficiencies, incomplete)
Congenital absence of radius and ulna (with or without absence of some [but not all] distal elements)
Distal phocomelia of upper limb

755.26 Longitudinal deficiency, radial, complete or partial (with or without distal deficiencies, incomplete)
Agenesis of radius
Congenital absence of radius (with or without absence of some [but not all] distal elements)

755.27 Longitudinal deficiency, ulnar, complete or partial (with or without distal deficiencies, incomplete)
Agenesis of ulna
Congenital absence of ulna (with or without absence of some [but not all] distal elements)

755.28 Longitudinal deficiency, carpals or metacarpals, complete or partial (with or without incomplete phalangeal deficiency)

755.29 Longitudinal deficiency, phalanges, complete or partial
Absence of finger, congenital
Aphalangia of upper limb, terminal, complete or partial

Excludes *terminal deficiency of all five digits (755.21)*
transverse deficiency of phalanges (755.21)

● **755.3 Reduction deformities of lower limb**

❑ **755.30 Unspecified reduction deformity of lower limb**
Ectromelia NOS of lower limb
Hemimelia NOS of lower limb
Shortening of leg, congenital

755.31 Transverse deficiency of lower limb
Amelia of lower limb
Congenital absence of:
foot
leg, including foot and toes
lower limb, complete
toes, all, complete
Transverse hemimelia of lower limb

755.32 Longitudinal deficiency of lower limb, NEC
Phocomelia NOS of lower limb

755.33 Longitudinal deficiency, combined, involving femur, tibia, and fibula (complete or incomplete)
Congenital absence of thigh and (lower) leg (complete or incomplete) with or without metacarpal deficiency and/or phalangeal deficiency, incomplete
Phocomelia, complete, of lower limb

755.34 Longitudinal deficiency, femoral, complete or partial (with or without distal deficiencies, incomplete)
Congenital absence of femur (with or without absence of some [but not all] distal elements)
Proximal phocomelia of lower limb

755.35 Longitudinal deficiency, tibiofibular, complete or partial (with or without distal deficiencies, incomplete)
Congenital absence of tibia and fibula (with or without absence of some [but not all] distal elements)
Distal phocomelia of lower limb

755.36 Longitudinal deficiency, tibia, complete or partial (with or without distal deficiencies, incomplete)
Agenesis of tibia
Congenital absence of tibia (with or without absence of some [but not all] distal elements)

755.37 Longitudinal deficiency, fibular, complete or partial (with or without distal deficiencies, incomplete)
Agenesis of fibula
Congenital absence of fibula (with or without absence of some [but not all] distal elements)

755.38 Longitudinal deficiency, tarsals or metatarsals, complete or partial (with or without incomplete phalangeal deficiency)

755.39 Longitudinal deficiency, phalanges, complete or partial
Absence of toe, congenital
Aphalangia of lower limb, terminal, complete or partial

Excludes *terminal deficiency of all five digits (755.31)*
transverse deficiency of phalanges (755.31)

❑ **755.4 Reduction deformities, unspecified limb**
Absence, congenital (complete or partial) of limb NOS
Amelia of unspecified limb
Ectromelia of unspecified limb
Hemimelia of unspecified limb
Phocomelia of unspecified limb

● **755.5 Other anomalies of upper limb, including shoulder girdle**

❑ **755.50 Unspecified anomaly of upper limb**

755.51 Congenital deformity of clavicle

755.52 Congenital elevation of scapula
Sprengel's deformity

755.53 Radioulnar synostosis

755.54 Madelung's deformity

755.55 Acrocephalosyndactyly
Apert's syndrome

755.56 Accessory carpal bones

755.57 Macrodactylia (fingers)

755.58 Cleft hand, congenital
Lobster-claw hand

❑ **755.59 Other**
Cleidocranial dysostosis
Cubitus:
valgus, congenital
varus, congenital

Excludes *club hand (congenital) (754.89)*
congenital dislocation of elbow (754.89)

● **755.6 Other anomalies of lower limb, including pelvic girdle**

❑ **755.60 Unspecified anomaly of lower limb**

755.61 Coxa valga, congenital

755.62 Coxa vara, congenital

❑ **755.63 Other congenital deformity of hip (joint)**
Congenital anteversion of femur (neck)

Excludes *congenital dislocation of hip (754.30–754.35)*

755.64 Congenital deformity of knee (joint)
Congenital:
absence of patella
genu valgum [knock-knee]
genu varum [bowleg]
Rudimentary patella

755.65 Macrodactylia of toes

❑ **755.66 Other anomalies of toes**
Congenital:
hallux valgus
hallux varus
hammer toe

755.67 Anomalies of foot, NEC
Astragaloscaphoid synostosis
Calcaneonavicular bar
Coalition of calcaneus
Talonavicular synostosis
Tarsal coalitions

❑ **755.69 Other**
Congenital:
angulation of tibia
deformity (of):
ankle (joint)
sacroiliac (joint)
fusion of sacroiliac joint

❑ **755.8 Other specified anomalies of unspecified limb**

❑ **755.9 Unspecified anomaly of unspecified limb**
Congenital:
anomaly NOS of unspecified limb
deformity NOS of unspecified limb

Excludes *reduction deformity of unspecified limb (755.4)*

● **756 Other congenital musculoskeletal anomalies**

Excludes *those deformities classifiable to 754.0–754.8*

756.0 Anomalies of skull and face bones
Absence of skull bones
Acrocephaly
Congenital deformity of forehead
Craniosynostosis
Crouzon's disease
Hypertelorism
Imperfect fusion of skull
Oxycephaly
Platybasia
Premature closure of cranial sutures
Tower skull
Trigonocephaly

Excludes *acrocephalosyndactyly [Apert's syndrome] (755.55)*
dentofacial anomalies (524.0–524.9)
skull defects associated with brain anomalies, such as:
anencephalus (740.0)
encephalocele (742.0)
hydrocephalus (742.3)
microcephalus (742.1)

● **756.1 Anomalies of spine**

❑ **756.10 Anomaly of spine, unspecified**

756.11 Spondylolysis, lumbosacral region
Prespondylolisthesis (lumbosacral)

756.12 Spondylolisthesis

756.13 Absence of vertebra, congenital

756.14 Hemivertebra

756.15 Fusion of spine [vertebra], congenital

756.16 Klippel-Feil syndrome

756.17 Spina bifida occulta

Excludes *spina bifida (aperta) (741.0–741.9)*

❑ **756.19 Other**
Platyspondylia
Supernumerary vertebra

756.2 Cervical rib
Supernumerary rib in the cervical region

❑756.3 **Other anomalies of ribs and sternum**
Congenital absence of:
rib
sternum
Congenital:
fissure of sternum
fusion of ribs
Sternum bifidum
Excludes *nonteratogenic deformity of chest wall (754.81–754.89)*

756.4 **Chondrodystrophy**
Achondroplasia
Chondrodystrophia (fetalis)
Dyschondroplasia
Enchondromatosis
Ollier's disease
Excludes *lipochondrodystrophy [Hurler's syndrome] (277.5)*
Morquio's disease (277.5)

●756.5 **Osteodystrophies**
❑756.50 **Osteodystrophy, unspecified**
756.51 **Osteogenesis imperfecta**
Fragilitas ossium
Osteopsathyrosis
756.52 **Osteopetrosis**
756.53 **Osteopoikilosis**
756.54 **Polyostotic fibrous dysplasia of bone**
756.55 **Chondroectodermal dysplasia**
Ellis-van Creveld syndrome
756.56 **Multiple epiphyseal dysplasia**
❑756.59 **Other**
Albright (-McCune)-Sternberg syndrome

756.6 **Anomalies of diaphragm**
Absence of diaphragm
Congenital hernia:
diaphragmatic
foramen of Morgagni
Eventration of diaphragm
Excludes *congenital hiatus hernia (750.6)*

●756.7 **Anomalies of abdominal wall**
❑756.70 **Anomaly of abdominal wall, unspecified**
756.71 **Prune belly syndrome**
Eagle-Barrett syndrome
Prolapse of bladder mucosa
❑756.79 **Other congenital anomalies of abdominal wall**
Exomphalos
Gastroschisis
Omphalocele
Excludes *umbilical hernia (551–553 with .1)*

●756.8 **Other specified anomalies of muscle, tendon, fascia, and connective tissue**
756.81 **Absence of muscle and tendon**
Absence of muscle (pectoral)
756.82 **Accessory muscle**
756.83 **Ehlers-Danlos syndrome**
❑756.89 **Other**
Amyotrophia congenita
Congenital shortening of tendon

❑756.9 **Other and unspecified anomalies of musculoskeletal system**
Congenital:
anomaly NOS of musculoskeletal system, NEC
deformity NOS of musculoskeletal system, NEC

●757 **Congenital anomalies of the integument**
Includes: anomalies of skin, subcutaneous tissue, hair, nails, and breast
Excludes *hemangioma (228.00–228.09)*
pigmented nevus (216.0–216.9)

757.0 **Hereditary edema of legs**
Congenital lymphedema
Hereditary trophedema
Milroy's disease

757.1 **Ichthyosis congenita**
Congenital ichthyosis
Harlequin fetus
Ichthyosiform erythroderma

757.2 **Dermatoglyphic anomalies**
Abnormal palmar creases

●757.3 **Other specified anomalies of skin**
757.31 **Congenital ectodermal dysplasia**
757.32 **Vascular hamartomas**
Birthmarks
Port-wine stain
Strawberry nevus
757.33 **Congenital pigmentary anomalies of skin**
Congenital poikiloderma
Urticaria pigmentosa
Xeroderma pigmentosum
Excludes *albinism (270.2)*
❑757.39 **Other**
Accessory skin tags, congenital
Congenital scar
Epidermolysis bullosa
Keratoderma (congenital)
Excludes *pilonidal cyst (685.0–685.1)*

❑757.4 **Specified anomalies of hair**
Congenital:
alopecia
atrichosis
beaded hair
hypertrichosis
monilethrix
Persistent lanugo

❑757.5 **Specified anomalies of nails**
Anonychia
Congenital:
clubnail
koilonychia
leukonychia
onychauxis
pachyonychia

❑757.6 **Specified anomalies of breast**
Absent breast or nipple
Accessory breast or nipple
Supernumerary breast or nipple
Hypoplasia of breast
Excludes *absence of pectoral muscle (756.81)*

❑757.8 **Other specified anomalies of the integument**

❑757.9 **Unspecified anomaly of the integument**
Congenital:
anomaly NOS of integument
deformity NOS of integument

758 Chromosomal anomalies

Use additional codes for conditions associated with the chromosomal anomalies

Includes: syndromes associated with anomalies in the number and form of chromosomes

758.0 Down's syndrome
Mongolism
Translocation Down's syndrome
Trisomy:
21 or 22
G

758.1 Patau's syndrome
Trisomy:
13
D_1

758.2 Edwards's syndrome
Trisomy:
18
E_3

758.3 Autosomal deletion syndromes

758.31 Cri-du-chat syndrome
Deletion 5p

758.32 Velo-cardio-facial syndrome
Deletion 22q11.2

758.33 Other microdeletions
Miller-Dieker syndrome
Smith-Magenis syndrome

758.39 Other autosomal deletions

758.4 Balanced autosomal translocation in normal individual

758.5 Other conditions due to autosomal anomalies
Accessory autosomes, NEC

758.6 Gonadal dysgenesis
Ovarian dysgenesis
Turner's syndrome
XO syndrome

Excludes *pure gonadal dysgenesis (752.7)*

758.7 Klinefelter's syndrome
XXY syndrome

758.8 Other conditions due to chromosome anomalies

758.81 Other conditions due to sex chromosome anomalies

758.89 Other

758.9 Conditions due to anomaly of unspecified chromosome

759 Other and unspecified congenital anomalies

759.0 Anomalies of spleen
Aberrant spleen
Absent spleen
Accessory spleen
Congenital splenomegaly
Ectopic spleen
Lobulation of spleen

759.1 Anomalies of adrenal gland
Aberrant adrenal gland
Absent adrenal gland
Accessory adrenal gland

Excludes *adrenogenital disorders (255.2)*
congenital disorders of steroid metabolism (255.2)

759.2 Anomalies of other endocrine glands
Absent parathyroid gland
Accessory thyroid gland
Persistent thyroglossal or thyrolingual duct
Thyroglossal (duct) cyst

Excludes *congenital:*
goiter (246.1)
hypothyroidism (243)

759.3 Situs inversus
Situs inversus or transversus:
abdominalis
thoracis
Transposition of viscera:
abdominal
thoracic

Excludes *dextrocardia without mention of complete transposition (746.87)*

759.4 Conjoined twins
Craniopagus
Dicephalus
Pygopagus
Thoracopagus
Xiphopagus

759.5 Tuberous sclerosis
Bourneville's disease
Epiloia

759.6 Other hamartoses, NEC
Syndrome:
Peutz-Jeghers
Sturge-Weber (-Dimitri)
von Hippel-Lindau

Excludes *neurofibromatosis (237.7)*

759.7 Multiple congenital anomalies, so described
Congenital:
anomaly, multiple NOS
deformity, multiple NOS

759.8 Other specified anomalies

759.81 Prader-Willi syndrome

759.82 Marfan syndrome

759.83 Fragile X syndrome

759.89 Other
Congenital malformation syndromes affecting multiple systems, NEC
Laurence-Moon-Biedl syndrome

759.9 Congenital anomaly, unspecified

15. CERTAIN CONDITIONS ORIGINATING IN THE PERINATAL PERIOD (760–779)

Includes: conditions which have their origin in the perinatal period, before birth through the first 28 days after birth, even though death or morbidity occurs later

Use additional code(s) to further specify condition

MATERNAL CAUSES OF PERINATAL MORBIDITY AND MORTALITY (760–763)

● **760 Fetus or newborn affected by maternal conditions which may be unrelated to present pregnancy**

Includes: the listed maternal conditions only when specified as a cause of mortality or morbidity of the fetus or newborn

Excludes *maternal endocrine and metabolic disorders affecting fetus or newborn (775.0–775.9)*

760.0 Maternal hypertensive disorders
Fetus or newborn affected by maternal conditions classifiable to 642

760.1 Maternal renal and urinary tract diseases
Fetus or newborn affected by maternal conditions classifiable to 580–599

760.2 Maternal infections
Fetus or newborn affected by maternal infectious disease classifiable to 001–136 and 487, but fetus or newborn not manifesting that disease

Excludes *congenital infectious diseases (771.0–771.8)*
maternal genital tract and other localized infections (760.8)

❑**760.3 Other chronic maternal circulatory and respiratory diseases**
Fetus or newborn affected by chronic maternal conditions classifiable to 390–459, 490–519, 745–748

760.4 Maternal nutritional disorders
Fetus or newborn affected by:
maternal disorders classifiable to 260–269
maternal malnutrition NOS

Excludes *fetal malnutrition (764.10–764.29)*

760.5 Maternal injury
Fetus or newborn affected by maternal conditions classifiable to 800–995

760.6 Surgical operation on mother

Excludes *cesarean section for present delivery (763.4)*
damage to placenta from amniocentesis, cesarean section, or surgical induction (762.1)
previous surgery to uterus or pelvic organs (763.89)

● **760.7 Noxious influences affecting fetus or newborn via placenta or breast milk**
Fetus or newborn affected by noxious substance transmitted via placenta or breast milk

Excludes *anesthetic and analgesic drugs administered during labor and delivery (763.5)*
drug withdrawal syndrome in newborn (779.5)

❑**760.70 Unspecified noxious substance**
Fetus or newborn affected by:
Drug, NEC

760.71 Alcohol
Fetal alcohol syndrome

760.72 Narcotics

760.73 Hallucinogenic agents

760.74 Anti-infectives
Antibiotics
Antifungals

760.75 Cocaine

760.76 Diethylstilbestrol [DES]

760.77 Anticonvulsants
Carbamazepine
Phenobarbital
Phenytoin
Valproic acid

760.78 Antimetabolic agents
Methotrexate
Retinoic acid
Statins

❑**760.79 Other**
Fetus or newborn affected by:
immune sera transmitted via placenta or breast milk
medicinal agents, NEC, transmitted via placenta or breast milk
toxic substance, NEC, transmitted via placenta or breast milk

❑**760.8 Other specified maternal conditions affecting fetus or newborn**
Maternal genital tract and other localized infection affecting fetus or newborn, but fetus or newborn not manifesting that disease

Excludes *maternal urinary tract infection affecting fetus or newborn (760.1)*

760.9 Unspecified maternal condition affecting fetus or newborn

● **761 Fetus or newborn affected by maternal complications of pregnancy**

Includes: the listed maternal conditions only when specified as a cause of mortality or morbidity of the fetus or newborn

761.0 Incompetent cervix

761.1 Premature rupture of membranes

761.2 Oligohydramnios

Excludes *that due to premature rupture of membranes (761.1)*

761.3 Polyhydramnios
Hydramnios (acute) (chronic)

761.4 Ectopic pregnancy
Pregnancy:
abdominal
intraperitoneal
tubal

761.5 Multiple pregnancy
Triplet (pregnancy)
Twin (pregnancy)

761.6 Maternal death

761.7 Malpresentation before labor
Breech presentation before labor
External version before labor
Oblique lie before labor
Transverse lie before labor
Unstable lie before labor

❑**761.8 Other specified maternal complications of pregnancy affecting fetus or newborn**
Spontaneous abortion, fetus

❑**761.9 Unspecified maternal complication of pregnancy affecting fetus or newborn**

● **762 Fetus or newborn affected by complications of placenta, cord, and membranes**

Includes: the listed maternal conditions only when specified as a cause of mortality or morbidity in the fetus or newborn

762.0 Placenta previa

❑762.1 **Other forms of placental separation and hemorrhage**
Abruptio placentae
Antepartum hemorrhage
Damage to placenta from amniocentesis, cesarean section, or surgical induction
Maternal blood loss
Premature separation of placenta
Rupture of marginal sinus

❑762.2 **Other and unspecified morphological and functional abnormalities of placenta**
Placental:
dysfunction
infarction
insufficiency

762.3 **Placental transfusion syndromes**
Placental and cord abnormality resulting in twin-to-twin or other transplacental transfusion

Use additional code to indicate resultant condition in fetus or newborn:
fetal blood loss (772.0)
polycythemia neonatorum (776.4)

762.4 **Prolapsed cord**
Cord presentation

❑762.5 **Other compression of umbilical cord**
Cord around neck
Entanglement of cord
Knot in cord
Torsion of cord

❑762.6 **Other and unspecified conditions of umbilical cord**
Short cord
Thrombosis of umbilical cord
Varices of umbilical cord
Velamentous insertion of umbilical cord
Vasa previa

Excludes *infection of umbilical cord (771.4)*
single umbilical artery (747.5)

762.7 **Chorioamnionitis**
Amnionitis
Membranitis
Placentitis

❑762.8 **Other specified abnormalities of chorion and amnion**

❑762.9 **Unspecified abnormality of chorion and amnion**

● 763 **Fetus or newborn affected by other complications of labor and delivery**

Includes: the listed conditions only when specified as a cause of mortality or morbidity in the fetus or newborn

763.0 **Breech delivery and extraction**

❑763.1 **Other malpresentation, malposition, and disproportion during labor and delivery**
Fetus or newborn affected by:
abnormality of bony pelvis
contracted pelvis
persistent occipitoposterior position
shoulder presentation
transverse lie
conditions classifiable to 652, 653, and 660

763.2 **Forceps delivery**
Fetus or newborn affected by forceps extraction

763.3 **Delivery by vacuum extractor**

763.4 **Cesarean delivery**

Excludes *placental separation or hemorrhage from cesarean section (762.1)*

763.5 **Maternal anesthesia and analgesia**
Reactions and intoxications from maternal opiates and tranquilizers during labor and delivery

Excludes *drug withdrawal syndrome in newborn (779.5)*

763.6 **Precipitate delivery**
Rapid second stage

763.7 **Abnormal uterine contractions**
Fetus or newborn affected by:
contraction ring
hypertonic labor
hypotonic uterine dysfunction
uterine inertia or dysfunction
conditions classifiable to 661, except 661.3

● 763.8 **Other specified complications of labor and delivery affecting fetus or newborn**

763.81 **Abnormality in fetal heart rate or rhythm before the onset of labor**

763.82 **Abnormality in fetal heart rate or rhythm during labor**

❑763.83 **Abnormality in fetal heart rate or rhythm, unspecified as to time of onset**

763.84 **Meconium passage during delivery**

Excludes *meconium aspiration (770.11, 770.12)*
meconium staining (779.84)

763.89 **Other specified complications of labor and delivery affecting fetus or newborn**
Fetus or newborn affected by:
abnormality of maternal soft tissues
destructive operation on live fetus to facilitate delivery
induction of labor (medical)
previous surgery to uterus or pelvic organs
other conditions classifiable to 650–669
other procedures used in labor and delivery

❑763.9 **Unspecified complication of labor and delivery affecting fetus or newborn**

OTHER CONDITIONS ORIGINATING IN THE PERINATAL PERIOD (764–779)

The following fifth-digit subclassification is for use with category 764 and codes 765.0 and 765.1 to denote birthweight:

❑ 0 **unspecified [weight]**
1 **less than 500 grams**
2 **500–749 grams**
3 **750–999 grams**
4 **1,000–1,249 grams**
5 **1,250–1,499 grams**
6 **1,500–1,749 grams**
7 **1,750–1,999 grams**
8 **2,000–2,499 grams**
9 **2,500 grams and over**

● 764 **Slow fetal growth and fetal malnutrition**

Requires fifth digit. See beginning of section 764–779 for codes and definitions.

● 764.0 **"Light-for-dates" without mention of fetal malnutrition**
Infants underweight for gestational age
"Small-for-dates"

● 764.1 **"Light-for-dates" with signs of fetal malnutrition**
Infants "light-for-dates" classifiable to 764.0, who in addition show signs of fetal malnutrition, such as dry peeling skin and loss of subcutaneous tissue

● 764.2 **Fetal malnutrition without mention of "light-for-dates"**
Infants, not underweight for gestational age, showing signs of fetal malnutrition, such as dry peeling skin and loss of subcutaneous tissue
Intrauterine malnutrition

● ❑764.9 **Fetal growth retardation, unspecified**
Intrauterine growth retardation

● 765 **Disorders relating to short gestation and low birthweight**

Requires fifth digit. See beginning of section 764–779 for codes and definitions.

Includes: the listed conditions, without further specification, as causes of mortality, morbidity, or additional care, in fetus or newborn

● 765.0 **Extreme immaturity**

Note: Usually implies a birthweight of less than 1,000 grams

Use additional code for weeks of gestation (765.20–765.29)

● ❑765.1 **Other preterm infants**

Note: Usually implies birthweight of 1,000–2,499 grams
Prematurity NOS
Prematurity or small size, not classifiable to 765.0 or as "light-for-dates" in 764

Use additional code for weeks of gestation (765.20–765.29)

● 765.2 **Weeks of gestation**

❑765.20 **Unspecified weeks of gestation**

765.21 **Less than 24 completed weeks of gestation**

765.22 **24 completed weeks of gestation**

765.23 **25–26 completed weeks of gestation**

765.24 **27–28 completed weeks of gestation**

765.25 **29–30 completed weeks of gestation**

765.26 **31–32 completed weeks of gestation**

765.27 **33–34 completed weeks of gestation**

765.28 **35–36 completed weeks of gestation**

765.29 **37 or more completed weeks of gestation**

● 766 **Disorders relating to long gestation and high birthweight**

Includes: the listed conditions, without further specification, as causes of mortality, morbidity, or additional care, in fetus or newborn

766.0 **Exceptionally large baby**

Note: Usually implies a birthweight of 4,500 grams or more.

❑766.1 **Other "heavy-for-dates" infants**

Other fetus or infant "heavy-" or "large-for-dates" regardless of period of gestation

● 766.2 **Late infant, not "heavy-for-dates"**

766.21 **Post-term infant**

Infant with gestation period over 40 completed weeks to 42 completed weeks

766.22 **Prolonged gestation of infant**

Infant with gestation period over 42 completed weeks
Postmaturity NOS

● 767 **Birth trauma**

767.0 **Subdural and cerebral hemorrhage**

Subdural and cerebral hemorrhage, whether described as due to birth trauma or to intrapartum anoxia or hypoxia
Subdural hematoma (localized)
Tentorial tear

Use additional code to identify cause

Excludes *intraventricular hemorrhage (772.10–772.14)*
subarachnoid hemorrhage (772.2)

● 767.1 **Injuries to scalp**

767.11 **Epicranial subaponeurotic hemorrhage (massive)**

Subgaleal hemorrhage

❑767.19 **Other injuries to scalp**

Caput succedaneum
Cephalhematoma
Chignon (from vacuum extraction)

767.2 **Fracture of clavicle**

❑767.3 **Other injuries to skeleton**

Fracture of:
long bones
skull

Excludes *congenital dislocation of hip (754.30–754.35)*
fracture of spine, congenital (767.4)

767.4 **Injury to spine and spinal cord**

Dislocation of spine or spinal cord due to birth trauma
Fracture of spine or spinal cord due to birth trauma
Laceration of spine or spinal cord due to birth trauma
Rupture of spine or spinal cord due to birth trauma

767.5 **Facial nerve injury**

Facial palsy

767.6 **Injury to brachial plexus**

Palsy or paralysis:
brachial
Erb (-Duchenne)
Klumpke (-Déjérine)

❑767.7 **Other cranial and peripheral nerve injuries**

Phrenic nerve paralysis

❑767.8 **Other specified birth trauma**

Eye damage
Hematoma of:
liver (subcapsular)
testes
vulva
Rupture of:
liver
spleen
Scalpel wound
Traumatic glaucoma

Excludes *hemorrhage classifiable to 772.0–772.9*

❑767.9 **Birth trauma, unspecified**

Birth injury NOS

● 768 **Intrauterine hypoxia and birth asphyxia**

Use only when associated with newborn morbidity classifiable elsewhere

Excludes *acidemia NOS of newborn (775.81)* ◀
acidosis NOS of newborn (775.81) ◀
cerebral ischemia NOS (779.2) ◀
hypoxia NOS of newborn (770.88) ◀
mixed metabolic and respiratory acidosis of newborn (775.81) ◀
respiratory arrest of newborn (770.87) ◀

❑768.0 **Fetal death from asphyxia or anoxia before onset of labor or at unspecified time**

768.1 **Fetal death from asphyxia or anoxia during labor**

768.2 **Fetal distress before onset of labor, in liveborn infant**

Fetal metabolic acidemia before onset of labor, in liveborn infant

768.3 **Fetal distress first noted during labor and delivery, in liveborn infant** ⬅

Fetal metabolic acidemia first noted during labor and delivery, in liveborn infant ⬅

❑768.4 **Fetal distress, unspecified as to time of onset, in liveborn infant**
Fetal metabolic acidemia unspecified as to time of onset, in liveborn infant

768.5 **Severe birth asphyxia**
Birth asphyxia with neurologic involvement
Excludes *hypoxic-ischemic encephalopathy (HIE) (768.7)* ◀

768.6 **Mild or moderate birth asphyxia**
Other specified birth asphyxia (without mention of neurologic involvement)
Excludes *hypoxic-ischemic encephalopathy (HIE) (768.7)* ◀

768.7 **Hypoxic-ischemic encephalopathy (HIE)** ◀

❑768.9 **Unspecified birth asphyxia in liveborn infant** ⇐
Anoxia NOS, in liveborn infant
Asphyxia NOS, in liveborn infant

769 **Respiratory distress syndrome**
Cardiorespiratory distress syndrome of newborn
Hyaline membrane disease (pulmonary)
Idiopathic respiratory distress syndrome [IRDS or RDS] of newborn
Pulmonary hypoperfusion syndrome
Excludes *transient tachypnea of newborn (770.6)*

● 770 **Other respiratory conditions of fetus and newborn**

770.0 **Congenital pneumonia**
Infective pneumonia acquired prenatally
Excludes *pneumonia from infection acquired after birth (480.0–486)*

● 770.1 **Fetal and newborn aspiration**
Excludes *aspiration of postnatal stomach contents (770.85, 770.86)*
meconium passage during delivery (763.84)
meconium staining (779.84)

770.10 **Fetal and newborn aspiration, unspecified**

770.11 **Meconium aspiration without respiratory symptoms**
Meconium aspiration NOS

770.12 **Meconium aspiration with respiratory symptoms**
Meconium aspiration pneumonia
Meconium aspiration pneumonitis
Meconium aspiration syndrome NOS
Use additional code to identify any secondary pulmonary hypertension (416.8), if applicable

770.13 **Aspiration of clear amniotic fluid without respiratory symptoms**
Aspiration of clear amniotic fluid NOS

770.14 **Aspiration of clear amniotic fluid with respiratory symptoms**
Aspiration of clear amniotic fluid with pneumonia
Aspiration of clear amniotic fluid with pneumonitis
Use additional code to identify any secondary pulmonary hypertension (416.8), if applicable

770.15 **Aspiration of blood without respiratory symptoms**
Aspiration of blood NOS

770.16 **Aspiration of blood with respiratory symptoms**
Aspiration of blood with pneumonia
Aspiration of blood with pneumonitis
Use additional code to identify any secondary pulmonary hypertension (416.8), if applicable

770.17 **Other fetal and newborn aspiration without respiratory symptoms**

770.18 **Other fetal and newborn aspiration with respiratory symptoms**
Other aspiration pneumonia
Other aspiration pneumonitis
Use additional code to identify any secondary pulmonary hypertension (416.8), if applicable

770.2 **Interstitial emphysema and related conditions**
Pneumomediastinum originating in the perinatal period
Pneumopericardium originating in the perinatal period
Pneumothorax originating in the perinatal period

770.3 **Pulmonary hemorrhage**
Hemorrhage:
alveolar (lung) originating in the perinatal period
intra-alveolar (lung) originating in the perinatal period
massive pulmonary originating in the perinatal period

770.4 **Primary atelectasis**
Pulmonary immaturity NOS

❑770.5 **Other and unspecified atelectasis**
Atelectasis:
NOS originating in the perinatal period
partial originating in the perinatal period
secondary originating in the perinatal period
Pulmonary collapse originating in the perinatal period

770.6 **Transitory tachypnea of newborn**
Idiopathic tachypnea of newborn
Wet lung syndrome
Excludes *respiratory distress syndrome (769)*

770.7 **Chronic respiratory disease arising in the perinatal period**
Bronchopulmonary dysplasia
Interstitial pulmonary fibrosis of prematurity
Wilson-Mikity syndrome

● ❑770.8 **Other respiratory problems after birth**
Excludes *mixed metabolic and respiratory acidosis of newborn (775.81)* ◀

770.81 **Primary apnea of newborn**
Apneic spells of newborn NOS
Essential apnea of newborn
Sleep apnea of newborn

770.82 **Other apnea of newborn**
Obstructive apnea of newborn

770.83 **Cyanotic attacks of newborn**

770.84 **Respiratory failure of newborn**
Excludes *respiratory distress syndrome (769)*

770.85 **Aspiration of postnatal stomach contents without respiratory symptoms**
Aspiration of postnatal stomach contents NOS

770.86 **Aspiration of postnatal stomach contents with respiratory symptoms**
Aspiration of postnatal stomach contents with pneumonia
Aspiration of postnatal stomach contents with pneumonitis
Use additional code to identify any secondary pulmonary hypertension (416.8), if applicable

770.87 **Respiratory arrest of newborn** ◀

770.88 **Hypoxemia of newborn** ◀
Hypoxia NOS of newborn ◀

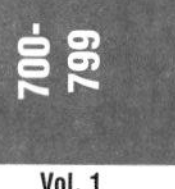

ICD-9-CM
700-799
Vol. 1

770.89 **Other respiratory problems after birth**

770.9 **Unspecified respiratory condition of fetus and newborn**

771 **Infections specific to the perinatal period**

Includes: infections acquired before or during birth or via the umbilicus or during the first 28 days after birth

Excludes *congenital pneumonia (770.0)*
congenital syphilis (090.0–090.9)
maternal infectious disease as a cause of mortality or morbidity in fetus or newborn, but fetus or newborn not manifesting the disease (760.2)
ophthalmia neonatorum due to gonococcus (098.40)
other infections not specifically classified to this category

771.0 **Congenital rubella**
Congenital rubella pneumonitis

771.1 **Congenital cytomegalovirus infection**
Congenital cytomegalic inclusion disease

771.2 **Other congenital infections**
Congenital:
herpes simplex
listeriosis
malaria
Congenital:
toxoplasmosis
tuberculosis

771.3 **Tetanus neonatorum**
Tetanus omphalitis

Excludes *hypocalcemic tetany (775.4)*

771.4 **Omphalitis of the newborn**
Infection:
navel cord
Infection:
umbilical stump

Excludes *tetanus omphalitis (771.3)*

771.5 **Neonatal infective mastitis**

Excludes *noninfective neonatal mastitis (778.7)*

771.6 **Neonatal conjunctivitis and dacryocystitis**
Ophthalmia neonatorum NOS

Excludes *ophthalmia neonatorum due to gonococcus (098.40)*

771.7 **Neonatal Candida infection**
Neonatal moniliasis
Thrush in newborn

771.8 **Other infections specific to the perinatal period**
Use additional code to identify organism (041.00–041.9)

771.81 **Septicemia [sepsis] of newborn**

771.82 **Urinary tract infection of newborn**

771.83 **Bacteremia of newborn**

771.89 **Other infections specific to the perinatal period**
Intra-amniotic infection of fetus NOS
Infection of newborn NOS

772 **Fetal and neonatal hemorrhage**

Excludes *hematological disorders of fetus and newborn (776.0–776.9)*

772.0 **Fetal blood loss**
Fetal blood loss from:
cut end of co-twin's cord
placenta
ruptured cord
vasa previa
Fetal exsanguination
Fetal hemorrhage into:
co-twin
mother's circulation

772.1 **Intraventricular hemorrhage**
Intraventricular hemorrhage from any perinatal cause

772.10 **Unspecified grade**

772.11 **Grade I**
Bleeding into germinal matrix

772.12 **Grade II**
Bleeding into ventricle

772.13 **Grade III**
Bleeding with enlargement of ventricle

772.14 **Grade IV**
Bleeding into cerebral cortex

772.2 **Subarachnoid hemorrhage**
Subarachnoid hemorrhage from any perinatal cause

Excludes *subdural and cerebral hemorrhage (767.0)*

772.3 **Umbilical hemorrhage after birth**
Slipped umbilical ligature

772.4 **Gastrointestinal hemorrhage**

Excludes *swallowed maternal blood (777.3)*

772.5 **Adrenal hemorrhage**

772.6 **Cutaneous hemorrhage**
Bruising in fetus or newborn
Ecchymoses in fetus or newborn
Petechiae in fetus or newborn
Superficial hematoma in fetus or newborn

772.8 **Other specified hemorrhage of fetus or newborn**

Excludes *hemorrhagic disease of newborn (776.0)*
pulmonary hemorrhage (770.3)

772.9 **Unspecified hemorrhage of newborn**

773 **Hemolytic disease of fetus or newborn, due to isoimmunization**

773.0 **Hemolytic disease due to Rh isoimmunization**
Anemia due to RH:
antibodies
isoimmunization
maternal/fetal incompatibility
Erythroblastosis (fetalis) due to RH:
antibodies
isoimmunization
maternal/fetal incompatibility
Hemolytic disease (fetus) (newborn) due to RH:
antibodies
isoimmunization
maternal/fetal incompatibility
Jaundice due to RH:
antibodies
isoimmunization
maternal/fetal incompatibility
Rh hemolytic disease
Rh isoimmunization

773.1 **Hemolytic disease due to ABO isoimmunization**
ABO hemolytic disease
ABO isoimmunization
Anemia due to ABO:
antibodies
isoimmunization
maternal/fetal incompatibility
Erythroblastosis (fetalis) due to ABO:
antibodies
isoimmunization
maternal/fetal incompatibility
Hemolytic disease (fetus) (newborn) due to ABO:
antibodies
isoimmunization
maternal/fetal incompatibility
Jaundice due to ABO:
antibodies
isoimmunization
maternal/fetal incompatibility

❑773.2 **Hemolytic disease due to other and unspecified isoimmunization**
Erythroblastosis (fetalis) (neonatorum) NOS
Hemolytic disease (fetus) (newborn) NOS
Jaundice or anemia due to other and unspecified blood-group incompatibility

773.3 **Hydrops fetalis due to isoimmunization**
Use additional code, if desired, to identify type of isoimmunization (773.0–773.2)

773.4 **Kernicterus due to isoimmunization**
Use additional code, if desired, to identify type of isoimmunization (773.0–773.2)

773.5 **Late anemia due to isoimmunization**

● 774 **Other perinatal jaundice**

● 774.0 ***Perinatal jaundice from hereditary hemolytic anemias***
Code first underlying disease (282.0–282.9)

❑774.1 **Perinatal jaundice from other excessive hemolysis**
Fetal or neonatal jaundice from:
- bruising
- drugs or toxins transmitted from mother
- infection
- polycythemia
- swallowed maternal blood

Use additional code to identify cause

Excludes *jaundice due to isoimmunization (773.0–773.2)*

774.2 **Neonatal jaundice associated with preterm delivery**
Hyperbilirubinemia of prematurity
Jaundice due to delayed conjugation associated with preterm delivery

● 774.3 **Neonatal jaundice due to delayed conjugation from other causes**

❑774.30 **Neonatal jaundice due to delayed conjugation, cause unspecified**

● 774.31 ***Neonatal jaundice due to delayed conjugation in diseases classified elsewhere***
Code first underlying diseases, as:
- congenital hypothyroidism (243)
- Crigler-Najjar syndrome (277.4)
- Gilbert's syndrome (277.4)

❑774.39 **Other**
Jaundice due to delayed conjugation from causes, such as:
- breast milk inhibitors
- delayed development of conjugating system

774.4 **Perinatal jaundice due to hepatocellular damage**
Fetal or neonatal hepatitis
Giant cell hepatitis
Inspissated bile syndrome

● ❑774.5 ***Perinatal jaundice from other causes***
Code first underlying cause, as:
- congenital obstruction of bile duct (751.61)
- galactosemia (271.1)
- mucoviscidosis (277.00–277.09)

❑774.6 **Unspecified fetal and neonatal jaundice**
Icterus neonatorum
Neonatal hyperbilirubinemia (transient)
Physiologic jaundice NOS in newborn

Excludes *that in preterm infants (774.2)*

774.7 **Kernicterus not due to isoimmunization**
Bilirubin encephalopathy
Kernicterus of newborn NOS

Excludes *kernicterus due to isoimmunization (773.4)*

● 775 **Endocrine and metabolic disturbances specific to the fetus and newborn**

Includes: transitory endocrine and metabolic disturbances caused by the infant's response to maternal endocrine and metabolic factors, its removal from them, or its adjustment to extrauterine existence

775.0 **Syndrome of "infant of a diabetic mother"**
Maternal diabetes mellitus affecting fetus or newborn (with hypoglycemia)

775.1 **Neonatal diabetes mellitus**
Diabetes mellitus syndrome in newborn infant

775.2 **Neonatal myasthenia gravis**

775.3 **Neonatal thyrotoxicosis**
Neonatal hyperthyroidism (transient)

775.4 **Hypocalcemia and hypomagnesemia of newborn**
Cow's milk hypocalcemia
Hypocalcemic tetany, neonatal
Neonatal hypoparathyroidism
Phosphate-loading hypocalcemia

❑775.5 **Other neonatal electrolyte disturbances**
Dehydration, neonatal

775.6 **Neonatal hypoglycemia**

Excludes *infant of mother with diabetes mellitus (775.0)*

775.7 **Late metabolic acidosis of newborn**

● 775.8 **Other neonatal endocrine and metabolic disturbances** ⇐

❑775.81 **Other acidosis of newborn** ◀
Acidemia NOS of newborn ◀
Acidosis of newborn NOS ◀
Mixed metabolic and respiratory acidosis of newborn ◀

❑775.89 **Other neonatal endocrine and metabolic disturbances** ◀
Amino-acid metabolic disorders described as transitory ◀

❑775.9 **Unspecified endocrine and metabolic disturbances specific to the fetus and newborn**

● 776 **Hematological disorders of fetus and newborn**

Includes: disorders specific to the fetus or newborn

776.0 **Hemorrhagic disease of newborn**
Hemorrhagic diathesis of newborn
Vitamin K deficiency of newborn

Excludes *fetal or neonatal hemorrhage (772.0–772.9)*

776.1 **Transient neonatal thrombocytopenia**
Neonatal thrombocytopenia due to:
- exchange transfusion
- idiopathic maternal thrombocytopenia
- isoimmunization

776.2 **Disseminated intravascular coagulation in newborn**

❑776.3 **Other transient neonatal disorders of coagulation**
Transient coagulation defect, newborn

776.4 **Polycythemia neonatorum**
Plethora of newborn
Polycythemia due to:
- donor twin transfusion
- maternal-fetal transfusion

776.5 **Congenital anemia**
Anemia following fetal blood loss

Excludes *anemia due to isoimmunization (773.0–773.2, 773.5)*
hereditary hemolytic anemias (282.0–282.9)

776.6 **Anemia of prematurity**

776.7 **Transient neonatal neutropenia**
Isoimmune neutropenia
Maternal transfer neutropenia
Excludes *congenital neutropenia (nontransient) (288.01)* ◀

❑776.8 **Other specified transient hematological disorders**

❑776.9 **Unspecified hematological disorder specific to fetus or newborn**

● 777 **Perinatal disorders of digestive system**
Includes: disorders specific to the fetus and newborn
Excludes *intestinal obstruction classifiable to 560.0–560.9*

777.1 **Meconium obstruction**
Congenital fecaliths
Delayed passage of meconium
Meconium ileus NOS
Meconium plug syndrome
Excludes *meconium ileus in cystic fibrosis (277.01)*

777.2 **Intestinal obstruction due to inspissated milk**

777.3 **Hematemesis and melena due to swallowed maternal blood**
Swallowed blood syndrome in newborn
Excludes *that not due to swallowed maternal blood (772.4)*

777.4 **Transitory ileus of newborn**
Excludes *Hirschsprung's disease (751.3)*

777.5 **Necrotizing enterocolitis in fetus or newborn**
Pseudomembranous enterocolitis in newborn

777.6 **Perinatal intestinal perforation**
Meconium peritonitis

❑777.8 **Other specified perinatal disorders of digestive system**

❑777.9 **Unspecified perinatal disorder of digestive system**

● 778 **Conditions involving the integument and temperature regulation of fetus and newborn**

778.0 **Hydrops fetalis not due to isoimmunization**
Idiopathic hydrops
Excludes *hydrops fetalis due to isoimmunization (773.3)*

778.1 **Sclerema neonatorum**

778.2 **Cold injury syndrome of newborn**

❑778.3 **Other hypothermia of newborn**

❑778.4 **Other disturbances of temperature regulation of newborn**
Dehydration fever in newborn
Environmentally induced pyrexia
Hyperthermia in newborn
Transitory fever of newborn

❑778.5 **Other and unspecified edema of newborn**
Edema neonatorum

778.6 **Congenital hydrocele**
Congenital hydrocele of tunica vaginalis

778.7 **Breast engorgement in newborn**
Noninfective mastitis of newborn
Excludes *infective mastitis of newborn (771.5)*

❑778.8 **Other specified conditions involving the integument of fetus and newborn**
Urticaria neonatorum
Excludes *impetigo neonatorum (684)*
pemphigus neonatorum (684)

❑778.9 **Unspecified condition involving the integument and temperature regulation of fetus and newborn**

● 779 **Other and ill-defined conditions originating in the perinatal period**

779.0 **Convulsions in newborn**
Fits in newborn
Seizures in newborn

❑779.1 **Other and unspecified cerebral irritability in newborn**

779.2 **Cerebral depression, coma, and other abnormal cerebral signs**
Cerebral ischemia NOS of newborn ◀
CNS dysfunction in newborn NOS
Excludes *cerebral ischemia due to birth trauma (767.0)* ◀
intrauterine cerebral ischemia (768.2–768.9) ◀
intraventricular hemorrhage (772.10–772.14) ◀

779.3 **Feeding problems in newborn**
Regurgitation of food in newborn
Slow feeding in newborn
Vomiting in newborn

779.4 **Drug reactions and intoxications specific to newborn**
Gray syndrome from chloramphenicol administration in newborn
Excludes *fetal alcohol syndrome (760.71)*
reactions and intoxications from maternal opiates and tranquilizers (763.5)

779.5 **Drug withdrawal syndrome in newborn**
Drug withdrawal syndrome in infant of dependent mother
Excludes *fetal alcohol syndrome (760.71)*

779.6 **Termination of pregnancy (fetus)**
Fetal death due to:
induced abortion
termination of pregnancy
Excludes *spontaneous abortion (fetus) (761.8)*

779.7 **Periventricular leukomalacia**

● ❑779.8 **Other specified conditions originating in the perinatal period**

779.81 **Neonatal bradycardia**
Excludes *abnormality in fetal heart rate or rhythm complicating labor and delivery (763.81–763.83)*
bradycardia due to birth asphyxia (768.5–768.9)

779.82 **Neonatal tachycardia**
Excludes *abnormality in fetal heart rate or rhythm complicating labor and delivery (763.81–763.83)*

779.83 **Delayed separation of umbilical cord**

779.84 **Meconium staining**
Excludes *meconium aspiration (770.11, 770.12)*
meconium passage during delivery (763.84)

779.85 **Cardiac arrest of newborn** ◀

❑779.89 **Other specified conditions originating in the perinatal period**
Use additional code to specify condition

❑779.9 **Unspecified condition originating in the perinatal period**
Congenital debility NOS
Stillbirth, NEC

16. SYMPTOMS, SIGNS, AND ILL-DEFINED CONDITIONS (780–799)

This section includes symptoms, signs, abnormal results of laboratory or other investigative procedures, and ill-defined conditions regarding which no diagnosis classifiable elsewhere is recorded.

Signs and symptoms that point rather definitely to a given diagnosis are assigned to some category in the preceding part of the classification. In general, categories 780–796 include the more ill-defined conditions and symptoms that point with perhaps equal suspicion to two or more diseases or to two or more systems of the body, and without the necessary study of the case to make a final diagnosis. Practically all categories in this group could be designated as "not otherwise specified," or as "unknown etiology," or as "transient." The Alphabetic Index should be consulted to determine which symptoms and signs are to be allocated here and which to more specific sections of the classification; the residual subcategories numbered .9 are provided for other relevant symptoms which cannot be allocated elsewhere in the classification.

The conditions and signs or symptoms included in categories 780–796 consist of: (a) cases for which no more specific diagnosis can be made even after all facts bearing on the case have been investigated; (b) signs or symptoms existing at the time of initial encounter that proved to be transient and whose causes could not be determined; (c) provisional diagnoses in a patient who failed to return for further investigation or care; (d) cases referred elsewhere for investigation or treatment before the diagnosis was made; (e) cases in which a more precise diagnosis was not available for any other reason; (f) certain symptoms which represent important problems in medical care and which it might be desired to classify in addition to a known cause.

SYMPTOMS (780–789)

● **780 General symptoms**

● **780.0 Alteration of consciousness**

Excludes *coma:*
diabetic (250.2–250.3)
hepatic (572.2)
originating in the perinatal period (779.2)

780.01 Coma

780.02 Transient alteration of awareness

780.03 Persistent vegetative state

❑ **780.09 Other**
Drowsiness
Semicoma
Somnolence
Stupor
Unconsciousness

780.1 Hallucinations
Hallucinations:
NOS
auditory
gustatory
olfactory
tactile

Excludes *those associated with mental disorders, as functional psychoses (295.0–298.9)*
organic brain syndromes (290.0–294.9, 310.0–310.9)
visual hallucinations (368.16)

780.2 Syncope and collapse
Blackout
Fainting
(Near) (Pre)syncope
Vasovagal attack

Excludes *carotid sinus syncope (337.0)*
heat syncope (992.1)
neurocirculatory asthenia (306.2)
orthostatic hypotension (458.0)
shock NOS (785.50)

● **780.3 Convulsions**

Excludes *convulsions:*
epileptic (345.10–345.91)
in newborn (779.0)

780.31 Febrile convulsions (simple), unspecified ⬅
Febrile seizures NOS ⬅

780.32 Complex febrile convulsions ◀
Febrile seizure: ◀
atypical ◀
complex ◀
complicated ◀

Excludes *status epilepticus (345.3)* ◀

❑ **780.39 Other convulsions**
Convulsive disorder NOS
Fits NOS
Recurrent convulsions NOS ◀
Seizures NOS

780.4 Dizziness and giddiness
Light-headedness
Vertigo NOS

Excludes *Ménière's disease and other specified vertiginous syndromes (386.0–386.9)*

● **780.5 Sleep disturbances**

Excludes *circ adian rhythm sleep disorders (327.30–327.39)*
organic hypersomnia (327.10–327.19)
organic insomnia (327.00–327.09)
organic sleep apnea (327.20–327.29)
organic sleep related movement disorders (327.51–327.59)
parasomnias (327.40–327.49)
that of nonorganic origin (307.40–307.49)

❑ **780.50 Sleep disturbance, unspecified**

❑ **780.51 Insomnia with sleep apnea, unspecified**

❑ **780.52 Insomnia, unspecified**

❑ **780.53 Hypersomnia with sleep apnea, unspecified**

❑ **780.54 Hypersomnia, unspecified**

780.55 Disruptions of 24 hour sleep wake cycle, unspecified

780.56 Dysfunctions associated with sleep stages or arousal from sleep

❑ **780.57 Unspecified sleep apnea**

❑ **780.58 Sleep related movement disorder, unspecified**

Excludes *restless legs syndrome (333.94)* ⬅

❑ **780.59 Other**

780.6 Fever
Chills with fever
Fever NOS
Fever of unknown origin (FUO)
Hyperpyrexia NOS
Pyrexia NOS
Pyrexia of unknown origin

Code first underlying condition when associated fever is present, such as with: ◀
leukemia (codes from categories 204–208) ◀
neutropenia (288.00–288.09) ◀
sickle-cell disease (282.60–282.69) ◀

Excludes *pyrexia of unknown origin (during):*
in newborn (778.4)
labor (659.2)
the puerperium (672)

● **780.7 Malaise and fatigue**

Excludes *debility, unspecified (799.3)*
fatigue (during):
combat (308.0–308.9)
heat (992.6)
pregnancy (646.8)
neurasthenia (300.5)
senile asthenia (797)

780.71 Chronic fatigue syndrome

❑**780.79 Other malaise and fatigue**
Asthenia NOS
Lethargy
Postviral (asthenic) syndrome
Tiredness

780.8 Generalized hyperhidrosis
Diaphoresis
Excessive sweating
Secondary hyperhidrosis

Excludes *focal (localized) (primary) (secondary) hyperhidrosis (705.21–705.22)*
Frey's syndrome (705.22)

● **780.9 Other general symptoms**

Excludes *hypothermia:*
NOS (accidental) (991.6)
due to anesthesia (995.89)
memory disturbance as part of a pattern of mental disorder
of newborn (778.2–778.3)

780.91 Fussy infant (baby)

780.92 Excessive crying of infant (baby)

Excludes *excessive crying of child, adolescent, or adult (780.95)*

780.93 Memory loss
Amnesia (retrograde)
Memory loss NOS

Excludes *mild memory disturbance due to organic brain damage (310.1)*
transient global amnesia (437.7)

780.94 Early satiety

780.95 Excessive crying of child, adolescent, or adult ⬅

Excludes *excessive crying of infant (baby) (780.92)*

780.96 Generalized pain ◀
Pain NOS ◀

780.97 Altered mental status ◀
Change in mental status ◀

Excludes *altered level of consciousness (780.01–780.09)* ◀
altered mental status due to known condition-code to condition ◀
delirium NOS (780.09) ◀

780.99 Other general symptoms ⬅
Chill(s) NOS
Hypothermia, not associated with low environmental temperature

● **781 Symptoms involving nervous and musculoskeletal systems**

Excludes *depression NOS (311)*
disorders specifically relating to:
back (724.0–724.9)
hearing (388.0–389.9)
joint (718.0–719.9)
limb (729.0–729.9)
neck (723.0–723.9)
vision (368.0–369.9)
pain in limb (729.5)

781.0 Abnormal involuntary movements
Abnormal head movements
Fasciculation
Spasms NOS
Tremor NOS

Excludes *abnormal reflex (796.1)*
chorea NOS (333.5)
infantile spasms (345.60–345.61)
spastic paralysis (342.1, 343.0–344.9)
specified movement disorders classifiable to 333 (333.0–333.9)
that of nonorganic origin (307.2–307.3)

781.1 Disturbances of sensation of smell and taste
Anosmia
Parosmia
Parageusia

781.2 Abnormality of gait
Gait:
ataxic
paralytic
spastic
staggering

Excludes *ataxia:*
NOS (781.3)
locomotor (progressive) (094.0)
difficulty in walking (719.7) ◀

781.3 Lack of coordination
Ataxia NOS
Muscular incoordination

Excludes *ataxic gait (781.2)*
cerebellar ataxia (334.0–334.9)
difficulty in walking (719.7)
vertigo NOS (780.4)

781.4 Transient paralysis of limb
Monoplegia, transient NOS

Excludes *paralysis (342.0–344.9)*

781.5 Clubbing of fingers

781.6 Meningismus
Dupré's syndrome
Meningism

781.7 Tetany
Carpopedal spasm

Excludes *tetanus neonatorum (771.3)*
tetany:
hysterical (300.11)
newborn (hypocalcemic) (775.4)
parathyroid (252.1)
psychogenic (306.0)

781.8 Neurologic neglect syndrome
Asomatognosia
Hemi-akinesia
Hemi-inattention
Hemispatial neglect
Left-sided neglect
Sensory extinction
Sensory neglect
Visuospatial neglect

● **781.9 Other symptoms involving nervous and musculoskeletal systems**

781.91 Loss of height

Excludes *osteoporosis (733.00–733.09)*

781.92 Abnormal posture

781.93 Ocular torticollis

781.94 Facial weakness
Facial droop

Excludes *facial weakness due to late effect of cerebrovascular accident (438.83)*

781.99 Other symptoms involving nervous and musculoskeletal system

● **782 Symptoms involving skin and other integumentary tissue**

Excludes *symptoms relating to breast (611.71–611.79)*

782.0 Disturbance of skin sensation
Anesthesia of skin
Burning or prickling sensation
Hyperesthesia
Hypoesthesia
Numbness
Paresthesia
Tingling

❑**782.1 Rash and other nonspecific skin eruption**
Exanthem

Excludes *vesicular eruption (709.8)*

782.2 Localized superficial swelling, mass, or lump
Subcutaneous nodules

Excludes *localized adiposity (278.1)*

782.3 Edema
Anasarca
Dropsy
Localized edema NOS

Excludes *ascites (789.5)*
edema of:
newborn NOS (778.5)
pregnancy (642.0–642.9, 646.1)
fluid retention (276.6)
hydrops fetalis (773.3, 778.0)
hydrothorax (511.8)
nutritional edema (260, 262)

❑**782.4 Jaundice, unspecified, not of newborn**
Cholemia NOS
Icterus NOS

Excludes *due to isoimmunization (773.0–773.2, 773.4)*
jaundice in newborn (774.0–774.7)

782.5 Cyanosis

Excludes *newborn (770.83)*

● **782.6 Pallor and flushing**

❑**782.61 Pallor**

❑**782.62 Flushing**
Excessive blushing

782.7 Spontaneous ecchymoses
Petechiae

Excludes *ecchymosis in fetus or newborn (772.6)*
purpura (287.0–287.9)

782.8 Changes in skin texture
Induration of skin
Thickening of skin

❑**782.9 Other symptoms involving skin and integumentary tissues**

● **783 Symptoms concerning nutrition, metabolism, and development**

783.0 Anorexia
Loss of appetite

Excludes *anorexia nervosa (307.1)*
loss of appetite of nonorganic origin (307.59)

783.1 Abnormal weight gain

Excludes *excessive weight gain in pregnancy (646.1)*
obesity (278.00)
morbid (278.01)

● **783.2 Abnormal loss of weight and underweight**
Use additional code to identify Body Mass Index (BMI), if known (V85.0–V85.54) ⬅

783.21 Loss of weight

783.22 Underweight

783.3 Feeding difficulties and mismanagement
Feeding problem (elderly) (infant)

Excludes *feeding disturbance or problems:*
in newborn (779.3)
of nonorganic origin (307.50–307.59)

● **783.4 Lack of expected normal physiological development in childhood**

Excludes *delay in sexual development and puberty (259.0)*
gonadal dysgenesis (758.6)
pituitary dwarfism (253.3)
slow fetal growth and fetal malnutrition (764.00–764.99)
specific delays in mental development (315.0–315.9)

❑**783.40 Lack of normal physiological development, unspecified**
Inadequate development
Lack of development

783.41 Failure to thrive
Failure to gain weight

783.42 Delayed milestones
Late talker
Late walker

783.43 Short stature
Growth failure
Growth retardation
Lack of growth
Physical retardation

783.5 Polydipsia
Excessive thirst

783.6 Polyphagia
Excessive eating
Hyperalimentation NOS

Excludes *disorders of eating of nonorganic origin (307.50–307.59)*

783.7 Adult failure to thrive

❑**783.9 Other symptoms concerning nutrition, metabolism, and development**
Hypometabolism

Excludes *abnormal basal metabolic rate (794.7)*
dehydration (276.51)
other disorders of fluid, electrolyte, and acid-base balance (276.0–276.9)

● **784 Symptoms involving head and neck**

Excludes *encephalopathy NOS (348.30)*
specific symptoms involving neck classifiable to 723 (723.0–723.9)

784.0 Headache
Facial pain
Pain in head NOS

Excludes *atypical face pain (350.2)*
migraine (346.0–346.9)
tension headache (307.81)

784.1 Throat pain

Excludes *dysphagia (787.2)*
neck pain (723.1)
sore throat (462)
chronic (472.1)

784.2 Swelling, mass, or lump in head and neck
Space-occupying lesion, intracranial NOS

784.3 Aphasia

Excludes *aphasia due to late effects of cerebrovascular disease (438.11)* ◀
developmental aphasia (315.31)

● **784.4 Voice disturbance**

❑**784.40 Voice disturbance, unspecified**

784.41 Aphonia
Loss of voice

❑**784.49 Other**
Change in voice
Dysphonia
Hoarseness
Hypernasality
Hyponasality

❑**784.5 Other speech disturbance**
Dysarthria
Dysphasia
Slurred speech

Excludes *stammering and stuttering (307.0)*
that of nonorganic origin (307.0, 307.9)

● **784.6 Other symbolic dysfunction**

Excludes *developmental learning delays (315.0–315.9)*

❑**784.60 Symbolic dysfunction, unspecified**

784.61 Alexia and dyslexia
Alexia (with agraphia)

ICD-9-CM 700-799 Vol. 1

❑784.69 Other
Acalculia
Agnosia
Agraphia NOS
Apraxia

784.7 Epistaxis
Hemorrhage from nose
Nosebleed

784.8 Hemorrhage from throat
Excludes *hemoptysis (786.3)*

● 784.9 Other symptoms involving head and neck ⬅

784.91 Postnasal drip ◀

❑784.99 Other symptoms involving head and neck ◀
Choking sensation ◀
Halitosis ◀
Mouth breathing ◀
Sneezing ◀

● 785 Symptoms involving cardiovascular system
Excludes *heart failure NOS (428.9)*

❑785.0 Tachycardia, unspecified
Rapid heart beat
Excludes *neonatal tachycardia (779.82)*
paroxysmal tachycardia (427.0–427.2)

785.1 Palpitations
Awareness of heart beat
Excludes *specified dysrhythmias (427.0–427.9)*

785.2 Undiagnosed cardiac murmurs
Heart murmur NOS

❑785.3 Other abnormal heart sounds
Cardiac dullness, increased or decreased
Friction fremitus, cardiac
Precordial friction

785.4 Gangrene
Gangrene:
NOS
spreading cutaneous
Gangrenous cellulitis
Phagedena
Code first any associated underlying condition
Excludes *gangrene of certain sites—see Alphabetic Index*
gangrene with atherosclerosis of the extremities (440.24)
gas gangrene (040.0)

● 785.5 Shock without mention of trauma

❑785.50 Shock, unspecified
Failure of peripheral circulation

785.51 Cardiogenic shock

● *785.52 Septic shock* ⬅
Endotoxic
Gram-negative
Code first:
systemic inflammatory response syndrome due to infectious process with organ dysfunction (995.92)

❑785.59 Other
Shock:
hypovolemic
Excludes *shock (due to):*
anesthetic (995.4)
anaphylactic (995.0)
due to serum (999.4)
electric (994.8)
following abortion (639.5)
lightning (994.0)
obstetrical (669.1)
postoperative (998.0)
traumatic (958.4)

785.6 Enlargement of lymph nodes
Lymphadenopathy
"Swollen glands"
Excludes *lymphadenitis (chronic) (289.1–289.3)*
acute (683)

❑785.9 Other symptoms involving cardiovascular system
Bruit (arterial)
Weak pulse

● 786 Symptoms involving respiratory system and other chest symptoms

● 786.0 Dyspnea and respiratory abnormalities

❑786.00 Respiratory abnormality, unspecified

786.01 Hyperventilation
Excludes *hyperventilation, psychogenic (306.1)*

786.02 Orthopnea

786.03 Apnea
Excludes *apnea of newborn (770.81, 770.82)*
sleep apnea (780.51, 780.53, 780.57)

786.04 Cheyne-Stokes respiration

786.05 Shortness of breath

786.06 Tachypnea
Excludes *transitory tachypnea of newborn (770.6)*

786.07 Wheezing
Excludes *asthma (493.00–493.92)*

❑786.09 Other
Respiratory:
distress
insufficiency
Excludes *respiratory distress:*
following trauma and surgery (518.5)
newborn (770.89)
respiratory failure (518.81, 518.83–518.84)
newborn (770.84)
syndrome (newborn) (769)
adult (518.5)

786.1 Stridor
Excludes *congenital laryngeal stridor (748.3)*

786.2 Cough
Excludes *cough:*
psychogenic (306.1)
smokers' (491.0)
with hemorrhage (786.3)

786.3 Hemoptysis
Cough with hemorrhage
Pulmonary hemorrhage NOS
Excludes *pulmonary hemorrhage of newborn (770.3)*

786.4 Abnormal sputum
Abnormal:
amount of sputum
color of sputum
odor of sputum
Excessive sputum

● 786.5 Chest pain

❑786.50 Chest pain, unspecified

786.51 Precordial pain

786.52 Painful respiration
Pain:
anterior chest wall
pleuritic
pleurodynia
Excludes *epidemic pleurodynia (074.1)*

❑786.59 Other
Discomfort in chest
Pressure in chest
Tightness in chest
Excludes *pain in breast (611.71)*

786.6 Swelling, mass, or lump in chest
Excludes *lump in breast (611.72)*

786.7 Abnormal chest sounds
Abnormal percussion, chest
Friction sounds, chest
Rales
Tympany, chest
Excludes *wheezing (786.07)*

786.8 Hiccough
Excludes *psychogenic hiccough (306.1)*

❑ **786.9 Other symptoms involving respiratory system and chest**
Breath-holding spell

● **787 Symptoms involving digestive system**
Excludes *constipation (564.00–564.09)*
pylorospasm (537.81)
congenital (750.5)

● **787.0 Nausea and vomiting**
Emesis
Excludes *hematemesis NOS (578.0)*
vomiting:
bilious, following gastrointestinal surgery (564.3)
cyclical (536.2)
psychogenic (306.4)
excessive, in pregnancy (643.0–643.9)
habit (536.2)
of newborn (779.3)
psychogenic NOS (307.54)

787.01 Nausea with vomiting

787.02 Nausea alone

787.03 Vomiting alone

787.1 Heartburn
Pyrosis
Waterbrash
Excludes *dyspepsia or indigestion (536.8)*

787.2 Dysphagia
Difficulty in swallowing

787.3 Flatulence, eructation, and gas pain
Abdominal distention (gaseous)
Bloating
Tympanites (abdominal) (intestinal)
Excludes *aerophagy (306.4)*

787.4 Visible peristalsis
Hyperperistalsis

787.5 Abnormal bowel sounds
Absent bowel sounds
Hyperactive bowel sounds

787.6 Incontinence of feces
Encopresis NOS
Incontinence of sphincter ani
Excludes *that of nonorganic origin (307.7)*

787.7 Abnormal feces
Bulky stools
Excludes *abnormal stool content (792.1)*
melena:
NOS (578.1)
newborn (772.4, 777.3)

● **787.9 Other symptoms involving digestive system**
Excludes *gastrointestinal hemorrhage (578.0–578.9)*
intestinal obstruction (560.0–560.9)
specific functional digestive disorders:
esophagus (530.0–530.9)
stomach and duodenum (536.0–536.9)
those not elsewhere classified (564.00–564.9)

787.91 Diarrhea
Diarrhea NOS

787.99 Other
Change in bowel habits
Tenesmus (rectal)

● **788 Symptoms involving urinary system**
Excludes *hematuria (599.7)*
nonspecific findings on examination of the urine (791.0–791.9)
small kidney of unknown cause (589.0–589.9)
uremia NOS (586)
urinary obstruction (599.60, 599.69) ◄

788.0 Renal colic
Colic (recurrent) of:
kidney
ureter

788.1 Dysuria
Painful urination
Strangury

● **788.2 Retention of urine** ◄▮▮▮
Code if applicable, any causal condition first, such as: ◄
hyperplasia of prostate (600.0–600.9 with fifth-digit 1) ◄

❑ **788.20 Retention of urine, unspecified**

788.21 Incomplete bladder emptying

❑ **788.29 Other specified retention of urine**

● **788.3 Urinary incontinence**
Excludes *that of nonorganic origin (307.6)*
Code, if applicable, any causal condition first, such as:
congenital ureterocele (753.23)
genital prolapse (618.00–618.9)
hyperplasia of prostate (600.0–600.9 with fifth-digit 1) ◄

❑ **788.30 Urinary incontinence, unspecified**
Enuresis NOS

788.31 Urge incontinence

788.32 Stress incontinence, male
Excludes *stress incontinence, female (625.6)*

788.33 Mixed incontinence (female) (male)
Urge and stress

788.34 Incontinence without sensory awareness

788.35 Post-void dribbling

788.36 Nocturnal enuresis

788.37 Continuous leakage

788.38 Overflow incontinence

❑ **788.39 Other urinary incontinence**

● **788.4 Frequency of urination and polyuria**
Code, if applicable, any causal condition first, such as: ◄
hyperplasia of prostate (600.0–600.9 with fifth-digit 1) ◄

788.41 Urinary frequency
Frequency of micturition

788.42 Polyuria

788.43 Nocturia

788.5 Oliguria and anuria
Deficient secretion of urine
Suppression of urinary secretion
Excludes *that complicating:*
abortion (634–638 with .3, 639.3)
ectopic or molar pregnancy (639.3)
pregnancy, childbirth, or the puerperium (642.0–642.9, 646.2)

● **788.6 Other abnormality of urination**
Code, if applicable, any causal condition first, such as: ◄
hyperplasia of prostate (600.0–600.9 with fifth-digit 1) ◄

788.61 **Splitting of urinary stream**
Intermittent urinary stream

788.62 **Slowing of urinary stream**
Weak stream

788.63 **Urgency of urination**

Excludes *urge incontinence (788.31, 788.33)*

788.64 **Urinary hesitancy** ◀

788.65 **Straining on urination** ◀

❑788.69 **Other**

788.7 **Urethral discharge**
Penile discharge
Urethrorrhea

788.8 **Extravasation of urine**

❑788.9 **Other symptoms involving urinary system**
Extrarenal uremia
Vesical:
pain
tenesmus

● 789 **Other symptoms involving abdomen and pelvis**

The following fifth-digit subclassification is to be used for codes 789.0, 789.3, 789.4, 789.6
❑ 0 **unspecified site**
1 **right upper quadrant**
2 **left upper quadrant**
3 **right lower quadrant**
4 **left lower quadrant**
5 **periumbilic**
6 **epigastric**
❑ 7 **generalized**
❑ 9 **other specified site**
multiple sites

Excludes *symptoms referable to genital organs:*
female (625.0–625.9)
male (607.0–608.9)
psychogenic (302.70–302.79)

● 789.0 **Abdominal pain**
Colic:
NOS
infantile
Cramps, abdominal

Excludes *renal colic (788.0)*

789.1 **Hepatomegaly**
Enlargement of liver

789.2 **Splenomegaly**
Enlargement of spleen

● 789.3 **Abdominal or pelvic swelling, mass, or lump**
Diffuse or generalized swelling or mass:
abdominal NOS
umbilical

Excludes *abdominal distention (gaseous) (787.3)*
ascites (789.5)

● 789.4 **Abdominal rigidity**

789.5 **Ascites**
Fluid in peritoneal cavity

● 789.6 **Abdominal tenderness**
Rebound tenderness

❑789.9 **Other symptoms involving abdomen and pelvis**
Umbilical:
bleeding
Umbilical:
discharge

NONSPECIFIC ABNORMAL FINDINGS (790–796)

● 790 **Nonspecific findings on examination of blood**

Excludes *abnormality of:*
platelets (287.0–287.9)
thrombocytes (287.0–287.9)
white blood cells (288.00–288.9) ⬅

● 790.0 **Abnormality of red blood cells**

Excludes *anemia:*
congenital (776.5)
newborn, due to isoimmunization (773.0–773.2, 773.5)
of premature infant (776.6)
other specified types (280.0–285.9)
hemoglobin disorders (282.5–282.7)
polycythemia:
familial (289.6)
neonatorum (776.4)
secondary (289.0)
vera (238.4)

790.01 **Precipitous drop in hematocrit**
Drop in hematocrit

❑790.09 **Other abnormality of red blood cells**
Abnormal red cell morphology NOS
Abnormal red cell volume NOS
Anisocytosis
Poikilocytosis

❑790.1 **Elevated sedimentation rate**

● 790.2 **Abnormal glucose**

Excludes *diabetes mellitus (250.00–250.93)*
dysmetabolic syndrome X (277.7)
gestational diabetes (648.8)
glycosuria (791.5)
hypoglycemia (251.2)
that complicating pregnancy, childbirth, or the puerperium (648.8)

790.21 **Impaired fasting glucose**
Elevated fasting glucose

790.22 **Impaired glucose tolerance test (oral)**
Elevated glucose tolerance test

790.29 **Other abnormal glucose**
Abnormal glucose NOS
Abnormal non-fasting glucose
Hyperglycemia NOS ◀
Pre-diabetes NOS

790.3 **Excessive blood level of alcohol**
Elevated blood-alcohol

❑790.4 **Nonspecific elevation of levels of transaminase or lactic acid dehydrogenase [LDH]**

❑790.5 **Other nonspecific abnormal serum enzyme levels**
Abnormal serum level of:
acid phosphatase
alkaline phosphatase
amylase
lipase

Excludes *deficiency of circulating enzymes (277.6)*

❑790.6 **Other abnormal blood chemistry**
Abnormal blood levels of:
cobalt
copper
iron
lead ◀
lithium
magnesium
mineral
zinc

Excludes *abnormality of electrolyte or acid-base balance (276.0–276.9)*
hypoglycemia NOS (251.2)
lead poisoning (984.0–984.9) ◀
specific finding indicating abnormality of:
amino-acid transport and metabolism (270.0–270.9)
carbohydrate transport and metabolism (271.0–271.9)
lipid metabolism (272.0–272.9)
uremia NOS (586)

790.7 **Bacteremia**

Excludes *bacteremia of newborn (771.83)*
septicemia (038)

Use additional code to identify organism (041)

790.8 **Viremia, unspecified**

790.9 **Other nonspecific findings on examination of blood**

790.91 **Abnormal arterial blood gases**

790.92 **Abnormal coagulation profile**

Abnormal or prolonged:
bleeding time
coagulation time
partial thromboplastin time [PTT]
prothrombin time [PT]

Excludes *coagulation (hemorrhagic) disorders (286.0–286.9)*

790.93 **Elevated prostate specific antigen [PSA]**

790.94 **Euthyroid sick syndrome**

790.95 **Elevated C-reactive protein (CRP)**

790.99 **Other**

791 **Nonspecific findings on examination of urine**

Excludes *hematuria NOS (599.7)*
specific findings indicating abnormality of:
amino-acid transport and metabolism (270.0–270.9)
carbohydrate transport and metabolism (271.0–271.9)

791.0 **Proteinuria**

Albuminuria
Bence-Jones proteinuria

Excludes *postural proteinuria (593.6)*
that arising during pregnancy or the puerperium (642.0–642.9, 646.2)

791.1 **Chyluria**

Excludes *filarial (125.0–125.9)*

791.2 **Hemoglobinuria**

791.3 **Myoglobinuria**

791.4 **Biliuria**

791.5 **Glycosuria**

Excludes *renal glycosuria (271.4)*

791.6 **Acetonuria**

Ketonuria

791.7 **Other cells and casts in urine**

791.9 **Other nonspecific findings on examination of urine**

Crystalluria
Elevated urine levels of:
17-ketosteroids
catecholamines
indolacetic acid
vanillylmandelic acid [VMA]
Melanuria

792 **Nonspecific abnormal findings in other body substances**

Excludes *that in chromosomal analysis (795.2)*

792.0 **Cerebrospinal fluid**

792.1 **Stool contents**

Abnormal stool color
Fat in stool
Mucus in stool
Occult blood
Pus in stool

Excludes *blood in stool [melena] (578.1)*
newborn (772.4, 777.3)

792.2 **Semen**

Abnormal spermatozoa

Excludes *azoospermia (606.0)*
oligospermia (606.1)

792.3 **Amniotic fluid**

792.4 **Saliva**

Excludes *that in chromosomal analysis (795.2)*

792.5 **Cloudy (hemodialysis) (peritoneal) dialysis effluent**

792.9 **Other nonspecific abnormal findings in body substances**

Peritoneal fluid
Pleural fluid
Synovial fluid
Vaginal fluids

793 **Nonspecific abnormal findings on radiological and other examination of body structure**

Includes: nonspecific abnormal findings of:
thermography
ultrasound examination [echogram]
x-ray examination

Excludes *abnormal results of function studies and radioisotope scans (794.0–794.9)*

793.0 **Skull and head**

Excludes *nonspecific abnormal echoencephalogram (794.01)*

793.1 **Lung field**

Coin lesion lung
Shadow, lung

793.2 **Other intrathoracic organ**

Abnormal:
echocardiogram
heart shadow
ultrasound cardiogram
Mediastinal shift

793.3 **Biliary tract**

Nonvisualization of gallbladder

793.4 **Gastrointestinal tract**

793.5 **Genitourinary organs**

Filling defect:
bladder
kidney
ureter

793.6 **Abdominal area, including retroperitoneum**

793.7 **Musculoskeletal system**

793.8 **Breast**

793.80 **Abnormal mammogram, unspecified**

793.81 **Mammographic microcalcification**

Excludes *mammographic calcification (793.89)*
mammographic calculus (793.89)

793.89 **Other abnormal findings on radiological examination of breast**

Mammographic calcification
Mammographic calculus

793.9 **Other**

Excludes *abnormal finding by radioisotope localization of placenta (794.9)*

793.91 **Image test inconclusive due to excess body fat**

Use additional code to identify Body Mass Index (BMI), if known (V85.0–V85.54)

793.99 **Other nonspecific abnormal findings on radiological and other examinations of body structure**

Abnormal:
placental finding by x-ray or ultrasound method
radiological findings in skin and subcutaneous tissue

794 **Nonspecific abnormal results of function studies**

Includes: radioisotope:
scans
uptake studies
scintiphotography

ICD-9-CM 700-799 Vol. 1

● 794.0 Brain and central nervous system

❑ 794.00 Abnormal function study, unspecified

794.01 Abnormal echoencephalogram

794.02 Abnormal electroencephalogram [EEG]

794.09 Other
Abnormal brain scan

● 794.1 Peripheral nervous system and special senses

❑ 794.10 Abnormal response to nerve stimulation, unspecified

794.11 Abnormal retinal function studies
Abnormal electroretinogram [ERG]

794.12 Abnormal electro-oculogram [EOG]

794.13 Abnormal visually evoked potential

794.14 Abnormal oculomotor studies

794.15 Abnormal auditory function studies

794.16 Abnormal vestibular function studies

794.17 Abnormal electromyogram [EMG]

Excludes *that of eye (794.14)*

❑ 794.19 Other

794.2 Pulmonary
Abnormal lung scan
Reduced:
ventilatory capacity
vital capacity

● 794.3 Cardiovascular

❑ 794.30 Abnormal function study, unspecified

794.31 Abnormal electrocardiogram [ECG] [EKG]

Excludes *long QT syndrome (426.82)*

❑ 794.39 Other
Abnormal:
ballistocardiogram
phonocardiogram
vectorcardiogram

794.4 Kidney
Abnormal renal function test

794.5 Thyroid
Abnormal thyroid:
scan
uptake

❑ 794.6 Other endocrine function study

794.7 Basal metabolism
Abnormal basal metabolic rate [BMR]

794.8 Liver
Abnormal liver scan

❑ 794.9 Other
Bladder
Pancreas
Placenta
Spleen

● 795 Other and nonspecific abnormal cytological, histological, immunological, and DNA test findings

Excludes *nonspecific abnormalities of red blood cells (790.01–790.09)*

● 795.0 Abnormal Papanicolaou smear of cervix and cervical HPV
Abnormal thin preparation smear of cervix
Abnormal cervical cytology

Excludes *carcinoma in-situ of cervix (233.1)*
cervical intraepithelial neoplasia I (CIN I) (622.11)
cervical intraepithelial neoplasia II (CIN II) (622.12)
cervical intraepithelial neoplasia III (CIN III) (233.1)
dysplasia (histologically confirmed) of cervix (uteri) NOS (622.10)
mild dysplasia (histologically confirmed) (622.11)
moderate dysplasia (histologically confirmed) (622.12)
severe dysplasia (histological confirmed) (233.1)

❑ 795.00 Abnormal glandular Papanicolaou smear of cervix
Atypical endocervical cells NOS
Atypical endometrial cells NOS
Atypical glandular cells NOS

795.01 Papanicolaou smear of cervix with atypical squamous cells of undetermined significance (ASC-US)

795.02 Papanicolaou smear of cervix with atypical squamous cells cannot exclude high grade squamous intraepithelial lesion (ASC-H)

795.03 Papanicolaou smear of cervix with low grade sqaumous intraepithelial lesion (LGSIL)

795.04 Papanicolaou smear of cervix with high grade squamous intraepithelial lesion (HGSIL) ⇐

795.05 Cervical high risk human papillomavirus (HPV) DNA test positive

795.06 Papanicolaou smear of cervix with cytologic evidence of malignancy ◄

795.08 Unsatisfactory smear
Inadequate sample

❑ 795.09 Other abnormal Papanicolaou smear of cervix and cervical HVP
Cervical low risk human papillomavirus (HPV) DNA test positive

Use additional code for associated human papillomavirus (079.4)

Excludes *encounter for Papanicolaou cervical smear to confirm findings of recent normal smear following initial abnormal smear (V72.32)*

❑ 795.1 Nonspecific abnormal Papanicolaou smear of other site

❑ 795.2 Nonspecific abnormal findings on chromosomal analysis
Abnormal karyotype

● ❑ 795.3 Nonspecific positive culture findings
Positive culture findings in:
nose
sputum
throat
wound

Excludes *that of:*
blood (790.7–790.8)
urine (791.9)

795.31 Nonspecific positive findings for anthrax
Positive findings by nasal swab

❑ 795.39 Other nonspecific positive culture findings

❑ 795.4 Other nonspecific abnormal histological findings

❑ 795.5 Nonspecific reaction to tuberculin skin test without active tuberculosis
Abnormal result of Mantoux test
PPD positive
Tuberculin (skin test):
positive
reactor

795.6 False positive serological test for syphilis
False positive Wassermann reaction

● 795.7 Other nonspecific immunological findings

Excludes *abnormal tumor markers (795.81–795.89)* ◄
elevated prostate specific antigen [PSA] (790.93) ◄
elevated tumor associated antigens (795.81–795.89) ◄
isoimmunization, in pregnancy (656.1–656.2)
affecting fetus or newborn (773.0–773.2)

❑795.71 **Nonspecific serologic evidence of human immunodeficiency virus [HIV]**
Inconclusive human immunodeficiency virus [HIV] test (adult) (infant)

Note: This code is ONLY to be used when a test finding is reported as nonspecific. Asymptomatic positive findings are coded to V08. If any HIV infection symptom or condition is present, see code 042. Negative findings are not coded.

Excludes *acquired immunodeficiency syndrome [AIDS] (042)*
asymptomatic human immunodeficiency virus [HIV] infection status (V08)
HIV infection, symptomatic (042)
human immunodeficiency virus [HIV] disease (042)
positive (status) NOS (V08)

❑795.79 **Other and unspecified nonspecific immunological findings**
Raised antibody titer
Raised level of immunoglobulins

● 795.8 **Abnormal tumor markers** ◀
Elevated tumor associated antigens [TAA] ◀
Elevated tumor specific antigens [TSA] ◀

Excludes *elevated prostate specific antigen [PSA] (790.93)* ◀

795.81 **Elevated carcinoembryonic antigen [CEA]** ◀

795.82 **Elevated cancer antigen 125 [CA 125]** ◀

❑795.89 **Other abnormal tumor markers** ◀

● 796 **Other nonspecific abnormal findings**

❑796.0 **Nonspecific abnormal toxicological findings**
Abnormal levels of heavy metals or drugs in blood, urine, or other tissue

Excludes *excessive blood level of alcohol (790.3)*

796.1 **Abnormal reflex**

796.2 **Elevated blood pressure reading without diagnosis of hypertension**

Note: This category is to be used to record an episode of elevated blood pressure in a patient in whom no formal diagnosis of hypertension has been made, or as an incidental finding.

❑796.3 **Nonspecific low blood pressure reading**

❑796.4 **Other abnormal clinical findings**

❑796.5 **Abnormal finding on antenatal screening**

❑796.6 **Abnormal findings on neonatal screening**

Excludes *nonspecific serologic evidence of human immunodeficiency virus [HIV] (795.71)*

❑796.9 **Other**

ILL-DEFINED AND UNKNOWN CAUSES OF MORBIDITY AND MORTALITY (797–799)

797 **Senility without mention of psychosis**
Old age
Senescence
Senile asthenia
Senile:
debility
exhaustion

Excludes *senile psychoses (290.0–290.9)*

● 798 **Sudden death, cause unknown**

798.0 **Sudden infant death syndrome**
Cot death
Crib death
Sudden death of nonspecific cause in infancy

● 798.1 **Instantaneous death**

● 798.2 **Death occurring in less than 24 hours from onset of symptoms, not otherwise explained**
Death known not to be violent or instantaneous, for which no cause could be discovered
Died without sign of disease

● 798.9 **Unattended death**
Death in circumstances where the body of the deceased was found and no cause could be discovered
Found dead

● 799 **Other ill-defined and unknown causes of morbidity and mortality**

● 799.0 **Asphyxia and hypoxemia**

Excludes *asphyxia and hypoxemia (due to):*
carbon monoxide (986)
hypercapnia (786.09)
inhalation of food or foreign body (932–934.9)
newborn (768.0–768.9)
traumatic (994.7)

799.01 **Asphyxia**

799.02 **Hypoxemia**

799.1 **Respiratory arrest**
Cardiorespiratory failure

Excludes *cardiac arrest (427.5)*
failure of peripheral circulation (785.50)
respiratory distress:
NOS (786.09)
acute (518.82)
following trauma or surgery (518.5)
newborn (770.89)
syndrome (newborn) (769)
adult (following trauma or surgery) (518.5)
other (518.82)
respiratory failure (518.81, 518.83–518.84)
newborn (770.84)
respiratory insufficiency (786.09)
acute (518.82)

799.2 **Nervousness**
"Nerves"

❑799.3 **Debility, unspecified**

Excludes *asthenia (780.79)*
nervous debility (300.5)
neurasthenia (300.5)
senile asthenia (797)

799.4 **Cachexia** ⬅
Wasting disease

Code first underlying condition, if known ◀

● 799.8 **Other ill-defined conditions**

799.81 **Decreased libido**
Decreased sexual desire

Excludes *psychosexual dysfunction with inhibited sexual desire (302.71)*

❑799.89 **Other ill-defined conditions**

❑799.9 **Other unknown and unspecified cause**
Undiagnosed disease, not specified as to site or system involved
Unknown cause of morbidity or mortality

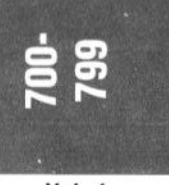
ICD-9-CM
700-799
Vol. 1

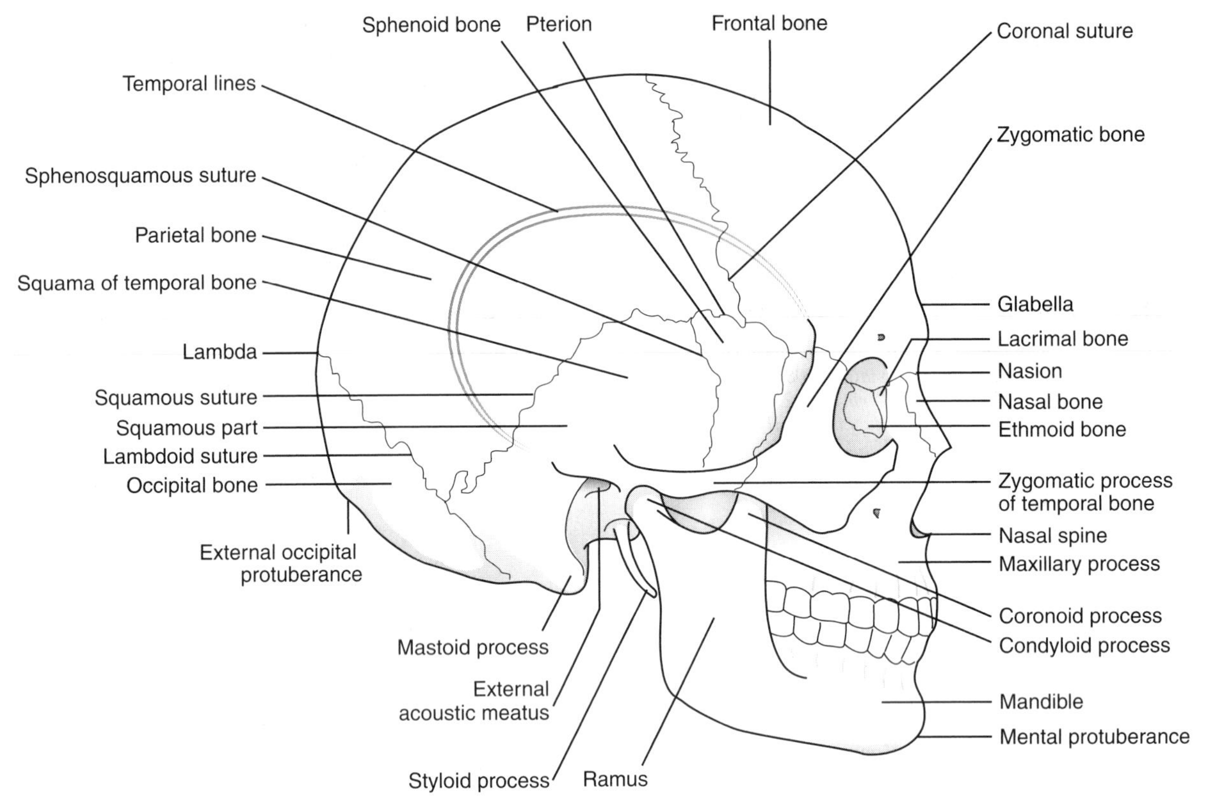
Sphenoid bone
Pterion
Frontal bone
Coronal suture
Temporal lines
Zygomatic bone
Sphenosquamous suture
Parietal bone
Squama of temporal bone
Glabella
Lacrimal bone
Lambda
Nasion
Squamous suture
Nasal bone
Squamous part
Ethmoid bone
Lambdoid suture
Occipital bone
Zygomatic process of temporal bone
Nasal spine
External occipital protuberance
Maxillary process
Coronoid process
Mastoid process
Condyloid process
External acoustic meatus
Mandible
Mental protuberance
Styloid process
Ramus

Figure 17–1 Lateral view of skull.

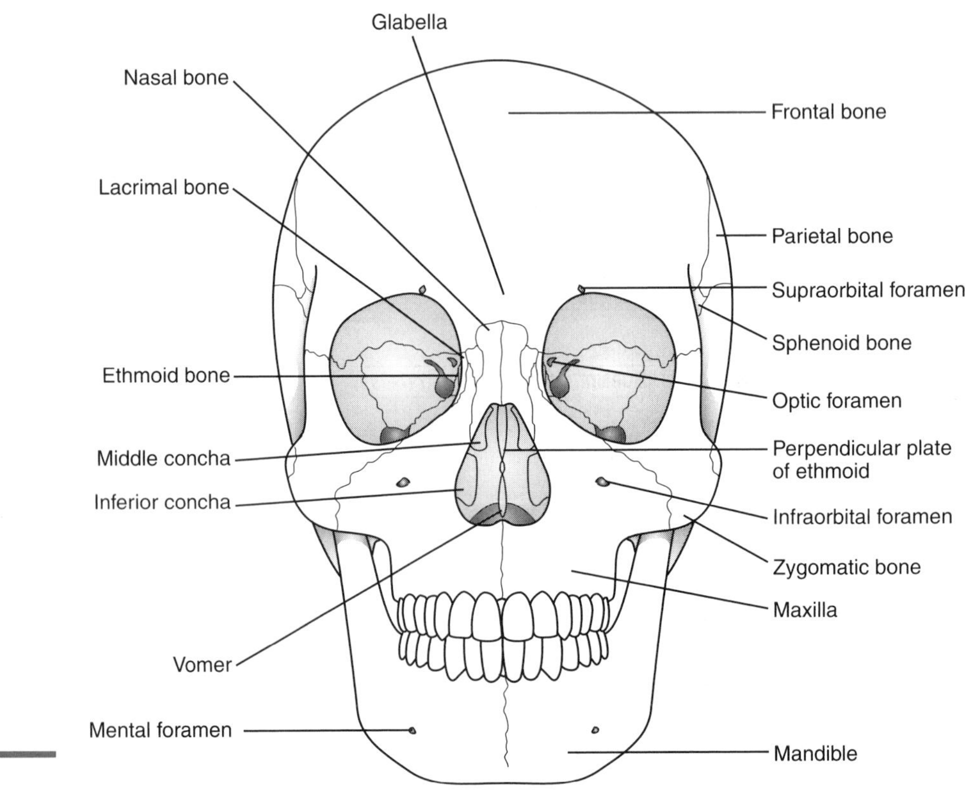
Glabella
Nasal bone
Frontal bone
Lacrimal bone
Parietal bone
Supraorbital foramen
Sphenoid bone
Ethmoid bone
Optic foramen
Middle concha
Perpendicular plate of ethmoid
Inferior concha
Infraorbital foramen
Zygomatic bone
Maxilla
Vomer
Mental foramen
Mandible

Figure 17–2 Frontal view of skull.

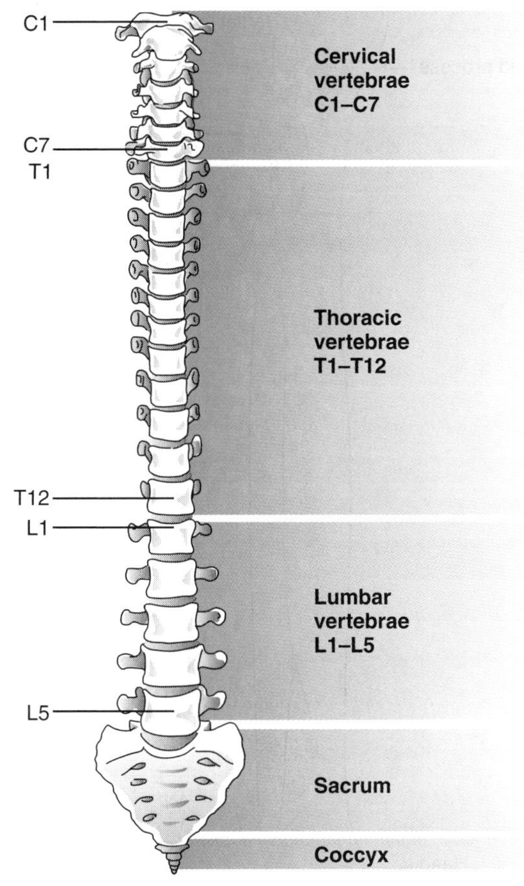
C1
C7
T1
T12
L1
L5
Cervical vertebrae C1–C7
Thoracic vertebrae T1–T12
Lumbar vertebrae L1–L5
Sacrum
Coccyx

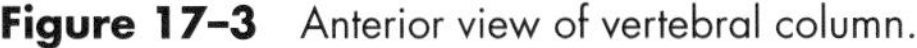

Figure 17–3 Anterior view of vertebral column.

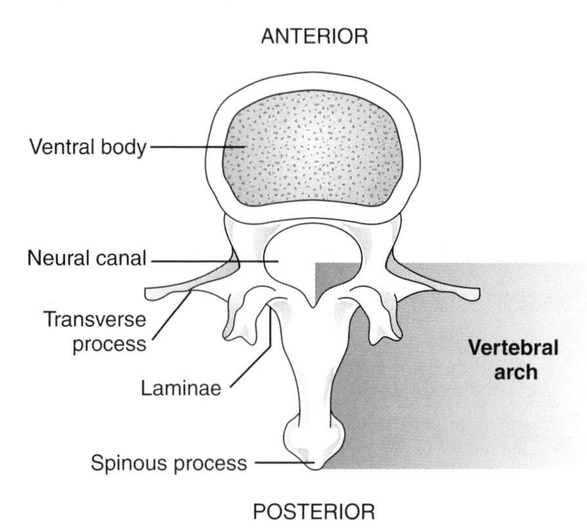
ANTERIOR
Ventral body
Neural canal
Transverse process
Laminae
Spinous process
Vertebral arch
POSTERIOR

Figure 17–4 Vertebra viewed from above.

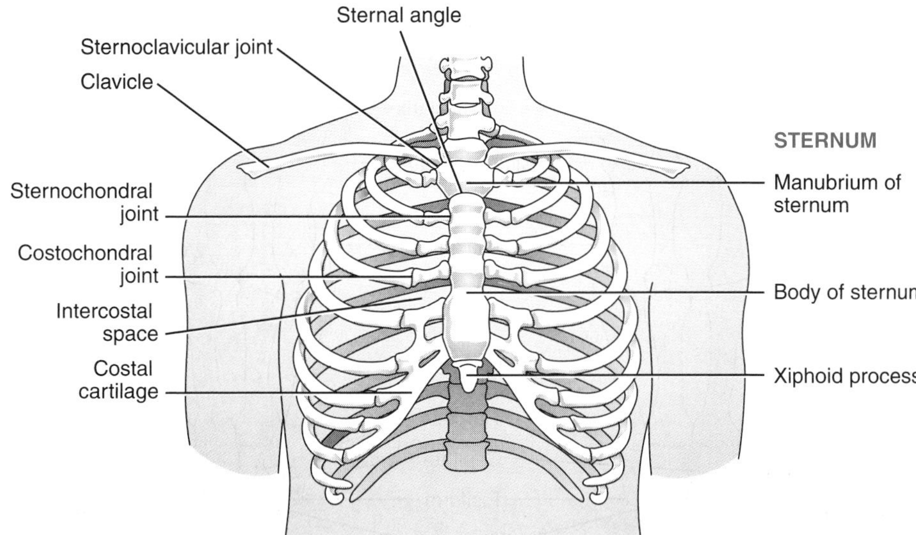
Sternal angle
Sternoclavicular joint
Clavicle
Sternochondral joint
Costochondral joint
Intercostal space
Costal cartilage
STERNUM
Manubrium of sternum
Body of sternum
Xiphoid process

Figure 17–5 Anterior view of rib cage.

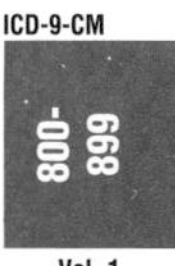
ICD-9-CM
800-999
Vol. 1

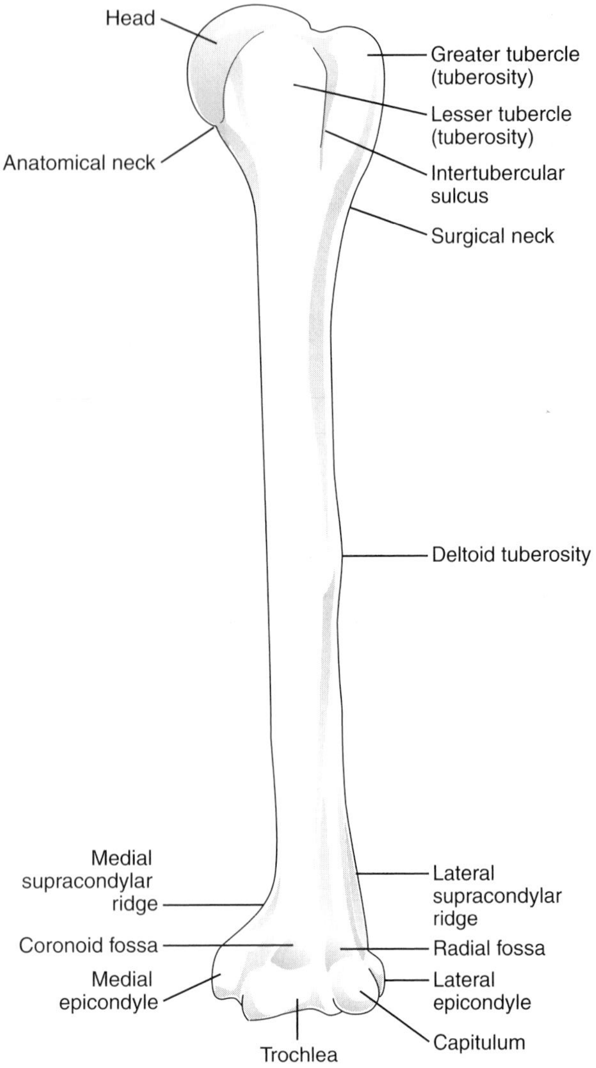

Head
Greater tubercle (tuberosity)
Lesser tubercle (tuberosity)
Anatomical neck
Intertubercular sulcus
Surgical neck
Deltoid tuberosity
Medial supracondylar ridge
Lateral supracondylar ridge
Coronoid fossa
Radial fossa
Medial epicondyle
Lateral epicondyle
Capitulum
Trochlea

Figure 17–6 Anterior aspect of left humerus.

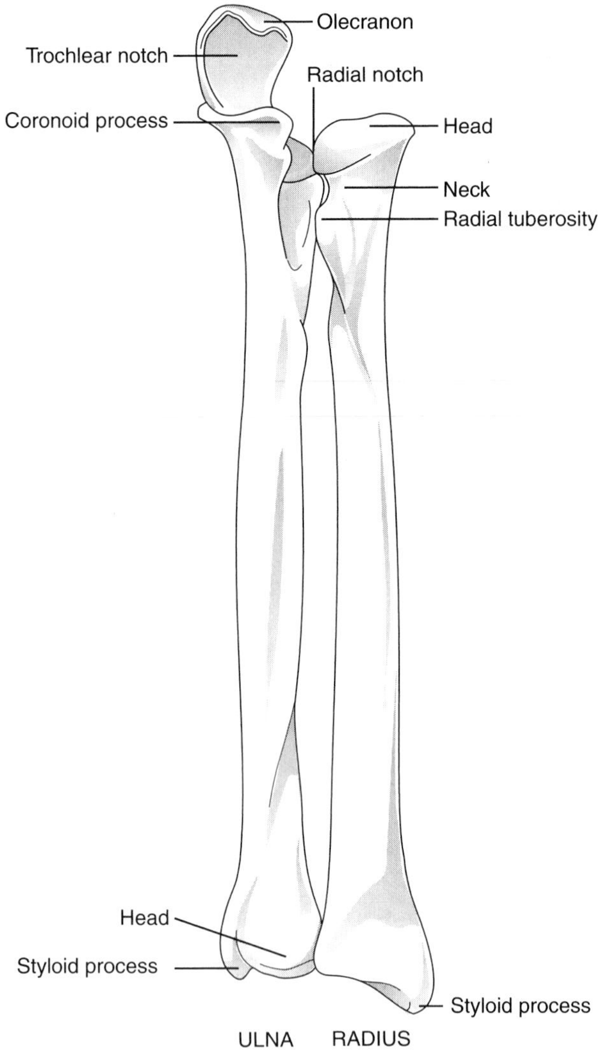

Olecranon
Trochlear notch
Radial notch
Coronoid process
Head
Neck
Radial tuberosity
Head
Styloid process
Styloid process
ULNA
RADIUS

Figure 17–7 Anterior aspect of left radius and ulna.

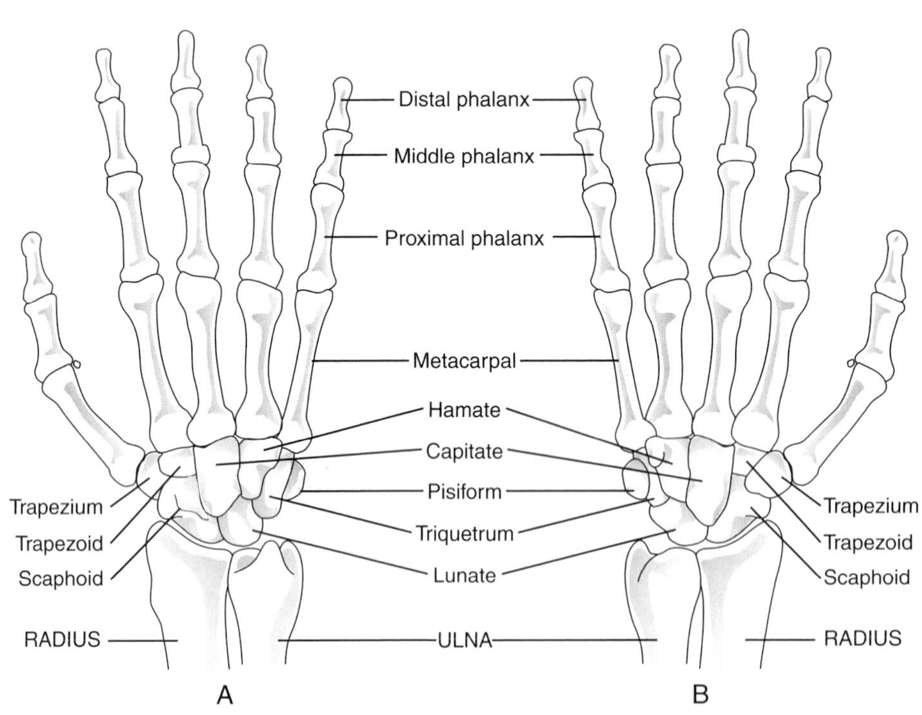
Distal phalanx
Middle phalanx
Proximal phalanx
Metacarpal
Hamate
Capitate
Pisiform
Triquetrum
Lunate
Trapezium
Trapezoid
Scaphoid
Trapezium
Trapezoid
Scaphoid
RADIUS
ULNA
RADIUS
A
B

Figure 17–8 Right hand and wrist: **A.** Dorsal surface. **B.** Palmar surface.

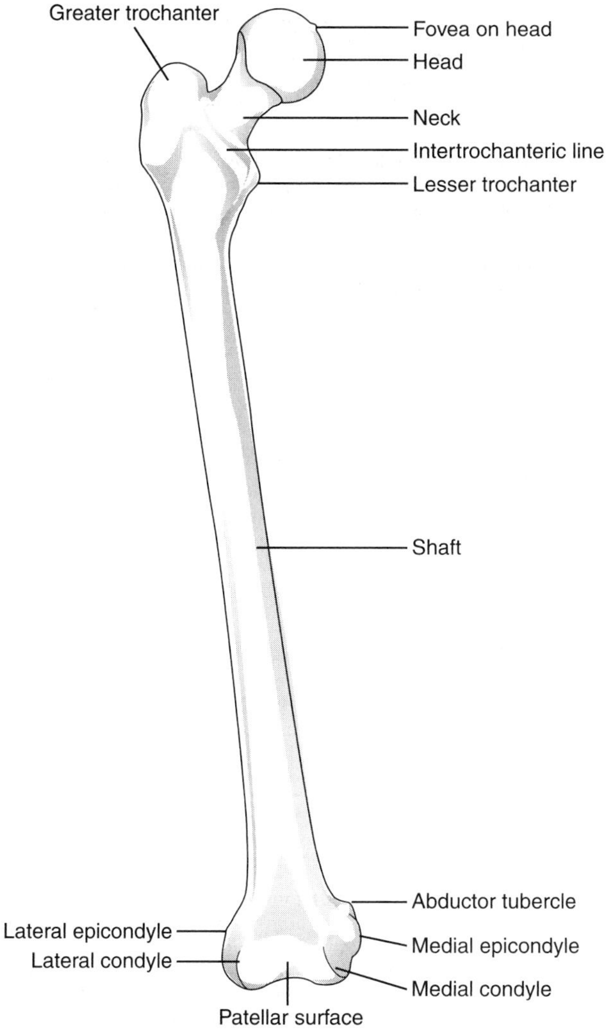

Greater trochanter
Fovea on head
Head
Neck
Intertrochanteric line
Lesser trochanter
Shaft
Abductor tubercle
Lateral epicondyle
Lateral condyle
Medial epicondyle
Medial condyle
Patellar surface

Figure 17–9 Anterior aspect of right femur.

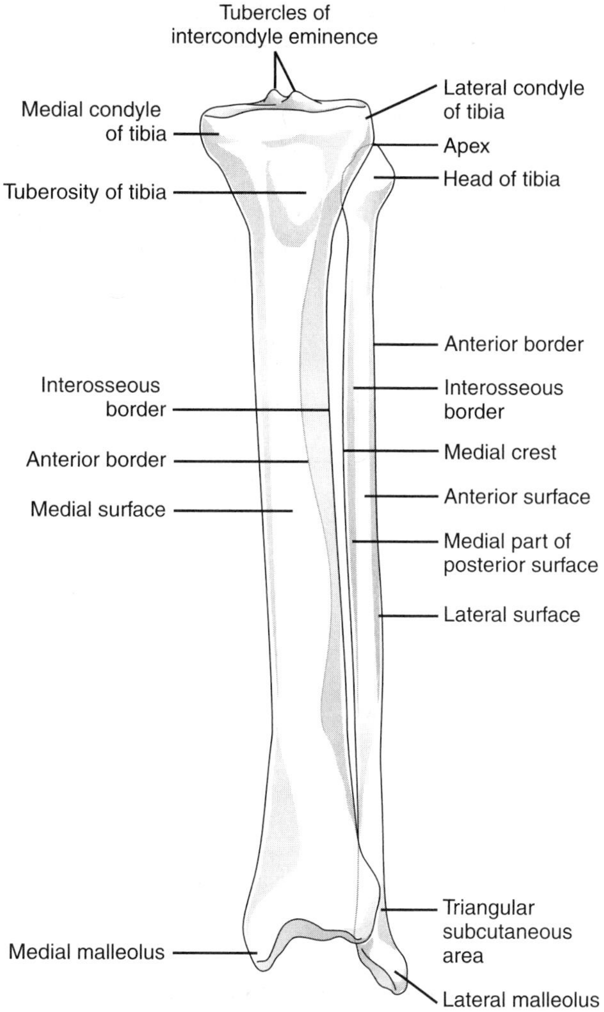

Tubercles of intercondyle eminence
Medial condyle of tibia
Lateral condyle of tibia
Apex
Head of tibia
Tuberosity of tibia
Anterior border
Interosseous border
Interosseous border
Medial crest
Anterior border
Anterior surface
Medial surface
Medial part of posterior surface
Lateral surface
Triangular subcutaneous area
Medial malleolus
Lateral malleolus

Figure 17–10 Anterior aspect of left tibia and fibula.

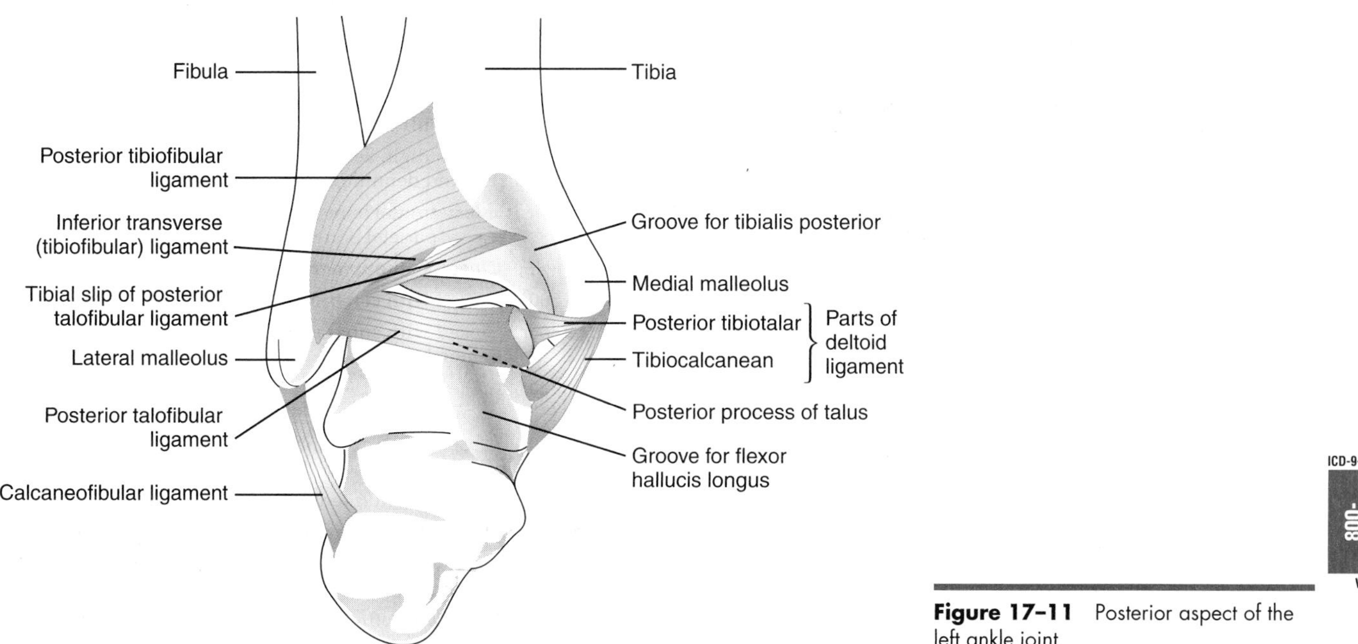
Fibula
Tibia
Posterior tibiofibular ligament
Inferior transverse (tibiofibular) ligament
Groove for tibialis posterior
Medial malleolus
Tibial slip of posterior talofibular ligament
Posterior tibiotalar
Tibiocalcanean
Parts of deltoid ligament
Lateral malleolus
Posterior talofibular ligament
Posterior process of talus
Groove for flexor hallucis longus
Calcaneofibular ligament

Figure 17–11 Posterior aspect of the left ankle joint.

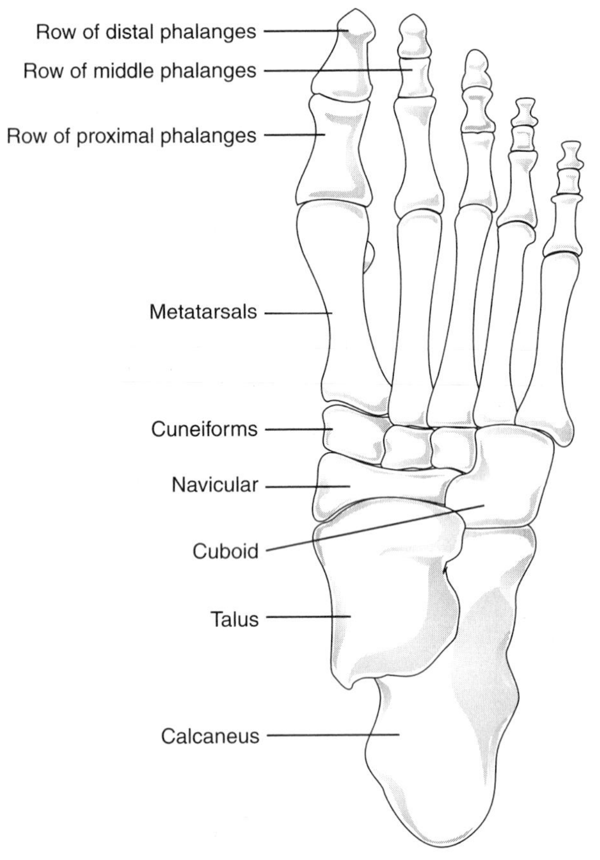
Row of distal phalanges
Row of middle phalanges
Row of proximal phalanges
Metatarsals
Cuneiforms
Navicular
Cuboid
Talus
Calcaneus

Figure 17–12 Right foot viewed from above.

17. INJURY AND POISONING (800–999)

Use E code(s) to identify the cause and intent of the injury or poisoning (E800-E999)

Note:

1. The principle of multiple coding of injuries should be followed wherever possible. Combination categories for multiple injuries are provided for use when there is insufficient detail as to the nature of the individual conditions, or for primary tabulation purposes when it is more convenient to record a single code; otherwise, the component injuries should be coded separately.

   Where multiple sites of injury are specified in the titles, the word "with" indicates involvement of both sites, and the word "and" indicates involvement of either or both sites. The word "finger" includes thumb.

2. Categories for "late effect" of injuries are to be found at 905–909.

FRACTURES (800–829)

Excludes *malunion (733.81)*
nonunion (733.82)
pathologic or spontaneous fracture (733.10–733.19)
stress fractures (733.93–733.95)

The terms "condyle," "coronoid process," "ramus," and "symphysis" indicate the portion of the bone fractured, not the name of the bone involved.

The descriptions "closed" and "open" used in the fourth-digit subdivisions include the following terms:

closed (with or without delayed healing):
- comminuted
- depressed
- elevated
- fissured
- fracture NOS
- greenstick
- impacted
- linear
- simple
- slipped epiphysis
- spiral

open (with or without delayed healing):
- compound
- infected
- missile
- puncture
- with foreign body

Note: A fracture not indicated as closed or open should be classified as closed.

FRACTURE OF SKULL (800–804)

The following fifth-digit subclassification is for use with the appropriate codes in categories 800, 801, 803, and 804:

❑ **0 unspecified state of consciousness**
1 with no loss of consciousness
2 with brief [less than one hour] loss of consciousness
3 with moderate [1–24 hours] loss of consciousness
4 with prolonged [more than 24 hours] loss of consciousness and return to pre-existing conscious level
5 with prolonged [more than 24 hours] loss of consciousness, without return to pre-existing conscious

Use fifth-digit 5 to designate when a patient is unconscious and dies before regaining consciousness, regardless of the duration of the loss of consciousness

❑ **6 with loss of consciousness of unspecified duration**
❑ **9 with concussion, unspecified**

● **800 Fracture of vault of skull**

Requires fifth digit. See beginning of section 800–804 for codes and definitions.

Includes: frontal bone
parietal bone

● **800.0 Closed without mention of intracranial injury**
● **800.1 Closed with cerebral laceration and contusion**
● **800.2 Closed with subarachnoid, subdural, and extradural hemorrhage**
● ❑ **800.3 Closed with other and unspecified intracranial hemorrhage**
● ❑ **800.4 Closed with intracranial injury of other and unspecified nature**
● **800.5 Open without mention of intracranial injury**
● **800.6 Open with cerebral laceration and contusion**
● **800.7 Open with subarachnoid, subdural, and extradural hemorrhage**
● ❑ **800.8 Open with other and unspecified intracranial hemorrhage**

800.9 Open with intracranial injury of other and unspecified nature

801 Fracture of base of skull

Requires fifth digit. See beginning of section 800–804 for codes and definitions.

Includes: fossa:
- anterior
- middle
- posterior

occiput bone
orbital roof
sinus:
- ethmoid
- frontal

sphenoid bone
temporal bone

801.0 Closed without mention of intracranial injury

801.1 Closed with cerebral laceration and contusion

801.2 Closed with subarachnoid, subdural, and extradural hemorrhage

801.3 Closed with other and unspecified intracranial hemorrhage

801.4 Closed with intracranial injury of other and unspecified nature

801.5 Open without mention of intracranial injury

801.6 Open with cerebral laceration and contusion

801.7 Open with subarachnoid, subdural, and extradural hemorrhage

801.8 Open with other and unspecified intracranial hemorrhage

801.9 Open with intracranial injury of other and unspecified nature

802 Fracture of face bones

802.0 Nasal bones, closed

802.1 Nasal bones, open

802.2 Mandible, closed
Inferior maxilla
Lower jaw (bone)

802.20 Unspecified site

802.21 Condylar process

802.22 Subcondylar

802.23 Coronoid process

802.24 Ramus, unspecified

802.25 Angle of jaw

802.26 Symphysis of body

802.27 Alveolar border of body

802.28 Body, other and unspecified

802.29 Multiple sites

802.3 Mandible, open

802.30 Unspecified site

802.31 Condylar process

802.32 Subcondylar

802.33 Coronoid process

802.34 Ramus, unspecified

802.35 Angle of jaw

802.36 Symphysis of body

802.37 Alveolar border of body

802.38 Body, other and unspecified

802.39 Multiple sites

802.4 Malar and maxillary bones, closed
Superior maxilla
Upper jaw (bone)
Zygoma
Zygomatic arch

802.5 Malar and maxillary bones, open

802.6 Orbital floor (blow-out), closed

802.7 Orbital floor (blow-out), open

802.8 Other facial bones, closed
Alveolus
Orbit:
- NOS
- part other than roof or floor

Palate

Excludes *orbital:*
- *floor (802.6)*
- *roof (801.0–801.9)*

802.9 Other facial bones, open

803 Other and unqualified skull fractures

Requires fifth digit. See beginning of section 800–804 for codes and definitions.

Includes: skull NOS
skull multiple NOS

803.0 Closed without mention of intracranial injury

803.1 Closed with cerebral laceration and contusion

803.2 Closed with subarachnoid, subdural, and extradural hemorrhage

803.3 Closed with other and unspecified intracranial hemorrhage

803.4 Closed with intracranial injury of other and unspecified nature

803.5 Open without mention of intracranial injury

803.6 Open with cerebral laceration and contusion

803.7 Open with subarachnoid, subdural, and extradural hemorrhage

803.8 Open with other and unspecified intracranial hemorrhage

803.9 Open with intracranial injury of other and unspecified nature

804 Multiple fractures involving skull or face with other bones

Requires fifth digit. See beginning of section 800–804 for codes and definitions.

804.0 Closed without mention of intracranial injury

804.1 Closed with cerebral laceration and contusion

804.2 Closed with subarachnoid, subdural, and extradural hemorrhage

804.3 Closed with other and unspecified intracranial hemorrhage

804.4 Closed with intracranial injury of other and unspecified nature

804.5 Open without mention of intracranial injury

804.6 Open with cerebral laceration and contusion

804.7 Open with subarachnoid, subdural, and extradural hemorrhage

804.8 Open with other and unspecified intracranial hemorrhage

804.9 Open with intracranial injury of other and unspecified nature

FRACTURE OF NECK AND TRUNK (805–809)

805 Fracture of vertebral column without mention of spinal cord injury

Includes: neural arch
spine
spinous process
transverse process
vertebra

The following fifth-digit subclassification is for use with codes 805.0–805.1:

- 0 **cervical vertebra, unspecified level**
- 1 **first cervical vertebra**
- 2 **second cervical vertebra**
- 3 **third cervical vertebra**
- 4 **fourth cervical vertebra**
- 5 **fifth cervical vertebra**
- 6 **sixth cervical vertebra**
- 7 **seventh cervical vertebra**
- 8 **multiple cervical vertebrae**

805.0 Cervical, closed
Atlas
Axis

805.1 Cervical, open

805.2 Dorsal [thoracic], closed

805.3 Dorsal [thoracic], open

805.4 Lumbar, closed

805.5 Lumbar, open

805.6 Sacrum and coccyx, closed

805.7 Sacrum and coccyx, open

805.8 Unspecified, closed

805.9 Unspecified, open

806 Fracture of vertebral column with spinal cord injury

Includes: any condition classifiable to 805 with:
complete or incomplete transverse lesion (of cord)
hematomyelia
injury to:
cauda equina
nerve
paralysis
paraplegia
quadriplegia
spinal concussion

806.0 Cervical, closed

806.00 C_1-C_4 level with unspecified spinal cord injury
Cervical region NOS with spinal cord injury NOS

806.01 C_1-C_4 level with complete lesion of cord

806.02 C_1-C_4 level with anterior cord syndrome

806.03 C_1-C_4 level with central cord syndrome

806.04 C_1-C_4 level with other specified spinal cord injury
C_1-C_4 level with:
incomplete spinal cord lesion NOS
posterior cord syndrome

806.05 C_5-C_7 level with unspecified spinal cord injury

806.06 C_5-C_7 level with complete lesion of cord

806.07 C_5-C_7 level with anterior cord syndrome

806.08 C_5-C_7 level with central cord syndrome

806.09 C_5-C_7 level with other specified spinal cord injury
C_5-C_7 level with:
incomplete spinal cord lesion NOS
posterior cord syndrome

806.1 Cervical, open

806.10 C_1-C_4 level with unspecified spinal cord injury

806.11 C_1-C_4 level with complete lesion of cord

806.12 C_1-C_4 level with anterior cord syndrome

806.13 C_1-C_4 level with central cord syndrome

806.14 C_1-C_4 level with other specified spinal cord injury
C_1-C_4 level with:
incomplete spinal cord lesion NOS
posterior cord syndrome

806.15 C_5-C_7 level with unspecified spinal cord injury

806.16 C_5-C_7 level with complete lesion of cord

806.17 C_5-C_7 level with anterior cord syndrome

806.18 C_5-C_7 level with central cord syndrome

806.19 C_5-C_7 level with other specified spinal cord injury
C_5-C_7 level with:
incomplete spinal cord lesion NOS
posterior cord syndrome

806.2 Dorsal [thoracic], closed

806.20 T_1-T_6 level with unspecified spinal cord injury
Thoracic region NOS with spinal cord injury NOS

806.21 T_1-T_6 level with complete lesion of cord

806.22 T_1-T_6 level with anterior cord syndrome

806.23 T_1-T_6 level with central cord syndrome

806.24 T_1-T_6 level with other specified spinal cord injury
T_1-T_6 level with:
incomplete spinal cord lesion NOS
posterior cord syndrome

806.25 T_7-T_{12} level with unspecified spinal cord injury

806.26 T_7-T_{12} level with complete lesion of cord

806.27 T_7-T_{12} level with anterior cord syndrome

806.28 T_7-T_{12} level with central cord syndrome

806.29 T_7-T_{12} level with other specified spinal cord injury
T_7-T_{12} level with:
incomplete spinal cord lesion NOS
posterior cord syndrome

806.3 Dorsal [thoracic], open

806.30 T_1-T_6 level with unspecified spinal cord injury

806.31 T_1-T_6 level with complete lesion of cord

806.32 T_1-T_6 level with anterior cord syndrome

806.33 T_1-T_6 level with central cord syndrome

806.34 T_1-T_6 level with other specified spinal cord injury
T_1-T_6 level with:
incomplete spinal cord lesion NOS
posterior cord syndrome

806.35 T_7-T_{12} level with unspecified spinal cord injury

806.36 T_7-T_{12} level with complete lesion of cord

806.37 T_7-T_{12} level with anterior cord syndrome

806.38 T_7-T_{12} level with central cord syndrome

806.39 T_7-T_{12} level with other specified spinal cord injury
T_7-T_{12} level with:
incomplete spinal cord lesion NOS
posterior cord syndrome

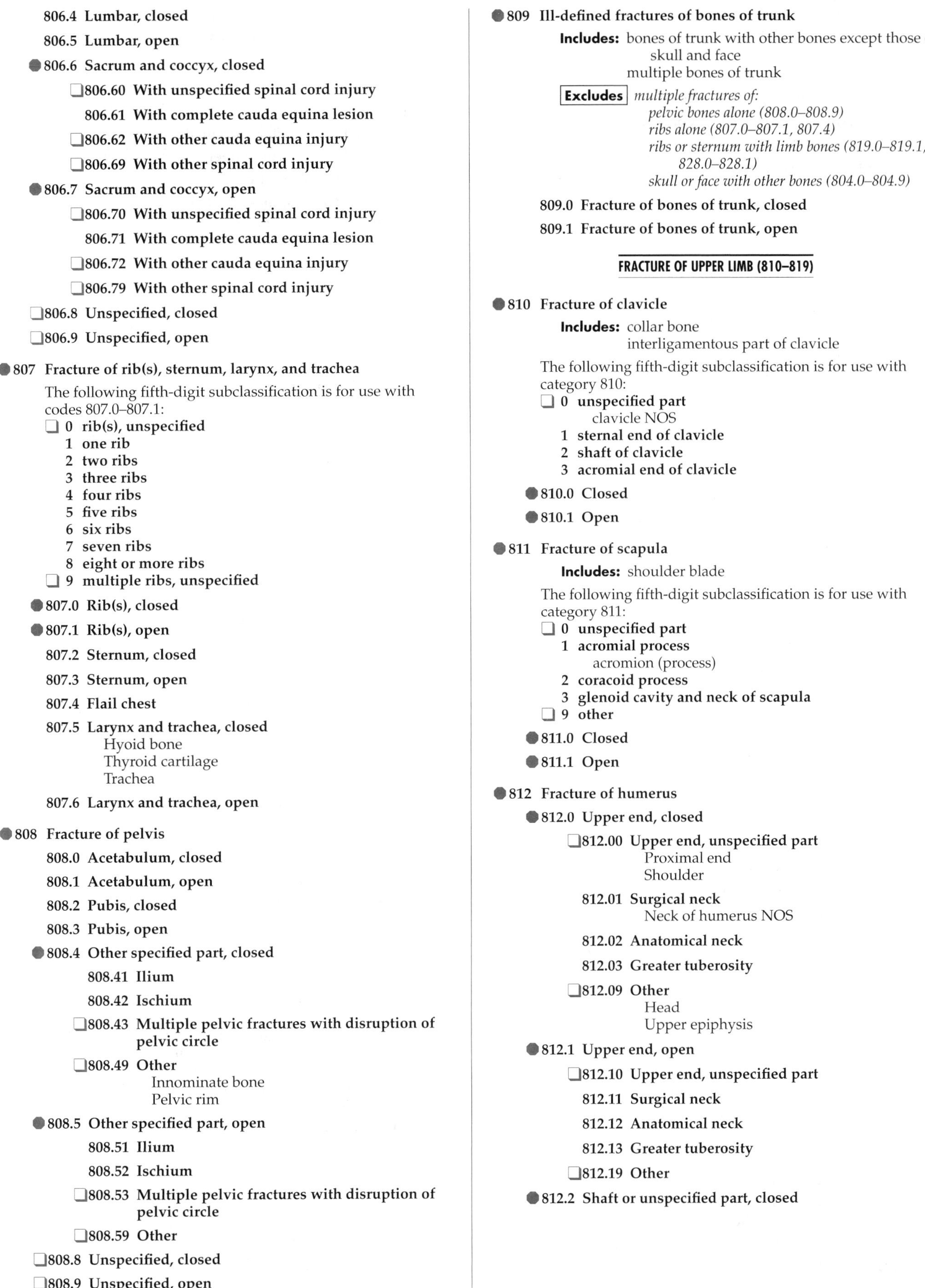

806.4 **Lumbar, closed**

806.5 **Lumbar, open**

● 806.6 **Sacrum and coccyx, closed**

❑ 806.60 **With unspecified spinal cord injury**

806.61 **With complete cauda equina lesion**

❑ 806.62 **With other cauda equina injury**

❑ 806.69 **With other spinal cord injury**

● 806.7 **Sacrum and coccyx, open**

❑ 806.70 **With unspecified spinal cord injury**

806.71 **With complete cauda equina lesion**

❑ 806.72 **With other cauda equina injury**

❑ 806.79 **With other spinal cord injury**

❑ 806.8 **Unspecified, closed**

❑ 806.9 **Unspecified, open**

● 807 **Fracture of rib(s), sternum, larynx, and trachea**

The following fifth-digit subclassification is for use with codes 807.0–807.1:

❑ 0 **rib(s), unspecified**
1 **one rib**
2 **two ribs**
3 **three ribs**
4 **four ribs**
5 **five ribs**
6 **six ribs**
7 **seven ribs**
8 **eight or more ribs**
❑ 9 **multiple ribs, unspecified**

● 807.0 **Rib(s), closed**

● 807.1 **Rib(s), open**

807.2 **Sternum, closed**

807.3 **Sternum, open**

807.4 **Flail chest**

807.5 **Larynx and trachea, closed**
Hyoid bone
Thyroid cartilage
Trachea

807.6 **Larynx and trachea, open**

● 808 **Fracture of pelvis**

808.0 **Acetabulum, closed**

808.1 **Acetabulum, open**

808.2 **Pubis, closed**

808.3 **Pubis, open**

● 808.4 **Other specified part, closed**

808.41 **Ilium**

808.42 **Ischium**

❑ 808.43 **Multiple pelvic fractures with disruption of pelvic circle**

❑ 808.49 **Other**
Innominate bone
Pelvic rim

● 808.5 **Other specified part, open**

808.51 **Ilium**

808.52 **Ischium**

❑ 808.53 **Multiple pelvic fractures with disruption of pelvic circle**

❑ 808.59 **Other**

❑ 808.8 **Unspecified, closed**

❑ 808.9 **Unspecified, open**

● 809 **Ill-defined fractures of bones of trunk**

Includes: bones of trunk with other bones except those of skull and face
multiple bones of trunk

Excludes *multiple fractures of:*
pelvic bones alone (808.0–808.9)
ribs alone (807.0–807.1, 807.4)
ribs or sternum with limb bones (819.0–819.1, 828.0–828.1)
skull or face with other bones (804.0–804.9)

809.0 **Fracture of bones of trunk, closed**

809.1 **Fracture of bones of trunk, open**

FRACTURE OF UPPER LIMB (810–819)

● 810 **Fracture of clavicle**

Includes: collar bone
interligamentous part of clavicle

The following fifth-digit subclassification is for use with category 810:

❑ 0 **unspecified part**
clavicle NOS
1 **sternal end of clavicle**
2 **shaft of clavicle**
3 **acromial end of clavicle**

● 810.0 **Closed**

● 810.1 **Open**

● 811 **Fracture of scapula**

Includes: shoulder blade

The following fifth-digit subclassification is for use with category 811:

❑ 0 **unspecified part**
1 **acromial process**
acromion (process)
2 **coracoid process**
3 **glenoid cavity and neck of scapula**
❑ 9 **other**

● 811.0 **Closed**

● 811.1 **Open**

● 812 **Fracture of humerus**

● 812.0 **Upper end, closed**

❑ 812.00 **Upper end, unspecified part**
Proximal end
Shoulder

812.01 **Surgical neck**
Neck of humerus NOS

812.02 **Anatomical neck**

812.03 **Greater tuberosity**

❑ 812.09 **Other**
Head
Upper epiphysis

● 812.1 **Upper end, open**

❑ 812.10 **Upper end, unspecified part**

812.11 **Surgical neck**

812.12 **Anatomical neck**

812.13 **Greater tuberosity**

❑ 812.19 **Other**

● 812.2 **Shaft or unspecified part, closed**

❑812.20 Unspecified part of humerus
Humerus NOS
Upper arm NOS

812.21 Shaft of humerus

● 812.3 Shaft or unspecified part, open

❑812.30 Unspecified part of humerus

812.31 Shaft of humerus

● 812.4 Lower end, closed
Distal end of humerus
Elbow

❑812.40 Lower end, unspecified part

812.41 Supracondylar fracture of humerus

812.42 Lateral condyle
External condyle

812.43 Medial condyle
Internal epicondyle

❑812.44 Condyle(s), unspecified
Articular process NOS
Lower epiphysis

❑812.49 Other
Multiple fractures of lower end
Trochlea

● 812.5 Lower end, open

❑812.50 Lower end, unspecified part

812.51 Supracondylar fracture of humerus

812.52 Lateral condyle

812.53 Medial condyle

❑812.54 Condyle(s), unspecified

❑812.59 Other

● 813 Fracture of radius and ulna

● 813.0 Upper end, closed
Proximal end

❑813.00 Upper end of forearm, unspecified

813.01 Olecranon process of ulna

813.02 Coronoid process of ulna

813.03 Monteggia's fracture

❑813.04 Other and unspecified fractures of proximal end of ulna (alone)
Multiple fractures of ulna, upper end

813.05 Head of radius

813.06 Neck of radius

❑813.07 Other and unspecified fractures of proximal end of radius (alone)
Multiple fractures of radius, upper end

813.08 Radius with ulna, upper end [any part]

● 813.1 Upper end, open

❑813.10 Upper end of forearm, unspecified

813.11 Olecranon process of ulna

813.12 Coronoid process of ulna

813.13 Monteggia's fracture

❑813.14 Other and unspecified fractures of proximal end of ulna (alone)

813.15 Head of radius

813.16 Neck of radius

❑813.17 Other and unspecified fractures of proximal end of radius (alone)

813.18 Radius with ulna, upper end [any part]

● 813.2 Shaft, closed

❑813.20 Shaft, unspecified

813.21 Radius (alone)

813.22 Ulna (alone)

813.23 Radius with ulna

● 813.3 Shaft, open

❑813.30 Shaft, unspecified

813.31 Radius (alone)

813.32 Ulna (alone)

813.33 Radius with ulna

● 813.4 Lower end, closed
Distal end

❑813.40 Lower end of forearm, unspecified

813.41 Colles' fracture
Smith's fracture

❑813.42 Other fractures of distal end of radius (alone)
Dupuytren's fracture, radius
Radius, lower end

813.43 Distal end of ulna (alone)
Ulna:
head
lower end
Ulna:
lower epiphysis
styloid process

813.44 Radius with ulna, lower end

813.45 Torus fracture of radius

● 813.5 Lower end, open

❑813.50 Lower end of forearm, unspecified

813.51 Colles' fracture

❑813.52 Other fractures of distal end of radius (alone)

813.53 Distal end of ulna (alone)

813.54 Radius with ulna, lower end

● 813.8 Unspecified part, closed

❑813.80 Forearm, unspecified

❑813.81 Radius (alone)

❑813.82 Ulna (alone)

❑813.83 Radius with ulna

● 813.9 Unspecified part, open

❑813.90 Forearm, unspecified

❑813.91 Radius (alone)

❑813.92 Ulna (alone)

❑813.93 Radius with ulna

● 814 Fracture of carpal bone(s)

The following fifth-digit subclassification is for use with category 814:

❑ 0 carpal bone, unspecified
Wrist NOS
1 navicular [scaphoid] of wrist
2 lunate [semilunar] bone of wrist
3 triquetral [cuneiform] bone of wrist
4 pisiform
5 trapezium bone [larger multangular]
6 trapezoid bone [smaller multangular]
7 capitate bone [os magnum]
8 hamate [unciform] bone
❑ 9 other

● 814.0 Closed

● 814.1 Open

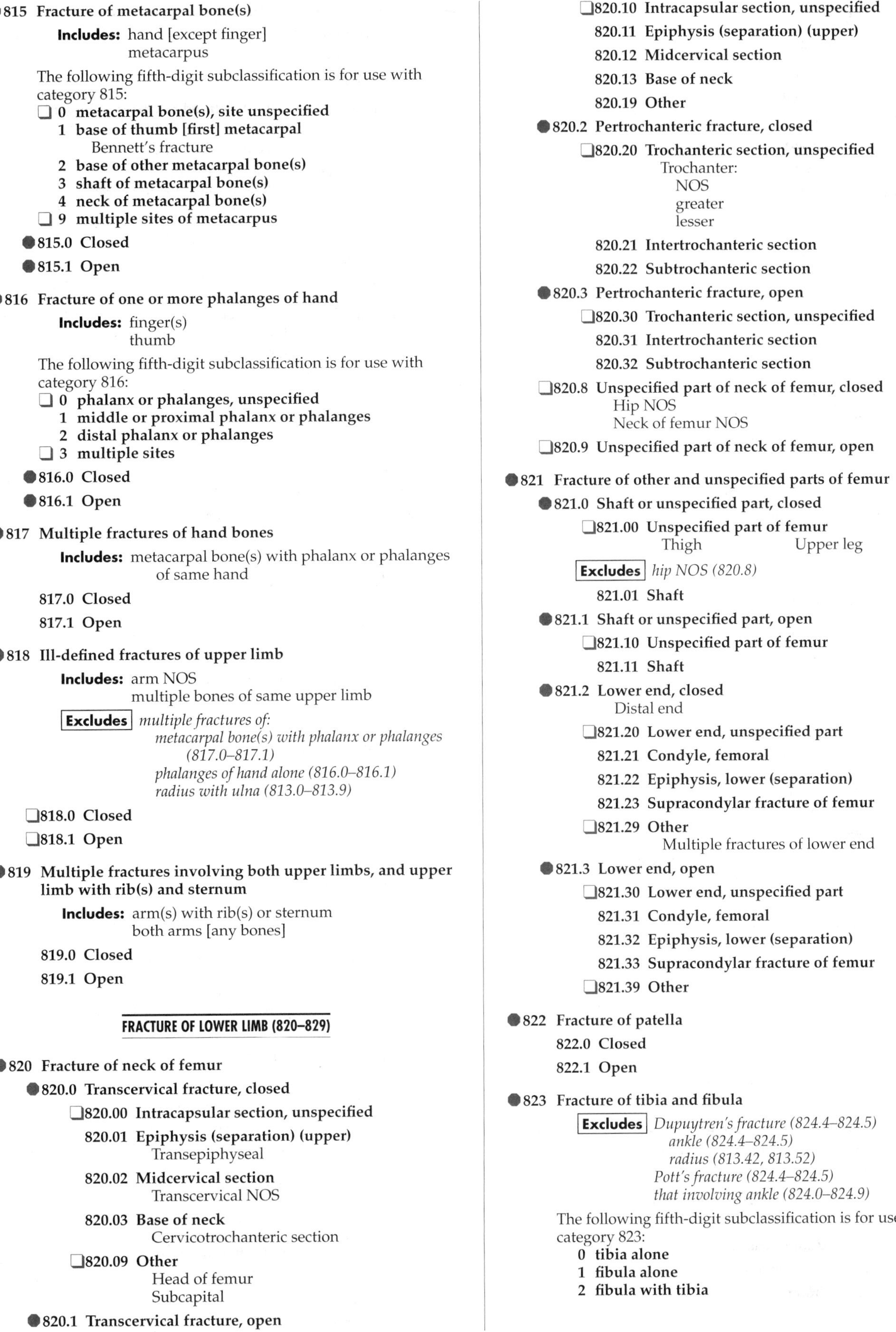

● 815 **Fracture of metacarpal bone(s)**

Includes: hand [except finger]
metacarpus

The following fifth-digit subclassification is for use with category 815:
❑ 0 **metacarpal bone(s), site unspecified**
1 **base of thumb [first] metacarpal**
Bennett's fracture
2 **base of other metacarpal bone(s)**
3 **shaft of metacarpal bone(s)**
4 **neck of metacarpal bone(s)**
❑ 9 **multiple sites of metacarpus**

● 815.0 **Closed**

● 815.1 **Open**

● 816 **Fracture of one or more phalanges of hand**

Includes: finger(s)
thumb

The following fifth-digit subclassification is for use with category 816:
❑ 0 **phalanx or phalanges, unspecified**
1 **middle or proximal phalanx or phalanges**
2 **distal phalanx or phalanges**
❑ 3 **multiple sites**

● 816.0 **Closed**

● 816.1 **Open**

● 817 **Multiple fractures of hand bones**

Includes: metacarpal bone(s) with phalanx or phalanges of same hand

817.0 **Closed**

817.1 **Open**

● 818 **Ill-defined fractures of upper limb**

Includes: arm NOS
multiple bones of same upper limb

Excludes *multiple fractures of:*
metacarpal bone(s) with phalanx or phalanges (817.0–817.1)
phalanges of hand alone (816.0–816.1)
radius with ulna (813.0–813.9)

❑ 818.0 **Closed**

❑ 818.1 **Open**

● 819 **Multiple fractures involving both upper limbs, and upper limb with rib(s) and sternum**

Includes: arm(s) with rib(s) or sternum
both arms [any bones]

819.0 **Closed**

819.1 **Open**

FRACTURE OF LOWER LIMB (820–829)

● 820 **Fracture of neck of femur**

● 820.0 **Transcervical fracture, closed**

❑ 820.00 **Intracapsular section, unspecified**

820.01 **Epiphysis (separation) (upper)**
Transepiphyseal

820.02 **Midcervical section**
Transcervical NOS

820.03 **Base of neck**
Cervicotrochanteric section

❑ 820.09 **Other**
Head of femur
Subcapital

● 820.1 **Transcervical fracture, open**

❑ 820.10 **Intracapsular section, unspecified**

820.11 **Epiphysis (separation) (upper)**

820.12 **Midcervical section**

820.13 **Base of neck**

820.19 **Other**

● 820.2 **Pertrochanteric fracture, closed**

❑ 820.20 **Trochanteric section, unspecified**
Trochanter:
NOS
greater
lesser

820.21 **Intertrochanteric section**

820.22 **Subtrochanteric section**

● 820.3 **Pertrochanteric fracture, open**

❑ 820.30 **Trochanteric section, unspecified**

820.31 **Intertrochanteric section**

820.32 **Subtrochanteric section**

❑ 820.8 **Unspecified part of neck of femur, closed**
Hip NOS
Neck of femur NOS

❑ 820.9 **Unspecified part of neck of femur, open**

● 821 **Fracture of other and unspecified parts of femur**

● 821.0 **Shaft or unspecified part, closed**

❑ 821.00 **Unspecified part of femur**
Thigh Upper leg

Excludes *hip NOS (820.8)*

821.01 **Shaft**

● 821.1 **Shaft or unspecified part, open**

❑ 821.10 **Unspecified part of femur**

821.11 **Shaft**

● 821.2 **Lower end, closed**
Distal end

❑ 821.20 **Lower end, unspecified part**

821.21 **Condyle, femoral**

821.22 **Epiphysis, lower (separation)**

821.23 **Supracondylar fracture of femur**

❑ 821.29 **Other**
Multiple fractures of lower end

● 821.3 **Lower end, open**

❑ 821.30 **Lower end, unspecified part**

821.31 **Condyle, femoral**

821.32 **Epiphysis, lower (separation)**

821.33 **Supracondylar fracture of femur**

❑ 821.39 **Other**

● 822 **Fracture of patella**

822.0 **Closed**

822.1 **Open**

● 823 **Fracture of tibia and fibula**

Excludes *Dupuytren's fracture (824.4–824.5)*
ankle (824.4–824.5)
radius (813.42, 813.52)
Pott's fracture (824.4–824.5)
that involving ankle (824.0–824.9)

The following fifth-digit subclassification is for use with category 823:
0 **tibia alone**
1 **fibula alone**
2 **fibula with tibia**

ICD-9-CM 800–899 Vol. 1

823.0 Upper end, closed
Head
Proximal end
Tibia:
condyles
tuberosity

823.1 Upper end, open

823.2 Shaft, closed

823.3 Shaft, open

823.4 Torus fracture

823.8 Unspecified part, closed
Lower leg NOS

823.9 Unspecified part, open

824 Fracture of ankle

824.0 Medial malleolus, closed
Tibia involving:
ankle
malleolus

824.1 Medial malleolus, open

824.2 Lateral malleolus, closed
Fibula involving:
ankle
malleolus

824.3 Lateral malleolus, open

824.4 Bimalleolar, closed
Dupuytren's fracture, fibula
Pott's fracture

824.5 Bimalleolar, open

824.6 Trimalleolar, closed
Lateral and medial malleolus with anterior or posterior lip of tibia

824.7 Trimalleolar, open

824.8 Unspecified, closed
Ankle NOS

824.9 Unspecified, open

825 Fracture of one or more tarsal and metatarsal bones

825.0 Fracture of calcaneus, closed
Heel bone
Os calcis

825.1 Fracture of calcaneus, open

825.2 Fracture of other tarsal and metatarsal bones, closed

825.20 Unspecified bone(s) of foot [except toes]
Instep

825.21 Astragalus
Talus

825.22 Navicular [scaphoid], foot

825.23 Cuboid

825.24 Cuneiform, foot

825.25 Metatarsal bone(s)

825.29 Other
Tarsal with metatarsal bone(s) only

Excludes *calcaneus (825.0)*

825.3 Fracture of other tarsal and metatarsal bones, open

825.30 Unspecified bone(s) of foot [except toes]

825.31 Astragalus

825.32 Navicular [scaphoid], foot

825.33 Cuboid

825.34 Cuneiform, foot

825.35 Metatarsal bone(s)

825.39 Other

826 Fracture of one or more phalanges of foot

Includes: toe(s)

826.0 Closed

826.1 Open

827 Other, multiple, and ill-defined fractures of lower limb

Includes: leg NOS
multiple bones of same lower limb

Excludes *multiple fractures of:*
ankle bones alone (824.4–824.9)
phalanges of foot alone (826.0–826.1)
tarsal with metatarsal bones (825.29, 825.39)
tibia with fibula (823.0–823.9 with fifth-digit 2)

827.0 Closed

827.1 Open

828 Multiple fractures involving both lower limbs, lower with upper limb, and lower limb(s) with rib(s) and sternum

Includes: arm(s) with leg(s) [any bones]
both legs [any bones]
leg(s) with rib(s) or sternum

828.0 Closed

828.1 Open

829 Fracture of unspecified bones

829.0 Unspecified bone, closed

829.1 Unspecified bone, open

DISLOCATION (830–839)

Includes: displacement
subluxation

Excludes *congenital dislocation (754.0–755.8)*
pathological dislocation (718.2)
recurrent dislocation (718.3)

The descriptions "closed" and "open," used in the fourth-digit subdivisions, include the following terms:
closed:
complete
dislocation NOS
partial
simple
uncomplicated
open:
compound
infected
with foreign body

Note: A dislocation not indicated as closed or open should be classified as closed.

830 Dislocation of jaw

Includes: jaw (cartilage) (meniscus)
mandible
maxilla (inferior)
temporomandibular (joint)

830.0 Closed dislocation

830.1 Open dislocation

831 Dislocation of shoulder

Excludes *sternoclavicular joint (839.61, 839.71)*
sternum (839.61, 839.71)

The following fifth-digit subclassification is for use with category 831:
0 shoulder, unspecified
humerus NOS
1 anterior dislocation of humerus
2 posterior dislocation of humerus
3 inferior dislocation of humerus
4 acromioclavicular (joint)
clavicle
9 other
Scapula

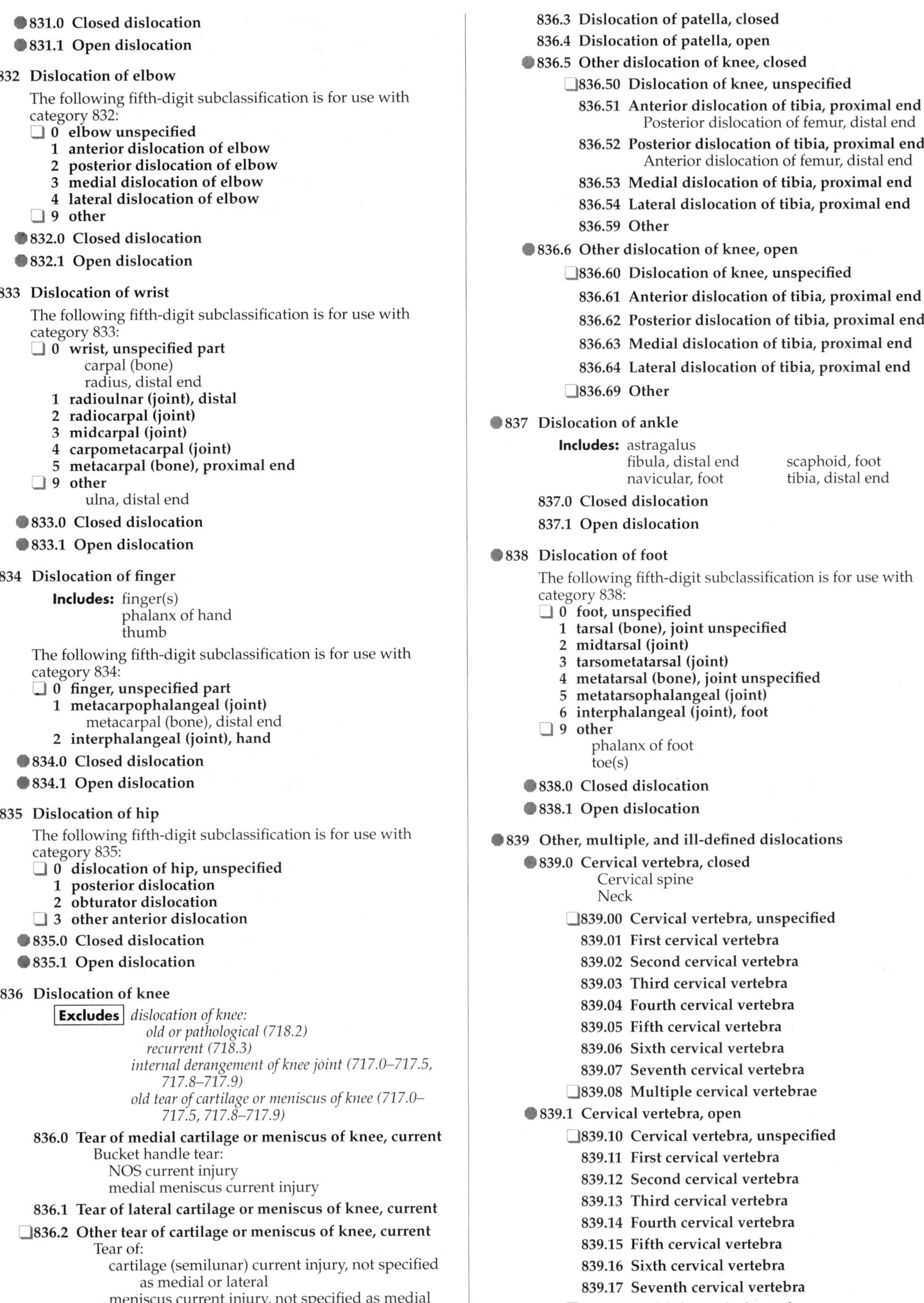

● 831.0 Closed dislocation

● 831.1 Open dislocation

● **832 Dislocation of elbow**

The following fifth-digit subclassification is for use with category 832:
- ❑ 0 elbow unspecified
- 1 anterior dislocation of elbow
- 2 posterior dislocation of elbow
- 3 medial dislocation of elbow
- 4 lateral dislocation of elbow
- ❑ 9 other

● 832.0 Closed dislocation

● 832.1 Open dislocation

● **833 Dislocation of wrist**

The following fifth-digit subclassification is for use with category 833:
- ❑ 0 wrist, unspecified part
  - carpal (bone)
  - radius, distal end
- 1 radioulnar (joint), distal
- 2 radiocarpal (joint)
- 3 midcarpal (joint)
- 4 carpometacarpal (joint)
- 5 metacarpal (bone), proximal end
- ❑ 9 other
  - ulna, distal end

● 833.0 Closed dislocation

● 833.1 Open dislocation

● **834 Dislocation of finger**

Includes: finger(s)
phalanx of hand
thumb

The following fifth-digit subclassification is for use with category 834:
- ❑ 0 finger, unspecified part
- 1 metacarpophalangeal (joint)
  - metacarpal (bone), distal end
- 2 interphalangeal (joint), hand

● 834.0 Closed dislocation

● 834.1 Open dislocation

● **835 Dislocation of hip**

The following fifth-digit subclassification is for use with category 835:
- ❑ 0 dislocation of hip, unspecified
- 1 posterior dislocation
- 2 obturator dislocation
- ❑ 3 other anterior dislocation

● 835.0 Closed dislocation

● 835.1 Open dislocation

● **836 Dislocation of knee**

Excludes *dislocation of knee:*
old or pathological (718.2)
recurrent (718.3)
internal derangement of knee joint (717.0–717.5, 717.8–717.9)
old tear of cartilage or meniscus of knee (717.0–717.5, 717.8–717.9)

836.0 Tear of medial cartilage or meniscus of knee, current
Bucket handle tear:
NOS current injury
medial meniscus current injury

836.1 Tear of lateral cartilage or meniscus of knee, current

❑ 836.2 Other tear of cartilage or meniscus of knee, current
Tear of:
cartilage (semilunar) current injury, not specified as medial or lateral
meniscus current injury, not specified as medial or lateral

836.3 Dislocation of patella, closed

836.4 Dislocation of patella, open

● 836.5 Other dislocation of knee, closed

❑ 836.50 Dislocation of knee, unspecified

836.51 Anterior dislocation of tibia, proximal end
Posterior dislocation of femur, distal end

836.52 Posterior dislocation of tibia, proximal end
Anterior dislocation of femur, distal end

836.53 Medial dislocation of tibia, proximal end

836.54 Lateral dislocation of tibia, proximal end

836.59 Other

● 836.6 Other dislocation of knee, open

❑ 836.60 Dislocation of knee, unspecified

836.61 Anterior dislocation of tibia, proximal end

836.62 Posterior dislocation of tibia, proximal end

836.63 Medial dislocation of tibia, proximal end

836.64 Lateral dislocation of tibia, proximal end

❑ 836.69 Other

● **837 Dislocation of ankle**

Includes: astragalus
fibula, distal end
navicular, foot
scaphoid, foot
tibia, distal end

837.0 Closed dislocation

837.1 Open dislocation

● **838 Dislocation of foot**

The following fifth-digit subclassification is for use with category 838:
- ❑ 0 foot, unspecified
- 1 tarsal (bone), joint unspecified
- 2 midtarsal (joint)
- 3 tarsometatarsal (joint)
- 4 metatarsal (bone), joint unspecified
- 5 metatarsophalangeal (joint)
- 6 interphalangeal (joint), foot
- ❑ 9 other
  - phalanx of foot
  - toe(s)

● 838.0 Closed dislocation

● 838.1 Open dislocation

● **839 Other, multiple, and ill-defined dislocations**

● 839.0 Cervical vertebra, closed
Cervical spine
Neck

❑ 839.00 Cervical vertebra, unspecified

839.01 First cervical vertebra

839.02 Second cervical vertebra

839.03 Third cervical vertebra

839.04 Fourth cervical vertebra

839.05 Fifth cervical vertebra

839.06 Sixth cervical vertebra

839.07 Seventh cervical vertebra

❑ 839.08 Multiple cervical vertebrae

● 839.1 Cervical vertebra, open

❑ 839.10 Cervical vertebra, unspecified

839.11 First cervical vertebra

839.12 Second cervical vertebra

839.13 Third cervical vertebra

839.14 Fourth cervical vertebra

839.15 Fifth cervical vertebra

839.16 Sixth cervical vertebra

839.17 Seventh cervical vertebra

❑ 839.18 Multiple cervical vertebrae

- 839.2 Thoracic and lumbar vertebra, closed
  - 839.20 Lumbar vertebra
  - 839.21 Thoracic vertebra
    Dorsal [thoracic] vertebra
- 839.3 Thoracic and lumbar vertebra, open
  - 839.30 Lumbar vertebra
  - 839.31 Thoracic vertebra
- 839.4 Other vertebra, closed
  - 839.40 Vertebra, unspecified site
    Spine NOS
  - 839.41 Coccyx
  - 839.42 Sacrum
    Sacroiliac (joint)
  - 839.49 Other
- 839.5 Other vertebra, open
  - 839.50 Vertebra, unspecified site
  - 839.51 Coccyx
  - 839.52 Sacrum
  - 839.59 Other
- 839.6 Other location, closed
  - 839.61 Sternum
    Sternoclavicular joint
  - 839.69 Other
    Pelvis
- 839.7 Other location, open
  - 839.71 Sternum
  - 839.79 Other
- 839.8 Multiple and ill-defined, closed
  Arm
  Back
  Hand
  Multiple locations, except fingers or toes alone
  Other ill-defined locations
  Unspecified location
- 839.9 Multiple and ill-defined, open

SPRAINS AND STRAINS OF JOINTS AND ADJACENT MUSCLES (840–848)

Includes: avulsion of joint capsule, ligament, muscle, tendon
hemarthrosis of joint capsule, ligament, muscle, tendon
laceration of joint capsule, ligament, muscle, tendon
rupture of joint capsule, ligament, muscle, tendon
sprain of joint capsule, ligament, muscle, tendon
strain of joint capsule, ligament, muscle, tendon
tear of joint capsule, ligament, muscle, tendon

Excludes *laceration of tendon in open wounds (880–884 and 890–894 with .2)*

- 840 Sprains and strains of shoulder and upper arm
  - 840.0 Acromioclavicular (joint) (ligament)
  - 840.1 Coracoclavicular (ligament)
  - 840.2 Coracohumeral (ligament)
  - 840.3 Infraspinatus (muscle) (tendon)
  - 840.4 Rotator cuff (capsule)
    Excludes *complete rupture of rotator cuff, nontraumatic (727.61)*
  - 840.5 Subscapularis (muscle)
  - 840.6 Supraspinatus (muscle) (tendon)
  - 840.7 Superior glenoid labrum lesion
    SLAP lesion
  - 840.8 Other specified sites of shoulder and upper arm
  - 840.9 Unspecified site of shoulder and upper arm
    Arm NOS
    Shoulder NOS
- 841 Sprains and strains of elbow and forearm
  - 841.0 Radial collateral ligament
  - 841.1 Ulnar collateral ligament
  - 841.2 Radiohumeral (joint)
  - 841.3 Ulnohumeral (joint)
  - 841.8 Other specified sites of elbow and forearm
  - 841.9 Unspecified site of elbow and forearm
    Elbow NOS
- 842 Sprains and strains of wrist and hand
  - 842.0 Wrist
    - 842.00 Unspecified site
    - 842.01 Carpal (joint)
    - 842.02 Radiocarpal (joint) (ligament)
    - 842.09 Other
      Radioulnar joint, distal
  - 842.1 Hand
    - 842.10 Unspecified site
    - 842.11 Carpometacarpal (joint)
    - 842.12 Metacarpophalangeal (joint)
    - 842.13 Interphalangeal (joint)
    - 842.19 Other
      Midcarpal (joint)
- 843 Sprains and strains of hip and thigh
  - 843.0 Iliofemoral (ligament)
  - 843.1 Ischiocapsular (ligament)
  - 843.8 Other specified sites of hip and thigh
  - 843.9 Unspecified site of hip and thigh
    Hip NOS
    Thigh NOS
- 844 Sprains and strains of knee and leg
  - 844.0 Lateral collateral ligament of knee
  - 844.1 Medial collateral ligament of knee
  - 844.2 Cruciate ligament of knee
  - 844.3 Tibiofibular (joint) (ligament), superior
  - 844.8 Other specified sites of knee and leg
  - 844.9 Unspecified site of knee and leg
    Knee NOS
    Leg NOS
- 845 Sprains and strains of ankle and foot
  - 845.0 Ankle
    - 845.00 Unspecified site
    - 845.01 Deltoid (ligament), ankle
      Internal collateral (ligament), ankle
    - 845.02 Calcaneofibular (ligament)
    - 845.03 Tibiofibular (ligament), distal
    - 845.09 Other
      Achilles tendon
  - 845.1 Foot
    - 845.10 Unspecified site
    - 845.11 Tarsometatarsal (joint) (ligament)

845.12 **Metatarsophalangeal (joint)**

845.13 **Interphalangeal (joint), toe**

❑845.19 **Other**

● 846 **Sprains and strains of sacroiliac region**

846.0 **Lumbosacral (joint) (ligament)**

846.1 **Sacroiliac ligament**

846.2 **Sacrospinatus (ligament)**

846.3 **Sacrotuberous (ligament)**

❑846.8 **Other specified sites of sacroiliac region**

❑846.9 **Unspecified site of sacroiliac region**

● 847 **Sprains and strains of other and unspecified parts of back**

Excludes *lumbosacral (846.0)*

847.0 **Neck**

Anterior longitudinal (ligament), cervical
Atlanto-axial (joints)
Atlanto-occipital (joints)
Whiplash injury

Excludes *neck injury NOS (959.09)*
thyroid region (848.2)

847.1 **Thoracic**

847.2 **Lumbar**

847.3 **Sacrum**

Sacrococcygeal (ligament)

847.4 **Coccyx**

❑847.9 **Unspecified site of back**

Back NOS

● 848 **Other and ill-defined sprains and strains**

848.0 **Septal cartilage of nose**

848.1 **Jaw**

Temporomandibular (joint) (ligament)

848.2 **Thyroid region**

Cricoarytenoid (joint) (ligament)
Cricothyroid (joint) (ligament)
Thyroid cartilage

848.3 **Ribs**

Chondrocostal (joint) without mention of injury to sternum
Costal cartilage without mention of injury to sternum

● 848.4 **Sternum**

❑848.40 **Unspecified site**

848.41 **Sternoclavicular (joint) (ligament)**

848.42 **Chondrosternal (joint)**

❑848.49 **Other**

Xiphoid cartilage

848.5 **Pelvis**

Symphysis pubis

Excludes *that in childbirth (665.6)*

❑848.8 **Other specified sites of sprains and strains**

❑848.9 **Unspecified site of sprain and strain**

INTRACRANIAL INJURY, EXCLUDING THOSE WITH SKULL FRACTURE (850–854)

Excludes *intracranial injury with skull fracture (800–801 and 803–804, except .0 and .5)*
open wound of head without intracranial injury (870.0–873.9)
skull fracture alone (800–801 and 803–804 with .0, .5)

Note: The description "with open intracranial wound," used in the fourth-digit subdivisions, includes those specified as open or with mention of infection or foreign body.

The following fifth-digit subclassification is for use with categories 851–854:

❑ 0 **unspecified state of consciousness**
1 **with no loss of consciousness**
2 **with brief [less than one hour] loss of consciousness**
3 **with moderate [1–24 hours] loss of consciousness**
4 **with prolonged [more than 24 hours] loss of consciousness and return to pre-existing conscious level**
5 **with prolonged [more than 24 hours] loss of consciousness without return to pre-existing conscious level**

Use fifth-digit 5 to designate when a patient is unconscious and dies before regaining consciousness, regardless of the duration of the loss of consciousness

❑ 6 **with loss of consciousness of unspecified duration**
❑ 9 **with concussion, unspecified**

● 850 **Concussion**

Includes: commotio cerebri

Excludes *concussion with:*
cerebral laceration or contusion (851.0–851.9)
cerebral hemorrhage (852–853)
head injury NOS (959.01)

850.0 **With no loss of consciousness**

Concussion with mental confusion or disorientation, without loss of consciousness

● 850.1 **With brief loss of consciousness**

Loss of consciousness for less than one hour

850.11 **with loss of consciousness of 30 minutes or less**

850.12 **with loss of consciousness from 31 to 59 minutes**

850.2 **With moderate loss of consciousness**

Loss of consciousness for 1–24 hours

850.3 **With prolonged loss of consciousness and return to pre-existing conscious level**

Loss of consciousness for more than 24 hours with complete recovery

850.4 **With prolonged loss of consciousness, without return to pre-existing conscious level**

❑850.5 **With loss of consciousness of unspecified duration**

❑850.9 **Concussion, unspecified**

● 851 **Cerebral laceration and contusion**

Requires fifth digit. See beginning of section 850–854 for codes and definitions.

● 851.0 **Cortex (cerebral) contusion without mention of open intracranial wound**

● 851.1 **Cortex (cerebral) contusion with open intracranial wound**

● 851.2 **Cortex (cerebral) laceration without mention of open intracranial wound**

● 851.3 **Cortex (cerebral) laceration with open intracranial wound**

● 851.4 **Cerebellar or brain stem contusion without mention of open intracranial wound**

● 851.5 **Cerebellar or brain stem contusion with open intracranial wound**

● 851.6 **Cerebellar or brain stem laceration without mention of open intracranial wound**

● 851.7 **Cerebellar or brain stem laceration with open intracranial wound**

● ❑851.8 **Other and unspecified cerebral laceration and contusion, without mention of open intracranial wound**
Brain (membrane) NOS

● ❑851.9 **Other and unspecified cerebral laceration and contusion, with open intracranial wound**

● 852 **Subarachnoid, subdural, and extradural hemorrhage, following injury**

Requires fifth digit. See beginning of section 850–854 for codes and definitions.

Excludes *cerebral contusion or laceration (with hemorrhage) (851.0–851.9)*

● 852.0 **Subarachnoid hemorrhage following injury without mention of open intracranial wound**
Middle meningeal hemorrhage following injury

● 852.1 **Subarachnoid hemorrhage following injury with open intracranial wound**

● 852.2 **Subdural hemorrhage following injury without mention of open intracranial wound**

● 852.3 **Subdural hemorrhage following injury with open intracranial wound**

● 852.4 **Extradural hemorrhage following injury without mention of open intracranial wound**
Epidural hematoma following injury

● 852.5 **Extradural hemorrhage following injury with open intracranial wound**

● 853 **Other and unspecified intracranial hemorrhage following injury**

Requires fifth digit. See beginning of section 850–854 for codes and definitions.

● ❑853.0 **Without mention of open intracranial wound**
Cerebral compression due to injury
Intracranial hematoma following injury
Traumatic cerebral hemorrhage

● ❑853.1 **With open intracranial wound**

● 854 **Intracranial injury of other and unspecified nature**

Includes: injury:
brain NOS
cavernous sinus
intracranial

Excludes *any condition classifiable to 850–853*
head injury NOS (959.01)

● ❑854.0 **Without mention of open intracranial wound**

● ❑854.1 **With open intracranial wound**

INTERNAL INJURY OF THORAX, ABDOMEN, AND PELVIS (860–869)

Includes: blast injuries of internal organs
blunt trauma of internal organs
bruise of internal organs
concussion injuries (except cerebral) of internal organs
crushing of internal organs
hematoma of internal organs
laceration of internal organs
puncture of internal organs
tear of internal organs
traumatic rupture of internal organs

Excludes *concussion NOS (850.0–850.9)*
flail chest (807.4)
foreign body entering through orifice (930.0–939.9)
injury to blood vessels (901.0–902.9)

Note: The description "with open wound," used in the fourth-digit subdivisions, includes those with mention of infection or foreign body.

● 860 **Traumatic pneumothorax and hemothorax**

860.0 **Pneumothorax without mention of open wound into thorax**

860.1 **Pneumothorax with open wound into thorax**

860.2 **Hemothorax without mention of open wound into thorax**

860.3 **Hemothorax with open wound into thorax**

860.4 **Pneumohemothorax without mention of open wound into thorax**

860.5 **Pneumohemothorax with open wound into thorax**

● 861 **Injury to heart and lung**

Excludes *injury to blood vessels of thorax (901.0–901.9)*

● 861.0 **Heart, without mention of open wound into thorax**

❑861.00 **Unspecified injury**

861.01 **Contusion**
Cardiac contusion
Myocardial contusion

861.02 **Laceration without penetration of heart chambers**

861.03 **Laceration with penetration of heart chambers**

● 861.1 **Heart, with open wound into thorax**

❑861.10 **Unspecified injury**

861.11 **Contusion**

861.12 **Laceration without penetration of heart chambers**

861.13 **Laceration with penetration of heart chambers**

● 861.2 **Lung, without mention of open wound into thorax**

❑861.20 **Unspecified injury**

861.21 **Contusion**

861.22 **Laceration**

● 861.3 **Lung, with open wound into thorax**

❑861.30 **Unspecified injury**

861.31 **Contusion**

861.32 **Laceration**

● 862 **Injury to other and unspecified intrathoracic organs**

Excludes *injury to blood vessels of thorax (901.0–901.9)*

862.0 **Diaphragm, without mention of open wound into cavity**

862.1 **Diaphragm, with open wound into cavity**

● 862.2 Other specified intrathoracic organs, without mention of open wound into cavity

862.21 Bronchus

862.22 Esophagus

❑ 862.29 Other
Pleura
Thymus gland

● 862.3 Other specified intrathoracic organs, with open wound into cavity

862.31 Bronchus

862.32 Esophagus

❑ 862.39 Other

❑ 862.8 Multiple and unspecified intrathoracic organs, without mention of open wound into cavity
Crushed chest
Multiple intrathoracic organs

❑ 862.9 Multiple and unspecified intrathoracic organs, with open wound into cavity

● 863 Injury to gastrointestinal tract

Excludes *anal sphincter laceration during delivery (664.2)*
bile duct (868.0–868.1 with fifth-digit 2)
gallbladder (868.0–868.1 with fifth-digit 2)

863.0 Stomach, without mention of open wound into cavity

863.1 Stomach, with open wound into cavity

● 863.2 Small intestine, without mention of open wound into cavity

❑ 863.20 Small intestine, unspecified site

863.21 Duodenum

❑ 863.29 Other

● 863.3 Small intestine, with open wound into cavity

❑ 863.30 Small intestine, unspecified site

863.31 Duodenum

❑ 863.39 Other

● 863.4 Colon or rectum, without mention of open wound into cavity

❑ 863.40 Colon, unspecified site

863.41 Ascending [right] colon

863.42 Transverse colon

863.43 Descending [left] colon

863.44 Sigmoid colon

863.45 Rectum

❑ 863.46 Multiple sites in colon and rectum

❑ 863.49 Other

● 863.5 Colon or rectum, with open wound into cavity

❑ 863.50 Colon, unspecified site

863.51 Ascending [right] colon

863.52 Transverse colon

863.53 Descending [left] colon

863.54 Sigmoid colon

863.55 Rectum

❑ 863.56 Multiple sites in colon and rectum

❑ 863.59 Other

● 863.8 Other and unspecified gastrointestinal sites, without mention of open wound into cavity

❑ 863.80 Gastrointestinal tract, unspecified site

863.81 Pancreas, head

863.82 Pancreas, body

863.83 Pancreas, tail

❑ 863.84 Pancreas, multiple and unspecified sites

863.85 Appendix

❑ 863.89 Other
Intestine NOS

● 863.9 Other and unspecified gastrointestinal sites, with open wound into cavity

❑ 863.90 Gastrointestinal tract, unspecified site

863.91 Pancreas, head

863.92 Pancreas, body

863.93 Pancreas, tail

❑ 863.94 Pancreas, multiple and unspecified sites

863.95 Appendix

❑ 863.99 Other

● 864 Injury to liver

The following fifth-digit subclassification is for use with category 864:

❑ 0 unspecified injury
1 hematoma and contusion
2 laceration, minor
Laceration involving capsule only, or without significant involvement of hepatic parenchyma [i.e., less than 1 cm deep]
3 laceration, moderate
Laceration involving parenchyma but without major disruption of parenchyma [i.e., less than 10 cm long and less than 3 cm deep]
4 laceration, major
Laceration with significant disruption of hepatic parenchyma [i.e., 10 cm long and 3 cm deep]
Multiple moderate lacerations, with or without hematoma
Stellate lacerations of liver
❑ 5 laceration, unspecified
❑ 9 other

● 864.0 Without mention of open wound into cavity

● 864.1 With open wound into cavity

● 865 Injury to spleen

The following fifth-digit subclassification is for use with category 865:

❑ 0 unspecified injury
1 hematoma without rupture of capsule
2 capsular tears, without major disruption of parenchyma
3 laceration extending into parenchyma
4 massive parenchymal disruption
❑ 9 other

● 865.0 Without mention of open wound into cavity

● 865.1 With open wound into cavity

● 866 Injury to kidney

The following fifth-digit subclassification is for use with category 866:

❑ 0 unspecified injury
1 hematoma without rupture of capsule
2 laceration
3 complete disruption of kidney parenchyma

● 866.0 Without mention of open wound into cavity

● 866.1 With open wound into cavity

● 867 Injury to pelvic organs

Excludes *injury during delivery (664.0–665.9)*

867.0 Bladder and urethra, without mention of open wound into cavity

867.1 Bladder and urethra, with open wound into cavity

867.2 Ureter, without mention of open wound into cavity

867.3 Ureter, with open wound into cavity

867.4 Uterus, without mention of open wound into cavity

867.5 Uterus, with open wound into cavity

❑867.6 Other specified pelvic organs, without mention of open wound into cavity
Fallopian tube
Ovary
Prostate
Seminal vesicle
Vas deferens

❑867.7 Other specified pelvic organs, with open wound into cavity

❑867.8 Unspecified pelvic organ, without mention of open wound into cavity

❑867.9 Unspecified pelvic organ, with open wound into cavity

● 868 Injury to other intra-abdominal organs

The following fifth-digit subclassification is for use with category 868:
❑ 0 unspecified intra-abdominal organ
1 adrenal gland
2 bile duct and gallbladder
3 peritoneum
4 retroperitoneum
❑ 9 other and multiple intra-abdominal organs

● 868.0 Without mention of open wound into cavity

● 868.1 With open wound into cavity

● 869 Internal injury to unspecified or ill-defined organs

Includes: internal injury NOS
multiple internal injury NOS

❑869.0 Without mention of open wound into cavity

❑869.1 With open wound into cavity

OPEN WOUNDS (870–897)

Note: The description "complicated" used in the fourth-digit subdivisions includes those with mention of delayed healing, delayed treatment, foreign body, or infection.

Includes: animal bite
avulsion
cut
laceration
puncture wound
traumatic amputation

Excludes *burn (940.0–949.5)*
crushing (925–929.9)
puncture of internal organs (860.0–869.1)
superficial injury (910.0–919.9)
that incidental to:
dislocation (830.0–839.9)
fracture (800.0–829.1)
internal injury (860.0–869.1)
intracranial injury (851.0–854.1)

Use additional code to identify infection

OPEN WOUND OF HEAD, NECK, AND TRUNK (870–879)

● 870 Open wound of ocular adnexa

870.0 Laceration of skin of eyelid and periocular area

870.1 Laceration of eyelid, full-thickness, not involving lacrimal passages

870.2 Laceration of eyelid involving lacrimal passages

870.3 Penetrating wound of orbit, without mention of foreign body

870.4 Penetrating wound of orbit with foreign body

Excludes *retained (old) foreign body in orbit (376.6)*

❑870.8 Other specified open wounds of ocular adnexa

❑870.9 Unspecified open wound of ocular adnexa

● 871 Open wound of eyeball

Excludes *2nd cranial nerve [optic] injury (950.0–950.9)*
3rd cranial nerve [oculomotor] injury (951.0)

871.0 Ocular laceration without prolapse of intraocular tissue

871.1 Ocular laceration with prolapse or exposure of intraocular tissue

871.2 Rupture of eye with partial loss of intraocular tissue

871.3 Avulsion of eye
Traumatic enucleation

❑871.4 Unspecified laceration of eye

871.5 Penetration of eyeball with magnetic foreign body

Excludes *retained (old) magnetic foreign body in globe (360.50–360.59)*

871.6 Penetration of eyeball with (nonmagnetic) foreign body

Excludes *retained (old) (nonmagnetic) foreign body in globe (360.60–360.69)*

❑871.7 Unspecified ocular penetration

❑871.9 Unspecified open wound of eyeball

● 872 Open wound of ear

● 872.0 External ear, without mention of complication

❑872.00 External ear, unspecified site

872.01 Auricle, ear
Pinna

872.02 Auditory canal

● 872.1 External ear, complicated

❑872.10 External ear, unspecified site

872.11 Auricle, ear

872.12 Auditory canal

● 872.6 Other specified parts of ear, without mention of complication

872.61 Ear drum
Drumhead
Tympanic membrane

872.62 Ossicles

872.63 Eustachian tube

872.64 Cochlea

❑872.69 Other and multiple sites

● 872.7 Other specified parts of ear, complicated

872.71 Ear drum

872.72 Ossicles

872.73 Eustachian tube

872.74 Cochlea

❑872.79 Other and multiple sites

❑872.8 Ear, part unspecified, without mention of complication
Ear NOS

❑872.9 Ear, part unspecified, complicated

● 873 Other open wound of head

873.0 Scalp, without mention of complication

873.1 Scalp, complicated

● 873.2 Nose, without mention of complication

❑873.20 Nose, unspecified site

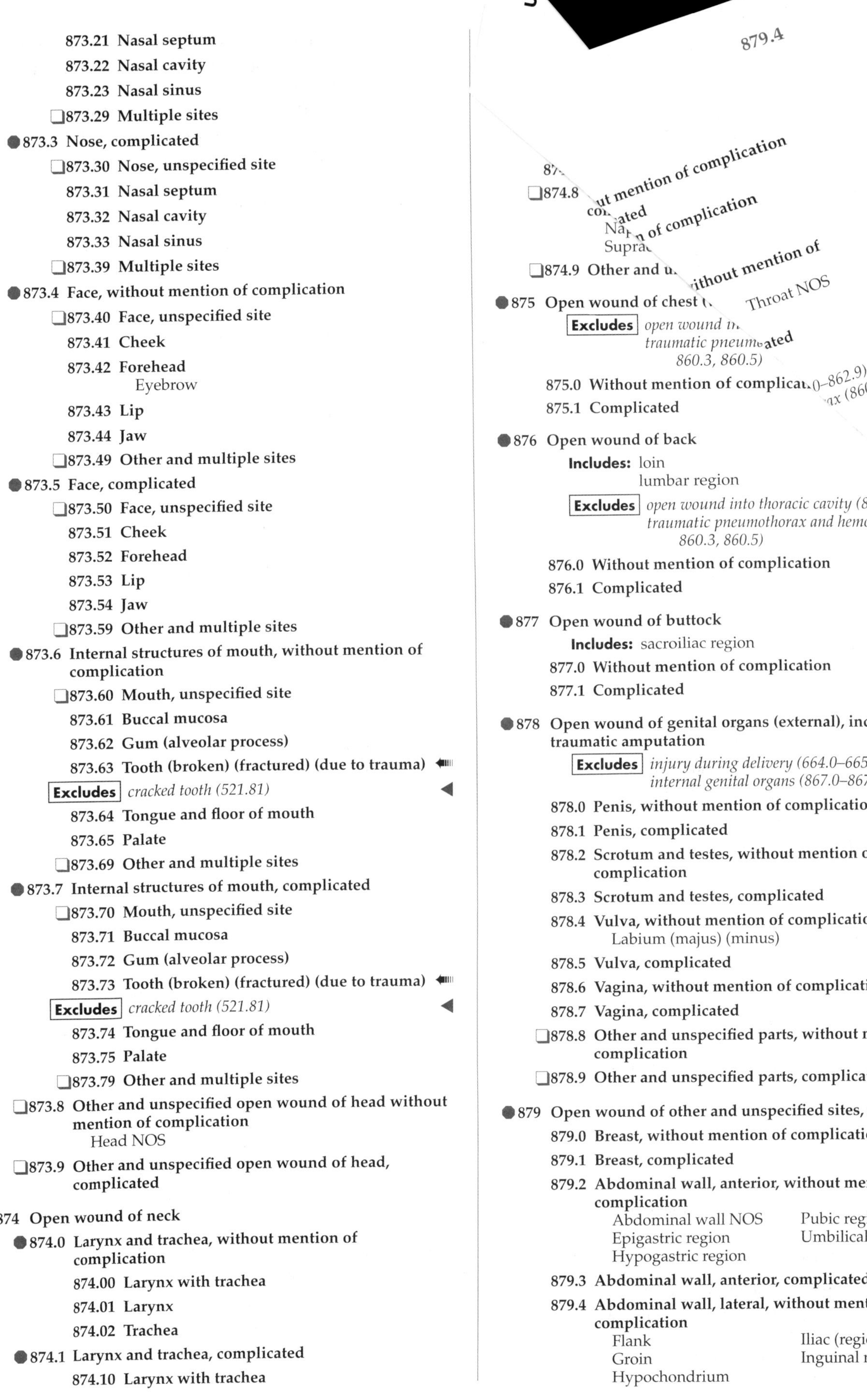

873.21 Nasal septum
873.22 Nasal cavity
873.23 Nasal sinus
❑873.29 Multiple sites

● 873.3 Nose, complicated
❑873.30 Nose, unspecified site
873.31 Nasal septum
873.32 Nasal cavity
873.33 Nasal sinus
❑873.39 Multiple sites

● 873.4 Face, without mention of complication
❑873.40 Face, unspecified site
873.41 Cheek
873.42 Forehead
Eyebrow
873.43 Lip
873.44 Jaw
❑873.49 Other and multiple sites

● 873.5 Face, complicated
❑873.50 Face, unspecified site
873.51 Cheek
873.52 Forehead
873.53 Lip
873.54 Jaw
❑873.59 Other and multiple sites

● 873.6 Internal structures of mouth, without mention of complication
❑873.60 Mouth, unspecified site
873.61 Buccal mucosa
873.62 Gum (alveolar process)
873.63 Tooth (broken) (fractured) (due to trauma)
Excludes *cracked tooth (521.81)* ◀
873.64 Tongue and floor of mouth
873.65 Palate
❑873.69 Other and multiple sites

● 873.7 Internal structures of mouth, complicated
❑873.70 Mouth, unspecified site
873.71 Buccal mucosa
873.72 Gum (alveolar process)
873.73 Tooth (broken) (fractured) (due to trauma)
Excludes *cracked tooth (521.81)* ◀
873.74 Tongue and floor of mouth
873.75 Palate
❑873.79 Other and multiple sites

❑873.8 Other and unspecified open wound of head without mention of complication
Head NOS

❑873.9 Other and unspecified open wound of head, complicated

● 874 Open wound of neck

● 874.0 Larynx and trachea, without mention of complication
874.00 Larynx with trachea
874.01 Larynx
874.02 Trachea

● 874.1 Larynx and trachea, complicated
874.10 Larynx with trachea

879.4

87...
❑874.8 ...ut mention of complication
co...ated
Na...n of complication
Supra...
❑874.9 Other and u...ithout mention of
Throat NOS

● 875 Open wound of chest ...
Excludes *open wound in... traumatic pneum...ated 860.3, 860.5)*
875.0 Without mention of complica...0–862.9) ...ax (860.1,
875.1 Complicated

● 876 Open wound of back
Includes: loin
lumbar region
Excludes *open wound into thoracic cavity (860.0–862.9), traumatic pneumothorax and hemothorax (860.1, 860.3, 860.5)*
876.0 Without mention of complication
876.1 Complicated

● 877 Open wound of buttock
Includes: sacroiliac region
877.0 Without mention of complication
877.1 Complicated

● 878 Open wound of genital organs (external), including traumatic amputation
Excludes *injury during delivery (664.0–665.9)*
internal genital organs (867.0–867.9)
878.0 Penis, without mention of complication
878.1 Penis, complicated
878.2 Scrotum and testes, without mention of complication
878.3 Scrotum and testes, complicated
878.4 Vulva, without mention of complication
Labium (majus) (minus)
878.5 Vulva, complicated
878.6 Vagina, without mention of complication
878.7 Vagina, complicated
❑878.8 Other and unspecified parts, without mention of complication
❑878.9 Other and unspecified parts, complicated

● 879 Open wound of other and unspecified sites, except limbs
879.0 Breast, without mention of complication
879.1 Breast, complicated
879.2 Abdominal wall, anterior, without mention of complication
Abdominal wall NOS — Pubic region
Epigastric region — Umbilical region
Hypogastric region
879.3 Abdominal wall, anterior, complicated
879.4 Abdominal wall, lateral, without mention of complication
Flank — Iliac (region)
Groin — Inguinal region
Hypochondrium

879.5

without

NOS

879.5 Abdom of trunk, complicated

879.6 Other ment of unspecified site(s), plication
ds NOS

879.7 O

879.8 multiple) of unspecified site(s),

870 OUND OF UPPER LIMB (880–887)

d of shoulder and upper arm

ving fifth-digit subclassification is for use with
88y 880:
shoulder region
1 scapular region
2 axillary region
3 upper arm
9 multiple sites

880.0 Without mention of complication

880.1 Complicated

880.2 With tendon involvement

881 Open wound of elbow, forearm, and wrist

The following fifth-digit subclassification is for use with category 881:
0 forearm
1 elbow
2 wrist

881.0 Without mention of complication

881.1 Complicated

881.2 With tendon involvement

882 Open wound of hand except finger(s) alone

882.0 Without mention of complication

882.1 Complicated

882.2 With tendon involvement

883 Open wound of finger(s)

Includes: fingernail
thumb (nail)

883.0 Without mention of complication

883.1 Complicated

883.2 With tendon involvement

884 Multiple and unspecified open wound of upper limb

Includes: arm NOS
multiple sites of one upper limb
upper limb NOS

884.0 Without mention of complication

884.1 Complicated

884.2 With tendon involvement

885 Traumatic amputation of thumb (complete) (partial)

Includes: thumb(s) (with finger(s) of either hand)

885.0 Without mention of complication

885.1 Complicated

886 Traumatic amputation of other finger(s) (complete) (partial)

Includes: finger(s) of one or both hands, without mention of thumb(s)

886.0 Without mention of complication

886.1 Complicated

887 Traumatic amputation of arm and hand (complete) (partial)

887.0 Unilateral, below elbow, without mention of complication

887.1 Unilateral, below elbow, complicated

887.2 Unilateral, at or above elbow, without mention of complication

887.3 Unilateral, at or above elbow, complicated

887.4 Unilateral, level not specified, without mention of complication

887.5 Unilateral, level not specified, complicated

887.6 Bilateral [any level], without mention of complication
One hand and other arm

887.7 Bilateral [any level], complicated

OPEN WOUND OF LOWER LIMB (890–897)

890 Open wound of hip and thigh

890.0 Without mention of complication

890.1 Complicated

890.2 With tendon involvement

891 Open wound of knee, leg [except thigh], and ankle

Includes: leg NOS
multiple sites of leg, except thigh

Excludes *that of thigh (890.0–890.2)*
with multiple sites of lower limb (894.0–894.2)

891.0 Without mention of complication

891.1 Complicated

891.2 With tendon involvement

892 Open wound of foot except toe(s) alone

Includes: heel

892.0 Without mention of complication

892.1 Complicated

892.2 With tendon involvement

893 Open wound of toe(s)

Includes: toenail

893.0 Without mention of complication

893.1 Complicated

893.2 With tendon involvement

894 Multiple and unspecified open wound of lower limb

Includes: lower limb NOS
multiple sites of one lower limb, with thigh

894.0 Without mention of complication

894.1 Complicated

894.2 With tendon involvement

895 Traumatic amputation of toe(s) (complete) (partial)

Includes: toe(s) of one or both feet

895.0 Without mention of complication

895.1 Complicated

896 Traumatic amputation of foot (complete) (partial)

896.0 Unilateral, without mention of complication

896.1 Unilateral, complicated

896.2 Bilateral, without mention of complication

Excludes *one foot and other leg (897.6–897.7)*

896.3 Bilateral, complicated

897 Traumatic amputation of leg(s) (complete) (partial)

897.0 Unilateral, below knee, without mention of complication

897.1 Unilateral, below knee, complicated

897.2 Unilateral, at or above knee, without mention of complication

897.3 Unilateral, at or above knee, complicated

897.4 Unilateral, level not specified, without mention of complication

897.5 Unilateral, level not specified, complicated

897.6 Bilateral [any level], without mention of complication
One foot and other leg

897.7 Bilateral [any level], complicated

INJURY TO BLOOD VESSELS (900–904)

Includes: arterial hematoma of blood vessel, secondary to other injuries, e.g., fracture or open wound
avulsion of blood vessel, secondary to other injuries, e.g., fracture or open wound
cut of blood vessel, secondary to other injuries, e.g., fracture or open wound
laceration of blood vessel, secondary to other injuries, e.g., fracture or open wound
rupture of blood vessel, secondary to other injuries, e.g., fracture or open wound
traumatic aneurysm or fistula (arteriovenous) of blood vessel, secondary to other injuries, e.g., fracture or open wound

Excludes *accidental puncture or laceration during medical procedure (998.2)*
intracranial hemorrhage following injury (851.0–854.1)

900 Injury to blood vessels of head and neck

900.0 Carotid artery

900.00 Carotid artery, unspecified

900.01 Common carotid artery

900.02 External carotid artery

900.03 Internal carotid artery

900.1 Internal jugular vein

900.8 Other specified blood vessels of head and neck

900.81 External jugular vein
Jugular vein NOS

900.82 Multiple blood vessels of head and neck

900.89 Other

900.9 Unspecified blood vessel of head and neck

901 Injury to blood vessels of thorax

Excludes *traumatic hemothorax (860.2–860.5)*

901.0 Thoracic aorta

901.1 Innominate and subclavian arteries

901.2 Superior vena cava

901.3 Innominate and subclavian veins

901.4 Pulmonary blood vessels

901.40 Pulmonary vessel(s), unspecified

901.41 Pulmonary artery

901.42 Pulmonary vein

901.8 Other specified blood vessels of thorax

901.81 Intercostal artery or vein

901.82 Internal mammary artery or vein

901.83 Multiple blood vessels of thorax

901.89 Other
Azygos vein
Hemiazygos vein

901.9 Unspecified blood vessel of thorax

902 Injury to blood vessels of abdomen and pelvis

902.0 Abdominal aorta

902.1 Inferior vena cava

902.10 Inferior vena cava, unspecified

902.11 Hepatic veins

902.19 Other

902.2 Celiac and mesenteric arteries

902.20 Celiac and mesenteric arteries, unspecified

902.21 Gastric artery

902.22 Hepatic artery

902.23 Splenic artery

902.24 Other specified branches of celiac axis

902.25 Superior mesenteric artery (trunk)

902.26 Primary branches of superior mesenteric artery
Ileo-colic artery

902.27 Inferior mesenteric artery

902.29 Other

902.3 Portal and splenic veins

902.31 Superior mesenteric vein and primary subdivisions
Ileo-colic vein

902.32 Inferior mesenteric vein

902.33 Portal vein

902.34 Splenic vein

902.39 Other
Cystic vein
Gastric vein

902.4 Renal blood vessels

902.40 Renal vessel(s), unspecified

902.41 Renal artery

902.42 Renal vein

902.49 Other
Suprarenal arteries

902.5 Iliac blood vessels

902.50 Iliac vessel(s), unspecified

902.51 Hypogastric artery

902.52 Hypogastric vein

902.53 Iliac artery

902.54 Iliac vein

902.55 Uterine artery

902.56 Uterine vein

902.59 Other

902.8 Other specified blood vessels of abdomen and pelvis

902.81 Ovarian artery

902.82 Ovarian vein

902.87 Multiple blood vessels of abdomen and pelvis

902.89 Other

902.9 Unspecified blood vessel of abdomen and pelvis

903 Injury to blood vessels of upper extremity

903.0 Axillary blood vessels

903.00 Axillary vessel(s), unspecified

903.01 Axillary artery

903.02 Axillary vein

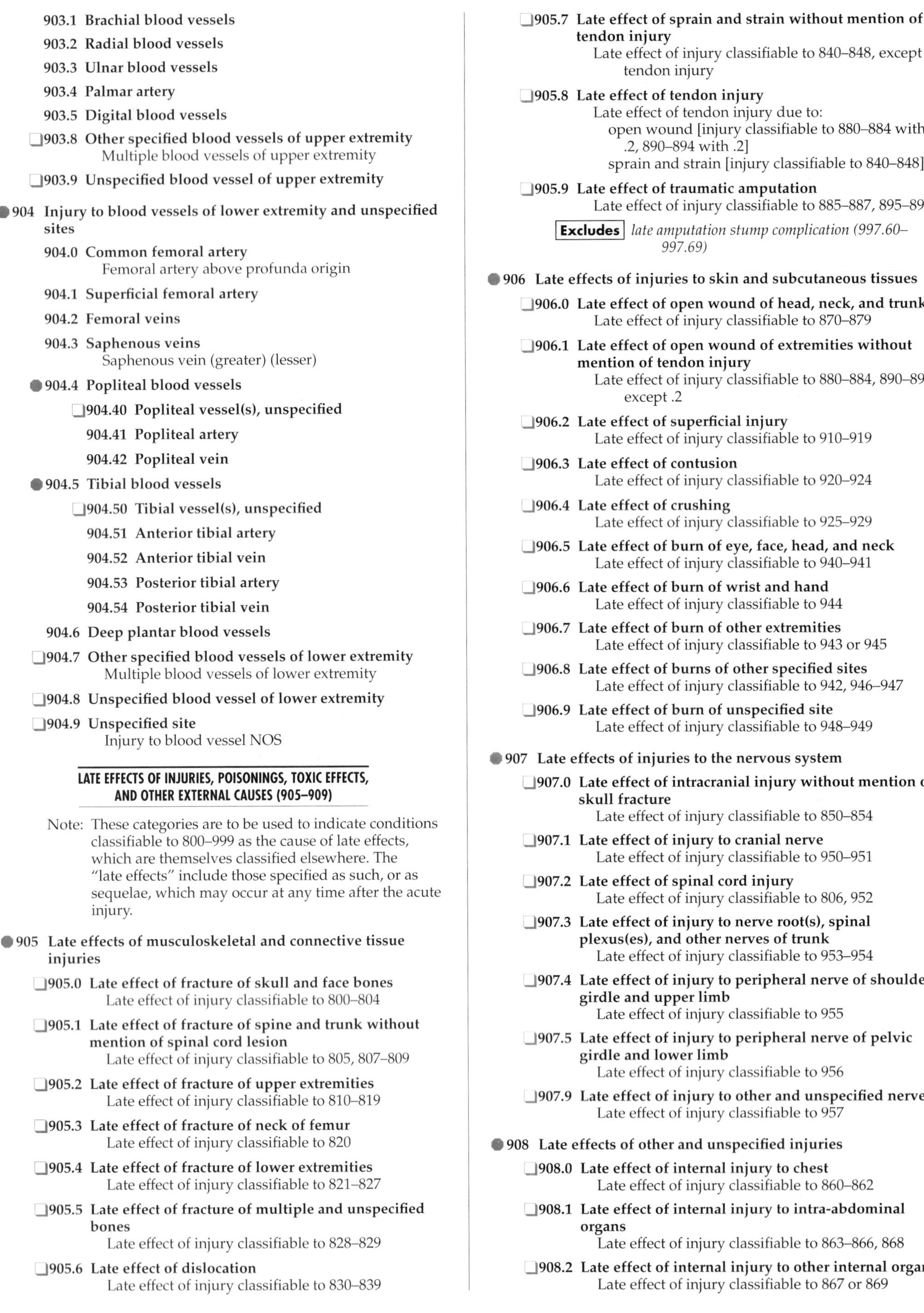

903.1 **Brachial blood vessels**

903.2 **Radial blood vessels**

903.3 **Ulnar blood vessels**

903.4 **Palmar artery**

903.5 **Digital blood vessels**

❑903.8 **Other specified blood vessels of upper extremity**
Multiple blood vessels of upper extremity

❑903.9 **Unspecified blood vessel of upper extremity**

● 904 **Injury to blood vessels of lower extremity and unspecified sites**

904.0 **Common femoral artery**
Femoral artery above profunda origin

904.1 **Superficial femoral artery**

904.2 **Femoral veins**

904.3 **Saphenous veins**
Saphenous vein (greater) (lesser)

● 904.4 **Popliteal blood vessels**

❑904.40 **Popliteal vessel(s), unspecified**

904.41 **Popliteal artery**

904.42 **Popliteal vein**

● 904.5 **Tibial blood vessels**

❑904.50 **Tibial vessel(s), unspecified**

904.51 **Anterior tibial artery**

904.52 **Anterior tibial vein**

904.53 **Posterior tibial artery**

904.54 **Posterior tibial vein**

904.6 **Deep plantar blood vessels**

❑904.7 **Other specified blood vessels of lower extremity**
Multiple blood vessels of lower extremity

❑904.8 **Unspecified blood vessel of lower extremity**

❑904.9 **Unspecified site**
Injury to blood vessel NOS

LATE EFFECTS OF INJURIES, POISONINGS, TOXIC EFFECTS, AND OTHER EXTERNAL CAUSES (905–909)

Note: These categories are to be used to indicate conditions classifiable to 800–999 as the cause of late effects, which are themselves classified elsewhere. The "late effects" include those specified as such, or as sequelae, which may occur at any time after the acute injury.

● 905 **Late effects of musculoskeletal and connective tissue injuries**

❑905.0 **Late effect of fracture of skull and face bones**
Late effect of injury classifiable to 800–804

❑905.1 **Late effect of fracture of spine and trunk without mention of spinal cord lesion**
Late effect of injury classifiable to 805, 807–809

❑905.2 **Late effect of fracture of upper extremities**
Late effect of injury classifiable to 810–819

❑905.3 **Late effect of fracture of neck of femur**
Late effect of injury classifiable to 820

❑905.4 **Late effect of fracture of lower extremities**
Late effect of injury classifiable to 821–827

❑905.5 **Late effect of fracture of multiple and unspecified bones**
Late effect of injury classifiable to 828–829

❑905.6 **Late effect of dislocation**
Late effect of injury classifiable to 830–839

❑905.7 **Late effect of sprain and strain without mention of tendon injury**
Late effect of injury classifiable to 840–848, except tendon injury

❑905.8 **Late effect of tendon injury**
Late effect of tendon injury due to:
open wound [injury classifiable to 880–884 with .2, 890–894 with .2]
sprain and strain [injury classifiable to 840–848]

❑905.9 **Late effect of traumatic amputation**
Late effect of injury classifiable to 885–887, 895–897

Excludes *late amputation stump complication (997.60–997.69)*

● 906 **Late effects of injuries to skin and subcutaneous tissues**

❑906.0 **Late effect of open wound of head, neck, and trunk**
Late effect of injury classifiable to 870–879

❑906.1 **Late effect of open wound of extremities without mention of tendon injury**
Late effect of injury classifiable to 880–884, 890–894 except .2

❑906.2 **Late effect of superficial injury**
Late effect of injury classifiable to 910–919

❑906.3 **Late effect of contusion**
Late effect of injury classifiable to 920–924

❑906.4 **Late effect of crushing**
Late effect of injury classifiable to 925–929

❑906.5 **Late effect of burn of eye, face, head, and neck**
Late effect of injury classifiable to 940–941

❑906.6 **Late effect of burn of wrist and hand**
Late effect of injury classifiable to 944

❑906.7 **Late effect of burn of other extremities**
Late effect of injury classifiable to 943 or 945

❑906.8 **Late effect of burns of other specified sites**
Late effect of injury classifiable to 942, 946–947

❑906.9 **Late effect of burn of unspecified site**
Late effect of injury classifiable to 948–949

● 907 **Late effects of injuries to the nervous system**

❑907.0 **Late effect of intracranial injury without mention of skull fracture**
Late effect of injury classifiable to 850–854

❑907.1 **Late effect of injury to cranial nerve**
Late effect of injury classifiable to 950–951

❑907.2 **Late effect of spinal cord injury**
Late effect of injury classifiable to 806, 952

❑907.3 **Late effect of injury to nerve root(s), spinal plexus(es), and other nerves of trunk**
Late effect of injury classifiable to 953–954

❑907.4 **Late effect of injury to peripheral nerve of shoulder girdle and upper limb**
Late effect of injury classifiable to 955

❑907.5 **Late effect of injury to peripheral nerve of pelvic girdle and lower limb**
Late effect of injury classifiable to 956

❑907.9 **Late effect of injury to other and unspecified nerve**
Late effect of injury classifiable to 957

● 908 **Late effects of other and unspecified injuries**

❑908.0 **Late effect of internal injury to chest**
Late effect of injury classifiable to 860–862

❑908.1 **Late effect of internal injury to intra-abdominal organs**
Late effect of injury classifiable to 863–866, 868

❑908.2 **Late effect of internal injury to other internal organs**
Late effect of injury classifiable to 867 or 869

❏908.3 **Late effect of injury to blood vessel of head, neck, and extremities**
Late effect of injury classifiable to 900, 903–904

❏908.4 **Late effect of injury to blood vessel of thorax, abdomen, and pelvis**
Late effect of injury classifiable to 901–902

❏908.5 **Late effect of foreign body in orifice**
Late effect of injury classifiable to 930–939

❏908.6 **Late effect of certain complications of trauma**
Late effect of complications classifiable to 958

❏908.9 **Late effect of unspecified injury**
Late effect of injury classifiable to 959

● 909 **Late effects of other and unspecified external causes**

❏909.0 **Late effect of poisoning due to drug, medicinal or biological substance**
Late effect of conditions classifiable to 960–979
Excludes *Late effect of adverse effect of drug, medicinal or biological substance (909.5)*

❏909.1 **Late effect of toxic effects of nonmedical substances**
Late effect of conditions classifiable to 980–989

❏909.2 **Late effect of radiation**
Late effect of conditions classifiable to 990

❏909.3 **Late effect of complications of surgical and medical care**
Late effect of conditions classifiable to 996–999

❏909.4 **Late effect of certain other external causes**
Late effect of conditions classifiable to 991–994

❏909.5 **Late effect of adverse effect of drug, medicinal or biological substance**
Excludes *late effect of poisoning due to drug, medicinal or biological substances (909.0)*

❏909.9 **Late effect of other and unspecified external causes**

SUPERFICIAL INJURY (910–919)

Excludes *burn (blisters) (940.0–949.5)*
contusion (920–924.9)
foreign body:
granuloma (728.82)
inadvertently left in operative wound (998.4)
residual, in soft tissue (729.6)
insect bite, venomous (989.5)
open wound with incidental foreign body (870.0–897.7)

● 910 **Superficial injury of face, neck, and scalp except eye**
Includes: cheek, ear, gum, lip, nose, throat
Excludes *eye and adnexa (918.0–918.9)*

910.0 **Abrasion or friction burn without mention of infection**

910.1 **Abrasion or friction burn, infected**

910.2 **Blister without mention of infection**

910.3 **Blister, infected**

910.4 **Insect bite, nonvenomous, without mention of infection**

910.5 **Insect bite, nonvenomous, infected**

910.6 **Superficial foreign body (splinter) without major open wound and without mention of infection**

910.7 **Superficial foreign body (splinter) without major open wound, infected**

❏910.8 **Other and unspecified superficial injury of face, neck, and scalp without mention of infection**

❏910.9 **Other and unspecified superficial injury of face, neck, and scalp, infected**

● 911 **Superficial injury of trunk**
Includes: abdominal wall, anus, back, breast, buttock, chest wall, flank, groin, interscapular region, labium (majus) (minus), penis, perineum, scrotum, testis, vagina, vulva
Excludes *hip (916.0–916.9)*
scapular region (912.0–912.9)

911.0 **Abrasion or friction burn without mention of infection**

911.1 **Abrasion or friction burn, infected**

911.2 **Blister without mention of infection**

911.3 **Blister, infected**

911.4 **Insect bite, nonvenomous, without mention of infection**

911.5 **Insect bite, nonvenomous, infected**

911.6 **Superficial foreign body (splinter) without major open wound and without mention of infection**

911.7 **Superficial foreign body (splinter) without major open wound, infected**

❏911.8 **Other and unspecified superficial injury of trunk without mention of infection**

❏911.9 **Other and unspecified superficial injury of trunk, infected**

● 912 **Superficial injury of shoulder and upper arm**
Includes: axilla
scapular region

912.0 **Abrasion or friction burn without mention of infection**

912.1 **Abrasion or friction burn, infected**

912.2 **Blister without mention of infection**

912.3 **Blister, infected**

912.4 **Insect bite, nonvenomous, without mention of infection**

912.5 **Insect bite, nonvenomous, infected**

912.6 **Superficial foreign body (splinter) without major open wound and without mention of infection**

912.7 **Superficial foreign body (splinter) without major open wound, infected**

❏912.8 **Other and unspecified superficial injury of shoulder and upper arm without mention of infection**

❏912.9 **Other and unspecified superficial injury of shoulder and upper arm, infected**

● 913 **Superficial injury of elbow, forearm, and wrist**

913.0 **Abrasion or friction burn without mention of infection**

913.1 **Abrasion or friction burn, infected**

913.2 **Blister without mention of infection**

913.3 **Blister, infected**

913.4 **Insect bite, nonvenomous, without mention of infection**

913.5 **Insect bite, nonvenomous, infected**

913.6 **Superficial foreign body (splinter) without major open wound and without mention of infection**

913.7 **Superficial foreign body (splinter) without major open wound, infected**

❏913.8 **Other and unspecified superficial injury of elbow, forearm, and wrist without mention of infection**

❏913.9 **Other and unspecified superficial injury of elbow, forearm, and wrist, infected**

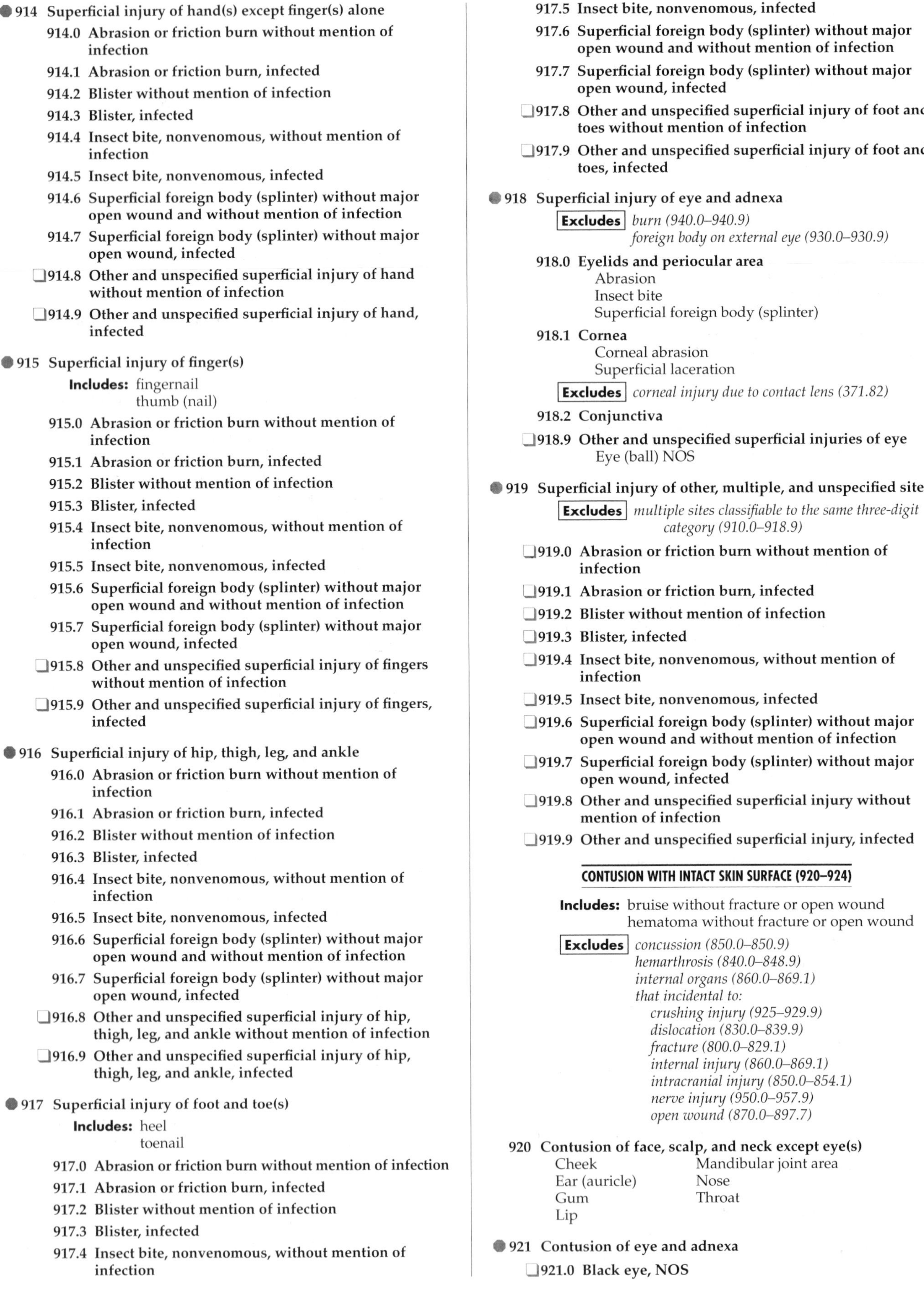

● 914 Superficial injury of hand(s) except finger(s) alone

914.0 Abrasion or friction burn without mention of infection

914.1 Abrasion or friction burn, infected

914.2 Blister without mention of infection

914.3 Blister, infected

914.4 Insect bite, nonvenomous, without mention of infection

914.5 Insect bite, nonvenomous, infected

914.6 Superficial foreign body (splinter) without major open wound and without mention of infection

914.7 Superficial foreign body (splinter) without major open wound, infected

❑914.8 Other and unspecified superficial injury of hand without mention of infection

❑914.9 Other and unspecified superficial injury of hand, infected

● 915 Superficial injury of finger(s)

Includes: fingernail
thumb (nail)

915.0 Abrasion or friction burn without mention of infection

915.1 Abrasion or friction burn, infected

915.2 Blister without mention of infection

915.3 Blister, infected

915.4 Insect bite, nonvenomous, without mention of infection

915.5 Insect bite, nonvenomous, infected

915.6 Superficial foreign body (splinter) without major open wound and without mention of infection

915.7 Superficial foreign body (splinter) without major open wound, infected

❑915.8 Other and unspecified superficial injury of fingers without mention of infection

❑915.9 Other and unspecified superficial injury of fingers, infected

● 916 Superficial injury of hip, thigh, leg, and ankle

916.0 Abrasion or friction burn without mention of infection

916.1 Abrasion or friction burn, infected

916.2 Blister without mention of infection

916.3 Blister, infected

916.4 Insect bite, nonvenomous, without mention of infection

916.5 Insect bite, nonvenomous, infected

916.6 Superficial foreign body (splinter) without major open wound and without mention of infection

916.7 Superficial foreign body (splinter) without major open wound, infected

❑916.8 Other and unspecified superficial injury of hip, thigh, leg, and ankle without mention of infection

❑916.9 Other and unspecified superficial injury of hip, thigh, leg, and ankle, infected

● 917 Superficial injury of foot and toe(s)

Includes: heel
toenail

917.0 Abrasion or friction burn without mention of infection

917.1 Abrasion or friction burn, infected

917.2 Blister without mention of infection

917.3 Blister, infected

917.4 Insect bite, nonvenomous, without mention of infection

917.5 Insect bite, nonvenomous, infected

917.6 Superficial foreign body (splinter) without major open wound and without mention of infection

917.7 Superficial foreign body (splinter) without major open wound, infected

❑917.8 Other and unspecified superficial injury of foot and toes without mention of infection

❑917.9 Other and unspecified superficial injury of foot and toes, infected

● 918 Superficial injury of eye and adnexa

Excludes *burn (940.0–940.9)*
foreign body on external eye (930.0–930.9)

918.0 Eyelids and periocular area
Abrasion
Insect bite
Superficial foreign body (splinter)

918.1 Cornea
Corneal abrasion
Superficial laceration

Excludes *corneal injury due to contact lens (371.82)*

918.2 Conjunctiva

❑918.9 Other and unspecified superficial injuries of eye
Eye (ball) NOS

● 919 Superficial injury of other, multiple, and unspecified sites

Excludes *multiple sites classifiable to the same three-digit category (910.0–918.9)*

❑919.0 Abrasion or friction burn without mention of infection

❑919.1 Abrasion or friction burn, infected

❑919.2 Blister without mention of infection

❑919.3 Blister, infected

❑919.4 Insect bite, nonvenomous, without mention of infection

❑919.5 Insect bite, nonvenomous, infected

❑919.6 Superficial foreign body (splinter) without major open wound and without mention of infection

❑919.7 Superficial foreign body (splinter) without major open wound, infected

❑919.8 Other and unspecified superficial injury without mention of infection

❑919.9 Other and unspecified superficial injury, infected

CONTUSION WITH INTACT SKIN SURFACE (920–924)

Includes: bruise without fracture or open wound
hematoma without fracture or open wound

Excludes *concussion (850.0–850.9)*
hemarthrosis (840.0–848.9)
internal organs (860.0–869.1)
that incidental to:
crushing injury (925–929.9)
dislocation (830.0–839.9)
fracture (800.0–829.1)
internal injury (860.0–869.1)
intracranial injury (850.0–854.1)
nerve injury (950.0–957.9)
open wound (870.0–897.7)

920 Contusion of face, scalp, and neck except eye(s)
Cheek
Ear (auricle)
Gum
Lip
Mandibular joint area
Nose
Throat

● 921 Contusion of eye and adnexa

❑921.0 Black eye, NOS

921.1 **Contusion of eyelids and periocular area**

921.2 **Contusion of orbital tissues**

921.3 **Contusion of eyeball**

❑921.9 **Unspecified contusion of eye**
Injury of eye NOS

● 922 **Contusion of trunk**

922.0 **Breast**

922.1 **Chest wall**

922.2 **Abdominal wall**

Flank
Groin

● 922.3 **Back**

922.31 **Back**

Excludes *interscapular region (922.33)*

922.32 **Buttock**

922.33 **Interscapular region**

Excludes *scapular region (923.01)*

922.4 **Genital organs**

Labium (majus) (minus)
Penis
Perineum
Scrotum
Testis
Vagina
Vulva

❑922.8 **Multiple sites of trunk**

❑922.9 **Unspecified part**
Trunk NOS

● 923 **Contusion of upper limb**

● 923.0 **Shoulder and upper arm**

923.00 **Shoulder region**

923.01 **Scapular region**

923.02 **Axillary region**

923.03 **Upper arm**

❑923.09 **Multiple sites**

● 923.1 **Elbow and forearm**

923.10 **Forearm**

923.11 **Elbow**

● 923.2 **Wrist and hand(s), except finger(s) alone**

923.20 **Hand(s)**

923.21 **Wrist**

923.3 **Finger**
Fingernail
Thumb (nail)

❑923.8 **Multiple sites of upper limb**

❑923.9 **Unspecified part of upper limb**
Arm NOS

● 924 **Contusion of lower limb and of other and unspecified sites**

● 924.0 **Hip and thigh**

924.00 **Thigh**

924.01 **Hip**

● 924.1 **Knee and lower leg**

924.10 **Lower leg**

924.11 **Knee**

● 924.2 **Ankle and foot, excluding toe(s)**

924.20 **Foot**
Heel

924.21 **Ankle**

924.3 **Toe**
Toenail

❑924.4 **Multiple sites of lower limb**

❑924.5 **Unspecified part of lower limb**
Leg NOS

❑924.8 **Multiple sites, not elsewhere classified**

❑924.9 **Unspecified site**

CRUSHING INJURY (925–929)

Use additional code to identify any associated injuries, such as:
fractures (800–829)
internal injuries (860.0–869.1)
intracranial injury (850.0–854.1)

● 925 **Crushing injury of face, scalp, and neck**
Cheek
Ear
Larynx
Pharynx
Throat

925.1 **Crushing injury of face and scalp**
Cheek
Ear

925.2 **Crushing injury of neck**
Larynx
Throat
Pharynx

● 926 **Crushing injury of trunk**

926.0 **External genitalia**
Labium (majus) (minus)
Penis
Scrotum
Testis
Vulva

● 926.1 **Other specified sites**

926.11 **Back**

926.12 **Buttock**

❑926.19 **Other**
Breast

❑926.8 **Multiple sites of trunk**

❑926.9 **Unspecified site**
Trunk NOS

● 927 **Crushing injury of upper limb**

● 927.0 **Shoulder and upper arm**

927.00 **Shoulder region**

927.01 **Scapular region**

927.02 **Axillary region**

927.03 **Upper arm**

❑927.09 **Multiple sites**

● 927.1 **Elbow and forearm**

927.10 **Forearm**

927.11 **Elbow**

● 927.2 **Wrist and hand(s), except finger(s) alone**

927.20 **Hand(s)**

927.21 **Wrist**

927.3 **Finger(s)**

❑927.8 **Multiple sites of upper limb**

❑927.9 **Unspecified site**
Arm NOS

● 928 Crushing injury of lower limb
● 928.0 Hip and thigh
928.00 Thigh
928.01 Hip
● 928.1 Knee and lower leg
928.10 Lower leg
928.11 Knee
● 928.2 Ankle and foot, excluding toe(s) alone
928.20 Foot
Heel
928.21 Ankle
928.3 Toe(s)
❑928.8 Multiple sites of lower limb
❑928.9 Unspecified site
Leg NOS

● 929 Crushing injury of multiple and unspecified sites
❑929.0 Multiple sites, not elsewhere classified
❑929.9 Unspecified site

EFFECTS OF FOREIGN BODY ENTERING THROUGH ORIFICE (930–939)

Excludes *foreign body:*
granuloma (728.82)
inadvertently left in operative wound (998.4, 998.7)
in open wound (800–839, 851–897)
residual, in soft tissues (729.6)
superficial without major open wound (910–919 with .6 or .7)

● 930 Foreign body on external eye
Excludes *foreign body in penetrating wound of:*
eyeball (871.5–871.6)
retained (old) (360.5–360.6)
ocular adnexa (870.4)
retained (old) (376.6)
930.0 Corneal foreign body
930.1 Foreign body in conjunctival sac
930.2 Foreign body in lacrimal punctum
❑930.8 Other and combined sites
❑930.9 Unspecified site
External eye NOS

931 Foreign body in ear
Auditory canal
Auricle

932 Foreign body in nose
Nasal sinus
Nostril

● 933 Foreign body in pharynx and larynx
933.0 Pharynx
Nasopharynx
Throat NOS
933.1 Larynx
Asphyxia due to foreign body
Choking due to:
food (regurgitated)
phlegm

● 934 Foreign body in trachea, bronchus, and lung
934.0 Trachea
934.1 Main bronchus
❑934.8 Other specified parts
Bronchioles
Lung
❑934.9 Respiratory tree, unspecified
Inhalation of liquid or vomitus, lower respiratory tract NOS

● 935 Foreign body in mouth, esophagus, and stomach
935.0 Mouth
935.1 Esophagus
935.2 Stomach

936 Foreign body in intestine and colon

937 Foreign body in anus and rectum
Rectosigmoid (junction)

❑938 Foreign body in digestive system, unspecified
Alimentary tract NOS
Swallowed foreign body

● 939 Foreign body in genitourinary tract
939.0 Bladder and urethra
939.1 Uterus, any part
Excludes *intrauterine contraceptive device:*
complications from (996.32, 996.65)
presence of (V45.51)
939.2 Vulva and vagina
939.3 Penis
❑939.9 Unspecified site

BURNS (940–949)

Includes: burns from:
electrical heating appliance
electricity
flame
hot object
lightning
radiation
chemical burns (external) (internal)
scalds

Excludes *friction burns (910–919 with .0, .1)*
sunburn (692.71, 692.76–692.77)

● 940 Burn confined to eye and adnexa
940.0 Chemical burn of eyelids and periocular area
❑940.1 Other burns of eyelids and periocular area
940.2 Alkaline chemical burn of cornea and conjunctival sac
940.3 Acid chemical burn of cornea and conjunctival sac
❑940.4 Other burn of cornea and conjunctival sac
940.5 Burn with resulting rupture and destruction of eyeball
❑940.9 Unspecified burn of eye and adnexa

● 941 Burn of face, head, and neck
Excludes *mouth (947.0)*
The following fifth-digit subclassification is for use with category 941:
❑ 0 face and head, unspecified site
1 ear [any part]
2 eye (with other parts of face, head, and neck)
3 lip(s)
4 chin
5 nose (septum)
6 scalp [any part]
temple (region)
7 forehead and cheek
8 neck
❑ 9 multiple sites [except with eye] of face, head, and neck

- 941.0 Unspecified degree
- 941.1 Erythema [first degree]
- 941.2 Blisters, epidermal loss [second degree]
- 941.3 Full-thickness skin loss [third degree NOS]
- 941.4 Deep necrosis of underlying tissues [deep third degree] without mention of loss of a body part
- 941.5 Deep necrosis of underlying tissues [deep third degree] with loss of a body part

942 Burn of trunk

Excludes *scapular region (943.0–943.5 with fifth-digit 6)*

The following fifth-digit subclassification is for use with category 942:

- 0 trunk, unspecified site
- 1 breast
- 2 chest wall, excluding breast and nipple
- 3 abdominal wall
  - flank
  - groin
- 4 back [any part]
  - buttock
  - interscapular region
- 5 genitalia
  - labium (majus) (minus)
  - penis
  - perineum
  - scrotum
  - testis
  - vulva
- 9 other and multiple sites of trunk

- 942.0 Unspecified degree
- 942.1 Erythema [first degree]
- 942.2 Blisters, epidermal loss [second degree]
- 942.3 Full-thickness skin loss [third degree NOS]
- 942.4 Deep necrosis of underlying tissues [deep third degree] without mention of loss of a body part
- 942.5 Deep necrosis of underlying tissues [deep third degree] with loss of a body part

943 Burn of upper limb, except wrist and hand

The following fifth-digit subclassification is for use with category 943:

- 0 upper limb, unspecified site
- 1 forearm
- 2 elbow
- 3 upper arm
- 4 axilla
- 5 shoulder
- 6 scapular region
- 9 multiple sites of upper limb, except wrist and hand

- 943.0 Unspecified degree
- 943.1 Erythema [first degree]
- 943.2 Blisters, epidermal loss [second degree]
- 943.3 Full-thickness skin loss [third degree NOS]
- 943.4 Deep necrosis of underlying tissues [deep third degree] without mention of loss of a body part
- 943.5 Deep necrosis of underlying tissues [deep third degree] with loss of a body part

944 Burn of wrist(s) and hand(s)

The following fifth-digit subclassification is for use with category 944:

- 0 hand, unspecified site
- 1 single digit [finger (nail)] other than thumb
- 2 thumb (nail)
- 3 two or more digits, not including thumb
- 4 two or more digits including thumb
- 5 palm
- 6 back of hand
- 7 wrist
- 8 multiple sites of wrist(s) and hand(s)

- 944.0 Unspecified degree
- 944.1 Erythema [first degree]
- 944.2 Blisters, epidermal loss [second degree]
- 944.3 Full-thickness skin loss [third degree NOS]
- 944.4 Deep necrosis of underlying tissues [deep third degree] without mention of loss of a body part
- 944.5 Deep necrosis of underlying tissues [deep third degree] with loss of a body part

945 Burn of lower limb(s)

The following fifth-digit subclassification is for use with category 945:

- 0 lower limb [leg], unspecified site
- 1 toe(s) (nail)
- 2 foot
- 3 ankle
- 4 lower leg
- 5 knee
- 6 thigh [any part]
- 9 multiple sites of lower limb(s)

- 945.0 Unspecified degree
- 945.1 Erythema [first degree]
- 945.2 Blisters, epidermal loss [second degree]
- 945.3 Full-thickness skin loss [third degree NOS]
- 945.4 Deep necrosis of underlying tissues [deep third degree] without mention of loss of a body part
- 945.5 Deep necrosis of underlying tissues [deep third degree] with loss of a body part

946 Burns of multiple specified sites

Includes: burns of sites classifiable to more than one three-digit category in 940–945

Excludes *multiple burns NOS (949.0–949.5)*

- 946.0 Unspecified degree
- 946.1 Erythema [first degree]
- 946.2 Blisters, epidermal loss [second degree]
- 946.3 Full-thickness skin loss [third degree NOS]
- 946.4 Deep necrosis of underlying tissues [deep third degree] without mention of loss of a body part
- 946.5 Deep necrosis of underlying tissues [deep third degree] with loss of a body part

947 Burn of internal organs

Includes: burns from chemical agents (ingested)

- 947.0 Mouth and pharynx
  - Gum
  - Tongue
- 947.1 Larynx, trachea, and lung
- 947.2 Esophagus
- 947.3 Gastrointestinal tract
  - Colon
  - Rectum
  - Small intestine
  - Stomach
- 947.4 Vagina and uterus
- 947.8 Other specified sites
- 947.9 Unspecified site

● **948 Burns classified according to extent of body surface involved**

Note: This category is to be used when the site of the burn is unspecified, or with categories 940–947 when the site is specified.

Excludes *sunburn (692.71, 692.76–692.77)*

The following fifth-digit subclassification is for use with category 948 to indicate the percent of body surface with third degree burn; valid digits are in [brackets] under each code:

0 **less than 10 percent or unspecified**
1 **10–19%**
2 **20–29%**
3 **30–39%**
4 **40–49%**
5 **50–59%**
6 **60–69%**
7 **70–79%**
8 **80–89%**
9 **90% or more of body surface**

● **948.0 Burn [any degree] involving less than 10 percent of body surface**
[0]

● **948.1 10–19 percent of body surface**
[0–1]

● **948.2 20–29 percent of body surface**
[0–2]

● **948.3 30–39 percent of body surface**
[0–3]

● **948.4 40–49 percent of body surface**
[0–4]

● **948.5 50–59 percent of body surface**
[0–5]

● **948.6 60–69 percent of body surface**
[0–6]

● **948.7 70–79 percent of body surface**
[0–7]

● **948.8 80–89 percent of body surface**
[0–8]

● **948.9 90 percent or more of body surface**
[0–9]

● **949 Burn, unspecified**

Includes: burn NOS
multiple burns NOS

Excludes *burn of unspecified site but with statement of the extent of body surface involved (948.0–948.9)*

❑ **949.0 Unspecified degree**

❑ **949.1 Erythema [first degree]**

❑ **949.2 Blisters, epidermal loss [second degree]**

❑ **949.3 Full-thickness skin loss [third degree NOS]**

❑ **949.4 Deep necrosis of underlying tissues [deep third degree] without mention of loss of a body part**

❑ **949.5 Deep necrosis of underlying tissues [deep third degree] with loss of a body part**

INJURY TO NERVES AND SPINAL CORD (950–957)

Includes: division of nerve
lesion in continuity (with open wound)
traumatic neuroma (with open wound)
traumatic transient paralysis (with open wound)

Excludes *accidental puncture or laceration during medical procedure (998.2)*

● **950 Injury to optic nerve and pathways**

950.0 Optic nerve injury
Second cranial nerve

950.1 Injury to optic chiasm

950.2 Injury to optic pathways

950.3 Injury to visual cortex

❑ **950.9 Unspecified**
Traumatic blindness NOS

● **951 Injury to other cranial nerve(s)**

951.0 Injury to oculomotor nerve
Third cranial nerve

951.1 Injury to trochlear nerve
Fourth cranial nerve

951.2 Injury to trigeminal nerve
Fifth cranial nerve

951.3 Injury to abducens nerve
Sixth cranial nerve

951.4 Injury to facial nerve
Seventh cranial nerve

951.5 Injury to acoustic nerve
Auditory nerve
Eighth cranial nerve
Traumatic deafness NOS

951.6 Injury to accessory nerve
Eleventh cranial nerve

951.7 Injury to hypoglossal nerve
Twelfth cranial nerve

❑ **951.8 Injury to other specified cranial nerves**
Glossopharyngeal [9th cranial] nerve
Olfactory [1st cranial] nerve
Pneumogastric [10th cranial] nerve
Traumatic anosmia NOS
Vagus [10th cranial] nerve

❑ **951.9 Injury to unspecified cranial nerve**

● **952 Spinal cord injury without evidence of spinal bone injury**

● **952.0 Cervical**

❑ **952.00 C_1-C_4 level with unspecified spinal cord injury**
Spinal cord injury, cervical region NOS

952.01 C_1-C_4 level with complete lesion of spinal cord

952.02 C_1-C_4 level with anterior cord syndrome

952.03 C_1-C_4 level with central cord syndrome

❑ **952.04 C_1-C_4 level with other specified spinal cord injury**
Incomplete spinal cord lesion at C_1-C_4 level:
NOS
with posterior cord syndrome

❑ **952.05 C_5-C_7 level with unspecified spinal cord injury**

952.06 C_5-C_7 level with complete lesion of spinal cord

952.07 C_5-C_7 level with anterior cord syndrome

952.08 C_5-C_7 level with central cord syndrome

❑952.09 **C_5-C_7 level with other specified spinal cord injury**
Incomplete spinal cord lesion at C_5-C_7 level:
NOS
with posterior cord syndrome

● 952.1 **Dorsal [thoracic]**

❑952.10 **T_1-T_6 level with unspecified spinal cord injury**
Spinal cord injury, thoracic region NOS

952.11 **T_1-T_6 level with complete lesion of spinal cord**

952.12 **T_1-T_6 level with anterior cord syndrome**

952.13 **T_1-T_6 level with central cord syndrome**

❑952.14 **T_1-T_6 level with other specified spinal cord injury**
Incomplete spinal cord lesion at T_1-T_6 level:
NOS
with posterior cord syndrome

❑952.15 **T_7-T_{12} level with unspecified spinal cord injury**

952.16 **T_7-T_{12} level with complete lesion of spinal cord**

952.17 **T_7-T_{12} level with anterior cord syndrome**

952.18 **T_7-T_{12} level with central cord syndrome**

❑952.19 **T_7-T_{12} level with other specified spinal cord injury**
Incomplete spinal cord lesion at T_7-T_{12} level:
NOS
with posterior cord syndrome

952.2 **Lumbar**

952.3 **Sacral**

952.4 **Cauda equina**

❑952.8 **Multiple sites of spinal cord**

❑952.9 **Unspecified site of spinal cord**

● 953 **Injury to nerve roots and spinal plexus**

953.0 **Cervical root**

953.1 **Dorsal root**

953.2 **Lumbar root**

953.3 **Sacral root**

953.4 **Brachial plexus**

953.5 **Lumbosacral plexus**

❑953.8 **Multiple sites**

❑953.9 **Unspecified site**

● 954 **Injury to other nerve(s) of trunk, excluding shoulder and pelvic girdles**

954.0 **Cervical sympathetic**

❑954.1 **Other sympathetic**
Celiac ganglion or plexus
Inferior mesenteric plexus
Splanchnic nerve(s)
Stellate ganglion

❑954.8 **Other specified nerve(s) of trunk**

❑954.9 **Unspecified nerve of trunk**

● 955 **Injury to peripheral nerve(s) of shoulder girdle and upper limb**

955.0 **Axillary nerve**

955.1 **Median nerve**

955.2 **Ulnar nerve**

955.3 **Radial nerve**

955.4 **Musculocutaneous nerve**

955.5 **Cutaneous sensory nerve, upper limb**

955.6 **Digital nerve**

❑955.7 **Other specified nerve(s) of shoulder girdle and upper limb**

❑955.8 **Multiple nerves of shoulder girdle and upper limb**

❑955.9 **Unspecified nerve of shoulder girdle and upper limb**

● 956 **Injury to peripheral nerve(s) of pelvic girdle and lower limb**

956.0 **Sciatic nerve**

956.1 **Femoral nerve**

956.2 **Posterior tibial nerve**

956.3 **Peroneal nerve**

956.4 **Cutaneous sensory nerve, lower limb**

❑956.5 **Other specified nerve(s) of pelvic girdle and lower limb**

❑956.8 **Multiple nerves of pelvic girdle and lower limb**

❑956.9 **Unspecified nerve of pelvic girdle and lower limb**

● 957 **Injury to other and unspecified nerves**

957.0 **Superficial nerves of head and neck**

❑957.1 **Other specified nerve(s)**

❑957.8 **Multiple nerves in several parts**
Multiple nerve injury NOS

❑957.9 **Unspecified site**
Nerve injury NOS

CERTAIN TRAUMATIC COMPLICATIONS AND UNSPECIFIED INJURIES (958–959)

● 958 **Certain early complications of trauma**

Excludes *adult respiratory distress syndrome (518.5)*
flail chest (807.4)
shock lung (518.5)
that occurring during or following medical procedures (996.0–999.9)

958.0 **Air embolism**
Pneumathemia

Excludes *that complicating:*
abortion (634–638 with .6, 639.6)
ectopic or molar pregnancy (639.6)
pregnancy, childbirth, or the puerperium (673.0)

958.1 **Fat embolism**

Excludes *that complicating:*
abortion (634–638 with .6, 639.6)
pregnancy, childbirth, or the puerperium (673.8)

958.2 **Secondary and recurrent hemorrhage**

958.3 **Posttraumatic wound infection, not elsewhere classified**

Excludes *infected open wounds—code to complicated open wound of site*

958.4 **Traumatic shock**
Shock (immediate) (delayed) following injury

Excludes *shock:*
anaphylactic (995.0)
due to serum (999.4)
anesthetic (995.4)
electric (994.8)
following abortion (639.5)
lightning (994.0)
nontraumatic NOS (785.50)
obstetric (669.1)
postoperative (998.0)

958.5 **Traumatic anuria**
Crush syndrome
Renal failure following crushing

Excludes *that due to a medical procedure (997.5)*

958.6 Volkmann's ischemic contracture
Posttraumatic muscle contracture

958.7 Traumatic subcutaneous emphysema
Excludes *subcutaneous emphysema resulting from a procedure (998.81)*

❑ **958.8 Other early complications of trauma**

● **958.9 Traumatic compartment syndrome** ◄
Excludes *nontraumatic compartment syndrome (729.71–729.79)* ◄

❑ **958.90 Compartment syndrome, unspecified** ◄

958.91 Traumatic compartment syndrome of upper extremity ◄
Traumatic compartment syndrome of shoulder, arm, forearm, wrist, hand, and fingers ◄

958.92 Traumatic compartment syndrome of lower extremity ◄
Traumatic compartment syndrome of hip, buttock, thigh, leg, foot, and toes ◄

958.93 Traumatic compartment syndrome of abdomen ◄

❑ **958.99 Traumatic compartment syndrome of other sites** ◄

● **959 Injury, other and unspecified**
Includes: injury NOS
Excludes *injury NOS of:*
blood vessels (900.0–904.9)
eye (921.0–921.9)
internal organs (860.0–869.1)
intracranial sites (854.0–854.1)
nerves (950.0–951.9, 953.0–957.9)
spinal cord (952.0–952.9)

● **959.0 Head, face, and neck**

❑ **959.01 Head injury, unspecified**
Excludes *concussion (850.0–850.9)*
with head injury NOS (850.0–850.9)
head injury NOS with loss of consciousness (850.1–850.5)
specified head injuries (850.0–854.1)

959.09 Injury of face and neck

● **959.1 Trunk**
Excludes *scapular region (959.2)*

❑ **959.11 Other injury of chest wall**

❑ **959.12 Other injury of abdomen**

959.13 Fracture of corpus cavernosum penis

959.14 Other injury of external genitals

❑ **959.19 Other injury of other sites of trunk**
Injury of trunk NOS

959.2 Shoulder and upper arm
Axilla
Scapular region

959.3 Elbow, forearm, and wrist

959.4 Hand, except finger

959.5 Finger
Fingernail
Thumb (nail)

959.6 Hip and thigh
Upper leg

959.7 Knee, leg, ankle, and foot

❑ **959.8 Other specified sites, including multiple**
Excludes *multiple sites classifiable to the same four-digit category (959.0–959.7)*

❑ **959.9 Unspecified site**

POISONING BY DRUGS, MEDICINAL AND BIOLOGICAL SUBSTANCES (960–979)

Includes: overdose of these substances
wrong substance given or taken in error

Excludes *adverse effects ["hypersensitivity," "reaction," etc.] of correct substance properly administered. Such cases are to be classified according to the nature of the adverse effect, such as:*
adverse effect NOS (995.20) ⬅
allergic lymphadenitis (289.3)
aspirin gastritis (535.4)
blood disorders (280.0–289.9)
dermatitis:
contact (692.0–692.9)
due to ingestion (693.0–693.9)
nephropathy (583.9)
[The drug giving rise to the adverse effect may be identified by use of categories E930–E949.]
drug dependence (304.0–304.9)
drug reaction and poisoning affecting the newborn (760.0–779.9)
nondependent abuse of drugs (305.0–305.9)
pathological drug intoxication (292.2)

Use additional code to specify the effects of the poisoning

● **960 Poisoning by antibiotics**
Excludes *antibiotics:*
ear, nose, and throat (976.6)
eye (976.5)
local (976.0)

960.0 Penicillins
Ampicillin
Carbenicillin
Cloxacillin
Penicillin G

960.1 Antifungal antibiotics
Amphotericin B
Griseofulvin
Nystatin
Trichomycin
Excludes *preparations intended for topical use (976.0–976.9)*

960.2 Chloramphenicol group
Chloramphenicol
Thiamphenicol

960.3 Erythromycin and other macrolides
Oleandomycin
Spiramycin

960.4 Tetracycline group
Doxycycline
Minocycline
Oxytetracycline

960.5 Cephalosporin group
Cephalexin
Cephaloglycin
Cephaloridine
Cephalothin

960.6 Antimycobacterial antibiotics
Cycloserine
Kanamycin
Rifampin
Streptomycin

960.7 Antineoplastic antibiotics
Actinomycin such as:
Bleomycin
Cactinomycin
Dactinomycin
Daunorubicin
Mitomycin

❑ **960.8 Other specified antibiotics**

❑ **960.9 Unspecified antibiotic**

● **961 Poisoning by other anti-infectives**
Excludes *anti-infectives:*
ear, nose, and throat (976.6)
eye (976.5)
local (976.0)

961.0 Sulfonamides
Sulfadiazine
Sulfafurazole
Sulfamethoxazole

961.1 Arsenical anti-infectives

961.2 Heavy metal anti-infectives
Compounds of:
antimony
bismuth
Compounds of:
lead
mercury

Excludes *mercurial diuretics (974.0)*

961.3 Quinoline and hydroxyquinoline derivatives
Chiniofon
Diiodohydroxyquin

Excludes *antimalarial drugs (961.4)*

961.4 Antimalarials and drugs acting on other blood protozoa
Chloroquine
Cycloguanil
Primaquine
Proguanil [chloroguanide]
Pyrimethamine
Quinine

❑ **961.5 Other antiprotozoal drugs**
Emetine

961.6 Anthelmintics
Hexylresorcinol
Piperazine
Thiabendazole

961.7 Antiviral drugs
Methisazone

Excludes *amantadine (966.4)*
cytarabine (963.1)
idoxuridine (976.5)

❑ **961.8 Other antimycobacterial drugs**
Ethambutol
Ethionamide
Isoniazid
Para-aminosalicylic acid derivatives
Sulfones

❑ **961.9 Other and unspecified anti-infectives**
Flucytosine
Nitrofuran derivatives

● **962 Poisoning by hormones and synthetic substitutes**

Excludes *oxytocic hormones (975.0)*

962.0 Adrenal cortical steroids
Cortisone derivatives
Desoxycorticosterone derivatives
Fluorinated corticosteroids

962.1 Androgens and anabolic congeners
Methandriol
Nandrolone
Oxymetholone
Testosterone

962.2 Ovarian hormones and synthetic substitutes
Contraceptives, oral
Estrogens
Estrogens and progestogens, combined
Progestogens

962.3 Insulins and antidiabetic agents
Acetohexamide
Biguanide derivatives, oral
Chlorpropamide
Glucagon
Insulin
Phenformin
Sulfonylurea derivatives, oral
Tolbutamide

962.4 Anterior pituitary hormones
Corticotropin
Gonadotropin
Somatotropin [growth hormone]

962.5 Posterior pituitary hormones
Vasopressin

Excludes *oxytocic hormones (975.0)*

962.6 Parathyroid and parathyroid derivatives

962.7 Thyroid and thyroid derivatives
Dextrothyroxin
Levothyroxine sodium
Liothyronine
Thyroglobulin

962.8 Antithyroid agents
Iodides
Thiouracil
Thiourea

❑ **962.9 Other and unspecified hormones and synthetic substitutes**

● **963 Poisoning by primarily systemic agents**

963.0 Antiallergic and antiemetic drugs
Antihistamines
Chlorpheniramine
Diphenhydramine
Diphenylpyraline
Thonzylamine
Tripelennamine

Excludes *phenothiazine-based tranquilizers (969.1)*

963.1 Antineoplastic and immunosuppressive drugs
Azathioprine
Busulfan
Chlorambucil
Cyclophosphamide
Cytarabine
Fluorouracil
Mercaptopurine
thio-TEPA

Excludes *antineoplastic antibiotics (960.7)*

963.2 Acidifying agents

963.3 Alkalizing agents

963.4 Enzymes, not elsewhere classified
Penicillinase

963.5 Vitamins, not elsewhere classified
Vitamin A
Vitamin D

Excludes *nicotinic acid (972.2)*
vitamin K (964.3)

❑ **963.8 Other specified systemic agents**
Heavy metal antagonists

❑ **963.9 Unspecified systemic agent**

● **964 Poisoning by agents primarily affecting blood constituents**

964.0 Iron and its compounds
Ferric salts
Ferrous sulfate and other ferrous salts

964.1 Liver preparations and other antianemic agents
Folic acid

964.2 Anticoagulants
Coumarin
Heparin
Phenindione
Warfarin sodium

964.3 Vitamin K [phytonadione]

964.4 Fibrinolysis-affecting drugs
Aminocaproic acid
Streptodornase
Streptokinase
Urokinase

964.5 Anticoagulant antagonists and other coagulants
Hexadimethrine
Protamine sulfate

964.6 Gamma globulin

964.7 Natural blood and blood products
Blood plasma
Human fibrinogen
Packed red cells
Whole blood

Excludes *transfusion reactions (999.4–999.8)*

❑**964.8 Other specified agents affecting blood constituents**
Macromolecular blood substitutes
Plasma expanders

❑**964.9 Unspecified agents affecting blood constituents**

● **965 Poisoning by analgesics, antipyretics, and antirheumatics**
Use additional code to identify:
drug dependence (304.0–304.9)
nondependent abuse (305.0–305.9)

● **965.0 Opiates and related narcotics**

❑**965.00 Opium (alkaloids), unspecified**

965.01 Heroin
Diacetylmorphine

965.02 Methadone

❑**965.09 Other**
Codeine [methylmorphine]
Meperidine [pethidine]
Morphine

965.1 Salicylates
Acetylsalicylic acid [aspirin]
Salicylic acid salts

965.4 Aromatic analgesics, not elsewhere classified
Acetanilid
Paracetamol [acetaminophen]
Phenacetin [acetophenetidin]

965.5 Pyrazole derivatives
Aminophenazone [aminopyrine]
Phenylbutazone

● **965.6 Antirheumatics [antiphlogistics]**

Excludes *salicylates (965.1)*
steroids (962.0–962.9)

965.61 Propionic acid derivatives
Fenoprofen
Flurbiprofen
Ibuprofen
Ketoprofen
Naproxen
Oxaprozin

❑**965.69 Other antirheumatics**
Gold salts
Indomethacin

❑**965.7 Other non-narcotic analgesics**
Pyrabital

❑**965.8 Other specified analgesics and antipyretics**
Pentazocine

❑**965.9 Unspecified analgesic and antipyretic**

● **966 Poisoning by anticonvulsants and anti-Parkinsonism drugs**

966.0 Oxazolidine derivatives
Paramethadione
Trimethadione

966.1 Hydantoin derivatives
Phenytoin

966.2 Succinimides
Ethosuximide
Phensuximide

❑**966.3 Other and unspecified anticonvulsants**
Primidone

Excludes *barbiturates (967.0)*
sulfonamides (961.0)

966.4 Anti-Parkinsonism drugs
Amantadine
Ethopropazine [profenamine]
Levodopa [L-dopa]

● **967 Poisoning by sedatives and hypnotics**
Use additional code to identify:
drug dependence (304.0–304.9)
nondependent abuse (305.0–305.9)

967.0 Barbiturates
Amobarbital [amylobarbitone]
Barbital [barbitone]
Butabarbital [butabarbitone]
Pentobarbital [pentobarbitone]
Phenobarbital [phenobarbitone]
Secobarbital [quinalbarbitone]

Excludes *thiobarbiturate anesthetics (968.3)*

967.1 Chloral hydrate group

967.2 Paraldehyde

967.3 Bromine compounds
Bromide
Carbromal (derivatives)

967.4 Methaqualone compounds

967.5 Glutethimide group

967.6 Mixed sedatives, not elsewhere classified

❑**967.8 Other sedatives and hypnotics**

❑**967.9 Unspecified sedative or hypnotic**
Sleeping:
drug NOS
pill NOS
Sleeping:
tablet NOS

● **968 Poisoning by other central nervous system depressants and anesthetics**

Excludes *drug dependence (304.0–304.9)*
nondependent abuse (305.0–305.9)

968.0 Central nervous system muscle-tone depressants
Chlorphenesin (carbamate)
Mephenesin
Methocarbamol

968.1 Halothane

❑**968.2 Other gaseous anesthetics**
Ether
Halogenated hydrocarbon derivatives, except halothane
Nitrous oxide

968.3 Intravenous anesthetics
Ketamine
Methohexital [methohexitone]
Thiobarbiturates, such as thiopental sodium

❑**968.4 Other and unspecified general anesthetics**

968.5 Surface [topical] and infiltration anesthetics
Cocaine
Lidocaine [lignocaine]
Procaine
Tetracaine

968.6 Peripheral nerve- and plexus-blocking anesthetics

968.7 Spinal anesthetics

❑**968.9 Other and unspecified local anesthetics**

● **969 Poisoning by psychotropic agents**

Excludes *drug dependence (304.0–304.9)*
nondependent abuse (305.0–305.9)

969.0 Antidepressants
Amitriptyline
Imipramine
Monoamine oxidase [MAO] inhibitors

969.1 **Phenothiazine-based tranquilizers**
Chlorpromazine
Fluphenazine
Prochlorperazine
Promazine

969.2 **Butyrophenone-based tranquilizers**
Haloperidol
Trifluperidol
Spiperone

❑969.3 **Other antipsychotics, neuroleptics, and major tranquilizers**

969.4 **Benzodiazepine-based tranquilizers**
Chlordiazepoxide
Lorazepam
Diazepam
Medazepam
Flurazepam
Nitrazepam

❑969.5 **Other tranquilizers**
Hydroxyzine
Meprobamate

969.6 **Psychodysleptics [hallucinogens]**
Cannabis (derivatives)
Lysergide [LSD]
Marijuana (derivatives)
Mescaline
Psilocin
Psilocybin

969.7 **Psychostimulants**
Amphetamine
Caffeine

Excludes *central appetite depressants (977.0)*

❑969.8 **Other specified psychotropic agents**

❑969.9 **Unspecified psychotropic agent**

● 970 **Poisoning by central nervous system stimulants**

970.0 **Analeptics**
Lobeline
Nikethamide

970.1 **Opiate antagonists**
Levallorphan
Nalorphine
Naloxone

❑970.8 **Other specified central nervous system stimulants**

❑970.9 **Unspecified central nervous system stimulant**

● 971 **Poisoning by drugs primarily affecting the autonomic nervous system**

971.0 **Parasympathomimetics [cholinergics]**
Acetylcholine
Anticholinesterase:
organophosphorus
reversible
Pilocarpine

971.1 **Parasympatholytics [anticholinergics and antimuscarinics] and spasmolytics**
Atropine
Homatropine
Hyoscine [scopolamine]
Quaternary ammonium derivatives

Excludes *papaverine (972.5)*

971.2 **Sympathomimetics [adrenergics]**
Epinephrine [adrenalin]
Levarterenol [noradrenalin]

971.3 **Sympatholytics [antiadrenergics]**
Phenoxybenzamine
Tolazoline hydrochloride

❑971.9 **Unspecified drug primarily affecting autonomic nervous system**

● 972 **Poisoning by agents primarily affecting the cardiovascular system**

972.0 **Cardiac rhythm regulators**
Practolol
Procainamide
Propranolol
Quinidine

Excludes *lidocaine (968.5)*

972.1 **Cardiotonic glycosides and drugs of similar action**
Digitalis glycosides
Digoxin
Strophanthins

972.2 **Antilipemic and antiarteriosclerotic drugs**
Clofibrate
Nicotinic acid derivatives

972.3 **Ganglion-blocking agents**
Pentamethonium bromide

972.4 **Coronary vasodilators**
Dipyridamole
Nitrates [nitroglycerin]
Nitrites

❑972.5 **Other vasodilators**
Cyclandelate
Diazoxide
Papaverine

Excludes *nicotinic acid (972.2)*

❑972.6 **Other antihypertensive agents**
Clonidine
Guanethidine
Rauwolfia alkaloids
Reserpine

972.7 **Antivaricose drugs, including sclerosing agents**
Sodium morrhuate
Zinc salts

972.8 **Capillary-active drugs**
Adrenochrome derivatives
Metaraminol

❑972.9 **Other and unspecified agents primarily affecting the cardiovascular system**

● 973 **Poisoning by agents primarily affecting the gastrointestinal system**

973.0 **Antacids and antigastric secretion drugs**
Aluminum hydroxide
Magnesium trisilicate

973.1 **Irritant cathartics**
Bisacodyl
Castor oil
Phenolphthalein

973.2 **Emollient cathartics**
Dioctyl sulfosuccinates

❑973.3 **Other cathartics, including intestinal atonia drugs**
Magnesium sulfate

973.4 **Digestants**
Pancreatin
Pepsin
Papain

973.5 **Antidiarrheal drugs**
Kaolin
Pectin

Excludes *anti-infectives (960.0–961.9)*

973.6 **Emetics**

❑973.8 **Other specified agents primarily affecting the gastro-intestinal system**

❑973.9 **Unspecified agent primarily affecting the gastro-intestinal system**

● 974 **Poisoning by water, mineral, and uric acid metabolism drugs**

974.0 **Mercurial diuretics**
Chlormerodrin
Mercaptomerin
Mersalyl

974.1 Purine derivative diuretics
Theobromine
Theophylline
Excludes *aminophylline [theophylline ethylenediamine] (975.7)*
caffeine (969.7)

974.2 Carbonic acid anhydrase inhibitors
Acetazolamide

974.3 Saluretics
Benzothiadiazides
Chlorothiazide group

❑**974.4 Other diuretics**
Ethacrynic acid
Furosemide

974.5 Electrolytic, caloric, and water-balance agents

❑**974.6 Other mineral salts, not elsewhere classified**

974.7 Uric acid metabolism drugs
Allopurinol
Colchicine
Probenecid

● **975 Poisoning by agents primarily acting on the smooth and skeletal muscles and respiratory system**

975.0 Oxytocic agents
Ergot alkaloids
Oxytocin
Prostaglandins

975.1 Smooth muscle relaxants
Adiphenine
Metaproterenol [orciprenaline]
Excludes *papaverine (972.5)*

975.2 Skeletal muscle relaxants

❑**975.3 Other and unspecified drugs acting on muscles**

975.4 Antitussives
Dextromethorphan
Pipazethate

975.5 Expectorants
Acetylcysteine
Guaifenesin
Terpin hydrate

975.6 Anti-common cold drugs

975.7 Antiasthmatics
Aminophylline [theophylline ethylenediamine]

❑**975.8 Other and unspecified respiratory drugs**

● **976 Poisoning by agents primarily affecting skin and mucous membrane, ophthalmological, otorhinolaryngological, and dental drugs**

976.0 Local anti-infectives and anti-inflammatory drugs

976.1 Antipruritics

976.2 Local astringents and local detergents

976.3 Emollients, demulcents, and protectants

976.4 Keratolytics, keratoplastics, other hair treatment drugs and preparations

976.5 Eye anti-infectives and other eye drugs
Idoxuridine

976.6 Anti-infectives and other drugs and preparations for ear, nose, and throat

976.7 Dental drugs topically applied
Excludes *anti-infectives (976.0)*
local anesthetics (968.5)

❑**976.8 Other agents primarily affecting skin and mucous membrane**
Spermicides [vaginal contraceptives]

❑**976.9 Unspecified agent primarily affecting skin and mucous membrane**

● **977 Poisoning by other and unspecified drugs and medicinal substances**

977.0 Dietetics
Central appetite depressants

977.1 Lipotropic drugs

977.2 Antidotes and chelating agents, not elsewhere classified

977.3 Alcohol deterrents

977.4 Pharmaceutical excipients
Pharmaceutical adjuncts

❑**977.8 Other specified drugs and medicinal substances**
Contrast media used for diagnostic x-ray procedures
Diagnostic agents and kits

❑**977.9 Unspecified drug or medicinal substance**

● **978 Poisoning by bacterial vaccines**

978.0 BCG

978.1 Typhoid and paratyphoid

978.2 Cholera

978.3 Plague

978.4 Tetanus

978.5 Diphtheria

978.6 Pertussis vaccine, including combinations with a pertussis component

❑**978.8 Other and unspecified bacterial vaccines**

978.9 Mixed bacterial vaccines, except combinations with a pertussis component

● **979 Poisoning by other vaccines and biological substances**
Excludes *gamma globulin (964.6)*

979.0 Smallpox vaccine

979.1 Rabies vaccine

979.2 Typhus vaccine

979.3 Yellow fever vaccine

979.4 Measles vaccine

979.5 Poliomyelitis vaccine

❑**979.6 Other and unspecified viral and rickettsial vaccines**
Mumps vaccine

979.7 Mixed viral-rickettsial and bacterial vaccines, except combinations with a pertussis component
Excludes *combinations with a pertussis component (978.6)*

❑**979.9 Other and unspecified vaccines and biological substances**

TOXIC EFFECTS OF SUBSTANCES CHIEFLY NONMEDICINAL AS TO SOURCE (980–989)

Excludes *burns from chemical agents (ingested) (947.0–947.9)*
localized toxic effects indexed elsewhere (001.0–799.9)
respiratory conditions due to external agents (506.0–508.9)

Use additional code to specify the nature of the toxic effect

● **980 Toxic effect of alcohol**

980.0 Ethyl alcohol
Denatured alcohol
Ethanol
Grain alcohol

Use additional code to identify any associated:
acute alcohol intoxication (305.0)
in alcoholism (303.0)
drunkenness (simple) (305.0)
pathological (291.4)

980.1 Methyl alcohol
Methanol
Wood alcohol

980.2 Isopropyl alcohol
Dimethyl carbinol
Isopropanol
Rubbing alcohol

980.3 Fusel oil
Alcohol:
amyl
butyl
propyl

❑**980.8 Other specified alcohols**

❑**980.9 Unspecified alcohol**

981 Toxic effect of petroleum products
Benzine
Gasoline
Kerosene
Paraffin wax
Petroleum:
ether
naphtha
spirit

● **982 Toxic effect of solvents other than petroleum based**

982.0 Benzene and homologues

982.1 Carbon tetrachloride

982.2 Carbon disulfide
Carbon bisulfide

❑**982.3 Other chlorinated hydrocarbon solvents**
Tetrachloroethylene
Trichloroethylene

Excludes *chlorinated hydrocarbon preparations other than solvents (989.2)*

982.4 Nitroglycol

❑**982.8 Other nonpetroleum-based solvents**
Acetone

● **983 Toxic effect of corrosive aromatics, acids, and caustic alkalis**

983.0 Corrosive aromatics
Carbolic acid or phenol
Cresol

983.1 Acids
Acid:
hydrochloric
nitric
sulfuric

983.2 Caustic alkalis
Lye
Potassium hydroxide
Sodium hydroxide

❑**983.9 Caustic, unspecified**

● **984 Toxic effect of lead and its compounds (including fumes)**

Includes: that from all sources except medicinal substances

984.0 Inorganic lead compounds
Lead dioxide
Lead salts

984.1 Organic lead compounds
Lead acetate
Tetraethyl lead

❑**984.8 Other lead compounds**

❑**984.9 Unspecified lead compound**

● **985 Toxic effect of other metals**

Includes: that from all sources except medicinal substances

985.0 Mercury and its compounds
Minamata disease

985.1 Arsenic and its compounds

985.2 Manganese and its compounds

985.3 Beryllium and its compounds

985.4 Antimony and its compounds

985.5 Cadmium and its compounds

985.6 Chromium

❑**985.8 Other specified metals**
Brass fumes
Copper salts
Iron compounds
Nickel compounds

❑**985.9 Unspecified metal**

986 Toxic effect of carbon monoxide

● **987 Toxic effect of other gases, fumes, or vapors**

987.0 Liquefied petroleum gases
Butane
Propane

❑**987.1 Other hydrocarbon gas**

987.2 Nitrogen oxides
Nitrogen dioxide
Nitrous fumes

987.3 Sulfur dioxide

987.4 Freon
Dichloromonofluoromethane

987.5 Lacrimogenic gas
Bromobenzyl cyanide
Chloroacetophenone
Ethyliodoacetate

987.6 Chlorine gas

987.7 Hydrocyanic acid gas

❑**987.8 Other specified gases, fumes, or vapors**
Phosgene
Polyester fumes

❑**987.9 Unspecified gas, fume, or vapor**

● **988 Toxic effect of noxious substances eaten as food**

Excludes *allergic reaction to food, such as:*
gastroenteritis (558.3)
rash (692.5, 693.1)
food poisoning (bacterial) (005.0–005.9)
toxic effects of food contaminants, such as:
aflatoxin and other mycotoxin (989.7)
mercury (985.0)

988.0 Fish and shellfish

988.1 Mushrooms

988.2 Berries and other plants

❑**988.8 Other specified noxious substances eaten as food**

❑**988.9 Unspecified noxious substance eaten as food**

● **989 Toxic effect of other substances, chiefly nonmedicinal as to source**

989.0 Hydrocyanic acid and cyanides
Potassium cyanide
Sodium cyanide

Excludes *gas and fumes (987.7)*

989.1 Strychnine and salts

989.2 Chlorinated hydrocarbons
Aldrin
Chlordane
DDT
Dieldrin

Excludes *chlorinated hydrocarbon solvents (982.0–982.3)*

989.3 Organophosphate and carbamate
Carbaryl
Dichlorvos
Malathion
Parathion
Phorate
Phosdrin

❑**989.4 Other pesticides, not elsewhere classified**
Mixtures of insecticides

989.5 Venom
Bites of venomous snakes, lizards, and spiders
Tick paralysis

989.6 Soaps and detergents

989.7 Aflatoxin and other mycotoxin [food contaminants]

● **989.8 Other substances, chiefly nonmedicinal as to source**

989.81 Asbestos

Excludes *asbestosis (501)*
exposure to asbestos (V15.84)

989.82 Latex

989.83 Silicone

Excludes *silicone used in medical devices, implants, and grafts (996.00–996.79)*

989.84 Tobacco

989.89 Other

❑**989.9 Unspecified substance, chiefly nonmedicinal as to source**

OTHER AND UNSPECIFIED EFFECTS OF EXTERNAL CAUSES (990–995)

❑**990 Effects of radiation, unspecified**
Complication of:
phototherapy
radiation therapy
Radiation sickness

Excludes *specified adverse effects of radiation. Such conditions are to be classified according to the nature of the adverse effect, as:*
burns (940.0–949.5)
dermatitis (692.7–692.8)
leukemia (204.0–208.9)
pneumonia (508.0)
sunburn (692.71, 692.76–692.77)

[The type of radiation giving rise to the adverse effect may be identified by use of the E codes.]

● **991 Effects of reduced temperature**

991.0 Frostbite of face

991.1 Frostbite of hand

991.2 Frostbite of foot

❑**991.3 Frostbite of other and unspecified sites**

991.4 Immersion foot
Trench foot

991.5 Chilblains
Erythema pernio
Perniosis

991.6 Hypothermia
Hypothermia (accidental)

Excludes *hypothermia following anesthesia (995.89)*
hypothermia not associated with low environmental temperature (780.99)

❑**991.8 Other specified effects of reduced temperature**

❑**991.9 Unspecified effect of reduced temperature**
Effects of freezing or excessive cold NOS

● **992 Effects of heat and light**

Excludes *burns (940.0–949.5)*
diseases of sweat glands due to heat (705.0–705.9)
malignant hyperpyrexia following anesthesia (995.86)
sunburn (692.71, 692.76–692.77)

992.0 Heat stroke and sunstroke
Heat apoplexy
Heat pyrexia
Ictus solaris
Siriasis
Thermoplegia

992.1 Heat syncope
Heat collapse

992.2 Heat cramps

992.3 Heat exhaustion, anhydrotic
Heat prostration due to water depletion

Excludes *that associated with salt depletion (992.4)*

992.4 Heat exhaustion due to salt depletion
Heat prostration due to salt (and water) depletion

❑**992.5 Heat exhaustion, unspecified**
Heat prostration NOS

992.6 Heat fatigue, transient

992.7 Heat edema

❑**992.8 Other specified heat effects**

❑**992.9 Unspecified**

● **993 Effects of air pressure**

993.0 Barotrauma, otitic
Aero-otitis media
Effects of high altitude on ears

993.1 Barotrauma, sinus
Aerosinusitis
Effects of high altitude on sinuses

❑**993.2 Other and unspecified effects of high altitude**
Alpine sickness
Andes disease
Anoxia due to high altitude
Hypobaropathy
Mountain sickness

993.3 Caisson disease
Bends
Compressed-air disease
Decompression sickness
Divers' palsy or paralysis

993.4 Effects of air pressure caused by explosion

❑**993.8 Other specified effects of air pressure**

❑**993.9 Unspecified effect of air pressure**

● **994 Effects of other external causes**

Excludes *certain adverse effects not elsewhere classified (995.0–995.8)*

994.0 Effects of lightning
Shock from lightning
Struck by lightning NOS

Excludes *burns (940.0–949.5)*

994.1 Drowning and nonfatal submersion
Bathing cramp
Immersion

994.2 Effects of hunger
Deprivation of food
Starvation

994.3 Effects of thirst
Deprivation of water

994.4 Exhaustion due to exposure

994.5 Exhaustion due to excessive exertion
Overexertion

994.6 Motion sickness
Air sickness
Seasickness
Travel sickness

994.7 Asphyxiation and strangulation
Suffocation (by):
bedclothes
cave-in
constriction
mechanical
plastic bag
pressure
strangulation

Excludes *asphyxia from:*
carbon monoxide (986)
inhalation of food or foreign body (932–934.9)
other gases, fumes, and vapors (987.0–987.9)

994.8 Electrocution and nonfatal effects of electric current
Shock from electric current

Excludes *electric burns (940.0–949.5)*

❑**994.9 Other effects of external causes**
Effects of:
abnormal gravitational [G] forces or states
weightlessness

● **995 Certain adverse effects not elsewhere classified**

Excludes *complications of surgical and medical care (996.0–999.9)*

❑**995.0 Other anaphylactic shock**
Allergic shock NOS or due to adverse effect of correct medicinal substance properly administered
Anaphylactic reaction NOS or due to adverse effect of correct medicinal substance properly administered
Anaphylaxis NOS or due to adverse effect of correct medicinal substance properly administered

Excludes *anaphylactic reaction to serum (999.4)*
anaphylactic shock due to adverse food reaction (995.60–995.69)

Use additional E code to identify external cause, such as:
adverse effects of correct medicinal substance properly administered [E930–E949]

995.1 Angioneurotic edema
Giant urticaria

Excludes *urticaria:*
due to serum (999.5)
other specified (698.2, 708.0–708.9, 757.33)

● **995.2 Other and unspecified adverse effect of drug, medicinal and biological substance** (Revised)
Adverse effect to correct medicinal substance properly administered
Allergic reaction to correct medicinal substance properly administered
Hypersensitivity to correct medicinal substance properly administered
Idiosyncrasy due to correct medicinal substance properly administered
Drug:
hypersensitivity NOS
reaction NOS

Excludes *pathological drug intoxication (292.2)*

❑**995.20 Unspecified adverse effect of unspecified drug, medicinal and biological substance** ◀

995.21 Arthus phenomenon ◀
Arthus reaction ◀

❑**995.22 Unspecified adverse effect of anesthesia** ◀

❑**995.23 Unspecified adverse effect of insulin** ◀

❑**995.27 Other drug allergy** ◀
Drug allergy NOS ◀
Drug hypersensitivity NOS ◀

❑**995.29 Unspecified adverse effect of other drug, medicinal and biological substance** ◀

❑**995.3 Allergy, unspecified**
Allergic reaction NOS
Hypersensitivity NOS
Idiosyncrasy NOS

Excludes *allergic reaction NOS to correct medicinal substance properly administered (995.27)* (Revised)
allergy to existing dental restorative materials (525.66) ◀
specific types of allergic reaction, such as:
allergic diarrhea (558.3)
dermatitis (691.0–693.9)
hayfever (477.0–477.9)

995.4 Shock due to anesthesia
Shock due to anesthesia in which the correct substance was properly administered

Excludes *complications of anesthesia in labor or delivery (668.0–668.9)*
overdose or wrong substance given (968.0–969.9)
postoperative shock NOS (998.0)
specified adverse effects of anesthesia classified elsewhere, such as:
anoxic brain damage (348.1)
hepatitis (070.0–070.9), etc.
unspecified adverse effect of anesthesia (995.22) (Revised)

● **995.5 Child maltreatment syndrome**
Use additional code(s), if applicable, to identify any associated injuries

Use additional E code to identify:
nature of abuse (E960–E968)
perpetrator (E967.0–E967.9)

❑**995.50 Child abuse, unspecified**

995.51 Child emotional/psychological abuse
Use additional code to identify intent of neglect (E904.0–E968.4)

995.52 Child neglect (nutritional)
Use additional code to identify intent of neglect (E904.0–E968.4)

995.53 Child sexual abuse

995.54 Child physical abuse
Battered baby or child syndrome

Excludes *Shaken infant syndrome (995.55)*

995.55 Shaken infant syndrome
Use additional code(s) to identify any associated injuries

❑**995.59 Other child abuse and neglect**
Multiple forms of abuse
Use additional code to identify intent of neglect (E904.0–E968.4)

● **995.6 Anaphylactic shock due to adverse food reaction**
Anaphylactic shock due to nonpoisonous foods

❑**995.60 Due to unspecified food**

995.61 Due to peanuts

995.62 Due to crustaceans

995.63 Due to fruits and vegetables

995.64 Due to tree nuts and seeds

995.65 Due to fish

995.66 Due to food additives

995.67 Due to milk products

995.68 Due to eggs

❑ **995.69 Due to other specified food**

995.7 Other adverse food reactions, not elsewhere classified

Use additional code to identify the type of reaction, such as:
hives (708.0)
wheezing (786.07)

Excludes *anaphylactic shock due to adverse food reaction (995.60–995.69)*
asthma (493.0, 493.9)
dermatitis due to food (693.1)
in contact with the skin (692.5)
gastroenteritis and colitis due to food (558.3)
rhinitis due to food (477.1)

● **995.8 Other specified adverse effects, not elsewhere classified**

❑ **995.80 Adult maltreatment, unspecified**
Abused person NOS

Use additional code to identify:
any associated injury
perpetrator (E967.0–E967.9)

995.81 Adult physical abuse
Battered:
person syndrome, NEC
man
spouse
woman

Use additional code to identify:
any associated injury
nature of abuse (E960–E968)
perpetrator (E967.0–E967.9)

995.82 Adult emotional/psychological abuse

Use additional E code to identify perpetrator (E967.0–E967.9)

995.83 Adult sexual abuse

Use additional code to identify:
any associated injury
perpetrator (E967.0–E967.9)

995.84 Adult neglect (nutritional)

Use additional code to identify:
intent of neglect (E904.0–E968.4)
perpetrator (E967.0–E967.9)

❑ **995.85 Other adult abuse and neglect**
Multiple forms of abuse and neglect

Use additional code to identify any associated injury
intent of neglect (E904.0, E968.4)
nature of abuse (E960–E968)
perpetrator (E967.0–E967.9)

995.86 Malignant hyperthermia
Malignant hyperpyrexia due to anesthesia

❑ **995.89 Other**
Hypothermia due to anesthesia

● **995.9 Systemic inflammatory response syndrome (SIRS)** ⬅

❑ **995.90 Systemic inflammatory response syndrome, unspecified SIRS NOS**

● *995.91 Sepsis* ⬅
Systemic inflammatory response syndrome due to infectious process with acute organ dysfunction ◀

Code first underlying infection ◀

Excludes *sepsis with acute organ dysfunction (995.92)* ◀
sepsis with multiple organ dysfunction (995.92) ◀
severe sepsis (995.92) ◀

● *995.92 Severe sepsis* ⬅
Sepsis with acute organ dysfunction ◀
Sepsis with multiple organ dysfunction (MOD) ◀
Systemic inflammatory response syndrome due to infectious process with acute organ dysfunction ◀

Code first underlying infection ◀

Use additional code to specify acute organ dysfunction, such as: ⬅
acute renal failure (584.5–584.9)
acute respiratory failure (518.81)
critical illness myopathy (359.81)
critical illness polyneuropathy (357.82)
disseminated intravascular coagulopathy (DIC) syndrome (286.6) ◀
encephalopathy (348.31)
hepatic failure (570)
septic shock (785.52)

● *995.93 Systemic inflammatory response syndrome due to noninfectious process without acute organ dysfunction* ⬅
Code first underlying conditions, such as: ◀
acute pancreatitis (577.0) ◀
trauma ◀

Excludes *systemic inflammatory response syndrome due to noninfectious process with acute organ dysfunction (995.94)* ◀

● *995.94 Systemic inflammatory response syndrome due to noninfectious process with acute organ dysfunction* ⬅
Code first underlying conditions, such as: ◀
acute pancreatitis (577.0) ◀
trauma ◀

Use additional code to specify acute organ dysfunction, such as: ⬅
acute renal failure (584.5–584.9)
acute respiratory failure (518.81)
critical illness myopathy (359.81)
critical illness polyneuropathy (357.82)
disseminated intravascular coagulopathy (DIC) syndrome (286.6) ◀
encephalopathy (348.31)
hepatic failure (570)

Excludes *severe sepsis (995.92)* ◀

COMPLICATIONS OF SURGICAL AND MEDICAL CARE, NOT ELSEWHERE CLASSIFIED (996–999)

Excludes *adverse effects of medicinal agents (001.0–799.9, 995.0–995.8)*
burns from local applications and irradiation (940.0–949.5)
complications of:
conditions for which the procedure was performed
surgical procedures during abortion, labor, and delivery (630–676.9)
poisoning and toxic effects of drugs and chemicals (960.0–989.9)
postoperative conditions in which no complications are present, such as:
artificial opening status (V44.0–V44.9)
closure of external stoma (V55.0–V55.9)
fitting of prosthetic device (V52.0–V52.9)
specified complications classified elsewhere:
anesthetic shock (995.4)
electrolyte imbalance (276.0–276.9)
postlaminectomy syndrome (722.80–722.83)
postmastectomy lymphedema syndrome (457.0)
postoperative psychosis (293.0–293.9)
any other condition classified elsewhere in the Alphabetic Index when described as due to a procedure

● 996 Complications peculiar to certain specified procedures

Includes: complications, not elsewhere classified, in the use of artificial substitutes [e.g., Dacron, metal, Silastic, Teflon] or natural sources [e.g., bone] involving:
anastomosis (internal)
graft (bypass) (patch)
implant
internal device:
catheter
electronic
fixation
prosthetic
reimplant
transplant

Excludes *accidental puncture or laceration during procedure (998.2)*
complications of internal anastomosis of:
gastrointestinal tract (997.4)
urinary tract (997.5)
mechanical complication of respirator (V46.14)
other specified complications classified elsewhere, such as:
hemolytic anemia (283.1)
functional cardiac disturbances (429.4)
serum hepatitis (070.2–070.3)

● 996.0 Mechanical complication of cardiac device, implant, and graft

Breakdown (mechanical)
Displacement
Leakage
Obstruction, mechanical
Perforation
Protrusion

❑996.00 Unspecified device, implant, and graft

996.01 Due to cardiac pacemaker (electrode)

996.02 Due to heart valve prosthesis

996.03 Due to coronary bypass graft

Excludes *atherosclerosis of graft (414.02, 414.03)*
embolism [occlusion NOS] [thrombus] of graft (996.72)

996.04 Due to automatic implantable cardiac defibrillator

❑996.09 Other

❑996.1 Mechanical complication of other vascular device, implant, and graft

Mechanical complications involving:
aortic (bifurcation) graft (replacement)
arteriovenous:
dialysis catheter
fistula surgically created
shunt surgically created
balloon (counterpulsation) device, intra-aortic
carotid artery bypass graft
femoral-popliteal bypass graft
umbrella device, vena cava

Excludes *atherosclerosis of biological graft (440.30–440.32)*
embolism [occlusion NOS] [thrombus] of (biological) (synthetic) graft (996.74)
peritoneal dialysis catheter (996.56)

996.2 Mechanical complication of nervous system device, implant, and graft

Mechanical complications involving:
dorsal column stimulator
electrodes implanted in brain [brain "pacemaker"]
peripheral nerve graft
ventricular (communicating) shunt

● 996.3 Mechanical complication of genitourinary device, implant, and graft

❑996.30 Unspecified device, implant, and graft

996.31 Due to urethral [indwelling] catheter

996.32 Due to intrauterine contraceptive device

❑996.39 Other

Cystostomy catheter
Prosthetic reconstruction of vas deferens
Repair (graft) of ureter without mention of resection

Excludes *complications due to:*
external stoma of urinary tract (997.5)
internal anastomosis of urinary tract (997.5)

● 996.4 Mechanical complication of internal orthopedic device, implant, and graft

Mechanical complications involving:
external (fixation) device utilizing internal screw(s), pin(s), or other methods of fixation
grafts of bone, cartilage, muscle, or tendon
internal (fixation) device such as nail, plate, rod, etc.

Use additional code to identify prosthetic joint with mechanical complication (V43.60–V43.69)

Excludes *complications of external orthopedic device, such as:*
pressure ulcer due to cast (707.00–707.09)

996.40 Unspecified mechanical complication of internal orthopedic device, implant, and graft

996.41 Mechanical loosening of prosthetic joint

Aseptic loosening

996.42 Dislocation of prosthetic joint

Instability of prosthetic joint
Subluxation of prosthetic joint

996.43 Prosthetic joint implant failure

Breakage (fracture) of prosthetic joint

996.44 Peri-prosthetic fracture around prosthetic joint

996.45 Peri-prosthetic osteolysis

Use additional code to identify major osseous defect, if applicable (731.3) ◄

996.46 Articular bearing surface wear of prosthetic joint

❑996.47 Other mechanical complication of prosthetic joint implant

Mechanical complication of prosthetic joint NOS

❑996.49 Other mechanical complication of other internal orthopedic device, implant, and graft

Excludes *mechanical complication of prosthetic joint implant (996.41–996.47)*

● 996.5 Mechanical complication of other specified prosthetic device, implant, and graft

Mechanical complications involving:
prosthetic implant in:
bile duct
breast
chin
orbit of eye
nonabsorbable surgical material NOS
other graft, implant, and internal device, not elsewhere classified

996.51 Due to corneal graft

❑996.52 Due to graft of other tissue, not elsewhere classified

Skin graft failure or rejection

Excludes *failure of artificial skin graft (996.55)*
failure of decellularized allodermis (996.55)
sloughing of temporary skin allografts or xenografts (pigskin)-omit code

996.53 Due to ocular lens prosthesis

Excludes *contact lenses—code to condition*

996.54 Due to breast prosthesis
Breast capsule (prosthesis)
Mammary implant

996.55 Due to artificial skin graft and decellularized allodermis
Dislodgement
Displacement
Failure
Non-adherence
Poor incorporation
Shearing

996.56 Due to peritoneal dialysis catheter

Excludes *mechanical complication of arteriovenous dialysis catheter (996.1)*

996.57 Due to insulin pump

❑**996.59 Due to other implant and internal device, not elsewhere classified**
Nonabsorbable surgical material NOS
Prosthetic implant in:
bile duct
chin
orbit of eye

● **996.6 Infection and inflammatory reaction due to internal prosthetic device, implant, and graft**
Infection (causing obstruction) due to (presence of) any device, implant, and graft classifiable to 996.0–996.5
Inflammation due to (presence of) any device, implant, and graft classifiable to 996.0–996.5

Use additional code to identify specified infections

❑**996.60 Due to unspecified device, implant, and graft**

996.61 Due to cardiac device, implant, and graft
Cardiac pacemaker or defibrillator:
electrode(s), lead(s)
pulse generator
subcutaneous pocket
Coronary artery bypass graft
Heart valve prosthesis

❑**996.62 Due to vascular device, implant, and graft**
Arterial graft
Arteriovenous fistula or shunt
Infusion pump
Vascular catheter (arterial) (dialysis) (venous)

996.63 Due to nervous system device, implant and graft
Electrodes implanted in brain
Peripheral nerve graft
Spinal canal catheter
Ventricular (communicating) shunt (catheter)

996.64 Due to indwelling urinary catheter

Use additional code to identify specified infections, such as:
Cystitis (595.0–595.9)
Sepsis (038.0–038.9)

❑**996.65 Due to other genitourinary device, implant and graft**
Intrauterine contraceptive device

996.66 Due to internal joint prosthesis

Use additional code to identify infected prosthetic joint (V43.60–V43.69)

❑**996.67 Due to other internal orthopedic device, implant and graft**
Bone growth stimulator (electrode)
Internal fixation device (pin) (rod) (screw)

996.68 Due to peritoneal dialysis catheter
Exit-site infection or inflammation

❑**996.69 Due to other internal prosthetic device, implant, and graft**
Breast prosthesis
Ocular lens prosthesis
Prosthetic orbital implant

● **996.7 Other complications of internal (biological) (synthetic) prosthetic device, implant, and graft**
Complication NOS due to (presence of) any device, implant, and graft classifiable to 996.0–996.5
occlusion NOS
Embolism due to (presence of) any device, implant, and graft classifiable to 996.0–996.5
Fibrosis due to (presence of) any device, implant, and graft classifiable to 996.0–996.5
Hemorrhage due to (presence of) any device, implant, and graft classifiable to 996.0–996.5
Pain due to (presence of) any device, implant, and graft classifiable to 996.0–996.5
Stenosis due to (presence of) any device, implant, and graft classifiable to 996.0–996.5
Thrombus due to (presence of) any device, implant, and graft classifiable to 996.0–996.5
Use additional code to identify complication, such as: ◀
pain due to presence of device, implant, or graft (338.18–338.19, 338.28–338.29) ◀

Excludes *transplant rejection (996.8)*

❑**996.70 Due to unspecified device, implant, and graft**

996.71 Due to heart valve prosthesis

996.72 Due to other cardiac device, implant, and graft
Cardiac pacemaker or defibrillator:
electrode(s), lead(s)
subcutaneous pocket
Coronary artery bypass (graft)

Excludes *occlusion due to atherosclerosis (414.00–414.07)*

996.73 Due to renal dialysis device, implant, and graft

❑**996.74 Due to vascular device, implant, and graft**

Excludes *occlusion of biological graft due to atherosclerosis (440.30–440.32)*

996.75 Due to nervous system device, implant, and graft

996.76 Due to genitourinary device, implant, and graft

996.77 Due to internal joint prosthesis

❑**996.78 Due to other internal orthopedic device, implant, and graft**

❑**996.79 Due to other internal prosthetic device, implant, and graft**

● **996.8 Complications of transplanted organ**
Transplant failure or rejection

Use additional code to identify nature of complication, such as:
Cytomegalovirus [CMV] infection (078.5)

❑**996.80 Transplanted organ, unspecified**

996.81 Kidney

996.82 Liver

996.83 Heart

996.84 Lung

996.85 Bone marrow
Graft-versus-host disease (acute) (chronic)

996.86 Pancreas

996.87 Intestine

❑**996.89 Other specified transplanted organ**

● 996.9 **Complications of reattached extremity or body part**

❑ 996.90 **Unspecified extremity**

996.91 **Forearm**

996.92 **Hand**

996.93 **Finger(s)**

❑ 996.94 **Upper extremity, other and unspecified**

996.95 **Foot and toe(s)**

❑ 996.96 **Lower extremity, other and unspecified**

❑ 996.99 **Other specified body part**

● 997 **Complications affecting specified body systems, not elsewhere classified**

Use additional code to identify complication

Excludes *the listed conditions when specified as:*
causing shock (998.0)
complications of:
anesthesia:
adverse effect (001.0–799.9, 995.0–995.8)
in labor or delivery (668.0–668.9)
poisoning (968.0–968.9)
implanted device or graft (996.0–996.9)
obstetrical procedures (669.0–669.4)
reattached extremity (996.90–996.96)
transplanted organ (996.80–996.89)

● 997.0 **Nervous system complications**

❑ 997.00 **Nervous system complication, unspecified**

997.01 **Central nervous system complication**
Anoxic brain damage
Cerebral hypoxia

Excludes *Cerebrovascular hemorrhage or infarction (997.02)*

997.02 **Iatrogenic cerebrovascular infarction or hemorrhage**
Postoperative stroke

❑ 997.09 **Other nervous system complications**

997.1 **Cardiac complications**
Cardiac:
arrest during or resulting from a procedure
insufficiency during or resulting from a procedure
Cardiorespiratory failure during or resulting from a procedure
Heart failure during or resulting from a procedure

Excludes *the listed conditions as long-term effects of cardiac surgery or due to the presence of cardiac prosthetic device (429.4)*

997.2 **Peripheral vascular complications**
Phlebitis or thrombophlebitis during or resulting from a procedure

Excludes *the listed conditions due to:*
implant or catheter device (996.62)
infusion, perfusion, or transfusion (999.2)
complications affecting blood vessels (997.71–997.79)

997.3 **Respiratory complications**
Mendelson's syndrome resulting from a procedure
Pneumonia (aspiration) resulting from a procedure

Excludes *iatrogenic [postoperative] pneumothorax (512.1)*
iatrogenic pulmonary embolism (415.11)
Mendelson's syndrome in labor and delivery (668.0)
specified complications classified elsewhere, such as:
adult respiratory distress syndrome (518.5)
pulmonary edema, postoperative (518.4)
respiratory insufficiency, acute, postoperative (518.5)
shock lung (518.5)
tracheostomy complication (519.00–519.09)
transfusion related acute lung injury (TRALI) (518.7) ◄

997.4 **Digestive system complications**
Complications of:
Intestinal (internal) anastomosis and bypass, not elsewhere classified, except that involving urinary tract
Hepatic failure specified as due to a procedure
Hepatorenal syndrome specified as due to a procedure
Intestinal obstruction NOS specified as due to a procedure

Excludes *specified gastrointestinal complications classified elsewhere, such as:*
blind loop syndrome (579.2)
colostomy or enterostomy complications (569.60–569.69)
gastrojejunal ulcer (534.0–534.9)
gastrostomy complications (536.40–536.49)
infection of esophagostomy (530.86)
infection of external stoma (569.61)
mechanical complication of esophagostomy (530.87)
pelvic peritoneal adhesions, female (614.6)
peritoneal adhesions (568.0)
peritoneal adhesions with obstruction (560.81)
postcholecystectomy syndrome (576.0)
postgastric surgery syndromes (564.2)
vomiting following gastrointestinal surgery (564.3)

997.5 **Urinary complications**
Complications of:
external stoma of urinary tract
internal anastomosis and bypass of urinary tract, including that involving intestinal tract
Oliguria or anuria specified as due to procedure
Renal:
failure (acute) specified as due to procedure
insufficiency (acute) specified as due to procedure
Tubular necrosis (acute) specified as due to procedure

Excludes *specified complications classified elsewhere, such as:*
postoperative stricture of:
ureter (593.3)
urethra (598.2)

● 997.6 **Amputation stump complication**

Excludes *admission for treatment for a current traumatic amputation—code to complicated traumatic amputation*
phantom limb (syndrome) (353.6)

❑ 997.60 **Unspecified complication**

997.61 **Neuroma of amputation stump**

997.62 **Infection (chronic)**
Use additional code to identify the organism

❑ 997.69 **Other**

● 997.7 **Vascular complications of other vessels**

Excludes *peripheral vascular complications (997.2)*

997.71 **Vascular complications of mesenteric artery**

997.72 **Vascular complications of renal artery**

❑ 997.79 **Vascular complications of other vessels**

● 997.9 **Complications affecting other specified body systems, not elsewhere classified**

Excludes *specified complications classified elsewhere, such as:*
broad ligament laceration syndrome (620.6)
postartificial menopause syndrome (627.4)
postoperative stricture of vagina (623.2)

997.91 **Hypertension**

Excludes *Essential hypertension (401.0–401.9)*

❑ 997.99 **Other**
Vitreous touch syndrome

● 998 **Other complications of procedures, NEC**

998.0 **Postoperative shock**
Collapse NOS during or resulting from a surgical procedure
Shock (endotoxic) (hypovolemic) (septic) during or resulting from a surgical procedure

Excludes *shock:*
anaphylactic due to serum (999.4)
anesthetic (995.4)
electric (994.8)
following abortion (639.5)
obstetric (669.1)
traumatic (958.4)

● 998.1 **Hemorrhage or hematoma or seroma complicating a procedure**

Excludes *hemorrhage, hematoma, or seroma:*
complicating cesarean section or puerperal perineal wound (674.3)
due to implant device or graft (996.70–996.79)

998.11 **Hemorrhage complicating a procedure**

998.12 **Hematoma complicating a procedure**

998.13 **Seroma complicating a procedure**

998.2 **Accidental puncture or laceration during a procedure**
Accidental perforation by catheter or other instrument during a procedure on:
blood vessel
nerve
organ

Excludes *iatrogenic [postoperative] pneumothorax (512.1)*
puncture or laceration caused by implanted device intentionally left in operation wound (996.0–996.5)
specified complications classified elsewhere, such as:
broad ligament laceration syndrome (620.6)
trauma from instruments during delivery (664.0–665.9)

● 998.3 **Disruption of operation wound**
Dehiscence of operation wound
Rupture of operation wound

Excludes *disruption of:*
amputation of stump (997.6)
cesarean wound (674.1)
perineal wound, puerperal (674.2)

998.31 **Disruption of internal operation wound**

998.32 **Disruption of external operation wound**
Disruption of operation wound NOS

998.4 **Foreign body accidentally left during a procedure**
Adhesions due to foreign body accidentally left in operative wound or body cavity during a procedure
Obstruction due to foreign body accidentally left in operative wound or body cavity during a procedure
Perforation due to foreign body accidentally left in operative wound or body cavity during a procedure

Excludes *obstruction or perforation caused by implanted device intentionally left in body (996.0–996.5)*

● 998.5 **Postoperative infection**

Excludes *bleb associated endophthalmitis (379.63)* ◄
infection due to:
implanted device (996.60–996.69)
infusion, perfusion, or transfusion (999.3)
postoperative obstetrical wound infection (674.3)

998.51 **Infected postoperative seroma**
Use additional code to identify organism

❑ 998.59 **Other postoperative infection**
Abscess: postoperative
intra-abdominal postoperative
stitch postoperative
subphrenic postoperative
wound postoperative
Septicemia postoperative

Use additional code to identify infection

998.6 **Persistent postoperative fistula**

998.7 **Acute reaction to foreign substance accidentally left during a procedure**
Peritonitis:
aseptic
chemical

● 998.8 **Other specified complications of procedures, not elsewhere classified**

998.81 **Emphysema (subcutaneous) (surgical) resulting from a procedure**

998.82 **Cataract fragments in eye following cataract surgery**

998.83 **Non-healing surgical wound**

❑ 998.89 **Other specified complications**

❑ 998.9 **Unspecified complication of procedure, not elsewhere classified**
Postoperative complication NOS

Excludes *complication NOS of obstetrical surgery or procedure (669.4)*

● 999 Complications of medical care, not elsewhere classified

Includes: complications, not elsewhere classified, of:
dialysis (hemodialysis) (peritoneal) (renal)
extracorporeal circulation
hyperalimentation therapy
immunization
infusion
inhalation therapy
injection
inoculation
perfusion
transfusion
vaccination
ventilation therapy

Excludes *specified complications classified elsewhere such as:*
complications of implanted device (996.0–996.9)
contact dermatitis due to drugs (692.3)
dementia dialysis (294.8)
transient (293.9)
dialysis disequilibrium syndrome (276.0–276.9)
poisoning and toxic effects of drugs and chemicals (960.0–989.9)
postvaccinal encephalitis (323.51) ◄Revised
water and electrolyte imbalance (276.0–276.9)

999.0 Generalized vaccinia

999.1 Air embolism
Air embolism to any site following infusion, perfusion, or transfusion

Excludes *embolism specified as:*
complicating:
abortion (634–638 with .6, 639.6)
ectopic or molar pregnancy (639.6)
pregnancy, childbirth, or the puerperium (673.0)
due to implanted device (996.7)
traumatic (958.0)

❑ 999.2 Other vascular complications
Phlebitis following infusion, perfusion, or transfusion
Thromboembolism following infusion, perfusion, or transfusion
Thrombophlebitis following infusion, perfusion, or transfusion

Excludes *the listed conditions when specified as:*
due to implanted device (996.61–996.62, 996.72–996.74)
postoperative NOS (997.2, 997.71–997.79)

❑ 999.3 Other infection
Infection following infusion, injection, transfusion, or vaccination
Sepsis following infusion, injection, transfusion, or vaccination
Septicemia following infusion, injection, transfusion, or vaccination

Excludes *the listed conditions when specified as:*
due to implanted device (996.60–996.69)
postoperative NOS (998.51–998.59)

999.4 Anaphylactic shock due to serum

Excludes *shock:*
allergic NOS (995.0)
anaphylactic:
NOS (995.0)
due to drugs and chemicals (995.0)

❑ 999.5 Other serum reaction
Intoxication by serum
Protein sickness
Serum rash
Serum sickness
Urticaria due to serum

Excludes *serum hepatitis (070.2–070.3)*

999.6 ABO incompatibility reaction
Incompatible blood transfusion
Reaction to blood group incompatibility in infusion or transfusion

999.7 Rh incompatibility reaction
Reactions due to Rh factor in infusion or transfusion

❑ 999.8 Other transfusion reaction
Septic shock due to transfusion
Transfusion reaction NOS

Excludes *postoperative shock (998.0)*
transfusion related acute lung injury (TRALI) (518.7) ◄New

❑ 999.9 Other and unspecified complications of medical care, not elsewhere classified
Complications, not elsewhere classified, of:
electroshock therapy
inhalation therapy
ultrasound therapy
ventilation therapy
Unspecified misadventure of medical care

Excludes *unspecified complication of:*
phototherapy (990)
radiation therapy (990)

V-Codes—SUPPLEMENTARY CLASSIFICATION OF FACTORS INFLUENCING HEALTH STATUS AND CONTACT WITH HEALTH SERVICES (V01–V86)

This classification is provided to deal with occasions when circumstances other than a disease or injury classifiable to categories 001–999 (the main part of ICD) are recorded as "diagnoses" or "problems." This can arise mainly in three ways:

a) When a person who is not currently sick encounters the health services for some specific purpose, such as to act as a donor of an organ or tissue, to receive prophylactic vaccination, or to discuss a problem which is in itself not a disease or injury. This will be a fairly rare occurrence among hospital inpatients, but will be relatively more common among hospital outpatients and patients of family practitioners, health clinics, etc.

b) When a person with a known disease or injury, whether it is current or resolving, encounters the health care system for a specific treatment of that disease or injury (e.g., dialysis for renal disease; chemotherapy for malignancy; cast change).

c) When some circumstance or problem is present which influences the person's health status but is not in itself a current illness or injury. Such factors may be elicited during population surveys, when the person may or may not be currently sick, or be recorded as an additional factor to be borne in mind when the person is receiving care for some current illness or injury classifiable to categories 001–999.

In the latter circumstances the V code should be used only as a supplementary code and should not be the one selected for use in primary, single cause tabulations. Examples of these circumstances are a personal history of certain diseases, or a person with an artificial heart valve in situ.

PERSONS WITH POTENTIAL HEALTH HAZARDS RELATED TO COMMUNICABLE DISEASES (V01–V06)

Excludes *family history of infectious and parasitic diseases (V18.8)*
personal history of infectious and parasitic diseases (V12.0)

● **V01 Contact with or exposure to communicable diseases**

- 1/2 **V01.0 Cholera**
  Conditions classifiable to 001
- 1/2 **V01.1 Tuberculosis**
  Conditions classifiable to 010–018
- 1/2 **V01.2 Poliomyelitis**
  Conditions classifiable to 045
- 1/2 **V01.3 Smallpox**
  Conditions classifiable to 050
- 1/2 **V01.4 Rubella**
  Conditions classifiable to 056
- 1/2 **V01.5 Rabies**
  Conditions classifiable to 071
- 1/2 **V01.6 Venereal diseases**
  Conditions classifiable to 090–099
- ● **V01.7 Other viral diseases**
  Conditions classifiable to 042–078, and V08, except as above
  - 1/2 **V01.71 Varicella**
  - 1/2 **V01.79 Other viral diseases**
- ● **V01.8 Other communicable diseases**
  Conditions classifiable to 001–136, except as above
  - 1/2 **V01.81 Anthrax**
  - 1/2 **V01.82 Exposure to SARS-associated coronavirus**
  - 1/2 **V01.83 Escherichia coli (E. coli)**
  - 1/2 **V01.84 Meningococcus**
  - 1/2 **V01.89 Other communicable diseases**
- 1/2 **V01.9 Unspecified communicable disease**

● **V02 Carrier or suspected carrier of infectious diseases**

- 1/2 **V02.0 Cholera**
- 1/2 **V02.1 Typhoid**
- 1/2 **V02.2 Amebiasis**
- 1/2 **V02.3 Other gastrointestinal pathogens**
- 1/2 **V02.4 Diphtheria**
- ● **V02.5 Other specified bacterial diseases**
  - 1/2 **V02.51 Group B streptococcus**
  - 1/2 **V02.52 Other streptococcus**
  - 1/2 **V02.59 Other specified bacterial diseases**
    Meningococcal
    Staphylococcal
- ● **V02.6 Viral hepatitis**
  - 1/2 **V02.60 Viral hepatitis carrier, unspecified**
  - 1/2 **V02.61 Hepatitis B carrier**
  - 1/2 **V02.62 Hepatitis C carrier**
  - 1/2 **V02.69 Other viral hepatitis carrier**
- 1/2 **V02.7 Gonorrhea**
- 1/2 **V02.8 Other venereal diseases**
- 1/2 **V02.9 Other specified infectious organism**

● **V03 Need for prophylactic vaccination and inoculation against bacterial diseases**

Excludes *vaccination not carried out (V64.00–V64.09)*
vaccines against combinations of diseases (V06.0–V06.9)

- 1/2 **V03.0 Cholera alone**
- 1/2 **V03.1 Typhoid-paratyphoid alone [TAB]**
- 1/2 **V03.2 Tuberculosis [BCG]**
- 1/2 **V03.3 Plague**
- 1/2 **V03.4 Tularemia**
- 1/2 **V03.5 Diphtheria alone**
- 1/2 **V03.6 Pertussis alone**
- 1/2 **V03.7 Tetanus toxoid alone**
- ● **V03.8 Other specified vaccinations against single bacterial diseases**
  - 1/2 **V03.81 Haemophilus influenzae, type B [Hib]**
  - 1/2 **V03.82 Streptococcus pneumoniae [pneumococcus]**
  - 1/2 **V03.89 Other specified vaccination**
- 1/2 **V03.9 Unspecified single bacterial disease**

● **V04 Need for prophylactic vaccination and inoculation against certain diseases**

Excludes *vaccines against combinations of diseases (V06.0–V06.9)*

- 1/2 **V04.0 Poliomyelitis**
- 1/2 **V04.1 Smallpox**
- 1/2 **V04.2 Measles alone**
- 1/2 **V04.3 Rubella alone**
- 1/2 **V04.4 Yellow fever**
- 1/2 **V04.5 Rabies**
- 1/2 **V04.6 Mumps alone**
- 1/2 **V04.7 Common cold**

● V04.8 Other viral diseases
1/2 V04.81 Influenza
1/2 V04.82 Respiratory syncytial virus (RSV)
1/2 V04.89 Other viral disease

● V05 Need for prophylactic vaccination and inoculation against single diseases
Excludes *vaccines against combinations of diseases (V06.0–V06.9)*

1/2 V05.0 Arthropod-borne viral encephalitis
1/2 V05.1 Other arthropod-borne viral diseases
1/2 V05.2 Leishmaniasis
1/2 V05.3 Viral hepatitis
1/2 V05.4 Varicella
Chicken pox
1/2 V05.8 Other specified disease
1/2 V05.9 Unspecified single disease

● V06 Need for prophylactic vaccination and inoculation against combinations of diseases
Note: Use additional single vaccination codes from categories V03–V05 to identify any vaccinations not included in a combination code.

1/2 V06.0 Cholera with typhoid-paratyphoid [cholera TAB]
1/2 V06.1 Diphtheria-tetanus-pertussis, combined [DTP] [DTaP]
1/2 V06.2 Diphtheria-tetanus-pertussis with typhoid-paratyphoid [DTP TAB]
1/2 V06.3 Diphtheria-tetanus-pertussis with poliomyelitis [DTP+polio]
1/2 V06.4 Measles-mumps-rubella [MMR]
1/2 V06.5 Tetanus-diphtheria [Td] [DT]
1/2 V06.6 Streptococcus pneumoniae [pneumococcus] and influenza
1/2 V06.8 Other combinations
Excludes *multiple single vaccination codes (V03.0–V05.9)*
1/2 V06.9 Unspecified combined vaccine

PERSONS WITH NEED FOR ISOLATION, OTHER POTENTIAL HEALTH HAZARDS AND PROPHYLACTIC MEASURES (V07–V09)

● V07 Need for isolation and other prophylactic measures
Excludes *prophylactic organ removal (V50.41–V50.49)*

1/2 V07.0 Isolation
Admission to protect the individual from his surroundings or for isolation of individual after contact with infectious diseases
1/2 V07.1 Desensitization to allergens
1/2 V07.2 Prophylactic immunotherapy
Administration of:
antivenin
immune sera [gamma globulin]
RhoGAM
tetanus antitoxin
● V07.3 Other prophylactic chemotherapy
1/2 V07.31 Prophylactic fluoride administration
1/2 V07.39 Other prophylactic chemotherapy
Excludes *maintenance chemotherapy following disease (V58.11)*
1/2 V07.4 Hormone replacement therapy (post menopausal)
1/2 V07.8 Other specified prophylactic measure
1/2 V07.9 Unspecified prophylactic measure

1/2 V08 Asymptomatic human immunodeficiency virus [HIV] infection status
HIV positive NOS
Note: This code is ONLY to be used when NO HIV infection symptoms or conditions are present. If any HIV infection symptoms or conditions are present, see code 042.
Excludes *AIDS (042)*
human immunodeficiency virus [HIV] disease (042)
exposure to HIV (V01.79)
nonspecific serologic evidence of HIV (795.71)
symptomatic human immunodeficiency virus [HIV] infection (042)

● V09 Infection with drug-resistant microorganisms
Note: This category is intended for use as an additional code for infectious conditions classified elsewhere to indicate the presence of drug-resistance of the infectious organism.

❷ V09.0 Infection with microorganisms resistant to penicillins
Methicillin-resistant staphylococcus aureus (MRSA)
❷ V09.1 Infection with microorganisms resistant to cephalosporins and other B-lactam antibiotics
❷ V09.2 Infection with microorganisms resistant to macrolides
❷ V09.3 Infection with microorganisms resistant to tetracyclines
❷ V09.4 Infection with microorganisms resistant to aminoglycosides
● V09.5 Infection with microorganisms resistant to quinolones and fluoroquinolones
❷ V09.50 Without mention of resistance to multiple quinolones and fluoroquinoles
❷ V09.51 With resistance to multiple quinolones and fluoroquinoles
❷ V09.6 Infection with microorganisms resistant to sulfonamides
● V09.7 Infection with microorganisms resistant to other specified antimycobacterial agents
Excludes *amikacin (V09.4)*
kanamycin (V09.4)
streptomycin [SM] (V09.4)
❷ V09.70 Without mention of resistance to multiple antimycobacterial agents
❷ V09.71 With resistance to multiple antimycobacterial agents
● V09.8 Infection with microorganisms resistant to other specified drugs
Vancomycin (glycopeptide) intermediate staphylococcus aureus (VISA/GISA)
Vancomycin (glycopeptide) resistant enterococcus (VRE)
Vancomycin (glycopeptide) resistant staphylococcus aureus (VRSA/GRSA)
❷ V09.80 Without mention of resistance to multiple drugs
❷ V09.81 With resistance to multiple drugs
● V09.9 Infection with drug-resistant microorganisms, unspecified
Drug resistance NOS
❷ V09.90 Without mention of multiple drug resistance
❷ V09.91 With multiple drug resistance
Multiple drug resistance NOS

PERSONS WITH POTENTIAL HEALTH HAZARDS RELATED TO PERSONAL AND FAMILY HISTORY (V10–V19)

Excludes *obstetric patients where the possibility that the fetus might be affected is the reason for observation or management during pregnancy (655.0–655.9)*

● **V10 Personal history of malignant neoplasm**

● **V10.0 Gastrointestinal tract**
History of conditions classifiable to 140–159

1/2 **V10.00 Gastrointestinal tract, unspecified**
1/2 **V10.01 Tongue**
1/2 **V10.02 Other and unspecified oral cavity and pharynx**
1/2 **V10.03 Esophagus**
1/2 **V10.04 Stomach**
1/2 **V10.05 Large intestine**
1/2 **V10.06 Rectum, rectosigmoid junction, and anus**
1/2 **V10.07 Liver**
1/2 **V10.09 Other**

● **V10.1 Trachea, bronchus, and lung**
History of conditions classifiable to 162

1/2 **V10.11 Bronchus and lung**
1/2 **V10.12 Trachea**

● **V10.2 Other respiratory and intrathoracic organs**
History of conditions classifiable to 160, 161, 163–165

1/2 **V10.20 Respiratory organ, unspecified**
1/2 **V10.21 Larynx**
1/2 **V10.22 Nasal cavities, middle ear, and accessory sinuses**
1/2 **V10.29 Other**

1/2 **V10.3 Breast**
History of conditions classifiable to 174 and 175

● **V10.4 Genital organs**
History of conditions classifiable to 179–187

1/2 **V10.40 Female genital organ, unspecified**
1/2 **V10.41 Cervix uteri**
1/2 **V10.42 Other parts of uterus**
1/2 **V10.43 Ovary**
1/2 **V10.44 Other female genital organs**
1/2 **V10.45 Male genital organ, unspecified**
1/2 **V10.46 Prostate**
1/2 **V10.47 Testis**
1/2 **V10.48 Epididymis**
1/2 **V10.49 Other male genital organs**

● **V10.5 Urinary organs**
History of conditions classifiable to 188 and 189

1/2 **V10.50 Urinary organ, unspecified**
1/2 **V10.51 Bladder**
1/2 **V10.52 Kidney**

Excludes *renal pelvis (V10.53)*

1/2 **V10.53 Renal pelvis**
1/2 **V10.59 Other**

● **V10.6 Leukemia**
Conditions classifiable to 204–208

Excludes *leukemia in remission (204–208)*

1/2 **V10.60 Leukemia, unspecified**
1/2 **V10.61 Lymphoid leukemia**
1/2 **V10.62 Myeloid leukemia**
1/2 **V10.63 Monocytic leukemia**
1/2 **V10.69 Other**

● **V10.7 Other lymphatic and hematopoietic neoplasms**
Conditions classifiable to 200–203

Excludes *listed conditions in 200–203 in remission*

1/2 **V10.71 Lymphosarcoma and reticulosarcoma**
1/2 **V10.72 Hodgkin's disease**
1/2 **V10.79 Other**

● **V10.8 Personal history of malignant neoplasm of other site**
History of conditions classifiable to 170–173, 190–195

1/2 **V10.81 Bone**
1/2 **V10.82 Malignant melanoma of skin**
1/2 **V10.83 Other malignant neoplasm of skin**
1/2 **V10.84 Eye**
1/2 **V10.85 Brain**
1/2 **V10.86 Other parts of nervous system**

Excludes *peripheral, sympathetic, and parasympathetic nerves (V10.89)*

1/2 **V10.87 Thyroid**
1/2 **V10.88 Other endocrine glands and related structures**
1/2 **V10.89 Other**

1/2 **V10.9 Unspecified personal history of malignant neoplasm**

● **V11 Personal history of mental disorder**

❑ **V11.0 Schizophrenia**

Excludes *that in remission (295.0–295.9 with fifth-digit 5)*

❑ **V11.1 Affective disorders**
Personal history of manic-depressive psychosis

Excludes *that in remission (296.0–296.6 with fifth-digit 5, 6)*

❑ **V11.2 Neurosis**
❑ **V11.3 Alcoholism**
❑ **V11.8 Other mental disorders**
❑ **V11.9 Unspecified mental disorder**

● **V12 Personal history of certain other diseases**

● **V12.0 Infectious and parasitic diseases**

Excludes *personal history of infectious diseases specific to a body system*

1/2 **V12.00 Unspecified infectious and parasitic disease**
1/2 **V12.01 Tuberculosis**
1/2 **V12.02 Poliomyelitis**
1/2 **V12.03 Malaria**
1/2 **V12.09 Other**

1/2 **V12.1 Nutritional deficiency**
1/2 **V12.2 Endocrine, metabolic, and immunity disorders**

Excludes *history of allergy (V14.0–V14.9, V15.01–V15.09)*

1/2 **V12.3 Diseases of blood and blood-forming organs**

● **V12.4 Disorders of nervous system and sense organs**

1/2 **V12.40 Unspecified disorder of nervous system and sense organs**
1/2 **V12.41 Benign neoplasm of the brain**
1/2 **V12.42 Infections of the central nervous system**
Encephalitis
Meningitis
1/2 **V12.49 Other disorders of nervous system and sense organs**

◀ New ⟸ Revised ❶ First Listed 1/2 First Listed or Additional ❷ Additional Only ● Use Additional Digit(s) ❑ Nonspecific Code

● V12.5 **Diseases of circulatory system**
Excludes *old myocardial infarction (412)*
postmyocardial infarction syndrome (411.0)

1/2 V12.50 **Unspecified circulatory disease**

1/2 V12.51 **Venous thrombosis and embolism**
Pulmonary embolism

1/2 V12.52 **Thrombophlebitis**

1/2 V12.59 **Other**

● V12.6 **Diseases of respiratory system**
Excludes *tuberculosis (V12.01)*

1/2 V12.60 **Unspecified disease of respiratory system**

1/2 V12.61 **Pneumonia (recurrent)**

1/2 V12.69 **Other diseases of respiratory system**

● V12.7 **Diseases of digestive system**

1/2 V12.70 **Unspecified digestive disease**

1/2 V12.71 **Peptic ulcer disease**

1/2 V12.72 **Colonic polyps**

1/2 V12.79 **Other**

● V13 **Personal history of other diseases**

● V13.0 **Disorders of urinary system**

1/2 V13.00 **Unspecified urinary disorder**

1/2 V13.01 **Urinary calculi**

1/2 V13.02 **Urinary (tract) infection**

1/2 V13.03 **Nephrotic syndrome**

1/2 V13.09 **Other**

1/2 V13.1 **Trophoblastic disease**
Excludes *supervision during a current pregnancy (V23.1)*

● V13.2 **Other genital system and obstetric disorders**
Excludes *supervision during a current pregnancy of a woman with poor obstetric history (V23.0–V23.9)*
habitual aborter (646.3)
without current pregnancy (629.9)

1/2 V13.21 **Personal history of pre-term labor**
Excludes *current pregnancy with history of pre-term labor (V23.41)*

1/2 V13.29 **Other genital system and obstetric disorders**

1/2 V13.3 **Diseases of skin and subcutaneous tissue**

❑ V13.4 **Arthritis**

1/2 V13.5 **Other musculoskeletal disorders**

● V13.6 **Congenital malformations**

1/2 V13.61 **Hypospadias**
Note: According to the Guidelines, this code is both a First/Additional and Additional Only code.

❑ V13.69 **Other congenital malformations**

1/2 V13.7 **Perinatal problems**
Excludes *low birth weight status (V21.30–V21.35)*

1/2 V13.8 **Other specified diseases**

1/2 V13.9 **Unspecified disease**

● V14 **Personal history of allergy to medicinal agents**

2 V14.0 **Penicillin**

2 V14.1 **Other antibiotic agent**

2 V14.2 **Sulfonamides**

2 V14.3 **Other anti-infective agent**

2 V14.4 **Anesthetic agent**

2 V14.5 **Narcotic agent**

2 V14.6 **Analgesic agent**

2 V14.7 **Serum or vaccine**

2 V14.8 **Other specified medicinal agents**

2 V14.9 **Unspecified medicinal agent**

● V15 **Allergy, other than to medicinal agents**

● V15.0 **Allergy, other than to medicinal agents**
Excludes *allergy to food substance used as base for medicinal agent (V14.0–V14.9)*

2 V15.01 **Allergy to peanuts**

2 V15.02 **Allergy to milk products**
Excludes *lactose intolerance (271.3)*

2 V15.03 **Allergy to eggs**

2 V15.04 **Allergy to seafood**
Seafood (octopus) (squid) ink
Shellfish

2 V15.05 **Allergy to other foods**
Food additives
Nuts other than peanuts

2 V15.06 **Allergy to insects**
Bugs
Insect bites and stings
Spiders

2 V15.07 **Allergy to latex**
Latex sensitivity

2 V15.08 **Allergy to radiographic dye**
Contrast media used for diagnostic x-ray procedures

2 V15.09 **Other allergy, other than to medicinal agents**

2 V15.1 **Surgery to heart and great vessels**
Excludes *replacement by transplant or other means (V42.1–V42.2, V43.2–V43.4)*

2 V15.2 **Surgery to other major organs**
Excludes *replacement by transplant or other means (V42.0–V43.8)*

2 V15.3 **Irradiation**
Previous exposure to therapeutic or other ionizing radiation

● V15.4 **Psychological trauma**
Excludes *history of condition classifiable to 290–316 (V11.0–V11.9)*

2 V15.41 **History of physical abuse**
Rape

2 V15.42 **History of emotional abuse**
Neglect

2 V15.49 **Other**

2 V15.5 **Injury**

2 V15.6 **Poisoning**

❑ V15.7 **Contraception**
Excludes *current contraceptive management (V25.0–V25.4)*
presence of intrauterine contraceptive device as incidental finding (V45.5)

● V15.8 **Other specified personal history presenting hazards to health**

2 V15.81 **Noncompliance with medical treatment**

2 V15.82 **History of tobacco use**
Excludes *tobacco dependence (305.1)*

2 V15.84 **Exposure to asbestos**

2 V15.85 **Exposure to potentially hazardous body fluids**

❷ V15.86 Exposure to lead

❷ V15.87 History of Extracorporeal Membrane Oxygenation [ECMO]

1/2 V15.88 History of fall
At risk for falling

❷ V15.89 Other

❷ V15.9 **Unspecified personal history presenting hazards to health**

● **V16 Family history of malignant neoplasm**

1/2 V16.0 **Gastrointestinal tract**
Family history of condition classifiable to 140–159

1/2 V16.1 **Trachea, bronchus, and lung**
Family history of condition classifiable to 162

1/2 V16.2 **Other respiratory and intrathoracic organs**
Family history of condition classifiable to 160–161, 163–165

1/2 V16.3 **Breast**
Family history of condition classifiable to 174

● V16.4 **Genital organs**
Family history of condition classifiable to 179–187

1/2 V16.40 Genital organ, unspecified

1/2 V16.41 Ovary

1/2 V16.42 Prostate

1/2 V16.43 Testis

1/2 V16.49 Other

● V16.5 **Urinary organs**
Family history of condition classifiable to 189

1/2 V16.51 Kidney

1/2 V16.59 Other

1/2 V16.6 **Leukemia**
Family history of condition classifiable to 204–208

1/2 V16.7 **Other lymphatic and hematopoietic neoplasms**
Family history of condition classifiable to 200–203

1/2 V16.8 **Other specified malignant neoplasm**
Family history of other condition classifiable to 140–199

1/2 V16.9 **Unspecified malignant neoplasm**

● **V17 Family history of certain chronic disabling diseases**

1/2 V17.0 **Psychiatric condition**
Excludes *family history of mental retardation (V18.4)*

1/2 V17.1 **Stroke (cerebrovascular)**

1/2 V17.2 **Other neurological diseases**
Epilepsy
Huntington's chorea

1/2 V17.3 **Ischemic heart disease**

1/2 V17.4 **Other cardiovascular diseases**

1/2 V17.5 **Asthma**

1/2 V17.6 **Other chronic respiratory conditions**

1/2 V17.7 **Arthritis**

● V17.8 **Other musculoskeletal diseases**

1/2 V17.81 Osteoporosis

1/2 V17.89 Other musculoskeletal diseases

● **V18 Family history of certain other specific conditions**

1/2 V18.0 **Diabetes mellitus**

1/2 V18.1 **Other endocrine and metabolic diseases**

1/2 V18.2 **Anemia**

1/2 V18.3 **Other blood disorders**

1/2 V18.4 **Mental retardation**

● V18.5 **Digestive disorders**

1/2 V18.51 Colonic polyps ◀

Excludes *family history of malignant neoplasm of gastrointestinal tract (V16.0)* ◀

1/2 V18.59 Other digestive disorders ◀

● V18.6 **Kidney diseases**

1/2 V18.61 Polycystic kidney

1/2 V18.69 Other kidney diseases

1/2 V18.7 **Other genitourinary diseases**

1/2 V18.8 **Infectious and parasitic diseases**

1/2 V18.9 **Genetic disease carrier**

● **V19 Family history of other conditions**

1/2 V19.0 **Blindness or visual loss**

1/2 V19.1 **Other eye disorders**

1/2 V19.2 **Deafness or hearing loss**

1/2 V19.3 **Other ear disorders**

1/2 V19.4 **Skin conditions**

1/2 V19.5 **Congenital anomalies**

1/2 V19.6 **Allergic disorders**

1/2 V19.7 **Consanguinity**

1/2 V19.8 **Other condition**

PERSONS ENCOUNTERING HEALTH SERVICES IN CIRCUMSTANCES RELATED TO REPRODUCTION AND DEVELOPMENT (V20–V29)

● **V20 Health supervision of infant or child**

❶ V20.0 **Foundling**

❶ V20.1 **Other healthy infant or child receiving care**
Medical or nursing care supervision of healthy infant in cases of:
maternal illness, physical or psychiatric
socioeconomic adverse condition at home
too many children at home preventing or interfering with normal care

❶ V20.2 **Routine infant or child health check**
Developmental testing of infant or child
Immunizations appropriate for age
Initial and subsequent routine newborn check ◀
Routine vision and hearing testing

Excludes *special screening for developmental handicaps (V79.3)*

Use additional code(s) to identify:
Special screening examination(s) performed (V73.0–V82.9)

● **V21 Constitutional states in development**

❷ V21.0 **Period of rapid growth in childhood**

❷ V21.1 **Puberty**

❷ V21.2 **Other adolescence**

● V21.3 **Low birth weight status**

Excludes *history of perinatal problems (V13.7)*

❷ V21.30 Low birth weight status, unspecified

❷ V21.31 Low birth weight status, less than 500 grams

❷ V21.32 Low birth weight status, 500–999 grams

❷ V21.33 Low birth weight status, 1000–1499 grams

❷ V21.34 Low birth weight status, 1500–1999 grams

❷ V21.35 Low birth weight status, 2000–2500 grams

❷ V21.8 **Other specified constitutional states in development**

❷ V21.9 **Unspecified constitutional state in development**

● **V22 Normal pregnancy**
Excludes *pregnancy examination or test, pregnancy unconfirmed (V72.40)*

❶ **V22.0 Supervision of normal first pregnancy**

❶ **V22.1 Supervision of other normal pregnancy**

❷ **V22.2 Pregnant state, incidental**
Pregnant state NOS

● **V23 Supervision of high-risk pregnancy**

1/2 **V23.0 Pregnancy with history of infertility**

1/2 **V23.1 Pregnancy with history of trophoblastic disease**
Pregnancy with history of:
hydatidiform mole
vesicular mole
Excludes *that without current pregnancy (V13.1)*

1/2 **V23.2 Pregnancy with history of abortion**
Pregnancy with history of conditions classifiable to 634–638
Excludes *habitual aborter:*
care during pregnancy (646.3)
that without current pregnancy (629.9)

1/2 **V23.3 Grand multiparity**
Excludes *care in relation to labor and delivery (659.4)*
that without current pregnancy (V61.5)

● **V23.4 Pregnancy with other poor obstetric history**
Pregnancy with history of other conditions classifiable to 630–676

1/2 **V23.41 Pregnancy with history of pre-term labor**

1/2 **V23.49 Pregnancy with other poor obstetric history**

1/2 **V23.5 Pregnancy with other poor reproductive history**
Pregnancy with history of stillbirth or neonatal death

1/2 **V23.7 Insufficient prenatal care**
History of little or no prenatal care

● **V23.8 Other high-risk pregnancy**

1/2 **V23.81 Elderly primigravida**
First pregnancy in a woman who will be 35 years of age or older at expected date of delivery
Excludes *elderly primigravida complcating pregnancy (659.5)*

1/2 **V23.82 Elderly multigravida**
Second or more pregnancy in a woman who will be 35 years of age or older at expected date of delivery
Excludes *elderly multigravida complicating pregnancy (659.6)*

1/2 **V23.83 Young primigravida**
First pregnancy in a female less than 16 years old at expected date of delivery
Excludes *young primigravida complicating pregnancy (659.8)*

1/2 **V23.84 Young multigravida**
Second or more pregnancy in a female less than 16 years old at expected date of delivery
Excludes *young multigravida complicating pregnancy (659.8)*

1/2 **V23.89 Other high-risk pregnancy**

1/2 **V23.9 Unspecified high-risk pregnancy**

● **V24 Postpartum care and examination**

❶ **V24.0 Immediately after delivery**
Care and observation in uncomplicated cases

❶ **V24.1 Lactating mother**
Supervision of lactation

❶ **V24.2 Routine postpartum follow-up**

● **V25 Encounter for contraceptive management**

● **V25.0 General counseling and advice**

1/2 **V25.01 Prescription of oral contraceptives**

1/2 **V25.02 Initiation of other contraceptive measures**
Fitting of diaphragm
Prescription of foams, creams, or other agents

1/2 **V25.03 Encounter for emergency contraceptive counseling and prescription**
Encounter for postcoital contraceptive counseling and prescription

1/2 **V25.09 Other**
Family planning advice

1/2 **V25.1 Insertion of intrauterine contraceptive device**

1/2 **V25.2 Sterilization**
Admission for interruption of fallopian tubes or vas deferens

1/2 **V25.3 Menstrual extraction**
Menstrual regulation

● **V25.4 Surveillance of previously prescribed contraceptive methods**
Checking, reinsertion, or removal of contraceptive device
Repeat prescription for contraceptive method
Routine examination in connection with contraceptive maintenance
Excludes *presence of intrauterine contraceptive device as incidental finding (V45.5)*

1/2 **V25.40 Contraceptive surveillance, unspecified**

1/2 **V25.41 Contraceptive pill**

1/2 **V25.42 Intrauterine contraceptive device**
Checking, reinsertion, or removal of intrauterine device

1/2 **V25.43 Implantable subdermal contraceptive**

1/2 **V25.49 Other contraceptive method**

1/2 **V25.5 Insertion of implantable subdermal contraceptive**

1/2 **V25.8 Other specified contraceptive management**
Postvasectomy sperm count
Excludes *sperm count following sterilization reversal (V26.22)*
sperm count for fertility testing (V26.21)

1/2 **V25.9 Unspecified contraceptive management**

● **V26 Procreative management**

1/2 **V26.0 Tuboplasty or vasoplasty after previous sterilization**

1/2 **V26.1 Artificial insemination**

● **V26.2 Investigation and testing**
Excludes *postvasectomy sperm count (V25.8)*

1/2 **V26.21 Fertility testing**
Fallopian insufflation
Sperm count for fertility testing
Excludes *genetic counseling and testing (V26.31–V26.39)* ◂

1/2 **V26.22 Aftercare following sterilization reversal**
Fallopian insufflation following sterilization reversal
Sperm count following sterilization reversal

1/2 **V26.29 Other investigation and testing**

● **V26.3 Genetic counseling and testing**

Excludes *fertility testing (V26.21)*
nonprocreative genetic screening (V82.71, V82.79) ◀

1/2 **V26.31 Testing of female for genetic disease carrier status** (Revised)

1/2 **V26.32 Other genetic testing of female** (Revised)
Use additional code to identify habitual aborter (629.81, 646.3) ◀

1/2 **V26.33 Genetic counseling**

1/2 **V26.34 Testing of male for genetic disease carrier status** ◀

1/2 **V26.35 Encounter for testing of male partner of habitual aborter** ◀

1/2 **V26.39 Other genetic testing of male** ◀

1/2 **V26.4 General counseling and advice**

● **V26.5 Sterilization status**

❷ **V26.51 Tubal ligation status**

Excludes *infertility not due to previous tubal ligation (628.0–628.9)*

❷ **V26.52 Vasectomy status**

1/2 **V26.8 Other specified procreative management**

1/2 **V26.9 Unspecified procreative management**

● **V27 Outcome of delivery**

Note: This category is intended for the coding of the outcome of delivery on the mother's record.

❷ **V27.0 Single liveborn**

❷ **V27.1 Single stillborn**

❷ **V27.2 Twins, both liveborn**

❷ **V27.3 Twins, one liveborn and one stillborn**

❷ **V27.4 Twins, both stillborn**

❷ **V27.5 Other multiple birth, all liveborn**

❷ **V27.6 Other multiple birth, some liveborn**

❷ **V27.7 Other multiple birth, all stillborn**

❷ **V27.9 Unspecified outcome of delivery**
Single birth, outcome to infant unspecified
Multiple birth, outcome to infant unspecified

● **V28 Encounter for antenatal screening of mother** (Revised)

Excludes *abnormal findings on screening—code to findings*
routine prenatal care (V22.0–V23.9)

1/2 **V28.0 Screening for chromosomal anomalies by amniocentesis**

1/2 **V28.1 Screening for raised alpha-fetoprotein levels in amniotic fluid**

1/2 **V28.2 Other screening based on amniocentesis**

1/2 **V28.3 Screening for malformation using ultrasonics**

1/2 **V28.4 Screening for fetal growth retardation using ultrasonics**

1/2 **V28.5 Screening for isoimmunization**

1/2 **V28.6 Screening for Streptococcus B**

1/2 **V28.8 Other specified antenatal screening**

1/2 **V28.9 Unspecified antenatal screening**

● **V29 Observation and evaluation of newborns for suspected condition not found**

Note: This category is to be used for newborns, within the neonatal period (the first 28 days of life), who are suspected of having an abnormal condition resulting from exposure from the mother or the birth process, but without signs or symptoms, and which, after examination and observation, is found not to exist.

❶ **V29.0 Observation for suspected infectious condition**

❶ **V29.1 Observation for suspected neurological condition**

❶ **V29.2 Observation for suspected respiratory condition**

❶ **V29.3 Observation for suspected genetic or metabolic condition**

❶ **V29.8 Observation for other specified suspected condition**

❶ **V29.9 Observation for unspecified suspected condition**

LIVEBORN INFANTS ACCORDING TO TYPE OF BIRTH (V30–V39)

Note: These categories are intended for the coding of liveborn infants who are consuming health care [e.g., crib or bassinet occupancy].

The following fourth-digit subdivisions are for use with categories V30–V39:
.0 Born in hospital
.1 Born before admission to hospital
.2 Born outside hospital and not hospitalized

The following two fifth-digits are for use with the fourth-digit .0, born in hospital:
0 delivered without mention of cesarean delivery
1 delivered by cesarean delivery

❶ ● **V30 Single liveborn**

❶ ● **V31 Twin, mate liveborn**

❶ ● **V32 Twin, mate stillborn**

❶ ● **V33 Twin, unspecified**

❶ ● **V34 Other multiple, mates all liveborn**

❶ ● **V35 Other multiple, mates all stillborn**

❶ ● **V36 Other multiple, mates live- and stillborn**

❶ ● **V37 Other multiple, unspecified**

❶ ● **V39 Unspecified**

PERSONS WITH A CONDITION INFLUENCING THEIR HEALTH STATUS (V40–V49)

Note: These categories are intended for use when these conditions are recorded as "diagnoses" or "problems."

● **V40 Mental and behavioral problems**

❑ **V40.0 Problems with learning**

❑ **V40.1 Problems with communication [including speech]**

❑ **V40.2 Other mental problems**

❑ **V40.3 Other behavioral problems**

❑ **V40.9 Unspecified mental or behavioral problem**

● **V41 Problems with special senses and other special functions**

❑ **V41.0 Problems with sight**

❑V41.1 Other eye problems
❑V41.2 Problems with hearing
❑V41.3 Other ear problems
❑V41.4 Problems with voice production
❑V41.5 Problems with smell and taste
❑V41.6 Problems with swallowing and mastication
❑V41.7 Problems with sexual function
Excludes *marital problems (V61.10)*
psychosexual disorders (302.0–302.9)
❑V41.8 Other problems with special functions
❑V41.9 Unspecified problem with special functions

● **V42 Organ or tissue replaced by transplant**
Includes: homologous or heterologous (animal) (human) transplant organ status
❷ V42.0 Kidney
❷ V42.1 Heart
❷ V42.2 Heart valve
❷ V42.3 Skin
❷ V42.4 Bone
❷ V42.5 Cornea
❷ V42.6 Lung
❷ V42.7 Liver
● V42.8 Other specified organ or tissue
❷ V42.81 Bone marrow
❷ V42.82 Peripheral stem cells
❷ V42.83 Pancreas
❷ V42.84 Intestines
❷ V42.89 Other
❷ V42.9 Unspecified organ or tissue

● **V43 Organ or tissue replaced by other means**
Includes: organ or tissue assisted by other means
replacement of organ by:
artificial device
mechanical device
prosthesis
Excludes *cardiac pacemaker in situ (V45.01)*
fitting and adjustment of prosthetic device (V52.0–V52.9)
renal dialysis status (V45.1)
❷ V43.0 Eye globe
❷ V43.1 Lens
Pseudophakos
● V43.2 Heart
❷ V43.21 Heart assist device
1/2 V43.22 Fully implantable artificial heart
❷ V43.3 Heart valve
❷ V43.4 Blood vessel
❷ V43.5 Bladder
● V43.6 Joint
❷ V43.60 Unspecified joint
❷ V43.61 Shoulder
❷ V43.62 Elbow
❷ V43.63 Wrist
❷ V43.64 Hip
❷ V43.65 Knee
❷ V43.66 Ankle
❷ ❑ V43.69 Other
❷ V43.7 Limb
● V43.8 Other organ or tissue
❷ V43.81 Larynx
❷ V43.82 Breast
❷ V43.83 Artificial skin
❷ V43.89 Other

● **V44 Artificial opening status**
Excludes *artificial openings requiring attention or management (V55.0–V55.9)*
❷ V44.0 Tracheostomy
❷ V44.1 Gastrostomy
❷ V44.2 Ileostomy
❷ V44.3 Colostomy
❷ V44.4 Other artificial opening of gastrointestinal tract
● V44.5 Cystostomy
❷ V44.50 Cystostomy, unspecified
❷ V44.51 Cutaneous-vesicostomy
❷ V44.52 Appendico-vesicostomy
❷ V44.59 Other cystostomy
❷ V44.6 Other artificial opening of urinary tract
Nephrostomy
Ureterostomy
Urethrostomy
❷ V44.7 Artificial vagina
❷ V44.8 Other artificial opening status
❷ V44.9 Unspecified artificial opening status

● **V45 Other postprocedural states**
Excludes *aftercare management (V51–V58.9)*
malfunction or other complication—code to condition
● V45.0 Cardiac device in situ
Excludes *artificial heart (V43.22)*
heart assist device (V43.21)
❷ V45.00 Unspecified cardiac device
❷ V45.01 Cardiac pacemaker
❷ V45.02 Automatic implantable cardiac defibrillator
❷ V45.09 Other specified cardiac device
Carotid sinus pacemaker in situ
❷ V45.1 Renal dialysis status
Hemodialysis status
Patient requiring intermittent renal dialysis
Peritoneal dialysis status
Presence of arterial-venous shunt (for dialysis)
Excludes *admission for dialysis treatment or session (V56.0)*
❷ V45.2 Presence of cerebrospinal fluid drainage device
Cerebral ventricle (communicating) shunt, valve, or device in situ
Excludes *malfunction (996.2)*
❷ V45.3 Intestinal bypass or anastomosis status
Excludes *bariatric surgery status (V45.86)* ◀
gastric bypass status (V45.86) ◀
obesity surgery status (V45.86) ◀
❷ V45.4 Arthrodesis status
● V45.5 Presence of contraceptive device
Excludes *checking, reinsertion, or removal of device (V25.42)*
complication from device (996.32)
insertion of device (V25.1)
❷ V45.51 Intrauterine contraceptive device
❷ V45.52 Subdermal contraceptive implant
❷ V45.59 Other

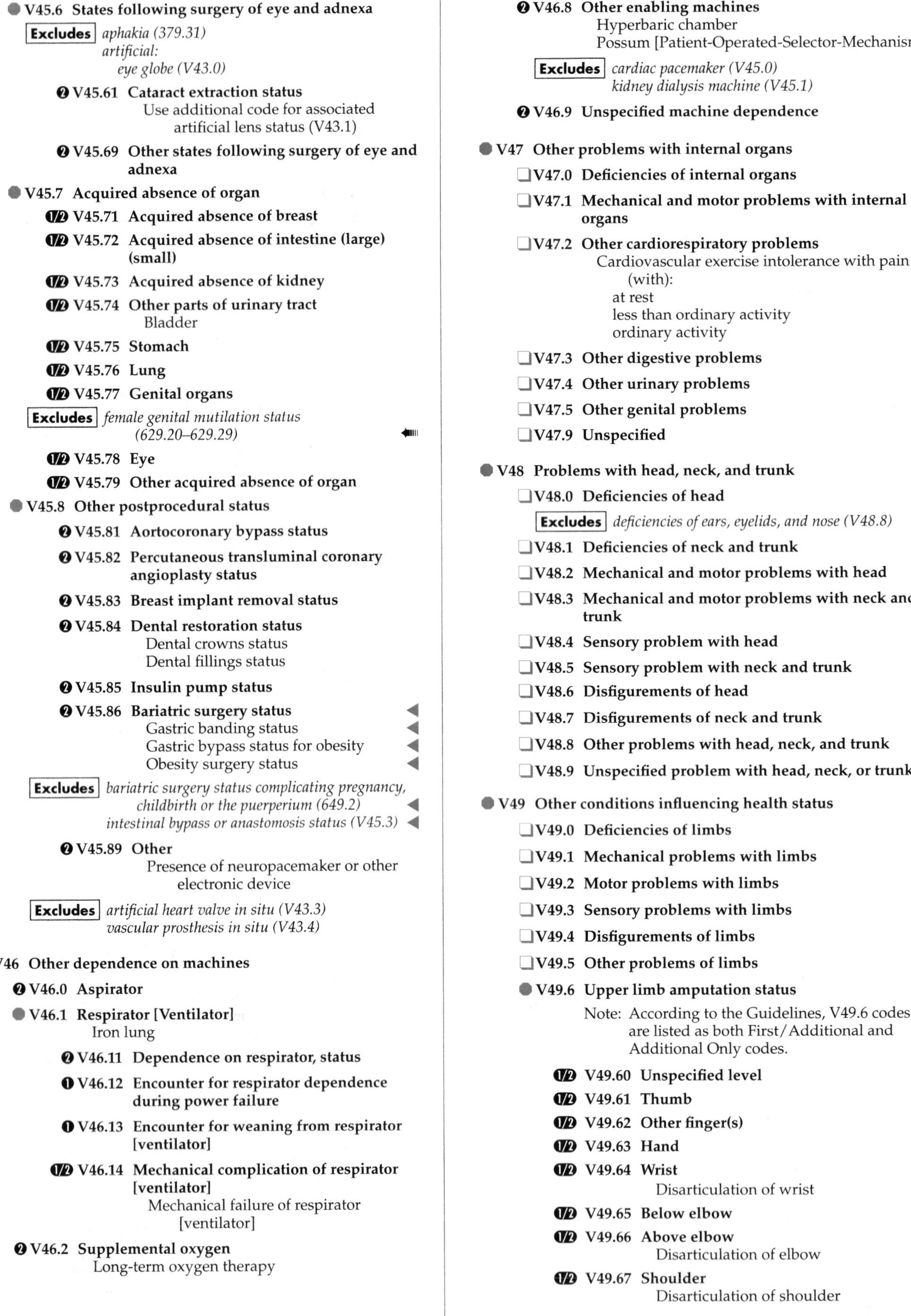

● **V45.6 States following surgery of eye and adnexa**

Excludes *aphakia (379.31)*
artificial:
eye globe (V43.0)

❷ **V45.61 Cataract extraction status**
Use additional code for associated artificial lens status (V43.1)

❷ **V45.69 Other states following surgery of eye and adnexa**

● **V45.7 Acquired absence of organ**

1/2 **V45.71 Acquired absence of breast**

1/2 **V45.72 Acquired absence of intestine (large) (small)**

1/2 **V45.73 Acquired absence of kidney**

1/2 **V45.74 Other parts of urinary tract**
Bladder

1/2 **V45.75 Stomach**

1/2 **V45.76 Lung**

1/2 **V45.77 Genital organs**

Excludes *female genital mutilation status (629.20–629.29)* ⇐

1/2 **V45.78 Eye**

1/2 **V45.79 Other acquired absence of organ**

● **V45.8 Other postprocedural status**

❷ **V45.81 Aortocoronary bypass status**

❷ **V45.82 Percutaneous transluminal coronary angioplasty status**

❷ **V45.83 Breast implant removal status**

❷ **V45.84 Dental restoration status**
Dental crowns status
Dental fillings status

❷ **V45.85 Insulin pump status**

❷ **V45.86 Bariatric surgery status** ◀
Gastric banding status ◀
Gastric bypass status for obesity ◀
Obesity surgery status ◀

Excludes *bariatric surgery status complicating pregnancy, childbirth or the puerperium (649.2)* ◀
intestinal bypass or anastomosis status (V45.3) ◀

❷ **V45.89 Other**
Presence of neuropacemaker or other electronic device

Excludes *artificial heart valve in situ (V43.3)*
vascular prosthesis in situ (V43.4)

● **V46 Other dependence on machines**

❷ **V46.0 Aspirator**

● **V46.1 Respirator [Ventilator]**
Iron lung

❷ **V46.11 Dependence on respirator, status**

❶ **V46.12 Encounter for respirator dependence during power failure**

❶ **V46.13 Encounter for weaning from respirator [ventilator]**

1/2 **V46.14 Mechanical complication of respirator [ventilator]**
Mechanical failure of respirator [ventilator]

❷ **V46.2 Supplemental oxygen**
Long-term oxygen therapy

❷ **V46.8 Other enabling machines**
Hyperbaric chamber
Possum [Patient-Operated-Selector-Mechanism]

Excludes *cardiac pacemaker (V45.0)*
kidney dialysis machine (V45.1)

❷ **V46.9 Unspecified machine dependence**

● **V47 Other problems with internal organs**

❑ **V47.0 Deficiencies of internal organs**

❑ **V47.1 Mechanical and motor problems with internal organs**

❑ **V47.2 Other cardiorespiratory problems**
Cardiovascular exercise intolerance with pain (with):
at rest
less than ordinary activity
ordinary activity

❑ **V47.3 Other digestive problems**

❑ **V47.4 Other urinary problems**

❑ **V47.5 Other genital problems**

❑ **V47.9 Unspecified**

● **V48 Problems with head, neck, and trunk**

❑ **V48.0 Deficiencies of head**

Excludes *deficiencies of ears, eyelids, and nose (V48.8)*

❑ **V48.1 Deficiencies of neck and trunk**

❑ **V48.2 Mechanical and motor problems with head**

❑ **V48.3 Mechanical and motor problems with neck and trunk**

❑ **V48.4 Sensory problem with head**

❑ **V48.5 Sensory problem with neck and trunk**

❑ **V48.6 Disfigurements of head**

❑ **V48.7 Disfigurements of neck and trunk**

❑ **V48.8 Other problems with head, neck, and trunk**

❑ **V48.9 Unspecified problem with head, neck, or trunk**

● **V49 Other conditions influencing health status**

❑ **V49.0 Deficiencies of limbs**

❑ **V49.1 Mechanical problems with limbs**

❑ **V49.2 Motor problems with limbs**

❑ **V49.3 Sensory problems with limbs**

❑ **V49.4 Disfigurements of limbs**

❑ **V49.5 Other problems of limbs**

● **V49.6 Upper limb amputation status**

Note: According to the Guidelines, V49.6 codes are listed as both First/Additional and Additional Only codes.

1/2 **V49.60 Unspecified level**

1/2 **V49.61 Thumb**

1/2 **V49.62 Other finger(s)**

1/2 **V49.63 Hand**

1/2 **V49.64 Wrist**
Disarticulation of wrist

1/2 **V49.65 Below elbow**

1/2 **V49.66 Above elbow**
Disarticulation of elbow

1/2 **V49.67 Shoulder**
Disarticulation of shoulder

◀ **New** ⇐ **Revised** ❶ **First Listed** 1/2 **First Listed or Additional** ❷ **Additional Only**
● **Use Additional Digit(s)** ❑ **Nonspecific Code**

● **V49.7 Lower limb amputation status**

Note: According to the Guidelines, V49.7 codes are listed as both First/Additional and Additional Only codes.

1/2 **V49.70 Unspecified level**

1/2 **V49.71 Great toe**

1/2 **V49.72 Other toe(s)**

1/2 **V49.73 Foot**

1/2 **V49.74 Ankle**

Disarticulation of ankle

1/2 **V49.75 Below knee**

1/2 **V49.76 Above knee**

Disarticulation of knee

1/2 **V49.77 Hip**

Disarticulation of hip

● **V49.8 Other specified conditions influencing health status**

1/2 **V49.81 Asymptomatic postmenopausal status (age-related) (natural)**

Excludes *menopausal and premenopausal disorders (627.0–627.9)*
postsurgical menopause (256.2)
premature menopause (256.31)
symptomatic menopause (627.0–627.9)

❷ **V49.82 Dental sealant status**

❷ **V49.83 Awaiting organ transplant status**

1/2 **V49.84 Bed confinement status**

1/2 **V49.89 Other specified conditions influencing health status**

❑ **V49.9 Unspecified**

PERSONS ENCOUNTERING HEALTH SERVICES FOR SPECIFIC PROCEDURES AND AFTERCARE (V50–V59)

Note: Categories V51–V58 are intended for use to indicate a reason for care in patients who may have already been treated for some disease or injury not now present, or who are receiving care to consolidate the treatment, to deal with residual states, or to prevent recurrence.

Excludes *follow-up examination for medical surveillance following treatment (V67.0–V67.9)*

● **V50 Elective surgery for purposes other than remedying health states**

1/2 **V50.0 Hair transplant**

1/2 **V50.1 Other plastic surgery for unacceptable cosmetic appearance**

Breast augmentation or reduction
Face-lift

Excludes *plastic surgery following healed injury or operation (V51)*

1/2 **V50.2 Routine or ritual circumcision**

Circumcision in the absence of significant medical indication

1/2 **V50.3 Ear piercing**

● **V50.4 Prophylactic organ removal**

Excludes *organ donations (V59.0–V59.9)*
therapeutic organ removal—code to condition

1/2 **V50.41 Breast**

1/2 **V50.42 Ovary**

1/2 **V50.49 Other**

1/2 **V50.8 Other**

1/2 **V50.9 Unspecified**

❑ **V51 Aftercare involving the use of plastic surgery**

Plastic surgery following healed injury or operation

Excludes *cosmetic plastic surgery (V50.1)*
plastic surgery as treatment for current injury—code to condition
repair of scar tissue—code to scar

● **V52 Fitting and adjustment of prosthetic device and implant**

Includes: removal of device

Excludes *malfunction or complication of prosthetic device (996.0–996.7)*
status only, without need for care (V43.0–V43.8)

1/2 **V52.0 Artificial arm (complete) (partial)**

1/2 **V52.1 Artificial leg (complete) (partial)**

1/2 **V52.2 Artificial eye**

1/2 **V52.3 Dental prosthetic device**

1/2 **V52.4 Breast prosthesis and implant**

Excludes *admission for breast implant insertion (V50.1)*

1/2 **V52.8 Other specified prosthetic device**

1/2 **V52.9 Unspecified prosthetic device**

● **V53 Fitting and adjustment of other device**

Includes: removal of device
replacement of device

Excludes *status only, without need for care (V45.0–V45.8)*

● **V53.0 Devices related to nervous system and special senses**

1/2 **V53.01 Fitting and adjustment of cerebral ventricle (communicating) shunt**

1/2 **V53.02 Neuropacemaker (brain) (peripheral nerve) (spinal cord)**

1/2 **V53.09 Fitting and adjustment of other devices related to nervous system and special senses**

Auditory substitution device
Visual substitution device

1/2 **V53.1 Spectacles and contact lenses**

1/2 **V53.2 Hearing aid**

● **V53.3 Cardiac device**

Reprogramming

1/2 **V53.31 Cardiac pacemaker**

Excludes *mechanical complication of cardiac pacemaker (996.01)*

1/2 **V53.32 Automatic implantable cardiac defibrillator**

1/2 **V53.39 Other cardiac device**

1/2 **V53.4 Orthodontic devices**

1/2 **V53.5 Other intestinal appliance**

Excludes *colostomy (V55.3)*
ileostomy (V55.2)
other artifical opening of digestive tract (V55.4)

1/2 **V53.6 Urinary devices**

Urinary catheter

Excludes *cystostomy (V55.5)*
nephrostomy (V55.6)
ureterostomy (V55.6)
urethrostomy (V55.6)

1/2 **V53.7 Orthopedic devices**

Orthopedic:
brace
cast
corset
shoes

Excludes *other orthopedic aftercare (V54)*

ICD-9-CM V01-V99 Vol. 1

1/2 V53.8 **Wheelchair**

● V53.9 **Other and unspecified device**

1/2 V53.90 **Unspecified device**

1/2 V53.91 **Fitting and adjustment of insulin pump**
Insulin pump titration

1/2 V53.99 **Other device**

● V54 **Other orthopedic aftercare**

Excludes *fitting and adjustment of orthopedic devices (V53.7)*
malfunction of internal orthopedic device (996.40–996.49)
other complication of nonmechanical nature (996.60–996.79)

● V54.0 **Aftercare involving internal fixation device**

Excludes *malfunction of internal orthopedic device (996.40–996.49)*
other complication of nonmechanical nature (996.60–996.79)
removal of external fixation device (V54.89)

1/2 V54.01 **Encounter for removal of internal fixation device**

1/2 V54.02 **Encounter for lengthening/adjustment of growth rod**

1/2 V54.09 **Other aftercare involving internal fixation device**

● V54.1 **Aftercare for healing traumatic fracture**

Excludes *aftercare for amputation stump (V54.89)* ◀

1/2 V54.10 **Aftercare for healing traumatic fracture of arm, unspecified**

1/2 V54.11 **Aftercare for healing traumatic fracture of upper arm**

1/2 V54.12 **Aftercare for healing traumatic fracture of lower arm**

1/2 V54.13 **Aftercare for healing traumatic fracture of hip**

1/2 V54.14 **Aftercare for healing traumatic fracture of leg, unspecified**

1/2 V54.15 **Aftercare for healing traumatic fracture of upper leg**

Excludes *aftercare for healing traumatic fracture of hip (V54.13)*

1/2 V54.16 **Aftercare for healing traumatic fracture of lower leg**

1/2 V54.17 **Aftercare for healing traumatic fracture of vertebrae**

1/2 V54.19 **Aftercare for healing traumatic fracture of other bone**

● V54.2 **Aftercare for healing pathologic fracture**

1/2 V54.20 **Aftercare for healing pathologic fracture of arm, unspecified**

1/2 V54.21 **Aftercare for healing pathologic fracture of upper arm**

1/2 V54.22 **Aftercare for healing pathologic fracture of lower arm**

1/2 V54.23 **Aftercare for healing pathologic fracture of hip**

1/2 V54.24 **Aftercare for healing pathologic fracture of leg, unspecified**

1/2 V54.25 **Aftercare for healing pathologic fracture of upper leg**

Excludes *aftercare for healing pathologic fracture of hip (V54.23)*

1/2 V54.26 **Aftercare for healing pathologic fracture of lower leg**

1/2 V54.27 **Aftercare for healing pathologic fracture of vertebrae**

1/2 V54.29 **Aftercare for healing pathologic fracture of other bone**

● V54.8 **Other orthopedic aftercare**

1/2 V54.81 **Aftercare following joint replacement**

Use additional code to identify joint replacement site (V43.60–V43.69)

1/2 V54.89 **Other orthopedic aftercar**
Aftercare for healing fracture NOS

1/2 V54.9 **Unspecified orthopedic aftercare**

● V55 **Attention to artificial openings**

Includes: adjustment or repositioning of catheter
closure
passage of sounds or bougies
reforming
removal or replacement of catheter
toilet or cleansing

Excludes *complications of external stoma (519.00–519.09, 569.60–569.69, 997.4, 997.5)*
status only, without need for care (V44.0–V44.9)

1/2 V55.0 **Tracheostomy**

1/2 V55.1 **Gastrostomy**

1/2 V55.2 **Ileostomy**

1/2 V55.3 **Colostomy**

1/2 V55.4 **Other artificial opening of digestive tract**

1/2 V55.5 **Cystostomy**

1/2 V55.6 **Other artificial opening of urinary tract**
Nephrostomy
Ureterostomy
Urethrostomy

1/2 V55.7 **Artificial vagina**

1/2 V55.8 **Other specified artificial opening**

1/2 V55.9 **Unspecified artificial opening**

● V56 **Encounter for dialysis and dialysis catheter care**

Use additional code to identify the associated condition

Excludes *dialysis preparation—code to condition*

❶ V56.0 **Extracorporeal dialysis**

Dialysis (renal) NOS

Excludes *dialysis status (V45.1)*

1/2 V56.1 **Fitting and adjustment of extracorporeal dialysis catheter**
Removal or replacement of catheter
Toilet or cleansing

Use additional code for any concurrent extracorporeal dialysis (V56.0)

1/2 V56.2 **Fitting and adjustment of peritoneal dialysis catheter**

Use additional code for any concurrent peritoneal dialysis (V56.8)

● V56.3 **Encounter for adequacy testing for dialysis**

1/2 V56.31 **Encounter for adequacy testing for hemodialysis**

1/2 V56.32 **Encounter for adequacy testing for peritoneal dialysis**
Peritoneal equilibration test

1/2 V56.8 **Other dialysis**
Peritoneal dialysis

● V57 **Care involving use of rehabilitation procedures**

Use additional code to identify underlying condition

❶ V57.0 **Breathing exercises**

◀ New ⇐ Revised ❶ First Listed 1/2 First Listed or Additional ❷ Additional Only ● Use Additional Digit(s) ❑ Nonspecific Code

➊ V57.1 **Other physical therapy**
Therapeutic and remedial exercises, except breathing

● V57.2 **Occupational therapy and vocational rehabilitation**

➊ V57.21 **Encounter for occupational therapy**

➊ V57.22 **Encounter for vocational therapy**

➊ V57.3 **Speech therapy**

➊ V57.4 **Orthoptic training**

● V57.8 **Other specified rehabilitation procedure**

➊ V57.81 **Orthotic training**
Gait training in the use of artificial limbs

➊ V57.89 **Other**
Multiple training or therapy

➊ V57.9 **Unspecified rehabilitation procedure**

● V58 **Encounter for other and unspecified procedures and aftercare**

Excludes *convalescence and palliative care (V66.0–V66.9)*

➊ V58.0 **Radiotherapy**
Encounter or admission for radiotherapy

Excludes *encounter for radioactive implant—code to condition*
radioactive iodine therapy—code to condition

● V58.1 **Encounter for antineoplastic chemotherapy and immunotherapy**
Encounter or admission for chemotherapy

Excludes *chemotherapy and immunotherapy for nonneoplastic conditions-code to condition*
prophylactic chemotherapy against disease which has never been present (V03.0–V07.9)

➊ V58.11 **Encounter for antineoplastic chemotherapy**

➊ V58.12 **Encounter for antineoplastic immunotherapy**

❑ V58.2 **Blood transfusion, without reported diagnosis**

● V58.3 **Attention to dressings and sutures** ⇐
Change or removal of wound packing ◀

Excludes *attention to drains (V58.49)* ◀
planned postoperative wound closure (V58.41) ◀

1/2 V58.30 **Encounter for change or removal of nonsurgical wound dressing** ◀
Encounter for change or removal of wound dressing NOS ◀

1/2 V58.31 **Encounter for change or removal of surgical wound dressing** ◀

1/2 V58.32 **Encounter for removal of sutures** ◀
Encounter for removal of staples ◀

● V58.4 **Other aftercare following surgery**

Note: Codes from this subcategory should be used in conjunction with other aftercare codes to fully identify the reason for the aftercare encounter.

Excludes *aftercare following sterilization reversal surgery (V26.22)*
attention to artificial openings (V55.0–V55.9)
orthopedic aftercare (V54.0–V54.9)

1/2 V58.41 **Encounter for planned post-operative wound closure**

Excludes *disruption of operative wound (998.3)*
encounter for dressings and suture aftercare (V58.30–V58.32) ◀

1/2 V58.42 **Aftercare following surgery for neoplasm**
Conditions classifiable to 140–239

1/2 V58.43 **Aftercare following surgery for injury and trauma**
Conditions classifiable to 800–999

Excludes *aftercare for healing traumatic fracture (V54.10–V54.19)*

1/2 V58.44 **Aftercare following organ transplant**
Use additional code to identify the organ transplanted (V42.0–V42.9)

1/2 V58.49 **Other specified aftercare following surgery**
Change or removal of drains ◀

❑ V58.5 **Orthodontics**

Excludes *fitting and adjustment of orthodontic device (V53.4)*

● V58.6 **Long-term (current) drug use**

Excludes *drug abuse (305.00–305.93)*
drug dependence (304.00–304.93)
hormone replacement therapy (postmenopausal) (V07.4)

➋ V58.61 **Long-term (current) use of anticoagulants**

Excludes *long-term (current) use of aspirin (V58.66)*

➋ V58.62 **Long-term (current) use of antibiotics**

➋ V58.63 **Long-term (current) use of antiplatelet/antithrombotic**

Excludes *long-term (current) use of aspirin (V58.66)*

➋ V58.64 **Long-term (current) use of non-steroidal anti-inflammatories (NSAID)**

Excludes *long-term (current) use of aspirin (V58.66)*

➋ V58.65 **Long-term (current) use of steroids**

➋ V58.66 **Long-term (current) use of aspirin**

➋ V58.67 **Long-term (current) use of insulin**

➋ V58.69 **Long-term (current) use of other medications**
High-risk medications

● V58.7 **Aftercare following surgery to specified body systems, not elsewhere classified**

Note: Codes from this subcategory should be used in conjunction with other aftercare codes to fully identify the reason for the aftercare encounter.

Excludes *aftercare following organ transplant (V58.44)*
aftercare following surgery for neoplasm (V58.42)

1/2 V58.71 **Aftercare following surgery of the sense organs, NEC**
Conditions classifiable to 360–379, 380–389

1/2 V58.72 **Aftercare following surgery of the nervous system, NEC**
Conditions classifiable to 320–359

Excludes *aftercare following surgery of the sense organs, NEC (V58.71)*

1/2 V58.73 **Aftercare following surgery of the circulatory system, NEC**
Conditions classifiable to 390–459

1/2 V58.74 **Aftercare following surgery of the respiratory system, NEC**
Conditions classifiable to 460–519

1/2 V58.75 **Aftercare following surgery of the teeth, oral cavity and digestive system, NEC**
Conditions classifiable to 520–579

ICD-9-CM V01-V99 Vol. 1

[1/2] V58.76 Aftercare following surgery of the genitourinary system, NEC
Conditions classifiable to 580–629

Excludes *aftercare following sterilization reversal (V26.22)*

[1/2] V58.77 Aftercare following surgery of the skin and subcutaneous tissue, NEC
Conditions classifiable to 680–709

[1/2] V58.78 Aftercare following surgery of the musculoskeletal system, NEC
Conditions classifiable to 710–739

● **V58.8 Other specified procedures and aftercare**

[1/2] V58.81 Fitting and adjustment of vascular catheter
Removal or replacement of catheter
Toilet or cleansing

Excludes *complications of renal dialysis (996.73)*
complications of vascular catheter (996.74)
dialysis preparation—code to condition
encounter for dialysis (V56.0–V56.8)
fitting and adjustment of dialysis catheter (V56.1)

[1/2] V58.82 Fitting and adjustment of non-vascular catheter, NEC
Removal or replacement of catheter
Toilet or cleansing

Excludes *fitting and adjustment of peritoneal dialysis catheter (V56.2)*
fitting and adjustment of urinary catheter (V53.6)

[1/2] V58.83 Encounter for therapeutic drug monitoring
Use additional code for any associated long-term (current) drug use (V58.61–V58.69)

Excludes *blood-drug testing for medicolegal reasons (V70.4)*

[1/2] V58.89 Other specified aftercare

❏ **V58.9 Unspecified aftercare**

● **V59 Donors**

Excludes *examination of potential donor (V70.8)*
self-donation of organ or tissue—code to condition

● **V59.0 Blood**

➊ V59.01 Whole blood

➊ V59.02 Stem cells

➊ V59.09 Other

➊ V59.1 Skin

➊ V59.2 Bone

➊ V59.3 Bone marrow

➊ V59.4 Kidney

➊ V59.5 Cornea

➊ V59.6 Liver

● **V59.7 Egg (oocyte) (ovum)**

➊ V59.70 Egg (oocyte) (ovum) donor, unspecified

➊ V59.71 Egg (oocyte) (ovum) donor, under age 35, anonymous recipient
Egg donor, under age 35 NOS

➊ V59.72 Egg (oocyte) (ovum) donor, under age 35, designated recipient

➊ V59.73 Egg (oocyte) (ovum) donor, age 35 and over, anonymous recipient
Egg donor, age 35 and over NOS

➊ V59.74 Egg (oocyte) (ovum) donor, age 35 and over, designated recipient

➊ V59.8 Other specified organ or tissue

➊ V59.9 Unspecified organ or tissue

PERSONS ENCOUNTERING HEALTH SERVICES IN OTHER CIRCUMSTANCES (V60–V69)

● **V60 Housing, household, and economic circumstances**

➋ V60.0 Lack of housing
Hobos
Social migrants
Tramps
Transients
Vagabonds

➋ V60.1 Inadequate housing
Lack of heating
Restriction of space
Technical defects in home preventing adequate care

➋ V60.2 Inadequate material resources
Economic problem
Poverty NOS

➋ V60.3 Person living alone

➋ V60.4 No other household member able to render care
Person requiring care (has) (is):
family member too handicapped, ill, or otherwise unsuited to render care
partner temporarily away from home
temporarily away from usual place of abode

Excludes *holiday relief care (V60.5)*

➋ V60.5 Holiday relief care
Provision of health care facilities to a person normally cared for at home, to enable relatives to take a vacation

➋ V60.6 Person living in residential institution
Boarding school resident

➋ V60.8 Other specified housing or economic circumstances

➋ V60.9 Unspecified housing or economic circumstance

● **V61 Other family circumstances**

Includes: when these circumstances or fear of them, affecting the person directly involved or others, are mentioned as the reason, justified or not, for seeking or receiving medical advice or care

[1/2] V61.0 Family disruption
Divorce
Estrangement

● **V61.1 Counseling for marital and partner problems**

Excludes *problems related to:*
psychosexual disorders (302.0–302.9)
sexual function (V41.7)

[1/2] V61.10 Counseling for marital and partner problems, unspecified
Marital conflict
Marital relationship problem
Partner conflict
Partner relationship problem

[1/2] V61.11 Counseling for victim of spousal and partner abuse

Excludes *encounter for treatment of current injuries due to abuse (995.80–995.85)*

[1/2] V61.12 Counseling for perpetrator of spousal and partner abuse

● **V61.2 Parent-child problems**

[1/2] V61.20 Counseling for parent-child problem, unspecified
Concern about behavior of child
Parent-child conflict
Parent-child relationship problem

◀ New ⬅ Revised ➊ First Listed [1/2] First Listed or Additional ➋ Additional Only
● Use Additional Digit(s) ❏ Nonspecific Code

1/2 **V61.21 Counseling for victim of child abuse**
Child battering
Child neglect

Excludes *current injuries due to abuse (995.50–995.59)*

1/2 **V61.22 Counseling for perpetrator of parental child abuse**

Excludes *counseling for non-parental abuser (V62.83)*

1/2 **V61.29 Other**
Problem concerning adopted or foster child

1/2 **V61.3 Problems with aged parents or in-laws**

● **V61.4 Health problems within family**

1/2 **V61.41 Alcoholism in family**

1/2 **V61.49 Other**
Care of sick or handicapped person in family or household
Presence of sick or handicapped person in family or household

1/2 **V61.5 Multiparity**

1/2 **V61.6 Illegitimacy or illegitimate pregnancy**

1/2 **V61.7 Other unwanted pregnancy**

1/2 **V61.8 Other specified family circumstances**
Problems with family members, NEC
Sibling relationship problems

1/2 **V61.9 Unspecified family circumstance**

● **V62 Other psychosocial circumstances**

Includes: those circumstances or fear of them, affecting the person directly involved or others, mentioned as the reason, justified or not, for seeking or receiving medical advice or care

Excludes *previous psychological trauma (V15.41–V15.49)*

❷ **V62.0 Unemployment**

Excludes *circumstances when main problem is economic inadequacy or poverty (V60.2)*

❷ **V62.1 Adverse effects of work environment**

❷ **V62.2 Other occupational circumstances or maladjustment**
Career choice problem
Dissatisfaction with employment
Occupational problem

❷ **V62.3 Educational circumstances**
Academic problem
Dissatisfaction with school environment
Educational handicap

❷ **V62.4 Social maladjustment**
Acculturation problem
Cultural deprivation
Political, religious, or sex discrimination
Social:
isolation
persecution

❷ **V62.5 Legal circumstances**
Imprisonment
Legal investigation
Litigation
Prosecution

❷ **V62.6 Refusal of treatment for reasons of religion or conscience**

● **V62.8 Other psychological or physical stress, not elsewhere classified**

❷ **V62.81 Interpersonal problems, not elsewhere classified**
Relational problem NOS

❷ **V62.82 Bereavement, uncomplicated**

Excludes *bereavement as adjustment reaction (309.0)*

❷ **V62.83 Counseling for perpetrator of physical/sexual abuse**

Excludes *counseling for perpetrator of parental child abuse (V61.22)*
counseling for perpetrator of spousal and partner abuse (V61.12)

❷ **V62.84 Suicidal ideation**

Excludes *suicidal tendencies (300.9)*

❷ **V62.89 Other**
Borderline intellectual functioning
Life circumstance problems
Phase of life problems
Religious or spiritual problem

❷ **V62.9 Unspecified psychosocial circumstance**

● **V63 Unavailability of other medical facilities for care**

1/2 **V63.0 Residence remote from hospital or other health care facility**

1/2 **V63.1 Medical services in home not available**

Excludes *no other household member able to render care (V60.4)*

1/2 **V63.2 Person awaiting admission to adequate facility elsewhere**

1/2 **V63.8 Other specified reasons for unavailability of medical facilities**
Person on waiting list undergoing social agency investigation

1/2 **V63.9 Unspecified reason for unavailability of medical facilities**

● **V64 Persons encountering health services for specific procedures, not carried out**

● **V64.0 Vaccination not carried out**

❷ **V64.00 Vaccination not carried out, unspecified reason**

❷ **V64.01 Vaccination not carried out because of acute illness**

❷ **V64.02 Vaccination not carried out because of chronic illness or condition**

❷ **V64.03 Vaccination not carried out because of immune compromised state**

❷ **V64.04 Vaccination not carried out because of allergy to vaccine or component**

❷ **V64.05 Vaccination not carried out because of caregiver refusal**

❷ **V64.06 Vaccination not carried out because of patient refusal**

❷ **V64.07 Vaccination not carried out for religious reasons**

❷ **V64.08 Vaccination not carried out because patient had disease being vaccinated against**

❷ **V64.09 Vaccination not carried out for other reason**

❷ **V64.1 Surgical or other procedure not carried out because of contraindication**

❷ **V64.2 Surgical or other procedure not carried out because of patient's decision**

❷ **V64.3 Procedure not carried out for other reasons**

● **V64.4 Closed surgical procedure converted to open procedure**

❷ V64.41 Laparoscopic surgical procedure converted to open procedure

❷ V64.42 Thoracoscopic surgical procedure converted to open procedure

❷ V64.43 Arthroscopic surgical procedure converted to open procedure

● **V65 Other persons seeking consultation**

1/2 **V65.0 Healthy person accompanying sick person**
Boarder

● **V65.1 Person consulting on behalf of another person**
Advice or treatment for nonattending third party

Excludes *concern (normal) about sick person in family (V61.41–V61.49)*

1/2 **V65.11 Pediatric pre-birth visit for expecting mother**

1/2 **V65.19 Other person consulting on behalf of another person**

1/2 **V65.2 Person feigning illness**
Malingerer
Peregrinating patient

1/2 **V65.3 Dietary surveillance and counseling**
Dietary surveillance and counseling (in):
NOS
colitis
diabetes mellitus
food allergies or intolerance
gastritis
hypercholesterolemia
hypoglycemia
obesity

Use additional code to identify Body Mass Index (BMI), if known (V85.0–V85.54) ◀

● **V65.4 Other counseling, not elsewhere classified**
Health:
advice
education
instruction

Excludes *counseling (for):*
contraception (V25.40–V25.49)
genetic (V26.31–V26.39) ⬅
on behalf of third party (V65.11–V65.19)
procreative management (V26.4)

1/2 **V65.40 Counseling NOS**

1/2 **V65.41 Exercise counseling**

1/2 **V65.42 Counseling on substance use and abuse**

1/2 **V65.43 Counseling on injury prevention**

1/2 **V65.44 Human immunodeficiency virus [HIV] counseling**

1/2 **V65.45 Counseling on other sexually transmitted diseases**

1/2 **V65.46 Encounter for insulin pump training**

1/2 **V65.49 Other specified counseling**

1/2 **V65.5 Person with feared complaint in whom no diagnosis was made**
Feared condition not demonstrated
Problem was normal state
"Worried well"

1/2 **V65.8 Other reasons for seeking consultation**

Excludes *specified symptoms*

1/2 **V65.9 Unspecified reason for consultation**

● **V66 Convalescence and palliative care**

❶ **V66.0 Following surgery**

❶ **V66.1 Following radiotherapy**

❶ **V66.2 Following chemotherapy**

❶ **V66.3 Following psychotherapy and other treatment for mental disorder**

❶ **V66.4 Following treatment of fracture**

❶ **V66.5 Following other treatment**

❶ **V66.6 Following combined treatment**

❷ **V66.7 Encounter for palliative care**
End-of-life care
Hospice care
Terminal care

Code first underlying disease

❶ **V66.9 Unspecified convalescence**

● **V67 Follow-up examination**

Includes: surveillance only following completed treatment

Excludes *surveillance of contraception (V25.40–V25.49)*

● **V67.0 Following surgery**

1/2 **V67.00 Following surgery, unspecified**

1/2 **V67.01 Follow-up vaginal pap smear**
Vaginal pap smear, status-post hysterectomy for malignant condition

Use additional code to identify:
acquired absence of uterus (V45.77)
personal history of malignant neoplasm (V10.40–V10.44)

Excludes *vaginal pap smear status-post hysterectomy for non-malignant condition (V76.47)*

1/2 **V67.09 Following other surgery**

Excludes *sperm count following sterilization reversal (V26.22)*
sperm count for fertility testing (V26.21)

1/2 **V67.1 Following radiotherapy**

1/2 **V67.2 Following chemotherapy**
Cancer chemotherapy follow-up

1/2 **V67.3 Following psychotherapy and other treatment for mental disorder**

1/2 **V67.4 Following treatment of healed fracture**

Excludes *current (healing) fracture aftercare (V54.0–V54.9)*

● **V67.5 Following other treatment**

1/2 **V67.51 Following completed treatment with high-risk medication, not elsewhere classified**

Excludes *Long-term (current) drug use (V58.61–V58.69)*

1/2 **V67.59 Other**

1/2 **V67.6 Following combined treatment**

1/2 **V67.9 Unspecified follow-up examination**

● **V68 Encounters for administrative purposes**

❶ **V68.0 Issue of medical certificates**
Issue of medical certificate of:
cause of death
fitness
incapacity

Excludes *encounter for general medical examination (V70.0–V70.9)*

❶ **V68.1 Issue of repeat prescriptions**
Issue of repeat prescription for:
appliance
glasses
medications

Excludes *repeat prescription for contraceptives (V25.41–V25.49)*

V68.2 Request for expert evidence

V68.8 Other specified administrative purpose

V68.81 Referral of patient without examination or treatment

V68.89 Other

V68.9 Unspecified administrative purpose

V69 Problems related to lifestyle

V69.0 Lack of physical exercise

V69.1 Inappropriate diet and eating habits

Excludes *anorexia nervosa (307.1)*
bulimia (783.6)
malnutrition and other nutritional deficiencies (260–269.9)
other and unspecified eating disorders (307.50–307.59)

V69.2 High-risk sexual behavior

V69.3 Gambling and betting

Excludes *pathological gambling (312.31)*

V69.4 Lack of adequate sleep
Sleep deprivation

Excludes *insomnia (780.52)*

V69.5 Behavioral insomnia of childhood

V69.8 Other problems related to lifestyle
Self-damaging behavior

V69.9 Problem related to lifestyle, unspecified

PERSONS WITHOUT REPORTED DIAGNOSIS ENCOUNTERED DURING EXAMINATION AND INVESTIGATION OF INDIVIDUALS AND POPULATIONS (V70–V82)

Note: Nonspecific abnormal findings disclosed at the time of these examinations are classifiable to categories 790–796.

V70 General medical examination

Use additional code(s) to identify any special screening examination(s) performed (V73.0–V82.9)

V70.0 Routine general medical examination at a health care facility
Health checkup

Excludes *health checkup of infant or child (V20.2)*
pre-procedural general physical examination (V72.83)

V70.1 General psychiatric examination, requested by the authority

V70.2 General psychiatric examination, other and unspecified

V70.3 Other medical examination for administrative purposes
General medical examination for:
admission to old age home
adoption
camp
driving license
immigration and naturalization
insurance certification
marriage
prison
school admission
sports competition

Excludes *attendance for issue of medical certificates (V68.0)*
pre-employment screening (V70.5)

V70.4 Examination for medicolegal reasons
Blood-alcohol tests
Blood-drug tests
Paternity testing

Excludes *examination and observation following:*
accidents (V71.3, V71.4)
assault (V71.6)
rape (V71.5)

V70.5 Health examination of defined subpopulations
Armed forces personnel
Inhabitants of institutions
Occupational health examinations
Pre-employment screening
Preschool children
Prisoners
Prostitutes
Refugees
School children
Students

V70.6 Health examination in population surveys

Excludes *special screening (V73.0–V82.9)*

V70.7 Examination of participant in clinical trial
Examination of participant or control in clinical research

V70.8 Other specified general medical examinations
Examination of potential donor of organ or tissue

V70.9 Unspecified general medical examination

V71 Observation and evaluation for suspected conditions not found

Note: This category is to be used when persons without a diagnosis are suspected of having an abnormal condition, without signs or symptoms, which requires study, but after examination and observation, is found not to exist. This category is also for use for administrative and legal observation status.

V71.0 Observation for suspected mental condition

V71.01 Adult antisocial behavior
Dyssocial behavior or gang activity in adult without manifest psychiatric disorder

V71.02 Childhood or adolescent antisocial behavior
Dyssocial behavior or gang activity in child or adolescent without manifest psychiatric disorder

V71.09 Other suspected mental condition

V71.1 Observation for suspected malignant neoplasm

V71.2 Observation for suspected tuberculosis

V71.3 Observation following accident at work

V71.4 Observation following other accident
Examination of individual involved in motor vehicle traffic accident

V71.5 Observation following alleged rape or seduction
Examination of victim or culprit

V71.6 Observation following other inflicted injury
Examination of victim or culprit

V71.7 Observation for suspected cardiovascular disease

V71.8 Observation and evaluation for other specified suspected conditions

V71.81 Abuse and neglect

Excludes *adult abuse and neglect (995.80–995.85)*
child abuse and neglect (995.50–995.59)

V71.82 Observation and evaluation for suspected exposure to anthrax

➊ V71.83 **Observation and evaluation for suspected exposure to other biological agent**

➊ V71.89 **Other specified suspected conditions**

➊ V71.9 **Observation for unspecified suspected condition**

● V72 **Special investigations and examinations**

Includes: routine examination of specific system

Excludes *general medical examination (V70.0–70.4)*
general screening examination of defined populaiton groups (V70.5, V70.6, V70.7)
routine examination of infant or child (V20.2)

Use additional code(s) to identify any special screening examination(s) performed (V73.0–V82.9)

➊ V72.0 **Examination of eyes and vision**

● V72.1 **Examination of ears and hearing**

➊ V72.11 **Encounter for hearing examination following failed hearing screening** ◀

➊ V72.19 **Other examination of ears and hearing** ◀

➊ V72.2 **Dental examination**

➊ V72.3 **Gynecological examination**

Excludes *cervical Papanicolaou smear without general gynecological examination (V76.2)*
routine examination in contraceptive management (V25.40–V25.49)

➊ V72.31 **Routine gynecological examination**
General gynecological examination with or without Papanicolaou cervical smear
Pelvic examination (annual) (periodic)

Use additional code to identify routine vaginal Papanicolaou smear (V76.47)

➊ V72.32 **Encounter for Papanicolaou cervical smear to confirm findings of recent normal smear following initial abnormal smear**

● V72.4 **Pregnancy examination or test**

1/2 V72.40 **Pregnancy examination or test, pregnancy unconfirmed**
Possible pregnancy, not (yet) confirmed

1/2 V72.41 **Pregnancy examination or test, negative result**

1/2 V72.42 **Pregnancy examination or test, positive result**

1/2 ❑ V72.5 **Radiological examination, not elsewhere classified**
Routine chest x-ray

Excludes *examination for suspected tuberculosis (V71.2)*

1/2 ❑ V72.6 **Laboratory examination**

Excludes *that for suspected disorder (V71.0–V71.9)*

➊ V72.7 **Diagnostic skin and sensitization tests**
Allergy tests
Skin tests for hypersensitivity

Excludes *diagnostic skin tests for bacterial diseases (V74.0–V74.9)*

● V72.8 **Other specified examinations**

➊ V72.81 **Preoperative cardiovascular examination**
Pre-procedural cardiovascular examination

➊ V72.82 **Preoperative respiratory examination**
Pre-procedural respiratory examination

➊ V72.83 **Other specified preoperative examination**
Other pre-procedural examination
Pre-procedural general physical examination

Excludes *routine general medical examination (V70.0)*

➊ V72.84 **Preoperative examination, unspecified**
Pre-procedural examination, unspecified

➊ V72.85 **Other specified examination**

1/2 V72.86 **Encounter for blood typing**

➊ V72.9 **Unspecified examination**

● V73 **Special screening examination for viral and chlamydial diseases**

1/2 V73.0 **Poliomyelitis**

1/2 V73.1 **Smallpox**

1/2 V73.2 **Measles**

1/2 V73.3 **Rubella**

1/2 V73.4 **Yellow fever**

1/2 V73.5 **Other arthropod-borne viral diseases**
Dengue fever
Hemorrhagic fever
Viral encephalitis:
mosquito-borne
tick-borne

1/2 V73.6 **Trachoma**

● V73.8 **Other specified viral and chlamydial diseases**

1/2 V73.88 **Other specified chlamydial diseases**

1/2 V73.89 **Other specified viral diseases**

● V73.9 **Unspecified viral and chlamydial disease**

1/2 V73.98 **Unspecified chlamydial disease**

1/2 V73.99 **Unspecified viral disease**

● V74 **Special screening examination for bacterial and spirochetal diseases**

Includes: diagnostic skin tests for these diseases

1/2 V74.0 **Cholera**

1/2 V74.1 **Pulmonary tuberculosis**

1/2 V74.2 **Leprosy [Hansen's disease]**

1/2 V74.3 **Diphtheria**

1/2 V74.4 **Bacterial conjunctivitis**

1/2 V74.5 **Venereal disease**

1/2 V74.6 **Yaws**

1/2 V74.8 **Other specified bacterial and spirochetal diseases**
Brucellosis
Leptospirosis
Plague
Tetanus
Whooping cough

1/2 V74.9 **Unspecified bacterial and spirochetal disease**

● V75 **Special screening examination for other infectious diseases**

1/2 V75.0 **Rickettsial diseases**

1/2 V75.1 **Malaria**

1/2 V75.2 **Leishmaniasis**

1/2 V75.3 **Trypanosomiasis**
Chagas' disease
Sleeping sickness

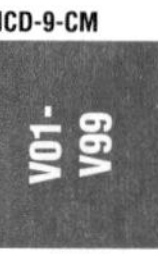
ICD-9-CM
V01-V99
Vol. 1

1/2 V75.4 Mycotic infections

1/2 V75.5 Schistosomiasis

1/2 V75.6 Filariasis

1/2 V75.7 Intestinal helminthiasis

1/2 V75.8 Other specified parasitic infections

1/2 V75.9 Unspecified infectious disease

● V76 Special screening for malignant neoplasms

1/2 V76.0 Respiratory organs

● V76.1 Breast

1/2 V76.10 Breast screening, unspecified

1/2 V76.11 Screening mammogram for high-risk patient

1/2 V76.12 Other screening mammogram

1/2 V76.19 Other screening breast examination

1/2 V76.2 Cervix

Routine cervical Papanicolaou smear

Excludes *that as part of a general gynecological examination (V72.31)*

1/2 V76.3 Bladder

● V76.4 Other sites

1/2 V76.41 Rectum

1/2 V76.42 Oral cavity

1/2 V76.43 Skin

1/2 V76.44 Prostate

1/2 V76.45 Testis

1/2 V76.46 Ovary

1/2 V76.47 Vagina

Vaginal pap smear status-post hysterectomy for nonmalignant condition

Use additional code to identify acquired absence of uterus (V45.77)

Excludes *vaginal pap smear status-post hysterectomy for malignant condition (V67.01)*

1/2 V76.49 Other sites

● V76.5 Intestine

1/2 V76.50 Intestine, unspecified

1/2 V76.51 Colon

Excludes *rectum (V76.41)*

1/2 V76.52 Small intestine

● V76.8 Other neoplasm

1/2 V76.81 Nervous system

1/2 V76.89 Other neoplasm

1/2 V76.9 Unspecified

● V77 Special screening for endocrine, nutritional, metabolic, and immunity disorders

1/2 V77.0 Thyroid disorders

1/2 V77.1 Diabetes mellitus

1/2 V77.2 Malnutrition

1/2 V77.3 Phenylketonuria [PKU]

1/2 V77.4 Galactosemia

1/2 V77.5 Gout

1/2 V77.6 Cystic fibrosis

Screening for mucoviscidosis

1/2 V77.7 Other inborn errors of metabolism

1/2 V77.8 Obesity

● V77.9 Other and unspecified endocrine, nutritional, metabolic, and immunity disorders

1/2 V77.91 Screening for lipoid disorders

Screening cholesterol level
Screening for hypercholesterolemia
Screening for hyperlipidemia

1/2 V77.99 Other and unspecified endocrine, nutritional, metabolic, and immunity disorders

● V78 Special screening for disorders of blood and blood-forming organs

1/2 V78.0 Iron deficiency anemia

1/2 V78.1 Other and unspecified deficiency anemia

1/2 V78.2 Sickle-cell disease or trait

1/2 V78.3 Other hemoglobinopathies

1/2 V78.8 Other disorders of blood and blood-forming organs

1/2 V78.9 Unspecified disorder of blood and blood-forming organs

● V79 Special screening for mental disorders and developmental handicaps

1/2 V79.0 Depression

1/2 V79.1 Alcoholism

1/2 V79.2 Mental retardation

1/2 V79.3 Developmental handicaps in early childhood

1/2 V79.8 Other specified mental disorders and developmental handicaps

1/2 V79.9 Unspecified mental disorder and developmental handicap

● V80 Special screening for neurological, eye, and ear diseases

1/2 V80.0 Neurological conditions

1/2 V80.1 Glaucoma

1/2 V80.2 Other eye conditions

Screening for:
cataract
congenital anomaly of eye
senile macular lesions

Excludes *general vision examination (V72.0)*

1/2 V80.3 Ear diseases

Excludes *general hearing examination (V72.1)*

● V81 Special screening for cardiovascular, respiratory, and genitourinary diseases

1/2 V81.0 Ischemic heart disease

1/2 V81.1 Hypertension

1/2 V81.2 Other and unspecified cardiovascular conditions

1/2 V81.3 Chronic bronchitis and emphysema

1/2 V81.4 Other and unspecified respiratory conditions

Excludes *screening for:*
lung neoplasm (V76.0)
pulmonary tuberculosis (V74.1)

1/2 V81.5 Nephropathy

Screening for asymptomatic bacteriuria

1/2 V81.6 Other and unspecified genitourinary conditions

● V82 Special screening for other conditions

1/2 V82.0 Skin conditions

1/2 V82.1 Rheumatoid arthritis

1/2 V82.2 Other rheumatic disorders

1/2 V82.3 **Congenital dislocation of hip**

1/2 V82.4 **Maternal screening for chromosomal anomalies**

Excludes *antenatal screening by amniocentesis (V28.0)*

1/2 V82.5 **Chemical poisoning and other contamination**
Screening for:
heavy metal poisoning
ingestion of radioactive substance
poisoning from contaminated water supply
radiation exposure

1/2 V82.6 **Multiphasic screening**

● V82.7 **Genetic screening** ◄

Excludes *genetic testing for procreative management (V26.31–V26.32)* ◄

1/2 V82.71 **Screening for genetic disease carrier status** ◄

1/2 V82.79 **Other genetic screening** ◄

● V82.8 **Other specified conditions**

1/2 V82.81 **Osteoporosis**
Use additional code to identify:
hormone replacement therapy (postmenopausal) status (V07.4)
postmenopausal (natural) status (V49.81)

1/2 V82.89 **Other specified conditions**

1/2 V82.9 **Unspecified condition**

GENETICS (V83–V84) ◄

● V83 **Generic carrier status**

● V83.0 **Hemophilia A carrier**

1/2 V83.01 **Asymptomatic hemophilia A carrier**

1/2 V83.02 **Symptomatic hemophilia A carrier**

● V83.8 **Other genetic carrier status**

1/2 V83.81 **Cystic fibrosis gene carrier**

1/2 V83.89 **Other genetic carrier status**

● V84 **Genetic susceptibility to disease**

Includes: Confirmed abnormal gene

Use additional code, if applicable, for any associated family history of the disease (V16–V19)

● V84.0 **Genetic susceptibility to malignant neoplasm**

Code first, if applicable, any current malignant neoplasms (140.0–195.8, 200.0–208.9, 230.0–234.9)

Use additional code, if applicable, for any personal history of malignant neoplasm (V10.0–V10.9)

❷ V84.01 **Genetic susceptibility to malignant neoplasm of breast**

❷ V84.02 **Genetic susceptibility to malignant neoplasm of ovary**

❷ V84.03 **Genetic susceptibility to malignant neoplasm of prostate**

❷ V84.04 **Genetic susceptibility to malignant neoplasm of endometrium**

❷ V84.09 **Genetic susceptibility to other malignant neoplasm**

❷ V84.8 **Genetic susceptibility to other disease**

BODY MASS INDEX (V85) ◄

● V85 **Body Mass Index [BMI]** ⟵
Kilograms per meters squared

Note: BMI adult codes are for use for persons over 20 years old.

❷ V85.0 **Body Mass Index less than 19, adult**

❷ V85.1 **Body Mass Index between 19–24, adult**

● V85.2 **Body Mass Index between 25–29, adult**

❷ V85.21 **Body Mass Index 25.0–25.9, adult**

❷ V85.22 **Body Mass Index 26.0–26.9, adult**

❷ V85.23 **Body Mass Index 27.0–27.9, adult**

❷ V85.24 **Body Mass Index 28.0–28.9, adult**

❷ V85.25 **Body Mass Index 29.0–29.9, adult**

● V85.3 **Body Mass Index between 30–39, adult**

❷ V85.30 **Body Mass Index 30.0–30.9, adult**

❷ V85.31 **Body Mass Index 31.0–31.9, adult**

❷ V85.32 **Body Mass Index 32.0–32.9, adult**

❷ V85.33 **Body Mass Index 33.0–33.9, adult**

❷ V85.34 **Body Mass Index 34.0–34.9, adult**

❷ V85.35 **Body Mass Index 35.0–35.9, adult**

❷ V85.36 **Body Mass Index 36.0–36.9, adult**

❷ V85.37 **Body Mass Index 37.0–37.9, adult**

❷ V85.38 **Body Mass Index 38.0–38.9, adult**

❷ V85.39 **Body Mass Index 39.0–39.9, adult**

❷ V85.4 **Body Mass Index 40 and over, adult**

● V85.5 **Body Mass Index, pediatric** ◄

Note: BMI pediatric codes are for use for persons age 2–20 years old. These percentiles are based on the growth charts published by the Centers for Disease Control and Prevention (CDC) ◄

❷ V85.51 **Body Mass Index, pediatric, less than 5th percentile for age** ◄

❷ V85.52 **Body Mass Index, pediatric, 5th percentile to less than 85th percentile for age** ◄

❷ V85.53 **Body Mass Index, pediatric, 85th percentile to less than 95th percentile for age** ◄

❷ V85.54 **Body Mass Index, pediatric, greater than or equal to 95th percentile for age** ◄

ESTROGEN RECEPTOR STATUS (V86) ◄

● V86 **Estrogen receptor status** ◄

Code first malignant neoplasm of breast (174.0–174.9, 175.0–175.9) ◄

❷ V86.0 **Estrogen receptor positive status [ER+]** ◄

❷ V86.1 **Estrogen receptor negative status [ER-]** ◄

◄ New ⟵ Revised ❶ First Listed 1/2 First Listed or Additional ❷ Additional Only
● Use Additional Digit(s) ❑ Nonspecific Code

E-Codes—SUPPLEMENTARY CLASSIFICATION OF EXTERNAL CAUSES OF INJURY AND POISONING (E800-E999)

This section is provided to permit the classification of environmental events, circumstances, and conditions as the cause of injury, poisoning, and other adverse effects. Where a code from this section is applicable, it is intended that it shall be used in addition to a code from one of the main chapters of ICD-9-CM, indicating the nature of the condition. Certain other conditions which may be stated to be due to external causes are classified in Chapters 1 to 16 of ICD-9-CM. For these, the "E" code classification should be used as an additional code for more detailed analysis.

Machinery accidents [other than those connected with transport] are classifiable to category E919, in which the fourth digit allows a broad classification of the type of machinery involved. If a more detailed classification of type of machinery is required, it is suggested that the "Classification of Industrial Accidents according to Agency," prepared by the International Labor Office, be used in addition; it is included in this publication.

Categories for "late effects" of accidents and other external causes are to be found at E929, E959, E969, E977, E989, and E999.

Definitions and examples related to transport accidents:

(a) A transport accident (E800–E848) is any accident involving a device designed primarily for, or being used at the time primarily for, conveying persons or goods from one place to another.

Includes: accidents involving:
aircraft and spacecraft (E840–E845)
watercraft (E830–E838)
motor vehicle (E810–E825)
railway (E800–E807)
other road vehicles (E826–E829)

In classifying accidents which involve more than one kind of transport, the above order of precedence of transport accidents should be used.

Accidents involving agricultural and construction machines, such as tractors, cranes, and bulldozers, are regarded as transport accidents only when these vehicles are under their own power on a highway [otherwise the vehicles are regarded as machinery]. Vehicles which can travel on land or water, such as hovercraft and other amphibious vehicles, are regarded as watercraft when on the water, as motor vehicles when on the highway, and as off-road motor vehicles when on land, but off the highway.

Excludes *accidents:*
in sports which involve the use of transport but where the transport vehicle itself was not involved in the accident
involving vehicles which are part of industrial equipment used entirely on industrial premises
occurring during transportation but unrelated to the hazards associated with the means of transportation [e.g., injuries received in a fight on board ship; transport vehicle involved in a cataclysm such as an earthquake]
to persons engaged in the maintenance or repair of transport equipment or vehicle not in motion, unless injured by another vehicle in motion

(b) A railway accident is a transport accident involving a railway train or other railway vehicle operated on rails, whether in motion or not.

Excludes *accidents:*
in repair shops
in roundhouse or on turntable
on railway premises but not involving a train or other railway vehicle

(c) A railway train or railway vehicle is any device with or without cars coupled to it, designed for traffic on a railway.

Includes: interurban:
electric car (operated chiefly on its own right-of-way, not open to other traffic)
streetcar (operated chiefly on its own right-of-way, not open to other traffic)
railway train, any power [diesel] [electric] [steam]
funicular
monorail or two-rail
subterranean or elevated
other vehicle designed to run on a railway track

Excludes *interurban electric cars [streetcars] specified to be operating on a right-of-way that forms part of the public street or highway [definition (n)]*

(d) A railway or railroad is a right-of-way designed for traffic on rails, which is used by carriages or wagons transporting passengers or freight, and by other rolling stock, and which is not open to other public vehicular traffic

(e) A motor vehicle accident is a transport accident involving a motor vehicle. It is defined as a motor vehicle traffic accident or as a motor vehicle nontraffic accident according to whether the accident occurs on a public highway or elsewhere.

Excludes *injury or damage due to cataclysm*
injury or damage while a motor vehicle, not under its own power, is being loaded on, or unloaded from, another conveyance

(f) A motor vehicle traffic accident is any motor vehicle accident occurring on a public highway [i.e., originating, terminating, or involving a vehicle partially on the highway]. A motor vehicle accident is assumed to have occurred on the highway unless another place is specified, except in the case of accidents involving only off-road motor vehicles which are classified as nontraffic accidents unless the contrary is stated.

(g) A motor vehicle nontraffic accident is any motor vehicle accident which occurs entirely in any place other than a public highway.

(h) A public highway [trafficway] or street is the entire width between property lines [or other boundary lines] of every way or place, of which any part is open to the use of the public for purposes of vehicular traffic as a matter of right or custom. A roadway is that part of the public highway designed, improved, and ordinarily used, for vehicular travel.

Includes: approaches (public) to:
docks
public building
station

Excludes *driveway (private)*
parking lot
ramp
roads in:
airfield
farm
industrial premises
mine
private grounds
quarry

(i) A motor vehicle is any mechanically or electrically powered device, not operated on rails, upon which any person or property may be transported or drawn upon a highway. Any object such as a trailer, coaster, sled, or wagon being towed by a motor vehicle is considered a part of the motor vehicle.

Includes: automobile [any type]
bus
construction machinery, farm and industrial machinery, steam roller, tractor, army tank, highway grader, or similar vehicle on wheels or treads, while in transport under own power
fire engine (motorized)
motorcycle
motorized bicycle [moped] or scooter
trolley bus not operating on rails
truck
van

Excludes *devices used solely to move persons or materials within the confines of a building and its premises, such as:*
building elevator
coal car in mine
electric baggage or mail truck used solely within a railroad station
electric truck used solely within an industrial plant
moving overhead crane

(j) A motorcycle is a two-wheeled motor vehicle having one or two riding saddles and sometimes having a third wheel for the support of a sidecar. The sidecar is considered part of the motorcycle.

Includes: motorized:
bicycle [moped]
scooter
tricycle

(k) An off-road motor vehicle is a motor vehicle of special design, to enable it to negotiate rough or soft terrain or snow. Examples of special design are high construction, special wheels and tires, driven by treads, or support on a cushion of air.

Includes: all terrain vehicle [ATV]
army tank
hovercraft, on land or swamp
snowmobile

(l) A driver of a motor vehicle is the occupant of the motor vehicle operating it or intending to operate it. A motorcyclist is the driver of a motorcycle. Other authorized occupants of a motor vehicle are passengers.

(m) An other road vehicle is any device, except a motor vehicle, in, on, or by which any person or property may be transported on a highway.

Includes: animal carrying a person or goods
animal-drawn vehicle
animal harnessed to conveyance
bicycle [pedal cycle]
streetcar
tricycle (pedal)

Excludes *pedestrian conveyance [definition (q)]*

(n) A streetcar is a device designed and used primarily for transporting persons within a municipality, running on rails, usually subject to normal traffic control signals, and operated principally on a right-of-way that forms part of the traffic way. A trailer being towed by a streetcar is considered a part of the streetcar.

Includes: interurban or intraurban electric or streetcar, when specified to be operating on a street or public highway
tram (car)
trolley (car)

(o) A pedal cycle is any road transport vehicle operated solely by pedals.

Includes: bicycle
pedal cycle
tricycle

Excludes *motorized bicycle [definition (i)]*

(p) A pedal cyclist is any person riding on a pedal cycle or in a sidecar attached to such a vehicle.

(q) A pedestrian conveyance is any human powered device by which a pedestrian may move other than by walking or by which a walking person may move another pedestrian.

Includes: baby carriage
coaster wagon
ice skates
perambulator
pushcart
pushchair
roller skates
scooter
skateboard
skis
sled
wheelchair

(r) A pedestrian is any person involved in an accident who was not at the time of the accident riding in or on a motor vehicle, railroad train, streetcar, animal-drawn or other vehicle, or on a bicycle or animal.

Includes: person:
changing tire of vehicle
in or operating a pedestrian conveyance
making adjustment to motor of vehicle
on foot

(s) A watercraft is any device for transporting passengers or goods on the water.

(t) A small boat is any watercraft propelled by paddle, oars, or small motor, with a passenger capacity of less than ten.

Includes: boat NOS
canoe
coble
dinghy
punt
raft
rowboat
rowing shell
scull
skiff
small motorboat

Excludes *barge*
lifeboat (used after abandoning ship)
raft (anchored) being used as a diving platform
yacht

(u) An aircraft is any device for transporting passengers or goods in the air.

Includes: airplane [any type]
balloon
bomber
dirigible
glider (hang)
military aircraft
parachute

(v) A commercial transport aircraft is any device for collective passenger or freight transportation by air, whether run on commercial lines for profit or by government authorities, with the exception of military craft.

RAILWAY ACCIDENTS (E800-E807)

Note: For definitions of railway accident and related terms see definitions (a) to (d).

Excludes *accidents involving railway train and:*
aircraft (E840.0-E845.9)
motor vehicle (E810.0-E825.9)
watercraft (E830.0-E838.9)

The following fourth-digit subdivisions are for use with categories E800-E807 to identify the injured person:

.0 Railway employee
Any person who by virtue of his employment in connection with a railway, whether by the railway company or not, is at increased risk of involvement in a railway accident, such as:
catering staff of train
driver
guard
porter
postal staff on train
railway fireman
shunter
sleeping car attendant

.1 Passenger on railway
Any authorized person traveling on a train, except a railway employee.

Excludes *intending passenger waiting at station (8)*
unauthorized rider on railway vehicle (8)

.2 Pedestrian
See definition (r)

.3 Pedal cyclist
See definition (p)

❑ **.8 Other specified person**
Intending passenger or bystander waiting at station
Unauthorized rider on railway vehicle

❑ **.9 Unspecified person**

● **E800 Railway accident involving collision with rolling stock**

Requires fourth digit. See beginning of section E800-E845 for codes and definitions.

Includes: collision between railway trains or railway vehicles, any kind
collision NOS on railway
derailment with antecedent collision with rolling stock or NOS

● ❑**E801 Railway accident involving collision with other object**

Requires fourth digit. See beginning of section E800-E845 for codes and definitions.

Includes: collision of railway train with:
buffers
fallen tree on railway
gates
platform
rock on railway
streetcar
other nonmotor vehicle
other object

Excludes *collision with:*
aircraft (E840.0-E842.9)
motor vehicle (E810.0-E810.9, E820.0-E822.9)

● **E802 Railway accident involving derailment without antecedent collision**

Requires fourth digit. See beginning of section E800-E845 for codes and definitions.

● **E803 Railway accident involving explosion, fire, or burning**

Requires fourth digit. See beginning of section E800-E845 for codes and definitions.

Excludes *explosion or fire, with antecedent derailment (E802.0-E802.9)*
explosion or fire, with mention of antecedent collision (E800.0-E801.9)

● **E804 Fall in, on, or from railway train**

Requires fourth digit. See beginning of section E800-E845 for codes and definitions.

Includes: fall while alighting from or boarding railway train

Excludes *fall related to collision, derailment, or explosion of railway train (E800.0-E803.9)*

● **E805 Hit by rolling stock**

Requires fourth digit. See beginning of section E800-E845 for codes and definitions.

Includes: crushed by railway train or part
injured by railway train or part
killed by railway train or part
knocked down by railway train or part
run over by railway train or part

Excludes *pedestrian hit by object set in motion by railway train (E806.0-E806.9)*

● ❑**E806 Other specified railway accident**

Requires fourth digit. See beginning of section E800-E845 for codes and definitions.

Includes: hit by object falling in railway train
injured by door or window on railway train
nonmotor road vehicle or pedestrian hit by object set in motion by railway train
railway train hit by falling:
earth NOS
rock
tree
other object

Excludes *railway accident due to cataclysm (E908-E909)*

● ❑**E807 Railway accident of unspecified nature**

Requires fourth digit. See beginning of section E800-E845 for codes and definitions.

Includes: found dead on railway right-of-way NOS
injured on railway right-of-way NOS
railway accident NOS

MOTOR VEHICLE TRAFFIC ACCIDENTS (E810-E819)

Note: For definitions of motor vehicle traffic accident, and related terms, see definitions (e) to (k).

Excludes *accidents involving motor vehicle and aircraft (E840.0-E845.9)*

The following fourth-digit subdivisions are for use with categories E810-E819 to identify the injured person:

.0 **Driver of motor vehicle other than motorcycle**
See definition (l)
.1 **Passenger in motor vehicle other than motorcycle**
See definition (l)
.2 **Motorcyclist**
See definition (l)
.3 **Passenger on motorcycle**
See definition (l)
.4 **Occupant of streetcar**
.5 **Rider of animal; occupant of animal-drawn vehicle**
.6 **Pedal cyclist**
See definition (p)
.7 **Pedestrian**
See definition (r)
❑ .8 **Other specified person**
Occupant of vehicle other than above
Person in railway train involved in accident
Unauthorized rider of motor vehicle
❑ .9 **Unspecified person**

● **E810 Motor vehicle traffic accident involving collision with train**

Requires fourth digit. See beginning of section E800-E845 for codes and definitions.

Excludes *motor vehicle collision with object set in motion by railway train (E815.0-E815.9)*
railway train hit by object set in motion by motor vehicle (E818.0-E818.9)

● **E811 Motor vehicle traffic accident involving re-entrant collision with another motor vehicle**

Requires fourth digit. See beginning of section E800-E845 for codes and definitions.

Includes: collision between motor vehicle which accidentally leaves the roadway then re-enters the same roadway, or the opposite roadway on a divided highway, and another motor vehicle

Excludes *collision on the same roadway when none of the motor vehicles involved have left and re-entered the roadway (E812.0-E812.9)*

● ❑ **E812 Other motor vehicle traffic accident involving collision with motor vehicle**

Requires fourth digit. See beginning of section E800-E845 for codes and definitions.

Includes: collision with another motor vehicle parked, stopped, stalled, disabled, or abandoned on the highway
motor vehicle collision NOS

Excludes *collision with object set in motion by another motor vehicle (E815.0-E815.9)*
re-entrant collision with another motor vehicle (E811.0-E811.9)

● ❑ **E813 Motor vehicle traffic accident involving collision with other vehicle**

Requires fourth digit. See beginning of section E800-E845 for codes and definitions.

Includes: collision between motor vehicle, any kind, and:
other road (nonmotor transport) vehicle, such as:
animal carrying a person
animal-drawn vehicle
pedal cycle
streetcar

Excludes *collision with:*
object set in motion by nonmotor road vehicle (E815.0-E815.9)
pedestrian (E814.0-E814.9)
nonmotor road vehicle hit by object set in motion by motor vehicle (E818.0-E818.9)

● **E814 Motor vehicle traffic accident involving collision with pedestrian**

Requires fourth digit. See beginning of section E800-E845 for codes and definitions.

Includes: collision between motor vehicle, any kind, and pedestrian
pedestrian dragged, hit, or run over by motor vehicle, any kind

Excludes *pedestrian hit by object set in motion by motor vehicle (E818.0-E818.9)*

● ❑ **E815 Other motor vehicle traffic accident involving collision on the highway**

Requires fourth digit. See beginning of section E800-E845 for codes and definitions.

Includes: collision (due to loss of control) (on highway) between motor vehicle, any kind, and:
abutment (bridge) (overpass)
animal (herded) (unattended)
fallen stone, traffic sign, tree, utility pole
guard rail or boundary fence
interhighway divider
landslide (not moving)
object set in motion by railway train or road vehicle (motor) (nonmotor)
object thrown in front of motor vehicle
safety island
temporary traffic sign or marker
wall of cut made for road
other object, fixed, movable, or moving

Excludes *collision with:*
any object off the highway (resulting from loss of control) (E816.0-E816.9)
any object which normally would have been off the highway and is not stated to have been on it (E816.0-E816.9)
motor vehicle parked, stopped, stalled, disabled, or abandoned on highway (E812.0-E812.9)
moving landslide (E909.2)
motor vehicle hit by object:
set in motion by railway train or road vehicle (motor) (nonmotor) (E818.0-E818.9)
thrown into or on vehicle (E818.0-E818.9)

● E816 Motor vehicle traffic accident due to loss of control, without collision on the highway

Requires fourth digit. See beginning of section E800-E845 for codes and definitions.

Includes: motor vehicle:
- failing to make curve and:
  - colliding with object off the highway
  - overturning
  - stopping abruptly off the highway
- going out of control (due to)
  - blowout and:
    - colliding with object off the highway
    - overturning
    - stopping abruptly off the highway
  - burst tire and:
    - colliding with object off the highway
    - overturning
    - stopping abruptly off the highway
  - driver falling asleep and:
    - colliding with object off the highway
    - overturning
    - stopping abruptly off the highway
  - driver inattention and:
    - colliding with object off the highway
    - overturning
    - stopping abruptly off the highway
  - excessive speed and:
    - colliding with object off the highway
    - overturning
    - stopping abruptly off the highway
  - failure of mechanical part and:
    - colliding with object off the highway
    - overturning
    - stopping abruptly off the highway

Excludes *collision on highway following loss of control (E810.0-E815.9)*
loss of control of motor vehicle following collision on the highway (E810.0-E815.9)

● E817 Noncollision motor vehicle traffic accident while boarding or alighting

Requires fourth digit. See beginning of section E800-E845 for codes and definitions.

Includes: fall down stairs of motor bus while boarding or alighting
fall from car in street while boarding or alighting
injured by moving part of the vehicle while boarding or alighting
trapped by door of motor bus while boarding or alighting

● ❑ E818 Other noncollision motor vehicle traffic accident

Requires fourth digit. See beginning of section E800-E845 for codes and definitions.

Includes: accidental poisoning from exhaust gas generated by motor vehicle while in motion
breakage of any part of motor vehicle while in motion
explosion of any part of motor vehicle while in motion
fall, jump, or being accidentally pushed from motor vehicle while in motion
fire starting in motor vehicle while in motion
hit by object thrown into or on motor vehicle while in motion
injured by being thrown against some part of, or object in, motor vehicle while in motion
injury from moving part of motor vehicle while in motion
object falling in or on motor vehicle while in motion
object thrown on motor vehicle while in motion
collision of railway train or road vehicle except motor vehicle, with object set in motion by motor vehicle
motor vehicle hit by object set in motion by railway train or road vehicle (motor) (nonmotor)
pedestrian, railway train, or road vehicle (motor) (nonmotor) hit by object set in motion by motor vehicle

Excludes *collision between motor vehicle and:*
object set in motion by railway train or road vehicle (motor) (nonmotor) (E815.0-E815.9)
object thrown towards the motor vehicle (E815.0-E815.9)
person overcome by carbon monoxide generated by stationary motor vehicle off the roadway with motor running (E868.2)

● ❑ E819 Motor vehicle traffic accident of unspecified nature

Requires fourth digit. See beginning of section E800-E845 for codes and definitions.

Includes: motor vehicle traffic accident NOS
traffic accident NOS

ICD-9-CM E800-E899 Vol. 1

MOTOR VEHICLE NONTRAFFIC ACCIDENTS (E820-E825)

Note: For definitions of motor vehicle nontraffic accident and related terms see definitions (a) to (k).

Includes: accidents involving motor vehicles being used in recreational or sporting activities off the highway
collision and noncollision motor vehicle accidents occurring entirely off the highway

Excludes *accidents involving motor vehicle and:*
aircraft (E840.0-E845.9)
watercraft (E830.0-E838.9)
accidents, not on the public highway, involving agricultural and construction machinery but not involving another motor vehicle (E919.0, E919.2, E919.7)

The following fourth-digit subdivisions are for use with categories E820-E825 to identify the injured person:

.0 Driver of motor vehicle other than motorcycle
See definition (l)
.1 Passenger in motor vehicle other than motorcycle
See definition (l)
.2 Motorcyclist
See definition (l)
.3 Passenger on motorcycle
See definition (l)
.4 Occupant of streetcar
.5 Rider of animal; occupant of animal-drawn vehicle
.6 Pedal cyclist
See definition (p)
.7 Pedestrian
See definition (r)
❑ **.8 Other specified person**
Occupant of vehicle other than above
Person on railway train involved in accident
Unauthorized rider of motor vehicle
❑ **.9 Unspecified person**

● **E820 Nontraffic accident involving motor-driven snow vehicle**

Requires fourth digit. See beginning of section E800-E845 for codes and definitions.

Includes: breakage of part of motor-driven snow vehicle (not on public highway)
fall from motor-driven snow vehicle (not on public highway)
hit by motor-driven snow vehicle (not on public highway)
overturning of motor-driven snow vehicle (not on public highway)
run over or dragged by motor-driven snow vehicle (not on public highway)
collision of motor-driven snow vehicle with:
animal (being ridden) (-drawn vehicle)
another off-road motor vehicle
other motor vehicle, not on public highway
railway train
other object, fixed or movable
injury caused by rough landing of motor-driven snow vehicle (after leaving ground on rough terrain)

Excludes *accident on the public highway involving motor driven snow vehicle (E810.0-E819.9)*

● ❑ **E821 Nontraffic accident involving other off-road motor vehicle**

Requires fourth digit. See beginning of section E800-E845 for codes and definitions.

Includes: breakage of part of off-road motor vehicle, except snow vehicle (not on public highway)
fall from off-road motor vehicle, except snow vehicle (not on public highway)
hit by off-road motor vehicle, except snow vehicle (not on public highway)
overturning of off-road motor vehicle, except snow vehicle (not on public highway)
run over or dragged by off-road motor vehicle, except snow vehicle (not on public highway)
thrown against some part of or object in off-road motor vehicle, except snow vehicle (not on public highway)
collision with:
animal (being ridden) (-drawn vehicle)
another off-road motor vehicle, except snow vehicle
other motor vehicle, not on public highway
other object, fixed or movable

Excludes *accident on public highway involving off-road motor vehicle (E810.0-E819.9)*
collision between motor driven snow vehicle and other off-road motor vehicle (E820.0-E820.9)
hovercraft accident on water (E830.0-E838.9)

● ❑ **E822 Other motor vehicle nontraffic accident involving collision with moving object**

Requires fourth digit. See beginning of section E800-E845 for codes and definitions.

Includes: collision, not on public highway, between motor vehicle, except off-road motor vehicle and:
animal
nonmotor vehicle
other motor vehicle, except off-road motor vehicle
pedestrian
railway train
other moving object

Excludes *collision with:*
motor-driven snow vehicle (E820.0-E820.9)
other off-road motor vehicle (E821.0-E821.9)

● ❑ **E823 Other motor vehicle nontraffic accident involving collision with stationary object**

Requires fourth digit. See beginning of section E800-E845 for codes and definitions.

Includes: collision, not on public highway, between motor vehicle, except off-road motor vehicle, and any object, fixed or movable, but not in motion

● ❑ **E824 Other motor vehicle nontraffic accident while boarding and alighting**

Requires fourth digit. See beginning of section E800-E845 for codes and definitions.

Includes: fall while boarding or alighting from motor vehicle except off-road motor vehicle, not on public highway
injury from moving part of motor vehicle while boarding or alighting from motor vehicle except off-road motor vehicle, not on public highway
trapped by door of motor vehicle while boarding or alighting from motor vehicle except off-road motor vehicle, not on public highway

E825 Other motor vehicle nontraffic accident of other and unspecified nature

Requires fourth digit. See beginning of section E800-E845 for codes and definitions.

Includes: accidental poisoning from carbon monoxide generated by motor vehicle while in motion, not on public highway
breakage of any part of motor vehicle while in motion, not on public highway
explosion of any part of motor vehicle while in motion, not on public highway
fall, jump, or being accidentally pushed from motor vehicle while in motion, not on public highway
fire starting in motor vehicle while in motion, not on public highway
hit by object thrown into, towards, or on motor vehicle while in motion, not on public highway
injured by being thrown against some part of, or object in, motor vehicle while in motion, not on public highway
injury from moving part of motor vehicle while in motion, not on public highway
object falling in or on motor vehicle while in motion, not on public highway
motor vehicle nontraffic accident NOS

Excludes *fall from or in stationary motor vehicle (E884.9, E885.9)*
overcome by carbon monoxide or exhaust gas generated by stationary motor vehicle off the roadway with motor running (E868.2)
struck by falling object from or in stationary motor vehicle (E916)

OTHER ROAD VEHICLE ACCIDENTS (E826-E829)

Note: Other road vehicle accidents are transport accidents involving road vehicles other than motor vehicles. For definitions of other road vehicle and related terms see definitions (m) to (o).

Includes: accidents involving other road vehicles being used in recreational or sporting activities

Excludes *collision of other road vehicle [any] with:*
aircraft (E840.0-E845.9)
motor vehicle (E813.0-E813.9, E820.0-E822.9)
railway train (E801.0-E801.9)

The following fourth-digit subdivisions are for use with categories E826-E829 to identify the injured person:

.0 Pedestrian
See definition (r)
.1 Pedal cyclist
See definition (p)
.2 Rider of animal
.3 Occupant of animal-drawn vehicle
.4 Occupant of streetcar
.8 Other specified person
.9 Unspecified person

E826 Pedal cycle accident
[0–9]
Requires fourth digit. See beginning of section E800-E845 for codes and definitions.

Includes: breakage of any part of pedal cycle
collision between pedal cycle and:
animal (being ridden) (herded) (unattended)
another pedal cycle
nonmotor road vehicle, any
pedestrian
other object, fixed, movable, or moving, not set in motion by motor vehicle, railway train, or aircraft
entanglement in wheel of pedal cycle
fall from pedal cycle
hit by object falling or thrown on the pedal cycle
pedal cycle accident NOS
pedal cycle overturned

E827 Animal-drawn vehicle accident
[0,2–4,8,9]
Requires fourth digit. See beginning of section E800-E845 for codes and definitions.

Includes: breakage of any part of vehicle
collision between animal-drawn vehicle and:
animal (being ridden) (herded) (unattended)
nonmotor road vehicle, except pedal cycle
pedestrian, pedestrian conveyance, or pedestrian vehicle
other object, fixed, movable, or moving, not set in motion by motor vehicle, railway train, or aircraft
fall from animal-drawn vehicle
knocked down by animal-drawn vehicle
overturning of animal-drawn vehicle
run over by animal-drawn vehicle
thrown from animal-drawn vehicle

Excludes *collision of animal-drawn vehicle with pedal cycle (E826.0-E826.9)*

ICD-9-CM E800-E899 Vol. 1

E828 Accident involving animal being ridden

[0,2,4,8,9] Requires fourth digit. See beginning of section E800-E845 for codes and definitions.

Includes: collision between animal being ridden and:
- another animal
- nonmotor road vehicle, except pedal cycle, and animal-drawn vehicle
- pedestrian, pedestrian conveyance, or pedestrian vehicle
- other object, fixed, movable, or moving, not set in motion by motor vehicle, railway train, or aircraft

fall from animal being ridden
knocked down by animal being ridden
thrown from animal being ridden
trampled by animal being ridden
ridden animal stumbled and fell

Excludes *collision of animal being ridden with:*
- *animal-drawn vehicle (E827.0-E827.9)*
- *pedal cycle (E826.0-E826.9)*

E829 Other road vehicle accidents

[0,4,8,9] Requires fourth digit. See beginning of section E800-E845 for codes and definitions.

Includes: accident while boarding or alighting from
- streetcar
- nonmotor road vehicle not classifiable to E826-E828

blow from object in
- streetcar
- nonmotor road vehicle not classifiable to E826-E828

breakage of any part of
- streetcar
- nonmotor road vehicle not classifiable to E826-E828

caught in door of
- streetcar
- nonmotor road vehicle not classifiable to E826-E828

derailment of
- streetcar
- nonmotor road vehicle not classifiable to E826-E828

fall in, on, or from
- streetcar
- nonmotor road vehicle not classifiable to E826-E828

fire in
- streetcar
- nonmotor road vehicle not classifiable to E826-E828

collision between streetcar or nonmotor road vehicle, except as in E826-E828, and:
- animal (not being ridden)
- another nonmotor road vehicle not classifiable to E826-E828
- pedestrian
- other object, fixed, movable, or moving, not set in motion by motor vehicle, railway train, or aircraft

nonmotor road vehicle accident NOS
streetcar accident NOS

Excludes *collision with:*
- *animal being ridden (E828.0-E828.9)*
- *animal-drawn vehicle (E827.0-E827.9)*
- *pedal cycle (E826.0-E826.9)*

WATER TRANSPORT ACCIDENTS (E830-E838)

Note: For definitions of water transport accident and related terms see definitions (a), (s), and (t).

Includes: watercraft accidents in the course of recreational activities

Excludes *accidents involving both aircraft, including objects set in motion by aircraft, and watercraft (E840.0-E845.9)*

The following fourth-digit subdivisions are for use with categories E830-E838 to identify the injured person:

.0 Occupant of small boat, unpowered

.1 Occupant of small boat, powered
See definition (t)

Excludes *water skier (4)*

.2 Occupant of other watercraft-crew
Persons:
- engaged in operation of watercraft
- providing passenger services [cabin attendants, ship's physician, catering personnel]
- working on ship during voyage in other capacity [musician in band, operators of shops and beauty parlors]

.3 Occupant of other watercraft—other than crew
Passenger
Occupant of lifeboat, other than crew, after abandoning ship

.4 Water skier

.5 Swimmer

.6 Dockers, stevedores
Longshoreman employed on the dock in loading and unloading ships

.8 Other specified person
Immigration and customs officials on board ship
Person:
- accompanying passenger or member of crew visiting boat

Pilot (guiding ship into port)

.9 Unspecified person

E830 Accident to watercraft causing submersion

Requires fourth digit. See beginning of section E800-E845 for codes and definitions.

Includes: submersion and drowning due to:
- boat overturning
- boat submerging
- falling or jumping from burning ship
- falling or jumping from crushed watercraft
- ship sinking
- other accident to watercraft

E831 Accident to watercraft causing other injury

Requires fourth digit. See beginning of section E800-E845 for codes and definitions.

Includes: any injury, except submersion and drowning, as a result of an accident to watercraft
burned while ship on fire
crushed between ships in collision
crushed by lifeboat after abandoning ship
fall due to collision or other accident to watercraft
hit by falling object due to accident to watercraft
injured in watercraft accident involving collision
struck by boat or part thereof after fall or jump from damaged boat

Excludes *burns from localized fire or explosion on board ship (E837.0-E837.9)*

E832 Other accidental submersion or drowning in water transport accident

Requires fourth digit. See beginning of section E800-E845 for codes and definitions.

Includes: submersion or drowning as a result of an accident other than accident to the watercraft, such as:
fall:
from gangplank
from ship
overboard
thrown overboard by motion of ship
washed overboard

Excludes *submersion or drowning of swimmer or diver who voluntarily jumps from boat not involved in an accident (E910.0-E910.9)*

E833 Fall on stairs or ladders in water transport

Requires fourth digit. See beginning of section E800-E845 for codes and definitions.

Excludes *fall due to accident to watercraft (E831.0-E831.9)*

E834 Other fall from one level to another in water transport

Requires fourth digit. See beginning of section E800-E845 for codes and definitions.

Excludes *fall due to accident to watercraft (E831.0-E831.9)*

E835 Other and unspecified fall in water transport

Requires fourth digit. See beginning of section E800-E845 for codes and definitions.

Excludes *fall due to accident to watercraft (E831.0-E831.9)*

E836 Machinery accident in water transport

Requires fourth digit. See beginning of section E800-E845 for codes and definitions.

Includes: injuries in water transport caused by:
deck machinery
engine room machinery
galley machinery
laundry machinery
loading machinery

E837 Explosion, fire, or burning in watercraft

Requires fourth digit. See beginning of section E800-E845 for codes and definitions.

Includes: explosion of boiler on steamship
localized fire on ship

Excludes *burning ship (due to collision or explosion) resulting in:*
submersion or drowning (E830.0-E830.9)
other injury (E831.0-E831.9)

E838 Other and unspecified water transport accident

Requires fourth digit. See beginning of section E800-E845 for codes and definitions.

Includes: accidental poisoning by gases or fumes on ship
atomic power plant malfunction in watercraft
crushed between ship and stationary object [wharf]
crushed between ships without accident to watercraft
crushed by falling object on ship or while loading or unloading
hit by boat while water skiing
struck by boat or part thereof (after fall from boat)
watercraft accident NOS

AIR AND SPACE TRANSPORT ACCIDENTS (E840-E845)

Note: For definition of aircraft and related terms see definitions (u) and (v).

The following fourth-digit subdivisions are for use with categories E840-E845 to identify the injured person:

.0 Occupant of spacecraft

.1 Occupant of military aircraft, any
Crew in military aircraft [air force] [army] [national guard] [navy]
Passenger (civilian) (military) in military aircraft [air force] [army] [national guard] [navy]
Troops in military aircraft [air force] [army] [national guard] [navy]

Excludes *occupants of aircraft operated under jurisdiction of police departments (5)*
parachutist (7)

.2 Crew of commercial aircraft (powered) in surface-to-surface transport

.3 Other occupant of commercial aircraft (powered) in surface-to-surface transport
Flight personnel:
not part of crew
on familiarization flight
Passenger on aircraft (powered) NOS

.4 Occupant of commercial aircraft (powered) in surface-to-air transport
Occupant [crew] [passenger] of aircraft (powered) engaged in activities, such as:
aerial spraying (crops) (fire retardants)
air drops of emergency supplies
air drops of parachutists, except from military craft
crop dusting
lowering of construction material [bridge or telephone pole]
sky writing

.5 Occupant of other powered aircraft
Occupant [crew] [passenger] of aircraft [powered] engaged in activities, such as:
aerobatic flying
aircraft racing
rescue operation
storm surveillance
traffic surveillance
Occupant of private plane NOS

.6 Occupant of unpowered aircraft, except parachutist
Occupant of aircraft classifiable to E842

.7 Parachutist (military) (other)
Person making voluntary descent

Excludes *person making descent after accident to aircraft (.1–.6)*

.8 Ground crew, airline employee
Persons employed at airfields (civil) (military) or launching pads, not occupants of aircraft

.9 Other person

E840 Accident to powered aircraft at takeoff or landing

Requires fourth digit. See beginning of section E800-E845 for codes and definitions.

Includes: collision of aircraft with any object, fixed, movable, or moving while taking off or landing
crash while taking off or landing
explosion on aircraft while taking off or landing
fire on aircraft while taking off or landing
forced landing

ICD-9-CM E800-E899 Vol. 1

● ❑**E841 Accident to powered aircraft, other and unspecified**

Requires fourth digit. See beginning of section E800-E845 for codes and definitions.

Includes: aircraft accident NOS
aircraft crash or wreck NOS
any accident to powered aircraft while in transit or when not specified whether in transit, taking off, or landing
collision of aircraft with another aircraft, bird, or any object, while in transit
explosion on aircraft while in transit
fire on aircraft while in transit

● **E842 Accident to unpowered aircraft**

[6–9] Requires fourth digit. See beginning of section E800-E845 for codes and definitions.

Includes: any accident, except collision with powered aircraft, to:
balloon
glider
hang glider
kite carrying a person
hit by object falling from unpowered aircraft

● **E843 Fall in, on, or from aircraft**

[0–9] Requires fourth digit. See beginning of section E800-E845 for codes and definitions.

Includes: accident in boarding or alighting from aircraft, any kind
fall in, on, or from aircraft [any kind], while in transit, taking off, or landing, except when as a result of an accident to aircraft

● ❑**E844 Other specified air transport accidents**

[0–9] Requires fourth digit. See beginning of section E800-E845 for codes and definitions.

Includes: hit by aircraft without accident to aircraft
hit by object falling from aircraft without accident to aircraft
injury by or from machinery on aircraft without accident to aircraft
injury by or from rotating propeller without accident to aircraft
injury by or from voluntary parachute descent without accident to aircraft
poisoning by carbon monoxide from aircraft while in transit without accident to aircraft
sucked into jet without accident to aircraft
any accident involving other transport vehicle (motor) (nonmotor) due to being hit by object set in motion by aircraft (powered)

Excludes *air sickness (E903)*
effects of:
high altitude (E902.0-E902.1)
pressure change (E902.0-E902.1)
injury in parachute descent due to accident to aircraft (E840.0-E842.9)

● **E845 Accident involving spacecraft**

[0,8,9] Requires fourth digit. See beginning of section E800-E845 for codes and definitions.

Includes: launching pad accident

Excludes *effects of weightlessness in spacecraft (E928.0)*

VEHICLE ACCIDENTS NOT ELSEWHERE CLASSIFIABLE (E846-E848)

E846 Accidents involving powered vehicles used solely within the buildings and premises of industrial or commercial establishment

Accident to, on, or involving:
battery-powered airport passenger vehicle
battery-powered trucks (baggage) (mail)
coal car in mine
logging car
self-propelled truck, industrial
station baggage truck (powered)
tram, truck, or tub (powered) in mine or quarry
Breakage of any part of vehicle
Collision with:
pedestrian
other vehicle or object within premises
Explosion of powered vehicle, industrial or commercial
Fall from powered vehicle, industrial or commercial
Overturning of powered vehicle, industrial or commercial
Struck by powered vehicle, industrial or commercial

Excludes *accidental poisoning by exhaust gas from vehicle not elsewhere classifiable (E868.2)*
injury by crane, lift (fork), or elevator (E919.2)

E847 Accidents involving cable cars not running on rails

Accident to, on, or involving:
cable car, not on rails
ski chair-lift
ski-lift with gondola
teleferique
Breakage of cable
Caught or dragged by cable car, not on rails
Fall or jump from cable car, not on rails
Object thrown from or in cable car not on rails

❑**E848 Accidents involving other vehicles, not elsewhere classifiable**

Accident to, on, or involving:
ice yacht
land yacht
nonmotor, nonroad vehicle NOS

● ***E849 Place of occurrence***

Note: *The following category is for use to denote the place where the injury or poisoning occurred.*

E849.0 Home

Apartment
Boarding house
Farm house
Home premises
House (residential)
Noninstitutional place of residence
Private:
driveway
garage
garden
home
walk
Swimming pool in private house or garden
Yard of home

Excludes *home under construction but not yet occupied (E849.3)*
institutional place of residence (E849.7)

E849.1 Farm

buildings
land under cultivation

Excludes *farm house and home premises of farm (E849.0)*

E849.2 Mine and quarry
Gravel pit
Sand pit
Tunnel under construction

E849.3 Industrial place and premises
Building under construction
Dockyard
Dry dock
Factory
building
premises
Garage (place of work)
Industrial yard
Loading platform (factory) (store)
Plant, industrial
Railway yard
Shop (place of work)
Warehouse
Workhouse

E849.4 Place for recreation and sport

Amusement park	*Playground, including school playground*
Baseball field	*Public park*
Basketball court	*Racecourse*
Beach resort	*Resort NOS*
Cricket ground	*Riding school*
Fives court	*Rifle range*
Football field	*Seashore resort*
Golf course	*Skating rink*
Gymnasium	*Sports palace*
Hockey field	*Stadium*
Holiday camp	*Swimming pool, public*
Ice palace	*Tennis court*
Lake resort	*Vacation resort*
Mountain resort	

Excludes *that in private house or garden (E849.0)*

E849.5 Street and highway

E849.6 Public building
Building (including adjacent grounds) used by the general public or by a particular group of the public, such as:
airport
bank
cafe
casino
church
cinema
clubhouse
courthouse
dance hall
garage building (for car storage)
hotel
market (grocery or other commodity)
movie house
music hall
nightclub
office
office building
opera house
post office
public hall
radio broadcasting station
restaurant
school (state) (public) (private)
shop, commercial
station (bus) (railway)
store
theater

Excludes *home garage (E849.0)*
industrial building or workplace (E849.3)

E849.7 Residential institution
Children's home
Dormitory
Hospital
Jail
Old people's home
Orphanage
Prison
Reform school

❑ *E849.8 Other specified places*
Beach NOS
Canal
Caravan site NOS
Derelict house
Desert
Dock
Forest
Harbor
Hill
Lake NOS
Mountain
Parking lot
Parking place
Pond or pool (natural)
Prairie
Public place NOS
Railway line
Reservoir
River
Sea
Seashore NOS
Stream
Swamp
Trailer court
Woods

❑ *E849.9 Unspecified place*

ACCIDENTAL POISONING BY DRUGS, MEDICINAL SUBSTANCES, AND BIOLOGICALS (E850-E858)

Includes: accidental overdose of drug, wrong drug given or taken in error, and drug taken inadvertently
accidents in the use of drugs and biologicals in medical and surgical procedures

Excludes *administration with suicidal or homicidal intent or intent to harm, or in circumstances classifiable to E980-E989 (E950.0-E950.5, E962.0, E980.0-E980.5)*
correct drug properly administered in therapeutic or prophylactic dosage, as the cause of adverse effect (E930.0-E949.9)

Note: See Alphabetic Index for more complete list of specific drugs to be classified under the fourth-digit subdivisions. The American Hospital Formulary numbers can be used to classify new drugs listed by the American Hospital Formulary Service (AHFS). See appendix C.

● **E850 Accidental poisoning by analgesics, antipyretics, and antirheumatics**

E850.0 Heroin
Diacetylmorphine

E850.1 Methadone

❑ **E850.2 Other opiates and related narcotics**
Codeine [methylmorphine]
Meperidine [pethidine]
Morphine
Opium (alkaloids)

ICD-9-CM E800-E899 Vol. 1

E850.3 Salicylates
Acetylsalicylic acid [aspirin]
Amino derivatives of salicylic acid
Salicylic acid salts

E850.4 Aromatic analgesics, not elsewhere classified
Acetanilid
Paracetamol [acetaminophen]
Phenacetin [acetophenetidin]

E850.5 Pyrazole derivatives
Aminophenazone [amidopyrine]
Phenylbutazone

E850.6 Antirheumatics [antiphlogistics]
Gold salts
Indomethacin

Excludes *salicylates (E850.3)*
steroids (E858.0)

❑ **E850.7 Other non-narcotic analgesics**
Pyrabital

❑ **E850.8 Other specified analgesics and antipyretics**
Pentazocine

❑ **E850.9 Unspecified analgesic or antipyretic**

E851 Accidental poisoning by barbiturates
Amobarbital [amylobarbitone]
Barbital [barbitone]
Butabarbital [butabarbitone]
Pentobarbital [pentobarbitone]
Phenobarbital [phenobarbitone]
Secobarbital [quinalbarbitone]

Excludes *thiobarbiturates (E855.1)*

● **E852 Accidental poisoning by other sedatives and hypnotics**

E852.0 Chloral hydrate group

E852.1 Paraldehyde

E852.2 Bromine compounds
Bromides
Carbromal (derivatives)

E852.3 Methaqualone compounds

E852.4 Glutethimide group

E852.5 Mixed sedatives, not elsewhere classified

❑ **E852.8 Other specified sedatives and hypnotics**

❑ **E852.9 Unspecified sedative or hypnotic**
Sleeping:
drug NOS
pill NOS
tablet NOS

● **E853 Accidental poisoning by tranquilizers**

E853.0 Phenothiazine-based tranquilizers
Chlorpromazine
Fluphenazine
Prochlorperazine
Promazine

E853.1 Butyrophenone-based tranquilizers
Haloperidol
Spiperone
Trifluperidol

E853.2 Benzodiazepine-based tranquilizers
Chlordiazepoxide
Diazepam
Flurazepam
Lorazepam
Medazepam
Nitrazepam

❑ **E853.8 Other specified tranquilizers**
Hydroxyzine
Meprobamate

❑ **E853.9 Unspecified tranquilizer**

● **E854 Accidental poisoning by other psychotropic agents**

E854.0 Antidepressants
Amitriptyline
Imipramine
Monoamine oxidase [MAO] inhibitors

E854.1 Psychodysleptics [hallucinogens]
Cannabis derivatives
Lysergide [LSD]
Marihuana (derivatives)
Mescaline
Psilocin
Psilocybin

E854.2 Psychostimulants
Amphetamine
Caffeine

Excludes *central appetite depressants (E858.8)*

E854.3 Central nervous system stimulants
Analeptics
Opiate antagonists

E854.8 Other psychotropic agents

● **E855 Accidental poisoning by other drugs acting on central and autonomic nervous system**

E855.0 Anticonvulsant and anti-Parkinsonism drugs
Amantadine
Hydantoin derivatives
Levodopa [L-dopa]
Oxazolidine derivatives [paramethadione] [trimethadione]
Succinimides

❑ **E855.1 Other central nervous system depressants**
Ether
Gaseous anesthetics
Halogenated hydrocarbon derivatives
Intravenous anesthetics
Thiobarbiturates, such as thiopental sodium

E855.2 Local anesthetics
Cocaine
Lidocaine [lignocaine]
Procaine
Tetracaine

E855.3 Parasympathomimetics [cholinergics]
Acetylcholine
Anticholinesterase:
organophosphorus
reversible
Pilocarpine

E855.4 Parasympatholytics [anticholinergics and antimuscarinics] and spasmolytics
Atropine
Homatropine
Hyoscine [scopolamine]
Quaternary ammonium derivatives

E855.5 Sympathomimetics [adrenergics]
Epinephrine [adrenalin]
Levarterenol [noradrenalin]

E855.6 Sympatholytics [antiadrenergics]
Phenoxybenzamine
Tolazoline hydrochloride

❑ **E855.8 Other specified drugs acting on central and autonomic nervous systems**

❑ **E855.9 Unspecified drug acting on central and autonomic nervous systems**

E856 Accidental poisoning by antibiotics

❑ **E857 Accidental poisoning by other anti-infectives**

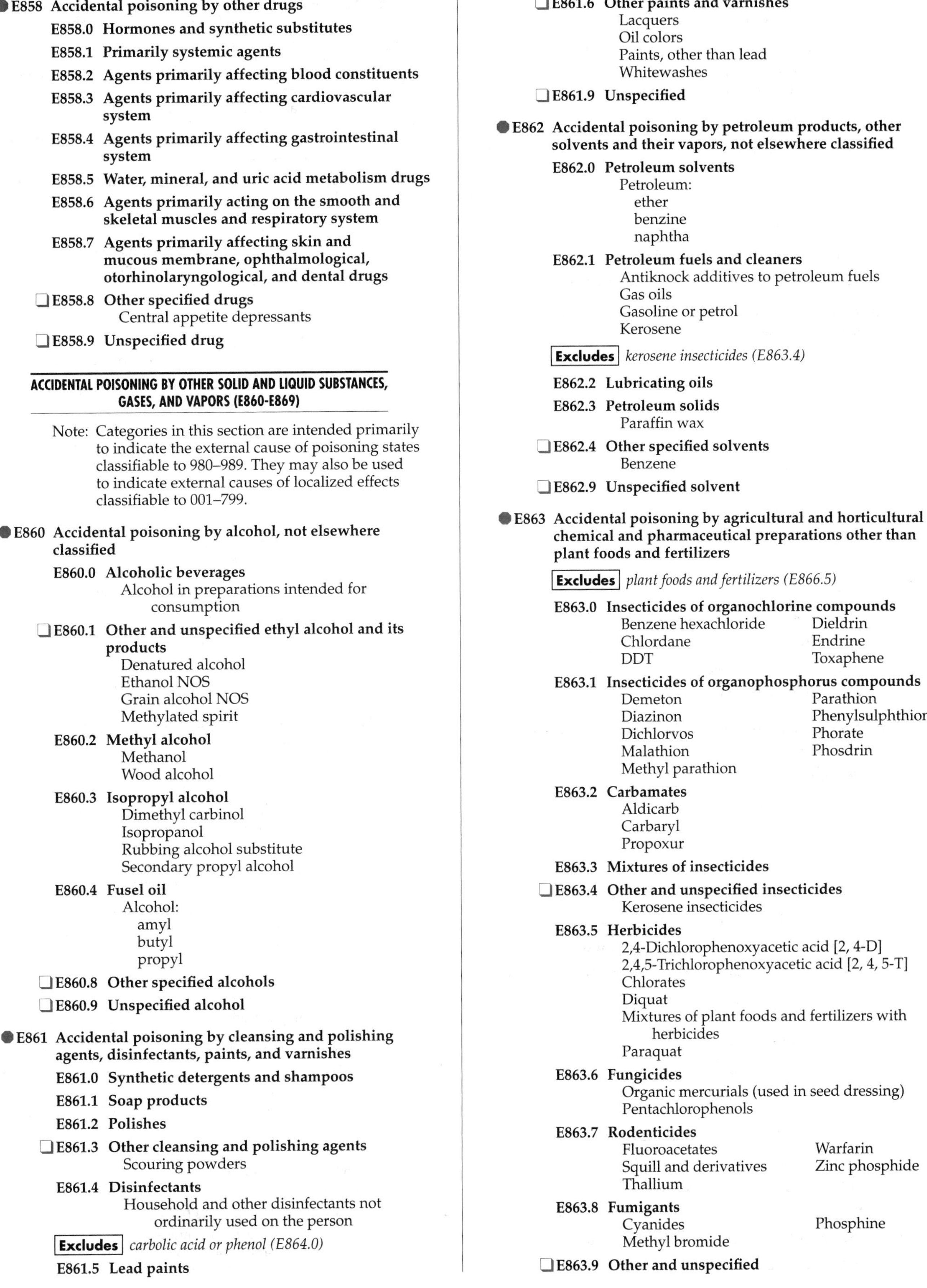

● **E858 Accidental poisoning by other drugs**

E858.0 Hormones and synthetic substitutes

E858.1 Primarily systemic agents

E858.2 Agents primarily affecting blood constituents

E858.3 Agents primarily affecting cardiovascular system

E858.4 Agents primarily affecting gastrointestinal system

E858.5 Water, mineral, and uric acid metabolism drugs

E858.6 Agents primarily acting on the smooth and skeletal muscles and respiratory system

E858.7 Agents primarily affecting skin and mucous membrane, ophthalmological, otorhinolaryngological, and dental drugs

❑ **E858.8 Other specified drugs**
Central appetite depressants

❑ **E858.9 Unspecified drug**

ACCIDENTAL POISONING BY OTHER SOLID AND LIQUID SUBSTANCES, GASES, AND VAPORS (E860-E869)

Note: Categories in this section are intended primarily to indicate the external cause of poisoning states classifiable to 980–989. They may also be used to indicate external causes of localized effects classifiable to 001–799.

● **E860 Accidental poisoning by alcohol, not elsewhere classified**

E860.0 Alcoholic beverages
Alcohol in preparations intended for consumption

❑ **E860.1 Other and unspecified ethyl alcohol and its products**
Denatured alcohol
Ethanol NOS
Grain alcohol NOS
Methylated spirit

E860.2 Methyl alcohol
Methanol
Wood alcohol

E860.3 Isopropyl alcohol
Dimethyl carbinol
Isopropanol
Rubbing alcohol substitute
Secondary propyl alcohol

E860.4 Fusel oil
Alcohol:
amyl
butyl
propyl

❑ **E860.8 Other specified alcohols**

❑ **E860.9 Unspecified alcohol**

● **E861 Accidental poisoning by cleansing and polishing agents, disinfectants, paints, and varnishes**

E861.0 Synthetic detergents and shampoos

E861.1 Soap products

E861.2 Polishes

❑ **E861.3 Other cleansing and polishing agents**
Scouring powders

E861.4 Disinfectants
Household and other disinfectants not ordinarily used on the person

Excludes *carbolic acid or phenol (E864.0)*

E861.5 Lead paints

❑ **E861.6 Other paints and varnishes**
Lacquers
Oil colors
Paints, other than lead
Whitewashes

❑ **E861.9 Unspecified**

● **E862 Accidental poisoning by petroleum products, other solvents and their vapors, not elsewhere classified**

E862.0 Petroleum solvents
Petroleum:
ether
benzine
naphtha

E862.1 Petroleum fuels and cleaners
Antiknock additives to petroleum fuels
Gas oils
Gasoline or petrol
Kerosene

Excludes *kerosene insecticides (E863.4)*

E862.2 Lubricating oils

E862.3 Petroleum solids
Paraffin wax

❑ **E862.4 Other specified solvents**
Benzene

❑ **E862.9 Unspecified solvent**

● **E863 Accidental poisoning by agricultural and horticultural chemical and pharmaceutical preparations other than plant foods and fertilizers**

Excludes *plant foods and fertilizers (E866.5)*

E863.0 Insecticides of organochlorine compounds
Benzene hexachloride
Chlordane
DDT
Dieldrin
Endrine
Toxaphene

E863.1 Insecticides of organophosphorus compounds
Demeton
Diazinon
Dichlorvos
Malathion
Methyl parathion
Parathion
Phenylsulphthion
Phorate
Phosdrin

E863.2 Carbamates
Aldicarb
Carbaryl
Propoxur

E863.3 Mixtures of insecticides

❑ **E863.4 Other and unspecified insecticides**
Kerosene insecticides

E863.5 Herbicides
2,4-Dichlorophenoxyacetic acid [2, 4-D]
2,4,5-Trichlorophenoxyacetic acid [2, 4, 5-T]
Chlorates
Diquat
Mixtures of plant foods and fertilizers with herbicides
Paraquat

E863.6 Fungicides
Organic mercurials (used in seed dressing)
Pentachlorophenols

E863.7 Rodenticides
Fluoroacetates
Squill and derivatives
Thallium
Warfarin
Zinc phosphide

E863.8 Fumigants
Cyanides
Methyl bromide
Phosphine

❑ **E863.9 Other and unspecified**

● **E864 Accidental poisoning by corrosives and caustics, not elsewhere classified**

Excludes *those as components of disinfectants (E861.4)*

E864.0 Corrosive aromatics
Carbolic acid or phenol

E864.1 Acids
Acid:
hydrochloric
nitric
sulfuric

E864.2 Caustic alkalis
Lye

❑ **E864.3 Other specified corrosives and caustics**

❑ **E864.4 Unspecified corrosives and caustics**

● **E865 Accidental poisoning from poisonous foodstuffs and poisonous plants**

Includes: any meat, fish, or shellfish
plants, berries, and fungi eaten as, or in mistake for food, or by a child

Excludes *anaphlyactic shock due to adverse food reaction (995.60–995.69)*
food poisoning (bacterial) (005.0–005.9)
poisoning and toxic reactions to venomous plants (E905.6–E905.7)

E865.0 Meat

E865.1 Shellfish

❑ **E865.2 Other fish**

E865.3 Berries and seeds

❑ **E865.4 Other specified plants**

E865.5 Mushrooms and other fungi

❑ **E865.8 Other specified foods**

❑ **E865.9 Unspecified foodstuff or poisonous plant**

● **E866 Accidental poisoning by other and unspecified solid and liquid substances**

Excludes *these substances as a component of:*
medicines (E850.0-E858.9)
paints (E861.5-E861.6)
pesticides (E863.0-E863.9)
petroleum fuels (E862.1)

E866.0 Lead and its compounds and fumes

E866.1 Mercury and its compounds and fumes

E866.2 Antimony and its compounds and fumes

E866.3 Arsenic and its compounds and fumes

❑ **E866.4 Other metals and their compounds and fumes**
Beryllium (compounds)
Brass fumes
Cadmium (compounds)
Copper salts
Iron (compounds)
Manganese (compounds)
Nickel (compounds)
Thallium (compounds)

E866.5 Plant foods and fertilizers

Excludes *mixtures with herbicides (E863.5)*

E866.6 Glues and adhesives

E866.7 Cosmetics

❑ **E866.8 Other specified solid or liquid substances**

❑ **E866.9 Unspecified solid or liquid substance**

E867 Accidental poisoning by gas distributed by pipeline
Carbon monoxide from incomplete combustion of piped gas
Coal gas NOS
Liquefied petroleum gas distributed through pipes (pure or mixed with air)
Piped gas (natural) (manufactured)

● **E868 Accidental poisoning by other utility gas and other carbon monoxide**

E868.0 Liquefied petroleum gas distributed in mobile containers
Butane or carbon monoxide from incomplete combustion of these gases
Liquefied hydrocarbon gas NOS or carbon monoxide from incomplete combustion of these gases
Propane or carbon monoxide from incomplete combustion of these gases

❑ **E868.1 Other and unspecified utility gas**
Acetylene or carbon monoxide from incomplete combustion of these gases
Gas NOS used for lighting, heating, or cooking or carbon monoxide from incomplete combustion of these gases
Water gas or carbon monoxide from incomplete combustion of these gases

E868.2 Motor vehicle exhaust gas
Exhaust gas from:
farm tractor, not in transit
gas engine
motor pump
motor vehicle, not in transit
any type of combustion engine not in watercraft

Excludes *poisoning by carbon monoxide from:*
aircraft while in transit (E844.0-E844.9)
motor vehicle while in transit (E818.0-E818.9)
watercraft whether or not in transit (E838.0-E838.9)

❑ **E868.3 Carbon monoxide from incomplete combustion of other domestic fuels**
Carbon monoxide from incomplete combustion of:
coal in domestic stove or fireplace
coke in domestic stove or fireplace
kerosene in domestic stove or fireplace
wood in domestic stove or fireplace

Excludes *carbon monoxide from smoke and fumes due to conflagration (E890.0-E893.9)*

❑ **E868.8 Carbon monoxide from other sources**
Carbon monoxide from:
blast furnace gas
incomplete combustion of fuels in industrial use
kiln vapor

❑ **E868.9 Unspecified carbon monoxide**

● **E869 Accidental poisoning by other gases and vapors**

Excludes *effects of gases used as anesthetics (E855.1, E938.2)*
fumes from heavy metals (E866.0-E866.4)
smoke and fumes due to conflagration or explosion (E890.0-E899)

E869.0 Nitrogen oxides

E869.1 Sulfur dioxide

E869.2 Freon

E869.3 Lacrimogenic gas [tear gas]
Bromobenzyl cyanide
Chloroacetophenone
Ethyliodoacetate

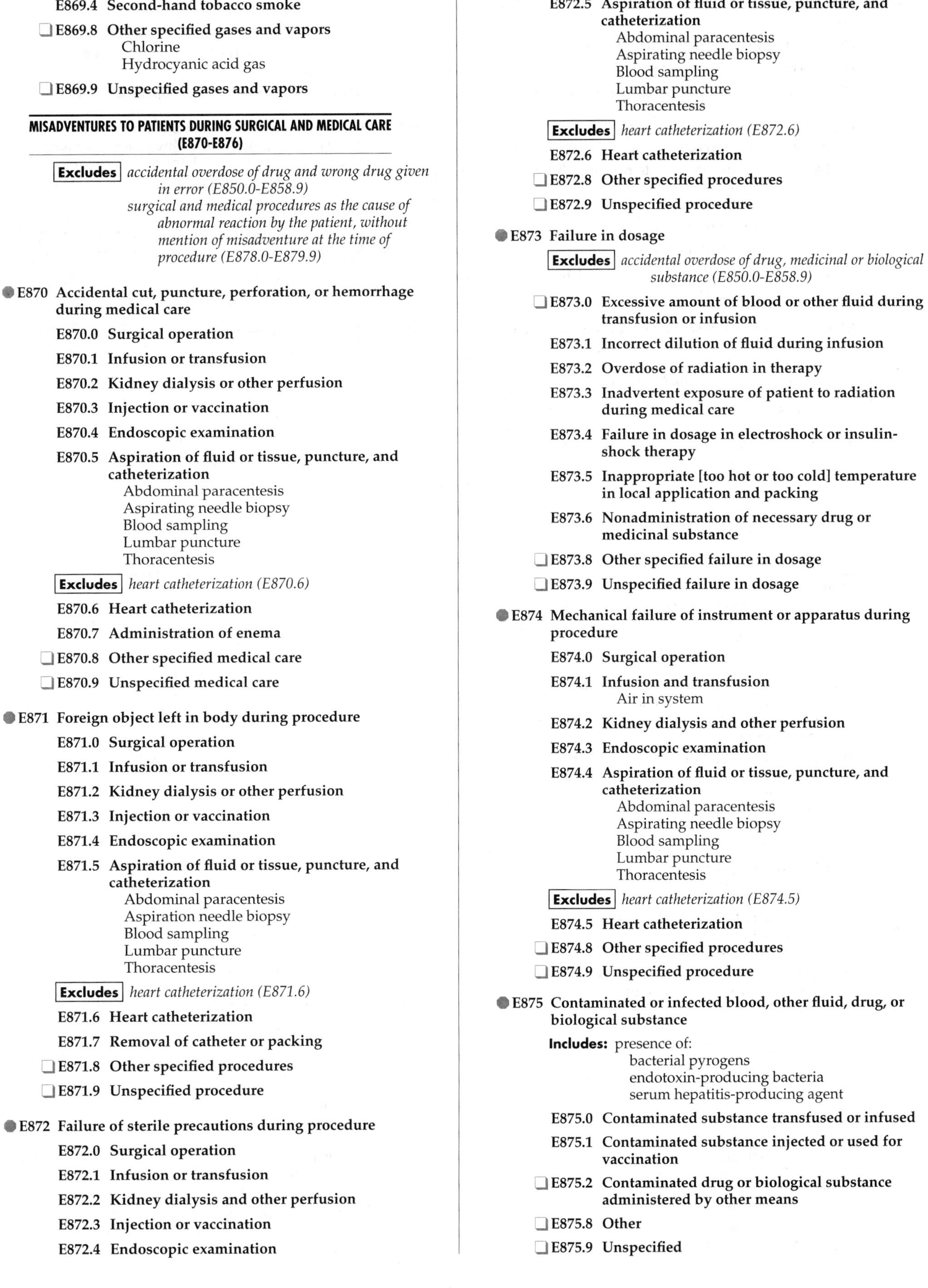

E869.4 Second-hand tobacco smoke

❑ E869.8 Other specified gases and vapors
Chlorine
Hydrocyanic acid gas

❑ E869.9 Unspecified gases and vapors

MISADVENTURES TO PATIENTS DURING SURGICAL AND MEDICAL CARE (E870-E876)

Excludes *accidental overdose of drug and wrong drug given in error (E850.0-E858.9)*
surgical and medical procedures as the cause of abnormal reaction by the patient, without mention of misadventure at the time of procedure (E878.0-E879.9)

● E870 Accidental cut, puncture, perforation, or hemorrhage during medical care

E870.0 Surgical operation

E870.1 Infusion or transfusion

E870.2 Kidney dialysis or other perfusion

E870.3 Injection or vaccination

E870.4 Endoscopic examination

E870.5 Aspiration of fluid or tissue, puncture, and catheterization
Abdominal paracentesis
Aspirating needle biopsy
Blood sampling
Lumbar puncture
Thoracentesis

Excludes *heart catheterization (E870.6)*

E870.6 Heart catheterization

E870.7 Administration of enema

❑ E870.8 Other specified medical care

❑ E870.9 Unspecified medical care

● E871 Foreign object left in body during procedure

E871.0 Surgical operation

E871.1 Infusion or transfusion

E871.2 Kidney dialysis or other perfusion

E871.3 Injection or vaccination

E871.4 Endoscopic examination

E871.5 Aspiration of fluid or tissue, puncture, and catheterization
Abdominal paracentesis
Aspiration needle biopsy
Blood sampling
Lumbar puncture
Thoracentesis

Excludes *heart catheterization (E871.6)*

E871.6 Heart catheterization

E871.7 Removal of catheter or packing

❑ E871.8 Other specified procedures

❑ E871.9 Unspecified procedure

● E872 Failure of sterile precautions during procedure

E872.0 Surgical operation

E872.1 Infusion or transfusion

E872.2 Kidney dialysis and other perfusion

E872.3 Injection or vaccination

E872.4 Endoscopic examination

E872.5 Aspiration of fluid or tissue, puncture, and catheterization
Abdominal paracentesis
Aspirating needle biopsy
Blood sampling
Lumbar puncture
Thoracentesis

Excludes *heart catheterization (E872.6)*

E872.6 Heart catheterization

❑ E872.8 Other specified procedures

❑ E872.9 Unspecified procedure

● E873 Failure in dosage

Excludes *accidental overdose of drug, medicinal or biological substance (E850.0-E858.9)*

❑ E873.0 Excessive amount of blood or other fluid during transfusion or infusion

E873.1 Incorrect dilution of fluid during infusion

E873.2 Overdose of radiation in therapy

E873.3 Inadvertent exposure of patient to radiation during medical care

E873.4 Failure in dosage in electroshock or insulin-shock therapy

E873.5 Inappropriate [too hot or too cold] temperature in local application and packing

E873.6 Nonadministration of necessary drug or medicinal substance

❑ E873.8 Other specified failure in dosage

❑ E873.9 Unspecified failure in dosage

● E874 Mechanical failure of instrument or apparatus during procedure

E874.0 Surgical operation

E874.1 Infusion and transfusion
Air in system

E874.2 Kidney dialysis and other perfusion

E874.3 Endoscopic examination

E874.4 Aspiration of fluid or tissue, puncture, and catheterization
Abdominal paracentesis
Aspirating needle biopsy
Blood sampling
Lumbar puncture
Thoracentesis

Excludes *heart catheterization (E874.5)*

E874.5 Heart catheterization

❑ E874.8 Other specified procedures

❑ E874.9 Unspecified procedure

● E875 Contaminated or infected blood, other fluid, drug, or biological substance

Includes: presence of:
bacterial pyrogens
endotoxin-producing bacteria
serum hepatitis-producing agent

E875.0 Contaminated substance transfused or infused

E875.1 Contaminated substance injected or used for vaccination

❑ E875.2 Contaminated drug or biological substance administered by other means

❑ E875.8 Other

❑ E875.9 Unspecified

ICD-9-CM E800-E899 Vol. 1

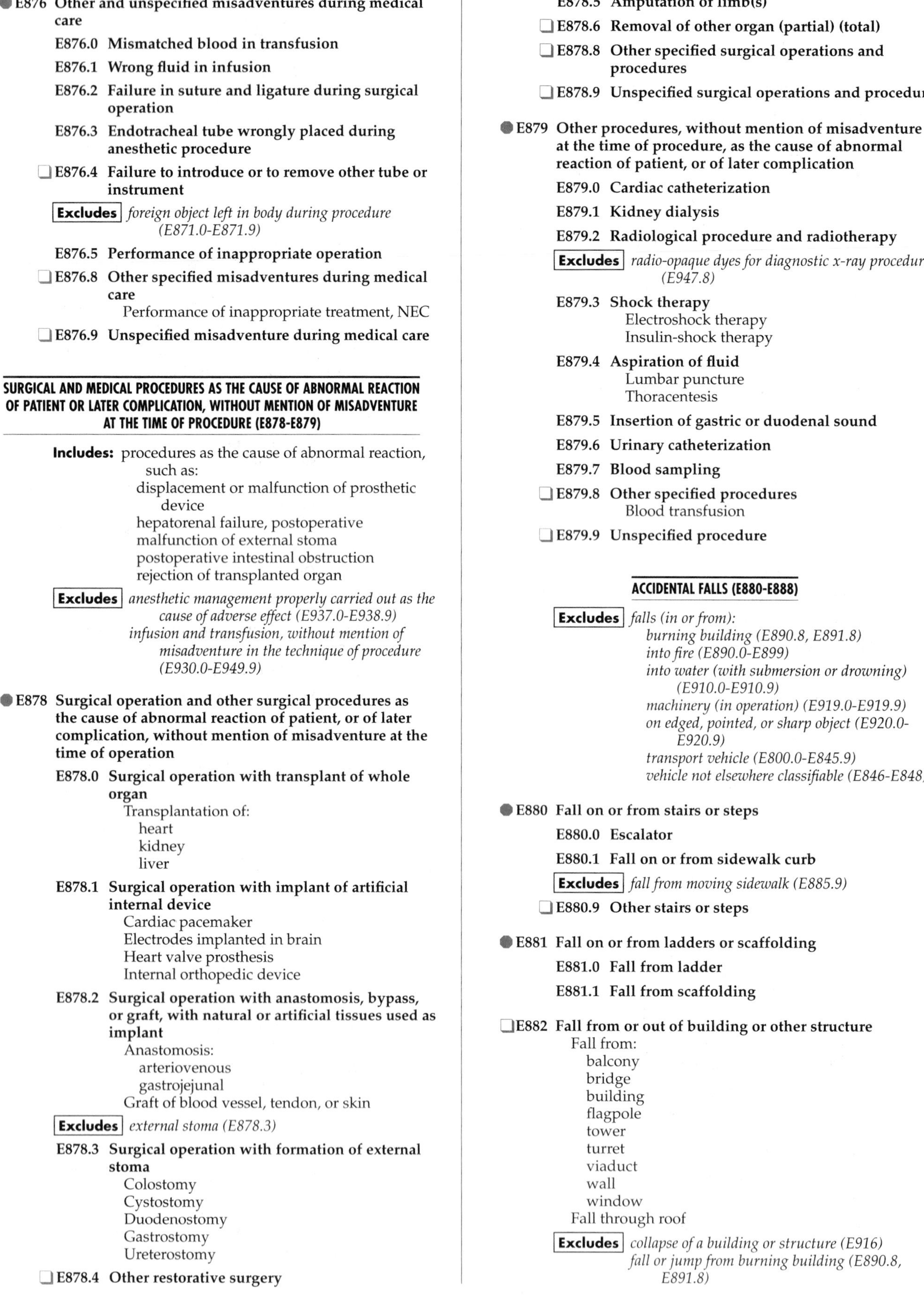

● **E876 Other and unspecified misadventures during medical care**

E876.0 Mismatched blood in transfusion

E876.1 Wrong fluid in infusion

E876.2 Failure in suture and ligature during surgical operation

E876.3 Endotracheal tube wrongly placed during anesthetic procedure

❑ **E876.4 Failure to introduce or to remove other tube or instrument**

Excludes *foreign object left in body during procedure (E871.0-E871.9)*

E876.5 Performance of inappropriate operation

❑ **E876.8 Other specified misadventures during medical care**

Performance of inappropriate treatment, NEC

❑ **E876.9 Unspecified misadventure during medical care**

SURGICAL AND MEDICAL PROCEDURES AS THE CAUSE OF ABNORMAL REACTION OF PATIENT OR LATER COMPLICATION, WITHOUT MENTION OF MISADVENTURE AT THE TIME OF PROCEDURE (E878-E879)

Includes: procedures as the cause of abnormal reaction, such as:
displacement or malfunction of prosthetic device
hepatorenal failure, postoperative
malfunction of external stoma
postoperative intestinal obstruction
rejection of transplanted organ

Excludes *anesthetic management properly carried out as the cause of adverse effect (E937.0-E938.9)*
infusion and transfusion, without mention of misadventure in the technique of procedure (E930.0-E949.9)

● **E878 Surgical operation and other surgical procedures as the cause of abnormal reaction of patient, or of later complication, without mention of misadventure at the time of operation**

E878.0 Surgical operation with transplant of whole organ

Transplantation of:
heart
kidney
liver

E878.1 Surgical operation with implant of artificial internal device

Cardiac pacemaker
Electrodes implanted in brain
Heart valve prosthesis
Internal orthopedic device

E878.2 Surgical operation with anastomosis, bypass, or graft, with natural or artificial tissues used as implant

Anastomosis:
arteriovenous
gastrojejunal
Graft of blood vessel, tendon, or skin

Excludes *external stoma (E878.3)*

E878.3 Surgical operation with formation of external stoma

Colostomy
Cystostomy
Duodenostomy
Gastrostomy
Ureterostomy

❑ **E878.4 Other restorative surgery**

E878.5 Amputation of limb(s)

❑ **E878.6 Removal of other organ (partial) (total)**

❑ **E878.8 Other specified surgical operations and procedures**

❑ **E878.9 Unspecified surgical operations and procedures**

● **E879 Other procedures, without mention of misadventure at the time of procedure, as the cause of abnormal reaction of patient, or of later complication**

E879.0 Cardiac catheterization

E879.1 Kidney dialysis

E879.2 Radiological procedure and radiotherapy

Excludes *radio-opaque dyes for diagnostic x-ray procedures (E947.8)*

E879.3 Shock therapy

Electroshock therapy
Insulin-shock therapy

E879.4 Aspiration of fluid

Lumbar puncture
Thoracentesis

E879.5 Insertion of gastric or duodenal sound

E879.6 Urinary catheterization

E879.7 Blood sampling

❑ **E879.8 Other specified procedures**

Blood transfusion

❑ **E879.9 Unspecified procedure**

ACCIDENTAL FALLS (E880-E888)

Excludes *falls (in or from):*
burning building (E890.8, E891.8)
into fire (E890.0-E899)
into water (with submersion or drowning) (E910.0-E910.9)
machinery (in operation) (E919.0-E919.9)
on edged, pointed, or sharp object (E920.0-E920.9)
transport vehicle (E800.0-E845.9)
vehicle not elsewhere classifiable (E846-E848)

● **E880 Fall on or from stairs or steps**

E880.0 Escalator

E880.1 Fall on or from sidewalk curb

Excludes *fall from moving sidewalk (E885.9)*

❑ **E880.9 Other stairs or steps**

● **E881 Fall on or from ladders or scaffolding**

E881.0 Fall from ladder

E881.1 Fall from scaffolding

❑ **E882 Fall from or out of building or other structure**

Fall from:
balcony
bridge
building
flagpole
tower
turret
viaduct
wall
window
Fall through roof

Excludes *collapse of a building or structure (E916)*
fall or jump from burning building (E890.8, E891.8)

E883 Fall into hole or other opening in surface

Includes: fall into:
cavity
dock
hole
pit
quarry
shaft
swimming pool
tank
well

Excludes *fall into water NOS (E910.9)*
that resulting in drowning or submersion without mention of injury (E910.0-E910.9)

E883.0 Accident from diving or jumping into water [swimming pool]
Strike or hit:
against bottom when jumping or diving into water
wall or board of swimming pool
water surface

Excludes *diving with insufficient air supply (E913.2)*
effects of air pressure from diving (E902.2)

E883.1 Accidental fall into well

E883.2 Accidental fall into storm drain or manhole

E883.9 Fall into other hole or other opening in surface

E884 Other fall from one level to another

E884.0 Fall from playground equipment

Excludes *recreational machinery (E919.8)*

E884.1 Fall from cliff

E884.2 Fall from chair

E884.3 Fall from wheelchair

E884.4 Fall from bed

E884.5 Fall from other furniture

E884.6 Fall from commode
Toilet

E884.9 Other fall from one level to another
Fall from:
embankment
haystack
stationary vehicle
tree

E885 Fall on same level from slipping, tripping, or stumbling

E885.0 Fall from (nonmotorized) scooter

E885.1 Fall from roller skates
In-line skates

E885.2 Fall from skateboard

E885.3 Fall from skis

E885.4 Fall from snowboard

E885.9 Fall from other slipping, tripping, or stumbling
Fall on moving sidewalk

E886 Fall on same level from collision, pushing, or shoving, by or with other person

Excludes *crushed or pushed by a crowd or human stampede (E917.1, E917.6)*

E886.0 In sports
Tackles in sports

Excludes *kicked, stepped on, struck by object, in sports (E917.0, E917.5)*

E886.9 Other and unspecified
Fall from collision of pedestrian (conveyance) with another pedestrian (conveyance)

E887 Fracture, cause unspecified

E888 Other and unspecified fall
Accidental fall NOS

E888.0 Fall resulting in striking against sharp object
Use additional external cause code to identify object (E920)

E888.1 Fall resulting in striking against other object

E888.8 Other fall

E888.9 Unspecified fall
Fall NOS

ICD-9-CM E800-E899 Vol. 1

ACCIDENTS CAUSED BY FIRE AND FLAMES (E890-E899)

Includes: asphyxia or poisoning due to conflagration or ignition
burning by fire
secondary fires resulting from explosion

Excludes *arson (E968.0)*
fire in or on:
machinery (in operation) (E919.0-E919.9)
transport vehicle other than stationary vehicle (E800.0-E845.9)
vehicle not elsewhere classifiable (E846-E848)

E890 Conflagration in private dwelling

Includes: conflagration in:
apartment
boarding house
camping place
caravan
farmhouse
house
conflagration in:
lodging house
mobile home
private garage
rooming house
tenement
conflagration originating from sources classifiable to E893-E898 in the above buildings

E890.0 Explosion caused by conflagration

E890.1 Fumes from combustion of polyvinylchloride [PVC] and similar material in conflagration

E890.2 Other smoke and fumes from conflagration
Carbon monoxide from conflagration in private building
Fumes NOS from conflagration in private building
Smoke NOS from conflagration in private building

E890.3 Burning caused by conflagration

E890.8 Other accident resulting from conflagration
Collapse of burning private building
Fall from burning private building
Hit by object falling from burning private building
Jump from burning private building

E890.9 Unspecified accident resulting from conflagration in private dwelling

E891 Conflagration in other and unspecified building or structure
Conflagration in:
barn
church
convalescent and other residential home
dormitory of educational institution
factory
farm outbuildings
hospital
hotel
school
store
theater
Conflagration originating from sources classifiable to E893-E898, in the above buildings

E891.0 Explosion caused by conflagration

E891.1 Fumes from combustion of polyvinylchloride [PVC] and similar material in conflagration

❑ **E891.2 Other smoke and fumes from conflagration**
Carbon monoxide from conflagration in building or structure
Fumes NOS from conflagration in building or structure
Smoke NOS from conflagration in building or structure

E891.3 Burning caused by conflagration

❑ **E891.8 Other accident resulting from conflagration**
Collapse of burning building or structure
Fall from burning building or structure
Hit by object falling from burning building or structure
Jump from burning building or structure

❑ **E891.9 Unspecified accident resulting from conflagration of other and unspecified building or structure**

E892 Conflagration not in building or structure
Fire (uncontrolled) (in) (of):
- forest
- grass
- hay
- lumber
- mine
- prairie
- transport vehicle [any], except while in transit
- tunnel

● **E893 Accident caused by ignition of clothing**

Excludes *ignition of clothing:*
from highly inflammable material (E894)
with conflagration (E890.0-E892)

E893.0 From controlled fire in private dwelling
Ignition of clothing from:
normal fire (charcoal) (coal) (electric) (gas) (wood) in:
- brazier in private dwelling (as listed in E890)
- fireplace in private dwelling (as listed in E890)
- furnace in private dwelling (as listed in E890)
- stove in private dwelling (as listed in E890)

❑ **E893.1 From controlled fire in other building or structure**
Ignition of clothing from:
normal fire (charcoal) (coal) (electric) (gas) (wood) in:
- brazier in other building or structure (as listed in E891)
- fireplace in other building or structure (as listed in E891)
- furnace in other building or structure (as listed in E891)
- stove in other building or structure (as listed in E891)

E893.2 From controlled fire not in building or structure
Ignition of clothing from:
- bonfire (controlled)
- brazier fire (controlled), not in building or structure
- trash fire (controlled)

Excludes *conflagration not in building (E892)*
trash fire out of control (E892)

❑ **E893.8 From other specified sources**
Ignition of clothing from:
- blowlamp
- blowtorch
- burning bedspread
- candle
- cigar
- cigarette
- lighter
- matches
- pipe
- welding torch

❑ **E893.9 Unspecified source**
Ignition of clothing (from controlled fire NOS) (in building NOS) NOS

E894 Ignition of highly inflammable material
Ignition of:
- benzine (with ignition of clothing)
- gasoline (with ignition of clothing)
- fat (with ignition of clothing)
- kerosene (with ignition of clothing)
- paraffin (with ignition of clothing)
- petrol (with ignition of clothing)

Excludes *ignition of highly inflammable material with:*
conflagration (E890.0-E892)
explosion (E923.0-E923.9)

E895 Accident caused by controlled fire in private dwelling
Burning by (flame of) normal fire (charcoal) (coal) (electric) (gas) (wood) in:
- brazier in private dwelling (as listed in E890)
- fireplace in private dwelling (as listed in E890)
- furnace in private dwelling (as listed in E890)
- stove in private dwelling (as listed in E890)

Excludes *burning by hot objects not producing fire or flames (E924.0-E924.9)*
ignition of clothing from these sources (E893.0)
poisoning by carbon monoxide from incomplete combustion of fuel (E867-E868.9)
that with conflagration (E890.0-E890.9)

❑ **E896 Accident caused by controlled fire in other and unspecified building or structure**
Burning by (flame of) normal fire (charcoal) (coal) (electric) (gas) (wood) in:
- brazier in other building or structure (as listed in E891)
- fireplace in other building or structure (as listed in E891)
- furnace in other building or structure (as listed in E891)
- stove in other building or structure (as listed in E891)

Excludes *burning by hot objects not producing fire or flames (E924.0-E924.9)*
ignition of clothing from these sources (E893.1)
poisoning by carbon monoxide from incomplete combustion of fuel (E867-E868.9)
that with conflagration (E891.0-E891.9)

E897 Accident caused by controlled fire not in building or structure
Burns from flame of:
- bonfire (controlled)
- brazier fire (controlled), not in building or structure
- trash fire (controlled)

Excludes *ignition of clothing from these sources (E893.2)*
trash fire out of control (E892)
that with conflagration (E892)

● **E898 Accident caused by other specified fire and flames**

Excludes *conflagration (E890.0-E892)*
that with ignition of:
clothing (E893.0-E893.9)
highly inflammable material (E894)

E898.0 Burning bedclothes
Bed set on fire NOS

❑ **E898.1 Other**
Burning by:
blowlamp
blowtorch
candle
cigar
cigarette
fire in room NOS
Burning by:
lamp
lighter
matches
pipe
welding torch

❑ **E899 Accident caused by unspecified fire**
Burning NOS

ACCIDENTS DUE TO NATURAL AND ENVIRONMENTAL FACTORS (E900-E909)

● **E900 Excessive heat**

E900.0 Due to weather conditions
Excessive heat as the external cause of:
ictus solaris
siriasis
sunstroke

E900.1 Of man-made origin
Heat (in):
boiler room
drying room
factory
furnace room
generated in transport vehicle
kitchen

❑ **E900.9 Of unspecified origin**

● **E901 Excessive cold**

E901.0 Due to weather conditions
Excessive cold as the cause of:
chilblains NOS
immersion foot

E901.1 Of man-made origin
Contact with or inhalation of:
dry ice
liquid air
liquid hydrogen
liquid nitrogen
Prolonged exposure in:
deep freeze unit
refrigerator

❑ **E901.8 Other specified origin**

❑ **E901.9 Of unspecified origin**

● **E902 High and low air pressure and changes in air pressure**

E902.0 Residence or prolonged visit at high altitude
Residence or prolonged visit at high altitude as the cause of:
Acosta syndrome
Alpine sickness
altitude sickness
Andes disease
anoxia, hypoxia
barotitis, barodontalgia, barosinusitis, otitic barotrauma
hypobarism, hypobaropathy
mountain sickness
range disease

E902.1 In aircraft
Sudden change in air pressure in aircraft during ascent or descent as the cause of:
aeroneurosis
aviators' disease

E902.2 Due to diving
High air pressure from rapid descent in water as the cause of:
caisson disease
divers' disease
divers' palsy or paralysis
Reduction in atmospheric pressure while surfacing from deep water diving as the cause of:
caisson disease
divers' disease
divers' palsy or paralysis

❑ **E902.8 Due to other specified causes**
Reduction in atmospheric pressure while surfacing from under ground

❑ **E902.9 Unspecified cause**

E903 Travel and motion

● **E904 Hunger, thirst, exposure, and neglect**

Excludes *any condition resulting from homicidal intent (E968.0-E968.9)*
hunger, thirst, and exposure resulting from accidents connected with transport (E800.0-E848)

E904.0 Abandonment or neglect of infants and helpless persons
Exposure to weather conditions resulting from abandonment or neglect
Hunger or thirst resulting from abandonment or neglect
Desertion of newborn
Inattention at or after birth
Lack of care (helpless person) (infant)

Excludes *criminal [purposeful] neglect (E968.4)*

E904.1 Lack of food
Lack of food as the cause of:
inanition
insufficient nourishment
starvation

Excludes *hunger resulting from abandonment or neglect (E904.0)*

E904.2 Lack of water
Lack of water as the cause of:
dehydration
inanition

Excludes *dehydration due to acute fluid loss (276.51)*

E904.3 Exposure (to weather conditions), not elsewhere classifiable
Exposure NOS
Humidity
Struck by hailstones

Excludes *struck by lightning (E907)*

E904.9 Privation, unqualified
Destitution

● **E905 Venomous animals and plants as the cause of poisoning and toxic reactions**

Includes: chemical released by animal
insects
release of venom through fangs, hairs, spines, tentacles, and other venom apparatus

Excludes *eating of poisonous animals or plants (E865.0-E865.9)*

E905.0 Venomous snakes and lizards
Cobra
Copperhead snake
Coral snake
Fer de lance
Gila monster
Krait
Mamba
Rattlesnake
Sea snake
Snake (venomous)
Viper
Water moccasin

Excludes *bites of snakes and lizards known to be nonvenomous (E906.2)*

E905.1 Venomous spiders
Black widow spider
Brown spider
Tarantula (venomous)

E905.2 Scorpion

E905.3 Hornets, wasps, and bees
Yellow jacket

E905.4 Centipede and venomous millipede (tropical)

❑ **E905.5 Other venomous arthropods**
Sting of:
ant
caterpillar

E905.6 Venomous marine animals and plants
Puncture by sea urchin spine
Sting of:
coral
jelly fish
nematocysts
sea anemone
sea cucumber
other marine animal or plant

Excludes *bites and other injuries caused by nonvenomous marine animal (E906.2-E906.8)*
bite of sea snake (venomous) (E905.0)

❑ **E905.7 Poisoning and toxic reactions caused by other plants**
Injection of poisons or toxins into or through skin by plant thorns, spines, or other mechanisms

Excludes *puncture wound NOS by plant thorns or spines (E920.8)*

❑ **E905.8 Other specified**

❑ **E905.9 Unspecified**
Sting NOS
Venomous bite NOS

● **E906 Other injury caused by animals**

Excludes *poisoning and toxic reactions caused by venomous animals and insects (E905.0-E905.9)*
road vehicle accident involving animals (E827.0-E828.9)
tripping or falling over an animal (E885.9)

E906.0 Dog bite

E906.1 Rat bite

E906.2 Bite of nonvenomous snakes and lizards

❑ **E906.3 Bite of other animal except arthropod**
Cats
Moray eel
Rodents, except rats
Shark

E906.4 Bite of nonvenomous arthropod
Insect bite NOS

E906.5 Bite by unspecified animal
Animal bite NOS

❑ **E906.8 Other specified injury caused by animal**
Butted by animal
Fallen on by horse or other animal, not being ridden
Gored by animal
Implantation of quills of porcupine
Pecked by bird
Run over by animal, not being ridden
Stepped on by animal, not being ridden

Excludes *injury by animal being ridden (E828.0-E828.9)*

❑ **E906.9 Unspecified injury caused by animal**

E907 Lightning

Excludes *injury from:*
fall of tree or other object caused by lightning (E916)
fire caused by lightning (E890.0-E892)

● **E908 Cataclysmic storms, and floods resulting from storms**

Excludes *collapse of dam or man-made structure causing flood (E909.3)*

E908.0 Hurricane
Storm surge
"Tidal wave" caused by storm action
Typhoon

E908.1 Tornado
Cyclone
Twisters

E908.2 Floods
Torrential rainfall
Flash flood

Excludes *collapse of dam or man-made structure causing flood (E909.3)*

E908.3 Blizzard (snow) (ice)

E908.4 Dust storm

E908.8 Other cataclysmic storms

E908.9 Unspecified cataclysmic storms, and floods resulting from storms
Storm NOS

E909 Cataclysmic earth surface movements and eruptions

E909.0 Earthquakes

E909.1 Volcanic eruptions
Burns from lava
Ash inhalation

E909.2 Avalanche, landslide, or mudslide

E909.3 Collapse of dam or man-made structure

E909.4 Tidal wave caused by earthquake
Tidal wave NOS
Tsunami

Excludes *tidal wave caused by tropical storm (E908.0)*

E909.8 Other cataclysmic earth surface movements and eruptions

E909.9 Unspecified cataclysmic earth surface movements and eruptions

ACCIDENTS CAUSED BY SUBMERSION, SUFFOCATION, AND FOREIGN BODIES (E910-E915)

● **E910 Accidental drowning and submersion**

Includes: immersion
swimmers' cramp

Excludes *diving accident (NOS) (resulting in injury except drowning) (E883.0)*
diving with insufficient air supply (E913.2)
drowning and submersion due to:
cataclysm (E908-E909)
machinery accident (E919.0-E919.9)
transport accident (E800.0-E845.9)
effect of high and low air pressure (E902.2)
injury from striking against objects while in running water (E917.2)

E910.0 While water-skiing
Fall from water skis with submersion or drowning

Excludes *accident to water-skier involving a watercraft and resulting in submersion or other injury (E830.4, E831.4)*

❑ **E910.1 While engaged in other sport or recreational activity with diving equipment**
Scuba diving NOS
Skin diving NOS
Underwater spear fishing NOS

❑ **E910.2 While engaged in other sport or recreational activity without diving equipment**
Fishing or hunting, except from boat or with diving equipment
Ice skating
Playing in water
Surfboarding
Swimming NOS
Voluntarily jumping from boat, not involved in accident, for swim NOS
Wading in water

Excludes *jumping into water to rescue another person (E910.3)*

E910.3 While swimming or diving for purposes other than recreation or sport
Marine salvage (with diving equipment)
Pearl diving (with diving equipment)
Placement of fishing nets (with diving equipment)
Rescue (attempt) of another person (with diving equipment)
Underwater construction or repairs (with diving equipment)

E910.4 In bathtub

❑ **E910.8 Other accidental drowning or submersion**
Drowning in:
quenching tank
swimming pool

❑ **E910.9 Unspecified accidental drowning or submersion**
Accidental fall into water NOS
Drowning NOS

E911 Inhalation and ingestion of food causing obstruction of respiratory tract or suffocation
Aspiration and inhalation of food [any] (into respiratory tract) NOS
Asphyxia by food [including bone, seed in food, regurgitated food]
Choked on food [including bone, seed in food, regurgitated food]
Suffocation by food [including bone, seed in food, regurgitated food]
Compression of trachea by food lodged in esophagus
Interruption of respiration by food lodged in esophagus
Obstruction of respiration by food lodged in esophagus
Obstruction of pharynx by food (bolus)

Excludes *injury, except asphyxia and obstruction of respiratory passage, caused by food (E915)*
obstruction of esophagus by food without mention of asphyxia or obstruction of respiratory passage (E915)

❑ **E912 Inhalation and ingestion of other object causing obstruction of respiratory tract or suffocation**
Aspiration and inhalation of foreign body except food (into respiratory tract) NOS
Foreign object [bean] in nose
Obstruction of pharynx by foreign body
Compression by foreign body in esophagus
Interruption of respiration by foreign body in esophagus
Obstruction of respiration by foreign body in esophagus

Excludes *injury, except asphyxia and obstruction of respiratory passage, caused by foreign body (E915)*
obstruction of esophagus by foreign body without mention of asphyxia or obstruction in respiratory passage (E915)

ICD-9-CM E900-E999 Vol. 1

● **E913 Accidental mechanical suffocation**

Excludes *mechanical suffocation from or by:*
accidental inhalation or ingestion of:
food (E911)
foreign object (E912)
cataclysm (E908-E909)
explosion (E921.0-E921.9, E923.0-E923.9)
machinery accident (E919.0-E919.9)

E913.0 In bed or cradle

Excludes *suffocation by plastic bag (E913.1)*

E913.1 By plastic bag

E913.2 Due to lack of air (in closed place)
Accidentally closed up in refrigerator or other airtight enclosed space
Diving with insufficient air supply

Excludes *suffocation by plastic bag (E913.1)*

E913.3 By falling earth or other substance
Cave-in NOS

Excludes *cave-in caused by cataclysmic earth surface movements and eruptions (E909.8)*
struck by cave-in without asphyxiation or suffocation (E916)

❑ **E913.8 Other specified means**
Accidental hanging, except in bed or cradle

❑ **E913.9 Unspecified means**
Asphyxia, mechanical NOS
Strangulation NOS
Suffocation NOS

E914 Foreign body accidentally entering eye and adnexa

Excludes *corrosive liquid (E924.1)*

❑ **E915 Foreign body accidentally entering other orifice**

Excludes *aspiration and inhalation of foreign body, any, (into respiratory tract) NOS (E911-E912)*

OTHER ACCIDENTS (E916-E928)

E916 Struck accidentally by falling object
Collapse of building, except on fire
Falling:
rock
snowslide NOS
stone
tree
Object falling from:
machine, not in operation
stationary vehicle

Code first: collapse of building on fire (E890.0-E891.9)
falling object in:
cataclysm (E908-E909)
machinery accidents (E919.0-E919.9)
transport accidents (E800.0-E845.9)
vehicle accidents not elsewhere classifiable (E846-E848)
object set in motion by:
explosion (E921.0-E921.9, E923.0-E923.9)
firearm (E922.0-E922.9)
projected object (E917.0-E917.9)

● **E917 Striking against or struck accidentally by objects or persons**

Includes: bumping into or against
object (moving) (projected) (stationary)
pedestrian conveyance
person
colliding with
object (moving) (projected) (stationary)
pedestrian conveyance
person
kicking against
object (moving) (projected) (stationary)
pedestrian conveyance
person
stepping on
object (moving) (projected) (stationary)
pedestrian conveyance
person
struck by
object (moving) (projected) (stationary)
pedestrian conveyance
person

Excludes *fall from:*
collision with another person, except when caused by a crowd (E886.0-E886.9)
stumbling over object (E885.9)
fall resulting in striking against object (E888.0, E888.1)
injury caused by:
assault (E960.0-E960.1, E967.0-E967.9)
cutting or piercing instrument (E920.0-E920.9)
explosion (E921.0-E921.9, E923.0-E923.9)
firearm (E922.0-E922.9)
machinery (E919.0-E919.9)
transport vehicle (E800.0-E845.9)
vehicle not elsewhere classifiable (E846-E848)

E917.0 In sports without subsequent fall
Kicked or stepped on during game (football) (rugby)
Struck by hit or thrown ball
Struck by hockey stick or puck

E917.1 Caused by a crowd, by collective fear or panic without subsequent fall
Crushed by crowd or human stampede
Pushed by crowd or human stampede
Stepped on by crowd or human stampede

E917.2 In running water without subsequent fall

Excludes *drowning or submersion (E910.0-E910.9) that in sports (E917.0, E917.5)*

E917.3 Furniture without subsequent fall

Excludes *fall from furniture (E884.2, E884.4–E884.5)*

E917.4 Other stationary object without subsequent fall
Bath tub
Fence
Lamp-post

E917.5 Object in sports with subsequent fall
Knocked down while boxing

E917.6 Caused by a crowd, by collective fear or panic with subsequent fall

E917.7 Furniture with subsequent fall

Excludes *fall from furniture (E884.2, E884.4–E884.5)*

❑ **E917.8 Other stationary object with subsequent fall**
Bath tub
Fence
Lamp-post

❑ **E917.9 Other striking against with or without subsequent fall**

E918 Caught accidentally in or between objects
Caught, crushed, jammed, or pinched in or between moving or stationary objects, such as:
escalator
folding object
hand tools, appliances, or implements
sliding door and door frame
under packing crate
washing machine wringer

Excludes *injury caused by:*
cutting or piercing instrument (E920.0-E920.9)
machinery (E919.0-E919.9)
transport vehicle (E800.0-E845.9)
vehicle not elsewhere classifiable (E846-E848)
struck accidentally by:
falling object (E916)
object (moving) (projected) (E917.0-E917.9)

● **E919 Accidents caused by machinery**

Includes: burned by machinery (accident)
caught in (moving parts of) machinery (accident)
collapse of machinery (accident)
crushed by machinery (accident)
cut or pierced by machinery (accident)
drowning or submersion caused by machinery (accident)
explosion of, on, in machinery (accident)
fall from or into moving part of machinery (accident)
fire starting in or on machinery (accident)
mechanical suffocation caused by machinery (accident)
object falling from, on, in motion by machinery (accident)
overturning of machinery (accident)
pinned under machinery (accident)
run over by machinery (accident)
struck by machinery (accident)
thrown from machinery (accident)
caught between machinery and other object
machinery accident NOS

Excludes *accidents involving machinery, not in operation (E884.9, E916-E918)*
injury caused by:
electric current in connection with machinery (E925.0-E925.9)
escalator (E880.0, E918)
explosion of pressure vessel in connection with machinery (E921.0-E921.9)
moving sidewalk (E885.9)
powered hand tools, appliances, and implements (E916-E918, E920.0-E921.9, E923.0-E926.9)
transport vehicle accidents involving machinery (E800.0-E848.9)
poisoning by carbon monoxide generated by machine (E868.8)

E919.0 Agricultural machines
Animal-powered agricultural machine
Combine
Derrick, hay
Farm machinery NOS
Farm tractor
Harvester
Hay mower or rake
Reaper
Thresher

Excludes *that in transport under own power on the highway (E810.0-E819.9)*
that being towed by another vehicle on the highway (E810.0-E819.9, E827.0-E827.9, E829.0-E829.9)
that involved in accident classifiable to E820-E829 (E820.0-E829.9)

E919.1 Mining and earth-drilling machinery
Bore or drill (land) (seabed)
Shaft hoist
Shaft lift
Under-cutter

Excludes *coal car, tram, truck, and tub in mine (E846)*

E919.2 Lifting machines and appliances
Chain hoist except in agricultural or mining operations
Crane except in agricultural or mining operations
Derrick except in agricultural or mining operations
Elevator (building) (grain) except in agricultural or mining operations
Forklift truck except in agricultural or mining operations
Lift except in agricultural or mining operations
Pulley block except in agricultural or mining operations
Winch except in agricultural or mining operations

Excludes *that being towed by another vehicle on the highway (E810.0-E819.9, E827.0-E827.9, E829.0-E829.9)*
that in transport under own power on the highway (E810.0-E819.9)
that involved in accident classifiable to E820-E829 (E820.0-E829.9)

E919.3 Metalworking machines
Abrasive wheel
Forging machine
Lathe
Mechanical shears
Metal:
drilling machine
Metal:
milling machine
power press
rolling-mill
sawing machine

E919.4 Woodworking and forming machines
Band saw
Bench saw
Circular saw
Molding machine
Overhead plane
Powered saw
Radial saw
Sander

Excludes *hand saw (E920.1)*

E919.5 Prime movers, except electrical motors
Gas turbine
Internal combustion engine
Steam engine
Water driven turbine

Excludes *that being towed by other vehicle on the highway (E810.0-E819.9, E827.0-E827.9, E829.0-E829.9)*
that in transport under own power on the highway (E810.0-E819.9)

E919.6 Transmission machinery
Transmission:
belt
cable
chain
gear
Transmission:
pinion
pulley
shaft

E919.7 Earth moving, scraping, and other excavating machines
Bulldozer
Road scraper
Steam shovel

Excludes *that being towed by other vehicle on the highway (E810.0-E819.9)*
that in transport under own power on the highway (E810.0-E819.9)

❑ **E919.8 Other specified machinery**
Machines for manufacture of:
clothing
foodstuffs and beverages
paper
Printing machine
Recreational machinery
Spinning, weaving, and textile machines

❑ **E919.9 Unspecified machinery**

● **E920 Accidents caused by cutting and piercing instruments or objects**

Includes: accidental injury (by) object:
edged
pointed
sharp

E920.0 Powered lawn mower

❑ **E920.1 Other powered hand tools**
Any powered hand tool [compressed air] [electric] [explosive cartridge] [hydraulic power], such as:
drill
hand saw
hedge clipper
rivet gun
snow blower
staple gun

Excludes *band saw (E919.4)*
bench saw (E919.4)

E920.2 Powered household appliances and implements
Blender
Electric:
beater or mixer
can opener
fan
knife
sewing machine
Garbage disposal appliance

E920.3 Knives, swords, and daggers

❑ **E920.4 Other hand tools and implements**
Axe
Can opener NOS
Chisel
Fork
Hand saw
Hoe
Ice pick
Needle (sewing)
Paper cutter
Pitchfork
Rake
Scissors
Screwdriver
Sewing machine, not powered
Shovel

E920.5 Hypodermic needle
Contaminated needle
Needle stick

❑ **E920.8 Other specified cutting and piercing instruments or objects**
Arrow
Broken glass
Dart
Edge of stiff paper
Lathe turnings
Nail
Plant thorn
Splinter
Tin can lid

Excludes *animal spines or quills (E906.8)*
flying glass due to explosion (E921.0-E923.9)

❑ **E920.9 Unspecified cutting and piercing instrument or object**

● **E921 Accident caused by explosion of pressure vessel**

Includes: accidental explosion of pressure vessels, whether or not part of machinery

Excludes *explosion of pressure vessel on transport vehicle (E800.0-E845.9)*

E921.0 Boilers

E921.1 Gas cylinders
Air tank
Pressure gas tank

❑ **E921.8 Other specified pressure vessels**
Aerosol can
Automobile tire
Pressure cooker

❑ **E921.9 Unspecified pressure vessel**

● **E922 Accident caused by firearm and air gun missile**

E922.0 Handgun
Pistol
Revolver

Excludes *Very pistol (E922.8)*

E922.1 Shotgun (automatic)

E922.2 Hunting rifle

E922.3 Military firearms
Army rifle
Machine gun

E922.4 Air gun
BB gun
Pellet gun

E922.5 Paintball gun

❑ **E922.8 Other specified firearm missile**
Very pistol [flare]

❑ **E922.9 Unspecified firearm missile**
Gunshot wound NOS
Shot NOS

● **E923 Accident caused by explosive material**

Includes: flash burns and other injuries resulting from explosion of explosive material
ignition of highly explosive material with explosion

Excludes *explosion:*
in or on machinery (E919.0-E919.9)
on any transport vehicle, except stationary motor vehicle (E800.0-E848)
with conflagration (E890.0, E891.0, E892)
secondary fires resulting from explosion (E890.0-E899)

E923.0 Fireworks

E923.1 Blasting materials
Blasting cap
Detonator
Dynamite
Explosive [any] used in blasting operations

E923.2 Explosive gases
Acetylene
Butane
Coal gas
Explosion in mine NOS
Fire damp
Gasoline fumes
Methane
Propane

❑ **E923.8 Other explosive materials**
Bomb
Explosive missile
Grenade
Mine
Shell
Torpedo
Explosion in munitions:
dump
factory

❑ **E923.9 Unspecified explosive material**
Explosion NOS

● **E924 Accident caused by hot substance or object, caustic or corrosive material, and steam**

Excludes *burning NOS (E899)*
chemical burn resulting from swallowing a corrosive substance (E860.0-E864.4)
fire caused by these substances and objects (E890.0-E894)
radiation burns (E926.0-E926.9)
therapeutic misadventures (E870.0-E876.9)

E924.0 Hot liquids and vapors, including steam
Burning or scalding by:
boiling water
hot or boiling liquids not primarily caustic or corrosive
liquid metal
steam
other hot vapor

Excludes *hot (boiling) tap water (E924.2)*

E924.1 Caustic and corrosive substances
Burning by:
acid [any kind]
ammonia
caustic oven cleaner or other substance
corrosive substance
lye
vitriol

E924.2 Hot (boiling) tap water

❑ **E924.8 Other**
Burning by:
heat from electric heating appliance
hot object NOS
light bulb
steam pipe

❑ **E924.9 Unspecified**

● **E925 Accident caused by electric current**

Includes: electric current from exposed wire, faulty appliance, high voltage cable, live rail, or open electric socket as the cause of:
burn
cardiac fibrillation
convulsion
electric shock
electrocution
puncture wound
respiratory paralysis

Excludes *burn by heat from electrical appliance (E924.8)*
lightning (E907)

E925.0 Domestic wiring and appliances

E925.1 Electric power generating plants, distribution stations, transmission lines
Broken power line

E925.2 Industrial wiring, appliances, and electrical machinery
Conductors
Control apparatus
Electrical equipment and machinery
Transformers

❑ **E925.8 Other electric current**
Wiring and appliances in or on:
farm [not farmhouse]
outdoors
public building
residential institutions
schools

❑ **E925.9 Unspecified electric current**
Burns or other injury from electric current NOS
Electric shock NOS
Electrocution NOS

● **E926 Exposure to radiation**

Excludes *abnormal reaction to or complication of treatment without mention of misadventure (E879.2)*
atomic power plant malfunction in water transport (E838.0-E838.9)
misadventure to patient in surgical and medical procedures (E873.2-E873.3)
use of radiation in war operations (E996-E997.9)

E926.0 Radiofrequency radiation
Overexposure to:
microwave radiation from:
high-powered radio and television transmitters
industrial radiofrequency induction heaters
radar installations
radar radiation from:
high-powered radio and television transmitters
industrial radiofrequency induction heaters
radar installations
radiofrequency from:
high-powered radio and television transmitters
industrial radiofrequency induction heaters
radar installations
radiofrequency radiation [any] from:
high-powered radio and television transmitters
industrial radiofrequency induction heaters
radar installations

E926.1 Infra-red heaters and lamps
Exposure to infra-red radiation from heaters and lamps as the cause of:
blistering
burning
charring
inflammatory change

Excludes *physical contact with heater or lamp (E924.8)*

E926.2 Visible and ultraviolet light sources
Arc lamps
Black light sources
Electrical welding arc
Oxygas welding torch
Sun rays
Tanning bed

Excludes *excessive heat from these sources (E900.1-E900.9)*

E926.3 X-rays and other electromagnetic ionizing radiation
Gamma rays
X-rays (hard) (soft)

E926.4 Lasers

E926.5 Radioactive isotopes
Radiobiologicals
Radiopharmaceuticals

❑ **E926.8 Other specified radiation**
Artificially accelerated beams of ionized particles generated by:
betatrons
synchrotrons

❑ **E926.9 Unspecified radiation**
Radiation NOS

E927 Overexertion and strenuous movements
Excessive physical exercise
Overexertion (from):
lifting
pulling
pushing
Strenuous movements in:
recreational activities
other activities

● **E928 Other and unspecified environmental and accidental causes**

E928.0 Prolonged stay in weightless environment
Weightlessness in spacecraft (simulator)

E928.1 Exposure to noise
Noise (pollution)
Sound waves
Supersonic waves

E928.2 Vibration

E928.3 Human bite

E928.4 External constriction caused by hair

E928.5 External constriction caused by other object

❑ **E928.8 Other**

❑ **E928.9 Unspecified accident**
Accident NOS stated as accidentally inflicted
Blow NOS stated as accidentally inflicted
Casualty (not due to war) stated as accidentally inflicted
Decapitation stated as accidentally inflicted
Injury [any part of body, or unspecified] stated as accidentally inflicted, but not otherwise specified
Killed stated as accidentally inflicted, but not otherwise specified
Knocked down stated as accidentally inflicted, but not otherwise specified
Mangled stated as accidentally inflicted, but not otherwise specified
Wound stated as accidentally inflicted, but not otherwise specified

Excludes *fracture, cause unspecified (E887)*
injuries undetermined whether accidentally or purposely inflicted (E980.0-E989)

LATE EFFECTS OF ACCIDENTAL INJURY (E929)

Note: This category is to be used to indicate accidental injury as the cause of death or disability from late effects, which are themselves classifiable elsewhere. The "late effects" include conditions reported as such or as sequelae, which may occur at any time after the acute accidental injury.

● **E929 Late effects of accidental injury**

Excludes *late effects of:*
surgical and medical procedures (E870.0-E879.9)
therapeutic use of drugs and medicines (E930.0-E949.9)

E929.0 Late effects of motor vehicle accident
Late effects of accidents classifiable to E810-E825

❑ **E929.1 Late effects of other transport accident**
Late effects of accidents classifiable to E800-E807, E826-E838, E840-E848

E929.2 Late effects of accidental poisoning
Late effects of accidents classifiable to E850-E858, E860-E869

E929.3 Late effects of accidental fall
Late effects of accidents classifiable to E880-E888

E929.4 Late effects of accident caused by fire
Late effects of accidents classifiable to E890-E899

E929.5 Late effects of accident due to natural and environmental factors
Late effects of accidents classifiable to E900-E909

❑ **E929.8 Late effects of other accidents**
Late effects of accidents classifiable to E910-E928.8

❑ **E929.9 Late effects of unspecified accident**
Late effects of accidents classifiable to E928.9

DRUGS, MEDICINAL AND BIOLOGICAL SUBSTANCES CAUSING ADVERSE EFFECTS IN THERAPEUTIC USE (E930-E949)

Includes: correct drug properly administered in therapeutic or prophylactic dosage, as the cause of any adverse effect including allergic or hypersensitivity reactions

Excludes *accidental overdose of drug and wrong drug given or taken in error (E850.0-E858.9)*
accidents in the technique of administration of drug or biological substance such as accidental puncture during injection, or contamination of drug (E870.0-E876.9)
administration with suicidal or homicidal intent or intent to harm, or in circumstances classifiable to E980-E989 (E950.0-E950.5, E962.0, E980.0-E980.5)
See Alphabetic Index for more complete list of specific drugs to be classified under the fourth-digit subdivisions. The American Hospital Formulary numbers can be used to classify new drugs listed by the American Hospital Formulary Service (AHFS). See appendix C.

● **E930 Antibiotics**

Excludes *that used as eye, ear, nose, and throat [ENT], and local anti-infectives (E946.0-E946.9)*

E930.0 Penicillins
Natural
Synthetic
Semisynthetic, such as:
ampicillin
cloxacillin
nafcillin
oxacillin

E930.1 Antifungal antibiotics
Amphotericin B
Griseofulvin
Hachimycin [trichomycin]
Nystatin

E930.2 Chloramphenicol group
Chloramphenicol
Thiamphenicol

E930.3 Erythromycin and other macrolides
Oleandomycin
Spiramycin

E930.4 Tetracycline group
Doxycycline
Minocycline
Oxytetracycline

E930.5 Cephalosporin group
Cephalexin
Cephaloglycin
Cephaloridine
Cephalothin

E930.6 Antimycobacterial antibiotics
Cycloserine
Kanamycin
Rifampin
Streptomycin

E930.7 Antineoplastic antibiotics
Actinomycins, such as:
Bleomycin
Cactinomycin
Dactinomycin
Daunorubicin
Mitomycin

Excludes *other antineoplastic drugs (E933.1)*

❑ E930.8 **Other specified antibiotics**

❑ E930.9 **Unspecified antibiotic**

● E931 **Other anti-infectives**

Excludes *ENT, and local anti-infectives (E946.0-E946.9)*

E931.0 **Sulfonamides**
Sulfadiazine
Sulfafurazole
Sulfamethoxazole

E931.1 **Arsenical anti-infectives**

E931.2 **Heavy metal anti-infectives**
Compounds of:
antimony
bismuth
lead
mercury

Excludes *mercurial diuretics (E944.0)*

E931.3 **Quinoline and hydroxyquinoline derivatives**
Chiniofon
Diiodohydroxyquin

Excludes *antimalarial drugs (E931.4)*

E931.4 **Antimalarials and drugs acting on other blood protozoa**
Chloroquine phosphate
Cycloguanil
Primaquine
Proguanil [chloroguanide]
Pyrimethamine
Quinine (sulphate)

❑ E931.5 **Other antiprotozoal drugs**
Emetine

E931.6 **Anthelmintics**
Hexylresorcinol
Male fern oleoresin
Piperazine
Thiabendazole

E931.7 **Antiviral drugs**
Methisazone

Excludes *amantadine (E936.4)*
cytarabine (E933.1)
idoxuridine (E946.5)

❑ E931.8 **Other antimycobacterial drugs**
Ethambutol
Ethionamide
Isoniazid
Para-aminosalicylic acid derivatives
Sulfones

❑ E931.9 **Other and unspecified anti-infectives**
Flucytosine
Nitrofuran derivatives

● E932 **Hormones and synthetic substitutes**

E932.0 **Adrenal cortical steroids**
Cortisone derivatives
Desoxycorticosterone derivatives
Fluorinated corticosteroids

E932.1 **Androgens and anabolic congeners**
Nandrolone phenpropionate
Oxymetholone
Testosterone and preparations

E932.2 **Ovarian hormones and synthetic substitutes**
Contraceptives, oral
Estrogens
Estrogens and progestogens combined
Progestogens

E932.3 **Insulins and antidiabetic agents**
Acetohexamide
Biguanide derivatives, oral
Chlorpropamide
Glucagon
Insulin
Phenformin
Sulfonylurea derivatives, oral
Tolbutamide

Excludes *adverse effect of insulin administered for shock therapy (E879.3)*

E932.4 **Anterior pituitary hormones**
Corticotropin
Gonadotropin
Somatotropin [growth hormone]

E932.5 **Posterior pituitary hormones**
Vasopressin

Excludes *oxytocic agents (E945.0)*

E932.6 **Parathyroid and parathyroid derivatives**

E932.7 **Thyroid and thyroid derivatives**
Dextrothyroxine
Levothyroxine sodium
Liothyronine
Thyroglobulin

E932.8 **Antithyroid agents**
Iodides
Thiouracil
Thiourea

❑ E932.9 **Other and unspecified hormones and synthetic substitutes**

● E933 **Primarily systemic agents**

E933.0 **Antiallergic and antiemetic drugs**
Antihistamines
Chlorpheniramine
Diphenhydramine
Diphenylpyraline
Thonzylamine
Tripelennamine

Excludes *phenothiazine-based tranquilizers (E939.1)*

E933.1 **Antineoplastic and immunosuppressive drugs**
Azathioprine
Busulfan
Chlorambucil
Cyclophosphamide
Cytarabine
Fluorouracil
Mechlorethamine hydrochloride
Mercaptopurine
Triethylenethiophosphoramide [thio-TEPA]

Excludes *antineoplastic antibiotics (E930.7)*

E933.2 **Acidifying agents**

E933.3 **Alkalizing agents**

E933.4 **Enzymes, not elsewhere classified**
Penicillinase

E933.5 **Vitamins, not elsewhere classified**
Vitamin A
Vitamin D

Excludes *nicotinic acid (E942.2)*
vitamin K (E934.3)

❑ E933.8 **Other systemic agents, not elsewhere classified**
Heavy metal antagonists

❑ E933.9 **Unspecified systemic agent**

● E934 **Agents primarily affecting blood constituents**

E934.0 **Iron and its compounds**
Ferric salts
Ferrous sulphate and other ferrous salts

❑ **E934.1 Liver preparations and other antianemic agents**
Folic acid

E934.2 Anticoagulants
Coumarin
Heparin
Phenindione
Prothrombin synthesis inhibitor
Warfarin sodium

E934.3 Vitamin K [phytonadione]

E934.4 Fibrinolysis-affecting drugs
Aminocaproic acid
Streptodornase
Streptokinase
Urokinase

❑ **E934.5 Anticoagulant antagonists and other coagulants**
Hexadimethrine bromide
Protamine sulfate

E934.6 Gamma globulin

E934.7 Natural blood and blood products
Blood plasma
Human fibrinogen
Packed red cells
Whole blood

❑ **E934.8 Other agents affecting blood constituents**
Macromolecular blood substitutes

❑ **E934.9 Unspecified agent affecting blood constituents**

● **E935 Analgesics, antipyretics, and antirheumatics**

E935.0 Heroin
Diacetylmorphine

E935.1 Methadone

❑ **E935.2 Other opiates and related narcotics**
Codeine [methylmorphine]
Morphine
Opium (alkaloids)
Meperidine [pethidine]

E935.3 Salicylates
Acetylsalicylic acid [aspirin]
Amino derivatives of salicylic acid
Salicylic acid salts

E935.4 Aromatic analgesics, not elsewhere classified
Acetanilid
Paracetamol [acetaminophen]
Phenacetin [acetophenetidin]

E935.5 Pyrazole derivatives
Aminophenazone [aminopyrine]
Phenylbutazone

E935.6 Antirheumatics [antiphlogistics]
Gold salts
Indomethacin

Excludes *salicylates (E935.3)*
steroids (E932.0)

❑ **E935.7 Other non-narcotic analgesics**
Pyrabital

❑ **E935.8 Other specified analgesics and antipyretics**
Pentazocine

❑ **E935.9 Unspecified analgesic and antipyretic**

● **E936 Anticonvulsants and anti-Parkinsonism drugs**

E936.0 Oxazolidine derivatives
Paramethadione
Trimethadione

E936.1 Hydantoin derivatives
Phenytoin

E936.2 Succinimides
Ethosuximide
Phensuximide

❑ **E936.3 Other and unspecified anticonvulsants**
Beclamide
Primidone

E936.4 Anti-Parkinsonism drugs
Amantadine
Ethopropazine [profenamine]
Levodopa [L-dopa]

● **E937 Sedatives and hypnotics**

E937.0 Barbiturates
Amobarbital [amylobarbitone]
Barbital [barbitone]
Butabarbital [butabarbitone]
Pentobarbital [pentobarbitone]
Phenobarbital [phenobarbitone]
Secobarbital [quinalbarbitone]

Excludes *thiobarbiturates (E938.3)*

E937.1 Chloral hydrate group

E937.2 Paraldehyde

E937.3 Bromine compounds
Bromide
Carbromal (derivatives)

E937.4 Methaqualone compounds

E937.5 Glutethimide group

E937.6 Mixed sedatives, not elsewhere classified

❑ **E937.8 Other sedatives and hypnotics**

❑ **E937.9 Unspecified**
Sleeping:
drug NOS
pill NOS
tablet NOS

● **E938 Other central nervous system depressants and anesthetics**

E938.0 Central nervous system muscle-tone depressants
Chlorphenesin (carbamate)
Mephenesin
Methocarbamol

E938.1 Halothane

❑ **E938.2 Other gaseous anesthetics**
Ether
Halogenated hydrocarbon derivatives, except halothane
Nitrous oxide

E938.3 Intravenous anesthetics
Ketamine
Methohexital [methohexitone]
Thiobarbiturates, such as thiopental sodium

❑ **E938.4 Other and unspecified general anesthetics**

E938.5 Surface and infiltration anesthetics
Cocaine
Lidocaine [lignocaine]
Procaine
Tetracaine

E938.6 Peripheral nerve- and plexus-blocking anesthetics

E938.7 Spinal anesthetics

❑ **E938.9 Other and unspecified local anesthetics**

● **E939 Psychotropic agents**

E939.0 Antidepressants
Amitriptyline
Imipramine
Monoamine oxidase [MAO] inhibitors

E939.1 Phenothiazine-based tranquilizers
Chlorpromazine
Fluphenazine
Phenothiazine
Prochlorperazine
Promazine

E939.2 Butyrophenone-based tranquilizers
Haloperidol
Spiperone
Trifluperidol

❑ **E939.3 Other antipsychotics, neuroleptics, and major tranquilizers**

E939.4 Benzodiazepine-based tranquilizers
Chlordiazepoxide
Diazepam
Flurazepam
Lorazepam
Medazepam
Nitrazepam

❑ **E939.5 Other tranquilizers**
Hydroxyzine
Meprobamate

E939.6 Psychodysleptics [hallucinogens]
Cannabis (derivatives)
Lysergide [LSD]
Marihuana (derivatives)
Mescaline
Psilocin
Psilocybin

E939.7 Psychostimulants
Amphetamine
Caffeine

Excludes *central appetite depressants (E947.0)*

❑ **E939.8 Other psychotropic agents**

❑ **E939.9 Unspecified psychotropic agent**

● **E940 Central nervous system stimulants**

E940.0 Analeptics
Lobeline
Nikethamide

E940.1 Opiate antagonists
Levallorphan
Nalorphine
Naloxone

❑ **E940.8 Other specified central nervous system stimulants**

❑ **E940.9 Unspecified central nervous system stimulant**

● **E941 Drugs primarily affecting the autonomic nervous system**

E941.0 Parasympathomimetics [cholinergics]
Acetylcholine
Anticholinesterase:
  organophosphorus
  reversible
Pilocarpine

E941.1 Parasympatholytics [anticholinergics and antimuscarinics] and spasmolytics
Atropine
Homatropine
Hyoscine [scopolamine]
Quaternary ammonium derivatives

Excludes *papaverine (E942.5)*

E941.2 Sympathomimetics [adrenergics]
Epinephrine [adrenalin]
Levarterenol [noradrenalin]

E941.3 Sympatholytics [antiadrenergics]
Phenoxybenzamine
Tolazoline hydrochloride

❑ **E941.9 Unspecified drug primarily affecting the autonomic nervous system**

● **E942 Agents primarily affecting the cardiovascular system**

E942.0 Cardiac rhythm regulators
Practolol
Procainamide
Propranolol
Quinidine

E942.1 Cardiotonic glycosides and drugs of similar action
Digitalis glycosides
Digoxin
Strophanthins

E942.2 Antilipemic and antiarteriosclerotic drugs
Cholestyramine
Clofibrate
Nicotinic acid derivatives
Sitosterols

Excludes *dextrothyroxine (E932.7)*

E942.3 Ganglion-blocking agents
Pentamethonium bromide

E942.4 Coronary vasodilators
Dipyridamole
Nitrates [nitroglycerin]
Nitrites
Prenylamine

❑ **E942.5 Other vasodilators**
Cyclandelate
Diazoxide
Hydralazine
Papaverine

❑ **E942.6 Other antihypertensive agents**
Clonidine
Guanethidine
Rauwolfia alkaloids
Reserpine

E942.7 Antivaricose drugs, including sclerosing agents
Monoethanolamine
Zinc salts

E942.8 Capillary-active drugs
Adrenochrome derivatives
Bioflavonoids
Metaraminol

❑ **E942.9 Other and unspecified agents primarily affecting the cardiovascular system**

● **E943 Agents primarily affecting gastrointestinal system**

E943.0 Antacids and antigastric secretion drugs
Aluminum hydroxide
Magnesium trisilicate

E943.1 Irritant cathartics
Bisacodyl
Castor oil
Phenolphthalein

E943.2 Emollient cathartics
Sodium dioctyl sulfosuccinate

❑ **E943.3 Other cathartics, including intestinal atonia drugs**
Magnesium sulfate

E943.4 Digestants
Pancreatin
Papain
Pepsin

E943.5 Antidiarrheal drugs
Bismuth subcarbonate
Kaolin
Pectin

Excludes *anti-infectives (E930.0-E931.9)*

E943.6 Emetics

❑ **E943.8 Other specified agents primarily affecting the gastrointestinal system**

❑ **E943.9 Unspecified agent primarily affecting the gastrointestinal system**

● **E944 Water, mineral, and uric acid metabolism drugs**

E944.0 Mercurial diuretics
Chlormerodrin
Mercaptomerin
Mercurophylline
Mersalyl

E944.1 Purine derivative diuretics
Theobromine
Theophylline

Excludes *aminophylline [theophylline ethylenediamine] (E945.7)*

E944.2 Carbonic acid anhydrase inhibitors
Acetazolamide

E944.3 Saluretics
Benzothiadiazides
Chlorothiazide group

❑ **E944.4 Other diuretics**
Ethacrynic acid
Furosemide

E944.5 Electrolytic, caloric, and water-balance agents

❑ **E944.6 Other mineral salts, not elsewhere classified**

E944.7 Uric acid metabolism drugs
Cinchophen and congeners
Colchicine
Phenoquin
Probenecid

● **E945 Agents primarily acting on the smooth and skeletal muscles and respiratory system**

E945.0 Oxytocic agents
Ergot alkaloids
Prostaglandins

E945.1 Smooth muscle relaxants
Adiphenine
Metaproterenol [orciprenaline]

Excludes *papaverine (E942.5)*

E945.2 Skeletal muscle relaxants
Alcuronium chloride
Suxamethonium chloride

❑ **E945.3 Other and unspecified drugs acting on muscles**

E945.4 Antitussives
Dextromethorphan
Pipazethate hydrochloride

E945.5 Expectorants
Acetylcysteine
Cocillana
Guaifenesin [glyceryl guaiacolate]
Ipecacuanha
Terpin hydrate

E945.6 Anti-common cold drugs

E945.7 Antiasthmatics
Aminophylline [theophylline ethylenediamine]

❑ **E945.8 Other and unspecified respiratory drugs**

● **E946 Agents primarily affecting skin and mucous membrane, ophthalmological, otorhinolaryngological, and dental drugs**

E946.0 Local anti-infectives and anti-inflammatory drugs

E946.1 Antipruritics

E946.2 Local astringents and local detergents

E946.3 Emollients, demulcents, and protectants

E946.4 Keratolytics, keratoplastics, other hair treatment drugs and preparations

E946.5 Eye anti-infectives and other eye drugs
Idoxuridine

E946.6 Anti-infectives and other drugs and preparations for ear, nose, and throat

E946.7 Dental drugs topically applied

❑ **E946.8 Other agents primarily affecting skin and mucous membrane**
Spermicides

❑ **E946.9 Unspecified agent primarily affecting skin and mucous membrane**

● **E947 Other and unspecified drugs and medicinal substances**

E947.0 Dietetics

E947.1 Lipotropic drugs

E947.2 Antidotes and chelating agents, not elsewhere classified

E947.3 Alcohol deterrents

E947.4 Pharmaceutical excipients

❑ **E947.8 Other drugs and medicinal substances**
Contrast media used for diagnostic x-ray procedures
Diagnostic agents and kits

❑ **E947.9 Unspecified drug or medicinal substance**

● **E948 Bacterial vaccines**

E948.0 BCG vaccine

E948.1 Typhoid and paratyphoid

E948.2 Cholera

E948.3 Plague

E948.4 Tetanus

E948.5 Diphtheria

E948.6 Pertussis vaccine, including combinations with a pertussis component

❑ **E948.8 Other and unspecified bacterial vaccines**

E948.9 Mixed bacterial vaccines, except combinations with a pertussis component

● **E949 Other vaccines and biological substances**

Excludes *gamma globulin (E934.6)*

E949.0 Smallpox vaccine

E949.1 Rabies vaccine

E949.2 Typhus vaccine

E949.3 Yellow fever vaccine

E949.4 Measles vaccine

E949.5 Poliomyelitis vaccine

❑ **E949.6 Other and unspecified viral and rickettsial vaccines**
Mumps vaccine

E949.7 Mixed viral-rickettsial and bacterial vaccines, except combinations with a pertussis component

Excludes *combinations with a pertussis component (E948.6)*

❑ **E949.9 Other and unspecified vaccines and biological substances**

SUICIDE AND SELF-INFLICTED INJURY (E950-E959)

Includes: injuries in suicide and attempted suicide
self-inflicted injuries specified as intentional

● **E950 Suicide and self-inflicted poisoning by solid or liquid substances**

E950.0 Analgesics, antipyretics, and antirheumatics

E950.1 Barbiturates

❑ **E950.2 Other sedatives and hypnotics**

E950.3 Tranquilizers and other psychotropic agents

❑ E950.4 **Other specified drugs and medicinal substances**

❑ E950.5 **Unspecified drug or medicinal substance**

E950.6 **Agricultural and horticultural chemical and pharmaceutical preparations other than plant foods and fertilizers**

E950.7 **Corrosive and caustic substances**
Suicide and self-inflicted poisoning by substances classifiable to E864

E950.8 **Arsenic and its compounds**

❑ E950.9 **Other and unspecified solid and liquid substances**

● E951 **Suicide and self-inflicted poisoning by gases in domestic use**

E951.0 **Gas distributed by pipeline**

E951.1 **Liquefied petroleum gas distributed in mobile containers**

❑ E951.8 **Other utility gas**

● E952 **Suicide and self-inflicted poisoning by other gases and vapors**

E952.0 **Motor vehicle exhaust gas**

❑ E952.1 **Other carbon monoxide**

❑ E952.8 **Other specified gases and vapors**

❑ E952.9 **Unspecified gases and vapors**

● E953 **Suicide and self-inflicted injury by hanging, strangulation, and suffocation**

E953.0 **Hanging**

E953.1 **Suffocation by plastic bag**

❑ E953.8 **Other specified means**

❑ E953.9 **Unspecified means**

E954 **Suicide and self-inflicted injury by submersion [drowning]**

● E955 **Suicide and self-inflicted injury by firearms, air guns, and explosives**

E955.0 **Handgun**

E955.1 **Shotgun**

E955.2 **Hunting rifle**

E955.3 **Military firearms**

❑ E955.4 **Other and unspecified firearm**
Gunshot NOS
Shot NOS

E955.5 **Explosives**

E955.6 **Air gun**
BB gun
Pellet gun

E955.7 **Paintball gun**

❑ E955.9 **Unspecified**

E956 **Suicide and self-inflicted injury by cutting and piercing instrument**

● E957 **Suicide and self-inflicted injuries by jumping from high place**

E957.0 **Residential premises**

❑ E957.1 **Other man-made structures**

E957.2 **Natural sites**

❑ E957.9 **Unspecified**

● E958 **Suicide and self-inflicted injury by other and unspecified means**

E958.0 **Jumping or lying before moving object**

E958.1 **Burns, fire**

E958.2 **Scald**

E958.3 **Extremes of cold**

E958.4 **Electrocution**

E958.5 **Crashing of motor vehicle**

E958.6 **Crashing of aircraft**

E958.7 **Caustic substances, except poisoning**

Excludes *poisoning by caustic substance (E950.7)*

❑ E958.8 **Other specified means**

❑ E958.9 **Unspecified means**

E959 **Late effects of self-inflicted injury**

Note: This category is to be used to indicate circumstances classifiable to E950-E958 as the cause of death or disability from late effects, which are themselves classifiable elsewhere. The "late effects" include conditions reported as such or as sequelae which may occur at any time after the attempted suicide or self-inflicted injury.

HOMICIDE AND INJURY PURPOSELY INFLICTED BY OTHER PERSONS (E960-E969)

Includes: injuries inflicted by another person with intent to injure or kill, by any means

Excludes *injuries due to:*
legal intervention (E970-E978)
operations of war (E990-E999)
terrorism (E979)

● E960 **Fight, brawl, rape**

E960.0 **Unarmed fight or brawl**
Beatings NOS
Brawl or fight with hands, fists, feet
Injured or killed in fight NOS

Excludes *homicidal:*
injury by weapons (E965.0-E966, E969)
strangulation (E963)
submersion (E964)

E960.1 **Rape**

E961 **Assault by corrosive or caustic substance, except poisoning**
Injury or death purposely caused by corrosive or caustic substance, such as:
acid [any]
corrosive substance
vitriol

Excludes *burns from hot liquid (E968.3)*
chemical burns from swallowing a corrosive substance (E962.0-E962.9)

● E962 **Assault by poisoning**

E962.0 **Drugs and medicinal substances**
Homicidal poisoning by any drug or medicinal substance

❑ E962.1 **Other solid and liquid substances**

❑ E962.2 **Other gases and vapors**

❑ E962.9 **Unspecified poisoning**

E963 **Assault by hanging and strangulation**
Homicidal (attempt):
garrotting or ligature
hanging
strangulation
suffocation

E964 **Assault by submersion [drowning]**

E965 Assault by firearms and explosives

E965.0 Handgun
Pistol
Revolver

E965.1 Shotgun

E965.2 Hunting rifle

E965.3 Military firearms

E965.4 Other and unspecified firearm

E965.5 Antipersonnel bomb

E965.6 Gasoline bomb

E965.7 Letter bomb

E965.8 Other specified explosive
Bomb NOS (placed in):
car
house
Dynamite

E965.9 Unspecified explosive

E966 Assault by cutting and piercing instrument
Assassination (attempt), homicide (attempt) by any instrument classifiable under E920
Homicidal:
cut any part of body
puncture any part of body
stab any part of body
Stabbed any part of body

E967 Perpetrator of child and adult abuse

Note: selection of the correct perpetrator code is based on the relationship between the perpetrator and the victim

E967.0 By father, stepfather, or boyfriend
Male partner of child's parent or guardian

E967.1 By other specified person

E967.2 By mother, stepmother, or girlfriend
Female partner of child's parent or guardian

E967.3 By spouse or partner
Abuse of spouse or partner by ex-spouse or ex-partner

E967.4 By child

E967.5 By sibling

E967.6 By grandparent

E967.7 By other relative

E967.8 By non-related caregiver

E967.9 By unspecified person

E968 Assault by other and unspecified means

E968.0 Fire
Arson
Homicidal burns NOS

Excludes *burns from hot liquid (E968.3)*

E968.1 Pushing from a high place

E968.2 Striking by blunt or thrown object

E968.3 Hot liquid
Homicidal burns by scalding

E968.4 Criminal neglect
Abandonment of child, infant, or other helpless person with intent to injure or kill

E968.5 Transport vehicle
Being struck by other vehicle or run down with intent to injure
Pushed in front of, thrown from, or dragged by moving vehicle with intent to injure

E968.6 Air gun
BB gun
Pellet gun

E968.7 Human bite

E968.8 Other specified means

E968.9 Unspecified means
Assassination (attempt) NOS
Homicidal (attempt):
injury NOS
wound NOS
Manslaughter (nonaccidental)
Murder (attempt) NOS
Violence, non-accidental

E969 Late effects of injury purposely inflicted by other person

Note: This category is to be used to indicate circumstances classifiable to E960-E968 as the cause of death or disability from late effects, which are themselves classifiable elsewhere. The "late effects" include conditions reported as such, or as sequelae which may occur at any time after the injury purposely inflicted by another person.

LEGAL INTERVENTION (E970-E978)

Includes: injuries inflicted by the police or other law-enforcing agents, including military on duty, in the course of arresting or attempting to arrest lawbreakers, suppressing disturbances, maintaining order, and other legal action
legal execution

Excludes *injuries caused by civil insurrections (E990.0-E999)*

E970 Injury due to legal intervention by firearms
Gunshot wound
Injury by:
machine gun
revolver
rifle pellet or rubber bullet
shot NOS

E971 Injury due to legal intervention by explosives
Injury by:
dynamite
explosive shell
grenade
motor bomb

E972 Injury due to legal intervention by gas
Asphyxiation by gas
Injury by tear gas
Poisoning by gas

E973 Injury due to legal intervention by blunt object
Hit, struck by:
baton (nightstick)
blunt object
stave

E974 Injury due to legal intervention by cutting and piercing instrument
Cut
Incised wound
Injured by bayonet
Stab wound

E975 Injury due to legal intervention by other specified means
Blow
Manhandling

E976 Injury due to legal intervention by unspecified means

E977 Late effects of injuries due to legal intervention

Note: This category is to be used to indicate circumstances classifiable to E970-E976 as the cause of death or disability from late effects, which are themselves classifiable elsewhere. The "late effects" include conditions reported as such, or as sequelae which may occur at any time after the injury due to legal intervention.

E978 Legal execution

All executions performed at the behest of the judiciary or ruling authority [whether permanent or temporary] as:
- asphyxiation by gas
- beheading, decapitation (by guillotine)
- capital punishment
- electrocution
- hanging
- poisoning
- shooting
- other specified means

TERRORISM (E979)

E979 Terrorism

Injuries resulting from the unlawful use of force or violence against persons or property to intimidate or coerce a Government, the civilian population, or any segment thereof, in furtherance of political or social objective

E979.0 Terrorism involving explosion of marine weapons
- Depth-charge
- Marine mine
  - mine NOS, at sea or in harbour
- Sea-based artillery shell
- Torpedo
- Underwater blast

E979.1 Terrorism involving destruction of aircraft
- Aircraft used as a weapon
- Aircraft:
  - burned
  - exploded
  - shot down
- Crushed by falling aircraft

E979.2 Terrorism involving other explosions and fragments
- Antipersonnel bomb (fragments)
- Blast NOS
- Explosion (of):
  - artillery shell
  - breech-block
  - cannon block
  - mortar bomb
  - munitions being used in terrorism
  - NOS
- Fragments from:
  - artillery shell
  - bomb
  - grenade
  - guided missile
  - land-mine
  - rocket
  - shell
  - shrapnel
- Mine NOS

E979.3 Terrorism involving fires, conflagration, and hot substances
- Burning building or structure
  - collapse of
  - fall from
  - hit by falling object in
  - jump from
- Conflagration NOS
- Fire (causing)
  - Asphyxia
  - Burns
  - NOS
  - Other injury
- Melting of fittings and furniture in burning
- Petrol bomb
- Smouldering building or structure

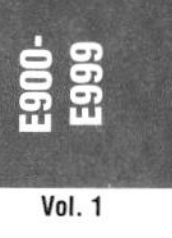
ICD-9-CM
E900-
E999
Vol. 1

E979.4 Terrorism involving firearms
- Bullet:
  - carbine
  - machine gun
  - pistol
  - rifle
  - rubber (rifle)
- Pellets (shotgun)

E979.5 Terrorism involving nuclear weapons
- Blast effects
- Exposure to ionizing radiation from nuclear weapon
- Fireball effects
- Heat from nuclear weapon
- Other direct and secondary effects of nuclear weapons

E979.6 Terrorism involving biological weapons
- Anthrax
- Cholera
- Smallpox

E979.7 Terrorism involving chemical weapons
- Gases, fumes, chemicals
- Hydrogen cyanide
- Phosgene
- Sarin

E979.8 Terrorism involving other means
- Drowning and submersion
- Lasers
- Piercing or stabbing instruments
- Terrorism NOS

E979.9 Terrorism secondary effects

Note: This code is for use to identify conditions occurring subsequent to a terrorist attack not those that are due to the initial terrorist act.

Excludes *late effect of terrorist attack (E999.1)*

INJURY UNDETERMINED WHETHER ACCIDENTALLY OR PURPOSELY INFLICTED (E980-E989)

Note: Categories E980-E989 are for use when it is unspecified or it cannot be determined whether the injuries are accidental (unintentional), suicide (attempted), or assault.

E980 Poisoning by solid or liquid substances, undetermined whether accidentally or purposely inflicted

E980.0 Analgesics, antipyretics, and antirheumatics

E980.1 Barbiturates

E980.2 Other sedatives and hypnotics

E980.3 Tranquilizers and other psychotropic agents

E980.4 Other specified drugs and medicinal substances

E980.5 Unspecified drug or medicinal substance

E980.6 **Corrosive and caustic substances**
Poisoning, undetermined whether accidental or purposeful, by substances classifiable to E864

E980.7 **Agricultural and horticultural chemical and pharmaceutical preparations other than plant foods and fertilizers**

E980.8 **Arsenic and its compounds**

❑ E980.9 **Other and unspecified solid and liquid substances**

● E981 **Poisoning by gases in domestic use, undetermined whether accidentally or purposely inflicted**

E981.0 **Gas distributed by pipeline**

E981.1 **Liquefied petroleum gas distributed in mobile containers**

❑ E981.8 **Other utility gas**

● E982 **Poisoning by other gases, undetermined whether accidentally or purposely inflicted**

E982.0 **Motor vehicle exhaust gas**

❑ E982.1 **Other carbon monoxide**

❑ E982.8 **Other specified gases and vapors**

❑ E982.9 **Unspecified gases and vapors**

● E983 **Hanging, strangulation, or suffocation, undetermined whether accidentally or purposely inflicted**

E983.0 **Hanging**

E983.1 **Suffocation by plastic bag**

❑ E983.8 **Other specified means**

❑ E983.9 **Unspecified means**

E984 **Submersion [drowning], undetermined whether accidentally or purposely inflicted**

● E985 **Injury by firearms, air guns, and explosives, undetermined whether accidentally or purposely inflicted**

E985.0 **Handgun**

E985.1 **Shotgun**

E985.2 **Hunting rifle**

E985.3 **Military firearms**

❑ E985.4 **Other and unspecified firearm**

E985.5 **Explosives**

E985.6 **Air gun**
BB gun
Pellet gun

E985.7 **Paintball gun**

E986 **Injury by cutting and piercing instruments, undetermined whether accidentally or purposely inflicted**

● E987 **Falling from high place, undetermined whether accidentally or purposely inflicted**

E987.0 **Residential premises**

❑ E987.1 **Other man-made structures**

E987.2 **Natural sites**

❑ E987.9 **Unspecified site**

● E988 **Injury by other and unspecified means, undetermined whether accidentally or purposely inflicted**

E988.0 **Jumping or lying before moving object**

E988.1 **Burns, fire**

E988.2 **Scald**

E988.3 **Extremes of cold**

E988.4 **Electrocution**

E988.5 **Crashing of motor vehicle**

E988.6 **Crashing of aircraft**

E988.7 **Caustic substances, except poisoning**

❑ E988.8 **Other specified means**

❑ E988.9 **Unspecified means**

E989 **Late effects of injury, undetermined whether accidentally or purposely inflicted**

Note: This category is to be used to indicate circumstances classifiable to E980-E988 as the cause of death or disability from late effects, which are themselves classifiable elsewhere. The "late effects" include conditions reported as such or as sequelae which may occur at any time after injury, undetermined whether accidentally or purposely inflicted.

INJURY RESULTING FROM OPERATIONS OF WAR (E990-E999)

Includes: injuries to military personnel and civilians caused by war and civil insurrections and occurring during the time of war and insurrection

Excludes *accidents during training of military personnel, manufacture of war material and transport, unless attributable to enemy action*

● E990 **Injury due to war operations by fires and conflagrations**

Includes: asphyxia, burns, or other injury originating from fire caused by a fire-producing device or indirectly by any conventional weapon

E990.0 **From gasoline bomb**

❑ E990.9 **From other and unspecified source**

● E991 **Injury due to war operations by bullets and fragments**

E991.0 **Rubber bullets (rifle)**

E991.1 **Pellets (rifle)**

❑ E991.2 **Other bullets**
Bullet [any, except rubber bullets and pellets]
carbine
machine gun
pistol
rifle
shotgun

E991.3 **Antipersonnel bomb (fragments)**

❑ E991.9 **Other and unspecified fragments**
Fragments from:
artillery shell
bombs, except antipersonnel
grenade
guided missile
land mine
rockets
shell
Shrapnel

E992 **Injury due to war operations by explosion of marine weapons**
Depth charge
Marine mines
Mine NOS, at sea or in harbor
Sea-based artillery shell
Torpedo
Underwater blast

❑ **E993 Injury due to war operations by other explosion**
Accidental explosion of munitions being used in war
Accidental explosion of own weapons
Air blast NOS
Blast NOS
Explosion NOS
Explosion of:
artillery shell
breech block
cannon block
mortar bomb
Injury by weapon burst

E994 Injury due to war operations by destruction of aircraft
Airplane:
burned
exploded
shot down
Crushed by falling airplane

❑ **E995 Injury due to war operations by other and unspecified forms of conventional warfare**
Battle wounds
Bayonet injury
Drowned in war operations

E996 Injury due to war operations by nuclear weapons
Blast effects
Exposure to ionizing radiation from nuclear weapons
Fireball effects
Heat
Other direct and secondary effects of nuclear weapons

● **E997 Injury due to war operations by other forms of unconventional warfare**

E997.0 Lasers

E997.1 Biological warfare

E997.2 Gases, fumes, and chemicals

❑ **E997.8 Other specified forms of unconventional warfare**

❑ **E997.9 Unspecified form of unconventional warfare**

E998 Injury due to war operations but occurring after cessation of hostilities
Injuries due to operations of war but occurring after cessation of hostilities by any means classifiable under E990-E997
Injuries by explosion of bombs or mines placed in the course of operations of war, if the explosion occurred after cessation of hostilities

● **E999 Late effect of injury due to war operations and terrorism**

Note: This category is to be used to indicate circumstances classifiable to E979, E990-E998 as the cause of death or disability from late effects, which are themselves classifiable elsewhere. The "late effects" include conditions reported as such or as sequelae which may occur at any time after injury resulting from operations of war or terrorism.

E999.0 Late effect of injury due to war operations

E999.1 Late effect of injury due to terrorism

APPENDIX A

MORPHOLOGY OF NEOPLASMS

The World Health Organization has published an adaptation of the International Classification of Diseases for Oncology (ICD-O). It contains a coded nomenclature for the morphology of neoplasms, which is reproduced here for those who wish to use it in conjunction with Chapter 2 of the International Classification of Diseases, 9th Revision, Clinical Modification.

The morphology code numbers consist of five digits; the first four identify the histological type of the neoplasm and the fifth indicates its behavior. The one-digit behavior code is as follows:

/0 Benign
/1 Uncertain whether benign or malignant
  Borderline malignancy
/2 Carcinoma in situ
  Intraepithelial
  Noninfiltrating
  Noninvasive
/3 Malignant, primary site
/6 Malignant, metastatic site
  Secondary site
/9 Malignant, uncertain whether primary or metastatic site

In the nomenclature below, the morphology code numbers include the behavior code appropriate to the histological type of neoplasm, but this behavior code should be changed if other reported information makes this necessary. For example, "chordoma (M9370/3)" is assumed to be malignant; the term "benign chordoma" should be coded M9370/0. Similarly, "superficial spreading adenocarcinoma (M8143/3)" described as "noninvasive" should be coded M8143/2 and "melanoma (M8720/3)" described as "secondary" should be coded M8720/6.

The following table shows the correspondence between the morphology code and the different sections of Chapter 2:

Morphology Code Histology/Behavior		ICD-9-CM Chapter 2	
Any	0	210-229	Benign neoplasms
M800-M8004	1	239	Neoplasms of unspecified nature
M8010+	1	235-238	Neoplasms of uncertain behavior
Any	2	230-234	Carcinoma in situ
Any	3	140-195 200-208	Malignant neoplasms, stated or presumed to be primary
Any	6	196-198	Malignant neoplasms, stated or presumed to be secondary

The ICD-O behavior digit /9 is inapplicable in an ICD context, since all malignant neoplasms are presumed to be primary (/3) or secondary (/6) according to other information on the medical record.

Only the first-listed term of the full ICD-O morphology nomenclature appears against each code number in the list below. The ICD-9-CM Alphabetical Index (Volume 2), however, includes all the ICD-O synonyms as well as a number of other morphological names still likely to be encountered on medical records but omitted from ICD-O as outdated or otherwise undesirable.

A coding difficulty sometimes arises where a morphological diagnosis contains two qualifying adjectives that have different code numbers. An example is "transitional cell epidermoid carcinomas." "Transitional cell carcinoma NOS" is M8120/3 and "epidermoid carcinoma NOS" is M8070/3. In such circumstances, the higher number (M8120/3 in this example) should be used, as it is usually more specific.

CODED NOMENCLATURE FOR MORPHOLOGY OF NEOPLASMS

M800 **Neoplasms NOS**
M8000/0 *Neoplasm, benign*
M8000/1 *Neoplasm, uncertain whether benign or malignant*
M8000/3 *Neoplasm, malignant*
M8000/6 *Neoplasm, metastatic*
M8000/9 *Neoplasm, malignant, uncertain whether primary or metastatic*
M8001/0 *Tumor cells, benign*
M8001/1 *Tumor cells, uncertain whether benign or malignant*
M8001/3 *Tumor cells, malignant*
M8002/3 *Malignant tumor, small cell type*
M8003/3 *Malignant tumor, giant cell type*
M8004/3 *Malignant tumor, fusiform cell type*

M801-M804 **Epithelial neoplasms NOS**
M8010/0 *Epithelial tumor, benign*
M8010/2 *Carcinoma in situ NOS*
M8010/3 *Carcinoma NOS*
M8010/6 *Carcinoma, metastatic NOS*
M8010/9 *Carcinomatosis*
M8011/0 *Epithelioma, benign*
M8011/3 *Epithelioma, malignant*
M8012/3 *Large cell carcinoma NOS*
M8020/3 *Carcinoma, undifferentiated type NOS*
M8021/3 *Carcinoma, anaplastic type NOS*
M8022/3 *Pleomorphic carcinoma*
M8030/3 *Giant cell and spindle cell carcinoma*
M8031/3 *Giant cell carcinoma*
M8032/3 *Spindle cell carcinoma*
M8033/3 *Pseudosarcomatous carcinoma*
M8034/3 *Polygonal cell carcinoma*
M8035/3 *Spheroidal cell carcinoma*
M8040/1 *Tumorlet*
M8041/3 *Small cell carcinoma NOS*
M8042/3 *Oat cell carcinoma*
M8043/3 *Small cell carcinoma, fusiform cell type*

M805-M808 **Papillary and squamous cell neoplasms**
M8050/0 *Papilloma NOS (except Papilloma of urinary bladder M8120/1)*
M8050/2 *Papillary carcinoma in situ*
M8050/3 *Papillary carcinoma NOS*
M8051/0 *Verrucous papilloma*
M8051/3 *Verrucous carcinoma NOS*
M8052/0 *Squamous cell papilloma*
M8052/3 *Papillary squamous cell carcinoma*
M8053/0 *Inverted papilloma*
M8060/0 *Papillomatosis NOS*
M8070/2 *Squamous cell carcinoma in situ NOS*
M8070/3 *Squamous cell carcinoma NOS*
M8070/6 *Squamous cell carcinoma, metastatic NOS*
M8071/3 *Squamous cell carcinoma, keratinizing type NOS*
M8072/3 *Squamous cell carcinoma, large cell, nonkeratinizing type*
M8073/3 *Squamous cell carcinoma, small cell, nonkeratinizing type*
M8074/3 *Squamous cell carcinoma, spindle cell type*
M8075/3 *Adenoid squamous cell carcinoma*
M8076/2 *Squamous cell carcinoma in situ with questionable stromal invasion*
M8076/3 *Squamous cell carcinoma, microinvasive*
M8080/2 *Queyrat's erythroplasia*
M8081/2 *Bowen's disease*
M8082/3 *Lymphoepithelial carcinoma*

M809-M811 **Basal cell neoplasms**
M8090/1 *Basal cell tumor*
M8090/3 *Basal cell carcinoma NOS*
M8091/3 *Multicentric basal cell carcinoma*
M8092/3 *Basal cell carcinoma, morphea type*
M8093/3 *Basal cell carcinoma, fibroepithelial type*
M8094/3 *Basosquamous carcinoma*
M8095/3 *Metatypical carcinoma*
M8096/0 *Intraepidermal epithelioma of Jadassohn*
M8100/0 *Trichoepithelioma*
M8101/0 *Trichofolliculoma*
M8102/0 *Tricholemmoma*
M8110/0 *Pilomatrixoma*

M812-M813 Transitional cell papillomas and carcinomas
M8120/0 *Transitional cell papilloma NOS*
M8120/1 *Urothelial papilloma*
M8120/2 *Transitional cell carcinoma in situ*
M8120/3 *Transitional cell carcinoma NOS*
M8121/0 *Schneiderian papilloma*
M8121/1 *Transitional cell papilloma, inverted type*
M8121/3 *Schneiderian carcinoma*
M8122/3 *Transitional cell carcinoma, spindle cell type*
M8123/3 *Basaloid carcinoma*
M8124/3 *Cloacogenic carcinoma*
M8130/3 *Papillary transitional cell carcinoma*

M814-M838 Adenomas and adenocarcinomas
M8140/0 *Adenoma NOS*
M8140/1 *Bronchial adenoma NOS*
M8140/2 *Adenocarcinoma in situ*
M8140/3 *Adenocarcinoma NOS*
M8140/6 *Adenocarcinoma, metastatic NOS*
M8141/3 *Scirrhous adenocarcinoma*
M8142/3 *Linitis plastica*
M8143/3 *Superficial spreading adenocarcinoma*
M8144/3 *Adenocarcinoma, intestinal type*
M8145/3 *Carcinoma, diffuse type*
M8146/0 *Monomorphic adenoma*
M8147/0 *Basal cell adenoma*
M8150/0 *Islet cell adenoma*
M8150/3 *Islet cell carcinoma*
M8151/0 *Insulinoma NOS*
M8151/3 *Insulinoma, malignant*
M8152/0 *Glucagonoma NOS*
M8152/3 *Glucagonoma, malignant*
M8153/1 *Gastrinoma NOS*
M8153/3 *Gastrinoma, malignant*
M8154/3 *Mixed islet cell and exocrine adenocarcinoma*
M8160/0 *Bile duct adenoma*
M8160/3 *Cholangiocarcinoma*
M8161/0 *Bile duct cystadenoma*
M8161/3 *Bile duct cystadenocarcinoma*
M8170/0 *Liver cell adenoma*
M8170/3 *Hepatocellular carcinoma NOS*
M8180/0 *Hepatocholangioma, benign*
M8180/3 *Combined hepatocellular carcinoma and cholangiocarcinoma*
M8190/0 *Trabecular adenoma*
M8190/3 *Trabecular adenocarcinoma*
M8191/0 *Embryonal adenoma*
M8200/0 *Eccrine dermal cylindroma*
M8200/3 *Adenoid cystic carcinoma*
M8201/3 *Cribriform carcinoma*
M8210/0 *Adenomatous polyp NOS*
M8210/3 *Adenocarcinoma in adenomatous polyp*
M8211/0 *Tubular adenoma NOS*
M8211/3 *Tubular adenocarcinoma*
M8220/0 *Adenomatous polyposis coli*
M8220/3 *Adenocarcinoma in adenomatous polyposis coli*
M8221/0 *Multiple adenomatous polyps*
M8230/3 *Solid carcinoma NOS*
M8231/3 *Carcinoma simplex*
M8240/1 *Carcinoid tumor NOS*
M8240/3 *Carcinoid tumor, malignant*
M8241/1 *Carcinoid tumor, argentaffin NOS*
M8241/3 *Carcinoid tumor, argentaffin, malignant*
M8242/1 *Carcinoid tumor, nonargentaffin NOS*
M8242/3 *Carcinoid tumor, nonargentaffin, malignant*
M8243/3 *Mucocarcinoid tumor, malignant*
M8244/3 *Composite carcinoid*
M8250/1 *Pulmonary adenomatosis*
M8250/3 *Bronchiolo-alveolar adenocarcinoma*
M8251/0 *Alveolar adenoma*
M8251/3 *Alveolar adenocarcinoma*
M8260/0 *Papillary adenoma NOS*
M8260/3 *Papillary adenocarcinoma NOS*
M8261/1 *Villous adenoma NOS*
M8261/3 *Adenocarcinoma in villous adenoma*
M8262/3 *Villous adenocarcinoma*
M8263/0 *Tubulovillous adenoma*
M8270/0 *Chromophobe adenoma*
M8270/3 *Chromophobe carcinoma*
M8280/0 *Acidophil adenoma*
M8280/3 *Acidophil carcinoma*
M8281/0 *Mixed acidophil-basophil adenoma*
M8281/3 *Mixed acidophil-basophil carcinoma*
M8290/0 *Oxyphilic adenoma*
M8290/3 *Oxyphilic adenocarcinoma*
M8300/0 *Basophil adenoma*
M8300/3 *Basophil carcinoma*
M8310/0 *Clear cell adenoma*
M8310/3 *Clear cell adenocarcinoma NOS*
M8311/1 *Hypernephroid tumor*
M8312/3 *Renal cell carcinoma*
M8313/0 *Clear cell adenofibroma*
M8320/3 *Granular cell carcinoma*
M8321/0 *Chief cell adenoma*
M8322/0 *Water-clear cell adenoma*
M8322/3 *Water-clear cell adenocarcinoma*
M8323/0 *Mixed cell adenoma*
M8323/3 *Mixed cell adenocarcinoma*
M8324/0 *Lipoadenoma*
M8330/0 *Follicular adenoma*
M8330/3 *Follicular adenocarcinoma NOS*
M8331/3 *Follicular adenocarcinoma, well differentiated type*
M8332/3 *Follicular adenocarcinoma, trabecular type*
M8333/0 *Microfollicular adenoma*
M8334/0 *Macrofollicular adenoma*
M8340/3 *Papillary and follicular adenocarcinoma*
M8350/3 *Nonencapsulated sclerosing carcinoma*
M8360/1 *Multiple endocrine adenomas*
M8361/1 *Juxtaglomerular tumor*
M8370/0 *Adrenal cortical adenoma NOS*
M8370/3 *Adrenal cortical carcinoma*
M8371/0 *Adrenal cortical adenoma, compact cell type*
M8372/0 *Adrenal cortical adenoma, heavily pigmented variant*
M8373/0 *Adrenal cortical adenoma, clear cell type*
M8374/0 *Adrenal cortical adenoma, glomerulosa cell type*
M8375/0 *Adrenal cortical adenoma, mixed cell type*
M8380/0 *Endometrioid adenoma NOS*
M8380/1 *Endometrioid adenoma, borderline malignancy*
M8380/3 *Endometrioid carcinoma*
M8381/0 *Endometrioid adenofibroma NOS*
M8381/1 *Endometrioid adenofibroma, borderline malignancy*
M8381/3 *Endometrioid adenofibroma, malignant*

M839-M842 Adnexal and skin appendage neoplasms
M8390/0 *Skin appendage adenoma*
M8390/3 *Skin appendage carcinoma*
M8400/0 *Sweat gland adenoma*
M8400/1 *Sweat gland tumor NOS*
M8400/3 *Sweat gland adenocarcinoma*
M8401/0 *Apocrine adenoma*
M8401/3 *Apocrine adenocarcinoma*
M8402/0 *Eccrine acrospiroma*
M8403/0 *Eccrine spiradenoma*
M8404/0 *Hidrocystoma*
M8405/0 *Papillary hydradenoma*
M8406/0 *Papillary syringadenoma*
M8407/0 *Syringoma NOS*
M8410/0 *Sebaceous adenoma*
M8410/3 *Sebaceous adenocarcinoma*
M8420/0 *Ceruminous adenoma*
M8420/3 *Ceruminous adenocarcinoma*

M843 Mucoepidermoid neoplasms
M8430/1 *Mucoepidermoid tumor*
M8430/3 *Mucoepidermoid carcinoma*

M844-M849 Cystic, mucinous, and serous neoplasms
M8440/0 *Cystadenoma NOS*
M8440/3 *Cystadenocarcinoma NOS*
M8441/0 *Serous cystadenoma NOS*
M8441/1 *Serous cystadenoma, borderline malignancy*
M8441/3 *Serous cystadenocarcinoma NOS*

M8450/0 *Papillary cystadenoma NOS*
M8450/1 *Papillary cystadenoma, borderline malignancy*
M8450/3 *Papillary cystadenocarcinoma NOS*
M8460/0 *Papillary serous cystadenoma NOS*
M8460/1 *Papillary serous cystadenoma, borderline malignancy*
M8460/3 *Papillary serous cystadenocarcinoma*
M8461/0 *Serous surface papilloma NOS*
M8461/1 *Serous surface papilloma, borderline malignancy*
M8461/3 *Serous surface papillary carcinoma*
M8470/0 *Mucinous cystadenoma NOS*
M8470/1 *Mucinous cystadenoma, borderline malignancy*
M8470/3 *Mucinous cystadenocarcinoma NOS*
M8471/0 *Papillary mucinous cystadenoma NOS*
M8471/1 *Papillary mucinous cystadenoma, borderline malignancy*
M8471/3 *Papillary mucinous cystadenocarcinoma*
M8480/0 *Mucinous adenoma*
M8480/3 *Mucinous adenocarcinoma*
M8480/6 *Pseudomyxoma peritonei*
M8481/3 *Mucin-producing adenocarcinoma*
M8490/3 *Signet ring cell carcinoma*
M8490/6 *Metastatic signet ring cell carcinoma*

M850-M854 Ductal, lobular, and medullary neoplasms
M8500/2 *Intraductal carcinoma, noninfiltrating NOS*
M8500/3 *Infiltrating duct carcinoma*
M8501/2 *Comedocarcinoma, noninfiltrating*
M8501/3 *Comedocarcinoma NOS*
M8502/3 *Juvenile carcinoma of the breast*
M8503/0 *Intraductal papilloma*
M8503/2 *Noninfiltrating intraductal papillary adenocarcinoma*
M8504/0 *Intracystic papillary adenoma*
M8504/2 *Noninfiltrating intracystic carcinoma*
M8505/0 *Intraductal papillomatosis NOS*
M8506/0 *Subareolar duct papillomatosis*
M8510/3 *Medullary carcinoma NOS*
M8511/3 *Medullary carcinoma with amyloid stroma*
M8512/3 *Medullary carcinoma with lymphoid stroma*
M8520/2 *Lobular carcinoma in situ*
M8520/3 *Lobular carcinoma NOS*
M8521/3 *Infiltrating ductular carcinoma*
M8530/3 *Inflammatory carcinoma*
M8540/3 *Paget's disease, mammary*
M8541/3 *Paget's disease and infiltrating duct carcinoma of breast*
M8542/3 *Paget's disease, extramammary (except Paget's disease of bone)*

M855 Acinar cell neoplasms
M8550/0 *Acinar cell adenoma*
M8550/1 *Acinar cell tumor*
M8550/3 *Acinar cell carcinoma*

M856-M858 Complex epithelial neoplasms
M8560/3 *Adenosquamous carcinoma*
M8561/0 *Adenolymphoma*
M8570/3 *Adenocarcinoma with squamous metaplasia*
M8571/3 *Adenocarcinoma with cartilaginous and osseous metaplasia*
M8572/3 *Adenocarcinoma with spindle cell metaplasia*
M8573/3 *Adenocarcinoma with apocrine metaplasia*
M8580/0 *Thymoma, benign*
M8580/3 *Thymoma, malignant*

M859-M867 Specialized gonadal neoplasms
M8590/1 *Sex cord-stromal tumor*
M8600/0 *Thecoma NOS*
M8600/3 *Theca cell carcinoma*
M8610/0 *Luteoma NOS*
M8620/1 *Granulosa cell tumor NOS*
M8620/3 *Granulosa cell tumor, malignant*
M8621/1 *Granulosa cell-theca cell tumor*
M8630/0 *Androblastoma, benign*
M8630/1 *Androblastoma NOS*
M8630/3 *Androblastoma, malignant*
M8631/0 *Sertoli-Leydig cell tumor*
M8632/1 *Gynandroblastoma*
M8640/0 *Tubular androblastoma NOS*
M8640/3 *Sertoli cell carcinoma*
M8641/0 *Tubular androblastoma with lipid storage*
M8650/0 *Leydig cell tumor, benign*
M8650/1 *Leydig cell tumor NOS*
M8650/3 *Leydig cell tumor, malignant*
M8660/0 *Hilar cell tumor*
M8670/0 *Lipid cell tumor of ovary*
M8671/0 *Adrenal rest tumor*

M868-M871 Paragangliomas and glomus tumors
M8680/1 *Paraganglioma NOS*
M8680/3 *Paraganglioma, malignant*
M8681/1 *Sympathetic paraganglioma*
M8682/1 *Parasympathetic paraganglioma*
M8690/1 *Glomus jugulare tumor*
M8691/1 *Aortic body tumor*
M8692/1 *Carotid body tumor*
M8693/1 *Extra-adrenal paraganglioma NOS*
M8693/3 *Extra-adrenal paraganglioma, malignant*
M8700/0 *Pheochromocytoma NOS*
M8700/3 *Pheochromocytoma, malignant*
M8710/3 *Glomangiosarcoma*
M8711/0 *Glomus tumor*
M8712/0 *Glomangioma*

M872-M879 Nevi and melanomas
M8720/0 *Pigmented nevus NOS*
M8720/3 *Malignant melanoma NOS*
M8721/3 *Nodular melanoma*
M8722/0 *Balloon cell nevus*
M8722/3 *Balloon cell melanoma*
M8723/0 *Halo nevus*
M8724/0 *Fibrous papule of the nose*
M8725/0 *Neuronevus*
M8726/0 *Magnocellular nevus*
M8730/0 *Nonpigmented nevus*
M8730/3 *Amelanotic melanoma*
M8740/0 *Junctional nevus*
M8740/3 *Malignant melanoma in junctional nevus*
M8741/2 *Precancerous melanosis NOS*
M8741/3 *Malignant melanoma in precancerous melanosis*
M8742/2 *Hutchinson's melanotic freckle*
M8742/3 *Malignant melanoma in Hutchinson's melanotic freckle*
M8743/3 *Superficial spreading melanoma*
M8750/0 *Intradermal nevus*
M8760/0 *Compound nevus*
M8761/1 *Giant pigmented nevus*
M8761/3 *Malignant melanoma in giant pigmented nevus*
M8770/0 *Epithelioid and spindle cell nevus*
M8771/3 *Epithelioid cell melanoma*
M8772/3 *Spindle cell melanoma NOS*
M8773/3 *Spindle cell melanoma, type A*
M8774/3 *Spindle cell melanoma, type B*
M8775/3 *Mixed epithelioid and spindle cell melanoma*
M8780/0 *Blue nevus NOS*
M8780/3 *Blue nevus, malignant*
M8790/0 *Cellular blue nevus*

M880 Soft tissue tumors and sarcomas NOS
M8800/0 *Soft tissue tumor, benign*
M8800/3 *Sarcoma NOS*
M8800/9 *Sarcomatosis NOS*
M8801/3 *Spindle cell sarcoma*
M8802/3 *Giant cell sarcoma (except of bone M9250/3)*
M8803/3 *Small cell sarcoma*
M8804/3 *Epithelioid cell sarcoma*

M881-M883 Fibromatous neoplasms
M8810/0 *Fibroma NOS*
M8810/3 *Fibrosarcoma NOS*
M8811/0 *Fibromyxoma*
M8811/3 *Fibromyxosarcoma*
M8812/0 *Periosteal fibroma*
M8812/3 *Periosteal fibrosarcoma*
M8813/0 *Fascial fibroma*
M8813/3 *Fascial fibrosarcoma*
M8814/3 *Infantile fibrosarcoma*
M8820/0 *Elastofibroma*

M8821/1 *Aggressive fibromatosis*
M8822/1 *Abdominal fibromatosis*
M8823/1 *Desmoplastic fibroma*
M8830/0 *Fibrous histiocytoma NOS*
M8830/1 *Atypical fibrous histiocytoma*
M8830/3 *Fibrous histiocytoma, malignant*
M8831/0 *Fibroxanthoma NOS*
M8831/1 *Atypical fibroxanthoma*
M8831/3 *Fibroxanthoma, malignant*
M8832/0 *Dermatofibroma NOS*
M8832/1 *Dermatofibroma protuberans*
M8832/3 *Dermatofibrosarcoma NOS*

M884 Myxomatous neoplasms
M8840/0 *Myxoma NOS*
M8840/3 *Myxosarcoma*

M885-M888 Lipomatous neoplasms
M8850/0 *Lipoma NOS*
M8850/3 *Liposarcoma NOS*
M8851/0 *Fibrolipoma*
M8851/3 *Liposarcoma, well differentiated type*
M8852/0 *Fibromyxolipoma*
M8852/3 *Myxoid liposarcoma*
M8853/3 *Round cell liposarcoma*
M8854/3 *Pleomorphic liposarcoma*
M8855/3 *Mixed type liposarcoma*
M8856/0 *Intramuscular lipoma*
M8857/0 *Spindle cell lipoma*
M8860/0 *Angiomyolipoma*
M8860/3 *Angiomyoliposarcoma*
M8861/0 *Angiolipoma NOS*
M8861/1 *Angiolipoma, infiltrating*
M8870/0 *Myelolipoma*
M8880/0 *Hibernoma*
M8881/0 *Lipoblastomatosis*

M889-M892 Myomatous neoplasms
M8890/0 *Leiomyoma NOS*
M8890/1 *Intravascular leiomyomatosis*
M8890/3 *Leiomyosarcoma NOS*
M8891/1 *Epithelioid leiomyoma*
M8891/3 *Epithelioid leiomyosarcoma*
M8892/1 *Cellular leiomyoma*
M8893/0 *Bizarre leiomyoma*
M8894/0 *Angiomyoma*
M8894/3 *Angiomyosarcoma*
M8895/0 *Myoma*
M8895/3 *Myosarcoma*
M8900/0 *Rhabdomyoma NOS*
M8900/3 *Rhabdomyosarcoma NOS*
M8901/3 *Pleomorphic rhabdomyosarcoma*
M8902/3 *Mixed type rhabdomyosarcoma*
M8903/0 *Fetal rhabdomyoma*
M8904/0 *Adult rhabdomyoma*
M8910/3 *Embryonal rhabdomyosarcoma*
M8920/3 *Alveolar rhabdomyosarcoma*

M893-M899 Complex mixed and stromal neoplasms
M8930/3 *Endometrial stromal sarcoma*
M8931/1 *Endolymphatic stromal myosis*
M8932/0 *Adenomyoma*
M8940/0 *Pleomorphic adenoma*
M8940/3 *Mixed tumor, malignant NOS*
M8950/3 *Mullerian mixed tumor*
M8951/3 *Mesodermal mixed tumor*
M8960/1 *Mesoblastic nephroma*
M8960/3 *Nephroblastoma NOS*
M8961/3 *Epithelial nephroblastoma*
M8962/3 *Mesenchymal nephroblastoma*
M8970/3 *Hepatoblastoma*
M8980/3 *Carcinosarcoma NOS*
M8981/3 *Carcinosarcoma, embryonal type*
M8982/0 *Myoepithelioma*
M8990/0 *Mesenchymoma, benign*
M8990/1 *Mesenchymoma NOS*
M8990/3 *Mesenchymoma, malignant*
M8991/3 *Embryonal sarcoma*

M900-M903 Fibroepithelial neoplasms
M9000/0 *Brenner tumor NOS*
M9000/1 *Brenner tumor, borderline malignancy*
M9000/3 *Brenner tumor, malignant*
M9010/0 *Fibroadenoma NOS*
M9011/0 *Intracanalicular fibroadenoma NOS*
M9012/0 *Pericanalicular fibroadenoma*
M9013/0 *Adenofibroma NOS*
M9014/0 *Serous adenofibroma*
M9015/0 *Mucinous adenofibroma*
M9020/0 *Cellular intracanalicular fibroadenoma*
M9020/1 *Cystosarcoma phyllodes NOS*
M9020/3 *Cystosarcoma phyllodes, malignant*
M9030/0 *Juvenile fibroadenoma*

M904 Synovial neoplasms
M9040/0 *Synovioma, benign*
M9040/3 *Synovial sarcoma NOS*
M9041/3 *Synovial sarcoma, spindle cell type*
M9042/3 *Synovial sarcoma, epithelioid cell type*
M9043/3 *Synovial sarcoma, biphasic type*
M9044/3 *Clear cell sarcoma of tendons and aponeuroses*

M905 Mesothelial neoplasms
M9050/0 *Mesothelioma, benign*
M9050/3 *Mesothelioma, malignant*
M9051/0 *Fibrous mesothelioma, benign*
M9051/3 *Fibrous mesothelioma, malignant*
M9052/0 *Epithelioid mesothelioma, benign*
M9052/3 *Epithelioid mesothelioma, malignant*
M9053/0 *Mesothelioma, biphasic type, benign*
M9053/3 *Mesothelioma, biphasic type, malignant*
M9054/0 *Adenomatoid tumor NOS*

M906-M909 Germ cell neoplasms
M9060/3 *Dysgerminoma*
M9061/3 *Seminoma NOS*
M9062/3 *Seminoma, anaplastic type*
M9063/3 *Spermatocytic seminoma*
M9064/3 *Germinoma*
M9070/3 *Embryonal carcinoma NOS*
M9071/3 *Endodermal sinus tumor*
M9072/3 *Polyembryoma*
M9073/1 *Gonadoblastoma*
M9080/0 *Teratoma, benign*
M9080/1 *Teratoma NOS*
M9080/3 *Teratoma, malignant NOS*
M9081/3 *Teratocarcinoma*
M9082/3 *Malignant teratoma, undifferentiated type*
M9083/3 *Malignant teratoma, intermediate type*
M9084/0 *Dermoid cyst*
M9084/3 *Dermoid cyst with malignant transformation*
M9090/0 *Struma ovarii NOS*
M9090/3 *Struma ovarii, malignant*
M9091/1 *Strumal carcinoid*

M910 Trophoblastic neoplasms
M9100/0 *Hydatidiform mole NOS*
M9100/1 *Invasive hydatidiform mole*
M9100/3 *Choriocarcinoma*
M9101/3 *Choriocarcinoma combined with teratoma*
M9102/3 *Malignant teratoma, trophoblastic*

M911 Mesonephromas
M9110/0 *Mesonephroma, benign*
M9110/1 *Mesonephric tumor*
M9110/3 *Mesonephroma, malignant*
M9111/1 *Endosalpingioma*

M912-M916 Blood vessel tumors
M9120/0 *Hemangioma NOS*
M9120/3 *Hemangiosarcoma*
M9121/0 *Cavernous hemangioma*
M9122/0 *Venous hemangioma*
M9123/0 *Racemose hemangioma*
M9124/3 *Kupffer cell sarcoma*

M9130/0 *Hemangioendothelioma, benign*
M9130/1 *Hemangioendothelioma NOS*
M9130/3 *Hemangioendothelioma, malignant*
M9131/0 *Capillary hemangioma*
M9132/0 *Intramuscular hemangioma*
M9140/3 *Kaposi's sarcoma*
M9141/0 *Angiokeratoma*
M9142/0 *Verrucous keratotic hemangioma*
M9150/0 *Hemangiopericytoma, benign*
M9150/1 *Hemangiopericytoma NOS*
M9150/3 *Hemangiopericytoma, malignant*
M9160/0 *Angiofibroma NOS*
M9161/1 *Hemangioblastoma*

M917 Lymphatic vessel tumors
M9170/0 *Lymphangioma NOS*
M9170/3 *Lymphangiosarcoma*
M9171/0 *Capillary lymphangioma*
M9172/0 *Cavernous lymphangioma*
M9173/0 *Cystic lymphangioma*
M9174/0 *Lymphangiomyoma*
M9174/1 *Lymphangiomyomatosis*
M9175/0 *Hemolymphangioma*

M918-M920 Osteomas and osteosarcomas
M9180/0 *Osteoma NOS*
M9180/3 *Osteosarcoma NOS*
M9181/3 *Chondroblastic osteosarcoma*
M9182/3 *Fibroblastic osteosarcoma*
M9183/3 *Telangiectatic osteosarcoma*
M9184/3 *Osteosarcoma in Paget's disease of bone*
M9190/3 *Juxtacortical osteosarcoma*
M9191/0 *Osteoid osteoma NOS*
M9200/0 *Osteoblastoma*

M921-M924 Chondromatous neoplasms
M9210/0 *Osteochondroma*
M9210/1 *Osteochondromatosis NOS*
M9220/0 *Chondroma NOS*
M9220/1 *Chondromatosis NOS*
M9220/3 *Chondrosarcoma NOS*
M9221/0 *Juxtacortical chondroma*
M9221/3 *Juxtacortical chondrosarcoma*
M9230/0 *Chondroblastoma NOS*
M9230/3 *Chondroblastoma, malignant*
M9240/3 *Mesenchymal chondrosarcoma*
M9241/0 *Chondromyxoid fibroma*

M925 Giant cell tumors
M9250/1 *Giant cell tumor of bone NOS*
M9250/3 *Giant cell tumor of bone, malignant*
M9251/1 *Giant cell tumor of soft parts NOS*
M9251/3 *Malignant giant cell tumor of soft parts*

M926 Miscellaneous bone tumors
M9260/3 *Ewing's sarcoma*
M9261/3 *Adamantinoma of long bones*
M9262/0 *Ossifying fibroma*

M927-M934 Odontogenic tumors
M9270/0 *Odontogenic tumor, benign*
M9270/1 *Odontogenic tumor NOS*
M9270/3 *Odontogenic tumor, malignant*
M9271/0 *Dentinoma*
M9272/0 *Cementoma NOS*
M9273/0 *Cementoblastoma, benign*
M9274/0 *Cementifying fibroma*
M9275/0 *Gigantiform cementoma*
M9280/0 *Odontoma NOS*
M9281/0 *Compound odontoma*
M9282/0 *Complex odontoma*
M9290/0 *Ameloblastic fibro-odontoma*
M9290/3 *Ameloblastic odontosarcoma*
M9300/0 *Adenomatoid odontogenic tumor*
M9301/0 *Calcifying odontogenic cyst*
M9310/0 *Ameloblastoma NOS*
M9310/3 *Ameloblastoma, malignant*
M9311/0 *Odontoameloblastoma*
M9312/0 *Squamous odontogenic tumor*
M9320/0 *Odontogenic myxoma*
M9321/0 *Odontogenic fibroma NOS*
M9330/0 *Ameloblastic fibroma*
M9330/3 *Ameloblastic fibrosarcoma*
M9340/0 *Calcifying epithelial odontogenic tumor*

M935-M937 Miscellaneous tumors
M9350/1 *Craniopharyngioma*
M9360/1 *Pinealoma*
M9361/1 *Pineocytoma*
M9362/3 *Pineoblastoma*
M9363/0 *Melanotic neuroectodermal tumor*
M9370/3 *Chordoma*

M938-M948 Gliomas
M9380/3 *Glioma, malignant*
M9381/3 *Gliomatosis cerebri*
M9382/3 *Mixed glioma*
M9383/1 *Subependymal glioma*
M9384/1 *Subependymal giant cell astrocytoma*
M9390/0 *Choroid plexus papilloma NOS*
M9390/3 *Choroid plexus papilloma, malignant*
M9391/3 *Ependymoma NOS*
M9392/3 *Ependymoma, anaplastic type*
M9393/1 *Papillary ependymoma*
M9394/1 *Myxopapillary ependymoma*
M9400/3 *Astrocytoma NOS*
M9401/3 *Astrocytoma, anaplastic type*
M9410/3 *Protoplasmic astrocytoma*
M9411/3 *Gemistocytic astrocytoma*
M9420/3 *Fibrillary astrocytoma*
M9421/3 *Pilocytic astrocytoma*
M9422/3 *Spongioblastoma NOS*
M9423/3 *Spongioblastoma polare*
M9430/3 *Astroblastoma*
M9440/3 *Glioblastoma NOS*
M9441/3 *Giant cell glioblastoma*
M9442/3 *Glioblastoma with sarcomatous component*
M9443/3 *Primitive polar spongioblastoma*
M9450/3 *Oligodendroglioma NOS*
M9451/3 *Oligodendroglioma, anaplastic type*
M9460/3 *Oligodendroblastoma*
M9470/3 *Medulloblastoma NOS*
M9471/3 *Desmoplastic medulloblastoma*
M9472/3 *Medullomyoblastoma*
M9480/3 *Cerebellar sarcoma NOS*
M9481/3 *Monstrocellular sarcoma*

M949-M952 Neuroepitheliomatous neoplasms
M9490/0 *Ganglioneuroma*
M9490/3 *Ganglioneuroblastoma*
M9491/0 *Ganglioneuromatosis*
M9500/3 *Neuroblastoma NOS*
M9501/3 *Medulloepithelioma NOS*
M9502/3 *Teratoid medulloepithelioma*
M9503/3 *Neuroepithelioma NOS*
M9504/3 *Spongioneuroblastoma*
M9505/1 *Ganglioglioma*
M9506/0 *Neurocytoma*
M9507/0 *Pacinian tumor*
M9510/3 *Retinoblastoma NOS*
M9511/3 *Retinoblastoma, differentiated type*
M9512/3 *Retinoblastoma, undifferentiated type*
M9520/3 *Olfactory neurogenic tumor*
M9521/3 *Esthesioneurocytoma*
M9522/3 *Esthesioneuroblastoma*
M9523/3 *Esthesioneuroepithelioma*

M953 Meningiomas
M9530/0 *Meningioma NOS*
M9530/1 *Meningiomatosis NOS*
M9530/3 *Meningioma, malignant*
M9531/0 *Meningotheliomatous meningioma*
M9532/0 *Fibrous meningioma*
M9533/0 *Psammomatous meningioma*
M9534/0 *Angiomatous meningioma*

M9535/0 *Hemangioblastic meningioma*
M9536/0 *Hemangiopericytic meningioma*
M9537/0 *Transitional meningioma*
M9538/1 *Papillary meningioma*
M9539/3 *Meningeal sarcomatosis*

M954-M957 Nerve sheath tumor
M9540/0 *Neurofibroma NOS*
M9540/1 *Neurofibromatosis NOS*
M9540/3 *Neurofibrosarcoma*
M9541/0 *Melanotic neurofibroma*
M9550/0 *Plexiform neurofibroma*
M9560/0 *Neurilemmoma NOS*
M9560/1 *Neurinomatosis*
M9560/3 *Neurilemmoma, malignant*
M9570/0 *Neuroma NOS*

M958 Granular cell tumors and alveolar soft part sarcoma
M9580/0 *Granular cell tumor NOS*
M9580/3 *Granular cell tumor, malignant*
M9581/3 *Alveolar soft part sarcoma*

M959-M963 Lymphomas, NOS or diffuse
M9590/0 *Lymphomatous tumor, benign*
M9590/3 *Malignant lymphoma NOS*
M9591/3 *Malignant lymphoma, non Hodgkin's type*
M9600/3 *Malignant lymphoma, undifferentiated cell type NOS*
M9601/3 *Malignant lymphoma, stem cell type*
M9602/3 *Malignant lymphoma, convoluted cell type NOS*
M9610/3 *Lymphosarcoma NOS*
M9611/3 *Malignant lymphoma, lymphoplasmacytoid type*
M9612/3 *Malignant lymphoma, immunoblastic type*
M9613/3 *Malignant lymphoma, mixed lymphocytic-histiocytic NOS*
M9614/3 *Malignant lymphoma, centroblastic-centrocytic, diffuse*
M9615/3 *Malignant lymphoma, follicular center cell NOS*
M9620/3 *Malignant lymphoma, lymphocytic, well differentiated NOS*
M9621/3 *Malignant lymphoma, lymphocytic, intermediate differentiation NOS*
M9622/3 *Malignant lymphoma, centrocytic*
M9623/3 *Malignant lymphoma, follicular center cell, cleaved NOS*
M9630/3 *Malignant lymphoma, lymphocytic, poorly differentiated NOS*
M9631/3 *Prolymphocytic lymphosarcoma*
M9632/3 *Malignant lymphoma, centroblastic type NOS*
M9633/3 *Malignant lymphoma, follicular center cell, noncleaved NOS*

M964 Reticulosarcomas
M9640/3 *Reticulosarcoma NOS*
M9641/3 *Reticulosarcoma, pleomorphic cell type*
M9642/3 *Reticulosarcoma, nodular*

M965-M966 Hodgkin's disease
M9650/3 *Hodgkin's disease NOS*
M9651/3 *Hodgkin's disease, lymphocytic predominance*
M9652/3 *Hodgkin's disease, mixed cellularity*
M9653/3 *Hodgkin's disease, lymphocytic depletion NOS*
M9654/3 *Hodgkin's disease, lymphocytic depletion, diffuse fibrosis*
M9655/3 *Hodgkin's disease, lymphocytic depletion, reticular type*
M9656/3 *Hodgkin's disease, nodular sclerosis NOS*
M9657/3 *Hodgkin's disease, nodular sclerosis, cellular phase*
M9660/3 *Hodgkin's paragranuloma*
M9661/3 *Hodgkin's granuloma*
M9662/3 *Hodgkin's sarcoma*

M969 Lymphomas, nodular or follicular
M9690/3 *Malignant lymphoma, nodular NOS*
M9691/3 *Malignant lymphoma, mixed lymphocytic-histiocytic, nodular*
M9692/3 *Malignant lymphoma, centroblastic-centrocytic, follicular*
M9693/3 *Malignant lymphoma, lymphocytic, well differentiated, nodular*
M9694/3 *Malignant lymphoma, lymphocytic, intermediate differentiation, nodular*
M9695/3 *Malignant lymphoma, follicular center cell, cleaved, follicular*
M9696/3 *Malignant lymphoma, lymphocytic, poorly differentiated, nodular*
M9697/3 *Malignant lymphoma, centroblastic type, follicular*
M9698/3 *Malignant lymphoma, follicular center cell, noncleaved, follicular*

M970 Mycosis fungoides
M9700/3 *Mycosis fungoides*
M9701/3 *Sezary's disease*

M971-M972 Miscellaneous reticuloendothelial neoplasms
M9710/3 *Microglioma*
M9720/3 *Malignant histiocytosis*
M9721/3 *Histiocytic medullary reticulosis*
M9722/3 *Letterer-Siwe's disease*

M973 Plasma cell tumors
M9730/3 *Plasma cell myeloma*
M9731/0 *Plasma cell tumor, benign*
M9731/1 *Plasmacytoma NOS*
M9731/3 *Plasma cell tumor, malignant*

M974 Mast cell tumors
M9740/1 *Mastocytoma NOS*
M9740/3 *Mast cell sarcoma*
M9741/3 *Malignant mastocytosis*

M975 Burkitt's tumor
M9750/3 *Burkitt's tumor*

M980-M994 Leukemias

M980 Leukemias NOS
M9800/3 *Leukemia NOS*
M9801/3 *Acute leukemia NOS*
M9802/3 *Subacute leukemia NOS*
M9803/3 *Chronic leukemia NOS*
M9804/3 *Aleukemic leukemia NOS*

M981 Compound leukemias
M9810/3 *Compound leukemia*

M982 Lymphoid leukemias
M9820/3 *Lymphoid leukemia NOS*
M9821/3 *Acute lymphoid leukemia*
M9822/3 *Subacute lymphoid leukemia*
M9823/3 *Chronic lymphoid leukemia*
M9824/3 *Aleukemic lymphoid leukemia*
M9825/3 *Prolymphocytic leukemia*

M983 Plasma cell leukemias
M9830/3 *Plasma cell leukemia*

M984 Erythroleukemias
M9840/3 *Erythroleukemia*
M9841/3 *Acute erythremia*
M9842/3 *Chronic erythremia*

M985 Lymphosarcoma cell leukemias
M9850/3 *Lymphosarcoma cell leukemia*

M986 Myeloid leukemias
M9860/3 *Myeloid leukemia NOS*
M9861/3 *Acute myeloid leukemia*
M9862/3 *Subacute myeloid leukemia*
M9863/3 *Chronic myeloid leukemia*
M9864/3 *Aleukemic myeloid leukemia*
M9865/3 *Neutrophilic leukemia*
M9866/3 *Acute promyelocytic leukemia*

M987 Basophilic leukemias
M9870/3 *Basophilic leukemia*

M988 Eosinophilic leukemias
M9880/3 *Eosinophilic leukemia*

M989 Monocytic leukemias
M9890/3 *Monocytic leukemia NOS*
M9891/3 *Acute monocytic leukemia*
M9892/3 *Subacute monocytic leukemia*

M9893/3 *Chronic monocytic leukemia*
M9894/3 *Aleukemic monocytic leukemia*

M990-M994 Miscellaneous leukemias

M9900/3 *Mast cell leukemia*
M9910/3 *Megakaryocytic leukemia*
M9920/3 *Megakaryocytic myelosis*
M9930/3 *Myeloid sarcoma*
M9940/3 *Hairy cell leukemia*

M995-M997 Miscellaneous myeloproliferative and lymphoproliferative disorders

M9950/1 *Polycythemia vera*
M9951/1 *Acute panmyelosis*
M9960/1 *Chronic myeloproliferative disease*
M9961/1 *Myelosclerosis with myeloid metaplasia*
M9962/1 *Idiopathic thrombocythemia*
M9970/1 *Chronic lymphoproliferative disease*

APPENDIX B

GLOSSARY OF MENTAL DISORDERS

Deleted as of October 1, 2004

APPENDIX C

CLASSIFICATION OF DRUGS BY AMERICAN HOSPITAL FORMULARY SERVICES LIST NUMBER AND THEIR ICD-9-CM EQUIVALENTS

The coding of adverse effects of drugs is keyed to the continually revised Hospital Formulary of the American Hospital Formulary Service (AHFS) published under the direction of the American Society of Hospital Pharmacists.

The following section gives the ICD-9-CM diagnosis code for each AHFS list.

AHFS List		ICD-9-CM Diagnosis Code
4:00	**ANTIHISTAMINE DRUGS**	**963.0**
8:00	**ANTI-INFECTIVE AGENTS**	
8:04	Amebicides	961.5
	hydroxyquinoline derivatives	961.3
	arsenical anti-infectives	961.1
8:08	Anthelmintics	961.6
	quinoline derivatives	961.3
8:12.04	Antifungal Antibiotics	960.1
	nonantibiotics	961.9
8:12.06	Cephalosporins	960.5
8:12.08	Chloramphenicol	960.2
8:12.12	The Erythromycins	960.3
8:12.16	The Penicillins	960.0
8:12.20	The Streptomycins	960.6
8:12.24	The Tetracyclines	960.4
8:12.28	Other Antibiotics	960.8
	antimycobacterial antibiotics	960.6
	macrolides	960.3
8:16	Antituberculars	961.8
	antibiotics	960.6
8:18	Antivirals	961.7
8:20	Plasmodicides (antimalarials)	961.4
8:24	Sulfonamides	961.0
8:26	The Sulfones	961.8
8:28	Treponemicides	961.2
8:32	Trichomonacides	961.5
	hydroxyquinoline derivatives	961.3
	nitrofuran derivatives	961.9
8:36	Urinary Germicides	961.9
	quinoline derivatives	961.3
8:40	Other Anti-Infectives	961.9
10:00	**ANTINEOPLASTIC AGENTS**	**963.1**
	antibiotics	960.7
	progestogens	962.2
12:00	**AUTONOMIC DRUGS**	
12:04	Parasympathomimetic (Cholinergic) Agents	971.0
12:08	Parasympatholytic (Cholinergic Blocking) Agents	971.1
12:12	Sympathomimetic (Adrenergic) Agents	971.2
12:16	Sympatholytic (Adrenergic Blocking) Agents	971.3
12:20	Skeletal Muscle Relaxants	975.2
	central nervous system muscle-tone depressants	968.0
16:00	**BLOOD DERIVATIVES**	**964.7**
20:00	**BLOOD FORMATION AND COAGULATION**	
20:04	Antianemia Drugs	964.1
20:04.04	Iron Preparations	964.0
20:04.08	Liver and Stomach Preparations	964.1
20:12.04	Anticoagulants	964.2
20:12.08	Antiheparin agents	964.5
20:12.12	Coagulants	964.5
20.12.16	Hemostatics	964.5
	capillary-active drugs	972.8
	fibrinolysis-affecting agents	964.4
	natural products	964.7
24:00	**CARDIOVASCULAR DRUGS**	
24:04	Cardiac Drugs	972.9
	cardiotonic agents	972.1
	rhythm regulators	972.0
24:06	Antilipemic Agents	972.2
	thyroid derivatives	962.7
24:08	Hypotensive Agents	972.6
	adrenergic blocking agents	971.3
	ganglion-blocking agents	972.3
	vasodilators	972.5
24:12	Vasodilating Agents	972.5
	coronary	972.4
	nicotinic acid derivatives	972.2
24:16	Sclerosing Agents	972.7
28:00	**CENTRAL NERVOUS SYSTEM DRUGS**	
28:04	General Anesthetics	968.4
	gaseous anesthetics	968.2
	halothane	968.1
	intravenous anesthetics	968.3
28:08	Analgesics and Antipyretics	965.9
	antirheumatics	965.6
	aromatic analgesics	965.4
	non-narcotics NEC	965.7
	opium alkaloids	965.00
	heroin	965.01
	methadone	965.02
	specified type NEC	965.09
	pyrazole derivatives	965.5
	salicylates	965.1
	specified type NEC	965.8
28:10	Narcotic Antagonists	970.1
28:12	Anticonvulsants	966.3
	barbiturates	967.0
	benzodiazepine-based tranquilizers	969.4
	bromides	967.3
	hydantoin derivatives	966.1
	oxazolidine derivative	966.0
	succinimides	966.2
28:16.04	Antidepressants	969.0
28:16.08	Tranquilizers	969.5
	benzodiazepine-based	969.4
	butyrophenone-based	969.2
	major NEC	969.3
	phenothiazine-based	969.1
28:16.12	Other Psychotherapeutic Agents	969.8
28:20	Respiratory and Cerebral Stimulants	970.9
	analeptics	970.0
	anorexigenic agents	977.0
	psychostimulants	969.7
	specified type NEC	970.8
28:24	Sedatives and Hypnotics	967.9
	barbiturates	967.0
	benzodiazepine-based tranquilizers	969.4
	chloral hydrate group	967.1
	glutethimide group	967.5
	intravenous anesthetics	968.3
	methaqualone	967.4
	paraldehyde	967.2
	phenothiazine-based tranquilizers	969.1
	specified type NEC	967.8
	thiobarbiturates	968.3
	tranquilizer NEC	969.5
36:00	**DIAGNOSTIC AGENTS**	**977.8**
40:00	**ELECTROLYTE, CALORIC, AND WATER BALANCE AGENTS NEC**	**974.5**
40:04	Acidifying Agents	963.2

Code	Class	ICD-9-CM
40:08	Alkalinizing Agents	963.3
40:10	Ammonia Detoxicants	974.5
40:12	Replacement Solutions NEC	974.5
	plasma volume expanders	964.8
40:16	Sodium-Removing Resins	974.5
40:18	Potassium-Removing Resins	974.5
40:20	Caloric Agents	974.5
40:24	Salt and Sugar Substitutes	974.5
40:28	Diuretics NEC	974.4
	carbonic acid anhydrase inhibitors	974.2
	mercurials	974.0
	purine derivatives	974.1
	saluretics	974.3
40:36	Irrigating Solutions	974.5
40:40	Uricosuric Agents	974.7
44:00	**ENZYMES NEC**	**963.4**
	fibrinolysis-affecting agents	964.4
	gastric agents	973.4
48:00	**EXPECTORANTS AND COUGH PREPARATIONS**	
	antihistamine agents	963.0
	antitussives	975.4
	codeine derivatives	965.09
	expectorants	975.5
	narcotic agents NEC	965.09
52:00	**EYE, EAR, NOSE, AND THROAT PREPARATIONS**	
52:04	Anti-Infectives	
	ENT	976.6
	ophthalmic	976.5
52:04.04	Antibiotics	
	ENT	976.6
	ophthalmic	976.5
52:04.06	Antivirals	
	ENT	976.6
	ophthalmic	976.5
52:04.08	Sulfonamides	
	ENT	976.6
	ophthalmic	976.5
52:04.12	Miscellaneous Anti-Infectives	
	ENT	976.6
	ophthalmic	976.5
52:08	Anti-Inflammatory Agents	
	ENT	976.6
	ophthalmic	976.5
52:10	Carbonic Anhydrase Inhibitors	974.2
52:12	Contact Lens Solutions	976.5
52:16	Local Anesthetics	968.5
52:20	Miotics	971.0
52:24	Mydriatics	
	adrenergics	971.2
	anticholinergics	971.1
	antimuscarinics	971.1
	parasympatholytics	971.1
	spasmolytics	971.1
	sympathomimetics	971.2
52:28	Mouth Washes and Gargles	976.6
52:32	Vasoconstrictors	971.2
52:36	Unclassified Agents	
	ENT	976.6
	ophthalmic	976.5
56:00	**GASTROINTESTINAL DRUGS**	
56:04	Antacids and Absorbents	973.0
56:08	Anti-Diarrhea Agents	973.5
56:10	Antiflatulents	973.8
56:12	Cathartics NEC	973.3
	emollients	973.2
	irritants	973.1
56:16	Digestants	973.4
56:20	Emetics and Antiemetics	
	antiemetics	963.0
	emetics	973.6
56:24	Lipotropic Agents	977.1
60:00	**GOLD COMPOUNDS**	**965.6**
64:00	**HEAVY METAL ANTAGONISTS**	**963.8**
68:00	**HORMONES AND SYNTHETIC SUBSTITUTES**	
68:04	Adrenals	962.0
68:08	Androgens	962.1
68:12	Contraceptives	962.2
68:16	Estrogens	962.2
68:18	Gonadotropins	962.4
68:20	Insulins and Antidiabetic Agents	962.3
68:20.08	Insulins	962.3
68:24	Parathyroid	962.6
68:28	Pituitary	
	anterior	962.4
	posterior	962.5
68:32	Progestogens	962.2
68:34	Other Corpus Luteum Hormones	962.2
68:36	Thyroid and Antithyroid	
	antithyroid	962.8
	thyroid	962.7
72:00	**LOCAL ANESTHETICS NEC**	**968.9**
	topical (surface) agents	968.5
	infiltrating agents (intradermal) (subcutaneous) (submucosal)	968.5
	nerve blocking agents (peripheral) (plexus) (regional)	968.6
	spinal	968.7
76:00	**OXYTOCICS**	**975.0**
78:00	**RADIOACTIVE AGENTS**	**990**
80:00	**SERUMS, TOXOIDS, AND VACCINE**	
80:04	Serums	979.9
	immune globulin (gamma) (human)	964.6
80:08	Toxoids NEC	978.8
	diphtheria	978.5
	and tetanus	978.9
	with pertussis component	978.6
	tetanus	978.4
	and diphtheria	978.9
	with pertussis component	978.6
80:12	Vaccines NEC	979.9
	bacterial NEC	978.8
	with	
	other bacterial component	978.9
	pertussis component	978.6
	viral and rickettsial component	979.7
	rickettsial NEC	979.6
	with	
	bacterial component	979.7
	pertussis component	978.6
	viral component	979.7
	viral NEC	979.6
	with	
	bacterial component	979.7
	pertussis component	978.6
	rickettsial component	979.7
84:00	**SKIN AND MUCOUS MEMBRANE PREPARATIONS**	
84:04	Anti-Infectives	976.0
84:04.04	Antibiotics	976.0
84:04.08	Fungicides	976.0
84:04.12	Scabicides and Pediculicides	976.0
84:04.16	Miscellaneous Local Anti-Infectives	976.0
84:06	Anti-Inflammatory Agents	976.0
84:08	Antipruritics and Local Anesthetics	
	antipruritics	976.1
	local anesthetics	968.5
84:12	Astringents	976.2
84:16	Cell Stimulants and Proliferants	976.8
84:20	Detergents	976.2
84:24	Emollients, Demulcents, and Protectants	976.3
84:28	Keratolytic Agents	976.4

84:32	Keratoplastic Agents	976.4
84:36	Miscellaneous Agents	976.8
86:00	**SPASMOLYTIC AGENTS**	**975.1**
	antiasthmatics	975.7
	papaverine	972.5
	theophylline	974.1
88:00	**VITAMINS**	
88:04	Vitamin A	963.5
88:08	Vitamin B Complex	963.5
	hematopoietic vitamin	964.1
	nicotinic acid derivatives	972.2
88:12	Vitamin C	963.5
88:16	Vitamin D	963.5
88:20	Vitamin E	963.5
88:24	Vitamin K Activity	964.3
88:28	Multivitamin Preparations	963.5
92:00	**UNCLASSIFIED THERAPEUTIC AGENTS**	**977.8**

APPENDIX D

CLASSIFICATION OF INDUSTRIAL ACCIDENTS ACCORDING TO AGENCY

Annex B to the Resolution concerning Statistics of Employment Injuries adopted by the Tenth International Conference of Labor Statisticians on 12 October 1962

1 MACHINES

11 **Prime-Movers, except Electrical Motors**
- 111 *Steam engines*
- 112 *Internal combustion engines*
- 119 *Others*

12 **Transmission Machinery**
- 121 *Transmission shafts*
- 122 *Transmission belts, cables, pulleys, pinions, chains, gears*
- 129 *Others*

13 **Metalworking Machines**
- 131 *Power presses*
- 132 *Lathes*
- 133 *Milling machines*
- 134 *Abrasive wheels*
- 135 *Mechanical shears*
- 136 *Forging machines*
- 137 *Rolling-mills*
- 139 *Others*

14 **Wood and Assimilated Machines**
- 141 *Circular saws*
- 142 *Other saws*
- 143 *Molding machines*
- 144 *Overhand planes*
- 149 *Others*

15 **Agricultural Machines**
- 151 *Reapers (including combine reapers)*
- 152 *Threshers*
- 159 *Others*

16 **Mining Machinery**
- 161 *Under-cutters*
- 169 *Others*

19 **Other Machines Not Elsewhere Classified**
- 191 *Earth-moving machines, excavating and scraping machines, except means of transport*
- 192 *Spinning, weaving and other textile machines*
- 193 *Machines for the manufacture of foodstuffs and beverages*
- 194 *Machines for the manufacture of paper*
- 195 *Printing machines*
- 199 *Others*

2 MEANS OF TRANSPORT AND LIFTING EQUIPMENT

21 **Lifting Machines and Appliances**
- 211 *Cranes*
- 212 *Lifts and elevators*
- 213 *Winches*
- 214 *Pulley blocks*
- 219 *Others*

22 **Means of Rail Transport**
- 221 *Inter-urban railways*
- 222 *Rail transport in mines, tunnels, quarries, industrial establishments, docks, etc.*
- 229 *Others*

23 **Other Wheeled Means of Transport, Excluding Rail Transport**
- 231 *Tractors*
- 232 *Lorries*
- 233 *Trucks*
- 234 *Motor vehicles, not elsewhere classified*
- 235 *Animal-drawn vehicles*
- 236 *Hand-drawn vehicles*
- 239 *Others*

24 **Means of Air Transport**

25 **Means of Water Transport**
- 251 *Motorized means of water transport*
- 252 *Non-motorized means of water transport*

26 **Other Means of Transport**
- 261 *Cable-cars*
- 262 *Mechanical conveyors, except cable-cars*
- 269 *Others*

3 OTHER EQUIPMENT

31 **Pressure Vessels**
- 311 *Boilers*
- 312 *Pressurized containers*
- 313 *Pressurized piping and accessories*
- 314 *Gas cylinders*
- 315 *Caissons, diving equipment*
- 319 *Others*

32 **Furnaces, Ovens, Kilns**
- 321 *Blast furnaces*
- 322 *Refining furnaces*
- 323 *Other furnaces*
- 324 *Kilns*
- 325 *Ovens*

33 **Refrigerating Plants**

34 **Electrical Installations, Including Electric Motors, but Excluding Electric Hand Tools**
- 341 *Rotating machines*
- 342 *Conductors*
- 343 *Transformers*
- 344 *Control apparatus*
- 349 *Others*

35 **Electric Hand Tools**

36 **Tools, Implements, and Appliances, Except Electric Hand Tools**
- 361 *Power-driven hand tools, except electric hand tools*
- 362 *Hand tools, not power-driven*
- 369 *Others*

37 **Ladders, Mobile Ramps**

38 **Scaffolding**

39 **Other Equipment, Not Elsewhere Classified**

4 MATERIALS, SUBSTANCES, AND RADIATIONS

41 **Explosives**

42 **Dusts, Gases, Liquids and Chemicals, Excluding Explosives**
- 421 *Dusts*
- 422 *Gases, vapors, fumes*
- 423 *Liquids, not elsewhere classified*
- 424 *Chemicals, not elsewhere classified*

43 **Flying Fragments**

44 **Radiations**
- 441 *Ionizing radiations*
- 449 *Others*

49 **Other Materials and Substances Not Elsewhere Classified**

5 WORKING ENVIRONMENT

51 **Outdoor**
511 *Weather*
512 *Traffic and working surfaces*
513 *Water*
519 *Others*

52 **Indoor**
521 *Floors*
522 *Confined quarters*
523 *Stairs*
524 *Other traffic and working surfaces*
525 *Floor openings and wall openings*
526 *Environmental factors (lighting, ventilation, temperature, noise, etc.)*
529 *Others*

53 **Underground**
531 *Roofs and faces of mine roads and tunnels, etc.*
532 *Floors of mine roads and tunnels, etc.*
533 *Working-faces of mines, tunnels, etc.*
534 *Mine shafts*
535 *Fire*
536 *Water*
539 *Others*

6 OTHER AGENCIES, NOT ELSEWHERE CLASSIFIED

61 **Animals**
611 *Live animals*
612 *Animals products*

69 **Other Agencies, Not Elsewhere Classified**

7 AGENCIES NOT CLASSIFIED FOR LACK OF SUFFICIENT DATA

APPENDIX E

LIST OF THREE-DIGIT CATEGORIES

1. INFECTIOUS AND PARASITIC DISEASES

Intestinal infectious diseases (001–009)

001 Cholera
002 Typhoid and paratyphoid fevers
003 Other salmonella infections
004 Shigellosis
005 Other food poisoning (bacterial)
006 Amebiasis
007 Other protozoal intestinal diseases
008 Intestinal infections due to other organisms
009 Ill-defined intestinal infections

Tuberculosis (010–018)

010 Primary tuberculous infection
011 Pulmonary tuberculosis
012 Other respiratory tuberculosis
013 Tuberculosis of meninges and central nervous system
014 Tuberculosis of intestines, peritoneum, and mesenteric glands
015 Tuberculosis of bones and joints
016 Tuberculosis of genitourinary system
017 Tuberculosis of other organs
018 Miliary tuberculosis

Zoonotic bacterial diseases (020–027)

020 Plague
021 Tularemia
022 Anthrax
023 Brucellosis
024 Glanders
025 Melioidosis
026 Rat-bite fever
027 Other zoonotic bacterial diseases

Other bacterial diseases (030–041)

030 Leprosy
031 Diseases due to other mycobacteria
032 Diphtheria
033 Whooping cough
034 Streptococcal sore throat and scarlet fever
035 Erysipelas
036 Meningococcal infection
037 Tetanus
038 Septicemia
039 Actinomycotic infections
040 Other bacterial diseases
041 Bacterial infection in conditions classified elsewhere and of unspecified site

Human immunodeficiency virus (042)

042 Human immunodeficiency virus [HIV] disease

Poliomyelitis and other non-arthropod-borne viral diseases of central nervous system (045–049)

045 Acute poliomyelitis
046 Slow virus infection of central nervous system
047 Meningitis due to enterovirus
048 Other enterovirus diseases of central nervous system
049 Other non-arthropod-borne viral diseases of central nervous system

Viral diseases accompanied by exanthem (050–057)

050 Smallpox
051 Cowpox and paravaccinia
052 Chickenpox
053 Herpes zoster
054 Herpes simplex
055 Measles
056 Rubella
057 Other viral exanthemata

Arthropod-borne viral diseases (060–066)

060 Yellow fever
061 Dengue
062 Mosquito-borne viral encephalitis
063 Tick-borne viral encephalitis
064 Viral encephalitis transmitted by other and unspecified arthropods
065 Arthropod-borne hemorrhagic fever
066 Other arthropod-borne viral diseases

Other diseases due to viruses and Chlamydiae (070–079)

070 Viral hepatitis
071 Rabies
072 Mumps
073 Ornithosis
074 Specific diseases due to Coxsackie virus
075 Infectious mononucleosis
076 Trachoma
077 Other diseases of conjunctiva due to viruses and Chlamydiae
078 Other diseases due to viruses and Chlamydiae
079 Viral infection in conditions classified elsewhere and of unspecified site

Rickettsioses and other arthropod-borne diseases (080–088)

080 Louse-borne [epidemic] typhus
081 Other typhus
082 Tick-borne rickettsioses
083 Other rickettsioses
084 Malaria
085 Leishmaniasis
086 Trypanosomiasis
087 Relapsing fever
088 Other arthropod-borne diseases

Syphilis and other venereal diseases (090–099)

090 Congenital syphilis
091 Early syphilis, symptomatic
092 Early syphilis, latent
093 Cardiovascular syphilis
094 Neurosyphilis
095 Other forms of late syphilis, with symptoms
096 Late syphilis, latent
097 Other and unspecified syphilis
098 Gonococcal infections
099 Other venereal diseases

Other spirochetal diseases (100–104)

100 Leptospirosis
101 Vincent's angina
102 Yaws
103 Pinta
104 Other spirochetal infection

Mycoses (110–118)

110 Dermatophytosis
111 Dermatomycosis, other and unspecified
112 Candidiasis
114 Coccidioidomycosis
115 Histoplasmosis
116 Blastomycotic infection
117 Other mycoses
118 Opportunistic mycoses

Helminthiases (120–129)

120 Schistosomiasis [bilharziasis]
121 Other trematode infections
122 Echinococcosis
123 Other cestode infection
124 Trichinosis
125 Filarial infection and dracontiasis
126 Ancylostomiasis and necatoriasis
127 Other intestinal helminthiases
128 Other and unspecified helminthiases
129 Intestinal parasitism, unspecified

Other infectious and parasitic diseases (130–136)
130 Toxoplasmosis
131 Trichomoniasis
132 Pediculosis and phthirus infestation
133 Acariasis
134 Other infestation
135 Sarcoidosis
136 Other and unspecified infectious and parasitic diseases

Late effects of infectious and parasitic diseases (137–139)
137 Late effects of tuberculosis
138 Late effects of acute poliomyelitis
139 Late effects of other infectious and parasitic diseases

2. NEOPLASMS

Malignant neoplasm of lip, oral cavity, and pharynx (140–149)
140 Malignant neoplasm of lip
141 Malignant neoplasm of tongue
142 Malignant neoplasm of major salivary glands
143 Malignant neoplasm of gum
144 Malignant neoplasm of floor of mouth
145 Malignant neoplasm of other and unspecified parts of mouth
146 Malignant neoplasm of oropharynx
147 Malignant neoplasm of nasopharynx
148 Malignant neoplasm of hypopharynx
149 Malignant neoplasm of other and ill-defined sites within the lip, oral cavity, and pharynx

Malignant neoplasm of digestive organs and peritoneum (150–159)
150 Malignant neoplasm of esophagus
151 Malignant neoplasm of stomach
152 Malignant neoplasm of small intestine, including duodenum
153 Malignant neoplasm of colon
154 Malignant neoplasm of rectum, rectosigmoid junction, and anus
155 Malignant neoplasm of liver and intrahepatic bile ducts
156 Malignant neoplasm of gallbladder and extrahepatic bile ducts
157 Malignant neoplasm of pancreas
158 Malignant neoplasm of retroperitoneum and peritoneum
159 Malignant neoplasm of other and ill-defined sites within the digestive organs and peritoneum

Malignant neoplasm of respiratory and intrathoracic organs (160–165)
160 Malignant neoplasm of nasal cavities, middle ear, and accessory sinuses
161 Malignant neoplasm of larynx
162 Malignant neoplasm of trachea, bronchus, and lung
163 Malignant neoplasm of pleura
164 Malignant neoplasm of thymus, heart, and mediastinum
165 Malignant neoplasm of other and ill-defined sites within the respiratory system and intrathoracic organs

Malignant neoplasm of bone, connective tissue, skin, and breast (170–176)
170 Malignant neoplasm of bone and articular cartilage
171 Malignant neoplasm of connective and other soft tissue
172 Malignant melanoma of skin
173 Other malignant neoplasm of skin
174 Malignant neoplasm of female breast
175 Malignant neoplasm of male breast

Kaposi's sarcoma (176)
176 Kaposi's sarcoma

Malignant neoplasm of genitourinary organs (179–189)
179 Malignant neoplasm of uterus, part unspecified
180 Malignant neoplasm of cervix uteri
181 Malignant neoplasm of placenta
182 Malignant neoplasm of body of uterus
183 Malignant neoplasm of ovary and other uterine adnexa
184 Malignant neoplasm of other and unspecified female genital organs
185 Malignant neoplasm of prostate
186 Malignant neoplasm of testis
187 Malignant neoplasm of penis and other male genital organs
188 Malignant neoplasm of bladder
189 Malignant neoplasm of kidney and other and unspecified urinary organs

Malignant neoplasm of other and unspecified sites (190–199)
190 Malignant neoplasm of eye
191 Malignant neoplasm of brain
192 Malignant neoplasm of other and unspecified parts of nervous system
193 Malignant neoplasm of thyroid gland
194 Malignant neoplasm of other endocrine glands and related structures
195 Malignant neoplasm of other and ill-defined sites
196 Secondary and unspecified malignant neoplasm of lymph nodes
197 Secondary malignant neoplasm of respiratory and digestive systems
198 Secondary malignant neoplasm of other specified sites
199 Malignant neoplasm without specification of site

Malignant neoplasm of lymphatic and hematopoietic tissue (200–208)
200 Lymphosarcoma and reticulosarcoma
201 Hodgkin's disease
202 Other malignant neoplasm of lymphoid and histiocytic tissue
203 Multiple myeloma and immunoproliferative neoplasms
204 Lymphoid leukemia
205 Myeloid leukemia
206 Monocytic leukemia
207 Other specified leukemia
208 Leukemia of unspecified cell type

Benign neoplasms (210–229)
210 Benign neoplasm of lip, oral cavity, and pharynx
211 Benign neoplasm of other parts of digestive system
212 Benign neoplasm of respiratory and intrathoracic organs
213 Benign neoplasm of bone and articular cartilage
214 Lipoma
215 Other benign neoplasm of connective and other soft tissue
216 Benign neoplasm of skin
217 Benign neoplasm of breast
218 Uterine leiomyoma
219 Other benign neoplasm of uterus
220 Benign neoplasm of ovary
221 Benign neoplasm of other female genital organs
222 Benign neoplasm of male genital organs
223 Benign neoplasm of kidney and other urinary organs
224 Benign neoplasm of eye
225 Benign neoplasm of brain and other parts of nervous system
226 Benign neoplasm of thyroid gland
227 Benign neoplasm of other endocrine glands and related structures
228 Hemangioma and lymphangioma, any site
229 Benign neoplasm of other and unspecified sites

Carcinoma in situ (230–234)
230 Carcinoma in situ of digestive organs
231 Carcinoma in situ of respiratory system
232 Carcinoma in situ of skin
233 Carcinoma in situ of breast and genitourinary system
234 Carcinoma in situ of other and unspecified sites

Neoplasms of uncertain behavior (235–238)
235 Neoplasm of uncertain behavior of digestive and respiratory systems
236 Neoplasm of uncertain behavior of genitourinary organs
237 Neoplasm of uncertain behavior of endocrine glands and nervous system
238 Neoplasm of uncertain behavior of other and unspecified sites and tissues

Neoplasms of unspecified nature (239)
239 Neoplasm of unspecified nature

3. ENDOCRINE, NUTRITIONAL AND METABOLIC DISEASES, AND IMMUNITY DISORDERS

Disorders of thyroid gland (240–246)
240 Simple and unspecified goiter
241 Nontoxic nodular goiter
242 Thyrotoxicosis with or without goiter
243 Congenital hypothyroidism
244 Acquired hypothyroidism
245 Thyroiditis
246 Other disorders of thyroid

Diseases of other endocrine glands (250–259)
250 Diabetes mellitus
251 Other disorders of pancreatic internal secretion
252 Disorders of parathyroid gland
253 Disorders of the pituitary gland and its hypothalamic control
254 Diseases of thymus gland
255 Disorders of adrenal glands
256 Ovarian dysfunction
257 Testicular dysfunction
258 Polyglandular dysfunction and related disorders
259 Other endocrine disorders

Nutritional deficiencies (260–269)
260 Kwashiorkor
261 Nutritional marasmus
262 Other severe protein-calorie malnutrition
263 Other and unspecified protein-calorie malnutrition
264 Vitamin A deficiency
265 Thiamine and niacin deficiency states
266 Deficiency of B-complex components
267 Ascorbic acid deficiency
268 Vitamin D deficiency
269 Other nutritional deficiencies

Other metabolic disorders and immunity disorders (270–279)
270 Disorders of amino-acid transport and metabolism
271 Disorders of carbohydrate transport and metabolism
272 Disorders of lipid metabolism
273 Disorders of plasma protein metabolism
274 Gout
275 Disorders of mineral metabolism
276 Disorders of fluid, electrolyte, and acid-base balance
277 Other and unspecified disorders of metabolism
278 Obesity and other hyperalimentation
279 Disorders involving the immune mechanism

4. DISEASES OF BLOOD AND BLOOD-FORMING ORGANS

Diseases of the blood and blood-forming organs (280–289)
280 Iron deficiency anemias
281 Other deficiency anemias
282 Hereditary hemolytic anemias
283 Acquired hemolytic anemias
284 Aplastic anemia
285 Other and unspecified anemias
286 Coagulation defects
287 Purpura and other hemorrhagic conditions
288 Diseases of white blood cells
289 Other diseases of blood and blood-forming organs

5. MENTAL DISORDERS

Organic psychotic conditions (290–294)
290 Senile and presenile organic psychotic conditions
291 Alcoholic psychoses
292 Drug psychoses
293 Transient organic psychotic conditions
294 Other organic psychotic conditions (chronic)

Other psychoses (295–299)
295 Schizophrenic psychoses
296 Affective psychoses
297 Paranoid states
298 Other nonorganic psychoses
299 Psychoses with origin specific to childhood

Neurotic disorders, personality disorders, and other nonpsychotic mental disorders (300–316)
300 Neurotic disorders
301 Personality disorders
302 Sexual deviations and disorders
303 Alcohol dependence syndrome
304 Drug dependence
305 Nondependent abuse of drugs
306 Physiological malfunction arising from mental factors
307 Special symptoms or syndromes, not elsewhere classified
308 Acute reaction to stress
309 Adjustment reaction
310 Specific nonpsychotic mental disorders following organic brain damage
311 Depressive disorder, not elsewhere classified
312 Disturbance of conduct, not elsewhere classified
313 Disturbance of emotions specific to childhood and adolescence
314 Hyperkinetic syndrome of childhood
315 Specific delays in development
316 Psychic factors associated with diseases classified elsewhere

Mental retardation (317–319)
317 Mild mental retardation
318 Other specified mental retardation
319 Unspecified mental retardation

6. DISEASES OF THE NERVOUS SYSTEM AND SENSE ORGANS

Inflammatory diseases of the central nervous system (320–326)
320 Bacterial meningitis
321 Meningitis due to other organisms
322 Meningitis of unspecified cause
323 Encephalitis, myelitis, and encephalomyelitis
324 Intracranial and intraspinal abscess
325 Phlebitis and thrombophlebitis of intracranial venous sinuses
326 Late effects of intracranial abscess or pyogenic infection

Hereditary and degenerative diseases of the central nervous system (330–337)
330 Cerebral degenerations usually manifest in childhood
331 Other cerebral degenerations
332 Parkinson's disease
333 Other extrapyramidal disease and abnormal movement disorders
334 Spinocerebellar disease
335 Anterior horn cell disease
336 Other diseases of spinal cord
337 Disorders of the autonomic nervous system

Other disorders of the central nervous system (340–349)
340 Multiple sclerosis
341 Other demyelinating diseases of central nervous system
342 Hemiplegia and hemiparesis
343 Infantile cerebral palsy
344 Other paralytic syndromes
345 Epilepsy
346 Migraine
347 Cataplexy and narcolepsy
348 Other conditions of brain
349 Other and unspecified disorders of the nervous system

Disorders of the peripheral nervous system (350–359)
350 Trigeminal nerve disorders
351 Facial nerve disorders
352 Disorders of other cranial nerves
353 Nerve root and plexus disorders
354 Mononeuritis of upper limb and mononeuritis multiplex
355 Mononeuritis of lower limb

356 Hereditary and idiopathic peripheral neuropathy
357 Inflammatory and toxic neuropathy
358 Myoneural disorders
359 Muscular dystrophies and other myopathies

Disorders of the eye and adnexa (360–379)
360 Disorders of the globe
361 Retinal detachments and defects
362 Other retinal disorders
363 Chorioretinal inflammations and scars and other disorders of choroid
364 Disorders of iris and ciliary body
365 Glaucoma
366 Cataract
367 Disorders of refraction and accommodation
368 Visual disturbances
369 Blindness and low vision
370 Keratitis
371 Corneal opacity and other disorders of cornea
372 Disorders of conjunctiva
373 Inflammation of eyelids
374 Other disorders of eyelids
375 Disorders of lacrimal system
376 Disorders of the orbit
377 Disorders of optic nerve and visual pathways
378 Strabismus and other disorders of binocular eye movements
379 Other disorders of eye

Diseases of the ear and mastoid process (380–389)
380 Disorders of external ear
381 Nonsuppurative otitis media and eustachian tube disorders
382 Suppurative and unspecified otitis media
383 Mastoiditis and related conditions
384 Other disorders of tympanic membrane
385 Other disorders of middle ear and mastoid
386 Vertiginous syndromes and other disorders of vestibular system
387 Otosclerosis
388 Other disorders of ear
389 Hearing loss

7. DISEASES OF THE CIRCULATORY SYSTEM

Acute rheumatic fever (390–392)
390 Rheumatic fever without mention of heart involvement
391 Rheumatic fever with heart involvement
392 Rheumatic chorea

Chronic rheumatic heart disease (393–398)
393 Chronic rheumatic pericarditis
394 Diseases of mitral valve
395 Diseases of aortic valve
396 Diseases of mitral and aortic valves
397 Diseases of other endocardial structures
398 Other rheumatic heart disease

Hypertensive disease (401–405)
401 Essential hypertension
402 Hypertensive heart disease
403 Hypertensive renal disease
404 Hypertensive heart and renal disease
405 Secondary hypertension

Ischemic heart disease (410–414)
410 Acute myocardial infarction
411 Other acute and subacute form of ischemic heart disease
412 Old myocardial infarction
413 Angina pectoris
414 Other forms of chronic ischemic heart disease

Diseases of pulmonary circulation (415–417)
415 Acute pulmonary heart disease
416 Chronic pulmonary heart disease
417 Other diseases of pulmonary circulation

Other forms of heart disease (420–429)
420 Acute pericarditis
421 Acute and subacute endocarditis
422 Acute myocarditis
423 Other diseases of pericardium
424 Other diseases of endocardium
425 Cardiomyopathy
426 Conduction disorders
427 Cardiac dysrhythmias
428 Heart failure
429 Ill-defined descriptions and complications of heart disease

Cerebrovascular disease (430–438)
430 Subarachnoid hemorrhage
431 Intracerebral hemorrhage
432 Other and unspecified intracranial hemorrhage
433 Occlusion and stenosis of precerebral arteries
434 Occlusion of cerebral arteries
435 Transcient cerebral ischemia
436 Acute but ill-defined cerebrovascular disease
437 Other and ill-defined cerebrovascular disease
438 Late effects of cerebrovascular disease

Diseases of arteries, arterioles, and capillaries (440–448)
440 Atherosclerosis
441 Aortic aneurysm and dissection
442 Other aneurysm
443 Other peripheral vascular disease
444 Arterial embolism and thrombosis
446 Polyarteritis nodosa and allied conditions
447 Other disorders of arteries and arterioles
448 Diseases of capillaries

Diseases of veins and lymphatics, and other diseases of circulatory system (451–459)
451 Phlebitis and thrombophlebitis
452 Portal vein thrombosis
453 Other venous embolism and thrombosis
454 Varicose veins of lower extremities
455 Hemorrhoids
456 Varicose veins of other sites
457 Noninfective disorders of lymphatic channels
458 Hypotension
459 Other disorders of circulatory system

8. DISEASES OF THE RESPIRATORY SYSTEM

Acute respiratory infections (460–466)
460 Acute nasopharyngitis [common cold]
461 Acute sinusitis
462 Acute pharyngitis
463 Acute tonsillitis
464 Acute laryngitis and tracheitis
465 Acute upper respiratory infections of multiple or unspecified sites
466 Acute bronchitis and bronchiolitis

Other diseases of upper respiratory tract (470–478)
470 Deviated nasal septum
471 Nasal polyps
472 Chronic pharyngitis and nasopharyngitis
473 Chronic sinusitis
474 Chronic disease of tonsils and adenoids
475 Peritonsillar abscess
476 Chronic laryngitis and laryngotracheitis
477 Allergic rhinitis
478 Other diseases of upper respiratory tract

Pneumonia and influenza (480–487)
480 Viral pneumonia
481 Pneumococcal pneumonia [*Streptococcus pneumoniae* pneumonia]
482 Other bacterial pneumonia
483 Pneumonia due to other specified organism
484 Pneumonia in infectious diseases classified elsewhere
485 Bronchopneumonia, organism unspecified

486 Pneumonia, organism unspecified
487 Influenza

Chronic obstructive pulmonary disease and allied conditions (490–496)
490 Bronchitis, not specified as acute or chronic
491 Chronic bronchitis
492 Emphysema
493 Asthma
494 Bronchiectasis
495 Extrinsic allergic alveolitis
496 Chronic airways obstruction, not elsewhere classified

Pneumoconioses and other lung diseases due to external agents (500–508)
500 Coalworkers' pneumoconiosis
501 Asbestosis
502 Pneumoconiosis due to other silica or silicates
503 Pneumoconiosis due to other inorganic dust
504 Pneumopathy due to inhalation of other dust
505 Pneumoconiosis, unspecified
506 Respiratory conditions due to chemical fumes and vapors
507 Pneumonitis due to solids and liquids
508 Respiratory conditions due to other and unspecified external agents

Other diseases of respiratory system (510–519)
510 Empyema
511 Pleurisy
512 Pneumothorax
513 Abscess of lung and mediastinum
514 Pulmonary congestion and hypostasis
515 Postinflammatory pulmonary fibrosis
516 Other alveolar and parietoalveolar pneumopathy
517 Lung involvement in conditions classified elsewhere
518 Other diseases of lung
519 Other diseases of respiratory system

9. DISEASES OF THE DIGESTIVE SYSTEM

Diseases of oral cavity, salivary glands, and jaws (520–529)
520 Disorders of tooth development and eruption
521 Diseases of hard tissues of teeth
522 Diseases of pulp and periapical tissues
523 Gingival and periodontal diseases
524 Dentofacial anomalies, including malocclusion
525 Other diseases and conditions of the teeth and supporting structures
526 Diseases of the jaws
527 Diseases of the salivary glands
528 Diseases of the oral soft tissues, excluding lesions specific for gingiva and tongue
529 Diseases and other conditions of the tongue

Diseases of esophagus, stomach, and duodenum (530–537)
530 Diseases of esophagus
531 Gastric ulcer
532 Duodenal ulcer
533 Peptic ulcer, site unspecified
534 Gastrojejunal ulcer
535 Gastritis and duodenitis
536 Disorders of function of stomach
537 Other disorders of stomach and duodenum

Appendicitis (540–543)
540 Acute appendicitis
541 Appendicitis, unqualified
542 Other appendicitis
543 Other diseases of appendix

Hernia of abdominal cavity (550–553)
550 Inguinal hernia
551 Other hernia of abdominal cavity, with gangrene
552 Other hernia of abdominal cavity, with obstruction, but without mention of gangrene
553 Other hernia of abdominal cavity without mention of obstruction or gangrene

Noninfective enteritis and colitis (555–558)
555 Regional enteritis
556 Ulcerative colitis
557 Vascular insufficiency of intestine
558 Other noninfective gastroenteritis and colitis

Other diseases of intestines and peritoneum (560–569)
560 Intestinal obstruction without mention of hernia
562 Diverticula of intestine
564 Functional digestive disorders, not elsewhere classified
565 Anal fissure and fistula
566 Abscess of anal and rectal regions
567 Peritonitis
568 Other disorders of peritoneum
569 Other disorders of intestine

Other diseases of digestive system (570–579)
570 Acute and subacute necrosis of liver
571 Chronic liver disease and cirrhosis
572 Liver abscess and sequelae of chronic liver disease
573 Other disorders of liver
574 Cholelithiasis
575 Other disorders of gallbladder
576 Other disorders of biliary tract
577 Diseases of pancreas
578 Gastrointestinal hemorrhage
579 Intestinal malabsorption

10. DISEASES OF THE GENITOURINARY SYSTEM

Nephritis, nephrotic syndrome, and nephrosis (580–589)
580 Acute glomerulonephritis
581 Nephrotic syndrome
582 Chronic glomerulonephritis
583 Nephritis and nephropathy, not specified as acute or chronic
584 Acute renal failure
585 Chronic renal failure
586 Renal failure, unspecified
587 Renal sclerosis, unspecified
588 Disorders resulting from impaired renal function
589 Small kidney of unknown cause

Other diseases of urinary system (590–599)
590 Infections of kidney
591 Hydronephrosis
592 Calculus of kidney and ureter
593 Other disorders of kidney and ureter
594 Calculus of lower urinary tract
595 Cystitis
596 Other disorders of bladder
597 Urethritis, not sexually transmitted, and urethral syndrome
598 Urethral stricture
599 Other disorders of urethra and urinary tract

Diseases of male genital organs (600–608)
600 Hyperplasia of prostate
601 Inflammatory diseases of prostate
602 Other disorders of prostate
603 Hydrocele
604 Orchitis and epididymitis
605 Redundant prepuce and phimosis
606 Infertility, male
607 Disorders of penis
608 Other disorders of male genital organs

Disorders of breast (610–611)
610 Benign mammary dysplasias
611 Other disorders of breast

Inflammatory disease of female pelvic organs (614–616)
614 Inflammatory disease of ovary, fallopian tube, pelvic cellular tissue, and peritoneum
615 Inflammatory diseases of uterus, except cervix
616 Inflammatory disease of cervix, vagina, and vulva

Other disorders of female genital tract (617–629)
617 Endometriosis
618 Genital prolapse
619 Fistula involving female genital tract
620 Noninflammatory disorders of ovary, fallopian tube, and broad ligament
621 Disorders of uterus, not elsewhere classified
622 Noninflammatory disorders of cervix
623 Noninflammatory disorders of vagina
624 Noninflammatory disorders of vulva and perineum
625 Pain and other symptoms associated with female genital organs
626 Disorders of menstruation and other abnormal bleeding from female genital tract
627 Menopausal and postmenopausal disorders
628 Infertility, female
629 Other disorders of female genital organs

11. COMPLICATIONS OF PREGNANCY, CHILDBIRTH, AND THE PUERPERIUM

Ectopic and molar pregnancy and other pregnancy with abortive outcome (630–639)
630 Hydatidiform mole
631 Other abnormal product of conception
632 Missed abortion
633 Ectopic pregnancy
634 Spontaneous abortion
635 Legally induced abortion
636 Illegally induced abortion
637 Unspecified abortion
638 Failed attempted abortion
639 Complications following abortion and ectopic and molar pregnancies

Complications mainly related to pregnancy (640–648)
640 Hemorrhage in early pregnancy
641 Antepartum hemorrhage, abruptio placentae, and placenta previa
642 Hypertension complicating pregnancy, childbirth, and the puerperium
643 Excessive vomiting in pregnancy
644 Early or threatened labor
645 Prolonged pregnancy
646 Other complications of pregnancy, not elsewhere classified
647 Infective and parasitic conditions in the mother classifiable elsewhere but complicating pregnancy, childbirth, and the puerperium
648 Other current conditions in the mother classifiable elsewhere but complicating pregnancy, childbirth, and the puerperium

Normal delivery, and other indications for care in pregnancy, labor, and delivery (650–659)
650 Normal delivery
651 Multiple gestation
652 Malposition and malpresentation of fetus
653 Disproportion
654 Abnormality of organs and soft tissues of pelvis
655 Known or suspected fetal abnormality affecting management of mother
656 Other fetal and placental problems affecting management of mother
657 Polyhydramnios
658 Other problems associated with amniotic cavity and membranes
659 Other indications for care or intervention related to labor and delivery and not elsewhere classified

Complications occurring mainly in the course of labor and delivery (660–669)
660 Obstructed labor
661 Abnormality of forces of labor
662 Long labor
663 Umbilical cord complications
664 Trauma to perineum and vulva during delivery
665 Other obstetrical trauma
666 Postpartum hemorrhage
667 Retained placenta or membranes, without hemorrhage
668 Complications of the administration of anesthetic or other sedation in labor and delivery
669 Other complications of labor and delivery, not elsewhere classified

Complications of the puerperium (670–677)
670 Major puerperal infection
671 Venous complications in pregnancy and the puerperium
672 Pyrexia of unknown origin during the puerperium
673 Obstetrical pulmonary embolism
674 Other and unspecified complications of the puerperium, not elsewhere classified
675 Infections of the breast and nipple associated with childbirth
676 Other disorders of the breast associated with childbirth, and disorders of lactation
677 Late effect of complication of pregnancy, childbirth, and the puerperium

12. DISEASES OF THE SKIN AND SUBCUTANEOUS TISSUE

Infections of skin and subcutaneous tissue (680–686)
680 Carbuncle and furuncle
681 Cellulitis and abscess of finger and toe
682 Other cellulitis and abscess
683 Acute lymphadenitis
684 Impetigo
685 Pilonidal cyst
686 Other local infections of skin and subcutaneous tissue

Other inflammatory conditions of skin and subcutaneous tissue (690–698)
690 Erythematosquamous dermatosis
691 Atopic dermatitis and related conditions
692 Contact dermatitis and other eczema
693 Dermatitis due to substances taken internally
694 Bullous dermatoses
695 Erythematous conditions
696 Psoriasis and similar disorders
697 Lichen
698 Pruritus and related conditions

Other diseases of skin and subcutaneous tissue (700–709)
700 Corns and callosities
701 Other hypertrophic and atrophic conditions of skin
702 Other dermatoses
703 Diseases of nail
704 Diseases of hair and hair follicles
705 Disorders of sweat glands
706 Diseases of sebaceous glands
707 Chronic ulcer of skin
708 Urticaria
709 Other disorders of skin and subcutaneous tissue

13. DISEASES OF THE MUSCULOSKELETAL SYSTEM AND CONNECTIVE TISSUE

Arthropathies and related disorders (710–719)
710 Diffuse diseases of connective tissue
711 Arthropathy associated with infections
712 Crystal arthropathies
713 Arthropathy associated with other disorders classified elsewhere
714 Rheumatoid arthritis and other inflammatory polyarthropathies
715 Osteoarthrosis and allied disorders
716 Other and unspecified arthropathies
717 Internal derangement of knee
718 Other derangement of joint
719 Other and unspecified disorder of joint

Dorsopathies (720–724)
720 Ankylosing spondylitis and other inflammatory spondylopathies
721 Spondylosis and allied disorders
722 Intervertebral disc disorders
723 Other disorders of cervical region
724 Other and unspecified disorders of back

Rheumatism, excluding the back (725–729)
725 Polymyalgia rheumatica
726 Peripheral enthesopathies and allied syndromes
727 Other disorders of synovium, tendon, and bursa
728 Disorders of muscle, ligament, and fascia
729 Other disorders of soft tissues

Osteopathies, chondropathies, and acquired musculoskeletal deformities (730–739)
730 Osteomyelitis, periostitis, and other infections involving bone
731 Osteitis deformans and osteopathies associated with other disorders classified elsewhere
732 Osteochondropathies
733 Other disorders of bone and cartilage
734 Flat foot
735 Acquired deformities of toe
736 Other acquired deformities of limbs
737 Curvature of spine
738 Other acquired deformity
739 Nonallopathic lesions, not elsewhere classified

14. CONGENITAL ANOMALIES

Congential anomalies (740–759)
740 Anencephalus and similar anomalies
741 Spina bifida
742 Other congenital anomalies of nervous system
743 Congenital anomalies of eye
744 Congenital anomalies of ear, face, and neck
745 Bulbus cordis anomalies and anomalies of cardiac septal closure
746 Other congenital anomalies of heart
747 Other congenital anomalies of circulatory system
748 Congenital anomalies of respiratory system
749 Cleft palate and cleft lip
750 Other congenital anomalies of upper alimentary tract
751 Other congenital anomalies of digestive system
752 Congenital anomalies of genital organs
753 Congenital anomalies of urinary system
754 Certain congenital musculoskeletal deformities
755 Other congenital anomalies of limbs
756 Other congenital musculoskeletal anomalies
757 Congenital anomalies of the integument
758 Chromosomal anomalies
759 Other and unspecified congenital anomalies

15. CERTAIN CONDITIONS ORIGINATING IN THE PERINATAL PERIOD

Maternal causes of perinatal morbidity and mortality (760–763)
760 Fetus or newborn affected by maternal conditions which may be unrelated to present pregnancy
761 Fetus or newborn affected by maternal complications of pregnancy
762 Fetus or newborn affected by complications of placenta, cord, and membranes
763 Fetus or newborn affected by other complications of labor and delivery

Other conditions originating in the perinatal period (764–779)
764 Slow fetal growth and fetal malnutrition
765 Disorders relating to short gestation and unspecified low birthweight
766 Disorders relating to long gestation and high birthweight
767 Birth trauma
768 Intrauterine hypoxia and birth asphyxia
769 Respiratory distress syndrome
770 Other respiratory conditions of fetus and newborn
771 Infections specific to the perinatal period
772 Fetal and neonatal hemorrhage
773 Hemolytic disease of fetus or newborn, due to isoimmunization
774 Other perinatal jaundice
775 Endocrine and metabolic disturbances specific to the fetus and newborn
776 Hematological disorders of fetus and newborn
777 Perinatal disorders of digestive system
778 Conditions involving the integument and temperature regulation of fetus and newborn
779 Other and ill-defined conditions originating in the perinatal period

16. SYMPTOMS, SIGNS, AND ILL-DEFINED CONDITIONS

Symptoms (780–789)
780 General symptoms
781 Symptoms involving nervous and musculoskeletal systems
782 Symptoms involving skin and other integumentary tissue
783 Symptoms concerning nutrition, metabolism, and development
784 Symptoms involving head and neck
785 Symptoms involving cardiovascular system
786 Symptoms involving respiratory system and other chest symptoms
787 Symptoms involving digestive system
788 Symptoms involving urinary system
789 Other symptoms involving abdomen and pelvis

Nonspecific abnormal findings (790–796)
790 Nonspecific findings on examination of blood
791 Nonspecific findings on examination of urine
792 Nonspecific abnormal findings in other body substances
793 Nonspecific abnormal findings on radiological and other examination of body structure
794 Nonspecific abnormal results of function studies
795 Nonspecific abnormal histological and immunological findings
796 Other nonspecific abnormal findings

Ill-defined and unknown causes of morbidity and mortality (797–799)
797 Senility without mention of psychosis
798 Sudden death, cause unknown
799 Other ill-defined and unknown causes of morbidity and mortality

17. INJURY AND POISONING

Fracture of skull (800–804)
800 Fracture of vault of skull
801 Fracture of base of skull
802 Fracture of face bones
803 Other and unqualified skull fractures
804 Multiple fractures involving skull or face with other bones

Fracture of spine and trunk (805–809)
805 Fracture of vertebral column without mention of spinal cord lesion
806 Fracture of vertebral column with spinal cord lesion
807 Fracture of rib(s), sternum, larynx, and trachea
808 Fracture of pelvis
809 Ill-defined fractures of bones of trunk

Fracture of upper limb (810–819)
810 Fracture of clavicle
811 Fracture of scapula
812 Fracture of humerus
813 Fracture of radius and ulna
814 Fracture of carpal bone(s)
815 Fracture of metacarpal bone(s)
816 Fracture of one or more phalanges of hand
817 Multiple fractures of hand bones
818 Ill-defined fractures of upper limb
819 Multiple fractures involving both upper limbs, and upper limb with rib(s) and sternum

Fracture of lower limb (820–829)
820 Fracture of neck of femur
821 Fracture of other and unspecified parts of femur
822 Fracture of patella
823 Fracture of tibia and fibula
824 Fracture of ankle
825 Fracture of one or more tarsal and metatarsal bones
826 Fracture of one or more phalanges of foot
827 Other, multiple, and ill-defined fractures of lower limb
828 Multiple fractures involving both lower limbs, lower with upper limb, and lower limb(s) with rib(s) and sternum
829 Fracture of unspecified bones

Dislocation (830–839)
830 Dislocation of jaw
831 Dislocation of shoulder
832 Dislocation of elbow
833 Dislocation of wrist
834 Dislocation of finger
835 Dislocation of hip
836 Dislocation of knee
837 Dislocation of ankle
838 Dislocation of foot
839 Other, multiple, and ill-defined dislocations

Sprains and strains of joints and adjacent muscles (840–848)
840 Sprains and strains of shoulder and upper arm
841 Sprains and strains of elbow and forearm
842 Sprains and strains of wrist and hand
843 Sprains and strains of hip and thigh
844 Sprains and strains of knee and leg
845 Sprains and strains of ankle and foot
846 Sprains and strains of sacroiliac region
847 Sprains and strains of other and unspecified parts of back
848 Other and ill-defined sprains and strains

Intracranial injury, excluding those with skull fracture (850–854)
850 Concussion
851 Cerebral laceration and contusion
852 Subarachnoid, subdural, and extradural hemorrhage, following injury
853 Other and unspecified intracranial hemorrhage following injury
854 Intracranial injury of other and unspecified nature

Internal injury of chest, abdomen, and pelvis (860–869)
860 Traumatic pneumothorax and hemothorax
861 Injury to heart and lung
862 Injury to other and unspecified intrathoracic organs
863 Injury to gastrointestinal tract
864 Injury to liver
865 Injury to spleen
866 Injury to kidney
867 Injury to pelvic organs
868 Injury to other intra-abdominal organs
869 Internal injury to unspecified or ill-defined organs

Open wound of head, neck, and trunk (870–879)
870 Open wound of ocular adnexa
871 Open wound of eyeball
872 Open wound of ear
873 Other open wound of head
874 Open wound of neck
875 Open wound of chest (wall)
876 Open wound of back
877 Open wound of buttock
878 Open wound of genital organs (external), including traumatic amputation
879 Open wound of other and unspecified sites, except limbs

Open wound of upper limb (880–887)
880 Open wound of shoulder and upper arm
881 Open wound of elbow, forearm, and wrist
882 Open wound of hand except finger(s) alone
883 Open wound of finger(s)
884 Multiple and unspecified open wound of upper limb
885 Traumatic amputation of thumb (complete) (partial)
886 Traumatic amputation of other finger(s) (complete) (partial)
887 Traumatic amputation of arm and hand (complete) (partial)

Open wound of lower limb (890–897)
890 Open wound of hip and thigh
891 Open wound of knee, leg [except thigh], and ankle
892 Open wound of foot except toe(s) alone
893 Open wound of toe(s)
894 Multiple and unspecified open wound of lower limb
895 Traumatic amputation of toe(s) (complete) (partial)
896 Traumatic amputation of foot (complete) (partial)
897 Traumatic amputation of leg(s) (complete) (partial)

Injury to blood vessels (900–904)
900 Injury to blood vessels of head and neck
901 Injury to blood vessels of thorax
902 Injury to blood vessels of abdomen and pelvis
903 Injury to blood vessels of upper extremity
904 Injury to blood vessels of lower extremity and unspecified sites

Late effects of injuries, poisonings, toxic effects, and other external causes (905–909)
905 Late effects of musculoskeletal and connective tissue injuries
906 Late effects of injuries to skin and subcutaneous tissues
907 Late effects of injuries to the nervous system
908 Late effects of other and unspecified injuries
909 Late effects of other and unspecified external causes

Superficial injury (910–919)
910 Superficial injury of face, neck, and scalp except eye
911 Superficial injury of trunk
912 Superficial injury of shoulder and upper arm
913 Superficial injury of elbow, forearm, and wrist
914 Superficial injury of hand(s) except finger(s) alone
915 Superficial injury of finger(s)
916 Superficial injury of hip, thigh, leg, and ankle
917 Superficial injury of foot and toe(s)
918 Superficial injury of eye and adnexa
919 Superficial injury of other, multiple, and unspecified sites

Contusion with intact skin surface (920–924)
920 Contusion of face, scalp, and neck except eye(s)
921 Contusion of eye and adnexa
922 Contusion of trunk
923 Contusion of upper limb
924 Contusion of lower limb and of other and unspecified sites

Crushing injury (925–929)
925 Crushing injury of face, scalp, and neck
926 Crushing injury of trunk
927 Crushing injury of upper limb
928 Crushing injury of lower limb
929 Crushing injury of multiple and unspecified sites

Effects of foreign body entering through orifice (930–939)
930 Foreign body on external eye
931 Foreign body in ear
932 Foreign body in nose
933 Foreign body in pharynx and larynx
934 Foreign body in trachea, bronchus, and lung
935 Foreign body in mouth, esophagus, and stomach
936 Foreign body in intestine and colon
937 Foreign body in anus and rectum
938 Foreign body in digestive system, unspecified
939 Foreign body in genitourinary tract

Burns (940–949)
940 Burn confined to eye and adnexa
941 Burn of face, head, and neck
942 Burn of trunk
943 Burn of upper limb, except wrist and hand
944 Burn of wrist(s) and hand(s)
945 Burn of lower limb(s)
946 Burns of multiple specified sites
947 Burn of internal organs

948 Burns classified according to extent of body surface involved
949 Burn, unspecified

Injury to nerves and spinal cord (950–957)
950 Injury to optic nerve and pathways
951 Injury to other cranial nerve(s)
952 Spinal cord injury without evidence of spinal bone injury
953 Injury to nerve roots and spinal plexus
954 Injury to other nerve(s) of trunk excluding shoulder and pelvic girdles
955 Injury to peripheral nerve(s) of shoulder girdle and upper limb
956 Injury to peripheral nerve(s) of pelvic girdle and lower limb
957 Injury to other and unspecified nerves

Certain traumatic complications and unspecified injuries (958–959)
958 Certain early complications of trauma
959 Injury, other and unspecified

Poisoning by drugs, medicinals, and biological substances (960–979)
960 Poisoning by antibiotics
961 Poisoning by other anti-infectives
962 Poisoning by hormones and synthetic substitutes
963 Poisoning by primarily systemic agents
964 Poisoning by agents primarily affecting blood constituents
965 Poisoning by analgesics, antipyretics, and antirheumatics
966 Poisoning by anticonvulsants and anti-parkinsonism drugs
967 Poisoning by sedatives and hypnotics
968 Poisoning by other central nervous system depressants and anesthetics
969 Poisoning by psychotropic agents
970 Poisoning by central nervous system stimulants
971 Poisoning by drugs primarily affecting the autonomic nervous system
972 Poisoning by agents primarily affecting the cardiovascular system
973 Poisoning by agents primarily affecting the gastrointestinal system
974 Poisoning by water, mineral, and uric acid metabolism drugs
975 Poisoning by agents primarily acting on the smooth and skeletal muscles and respiratory system
976 Poisoning by agents primarily affecting skin and mucous membrane, ophthalmological, otorhinolaryngological, and dental drugs
977 Poisoning by other and unspecified drugs and medicinals
978 Poisoning by bacterial vaccines
979 Poisoning by other vaccines and biological substances

Toxic effects of substances chiefly nonmedicinal as to source (980–989)
980 Toxic effect of alcohol
981 Toxic effect of petroleum products
982 Toxic effect of solvents other than petroleum-based
983 Toxic effect of corrosive aromatics, acids, and caustic alkalis
984 Toxic effect of lead and its compounds (including fumes)
985 Toxic effect of other metals
986 Toxic effect of carbon monoxide
987 Toxic effect of other gases, fumes, or vapors
988 Toxic effect of noxious substances eaten as food
989 Toxic effect of other substances, chiefly nonmedicinal as to source

Other and unspecified effects of external causes (990–995)
990 Effects of radiation, unspecified
991 Effects of reduced temperature
992 Effects of heat and light
993 Effects of air pressure
994 Effects of other external causes
995 Certain adverse effects, not elsewhere classified

Complications of surgical and medical care, not elsewhere classified (996–999)
996 Complications peculiar to certain specified procedures
997 Complications affecting specified body systems, not elsewhere classified
998 Other complications of procedures, not elsewhere classified
999 Complications of medical care, not elsewhere classified

SUPPLEMENTARY CLASSIFICATION OF FACTORS INFLUENCING HEALTH STATUS AND CONTACT WITH HEALTH SERVICES

Persons with potential health hazards related to communicable diseases (V01–V09)
V01 Contact with or exposure to communicable diseases
V02 Carrier or suspected carrier of infectious diseases
V03 Need for prophylactic vaccination and inoculation against bacterial diseases
V04 Need for prophylactic vaccination and inoculation against certain viral diseases
V05 Need for other prophylactic vaccination and inoculation against single diseases
V06 Need for prophylactic vaccination and inoculation against combinations of diseases
V07 Need for isolation and other prophylactic measures
V08 Asymptomatic human immunodeficiency virus [HIV] infection status
V09 Infection with drug-resistant microorganisms

Persons with potential health hazards related to personal and family history (V10–V19)
V10 Personal history of malignant neoplasm
V11 Personal history of mental disorder
V12 Personal history of certain other diseases
V13 Personal history of other diseases
V14 Personal history of allergy to medicinal agents
V15 Other personal history presenting hazards to health
V16 Family history of malignant neoplasm
V17 Family history of certain chronic disabling diseases
V18 Family history of certain other specific conditions
V19 Family history of other conditions

Persons encountering health services in circumstances related to reproduction and development (V20–V29)
V20 Health supervision of infant or child
V21 Constitutional states in development
V22 Normal pregnancy
V23 Supervision of high-risk pregnancy
V24 Postpartum care and examination
V25 Encounter for contraceptive management
V26 Procreative management
V27 Outcome of delivery
V28 Antenatal screening
V29 Observation and evaluation of newborns and infants for suspected condition not found

Liveborn infants according to type of birth (V30–V39)
V30 Single liveborn
V31 Twin, mate liveborn
V32 Twin, mate stillborn
V33 Twin, unspecified
V34 Other multiple, mates all liveborn
V35 Other multiple, mates all stillborn
V36 Other multiple, mates live- and stillborn
V37 Other multiple, unspecified
V39 Unspecified

Persons with a condition influencing their health status (V40–V49)
V40 Mental and behavioral problems
V41 Problems with special senses and other special functions
V42 Organ or tissue replaced by transplant
V43 Organ or tissue replaced by other means
V44 Artificial opening status
V45 Other postsurgical states
V46 Other dependence on machines
V47 Other problems with internal organs
V48 Problems with head, neck, and trunk
V49 Problems with limbs and other problems

Persons encountering health services for specific procedures and aftercare (V50–V59)

V50 Elective surgery for purposes other than remedying health states
V51 Aftercare involving the use of plastic surgery
V52 Fitting and adjustment of prosthetic device
V53 Fitting and adjustment of other device
V54 Other orthopedic aftercare
V55 Attention to artificial openings
V56 Encounter for dialysis and dialysis catheter care
V57 Care involving use of rehabilitation procedures
V58 Other and unspecified aftercare
V59 Donors

Persons encountering health services in other circumstances (V60–V69)

V60 Housing, household, and economic circumstances
V61 Other family circumstances
V62 Other psychosocial circumstances
V63 Unavailability of other medical facilities for care
V64 Persons encountering health services for specific procedures, not carried out
V65 Other persons seeking consultation without complaint or sickness
V66 Convalescence and palliative care
V67 Follow-up examination
V68 Encounters for administrative purposes
V69 Problems related to lifestyle

Persons without reported diagnosis encountered during examination and investigation of individuals and populations (V70–V82)

V70 General medical examination
V71 Observation and evaluation for suspected conditions
V72 Special investigations and examinations
V73 Special screening examination for viral and chlamydial diseases
V74 Special screening examination for bacterial and spirochetal diseases
V75 Special screening examination for other infectious diseases
V76 Special screening for malignant neoplasms
V77 Special screening for endocrine, nutritional, metabolic, and immunity disorders
V78 Special screening for disorders of blood and blood-forming organs
V79 Special screening for mental disorders and developmental handicaps
V80 Special screening for neurological, eye, and ear diseases
V81 Special screening for cardiovascular, respiratory, and genitourinary diseases
V82 Special screening for other conditions

SUPPLEMENTARY CLASSIFICATION OF EXTERNAL CAUSES OF INJURY AND POISONING

Railway accidents (E800–E807)

E800 Railway accident involving collision with rolling stock
E801 Railway accident involving collision with other object
E802 Railway accident involving derailment without antecedent collision
E803 Railway accident involving explosion, fire, or burning
E804 Fall in, on, or from railway train
E805 Hit by rolling stock
E806 Other specified railway accident
E807 Railway accident of unspecified nature

Motor vehicle traffic accidents (E810–E819)

E810 Motor vehicle traffic accident involving collision with train
E811 Motor vehicle traffic accident involving re-entrant collision with another motor vehicle
E812 Other motor vehicle traffic accident involving collision with another motor vehicle
E813 Motor vehicle traffic accident involving collision with other vehicle
E814 Motor vehicle traffic accident involving collision with pedestrian
E815 Other motor vehicle traffic accident involving collision on the highway
E816 Motor vehicle traffic accident due to loss of control, without collision on the highway
E817 Noncollision motor vehicle traffic accident while boarding or alighting
E818 Other noncollision motor vehicle traffic accident
E819 Motor vehicle traffic accident of unspecified nature

Motor vehicle nontraffic accidents (E820–E825)

E820 Nontraffic accident involving motor-driven snow vehicle
E821 Nontraffic accident involving other off-road motor vehicle
E822 Other motor vehicle nontraffic accident involving collision with moving object
E823 Other motor vehicle nontraffic accident involving collision with stationary object
E824 Other motor vehicle nontraffic accident while boarding and alighting
E825 Other motor vehicle nontraffic accident of other and unspecified nature

Other road vehicle accidents (E826–E829)

E826 Pedal cycle accident
E827 Animal-drawn vehicle accident
E828 Accident involving animal being ridden
E829 Other road vehicle accidents

Water transport accidents (E830–E838)

E830 Accident to watercraft causing submersion
E831 Accident to watercraft causing other injury
E832 Other accidental submersion or drowning in water transport accident
E833 Fall on stairs or ladders in water transport
E834 Other fall from one level to another in water transport
E835 Other and unspecified fall in water transport
E836 Machinery accident in water transport
E837 Explosion, fire, or burning in watercraft
E838 Other and unspecified water transport accident

Air and space transport accidents (E840–E845)

E840 Accident to powered aircraft at takeoff or landing
E841 Accident to powered aircraft, other and unspecified
E842 Accident to unpowered aircraft
E843 Fall in, on, or from aircraft
E844 Other specified air transport accidents
E845 Accident involving spacecraft

Vehicle accidents, not elsewhere classifiable (E846–E849)

E846 Accidents involving powered vehicles used solely within the buildings and premises of an industrial or commercial establishment
E847 Accidents involving cable cars not running on rails
E848 Accidents involving other vehicles, not elsewhere classifiable
E849 Place of occurrence

Accidental poisoning by drugs, medicinal substances, and biologicals (E850–E858)

E850 Accidental poisoning by analgesics, antipyretics, and antirheumatics
E851 Accidental poisoning by barbiturates
E852 Accidental poisoning by other sedatives and hypnotics
E853 Accidental poisoning by tranquilizers
E854 Accidental poisoning by other psychotropic agents
E855 Accidental poisoning by other drugs acting on central and autonomic nervous systems
E856 Accidental poisoning by antibiotics
E857 Accidental poisoning by anti-infectives
E858 Accidental poisoning by other drugs

Accidental poisoning by other solid and liquid substances, gases, and vapors (E860–E869)

E860 Accidental poisoning by alcohol, not elsewhere classified
E861 Accidental poisoning by cleansing and polishing agents, disinfectants, paints, and varnishes
E862 Accidental poisoning by petroleum products, other solvents and their vapors, not elsewhere classified

E863 Accidental poisoning by agricultural and horticultural chemical and pharmaceutical preparations other than plant foods and fertilizers
E864 Accidental poisoning by corrosives and caustics, not elsewhere classified
E865 Accidental poisoning from poisonous foodstuffs and poisonous plants
E866 Accidental poisoning by other and unspecified solid and liquid substances
E867 Accidental poisoning by gas distributed by pipeline
E868 Accidental poisoning by other utility gas and other carbon monoxide
E869 Accidental poisoning by other gases and vapors

Misadventures to patients during surgical and medical care (E870–E876)
E870 Accidental cut, puncture, perforation, or hemorrhage during medical care
E871 Foreign object left in body during procedure
E872 Failure of sterile precautions during procedure
E873 Failure in dosage
E874 Mechanical failure of instrument or apparatus during procedure
E875 Contaminated or infected blood, other fluid, drug, or biological substance
E876 Other and unspecified misadventures during medical care

Surgical and medical procedures as the cause of abnormal reaction of patient or later complication, without mention of misadventure at the time of procedure (E878–E879)
E878 Surgical operation and other surgical procedures as the cause of abnormal reaction of patient, or of later complication, without mention of misadventure at the time of operation
E879 Other procedures, without mention of misadventure at the time of procedure, as the cause of abnormal reaction of patient, or of later complication

Accidental falls (E880–E888)
E880 Fall on or from stairs or steps
E881 Fall on or from ladders or scaffolding
E882 Fall from or out of building or other structure
E883 Fall into hole or other opening in surface
E884 Other fall from one level to another
E885 Fall on same level from slipping, tripping, or stumbling
E886 Fall on same level from collision, pushing, or shoving, by or with other person
E887 Fracture, cause unspecified
E888 Other and unspecified fall

Accidents caused by fire and flames (E890–E899)
E890 Conflagration in private dwelling
E891 Conflagration in other and unspecified building or structure
E892 Conflagration not in building or structure
E893 Accident caused by ignition of clothing
E894 Ignition of highly inflammable material
E895 Accident caused by controlled fire in private dwelling
E896 Accident caused by controlled fire in other and unspecified building or structure
E897 Accident caused by controlled fire not in building or structure
E898 Accident caused by other specified fire and flames
E899 Accident caused by unspecified fire

Accidents due to natural and environmental factors (E900–E909)
E900 Excessive heat
E901 Excessive cold
E902 High and low air pressure and changes in air pressure
E903 Travel and motion
E904 Hunger, thirst, exposure, and neglect
E905 Venomous animals and plants as the cause of poisoning and toxic reactions
E906 Other injury caused by animals
E907 Lightning
E908 Cataclysmic storms, and floods resulting from storms
E909 Cataclysmic earth surface movements and eruptions

Accidents caused by submersion, suffocation, and foreign bodies (E910–E915)
E910 Accidental drowning and submersion
E911 Inhalation and ingestion of food causing obstruction of respiratory tract or suffocation
E912 Inhalation and ingestion of other object causing obstruction of respiratory tract or suffocation
E913 Accidental mechanical suffocation
E914 Foreign body accidentally entering eye and adnexa
E915 Foreign body accidentally entering other orifice

Other accidents (E916–E928)
E916 Struck accidentally by falling object
E917 Striking against or struck accidentally by objects or persons
E918 Caught accidentally in or between objects
E919 Accidents caused by machinery
E920 Accidents caused by cutting and piercing instruments or objects
E921 Accident caused by explosion of pressure vessel
E922 Accident caused by firearm missile
E923 Accident caused by explosive material
E924 Accident caused by hot substance or object, caustic or corrosive material, and steam
E925 Accident caused by electric current
E926 Exposure to radiation
E927 Overexertion and strenuous movements
E928 Other and unspecified environmental and accidental causes

Late effects of accidental injury (E929)
E929 Late effects of accidental injury

Drugs, medicinal and biological substances causing adverse effects in therapeutic use (E930–E949)
E930 Antibiotics
E931 Other anti-infectives
E932 Hormones and synthetic substitutes
E933 Primarily systemic agents
E934 Agents primarily affecting blood constituents
E935 Analgesics, antipyretics, and antirheumatics
E936 Anticonvulsants and anti-parkinsonism drugs
E937 Sedatives and hypnotics
E938 Other central nervous system depressants and anesthetics
E939 Psychotropic agents
E940 Central nervous system stimulants
E941 Drugs primarily affecting the autonomic nervous system
E942 Agents primarily affecting the cardiovascular system
E943 Agents primarily affecting gastrointestinal system
E944 Water, mineral, and uric acid metabolism drugs
E945 Agents primarily acting on the smooth and skeletal muscles and respiratory system
E946 Agents primarily affecting skin and mucous membrane, ophthalmological, otorhinolaryngological, and dental drugs
E947 Other and unspecified drugs and medicinal substances
E948 Bacterial vaccines
E949 Other vaccines and biological substances

Suicide and self-inflicted injury (E950–E959)
E950 Suicide and self-inflicted poisoning by solid or liquid substances
E951 Suicide and self-inflicted poisoning by gases in domestic use
E952 Suicide and self-inflicted poisoning by other gases and vapors
E953 Suicide and self-inflicted injury by hanging, strangulation, and suffocation
E954 Suicide and self-inflicted injury by submersion [drowning]
E955 Suicide and self-inflicted injury by firearms and explosives
E956 Suicide and self-inflicted injury by cutting and piercing instruments
E957 Suicide and self-inflicted injuries by jumping from high place
E958 Suicide and self-inflicted injury by other and unspecified means
E959 Late effects of self-inflicted injury

Homicide and injury purposely inflicted by other persons (E960–E969)

E960 Fight, brawl, and rape
E961 Assault by corrosive or caustic substance, except poisoning
E962 Assault by poisoning
E963 Assault by hanging and strangulation
E964 Assault by submersion [drowning]
E965 Assault by firearms and explosives
E966 Assault by cutting and piercing instrument
E967 Child and adult battering and other maltreatment
E968 Assault by other and unspecified means
E969 Late effects of injury purposely inflicted by other person

Legal intervention (E970–E978)

E970 Injury due to legal intervention by firearms
E971 Injury due to legal intervention by explosives
E972 Injury due to legal intervention by gas
E973 Injury due to legal intervention by blunt object
E974 Injury due to legal intervention by cutting and piercing instruments
E975 Injury due to legal intervention by other specified means
E976 Injury due to legal intervention by unspecified means
E977 Late effects of injuries due to legal intervention
E978 Legal execution

Injury undetermined whether accidentally or purposely inflicted (E980–E989)

E980 Poisoning by solid or liquid substances, undetermined whether accidentally or purposely inflicted
E981 Poisoning by gases in domestic use, undetermined whether accidentally or purposely inflicted
E982 Poisoning by other gases, undetermined whether accidentally or purposely inflicted
E983 Hanging, strangulation, or suffocation, undetermined whether accidentally or purposely inflicted
E984 Submersion [drowning], undetermined whether accidentally or purposely inflicted
E985 Injury by firearms and explosives, undetermined whether accidentally or purposely inflicted
E986 Injury by cutting and piercing instruments, undetermined whether accidentally or purposely inflicted
E987 Falling from high place, undetermined whether accidentally or purposely inflicted
E988 Injury by other and unspecified means, undetermined whether accidentally or purposely inflicted
E989 Late effects of injury, undetermined whether accidentally or purposely inflicted

Injury resulting from operations of war (E990–E999)

E990 Injury due to war operations by fires and conflagrations
E991 Injury due to war operations by bullets and fragments
E992 Injury due to war operations by explosion of marine weapons
E993 Injury due to war operations by other explosion
E994 Injury due to war operations by destruction of aircraft
E995 Injury due to war operations by other and unspecified forms of conventional warfare
E996 Injury due to war operations by nuclear weapons
E997 Injury due to war operations by other forms of unconventional warfare
E998 Injury due to war operations but occurring after cessation of hostilities
E999 Late effects of injury due to war operations

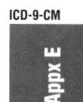
Appx E

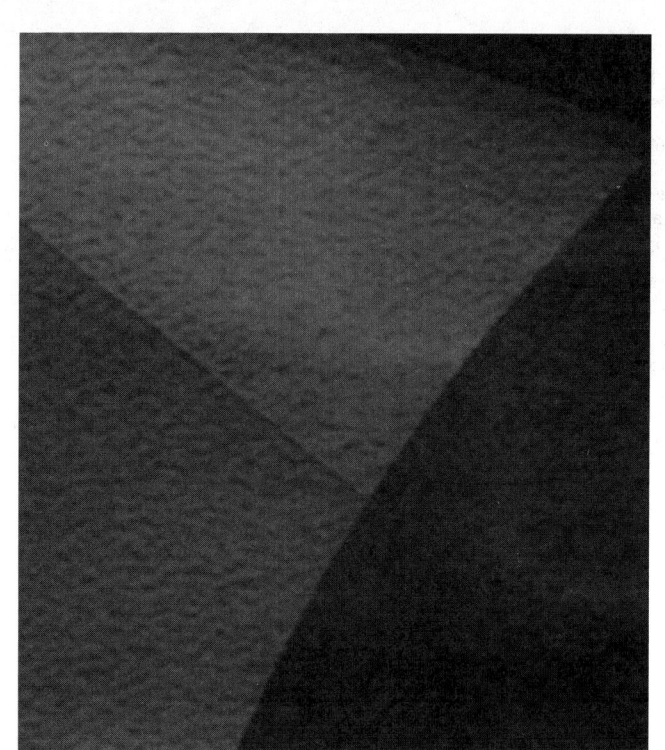

PART IV

Procedures Volume 3

A

Abbe operation
construction of vagina 70.61
intestinal anastomosis - *see* Anastomosis, intestine
Abciximab, infusion 99.20
Abdominocentesis 54.91
Abdominohysterectomy 68.49
laparoscopic 68.41
Abdominoplasty 86.83
Abdominoscopy 54.21
Abdominouterotomy 68.0
obstetrical 74.99
Abduction, arytenoid 31.69
Ablation
biliary tract (lesion) by ERCP 51.64
endometrial (hysteroscopic) 68.23
inner ear (cryosurgery) (ultrasound) 20.79
by injection 20.72
lesion
esophagus 42.39
endoscopic 42.33
heart
by peripherally inserted catheter 37.34
endovascular approach 37.34
Maze procedure (Cox-maze)
endovascular approach 37.34
open (trans-thoracic) approach 37.33
trans-thoracic approach 37.33
intestine
large 45.49
endoscopic 45.43
large intestine 45.49
endoscopic 45.43
liver 50.26
laparoscopic 50.25
open 50.23
percutaneous 50.24
lung 32.26
open 32.23
percutaneous 32.24
thoracoscopic 32.25
renal 55.35
laparoscopic 55.34
open 55.32
percutaneous 55.33
pituitary 07.69
by
Cobalt-60 92.32
implantation (strontium-yttrium) (Y) NEC 07.68
transfrontal approach 07.64
transsphenoidal approach 07.65
proton beam (Bragg peak) 92.33
prostate
by
cryoablation 60.62
laser, transurethral 60.21
radical cryosurgical ablation (RCSA) 60.62
radiofrequency thermotherapy 60.97
transurethral needle ablation (TUNA) 60.97
tissue
heart - *see* Ablation, lesion, heart
liver – *see* Ablation, lesion, liver
lung – *see* Ablation, lesion, lung
renal – *see* Ablation, lesion, renal
Abortion, therapeutic 69.51
by
aspiration curettage 69.51
dilation and curettage 69.01
hysterectomy - *see* Hysterectomy
hysterotomy 74.91
insertion
laminaria 69.93
prostaglandin suppository 96.49
intra-amniotic injection (saline) 75.0
Abrasion
corneal epithelium 11.41
for smear or culture 11.21
epicardial surface 36.39
pleural 34.6
skin 86.25
Abscission, cornea 11.49
Absorptiometry
photon (dual) (single) 88.98
Aburel operation (intra-amniotic injection for abortion) 75.0
Accouchement forcé 73.99
Acetabulectomy 77.85
Acetabuloplasty NEC 81.40
with prosthetic implant 81.52
Achillorrhaphy 83.64
delayed 83.62
Achillotenotomy 83.11
plastic 83.85
Achillotomy 83.11
plastic 83.85
Acid peel, skin 86.24
Acromionectomy 77.81
Acromioplasty 81.83
for recurrent dislocation of shoulder 81.82
partial replacement 81.81
total replacement 81.80
Actinotherapy 99.82
Activities of daily living (ADL)
therapy 93.83
training for the blind 93.78
Acupuncture 99.92
with smouldering moxa 93.35
for anesthesia 99.91
Adams operation
advancement of round ligament 69.22
crushing of nasal septum 21.88
excision of palmar fascia 82.35
Adenectomy - *see also* Excision, by site
prostate NEC 60.69
retropubic 60.4
Adenoidectomy (without tonsillectomy) 28.6
with tonsillectomy 28.3
Adhesiolysis - *see also* Lysis, adhesions
for collapse of lung 33.39
middle ear 20.23
Adipectomy 86.83
Adjustment
cardiac pacemaker program (reprogramming) - *omit code*
cochlear prosthetic device (external components) 95.49
dental 99.97
gastric restrictive device (laparoscopic) 44.98
occlusal 24.8
spectacles 95.31
Administration (of) - *see also* Injection
Activase® 99.10
adhesion barrier substance 99.77
Alteplase (tPA, generic) 99.10
Administration (of) *(Continued)*
Anistreplase (tPA, generic) 99.10
antitoxins NEC 99.58
botulism 99.57
diphtheria 99.58
gas gangrene 99.58
scarlet fever 99.58
tetanus 99.56
Bender Visual-Motor Gestalt test 94.02
Benton Visual Retention test 94.02
DrotAA 00.11
Eminase® 99.10
inhaled nitric oxide 00.12
intelligence test or scale (Stanford-Binet) (Wechsler) (adult) (children) 94.01
Minnesota Multiphasic Personality Inventory (MMPI) 94.02
MMPI (Minnesota Multiphasic Personality Inventory) 94.02
neuroprotective agent 99.75
psychologic test 94.02
Retavase® 99.10
Reteplase (tPA, generic) 99.10
Stanford-Binet test 94.01
Streptase® 99.10
Streptokinase (tPA, generic) 99.10
Tenecteplase (tPA, generic) 99.10
TNKase™ 99.10
toxoid
diphtheria 99.36
with tetanus and pertussis, combined (DTP) 99.39
tetanus 99.38
with diphtheria and pertussis, combined (DTP) 99.39
vaccine - *see also* Vaccination
BCG 99.33
measles-mumps-rubella (MMR) 99.48
poliomyelitis 99.41
TAB 99.32
Wechsler
Intelligence Scale (adult) (children) 94.01
Memory Scale 94.02
Xigris® 00.11
Adrenalectomy (unilateral) 07.22
with partial removal of remaining gland 07.29
bilateral 07.3
partial 07.29
subtotal 07.29
complete 07.3
partial NEC 07.29
remaining gland 07.3
subtotal NEC 07.29
total 07.3
Adrenalorrhaphy 07.44
Adrenalotomy (with drainage) 07.41
Advancement
extraocular muscle 15.12
multiple (with resection or recession) 15.3
eyelid muscle 08.59
eye muscle 15.12
multiple (with resection or recession) 15.3
graft - *see* Graft
leaflet (heart) 35.10
pedicle (flap) 86.72
profundus tendon (Wagner) 82.51
round ligament 69.22
tendon 83.71

New Revised

Advancement *(Continued)*
tendon *(Continued)*
hand 82.51
profundus (Wagner) 82.51
Wagner (profundus tendon) 82.51
Albee operation
bone peg, femoral neck 78.05
graft for slipping patella 78.06
sliding inlay graft, tibia 78.07
Albert operation (arthrodesis of knee) 81.22
Aldridge (-Studdiford) operation (urethral sling) 59.5
Alexander operation
prostatectomy
perineal 60.62
suprapubic 60.3
shortening of round ligaments 69.22
Alexander-Adams operation (shortening of round ligaments) 69.22
Alimentation, parenteral 99.29
Allograft - *see* Graft
Almoor operation (extrapetrosal drainage) 20.22
Altemeier operation (perineal rectal pull-through) 48.49
Alveolectomy (interradicular) (intraseptal) (radical) (simple) (with graft) (with implant) 24.5
Alveoloplasty (with graft or implant) 24.5
Alveolotomy (apical) 24.0
Ambulatory cardiac monitoring (ACM) 89.50
Ammon operation (dacryocystotomy) 09.53
Amniocentesis (transuterine) (diagnostic) 75.1
with intra-amniotic injection of saline 75.0
Amniography 87.81
Amnioinfusion 75.37
Amnioscopy, internal 75.31
Amniotomy 73.09
to induce labor 73.01
Amputation (cineplastic) (closed flap) (guillotine) (kineplastic) (open) 84.91
abdominopelvic 84.19
above-elbow 84.07
above-knee (AK) 84.17
ankle (disarticulation) 84.13
through malleoli of tibia and fibula 84.14
arm NEC 84.00
through
carpals 84.03
elbow (disarticulation) 84.06
forearm 84.05
humerus 84.07
shoulder (disarticulation) 84.08
wrist (disarticulation) 84.04
upper 84.07
Batch-Spittler-McFaddin (knee disarticulation) 84.16
below-knee (BK) NEC 84.15
conversion into above-knee amputation 84.17
Boyd (hip disarticulation) 84.18
Callander's (knee disarticulation) 84.16
carpals 84.03
cervix 67.4
Chopart's (midtarsal) 84.12
clitoris 71.4
Dieffenbach (hip disarticulation) 84.18

Amputation *(Continued)*
Dupuytren's (shoulder disarticulation) 84.08
ear, external 18.39
elbow (disarticulation) 84.06
finger, except thumb 84.01
thumb 84.02
foot (middle) 84.12
forearm 84.05
forefoot 84.12
forequarter 84.09
Gordon-Taylor (hindquarter) 84.19
Gritti-Stokes (knee disarticulation) 84.16
Guyon (ankle) 84.13
hallux 84.11
hand 84.03
Hey's (foot) 84.12
hindquarter 84.19
hip (disarticulation) 84.18
humerus 84.07
interscapulothoracic 84.09
interthoracoscapular 84.09
King-Steelquist (hindquarter) 84.19
Kirk (thigh) 84.17
knee (disarticulation) 84.16
Kutler (revision of current traumatic amputation of finger) 84.01
Larry (shoulder disarticulation) 84.08
leg NEC 84.10
above knee (AK) 84.17
below knee (BK) 84.15
through
ankle (disarticulation) 84.13
femur (AK) 84.17
foot 84.12
hip (disarticulation) 84.18
tibia and fibula (BK) 84.15
Lisfranc
foot 84.12
shoulder (disarticulation) 84.08
Littlewood (forequarter) 84.09
lower limb NEC (*see also* Amputation, leg) 84.10
Mazet (knee disarticulation) 84.16
metacarpal 84.03
metatarsal 84.11
head (bunionectomy) 77.59
metatarsophalangeal (joint) 84.11
midtarsal 84.12
nose 21.4
penis (circle) (complete) (flap) (partial) (radical) 64.3
Pirogoff's (ankle amputation through malleoli of tibia and fibula) 84.14
ray
finger 84.01
foot 84.11
toe (metatarsal head) 84.11
root (tooth) (apex) 23.73
with root canal therapy 23.72
shoulder (disarticulation) 84.08
Sorondo-Ferre (hindquarter) 84.19
S. P. Rogers (knee disarticulation) 84.16
supracondylar, above-knee 84.17
supramalleolar, foot 84.14
Syme's (ankle amputation through malleoli of tibia and fibula) 84.14
thigh 84.17
thumb 84.02
toe (through metatarsophalangeal joint) 84.11

Amputation *(Continued)*
transcarpal 84.03
transmetatarsal 84.12
upper limb NEC (*see also* Amputation, arm) 84.00
wrist (disarticulation) 84.04
Amygdalohippocampotomy 01.39
Amygdalotomy 01.39
Analysis
cardiac rhythm device (CRT-D) (CRT-P) (AICD) (pacemaker) - *see* Interrogation
character 94.03
gastric 89.39
psychologic 94.31
transactional
group 94.44
individual 94.39
Anastomosis
abdominal artery to coronary artery 36.17
accessory-facial nerve 04.72
accessory-hypoglossal nerve 04.73
anus (with formation of endorectal ileal pouch) 45.95
aorta (descending)-pulmonary (artery) 39.0
aorta-renal artery 39.24
aorta-subclavian artery 39.22
aortoceliac 39.26
aorto(ilio)femoral 39.25
aortomesenteric 39.26
appendix 47.99
arteriovenous NEC 39.29
for renal dialysis 39.27
artery (suture of distal to proximal end) 39.31
with
bypass graft 39.29
extracranial-intracranial [EC-IC] 39.28
excision or resection of vessel - *see* Arteriectomy, with anastomosis, by site
revision 39.49
bile ducts 51.39
bladder NEC 57.88
with
isolated segment of intestine 57.87 *[45.50]*
colon (sigmoid) 57.87 *[45.52]*
ileum 57.87 *[45.51]*
open loop of ileum 57.87 *[45.51]*
to intestine 57.88
ileum 57.87 *[45.51]*
bowel - *see also* Anastomosis, intestine 45.90
bronchotracheal 33.48
bronchus 33.48
carotid-subclavian artery 39.22
caval-mesenteric vein 39.1
caval-pulmonary artery 39.21
cervicoesophageal 42.59
colohypopharyngeal (intrathoracic) 42.55
antesternal or antethoracic 42.65
common bile duct 51.39
common pulmonary trunk and left atrium (posterior wall) 35.82
cystic bile duct 51.39
cystocolic 57.88
epididymis to vas deferens 63.83
esophagocolic (intrathoracic) NEC 42.56
with interposition 42.55

Anastomosis *(Continued)*
esophagocolic *(Continued)*
antesternal or antethoracic NEC 42.66
with interposition 42.65
esophagocologastric (intrathoracic) 42.55
antesternal or antethoracic 42.65
esophagoduodenal (intrathoracic) NEC 42.54
with interposition 42.53
esophagoenteric (intrathoracic) NEC - *see also* Anastomosis, esophagus, to intestinal segment 42.54
antesternal or antethoracic NEC - *see also* Anastomosis, esophagus, antesternal, to intestinal segment 42.64
esophagoesophageal (intrathoracic) 42.51
antesternal or antethoracic 42.61
esophagogastric (intrathoracic) 42.52
antesternal or antethoracic 42.62
esophagus (intrapleural) (intrathoracic) (retrosternal) NEC 42.59
with
gastrectomy (partial) 43.5
complete or total 43.99
interposition (of) NEC 42.58
colon 42.55
jejunum 42.53
small bowel 42.53
antesternal or antethoracic NEC 42.69
antesternal or antethoracic NEC
with
interposition (of) NEC 42.68
colon 42.65
jejunal loop 42.63
small bowel 42.63
rubber tube 42.68
to intestinal segment NEC 42.64
with interposition 42.68
colon NEC 42.66
with interposition 42.65
small bowel NEC 42.64
with interposition 42.63
to intestinal segment (intrathoracic) NEC 42.54
with interposition 42.58
antesternal or antethoracic NEC 42.64
with interposition 42.68
colon (intrathoracic) NEC 42.56
with interposition 42.55
antesternal or antethoracic 42.66
with interposition 42.65
small bowel NEC 42.54
with interposition 42.53
antesternal or antethoracic 42.64
with interposition 42.63
facial-accessory nerve 04.72
facial-hypoglossal nerve 04.71
fallopian tube 66.73
by reanastomosis 66.79
gallbladder 51.35
to
hepatic ducts 51.31
intestine 51.32
pancreas 51.33
stomach 51.34
gastroepiploic artery to coronary artery 36.17

Anastomosis *(Continued)*
hepatic duct 51.39
hypoglossal-accessory nerve 04.73
hypoglossal-facial nerve 04.71
ileal loop to bladder 57.87 *[45.51]*
ileoanal 45.95
ileorectal 45.93
inferior vena cava and portal vein 39.1
internal mammary artery (to)
coronary artery (single vessel) 36.15
double vessel 36.16
myocardium 36.2
intestine 45.90
large-to-anus 45.95
large-to-large 45.94
large-to-rectum 45.94
large-to-small 45.93
small-to-anus 45.95
small-to-large 45.93
small-to-rectal stump 45.92
small-to-small 45.91
intrahepatic 51.79
intrathoracic vessel NEC 39.23
kidney (pelvis) 55.86
lacrimal sac to conjunctiva 09.82
left-to-right (systemic-pulmonary artery) 39.0
lymphatic (channel) (peripheral) 40.9
mesenteric-caval 39.1
mesocaval 39.1
nasolacrimal 09.81
nerve (cranial) (peripheral) NEC 04.74
accessory-facial 04.72
accessory-hypoglossal 04.73
hypoglossal-facial 04.71
pancreas (duct) (to) 52.96
bile duct 51.39
gall bladder 51.33
intestine 52.96
jejunum 52.96
stomach 52.96
pleurothecal (with valve) 03.79
portacaval 39.1
portal vein to inferior vena cava 39.1
pulmonary-aortic (Pott's) 39.0
pulmonary artery and superior vena cava 39.21
pulmonary-innominate artery (Blalock) 39.0
pulmonary-subclavian artery (Blalock-Taussig) 39.0
pulmonary vein and azygos vein 39.23
pyeloileocutaneous 56.51
pyeloureterovesical 55.86
radial artery 36.19
rectum, rectal NEC 48.74
stump to small intestine 45.92
renal (pelvis) 55.86
vein and splenic vein 39.1
renoportal 39.1
salpingothecal (with valve) 03.79
splenic to renal veins 39.1
splenorenal (venous) 39.1
arterial 39.26
subarachnoid-peritoneal (with valve) 03.71
subarachnoid-ureteral (with valve) 03.72
subclavian-aortic 39.22
superior vena cava to pulmonary artery 39.21
systemic-pulmonary artery 39.0

Anastomosis *(Continued)*
thoracic artery (to)
coronary artery (single) 36.15
double 36.16
myocardium 36.2
ureter (to) NEC 56.79
bladder 56.74
colon 56.71
ileal pouch (bladder) 56.51
ileum 56.71
intestine 56.71
skin 56.61
ureterocalyceal 55.86
ureterocolic 56.71
ureterovesical 56.74
urethra (end-to-end) 58.44
vas deferens 63.82
veins (suture of proximal to distal end) (with bypass graft) 39.29
with excision or resection of vessel - *see* Phlebectomy, with anastomosis, by site
mesenteric to vena cava 39.1
portal to inferior vena cava 39.1
revision 39.49
splenic and renal 39.1
ventricle, ventricular (intracerebral) (with valve) (*see also* Shunt, ventricular) 02.2
ventriculoatrial (with valve) 02.32
ventriculocaval (with valve) 02.32
ventriculomastoid (with valve) 02.31
ventriculopleural (with valve) 02.33
vesicle - *see* Anastomosis, bladder
Anderson operation (tibial lengthening) 78.37
Anel operation (dilation of lacrimal duct) 09.42
Anesthesia
acupuncture for 99.91
cryoanalgesia nerve (cranial) (peripheral) 04.2
spinal - *omit code*
Aneurysmectomy 38.60
with
anastomosis 38.30
abdominal
artery 38.36
vein 38.37
aorta (arch) (ascending) (descending) 38.34
head and neck NEC 38.32
intracranial NEC 38.31
lower limb
artery 38.38
vein 38.39
thoracic NEC 38.35
upper limb (artery) (vein) 38.33
graft replacement (interposition) 38.40
abdominal
aorta 38.44
artery 38.46
vein 38.47
aorta (arch) (ascending) (descending thoracic)
abdominal 38.44
thoracic 38.45
thoracoabdominal 38.45 *[38.44]*
head and neck NEC 38.42
intracranial NEC 38.41
lower limb
artery 38.48
vein 38.49

Aneurysmectomy *(Continued)*
with *(Continued)*
graft replacement *(Continued)*
thoracic NEC 38.45
upper limb (artery) (vein) 38.43
abdominal
artery 38.66
vein 38.67
aorta (arch) (ascending) (descending) 38.64
atrial, auricular 37.32
head and neck NEC 38.62
heart 37.32
intracranial NEC 38.61
lower limb
artery 38.68
vein 38.69
sinus of Valsalva 35.39
thoracic NEC 38.65
upper limb (artery) (vein) 38.63
ventricle (myocardium) 37.32
Aneurysmoplasty - *see* Aneurysmorrhaphy
Aneurysmorrhaphy NEC 39.52
by or with
anastomosis - *see* Aneurysmectomy, with anastomosis, by site
clipping 39.51
coagulation 39.52
electrocoagulation 39.52
endovascular graft
abdominal aorta 39.71
lower extremity artery(ies) 39.79
thoracic aorta 39.73
upper extremity artery(ies) 39.79
excision or resection - *see also* Aneurysmectomy, by site
with
anastomosis - *see* Aneurysmectomy, with anastomosis, by site
graft replacement - *see* Aneurysmectomy, with graft replacement, by site
filipuncture 39.52
graft replacement - *see* Aneurysmectomy, with graft replacement, by site
methyl methacrylate 39.52
suture 39.52
wiring 39.52
wrapping 39.52
Matas' 39.52
Aneurysmotomy - *see* Aneurysmectomy
Angiectomy
with
anastomosis 38.30
abdominal
artery 38.36
vein 38.37
aorta (arch) (ascending) (descending) 38.34
head and neck NEC 38.32
intracranial NEC 38.31
lower limb
artery 38.38
vein 38.39
thoracic vessel NEC 38.35
upper limb (artery) (vein) 38.33
graft replacement (interposition) 38.40
abdominal
aorta 38.44
Angiectomy *(Continued)*
with *(Continued)*
graft replacement *(Continued)*
abdominal *(Continued)*
artery 38.46
vein 38.47
aorta (arch) (ascending) (descending thoracic)
abdominal 38.44
thoracic 38.45
thoracoabdominal 38.45 *[38.44]*
head and neck NEC 38.42
intracranial NEC 38.41
lower limb
artery 38.48
vein 38.49
thoracic vessel NEC 38.45
upper limb (artery) (vein) 38.43
Angiocardiography (selective) 88.50
carbon dioxide (negative contrast) 88.58
combined right and left heart 88.54
left heart (aortic valve) (atrium) (ventricle) (ventricular outflow tract) 88.53
combined with right heart 88.54
right heart (atrium) (pulmonary valve) (ventricle) (ventricular outflow tract) 88.52
combined with left heart 88.54
vena cava (inferior) (superior) 88.51
Angiography (arterial) - *see also* Arteriography 88.40
by radioisotope - *see* Scan, radioisotope, by site
by ultrasound - *see* Ultrasonography, by site
basilar 88.41
brachial 88.49
carotid (internal) 88.41
celiac 88.47
cerebral (posterior circulation) 88.41
coronary NEC 88.57
eye (fluorescein) 95.12
femoral 88.48
heart 88.50
intra-abdominal NEC 88.47
intracranial 88.41
intrathoracic vessels NEC 88.44
lower extremity NEC 88.48
neck 88.41
placenta 88.46
pulmonary 88.43
renal 88.45
specified artery NEC 88.49
transfemoral 88.48
upper extremity NEC 88.49
veins - *see* Phlebography
vertebral 88.41
Angioplasty (laser) - *see also* Repair, blood vessel

> Note: Also use 00.40, 00.41, 00.42, or 00.43 to show the total number of vessels treated. Use code 00.44 once to show procedure on a bifurcated vessel. In addition, use 00.45, 00.46, 00.47, or 00.48 to show the number of vascular stents inserted. ⬅

balloon (percutaneous transluminal) NEC 39.50
coronary artery 00.66
coronary 36.09
Angioplasty *(Continued)*
coronary *(Continued)*
open chest approach 36.03
percutaneous transluminal (balloon) 00.66
percutaneous transluminal (balloon) (single vessel) 00.66
basilar 00.61
carotid 00.61
cerebral (intracranial) 00.62
cerebrovascular
cerebral (intracranial) 00.62
precerebral (extracranial) 00.61
carotid 00.61
coronary (balloon) 00.66
femoropopliteal 39.50
iliac 39.50
lower extremity NOS 39.50
mesenteric 39.50
peripheral NEC 39.50
precerebral (extracranial) 00.61
carotid 00.61
renal 39.50
subclavian 39.50
upper extremity NOS 39.50
vertebral 00.61
specified site NEC 39.50
cerebrovascular
cerebral (intracranial) 00.62
precerebral (extracranial) 00.61
peripheral 39.50
Angiorrhaphy 39.30
artery 39.31
vein 39.32
Angioscopy, percutaneous 38.22
eye (fluorescein) 95.12
Angiotomy 38.00
abdominal
artery 38.06
vein 38.07
aorta (arch) (ascending) (descending) 38.04
head and neck NEC 38.02
intracranial NEC 38.01
lower limb
artery 38.08
vein 38.09
thoracic NEC 38.05
upper limb (artery) (vein) 38.03
Angiotripsy 39.98
Ankylosis, production of - *see* Arthrodesis
Annuloplasty (heart) (posteromedial) 35.33
Anoplasty 49.79
with hemorrhoidectomy 49.46
Anoscopy 49.21
Antibiogram - *see* Examination, microscopic
Antiembolic filter, vena cava 38.7
Antiphobic treatment 94.39
Antrectomy
mastoid 20.49
maxillary 22.39
radical 22.31
pyloric 43.6
Antrostomy - *see* Antrotomy
Antrotomy (exploratory) (nasal sinus) 22.2
Caldwell-Luc (maxillary sinus) 22.39
with removal of membrane lining 22.31
intranasal 22.2

Antrotomy *(Continued)*
intranasal *(Continued)*
with external approach (Caldwell-Luc) 22.39
radical 22.31
maxillary (simple) 22.2
with Caldwell-Luc approach 22.39
with removal of membrane lining 22.31
external (Caldwell-Luc approach) 22.39
with removal of membrane lining 22.31
radical (with removal of membrane lining) 22.31
Antrum window operation - *see* Antrotomy, maxillary
Aorticopulmonary window operation 39.59
Aortogram, aortography (abdominal) (retrograde) (selective) (translumbar) 88.42
Aortoplasty (aortic valve) (gusset type) 35.11
Aortotomy 38.04
Apexcardiogram (with ECG lead) 89.57
Apheresis, therapeutic - *see* category 99.7
Apicectomy
lung 32.3
petrous pyramid 20.59
tooth (root) 23.73
with root canal therapy 23.72
Apicoectomy 23.73
with root canal therapy 23.72
Apicolysis (lung) 33.39
Apicostomy, alveolar 24.0
Aponeurectomy 83.42
hand 82.33
Aponeurorrhaphy - *see also* Suture, tendon 83.64
hand - *see also* Suture, tendon, hand 82.45
Aponeurotomy 83.13
hand 82.11
Appendectomy (with drainage) 47.09
incidental 47.19
laparoscopic 47.11
laparoscopic 47.01
Appendicectomy (with drainage) 47.09
incidental 47.19
laparoscopic 47.11
laparoscopic 47.01
Appendicocecostomy 47.91
Appendicoenterostomy 47.91
Appendicolysis 54.59
with appendectomy 47.09
laparoscopic 47.01
other 47.09
laparoscopic 54.51
Appendicostomy 47.91
closure 47.92
Appendicotomy 47.2
Application
adhesion barrier substance 99.77
anti-shock trousers 93.58
arch bars (orthodontic) 24.7
for immobilization (fracture) 93.55
barrier substance, adhesion 99.77
Barton's tongs (skull) (with synchronous skeletal traction) 02.94
bone growth stimulator (surface) (transcutaneous) 99.86

Application *(Continued)*
bone morphogenetic protein (Infuse™) (OP-1™) (recombinant) (rhBMP) 84.52
Bryant's traction 93.44
with reduction of fracture or dislocation - *see* Reduction, fracture *and* Reduction, dislocation
Buck's traction 93.46
caliper tongs (skull) (with synchronous skeletal traction) 02.94
cast (fiberglass) (plaster) (plastic) NEC 93.53
with reduction of fracture or dislocation - *see* Reduction, fracture *and* Reduction, dislocation
spica 93.51
cervical collar 93.52
with reduction of fracture or dislocation - *see* Reduction, fracture *and* Reduction, dislocation
clamp, cerebral aneurysm (Crutchfield) (Silverstone) 39.51
croupette, croup tent 93.94
crown (artificial) 23.41
Crutchfield tongs (skull) (with synchronous skeletal traction) 02.94
Dunlop's traction 93.44
with reduction of fracture or dislocation - *see* Reduction, fracture *and* Reduction, dislocation
elastic stockings 93.59
electronic gaiter 93.59
external fixator device (bone) 78.10
carpal, metacarpal 78.14
clavicle 78.11
computer assisted (dependent) 84.73 ◀
femur 78.15
fibula 78.17
humerus 78.12
hybrid device or system 84.73
Ilizarov type 84.72
monoplanar system or device 84.71
patella 78.16
pelvic 78.19
phalanges (foot) (hand) 78.19
radius 78.13
ring device or system 84.72
scapula 78.11
Sheffield type 84.72
specified site NEC 78.19
tarsal, metatarsal 78.18
thorax (ribs) (sternum) 78.11
tibia 78.17
ulna 78.13
vertebrae 78.19
forceps, with delivery - *see* Delivery, forceps
graft - *see* Graft
gravity (G-) suit 93.59
hybrid device or system 84.73
Ilizarov type 84.72
intermittent pressure device 93.59
Jewett extension brace 93.59
Jobst pumping unit (reduction of edema) 93.59
Lyman Smith traction 93.44
with reduction of fracture or dislocation - *see* Reduction, fracture *and* Reduction, dislocation
MAST (military anti-shock trousers) 93.58
Minerva jacket 93.52

Application *(Continued)*
minifixator device (bone) - *see* category 78.1
monoplanar system or device 84.71
neck support (molded) 93.52
obturator (orthodontic) 24.7
orthodontic appliance (obturator) (wiring) 24.7
pelvic sling 93.44
with reduction of fracture or dislocation - *see* Reduction, fracture *and* Reduction, dislocation
peridontal splint (orthodontic) 24.7
plaster jacket 93.51
Minerva 93.52
pressure
dressing (bandage) (Gibney) (Robert Jones') (Shanz) 93.56
trousers (anti-shock) (MAST) 93.58
prosthesis for missing ear 18.71
ring device or sytem 84.72
Russell's traction 93.44
with reduction of fracture or dislocation - *see* Reduction, fracture *and* Reduction, dislocation
Sheffield type 84.72
splint, for immobilization (plaster) (pneumatic) (tray) 93.54
with fracture reduction - *see* Reduction, fracture
stereotactic head frame 93.59
strapping (non-traction) 93.59 ◀
substance, adhesion barrier 99.77
Thomas' collar 93.52
with reduction of fracture or dislocation - *see* Reduction, fracture *and* Reduction, dislocation
traction
with reduction of fracture or dislocation - *see* Reduction, fracture *and* Reduction, dislocation
adhesive tape (skin) 93.46
boot 93.46
Bryant's 93.44
Buck's 93.46
Cotrel's 93.42
Dunlop's 93.44
gallows 93.46
Lyman Smith 93.44
Russell's 93.44
skeletal NEC 93.44
intermittent 93.43
skin, limbs NEC 93.46
spinal NEC 93.42
with skull device (halo) (caliper) (Crutchfield) (Gardner-Wells) (Vinke) (tongs) 93.41
with synchronous insertion 02.94
Thomas' splint 93.45
Unna's paste boot 93.53
vasopneumatic device 93.58
Velpeau dressing 93.59
Vinke tongs (skull) (with synchronous skeletal traction) 02.94
wound dressing NEC 93.57
Aquapheresis 99.78
Arc lamp - *see* Photocoagulation
Arrest
bone growth (epiphyseal) 78.20
by stapling - *see* Stapling, epiphyseal plate
femur 78.25
fibula 78.27
humerus 78.22

Arrest *(Continued)*
bone growth *(Continued)*
radius 78.23
tibia 78.27
ulna 78.23
cardiac, induced (anoxic) (circulatory) 39.63
circulatory, induced (anoxic) 39.63
hemorrhage - *see* Control, hemorrhage
Arslan operation (fenestration of inner ear) 20.61
Arteriectomy 38.60
with
anastomosis 38.30
abdominal 38.36
aorta (arch) (ascending) (descending) (thoracic) 38.34
head and neck NEC 38.32
intracranial NEC 38.31
lower limb 38.38
thoracic NEC 38.35
upper limb 38.33
graft replacement (interposition) 38.40
abdominal 38.36
aorta 38.44
aorta (arch) (ascending) (descending thoracic)
abdominal 38.44
thoracic 38.45
thoracoabdominal 38.45 [38.44]
head and neck NEC 38.42
intracranial NEC 38.41
lower limb 38.48
thoracic NEC 38.45
upper limb 38.43
abdominal 38.66
aorta (arch) (ascending) (descending) 38.64
head and neck NEC 38.62
intracranial NEC 38.61
lower-limb 38.68
thoracic NEC 38.65
upper limb 38.63
Arteriography (contrast) (fluoroscopic) (retrograde) 88.40
by
radioisotope - *see* Scan, radioisotope
ultrasound (Doppler) - *see* Ultrasonography, by site
aorta (arch) (ascending) (descending) 88.42
basilar 88.41
brachial 88.49
carotid (internal) 88.41
cerebral (posterior circulation) 88.41
coronary (direct) (selective) NEC 88.57
double catheter technique (Judkins) (Ricketts and Abrams) 88.56
single catheter technique (Sones) 88.55
Doppler (ultrasonic) - *see* Ultrasonography, by site
femoral 88.48
head and neck 88.41
intra-abdominal NEC 88.47
intrathoracic NEC 88.44
lower extremity 88.48
placenta 88.46
pulmonary 88.43
radioisotope - *see* Scan, radioisotope
renal 88.45
specified site NEC 88.49
superior mesenteric artery 88.47
transfemoral 88.48
Arteriography *(Continued)*
ultrasound - *see* Ultrasonography, by site
upper extremity 88.49
Arterioplasty - *see* Repair, artery
Arteriorrhaphy 39.31
Arteriotomy 38.00
abdominal 38.06
aorta (arch) (ascending) (descending) 38.04
head and neck NEC 38.02
intracranial NEC 38.01
lower limb 38.08
thoracic NEC 38.05
upper limb 38.03
Arteriovenostomy 39.29
for renal dialysis 39.27
Arthrectomy 80.90
ankle 80.97
elbow 80.92
foot and toe 80.98
hand and finger 80.94
hip 80.95
intervertebral disc - *see* category 80.5
knee 80.96
semilunar cartilage 80.6
shoulder 80.91
specified site NEC 80.99
spine NEC 80.99
wrist 80.93
Arthrocentesis 81.91
for arthrography - *see* Arthrogram
Arthrodesis (compression) (extra-articular) (intra-articular) (with bone graft) (with fixation device) 81.20
ankle 81.11
carporadial 81.25
cricoarytenoid 31.69
elbow 81.24
finger 81.28
foot NEC 81.17
hip 81.21
interphalangeal
finger 81.28
toe NEC 77.58
claw toe repair 77.57
hammer toe repair 77.56
ischiofemoral 81.21
knee 81.22
lumbosacral, lumbar NEC 81.08
ALIF (anterior lumbar interbody fusion) 81.06
anterior (interbody), anterolateral technique 81.06
lateral transverse process technique 81.07
PLIF (posterior lumbar interbody fusion) 81.08
posterior (interbody), posterolateral technique 81.08
TLIF (transforaminal lumbar interbody fusion) 81.08
McKeever (metatarsophalangeal) 81.16
metacarpocarpal 81.26
metacarpophalangeal 81.27
metatarsophalangeal 81.16
midtarsal 81.14
PLIF (posterior lumbar interbody fusion) 81.08
plantar 81.11
sacroiliac 81.08
shoulder 81.23
specified joint NEC 81.29
Arthrodesis *(Continued)*
spinal - *see also* Fusion, spinal 81.00
subtalar 81.13
tarsometatarsal 81.15
tibiotalar 81.11
TLIF (transforaminal lumbar interbody fusion) 81.08
toe NEC 77.58
claw toe repair 77.57
hammer toe repair 77.56
triple 81.12
wrist 81.26
Arthroendoscopy - *see* Arthroscopy
Arthroereisis, subtalar joint 81.18
Arthrogram, arthrography 88.32
temporomandibular 87.13
Arthrolysis 93.26
Arthroplasty (with fixation device) (with traction) 81.96
ankle 81.49
carpals 81.75
with prosthetic implant 81.74
carpocarpal, carpometacarpal 81.75
with prosthetic implant 81.74
Carroll and Taber (proximal interphalangeal joint) 81.72
cup (partial hip) 81.52
Curtis (interphalangeal joint) 81.72
elbow 81.85
with prosthetic replacement (total) 81.84
femoral head NEC 81.40
with prosthetic implant 81.52
finger(s) 81.72
with prosthetic implant 81.71
foot (metatarsal) with joint replacement 81.57
Fowler (metacarpophalangeal joint) 81.72
hand (metacarpophalangeal) (interphalangeal) 81.72
with prosthetic implant 81.71
hip (with bone graft) 81.40
cup (partial hip) 81.52
femoral head NEC 81.40
with prosthetic implant 81.52
with total replacement 81.51
partial replacement 81.52
total replacement 81.51
interphalangeal joint 81.72
with prosthetic implant 81.71
Kessler (carpometacarpal joint) 81.74
knee (*see also* Repair, knee) 81.47
prosthetic replacement (bicompartmental) (hemijoint) (partial) (total) (tricompartmental) (unicompartmental) 81.54
revision 81.55
metacarpophalangeal joint 81.72
with prosthetic implant 81.71
shoulder 81.83
prosthetic replacement (partial) 81.81
total 81.80
for recurrent dislocation 81.82
temporomandibular 76.5
toe NEC 77.58
with prosthetic replacement 81.57
for hallux valgus repair 77.59
wrist 81.75
with prosthetic implant 81.74
total replacement 81.73
Arthroscopy 80.20
ankle 80.27
elbow 80.22

Arthroscopy *(Continued)*
finger 80.24
foot 80.28
hand 80.24
hip 80.25
knee 80.26
shoulder 80.21
specified site NEC 80.29
toe 80.28
wrist 80.23
Arthrostomy - *see also* Arthrotomy 80.10
Arthrotomy 80.10
as operative approach - *omit code*
with
arthrography - *see* Arthrogram
arthroscopy - *see* Arthroscopy
injection of drug 81.92
removal of prosthesis (*see also* Removal, prosthesis, joint structures) 80.00
ankle 80.17
elbow 80.12
foot and toe 80.18
hand and finger 80.14
hip 80.15
knee 80.16
shoulder 80.11
specified site NEC 80.19
spine 80.19
wrist 80.13
Artificial
insemination 69.92
kidney 39.95
rupture of membranes 73.09
Arytenoidectomy 30.29
Arytenoidopexy 31.69
Asai operation (larynx) 31.75
Aspiration
abscess - *see* Aspiration, by site
anterior chamber, eye (therapeutic) 12.91
diagnostic 12.21
aqueous (eye) (humor) (therapeutic) 12.91
diagnostic 12.21
ascites 54.91
Bartholin's gland (cyst) (percutaneous) 71.21
biopsy - *see* Biopsy, by site
bladder (catheter) 57.0
percutaneous (needle) 57.11
bone marrow (for biopsy) 41.31
from donor for transplant 41.91
stem cell 99.79
branchial cleft cyst 29.0
breast 85.91
bronchus 96.05
with lavage 96.56
bursa (percutaneous) 83.94
hand 82.92
calculus, bladder 57.0
cataract 13.3
with
phacoemulsification 13.41
phacofragmentation 13.43
posterior route 13.42
chest 34.91
cisternal 01.01
cranial (puncture) 01.09
craniobuccal pouch 07.72
craniopharyngioma 07.72
cul-de-sac (abscess) 70.0
curettage, uterus 69.59
after abortion or delivery 69.52

Aspiration *(Continued)*
curettage, uterus *(Continued)*
diagnostic 69.59
to terminate pregnancy 69.51
cyst - *see* Aspiration, by site
diverticulum, pharynx 29.0
endotracheal 96.04
with lavage 96.56
extradural 01.09
eye (anterior chamber) (therapeutic) 12.91
diagnostic 12.21
fallopian tube 66.91
fascia 83.95
hand 82.93
gallbladder (percutaneous) 51.01
hematoma - *see also* Aspiration, by site
obstetrical 75.92
incisional 75.91
hydrocele, tunica vaginalis 61.91
hygroma - *see* Aspiration, by site
hyphema 12.91
hypophysis 07.72
intracranial space (epidural) (extradural) (subarachnoid) (subdural) (ventricular) 01.09
through previously implanted catheter or reservoir (Ommaya) (Rickham) 01.02
joint 81.91
for arthrography - *see* Arthrogram
kidney (cyst) (pelvis) (percutaneous) (therapeutic) 55.92
diagnostic 55.23
liver (percutaneous) 50.91
lung (percutaneous) (puncture) (needle) (trocar) 33.93
middle ear 20.09
with intubation 20.01
muscle 83.95
hand 82.93
nail 86.01
nasal sinus 22.00
by puncture 22.01
through natural ostium 22.02
nasotracheal 96.04
with lavage 96.56
orbit, diagnostic 16.22
ovary 65.91
percutaneous - *see* Aspiration, by site
pericardium (wound) 37.0
pituitary gland 07.72
pleural cavity 34.91
prostate (percutaneous) 60.91
Rathke's pouch 07.72
seminal vesicles 60.71
seroma - *see* Aspiration, by site
skin 86.01
soft tissue NEC 83.95
hand 82.93
spermatocele 63.91
spinal (puncture) 03.31
spleen (cyst) 41.1
stem cell 99.79
subarachnoid space (cerebral) 01.09
subcutaneous tissue 86.01
subdural space (cerebral) 01.09
tendon 83.95
hand 82.93
testis 62.91
thymus 07.92
thyroid (field) (gland) 06.01
postoperative 06.02
trachea 96.04

Aspiration *(Continued)*
trachea *(Continued)*
with lavage 96.56
percutaneous 31.99
tunica vaginalis (hydrocele) (percutaneous) 61.91
vitreous (and replacement) 14.72
diagnostic 14.11
Assessment
fitness to testify 94.11
mental status 94.11
nutritional status 89.39
personality 94.03
temperament 94.02
vocational 93.85
Assistance
cardiac - *see also* Resuscitation, cardiac
extracorporeal circulation 39.61
endotracheal respiratory - *see* category 96.7
hepatic, extracorporeal 50.92
respiratory (endotracheal) (mechanical) - *see* Ventilation, mechanical
Astragalectomy 77.98
Asymmetrogammagram - *see* Scan, radioisotope
Atherectomy
cerebrovascular - *see* Angioplasty
coronary - *see* Angioplasty
peripheral 39.50
Atriocommissuropexy (mitral valve) 35.12
Atrioplasty NEC 37.99
combined with repair of valvular and ventricular septal defects - *see* Repair, endocardial cushion defect
septum (heart) NEC 35.71
Atrioseptopexy - *see also* Repair, atrial septal defect 35.71
Atrioseptoplasty - *see also* Repair, atrial septal defect 35.71
Atrioseptostomy (balloon) 35.41
Atriotomy 37.11
Atrioventriculostomy (cerebral-heart) 02.32
Attachment
eye muscle
orbicularis oculi to eyebrow 08.36
rectus to frontalis 15.9
pedicle (flap) graft 86.74
hand 86.73
lip 27.57
mouth 27.57
pharyngeal flap (for cleft palate repair) 27.62
secondary or subsequent 27.63
retina - *see* Reattachment, retina
Atticoantrostomy (ear) 20.49
Atticoantrotomy (ear) 20.49
Atticotomy (ear) 20.23
Audiometry (Bekesy 5-tone) (impedance) (stapedial reflex response) (subjective) 95.41
Augmentation
bladder 57.87
breast - *see* Mammoplasty, augmentation
buttock ("fanny-lift") 86.89
chin 76.68
genioplasty 76.68
mammoplasty - *see* Mammoplasty, augmentation
outflow tract (pulmonary valve) (gusset type) 35.26

Augmentation *(Continued)*
outflow tract *(Continued)*
in total repair of tetralogy of Fallot 35.81
vocal cord(s) 31.0
Auriculectomy 18.39
Autograft - *see* Graft
Autologous - *see* Blood, transfusion
Autopsy 89.8
Autotransfusion (whole blood) 99.02 - *see* Blood, transfusion
Autotransplant, autotransplantation - *see also* Reimplantation
adrenal tissue (heterotopic) (orthotopic) 07.45
kidney 55.61
lung - *see* Transplant, transplantation, lung
ovary 65.72
laparoscopic 65.75
pancreatic tissue 52.81
parathyroid tissue (heterotopic) (orthotopic) 06.95
thyroid tissue (heterotopic) (orthotopic) 06.94
tooth 23.5
Avulsion, nerve (cranial) (peripheral) NEC 04.07
acoustic 04.01
phrenic 33.31
sympathetic 05.29
Azygography 88.63

B

Bacterial smear - *see* Examination, microscopic
Baffes operation (interatrial transposition of venous return) 35.91
Baffle, atrial or interatrial 35.91
Balanoplasty 64.69
Baldy-Webster operation (uterine suspension) 69.22
Ballistocardiography 89.59
Balloon
  angioplasty - *see* Angioplasty, balloon
  pump, intra-aortic 37.61
  systostomy (atrial) 35.41
Ball operation
  herniorrhaphy - *see* Repair, hernia, inguinal
  undercutting 49.02
Bandage 93.37
  elastic 93.56
Banding
  gastric 44.68
    vertical 44.68
  pulmonary artery 38.85
Bankhart operation (capsular repair into glenoid, for shoulder dislocation) 81.82
Bardenheurer operation (ligation of innominate artery) 38.85
Barium swallow 87.61
Barkan operation (goniotomy) 12.52
  with goniopuncture 12.53
Barr operation (transfer of tibialis posterior tendon) 83.75
Barsky operation (closure of cleft hand) 82.82
Basal metabolic rate 89.39
Basiotripsy 73.8
Bassett operation (vulvectomy with inguinal lymph node dissection) 71.5 *[40.3]*
Bassini operation - *see* Repair, hernia, inguinal
Batch-Spittler-McFaddin operation (knee disarticulation) 84.16
Batista operation (partial ventriculectomy) (ventricular reduction) (ventricular remodeling) 37.35
Bearing surface, hip replacement
  ceramic-on-ceramic 00.76
  ceramic-on-polyethylene 00.77 ◄
  metal-on-metal 00.75
  metal on polyethylene 00.74
Beck operation
  aorta-coronary sinus shunt 36.39
  epicardial poudrage 36.39
Beck-Jianu operation (permanent gastrostomy) 43.19
Behavior modification 94.33
Bell-Beuttner operation (subtotal abdominal hysterectomy) 68.39
  laparoscopic 68.31
Belsey operation (esophagogastric sphincter) 44.65
Benenenti operation (rotation of bulbous urethra) 58.49
Berke operation (levator resection of eyelid) 08.33
Bicuspidization of heart valve 35.10
  aortic 35.11
  mitral 35.12
Bicycle dynamometer 93.01
Biesenberger operation (size reduction of breast, bilateral) 85.32
  unilateral 85.31
Bifurcation, bone - *see also* Osteotomy 77.30
Bigelow operation (litholapaxy) 57.0
Bililite therapy (ultraviolet) 99.82
Billroth I operation (partial gastrectomy with gastroduodenostomy) 43.6
Billroth II operation (partial gastrectomy with gastrojejunostomy) 43.7
Binnie operation (hepatopexy) 50.69
Biofeedback, psychotherapy 94.39
Biopsy
  abdominal wall 54.22
  adenoid 28.11
  adrenal gland NEC 07.11
    closed 07.11
    open 07.12
    percutaneous (aspiration) (needle) 07.11
  alveolus 24.12
  anus 49.23
  appendix 45.26
  artery (any site) 38.21
  aspiration - *see* Biopsy, by site
  bile ducts 51.14
    closed (endoscopic) 51.14
    open 51.13
    percutaneous (needle) 51.12
  bladder 57.33
    closed 57.33
    open 57.34
    transurethral 57.33
  blood vessel (any site) 38.21
  bone 77.40
    carpal, metacarpal 77.44
    clavicle 77.41
    facial 76.11
    femur 77.45
    fibula 77.47
    humerus 77.42
    marrow 41.31
    patella 77.46
    pelvic 77.49
    phalanges (foot) (hand) 77.49
    radius 77.43
    scapula 77.41
    specified site NEC 77.49
    tarsal, metatarsal 77.48
    thorax (ribs) (sternum) 77.41
    tibia 77.47
    ulna 77.43
    vertebrae 77.49
  bowel - *see* Biopsy, intestine
  brain NEC 01.13
    closed 01.13
    open 01.14
    percutaneous (needle) 01.13
  breast 85.11
    blind 85.11
    closed 85.11
    open 85.12
    percutaneous (needle) (Vimm-Silverman) 85.11
  bronchus NEC 33.24
    brush 33.24
    closed (endoscopic) 33.24
    open 33.25
    washings 33.24
  bursa 83.21
  cardioesophageal (junction) 44.14
    closed (endoscopic) 44.14
    open 44.15
Biopsy *(Continued)*
  cecum 45.25
    brush 45.25
    closed (endoscopic) 45.25
    open 45.26
  cerebral meninges NEC 01.11
    closed 01.11
    open 01.12
    percutaneous (needle) 01.11
  cervix (punch) 67.12
    conization (sharp) 67.2
  chest wall 34.23
  clitoris 71.11
  colon 45.25
    brush 45.25
    closed (endoscopic) 45.25
    open 45.26
  conjunctiva 10.21
  cornea 11.22
  cul-de-sac 70.23
  diaphragm 34.27
  duodenum 45.14
    brush 45.14
    closed (endoscopic) 45.14
    open 45.15
  ear (external) 18.12
    middle or inner 20.32
  endocervix 67.11
  endometrium NEC 68.16
    by
      aspiration curettage 69.59
      dilation and curettage 69.09
    closed (endoscopic) 68.16
    open 68.13
  epididymis 63.01
  esophagus 42.24
    closed (endoscopic) 42.24
    open 42.25
  extraocular muscle or tendon 15.01
  eye 16.23
    muscle (oblique) (rectus) 15.01
  eyelid 08.11
  fallopian tube 66.11
  fascia 83.21
  fetus 75.33
  gallbladder 51.12
    closed (endoscopic) 51.14
    open 51.13
    percutaneous (needle) 51.12
  ganglion (cranial) (peripheral) NEC 04.11
    closed 04.11
    open 04.12
    percutaneous (needle) 04.11
    sympathetic nerve 05.11
  gum 24.11
  heart 37.25
  hypophysis - *see also* Biopsy, pituitary gland 07.15
  ileum 45.14
    brush 45.14
    closed (endoscopic) 45.14
    open 45.15
  intestine NEC 45.27
    large 45.25
      brush 45.25
      closed (endoscopic) 45.25
      open 45.26
    small 45.14
      brush 45.14
      closed (endoscopic) 45.14
      open 45.15
  intra-abdominal mass 54.24

◄ New   ⟸ Revised

Biopsy *(Continued)*
intra-abdominal mass *(Continued)*
closed 54.24
percutaneous (needle) 54.24
iris 12.22
jejunum 45.14
brush 45.14
closed (endoscopic) 45.14
open 45.15
joint structure (aspiration) 80.30
ankle 80.37
elbow 80.32
foot and toe 80.38
hand and finger 80.34
hip 80.35
knee 80.36
shoulder 80.31
specified site NEC 80.39
spine 80.39
wrist 80.33
kidney 55.23
closed 55.23
open 55.24
percutaneous (aspiration) (needle) 55.23
labia 71.11
lacrimal
gland 09.11
sac 09.12
larynx 31.43
brush 31.43
closed (endoscopic) 31.43
open 31.45
lip 27.23
liver 50.11
closed 50.11
laparoscopic 50.19
open 50.12
percutaneous (aspiration) (needle) 50.11
lung NEC 33.27
brush 33.24
closed (percutaneous) (needle) 33.26
brush 33.24
endoscopic 33.27
brush 33.24
endoscopic 33.27
brush 33.24
open 33.28
transbronchial 33.27
lymphatic structure (channel) (node) (vessel) 40.11
mediastinum NEC 34.25
closed 34.25
open 34.26
percutaneous (needle) 34.25
meninges (cerebral) NEC 01.11
closed 01.11
open 01.12
percutaneous (needle) 01.11
spinal 03.32
mesentery 54.23
mouth NEC 27.24
muscle 83.21
extraocular 15.01
ocular 15.01
nasopharynx 29.12
nerve (cranial) (peripheral) NEC 04.11
closed 04.11
open 04.12
percutaneous (needle) 04.11
sympathetic 05.11
nose, nasal 21.22
sinus 22.11

Biopsy *(Continued)*
nose, nasal *(Continued)*
sinus *(Continued)*
closed (endoscopic) (needle) 22.11
open 22.12
ocular muscle or tendon 15.01
omentum
closed 54.24
open 54.23
percutaneous (needle) 54.24
orbit 16.23
by aspiration 16.22
ovary 65.12
by aspiration 65.11
laparoscopic 65.13
palate (bony) 27.21
soft 27.22
pancreas 52.11
closed (endoscopic) 52.11
open 52.12
percutaneous (aspiration) (needle) 52.11
pancreatic duct 52.14
closed (endoscopic) 52.14
parathyroid gland 06.13
penis 64.11
perianal tissue 49.22
pericardium 37.24
periprostatic 60.15
perirectal tissue 48.26
perirenal tissue 59.21
peritoneal implant
closed 54.24
open 54.23
percutaneous (needle) 54.24
peritoneum
closed 54.24
open 54.23
percutaneous (needle) 54.24
periurethral tissue 58.24
perivesical tissue 59.21
pharynx, pharyngeal 29.12
pineal gland 07.17
pituitary gland 07.15
transfrontal approach 07.13
transsphenoidal approach 07.14
pleura, pleural 34.24
prostate NEC 60.11
closed (transurethral) 60.11
open 60.12
percutaneous (needle) 60.11
transrectal 60.11
rectum 48.24
brush 48.24
closed (endoscopic) 48.24
open 48.25
retroperitoneal tissue 54.24
salivary gland or duct 26.11
closed (needle) 26.11
open 26.12
scrotum 61.11
seminal vesicle NEC 60.13
closed 60.13
open 60.14
percutaneous (needle) 60.13
sigmoid colon 45.25
brush 45.25
closed (endoscopic) 45.25
open 45.26
sinus, nasal 22.11
closed (endoscopic) (needle) 22.11
open 22.12
skin (punch) 86.11
skull 01.15
soft palate 27.22

Biopsy *(Continued)*
soft tissue NEC 83.21
spermatic cord 63.01
sphincter of Oddi 51.14
closed (endoscopic) 51.14
open 51.13
spinal cord (meninges) 03.32
spleen 41.32
closed 41.32
open 41.33
percutaneous (aspiration) (needle) 41.32
stomach 44.14
brush 44.14
closed (endoscopic) 44.14
open 44.15
subcutaneous tissue (punch) 86.11
supraglottic mass 29.12
sympathetic nerve 05.11
tendon 83.21
extraocular 15.01
ocular 15.01
testis NEC 62.11
closed 62.11
open 62.12
percutaneous (needle) 62.11
thymus 07.16
thyroid gland NEC 06.11
closed 06.11
open 06.12
percutaneous (aspiration) (needle) 06.11
tongue 25.01
closed (needle) 25.01
open 25.02
tonsil 28.11
trachea 31.44
brush 31.44
closed (endoscopic) 31.44
open 31.45
tunica vaginalis 61.11
umbilicus 54.22
ureter 56.33
closed (percutaneous) 56.32
endoscopic 56.33
open 56.34
transurethral 56.33
urethra 58.23
uterus, uterine (endometrial) 68.16
by
aspiration curettage 69.59
dilation and curettage 69.09
closed (endoscopic) 68.16
ligaments 68.15
closed (endoscopic) 68.15
open 68.14
open 68.13
uvula 27.22
vagina 70.24
vas deferens 63.01
vein (any site) 38.21
vulva 71.11
Bischoff operation (ureteroneocystostomy) 56.74
Bisection - *see also* Excision
hysterectomy 68.39
laparoscopic 68.31
ovary 65.29
laparoscopic 65.25
stapes foot plate 19.19
with incus replacement 19.11
Bischoff operation (spinal myelotomy) 03.29

Blalock operation (systemic-pulmonary anastomosis) 39.0
Blalock-Hanlon operation (creation of atrial septal defect) 35.42
Blalock-Taussig operation (subclavian-pulmonary anastomosis) 39.0
Blascovic operation (resection and advancement of levator palpebrae superioris) 08.33
Blepharectomy 08.20
Blepharoplasty - *see also* Reconstruction, eyelid 08.70
  extensive 08.44
Blepharorrhaphy 08.52
  division or severing 08.02
Blepharotomy 08.09
Blind rehabilitation therapy NEC 93.78
Block
  caudal - *see* Injection, spinal celiac ganglion or plexus 05.31
  dissection
    breast
      bilateral 85.46
      unilateral 85.45
    bronchus 32.6
    larynx 30.3
    lymph nodes 40.50
    neck 40.40
    vulva 71.5
  epidural, spinal - *see* Injection, spinal
  gasserian ganglion 04.81
  intercostal nerves 04.81
  intrathecal - *see* Injection, spinal
  nerve (cranial) (peripheral) NEC 04.81
  paravertebral stellate ganglion 05.31
  peripheral nerve 04.81
  spinal nerve root (intrathecal) - *see* Injection, spinal
  stellate (ganglion) 05.31
  subarachnoid, spinal - *see* Injection, spinal
  sympathetic nerve 05.31
  trigeminal nerve 04.81
Blood
  flow study, Doppler-type (ultrasound) - *see* Ultrasonography
  patch, spine (epidural) 03.95
  transfusion
    antihemophilic factor 99.06
    autologous
      collected prior to surgery 99.02
      intraoperative 99.00
      perioperative 99.00
      postoperative 99.00
      previously collected 99.02
      salvage 99.00
    blood expander 99.08
    blood surrogate 99.09
    coagulation factors 99.06
    exchange 99.01
    granulocytes 99.09
    hemodilution 99.03
    other substance 99.09
    packed cells 99.04
    plasma 99.07
    platelets 99.05
    serum, other 99.07
    thrombocytes 99.05
Blount operation
  femoral shortening (with blade plate) 78.25
    by epiphyseal stapling 78.25
Boari operation (bladder flap) 56.74
Bobb operation (cholelithotomy) 51.04
Bone
  age studies 88.33
  mineral density study 88.98
Bonney operation (abdominal hysterectomy) 68.49
  laparoscopic 68.41
Borthen operation (iridotasis) 12.63
Bost operation
  plantar dissection 80.48
  radiocarpal fusion 81.26
Bosworth operation
  arthroplasty for acromioclavicular separation 81.83
  fusion of posterior lumbar and lumbosacral spine 81.08
    for pseudarthrosis 81.38
  resection of radial head ligaments (for tennis elbow) 80.92
  shelf procedure, hip 81.40
Bottle repair of hydrocele, tunica-vaginalis 61.2
Boyd operation (hip disarticulation) 84.18
Brachytherapy
  intravascular 92.27
Brauer operation (cardiolysis) 37.10
Breech extraction - *see* Extraction, breech
Bricker operation (ileoureterostomy) 56.51
Brisement (forcé) 93.26
Bristow operation (repair of shoulder dislocation) 81.82
Brock operation (pulmonary valvotomy) 35.03
Brockman operation (soft tissue release for clubfoot) 83.84
Bronchogram, bronchography 87.32
  endotracheal 87.31
  transcricoid 87.32
Bronchoplasty 33.48
Bronchorrhaphy 33.41
Bronchoscopy NEC 33.23
  with biopsy 33.24
    lung 33.27
      brush 33.24
  fiberoptic 33.22
    with biopsy 33.24
      lung 33.27
        brush 33.24
  through tracheostomy 33.21
    with biopsy 33.24
      lung 33.27
        brush 33.24
Bronchospirometry 89.38
Bronchostomy 33.0
  closure 33.42
Bronchotomy 33.0
Browne (-Denis) operation (hypospadias repair) 58.45
Brunschwig operation (temporary gastrostomy) 43.19
Buckling, scleral 14.49
  with
    air tamponade 14.49
    implant (silicone) (vitreous) 14.41
    resection of sclera 14.49
    vitrectomy 14.49
    vitreous implant (silicone) 14.41
Bunionectomy (radical) 77.59
  with
    arthrodesis 77.52
    osteotomy of first metatarsal 77.51
    resection of joint with prosthetic implant 77.59
    soft tissue correction NEC 77.53
Bunnell operation (tendon transfer) 82.56
Burch procedure (retropubic urethral suspension for urinary stress incontinence) 59.5
Burgess operation (amputation of ankle) 84.14
Burn dressing 93.57
Burr holes 01.24
Bursectomy 83.5
  hand 82.31
Bursocentesis 83.94
  hand 82.92
Bursotomy 83.03
  hand 82.03
Burying of fimbriae in uterine wall 66.97
Bypass
  abdominal - coronary artery 36.17
  aortocoronary (catheter stent) (with prosthesis) (with saphenous vein graft) (with vein graft) 36.10
    one coronary vessel 36.11
    two coronary vessels 36.12
    three coronary vessels 36.13
    four coronary vessels 36.14
  arterial (graft) (mandril grown graft) (vein graft) NEC 39.29
    carotid-cerebral 39.28
    carotid-vertebral 39.28
    extracranial-intracranial [EC-IC] 39.28
    intra-abdominal NEC 39.26
    intrathoracic NEC 39.23
    peripheral NEC 39.29
  cardiopulmonary 39.61
    open 39.61
    percutaneous (closed) 39.66
  carotid-cerebral 39.28
  carotid-vertebral 39.28
  coronary - *see also* Bypass, aortocoronary 36.10
  extracranial-intracranial [EC-IC] 39.28
  gastric 44.39
    high 44.31
    laparoscopic 44.38
    Printen and Mason 44.31
  gastroduodenostomy (Jaboulay's) 44.39
    laparoscopic 44.38
  gastroenterostomy 44.39
    laparoscopic 44.38
  gastroepiploic - coronary artery 36.17
  gastrogastrostomy 44.39
    laparoscopic 44.38
  graft, pressurized treatment 00.16
  heart-lung (complete) (partial) 39.61
    open 39.61
    percutaneous (closed) 39.66
  high gastric 44.31
  ileo-jejunal 45.91
  internal mammary-coronary artery (single) 36.15
    double vessel 36.16
  jejunal-ileum 45.91
  pulmonary 39.61
    open 39.61
    percutaneous (closed) 39.66
  shunt
    intestine
      large-to-large 45.94
      small-to-large 45.93
      small-to-small 45.91
    stomach 44.39
      high gastric 44.31
      laparoscopic 44.38
  terminal ileum 45.93

Bypass *(Continued)*
vascular (arterial) (graft) (mandril grown graft) (vein graft) NEC 39.29
aorta-carotid-brachial 39.22
aorta-iliac-femoral 39.25
aorta-renal 39.24
aorta-subclavian-carotid 39.22
aortic-superior mesenteric 39.26
aortocarotid 39.22
aortoceliac 39.26
aortocoronary - *see also* Bypass, aortocoronary 36.10
aortofemoral 39.25
aortofemoral-popliteal 39.25
aortoiliac 39.25
to popliteal 39.25
aortoiliofemoral 39.25
aortomesenteric 39.26
aortopopliteal 39.25

Bypass *(Continued)*
vascular NEC *(Continued)*
aortorenal 39.24
aortosubclavian 39.22
axillary-brachial 39.29
axillary-femoral (superficial) 39.29
axillofemoral (superficial) 39.29
carotid-cerebral 39.28
carotid-vertebral 39.28
carotid to subclavian artery 39.22
common hepatic-common iliac-renal 39.26
coronary - *see also* Bypass, aortocoronary 36.10
extracranial-intracranial [EC-IC] 39.28
femoral-femoral 39.29
femoroperoneal 39.29
femoropopliteal (reversed saphenous vein) (saphenous) 39.29

Bypass *(Continued)*
vascular NEC *(Continued)*
femorotibial (anterior) (posterior) 39.29
iliofemoral 39.25
ilioiliac 39.26
internal mammary-coronary artery (single) 36.15
double vessel 36.16
intra-abdominal (arterial) NEC 39.26
venous NEC 39.1
intrathoracic NEC 39.23
peripheral artery NEC 39.29
popliteal-tibial 39.29
renal artery 39.24
splenorenal (venous) 39.1
arterial 39.26
subclavian-axillary 39.29
subclavian-carotid 39.22
subclavian-subclavian 39.22
Y graft to renal arteries 39.24

C

Caldwell operation (sulcus extension) 24.91
Caldwell-Luc operation (maxillary sinusotomy) 22.39
with removal of membrane lining 22.31
Calibration, urethra 89.29
Calicectomy (renal) 55.4
Callander operation (knee disarticulation) 84.16
Caloric test, vestibular function 95.44
Calycectomy (renal) 55.4
Calyco-ileoneocystostomy 55.86
Calycotomy (renal) 55.11
Campbell operation
bone block, ankle 81.11
fasciotomy (iliac crest) 83.14
reconstruction of anterior cruciate ligament 81.45
Campimetry 95.05
Canaliculodacryocystorhinostomy 09.81
Canaliculoplasty 09.73
Canaliculorhinostomy 09.81
Canaloplasty, external auditory meatus 18.6
Cannulation - *see also* Insertion, catheter
ampulla of Vater 51.99
antrum 22.01
arteriovenous 39.93
artery 38.91
caval-mesenteric vein 39.1
cisterna chyli 40.61
Eustachian tube 20.8
lacrimal apparatus 09.42
lymphatic duct, left (thoracic) 40.61
nasal sinus (by puncture) 22.01
through natural ostium 22.02
pancreatic duct 52.92
by retrograde endoscopy (ERP) 52.93
renoportal 39.1
sinus (nasal) (by puncture) 22.01
through natural ostium 22.02
splenorenal (venous) 39.1
arterial 39.26
thoracic duct (cervical approach) (thoracic approach) 40.61
Cannulization - *see* Cannulation
Canthocystostomy 09.82
Canthoplasty 08.59
Canthorrhaphy 08.52
division or severing 08.02
Canthotomy 08.51
Capsulectomy
joint - *see also* Arthrectomy 80.90
kidney 55.91
lens 13.65
with extraction of lens 13.51
ovary 65.29
laparoscopic 65.25
Capsulo-iridectomy 13.65
Capsuloplasty - *see* Arthroplasty
Capsulorrhaphy 81.96
with arthroplasty - *see* Arthroplasty
ankle 81.94
foot 81.94
lower extremity NEC 81.95
upper extremity 81.93
Capsulotomy
joint - *see also* Division, joint capsule 80.40
for claw toe repair 77.57

Capsulotomy *(Continued)*
lens 13.64
with
discission of lens 13.2
removal of foreign body 13.02
by magnet extraction 13.01
Cardiac
mapping 37.27
massage (external) (closed chest) 99.63
open chest 37.91
retraining 93.36
Cardiac support device (CSD) 37.41
Cardiectomy (stomach) 43.5
Cardiocentesis 37.0
Cardiography - *see also* Angiocardiography 88.50
Cardiolysis 37.10
Cardiomyopexy 36.39
Cardiomyotomy 42.7
Cardio-omentopexy 36.39
Cardiopericardiopexy 36.39
Cardioplasty (stomach and esophagus) 44.65
stomach alone 44.66
laparoscopic 44.67
Cardioplegia 39.63
Cardiopneumopexy 36.39
Cardiorrhaphy 37.49
Cardioschisis 37.12
Cardiosplenopexy 36.39
Cardiotomy (exploratory) 37.11
Cardiovalvulotomy - *see* Valvulotomy, heart
Cardioversion (external) 99.62
atrial 99.61
Carotid pulse tracing with ECG lead 89.56
Carpectomy (partial) 77.84
total 77.94
Carroll and Taber arthroplasty (proximal interphalangeal joint) 81.72
Casting (for immobilization) NEC 93.53
with fracture-reduction - *see* Reduction, fracture
Castration
female (oophorectomy, bilateral) 65.51
laparoscopic 65.53
male 62.41
C.A.T. (computerized axial tomography) - *see also* Scan, C.A.T. 88.38
Catheterization - *see also* Insertion, catheter
arteriovenous 39.93
artery 38.91
bladder, indwelling 57.94
percutaneous (cystostomy) 57.17
suprapubic NEC 57.18
bronchus 96.05
with lavage 96.56
cardiac (right) 37.21
combined left and right 37.23
left 37.22
combined with right heart 37.23
right 37.21
combined with left heart 37.23
central venous NEC 38.93
peripherally inserted central catheter (PICC) 38.93
chest 34.04
revision (with lysis of adhesions) 34.04
Eustachian tube 20.8
heart (right) 37.21
combined left and right 37.23

Catheterization *(Continued)*
heart *(Continued)*
left 37.22
combined with right heart 37.23
right 37.21
combined with left heart 37.23
hepatic vein 38.93
inferior vena cava 38.93
intercostal space (with water seal), for drainage 34.04
revision (with lysis of adhesions) 34.04
lacrimonasal duct 09.44
laryngeal 96.05
nasolacrimal duct 09.44
pancreatic cyst 52.01
renal vein 38.93
Swan-Ganz (pulmonary) 89.64
transtracheal for oxygenation 31.99
umbilical vein 38.92
ureter (to kidney) 59.8
for retrograde pyelogram 87.74
urethra, indwelling 57.94
vein NEC 38.93
for renal dialysis 38.95
Cattell operation (herniorrhaphy) 53.51
Cauterization - *see also* Destruction, lesion, by site
anus NEC 49.39
endoscopic 49.31
Bartholin's gland 71.24
broad ligament 69.19
bronchus 32.09
endoscopic 32.01
canaliculi 09.73
cervix 67.32
chalazion 08.25
choroid plexus 02.14
conjunctiva 10.33
lesion 10.32
cornea (fistula) (ulcer) 11.42
ear, external 18.29
endometrial implant - *see* Excision, lesion, by site
entropion 08.41
esophagus 42.39
endoscopic 42.33
eyelid 08.25
for entropion or ectropion 08.41
fallopian tube 66.61
by endoscopy (hysteroscopy) (laparoscopy) 66.29
hemorrhoids 49.43
iris 12.41
lacrimal
gland 09.21
punctum 09.72
for eversion 09.71
sac 09.6
larynx 30.09
liver 50.29
lung 32.29
endoscopic 32.28
meibomian gland 08.25
nose, for epistaxis (with packing) 21.03
ovary 65.29
laparoscopic 65.25
palate (bony) 27.31
pannus (superficial) 11.42
pharynx 29.39
punctum, lacrimal 09.72
for eversion 09.71
rectum 48.32
radical 48.31

Cauterization *(Continued)*
round ligament 69.19
sclera 12.84
with iridectomy 12.62
skin 86.3
subcutaneous tissue 86.3
tonsillar fossa 28.7
urethra 58.39
endoscopic 58.31
uterosacral ligament 69.19
uterotubal ostia 66.61
uterus 68.29
vagina 70.33
vocal cords 30.09
vulva 71.3
Cavernoscopy 34.21
Cavernostomy 33.1
Cavernotomy, kidney 55.39
Cavography (inferior vena cava) 88.51
Cecectomy (with resection of terminal ileum) 45.72
Cecil operation (urethral reconstruction) 58.46
Cecocoloplicopexy 46.63
Cecocolostomy 45.94
Cecofixation 46.64
Ceco-ileostomy 45.93
Cecopexy 46.64
Cecoplication 46.62
Cecorrhaphy 46.75
Cecosigmoidostomy 45.94
Cecostomy (tube) - *see also* Colostomy 46.10
Cecotomy 45.03
Celiocentesis 54.91
Celioscopy 54.21
Celiotomy, exploratory 54.11
Cell block and Papanicolaou smear - *see* Examination, microscopic
Cephalogram 87.17
dental 87.12
orthodontic 87.12
Cephalometry, cephalometrics 87.17
echo 88.78
orthodontic 87.12
ultrasound (sonar) 88.78
x-ray 87.81
Cephalotomy, fetus 73.8
Cerclage
anus 49.72
cervix 67.5
transabdominal 67.51
transvaginal 67.59
isthmus uteri (cervix) 67.59
retinal reattachment - *see also* Buckling, scleral 14.49
sclera - *see also* Buckling, scleral 14.49
Cervicectomy (with synchronous colporrhaphy) 67.4
Cervicoplasty 67.69
Cesarean section 74.99
classical 74.0
corporeal 74.0
extraperitoneal 74.2
fundal 74.0
laparotrachelotomy 74.1
Latzko 74.2
low cervical 74.1
lower uterine segment 74.1
peritoneal exclusion 74.4
specified type NEC 74.4
supravesical 74.2
transperitoneal 74.4
classical 74.0
low cervical 74.1

Cesarean section *(Continued)*
upper uterine segment 74.0
vaginal 74.4
Waters 74.2
Chandler operation (hip fusion) 81.21
Change - *see also* Replacement
cast NEC 97.13
lower limb 97.12
upper limb 97.11
cystostomy catheter or tube 59.94
gastrostomy tube 97.02
length
bone - *see either category* 78.2 Shortening, bone *or* category 78.3 Lengthening, bone
muscle 83.85
hand 82.55
tendon 83.85
hand 82.55
nephrostomy catheter or tube 55.93
pyelostomy catheter or tube 55.94
tracheostomy tube 97.23
ureterostomy catheter or tube 59.93
urethral catheter, indwelling 57.95
Character analysis, psychologic 94.03
Charles operation (correction of lymphedema) 40.9
Charnley operation (compression arthrodesis)
ankle 81.11
hip 81.21
knee 81.22
Cheatle-Henry operation - *see* Repair, hernia, femoral
Check
automatic implantable cardioverter/defibrillator (AICD) (interrogation only) 89.49
CRT-D (cardiac resynchronization defibrillator) (interrogation only) 89.49
CRT-P (cardiac resynchronization pacemaker) (interrogation only) 89.45
pacemaker, artificial (cardiac) (function) (interrogation only) (rate) 89.45
amperage threshold 89.48
artifact wave form 89.46
electrode impedance 89.47
voltage threshold 89.48
vision NEC 95.09
Cheiloplasty 27.59
Cheilorrhaphy 27.51
Cheilostomatoplasty 27.59
Cheilotomy 27.0
Chemical peel, skin 86.24
Chemocauterization - *see also* Destruction, lesion, by site
corneal epithelium 11.41
palate 27.31
Chemodectomy 39.8
Chemoembolization 99.25
Chemolysis
nerve (peripheral) 04.2
spinal canal structure 03.8
Chemoneurolysis 04.2
Chemonucleolysis (nucleus pulposus) 80.52
Chemopallidectomy 01.42
Chemopeel (skin) 86.24
Chemosurgery
esophagus 42.39
endoscopic 42.33
Mohs' 86.24
skin (superficial) 86.24

Chemosurgery *(Continued)*
stomach 43.49
endoscopic 43.41
Chemothalamectomy 01.41
Chemotherapy - *see also* Immunotherapy
Antabuse 94.25
for cancer NEC 99.25
brain wafer implantation 00.10
implantation of chemotherapeutic agent 00.10
interstitial implantation 00.10
intracavitary implantation 00.10
wafer chemotherapy 00.10
lithium 94.22
methadone 94.25
palate (bony) 27.31
Chevalier-Jackson operation (partial laryngectomy) 30.29
Child operation (radical subtotal pancreatectomy) 52.53
Cholangiocholangiostomy 51.39
Cholangiocholecystocholedochectomy 51.22
Cholangio-enterostomy 51.39
Cholangiogastrostomy 51.39
Cholangiogram 87.54
endoscopic retrograde (ERC) 51.11
intraoperative 87.53
intravenous 87.52
percutaneous hepatic 87.51
transhepatic 87.53
Cholangiography - *see also* Cholangiogram 87.54
Cholangiojejunostomy (intrahepatic) 51.39
Cholangiopancreatography, endoscopic retrograde (ERCP) 51.10
Cholangiostomy 51.59
Cholangiotomy 51.59
Cholecystectomy (total) 51.22
partial 51.21
laparoscopic 51.24
total 51.22
laparoscopic 51.23
Cholecystenterorrhaphy 51.91
Cholecystocecostomy 51.32
Cholecystocholangiogram 87.59
Cholecystocolostomy 51.32
Cholecystoduodenostomy 51.32
Cholecystoenterostomy (Winiwater) 51.32
Cholecystogastrostomy 51.34
Cholecystogram 87.59
Cholecystoileostomy 51.32
Cholecystojejunostomy (Roux-en-Y) (with jejunojejunostomy) 51.32
Cholecystopancreatostomy 51.33
Cholecystopexy 51.99
Cholecystorrhaphy 51.91
Cholecystostomy NEC 51.03
by trocar 51.02
Cholecystotomy 51.04
percutaneous 51.01
Choledochectomy 51.63
Choledochoduodenostomy 51.36
Choledochoenterostomy 51.36
Choledochojejunostomy 51.36
Choledocholithotomy 51.41
endoscopic 51.88
Choledocholithotripsy 51.41
endoscopic 51.88
Choledochopancreatostomy 51.39
Choledochoplasty 51.72
Choledochorrhaphy 51.71
Choledochoscopy 51.11

Choledochostomy 51.51
Choledochotomy 51.51
Cholelithotomy 51.04
Chondrectomy 80.90
ankle 80.97
elbow 80.92
foot and toe 80.98
hand and finger 80.94
hip 80.95
intervertebral cartilage - *see* category 80.5
knee (semilunar cartilage) 80.6
nasal (submucous) 21.5
semilunar cartilage (knee) 80.6
shoulder 80.91
specified site NEC 80.99
spine - *see* category 80.5
wrist 80.93
Chondroplasty - *see* Arthroplasty
Chondrosternoplasty (for pectus excavatum repair) 34.74
Chondrotomy - *see also* Division, cartilage 80.40
nasal 21.1
Chopart operation (midtarsal amputation) 84.12
Chordectomy, vocal 30.22
Chordotomy (spinothalamic) (anterior) (posterior) NEC 03.29
percutaneous 03.21
stereotactic 03.21
Ciliarotomy 12.55
Ciliectomy (ciliary body) 12.44
eyelid margin 08.20
Cinch, cinching
for scleral buckling - *see also* Buckling, scleral 14.49
ocular muscle (oblique) (rectus) 15.22
multiple (two or more muscles) 15.4
Cineangiocardiography - *see also* Angiocardiography 88.50
Cineplasty, cineplastic prosthesis
amputation - *see* Amputation
arm 84.44
biceps 84.44
extremity 84.40
lower 84.48
upper 84.44
leg 84.48
Cineradiograph - *see* Radiography
Cingulumotomy (brain) (percutaneous radiofrequency) 01.32
Circumcision (male) 64.0
female 71.4
CISH [classic infrafascial SEMM hysterectomy] 68.31
Clagett operation (closure of chest wall following open flap drainage) 34.72
Clamp and cautery, hemorrhoids 49.43
Clamping
aneurysm (cerebral) 39.51
blood vessel - *see* Ligation, blood vessel
ventricular shunt 02.43
Clavicotomy 77.31
fetal 73.8
Claviculectomy (partial) 77.81
total 77.91
Clayton operation (resection of metatarsal heads and bases of phalanges) 77.88
Cleaning, wound 96.59
Clearance
bladder (transurethral) 57.0

Clearance *(Continued)*
pelvic
female 68.8
male 57.71
prescalene fat pad 40.21
renal pelvis (transurethral) 56.0
ureter (transurethral) 56.0
Cleidotomy 77.31
fetal 73.8
Clipping
aneurysm (basilar) (carotid) (cerebellar) (cerebellopontine) (communicating artery) (vertebral) 39.51
arteriovenous fistula 39.53
frenulum, frenum
labia (lips) 27.91
lingual (tongue) 25.91
tip of uvula 27.72
Clitoridectomy 71.4
Clitoridotomy 71.4
Clivogram 87.02
Closure - *see also* Repair
abdominal wall 54.63
delayed (granulating wound) 54.62
secondary 54.61
tertiary 54.62
amputation stump, secondary 84.3
aorticopulmonary fenestration (fistula) 39.59
appendicostomy 47.92
artificial opening
bile duct 51.79
bladder 57.82
bronchus 33.42
common duct 51.72
esophagus 42.83
gallbladder 51.92
hepatic duct 51.79
intestine 46.50
large 46.52
small 46.51
kidney 55.82
larynx 31.62
rectum 48.72
stomach 44.62
thorax 34.72
trachea 31.72
ureter 56.83
urethra 58.42
atrial septal defect - *see also* Repair, atrial septal defect 35.71
with umbrella device (King-Mills type) 35.52
combined with repair of valvular and ventricular septal defects - *see* Repair, endocardial cushion defect
bronchostomy 33.42
cecostomy 46.52
cholecystostomy 51.92
cleft hand 82.82
colostomy 46.52
cystostomy 57.82
diastema (alveolar) (dental) 24.8
disrupted abdominal wall (postoperative) 54.61
duodenostomy 46.51
encephalocele 02.12
endocardial cushion defect - *see also* Repair, endocardial cushion defect 35.73
enterostomy 46.50
esophagostomy 42.83

Closure *(Continued)*
fenestration
aorticopulmonary 39.59
septal, heart - *see also* Repair, heart, septum 35.70
filtering bleb, corneoscleral (postglaucoma) 12.66
fistula
abdominothoracic 34.83
anorectal 48.73
anovaginal 70.73
antrobuccal 22.71
anus 49.73
aorticopulmonary (fenestration) 39.59
aortoduodenal 39.59
appendix 47.92
biliary tract 51.79
bladder NEC 57.84
branchial cleft 29.52
bronchocutaneous 33.42
bronchoesophageal 33.42
bronchomediastinal 34.73
bronchopleural 34.73
bronchopleurocutaneous 34.73
bronchopleuromediastinal 34.73
bronchovisceral 33.42
bronchus 33.42
cecosigmoidal 46.76
cerebrospinal fluid 02.12
cervicoaural 18.79
cervicosigmoidal 67.62
cervicovesical 57.84
cervix 67.62
cholecystocolic 51.93
cholecystoduodenal 51.93
cholecystoenteric 51.93
cholecystogastric 51.93
cholecystojejunal 51.93
cisterna chyli 40.63
colon 46.76
colovaginal 70.72
common duct 51.72
cornea 11.49
with lamellar graft (homograft) 11.62
autograft 11.61
diaphragm 34.83
duodenum 46.72
ear, middle 19.9
ear drum 19.4
enterocolic 46.74
enterocutaneous 46.74
enterouterine 69.42
enterovaginal 70.74
enterovesical 57.83
esophagobronchial 33.42
esophagocutaneous 42.84
esophagopleurocutaneous 34.73
esophagotracheal 31.73
esophagus NEC 42.84
fecal 46.79
gallbladder 51.93
gastric NEC 44.63
gastrocolic 44.63
gastroenterocolic 44.63
gastroesophageal 42.84
gastrojejunal 44.63
gastrojejunocolic 44.63
heart valve - *see* Repair, heart, valve
hepatic duct 51.79
hepatopleural 34.73
hepatopulmonary 34.73
ileorectal 46.74
ileosigmoidal 46.74

Closure *(Continued)*
fistula *(Continued)*
ileovesical 57.83
ileum 46.74
in ano 49.73
intestine 46.79
large 46.76
small NEC 46.74
intestinocolonic 46.74
intestinoureteral 56.84
intestinouterine 69.42
intestinovaginal 70.74
intestinovesical 57.83
jejunum 46.74
kidney 55.83
lacrimal 09.99
laryngotracheal 31.62
larynx 31.62
lymphatic duct, left (thoracic) 40.63
mastoid (antrum) 19.9
mediastinobronchial 34.73
mediastinocutaneous 34.73
mouth (external) 27.53
nasal 21.82
sinus 22.71
nasolabial 21.82
nasopharyngeal 21.82
oroantral 22.71
oronasal 21.82
oval window (ear) 20.93
pancreaticoduodenal 52.95
perilymph 20.93
perineorectal 48.73
perineosigmoidal 46.76
perineourethroscrotal 58.43
perineum 71.72
perirectal 48.93
pharyngoesophageal 29.53
pharynx NEC 29.53
pleura, pleural NEC 34.93
pleurocutaneous 34.73
pleuropericardial 37.49
pleuroperitoneal 34.83
pulmonoperitoneal 34.83
rectolabial 48.73
rectoureteral 56.84
rectourethral 58.43
rectovaginal 70.73
rectovesical 57.83
rectovesicovaginal 57.83
rectovulvar 48.73
rectum NEC 48.73
renal 55.83
reno-intestinal 55.83
round window 20.93
salivary (gland) (duct) 26.42
scrotum 61.42
sigmoidovaginal 70.74
sigmoidovesical 57.83
splenocolic 41.95
stomach NEC 44.63
thoracic duct 40.63
thoracoabdominal 34.83
thoracogastric 34.83
thoracointestinal 34.83
thorax NEC 34.73
trachea NEC 31.73
tracheoesophageal 31.73
tympanic membrane - *see also* Tympanoplasty 19.4
umbilicourinary 57.51
ureter 56.84
ureterocervical 56.84
ureterorectal 56.84

Closure *(Continued)*
fistula *(Continued)*
ureterosigmoidal 56.84
ureterovaginal 56.84
ureterovesical 56.84
urethra 58.43
urethroperineal 58.43
urethroperineovesical 57.84
urethrorectal 58.43
urethroscrotal 58.43
urethrovaginal 58.43
uteroenteric 69.42
uterointestinal 69.42
uterorectal 69.42
uteroureteric 56.84
uterovaginal 69.42
uterovesical 57.84
vagina 70.75
vaginocutaneous 70.75
vaginoenteric 70.74
vaginoperineal 70.75
vaginovesical 57.84
vesicocervicovaginal 57.84
vesicocolic 57.83
vesicocutaneous 57.84
vesicoenteric 57.83
vesicometrorectal 57.83
vesicoperineal 57.84
vesicorectal 57.83
vesicosigmoidal 57.83
vesicosigmoidovaginal 57.83
vesicoureteral 56.84
vesicoureterovaginal 56.84
vesicourethral 57.84
vesicourethrorectal 57.83
vesicouterine 57.84
vesicovaginal 57.84
vulva 71.72
vulvorectal 48.73
foramen ovale (patent) 35.71
with
prosthesis (open heart technique) 35.51
closed heart technique 35.52
tissue graft 35.61
gastroduodenostomy 44.5
gastrojejunostomy 44.5
gastrostomy 44.62
ileostomy 46.51
jejunostomy 46.51
laceration - *see also* Suture, by site
liver 50.61
laparotomy, delayed 54.62
meningocele (spinal) 03.51
cerebral 02.12
myelomeningocele 03.52
nephrostomy 55.82
palmar cleft 82.82
patent ductus arteriosus 38.85
pelviostomy 55.82
peptic ulcer (bleeding) (perforated) 44.40
perforation
ear drum - *see also* Tympanoplasty 19.4
esophagus 42.82
nasal septum 21.88
tympanic membrane - *see also* Tympanoplasty 19.4
proctostomy 48.72
punctum, lacrimal (papilla) 09.91
pyelostomy 55.82
rectostomy 48.72
septum defect (heart) - *see also* Repair, heart, septum 35.70

Closure *(Continued)*
sigmoidostomy 46.52
skin (V-Y type) 86.59
stoma
bile duct 51.79
bladder 57.82
bronchus 33.42
common duct 51.72
esophagus 42.83
gallbladder 51.92
hepatic duct 51.79
intestine 46.50
large 46.52
small 46.51
kidney 55.82
larynx 31.62
rectum 48.72
stomach 44.62
thorax 34.72
trachea 31.72
ureter 56.83
urethra 58.42
thoracostomy 34.72
tracheostomy 31.72
ulcer (bleeding) (peptic) (perforated) 44.40
duodenum 44.42
gastric 44.41
intestine (perforated) 46.79
skin 86.59
stomach 44.41
ureterostomy 56.83
urethrostomy 58.42
vagina 70.8
vascular percutaneous puncture - *omit code* vesicostomy 57.22
wound - *see also* Suture, by site
with graft - *see* Graft
with tissue adhesive 86.59
Coagulation, electrocoagulation - *see also* Destruction, lesion, by site
aneurysm (cerebral) (peripheral vessel) 39.52
arteriovenous fistula 39.53
brain tissue (incremental) (radiofrequency) 01.59
broad ligament 69.19
cervix 67.32
ear
external 18.29
inner 20.79
middle 20.51
fallopian tube 66.61
gasserian ganglion 04.05
nose, for epistaxis (with packing) 21.03
ovary 65.29
laparoscopic 65.25
pharynx (by diathermy) 29.39
prostatic bed 60.94
rectum (polyp) 48.32
radical 48.31
retina (for)
destruction of lesion 14.21
reattachment 14.51
repair for tear 14.31
round ligament 69.19
semicircular canals 20.79
spinal cord (lesion) 03.4
urethrovesical junction, transurethral 57.49
uterosacral ligament 69.19
uterus 68.29
vagina 70.33
vulva 71.3

ICD-9-CM C Vol. 3

Coating, aneurysm of brain 39.52
Cobalt-60 therapy (treatment) 92.23
Coccygectomy (partial) 77.89
  total 77.99
Coccygotomy 77.39
"Cocked hat" procedure (metacarpal lengthening and transfer of local flap) 82.69
Cockett operation (varicose vein)
  lower limb 38.59
  upper limb 38.53
Cody tack (perforation of footplate) 19.0
Coffey operation (uterine suspension) (Meig's modification) 69.22
Cole operation (anterior tarsal wedge osteotomy) 77.28
Colectomy (partial) (segmental) (subtotal) 45.79
  cecum (with terminal ileum) 45.72
  left (Hartmann) (lower) (radical) 45.75
  multiple segmental 45.71
  right (radical) 45.73
  sigmoid 45.76
  terminal ileum with cecum 45.72
  total 45.8
  transverse 45.74
Collapse, lung, surgical 33.39
  by
    destruction of phrenic nerve 33.31
    pneumoperitoneum 33.33
    pneumothorax, artificially-induced 33.32
    thoracoplasty 33.34
Collection, sperm for artificial insemination 99.96
Collis-Nissen operation (hiatal hernia repair with esophagogastroplasty) 53.80
Colocentesis 45.03
Colocolostomy 45.94
  proximal to distal segment 45.79
Colocystoplasty 57.87 [45.52]
Colofixation 46.64
Coloileotomy 45.00
Colonna operation
  adductor tenotomy (first stage) 83.12
  hip arthroplasty (second stage) 81.40
  reconstruction of hip (second stage) 81.40
Colonoscopy 45.23
  with biopsy 45.25
    rectum 48.24
  fiberoptic (flexible) 45.23
  intraoperative 45.21
  through stoma (artificial) 45.22
  transabdominal 45.21
Colopexy 46.63
Coloplication 46.64
Coloproctostomy 45.94
Colorectosigmoidostomy 45.94
Colorectostomy 45.94
Colorrhaphy 46.75
Coloscopy - *see* Colonoscopy
Colosigmoidostomy 45.94
Colostomy (ileo-ascending) (ileotransverse) (perineal) (transverse) 46.10
  with anterior rectal resection 48.62
  delayed opening 46.14
  loop 46.03
  permanent (magnetic) 46.13
  temporary 46.11
Colotomy 45.03
Colpectomy 70.4
Colpoceliocentesis 70.0
Colpocentesis 70.0
Colpocleisis (complete) (partial) 70.8
Colpohysterectomy 68.59
  laparoscopically assisted (LAVH) 68.51
Colpoperineoplasty 70.79
  with repair of urethrocele 70.50
Colpoperineorrhaphy 70.71
  following delivery 75.69
Colpopexy 70.77
Colpoplasty 70.79
Colpopoiesis 70.61
Colporrhaphy 70.71
  anterior (cystocele repair) 70.51
  for repair of
    cystocele 70.51
      with rectocele 70.50
    enterocele 70.92
    rectocele 70.52
      with cystocele 70.50
    urethrocele 70.51
  posterior (rectocele repair) 70.52
Colposcopy 70.21
Colpotomy 70.14
  for pelvic peritoneal drainage 70.12
Commando operation (radical glossectomy) 25.4
Commissurotomy
  closed heart technique - *see* Valvulotomy, heart
  open heart technique - *see* Valvuloplasty, heart
Compression, trigeminal nerve 04.02
Conchectomy 21.69
Conchotomy 21.1
Conduction study, nerve 89.15
Conduitogram, ileum 87.78
Condylectomy - *see* category 77.8
  mandible 76.5
Condylotomy NEC - *see also* Division, joint capsule 80.40
  mandible (open) 76.62
    closed 76.61
Conization
  cervix (knife) (sharp) (biopsy) 67.2
    by
      cryosurgery 67.33
      electroconization 67.32
Conjunctivocystorhinostomy 09.82
  with insertion of tube or stent 09.83
Conjunctivodacryocystorhinostomy (CDCR) 09.82
  with insertion of tube or stent 09.83
Conjunctivodacryocystostomy 09.82
  with insertion of tube or stent 09.83
Conjunctivoplasty 10.49
Conjunctivorhinostomy 09.82
  with insertion of tube or stent 09.83
Constriction of globe, for scleral buckling - *see also* Buckling, scleral 14.49
Construction
  auricle, ear (with graft) (with implant) 18.71
  ear
    auricle (with graft) (with implant) 18.71
    meatus (osseous) (skin-lined) 18.6
  endorectal ileal pouch (H-pouch) (J-pouch) (S-pouch) (with anastomosis to anus) 45.95
  esophagus, artificial - *see* Anastomosis, esophagus
  ileal bladder (open) 56.51
    closed 57.87 *[45.51]*
  ileal conduit 56.51
Construction *(Continued)*
  larynx, artificial 31.75
  patent meatus (ear) 18.6
  penis (rib graft) (skin graft) (myocutaneous flap) 64.43
  pharyngeal valve, artificial 31.75
  urethra 58.46
  vagina, artificial 70.61
  venous valves (peripheral) 39.59
Consultation 89.09
  comprehensive 89.07
  limited (single organ system) 89.06
  specified type NEC 89.08
Continuous positive airway pressure (CPAP) 93.90
Control
  atmospheric pressure and composition NEC 93.98
    antigen-free air conditioning 93.98
    decompression chamber 93.97
    mountain sanatorium 93.98
  epistaxis 21.00
    by
      cauterization (and packing) 21.03
      coagulation (with packing) 21.03
      electrocoagulation (with packing) 21.03
      excision of nasal mucosa with grafting 21.07
      ligation of artery 21.09
        ethmoidal 21.04
        external carotid 21.06
        maxillary (transantral) 21.05
      packing (nasal) (anterior) 21.01
        posterior (and anterior) 21.02
      specified means NEC 21.09
  hemorrhage 39.98
    abdominal cavity 54.19
    adenoids (postoperative) 28.7
    anus (postoperative) 49.95
    bladder (postoperative) 57.93
    chest 34.09
    colon 45.49
      endoscopic 45.43
    duodenum (ulcer) 44.49
      by
        embolization (transcatheter) 44.44
        suture (ligation) 44.42
      endoscopic 44.43
    esophagus 42.39
      endoscopic 42.33
    gastric (ulcer) 44.49
      by
        embolization (transcatheter) 44.44
        suture (ligation) 44.41
      endoscopic 44.43
    intrapleural 34.09
      postoperative (recurrent) 34.03
    laparotomy site 54.12
    nose - *see also* Control, epistaxis 21.00
    peptic (ulcer) 44.49
      by
        embolization (transcatheter) 44.44
        suture (ligation) 44.40
      endoscopic 44.43
    pleura, pleural cavity 34.09
      postoperative (recurrent) 34.03
    postoperative NEC 39.98
    postvascular surgery 39.41
    prostate 60.94
    specified site NEC 39.98
    stomach - *see* Control, hemorrhage, gastric

Control *(Continued)*
hemorrhage *(Continued)*
thorax NEC 34.09
postoperative (recurrent) 34.03
thyroid (postoperative) 06.02
tonsils (postoperative) 28.7
Conversion
anastomosis - *see* Revision, anastomosis
cardiac rhythm NEC 99.69
to sinus rhythm 99.62
gastrostomy to jejunostomy (endoscopic) 44.32
obstetrical position - *see* Version
Cooling, gastric 96.31
Cordectomy, vocal 30.22
CorCap™ 37.41
Cordopexy, vocal 31.69
Cordotomy
spinal (bilateral) NEC 03.29
percutaneous 03.21
vocal 31.3
Corectomy 12.12
Corelysis 12.35
Coreoplasty 12.35
Corneoconjunctivoplasty 11.53
Corpectomy (vertebral) 80.99 ◄
with diskectomy 80.99 ◄
Correction - *see also* Repair
atresia
esophageal 42.85
by magnetic forces 42.99
external meatus (ear) 18.6
nasopharynx, nasopharyngeal 29.4
rectum 48.0
tricuspid 35.94
atrial septal defect - *see also* Repair, atrial septal defect 35.71
combined with repair of valvular and ventricular septal defects - *see* Repair, endocardial cushion defect
blepharoptosis - *see also* Repair, blepharoptosis 08.36
bunionette (with osteotomy) 77.54
chordee 64.42
claw toe 77.57
cleft
lip 27.54
palate 27.62
clubfoot NEC 83.84
coarctation of aorta
with
anastomosis 38.34
graft replacement 38.44
cornea NEC 11.59
refractive NEC 11.79
epikeratophakia 11.76
keratomileusis 11.71
keratophakia 11.72
radial keratotomy 11.75
esophageal atresia 42.85
by magnetic forces 42.99
everted lacrimal punctum 09.71
eyelid
ptosis - *see also* Repair, blepharoptosis 08.36
retraction 08.38
fetal defect 75.36
forcible, of musculoskeletal deformity NEC 93.29
hammer toe 77.56
hydraulic pressure, open surgery for penile inflatable prosthesis 64.99
urinary artificial sphincter 58.99
intestinal malrotation 46.80

Correction *(Continued)*
intestinal malrotation *(Continued)*
large 46.82
small 46.81
inverted uterus - *see* Repair, inverted uterus
lymphedema (of limb) 40.9
excision with graft 40.9
obliteration of lymphatics 40.9
transplantation of autogenous lymphatics 40.9
nasopharyngeal atresia 29.4
overlapping toes 77.58
palate (cleft) 27.62
prognathism NEC 76.64
prominent ear 18.5
punctum (everted) 09.71
spinal pseudarthrosis - *see* Refusion, spinal
syndactyly 86.85
tetralogy of Fallot
one-stage 35.81
partial - *see* specific procedure
total 35.81
total anomalous pulmonary venous connection
one-stage 35.82
partial - *see* specific procedure
total 35.82
transposition, great arteries, total 35.84
tricuspid atresia 35.94
truncus arteriosus
one-stage 35.83
partial - *see* specific procedure
total 35.83
ureteropelvic junction 55.87
ventricular septal defect - *see also* Repair, ventricular septal defect 35.72
combined with repair of valvular and atrial septal defects - *see* Repair, endocardial cushion defect
Costectomy 77.91
with lung excision - *see* Excision, lung
associated with thoracic operation - *omit code*
Costochondrectomy 77.91
associated with thoracic operation - *omit code*
Costosternoplasty (pectus excavatum repair) 34.74
Costotomy 77.31
Costotransversectomy 77.91
associated with thoracic operation - *omit code*
Counseling (for) NEC 94.49
alcoholism 94.46
drug addiction 94.45
employers 94.49
family (medical) (social) 94.49
marriage 94.49
ophthalmologic (with instruction) 95.36
pastoral 94.49
Countershock, cardiac NEC 99.62
Coventry operation (tibial wedge osteotomy) 77.27
CPAP (continuous positive airway pressure) 93.90
Craniectomy 01.25
linear (opening of cranial suture) 02.01
reopening of site 01.23
strip (opening of cranial suture) 02.01
Cranioclasis, fetal 73.8

Cranioplasty 02.06
with synchronous repair of encephalocele 02.12
Craniotomy 01.24
as operative approach - *omit code*
fetal 73.8
for decompression of fracture 02.02
reopening of site 01.23
Craterization, bone - *see also* Excision, lesion, bone 77.60
Crawford operation (tarso-frontalis sling of eyelid) 08.32
Creation - *see also* Formation
cardiac device (defibrillator) (pacemaker) pocket
with initial insertion of cardiac device - *omit code*
new site (skin) (subcutaneous) 37.79
conduit
ileal (urinary) 56.51
left ventricle and aorta 35.93
right atrium and pulmonary artery 35.94
right ventricle and pulmonary (distal) artery 35.92
in repair of
pulmonary artery atresia 35.92
transposition of great vessels 35.92
truncus arteriosus 35.83
endorectal ileal pouch (H-pouch) (J-pouch) (S-pouch) (with anastomosis to anus) 45.95
esophagogastric sphincteric competence NEC 44.66
laparoscopic 44.67
Hartmann pouch - *see* Colectomy, by site
interatrial fistula 35.42
pericardial window 37.12
pleural window, for drainage 34.09
pocket
cardiac device (defibrillator) (pacemaker)
with initial insertion of cardiac device - *omit code*
new site (skin) (subcutaneous) 37.79
loop recorder 37.79
thalamic stimulator pulse generator
with initial insertion of battery package - *omit code*
new site (skin) (subcutaneous) 86.09
shunt - *see also* Shunt
arteriovenous fistula, for dialysis 39.93
left-to-right (systemic to pulmonary circulation) 39.0
subcutaneous tunnel for esophageal anastomosis 42.86
with anastomosis - *see* Anastomosis, esophagus, antesternal
syndactyly (finger) (toe) 86.89
thalamic stimulator pulse generator
with initial insertion of battery package - *omit code*
new site (skin) (subcutaneous) 86.09
tracheoesophageal fistula 31.95
window
pericardial 37.12
pleura, for drainage 34.09
Credé maneuver 73.59
Cricoidectomy 30.29
Cricothyreotomy (for assistance in breathing) 31.1
Cricothyroidectomy 30.29

ICD-9-CM C Vol. 3

Cricothyrostomy 31.1
Cricothyrotomy (for assistance in breathing) 31.1
Cricotomy (for assistance in breathing) 31.1
Cricotracheotomy (for assistance in breathing) 31.1
Crisis intervention 94.35
Croupette, croup tent 93.94
Crown, dental (ceramic) (gold) 23.41
Crushing
  bone - *see* category 78.4
  calculus
    bile (hepatic) passage 51.49
      endoscopic 51.88
    bladder (urinary) 57.0
    pancreatic duct 52.09
      endoscopic 52.94
  fallopian tube - *see also* Ligation, fallopian tube 66.39
  ganglion - *see* Crushing, nerve
  hemorrhoids 49.45
  nasal septum 21.88
  nerve (cranial) (peripheral) NEC 04.03
    acoustic 04.01
    auditory 04.01
    phrenic 04.03
      for collapse of lung 33.31
    sympathetic 05.0
    trigeminal 04.02
    vestibular 04.01
  vas deferens 63.71
Cryoablation - *see* Ablation
Cryoanalgesia, nerve (cranial) (peripheral) 04.2
Cryoconization, cervix 67.33
Cryodestruction - *see* Destruction, lesion, by site
Cryoextraction, lens - *see also* Extraction, cataract, intracapsular 13.19
Cryohypophysectomy (complete) (total) - *see also* Hypophysectomy 07.69
Cryoleucotomy 01.32
Cryopexy, retinal - *see* Cryotherapy, retina
Cryoprostatectomy 60.62
Cryoretinopexy (for)
  reattachment 14.52
  repair of tear or defect 14.32
Cryosurgery - *see* Cryotherapy
Cryothalamectomy 01.41
Cryotherapy - *see also* Destruction, lesion, by site
  bladder 57.59
  brain 01.59
  cataract 13.19
  cervix 67.33
  choroid - *see* Cryotherapy, retina
  ciliary body 12.72
  corneal lesion (ulcer) 11.43
    to reshape cornea 11.79
  ear
    external 18.29
    inner 20.79
  esophagus 42.39
    endoscopic 42.33
  eyelid 08.25
  hemorrhoids 49.44
  iris 12.41
  nasal turbinates 21.61
  palate (bony) 27.31
  prostate 60.62
  retina (for)
    destruction of lesion 14.22
    reattachment 14.52
    repair of tear 14.32
  skin 86.3

Cryotherapy *(Continued)*
  stomach 43.49
    endoscopic 43.41
  subcutaneous tissue 86.3
  turbinates (nasal) 21.61
  warts 86.3
    genital 71.3
Cryptectomy (anus) 49.39
  endoscopic 49.31
Cryptorchidectomy (unilateral) 62.3
  bilateral 62.41
Cryptotomy (anus) 49.39
  endoscopic 49.31
Cuirass 93.99
Culdocentesis 70.0
Culdoplasty 70.92
Culdoscopy (exploration) (removal of foreign body or lesion) 70.22
Culdotomy 70.12
Culp-Deweerd operation (spiral flap pyeloplasty) 55.87
Culp-Scardino operation (ureteral flap pyeloplasty) 55.87
Culture (and sensitivity) - *see* Examination, microscopic
Curettage (with packing) (with secondary closure) - *see also* Dilation and curettage
  adenoids 28.6
  anus 49.39
    endoscopic 49.31
  bladder 57.59
    transurethral 57.49
  bone - *see also* Excision, lesion, bone 77.60
  brain 01.59
  bursa 83.39
    hand 82.29
  cartilage - *see also* Excision, lesion, joint 80.80
  cerebral meninges 01.51
  chalazion 08.25
  conjunctiva (trachoma follicles) 10.33
  corneal epithelium 11.41
    for smear or culture 11.21
  ear, external 18.29
  eyelid 08.25
  joint - *see also* Excision, lesion, joint 80.80
  meninges (cerebral) 01.51
    spinal 03.4
  muscle 83.32
    hand 82.22
  nerve (peripheral) 04.07
    sympathetic 05.29
  sclera 12.84
  skin 86.3
  spinal cord (meninges) 03.4
  subgingival 24.31
  tendon 83.39
    sheath 83.31
      hand 82.21
  uterus (with dilation) 69.09
    aspiration (diagnostic) NEC 69.59
      after abortion or delivery 69.52
      to terminate pregnancy 69.51
    following delivery or abortion 69.02
Curette evacuation, lens 13.2
Curtis operation (interphalangeal joint arthroplasty) 81.72
Cutaneolipectomy 86.83
Cutdown, venous 38.94
Cutting
  nerve (cranial) (peripheral) NEC 04.03
    acoustic 04.01
    auditory 04.01
    root, spinal 03.1

Cutting *(Continued)*
  nerve NEC *(Continued)*
    sympathetic 05.0
    trigeminal 04.02
    vestibular 04.01
  pedicle (flap) graft 86.71
  pylorus (with wedge resection) 43.3
  spinal nerve root 03.1
  ureterovesical orifice 56.1
  urethral sphincter 58.5
CVP (central venous pressure monitoring) 89.62
Cyclectomy (ciliary body) 12.44
  eyelid margin 08.20
Cyclicotomy 12.55
Cycloanemization 12.74
Cyclocryotherapy 12.72
Cyclodialysis (initial) (subsequent) 12.55
Cyclodiathermy (penetrating) (surface) 12.71
Cycloelectrolysis 12.71
Cyclophotocoagulation 12.73
Cyclotomy 12.55
Cystectomy - *see also* Excision, lesion, by site
  gallbladder - *see* Cholecystectomy
  urinary (partial) (subtotal) 57.6
    complete (with urethrectomy) 57.79
    radical 57.71
      with pelvic exenteration (female) 68.8
    total (with urethrectomy) 57.79
Cystocolostomy 57.88
Cystogram, cystography NEC 87.77
Cystolitholapaxy 57.0
Cystolithotomy 57.19
Cystometrogram 89.22
Cystopexy NEC 57.89
Cystoplasty NEC 57.89
Cystoproctostomy 57.88
Cystoprostatectomy, radical 57.71
Cystopyelography 87.74
Cystorrhaphy 57.81
Cystoscopy (transurethral) 57.32
  with biopsy 57.33
  for
    control of hemorrhage
      bladder 57.93
      prostate 60.94
    retrograde pyelography 87.74
  ileal conduit 56.35
  through stoma (artificial) 57.31
Cystostomy
  closed (suprapubic) (percutaneous) 57.17
  open (suprapubic) 57.18
  percutaneous (closed) (suprapubic) 57.17
  suprapubic
    closed 57.17
    open 57.18
Cystotomy (open) (for removal of calculi) 57.19
Cystourethrogram (retrograde) (voiding) 87.76
Cystourethropexy (by) 59.79
  levator muscle sling 59.71
  retropubic suspension 59.5
  suprapubic suspension 59.4
Cystourethroplasty 57.85
Cystourethroscopy 57.32
  with biopsy
    bladder 57.33
    ureter 56.33
Cytology - *see* Examination, microscopic

D

Dacryoadenectomy 09.20
  partial 09.22
  total 09.23
Dacryoadenotomy 09.0
Dacryocystectomy (complete) (partial) 09.6
Dacryocystogram 87.05
Dacryocystorhinostomy (DCR) (by intubation) (external) (intranasal) 09.81
Dacryocystostomy 09.53
Dacryocystosyringotomy 09.53
Dacryocystotomy 09.53
Dahlman operation (excision of esophageal diverticulum) 42.31
Dana operation (posterior rhizotomy) 03.1
Danforth operation (fetal) 73.8
Darrach operation (ulnar resection) 77.83
Davis operation (intubated ureterotomy) 56.2
Deaf training 95.49
Debridement
  abdominal wall 54.3
  bone - *see also* Excision, lesion, bone 77.60
    fracture - *see* Debridement, open fracture
  brain 01.59
  burn (skin) 86.28
    excisional 86.22
    nonexcisional 86.28
  bursa 83.5
  cerebral meninges 01.51
  dental 96.54
  fascia 83.39
  flap graft 86.75
  graft (flap) (pedicle) 86.75
  heart valve (calcified) - *see* Valvuloplasty, heart
  infection (skin) 86.28
    excisional 86.22
    nail (bed) (fold) 86.27
    nonexcisional 86.28
  joint - *see* Excision, lesion, joint
  meninges (cerebral) 01.51
    spinal 03.4
  muscle 83.45
    hand 82.36
  nail (bed) (fold) 86.27
  nerve (peripheral) 04.07
  open fracture (compound) 79.60
    arm NEC 79.62
    carpal, metacarpal 79.63
    facial bone 76.2
    femur 79.65
    fibula 79.66
    foot NEC 79.67
    hand NEC 79.63
    humerus 79.61
    leg NEC 79.66
    phalanges
      foot 79.68
      hand 79.64
    radius 79.62
    specified site NEC 79.69
    tarsal, metatarsal 79.67
    tibia 79.66
    ulna 79.62
  patella 77.66
  pedicle graft 86.75
  skin or subcutaneous tissue (burn) (infection) (wound) 86.28

Debridement *(Continued)*
  skin or subcutaneous tissue *(Continued)*
    cardioverter/defibrillator (automatic) pocket 37.79 (Revised)
    excisional 86.22
    graft 86.75
    nail, nail bed, or nail fold 86.27
    nonexcisional 86.28
    pacemaker pocket 37.79
    pocket
      cardiac device NEC 37.79 (New)
      cardiac pacemaker 37.79
      cardioverter/defibrillator (automatic) 37.79 (Revised)
  skull 01.25
    compound fracture 02.02
  spinal cord (meninges) 03.4
  VersaJet™ 86.28 (New)
  wound (skin) 86.28
    excisional 86.22
    nonexcisional 86.28
Decapitation, fetal 73.8
Decapsulation, kidney 55.91
Declotting - *see also* Removal, thrombus
  arteriovenous cannula or shunt 39.49
Decompression
  anus (imperforate) 48.0
  biliary tract 51.49
    by intubation 51.43
      endoscopic 51.87
      percutaneous 51.98
  brain 01.24
  carpal tunnel 04.43
  cauda equina 03.09
  chamber 93.97
  colon 96.08
    by incision 45.03
    endoscopic (balloon) 46.85
  common bile duct 51.42
    by intubation 51.43
      endoscopic 51.87
      percutaneous 51.98
  cranial 01.24
    for skull fracture 02.02
  endolymphatic sac 20.79
  ganglion (peripheral) NEC 04.49
    cranial NEC 04.42
  gastric 96.07
  heart 37.0
  intestine 96.08
    by incision 45.00
    endoscopic (balloon) 46.85
  intracranial 01.24
  labyrinth 20.79
  laminectomy 03.09
  laminotomy 03.09
  median nerve 04.43
  muscle 83.02
    hand 82.02
  nerve (peripheral) NEC 04.49
    auditory 04.42
    cranial NEC 04.42
    median 04.43
    trigeminal (root) 04.41
  orbit - *see also* Orbitotomy 16.09
  pancreatic duct 52.92
    endoscopic 52.93
  pericardium 37.0
  rectum 48.0
  skull fracture 02.02
  spinal cord (canal) 03.09
  tarsal tunnel 04.44
  tendon (sheath) 83.01
    hand 82.01

Decompression *(Continued)*
  thoracic outlet
    by
      myotomy (division of scalenus anticus muscle) 83.19
      tenotomy 83.13
  trigeminal (nerve root) 04.41
Decortication
  arterial 05.25
  brain 01.51
  cerebral meninges 01.51
  heart 37.31
  kidney 55.91
  lung (partial) (total) 34.51
  nasal turbinates - *see* Turbinectomy
  nose 21.89
  ovary 65.29
    laparoscopic 65.25
  periarterial 05.25
  pericardium 37.31
  ventricle, heart (complete) 37.31
Decoy, E2F 00.16
Deepening
  alveolar ridge 24.5
  buccolabial sulcus 24.91
  lingual sulcus 24.91
Defatting, flap or pedicle graft 86.75
Defibrillation, electric (external) (internal) 99.62
  automatic cardioverter/defibrillator - *see* category 37.9
de Grandmont operation (tarsectomy) 08.35
Delaying of pedicle graft 86.71
Delivery (with)
  assisted spontaneous 73.59
  breech extraction (assisted) 72.52
    partial 72.52
      with forceps to aftercoming head 72.51
    total 72.54
      with forceps to aftercoming head 72.53
    unassisted (spontaneous delivery) - *omit code*
  cesarean section - *see* Cesarean section
  Credé maneuver 73.59
  De Lee maneuver 72.4
  forceps 72.9
    application to aftercoming head (Piper) 72.6
      with breech extraction
        partial 72.51
        total 72.53
    Barton's 72.4
    failed 73.3
    high 72.39
      with episiotomy 72.31
    low (outlet) 72.0
      with episiotomy 72.1
    mid- 72.29
      with episiotomy 72.21
    outlet (low) 72.0
      with episiotomy 72.1
    rotation of fetal head 72.4
    trial 73.3
    instrumental NEC 72.9
      specified NEC 72.8
  key-in-lock rotation 72.4
  Kielland rotation 72.4
  Malstrom's extraction 72.79
    with episiotomy 72.71
  manually assisted (spontaneous) 73.59

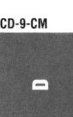

ICD-9-CM D Vol. 3

Delivery *(Continued)*
spontaneous (unassisted) 73.59
assisted 73.59
vacuum extraction 72.79
with episiotomy 72.71
Delorme operation
pericardiectomy 37.31
proctopexy 48.76
repair of prolapsed rectum 48.76
thoracoplasty 33.34
Denervation
aortic body 39.8
carotid body 39.8
facet, percutaneous (radiofrequency) 03.96
ovarian 65.94
paracervical uterine 69.3
uterosacral 69.3
Denker operation (radical maxillary antrotomy) 22.31
Dennis-Barco operation - *see* Repair, hernia, femoral
Denonvilliers operation (limited rhinoplasty) 21.86
Densitometry, bone (serial) (radiographic) 88.98
Depilation, skin 86.92
Derlacki operation (tympanoplasty) 19.4
Dermabond 86.59
Dermabrasion (laser) 86.25
for wound debridement 86.28
Derotation - *see* Reduction, torsion
Desensitization
allergy 99.12
psychologic 94.33
Desmotomy - *see also* Division, ligament 80.40
Destruction
breast 85.20
chorioretinopathy - *see also* Destruction, lesion, choroid 14.29
ciliary body 12.74
epithelial downgrowth, anterior chamber 12.93
fallopian tube 66.39
with
crushing (and ligation) 66.31
by endoscopy (laparoscopy) 66.21
division (and ligation) 66.32
by endoscopy (culdoscopy) (hysteroscopy) (laparoscopy) (peritoneoscopy) 66.22
ligation 66.39
with
crushing 66.31
by endoscopy (laparoscopy) 66.21
division 66.32
by endoscopy (culdoscopy) (hysteroscopy) (laparoscopy) (peritoneoscopy) 66.22
fetus 73.8
hemorrhoids 49.49
by
cryotherapy 49.44
sclerotherapy 49.42
inner ear NEC 20.79
by injection 20.72
intervertebral disc (NOS) 80.50
by injection 80.52
by other specified method 80.59
herniated (nucleus pulposus) 80.51

Destruction *(Continued)*
lacrimal sac 09.6
lesion (local)
anus 49.39
endoscopic 49.31
Bartholin's gland 71.24
by
aspiration 71.21
excision 71.24
incision 71.22
marsupialization 71.23
biliary ducts 51.69
endoscopic 51.64
bladder 57.59
transurethral 57.49
bone - *see* Excision, lesion, bone
bowel - *see* Destruction, lesion, intestine
brain (transtemporal approach) NEC 01.59
by stereotactic radiosurgery 92.30
cobalt 60 92.32
linear accelerator (LINAC) 92.31
multi-source 92.32
particle beam 92.33
particulate 92.33
radiosurgery NEC 92.39
single source photon 92.31
breast NEC 85.20
bronchus NEC 32.09
endoscopic 32.01
cerebral NEC 01.59
meninges 01.51
cervix 67.39
by
cauterization 67.32
cryosurgery, cryoconization 67.33
electroconization 67.32
choroid 14.29
by
cryotherapy 14.22
diathermy 14.21
implantation of radiation source 14.27
photocoagulation 14.25
laser 14.24
xenon arc 14.23
radiation therapy 14.26
ciliary body (nonexcisional) 12.43
by excision 12.44
conjunctiva 10.32
by excision 10.31
cornea NEC 11.49
by
cryotherapy 11.43
electrocauterization 11.42
thermocauterization 11.42
cul-de-sac 70.32
duodenum NEC 45.32
by excision 45.31
endoscopic 45.30
endoscopic 45.30
esophagus (chemosurgery) (cryosurgery) (electroresection) (fulguration) NEC 42.39
by excision 42.32
endoscopic 42.33
endoscopic 42.33
eye NEC 16.93
eyebrow 08.25
eyelid 08.25
excisional - *see* Excision, lesion, eyelid

Destruction *(Continued)*
lesion *(Continued)*
heart 37.33
by catheter ablation 37.34
intestine (large) 45.49
by excision 45.41
endoscopic 45.43
polypectomy 45.42
endoscopic 45.43
polypectomy 45.42
small 45.34
by excision 45.33
intranasal 21.31
iris (nonexcisional) NEC 12.41
by excision 12.42
kidney 55.39
by marsupialization 55.31
lacrimal sac 09.6
larynx 30.09
liver 50.29
lung 32.29
endoscopic 32.28
meninges (cerebral) 01.51
spinal 03.4
nerve (peripheral) 04.07
sympathetic 05.29
nose 21.30
intranasal 21.31
specified NEC 21.32
ovary
by
aspiration 65.91
excision 65.29
laparoscopic 65.25
cyst by rupture (manual) 65.93
palate (bony) (local) 27.31
wide 27.32
pancreas 52.22
by marsupialization 52.3
endoscopic 52.21
pancreatic duct 52.22
endoscopic 52.21
penis 64.2
pharynx (excisional) 29.39
pituitary gland
by stereotactic radiosurgery 92.30
cobalt 60 92.32
linear accelerator (LINAC) 92.31
multi-source 92.32
particle beam 92.33
particulate 92.33
radiosurgery NEC 92.39
single source photon 92.31
rectum (local) 48.32
by
cryosurgery 48.34
electrocoagulation 48.32
excision 48.35
fulguration 48.32
laser (Argon) 48.33
polyp 48.36
radical 48.31
retina 14.29
by
cryotherapy 14.22
diathermy 14.21
implantation of radiation source 14.27
photocoagulation 14.25
laser 14.24
xenon arc 14.23
radiation therapy 14.26
salivary gland NEC 26.29
by marsupialization 26.21

Destruction *(Continued)*
lesion *(Continued)*
sclera 12.84
scrotum 61.3
skin NEC 86.3
sphincter of Oddi 51.69
endoscopic 51.64
spinal cord (meninges) 03.4
spleen 41.42
by marsupialization 41.41
stomach NEC 43.49
by excision 43.42
endoscopic 43.41
endoscopic 43.41
subcutaneous tissue NEC 86.3
testis 62.2
tongue 25.1
urethra (excisional) 58.39
endoscopic 58.31
uterus 68.29
nerve (cranial) (peripheral) (by cryoanalgesia) (by radiofrequency) 04.2
sympathetic, by injection of neurolytic agent 05.32
neuroma
acoustic 04.01
by craniotomy 04.01
by stereotactic radiosurgery 92.30
cobalt 60 92.32
linear accelerator (LINAC) 92.31
multi-source 92.32
particle beam 92.33
particulate 92.33
radiosurgery NEC 92.39
single source photon 92.31
cranial 04.07
Morton's 04.07
peripheral
Morton's 04.07
prostate (prostatic tissue)
by
cryotherapy 60.62
microwave 60.96
radiofrequency 60.97
transurethral microwave thermotherapy (TUMT) 60.96
transurethral needle ablation (TUNA) 60.97
TULIP (transurethral (ultrasound) guided laser induced prostatectomy) 60.21
TUMT (transurethral microwave thermotherapy) 60.96
TUNA (transurethral needle ablation) 60.97
semicircular canals, by injection 20.72
vestibule, by injection 20.72
Detachment, uterosacral ligaments 69.3
Determination
mental status (clinical) (medicolegal) (psychiatric) NEC 94.11
psychologic NEC 94.09
vital capacity (pulmonary) 89.37
Detorsion
intestine (twisted) (volvulus) 46.80
large 46.82
endoscopic (balloon) 46.85
small 46.81
kidney 55.84
ovary 65.95
spermatic cord 63.52
with orchiopexy 62.5
testis 63.52
with orchiopexy 62.5
Detorsion *(Continued)*
volvulus 46.80
endoscopic (balloon) 46.85
Detoxification therapy 94.25
alcohol 94.62
with rehabilitation 94.63
combined alcohol and drug 94.68
with rehabilitation 94.69
drug 94.65
with rehabilitation 94.66
combined alcohol and drug 94.68
with rehabilitation 94.69
Devascularization, stomach 44.99
Device
CorCap™ 37.41
external fixator - *see* Fixator, external
Dewebbing
esophagus 42.01
syndactyly (fingers) (toes) 86.85
Dextrorotation - *see* Reduction, torsion
Dialysis
hemodiafiltration, hemofiltration (extracorporeal) 39.95
kidney (extracorporeal) 39.95
liver 50.92
peritoneal 54.98
renal (extracorporeal) 39.95
Diaphanoscopy
nasal sinuses 89.35
skull (newborn) 89.16
Diaphysectomy - *see* category 77.8
Diathermy 93.34
choroid - *see* Diathermy, retina
nasal turbinates 21.61
retina
for
destruction of lesion 14.21
reattachment 14.51
repair of tear 14.31
surgical - *see* Destruction, lesion, by site
turbinates (nasal) 21.61
Dickson operation (fascial transplant) 83.82
Dickson-Diveley operation (tendon transfer and arthrodesis to correct claw toe) 77.57
Dieffenbach operation (hip disarticulation) 84.18
Dilation
achalasia 42.92
ampulla of Vater 51.81
endoscopic 51.84
anus, anal (sphincter) 96.23
biliary duct
endoscopic 51.84
pancreatic duct 52.99
endoscopic 52.98
percutaneous (endoscopy) 51.98
sphincter
of Oddi 51.81
endoscopic 51.84
pancreatic 51.82
endoscopic 51.85
bladder 96.25
neck 57.92
bronchus 33.91
cervix (canal) 67.0
obstetrical 73.1
to assist delivery 73.1
choanae (nasopharynx) 29.91
colon (endoscopic) (balloon) 46.85
colostomy stoma 96.24
duodenum (endoscopic) (balloon) 46.85
endoscopic - *see* Dilation, by site
Dilation *(Continued)*
enterostomy stoma 96.24
esophagus (by bougie) (by sound) 42.92
fallopian tube 66.96
foreskin (newborn) 99.95
frontonasal duct 96.21
gastrojejunostomy site, endoscopic 44.22
heart valve - *see* Valvulotomy, heart
ileostomy stoma 96.24
ileum (endoscopic) (balloon) 46.85
intestinal stoma (artificial) 96.24
intestine (endoscopic) (balloon) 46.85
jejunum (endoscopic) (balloon) 46.85
lacrimal
duct 09.42
punctum 09.41
larynx 31.98
lymphatic structure(s) (peripheral) 40.9
nares 21.99
nasolacrimal duct (retrograde) 09.43
with insertion of tube or stent 09.44
nasopharynx 29.91
pancreatic duct 52.99
endoscopic 52.98
pharynx 29.91
prostatic urethra (transurethral) (balloon) 60.95
punctum, lacrimal papilla 09.41
pylorus
by incision 44.21
endoscopic 44.22
rectum 96.22
salivary duct 26.91
sphenoid ostia 22.52
sphincter
anal 96.23
cardiac 42.92
of Oddi 51.81
endoscopic 51.84
pancreatic 51.82
endoscopic 51.85
pylorus, endoscopic 44.22
by incision 44.21
Stenson's duct 26.91
trachea 31.99
ureter 59.8
meatus 56.91
ureterovesical orifice 59.8
urethra 58.6
prostatic (transurethral) (balloon) 60.95
urethrovesical junction 58.6
vagina (instrumental) (manual) NEC 96.16
vesical neck 57.92
Wharton's duct 26.91
Wirsung's duct 52.99
endoscopic 52.98
Dilation and curettage, uterus (diagnostic) 69.09
after
abortion 69.02
delivery 69.02
to terminate pregnancy 69.01
Diminution, ciliary body 12.74
Disarticulation 84.91
ankle 84.13
elbow 84.06
finger, except thumb 84.01
thumb 84.02
hip 84.18
knee 84.16
shoulder 84.08

Disarticulation *(Continued)*
thumb 84.02
toe 84.11
wrist 84.04
Discectomy - *see* Diskectomy
Discission
capsular membrane 13.64
cataract (Wheeler knife) (Ziegler knife) 13.2
congenital 13.69
secondary membrane 13.64
iris 12.12
lens (capsule) (Wheeler knife) (Ziegler knife) (with capsulotomy) 13.2
orbitomaxillary, radical 16.51
pupillary 13.2
secondary membrane (after cataract) 13.64
vitreous strands (posterior approach) 14.74
anterior approach 14.73
Discogram, diskogram 87.21
Discolysis (by injection) 80.52
Diskectomy, (discectomy) intervertebral 80.51
with corpectomy 80.99 ◀
herniated (nucleus pulposus) 80.51
percutaneous 80.59
Dispensing (with fitting)
contact lens 95.32
low vision aids NEC 95.33
spectacles 95.31
Dissection - *see also* Excision
aneurysm 38.60
artery-vein-nerve bundle 39.91
branchial cleft fistula or sinus 29.52
bronchus 32.1
femoral hernia 53.29
groin, radical 40.54
larynx block (en bloc) 30.3
mediastinum with pneumonectomy 32.5
neck, radical 40.40
with laryngectomy 30.4
bilateral 40.42
unilateral 40.41
orbital fibrous bands 16.92
pterygium (with reposition) 11.31
radical neck - *see* Dissection, neck, radical
retroperitoneal NEC 59.00
thoracic structures (block) (brachial plexus, bronchus, lobe of lung, ribs, and sympathetic nerves) (en bloc) (radical) 32.6
vascular bundle 39.91
Distention, bladder (therapeutic) (intermittent) 96.25
Diversion
biliopancreatic (BPD) 43.7 *[45.51] [45.91]*
with duodenal switch 43.89 *[45.51] [45.91]*
urinary
cutaneous 56.61
ileal conduit 56.51
internal NEC 56.71
ureter to
intestine 56.71
skin 56.61
uretero-ileostomy 56.51
Diversional therapy 93.81
Diverticulectomy
bladder (suprapubic) 57.59
transurethral approach 57.49

Diverticulectomy *(Continued)*
duodenum 45.31
endoscopic 45.30
esophagus 42.31
endoscopic 42.33
esophagomyotomy 42.7
hypopharyngeal (by cricopharyngeal myotomy) 29.32
intestine
large 45.41
endoscopic 45.43
small 45.33
kidney 55.39
Meckel's 45.33
pharyngeal (by cricopharyngeal myotomy) 29.32
pharyngoesophageal (by cricopharyngeal myotomy) 29.32
stomach 43.42
endoscopic 43.41
urethra 58.39
endoscopic 58.31
Division
Achilles tendon 83.11
adductor tendon (hip) 83.12
adhesions - *see* Lysis, adhesions
angle of mandible (open) 76.62
closed 76.61
anterior synechiae 12.32
aponeurosis 83.13
arcuate ligament (spine) - *omit code*
arteriovenous fistula (with ligation) 39.53
artery (with ligation) 38.80
abdominal 38.86
aorta (arch) (ascending) (descending) 38.84
head and neck NEC 38.82
intracranial NEC 38.81
lower limb 38.88
thoracic NEC 38.85
upper limb 38.83
bladder neck 57.91
blepharorrhaphy 08.02
blood vessels, cornea 10.1
bone - *see also* Osteotomy 77.30
brain tissue 01.32
cortical adhesions 02.91
canaliculus 09.52
canthorrhaphy 08.02
cartilage 80.40
ankle 80.47
elbow 80.42
foot and toe 80.48
hand and finger 80.44
hip 80.45
knee 80.46
shoulder 80.41
specified site NEC 80.49
spine 80.49
wrist 80.43
cerebral tracts 01.32
chordae tendineae 35.32
common wall between posterior left atrium and coronary sinus (with roofing of resultant defect with patch graft) 35.82
congenital web
larynx 31.98
pharynx 29.54
endometrial synechiae 68.21
fallopian tube - *see* Ligation, fallopian tube
fascia 83.14
hand 82.12

Division *(Continued)*
frenulum, frenum
labial 27.91
lingual 25.91
tongue 25.91
ganglion, sympathetic 05.0
glossopharyngeal nerve 29.92
goniosynechiae 12.31
hypophyseal stalk - *see also* Hypophysectomy, partial 07.63
iliotibial band 83.14
isthmus
horseshoe kidney 55.85
thyroid 06.91
joint capsule 80.40
ankle 80.47
elbow 80.42
foot and toe 80.48
hand and finger 80.44
hip 80.45
knee 80.46
shoulder 80.41
specified site NEC 80.49
wrist 80.43
labial frenum 27.91
lacrimal ductules 09.0
laryngeal nerve (external) (recurrent) (superior) 31.91
ligament 80.40
ankle 80.47
arcuate (spine) - *omit code*
canthal 08.36
elbow 80.42
foot and toe 80.48
hand and finger 80.44
hip 80.45
knee 80.46
palpebrae 08.36
shoulder 80.41
specified site NEC 80.49
spine 80.49
arcuate - *omit code*
flavum - *omit code*
uterosacral 69.3
wrist 80.43
ligamentum flavum (spine) - *omit code*
meninges (cerebral) 01.31
muscle 83.19
hand 82.19
nasolacrimal duct stricture (with drainage) 09.59
nerve (cranial) (peripheral) NEC 04.03
acoustic 04.01
adrenal gland 07.42
auditory 04.01
glossopharyngeal 29.92
lacrimal branch 05.0
laryngeal (external) (recurrent) (superior) 31.91
phrenic 04.03
for collapse of lung 33.31
root, spinal or intraspinal 03.1
sympathetic 05.0
tracts
cerebral 01.32
spinal cord 03.29
percutaneous 03.21
trigeminal 04.02
vagus - *see also* Vagotomy 44.00
vestibular 04.01
otosclerotic process or material, middle ear 19.0
papillary muscle (heart) 35.31
patent ductus arteriosus 38.85

◀ New ⟵ Revised

Division *(Continued)*
penile adhesions 64.93
posterior synechiae 12.33
pylorus (with wedge resection) 43.3
rectum (stricture) 48.91
scalenus anticus muscle 83.19
Skene's gland 71.3
soft tissue NEC 83.19
hand 82.19
sphincter
anal (external) (internal) 49.59
left lateral 49.51
posterior 49.52
cardiac 42.7
of Oddi 51.82
endoscopic 51.85
pancreatic 51.82
endoscopic 51.85
spinal
cord tracts 03.29
percutaneous 03.21
nerve root 03.1
symblepharon (with insertion of conformer) 10.5
synechiae
endometrial 68.21
iris (posterior) 12.33
anterior 12.32
tarsorrhaphy 08.02
tendon 83.13
Achilles 83.11
adductor (hip) 83.12
hand 82.11
trabeculae carneae cordis (heart) 35.35
tympanum 20.23
uterosacral ligaments 69.3
vaginal septum 70.14
vas deferens 63.71
vein (with ligation) 38.80
abdominal 38.87
head and neck NEC 38.82
intracranial NEC 38.81
lower limb 38.89
varicose 38.59
thoracic NEC 38.85
upper limb 38.83
varicose 38.50
abdominal 38.57
head and neck NEC 38.52
intracranial NEC 38.51
lower limb 38.59
thoracic NEC 38.55
upper limb 38.53
vitreous, cicatricial bands (posterior approach) 14.74
anterior approach 14.73
Doleris operation (shortening of round ligaments) 69.22
D'Ombrain operation (excision of pterygium with corneal graft) 11.32
Domestic tasks therapy 93.83
Dopplergram, Doppler flow mapping - *see also* Ultrasonography
aortic arch 88.73
head and neck 88.71
heart 88.72
thorax NEC 88.73
Dorrance operation (push-back operation for cleft palate) 27.62
Dotter operation (transluminal angioplasty) 39.59
Douche, vagina 96.44
Douglas' operation (suture of tongue to lip for micrognathia) 25.59
Doyle operation (paracervical uterine denervation) 69.3
Drainage
by
anastomosis - *see* Anastomosis
aspiration - *see* Aspiration
incision - *see* Incision
abdomen 54.19
percutaneous 54.91
abscess - *see also* Drainage, by site and Incision, by site
appendix 47.2
with appendectomy 47.09
laparoscopic 47.01
parapharyngeal (oral) (transcervical) 28.0
peritonsillar (oral) (transcervical) 28.0
retropharyngeal (oral) (transcervical) 28.0
thyroid (field) (gland) 06.09
percutaneous (needle) 06.01
postoperative 06.02
tonsil, tonsillar (oral) (transcervical) 28.0
antecubital fossa 86.04
appendix 47.91
with appendectomy 47.09
laparoscopic 47.01
abscess 47.2
with appendectomy 47.09
laparoscopic 47.01
axilla 86.04
bladder (without incision) 57.0
by indwelling catheter 57.94
percutaneous suprapubic (closed) 57.17
suprapubic NEC 57.18
buccal space 27.0
bursa 83.03
by aspiration 83.94
hand 82.92
hand 82.03
by aspiration 82.92
radial 82.03
ulnar 82.03
cerebrum, cerebral (meninges) (ventricle) (incision) (trephination) 01.39
by
anastomosis - *see* Shunt, ventricular
aspiration 01.09
through previously implanted catheter 01.02
chest (closed) 34.04
open (by incision) 34.09
cranial sinus (incision) (trephination) 01.21
by aspiration 01.09
cul-de-sac 70.12
by aspiration 70.0
cyst - *see also* Drainage, by site and Incision, by site
pancreas (by catheter) 52.01
by marsupialization 52.3
internal (anastomosis) 52.4
pilonidal 86.03
spleen, splenic (by marsupialization) 41.41
duodenum (tube) 46.39
by incision 45.01
ear
external 18.09
inner 20.79
middle (by myringotomy) 20.09
with intubation 20.01
Drainage *(Continued)*
epidural space, cerebral (incision) (trephination) 01.24
by aspiration 01.09
extradural space, cerebral (incision) (trephination) 01.24
by aspiration 01.09
extraperitoneal 54.0
facial region 27.0
fascial compartments, head and neck 27.0
fetal hydrocephalic head (needling) (trocar) 73.8
gallbladder 51.04
by
anastomosis 51.35
aspiration 51.01
incision 51.04
groin region (abdominal wall) (inguinal) 54.0
skin 86.04
subcutaneous tissue 86.04
hematoma - *see* Drainage, by site and Incision, by site
hydrocephalic head (needling) (trocar) 73.8
hypochondrium 54.0
intra-abdominal 54.19
iliac fossa 54.0
infratemporal fossa 27.0
intracranial space (epidural) (extradural) (incision) (trephination) 01.24
by aspiration 01.09
subarachnoid or subdural (incision) (trephination) 01.31
by aspiration 01.09
intraperitoneal 54.19
percutaneous 54.91
kidney (by incision) 55.01
by
anastomosis 55.86
catheter 59.8
pelvis (by incision) 55.11
liver 50.0
by aspiration 50.91
Ludwig's angina 27.0
lung (by incision) 33.1
by punch (needle) (trocar) 33.93
midpalmar space 82.04
mouth floor 27.0
mucocele, nasal sinus 22.00
by puncture 22.01
through natural ostium 22.02
omentum 54.19
percutaneous 54.91
ovary (aspiration) 65.91
by incision 65.09
laparoscopic 65.01
palmar space (middle) 82.04
pancreas (by catheter) 52.01
by anastomosis 52.96
parapharyngeal 28.0
paronychia 86.04
parotid space 27.0
pelvic peritoneum (female) 70.12
male 54.19
pericardium 37.0
perigastric 54.19
percutaneous 54.91
perineum
female 71.09
male 86.04
perisplenic tissue 54.19
percutaneous 54.91

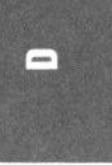

Drainage *(Continued)*
peritoneum 54.19
pelvic (female) 70.12
percutaneous 54.91
peritonsillar 28.0
pharyngeal space, lateral 27.0
pilonidal cyst or sinus 86.03
pleura (closed) 34.04
open (by incision) 34.09
popliteal space 86.04
postural 93.99
postzygomatic space 27.0
pseudocyst, pancreas 52.3
by anastomosis 52.4
pterygopalatine fossa 27.0
retropharyngeal 28.0
scrotum 61.0
skin 86.04
spinal (canal) (cord) 03.09
by anastomosis - *see* Shunt, spinal
diagnostic 03.31
spleen 41.2
cyst (by marsupialization) 41.41
subarachnoid space, cerebral (incision) (trephination) 01.31
by aspiration 01.09
subcutaneous tissue 86.04
subdiaphragmatic 54.19
percutaneous 54.91
subdural space, cerebral (incision) (trephination) 01.31
by aspiration 01.09
subhepatic space 54.19
percutaneous 54.91
sublingual space 27.0
submental space 27.0
subphrenic space 54.19
percutaneous 54.91
supraclavicular fossa 86.04

Drainage *(Continued)*
temporal pouches 27.0
tendon (sheath) 83.01
hand 82.01
thenar space 82.04
thorax (closed) 34.04
open (by incision) 34.09
thyroglossal tract (by incision) 06.09
by aspiration 06.01
thyroid (field) (gland) (by incision) 06.09
by aspiration 06.01
postoperative 06.02
tonsil 28.0
tunica vaginalis 61.0
ureter (by catheter) 59.8
by
anastomosis NEC - *see also* Anastomosis, ureter 56.79
incision 56.2
ventricle (cerebral) (incision) NEC 02.39
by
anastomosis - *see* Shunt, ventricular
aspiration 01.09
through previously implanted catheter 01.02
vertebral column 03.09
Drawing test 94.08
Dressing
burn 93.57
ulcer 93.56
wound 93.57
Drilling
bone - *see also* Incision, bone 77.10
ovary 65.99
Drotrecogin alfa (activated) infusion 00.11
Ductogram, mammary 87.35
Duhamel operation (abdominoperineal pull-through) 48.65

Duhrssen's
incisions (cervix, to assist delivery) 73.93
operation (vaginofixation of uterus) 69.22
Dunn operation (triple arthrodesis) 81.12
Duodenectomy 45.62
with
gastrectomy - *see* Gastrectomy
pancreatectomy - *see* Pancreatectomy
Duodenocholedochotomy 51.51
Duodenoduodenostomy 45.91
proximal to distal segment 45.62
Duodenoileostomy 45.91
Duodenojejunostomy 45.91
Duodenoplasty 46.79
Duodenorrhaphy 46.71
Duodenoscopy 45.13
through stoma (artificial) 45.12
transabdominal (operative) 45.11
Duodenostomy 46.39
Duodenotomy 45.01
Dupuytren operation
fasciectomy 82.35
fasciotomy 82.12
with excision 82.35
shoulder disarticulation 84.08
Durabond 86.59
Duraplasty 02.12
Durham (-Caldwell) operation (transfer of biceps femoris tendon) 83.75
DuToit and Roux operation (staple capsulorrhaphy of shoulder) 81.82
DuVries operation (tenoplasty) 83.88
Dwyer operation
fasciotomy 83.14
soft tissue release NEC 83.84
wedge osteotomy, calcaneus 77.28

E

E2F decoy 00.16
Eagleton operation (extrapetrosal drainage) 20.22
ECG - *see* Electrocardiogram
Echocardiography 88.72
  intracardiac (heart chambers) (ICE) 37.28
  intravascular (coronary vessels) 00.24
  transesophageal 88.72
    monitoring (Doppler) (ultrasound) 89.68
Echoencephalography 88.71
Echography - *see* Ultrasonography
Echogynography 88.79
Echoplacentogram 88.78
ECMO (extracorporeal membrane oxygenation) 39.65
Eden-Hybinette operation (glenoid bone block) 78.01
Educational therapy (bed-bound children) (handicapped) 93.82
EEG (electroencephalogram) 89.14
  monitoring (radiographic) (video) 89.19
Effler operation (heart) 36.2
Effleurage 93.39
EGD (esophagogastroduodenoscopy) 45.13
  with closed biopsy 45.16
Eggers operation
  tendon release (patellar retinacula) 83.13
  tendon transfer (biceps femoris tendon) (hamstring tendon) 83.75
EKG - *see also* Electrocardiogram 89.52
Elastic hosiery 93.59
Electrocardiogram (with 12 or more leads) 89.52
  with vectorcardiogram 89.53
  fetal (scalp), intrauterine 75.32
  rhythm (with one to three leads) 89.51
Electrocautery - *see also* Cauterization
  cervix 67.32
  corneal lesion (ulcer) 11.42
  esophagus 42.39
    endoscopic 42.33
Electrocoagulation - *see also* Destruction, lesion, by site
  aneurysm (cerebral) (peripheral vessels) 39.52
  cervix 67.32
  cystoscopic 57.49
  ear
    external 18.29
    inner 20.79
    middle 20.51
  fallopian tube (lesion) 66.61
    for tubal ligation - *see* Ligation, fallopian tube
  gasserian ganglion 04.02
  nasal turbinates 21.61
  nose, for epistaxis (with packing) 21.03
  ovary 65.29
    laparoscopic 65.25
  prostatic bed 60.94
  rectum (polyp) 48.32
    radical 48.31
  retina (for)
    destruction of lesion 14.21
    reattachment 14.51
    repair of tear 14.31
  round ligament 69.19
  semicircular canals 20.79

Electrocoagulation *(Continued)*
  urethrovesical junction, transurethral 57.49
  uterine ligament 69.19
  uterosacral ligament 69.19
  uterus 68.29
  vagina 70.33
  vulva 71.3
Electrocochleography 20.31
Electroconization, cervix 67.32
Electroconvulsive therapy (ECT) 94.27
Electroencephalogram (EEG) 89.14
  monitoring (radiographic) (video) 89.19
Electrogastrogram 44.19
Electrokeratotomy 11.49
Electrolysis
  ciliary body 12.71
  hair follicle 86.92
  retina (for)
    destruction of lesion 14.21
    reattachment 14.51
    repair of tear 14.31
  skin 86.92
  subcutaneous tissue 86.92
Electromyogram, electromyography (EMG) (muscle) 93.08
  eye 95.25
  urethral sphincter 89.23
Electronarcosis 94.29
Electronic gaiter 93.59
Electronystagmogram (ENG) 95.24
Electro-oculogram (EOG) 95.22
Electroresection - *see also* Destruction, lesion, by site
  bladder neck (transurethral) 57.49
  esophagus 42.39
    endoscopic 42.33
  prostate (transurethral) 60.29
  stomach 43.49
    endoscopic 43.41
Electroretinogram (ERG) 95.21
Electroshock therapy (EST) 94.27
  subconvulsive 94.26
Elevation
  bone fragments (fractured)
  orbit 76.79
    sinus (nasal)
      frontal 22.79
      maxillary 22.79
    skull (with debridement) 02.02
    spinal 03.53
  pedicle graft 86.71
Elliot operation (scleral trephination with iridectomy) 12.61
Ellis Jones operation (repair of peroneal tendon) 83.88
Ellison operation (reinforcement of collateral ligament) 81.44
Elmslie-Cholmeley operation (tarsal wedge osteotomy) 77.28
Eloesser operation
  thoracoplasty 33.34
  thoracostomy 34.09
Elongation - *see* Lengthening
Embolectomy 38.00
  with endarterectomy - *see* Endarterectomy
  abdominal
    artery 38.06
    vein 38.07
  aorta (arch) (ascending) (descending) 38.04
  arteriovenous shunt or cannula 39.49 ◀

Embolectomy *(Continued)*
  bovine graft 39.49 ◀
  head and neck NEC 38.02
  intracranial NEC 38.01
  lower limb
    artery 38.08
    vein 38.09
  mechanical ◀
    endovascular ◀
      head and neck 39.74 ◀
  pulmonary (artery) (vein) 38.05 ◀
  thoracic NEC 38.05
  upper limb (artery) (vein) 38.03
Embolization (transcatheter)
  adhesive (glue) 39.79
    head and neck 39.72
  arteriovenous fistula 39.53
    endovascular 39.72
  artery (selective) 38.80
    by
      endovascular approach 39.79
        head and neck vessels 39.72
      percutaneous transcatheter infusion 99.29
    abdominal NEC 38.86
      duodenal (transcatheter) 44.44
      gastric (transcatheter) 44.44
      renal (transcatheter) 38.86
    aorta (arch) (ascending) (descending) 38.84
    duodenal (transcatheter) 44.44
    gastric (transcatheter) 44.44
    head and neck NEC 38.82
    intracranial NEC 38.81
    lower limb 38.88
    renal (transcatheter) 38.86
    thoracic NEC 38.85
    upper limb 38.83
  AVM intracranial, endovascular approach 39.72
  carotid cavernous fistula 39.53
  chemoembolization 99.25
  coil, endovascular 39.79
    head and neck 39.72
  vein (selective) 38.80
    by
      endovascular approach 39.79
        head and neck 39.72
    abdominal NEC 38.87
      duodenal (transcatheter) 44.44
      gastric (transcatheter) 44.44
    duodenal (transcatheter) 44.44
    gastric (transcatheter) 44.44
Embryotomy 73.8
EMG - *see* Electromyogram
Emmet operation (cervix) 67.61
Encephalocentesis - *see also* Puncture 01.09
  fetal head, transabdominal 73.8
Encephalography (cisternal puncture) (fractional) (lumbar) (pneumoencephalogram) 87.01
Encephalopuncture 01.09
Encircling procedure - *see also* Cerclage
  sclera, for buckling 14.49
    with implant 14.41
Endarterectomy (gas) (with patch graft) 38.10
  abdominal 38.16
  aorta (arch) (ascending) (descending) 38.14
  coronary artery - *see* category 36.0
    open chest approach 36.03

Endarterectomy *(Continued)*
head and neck (open) NEC 38.12

Note: Also use 00.40, 00.41, 00.42, or 00.43 to show the total number of vessels treated. Use code 00.44 once to show procedure on a bifurcated vessel. In addition, use 00.45, 00.46, 00.47, or 00.48 to show the number of vascular stents inserted.

percutaneous approach, intracranial vessel(s) 00.62
percutaneous approach, precerebral (extracranial) vessel(s) 00.61
intracranial (open) NEC 38.11

Note: Also use 00.40, 00.41, 00.42, or 00.43 to show the total number of vessels treated. Use code 00.44 once to show procedure on a bifurcated vessel. In addition, use 00.45, 00.46, 00.47, or 00.48 to show the number of vascular stents inserted.

percutaneous approach, intracranial vessel(s) 00.62
lower limb 38.18
thoracic NEC 38.15
upper limb 38.13
Endoaneurysmorrhaphy - *see also* Aneurysmorrhaphy 39.52
by or with
endovascular graft
abdominal aorta 39.71
lower extremity artery(ies) 39.79
thoracic aorta 39.73
upper extremity artery(ies) 39.79
Endolymphatic (-subarachnoid) shunt 20.71
Endometrectomy (uterine) (internal) 68.29
bladder 57.59
cul-de-sac 70.32
Endoprosthesis
bile duct 51.87
femoral head (bipolar) 81.52
Endoscopy
with biopsy - *see* Biopsy, by site, closed
anus 49.21
biliary tract (operative) 51.11
by retrograde cholangiography (ERC) 51.11
by retrograde cholangiopancreatography (ERCP) 51.10
intraoperative 51.11
percutaneous (via T-tube or other tract) 51.98
with removal of common duct stones 51.96
bladder 57.32
through stoma (artificial) 57.31
bronchus NEC 33.23
with biopsy 33.24
fiberoptic 33.22
through stoma (artificial) 33.21
colon 45.23
through stoma (artificial) 45.22
transabdominal (operative) 45.21
cul-de-sac 70.22
ear 18.11
esophagus NEC 42.23
through stoma (artificial) 42.22
transabdominal (operative) 42.21
ileum 45.13

Endoscopy *(Continued)*
ileum *(Continued)*
through stoma (artificial) 45.12
transabdominal (operative) 45.11
intestine NEC 45.24
large 45.24
fiberoptic (flexible) 45.23
through stoma (artificial) 45.22
transabdominal (intraoperative) 45.21
small 45.13
esophagogastroduodenoscopy (EGD) 45.13
with closed biopsy 45.16
through stoma (artificial) 45.12
transabdominal (operative) 45.11
jejunum 45.13
through stoma (artificial) 45.12
transabdominal (operative) 45.11
kidney 55.21
larynx 31.42
through stoma (artificial) 31.41
lung - *see* Bronchoscopy
mediastinum (transpleural) 34.22
nasal sinus 22.19
nose 21.21
pancreatic duct 52.13
pelvis 55.22
peritoneum 54.21
pharynx 29.11
rectum 48.23
through stoma (artificial) 48.22
transabdominal (operative) 48.21
sinus, nasal 22.19
stomach NEC 44.13
through stoma (artificial) 44.12
transabdominal (operative) 44.11
thorax (transpleural) 34.21
trachea NEC 31.42
through stoma (artificial) 31.41
transpleural
mediastinum 34.22
thorax 34.21
ureter 56.31
urethra 58.22
uterus 68.12
vagina 70.21
Enema (transanal) NEC 96.39
for removal of impacted feces 96.38
ENG (electronystagmogram) 95.24
Enlargement
aortic lumen, thoracic 38.14
atrial septal defect (pre-existing) 35.41
in repair of total anomalous pulmonary venous connection 35.82
eye socket 16.64
foramen ovale (pre-existing) 35.41
in repair of total anomalous pulmonary venous connection 35.82
intestinal stoma 46.40
large intestine 46.43
small intestine 46.41
introitus 96.16
orbit (eye) 16.64
palpebral fissure 08.51
punctum 09.41
sinus tract (skin) 86.89
Enterectomy NEC 45.63
Enteroanastomosis
large-to-large intestine 45.94
small-to-large intestine 45.93
small-to-small intestine 45.91

Enterocelectomy 53.9
female 70.92
vaginal 70.92
Enterocentesis 45.00
duodenum 45.01
large intestine 45.03
small intestine NEC 45.02
Enterocholecystostomy 51.32
Enteroclysis (small bowel) 96.43
Enterocolectomy NEC 45.79
Enterocolostomy 45.93
Enteroentectropy 46.99
Enteroenterostomy 45.90
small-to-large intestine 45.93
small-to-small intestine 45.91
Enterogastrostomy 44.39
laparoscopic 44.38
Enterolithotomy 45.00
Enterolysis 54.59
laparoscopic 54.51
Enteropancreatostomy 52.96
Enterorrhaphy 46.79
large intestine 46.75
small intestine 46.73
Enterostomy NEC 46.39
cecum - *see also* Colostomy 46.10
colon (transverse) - *see also* Colostomy 46.10
loop 46.03
delayed opening 46.31
duodenum 46.39
loop 46.01
feeding NEC 46.39
percutaneous (endoscopic) 46.32
ileum (Brooke) (Dragstedt) 46.20
loop 46.01
jejunum (feeding) 46.39
loop 46.01
percutaneous (endoscopic) 46.32
sigmoid colon - *see also* Colostomy 46.10
loop 46.03
transverse colon - *see also* Colostomy 46.10
loop 46.03
Enterotomy 45.00
large intestine 45.03
small intestine 45.02
Enucleation - *see also* Excision, lesion, by site
cyst
broad ligament 69.19
dental 24.4
liver 50.29
ovarian 65.29
laparoscopic 65.25
parotid gland 26.29
salivary gland 26.29
skin 86.3
subcutaneous tissue 86.3
eyeball 16.49
with implant (into Tenon's capsule) 16.42
with attachment of muscles 16.41
EOG (electro-oculogram) 95.22
Epicardiectomy 36.39
Epididymectomy 63.4
with orchidectomy (unilateral) 62.3
bilateral 62.41
Epididymogram 87.93
Epididymoplasty 63.59
Epididymorrhaphy 63.81
Epididymotomy 63.92
Epididymovasostomy 63.83

Epiglottidectomy 30.21
Epikeratophakia 11.76
Epilation
eyebrow (forceps) 08.93
cryosurgical 08.92
electrosurgical 08.91
eyelid (forceps) NEC 08.93
cryosurgical 08.92
electrosurgical 08.91
skin 86.92
Epiphysiodesis - *see also* Arrest, bone growth - *see* category 78.2
Epiphysiolysis - *see also* Arrest, bone growth - *see* category 78.2
Epiploectomy 54.4
Epiplopexy 54.74
Epiplorrhaphy 54.74
Episioperineoplasty 71.79
Episioperineorrhaphy 71.71
obstetrical 75.69
Episioplasty 71.79
Episioproctotomy 73.6
Episiorrhaphy 71.71
following routine episiotomy - *see* Episiotomy for obstetrical laceration 75.69
Episiotomy (with subsequent episiorrhaphy) 73.6
high forceps 72.31
low forceps 72.1
mid forceps 72.21
nonobstetrical 71.09
outlet forceps 72.1
EPS (electrophysiologic stimulation)
as part of intraoperative testing – *omit code*
catheter based invasive electrophysiologic testing 37.26
device interrogation only without arrhythmia induction (bedside check) 89.45-89.49
noninvasive programmed electrical stimulation (NIPS) 37.20
Eptifibatide, infusion 99.20
Equalization, leg
lengthening - *see* category 78.3
shortening - *see* category 78.2
Equilibration (occlusal) 24.8
Equiloudness balance 95.43
ERC (endoscopic retrograde cholangiography) 51.11
ERCP (endoscopic retrograde cholangiopancreatography) 51.10
cannulation of pancreatic duct 52.93
ERG (electroretinogram) 95.21
ERP (endoscopic retrograde pancreatography) 52.13
Eruption, tooth, surgical 24.6
Erythrocytapheresis, therapeutic 99.73
Escharectomy 86.22
Escharotomy 86.09
Esophageal voice training (postlaryngectomy) 93.73
Esophagectomy 42.40
abdominothoracocervical (combined) (synchronous) 42.42
partial or subtotal 42.41
total 42.42
Esophagocologastrostomy (intrathoracic) 42.55
antesternal or antethoracic 42.65
Esophagocolostomy (intrathoracic) **NEC** 42.56
with interposition of colon 42.55
Esophagocolostomy NEC *(Continued)*
antesternal or antethoracic NEC 42.66
with interposition of colon 42.65
Esophagoduodenostomy (intrathoracic) **NEC** 42.54
with
complete gastrectomy 43.99
interposition of small bowel 42.53
Esophagoenterostomy (intrathoracic) **NEC** - *see also* Anastomosis, esophagus, to intestinal segment 42.54
antesternal or antethoracic - *see also* Anastomosis, esophagus, antesternal, to intestinal segment 42.64
Esophagoesophagostomy (intrathoracic) 42.51
antesternal or antethoracic 42.61
Esophagogastrectomy 43.99
Esophagogastroduodenoscopy (EGD) 45.13
with closed biopsy 45.16
through stoma (artificial) 45.12
transabdominal (operative) 45.11
Esophagogastromyotomy 42.7
Esophagogastropexy 44.65
Esophagogastroplasty 44.65
Esophagogastroscopy NEC 44.13
through stoma (artificial) 44.12
transabdominal (operative) 44.11
Esophagogastrostomy (intrathoracic) 42.52
with partial gastrectomy 43.5
antesternal or antethoracic 42.62
Esophagoileostomy (intrathoracic) NEC 42.54
with interposition of small bowel 42.53
antesternal or antethoracic NEC 42.64
with interposition of small bowel 42.63
Esophagojejunostomy (intrathoracic) NEC 42.54
with
complete gastrectomy 43.99
interposition of small bowel 42.53
antesternal or antethoracic NEC 42.64
with interposition of small bowel 42.63
Esophagomyotomy 42.7
Esophagoplasty NEC 42.89
Esophagorrhaphy 42.82
Esophagoscopy NEC 42.23
by incision (operative) 42.21
with closed biopsy 42.24
through stoma (artificial) 42.22
transabdominal (operative) 42.21
Esophagostomy 42.10
cervical 42.11
thoracic 42.19
Esophagotomy NEC 42.09
Estes operation (ovary) 65.72
laparoscopic 65.75
Estlander operation (thoracoplasty) 33.34
ESWL (extracorporeal shock wave lithotripsy) NEC 98.59
bile duct 98.52
bladder 98.51
gallbladder 98.52
kidney 98.51
Kock pouch (urinary diversion) 98.51
renal pelvis 98.51
specified site NEC 98.59
ureter 98.51
Ethmoidectomy 22.63
Ethmoidotomy 22.51
Evacuation
abscess - *see* Drainage, by site
Evacuation *(Continued)*
anterior chamber (eye) (aqueous) (hyphema) 12.91
cyst - *see also* Excision, lesion, by site
breast 85.91
kidney 55.01
liver 50.29
hematoma - *see also* Incision, hematoma
obstetrical 75.92
incisional 75.91
hemorrhoids (thrombosed) 49.47
pelvic blood clot (by incision) 54.19
by
culdocentesis 70.0
culdoscopy 70.22
retained placenta
with curettage 69.02
manual 75.4
streptothrix from lacrimal duct 09.42
Evaluation (of)
audiological 95.43
cardiac rhythm device (CRT-D) (CRT-P) (AICD) (pacemaker) - *see* Interrogation
criminal responsibility, psychiatric 94.11
functional (physical therapy) 93.01
hearing NEC 95.49
orthotic (for brace fitting) 93.02
prosthetic (for artificial limb fitting) 93.03
psychiatric NEC 94.19
commitment 94.13
psychologic NEC 94.08
testimentary capacity, psychiatric 94.11
Evans operation (release of clubfoot) 83.84
Evisceration
eyeball 16.39
with implant (into scleral shell) 16.31
ocular contents 16.39
with implant (into scleral shell) 16.31
orbit - *see also* Exenteration, orbit 16.59
pelvic (anterior) (posterior) (partial) (total) (female) 68.8
male 57.71
Evulsion
nail (bed) (fold) 86.23
skin 86.3
subcutaneous tissue 86.3
Examination (for)
breast
manual 89.36
radiographic NEC 87.37
thermographic 88.85
ultrasonic 88.73
cervical rib (by x-ray) 87.43
colostomy stoma (digital) 89.33
dental (oral mucosa) (periodontal) 89.31
radiographic NEC 87.12
enterostomy stoma (digital) 89.33
eye 95.09
color vision 95.06
comprehensive 95.02
dark adaptation 95.07
limited (with prescription of spectacles) 95.01
under anesthesia 95.04
fetus, intrauterine 75.35
general physical 89.7
glaucoma 95.03
gynecological 89.26
hearing 95.47
microscopic (specimen) (of) 91.9

ICD-9-CM E Vol. 3

Examination *(Continued)*
microscopic *(Continued)*

Note: Use the following fourth-digit subclassification with categories 90-91 to identify type of examination:

1 bacterial smear
2 culture
3 culture and sensitivity
4 parasitology
5 toxicology
6 cell block and Papanicolaou smear
9 other microscopic examination

adenoid 90.3
adrenal gland 90.1
amnion 91.4
anus 90.9
appendix 90.9
bile ducts 91.0
bladder 91.3
blood 90.5
bone 91.5
marrow 90.6
brain 90.0
breast 91.6
bronchus 90.4
bursa 91.5
cartilage 91.5
cervix 91.4
chest wall 90.4
chorion 91.4
colon 90.9
cul-de-sac 91.1
dental 90.8
diaphragm 90.4
duodenum 90.8
ear 90.3
endocrine gland NEC 90.1
esophagus 90.8
eye 90.2
fallopian tube 91.4
fascia 91.5
female genital tract 91.4
fetus 91.4
gallbladder 91.0
hair 91.6
ileum 90.9
jejunum 90.9
joint fluid 91.5
kidney 91.2
large intestine 90.9
larynx 90.3
ligament 91.5
liver 91.0
lung 90.4
lymph (node) 90.7
meninges 90.0
mesentery 91.1
mouth 90.8
muscle 91.5
musculoskeletal system 91.5
nails 91.6
nerve 90.0
nervous system 90.0
nose 90.3
omentum 91.1
operative wound 91.7
ovary 91.4
pancreas 91.0
parathyroid gland 90.1
penis 91.3
perirenal tissue 91.2
peritoneum (fluid) 91.1

Examination *(Continued)*
microscopic *(Continued)*
periureteral tissue 91.2
perivesical (tissue) 91.3
pharynx 90.3
pineal gland 90.1
pituitary gland 90.1
placenta 91.4
pleura (fluid) 90.4
prostate 91.3
rectum 90.9
retroperitoneum 91.1
semen 91.3
seminal vesicle 91.3
sigmoid 90.9
skin 91.6
small intestine 90.9
specified site NEC 91.8
spinal fluid 90.0
spleen 90.6
sputum 90.4
stomach 90.8
stool 90.9
synovial membrane 91.5
tendon 91.5
thorax NEC 90.4
throat 90.3
thymus 90.1
thyroid gland 90.1
tonsil 90.3
trachea 90.4
ureter 91.2
urethra 91.3
urine 91.3
uterus 91.4
vagina 91.4
vas deferens 91.3
vomitus 90.8
vulva 91.4
neurologic 89.13
neuro-ophthalmology 95.03
ophthalmoscopic 16.21
panorex, mandible 87.12
pelvic (manual) 89.26
instrumental (by pelvimeter) 88.25
pelvimetric 88.25
physical, general 89.7
postmortem 89.8
rectum (digital) 89.34
endoscopic 48.23
through stoma (artificial) 48.22
transabdominal 48.21
retinal disease 95.03
specified type (manual) NEC 89.39
thyroid field, postoperative 06.02
uterus (digital) 68.11
endoscopic 68.12
vagina 89.26
endoscopic 70.21
visual field 95.05
Exchange transfusion 99.01
intrauterine 75.2
Excision
aberrant tissue - *see* Excision, lesion, by site of tissue origin
abscess - *see* Excision, lesion, by site
accessory tissue - *see also* Excision, lesion, by site of tissue origin
lung 32.29
endoscopic 32.28
spleen 41.93
adenoids (tag) 28.6
with tonsillectomy 28.3
adenoma - *see* Excision, lesion, by site

Excision *(Continued)*
adrenal gland - *see also* Adrenalectomy 07.22
ampulla of Vater (with reimplantation of common duct) 51.62
anal papilla 49.39
endoscopic 49.31
aneurysm (arteriovenous) - *see also* Aneurysmectomy 38.60
coronary artery 36.91
heart 37.32
myocardium 37.32
sinus of Valsalva 35.39
ventricle (heart) 37.32
anus (complete) (partial) 49.6
aortic subvalvular ring 35.35
apocrine gland 86.3
aponeurosis 83.42
hand 82.33
appendiceal stump 47.09
laparoscopic 47.01
appendices epiploicae 54.4
appendix - *see also* Appendectomy
epididymis 63.3
testis 62.2
arcuate ligament (spine) - *omit code*
arteriovenous fistula - *see also* Aneurysmectomy 38.60
artery - *see also* Arteriectomy 38.60
Baker's cyst, knee 83.39
Bartholin's gland 71.24
basal ganglion 01.59
bile duct 51.69
endoscopic 51.64
bladder - *see also* Cystectomy
bleb (emphysematous), lung 32.29
endoscopic 32.28
blood vessel - *see also* Angiectomy 38.60
bone (ends) (partial), except facial - *see* category 77.8
facial NEC 76.39
total 76.45
with reconstruction 76.44
for graft (autograft) (homograft) - *see* category 77.7
fragments (chips) - *see also* Incision, bone 77.10
joint - *see also* Arthrotomy 80.10
necrotic - *see also* Sequestrectomy, bone 77.00
heterotopic, from
muscle 83.32
hand 82.22
skin 86.3
tendon 83.31
hand 82.21
mandible 76.31
with arthrodesis - *see* Arthrodesis
total 76.42
with reconstruction 76.41
spur - *see* Excision, lesion, bone
total, except facial - *see* category 77.9
facial NEC 76.45
with reconstruction 76.44
mandible 76.42
with reconstruction 76.41
brain 01.59
hemisphere 01.52
lobe 01.53
branchial cleft cyst or vestige 29.2
breast - *see also* Mastectomy 85.41
aberrant tissue 85.24
accessory 85.24
ectopic 85.24
nipple 85.25

Excision *(Continued)*
breast *(Continued)*
nipple *(Continued)*
accessory 85.24
segmental 85.23
supernumerary 85.24
wedge 85.21
broad ligament 69.19
bronchogenic cyst 32.09
endoscopic 32.01
bronchus (wide sleeve) NEC 32.1
buccal mucosa 27.49
bulbourethral gland 58.92
bulbous tuberosities (mandible) (maxilla) (fibrous) (osseous) 24.31
bunion - *see also* Bunionectomy 77.59
bunionette (with osteotomy) 77.54
bursa 83.5
hand 82.31
canal of Nuck 69.19
cardioma 37.33
carotid body (lesion) (partial) (total) 39.8
cartilage - *see also* Chondrectomy 80.90
intervertebral - *see* category 80.5
knee (semilunar) 80.6
larynx 30.29
nasal (submucous) 21.5
caruncle, urethra 58.39
endoscopic 58.31
cataract - *see also* Extraction, cataract 13.19
secondary membrane (after cataract) 13.65
cervical
rib 77.91
stump 67.4
cervix (stump) NEC 67.4
cold (knife) 67.2
conization 67.2
cryoconization 67.33
electroconization 67.32
chalazion (multiple) (single) 08.21
cholesteatoma - *see* Excision, lesion, by site
choroid plexus 02.14
cicatrix (skin) 86.3
cilia base 08.20
ciliary body, prolapsed 12.98
clavicle (head) (partial) 77.81
total (complete) 77.91
clitoris 71.4
coarctation of aorta (end-to-end anastomosis) 38.64
with
graft replacement (interposition)
abdominal 38.44
thoracic 38.45
thoracoabdominal 38.45 *[38.44]*
common
duct 51.63
wall between posterior and coronary sinus (with roofing or resultant defect with patch graft) 35.82
condyle - *see* category 77.8
mandible 76.5
conjunctival ring 10.31
cornea 11.49
epithelium (with chemocauterization) 11.41
for smear or culture 11.21
costal cartilage 80.99
cul-de-sac (Douglas') 70.92
cusp, heart valve 35.10
aortic 35.11

Excision *(Continued)*
cusp, heart valve *(Continued)*
mitral 35.12
tricuspid 35.14
cyst - *see also* Excision, lesion, by site
apical (tooth) 23.73
with root canal therapy 23.72
Baker's (popliteal) 83.39
breast 85.21
broad ligament 69.19
bronchogenic 32.09
endoscopic 32.01
cervix 67.39
dental 24.4
dentigerous 24.4
epididymis 63.2
fallopian tube 66.61
Gartner's duct 70.33
hand 82.29
labia 71.3
lung 32.29
endoscopic 32.28
mesonephric duct 69.19
Morgagni
female 66.61
male 62.2
mullerian duct 60.73
nasolabial 27.49
nasopalatine 27.31
by wide excision 27.32
ovary 65.29
laparoscopic 65.25
parovarian 69.19
pericardium 37.31
periodontal (apical) (lateral) 24.4
popliteal (Baker's), knee 83.39
radicular 24.4
spleen 41.42
synovial (membrane) 83.39
thyroglossal (with resection of hyoid bone) 06.7
urachal (bladder) 57.51
abdominal wall 54.3
vagina (Gartner's duct) 70.33
cystic
duct remnant 51.61
hygroma 40.29
dentinoma 24.4
diaphragm 34.81
disc, intervertebral NOS 80.50
herniated (nucleus pulposus) 80.51
other specified (diskectomy) 80.51
diverticulum
ampulla of Vater 51.62
anus 49.39
endoscopic 49.31
bladder 57.59
transurethral 57.49
duodenum 45.31
endoscopic 45.30
esophagus (local) 42.31
endoscopic 42.33
hypopharyngeal (by cricopharyngeal myotomy) 29.32
intestine
large 45.41
endoscopic 45.43
small NEC 45.33
Meckel's 45.33
pharyngeal (by cricopharyngeal myotomy) 29.32
pharyngoesophageal (by cricopharyngeal myotomy) 29.32

Excision *(Continued)*
diverticulum *(Continued)*
stomach 43.42
endoscopic 43.41
urethra 58.39
endoscopic 58.31
ventricle, heart 37.33
duct
mullerian 69.19
paramesonephric 69.19
thyroglossal (with resection of hyoid bone) 06.7
ear, external (complete) NEC 18.39
partial 18.29
radical 18.31
ectopic
abdominal fetus 74.3
tissue - *see also* Excision, lesion, by site of tissue origin
bone, from muscle 83.32
breast 85.24
lung 32.29
endoscopic 32.28
spleen 41.93
empyema pocket, lung 34.09
epididymis 63.4
epiglottis 30.21
epithelial downgrowth, anterior chamber (eye) 12.93
epulis (gingiva) 24.31
esophagus - *see also* Esophagectomy 42.40
exostosis - *see also* Excision, lesion, bone 77.60
auditory canal, external 18.29
facial bone 76.2
first metatarsal (hallux valgus repair) - *see* Bunionectomy
eye 16.49
with implant (into Tenon's capsule) 16.42
with attachment of muscles 16.41
eyelid 08.20
redundant skin 08.86
falciform ligament 54.4
fallopian tube - *see* Salpingectomy
fascia 83.44
for graft 83.43
hand 82.34
hand 82.35
for graft 82.34
fat pad NEC 86.3
knee (infrapatellar) (prepatellar) 86.3
scalene 40.21
fibroadenoma, breast 85.21
fissure, anus 49.39
endoscopic 49.31
fistula - *see also* Fistulectomy
anal 49.12
arteriovenous - *see also* Aneurysmectomy 38.60
ileorectal 46.74
lacrimal
gland 09.21
sac 09.6
rectal 48.73
vesicovaginal 57.84
frenulum, frenum
labial (lip) 27.41
lingual (tongue) 25.92
ganglion (hand) (tendon sheath) (wrist) 82.21
gasserian 04.05
site other than hand or nerve 83.31

ICD-9-CM

E

Vol. 3

Excision *(Continued)*
ganglion *(Continued)*
sympathetic nerve 05.29
trigeminal nerve 04.05
gastrocolic ligament 54.4
gingiva 24.31
glomus jugulare tumor 20.51
goiter - *see* Thyroidectomy
gum 24.31
hallux valgus - *see also* Bunionectomy
with prosthetic implant 77.59
hamartoma, mammary 85.21
heart assist system - *see* Removal
hematocele, tunica vaginalis 61.92
hematoma - *see* Drainage, by site
hemorrhoids (external) (internal) (tag) 49.46
heterotopic bone, from
muscle 83.32
hand 82.22
skin 86.3
tendon 83.31
hand 82.21
hydatid of Morgagni
female 66.61
male 62.2
hydatid cyst, liver 50.29
hydrocele
canal of Nuck (female) 69.19
male 63.1
round ligament 69.19
spermatic cord 63.1
tunica vaginalis 61.2
hygroma, cystic 40.29
hymen (tag) 70.31
hymeno-urethral fusion 70.31
intervertebral disc - *see* Excision, disc, intervertebral (NOS) 80.50
intestine - *see also* Resection, intestine 45.8
for interposition 45.50
large 45.52
small 45.51
large (total) 45.8
for interposition 45.52
local 45.41
endoscopic 45.43
segmental 45.79
multiple 45.71
small (total) 45.63
for interposition 45.51
local 45.33
partial 45.62
segmental 45.62
multiple 45.61
intraductal papilloma 85.21
iris prolapse 12.13
joint - *see also* Arthrectomy 80.90
keloid (scar), skin 86.3
labia - *see* Vulvectomy
lacrimal
gland 09.20
partial 09.22
total 09.23
passage 09.6
sac 09.6
lesion (local)
abdominal wall 54.3
accessory sinus - *see* Excision, lesion, nasal sinus
adenoids 28.92
adrenal gland(s) 07.21
alveolus 24.4
ampulla of Vater 51.62

Excision *(Continued)*
lesion *(Continued)*
anterior chamber (eye) NEC 12.40
anus 49.39
endoscopic 49.31
apocrine gland 86.3
artery 38.60
abdominal 38.66
aorta (arch) (ascending) (descending thoracic) 38.64
with end-to-end anastomosis 38.45
abdominal 38.44
thoracic 38.45
thoracoabdominal 38.45 *[38.44]*
with graft interposition graft replacement 38.45
abdominal 38.44
thoracic 38.45
thoracoabdominal 38.45 *[38.44]*
head and neck NEC 38.62
intracranial NEC 38.61
lower limb 38.68
thoracic NEC 38.65
upper limb 38.63
atrium 37.33
auditory canal or meatus, external 18.29
radical 18.31
auricle, ear 18.29
radical 18.31
biliary ducts 51.69
endoscopic 51.64
bladder (transurethral) 57.49
open 57.59
suprapubic 57.59
blood vessel 38.60
abdominal
artery 38.66
vein 38.67
aorta (arch) (ascending) (descending) 38.64
head and neck NEC 38.62
intracranial NEC 38.61
lower limb
artery 38.68
vein 38.69
thoracic NEC 38.65
upper limb (artery) (vein) 38.63
bone 77.60
carpal, metacarpal 77.64
clavicle 77.61
facial 76.2
femur 77.65
fibula 77.67
humerus 77.62
jaw 76.2
dental 24.4
patella 77.66
pelvic 77.69
phalanges (foot) (hand) 77.69
radius 77.63
scapula 77.61
skull 01.6
specified site NEC 77.69
tarsal, metatarsal 77.68
thorax (ribs) (sternum) 77.61
tibia 77.67
ulna 77.63
vertebrae 77.69
brain (transtemporal approach) NEC 01.59
by stereotactic radiosurgery 92.30
cobalt 60 92.32

Excision *(Continued)*
lesion *(Continued)*
brain *(Continued)*
by stereotactic radiosurgery *(Continued)*
linear accelerator (LINAC) 92.31
multi-source 92.32
particle beam 92.33
particulate 92.33
radiosurgery NEC 92.39
single source photon 92.31
breast (segmental) (wedge) 85.21
broad ligament 69.19
bronchus NEC 32.09
endoscopic 32.01
cerebral (cortex) NEC 01.59
meninges 01.51
cervix (myoma) 67.39
chest wall 34.4
choroid plexus 02.14
ciliary body 12.44
colon 45.41
endoscopic NEC 45.43
polypectomy 45.42
conjunctiva 10.31
cornea 11.49
cranium 01.6
cul-de-sac (Douglas') 70.32
dental (jaw) 24.4
diaphragm 34.81
duodenum (local) 45.31
endoscopic 45.30
ear, external 18.29
radical 18.31
endometrium 68.29
epicardium 37.31
epididymis 63.3
epiglottis 30.09
esophagus NEC 42.32
endoscopic 42.33
eye, eyeball 16.93
anterior segment NEC 12.40
eyebrow (skin) 08.20
eyelid 08.20
by
halving procedure 08.24
wedge resection 08.24
major
full-thickness 08.24
partial-thickness 08.23
minor 08.22
fallopian tube 66.61
fascia 83.39
hand 82.29
groin region (abdominal wall) (inguinal) 54.3
skin 86.3
subcutaneous tissue 86.3
gum 24.31
heart 37.33
hepatic duct 51.69
inguinal canal 54.3
intestine
large 45.41
endoscopic NEC 45.43
polypectomy 45.42
small NEC 45.33
intracranial NEC 01.59
intranasal 21.31
intraspinal 03.4
iris 12.42
jaw 76.2
dental 24.4
joint 80.80
ankle 80.87

Excision *(Continued)*
lesion *(Continued)*
joint *(Continued)*
elbow 80.82
foot and toe 80.88
hand and finger 80.84
hip 80.85
knee 80.86
shoulder 80.81
specified site NEC 80.89
spine 80.89
wrist 80.83
kidney 55.39
with partial nephrectomy 55.4
labia 71.3
lacrimal
gland (frontal approach) 09.21
passage 09.6
sac 09.6
larynx 30.09
ligament (joint) - *see also* Excision, lesion, joint 80.80
broad 69.19
round 69.19
uterosacral 69.19
lip 27.43
by wide excision 27.42
liver 50.29
lung NEC 32.29
by lung volume reduction surgery 32.22
by wide excision 32.3
endoscopic 32.28
lymph structure(s) (channel) (vessel) NEC 40.29
node - *see* Excision, lymph, node
mammary duct 85.21
mastoid (bone) 20.49
mediastinum 34.3
meninges (cerebral) 01.51
spinal 03.4
mesentery 54.4
middle ear 20.51
mouth NEC 27.49
muscle 83.32
hand 82.22
ocular 15.13
myocardium 37.33
nail 86.23
nasal sinus 22.60
antrum 22.62
with Caldwell-Luc approach 22.61
specified approach NEC 22.62
ethmoid 22.63
frontal 22.42
maxillary 22.62
with Caldwell-Luc approach 22.61
specified approach NEC 22.62
sphenoid 22.64
nasopharynx 29.3
nerve (cranial) (peripheral) 04.07
sympathetic 05.29
nonodontogenic 24.31
nose 21.30
intranasal 21.31
polyp 21.31
skin 21.32
specified site NEC 21.32
odontogenic 24.4
omentum 54.4
orbit 16.92
ovary 65.29

Excision *(Continued)*
lesion *(Continued)*
ovary *(Continued)*
by wedge resection 65.22
laparoscopic 65.24
that by laparoscope 65.25
palate (bony) 27.31
by wide excision 27.32
soft 27.49
pancreas (local) 52.22
endoscopic 52.21
parathyroid 06.89
parotid gland or duct NEC 26.29
pelvic wall 54.3
pelvirectal tissue 48.82
penis 64.2
pericardium 37.31
perineum (female) 71.3
male 86.3
periprostatic tissue 60.82
perirectal tissue 48.82
perirenal tissue 59.91
peritoneum 54.4
perivesical tissue 59.91
pharynx 29.3
diverticulum 29.32
pineal gland 07.53
pinna 18.29
radical 18.31
pituitary (gland) - *see also* Hypophysectomy, partial 07.63
by stereotactic radiosurgery 92.30
cobalt 60 92.32
linear accelerator (LINAC) 92.31
multi-source 92.32
particle beam 92.33
particulate 92.33
radiosurgery NEC 92.39
single source photon 92.31
pleura 34.59
pouch of Douglas 70.32
preauricular (ear) 18.21
presacral 54.4
prostate (transurethral) 60.61
pulmonary (fibrosis) 32.29
endoscopic 32.28
rectovaginal septum 48.82
rectum 48.35
polyp (endoscopic) 48.36
retroperitoneum 54.4
salivary gland or duct NEC 26.29
en bloc 26.32
sclera 12.84
scrotum 61.3
sinus (nasal) - *see* Excision, lesion, nasal sinus
Skene's gland 71.3
skin 86.3
breast 85.21
nose 21.32
radical (wide) (involving underlying or adjacent structure) (with flap closure) 86.4
scrotum 61.3
skull 01.6
soft tissue NEC 83.39
hand 82.29
spermatic cord 63.3
sphincter of Oddi 51.62
endoscopic 51.64
spinal cord (meninges) 03.4
spleen (cyst) 41.42

Excision *(Continued)*
lesion *(Continued)*
stomach NEC 43.42
endoscopic 43.41
polyp 43.41
polyp (endoscopic) 43.41
subcutaneous tissue 86.3
breast 85.21
subgingival 24.31
sweat gland 86.3
tendon 83.39
hand 82.29
ocular 15.13
sheath 83.31
hand 82.21
testis 62.2
thorax 34.4
thymus 07.81
thyroid 06.31
substernal or transsternal route 06.51
tongue 25.1
tonsil 28.92
trachea 31.5
tunica vaginalis 61.92
ureter 56.41
urethra 58.39
endoscopic 58.31
uterine ligament 69.19
uterosacral ligament 69.19
uterus 68.29
vagina 70.33
vein 38.60
abdominal 38.67
head and neck NEC 38.62
intracranial NEC 38.61
lower limb 38.69
thoracic NEC 38.65
upper limb 38.63
ventricle (heart) 37.33
vocal cords 30.09
vulva 71.3
ligament - *see also* Arthrectomy 80.90
broad 69.19
round 69.19
uterine 69.19
uterosacral 69.19
ligamentum flavum (spine) - *omit code*
lingual tonsil 28.5
lip 27.43
liver (partial) 50.22
loose body
bone - *see* Sequestrectomy, bone
joint 80.10
lung (complete) (with mediastinal dissection) 32.5
accessory or ectopic tissue 32.29
endoscopic 32.28
segmental 32.3
specified type NEC 32.29
endoscopic 32.28
volume reduction surgery 32.22
biologic lung volume reduction (BLVR) – *see* category 33.7 ◀
wedge 32.29
lymph, lymphatic
drainage area 40.29
radical - *see* Excision, lymph, node, radical
regional (with lymph node, skin, subcutaneous tissue, and fat) 40.3
node (simple) NEC 40.29

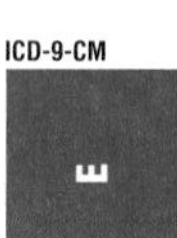
ICD-9-CM
E
Vol. 3

Excision *(Continued)*
lymph, lymphatic *(Continued)*
node NEC *(Continued)*
with
lymphatic drainage area (including skin, subcutaneous tissue, and fat) 40.3
mastectomy - *see* Mastectomy, radical
muscle and deep fascia - *see* Excision, lymph, node, radical
axillary 40.23
radical 40.51
regional (extended) 40.3
cervical (deep) (with excision of scalene fat pad) 40.21
with laryngectomy 30.4
radical (including muscle and deep fascia) 40.40
bilateral 40.42
unilateral 40.41
regional (extended) 40.3
superficial 40.29
groin 40.24
radical 40.54
regional (extended) 40.3
iliac 40.29
radical 40.53
regional (extended) 40.3
inguinal (deep) (superficial) 40.24
radical 40.54
regional (extended) 40.3
jugular - *see* Excision, lymph, node, cervical
mammary (internal) 40.22
external 40.29
radical 40.59
regional (extended) 40.3
radical 40.59
regional (extended) 40.3
paratracheal - *see* Excision, lymph, node, cervical
periaortic 40.29
radical 40.52
regional (extended) 40.3
radical 40.50
with mastectomy - *see* Mastectomy, radical
specified site NEC 40.59
regional (extended) 40.3
sternal - *see* Excision, lymph, node, mammary
structure(s) (simple) NEC 40.29
radical 40.59
regional (extended) 40.3
lymphangioma (simple) - *see also* Excision, lymph, lymphatic, node, 40.29
lymphocele 40.29
mastoid - *see also* Mastoidectomy 20.49
median bar, transurethral approach 60.29
meibomian gland 08.20
meniscus (knee) 80.6
acromioclavicular 80.91
jaw 76.5
sternoclavicular 80.91
temporomandibular (joint) 76.5
wrist 80.93
mullerian duct cyst 60.73
muscle 83.45
for graft 83.43
hand 82.34

Excision *(Continued)*
muscle *(Continued)*
hand 82.36
for graft 82.34
myositis ossificans 83.32
hand 82.22
nail (bed) (fold) 86.23
nasolabial cyst 27.49
nasopalatine cyst 27.31
by wide excision 27.32
neoplasm - *see* Excision, lesion, by site
nerve (cranial) (peripheral) NEC 04.07
sympathetic 05.29
neuroma (Morton's) (peripheral nerve) 04.07
acoustic
by craniotomy 04.01
by stereotactic radiosurgery 92.30
cobalt 60 92.32
linear accelerator (LINAC) 92.31
multi-source 92.32
particle beam 92.33
particulate 92.33
radiosurgery NEC 92.39
single source photon 92.31
sympathetic nerve 05.29
nipple 85.25
accessory 85.24
odontoma 24.4
orbital contents - *see also* Exenteration, orbit 16.59
osteochondritis dissecans - *see also* Excision, lesion, joint 80.80
ovary - *see also* Oophorectomy
partial 65.29
by wedge resection 65.22
laparoscopic 65.24
that by laparoscope 65.25
Pancoast tumor (lung) 32.6
pancreas (total) (with synchronous duodenectomy) 52.6
partial NEC 52.59
distal (tail) (with part of body) 52.52
proximal (head) (with part of body) (with synchronous duodenectomy) 52.51
radical subtotal 52.53
radical (one-stage) (two-stage) 52.7
subtotal 52.53
paramesonephric duct 69.19
parathyroid gland (partial) (subtotal) NEC - *see also* Parathyroidectomy 06.89
parotid gland - *see also* Excision, salivary gland 26.30
parovarian cyst 69.19
patella (complete) 77.96
partial 77.86
pelvirectal tissue 48.82
perianal tissue 49.04
skin tags 49.03
pericardial adhesions 37.31
periprostatic tissue 60.82
perirectal tissue 48.82
perirenal tissue 59.91
periurethral tissue 58.92
perivesical tissue 59.91
petrous apex cells 20.59
pharyngeal bands 29.54
pharynx (partial) 29.33

Excision *(Continued)*
pilonidal cyst or sinus (open) (with partial closure) 86.21
pineal gland (complete) (total) 07.54
partial 07.53
pituitary gland (complete) (total) - *see also* Hypophysectomy 07.69
pleura NEC 34.59
polyp - *see also* Excision, lesion, by site
esophagus 42.32
endoscopic 42.33
large intestine 45.41
endoscopic 45.42
nose 21.31
rectum (endoscopic) 48.36
stomach (endoscopic) 43.41
preauricular
appendage (remnant) 18.29
cyst, fistula, or sinus (congenital) 18.21
remnant 18.29
prolapsed iris (in wound) 12.13
prostate - *see* Prostatectomy
pterygium (simple) 11.39
with corneal graft 11.32
radius (head) (partial) 77.83
total 77.93
ranula, salivary gland NEC 26.29
rectal mucosa 48.35
rectum - *see* Resection, rectum
redundant mucosa
colostomy 45.41
endoscopic 45.43
duodenostomy 45.31
endoscopic 45.30
ileostomy 45.33
jejunostomy 45.33
perineum 71.3
rectum 48.35
vulva 71.3
renal vessel, aberrant 38.66
rib (cervical) 77.91
ring of conjunctiva around cornea 10.31
round ligament 69.19
salivary gland 26.30
complete 26.32
partial 26.31
radical 26.32
scalene fat pad 40.21
scar - *see also* Excision, lesion, by site
epicardium 37.31
mastoid 20.92
pericardium 37.31
pleura 34.59
skin 86.3
thorax 34.4
secondary membrane, lens 13.65
seminal vesicle 60.73
with radical prostatectomy 60.5
septum - *see also* Excision, by site
uterus (congenital) 68.22
vagina 70.33
sinus - *see also* Excision, lesion, by site
nasal - *see* Sinusectomy
pilonidal 86.21
preauricular (ear) (radical) 18.21
tarsi 80.88
thyroglossal (with resection of hyoid bone) 06.7
urachal (bladder) 57.51
abdominal wall 54.3
Skene's gland 71.3
skin (local) 86.3

Excision *(Continued)*
skin *(Continued)*
for graft (with closure of donor site) 86.91
radical (wide) (involving underlying or adjacent structure) (with flap closure) 86.4
tags
perianal 49.03
periauricular 18.29
soft tissue NEC 83.49
hand 82.39
spermatocele 63.2
spinous process 77.89
spleen (total) 41.5
accessory 41.93
partial 41.43
stomach - *see* Gastrectomy
sublingual gland (salivary) - *see also* Excision, salivary gland 26.30
submaxillary gland - *see also* Excision, salivary gland 26.30
supernumerary
breast 85.24
digits 86.26
sweat gland 86.3
synechiae - *see also* Lysis, synechiae
endometrial 68.21
tarsal plate (eyelid) 08.20
by wedge resection 08.24
tattoo 86.3
by dermabrasion 86.25
tendon (sheath) 83.42
for graft 83.41
hand 82.32
hand 82.33
for graft 82.32
thymus - *see also* Thymectomy 07.80
thyroglossal duct or tract (with resection of hyoid bone) 06.7
thyroid NEC - *see also* Thyroidectomy 06.39
tongue (complete) (total) 25.3
partial or subtotal 25.2
radical 25.4
tonsil 28.2
with adenoidectomy 28.3
lingual 28.5
tag 28.4
tooth NEC - *see also* Removal, tooth, surgical 23.19
from nasal sinus 22.60
torus
lingual 76.2
mandible, mandibularis 76.2
palate, palatinus 27.31
by wide excision 27.32
trabeculae carneae cordis (heart) 35.35
trochanteric lipomatosis 86.83
tumor - *see* Excision, lesion, by site
ulcer - *see also* Excision, lesion, by site
duodenum 45.31
endoscopic 45.30
stomach 43.42
endoscopic 43.41
umbilicus 54.3
urachus, urachal (cyst) (bladder) 57.51
abdominal wall 54.3
ureter, ureteral 56.40
with nephrectomy - *see* Nephrectomy
partial 56.41
stricture 56.41
total 56.42
ureterocele 56.41

Excision *(Continued)*
urethra, urethral 58.39
with complete cystectomy 57.79
endoscopic 58.31
septum 58.0
stricture 58.39
endoscopic 58.31
valve (congenital) 58.39
endoscopic (transurethral) (transvesical) 58.31
urethrovaginal septum 70.33
uterus (corpus) - *see also* Hysterectomy 68.9
cervix 67.4
lesion 67.39
lesion 68.29
septum 68.22
uvula 27.72
vagina (total) 70.4
varicocele, spermatic cord 63.1
vein - *see also* Phlebectomy 38.60
varicose 38.50
abdominal 38.57
head and neck NEC 38.52
intracranial NEC 38.51
lower limb 38.59
ovarian 38.67
thoracic NEC 38.55
upper limb 38.53
verucca - *see also* Excision, lesion, by site
eyelid 08.22
vesicovaginal septum 70.33
vitreous opacity 14.74
anterior approach 14.73
vocal cord(s) (submucous) 30.22
vulva (bilateral) (simple) - *see also* Vulvectomy 71.62
wart - *see also* Excision, lesion, by site
eyelid 08.22
wolffian duct 69.19
xanthoma (tendon sheath, hand) 82.21
site other than hand 83.31
Excisional biopsy - *see* Biopsy
Exclusion, pyloric 44.39
laparoscopic 44.38
Exenteration
ethmoid air cells 22.63
orbit 16.59
with
removal of adjacent structures 16.51
temporalis muscle transplant 16.59
therapeutic removal of bone 16.52
pelvic (organs) (female) 68.8
male 57.71
petrous pyramid air cells 20.59
Exercise (physical therapy) NEC 93.19
active musculoskeletal NEC 93.12
assisting 93.11
in pool 93.31
breathing 93.18
musculoskeletal
active NEC 93.12
passive NEC 93.17
neurologic 89.13
passive musculoskeletal NEC 93.17
resistive 93.13
Exfoliation, skin, by chemical 86.24
Exostectomy - *see also* Excision, lesion, bone 77.60
first metatarsal (hallux valgus repair) - *see* Bunionectomy
hallux valgus repair (with wedge osteotomy) - *see* Bunionectomy

Expiratory flow rate 89.38
Explant, explanation - *see* Removal
Exploration - *see also* Incision
abdomen 54.11
abdominal wall 54.0
adrenal (gland) 07.41
field 07.00
bilateral 07.02
unilateral 07.01
artery 38.00
abdominal 38.06
aorta (arch) (ascending) (descending) 38.04
head and neck NEC 38.02
intracranial NEC 38.01
lower limb 38.08
thoracic NEC 38.05
upper limb 38.03
auditory canal, external 18.02
axilla 86.09
bile duct(s) 51.59
common duct 51.51
endoscopic 51.11
for
relief of obstruction 51.42
endoscopic 51.84
removal of calculus 51.41
endoscopic 51.88
laparoscopic 51.11
for relief of obstruction 51.49
endoscopic 51.84
bladder (by incision) 57.19
endoscopic 57.32
through stoma (artificial) 57.31
bone - *see also* Incision, bone 77.10
brain (tissue) 01.39
breast 85.0
bronchus 33.0
endoscopic - *see* Bronchoscopy
bursa 83.03
hand 82.03
carotid body 39.8
carpal tunnel 04.43
choroid 14.9
ciliary body 12.44
colon 45.03
common bile duct 51.51
endoscopic 51.11
for
relief of obstruction 51.42
endoscopic 51.84
removal of calculus 51.41
endoscopic 51.88
coronary artery 36.99
cranium 01.24
cul-de-sac 70.12
endoscopic 70.22
disc space 03.09
duodenum 45.01
endoscopic - *see* Endoscopy, by site
epididymis 63.92
esophagus (by incision) NEC 42.09
endoscopic - *see* Esophagoscopy
ethmoid sinus 22.51
eyelid 08.09
fallopian tube 66.01
fascia 83.09
hand 82.09
flank 54.0
fossa (superficial) NEC 86.09
pituitary 07.71
frontal sinus 22.41
frontonasal duct 96.21
gallbladder 51.04

Exploration *(Continued)*
groin (region) (abdominal wall) (inguinal) 54.0
skin and subcutaneous tissue 86.09
heart 37.11
hepatic duct 51.59
hypophysis 07.72
ileum 45.02
inguinal canal (groin) 54.0
intestine (by incision) NEC 45.00
large 45.03
small 45.02
intrathoracic 34.02
jejunum 45.02
joint structures - *see also* Arthrotomy 80.10
kidney 55.01
pelvis 55.11
labia 71.09
lacrimal
gland 09.0
sac 09.53
laparotomy site 54.12
larynx (by incision) 31.3
endoscopic 31.42
liver 50.0
lung (by incision) 33.1
lymphatic structure(s) (channel) (node) (vessel) 40.0
mastoid 20.21
maxillary antrum or sinus (Caldwell-Luc approach) 22.39
mediastinum 34.1
endoscopic 34.22
middle ear (transtympanic) 20.23
muscle 83.02
hand 82.02
neck - *see also* Exploration, thyroid 06.09
nerve (cranial) (peripheral) NEC 04.04
auditory 04.01
root (spinal) 03.09
nose 21.1
orbit - *see also* Orbitotomy 16.09
pancreas 52.09
endoscopic 52.13
pancreatic duct 52.09
endoscopic 52.13
pelvis (by laparotomy) 54.11
by colpotomy 70.12
penis 64.92
perinephric area 59.09
perineum (female) 71.09
male 86.09
peripheral vessels
lower limb
artery 38.08
vein 38.09
upper limb (artery) (vein) 38.03
periprostatic tissue 60.81
perirenal tissue 59.09
perivesical tissue 59.19
petrous pyramid air cells 20.22
pilonidal sinus 86.03
pineal (gland) 07.52
field 07.51
pituitary (gland) 07.72
fossa 07.71
pleura 34.09
popliteal space 86.09
prostate 60.0
rectum - *see also* Proctoscopy 48.23
by incision 48.0
retroperitoneum 54.0
retropubic 59.19

Exploration *(Continued)*
salivary gland 26.0
sclera (by incision) 12.89
scrotum 61.0
shunt
ventriculoperitoneal at
peritoneal site 54.95
ventricular site 02.41
sinus
ethmoid 22.51
frontal 22.41
maxillary (Caldwell-Luc approach) 22.39
sphenoid 22.52
tract, skin and subcutaneous tissue 86.09
skin 86.09
soft tissue NEC 83.09
hand 82.09
spermatic cord 63.93
sphenoidal sinus 22.52
spinal (canal) (nerve root) 03.09
spleen 41.2
stomach (by incision) 43.0
endoscopic - *see* Gastroscopy
subcutaneous tissue 86.09
subdiaphragmatic space 54.11
superficial fossa 86.09
tarsal tunnel 04.44
tendon (sheath) 83.01
hand 82.01
testes 62.0
thymus (gland) 07.92
field 07.91
thyroid (field) (gland) (by incision) 06.09
postoperative 06.02
trachea (by incision) 31.3
endoscopic - *see* Tracheoscopy
tunica vaginalis 61.0
tympanum 20.09
transtympanic route 20.23
ureter (by incision) 56.2
endoscopic 56.31
urethra (by incision) 58.0
endoscopic 58.22
uterus (corpus) 68.0
cervix 69.95
digital 68.11
postpartal, manual 75.7
vagina (by incision) 70.14
endoscopic 70.21
vas deferens 63.6
vein 38.00
abdominal 38.07
head and neck NEC 38.02
intracranial NEC 38.01
lower limb 38.09
thoracic NEC 38.05
upper limb 38.03
vulva (by incision) 71.09
Exposure - *see also* Incision, by site
tooth (for orthodontic treatment) 24.6
Expression, trachoma follicles 10.33
Exsanguination transfusion 99.01
Extension
buccolabial sulcus 24.91
limb, forced 93.25
lingual sulcus 24.91
mandibular ridge 76.43
Exteriorization
esophageal pouch 42.12
intestine 46.03
large 46.03
small 46.01

Exteriorization *(Continued)*
maxillary sinus 22.9
pilonidal cyst or sinus (open excision) (with partial closure) 86.21
Extirpation - *see also* Excision, by site
aneurysm - *see* Aneurysmectomy
arteriovenous fistula - *see* Aneurysmectomy
lacrimal sac 09.6
larynx 30.3
with radical neck dissection (with synchronous thyroidectomy) (with synchronous tracheostomy) 30.4
nerve, tooth - *see also* Therapy, root canal 23.70
varicose vein (peripheral) (lower limb) 38.59
upper limb 38.53
Extracorporeal
circulation (regional), except hepatic 39.61
hepatic 50.92
percutaneous 39.66
hemodialysis 39.95
membrane oxygenation (ECMO) 39.65
photopheresis, therapeutic 99.88
shock wave lithotripsy (ESWL) NEC 98.59
bile duct 98.52
bladder 98.51
gallbladder 98.52
kidney 98.51
renal pelvis 98.51
specified site NEC 98.59
ureter 98.51
Extracranial-intracranial bypass [EC-IC] 39.28
Extraction
breech (partial) 72.52
with forceps to aftercoming head 72.51
total 72.54
with forceps to aftercoming head 72.53
cataract 13.19
after cataract (by)
capsulectomy 13.65
capsulotomy 13.64
discission 13.64
excision 13.65
iridocapsulectomy 13.65
mechanical fragmentation 13.66
needling 13.64
phacofragmentation (mechanical) 13.66
aspiration (simple) (with irrigation) 13.3
cryoextraction (intracapsular approach) 13.19
temporal inferior route (in presence of fistulization bleb) 13.11
curette evacuation (extracapsular approach) 13.2
emulsification (and aspiration) 13.41
erysiphake (intracapsular approach) 13.19
temporal inferior route (in presence of fistulization bleb) 13.11
extracapsular approach (with iridectomy) NEC 13.59
by temporal inferior route (in presence of fistulization bleb) 13.51

Extraction *(Continued)*
cataract *(Continued)*
extracapsular approach NEC *(Continued)*
aspiration (simple) (with irrigation) 13.3
curette evacuation 13.2
emulsification (and aspiration) 13.41
linear extraction 13.2
mechanical fragmentation with aspiration by
posterior route 13.42
specified route NEC 13.43
phacoemulsification (ultrasonic) (with aspiration) 13.41
phacofragmentation (mechanical) with aspiration by
posterior route 13.42
specified route NEC 13.43
ultrasonic (with aspiration) 13.41
rotoextraction (mechanical) with aspiration by
posterior route 13.42
specified route NEC 13.43
intracapsular (combined) (simple) (with iridectomy) (with suction) (with zonulolysis) 13.19

Extraction *(Continued)*
cataract *(Continued)*
intracapsular *(Continued)*
by temporal inferior route (in presence of fistulization bleb) 13.11
linear extraction (extracapsular approach) 13.2
phacoemulsification (and aspiration) 13.41
phacofragmentation (mechanical)
with aspiration by
posterior route 13.42
specified route NEC 13.43
ultrasonic 13.41
rotoextraction (mechanical)
with aspiration by
posterior route 13.42
specified route NEC 13.43
secondary membranous (after cataract) (by)
capsulectomy 13.65
capsulotomy 13.64
discission 13.64
excision 13.65
iridocapsulectomy 13.65
mechanical fragmentation 13.66
needling 13.64

Extraction *(Continued)*
cataract *(Continued)*
secondary membranous *(Continued)*
phacofragmentation (mechanical) 13.66
common duct stones (percutaneous) (through sinus tract) (with basket) 51.96
foreign body - *see* Removal, foreign body
kidney stone(s), percutaneous 55.03
with fragmentation procedure 55.04
lens (eye) - *see also* Extraction, cataract 13.19
Malstrom's 72.79
with episiotomy 72.71
menstrual, menses 69.6
milk from lactating breast (manual) (pump) 99.98
tooth (by forceps) (multiple) (single) NEC 23.09
with mucoperiosteal flap elevation 23.19
deciduous 23.01
surgical NEC - *see also* Removal, tooth, surgical 23.19
vacuum, fetus 72.79
with episiotomy 72.71
vitreous - *see also* Removal, vitreous 14.72

F

Face lift 86.82
Facetectomy 77.89
Facilitation, intraocular circulation NEC 12.59
Failed (trial) forceps 73.3
Family
counselling (medical) (social) 94.49
therapy 94.42
Farabeuf operation (ischiopubiotomy) 77.39
Fasanella-Servatt operation (blepharoptosis repair) 08.35
Fasciaplasty - *see* Fascioplasty
Fascia sling operation - *see* Operation, sling
Fasciectomy 83.44
for graft 83.43
hand 82.34
hand 82.35
for graft 82.34
palmar (release of Dupuytren's contracture) 82.35
Fasciodesis 83.89
hand 82.89
Fascioplasty - *see also* Repair, fascia 83.89
hand - *see also* Repair, fascia, hand 82.89
Fasciorrhaphy - *see* Suture, fascia
Fasciotomy 83.14
Dupuytren's 82.12
with excision 82.35
Dwyer 83.14
hand 82.12
Ober-Yount 83.14
orbital - *see also* Orbitotomy 16.09
palmar (release of Dupuytren's contracture) 82.12
with excision 82.35
Fenestration
aneurysm (dissecting), thoracic aorta 39.54
aortic aneurysm 39.54
cardiac valve 35.10
chest wall 34.01
ear
inner (with graft) 20.61
revision 20.62
tympanic 19.55
labyrinth (with graft) 20.61
Lempert's (endaural) 19.9
operation (aorta) 39.54
oval window, ear canal 19.55
palate 27.1
pericardium 37.12
semicircular canals (with graft) 20.61
stapes foot plate (with vein graft) 19.19
with incus replacement 19.11
tympanic membrane 19.55
vestibule (with graft) 20.61
Ferguson operation (hernia repair) 53.00
Fetography 87.81
Fetoscopy 75.31
Fiberoscopy - *see* Endoscopy, by site
Fibroidectomy, uterine 68.29
Fick operation (perforation of foot plate) 19.0
Filipuncture (aneurysm) (cerebral) 39.52
Filleting
hammer toe 77.56
pancreas 52.3
Filling, tooth (amalgam) (plastic) (silicate) 23.2
Filling, tooth *(Continued)*
root canal - *see also* Therapy, root canal 23.70
Fimbriectomy - *see also* Salpingectomy, partial 66.69
Uchida (with tubal ligation) 66.32
Finney operation (pyloroplasty) 44.29
Fissurectomy, anal 49.39
endoscopic 49.31
skin (subcutaneous tissue) 49.04
Fistulectomy - *see also* Closure, fistula, by site
abdominothoracic 34.83
abdominouterine 69.42
anus 49.12
appendix 47.92
bile duct 51.79
biliary tract NEC 51.79
bladder (transurethral approach) 57.84
bone - *see also* Excision, lesion, bone 77.60
branchial cleft 29.52
bronchocutaneous 33.42
bronchoesophageal 33.42
bronchomediastinal 34.73
bronchopleural 34.73
bronchopleurocutaneous 34.73
bronchopleuromediastinal 34.73
bronchovisceral 33.42
cervicosigmoidal 67.62
cholecystogastroenteric 51.93
cornea 11.49
diaphragm 34.83
enterouterine 69.42
esophagopleurocutaneous 34.73
esophagus NEC 42.84
fallopian tube 66.73
gallbladder 51.93
gastric NEC 44.63
hepatic duct 51.79
hepatopleural 34.73
hepatopulmonary 34.73
intestine
large 46.76
small 46.74
intestinouterine 69.42
joint - *see also* Excision, lesion, joint 80.80
lacrimal
gland 09.21
sac 09.6
laryngotracheal 31.62
larynx 31.62
mediastinocutaneous 34.73
mouth NEC 27.53
nasal 21.82
sinus 22.71
nasolabial 21.82
nasopharyngeal 21.82
oroantral 22.71
oronasal 21.82
pancreas 52.95
perineorectal 71.72
perineosigmoidal 71.72
perirectal, not opening into rectum 48.93
pharyngoesophageal 29.53
pharynx NEC 29.53
pleura 34.73
rectolabial 71.72
rectourethral 58.43
rectouterine 69.42
rectovaginal 70.73
rectovesical 57.83
rectovulvar 71.72
Fistulectomy *(Continued)*
rectum 48.73
salivary (duct) (gland) 26.42
scrotum 61.42
skin 86.3
stomach NEC 44.63
subcutaneous tissue 86.3
thoracoabdominal 34.83
thoracogastric 34.83
thoracointestinal 34.83
thorax NEC 34.73
trachea NEC 31.73
tracheoesophageal 31.73
ureter 56.84
urethra 58.43
uteroenteric 69.42
uterointestinal 69.42
uterorectal 69.42
uterovaginal 69.42
vagina 70.75
vesicosigmoidovaginal 57.83
vocal cords 31.62
vulvorectal 71.72
Fistulization
appendix 47.91
arteriovenous 39.27
cisterna chyli 40.62
endolymphatic sac (for decompression) 20.79
esophagus, external 42.10
cervical 42.11
specified technique NEC 42.19
interatrial 35.41
labyrinth (for decompression) 20.79
lacrimal sac into nasal cavity 09.81
larynx 31.29
lymphatic duct, left (thoracic) 40.62
orbit 16.09
peritoneal 54.93
salivary gland 26.49
sclera 12.69
by trephination 12.61
with iridectomy 12.65
sinus, nasal NEC 22.9
subarachnoid space 02.2
thoracic duct 40.62
trachea 31.29
tracheoesophageal 31.95
urethrovaginal 58.0
ventricle, cerebral - *see also* Shunt, ventricular 02.2
Fistulogram
abdominal wall 88.03
chest wall 87.38
retroperitoneum 88.14
specified site NEC 88.49 ◄
Fistulotomy, anal 49.11
Fitting
arch bars (orthodontic) 24.7
for immobilization (fracture) 93.55
artificial limb 84.40
contact lens 95.32
denture (total) 99.97
bridge (fixed) 23.42
removable 23.43
partial (fixed) 23.42
removable 23.43
hearing aid 95.48
obturator (orthodontic) 24.7
ocular prosthetics 95.34
orthodontic
appliance 24.7
obturator 24.7
wiring 24.7

Fitting *(Continued)*
orthotic device 93.23
periodontal splint (orthodontic) 24.7
prosthesis, prosthetic device
above knee 84.45
arm 84.43
lower (and hand) 84.42
upper (and shoulder) 84.41
below knee 84.46
hand (and lower arm) 84.42
leg 84.47
above knee 84.45
below knee 84.46
limb NEC 84.40
ocular 95.34
penis (external) 64.94
shoulder (and upper arm) 84.41
spectacles 95.31
Five-in-one repair, knee 81.42
Fixation
bone
external, without reduction 93.59
with fracture reduction - *see* Reduction, fracture
external fixator - *see* Fixator, external
cast immobilization NEC 93.53
splint 93.54
traction (skeletal) NEC 93.44
intermittent 93.43
internal (without fracture reduction) 78.50
with fracture reduction - *see* Reduction, fracture
carpal, metacarpal 78.54
clavicle 78.51
femur 78.55
fibula 78.57
humerus 78.52
patella 78.56
pelvic 78.59
phalanges (foot) (hand) 78.59
radius 78.53
scapula 78.51
specified site NEC 78.59
tarsal, metatarsal 78.58
thorax (ribs) (sternum) 78.51
tibia 78.57
ulna 78.53
vertebrae 78.59
breast (pendulous) 85.6
cardinal ligaments 69.22
cervical collar 93.52
duodenum 46.62
to abdominal wall 46.61
external (without manipulation for reduction) 93.59
with fracture reduction - *see* Reduction, fracture
cast immobilization NEC 93.53
pressure dressing 93.56
splint 93.54
strapping (non-traction) 93.59 ◀
traction (skeletal) NEC 93.44
intermittent 93.43
hip 81.40
ileum 46.62
to abdominal wall 46.61
internal
with fracture reduction - *see* Reduction, fracture
without fracture reduction - *see* Fixation, bone, internal
intestine 46.60

Fixation *(Continued)*
intestine *(Continued)*
large 46.64
to abdominal wall 46.63
small 46.62
to abdominal wall 46.61
to abdominal wall 46.60
iris (bombé) 12.11
jejunum 46.62
to abdominal wall 46.61
joint - *see* Arthroplasty
kidney 55.7
ligament
cardinal 69.22
palpebrae 08.36
omentum 54.74
parametrial 69.22
plaster jacket 93.51
other cast 93.53
rectum (sling) 48.76
spine, with fusion - *see also* Fusion, spinal 81.00
spleen 41.95
splint 93.54
tendon 83.88
hand 82.85
testis in scrotum 62.5
tongue 25.59
urethrovaginal (to Cooper's ligament) 70.77
uterus (abdominal) (vaginal) (ventrofixation) 69.22
vagina 70.77
Fixator, external
computer assisted (dependent) 84.73 ◀
hybrid device or sytem 84.73
Ilizarov type 84.72
monoplanar system 84.71
ring device or system 84.72
Sheffield type 84.72
Flooding (psychologic desensitization) 94.33
Flowmetry, Doppler (ultrasonic) - *see also* Ultrasonography
aortic arch 88.73
head and neck 88.71
heart 88.72
thorax NEC 88.73
Fluoroscopy - *see* Radiography
Fog therapy (respiratory) 93.94
Folding, eye muscle 15.22
multiple (two or more muscles) 15.4
Foley operation (pyeloplasty) 55.87
Fontan operation (creation of conduit between right atrium and pulmonary artery) 35.94
Foraminotomy 03.09
Forced extension, limb 93.25
Forceps delivery - *see* Delivery, forceps
Formation
adhesions
pericardium 36.39
pleura 34.6
anus, artificial - *see also* Colostomy 46.13
duodenostomy 46.39
ileostomy - *see also* Ileostomy 46.23
jejunostomy 46.39
percutaneous (endoscopic) (PEJ) 46.32
arteriovenous fistula (for kidney dialysis) (peripheral) (shunt) 39.27
external cannula 39.93
bone flap, cranial 02.03

Formation *(Continued)*
cardiac device (defibrillator) (pacemaker) pocket
with initial insertion of cardiac device - *omit code*
new site (skin) (subcutaneous) 37.79
colostomy - *see also* Colostomy 46.13
conduit
ileal (urinary) 56.51
left ventricle and aorta 35.93
right atrium and pulmonary artery 35.94
right ventricle and pulmonary (distal) artery 35.92
in repair of
pulmonary artery atresia 35.92
transposition of great vessels 35.92
truncus arteriosus 35.83
endorectal ileal pouch (H-pouch) (J-pouch) (S-pouch) (with anastomosis to anus) 45.95
fistula
arteriovenous (for kidney dialysis) (peripheral shunt) 39.27
external cannula 39.93
bladder to skin NEC 57.18
with bladder flap 57.21
percutaneous 57.17
cutaneoperitoneal 54.93
gastric 43.19
percutaneous (endoscopic) (transabdominal) 43.11
mucous - *see also* Colostomy 46.13
rectovaginal 48.99
tracheoesophageal 31.95
tubulovalvular (Beck-Jianu) (Frank's) (Janeway) (Spivack's) (Ssabanejew-Frank) 43.19
urethrovaginal 58.0
ileal
bladder
closed 57.87 *[45.51]*
open 56.51
conduit 56.51
interatrial fistula 35.42
mucous fistula - *see also* Colostomy 46.13
pericardial
baffle, interatrial 35.91
window 37.12
pleural window (for drainage) 34.09
pocket
cardiac device (defibrillator) (pacemaker)
with initial insertion of cardiac device - *omit code*
new site (skin) (subcutaneous) 37.79
loop recorder 37.79
thalamic stimulator pulse generator
with initial insertion of battery package - *omit code*
new site (skin) (subcutaneous) 86.09
pupil 12.39
by iridectomy 12.14
rectovaginal fistula 48.99
reversed gastric tube (intrathoracic) (retrosternal) 42.58
antesternal or antethoracic 42.68
septal defect, interatrial 35.42
shunt
abdominovenous 54.94

Formation *(Continued)*
shunt *(Continued)*
arteriovenous 39.93
peritoneojugular 54.94
peritoneo-vascular 54.94
pleuroperitoneal 34.05
transjugular intrahepatic portosystemic (TIPS) 39.1
subcutaneous tunnel
esophageal 42.86
with anastomosis - *see* Anastomosis, esophagus, antesternal
pulse generator lead wire 86.99
with initial procedure - *omit code*
thalamic stimulator pulse generator pocket
with initial insertion of battery package - *omit code*
new site (skin) (subcutaneous) 86.09
syndactyly (finger) (toe) 86.89
tracheoesophageal 31.95
tubulovalvular fistula (Beck-Jianu) (Frank's) (Janeway) (Spivak's) (Ssabanejew-Frank) 43.19
uretero-ileostomy, cutaneous 56.51
ureterostomy, cutaneous 56.61
ileal 56.51
urethrovaginal fistula 58.0
window
pericardial 37.12
pleural (for drainage) 34.09
Fothergill (-Donald) operation (uterine suspension) 69.22
Fowler operation
arthroplasty of metacarpophalangeal joint 81.72
release (mallet finger repair) 82.84
tenodesis (hand) 82.85
thoracoplasty 33.34
Fox operation (entropion repair with wedge resection) 08.43
Fracture, surgical - *see also* Osteoclasis 78.70
turbinates (nasal) 21.62
Fragmentation
lithotriptor - *see* Lithotripsy
mechanical
cataract (with aspiration) 13.43
posterior route 13.42
secondary membrane 13.66
secondary membrane (after cataract) 13.66
ultrasonic
cataract (with aspiration) 13.41
stones, urinary (Kock pouch) 59.95
urinary stones 59.95
percutaneous nephrostomy 55.04
Franco operation (suprapubic cystotomy) 57.18
Frank operation (permanent gastrostomy) 43.19
Frazier (-Spiller) operation (subtemporal trigeminal rhizotomy) 04.02
Fredet-Ramstedt operation (pyloromyotomy) (with wedge resection) 43.3
Freeing
adhesions - *see* Lysis, adhesions
anterior synechiae (with injection of air or liquid) 12.32
artery-vein-nerve bundle 39.91
extraocular muscle, entrapped 15.7
goniosynechiae (with injection of air or liquid) 12.31

Freeing *(Continued)*
intestinal segment for interposition 45.50
large 45.52
small 45.51
posterior synechiae 12.33
synechiae (posterior) 12.33
anterior (with injection of air or liquid) 12.32
vascular bundle 39.91
vessel 39.91
Freezing
gastric 96.32
prostate 60.62
Frenckner operation (intrapetrosal drainage) 20.22
Frenectomy
labial 27.41
lingual 25.92
lip 27.41
maxillary 27.41
tongue 25.92
Frenotomy
labial 27.91
lingual 25.91
Frenulumectomy - *see* Frenectomy
Frickman operation (abdominal proctopexy) 48.75
Frommel operation (shortening of uterosacral ligaments) 69.22
Fulguration - *see also* Electrocoagulation and Destruction, lesion, by site
adenoid fossa 28.7
anus 49.39
endoscopic 49.31
bladder (transurethral) 57.49
suprapubic 57.59
choroid 14.21
duodenum 45.32
endoscopic 45.30
esophagus 42.39
endoscopic 42.33
large intestine 45.49
endoscopic 45.43
polypectomy 45.42
penis 64.2
perineum, female 71.3
prostate, transurethral 60.29
rectum 48.32
radical 48.31
retina 14.21
scrotum 61.3
Skene's gland 71.3
skin 86.3
small intestine NEC 45.34
duodenum 45.32
endoscopic 45.30
stomach 43.49
endoscopic 43.41
subcutaneous tissue 86.3
tonsillar fossa 28.7
urethra 58.39
endoscopic 58.31
vulva 71.3
Function
study - *see also* Scan, radioisotope
gastric 89.39
muscle 93.08
ocular 95.25
nasal 89.12
pulmonary - *see* categories 89.37-89.38
renal 92.03
thyroid 92.01
urethral sphincter 89.23

Fundectomy, uterine 68.39
Fundoplication (esophageal) (Nissen's) 44.66
laparoscopic 44.67
Fundusectomy, gastric 43.89
Fusion
atlas-axis (spine) - *see* Fusion, spinal, atlas-axis
bone - *see also* Osteoplasty 78.40
cervical (spine) (C2 level or below) - *see* Fusion, spinal, cervical
claw toe 77.57
craniocervical - *see* Fusion, spinal, craniocervical
dorsal, dorsolumbar - *see* Fusion, spinal, dorsal, dorsolumbar
epiphyseal-diaphyseal - *see also* Arrest, bone growth 78.20
epiphysiodesis - *see also* Arrest, bone growth 78.20
hammer toe 77.56
joint (with bone graft) - *see also* Arthrodesis 81.20
ankle 81.11
claw toe 77.57
foot NEC 81.17
hammer toe 77.56
hip 81.21
interphalangeal, finger 81.28
ischiofemoral 81.21
metatarsophalangeal 81.16
midtarsal 81.14
overlapping toe(s) 77.58
pantalar 81.11
spinal - *see also* Fusion, spinal 81.00
subtalar 81.13
tarsal joints NEC 81.17
tarsometatarsal 81.15
tibiotalar 81.11
toe NEC 77.58
claw toe 77.57
hammer toe 77.56
overlapping toe(s) 77.58
lip to tongue 25.59
lumbar, lumbosacral - *see* Fusion, spinal, lumbar, lumbosacral
occiput-C2 (spinal) - *see* Fusion, spinal, occiput
spinal (with graft) (with internal fixation) (with instrumentation) 81.00
anterior lumbar interbody fusion (ALIF) 81.06
atlas-axis (anterior transoral) (posterior) 81.01
for pseudarthrosis 81.31
cervical (C2 level or below) NEC 81.02
anterior (interbody), anterolateral technique 81.02
for pseudarthrosis 81.32
C1-C2 level (anterior) (posterior) 81.01
for pseudarthrosis 81.31
for pseudarthrosis 81.32
posterior (interbody), posterolateral technique 81.03
for pseudarthrosis 81.33
craniocervical (anterior transoral) (posterior) 81.01
for pseudarthrosis NEC 81.31
dorsal, dorsolumbar NEC 81.05
anterior (interbody), anterolateral technique 81.04
for pseudarthrosis 81.34

Fusion *(Continued)*
spinal *(Continued)*
dorsal *(Continued)*
for pseudarthrosis 81.35
posterior (interbody), posterolateral technique 81.05
for pseudarthrosis 81.35
lumbar, lumbosacral NEC 81.08
anterior (interbody), anterolateral technique 81.06
for pseudarthrosis 81.36
for pseudarthrosis 81.38
lateral transverse process technique 81.07
for pseudarthrosis 81.37

Fusion *(Continued)*
spinal *(Continued)*
lumbar *(Continued)*
posterior (interbody), posterolateral technique 81.08
for pseudarthrosis 81.38
number of vertebrae - *see* codes 81.62-81.64
occiput-C2 (anterior transoral) (posterior) 81.01
for pseudarthrosis 81.31

Note: Also use either 81.62, 81.63, or 81.64 as an additional code to show the total number of vertebrae fused

Fusion *(Continued)*
spinal *(Continued)*
posterior lumbar interbody fusion (PLIF) 81.08
transforaminal lumbar interbody fusion (TLIF) 81.08
tongue (to lip) 25.59

G

Gait training 93.22
Galeaplasty 86.89
Galvanoionization 99.27
Games
  competitive 94.39
  organized 93.89
Gamma irradiation, stereotactic 92.32
Ganglionectomy
  gasserian 04.05
  lumbar sympathetic 05.23
  nerve (cranial) (peripheral) NEC 04.06
    sympathetic 05.29
  sphenopalatine (Meckel's) 05.21
  tendon sheath (wrist) 82.21
    site other than hand 83.31
  trigeminal 04.05
Ganglionotomy, trigeminal (radiofrequency) 04.02
Gant operation (wedge osteotomy of trochanter) 77.25
Garceau operation (tibial tendon transfer) 83.75
Gardner operation (spinal meningocele repair) 03.51
Gas endarterectomy 38.10
  abdominal 38.16
  aorta (arch) (ascending) (descending) 38.14
  coronary artery 36.09
  head and neck NEC 38.12
  intracranial NEC 38.11
  lower limb 38.18
  thoracic NEC 38.15
  upper limb 38.13
Gastrectomy (partial) (subtotal) NEC 43.89
  with
    anastomosis (to) NEC 43.89
      duodenum 43.6
      esophagus 43.5
      gastrogastric 43.89
      jejunum 43.7
    esophagogastrostomy 43.5
    gastroduodenostomy (bypass) 43.6
    gastroenterostomy (bypass) 43.7
    gastrogastrostomy (bypass) 43.89
    gastrojejunostomy (bypass) 43.7
    jejunal transposition 43.81
  complete NEC 43.99
    with intestinal interposition 43.91
  distal 43.6
  Hofmeister 43.7
  Polya 43.7
  proximal 43.5
  radical NEC 43.99
    with intestinal interposition 43.91
  total NEC 43.99
    with intestinal interposition 43.91
Gastrocamera 44.19
Gastroduodenectomy - *see* Gastrectomy
Gastroduodenoscopy 45.13
  through stoma (artificial) 45.12
  transabdominal (operative) 45.11
Gastroduodenostomy (bypass) (Jaboulay's) 44.39
  with partial gastrectomy 43.6
  laparoscopic 44.38
Gastroenterostomy (bypass) NEC 44.39
  with partial gastrectomy 43.7
  laparoscopic 44.38
Gastrogastrostomy (bypass) 44.39
  with partial gastrectomy 43.89
  laparoscopic 44.38
Gastrojejunostomy (bypass) 44.39
  with partial gastrectomy 43.7
  laparoscopic 44.38
  percutaneous (endoscopic) 44.32
Gastrolysis 54.59
  laparoscopic 54.51
Gastropexy 44.64
Gastroplasty NEC 44.69
  laparoscopic 44.68
  vertical banded gastroplasty (VBG) 44.68
Gastroplication 44.69
  laparoscopic 44.68
Gastropylorectomy 43.6
Gastrorrhaphy 44.61
Gastroscopy NEC 44.13
  through stoma (artificial) 44.12
  transabdominal (operative) 44.11
Gastrostomy (Brunschwig's) (decompression) (fine caliber tube) (Kader) (permanent) (Stamm) (Stamm- Kader) (temporary) (tube) (Witzel) 43.19
  Beck-Jianu 43.19
  Frank's 43.19
  Janeway 43.19
  percutaneous (endoscopic) (PEG) 43.11
  Spivack's 43.19
  Ssabanejew-Frank 43.19
Gastrotomy 43.0
  for control of hemorrhage 44.49
Gavage, gastric 96.35
Gelman operation (release of clubfoot) 83.84
Genioplasty (augmentation) (with graft) (with implant) 76.68
  reduction 76.67
Ghormley operation (hip fusion) 81.21
Gifford operation
  destruction of lacrimal sac 09.6
  keratotomy (delimiting) 11.1
    radial (refractive) 11.75
Gill operation
  arthrodesis of shoulder 81.23
  laminectomy 03.09
Gill-Stein operation (carporadial arthrodesis) 81.25
Gilliam operation (uterine suspension) 69.22
Gingivectomy 24.31
Gingivoplasty (with bone graft) (with soft tissue graft) 24.2
Girdlestone operation
  laminectomy with spinal fusion 81.00
  muscle transfer for claw toe repair 77.57
  resection of femoral head and neck (without insertion of joint prosthesis) 77.85
    with replacement prosthesis - *see* Implant, joint, hip
  resection of hip prosthesis 80.05
    with replacement prosthesis - *see* Implant, joint, hip
Girdlestone-Taylor operation (muscle transfer for claw toe repair) 77.57
Glenn operation (anastomosis of superior vena cava to right pulmonary artery) 39.21
Glenoplasty, shoulder 81.83
  with
    partial replacement 81.81
    total replacement 81.80
  for recurrent dislocation 81.82
Glomectomy
  carotid 39.8
  jugulare 20.51
Glossectomy (complete) (total) 25.3
  partial or subtotal 25.2
  radical 25.4
Glossopexy 25.59
Glossoplasty NEC 25.59
Glossorrhaphy 25.51
Glossotomy NEC 25.94
  for tongue tie 25.91
Glycoprotein IIB/IIIa inhibitor 99.20
Goebel-Frangenheim-Stoeckel operation (urethrovesical suspension) 59.4
Goldner operation (clubfoot release) 80.48
Goldthwaite operation
  ankle stabilization 81.11
  patellar stabilization 81.44
  tendon transfer for stabilization patella 81.44
Gonadectomy
  ovary
    bilateral 65.51
      laparoscopic 65.53
    unilateral 65.39
      laparoscopic 65.31
  testis
    bilateral 62.41
    unilateral 62.3
Goniopuncture 12.51
  with goniotomy 12.53
Gonioscopy 12.29
Goniospasis 12.59
Goniotomy (Barkan's) 12.52
  with goniopuncture 12.53
Goodal-Power operation (vagina) 70.8
Gordon-Taylor operation (hindquarter amputation) 84.19
GP IIB/IIIa inhibitor, infusion 99.20
Graber-Duvernay operation (drilling femoral head) 77.15
Graft, grafting
  aneurysm 39.52
    endovascular
      abdominal aorta 39.71
      lower extremity artery(ies)
      thoracic aorta 39.73
      upper extremity artery(ies)
  artery, arterial (patch) 39.58
    with
      excision or resection of vessel - *see* Arteriectomy, with graft replacement
      synthetic patch (Dacron) (Teflon) 39.57
      tissue patch (vein) (autogenous) (homograft) 39.56
  blood vessel (patch) 39.58
    with
      excision or resection of vessel - *see* Angiectomy, with graft replacement
      synthetic patch (Dacron) (Teflon) 39.57
      tissue patch (vein) (autogenous) (homograft) 39.56
  bone (autogenous) (bone bank) (dual onlay) (heterogeneous) (inlay) (massive onlay) (multiple) (osteoperiosteal) (peg) (subperiosteal) (with metallic fixation) 78.00
    with
      arthrodesis - *see* Arthrodesis

Graft, grafting *(Continued)*
bone *(Continued)*
with *(Continued)*
arthroplasty - *see* Arthroplasty
gingivoplasty 24.2
lengthening - *see* Lengthening, bone
carpals, metacarpals 78.04
clavicle 78.01
facial NEC 76.91
with total ostectomy 76.44
femur 78.05
fibula 78.07
humerus 78.02
joint - *see* Arthroplasty
mandible 76.91
with total mandibulectomy 76.41
marrow - *see* Transplant, bone, marrow
nose - *see* Graft, nose
patella 78.06
pelvic 78.09
pericranial 02.04
phalanges (foot) (hand) 78.09
radius 78.03
scapula 78.01
skull 02.04
specified site NEC 78.09
spine 78.09
with fusion - *see* Fusion, spinal
tarsal, metatarsal 78.08
thorax (ribs) (sternum) 78.01
thumb (with transfer of skin flap) 82.69
tibia 78.07
ulna 78.03
vertebrae 78.09
with fusion - *see* Fusion, spinal
breast - *see* also Mammoplasty 85.89
buccal sulcus 27.99
cartilage (joint) - *see* also Arthroplasty
nose - *see* Graft, nose
chest wall (mesh) (silastic) 34.79
conjunctiva (free) (mucosa) 10.44
for symblepharon repair 10.41
cornea - *see* also Keratoplasty 11.60
dermal-fat 86.69
dermal regenerative 86.67
dura 02.12
ear
auricle 18.79
external auditory meatus 18.6
inner 20.61
pedicle preparation 86.71
esophagus NEC 42.87
with interposition (intrathoracic) NEC 42.58
antesternal or antethoracic NEC 42.68
colon (intrathoracic) 42.55
antesternal or antethoracic 42.65
small bowel (intrathoracic) 42.53
antesternal or antethoracic 42.63
eyebrow - *see* also Reconstruction, eyelid, with graft 08.69
eyelid - *see* also Reconstruction, eyelid, with graft 08.69
free mucous membrane 08.62
eye socket (bone) (cartilage) (skin) 16.63
fallopian tube 66.79
fascia 83.82
with hernia repair - *see* Repair, hernia
eyelid 08.32

Graft, grafting *(Continued)*
fascia *(Continued)*
hand 82.72
tarsal cartilage 08.69
fat pad NEC 86.89
with skin graft - *see* Graft, skin, fullthickness
flap (advanced) (rotating) (sliding) - *see* also Graft, skin, pedicle
tarsoconjunctival 08.64
hair-bearing skin 86.64
hand
fascia 82.72
free skin 86.62
muscle 82.72
pedicle (flap) 86.73
tendon 82.79
heart, for revascularization, *see* category 36.3
joint - *see* Arthroplasty
larynx 31.69
lip 27.56
full-thickness 27.55
lymphatic structure(s) (channel) (node) (vessel) 40.9
mediastinal fat to myocardium 36.39
meninges (cerebral) 02.12
mouth, except palate 27.56
full-thickness 27.55
muscle 83.82
hand 82.72
myocardium, for revascularization 36.39
nasolabial flaps 21.86
nerve (cranial) (peripheral) 04.5
nipple 85.86
nose 21.89
with
augmentation 21.85
rhinoplasty - *see* Rhinoplasty
total reconstruction 21.83
septum 21.88
tip 21.86
omentum 54.74
to myocardium 36.39
orbit (bone) (cartilage) (skin) 16.63
outflow tract (patch) (pulmonary valve) 35.26
in total repair of tetralogy of Fallot 35.81
ovary 65.92
palate 27.69
for cleft palate repair 27.62
pedicle - *see* Graft, skin, pedicle
penis (rib) (skin) 64.49
pigskin 86.65
pinch - *see* Graft, skin, free
pocket - *see* Graft, skin, pedicle
porcine 86.65
postauricular (Wolff) 18.79
razor - *see* Graft, skin, free
rope - *see* Graft, skin, pedicle
saphenous vein in aortocoronary bypass - *see* Bypass, aorto-coronary
scrotum 61.49
skin (partial-thickness) (split-thickness) 86.69
amnionic membrane 86.66
auditory meatus (ear) 18.6
dermal-fat 86.69
for breast augmentation 85.50
dermal regenerative 86.67
ear
auditory meatus 18.6
postauricular 18.79

Graft, grafting *(Continued)*
skin *(Continued)*
eyelid 08.61
flap - *see* Graft, skin, pedicle
free (autogenous) NEC 86.60
lip 27.56
thumb 86.62
for
pollicization 82.61
reconstruction 82.69
full-thickness 86.63
breast 85.83
hand 86.61
hair-bearing 86.64
eyelid or eyebrow 08.63
hand 86.62
full-thickness 86.61
heterograft 86.65
homograft 86.66
island flap 86.70
mucous membrane 86.69
eyelid 08.62
nose - *see* Graft, nose
pedicle (flap) (tube) 86.70
advancement 86.72
attachment to site (advanced) (double) (rotating) (sliding) 86.74
hand (cross finger) (pocket) 86.73
lip 27.57
mouth 27.57
thumb 86.73
for
pollicization 82.61
reconstruction NEC 82.69
breast 85.84
transverse rectus abdominis musculocutaneous (TRAM) 85.7
defatting 86.75
delayed 86.71
design and raising 86.71
elevation 86.71
preparation of (cutting) 86.71
revision 86.75
sculpturing 86.71
transection 86.71
transfer 86.74
trimming 86.71
postauricular 18.79
rotation flap 86.70
specified site NEC 86.69
full-thickness 86.63
tarsal cartilage 08.69
temporalis muscle to orbit 16.63
with exenteration of orbit 16.59
tendon 83.81
for joint repair - *see* Arthroplasty
hand 82.79
testicle 62.69
thumb (for reconstruction) NEC 82.69
tongue (mucosal) (skin) 25.59
trachea 31.79
tubular (tube) - *see* Graft, skin, pedicle
tunnel - *see* Graft, skin, pedicle
tympanum - *see* also Tympanoplasty 19.4
ureter 56.89
vein (patch) 39.58
with
excision or resection of vessel - *see* Phlebectomy, with graft replacement

ICD-9-CM
G
Vol. 3

Graft, grafting *(Continued)*
vein *(Continued)*
with *(Continued)*
synthetic patch (Dacron) (Teflon) 39.57
tissue patch (vein) (autogenous) (homograft) 39.56
vermilion border (lip) 27.56
Grattage, conjunctiva 10.31
Green operation (scapulopexy) 78.41
Grice operation (subtalar arthrodesis) 81.13
Grip, strength 93.04
Gritti-Stokes operation (knee disarticulation) 84.16
Gross operation (herniorrhaphy) 53.49
Group therapy 94.44
Guttering, bone - *see also* Excision, lesion, bone 77.60
Guyon operation (amputation of ankle) 84.13

H

Hagner operation (epididymotomy) 63.92
Halsted operation - *see* Repair, hernia, inguinal
Hampton operation (anastomosis small intestine to rectal stump) 45.92
Hanging hip operation (muscle release) 83.19
Harelip operation 27.54
Harrison-Richardson operation (vaginal suspension) 70.77
Hartmann resection (of intestine) (with pouch) - *see* Colectomy, by site
Harvesting
bone marrow 41.91
stem cells 99.79
Hauser operation
achillotenotomy 83.11
bunionectomy with adductor tendon transfer 77.53
stabilization of patella 81.44
Heaney operation (vaginal hysterectomy) 68.59
laparoscopically assisted (LAVH) 68.51
Hearing aid (with battery replacement) 95.49
Hearing test 95.47
Hegar operation (perineorrhaphy) 71.79
Heine operation (cyclodialysis) 12.55
Heineke-Mikulicz operation (pyloroplasty) 44.29
Heller operation (esophagomyotomy) 42.7
Hellström operation (transplantation of aberrant renal vessel) 39.55
Hemicolectomy
left 45.75
right (extended) 45.73
Hemicystectomy 57.6
Hemigastrectomy - *see* Gastrectomy
Hemiglossectomy 25.2
Hemilaminectomy (decompression) (exploration) 03.09
Hemilaryngectomy (anterior) (lateral) (vertical) 30.1
Hemimandibulectomy 76.31
Hemimastectomy (radical) 85.23
Hemimaxillectomy (with bone graft) (with prosthesis) 76.39
Heminephrectomy 55.4
Hemipelvectomy 84.19
Hemispherectomy (cerebral) 01.52
Hemithyroidectomy (with removal of isthmus) (with removal of portion of remaining lobe) 06.2
Hemodiafiltration (extracorporeal) 39.95
Hemodialysis (extracorporeal) 39.95
Hemodilution 99.03
Hemofiltration (extracorporeal) 39.95
Hemorrhage control - *see* Control, hemorrhage
Hemorrhoidectomy 49.46
by
cautery, cauterization 49.43
crushing 49.45
cryotherapy, cryosurgery 49.44
excision 49.46
injection 49.42
ligation 49.45
Hemostasis - *see* Control, hemorrhage
Henley operation (jejunal transposition) 43.81
Hepatectomy (complete) (total) 50.4
partial or subtotal 50.22
Hepatic assistance, extracorporeal 50.92
Hepaticocholangiojejunostomy 51.37
Hepaticocystoduodenostomy 51.37
Hepaticodochotomy 51.59
Hepaticoduodenostomy 51.37
Hepaticojejunostomy 51.37
Hepaticolithectomy 51.49
endoscopic 51.88
Hepaticolithotomy 51.49
endoscopic 51.88
Hepaticostomy 51.59
Hepaticotomy 51.59
Hepatocholangiocystoduodenostomy 51.37
Hepatocholedochostomy 51.43
endoscopic 51.87
Hepatoduodenostomy 50.69
Hepatogastrostomy 50.69
Hepatojejunostomy 50.69
Hepatolithotomy
hepatic duct 51.49
liver 50.0
Hepatopexy 50.69
Hepatorrhaphy 50.61
Hepatostomy (external) (internal) 50.69
Hepatotomy (with packing) 50.0
Hernioplasty - *see* Repair, hernia
Herniorrhaphy - *see* Repair, hernia
Herniotomy - *see* Repair, hernia
Heterograft - *see* Graft
Heterotransplant, heterotransplantation - *see* Transplant
Hey operation (amputation of foot) 84.12
Hey-Groves operation (reconstruction of anterior cruciate ligament) 81.45
Heyman operation (soft tissue release for clubfoot) 83.84
Heyman-Herndon (-Strong) operation (correction of metatarsus varus) 80.48
Hibbs operation (lumbar spinal fusion) - *see* Fusion, lumbar
Higgins operation - *see* Repair, hernia, femoral
High forceps delivery 72.39
with episiotomy 72.31
Hill-Allison operation (hiatal hernia repair, transpleural approach) 53.80
Hinging, mitral valve 35.12
His bundle recording 37.29
Hitchcock operation (anchoring tendon of biceps) 83.88
Hofmeister operation (gastrectomy) 43.7
Hoke operation
midtarsal fusion 81.14
triple arthrodesis 81.12
Holth operation
iridencleisis 12.63
sclerectomy 12.65
Homans operation (correction of lymphedema) 40.9
Homograft - *see* Graft
Homotransplant, homotransplantation - *see* Transplant
Hosiery, elastic 93.59
Hutch operation (ureteroneocystostomy) 56.74
Hybinette-Eden operation (glenoid bone block) 78.01
Hydrocelectomy
canal of Nuck (female) 69.19
male 63.1
round ligament 69.19
spermatic cord 63.1
tunica vaginalis 61.2
Hydrotherapy 93.33
assisted exercise in pool 93.31
whirlpool 93.32
Hymenectomy 70.31
Hymenoplasty 70.76
Hymenorrhaphy 70.76
Hymenotomy 70.11
Hyperalimentation (parenteral) 99.15
Hyperbaric oxygenation 93.95
wound 93.59
Hyperextension, joint 93.25
Hyperthermia NEC 93.35
for cancer treatment (interstitial) (local) (radiofrequency) (regional) (ultrasound) (whole-body) 99.85
Hypnodrama, psychiatric 94.32
Hypnosis (psychotherapeutic) 94.32
for anesthesia - *omit code*
Hypnotherapy 94.32
Hypophysectomy (complete) (total) 07.69
partial or subtotal 07.63
transfrontal approach 07.61
transsphenoidal approach 07.62
specified approach NEC 07.68
transfrontal approach (complete) (total) 07.64
partial 07.61
transsphenoidal approach (complete) (total) 07.65
partial 07.62
Hypothermia (central) (local) 99.81
gastric (cooling) 96.31
freezing 96.32
systemic (in open heart surgery) 39.62
Hypotympanotomy 20.23
Hysterectomy 68.9
abdominal 68.49 ⬅
laparoscopic (total) [TLH] 68.41 ◀
partial or subtotal (supracervical) (supravaginal) 68.39
radical (modified) (Wertheim's) 68.69 ⬅
laparoscopic (total) [TLRH] 68.61 ◀
supracervical 68.39
classic infrafasical SEMM hysterectomy [CISH] 68.31
laparoscopically assisted [LASH] 68.31
vaginal (complete) (partial) (subtotal) (total) 68.59
laparoscopically assisted (LAVH) 68.51

Hysterectomy *(Continued)*
vaginal *(Continued)*
radical (Schauta) 68.79
laparoscopic [LRVH] 68.71
Hysterocolpectomy (radical) (vaginal) 68.79
abdominal 68.69
laparoscopic 68.61
laparoscopic 68.71
Hysterogram NEC 87.85
percutaneous 87.84
Hysterolysis 54.59
laparoscopic 54.51
Hysteromyomectomy 68.29
Hysteropexy 69.22
Hysteroplasty 69.49
Hysterorrhaphy 69.41
Hysterosalpingography gas (contrast) 87.82
opaque dye (contrast) 87.83
Hysterosalpingostomy 66.74
Hysteroscopy 68.12
with
ablation
endometrial 68.23
biopsy 68.16
Hysterotomy (with removal of foreign body) (with removal of hydatidiform mole) 68.0
for intrauterine transfusion 75.2
obstetrical 74.99
for termination of pregnancy 74.91
Hysterotrachelectomy 67.4
Hysterotracheloplasty 69.49
Hysterotrachelorrhaphy 69.41
Hysterotrachelotomy 69.95

I

ICCE (intracapsular cataract extraction) 13.19
Ileal
bladder
closed 57.87 *[45.51]*
open (ileoureterostomy) 56.51
conduit (ileoureterostomy) 56.51
Ileocecostomy 45.93
Ileocolectomy 45.73
Ileocolostomy 45.93
Ileocolotomy 45.00
Ileocystoplasty (isolated segment anastomosis) (open loop) 57.87 [45.51]
Ileoduodenotomy 45.01
Ileoectomy (partial) 45.62
with cecectomy 45.72
Ileoentectropy 46.99
Ileoesophagostomy 42.54
Ileoileostomy 45.91
proximal to distal segment 45.62
Ileoloopogram 87.78
Ileopancreatostomy 52.96
Ileopexy 46.61
Ileoproctostomy 45.95
Ileorectostomy 45.93
Ileorrhaphy 46.73
Ileoscopy 45.13
through stoma (artificial) 45.12
transabdominal (operative) 45.11
Ileosigmoidostomy 45.93
Ileostomy 46.20
continent (permanent) 46.22
for urinary diversion 56.51
delayed opening 46.24
Ileostomy *(Continued)*
Hendon (temporary) 46.21
loop 46.01
Paul (temporary) 46.21
permanent 46.23
continent 46.22
repair 46.41
revision 46.41
tangential (temporary) 46.21
temporary 46.21
transplantation to new site 46.23
tube (temporary) 46.21
ureteral
external 56.51
internal 56.71
Ileotomy 45.02
Ileotransversostomy 45.93
Ileoureterostomy (Bricker's) (ileal bladder) 56.51
Imaging (diagnostic)
diagnostic, not elsewhere classified 88.90
endovascular ultrasound - *see* Imaging, intravascular ultrasound
intraoperative
iMRI - *see* Imaging, magnetic resonance
intravascular - *see* Imaging, intravascular ultrasound
intravascular ultrasound (IVUS) 00.29
aorta 00.22
aortic arch 00.22
carotid vessel 00.21
cerebral vessel, extracranial 00.21
coronary vessel 00.24
intrathoracic vessel 00.22
other specified vessel 00.28
peripheral vessel 00.23
renal vessel 00.25
vena cava (inferior) (superior) 00.22
magnetic resonance (nuclear) (proton) NEC 88.97
abdomen 88.97
bladder (urinary) 88.95
bone marrow blood supply 88.94
brain (brain stem) 88.91
intraoperative (iMRI) 88.96
real-time 88.96
chest (hilar) (mediastinal) 88.92
computer assisted surgery (CAS) with MR/MRA 00.32
extremity (lower) (upper) 88.94
eye orbit 88.97
face 88.97
head NEC 88.97
musculoskeletal 88.94
myocardium 88.92
neck 88.97
orbit of eye 88.97
prostate 88.95
specified site NEC 88.97
spinal canal (cord) (spine) 88.93
Immobilization (by)
with fracture-reduction - *see* Reduction, fracture
bandage 93.59
bone 93.53
cast NEC 93.53
with reduction of fracture or dislocation - *see* Reduction, fracture, *and* Reduction, dislocation
device NEC 93.59
pressure dressing 93.56
splint (plaster) (tray) 93.54
Immobilization *(Continued)*
splint *(Continued)*
with reduction of fracture or dislocation - *see* Reduction, fracture, *and* Reduction, dislocation
stereotactic head frame 93.59
strapping (non-traction) 93.59
Immunization - *see also* Vaccination
allergy 99.12
autoimmune disease 99.13
BCG 99.33
brucellosis 99.55
cholera 99.31
diphtheria 99.36
DPT 99.39
epidemic parotitis 99.46
German measles 99.47
Hemophilus influenzae 99.52
influenza 99.52
measles 99.45
meningococcus 99.55
mumps 99.46
pertussis 99.37
plague 99.34
poliomyelitis 99.41
rabies 99.44
rubella 99.47
salmonella 99.55
smallpox 99.42
staphylococcus 99.55
TAB 99.32
tetanus 99.38
triple vaccine 99.48
tuberculosis 99.33
tularemia 99.35
typhoid-paratyphoid 99.32
typhus 99.55
viral NEC 99.55
whooping cough 99.37
yellow fever 99.43
Immunoadsorption
extracorporeal (ECI) 99.76
Immunotherapy, antineoplastic 99.28
C-Parvum 99.28
Interferon 99.28
Interleukin-2 (low-dose) 99.28
high-dose 00.15
Levamisole 99.28
Proleukin (low-dose) 99.28
high-dose 00.15
Thymosin 99.28
Implant, implantation
abdominal artery to coronary artery 36.17
artery
aortic branches to heart muscle 36.2
mammary to ventricular wall (Vineberg) 36.2
baffle, atrial or interatrial 35.91
biliary fistulous tract into stomach or intestine 51.39
bipolar endoprosthesis (femoral head) 81.52
bladder sphincter, artificial (inflatable) 58.93
blood vessels to myocardium 36.2
bone growth stimulator (invasive) (percutaneous) (semi-invasive) - *see* category 78.9
bone morphogenetic protein (Infuse™ (OP-1™) (recombinant) (rhBMP) 84.52
bone void filler 84.55
that with kyphoplasty 81.66
that with vertebroplasty 81.65

ICD-9-CM
H, I
Vol. 3

◀ New ⇐ Revised

Implant, implantation *(Continued)*
breast (for augmentation) (bilateral) 85.54
unilateral 85.53
cardiac resynchronization device
defibrillator (biventricular) (BiV ICD) (BiV pacemaker with defibrillator) (BiV pacing with defibrillator) (CRT-D) (device and one or more leads) (total system) 00.51 ⟸ Revised
left ventricular coronary venous lead only 00.52
pulse generator only 00.54
pacemaker (BiV) (biventricular) (CRT-P) (device and one or more leads) (total system) 00.50 ⟸ Revised
left ventricular coronary venous lead only 00.52
pulse generator only 00.53
cardiac support device (CSD) 37.41
cardiomyostimulation system 37.67
cardioverter/defibrillator (automatic) 37.94
leads only (patch electrode) (pacing) (sensing) 37.95
pulse generator only 37.96
total system 37.94
chest wall (mesh) (silastic) 34.79
chin (polyethylene) (silastic) 76.68
cochlear (electrode) 20.96
prosthetic device (electrode and receiver) 20.96
channel (single) 20.97
multiple 20.98
electrode only 20.99
internal coil only 20.99
CorCap™ 37.41
cornea 11.73
CRT-D (biventricular defibrillator) (BiV ICD) (BiV pacemaker with defibrillator) (BiV pacing with defibrillator) (cardiac resynchronization defibrillator) (device and one or more leads) 00.51 ⟸ Revised
left ventricular coronary venous lead only 00.52
pulse generator only 00.54
CRT-P (biventricular pacemaker) (BiV pacemaker) (cardiac resynchronization pacemaker) (device and one or more leads) 00.50 ⟸ Revised
left ventricular coronary venous lead only 00.52
pulse generator only 00.53
custodis eye 14.41
dental (endosseous) (prosthetic) 23.6
device
adjustable gastric band and port 44.95
bronchial device NOS 33.79 ◀ New
bronchial substance NOS 33.79 ◀ New
bronchial valve 33.71 ◀ New
cardiac support device (CSD) 37.41
CorCap™ 37.41
epicardial support device 37.41
prosthetic cardiac support device 37.41
Lap-Band™ 44.95
left atrial appendage 37.90
left atrial filter 37.90
left atrial occluder 37.90
subcutaneous for intracardiac hemodynamic monitoring 00.57 ◀ New

Implant, implantation *(Continued)*
device *(Continued)*
vascular access 86.07
ventricular support device 37.41
diaphragmatic pacemaker 34.85
Dynesys® 84.59 ◀ New
electrode(s)
brain 02.93
depth 02.93
foramen ovale 02.93
sphenoidal 02.96
cardiac (initial) (transvenous) 37.70
atrium (initial) 37.73
replacement 37.76
atrium and ventricle (initial) 37.72
replacement 37.76
epicardium (sternotomy or thoracotomy approach) 37.74
left ventricular coronary venous system 00.52
temporary transvenous pacemaker system 37.78
during and immediately following cardiac surgery 39.64
ventricle (initial) 37.71
replacement 37.76
depth 02.93
foramen ovale 02.93
gastric 04.92 ◀ New
heart - *see also* Implant, electrode(s), cardiac 37.70
intracranial 02.93
osteogenic (invasive) for bone growth stimulation - *see* category 78.9
peripheral nerve 04.92
sacral nerve 04.92
sphenoidal 02.96
spine 03.93
electroencephalographic receiver
brain 02.93
intracranial 02.93
electronic stimulator
anus (subcutaneous) 49.92
bladder 57.96
bone growth (invasive) (percutaneous) (semi-invasive) 78.9
brain - *see* Implant, neurostimulator, brain
carotid sinus 39.8
cochlear 20.96
channel (single) 20.97
multiple 20.98
gastric 04.92 ◀ New
intracranial - *see* Implant, neurostimulator, intracranial
peripheral nerve - *see* Implant, neurostimulator, peripheral nerve
phrenic nerve 34.85
skeletal muscle 83.92
spine - *see* Implant, neurostimulator, spine
ureter 56.92
electrostimulator - *see* Implant, electronic stimulator, by site
endoprosthesis
bile duct 51.87
femoral head (bipolar) 81.52
pancreatic duct 52.93
endosseous (dental) 23.6
epidural pegs 02.93
epikeratoprosthesis 11.73
estradiol (pellet) 99.23
eye (Iowa type) 16.61
integrated 16.41

Implant, implantation *(Continued)*
facial bone, synthetic (alloplastic) 76.92
fallopian tube (Mulligan hood) (silastic tube) (stent) 66.93
into uterus 66.74
gastroepiploic artery to coronary artery 36.17
half-heart 37.62
hearing device, electromagnetic 20.95
heart
artificial 37.52
total replacement system 37.52
assist system NEC 37.62
external 37.65
extrinsic 37.68
implantable 37.66
non-implantable 37.62
percutaneous external 37.68
pVAD 37.68
auxiliary ventricle 37.62
cardiac support device (CSD) 37.41
circulatory assist system - *see* Implant, heart, assist system
CorCap™ 37.41
epicardial support device 37.41
pacemaker - *see also* Implant, pacemaker, cardiac 37.80
prosthetic cardiac support device 37.41
total replacement system 37.52
valve(s)
prosthesis or synthetic device (partial) (synthetic) (total) 35.20
aortic 35.22
mitral 35.24
pulmonary 35.26
tricuspid 35.28
tissue graft 35.20
aortic 35.21
mitral 35.23
pulmonary 35.25
tricuspid 35.27
ventricular support device 37.41
inert material
breast (for augmentation) (bilateral) 85.54
unilateral 85.53
larynx 31.0
nose 21.85
orbit (eye socket) 16.69
reinsertion 16.62
scleral shell (cup) (with evisceration of eyeball) 16.31
reinsertion 16.62
Tenon's capsule (with enucleation of eyeball) 16.42
with attachment of muscles 16.41
reinsertion 16.62
urethra 59.79
vocal cord(s) 31.0
infusion pump 86.06
interbody spinal fusion device 84.51
intracardiac hemodynamic monitor, subcutaneous 00.57 ◀ New
joint (prosthesis) (silastic) (Swanson type) NEC 81.96
ankle (total) 81.56
revision 81.59
carpocarpal, carpometacarpal 81.74
elbow (total) 81.84
revision 81.97
extremity (bioelectric) (cineplastic) (kineplastic) 84.40

◀ New ⟸ Revised

Implant, implantation *(Continued)*
joint NEC *(Continued)*
extremity *(Continued)*
lower 84.48
revision 81.59
upper 84.44
revision 81.97
femoral (bipolar endoprosthesis) 81.52
revision NOS 81.53
acetabular and femoral components (total) 00.70
acetabular component only 00.71
acetabular liner and/or femoral head only 00.73
femoral component only 00.72
femoral head only and/or acetabular liner 00.73
total (acetabular and femoral components) 00.70
finger 81.71
hand (metacarpophalangeal) (interphalangeal) 81.71
revision 81.97
hip (partial) 81.52
revision NOS 81.53
acetabular and femoral components (total) 00.70
acetabular component only 00.71
acetabular liner and/or femoral head only 00.73
femoral component only 00.72
femoral head only and/or acetabular liner 00.73
partial
acetabular component only 00.71
acetabular liner and/or femoral head only 00.73
femoral component only 00.72
femoral head only and/or acetabular liner 00.73
total (acetabular and femoral components) 00.70
total 81.51
total 81.51
revision (acetabular and femoral components) 00.70
interphalangeal 81.71
revision 81.97
knee (partial) (total) 81.54
revision NOS 81.55
femoral component 00.82
partial
femoral component 00.82
patellar component 00.83
tibial component 00.81
tibial insert 00.84
patellar component 00.83
tibial component 00.81
tibial insert 00.84
total (all components) 00.80
metacarpophalangeal 81.71
revision 81.97
shoulder (partial) 81.81
revision 81.97
total replacement 81.80
toe 81.57
for hallux valgus repair 77.59
revision 81.59
wrist (partial) 81.74
revision 81.97
total replacement 81.73
kidney, mechanical 55.97

Implant, implantation *(Continued)*
Lap-Band™ 44.95
larynx 31.0
leads (cardiac) - *see* Implant, electrode(s), cardiac
limb lengthening device, internal (NOS) 84.54
with kinetic distraction 84.53
mammary artery
in ventricle (Vineberg) 36.2
to coronary artery (single vessel) 36.15
double vessel 36.16
M-Brace™ 84.59 ◄
Mulligan hood, fallopian tube 66.93
nerve (peripheral) 04.79
neuropacemaker - *see* Implant, neurostimulator, by site
neurostimulator
electrodes
brain 02.93
gastric 04.92 ◄
intracranial 02.93
peripheral nerve 04.92
sacral nerve 04.92
spine 03.93
pulse generator 86.96
dual array 86.95
rechargeable 86.98
single array 86.94
rechargeable 86.97
nose 21.85
Ommaya reservoir 02.2
orbit 16.69
reinsertion 16.62
outflow tract prosthesis (heart) (gusset type)
in
pulmonary valvuloplasty 35.26
total repair of tetralogy of Fallot 35.81
ovary into uterine cavity 65.72
laparoscopic 65.75
pacemaker
brain - *see* Implant, neurostimulator, brain
cardiac (device) (initial) (permanent) (replacement) 37.80
dual-chamber device (initial) 37.83
replacement 37.87
resynchronization device (biventricular pacemaker) (BiV pacemaker) (CRT-P) ⇐
device only (initial) (replacement) 00.53
total system (device and one or more leads) 00.50
transvenous lead into left ventricular coronary venous system 00.52
single-chamber device (initial) 37.81
rate responsive 37.82
replacement 37.85
rate responsive 37.86
temporary transvenous pacemaker system 37.78
during and immediately following cardiac surgery 39.64
carotid sinus 39.8
diaphragm 34.85
gastric 04.92 ◄
intracranial - *see* Implant, neurostimulator, intracranial

Implant, implantation *(Continued)*
pacemaker *(Continued)*
neural - *see* Implant, neurostimulator, by site
peripheral nerve - *see* Implant, neurostimulator, peripheral nerve
spine - *see* Implant, neurostimulator, spine
pancreas (duct) 52.96
penis, prosthesis (internal)
inflatable 64.97
non-inflatable 64.95
port, vascular access device 86.07
premaxilla 76.68
progesterone (subdermal) 99.23
prosthesis, prosthetic device
acetabulum (Aufranc-Turner) 81.52
ankle (total) 81.56
arm (bioelectric) (cineplastic) (kineplastic) 84.44
breast (bilateral) (Cronin) (Dow-Corning) (Perras-Pappillon) 85.54
unilateral 85.53
cardiac support device (CSD) (CorCap™) 37.41
cochlear 20.96
channel (single) 20.97
multiple 20.98
extremity (bioelectric) (cineplastic) (kineplastic) 84.40
lower 84.48
upper 84.44
fallopian tube (Mulligan hood) (stent) 66.93
femoral head (Austin-Moore) (bipolar) (Eicher) (Thompson) 81.52
revision NOS 81.53
acetabular and femoral components (total) 00.70
acetabular component only 00.71
acetabular liner and/or femoral head only 00.73
femoral component only 00.72
femoral head only and/or acetabular liner 00.73
partial
acetabular component only 00.71
acetabular liner and/or femoral head only 00.73
femoral component only 00.72
femoral head only and/or acetabular liner 00.73
total (acetabular and femoral components) 00.70
joint (Swanson type) NEC 81.96
ankle (total) 81.56
carpocarpal, carpometacarpal 81.74
elbow (total) 81.84
finger 81.71
hand (metacarpophalangeal) (interphalangeal) 81.71
hip (partial) 81.52
revision NOS 81.53
acetabular and femoral components (total) 00.70
acetabular component only 00.71
acetabular liner and/or femoral head only 00.73
femoral component only 00.72

ICD-9-CM
I
Vol. 3

Implant, implantation *(Continued)*
prosthesis, prosthetic device *(Continued)*
joint NEC *(Continued)*
hip *(Continued)*
revision NOS *(Continued)*
femoral head only and/or acetabular liner 00.73
partial
acetabular component only 00.71
acetabular liner and/or femoral head only 00.73
femoral component only 00.72
femoral head only and/or acetabular liner 00.73
total (acetabular and femoral components) 00.70
total 81.51
revision (acetabular and femoral components) 00.70
interphalangeal 81.71
knee (partial) (total) 81.54
revision NOS 81.55
femoral component 00.82
partial
femoral component 00.82
patellar component 00.83
tibial component 00.81
tibial insert 00.84
patellar component 00.83
tibial component 00.81
tibial insert 00.84
total (all components) 00.80
metacarpophalangeal 81.71
shoulder (partial) 81.81
total 81.80
toe 81.57
for hallux valgus repair 77.59
wrist (partial) 81.74
total 81.73
leg (bioelectric) (cineplastic) (kineplastic) 84.48
lens 13.91 ◀
outflow tract (heart) (gusset type)
in
pulmonary valvuloplasty 35.26
total repair of tetralogy of Fallot 35.81
penis (internal) (non-inflatable) 64.95
inflatable (internal) 64.97
skin (dermal regenerative) (matrix) 86.67
testicular (bilateral) (unilateral) 62.7
pulsation balloon (phase-shift) 37.61
pump, infusion 86.06
radial artery 36.19
radioactive isotope 92.27
radium (radon) 92.27
retinal attachment 14.41
with buckling 14.41
Rickham reservoir 02.2
silicone
breast (bilateral) 85.54
unilateral 85.53
skin (for filling of defect) 86.02
for augmentation NEC 86.89
spine NEC 84.59
interspinous process decompression device 84.58
stimoceiver - *see* Implant, neurostimulator, by site

Implant, implantation *(Continued)*
sudural
grids 02.93
strips 02.93
Swanson prosthesis (joint) (silastic) NEC 81.96
carpocarpal, carpometacarpal 81.74
finger 81.71
hand (interphalangeal) (metacarpophalangeal) 81.71
interphalangeal 81.71
knee (partial) (total) 81.54
revision 81.55
metacarpophalangeal 81.71
toe 81.57
for hallux valgus repair 77.59
wrist (partial) 81.74
total 81.73
systemic arteries into myocardium (Vineberg type operation) 36.2
Tandem™ heart 37.68
telescope (IMT) (miniature) 13.91 ◀
testicular prosthesis (bilateral) (unilateral) 62.7
tissue expander (skin) NEC 86.93
breast 85.95
tissue mandril (for vascular graft) 39.99
with
blood vessel repair 39.56
vascular bypass or shunt - *see* Bypass, vascular
tooth (bud) (germ) 23.5
prosthetic 23.6
umbrella, vena cava 38.7
ureters into
bladder 56.74
intestine 56.71
external diversion 56.51
skin 56.61
urethra
for repair of urinary stress incontinence
collagen 59.72
fat 59.72
polytef 59.72
urethral sphincter, artificial (inflatable) 58.93
urinary sphincter, artificial (inflatable) 58.93
vascular access device 86.07
vitreous (silicone) 14.75
for retinal reattachment 14.41
with buckling 14.41
vocal cord(s) (paraglottic) 31.98
X Stop™ 84.58 ◀
Implosion (psychologic desensitization) 94.33
Incision (and drainage)
with
exploration - *see* Exploration
removal of foreign body - *see* Removal, foreign body
abdominal wall 54.0
as operative approach - *omit code*
abscess - *see also* Incision, by site
appendix 47.2
with appendectomy 47.09
laparoscopic 47.01
extraperitoneal 54.0
ischiorectal 49.01
lip 27.0
omental 54.19
perianal 49.01
perigastric 54.19

Incision *(Continued)*
abscess *(Continued)*
perisplenic 54.19
peritoneal NEC 54.19
pelvic (female) 70.12
retroperitoneal 54.0
sclera 12.89
skin 86.04
subcutaneous tissue 86.04
subdiaphragmatic 54.19
subhepatic 54.19
subphrenic 54.19
vas deferens 63.6
adrenal gland 07.41
alveolus, alveolar bone 24.0
antecubital fossa 86.09
anus NEC 49.93
fistula 49.11
septum 49.91
appendix 47.2
artery 38.00
abdominal 38.06
aorta (arch) (ascending) (descending) 38.04
head and neck NEC 38.02
intracranial NEC 38.01
lower limb 38.08
thoracic NEC 38.05
upper limb 38.03
atrium (heart) 37.11
auditory canal or meatus, external 18.02
auricle 18.09
axilla 86.09
Bartholin's gland or cyst 71.22
bile duct (with T or Y tube insertion) NEC 51.59
common (exploratory) 51.51
for
relief of obstruction NEC 51.42
removal of calculus 51.41
for
exploration 51.59
relief of obstruction 51.49
bladder 57.19
neck (transurethral) 57.91
percutaneous suprapubic (closed) 57.17
suprapubic NEC 57.18
blood vessel - *see also* Angiotomy 38.00
bone 77.10
alveolus, alveolar 24.0
carpals, metacarpals 77.14
clavicle 77.11
facial 76.09
femur 77.15
fibula 77.17
humerus 77.12
patella 77.16
pelvic 77.19
phalanges (foot) (hand) 77.19
radius 77.13
scapula 77.11
skull 01.24
specified site NEC 77.19
tarsals, metatarsals 77.18
thorax (ribs) (sternum) 77.11
tibia 77.17
ulna 77.13
vertebrae 77.19
brain 01.39
cortical adhesions 02.91
breast (skin) 85.0
with removal of tissue expander 85.96
bronchus 33.0

Incision *(Continued)*
  buccal space 27.0
  bulbourethral gland 58.91
  bursa 83.03
    hand 82.03
    pharynx 29.0
  carotid body 39.8
  cerebral (meninges) 01.39
    epidural or extradural space 01.24
    subarachnoid or subdural space 01.31
  cerebrum 01.39
  cervix 69.95
    to
      assist delivery 73.93
      replace inverted uterus 75.93
  chalazion 08.09
    with removal of capsule 08.21
  cheek 86.09
  chest wall (for extrapleural drainage) (for removal of foreign body) 34.01
    as operative approach - *omit code*
  common bile duct (for exploration) 51.51
    for
      relief of obstruction 51.42
      removal of calculus 51.41
  common wall between posterior left atrium and coronary sinus (with roofing of resultant defect with patch graft) 35.82
  conjunctiva 10.1
  cornea 11.1
    radial (refractive) 11.75
  cranial sinus 01.21
  craniobuccal pouch 07.72
  cul-de-sac 70.12
  cyst
    dentigerous 24.0
    radicular (apical) (periapical) 24.0
  Duhrssen's (cervix, to assist delivery) 73.93
  duodenum 45.01
  ear
    external 18.09
    inner 20.79
    middle 20.23
  endocardium 37.11
  endolymphatic sac 20.79
  epididymis 63.92
  epidural space, cerebral 01.24
  epigastric region 54.0
    intra-abdominal 54.19
  esophagus, esophageal NEC 42.09
    web 42.01
  exploratory - *see* Exploration
  extradural space (cerebral) 01.24
  extrapleural 34.01
  eyebrow 08.09
  eyelid 08.09
    margin (trichiasis) 08.01
  face 86.09
  fallopian tube 66.01
  fascia 83.09
    with division 83.14
      hand 82.12
    hand 82.09
      with division 82.12
  fascial compartments, head and neck 27.0
  fistula, anal 49.11
  flank 54.0
  furuncle - *see* Incision, by site
  gallbladder 51.04
  gingiva 24.0
  gluteal 86.09

Incision *(Continued)*
  groin region (abdominal wall) (inguinal) 54.0
    skin 86.09
    subcutaneous tissue 86.09
  gum 24.0
  hair follicles 86.09
  heart 37.10
    valve - *see* Valvulotomy
  hematoma - *see also* Incision, by site
    axilla 86.04
    broad ligament 69.98
    ear 18.09
    episiotomy site 75.91
    fossa (superficial) NEC 86.04
    groin region (abdominal wall) (inguinal) 54.0
      skin 86.04
      subcutaneous tissue 86.04
    laparotomy site 54.12
    mediastinum 34.1
    perineum (female) 71.09
      male 86.04
    popliteal space 86.04
    scrotum 61.0
    skin 86.04
    space of Retzius 59.19
    subcutaneous tissue 86.04
    vagina (cuff) 70.14
      episiotomy site 75.91
      obstetrical NEC 75.92
  hepatic ducts 51.59
  hordeolum 08.09
  hygroma - *see also* Incision, by site
    cystic 40.0
  hymen 70.11
  hypochondrium 54.0
    intra-abdominal 54.19
  hypophysis 07.72
  iliac fossa 54.0
  infratemporal fossa 27.0
  ingrown nail 86.09
  intestine 45.00
    large 45.03
    small 45.02
  intracerebral 01.39
  intracranial (epidural space) (extradural space) 01.24
    subarachnoid or subdural space 01.31
  intraperitoneal 54.19
  ischiorectal tissue 49.02
    abscess 49.01
  joint structures - *see also* Arthrotomy 80.10
  kidney 55.01
    pelvis 55.11
  labia 71.09
  lacrimal
    canaliculus 09.52
    gland 09.0
    passage NEC 09.59
    punctum 09.51
    sac 09.53
  larynx NEC 31.3
  ligamentum flavum (spine) - *omit code*
  liver 50.0
  lung 33.1
  lymphangioma 40.0
  lymphatic structure (channel) (node) (vessel) 40.0
  mastoid 20.21
  mediastinum 34.1
  meibomian gland 08.09

Incision *(Continued)*
  meninges (cerebral) 01.31
    spinal 03.09
  midpalmar space 82.04
  mouth NEC 27.92
    floor 27.0
  muscle 83.02
    with division 83.19
      hand 82.19
    hand 82.02
      with division 82.19
  myocardium 37.11
  nailbed or nailfold 86.09
  nasolacrimal duct (stricture) 09.59
  neck 86.09
  nerve (cranial) (peripheral) NEC 04.04
    root (spinal) 03.1
  nose 21.1
  omentum 54.19
  orbit - *see also* Orbitotomy 16.09
  ovary 65.09
    laparoscopic 65.01
  palate 27.1
  palmar space (middle) 82.04
  pancreas 52.09
  pancreatic sphincter 51.82
    endoscopic 51.85
  parapharyngeal (oral) (transcervical) 28.0
  paronychia 86.09
  parotid
    gland or duct 26.0
    space 27.0
  pelvirectal tissue 48.81
  penis 64.92
  perianal (skin) (tissue) 49.02
    abscess 49.01
  perigastric 54.19
  perineum (female) 71.09
    male 86.09
  peripheral vessels
    lower limb
      artery 38.08
      vein 38.09
    upper limb (artery) (vein) 38.03
  periprostatic tissue 60.81
  perirectal tissue 48.81
  perirenal tissue 59.09
  perisplenic 54.19
  peritoneum 54.95
    by laparotomy 54.19
    pelvic (female) 70.12
      male 54.19
  periureteral tissue 59.09
  periurethral tissue 58.91
  perivesical tissue 59.19
  petrous pyramid (air cells) (apex) (mastoid) 20.22
  pharynx, pharyngeal (bursa) 29.0
    space, lateral 27.0
  pilonidal sinus (cyst) 86.03
  pineal gland 07.52
  pituitary (gland) 07.72
  pleura NEC 34.09
  popliteal space 86.09
  postzygomatic space 27.0
  pouch of Douglas 70.12
  prostate (perineal approach) (transurethral approach) 60.0
  pterygopalatine fossa 27.0
  pulp canal (tooth) 24.0
  Rathke's pouch 07.72
  rectovaginal septum 48.81

Incision *(Continued)*
rectum 48.0
stricture 48.91
renal pelvis 55.11
retroperitoneum 54.0
retropharyngeal (oral) (transcervical) 28.0
salivary gland or duct 26.0
sclera 12.89
scrotum 61.0
sebaceous cyst 86.04
seminal vesicle 60.72
sinus - *see* Sinusotomy
Skene's duct or gland 71.09
skin 86.09
with drainage 86.04
breast 85.0
cardiac pacemaker pocket, new site 37.79
ear 18.09
nose 21.1
subcutaneous tunnel for pulse generator lead wire 86.99
with initial procedure - *omit code*
thalamic stimulator pulse generator pocket, new site 86.09
with initial insertion of battery package - *omit code*
tunnel, subcutaneous, for pulse generator lead wire 86.99
with initial procedure - *omit code*
skull (bone) 01.24
soft tissue NEC 83.09
with division 83.19
hand 82.19
hand 82.09
with division 82.19
space of Retzius 59.19
spermatic cord 63.93
sphincter of Oddi 51.82
endoscopic 51.85
spinal
cord 03.09
nerve root 03.1
spleen 41.2
stomach 43.0
stye 08.09
subarachnoid space, cerebral 01.31
subcutaneous tissue 86.09
with drainage 86.04
tunnel
esophageal 42.86
with anastomosis - *see* Anastomosis, esophagus, antesternal
pulse generator lead wire 86.99
with initial procedure - *omit code*
subdiaphragmatic space 54.19
subdural space, cerebral 01.31
sublingual space 27.0
submandibular space 27.0
submaxillary 86.09
with drainage 86.04
submental space 27.0
subphrenic space 54.19
supraclavicular fossa 86.09
with drainage 86.04
sweat glands, skin 86.04
temporal pouches 27.0
tendon (sheath) 83.01
with division 83.13
hand 82.11
hand 82.01
with division 82.11

Incision *(Continued)*
testis 62.0
thenar space 82.04
thymus 07.92
thyroid (field) (gland) NEC 06.09
postoperative 06.02
tongue NEC 25.94
for tongue tie 25.91
tonsil 28.0
trachea NEC 31.3
tunica vaginalis 61.0
umbilicus 54.0
urachal cyst 54.0
ureter 56.2
urethra 58.0
uterus (corpus) 68.0
cervix 69.95
for termination of pregnancy 74.91
septum (congenital) 68.22
uvula 27.71
vagina (cuff) (septum) (stenosis) 70.14
for
incisional hematoma (episiotomy) 75.91
obstetrical hematoma NEC 75.92
pelvic abscess 70.12
vas deferens 63.6
vein 38.00
abdominal 38.07
head and neck NEC 38.02
intracranial NEC 38.01
lower limb 38.09
thoracic NEC 38.05
upper limb 38.03
vertebral column 03.09
vulva 71.09
obstetrical 75.92
web, esophageal 42.01
Incudectomy NEC 19.3
with
stapedectomy - *see also* Stapedectomy 19.19
tympanoplasty - *see* Tympanoplasty
Incudopexy 19.19
Incudostapediopexy 19.19
with incus replacement 19.11
Indentation, sclera, for buckling - *see also* Buckling, scleral 14.49
Indicator dilution flow measurement 89.68
Induction
abortion
by
D and C 69.01
insertion of prostaglandin suppository 96.49
intra-amniotic injection (prostaglandin) (saline) 75.0
labor
medical 73.4
surgical 73.01
intra- and extra-amniotic injection 73.1
stripping of membranes 73.1
Inflation
belt wrap 93.99
Eustachian tube 20.8
fallopian tube 66.8
with injection of therapeutic agent 66.95
Infolding, sclera, for buckling - *see also* Buckling, scleral 14.49
Infraction, turbinates (nasal) 21.62

Infundibulectomy
hypophyseal - *see also* Hypophysectomy, partial 07.63
ventricle (heart) (right) 35.34
in total repair of tetralogy of Fallot 35.81
Infusion (intra-arterial) (intravenous)
Abciximab 99.20
antibiotic
oxazolidinone class 00.14
antineoplastic agent (chemotherapeutic) 99.25
biological response modifier [BRM] 99.28
cintredekin besudotox 99.28 ◀
high-dose interleukin-2 00.15
low-dose interleukin-2 99.28
biological response modifier [BRM], antineoplastic agent 99.28
cintredekin besudotox 99.28 ◀
high-dose interleukin-2 00.15
low-dose interleukin-2 99.28
cancer chemotherapy agent NEC 99.25
cintredekin besudotox 99.28 ◀
drotrecogin alfa (activated) 00.11
electrolytes 99.18
enzymes, thrombolytic (streptokinase) (tissue plasminogen activator) (TPA) (urokinase)
direct coronary artery 36.04
intravenous 99.10
Eptifibatide 99.20
GP IIB/IIIa inhibitor 99.20
hormone substance NEC 99.24
human B-type natriuretic peptide (hBNP) 00.13
immunosuppressive antibody therapy 00.18
nesiritide 00.13
neuroprotective agent 99.75
nimodipine 99.75
nutritional substance - *see* Nutrition
platelet inhibitor
direct coronary artery 36.04
intravenous 99.20
Proleukin (low-dose) 99.28
high-dose 00.15
prophylactic substance NEC 99.29
radioimmunoconjugate 92.28
radioimmunotherapy 92.28
radioisotope (liquid brachytherapy) (liquid I-125) 92.20
recombinant protein 00.11
reteplase 99.10
therapeutic substance NEC 99.29
thrombolytic agent (enzyme) (streptokinase) 99.10
with percutaneous transluminal angioplasty

Note: Also use 00.40, 00.41, 00.42, or 00.43 to show the total number of vessels treated.

coronary 00.66
non-coronary vessel(s) 39.50
specified site NEC 39.50
direct intracoronary artery 36.04
tirofiban (HCl) 99.20
vaccine
tumor 99.28
vasopressor 00.17

Injection (into) (hypodermically) (intramuscularly) (intravenously) (acting locally or systemically)
Actinomycin D, for cancer chemotherapy 99.25
adhesion barrier substance 99.77
alcohol
nerve - *see* Injection, nerve
spinal 03.8
anterior chamber, eye (air) (liquid) (medication) 12.92
antibiotic 99.21
oxazolidinone class 00.14
anticoagulant 99.19
anti-D (Rhesus) globulin 99.11
antidote NEC 99.16
anti-infective NEC 99.22
antineoplastic agent (chemotherapeutic) NEC 99.25
biological response modifier [BRM] 99.28
cintredekin besudotox 99.28 ◀
high-dose interleukin-2 00.15
low-dose interleukin-2 99.28
antivenin 99.16
barrier substance, adhesion 99.77
BCG
for chemotherapy 99.25
vaccine 99.33
biological response modifier [BRM], antineoplastic agent 99.28
cintredekin besudotox 99.28 ◀
high-dose interleukin-2 00.15
low-dose interleukin-2 99.28
bone marrow 41.92
transplant - *see* Transplant, bone, marrow
breast (therapeutic agent) 85.92
inert material (silicone) (bilateral) 85.52
unilateral 85.51
bursa (therapeutic agent) 83.96
hand 82.94
cancer chemotherapeutic agent 99.25
caudal - *see* Injection, spinal
cintredekin besudotox 99.28 ◀
cortisone 99.23
costochondral junction 81.92
dinoprost-tromethine, intra-amniotic 75.0
disc, intervertebral (herniated) 80.52
ear, with alcohol 20.72
electrolytes 99.18
enzymes, thrombolytic (streptokinase) (tissue plasminogen activator) (TPA) (urokinase)
direct coronary artery 36.04
intravenous 99.10
epidural, spinal - *see* Injection, spinal
esophageal varices or blood vessel (endoscopic) (sclerosing agent) 42.33
Eustachian tube (inert material) 20.8
eye (orbit) (retrobulbar) 16.91
anterior chamber 12.92
subconjunctival 10.91
fascia 83.98
hand 82.96
gamma globulin 99.14
ganglion, sympathetic 05.39
ciliary 12.79
paravertebral stellate 05.39
gel, adhesion barrier - *see* Injection, adhesion barrier substances

Injection *(Continued)*
globulin
anti-D (Rhesus) 99.11
gamma 99.14
Rh immune 99.11
heart 37.92
heavy metal antagonist 99.16
hemorrhoids (sclerosing agent) 49.42
hormone NEC 99.24
human B-type natriuretic peptide (hBNP) 00.13
immune sera 99.14
inert material - *see* Implant, inert material
inner ear, for destruction 20.72
insulin 99.17
intervertebral space for herniated disc 80.52
intra-amniotic
for induction of
abortion 75.0
labor 73.1
intrathecal - *see* Injection, spinal
joint (therapeutic agent) 81.92
temporomandibular 76.96
kidney (cyst) (therapeutic substance) NEC 55.96
larynx 31.0
ligament (joint) (therapeutic substance) 81.92
liver 50.94
lung, for surgical collapse 33.32
Methotrexate, for cancer chemotherapy 99.25
nerve (cranial) (peripheral) 04.80
agent NEC 04.89
alcohol 04.2
anesthetic for analgesia 04.81
for operative anesthesia - *omit code*
neurolytic 04.2
phenol 04.2
laryngeal (external) (recurrent) (superior) 31.91
optic 16.91
sympathetic 05.39
alcohol 05.32
anesthetic for analgesia 05.31
neurolytic agent 05.32
phenol 05.32
nesiritide 00.13
neuroprotective agent 99.75
nimodipine 99.75
orbit 16.91
pericardium 37.93
peritoneal cavity
air 54.96
locally-acting therapeutic substance 54.97
platelet inhibitor
direct coronary artery 36.04
intravenous 99.20
prophylactic substance NEC 99.29
prostate 60.92
radioimmunoconjugate 92.28
radioimmunotherapy 92.28
radioisotopes (intracavitary) (intravenous) 92.28
renal pelvis (cyst) 55.96
retrobulbar (therapeutic substance) 16.91
for anesthesia - *omit code*
Rh immune globulin 99.11
RhoGAM 99.11
sclerosing agent NEC 99.29

Injection *(Continued)*
sclerosing agent NEC *(Continued)*
esophageal varices (endoscopic) 42.33
hemorrhoids 49.42
pleura 34.92
treatment of malignancy (cytotoxic agent) 34.92 *[99.25]*
with tetracycline 34.92 *[99.21]*
varicose vein 39.92
vein NEC 39.92
semicircular canals, for destruction 20.72
silicone - *see* Implant, inert material
skin (sclerosing agent) (filling material) 86.02
soft tissue 83.98
hand 82.96
spinal (canal) NEC 03.92
alcohol 03.8
anesthetic agent for analgesia 03.91
for operative anesthesia - *omit code*
contrast material (for myelogram) 87.21
destructive agent NEC 03.8
neurolytic agent NEC 03.8
phenol 03.8
proteolytic enzyme (chymodiactin) (chymopapain) 80.52
saline (hypothermic) 03.92
steroid NEC 03.92
spinal nerve root (intrathecal) - *see* Injection, spinal
steroid NEC 99.23
subarachnoid, spinal - *see* Injection, spinal
subconjunctival 10.91
tendon 83.97
hand 82.95
testis 62.92
therapeutic agent NEC 99.29
thoracic cavity 34.92
thrombolytic agent (enzyme) (streptokinase) 99.10
with percutaneous transluminal angioplasty

Note: Also use 00.40, 00.41, 00.42, or 00.43 to show the total number of vessels treated.

coronary 00.66
non-coronary vessels 39.50
specified site NEC 39.50
direct intracoronary artery 36.04
trachea 31.94
tranquilizer 99.26
tunica vaginalis (with aspiration) 61.91
tympanum 20.94
urethra (inert material)
for repair of urinary stress incontinence
collagen implant 59.72
endoscopic injection of implant 59.72
fat implant 59.72
polytef implant 59.72
vaccine
tumor 99.28
varices, esophagus (endoscopic) (sclerosing agent) 42.33
varicose vein (sclerosing agent) 39.92
esophagus (endoscopic) 42.33
vestibule, for destruction 20.72

Injection *(Continued)*
vitreous substitute (silicone) 14.75
for reattachment of retina 14.59
vocal cords 31.0
Inlay, tooth 23.3
Inoculation
antitoxins - *see* Administration, antitoxins
toxoids - *see* Administration, toxoids
vaccine - *see* Administration, vaccine
Insemination, artificial 69.92
Insertion
airway
esophageal obturator 96.03
nasopharynx 96.01
oropharynx 96.02
Allen-Brown cannula 39.93
arch bars (orthodontic) 24.7
for immobilization (fracture) 93.55
atrial septal umbrella 35.52
Austin-Moore prosthesis 81.52
baffle, heart (atrial) (interatrial) (intra-atrial) 35.91
bag, cervix (nonobstetrical) 67.0
after delivery or abortion 75.8
to assist delivery or induce labor 73.1
Baker's (tube) (for stenting) 46.85
balloon
gastric 44.93
heart (pulsation-type) (Kantrowitz) 37.61
intestine (for decompression) (for dilation) 46.85
band (adjustable)
gastric, laparoscopic 44.95
Lap-Band™ 44.95
Barton's tongs (skull) (with synchronous skeletal traction) 02.94
bipolar endoprosthesis (femoral head) 81.52
Blakemore-Sengstaken tube 96.06
bone growth stimulator (invasive) (percutaneous) (semi-invasive) - *see* category 78.9
bone morphogenetic protein (Infuse™) (OP-1™) (recombinant) (rhBMP) 84.52
bone void filler 84.55
that with kyphoplasty 81.66
that with vertebroplasty 81.65
bougie, cervix, nonobstetrical 67.0
to assist delivery or induce labor 73.1
breast implant (for augmentation) (bilateral) 85.54
unilateral 85.53
bridge (dental) (fixed) 23.42
removable 23.43
bubble (balloon), stomach 44.93
caliper tongs (skull) (with synchronous skeletal traction) 02.94
cannula
Allen-Brown 39.93
for extracorporeal membrane oxygenation (ECMO) - *omit code*
nasal sinus (by puncture) 22.01
through natural ostium 22.02
pancreatic duct 52.92
endoscopic 52.93
vessel to vessel 39.93
cardiac resynchronization device
defibrillator (biventricular defibrillator) (BiV ICD) (BiV pacemaker with defibrillator) (BiV pacing with defibrillator) (CRT- D) (device and one or more leads) (total system) 00.51 ⇐

Insertion *(Continued)*
cardiac resynchronization device *(Continued)*
defibrillator *(Continued)*
left ventricular coronary venous lead only 00.52
pulse generator only 00.54
pacemaker (biventricular pacemaker) (BiV pacemaker) (CRT-P) (device and one or more leads) (total system) 00.50 ⇐
left ventricular coronary venous lead only 00.52
pulse generator only 00.53
cardiac support device (CSD) (CorCap™) 37.41
carotid artery stent(s) (stent graft) (00.63)

Note: Also use 00.40, 00.41, 00.42, or 00.43 to show the total number of vessels treated. Use code 00.44 once to show procedure on a bifurcated vessel. In addition, use 00.45, 00.46, 00.47, or 00.48 to show the number of vascular stents inserted. ⇐

catheter
abdomen of fetus, for intrauterine transfusion 75.2
anterior chamber (eye), for permanent drainage (glaucoma) 12.79
artery 38.91
bile duct(s) 51.59
common 51.51
endoscopic 51.87
endoscopic 51.87
bladder, indwelling 57.94
suprapubic 57.18
percutaneous (closed) 57.17
bronchus 96.05
with lavage 96.56
central venous NEC 38.93
for
hemodialysis 38.95
pressure monitoring 89.62
peripherally inserted central catheter (PICC) 38.93
chest 34.04
revision (with lysis of adhesions) 34.04
cranial cavity 01.26
placement via burr hole(s) 01.28 ◀
esophagus (nonoperative) 96.06
permanent tube 42.81
intercostal (with water seal), for drainage 34.04
revision (with lysis of adhesions) 34.04
intracerebral 01.26 ◀
placement via burr hole(s) 01.28 ◀
spinal canal space (epidural) (subarachnoid) (subdural) for infusion of therapeutic or palliative substances 03.90
Swan-Ganz (pulmonary) 89.64
transtracheal for oxygenation 31.99
vein NEC 38.93
for renal dialysis 38.95
chest tube 34.04
choledochohepatic tube (for decompression) 51.43
endoscopic 51.87

Insertion *(Continued)*
cochlear prosthetic device - *see* Implant, cochlear prosthetic device
contraceptive device (intrauterine) 69.7
CorCap™ 37.41
cordis cannula 54.98
coronary (artery)

Note: Also use 00.40, 00.41, 00.42, or 00.43 to show the total number of vessels treated. Use code 00.44 once to show procedure on a bifurcated vessel. In addition, use 00.45, 00.46, 00.47, or 00.48 to show the number of vascular stents inserted. ⇐

stent, drug-eluting 36.07
stent, non-drug-eluting 36.06
Crosby-Cooney button 54.98
CRT-D (biventricular defibrillator) (BiV ICD) (BiV pacemaker with defibrillator) (BiV pacing with defibrillator) (cardiac resynchronization defibrillator) (device and one or more leads) 00.51 ⇐
left ventricular coronary venous lead only 00.52
pulse generator only 00.54
CRT-P (biventricular pacemaker) (BiV pacemaker) (cardiac resynchronization pacemaker) (device and one or more leads) 00.50 ⇐
left ventricular coronary venous lead only 00.52
pulse generator only 00.53
Crutchfield tongs (skull) (with synchronous skeletal traction) 02.94
Davidson button 54.98
denture (total) 99.97
device
adjustable gastric band and port 44.95
bronchial device NOS 33.79 ◀
bronchial substance NOS 33.79 ◀
bronchial valve 33.71 ◀
cardiac resynchronization – *see* Insertion, cardiac resynchronization device ◀
cardiac support device (CSD) 37.41
CorCap™ 37.41
epicardial support device 37.41
Lap-Band™ 44.95
left atrial appendage 37.90
left atrial filter 37.90
left atrial occluder 37.90
prosthetic cardiac support device 37.41
vascular access 86.07
ventricular support device 37.41
diaphragm, vagina 96.17
drainage tube
kidney 55.02
pelvis 55.12
renal pelvis 55.12
Dynesys® 84.59 ◀
elbow prosthesis (total) 81.84
revision 81.97
electrode(s)
bone growth stimulator (invasive) (percutaneous) (semi-invasive) - *see* category 78.9
brain 02.93
depth 02.93
foramen ovale 02.93
sphenoidal 02.96
depth 02.93

◀ **New** ⇐ **Revised**

Insertion *(Continued)*
electrode(s) *(Continued)*
foramen ovale 02.93
sacral nerve 04.92
gastric 04.92 ◀
heart (initial) (transvenous) 37.70
atrium (initial) 37.73
replacement 37.76
atrium and ventricle (initial) 37.72
replacement 37.76
epicardium (sternotomy or thoracotomy approach) 37.74
left ventricular coronary venous system 00.52
temporary transvenous pacemaker system 37.78
during and immediately following cardiac surgery 39.64
ventricle (initial) 37.71
replacement 37.76
intracranial 02.93
osteogenic (for bone growth stimulation) - *see* category 78.9
peripheral nerve 04.92
sphenoidal 02.96
spine 03.93
electroencephalographic receiver - *see* Implant, electroencephalographic receiver, by site
electronic stimulator - *see* Implant, electronic stimulator, by site
electrostimulator - *see* Implant, electronic stimulator, by site
endograft(s), endovascular graft(s)
endovascular, abdominal aorta 39.71
endovascular, head and neck vessels 39.72
endovascular, other vessels (for aneurysm) 39.79
endovascular, thoracic aorta 39.73
endoprosthesis
bile duct 51.87
femoral head (bipolar) 81.52
pancreatic duct 52.93
epidural pegs 02.93
external fixation device (bone) - *see* category 78.1
facial bone implant (alloplastic) (synthetic) 76.92
filling material, skin (filling of defect) 86.02
filter
vena cava (inferior) (superior) (transvenous) 38.7
fixator, mini device (bone) - *see* category 78.1
frame (stereotactic)
for radiosurgery 93.59
Gardner Wells tongs (skull) (with synchronous skeletal traction) 02.94
gastric bubble (balloon) 44.93
globe, into eye socket 16.69
Greenfield filter 38.7
halo device (skull) (with synchronous skeletal traction) 02.94
Harrington rod - *see also* Fusion, spinal, by level
with dorsal, dorsolumbar fusion 81.05
Harris pin 79.15
heart
assist system - *see* Implant, heart assist system
cardiac support device (CSD) 37.41

Insertion *(Continued)*
heart *(Continued)*
circulatory assist system - *see* Implant, heart assist system
CorCap™ 37.41
epicardial support device 37.41
pacemaker - *see* Insertion, pacemaker, cardiac
prosthetic cardiac support device 37.41
pump (Kantrowitz) 37.62
valve - *see* Replacement, heart valve
ventricular support device 37.41
hip prosthesis (partial) 81.52
revision NOS 81.53
acetabular and femoral components (total) 00.70
acetabular component only 00.71
acetabular liner and/or femoral head only 00.73
femoral component only 00.72
femoral head only and/or acetabular liner 00.73
partial
acetabular component only 00.71
acetabular liner and/or femoral head only 00.73
femoral component only 00.72
femoral head only and/or acetabular liner 00.73
total (acetabular and femoral components) 00.70
total 81.51
revision
acetabular and femoral components (total) 00.70
total (acetabular and femoral components) 00.70
Holter valve 02.2
Hufnagel valve - *see* Replacement, heart valve
implant - *see* Insertion, prosthesis
infusion pump 86.06
interbody spinal fusion device 84.51
intercostal catheter (with water seal) for drainage 34.04
intra-arterial blood gas monitoring system 89.60
intrauterine
contraceptive device 69.7
radium (intracavitary) 69.91
tamponade (nonobstetric) 69.91
Kantrowitz
heart pump 37.62
pulsation balloon (phase-shift) 37.61
keratoprosthesis 11.73
King-Mills umbrella device (heart) 35.52
Kirschner wire 93.44
with reduction of fracture or dislocation - *see* Reduction, fracture *and* Reduction, dislocation
knee prosthesis (partial (total) 81.54
revision NOS 81.55
femoral component 00.82
partial
femoral component 00.82
patellar component 00.83
tibial component 00.81
tibial insert 00.84
patellar component 00.83
tibial component 00.81
tibial insert 00.84
total (all components) 00.80
laminaria, cervix 69.93

Insertion *(Continued)*
Lap-Band™ 44.95
larynx, valved tube 31.75
leads - *see* Insertion, electrode(s)
lens, prosthetic (intraocular) 13.70
with cataract extraction, one-stage 13.71
secondary (subsequent to cataract extraction) 13.72
limb lengthening device, internal, NOS 84.54
with kinetic distraction 84.53
loop recorder 37.79
metal staples into epiphyseal plate - *see also* Stapling, epiphyseal plate 78.20
minifixator device (bone) - *see* category 78.1
M-Brace™ 84.59 ◀
Mobitz-Uddin umbrella, vena cava 38.7
mold, vagina 96.15
Moore (cup) 81.52
myringotomy device (button) (tube) 20.01
with intubation 20.01
nasobiliary drainage tube (endoscopic) 51.86
nasogastric tube
for
decompression, intestinal 96.07
feeding 96.6
naso-intestinal tube 96.08
nasolacrimal tube or stent 09.44
nasopancreatic drainage tube (endoscopic) 52.97
neuropacemaker - *see* Implant, neurostimulator, by site
neurostimulator - *see* Implant, neurostimulator, by site
non-coronary vessel
stent(s) (stent graft)

Note: Also use 00.40, 00.41, 00.42, or 00.43 to show the total number of vessels treated. Use code 00.44 once to show procedure on a bifurcated vessel. In addition, use 00.45, 00.46, 00.47, or 00.48 to show the number of vascular stents inserted. ⬅

with angioplasty or atherectomy 39.50
with bypass - *omit code*
basilar 00.64
carotid 00.63
extracranial 00.64
intracranial 00.65
peripheral 39.90
bare, drug-coated 39.90
drug-eluting 00.55
vertebral 00.64
non-invasive (surface) (transcutaneous) stimulator 99.86
obturator (orthodontic) 24.7
ocular implant
with synchronous
enucleation 16.42
with muscle attachment to implant 16.41
evisceration 16.31
following or secondary to
enucleation 16.61
evisceration 16.61
Ommaya reservoir 02.2

ICD-9-CM
I
Vol. 3

Insertion *(Continued)*
orbital implant (stent) (outside muscle cone) 16.69
with orbitotomy 16.02
orthodontic appliance (obturator) (wiring) 24.7
outflow tract prosthesis (heart) (gusset type)
in
pulmonary valvuloplasty 35.26
total repair of tetralogy of Fallot 35.81
pacemaker
brain - *see* Implant, neurostimulator, brain
cardiac (device) (initial) (permanent) (replacement) 37.80
dual-chamber device (initial) 37.83
replacement 37.87
during and immediately following cardiac surgery 39.64
resynchronization (biventricular pacemaker) (BiV pacemaker) (CRT-P) (device)
device only (initial) (replacement) 00.53
total system (device and one or more leads) 00.50
transvenous lead into left ventricular coronary venous system 00.52
single-chamber device (initial) 37.81
rate responsive 37.82
replacement 37.85
rate responsive 37.86
temporary transvenous pacemaker system 37.78
during and immediately following cardiac surgery 39.64
carotid 39.8
gastric 04.92
heart - *see* Insertion, pacemaker, cardiac
intracranial - *see* Implant, neurostimulator, intracranial
neural - *see* Implant, neurostimulator, by site
peripheral nerve - *see* Implant, neurostimulator, peripheral nerve
spine - *see* Implant, neurostimulator, spine
pacing catheter - *see* Insertion, pacemaker, cardiac
pack
auditory canal, external 96.11
cervix (nonobstetrical) 67.0
after delivery or abortion 75.8
to assist delivery or induce labor 73.1
rectum 96.19
sella turcica 07.79
vagina (nonobstetrical) 96.14
after delivery or abortion 75.8
palatal implant 27.64
penile prosthesis (internal) (non-inflatable) 64.95
inflatable (internal) 64.97
periodontal splint (orthodontic) 24.7
peripheral blood vessel - *see* non-coronary
pessary
cervix 96.18

Insertion *(Continued)*
pessary *(Continued)*
cervix *(Continued)*
to assist delivery or induce labor 73.1
vagina 96.18
pharyngeal valve, artificial 31.75
port, vascular access 86.07
prostaglandin suppository (for abortion) 96.49
prosthesis, prosthetic device
acetabulum (partial) 81.52
hip 81.52
revision NOS 81.53
acetabular and femoral components (total) 00.70
acetabular component only 00.71
acetabular liner and/or femoral head only 00.73
femoral component only 00.72
femoral head only and/or acetabular liner 00.73
partial
acetabular component only 00.71
acetabular liner and/or femoral head only 00.73
femoral component only 00.72
femoral head only and/or acetabular liner 00.73
total (acetabular and femoral components) 00.70
revision 81.53
ankle (total) 81.56
arm (bioelectric) (cineplastic) (kineplastic) 84.44
biliary tract 51.99
breast (bilateral) 85.54
unilateral 85.53
cardiac support device (CSD) (CorCap™) 37.41
chin (polyethylene) (silastic) 76.68
elbow (total) 81.84
revision 81.97
extremity (bioelectric) (cineplastic) (kineplastic) 84.40
lower 84.48
upper 84.44
fallopian tube 66.93
femoral head (Austin-Moore) (bipolar) (Eicher) (Thompson) 81.52
hip (partial) 81.52
revision NOS 81.53
acetabular and femoral components (total) 00.70
acetabular component only 00.71
acetabular liner and/or femoral head only 00.73
femoral component only 00.72
femoral head only and/or acetabular liner 00.73
partial
acetabular component only 00.71
acetabular liner and/or femoral head only 00.73
femoral component only 00.72
femoral head only and/or acetabular liner 00.73
total (acetabular and femoral components) 00.70
total 81.51

Insertion *(Continued)*
prosthesis, prosthetic device *(Continued)*
hip *(Continued)*
total *(Continued)*
revision
acetabular and femoral components (total) 00.70
total (acetabular and femoral components) 00.70
joint - *see* Arthroplasty
knee (partial) (total) 81.54
revision NOS 81.55
femoral component 00.82
partial
femoral component 00.82
patellar component 00.83
tibial component 00.81
tibial insert 00.84
patellar component 00.83
tibial component 00.81
tibial insert 00.84
total (all components) 00.80
leg (bioelectric) (cineplastic) (kineplastic) 84.48
lens 13.91
ocular (secondary) 16.61
with orbital exenteration 16.42
outflow tract (heart) (gusset type)
in
pulmonary valvuloplasty 35.26
total repair of tetralogy of Fallot 35.81
penis (internal) (noninflatable) 64.95
with
construction 64.43
reconstruction 64.44
inflatable (internal) 64.97
Rosen (for urinary incontinence) 59.79
shoulder
partial 81.81
revision 81.97
total 81.80
spine
artificial, NOS 84.60
cervical 84.62
nucleus 84.61
partial 84.61
total 84.62
lumbar, lumbosacral 84.65
nucleus 84.64
partial 84.64
total 84.65
thoracic (partial) (total) 84.63
other device 84.59
testicular (bilateral) (unilateral) 62.7
toe 81.57
hallux valgus repair 77.59
pseudophakos - *see also* Insertion, lens 13.70
pump, infusion 86.06
radioactive isotope 92.27
radium 92.27
radon seeds 92.27
Reuter bobbin (with intubation) 20.01
Rickham reservoir 02.2
Rosen prosthesis (for urinary incontinence) 59.79
Scribner shunt 39.93
Sengstaken-Blakemore tube 96.06
sensor (lead)
intra-arterial, for continuous blood gas monitoring 89.60
intracardiac hemodynamic monitoring 00.56

Insertion *(Continued)*
sieve, vena cava 38.7
skeletal muscle stimulator 83.92
skull
plate 02.05
stereotactic frame 93.59
tongs (Barton) (caliper) (Gardner Wells) (Vinke) (with synchronous skeletal traction) 02.94
spacer (cement) (joint) 84.56
spine 84.51
sphenoidal electrodes 02.96
spine
bone void filler
that with kyphoplasty 81.66
that with vertebroplasty 81.65
cage (BAK) 84.51
interbody spinal fusion device 84.51
interspinous process decompression device 84.58
non-fusion stabilization device 84.59 ◀
spacer 84.51
Spitz-Holter valve 02.2
Steinmann pin 93.44
with reduction of fracture or dislocation - *see* Reduction, fracture *and* Reduction, dislocation
stent(s) (stent graft)
artery (bare) (bonded) (drug coated) (non-drug-eluting)

Note: Also use 00.40, 00.41, 00.42, or 00.43 to show the total number of vessels treated. Use code 00.44 once to show procedure on a bifurcated vessel. In addition, use 00.45, 00.46, 00.47, or 00.48 to show the number of vascular stents inserted.

basilar 00.64
carotid 00.63
cerebrovascular
cerebral (intracranial) 00.65
precerebral (extracranial) 00.64
carotid 00.63
coronary (bare) (bonded) (drug coated) (non-drug-eluting) 36.06
extracranial 00.64
carotid 00.63
intracranial 00.65
non-coronary vessel
basilar 00.64
carotid 00.63
extracranial 00.64
intracranial 00.65
peripheral 39.90
bare, drug-coated 39.90
drug-eluting 00.55
vertebral 00.64
bile duct 51.43
endoscopic 51.87
percutaneous transhepatic 51.98
coronary (artery) (bare) (bonded) (drug-coated) (non-drug-eluting) 36.06

Note: Also use 00.40, 00.41, 00.42, or 00.43 to show the total number of vessels treated. Use code 00.44 once to show procedure on a bifurcated vessel. In addition, use 00.45, 00.46, 00.47, or 00.48 to show the number of vascular stents inserted.

Insertion *(Continued)*
stent(s) *(Continued)*
coronary *(Continued)*
drug-eluting 36.07
esophagus (endoscopic) (fluoroscopic) 42.81
mesenteric 39.90 ◀
bare, drug-coated 39.90 ◀
drug-eluting 00.55 ◀
non-coronary vessel

Note: Also use 00.40, 00.41, 00.42, or 00.43 to show the total number of vessels treated. Use code 00.44 once to show procedure on a bifurcated vessel. In addition, use 00.45, 00.46, 00.47, or 00.48 to show the number of vascular stents inserted.

with angioplasty or atherectomy 39.50
with bypass - *omit code*
basilar 00.64
carotid 00.63
extracranial 00.64
intracranial 00.65
mesenteric 39.90 ◀
bare, drug-coated 39.90 ◀
drug-eluting 00.55 ◀
peripheral 39.90
bare, drug-coated 39.90
drug-eluting 00.55
renal 39.90 ◀
bare, drug-coated 39.90 ◀
drug-eluting 00.55 ◀
vertebral 00.64
pancreatic duct 52.92
endoscopic 52.93
peripheral 39.90

Note: Also use 00.40, 00.41, 00.42, or 00.43 to show the total number of vessels treated. Use code 00.44 once to show procedure on a bifurcated vessel. In addition, use 00.45, 00.46, 00.47, or 00.48 to show the number of vascular stents inserted.

bare, drug-coated 39.90
drug-eluting 00.55
precerebral 00.64

Note: Also use 00.40, 00.41, 00.42 or 00.43 to show the total number of vessels treated. Use code 00.44 once to show procedure on a bifurcated vessel. In addition, use 00.45, 00.46, 00.47, or 00.48 to show the number of vascular stents inserted.

renal 39.90 ◀
bare, drug-coated 39.90 ◀
drug-eluting 00.55 ◀
subclavian 39.90

Note: Also use 00.40, 00.41, 00.42, or 00.43 to show the total number of vessels treated. Use code 00.44 once to show procedure on a bifurcated vessel. In addition, use 00.45, 00.46, 00.47, or 00.48 to show the number of vascular stents inserted.

bare, drug-coated 39.90
drug-eluting 00.55

Insertion *(Continued)*
stent(s) *(Continued)*
tracheobronchial 96.05
vertebral 00.64

Note: Also use 00.40, 00.41, 00.42, or 00.43 to show the total number of vessels treated. Use code 00.44 once to show procedure on a bifurcated vessel. In addition, use 00.45, 00.46, 00.47, or 00.48 to show the number of vascular stents inserted.

stimoceiver - *see* Implant, neurostimulator, by site
stimulator for bone growth - *see* category 78.9
subdural
grids 02.93
strips 02.93
suppository
prostaglandin (for abortion) 96.49
vagina 96.49
Swan-Ganz catheter (pulmonary) 89.64
tampon
esophagus 96.06
uterus 69.91
vagina 96.14
after delivery or abortion 75.8
Tandem™ heart 37.68
telescope (IMT) (miniature) 13.91 ◀
testicular prosthesis (bilateral) (unilateral) 62.7
tissue expander (skin) NEC 86.93
breast 85.95
tissue mandril (peripheral vessel) (Dacron) (Spark's type) 39.99
with
blood vessel repair 39.56
vascular bypass or shunt - *see* Bypass, vascular
tongs, skull (with synchronous skeletal traction) 02.94
totally implanted device for bone growth (invasive) - *see* category 78.9
tube - *see also* Catheterization and Intubation
bile duct 51.43
endoscopic 51.87
chest 34.04
revision (with lysis of adhesions) 34.04
endotracheal 96.04
esophagus (nonoperative) (Sengstaken) 96.06
permanent (silicone) (Souttar) 42.81
feeding
esophageal 42.81
gastric 96.6
nasogastric 96.6
gastric
by gastrostomy - *see* category 43.1
for
decompression, intestinal 96.07
feeding 96.6
intercostal (with water seal), for drainage 34.04
revision (with lysis of adhesions) 34.04
Miller-Abbott (for intestinal decompression) 96.08
nasobiliary (drainage) 51.86

Insertion *(Continued)*
tube *(Continued)*
nasogastric (for intestinal decompression) NEC 96.07
naso-intestinal 96.08
nasopancreatic drainage (endoscopic) 52.97
pancreatic duct 52.92
endoscopic 52.93
rectum 96.09
stomach (nasogastric) (for intestinal decompression) NEC 96.07
for feeding 96.6
tracheobronchial 96.05
umbrella device
atrial septum (King-Mills) 35.52
vena cava (Mobitz-Uddin) 38.7
ureteral stent (transurethral) 59.8
with ureterotomy 59.8 *[56.2]*
urinary sphincter, artificial (AUS) (inflatable) 58.93
vaginal mold 96.15
valve
bronchus 33.71 ◀
Holter 02.2
Hufnagel - *see* Replacement, heart valve
pharyngeal (artificial) 31.75
Spitz-Holter 02.2
vas deferens 63.95
vascular access device, totally implantable 86.07
vena cava sieve or umbrella 38.7
Vinke tongs (skull) (with synchronous skeletal traction) 02.94
X Stop™ 84.58 ◀

Instillation
bladder 96.49
digestive tract, except gastric gavage 96.43
genitourinary NEC 96.49
radioisotope (intracavitary) (intravenous) 92.28
thoracic cavity 34.92 ◀

Insufflation
Eustachian tube 20.8
fallopian tube (air) (dye) (gas) (saline) 66.8
for radiography - *see* Hysterosalpingography
therapeutic substance 66.95
lumbar retroperitoneal, bilateral 88.15

Intercricothyroidotomy (for assistance in breathing) 31.1

Intermittent positive pressure breathing (IPPB) 93.91

Interposition operation
esophageal reconstruction (intrathoracic) (retrosternal) NEC - *see also* Anastomosis, esophagus, with, interposition 42.58
antesternal or antethoracic NEC - *see also* Anastomosis, esophagus, antesternal, with, interposition 42.68
uterine suspension 69.21

Interrogation
cardioverter-defibrillator, automatic (AICD)
with catheter based invasive electrophysiologic testing 37.26 ◀
with NIPS (arrhythmia induction) 37.20 ⬅
interrogation only (bedside device check) 89.49

Interrogation *(Continued)*
CRT-D (cardiac resynchronization defibrillator)
with catheter based invasive electrophysiologic testing 37.26 ◀
with NIPS (arrhythmia induction) 37.20 ⬅
interrogation only (bedside device check) 89.49
CRT-P (cardiac resynchronization pacemaker)
with catheter based invasive electrophysiologic testing 37.26 ◀
with NIPS (arrhythmia induction) 37.20 ⬅
interrogation only (bedside device check) 89.45
pacemaker
with catheter based invasive electrophysiologic testing 37.26 ◀
with NIPS (arrhythmia induction) 37.20 ⬅
interrogation only (bedside device check) 89.45

Interruption
vena cava (inferior) (superior) 38.7

Interview (evaluation) (diagnostic)
medical, except psychiatric 89.05
brief (abbreviated history) 89.01
comprehensive (history and evaluation of new problem) 89.03
limited (interval history) 89.02
specified type NEC 89.04
psychiatric NEC 94.19
follow-up 94.19
initial 94.19
pre-commitment 94.13

Intimectomy 38.10
abdominal 38.16
aorta (arch) (ascending) (descending) 38.14
head and neck NEC 38.12
intracranial NEC 38.11
lower limb 38.18
thoracic NEC 38.15
upper limb 38.13

Introduction
orthodontic appliance 24.7
therapeutic substance (acting locally or systemically) NEC 99.29
bursa 83.96
hand 82.94
fascia 83.98
hand 82.96
heart 37.92
joint 81.92
temporomandibular 76.96
ligament (joint) 81.92
pericardium 37.93
soft tissue NEC 83.98
hand 82.96
tendon 83.97
hand 82.95
vein 39.92

Intubation - *see also* Catheterization and Insertion
bile duct(s) 51.59
common 51.51
endoscopic 51.87
endoscopic 51.87
esophagus (nonoperative) (Sengstaken) 96.06
permanent tube (silicone) (Souttar) 42.81

Intubation *(Continued)*
Eustachian tube 20.8
intestine (for decompression) 96.08
lacrimal for
dilation 09.42
tear drainage, intranasal 09.81
larynx 96.05
nasobiliary (drainage) 51.86
nasogastric
for
decompression, intestinal 96.07
feeding 96.6
naso-intestinal 96.08
nasolacrimal (duct) (with irrigation) 09.44
nasopancreatic drainage (endoscopic) 52.97
respiratory tract NEC 96.05
small intestine (Miller-Abbott) 96.08
stomach (nasogastric) (for intestinal decompression) NEC 96.07
for feeding 96.6
trachea 96.04
ventriculocisternal 02.2

Invagination, diverticulum
gastric 44.69
laparoscopic 44.68
pharynx 29.59
stomach 44.69
laparoscopic 44.68

Inversion
appendix 47.99
diverticulum
gastric 44.69
laparoscopic 44.68
intestine
large 45.49
endoscopic 45.43
small 45.34
stomach 44.69
laparoscopic 44.68
tunica vaginalis 61.49

Ionization, medical 99.27
Iontherapy 99.27
Iontophoresis 99.27
Iridectomy (basal) (buttonhole) (optical) (peripheral) (total) 12.14
with
capsulectomy 13.65
cataract extraction - *see* Extraction, cataract
filtering operation (for glaucoma) NEC 12.65
scleral
fistulization 12.65
thermocauterization 12.62
trephination 12.61

Iridencleisis 12.63
Iridesis 12.63
Irido-capsulectomy 13.65
Iridocyclectomy 12.44
Iridocystectomy 12.42
Iridodesis 12.63
Iridoplasty NEC 12.39
Iridosclerectomy 12.65
Iridosclerotomy 12.69
Iridotasis 12.63
Iridotomy 12.12
by photocoagulation 12.12
with transfixion 12.11
for iris bombé 12.11
specified type NEC 12.12

Iron lung 93.99

Irradiation
gamma, stereotactic 92.32
Irrigation
anterior chamber (eye) 12.91
bronchus NEC 96.56
canaliculus 09.42
catheter
ureter 96.46
urinary, indwelling NEC 96.48
vascular 96.57
ventricular 02.41
wound 96.58
cholecystostomy 96.41
cornea 96.51
with removal of foreign body 98.21
corpus cavernosum 64.98
cystostomy 96.47
ear (removal of cerumen) 96.52
enterostomy 96.36
eye 96.51
with removal of foreign body 98.21
gastrostomy 96.36
lacrimal
canaliculi 09.42
punctum 09.41
muscle 83.02
hand 82.02
nasal
passages 96.53
sinus 22.00
nasolacrimal duct 09.43
with insertion of tube or stent 09.44
nephrostomy 96.45
peritoneal 54.25
pyelostomy 96.45
rectal 96.39
stomach 96.33
tendon (sheath) 83.01
hand 82.01
trachea NEC 96.56
traumatic cataract 13.3
tube
biliary NEC 96.41
nasogastric NEC 96.34
pancreatic 96.42
ureterostomy 96.46
ventricular shunt 02.41
wound (cleaning) NEC 96.59
Irving operation (tubal ligation) 66.32
Irwin operation - *see also* Osteotomy 77.30
Ischiectomy (partial) 77.89
total 77.99
Ischiopubiotomy 77.39
Isolation
after contact with infectious disease 99.84
ileal loop 45.51
intestinal segment or pedicle flap
large 45.52
small 45.51
Isthmectomy, thyroid - *see also* Thyroidectomy, partial 06.39

J

Jaboulay operation (gastroduodenostomy) 44.39
laparoscopic 44.38
Janeway operation (permanent gastrostomy) 43.19
Jatene operation (arterial switch) 35.84
Jejunectomy 45.62
Jejunocecostomy 45.93
Jejunocholecystostomy 51.32
Jejunocolostomy 45.93
Jejunoileostomy 45.91
Jejunojejunostomy 45.91
Jejunopexy 46.61
Jejunorrhaphy 46.73
Jejunostomy (feeding) 46.39
delayed opening 46.31
loop 46.01
percutaneous (endoscopic) (PEJ) 46.32
revision 46.41
Jejunotomy 45.02
Johanson operation (urethral reconstruction) 58.46
Jones operation
claw toe (transfer of extensor hallucis longus tendon) 77.57
modified (with arthrodesis) 77.57
dacryocystorhinostomy 09.81
hammer toe (interphalangeal fusion) 77.56
modified (tendon transfer with arthrodesis) 77.57
repair of peroneal tendon 83.88
Joplin operation (exostectomy with tendon transfer) 77.53

K

Kader operation (temporary gastrostomy) 43.19
Kasai portoenterostomy 51.37
Kaufman operation (for urinary stress incontinence) 59.79
Kazanjian operation (buccal vestibular sulcus extension) 24.91
Kehr operation (hepatopexy) 50.69
Keller operation (bunionectomy) 77.59
Kelly (-Kennedy) operation (urethrovesical plication) 59.3
Kelly-Stoeckel operation (urethrovesical plication) 59.3
Kelotomy 53.9
Keratectomy (complete) (partial) (superficial) 11.49
for pterygium 11.39
with corneal graft 11.32
Keratocentesis (for hyphema) 12.91
Keratomileusis 11.71
Keratophakia 11.72
Keratoplasty (tectonic) (with autograft) (with homograft) 11.60
lamellar (nonpenetrating) (with homograft) 11.62
with autograft 11.61
penetrating (full-thickness) (with homograft) 11.64
with autograft 11.63
perforating - *see* Keratoplasty, penetrating
refractive 11.71
specified type NEC 11.69
Keratoprosthesis 11.73
Keratotomy (delimiting) (posterior) 11.1
radial (refractive) 11.75
Kerr operation (low cervical cesarean section) 74.1
Kessler operation (arthroplasty, carpometacarpal joint) 81.74
Kidner operation (excision of accessory navicular bone) (with tendon transfer) 77.98
Killian operation (frontal sinusotomy) 22.41
Kineplasty - *see* Cineplasty
King-Steelquist operation (hindquarter amputation) 84.19
Kirk operation (amputation through thigh) 84.17
Kock pouch
bowel anastomosis - *omit code*
continent ileostomy 46.22
cutaneous uretero-ileostomy 56.51
ESWL (electrocorporeal shock wave lithotripsy) 98.51
Kock pouch *(Continued)*
removal, calculus 57.19
revision, cutaneous uretero-ileostomy 56.52
urinary diversion procedure 56.51
Kockogram (ileal conduitogram) 87.78
Kockoscopy 45.12
Kondoleon operation (correction of lymphedema) 40.9
Krause operation (sympathetic denervation) 05.29
Kroener operation (partial salpingectomy) 66.69
Kroenlein operation (lateral orbitotomy) 16.01
Krönig operation (low cervical cesarean section) 74.1
Krunkenberg operation (reconstruction of below-elbow amputation) 82.89
Kuhnt-Szymanowski operation (ectropion repair with lid reconstruction) 08.44
Kyphoplasty 81.66

L

Labbe operation (gastrotomy) 43.0
Labiectomy (bilateral) 71.62
unilateral 71.61
Labyrinthectomy (transtympanic) 20.79
Labyrinthotomy (transtympanic) 20.79
Ladd operation (mobilization of intestine) 54.95
Lagrange operation (iridosclerectomy) 12.65
Lambrinudi operation (triple arthrodesis) 81.12
Laminectomy (decompression) (for exploration) 03.09
as operative approach - *omit code*
with
excision of herniated intervertebral disc (nucleus pulposus) 80.51
excision of other intraspinal lesion (tumor) 03.4
reopening of site 03.02
Laminography - *see* Radiography
Laminoplasty, expansile 03.09
Laminotomy (decompression) (for exploration) 03.09
as operative approach - *omit code*
reopening of site 03.02
Langenbeck operation (cleft palate repair) 27.62
Laparoamnioscopy 75.31
Laparorrhaphy 54.63
Laparoscopy 54.21
with
biopsy (intra-abdominal) 54.24
uterine ligaments 68.15
uterus 68.16
destruction of fallopian tubes - *see* Destruction, fallopian tube
Laparotomy NEC 54.19
as operative approach - *omit code*
exploratory (pelvic) 54.11
reopening of recent operative site (for control of hemorrhage) (for exploration) (for incision of hematoma) 54.12
Laparotrachelotomy 74.1
Lapidus operation (bunionectomy with metatarsal osteotomy) 77.51
Larry operation (shoulder disarticulation) 84.08
Laryngectomy
with radical neck dissection (with synchronous thyroidectomy) (with synchronous tracheostomy) 30.4
complete (with partial laryngectomy) (with synchronous tracheostomy) 30.3
with radical neck dissection (with synchronous thyroidectomy) (with synchronous tracheostomy) 30.4
frontolateral partial (extended) 30.29
glottosupraglottic partial 30.29
lateral partial 30.29
partial (frontolateral) (glottosupraglottic) (lateral) (submucous) (supraglottic) (vertical) 30.29
radical (with synchronous thyroidectomy) (with synchronous tracheostomy) 30.4
submucous (partial) 30.29
supraglottic partial 30.29
Laryngectomy *(Continued)*
total (with partial pharyngectomy) (with synchronous tracheostomy) 30.3
with radical neck dissection (with synchronous thyroidectomy) (with synchronous tracheostomy) 30.4
vertical partial 30.29
wide field 30.3
Laryngocentesis 31.3
Laryngoesophagectomy 30.4
Laryngofissure 30.29
Laryngogram 87.09
contrast 87.07
Laryngopharyngectomy (with synchronous tracheostomy) 30.3
radical (with synchronous thyroidectomy) 30.4
Laryngopharyngoesophagectomy (with synchronous tracheostomy) 30.3
with radical neck dissection (with synchronous thyroidectomy) 30.4
Laryngoplasty 31.69
Laryngorrhaphy 31.61
Laryngoscopy (suspension) (through artificial stoma) 31.42
Laryngostomy (permanent) 31.29
revision 31.63
temporary (emergency) 31.1
Laryngotomy 31.3
Laryngotracheobronchoscopy 33.23
with biopsy 33.24
Laryngotracheoscopy 31.42
Laryngotracheostomy (permanent) 31.29
temporary (emergency) 31.1
Laryngotracheotomy (temporary) 31.1
permanent 31.29
Laser - *see also* Coagulation, Destruction, *and* Photocoagulation, by site
angioplasty, percutaneous transluminal 39.59
coronary - *see* Angioplasty, coronary
Lash operation
internal cervical os repair 67.59
laparoscopic supracervical hysterectomy 68.31
LASIK (Laser-assisted in situ keratomileusis) 11.71
Latzko operation
cesarean section 74.2
colpocleisis 70.8
Lavage
antral 22.00
bronchus NEC 96.56
diagnostic (endoscopic) bronchoalveolar lavage (BAL) 33.24
endotracheal 96.56
gastric 96.33
lung (total) (whole) 33.99
diagnostic (endoscopic) bronchoalveolar lavage (BAL) 33.24
nasal sinus(es) 22.00
by puncture 22.01
through natural ostium 22.02
peritoneal (diagnostic) 54.25
trachea NEC 96.56
Leadbetter operation (urethral reconstruction) 58.46
Leadbetter-Politano operation (ureteroneocystostomy) 56.74
LEEP (loop electrosurgical excision procedure) of cervix 67.32
Le Fort operation (colpocleisis) 70.8
LeMesurier operation (cleft lip repair) 27.54
Lengthening
bone (with bone graft) 78.30
femur 78.35
for reconstruction of thumb 82.69
specified site NEC - *see also* category 78.3, 78.39
tibia 78.37
ulna 78.33
extraocular muscle NEC 15.21
multiple (two or more muscles) 15.4
fascia 83.89
hand 82.89
hamstring NEC 83.85
heel cord 83.85
leg
femur 78.35
tibia 78.37
levator palpebrae muscle 08.38
muscle 83.85
extraocular 15.21
multiple (two or more muscles) 15.4
hand 82.55
palate 27.62
secondary or subsequent 27.63
tendon 83.85
for claw toe repair 77.57
hand 82.55
Leriche operation (periarterial sympathectomy) 05.25
Leucotomy, leukotomy 01.32
Leukopheresis, therapeutic 99.72
Lid suture operation (blepharoptosis) 08.31
Ligation
adrenal vessel (artery) (vein) 07.43
aneurysm 39.52
appendages, dermal 86.26
arteriovenous fistula 39.53
coronary artery 36.99
artery 38.80
abdominal 38.86
adrenal 07.43
aorta (arch) (ascending) (descending) 38.84
coronary (anomalous) 36.99
ethmoidal 21.04
external carotid 21.06
for control of epistaxis - *see* Control, epistaxis
head and neck NEC 38.82
intracranial NEC 38.81
lower limb 38.88
maxillary (transantral) 21.05
middle meningeal 02.13
thoracic NEC 38.85
thyroid 06.92
upper limb 38.83
atrium, heart 37.99
auricle, heart 37.99
bleeding vessel - *see* Control, hemorrhage
blood vessel 38.80
abdominal
artery 38.86
vein 38.87
adrenal 07.43
aorta (arch) (ascending) (descending) 38.84
esophagus 42.91
endoscopic 42.33
head and neck 38.82

Ligation *(Continued)*
blood vessel *(Continued)*
intracranial NEC 38.81
lower limb
artery 38.88
vein 38.89
meningeal (artery) (longitudinal sinus) 02.13
thoracic NEC 38.85
thyroid 06.92
upper limb (artery) (vein) 38.83
bronchus 33.92
cisterna chyli 40.64
coronary
artery (anomalous) 36.99
sinus 36.39
dermal appendage 86.26
ductus arteriosus, patent 38.85
esophageal vessel 42.91
endoscopic 42.33
ethmoidal artery 21.04
external carotid artery 21.06
fallopian tube (bilateral) (remaining) (solitary) 66.39
by endoscopy (culdoscopy) (hysteroscopy) (laparoscopy) (peritoneoscopy) 66.29
with
crushing 66.31
by endoscopy (laparoscopy) 66.21
division 66.32
by endoscopy (culdoscopy) (laparoscopy) (peritoneoscopy) 66.22
Falope ring 66.39
by endoscopy (laparoscopy) 66.29
unilateral 66.92
fistula, arteriovenous 39.53
coronary artery 36.99
gastric
artery 38.86
varices 44.91
endoscopic 43.41
hemorrhoids 49.45
longitudinal sinus (superior) 02.13
lymphatic (channel) (peripheral) 40.9
thoracic duct 40.64
maxillary artery 21.05
meningeal vessel 02.13
spermatic
cord 63.72
varicocele 63.1
vein (high) 63.1
splenic vessels 38.86
subclavian artery 38.85
superior longitudinal sinus 02.13
supernumerary digit 86.26
thoracic duct 40.64
thyroid vessel (artery) (vein) 06.92
toes (supernumerary) 86.26
tooth 93.55
impacted 24.6
ulcer (peptic) (base) (bed) (bleeding vessel) 44.40
duodenal 44.42
gastric 44.41
ureter 56.95
varices
esophageal 42.91
endoscopic 42.33
gastric 44.91
endoscopic 43.41

Ligation *(Continued)*
varices *(Continued)*
peripheral vein (lower limb) 38.59
upper limb 38.53
varicocele 63.1
vas deferens 63.71
vein 38.80
abdominal 38.87
adrenal 07.43
head and neck NEC 38.82
intracranial NEC 38.81
lower limb 38.89
spermatic, high 63.1
thoracic NEC 38.85
thyroid 06.92
upper limb 38.83
varicose 38.50
abdominal 38.57
esophagus 42.91
endoscopic 42.33
gastric 44.91
endoscopic 43.41
head and neck 38.52
intracranial NEC 38.51
lower limb 38.59
stomach 44.91
thoracic NEC 38.55
upper limb 38.53
vena cava, inferior 38.7
venous connection between anomalous vein to
left innominate vein 35.82
superior vena cava 35.82
wart 86.26
Light coagulation - *see* Photocoagulation
Lindholm operation (repair of ruptured tendon) 83.88
Lingulectomy, lung 32.3
Linton operation (varicose vein) 38.59
Lipectomy (subcutaneous tissue) (abdominal) (submental) 86.83
Liposuction 86.83
Lip reading training 95.49
Lip shave 27.43
Lisfranc operation
foot amputation 84.12
shoulder disarticulation 84.08
Litholapaxy, bladder 57.0
by incision 57.19
Lithotomy
bile passage 51.49
bladder (urinary) 57.19
common duct 51.41
percutaneous 51.96
gallbladder 51.04
hepatic duct 51.49
kidney 55.01
percutaneous 55.03
ureter 56.2
Lithotripsy
bile duct NEC 51.49
extracorporeal shock wave (ESWL) 98.52
bladder 57.0
with ultrasonic fragmentation 57.0 *[59.95]*
extracorporeal shock wave (ESWL) 98.51
extracorporeal shock wave (ESWL) NEC 98.59
bile duct 98.52
bladder (urinary) 98.51
gallbladder 98.52
kidney 98.51

Lithotripsy *(Continued)*
extracorporeal shock wave NEC *(Continued)*
Kock pouch 98.51
renal pelvis 98.51
specified site NEC 98.59
ureter 98.51
gallbladder NEC 51.04
endoscopic 51.88
extracorporeal shock wave (ESWL) 98.52
kidney 56.0
extracorporeal shock wave (ESWL) 98.51
percutaneous nephrostomy with fragmentation (laser) (ultrasound) 55.04
renal pelvis 56.0
extracorporeal shock wave (ESWL) 98.51
percutaneous nephrostomy with fragmentation (laser) (ultrasound) 55.04
ureter 56.0
extracorporeal shock wave (ESWL) 98.51
Littlewood operation (forequarter amputation) 84.09
LLETZ (large loop excision of the transformation zone) of cervix 67.32
Lloyd-Davies operation (abdominoperineal resection) 48.5
Lobectomy
brain 01.53
partial 01.59
liver (with partial excision of adjacent lobes) 50.3
lung (complete) 32.4
partial 32.3
segmental (with resection of adjacent lobes) 32.4
thyroid (total) (unilateral) (with removal of isthmus) (with removal of portion of remaining lobe) 06.2
partial - *see also* Thyroidectomy, partial 06.39
substernal 06.51
subtotal - *see also* Thyroidectomy, partial 06.39
Lobotomy, brain 01.32
Localization, placenta 88.78
by RISA injection 92.17
Longmire operation (bile duct anastomosis) 51.39
Loop ileal stoma (*see also* Ileostomy) 46.01
Loopogram 87.78
Looposcopy (ileal conduit) 56.35
Lord operation
dilation of anal canal for hemorrhoids 49.49
hemorrhoidectomy 49.49
orchidopexy 62.5
Lower GI series (x-ray) 87.64
Lucas and Murray operation (knee arthrodesis with plate) 81.22
Lumpectomy
breast 85.21
specified site - *see* Excision, lesion, by site
Lymphadenectomy (simple) - *see also* Excision, lymph, node 40.29
Lymphadenotomy 40.0
Lymphangiectomy (radical) - *see also* Excision, lymph, node, by site, radical 40.50

Lymphangiogram
abdominal 88.04
cervical 87.08
intrathoracic 87.34
lower limb 88.36
pelvic 88.04
upper limb 88.34
Lymphangioplasty 40.9
Lymphangiorrhaphy 40.9
Lymphangiotomy 40.0
Lymphaticostomy 40.9
thoracic duct 40.62
Lysis
adhesions

Note: blunt - *omit code*
digital - *omit code*
manual - *omit code*
mechanical - *omit code*
without instrumentation - *omit code*

abdominal 54.59
laparoscopic 54.51
appendiceal 54.59
laparoscopic 54.51
artery-vein-nerve bundle 39.91
biliary tract 54.59
laparoscopic 54.51
bladder (neck) (intraluminal) 57.12
external 59.11
laparoscopic 59.12
transurethral 57.41
blood vessels 39.91
bone - *see* category 78.4
bursa 83.91
by stretching or manipulation 93.28
hand 82.91
cartilage of joint 93.26
chest wall 33.99
choanae (nasopharynx) 29.54
conjunctiva 10.5
corneovitreal 12.34
cortical (brain) 02.91
ear, middle 20.23
Eustachian tube 20.8
extraocular muscle 15.7
extrauterine 54.59
laparoscopic 54.51
eyelid 08.09
and conjunctiva 10.5

Lysis *(Continued)*
adhesions *(Continued)*
eye muscle 15.7
fallopian tube 65.89
laparoscopic 65.81
fascia 83.91
hand 82.91
by stretching or manipulation 93.26
gallbladder 54.59
laparoscopic 54.51
ganglion (peripheral) NEC 04.49
cranial NEC 04.42
hand 82.91
by stretching or manipulation 93.26
heart 37.10
intestines 54.59
laparoscopic 54.51
iris (posterior) 12.33
anterior 12.32
joint (capsule) (structure) - *see also* Division, joint capsule 80.40
kidney 59.02
laparoscopic 59.03
labia (vulva) 71.01
larynx 31.92
liver 54.59
laparoscopic 54.51
lung (for collapse of lung) 33.39
mediastinum 34.99
meninges (spinal) 03.6
cortical 02.91
middle ear 20.23
muscle 83.91
by stretching or manipulation 93.27
extraocular 15.7
hand 82.91
by stretching or manipulation 93.26
nasopharynx 29.54
nerve (peripheral) NEC 04.49
cranial NEC 04.42
roots, spinal 03.6
trigeminal 04.41
nose, nasal 21.91
ocular muscle 15.7
ovary 65.89
laparoscopic 65.81
pelvic 54.59
laparoscopic 54.51
penile 64.93

Lysis *(Continued)*
adhesions *(Continued)*
pericardium 37.12
perineal (female) 71.01
peripheral vessels 39.91
perirectal 48.81
perirenal 59.02
laparoscopic 59.03
peritoneum (pelvic) 54.59
laparoscopic 54.51
periureteral 59.02
laparoscopic 59.03
perivesical 59.11
laparoscopic 59.12
pharynx 29.54
pleura (for collapse of lung) 33.39
spermatic cord 63.94
spinal (cord) (meninges) (nerve roots) 03.6
spleen 54.59
laparoscopic 54.51
tendon 83.91
by stretching or manipulation 93.27
hand 82.91
by stretching or manipulation 93.26
thorax 34.99
tongue 25.93
trachea 31.92
tubo-ovarian 65.89
laparoscopic 65.81
ureter 59.02
with freeing or repositioning of ureter 59.02
intraluminal 56.81
laparoscopic 59.03
urethra (intraluminal) 58.5
uterus 54.59
intraluminal 68.21
laparoscopic 54.51
peritoneal 54.59
laparoscopic 54.51
vagina (intraluminal) 70.13
vitreous (posterior approach) 14.74
anterior approach 14.73
vulva 71.01
goniosynechiae (with injection of air or liquid) 12.31
synechiae (posterior) 12.33
anterior (with injection of air or liquid) 12.32

M

Madlener operation (tubal ligation) 66.31
Magnet extraction
foreign body
anterior chamber, eye 12.01
choroid 14.01
ciliary body 12.01
conjunctiva 98.22
cornea 11.0
eye, eyeball NEC 98.21
anterior segment 12.01
posterior segment 14.01
intraocular (anterior segment) 12.01
iris 12.01
lens 13.01
orbit 98.21
retina 14.01
sclera 12.01
vitreous 14.01
Magnetic resonance imaging (nuclear) - *see* Imaging, magnetic resonance
Magnuson (-Stack) operation (arthroplasty for recurrent shoulder dislocation) 81.82
Malleostapediopexy 19.19
with incus replacement 19.11
Malström's vacuum extraction 72.79
with episiotomy 72.71
Mammaplasty - *see* Mammoplasty
Mammectomy - *see also* Mastectomy
subcutaneous (unilateral) 85.34
with synchronous implant 85.33
bilateral 85.36
with synchronous implant 85.35
Mammilliplasty 85.87
Mammography NEC 87.37
Mammoplasty 85.89
with
full-thickness graft 85.83
muscle flap 85.85
pedicle graft 85.84
split-thickness graft 85.82
amputative (reduction) (bilateral) 85.32
unilateral 85.31
augmentation 85.50
with
breast implant (bilateral) 85.54
unilateral 85.53
injection into breast (bilateral) 85.52
unilateral 85.51
reduction (bilateral) 85.32
unilateral 85.31
revision 85.89
size reduction (gynecomastia) (bilateral) 85.32
unilateral 85.31
Mammotomy 85.0
Manchester (-Donald) (-Fothergill) operation (uterine suspension) 69.22
Mandibulectomy (partial) 76.31
total 76.42
with reconstruction 76.41
Maneuver (method)
Bracht 72.52
Credé 73.59
De Lee (key-in-lock) 72.4
Kristeller 72.54
Loveset's (extraction of arms in breech birth) 72.52
Mauriceau (-Smellie-Veit) 72.52
Pinard (total breech extraction) 72.54
Prague 72.52
Ritgen 73.59
Maneuver *(Continued)*
Scanzoni (rotation) 72.4
Van Hoorn 72.52
Wigand-Martin 72.52
Manipulation
with reduction of fracture or dislocation - *see* Reduction, fracture *and* Reduction, dislocation
enterostomy stoma (with dilation) 96.24
intestine (intra-abdominal) 46.80
large 46.82
small 46.81
joint
adhesions 93.26
temporomandibular 76.95
dislocation - *see* Reduction, dislocation
lacrimal passage (tract) NEC 09.49
muscle structures 93.27
musculoskeletal (physical therapy) NEC 93.29
nasal septum, displaced 21.88
osteopathic NEC 93.67
for general mobilization (general articulation) 93.61
high-velocity, low-amplitude forces (thrusting) 93.62
indirect forces 93.65
isotonic, isometric forces 93.64
low-velocity, high-amplitude forces (springing) 93.63
to move tissue fluids 93.66
rectum 96.22
salivary duct 26.91
stomach, intraoperative 44.92
temporomandibular joint NEC 76.95
ureteral calculus by catheter
with removal 56.0
without removal 59.8
uterus NEC 69.98
gravid 75.99
inverted
manual replacement (following delivery) 75.94
surgical - *see* Repair, inverted uterus
Manometry
esophageal 89.32
spinal fluid 89.15
urinary 89.21
Manual arts therapy 93.81
Mapping
cardiac (electrophysiologic) 37.27
doppler (flow) 88.72
electrocardiogram only 89.52
Marckwald operation (cervical os repair) 67.59
Marshall-Marchetti (-Krantz) operation (retropubic urethral suspension) 59.5
Marsupialization - *see also* Destruction, lesion, by site
cyst
Bartholin's 71.23
brain 01.59
cervical (nabothian) 67.31
dental 24.4
dentigerous 24.4
kidney 55.31
larynx 30.01
liver 50.21
ovary 65.21
laparoscopic 65.23
pancreas 52.3
pilonidal (open excision) (with partial closure) 86.21
Marsupialization *(Continued)*
cyst *(Continued)*
salivary gland 26.21
spinal (intraspinal) (meninges) 03.4
spleen, splenic 41.41
lesion
brain 01.59
cerebral 01.59
liver 50.21
pilonidal cyst or sinus (open excision) (with partial closure) 86.21
pseudocyst, pancreas 52.3
ranula, salivary gland 26.21
Massage
cardiac (external) (manual) (closed) 99.63
open 37.91
prostatic 99.94
rectal (for levator spasm) 99.93
MAST (military anti-shock trousers) 93.58
Mastectomy (complete) (prophylactic) (simple) (unilateral) 85.41
with
excision of regional lymph nodes 85.43
bilateral 85.44
preservation of skin and nipple 85.34
with synchronous implant 85.33
bilateral 85.36
with synchronous implant 85.35
bilateral 85.42
extended
radical (Urban) (unilateral) 85.47
bilateral 85.48
simple (with regional lymphadenectomy) (unilateral) 85.43
bilateral 85.44
modified radical (unilateral) 85.43
bilateral 85.44
partial 85.23
radical (Halsted) (Meyer) (unilateral) 85.45
bilateral 85.46
extended (Urban) (unilateral) 85.47
bilateral 85.48
modified (unilateral) 85.43
bilateral 85.44
subcutaneous 85.34
with synchronous implant 85.33
bilateral 85.36
with synchronous implant 85.35
subtotal 85.23
Masters' stress test (two-step) 89.42
Mastoidectomy (cortical) (conservative) 20.49
complete (simple) 20.41
modified radical 20.49
radical 20.42
modified 20.49
simple (complete) 20.41
Mastoidotomy 20.21
Mastoidotympanectomy 20.42
Mastopexy 85.6
Mastoplasty - *see* Mammoplasty
Mastorrhaphy 85.81
Mastotomy 85.0
Matas operation (aneurysmorrhaphy) 39.52
Mayo operation
bunionectomy 77.59
herniorrhaphy 53.49
vaginal hysterectomy 68.59
laparoscopically assisted (LAVH) 68.51

Mazet operation (knee disarticulation) 84.16
McBride operation (bunionectomy with soft tissue correction) 77.53
McBurney operation - *see* Repair, hernia, inguinal
McCall operation (enterocele repair) 70.92
McCauley operation (release of clubfoot) 83.84
McDonald operation (encirclement suture, cervix) 67.59
McIndoe operation (vaginal construction) 70.61
McKeever operation (fusion of first metatarsophalangeal joint for hallux valgus repair) 77.52
McKissock operation (breast reduction) 85.33
McReynolds operation (transposition of pterygium) 11.31
McVay operation
  femoral hernia - *see* Repair, hernia, femoral
  inguinal hernia - *see* Repair, hernia, inguinal
Measurement
  airway resistance 89.38
  anatomic NEC 89.39
  arterial blood gases 89.65
    basal metabolic rate (BMR) 89.39
    blood gases
      arterial 89.65
        continuous intra-arterial 89.60
      venous 89.66
  body 93.07
  cardiac output (by)
    Fick method 89.67
    indicator dilution technique 89.68
    oxygen consumption technique 89.67
    thermodilution indicator 89.68
  cardiovascular NEC 89.59
  central venous pressure 89.62
  coronary blood flow 89.69
  gastric function NEC 89.39
  girth 93.07
  intelligence 94.01
  intracranial pressure 01.18
  intraocular tension or pressure 89.11
    as part of extended ophthalmologic work-up 95.03
  intrauterine pressure 89.62
  limb length 93.06
  lung volume 89.37
  mixed venous blood gases 89.66
  physiologic NEC 89.39
  portovenous pressure 89.62
  range of motion 93.05
  renal clearance 89.29
  respiratory NEC 89.38
  skin fold thickness 93.07
  skull circumference 93.07
  sphincter of Oddi pressure 51.15
  systemic arterial
    blood gases 89.65
      continuous intra-arterial 89.60
    pressure 89.61
  urine (bioassay) (chemistry) 89.29
  vascular 89.59
  venous blood gases 89.66
  vital capacity (pulmonary) 89.37
Meatoplasty
  ear 18.6
  urethra 58.47
Meatotomy
  ureter 56.1
  urethra 58.1
    internal 58.5
Mechanical ventilation - *see* Ventilation
Mediastinectomy 34.3
Mediastinoscopy (transpleural) 34.22
Mediastinotomy 34.1
  with pneumonectomy 32.5
Meloplasty, facial 86.82
Meningeorrhaphy (cerebral) 02.12
  spinal NEC 03.59
    for
      meningocele 03.51
      myelomeningocele 03.52
Meniscectomy (knee) NEC 80.6
  acromioclavicular 80.91
  sternoclavicular 80.91
  temporomandibular (joint) 76.5
  wrist 80.93
Menstrual extraction or regulation 69.6
Mentoplasty (augmentation) (with graft) (with implant) 76.68
  reduction 76.67
Mesenterectomy 54.4
Mesenteriopexy 54.75
Mesenteriplication 54.75
Mesocoloplication 54.75
Mesopexy 54.75
Metatarsectomy 77.98
Metroplasty 69.49
Mid-forceps delivery 72.29
Mikulicz operation (exteriorization of intestine) (first stage) 46.03
  second stage 46.04
Miles operation (proctectomy) 48.5
Military anti-shock trousers (MAST) 93.58
Millard operation (cheiloplasty) 27.54
Miller operation
  midtarsal arthrodesis 81.14
  urethrovesical suspension 59.4
Millin-Read operation (urethrovesical suspension) 59.4
Mist therapy 93.94
Mitchell operation (hallux valgus repair) 77.51
Mobilization
  joint NEC 93.16
  mandible 76.95
  neostrophingic (mitral valve) 35.12
  spine 93.15
  stapes (transcrural) 19.0
  testis in scrotum 62.5
Mohs operation (chemosurgical excision of skin) 86.24
Molegraphy 87.81
Monitoring
  cardiac output (by)
    ambulatory (ACM) 89.50
    electrographic 89.54
      during surgery - *omit code*
    Fick method 89.67
    Holter-type device 89.50
    indicator dilution technique 89.68
    intracardiac hemodynamic ◀
      sensor (lead) 00.56 ◀
      subcutaneous device 00.57 ◀
    oxygen consumption technique 89.67
    specified technique NEC 89.68
    telemetry (cardiac) 89.54
    thermodilution indicator 89.68
    transesophageal (Doppler) (ultrasound) 89.68
  central venous pressure 89.62
Monitoring *(Continued)*
  circulatory NEC 89.69
  continuous intra-arterial blood gas 89.60
  coronary blood flow (coincidence counting technique) 89.69
  electroencephalographic 89.19
    radio-telemetered 89.19
    video 89.19
  fetus (fetal heart)
    antepartum
      nonstress (fetal activity acceleration determinations) 75.34
      oxytocin challenge (contraction stress test) 75.35
      ultrasonography (early pregnancy) (Doppler) 88.78
    intrapartum (during labor) (extrauterine) (external) 75.34
      auscultatory (stethoscopy) - *omit code*
      internal (with contraction measurements) (ECG) 75.32
      intrauterine (direct) (ECG) 75.32
      phonocardiographic (extrauterine) 75.34
      pulsed ultrasound (Doppler) 88.78
      transcervical fetal oxygen saturation monitoring 75.38
      transcervical fetal SpO_2 monitoring 75.38
  Holter-type device (cardiac) 89.50
  intracranial pressure 01.18
  pulmonary artery
    pressure 89.63
    wedge 89.64
  sleep (recording) - *see* categories 89.17–89.18
  systemic arterial pressure 89.61
  telemetry (cardiac) 89.54
  transesophageal cardiac output (Doppler) 89.68
  ventricular pressure (cardiac) 89.62
Moore operation (arthroplasty) 81.52
Moschowitz
  enterocele repair 70.92
  herniorrhaphy - *see* Repair, hernia, femoral
  sigmoidopexy 46.63
Mountain resort sanitarium 93.98
Mouth-to-mouth resuscitation 93.93
Moxibustion 93.35
MRI - *see* Imaging, magnetic resonance
Muller operation (banding of pulmonary artery) 38.85
Multiple sleep latency test (MSLT) 89.18
Mumford operation (partial claviculectomy) 77.81
Musculoplasty - *see also* Repair, muscle 83.87
  hand - *see also* Repair, muscle, hand 82.89
Music therapy 93.84
Mustard operation (interatrial transposition of venous return) 35.91
Myectomy 83.45
  anorectal 48.92
  eye muscle 15.13
    multiple 15.3
  for graft 83.43
    hand 82.34
  hand 82.36
    for graft 82.34
  levator palpebrae 08.33
  rectal 48.92

Myelogram, myelography (air) (gas) 87.21
posterior fossa 87.02
Myelotomy
spine, spinal (cord) (tract) (one-stage) (two-stage) 03.29
percutaneous 03.21
Myocardiectomy (infarcted area) 37.33
Myocardiotomy 37.11
Myoclasis 83.99
hand 82.99
Myomectomy (uterine) 68.29
broad ligament 69.19
Myoplasty - *see also* Repair, muscle 83.87
hand - *see also* Repair, muscle, hand 82.89
mastoid 19.9
Myorrhaphy 83.65
hand 82.46
Myosuture 83.65
hand 82.46
Myotasis 93.27
Myotenontoplasty - *see also* Repair, tendon 83.88
hand 82.86
Myotenoplasty - *see also* Repair, tendon 83.88
hand 82.86
Myotenotomy 83.13
hand 82.11
Myotomy 83.02
with division 83.19
hand 82.19
colon NEC 46.92
sigmoid 46.91
cricopharyngeal 29.31
that for pharyngeal (pharyngoesophageal) diverticulectomy 29.32
esophagus 42.7
eye (oblique) (rectus) 15.21
multiple (two or more muscles) 15.4
hand 82.02
with division 82.19
levator palpebrae 08.38
sigmoid (colon) 46.91
Myringectomy 20.59
Myringodectomy 20.59
Myringomalleolabyrinthopexy 19.52
Myringoplasty (epitympanic, type I) (by cauterization) (by graft) 19.4
revision 19.6
Myringostapediopexy 19.53
Myringostomy 20.01
Myringotomy (with aspiration) (with drainage) 20.09
with insertion of tube or drainage device (button) (grommet) 20.01

N

Nailing, intramedullary - *see* Reduction, fracture with internal fixation
with fracture reduction - *see* Reduction, fracture with internal fixation ◄
internal (without fracture reduction) 78.50 ◄
Narcoanalysis 94.21
Narcosynthesis 94.21
Narrowing, palpebral fissure 08.51
Nasopharyngogram 87.09
contrast 87.06
Necropsy 89.8
Needleoscopy (fetus) 75.31
Needling
Bartholin's gland (cyst) 71.21
cataract (secondary) 13.64
fallopian tube 66.91
hydrocephalic head 73.8
lens (capsule) 13.2
pupillary membrane (iris) 12.35
Nephrectomy (complete) (total) (unilateral) 55.51
bilateral 55.54
partial (wedge) 55.4
remaining or solitary kidney 55.52
removal, transplanted kidney 55.53
Nephrocolopexy 55.7
Nephrocystanastomosis NEC 56.73
Nephrolithotomy 55.01
Nephrolysis 59.02
laparoscopic 59.03
Nephropexy 55.7
Nephroplasty 55.89
Nephropyeloplasty 55.87
Nephropyeloureterostomy 55.86
Nephrorrhaphy 55.81
Nephroscopy 55.21
Nephrostolithotomy, percutaneous 55.03
Nephrostomy (with drainage tube) 55.02
closure 55.82
percutaneous 55.03
with fragmentation (ultrasound) 55.04
Nephrotomogram, nephrotomography NEC 87.72
Nephrotomy 55.01
Nephroureterectomy (with bladder cuff) 55.51
Nephroureterocystectomy 55.51 *[57.79]*
Nerve block (cranial) (peripheral) NEC - *see also* Block, by site 04.81
Neurectasis (cranial) (peripheral) 04.91
Neurectomy (cranial) (infraorbital) (occipital) (peripheral) (spinal) NEC 04.07
gastric (vagus) - *see also* Vagotomy 44.00
opticociliary 12.79
Neurectomy *(Continued)*
paracervical 05.22
presacral 05.24
retrogasserian 04.07
sympathetic - *see* Sympathectomy
trigeminal 04.07
tympanic 20.91
Neurexeresis NEC 04.07
Neuroablation
radiofrequency 04.2
Neuroanastomosis (cranial) (peripheral) NEC 04.74
accessory-facial 04.72
accessory-hypoglossal 04.73
hypoglossal-facial 04.71
Neurolysis (peripheral nerve) NEC 04.49
carpal tunnel 04.43
cranial nerve NEC 04.42
spinal (cord) (nerve roots) 03.6
tarsal tunnel 04.44
trigeminal nerve 04.41
Neuroplasty (cranial) (peripheral) NEC 04.79
of old injury (delayed repair) 04.76
revision 04.75
Neurorrhaphy (cranial) (peripheral) 04.3
Neurotomy (cranial) (peripheral) (spinal) NEC 04.04
acoustic 04.01
glossopharyngeal 29.92
lacrimal branch 05.0
retrogasserian 04.02
sympathetic 05.0
vestibular 04.01
Neurotripsy (peripheral) NEC 04.03
trigeminal 04.02
Nicola operation (tenodesis for recurrent dislocation of shoulder) 81.82
Nimodipine, infusion 99.75
NIPS (non-invasive programmed electrical stimulation) 37.20 ⬅
Nissen operation (fundoplication of stomach) 44.66
laparoscopic 44.67
Noble operation (plication of small intestine) 46.62
Norman Miller operation (vaginopexy) 70.77
Norton operation (extraperitoneal cesarean section) 74.2
Nuclear magnetic resonance imaging - *see* Imaging, magnetic resonance
Nutrition, concentrated substances
enteral infusion (of) 96.6
parenteral (total) 99.15
peripheral parenteral 99.15

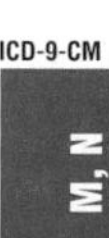

O

Ober (-Yount) operation (gluteal-iliotibial fasciotomy) 83.14
Obliteration
  bone cavity - *see also* Osteoplasty 78.40
  calyceal diverticulum 55.39
  canaliculi 09.6
  cerebrospinal fistula 02.12
  cul-de-sac 70.92
  frontal sinus (with fat) 22.42
  lacrimal punctum 09.91
  lumbar pseudomeningocele 03.51
  lymphatic structure(s) (peripheral) 40.9
  maxillary sinus 22.31
  meningocele (sacral) 03.51
  pelvic 68.8
  pleural cavity 34.6
  sacral meningocele 03.51
  Skene's gland 71.3
  tympanomastoid cavity 19.9
  vagina, vaginal (partial) (total) 70.4
    vault 70.8
Occlusal molds (dental) 89.31
Occlusion
  artery
    by embolization - *see* Embolization, artery
    by endovascular approach - *see* Embolization, artery
    by ligation - *see* Ligation, artery
  fallopian tube - *see* Ligation, fallopian tube
  patent ductus arteriosus (PDA) 38.85
  vein
    by embolization - *see* Embolization, vein
    by endovascular approach - *see* Embolization, vein
    by ligation - *see* Ligation, vein
  vena cava (surgical) 38.7
Occupational therapy 93.83
O'Donoghue operation (triad knee repair) 81.43
Odontectomy NEC - *see also* Removal, tooth, surgical 23.19
Oleothorax 33.39
Olshausen operation (uterine suspension) 69.22
Omentectomy 54.4
Omentofixation 54.74
Omentopexy 54.74
Omentoplasty 54.74
Omentorrhaphy 54.74
Omentotomy 54.19
Omphalectomy 54.3
Onychectomy 86.23
Onychoplasty 86.86
Onychotomy 86.09
  with drainage 86.04
Oophorectomy (unilateral) 65.39
  with salpingectomy 65.49
    laparoscopic 65.41
  bilateral (same operative episode) 65.51
    laparoscopic 65.53
    with salpingectomy 65.61
      laparoscopic 65.63
  laparoscopic 65.31
  partial 65.29
    laparoscopic 65.25
    wedge 65.22
      that by laparoscope 65.24
  remaining ovary 65.52
    laparoscopic 65.54
Oophorectomy *(Continued)*
  remaining ovary *(Continued)*
    with tube 65.62
      laparoscopic 65.64
Oophorocystectomy 65.29
  laparoscopic 65.25
Oophoropexy 65.79
Oophoroplasty 65.79
Oophororrhaphy 65.71
  laparoscopic 65.74
Oophorostomy 65.09
  laparoscopic 65.01
Oophorotomy 65.09
  laparoscopic 65.01
Opening
  bony labyrinth (ear) 20.79
  cranial suture 02.01
  heart valve
    closed heart technique - *see* Valvulotomy, by site
    open heart technique - *see* Valvuloplasty, by site
  spinal dura 03.09
Operation
  Abbe
    construction of vagina 70.61
    intestinal anastomosis - *see* Anastomosis, intestine
  abdominal (region) NEC 54.99
  abdominoperineal NEC 48.5
  Aburel (intra-amniotic injection for abortion) 75.0
  Adams
    advancement of round ligament 69.22
    crushing of nasal septum 21.88
    excision of palmar fascia 82.35
  adenoids NEC 28.99
  adrenal (gland) (nerve) (vessel) NEC 07.49
  Albee
    bone peg, femoral neck 78.05
    graft for slipping patella 78.06
    sliding inlay graft, tibia 78.07
  Albert (arthrodesis, knee) 81.22
  Aldridge (-Studdiford) (urethral sling) 59.5
  Alexander
    prostatectomy
      perineal 60.62
      suprapubic 60.3
    shortening of round ligaments of uterus 69.22
  Alexander-Adams (shortening of round ligaments of uterus) 69.22
  Almoor (extrapetrosal drainage) 20.22
  Altemeier (perineal rectal pull-through) 48.49
  Ammon (dacryocystotomy) 09.53
  Anderson (tibial lengthening) 78.37
  Anel (dilation of lacrimal duct) 09.42
  anterior chamber (eye) NEC 12.99
  anti-incontinence NEC 59.79
  antrum window (nasal sinus) 22.2
    with Caldwell-Luc approach 22.39
  anus NEC 49.99
  aortic body NEC 39.8
  aorticopulmonary window 39.59
  appendix NEC 47.99
  Arslan (fenestration of inner ear) 20.61
  artery NEC 39.99
  Asai (larynx) 31.75
  Baffes (interatrial transposition of venous return) 35.91
Operation *(Continued)*
  Baldy-Webster (uterine suspension) 69.22
  Ball
    herniorrhaphy - *see* Repair, hernia, inguinal
    undercutting 49.02
  Bankhart (capsular repair into glenoid, for shoulder dislocation) 81.82
  Bardenheurer (ligation of innominate artery) 38.85
  Barkan (goniotomy) 12.52
    with goniopuncture 12.53
  Barr (transfer of tibialis posterior tendon) 83.75
  Barsky (closure of cleft hand) 82.82
  Bassett (vulvectomy with inguinal lymph node dissection) 71.5 *[40.3]*
  Bassini (herniorrhaphy) - *see* Repair, hernia, inguinal
  Batch-Spittler-McFaddin (knee disarticulation) 84.16
  Batista (partial ventriculectomy) (ventricular reduction) (ventricular remodeling) 37.35
  Beck I (epicardial poudrage) 36.39
  Beck II (aorta-coronary sinus shunt) 36.39
  Beck-Jianu (permanent gastrostomy) 43.19
  Bell-Beuttner (subtotal abdominal hysterectomy) 68.39
  Belsey (esophagogastric sphincter) 44.65
  Benenenti (rotation of bulbous urethra) 58.49
  Berke (levator resection, eyelid) 08.33
  Biesenberger (size reduction of breast, bilateral) 85.32
    unilateral 85.31
  Bigelow (litholapaxy) 57.0
  biliary (duct) (tract) NEC 51.99
  Billroth I (partial gastrectomy with gastroduodenostomy) 43.6
  Billroth II (partial gastrectomy with gastrojejunostomy) 43.7
  Binnie (hepatopexy) 50.69
  Bischoff (ureteroneocystostomy) 56.74
  bisection hysterectomy 68.39
    laparoscopic 68.31
  Bishoff (spinal myelotomy) 03.29
  bladder NEC 57.99
    flap 56.74
  Blalock (systemic-pulmonary anastomosis) 39.0
  Blalock-Hanlon (creation of atrial septal defect) 35.42
  Blalock-Taussig (subclavian-pulmonary anastomosis) 39.0
  Blascovic (resection and advancement of levator palpebrae superioris) 08.33
  blood vessel NEC 39.99
  Blount
    femoral shortening (with blade plate) 78.25
      by epiphyseal stapling 78.25
  Boari (bladder flap) 56.74
  Bobb (cholelithotomy) 51.04
  bone NEC - *see* category 78.4
    facial 76.99
    injury NEC - *see* category 79.9
    marrow NEC 41.98
    skull NEC 02.99

Operation *(Continued)*
Bonney (abdominal hysterectomy) 68.49
laparoscopic 68.41
Borthen (iridotasis) 12.63
Bost
plantar dissection 80.48
radiocarpal fusion 81.26
Bosworth
arthroplasty for acromioclavicular separation 81.83
fusion of posterior lumbar spine 81.08
for pseudarthrosis 81.38
resection of radial head ligaments (for tennis elbow) 80.92
shelf procedure, hip 81.40
Bottle (repair of hydrocele of tunica vaginalis) 61.2
Boyd (hip disarticulation) 84.18
brain NEC 02.99
Brauer (cardiolysis) 37.10
breast NEC 85.99
Bricker (ileoureterostomy) 56.51
Bristow (repair of shoulder dislocation) 81.82
Brock (pulmonary valvulotomy) 35.03
Brockman (soft tissue release for clubfoot) 83.84
bronchus NEC 33.98
Browne (-Denis) (hypospadias repair) 58.45
Brunschwig (temporary gastrostomy) 43.19
buccal cavity NEC 27.99
Bunnell (tendon transfer) 82.56
Burch procedure (retropubic urethral suspension for urinary stress incontinence) 59.5
Burgess (amputation of ankle) 84.14
bursa NEC 83.99
hand 82.99
bypass - *see* Bypass
Caldwell (sulcus extension) 24.91
Caldwell-Luc (maxillary sinusotomy) 22.39
with removal of membrane lining 22.31
Callander (knee disarticulation) 84.16
Campbell
bone block, ankle 81.11
fasciotomy (iliac crest) 83.14
reconstruction of anterior cruciate ligaments 81.45
canthus NEC 08.99
cardiac NEC 37.99
septum NEC 35.98
valve NEC 35.99
carotid body or gland NEC 39.8
Carroll and Taber (arthroplasty, proximal interphalangeal joint) 81.72
Cattell (herniorrhaphy) 53.51
Cecil (urethral reconstruction) 58.46
cecum NEC 46.99
cerebral (meninges) NEC 02.99
cervix NEC 69.99
Chandler (hip fusion) 81.21
Charles (correction of lymphedema) 40.9
Charnley (compression arthrodesis)
ankle 81.11
hip 81.21
knee 81.22
Cheatle-Henry - *see* Repair, hernia, femoral
chest cavity NEC 34.99

Operation *(Continued)*
Chevalier-Jackson (partial laryngectomy) 30.29
Child (radical subtotal pancreatectomy) 52.53
Chopart (midtarsal amputation) 84.12
chordae tendineae NEC 35.32
choroid NEC 14.9
ciliary body NEC 12.98
cisterna chyli NEC 40.69
Clagett (closure of chest wall following open flap drainage) 34.72
Clayton (resection of metatarsal heads and bases of phalanges) 77.88
clitoris NEC 71.4
cocked hat (metacarpal lengthening and transfer of local flap) 82.69
Cockett (varicose vein)
lower limb 38.59
upper limb 38.53
Cody tack (perforation of footplate) 19.0
Coffey (uterine suspension) (Meig's modification) 69.22
Cole (anterior tarsal wedge osteotomy) 77.28
Collis-Nissen (hiatal hernia repair) 53.80
colon NEC 46.99
Colonna
adductor tenotomy (first stage) 83.12
hip arthroplasty (second stage) 81.40
reconstruction of hip (second stage) 81.40
commando (radical glossectomy) 25.4
conjunctiva NEC 10.99
destructive NEC 10.33
Cox-maze procedure (ablation or destruction of heart tissue) - *see* maze procedure
cornea NEC 11.99
Coventry (tibial wedge osteotomy) 77.27
Crawford (tarso-frontalis sling of eyelid) 08.32
cul-de-sac NEC 70.92
Culp-Deweerd (spiral flap pyeloplasty) 55.87
Culp-Scardino (ureteral flap pyeloplasty) 55.87
Curtis (interphalangeal joint arthroplasty) 81.72
cystocele NEC 70.51
Dahlman (excision of esophageal diverticulum) 42.31
Dana (posterior rhizotomy) 03.1
Danforth (fetal) 73.8
Darrach (ulnar resection) 77.83
Davis (intubated ureterotomy) 56.2
de Grandmont (tarsectomy) 08.35
Delorme
pericardiectomy 37.31
proctopexy 48.76
repair of prolapsed rectum 48.76
thoracoplasty 33.34
Denker (radical maxillary antrotomy) 22.31
Dennis-Varco (herniorrhaphy) - *see* Repair, hernia, femoral
Denonvilliers (limited rhinoplasty) 21.86
dental NEC 24.99
orthodontic NEC 24.8
Derlacki (tympanoplasty) 19.4
diaphragm NEC 34.89

Operation *(Continued)*
Dickson (fascial transplant) 83.82
Dickson-Diveley (tendon transfer and arthrodesis to correct claw toe) 77.57
Dieffenbach (hip disarticulation) 84.18
digestive tract NEC 46.99
Doléris (shortening of round ligaments) 69.22
D'Ombrain (excision of pterygium with corneal graft) 11.32
Dorrance (push-back operation for cleft palate) 27.62
Dotter (transluminal angioplasty) 39.59
Douglas (suture of tongue to lip for micrognathia) 25.59
Doyle (paracervical uterine denervation) 69.3
Dühamel (abdominoperineal pull-through) 48.65
Duhrssen's (vaginofixation of uterus) 69.22
Dunn (triple arthrodesis) 81.12
duodenum NEC 46.99
Dupuytren
fasciectomy 82.35
fasciotomy 82.12
with excision 82.35
shoulder disarticulation 84.08
Durham (-Caldwell) (transfer of biceps femoris tendon) 83.75
DuToit and Roux (staple capsulorrhaphy of shoulder) 81.82
DuVries (tenoplasty) 83.88
Dwyer
fasciotomy 83.14
soft tissue release NEC 83.84
wedge osteotomy, calcaneus 77.28
Eagleton (extrapetrosal drainage) 20.22
ear (external) NEC 18.9
middle or inner NEC 20.99
Eden-Hybinette (glenoid bone block) 78.01
Effler (heart) 36.2
Eggers
tendon release (patellar retinacula) 83.13
tendon transfer (biceps femoris tendon) (hamstring tendon) 83.75
Elliot (scleral trephination with iridectomy) 12.61
Ellis Jones (repair of peroneal tendon) 83.88
Ellison (reinforcement of collateral ligament) 81.44
Elmslie-Cholmeley (tarsal wedge osteotomy) 77.28
Eloesser
thoracoplasty 33.34
thoracostomy 34.09
Emmet (cervix) 67.61
endorectal pull-through 48.41
epididymis NEC 63.99
esophagus NEC 42.99
Estes (ovary) 65.72
laparoscopic 65.75
Estlander (thoracoplasty) 33.34
Evans (release of clubfoot) 83.84
extraocular muscle NEC 15.9
multiple (two or more muscles) 15.4
with temporary detachment from globe 15.3
revision 15.6

Operation *(Continued)*
extraocular muscle NEC *(Continued)*
single 15.29
with temporary detachment from globe 15.19
eyeball NEC 16.99
eyelid(s) NEC 08.99
face NEC 27.99
facial bone or joint NEC 76.99
fallopian tube NEC 66.99
Farabeuf (ischiopubiotomy) 77.39
Fasanella-Servatt (blepharoptosis repair) 08.35
fascia NEC 83.99
hand 82.99
female (genital organs) NEC 71.9
hysterectomy NEC 68.9
fenestration (aorta) 39.54
Ferguson (hernia repair) 53.00
Fick (perforation of footplate) 19.0
filtering (for glaucoma) 12.79
with iridectomy 12.65
Finney (pyloroplasty) 44.2
fistulizing, sclera NEC 12.69
Foley (pyeloplasty) 55.87
Fontan (creation of conduit between right atrium and pulmonary artery) 35.94
Fothergill (-Donald) (uterine suspension) 69.22
Fowler
arthroplasty of metacarpophalangeal joint 81.72
release (mallet finger repair) 82.84
tenodesis (hand) 82.85
thoracoplasty 33.34
Fox (entropion repair with wedge resection) 08.43
Franco (suprapubic cystotomy) 57.19
Frank (permanent gastrostomy) 43.19
Frazier (-Spiller) (subtemporal trigeminal rhizotomy) 04.02
Fredet-Ramstedt (pyloromyotomy) (with wedge resection) 43.3
Frenckner (intrapetrosal drainage) 20.22
Frickman (abdominal proctopexy) 48.75
Frommel (shortening of uterosacral ligaments) 69.22
Gabriel (abdominoperineal resection of rectum) 48.5
gallbladder NEC 51.99
ganglia NEC 04.99
sympathetic 05.89
Gant (wedge osteotomy of trochanter) 77.25
Garceau (tibial tendon transfer) 83.75
Gardner (spinal meningocele repair) 03.51
gastric NEC 44.99
Gelman (release of clubfoot) 83.84
genital organ NEC
female 71.9
male 64.99
Ghormley (hip fusion) 81.21
Giffod
destruction of lacrimal sac 09.6
keratotomy (delimiting) 11.1
Gill
arthrodesis of shoulder 81.23
laminectomy 03.09
Gill-Stein (carporadial arthrodesis) 81.25
Gilliam (uterine suspension) 69.22
Girdlestone
laminectomy with spinal fusion 81.00

Operation *(Continued)*
Girdlestone *(Continued)*
muscle transfer for claw toe 77.57
resection of femoral head and neck (without insertion of joint prosthesis) 77.85
with replacement prosthesis - *see* Implant, joint, hip
resection of hip prosthesis 80.05
with replacement prosthesis - *see* Implant, joint, hip
Girdlestone-Taylor (muscle transfer for claw toe repair) 77.57
glaucoma NEC 12.79
Glenn (anastomosis of superior vena cava to right pulmonary artery) 39.21
globus pallidus NEC 01.42
Goebel-Frangenheim-Stoeckel (urethrovesical suspension) 59.4
Goldner (clubfoot release) 80.48
Goldthwaite
ankle stabilization 81.11
patella stabilization 81.44
tendon transfer for patella dislocation 81.44
Goodall-Power (vagina) 70.4
Gordon-Taylor (hindquarter amputation) 84.19
Graber-Duvernay (drilling femoral head) 77.15
Green (scapulopexy) 78.41
Grice (subtalar arthrodesis) 81.13
Gritti-Stokes (knee disarticulation) 84.16
Gross (herniorrhaphy) 53.49
gum NEC 24.39
Guyon (amputation of ankle) 84.13
Hagner (epididymotomy) 63.92
Halsted - *see* Repair, hernia, inguinal
Hampton (anastomosis, small intestine to rectal stump) 45.92
hanging hip (muscle release) 83.19
harelip 27.54
Harrison-Richardson (vaginal suspension) 70.77
Hartmann - *see* Colectomy, by site
Hauser
achillotenotomy 83.11
bunionectomy with adductor tendon transfer 77.53
stabilization of patella 81.44
Heaney (vaginal hysterectomy) 68.59
laparoscopically assisted (LAVH) 68.51
heart NEC 37.99
valve NEC 35.99
adjacent structure NEC 35.39
Hegar (perineorrhaphy) 71.79
Heine (cyclodialysis) 12.55
Heineke-Mikulicz (pyloroplasty) - *see* category 44.2
Heller (esophagomyotomy) 42.7
Hellström (transplantation of aberrant renal vessel) 39.55
hemorrhoids NEC 49.49
Henley (jejunal transposition) 43.81
hepatic NEC 50.99
hernia - *see* Repair, hernia
Hey (amputation of foot) 84.12
Hey-Groves (reconstruction of anterior cruciate ligament) 81.45
Heyman (soft tissue release for clubfoot) 83.84
Heyman-Herndon (-Strong) (correction of metatarsus varus) 80.48

Operation *(Continued)*
Hibbs (lumbar spinal fusion) - *see* Fusion, lumbar
Higgins - *see* Repair, hernia, femoral
Hill-Allison (hiatal hernia repair, transpleural approach) 53.80
Hitchcock (anchoring tendon of biceps) 83.88
Hofmeister (gastrectomy) 43.7
Hoke
midtarsal fusion 81.14
triple arthrodesis 81.12
Holth
iridencleisis 12.63
sclerectomy 12.65
Homans (correction of lymphedema) 40.9
Hutch (ureteroneocystostomy) 56.74
Hybinette-Eden (glenoid bone block) 78.01
hymen NEC 70.91
hypopharynx NEC 29.99
hypophysis NEC 07.79
ileal loop 56.51
ileum NEC 46.99
intestine NEC 46.99
iris NEC 12.97
inclusion 12.63
Irving (tubal ligation) 66.32
Irwin - *see also* Osteotomy 77.30
Jaboulay (gastroduodenostomy) 44.39
laparoscopic 44.38
Janeway (permanent gastrostomy) 43.19
Jatene (arterial switch) 35.84
jejunum NEC 46.99
Johanson (urethral reconstruction) 58.46
joint (capsule) (ligament) (structure) NEC 81.99
facial NEC 76.99
Jones
claw toe (transfer of extensor hallucis longus tendon) 77.57
modified (with arthrodesis) 77.57
dacryocystorhinostomy 09.81
hammer toe (interphalangeal fusion) 77.56
modified (tendon transfer with arthrodesis) 77.57
repair of peroneal tendon 83.88
Joplin (exostectomy with tendon transfer) 77.53
Kader (temporary gastrostomy) 43.19
Kaufman (for urinary stress incontinence) 59.79
Kazanjian (buccal vestibular sulcus extension) 24.91
Kehr (hepatopexy) 50.69
Keller (bunionectomy) 77.59
Kelly (-Kennedy) (urethrovesical plication) 59.3
Kelly-Stoeckel (urethrovesical plication) 59.3
Kerr (cesarean section) 74.1
Kessler (arthroplasty, carpometacarpal joint) 81.74
Kidner (excision of accessory navicular bone) (with tendon transfer) 77.98
kidney NEC 55.99
Killian (frontal sinusotomy) 22.41
King-Steelquist (hindquarter amputation) 84.19
Kirk (amputation through thigh) 84.17
Kock pouch
bowel anastomosis - *omit code*

Operation *(Continued)*
Kock pouch *(Continued)*
continent ileostomy 46.22
cutaneous uretero-ileostomy 56.51
ESWL (electrocorporeal shock wave lithotripsy) 98.51
removal, calculus 57.19
revision, cutaneous uretero-ileostomy 56.52
urinary diversion procedure 56.51
Kondoleon (correction of lymphedema) 40.9
Krause (sympathetic denervation) 05.29
Kroener (partial salpingectomy) 66.69
Kroenlein (lateral orbitotomy) 16.01
Krönig (low cervical cesarean section) 74.1
Krukenberg (reconstruction of below-elbow amputation) 82.89
Kuhnt-Szymanowski (ectropion repair with lid reconstruction) 08.44
Labbe (gastrotomy) 43.0
labia NEC 71.8
lacrimal
gland 09.3
system NEC 09.99
Ladd (mobilization of intestine) 54.95
Lagrange (iridosclerectomy) 12.65
Lambrinudi (triple arthrodesis) 81.12
Langenbeck (cleft palate repair) 27.62
Lapidus (bunionectomy with metatarsal osteotomy) 77.51
Larry (shoulder disarticulation) 84.08
larynx NEC 31.98
Lash
internal cervical os repair 67.59
laparoscopic supracervical hysterectomy 68.31
Latzko
cesarean section, extraperitoneal 74.2
colpocleisis 70.8
Leadbetter (urethral reconstruction) 58.46
Leadbetter-Politano (ureteroneocystostomy) 56.74
Le Fort (colpocleisis) 70.8
LeMesurier (cleft lip repair) 27.54
lens NEC 13.90 ⇐
Leriche (periarterial sympathectomy) 05.25
levator muscle sling
eyelid ptosis repair 08.33
urethrovesical suspension 59.71
urinary stress incontinence 59.71
lid suture (blepharoptosis) 08.31
ligament NEC 81.99
broad NEC 69.98
round NEC 69.98
uterine NEC 69.98
Lindholm (repair of ruptured tendon) 83.88
Linton (varicose vein) 38.59
lip NEC 27.99
Lisfranc
foot amputation 84.12
shoulder disarticulation 84.08
Littlewood (forequarter amputation) 84.09
liver NEC 50.99
Lloyd-Davies (abdominoperineal resection) 48.5
Longmire (bile duct anastomosis) 51.39

Operation *(Continued)*
Lord
dilation of anal canal for hemorrhoids 49.49
hemorrhoidectomy 49.49
orchidopexy 62.5
Lucas and Murray (knee arthrodesis with plate) 81.22
lung NEC 33.99
lung volume reduction 32.22
biologic lung volume reduction (BLVR) - *see* category 33.7 ◀
lymphatic structure(s) NEC 40.9
duct, left (thoracic) NEC 40.69
Madlener (tubal ligation) 66.31
Magnuson (-Stack) (arthroplasty for recurrent shoulder dislocation) 81.82
male genital organs NEC 64.99
Manchester (-Donald) (-Fothergill) (uterine suspension) 69.22
mandible NEC 76.99
orthognathic 76.64
Marckwald (cervical os repair) 67.59
Marshall-Marchetti (-Krantz) (retropubic urethral suspension) 59.5
Matas (aneurysmorrhaphy) 39.52
Mayo
bunionectomy 77.59
herniorrhaphy 53.49
vaginal hysterectomy 68.59
laparoscopically assisted (LAVH) 68.51
Maze procedure (ablation or destruction of heart tissue)
by incision (open) 37.33
by peripherally inserted catheter 37.34
endovascular approach 37.34
trans-thoracic approach 37.33
Mazet (knee disarticulation) 84.16
McBride (bunionectomy with soft tissue correction) 77.53
McBurney - *see* Repair, hernia, inguinal
McCall (enterocele repair) 70.92
McCauley (release of clubfoot) 83.84
McDonald (encirclement suture, cervix) 67.59
McIndoe (vaginal construction) 70.61
McKeever (fusion of first metatarsophalangeal joint for hallux valgus repair) 77.52
McKissock (breast reduction) 85.33
McReynolds (transposition of pterygium) 11.31
McVay
femoral hernia - *see* Repair, hernia, femoral
inguinal hernia - *see* Repair, hernia, inguinal
meninges (spinal) NEC 03.99
cerebral NEC 02.99
mesentery NEC 54.99
Mikulicz (exteriorization of intestine) (first stage) 46.03
second stage 46.04
Miles (complete proctectomy) 48.5
Millard (cheiloplasty) 27.54
Miller
midtarsal arthrodesis 81.14
urethrovesical suspension 59.4
Millin-Read (urethrovesical suspension) 59.4
Mitchell (hallux valgus repair) 77.51

Operation *(Continued)*
Mohs (chemosurgical excision of skin) 86.24
Moore (arthroplasty) 81.52
Moschowitz
enterocele repair 70.92
herniorrhaphy - *see* Repair, hernia, femoral
sigmoidopexy 46.63
mouth NEC 27.99
Muller (banding of pulmonary artery) 38.85
Mumford (partial claviculectomy) 77.81
muscle NEC 83.99
extraocular - *see* Operation, extraocular
hand NEC 82.99
papillary heart NEC 35.31
musculoskeletal system NEC 84.99
Mustard (interatrial transposition of venous return) 35.91
nail (finger) (toe) NEC 86.99
nasal sinus NEC 22.9
nasopharynx NEC 29.99
nerve (cranial) (peripheral) NEC 04.99
adrenal NEC 07.49
sympathetic NEC 05.89
nervous system NEC 05.9
Nicola (tenodesis for recurrent dislocation of shoulder) 81.82
nipple NEC 85.99
Nissen (fundoplication of stomach) 44.66
laparoscopic 44.67
Noble (plication of small intestine) 46.62
node (lymph) NEC 40.9
Norman Miller (vaginopexy) 70.77
Norton (extraperitoneal cesarean operation) 74.2
nose, nasal NEC 21.99
sinus NEC 22.9
Ober (-Yount) (gluteal-iliotibial fasciotomy) 83.14
obstetric NEC 75.99
ocular NEC 16.99
muscle - *see* Operation, extraocular muscle
O'Donoghue (triad knee repair) 81.43
Olshausen (uterine suspension) 69.22
omentum NEC 54.99
ophthalmologic NEC 16.99
oral cavity NEC 27.99
orbicularis muscle sling 08.36
orbit NEC 16.98
oropharynx NEC 29.99
orthodontic NEC 24.8
orthognathic NEC 76.69
Oscar Miller (midtarsal arthrodesis) 81.14
Osmond-Clark (soft tissue release with peroneus brevis tendon transfer) 83.75
ovary NEC 65.99
Oxford (for urinary incontinence) 59.4
palate NEC 27.99
palpebral ligament sling 08.36
Panas (linear proctotomy) 48.0
Pancoast (division of trigeminal nerve at foramen ovale) 04.02
pancreas NEC 52.99
pantaloon (revision of gastric anastomosis) 44.5
papillary muscle (heart) NEC 35.31

Operation *(Continued)*
Paquin (ureteroneocystostomy) 56.74
parathyroid gland(s) NEC 06.99
parotid gland or duct NEC 26.99
Partsch (marsupialization of dental cyst) 24.4
Pattee (auditory canal) 18.6
Peet (splanchnic resection) 05.29
Pemberton
  osteotomy of ilium 77.39
  rectum (mobilization and fixation for prolapse repair) 48.76
penis NEC 64.98
Pereyra (paraurethral suspension) 59.6
pericardium NEC 37.99
perineum (female) NEC 71.8
  male NEC 86.99
perirectal tissue NEC 48.99
perirenal tissue NEC 59.92
peritoneum NEC 54.99
periurethral tissue NEC 58.99
perivesical tissue NEC 59.92
pharyngeal flap (cleft palate repair) 27.62
  secondary or subsequent 27.63
pharynx, pharyngeal (pouch) NEC 29.99
pineal gland NEC 07.59
Pinsker (obliteration of nasoseptal telangiectasia) 21.07
Piper (forceps) 72.6
Pirogoff (ankle amputation through malleoli of tibia and fibula) 84.14
pituitary gland NEC 07.79
plastic - *see* Repair, by site
pleural cavity NEC 34.99
Politano-Leadbetter (ureteroneocystostomy) 56.74
pollicization (with nerves and blood supply) 82.61
Polya (gastrectomy) 43.7
Pomeroy (ligation and division of fallopian tubes) 66.32
Poncet
  lengthening of Achilles tendon 83.85
  urethrostomy, perineal 58.0
Porro (cesarean section) 74.99
posterior chamber (eye) NEC 14.9
Potts-Smith (descending aorta-left pulmonary artery anastomosis) 39.0
Printen and Mason (high gastric bypass) 44.31
prostate NEC - *see also* Prostatectomy 60.69
  specified type 60.99
pterygium 11.39
  with corneal graft 11.32
Puestow (pancreaticojejunostomy) 52.96
pull-through NEC 48.49
pulmonary NEC 33.99
push-back (cleft palate repair) 27.62
Putti-Platt (capsulorrhaphy of shoulder for recurrent dislocation) 81.82
pyloric exclusion 44.39
  laparoscopic 44.38
pyriform sinus NEC 29.99
"rabbit ear" (anterior urethropexy) (Tudor) 59.79
Ramadier (intrapetrosal drainage) 20.22
Ramstedt (pyloromyotomy) (with wedge resection) 43.3
Rankin
  exteriorization of intestine 46.03
  proctectomy (complete) 48.5
Rashkind (balloon septostomy) 35.41

Operation *(Continued)*
Rastelli (creation of conduit between right ventricle and pulmonary artery) 35.92
  in repair of
    pulmonary artery atresia 35.92
    transposition of great vessels 35.92
    truncus arteriosus 35.83
Raz-Pereyra procedure (bladder neck suspension) 59.79
rectal NEC 48.99
rectocele NEC 70.52
re-entry (aorta) 39.54
renal NEC 55.99
respiratory (tract) NEC 33.99
retina NEC 14.9
Ripstein (repair of rectal prolapse) 48.75
Rodney Smith (radical subtotal pancreatectomy) 52.53
Roux-en-Y
  bile duct 51.36
  cholecystojejunostomy 51.32
  esophagus (intrathoracic) 42.54
  gastroenterostomy 44.39
    laparoscopic 44.38
  gastrojenunostomy 44.39
    laparoscopic 44.38
  pancreaticojejunostomy 52.96
Roux-Goldthwait (repair of patellar dislocation) 81.44
Roux-Herzen-Judine (jejunal loop interposition) 42.63
Ruiz-Mora (proximal phalangectomy for hammer toe) 77.99
Russe (bone graft of scaphoid) 78.04
Saemisch (corneal section) 11.1
salivary gland or duct NEC 26.99
Salter (innominate osteotomy) 77.39
Sauer-Bacon (abdominoperineal resection) 48.5
Schanz (femoral osteotomy) 77.35
Schauta (-Amreich) (radical vaginal hysterectomy) 68.79 ⬅
  laparoscopic 68.71 ◀
Schede (thoracoplasty) 33.34
Scheie
  cautery of sclera 12.62
  sclerostomy 12.62
Schlatter (total gastrectomy) 43.99
Schroeder (endocervical excision) 67.39
Schuchardt (nonobstetrical episiotomy) 71.09
Schwartze (simple mastoidectomy) 20.41
sclera NEC 12.89
Scott
  intestinal bypass for obesity 45.93
  jejunocolostomy (bypass) 45.93
scrotum NEC 61.99
Seddon-Brooks (transfer of pectoralis major tendon) 83.75
Semb (apicolysis of lung) 33.39
seminal vesicle NEC 60.79
Senning (correction of transposition of great vessels) 35.91
Sever (division of soft tissue of arm) 83.19
Sewell (heart) 36.2
sex transformation NEC 64.5
Sharrard (iliopsoas muscle transfer) 83.77
shelf (hip arthroplasty) 81.40
Shirodkar (encirclement suture, cervix) 67.59
sigmoid NEC 46.99
Silver (bunionectomy) 77.59

Operation *(Continued)*
Sistrunk (excision of thyroglossal cyst) 06.7
Skene's gland NEC 71.8
skin NEC 86.99
skull NEC 02.99
sling
  eyelid
    fascia lata, palpebral 08.36
    frontalis fascial 08.32
    levator muscle 08.33
    orbicularis muscle 08.36
    palpebrae ligament, fascia lata 08.36
    tarsus muscle 08.35
  fascial (fascia lata)
    eye 08.32
    for facial weakness (trigeminal nerve paralysis) 86.81
    palpebral ligament 08.36
    tongue 25.59
  tongue (fascial) 25.59
  urethra (suprapubic) 59.4
    retropubic 59.5
  urethrovesical 59.5
Slocum (pes anserinus transfer) 81.47
Sluder (tonsillectomy) 28.2
Smith (open osteotomy of mandible) 76.62
Smith-Peterson (radiocarpal arthrodesis) 81.25
Smithwick (sympathectomy) 05.29
Soave (endorectal pull-through) 48.41
soft tissue NEC 83.99
  hand 82.99
Sonneberg (inferior maxillary neurectomy) 04.07
Sorondo-Ferré (hindquarter amputation) 84.19
Soutter (iliac crest fasciotomy) 83.14
Spalding-Richardson (uterine suspension) 69.22
spermatic cord NEC 63.99
sphincter of Oddi NEC 51.89
spinal (canal) (cord) (structures) NEC 03.99
Spinelli (correction of inverted uterus) 75.93
Spivack (permanent gastrostomy) 43.19
spleen NEC 41.99
S.P. Rogers (knee disarticulation) 84.16
Ssabanejew-Frank (permanent gastrostomy) 43.19
Stacke (simple mastoidectomy) 20.41
Stallard (conjunctivocystorhinostomy) 09.82
  with insertion of tube or stent 09.83
Stamm (-Kader) (temporary gastrostomy) 43.19
Steinberg 44.5
Steindler
  fascia stripping (for cavus deformity) 83.14
  flexorplasty (elbow) 83.77
  muscle transfer 83.77
sterilization NEC
  female - *see also* specific operation 66.39
  male - *see also* Ligation, vas deferens 63.70
Stewart (renal plication with pyeloplasty) 55.87
stomach NEC 44.99
Stone (anoplasty) 49.79
Strassman (metroplasty) 69.49

Operation *(Continued)*
Strassman *(Continued)*
metroplasty (Jones modification) 69.49
uterus 68.22
Strayer (gastrocnemius recession) 83.72
stress incontinence - *see* Repair, stress incontinence
Stromeyer-Little (hepatotomy) 50.0
Strong (unbridling of celiac artery axis) 39.91
Sturmdorf (conization of cervix) 67.2
subcutaneous tissue NEC 86.99
sublingual gland or duct NEC 26.99
submaxillary gland or duct NEC 26.99
Summerskill (dacryocystorhinostomy by intubation) 09.81
Surmay (jejunostomy) 46.39
Swenson
bladder reconstruction 57.87
proctectomy 48.49
Swinney (urethral reconstruction) 58.46
Syme
ankle amputation through malleoli of tibia and fibula 84.14
urethrotomy, external 58.0
sympathetic nerve NEC 05.89
Taarnhoj (trigeminal nerve root decompression) 04.41
Tack (sacculotomy) 20.79
Talma-Morison (omentopexy) 54.74
Tanner (devascularization of stomach) 44.99
TAPVC NEC 35.82
tarsus NEC 08.99
muscle sling 08.35
tendon NEC 83.99
extraocular NEC 15.9
hand NEC 82.99
testis NEC 62.99
tetralogy of Fallot
partial repair - *see* specific procedure
total (one-stage) 35.81
Thal (repair of esophageal stricture) 42.85
thalamus 01.41
by stereotactic radiosurgery 92.32
cobalt 60 92.32
linear accelerator (LINAC) 92.31
multi-source 92.32
particle beam 92.33
particulate 92.33
radiosurgery NEC 92.39
single source photon 92.31
Thiersch
anus 49.79
skin graft 86.69
hand 86.62
Thompson
cleft lip repair 27.54
correction of lymphedema 40.9
quadricepsplasty 83.86
thumb apposition with bone graft 82.69
thoracic duct NEC 40.69
thorax NEC 34.99
Thorek (partial cholecystectomy) 51.21
three-snip, punctum 09.51
thymus NEC 07.99
thyroid gland NEC 06.98
TKP (thermokeratoplasty) 11.74
Tomkins (metroplasty) 69.49
tongue NEC 25.99

Operation *(Continued)*
tongue NEC *(Continued)*
flap, palate 27.62
tie 25.91
tonsil NEC 28.99
Torek (-Bevan) (orchidopexy) (first stage) (second stage) 62.5
Torkildsen (ventriculocisternal shunt) 02.2
Torpin (cul-de-sac resection) 70.92
Toti (dacryocystorhinostomy) 09.81
Touchas 86.83
Touroff (ligation of subclavian artery) 38.85
trabeculae corneae cordis (heart) NEC 35.35
trachea NEC 31.99
Trauner (lingual sulcus extension) 24.91
truncus arteriosus NEC 35.83
Tsuge (macrodactyly repair) 82.83
Tudor "rabbit ear" (anterior urethropexy) 59.79
Tuffier
apicolysis of lung 33.39
vaginal hysterectomy 68.59
laparoscopically assisted (LAVH) 68.51
tunica vaginalis NEC 61.99
Turco (release of joint capsules in clubfoot) 80.48
Uchida (tubal ligation with or without fimbriectomy) 66.32
umbilicus NEC 54.99
urachus NEC 57.51
Urban (mastectomy) (unilateral) 85.47
bilateral 85.48
ureter NEC 56.99
urethra NEC 58.99
urinary system NEC 59.99
uterus NEC 69.99
supporting structures NEC 69.98
uvula NEC 27.79
vagina NEC 70.91
vascular NEC 39.99
vas deferens NEC 63.99
ligation NEC 63.71
vein NEC 39.99
vena cava sieve 38.7
vertebra NEC 78.49
vesical (bladder) NEC 57.99
vessel NEC 39.99
cardiac NEC 36.99
Vicq d'Azyr (larynx) 31.1
Vidal (varicocele ligation) 63.1
Vineberg (implantation of mammary artery into ventricle) 36.2
vitreous NEC 14.79
vocal cord NEC 31.98
von Kraske (proctectomy) 48.64
Voss (hanging hip operation) 83.19
Vulpius (-Compere) (lengthening of gastrocnemius muscle) 83.85
vulva NEC 71.8
Ward-Mayo (vaginal hysterectomy) 68.59
laparoscopically assisted (LAVH) 68.51
Wardill (cleft palate) 27.62
Waters (extraperitoneal cesarean section) 74.2
Waterston (aorta-right pulmonary artery anastomosis) 39.0
Watkins (-Wertheim) (uterus interposition) 69.21

Operation *(Continued)*
Watson-Jones
hip arthrodesis 81.21
reconstruction of lateral ligaments, ankle 81.49
shoulder arthrodesis (extra-articular) 81.23
tenoplasty 83.88
Weir
appendicostomy 47.91
correction of nostrils 21.86
Wertheim (radical hysterectomy) 68.69 ⇐ Revised
laparoscopic 68.61 ◀ New
West (dacryocystorhinostomy) 09.81
Wheeler
entropion repair 08.44
halving procedure (eyelid) 08.24
Whipple (radical pancreaticoduodenectomy) 52.7
Child modification (radical subtotal pancreatectomy) 52.53
Rodney Smith modification (radical subtotal pancreatectomy) 52.53
White (lengthening of tendo calcaneus by incomplete tenotomy) 83.11
Whitehead
glossectomy, radical 25.4
hemorrhoidectomy 49.46
Whitman
foot stabilization (talectomy) 77.98
hip reconstruction 81.40
repair of serratus anterior muscle 83.87
talectomy 77.98
trochanter wedge osteotomy 77.25
Wier (entropion repair) 08.44
Williams-Richardson (vaginal construction) 70.61
Wilms (thoracoplasty) 33.34
Wilson (angulation osteotomy for hallux valgus) 77.51
window
antrum (nasal sinus) - *see* Antrotomy, maxillary
aorticopulmonary 39.59
bone cortex - *see also* Incision, bone 77.10
facial 76.09
nasoantral - *see* Antrotomy, maxillary
pericardium 37.12
pleural 34.09
Winiwarter (cholecystoenterostomy) 51.32
Witzel (temporary gastrostomy) 43.19
Woodward (release of high riding scapula) 81.83
Young
epispadias repair 58.45
tendon transfer (anterior tibialis) (repair of flat foot) 83.75
Yount (division of iliotibial band) 83.14
Zancolli
capsuloplasty 81.72
tendon transfer (biceps) 82.56
Ziegler (iridectomy) 12.14
Operculectomy 24.6
Ophthalmectomy 16.49
with implant (into Tenon's capsule) 16.42
with attachment of muscles 16.41
Ophthalmoscopy 16.21
Opponensplasty (hand) 82.56
Orbitomaxillectomy, radical 16.51

Orbitotomy (anterior) (frontal) (temporofrontal) (transfrontal) NEC 16.09
  with
    bone flap 16.01
    insertion of implant 16.02
  Kroenlein (lateral) 16.01
  lateral 16.01
Orchidectomy (with epididymectomy) (unilateral) 62.3
  bilateral (radical) 62.41
  remaining or solitary testis 62.42
Orchidopexy 62.5
Orchidoplasty 62.69
Orchidorrhaphy 62.61
Orchidotomy 62.0
Orchiectomy (with epididymectomy) (unilateral) 62.3
  bilateral (radical) 62.41
  remaining or solitary testis 62.42
Orchiopexy 62.5
Orchioplasty 62.69
Orthoroentgenography - *see* Radiography
Oscar Miller operation (midtarsal arthrodesis) 81.14
Osmond-Clark operation (soft tissue release with peroneus brevis tendon transfer) 83.75
Ossiculectomy NEC 19.3
  with
    stapedectomy - *see also* Stapedectomy 19.19
    stapes mobilization 19.0
    tympanoplasty 19.53
      revision 19.6
Ossiculotomy NEC 19.3
Ostectomy (partial), except facial - *see also* category 77.8
  facial NEC 76.39
    total 76.45
      with reconstruction 76.44
  first metatarsal head - *see* Bunionectomy
  for graft (autograft) (homograft) - *see also* category 77.7
    mandible 76.31
      total 76.42
        with reconstruction 76.41
  total, except facial - *see also* category 77.9
    facial NEC 76.45
      with reconstruction 76.44
    mandible 76.42
      with reconstruction 76.41
Osteoarthrotomy - *see also* Osteotomy 77.30
Osteoclasis 78.70
  carpal, metacarpal 78.74
  clavicle 78.71
  ear 20.79
  femur 78.75
  fibula 78.77
  humerus 78.72
  patella 78.76
  pelvic 78.79
  phalanges (foot) (hand) 78.79
  radius 78.73
  scapula 78.71
  specified site NEC 78.79
  tarsal, metatarsal 78.78
  thorax (ribs) (sternum) 78.71
  tibia 78.77
  ulna 78.73
  vertebrae 78.79
Osteolysis - *see* category 78.4
Osteopathic manipulation - *see also* Manipulation, osteopathic 93.67
Osteoplasty NEC - *see* category 78.4
  with bone graft - *see* Graft, bone
  for
    bone lengthening - *see* Lengthening, bone
    bone shortening - *see* Shortening, bone
    repair of malunion or nonunion of fracture - *see* Repair, fracture, malunion or nonunion
  carpal, metacarpal 78.44
  clavicle 78.41
  cranium NEC 02.06
    with
      flap (bone) 02.03
      graft (bone) 02.04
  facial bone NEC 76.69
  femur 78.45
  fibula 78.47
  humerus 78.42
  mandible, mandibular NEC 76.64
    body 76.63
    ramus (open) 76.62
      closed 76.61
  maxilla (segmental) 76.65
    total 76.66
  nasal bones 21.89
  patella 78.46
  pelvic 78.49
  phalanges (foot) (hand) 78.49
  radius 78.43
  scapula 78.41
  skull NEC 02.06
    with
      flap (bone) 02.03
      graft (bone) 02.04
  specified site NEC 78.49
  tarsal, metatarsal 78.48
  thorax (ribs) (sternum) 78.41
  tibia 78.47
  ulna 78.43
  vertebrae 78.49
Osteorrhaphy - *see also* Osteoplasty 78.40
Osteosynthesis (fracture) - *see* Reduction, fracture
Osteotomy (adduction) (angulation) (block) (derotational) (displacement) (partial) (rotational) 77.30
  carpals, metacarpals 77.34
    wedge 77.24
  clavicle 77.31
    wedge 77.21
  facial bone NEC 76.69
  femur 77.35
    wedge 77.25
  fibula 77.37
    wedge 77.27
  humerus 77.32
    wedge 77.22
  mandible (segmental) (subapical) 76.64
    angle (open) 76.62
      closed 76.61
    body 76.63
    Gigli saw 76.61
    ramus (open) 76.62
      closed 76.61
  maxilla (segmental) 76.65
    total 76.66
  metatarsal 77.38
    wedge 77.28
      for hallux valgus repair 77.51
Osteotomy *(Continued)*
  patella 77.36
    wedge 77.26
  pelvic 77.39
    wedge 77.29
  phalanges (foot) (hand) 77.39
    for repair of
      bunion - *see* Bunionectomy
      bunionette 77.54
      hallux valgus - *see* Bunionectomy
    wedge 77.29
      for repair of
        bunion - *see* Bunionectomy
        bunionette 77.54
        hallux valgus - *see* Bunionectomy
  radius 77.33
    wedge 77.23
  scapula 77.31
    wedge 77.21
  specified site NEC 77.39
    wedge 77.29
  tarsal 77.38
    wedge 77.28
  thorax (ribs) (sternum) 77.31
    wedge 77.21
  tibia 77.37
    wedge 77.27
  toe 77.39
    for repair of
      bunion - *see* Bunionectomy
      bunionette 77.54
      hallux valgus - *see* Bunionectomy
    wedge 77.29
      for repair of
        bunion - *see* Bunionectomy
        bunionette 77.54
        hallux valgus - *see* Bunionectomy
  ulna 77.33
    wedge 77.23
  vertebrae 77.39
    wedge 77.29
Otonecrectomy (inner ear) 20.79
Otoplasty (external) 18.79
  auditory canal or meatus 18.6
  auricle 18.79
  cartilage 18.79
    reconstruction 18.71
  prominent or protruding 18.5
Otoscopy 18.11
Outfolding, sclera, for buckling - *see also* Buckling, scleral 14.49
Outfracture, turbinates (nasal) 21.62
Output and clearance, circulatory 92.05
Overdistension, bladder (therapeutic) 96.25
Overlapping, sclera, for buckling - *see also* Buckling, scleral 14.49
Oversewing
  pleural bleb 32.21
  ulcer crater (peptic) 44.40
    duodenum 44.42
    stomach 44.41
Oxford operation (for urinary incontinence) 59.4
Oximetry
  fetal pulse 75.38
Oxygenation 93.96
  extracorporeal membrane (ECMO) 39.65
  hyperbaric 93.95
    wound 93.59
Oxygen therapy (catalytic) (pump) 93.96
  hyperbaric 93.95

P

Pacemaker
cardiac - *see also* Insertion, pacemaker, cardiac
intraoperative (temporary) 39.64
temporary (during and immediately following cardiac surgery) 39.64
Packing - *see also* Insertion, pack
auditory canal 96.11
nose, for epistaxis (anterior) 21.01
posterior (and anterior) 21.02
rectal 96.19
sella turcica 07.79
vaginal 96.14
Palatoplasty 27.69
for cleft palate 27.62
secondary or subsequent 27.63
Palatorrhaphy 27.61
for cleft palate 27.62
Pallidectomy 01.42
Pallidoansotomy 01.42
Pallidotomy 01.42
by stereotactic radiosurgery 92.32
cobalt 60 92.32
linear accelerator (LINAC) 92.31
multi-source 92.32
particle beam 92.33
particulate 92.33
radiosurgery NEC 92.39
single source photon 92.31
Panas operation (linear proctotomy) 48.0
Pancoast operation (division of trigeminal nerve at foramen ovale) 04.02
Pancreatectomy (total) (with synchronous duodenectomy) 52.6
partial NEC 52.59
distal (tail) (with part of body) 52.52
proximal (head) (with part of body) (with synchronous duodenectomy) 52.51
radical 52.53
subtotal 52.53
radical 52.7
subtotal 52.53
Pancreaticocystoduodenostomy 52.4
Pancreaticocystoenterostomy 52.4
Pancreaticocystogastrostomy 52.4
Pancreaticocystojejunostomy 52.4
Pancreaticoduodenectomy (total) 52.6
partial NEC 52.59
proximal 52.51
radical subtotal 52.53
radical (one-stage) (two-stage) 52.7
subtotal 52.53
Pancreaticoduodenostomy 52.96
Pancreaticoenterostomy 52.96
Pancreaticogastrostomy 52.96
Pancreaticoileostomy 52.96
Pancreaticojejunostomy 52.96
Pancreatoduodenectomy (total) 52.6
partial NEC 52.59
radical (one-stage) (two-stage) 52.7
subtotal 52.53
Pancreatogram 87.66
endoscopic retrograde (ERP) 52.13
Pancreatolithotomy 52.09
endoscopic 52.94
Pancreatotomy 52.09
Pancreolithotomy 52.09
endoscopic 52.94
Panendoscopy 57.32
specified site, other than bladder - *see* Endoscopy, by site
through artificial stoma 57.31
Panhysterectomy (abdominal) 68.49 (Revised)
laparoscopic 68.41 (New)
vaginal 68.59
laparoscopically assisted (LAVH) 68.51
Panniculectomy 86.83
Panniculotomy 86.83
Pantaloon operation (revision of gastric anastomosis) 44.5
Papillectomy, anal 49.39
endoscopic 49.31
Papillotomy (pancreas) 51.82
endoscopic 51.85
Paquin operation (ureteroneocystostomy) 56.74
Paracentesis
abdominal (percutaneous) 54.91
anterior chamber, eye 12.91
bladder 57.11
cornea 12.91
eye (anterior chamber) 12.91
thoracic, thoracis 34.91
tympanum 20.09
with intubation 20.01
Parasitology - *see* Examination, microscopic
Parathyroidectomy (partial) (subtotal) NEC 06.89
complete 06.81
ectopic 06.89
global removal 06.81
mediastinal 06.89
total 06.81
Parenteral nutrition, total 99.15
peripheral 99.15
Parotidectomy 26.30
complete 26.32
partial 26.31
radical 26.32
Partsch operation (marsupialization of dental cyst) 24.4
Passage - *see* Insertion and Intubation
Passage of sounds, urethra 58.6
Patch
blood, spinal (epidural) 03.95
graft - *see* Graft
spinal, blood (epidural) 03.95
subdural, brain 02.12
Patellapexy 78.46
Patellaplasty NEC 78.46
Patellectomy 77.96
partial 77.86
Pattee operation (auditory canal) 18.6
Pectenotomy - *see also* Sphincterotomy, anal 49.59
Pedicle flap - *see* Graft, skin, pedicle
Peet operation (splanchnic resection) 05.29
PEG (percutaneous endoscopic gastrostomy) 43.11
PEJ (percutaneous endoscopic jejunostomy) 46.32
Pelvectomy, kidney (partial) 55.4
Pelvimetry 88.25
gynecological 89.26
Pelviolithotomy 55.11
Pelvioplasty, kidney 55.87
Pelviostomy 55.12
closure 55.82
Pelviotomy 77.39
to assist delivery 73.94
Pelvi-ureteroplasty 55.87
Pemberton operation
osteotomy of ilium 77.39
rectum (mobilization and fixation for prolapse repair) 48.76
Penectomy 64.3
Pereyra operation (paraurethral suspension) 59.6
Perforation
stapes footplate 19.0
Perfusion NEC 39.97
carotid artery 39.97
coronary artery 39.97
for
chemotherapy NEC 99.25
hormone therapy NEC 99.24
head 39.97
hyperthermic (lymphatic), localized region or site 93.35
intestine (large) (local) 46.96
small 46.95
kidney, local 55.95
limb (lower) (upper) 39.97
liver, localized 50.93
neck 39.97
subarachnoid (spinal cord) (refrigerated saline) 03.92
total body 39.96
Pericardiectomy 37.31
Pericardiocentesis 37.0
Pericardiolysis 37.12
Pericardioplasty 37.49
Pericardiorrhaphy 37.49
Pericardiostomy (tube) 37.12
Pericardiotomy 37.12
Peridectomy 10.31
Perilimbal suction 89.11
Perimetry 95.05
Perineoplasty 71.79
Perineorrhaphy 71.71
obstetrical laceration (current) 75.69
Perineotomy (nonobstetrical) 71.09
to assist delivery - *see* Episiotomy
Periosteotomy - *see also* Incision, bone 77.10
facial bone 76.09
Perirectofistulectomy 48.93
Peritectomy 10.31
Peritomy 10.1
Peritoneocentesis 54.91
Peritoneoscopy 54.21
Peritoneotomy 54.19
Peritoneumectomy 54.4
Phacoemulsification (ultrasonic) (with aspiration) 13.41
Phacofragmentation (mechanical) (with aspiration) 13.43
posterior route 13.42
ultrasonic 13.41
Phalangectomy (partial) 77.89
claw toe 77.57
cockup toe 77.58
hammer toe 77.56
overlapping toe 77.58
total 77.99
Phalangization (fifth metacarpal) 82.81
Pharyngeal flap operation (cleft palate repair) 27.62
secondary or subsequent 27.63
Pharyngectomy (partial) 29.33
with laryngectomy 30.3
Pharyngogram 87.09
contrast 87.06
Pharyngolaryngectomy 30.3

Pharyngoplasty (with silastic implant) 29.4
for cleft palate 27.62
secondary or subsequent 27.63
Pharyngorrhaphy 29.51
for cleft palate 27.62
Pharyngoscopy 29.11
Pharyngotomy 29.0
Phenopeel (skin) 86.24
Phlebectomy 38.60
with
anastomosis 38.30
abdominal 38.37
head and neck NEC 38.32
intracranial NEC 38.31
lower limb 38.39
thoracic NEC 38.35
upper limb 38.33
graft replacement 38.40
abdominal 38.47
head and neck NEC 38.42
intracranial NEC 38.41
lower limb 38.49
thoracic NEC 38.45
upper limb 38.43
abdominal 38.67
head and neck NEC 38.62
intracranial NEC 38.61
lower limb 38.69
thoracic NEC 38.65
upper limb 38.63
varicose 38.50
abdominal 38.57
head and neck NEC 38.52
intracranial NEC 38.51
lower limb 38.59
thoracic NEC 38.55
upper limb 38.53
Phlebogoniostomy 12.52
Phlebography (contrast) (retrograde) 88.60
by radioisotope - *see* Scan, radioisotope, by site
adrenal 88.65
femoral 88.66
head 88.61
hepatic 88.64
impedance 88.68
intra-abdominal NEC 88.65
intrathoracic NEC 88.63
lower extremity NEC 88.66
neck 88.61
portal system 88.64
pulmonary 88.62
specified site NEC 88.67
vena cava (inferior) (superior) 88.51
Phleborrhaphy 39.32
Phlebotomy 38.99
Phonocardiogram, with ECG lead 89.55
Photochemotherapy NEC 99.83
extracorporeal 99.88
Photocoagulation
ciliary body 12.73
eye, eyeball 16.99
iris 12.41
macular hole - *see* Photocoagulation, retina
orbital lesion 16.92
retina
for
destruction of lesion 14.25
reattachment 14.55
repair of tear or defect 14.35
Photocoagulation *(Continued)*
retina *(Continued)*
laser (beam)
for
destruction of lesion 14.24
reattachment 14.54
repair of tear or defect 14.34
xenon arc
for
destruction of lesion 14.23
reattachment 14.53
repair of tear or defect 14.33
Photography 89.39
fundus 95.11
Photopheresis, therapeutic 99.88
Phototherapy NEC 99.83
newborn 99.83
ultraviolet 99.82
Phrenemphraxis 04.03
for collapse of lung 33.31
Phrenicectomy 04.03
for collapse of lung 33.31
Phrenicoexeresis 04.03
for collapse of lung 33.31
Phrenicotomy 04.03
for collapse of lung 33.31
Phrenicotripsy 04.03
for collapse of lung 33.31
Phrenoplasty 34.84
Physical medicine - *see* Therapy, physical
Physical therapy - *see* Therapy, physical
Physiotherapy, chest 93.99
PICC (peripherally inserted central catheter) 38.93
Piercing ear, external (pinna) 18.01
Pigmenting, skin 86.02
Pilojection (aneurysm) (Gallagher) 39.52
Pinealectomy (complete) (total) 07.54
partial 07.53
Pinealotomy (with drainage) 07.52
Pinning
bone - *see* Fixation, bone, internal
ear 18.5
Pinsker operation (obliteration of nasoseptal telangiectasia) 21.07
Piper operation (forceps) 72.6
Pirogoff operation (ankle amputation through malleoli of tibia and fibula) 84.14
Pituitectomy (complete) (total) - *see also* Hypophysectomy 07.69
Placentogram, placentography 88.46
with radioisotope (RISA) 92.17
Planing, skin 86.25
Plantation, tooth (bud) (germ) 23.5
prosthetic 23.6
Plasma exchange 99.07
Plasmapheresis, therapeutic 99.71
Plastic repair - *see* Repair, by site
Plasty - *see also* Repair, by site
bladder neck (V-Y) 57.85
skin (without graft) 86.89
subcutaneous tissue 86.89
Platelet inhibitor (GP IIB/IIIa inhibitor only), infusion 99.20
Plateletpheresis, therapeutic 99.74
Play
psychotherapy 94.36
therapy 93.81
Pleating
eye muscle 15.22
multiple (two or more muscles) 15.4
sclera, for buckling - *see also* Buckling, scleral 14.49
Plethysmogram (carotid) 89.58
air-filled (pneumatic) 89.58
capacitance 89.58
cerebral 89.58
differential 89.58
oculoplethysmogram 89.58
penile 89.58
photoelectric 89.58
regional 89.58
respiratory function measurement (body) 89.38
segmental 89.58
strain-gauge 89.58
thoracic impedance 89.38
venous occlusion 89.58
water-filled 89.58
Plethysmography
CaverMap™ 89.58 ◀
penile 89.58
Pleurectomy NEC 34.59
Pleurocentesis 34.91
Pleurodesis 34.6
chemical 34.92
with cancer chemotherapy substance 34.92 *[99.25]*
tetracycline 34.92 *[99.21]*
Pleurolysis (for collapse of lung) 33.39
Pleuropexy 34.99
Pleurosclerosis 34.6
chemical 34.92
with cancer chemotherapy substance 34.92 *[99.25]*
tetracycline 34.92 *[99.21]*
Pleurotomy 34.09
Plexectomy
choroid 02.14
hypogastric 05.24
Plication
aneurysm
heart 37.32
annulus, heart valve 35.33
bleb (emphysematous), lung 32.21
broad ligament 69.22
diaphragm (for hernia repair) (thoracic approach) (thoracoabdominal approach) 53.81
eye muscle (oblique) (rectus) 15.22
multiple (two or more muscles) 15.4
fascia 83.89
hand 82.89
inferior vena cava 38.7
intestine (jejunum) (Noble) 46.62
Kelly (-Stoeckel) (urethrovesical junction) 59.3
levator, for blepharoptosis 08.34
ligament - *see also* Arthroplasty 81.96
broad 69.22
round 69.22
uterosacral 69.22
mesentery 54.75
round ligament 69.22
sphincter, urinary bladder 57.85
stomach 44.69
laparoscopic 44.68
superior vena cava 38.7
tendon 83.85
hand 82.55
tricuspid valve (with repositioning) 35.14
ureter 56.89
urethra 58.49
urethrovesical junction 59.3
vein (peripheral) 39.59
vena cava (inferior) (superior) 38.7

Plication *(Continued)*
ventricle (heart)
aneurysm 37.32
Plicotomy, tympanum 20.23
Plombage, lung 33.39
Pneumocentesis 33.93
Pneumocisternogram 87.02
Pneumoencephalogram 87.01
Pneumogram, pneumography
extraperitoneal 88.15
mediastinal 87.33
orbit 87.14
pelvic 88.13
peritoneum NEC 88.13
presacral 88.15
retroperitoneum 88.15
Pneumogynecography 87.82
Pneumomediastinography 87.33
Pneumonectomy (complete) (extended) (radical) (standard) (total) (with mediastinal dissection) 32.5
partial
complete excision, one lobe 32.4
resection (wedge), one lobe 32.3
Pneumonolysis (for collapse of lung) 33.39
Pneumonotomy (with exploration) 33.1
Pneumoperitoneum (surgically-induced) 54.96
for collapse of lung 33.33
pelvic 88.12
Pneumothorax (artificial) (surgical) 33.32
intrapleural 33.32
Pneumoventriculogram 87.02
Politano-Leadbetter operation (ureteroneocystostomy) 56.74
Politzerization, Eustachian tube 20.8
Pollicization (with carry over of nerves and blood supply) 82.61
Polya operation (gastrectomy) 43.7
Polypectomy - *see also* Excision, lesion, by site
esophageal 42.32
endoscopic 42.33
gastric (endoscopic) 43.41
large intestine (colon) 45.42
nasal 21.31
rectum (endoscopic) 48.36
Polysomnogram 89.17
Pomeroy operation (ligation and division of fallopian tubes) 66.32
Poncet operation
lengthening of Achilles tendon 83.85
urethrostomy, perineal 58.0
Porro operation (cesarean section) 74.99
Portoenterostomy (Kasai) 51.37
Positrocephalogram 92.11
Positron emission tomography (PET) - *see* Scan, radioisotope
Postmortem examination 89.8
Potts-Smith operation (descending aorta-left pulmonary artery anastomosis) 39.0
Poudrage
intrapericardial 36.39
pleural 34.6
PPN (peripheral parenteral nutrition) 99.15
Preparation (cutting), pedicle (flap) graft 86.71
Preputiotomy 64.91
Prescription for glasses 95.31
Pressure support
ventilation [PSV] - *see* category 96.7
Pressurized
graft treatment 00.16
Printen and Mason operation (high gastric bypass) 44.31
Probing
canaliculus, lacrimal (with irrigation) 09.42
lacrimal
canaliculi 09.42
punctum (with irrigation) 09.41
nasolacrimal duct (with irrigation) 09.43
with insertion of tube or stent 09.44
salivary duct (for dilation of duct) (for removal of calculus) 26.91
with incision 26.0
Procedure - *see also* specific procedure
diagnostic NEC
abdomen (region) 54.29
adenoid 28.19
adrenal gland 07.19
alveolus 24.19
amnion 75.35
anterior chamber, eye 12.29
anus 49.29
appendix 45.28
biliary tract 51.19
bladder 57.39
blood vessel (any site) 38.29
bone 78.80
carpal, metacarpal 78.84
clavicle 78.81
facial 76.19
femur 78.85
fibula 78.87
humerus 78.82
marrow 41.38
patella 78.86
pelvic 78.89
phalanges (foot) (hand) 78.89
radius 78.83
scapula 78.81
specified site NEC 78.89
tarsal, metatarsal 78.88
thorax (ribs) (sternum) 78.81
tibia 78.87
ulna 78.83
vertebrae 78.89
brain 01.18
breast 85.19
bronchus 33.29
buccal 27.24
bursa 83.29
canthus 08.19
cecum 45.28
cerebral meninges 01.18
cervix 67.19
chest wall 34.28
choroid 14.19
ciliary body 12.29
clitoris 71.19
colon 45.28
conjunctiva 10.29
cornea 11.29
cul-de-sac 70.29
dental 24.19
diaphragm 34.28
duodenum 45.19
ear
external 18.19
inner and middle 20.39
epididymis 63.09
esophagus 42.29
eustachian tube 20.39
extraocular muscle or tendon 15.09
Procedure *(Continued)*
diagnostic NEC *(Continued)*
eye 16.29
anterior chamber 12.29
posterior chamber 14.19
eyeball 16.29
eyelid 08.19
fallopian tube 66.19
fascia (any site) 83.29
fetus 75.35
gallbladder 51.19
ganglion (cranial) (peripheral) 04.19
sympathetic 05.19
gastric 44.19
globus pallidus 01.18
gum 24.19
heart 37.29
hepatic 50.19
hypophysis 07.19
ileum 45.19
intestine 45.29
large 45.28
small 45.19
iris 12.29
jejunum 45.19
joint (capsule) (ligament) (structure) NEC 81.98
facial 76.19
kidney 55.29
labia 71.19
lacrimal (system) 09.19
large intestine 45.28
larynx 31.48
ligament 81.98
uterine 68.19
liver 50.19
lung 33.29
lymphatic structure (channel) (gland) (node) (vessel) 40.19
mediastinum 34.29
meninges (cerebral) 01.18
spinal 03.39
mouth 27.29
muscle 83.29
extraocular (oblique) (rectus) 15.09
papillary (heart) 37.29
nail 86.19
nasopharynx 29.19
nerve (cranial) (peripheral) NEC 04.19
sympathetic 05.19
nipple 85.19
nose, nasal 21.29
sinus 22.19
ocular 16.29
muscle 15.09
omentum 54.29
ophthalmologic 16.29
oral (cavity) 27.29
orbit 16.29
orthodontic 24.19
ovary 65.19
laparoscopic 65.14
palate 27.29
pancreas 52.19
papillary muscle (heart) 37.29
parathyroid gland 06.19
penis 64.19
perianal tissue 49.29
pericardium 37.29
periprostatic tissue 60.18
perirectal tissue 48.29
perirenal tissue 59.29
peritoneum 54.29

Procedure *(Continued)*
diagnostic NEC *(Continued)*
periurethral tissue 58.29
perivesical tissue 59.29
pharynx 29.19
pineal gland 07.19
pituitary gland 07.19
pleura 34.28
posterior chamber, eye 14.19
prostate 60.18
pulmonary 33.29
rectosigmoid 48.29
rectum 48.29
renal 55.29
respiratory 33.29
retina 14.19
retroperitoneum 59.29
salivary gland or duct 26.19
sclera 12.29
scrotum 61.19
seminal vesicle 60.19
sigmoid 45.28
sinus, nasal 22.19
skin 86.19
skull 01.19
soft tissue 83.29
spermatic cord 63.09
sphincter of Oddi 51.19
spine, spinal (canal) (cord) (meninges) (structure) 03.39
spleen 41.39
stomach 44.19
subcutaneous tissue 86.19
sympathetic nerve 05.19
tarsus 09.19
tendon NEC 83.29
extraocular 15.09
testicle 62.19
thalamus 01.18
thoracic duct 40.19
thorax 34.28
thymus 07.19
thyroid gland 06.19
tongue 25.09
tonsils 28.19
tooth 24.19
trachea 31.49
tunica vaginalis 61.19
ureter 56.39
urethra 58.29
uterus and supporting structures 68.19
uvula 27.29
vagina 70.29
vas deferens 63.09
vesical 57.39
vessel (blood) (any site) 38.2
vitreous 14.19
vulva 71.19
fistulizing, sclera NEC 12.69
miscellaneous (nonoperative) NEC 99.99
respiratory (nonoperative) NEC 93.99
surgical - *see* Operation
Proctectasis 96.22
Proctectomy (partial) - *see also* Resection, rectum 48.69
abdominoperineal 48.5
complete (Miles) (Rankin) 48.5
pull-through 48.49
Proctoclysis 96.37
Proctolysis 48.99
Proctopexy (Delorme) 48.76
abdominal (Ripstein) 48.75
Proctoplasty 48.79
Proctorrhaphy 48.71
Proctoscopy 48.23
with biopsy 48.24
through stoma (artificial) 48.22
transabdominal approach 48.21
Proctosigmoidectomy - *see also* Resection, rectum 48.69
Proctosigmoidopexy 48.76
Proctosigmoidoscopy (rigid) 48.23
with biopsy 48.24
flexible 45.24
through stoma (artificial) 48.22
transabdominal approach 48.21
Proctostomy 48.1
Proctotomy (decompression) (linear) 48.0
Production - *see also* Formation *and* Creation
atrial septal defect 35.42
subcutaneous tunnel for esophageal anastomosis 42.86
with anastomosis - *see* Anastomosis, esophagus, antesternal
Prognathic recession 76.64
Prophylaxis, dental (scaling) (polishing) 96.54
Prostatectomy (complete) (partial) NEC 60.69
loop 60.29
perineal 60.62
radical (any approach) 60.5
retropubic (punch) (transcapsular) 60.4
suprapubic (punch) (transvesical) 60.3
transcapsular NEC 60.69
retropubic 60.4
transperineal 60.62
transurethral 60.29
ablation (contact) (noncontact) by laser 60.21
electrovaporization 60.29
enucleative 60.29
resection of prostate (TURP) 60.29
ultrasound guided, laser induced (TULIP) 60.21
transvesical punch (suprapubic) 60.3
Prostatocystotomy 60.0
Prostatolithotomy 60.0
Prostatotomy (perineal) 60.0
Prostatovesiculectomy 60.5
Protection (of)
individual from his surroundings 99.84
surroundings from individual 99.84
Psychoanalysis 94.31
Psychodrama 94.43
Psychotherapy NEC 94.39
biofeedback 94.39
exploratory verbal 94.37
group 94.44
for psychosexual dysfunctions 94.41
play 94.36
psychosexual dysfunctions 94.34
supportive verbal 94.38
PTCA (percutaneous transluminal coronary angioplasty) - *see* Angioplasty, balloon, coronary
Ptyalectasis 26.91
Ptyalithotomy 26.0
Ptyalolithotomy 26.0
Pubiotomy 77.39
assisting delivery 73.94
Pubococcygeoplasty 59.71
Puestow operation (pancreaticojejunostomy) 52.96
Pull-through
abdomino-anal 48.49
abdominoperineal 48.49
Duhamel type 48.65
endorectal 48.41
Pulmowrap 93.99
Pulpectomy - *see also* Therapy, root canal 23.70
Pulpotomy - *see also* Therapy, root canal 23.70
Pump-oxygenator, for extracorporeal circulation 39.61
percutaneous 39.66
Punch
operation
bladder neck, transurethral 57.49
prostate - *see* Prostatectomy
resection, vocal cords 30.22
Puncture
antrum (nasal) (bilateral) (unilateral) 22.01
artery NEC 38.98
for
arteriography - *see also* Arteriography 88.40
for
coronary arteriography - *see also* Arteriography, coronary 88.57
percutaneous vascular closure - *omit code*
bladder, suprapubic (for drainage) NEC 57.18
needle 57.11
percutaneous (suprapubic) 57.17
bursa 83.94
hand 82.92
cisternal 01.01
with contrast media 87.02
cranial 01.09
with contrast media 87.02
craniobuccal pouch 07.72
craniopharyngioma 07.72
fallopian tube 66.91
fontanel, anterior 01.09
heart 37.0
for intracardiac injection 37.92
hypophysis 07.72
iris 12.12
joint 81.91
kidney (percutaneous) 55.92
larynx 31.98
lumbar (diagnostic) (removal of dye) 03.31
lung (for aspiration) 33.93
nasal sinus 22.01
pericardium 37.0
pituitary gland 07.72
pleural cavity 34.91
Rathke's pouch 07.72
spinal 03.31
spleen 41.1
for biopsy 41.32
sternal (for bone marrow biopsy) 41.31
donor for bone marrow transplant 41.91
vein NEC 38.99
for
phlebography - *see also* Phlebography 88.60
transfusion - *see* Transfusion
ventricular shunt tubing 01.02
Pupillotomy 12.35

Push-back operation (cleft palate repair) 27.62
Putti-Platt operation (capsulorrhaphy of shoulder for recurrent dislocation) 81.82
pVAD (percutaneous ventricular assist device) 37.68
Pyelogram (intravenous) 87.73
  infusion (continuous) (diuretic) 87.73
  percutaneous 87.75
  retrograde 87.74
Pyeloileostomy 56.71
Pyelolithotomy 55.11
Pyeloplasty 55.87
Pyelorrhaphy 55.81
Pyeloscopy 55.22
Pyelostolithotomy, percutaneous 55.03
Pyelostomy 55.12
  closure 55.82
Pyelotomy 55.11
Pyeloureteroplasty 55.87
Pylorectomy 43.6
Pyloroduodenotomy - *see* category 44.2
Pyloromyotomy (Ramstedt) (with wedge resection) 43.3
Pyloroplasty (Finney) (Heineke-Mikulicz) 44.29
Pyloroplasty *(Continued)*
  dilation, endoscopic 44.22
    by incision 44.21
  not elsewhere classified 44.29
  revision 44.29
Pylorostomy - *see* Gastrostomy

Quadrant resection of breast 85.22
Quadricepsplasty (Thompson) 83.86
Quarantine 99.84
Quenuthoracoplasty 77.31
Quotient, respiratory 89.38

R

Rachicentesis 03.31
Rachitomy 03.09
Radiation therapy - *see also* Therapy, radiation
  teleradiotherapy - *see* Teleradiotherapy
Radical neck dissection - *see* Dissection, neck
Radicotomy 03.1
Radiculectomy 03.1
Radiculotomy 03.1
Radiography (diagnostic) **NEC** 88.39
  abdomen, abdominal (flat plate) NEC 88.19
    wall (soft tissue) NEC 88.09
  adenoid 87.09
  ankle (skeletal) 88.28
    soft tissue 88.37
  bone survey 88.31
  bronchus 87.49
  chest (routine) 87.44
    wall NEC 87.39
  clavicle 87.43
  computer assisted surgery (CAS) with fluoroscopy 00.33
  contrast (air) (gas) (radio-opaque substance) NEC
    abdominal wall 88.03
    arteries (by fluoroscopy) - *see* Arteriography
    bile ducts NEC 87.54
    bladder NEC 87.77
    brain 87.02
    breast 87.35
    bronchus NEC (transcricoid) 87.32
      endotracheal 87.31
    epididymis 87.93
    esophagus 87.61
    fallopian tubes
      gas 87.82
      opaque dye 87.83
    fistula (sinus tract) - *see also* Radiography, contrast, by site
      abdominal wall 88.03
      chest wall 87.38
    gallbladder NEC 87.59
    intervertebral disc(s) 87.21
    joints 88.32
    larynx 87.07
    lymph - *see* Lymphangiogram
    mammary ducts 87.35
    mediastinum 87.33
    nasal sinuses 87.15
    nasolacrimal ducts 87.05
    nasopharynx 87.06
    orbit 87.14
    pancreas 87.66
    pelvis
      gas 88.12
      opaque dye 88.11
    peritoneum NEC 88.13
    retroperitoneum NEC 88.15
    seminal vesicles 87.91
    sinus tract - *see also* Radiography, contrast, by site
      abdominal wall 88.03
      chest wall 87.38
      nose 87.15
    skull 87.02
    spinal disc(s) 87.21
    trachea 87.32
    uterus
      gas 87.82
      opaque dye 87.83

Radiography NEC *(Continued)*
  contrast *(Continued)*
    vas deferens 87.94
    veins (by fluoroscopy) - *see* Phlebography
    vena cava (inferior) (superior) 88.51
  dental NEC 87.12
  diaphragm 87.49
  digestive tract NEC 87.69
    barium swallow 87.61
    lower GI series 87.64
    small bowel series 87.63
    upper GI series 87.62
  elbow (skeletal) 88.22
    soft tissue 88.35
  epididymis NEC 87.95
  esophagus 87.69
    barium-swallow 87.61
  eye 95.14
  face, head, and neck 87.09
  facial bones 87.16
  fallopian tubes 87.85
  foot 88.28
  forearm (skeletal) 88.22
    soft tissue 88.35
  frontal area, facial 87.16
  genital organs
    female NEC 87.89
    male NEC 87.99
  hand (skeletal) 88.23
    soft tissue 88.35
  head NEC 87.09
  heart 87.49
  hip (skeletal) 88.26
    soft tissue 88.37
  intestine NEC 87.65
  kidney-ureter-bladder (KUB) 87.79
  knee (skeletal) 88.27
    soft tissue 88.37
  KUB (kidney-ureter-bladder) 87.79
  larynx 87.09
  lower leg (skeletal) 88.27
    soft tissue 88.37
  lower limb (skeletal) NEC 88.29
    soft tissue NEC 88.37
  lung 87.49
  mandible 87.16
  maxilla 87.16
  mediastinum 87.49
  nasal sinuses 87.16
  nasolacrimal duct 87.09
  nasopharynx 87.09
  neck NEC 87.09
  nose 87.16
  orbit 87.16
  pelvis (skeletal) 88.26
    pelvimetry 88.25
    soft tissue 88.19
  prostate NEC 87.92
  retroperitoneum NEC 88.16
  ribs 87.43
  root canal 87.12
  salivary gland 87.09
  seminal vesicles NEC 87.92
  shoulder (skeletal) 88.21
    soft tissue 88.35
  skeletal NEC 88.33
    series (whole or complete) 88.31
  skull (lateral, sagittal, or tangential projection) NEC 87.17
  spine NEC 87.29
    cervical 87.22
    lumbosacral 87.24
    sacrococcygeal 87.24
    thoracic 87.23

Radiography NEC *(Continued)*
  sternum 87.43
  supraorbital area 87.16
  symphysis menti 87.16
  teeth NEC 87.12
    full-mouth 87.11
  thigh (skeletal) 88.27
    soft tissue 88.37
  thyroid region 87.09
  tonsils and adenoids 87.09
  trachea 87.49
  ultrasonic - *see* Ultrasonography
  upper arm (skeletal) 88.21
    soft tissue 88.35
  upper limb (skeletal) NEC 88.24
    soft tissue NEC 88.35
  urinary system NEC 87.79
  uterus NEC 87.85
    gravid 87.81
  uvula 87.09
  vas deferens NEC 87.95
  wrist 88.23
  zygomaticomaxillary complex 87.16
Radioimmunotherapy 92.28
Radioisotope
  scanning - *see* Scan, radioisotope
  therapy - *see* Therapy, radioisotope
Radiology
  diagnostic - *see* Radiography
  therapeutic - *see* Therapy, radiation
Radiosurgery, stereotactic 92.30
  cobalt 60 92.32
  linear accelerator (LINAC) 92.31
  multi-source 92.32
  particle beam 92.33
  particulate 92.33
  radiosurgery NEC 92.39
  single source photon 92.31
Raising, pedicle graft 86.71
Ramadier operation (intrapetrosal drainage) 20.22
Ramisection (sympathetic) 05.0
Ramstedt operation (pyloromyotomy) (with wedge resection) 43.3
Range of motion testing 93.05
Rankin operation
  exteriorization of intestine 46.03
  proctectomy (complete) 48.5
Rashkind operation (balloon septostomy) 35.41
Rastelli operation (creation of conduit between right ventricle and pulmonary artery) 35.92
  in repair of
    pulmonary artery atresia 35.92
    transposition of great vessels 35.92
    truncus arteriosus 35.83
Raz-Pereyra procedure (bladder neck suspension) 59.79
RCSA (radical cryosurgical ablation) of prostate 60.62
Readjustment - *see* Adjustment
Reamputation, stump 84.3
Reanastomosis - *see* Anastomosis
Reattachment
  amputated ear 18.72
  ankle 84.27
  arm (upper) NEC 84.24
  choroid and retina NEC 14.59
    by
      cryotherapy 14.52
      diathermy 14.51
      electrocoagulation 14.51
      photocoagulation 14.55
        laser 14.54
        xenon arc 14.53

◀ New ⟸ Revised

Reattachment *(Continued)*
ear (amputated) 18.72
extremity 84.29
ankle 84.27
arm (upper) NEC 84.24
fingers, except thumb 84.22
thumb 84.21
foot 84.26
forearm 84.23
hand 84.23
leg (lower) NEC 84.27
thigh 84.28
thumb 84.21
toe 84.25
wrist 84.23
finger 84.22
thumb 84.21
foot 84.26
forearm 84.23
hand 84.23
joint capsule - *see also* Arthroplasty 81.96
leg (lower) NEC 84.27
ligament - *see also* Arthroplasty
uterosacral 69.22
muscle 83.74
hand 82.54
papillary (heart) 35.31
nerve (peripheral) 04.79
nose (amputated) 21.89
papillary muscle (heart) 35.31
penis (amputated) 64.45
retina (and choroid) NEC 14.59
by
cryotherapy 14.52
diathermy 14.51
electrocoagulation 14.51
photocoagulation 14.55
laser 14.54
xenon arc 14.53
tendon (to tendon) 83.73
hand 82.53
to skeletal attachment 83.88
hand 82.85
thigh 84.28
thumb 84.21
toe 84.25
tooth 23.5
uterosacral ligament(s) 69.22
vessels (peripheral) 39.59
renal, aberrant 39.55
wrist 84.23
Recession
extraocular muscle 15.11
multiple (two or more muscles) (with advancement or resection) 15.3
gastrocnemius tendon (Strayer operation) 83.72
levator palpebrae (superioris) muscle 08.38
prognathic jaw 76.64
tendon 83.72
hand 82.52
Reclosure - *see also* Closure
disrupted abdominal wall (postoperative) 54.61
Reconstruction (plastic) - *see also* Construction and Repair, by site
alveolus, alveolar (process) (ridge) (with graft or implant) 24.5
artery (graft) - *see* Graft, artery
artificial stoma, intestine 46.40
auditory canal (external) 18.6
auricle (ear) 18.71

Reconstruction *(Continued)*
bladder 57.87
with
ileum 57.87 *[45.51]*
sigmoid 57.87 *[45.52]*
bone, except facial - *see also* Osteoplasty 78.40
facial NEC 76.46
with total ostectomy 76.44
mandible 76.43
with total mandibulectomy 76.41
breast, total 85.7
bronchus 33.48
canthus (lateral) 08.59
cardiac annulus 35.33
chest wall (mesh) (silastic) 34.79
cleft lip 27.54
conjunctival cul-de-sac 10.43
with graft (buccal mucous membrane) (free) 10.42
cornea NEC 11.79
diaphragm 34.84
ear (external) (auricle) 18.71
external auditory canal 18.6
meatus (new) (osseous skin-lined) 18.6
ossicles 19.3
prominent or protruding 18.5
eyebrow 08.70
eyelid 08.70
with graft or flap 08.69
hair follicle 08.63
mucous membrane 08.62
skin 08.61
tarsoconjunctival (one-stage) (two-stage) 08.64
full-thickness 08.74
involving lid margin 08.73
partial-thickness 08.72
involving lid margin 08.71
eye socket 16.64
with graft 16.63
fallopian tube 66.79
foot and toes (with fixation device) 81.57
with prosthetic implant 81.57
frontonasal duct 22.79
hip (total) (with prosthesis) 81.51
intraoral 27.59
joint - *see* Arthroplasty
lymphatic (by transplantation) 40.9
mandible 76.43
with total mandibulectomy 76.41
mastoid cavity 19.9
mouth 27.59
nipple NEC 85.87
nose (total) (with arm flap) (with forehead flap) 21.83
ossicles (graft) (prosthesis) NEC 19.3
with
stapedectomy 19.19
tympanoplasty 19.53
pelvic floor 71.79
penis (rib graft) (skin graft) (myocutaneous flap) 64.44
pharynx 29.4
scrotum (with pedicle flap) (with rotational flap) 61.49
skin (plastic) (without graft) NEC 86.89
with graft - *see* Graft, skin
subcutaneous tissue (plastic) (without skin graft) NEC 86.89
with graft - *see* Graft, skin

Reconstruction *(Continued)*
tendon pulley (with graft) (with local tissue) 83.83
for opponensplasty 82.71
hand 82.71
thumb (osteoplastic) (with bone graft) (with skin graft) 82.69
trachea (with graft) 31.75
umbilicus 53.49
ureteropelvic junction 55.87
urethra 58.46
vagina 70.62
vas deferens, surgically divided 63.82
Recontour, gingiva 24.2
Recreational therapy 93.81
Rectectomy - *see also* Resection, rectum 48.69
Rectopexy (Delorme) 48.76
abdominal (Ripstein) 48.75
Rectoplasty 48.79
Rectorectostomy 48.74
Rectorrhaphy 48.71
Rectosigmoidectomy - *see also* Resection, rectum 48.69
transsacral 48.61
Rectosigmoidostomy 45.94
Rectostomy 48.1
closure 48.72
Red cell survival studies 92.05
Reduction – *see also* Excision, by site
adipose tissue 86.83
batwing arms 86.83
breast (bilateral) 85.32
unilateral 85.31
bulbous tuberosities (mandible) (maxilla) (fibrous) (osseous) 24.31
buttocks 86.83
diastasis, ankle mortise (closed) 79.77
open 79.87
dislocation (of joint) (manipulation) (with cast) (with splint) (with traction device) (closed) 79.70
with fracture - *see* Reduction, fracture, by site
ankle (closed) 79.77
open 79.87
elbow (closed) 79.72
open 79.82
finger (closed) 79.74
open 79.84
foot (closed) 79.78
open 79.88
hand (closed) 79.74
open 79.84
hip (closed) 79.75
open 79.85
knee (closed) 79.76
open 79.86
open (with external fixation) (with internal fixation) 79.80
specified site NEC 79.89
shoulder (closed) 79.71
open 79.81
specified site (closed) NEC 79.79
open 79.89
temporomandibular (closed) 76.93
open 76.94
toe (closed) 79.78
open 79.88
wrist (closed) 79.73
open 79.83
elephantiasis, scrotum 61.3
epistaxis - *see also* Control, epistaxis 21.00

Reduction *(Continued)*
fracture (bone) (with cast) (with splint) (with traction device) (closed) 79.00
with internal fixation 79.10
alveolar process (with stabilization of teeth)
mandible (closed) 76.75
open 76.77
maxilla (closed) 76.73
open 76.77
open 76.77
ankle - *see* Reduction, fracture, leg
arm (closed) NEC 79.02
with internal fixation 79.12
open 79.22
with internal fixation 79.32
blow-out - *see* Reduction, fracture, orbit
carpal, metacarpal (closed) 79.03
with internal fixation 79.13
open 79.23
with internal fixation 79.33
epiphysis - *see* Reduction, separation
facial (bone) NEC 76.70
closed 76.78
open 76.79
femur (closed) 79.05
with internal fixation 79.15
open 79.25
with internal fixation 79.35
fibula (closed) 79.06
with internal fixation 79.16
open 79.26
with internal fixation 79.36
foot (closed) NEC 79.07
with internal fixation 79.17
open 79.27
with internal fixation 79.37
hand (closed) NEC 79.03
with internal fixation 79.13
open 79.23
with internal fixation 79.33
humerus (closed) 79.01
with internal fixation 79.11
open 79.21
with internal fixation 79.31
jaw (lower) - *see also* Reduction, fracture, mandible
upper - *see* Reduction, fracture, maxilla
larynx 31.64
leg (closed) NEC 79.06
with internal fixation 79.16
open 79.26
with internal fixation 79.36
malar (closed) 76.71
open 76.72
mandible (with dental wiring) (closed) 76.75
open 76.76
maxilla (with dental wiring) (closed) 76.73
open 76.74
nasal (closed) 21.71
open 21.72
open 79.20
with internal fixation 79.30
specified site NEC 79.29
with internal fixation 79.39
orbit (rim) (wall) (closed) 76.78
open 76.79
patella (open) (with internal fixation) 79.36

Reduction *(Continued)*
fracture *(Continued)*
phalanges
foot (closed) 79.08
with internal fixation 79.18
open 79.28
with internal fixation 79.38
hand (closed) 79.04
with internal fixation 79.14
open 79.24
with internal fixation 79.34
radius (closed) 79.02
with internal fixation 79.12
open 79.22
with internal fixation 79.32
skull 02.02
specified site (closed) NEC 79.09
with internal fixation 79.19
open 79.29
with internal fixation 79.39
spine 03.53
tarsal, metatarsal (closed) 79.07
with internal fixation 79.17
open 79.27
with internal fixation 79.37
tibia (closed) 79.06
with internal fixation 79.16
open 79.26
with internal fixation 79.36
ulna (closed) 79.02
with internal fixation 79.12
open 79.22
with internal fixation 79.32
vertebra 03.53
zygoma, zygomatic arch (closed) 76.71
open 76.72
fracture dislocation - *see* Reduction, fracture
heart volume 37.35
hemorrhoids (manual) 49.41
hernia - *see also* Repair, hernia
manual 96.27
intussusception (open) 46.80
with
fluoroscopy 96.29
ionizing radiation enema 96.29
ultrasonography guidance 96.29
hydrostatic 96.29
large intestine 46.82
endoscopic (balloon) 46.85
pneumatic 96.29
small intestine 46.81
lung volume 32.22
biologic lung volume reduction (BLVR) – *see* category 33.7 ◄
malrotation, intestine (manual) (surgical) 46.80
large 46.82
endoscopic (balloon) 46.85
small 46.81
mammoplasty (bilateral) 85.32
unilateral 85.31
prolapse
anus (operative) 49.94
colostomy (manual) 96.28
enterostomy (manual) 96.28
ileostomy (manual) 96.28
rectum (manual) 96.26
uterus
by pessary 96.18
surgical 69.22
ptosis overcorrection 08.37
retroversion, uterus by pessary 96.18

Reduction *(Continued)*
separation, epiphysis (with internal fixation) (closed) 79.40
femur (closed) 79.45
open 79.55
fibula (closed) 79.46
open 79.56
humerus (closed) 79.41
open 79.51
open 79.50
specified site (closed) NEC - *see also* category 79.4
open - *see* category 79.5
tibia (closed) 79.46
open 79.56
size
abdominal wall (adipose) (pendulous) 86.83
arms (adipose) (batwing) 86.83
breast (bilateral) 85.32
unilateral 85.31
buttocks (adipose) 86.83
finger (macrodactyly repair) 82.83
skin 86.83
subcutaneous tissue 86.83
thighs (adipose) 86.83
torsion
intestine (manual) (surgical) 46.80
large 46.82
endoscopic (balloon) 46.85
small 46.81
kidney pedicle 55.84
omentum 54.74
spermatic cord 63.52
with orchiopexy 62.5
testis 63.52
with orchiopexy 62.5
uterus NEC 69.98
gravid 75.99
ventricular 37.35
volvulus
intestine 46.80
large 46.82
endoscopic (balloon) 46.85
small 46.81
stomach 44.92
Reefing, joint capsule - *see also* Arthroplasty 81.96
Re-entry operation (aorta) 39.54
Re-establishment, continuity - *see also* Anastomosis
bowel 46.50
fallopian tube 66.79
vas deferens 63.82
Referral (for)
psychiatric aftercare (halfway house) (outpatient clinic) 94.52
psychotherapy 94.51
rehabilitation
alcoholism 94.53
drug addiction 94.54
psychologic NEC 94.59
vocational 94.55
Reformation
cardiac pacemaker pocket, new site (skin) (subcutaneous) 37.79
cardioverter/defibrillator (automatic) pocket, new site (skin) (subcutaneous) 37.99
chamber of eye 12.99
Refracture
bone (for faulty union) - *see also* Osteoclasis 78.70
nasal bones 21.88

Refusion
spinal, NOS 81.30
atlas-axis (anterior) (transoral) (posterior) 81.31
cervical (C2 level or below) NEC 81.32
anterior (interbody), anterolateral technique 81.32
C1-C2 level (anterior) (posterior) 81.31
posterior (interbody), posterolateral technique 81.33
craniocervical (anterior) (transoral) (posterior) 81.31
dorsal, dorsolumbar NEC 81.35
anterior (interbody), anterolateral technique 81.34
posterior (interbody), posterolateral technique 81.35
lumbar, lumbosacral NEC 81.38
anterior (interbody), anterolateral technique 81.36
anterior lumbar interbody fusion (ALIF) 81.36
lateral transverse process technique 81.37
posterior lumbar interbody fusion (PLIF) 81.38
posterior (interbody), posterolateral technique 81.38
transforaminal lumbar interbody fusion (TLIF) 81.38
number of vertebrae - *see* codes 81.62–81.64
occiput–C2 (anterior) (transoral) (posterior) 81.31
refusion NEC 81.39

Note: Also use either 81.62, 81.63, or 81.64 as an additional code to show the total number of vertebrae fused

Regional blood flow study 92.05
Regulation, menstrual 69.6
Rehabilitation programs NEC 93.89
alcohol 94.61
with detoxification 94.63
combined alcohol and drug 94.67
with detoxification 94.69
drug 94.64
with detoxification 94.66
combined drug and alcohol 94.67
with detoxification 94.69
sheltered employment 93.85
vocational 93.85
Reimplantation
adrenal tissue (heterotopic) (orthotopic) 07.45
artery 39.59
renal, aberrant 39.55
bile ducts following excision of ampulla of Vater 51.62
extremity - *see* Reattachment, extremity
fallopian tube into uterus 66.74
kidney 55.61
lung 33.5
ovary 65.72
laparoscopic 65.75
pancreatic tissue 52.81
parathyroid tissue (heterotopic) (orthotopic) 06.95
pulmonary artery for hemitruncus repair 35.83
renal vessel, aberrant 39.55

Reimplantation *(Continued)*
testis in scrotum 62.5
thyroid tissue (heterotopic) (orthotopic) 06.94
tooth 23.5
ureter into bladder 56.74
Reinforcement - *see also* Repair, by site
sclera NEC 12.88
with graft 12.87
Reinsertion - *see also* Insertion or Revision
cystostomy tube 59.94
fixation device (internal) - *see also* Fixation, bone, internal 78.50
heart valve (prosthetic) 35.95
Holter (-Spitz) valve 02.42
implant (expelled) (extruded)
eyeball (with conjunctival graft) 16.62
orbital 16.62
nephrostomy tube 55.93
pyelostomy tube 55.94
ureteral stent (transurethral) 59.8
with ureterotomy 59.8 *[56.2]*
ureterostomy tube 59.93
valve
heart (prosthetic) 35.95
ventricular (cerebral) 02.42
Relaxation - *see also* Release training 94.33
Release
carpal tunnel (for nerve decompression) 04.43
celiac artery axis 39.91
central slip, extensor tendon, hand (mallet finger repair) 82.84
chordee 64.42
clubfoot NEC 83.84
de Quervain's tenosynovitis 82.01
Dupuytren's contracture (by palmar fasciectomy) 82.35
by fasciotomy (subcutaneous) 82.12
with excision 82.35
Fowler (mallet finger repair) 82.84
joint (capsule) (adherent) (constrictive) - *see also* Division, joint capsule 80.40
laryngeal 31.92
ligament - *see also* Division, ligament 80.40
median arcuate 39.91
median arcuate ligament 39.91
muscle (division) 83.19
hand 82.19
nerve (peripheral) NEC 04.49
cranial NEC 04.42
trigeminal 04.41
pressure, intraocular 12.79
scar tissue
skin 86.84
stoma - *see* Revision, stoma
tarsal tunnel 04.44
tendon 83.13
hand 82.11
extensor, central slip (mallet finger repair) 82.84
sheath 83.01
hand 82.01
tenosynovitis 83.01
abductor pollicis longus 82.01
de Quervain's 82.01
external pollicis brevis 82.01
hand 82.01
torsion
intestine 46.80
large 46.82
endoscopic (balloon) 46.85
small 46.81

Release *(Continued)*
torsion *(Continued)*
kidney pedicle 55.84
ovary 65.95
testes 63.52
transverse carpal ligament (for nerve decompression) 04.43
trigger finger or thumb 82.01
urethral stricture 58.5
Volkmann's contracture
excision of scar, muscle 83.32
fasciotomy 83.14
muscle transplantation 83.77
web contracture (skin) 86.84
Relief - *see* Release
Relocation - *see also* Revision
cardiac device (CRT-D) (CRT-P) (defibrillator) (pacemaker) pocket, new site (skin) (subcutaneous) 37.79
CRT-D pocket 37.79
CRT-P pocket 37.79
subcutaneous device pocket NEC 86.09
Remobilization
joint 93.16
stapes 19.0
Remodel
ventricle 37.35
Removal - *see also* Excision
Abrams bar (chest wall) 34.01
abscess - *see* Incision, by site
adenoid tag(s) 28.6
anal sphincter
with revision 49.75
without revision 49.76
arch bars (orthodontic) 24.8
immobilization device 97.33
arterial graft or prosthesis 39.49
arteriovenous shunt (device) 39.43
with creation of new shunt 39.42
Barton's tongs (skull) 02.95
with synchronous replacement 02.94
bladder sphincter, artificial 58.99
with replacement 58.93
blood clot - *see also* Incision, by site
bladder (by incision) 57.19
without incision 57.0
kidney (without incision) 56.0
by incision 55.01
ureter
by incision 56.2
bone fragment (chip) - *see also* Incision, bone 77.10
joint - *see also* Arthrotomy 80.10
necrotic - *see also* Sequestrectomy, bone 77.00
joint - *see also* Arthrotomy 80.10
skull 01.25
with debridement of compound fracture 02.02
bone growth stimulator - *see* category 78.6
bony spicules, spinal canal 03.53
brace 97.88
breast implant 85.94
tissue expander 85.96
bronchial device or substance ◀
endoscopic 33.78 ◀
calcareous deposit
bursa 83.03
hand 82.03
tendon, intratendinous 83.39
hand 82.29
calcification, heart valve leaflets - *see* Valvuloplasty, heart

ICD-9-CM R Vol. 3

Removal *(Continued)*
calculus
bile duct (by incision) 51.49
endoscopic 51.88
laparoscopic 51.88
percutaneous 51.98
bladder (by incision) 57.19
without incision 57.0
common duct (by incision) 51.41
endoscopic 51.88
laparoscopic 51.88
percutaneous 51.96
gallbladder 51.04
endoscopic 51.88
laparoscopic 51.88
kidney (by incision) 55.01
without incision (transurethral) 56.0
percutaneous 55.03
with fragmentation (ultrasound) 55.04
renal pelvis (by incision) 55.11
percutaneous nephrostomy 55.03
with fragmentation 55.04
transurethral 56.0
lacrimal
canaliculi 09.42
by incision 09.52
gland 09.3
by incision 09.0
passage(s) 09.49
by incision 09.59
punctum 09.41
by incision 09.51
sac 09.49
by incision 09.53
pancreatic duct (by incision) 52.09
endoscopic 52.94
perirenal tissue 59.09
pharynx 29.39
prostate 60.0
salivary gland (by incision) 26.0
by probe 26.91
ureter (by incision) 56.2
without incision 56.0
urethra (by incision) 58.0
without incision 58.6
caliper tongs (skull) 02.95
cannula
for extracorporeal membrane oxygenation (ECMO) - *omit code*
cardiac pacemaker (device) (initial) (permanent) (cardiac resynchronization device, CRT-P) 37.89
with replacement (by)
cardiac resynchronization pacemaker (CRT-P)
device only 00.53
total system 00.50
dual chamber device 37.87
single-chamber device 37.85
rate responsive 37.86
cardioverter/defibrillator pulse generator without replacement (cardiac resynchronization defibrillator device (CRT-D) 37.79 ⬅
cast 97.88
with reapplication 97.13
lower limb 97.12
upper limb 97.11
catheter (indwelling) - *see also* Removal, tube
bladder 97.64
cranial cavity 01.27

Removal *(Continued)*
catheter *(Continued)*
middle ear (tympanum) 20.1
ureter 97.62
urinary 97.64
ventricular (cerebral) 02.43
with synchronous replacement 02.42
cerclage material, cervix 69.96
cerumen, ear 96.52
corneal epithelium 11.41
for smear or culture 11.21
coronary artery obstruction (thrombus) 36.09
direct intracoronary artery infusion 36.04
open chest approach 36.03
percutaneous transluminal (balloon) 00.66

Note: Also use 00.40, 00.41, 00.42, or 00.43 to show the total number of vessels treated. Use code 00.44 once to show procedure on a bifurcated vessel. In addition, use 00.45, 00.46, 00.47, or 00.48 to show the number of vascular stents inserted. ⬅

Crutchfield tongs (skull) 02.95
with synchronous replacement 02.94
cyst - *see also* Excision, lesion, by site
dental 24.4
lung 32.29
endoscopic 32.28
cystic duct remnant 51.61
decidua (by)
aspiration curettage 69.52
curettage (D and C) 69.02
manual 75.4
dental wiring (immobilization device) 97.33
orthodontic 24.8
device (therapeutic) NEC 97.89
abdomen NEC 97.86
bronchus 33.78 ◀
valve 33.78 ◀
digestive system NEC 97.59
drainage - *see* Removal, tube
external fixation device 97.88
mandibular NEC 97.36
minifixator (bone) - *see* category 78.6
for musculoskeletal immobilization NEC 97.88
genital tract NEC 97.79
head and neck NEC 97.39
intrauterine contraceptive 97.71
spine 80.09
thorax NEC 97.49
trunk NEC 97.87
urinary system NEC 97.69
diaphragm, vagina 97.73
drainage device - *see* Removal, tube
dye, spinal canal 03.31
ectopic fetus (from) 66.02
abdominal cavity 74.3
extraperitoneal (intraligamentous) 74.3
fallopian tube (by salpingostomy) 66.02
by salpingotomy 66.01
with salpingectomy 66.62
intraligamentous 74.3
ovarian 74.3

Removal *(Continued)*
ectopic fetus *(Continued)*
peritoneal (following uterine or tubal rupture) 74.3
site NEC 74.3
tubal (by salpingostomy) 66.02
by salpingotomy 66.01
with salpingectomy 66.62
electrodes
bone growth stimulator - *see* category 78.6
brain 01.22
depth 01.22
with synchronous replacement 02.93
foramen ovale 01.22
with synchronous replacement 02.93
sphenoidal - *omit code*
with synchronous replacement 02.96
cardiac pacemaker (atrial) (transvenous) (ventricular) 37.77
with replacement 37.76
depth 01.22
with synchronous replacement 02.93
epicardial (myocardial) 37.77
with replacement (by)
atrial and/or ventricular lead(s) (electrode) 37.76
epicardial lead 37.74
epidural pegs 01.22
with synchronous replacement 02.93
foramen ovale 01.22
with synchronous replacement 02.93
gastric 04.93 ◀
with synchronous replacement 04.92 ◀
intracranial 01.22
with synchronous replacement 02.93
peripheral nerve 04.93
with synchronous replacement 04.92
sacral nerve 04.93
sphenoidal - *omit code*
with synchronous replacement 02.96
spinal 03.94
with synchronous replacement 03.93
temporary transvenous pacemaker system - *omit code*
electroencephalographic receiver (brain) (intracranial) 01.22
with synchronous replacement 02.93
electronic
stimulator - *see* Removal, neurostimulator, by site
bladder 57.98
bone 78.6
skeletal muscle 83.93
with synchronous replacement 83.92
ureter 56.94
electrostimulator - *see* Removal, electronic, stimulator, by site
embolus 38.00
with endarterectomy - *see* Endarterectomy
abdominal
artery 38.06
vein 38.07

- **Removal** *(Continued)*
  - embolus *(Continued)*
    - aorta (arch) (ascending) (descending) 38.04
    - arteriovenous shunt or cannula 39.49
    - bovine graft 39.49
    - head and neck vessel
      - endovascular approach 39.74
      - open approach, intracranial vessels 38.01
      - open approach, other vessels of head and neck 38.02
    - intracranial vessel
      - endovascular approach 39.74
      - open approach, intracranial vessels 38.01
      - open approach, other vessels of head and neck 38.02
    - lower limb
      - artery 38.08
      - vein 38.09
    - pulmonary (artery) (vein) 38.05
    - thoracic vessel NEC 38.05
    - upper limb (artery) (vein) 38.03
  - embryo - *see* Removal, ectopic fetus
  - encircling tube, eye (episcleral) 14.6
  - epithelial downgrowth, anterior chamber 12.93
  - external fixation device 97.88
    - mandibular NEC 97.36
    - minifixator (bone) - *see* category 78.6
  - extrauterine embryo - *see* Removal, ectopic fetus
  - eyeball 16.49
    - with implant 16.42
      - with attachment of muscles 16.41
  - fallopian tube - *see* Salpingectomy
  - feces (impacted) (by flushing) (manual) 96.38
  - fetus, ectopic - *see* Removal, ectopic fetus
  - fingers, supernumerary 86.26
  - fixation device
    - external 97.88
      - mandibular NEC 97.36
      - minifixator (bone) - *see* category 78.6
    - internal 78.60
      - carpal, metacarpal 78.64
      - clavicle 78.61
      - facial (bone) 76.97
      - femur 78.65
      - fibula 78.67
      - humerus 78.62
      - patella 78.66
      - pelvic 78.69
      - phalanges (foot) (hand) 78.69
      - radius 78.63
      - scapula 78.61
      - specified site NEC 78.69
      - tarsal, metatarsal 78.68
      - thorax (ribs) (sternum) 78.61
      - tibia 78.67
      - ulna 78.63
      - vertebrae 78.69
  - foreign body NEC - *see also* Incision, by site 98.20
    - abdominal (cavity) 54.92
      - wall 54.0
    - adenoid 98.13
      - by incision 28.91
    - alveolus, alveolar bone 98.22
      - by incision 24.0

- **Removal** *(Continued)*
  - foreign body NEC *(Continued)*
    - antecubital fossa 98.27
      - by incision 86.05
    - anterior chamber 12.00
      - by incision 12.02
        - with use of magnet 12.01
    - anus (intraluminal) 98.05
      - by incision 49.93
    - artificial stoma (intraluminal) 98.18
    - auditory canal, external 18.02
    - axilla 98.27
      - by incision 86.05
    - bladder (without incision) 57.0
      - by incision 57.19
    - bone, except fixation device - *see also* Incision, bone 77.10
      - alveolus, alveolar 98.22
        - by incision 24.0
    - brain 01.39
      - without incision into brain 01.24
    - breast 85.0
    - bronchus (intraluminal) 98.15
      - by incision 33.0
    - bursa 83.03
      - hand 82.03
    - canthus 98.22
      - by incision 08.51
    - cerebral meninges 01.31
    - cervix (intraluminal) NEC 98.16
      - penetrating 69.97
    - choroid (by incision) 14.00
      - with use of magnet 14.01
      - without use of magnet 14.02
    - ciliary body (by incision) 12.00
      - with use of magnet 12.01
      - without use of magnet 12.02
    - conjunctiva (by magnet) 98.22
      - by incision 10.0
    - cornea 98.21
      - by
        - incision 11.1
        - magnet 11.0
    - duodenum 98.03
      - by incision 45.01
    - ear (intraluminal) 98.11
      - with incision 18.09
    - epididymis 63.92
    - esophagus (intraluminal) 98.02
      - by incision 42.09
    - extrapleural (by incision) 34.01
    - eye, eyeball (by magnet) 98.21
      - anterior segment (by incision) 12.00
        - with use of magnet 12.01
        - without use of magnet 12.02
      - posterior segment (by incision) 14.00
        - with use of magnet 14.01
        - without use of magnet 14.02
      - superficial 98.21
    - eyelid 98.22
      - by incision 08.09
    - fallopian tube
      - by salpingostomy 66.02
      - by salpingotomy 66.01
    - fascia 83.09
      - hand 82.09
    - foot 98.28
    - gallbladder 51.04
    - groin region (abdominal wall) (inguinal) 54.0
    - gum 98.22
      - by incision 24.0

- **Removal** *(Continued)*
  - foreign body NEC *(Continued)*
    - hand 98.26
    - head and neck NEC 98.22
    - heart 37.11
    - internal fixation device - *see* Removal, fixation device, internal
    - intestine
      - by incision 45.00
      - large (intraluminal) 98.04
        - by incision 45.03
      - small (intraluminal) 98.03
        - by incision 45.02
    - intraocular (by incision) 12.00
      - with use of magnet 12.01
      - without use of magnet 12.02
    - iris (by incision) 12.00
      - with use of magnet 12.01
      - without use of magnet 12.02
    - joint structures - *see also* Arthrotomy 80.10
    - kidney (transurethral) (by endoscopy) 56.0
      - by incision 55.01
      - pelvis (transurethral) 56.0
        - by incision 55.11
    - labia 98.23
      - by incision 71.09
    - lacrimal
      - canaliculi 09.42
        - by incision 09.52
      - gland 09.3
        - by incision 09.0
      - passage(s) 09.49
        - by incision 09.59
      - punctum 09.41
        - by incision 09.51
      - sac 09.49
        - by incision 09.53
    - large intestine (intraluminal) 98.04
      - by incision 45.03
    - larynx (intraluminal) 98.14
      - by incision 31.3
    - lens 13.00
      - by incision 13.02
        - with use of magnet 13.01
    - liver 50.0
    - lower limb, except foot 98.29
      - foot 98.28
    - lung 33.1
    - mediastinum 34.1
    - meninges (cerebral) 01.31
      - spinal 03.01
    - mouth (intraluminal) 98.01
      - by incision 27.92
    - muscle 83.02
      - hand 82.02
    - nasal sinus 22.50
      - antrum 22.2
        - with Caldwell-Luc approach 22.39
      - ethmoid 22.51
      - frontal 22.41
      - maxillary 22.2
        - with Caldwell-Luc approach 22.39
      - sphenoid 22.52
    - nerve (cranial) (peripheral) NEC 04.04
      - root 03.01
    - nose (intraluminal) 98.12
      - by incision 21.1
    - oral cavity (intraluminal) 98.01
      - by incision 27.92

ICD-9-CM R Vol. 3

Removal *(Continued)*
foreign body NEC *(Continued)*
orbit (by magnet) 98.21
by incision 16.1
palate (penetrating) 98.22
by incision 27.1
pancreas 52.09
penis 98.24
by incision 64.92
pericardium 37.12
perineum (female) 98.23
by incision 71.09
male 98.25
by incision 86.05
perirenal tissue 59.09
peritoneal cavity 54.92
perivesical tissue 59.19
pharynx (intraluminal) 98.13
by pharyngotomy 29.0
pleura (by incision) 34.09
popliteal space 98.29
by incision 86.05
rectum (intraluminal) 98.05
by incision 48.0
renal pelvis (transurethral) 56.0
by incision 56.1
retina (by incision) 14.00
with use of magnet 14.01
without use of magnet 14.02
retroperitoneum 54.92
sclera (by incision) 12.00
with use of magnet 12.01
without use of magnet 12.02
scrotum 98.24
by incision 61.0
sinus (nasal) 22.50
antrum 22.2
with Caldwell-Luc approach 22.39
ethmoid 22.51
frontal 22.41
maxillary 22.2
with Caldwell-Luc approach 22.39
sphenoid 22.52
skin NEC 98.20
by incision 86.05
skull 01.24
with incision into brain 01.39
small intestine (intraluminal) 98.03
by incision 45.02
soft tissue NEC 83.09
hand 82.09
spermatic cord 63.93
spinal (canal) (cord) (meninges) 03.01
stomach (intraluminal) 98.03
bubble (balloon) 44.94
by incision 43.0
subconjunctival (by magnet) 98.22
by incision 10.0
subcutaneous tissue NEC 98.20
by incision 86.05
supraclavicular fossa 98.27
by incision 86.05
tendon (sheath) 83.01
hand 82.01
testis 62.0
thorax (by incision) 34.09
thyroid (field) (gland) (by incision) 06.09
tonsil 98.13
by incision 28.91
trachea (intraluminal) 98.15
by incision 31.3
trunk NEC 98.25

Removal *(Continued)*
foreign body NEC *(Continued)*
tunica vaginalis 98.24
upper limb, except hand 98.27
hand 98.26
ureter (transurethral) 56.0
by incision 56.2
urethra (intraluminal) 98.19
by incision 58.0
uterus (intraluminal) 98.16
vagina (intraluminal) 98.17
by incision 70.14
vas deferens 63.6
vitreous (by incision) 14.00
with use of magnet 14.01
without use of magnet 14.02
vulva 98.23
by incision 71.09
gallstones
bile duct (by incision) NEC 51.49
endoscopic 51.88
common duct (by incision) 51.41
endoscopic 51.88
percutaneous 51.96
duodenum 45.01
gallbladder 51.04
endoscopic 51.88
laparoscopic 51.88
hepatic ducts 51.49
endoscopic 51.88
intestine 45.00
large 45.03
small NEC 45.02
liver 50.0
Gardner Wells tongs (skull) 02.95
with synchronous replacement 02.94
gastric band (adjustable), laparoscopic 44.97
gastric bubble (balloon) 44.94
granulation tissue - *see also* Excision, lesion, by site
with repair - *see* Repair, by site
cranial 01.6
skull 01.6
halo traction device (skull) 02.95
with synchronous replacement 02.94
heart assist system
with replacement 37.63
intra-aortic balloon pump (IABP) 97.44
nonoperative 97.44
open removal 37.64
percutaneous external device 97.44
hematoma - *see* Drainage, by site
Hoffman minifixator device (bone) - *see* category 78.6
hydatidiform mole 68.0
impacted
feces (rectum) (by flushing) (manual) 96.38
tooth 23.19
from nasal sinus (maxillary) 22.61
implant
breast 85.94
cochlear prosthetic device 20.99
cornea 11.92
lens (prosthetic) 13.8
middle ear NEC 20.99
ocular 16.71
posterior segment 14.6
orbit 16.72
retina 14.6
tympanum 20.1

Removal *(Continued)*
implantable hemodynamic sensor (lead) and monitor device 37.79 ◀
internal fixation device - *see* Removal, fixation device, internal
intra-aortic balloon pump (IABP) 97.44
intrauterine contraceptive device (IUD) 97.71
joint (structure) NOS 80.90
ankle 80.97
elbow 80.92
foot and toe 80.98
hand and finger 80.94
hip 80.95
knee 80.96
other specified sites 80.99
shoulder 80.91
spine 80.99
toe 80.98
wrist 80.93
Kantrowitz heart pump 37.64
nonoperative 97.44
keel (tantalum plate), larynx 31.98
kidney - *see also* Nephrectomy
mechanical 55.98
transplanted or rejected 55.53
laminaria (tent), uterus 97.79
leads (cardiac) - *see* Removal, electrodes, cardiac pacemaker
lesion - *see* Excision, lesion, by site
ligamentum flavum (spine) - *omit code*
ligature
fallopian tube 66.79
ureter 56.86
vas deferens 63.84
limb lengthening device, internal - *see* category 78.6
loop recorder 86.05
loose body
bone - *see* Sequestrectomy, bone
joint 80.10
mesh (surgical) - *see* Removal, foreign body, by site
lymph node - *see* Excision, lymph, node
minifixator device (bone) - *see* category 78.6
external fixation device 97.88
Mulligan hood, fallopian tube 66.94
with synchronous replacement 66.93
muscle stimulator (skeletal) 83.93
with replacement 83.92
myringotomy device or tube 20.1
nail (bed) (fold) 86.23
internal fixation device - *see* Removal, fixation device, internal
necrosis
skin 86.28
excisional 86.22
neuropacemaker - *see* Removal, neurostimulator, by site
neurostimulator
brain 01.22
with synchronous replacement 02.93
electrodes
brain 01.22
with synchronous replacement 02.93
gastric 04.93 ◀
with synchronous replacement 04.92 ◀
intracranial 01.22
with synchronous replacement 02.93

Removal *(Continued)*
neurostimulator *(Continued)*
electrodes *(Continued)*
peripheral nerve 04.93
with synchronous replacement 04.92
sacral nerve 04.93
with synchronous replacement 04.92
spinal 03.94
with synchronous replacement 03.93
pulse generator (single array, dual array) 86.05
with synchronous replacement 86.96
dual array 86.95
rechargeable 86.98
single array 86.94
rechargeable 86.97
nonabsorbable surgical material NEC - *see* Removal, foreign body, by site
odontoma (tooth) 24.4
orbital implant 16.72
osteocartilaginous loose body, joint structures - *see also* Arthrotomy 80.10
outer attic wall (middle ear) 20.59
ovo-testis (unilateral) 62.3
bilateral 62.41
pacemaker
brain (intracranial) - *see* Removal, neurostimulator
cardiac (device) (initial) (permanent) 37.89
with replacement
dual-chamber device 37.87
single-chamber device 37.85
rate responsive 37.86
electrodes (atrial) (transvenous) (ventricular) 37.77
with replacement 37.76
epicardium (myocardium) 37.77
with replacement (by)
atrial and/or ventricular lead(s) (electrode) 37.76
epicardial lead 37.74
temporary transvenous pacemaker system - *omit code*
intracranial - *see* Removal, neurostimulator
neural - *see* Removal, neurostimulator
peripheral nerve - *see* Removal, neurostimulator
spinal - *see* Removal, neurostimulator
pack, packing
dental 97.34
intrauterine 97.72
nasal 97.32
rectum 97.59
trunk NEC 97.85
vagina 97.75
vulva 97.75
pantopaque dye, spinal canal 03.31
patella (complete) 77.96
partial 77.86
pectus deformity implant device 34.01
pelvic viscera, en masse (female) 68.8
male 57.71
pessary, vagina NEC 97.74
pharynx (partial) 29.33
phlebolith - *see* Removal, embolus

Removal *(Continued)*
placenta (by)
aspiration curettage 69.52
D and C 69.02
manual 75.4
plaque, dental 96.54
plate, skull 02.07
with synchronous replacement 02.05
polyp - *see also* Excision, lesion, by site
esophageal 42.32
endoscopic 42.33
gastric (endoscopic) 43.41
intestine 45.41
endoscopic 45.42
nasal 21.31
prosthesis
bile duct 51.95
nonoperative 97.55
cochlear prosthetic device 20.99
dental 97.35
eye 97.31
facial bone 76.99
fallopian tube 66.94
with synchronous replacement 66.93
joint structures 80.00
ankle 80.07
elbow 80.02
foot and toe 80.08
hand and finger 80.04
hip 80.05
knee 80.06
shoulder 80.01
specified site NEC 80.09
spine 80.09
wrist 80.03
lens 13.8
penis (internal), without replacement 64.96
Rosen (urethra) 59.99
testicular, by incision 62.0
urinary sphincter, artificial 58.99
with replacement 58.93
pseudophakos 13.8
pterygium 11.39
with corneal graft 11.32
pulse generator
cardiac pacemaker 37.86
cardioverter/defibrillator 37.79 ⬅
neurostimulator - *see* Removal, neurostimulator, pulse generator
pump assist device, heart 37.64
with replacement 37.63
nonoperative 97.44
radioactive material - *see* Removal, foreign body, by site
redundant skin, eyelid 08.86
rejected organ
kidney 55.53
testis 62.42
reservoir, ventricular (Ommaya) (Rickham) 02.43
with synchronous replacement 02.42
retained placenta (by)
aspiration curettage 69.52
D and C 69.02
manual 75.4
retinal implant 14.6
rhinolith 21.31
rice bodies, tendon sheaths 83.01
hand 82.01
Roger-Anderson minifixator device (bone) - *see* category 78.6
root, residual (tooth) (buried) (retained) 23.11

Removal *(Continued)*
Rosen prosthesis (urethra) 59.99
scleral buckle or implant 14.6
Scribner shunt 39.43
secondary membranous cataract (with iridectomy) 13.65
secundines (by)
aspiration curettage 69.52
D and C 69.02
manual 75.4
sequestrum - *see* Sequestrectomy
seton, anus 49.93
Shepard's tube (ear) 20.1
Shirodkar suture, cervix 69.96
shunt
arteriovenous 39.43
with creation of new shunt 39.42
lumbar-subarachnoid NEC 03.98
pleurothecal 03.98
salpingothecal 03.98
spinal (thecal) NEC 03.98
subarachnoid-peritoneal 03.98
subarachnoid-ureteral 03.98
silastic tubes
ear 20.1
fallopian tubes 66.94
with synchronous replacement 66.93
skin
necrosis or slough 86.28
excisional 86.22
superficial layer (by dermabrasion) 86.25
skull tongs 02.95
with synchronous replacement 02.94
spacer (cement) (joint) 84.57
splint 97.88
stent
bile duct 97.55
larynx 31.98
ureteral 97.62
urethral 97.65
stimoceiver - *see* Removal, neurostimulator
subdural
grids 01.22
strips 01.22
supernumerary digit(s) 86.26
suture(s) NEC 97.89
abdominal wall 97.83
by incision - *see* Incision, by site
genital tract 97.79
head and neck 97.38
thorax 97.43
trunk NEC 97.84
symblepharon - *see* Repair, symblepharon
temporary transvenous pacemaker system - *omit code*
testis (unilateral) 62.3
bilateral 62.41
remaining or solitary 62.42
thrombus 38.00
with endarterectomy - *see* Endarterectomy
abdominal
artery 38.06
vein 38.07
aorta (arch) (ascending) (descending) 38.04
arteriovenous shunt or cannula 39.49
bovine graft 39.49
coronary artery 36.09
head and neck vessel NEC 38.02

Removal *(Continued)*
thrombus *(Continued)*
intracranial vessel NEC 38.01
lower limb
artery 38.08
vein 38.09
pulmonary (artery) (vein) 38.05
thoracic vessel NEC 38.05
upper limb (artery) (vein) 38.03
tissue expander (skin) NEC 86.05
breast 85.96
toes, supernumerary 86.26
tongs, skull 02.95
with synchronous replacement 02.94
tonsil tag 28.4
tooth (by forceps) (multiple) (single) NEC 23.09
deciduous 23.01
surgical NEC 23.19
impacted 23.19
surgical NEC *(Continued)*
residual root 23.11
root apex 23.73
with root canal therapy 23.72
trachoma follicles 10.33
T-tube (bile duct) 97.55
tube
appendix 97.53
bile duct (T-tube) NEC 97.55
cholecystostomy 97.54
cranial cavity 01.27
cystostomy 97.63
ear (button) 20.1
gastrostomy 97.51
large intestine 97.53
liver 97.55
mediastinum 97.42
nephrostomy 97.61
pancreas 97.56
peritoneum 97.82
pleural cavity 97.41
pyelostomy 97.61
retroperitoneum 97.81
small intestine 97.52
thoracotomy 97.41
tracheostomy 97.37
tympanostomy 20.1
tympanum 20.1
ureterostomy 97.62
ureteral splint (stent) 97.62
urethral sphincter, artificial 58.99
with replacement 58.93
urinary sphincter, artificial 58.99
with replacement 58.93
utricle 20.79
valve
vas deferens 63.85
ventricular (cerebral) 02.43
vascular graft or prosthesis 39.49
ventricular shunt or reservoir 02.43
with synchronous replacement 02.42
Vinke tongs (skull) 02.95
with synchronous replacement 02.94
vitreous (with replacement) 14.72
anterior approach (partial) 14.71
open sky technique 14.71
Wagner-Brooker minifixator device (bone) - *see* category 78.6
wiring, dental (immobilization device) 97.33
orthodontic 24.8

Renipuncture (percutaneous) 55.92
Renogram 92.03
Renotransplantation NEC 55.69

Note: To report donor source:
cadaver 00.93
live non-related donor 00.92
live related donor 00.91
live unrelated donor 00.92

Reopening - *see also* Incision, by site
blepharorrhaphy 08.02
canthorrhaphy 08.02
cilia base 08.71
craniotomy or craniectomy site 01.23
fallopian tube (divided) 66.79
iris in anterior chambers 12.97
laminectomy or laminotomy site 03.02
laparotomy site 54.12
osteotomy site - *see also* Incision, bone 77.10
facial bone 76.09
tarsorrhaphy 08.02
thoracotomy site (for control of hemorrhage) (for examination) (for exploration) 34.03
thyroid field wound (for control of hemorrhage) (for examination) (for exploration) (for removal of hematoma) 06.02
Repacking - *see* Replacement, pack, by site
Repair
abdominal wall 54.72
adrenal gland 07.44
alveolus, alveolar (process) (ridge) (with graft) (with implant) 24.5
anal sphincter 49.79
artificial sphincter
implantation 49.75
revision 49.75
laceration (by suture) 49.71
obstetric (current) 75.62
old 49.79
aneurysm (false) (true) 39.52
by or with
clipping 39.51
coagulation 39.52
coil (endovascular approach) 39.79
head and neck 39.72
electrocoagulation 39.52
excision or resection of vessel - *see also* Aneurysmectomy, by site
with
anastomosis - *see* Aneurysmectomy, with anastomosis, by site
graft replacement - *see* Aneurysmectomy, with graft replacement, by site
endovascular graft 39.79
abdominal aorta 39.71
head and neck 39.72
lower extremity artery(ies) 39.79
thoracic aorta 39.73
upper extremity artery(ies) 39.79
filipuncture 39.52
graft replacement - *see* Aneurysmectomy, with graft replacement, by site
ligation 39.52

Repair *(Continued)*
aneurysm *(Continued)*
by or with *(Continued)*
liquid tissue adhesive (glue) 39.79
endovascular approach 39.79
head and neck 39.72
methyl methacrylate 39.52
endovascular approach 39.79
head and neck 39.72
occlusion 39.52
endovascular approach 39.79
head and neck 39.72
suture 39.52
trapping 39.52
wiring 39.52
wrapping (gauze) (methyl methacrylate) (plastic) 39.52
coronary artery 36.91
heart 37.32
sinus of Valsalva 35.39
thoracic aorta (dissecting), by fenestration 39.54
anomalous pulmonary venous connection (total)
one-stage 35.82
partial - *see* specific procedure
total 35.82
anus 49.79
laceration (by suture) 49.71
obstetric (current) 75.62
old 49.79
aorta 39.31
aorticopulmonary window 39.59
arteriovenous fistula 39.53
by or with
clipping 39.53
coagulation 39.53
coil (endovascular approach) 39.79
head and neck vessels 39.72
division 39.53
excision or resection - *see also* Aneurysmectomy, by site
with
anastomosis - *see* Aneurysmectomy, with anastomosis, by site
graft replacement - *see* Aneurysmectomy, with graft replacement, by site
ligation 39.53
coronary artery 36.99
occlusion 39.53
endovascular approach 39.79
head and neck 39.72
suture 39.53
artery NEC 39.59
by
endovascular approach
abdominal aorta 39.71
head and neck (embolization or occlusion) 39.72
other repair (of aneurysms) 39.79
percutaneous repair of intracranial vessel(s) (for stent insertion) 00.62

Note: Also use 00.40, 00.41, 00.42, or 00.43 to show the total number of vessels treated. Use code 00.44 once to show procedure on a bifurcated vessel. In addition, use 00.45, 00.46, 00.47, or 00.48 to show the number of vascular stents inserted.

Repair *(Continued)*
artery NEC *(Continued)*
by *(Continued)*
endovascular approach *(Continued)*
percutaneous repair of precerebral (extracranial) vessel(s) (for stent insertion) 00.61

Note: Also use 00.40, 00.41, 00.42, or 00.43 to show the total number of vessels treated. Use code 00.44 once to show procedure on a bifurcated vessel. In addition, use 00.45, 00.46, 00.47, or 00.48 to show the number of vascular stents inserted.

non-coronary percutaneous transluminal angioplasty or atherectomy

Note: Also use 00.40, 00.41, 00.42, or 00.43 to show the total number of vessels treated. Use code 00.44 once to show procedure on a bifurcated vessel. In addition, use 00.45, 00.46, 00.47, or 00.48 to show the number of vascular stents inserted.

basilar 00.61
carotid 00.61
femoropopliteal 39.50
iliac 39.50
lower extremity NOS 39.50
mesenteric 39.50
renal 39.50
upper extremity NOS 39.50
vertebral 00.61
with
patch graft 39.58
with excision or resection of vessel - *see* Arteriectomy, with graft replacement, by site
synthetic (Dacron) (Teflon) 39.57
tissue (vein) (autogenous) (homograft) 39.56
suture 39.31
coronary NEC 36.99
by angioplasty - *see* Angioplasty, coronary
by atherectomy - *see* Angioplasty, coronary
artificial opening - *see* Repair, stoma
atrial septal defect 35.71
with
prosthesis (open heart technique) 35.51
closed heart technique 35.52
tissue graft 35.61
combined with repair of valvular and ventricular septal defects - *see* Repair, endocardial cushion defect
in total repair of total anomalous pulmonary venous connection 35.82
atrioventricular canal defect (any type) 35.73
with
prosthesis 35.54
tissue graft 35.63
bifid digit (finger) 82.89
bile duct NEC 51.79
laceration (by suture) NEC 51.79
common bile duct 51.71
bladder NEC 57.89
exstrophy 57.86

Repair *(Continued)*
bladder NEC *(Continued)*
for stress incontinence - *see* Repair, stress incontinence
laceration (by suture) 57.81
obstetric (current) 75.61
old 57.89
neck 57.85
blepharophimosis 08.59
blepharoptosis 08.36
by
frontalis muscle technique (with)
fascial sling 08.32
suture 08.31
levator muscle technique 08.34
with resection or advancement 08.33
orbicularis oculi muscle sling 08.36
tarsal technique 08.35
blood vessel NEC 39.59
patch graft 39.58
with excision or resection - *see* Angiectomy, with graft replacement
synthetic (Dacron) (Teflon) 39.57
tissue (vein) (autogenous) (homograft) 39.56
resection - *see* Angiectomy
suture 39.30
coronary artery NEC 36.99
by angioplasty - *see* Angioplasty, coronary
by atherectomy - *see* Angioplasty, coronary
peripheral vessel NEC 39.59
by angioplasty 39.50

Note: Also use 00.40, 00.41, 00.42, or 00.43 to show the total number of vessels treated. Use code 00.44 once to show procedure on a bifurcated vessel. In addition, use 00.45, 00.46, 00.47, or 00.48 to show the number of vascular stents inserted.

by atherectomy 39.50

Note: Also use 00.40, 00.41, 00.42, or 00.43 to show the total number of vessels treated. Use code 00.44 once to show procedure on a bifurcated vessel. In addition, use 00.45, 00.46, 00.47, or 00.48 to show the number of vascular stents inserted.

by endovascular approach 39.79
bone NEC - *see also* Osteoplasty - *see* category 78.4
by synostosis technique - *see* Arthrodesis
accessory sinus 22.79
cranium NEC 02.06
with
flap (bone) 02.03
graft (bone) 02.04
for malunion, nonunion, or delayed union of fracture - *see* Repair, fracture, malunion or nonunion
nasal 21.89
skull NEC 02.06
with
flap (bone) 02.03
graft (bone) 02.04
bottle, hydrocele of tunica vaginalis 61.2
brain (trauma) NEC 02.92

Repair *(Continued)*
breast (plastic) - *see also* Mammoplasty 85.89
broad ligament 69.29
bronchus NEC 33.48
laceration (by suture) 33.41
bunionette (with osteotomy) 77.54
canaliculus, lacrimal 09.73
canthus (lateral) 08.59
cardiac pacemaker NEC 37.89
electrode(s) (lead) NEC 37.75
cardioverter/defibrillator (automatic) pocket (skin) (subcutaneous) 37.99
cerebral meninges 02.12
cervix 67.69
internal os 67.59
transabdominal 67.51
transvaginal 67.59
laceration (by suture) 67.61
obstetric (current) 75.51
old 67.69
chest wall (mesh) (silastic) NEC 34.79
chordae tendineae 35.32
choroid NEC 14.9
with retinal repair - *see* Repair, retina
cisterna chyli 40.69
claw toe 77.57
cleft
hand 82.82
laryngotracheal 31.69
lip 27.54
palate 27.62
secondary or subsequent 27.63
coarctation of aorta - *see* Excision, coarctation of aorta
cochlear prosthetic device 20.99
external components only 95.49
cockup toe 77.58
colostomy 46.43
conjunctiva NEC 10.49
with scleral repair 12.81
laceration 10.6
with repair of sclera 12.81
late effect of trachoma 10.49
cornea NEC 11.59
with
conjunctival flap 11.53
transplant - *see* Keratoplasty
postoperative dehiscence 11.52
coronary artery NEC 36.99
by angioplasty - *see* Angioplasty, coronary
by atherectomy - *see* Angioplasty, coronary
cranium NEC 02.06
with
flap (bone) 02.03
graft (bone) 02.04
cusp, valve - *see* Repair, heart, valve
cystocele 70.51
and rectocele 70.50
dental arch 24.8
diaphragm NEC 34.84
diastasis recti 83.65
diastematomyelia 03.59
ear (external) 18.79
auditory canal or meatus 18.6
auricle NEC 18.79
cartilage NEC 18.79
laceration (by suture) 18.4
lop ear 18.79
middle NEC 19.9
prominent or protruding 18.5
ectropion 08.49

Repair *(Continued)*
ectropion *(Continued)*
by or with
lid reconstruction 08.44
suture (technique) 08.42
thermocauterization 08.41
wedge resection 08.43
encephalocele (cerebral) 02.12
endocardial cushion defect 35.73
with
prosthesis (grafted to septa) 35.54
tissue graft 35.63
enterocele (female) 70.92
male 53.9
enterostomy 46.40
entropion 08.49
by or with
lid reconstruction 08.44
suture (technique) 08.42
thermocauterization 08.41
wedge resection 08.43
epicanthus (fold) 08.59
epididymis (and spermatic cord) NEC 63.59
with vas deferens 63.89
epiglottis 31.69
episiotomy
routine following delivery - *see* Episiotomy
secondary 75.69
epispadias 58.45
esophagus, esophageal NEC 42.89
fistula NEC 42.84
stricture 42.85
exstrophy of bladder 57.86
eye, eyeball 16.89
multiple structures 16.82
rupture 16.82
socket 16.64
with graft 16.63
eyebrow 08.89
linear 08.81
eyelid 08.89
full-thickness 08.85
involving lid margin 08.84
laceration 08.81
full-thickness 08.85
involving lid margin 08.84
partial-thickness 08.83
involving lid margin 08.82
linear 08.81
partial-thickness 08.83
involving lid margin 08.82
retraction 08.38
fallopian tube (with prosthesis) 66.79
by
anastomosis 66.73
reanastomosis 66.79
reimplantation into
ovary 66.72
uterus 66.74
suture 66.71
false aneurysm - *see* Repair, aneurysm
fascia 83.89
by or with
arthroplasty - *see* Arthroplasty
graft (fascial) (muscle) 83.82
hand 82.72
tendon 83.81
hand 82.79
suture (direct) 83.65
hand 82.46
hand 82.89
by
graft NEC 82.79

Repair *(Continued)*
fascia *(Continued)*
hand *(Continued)*
by *(Continued)*
graft NEC *(Continued)*
fascial 82.72
muscle 82.72
suture (direct) 82.46
joint - *see* Arthroplasty
filtering bleb (corneal) (scleral) (by excision) 12.82
by
corneal graft - *see also* Keratoplasty 11.60
scleroplasty 12.82
suture 11.51
with conjunctival flap 11.53
fistula - *see also* Closure, fistula
anovaginal 70.73
arteriovenous 39.53
clipping 39.53
coagulation 39.53
endovascular approach 39.79
head and neck 39.72
division 39.53
excision or resection - *see also* Aneurysmectomy, by site
with
anastomosis - *see* Aneurysmectomy, with anastomosis, by site
graft replacement - *see* Aneurysmectomy, with graft replacement, by site
ligation 39.53
coronary artery 36.99
occlusion 39.53
endovascular approach 39.79
head and neck 39.72
suture 39.53
cervicovesical 57.84
cervix 67.62
choledochoduodenal 51.72
colovaginal 70.72
enterovaginal 70.74
enterovesical 57.83
esophagocutaneous 42.84
ileovesical 57.83
intestinovaginal 70.74
intestinovesical 57.83
oroantral 22.71
perirectal 48.93
pleuropericardial 37.49
rectovaginal 70.73
rectovesical 57.83
rectovesicovaginal 57.83
scrotum 61.42
sigmoidovaginal 70.74
sinus
nasal 22.71
of Valsalva 35.39
splenocolic 41.95
urethroperineovesical 57.84
urethrovesical 57.84
urethrovesicovaginal 57.84
uterovesical 57.84
vagina NEC 70.75
vaginocutaneous 70.75
vaginoenteric NEC 70.74
vaginoileal 70.74
vaginoperineal 70.75
vaginovesical 57.84
vesicocervicovaginal 57.84
vesicocolic 57.83

Repair *(Continued)*
fistula *(Continued)*
vesicocutaneous 57.84
vesicoenteric 57.83
vesicointestinal 57.83
vesicometrorectal 57.83
vesicoperineal 57.84
vesicorectal 57.83
vesicosigmoidal 57.83
vesicosigmoidovaginal 57.83
vesicourethral 57.84
vesicourethrorectal 57.83
vesicouterine 57.84
vesicovaginal 57.84
vulva 71.72
vulvorectal 48.73
foramen ovale (patent) 35.71
with
prosthesis (open heart technique) 35.51
closed heart technique 35.52
tissue graft 35.61
fracture - *see also* Reduction, fracture
larynx 31.64
malunion or nonunion (delayed) NEC - *see* category 78.4
with
graft - *see* Graft, bone
insertion (of)
bone growth stimulator (invasive) - *see* category 78.9
internal fixation device 78.5
manipulation for realignment - *see* Reduction, fracture, by site, closed
osteotomy
with
correction of alignment - *see* category 77.3
with internal fixation device - *see* categories 77.3 *[78.5]*
with intramedullary rod - *see* categories 77.3 *[78.5]*
replacement arthroplasty - *see* Arthroplasty
sequestrectomy - *see* category 77.0
Sofield type procedure - *see* categories 77.3 *[78.5]*
synostosis technique - *see* Arthrodesis
vertebra 03.53
funnel chest (with implant) 34.74
gallbladder 51.91
gastroschisis 54.71
great vessels NEC 39.59
laceration (by suture) 39.30
artery 39.31
vein 39.32
hallux valgus NEC 77.59
resection of joint with prosthetic implant 77.59
hammer toe 77.56
hand 82.89
with graft or implant 82.79
fascia 82.72
muscle 82.72
tendon 82.79
heart 37.49
assist system 37.63
septum 35.70

Repair *(Continued)*
heart *(Continued)*
septum *(Continued)*
with
prosthesis 35.50
tissue graft 35.60
atrial 35.71
with
prosthesis (open heart technique) 35.51
closed heart technique 35.52
tissue graft 35.61
combined with repair of valvular and ventricular septal defects - *see* Repair, endocardial cushion defect
in total repair of
tetralogy of Fallot 35.81
total anomalous pulmonary venous connection 35.82
truncus arteriosus 35.83
combined with repair of valvular defect - *see* Repair, endocardial cushion defect
ventricular 35.72
with
prosthesis (open heart technique) 35.53
closed heart technique 35.55
tissue graft 35.62
combined with repair of valvular and atrial septal defects - *see* Repair, endocardial cushion defect
in total repair of
tetralogy of Fallot 35.81
total anomalous pulmonary venous connection 35.82
truncus arteriosus 35.83
total replacement system 37.52
implantable battery 37.54
implantable controller 37.54
thoracic unit 37.53
transcutaneous energy transfer [TET] device 37.54
valve (cusps) (open heart technique) 35.10
with prosthesis or tissue graft 35.20
aortic (without replacement) 35.11
with
prosthesis 35.22
tissue graft 35.21
combined with repair of atrial and ventricular septal defects - *see* Repair, endocardial cushion defect
mitral (without replacement) 35.12
with
prosthesis 35.24
tissue graft 35.23
pulmonary (without replacement) 35.13
with
prosthesis 35.26
in total repair of tetralogy of Fallot 35.81
tissue graft 35.25
tricuspid (without replacement) 35.14
with
prosthesis 35.28
tissue graft 35.27

Repair *(Continued)*
hepatic duct 51.79
hernia NEC 53.9
anterior abdominal wall NEC 53.59
with prosthesis or graft 53.69
colostomy 46.42
crural 53.29
cul-de-sac (Douglas') 70.92
diaphragmatic
abdominal approach 53.7
thoracic, thoracoabdominal approach 53.80
epigastric 53.59
with prosthesis or graft 53.69
esophageal hiatus
abdominal approach 53.7
thoracic, thoracoabdominal approach 53.80
fascia 83.89
hand 82.89
femoral (unilateral) 53.29
with prosthesis or graft 53.21
bilateral 53.39
with prosthesis or graft 53.31
Ferguson 53.00
Halsted 53.00
Hill-Allison (hiatal hernia repair, transpleural approach) 53.80
hypogastric 53.59
with prosthesis or graft 53.69
incisional 53.51
with prosthesis or graft 53.61
inguinal (unilateral) 53.00
with prosthesis or graft 53.05
bilateral 53.10
with prosthesis or graft 53.17
direct 53.11
with prosthesis or graft 53.14
direct and indirect 53.13
with prosthesis or graft 53.16
indirect 53.12
with prosthesis or graft 53.15
direct (unilateral) 53.01
with prosthesis or graft 53.03
and indirect (unilateral) 53.01
with prosthesis or graft 53.03
bilateral 53.13
with prosthesis or graft 53.16
bilateral 53.11
with prosthesis or graft 53.14
indirect (unilateral) 53.02
with prosthesis or graft 53.04
and direct (unilateral) 53.01
with prosthesis or graft 53.03
bilateral 53.13
with prosthesis or graft 53.16
bilateral 53.12
with prosthesis or graft 53.15
internal 53.9
ischiatic 53.9
ischiorectal 53.9
lumbar 53.9
manual 96.27
obturator 53.9
omental 53.9
paraesophageal 53.7
parahiatal 53.7
paraileostomy 46.41
parasternal 53.82
paraumbilical 53.49
with prosthesis 53.41
pericolostomy 46.42
perineal (enterocele) 53.9
preperitoneal 53.29

Repair *(Continued)*
hernia NEC *(Continued)*
pudendal 53.9
retroperitoneal 53.9
sciatic 53.9
scrotal - *see* Repair, hernia, inguinal
spigelian 53.59
with prosthesis or graft 53.69
umbilical 53.49
with prosthesis 53.41
uveal 12.39
ventral 53.59
incisional 53.51
with prosthesis or graft 53.61
hydrocele
round ligament 69.19
spermatic cord 63.1
tunica vaginalis 61.2
hymen 70.76
hypospadias 58.45
ileostomy 46.41
ingrown toenail 86.23
intestine, intestinal NEC 46.79
fistula - *see* Closure, fistula, intestine
laceration
large intestine 46.75
small intestine NEC 46.73
stoma - *see* Repair, stoma
inverted uterus NEC 69.29
manual
nonobstetric 69.94
obstetric 75.94
obstetrical
manual 75.94
surgical 75.93
vaginal approach 69.23
iris (rupture) NEC 12.39
jejunostomy 46.41
joint (capsule) (cartilage) NEC - *see also* Arthroplasty 81.96
kidney NEC 55.89
knee (joint) NEC 81.47
collateral ligaments 81.46
cruciate ligaments 81.45
five-in-one 81.42
triad 81.43
labia - *see* Repair, vulva
laceration - *see* Suture, by site
lacrimal system NEC 09.99
canaliculus 09.73
punctum 09.72
for eversion 09.71
laryngostomy 31.62
laryngotracheal cleft 31.69
larynx 31.69
fracture 31.64
laceration 31.61
leads (cardiac) NEC 37.75
ligament - *see also* Arthroplasty 81.96
broad 69.29
collateral, knee NEC 81.46
cruciate, knee NEC 81.45
round 69.29
uterine 69.29
lip NEC 27.59
cleft 27.54
laceration (by suture) 27.51
liver NEC 50.69
laceration 50.61
lop ear 18.79
lung NEC 33.49
lymphatic (channel) (peripheral) NEC 40.9
duct, left (thoracic) NEC 40.69
macrodactyly 82.83

ICD-9-CM R Vol. 3

Repair *(Continued)*
mallet finger 82.84
mandibular ridge 76.64
mastoid (antrum) (cavity) 19.9
meninges (cerebral) NEC 02.12
spinal NEC 03.59
meningocele 03.51
myelomeningocele 03.52
meningocele (spinal) 03.51
cranial 02.12
mesentery 54.75
mouth NEC 27.59
laceration NEC 27.52
muscle NEC 83.87
by
graft or implant (fascia) (muscle) 83.82
hand 82.72
tendon 83.81
hand 82.79
suture (direct) 83.65
hand 82.46
transfer or transplantation (muscle) 83.77
hand 82.58
hand 82.89
by
graft or implant NEC 82.79
fascia 82.72
suture (direct) 82.46
transfer or transplantation (muscle) 82.58
musculotendinous cuff, shoulder 83.63
myelomeningocele 03.52
nasal
septum (perforation) NEC 21.88
sinus NEC 22.79
fistula 22.71
nasolabial flaps (plastic) 21.86
nasopharyngeal atresia 29.4
nerve (cranial) (peripheral) NEC 04.79
old injury 04.76
revision 04.75
sympathetic 05.81
nipple NEC 85.87
nose (external) (internal) (plastic) NEC - *see also* Rhinoplasty 21.89
laceration (by suture) 21.81
notched lip 27.59
omentum 54.74
omphalocele 53.49
with prosthesis 53.41
orbit 16.89
wound 16.81
ostium
primum defect 35.73
with
prosthesis 35.54
tissue graft 35.63
secundum defect 35.71
with
prosthesis (open heart technique) 35.51
closed heart technique 35.52
tissue graft 35.61
ovary 65.79
with tube 65.73
laparoscopic 65.76
overlapping toe 77.58
pacemaker
cardiac
device (permanent) 37.89
electrodes (leads) NEC 37.75
pocket (skin) (subcutaneous) 37.79

Repair *(Continued)*
palate NEC 27.69
cleft 27.62
secondary or subsequent 27.63
laceration (by suture) 27.61
pancreas NEC 52.95
Wirsung's duct 52.99
papillary muscle (heart) 35.31
patent ductus arteriosus 38.85
pectus deformity (chest) (carinatum) (excavatum) 34.74
pelvic floor NEC 70.79
obstetric laceration (current) 75.69
old 70.79
penis NEC 64.49
for epispadias or hypospadias 58.45
inflatable prosthesis 64.99
laceration 64.41
pericardium 37.49
perineum (female) 71.79
laceration (by suture) 71.71
obstetric (current) 75.69
old 71.79
male NEC 86.89
laceration (by suture) 86.59
peritoneum NEC 54.73
by suture 54.64
pharynx NEC 29.59
laceration (by suture) 29.51
plastic 29.4
pleura NEC 34.93
postcataract wound dehiscence 11.52
with conjunctival flap 11.53
pouch of Douglas 70.52
primum ostium defect 35.73
with
prosthesis 35.54
tissue graft 35.63
prostate 60.93
ptosis, eyelid - *see* Repair, blepharoptosis
punctum, lacrimal NEC 09.72
for correction of eversion 09.71
quadriceps (mechanism) 83.86
rectocele (posterior colporrhaphy) 70.52
and cystocele 70.50
rectum NEC 48.79
laceration (by suture) 48.71
prolapse NEC 48.76
abdominal approach 48.75
retina, retinal
detachment 14.59
by
cryotherapy 14.52
diathermy 14.51
photocoagulation 14.55
laser 14.54
xenon arc 14.53
scleral buckling - *see also* Buckling, scleral 14.49
tear or defect 14.39
by
cryotherapy 14.32
diathermy 14.31
photocoagulation 14.35
laser 14.34
xenon arc 14.33
retroperitoneal tissue 54.73
rotator cuff (graft) (suture) 83.63 ⬅
round ligament 69.29
ruptured tendon NEC 83.88
hand 82.86
salivary gland or duct NEC 26.49
sclera, scleral 12.89

Repair *(Continued)*
sclera, scleral *(Continued)*
fistula 12.82
staphyloma NEC 12.86
with graft 12.85
scrotum 61.49
sinus
nasal NEC 22.79
of Valsalva (aneurysm) 35.39
skin (plastic) (without graft) 86.89
laceration (by suture) 86.59
skull NEC 02.06
with
flap (bone) 02.03
graft (bone) 02.04
spermatic cord NEC 63.59
laceration (by suture) 63.51
sphincter ani 49.79
laceration (by suture) 49.71
obstetric (current) 75.62
old 49.79
spina bifida NEC 03.59
meningocele 03.51
myelomeningocele 03.52
spinal (cord) (meninges) (structures) NEC 03.59
meningocele 03.51
myelomeningocele 03.52
spleen 41.95
sternal defect 78.41
stoma
bile duct 51.79
bladder 57.22
bronchus 33.42
common duct 51.72
esophagus 42.89
gallbladder 51.99
hepatic duct 51.79
intestine 46.40
large 46.43
small 46.41
kidney 55.89
larynx 31.63
rectum 48.79
stomach 44.69
laparoscopic 44.68
thorax 34.79
trachea 31.74
ureter 56.62
urethra 58.49
stomach NEC 44.69
laceration (by suture) 44.61
laparoscopic 44.68
stress incontinence (urinary) NEC 59.79
by
anterior urethropexy 59.79
Burch 59.5
cystourethropexy (with levator muscle sling) 59.71
injection of implant (fat) (collagen) (polytef) 59.72
paraurethral suspension (Pereyra) 59.6
periurethral suspension 59.6
plication of urethrovesical junction 59.3
pubococcygeal sling 59.71
retropubic urethral suspension 59.5
suprapubic sling 59.4
tension free vaginal tape 59.79
urethrovesical suspension 59.4
gracilis muscle transplant 59.71
levator muscle sling 59.71

Repair *(Continued)*
stress incontinence NEC *(Continued)*
subcutaneous tissue (plastic) (without skin graft) 86.89
laceration (by suture) 86.59
supracristal defect (heart) 35.72
with
prosthesis (open heart technique) 35.53
closed heart technique 35.55
tissue graft 35.62
symblepharon NEC 10.49
by division (with insertion of conformer) 10.5
with free graft 10.41
syndactyly 86.85
synovial membrane, joint - *see* Arthroplasty
telecanthus 08.59
tendon 83.88
by or with
arthroplasty - *see* Arthroplasty
graft or implant (tendon) 83.81
fascia 83.82
hand 82.72
hand 82.79
muscle 83.82
hand 82.72
suture (direct) (immediate) (primary) - *see also* Suture, tendon 83.64
hand 82.45
transfer for transplantation (tendon) 83.75
hand 82.56
hand 82.86
by
graft or implant (tendon) 82.79
suture (direct) (immediate) (primary) - *see also* Suture, tendon, hand 82.45
transfer or transplantation (tendon) 82.56
rotator cuff (direct suture) 83.63
ruptured NEC 83.88
hand 82.86
sheath (direct suture) 83.61
hand 82.41
testis NEC 62.69
tetralogy of Fallot
partial - *see* specific procedure
total (one-stage) 35.81
thoracic duct NEC 40.69
thoracostomy 34.72
thymus (gland) 07.93
tongue NEC 25.59
tooth NEC 23.2
by
crown (artificial) 23.41
filling (amalgam) (plastic) (silicate) 23.2
inlay 23.3
total anomalous pulmonary venous connection
partial - *see* specific procedure
total (one-stage) 35.82
trachea NEC 31.79
laceration (by suture) 31.71
tricuspid atresia 35.94
truncus arteriosus
partial - *see* specific procedure
total (one-stage) 35.83
tunica vaginalis 61.49
laceration (by suture) 61.41

Repair *(Continued)*
tympanum - *see* Tympanoplasty
ureter NEC 56.89
laceration (by suture) 56.82
ureterocele 56.89
urethra NEC 58.49
laceration (by suture) 58.41
obstetric (current) 75.61
old 58.49
meatus 58.47
urethrocele (anterior colporrhaphy) (female) 70.51
and rectocele 70.50
urinary sphincter, artificial (component) 58.99
urinary stress incontinence - *see* Repair, stress incontinence
uterus, uterine 69.49
inversion - *see* Repair, inverted uterus
laceration (by suture) 69.41
obstetric (current) 75.50
old 69.49
ligaments 69.29
by
interposition 69.21
plication 69.22
uvula 27.73
with synchronous cleft palate repair 27.62
vagina, vaginal (cuff) (wall) NEC 70.79
anterior 70.51
with posterior repair 70.50
cystocele 70.51
and rectocele 70.50
enterocele 70.92
laceration (by suture) 70.71
obstetric (current) 75.69
old 70.79
posterior 70.52
with anterior repair 70.50
rectocele 70.52
and cystocele 70.50
urethrocele 70.51
and rectocele 70.50
varicocele 63.1
vas deferens 63.89
by
anastomosis 63.82
to epididymis 63.83
reconstruction 63.82
laceration (by suture) 63.81
vein NEC 39.59
with
patch graft 39.58
with excision or resection of vessel - *see* Phlebectomy, with graft replacement, by site
synthetic (Dacron) (Teflon) 39.57
tissue (vein) (autogenous) (homograft) 39.56
suture 39.32
by
endovascular approach
head and neck (embolization or occlusion) 39.72
ventricular septal defect 35.72
with
prosthesis (open heart technique) 35.53
closed heart technique 35.55
in total repair of tetralogy of Fallot 35.81
tissue graft 35.62

Repair *(Continued)*
ventricular septal defect *(Continued)*
combined with repair of valvular and atrial septal defects - *see* Repair, endocardial cushion defect
in total repair of
tetralogy of Fallot 35.81
truncus arteriosus 35.83
vertebral arch defect (spina bifida) 03.59
vulva NEC 71.79
laceration (by suture) 71.71
obstetric (current) 75.69
old 71.79
Wirsung's duct 52.99
wound (skin) (without graft) 86.59
abdominal wall 54.63
dehiscence 54.61
postcataract dehiscence (corneal) 11.52

Replacement
acetabulum (with prosthesis) 81.52
ankle, total 81.56
revision 81.59
aortic valve (with prosthesis) 35.22
with tissue graft 35.21
artery - *see* Graft, artery
bag - *see* Replacement, pack or bag
Barton's tongs (skull) 02.94
bladder
with
ileal loop 57.87 *[45.51]*
sigmoid 57.87 *[45.52]*
sphincter, artificial 58.93
bronchial device NOS 33.79
bronchial substance NOS 33.79
bronchial valve 33.71
caliper tongs (skull) 02.94
cannula
arteriovenous shunt 39.94
pancreatic duct 97.05
vessel-to-vessel (arteriovenous) 39.94
cardiac resynchronization device
defibrillator (biventricular defibrillator) (BiV ICD) (BiV pacemaker with defibrillator) (BiV pacing with defibrillator) (CRT-D) (device and one or more leads) (total system) 00.51
left ventricular coronary venous lead only 00.52
pulse generator only 00.52
pacemaker (biventricular pacemaker) (BiV pacemaker) (CRT-P) (device and one or more leads) (total system) 00.50
left ventricular coronary venous lead only 00.52
pulse generator only 00.53
cardioverter/defibrillator (total system) 37.94
leads only (electrodes) (sensing) (pacing) 37.97
pulse generator only 37.98
cast NEC 97.13
lower limb 97.12
upper limb 97.11
catheter
bladder (indwelling) 57.95
cystostomy 59.94
ventricular shunt (cerebral) 02.42
wound 97.15

ICD-9-CM

R

Vol. 3

Replacement *(Continued)*
CRT-D (biventricular defibrillator) (BiV ICD) (BiV pacemaker with defibrillator) (BiV pacing with defibrillator) (cardiac resynchronization defibrillator) (device and one or more leads) 00.51
left ventricular coronary venous lead only 00.52
pulse generator only 00.54
CRT-P (biventricular pacemaker) (BiV pacemaker) (cardiac resynchronization pacemaker) (device and one or more leads) 00.50
left ventricular coronary venous lead only 00.52
pulse generator only 00.53
Crutchfield tongs (skull) 02.94
cystostomy tube (catheter) 59.94
device
subcutaneous for intracardiac hemodynamic monitoring 00.57
diaphragm, vagina 97.24
disc - *see* Replacement, intervertebral disc
drain - *see also* Replacement, tube
vagina 97.26
vulva 97.26
wound, musculoskeletal or skin 97.16
ear (prosthetic) 18.71
elbow (joint), total 81.84
electrode(s) - *see* Implant, electrode or lead, by site or name of device
brain
depth 02.93
foramen ovale 02.93
sphenoidal 02.96
depth 02.93
foramen ovale 02.93
gastric 04.92
intracranial 02.93
pacemaker - *see* Replacement, pacemaker, electrode(s)
peripheral nerve 04.92
sacral nerve 04.92
sphenoidal 02.96
spine 03.93
electroencephalographic receiver (brain) (intracranial) 02.93
electronic
cardioverter/defibrillator - *see* Replacement, cardioverter/defibrillator
leads (electrode)(s) - *see* Replacement, electrode(s)
stimulator - *see also* Implant, electronic stimulator, by site
bladder 57.97
muscle (skeletal) 83.92
ureter 56.93
electrostimulator - *see* Implant, electronic stimulator, by site
enterostomy device (tube)
large intestine 97.04
small intestine 97.03
epidural pegs 02.93
femoral head, by prosthesis 81.52
revision 81.53
Gardner Wells tongs (skull) 02.94
gastric band, laparoscopic 44.96
gastric port device (subcutaneous) 44.96
graft - *see* Graft
halo traction device (skull) 02.94

Replacement *(Continued)*
Harrington rod (with refusion of spine) - *see* Refusion, spinal
heart
artificial
total replacement system 37.52
implantable battery 37.54
implantable controller 37.54
thoracic unit 37.53
transcutaneous energy transfer [TET] device 37.54
total replacement system 37.52
implantable battery 37.54
implantable controller 37.54
thoracic unit 37.53
transcutaneous energy transfer [TET] device 37.54
valve (with prosthesis) (with tissue graft) 35.20
aortic (with prosthesis) 35.22
with tissue graft 35.21
mitral (with prosthesis) 35.24
with tissue graft 35.23
poppet (prosthetic) 35.95
pulmonary (with prosthesis) 35.26
with tissue graft 35.25
in total repair of tetralogy of Fallot 35.81
tricuspid (with prosthesis) 35.28
with tissue graft 35.27
hip (partial) (with fixation device) (with prosthesis) (with traction) 81.52
acetabulum 81.52
revision 81.53
femoral head 81.52
revision 81.53
total 81.51
revision 81.53
intervertebral disc
artificial, NOS 84.60
cervical 84.62
nucleus 84.61
partial 84.61
total 84.62
lumbar, lumbosacral 84.65
nucleus 84.64
partial 84.64
total 84.65
thoracic (partial) (total) 84.63
inverted uterus - *see* Repair, inverted uterus
iris NEC 12.39
kidney, mechanical 55.97
knee (bicompartmental) (hemijoint) (partial) (total) (tricompartmental) (unicompartmental) 81.54
revision 81.55
laryngeal stent 31.93
leads (electrode)(s) - *see* Replacement, electrode(s)
mechanical kidney 55.97
mitral valve (with prosthesis) 35.24
with tissue graft 35.23
Mulligan hood, fallopian tube 66.93
muscle stimulator (skeletal) 83.92
nephrostomy tube 55.93
neuropacemaker - *see* Implant, neurostimulator by site
neurostimulator - *see* Implant, neurostimulator, by site
skeletal muscle 83.92
pacemaker
brain - *see* Implant, neurostimulator, brain

Replacement *(Continued)*
pacemaker *(Continued)*
cardiac device (initial) (permanent)
dual-chamber device 37.87
resynchronization - *see* Replacement, CRT-P
single-chamber device 37.85
rate responsive 37.86
electrode(s), cardiac (atrial) (transvenous) (ventricular) 37.76
epicardium (myocardium) 37.74
left ventricular coronary venous system 00.52
gastric – *see* Implant, neurostimulator, gastric
intracranial - *see* Implant, neurostimulator, intracranial
neural - *see* Implant, neurostimulator, by site
peripheral nerve - *see* Implant, neurostimulator, peripheral nerve
sacral nerve - *see* Implant, neurostimulator, sacral nerve
spine - *see* Implant, neurostimulator, spine
temporary transvenous pacemaker system 37.78
pack or bag
nose 97.21
teeth, tooth 97.22
vagina 97.26
vulva 97.26
wound 97.16
pessary, vagina NEC 97.25
prosthesis
acetabulum 81.53
arm (bioelectric) (cineplastic) (kineplastic) 84.44
biliary tract 51.99
cochlear 20.96
channel (single) 20.97
multiple 20.98
elbow 81.97
extremity (bioelectric) (cineplastic) (kineplastic) 84.40
lower 84.48
upper 84.44
fallopian tube (Mulligan hood) (stent) 66.93
femur 81.53
knee 81.55
leg (bioelectric) (cineplastic) (kineplastic) 84.48
penis (internal) (non-inflatable) 64.95
inflatable (internal) 64.97
pulmonary valve (with prosthesis) 35.26
with tissue graft 35.25
in total repair of tetralogy of Fallot 35.81
pyelostomy tube 55.94
rectal tube 96.09
sensor (lead)
intracardiac hemodynamic monitoring 00.56
shoulder NEC 81.83
partial 81.81
total 81.80
skull
plate 02.05
tongs 02.94
specified appliance or device NEC 97.29
stent
bile duct 97.05
fallopian tube 66.93

◀ New ⬅ Revised

Replacement *(Continued)*
- stent *(Continued)*
  - larynx 31.93
  - pancreatic duct 97.05
  - trachea 31.93
- stimoceiver - *see* Implant, stimoceiver, by site
- subdural
  - grids 02.93
  - strips 02.93
- testis in scrotum 62.5
- tongs, skull 02.94
- tracheal stent 31.93
- tricuspid valve (with prosthesis) 35.28
  - with tissue graft 35.27
- tube
  - bile duct 97.05
  - bladder 57.95
  - cystostomy 59.94
  - esophagostomy 97.01
  - gastrostomy 97.02
  - large intestine 97.04
  - nasogastric 97.01
  - nephrostomy 55.93
  - pancreatic duct 97.05
  - pyelostomy 55.94
  - rectal 96.09
  - small intestine 97.03
  - tracheostomy 97.23
  - ureterostomy 59.93
  - ventricular (cerebral) 02.42
- umbilical cord, prolapsed 73.92
- ureter (with)
  - bladder flap 56.74
  - ileal segment implanted into bladder 56.89 *[45.51]*
- ureterostomy tube 59.93
- urethral sphincter, artificial 58.93
- urinary sphincter, artificial 58.93
- valve
  - heart - *see also* Replacement, heart valve, poppet (prosthetic) 35.95
  - ventricular (cerebral) 02.42
- ventricular shunt (catheter) (valve) 02.42
- Vinke tongs (skull) 02.94
- vitreous (silicone) 14.75
  - for retinal reattachment 14.59

Replant, replantation - *see also* Reattachment
- extremity - *see* Reattachment, extremity
- penis 64.45
- scalp 86.51
- tooth 23.5

Reposition
- cardiac pacemaker
  - electrode(s) (atrial) (transvenous) (ventricular) 37.75
  - pocket 37.79
- cardiac resynchronization defibrillator (CRT-D) – *see* Revision, cardiac resynchronization defibrillator ◀
- cardiac resynchronization pacemaker (CRT-P) – *see* Revision, cardiac resynchronization pacemaker ◀
- cardioverter/defibrillator (automatic)
  - lead(s) (epicardial patch) (pacing) (sensing) 37.75 ⇐
  - pocket 37.79 ⇐
  - pulse generator 37.79 ⇐
- cilia base 08.71
- implantable hemodynamic sensor (lead) and monitor device 37.79 ◀
- iris 12.39

Reposition *(Continued)*
- neurostimulator
  - leads
    - subcutaneous, without device replacement 86.09
    - within brain 02.93
    - within or over gastric nerve 04.92 ◀
    - within or over peripheral nerve 04.92
    - within or over sacral nerve 04.92
    - within spine 03.93
  - pulse generator
    - subcutaneous, without device replacement 86.09
- renal vessel, aberrant 39.55
- subcutaneous device pocket NEC 86.09
- thyroid tissue 06.94
- tricuspid valve (with plication) 35.14

Resection - *see also* Excision, by site
- abdominoendorectal (combined) 48.5
- abdominoperineal (rectum) 48.5
  - pull-through (Altemeier) (Swenson) NEC 48.49
    - Duhamel type 48.65
- alveolar process and palate (en bloc) 27.32
- aneurysm - *see* Aneurysmectomy
- aortic valve (for subvalvular stenosis) 35.11
- artery - *see* Arteriectomy
- bile duct NEC 51.69
  - common duct NEC 51.63
- bladder (partial) (segmental) (transvesical) (wedge) 57.6
  - complete or total 57.79
  - lesion NEC 57.59
    - transurethral approach 57.49
  - neck 57.59
    - transurethral approach 57.49
- blood vessel - *see* Angiectomy
- brain 01.59
  - by
    - stereotactic radiosurgery 92.30
      - cobalt 60 92.32
      - linear accelerator (LINAC) 92.31
      - multi-source 92.32
      - particle beam 92.33
      - particulate 92.33
      - radiosurgery NEC 92.39
      - single source photon 92.31
  - hemisphere 01.52
  - lobe 01.53
- breast - *see also* Mastectomy
  - quadrant 85.22
  - segmental 85.23
- broad ligament 69.19
- bronchus (sleeve) (wide sleeve) 32.1
  - block (en bloc) (with radical dissection of brachial plexus, bronchus, lobe of lung, ribs, and sympathetic nerves) 32.6
- bursa 83.5
  - hand 82.31
- cecum (and terminal ileum) 45.72
- cerebral meninges 01.51
- chest wall 34.4
- clavicle 77.81
- clitoris 71.4
- colon (partial) (segmental) 45.79
  - ascending (cecum and terminal ileum) 45.72
  - cecum (and terminal ileum) 45.72
  - complete 45.8
  - descending (sigmoid) 45.76

Resection *(Continued)*
- colon *(Continued)*
  - for interposition 45.52
  - Hartmann 45.75
  - hepatic flexure 45.73
  - left radical (hemicolon) 45.75
  - multiple segmental 45.71
  - right radical (hemicolon) (ileocolectomy) 45.73
  - segmental NEC 45.79
    - multiple 45.71
  - sigmoid 45.76
  - splenic flexure 45.75
  - total 45.8
  - transverse 45.74
- conjunctiva, for pterygium 11.39
  - corneal graft 11.32
- cornual (fallopian tube) (unilateral) 66.69
  - bilateral 66.63
- diaphragm 34.81
- endaural 20.79
- endorectal (pull-through) (Soave) 48.41
  - combined abdominal 48.5
- esophagus (partial) (subtotal) - *see also* Esophagectomy 42.41
  - total 42.42
- exteriorized intestine - *see* Resection, intestine, exteriorized
- fascia 83.44
  - for graft 83.43
    - hand 82.34
  - hand 82.35
    - for graft 82.34
- gallbladder (total) 51.22
- gastric (partial) (sleeve) (subtotal) NEC - *see also* Gastrectomy 43.89
  - with anastomosis NEC 43.89
    - esophagogastric 43.5
    - gastroduodenal 43.6
    - gastrogastric 43.89
    - gastrojejunal 43.7
  - complete or total NEC 43.99
    - with intestinal interposition 43.91
  - radical NEC 43.99
    - with intestinal interposition 43.91
  - wedge 43.42
    - endoscopic 43.41
- hallux valgus (joint) - *see also* Bunionectomy with prosthetic implant 77.59
- hepatic
  - duct 51.69
  - flexure (colon) 45.73
- infundibula, heart (right) 35.34
- intestine (partial) NEC 45.79
  - cecum (with terminal ileum) 45.72
  - exteriorized (large intestine) 46.04
    - small intestine 46.02
  - for interposition 45.50
    - large intestine 45.52
    - small intestine 45.51
  - hepatic flexure 45.73
  - ileum 45.62
    - with cecum 45.72
  - large (partial) (segmental) NEC 45.79
    - for interposition 45.52
    - multiple segmental 45.71
    - total 45.8
  - left hemicolon 45.75
  - multiple segmental (large intestine) 45.71
    - small intestine 45.61
  - right hemicolon 45.73
  - segmental (large intestine) 45.79

ICD-9-CM R Vol. 3

Resection *(Continued)*
intestine NEC *(Continued)*
segmental *(Continued)*
multiple 45.71
small intestine 45.62
multiple 45.61
sigmoid 45.76
small (partial) (segmental) NEC 45.62
for interposition 45.51
multiple segmental 45.61
total 45.63
total
large intestine 45.8
small intestine 45.63
joint structure NEC - *see also* Arthrectomy 80.90
kidney (segmental) (wedge) 55.4
larynx - *see also* Laryngectomy
submucous 30.29
lesion - *see* Excision, lesion, by site
levator palpebrae muscle 08.33
ligament - *see also* Arthrectomy 80.90
broad 69.19
round 69.19
uterine 69.19
lip (wedge) 27.43
liver (partial) (wedge) 50.22
lobe (total) 50.3
total 50.4
lung (wedge) NEC 32.29
endoscopic 32.28
segmental (any part) 32.3
volume reduction 32.22
biologic lung volume reduction (BLVR) – *see* category 33.7 ◀
meninges (cerebral) 01.51
spinal 03.4
mesentery 54.4
muscle 83.45
extraocular 15.13
with
advancement or recession of other eye muscle 15.3
suture of original insertion 15.13
levator palpebrae 08.33
Muller's, for blepharoptosis 08.35
orbicularis oculi 08.20
tarsal, for blepharoptosis 08.35
for graft 83.43
hand 82.34
hand 82.36
for graft 82.34
ocular - *see* Resection, muscle, extraocular
myocardium 37.33
nasal septum (submucous) 21.5
nerve (cranial) (peripheral) NEC 04.07
phrenic 04.03
for collapse of lung 33.31
sympathetic 05.29
vagus - *see* Vagotomy
nose (complete) (extended) (partial) (radical) 21.4
omentum 54.4
orbitomaxillary, radical 16.51
ovary - *see also* Oophorectomy
wedge 65.22
laparoscopic 65.24
palate (bony) (local) 27.31
by wide excision 27.32
soft 27.49
pancreas (total) (with synchronous duodenectomy) 52.6

Resection *(Continued)*
pancreas *(Continued)*
partial NEC 52.59
distal (tail) (with part of body) 52.52
proximal (head) (with part of body) (with synchronous duodenectomy) 52.51
radical subtotal 52.53
radical (one-stage) (two-stage) 52.7
subtotal 52.53
pancreaticoduodenal - *see also* Pancreatectomy 52.6
pelvic viscera (en masse) (female) 68.8
male 57.71
penis 64.3
pericardium (partial) (for)
chronic constrictive pericarditis 37.31
drainage 37.12
removal of adhesions 37.31
peritoneum 54.4
pharynx (partial) 29.33
phrenic nerve 04.03
for collapse of lung 33.31
prostate - *see also* Prostatectomy
transurethral (punch) 60.29
pterygium 11.39
radial head 77.83
rectosigmoid - *see also* Resection, rectum 48.69
rectum (partial) NEC 48.69
with
pelvic exenteration 68.8
transsacral sigmoidectomy 48.61
abdominoendorectal (combined) 48.5
abdominoperineal 48.5
pull-through NEC 48.49
Duhamel type 48.65
anterior 48.63
with colostomy (synchronous) 48.62
Duhamel 48.65
endorectal 48.41
combined abdominal 48.5
posterior 48.64
pull-through NEC 48.49
endorectal 48.41
submucosal (Soave) 48.41
combined abdominal 48.5
rib (transaxillary) 77.91
as operative approach - *omit code*
incidental to thoracic operation - *omit code*
right ventricle (heart), for infundibular stenosis 35.34
root (tooth) (apex) 23.73
with root canal therapy 23.72
residual or retained 23.11
round ligament 69.19
sclera 12.65
with scleral buckling - *see also* Buckling, scleral 14.49
lamellar (for retinal reattachment) 14.49
with implant 14.41
scrotum 61.3
soft tissue NEC 83.49
hand 82.39
sphincter of Oddi 51.89
spinal cord (meninges) 03.4
splanchnic 05.29
splenic flexure (colon) 45.75
sternum 77.81

Resection *(Continued)*
stomach (partial) (sleeve) (subtotal) NEC - *see also* Gastrectomy 43.89
with anastomosis NEC 43.89
esophagogastric 43.5
gastroduodenal 43.6
gastrogastric 43.89
gastrojejunal 43.7
complete or total NEC 43.99
with intestinal interposition 43.91
fundus 43.89
radical NEC 43.99
with intestinal interposition 43.91
wedge 43.42
endoscopic 43.41
submucous
larynx 30.29
nasal septum 21.5
vocal cords 30.22
synovial membrane (complete) (partial) - *see also* Synovectomy 80.70
tarsolevator 08.33
tendon 83.42
hand 82.33
thoracic structures (block) (en bloc) (radical) (brachial plexus, bronchus, lobes of lung, ribs, and sympathetic nerves) 32.6
thorax 34.4
tongue 25.2
wedge 25.1
tooth root 23.73
with root canal therapy 23.72
apex (abscess) 23.73
with root canal therapy 23.72
residual or retained 23.11
trachea 31.5
transurethral
bladder NEC 57.49
prostate 60.29
transverse colon 45.74
turbinates - *see* Turbinectomy
ureter (partial) 56.41
total 56.42
uterus - *see* Hysterectomy
vein - *see* Phlebectomy
ventricle (heart) 37.35
infundibula 35.34
vesical neck 57.59
transurethral 57.49
vocal cords (punch) 30.22
Respirator, volume-controlled (Bennett) (Byrd) - *see* Ventilation
Restoration
cardioesophageal angle 44.66
laparoscopic 44.67
dental NEC 23.49
by
application of crown (artificial) 23.41
insertion of bridge (fixed) 23.42
removable 23.43
extremity - *see* Reattachment, extremity
eyebrow 08.70
with graft 08.63
eye socket 16.64
with graft 16.63
tooth NEC 23.2
by
crown (artificial) 23.41
filling (amalgam) (plastic) (silicate) 23.2
inlay 23.3

Restrictive
gastric band, laparoscopic 44.95
Resurfacing, hip 00.86 ◀
acetabulum 00.87 ◀
with femoral head 00.85 ◀
femoral head 00.86 ◀
with acetabulum 00.85 ◀
partial NOS 00.85 ◀
acetabulum 00.87 ◀
femoral head 00.86 ◀
total (acetabulum and femoral head) 00.85 ◀
Resuscitation
artificial respiration 93.93
cardiac 99.60
cardioversion 99.62
atrial 99.61
defibrillation 99.62
external massage 99.63
open chest 37.91
intracardiac injection 37.92
cardiopulmonary 99.60
endotracheal intubation 96.04
manual 93.93
mouth-to-mouth 93.93
pulmonary 93.93
Resuture
abdominal wall 54.61
cardiac septum prosthesis 35.95
chest wall 34.71
heart valve prosthesis (poppet) 35.95
wound (skin and subcutaneous tissue) (without graft) NEC 86.59
Retavase, infusion 99.10
Reteplase, infusion 99.10
Retinaculotomy NEC - *see also* Division, ligament 80.40
carpal tunnel (flexor) 04.43
Retraining
cardiac 93.36
vocational 93.85
Retrogasserian neurotomy 04.02
Revascularization
cardiac (heart muscle) (myocardium) (direct) 36.10
with
bypass anastomosis
abdominal artery to coronary artery 36.17
aortocoronary (catheter stent) (homograft) (prosthesis) (saphenous vein graft) 36.10
one coronary vessel 36.11
two coronary vessels 36.12
three coronary vessels 36.13
four coronary vessels 36.14
gastroepiploic artery to coronary artery 36.17
internal mammary-coronary artery (single vessel) 36.15
double vessel 36.16
specified type NEC 36.19
thoracic artery-coronary artery (single vessel) 36.15
double vessel 36.16
implantation of artery into heart (muscle) (myocardium) (ventricle) 36.2
indirect 36.2
specified type NEC 36.39
transmyocardial
endoscopic 36.33 ◀
endovascular 36.34 ◀
open chest 36.31

Revascularization *(Continued)*
cardiac *(Continued)*
transmyocardial *(Continued)*
percutaneous 36.34 (Revised)
specified type NEC 36.32
thoracoscopic 36.33 (Revised)
Reversal, intestinal segment 45.50
large 45.52
small 45.51
Revision
amputation stump 84.3
current traumatic - *see* Amputation
anastomosis
biliary tract 51.94
blood vessel 39.49
gastric, gastrointestinal (with jejunal interposition) 44.5
intestine (large) 46.94
small 46.93
pleurothecal 03.97
pyelointestinal 56.72
salpingothecal 03.97
subarachnoid-peritoneal 03.97
subarachnoid-ureteral 03.97
ureterointestinal 56.72
ankle replacement (prosthesis) 81.59
anterior segment (eye) wound (operative) NEC 12.83
arteriovenous shunt (cannula) (for dialysis) 39.42
arthroplasty - *see* Arthroplasty
bone flap, skull 02.06
breast implant 85.93
bronchostomy 33.42
bypass graft (vascular) 39.49
abdominal - coronary artery 36.17
aortocoronary (catheter stent) (with prosthesis) (with saphenous vein graft) (with vein graft) 36.10
one coronary vessel 36.11
two coronary vessels 36.12
three coronary vessels 36.13
four coronary vessels 36.14
CABG - *see* Revision, aortocoronary bypass graft
chest tube - *see* intercostal catheter
coronary artery bypass graft (CABG) *see* Revision, aortocoronary bypass graft, abdominal - coronary artery bypass, and internal mammary - coronary artery bypass
intercostal catheter (with lysis of adhesions) 34.04
internal mammary - coronary artery (single) 36.15
double vessel 36.16
cannula, vessel-to-vessel (arteriovenous) 39.94
canthus, lateral 08.59
cardiac pacemaker
device (permanent) 37.89
electrode(s) (atrial) (transvenous) (ventricular) 37.75
pocket 37.79
cardiac resynchronization defibrillator (CRT-D) (Revised)
device 37.79 ◀
electrode(s) 37.75 ◀
pocket 37.79 ◀
cardiac resynchronization pacemaker (CRT-P)
device (permanent) 37.89

Revision *(Continued)*
cardiac resynchronization pacemaker *(Continued)*
electrode(s) (atrial) (transvenous) (ventricular) 37.75
pocket 37.79
cardioverter/defibrillator (automatic)
pocket 37.79 (Revised)
cholecystostomy 51.99
cleft palate repair 27.63
colostomy 46.43
conduit, urinary 56.52
cystostomy (stoma) 57.22
disc - *see* Revision, intervertebral disc
elbow replacement (prosthesis) 81.97
enterostomy (stoma) 46.40
large intestine 46.43
small intestine 46.41
enucleation socket 16.64
with graft 16.63
esophagostomy 42.83
exenteration cavity 16.66
with secondary graft 16.65
extraocular muscle surgery 15.6
fenestration, inner ear 20.62
filtering bleb 12.66
fixation device (broken) (displaced) - *see also* Fixation, bone, internal 78.50
flap or pedicle graft (skin) 86.75
foot replacement (prosthesis) 81.59
gastric anastomosis (with jejunal interposition) 44.5
gastric band, laparoscopic 44.96
gastric port device
laparoscopic 44.96
gastroduodenostomy (with jejunal interposition) 44.5
gastrointestinal anastomosis (with jejunal interposition) 44.5
gastrojejunostomy 44.5
gastrostomy 44.69
laparoscopic 44.68
hand replacement (prosthesis) 81.97
heart procedure NEC 35.95
hip replacement NOS 81.53
acetabular and femoral components (total) 00.70
acetabular component only 00.71
acetabular liner and/or femoral head only 00.73
femoral component only 00.72
femoral head only and/or acetabular liner 00.73
partial
acetabular component only 00.71
acetabular liner and/or femoral head only 00.73
femoral component only 00.72
femoral head only and/or acetabular liner 00.73
total (acetabular and femoral components) 00.70
Holter (-Spitz) valve 02.42
ileal conduit 56.52
ileostomy 46.41
intervertebral disc, artificial (partial) (total) NOS 84.69
cervical 84.66
lumbar, lumbosacral 84.68
thoracic 84.67
jejunoileal bypass 46.93
jejunostomy 46.41

ICD-9-CM R Vol. 3

Revision *(Continued)*
joint replacement
acetabular and femoral components (total) 00.70
acetabular component only 00.71
acetabular liner and/or femoral head only 00.73
ankle 81.59
elbow 81.97
femoral component only 00.72
femoral head only and/or acetabular liner 00.73
foot 81.59
hand 81.97
hip 81.53
acetabular and femoral components (total) 00.70
acetabular component only 00.71
acetabular liner and/or femoral head only 00.73
femoral component only 00.72
femoral head only and/or acetabular liner 00.73
partial
acetabular component only 00.71
acetabular liner and/or femoral head only 00.73
femoral component only 00.72
femoral head only and/or acetabular liner 00.73
total (acetabular and femoral components) 00.70
knee replacement NOS 81.55
femoral component 00.82
partial
femoral component 00.82
patellar component 00.83
tibial component 00.81
tibial insert 00.84
patellar component 00.83
tibial component 00.81
tibial insert 00.84
total (all components) 00.80
lower extremity NEC 81.59
toe 81.59
upper extremity 81.97
wrist 81.97
knee replacement (prosthesis) NOS 81.55
femoral component 00.82
partial
femoral component 00.82
patellar component 00.83
tibial component 00.81
tibial insert 00.84
patellar component 00.83
tibial component 00.81
tibial insert 00.84
total (all components) 00.80
laryngostomy 31.63
lateral canthus 08.59
mallet finger 82.84
mastoid antrum 19.9
mastoidectomy 20.92
nephrostomy 55.89
neuroplasty 04.75
ocular implant 16.62
orbital implant 16.62
pocket
cardiac device (defibrillator) (pacemaker)
with initial insertion of cardiac device - *omit code*

Revision *(Continued)*
pocket *(Continued)*
cardiac device *(Continued)*
new site (cardiac device pocket) (skin) (subcutaneous) 37.79
intracardiac hemodynamic monitoring 37.79 ◀
subcutaneous device pocket NEC
with initial insertion of generator or device - *omit code*
new site 86.09
thalamic stimulator pulse generator
with initial insertion of battery package - *omit code*
new site (skin) (subcutaneous) 86.09
previous mastectomy site - *see* categories 85.0–85.99
proctostomy 48.79
prosthesis
acetabular and femoral components (total) 00.70
acetabular component only 00.71
acetabular liner and/or femoral head only 00.73
ankle 81.59
breast 85.93
elbow 81.97
femoral component only 00.72
femoral head only and/or acetabular liner 00.73
foot 81.59
hand 81.97
heart valve (poppet) 35.95
hip 81.53
acetabular and femoral components (total) 00.70
acetabular component only 00.71
acetabular liner and/or femoral head only 00.73
femoral component only 00.72
femoral head only and/or acetabular liner 00.73
partial
acetabular component only 00.71
acetabular liner and/or femoral head only 00.73
femoral component only 00.72
femoral head only and/or acetabular liner 00.73
total (acetabular and femoral components) 00.70
knee NOS 81.55
femoral component 00.82
partial
femoral component 00.82
patellar component 00.83
tibial component 00.81
tibial insert 00.84
patellar component 00.83
tibial component 00.81
tibial insert 00.84
total (all components) 00.80
lower extremity NEC 81.59
shoulder 81.97
toe 81.59
upper extremity 81.97
wrist 81.97
ptosis overcorrection 08.37
pyelostomy 55.12
pyloroplasty 44.29
rhinoplasty 21.84
scar
skin 86.84
with excision 86.3

Revision *(Continued)*
scleral fistulization 12.66
shoulder replacement (prosthesis) 81.97
shunt
arteriovenous (cannula) (for dialysis) 39.42
lumbar-subarachnoid NEC 03.97
peritoneojugular 54.99
peritoneovascular 54.99
pleurothecal 03.97
salpingothecal 03.97
spinal (thecal) NEC 03.97
subarachnoid-peritoneal 03.97
subarachnoid-ureteral 03.97
ventricular (cerebral) 02.42
ventriculoperitoneal
at peritoneal site 54.95
at ventricular site 02.42
stapedectomy NEC 19.29
with incus replacement (homograft) (prosthesis) 19.21
stoma
bile duct 51.79
bladder (vesicostomy) 57.22
bronchus 33.42
common duct 51.72
esophagus 42.89
gallbladder 51.99
hepatic duct 51.79
intestine 46.40
large 46.43
small 46.41
kidney 55.89
larynx 31.63
rectum 48.79
stomach 44.69
laparoscopic 44.68
thorax 34.79
trachea 31.74
ureter 56.62
urethra 58.49
tack operation 20.79
toe replacement (prosthesis) 81.59
tracheostomy 31.74
tunnel
pulse generator lead wire 86.99
with initial procedure - *omit code*
tympanoplasty 19.6
uretero-ileostomy, cutaneous 56.52
ureterostomy (cutaneous) (stoma) NEC 56.62
ileal 56.52
urethrostomy 58.49
urinary conduit 56.52
vascular procedure (previous) NEC 39.49
ventricular shunt (cerebral) 02.42
vesicostomy stoma 57.22
wrist replacement (prosthesis) 81.97
Rhinectomy 21.4
Rhinocheiloplasty 27.59
cleft lip 27.54
Rhinomanometry 89.12
Rhinoplasty (external) (internal) NEC 21.87
augmentation (with graft) (with synthetic implant) 21.85
limited 21.86
revision 21.84
tip 21.86
twisted nose 21.84
Rhinorrhaphy (external) (internal) 21.81
for epistaxis 21.09
Rhinoscopy 21.21
Rhinoseptoplasty 21.84

Rhinotomy 21.1
Rhizotomy (radiofrequency) (spinal) 03.1
  acoustic 04.01
  trigeminal 04.02
Rhytidectomy (facial) 86.82
  eyelid
    lower 08.86
    upper 08.87
Rhytidoplasty (facial) 86.82
Ripstein operation (repair of prolapsed rectum) 48.75
Rodney Smith operation (radical subtotal pancreatectomy) 52.53
Roentgenography - *see also* Radiography
  cardiac, negative contrast 88.58
Rolling of conjunctiva 10.33
Root
  canal (tooth) (therapy) 23.70
    with
      apicoectomy 23.72
      irrigation 23.71
    resection (tooth) (apex) 23.73
      with root canal therapy 23.72
      residual or retained 23.11
Rotation of fetal head
  forceps (instrumental) (Kielland) (Scanzoni) (key-in-lock) 72.4
  manual 73.51
Routine
  chest x-ray 87.44
  psychiatric visit 94.12
Roux-en-Y operation
  bile duct 51.36
  cholecystojejunostomy 51.32
  esophagus (intrathoracic) 42.54
  gastroenterostomy 44.39
    laparoscopic 44.38
  gastrojejunostomy 44.39
    laparoscopic 44.38
  pancreaticojejunostomy 52.96
Roux-Goldthwait operation (repair of recurrent patellar dislocation) 81.44
Roux-Herzen-Judine operation (jejunal loop interposition) 42.63
Rubin test (insufflation of fallopian tube) 66.8
Ruiz-Mora operation (proximal phalangectomy for hammer toe) 77.99
Rupture
  esophageal web 42.01
  joint adhesions, manual 93.26
  membranes, artificial 73.09
    for surgical induction of labor 73.01
  ovarian cyst, manual 65.93
Russe operation (bone graft of scaphoid) 78.04

S

Sacculotomy (tack) 20.79
Sacrectomy (partial) 77.89
  total 77.99
Saemisch operation (corneal section) 11.1
Salpingectomy (bilateral) (total) (transvaginal) 66.51
  with oophorectomy 65.61
    laparoscopic 65.63
  partial (unilateral) 66.69
    with removal of tubal pregnancy 66.62
    bilateral 66.63
      for sterilization 66.39
        by endoscopy 66.29
Salpingectomy *(Continued)*
  remaining or solitary tube 66.52
    with ovary 65.62
      laparoscopic 65.64
  unilateral (total) 66.4
    with
      oophorectomy 65.49
        laparoscopic 65.41
      removal of tubal pregnancy 66.62
    partial 66.69
Salpingography 87.85
Salpingohysterostomy 66.74
Salpingo-oophorectomy (unilateral) 65.49
  that by laparoscope 65.41
  bilateral (same operative episode) 65.61
    laparoscopic 65.63
  remaining or solitary tube and ovary 65.62
    laparoscopic 65.64
Salpingo-oophoroplasty 65.73
  laparoscopic 65.76
Salpingo-oophororrhaphy 65.79
Salpingo-oophorostomy 66.72
Salpingo-oophorotomy 65.09
  laparoscopic 65.01
Salpingoplasty 66.79
Salpingorrhaphy 66.71
Salpingosalpingostomy 66.73
Salpingostomy (for removal of non-ruptured ectopic pregnancy) 66.02
Salpingotomy 66.01
Salpingo-uterostomy 66.74
Salter operation (innominate osteotomy) 77.39
Salvage (autologous blood) (intraoperative) (perioperative) (postoperative) 99.00
Sampling, blood for genetic determination of fetus 75.33
Sandpapering (skin) 86.25
Saucerization
  bone - *see also* Excision, lesion, bone 77.60
  rectum 48.99
Sauer-Bacon operation (abdominoperineal resection) 48.5
Scalenectomy 83.45
Scalenotomy 83.19
Scaling and polishing, dental 96.54
Scan, scanning
  C.A.T. (computerized axial tomography) 88.38
    with computer assisted surgery (CAS) 00.31
    abdomen 88.01
    bone 88.38
      mineral density 88.98
    brain 87.03
    head 87.03
    kidney 87.71
    skeletal 88.38
      mineral density 88.98
    thorax 87.41
  computerized axial tomography (C.A.T.) - *see also* Scan, C.A.T. 88.38
  C.T. - *see* Scan, C.A.T.
  gallium - *see* Scan, radioisotope
  liver 92.02
  MUGA (multiple gated acquisition) - *see* Scan, radioiostope
  positron emission tomography (PET) - *see* Scan, radioisotope
  radioisotope
    adrenal 92.09
Scan, scanning *(Continued)*
  radioisotope *(Continued)*
    bone 92.14
      marrow 92.05
    bowel 92.04
    cardiac output 92.05
    cardiovascular 92.05
    cerebral 92.11
    circulation time 92.05
    eye 95.16
    gastrointestinal 92.04
    head NEC 92.12
    hematopoietic 92.05
    intestine 92.04
    iodine-131 92.01
    kidney 92.03
    liver 92.02
    lung 92.15
    lymphatic system 92.16
    myocardial infarction 92.05
    pancreatic 92.04
    parathyroid 92.13
    pituitary 92.11
    placenta 92.17
    protein-bound iodine 92.01
    pulmonary 92.15
    radio-iodine uptake 92.01
    renal 92.03
    specified site NEC 92.19
    spleen 92.05
    thyroid 92.01
    total body 92.18
    uterus 92.19
  renal 92.03
  thermal - *see* Thermography
Scapulectomy (partial) 77.81
  total 77.91
Scapulopexy 78.41
Scarification
  conjunctiva 10.33
  nasal veins (with packing) 21.03
  pericardium 36.39
  pleura 34.6
    chemical 34.92
      with cancer chemotherapy substance 34.92 *[99.25]*
        tetracycline 34.92 *[99.21]*
Schanz operation (femoral osteotomy) 77.35
Schauta (-Amreich) operation (radical vaginal hysterectomy) 68.79
  laparoscopic 68.71
Schede operation (thoracoplasty) 33.34
Scheie operation
  cautery of sclera 12.62
  sclerostomy 12.62
Schlatter operation (total gastrectomy) 43.99
Schroeder operation (endocervical excision) 67.39
Schuchardt operation (nonobstetrical episiotomy) 71.09
Schwartze operation (simple mastoidectomy) 20.41
Scintiphotography - *see* Scan, radioisotope
Scintiscan - *see* Scan, radioisotope
Sclerectomy (punch) (scissors) 12.65
  for retinal reattachment 14.49
  Holth's 12.65
  trephine 12.61
    with implant 14.41
Scleroplasty 12.89
Sclerosis - *see* Sclerotherapy

ICD-9-CM
R, S
Vol. 3

Sclerostomy (Scheie's) 12.62
Sclerotherapy
  esophageal varices (endoscopic) 42.33
  hemorrhoids 49.42
  pleura 34.92
    treatment of malignancy (cytotoxic agent) 34.92 *[99.25]*
      with tetracycline 34.92 *[99.21]*
  varicose vein 39.92
  vein NEC 39.92
Sclerotomy (exploratory) 12.89
  anterior 12.89
    with
      iridectomy 12.65
      removal of vitreous 14.71
  posterior 12.89
    with
      iridectomy 12.65
      removal of vitreous 14.72
Scott operation
  intestinal bypass for obesity 45.93
  jejunocolostomy (bypass) 45.93
Scraping
  corneal epithelium 11.41
    for smear or culture 11.21
  trachoma follicles 10.33
Scrotectomy (partial) 61.3
Scrotoplasty 61.49
Scrotorrhaphy 61.41
Scrototomy 61.0
Scrub, posterior nasal (adhesions) 21.91
Sculpturing, heart valve - *see* Valvuloplasty, heart
Section - *see also* Division and Incision
  cesarean - *see* Cesarean section
  ganglion, sympathetic 05.0
  hypophyseal stalk - *see also* Hypophysectomy, partial 07.63
  ligamentum flavum (spine) - *omit code*
  nerve (cranial) (peripheral) NEC 04.03
    acoustic 04.01
    spinal root (posterior) 03.1
    sympathetic 05.0
    trigeminal tract 04.02
  Saemisch (corneal) 11.1
  spinal ligament 80.49
    arcuate - *omit code*
    flavum - *omit code*
  tooth (impacted) 23.19
Seddon-Brooks operation (transfer of pectoralis major tendon) 83.75
Semb operation (apicolysis of lung) 33.39
Senning operation (correction of transposition of great vessels) 35.91
Separation
  twins (attached) (conjoined) (Siamese) 84.93
  asymmetrical (unequal) 84.93
  symmetrical (equal) 84.92
Septectomy
  atrial (closed) 35.41
    open 35.42
    transvenous method (balloon) 35.41
  submucous (nasal) 21.5
Septoplasty NEC 21.88
  with submucous resection of septum 21.5
Septorhinoplasty 21.84
Septostomy (atrial) (balloon) 35.41
Septotomy, nasal 21.1
Sequestrectomy
  bone 77.00
    carpals, metacarpals 77.04
Sequestrectomy *(Continued)*
  bone *(Continued)*
    clavicle 77.01
    facial 76.01
    femur 77.05
    fibula 77.07
    humerus 77.02
    nose 21.32
    patella 77.06
    pelvic 77.09
    phalanges (foot) (hand) 77.09
    radius 77.03
    scapula 77.01
    skull 01.25
    specified site NEC 77.09
    tarsals, metatarsals 77.08
    thorax (ribs) (sternum) 77.01
    tibia 77.07
    ulna 77.03
    vertebrae 77.09
  nose 21.32
  skull 01.25
Sesamoidectomy 77.98
Setback, ear 18.5
Sever operation (division of soft tissue of arm) 83.19
Severing of blepharorrhaphy 08.02
Sewell operation (heart) 36.2
Sharrard operation (iliopsoas muscle transfer) 83.77
Shaving
  bone - *see also* Excision, lesion, bone 77.60
  cornea (epithelium) 11.41
    for smear or culture 11.21
  patella 77.66
Shelf operation (hip arthroplasty) 81.40
Shirodkar operation (encirclement suture, cervix) 67.59
Shock therapy
  chemical 94.24
  electroconvulsive 94.27
  electrotonic 94.27
  insulin 94.24
  subconvulsive 94.26
Shortening
  bone (fusion) 78.20
    femur 78.25
    specified site NEC - *see* category 78.2
    tibia 78.27
    ulna 78.23
  endopelvic fascia 69.22
  extraocular muscle NEC 15.22
    multiple (two or more muscles) 15.4
  eyelid margin 08.71
  eye muscle NEC 15.22
    multiple (two or more muscles) (with lengthening) 15.4
  finger (macrodactyly repair) 82.83
  heel cord 83.85
  levator palpebrae muscle 08.33
  ligament - *see also* Arthroplasty
    round 69.22
    uterosacral 69.22
  muscle 83.85
    extraocular 15.22
      multiple (two or more muscles) 15.4
    hand 82.55
  sclera (for repair of retinal detachment) 14.59
    by scleral buckling - *see also* Buckling, scleral 14.49
Shortening *(Continued)*
  tendon 83.85
    hand 82.55
  ureter (with reimplantation) 56.41
Shunt - *see also* Anastomosis and Bypass, vascular
  abdominovenous 54.94
  aorta-coronary sinus 36.39
  aorta (descending)-pulmonary (artery) 39.0
  aortocarotid 39.22
  aortoceliac 39.26
  aortofemoral 39.25
  aortoiliac 39.25
  aortoiliofemoral 39.25
  aortomesenteric 39.26
  aorto-myocardial (graft) 36.2
  aortorenal 39.24
  aortosubclavian 39.22
  apicoaortic 35.93
  arteriovenous NEC 39.29
    for renal dialysis (by)
      anastomosis 39.27
      external cannula 39.93
  ascending aorta to pulmonary artery (Waterston) 39.0
  axillary-femoral 39.29
  carotid-carotid 39.22
  carotid-subclavian 39.22
  caval-mesenteric 39.1
  corpora cavernosa-corpus spongiosum 64.98
  corpora-saphenous 64.98
  descending aorta to pulmonary artery (Potts-Smith) 39.0
  endolymphatic (-subarachnoid) 20.71
  endolymph-perilymph 20.71
  extracranial-intracranial (EC-IC) 39.28
  femoroperoneal 39.29
  femoropopliteal 39.29
  iliofemoral 39.25
  ilioiliac 39.25
  intestinal
    large-to-large 45.94
    small-to-large 45.93
    small-to-small 45.91
  left subclavian to descending aorta (Blalock-Park) 39.0
  left-to-right (systemic-pulmonary artery) 39.0
  left ventricle (heart) (apex) and aorta 35.93
  lienorenal 39.1
  lumbar-subarachnoid (with valve) NEC 03.79
  mesocaval 39.1
  peritoneal-jugular 54.94
  peritoneo-vascular 54.94
  peritoneovenous 54.94
  pleuroperitoneal 34.05
  pleurothecal (with valve) 03.79
  portacaval (double) 39.1
  portal-systemic 39.1
  portal vein to vena cava 39.1
  pulmonary-innominate 39.0
  pulmonary vein to atrium 35.82
  renoportal 39.1
  right atrium and pulmonary artery 35.94
  right ventricle and pulmonary artery (distal) 35.92
    in repair of
      pulmonary artery atresia 35.92

Shunt *(Continued)*
right ventricle and pulmonary artery *(Continued)*
in repair of *(Continued)*
transposition of great vessels 35.92
truncus arteriosus 35.83
salpingothecal (with valve) 03.79
semicircular subarachnoid 20.71
spinal (thecal) (with valve) NEC 03.79
subarachnoid-peritoneal 03.71
subarachnoid-ureteral 03.72
splenorenal (venous) 39.1
arterial 39.26
subarachnoid-peritoneal (with valve) 03.71
subarachnoid-ureteral (with valve) 03.72
subclavian-pulmonary 39.0
subdural-peritoneal (with valve) 02.34
superior mesenteric-caval 39.1
systemic-pulmonary artery 39.0
transjugular intrahepatic portosystemic [TIPS] 39.1
vena cava to pulmonary artery (Green) 39.21
ventricular (cerebral) (with valve) 02.2
to
abdominal cavity or organ 02.34
bone marrow 02.39
cervical subarachnoid space 02.2
circulatory system 02.32
cisterna magna 02.2
extracranial site NEC 02.39
gallbladder 02.34
head or neck structure 02.31
intracerebral site NEC 02.2
lumbar site 02.39
mastoid 02.31
nasopharynx 02.31
thoracic cavity 02.33
ureter 02.35
urinary system 02.35
venous system 02.32
ventriculoatrial (with valve) 02.32
ventriculocaval (with valve) 02.32
ventriculocisternal (with valve) 02.2
ventriculolumbar (with valve) 02.39
ventriculomastoid (with valve) 02.31
ventriculonasopharyngeal 02.31
ventriculopleural (with valve) 02.33
Sialoadenectomy (parotid) (sublingual) (submaxillary) 26.30
complete 26.32
partial 26.31
radical 26.32
Sialoadenolithotomy 26.0
Sialoadenotomy 26.0
Sialodochoplasty NEC 26.49
Sialogram 87.09
Sialolithotomy 26.0
Sieve, vena cava 38.7
Sigmoid bladder 57.87 *[45.52]*
Sigmoidectomy 45.76
Sigmoidomyotomy 46.91
Sigmoidopexy (Moschowitz) 46.63
Sigmoidoproctectomy - *see also* Resection, rectum 48.69
Sigmoidoproctostomy 45.94
Sigmoidorectostomy 45.94
Sigmoidorrhaphy 46.75
Sigmoidoscopy (rigid) 48.23
with biopsy 45.25
flexible 45.24
Sigmoidoscopy *(Continued)*
through stoma (artificial) 45.22
transabdominal 45.21
Sigmoidosigmoidostomy 45.94
proximal to distal segment 45.76
Sigmoidostomy - *see also* Colostomy 46.10
Sigmoidotomy 45.03
Sign language 93.75
Silver operation (bunionectomy) 77.59
Sinogram
abdominal wall 88.03
chest wall 87.38
retroperitoneum 88.14
Sinusectomy (nasal) (complete) (partial) (with turbinectomy) 22.60
antrum 22.62
with Caldwell-Luc approach 22.61
ethmoid 22.63
frontal 22.42
maxillary 22.62
with Caldwell-Luc approach 22.61
sphenoid 22.64
Sinusotomy (nasal) 22.50
antrum (intranasal) 22.2
with external approach (Caldwell-Luc) 22.39
radical (with removal of membrane lining) 22.31
ethmoid 22.51
frontal 22.41
maxillary (intranasal) 22.2
external approach (Caldwell-Luc) 22.39
radical (with removal of membrane lining) 22.31
multiple 22.53
perinasal 22.50
sphenoid 22.52
Sistrunk operation (excision of thyroglossal cyst) 06.7
Size reduction
abdominal wall (adipose) (pendulous) 86.83
arms (adipose) (batwing) 86.83
breast (bilateral) 85.32
unilateral 85.31
buttocks (adipose) 86.83
skin 86.83
subcutaneous tissue 86.83
thighs (adipose) 86.83
Skeletal series (x-ray) 88.31
Sling - *see also* Operation, sling
fascial (fascia lata)
for facial weakness (trigeminal nerve paralysis) 86.81
mouth 86.81
orbicularis (mouth) 86.81
tongue 25.59
levator muscle (urethrocystopexy) 59.71
pubococcygeal 59.71
rectum (puborectalis) 48.76
tongue (fascial) 25.59
Slitting
canaliculus for
passage of tube 09.42
removal of streptothrix 09.42
lens 13.2
prepuce (dorsal) (lateral) 64.91
Slocum operation (pes anserinus transfer) 81.47
Sluder operation (tonsillectomy) 28.2
Small bowel series (x-ray) 87.63
Smith operation (open osteotomy of mandible) 76.62
Smith-Peterson operation (radiocarpal arthrodesis) 81.25
Smithwick operation (sympathectomy) 05.29
Snaring, polyp, colon (endoscopic) 45.42
Snip, punctum (with dilation) 09.51
Soave operation (endorectal pull-through) 48.41
Somatotherapy, psychiatric NEC 94.29
Sonneberg operation (inferior maxillary neurectomy) 04.07
Sorondo-Ferré operation (hindquarter amputation) 84.19
Soutter operation (iliac crest fasciotomy) 83.14
Spaulding-Richardson operation (uterine suspension) 69.22
Spectrophotometry NEC 89.39
blood 89.39
placenta 89.29
urine 89.29
Speech therapy NEC 93.75
Spermatocelectomy 63.2
Spermatocystectomy 60.73
Spermatocystotomy 60.72
Sphenoidectomy 22.64
Sphenoidotomy 22.52
Sphincterectomy, anal 49.6
Sphincteroplasty
anal 49.79
obstetrical laceration (current) 75.62
old 49.79
bladder neck 57.85
pancreas 51.83
sphincter of Oddi 51.83
Sphincterorrhaphy, anal 49.71
obstetrical laceration (current) 75.62
old 49.79
Sphincterotomy
anal (external) (internal) 49.59
left lateral 49.51
posterior 49.52
bladder (neck) (transurethral) 57.91
choledochal 51.82
endoscopic 51.85
iris 12.12
pancreatic 51.82
endoscopic 51.85
sphincter of Oddi 51.82
endoscopic 51.85
transduodenal ampullary 51.82
endoscopic 51.85
Spinal anesthesia - *omit code*
Spinelli operation (correction of inverted uterus) 75.93
Spirometry (incentive) (respiratory) 89.37
Spivack operation (permanent gastrostomy) 43.19
Splanchnicectomy 05.29
Splanchnicotomy 05.0
Splenectomy (complete) (total) 41.5
partial 41.43
Splenogram 88.64
radioisotope 92.05
Splenolysis 54.59
laparoscopic 54.51
Splenopexy 41.95
Splenoplasty 41.95
Splenoportogram (by splenic arteriography) 88.64
Splenorrhaphy 41.95
Splenotomy 41.2

- **Splinting**
  - dental (for immobilization) 93.55
    - orthodontic 24.7
  - musculoskeletal 93.54
  - ureteral 56.2
- **Splitting** - *see also* Division
  - canaliculus 09.52
  - lacrimal papilla 09.51
  - spinal cord tracts 03.29
    - percutaneous 03.21
  - tendon sheath 83.01
    - hand 82.01
- **Spondylosyndesis** - *see also* Fusion, spinal 81.00
- **S.P. Rogers operation** (knee disarticulation) 84.16
- **Ssabanejew-Frank operation** (permanent gastrostomy) 43.19
- **Stab, intercostal** 34.09
- **Stabilization, joint** - *see also* Arthrodesis
  - patella (for recurrent dislocation) 81.44
- **Stacke operation** (simple mastoidectomy) 20.41
- **Stallard operation** (conjunctivocystorhinostomy) 09.82
  - with insertion of tube or stent 09.83
- **Stamm (-Kader) operation** (temporary gastrostomy) 43.19
- **Stapedectomy** 19.19
  - with incus replacement (homograft) (prosthesis) 19.11
  - revision 19.29
    - with incus replacement 19.21
- **Stapediolysis** 19.0
- **Stapling**
  - artery 39.31
  - blebs, lung (emphysematous) 32.21
  - diaphysis - *see also* Stapling, epiphyseal plate 78.20
  - epiphyseal plate 78.20
    - femur 78.25
    - fibula 78.27
    - humerus 78.22
    - radius 78.23
    - specified site NEC 78.29
    - tibia 78.27
    - ulna 78.23
  - gastric varices 44.91
  - graft - *see* Graft
  - vein 39.32
- **STARR** (stapled transanal rectal resection) 70.52
- **Steinberg operation** 44.5
- **Steindler operation**
  - fascia stripping (for cavus deformity) 83.14
  - flexorplasty (elbow) 83.77
  - muscle transfer 83.77
- **Stereotactic head frame application** 93.59
- **Stereotactic radiosurgery** 92.30
  - cobalt 60 92.32
  - linear accelerator (LINAC) 92.31
  - multi-source 92.32
  - particle beam 92.33
  - particulate 92.33
  - radiosurgery NEC 92.39
  - single source photon 92.31
- **Sterilization**
  - female - *see also* specific operation 66.39
  - male NEC - *see also* Ligation, vas deferens 63.70
- **Sternotomy** 77.31
  - as operative approach - *omit code*
  - for bone marrow biopsy 41.31
- **Stewart operation** (renal plication with pyeloplasty) 55.87
- **Stimulation** (electronic) - *see also* Implant, electronic stimulator
  - bone growth (percutaneous) - *see* category 78.9
    - transcutaneous (surface) 99.86
  - cardiac (external) 99.62
    - internal 37.91
  - carotid sinus 99.64
  - CaverMap™ 89.58 ◀
  - defibrillator
    - as part of intraoperative testing – *omit code* ◀
    - catheter based invasive electrophysiologic testing 37.26 ◀
    - device interrogation only without arrhythmia induction (bedside check) 89.45–89.49 ◀
    - non-invasive programmed electrical stimulation (NIPS) 37.20 ⬅
  - electrophysiologic, cardiac ⬅
    - as part of intraoperative testing – *omit code* ◀
    - catheter based invasive electrophysiologic testing 37.26 ◀
    - device interrogation only without arrhythmia induction (bedside check) 89.45–89.49 ◀
    - noninvasive programmed electrical stimulation (NIPS) 37.20 ◀
  - nerve ⬅
    - CaverMap™ 89.58 ◀
    - penile 89.58 ◀
    - peripheral or spinal cord, transcutaneous 93.39 ◀
- **Stitch, Kelly-Stoeckel** (urethra) 59.3
- **Stomatoplasty** 27.59
- **Stomatorrhaphy** 27.52
- **Stone operation** (anoplasty) 49.79
- **Strapping** (non-traction) 93.59 ◀
- **Strassman operation** (metroplasty) 69.49
- **Strayer operation** (gastrocnemius recession) 83.72
- **Stretching**
  - eyelid (with elongation) 08.71
  - fascia 93.28
  - foreskin 99.95
  - iris 12.63
  - muscle 93.27
  - nerve (cranial) (peripheral) 04.91
  - tendon 93.27
- **Stripping**
  - bone - *see also* Incision, bone 77.10
  - carotid sinus 39.8
  - cranial suture 02.01
  - fascia 83.14
    - hand 82.12
  - membranes for surgical induction of labor 73.1
  - meninges (cerebral) 01.51
    - spinal 03.4
  - saphenous vein, varicose 38.59
  - subdural membrane (cerebral) 01.51
    - spinal 03.4
  - varicose veins (lower limb) 38.59
    - upper limb 38.53
  - vocal cords 30.09
- **Stromeyer-Little operation** (hepatotomy) 50.0
- **Strong operation** (unbridling of celiac artery axis) 39.91
- **Stryker frame** 93.59
- **Study**
  - bone mineral density 88.98
- **Study** *(Continued)*
  - bundle of His 37.29
  - color vision 95.06
  - conduction, nerve (median) 89.15
  - dark adaptation, eye 95.07
  - electrophysiologic stimulation and recording, cardiac ⬅
    - as part of intraoperative testing – *omit code* ◀
    - catheter based invasive electrophysiologic testing 37.26 ◀
    - device interrogation only without arrhythmia induction (bedside check) 89.45–89.49 ◀
    - noninvasive programmed electrical stimulation (NIPS) 37.20 ◀
  - function - *see also* Function, study
    - radioisotope - *see* Scan, radioisotope
  - lacrimal flow (radiographic) 87.05
  - ocular motility 95.15
  - pulmonary function - *see* categories 89.37–89.38
  - radiographic - *see* Radiography
  - radio-iodinated triolein 92.04
  - renal clearance 92.03
  - spirometer 89.37
  - tracer - *see also* Scan, radioisotope, eye (P32) 95.16
  - ultrasonic - *see* Ultrasonography
  - visual field 95.05
  - xenon flow NEC 92.19
    - cardiovascular 92.05
    - pulmonary 92.15
- **Sturmdorf operation** (conization of cervix) 67.2
- **Submucous resection**
  - larynx 30.29
  - nasal septum 21.5
- **Summerskill operation** (dacryocystorhinostomy by intubation) 09.81
- **Surgery**
  - computer assisted (CAS) 00.39
    - CAS with CT/CTA 00.31
    - CAS with fluoroscopy 00.33
    - CAS with MR/MRA 00.32
    - CAS with multiple datasets 00.35
      - imageless 00.34
      - other CAS 00.39
    - IGS - *see* Surgery, computer assisted
    - image guided - *see* Surgery, computer assisted
    - navigation (CT-free, IGN image guided, imageless) - *see* Surgery, computer assisted
- **Surmay operation** (jejunostomy) 46.39
- **Suspension**
  - balanced, for traction 93.45
  - bladder NEC 57.89
  - diverticulum, pharynx 29.59
  - kidney 55.7
  - Olshausen (uterus) 69.22
  - ovary 65.79
  - paraurethral (Pereyra) 59.6
  - periurethral 59.6
  - urethra (retropubic) (sling) 59.5
  - urethrovesical
    - Goebel-Frangenheim-Stoeckel 59.4
    - gracilis muscle transplant 59.71
    - levator muscle sling 59.71
    - Marshall-Marchetti (-Krantz) 59.5
    - Millin-Read 59.4
    - suprapubic 59.4
  - uterus (abdominal or vaginal approach) 69.22
  - vagina 70.77

Suture (laceration)
abdominal wall 54.63
secondary 54.61
adenoid fossa 28.7
adrenal (gland) 07.44
aneurysm (cerebral) (peripheral) 39.52
anus 49.71
obstetric laceration (current) 75.62
old 49.79
aorta 39.31
aponeurosis - *see also* Suture, tendon 83.64
arteriovenous fistula 39.53
artery 39.31
percutaneous puncture closure - *omit code*
bile duct 51.79
bladder 57.81
obstetric laceration (current) 75.61
blood vessel NEC 39.30
artery 39.31
percutaneous puncture closure - *omit code*
vein 39.32
breast (skin) 85.81
bronchus 33.41
bursa 83.99
hand 82.99
canaliculus 09.73
cecum 46.75
cerebral meninges 02.11
cervix (traumatic laceration) 67.61
internal os, encirclement 67.59
obstetric laceration (current) 75.51
old 67.69
chest wall 34.71
cleft palate 27.62
clitoris 71.4
colon 46.75
common duct 51.71
conjunctiva 10.6
cornea 11.51
with conjunctival flap 11.53
corneoscleral 11.51
with conjunctival flap 11.53
diaphragm 34.82
duodenum 46.71
ulcer (bleeding) (perforated) 44.42
endoscopic 44.43
dura mater (cerebral) 02.11
spinal 03.59
ear, external 18.4
enterocele 70.92
entropion 08.42
epididymis (and)
spermatic cord 63.51
vas deferens 63.81
episiotomy - *see* Episiotomy
esophagus 42.82
eyeball 16.89
eyebrow 08.81
eyelid 08.81
with entropion or ectropion repair 08.42
fallopian tube 66.71
fascia 83.65
hand 82.46
to skeletal attachment 83.89
hand 82.89
gallbladder 51.91
ganglion, sympathetic 05.81
gingiva 24.32
great vessel 39.30
artery 39.31
vein 39.32

Suture *(Continued)*
gum 24.32
heart 37.49
hepatic duct 51.79
hymen 70.76
ileum 46.73
intestine 46.79
large 46.75
small 46.73
jejunum 46.73
joint capsule 81.96
with arthroplasty - *see* Arthroplasty
ankle 81.94
foot 81.94
lower extremity NEC 81.95
upper extremity 81.93
kidney 55.81
labia 71.71
laceration - *see* Suture, by site
larynx 31.61
ligament 81.96
with arthroplasty - *see* Arthroplasty
ankle 81.94
broad 69.29
Cooper's 54.64
foot and toes 81.94
gastrocolic 54.73
knee 81.95
lower extremity NEC 81.95
sacrouterine 69.29
upper extremity 81.93
uterine 69.29
ligation - *see* Ligation
lip 27.51
liver 50.61
lung 33.43
meninges (cerebral) 02.11
spinal 03.59
mesentery 54.75
mouth 27.52
muscle 83.65
hand 82.46
ocular (oblique) (rectus) 15.7
nerve (cranial) (peripheral) 04.3
sympathetic 05.81
nose (external) (internal) 21.81
for epistaxis 21.09
obstetric laceration NEC 75.69
bladder 75.61
cervix 75.51
corpus uteri 75.52
pelvic floor 75.69
perineum 75.69
rectum 75.62
sphincter ani 75.62
urethra 75.61
uterus 75.50
vagina 75.69
vulva 75.69
omentum 54.64
ovary 65.71
laparoscopic 65.74
palate 27.61
cleft 27.62
palpebral fissure 08.59
pancreas 52.95
pelvic floor 71.71
obstetric laceration (current) 75.69
penis 64.41
peptic ulcer (bleeding) (perforated) 44.40
pericardium 37.49
perineum (female) 71.71
after delivery 75.69

Suture *(Continued)*
perineum *(Continued)*
after delivery *(Continued)*
episiotomy repair - *see* Episiotomy
male 86.59
periosteum 78.20
carpal, metacarpal 78.24
femur 78.25
fibula 78.27
humerus 78.22
pelvic 78.29
phalanges (foot) (hand) 78.29
radius 78.23
specified site NEC 78.29
tarsal, metatarsal 78.28
tibia 78.27
ulna 78.23
vertebrae 78.29
peritoneum 54.64
periurethral tissue to symphysis pubis 59.5
pharynx 29.51
pleura 34.93
rectum 48.71
obstetric laceration (current) 75.62
retina (for reattachment) 14.59
sacrouterine ligament 69.29
salivary gland 26.41
scalp 86.59
replantation 86.51
sclera (with repair of conjunctiva) 12.81
scrotum (skin) 61.41
secondary
abdominal wall 54.61
episiotomy 75.69
peritoneum 54.64
sigmoid 46.75
skin (mucous membrane) (without graft) 86.59
with graft - *see* Graft, skin
breast 85.81
ear 18.4
eyebrow 08.81
eyelid 08.81
nose 21.81
penis 64.41
scalp 86.59
replantation 86.51
scrotum 61.41
vulva 71.71
specified site NEC - *see* Repair, by site
spermatic cord 63.51
sphincter ani 49.71
obstetric laceration (current) 75.62
old 49.79
spinal meninges 03.59
spleen 41.95
stomach 44.61
ulcer (bleeding) (perforated) 44.41
endoscopic 44.43
subcutaneous tissue (without skin graft) 86.59
with graft - *see* Graft, skin
tendon (direct) (immediate) (primary) 83.64
delayed (secondary) 83.62
hand NEC 82.43
flexors 82.42
hand NEC 82.45
delayed (secondary) 82.43
flexors 82.44
delayed (secondary) 82.42
ocular 15.7
rotator cuff 83.63

Suture *(Continued)*
tendon *(Continued)*
sheath 83.61
hand 82.41
supraspinatus (rotator cuff repair) 83.63
to skeletal attachment 83.88
hand 82.85
Tenon's capsule 15.7
testis 62.61
thymus 07.93
thyroid gland 06.93
tongue 25.51
tonsillar fossa 28.7
trachea 31.71
tunica vaginalis 61.41
ulcer (bleeding) (perforated) (peptic) 44.40
duodenum 44.42
endoscopic 44.43
gastric 44.41
endoscopic 44.43
intestine 46.79
skin 86.59
stomach 44.41
endoscopic 44.43
ureter 56.82
urethra 58.41
obstetric laceration (current) 75.61
uterosacral ligament 69.29
uterus 69.41
obstetric laceration (current) 75.50
old 69.49
uvula 27.73
vagina 70.71
obstetric laceration (current) 75.69
old 70.79
vas deferens 63.81
vein 39.32
vulva 71.71
obstetric laceration (current) 75.69
old 71.79
Suture-ligation - *see also* Ligation
blood vessel - *see* Ligation, blood vessel
Sweep, anterior iris 12.97
Swenson operation
bladder reconstruction 57.87
proctectomy 48.49
Swinney operation (urethral reconstruction) 58.46
Switch, switching
coronary arteries 35.84
great arteries, total 35.84
Syme operation
ankle amputation through malleoli of tibia and fibula 84.14
urethrotomy, external 58.0
Sympathectomy NEC 05.29
cervical 05.22
cervicothoracic 05.22
lumbar 05.23
periarterial 05.25
presacral 05.24
renal 05.29
thoracolumbar 05.23
tympanum 20.91
Sympatheticotripsy 05.0
Symphysiotomy 77.39
assisting delivery (obstetrical) 73.94
kidney (horseshoe) 55.85
Symphysis, pleural 34.6
Synchondrotomy - *see also* Division, cartilage 80.40
Syndactylization 86.89
Syndesmotomy - *see also* Division, ligament 80.40
Synechiotomy
endometrium 68.21
iris (posterior) 12.33
anterior 12.32
Synovectomy (joint) (complete) (partial) 80.70
ankle 80.77
elbow 80.72
foot and toe 80.78
hand and finger 80.74
hip 80.75
knee 80.76
shoulder 80.71
specified site NEC 80.79
spine 80.79
tendon sheath 83.42
hand 82.33
wrist 80.73
Syringing
lacrimal duct or sac 09.43
nasolacrimal duct 09.43
with
dilation 09.43
insertion of tube or stent 09.44

T

Taarnhoj operation (trigeminal nerve root decompression) 04.41
Tack operation (sacculotomy) 20.79
Take-down
anastomosis
arterial 39.49
blood vessel 39.49
gastric, gastrointestinal 44.5
intestine 46.93
stomach 44.5
vascular 39.49
ventricular 02.43
arterial bypass 39.49
arteriovenous shunt 39.43
with creation of new shunt 39.42
cecostomy 46.52
colostomy 46.52
duodenostomy 46.51
enterostomy 46.50
esophagostomy 42.83
gastroduodenostomy 44.5
gastrojejunostomy 44.5
ileostomy 46.51
intestinal stoma 46.50
large 46.52
small 46.51
jejunoileal bypass 46.93
jejunostomy 46.51
laryngostomy 31.62
sigmoidostomy 46.52
stoma
bile duct 51.79
bladder 57.82
bronchus 33.42
common duct 51.72
esophagus 42.83
gallbladder 51.92
hepatic duct 51.79
intestine 46.50
large 46.52
small 46.51
kidney 55.82
larynx 31.62
rectum 48.72
Take-down *(Continued)*
stoma *(Continued)*
stomach 44.62
thorax 34.72
trachea 31.72
ureter 56.83
urethra 58.42
systemic-pulmonary artery anastomosis 39.49
in total repair of tetralogy of Fallot 35.81
tracheostomy 31.72
vascular anastomosis or bypass 39.49
ventricular shunt (cerebral) 02.43
Talectomy 77.98
Talma-Morison operation (omentopexy) 54.74
Tamponade
esophageal 96.06
intrauterine (nonobstetric) 69.91
after delivery or abortion 75.8
antepartum 73.1
vagina 96.14
after delivery or abortion 75.8
antepartum 73.1
Tanner operation (devascularization of stomach) 44.99
Tap
abdomen 54.91
chest 34.91
cisternal 01.01
cranial 01.09
joint 81.91
lumbar (diagnostic) (removal of dye) 03.31
perilymphatic 20.79
spinal (diagnostic) 03.31
subdural (through fontanel) 01.09
thorax 34.91
Tarsectomy 08.20
de Grandmont 08.35
Tarsoplasty - *see also* Reconstruction, eyelid 08.70
Tarsorrhaphy (lateral) 08.52
division or severing 08.02
Tattooing
cornea 11.91
skin 86.02
Tautening, eyelid for entropion 08.42
Telemetry (cardiac) 89.54
Teleradiotherapy
beta particles 92.25
Betatron 92.24
cobalt-60 92.23
electrons 92.25
iodine-125 92.23
linear accelerator 92.24
neutrons 92.26
particulate radiation NEC 92.26
photons 92.24
protons 92.26
radioactive cesium 92.23
radioisotopes NEC 92.23
Temperament assessment 94.02
Temperature gradient study - *see also* Thermography 88.89
Tendinoplasty - *see* Repair, tendon
Tendinosuture (immediate) (primary) - *see also* Suture, tendon 83.64
hand - *see also* Suture, tendon, hand 82.45
Tendolysis 83.91
hand 82.91
Tendoplasty - *see* Repair, tendon

Tenectomy 83.39
eye 15.13
levator palpebrae 08.33
multiple (two or more tendons) 15.3
hand 82.29
levator palpebrae 08.33
tendon sheath 83.31
hand 82.21
Tenodesis (tendon fixation to skeletal attachment) 83.88
Fowler 82.85
hand 82.85
Tenolysis 83.91
hand 82.91
Tenomyoplasty - *see also* Repair, tendon 83.88
hand - *see also* Repair, tendon, hand 82.86
Tenomyotomy - *see* Tenonectomy
Tenonectomy 83.42
for graft 83.41
hand 82.32
hand 82.33
for graft 82.32
Tenontomyoplasty - *see* Repair, tendon
Tenontoplasty - *see* Repair, tendon
Tenoplasty - *see also* Repair, tendon 83.88
hand - *see also* Repair, tendon, hand 82.86
Tenorrhaphy - *see also* Suture, tendon 83.64
hand - *see also* Suture, tendon, hand 82.45
to skeletal attachment 83.88
hand 82.85
Tenosuspension 83.88
hand 82.86
Tenosuture - *see also* Suture, tendon 83.64
hand - *see also* Suture, tendon, hand 82.45
to skeletal attachment 83.88
hand 82.85
Tenosynovectomy 83.42
hand 82.33
Tenotomy 83.13
Achilles tendon 83.11
adductor (hip) (subcutaneous) 83.12
eye 15.12
levator palpebrae 08.38
multiple (two or more tendons) 15.4
hand 82.11
levator palpebrae 08.38
pectoralis minor tendon (decompression, thoracic outlet) 83.13
stapedius 19.0
tensor tympani 19.0
Tenovaginotomy - *see* Tenotomy
Tensing, orbicularis oculi 08.59
Termination of pregnancy
by
aspiration curettage 69.51
dilation and curettage 69.01
hysterectomy - *see* Hysterectomy
hysterotomy 74.91
intra-amniotic injection (saline) 75.0
Test, testing (for)
14 C-Urea breath 89.39
auditory function NEC 95.46
Bender Visual-Motor Gestalt 94.02
Benton Visual Retention 94.02
cardiac (vascular)
function NEC 89.59
stress 89.44
bicycle ergometer 89.43
Masters' two-step 89.42
treadmill 89.41
Test, testing *(Continued)*
Denver developmental (screening) 94.02
fetus, fetal
nonstress (fetal activity acceleration determinations) 75.34
oxytocin challenge (contraction stress) 75.35
sensitivity (to oxytocin) - *omit code*
function
cardiac NEC 89.59
hearing NEC 95.46
muscle (by)
electromyography 93.08
manual 93.04
neurologic NEC 89.15
vestibular 95.46
clinical 95.44
glaucoma NEC 95.26
hearing 95.47
clinical NEC 95.42
intelligence 94.01
internal jugular-subclavian venous reflux 89.62
intracarotid amobarbital (Wada) 89.10
Masters' two-step stress (cardiac) 89.42
muscle function (by)
electromyography 93.08
manual 93.04
neurologic function NEC 89.15
nocturnal penile tumescence 89.29
provocative, for glaucoma 95.26
psychologic NEC 94.08
psychometric 94.01
radio-cobalt B12 Schilling 92.04
range of motion 93.05
rotation (Bárány chair) (hearing) 95.45
sleep disorder function - *see* categories 89.17–89.18
Stanford-Binet 94.01
Thallium stress (transesophageal pacing) 89.44
tuning fork (hearing) 95.42
urea breath (14 C) 89.39
vestibular function NEC 95.46
thermal 95.44
Wada (hemispheric function) 89.10
whispered speech (hearing) 95.42
TEVAP (transurethral electrovaporization of prostate) 60.29
Thalamectomy 01.41
Thalamotomy 01.41
by stereotactic radiosurgery 92.32
cobalt 60 92.32
linear accelerator (LINAC) 92.31
multi-source 92.32
particle beam 92.33
particulate 92.33
radiosurgery NEC 92.39
single source photon 92.31
Thal operation (repair of esophageal stricture) 42.85
Theleplasty 85.87
Therapy
Antabuse 94.25
art 93.89
aversion 94.33
behavior 94.33
Bennett respirator - *see* category 96.7
blind rehabilitation NEC 93.78
Byrd respirator - *see* category 96.7
carbon dioxide 94.25
cobalt-60 92.23
conditioning, psychiatric 94.33
Therapy *(Continued)*
continuous positive airway pressure (CPAP) 93.90
croupette, croup tent 93.94
daily living activities 93.83
for the blind 93.78
dance 93.89
desensitization 94.33
detoxification 94.25
diversional 93.81
domestic tasks 93.83
for the blind 93.78
educational (bed-bound children) (handicapped) 93.82
electroconvulsive (ECT) 94.27
electroshock (EST) 94.27
subconvulsive 94.26
electrotonic (ETT) 94.27
encounter group 94.44
extinction 94.33
family 94.42
fog (inhalation) 93.94
gamma ray 92.23
group NEC 94.44
for psychosexual dysfunctions 94.41
hearing NEC 95.49
heat NEC 93.35
for cancer treatment 99.85
helium 93.98
hot pack(s) 93.35
hyperbaric oxygen 93.95
wound 93.59
hyperthermia NEC 93.35
for cancer treatment 99.85
individual, psychiatric NEC 94.39
for psychosexual dysfunction 94.34
industrial 93.89
infrared irradiation 93.35
inhalation NEC 93.96
nitric oxide 00.12
insulin shock 94.24
intermittent positive pressure breathing (IPPB) 93.91
IPPB (intermittent positive pressure breathing) 93.91
leech 99.99
lithium 94.22
maggot 86.28
manipulative, osteopathic - *see also* Manipulation, osteopathic 93.67
manual arts 93.81
methadone 94.25
mist (inhalation) 93.94
music 93.84
nebulizer 93.94
neuroleptic 94.23
nitric oxide 00.12
occupational 93.83
oxygen 93.96
catalytic 93.96
hyperbaric 93.95
wound 93.59
wound (hyperbaric) 93.59
paraffin bath 93.35
physical NEC 93.39
combined (without mention of components) 93.38
diagnostic NEC 93.09
play 93.81
psychotherapeutic 94.36
positive and expiratory pressure - *see* category 96.7
psychiatric NEC 94.39

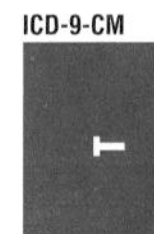
ICD-9-CM
T
Vol. 3

Therapy *(Continued)*
psychiatric NEC *(Continued)*
drug NEC 94.25
lithium 94.22
radiation 92.29
contact (150 KVP or less) 92.21
deep (200-300 KVP) 92.22
high voltage (200-300 KVP) 92.22
low voltage (150 KVP or less) 92.21
megavoltage 92.24
orthovoltage 92.22
particle source NEC 92.26
photon 92.24
radioisotope (teleradiotherapy) 92.23
retinal lesion 14.26
superficial (150 KVP or less) 92.21
supervoltage 92.24
radioisotope, radioisotopic NEC 92.29
implantation or insertion 92.27
injection or instillation 92.28
teleradiotherapy 92.23
radium (radon) 92.23
recreational 93.81
rehabilitation NEC 93.89
respiratory NEC 93.99
bi-level airway pressure 93.90
continuous positive airway pressure [CPAP] 93.90
endotracheal respiratory assistance - *see* category 96.7
intermittent mandatory ventilation [IMV] - *see* category 96.7
intermittent positive pressure breathing [IPPB] 93.91
negative pressure (continuous) [CNP] 93.99
nitric oxide 00.12
non-invasive positive pressure (NIPPV) 93.90
other continuous (unspecified duration) 96.70
for less than 96 consecutive hours 96.71
for 96 consecutive hours or more 96.72
positive end-expiratory pressure [PEEP] - *see* category 96.7
pressure support ventilation [PSV] - *see* category 96.7
root canal 23.70
with
apicoectomy 23.72
irrigation 23.71
shock
chemical 94.24
electric 94.27
subconvulsive 94.26
insulin 94.24
speech 93.75
for correction of defect 93.74
ultrasound
heat therapy 93.35
hyperthermia for cancer treatment 99.85
physical therapy 93.35
therapeutic - *see* Ultrasound
ultraviolet light 99.82
Thermocautery - *see* Cauterization
Thermography 88.89
blood vessel 88.86
bone 88.83
breast 88.85
cerebral 88.81
Thermography *(Continued)*
eye 88.82
lymph gland 88.89
muscle 88.84
ocular 88.82
osteoarticular 88.83
specified site NEC 88.89
vein, deep 88.86
Thermokeratoplasty 11.74
Thermosclerectomy 12.62
Thermotherapy (hot packs) (paraffin bath) NEC 93.35
prostate
by
microwave 60.96
radiofrequency 60.97
transurethral microwave thermotherapy (TUMT) 60.96
transurethral needle ablation (TUNA) 60.97
TUMT (transurethral microwave thermotherapy) 60.96
TUNA (transurethral needle ablation 60.97
Thiersch operation
anus 49.79
skin graft 86.69
hand 86.62
Thompson operation
cleft lip repair 27.54
correction of lymphedema 40.9
quadricepsplasty 83.86
thumb apposition with bone graft 82.69
Thoracectomy 34.09
for lung collapse 33.34
Thoracentesis 34.91
Thoracocentesis 34.91
Thoracolysis (for collapse of lung) 33.39
Thoracoplasty (anterior) (extrapleural) (paravertebral) (posterolateral) (complete) (partial) 33.34
Thoracoscopy, transpleural (for exploration) 34.21
Thoracostomy 34.09
for lung collapse 33.32
Thoracotomy (with drainage) 34.09
as operative approach - *omit code*
exploratory 34.02
Three-snip operation, punctum 09.51
Thrombectomy 38.00
with endarterectomy - *see* Endarterectomy
abdominal
artery 38.06
vein 38.07
aorta (arch) (ascending) (descending) 38.04
arteriovenous shunt or cannula 39.49 ◀
bovine graft 39.49 ◀
coronary artery 36.09
head and neck vessel NEC 38.02
intracranial vessel NEC 38.01
lower limb
artery 38.08
vein 38.09
mechanical ◀
endovascular ◀
head and neck 39.74 ◀
pulmonary vessel 38.05
thoracic vessel NEC 38.05
upper limb (artery) (vein) 38.03
Thromboendarterectomy 38.10
abdominal 38.16
Thromboendarterectomy *(Continued)*
aorta (arch) (ascending) (descending) 38.14
coronary artery 36.09
open chest approach 36.03
head and neck NEC 38.12
intracranial NEC 38.11
lower limb 38.18
thoracic NEC 38.15
upper limb 38.13
Thymectomy 07.80
partial 07.81
total 07.82
Thymopexy 07.99
Thyrochondrotomy 31.3
Thyrocricoidectomy 30.29
Thyrocricotomy (for assistance in breathing) 31.1
Thyroidectomy NEC 06.39
by mediastinotomy - *see also* Thyroidectomy, substernal 06.50
with laryngectomy - *see* Laryngectomy
complete or total 06.4
substernal (by mediastinotomy) (transsternal route) 06.52
transoral route (lingual) 06.6
lingual (complete) (partial) (subtotal) (total) 06.6
partial or subtotal NEC 06.39
with complete removal of remaining lobe 06.2
submental route (lingual) 06.6
substernal (by mediastinotomy) (transsternal route) 06.51
remaining tissue 06.4
submental route (lingual) 06.6
substernal (by mediastinotomy) (transsternal route) 06.50
complete or total 06.52
partial or subtotal 06.51
transoral route (lingual) 06.6
transsternal route - *see also* Thyroidectomy, substernal 06.50
unilateral (with removal of isthmus) (with removal of portion of other lobe) 06.2
Thyroidorrhaphy 06.93
Thyroidotomy (field) (gland) NEC 06.09
postoperative 06.02
Thyrotomy 31.3
with tantalum plate 31.69
Tirofiban (HCl), infusion 99.20
Toilette
skin - *see* Debridement, skin or subcutaneous tissue
tracheostomy 96.55
Token economy (behavior therapy) 94.33
Tomkins operation (metroplasty) 69.49
Tomography - *see also* Radiography
abdomen NEC 88.02
cardiac 87.42
computerized axial NEC 88.38
abdomen 88.01
bone 88.38
quantitative 88.98
brain 87.03
head 87.03
kidney 87.71
skeletal 88.38
quantitative 88.98
thorax 87.41
head NEC 87.04
kidney NEC 87.72

Tomography *(Continued)*
lung 87.42
thorax NEC 87.42
Tongue tie operation 25.91
Tonography 95.26
Tonometry 89.11
Tonsillectomy 28.2
with adenoidectomy 28.3
Tonsillotomy 28.0
Topectomy 01.32
Torek (-Bevan) operation (orchidopexy) (first stage) (second stage) 62.5
Torkildsen operation (ventriculocisternal shunt) 02.2
Torpin operation (cul-de-sac resection) 70.92
Toti operation (dacryocystorhinostomy) 09.81
Touchas operation 86.83
Touroff operation (ligation of subclavian artery) 38.85
Toxicology - *see* Examination, microscopic
TPN (total parenteral nutrition) 99.15
Trabeculectomy ab externo 12.64
Trabeculodialysis 12.59
Trabeculotomy ab externo 12.54
Trachelectomy 67.4
Trachelopexy 69.22
Tracheloplasty 67.69
Trachelorrhaphy (Emmet) (suture) 67.61
obstetrical 75.51
Trachelotomy 69.95
obstetrical 73.93
Tracheocricotomy (for assistance in breathing) 31.1
Tracheofissure 31.1
Tracheography 87.32
Tracheolaryngotomy (emergency) 31.1
permanent opening 31.29
Tracheoplasty 31.79
with artificial larynx 31.75
Tracheorrhaphy 31.71
Tracheoscopy NEC 31.42
through tracheotomy (stoma) 31.41
Tracheostomy (emergency) (temporary) (for assistance in breathing) 31.1
mediastinal 31.21
permanent NEC 31.29
revision 31.74
Tracheotomy (emergency) (temporary) (for assistance in breathing) 31.1
permanent 31.29
Tracing, carotid pulse with ECG lead 89.56
Traction
with reduction of fracture or dislocation - *see* Reduction, fracture, *and* Reduction, dislocation
adhesive tape (skin) 93.46
boot 93.46
Bryant's (skeletal) 93.44
Buck's 93.46
caliper tongs 93.41
with synchronous insertion of device 02.94
Cortel's (spinal) 93.42
Crutchfield tongs 93.41
with synchronous insertion of device 02.94
Dunlop's (skeletal) 93.44
gallows 93.46
Gardner Wells 93.41
with synchronous insertion of device 02.94

Traction *(Continued)*
halo device, skull 93.41
with synchronous insertion of device 02.94
Lyman Smith (skeletal) 93.44
manual, intermittent 93.21
mechanical, intermittent 93.21
Russell's (skeletal) 93.44
skeletal NEC 93.44
intermittent 93.43
skin, limbs NEC 93.46
spinal NEC 93.42
with skull device (halo) (caliper) (Crutchfield) (Gardner Wells) (Vinke) (tongs) 93.41
with synchronous insertion of device 02.94
Thomas' splint 93.45
Vinke tongs 93.41
with synchronous insertion of device 02.94
Tractotomy
brain 01.32
medulla oblongata 01.32
mesencephalon 01.32
percutaneous 03.21
spinal cord (one-stage) (two-stage) 03.29
trigeminal (percutaneous) (radiofrequency) 04.02
Training (for) (in)
ADL (activities of daily living) 93.83
for the blind 93.78
ambulation 93.22
braille 93.77
crutch walking 93.24
dyslexia 93.71
dysphasia 93.72
esophageal speech (postlaryngectomy) 93.73
gait 93.22
joint movements 93.14
lip reading 93.75
Moon (blind reading) 93.77
orthoptic 95.35
prenatal (natural childbirth) 93.37
prosthetic or orthotic device usage 93.24
relaxation 94.33
speech NEC 93.75
esophageal type 93.73
for correction of defect 93.74
use of lead dog for the blind 93.76
vocational 93.85
TRAM (transverse rectus abdominis musculocutaneous) flap of breast 85.7
Transactional analysis
group 94.44
individual 94.39
Transection - *see also* Division
artery (with ligation) - *see also* Division, artery 38.80
renal, aberrant (with reimplantation) 39.55
bone - *see also* Osteotomy 77.30
fallopian tube (bilateral) (remaining) (solitary) 66.39
by endoscopy 66.22
unilateral 66.92
isthmus, thyroid 06.91
muscle 83.19
eye 15.13
multiple (two or more muscles) 15.3
hand 82.19

Transection *(Continued)*
nerve (cranial) (peripheral) NEC 04.03
acoustic 04.01
root (spinal) 03.1
sympathetic 05.0
tracts in spinal cord 03.29
trigeminal 04.02
vagus (transabdominal) - *see also* Vagotomy 44.00
pylorus (with wedge resection) 43.3
renal vessel, aberrant (with reimplantation) 39.55
spinal
cord tracts 03.29
nerve root 03.1
tendon 83.13
hand 82.11
uvula 27.71
vas deferens 63.71
vein (with ligation) - *see also* Division, vein 38.80
renal, aberrant (with reimplantation) 39.55
varicose (lower limb) 38.59
Transfer, transference
bone shaft, fibula into tibia 78.47
digital (to replace absent thumb) 82.69
finger (to thumb) (same hand) 82.61
to
finger, except thumb 82.81
opposite hand (with amputation) 82.69 *[84.01]*
toe (to thumb) (with amputation) 82.69 *[84.11]*
to finger, except thumb 82.81 *[84.11]*
fat pad NEC 86.89
with skin graft - *see* Graft, skin, full-thickness
finger (to replace absent thumb) (same hand) 82.61
to
finger, except thumb 82.81
opposite hand (with amputation) 82.69 *[84.01]*
muscle origin 83.77
hand 82.58
nerve (cranial) (peripheral) (radial anterior) (ulnar) 04.6
pedicle graft 86.74
pes anserinus (tendon) (repair of knee) 81.47
tarsoconjunctival flap, from opposing lid 08.64
tendon 83.75
hand 82.56
pes anserinus (repair of knee) 81.47
toe-to-thumb (free) (pedicle) (with amputation) 82.69 *[84.11]*
Transfixion - *see also* Fixation
iris (bombé) 12.11
Transfusion (of) 99.03
antihemophilic factor 99.06
antivenin 99.16
autologous blood
collected prior to surgery 99.02
intraoperative 99.00
perioperative 99.00
postoperative 99.00
previously collected 99.02
salvage 99.00
blood (whole) NOS 99.03
expander 99.08
surrogate 99.09
bone marrow 41.00

ICD-9-CM
T
Vol. 3

Transfusion *(Continued)*
bone marrow *(Continued)*
allogeneic 41.03
with purging 41.02
allograft 41.03
with purging 41.02
autograft 41.01
with purging 41.09
autologous 41.01
with purging 41.09
coagulation factors 99.06
Dextran 99.08
exchange 99.01
intraperitoneal 75.2
in utero (with hysterotomy) 75.2
exsanguination 99.01
gamma globulin 99.14
granulocytes 99.09
hemodilution 99.03
intrauterine 75.2
packed cells 99.04
plasma 99.07
platelets 99.05
replacement, total 99.01
serum NEC 99.07
substitution 99.01
thrombocytes 99.05
Transillumination
nasal sinuses 89.35
skull (newborn) 89.16
Translumbar aortogram 88.42
Transplant, transplantation

Note: To report donor source:
cadaver 00.93
live non-related donor 00.92
live related donor 00.91
live unrelated donor 00.92

artery 39.59
renal, aberrant 39.55
autotransplant - *see* Reimplantation
blood vessel 39.59
renal, aberrant 39.55
bone - *see also* Graft, bone 78.00
marrow 41.00
allogeneic 41.03
with purging 41.02
allograft 41.03
with purging 41.02
autograft 41.01
with purging 41.09
autologous 41.01
with purging 41.09
stem cell
allogeneic (hematopoietic) 41.05
with purging 41.08
autologous (hematopoietic) 41.04
with purging 41.07
cord blood 41.06
stem cell
allogeneic (hematopoietic) 41.05
with purging 41.08
autologous (hematopoietic) 41.04
with purging 41.07
cord blood 41.06
combined heart-lung 33.6
conjunctiva, for pterygium 11.39
corneal - *see also* Keratoplasty 11.60
dura 02.12
fascia 83.82
hand 82.72
finger (replacing absent thumb) (same hand) 82.61

Transplant, transplantation *(Continued)*
finger *(Continued)*
to
finger, except thumb 82.81
opposite hand (with amputation) 82.69 *[84.01]*
gracilis muscle (for) 83.77
anal incontinence 49.74
urethrovesical suspension 59.71
hair follicles
eyebrow 08.63
eyelid 08.63
scalp 86.64
heart (orthotopic) 37.51
combined with lung 33.6
ileal stoma to new site 46.23
intestine 46.97
Islets of Langerhans (cells) 52.86
allotransplantation of cells 52.85
autotransplantation of cells 52.84
heterotransplantation 52.85
homotransplantation 52.84
kidney NEC 55.69
liver 50.59
auxiliary (permanent) (temporary) (recipient's liver in situ) 50.51
cells into spleen via percutaneous catheterization 38.91
lung 33.50
bilateral 33.52
combined with heart 33.6
double 33.52
single 33.51
unilateral 33.51
lymphatic structure(s) (peripheral) 40.9
mammary artery to myocardium or ventricular wall 36.2
muscle 83.77
gracilis (for) 83.77
anal incontinence 49.74
urethrovesical suspension 59.71
hand 82.58
temporalis 83.77
with orbital exenteration 16.59
nerve (cranial) (peripheral) 04.6
ovary 65.92
pancreas 52.80
heterotransplant 52.83
homotransplant 52.82
Islets of Langerhans (cells) 52.86
allotransplantation of cells 52.85
autotransplantation of cells 52.84
heterotransplantation 52.85
homotransplantation 52.84
reimplantation 52.81
pes anserinus (tendon) (repair of knee) 81.47
renal NEC 55.69
vessel, aberrant 39.55
salivary duct opening 26.49
skin - *see* Graft, skin
spermatic cord 63.53
spleen 41.94
stem cell(s)
allogeneic (hematopoietic) 41.05
with purging 41.08
autologous (hematopoietic) 41.04
with purging 41.07
cord blood 41.06
tendon 83.75
hand 82.56
pes anserinus (repair of knee) 81.47
superior rectus (blepharoptosis) 08.36

Transplant, transplantation *(Continued)*
testis to scrotum 62.5
thymus 07.94
thyroid tissue 06.94
toe (replacing absent thumb) (with amputation) 82.69 *[84.11]*
to finger, except thumb 82.81 *[84.11]*
tooth 23.5
ureter to
bladder 56.74
ileum (external diversion) 56.51
internal diversion only 56.71
intestine 56.71
skin 56.61
vein (peripheral) 39.59
renal, aberrant 39.55
vitreous 14.72
anterior approach 14.71
Transposition
extraocular muscles 15.5
eyelash flaps 08.63
eye muscle (oblique) (rectus) 15.5
finger (replacing absent thumb) (same hand) 82.61
to
finger, except thumb 82.81
opposite hand (with amputation) 82.69 *[84.01]*
interatrial venous return 35.91
jejunal (Henley) 43.81
joint capsule - *see also* Arthroplasty 81.96
muscle NEC 83.79
extraocular 15.5
hand 82.59
nerve (cranial) (peripheral) (radial anterior) (ulnar) 04.6
nipple 85.86
pterygium 11.31
tendon NEC 83.76
hand 82.57
vocal cords 31.69
Transureteroureterostomy 56.75
Transversostomy - *see also* Colostomy 46.10
Trapping, aneurysm (cerebral) 39.52
Trauner operation (lingual sulcus extension) 24.91
Trephination, trephining
accessory sinus - *see* Sinusotomy
corneoscleral 12.89
cranium 01.24
nasal sinus - *see* Sinusotomy
sclera (with iridectomy) 12.61
Trial (failed) forceps 73.3
Trigonectomy 57.6
Trimming, amputation stump 84.3
Triple arthrodesis 81.12
Trochanterplasty 81.40
Tsuge operation (macrodactyly repair) 82.83
Tuck, tucking - *see also* Plication
eye muscle 15.22
multiple (two or more muscles) 15.4
levator palpebrae, for blepharoptosis 08.34
Tudor "rabbit ear" operation (anterior urethropexy) 59.79
Tuffier operation
apicolysis of lung 33.39
vaginal hysterectomy 68.59
laparoscopically assisted (LAVH) 68.51
TULIP (transurethral ultrasound guided laser induced prostatectomy) 60.21

TUMT (transurethral microwave thermotherapy) of prostate 60.96
TUNA (transurethral needle ablation) of prostate 60.97
Tunnel, subcutaneous (antethoracic) 42.86
esophageal 42.68
with anastomosis - *see* Anastomosis, esophagus, antesternal 42.68
pulse generator lead wire 86.99
with initial procedure - *omit code*
Turbinectomy (complete) (partial) NEC 21.69
by
cryosurgery 21.61
diathermy 21.61
with sinusectomy - *see* Sinusectomy
Turco operation (release of joint capsules in clubfoot) 80.48
TURP (transurethral resection of prostate) 60.29
Tylectomy (breast) (partial) 85.21
Tympanectomy 20.59
with tympanoplasty - *see* Tympanoplasty
Tympanogram 95.41
Tympanomastoidectomy 20.42
Tympanoplasty (type I) (with graft) 19.4
with
air pocket over round window 19.54
fenestra in semicircular canal 19.55
graft against
incus or malleus 19.52
mobile and intact stapes 19.53
incudostapediopexy 19.52
epitympanic, type I 19.4
revision 19.6
type
II (graft against incus or malleus) 19.52
III (graft against mobile and intact stapes) 19.53
IV (air pocket over round window) 19.54
V (fenestra in semicircular canal) 19.55
Tympanosympathectomy 20.91
Tympanotomy 20.09
with intubation 20.01

U

Uchida operation (tubal ligation with or without fimbriectomy) 66.32
UFR (uroflowmetry) 89.24
Ultrafiltration 99.78
hemodiafiltration 39.95
hemodialysis (kidney) 39.95
removal, plasma water 99.78
therapeutic plasmapheresis 99.71
Ultrasonography
abdomen 88.76
aortic arch 88.73
biliary tract 88.74
breast 88.73
deep vein thrombosis 88.77
digestive system 88.74
eye 95.13
head and neck 88.71
heart 88.72
intestine 88.74
Ultrasonography *(Continued)*
intravascular - *see* Ultrasound, intravascular (IVUS)
lung 88.73
midline shift, brain 88.71
multiple sites 88.79
peripheral vascular system 88.77
retroperitoneum 88.76
therapeutic - *see* Ultrasound
thorax NEC 88.73
total body 88.79
urinary system 88.75
uterus 88.79
gravid 88.78
Ultrasound
diagnostic - *see* Ultrasonography
fragmentation (of)
cataract (with aspiration) 13.41
urinary calculus, stones (Kock pouch) 59.95
heart
intracardiac (heart chambers) (ICE) 37.28
intravascular (coronary vessels) (IVUS) 00.24
non-invasive 88.72
inner ear 20.79
intravascular (IVUS) 00.29
aorta 00.22
aortic arch 00.22
cerebral vessel, extracranial 00.21
coronary vessel 00.24
intrathoracic vessel 00.22
other specified vessel 00.28
peripheral vessel 00.23
renal vessel 00.25
vena cava (inferior) (superior) 00.22
therapeutic
head 00.01
heart 00.02
neck 00.01
other therapeutic ultrasound 00.09
peripheral vascular vessels 00.03
vessels of head and neck 00.01
therapy 93.35
Umbilectomy 54.3
Unbridling
blood vessel, peripheral 39.91
celiac artery axis 39.91
Uncovering - *see* Incision, by site
Undercutting
hair follicle 86.09
perianal tissue 49.02
Unroofing - *see also* Incision, by site
external
auditory canal 18.02
ear NEC 18.09
kidney cyst 55.39
UPP (urethral pressure profile) 89.25
Upper GI series (x-ray) 87.62
UPPP (uvulopalatopharyngoplasty) 27.69 *[29.4]*
Uranoplasty (for cleft palate repair) 27.62
Uranorrhaphy (for cleft palate repair) 27.62
Uranostaphylorrhaphy 27.62
Urban operation (mastectomy) (unilateral) 85.47
bilateral 85.48
Ureterectomy 56.40
with nephrectomy 55.51
partial 56.41
total 56.42
Ureterocecostomy 56.71
Ureterocelectomy 56.41
Ureterocolostomy 56.71
Ureterocystostomy 56.74
Ureteroenterostomy 56.71
Ureteroileostomy (internal diversion) 56.71
external diversion 56.51
Ureterolithotomy 56.2
Ureterolysis 59.02
with freeing or repositioning of ureter 59.02
laparoscopic 59.03
Ureteroneocystostomy 56.74
Ureteropexy 56.85
Ureteroplasty 56.89
Ureteroplication 56.89
Ureteroproctostomy 56.71
Ureteropyelography (intravenous) (diuretic infusion) 87.73
percutaneous 87.75
retrograde 87.74
Ureteropyeloplasty 55.87
Ureteropyelostomy 55.86
Ureterorrhaphy 56.82
Ureteroscopy 56.31
with biopsy 56.33
Ureterosigmoidostomy 56.71
Ureterostomy (cutaneous) (external) (tube) 56.61
closure 56.83
ileal 56.51
Ureterotomy 56.2
Ureteroureterostomy (crossed) 56.75
lumbar 56.41
resection with end-to-end anastomosis 56.41
spatulated 56.41
Urethral catheterization, indwelling 57.94
Urethral pressure profile (UPP) 89.25
Urethrectomy (complete) (partial) (radical) 58.39
with
complete cystectomy 57.79
pelvic exenteration 68.8
radical cystectomy 57.71
Urethrocystography (retrograde) (voiding) 87.76
Urethrocystopexy (by) 59.79
levator muscle sling 59.71
retropubic suspension 59.5
suprapubic suspension 59.4
Urethrolithotomy 58.0
Urethrolysis 58.5
Urethropexy 58.49
anterior 59.79
Urethroplasty 58.49
augmentation 59.79
collagen implant 59.72
fat implant 59.72
injection (endoscopic) of implant into urethra 59.72
polytef implant 59.72
Urethrorrhaphy 58.41
Urethroscopy 58.22
for control of hemorrhage of prostate 60.94
perineal 58.21
Urethrostomy (perineal) 58.0
Urethrotomy (external) 58.0
internal (endoscopic) 58.5
Uroflowmetry (UFR) 89.24
Urography (antegrade) (excretory) (intravenous) 87.73
retrograde 87.74

Uteropexy (abdominal approach) (vaginal approach) 69.22
UVP (uvulopalatopharyngoplasty) 27.69 *[29.4]*
Uvulectomy 27.72
Uvulopalatopharyngoplasty (UPPP) 27.69 *[29.4]*
Uvulotomy 27.71

V

Vaccination (prophylactic) (against) 99.59
  anthrax 99.55
  brucellosis 99.55
  cholera 99.31
  common cold 99.51
  disease NEC 99.55
    arthropod-borne viral NEC 99.54
  encephalitis, arthropod-borne viral 99.53
  German measles 99.47
  hydrophobia 99.44
  infectious parotitis 99.46
  influenza 99.52
  measles 99.45
  mumps 99.46
  paratyphoid fever 99.32
  pertussis 99.37
  plague 99.34
  poliomyelitis 99.41
  rabies 99.44
  Rocky Mountain spotted fever 99.55
  rubella 99.47
  rubeola 99.45
  smallpox 99.42
  Staphylococcus 99.55
  Streptococcus 99.55
  tuberculosis 99.33
  tularemia 99.35
  tumor 99.28
  typhoid 99.32
  typhus 99.55
  undulant fever 99.55
  yellow fever 99.43
Vacuum extraction, fetal head 72.79
  with episiotomy 72.71
VAD (vascular access device) - *see* Implant, heart assist system
Vagectomy (subdiaphragmatic) - *see also* Vagotomy 44.00
Vaginal douche 96.44
Vaginectomy 70.4
Vaginofixation 70.77
Vaginoperineotomy 70.14
Vaginoplasty 70.79
Vaginorrhaphy 70.71
  obstetrical 75.69
Vaginoscopy 70.21
Vaginotomy 70.14
  for
    culdocentesis 70.0
    pelvic abscess 70.12
Vagotomy (gastric) 44.00
  parietal cell 44.02
  selective NEC 44.03
    highly 44.02
    Holle's 44.02
    proximal 44.02
  truncal 44.01
Valvotomy - *see* Valvulotomy
Valvulectomy, heart - *see* Valvuloplasty, heart
Valvuloplasty
  heart (open heart technique) (without valve replacement) 35.10
    with prosthesis or tissue graft - *see* Replacement, heart, valve, by site
    aortic valve 35.11
      percutaneous (balloon) 35.96
    combined with repair of atrial and ventricular septal defects - *see* Repair, endocardial cushion defect
    mitral valve 35.12
    percutaneous (balloon) 35.96
    pulmonary valve 35.13
      in total repair of tetralogy of Fallot 35.81
      percutaneous (balloon) 35.96
    tricuspid valve 35.14
Valvulotomy
  heart (closed heart technique) (transatrial) (transventricular) 35.00
    aortic valve 35.01
    mitral valve 35.02
    open heart technique - *see* Valvuloplasty, heart
    pulmonary valve 35.03
      in total repair of tetralogy of Fallot 35.81
    tricuspid valve 35.04
Varicocelectomy, spermatic cord 63.1
Varicotomy, peripheral vessels (lower limb) 38.59
  upper limb 38.53
Vascular closure, percutaneous puncture - *omit code*
Vascularization - *see* Revascularization
Vasectomy (complete) (partial) 63.73
Vasogram 87.94
Vasoligation 63.71
  gastric 38.86
Vasorrhaphy 63.81
Vasostomy 63.6
Vasotomy 63.6
Vasotripsy 63.71
Vasovasostomy 63.82
Vectorcardiogram (VCG) (with ECG) 89.53
Venectomy - *see* Phlebectomy
Venipuncture NEC 38.99
  for injection of contrast material - *see* Phlebography
Venography - *see* Phlebography
Venorrhaphy 39.32
Venotomy 38.00
  abdominal 38.07
  head and neck NEC 38.02
  intracranial NEC 38.01
  lower limb 38.09
  thoracic NEC 38.05
  upper limb 38.03
Venotripsy 39.98
Venovenostomy 39.29
Ventilation
  bi-level airway pressure 93.90
  continuous positive airway pressure [CPAP] 93.90
  endotracheal respiratory assistance - *see* category 96.7
  intermittent mandatory ventilation [IMV] - *see* category 96.7
  intermittent positive pressure breathing [IPPB] 93.91
  mechanical
    endotracheal respiratory assistance - *see* category 96.7
Ventilation *(Continued)*
  mechanical *(Continued)*
    intermittent mandatory ventilation [IMV] - *see* category 96.7
    other continuous (unspecified duration) 96.70
      for less than 96 consecutive hours 96.71
      for 96 consecutive hours or more 96.72
    positive end-expiratory pressure [PEEP] - *see* category 96.7
    pressure support ventilation [PSV] - *see* category 96.7
  negative pressure (continuous) [CNP] 93.99
  non-invasive positive pressure (NIPPV) 93.90
Ventriculectomy, heart
  partial 37.35
Ventriculocholecystostomy 02.34
Ventriculocisternostomy 02.2
Ventriculocordectomy 30.29
Ventriculogram, ventriculography (cerebral) 87.02
  cardiac
    left ventricle (outflow tract) 88.53
      combined with right heart 88.54
    right ventricle (outflow tract) 88.52
      combined with left heart 88.54
  radionuclide cardiac 92.05
Ventriculomyocardiotomy 37.11
Ventriculoperitoneostomy 02.34
Ventriculopuncture 01.09
  through previously implanted catheter or reservoir (Ommaya) (Rickham) 01.02
Ventriculoseptopexy - *see also* Repair, ventricular septal defect 35.72
Ventriculoseptoplasty - *see also* Repair, ventricular septal defect 35.72
Ventriculostomy 02.2
Ventriculotomy
  cerebral 02.2
  heart 37.11
Ventriculoureterostomy 02.35
Ventriculovenostomy 02.32
Ventrofixation, uterus 69.22
Ventrohysteropexy 69.22
Ventrosuspension, uterus 69.22
VEP (visual evoked potential) 95.23
Version, obstetrical (bimanual) (cephalic) (combined) (internal) (podalic) 73.21
  with extraction 73.22
  Braxton Hicks 73.21
    with extraction 73.22
  external (bipolar) 73.91
  Potter's (podalic) 73.21
    with extraction 73.22
  Wigand's (external) 73.91
  Wright's (cephalic) 73.21
    with extraction 73.22
Vertebroplasty (percutaneous) 81.65
Vesicolithotomy (suprapubic) 57.19
Vesicostomy 57.21
Vesicourethroplasty 57.85
Vesiculectomy 60.73
  with radical prostatectomy 60.5
Vesiculogram, seminal 87.92
  contrast 87.91
Vesiculotomy 60.72
Vestibuloplasty (buccolabial) (lingual) 24.91
Vestibulotomy 20.79

Vicq D'Azyr operation (larynx) 31.1
Vidal operation (varicocele ligation) 63.1
Vidianectomy 05.21
Villusectomy - *see also* Synovectomy 80.70
Vision check 95.09
Visual evoked potential (VEP) 95.23
Vitrectomy (mechanical) (posterior approach) 14.74
with scleral buckling 14.49
anterior approach 14.73
Vocational
assessment 93.85
retraining 93.85
schooling 93.82
Voice training (postlaryngectomy) 93.73
von Kraske operation (proctectomy) 48.64
Voss operation (hanging hip operation) 83.19
Vulpius (-Compere) operation (lengthening of gastrocnemius muscle) 83.85
Vulvectomy (bilateral) (simple) 71.62
partial (unilateral) 71.61
radical (complete) 71.5
unilateral 71.61
V-Y operation (repair)
bladder 57.89
neck 57.85
ectropion 08.44
lip 27.59
skin (without graft) 86.89
subcutaneous tissue (without skin graft) 86.89
tongue 25.59

W

Wada test (hemispheric function) 89.10
Ward-Mayo operation (vaginal hysterectomy) 68.59
laparoscopically assisted (LAVH) 68.51
Washing - *see* Lavage and Irrigation
Waterston operation (aorta-right pulmonary artery anastomosis) 39.0
Watkins (-Wertheim) operation (uterus interposition) 69.21
Watson-Jones operation
hip arthrodesis 81.21
reconstruction of lateral ligaments, ankle 81.49
shoulder arthrodesis (extra-articular) 81.23
tenoplasty 83.88
Webbing (syndactylization) 86.89
Weir operation
appendicostomy 47.91
correction of nostrils 21.86
Wertheim operation (radical hysterectomy) 68.69
laparoscopic 68.61
West operation (dacryocystorhinostomy) 09.81
Wheeler operation
entropion repair 08.44
halving procedure (eyelid) 08.24
Whipple operation (radical pancreaticoduodenectomy) 52.7
Child modification (radical subtotal pancreatectomy) 52.53
Rodney Smith modification (radical subtotal pancreatectomy) 52.53
White operation (lengthening of tendo calcaneus by incomplete tenotomy) 83.11
Whitehead operation
glossectomy, radical 25.4
hemorrhoidectomy 49.46
Whitman operation
foot stabilization (talectomy) 77.98
hip reconstruction 81.40
repair of serratus anterior muscle 83.87
talectomy 77.98
trochanter wedge osteotomy 77.25
Wier operation (entropion repair) 08.44
Williams-Richardson operation (vaginal construction) 70.61
Wilms operation (thoracoplasty) 33.34
Wilson operation (angulation osteotomy for hallux valgus) 77.51
Window operation
antrum (nasal sinus) - *see* Antrotomy, maxillary
aorticopulmonary 39.59
bone cortex - *see also* Incision, bone 77.10
facial 76.09
nasoantral - *see* Antrotomy, maxillary
pericardium 37.12
pleura 34.09
Winiwarter operation (cholecystoenterostomy) 51.32
Wiring
aneurysm 39.52
dental (for immobilization) 93.55
with fracture-reduction - *see* Reduction, fracture
orthodontic 24.7
Wirsungojejunostomy 52.96
Witzel operation (temporary gastrostomy) 43.19
Woodward operation (release of high riding scapula) 81.83
Wrapping, aneurysm (gauze) (methyl methacrylate) (plastic) 39.52

X

Xenograft 86.65
Xerography, breast 87.36
Xeromammography 87.36
Xiphoidectomy 77.81
X-ray
chest (routine) 87.44
wall NEC 87.39
contrast - *see* Radiography, contrast
diagnostic - *see* Radiography
injection of radio-opaque substance - *see* Radiography, contrast
skeletal series, whole or complete 88.31
therapeutic - *see* Therapy, radiation

Y

Young operation
epispadias repair 58.45
tendon transfer (anterior tibialis) (repair of flat foot) 83.75
Yount operation (division of iliotibial band) 83.14

Z

Zancolli operation
capsuloplasty 81.72
tendon transfer (biceps) 82.56
Ziegler operation (iridectomy) 12.14
Zonulolysis (with lens extraction) - *see also* Extraction, cataract, intracapsular 13.19
Z-plasty
epicanthus 08.59
eyelid - *see also* Reconstruction, eyelid 08.70
hypopharynx 29.4
skin (scar) (web contracture) 86.84
with excision of lesion 86.3

Code also note: This instruction is used in the Tabular List for two purposes:

1) To code components of a procedure that are performed at the same time, and
2) To code the use of special adjunctive procedures or equipment.

Includes note: This note appears immediately under a two- or three-digit code title. The information further defines, or gives examples of, the contents of the category.

Excludes note: Terms following the word "Excludes" are to be coded elsewhere as indicated in each case.

TABULAR LIST OF PROCEDURES

0. PROCEDURES AND INTERVENTIONS, NOT ELSEWHERE CLASSIFIED (00)

● **00.0 Therapeutic ultrasound**

Excludes *diagnostic ultrasound (non-invasive) (88.71–88.79)*
intracardiac echocardiography [ICE] (heart chambers(s)) (37.28)
intravascular imaging (adjunctive) (00.21–00.29)

00.01 Therapeutic ultrasound of vessels of head and neck
Anti-restenotic ultrasound
Intravascular non-ablative ultrasound

Excludes *diagnostic ultrasound of:*
eye (95.13)
head and neck (88.71)
that of inner ear (20.79)
ultrasonic:
angioplasty of non-coronary vessel (39.50)
embolectomy (38.01, 38.02)
endarterectomy (38.11, 38.12)
thrombectomy (38.01, 38.02)

00.02 Therapeutic ultrasound of heart
Anti-restenotic ultrasound
Intravascular non-ablative ultrasound

Excludes *diagnostic ultrasound of heart (88.72)*
ultrasonic ablation of heart lesion (37.34)
ultrasonic angioplasty of coronary vessels (00.66, 36.09)

00.03 Therapeutic ultrasound of peripheral vascular vessels
Anti-restenotic ultrasound
Intravascular non-ablative ultrasound

Excludes *diagnostic ultrasound of peripheral vascular system (88.77)*
ultrasonic angioplasty of:
non-coronary vessel (39.50)

00.09 Other therapeutic ultrasound

Excludes *ultrasonic:*
fragmentation of urinary stones (59.95)
percutaneous nephrostomy with fragmentation (55.04)
physical therapy (93.35)
transurethral guided laser induced prostatectomy (TULIP) (60.21)

● **00.1 Pharmaceuticals**

00.10 Implantation of chemotherapeutic agent
Brain wafer chemotherapy
Interstitial/intracavitary

Excludes *injection or infusion of cancer chemotherapeutic substance (99.25)*

00.11 Infusion of drotrecogin alfa (activated)
Infusion of recombinant protein

00.12 Administration of inhaled nitric oxide
Nitric oxide therapy

00.13 Injection or infusion of nesiritide
Human B-type natriuretic peptide (hBNP)

00.14 Injection or infusion of oxazolidinone class of antibiotics
Linezolid injection

00.15 High-dose infusion interleukin-2 (IL-2)
Infusion (IV bolus, CIV) interleukin
Injection aldesleukin

Excludes *low-dose infusion interleukin-2 (99.28)*

00.16 Pressurized treatment of venous bypass graft [conduit] with pharmaceutical substance
Ex-vivo treatment of vessel
Hyperbaric pressurized graft [conduit]

00.17 Infusion of vasopressor agent

00.18 Infusion of immunosuppressive antibody therapy during induction phase of solid organ transplantation
Monoclonal antibody therapy
Polyclonal antibody therapy

● **00.2 Intravascular imaging of blood vessels**
Endovascular ultrasonography
Intravascular [ultrasound] imaging of blood vessels
Intravascular ultrasound (IVUS)

Code also any synchronous diagnostic or therapeutic procedures

Note: Real-time imaging of lumen of blood vessel(s) using sound waves

Excludes *adjunct vascular system procedures, number of vessels treated (00.40–00.43)*
diagnostic procedures on blood vessels (38.21–38.29)
diagnostic ultrasound of peripheral vascular system (88.77)
magnetic resonance imaging (MRI) (88.91–88.97)
therapeutic ultrasound (00.01–00.09)

00.21 Intravascular imaging of extracranial cerebral vessels
Common carotid vessels and branches
Intravascular ultrasound (IVUS), extracranial cerebral vessels

Excludes *diagnostic ultrasound (non-invasive) of head and neck (88.71)*

00.22 Intravascular imaging of intrathoracic vessels
Aorta and aortic arch
Intravascular ultrasound (IVUS), intrathoracic vessels
Vena cava (superior) (inferior)

Excludes *diagnostic ultrasound (non-invasive) of other sites of thorax (88.73)*

00.23 Intravascular imaging of peripheral vessels
Imaging of:
vessels of arm(s)
vessels of leg(s)
Intravascular ultrasound (IVUS), peripheral vessels

Excludes *diagnostic ultrasound (non-invasive) of peripheral vascular system (88.77)*

00.24 Intravascular imaging of coronary vessels
Intravascular ultrasound (IVUS), coronary vessels

Excludes *diagnostic ultrasound (non-invasive) of heart (88.72)*
intracardiac echocardiography [ICE] (ultrasound of heart chamber(s) (37.28)

00.25 Intravascular imaging, renal vessel(s)
Intravascular ultrasound (IVUS), renal vessels
Renal artery

Excludes *diagnostic ultrasound (non-invasive) of urinary system (88.75)*

00.28 Intravascular imaging, other specified vessel(s)

00.29 Intravascular imaging, unspecified vessels

● **00.3 Computer assisted surgery [CAS]**
CT-free navigation
Image guided navigation (IGN)
Image guided surgery (IGS)
Imageless navigation

Code also diagnostic or therapeutic procedure

Excludes *stereotactic frame application only (93.59)*

00.31 Computer assisted surgery with CT/CTA

00.32 Computer assisted surgery with MR/MRA

00.33 Computer assisted surgery with fluoroscopy

00.34 Imageless computer assisted surgery

00.35 Computer assisted surgery with multiple datasets

00.39 Other computer assisted surgery
Computer assisted surgery NOS

● **00.4 Adjunct vascular system procedures**

Note: These codes can apply to both coronary and peripheral vessels. These codes are to be used in conjunction with other therapeutic procedure codes to provide additional information on the number of vessels upon which a procedure was performed and/or the number of stents inserted. As appropriate, code both the number of vessels operated on (00.40–00.43), and the number of stents inserted (00.45–00.48).

Code also any:
angioplasty or atherectomy (00.61–00.62, 00.66, 39.50)
endarterectomy (38.10–38.18)
insertion of vascular stent(s) (00.55, 00.63–00.65, 36.06–36.07, 39.90)
other removal of coronary artery obstruction (36.09)

00.40 Procedure on single vessel
Number of vessels, unspecified

Excludes *(aorto)coronary bypass (36.10–36.19)*
intravascular imaging of blood vessels (00.21–00.29)

00.41 Procedure on two vessels

Excludes *(aorto)coronary bypass (36.10–36.19)*
intravascular imaging of blood vessels (00.21–00.29)

00.42 Procedure on three vessels

Excludes *(aorto)coronary bypass (36.10–36.19)*
intravascular imaging of blood vessels (00.21–00.29)

00.43 Procedure on four or more vessels

Excludes *(aorto)coronary bypass (36.10–36.19)*
intravascular imaging of blood vessels (00.21–00.29)

00.44 Procedure on vessel bifurcation ◄
Note: This code is to be used to identify the presence of a vessel bifurcation; it does not describe a specific bifurcation stent. Use this code only once per operative episode, irrespective of the number of bifurcations in vessels. ◄

00.45 Insertion of one vascular stent
Number of stents, unspecified

00.46 Insertion of two vascular stents

00.47 Insertion of three vascular stents

00.48 Insertion of four or more vascular stents

● **00.5 Other cardiovascular procedures**

✖ **00.50 Implantation of cardiac resynchronization pacemaker without mention of defibrillation, total system [CRT-P]**
BiV pacemaker ◄
Biventricular pacemaker ◄
Biventricular pacing without internal cardiac defibrillator
Implantation of cardiac resynchronization (biventricular) pulse generator pacing device, formation of pocket, transvenous leads including placement of lead into left ventricular coronary venous system, and intraoperative procedures for evaluation of lead signals.
That with CRT-P generator and one or more leads
Note: Device testing during procedure – *omit code* ◄

Excludes *implantation of cardiac resynchronization defibrillator, total system [CRT-D] (00.51)*
insertion or replacement of any type pacemaker device (37.80–37.87)
replacement of cardiac resynchronization defibrillator pulse generator only [CRT-D] (00.54)
replacement of cardiac resynchronization pacemaker pulse generator only [CRT-P] (00.53)

✖ **00.51 Implantation of cardiac resynchronization defibrillator, total system [CRT-D]**
BiV defibrillator ◄
BiV ICD ◄
BiV pacemaker with defibrillator ◄
BiV pacing with defibrillator ◄
Biventricular defibrillator ◄
Biventricular pacing with internal cardiac defibrillator
Implantation of a cardiac resynchronization (biventricular) pulse generator with defibrillator [AICD], formation of pocket, transvenous leads, including placement of lead into left ventricular coronary venous system, intraoperative procedures for evaluation of lead signals, and obtaining defibrillator threshold measurements.
That with CRT-D generator and one or more leads
Note: Device testing during procedure – *omit code* ◄

Excludes *implantation of cardiac resynchronization pacemaker, total system [CRT-P] (00.50)*
implantation or replacement of automatic cardioverter/defibrillator, total system [AICD] (37.94)
replacement of cardiac resynchronization defibrillator pulse generator, only [CRT-D] (00.54)

✖ **00.52 Implantation or replacement of transvenous lead [electrode] into left ventricular coronary venous system**

Excludes *implantation of cardiac resynchronization defibrillator, total system [CRT-D] (00.51)*
implantation of cardiac resynchronization pacemaker, total system [CRT-P] (00.50)
initial insertion of transvenous lead [electrode] (37.70–37.72)
replacement of transvenous atrial and/or ventricular lead(s) [electrodes] (37.76)

✖ **00.53 Implantation or replacement of cardiac resynchronization pacemaker pulse generator only [CRT-P]**

Implantation of CRT-P device with removal of any existing CRT-P or other pacemaker device

Note: Device testing during procedure – *omit code* ◀

Excludes *implantation of cardiac resynchronization pacemaker, total system [CRT-P] (00.50)*
implantation or replacement of cardiac resynchronization defibrillator pulse generator only [CRT-D] (00.54)
insertion or replacement of any type pacemaker device (37.80–37.87)

✖ **00.54 Implantation or replacement of cardiac resynchronization defibrillator pulse generator device only [CRT-D]**

Implantation of CRT-D device with removal of any existing CRT-D, CRT-P, pacemaker, or defibrillator device

Note: Device testing during procedure – *omit code* ◀

Excludes *implantation of automatic cardioverter/defibrillator pulse generator only (37.96)*
implantation of cardiac resynchronization defibrillator, total system [CRT-D] (00.51)
implantation or replacement of cardiac resynchronization pacemaker pulse generator only [CRT-P] (00.53)

00.55 Insertion of drug-eluting peripheral vessel stent(s)

Endograft(s)
Endovascular graft(s)
Stent grafts

Code also any:
angioplasty or atherectomy of other non-coronary vessel(s) (39.50)
number of vascular stents inserted (00.45–00.48)
number of vessels treated (00.40–00.43)
procedure on vessel bifurcation (00.44) ◀

Excludes *drug-coated peripheral stents, e.g., heparin coated (39.90)*
insertion of cerebrovascular stent(s) (00.63–00.65)
insertion of drug-eluting coronary artery stent (36.07)
insertion of non-drug-eluting stent(s):
coronary artery (36.06)
peripheral vessel (39.90)
that for aneurysm repair (39.71–39.79)

00.56 Insertion or replacement of implantable pressure sensor (lead) for intracardiac hemodynamic monitoring ◀

Code also any associated implantation or replacement of monitor (00.57) ◀

Excludes *circulatory monitoring (blood gas, arterial or venous pressure, cardiac output and coronary blood flow) (89.60–89.69)* ◀

00.57 Implantation or replacement of subcutaneous device for intracardiac hemodynamic monitoring ◀

Implantation of monitoring device with formation of subcutaneous pocket and connection to intracardiac pressure sensor (lead) ◀

Code also any associated insertion or replacement of implanted pressure sensor (lead) (00.56) ◀

● **00.6 Procedures on blood vessels**

00.61 Percutaneous angioplasty or atherectomy of precerebral (extracranial) vessel(s)

Basilar
Carotid
Vertebral

Code also any:
injection or infusion of thrombolytic agent (99.10)
number of vascular stents inserted (00.45–00.48)
number of vessels treated (00.40–00.43)
percutaneous insertion of carotid artery stent(s) (00.63)
percutaneous insertion of other precerebral artery stent(s) (00.64)
procedure on vessel bifurcation (00.44) ◀

Excludes *angioplasty or atherectomy of other non-coronary vessel(s) (39.50)*
removal of cerebrovascular obstruction of vessel(s) by open approach (38.01–38.02, 38.11–38.12, 38.31–38.32, 38.41–38.42)

00.62 Percutaneous angioplasty or atherectomy of intracranial vessel(s)

Code also any:
injection or infusion of thrombolytic agent (99.10)
number of vascular stents inserted (00.45–00.48)
number of vessels treated (00.40–00.43)
percutaneous insertion of intracranial stent(s) (00.65)
procedure on vessel bifurcation (00.44) ◀

Excludes *angioplasty or atherectomy of other non-coronary vessel(s) (39.50)*
removal of cerebrovascular obstruction of vessel(s) by open approach (38.01–38.02, 38.11–38.12, 38.31–38.32, 38.41–38.42)

00.63 Percutaneous insertion of carotid artery stent(s)

Includes the use of any embolic protection device, distal protection device, filter device, or stent delivery system

Non-drug-eluting stents

Code also any:
number of vascular stents inserted (00.45–00.48)
number of vessels treated (00.40–00.43)
percutaneous angioplasty or atherectomy of precerebral vessel(s) (00.61)
procedure on vessel bifurcation (00.44) ◀

Excludes *angioplasty or atherectomy of other non-coronary vessel(s) (39.50)*
insertion of drug-eluting peripheral vessel stent(s) (00.55)

00.64 Percutaneous insertion of other precerebral (extracranial) artery stent(s)

Includes the use of any embolic protection device, distal protection device, filter device, or stent delivery system
Basilar stent
Vertebral stent

Code also any:
number of vascular stents inserted (00.45–00.48)
number of vessels treated (00.40–00.43)
percutaneous angioplasty or atherectomy of intracranial vessel(s) (00.61)
procedure on vessel bifurcation (00.44) ◀

Excludes *angioplasty or atherectomy of other non-coronary vessel(s) (39.50)*
insertion of drug-eluting peripheral vessel stent(s) (00.55)

00.65 Percutaneous insertion of intracranial vascular stent(s)
Includes the use of any embolic protection device, distal protection device, filter device, or stent delivery system

Code also any:
number of vascular stents inserted (00.45–00.48)
number of vessels treated (00.40–00.43)
percutaneous angioplasty or atherectomy of precerebral vessel(s) (00.62)
procedure on vessel bifurcation (00.44) ◀

Excludes *angioplasty or atherectomy of other non-coronary vessel(s) (39.50)*
insertion of drug-eluting peripheral vessel stent(s) (00.55)

00.66 Percutaneous transluminal coronary angioplasty [PTCA] or coronary atherectomy
Balloon angioplasty of coronary artery
Coronary atherectomy
Percutaneous coronary angioplasty NOS
PTCA NOS

Code also any:
injection or infusion of thrombolytic agent (99.10)
insertion of coronary artery stent(s) (36.06–36.07)
intracoronary artery thrombolytic infusion (36.04)
number of vascular stents inserted (00.45–00.48)
number of vessels treated (00.40–00.43)
procedure on vessel bifurcation (00.44) ◀

● **00.7 Other hip procedures**

00.70 Revision of hip replacement, both acetabular and femoral components
Total hip revision

Code also any:
removal of (cement) (joint) spacer (84.57)
type of bearing surface, if known (00.74–00.77)

Excludes *revision of hip replacement, acetabular component only (00.71)*
revision of hip replacement, femoral component only (00.72)
revision of hip replacement, Not Otherwise Specified (81.53)
revision with replacement of acetabular liner and/or femoral head only (00.73)

00.71 Revision of hip replacement, acetabular component
Partial, acetabular component only
That with:
exchange of acetabular cup and liner
exchange of femoral head

Code also any type of bearing surface, if known (00.74–00.77)

Excludes *revision of hip replacement, both acetabular and femoral components (00.70)*
revision of hip replacement, femoral component (00.72)
revision of hip replacement, Not Otherwise Specified (81.53)
revision with replacement of acetabular liner and/or femoral head only (00.73)

00.72 Revision of hip replacement, femoral component
Partial, femoral component only
That with:
exchange of acetabular liner
exchange of femoral stem and head

Code also any type of bearing surface, if known (00.74–00.77)

Excludes *revision of hip replacement, acetabular component (00.71)*
revision of hip replacement, both acetabular and femoral components (00.70)
revision of hip replacement, not otherwise specified (81.53)
revision with replacement of acetabular liner and/or femoral head only (00.73)

00.73 Revision of hip replacement, acetabular liner and/or femoral head only

Code also any type of bearing surface, if known (00.74–00.77)

00.74 Hip replacement bearing surface, metal on polyethylene

00.75 Hip replacement bearing surface, metal-on-metal

00.76 Hip replacement bearing surface, ceramic-on-ceramic

00.77 Hip replacement bearing surface, ceramic-on-polyethylene ◀

● **00.8 Other knee and hip procedures**

Note: Report up to two components using 00.81–00.83 to describe revision of knee replacements. If all three components are revised, report 00.80.

00.80 Revision of knee replacement, total (all components)
Replacement of femoral, tibial, and patellar components (all components)

Code also any removal of (cement) (joint) spacer (84.57)

Excludes *revision of only one or two components (tibial, femoral or patellar component) (00.81–00.84)*

00.81 Revision of knee replacement, tibial component
Replacement of tibial baseplate and tibial insert (liner)

Excludes *revision of knee replacement, total (all components) (00.80)*

00.82 Revision of knee replacement, femoral component
That with replacement of tibial insert (liner)

Excludes *revision of knee replacement, total (all components) (00.80)*

00.83 Revision of knee replacement, patellar component

Excludes *revision of knee replacement, total (all components) (00.80)*

00.84 Revision of total knee replacement, tibial insert (liner)
Replacement of tibial insert (liner)

Excludes *that with replacement of tibial component (tibial baseplate and liner) (00.81)*

00.85 Resurfacing hip, total, acetabulum and femoral head ◀
Hip resurfacing arthroplasty, total ◀

00.86 Resurfacing hip, partial, femoral head ◀
Hip resurfacing arthroplasty, NOS ◀
Hip resurfacing arthroplasty, partial, femoral head ◀
Excludes *that with resurfacing of acetabulum (00.85)* ◀

00.87 Resurfacing hip, partial, acetabulum ◀
Hip resurfacing arthroplasty, partial, acetabulum ◀
Excludes *that with resurfacing of femoral head (00.85)* ◀

● **00.9 Other procedures and interventions**

00.91 Transplant from live related donor
Code also organ transplant procedure

00.92 Transplant from live non-related donor
Code also organ transplant procedure

00.93 Transplant from cadaver
Code also organ transplant procedure

1. OPERATIONS ON THE NERVOUS SYSTEM (01–05)

● **01 Incision and excision of skull, brain, and cerebral meninges**

● **01.0 Cranial puncture**

01.01 Cisternal puncture
Cisternal tap

Excludes *pneumocisternogram (87.02)*

01.02 Ventriculopuncture through previously implanted catheter
Puncture of ventricular shunt tubing

01.09 Other cranial puncture
Aspiration of:
subarachnoid space
subdural space
Cranial aspiration NOS
Puncture of anterior fontanel
Subdural tap (through fontanel)

● **01.1 Diagnostic procedures on skull, brain, and cerebral meninges**

01.11 Closed [percutaneous] [needle] biopsy of cerebral meninges
Burr hole approach

✖ **01.12 Open biopsy of cerebral meninges**

01.13 Closed [percutaneous] [needle] biopsy of brain
Burr hole approach
Stereotactic method

✖ **01.14 Open biopsy of brain**

✖ **01.15 Biopsy of skull**

✖ **01.18 Other diagnostic procedures on brain and cerebral meninges**

Excludes *cerebral:*
arteriography (88.41)
thermography (88.81)
contrast radiogram of brain (87.01–87.02)
echoencephalogram (88.71)
electroencephalogram (89.14)
microscopic examination of specimen from nervous system and of spinal fluid (90.01–90.09)
neurologic examination (89.13)
phlebography of head and neck (88.61)
pneumoencephalogram (87.01)
radioisotope scan:
cerebral (92.11)
head NEC (92.12)
tomography of head:
C.A.T. scan (87.03)
other (87.04)

✖ **01.19 Other diagnostic procedures on skull**

Excludes *transillumination of skull (89.16)*
x-ray of skull (87.17)

● **01.2 Craniotomy and craniectomy**

Excludes *decompression of skull fracture (02.02)*
exploration of orbit (16.01–16.09)
that as operative approach

✖ **01.21 Incision and drainage of cranial sinus**

✖ **01.22 Removal of intracranial neurostimulator lead(s)**

Code also any removal of neurostimulator pulse generator (86.05)

Excludes *removal with synchronous replacement (02.93)*

✖ **01.23 Reopening of craniotomy site**

✖ **01.24 Other craniotomy**
Cranial:
decompression
exploration
trephination
Craniotomy NOS
Craniotomy with removal of:
epidural abscess
extradural hematoma
foreign body of skull

Excludes *removal of foreign body with incision into brain (01.39)*

✖ **01.25 Other craniectomy**
Debridement of skull NOS
Sequestrectomy of skull

Excludes *debridement of compound fracture of skull (02.02)*
strip craniectomy (02.01)

✖ **01.26 Insertion of catheter(s) into cranial cavity or tissue** ⬅ Revised

Code also any concomitant procedure (e.g. resection (01.59))

Excludes *placement of intracerebral catheter(s) via burr hole(s) (01.28)* ◀ New

✖ **01.27 Removal of catheter(s) from cranial cavity or tissue** ⬅ Revised

✖ **01.28 Placement of intracerebral catheter(s) via burr hole(s)** ◀ New
Convection enhanced delivery ◀
Stereotactic placement of intracerebral catheter(s) ◀

Code also infusion of medication ◀

Excludes *insertion of catheter(s) into cranial cavity or tissue(s) (01.26)* ◀

● **01.3 Incision of brain and cerebral meninges**

✖ **01.31 Incision of cerebral meninges**
Drainage of:
intracranial hygroma
subarachnoid abscess (cerebral)
subdural empyema

✖ **01.32 Lobotomy and tractotomy**
Division of:
brain tissue
cerebral tracts
Percutaneous (radiofrequency) cingulotomy

✖ **01.39 Other incision of brain**
Amygdalohippocampotomy
Drainage of intracerebral hematoma
Incision of brain NOS

Excludes *division of cortical adhesions (02.91)*

● **01.4 Operations on thalamus and globus pallidus**

✖ **01.41 Operations on thalamus**
Chemothalamectomy
Thalamotomy

Excludes *that by stereotactic radiosurgery (92.30–92.39)*

✖ **01.42 Operations on globus pallidus**
Pallidoansectomy
Pallidotomy

Excludes *that by stereotactic radiosurgery (92.30–92.39)*

● **01.5 Other excision or destruction of brain and meninges**

✖ **01.51 Excision of lesion or tissue of cerebral meninges**
Decortication of (cerebral) meninges
Resection of (cerebral) meninges
Stripping of subdural membrane of (cerebral) meninges

Excludes *biopsy of cerebral meninges (01.11–01.12)*

✖01.52 **Hemispherectomy**

✖01.53 **Lobectomy of brain**

✖01.59 **Other excision or destruction of lesion or tissue of brain**
Curettage of brain
Debridement of brain
Marsupialization of brain cyst
Transtemporal (mastoid) excision of brain tumor

Excludes *biopsy of brain (01.13–01.14)*
that by stereotactic radiosurgery (92.30–92.39)

✖01.6 **Excision of lesion of skull**
Removal of granulation tissue of cranium

Excludes *biopsy of skull (01.15)*
sequestrectomy (01.25)

●02 **Other operations on skull, brain, and cerebral meninges**

●02.0 **Cranioplasty**

Excludes *that with synchronous repair of encephalocele (02.12)*

✖02.01 **Opening of cranial suture**
Linear craniectomy
Strip craniectomy

✖02.02 **Elevation of skull fracture fragments**
Debridement of compound fracture of skull
Decompression of skull fracture
Reduction of skull fracture

Code also any synchronous debridement of brain (01.59)

Excludes *debridement of skull NOS (01.25)*
removal of granulation tissue of cranium (01.6)

✖02.03 **Formation of cranial bone flap**
Repair of skull with flap

✖02.04 **Bone graft to skull**
Pericranial graft (autogenous) (heterogenous)

✖02.05 **Insertion of skull plate**
Replacement of skull plate

✖02.06 **Other cranial osteoplasty**
Repair of skull NOS
Revision of bone flap of skull

✖02.07 **Removal of skull plate**

Excludes *removal with synchronous replacement (02.05)*

●02.1 **Repair of cerebral meninges**

Excludes *marsupialization of cerebral lesion (01.59)*

✖02.11 **Simple suture of dura mater of brain**

✖02.12 **Other repair of cerebral meninges**
Closure of fistula of cerebrospinal fluid
Dural graft
Repair of encephalocele including synchronous cranioplasty
Repair of meninges NOS
Subdural patch

✖02.13 **Ligation of meningeal vessel**
Ligation of:
longitudinal sinus
middle meningeal artery

✖02.14 **Choroid plexectomy**
Cauterization of choroid plexus

✖02.2 **Ventriculostomy**
Anastomosis of ventricle to:
cervical subarachnoid space
cisterna magna
Insertion of Holter valve
Ventriculocisternal intubation

●02.3 **Extracranial ventricular shunt**

Includes: that with insertion of valve

✖02.31 **Ventricular shunt to structure in head and neck**
Ventricle to nasopharynx shunt
Ventriculomastoid anastomosis

✖02.32 **Ventricular shunt to circulatory system**
Ventriculoatrial anastomosis
Ventriculocaval shunt

✖02.33 **Ventricular shunt to thoracic cavity**
Ventriculopleural anastomosis

✖02.34 **Ventricular shunt to abdominal cavity and organs**
Ventriculocholecystostomy
Ventriculoperitoneostomy

✖02.35 **Ventricular shunt to urinary system**
Ventricle to ureter shunt

✖02.39 **Other operations to establish drainage of ventricle**
Ventricle to bone marrow shunt
Ventricular shunt to extracranial site NEC

●02.4 **Revision, removal, and irrigation of ventricular shunt**

Excludes *revision of distal catheter of ventricular shunt (54.95)*

02.41 **Irrigation and exploration of ventricular shunt**
Exploration of ventriculoperitoneal shunt at ventricular site
Re-programming of ventriculoperitoneal shunt

✖02.42 **Replacement of ventricular shunt**
Reinsertion of Holter valve
Replacement of ventricular catheter
Revision of ventriculoperitoneal shunt at ventricular site

✖02.43 **Removal of ventricular shunt**

●02.9 **Other operations on skull, brain, and cerebral meninges**

Excludes *operations on:*
pineal gland (07.17, 07.51–07.59)
pituitary gland [hypophysis] (07.13–07.15, 07.61–07.79)

✖02.91 **Lysis of cortical adhesions**

✖02.92 **Repair of brain**

✖02.93 **Implantation or replacement of intracranial neurostimulator lead(s)**
Implantation, insertion, placement, or replacement of intracranial:
brain pacemaker [neuropacemaker]
depth electrodes
epidural pegs
electroencephalographic receiver
foramen ovale electrodes
intracranial electrostimulator
subdural grids
subdural strips

Code also any insertion of neurostimulator pulse generator (86.94–86.98) ⬅

✖02.94 **Insertion or replacement of skull tongs or halo traction device**

02.95 **Removal of skull tongs or halo traction device**

02.96 **Insertion of sphenoidal electrodes**

✖02.99 **Other**

Excludes *chemical shock therapy (94.24)*
electroshock therapy:
subconvulsive (94.26)
other (94.27)

● 03 **Operations on spinal cord and spinal canal structures**
Code also any application or administration of an adhesion barrier substance (99.77)

● 03.0 **Exploration and decompression of spinal canal structures**

✖ 03.01 **Removal of foreign body from spinal canal**

✖ 03.02 **Reopening of laminectomy site**

✖ 03.09 **Other exploration and decompression of spinal canal**
Decompression:
laminectomy
laminotomy
Expansile laminoplasty
Exploration of spinal nerve root
Foraminotomy

Excludes *drainage of spinal fluid by anastomosis (03.71–03.79)*
laminectomy with excision of intervertebral disc (80.51)
spinal tap (03.31)
that as operative approach

✖ 03.1 **Division of intraspinal nerve root**
Rhizotomy

● 03.2 **Chordotomy**

✖ 03.21 **Percutaneous chordotomy**
Stereotactic chordotomy

✖ 03.29 **Other chordotomy**
Chordotomy NOS
Tractotomy (one-stage) (two-stage) of spinal cord
Transection of spinal cord tracts

● 03.3 **Diagnostic procedures on spinal cord and spinal canal structures**

03.31 **Spinal tap**
Lumbar puncture for removal of dye

Excludes *lumbar puncture for injection of dye [myelogram] (87.21)*

✖ 03.32 **Biopsy of spinal cord or spinal meninges**

✖ 03.39 **Other diagnostic procedures on spinal cord and spinal canal structures**

Excludes *microscopic examination of specimen from nervous system or of spinal fluid (90.01–90.09)*
x-ray of spine (87.21–87.29)

✖ 03.4 **Excision or destruction of lesion of spinal cord or spinal meninges**
Curettage of spinal cord or spinal meninges
Debridement of spinal cord or spinal meninges
Marsupialization of cyst of spinal cord or spinal meninges
Resection of spinal cord or spinal meninges

Excludes *biopsy of spinal cord or meninges (03.32)*

● 03.5 **Plastic operations on spinal cord structures**

✖ 03.51 **Repair of spinal meningocele**
Repair of meningocele NOS

✖ 03.52 **Repair of spinal myelomeningocele**

✖ 03.53 **Repair of vertebral fracture**
Elevation of spinal bone fragments
Reduction of fracture of vertebrae
Removal of bony spicules from spinal canal

Excludes *kyphoplasty (81.66)*
vertebroplasty (81.65)

✖ 03.59 **Other repair and plastic operations on spinal cord structures**
Repair of:
diastematomyelia
spina bifida NOS
spinal cord NOS
spinal meninges NOS
vertebral arch defect

✖ 03.6 **Lysis of adhesions of spinal cord and nerve roots**

● 03.7 **Shunt of spinal theca**
Includes: that with valve

✖ 03.71 **Spinal subarachnoid-peritoneal shunt**

✖ 03.72 **Spinal subarachnoid-ureteral shunt**

✖ 03.79 **Other shunt of spinal theca**
Lumbar-subarachnoid shunt NOS
Pleurothecal anastomosis
Salpingothecal anastomosis

03.8 **Injection of destructive agent into spinal canal**

● 03.9 **Other operations on spinal cord and spinal canal structures**

03.90 **Insertion of catheter into spinal canal for infusion of therapeutic or palliative substances**
Insertion of catheter into epidural, subarachnoid, or subdural space of spine with intermittent or continuous infusion of drug (with creation of any reservoir)
Code also any implantation of infusion pump (86.06)

03.91 **Injection of anesthetic into spinal canal for analgesia**

Excludes *that for operative anesthesia—omit code*

03.92 **Injection of other agent into spinal canal**
Intrathecal injection of steroid
Subarachnoid perfusion of refrigerated saline

Excludes *injection of:*
contrast material for myelogram (87.21)
destructive agent into spinal canal (03.8)

✖ 03.93 **Implantation or replacement of spinal neurostimulator lead(s)**
Code also any insertion of neurostimulator pulse generator (86.94–86.98) ⬅

✖ 03.94 **Removal of spinal neurostimulator lead(s)**
Code also any removal of neurostimulator pulse generator (86.05)

03.95 **Spinal blood patch**

03.96 **Percutaneous denervation of facet**

✖ 03.97 **Revision of spinal thecal shunt**

✖ 03.98 **Removal of spinal thecal shunt**

✖ 03.99 **Other**

● 04 **Operations on cranial and peripheral nerves**

● 04.0 **Incision, division, and excision of cranial and peripheral nerves**

Excludes *opticociliary neurectomy (12.79)*
sympathetic ganglionectomy (05.21–05.29)

✖ 04.01 **Excision of acoustic neuroma**
That by craniotomy

Excludes *that by stereotactic radiosurgery (92.30–92.39)*

✖ 04.02 **Division of trigeminal nerve**
Retrogasserian neurotomy

✖ **04.03 Division or crushing of other cranial and peripheral nerves**
Excludes *that of:*
glossopharyngeal nerve (29.92)
laryngeal nerve (31.91)
nerves to adrenal glands (07.42)
phrenic nerve for collapse of lung (33.31)
vagus nerve (44.00–44.03)

✖ **04.04 Other incision of cranial and peripheral nerves**

✖ **04.05 Gasserian ganglionectomy**

✖ **04.06 Other cranial or peripheral ganglionectomy**
Excludes *sympathetic ganglionectomy (05.21–05.29)*

✖ **04.07 Other excision or avulsion of cranial and peripheral nerves**
Curettage of peripheral nerve
Debridement of peripheral nerve
Resection of peripheral nerve
Excision of peripheral neuroma [Morton's]
Excludes *biopsy of cranial or peripheral nerve (04.11–04.12)*

● **04.1 Diagnostic procedures on peripheral nervous system**

04.11 Closed [percutaneous] [needle] biopsy of cranial or peripheral nerve or ganglion

✖ **04.12 Open biopsy of cranial or peripheral nerve or ganglion**

✖ **04.19 Other diagnostic procedures on cranial and peripheral nerves and ganglia**
Excludes *microscopic examination of specimen from nervous system (90.01–90.09)*
neurologic examination (89.13)

04.2 Destruction of cranial and peripheral nerves
Destruction of cranial or peripheral nerves by:
cryoanalgesia
injection of neurolytic agent
radiofrequency
Radiofrequency ablation

✖ **04.3 Suture of cranial and peripheral nerves**

● **04.4 Lysis of adhesions and decompression of cranial and peripheral nerves**

✖ **04.41 Decompression of trigeminal nerve root**

✖ **04.42 Other cranial nerve decompression**

✖ **04.43 Release of carpal tunnel**

✖ **04.44 Release of tarsal tunnel**

✖ **04.49 Other peripheral nerve or ganglion decompression or lysis of adhesions**
Peripheral nerve neurolysis NOS

✖ **04.5 Cranial or peripheral nerve graft**

✖ **04.6 Transposition of cranial and peripheral nerves**
Nerve transplantation

● **04.7 Other cranial or peripheral neuroplasty**

✖ **04.71 Hypoglossal-facial anastomosis**

✖ **04.72 Accessory-facial anastomosis**

✖ **04.73 Accessory-hypoglossal anastomosis**

✖ **04.74 Other anastomosis of cranial or peripheral nerve**

✖ **04.75 Revision of previous repair of cranial and peripheral nerves**

✖ **04.76 Repair of old traumatic injury of cranial and peripheral nerves**

✖ **04.79 Other neuroplasty**

● **04.8 Injection into peripheral nerve**
Excludes *destruction of nerve (by injection of neurolytic agent) (04.2)*

04.80 Peripheral nerve injection, not otherwise specified

04.81 Injection of anesthetic into peripheral nerve for analgesia
Excludes *that for operative anesthesia*

04.89 Injection of other agent, except neurolytic
Excludes *injection of neurolytic agent (04.2)*

● **04.9 Other operations on cranial and peripheral nerves**

✖ **04.91 Neurectasis**

✖ **04.92 Implantation or replacement of peripheral neurostimulator lead(s)**
Code also any insertion of neurostimulator pulse generator (86.94–86.98) ⬅

✖ **04.93 Removal of peripheral neurostimulator lead(s)**
Code also any removal of neurostimulator pulse generator (86.05)

✖ **04.99 Other**

● **05 Operations on sympathetic nerves or ganglia**
Excludes *paracervical uterine denervation (69.3)*

✖ **05.0 Division of sympathetic nerve or ganglion**
Excludes *that of nerves to adrenal glands (07.42)*

● **05.1 Diagnostic procedures on sympathetic nerves or ganglia**

✖ **05.11 Biopsy of sympathetic nerve or ganglion**

✖ **05.19 Other diagnostic procedures on sympathetic nerves or ganglia**

● **05.2 Sympathectomy**

✖ **05.21 Sphenopalatine ganglionectomy**

✖ **05.22 Cervical sympathectomy**

✖ **05.23 Lumbar sympathectomy**

✖ **05.24 Presacral sympathectomy**

✖ **05.25 Periarterial sympathectomy**

✖ **05.29 Other sympathectomy and ganglionectomy**
Excision or avulsion of sympathetic nerve NOS
Sympathetic ganglionectomy NOS
Excludes *biopsy of sympathetic nerve or ganglion (05.11)*
opticociliary neurectomy (12.79)
periarterial sympathectomy (05.25)
tympanosympathectomy (20.91)

● **05.3 Injection into sympathetic nerve or ganglion**
Excludes *injection of ciliary sympathetic ganglion (12.79)*

05.31 Injection of anesthetic into sympathetic nerve for analgesia

05.32 Injection of neurolytic agent into sympathetic nerve

05.39 Other injection into sympathetic nerve or ganglion

● **05.8 Other operations on sympathetic nerves or ganglia**

✖ **05.81 Repair of sympathetic nerve or ganglion**

✖ **05.89 Other**

✖ **05.9 Other operations on nervous system**

2. OPERATIONS ON THE ENDOCRINE SYSTEM (06–07)

● 06 Operations on thyroid and parathyroid glands

Includes: incidental resection of hyoid bone

06.0 Incision of thyroid field

Excludes *division of isthmus (06.91)*

06.01 Aspiration of thyroid field
Percutaneous or needle drainage of thyroid field

Excludes *aspiration biopsy of thyroid (06.11)*
drainage by incision (06.09)
postoperative aspiration of field (06.02)

✖ 06.02 Reopening of wound of thyroid field
Reopening of wound of thyroid field for:
control of (postoperative) hemorrhage
examination
exploration
removal of hematoma

✖ 06.09 Other incision of thyroid field
Drainage of hematoma by incision
Drainage of thyroglossal tract by incision
Exploration:
neck by incision
thyroid (field) by incision
Removal of foreign body by incision
Thyroidotomy NOS by incision

Excludes *postoperative exploration (06.02)*
removal of hematoma by aspiration (06.01)

● 06.1 Diagnostic procedures on thyroid and parathyroid glands

06.11 Closed [percutaneous] [needle] biopsy of thyroid gland
Aspiration biopsy of thyroid

✖ 06.12 Open biopsy of thyroid gland

✖ 06.13 Biopsy of parathyroid gland

✖ 06.19 Other diagnostic procedures on thyroid and parathyroid glands

Excludes *radioisotope scan of:*
parathyroid (92.13)
thyroid (92.01)
soft tissue x-ray of thyroid field (87.09)

✖ 06.2 Unilateral thyroid lobectomy
Complete removal of one lobe of thyroid (with removal of isthmus or portion of other lobe)
Hemithyroidectomy

Excludes *partial substernal thyroidectomy (06.51)*

● 06.3 Other partial thyroidectomy

✖ 06.31 Excision of lesion of thyroid

Excludes *biopsy of thyroid (06.11–06.12)*

✖ 06.39 Other
Isthmectomy
Partial thyroidectomy NOS

Excludes *partial substernal thyroidectomy (06.51)*

✖ 06.4 Complete thyroidectomy

Excludes *complete substernal thyroidectomy (06.52)*
that with laryngectomy (30.3–30.4)

● 06.5 Substernal thyroidectomy

✖ 06.50 Substernal thyroidectomy, not otherwise specified

✖ 06.51 Partial substernal thyroidectomy

✖ 06.52 Complete substernal thyroidectomy

✖ 06.6 Excision of lingual thyroid
Excision of thyroid by:
submental route
transoral route

✖ 06.7 Excision of thyroglossal duct or tract

● 06.8 Parathyroidectomy

✖ 06.81 Complete parathyroidectomy

✖ 06.89 Other parathyroidectomy
Parathyroidectomy NOS
Partial parathyroidectomy

Excludes *biopsy of parathyroid (06.13)*

● 06.9 Other operations on thyroid (region) and parathyroid

✖ 06.91 Division of thyroid isthmus
Transection of thyroid isthmus

✖ 06.92 Ligation of thyroid vessels

✖ 06.93 Suture of thyroid gland

✖ 06.94 Thyroid tissue reimplantation
Autotransplantation of thyroid tissue

✖ 06.95 Parathyroid tissue reimplantation
Autotransplantation of parathyroid tissue

✖ 06.98 Other operations on thyroid glands

✖ 06.99 Other operations on parathyroid glands

● 07 Operations on other endocrine glands

Includes: operations on:
adrenal glands
pineal gland
pituitary gland
thymus

Excludes *operations on:*
aortic and carotid bodies (39.8)
ovaries (65.0–65.99)
pancreas (52.01–52.99)
testes (62.0–62.99)

● 07.0 Exploration of adrenal field

Excludes *incision of adrenal (gland) (07.41)*

✖ 07.00 Exploration of adrenal field, not otherwise specified

✖ 07.01 Unilateral exploration of adrenal field

✖ 07.02 Bilateral exploration of adrenal field

● 07.1 Diagnostic procedures on adrenal glands, pituitary gland, pineal gland, and thymus

07.11 Closed [percutaneous] [needle] biopsy of adrenal gland

✖ 07.12 Open biopsy of adrenal gland

✖ 07.13 Biopsy of pituitary gland, transfrontal approach

✖ 07.14 Biopsy of pituitary gland, transsphenoidal approach

✖ 07.15 Biopsy of pituitary gland, unspecified approach

✖ 07.16 Biopsy of thymus

✖ 07.17 Biopsy of pineal gland

✖ 07.19 Other diagnostic procedures on adrenal glands, pituitary gland, pineal gland, and thymus

Excludes *microscopic examination of specimen from endocrine gland (90.11–90.19)*
radioisotope scan of pituitary gland (92.11)

● 07.2 Partial adrenalectomy

✖ 07.21 Excision of lesion of adrenal gland

Excludes *biopsy of adrenal gland (07.11–07.12)*

✖ 07.22 Unilateral adrenalectomy
Adrenalectomy NOS

Excludes *excision of remaining adrenal gland (07.3)*

✖ 07.29 Other partial adrenalectomy
Partial adrenalectomy NOS

✖07.3 **Bilateral adrenalectomy**
Excision of remaining adrenal gland
Excludes *bilateral partial adrenalectomy (07.29)*

●07.4 **Other operations on adrenal glands, nerves, and vessels**

✖07.41 **Incision of adrenal gland**
Adrenalotomy (with drainage)

✖07.42 **Division of nerves to adrenal glands**

✖07.43 **Ligation of adrenal vessels**

✖07.44 **Repair of adrenal gland**

✖07.45 **Reimplantation of adrenal tissue**
Autotransplantation of adrenal tissue

✖07.49 **Other**

●07.5 **Operations on pineal gland**

✖07.51 **Exploration of pineal field**
Excludes *that with incision of pineal gland (07.52)*

✖07.52 **Incision of pineal gland**

✖07.53 **Partial excision of pineal gland**
Excludes *biopsy of pineal gland (07.17)*

✖07.54 **Total excision of pineal gland**
Pinealectomy (complete) (total)

✖07.59 **Other operations on pineal gland**

●07.6 **Hypophysectomy**

✖07.61 **Partial excision of pituitary gland, transfrontal approach**
Cryohypophysectomy, partial transfrontal approach
Division of hypophyseal stalk transfrontal approach
Excision of lesion of pituitary [hypophysis] transfrontal approach
Hypophysectomy, subtotal transfrontal approach
Infundibulectomy, hypophyseal transfrontal approach
Excludes *biopsy of pituitary gland, transfrontal approach (07.13)*

✖07.62 **Partial excision of pituitary gland, transsphenoidal approach**
Excludes *biopsy of pituitary gland, transsphenoidal approach (07.14)*

✖07.63 **Partial excision of pituitary gland, unspecified approach**
Excludes *biopsy of pituitary gland NOS (07.15)*

✖07.64 **Total excision of pituitary gland, transfrontal approach**
Ablation of pituitary by implantation (strontium-yttrium) (Y) transfrontal approach
Cryohypophysectomy, complete transfrontal approach

✖07.65 **Total excision of pituitary gland, transsphenoidal approach**

✖07.68 **Total excision of pituitary gland, other specified approach**

✖07.69 **Total excision of pituitary gland, unspecified approach**
Hypophysectomy NOS
Pituitectomy NOS

●07.7 **Other operations on hypophysis**

✖07.71 **Exploration of pituitary fossa**
Excludes *exploration with incision of pituitary gland (07.72)*

✖07.72 **Incision of pituitary gland**
Aspiration of:
craniobuccal pouch
craniopharyngioma
hypophysis
pituitary gland
Rathke's pouch

✖07.79 **Other**
Insertion of pack into sella turcica

●07.8 **Thymectomy**

✖07.80 **Thymectomy, not otherwise specified**

✖07.81 **Partial excision of thymus**
Excludes *biopsy of thymus (07.16)*

✖07.82 **Total excision of thymus**

●07.9 **Other operations on thymus**

✖07.91 **Exploration of thymus field**
Excludes *exploration with incision of thymus (07.92)*

✖07.92 **Incision of thymus**

✖07.93 **Repair of thymus**

✖07.94 **Transplantation of thymus**

✖07.99 **Other**
Thymopexy

3. OPERATIONS ON THE EYE (08–16)

● **08 Operations on eyelids**

Includes: operations on the eyebrow

● **08.0 Incision of eyelid**

08.01 Incision of lid margin

08.02 Severing of blepharorrhaphy

08.09 Other incision of eyelid

● **08.1 Diagnostic procedures on eyelid**

✖ **08.11 Biopsy of eyelid**

08.19 Other diagnostic procedures on eyelid

● **08.2 Excision or destruction of lesion or tissue of eyelid**

Code also any synchronous reconstruction (08.61–08.74)

Excludes *biopsy of eyelid (08.11)*

✖ **08.20 Removal of lesion of eyelid, not otherwise specified**

Removal of meibomian gland NOS

✖ **08.21 Excision of chalazion**

✖ **08.22 Excision of other minor lesion of eyelid**

Excision of:
verucca
wart

✖ **08.23 Excision of major lesion of eyelid, partial-thickness**

Excision involving one-fourth or more of lid margin, partial-thickness

✖ **08.24 Excision of major lesion of eyelid, full-thickness**

Excision involving one-fourth or more of lid margin, full-thickness
Wedge resection of eyelid

✖ **08.25 Destruction of lesion of eyelid**

● **08.3 Repair of blepharoptosis and lid retraction**

✖ **08.31 Repair of blepharoptosis by frontalis muscle technique with suture**

✖ **08.32 Repair of blepharoptosis by frontalis muscle technique with fascial sling**

✖ **08.33 Repair of blepharoptosis by resection or advancement of levator muscle or aponeurosis**

✖ **08.34 Repair of blepharoptosis by other levator muscle techniques**

✖ **08.35 Repair of blepharoptosis by tarsal technique**

✖ **08.36 Repair of blepharoptosis by other techniques**

Correction of eyelid ptosis NOS
Orbicularis oculi muscle sling for correction of blepharoptosis

✖ **08.37 Reduction of overcorrection of ptosis**

✖ **08.38 Correction of lid retraction**

● **08.4 Repair of entropion or ectropion**

✖ **08.41 Repair of entropion or ectropion by thermocauterization**

✖ **08.42 Repair of entropion or ectropion by suture technique**

✖ **08.43 Repair of entropion or ectropion with wedge resection**

✖ **08.44 Repair of entropion or ectropion with lid reconstruction**

✖ **08.49 Other repair of entropion or ectropion**

● **08.5 Other adjustment of lid position**

✖ **08.51 Canthotomy**

Enlargement of palpebral fissure

✖ **08.52 Blepharorrhaphy**

Canthorrhaphy
Tarsorrhaphy

✖ **08.59 Other**

Canthoplasty NOS
Repair of epicanthal fold

● **08.6 Reconstruction of eyelid with flaps or grafts**

Excludes *that associated with repair of entropion and ectropion (08.44)*

✖ **08.61 Reconstruction of eyelid with skin flap or graft**

✖ **08.62 Reconstruction of eyelid with mucous membrane flap or graft**

✖ **08.63 Reconstruction of eyelid with hair follicle graft**

✖ **08.64 Reconstruction of eyelid with tarsoconjunctival flap**

Transfer of tarsoconjunctival flap from opposing lid

✖ **08.69 Other reconstruction of eyelid with flaps or grafts**

● **08.7 Other reconstruction of eyelid**

Excludes *that associated with repair of entropion and ectropion (08.44)*

✖ **08.70 Reconstruction of eyelid, not otherwise specified**

✖ **08.71 Reconstruction of eyelid involving lid margin, partial-thickness**

✖ **08.72 Other reconstruction of eyelid, partial-thickness**

✖ **08.73 Reconstruction of eyelid involving lid margin, full-thickness**

✖ **08.74 Other reconstruction of eyelid, full-thickness**

● **08.8 Other repair of eyelid**

08.81 Linear repair of laceration of eyelid or eyebrow

08.82 Repair of laceration involving lid margin, partial-thickness

08.83 Other repair of laceration of eyelid, partial-thickness

08.84 Repair of laceration involving lid margin, full-thickness

08.85 Other repair of laceration of eyelid, full-thickness

08.86 Lower eyelid rhytidectomy

08.87 Upper eyelid rhytidectomy

08.89 Other eyelid repair

● **08.9 Other operations on eyelids**

✖ **08.91 Electrosurgical epilation of eyelid**

✖ **08.92 Cryosurgical epilation of eyelid**

✖ **08.93 Other epilation of eyelid**

✖ **08.99 Other**

● **09 Operations on lacrimal system**

✖ **09.0 Incision of lacrimal gland**

Incision of lacrimal cyst (with drainage)

● **09.1 Diagnostic procedures on lacrimal system**

✖ **09.11 Biopsy of lacrimal gland**

✖ **09.12 Biopsy of lacrimal sac**

✖ **09.19 Other diagnostic procedures on lacrimal system**

Excludes *contrast dacryocystogram (87.05)*
soft tissue x-ray of nasolacrimal duct (87.09)

● **09.2 Excision of lesion or tissue of lacrimal gland**

✖ **09.20 Excision of lacrimal gland, not otherwise specified**

✖ **09.21 Excision of lesion of lacrimal gland**

Excludes *biopsy of lacrimal gland (09.11)*

✖ 09.22 Other partial dacryoadenectomy
Excludes *biopsy of lacrimal gland (09.11)*
✖ 09.23 Total dacryoadenectomy
✖ 09.3 Other operations on lacrimal gland
● 09.4 Manipulation of lacrimal passage
Includes: removal of calculus
that with dilation
Excludes *contrast dacryocystogram (87.05)*
✖ 09.41 Probing of lacrimal punctum
✖ 09.42 Probing of lacrimal canaliculi
✖ 09.43 Probing of nasolacrimal duct
Excludes *that with insertion of tube or stent (09.44)*
✖ 09.44 Intubation of nasolacrimal duct
Insertion of stent into nasolacrimal duct
✖ 09.49 Other manipulation of lacrimal passage
● 09.5 Incision of lacrimal sac and passages
✖ 09.51 Incision of lacrimal punctum
✖ 09.52 Incision of lacrimal canaliculi
✖ 09.53 Incision of lacrimal sac
✖ 09.59 Other incision of lacrimal passages
Incision (and drainage) of nasolacrimal duct NOS
✖ 09.6 Excision of lacrimal sac and passage
Excludes *biopsy of lacrimal sac (09.12)*
● 09.7 Repair of canaliculus and punctum
Excludes *repair of eyelid (08.81–08.89)*
✖ 09.71 Correction of everted punctum
✖ 09.72 Other repair of punctum
✖ 09.73 Repair of canaliculus
● 09.8 Fistulization of lacrimal tract to nasal cavity
✖ 09.81 Dacryocystorhinostomy [DCR]
✖ 09.82 Conjunctivocystorhinostomy
Conjunctivodacryocystorhinostomy [CDCR]
Excludes *that with insertion of tube or stent (09.83)*
✖ 09.83 Conjunctivorhinostomy with insertion of tube or stent
● 09.9 Other operations on lacrimal system
✖ 09.91 Obliteration of lacrimal punctum
✖ 09.99 Other

● 10 Operations on conjunctiva
✖ 10.0 Removal of embedded foreign body from conjunctiva by incision
Excludes *removal of:*
embedded foreign body without incision (98.22)
superficial foreign body (98.21)
✖ 10.1 Other incision of conjunctiva
● 10.2 Diagnostic procedures on conjunctiva
✖ 10.21 Biopsy of conjunctiva
✖ 10.29 Other diagnostic procedures on conjunctiva
● 10.3 Excision or destruction of lesion or tissue of conjunctiva
✖ 10.31 Excision of lesion or tissue of conjunctiva
Excision of ring of conjunctiva around cornea
Excludes *biopsy of conjunctiva (10.21)*
✖ 10.32 Destruction of lesion of conjunctiva
Excludes *excision of lesion (10.31)*
thermocauterization for entropion (08.41)
✖ 10.33 Other destructive procedures on conjunctiva
Removal of trachoma follicles
● 10.4 Conjunctivoplasty
✖ 10.41 Repair of symblepharon with free graft
✖ 10.42 Reconstruction of conjunctival cul-de-sac with free graft
Excludes *revision of enucleation socket with graft (16.63)*
✖ 10.43 Other reconstruction of conjunctival cul-de-sac
Excludes *revision of enucleation socket (16.64)*
✖ 10.44 Other free graft to conjunctiva
✖ 10.49 Other conjunctivoplasty
Excludes *repair of cornea with conjunctival flap (11.53)*
✖ 10.5 Lysis of adhesions of conjunctiva and eyelid
Division of symblepharon (with insertion of conformer)
✖ 10.6 Repair of laceration of conjunctiva
Excludes *that with repair of sclera (12.81)*
● 10.9 Other operations on conjunctiva
✖ 10.91 Subconjunctival injection
✖ 10.99 Other

● 11 Operations on cornea
✖ 11.0 Magnetic removal of embedded foreign body from cornea
Excludes *that with incision (11.1)*
✖ 11.1 Incision of cornea
Incision of cornea for removal of foreign body
● 11.2 Diagnostic procedures on cornea
✖ 11.21 Scraping of cornea for smear or culture
✖ 11.22 Biopsy of cornea
✖ 11.29 Other diagnostic procedures on cornea
● 11.3 Excision of pterygium
✖ 11.31 Transposition of pterygium
✖ 11.32 Excision of pterygium with corneal graft
✖ 11.39 Other excision of pterygium
● 11.4 Excision or destruction of tissue or other lesion of cornea
✖ 11.41 Mechanical removal of corneal epithelium
That by chemocauterization
Excludes *that for smear or culture (11.21)*
✖ 11.42 Thermocauterization of corneal lesion
✖ 11.43 Cryotherapy of corneal lesion
✖ 11.49 Other removal or destruction of corneal lesion
Excision of cornea NOS
Excludes *biopsy of cornea (11.22)*
● 11.5 Repair of cornea
✖ 11.51 Suture of corneal laceration
✖ 11.52 Repair of postoperative wound dehiscence of cornea
✖ 11.53 Repair of corneal laceration or wound with conjunctival flap
✖ 11.59 Other repair of cornea
● 11.6 Corneal transplant
Excludes *excision of pterygium with corneal graft (11.32)*
✖ 11.60 Corneal transplant, not otherwise specified
Keratoplasty NOS
Note: To report donor source - *see* codes 00.91–00.93)
✖ 11.61 Lamellar keratoplasty with autograft
✖ 11.62 Other lamellar keratoplasty
✖ 11.63 Penetrating keratoplasty with autograft
Perforating keratoplasty with autograft

✖11.64 Other penetrating keratoplasty
Perforating keratoplasty (with homograft)

✖11.69 Other corneal transplant

● 11.7 Other reconstructive and refractive surgery on cornea

✖11.71 Keratomileusis

✖11.72 Keratophakia

✖11.73 Keratoprosthesis

✖11.74 Thermokeratoplasty

✖11.75 Radial keratotomy

✖11.76 Epikeratophakia

✖11.79 Other

● 11.9 Other operations on cornea

✖11.91 Tattooing of cornea

✖11.92 Removal of artificial implant from cornea

✖11.99 Other

● 12 Operations on iris, ciliary body, sclera, and anterior chamber

Excludes *operations on cornea (11.0–11.99)*

● 12.0 Removal of intraocular foreign body from anterior segment of eye

✖12.00 Removal of intraocular foreign body from anterior segment of eye, not otherwise specified

✖12.01 Removal of intraocular foreign body from anterior segment of eye with use of magnet

✖12.02 Removal of intraocular foreign body from anterior segment of eye without use of magnet

● 12.1 Iridotomy and simple iridectomy

Excludes *iridectomy associated with:*
cataract extraction (13.11–13.69)
removal of lesion (12.41–12.42)
scleral fistulization (12.61–12.69)

✖12.11 Iridotomy with transfixion

✖12.12 Other iridotomy
Corectomy
Discission of iris
Iridotomy NOS

✖12.13 Excision of prolapsed iris

✖12.14 Other iridectomy
Iridectomy (basal) (peripheral) (total)

● 12.2 Diagnostic procedures on iris, ciliary body, sclera, and anterior chamber

✖12.21 Diagnostic aspiration of anterior chamber of eye

✖12.22 Biopsy of iris

✖12.29 Other diagnostic procedures on iris, ciliary body, sclera, and anterior chamber

● 12.3 Iridoplasty and coreoplasty

✖12.31 Lysis of goniosynechiae
Lysis of goniosynechiae by injection of air or liquid

✖12.32 Lysis of other anterior synechiae
Lysis of anterior synechiae:
NOS
by injection of air or liquid

✖12.33 Lysis of posterior synechiae
Lysis of iris adhesions NOS

✖12.34 Lysis of corneovitreal adhesions

✖12.35 Coreoplasty
Needling of pupillary membrane

✖12.39 Other iridoplasty

● 12.4 Excision or destruction of lesion of iris and ciliary body

✖12.40 Removal of lesion of anterior segment of eye, not otherwise specified

✖12.41 Destruction of lesion of iris, nonexcisional
Destruction of lesion of iris by:
cauterization
cryotherapy
photocoagulation

✖12.42 Excision of lesion of iris

Excludes *biopsy of iris (12.22)*

✖12.43 Destruction of lesion of ciliary body, nonexcisional

✖12.44 Excision of lesion of ciliary body

● 12.5 Facilitation of intraocular circulation

✖12.51 Goniopuncture without goniotomy

✖12.52 Goniotomy without goniopuncture

✖12.53 Goniotomy with goniopuncture

✖12.54 Trabeculotomy ab externo

✖12.55 Cyclodialysis

✖12.59 Other facilitation of intraocular circulation

● 12.6 Scleral fistulization

Excludes *exploratory sclerotomy (12.89)*

✖12.61 Trephination of sclera with iridectomy

✖12.62 Thermocauterization of sclera with iridectomy

✖12.63 Iridencleisis and iridotasis

✖12.64 Trabeculectomy ab externo

✖12.65 Other scleral fistulization with iridectomy

✖12.66 Postoperative revision of scleral fistulization procedure
Revision of filtering bleb

Excludes *repair of fistula (12.82)*

✖12.69 Other fistulizing procedure

● 12.7 Other procedures for relief of elevated intraocular pressure

✖12.71 Cyclodiathermy

✖12.72 Cyclocryotherapy

✖12.73 Cyclophotocoagulation

✖12.74 Diminution of ciliary body, not otherwise specified

✖12.79 Other glaucoma procedures

● 12.8 Operations on sclera

Excludes *those associated with:*
retinal reattachment (14.41–14.59)
scleral fistulization (12.61–12.69)

✖12.81 Suture of laceration of sclera
Suture of sclera with synchronous repair of conjunctiva

✖12.82 Repair of scleral fistula

Excludes *postoperative revision of scleral fistulization procedure (12.66)*

✖12.83 Revision of operative wound of anterior segment, not elsewhere classified

Excludes *postoperative revision of scleral fistulization procedure (12.66)*

✖12.84 Excision or destruction of lesion of sclera

✖12.85 Repair of scleral staphyloma with graft

✖12.86 Other repair of scleral staphyloma

✖12.87 Scleral reinforcement with graft

✖12.88 **Other scleral reinforcement**

✖12.89 **Other operations on sclera**
Exploratory sclerotomy

● 12.9 **Other operations on iris, ciliary body, and anterior chamber**

✖12.91 **Therapeutic evacuation of anterior chamber**
Paracentesis of anterior chamber

Excludes *diagnostic aspiration (12.21)*

✖12.92 **Injection into anterior chamber**
Injection of:
air into anterior chamber
liquid into anterior chamber
medication into anterior chamber

✖12.93 **Removal or destruction of epithelial downgrowth from anterior chamber**

Excludes *that with iridectomy (12.41–12.42)*

✖12.97 **Other operations on iris**

✖12.98 **Other operations on ciliary body**

✖12.99 **Other operations on anterior chamber**

● 13 **Operations on lens**

● 13.0 **Removal of foreign body from lens**

Excludes *removal of pseudophakos (13.8)*

✖13.00 **Removal of foreign body from lens, not otherwise specified**

✖13.01 **Removal of foreign body from lens with use of magnet**

✖13.02 **Removal of foreign body from lens without use of magnet**

● 13.1 **Intracapsular extraction of lens**

Code also any synchronous insertion of pseudophakos (13.71)

✖13.11 **Intracapsular extraction of lens by temporal inferior route**

✖13.19 **Other intracapsular extraction of lens**
Cataract extraction NOS
Cryoextraction of lens
Erysiphake extraction of cataract
Extraction of lens NOS

✖13.2 **Extracapsular extraction of lens by linear extraction technique**

✖13.3 **Extracapsular extraction of lens by simple aspiration (and irrigation) technique**
Irrigation of traumatic cataract

● 13.4 **Extracapsular extraction of lens by fragmentation and aspiration technique**

✖13.41 **Phacoemulsification and aspiration of cataract**

✖13.42 **Mechanical phacofragmentation and aspiration of cataract by posterior route**

Code also any synchronous vitrectomy (14.74)

✖13.43 **Mechanical phacofragmentation and other aspiration of cataract**

● 13.5 **Other extracapsular extraction of lens**

Code also any synchronous insertion of pseudophakos (13.71)

✖13.51 **Extracapsular extraction of lens by temporal inferior route**

✖13.59 **Other extracapsular extraction of lens**

● 13.6 **Other cataract extraction**

Code also any synchronous insertion of pseudophakos (13.71)

✖13.64 **Discission of secondary membrane [after cataract]**

✖13.65 **Excision of secondary membrane [after cataract]**
Capsulectomy

✖13.66 **Mechanical fragmentation of secondary membrane [after cataract]**

✖13.69 **Other cataract extraction**

● 13.7 **Insertion of prosthetic lens [pseudophakos]**

Excludes *implantation of intraocular telescope prosthesis (13.91)* ◀

✖13.70 **Insertion of pseudophakos, not otherwise specified**

✖13.71 **Insertion of intraocular lens prosthesis at time of cataract extraction, one-stage**

Code also synchronous extraction of cataract (13.11–13.69)

✖13.72 **Secondary insertion of intraocular lens prosthesis**

✖13.8 **Removal of implanted lens**
Removal of pseudophakos

● 13.9 **Other operations on lens** ⬅

13.90 **Operation on lens, NEC** ◀

13.91 **Implantation of intraocular telescope prosthesis** ◀
Removal of lens, any method ◀
Implantable miniature telescope ◀

Excludes *secondary insertion of ocular implant (16.61)* ◀

● 14 **Operations on retina, choroid, vitreous, and posterior chamber**

● 14.0 **Removal of foreign body from posterior segment of eye**

Excludes *removal of surgically implanted material (14.6)*

✖14.00 **Removal of foreign body from posterior segment of eye, not otherwise specified**

✖14.01 **Removal of foreign body from posterior segment of eye with use of magnet**

✖14.02 **Removal of foreign body from posterior segment of eye without use of magnet**

● 14.1 **Diagnostic procedures on retina, choroid, vitreous, and posterior chamber**

✖14.11 **Diagnostic aspiration of vitreous**

✖14.19 **Other diagnostic procedures on retina, choroid, vitreous, and posterior chamber**

● 14.2 **Destruction of lesion of retina and choroid**

Includes: destruction of chorioretinopathy or isolated chorioretinal lesion

Excludes *that for repair of retina (14.31–14.59)*

✖14.21 **Destruction of chorioretinal lesion by diathermy**

✖14.22 **Destruction of chorioretinal lesion by cryotherapy**

14.23 **Destruction of chorioretinal lesion by xenon arc photocoagulation**

14.24 **Destruction of chorioretinal lesion by laser photocoagulation**

14.25 **Destruction of chorioretinal lesion by photocoagulation of unspecified type**

✖14.26 **Destruction of chorioretinal lesion by radiation therapy**

✖14.27 **Destruction of chorioretinal lesion by implantation of radiation source**

✖14.29 **Other destruction of chorioretinal lesion**
Destruction of lesion of retina and choroid NOS

● 14.3 Repair of retinal tear

Includes: repair of retinal defect

Excludes *repair of retinal detachment (14.41–14.59)*

✖ 14.31 Repair of retinal tear by diathermy

✖ 14.32 Repair of retinal tear by cryotherapy

14.33 Repair of retinal tear by xenon arc photocoagulation

14.34 Repair of retinal tear by laser photocoagulation

14.35 Repair of retinal tear by photocoagulation of unspecified type

✖ 14.39 Other repair of retinal tear

● 14.4 Repair of retinal detachment with scleral buckling and implant

✖ 14.41 Scleral buckling with implant

✖ 14.49 Other scleral buckling

Scleral buckling with:
air tamponade
resection of sclera
vitrectomy

● 14.5 Other repair of retinal detachment

Includes: that with drainage

✖ 14.51 Repair of retinal detachment with diathermy

✖ 14.52 Repair of retinal detachment with cryotherapy

✖ 14.53 Repair of retinal detachment with xenon arc photocoagulation

✖ 14.54 Repair of retinal detachment with laser photocoagulation

✖ 14.55 Repair of retinal detachment with photocoagulation of unspecified type

✖ 14.59 Other

✖ 14.6 Removal of surgically implanted material from posterior segment of eye

● 14.7 Operations on vitreous

✖ 14.71 Removal of vitreous, anterior approach

Open sky technique
Removal of vitreous, anterior approach (with replacement)

✖ 14.72 Other removal of vitreous

Aspiration of vitreous by posterior sclerotomy

✖ 14.73 Mechanical vitrectomy by anterior approach

✖ 14.74 Other mechanical vitrectomy ◀

Posterior approach

✖ 14.75 Injection of vitreous substitute

Excludes *that associated with removal (14.71–14.72)*

✖ 14.79 Other operations on vitreous

✖ 14.9 Other operations on retina, choroid, and posterior chamber

● 15 Operations on extraocular muscles

● 15.0 Diagnostic procedures on extraocular muscles or tendons

✖ 15.01 Biopsy of extraocular muscle or tendon

✖ 15.09 Other diagnostic procedures on extraocular muscles and tendons

● 15.1 Operations on one extraocular muscle involving temporary detachment from globe

✖ 15.11 Recession of one extraocular muscle

✖ 15.12 Advancement of one extraocular muscle

✖ 15.13 Resection of one extraocular muscle

✖ 15.19 Other operations on one extraocular muscle involving temporary detachment from globe

Excludes *transposition of muscle (15.5)*

● 15.2 Other operations on one extraocular muscle

✖ 15.21 Lengthening procedure on one extraocular muscle

✖ 15.22 Shortening procedure on one extraocular muscle

✖ 15.29 Other

✖ 15.3 Operations on two or more extraocular muscles involving temporary detachment from globe, one or both eyes

✖ 15.4 Other operations on two or more extraocular muscles, one or both eyes

✖ 15.5 Transposition of extraocular muscles

Excludes *that for correction of ptosis (08.31–08.36)*

✖ 15.6 Revision of extraocular muscle surgery

✖ 15.7 Repair of injury of extraocular muscle

Freeing of entrapped extraocular muscle
Lysis of adhesions of extraocular muscle
Repair of laceration of extraocular muscle, tendon, or Tenon's capsule

✖ 15.9 Other operations on extraocular muscles and tendons

● 16 Operations on orbit and eyeball

Excludes *reduction of fracture of orbit (76.78–76.79)*

● 16.0 Orbitotomy

✖ 16.01 Orbitotomy with bone flap

Orbitotomy with lateral approach

✖ 16.02 Orbitotomy with insertion of orbital implant

Excludes *that with bone flap (16.01)*

✖ 16.09 Other orbitotomy

✖ 16.1 Removal of penetrating foreign body from eye, not otherwise specified

Excludes *removal of nonpenetrating foreign body (98.21)*

● 16.2 Diagnostic procedures on orbit and eyeball

16.21 Ophthalmoscopy

✖ 16.22 Diagnostic aspiration of orbit

✖ 16.23 Biopsy of eyeball and orbit

✖ 16.29 Other diagnostic procedures on orbit and eyeball

Excludes *examination of form and structure of eye (95.11–95.16)*
general and subjective eye examination (95.01–95.09)
microscopic examination of specimen from eye (90.21–90.29)
objective functional tests of eye (95.21–95.26)
ocular thermography (88.82)
tonometry (89.11)
x-ray of orbit (87.14, 87.16)

● 16.3 Evisceration of eyeball

✖ 16.31 Removal of ocular contents with synchronous implant into scleral shell

✖ 16.39 Other evisceration of eyeball

● 16.4 Enucleation of eyeball

✖ 16.41 Enucleation of eyeball with synchronous implant into Tenon's capsule with attachment of muscles

Integrated implant of eyeball

✖ 16.42 Enucleation of eyeball with other synchronous implant

✖ 16.49 Other enucleation of eyeball

Removal of eyeball NOS

● **16.5 Exenteration of orbital contents**

✖ **16.51 Exenteration of orbit with removal of adjacent structures**
Radical orbitomaxillectomy

✖ **16.52 Exenteration of orbit with therapeutic removal of orbital bone**

✖ **16.59 Other exenteration of orbit**
Evisceration of orbit NOS
Exenteration of orbit with temporalis muscle transplant

● **16.6 Secondary procedures after removal of eyeball**

Excludes *that with synchronous:*
enucleation of eyeball (16.41–16.42)
evisceration of eyeball (16.31)

✖ **16.61 Secondary insertion of ocular implant**

✖ **16.62 Revision and reinsertion of ocular implant**

✖ **16.63 Revision of enucleation socket with graft**

✖ **16.64 Other revision of enucleation socket**

✖ **16.65 Secondary graft to exenteration cavity**

✖ **16.66 Other revision of exenteration cavity**

✖ **16.69 Other secondary procedures after removal of eyeball**

● **16.7 Removal of ocular or orbital implant**

✖ **16.71 Removal of ocular implant**

✖ **16.72 Removal of orbital implant**

● **16.8 Repair of injury of eyeball and orbit**

✖ **16.81 Repair of wound of orbit**

Excludes *reduction of orbital fracture (76.78–76.79)*
repair of extraocular muscles (15.7)

✖ **16.82 Repair of rupture of eyeball**
Repair of multiple structures of eye

Excludes *repair of laceration of:*
cornea (11.51–11.59)
sclera (12.81)

✖ **16.89 Other repair of injury of eyeball or orbit**

● **16.9 Other operations on orbit and eyeball**

Excludes *irrigation of eye (96.51)*
prescription and fitting of low vision aids (95.31–95.33)
removal of:
eye prosthesis NEC (97.31)
nonpenetrating foreign body from eye without incision (98.21)

16.91 Retrobulbar injection of therapeutic agent

Excludes *injection of radiographic contrast material (87.14)*
opticociliary injection (12.79)

✖ **16.92 Excision of lesion of orbit**

Excludes *biopsy of orbit (16.23)*

✖ **16.93 Excision of lesion of eye, unspecified structure**

Excludes *biopsy of eye NOS (16.23)*

✖ **16.98 Other operations on orbit**

✖ **16.99 Other operations on eyeball**

4. OPERATIONS ON THE EAR (18–20)

● 18 **Operations on external ear**

Includes: operations on:
external auditory canal
skin and cartilage of:
auricle
meatus

● 18.0 **Incision of external ear**

Excludes *removal of intraluminal foreign body (98.11)*

18.01 **Piercing of ear lobe**
Piercing of pinna

18.02 **Incision of external auditory canal**

18.09 **Other incision of external ear**

● 18.1 **Diagnostic procedures on external ear**

18.11 **Otoscopy**

18.12 **Biopsy of external ear**

18.19 **Other diagnostic procedures on external ear**

Excludes *microscopic examination of specimen from ear (90.31–90.39)*

● 18.2 **Excision or destruction of lesion of external ear**

✖ 18.21 **Excision of preauricular sinus**
Radical excision of preauricular sinus or cyst

Excludes *excision of preauricular remnant [appendage] (18.29)*

18.29 **Excision or destruction of other lesion of external ear**
Cauterization of external ear
Coagulation of external ear
Cryosurgery of external ear
Curettage of external ear
Electrocoagulation of external ear
Enucleation of external ear
Excision of:
exostosis of external auditory canal
preauricular remnant [appendage]
Partial excision of ear

Excludes *biopsy of external ear (18.12)*
radical excision of lesion (18.31)
removal of cerumen (96.52)

● 18.3 **Other excision of external ear**

Excludes *biopsy of external ear (18.12)*

✖ 18.31 **Radical excision of lesion of external ear**

Excludes *radical excision of preauricular sinus (18.21)*

✖ 18.39 **Other**
Amputation of external ear

Excludes *excision of lesion (18.21–18.29, 18.31)*

18.4 **Suture of laceration of external ear**

✖ 18.5 **Surgical correction of prominent ear**
Ear:
pinning
setback

✖ 18.6 **Reconstruction of external auditory canal**
Canaloplasty of external auditory meatus
Construction [reconstruction] of external meatus of ear:
osseous portion
skin-lined portion (with skin graft)

● 18.7 **Other plastic repair of external ear**

✖ 18.71 **Construction of auricle of ear**
Prosthetic appliance for absent ear
Reconstruction:
auricle
ear

✖ 18.72 **Reattachment of amputated ear**

✖ 18.79 **Other plastic repair of external ear**
Otoplasty NOS
Postauricular skin graft
Repair of lop ear

✖ 18.9 **Other operations on external ear**

Excludes *irrigation of ear (96.52)*
packing of external auditory canal (96.11)
removal of:
cerumen (96.52)
foreign body (without incision) (98.11)

● 19 **Reconstructive operations on middle ear**

✖ 19.0 **Stapes mobilization**
Division, otosclerotic:
material
process
Remobilization of stapes
Stapediolysis
Transcrural stapes mobilization

Excludes *that with synchronous stapedectomy (19.11–19.19)*

● 19.1 **Stapedectomy**

Excludes *revision of previous stapedectomy (19.21–19.29)*
stapes mobilization only (19.0)

✖ 19.11 **Stapedectomy with incus replacement**
Stapedectomy with incus:
homograft
prosthesis

✖ 19.19 **Other stapedectomy**

19.2 **Revision of stapedectomy**

✖ 19.21 **Revision of stapedectomy with incus replacement**

✖ 19.29 **Other revision of stapedectomy**

✖ 19.3 **Other operations on ossicular chain**
Incudectomy NOS
Ossiculectomy NOS
Reconstruction of ossicles, second stage

✖ 19.4 **Myringoplasty**
Epitympanic, type I
Myringoplasty by:
cauterization
graft
Tympanoplasty (type I)

● 19.5 **Other tympanoplasty**

✖ 19.52 **Type II tympanoplasty**
Closure of perforation with graft against incus or malleus

✖ 19.53 **Type III tympanoplasty**
Graft placed in contact with mobile and intact stapes

✖ 19.54 **Type IV tympanoplasty**
Mobile footplate left exposed with air pocket between round window and graft

✖ 19.55 **Type V tympanoplasty**
Fenestra in horizontal semicircular canal covered by graft

✖ 19.6 **Revision of tympanoplasty**

✖ 19.9 **Other repair of middle ear**
Closure of mastoid fistula
Mastoid myoplasty
Obliteration of tympanomastoid cavity

● 20 **Other operations on middle and inner ear**

● 20.0 **Myringotomy**

✖ 20.01 **Myringotomy with insertion of tube**
Myringostomy

✖ 20.09 **Other myringotomy**
Aspiration of middle ear NOS

20.1 Removal of tympanostomy tube

● **20.2 Incision of mastoid and middle ear**

✖ **20.21 Incision of mastoid**

✖ **20.22 Incision of petrous pyramid air cells**

✖ **20.23 Incision of middle ear**
Atticotomy
Division of tympanum
Lysis of adhesions of middle ear

Excludes *division of otosclerotic process (19.0)*
stapediolysis (19.0)
that with stapedectomy (19.11–19.19)

● **20.3 Diagnostic procedures on middle and inner ear**

20.31 Electrocochleography

✖ **20.32 Biopsy of middle and inner ear**

✖ **20.39 Other diagnostic procedures on middle and inner ear**

Excludes *auditory and vestibular function tests (89.13, 95.41–95.49)*
microscopic examination of specimen from ear (90.31–90.39)

● **20.4 Mastoidectomy**
Code also any:
skin graft (18.79)
tympanoplasty (19.4–19.55)

Excludes *that with implantation of cochlear prosthetic device (20.96–20.98)*

✖ **20.41 Simple mastoidectomy**

✖ **20.42 Radical mastoidectomy**

✖ **20.49 Other mastoidectomy**
Atticoantrostomy
Mastoidectomy:
NOS
modified radical

● **20.5 Other excision of middle ear**

Excludes *that with synchronous mastoidectomy (20.41–20.49)*

✖ **20.51 Excision of lesion of middle ear**

Excludes *biopsy of middle ear (20.32)*

✖ **20.59 Other**
Apicectomy of petrous pyramid
Tympanectomy

● **20.6 Fenestration of inner ear**

✖ **20.61 Fenestration of inner ear (initial)**
Fenestration of:
labyrinth with graft (skin) (vein)
semicircular canals with graft (skin) (vein)
vestibule with graft (skin) (vein)

Excludes *that with tympanoplasty, type V (19.55)*

✖ **20.62 Revision of fenestration of inner ear**

● **20.7 Incision, excision, and destruction of inner ear**

✖ **20.71 Endolymphatic shunt**

✖ **20.72 Injection into inner ear**
Destruction by injection (alcohol):
inner ear
semicircular canals
vestibule

✖ **20.79 Other incision, excision, and destruction of inner ear**
Decompression of labyrinth
Drainage of inner ear
Fistulization:
endolymphatic sac
labyrinth
Incision of endolymphatic sac
Labyrinthectomy (transtympanic)
Opening of bony labyrinth
Perilymphatic tap

Excludes *biopsy of inner ear (20.32)*

20.8 Operations on Eustachian tube
Catheterization of eustachian tube
Inflation of eustachian tube
Injection (Teflon paste) of eustachian tube
Insufflation (boric acid-salicylic acid)
Intubation of eustachian tube
Politzerization of eustachian tube

● **20.9 Other operations on inner and middle ear**

✖ **20.91 Tympanosympathectomy**

✖ **20.92 Revision of mastoidectomy**

✖ **20.93 Repair of oval and round windows**
Closure of fistula:
oval window
perilymph
round window

20.94 Injection of tympanum

✖ **20.95 Implantation of electromagnetic hearing device**
Bone conduction hearing device

Excludes *cochlear prosthetic device (20.96–20.98)*

✖ **20.96 Implantation or replacement of cochlear prosthetic device, not otherwise specified**
Implantation of receiver (within skull) and insertion of electrode(s) in the cochlea

Includes: mastoidectomy

Excludes *electromagnetic hearing device (20.95)*

✖ **20.97 Implantation or replacement of cochlear prosthetic device, single channel**
Implantation of receiver (within skull) and insertion of electrode in the cochlea

Includes: mastoidectomy

Excludes *electromagnetic hearing device (20.95)*

✖ **20.98 Implantation or replacement of cochlear prosthetic device, multiple channel**
Implantation of receiver (within skull) and insertion of electrodes in the cochlea

Includes: mastoidectomy

Excludes *electromagnetic hearing device (20.95)*

✖ **20.99 Other operations on middle and inner ear**
Repair or removal of cochlear prosthetic device (receiver) (electrode)

Excludes *adjustment (external components) of cochlear prosthetic device (95.49)*
fitting of hearing aid (95.48)

5. OPERATIONS ON THE NOSE, MOUTH, AND PHARYNX (21–29)

● **21 Operations on nose**

Includes: operations on:
bone of nose
skin of nose

● **21.0 Control of epistaxis**

21.00 Control of epistaxis, not otherwise specified

21.01 Control of epistaxis by anterior nasal packing

21.02 Control of epistaxis by posterior (and anterior) packing

21.03 Control of epistaxis by cauterization (and packing)

✖ **21.04 Control of epistaxis by ligation of ethmoidal arteries**

✖ **21.05 Control of epistaxis by (transantral) ligation of the maxillary artery**

✖ **21.06 Control of epistaxis by ligation of the external carotid artery**

✖ **21.07 Control of epistaxis by excision of nasal mucosa and skin grafting of septum and lateral nasal wall**

✖ **21.09 Control of epistaxis by other means**

21.1 Incision of nose
Chondrotomy
Incision of skin of nose
Nasal septotomy

● **21.2 Diagnostic procedures on nose**

21.21 Rhinoscopy

21.22 Biopsy of nose

21.29 Other diagnostic procedures on nose

Excludes *microscopic examination of specimen from nose (90.31–90.39)*
nasal:
function study (89.12)
x-ray (87.16)
rhinomanometry (89.12)

● **21.3 Local excision or destruction of lesion of nose**

Excludes *biopsy of nose (21.22)*
nasal fistulectomy (21.82)

21.30 Excision or destruction of lesion of nose, not otherwise specified

21.31 Local excision or destruction of intranasal lesion
Nasal polypectomy

21.32 Local excision or destruction of other lesion of nose

✖ **21.4 Resection of nose**
Amputation of nose

✖ **21.5 Submucous resection of nasal septum**

● **21.6 Turbinectomy**

✖ **21.61 Turbinectomy by diathermy or cryosurgery**

✖ **21.62 Fracture of the turbinates**

✖ **21.69 Other turbinectomy**

Excludes *turbinectomy associated with sinusectomy (22.31–22.39, 22.42, 22.60–22.64)*

● **21.7 Reduction of nasal fracture**

21.71 Closed reduction of nasal fracture

✖ **21.72 Open reduction of nasal fracture**

● **21.8 Repair and plastic operations on the nose**

21.81 Suture of laceration of nose

✖ **21.82 Closure of nasal fistula**
Nasolabial fistulectomy
Nasopharyngeal fistulectomy
Oronasal fistulectomy

✖ **21.83 Total nasal reconstruction**
Reconstruction of nose with:
arm flap
forehead flap

✖ **21.84 Revision rhinoplasty**
Rhinoseptoplasty
Twisted nose rhinoplasty

✖ **21.85 Augmentation rhinoplasty**
Augmentation rhinoplasty with:
graft
synthetic implant

✖ **21.86 Limited rhinoplasty**
Plastic repair of nasolabial flaps
Tip rhinoplasty

✖ **21.87 Other rhinoplasty**
Rhinoplasty NOS

✖ **21.88 Other septoplasty**
Crushing of nasal septum
Repair of septal perforation

Excludes *septoplasty associated with submucous resection of septum (21.5)*

✖ **21.89 Other repair and plastic operations on nose**
Reattachment of amputated nose

● **21.9 Other operations on nose**

21.91 Lysis of adhesions of nose
Posterior nasal scrub

✖ **21.99 Other**

Excludes *dilation of frontonasal duct (96.21)*
irrigation of nasal passages (96.53)
removal of:
intraluminal foreign body without incision (98.12)
nasal packing (97.32)
replacement of nasal packing (97.21)

● **22 Operations on nasal sinuses**

● **22.0 Aspiration and lavage of nasal sinus**

22.00 Aspiration and lavage of nasal sinus, not otherwise specified

22.01 Puncture of nasal sinus for aspiration or lavage

22.02 Aspiration or lavage of nasal sinus through natural ostium

● **22.1 Diagnostic procedures on nasal sinus**

22.11 Closed [endoscopic] [needle] biopsy of nasal sinus

✖ **22.12 Open biopsy of nasal sinus**

22.19 Other diagnostic procedures on nasal sinuses
Endoscopy without biopsy

Excludes *transillumination of sinus (89.35)*
x-ray of sinus (87.15–87.16)

22.2 Intranasal antrotomy

Excludes *antrotomy with external approach (22.31–22.39)*

● **22.3 External maxillary antrotomy**

✖ **22.31 Radical maxillary antrotomy**
Removal of lining membrane of maxillary sinus using Caldwell-Luc approach

✖ **22.39 Other external maxillary antrotomy**
Exploration of maxillary antrum with Caldwell-Luc approach

● **22.4 Frontal sinusotomy and sinusectomy**

✖ **22.41 Frontal sinusotomy**

✖22.42 **Frontal sinusectomy**
Excision of lesion of frontal sinus
Obliteration of frontal sinus (with fat)
Excludes *biopsy of nasal sinus (22.11–22.12)*

●22.5 **Other nasal sinusotomy**

✖22.50 **Sinusotomy, not otherwise specified**

✖22.51 **Ethmoidotomy**

✖22.52 **Sphenoidotomy**

✖22.53 **Incision of multiple nasal sinuses**

●22.6 **Other nasal sinusectomy**
Includes: that with incidental turbinectomy
Excludes *biopsy of nasal sinus (22.11–22.12)*

✖22.60 **Sinusectomy, not otherwise specified**

✖22.61 **Excision of lesion of maxillary sinus with Caldwell-Luc approach**

✖22.62 **Excision of lesion of maxillary sinus with other approach**

✖22.63 **Ethmoidectomy**

✖22.64 **Sphenoidectomy**

●22.7 **Repair of nasal sinus**

✖22.71 **Closure of nasal sinus fistula**
Repair of oro-antral fistula

✖22.79 **Other repair of nasal sinus**
Reconstruction of frontonasal duct
Repair of bone of accessory sinus

✖22.9 **Other operations on nasal sinuses**
Exteriorization of maxillary sinus
Fistulization of sinus
Excludes *dilation of frontonasal duct (96.21)*

●23 **Removal and restoration of teeth**

●23.0 **Forceps extraction of tooth**

23.01 **Extraction of deciduous tooth**

23.09 **Extraction of other tooth**
Extraction of tooth NOS

●23.1 **Surgical removal of tooth**

23.11 **Removal of residual root**

23.19 **Other surgical extraction of tooth**
Odontectomy NOS
Removal of impacted tooth
Tooth extraction with elevation of muco-periosteal flap

23.2 **Restoration of tooth by filling**

23.3 **Restoration of tooth by inlay**

●23.4 **Other dental restoration**

23.41 **Application of crown**

23.42 **Insertion of fixed bridge**

23.43 **Insertion of removable bridge**

23.49 **Other**

23.5 **Implantation of tooth**

23.6 **Prosthetic dental implant**
Endosseous dental implant

●23.7 **Apicoectomy and root canal therapy**

23.70 **Root canal, not otherwise specified**

23.71 **Root canal therapy with irrigation**

23.72 **Root canal therapy with apicoectomy**

23.73 **Apicoectomy**

●24 **Other operations on teeth, gums, and alveoli**

24.0 **Incision of gum or alveolar bone**
Apical alveolotomy

●24.1 **Diagnostic procedures on teeth, gums, and alveoli**

24.11 **Biopsy of gum**

24.12 **Biopsy of alveolus**

24.19 **Other diagnostic procedures on teeth, gums, and alveoli**
Excludes *dental:*
examination (89.31)
x-ray:
full-mouth (87.11)
other (87.12)
microscopic examination of dental specimen (90.81–90.89)

24.2 **Gingivoplasty**
Gingivoplasty with bone or soft tissue graft

●24.3 **Other operations on gum**

24.31 **Excision of lesion or tissue of gum**
Excludes *biopsy of gum (24.11)*
excision of odontogenic lesion (24.4)

24.32 **Suture of laceration of gum**

24.39 **Other**

✖24.4 **Excision of dental lesion of jaw**
Excision of odontogenic lesion

✖24.5 **Alveoloplasty**
Alveolectomy (interradicular) (intraseptal) (radical) (simple) (with graft or implant)
Excludes *biopsy of alveolus (24.12)*
en bloc resection of alveolar process and palate (27.32)

24.6 **Exposure of tooth**

24.7 **Application of orthodontic appliance**
Application, insertion, or fitting of:
arch bars
orthodontic obturator
orthodontic wiring
periodontal splint
Excludes *nonorthodontic dental wiring (93.55)*

24.8 **Other orthodontic operation**
Closure of diastema (alveolar) (dental)
Occlusal adjustment
Removal of arch bars
Repair of dental arch
Excludes *removal of nonorthodontic wiring (97.33)*

●24.9 **Other dental operations**

24.91 **Extension or deepening of buccolabial or lingual sulcus**

24.99 **Other**
Excludes *dental:*
debridement (96.54)
examination (89.31)
prophylaxis (96.54)
scaling and polishing (96.54)
wiring (93.55)
fitting of dental appliance [denture] (99.97)
microscopic examination of dental specimen (90.81–90.89)
removal of dental:
packing (97.34)
prosthesis (97.35)
wiring (97.33)
replacement of dental packing (97.22)

●25 **Operations on tongue**

●25.0 **Diagnostic procedures on tongue**

25.01 **Closed [needle] biopsy of tongue**

✖25.02 **Open biopsy of tongue**
Wedge biopsy

25.09 **Other diagnostic procedures on tongue**

✖25.1 **Excision or destruction of lesion or tissue of tongue**

Excludes *biopsy of tongue (25.01–25.02)*
frenumectomy:
labial (27.41)
lingual (25.92)

✖25.2 **Partial glossectomy**

✖25.3 **Complete glossectomy**
Glossectomy NOS

Code also any neck dissection (40.40–40.42)

✖25.4 **Radical glossectomy**

Code also any:
neck dissection (40.40–40.42)
tracheostomy (31.1–31.29)

● 25.5 **Repair of tongue and glossoplasty**

25.51 **Suture of laceration of tongue**

✖25.59 **Other repair and plastic operations on tongue**
Fascial sling of tongue
Fusion of tongue (to lip)
Graft of mucosa or skin to tongue

Excludes *lysis of adhesions of tongue (25.93)*

● 25.9 **Other operations on tongue**

25.91 **Lingual frenotomy**

Excludes *labial frenotomy (27.91)*

25.92 **Lingual frenectomy**

Excludes *labial frenectomy (27.41)*

25.93 **Lysis of adhesions of tongue**

✖25.94 **Other glossotomy**

✖25.99 **Other**

● 26 **Operations on salivary glands and ducts**

Includes: operations on:
lesser salivary gland and duct
parotid gland and duct
sublingual gland and duct
submaxillary gland and duct

Code also any neck dissection (40.40–40.42)

26.0 **Incision of salivary gland or duct**

● 26.1 **Diagnostic procedures on salivary glands and ducts**

26.11 **Closed [needle] biopsy of salivary gland or duct**

✖26.12 **Open biopsy of salivary gland or duct**

26.19 **Other diagnostic procedures on salivary glands and ducts**

Excludes *x-ray of salivary gland (87.09)*

● 26.2 **Excision of lesion of salivary gland**

✖26.21 **Marsupialization of salivary gland cyst**

✖26.29 **Other excision of salivary gland lesion**

Excludes *biopsy of salivary gland (26.11–26.12)*
salivary fistulectomy (26.42)

● 26.3 **Sialoadenectomy**

✖26.30 **Sialoadenectomy, not otherwise specified**

✖26.31 **Partial sialoadenectomy**

✖26.32 **Complete sialoadenectomy**
En bloc excision of salivary gland lesion
Radical sialoadenectomy

● 26.4 **Repair of salivary gland or duct**

✖26.41 **Suture of laceration of salivary gland**

✖26.42 **Closure of salivary fistula**

✖26.49 **Other repair and plastic operations on salivary gland or duct**
Fistulization of salivary gland
Plastic repair of salivary gland or duct NOS
Transplantation of salivary duct opening

● 26.9 **Other operations on salivary gland or duct**

26.91 **Probing of salivary duct**

✖26.99 **Other**

● 27 **Other operations on mouth and face**

Includes: operations on:
lips
palate
soft tissue of face and mouth, except tongue and gingiva

Excludes *operations on:*
gingiva (24.0–24.99)
tongue (25.01–25.99)

✖27.0 **Drainage of face and floor of mouth**
Drainage of:
facial region (abscess)
fascial compartment of face
Ludwig's angina

Excludes *drainage of thyroglossal tract (06.09)*

✖27.1 **Incision of palate**

● 27.2 **Diagnostic procedures on oral cavity**

✖27.21 **Biopsy of bony palate**

✖27.22 **Biopsy of uvula and soft palate**

27.23 **Biopsy of lip**

27.24 **Biopsy of mouth, unspecified structure**

27.29 **Other diagnostic procedures on oral cavity**

Excludes *soft tissue x-ray (87.09)*

● 27.3 **Excision of lesion or tissue of bony palate**

✖27.31 **Local excision or destruction of lesion or tissue of bony palate**
Local excision or destruction of palate by:
cautery
chemotherapy
cryotherapy

Excludes *biopsy of bony palate (27.21)*

✖27.32 **Wide excision or destruction of lesion or tissue of bony palate**
En bloc resection of alveolar process and palate

● 27.4 **Excision of other parts of mouth**

27.41 **Labial frenectomy**

Excludes *division of labial frenum (27.91)*

✖27.42 **Wide excision of lesion of lip**

✖27.43 **Other excision of lesion or tissue of lip**

✖27.49 **Other excision of mouth**

Excludes *biopsy of mouth NOS (27.24)*
excision of lesion of:
palate (27.31–27.32)
tongue (25.1)
uvula (27.72)
fistulectomy of mouth (27.53)
frenectomy of:
lip (27.41)
tongue (25.92)

● 27.5 **Plastic repair of mouth**

Excludes *palatoplasty (27.61–27.69)*

27.51 **Suture of laceration of lip**

27.52 **Suture of laceration of other part of mouth**

✖27.53 **Closure of fistula of mouth**

Excludes *fistulectomy:*
nasolabial (21.82)
oro-antral (22.71)
oronasal (21.82)

✖27.54 **Repair of cleft lip**

✖27.55 **Full-thickness skin graft to lip and mouth**

✖ 27.56 **Other skin graft to lip and mouth**

✖ 27.57 **Attachment of pedicle or flap graft to lip and mouth**

✖ 27.59 **Other plastic repair of mouth**

● 27.6 **Palatoplasty**

✖ 27.61 **Suture of laceration of palate**

✖ 27.62 **Correction of cleft palate**
Correction of cleft palate by push-back operation

Excludes *revision of cleft palate repair (27.63)*

✖ 27.63 **Revision of cleft palate repair**
Secondary:
attachment of pharyngeal flap
lengthening of palate

✖ 27.64 **Insertion of palatal implant**

✖ 27.69 **Other plastic repair of palate**
Code also any insertion of palatal implant (27.64)

Excludes *fistulectomy of mouth (27.53)*

● 27.7 **Operations on uvula**

✖ 27.71 **Incision of uvula**

✖ 27.72 **Excision of uvula**

Excludes *biopsy of uvula (27.22)*

✖ 27.73 **Repair of uvula**

Excludes *that with synchronous cleft palate repair (27.62)*
uranostaphylorrhaphy (27.62)

✖ 27.79 **Other operations on uvula**

● 27.9 **Other operations on mouth and face**

27.91 **Labial frenotomy**
Division of labial frenum

Excludes *lingual frenotomy (25.91)*

✖ 27.92 **Incision of mouth, unspecified structure**

Excludes *incision of:*
gum (24.0)
palate (27.1)
salivary gland or duct (26.0)
tongue (25.94)
uvula (27.71)

✖ 27.99 **Other operations on oral cavity**
Graft of buccal sulcus

Excludes *removal of:*
intraluminal foreign body (98.01)
penetrating foreign body from mouth without incision (98.22)

● 28 **Operations on tonsils and adenoids**

28.0 **Incision and drainage of tonsil and peritonsillar structures**
Drainage (oral) (transcervical) of:
parapharyngeal abscess
peritonsillar abscess
retropharyngeal abscess
tonsillar abscess

● 28.1 **Diagnostic procedures on tonsils and adenoids**

✖ 28.11 **Biopsy of tonsils and adenoids**

✖ 28.19 **Other diagnostic procedures on tonsils and adenoids**

Excludes *soft tissue x-ray (87.09)*

✖ 28.2 **Tonsillectomy without adenoidectomy**

✖ 28.3 **Tonsillectomy with adenoidectomy**

✖ 28.4 **Excision of tonsil tag**

✖ 28.5 **Excision of lingual tonsil**

✖ 28.6 **Adenoidectomy without tonsillectomy**
Excision of adenoid tag

✖ 28.7 **Control of hemorrhage after tonsillectomy and adenoidectomy**

● 28.9 **Other operations on tonsils and adenoids**

✖ 28.91 **Removal of foreign body from tonsil and adenoid by incision**

Excludes *that without incision (98.13)*

✖ 28.92 **Excision of lesion of tonsil and adenoid**

Excludes *biopsy of tonsil and adenoid (28.11)*

✖ 28.99 **Other**

● 29 **Operations on pharynx**

Includes: operations on:
hypopharynx
nasopharynx
oropharynx
pharyngeal pouch
pyriform sinus

✖ 29.0 **Pharyngotomy**
Drainage of pharyngeal bursa

Excludes *incision and drainage of retropharyngeal abscess (28.0)*
removal of foreign body (without incision) (98.13)

● 29.1 **Diagnostic procedures on pharynx**

29.11 **Pharyngoscopy**

29.12 **Pharyngeal biopsy**
Biopsy of supraglottic mass

29.19 **Other diagnostic procedures on pharynx**

Excludes *x-ray of nasopharynx:*
contrast (87.06)
other (87.09)

✖ 29.2 **Excision of branchial cleft cyst or vestige**

Excludes *branchial cleft fistulectomy (29.52)*

● 29.3 **Excision or destruction of lesion or tissue of pharynx**

✖ 29.31 **Cricopharyngeal myotomy**

Excludes *that with pharyngeal diverticulectomy (29.32)*

✖ 29.32 **Pharyngeal diverticulectomy**

✖ 29.33 **Pharyngectomy (partial)**

Excludes *laryngopharyngectomy (30.3)*

✖ 29.39 **Other excision or destruction of lesion or tissue of pharynx**

✖ 29.4 **Plastic operation on pharynx**
Correction of nasopharyngeal atresia

Excludes *pharyngoplasty associated with cleft palate repair (27.62–27.63)*

● 29.5 **Other repair of pharynx**

✖ 29.51 **Suture of laceration of pharynx**

✖ 29.52 **Closure of branchial cleft fistula**

✖ 29.53 **Closure of other fistula of pharynx**
Pharyngoesophageal fistulectomy

✖ 29.54 **Lysis of pharyngeal adhesions**

✖ 29.59 **Other**

● 29.9 **Other operations on pharynx**

29.91 **Dilation of pharynx**
Dilation of nasopharynx

✖ 29.92 **Division of glossopharyngeal nerve**

✖ 29.99 **Other**

Excludes *insertion of radium into pharynx and nasopharynx (92.27)*
removal of intraluminal foreign body (98.13)

6. OPERATIONS ON THE RESPIRATORY SYSTEM (30–34)

● **30 Excision of larynx**

● **30.0 Excision or destruction of lesion or tissue of larynx**

✖ **30.01 Marsupialization of laryngeal cyst**

✖ **30.09 Other excision or destruction of lesion or tissue of larynx**
Stripping of vocal cords
Excludes *biopsy of larynx (31.43)*
laryngeal fistulectomy (31.62)
laryngotracheal fistulectomy (31.62)

✖ **30.1 Hemilaryngectomy**

● **30.2 Other partial laryngectomy**

✖ **30.21 Epiglottidectomy**

✖ **30.22 Vocal cordectomy**
Excision of vocal cords

✖ **30.29 Other partial laryngectomy**
Excision of laryngeal cartilage

✖ **30.3 Complete laryngectomy**
Block dissection of larynx (with thyroidectomy) (with synchronous tracheostomy)
Laryngopharyngectomy
Excludes *that with radical neck dissection (30.4)*

✖ **30.4 Radical laryngectomy**
Complete [total] laryngectomy with radical neck dissection (with thyroidectomy) (with synchronous tracheostomy)

● **31 Other operations on larynx and trachea**

31.0 Injection of larynx
Injection of inert material into larynx or vocal cords

31.1 Temporary tracheostomy
Tracheotomy for assistance in breathing

● **31.2 Permanent tracheostomy**

✖ **31.21 Mediastinal tracheostomy**

✖ **31.29 Other permanent tracheostomy**
Excludes *that with laryngectomy (30.3–30.4)*

✖ **31.3 Other incision of larynx or trachea**
Excludes *that for assistance in breathing (31.1–31.29)*

● **31.4 Diagnostic procedures on larynx and trachea**

31.41 Tracheoscopy through artificial stoma
Excludes *that with biopsy (31.43–31.44)*

31.42 Laryngoscopy and other tracheoscopy
Excludes *that with biopsy (31.43–31.44)*

31.43 Closed [endoscopic] biopsy of larynx

31.44 Closed [endoscopic] biopsy of trachea

✖ **31.45 Open biopsy of larynx or trachea**

31.48 Other diagnostic procedures on larynx
Excludes *contrast laryngogram (87.07)*
microscopic examination of specimen from larynx (90.31–90.39)
soft tissue x-ray of larynx NEC (87.09)

31.49 Other diagnostic procedures on trachea
Excludes *microscopic examination of specimen from trachea (90.41–90.49)*
x-ray of trachea (87.49)

✖ **31.5 Local excision or destruction of lesion or tissue of trachea**
Excludes *biopsy of trachea (31.44–31.45)*
laryngotracheal fistulectomy (31.62)
tracheoesophageal fistulectomy (31.73)

● **31.6 Repair of larynx**

✖ **31.61 Suture of laceration of larynx**

✖ **31.62 Closure of fistula of larynx**
Laryngotracheal fistulectomy
Take-down of laryngostomy

✖ **31.63 Revision of laryngostomy**

✖ **31.64 Repair of laryngeal fracture**

✖ **31.69 Other repair of larynx**
Arytenoidopexy
Graft of larynx
Transposition of vocal cords
Excludes *construction of artificial larynx (31.75)*

● **31.7 Repair and plastic operations on trachea**

✖ **31.71 Suture of laceration of trachea**

✖ **31.72 Closure of external fistula of trachea**
Closure of tracheotomy

✖ **31.73 Closure of other fistula of trachea**
Tracheoesophageal fistulectomy
Excludes *laryngotracheal fistulectomy (31.62)*

✖ **31.74 Revision of tracheostomy**

✖ **31.75 Reconstruction of trachea and construction of artificial larynx**
Tracheoplasty with artificial larynx

✖ **31.79 Other repair and plastic operations on trachea**

● **31.9 Other operations on larynx and trachea**

✖ **31.91 Division of laryngeal nerve**

✖ **31.92 Lysis of adhesions of trachea or larynx**

31.93 Replacement of laryngeal or tracheal stent

31.94 Injection of locally-acting therapeutic substance into trachea

31.95 Tracheoesophageal fistulization

✖ **31.98 Other operations on larynx**
Dilation of larynx
Division of congenital web of larynx
Removal of keel or stent of larynx
Excludes *removal of intraluminal foreign body from larynx without incision (98.14)*

✖ **31.99 Other operations on trachea**
Excludes *removal of:*
intraluminal foreign body from trachea without incision (98.15)
tracheostomy tube (97.37)
replacement of tracheostomy tube (97.23)
tracheostomy toilette (96.55)

● **32 Excision of lung and bronchus**

Includes: rib resection as operative approach
sternotomy as operative approach
sternum-splitting incision as operative approach
thoracotomy as operative approach

Code also any synchronous bronchoplasty (33.48)

● **32.0 Local excision or destruction of lesion or tissue of bronchus**
Excludes *biopsy of bronchus (33.24–33.25)*
bronchial fistulectomy (33.42)

32.01 Endoscopic excision or destruction of lesion or tissue of bronchus

✖ **32.09 Other local excision or destruction of lesion or tissue of bronchus**
Excludes *that by endoscopic approach (32.01)*

✖ **32.1 Other excision of bronchus**
Resection (wide sleeve) of bronchus
Excludes *radical dissection [excision] of bronchus (32.6)*

● 32.2 **Local excision or destruction of lesion or tissue of lung**

✖ 32.21 **Plication of emphysematous bleb**

✖ 32.22 **Lung volume reduction surgery**

✖ 32.23 **Open ablation of lung lesion or tissue** ◀

✖ 32.24 **Percutaneous ablation of lung lesion or tissue** ◀

✖ 32.25 **Thoracoscopic ablation of lung lesion or tissue** ◀

✖ 32.26 **Other and unspecified ablation of lung lesion or tissue** ◀

32.28 **Endoscopic excision or destruction of lesion or tissue of lung**

Excludes *ablation of lung lesion or tissue:* ◀
open (32.23) ◀
other (32.26) ◀
percutaneous (32.24) ◀
thoracoscopic (32.25) ◀
biopsy of lung (33.26–33.27)

✖ 32.29 **Other local excision or destruction of lesion or tissue of lung**
Resection of lung:
NOS
wedge

Excludes *ablation of lung lesion or tissue:* ◀
open (32.23) ◀
other (32.26) ◀
percutaneous (32.24) ◀
thoracoscopic (32.25) ◀
biopsy of lung (33.26–33.27)
that by endoscopic approach (32.28)
wide excision of lesion of lung (32.3)

✖ 32.3 **Segmental resection of lung**
Partial lobectomy

✖ 32.4 **Lobectomy of lung**
Lobectomy with segmental resection of adjacent lobes of lung

Excludes *that with radical dissection [excision] of thoracic structures (32.6)*

✖ 32.5 **Complete pneumonectomy**
Excision of lung NOS
Pneumonectomy (with mediastinal dissection)

✖ 32.6 **Radical dissection of thoracic structures**
Block [en bloc] dissection of bronchus, lobe of lung, brachial plexus, intercostal structure, ribs (transverse process), and sympathetic nerves

✖ 32.9 **Other excision of lung**

Excludes *biopsy of lung and bronchus (33.24–33.27)*
pulmonary decortication (34.51)

● 33 **Other operations on lung and bronchus**

Includes: rib resection as operative approach
sternotomy as operative approach
sternum-splitting incision as operative approach
thoracotomy as operative approach

✖ 33.0 **Incision of bronchus**

✖ 33.1 **Incision of lung**

Excludes *puncture of lung (33.93)*

● 33.2 **Diagnostic procedures on lung and bronchus**

33.21 **Bronchoscopy through artificial stoma**

Excludes *that with biopsy (33.24, 33.27)*

33.22 **Fiber-optic bronchoscopy**

Excludes *that with biopsy (33.24, 33.27)*

33.23 **Other bronchoscopy**

Excludes *that for:*
aspiration (96.05)
biopsy (33.24, 33.27)

✖ 33.24 **Closed [endoscopic] biopsy of bronchus**
Bronchoscopy (fiberoptic) (rigid) with:
brush biopsy of "lung"
brushing or washing for specimen collection
excision (bite) biopsy
Diagnostic bronchoalveolar lavage (BAL)

Excludes *closed biopsy of lung, other than brush biopsy of "lung" (33.26, 33.27)*
whole lung lavage (33.99)

✖ 33.25 **Open biopsy of bronchus**

Excludes *open biopsy of lung (33.28)*

33.26 **Closed [percutaneous] [needle] biopsy of lung**

Excludes *endoscopic biopsy of lung (33.27)*

✖ 33.27 **Closed endoscopic biopsy of lung**
Fiber-optic (flexible) bronchoscopy with fluoroscopic guidance with biopsy
Transbronchial lung biopsy

Excludes *brush biopsy of "lung" (33.24)*
percutaneous biopsy of lung (33.26)

✖ 33.28 **Open biopsy of lung**

✖ 33.29 **Other diagnostic procedures on lung and bronchus**

Excludes *contrast bronchogram:*
endotracheal (87.31)
other (87.32)
lung scan (92.15)
magnetic resonance imaging (88.92)
microscopic examination of specimen from bronchus or lung (90.41–90.49)
routine chest x-ray (87.44)
ultrasonography of lung (88.73)
vital capacity determination (89.37)
x-ray of bronchus or lung NOS (87.49)

● 33.3 **Surgical collapse of lung**

33.31 **Destruction of phrenic nerve for collapse of lung**

33.32 **Artificial pneumothorax for collapse of lung**
Thoracotomy for collapse of lung

33.33 **Pneumoperitoneum for collapse of lung**

✖ 33.34 **Thoracoplasty**

✖ 33.39 **Other surgical collapse of lung**
Collapse of lung NOS

● 33.4 **Repair and plastic operation on lung and bronchus**

✖ 33.41 **Suture of laceration of bronchus**

✖ 33.42 **Closure of bronchial fistula**
Closure of bronchostomy
Fistulectomy:
bronchocutaneous
bronchoesophageal
bronchovisceral

Excludes *closure of fistula:*
bronchomediastinal (34.73)
bronchopleural (34.73)
bronchopleuromediastinal (34.73)

✖ 33.43 **Closure of laceration of lung**

✖ 33.48 **Other repair and plastic operations on bronchus**

✖ 33.49 **Other repair and plastic operations on lung**

Excludes *closure of pleural fistula (34.73)*

✖ **33.5 Lung transplant**

Note: To report donor source - *see* codes 00.91–00.93

Excludes *combined heart-lung transplantation (33.6)*

Code also cardiopulmonary bypass [extracorporeal circulation] [heart-lung machine] (39.61)

✖ **33.50 Lung transplantation, not otherwise specified**

✖ **33.51 Unilateral lung transplantation**

✖ **33.52 Bilateral lung transplantation**
Double-lung transplantation
En bloc transplantation

Code also cardiopulmonary bypass [extracorporeal circulation] [heart-lung machine] (39.61)

✖ **33.6 Combined heart-lung transplantation**

Note: To report donor source - *see* codes 00.91–00.93

Code also cardiopulmonary bypass [extracorporeal circulation] [heart-lung machine] (39.61)

● **33.7 Endoscopic insertion, replacement and removal of therapeutic device or substances in bronchus or lung** ◀
Biologic Lung Volume Reduction (BLVR) ◀

Excludes *insertion of tracheobronchial stent (96.05)* ◀

✖ **33.71 Endoscopic insertion or replacement of bronchial valve(s)** ◀
Endobronchial airflow redirection valve ◀
Intrabronchial airflow redirection valve ◀

✖ **33.78 Endoscopic removal of bronchial device(s) or substances** ◀

✖ **33.79 Endoscopic insertion of other bronchial device or substances** ◀
Biologic Lung Volume Reduction NOS (BLVR) ◀

● **33.9 Other operations on lung and bronchus**

33.91 Bronchial dilation

✖ **33.92 Ligation of bronchus**

✖ **33.93 Puncture of lung**

Excludes *needle biopsy (33.26)*

✖ **33.98 Other operations on bronchus**

Excludes *bronchial lavage (96.56)*
removal of intraluminal foreign body from bronchus without incision (98.15)

✖ **33.99 Other operations on lung**
Whole lung lavage

Excludes *other continuous mechanical ventilation (96.70–96.72)*
respiratory therapy (93.90–93.99)

● **34 Operations on chest wall, pleura, mediastinum, and diaphragm**

Excludes *operations on breast (85.0–85.99)*

● **34.0 Incision of chest wall and pleura**

Excludes *that as operative approach—omit code*

34.01 Incision of chest wall
Extrapleural drainage

Excludes *incision of pleura (34.09)*

✖ **34.02 Exploratory thoracotomy**

✖ **34.03 Reopening of recent thoracotomy site**

34.04 Insertion of intercostal catheter for drainage
Chest tube
Closed chest drainage
Revision of intercostal catheter (chest tube) (with lysis of adhesions)

34.05 Creation of pleuroperitoneal shunt

34.09 Other incision of pleura
Creation of pleural window for drainage
Intercostal stab
Open chest drainage

Excludes *thoracoscopy (34.21)*
thoracotomy for collapse of lung (33.32)

✖ **34.1 Incision of mediastinum**

Excludes *mediastinoscopy (34.22)*
mediastinotomy associated with pneumonectomy (32.5)

● **34.2 Diagnostic procedures on chest wall, pleura, mediastinum, and diaphragm**

✖ **34.21 Transpleural thoracoscopy**

✖ **34.22 Mediastinoscopy**

Code also any lymph node biopsy (40.11)

34.23 Biopsy of chest wall

34.24 Pleural biopsy

34.25 Closed [percutaneous] [needle] biopsy of mediastinum

✖ **34.26 Open mediastinal biopsy**

✖ **34.27 Biopsy of diaphragm**

✖ **34.28 Other diagnostic procedures on chest wall, pleura, and diaphragm**

Excludes *angiocardiography (88.50–88.58)*
aortography (88.42)
arteriography of:
intrathoracic vessels NEC (88.44)
pulmonary arteries (88.43)
microscopic examination of specimen from chest wall, pleura, and diaphragm (90.41–90.49)
phlebography of:
intrathoracic vessels NEC (88.63)
pulmonary veins (88.62)
radiological examinations of thorax:
C.A.T. scan (87.41)
diaphragmatic x-ray (87.49)
intrathoracic lymphangiogram (87.34)
routine chest x-ray (87.44)
sinogram of chest wall (87.38)
soft tissue x-ray of chest wall NEC (87.39)
tomogram of thorax NEC (87.42)
ultrasonography of thorax 88.73)

✖ **34.29 Other diagnostic procedures on mediastinum**

Excludes *mediastinal:*
pneumogram (87.33)
x-ray NEC (87.49)

✖ **34.3 Excision or destruction of lesion or tissue of mediastinum**

Excludes *biopsy of mediastinum (34.25–34.26)*
mediastinal fistulectomy (34.73)

✖ **34.4 Excision or destruction of lesion of chest wall**
Excision of lesion of chest wall NOS (with excision of ribs)

Excludes *biopsy of chest wall (34.23)*
costectomy not incidental to thoracic procedure (77.91)
excision of lesion of:
breast (85.20–85.25)
cartilage (80.89)
skin (86.2–86.3)
fistulectomy (34.73)

● **34.5 Pleurectomy**

✖ **34.51 Decortication of lung**

✖ 34.59 **Other excision of pleura**
Excision of pleural lesion

Excludes *biopsy of pleura (34.24)*
pleural fistulectomy (34.73)

✖ 34.6 **Scarification of pleura**
Pleurosclerosis

Excludes *injection of sclerosing agent (34.92)*

● 34.7 **Repair of chest wall**

34.71 **Suture of laceration of chest wall**

Excludes *suture of skin and subcutaneous tissue alone (86.59)*

34.72 **Closure of thoracostomy**

✖ 34.73 **Closure of other fistula of thorax**
Closure of:
bronchopleural fistula
bronchopleurocutaneous fistula
bronchopleuromediastinal fistula

✖ 34.74 **Repair of pectus deformity**
Repair of:
pectus carinatum (with implant)
pectus excavatum (with implant)

✖ 34.79 **Other repair of chest wall**
Repair of chest wall NOS

● 34.8 **Operations on diaphragm**

✖ 34.81 **Excision of lesion or tissue of diaphragm**

Excludes *biopsy of diaphragm (34.27)*

✖ 34.82 **Suture of laceration of diaphragm**

✖ 34.83 **Closure of fistula of diaphragm**
Thoracicoabdominal fistulectomy
Thoracicogastric fistulectomy
Thoracicointestinal fistulectomy

✖ 34.84 **Other repair of diaphragm**

Excludes *repair of diaphragmatic hernia (53.7–53.82)*

✖ 34.85 **Implantation of diaphragmatic pacemaker**

✖ 34.89 **Other operations on diaphragm**

● 34.9 **Other operations on thorax**

34.91 **Thoracentesis**

34.92 **Injection into thoracic cavity**
Chemical pleurodesis
Injection of cytotoxic agent or tetracycline
Instillation into thoracic cavity ◀
Requires additional code for any cancer chemotherapeutic substance (99.25)

Excludes *that for collapse of lung (33.32)*

✖ 34.93 **Repair of pleura**

✖ 34.99 **Other**

Excludes *removal of:*
mediastinal drain (97.42)
sutures (97.43)
thoracotomy tube (97.41)

7. OPERATIONS ON THE CARDIOVASCULAR SYSTEM (35–39)

● **35 Operations on valves and septa of heart**

Includes: sternotomy (median) (transverse) as operative approach
thoracotomy as operative approach

Code also cardiopulmonary bypass [extracorporeal circulation] [heart-lung machine] (39.61)

● **35.0 Closed heart valvotomy**

Excludes *percutaneous (balloon) valvuloplasty (35.96)*

✖ **35.00 Closed heart valvotomy, unspecified valve**

✖ **35.01 Closed heart valvotomy, aortic valve**

✖ **35.02 Closed heart valvotomy, mitral valve**

✖ **35.03 Closed heart valvotomy, pulmonary valve**

✖ **35.04 Closed heart valvotomy, tricuspid valve**

● **35.1 Open heart valvuloplasty without replacement**

Includes: open heart valvotomy

Excludes *that associated with repair of:*
endocardial cushion defect (35.54, 35.63, 35.73)
percutaneous (balloon) valvuloplasty (35.96)
valvular defect associated with atrial and ventricular septal defects (35.54, 35.63, 35.73)

Code also cardiopulmonary bypass if performed [extracorporeal circulation] [heart-lung machine] (39.61)

✖ **35.10 Open heart valvuloplasty without replacement, unspecified valve**

✖ **35.11 Open heart valvuloplasty of aortic valve without replacement**

✖ **35.12 Open heart valvuloplasty of mitral valve without replacement**

✖ **35.13 Open heart valvuloplasty of pulmonary valve without replacement**

✖ **35.14 Open heart valvuloplasty of tricuspid valve without replacement**

● **35.2 Replacement of heart valve**

Includes: excision of heart valve with replacement

Code also cardiopulmonary bypass [extracorporeal circulation] [heart-lung machine] (39.61)

Excludes *that associated with repair of:*
endocardial cushion defect (35.54, 35.63, 35.73)
valvular defect associated with atrial and ventricular septal defects (35.54, 35.63, 35.73)

✖ **35.20 Replacement of unspecified heart valve**
Repair of unspecified heart valve with tissue graft or prosthetic implant

✖ **35.21 Replacement of aortic valve with tissue graft**
Repair of aortic valve with tissue graft (autograft) (heterograft) (homograft)

✖ **35.22 Other replacement of aortic valve**
Repair of aortic valve with replacement:
NOS
prosthetic (partial) (synthetic) (total)

✖ **35.23 Replacement of mitral valve with tissue graft**
Repair of mitral valve with tissue graft (autograft) (heterograft) (homograft)

✖ **35.24 Other replacement of mitral valve**
Repair of mitral valve with replacement:
NOS
prosthetic (partial) (synthetic) (total)

✖ **35.25 Replacement of pulmonary valve with tissue graft**
Repair of pulmonary valve with tissue graft (autograft) (heterograft) (homograft)

✖ **35.26 Other replacement of pulmonary valve**
Repair of pulmonary valve with replacement:
NOS
prosthetic (partial) (synthetic) (total)

✖ **35.27 Replacement of tricuspid valve with tissue graft**
Repair of tricuspid valve with tissue graft (autograft) (heterograft) (homograft)

✖ **35.28 Other replacement of tricuspid valve**
Repair of tricuspid valve with replacement:
NOS
prosthetic (partial) (synthetic) (total)

● **35.3 Operations on structures adjacent to heart valves**

Code also cardiopulmonary bypass [extracorporeal circulation] [heart-lung machine] (39.61)

✖ **35.31 Operations on papillary muscle**
Division of papillary muscle
Reattachment of papillary muscle
Repair of papillary muscle

✖ **35.32 Operations on chordae tendineae**
Division of chordae tendineae
Repair of chordae tendineae

✖ **35.33 Annuloplasty**
Plication of annulus

✖ **35.34 Infundibulectomy**
Right ventricular infundibulectomy

✖ **35.35 Operations on trabeculae carneae cordis**
Division of trabeculae carneae cordis
Excision of trabeculae carneae cordis
Excision of aortic subvalvular ring

✖ **35.39 Operations on other structures adjacent to valves of heart**
Repair of sinus of Valsalva (aneurysm)

● **35.4 Production of septal defect in heart**

35.41 Enlargement of existing atrial septal defect
Rashkind procedure
Septostomy (atrial) (balloon)

✖ **35.42 Creation of septal defect in heart**
Blalock-Hanlon operation

● **35.5 Repair of atrial and ventricular septa with prosthesis**

Includes: repair of septa with synthetic implant or patch

Code also cardiopulmonary bypass [extracorporeal circulation] [heart-lung machine] (39.61)

✖ **35.50 Repair of unspecified septal defect of heart with prosthesis**

Excludes *that associated with repair of:*
endocardial cushion defect (35.54)
septal defect associated with valvular defect (35.54)

✖ **35.51 Repair of atrial septal defect with prosthesis, open technique**
Atrioseptoplasty with prosthesis
Correction of atrial septal defect with prosthesis
Repair:
foramen ovale (patent)
with prosthesis ostium secundum defect with prosthesis

Excludes *that associated with repair of:*
atrial septal defect associated with valvular and ventricular septal defects (35.54)
endocardial cushion defect (35.54)

✖ **35.52 Repair of atrial septal defect with prosthesis, closed technique**
Insertion of atrial septal umbrella [King-Mills]

✖35.53 **Repair of ventricular septal defect with prosthesis, open technique** ⬅
Correction of ventricular septal defect with prosthesis
Repair of supracristal defect with prosthesis

Excludes *that associated with repair of:*
endocardial cushion defect (35.54)
ventricular defect associated with valvular and atrial septal defects (35.54)

✖35.54 **Repair of endocardial cushion defect with prosthesis**
Repair:
atrioventricular canal with prosthesis (grafted to septa)
ostium primum defect with prosthesis (grafted to septa)
valvular defect associated with atrial and ventricular septal defects with prosthesis (grafted to septa)

Excludes *repair of isolated:*
atrial septal defect (35.51–35.52)
valvular defect (35.20, 35.22, 35.24, 35.26, 35.28)
ventricular septal defect (35.53)

✖35.55 **Repair of ventricular septal defect with prosthesis, closed technique** ◀

●35.6 **Repair of atrial and ventricular septa with tissue graft**

Code also cardiopulmonary bypass [extracorporeal circulation] [heart-lung machine] (39.61)

✖35.60 **Repair of unspecified septal defect of heart with tissue graft**

Excludes *that associated with repair of:*
endocardial cushion defect (35.63)
septal defect associated with valvular defect (35.63)

✖35.61 **Repair of atrial septal defect with tissue graft**
Atrioseptoplasty with tissue graft
Correction of atrial septal defect with tissue graft
Repair:
foramen ovale (patent) with tissue graft
ostium secundum defect with tissue graft

Excludes *that associated with repair of:*
atrial septal defect associated with valvular and ventricular septal defects (35.63)
endocardial cushion defect (35.63)

✖35.62 **Repair of ventricular septal defect with tissue graft**
Correction of ventricular septal defect with tissue graft
Repair of supracristal defect with tissue graft

Excludes *that associated with repair of:*
endocardial cushion defect (35.63)
ventricular defect associate with valvular and atrial septal defects (35.63)

✖35.63 **Repair of endocardial cushion defect with tissue graft**
Repair of:
atrioventricular canal with tissue graft
ostium primum defect with tissue graft
valvular defect associated with atrial and ventricular septal defects with tissue graft

Excludes *repair of isolated:*
atrial septal defect (35.61)
valvular defect (35.20–35.21, 35.23, 35.25, 35.27)
ventricular septal defect (35.62)

●35.7 **Other and unspecified repair of atrial and ventricular septa**

Code also cardiopulmonary bypass [extracorporeal circulation] [heart-lung machine] (39.61)

✖35.70 **Other and unspecified repair of unspecified septal defect of heart**
Repair of septal defect NOS

Excludes *that associated with repair of:*
endocardial cushion defect (35.73)
septal defect associated with valvular defect (35.73)

✖35.71 **Other and unspecified repair of atrial septal defect**
Repair NOS:
atrial septum
foramen ovale (patent)
ostium secundum defect

Excludes *that associated with repair of:*
atrial septal defect associated with valvular ventricular septal defects (35.73)
endocardial cushion defect (35.73)

✖35.72 **Other and unspecified repair of ventricular septal defect**
Repair NOS:
supracristal defect
ventricular septum

Excludes *that associated with repair of:*
endocardial cushion defect (35.73)
ventricular septal defect associated with valvular and atrial septal defects (35.73)

✖35.73 **Other and unspecified repair of endocardial cushion defect**
Repair NOS:
atrioventricular canal
ostium primum defect
valvular defect associated with atrial and ventricular septal defects

Excludes *repair of isolated:*
atrial septal defect (35.71)
valvular defect (35.20, 35.22, 35.24, 35.26, 35.28)
ventricular septal defect (35.72)

●35.8 **Total repair of certain congenital cardiac anomalies**

Note: For partial repair of defect [e.g., repair of atrial septal defect in tetralogy of Fallot]

✖35.81 **Total repair of tetralogy of Fallot**
One-stage total correction of tetralogy of Fallot with or without:
commissurotomy of pulmonary valve
infundibulectomy
outflow tract prosthesis
patch graft of outflow tract
prosthetic tube for pulmonary artery
repair of ventricular septal defect (with prosthesis)
take-down of previous systemic-pulmonary artery anastomosis

✖ **35.82 Total repair of total anomalous pulmonary venous connection**
One-stage total correction of total anomalous pulmonary venous connection with or without:
anastomosis between (horizontal) common pulmonary trunk and posterior wall of left atrium (side-to-side)
enlargement of foramen ovale
incision [excision] of common wall between posterior left atrium and coronary sinus and roofing of resultant defect with patch graft (synthetic)
ligation of venous connection (descending anomalous vein) (to left innominate vein) (to superior vena cava)
repair of atrial septal defect (with prosthesis)

✖ **35.83 Total repair of truncus arteriosus**
One-stage total correction of truncus arteriosus with or without:
construction (with aortic homograft) (with prosthesis) of a pulmonary artery placed from right ventricle to arteries supplying the lung
ligation of connections between aorta and pulmonary artery
repair of ventricular septal defect (with prosthesis)

✖ **35.84 Total correction of transposition of great vessels, not elsewhere classified**
Arterial switch operation [Jatene]
Total correction of transposition of great arteries at the arterial level by switching the great arteries, including the left or both coronary arteries, implanted in the wall of the pulmonary artery

Excludes *baffle operation [Mustard] [Senning] (35.91)*
creation of shunt between right ventricle and pulmonary artery [Rastelli] (35.92)

● **35.9 Other operations on valves and septa of heart**
Code also cardiopulmonary bypass, if performed [extracorporeal circulation] [heart-lung machine] (39.61)

✖ **35.91 Interatrial transposition of venous return**
Baffle:
atrial
interatrial
Mustard's operation
Resection of atrial septum and insertion of patch to direct systemic venous return to tricuspid valve and pulmonary venous return to mitral valve

✖ **35.92 Creation of conduit between right ventricle and pulmonary artery**
Creation of shunt between right ventricle and (distal) pulmonary artery

Excludes *that associated with total repair of truncus arteriosus (35.83)*

✖ **35.93 Creation of conduit between left ventricle and aorta**
Creation of apicoaortic shunt
Shunt between apex of left ventricle and aorta

✖ **35.94 Creation of conduit between atrium and pulmonary artery**
Fontan procedure

✖ **35.95 Revision of corrective procedure on heart**
Replacement of prosthetic heart valve poppet
Resuture of prosthesis of:
septum
valve

Excludes *complete revision—code to specific procedure*
replacement of prosthesis or graft of:
septum (35.50–35.63)
valve (35.20–35.28)

✖ **35.96 Percutaneous valvuloplasty**
Percutaneous balloon valvuloplasty

✖ **35.98 Other operations on septa of heart**

✖ **35.99 Other operations on valves of heart**

● **36 Operations on vessels of heart**
Includes: sternotomy (median) (transverse) as operative approach
thoracotomy as operative approach

Code also any:
cardiopulmonary bypass, if performed [extracorporeal circulation] [heart-lung machine] (39.61)
injection or infusion of platelet inhibitor (99.20)
injection or infusion of thrombolytic agent (99.10)

● **36.0 Removal of coronary artery obstruction and insertion of stent(s)**

✖ **36.03 Open chest coronary artery angioplasty**
Coronary (artery):
endarterectomy (with patch graft)
thromboendarterectomy (with patch graft)
Open surgery for direct relief of coronary artery obstruction

Excludes *that with coronary artery bypass graft (36.10–36.19)*

Code also any:
insertion of drug-eluting coronary stent(s) (36.07)
insertion of non-drug-eluting coronary stent(s) (36.06)
number of vascular stents inserted (00.45–00.48)
number of vessels treated (00.40–00.43)
procedure on vessel bifurcation (00.44) ◀

36.04 Intracoronary artery thrombolytic infusion
That by direct coronary artery injection, infusion, or catheterization
enzyme infusion
platelet inhibitor

Excludes *infusion of platelet inhibitor (99.20)*
infusion of thrombolytic agent (99.10)
that associated with any procedure in 36.03 (Revised)

✖ **36.06 Insertion of non-drug-eluting coronary artery stent(s)**
Bare stent(s)
Bonded stent(s)
Drug-coated stent(s), i.e., heparin coated
Endograft(s)
Endovascular graft(s)
Stent graft(s)

Code also any:
number of vascular stents inserted (00.45–00.48)
number of vessels treated (00.40–00.43)
open chest coronary artery angioplasty (36.03)
percutaneous transluminal coronary angioplasty [PTCA] or coronary atherectomy (00.66)
procedure on vessel bifurcation (00.44) ◀

Excludes *insertion of drug-eluting coronary artery stent(s) (36.07)*

36.07 Insertion of drug-eluting coronary artery stent(s)
Endograft(s)
Endovascular graft(s)
Stent graft(s)

Code also any:
number of vascular stents inserted (00.45–00.48)
number of vessels treated (00.40–00.43)
open chest coronary artery angioplasty (36.03)
percutaneous transluminal coronary angioplasty [PTCA] or coronary atherectomy (00.66)
procedure on vessel bifurcation (00.44) ◀

Excludes *drug-coated stents, e.g., heparin coated (36.06)*
insertion of non-drug-eluting coronary artery stent(s) (36.06)

✖ **36.09 Other removal of coronary artery obstruction**
Coronary angioplasty NOS

Code also any:
number of vascular stents inserted (00.45–00.48)
number of vessels treated (00.40–00.43)
procedure on vessel bifurcation (00.44) ◀

Excludes *that by open angioplasty (36.03)*
that by percutaneous transluminal coronary angioplasty [PTCA] or coronary atherectomy (00.66)

● **36.1 Bypass anastomosis for heart revascularization**

Note: Do not assign codes from series 00.40–00.43 with codes from series 36.10–36.19

Code also cardiopulmonary bypass [extracorporeal circulation] [heart-lung machine] (39.61)

Code also pressurized treatment of venous bypass graft [conduit] with pharmaceutical substance, if performed (00.16)

✖ **36.10 Aortocoronary bypass for heart revascularization, not otherwise specified**
Direct revascularization:
cardiac with catheter stent, prosthesis, or vein graft
coronary with catheter stent, prosthesis, or vein graft
heart muscle with catheter stent, prosthesis, or vein graft
myocardial with catheter stent, prosthesis, or vein graft
Heart revascularization NOS

✖ **36.11 (Aorto)coronary bypass of one coronary artery**

✖ **36.12 (Aorto)coronary bypass of two coronary arteries**

✖ **36.13 (Aorto)coronary bypass of three coronary arteries**

✖ **36.14 (Aorto)coronary bypass of four or more coronary arteries**

✖ **36.15 Single internal mammary-coronary artery bypass**
Anastomosis (single):
mammary artery to coronary artery
thoracic artery to coronary artery

✖ **36.16 Double internal mammary-coronary artery bypass**
Anastomosis, double:
mammary artery to coronary artery
thoracic artery to coronary artery

✖ **36.17 Abdominal-coronary artery bypass**
Anastomosis:
Gastroepiploic-coronary artery

✖ **36.19 Other bypass anastomosis for heart revascularization**

✖ **36.2 Heart revascularization by arterial implant**
Implantation of:
aortic branches [ascending aortic branches] into heart muscle
blood vessels into myocardium
internal mammary artery [internal thoracic artery] into:
heart muscle
myocardium
ventricle
ventricular wall
indirect heart revascularization NOS

● **36.3 Other heart revascularization**

✖ **36.31 Open chest transmyocardial revascularization**

✖ **36.32 Other transmyocardial revascularization** ⇐

✖ **36.33 Endoscopic transmyocardial revascularization** ◀
Robot-assisted transmyocardial revascularization ◀
Thoracoscopic transmyocardial revascularization ◀

✖ **36.34 Percutaneous transmyocardial revascularization** ◀
Endovascular transmyocardial revascularization ◀

✖ **36.39 Other heart revascularization**
Abrasion of epicardium
Cardio-omentopexy
Intrapericardial poudrage
Myocardial graft:
mediastinal fat
omentum
pectoral muscles

● **36.9 Other operations on vessels of heart**

Code also cardiopulmonary bypass [extracorporeal circulation] [heart-lung machine] (39.61)

✖ **36.91 Repair of aneurysm of coronary vessel**

✖ **36.99 Other operations on vessels of heart**
Exploration of coronary artery
Incision of coronary artery
Ligation of coronary artery
Repair of arteriovenous fistula

● **37 Other operations on heart and pericardium**

Code also any injection or infusion of platelet inhibitor (99.20)

37.0 Pericardiocentesis

● **37.1 Cardiotomy and pericardiotomy**

Code also cardiopulmonary bypass [extracorporeal circulation] [heart-lung machine] (39.61)

✖ **37.10 Incision of heart, not otherwise specified**
Cardiolysis NOS

✖ **37.11 Cardiotomy**
Incision of:
atrium
endocardium
myocardium
ventricle

✖ **37.12 Pericardiotomy**
Pericardial window operation
Pericardiolysis
Pericardiotomy

● 37.2 **Diagnostic procedures on heart and pericardium**

37.20 **Noninvasive programmed electrical stimulation [NIPS]** ◀

Excludes *that as part of intraoperative testing – omit code* ◀
catheter based invasive electrophysiologic testing (37.26) ◀
device interrogation only without arrhythmia induction (bedside check) (89.45–89.49) ◀

37.21 **Right heart cardiac catheterization**
Cardiac catheterization NOS

Excludes *that with catheterization of left heart (37.23)*

37.22 **Left heart cardiac catheterization**

Excludes *that with catheterization of right heart (37.23)*

37.23 **Combined right and left heart cardiac catheterization**

✖ 37.24 **Biopsy of pericardium**

37.25 **Biopsy of heart**

37.26 **Catheter based invasive electrophysiologic testing** ⬅
Electrophysiologic studies [EPS]

Code also any concomitant procedure

Excludes *device interrogation only without arrhythmia induction (bedside check) (89.45–89.49)*
His bundle recording (37.29)
noninvasive programmed electrical stimulation (NIPS) (37.20) ◀
that as part of intraoperative testing – omit code ◀

37.27 **Cardiac mapping**

Code also any concomitant procedure

Excludes *electrocardiogram (89.52)*
His bundle recording (37.29)

37.28 **Intracardiac echocardiography**
Echocardiography of heart chambers
ICE

Code also any synchronous Doppler flow mapping (88.72)

Excludes *intravascular imaging of coronary vessels (intravascular ultrasound) (IVUS) (00.24)*

37.29 **Other diagnostic procedures on heart and pericardium**

Excludes *angiocardiography (88.50–88.58)*
cardiac function tests (89.41–89.69)
cardiovascular radioisotopic scan and function study (92.05)
coronary arteriography (88.55–88.57)
diagnostic pericardiocentesis (37.0)
diagnostic ultrasound of heart (88.72)
x-ray of heart (87.49)

● 37.3 **Pericardiectomy and excision of lesion of heart**

Code also cardiopulmonary bypass [extracorporeal circulation] [heart-lung machine] (39.61)

✖ 37.31 **Pericardiectomy**
Excision of:
adhesions of pericardium
constricting scar of:
epicardium
pericardium

✖ 37.32 **Excision of aneurysm of heart**
Repair of aneurysm of heart

✖ 37.33 **Excision or destruction of other lesion or tissue of heart, open approach**
Ablation of heart tissue (cryoablation) (electrocurrent) (laser) (microwave) (radiofrequency) (resection), open chest approach
Cox-maze procedure
Maze procedure
Modified maze procedure, trans-thoracic approach

Excludes *ablation, excision, or destruction of lesion or tissue of heart, endovascular approach (37.34)*

✖ 37.34 **Excision or destruction of other lesion or tissue of heart, other approach**
Ablation of heart tissue (cryoablation) (electrocurrent) (laser) (microwave) (radiofrequency) (resection), via peripherally inserted catheter
Modified maze procedure, endovascular approach

✖ 37.35 **Partial ventriculectomy**
Ventricular reduction surgery
Ventricular remodeling

Code also any synchronous:
mitral valve repair (35.02, 35.12)
mitral valve replacement (35.23–35.24)

● 37.4 **Repair of heart and pericardium**

✖ 37.41 **Implantation of prosthetic cardiac support device around the heart**
Cardiac support device (CSD)
Epicardial support device
Fabric (textile) (mesh) device
Ventricular support device on surface of heart

Code also any:
cardiopulmonary bypass [extracorporeal circulation] [heart-lung machine] if performed (39.61)
mitral valve repair (35.02, 35.12)
mitral valve replacement (35.23–35.24)
transesophageal echocardiography (88.72)

Excludes *circulatory assist systems (37.61–37.68)*

✖ 37.49 **Other repair of heart and pericardium**

● 37.5 **Heart replacement procedures**

Excludes *combined heart-lung transplantation (33.6)*

✖ 37.51 **Heart transplantation**

Excludes *combined heart-lung transplantation (33.6)*

✖ 37.52 **Implantation of total replacement heart system**
Artificial heart
Implantation of fully implantable total replacement heart system, including ventriculectomy

Excludes *implantation of heart assist system [VAD] (37.62, 37.65, 37.66)*

✖ 37.53 **Replacement or repair of thoracic unit of total replacement heart system**

Excludes *replacement and repair of heart assist system [VAD] (37.63)*

✖ 37.54 **Replacement or repair of other implantable component of total replacement heart system**
Implantable battery
Implantable controller
Transcutaneous energy transfer (TET) device

Excludes *replacement and repair of heart assist system [VAD] (37.63)*
replacement or repair of thoracic unit of total replacement heart system (37.53)

● **37.6 Implantation of heart circulatory assist system**

Excludes *implantation of prosthetic cardiac support system (37.41)*

✖ **37.61 Implant of pulsation balloon**

✖ **37.62 Insertion of non-implantable heart assist system**

Insertion of heart assist system, NOS
Insertion of heart pump

Excludes *implantation of total replacement heart system (37.52)*
insertion of percutaneous external heart assist device (37.68)

✖ **37.63 Repair of heart assist system**

Replacement of parts of an existing ventricular assist device (VAD)

Excludes *replacement or repair of other implantable component of total replacement heart system [artificial heart] (37.54)*
replacement or repair of thoracic unit of total replacement heart system [artificial heart] (37.53)

✖ **37.64 Removal of heart assist system**

Excludes *explanation [removal] of percutaneous external heart assist device (97.44)*
that with replacement of implant (37.63)

✖ **37.65 Implant of external heart assist system**

Note: Device (outside the body but connected to heart) with external circulation and pump. Includes open chest (sternotomy) procedure for cannulae attachments

Excludes *implant of pulsation balloon (37.61)*
implantation of total replacement heart system (37.52)
insertion of percutaneous external heart assist device (37.68)

✖ **37.66 Insertion of implantable heart assist system**

Axial flow heart assist system
Diagonal pump heart assist system
Left ventricular assist device (LVAD)
Pulsatile heart assist system
Right ventricular assist device (RVAD)
Rotary pump heart assist system
Transportable, implantable heart assist system
Ventricular assist device (VAD) not otherwise specified

Note: Device directly connected to the heart and implanted in the upper left quadrant of peritoneal cavity.

Note: This device can be used for either destination therapy (DT) or bridge-to-transplant (BTT) ◀

Excludes *implant of pulsation balloon (37.61)*
implantation of total replacement heart system [artificial heart] (37.52)
insertion of percutaneous external heart assist device (37.68)

✖ **37.67 Implantation of cardiomyostimulation system**

Note: Two-step open procedure consisting of transfer of one end of the latissimus dorsi muscle; wrapping it around the heart; rib resection; implantation of epicardial cardiac pacing leads into the right ventricle; tunneling and pocket creation for the cardiomyostimulator.

✖ **37.68 Insertion of percutaneous external heart assist device**

Includes percutaneous [femoral] insertion of cannulae attachments
Circulatory assist device
Extrinsic heart assist device
pVAD
Percutaneous heart assist device

● **37.7 Insertion, revision, replacement, and removal of leads; insertion of temporary pacemaker system; or revision of cardiac device pocket** (Revised)

Code also any insertion and replacement of pacemaker device (37.80–37.87)

Excludes *implantation or replacement of transvenous lead [electrode] into left ventricular cardiac venous system (00.52)*

37.70 Initial insertion of lead [electrode], not otherwise specified

Excludes *insertion of temporary transvenous pacemaker system (37.78)*
replacement of atrial and/or ventricular lead(s) (37.76)

37.71 Initial insertion of transvenous lead [electrode] into ventricle

Excludes *insertion of temporary transvenous pacemaker system (37.78)*
replacement of atrial and/or ventricular lead(s) (37.76)

37.72 Initial insertion of transvenous leads [electrodes] into atrium and ventricle

Excludes *insertion of temporary transvenous pacemaker system (37.78)*
replacement of atrial and/or ventricular lead(s) (37.76)

37.73 Initial insertion of transvenous lead [electrode] into atrium

Excludes *insertion of temporary transvenous pacemaker system (37.78)*
replacement of atrial and/or ventricular lead(s) (37.76)

✖ **37.74 Insertion or replacement of epicardial lead [electrode] into epicardium**

Insertion or replacement of epicardial by:
sternotomy
thoracotomy

Excludes *replacement of atrial and/or ventricular lead(s) (37.76)*

✖ **37.75 Revision of lead [electrode]**

Repair of electrode [removal with re-insertion]
Repositioning of lead(s) (AICD) (cardiac device) (CRT-D) (CRT-P) (defibrillator) (pacemaker) (pacing) (sensing) [electrode] (Revised)
Revision of lead NOS

Excludes *repositioning of temporary transvenous pacemaker system—omit code*

✖ **37.76 Replacement of transvenous atrial and/or ventricular lead(s) [electrode]**

Removal or abandonment of existing transvenous or epicardial lead(s) with transvenous lead(s) replacement

Excludes *replacement of epicardial lead [electrode] (37.74)*

✖ **37.77 Removal of lead(s) [electrode] without replacement**
Removal:
epicardial lead (transthoracic approach)
transvenous lead(s)

Excludes *removal of temporary transvenous pacemaker system—omit code*
that with replacement of:
atrial and/or ventricular lead(s) [electrode] (37.76)
epicardial lead [electrode] (37.74)

37.78 Insertion of temporary transvenous pacemaker system

Excludes *intraoperative cardiac pacemaker (39.64)*

✖ **37.79 Revision or relocation of cardiac device pocket**
Debridement and reforming pocket (skin and subcutaneous tissue)
Insertion of loop recorder ◀
Relocation of pocket [creation of new pocket] pacemaker or CRT-P
Removal of cardiac device/pulse generator without replacement ◀
Removal of the implantable hemodynamic pressure sensor (lead) and monitor device ◀
Removal without replacement of cardiac resynchronization defibrillator device ◀
Repositioning of implantable hemodynamic pressure sensor (lead) and monitor device ◀
Repositioning of pulse generator ◀
Revision of cardioverter/defibrillator (automatic) pocket ◀
Revision of pocket for intracardiac hemodynamic monitoring ◀
Revision or relocation of CRT-D pocket ◀
Revision or relocation of pacemaker, defibrillator, or other implanted cardiac device pocket

Excludes *removal of loop recorder (86.05)* ◀

● **37.8 Insertion, replacement, removal, and revision of pacemaker device**

Code also any lead insertion, lead replacement, lead removal, and/or lead revision (37.70–37.77)

Note: Device testing during procedure – *omit code* ◀

Excludes *implantation of cardiac resynchronization pacemaker [CRT-P] (00.50)*
implantation or replacement of cardiac resynchronization pacemaker pulse generator only [CRT-P] (00.53)

✖ **37.80 Insertion of permanent pacemaker, initial or replacement, type of device not specified**

37.81 Initial insertion of single-chamber device, not specified as rate responsive

Excludes *replacement of existing pacemaker device (37.85–37.87)*

37.82 Initial insertion of single-chamber device, rate responsive
Rate responsive to physiologic stimuli other than atrial rate

Excludes *replacement of existing pacemaker device (37.85–37.87)*

37.83 Initial insertion of dual-chamber device
Atrial ventricular sequential device

Excludes *replacement of existing pacemaker device (37.85–37.87)*

✖ **37.85 Replacement of any type pacemaker device with single-chamber device, not specified as rate responsive**

✖ **37.86 Replacement of any type of pacemaker device with single-chamber device, rate responsive**
Rate responsive to physiologic stimuli other than atrial rate

✖ **37.87 Replacement of any type pacemaker device with dual-chamber device**
Atrial ventricular sequential device

✖ **37.89 Revision or removal of pacemaker device**
Removal without replacement of cardiac resynchronization pacemaker device [CRT-P]
Repair of pacemaker device

Excludes *removal of temporary transvenous pacemaker system—omit code*
replacement of existing pacemaker device (37.85–37.87)
replacement of existing pacemaker device with CRT-P pacemaker device (00.53)

● **37.9 Other operations on heart and pericardium**

✖ **37.90 Insertion of left atrial appendage device**
Left atrial filter
Left atrial occluder
Transeptal catheter technique

✖ **37.91 Open chest cardiac massage**

Excludes *closed chest cardiac massage (99.63)*

37.92 Injection of therapeutic substance into heart

37.93 Injection of therapeutic substance into pericardium

✖ **37.94 Implantation or replacement of automatic cardioverter/defibrillator, total system [AICD]**
Implantation of defibrillator with leads (epicardial patches), formation of pocket (abdominal fascia) (subcutaneous), any transvenous leads, intraoperative procedures for evaluation of lead signals, and obtaining defibrillator threshold measurements ⬅
Techniques:
lateral thoracotomy
medial sternotomy
subxiphoid procedure

Code also extracorporeal circulation, if performed (39.61)

Code also any concomitant procedure [e.g., coronary bypass] (36.00–36.19)

Note: Device testing during procedure – *omit code* ◀

Excludes *implantation of cardiac resynchronization defibrillator, total system [CRT-D] (00.51)*

✖ **37.95 Implantation of automatic cardioverter/defibrillator lead(s) only**

✖ **37.96 Implantation of automatic cardioverter/defibrillator pulse generator only**

Note: Device testing during procedure – *omit code* ◀

Excludes *implantation or replacement of cardiac resynchronization defibrillator, pulse generator device only [CRT-D] (00.54)*

✖ **37.97 Replacement of automatic cardioverter/defibrillator lead(s) only**

Excludes *replacement of epicardial lead [electrode] into epicardium (37.74)* ◀
replacement of transvenous lead [electrode] into left ventricular coronary venous system (00.52) ◀

✖ **37.98 Replacement of automatic cardioverter/defibrillator pulse generator only**

Note: Device testing during procedure – *omit code* ◀

Excludes *replacement of cardiac resynchronization defibrillator, pulse generator device only [CRT-D] (00.54)*

✖ **37.99 Other** (Revised)

Excludes *cardiac retraining (93.36)*
conversion of cardiac rhythm (99.60–99.69)
implantation of prosthetic cardiac support device (37.41)
insertion of left atrial appendage device (37.90)
maze procedure (Cox-maze), open (37.33)
maze procedure, endovascular approach (37.34)
repositioning of pulse generator (37.79) ◀
revision of lead(s) (37.75) ◀
revision or relocation of pacemaker, defibrillator or other implanted cardiac device pocket (37.79) ◀

● **38 Incision, excision, and occlusion of vessels**

Code also any application or administration of an adhesion barrier substance (99.77)

Code also cardiopulmonary bypass [extracorporeal circulation] [heart-lung machine] (39.61)

Excludes *that of coronary vessels (00.66, 36.03, 36.04, 36.09, 36.10–36.99)* (Revised)

The following fourth-digit subclassification is for use with appropriate categories in section 38.0, 38.1, 38.3, 38.5, 38.6, 38.8, and 38.9 according to site. Valid fourth-digits are in [brackets] at the end of each code/description.

0 **unspecified site**
1 **intracranial vessels**
Cerebral (anterior) (middle)
Circle of Willis
Posterior communicating artery
2 **other vessels of head and neck**
Carotid artery (common) (external) (internal)
Jugular vein (external) (internal)
3 **upper limb vessels**
Axillary
Brachial
Radial
Ulnar
4 **aorta**
5 **other thoracic vessels**
Innominate
Pulmonary (artery) (vein)
Subclavian
Vena cava, superior
6 **abdominal arteries**
Celiac
Gastric
Hepatic
Iliac
Mesenteric
Renal
Splenic
Umbilical

Excludes *abdominal aorta (4)*

7 **abdominal veins**
Iliac
Portal
Renal
Splenic
Vena cava (inferior)
8 **lower limb arteries**
Femoral (common) (superficial)
Popliteal
Tibial
9 **lower limb veins**
Femoral
Popliteal
Saphenous
Tibial

✖● **38.0 Incision of vessel**
[0–9] Embolectomy
Thrombectomy

Excludes *endovascular removal of obstruction from head and neck vessel(s) (39.74)* ◀
puncture or catheterization of any:
artery (38.91, 38.98)
vein (38.92–38.95, 38.99)

✖● **38.1 Endarterectomy**
[0–6, 8] Endarterectomy with:
embolectomy
patch graft
temporary bypass during procedure
thrombectomy

Code also any:
number of vascular stents inserted (00.45–00.48)
number of vessels treated (00.40–00.43)
procedure on vessel bifurcation (00.44) ◀

● **38.2 Diagnostic procedures on blood vessels**

Excludes *adjunct vascular system procedures (00.40–00.43)*

✖ **38.21 Biopsy of blood vessel**

38.22 Percutaneous angioscopy

Excludes *angioscopy of eye (95.12)*

✖ **38.29 Other diagnostic procedures on blood vessels**

Excludes *blood vessel thermography (88.86)*
circulatory monitoring (89.61–89.69)
contrast:
angiocardiography (88.50–88.58)
arteriography (88.40–88.49)
phlebography (88.60–88.67)
impedance phlebography (88.68)
peripheral vascular ultrasonography (88.77)
plethysmogram (89.58)

✖● **38.3 Resection of vessel with anastomosis**
[0–9] Angiectomy
Excision of:
aneurysm (arteriovenous) with anastomosis
blood vessel (lesion) with anastomosis

✖● 38.4 Resection of vessel with replacement
[0–9] Angiectomy
Excision of:
aneurysm (arteriovenous) or blood vessel (lesion) with replacement
Partial resection with replacement ◀

Excludes *endovascular repair of aneurysm (39.71–39.79)*

Requires the use of one of the following fourth-digit subclassifications to identify site:

0 unspecified site
1 intracranial vessels
Cerebral (anterior) (middle)
Circle of Willis
Posterior communicating artery
2 other vessels of head and neck
Carotid artery (common) (external) (internal)
Jugular vein (external) (internal)
3 upper limb vessels
Axillary
Brachial
Radial
Ulnar
4 aorta, abdominal
Code also any thoracic vessel involvement (thoracoabdominal procedure) (38.45)
5 thoracic vessels
Aorta (thoracic)
Innominate
Pulmonary (artery) (vein)
Subclavian
Vena cava, superior
Code also any abdominal aorta involvement (thoracoabdominal procedure) (38.44)
6 abdominal arteries
Celiac
Gastric
Hepatic
Iliac
Mesenteric
Renal
Splenic
Umbilical

Excludes *abdominal aorta (4)*

7 abdominal veins
Iliac
Portal
Renal
Splenic
Vena cava (inferior)
8 lower limb arteries
Femoral (common) (superficial)
Popliteal
Tibial
9 lower limb veins
Femoral
Popliteal
Saphenous
Tibial

✖● 38.5 Ligation and stripping of varicose veins
[0–3, 5, 7, 9]

Excludes *ligation of varices:*
esophageal (42.91)
gastric (44.91)

✖● 38.6 Other excision of vessel
[0–9] Excision of blood vessel (lesion) NOS

Excludes *excision of vessel for aortocoronary bypass (36.10–36.14)*
excision with:
anastomosis (38.30–38.39)
graft replacement (38.40–38.49)
implant (38.40–38.49)

38.7 Interruption of the vena cava
Insertion of implant or sieve in vena cava
Ligation of vena cava (inferior) (superior)
Plication of vena cava

✖● 38.8 Other surgical occlusion of vessels
[0–9] Clamping of blood vessel
Division of blood vessel
Ligation of blood vessel
Occlusion of blood vessel

Excludes *adrenal vessels (07.43)*
esophageal varices (42.91)
gastric or duodenal vessel for ulcer (44.40–44.49)
gastric varices (44.91)
meningeal vessel (02.13)
percutaneous transcatheter infusion embolization (99.29)
spermatic vein for varicocele (63.1)
surgical occlusion of vena cava (38.7)
that for chemoembolization (99.25)
that for control of (postoperative) hemorrhage:
anus (49.95)
bladder (57.93)
following vascular procedure (39.41)
nose (21.00–21.09)
prostate (60.94)
tonsil (28.7)
thyroid vessel (06.92)
transcatheter (infusion) (99.29)

● 38.9 Puncture of vessel

Excludes *that for circulatory monitoring (89.60–89.69)*

38.91 Arterial catheterization

38.92 Umbilical vein catheterization

38.93 Venous catheterization, not elsewhere classified

Excludes *that for cardiac catheterization (37.21–37.23)*
that for renal dialysis (38.95)

38.94 Venous cutdown

38.95 Venous catheterization for renal dialysis

Excludes *insertion of totally implantable vascular access device [VAD] (86.07)*

38.98 Other puncture of artery

Excludes *that for:*
arteriography (88.40–88.49)
coronary arteriography (88.55–88.57)

38.99 Other puncture of vein
Phlebotomy

Excludes *that for:*
angiography (88.60–88.69)
extracorporeal circulation (39.61, 50.92)
injection or infusion of:
sclerosing solution (39.92)
therapeutic or prophylactic substance (99.11–99.29)
perfusion (39.96–39.97)
phlebography (88.60–88.69)
transfusion (99.01–99.09)

● 39 Other operations on vessels

Excludes *those on coronary vessels (36.00–36.99)*

✖ 39.0 Systemic to pulmonary artery shunt
Descending aorta-pulmonary artery anastomosis (graft)
Left to right anastomosis (graft)
Subclavian-pulmonary anastomosis (graft)

Code also cardiopulmonary bypass [extracorporeal circulation] [heart-lung machine] (39.61)

✖ 39.1 **Intra-abdominal venous shunt**
Anastomosis:
mesocaval
portacaval
portal vein to inferior vena cava
splenic and renal veins
transjugular intrahepatic portosystemic shunt (TIPS)

Excludes *peritoneovenous shunt (54.94)*

● 39.2 **Other shunt or vascular bypass**

Code also pressurized treatment of venous bypass graft [conduit] with pharmaceutical substance, if performed (00.16)

✖ 39.21 **Caval-pulmonary artery anastomosis**

Code also cardiopulmonary bypass (39.61)

✖ 39.22 **Aorta-subclavian-carotid bypass**
Bypass (arterial):
aorta to carotid and brachial
aorta to subclavian and carotid
carotid to subclavian

✖ 39.23 **Other intrathoracic vascular shunt or bypass**
Intrathoracic (arterial) bypass graft NOS

Excludes *coronary artery bypass (36.10–36.19)*

✖ 39.24 **Aorta-renal bypass**

✖ 39.25 **Aorta-iliac-femoral bypass**
Bypass:
aortofemoral
aortoiliac
aortoiliac to popliteal
aortopopliteal
iliofemoral [iliac-femoral]

✖ 39.26 **Other intra-abdominal vascular shunt or bypass**
Bypass:
aortoceliac
aortic-superior mesenteric
common hepatic-common iliac-renal
Intra-abdominal arterial bypass graft NOS

Excludes *peritoneovenous shunt (54.94)*

✖ 39.27 **Arteriovenostomy for renal dialysis**
Anastomosis for renal dialysis
Formation of (peripheral) arteriovenous fistula for renal [kidney] dialysis

Code also any renal dialysis (39.95)

✖ 39.28 **Extracranial-intracranial (EC-IC) vascular bypass**

✖ 39.29 **Other (peripheral) vascular shunt or bypass**
Bypass (graft):
axillary-brachial
axillary-femoral [axillofemoral] (superficial)
brachial
femoral-femoral
femoroperoneal
femoropopliteal (arteries)
femorotibial (anterior) (posterior)
popliteal
vascular NOS

Excludes *peritoneovenous shunt (54.94)*

● 39.3 **Suture of vessel**
Repair of laceration of blood vessel

Excludes *any other vascular puncture closure device—omit code*
suture of aneurysm (39.52)
that for control of hemorrhage (postoperative):
anus (49.95)
bladder (57.93)
following vascular procedure (39.41)
nose (21.00–21.09)
prostate (60.94)
tonsil (28.7)

✖ 39.30 **Suture of unspecified blood vessel**

✖ 39.31 **Suture of artery**

✖ 39.32 **Suture of vein**

● 39.4 **Revision of vascular procedure**

✖ 39.41 **Control of hemorrhage following vascular surgery**

Excludes *that for control of hemorrhage (post operative):*
anus (49.95)
bladder (57.93)
nose (21.00–21.09)
prostate (60.94)
tonsil (28.7)

✖ 39.42 **Revision of arteriovenous shunt for renal dialysis**
Conversion of renal dialysis:
end-to-end anastomosis to end-to-side
end-to-side anastomosis to end-to-end
vessel-to-vessel cannula to arteriovenous shunt
Removal of old arteriovenous shunt and creation of new shunt

Excludes *replacement of vessel-to-vessel cannula (39.94)*

✖ 39.43 **Removal of arteriovenous shunt for renal dialysis**

Excludes *that with replacement [revision] of shunt (39.42)*

✖ 39.49 **Other revision of vascular procedure**
Declotting (graft)
Revision of:
anastomosis of blood vessel
vascular procedure (previous)

● 39.5 **Other repair of vessels**

✖ 39.50 **Angioplasty or atherectomy of other non-coronary vessel(s)**
Percutaneous transluminal angioplasty (PTA) of non-coronary vessels:
Lower extremity vessels
Mesenteric artery
Renal artery
Upper extremity vessels

Code also any:
injection or infusion of thrombolytic agent (99.10)
insertion of non-coronary stent(s) or stent grafts(s) (39.90)
number of vascular stents inserted (00.45–00.48)
number of vessels treated (00.40–00.43)
procedure on vessel bifurcation (00.44) ◀

Excludes *percutaneous angioplasty or atherectomy of precerebral or cerebral vessel(s) (00.61–00.62)*

✖ 39.51 **Clipping of aneurysm**

Excludes *clipping of arteriovenous fistula (39.53)*

✖ 39.52 **Other repair of aneurysm**
Repair of aneurysm by:
coagulation
electrocoagulation
filipuncture
methyl methacrylate
suture
wiring
wrapping

Excludes *endovascular repair of aneurysm (39.71–39.79)*
re-entry operation (aorta) (39.54)
that with:
graft replacement (38.40–38.49)
resection (38.30–38.49, 38.60–38.69)

✖ **39.53 Repair of arteriovenous fistula**
Embolization of carotid cavernous fistula
Repair of arteriovenous fistula by:
clipping
coagulation
ligation and division

Excludes *repair of:*
arteriovenous shunt for renal dialysis (39.42)
head and neck vessels, endovascular approach (39.72)
that with:
graft replacement (38.40–38.49)
resection (38.30–38.49, 38.60–38.69)

✖ **39.54 Re-entry operation (aorta)**
Fenestration of dissecting aneurysm of thoracic aorta

Code also cardiopulmonary bypass [extracorporeal circulation] [heart-lung machine] (39.61)

✖ **39.55 Reimplantation of aberrant renal vessel**

✖ **39.56 Repair of blood vessel with tissue patch graft**

Excludes *that with resection (38.40–38.49)*

✖ **39.57 Repair of blood vessel with synthetic patch graft**

Excludes *that with resection (38.40–38.49)*

✖ **39.58 Repair of blood vessel with unspecified type of patch graft**

Excludes *that with resection (38.40–38.49)*

✖ **39.59 Other repair of vessel**
Aorticopulmonary window operation
Arterioplasty NOS
Construction of venous valves (peripheral)
Plication of vein (peripheral)
Reimplantation of artery

Code also cardiopulmonary bypass [extracorporeal circulation] [heart-lung machine] (39.61)

Excludes *interruption of the vena cava (38.7)*
reimplantation of renal artery (39.55)
that with:
graft (39.56–39.58)
resection (38.30–38.49, 38.60–38.69)

● **39.6 Extracorporeal circulation and procedures auxiliary to heart surgery**

39.61 Extracorporeal circulation auxiliary to open heart surgery
Artificial heart and lung
Cardiopulmonary bypass
Pump oxygenator

Excludes *extracorporeal hepatic assistance (50.92)*
extracorporeal membrane oxygenation [ECMO] (39.65)
hemodialysis (39.95)
percutaneous cardiopulmonary bypass (39.66)

39.62 Hypothermia (systemic) incidental to open heart surgery

39.63 Cardioplegia
Arrest:
anoxic
circulatory

39.64 Intraoperative cardiac pacemaker
Temporary pacemaker used during and immediately following cardiac surgery

39.65 Extracorporeal membrane oxygenation [ECMO]

Excludes *extracorporeal circulation auxiliary to open heart surgery (39.61)*
percutaneous cardiopulmonary bypass (39.66)

39.66 Percutaneous cardiopulmonary bypass
Closed chest

Excludes *extracorporeal circulation auxiliary to open heart surgery (39.61)*
extracorporeal hepatic assistance (50.92)
extracorporeal membrane oxygenation [ECMO] (39.65)
hemodialysis (39.95)

● **39.7 Endovascular repair of vessel**
Endoluminal repair

Excludes *angioplasty or atherectomy of other non-coronary vessel (39.50)*
insertion of non-drug-eluting peripheral vessel stent(s) (39.90)
other repair of aneurysm (39.52)
percutaneous insertion of carotid artery stent(s) (00.63)
percutaneous insertion of intracranial stent(s) (00.65)
percutaneous insertion of other precerebral artery stent(s) (00.64)
resection of abdominal aorta with replacement (38.44)
resection of lower limb arteries with replacement (38.48)
resection of thoracic aorta with replacement (38.45)
resection of upper limb vessels with replacement (38.43)

✖ **39.71 Endovascular implantation of graft in abdominal aorta**
Endovascular repair of abdominal aortic aneurysm with graft
Stent graft(s)

✖ **39.72 Endovascular repair or occlusion of head and neck vessels**
Coil embolization or occlusion
Endograft(s)
Endovascular graft(s)
Liquid tissue adhesive (glue) embolization or occlusion
Other implant or substance for repair, embolization or occlusion
That for repair of aneurysm, arteriovenous malformation [AVM], or fistula

Excludes *mechanical thrombectomy of pre-cerebral and cerebral vessels (39.74)* ◄

✖ **39.73 Endovascular implantation of graft in thoracic aorta**
Endograft(s)
Endovascular graft(s)
Endovascular repair of defect of thoracic aorta with graft(s) or device(s)
Stent graft(s) or device(s)
That for repair of aneurysm, dissection, or injury

Excludes *fenestration of dissecting aneurysm of thoracic aorta (39.54)*

✖ **39.74 Endovascular removal of obstruction from head and neck vessel(s)** ◀
Endovascular embolectomy ◀
Endovascular thrombectomy of pre-cerebral and cerebral vessels ◀
Mechanical embolectomy or thrombectomy ◀
Code also: ◀
any injection or infusion of thrombolytic agent (99.10) ◀
number of vessels treated (00.40–00.43) ◀
procedure on vessel bifurcation (00.44) ◀
Excludes *endarterectomy of intracranial vessels and other vessels of head and neck (38.11–38.12)* ◀
occlusive endovascular repair of head or neck vessels (39.72) ◀
open embolectomy or thrombectomy (38.01–38.02) ◀

✖ **39.79 Other endovascular repair (of aneurysm) of other vessels**
Coil embolization or occlusion
Endograft(s)
Endovascular graft(s)
Liquid tissue adhesive (glue) embolization or occlusion
Other implant or substance for repair, embolization or occlusion
Excludes *endovascular implantation of graft in thoracic aorta (39.73)*
endovascular repair or occlusion of head and neck vessels (39.72)
insertion of drug-eluting peripheral vessel stent(s) (00.55)
insertion of non-drug-eluting peripheral vessel stent(s) (for other than aneurysm repair) (39.90)
non-endovascular repair of arteriovenous fistula (39.53)
other surgical occlusion of vessels - see category *38.8*
percutaneous transcatheter infusion (99.29)
transcatheter embolization for gastric or duodenal bleeding (44.44)

✖ **39.8 Operations on carotid body and other vascular bodies**
Chemodectomy
Denervation of:
aortic body
carotid body
Glomectomy, carotid
Implantation into carotid body:
electronic stimulator
pacemaker
Excludes *excision of glomus jugulare (20.51)*

● **39.9 Other operations on vessels**

39.90 Insertion of non-drug-eluting, peripheral vessel stent(s)
Bare stent(s)
Bonded stent(s)
Drug-coated stent(s), i.e., heparin coated
Endograft(s)
Endovascular graft(s)
Endovascular recanalization techniques
Stent graft(s)
Excludes *insertion of drug-eluting, peripheral vessel stent(s) (00.55)*
percutaneous insertion of carotid artery stent(s) (00.63)
percutaneous insertion of intracranial stent(s) (00.65)
percutaneous insertion of other precerebral artery stent(s) (00.64)
that for aneurysm repair (39.71–39.79)
Code also any:
non-coronary angioplasty or atherectomy (39.50)
number of vascular stents inserted (00.45–00.48)
number of vessels treated (00.40–00.43)
procedure on vessel bifurcation (00.44) ◀

✖ **39.91 Freeing of vessel**
Dissection and freeing of adherent tissue:
artery-vein-nerve bundle
vascular bundle

✖ **39.92 Injection of sclerosing agent into vein**
Excludes *injection:*
esophageal varices (42.33)
hemorrhoids (49.42)

✖ **39.93 Insertion of vessel-to-vessel cannula**
Formation of:
arteriovenous:
fistula by external cannula
shunt by external cannula
Code also any renal dialysis (39.95)

✖ **39.94 Replacement of vessel-to-vessel cannula**
Revision of vessel-to-vessel cannula

39.95 Hemodialysis
Artificial kidney
Hemodiafiltration
Hemofiltration
Renal dialysis
Excludes *peritoneal dialysis (54.98)*

39.96 Total body perfusion
Code also substance perfused (99.21–99.29)

39.97 Other perfusion
Perfusion NOS
Perfusion, local [regional] of:
carotid artery
coronary artery
head
lower limb
neck
upper limb
Code also substance perfused (99.21–99.29)
Excludes *perfusion of:*
kidney (55.95)
large intestine (46.96)
liver (50.93)
small intestine (46.95)

✖ **39.98 Control of hemorrhage, not otherwise specified**
Angiotripsy
Control of postoperative hemorrhage NOS
Venotripsy
Excludes *control of hemorrhage (postoperative):*
anus (49.95)
bladder (57.93)
following vascular procedure (39.41)
nose (21.00–21.09)
prostate (60.94)
tonsil (28.7)
that by:
ligation (38.80–38.89)
suture (39.30–39.32)

✖ **39.99 Other operations on vessels**
Excludes *injection or infusion of therapeutic or prophylactic substance (99.11–99.29)*
transfusion of blood and blood components (99.01–99.09)

8. OPERATIONS ON THE HEMIC AND LYMPHATIC SYSTEM (40–41)

● 40 Operations on lymphatic system

✖ 40.0 Incision of lymphatic structures

● 40.1 Diagnostic procedures on lymphatic structures

✖ 40.11 Biopsy of lymphatic structure

✖ 40.19 Other diagnostic procedures on lymphatic structures

Excludes *lymphangiogram:*
abdominal (88.04)
cervical (87.08)
intrathoracic (87.34)
lower limb (88.36)
upper limb (88.34)
microscopic examination of specimen (90.71–90.79)
radioisotope scan (92.16)
thermography (88.89)

● 40.2 Simple excision of lymphatic structure

Excludes *biopsy of lymphatic structure (40.11)*

✖ 40.21 Excision of deep cervical lymph node

✖ 40.22 Excision of internal mammary lymph node

✖ 40.23 Excision of axillary lymph node

✖ 40.24 Excision of inguinal lymph node

✖ 40.29 Simple excision of other lymphatic structure
Excision of:
cystic hygroma
lymphangioma
Simple lymphadenectomy

✖ 40.3 Regional lymph node excision
Extended regional lymph node excision
Regional lymph node excision with excision of lymphatic drainage area including skin, subcutaneous tissue, and fat

● 40.4 Radical excision of cervical lymph nodes
Resection of cervical lymph nodes down to muscle and deep fascia

Excludes *that associated with radical laryngectomy (30.4)*

✖ 40.40 Radical neck dissection, not otherwise specified

✖ 40.41 Radical neck dissection, unilateral

✖ 40.42 Radical neck dissection, bilateral

● 40.5 Radical excision of other lymph nodes

Excludes *that associated with radical mastectomy (85.45–85.48)*

✖ 40.50 Radical excision of lymph nodes, not otherwise specified
Radical (lymph) node dissection NOS

✖ 40.51 Radical excision of axillary lymph nodes

✖ 40.52 Radical excision of periaortic lymph nodes

✖ 40.53 Radical excision of iliac lymph nodes

✖ 40.54 Radical groin dissection

✖ 40.59 Radical excision of other lymph nodes

Excludes *radical neck dissection (40.40–40.42)*

● 40.6 Operations on thoracic duct

✖ 40.61 Cannulation of thoracic duct

✖ 40.62 Fistulization of thoracic duct

✖ 40.63 Closure of fistula of thoracic duct

✖ 40.64 Ligation of thoracic duct

✖ 40.69 Other operations on thoracic duct

✖ 40.9 Other operations on lymphatic structures
Anastomosis of peripheral lymphatics
Dilation of peripheral lymphatics
Ligation of peripheral lymphatics
Obliteration of peripheral lymphatics
Reconstruction of peripheral lymphatics
Repair of peripheral lymphatics
Transplantation of peripheral lymphatics
Correction of lymphedema of limb, NOS

Excludes *reduction of elephantiasis of scrotum (61.3)*

● 41 Operations on bone marrow and spleen

● 41.0 Bone marrow or hematopoietic stem cell transplant

Note: To report donor source - *see* codes 00.91–00.93

Excludes *aspiration of bone marrow from donor (41.91)*

✖ 41.00 Bone marrow transplant, not otherwise specified

✖ 41.01 Autologous bone marrow transplant without purging

Excludes *that with purging (41.09)*

✖ 41.02 Allogeneic bone marrow transplant with purging
Allograft of bone marrow with in vitro removal (purging) of T-cells

✖ 41.03 Allogeneic bone marrow transplant without purging
Allograft of bone marrow NOS

✖ 41.04 Autologous hematopoietic stem cell transplant without purging

Excludes *that with purging (41.07)*

✖ 41.05 Allogeneic hematopoietic stem cell transplant without purging

Excludes *that with purging (41.08)*

✖ 41.06 Cord blood stem cell transplant

✖ 41.07 Autologous hematopoietic stem cell transplant with purging
Cell depletion

✖ 41.08 Allogeneic hematopoietic stem cell transplant with purging
Cell depletion

✖ 41.09 Autologous bone marrow transplant with purging
with extracorporeal purging of malignant cells from marrow
Cell depletion

41.1 Puncture of spleen

Excludes *aspiration biopsy of spleen (41.32)*

✖ 41.2 Splenotomy

● 41.3 Diagnostic procedures on bone marrow and spleen

41.31 Biopsy of bone marrow

41.32 Closed [aspiration] [percutaneous] biopsy of spleen

✖ 41.33 Open biopsy of spleen

41.38 Other diagnostic procedures on bone marrow

Excludes *microscopic examination of specimen from bone marrow (90.61–90.69)*
radioisotope scan (92.05)

41.39 Other diagnostic procedures on spleen

Excludes *microscopic examination of specimen from spleen (90.61–90.69)*
radioisotope scan (92.05)

● 41.4 Excision or destruction of lesion or tissue of spleen

Excludes *excision of accessory spleen (41.93)*

Code also any application or administration of an adhesion barrier substance (99.77)

✖41.41 **Marsupialization of splenic cyst**

✖41.42 **Excision of lesion or tissue of spleen**

Excludes *biopsy of spleen (41.32–41.33)*

✖41.43 **Partial splenectomy**

✖41.5 **Total splenectomy**
Splenectomy NOS

Code also any application or administration of an adhesion barrier substance (99.77)

●41.9 **Other operations on spleen and bone marrow**

Code also any application or administration of an adhesion barrier substance (99.77)

41.91 **Aspiration of bone marrow from donor for transplant**

Excludes *biopsy of bone marrow (41.31)*

41.92 **Injection into bone marrow**

Excludes *bone marrow transplant (41.00–41.03)*

✖41.93 **Excision of accessory spleen**

✖41.94 **Transplantation of spleen**

✖41.95 **Repair and plastic operations on spleen**

41.98 **Other operations on bone marrow**

✖41.99 **Other operations on spleen**

9. OPERATIONS ON THE DIGESTIVE SYSTEM (42–54)

● **42 Operations on esophagus**

● **42.0 Esophagotomy**

✖ **42.01 Incision of esophageal web**

✖ **42.09 Other incision of esophagus**
Esophagotomy NOS

Excludes *esophagomyotomy (42.7)*
esophagostomy (42.10–42.19)

● **42.1 Esophagostomy**

✖ **42.10 Esophagostomy, not otherwise specified**

✖ **42.11 Cervical esophagostomy**

✖ **42.12 Exteriorization of esophageal pouch**

✖ **42.19 Other external fistulization of esophagus**
Thoracic esophagostomy

Code also any resection (42.40–42.42)

● **42.2 Diagnostic procedures on esophagus**

✖ **42.21 Operative esophagoscopy by incision**

42.22 Esophagoscopy through artificial stoma

Excludes *that with biopsy (42.24)*

42.23 Other esophagoscopy

Excludes *that with biopsy (42.24)*

42.24 Closed [endoscopic] biopsy of esophagus
Brushing or washing for specimen collection
Esophagoscopy with biopsy
Suction biopsy of the esophagus

Excludes *esophagogastroduodenoscopy [EGD] with closed biopsy (45.16)*

✖ **42.25 Open biopsy of esophagus**

42.29 Other diagnostic procedures on esophagus

Excludes *barium swallow (87.61)*
esophageal manometry (89.32)
microscopic examination of specimen from esophagus (90.81–90.89)

● **42.3 Local excision or destruction of lesion or tissue of esophagus**

✖ **42.31 Local excision of esophageal diverticulum**

✖ **42.32 Local excision of other lesion or tissue of esophagus**

Excludes *biopsy of esophagus (42.24–42.25)*
esophageal fistulectomy (42.84)

42.33 Endoscopic excision or destruction of lesion or tissue of esophagus
Ablation of esophageal neoplasm by endoscopic approach
Control of esophageal bleeding by endoscopic approach
Esophageal polypectomy by endoscopic approach
Esophageal varices by endoscopic approach
Injection of esophageal varices by endoscopic approach

Excludes *biopsy of esophagus (42.24–42.25)*
fistulectomy (42.84)
open ligation of esophageal varices (42.91)

✖ **42.39 Other destruction of lesion or tissue of esophagus**

Excludes *that by endoscopic approach (42.33)*

● **42.4 Excision of esophagus**

Excludes *esophagogastrectomy NOS (43.99)*

✖ **42.40 Esophagectomy, not otherwise specified**

✖ **42.41 Partial esophagectomy**

Code also any synchronous:
anastomosis other than end-to-end (42.51–42.69)
esophagostomy (42.10–42.19)
gastrostomy (43.11–43.19)

✖ **42.42 Total esophagectomy**

Code also any synchronous:
gastrostomy (43.11–43.19)
interposition or anastomosis other than end-to-end (42.51–42.69)

Excludes *esophagogastrectomy (43.99)*

● **42.5 Intrathoracic anastomosis of esophagus**

Code also any synchronous:
esophagectomy (42.40–42.42)
gastrostomy (43.1)

✖ **42.51 Intrathoracic esophagoesophagostomy**

✖ **42.52 Intrathoracic esophagogastrostomy**

✖ **42.53 Intrathoracic esophageal anastomosis with interposition of small bowel**

✖ **42.54 Other intrathoracic esophagoenterostomy**
Anastomosis of esophagus to intestinal segment NOS

✖ **42.55 Intrathoracic esophageal anastomosis with interposition of colon**

✖ **42.56 Other intrathoracic esophagocolostomy**
Esophagocolostomy NOS

✖ **42.58 Intrathoracic esophageal anastomosis with other interposition**
Construction of artificial esophagus
Retrosternal formation of reversed gastric tube

✖ **42.59 Other intrathoracic anastomosis of esophagus**

● **42.6 Antesternal anastomosis of esophagus**

Code also any synchronous:
esophagectomy (42.40–42.42)
gastrostomy (43.1)

✖ **42.61 Antesternal esophagoesophagostomy**

✖ **42.62 Antesternal esophagogastrostomy**

✖ **42.63 Antesternal esophageal anastomosis with interposition of small bowel**

✖ **42.64 Other antesternal esophagoenterostomy**
Antethoracic:
esophagoenterostomy
esophagoileostomy
esophagojejunostomy

✖ **42.65 Antesternal esophageal anastomosis with interposition of colon**

✖ **42.66 Other antesternal esophagocolostomy**
Antethoracic esophagocolostomy

✖ **42.68 Other antesternal esophageal anastomosis with interposition**

✖ **42.69 Other antesternal anastomosis of esophagus**

✖ **42.7 Esophagomyotomy**

● **42.8 Other repair of esophagus**

42.81 Insertion of permanent tube into esophagus

✖ **42.82 Suture of laceration of esophagus**

✖ **42.83 Closure of esophagostomy**

✖ **42.84 Repair of esophageal fistula, not elsewhere classified**

Excludes *repair of fistula:*
bronchoesophageal (33.42)
esophagopleurocutaneous (34.73)
pharyngoesophageal (29.53)
tracheoesophageal (31.73)

✖ **42.85 Repair of esophageal stricture**

✖ **42.86 Production of subcutaneous tunnel without esophageal anastomosis**

✖ **42.87 Other graft of esophagus**

Excludes *antesternal esophageal anastomosis with interposition of:*
colon (42.65)
small bowel (42.63)
antesternal esophageal anastomosis with other interposition (42.68)
intrathoracic esophageal anastomosis with interposition of:
colon (42.55)
small bowel (42.53)
intrathoracic esophageal anastomosis with other interposition (42.58)

✖ **42.89 Other repair of esophagus**

● **42.9 Other operations on esophagus**

✖ **42.91 Ligation of esophageal varices**

Excludes *that by endoscopic approach (42.33)*

42.92 Dilation of esophagus
Dilation of cardiac sphincter

Excludes *intubation of esophagus (96.03, 96.06–96.08)*

42.99 Other

Excludes *insertion of Sengstaken tube (96.06)*
intubation of esophagus (96.03, 96.06–96.08)
removal of intraluminal foreign body from esophagus without incision (98.02)
tamponade of esophagus (96.06)

● **43 Incision and excision of stomach**

Code also any application or administration of an adhesion barrier substance (99.77)

✖ **43.0 Gastrotomy**

Excludes *gastrostomy (43.11–43.19)*
that for control of hemorrhage (44.49)

● **43.1 Gastrostomy**

43.11 Percutaneous [endoscopic] gastrostomy [PEG]
Percutaneous transabdominal gastrostomy

43.19 Other gastrostomy

Excludes *percutaneous [endoscopic] gastrostomy [PEG] (43.11)*

✖ **43.3 Pyloromyotomy**

● **43.4 Local excision or destruction of lesion or tissue of stomach**

43.41 Endoscopic excision or destruction of lesion or tissue of stomach
Gastric polypectomy by endoscopic approach
Gastric varices by endoscopic approach

Excludes *biopsy of stomach (44.14–44.15)*
control of hemorrhage (44.43)
open ligation of gastric varices (44.91)

✖ **43.42 Local excision of other lesion or tissue of stomach**

Excludes *biopsy of stomach (44.14–44.15)*
gastric fistulectomy (44.62–44.63)
partial gastrectomy (43.5–43.89)

✖ **43.49 Other destruction of lesion or tissue of stomach**

Excludes *that by endoscopic approach (43.41)*

✖ **43.5 Partial gastrectomy with anastomosis to esophagus**
Proximal gastrectomy

✖ **43.6 Partial gastrectomy with anastomosis to duodenum**
Billroth I operation
Distal gastrectomy
Gastropylorectomy

✖ **43.7 Partial gastrectomy with anastomosis to jejunum**
Billroth II operation

● **43.8 Other partial gastrectomy**

✖ **43.81 Partial gastrectomy with jejunal transposition**
Henley jejunal transposition operation

Code also any synchronous intestinal resection (45.51)

✖ **43.89 Other**
Partial gastrectomy with bypass gastrogastrostomy
Sleeve resection of stomach

● **43.9 Total gastrectomy**

✖ **43.91 Total gastrectomy with intestinal interposition**

✖ **43.99 Other total gastrectomy**
Complete gastroduodenectomy
Esophagoduodenostomy with complete gastrectomy
Esophagogastrectomy NOS
Esophagojejunostomy with complete gastrectomy
Radical gastrectomy

● **44 Other operations on stomach**

Code also any application or administration of an adhesion barrier substance (99.77)

● **44.0 Vagotomy**

✖ **44.00 Vagotomy, not otherwise specified**
Division of vagus nerve NOS

✖ **44.01 Truncal vagotomy**

✖ **44.02 Highly selective vagotomy**
Parietal cell vagotomy
Selective proximal vagotomy

✖ **44.03 Other selective vagotomy**

● **44.1 Diagnostic procedures on stomach**

✖ **44.11 Transabdominal gastroscopy**
Intraoperative gastroscopy

Excludes *that with biopsy (44.14)*

44.12 Gastroscopy through artificial stoma

Excludes *that with biopsy (44.14)*

44.13 Other gastroscopy

Excludes *that with biopsy (44.14)*

44.14 Closed [endoscopic] biopsy of stomach
Brushing or washing for specimen collection

Excludes *esophagogastroduodenoscopy [EGD] with closed biopsy (45.16)*

✖ **44.15 Open biopsy of stomach**

44.19 Other diagnostic procedures on stomach

Excludes *gastric lavage (96.33)*
microscopic examination of specimen from stomach (90.81–90.89)
upper GI series (87.62)

● **44.2 Pyloroplasty**

✖ **44.21 Dilation of pylorus by incision**

44.22 Endoscopic dilation of pylorus
Dilation with balloon endoscope
Endoscopic dilation of gastrojejunostomy site

✖ **44.29 Other pyloroplasty**
Pyloroplasty NOS
Revision of pylorus

● **44.3 Gastroenterostomy without gastrectomy**

✖ **44.31 High gastric bypass**
Printen and Mason gastric bypass

✖ **44.32 Percutaneous [endoscopic] gastrojejunostomy**
Endoscopic conversion of gastrostomy to jejunostomy

44.38 Laparoscopic gastroenterostomy
Bypass:
gastroduodenostomy
gastroenterostomy
gastrogastrostomy
Laparoscopic gastrojejunostomy without gastrectomy NEC

Excludes *gastroenterostomy, open approach (44.39)*

✖ **44.39 Other gastroenterostomy**
Bypass:
gastroduodenostomy
gastroenterostomy
gastrogastrostomy
Gastrojejunostomy without gastrectomy NOS

● **44.4 Control of hemorrhage and suture of ulcer of stomach or duodenum**

✖ **44.40 Suture of peptic ulcer, not otherwise specified**

✖ **44.41 Suture of gastric ulcer site**

Excludes *ligation of gastric varices (44.91)*

✖ **44.42 Suture of duodenal ulcer site**

44.43 Endoscopic control of gastric or duodenal bleeding

44.44 Transcatheter embolization for gastric or duodenal bleeding

Excludes *surgical occlusion of abdominal vessels (38.86–38.87)*

44.49 Other control of hemorrhage of stomach or duodenum
That with gastrotomy

✖ **44.5 Revision of gastric anastomosis**
Closure of:
gastric anastomosis
gastroduodenostomy
gastrojejunostomy
Pantaloon operation

● **44.6 Other repair of stomach**

✖ **44.61 Suture of laceration of stomach**

Excludes *that of ulcer site (44.41)*

44.62 Closure of gastrostomy

✖ **44.63 Closure of other gastric fistula**
Closure of:
gastrocolic fistula
gastrojejunocolic fistula

✖ **44.64 Gastropexy**

✖ **44.65 Esophagogastroplasty**
Belsey operation
Esophagus and stomach cardioplasty

✖ **44.66 Other procedures for creation of esophagogastric sphincteric competence**
Fundoplication
Gastric cardioplasty
Nissen's fundoplication
Restoration of cardio-esophageal angle

Excludes *that by laparoscopy (44.67)*

44.67 Laparoscopic procedures for creation of esophagogastric sphincteric competence
Fundoplication
Gastric cardioplasty
Nissen's fundoplication
Restoration of cardio-esophageal angle

44.68 Laparoscopic gastroplasty
Banding
Silastic vertical banding
Vertical banded gastroplasty (VBG)

Code also any synchronous laparoscopic gastroenterostomy (44.38)

Excludes *insertion, laparoscopic adjustable gastric band (restrictive procedure) (44.95)*
other repair of stomach, open approach (44.61–44.65, 44.69)

✖ **44.69 Other**
Inversion of gastric diverticulum
Repair of stomach NOS

● **44.9 Other operations on stomach**

✖ **44.91 Ligation of gastric varices**

Excludes *that by endoscopic approach (43.41)*

✖ **44.92 Intraoperative manipulation of stomach**
Reduction of gastric volvulus

44.93 Insertion of gastric bubble (balloon)

44.94 Removal of gastric bubble (balloon)

✖ **44.95 Laparoscopic gastric restrictive procedure**
Adjustable gastric band and port insertion

Excludes *laparoscopic gastroplasty (44.68)*
other repair of stomach (44.69)

✖ **44.96 Laparoscopic revision of gastric restrictive procedure**
Revision or replacement of:
adjustable gastric band
subcutaneous gastric port device

✖ **44.97 Laparoscopic removal of gastric restrictive device(s)**
Removal of either or both:
adjustable gastric band
subcutaneous port device

Excludes *nonoperative removal of gastric restrictive device(s) (97.86)*
open removal of gastric restrictive device(s) (44.99)

✖ **44.98 (Laparoscopic) adjustment of size of adjustable gastric restrictive device**
Infusion of saline for device tightening
Withdrawal of saline for device loosening

Code also any:
abdominal ultrasound (88.76)
abdominal wall fluoroscopy (88.09)
barium swallow (87.61)

✖ **44.99 Other**

Excludes *change of gastrostomy tube (97.02)*
dilation of cardiac sphincter (42.92)
gastric:
cooling (96.31)
freezing (96.32)
gavage (96.35)
hypothermia (96.31)
lavage (96.33)
insertion of nasogastric tube (96.07)
irrigation of gastrostomy (96.36)
irrigation of nasogastric tube (96.34)
removal of:
gastrostomy tube (97.51)
intraluminal foreign body from stomach without incision (98.03)
replacement of:
gastrostomy tube (97.02)
(naso-)gastric tube (97.01)

● **45 Incision, excision, and anastomosis of intestine**

Code also any application or administration of an adhesion barrier substance (99.77)

● **45.0 Enterotomy**

Excludes *duodenocholedochotomy (51.41–51.42, 51.51)*
that for destruction of lesion (45.30–45.34)
that of exteriorized intestine (46.14, 46.24, 46.31)

✖ **45.00 Incision of intestine, not otherwise specified**

✖ **45.01 Incision of duodenum**

✖ **45.02 Other incision of small intestine**

✖ **45.03 Incision of large intestine**

Excludes *proctotomy (48.0)*

● **45.1 Diagnostic procedures on small intestine**

Code also any laparotomy (54.11–54.19)

✖ **45.11 Transabdominal endoscopy of small intestine**
Intraoperative endoscopy of small intestine

Excludes *that with biopsy (45.14)*

45.12 Endoscopy of small intestine through artificial stoma

Excludes *that with biopsy (45.14)*

45.13 Other endoscopy of small intestine
Esophagogastroduodenoscopy [EGD]

Excludes *that with biopsy (45.14, 45.16)*

45.14 Closed [endoscopic] biopsy of small intestine
Brushing or washing for specimen collection

Excludes *esophagogastroduodenoscopy [EGD] with closed biopsy (45.16)*

✖ **45.15 Open biopsy of small intestine**

45.16 Esophagogastroduodenoscopy [EGD] with closed biopsy
Biopsy of one or more sites involving esophagus, stomach, and/or duodenum

45.19 Other diagnostic procedures on small intestine

Excludes *microscopic examination of specimen from small intestine (90.91–90.99)*
radioisotope scan (92.04)
ultrasonography (88.74)
x-ray (87.61–87.69)

● **45.2 Diagnostic procedures on large intestine**

Code also any laparotomy (54.11–54.19)

✖ **45.21 Transabdominal endoscopy of large intestine**
Intraoperative endoscopy of large intestine

Excludes *that with biopsy (45.25)*

45.22 Endoscopy of large intestine through artificial stoma

Excludes *that with biopsy (45.25)*

45.23 Colonoscopy
Flexible fiberoptic colonoscopy

Excludes *endoscopy of large intestine through artificial stoma (45.22)*
flexible sigmoidoscopy (45.24)
rigid proctosigmoidoscopy (48.23)
transabdominal endoscopy of large intestine (45.21)

45.24 Flexible sigmoidoscopy
Endoscopy of descending colon

Excludes *rigid proctosigmoidoscopy (48.23)*

45.25 Closed [endoscopic] biopsy of large intestine
Biopsy, closed, of unspecified intestinal site
Brushing or washing for specimen collection
Colonoscopy with biopsy

Excludes *proctosigmoidoscopy with biopsy (48.24)*

✖ **45.26 Open biopsy of large intestine**

45.27 Intestinal biopsy, site unspecified

45.28 Other diagnostic procedures on large intestine

45.29 Other diagnostic procedures on intestine, site unspecified

Excludes *microscopic examination of specimen (90.91–90.99)*
scan and radioisotope function study (92.04)
ultrasonography (88.74)
x-ray (87.61–87.69)

● **45.3 Local excision or destruction of lesion or tissue of small intestine**

45.30 Endoscopic excision or destruction of lesion of duodenum

Excludes *biopsy of duodenum (45.14–45.15)*
control of hemorrhage (44.43)
fistulectomy (46.72)

✖ **45.31 Other local excision of lesion of duodenum**

Excludes *biopsy of duodenum (45.14–45.15)*
fistulectomy (46.72)
multiple segmental resection (45.61)
that by endoscopic approach (45.30)

✖ **45.32 Other destruction of lesion of duodenum**

Excludes *that by endoscopic approach (45.30)*

✖ **45.33 Local excision of lesion or tissue of small intestine, except duodenum**
Excision of redundant mucosa of ileostomy

Excludes *biopsy of small intestine (45.14–45.15)*
fistulectomy (46.74)
multiple segmental resection (45.61)

✖ **45.34 Other destruction of lesion of small intestine, except duodenum**

● **45.4 Local excision or destruction of lesion or tissue of large intestine**

✖ **45.41 Excision of lesion or tissue of large intestine**
Excision of redundant mucosa of colostomy

Excludes *biopsy of large intestine (45.25–45.27)*
endoscopic polypectomy of large intestine (45.42)
fistulectomy (46.76)
multiple segmental resection (45.71)
that by endoscopic approach (45.42–45.43)

45.42 Endoscopic polypectomy of large intestine

Excludes *that by open approach (45.41)*

45.43 Endoscopic destruction of other lesion or tissue of large intestine
Endoscopic ablation of tumor of large intestine
Endoscopic control of colonic bleeding

Excludes *endoscopic polypectomy of large intestine (45.42)*

✖ **45.49 Other destruction of lesion of large intestine**

Excludes *that by endoscopic approach (45.43)*

● **45.5 Isolation of intestinal segment**

Code also any synchronous:
anastomosis other than end-to-end (45.90–45.94)
enterostomy (46.10–46.39)

✖ **45.50 Isolation of intestinal segment, not otherwise specified**
Isolation of intestinal pedicle flap
Reversal of intestinal segment

✖ **45.51 Isolation of segment of small intestine**
Isolation of ileal loop
Resection of small intestine for interposition

✖ **45.52 Isolation of segment of large intestine**
Resection of colon for interposition

● **45.6 Other excision of small intestine**

Code also any synchronous:
anastomosis other than end-to-end (45.90–45.93, 45.95)
colostomy (46.10–46.13)
enterostomy (46.10–46.39)

Excludes *cecectomy (45.72)*
enterocolectomy (45.79)
gastroduodenectomy (43.6–43.99)
ileocolectomy (45.73)
pancreatoduodenectomy (52.51–52.7)

✖ **45.61 Multiple segmental resection of small intestine**
Segmental resection for multiple traumatic lesions of small intestine

✖ **45.62 Other partial resection of small intestine**
Duodenectomy
Ileectomy
Jejunectomy

Excludes *duodenectomy with synchronous pancreatectomy (52.51–52.7)*
resection of cecum and terminal ileum (45.72)

✖ **45.63 Total removal of small intestine**

● **45.7 Partial excision of large intestine**

Code also any synchronous:
anastomosis other than end-to-end (45.92–45.94)
enterostomy (46.10–46.39)

✖ **45.71 Multiple segmental resection of large intestine**
Segmental resection for multiple traumatic lesions of large intestine

✖ **45.72 Cecectomy**
Resection of cecum and terminal ileum

✖ **45.73 Right hemicolectomy**
Ileocolectomy
Right radical colectomy

✖ **45.74 Resection of transverse colon**

✖ **45.75 Left hemicolectomy**

Excludes *proctosigmoidectomy (48.41–48.69)*
second stage Mikulicz operation (46.04)

✖ **45.76 Sigmoidectomy**

✖ **45.79 Other partial excision of large intestine**
Enterocolectomy NEC

✖ **45.8 Total intra-abdominal colectomy**
Excision of cecum, colon, and sigmoid

Excludes *coloproctectomy (48.41–48.69)*

● **45.9 Intestinal anastomosis**

Code also any synchronous resection (45.31–45.8, 48.41–48.69)

Excludes *end-to-end anastomosis—omit code*

✖ **45.90 Intestinal anastomosis, not otherwise specified**

✖ **45.91 Small-to-small intestinal anastomosis**

✖ **45.92 Anastomosis of small intestine to rectal stump**
Hampton procedure

✖ **45.93 Other small-to-large intestinal anastomosis**

✖ **45.94 Large-to-large intestinal anastomosis**

Excludes *rectorectostomy (48.74)*

✖ **45.95 Anastomosis to anus**
Formation of endorectal ileal pouch (H-pouch) (J-pouch) (S-pouch) with anastomosis of small intestine to anus

● **46 Other operations on intestine**

Code also any application or administration of an adhesion barrier substance (99.77)

● **46.0 Exteriorization of intestine**

Includes: loop enterostomy
multiple stage resection of intestine

✖ **46.01 Exteriorization of small intestine**
Loop ileostomy

✖ **46.02 Resection of exteriorized segment of small intestine**

✖ **46.03 Exteriorization of large intestine**
Exteriorization of intestine NOS
First stage Mikulicz exteriorization of intestine
Loop colostomy

✖ **46.04 Resection of exteriorized segment of large intestine**
Resection of exteriorized segment of intestine NOS
Second stage Mikulicz operation

● **46.1 Colostomy**

Code also any synchronous resection (45.49, 45.71–45.79, 45.8)

Excludes *loop colostomy (46.03)*
that with abdominoperineal resection of rectum (48.5)
that with synchronous anterior rectal resection (48.62)

✖ **46.10 Colostomy, not otherwise specified**

✖ **46.11 Temporary colostomy**

✖ **46.13 Permanent colostomy**

46.14 Delayed opening of colostomy

● **46.2 Ileostomy**

Code also any synchronous resection (45.34, 45.61–45.63)

Excludes *loop ileostomy (46.01)*

✖ **46.20 Ileostomy, not otherwise specified**

✖ **46.21 Temporary ileostomy**

✖ **46.22 Continent ileostomy**

✖ **46.23 Other permanent ileostomy**

46.24 Delayed opening of ileostomy

● **46.3 Other enterostomy**

Code also any synchronous resection (45.61–45.8)

46.31 Delayed opening of other enterostomy

46.32 Percutaneous (endoscopic) jejunostomy [PEJ]

46.39 Other
Duodenostomy
Feeding enterostomy

● **46.4 Revision of intestinal stoma**

✖ **46.40 Revision of intestinal stoma, not otherwise specified**
Plastic enlargement of intestinal stoma
Reconstruction of stoma of intestine
Release of scar tissue of intestinal stoma

Excludes *excision of redundant mucosa (45.41)*

✖ **46.41 Revision of stoma of small intestine**

Excludes *excision of redundant mucosa (45.33)*

✖ **46.42 Repair of pericolostomy hernia**

✖ **46.43 Other revision of stoma of large intestine**

Excludes *excision of redundant mucosa (45.41)*

● **46.5 Closure of intestinal stoma**

Code also any synchronous resection (45.34, 45.49, 45.61–45.8)

✖ **46.50 Closure of intestinal stoma, not otherwise specified**

✖ **46.51 Closure of stoma of small intestine**

✖ **46.52 Closure of stoma of large intestine**
Closure or take-down of:
cecostomy
colostomy
sigmoidostomy

● **46.6 Fixation of intestine**

✖ **46.60 Fixation of intestine, not otherwise specified**
Fixation of intestine to abdominal wall

✖ **46.61 Fixation of small intestine to abdominal wall**
Ileopexy

✖ **46.62 Other fixation of small intestine**
Noble plication of small intestine
Plication of jejunum

✖ **46.63 Fixation of large intestine to abdominal wall**
Cecocoloplicopexy
Sigmoidopexy (Moschowitz)

✖ **46.64 Other fixation of large intestine**
Cecofixation
Colofixation

● **46.7 Other repair of intestine**

Excludes *closure of:*
ulcer of duodenum (44.42)
vesicoenteric fistula (57.83)

✖ **46.71 Suture of laceration of duodenum**

✖ **46.72 Closure of fistula of duodenum**

✖ **46.73 Suture of laceration of small intestine, except duodenum**

✖ **46.74 Closure of fistula of small intestine, except duodenum**

Excludes *closure of:*
artificial stoma (46.51)
vaginal fistula (70.74)
repair of gastrojejunocolic fistula (44.63)

✖ **46.75 Suture of laceration of large intestine**

✖ **46.76 Closure of fistula of large intestine**

Excludes *closure of:*
gastrocolic fistula (44.63)
rectal fistula (48.73)
sigmoidovesical fistula (57.83)
stoma (46.52)
vaginal fistula (70.72–70.73)
vesicocolic fistula (57.83)
vesicosigmoidovaginal fistula (57.83)

✖ **46.79 Other repair of intestine**
Duodenoplasty

● **46.8 Dilation and manipulation of intestine**

✖ **46.80 Intra-abdominal manipulation of intestine, not otherwise specified**
Correction of intestinal malrotation
Reduction of:
intestinal torsion
intestinal volvulus
intussusception

Excludes *reduction of intussusception with:*
fluoroscopy (96.29)
ionizing radiation enema (96.29)
ultrasonography guidance (96.29)

✖ **46.81 Intra-abdominal manipulation of small intestine**

✖ **46.82 Intra-abdominal manipulation of large intestine**

46.85 Dilation of intestine
Dilation (balloon) of duodenum
Dilation (balloon) of jejunum
Endoscopic dilation (balloon) of large intestine
That through rectum or colostomy

● **46.9 Other operations on intestines**

✖ **46.91 Myotomy of sigmoid colon**

✖ **46.92 Myotomy of other parts of colon**

✖ **46.93 Revision of anastomosis of small intestine**

✖ **46.94 Revision of anastomosis of large intestine**

46.95 Local perfusion of small intestine

Code also substance perfused (99.21–99.29)

46.96 Local perfusion of large intestine

Code also substance perfused (99.21–99.29)

46.97 Transplant of intestine

Note: To report donor source - *see* codes 00.91–00.93

✖ **46.99 Other**
Ileoentectropy

Excludes *diagnostic procedures on intestine (45.11–45.29)*
dilation of enterostomy stoma (96.24)
intestinal intubation (96.08)
removal of:
intraluminal foreign body from large intestine without incision (98.04)
intraluminal foreign body from small intestine without incision (98.03)
tube from large intestine (97.53)
tube from small intestine (97.52)
replacement of:
large intestine tube or enterostomy device (97.04)
small intestine tube or enterostomy device (97.03)

● **47 Operations on appendix**

Code also any application or administration of an adhesion barrier substance (99.77)

Includes: appendiceal stump

✖ **47.0 Appendectomy**

Excludes *incidental appendectomy, so described*
laparoscopic (47.11)
other (47.19)

✖ **47.01 Laparoscopic appendectomy**

✖ **47.09 Other appendectomy**

● **47.1 Incidental appendectomy**

✖ **47.11 Laparoscopic incidental appendectomy**

✖ **47.19 Other incidental appendectomy**

✖ **47.2 Drainage of appendiceal abscess**

Excludes *that with appendectomy (47.0)*

● **47.9 Other operations on appendix**

✖ **47.91 Appendicostomy**

✖ **47.92 Closure of appendiceal fistula**

✖ **47.99 Other**
Anastomosis of appendix

Excludes *diagnostic procedures on appendix (45.21–45.29)*

● **48 Operations on rectum, rectosigmoid, and perirectal tissue**

Code also any application or administration of an adhesion barrier substance (99.77)

✖48.0 **Proctotomy**
Decompression of imperforate anus
Panas' operation [linear proctotomy]

Excludes *incision of perirectal tissue (48.81)*

✖48.1 **Proctostomy**

● 48.2 **Diagnostic procedures on rectum, rectosigmoid, and perirectal tissue**

✖48.21 **Transabdominal proctosigmoidoscopy**
Intraoperative proctosigmoidoscopy

Excludes *that with biopsy (48.24)*

48.22 **Proctosigmoidoscopy through artificial stoma**

Excludes *that with biopsy (48.24)*

48.23 **Rigid proctosigmoidoscopy**

Excludes *flexible sigmoidoscopy (45.24)*

48.24 **Closed [endoscopic] biopsy of rectum**
Brushing or washing for specimen collection
Proctosigmoidoscopy with biopsy

✖48.25 **Open biopsy of rectum**

48.26 **Biopsy of perirectal tissue**

48.29 **Other diagnostic procedures on rectum, rectosigmoid, and perirectal tissue**

Excludes *digital examination of rectum (89.34)*
lower GI series (87.64)
microscopic examination of specimen from rectum (90.91–90.99)

● 48.3 **Local excision or destruction of lesion or tissue of rectum**

48.31 **Radical electrocoagulation of rectal lesion or tissue**

48.32 **Other electrocoagulation of rectal lesion or tissue**

48.33 **Destruction of rectal lesion or tissue by laser**

48.34 **Destruction of rectal lesion or tissue by cryosurgery**

✖48.35 **Local excision of rectal lesion or tissue**

Excludes *biopsy of rectum (48.24–48.25)*
excision of perirectal tissue (48.82)
hemorrhoidectomy (49.46)
[endoscopic] polypectomy of rectum (48.36)
rectal fistulectomy (48.73)

48.36 **[Endoscopic] polypectomy of rectum**

● 48.4 **Pull-through resection of rectum**

Code also any synchronous anastomosis other than end-to-end (45.90, 45.92–45.95)

✖48.41 **Soave submucosal resection of rectum**
Endorectal pull-through operation

✖48.49 **Other pull-through resection of rectum**
Abdominoperineal pull-through
Altemeier operation
Swenson proctectomy

Excludes *Duhamel abdominoperineal pull-through (48.65)*

✖48.5 **Abdominoperineal resection of rectum**
Combined abdominoendorectal resection
Complete proctectomy

Includes: with synchronous colostomy

Code also any synchronous anastomosis other than end-to-end (45.90, 45.92–45.95)

Excludes *Duhamel abdominoperineal pull-through (48.65)*
that as part of pelvic exenteration (68.8)

● 48.6 **Other resection of rectum**

Code also any synchronous anastomosis other than end-to-end (45.90, 45.92–45.95)

✖48.61 **Transsacral rectosigmoidectomy**

✖48.62 **Anterior resection of rectum with synchronous colostomy**

✖48.63 **Other anterior resection of rectum**

Excludes *that with synchronous colostomy (48.62)*

✖48.64 **Posterior resection of rectum**

✖48.65 **Duhamel resection of rectum**
Duhamel abdominoperineal pull-through

✖48.69 **Other**
Partial proctectomy
Rectal resection NOS

● 48.7 **Repair of rectum**

Excludes *repair of:*
current obstetric laceration (75.62)
vaginal rectocele (70.50, 70.52)

✖48.71 **Suture of laceration of rectum**

✖48.72 **Closure of proctostomy**

✖48.73 **Closure of other rectal fistula**

Excludes *fistulectomy:*
perirectal (48.93)
rectourethral (58.43)
rectovaginal (70.73)
rectovesical (57.83)
rectovesicovaginal (57.83)

✖48.74 **Rectorectostomy**
Rectal anastomosis NOS

✖48.75 **Abdominal proctopexy**
Frickman procedure
Ripstein repair of rectal prolapse

✖48.76 **Other proctopexy**
Delorme repair of prolapsed rectum
Proctosigmoidopexy
Puborectalis sling operation

Excludes *manual reduction of rectal prolapse (96.26)*

✖48.79 **Other repair of rectum**
Repair of old obstetric laceration of rectum

Excludes *anastomosis to:*
large intestine (45.94)
small intestine (45.92–45.93)
repair of:
current obstetric laceration (75.62)
vaginal rectocele (70.50, 70.52)

● 48.8 **Incision or excision of perirectal tissue or lesion**

Includes: pelvirectal tissue
rectovaginal septum

✖48.81 **Incision of perirectal tissue**
Incision of rectovaginal septum

✖48.82 **Excision of perirectal tissue**

Excludes *perirectal biopsy (48.26)*
perirectofistulectomy (48.93)
rectal fistulectomy (48.73)

● 48.9 **Other operations on rectum and perirectal tissue**

✖48.91 **Incision of rectal stricture**

✖48.92 **Anorectal myectomy**

✖48.93 **Repair of perirectal fistula**

Excludes *that opening into rectum (48.73)*

✖48.99 **Other**

Excludes *digital examination of rectum (89.34)*
dilation of rectum (96.22)
insertion of rectal tube (96.09)
irrigation of rectum (96.38–96.39)
manual reduction of rectal prolapse (96.26)
proctoclysis (96.37)
rectal massage (99.93)
rectal packing (96.19)
removal of:
impacted feces (96.38)
intraluminal foreign body from rectum without incision (98.05)
rectal packing (97.59)
transanal enema (96.39)

● **49 Operations on anus**

Code also any application or administration of an adhesion barrier substance (99.77)

● **49.0 Incision or excision of perianal tissue**

✖49.01 **Incision of perianal abscess**

✖49.02 **Other incision of perianal tissue**
Undercutting of perianal tissue

Excludes *anal fistulotomy (49.11)*

49.03 **Excision of perianal skin tags**

✖49.04 **Other excision of perianal tissue**

Excludes *anal fistulectomy (49.12)*
biopsy of perianal tissue (49.22)

● **49.1 Incision or excision of anal fistula**

Excludes *closure of anal fistula (49.73)*

✖49.11 **Anal fistulotomy**

✖49.12 **Anal fistulectomy**

● **49.2 Diagnostic procedures on anus and perianal tissue**

49.21 **Anoscopy**

49.22 **Biopsy of perianal tissue**

49.23 **Biopsy of anus**

49.29 **Other diagnostic procedures on anus and perianal tissue**

Excludes *microscopic examination of specimen from anus (90.91–90.99)*

● **49.3 Local excision or destruction of other lesion or tissue of anus**
Anal cryptotomy
Cauterization of lesion of anus

Excludes *biopsy of anus (49.23)*
control of (postoperative) hemorrhage of anus (49.95)
hemorrhoidectomy (49.46)

49.31 **Endoscopic excision or destruction of lesion or tissue of anus**

✖49.39 **Other local excision or destruction of lesion or tissue of anus**

Excludes *that by endoscopic approach (49.31)*

● **49.4 Procedures on hemorrhoids**

49.41 **Reduction of hemorrhoids**

49.42 **Injection of hemorrhoids**

49.43 **Cauterization of hemorrhoids**
Clamp and cautery of hemorrhoids

✖49.44 **Destruction of hemorrhoids by cryotherapy**

✖49.45 **Ligation of hemorrhoids**

✖49.46 **Excision of hemorrhoids**
Hemorrhoidectomy NOS

49.47 **Evacuation of thrombosed hemorrhoids**

✖49.49 **Other procedures on hemorrhoids**
Lord procedure

● **49.5 Division of anal sphincter**

✖49.51 **Left lateral anal sphincterotomy**

✖49.52 **Posterior anal sphincterotomy**

✖49.59 **Other anal sphincterotomy**
Division of sphincter NOS

✖**49.6 Excision of anus**

● **49.7 Repair of anus**

Excludes *repair of current obstetric laceration (75.62)*

✖49.71 **Suture of laceration of anus**

✖49.72 **Anal cerclage**

✖49.73 **Closure of anal fistula**

Excludes *excision of anal fistula (49.12)*

✖49.74 **Gracilis muscle transplant for anal incontinence**

✖49.75 **Implantation or revision of artificial anal sphincter**
Removal with subsequent replacement
Replacement during same or subsequent operative episode

✖49.76 **Removal of artificial anal sphincter**
Explanation or removal without replacement

Excludes *revision with implantation during same operative episode (49.75)*

✖49.79 **Other repair of anal sphincter**
Repair of old obstetric laceration of anus

Excludes *anoplasty with synchronous hemorrhoidectomy (49.46)*
repair of current obstetric laceration (75.62)

● **49.9 Other operations on anus**

Excludes *dilation of anus (sphincter) (96.23)*

✖49.91 **Incision of anal septum**

✖49.92 **Insertion of subcutaneous electrical anal stimulator**

49.93 **Other incision of anus**
Removal of:
foreign body from anus with incision
seton from anus

Excludes *anal fistulotomy (49.11)*
removal of intraluminal foreign body without incision (98.05)

49.94 **Reduction of anal prolapse**

Excludes *manual reduction of rectal prolapse (96.26)*

49.95 **Control of (postoperative) hemorrhage of anus**

49.99 **Other**

● **50 Operations on liver**

Code also any application or administration of an adhesion barrier substance (99.77)

✖**50.0 Hepatotomy**
Incision of abscess of liver
Removal of gallstones from liver
Stromeyer-Little operation

● **50.1 Diagnostic procedures on liver**

50.11 **Closed (percutaneous) [needle] biopsy of liver**
Diagnostic aspiration of liver

✖50.12 **Open biopsy of liver**
Wedge biopsy

✖50.19 **Other diagnostic procedures on liver**
Laparoscopic liver biopsy

Excludes *liver scan and radioisotope function study (92.02)*
microscopic examination of specimen from liver (91.01–91.09)

● **50.2 Local excision or destruction of liver tissue or lesion**

✖ **50.21 Marsupialization of lesion of liver**

✖ **50.22 Partial hepatectomy**
Wedge resection of liver

Excludes *biopsy of liver (50.11–50.12)*
hepatic lobectomy (50.3)

✖ **50.23 Open ablation of liver lesion or tissue** ◀

✖ **50.24 Percutaneous ablation of liver lesion or tissue** ◀

✖ **50.25 Laparoscopic ablation of liver lesion or tissue** ◀

✖ **50.26 Other and unspecified ablation of liver lesion or tissue** ◀

✖ **50.29 Other destruction of lesion of liver**
Cauterization of hepatic lesion
Enucleation of hepatic lesion
Evacuation of hepatic lesion

Excludes *ablation of liver lesion or tissue:* ◀
laparoscopic (50.25) ◀
open (50.23) ◀
other (50.26) ◀
percutaneous (50.24) ◀
percutaneous aspiration of lesion (50.91)

● **50.3 Lobectomy of liver**
Total hepatic lobectomy with partial excision of other lobe

✖ **55.32 Open ablation of renal lesion or tissue** ◀

✖ **55.33 Percutaneous ablation of renal lesion or tissue** ◀

✖ **55.34 Laparoscopic ablation of renal lesion or tissue** ◀

✖ **55.35 Other and unspecified ablation of renal lesion or tissue** ◀

✖ **55.39 Other local excision or destruction of renal lesion or tissue** ◀

Excludes *ablation of renal lesion or tissue:* ◀
laparoscopic (55.34) ◀
open (55.32) ◀
other (55.35) ◀
percutaneous (55.33) ◀

✖ **50.4 Total hepatectomy**

● **50.5 Liver transplant**

Note: To report donor source - *see* codes 00.91–00.93

✖ **50.51 Auxiliary liver transplant**
Auxiliary hepatic transplantation leaving patient's own liver in situ

✖ **50.59 Other transplant of liver**

● **50.6 Repair of liver**

✖ **50.61 Closure of laceration of liver**

✖ **50.69 Other repair of liver**
Hepatopexy

● **50.9 Other operations on liver**

Excludes *lysis of adhesions (54.5)*

50.91 Percutaneous aspiration of liver

Excludes *percutaneous biopsy (50.11)*

50.92 Extracorporeal hepatic assistance

Includes: Liver dialysis

50.93 Localized perfusion of liver

50.94 Other injection of therapeutic substance into liver

50.99 Other

● **51 Operations on gallbladder and biliary tract**

Code also any application or administration of an adhesion barrier substance (99.77)

Includes: operations on:
ampulla of Vater
common bile duct
cystic duct
hepatic duct
intrahepatic bile duct
sphincter of Oddi

● **51.0 Cholecystotomy and cholecystostomy**

51.01 Percutaneous aspiration of gallbladder
Percutaneous cholecystotomy for drainage
That by: needle or catheter

Excludes *needle biopsy (51.12)*

✖ **51.02 Trocar cholecystostomy**

✖ **51.03 Other cholecystostomy**

✖ **51.04 Other cholecystotomy**
Cholelithotomy NOS

● **51.1 Diagnostic procedures on biliary tract**

Excludes *that for endoscopic procedures classifiable to 51.64, 51.84–51.88, 52.14, 52.21, 52.93–52.94, 52.97–52.98*

51.10 Endoscopic retrograde cholangiopancreatography [ERCP]

Excludes *endoscopic retrograde:*
cholangiography [ERC] (51.11)
pancreatography [ERP] (52.13)

51.11 Endoscopic retrograde cholangiography [ERC]
Laparoscopic exploration of common bile duct

Excludes *endoscopic retrograde:*
cholangiopancreatography [ERCP] (51.10)
pancreatography [ERP] (52.13)

51.12 Percutaneous biopsy of gallbladder or bile ducts
Needle biopsy of gallbladder

✖ **51.13 Open biopsy of gallbladder or bile ducts**

51.14 Other closed [endoscopic] biopsy of biliary duct or sphincter of Oddi
Brushing or washing for specimen collection
Closed biopsy of biliary duct or sphincter of Oddi by procedures classifiable to 51.10–51.11, 52.13

51.15 Pressure measurement of sphincter of Oddi
Pressure measurement of sphincter by procedures classifiable to 51.10–51.11, 52.13

✖ **51.19 Other diagnostic procedures on biliary tract**

Excludes *biliary tract x-ray (87.51–87.59)*
microscopic examination of specimen from biliary tract (91.01–91.09)

● **51.2 Cholecystectomy**

✖ **51.21 Other partial cholecystectomy**
Revision of prior cholecystectomy

Excludes *that by laparoscope (51.24)*

✖ **51.22 Cholecystectomy**

Excludes *laparoscopic cholecystectomy (51.23)*

✖ **51.23 Laparoscopic cholecystectomy**
That by laser

✖ **51.24 Laparoscopic partial cholecystectomy**

● **51.3 Anastomosis of gallbladder or bile duct**

Excludes *resection with end-to-end anastomosis (51.61–51.69)*

✖ **51.31 Anastomosis of gallbladder to hepatic ducts**

✖ **51.32 Anastomosis of gallbladder to intestine**

✖ 51.33 **Anastomosis of gallbladder to pancreas**

✖ 51.34 **Anastomosis of gallbladder to stomach**

✖ 51.35 **Other gallbladder anastomosis**
Gallbladder anastomosis NOS

✖ 51.36 **Choledochoenterostomy**

✖ 51.37 **Anastomosis of hepatic duct to gastrointestinal tract**
Kasai portoenterostomy

✖ 51.39 **Other bile duct anastomosis**
Anastomosis of bile duct NOS
Anastomosis of unspecified bile duct to:
intestine
liver
pancreas
stomach

● 51.4 **Incision of bile duct for relief of obstruction**

✖ 51.41 **Common duct exploration for removal of calculus**

Excludes *percutaneous extraction (51.96)*

✖ 51.42 **Common duct exploration for relief of other obstruction**

✖ 51.43 **Insertion of choledochohepatic tube for decompression**
Hepatocholedochostomy

✖ 51.49 **Incision of other bile ducts for relief of obstruction**

● 51.5 **Other incision of bile duct**

Excludes *that for relief of obstruction (51.41–51.49)*

✖ 51.51 **Exploration of common duct**
Incision of common bile duct

✖ 51.59 **Incision of other bile duct**

● 51.6 **Local excision or destruction of lesion or tissue of biliary ducts and sphincter of Oddi**

Code also anastomosis other than end-to-end (51.31, 51.36–51.39)

Excludes *biopsy of bile duct (51.12–51.13)*

✖ 51.61 **Excision of cystic duct remnant**

✖ 51.62 **Excision of ampulla of Vater (with reimplantation of common duct)**

✖ 51.63 **Other excision of common duct**
Choledochectomy

Excludes *fistulectomy (51.72)*

51.64 **Endoscopic excision or destruction of lesion of biliary ducts or sphincter of Oddi**
Excision or destruction of lesion of biliary duct by procedures classifiable to 51.10–51.11, 52.13

✖ 51.69 **Excision of other bile duct**
Excision of lesion of bile duct NOS

Excludes *fistulectomy (51.79)*

● 51.7 **Repair of bile ducts**

✖ 51.71 **Simple suture of common bile duct**

✖ 51.72 **Choledochoplasty**
Repair of fistula of common bile duct

✖ 51.79 **Repair of other bile ducts**
Closure of artificial opening of bile duct NOS
Suture of bile duct NOS

Excludes *operative removal of prosthetic device (51.95)*

● 51.8 **Other operations on biliary ducts and sphincter of Oddi**

✖ 51.81 **Dilation of sphincter of Oddi**
Dilation of ampulla of Vater

Excludes *that by endoscopic approach (51.84)*

✖ 51.82 **Pancreatic sphincterotomy**
Incision of pancreatic sphincter
Transduodenal ampullary sphincterotomy

Excludes *that by endoscopic approach (51.85)*

✖ 51.83 **Pancreatic sphincteroplasty**

51.84 **Endoscopic dilation of ampulla and biliary duct**
Dilation of ampulla and biliary duct by procedures classifiable to 51.10–51.11, 52.13

51.85 **Endoscopic sphincterotomy and papillotomy**
Sphincterotomy and papillotomy by procedures classifiable to 51.10–51.11, 52.13

51.86 **Endoscopic insertion of nasobiliary drainage tube**
Insertion of nasobiliary tube by procedures classifiable to 51.10–51.11, 52.13

51.87 **Endoscopic insertion of stent (tube) into bile duct**
Endoprosthesis of bile duct
Insertion of stent into bile duct by procedures classifiable to 51.10–51.11, 52.13

Excludes *nasobiliary drainage tube (51.86)*
replacement of stent (tube) (97.05)

51.88 **Endoscopic removal of stone(s) from biliary tract**
Laparoscopic removal of stone(s) from biliary tract
Removal of biliary tract stone(s) by procedures classifiable to 51.10–51.11, 52.13

Excludes *percutaneous extraction of common duct stones (51.96)*

✖ 51.89 **Other operations on sphincter of Oddi**

● 51.9 **Other operations on biliary tract**

✖ 51.91 **Repair of laceration of gallbladder**

✖ 51.92 **Closure of cholecystostomy**

✖ 51.93 **Closure of other biliary fistula**
Cholecystogastroenteric fistulectomy

✖ 51.94 **Revision of anastomosis of biliary tract**

✖ 51.95 **Removal of prosthetic device from bile duct**

Excludes *nonoperative removal (97.55)*

51.96 **Percutaneous extraction of common duct stones**

51.98 **Other percutaneous procedures on biliary tract**
Percutaneous biliary endoscopy via existing T-tube or other tract for:
dilation of biliary duct stricture
removal of stone(s) except common duct stone
exploration (postoperative)
Percutaneous transhepatic biliary drainage

Excludes *percutaneous aspiration of gallbladder (51.01)*
percutaneous biopsy and/or collection of specimen by brushing or washing (51.12)
percutaneous removal of common duct stone(s) (51.96)

✖ 51.99 **Other**
Insertion or replacement of biliary tract prosthesis

Excludes *biopsy of gallbladder (51.12–51.13)*
irrigation of cholecystostomy and other biliary tube (96.41)
lysis of peritoneal adhesions (54.5)
nonoperative removal of:
cholecystostomy tube (97.54)
tube from biliary tract or liver (97.55)

● 52 **Operations on pancreas**

Code also any application or administration of an adhesion barrier substance (99.77)

Includes: operations on pancreatic duct

● 52.0 **Pancreatotomy**

✖ 52.01 **Drainage of pancreatic cyst by catheter**

✖ 52.09 **Other pancreatotomy**
Pancreatolithotomy

Excludes *drainage by anastomosis (52.4, 52.96)*
incision of pancreatic sphincter (51.82)
marsupialization of cyst (52.3)

● 52.1 **Diagnostic procedures on pancreas**

52.11 **Closed [aspiration] [needle] [percutaneous] biopsy of pancreas**

✖ 52.12 **Open biopsy of pancreas**

52.13 **Endoscopic retrograde pancreatography [ERP]**

Excludes *endoscopic retrograde:*
cholangiography [ERC] (51.11)
cholangiopancreatography [ERCP] (51.10)
that for procedures classifiable to 51.14–51.15, 51.64, 51.84–51.88, 52.14, 52.21, 52.92–52.94, 52.97–52.98

52.14 **Closed [endoscopic] biopsy of pancreatic duct**
Closed biopsy of pancreatic duct by procedures classifiable to 51.10–51.11, 52.13

✖ 52.19 **Other diagnostic procedures on pancreas**

Excludes *contrast pancreatogram (87.66)*
endoscopic retrograde pancreatography [ERP] (52.13)
microscopic examination of specimen from pancreas (91.01–91.09)

● 52.2 **Local excision or destruction of pancreas and pancreatic duct**

Excludes *biopsy of pancreas (52.11–52.12, 52.14)*
pancreatic fistulectomy (52.95)

52.21 **Endoscopic excision or destruction of lesion or tissue of pancreatic duct**
Excision or destruction of lesion or tissue of pancreatic duct by procedures classifiable to 51.10–51.11, 52.13

✖ 52.22 **Other excision or destruction of lesion or tissue of pancreas or pancreatic duct**

✖ 52.3 **Marsupialization of pancreatic cyst**

Excludes *drainage of cyst by catheter (52.01)*

✖ 52.4 **Internal drainage of pancreatic cyst**
Pancreaticocystoduodenostomy
Pancreaticocystogastrostomy
Pancreaticocystojejunostomy

● 52.5 **Partial pancreatectomy**

Excludes *pancreatic fistulectomy (52.95)*

✖ 52.51 **Proximal pancreatectomy**
Excision of head of pancreas (with part of body)
Proximal pancreatectomy with synchronous duodenectomy

✖ 52.52 **Distal pancreatectomy**
Excision of tail of pancreas (with part of body)

✖ 52.53 **Radical subtotal pancreatectomy**

✖ 52.59 **Other partial pancreatectomy**

✖ 52.6 **Total pancreatectomy**
Pancreatectomy with synchronous duodenectomy

✖ 52.7 **Radical pancreaticoduodenectomy**
One-stage pancreaticoduodenal resection with choledochojejunal anastomosis, pancreaticojejunal anastomosis, and gastrojejunostomy
Two-stage pancreaticoduodenal resection (first stage) (second stage)
Radical resection of the pancreas
Whipple procedure

Excludes *radical subtotal pancreatectomy (52.53)*

● 52.8 **Transplant of pancreas**

Note: To report donor source - *see* codes 00.91–00.93

✖ 52.80 **Pancreatic transplant, not otherwise specified**

✖ 52.81 **Reimplantation of pancreatic tissue**

✖ 52.82 **Homotransplant of pancreas**

✖ 52.83 **Heterotransplant of pancreas**

52.84 **Autotransplantation of cells of Islets of Langerhans**
Homotransplantation of islet cells of pancreas

52.85 **Allotransplantation of cells of Islets of Langerhans**
Heterotransplantation of islet cells of pancreas

✖ 52.86 **Transplantation of cells of Islets of Langerhans, not otherwise specified**

● 52.9 **Other operations on pancreas**

✖ 52.92 **Cannulation of pancreatic duct**

Excludes *that by endoscopic approach (52.93)*

52.93 **Endoscopic insertion of stent (tube) into pancreatic duct**
Insertion of cannula or stent into pancreatic duct by procedures classifiable to 51.10–51.11, 52.13

Excludes *endoscopic insertion of nasopancreatic drainage tube (52.97)*
replacement of stent (tube) (97.05)

52.94 **Endoscopic removal of stone(s) from pancreatic duct**
Removal of stone(s) from pancreatic duct by procedures classifiable to 51.10–51.11, 52.13

✖ 52.95 **Other repair of pancreas**
Fistulectomy of pancreas
Simple suture of pancreas

✖ 52.96 **Anastomosis of pancreas**
Anastomosis of pancreas (duct) to:
intestine
jejunum
stomach

Excludes *anastomosis to:*
bile duct (51.39)
gallbladder (51.33)

52.97 **Endoscopic insertion of nasopancreatic drainage tube**
Insertion of nasopancreatic drainage tube by procedures classifiable to 51.10–51.11, 52.13

Excludes *drainage of pancreatic cyst by catheter (52.01)*
replacement of stent (tube) (97.05)

52.98 **Endoscopic dilation of pancreatic duct**
Dilation of Wirsung's duct by procedures classifiable to 51.10–51.11, 52.13

✖ 52.99 **Other**
Dilation of pancreatic [Wirsung's] duct by open approach
Repair of pancreatic [Wirsung's] duct by open approach

Excludes *irrigation of pancreatic tube (96.42)*
removal of pancreatic tube (97.56)

● 53 **Repair of hernia**

Code also any application or administration of an adhesion barrier substance (99.77)

Includes: hernioplasty
herniorrhaphy

Excludes *manual reduction of hernia (96.27)*

● 53.0 **Unilateral repair of inguinal hernia**

✖ 53.00 **Unilateral repair of inguinal hernia, not otherwise specified**
Inguinal herniorrhaphy NOS

✖ 53.01 **Repair of direct inguinal hernia**

✖ 53.02 **Repair of indirect inguinal hernia**

✖ 53.03 **Repair of direct inguinal hernia with graft or prosthesis**

✖ 53.04 **Repair of indirect inguinal hernia with graft or prosthesis**

✖ 53.05 **Repair of inguinal hernia with graft or prosthesis, not otherwise specified**

● 53.1 **Bilateral repair of inguinal hernia**

✖ 53.10 **Bilateral repair of inguinal hernia, not otherwise specified**

✖ 53.11 **Bilateral repair of direct inguinal hernia**

✖ 53.12 **Bilateral repair of indirect inguinal hernia**

✖ 53.13 **Bilateral repair of inguinal hernia, one direct and one indirect**

✖ 53.14 **Bilateral repair of direct inguinal hernia with graft or prosthesis**

✖ 53.15 **Bilateral repair of indirect inguinal hernia with graft or prosthesis**

✖ 53.16 **Bilateral repair of inguinal hernia, one direct and one indirect, with graft or prosthesis**

✖ 53.17 **Bilateral inguinal hernia repair with graft or prosthesis, not otherwise specified**

● 53.2 **Unilateral repair of femoral hernia**

✖ 53.21 **Unilateral repair of femoral hernia with graft or prosthesis**

✖ 53.29 **Other unilateral femoral herniorrhaphy**

● 53.3 **Bilateral repair of femoral hernia**

✖ 53.31 **Bilateral repair of femoral hernia with graft or prosthesis**

✖ 53.39 **Other bilateral femoral herniorrhaphy**

● 53.4 **Repair of umbilical hernia**

Excludes *repair of gastroschisis (54.71)*

✖ 53.41 **Repair of umbilical hernia with prosthesis**

✖ 53.49 **Other umbilical herniorrhaphy**

● 53.5 **Repair of other hernia of anterior abdominal wall (without graft or prosthesis)**

✖ 53.51 **Incisional hernia repair**

✖ 53.59 **Repair of other hernia of anterior abdominal wall**
Repair of hernia:
epigastric
hypogastric
spigelian
ventral

● 53.6 **Repair of other hernia of anterior abdominal wall with graft or prosthesis**

✖ 53.61 **Incisional hernia repair with prosthesis**

✖ 53.69 **Repair of other hernia of anterior abdominal wall with prosthesis**

✖ 53.7 **Repair of diaphragmatic hernia, abdominal approach**

● 53.8 **Repair of diaphragmatic hernia, thoracic approach**

✖ 53.80 **Repair of diaphragmatic hernia with thoracic approach, not otherwise specified**
Thoracoabdominal repair of diaphragmatic hernia

✖ 53.81 **Plication of the diaphragm**

✖ 53.82 **Repair of parasternal hernia**

✖ 53.9 **Other hernia repair**
Repair of hernia:
ischiatic
ischiorectal
lumbar
obturator
Repair of hernia:
omental
retroperitoneal
sciatic

Excludes *relief of strangulated hernia with exteriorization of intestine (46.01, 46.03)*
repair of pericolostomy hernia (46.42)
repair of vaginal enterocele (70.92)

● 54 **Other operations on abdominal region**

Code also any application or administration of an adhesion barrier substance (99.77)

Includes: operations on:
epigastric region
flank
groin region
hypochondrium
inguinal region
loin region
male pelvic cavity
mesentery
omentum
peritoneum
retroperitoneal tissue space

Excludes *female pelvic cavity (69.01–70.92)*
hernia repair (53.00–53.9)
obliteration of cul-de-sac (70.92)
retroperitoneal tissue dissection (59.00–59.09)
skin and subcutaneous tissue of abdominal wall (86.01–86.99)

✖ 54.0 **Incision of abdominal wall**
Drainage of:
abdominal wall
extraperitoneal abscess
retroperitoneal abscess

Excludes *incision of peritoneum (54.95)*
laparotomy (54.11–54.19)

● 54.1 **Laparotomy**

✖ 54.11 **Exploratory laparotomy**

Excludes *exploration incidental to intra-abdominal surgery—omit code*

✖ 54.12 **Reopening of recent laparotomy site**
Reopening of recent laparotomy site for:
control of hemorrhage
exploration
incision of hematoma

✖ 54.19 **Other laparotomy**
Drainage of intraperitoneal abscess or hematoma

Excludes *culdocentesis (70.0)*
drainage of appendiceal abscess (47.2)
exploration incidental to intra-abdominal surgery—omit code
Ladd operation (54.95)
percutaneous drainage of abdomen (54.91)
removal of foreign body (54.92)

● 54.2 **Diagnostic procedures of abdominal region**

✖ 54.21 **Laparoscopy**
Peritoneoscopy

Excludes *laparoscopic cholecystectomy (51.23)*
that incidental to destruction of fallopian tubes (66.21–66.29)

✖ 54.22 **Biopsy of abdominal wall or umbilicus**

✖ **54.23 Biopsy of peritoneum**
Biopsy of:
mesentery
omentum
peritoneal implant

Excludes *closed biopsy of:*
omentum (54.24)
peritoneum (54.24)

54.24 Closed [percutaneous] [needle] biopsy of intra-abdominal mass
Closed biopsy of:
omentum
peritoneal implant
peritoneum

Excludes *that of:*
fallopian tube (66.11)
ovary (65.11)
uterine ligaments (68.15)
uterus (68.16)

54.25 Peritoneal lavage
Diagnostic peritoneal lavage

Excludes *peritoneal dialysis (54.98)*

✖ **54.29 Other diagnostic procedures on abdominal region**

Excludes *abdominal lymphangiogram (88.04)*
abdominal x-ray NEC (88.19)
angiocardiography of venae cava (88.51)
C.A.T. scan of abdomen (88.01)
contrast x-ray of abdominal cavity (88.11–88.15)
intra-abdominal arteriography NEC (88.47)
microscopic examination of peritoneal and retroperitoneal specimen (91.11–91.19)
phlebography of:
intra-abdominal vessels NEC (88.65)
portal venous system (88.64)
sinogram of abdominal wall (88.03)
soft tissue x-ray of abdominal wall NEC (88.09)
tomography of abdomen NEC (88.02)
ultrasonography of abdomen and retroperitoneum (88.76)

✖ **54.3 Excision or destruction of lesion or tissue of abdominal wall or umbilicus**
Debridement of abdominal wall
Omphalectomy

Excludes *biopsy of abdominal wall or umbilicus (54.22)*
size reduction operation (86.83)
that of skin of abdominal wall (86.22, 86.26, 86.3)

✖ **54.4 Excision or destruction of peritoneal tissue**
Excision of:
appendices epiploicae
falciform ligament
gastrocolic ligament
lesion of:
mesentery
omentum
peritoneum
presacral lesion NOS
retroperitoneal lesion NOS

Excludes *biopsy of peritoneum (54.23)*
endometrectomy of cul-de-sac (70.32)

54.5 Lysis of peritoneal adhesions
Freeing of adhesions of:
biliary tract
intestines
liver
pelvic peritoneum
peritoneum
spleen
uterus

Excludes *lysis of adhesions of:*
bladder (59.11)
fallopian tube and ovary
laparoscopic (65.81)
other (65.89)
kidney (59.02)
ureter (59.02)

✖ **54.51 Laparoscopic lysis of peritoneal adhesions**

✖ **54.59 Other lysis of peritoneal adhesions**

● **54.6 Suture of abdominal wall and peritoneum**

✖ **54.61 Reclosure of postoperative disruption of abdominal wall**

✖ **54.62 Delayed closure of granulating abdominal wound**
Tertiary subcutaneous wound closure

✖ **54.63 Other suture of abdominal wall**
Suture of laceration of abdominal wall

Excludes *closure of operative wound—omit code*

✖ **54.64 Suture of peritoneum**
Secondary suture of peritoneum

Excludes *closure of operative wound—omit code*

● **54.7 Other repair of abdominal wall and peritoneum**

✖ **54.71 Repair of gastroschisis**

✖ **54.72 Other repair of abdominal wall**

✖ **54.73 Other repair of peritoneum**
Suture of gastrocolic ligament

✖ **54.74 Other repair of omentum**
Epiplorrhaphy
Graft of omentum
Omentopexy
Reduction of torsion of omentum

Excludes *cardio-omentopexy (36.39)*

✖ **54.75 Other repair of mesentery**
Mesenteric plication
Mesenteropexy

● **54.9 Other operations of abdominal region**

Excludes *removal of ectopic pregnancy (74.3)*

54.91 Percutaneous abdominal drainage
Paracentesis

Excludes *creation of cutaneoperitoneal fistula (54.93)*

✖ **54.92 Removal of foreign body from peritoneal cavity**

✖ **54.93 Creation of cutaneoperitoneal fistula**

✖ **54.94 Creation of peritoneovascular shunt**
Peritoneovenous shunt

✖ **54.95 Incision of peritoneum**
Exploration of ventriculoperitoneal shunt at peritoneal site
Ladd operation
Revision of distal catheter of ventricular shunt
Revision of ventriculoperitoneal shunt at peritoneal site

Excludes *that incidental to laparotomy (54.11–54.19)*

54.96 Injection of air into peritoneal cavity
Pneumoperitoneum

Excludes *that for:*
collapse of lung (33.33)
radiography (88.12–88.13, 88.15)

54.97 Injection of locally-acting therapeutic substance into peritoneal cavity

Excludes *peritoneal dialysis (54.98)*

54.98 Peritoneal dialysis

Excludes *peritoneal lavage (diagnostic) (54.25)*

54.99 Other

Excludes *removal of:*
abdominal wall suture (97.83)
peritoneal drainage device (97.82)
retroperitoneal drainage device (97.81)

10. OPERATIONS ON THE URINARY SYSTEM (55–59)

● 55 **Operations on kidney**

Code also any application or administration of an adhesion barrier substance (99.77)

Includes: operations on renal pelvis

Excludes *perirenal tissue (59.00–59.09, 59.21–59.29, 59.91–59.92)*

● 55.0 **Nephrotomy and nephrostomy**

Excludes *drainage by:*
anastomosis (55.86)
aspiration (55.92)
incision of kidney pelvis (55.11–55.12)

✖ 55.01 **Nephrotomy**
Evacuation of renal cyst
Exploration of kidney
Nephrolithotomy

✖ 55.02 **Nephrostomy**

✖ 55.03 **Percutaneous nephrostomy without fragmentation**
Nephrostolithotomy, percutaneous (nephroscopic)
Percutaneous removal of kidney stone(s) by:
basket extraction
forceps extraction (nephroscopic)
Pyelostolithotomy, percutaneous (nephroscopic)
With placement of catheter down ureter

Excludes *percutaneous removal by fragmentation (55.04)*
repeat nephroscopic removal during current episode (55.92)

✖ 55.04 **Percutaneous nephrostomy with fragmentation**
Percutaneous nephrostomy with disruption of kidney stone by ultrasonic energy and extraction (suction) through endoscope
With placement of catheter down ureter
With fluoroscopic guidance

Excludes *repeat fragmentation during current episode (59.95)*

● 55.1 **Pyelotomy and pyelostomy**

Excludes *drainage by anastomosis (55.86)*
percutaneous pyelostolithotomy (55.03)
removal of calculus without incision (56.0)

✖ 55.11 **Pyelotomy**
Exploration of renal pelvis
Pyelolithotomy

✖ 55.12 **Pyelostomy**
Insertion of drainage tube into renal pelvis

● 55.2 **Diagnostic procedures on kidney**

55.21 **Nephroscopy**

55.22 **Pyeloscopy**

55.23 **Closed [percutaneous] [needle] biopsy of kidney**
Endoscopic biopsy via existing nephrostomy, nephrotomy, pyelostomy, or pyelotomy

✖ 55.24 **Open biopsy of kidney**

✖ 55.29 **Other diagnostic procedures on kidney**

Excludes *microscopic examination of specimen from kidney (91.21–91.29)*
pyelogram:
intravenous (87.73)
percutaneous (87.75)
retrograde (87.74)
radioisotope scan (92.03)
renal arteriography (88.45)
tomography:
C.A.T. scan (87.71)
other (87.72)

● 55.3 **Local excision or destruction of lesion or tissue of kidney**

✖ 55.31 **Marsupialization of kidney lesion**

✖ 55.39 **Other local destruction or excision of renal lesion or tissue**
Obliteration of calyceal diverticulum

Excludes *biopsy of kidney (55.23–55.24)*
partial nephrectomy (55.4)
percutaneous aspiration of kidney (55.92)
wedge resection of kidney (55.4)

✖ 55.4 **Partial nephrectomy**
Calycectomy
Wedge resection of kidney

Code also any synchronous resection of ureter (56.40–56.42)

● 55.5 **Complete nephrectomy**

Code also any synchronous excision of:
adrenal gland (07.21–07.3)
bladder segment (57.6)
lymph nodes (40.3, 40.52–40.59)

✖ 55.51 **Nephroureterectomy**
Nephroureterectomy with bladder cuff
Total nephrectomy (unilateral)

Excludes *removal of transplanted kidney (55.53)*

✖ 55.52 **Nephrectomy of remaining kidney**
Removal of solitary kidney

Excludes *removal of transplanted kidney (55.53)*

✖ 55.53 **Removal of transplanted or rejected kidney**

✖ 55.54 **Bilateral nephrectomy**

Excludes *complete nephrectomy NOS (55.51)*

● 55.6 **Transplant of kidney**

Note: To report donor source - *see* codes 00.91–00.93

✖ 55.61 **Renal autotransplantation**

✖ 55.69 **Other kidney transplantation**

✖ 55.7 **Nephropexy**
Fixation or suspension of movable [floating] kidney

● 55.8 **Other repair of kidney**

✖ 55.81 **Suture of laceration of kidney**

✖ 55.82 **Closure of nephrostomy and pyelostomy**

✖ 55.83 **Closure of other fistula of kidney**

✖ 55.84 **Reduction of torsion of renal pedicle**

✖ 55.85 **Symphysiotomy for horseshoe kidney**

✖ 55.86 **Anastomosis of kidney**
Nephropyeloureterostomy
Pyeloureterovesical anastomosis
Ureterocalyceal anastomosis

Excludes *nephrocystanastomosis NOS (56.73)*

✖ 55.87 **Correction of ureteropelvic junction**

✖ 55.89 **Other**

● 55.9 **Other operations on kidney**

Excludes *lysis of perirenal adhesions (59.02)*

✖ 55.91 **Decapsulation of kidney**
Capsulectomy of kidney
Decortication of kidney

55.92 **Percutaneous aspiration of kidney (pelvis)**
Aspiration of renal cyst
Renipuncture

Excludes *percutaneous biopsy of kidney (55.23)*

55.93 **Replacement of nephrostomy tube**

55.94 **Replacement of pyelostomy tube**

55.95 **Local perfusion of kidney**

55.96 **Other injection of therapeutic substance into kidney**
Injection into renal cyst

✖55.97 **Implantation or replacement of mechanical kidney**

✖55.98 **Removal of mechanical kidney**

✖55.99 **Other**
Excludes *removal of pyelostomy or nephrostomy tube (97.61)*

● 56 **Operations on ureter**
Code also any application or administration of an adhesion barrier substance (99.77)

✖56.0 **Transurethral removal of obstruction from ureter and renal pelvis**
Removal of:
blood clot from ureter or renal pelvis without incision
calculus from ureter or renal pelvis without incision
foreign body from ureter or renal pelvis without incision
Excludes *manipulation without removal of obstruction (59.8)*
that by incision (55.11, 56.2)
transurethral insertion of ureteral stent for passage of calculus (59.8)

✖56.1 **Ureteral meatotomy**

✖56.2 **Ureterotomy**
Incision of ureter for:
drainage
exploration
removal of calculus
Excludes *cutting of ureterovesical orifice (56.1)*
removal of calculus without incision (56.0)
transurethral insertion of ureteral stent for passage of calculus (59.8)
urinary diversion (56.51–56.79)

● 56.3 **Diagnostic procedures on ureter**

56.31 **Ureteroscopy**

56.32 **Closed percutaneous biopsy of ureter**
Excludes *endoscopic biopsy of ureter (56.33)*

56.33 **Closed endoscopic biopsy of ureter**
Cystourethroscopy with ureteral biopsy
Transurethral biopsy of ureter
Ureteral endoscopy with biopsy through ureterotomy
Ureteroscopy with biopsy
Excludes *percutaneous biopsy of ureter (56.32)*

✖56.34 **Open biopsy of ureter**

56.35 **Endoscopy (cystoscopy) (looposcopy) of ileal conduit**

✖56.39 **Other diagnostic procedures on ureter**
Excludes *microscopic examination of specimen from ureter (91.21–91.29)*

● 56.4 **Ureterectomy**
Code also anastomosis other than end-to-end (56.51–56.79)
Excludes *fistulectomy (56.84)*
nephroureterectomy (55.51–55.54)

✖56.40 **Ureterectomy, not otherwise specified**

✖56.41 **Partial ureterectomy**
Excision of lesion of ureter
Shortening of ureter with reimplantation
Excludes *biopsy of ureter (56.32–56.34)*

✖56.42 **Total ureterectomy**

● 56.5 **Cutaneous uretero-ileostomy**

✖56.51 **Formation of cutaneous uretero-ileostomy**
Construction of ileal conduit
External ureteral ileostomy
Formation of open ileal bladder
Ileal loop operation
Ileoureterostomy (Bricker's) (ileal bladder)
Transplantation of ureter into ileum with external diversion
Excludes *closed ileal bladder (57.87)*
replacement of ureteral defect by ileal segment (56.89)

✖56.52 **Revision of cutaneous uretero-ileostomy**

● 56.6 **Other external urinary diversion**

✖56.61 **Formation of other cutaneous ureterostomy**
Anastomosis of ureter to skin
Ureterostomy NOS

✖56.62 **Revision of other cutaneous ureterostomy**
Revision of ureterostomy stoma
Excludes *nonoperative removal of ureterostomy tube (97.62)*

● 56.7 **Other anastomosis or bypass of ureter**
Excludes *ureteropyelostomy (55.86)*

✖56.71 **Urinary diversion to intestine**
Anastomosis of ureter to intestine
Internal urinary diversion NOS
Code also any synchronous colostomy (46.10–46.13)
Excludes *external ureteral ileostomy (56.51)*

✖56.72 **Revision of ureterointestinal anastomosis**
Excludes *revision of external ureteral ileostomy (56.52)*

✖56.73 **Nephrocystanastomosis, not otherwise specified**

✖56.74 **Ureteroneocystostomy**
Replacement of ureter with bladder flap
Ureterovesical anastomosis

✖56.75 **Transureteroureterostomy**
Excludes *ureteroureterostomy associated with partial resection (56.41)*

✖56.79 **Other**

● 56.8 **Repair of ureter**

✖56.81 **Lysis of intraluminal adhesions of ureter**
Excludes *lysis of periureteral adhesions (59.01–59.02)*
ureterolysis (59.01–59.02)

✖56.82 **Suture of laceration of ureter**

✖56.83 **Closure of ureterostomy**

✖56.84 **Closure of other fistula of ureter**

✖56.85 **Ureteropexy**

✖56.86 **Removal of ligature from ureter**

✖56.89 **Other repair of ureter**
Graft of ureter
Replacement of ureter with ileal segment implanted into bladder
Ureteroplication

● 56.9 **Other operations on ureter**

56.91 **Dilation of ureteral meatus**

✖56.92 **Implantation of electronic ureteral stimulator**

✖56.93 **Replacement of electronic ureteral stimulator**

✖56.94 **Removal of electronic ureteral stimulator**
Excludes *that with synchronous replacement (56.93)*

✖56.95 **Ligation of ureter**

✖56.99 **Other**
Excludes *removal of ureterostomy tube and ureteral catheter (97.62)*
ureteral catheterization (59.8)

● **57 Operations on urinary bladder**

Code also any application or administration of an adhesion barrier substance (99.77)

Excludes *perivesical tissue (59.11–59.29, 59.91–59.92)*
ureterovesical orifice (56.0–56.99)

57.0 Transurethral clearance of bladder
Drainage of bladder without incision
Removal of:
blood clots from bladder without incision
calculus from bladder without incision
foreign body from bladder without incision

Excludes *that by incision (57.19)*

● **57.1 Cystotomy and cystostomy**

Excludes *cystotomy and cystostomy as operative approach—omit code*

57.11 Percutaneous aspiration of bladder

✖ **57.12 Lysis of intraluminal adhesions with incision into bladder**

Excludes *transurethral lysis of intraluminal adhesions (57.41)*

57.17 Percutaneous cystostomy
Closed cystostomy
Percutaneous suprapubic cystostomy

Excludes *removal of cystostomy tube (97.63)*
replacement of cystostomy tube (59.94)

✖ **57.18 Other suprapubic cystostomy**

Excludes *percutaneous cystostomy (57.17)*
removal of cystostomy tube (97.63)
replacement of cystostomy tube (59.94)

✖ **57.19 Other cystotomy**
Cystolithotomy

Excludes *percutaneous cystostomy (57.17)*
suprapubic cystostomy (57.18)

● **57.2 Vesicostomy**

Excludes *percutaneous cystostomy (57.17)*
suprapubic cystostomy (57.18)

✖ **57.21 Vesicostomy**
Creation of permanent opening from bladder to skin using a bladder flap

✖ **57.22 Revision or closure of vesicostomy**

Excludes *closure of cystostomy (57.82)*

● **57.3 Diagnostic procedures on bladder**

57.31 Cystoscopy through artificial stoma

57.32 Other cystoscopy
Transurethral cystoscopy

Excludes *cystourethroscopy with ureteral biopsy (56.33)*
retrograde pyelogram (87.74)
that for control of hemorrhage (postoperative):
bladder (57.93)
prostate (60.94)

✖ **57.33 Closed [transurethral] biopsy of bladder**

✖ **57.34 Open biopsy of bladder**

✖ **57.39 Other diagnostic procedures on bladder**

Excludes *cystogram NEC (87.77)*
microscopic examination of specimen from bladder (91.31–91.39)
retrograde cystourethrogram (87.76)
therapeutic distention of bladder (96.25)

● **57.4 Transurethral excision or destruction of bladder tissue**

✖ **57.41 Transurethral lysis of intraluminal adhesions**

✖ **57.49 Other transurethral excision or destruction of lesion or tissue of bladder**
Endoscopic resection of bladder lesion

Excludes *transurethral biopsy of bladder (57.33)*
transurethral fistulectomy (57.83–57.84)

● **57.5 Other excision or destruction of bladder tissue**

Excludes *that with transurethral approach (57.41–57.49)*

✖ **57.51 Excision of urachus**
Excision of urachal sinus of bladder

Excludes *excision of urachal cyst of abdominal wall (54.3)*

✖ **57.59 Open excision or destruction of other lesion or tissue of bladder**
Endometrectomy of bladder
Suprapubic excision of bladder lesion

Excludes *biopsy of bladder (57.33–57.34)*
fistulectomy of bladder (57.83–57.84)

✖ **57.6 Partial cystectomy**
Excision of bladder dome
Trigonectomy
Wedge resection of bladder

● **57.7 Total cystectomy**

Includes: total cystectomy with urethrectomy

✖ **57.71 Radical cystectomy**
Pelvic exenteration in male
Removal of bladder, prostate, seminal vesicles, and fat
Removal of bladder, urethra, and fat in a female

Code also any:
lymph node dissection (40.3, 40.5)
urinary diversion (56.51–56.79)

Excludes *that as part of pelvic exenteration in female (68.8)*

✖ **57.79 Other total cystectomy**

● **57.8 Other repair of urinary bladder**

Excludes *repair of:*
current obstetric laceration (75.61)
cystocele (70.50–70.51)
that for stress incontinence (59.3–59.79)

✖ **57.81 Suture of laceration of bladder**

✖ **57.82 Closure of cystostomy**

✖ **57.83 Repair of fistula involving bladder and intestine**
Rectovesicovaginal fistulectomy
Vesicosigmoidovaginal fistulectomy

✖ **57.84 Repair of other fistula of bladder**
Cervicovesical fistulectomy
Urethroperineovesical fistulectomy
Uterovesical fistulectomy
Vaginovesical fistulectomy

Excludes *vesicoureterovaginal fistulectomy (56.84)*

✖ **57.85 Cystourethroplasty and plastic repair of bladder neck**
Plication of sphincter of urinary bladder
V-Y plasty of bladder neck

✖ **57.86 Repair of bladder exstrophy**

✖ **57.87 Reconstruction of urinary bladder**
Anastomosis of bladder with isolated segment of ileum
Augmentation of bladder
Replacement of bladder with ileum or sigmoid [closed ileal bladder]

Code also resection of intestine (45.50–45.52)

✖ **57.88 Other anastomosis of bladder**
Anastomosis of bladder to intestine NOS
Cystocolic anastomosis

Excludes *formation of closed ileal bladder (57.87)*

✖ **57.89 Other repair of bladder**
Bladder suspension, not elsewhere classified
Cystopexy NOS
Repair of old obstetric laceration of bladder

Excludes *repair of current obstetric laceration (75.61)*

● 57.9 **Other operations on bladder**

✖ 57.91 **Sphincterotomy of bladder**
Division of bladder neck

57.92 **Dilation of bladder neck**

✖ 57.93 **Control of (postoperative) hemorrhage of bladder**

57.94 **Insertion of indwelling urinary catheter**

57.95 **Replacement of indwelling urinary catheter**

✖ 57.96 **Implantation of electronic bladder stimulator**

✖ 57.97 **Replacement of electronic bladder stimulator**

✖ 57.98 **Removal of electronic bladder stimulator**

Excludes *that with synchronous replacement (57.97)*

✖ 57.99 **Other**

Excludes *irrigation of:*
cystostomy (96.47)
other indwelling urinary catheter (96.48)
lysis of external adhesions (59.11)
removal of:
cystostomy tube (97.63)
other urinary drainage device (97.64)
therapeutic distention of bladder (96.25)

● 58 **Operations on urethra**

Code also any application or administration of an adhesion barrier substance (99.77)

Includes: operations on:
bulbourethral gland [Cowper's gland]
periurethral tissue

✖ 58.0 **Urethrotomy**
Excision of urethral septum
Formation of urethrovaginal fistula
Perineal urethrostomy
Removal of calculus from urethra by incision

Excludes *drainage of bulbourethral gland or periurethral tissue (58.91)*
internal urethral meatotomy (58.5)
removal of urethral calculus without incision (58.6)

✖ 58.1 **Urethral meatotomy**

Excludes *internal urethral meatotomy (58.5)*

● 58.2 **Diagnostic procedures on urethra**

58.21 **Perineal urethroscopy**

58.22 **Other urethroscopy**

58.23 **Biopsy of urethra**

58.24 **Biopsy of periurethral tissue**

58.29 **Other diagnostic procedures on urethra and periurethral tissue**

Excludes *microscopic examination of specimen from urethra (91.31–91.39)*
retrograde cystourethrogram (87.76)
urethral pressure profile (89.25)
urethral sphincter electromyogram (89.23)

● 58.3 **Excision or destruction of lesion or tissue of urethra**

Excludes *biopsy of urethra (58.23)*
excision of bulbourethral gland (58.92)
fistulectomy (58.43)
urethrectomy as part of:
complete cystectomy (57.79)
pelvic evisceration (68.8)
radical cystectomy (57.71)

58.31 **Endoscopic excision or destruction of lesion or tissue of urethra**
Fulguration of urethral lesion

58.39 **Other local excision or destruction of lesion or tissue of urethra**
Excision of:
congenital valve of urethra
lesion of urethra
stricture of urethra
Urethrectomy

Excludes *that by endoscopic approach (58.31)*

● 58.4 **Repair of urethra**

Excludes *repair of current obstetric laceration (75.61)*

✖ 58.41 **Suture of laceration of urethra**

✖ 58.42 **Closure of urethrostomy**

✖ 58.43 **Closure of other fistula of urethra**

Excludes *repair of urethroperineovesical fistula (57.84)*

✖ 58.44 **Reanastomosis of urethra**
Anastomosis of urethra

✖ 58.45 **Repair of hypospadias or epispadias**

✖ 58.46 **Other reconstruction of urethra**
Urethral construction

✖ 58.47 **Urethral meatoplasty**

✖ 58.49 **Other repair of urethra**
Benenenti rotation of bulbous urethra
Repair of old obstetric laceration of urethra
Urethral plication

Excludes *repair of:*
current obstetric laceration (75.61)
urethrocele (70.50–70.51)

✖ 58.5 **Release of urethral stricture**
Cutting of urethral sphincter
Internal urethral meatotomy
Urethrolysis

58.6 **Dilation of urethra**
Dilation of urethrovesical junction
Passage of sounds through urethra
Removal of calculus from urethra without incision

Excludes *urethral calibration (89.29)*

● 58.9 **Other operations on urethra and periurethral tissue**

✖ 58.91 **Incision of periurethral tissue**
Drainage of bulbourethral gland

✖ 58.92 **Excision of periurethral tissue**

Excludes *biopsy of periurethral tissue (58.24)*
lysis of periurethral adhesions
laparoscopic (59.12)
other (59.11)

✖ 58.93 **Implantation of artificial urinary sphincter [AUS]**
Placement of inflatable:
bladder sphincter
urethral sphincter
Removal with replacement of sphincter device [AUS]
With pump and/or reservoir

✖ 58.99 **Other**
Removal of inflatable urinary sphincter without replacement
Repair of inflatable sphincter pump and/or reservoir
Surgical correction of hydraulic pressure of inflatable sphincter device

Excludes *removal of:*
intraluminal foreign body from urethra without incision (98.19)
urethral stent (97.65)

● 59 **Other operations on urinary tract**

Code also any application or administration of an adhesion barrier substance (99.77)

● 59.0 **Dissection of retroperitoneal tissue**

✖ 59.00 **Retroperitoneal dissection, not otherwise specified**

✖ 59.02 **Other lysis of perirenal or periureteral adhesions**

Excludes *that by laparoscope (59.03)*

✖ 59.03 **Laparoscopic lysis of perirenal or periureteral adhesions**

✖ 59.09 **Other incision of perirenal or periureteral tissue**
Exploration of perinephric area
Incision of perirenal abscess

● 59.1 **Incision of perivesical tissue**

✖ 59.11 **Other lysis of perivesical adhesions**

✖ 59.12 **Laparoscopic lysis of perivesical adhesions**

✖ 59.19 **Other incision of perivesical tissue**
Exploration of perivesical tissue
Incision of hematoma of space of Retzius
Retropubic exploration

● 59.2 **Diagnostic procedures on perirenal and perivesical tissue**

✖ 59.21 **Biopsy of perirenal or perivesical tissue**

✖ 59.29 **Other diagnostic procedures on perirenal tissue, perivesical tissue, and retroperitoneum**

Excludes *microscopic examination of specimen from:*
perirenal tissue (91.21–91.29)
perivesical tissue (91.31–91.39)
retroperitoneum NEC (91.11–91.19)
retroperitoneal x-ray (88.14–88.16)

✖ 59.3 **Plication of urethrovesical junction**
Kelly-Kennedy operation on urethra
Kelly-Stoeckel urethral plication

✖ 59.4 **Suprapubic sling operation**
Goebel-Frangenheim-Stoeckel urethrovesical suspension
Millin-Read urethrovesical suspension
Oxford operation for urinary incontinence
Urethrocystopexy by suprapubic suspension

✖ 59.5 **Retropubic urethral suspension**
Burch procedure
Marshall-Marchetti-Krantz operation
Suture of periurethral tissue to symphysis pubis
Urethral suspension NOS

✖ 59.6 **Paraurethral suspension**
Pereyra paraurethral suspension
Periurethral suspension

● 59.7 **Other repair of urinary stress incontinence**

✖ 59.71 **Levator muscle operation for urethrovesical suspension**
Cystourethropexy with levator muscle sling
Gracilis muscle transplant for urethrovesical suspension
Pubococcygeal sling

59.72 **Injection of implant into urethra and/or bladder neck**
Collagen implant
Endoscopic injection of implant
Fat implant
Polytef implant

✖ 59.79 **Other**
Anterior urethropexy
Repair of stress incontinence NOS
Tudor "rabbit ear" urethropexy

59.8 **Ureteral catheterization**
Drainage of kidney by catheter
Insertion of ureteral stent
Ureterovesical orifice dilation

Code also any ureterotomy (56.2)

Excludes *that for:*
retrograde pyelogram (87.74)
transurethral removal of calculus or clot from ureter and renal pelvis (56.0)

● 59.9 **Other operations on urinary system**

Excludes *nonoperative removal of therapeutic device (97.61–97.69)*

✖ 59.91 **Excision of perirenal or perivesical tissue**

Excludes *biopsy of perirenal or perivesical tissue (59.21)*

✖ 59.92 **Other operations on perirenal or perivesical tissue**

59.93 **Replacement of ureterostomy tube**
Change of ureterostomy tube
Reinsertion of ureterostomy tube

Excludes *nonoperative removal of ureterostomy tube (97.62)*

59.94 **Replacement of cystostomy tube**

Excludes *nonoperative removal of cystostomy tube (97.63)*

59.95 **Ultrasonic fragmentation of urinary stones**
Shattered urinary stones

Excludes *percutaneous nephrostomy with fragmentation (55.04)*
shock-wave disintegration (98.51)

59.99 **Other**

Excludes *instillation of medication into urinary tract (96.49)*
irrigation of urinary tract (96.45–96.48)

11. OPERATIONS ON THE MALE GENITAL ORGANS (60–64)

● 60 Operations on prostate and seminal vesicles

Code also any application or administration of an adhesion barrier substance (99.77)

Includes: operations on periprostatic tissue

Excludes *that associated with radical cystectomy (57.71)*

✖ 60.0 Incision of prostate
Drainage of prostatic abscess
Prostatolithotomy

Excludes *drainage of periprostatic tissue only (60.81)*

● 60.1 Diagnostic procedures on prostate and seminal vesicles

60.11 Closed [percutaneous] [needle] biopsy of prostate
Approach:
transrectal
transurethral
Punch biopsy

✖ 60.12 Open biopsy of prostate

60.13 Closed [percutaneous] biopsy of seminal vesicles
Needle biopsy of seminal vesicles

✖ 60.14 Open biopsy of seminal vesicles

✖ 60.15 Biopsy of periprostatic tissue

✖ 60.18 Other diagnostic procedures on prostate and periprostatic tissue

Excludes *microscopic examination of specimen from prostate (91.31–91.39)*
x-ray of prostate (87.92)

✖ 60.19 Other diagnostic procedures on seminal vesicles

Excludes *microscopic examination of specimen from seminal vesicles (91.31–91.39)*
x-ray:
contrast seminal vesiculogram (87.91)
other (87.92)

● 60.2 Transurethral prostatectomy

Excludes *local excision of lesion of prostate (60.61)*

✖ 60.21 Transurethral (ultrasound) guided laser induced prostatectomy (TULIP)
Ablation (contact) (noncontact) by laser

✖ 60.29 Other transurethral prostatectomy
Excision of median bar by transurethral approach
Transurethral electrovaporization of prostrate (TEVAP)
Transurethral enucleative procedure
Transurethral prostatectomy NOS
Transurethral resection of prostate (TURP)

✖ 60.3 Suprapubic prostatectomy
Transvesical prostatectomy

Excludes *local excision of lesion of prostate (60.61)*
radical prostatectomy (60.5)

✖ 60.4 Retropubic prostatectomy

Excludes *local excision of lesion of prostate (60.61)*
radical prostatectomy (60.5)

✖ 60.5 Radical prostatectomy
Prostatovesiculectomy
Radical prostatectomy by any approach

Excludes *cystoprostatectomy (57.71)*

● 60.6 Other prostatectomy

✖ 60.61 Local excision of lesion of prostate
Excision of prostatic lesion by any approach

Excludes *biopsy of prostate (60.11–60.12)*

✖ 60.62 Perineal prostatectomy
Cryoablation of prostate
Cryoprostatectomy
Cryosurgery of prostate
Radical cryosurgical ablation of prostate (RCSA)

Excludes *local excision of lesion of prostate (60.61)*

✖ 60.69 Other

● 60.7 Operations on seminal vesicles

60.71 Percutaneous aspiration of seminal vesicle

Excludes *needle biopsy of seminal vesicle (60.13)*

✖ 60.72 Incision of seminal vesicle

✖ 60.73 Excision of seminal vesicle
Excision of Müllerian duct cyst
Spermatocystectomy

Excludes *biopsy of seminal vesicle (60.13–60.14)*
prostatovesiculectomy (60.5)

✖ 60.79 Other operations on seminal vesicles

● 60.8 Incision or excision of periprostatic tissue

✖ 60.81 Incision of periprostatic tissue
Drainage of periprostatic abscess

✖ 60.82 Excision of periprostatic tissue
Excision of lesion of periprostatic tissue

Excludes *biopsy of periprostatic tissue (60.15)*

● 60.9 Other operations on prostate

60.91 Percutaneous aspiration of prostate

Excludes *needle biopsy of prostate (60.11)*

60.92 Injection into prostate

✖ 60.93 Repair of prostate

✖ 60.94 Control of (postoperative) hemorrhage of prostate
Coagulation of prostatic bed
Cystoscopy for control of prostatic hemorrhage

✖ 60.95 Transurethral balloon dilation of the prostatic urethra

60.96 Transurethral destruction of prostate tissue by microwave thermotherapy
Transurethral microwave thermotherapy (TUMT) of prostate

Excludes *prostatectomy:*
other (60.61–60.69)
radical (60.5)
retropubic (60.4)
suprapubic (60.3)
transurethral (60.21–60.29)

60.97 Other transurethral destruction of prostate tissue by other thermotherapy
Radiofrequency thermotherapy
Transurethral needle ablation (TUNA) of prostate

Excludes *prostatectomy:*
other (60.61–60.69)
radical (60.5)
retropubic (60.4)
suprapubic (60.3)
transurethral (60.21–60.29)

✖ 60.99 Other

Excludes *prostatic massage (99.94)*

● 61 Operations on scrotum and tunica vaginalis

61.0 Incision and drainage of scrotum and tunica vaginalis

Excludes *percutaneous aspiration of hydrocele (61.91)*

● 61.1 Diagnostic procedures on scrotum and tunica vaginalis

61.11 Biopsy of scrotum or tunica vaginalis

61.19 Other diagnostic procedures on scrotum and tunica vaginalis

✖ 61.2 **Excision of hydrocele (of tunica vaginalis)**
Bottle repair of hydrocele of tunica vaginalis

Excludes *percutaneous aspiration of hydrocele (61.91)*

61.3 **Excision or destruction of lesion or tissue of scrotum**
Fulguration of lesion of scrotum
Reduction of elephantiasis of scrotum
Partial scrotectomy of scrotum

Excludes *biopsy of scrotum (61.11)*
scrotal fistulectomy (61.42)

● 61.4 **Repair of scrotum and tunica vaginalis**

61.41 **Suture of laceration of scrotum and tunica vaginalis**

✖ 61.42 **Repair of scrotal fistula**

✖ 61.49 **Other repair of scrotum and tunica vaginalis**
Reconstruction with rotational or pedicle flaps

● 61.9 **Other operations on scrotum and tunica vaginalis**

61.91 **Percutaneous aspiration of tunica vaginalis**
Aspiration of hydrocele of tunica vaginalis

✖ 61.92 **Excision of lesion of tunica vaginalis other than hydrocele**
Excision of hematocele of tunica vaginalis

✖ 61.99 **Other**

Excludes *removal of foreign body from scrotum without incision (98.24)*

● 62 **Operations on testes**

✖ 62.0 **Incision of testis**

● 62.1 **Diagnostic procedures on testes**

62.11 **Closed [percutaneous] [needle] biopsy of testis**

✖ 62.12 **Open biopsy of testis**

✖ 62.19 **Other diagnostic procedures on testes**

✖ 62.2 **Excision or destruction of testicular lesion**
Excision of appendix testis
Excision of cyst of Morgagni in the male

Excludes *biopsy of testis (62.11–62.12)*

✖ 62.3 **Unilateral orchiectomy**
Orchidectomy (with epididymectomy) NOS

● 62.4 **Bilateral orchiectomy**
Male castration
Radical bilateral orchiectomy (with epididymectomy)

Code also any synchronous lymph node dissection (40.3, 40.5)

✖ 62.41 **Removal of both testes at same operative episode**
Bilateral orchidectomy NOS

✖ 62.42 **Removal of remaining testis**
Removal of solitary testis

✖ 62.5 **Orchiopexy**
Mobilization and replacement of testis in scrotum
Orchiopexy with detorsion of testis
Torek (-Bevan) operation (orchidopexy) (first stage) (second stage)
Transplantation to and fixation of testis in scrotum

● 62.6 **Repair of testes**

Excludes *reduction of torsion (63.52)*

✖ 62.61 **Suture of laceration of testis**

✖ 62.69 **Other repair of testis**
Testicular graft

✖ 62.7 **Insertion of testicular prosthesis**

● 62.9 **Other operations on testes**

62.91 **Aspiration of testis**

Excludes *percutaneous biopsy of testis (62.11)*

62.92 **Injection of therapeutic substance into testis**

✖ 62.99 **Other**

● 63 **Operations on spermatic cord, epididymis, and vas deferens**

● 63.0 **Diagnostic procedures on spermatic cord, epididymis, and vas deferens**

63.01 **Biopsy of spermatic cord, epididymis, or vas deferens**

✖ 63.09 **Other diagnostic procedures on spermatic cord, epididymis, and vas deferens**

Excludes *contrast epididymogram (87.93)*
contrast vasogram (87.94)
other x-ray of epididymis and vas deferens (87.95)

✖ 63.1 **Excision of varicocele and hydrocele of spermatic cord**
High ligation of spermatic vein
Hydrocelectomy of canal of Nuck

✖ 63.2 **Excision of cyst of epididymis**
Spermatocelectomy

✖ 63.3 **Excision of other lesion or tissue of spermatic cord and epididymis**
Excision of appendix epididymis

Excludes *biopsy of spermatic cord or epididymis (63.01)*

✖ 63.4 **Epididymectomy**

Excludes *that synchronous with orchiectomy (62.3–62.42)*

● 63.5 **Repair of spermatic cord and epididymis**

✖ 63.51 **Suture of laceration of spermatic cord and epididymis**

63.52 **Reduction of torsion of testis or spermatic cord**

Excludes *that associated with orchiopexy (62.5)*

✖ 63.53 **Transplantation of spermatic cord**

✖ 63.59 **Other repair of spermatic cord and epididymis**

63.6 **Vasotomy**
Vasostomy

● 63.7 **Vasectomy and ligation of vas deferens**

63.70 **Male sterilization procedure, not otherwise specified**

63.71 **Ligation of vas deferens**
Crushing of vas deferens
Division of vas deferens

63.72 **Ligation of spermatic cord**

63.73 **Vasectomy**

● 63.8 **Repair of vas deferens and epididymis**

✖ 63.81 **Suture of laceration of vas deferens and epididymis**

✖ 63.82 **Reconstruction of surgically divided vas deferens**

✖ 63.83 **Epididymovasostomy**

63.84 **Removal of ligature from vas deferens**

✖ 63.85 **Removal of valve from vas deferens**

✖ 63.89 **Other repair of vas deferens and epididymis**

● 63.9 **Other operations on spermatic cord, epididymis, and vas deferens**

63.91 **Aspiration of spermatocele**

✖ 63.92 **Epididymotomy**

✖ 63.93 **Incision of spermatic cord**

✖ 63.94 **Lysis of adhesions of spermatic cord**

✖ 63.95 **Insertion of valve in vas deferens**

✖ 63.99 **Other**

● 64 **Operations on penis**

Includes: operations on:
corpora cavernosa
glans penis
prepuce

✖ 64.0 **Circumcision**

● 64.1 **Diagnostic procedures on the penis**

✖64.11 **Biopsy of penis**

64.19 **Other diagnostic procedures on penis**

✖64.2 **Local excision or destruction of lesion of penis**

Excludes *biopsy of penis (64.11)*

✖64.3 **Amputation of penis**

●64.4 **Repair and plastic operation on penis**

✖64.41 **Suture of laceration of penis**

✖64.42 **Release of chordee**

✖64.43 **Construction of penis**

✖64.44 **Reconstruction of penis**

✖64.45 **Replantation of penis**
Reattachment of amputated penis

✖64.49 **Other repair of penis**

Excludes *repair of epispadias and hypospadias (58.45)*

✖64.5 **Operations for sex transformation, not elsewhere classified**

●64.9 **Other operations on male genital organs**

64.91 **Dorsal or lateral slit of prepuce**

✖64.92 **Incision of penis**

✖64.93 **Division of penile adhesions**

64.94 **Fitting of external prosthesis of penis**
Penile prosthesis NOS

✖64.95 **Insertion or replacement of non-inflatable penile prosthesis**
Insertion of semi-rigid rod prosthesis into shaft of penis

Excludes *external penile prosthesis (64.94)*
inflatable penile prosthesis (64.97)
plastic repair, penis (64.43–64.49)
that associated with:
construction (64.43)
reconstruction (64.44)

✖64.96 **Removal of internal prosthesis of penis**
Removal without replacement of non-inflatable or inflatable penile prosthesis

✖64.97 **Insertion or replacement of inflatable penile prosthesis**
Insertion of cylinders into shaft of penis and placement of pump and reservoir

Excludes *external penile prosthesis (64.94)*
non-inflatable penile prosthesis (64.95)
plastic repair, penis (64.43–64.49)

✖64.98 **Other operations on penis**
Corpora cavernosa-corpus spongiosum shunt
Corpora-saphenous shunt
Irrigation of corpus cavernosum

Excludes *removal of foreign body:*
intraluminal (98.19)
without incision (98.24)
stretching of foreskin (99.95)

✖64.99 **Other**

Excludes *collection of sperm for artificial insemination (99.96)*

12. OPERATIONS ON THE FEMALE GENITAL ORGANS (65–71)

● 65 Operations on ovary

Code also any application or administration of an adhesion barrier substance (99.77)

● 65.0 Oophorotomy
Salpingo-oophorotomy

✖ 65.01 Laparoscopic oophorotomy

✖ 65.09 Other oophorotomy

● 65.1 Diagnostic procedures on ovaries

✖ 65.11 Aspiration biopsy of ovary

✖ 65.12 Other biopsy of ovary

✖ 65.13 Laparoscopic biopsy of ovary

✖ 65.14 Other laparoscopic diagnostic procedures on ovaries

✖ 65.19 Other diagnostic procedures on ovaries

Excludes *microscopic examination of specimen from ovary (91.41–91.49)*

● 65.2 Local excision or destruction of ovarian lesion or tissue

✖ 65.21 Marsupialization of ovarian cyst

Excludes *that by laparoscope (65.23)*

✖ 65.22 Wedge resection of ovary

Excludes *that by laparoscope (65.24)*

✖ 65.23 Laparoscopic marsupialization of ovarian cyst

✖ 65.24 Laparoscopic wedge resection of ovary

✖ 65.25 Other laparoscopic local excision or destruction of ovary

✖ 65.29 Other local excision or destruction of ovary
Bisection of ovary
Cauterization of ovary
Partial excision of ovary

Excludes *biopsy of ovary (65.11–65.13)*
that by laparoscope (65.25)

● 65.3 Unilateral oophorectomy

✖ 65.31 Laparoscopic unilateral oophorectomy

✖ 65.39 Other unilateral oophorectomy

Excludes *that by laparoscope (65.31)*

● 65.4 Unilateral salpingo-oophorectomy

✖ 65.41 Laparoscopic unilateral salpingo-oophorectomy

✖ 65.49 Other unilateral salpingo-oophorectomy

● 65.5 Bilateral oophorectomy

✖ 65.51 Other removal of both ovaries at same operative episode
Female castration

Excludes *that by laparoscope (65.53)*

✖ 65.52 Other removal of remaining ovary
Removal of solitary ovary

Excludes *that by laparoscope (65.54)*

✖ 65.53 Laparoscopic removal of both ovaries at same operative episode

✖ 65.54 Laparoscopic removal of remaining ovary

● 65.6 Bilateral salpingo-oophorectomy

✖ 65.61 Other removal of both ovaries and tubes at same operative episode

Excludes *that by laparoscope (65.63)*

✖ 65.62 Other removal of remaining ovary and tube
Removal of solitary ovary and tube

Excludes *that by laparoscope (65.64)*

✖ 65.63 Laparoscopic removal of both ovaries and tubes at same operative episode

✖ 65.64 Laparoscopic removal of remaining ovary and tube

● 65.7 Repair of ovary

Excludes *salpingo-oophorostomy (66.72)*

✖ 65.71 Other simple suture of ovary

Excludes *that by laparoscope (65.74)*

✖ 65.72 Other reimplantation of ovary

Excludes *that by laparoscope (65.75)*

✖ 65.73 Other salpingo-oophoroplasty

Excludes *that by laparoscope (65.76)*

✖ 65.74 Laparoscopic simple suture of ovary

✖ 65.75 Laparoscopic reimplantation of ovary

✖ 65.76 Laparoscopic salpingo-oophoroplasty

✖ 65.79 Other repair of ovary
Oophoropexy

● 65.8 Lysis of adhesions of ovary and fallopian tube

✖ 65.81 Laparoscopic lysis of adhesions of ovary and fallopian tube

✖ 65.89 Other lysis of adhesions of ovary and fallopian tube

Excludes *that by laparoscope (65.81)*

● 65.9 Other operations on ovary

✖ 65.91 Aspiration of ovary

Excludes *aspiration biopsy of ovary (65.11)*

✖ 65.92 Transplantation of ovary

Excludes *reimplantation of ovary*
laparoscopic (65.75)
other (65.72)

✖ 65.93 Manual rupture of ovarian cyst

✖ 65.94 Ovarian denervation

✖ 65.95 Release of torsion of ovary

✖ 65.99 Other
Ovarian drilling

● 66 Operations on fallopian tubes

Code also any application or administration of an adhesion barrier substance (99.77)

● 66.0 Salpingotomy and salpingostomy

✖ 66.01 Salpingotomy

✖ 66.02 Salpingostomy

● 66.1 Diagnostic procedures on fallopian tubes

✖ 66.11 Biopsy of fallopian tube

✖ 66.19 Other diagnostic procedures on fallopian tubes

Excludes *microscopic examination of specimen from fallopian tubes (91.41–91.49)*
radiography of fallopian tubes (87.82–87.83, 87.85)
Rubin's test (66.8)

● 66.2 Bilateral endoscopic destruction or occlusion of fallopian tubes

Includes: bilateral endoscopic destruction or occlusion of fallopian tubes by:
culdoscopy
endoscopy
hysteroscopy
laparoscopy
peritoneoscopy
endoscopic destruction of solitary fallopian tube

✖ 66.21 Bilateral endoscopic ligation and crushing of fallopian tubes

✖ 66.22 **Bilateral endoscopic ligation and division of fallopian tubes**

✖ 66.29 **Other bilateral endoscopic destruction or occlusion of fallopian tubes**

● 66.3 **Other bilateral destruction or occlusion of fallopian tubes**

Includes: destruction of solitary fallopian tube

Excludes *endoscopic destruction or occlusion of fallopian tubes (66.21–66.29)*

✖ 66.31 **Other bilateral ligation and crushing of fallopian tubes**

✖ 66.32 **Other bilateral ligation and division of fallopian tubes**
Pomeroy operation

✖ 66.39 **Other bilateral destruction or occlusion of fallopian tubes**
Female sterilization operation NOS

✖ 66.4 **Total unilateral salpingectomy**

● 66.5 **Total bilateral salpingectomy**

Excludes *bilateral partial salpingectomy for sterilization (66.39)*
that with oophorectomy (65.61–65.64)

✖ 66.51 **Removal of both fallopian tubes at same operative episode**

✖ 66.52 **Removal of remaining fallopian tube**
Removal of solitary fallopian tube

● 66.6 **Other salpingectomy**

Includes: salpingectomy by:
cauterization
coagulation
electrocoagulation
excision

Excludes *fistulectomy (66.73)*

✖ 66.61 **Excision or destruction of lesion of fallopian tube**

Excludes *biopsy of fallopian tube (66.11)*

✖ 66.62 **Salpingectomy with removal of tubal pregnancy**
Code also any synchronous oophorectomy (65.31, 65.39)

✖ 66.63 **Bilateral partial salpingectomy, not otherwise specified**

✖ 66.69 **Other partial salpingectomy**

● 66.7 **Repair of fallopian tube**

✖ 66.71 **Simple suture of fallopian tube**

✖ 66.72 **Salpingo-oophorostomy**

✖ 66.73 **Salpingo-salpingostomy**

✖ 66.74 **Salpingo-uterostomy**

✖ 66.79 **Other repair of fallopian tube**
Graft of fallopian tube
Reopening of divided fallopian tube
Salpingoplasty

66.8 **Insufflation of fallopian tube**
Insufflation of fallopian tube with:
air
dye
gas
saline
Rubin's test

Excludes *insufflation of therapeutic agent (66.95)*
that for hysterosalpingography (87.82–87.83)

● 66.9 **Other operations on fallopian tubes**

66.91 **Aspiration of fallopian tube**

✖ 66.92 **Unilateral destruction or occlusion of fallopian tube**

Excludes *that of solitary tube (66.21–66.39)*

✖ 66.93 **Implantation or replacement of prosthesis of fallopian tube**

✖ 66.94 **Removal of prosthesis of fallopian tube**

✖ 66.95 **Insufflation of therapeutic agent into fallopian tubes**

✖ 66.96 **Dilation of fallopian tube**

✖ 66.97 **Burying of fimbriae in uterine wall**

✖ 66.99 **Other**

Excludes *lysis of adhesions of ovary and tube*
laparoscopic (65.81)
other (65.89)

● 67 **Operations on cervix**

Code also any application or administration of an adhesion barrier substance (99.77)

67.0 **Dilation of cervical canal**

Excludes *dilation and curettage (69.01–69.09)*
that for induction of labor (73.1)

● 67.1 **Diagnostic procedures on cervix**

✖ 67.11 **Endocervical biopsy**

Excludes *conization of cervix (67.2)*

✖ 67.12 **Other cervical biopsy**
Punch biopsy of cervix NOS

Excludes *conization of cervix (67.2)*

✖ 67.19 **Other diagnostic procedures on cervix**

Excludes *microscopic examination of specimen from cervix (91.41–91.49)*

✖ 67.2 **Conization of cervix**

Excludes *that by:*
cryosurgery (67.33)
electrosurgery (67.32)

● 67.3 **Other excision or destruction of lesion or tissue of cervix**

✖ 67.31 **Marsupialization of cervical cyst**

✖ 67.32 **Destruction of lesion of cervix by cauterization**
Electroconization of cervix
LEEP (loop electrosurgical excision procedure)
LLETZ (large loop excision of the transformation zone)

✖ 67.33 **Destruction of lesion of cervix by cryosurgery**
Cryoconization of cervix

✖ 67.39 **Other excision or destruction of lesion or tissue of cervix**

Excludes *biopsy of cervix (67.11–67.12)*
cervical fistulectomy (67.62)
conization of cervix (67.2)

✖ 67.4 **Amputation of cervix**
Cervicectomy with synchronous colporrhaphy

● 67.5 **Repair of internal cervical os**

✖ 67.51 **Transabdominal cerclage of cervix**

✖ 67.59 **Other repair of internal cervical os**
Cerclage of isthmus uteri
McDonald operation
Shirodkar operation
Transvaginal cerclage

Excludes *laparoscopically assisted supracervical hysterectomy [LASH] (68.31)*
transabdominal cerclage of cervix (67.51)

● 67.6 **Other repair of cervix**

Excludes *repair of current obstetric laceration (75.51)*

✖ **67.61 Suture of laceration of cervix**

✖ **67.62 Repair of fistula of cervix**
Cervicosigmoidal fistulectomy

Excludes *fistulectomy:*
cervicovesical (57.84)
ureterocervical (56.84)
vesicocervicovaginal (57.84)

✖ **67.69 Other repair of cervix**
Repair of old obstetric laceration of cervix

● **68 Other incision and excision of uterus**

Code also any application or administration of an adhesion barrier substance (99.77)

✖ **68.0 Hysterotomy**
Hysterotomy with removal of hydatidiform mole

Excludes *hysterotomy for termination of pregnancy (74.91)*

● **68.1 Diagnostic procedures on uterus and supporting structures**

68.11 Digital examination of uterus

Excludes *pelvic examination, so described (89.26)*
postpartal manual exploration of uterine cavity (75.7)

68.12 Hysteroscopy

Excludes *that with biopsy (68.16)*

✖ **68.13 Open biopsy of uterus**

Excludes *closed biopsy of uterus (68.16)*

✖ **68.14 Open biopsy of uterine ligaments**

Excludes *closed biopsy of uterine ligaments (68.15)*

✖ **68.15 Closed biopsy of uterine ligaments**
Endoscopic (laparoscopy) biopsy of uterine adnexa, except ovary and fallopian tube

✖ **68.16 Closed biopsy of uterus**
Endoscopic (laparoscopy) (hysteroscopy) biopsy of uterus

Excludes *open biopsy of uterus (68.13)*

✖ **68.19 Other diagnostic procedures on uterus and supporting structures**

Excludes *diagnostic:*
aspiration curettage (69.59)
dilation and curettage (69.09)
microscopic examination of specimen from uterus (91.41–91.49)
pelvic examination (89.26)
radioisotope scan of:
placenta (92.17)
uterus (92.19)
ultrasonography of uterus (88.78–88.79)
x-ray of uterus (87.81–87.89)

● **68.2 Excision or destruction of lesion or tissue of uterus**

✖ **68.21 Division of endometrial synechiae**
Lysis of intraluminal uterine adhesions

✖ **68.22 Incision or excision of congenital septum of uterus**

✖ **68.23 Endometrial ablation**
Dilation and curettage
Hysteroscopic endometrial ablation

✖ **68.29 Other excision or destruction of lesion of uterus**
Uterine myomectomy

Excludes *biopsy of uterus (68.13)*
uterine fistulectomy (69.42)

● **68.3 Subtotal abdominal hysterectomy**

✖ **68.31 Laparoscopic supracervical hysterectomy [LSH]**
Classic infrafascial SEMM hysterectomy [CISH]
Laparoscopically assisted supracervical hysterectomy [LASH]

✖ **68.39 Other and unspecified subtotal abdominal hysterectomy, NOS** ⬅
Supracervical hysterectomy

Excludes *classic infrafascial SEMM hysterectomy [CISH] (68.31)*
laparoscopic supracervical hysterectomy [LSH] (68.31)

● **68.4 Total abdominal hysterectomy**
Hysterectomy:
extended

Code also any synchronous removal of tubes and ovaries (65.31–65.64) ⬅

Excludes *laparoscopic total abdominal hysterectomy (68.41)* ◀
radical abdominal hysterectomy, any approach (68.61–68.69) ◀

✖ **68.41 Laparoscopic total abdominal hysterectomy** ◀
Total laparoscopic hysterectomy [TLH] ◀

✖ **68.49 Other and unspecified total abdominal hysterectomy** ◀
Hysterectomy: ◀
Extended ◀

● **68.5 Vaginal hysterectomy**

Code also any synchronous:
removal of tubes and ovaries (65.31–65.64)
repair of cystocele or rectocele (70.50–70.52)
repair of pelvic floor (70.79)

✖ **68.51 Laparoscopically assisted vaginal hysterectomy (LAVH)**

✖ **68.59 Other and unspecified vaginal hysterectomy** ⬅

Excludes *laparoscopically assisted vaginal hysterectomy (LAVH) (68.51)*
radical vaginal hysterectomy (68.7)

● **68.6 Radical abdominal hysterectomy** ⬅
Modified radical hysterectomy
Wertheim's operation

Code also any synchronous:
lymph gland dissection (40.3, 40.5)
removal of tubes and ovaries (65.31–65.64) ⬅

Excludes *pelvic evisceration (68.8)*

✖ **68.61 Laparoscopic radical abdominal hysterectomy** ◀
Laparoscopic modified radical hysterectomy ◀
Total laparoscopic radical hysterectomy [TLRH] ◀

✖ **68.69 Other and unspecified radical abdominal hysterectomy** ◀
Modified radical hysterectomy ◀
Wertheim's operation ◀

Excludes *laparoscopic total abdominal hysterectomy (68.41)* ◀
laparoscopic radical abdominal hysterectomy (68.61) ◀

● **68.7 Radical vaginal hysterectomy**
Schauta operation

Code also any synchronous:
lymph gland dissection (40.3, 40.5)
removal of tubes and ovaries (65.31–65.64) ⬅

Excludes *abdominal hysterectomy, any approach (68.31–68.39, 68.41–68.49, 68.61–68.69, 68.9)* ◀

✖ **68.71 Laparoscopic radical vaginal hysterectomy [LRVH]** ◀

✖ **68.79 Other and unspecified radical vaginal hysterectomy** ◀
Hysterocolpectomy ◀
Schauta operation ◀

✖68.8 **Pelvic evisceration**
Removal of ovaries, tubes, uterus, vagina, bladder, and urethra (with removal of sigmoid colon and rectum)
Code also any synchronous:
colostomy (46.12–46.13)
lymph gland dissection (40.3, 40.5)
urinary diversion (56.51–56.79)

✖68.9 **Other and unspecified hysterectomy**
Hysterectomy NOS
Excludes *abdominal hysterectomy, any approach (68.31–68.39, 68.41–68.49, 68.61–68.69)* ⬅
vaginal hysterectomy, any approach (68.51–68.59, 68.71–68.79) ⬅

● 69 **Other operations on uterus and supporting structures**
Code also any application or administration of an adhesion barrier substance (99.77)

● 69.0 **Dilation and curettage of uterus**
Excludes *aspiration curettage of uterus (69.51–69.59)*

✖69.01 **Dilation and curettage for termination of pregnancy**

✖69.02 **Dilation and curettage following delivery or abortion**

✖69.09 **Other dilation and curettage**
Diagnostic D and C

● 69.1 **Excision or destruction of lesion or tissue of uterus and supporting structures**

✖69.19 **Other excision or destruction of uterus and supporting structures**
Excludes *biopsy of uterine ligament (68.14)*

● 69.2 **Repair of uterine supporting structures**

✖69.21 **Interposition operation**
Watkins procedure

✖69.22 **Other uterine suspension**
Hysteropexy
Manchester operation
Plication of uterine ligament

✖69.23 **Vaginal repair of chronic inversion of uterus**

✖69.29 **Other repair of uterus and supporting structures**

✖69.3 **Paracervical uterine denervation**

● 69.4 **Uterine repair**
Excludes *repair of current obstetric laceration (75.50–75.52)*

✖69.41 **Suture of laceration of uterus**

✖69.42 **Closure of fistula of uterus**
Excludes *uterovesical fistulectomy (57.84)*

✖69.49 **Other repair of uterus**
Repair of old obstetric laceration of uterus

● 69.5 **Aspiration curettage of uterus**
Excludes *menstrual extraction (69.6)*

✖69.51 **Aspiration curettage of uterus for termination of pregnancy**
Therapeutic abortion NOS

✖69.52 **Aspiration curettage following delivery or abortion**

69.59 **Other aspiration curettage of uterus**

69.6 **Menstrual extraction or regulation**

69.7 **Insertion of intrauterine contraceptive device**

● 69.9 **Other operations on uterus, cervix, and supporting structures**
Excludes *obstetric dilation or incision of cervix (73.1, 73.93)*

69.91 **Insertion of therapeutic device into uterus**
Excludes *insertion of:*
intrauterine contraceptive device (69.7)
laminaria (69.93)
obstetric insertion of bag, bougie, or pack (73.1)

69.92 **Artificial insemination**

69.93 **Insertion of laminaria**

69.94 **Manual replacement of inverted uterus**
Excludes *that in immediate postpartal period (75.94)*

✖69.95 **Incision of cervix**
Excludes *that to assist delivery (73.93)*

69.96 **Removal of cerclage material from cervix**

✖69.97 **Removal of other penetrating foreign body from cervix**
Excludes *removal of intraluminal foreign body from cervix (98.16)*

✖69.98 **Other operations on supporting structures of uterus**
Excludes *biopsy of uterine ligament (68.14)*

✖69.99 **Other operations on cervix and uterus**
Excludes *removal of:*
foreign body (98.16)
intrauterine contraceptive device (97.71)
obstetric bag, bougie, or pack (97.72)
packing (97.72)

● 70 **Operations on vagina and cul-de-sac**
Code also any application or administration of an adhesion barrier substance (99.77)

70.0 **Culdocentesis**

70.1 **Incision of vagina and cul-de-sac**

70.11 **Hymenotomy**

✖70.12 **Culdotomy**

✖70.13 **Lysis of intraluminal adhesions of vagina**

✖70.14 **Other vaginotomy**
Division of vaginal septum
Drainage of hematoma of vaginal cuff

● 70.2 **Diagnostic procedures on vagina and cul-de-sac**

70.21 **Vaginoscopy**

70.22 **Culdoscopy**

✖70.23 **Biopsy of cul-de-sac**

✖70.24 **Vaginal biopsy**

✖70.29 **Other diagnostic procedures on vagina and cul-de-sac**

● 70.3 **Local excision or destruction of vagina and cul-de-sac**

✖70.31 **Hymenectomy**

✖70.32 **Excision or destruction of lesion of cul-de-sac**
Endometrectomy of cul-de-sac
Excludes *biopsy of cul-de-sac (70.23)*

✖70.33 **Excision or destruction of lesion of vagina**
Excludes *biopsy of vagina (70.24)*
vaginal fistulectomy (70.72–70.75)

✖70.4 **Obliteration and total excision of vagina**
Vaginectomy
Excludes *obliteration of vaginal vault (70.8)*

● 70.5 **Repair of cystocele and rectocele**

✖70.50 **Repair of cystocele and rectocele**

✖70.51 **Repair of cystocele**
Anterior colporrhaphy (with urethrocele repair)

✖70.52 **Repair of rectocele**
Posterior colporrhaphy

●70.6 **Vaginal construction and reconstruction**

✖70.61 **Vaginal construction**

✖70.62 **Vaginal reconstruction**

●70.7 **Other repair of vagina**

Excludes *lysis of intraluminal adhesions (70.13)*
repair of current obstetric laceration (75.69)
that associated with cervical amputation (67.4)

✖70.71 **Suture of laceration of vagina**

✖70.72 **Repair of colovaginal fistula**

✖70.73 **Repair of rectovaginal fistula**

✖70.74 **Repair of other vaginoenteric fistula**

✖70.75 **Repair of other fistula of vagina**

Excludes *repair of fistula:*
rectovesicovaginal (57.83)
ureterovaginal (56.84)
urethrovaginal (58.43)
uterovaginal (69.42)
vesicocervicovaginal (57.84)
vesicosigmoidovaginal (57.83)
vesicoureterovaginal (56.84)
vesicovaginal (57.84)

✖70.76 **Hymenorrhaphy**

✖70.77 **Vaginal suspension and fixation**

✖70.79 **Other repair of vagina**
Colpoperineoplasty
Repair of old obstetric laceration of vagina

✖70.8 **Obliteration of vaginal vault**
LeFort operation

●70.9 **Other operations on vagina and cul-de-sac**

✖70.91 **Other operations on vagina**

Excludes *insertion of:*
diaphragm (96.17)
mold (96.15)
pack (96.14)
pessary (96.18)
suppository (96.49)
removal of:
diaphragm (97.73)
foreign body (98.17)
pack (97.75)
pessary (97.74)
replacement of:
diaphragm (97.24)
pack (97.26)
pessary (97.25)
vaginal dilation (96.16)
vaginal douche (96.44)

✖70.92 **Other operations on cul-de-sac**
Obliteration of cul-de-sac
Repair of vaginal enterocele

●71 **Operations on vulva and perineum**

Code also any application or administration of an adhesion barrier substance (99.77)

●71.0 **Incision of vulva and perineum**

✖71.01 **Lysis of vulvar adhesions**

✖71.09 **Other incision of vulva and perineum**
Enlargement of introitus NOS

Excludes *removal of foreign body without incision (98.23)*

●71.1 **Diagnostic procedures on vulva**

✖71.11 **Biopsy of vulva**

✖71.19 **Other diagnostic procedures on vulva**

●71.2 **Operations on Bartholin's gland**

71.21 **Percutaneous aspiration of Bartholin's gland (cyst)**

✖71.22 **Incision of Bartholin's gland (cyst)**

✖71.23 **Marsupialization of Bartholin's gland (cyst)**

✖71.24 **Excision or other destruction of Bartholin's gland (cyst)**

✖71.29 **Other operations on Bartholin's gland**

✖71.3 **Other local excision or destruction of vulva and perineum**
Division of Skene's gland

Excludes *biopsy of vulva (71.11)*
vulvar fistulectomy (71.72)

✖71.4 **Operations on clitoris**
Amputation of clitoris
Clitoridotomy
Female circumcision

✖71.5 **Radical vulvectomy**

Code also any synchronous lymph gland dissection (40.3, 40.5)

●71.6 **Other vulvectomy**

✖71.61 **Unilateral vulvectomy**

✖71.62 **Bilateral vulvectomy**
Vulvectomy NOS

●71.7 **Repair of vulva and perineum**

Excludes *repair of current obstetric laceration (75.69)*

✖71.71 **Suture of laceration of vulva or perineum**

✖71.72 **Repair of fistula of vulva or perineum**

Excludes *repair of fistula:*
urethroperineal (58.43)
urethroperineovesical (57.84)
vaginoperineal (70.75)

✖71.79 **Other repair of vulva and perineum**
Repair of old obstetric laceration of vulva or perineum

✖71.8 **Other operations on vulva**

Excludes *removal of:*
foreign body without incision (98.23)
packing (97.75)
replacement of packing (97.26)

✖71.9 **Other operations on female genital organs**

13. OBSTETRICAL PROCEDURES (72–75)

● 72 **Forceps, vacuum, and breech delivery**

72.0 **Low forceps operation**
Outlet forceps operation

72.1 **Low forceps operation with episiotomy**
Outlet forceps operation with episiotomy

● 72.2 **Mid forceps operation**

72.21 **Mid forceps operation with episiotomy**

72.29 **Other mid forceps operation**

● 72.3 **High forceps operation**

72.31 **High forceps operation with episiotomy**

72.39 **Other high forceps operation**

72.4 **Forceps rotation of fetal head**
De Lee maneuver
Key-in-lock rotation
Kielland rotation
Scanzoni's maneuver

Code also any associated forceps extraction (72.0–72.39)

● 72.5 **Breech extraction**

72.51 **Partial breech extraction with forceps to aftercoming head**

72.52 **Other partial breech extraction**

72.53 **Total breech extraction with forceps to aftercoming head**

72.54 **Other total breech extraction**

72.6 **Forceps application to aftercoming head**
Piper forceps operation

Excludes *partial breech extraction with forceps to aftercoming head (72.51)*
total breech extraction with forceps to aftercoming head (72.53)

● 72.7 **Vacuum extraction**

Includes: Malström's extraction

72.71 **Vacuum extraction with episiotomy**

72.79 **Other vacuum extraction**

72.8 **Other specified instrumental delivery**

72.9 **Unspecified instrumental delivery**

● 73 **Other procedures inducing or assisting delivery**

● 73.0 **Artificial rupture of membranes**

73.01 **Induction of labor by artificial rupture of membranes**
Surgical induction NOS

Excludes *artificial rupture of membranes after onset of labor (73.09)*

73.09 **Other artificial rupture of membranes**
Artificial rupture of membranes at time of delivery

73.1 **Other surgical induction of labor**
Induction by cervical dilation

Excludes *injection for abortion (75.0)*
insertion of suppository for abortion (96.49)

● 73.2 **Internal and combined version and extraction**

73.21 **Internal and combined version without extraction**
Version NOS

73.22 **Internal and combined version with extraction**

73.3 **Failed forceps**
Application of forceps without delivery
Trial forceps

73.4 **Medical induction of labor**

Excludes *medication to augment active labor*

● 73.5 **Manually assisted delivery**

73.51 **Manual rotation of fetal head**

73.59 **Other manually assisted delivery**
Assisted spontaneous delivery
Credé maneuver

73.6 **Episiotomy**
Episioproctotomy
Episiotomy with subsequent episiorrhaphy

Excludes *that with:*
high forceps (72.31)
low forceps (72.1)
mid forceps (72.21)
outlet forceps (72.1)
vacuum extraction (72.71)

73.8 **Operations on fetus to facilitate delivery**
Clavicotomy on fetus
Destruction of fetus
Needling of hydrocephalic head

● 73.9 **Other operations assisting delivery**

73.91 **External version**

73.92 **Replacement of prolapsed umbilical cord**

73.93 **Incision of cervix to assist delivery**
Dührssen's incisions

✖ 73.94 **Pubiotomy to assist delivery**
Obstetric symphysiotomy

✖ 73.99 **Other**

Excludes *dilation of cervix, obstetrical to induce labor (73.1)*
insertion of bag or bougie to induce labor (73.1)
removal of cerclage material (69.96)

● 74 **Cesarean section and removal of fetus**

Code also any synchronous:
hysterectomy (68.3–68.4, 68.6, 68.8)
myomectomy (68.29)
sterilization (66.31–66.39, 66.63)

✖ 74.0 **Classical cesarean section**
Transperitoneal classical cesarean section

✖ 74.1 **Low cervical cesarean section**
Lower uterine segment cesarean section

✖ 74.2 **Extraperitoneal cesarean section**
Supravesical cesarean section

✖ 74.3 **Removal of extratubal ectopic pregnancy**
Removal of:
ectopic abdominal pregnancy
fetus from peritoneal or extraperitoneal cavity following uterine or tubal rupture

Excludes *that by salpingostomy (66.02)*
that by salpingotomy (66.01)
that with synchronous salpingectomy (66.62)

✖ 74.4 **Cesarean section of other specified type**
Peritoneal exclusion cesarean section
Transperitoneal cesarean section NOS
Vaginal cesarean section

● 74.9 **Cesarean section of unspecified type**

✖ 74.91 **Hysterotomy to terminate pregnancy**
Therapeutic abortion by hysterotomy

✖ 74.99 **Other cesarean section of unspecified type**
Cesarean section NOS
Obstetrical abdominouterotomy
Obstetrical hysterotomy

● **75 Other obstetric operations**

75.0 Intra-amniotic injection for abortion
Injection of:
prostaglandin for induction of abortion
saline for induction of abortion
Termination of pregnancy by intrauterine injection

Excludes *insertion of prostaglandin suppository for abortion (96.49)*

75.1 Diagnostic amniocentesis

75.2 Intrauterine transfusion
Exchange transfusion in utero
Insertion of catheter into abdomen of fetus for transfusion

Code also any hysterotomy approach (68.0)

● **75.3 Other intrauterine operations on fetus and amnion**

Code also any hysterotomy approach (68.0)

75.31 Amnioscopy
Fetoscopy
Laparoamnioscopy

75.32 Fetal EKG (scalp)

75.33 Fetal blood sampling and biopsy

75.34 Other fetal monitoring
Antepartum fetal nonstress test
Fetal monitoring, not otherwise specified

Excludes *fetal pulse oximetry (75.38)*

✖ **75.35 Other diagnostic procedures on fetus and amnion**
Intrauterine pressure determination

Excludes *amniocentesis (75.1)*
diagnostic procedures on gravid uterus and placenta (87.81, 88.46, 88.78, 92.17)

✖ **75.36 Correction of fetal defect**

75.37 Amnioinfusion

Code also injection of antibiotic (99.21)

75.38 Fetal pulse oximetry
Transcervical fetal oxygen saturation monitoring
Transcervical fetal SpO_2 monitoring

75.4 Manual removal of retained placenta

Excludes *aspiration curettage (69.52)*
dilation and curettage (69.02)

● **75.5 Repair of current obstetric laceration of uterus**

✖ **75.50 Repair of current obstetric laceration of uterus, not otherwise specified**

✖ **75.51 Repair of current obstetric laceration of cervix**

✖ **75.52 Repair of current obstetric laceration of corpus uteri**

● **75.6 Repair of other current obstetric laceration**

✖ **75.61 Repair of current obstetric laceration of bladder and urethra**

75.62 Repair of current obstetric laceration of rectum and sphincter ani

75.69 Repair of other current obstetric laceration
Episioperineorrhaphy
Repair of:
pelvic floor
perineum
vagina
vulva
Secondary repair of episiotomy

Excludes *repair of routine episiotomy (73.6)*

75.7 Manual exploration of uterine cavity, postpartum

75.8 Obstetric tamponade of uterus or vagina

Excludes *antepartum tamponade (73.1)*

● **75.9 Other obstetric operations**

75.91 Evacuation of obstetrical incisional hematoma of perineum
Evacuation of hematoma of:
episiotomy
perineorrhaphy

75.92 Evacuation of other hematoma of vulva or vagina

✖ **75.93 Surgical correction of inverted uterus**
Spintelli operation

Excludes *vaginal repair of chronic inversion of uterus (69.23)*

75.94 Manual replacement of inverted uterus

✖ **75.99 Other**

14. OPERATIONS ON THE MUSCULOSKELETAL SYSTEM (76–84)

● 76 **Operations on facial bones and joints**

Excludes *accessory sinuses (22.00–22.9)*
nasal bones (21.00–21.99)
skull (01.01–02.99)

● 76.0 **Incision of facial bone without division**

✖ 76.01 **Sequestrectomy of facial bone**
Removal of necrotic bone chip from facial bone

✖ 76.09 **Other incision of facial bone**
Reopening of osteotomy site of facial bone

Excludes *osteotomy associated with orthognathic surgery (76.61–76.69)*
removal of internal fixation device (76.97)

● 76.1 **Diagnostic procedures on facial bones and joints**

✖ 76.11 **Biopsy of facial bone**

✖ 76.19 **Other diagnostic procedures on facial bones and joints**

Excludes *contrast arthrogram of temporomandibular joint (87.13)*
other x-ray (87.11–87.12, 87.14–87.16)

76.2 **Local excision or destruction of lesion of facial bone**

Excludes *biopsy of facial bone (76.11)*
excision of odontogenic lesion (24.4)

● 76.3 **Partial ostectomy of facial bone**

✖ 76.31 **Partial mandibulectomy**
Hemimandibulectomy

Excludes *that associated with temporomandibular arthroplasty (76.5)*

✖ 76.39 **Partial ostectomy of other facial bone**
Hemimaxillectomy (with bone graft or prosthesis)

● 76.4 **Excision and reconstruction of facial bones**

✖ 76.41 **Total mandibulectomy with synchronous reconstruction**

✖ 76.42 **Other total mandibulectomy**

✖ 76.43 **Other reconstruction of mandible**

Excludes *genioplasty (76.67–76.68)*
that with synchronous total mandibulectomy (76.41)

✖ 76.44 **Total ostectomy of other facial bone with synchronous reconstruction**

✖ 76.45 **Other total ostectomy of other facial bone**

✖ 76.46 **Other reconstruction of other facial bone**

Excludes *that with synchronous total ostectomy (76.44)*

✖ 76.5 **Temporomandibular arthroplasty**

● 76.6 **Other facial bone repair and orthognathic surgery**

Code also any synchronous:
bone graft (76.91)
synthetic implant (76.92)

Excludes *reconstruction of facial bones (76.41–76.46)*

✖ 76.61 **Closed osteoplasty [osteotomy] of mandibular ramus**
Gigli saw osteotomy

✖ 76.62 **Open osteoplasty [osteotomy] of mandibular ramus**

✖ 76.63 **Osteoplasty [osteotomy] of body of mandible**

✖ 76.64 **Other orthognathic surgery on mandible**
Mandibular osteoplasty NOS
Segmental or subapical osteotomy

✖ 76.65 **Segmental osteoplasty [osteotomy] of maxilla**
Maxillary osteoplasty NOS

✖ 76.66 **Total osteoplasty [osteotomy] of maxilla**

✖ 76.67 **Reduction genioplasty**
Reduction mentoplasty

✖ 76.68 **Augmentation genioplasty**
Mentoplasty:
NOS
with graft or implant

✖ 76.69 **Other facial bone repair**
Osteoplasty of facial bone NOS

● 76.7 **Reduction of facial fracture**

Includes: internal fixation

Code also any synchronous:
bone graft (76.91)
synthetic implant (76.92)

Excludes *that of nasal bones (21.71–21.72)*

✖ 76.70 **Reduction of facial fracture, not otherwise specified**

76.71 **Closed reduction of malar and zygomatic fracture**

✖ 76.72 **Open reduction of malar and zygomatic fracture**

76.73 **Closed reduction of maxillary fracture**

✖ 76.74 **Open reduction of maxillary fracture**

76.75 **Closed reduction of mandibular fracture**

✖ 76.76 **Open reduction of mandibular fracture**

✖ 76.77 **Open reduction of alveolar fracture**
Reduction of alveolar fracture with stabilization of teeth

76.78 **Other closed reduction of facial fracture**
Closed reduction of orbital fracture

Excludes *nasal bone (21.71)*

✖ 76.79 **Other open reduction of facial fracture**
Open reduction of orbit rim or wall

Excludes *nasal bone (21.72)*

● 76.9 **Other operations on facial bones and joints**

✖ 76.91 **Bone graft to facial bone**
Autogenous graft to facial bone
Bone bank graft to facial bone
Heterogenous graft to facial bone

✖ 76.92 **Insertion of synthetic implant in facial bone**
Alloplastic implant to facial bone

76.93 **Closed reduction of temporomandibular dislocation**

✖ 76.94 **Open reduction of temporomandibular dislocation**

76.95 **Other manipulation of temporomandibular joint**

76.96 **Injection of therapeutic substance into temporomandibular joint**

✖ 76.97 **Removal of internal fixation device from facial bone**

Excludes *removal of:*
dental wiring (97.33)
external mandibular fixation device NEC (97.36)

✖ 76.99 **Other**

● **77 Incision, excision, and division of other bones**

Excludes *laminectomy for decompression (03.09)*
operations on:
accessory sinuses (22.00–22.9)
ear ossicles (19.0–19.55)
facial bones (76.01–76.99)
joint structures (80.00–81.99)
mastoid (19.9–20.99)
nasal bones (21.00–21.99)
skull (01.01–02.99)

The following fourth-digit subclassification is for use with appropriate categories in section 77 to identify the site. Valid fourth-digit categories are in brackets under each code.

0 **unspecified site**
1 **scapula, clavicle, and thorax [ribs and sternum]**
2 **humerus**
3 **radius and ulna**
4 **carpals and metacarpals**
5 **femur**
6 **patella**
7 **tibia and fibula**
8 **tarsals and metatarsals**
9 **other**
Pelvic bones
Phalanges (of foot) (of hand)
Vertebrae

✖● **77.0 Sequestrectomy**
[0–9]

✖● **77.1 Other incision of bone without division**
[0–9] Reopening of osteotomy site

Excludes *aspiration of bone marrow (41.31, 41.91)*
removal of internal fixation device (78.60–78.69)

✖● **77.2 Wedge osteotomy**
[0–9]

Excludes *that for hallux valgus (77.51)*

✖● **77.3 Other division of bone**
[0–9] Osteoarthrotomy

Excludes *clavicotomy of fetus (73.8)*
laminotomy or incision of vertebra (03.01–03.09)
pubiotomy to assist delivery (73.94)
sternotomy incidental to thoracic operation—omit code

✖● **77.4 Biopsy of bone**
[0–9]

● **77.5 Excision and repair of bunion and other toe deformities**

✖ **77.51 Bunionectomy with soft tissue correction and osteotomy of the first metatarsal**

✖ **77.52 Bunionectomy with soft tissue correction and arthrodesis**

✖ **77.53 Other bunionectomy with soft tissue correction**

✖ **77.54 Excision or correction of bunionette**
That with osteotomy

✖ **77.56 Repair of hammer toe**
Filleting of hammer toe
Fusion of hammer toe
Phalangectomy (partial) of hammer toe

✖ **77.57 Repair of claw toe**
Capsulotomy of claw toe
Fusion of claw toe
Phalangectomy (partial) of claw toe
Tendon lengthening of claw toe

✖ **77.58 Other excision, fusion, and repair of toes**
Cockup toe repair
Overlapping toe repair
That with use of prosthetic materials

✖ **77.59 Other bunionectomy**
Resection of hallux valgus joint with insertion of prosthesis

✖● **77.6 Local excision of lesion or tissue of bone**
[0–9]

Excludes *biopsy of bone (77.40–77.49)*
debridement of compound fracture (79.60–79.69)

✖● **77.7 Excision of bone for graft**
[0–9]

✖● **77.8 Other partial ostectomy**
[0–9] Condylectomy

Excludes *amputation (84.00–84.19, 84.91)*
arthrectomy (80.90–80.99)
excision of bone ends associated with:
arthrodesis (81.00–81.29)
arthroplasty (81.31–81.87)
excision of cartilage (80.5–80.6, 80.80–80.99)
excision of head of femur with synchronous replacement (00.70–00.73, 81.51–81.53)
hemilaminectomy (03.01–03.09)
laminectomy (03.01–03.09)
ostectomy for hallux valgus (77.51–77.59)
partial amputation:
finger (84.01)
thumb (84.02)
toe (84.11)
resection of ribs incidental to thoracic operation—omit code
that incidental to other operation—omit code

✖● **77.9 Total ostectomy**
[0–9]

Excludes *amputation of limb (84.00–84.19, 84.91)*
that incidental to other operation—omit code

● **78 Other operations on bones, except facial bones**

Excludes *operations on:*
accessory sinuses (22.00–22.9)
facial bones (76.01–76.99)
joint structures (80.00–81.99)
nasal bones (21.00–21.99)
skull (01.01–02.99)

The following fourth-digit subclassification is for use with categories in section 78 to identify the site. Valid fourth-digit categories are in [brackets] under each code.

0 **unspecified site**
1 **scapula, clavicle, and thorax [ribs and sternum]**
2 **humerus**
3 **radius and ulna**
4 **carpals and metacarpals**
5 **femur**
6 **patella**
7 **tibia and fibula**
8 **tarsals and metatarsals**
9 **other**
Pelvic bones
Phalanges (of foot) (of hand)
Vertebrae

✖● **78.0 Bone graft**
[0–9] Bone:
bank graft
graft (autogenous) (heterogenous)
That with debridement of bone graft site (removal of sclerosed, fibrous, or necrotic bone or tissue)
Transplantation of bone

Code also any excision of bone for graft (77.70–77.79)

Excludes *that for bone lengthening (78.30–78.39)*

✖● **78.1 Application of external fixator device**
[0–9] Fixator with insertion of pins/wires/screws into bone

Code also any type of fixator device, if known (84.71–84.73)

Excludes *other immobilization, pressure, and attention to wound (93.51–93.59)*

✖● **78.2 Limb shortening procedures**
[0, 2–5, 7–9] Epiphyseal stapling
Open epiphysiodesis
Percutaneous epiphysiodesis
Resection/osteotomy

✖● **78.3 Limb lengthening procedures**
[0, 2–5, 7–9] Bone graft with or without internal fixation devices or osteotomy
Distraction technique with or without corticotomy/osteotomy

Code also any application of an external fixation device (78.10–78.19)

✖● **78.4 Other repair or plastic operations on bone**
[0–9] Other operation on bone NEC
Repair of malunion or nonunion fracture NEC

Excludes *application of external fixation device (78.10–78.19)*
limb lengthening procedures (78.30–78.39)
limb shortening procedures (78.20–78.29)
osteotomy (77.3)
reconstruction of thumb (82.61–82.69)
repair of pectus deformity (34.74)
repair with bone graft (78.00–78.09)

✖● **78.5 Internal fixation of bone without fracture reduction**
[0–9] Internal fixation of bone (prophylactic)
Reinsertion of internal fixation device
Revision of displaced or broken fixation device

Excludes *arthroplasty and arthrodesis (81.00–81.85)*
bone graft (78.00–78.09)
limb shortening procedures (78.20–78.29)
that for fracture reduction (79.10–79.19, 79.30–79.59)

✖● **78.6 Removal of implanted devices from bone**
[0–9] External fixator device (invasive)
Internal fixation device
Removal of bone growth stimulator (invasive)
Removal of internal limb lengthening device

Excludes *removal of cast, splint, and traction device (Kirschner wire) (Steinmann pin) (97.88)*
removal of skull tongs or halo traction device (02.95)

✖● **78.7 Osteoclasis**
[0–9]

✖● **78.8 Diagnostic procedures on bone, not elsewhere**
[0–9] **classified**

Excludes *biopsy of bone (77.40–77.49)*
magnetic resonance imaging (88.94)
microscopic examination of specimen from bone (91.51–91.59)
radioisotope scan (92.14)
skeletal x-ray (87.21–87.29, 87.43, 88.21–88.33)
thermography (88.83)

✖● **78.9 Insertion of bone growth stimulator**
[0–9] Insertion of:
bone stimulator (electrical) to aid bone healing
osteogenic electrodes for bone growth stimulation
totally implanted device (invasive)

Excludes *non-invasive (transcutaneous) (surface) stimulator (99.86)*

● **79 Reduction of fracture and dislocation**

Includes: application of cast or splint
Reduction with insertion of traction device (Kirschner wire) (Steinmann pin)

Code also any:
application of external fixator device (78.10–78.19)
type of fixator device, if known (84.71–84.73)

Excludes *external fixation alone for immobilization of fracture (93.51–93.56, 93.59)*
internal fixation without reduction of fracture (78.50–78.59)
operations on:
facial bones (76.70–76.79)
nasal bones (21.71–21.72)
orbit (76.78–76.79)
skull (02.02)
vertebrae (03.53)
removal of cast or splint (97.88)
replacement of cast or splint (97.11–97.14)
traction alone for reduction of fracture (93.41–93.46)

The following fourth-digit subclassification is for use with appropriate categories in section 79 to identify the site. Valid fourth-digit categories are in [brackets] under each code.

0 unspecified site
1 humerus
2 radius and ulna
Arm NOS
3 carpals and metacarpals
Hand NOS
4 phalanges of hand
5 femur
6 tibia and fibula
Leg NOS
7 tarsals and metatarsals
Foot NOS
8 phalanges of foot
9 other specified bone

● **79.0 Closed reduction of fracture without internal fixation**

Excludes *that for separation of epiphysis (79.40–79.49)*

✖● **79.1 Closed reduction of fracture with internal fixation**

Excludes *that for separation of epiphysis (79.40–79.49)*

✖● **79.2 Open reduction of fracture without internal fixation**
[0–9]

Excludes *that for separation of epiphysis (79.50–79.59)*

✖● **79.3 Open reduction of fracture with internal fixation**
[0–9]

Excludes *that for separation of epiphysis (79.50–79.59)*

✖● **79.4 Closed reduction of separated epiphysis**
[0–2, 5, 6, 9] Reduction with or without internal fixation

✖● **79.5 Open reduction of separated epiphysis**
[0–2, 5, 6, 9] Reduction with or without internal fixation

✖● **79.6 Debridement of open fracture site**
[0–9] Debridement of compound fracture

● **79.7 Closed reduction of dislocation**

Includes: closed reduction (with external traction device)

Excludes *closed reduction of dislocation of temporomandibular joint (76.93)*

79.70 Closed reduction of dislocation of unspecified site

79.71 Closed reduction of dislocation of shoulder

79.72 Closed reduction of dislocation of elbow

79.73 Closed reduction of dislocation of wrist

79.74 **Closed reduction of dislocation of hand and finger**

79.75 **Closed reduction of dislocation of hip**

79.76 **Closed reduction of dislocation of knee**

79.77 **Closed reduction of dislocation of ankle**

79.78 **Closed reduction of dislocation of foot and toe**

79.79 **Closed reduction of dislocation of other specified sites**

● 79.8 **Open reduction of dislocation**

Includes: open reduction (with internal and external fixation devices)

Excludes *open reduction of dislocation of temporomandibular joint (76.94)*

✖ 79.80 **Open reduction of dislocation of unspecified site**

✖ 79.81 **Open reduction of dislocation of shoulder**

✖ 79.82 **Open reduction of dislocation of elbow**

✖ 79.83 **Open reduction of dislocation of wrist**

✖ 79.84 **Open reduction of dislocation of hand and finger**

✖ 79.85 **Open reduction of dislocation of hip**

✖ 79.86 **Open reduction of dislocation of knee**

✖ 79.87 **Open reduction of dislocation of ankle**

✖ 79.88 **Open reduction of dislocation of foot and toe**

✖ 79.89 **Open reduction of dislocation of other specified sites**

✖● 79.9 **Unspecified operation on bone injury**
[0–9]

● 80 **Incision and excision of joint structures**

Includes: operations on:
capsule of joint
cartilage
condyle
ligament
meniscus
synovial membrane

Excludes *cartilage of:*
ear (18.01–18.9)
nose (21.00–21.99)
temporomandibular joint (76.01–76.99)

The following fourth-digit subclassification is for use with appropriate categories in section 80 to identify the site:

0 **unspecified site**
1 **shoulder**
2 **elbow**
3 **wrist**
4 **hand and finger**
5 **hip**
6 **knee**
7 **ankle**
8 **foot and toe**
9 **other specified sites**
Spine

✖● 80.0 **Arthrotomy for removal of prosthesis**

Code also any:
insertion of (cement) (joint) spacer (84.56)
removal of (cement) (joint) spacer (84.57)

✖● 80.1 **Other arthrotomy**

Arthrostomy

Excludes *that for:*
arthrography (88.32)
arthroscopy (80.20–80.29)
injection of drug (81.92)
operative approach—omit code

✖● 80.2 **Arthroscopy**

● 80.3 **Biopsy of joint structure**

Aspiration biopsy

✖● 80.4 **Division of joint capsule, ligament, or cartilage**

Goldner clubfoot release
Heyman-Herndon(-Strong) correction of metatarsus varus
Release of:
adherent or constrictive joint capsule
joint
ligament

Excludes *symphysiotomy to assist delivery (73.94)*
that for:
carpal tunnel syndrome (04.43)
tarsal tunnel syndrome (04.44)

● 80.5 **Excision or destruction of intervertebral disc**

✖ 80.50 **Excision or destruction of intervertebral disc, unspecified**

Unspecified as to excision or destruction

✖ 80.51 **Excision of intervertebral disc**

Diskectomy
Removal of herniated nucleus pulposus
Level:
cervical
thoracic
lumbar (lumbosacral)
That by laminotomy or hemilaminectomy
That with decompression of spinal nerve root at same level
Requires additional code for any concomitant decompression of spinal nerve root at different level from excision site

Code also any concurrent spinal fusion (81.00–81.09)

Excludes *intervertebral chemonucleolysis (80.52)*
laminectomy for exploration of intraspinal canal (03.09)
laminotomy for decompression of spinal nerve root only (03.09)
that for insertion of (non-fusion) spinal disc replacement device (84.60–84.69)
that with corpectomy, (vertebral) (80.99) ◀

80.52 **Intervertebral chemonucleolysis**

With aspiration of disc fragments
With diskography
Injection of proteolytic enzyme into intervertebral space (chymopapain)

Excludes *injection of anesthetic substance (03.91)*
injection of other substances (03.92)

✖ 80.59 **Other destruction of intervertebral disc**

Destruction NEC
That by laser

✖ 80.6 **Excision of semilunar cartilage of knee**

Excision of meniscus of knee

✖● 80.7 **Synovectomy**

Complete or partial resection of synovial membrane

Excludes *excision of Baker's cyst (83.39)*

✖● 80.8 **Other local excision or destruction of lesion of joint**

✖● 80.9 **Other excision of joint**

Excludes *cheilectomy of joint (77.80–77.89)*
excision of bone ends (77.80–77.89)

● 81 **Repair and plastic operations on joint structures**

● 81.0 **Spinal fusion**

Code also the total number of vertebrae fused (81.62–81.64)

Code also any insertion of interbody spinal fusion device (84.51)

Code also any insertion of recombinant bone morphogenetic protein (84.52)

Includes: arthrodesis of spine with:
bone graft
internal fixation

Excludes *correction of pseudarthrosis of spine (81.30–81.39)*
refusion of spine (81.30–81.39)

✖ 81.00 **Spinal fusion, not otherwise specified**

✖ 81.01 **Atlas-axis spinal fusion**
Craniocervical fusion by anterior, transoral, or posterior technique
C1-C2 fusion by anterior, transoral, or posterior technique
Occiput C2 fusion by anterior, transoral, or posterior technique

✖ 81.02 **Other cervical fusion, anterior technique**
Arthrodesis of C2 level or below:
anterior (interbody) technique
anterolateral technique

✖ 81.03 **Other cervical fusion, posterior technique**
Arthrodesis of C2 level or below:
posterior (interbody) technique
posterolateral technique

✖ 81.04 **Dorsal and dorsolumbar fusion, anterior technique**
Arthrodesis of thoracic or thoracolumbar region:
anterior (interbody) technique
anterolateral technique

✖ 81.05 **Dorsal and dorsolumbar fusion, posterior technique**
Arthrodesis of thoracic or thoracolumbar region:
posterior (interbody) technique
posterolateral technique

✖ 81.06 **Lumbar and lumbosacral fusion, anterior technique**
Anterior lumbar interbody fusion (ALIF)
Arthrodesis of lumbar or lumbosacral region:
anterior (interbody) technique
anterolateral technique

✖ 81.07 **Lumbar and lumbosacral fusion, lateral transverse process technique**

✖ 81.08 **Lumbar and lumbosacral fusion, posterior technique**
Arthrodesis of lumbar or lumbosacral region:
posterior (interbody) technique
posterolateral technique
Posterior lumbar interbody fusion (PLIF)
Transforaminal lumbar interbody fusion (TLIF)

● 81.1 **Arthrodesis and arthroereisis of foot and ankle**

Includes: arthrodesis of foot and ankle with:
bone graft
external fixation device

✖ 81.11 **Ankle fusion**
Tibiotalar fusion

✖ 81.12 **Triple arthrodesis**
Talus to calcaneus and calcaneus to cuboid and navicular

✖ 81.13 **Subtalar fusion**

Excludes *arthroereisis (81.18)*

✖ 81.14 **Midtarsal fusion**

✖ 81.15 **Tarsometatarsal fusion**

✖ 81.16 **Metatarsophalangeal fusion**

✖ 81.17 **Other fusion of foot**

✖ 81.18 **Subtalar joint arthroereisis**

● 81.2 **Arthrodesis of other joint**

Includes: arthrodesis with:
bone graft
external fixation device
excision of bone ends and compression

✖ 81.20 **Arthrodesis of unspecified joint**

✖ 81.21 **Arthrodesis of hip**

✖ 81.22 **Arthrodesis of knee**

✖ 81.23 **Arthrodesis of shoulder**

✖ 81.24 **Arthrodesis of elbow**

✖ 81.25 **Carporadial fusion**

✖ 81.26 **Metacarpocarpal fusion**

✖ 81.27 **Metacarpophalangeal fusion**

✖ 81.28 **Interphalangeal fusion**

✖ 81.29 **Arthrodesis of other specified joints**

● 81.3 **Refusion of spine**

Includes: arthrodesis of spine with:
bone graft
internal fixation
correction of pseudarthrosis of spine

Code also any insertion of interbody spinal fusion device (84.51)

Code also any insertion of recombinant bone morphogenetic protein (84.52)

Code also the total number of vertebra fused (81.62–81.64)

✖ 81.30 **Refusion of spine, not otherwise specified**

✖ 81.31 **Refusion of atlas-axis spine**
Craniocervical fusion by anterior, transoral, or posterior technique
C1-C2 fusion by anterior, transoral, or posterior technique
Occiput C2 fusion by anterior, transoral, or posterior technique

✖ 81.32 **Refusion of other cervical spine, anterior technique**
Arthrodesis of C2 level or below:
anterior (interbody) technique
anterolateral technique

✖ 81.33 **Refusion of other cervical spine, posterior technique**
Arthrodesis of C2 level or below:
posterior (interbody) technique
posterolateral technique

✖ 81.34 **Refusion of dorsal and dorsolumbar spine, anterior technique**
Arthrodesis of thoracic or thoracolumbar region:
anterior (interbody) technique
anterolateral technique

✖ 81.35 **Refusion of dorsal and dorsolumbar spine, posterior technique**
Arthrodesis of thoracic or thoracolumbar region:
posterior (interbody) technique
posterolateral technique

✖ 81.36 **Refusion of lumbar and lumbosacral spine, anterior technique**
Anterior lumbar interbody fusion (ALIF)
Arthrodesis of lumbar or lumbosacral region:
anterior (interbody) technique
anterolateral technique

✖ 81.37 **Refusion of lumbar and lumbosacral spine, lateral transverse process technique**

✖81.38 **Refusion of lumbar and lumbosacral spine, posterior technique**
Arthrodesis of lumbar or lumbosacral region:
posterior (interbody) technique
posterolateral technique
Posterior lumbar interbody fusion (PLIF)
Transforaminal lumbar interbody fusion (TLIF)

✖81.39 **Refusion of spine, not elsewhere classified**

●81.4 **Other repair of joint of lower extremity**

Includes: arthroplasty of lower extremity with:
external traction or fixation
graft of bone (chips) or cartilage
internal fixation device

✖81.40 **Repair of hip, not elsewhere classified**

✖81.42 **Five-in-one repair of knee**
Medial meniscectomy, medial collateral ligament repair, vastus medialis advancement, semitendinosus advancement, and pes anserinus transfer

✖81.43 **Triad knee repair**
Medial meniscectomy with repair of the anterior cruciate ligament and the medial collateral ligament
O'Donoghue procedure

✖81.44 **Patellar stabilization**
Roux-Goldthwait operation for recurrent dislocation of patella

✖81.45 **Other repair of the cruciate ligaments**

✖81.46 **Other repair of the collateral ligaments**

✖81.47 **Other repair of knee**

✖81.49 **Other repair of ankle**

●81.5 **Joint replacement of lower extremity**

Includes: arthroplasty of lower extremity with:
external traction or fixation
graft of bone (chips) or cartilage
internal fixation device or prosthesis
removal of cement spacer

✖81.51 **Total hip replacement**
Replacement of both femoral head and acetabulum by prosthesis
Total reconstruction of hip

Code also any type of bearing surface, if known (00.74–00.76)

✖81.52 **Partial hip replacement**
Bipolar endoprosthesis

Code also any type of bearing surface, if known (00.74–00.76)

✖81.53 **Revision of hip replacement, not otherwise specified**
Revision of hip replacement, not specified as to components(s) replaced (acetabular, femoral, or both)

Code also any:
removal of (cement) (joint) spacer (84.57)
type of bearing surface, if known (00.74–00.76)

Excludes *revision of hip replacement, components specified (00.70–00.73)*

✖81.54 **Total knee replacement**
Bicompartmental
Tricompartmental
Unicompartmental (hemijoint)

✖81.55 **Revision of knee replacement not otherwise specified**

Code also any removal of (cement) spacer (84.57)

Excludes *arthrodesis of knee (81.22)*
revision of knee replacement, components specified (00.80–00.84)

✖81.56 **Total ankle replacement**

✖81.57 **Replacement of joint of foot and toe**

✖81.59 **Revision of joint replacement of lower extremity, not elsewhere classified**

●81.6 **Other procedures on spine**
Note: Number of vertebrae
The vertebral spine consists of 25 vertebrae in the following order and number:
Cervical: C1 (atlas), C2 (axis), C3, C4, C5, C6, C7
Thoracic or Dorsal: T1, T2, T3, T4, T5, T6, T7, T8, T9, T10, T11, T12
Lumbar and Sacral: L1, L2, L3, L4, L5, S1

Coders should report only one code from the series 81.62 or 81.63 or 81.64 to show the total number of vertebrae fused on the patient.

Code also the level and approach of the fusion or refusion (81.00–81.08, 81.30–81.39)

✖81.62 **Fusion or refusion of 2–3 vertebrae**

✖81.63 **Fusion or refusion of 4–8 vertebrae**

✖81.64 **Fusion or refusion of 9 or more vertebrae**

✖81.65 **Vertebroplasty**
Injection of bone void filler (cement) (polymethylmethacrylate) (PMMA) into the diseased or fractured vertebral body

Excludes *kyphoplasty (81.66)*

✖81.66 **Kyphoplasty**
Insertion of inflatable balloon, bone tamp, or other device to create a cavity for partial restoration of height of diseased or fractured vertebral body prior to injection of bone void filler (cement) (polymethylmethacrylate) (PMMA)

Excludes *vertebroplasty (81.65)*

●81.7 **Arthroplasty and repair of hand, fingers, and wrist**

Includes: arthroplasty of hand and finger with:
external traction or fixation
graft of bone (chips) or cartilage
internal fixation device or prosthesis

Excludes *operations on muscle, tendon, and fascia of hand (82.01–82.99)*

✖81.71 **Arthroplasty of metacarpophalangeal and interphalangeal joint with implant**

✖81.72 **Arthroplasty of metacarpophalangeal and interphalangeal joint without implant**

✖81.73 **Total wrist replacement**

✖81.74 **Arthroplasty of carpocarpal or carpometacarpal joint with implant**

✖81.75 **Arthroplasty of carpocarpal or carpometacarpal joint without implant**

✖81.79 **Other repair of hand, fingers, and wrist**

●81.8 **Arthroplasty and repair of shoulder and elbow**

Includes: arthroplasty of upper limb NEC with:
external traction or fixation
graft of bone (chips) or cartilage
internal fixation device or prosthesis

✖81.80 **Total shoulder replacement**

✖81.81 **Partial shoulder replacement**

✖81.82 **Repair of recurrent dislocation of shoulder**

✖ 81.83 **Other repair of shoulder**
Revision of arthroplasty of shoulder

✖ 81.84 **Total elbow replacement**

✖ 81.85 **Other repair of elbow**

● 81.9 **Other operations on joint structures**

81.91 **Arthrocentesis**
Joint aspiration

Excludes *that for:*
arthrography (88.32)
biopsy of joint structure (80.30–80.39)
injection of drug (81.92)

81.92 **Injection of therapeutic substance into joint or ligament**

✖ 81.93 **Suture of capsule or ligament of upper extremity**

Excludes *that associated with arthroplasty (81.71–81.75, 81.80–81.81, 81.84)*

✖ 81.94 **Suture of capsule or ligament of ankle and foot**

Excludes *that associated with arthroplasty (81.56–81.59)*

✖ 81.95 **Suture of capsule or ligament of other lower extremity**

Excludes *that associated with arthroplasty (81.51–81.55, 81.59)*

✖ 81.96 **Other repair of joint**

✖ 81.97 **Revision of joint replacement of upper extremity**
Partial
Removal of cement spacer
Total

✖ 81.98 **Other diagnostic procedures on joint structures**

Excludes *arthroscopy (80.20–80.29)*
biopsy of joint structure (80.30–80.39)
microscopic examination of specimen from joint (91.51–91.59)
thermography (88.83)
x-ray (87.21–87.29, 88.21–88.33)

✖ 81.99 **Other**

● 82 **Operations on muscle, tendon, and fascia of hand**

Includes: operations on:
aponeurosis
synovial membrane (tendon sheath)
tendon sheath

● 82.0 **Incision of muscle, tendon, fascia, and bursa of hand**

✖ 82.01 **Exploration of tendon sheath of hand**
Incision of tendon sheath of hand
Removal of rice bodies in tendon sheath of hand

Excludes *division of tendon (82.11)*

✖ 82.02 **Myotomy of hand**

Excludes *myotomy for division (82.19)*

✖ 82.03 **Bursotomy of hand**

82.04 **Incision and drainage of palmar or thenar space**

✖ 82.09 **Other incision of soft tissue of hand**

Excludes *incision of skin and subcutaneous tissue alone (86.01–86.09)*

● 82.1 **Division of muscle, tendon, and fascia of hand**

✖ 82.11 **Tenotomy of hand**
Division of tendon of hand

✖ 82.12 **Fasciotomy of hand**
Division of fascia of hand

✖ 82.19 **Other division of soft tissue of hand**
Division of muscle of hand

● 82.2 **Excision of lesion of muscle, tendon, and fascia of hand**

✖ 82.21 **Excision of lesion of tendon sheath of hand**
Ganglionectomy of tendon sheath (wrist)

✖ 82.22 **Excision of lesion of muscle of hand**

✖ 82.29 **Excision of other lesion of soft tissue of hand**

Excludes *excision of lesion of skin and subcutaneous tissue (86.21–86.3)*

● 82.3 **Other excision of soft tissue of hand**

Code also any skin graft (86.61–86.62, 86.73)

Excludes *excision of skin and subcutaneous tissue (86.21–86.3)*

✖ 82.31 **Bursectomy of hand**

✖ 82.32 **Excision of tendon of hand for graft**

✖ 82.33 **Other tenonectomy of hand**
Tenosynovectomy of hand

Excludes *excision of lesion of:*
tendon (82.29)
sheath (82.21)

✖ 82.34 **Excision of muscle or fascia of hand for graft**

✖ 82.35 **Other fasciectomy of hand**
Release of Dupuytren's contracture

Excludes *excision of lesion of fascia (82.29)*

✖ 82.36 **Other myectomy of hand**

Excludes *excision of lesion of muscle (82.22)*

✖ 82.39 **Other excision of soft tissue of hand**

Excludes *excision of skin (86.21–86.3)*
excision of soft tissue lesion (82.29)

● 82.4 **Suture of muscle, tendon, and fascia of hand**

✖ 82.41 **Suture of tendon sheath of hand**

✖ 82.42 **Delayed suture of flexor tendon of hand**

✖ 82.43 **Delayed suture of other tendon of hand**

✖ 82.44 **Other suture of flexor tendon of hand**

Excludes *delayed suture of flexor tendon of hand (82.42)*

✖ 82.45 **Other suture of other tendon of hand**

Excludes *delayed suture of other tendon of hand (82.43)*

✖ 82.46 **Suture of muscle or fascia of hand**

● 82.5 **Transplantation of muscle and tendon of hand**

✖ 82.51 **Advancement of tendon of hand**

✖ 82.52 **Recession of tendon of hand**

✖ 82.53 **Reattachment of tendon of hand**

✖ 82.54 **Reattachment of muscle of hand**

✖ 82.55 **Other change in hand muscle or tendon length**

✖ 82.56 **Other hand tendon transfer or transplantation**

Excludes *pollicization of thumb (82.61)*
transfer of finger, except thumb (82.81)

✖ 82.57 **Other hand tendon transposition**

✖ 82.58 **Other hand muscle transfer or transplantation**

✖ 82.59 **Other hand muscle transposition**

● 82.6 **Reconstruction of thumb**

Includes: digital transfer to act as thumb

Code also any amputation for digital transfer (84.01, 84.11)

✖ 82.61 **Pollicization operation carrying over nerves and blood supply**

✖ 82.69 **Other reconstruction of thumb**
"Cocked-hat" procedure [skin flap and bone]
Grafts:
bone to thumb skin (pedicle) to thumb

● 82.7 **Plastic operation on hand with graft or implant**

✖ 82.71 **Tendon pulley reconstruction**
Reconstruction for opponensplasty

✖82.72 **Plastic operation on hand with graft of muscle or fascia**

✖82.79 **Plastic operation on hand with other graft or implant**
Tendon graft to hand

●82.8 **Other plastic operations on hand**

✖82.81 **Transfer of finger, except thumb**
Excludes *pollicization of thumb (82.61)*

✖82.82 **Repair of cleft hand**

✖82.83 **Repair of macrodactyly**

✖82.84 **Repair of mallet finger**

✖82.85 **Other tenodesis of hand**
Tendon fixation of hand NOS

✖82.86 **Other tenoplasty of hand**
Myotenoplasty of hand

✖82.89 **Other plastic operations on hand**
Plication of fascia
Repair of fascial hernia
Excludes *that with graft or implant (82.71–82.79)*

●82.9 **Other operations on muscle, tendon, and fascia of hand**
Excludes *diagnostic procedures on soft tissue of hand (83.21–83.29)*

✖82.91 **Lysis of adhesions of hand**
Freeing of adhesions of fascia, muscle, and tendon of hand
Excludes *decompression of carpal tunnel (04.43)*
that by stretching or manipulation only (93.26)

82.92 **Aspiration of bursa of hand**

82.93 **Aspiration of other soft tissue of hand**
Excludes *skin and subcutaneous tissue (86.01)*

82.94 **Injection of therapeutic substance into bursa of hand**

82.95 **Injection of therapeutic substance into tendon of hand**

82.96 **Other injection of locally-acting therapeutic substance into soft tissue of hand**
Excludes *subcutaneous or intramuscular injection (99.11–99.29)*

✖82.99 **Other operations on muscle, tendon, and fascia of hand**

●83 **Operations on muscle, tendon, fascia, and bursa, except hand**
Includes: operations on:
aponeurosis
synovial membrane of bursa and tendon sheaths
tendon sheaths
Excludes *diaphragm (34.81–34.89)*
hand (82.01–82.99)
muscles of eye (15.01–15.9)

●83.0 **Incision of muscle, tendon, fascia, and bursa**

✖83.01 **Exploration of tendon sheath**
Incision of tendon sheath
Removal of rice bodies from tendon sheath

✖83.02 **Myotomy**
Excludes *cricopharyngeal myotomy (29.31)*

✖83.03 **Bursotomy**
Removal of calcareous deposit of bursa
Excludes *aspiration of bursa (percutaneous) (83.94)*

✖83.09 **Other incision of soft tissue**
Incision of fascia
Excludes *incision of skin and subcutaneous tissue alone (86.01–86.09)*

●83.1 **Division of muscle, tendon, and fascia**

✖83.11 **Achillotenotomy**

✖83.12 **Adductor tenotomy of hip**

✖83.13 **Other tenotomy**
Aponeurotomy
Division of tendon
Tendon release
Tendon transection
Tenotomy for thoracic outlet decompression

✖83.14 **Fasciotomy**
Division of fascia
Division of iliotibial band
Fascia stripping
Release of Volkmann's contracture by fasciotomy

✖83.19 **Other division of soft tissue**
Division of muscle
Muscle release
Myotomy for thoracic outlet decompression
Myotomy with division
Scalenotomy
Transection of muscle

●83.2 **Diagnostic procedures on muscle, tendon, fascia, and bursa, including that of hand**

✖83.21 **Biopsy of soft tissue**
Excludes *biopsy of chest wall (34.23)*
biopsy of skin and subcutaneous tissue (86.11)

✖83.29 **Other diagnostic procedures on muscle, tendon, fascia, and bursa, including that of hand**
Excludes *microscopic examination of specimen (91.51–91.59)*
soft tissue x-ray (87.09, 87.38–87.39, 88.09, 88.35, 88.37)
thermography of muscle (88.84)

●83.3 **Excision of lesion of muscle, tendon, fascia, and bursa**
Excludes *biopsy of soft tissue (83.21)*

✖83.31 **Excision of lesion of tendon sheath**
Excision of ganglion of tendon sheath, except of hand

✖83.32 **Excision of lesion of muscle**
Excision of:
heterotopic bone
muscle scar for release of Volkmann's contracture
myositis ossificans

✖83.39 **Excision of lesion of other soft tissue**
Excision of Baker's cyst
Excludes *bursectomy (83.5)*
excision of lesion of skin and subcutaneous tissue (86.3)
synovectomy (80.70–80.79)

●83.4 **Other excision of muscle, tendon, and fascia**

✖83.41 **Excision of tendon for graft**

✖83.42 **Other tenonectomy**
Excision of:
aponeurosis
tendon sheath
Tenosynovectomy

✖83.43 **Excision of muscle or fascia for graft**

✖83.44 **Other fasciectomy**

✖83.45 **Other myectomy**
Debridement of muscle NOS
Scalenectomy

✖83.49 **Other excision of soft tissue**

✖83.5 **Bursectomy**

●83.6 **Suture of muscle, tendon, and fascia**

✖83.61 **Suture of tendon sheath**

✖83.62 **Delayed suture of tendon**

✖83.63 **Rotator cuff repair**

✖83.64 **Other suture of tendon**
Achillorrhaphy
Aponeurorrhaphy

Excludes *delayed suture of tendon (83.62)*

✖83.65 **Other suture of muscle or fascia**
Repair of diastasis recti

●83.7 **Reconstruction of muscle and tendon**

Excludes *reconstruction of muscle and tendon associated with arthroplasty*

✖83.71 **Advancement of tendon**

✖83.72 **Recession of tendon**

✖83.73 **Reattachment of tendon**

✖83.74 **Reattachment of muscle**

✖83.75 **Tendon transfer or transplantation**

✖83.76 **Other tendon transposition**

✖83.77 **Muscle transfer or transplantation**
Release of Volkmann's contracture by muscle transplantation

✖83.79 **Other muscle transposition**

●83.8 **Other plastic operations on muscle, tendon, and fascia**

Excludes *plastic operations on muscle, tendon, and fascia associated with arthroplasty*

✖83.81 **Tendon graft**

✖83.82 **Graft of muscle or fascia**

✖83.83 **Tendon pulley reconstruction**

✖83.84 **Release of clubfoot, not elsewhere classified**
Evans operation on clubfoot

✖83.85 **Other change in muscle or tendon length**
Hamstring lengthening
Heel cord shortening
Plastic achillotenotomy
Tendon plication

✖83.86 **Quadricepsplasty**

✖83.87 **Other plastic operations on muscle**
Musculoplasty
Myoplasty

✖83.88 **Other plastic operations on tendon**
Myotenoplasty
Tendon fixation
Tenodesis
Tenoplasty

✖83.89 **Other plastic operations on fascia**
Fascia lengthening
Fascioplasty
Plication of fascia

●83.9 **Other operations on muscle, tendon, fascia, and bursa**

Excludes *nonoperative:*
manipulation (93.25–93.29)
stretching (93.27–93.29)

✖83.91 **Lysis of adhesions of muscle, tendon, fascia, and bursa**

Excludes *that for tarsal tunnel syndrome (04.44)*

✖83.92 **Insertion or replacement of skeletal muscle stimulator**
Implantation, insertion, placement, or replacement of skeletal muscle:
electrodes
stimulator

✖83.93 **Removal of skeletal muscle stimulator**

83.94 **Aspiration of bursa**

83.95 **Aspiration of other soft tissue**

Excludes *that of skin and subcutaneous tissue (86.01)*

83.96 **Injection of therapeutic substance into bursa**

83.97 **Injection of therapeutic substance into tendon**

83.98 **Injection of locally-acting therapeutic substance into other soft tissue**

Excludes *subcutaneous or intramuscular injection (99.11–99.29)*

✖83.99 **Other operations on muscle, tendon, fascia, and bursa**
Suture of bursa

●84 **Other procedures on musculoskeletal system**

●84.0 **Amputation of upper limb**

Excludes *revision of amputation stump (84.3)*

✖84.00 **Upper limb amputation, not otherwise specified**
Closed flap amputation of upper limb NOS
Kineplastic amputation of upper limb NOS
Open or guillotine amputation of upper limb NOS
Revision of current traumatic amputation of upper limb NOS

✖84.01 **Amputation and disarticulation of finger**

Excludes *ligation of supernumerary finger (86.26)*

✖84.02 **Amputation and disarticulation of thumb**

✖84.03 **Amputation through hand**
Amputation through carpals

✖84.04 **Disarticulation of wrist**

✖84.05 **Amputation through forearm**
Forearm amputation

✖84.06 **Disarticulation of elbow**

✖84.07 **Amputation through humerus**
Upper arm amputation

✖84.08 **Disarticulation of shoulder**

✖84.09 **Interthoracoscapular amputation**
Forequarter amputation

●84.1 **Amputation of lower limb**

Excludes *revision of amputation stump (84.3)*

✖84.10 **Lower limb amputation, not otherwise specified**
Closed flap amputation of lower limb NOS
Kineplastic amputation of lower limb NOS
Open or guillotine amputation of lower limb NOS
Revision of current traumatic amputation of lower limb NOS

✖84.11 **Amputation of toe**
Amputation through metatarsophalangeal joint
Disarticulation of toe
Metatarsal head amputation
Ray amputation of foot (disarticulation of the metatarsal head of the toe extending across the forefoot just proximal to the metatarsophalangeal crease)

Excludes *ligation of supernumerary toe (86.26)*

✖ 84.12 **Amputation through foot**
Amputation of forefoot
Amputation through middle of foot
Chopart's amputation
Midtarsal amputation
Transmetatarsal amputation (amputation of the forefoot, including all the toes)

Excludes *ray amputation of foot (84.11)*

✖ 84.13 **Disarticulation of ankle**

✖ 84.14 **Amputation of ankle through malleoli of tibia and fibula**

✖ 84.15 **Other amputation below knee**
Amputation of leg through tibia and fibula NOS

✖ 84.16 **Disarticulation of knee**
Batch, Spitler, and McFaddin amputation
Mazet amputation
S.P. Roger's amputation

✖ 84.17 **Amputation above knee**
Amputation of leg through femur
Amputation of thigh
Conversion of below-knee amputation into above-knee amputation
Supracondylar above-knee amputation

✖ 84.18 **Disarticulation of hip**

✖ 84.19 **Abdominopelvic amputation**
Hemipelvectomy
Hindquarter amputation

● 84.2 **Reattachment of extremity**

✖ 84.21 **Thumb reattachment**

✖ 84.22 **Finger reattachment**

✖ 84.23 **Forearm, wrist, or hand reattachment**

✖ 84.24 **Upper arm reattachment**
Reattachment of arm NOS

✖ 84.25 **Toe reattachment**

✖ 84.26 **Foot reattachment**

✖ 84.27 **Lower leg or ankle reattachment**
Reattachment of leg NOS

✖ 84.28 **Thigh reattachment**

✖ 84.29 **Other reattachment**

✖ 84.3 **Revision of amputation stump**
Reamputation of stump
Secondary closure of stump
Trimming of stump

Excludes *revision of current traumatic amputation [revision by further amputation of current injury] (84.00–84.19, 84.91)*

● 84.4 **Implantation or fitting of prosthetic limb device**

✖ 84.40 **Implantation or fitting of prosthetic limb device, not otherwise specified**

84.41 **Fitting of prosthesis of upper arm and shoulder**

84.42 **Fitting of prosthesis of lower arm and hand**

84.43 **Fitting of prosthesis of arm, not otherwise specified**

✖ 84.44 **Implantation of prosthetic device of arm**

84.45 **Fitting of prosthesis above knee**

84.46 **Fitting of prosthesis below knee**

84.47 **Fitting of prosthesis of leg, not otherwise specified**

✖ 84.48 **Implantation of prosthetic device of leg**

● 84.5 **Implantation of other musculoskeletal devices an substances**

Excludes *insertion of (non-fusion) spinal disc replacement device (84.60–84.69)*

84.51 **Insertion of interbody spinal fusion device**
Insertion of: cages (carbon, ceramic, metal, plastic, or titanium)
interbody fusion cage
synthetic cages or spacers
threaded bone dowels

Code also refusion of spine (81.30–81.39)

Code also spinal fusion (81.00–81.08)

84.52 **Insertion of recombinant bone morphogenetic protein rhBMP**
That via collagen sponge, coral, ceramic, and other carriers

Code also primary procedure performed:
fracture repair (79.00–79.99)
spinal fusion (81.00–81.08)
spinal refusion (81.30–81.39)

84.53 **Implantation of internal limb lengthening device with kinetic distraction**

Code also limb lengthening procedure (78.30–78.39)

84.54 **Implantation of other internal limb lengthening device**
Implantation of internal limb lengthening device Not Otherwise Specified (NOS)

Code also limb lengthening procedure (78.30–78.39)

84.55 **Insertion of bone void filler**
Insertion of:
acrylic cement (PMMA)
bone void cement
calcium based bone void filler
polymethylmethacrylate (PMMA)

Excludes *that with kyphoplasty (81.66)*
that with vertebroplasty (81.65)

84.56 **Insertion of (cement) spacer**
Insertion of joint spacer

84.57 **Removal of (cement) spacer**
Removal of joint spacer

84.58 **Implantation of interspinous process decompression device**

Excludes *fusion of spine (81.00–81.08, 81.30–81.39)*

84.59 **Insertion of other spinal devices**
Insertion of non-fusion spinal stabilization device ◀

84.6 **Replacement of spinal disc**

Includes: non-fusion arthroplasty of the spine with insertion of artificial disc prosthesis

84.60 **Insertion of spinal disc prosthesis, not otherwise specified**
Replacement of spinal disc, NOS

Includes: diskectomy (discectomy)

84.61 **Insertion of partial spinal disc prosthesis, cervical**
Nuclear replacement device, cervical
Partial artificial disc prosthesis (flexible), cervical
Replacement of nuclear disc (nucleus pulposus), cervical

Includes: diskectomy (discectomy)

84.62 Insertion of total spinal disc prosthesis, cervical
Replacement of cervical spinal disc, NOS
Replacement of total spinal disc, cervical
Total artificial disc prosthesis (flexible), cervical

Includes: diskectomy (discectomy)

84.63 Insertion of spinal disc prosthesis, thoracic
Artificial disc prosthesis (flexible), thoracic
Replacement of thoracic spinal disc, partial or total

Includes: diskectomy (discectomy)

84.64 Insertion of partial spinal disc prosthesis, lumbosacral
Nuclear replacement device, lumbar
Partial artificial disc prosthesis (flexible), lumbar
Replacement of nuclear disc (nucleus pulposus), lumbar

Includes: diskectomy (discectomy)

84.65 Insertion of total spinal disc prosthesis, lumbosacral
Replacement of lumbar spinal disc, NOS
Replacement of total spinal disc, lumbar
Total artificial disc prosthesis (flexible), lumbar

Includes: diskectomy (discectomy)

84.66 Revision or replacement of artificial spinal disc prosthesis, cervical
Removal of (partial) (total) spinal disc prosthesis with synchronous insertion of new (partial) (total) spinal disc prosthesis, cervical
Repair of previously inserted spinal disc prosthesis, cervical

84.67 Revision or replacement of artificial spinal disc prosthesis, thoracic
Removal of (partial) (total) spinal disc prosthesis with synchronous insertion of new (partial) (total) spinal disc prosthesis, thoracic
Repair of previously inserted spinal disc prosthesis, thoracic

84.68 Revision or replacement of artificial spinal disc prosthesis, lumbosacral
Removal of (partial) (total) spinal disc prosthesis with synchronous insertion of new (partial) (total) spinal disc prosthesis, lumbosacral
Repair of previously inserted spinal disc prosthesis, lumbosacral

❑ **84.69 Revision or replacement of artificial spinal disc prosthesis, not otherwise specified**
Removal of (partial) (total) spinal disc prosthesis with synchronous insertion of new (partial) (total) spinal disc prosthesis
Repair of previously inserted spinal disc prosthesis

● **84.7 Adjunct codes for external fixator devices**

Code also any primary procedure performed:
application of external fixator device (78.10, 78.12–78.13, 78.15, 78.17–78.19)
reduction of fracture and dislocation (79.00–79.89)

84.71 Application of external fixator device, monoplanar system

Excludes *other hybrid device or system (84.73)*
ring device or system (84.72)

84.72 Application of external fixator device, ring system
Ilizarov type
Sheffield type

Excludes *monoplanar device or system (84.71)*
other hybrid device or system (84.73)

84.73 Application of hybrid external fixator device
Computer (assisted) (dependent) external fixator device ◀
Hybrid system using both ring and monoplanar devices

Excludes *monoplanar device or system, when used alone (84.71)*
ring device or system, when used alone (84.72)

● **84.9 Other operations on musculoskeletal system**

Excludes *nonoperative manipulation (93.25–93.29)*

✖ **84.91 Amputation, not otherwise specified**

✖ **84.92 Separation of equal conjoined twins**

✖ **84.93 Separation of unequal conjoined twins**
Separation of conjoined twins NOS

✖ **84.99 Other**

15. OPERATIONS ON THE INTEGUMENTARY SYSTEM (85–86)

● 85 **Operations on the breast**

Includes: operations on the skin and subcutaneous tissue of:
breast female or male
previous mastectomy site female or male
revision of previous mastectomy site

85.0 **Mastotomy**
Incision of breast (skin)
Mammotomy
Excludes *aspiration of breast (85.91)*
removal of implant (85.94)

● 85.1 **Diagnostic procedures on breast**

85.11 **Closed [percutaneous] [needle] biopsy of breast**

✖ 85.12 **Open biopsy of breast**

85.19 **Other diagnostic procedures on breast**
Excludes *mammary ductogram (87.35)*
mammography NEC (87.37)
manual examination (89.36)
microscopic examination of specimen (91.61–91.69)
thermography (88.85)
ultrasonography (88.73)
xerography (87.36)

● 85.2 **Excision or destruction of breast tissue**
Excludes *mastectomy (85.41–85.48)*
reduction mammoplasty (85.31–85.32)

✖ 85.20 **Excision or destruction of breast tissue, not otherwise specified**

✖ 85.21 **Local excision of lesion of breast**
Lumpectomy
Removal of area of fibrosis from breast
Excludes *biopsy of breast (85.11–85.12)*

✖ 85.22 **Resection of quadrant of breast**

✖ 85.23 **Subtotal mastectomy**
Excludes *quadrant resection (85.22)*

✖ 85.24 **Excision of ectopic breast tissue**
Excision of accessory nipple

✖ 85.25 **Excision of nipple**
Excludes *excision of accessory nipple (85.24)*

● 85.3 **Reduction mammoplasty and subcutaneous mammectomy**

✖ 85.31 **Unilateral reduction mammoplasty**
Unilateral:
amputative mammoplasty
size reduction mammoplasty

✖ 85.32 **Bilateral reduction mammoplasty**
Amputative mammoplasty
Reduction mammoplasty (for gynecomastia)

✖ 85.33 **Unilateral subcutaneous mammectomy with synchronous implant**
Excludes *that without synchronous implant (85.34)*

✖ 85.34 **Other unilateral subcutaneous mammectomy**
Removal of breast tissue with preservation of skin and nipple
Subcutaneous mammectomy NOS

✖ 85.35 **Bilateral subcutaneous mammectomy with synchronous implant**
Excludes *that without synchronous implant (85.36)*

✖ 85.36 **Other bilateral subcutaneous mammectomy**

● 85.4 **Mastectomy**

✖ 85.41 **Unilateral simple mastectomy**
Mastectomy:
NOS
complete

✖ 85.42 **Bilateral simple mastectomy**
Bilateral complete mastectomy

✖ 85.43 **Unilateral extended simple mastectomy**
Extended simple mastectomy NOS
Modified radical mastectomy
Simple mastectomy with excision of regional lymph nodes

✖ 85.44 **Bilateral extended simple mastectomy**

✖ 85.45 **Unilateral radical mastectomy**
Excision of breast, pectoral muscles, and regional lymph nodes [axillary, clavicular, supraclavicular]
Radical mastectomy NOS

✖ 85.46 **Bilateral radical mastectomy**

✖ 85.47 **Unilateral extended radical mastectomy**
Excision of breast, muscles, and lymph nodes [axillary, clavicular, supraclavicular, internal mammary, and mediastinal]
Extended radical mastectomy NOS

✖ 85.48 **Bilateral extended radical mastectomy**

● 85.5 **Augmentation mammoplasty**
Excludes *that associated with subcutaneous mammectomy (85.33, 85.35)*

✖ 85.50 **Augmentation mammoplasty, not otherwise specified**

85.51 **Unilateral injection into breast for augmentation**

85.52 **Bilateral injection into breast for augmentation**
Injection into breast for augmentation NOS

✖ 85.53 **Unilateral breast implant**

✖ 85.54 **Bilateral breast implant**
Breast implant NOS

✖ 85.6 **Mastopexy**

✖ 85.7 **Total reconstruction of breast**

● 85.8 **Other repair and plastic operations on breast**
Excludes *that for:*
augmentation (85.50–85.54)
reconstruction (85.7)
reduction (85.31–85.32)

85.81 **Suture of laceration of breast**

✖ 85.82 **Split-thickness graft to breast**

✖ 85.83 **Full-thickness graft to breast**

✖ 85.84 **Pedicle graft to breast**

✖ 85.85 **Muscle flap graft to breast**

✖ 85.86 **Transposition of nipple**

✖ 85.87 **Other repair or reconstruction of nipple**

✖ 85.89 **Other mammoplasty**

● 85.9 **Other operations on the breast**

85.91 **Aspiration of breast**
Excludes *percutaneous biopsy of breast (85.11)*

85.92 **Injection of therapeutic agent into breast**
Excludes *that for augmentation of breast (85.51–85.52)*

✖ 85.93 **Revision of implant of breast**

✖ 85.94 **Removal of implant of breast**

✖ 85.95 **Insertion of breast tissue expander**
Insertion (soft tissue) of tissue expander (one or more) under muscle or platysma to develop skin flaps for donor use

✖ **85.96 Removal of breast tissue expander(s)**

✖ **85.99 Other**

● **86 Operations on skin and subcutaneous tissue**

Includes: operations on:
hair follicles
male perineum
nails
sebaceous glands
subcutaneous fat pads
sudoriferous glands
superficial fossae

Excludes *those on skin of:*
anus (49.01–49.99)
breast (mastectomy site) (85.0–85.99)
ear (18.01–18.9)
eyebrow (08.01–08.99)
eyelid (08.01–08.99)
female perineum (71.01–71.9)
lips (27.0–27.99)
nose (21.00–21.99)
penis (64.0–64.99)
scrotum (61.0–61.99)
vulva (71.01–71.9)

● **86.0 Incision of skin and subcutaneous tissue**

86.01 Aspiration of skin and subcutaneous tissue
Aspiration of:
abscess of nail, skin, or subcutaneous tissue
hematoma of nail, skin, or subcutaneous tissue
seroma of nail, skin, or subcutaneous tissue

86.02 Injection or tattooing of skin lesion or defect
Injection of filling material
Insertion of filling material
Pigmenting of skin of filling material

86.03 Incision of pilonidal sinus or cyst

Excludes *marsupialization (86.21)*

86.04 Other incision with drainage of skin and subcutaneous tissue

Excludes *drainage of:*
fascial compartments of face and mouth (27.0)
palmar or thenar space (82.04)
pilonidal sinus or cyst (86.03)

86.05 Incision with removal of foreign body or device from skin and subcutaneous tissue
Removal of loop recorder
Removal of neurostimulator pulse generator (single array, dual array)
Removal of tissue expander(s) from skin or soft tissue other than breast tissue

Excludes *removal of foreign body without incision (98.20–98.29)*

✖ **86.06 Insertion of totally implantable infusion pump**
Code also any associated catheterization

Excludes *insertion of totally implantable vascular access device (86.07)*

86.07 Insertion of totally implantable vascular access device [VAD]
Totally implanted port

Excludes *insertion of totally implantable infusion pump (86.06)*

86.09 Other incision of skin and subcutaneous tissue
Creation of thalamic stimulator pulse generator pocket, new site
Escharotomy
Exploration:
sinus tract, skin
superficial fossa
Relocation of subcutaneous device pocket NEC
Reopening subcutaneous pocket for device revision without replacement
Undercutting of hair follicle

Excludes *creation of loop recorder pocket, new site, and insertion/relocation of device (37.79)*
creation of pocket for implantable, patient-activated cardiac event recorder and insertion/relocation of device (37.79)
removal of catheter from cranial cavity (01.27)
that of:
cardiac pacemaker pocket, new site (37.79)
fascial compartments of face and mouth (27.0)

● **86.1 Diagnostic procedures on skin and subcutaneous tissue**

86.11 Biopsy of skin and subcutaneous tissue

86.19 Other diagnostic procedures on skin and subcutaneous tissue

Excludes *microscopic examination of specimen from skin and subcutaneous tissue (91.61–91.79)*

● **86.2 Excision or destruction of lesion or tissue of skin and subcutaneous tissue**

✖ **86.21 Excision of pilonidal cyst or sinus**
Marsupialization of cyst

Excludes *incision of pilonidal cyst or sinus (86.03)*

✖ **86.22 Excisional debridement of wound, infection, or burn**
Removal by excision of:
devitalized tissue
necrosis
slough

Excludes *debridement of:*
abdominal wall (wound) (54.3)
bone (77.60–77.69)
muscle (83.45)
of hand (82.36)
nail (bed) (fold) (86.27)
nonexcisional debridement of wound, infection, or burn (86.28)
open fracture site (79.60–79.69)
pedicle or flap graft (86.75)

86.23 Removal of nail, nail bed, or nail fold

86.24 Chemosurgery of skin
Chemical peel of skin

✖ **86.25 Dermabrasion**
That with laser

Excludes *dermabrasion of wound to remove embedded debris (86.28)*

86.26 Ligation of dermal appendage

Excludes *excision of preauricular appendage (18.29)*

86.27 Debridement of nail, nail bed, or nail fold
Removal of:
necrosis
slough

Excludes *removal of nail, nail bed, or nail fold (86.23)*

86.28 Nonexcisional debridement of wound, infection, or burn
Debridement NOS
Maggot therapy
Removal of devitalized tissue, necrosis, and slough by such methods as:
brushing
irrigation (under pressure)
scrubbing
washing
Water scalpel (jet) ◀

86.3 Other local excision or destruction of lesion or tissue of skin and subcutaneous tissue
Destruction of skin by:
cauterization cryosurgery
fulguration
laser beam
That with Z-plasty

Excludes *adipectomy (86.83)*
biopsy of skin (86.11)
wide or radical excision of skin (86.4)
Z-plasty without excision (86.84)

✖ **86.4 Radical excision of skin lesion**
Wide excision of skin lesion involving underlying or adjacent structure
Code also any lymph node dissection (40.3–40.5)

● **86.5 Suture or other closure of skin and subcutaneous tissue**

86.51 Replantation of scalp

86.59 Closure of skin and subcutaneous tissue of other sites
Adhesives (surgical) (tissue)
Staples
Sutures

Excludes *application of adhesive strips (butterfly)—omit code*

● **86.6 Free skin graft**

Includes: excision of skin for autogenous graft

Excludes *construction or reconstruction of:*
penis (64.43–64.44)
trachea (31.75)
vagina (70.61–70.62)

✖ **86.60 Free skin graft, not otherwise specified**

✖ **86.61 Full-thickness skin graft to hand**

Excludes *heterograft (86.65)*
homograft (86.66)

✖ **86.62 Other skin graft to hand**

Excludes *heterograft (86.65)*
homograft (86.66)

✖ **86.63 Full-thickness skin graft to other sites**

Excludes *heterograft (86.65)*
homograft (86.66)

86.64 Hair transplant

Excludes *hair follicle transplant to eyebrow or eyelash (08.63)*

✖ **86.65 Heterograft to skin**
Pigskin graft
Porcine graft

Excludes *application of dressing only (93.57)*

✖ **86.66 Homograft to skin**
Graft to skin of:
amnionic membrane from donor skin from donor

86.67 Dermal regenerative graft
Artificial skin, NOS
Creation of "neodermis"
Decellularized allodermis
Integumentary matrix implants
Prosthetic implant of dermal layer of skin
Regenerate dermal layer of skin

Excludes *heterograft to skin (86.65)*
homograft to skin (86.66)

✖ **86.69 Other skin graft to other sites**

Excludes *heterograft (86.65)*
homograft (86.66)

● **86.7 Pedicle grafts or flaps**

Excludes *construction or reconstruction of:*
penis (64.43–64.44)
trachea (31.75)
vagina (70.61–70.62)

✖ **86.70 Pedicle or flap graft, not otherwise specified**

✖ **86.71 Cutting and preparation of pedicle grafts or flaps**
Elevation of pedicle from its bed
Flap design and raising
Partial cutting of pedicle or tube
Pedicle delay

Excludes *pollicization or digital transfer (82.61, 82.81)*
revision of pedicle (86.75)

✖ **86.72 Advancement of pedicle graft**

✖ **86.73 Attachment of pedicle or flap graft to hand**

Excludes *pollicization or digital transfer (82.61, 82.81)*

✖ **86.74 Attachment of pedicle or flap graft to other sites**
Attachment by:
advanced flap
double pedicled flap
pedicle graft
rotating flap
sliding flap
tube graft

✖ **86.75 Revision of pedicle or flap graft**
Debridement of pedicle or flap graft
Defatting of pedicle or flap graft

● **86.8 Other repair and reconstruction of skin and subcutaneous tissue**

✖ **86.81 Repair for facial weakness**

✖ **86.82 Facial rhytidectomy**
Face lift

Excludes *rhytidectomy of eyelid (08.86–08.87)*

✖ **86.83 Size reduction plastic operation**
Reduction of adipose tissue of:
abdominal wall (pendulous)
arms (batwing)
buttock
liposuction
thighs (trochanteric lipomatosis)

Excludes *breast (85.31–85.32)*

✖ **86.84 Relaxation of scar or web contracture of skin**
Z-plasty of skin

Excludes *Z-plasty with excision of lesion (86.3)*

✖ **86.85 Correction of syndactyly**

✖ 86.86 **Onychoplasty**

✖ 86.89 **Other repair and reconstruction of skin and subcutaneous tissue**

Excludes *mentoplasty (76.67–76.68)*

● 86.9 **Other operations on skin and subcutaneous tissue**

✖ 86.91 **Excision of skin for graft**

Excision of skin with closure of donor site

Excludes *that with graft at same operative episode (86.60-86.69)*

86.92 **Electrolysis and other epilation of skin**

Excludes *epilation of eyelid (08.91–08.93)*

✖ 86.93 **Insertion of tissue expander**

Insertion (subcutaneous) (soft tissue) of expander (one or more) in scalp (subgaleal space), face, neck, trunk except breast, and upper and lower extremities for development of skin flaps for donor use

Excludes *flap graft preparation (86.71)*
tissue expander, breast (85.95)

86.94 **Insertion or replacement of single array neurostimulator pulse generator, not specified as rechargeable**

Pulse generator (single array, single channel) for intracranial, spinal, and peripheral neurostimulator

Excludes *insertion or replacement of single array rechargeable neurostimulator pulse generator (86.97)*

Code also any associated lead implantation (02.93, 03.93, 04.92)

86.95 **Insertion or replacement of dual array neurostimulator pulse generator, not specified as rechargeable**

Pulse generator (dual array, dual channel) for intracranial, spinal, and peripheral neurostimulator

Code also any associated lead implantation (02.93, 03.93, 04.92)

Excludes *insertion or replacement of dual array rechargeable neurostimulator pulse generator (86.98)*

86.96 **Insertion or replacement of other neurostimulator pulse generator**

Code also any associated lead implantation (02.93, 03.93, 04.92)

Excludes *insertion of dual array neurostimulator pulse generator (86.95, 86.98)*
insertion of single array neurostimulator pulse generator (86.94, 86.97)

86.97 **Insertion or replacement of single array rechargeable neurostimulator pulse generator**

Rechargeable pulse generator (single array, single channel) for intracranial, spinal, and peripheral neurostimulator

Code also any associated lead implantation (02.93, 03.93, 04.92)

86.98 **Insertion or replacement of dual array rechargeable neurostimulator pulse generator**

Rechargeable pulse generator (dual array, dual channel) for intracranial, spinal, and peripheral neurostimulator

Code also any associated lead implantation (02.93, 03.93, 04.92)

86.99 **Other**

Excludes *removal of sutures from:*
abdomen (97.83)
head and neck (97.38)
thorax (97.43)
trunk NEC (97.84)
wound catheter:
irrigation (96.58)
replacement (97.15)

16. MISCELLANEOUS DIAGNOSTIC AND THERAPEUTIC PROCEDURES (87–99)

● 87 Diagnostic Radiology

● 87.0 Soft tissue x-ray of face, head, and neck
Excludes *angiography (88.40–88.68)*

87.01 Pneumoencephalogram

87.02 Other contrast radiogram of brain and skull
Pneumocisternogram
Pneumoventriculogram
Posterior fossa myelogram

87.03 Computerized axial tomography of head
C.A.T. scan of head

87.04 Other tomography of head

87.05 Contrast dacryocystogram

87.06 Contrast radiogram of nasopharynx

87.07 Contrast laryngogram

87.08 Cervical lymphangiogram

87.09 Other soft tissue x-ray of face, head, and neck
Noncontrast x-ray of:
adenoid
larynx
nasolacrimal duct
nasopharynx
salivary gland
thyroid region
uvula
Excludes *x-ray study of eye (95.14)*

● 87.1 Other x-ray of face, head, and neck
Excludes *angiography (88.40–88.68)*

87.11 Full-mouth x-ray of teeth

87.12 Other dental x-ray
Orthodontic cephalogram or cephalometrics
Panorex examination of mandible
Root canal x-ray

87.13 Temporomandibular contrast arthrogram

87.14 Contrast radiogram of orbit

87.15 Contrast radiogram of sinus

87.16 Other x-ray of facial bones
X-ray of:
frontal area
mandible
maxilla
nasal sinuses
nose
orbit
supraorbital area
symphysis menti
zygomaticomaxillary complex

87.17 Other x-ray of skull
Lateral projection of skull
Sagittal projection of skull
Tangential projection of skull

● 87.2 X-ray of spine

87.21 Contrast myelogram

87.22 Other x-ray of cervical spine

87.23 Other x-ray of thoracic spine

87.24 Other x-ray of lumbosacral spine
Sacrococcygeal x-ray

87.29 Other x-ray of spine
Spinal x-ray NOS

● 87.3 Soft tissue x-ray of thorax
Excludes *angiocardiography (88.50–88.58)*
angiography (88.40–88.68)

87.31 Endotracheal bronchogram

87.32 Other contrast bronchogram
Transcricoid bronchogram

87.33 Mediastinal pneumogram

87.34 Intrathoracic lymphangiogram

87.35 Contrast radiogram of mammary ducts

87.36 Xerography of breast

87.37 Other mammography

87.38 Sinogram of chest wall
Fistulogram of chest wall

87.39 Other soft tissue x-ray of chest wall

● 87.4 Other x-ray of thorax
Excludes *angiocardiography (88.50–88.58)*
angiography (88.40–88.68)

87.41 Computerized axial tomography of thorax
C.A.T. scan of thorax
Crystal linear scan of x-ray beam of thorax
Electronic subtraction of thorax
Photoelectric response of thorax
Tomography with use of computer, x-rays, and camera of thorax

87.42 Other tomography of thorax
Cardiac tomogram

87.43 X-ray of ribs, sternum, and clavicle
Examination for:
cervical rib
fracture

87.44 Routine chest x-ray, so described
X-ray of chest NOS

87.49 Other chest x-ray
X-ray of:
bronchus NOS
diaphragm NOS
heart NOS
lung NOS
mediastinum NOS
trachea NOS

● 87.5 Biliary tract x-ray

87.51 Percutaneous hepatic cholangiogram

87.52 Intravenous cholangiogram

✖ 87.53 Intraoperative cholangiogram

87.54 Other cholangiogram

87.59 Other biliary tract x-ray
Cholecystogram

● 87.6 Other x-ray of digestive system

87.61 Barium swallow

87.62 Upper GI series

87.63 Small bowel series

87.64 Lower GI series

87.65 Other x-ray of intestine

87.66 Contrast pancreatogram

87.69 Other digestive tract x-ray

● 87.7 X-ray of urinary system
Excludes *angiography of renal vessels (88.45, 88.65)*

87.71 Computerized axial tomography of kidney
C.A.T. scan of kidney

87.72 Other nephrotomogram

87.73 Intravenous pyelogram
Diuretic infusion pyelogram

87.74 Retrograde pyelogram

87.75 Percutaneous pyelogram

87.76 **Retrograde cystourethrogram**

87.77 **Other cystogram**

87.78 **Ileal conduitogram**

87.79 **Other x-ray of the urinary system**
KUB x-ray

● 87.8 **X-ray of female genital organs**

87.81 **X-ray of gravid uterus**
Intrauterine cephalometry by x-ray

87.82 **Gas contrast hysterosalpingogram**

87.83 **Opaque dye contrast hysterosalpingogram**

87.84 **Percutaneous hysterogram**

87.85 **Other x-ray of fallopian tubes and uterus**

87.89 **Other x-ray of female genital organs**

● 87.9 **X-ray of male genital organs**

87.91 **Contrast seminal vesiculogram**

87.92 **Other x-ray of prostate and seminal vesicles**

87.93 **Contrast epididymogram**

87.94 **Contrast vasogram**

87.95 **Other x-ray of epididymis and vas deferens**

87.99 **Other x-ray of male genital organs**

● 88 **Other diagnostic radiology and related techniques**

● 88.0 **Soft tissue x-ray of abdomen**

Excludes *angiography (88.40–88.68)*

88.01 **Computerized axial tomography of abdomen**
C.A.T. scan of abdomen

Excludes *C.A.T. scan of kidney (87.71)*

88.02 **Other abdomen tomography**

Excludes *nephrotomogram (87.72)*

88.03 **Sinogram of abdominal wall**
Fistulogram of abdominal wall

88.04 **Abdominal lymphangiogram**

88.09 **Other soft tissue x-ray of abdominal wall**

● 88.1 **Other x-ray of abdomen**

88.11 **Pelvic opaque dye contrast radiography**

88.12 **Pelvic gas contrast radiography**
Pelvic pneumoperitoneum

88.13 **Other peritoneal pneumogram**

88.14 **Retroperitoneal fistulogram**

88.15 **Retroperitoneal pneumogram**

88.16 **Other retroperitoneal x-ray**

88.19 **Other x-ray of abdomen**
Flat plate of abdomen

● 88.2 **Skeletal x-ray of extremities and pelvis**

Excludes *contrast radiogram of joint (88.32)*

88.21 **Skeletal x-ray of shoulder and upper arm**

88.22 **Skeletal x-ray of elbow and forearm**

88.23 **Skeletal x-ray of wrist and hand**

88.24 **Skeletal x-ray of upper limb, not otherwise specified**

88.25 **Pelvimetry**

88.26 **Other skeletal x-ray of pelvis and hip**

88.27 **Skeletal x-ray of thigh, knee, and lower leg**

88.28 **Skeletal x-ray of ankle and foot**

88.29 **Skeletal x-ray of lower limb, not otherwise specified**

● 88.3 **Other x-ray**

88.31 **Skeletal series**
X-ray of whole skeleton

88.32 **Contrast arthrogram**

Excludes *that of temporomandibular joint (87.13)*

88.33 **Other skeletal x-ray**

Excludes *skeletal x-ray of:*
extremities and pelvis (88.21–88.29)
face, head, and neck (87.11–87.17)
spine (87.21–87.29)
thorax (87.43)

88.34 **Lymphangiogram of upper limb**

88.35 **Other soft tissue x-ray of upper limb**

88.36 **Lymphangiogram of lower limb**

88.37 **Other soft tissue x-ray of lower limb**

Excludes *femoral angiography (88.48, 88.66)*

88.38 **Other computerized axial tomography**
C.A.T. scan NOS

Excludes *C.A.T. scan of:*
abdomen (88.01)
head (87.03)
kidney (87.71)
thorax (87.41)

88.39 **X-ray, other and unspecified**

● 88.4 **Arteriography using contrast material**

Includes: angiography of arteries
arterial puncture for injection of contrast material
radiography of arteries (by fluoroscopy)
retrograde arteriography

Note: The fourth-digit subclassification identifies the site to be viewed, not the site of injection.

Excludes *arteriography using:*
radioisotopes or radionuclides (92.01–92.19)
ultrasound (88.71–88.79)
fluorescein angiography of eye (95.12)

88.40 **Arteriography using contrast material, unspecified site**

88.41 **Arteriography of cerebral arteries**
Angiography of:
basilar artery
carotid (internal)
posterior cerebral circulation
vertebral artery

88.42 **Aortography**
Arteriography of aorta and aortic arch

88.43 **Arteriography of pulmonary arteries**

88.44 **Arteriography of other intrathoracic vessels**

Excludes *angiocardiography (88.50–88.58)*
arteriography of coronary arteries (88.55–88.57)

88.45 **Arteriography of renal arteries**

88.46 **Arteriography of placenta**
Placentogram using contrast material

88.47 **Arteriography of other intra-abdominal arteries**

88.48 **Arteriography of femoral and other lower extremity arteries**

88.49 **Arteriography of other specified sites**

● 88.5 **Angiocardiography using contrast material**

Includes: arterial puncture and insertion of arterial catheter for injection of contrast material
cineangiocardiography
selective angiocardiography

Code also synchronous cardiac catheterization (37.21–37.23)

Excludes *angiography of pulmonary vessels (88.43, 88.62)*

88.50 **Angiocardiography, not otherwise specified**

88.51 Angiocardiography of venae cavae
Inferior vena cavography
Phlebography of vena cava (inferior) (superior)

88.52 Angiocardiography of right heart structures
Angiocardiography of:
pulmonary valve
right atrium
right ventricle (outflow tract)

Excludes *that combined with left heart angiocardiography (88.54)*

88.53 Angiocardiography of left heart structures
Angiocardiography of:
aortic valve
left atrium
left ventricle (outflow tract)

Excludes *that combined with right heart angiocardiography (88.54)*

88.54 Combined right and left heart angiocardiography

88.55 Coronary arteriography using a single catheter
Coronary arteriography by Sones technique
Direct selective coronary arteriography using a single catheter

88.56 Coronary arteriography using two catheters
Coronary arteriography by:
Judkins technique
Ricketts and Abrams technique
Direct selective coronary arteriography using two catheters

88.57 Other and unspecified coronary arteriography
Coronary arteriography NOS

88.58 Negative-contrast cardiac roentgenography
Cardiac roentgenography with injection of carbon dioxide

● **88.6 Phlebography**

Includes: angiography of veins
radiography of veins (by fluoroscopy)
retrograde phlebography
venipuncture for injection of contrast material
venography using contrast material

Note: The fourth-digit subclassification (88.60–88.67) identifies the site to be viewed, not the site of injection.

Excludes *angiography using:*
radioisotopes or radionuclides (92.01–92.19)
ultrasound (88.71–88.79)
fluorescein angiography of eye (95.12)

88.60 Phlebography using contrast material, unspecified site

88.61 Phlebography of veins of head and neck using contrast material

88.62 Phlebography of pulmonary veins using contrast material

88.63 Phlebography of other intrathoracic veins using contrast material

88.64 Phlebography of the portal venous system using contrast material
Splenoportogram (by splenic arteriography)

88.65 Phlebography of other intra-abdominal veins using contrast material

88.66 Phlebography of femoral and other lower extremity veins using contrast material

88.67 Phlebography of other specified sites using contrast material

88.68 Impedance phlebography

● **88.7 Diagnostic ultrasound**
Non-invasive ultrasound

Includes: echography
ultrasonic angiography
ultrasonography

Excludes *intravascular imaging (adjunctive) (IVUS) (00.21–00.29)*
therapeutic ultrasound (00.01–00.09)

88.71 Diagnostic ultrasound of head and neck
Determination of midline shift of brain
Echoencephalography

Excludes *eye (95.13)*

88.72 Diagnostic ultrasound of heart
Echocardiography
Transesophageal echocardiography

Excludes *echocardiography of heart chambers (37.28)*
intracardiac echocardiography (ICE) (37.28)
intravascular (IVUS) imaging of coronary vessels (00.24)

88.73 Diagnostic ultrasound of other sites of thorax
Aortic arch ultrasonography
Breast ultrasonography
Lung ultrasonography

88.74 Diagnostic ultrasound of digestive system

88.75 Diagnostic ultrasound of urinary system

88.76 Diagnostic ultrasound of abdomen and retroperitoneum

88.77 Diagnostic ultrasound of peripheral vascular system
Deep vein thrombosis ultrasonic scanning

Excludes *adjunct vascular system procedures (00.40–00.43)*

88.78 Diagnostic ultrasound of gravid uterus
Intrauterine cephalometry:
echo
ultrasonic
Placental localization by ultrasound

88.79 Other diagnostic ultrasound
Ultrasonography of:
multiple sites
nongravid uterus
total body

● **88.8 Thermography**

88.81 Cerebral thermography

88.82 Ocular thermography

88.83 Bone thermography
Osteoarticular thermography

88.84 Muscle thermography

88.85 Breast thermography

88.86 Blood vessel thermography
Deep vein thermography

88.89 Thermography of other sites
Lymph gland thermography
Thermography NOS

● **88.9 Other diagnostic imaging**

88.90 Diagnostic imaging, not elsewhere classified

88.91 Magnetic resonance imaging of brain and brain stem

Excludes *intraoperative magnetic resonance imaging (88.96)*
real-time magnetic resonance imaging (88.96)

88.92 Magnetic resonance imaging of chest and myocardium
For evaluation of hilar and mediastinal lymphadenopathy

88.93 Magnetic resonance imaging of spinal canal
Spinal cord levels:
cervical
thoracic
lumbar (lumbosacral)
Spinal cord
Spine

88.94 Magnetic resonance imaging of musculoskeletal
Bone marrow blood supply
Extremities (upper) (lower)

88.95 Magnetic resonance imaging of pelvis, prostate, and bladder

88.96 Other intraoperative magnetic resonance imaging
iMRI
Real-time magnetic resonance imaging

88.97 Magnetic resonance imaging of other and unspecified sites
Abdomen
Eye orbit
Face
Neck

88.98 Bone mineral density studies
Dual photon absorptiometry
Quantitative computed tomography (CT) studies
Radiographic densitometry
Single photon absorptiometry

● **89 Interview, evaluation, consultation, and examination**

● **89.0 Diagnostic interview, consultation, and evaluation**

Excludes *psychiatric diagnostic interview (94.11–94.19)*

89.01 Interview and evaluation, described as brief
Abbreviated history and evaluation

89.02 Interview and evaluation, described as limited
Interval history and evaluation

89.03 Interview and evaluation, described as comprehensive
History and evaluation of new problem

89.04 Other interview and evaluation

89.05 Diagnostic interview and evaluation, not otherwise specified

89.06 Consultation, described as limited
Consultation on a single organ system

89.07 Consultation, described as comprehensive

89.08 Other consultation

89.09 Consultation, not otherwise specified

● **89.1 Anatomic and physiologic measurements and manual examinations—nervous system and sense organs**

Excludes *ear examination (95.41–95.49)*
eye examination (95.01–95.26)
the listed procedures when done as part of a general physical examination (89.7)

89.10 Intracarotid amobarbital test
Wada test

89.11 Tonometry

89.12 Nasal function study
Rhinomanometry

89.13 Neurologic examination

89.14 Electroencephalogram

Excludes *that with polysomnogram (89.17)*

89.15 Other nonoperative neurologic function tests

89.16 Transillumination of newborn skull

89.17 Polysomnogram
Sleep recording

89.18 Other sleep disorder function tests
Multiple sleep latency test [MSLT]

89.19 Video and radio-telemetered electroencephalographic monitoring
Radiographic EEG monitoring
Video EEG monitoring

● **89.2 Anatomic and physiologic measurements and manual examinations—genitourinary system**

Excludes *the listed procedures when done as part of a general physical examination (89.7)*

89.21 Urinary manometry
Manometry through:
indwelling ureteral catheter
nephrostomy
pyelostomy
ureterostomy

89.22 Cystometrogram

89.23 Urethral sphincter electromyogram

89.24 Uroflowmetry [UFR]

89.25 Urethral pressure profile [UPP]

89.26 Gynecological examination
Pelvic examination

89.29 Other nonoperative genitourinary system measurements
Bioassay of urine
Renal clearance
Urine chemistry

● **89.3 Other anatomic and physiologic measurements and manual examinations**

Excludes *the listed procedures when done as part of a general physical examination (89.7)*

89.31 Dental examination
Oral mucosal survey
Periodontal survey

89.32 Esophageal manometry

89.33 Digital examination of enterostomy stoma
Digital examination of colostomy stoma

89.34 Digital examination of rectum

89.35 Transillumination of nasal sinuses

89.36 Manual examination of breast

89.37 Vital capacity determination

89.38 Other nonoperative respiratory measurements
Plethysmography for measurement of respiratory function
Thoracic impedance plethysmography

89.39 Other nonoperative measurements and examinations
14 C-Urea breath test
Basal metabolic rate [BMR]
Gastric:
analysis
function NEC

Excludes *body measurement (93.07)*
cardiac tests (89.41–89.69)
fundus photography (95.11)
limb length measurement (93.06)

● **89.4 Cardiac stress tests, pacemaker and defibrillator checks**

89.41 Cardiovascular stress test using treadmill

89.42 Masters' two-step stress test

89.43 Cardiovascular stress test using bicycle ergometer

89.44 Other cardiovascular stress test
Thallium stress test with or without transesophageal pacing

89.45 Artificial pacemaker rate check
Artificial pacemaker function check NOS
Bedside device check of pacemaker or cardiac resynchronization pacemaker [CRT-P]
Interrogation only without arrhythmia induction

Excludes *catheter based invasive electrophysiologic testing (37.26)* ◄
non-invasive programmed electrical stimulation [NIPS] (arrhythmia induction) (37.20) ◄

89.46 Artificial pacemaker artifact wave form check

89.47 Artificial pacemaker electrode impedance check

89.48 Artificial pacemaker voltage or amperage threshold check

89.49 Automatic implantable cardioverter/defibrillator (AICD) check
Bedside check of an AICD or cardiac resynchronization defibrillator [CRT-D]
Checking pacing thresholds of device
Interrogation only without arrhythmia induction

Excludes *catheter based invasive electrophysiologic testing (37.26)* ◄
non-invasive programmed electrical stimulation [NIPS] (arrhythmia induction) (37.20) ◄

● **89.5 Other nonoperative cardiac and vascular diagnostic procedures**

Excludes *fetal EKG (75.32)*

89.50 Ambulatory cardiac monitoring
Analog devices [Holter-type]

89.51 Rhythm electrocardiogram
Rhythm EKG (with one to three leads)

89.52 Electrocardiogram
ECG NOS
EKG (with 12 or more leads)

89.53 Vectorcardiogram (with ECG)

89.54 Electrographic monitoring
Telemetry

Excludes *ambulatory cardiac monitoring (89.50)*
electrographic monitoring during surgery—omit code

89.55 Phonocardiogram with ECG lead

89.56 Carotid pulse tracing with ECG lead

Excludes *oculoplethysmography (89.58)*

89.57 Apexcardiogram (with ECG lead)

89.58 Plethysmogram
Penile plethysmography with nerve stimulation

Excludes *plethysmography (for):*
measurement of respiratory function (89.38)
thoracic impedance (89.38)

89.59 Other nonoperative cardiac and vascular measurements

● **89.6 Circulatory monitoring**

Excludes *electrocardiographic monitoring during surgery—omit code*
implantation or replacement of subcutaneous device for intracardiac hemodynamic monitoring (00.57) ◄
insertion or replacement of implantable pressure sensor (lead) for intracardiac hemodynamic monitoring (00.56) ◄

89.60 Continuous intra-arterial blood gas monitoring
Insertion of blood gas monitoring system and continuous monitoring of blood gases through an intra-arterial sensor

89.61 Systemic arterial pressure monitoring

89.62 Central venous pressure monitoring

89.63 Pulmonary artery pressure monitoring

Excludes *pulmonary artery wedge monitoring (89.64)*

89.64 Pulmonary artery wedge monitoring
Pulmonary capillary wedge [PCW] monitoring
Swan-Ganz catheterization

89.65 Measurement of systemic arterial blood gases

Excludes *continuous intra-arterial blood gas monitoring (89.60)*

89.66 Measurement of mixed venous blood gases

89.67 Monitoring of cardiac output by oxygen consumption technique
Fick method

89.68 Monitoring of cardiac output by other technique
Cardiac output monitor by thermodilution indicator

89.69 Monitoring of coronary blood flow
Coronary blood flow monitoring by coincidence counting technique

89.7 General physical examination

89.8 Autopsy

● **90 Microscopic examination-I**

The following fourth-digit subclassification is for use with categories in section 90 to identify type of examination:

1 **bacterial smear**
2 **culture**
3 **culture and sensitivity**
4 **parasitology**
5 **toxicology**
6 **cell block and Papanicolaou smear**
9 **other microscopic examination**

● **90.0 Microscopic examination of specimen from nervous system and of spinal fluid**

● **90.1 Microscopic examination of specimen from endocrine gland, not elsewhere classified**

● **90.2 Microscopic examination of specimen from eye**

● **90.3 Microscopic examination of specimen from ear, nose, throat, and larynx**

● **90.4 Microscopic examination of specimen from trachea, bronchus, pleura, lung, and other thoracic specimen, and of sputum**

● **90.5 Microscopic examination of blood**

● **90.6 Microscopic examination of specimen from spleen and of bone marrow**

● **90.7 Microscopic examination of specimen from lymph node and of lymph**

● **90.8 Microscopic examination of specimen from upper gastrointestinal tract and of vomitus**

● **90.9 Microscopic examination of specimen from lower gastrointestinal tract and of stool**

● **91 Microscopic examination-II**

The following fourth-digit subclassification is for use with categories in section 91 to identify type of examination

1 **bacterial smear**
2 **culture**
3 **culture and sensitivity**
4 **parasitology**
5 **toxicology**
6 **cell block and Papanicolaou smear**
9 **other microscopic examination**

● **91.0 Microscopic examination of specimen from liver, biliary tract, and pancreas**

● 91.1 **Microscopic examination of peritoneal and retroperitoneal specimen**

● 91.2 **Microscopic examination of specimen from kidney, ureter, perirenal, and periureteral tissue**

● 91.3 **Microscopic examination of specimen from bladder, urethra, prostate, seminal vesicle, perivesical tissue, and of urine and semen**

● 91.4 **Microscopic examination of specimen from female genital tract**
Amnionic sac
Fetus

● 91.5 **Microscopic examination of specimen from musculoskeletal system and of joint fluid**
Microscopic examination of:
bone
bursa
cartilage
fascia
ligament
muscle
synovial membrane
tendon

● 91.6 **Microscopic examination of specimen from skin and other integument**
Microscopic examination of:
hair
nails
skin

Excludes *mucous membrane—code to organ site that of operative wound (91.70–91.79)*

● 91.7 **Microscopic examination of specimen from operative wound**

● 91.8 **Microscopic examination of specimen from other site**

● 91.9 **Microscopic examination of specimen from unspecified site**

● 92 Nuclear medicine

● 92.0 **Radioisotope scan and function study**

92.01 **Thyroid scan and radioisotope function studies**
Iodine-131 uptake
Protein-bound iodine
Radio-iodine uptake

92.02 **Liver scan and radioisotope function study**

92.03 **Renal scan and radioisotope function study**
Renal clearance study

92.04 **Gastrointestinal scan and radioisotope function study**
Radio-cobalt B12 Schilling test
Radio-iodinated triolein study

92.05 **Cardiovascular and hematopoietic scan and radioisotope function study**
Bone marrow scan or function study
Cardiac output scan or function study
Circulation time scan or function study
Radionuclide cardiac ventriculogram scan or function study
Spleen scan or function study

92.09 **Other radioisotope function studies**

● 92.1 **Other radioisotope scan**

92.11 **Cerebral scan**
Pituitary

92.12 **Scan of other sites of head**

Excludes *eye (95.16)*

92.13 **Parathyroid scan**

92.14 **Bone scan**

92.15 **Pulmonary scan**

92.16 **Scan of lymphatic system**

92.17 **Placental scan**

92.18 **Total body scan**

92.19 **Scan of other sites**

● 92.2 **Therapeutic radiology and nuclear medicine**

Excludes *that for:*
ablation of pituitary gland (07.64–07.69)
destruction of chorioretinal lesion (14.26–14.27)

92.20 **Infusion of liquid brachytherapy radioisotope**
I-125 radioisotope
Intracavitary brachytherapy

Includes: removal of radioisotope

92.21 **Superficial radiation**
Contact radiation [up to 150 KVP]

92.22 **Orthovoltage radiation**
Deep radiation [200–300 KVP]

92.23 **Radioisotopic teleradiotherapy**
Teleradiotherapy using:
Cobalt-60
Iodine-125
radioactive cesium

92.24 **Teleradiotherapy using photons**
Megavoltage NOS
Supervoltage NOS
Use of:
Betatron
linear accelerator

92.25 **Teleradiotherapy using electrons**
Beta particles

92.26 **Teleradiotherapy of other particulate radiation**
Neutrons
Protons NOS

✖ 92.27 **Implantation or insertion of radioactive elements**
Intravascular brachytherapy

Code also incision of site

Excludes *infusion of liquid brachytherapy radioisotope (92.20)*

92.28 **Injection or instillation of radioisotopes**
Injection or infusion of radioimmunoconjugate
Intracavitary injection or instillation
Intravenous injection or instillation
Iodine-131 [I-131] tositumomab
Radioimmunotherapy
Ytrium-90 [Y-90] ibritumomab tiuxetan

Excludes *infusion of liquid brachytherapy radioisotope (92.20)*

92.29 **Other radiotherapeutic procedure**

● 92.3 **Stereotactic radiosurgery**

Excludes *stereotactic biopsy*

Code also stereotactic head frame application (93.59)

92.30 **Stereotactic radiosurgery, not otherwise specified**

92.31 **Single source photon radiosurgery**
High energy x-rays
Linear accelerator (LINAC)

92.32 **Multi-source photon radiosurgery**
Cobalt 60 radiation
Gamma irradiation

92.33 **Particulate radiosurgery**
Particle beam radiation (cyclotron)
Proton accelerator

92.39 **Stereotactic radiosurgery, not elsewhere classified**

● 93 **Physical therapy, respiratory therapy, rehabilitation, and related procedures**

● 93.0 **Diagnostic physical therapy**

93.01 **Functional evaluation**

93.02 Orthotic evaluation

93.03 Prosthetic evaluation

93.04 Manual testing of muscle function

93.05 Range of motion testing

93.06 Measurement of limb length

93.07 Body measurement
Girth measurement
Measurement of skull circumference

93.08 Electromyography

Excludes *eye EMG (95.25)*
that with polysomnogram (89.17)
urethral sphincter EMG (89.23)

93.09 Other diagnostic physical therapy procedure

● **93.1 Physical therapy exercises**

93.11 Assisting exercise

Excludes *assisted exercise in pool (93.31)* (Revised)

93.12 Other active musculoskeletal exercise

93.13 Resistive exercise

93.14 Training in joint movements

93.15 Mobilization of spine

93.16 Mobilization of other joints

Excludes *manipulation of temporomandibular joint (76.95)*

93.17 Other passive musculoskeletal exercise

93.18 Breathing exercise

93.19 Exercise, not elsewhere classified

● **93.2 Other physical therapy musculoskeletal manipulation**

93.21 Manual and mechanical traction

Excludes *skeletal traction (93.43–93.44)*
skin traction (93.45–93.46)
spinal traction (93.41–93.42)

93.22 Ambulation and gait training

93.23 Fitting of orthotic device

93.24 Training in use of prosthetic or orthotic device
Training in crutch walking

93.25 Forced extension of limb

93.26 Manual rupture of joint adhesions

93.27 Stretching of muscle or tendon

93.28 Stretching of fascia

93.29 Other forcible correction of deformity

● **93.3 Other physical therapy therapeutic procedures**

93.31 Assisted exercise in pool

93.32 Whirlpool treatment

93.33 Other hydrotherapy

93.34 Diathermy

93.35 Other heat therapy
Acupuncture with smoldering moxa
Hot packs
Hyperthermia NEC
Infrared irradiation
Moxibustion
Paraffin bath

Excludes *hyperthermia for treatment of cancer (99.85)*

93.36 Cardiac retraining

93.37 Prenatal training
Training for natural childbirth

93.38 Combined physical therapy without mention of the components

93.39 Other physical therapy

● **93.4 Skeletal traction and other traction**

93.41 Spinal traction using skull device
Traction using:
caliper tongs
Crutchfield tongs
halo device
Vinke tongs

Excludes *insertion of tongs or halo traction device (02.94)*

93.42 Other spinal traction
Cotrel's traction

Excludes *cervical collar (93.52)*

93.43 Intermittent skeletal traction

93.44 Other skeletal traction
Bryant's traction
Dunlop's traction
Lyman Smith traction
Russell's traction

93.45 Thomas' splint traction

93.46 Other skin traction of limbs
Adhesive tape traction
Boot traction
Buck's traction
Gallows traction

● **93.5 Other immobilization, pressure, and attention to wound**

Excludes *external fixator device (84.71–84.73)*
wound cleansing (96.58–96.59)

93.51 Application of plaster jacket

Excludes *Minerva jacket (93.52)*

93.52 Application of neck support
Application of:
cervical collar
Minerva jacket
molded neck support

93.53 Application of other cast

93.54 Application of splint
Plaster splint
Tray splint

Excludes *periodontal splint (24.7)*

93.55 Dental wiring

Excludes *that for orthodontia (24.7)*

93.56 Application of pressure dressing
Application of:
Gibney bandage
Robert Jones' bandage
Shanz dressing

93.57 Application of other wound dressing
Porcine wound dressing

93.58 Application of pressure trousers
Application of:
anti-shock trousers
MAST trousers
vasopneumatic device

93.59 Other immobilization, pressure, and attention to wound
Elastic stockings
Electronic gaiter
Intermittent pressure device
Oxygenation of wound (hyperbaric)
Stereotactic head frame application (New)
Strapping (non-traction)
Velpeau dressing

● **93.6 Osteopathic manipulative treatment**

93.61 Osteopathic manipulative treatment for general mobilization
General articulatory treatment

93.62 Osteopathic manipulative treatment using high-velocity, low-amplitude forces
Thrusting forces

93.63 Osteopathic manipulative treatment using low-velocity, high-amplitude forces
Springing forces

93.64 Osteopathic manipulative treatment using isotonic, isometric forces

93.65 Osteopathic manipulative treatment using indirect forces

93.66 Osteopathic manipulative treatment to move tissue fluids
Lymphatic pump

93.67 Other specified osteopathic manipulative treatment

● **93.7 Speech and reading rehabilitation and rehabilitation of the blind**

93.71 Dyslexia training

93.72 Dysphasia training

93.73 Esophageal speech training

93.74 Speech defect training

93.75 Other speech training and therapy

93.76 Training in use of lead dog for the blind

93.77 Training in braille or Moon

93.78 Other rehabilitation for the blind

● **93.8 Other rehabilitation therapy**

93.81 Recreation therapy
Diversional therapy
Play therapy

Excludes *play psychotherapy (94.36)*

93.82 Educational therapy
Education of bed-bound children
Special schooling for the handicapped

93.83 Occupational therapy
Daily living activities therapy

Excludes *training in activities of daily living for the blind (93.78)*

93.84 Music therapy

93.85 Vocational rehabilitation
Sheltered employment
Vocational:
assessment
retraining
training

93.89 Rehabilitation, not elsewhere classified

● **93.9 Respiratory therapy**

Excludes *insertion of airway (96.01–96.05)*
other continuous mechanical ventilation (96.70–96.72)

93.90 Continuous positive airway pressure [CPAP]
Bi-level airway pressure
Non-invasive positive pressure (NIPPV)

93.91 Intermittent positive pressure breathing [IPPB]

93.93 Nonmechanical methods of resuscitation
Artificial respiration
Manual resuscitation
Mouth-to-mouth resuscitation

93.94 Respiratory medication administered by nebulizer
Mist therapy

93.95 Hyperbaric oxygenation

Excludes *oxygenation of wound (93.59)*

93.96 Other oxygen enrichment
Catalytic oxygen therapy
Cytoreductive effect
Oxygenators
Oxygen therapy

Excludes *oxygenation of wound (93.59)*

93.97 Decompression chamber

93.98 Other control of atmospheric pressure and composition
Antigen-free air conditioning
Helium therapy

Excludes *inhaled nitric oxide therapy (INO) (00.12)*

93.99 Other respiratory procedures
Continuous negative pressure ventilation [CNP]
Postural drainage

● **94 Procedures related to the psyche**

● **94.0 Psychologic evaluation and testing**

94.01 Administration of intelligence test
Administration of:
Stanford-Binet
Wechsler Adult Intelligence Scale
Wechsler Intelligence Scale for Children

94.02 Administration of psychologic test
Administration of:
Bender Visual-Motor Gestalt Test
Benton Visual Retention Test
Minnesota Multiphasic Personality Inventory
Wechsler Memory Scale

94.03 Character analysis

94.08 Other psychologic evaluation and testing

94.09 Psychologic mental status determination, not otherwise specified

● **94.1 Psychiatric interviews, consultations, and evaluations**

94.11 Psychiatric mental status determination
Clinical psychiatric mental status determination
Evaluation for criminal responsibility
Evaluation for testimentary capacity
Medicolegal mental status determination
Mental status determination NOS

94.12 Routine psychiatric visit, not otherwise specified

94.13 Psychiatric commitment evaluation
Pre-commitment interview

94.19 Other psychiatric interview and evaluation
Follow-up psychiatric interview NOS

● **94.2 Psychiatric somatotherapy**

94.21 Narcoanalysis
Narcosynthesis

94.22 Lithium therapy

94.23 Neuroleptic therapy

94.24 Chemical shock therapy

94.25 Other psychiatric drug therapy

94.26 Subconvulsive electroshock therapy

94.27 Other electroshock therapy
Electroconvulsive therapy (ECT)
EST

94.29 Other psychiatric somatotherapy

● **94.3 Individual psychotherapy**

94.31 Psychoanalysis

94.32 Hypnotherapy
Hypnodrome
Hypnosis

94.33 Behavior therapy
Aversion therapy
Behavior modification
Desensitization therapy
Extinction therapy
Relaxation training
Token economy

94.34 Individual therapy for psychosexual dysfunction
Excludes *that performed in group setting (94.41)*

94.35 Crisis intervention

94.36 Play psychotherapy

94.37 Exploratory verbal psychotherapy

94.38 Supportive verbal psychotherapy

94.39 Other individual psychotherapy
Biofeedback

● **94.4 Other psychotherapy and counseling**

94.41 Group therapy for psychosexual dysfunction

94.42 Family therapy

94.43 Psychodrama

94.44 Other group therapy

94.45 Drug addiction counseling

94.46 Alcoholism counseling

94.49 Other counseling

● **94.5 Referral for psychologic rehabilitation**

94.51 Referral for psychotherapy

94.52 Referral for psychiatric aftercare:
That in:
halfway house
outpatient (clinic) facility

94.53 Referral for alcoholism rehabilitation

94.54 Referral for drug addiction rehabilitation

94.55 Referral for vocational rehabilitation

94.59 Referral for other psychologic rehabilitation

● **94.6 Alcohol and drug rehabilitation and detoxification**

94.61 Alcohol rehabilitation

94.62 Alcohol detoxification

94.63 Alcohol rehabilitation and detoxification

94.64 Drug rehabilitation

94.65 Drug detoxification

94.66 Drug rehabilitation and detoxification

94.67 Combined alcohol and drug rehabilitation

94.68 Combined alcohol and drug detoxification

94.69 Combined alcohol and drug rehabilitation and detoxification

● **95 Ophthalmologic and otologic diagnosis and treatment**

● **95.0 General and subjective eye examination**

95.01 Limited eye examination
Eye examination with prescription of spectacles

95.02 Comprehensive eye examination
Eye examination covering all aspects of the visual system

95.03 Extended ophthalmologic work-up
Examination (for):
glaucoma
neuro-ophthalmology
retinal disease

95.04 Eye examination under anesthesia
Code also type of examination

95.05 Visual field study

95.06 Color vision study

95.07 Dark adaptation study

95.09 Eye examination, not otherwise specified
Vision check NOS

● **95.1 Examinations of form and structure of eye**

95.11 Fundus photography

95.12 Fluorescein angiography or angioscopy of eye

95.13 Ultrasound study of eye

95.14 X-ray study of eye

95.15 Ocular motility study

95.16 P32 and other tracer studies of eye

● **95.2 Objective functional tests of eye**
Excludes *that with polysomnogram (89.17)*

95.21 Electroretinogram [ERG]

95.22 Electro-oculogram [EOG]

95.23 Visual evoked potential [VEP]

95.24 Electronystagmogram [ENG]

95.25 Electromyogram of eye [EMG]

95.26 Tonography, provocative tests, and other glaucoma testing

● **95.3 Special vision services**

95.31 Fitting and dispensing of spectacles

95.32 Prescription, fitting, and dispensing of contact lens

95.33 Dispensing of other low vision aids

95.34 Ocular prosthetics

95.35 Orthoptic training

95.36 Ophthalmologic counseling and instruction
Counseling in:
adaptation to visual loss
use of low vision aids

● **95.4 Nonoperative procedures related to hearing**

95.41 Audiometry
Békésy 5-tone audiometry
Impedance audiometry
Stapedial reflex response
Subjective audiometry
Tympanogram

95.42 Clinical test of hearing
Tuning fork test
Whispered speech test

95.43 **Audiological evaluation**
Audiological evaluation by:
Bárány noise machine
blindfold test
delayed feedback
masking
Weber lateralization

95.44 **Clinical vestibular function tests**
Thermal test of vestibular function

95.45 **Rotation tests**
Bárány chair

95.46 **Other auditory and vestibular function tests**

95.47 **Hearing examination, not otherwise specified**

95.48 **Fitting of hearing aid**

Excludes *implantation of electromagnetic hearing device (20.95)*

95.49 **Other nonoperative procedures related to hearing**
Adjustment (external components) of cochlear prosthetic device

● 96 **Nonoperative intubation and irrigation**

● 96.0 **Nonoperative intubation of gastrointestinal and respiratory tracts**

96.01 **Insertion of nasopharyngeal airway**

96.02 **Insertion of oropharyngeal airway**

96.03 **Insertion of esophageal obturator airway**

96.04 **Insertion of endotracheal tube**

96.05 **Other intubation of respiratory tract**

Excludes *endoscopic insertion or replacement of bronchial device or substance (33.71, 33.79)* ◄

96.06 **Insertion of Sengstaken tube**
Esophageal tamponade

96.07 **Insertion of other (naso-)gastric tube**
Intubation for decompression

Excludes *that for enteral infusion of nutritional substance (96.6)*

96.08 **Insertion of (naso-)intestinal tube**
Miller-Abbott tube (for decompression)

96.09 **Insertion of rectal tube**
Replacement of rectal tube

● 96.1 **Other nonoperative insertion**

Excludes *nasolacrimal intubation (09.44)*

96.11 **Packing of external auditory canal**

96.14 **Vaginal packing**

96.15 **Insertion of vaginal mold**

96.16 **Other vaginal dilation**

96.17 **Insertion of vaginal diaphragm**

96.18 **Insertion of other vaginal pessary**

96.19 **Rectal packing**

● 96.2 **Nonoperative dilation and manipulation**

96.21 **Dilation of frontonasal duct**

96.22 **Dilation of rectum**

96.23 **Dilation of anal sphincter**

96.24 **Dilation and manipulation of enterostomy stoma**

96.25 **Therapeutic distention of bladder**
Intermittent distention of bladder

96.26 **Manual reduction of rectal prolapse**

96.27 **Manual reduction of hernia**

96.28 **Manual reduction of enterostomy prolapse**

96.29 **Reduction of intussusception of alimentary tract**
With:
Fluoroscopy
Ionizing radiation enema
Ultrasonography guidance
Hydrostatic reduction
Pneumatic reduction

Excludes *intra-abdominal manipulation of intestine, not otherwise specified (46.80)*

● 96.3 **Nonoperative alimentary tract irrigation, cleaning, and local instillation**

96.31 **Gastric cooling**
Gastric hypothermia

96.32 **Gastric freezing**

96.33 **Gastric lavage**

96.34 **Other irrigation of (naso-)gastric tube**

96.35 **Gastric gavage**

96.36 **Irrigation of gastrostomy or enterostomy**

96.37 **Proctoclysis**

96.38 **Removal of impacted feces**
Removal of impaction:
by flushing
manually

96.39 **Other transanal enema**
Rectal irrigation

Excludes *reduction of intussusception of alimentary tract by ionizing radiation enema (96.29)*

● 96.4 **Nonoperative irrigation, cleaning, and local instillation of other digestive and genitourinary organs**

96.41 **Irrigation of cholecystostomy and other biliary tube**

96.42 **Irrigation of pancreatic tube**

96.43 **Digestive tract instillation, except gastric gavage**

96.44 **Vaginal douche**

96.45 **Irrigation of nephrostomy and pyelostomy**

96.46 **Irrigation of ureterostomy and ureteral catheter**

96.47 **Irrigation of cystostomy**

96.48 **Irrigation of other indwelling urinary catheter**

96.49 **Other genitourinary instillation**
Insertion of prostaglandin suppository

● 96.5 **Other nonoperative irrigation and cleaning**

96.51 **Irrigation of eye**
Irrigation of cornea

Excludes *irrigation with removal of foreign body (98.21)*

96.52 **Irrigation of ear**
Irrigation with removal of cerumen

96.53 **Irrigation of nasal passages**

96.54 **Dental scaling, polishing, and debridement**
Dental prophylaxis
Plaque removal

96.55 **Tracheostomy toilette**

96.56 **Other lavage of bronchus and trachea**

Excludes *diagnostic bronchoalveolar lavage (BAL) (33.24)*
whole lung lavage (33.99)

96.57 **Irrigation of vascular catheter**

96.58 **Irrigation of wound catheter**

96.59 **Other irrigation of wound**
Wound cleaning NOS

Excludes *debridement (86.22, 86.27–86.28)*

96.6 Enteral infusion of concentrated nutritional substances

● **96.7 Other continuous mechanical ventilation**

Includes: endotracheal respiratory assistance
intermittent mandatory ventilation [IMV]
positive end expiratory pressure [PEEP]
pressure support ventilation [PSV]
that by tracheostomy
weaning of an intubated (endotracheal tube) patient

Excludes *bi-level airway pressure (93.90)*
continuous negative pressure ventilation [CNP] (iron lung) (cuirass) (93.99)
continuous positive airway pressure [CPAP] (93.90)
intermittent positive pressure breathing [IPPB] (93.91)
non-invasive positive pressure (NIPPV) (93.90)
that by face mask (93.90–93.99)
that by nasal cannula (93.90–93.99)
that by nasal catheter (93.90–93.99)

Code also any associated:
endotracheal tube insertion (96.04)
tracheostomy (31.1–31.29)

Note: Endotracheal Intubation

To calculate the number of hours (duration) of continuous mechanical ventilation during a hospitalization, begin the count from the start of the (endotracheal) intubation. The duration ends with (endotracheal) extubation.

If a patient is intubated prior to admission, begin counting the duration from the time of the admission. If a patient is transferred (discharged) while intubated, the duration would end at the time of transfer (discharge).

For patients who begin on (endotracheal) intubation and subsequently have a tracheostomy performed for mechanical ventilation, the duration begins with the (endotracheal) intubation and ends when the mechanical ventilation is turned off (after the weaning period).

Tracheostomy

To calculate the number of hours of continuous mechanical ventilation during a hospitalization, begin counting the duration when mechanical ventilation is started. The duration ends when the mechanical ventilator is turned off (after the weaning period).

If a patient has received a tracheostomy prior to admission and is on mechanical ventilation at the time of admission, begin counting the duration from the time of admission. If a patient is transferred (discharged) while still on mechanical ventilation via tracheostomy, the duration would end at the time of the transfer (discharge).

96.70 Continuous mechanical ventilation of unspecified duration
Mechanical ventilation NOS

96.71 Continuous mechanical ventilation for less than 96 consecutive hours

96.72 Continuous mechanical ventilation for 96 consecutive hours or more

● **97 Replacement and removal of therapeutic appliances**

● **97.0 Nonoperative replacement of gastrointestinal appliance**

97.01 Replacement of (naso-)gastric or esophagostomy tube

97.02 Replacement of gastrostomy tube

97.03 Replacement of tube or enterostomy device of small intestine

97.04 Replacement of tube or enterostomy device of large intestine

97.05 Replacement of stent (tube) in biliary or pancreatic duct

● **97.1 Nonoperative replacement of musculoskeletal and integumentary system appliance**

97.11 Replacement of cast on upper limb

97.12 Replacement of cast on lower limb

97.13 Replacement of other cast

97.14 Replacement of other device for musculoskeletal immobilization

97.15 Replacement of wound catheter

97.16 Replacement of wound packing or drain

Excludes *repacking of:*
dental wound (97.22)
vulvar wound (97.26)

● **97.2 Other nonoperative replacement**

97.21 Replacement of nasal packing

97.22 Replacement of dental packing

97.23 Replacement of tracheostomy tube

97.24 Replacement and refitting of vaginal diaphragm

97.25 Replacement of other vaginal pessary

97.26 Replacement of vaginal or vulvar packing or drain

97.29 Other nonoperative replacements

● **97.3 Nonoperative removal of therapeutic device from head and neck**

97.31 Removal of eye prosthesis

Excludes *removal of ocular implant (16.71)*
removal of orbital implant (16.72)

97.32 Removal of nasal packing

97.33 Removal of dental wiring

97.34 Removal of dental packing

97.35 Removal of dental prosthesis

97.36 Removal of other external mandibular fixation device

97.37 Removal of tracheostomy tube

97.38 Removal of sutures from head and neck

97.39 Removal of other therapeutic device from head and neck

Excludes *removal of skull tongs (02.94)*

● **97.4 Nonoperative removal of therapeutic device from thorax**

97.41 Removal of thoracotomy tube or pleural cavity drain

97.42 Removal of mediastinal drain

97.43 Removal of sutures from thorax

97.44 Nonoperative removal of heart assist system
Explantation [removal] of circulatory assist device
Explantation [removal] of percutaneous external heart assist device
Intra-aortic balloon pump [IABP]
Removal of extrinsic heart assist device
Removal of pVAD
Removal of percutaneous heart assist device

97.49 Removal of other device from thorax

● 97.5 Nonoperative removal of therapeutic device from digestive system
- 97.51 Removal of gastrostomy tube
- 97.52 Removal of tube from small intestine
- 97.53 Removal of tube from large intestine or appendix
- 97.54 Removal of cholecystostomy tube
- 97.55 Removal of T-tube, other bile duct tube, or liver tube
  Removal of bile duct stent
- 97.56 Removal of pancreatic tube or drain
- 97.59 Removal of other device from digestive system
  Removal of rectal packing

● 97.6 Nonoperative removal of therapeutic device from urinary system
- 97.61 Removal of pyelostomy and nephrostomy tube
- 97.62 Removal of ureterostomy tube and ureteral catheter
- 97.63 Removal of cystostomy tube
- 97.64 Removal of other urinary drainage device
  Removal of indwelling urinary catheter
- 97.65 Removal of urethral stent
- 97.69 Removal of other device from urinary system

● 97.7 Nonoperative removal of therapeutic device from genital system
- 97.71 Removal of intrauterine contraceptive device
- 97.72 Removal of intrauterine pack
- 97.73 Removal of vaginal diaphragm
- 97.74 Removal of other vaginal pessary
- 97.75 Removal of vaginal or vulvar packing
- 97.79 Removal of other device from genital tract
  Removal of sutures

● 97.8 Other nonoperative removal of therapeutic device
- 97.81 Removal of retroperitoneal drainage device
- 97.82 Removal of peritoneal drainage device
- 97.83 Removal of abdominal wall sutures
- 97.84 Removal of sutures from trunk, not elsewhere classified
- 97.85 Removal of packing from trunk, not elsewhere classified
- 97.86 Removal of other device from abdomen
- 97.87 Removal of other device from trunk
- 97.88 Removal of external immobilization device
  Removal of:
  brace
  cast
  splint
- 97.89 Removal of other therapeutic device

● 98 Nonoperative removal of foreign body or calculus

● 98.0 Removal of intraluminal foreign body from digestive system without incision

Excludes *removal of therapeutic device (97.51–97.59)*

- 98.01 Removal of intraluminal foreign body from mouth without incision
- 98.02 Removal of intraluminal foreign body from esophagus without incision
- 98.03 Removal of intraluminal foreign body from stomach and small intestine without incision
- 98.04 Removal of intraluminal foreign body from large intestine without incision
- 98.05 Removal of intraluminal foreign body from rectum and anus without incision

● 98.1 Removal of intraluminal foreign body from other sites without incision

Excludes *removal of therapeutic device (97.31–97.49, 97.61–97.89)*

- 98.11 Removal of intraluminal foreign body from ear without incision
- 98.12 Removal of intraluminal foreign body from nose without incision
- 98.13 Removal of intraluminal foreign body from pharynx without incision
- 98.14 Removal of intraluminal foreign body from larynx without incision
- 98.15 Removal of intraluminal foreign body from trachea and bronchus without incision
- 98.16 Removal of intraluminal foreign body from uterus without incision

Excludes *removal of intrauterine contraceptive device (97.71)*

- 98.17 Removal of intraluminal foreign body from vagina without incision
- 98.18 Removal of intraluminal foreign body from artificial stoma without incision
- 98.19 Removal of intraluminal foreign body from urethra without incision

● 98.2 Removal of other foreign body without incision

Excludes *removal of intraluminal foreign body (98.01–98.19)*

- 98.20 Removal of foreign body, not otherwise specified
- 98.21 Removal of superficial foreign body from eye without incision
- 98.22 Removal of other foreign body without incision from head and neck
  Removal of embedded foreign body from eyelid or conjunctiva without incision
- 98.23 Removal of foreign body from vulva without incision
- 98.24 Removal of foreign body from scrotum or penis without incision
- 98.25 Removal of other foreign body without incision from trunk except scrotum, penis, or vulva
- 98.26 Removal of foreign body from hand without incision
- 98.27 Removal of foreign body without incision from upper limb, except hand
- 98.28 Removal of foreign body from foot without incision
- 98.29 Removal of foreign body without incision from lower limb, except foot

● 98.5 Extracorporeal shockwave lithotripsy [ESWL]

Lithotriptor tank procedure
Disintegration of stones by extracorporeal induced shockwaves
That with insertion of stent

- 98.51 Extracorporeal shockwave lithotripsy [ESWL] of the kidney, ureter, and/or bladder
- 98.52 Extracorporeal shockwave lithotripsy [ESWL] of the gallbladder and/or bile duct
- 98.59 Extracorporeal shockwave lithotripsy of other sites

● 99 Other nonoperative procedures

● 99.0 Transfusion of blood and blood components

Use additional code for that done via catheter or cutdown (38.92–38.94)

99.00 Perioperative autologous transfusion of whole blood or blood components
Intraoperative blood collection
Postoperative blood collection
Salvage

99.01 Exchange transfusion
Transfusion:
exsanguination
replacement

99.02 Transfusion of previously collected autologous blood
Blood component

99.03 Other transfusion of whole blood
Transfusion:
blood NOS
hemodilution
NOS

99.04 Transfusion of packed cells

99.05 Transfusion of platelets
Transfusion of thrombocytes

99.06 Transfusion of coagulation factors
Transfusion of antihemophilic factor

99.07 Transfusion of other serum
Transfusion of plasma

Excludes *injection [transfusion] of:*
antivenin (99.16)
gamma globulin (99.14)

99.08 Transfusion of blood expander
Transfusion of Dextran

99.09 Transfusion of other substance
Transfusion of:
blood surrogate
granulocytes

Excludes *transplantation [transfusion] of bone marrow (41.0)*

● 99.1 Injection or infusion of therapeutic or prophylactic substance

Includes: injection or infusion given:
hypodermically acting locally or systemically
intramuscularly acting locally or systemically
intravenously acting locally or systemically

99.10 Injection or infusion of thrombolytic agent
Alteplase ◀
Anistreplase ◀
Reteplase ◀
Streptokinase
Tenecteplase ◀
Tissue plasminogen activator (TPA)
Urokinase

Excludes *aspirin—omit code*
GP IIB/IIIa platelet inhibitors (99.20)
heparin (99.19)
warfarin—omit code

99.11 Injection of Rh immune globulin
Injection of:
Anti-D (Rhesus) globulin
RhoGAM

99.12 Immunization for allergy
Desensitization

99.13 Immunization for autoimmune disease

99.14 Injection of gamma globulin
Injection of immune sera

99.15 Parenteral infusion of concentrated nutritional substances
Hyperalimentation
Total parenteral nutrition [TPN]
Peripheral parenteral nutrition [PPN]

99.16 Injection of antidote
Injection of:
antivenin
heavy metal antagonist

99.17 Injection of insulin

99.18 Injection or infusion of electrolytes

99.19 Injection of anticoagulant

Excludes *infusion of drotrecogin alfa (activated) (00.11)*

● 99.2 Injection or infusion of other therapeutic or prophylactic substance

Includes: injection or infusion given:
hypodermically acting locally or systemically
intramuscularly acting locally or systemically
intravenously acting locally or systemically

Use additional code for:
injection (into):
breast (85.92)
bursa (82.94, 83.96)
intraperitoneal (cavity) (54.97)
intrathecal (03.92)
joint (76.96, 81.92)
kidney (55.96)
liver (50.94)
orbit (16.91)
other sites—see Alphabetic Index
perfusion:
NOS (39.97)
intestine (46.95, 46.96)
kidney (55.95)
liver (50.93)
total body (39.96)

99.20 Injection or infusion of platelet inhibitor
Glycoprotein IIB/IIIa inhibitor
GP IIB/IIIa inhibitor
GP IIB/IIa inhibitor

Excludes *infusion of heparin (99.19)*
injection or infusion of thrombolytic agent (99.10)

99.21 Injection of antibiotic

Excludes *injection or infusion of oxazolidinone class of antibiotics (00.14)*

99.22 Injection of other anti-infective

Excludes *injection or infusion of oxazolidinone class of antibiotics (00.14)*

99.23 Injection of steroid
Injection of cortisone
Subdermal implantation of progesterone

99.24 Injection of other hormone

99.25 Injection or infusion of cancer chemotherapeutic substance
Chemoembolization
Injection or infusion of antineoplastic agent

Excludes *immunotherapy, antineoplastic (00.15, 99.28)*
implantation of chemotherapeutic agent (00.10)
injection of radioisotope (92.28)
injection or infusion of biological response modifier [BRM] as an antineoplastic agent (99.28)

99.26 **Injection of tranquilizer**

99.27 **Iontophoresis**

99.28 **Injection or infusion of biological response modifier [BRM] as an antineoplastic agent**
Low-dose interleukin-2 (IL-2) therapy
Immunotherapy, antineoplastic
Infusion of cintredekin besudotox ◀
Interleukin therapy
Tumor vaccine

Excludes *high-dose infusion interleukin-2 [IL-2] (00.15)*

99.29 **Injection or infusion of other therapeutic or prophylactic substance**

Excludes *administration of neuroprotective agent (99.75)*
immunization (99.31–99.59)
injection of sclerosing agent into:
esophageal varices (42.33)
hemorrhoids (49.42)
veins (39.92)
injection or infusion of human B-type natriuretic peptide (hBNP) (00.13)
injection or infusion of nesiritide (00.13)
injection or infusion of platelet inhibitor (99.20)
injection or infusion of thrombolytic agent (99.10)

● 99.3 **Prophylactic vaccination and inoculation against certain bacterial diseases**

99.31 **Vaccination against cholera**

99.32 **Vaccination against typhoid and paratyphoid fever**
Administration of TAB vaccine

99.33 **Vaccination against tuberculosis**
Administration of BCG vaccine

99.34 **Vaccination against plague**

99.35 **Vaccination against tularemia**

99.36 **Administration of diphtheria toxoid**

Excludes *administration of:*
diphtheria antitoxin (99.58)
diphtheria-tetanus-pertussis, combined (99.39)

99.37 **Vaccination against pertussis**

Excludes *administration of diphtheria-tetanus-pertussis, combined (99.39)*

99.38 **Administration of tetanus toxoid**

Excludes *administration of:*
diphtheria-tetanus-pertussis, combined (99.39)
tetanus antitoxin (99.56)

99.39 **Administration of diphtheria-tetanus-pertussis, combined**

● 99.4 **Prophylactic vaccination and inoculation against certain viral diseases**

99.41 **Administration of poliomyelitis vaccine**

99.42 **Vaccination against smallpox**

99.43 **Vaccination against yellow fever**

99.44 **Vaccination against rabies**

99.45 **Vaccination against measles**

Excludes *administration of measles-mumps-rubella vaccine (99.48)*

99.46 **Vaccination against mumps**

Excludes *administration of measles-mumps-rubella vaccine (99.48)*

99.47 **Vaccination against rubella**

Excludes *administration of measles-mumps-rubella vaccine (99.48)*

99.48 **Administration of measles-mumps-rubella vaccine**

● 99.5 **Other vaccination and inoculation**

99.51 **Prophylactic vaccination against the common cold**

99.52 **Prophylactic vaccination against influenza**

99.53 **Prophylactic vaccination against arthropod-borne viral encephalitis**

99.54 **Prophylactic vaccination against other arthropod-borne viral diseases**

99.55 **Prophylactic administration of vaccine against other diseases**
Vaccination against:
anthrax
brucellosis
Rocky Mountain spotted fever
Staphylococcus
Streptococcus
typhus

99.56 **Administration of tetanus antitoxin**

99.57 **Administration of botulism antitoxin**

99.58 **Administration of other antitoxins**
Administration of:
diphtheria antitoxin
gas gangrene antitoxin
scarlet fever antitoxin

99.59 **Other vaccination and inoculation**
Vaccination NOS

Excludes *injection of:*
gamma globulin (99.14)
Rh immune globulin (99.11)
immunization for:
allergy (99.12)
autoimmune disease (99.13)

● 99.6 **Conversion of cardiac rhythm**

Excludes *open chest cardiac:*
electric stimulation (37.91)
massage (37.91)

99.60 **Cardiopulmonary resuscitation, not otherwise specified**

99.61 **Atrial cardioversion**

99.62 **Other electric countershock of heart**
Cardioversion:
NOS
external
Conversion to sinus rhythm
Defibrillation
External electrode stimulation

99.63 **Closed chest cardiac massage**
Cardiac massage NOS
Manual external cardiac massage

99.64 **Carotid sinus stimulation**

99.69 **Other conversion of cardiac rhythm**

● 99.7 **Therapeutic apheresis or other injection, administration, or infusion of other therapeutic or prophylactic substance**

99.71 **Therapeutic plasmapheresis**

Excludes *extracorporeal immunoadsorption [ECI] (99.76)*

99.72 Therapeutic leukopheresis
Therapeutic leukocytapheresis

99.73 Therapeutic erythrocytapheresis
Therapeutic erythropheresis

99.74 Therapeutic plateletpheresis

99.75 Administration of neuroprotective agent

99.76 Extracorporeal immunoadsorption
Removal of antibodies from plasma with protein A columns

99.77 Application or administration of adhesion barrier substance

99.78 Aquapheresis
Plasma water removal
Ultrafiltration [for water removal]

Excludes *hemodiafiltration (39.95)*
hemodialysis (39.95)
therapeutic plasmapheresis (99.71)

99.79 Other
Apheresis (harvest) of stem cells

● **99.8 Miscellaneous physical procedures**

99.81 Hypothermia (central) (local)

Excludes *gastric cooling (96.31)*
gastric freezing (96.32)
that incidental to open heart surgery (39.62)

99.82 Ultraviolet light therapy
Actinotherapy

99.83 Other phototherapy
Phototherapy of the newborn

Excludes *extracorporeal photochemotherapy (99.88)*
photocoagulation of retinal lesion (14.23–14.25, 14.33–14.35, 14.53–14.55)

99.84 Isolation
Isolation after contact with infectious disease
Protection of individual from his surroundings
Protection of surroundings from individual

99.85 Hyperthermia for treatment of cancer
Hyperthermia (adjunct therapy) induced by microwave, ultrasound, low energy radio frequency, probes (interstitial), or other means in the treatment of cancer

Code also any concurrent chemotherapy or radiation therapy

99.86 Non-invasive placement of bone growth stimulator
Transcutaneous (surface) placement of pads or patches for stimulation to aid bone healing

Excludes *insertion of invasive or semi-invasive bone growth stimulators (device) (percutaneous electrodes) (78.90–78.99)*

99.88 Therapeutic photopheresis
Extracorporeal photochemotherapy
Extracorporeal photopheresis

Excludes *other phototherapy (99.83)*
ultraviolet light therapy (99.82)

● **99.9 Other miscellaneous procedures**

99.91 Acupuncture for anesthesia

99.92 Other acupuncture

Excludes *that with smoldering moxa (93.35)*

99.93 Rectal massage (for levator spasm)

99.94 Prostatic massage

99.95 Stretching of foreskin

99.96 Collection of sperm for artificial insemination

99.97 Fitting of denture

99.98 Extraction of milk from lactating breast

99.99 Other
Leech therapy

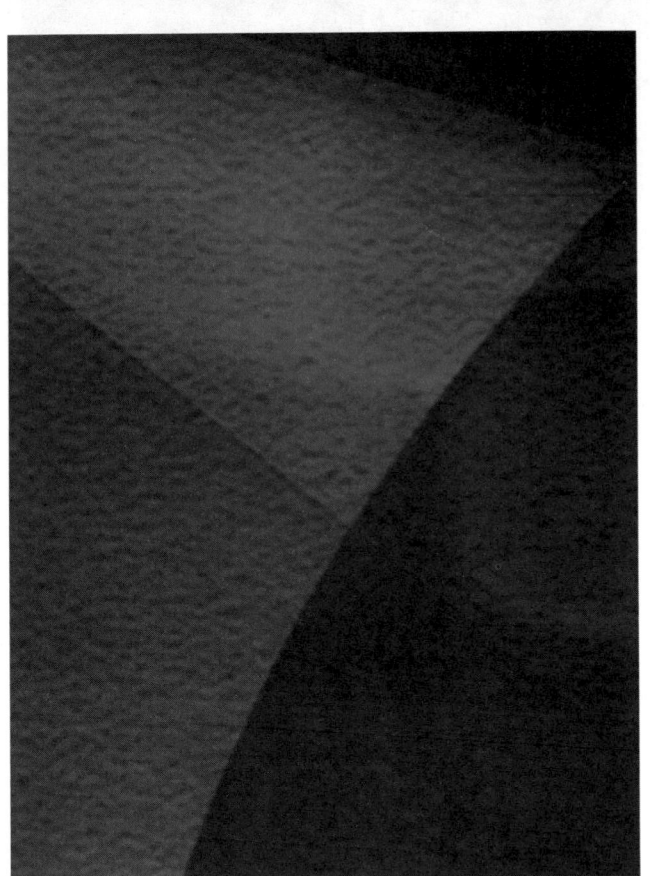

UNIT TWO

2006 INPATIENT PROCEDURES

For the 2007 updates, see the companion website in December 2006 at: http://evolve.elsevier.com/Buck/icd

2006 INPATIENT PROCEDURES

The following list is part of the changes to the Hospital Outpatient Prospective Payment System for Calendar Year 2006. Specifically, the file is Addendum E that lists the codes that are only payable as inpatient procedures (proposed) as displayed at http://a257.g.akamaitech.net/7/257/2422/01jan20051800/edocket.access.gpo.gov/2005/pdf/05-22136.pdf

00176	00882	20816	21423	22812	27076	27303	27888	32486
00192	00904	20824	21431	22818	27077	27365	28800	32488
00214	00908	20827	21432	22819	27078	27445	28805	32491
00215	00932	20838	21433	22830	27079	27447	31225	32500
0021T	00934	20930	21435	22840	27090	27448	31230	32501
0024T	00936	20931	21436	22841	27091	27450	31290	32520
0033T	00944	20936	21510	22842	27120	27454	31291	32522
0034T	01140	20937	21615	22843	27122	27455	31360	32525
0035T	01150	20938	21616	22844	27125	27457	31365	32540
0036T	01212	20955	21620	22845	27130	27465	31367	32650
0037T	01214	20956	21627	22846	27132	27466	31368	32651
0038T	01232	20957	21630	22847	27134	27468	31370	32652
0039T	01234	20962	21632	22848	27137	27470	31375	32653
00404	01272	20969	21705	22849	27138	27472	31380	32654
00406	01274	20970	21740	22850	27140	27477	31382	32655
0040T	01402	21045	21750	22851	27146	27479	31390	32656
00452	01404	21141	21810	22852	27147	27485	31395	32657
00474	01442	21142	21825	22855	27151	27486	31584	32658
0048T	01444	21143	22110	23200	27156	27487	31587	32659
0049T	01486	21145	22112	23210	27158	27488	31725	32660
0050T	01502	21146	22114	23220	27161	27495	31760	32661
0051T	01632	21147	22116	23221	27165	27506	31766	32662
00524	01634	21151	22210	23222	27170	27507	31770	32663
0052T	01636	21154	22212	23332	27175	27511	31775	32664
0053T	01638	21155	22214	23472	27176	27513	31780	32665
00540	01652	21159	22216	23900	27177	27514	31781	32800
00542	01654	21160	22220	23920	27178	27519	31786	32810
00546	01656	21172	22224	24900	27179	27535	31800	32815
00560	01756	21179	22226	24920	27181	27536	31805	32820
00561	01990	21180	22318	24930	27185	27540	32035	32850
00562	11004	21182	22319	24931	27187	27556	32036	32851
00580	11005	21183	22325	24940	27215	27557	32095	32852
00604	11006	21184	22326	25900	27217	27558	32100	32853
00622	11008	21188	22327	25905	27218	27580	32110	32854
00632	15756	21193	22328	25909	27222	27590	32120	32855
00670	15757	21194	22532	25915	27226	27591	32124	32856
0075T	15758	21196	22533	25920	27227	27592	32140	32900
0076T	16035	21247	22534	25924	27228	27596	32141	32905
0077T	16036	21255	22548	25927	27232	27598	32150	32906
0078T	19200	21256	22554	25931	27236	27645	32151	32940
00792	19220	21268	22556	26551	27240	27646	32160	32997
00794	19271	21343	22558	26553	27244	27702	32200	33015
00796	19272	21344	22585	26554	27245	27703	32215	33020
0079T	19361	21346	22590	26556	27248	27712	32220	33025
00802	19364	21347	22595	26992	27253	27715	32225	33030
0080T	19367	21348	22600	27005	27254	27720	32310	33031
0081T	19368	21360	22610	27006	27258	27722	32320	33050
00844	19369	21365	22630	27025	27259	27724	32402	33120
00846	20660	21366	22632	27030	27280	27725	32440	33130
00848	20661	21385	22800	27036	27282	27727	32442	33140
00864	20664	21386	22802	27054	27284	27880	32445	33141
00865	20802	21387	22804	27070	27286	27881	32480	33200
00866	20805	21395	22808	27071	27290	27882	32482	33201
00868	20808	21422	22810	27075	27295	27886	32484	33236

33237
33238
33243
33245
33246
33250
33251
33253
33261
33300
33305
33310
33315
33320
33321
33322
33330
33332
33335
33400
33401
33403
33404
33405
33406
33410
33411
33412
33413
33414
33415
33416
33417
33420
33422
33425
33426
33427
33430
33460
33463
33464
33465
33468
33470
33471
33472
33474
33475
33476
33478
33496
33500
33501
33502
33503
33504
33505
33506
33510
33511
33512
33513
33514
33516
33517
33518
33519
33521
33522
33523
33530
33533
33534
33535
33536
33542
33545
33572
33600
33602
33606
33608
33610
33611
33612
33615
33617
33619
33641
33645
33647
33660
33665
33670
33681
33684
33688
33690
33692
33694
33697
33702
33710
33720
33722
33730
33732
33735
33736
33737
33750
33755
33762
33764
33766
33767
33770
33771
33774
33775
33776
33777
33778
33779
33780
33781
33786
33788
33800
33802
33803
33813
33814
33820
33822
33824
33840
33845
33851
33852
33853
33860
33861
33863
33870
33875
33877
33910
33915
33916
33917
33918
33919
33920
33922
33924
33930
33933
33935
33940
33944
33945
33960
33961
33967
33968
33970
33971
33973
33974
33975
33976
33977
33978
33979
33980
34001
34051
34151
34401
34451
34502
34800
34802
34803
34804
34805
34808
34812
34813
34820
34825
34826
34830
34831
34832
34833
34834
34900
35001
35002
35005
35013
35021
35022
35045
35081
35082
35091
35092
35102
35103
35111
35112
35121
35122
35131
35132
35141
35142
35151
35152
35182
35189
35211
35216
35221
35241
35246
35251
35271
35276
35281
35301
35311
35331
35341
35351
35355
35361
35363
35371
35372
35381
35390
35400
35450
35452
35454
35456
35480
35481
35482
35483
35501
35506
35507
35508
35509
35510
35511
35512
35515
35516
35518
35521
35522
35525
35526
35531
35533
35536
35541
35546
35548
35549
35551
35556
35558
35560
35563
35565
35566
35571
35583
35585
35587
35600
35601
35606
35612
35616
35621
35623
35626
35631
35636
35641
35642
35645
35646
35647
35650
35651
35654
35656
35661
35663
35665
35666
35671
35681
35682
35683
35691
35693
35694
35695
35697
35700
35701
35721
35741
35800
35820
35840
35870
35901
35905
35907
36660
36822
36823
37140
37145
37160
37180
37181
37182
37215
37216
37616
37617
37618
37660
37788
38100
38101
38102
38115
38380
38381
38382
38562
38564
38724
38746
38747
38765
38770
38780
39000
39010
39200
39220
39499
39501
39502
39503
39520
39530
39531
39540
39541
39545
39560
39561
39599
41130
41135
41140
41145
41150
41153
41155
42426
42845
42894
42953
42961
42971
43045
43100
43101
43107
43108
43112
43113
43116
43117
43118
43121
43122
43123
43124
43135
43300
43305
43310
43312
43313
43314
43320
43324
43325
43326
43330
43331
43340
43341
43350
43351
43352
43360
43361
43400
43401
43405
43410
43415
43420
43425
43460
43496
43500
43501
43502
43520
43605
43610
43611
43620
43621
43622
43631
43632
43633
43634
43635
43638
43639
43640
43641
43644
43645
43800
43810
43820
43825
43832
43840
43842
43843
43845
43846
43847
43848
43850
43855
43860
43865
43880
44005
44010
44015
44020
44021
44025
44050
44055
44110
44111
44120
44121
44125
44126
44127
44128
44130
44132
44133
44135
44136
44137
44139
44140
44141
44143
44144
44145
44146
44147
44150
44151
44152
44153
44155
44156
44160
44202
44203
44204
44205
44210
44211
44212
44300
44310
44314
44316
44320
44322
44345
44346
44602
44603
44604
44605
44615
44620
44625
44626
44640
44650
44660
44661
44680
44700
44715
44720
44721
44800
44820
44850
44899
44900
44950
44955

44960
45110
45111
45112
45113
45114
45116
45119
45120
45121
45123
45126
45130
45135
45136
45540
45550
45562
45563
45800
45805
45820
45825
46705
46715
46716
46730
46735
46740
46742
46744
46746
46748
46751
47010
47015
47100
47120
47122
47125
47130
47133
47135
47136
47140
47141
47142
47143
47144
47145
47146
47147
47300
47350
47360
47361
47362
47380
47381
47400
47420
47425
47460
47480
47550
47570
47600
47605
47610
47612
47620
47700
47701
47711
47712
47715
47716
47720
47721
47740
47741
47760
47765
47780
47785
47800
47801
47802
47900
48000
48001
48005
48020
48100
48120
48140
48145
48146
48148
48150
48152
48153
48154
48155
48180
48400
48500
48510
48520
48540
48545
48547
48551
48552
48556
49000
49002
49010
49020
49040
49060
49062
49201
49215
49220
49255
49425
49428
49605
49606
49610
49611
49900
49904
49905
49906
50010
50040
50045
50060
50065
50070
50075
50100
50120
50125
50130
50135
50205
50220
50225
50230
50234
50236
50240
50280
50290
50300
50320
50323
50325
50327
50328
50329
50340
50360
50365
50370
50380
50400
50405
50500
50520
50525
50526
50540
50545
50546
50547
50548
50580
50600
50605
50610
50620
50630
50650
50660
50700
50715
50722
50725
50727
50728
50740
50750
50760
50770
50780
50782
50783
50785
50800
50810
50815
50820
50825
50830
50840
50845
50860
50900
50920
50930
50940
51060
51525
51530
51535
51550
51555
51565
51570
51575
51580
51585
51590
51595
51596
51597
51800
51820
51840
51841
51845
51860
51865
51900
51920
51925
51940
51960
51980
53415
53448
54125
54130
54135
54332
54336
54390
54411
54417
54430
54535
54650
55605
55650
55801
55810
55812
55815
55821
55831
55840
55842
55845
55862
55865
55866
56630
56631
56632
56633
56634
56637
56640
57110
57111
57112
57270
57280
57282
57283
57292
57305
57307
57308
57311
57335
57531
57540
57545
58140
58146
58150
58152
58180
58200
58210
58240
58260
58262
58263
58267
58270
58275
58280
58285
58290
58291
58292
58293
58294
58400
58410
58520
58540
58605
58611
58700
58720
58740
58750
58752
58760
58805
58822
58825
58940
58943
58950
58951
58952
58953
58954
58956
58960
59120
59121
59130
59135
59136
59140
59325
59350
59514
59525
59620
59830
59850
59851
59852
59855
59856
59857
60254
60270
60271
60502
60505
60520
60521
60522
60540
60545
60600
60605
60650
61105
61107
61108
61120
61140
61150
61151
61154
61156
61210
61250
61253
61304
61305
61312
61313
61314
61315
61316
61320
61321
61322
61323
61332
61333
61340
61343
61345
61440
61450
61458
61460
61470
61480
61490
61500
61501
61510
61512
61514
61516
61517
61518
61519
61520
61521
61522
61524
61526
61530
61531
61533
61534
61535
61536
61537
61538
61539
61540
61541
61542
61543
61544
61545
61546
61548
61550
61552
61556
61557
61558
61559
61563
61564
61566
61567
61570
61571
61575
61576
61580
61581
61582
61583
61584
61585
61586
61590
61591
61592
61595
61596
61597
61598
61600
61601
61605
61606
61607
61608
61609
61610
61611
61612
61613
61615
61616
61618
61619
61624
61680
61682
61684
61686
61690
61692
61697
61698
61700
61702
61703
61705
61708
61710
61711
61720
61735
61750
61751
61760
61770
61850
61860
61863
61864
61867
61868
61870
61875
62000
62005
62010
62100
62115
62116
62117
62120
62121
62140
62141
62142
62143
62145
62146
62147
62148
62161
62162
62163
62164
62165
62180
62190
62192
62200
62201
62220
62223
62256
62258
63043
63044
63050
63051
63075
63076
63077
63078
63081
63082

63085
63086
63087
63088
63090
63091
63101
63102
63103
63170
63172
63173
63180
63182
63185
63190
63191
63194
63195
63196
63197
63198
63199
63200
63250
63251
63252
63265
63266
63267
63268
63270
63271
63272
63273
63275
63276
63277
63278
63280
63281
63282
63283
63285
63286
63287
63290
63295
63300
63301
63302
63303
63304
63305
63306
63307
63308
63700
63702
63704
63706
63707
63709
63710
63740
64752
64755
64760
64804
64809
64818
64866
64868
65273
69155
69535
69554
69950
69970
75900
75952
75953
75954
92970
92971
92975
92992
92993
99190
99191
99192
99251
99252
99253
99254
99255
99261
99262
99263
99293
99294
99295
99296
99298
99299
99356
99357
99433
G0341
G0342
G0343

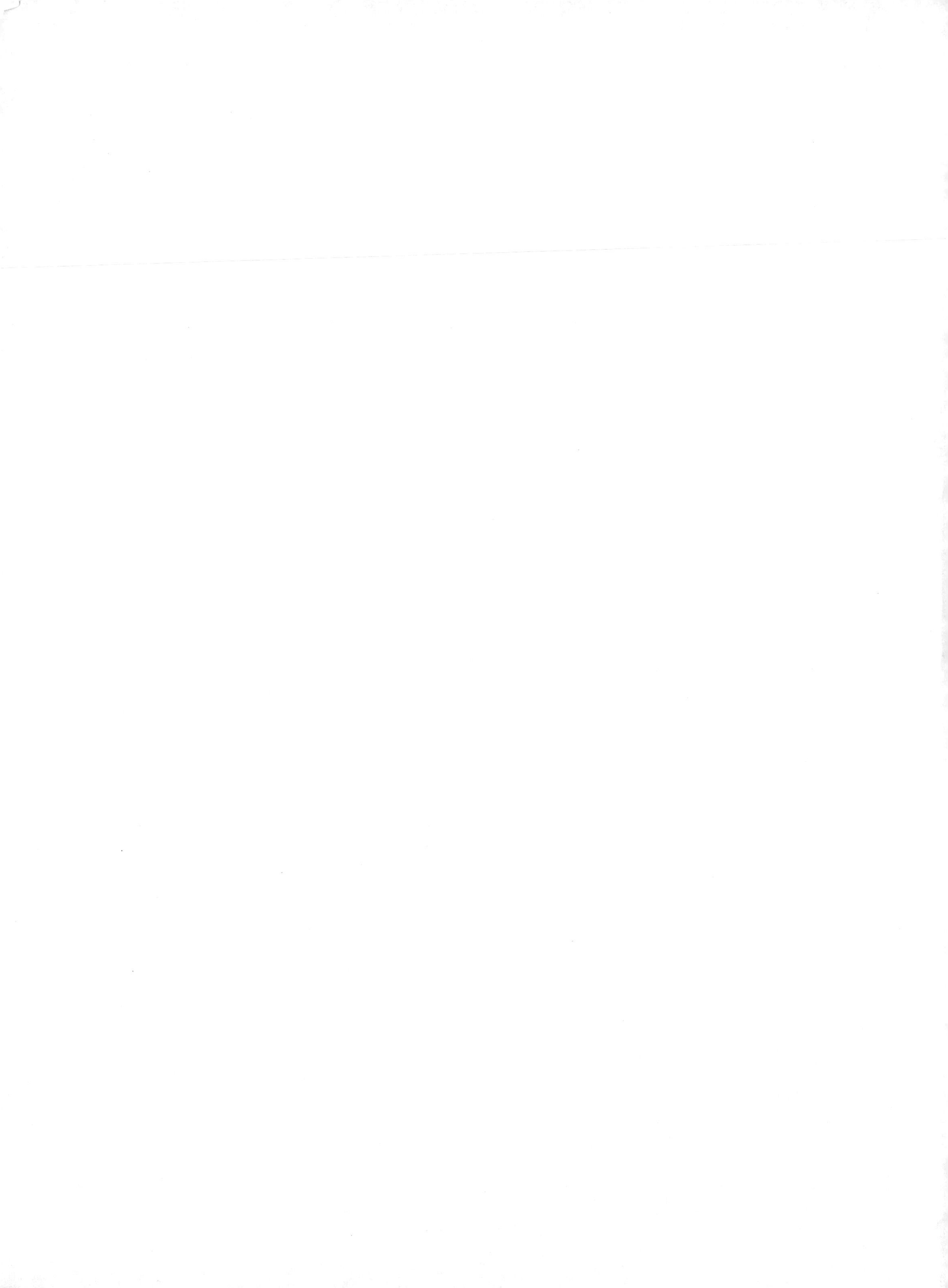